P9-DZZ-907

evolve

ELSEVIER

YOU'VE JUST PURCHASED
MORE THAN
A TEXTBOOK!

Evolve Student Resources for *Lewis: Medical-Surgical Nursing in Canada, Fourth Canadian Edition*, include the following:

- Key Points
- Review Questions
- Answer Guidelines for Textbook Case Studies
- Student Case Studies
- Nursing Care Plans
- Managing Multiple Patients Case Studies and Answers for RNs
- Conceptual Care Map Creator
- Audio Glossary
- Supporting Media
  - Animations
  - Audio
- Fluids and Electrolytes Tutorial

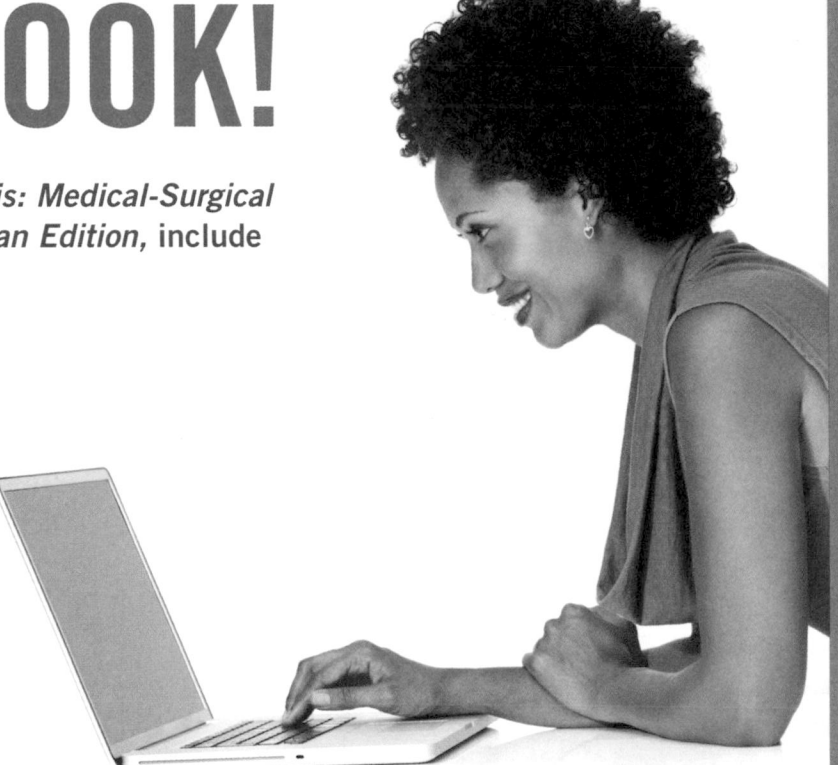

Activate the complete learning experience that comes with each textbook purchase by registering at

http://evolve.elsevier.com/Canada/Lewis/medsurg/

REGISTER TODAY!

You can now purchase Elsevier products on Evolve!
Go to evolve.elsevier.com/html/shop-promo.html to search and browse for products.

2015v1.0

Medical-Surgical Nursing in Canada

FOURTH CANADIAN EDITION

Assessment and Management of Clinical Problems

Sharon L. Lewis, RN, PhD, FAAN
Professor Emerita, University of New Mexico, Albuquerque, New Mexico;
Former Castella Distinguished Professor, School of Nursing, University of Texas Health Science Center at San Antonio, San Antonio, Texas;
Developer and Consultant, Stress-Busting Program for Family Caregivers

Linda Bucher, RN, PhD, CEN, CNE
Emerita Professor, School of Nursing, University of Delaware, Newark, Delaware;
Per Diem Staff Nurse, Emergency Department, Virtua Memorial Hospital, Mt. Holly, New Jersey

Margaret McLean Heitkemper, RN, PhD, FAAN
Professor and Chairperson, Biobehavioral Nursing and Health Systems, Elizabeth Sterling Soule Endowed Chair in Nursing, School of Nursing;
Adjunct Professor, Division of Gastroenterology, School of Medicine, University of Washington, Seattle, Washington

Mariann M. Harding, RN, PhD, CNE
Associate Professor of Nursing, Kent State University at Tuscarawas, New Philadelphia, Ohio

Maureen A. Barry, RN, MScN
Associate Professor, Teaching Stream, Lawrence S. Bloomberg Faculty of Nursing, University of Toronto, Toronto, Ontario

Jana Lok, RN, MN, PhD, ENC(C)
Assistant Professor, Teaching Stream, Lawrence S. Bloomberg Faculty of Nursing, University of Toronto, Toronto, Ontario

Jane Tyerman, RN, MScN, PhD
Nursing Professor, Trent/Fleming School of Nursing, Peterborough, Ontario

Sandra Goldsworthy, RN, MSc, PhD, CNCC(C), CMSN(C)
Associate Dean Teaching-Learning and Technology;
Associate Professor
Research Professorship in Simulation
Faculty of Nursing
University of Calgary
Calgary, Alberta

Section Editors for the US 10th Edition
Jeffrey Kwong, DNP, MPH, ANP-BC, FAANP
Associate Professor of Nursing at CUMC, Program Director, Adult-Gerontology Nurse Practitioner Program, Program Director, HIV Sub-Specialty, Program Director, Elder LGBT Interprofessional Collaborative Care Program (ENLINC), Program Director, Collaborative Access for LGBT Adults (CALA), Columbia University School of Nursing, New York, New York

Dottie Roberts, RN, EdD, MSN, MACI, OCNS-C, CMSRN, CNE
Executive Director, Orthopaedic Nurses Certification Board, Chicago, Illinois;
Editor, "MEDSURG Nursing," Official Journal of the Academy of Medical-Surgical Nurses, Pitman, New Jersey

ELSEVIER

ELSEVIER

Copyright © 2019 Elsevier Canada, a division of Reed Elsevier Canada, Ltd.

This adaptation of *Medical-Surgical Nursing: Assessment and Management of Clinical Problems*, 10th Edition, by Sharon L. Lewis, Linda Bucher, Margaret McLean Heitkemper, and Mariann M. Harding is published by arrangement with Elsevier Inc.

ISBN: 978-0-323-32852-4 (hardcover)
Copyright © 2017, Elsevier Inc. All Rights Reserved.
Previous editions copyrighted 2014, 2011, 2007, 2003, 2000, 1996, 1992, 19897, 1983 by Mosby, Inc., an affiliate of Elsevier, Inc.

All rights reserved. No part of this publication may be reproduced or transmitted in any form or by any means, electronic or mechanical, including photocopy, recording, or any information storage and retrieval system, without permission in writing from the publisher. Reproducing passages from this book without such written permission is an infringement of copyright law.

ISBN: 978-1-77172-048-9

Requests for permission to make copies of any part of the work should be mailed to: College Licensing Officer, access ©, 1 Yonge Street, Suite 1900, Toronto, ON M5E 1E5. Fax: (416) 868-1621. All other inquiries should be directed to the publisher.

Every reasonable effort has been made to acquire permission for copyrighted material used in this text and to acknowledge all such indebtedness accurately. Any errors and omissions called to the publisher's attention will be corrected in future printings.

Notices

Knowledge and best practice in this field are constantly changing. As new research and experience broaden our understanding, changes in research methods, professional practices, or medical treatment may become necessary.

Practitioners and researchers must always rely on their own experience and knowledge in evaluating and using any information, methods, compounds, or experiments described herein. In using such information or methods they should be mindful of their own safety and the safety of others, including parties for whom they have a professional responsibility.

With respect to any drug or pharmaceutical products identified, readers are advised to check the most current information provided (i) on procedures featured or (ii) by the manufacturer of each product to be administered, to verify the recommended dose or formula, the method and duration of administration, and contraindications. It is the responsibility of practitioners, relying on their own experience and knowledge of their patients, to make diagnoses, to determine dosages and the best treatment for each individual patient, and to take all appropriate safety precautions.

To the fullest extent of the law, neither the Publisher nor the authors, contributors, or editors, assume any liability for any injury and/or damage to persons or property as a matter of products liability, negligence or otherwise, or from any use or operation of any methods, products, instructions, or ideas contained in the material herein.

NANDA International, Inc.: Nursing Diagnoses --Definitions and Classification 2018–2020 © 2017 NANDA International, ISBN 978-1-62623-929-6. Used by arrangement with the Thieme Group, Stuttgart/New York.

Library and Archives Canada Cataloguing in Publication

Medical-surgical nursing in Canada : assessment and management of clinical problems / [American editors] Sharon L. Lewis, RN, PhD, FAAN, Professor Emerita, University of New Mexico, Albuquerque, New Mexico, Former Castella Distinguished Professor, School of Nursing, University of Texas Health Science Center at San Antonio, San Antonio, Texas, Developer and Consultant, Stress-Busting Program for Family Caregivers [and 3 others]; Canadian editors, Maureen A. Barry, RN, MScN, Associate Professor, Teaching Stream, Lawrence S. Bloomberg Faculty of Nursing, University of Toronto, Toronto, Ontario, Jana Lok, RN, MN, PhD, ENC(C), Assistant Professor, Teaching Stream, Lawrence S. Bloomberg Faculty of Nursing, University of Toronto, Toronto, Ontario, Jane Tyerman, RN, MScN, PhD, Professor, Trent/Fleming School of Nursing, Trent University, Peterborough, Ontario, Sandra Goldsworthy, RN, MSc, PhD, CNCC(C), CMSN(C), Associate Professor, Faculty of Nursing, University of Calgary, Calgary, Alberta.—Fourth Canadian edition.
Includes index.
Section editors, Jeffrey Kwong and Dottie Roberts.
ISBN 978-1-77172-048-9 (hardcover)

1. Nursing–Textbooks. 2. Surgical nursing—Textbooks. 3. Textbooks. I. Lewis, Sharon Lynette, editor II. Barry, Maureen, 1951-, editor III. Lok, Jana, editor IV. Tyerman, Jane, editor V. Goldsworthy, Sandra, 1961-, editor
RT41.L49 2018 610.73 C2017-906176-3

VP Medical and Canadian Education: Madelene J. Hyde
Content Strategist: Roberta A. Spinosa-Millman
Content Development Specialist: Dawn Slawecki
Publishing Services Manager: Julie Eddy
Senior Project Manager: Mary Stueck
Copy Editors: Anne Ostroff, Cathy Witlox, Sherry Hinman
Cover Design: Brett J. Miller, BJM Graphic Design & Communications
Cover Image: echo3005/Shutterstock.com
Design Direction: Ryan Cook, Ashley Miner

Elsevier Canada
420 Main Street East, Suite 636, Milton, ON Canada L9T 5G3
Phone: 416-644-7053

Printed in Canada
1 2 3 4 5   22 21 20 19 18

Ebook ISBN: 978-1-77172-050-2

Working together
to grow libraries in
developing countries

www.elsevier.com • www.bookaid.org

CONTENTS

**SECTION 2
Pathophysiological
Mechanisms
of Disease**

SECTION 3
Perioperative Care

SECTION 4
Problems Related to Altered Sensory Input

**SECTION 5
Problems of Oxygenation:
Ventilation**

SECTION 6
Problems of Oxygenation: Transport

SECTION 7
Problems of Oxygenation: Perfusion

SECTION 8
Problems of Ingestion, Digestion, Absorption, and Elimination

SECTION 9
Problems of Urinary Function

**SECTION 10
Problems Related to
Regulatory and Reproductive
Mechanisms**

SECTION 11
Problems Related to
Movement
and Coordination

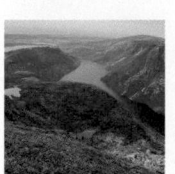

SECTION 12
Nursing Care in Specialized Settings

Appendices

SHARON L. LEWIS, RN, PhD, FAAN

Sharon Lewis received her Bachelor of Science in nursing from the University of Wisconsin–Madison, Master of Science in nursing with a minor in biological sciences from the University of Colorado–Denver, and PhD in immunology from the Department of Pathology at the University of New Mexico School of Medicine. She had a 2-year postdoctoral fellowship from the National Kidney Foundation. Her more than 45 years of teaching experience include inservice education and teaching in associate degree, baccalaureate, master's degree, and doctoral programs in Maryland, Illinois, Wisconsin, New Mexico, and Texas. Favourite teaching areas are pathophysiology, immunology, and family caregiving. She has been actively involved in clinical research for the past 35 years, investigating altered immune responses in various disorders and developing a stress management program for family caregivers. Her current primary professional responsibility is disseminating the Stress-Busting for Family Caregivers Program that she developed. Her free time is spent biking, landscaping, gardening, and being a grandmother.

LINDA BUCHER, RN, PhD, CEN, CNE

Linda Bucher is an Emerita Professor in the School of Nursing at the University of Delaware in Newark, Delaware. She received her Bachelor of Science in nursing from Thomas Jefferson University in Philadelphia, her Master of Science in adult health and illness from the University of Pennsylvania in Philadelphia, and her doctorate in nursing from Widener University in Chester, Pennsylvania. Her 40 years of nursing experience have spanned staff and patient education, acute and critical care nursing, and teaching in associate, baccalaureate, and graduate nursing programs in New Jersey, Pennsylvania, and Delaware. Her preferred teaching areas include emergency and cardiac nursing and evidence-based practice. She maintains her clinical practice by working as an emergency nurse, actively participates in the American Association of Critical Care Nurses, and volunteers as a postoperative nurse for Operation Smile. In her free time, she enjoys traveling and skiing with her family.

MARGARET MCLEAN HEITKEMPER, RN, PhD, FAAN

Margaret Heitkemper is Professor and Chairperson, Department of Biobehavioral Nursing and Health Systems at the School of Nursing, and Adjunct Professor, Division of Gastroenterology at the School of Medicine at the University of Washington. She is also Director of the National Institutes of Health-National Institute for Nursing Research–funded Center for Research on Management of Sleep Disturbances at the University of Washington. In the fall of 2006, Dr. Heitkemper was appointed the Elizabeth Sterling Soule Endowed Chair in Nursing. Dr. Heitkemper received her Bachelor of Science in nursing from Seattle University, a Master of Nursing in gerontologic nursing from the University of Washington, and a doctorate in Physiology and Biophysics from the University of Illinois–Chicago. She has been on faculty at the University of Washington since 1981 and has been the recipient of three School of Nursing Excellence in Teaching awards and the University of Washington Distinguished Teaching Award. In addition, in 2002 she received the Distinguished Nutrition Support Nurse Award from the American Society for Parenteral and Enteral Nutrition (ASPEN), in 2003 the American Gastroenterological Association and Janssen Award for Clinical Research in Gastroenterology, and in 2005 she was the first recipient of the Pfizer and Friends of the National Institutes for Nursing Research Award for Research in Women's Health.

MARIANN M. HARDING, RN, PhD, CNE

Mariann Harding is an Associate Professor of Nursing at Kent State University Tuscarawas, New Philadelphia, Ohio, where she has been on the faculty since 2005. She received her diploma in nursing from Mt. Carmel School of Nursing in Columbus, Ohio, her Bachelor of Science in nursing from Ohio University in Athens, Ohio, her Master of Science in Nursing as an adult nurse practitioner from the Catholic University of America in Washington D.C., and her doctorate in nursing from West Virginia University in Morgantown, West Virginia. Her 29 years of nursing experience has primarily been in critical care nursing, and teaching in licensed practical, associate, and baccalaureate nursing programs. She currently teaches medical-surgical nursing, health care policy, and evidence-based practice. Her research has focused on promoting student success and health promotion among individuals with gout and facing cancer. Free time is spent with her family or travelling, walking, and reading.

MAUREEN A. BARRY, RN, MScN

Maureen A. Barry is an Associate Professor, Teaching Stream, and Director, Undergraduate Program at the Lawrence S. Bloomberg Faculty of Nursing at the University of Toronto. She received her Bachelor of Science in Nursing from the University of Windsor and her Master of Science in Nursing from the University of Toronto. She has been involved in nursing education for over twenty-five years and has taught in Nova Scotia, Quebec, and Ontario. Her clinical background is adult medicine and surgery and critical care. She has extensive experience in global health, having worked for 5 years in clinics in rural Kenya and Ethiopia and taught medical English in China. More recently, she has done volunteer work while on sabbatical in Zimbabwe, South Africa, and Uganda. She currently teaches medical–surgical nursing and persistent illness. She has won the Teaching Innovation Award from the Council of

Ontario University Programs in Nursing (COUPN) as well as multiple teaching awards from the University of Toronto. Her primary areas of interest and expertise are clinical education, simulation, online learning and technology in nursing education, test theory and development, and global health issues.

JANA LOK, RN, MN, PhD, ENC(C)

Jana Lok is an Assistant Professor, Teaching Stream, for the undergraduate program at the Lawrence S. Bloomberg Faculty of Nursing at the University of Toronto. She completed her undergraduate and graduate nursing degrees at the University of Toronto. Her clinical background is in emergency and trauma nursing, as well as pre-hospital emergency care. She holds a national CNA credential in Emergency Nursing. Dr. Lok has been involved in nursing education for nearly 15 years. She has spent almost 20 years of service with the Canadian Armed Forces (CAF) as both a Medic and Nursing Officer. She has overseen the training of CAF medical service personnel who have served on national and international operations. She received the Canadian Forces Decoration and Queen's Golden Jubilee Medal in recognition for her exemplary military service. She currently teaches pathophysiology and persistent illness and is part of the simulation team for the Faculty of Nursing undergraduate program. Her areas of interest and expertise include emergency and trauma nursing, emergency preparedness and disaster management, complementary therapies, clinical teaching and simulation.

JANE TYERMAN, RN, MScN, PhD

Jane Tyerman is a nursing professor at the Trent/Fleming School of Nursing in Peterborough, Ontario. She has over 25 years of experience in acute care clinical practice and 15 years academic BScN teaching experience. She received her Bachelor of Arts from the University of Ottawa, Bachelor of Nursing from Athabasca University, and her Master of Science and PhD from Queen's University. She is an Advanced Cardiac Life Support (ACLS) and Pediatric Advanced Life Support (PALS) instructor with the Canadian Heart and Stroke Foundation. She is a Canadian Hesi Live Review Educator, in which capacity she delivers onsite personalized courses to further prepare new graduate nurses for their NCLEX board examination. Dr. Tyerman has been nominated for and received many awards for her teaching innovation and excellence. Her research and publications focus on nursing simulation design, development, curriculum implementation, and virtual simulation using serious games. She is currently the co-president of the Ontario Simulation Alliance (OSA) and the national Canadian Alliance of Nurse educators using Simulation (CAN-Sim). Other research interests include neurofeedback, the impact of shiftwork on nurses' mental health, and psychiatric nursing care practices of acute care nurses.

SANDRA GOLDSWORTHY, RN, MSc, PhD, CNCC(C), CMSN(C)

Sandra Goldsworthy is a recognized critical care expert, having worked in this field for more than 25 years. Dr. Goldsworthy received her Honours Bachelor of Science in Nursing from Lakehead University, her Masters of Science (Nursing) from Queen's University, and her doctorate in Nursing from the University of British Columbia. As an Associate Professor in the Faculty of Nursing at the University of Calgary, with a Research Professorship in Simulation Education, she is also an accomplished practitioner, researcher and author. Dr. Goldsworthy holds two national CNA credentials in Critical Care and Medical Surgical Nursing. Her research focus is simulation and transfer of learning, job readiness and transition of new graduates. She has conducted and published research involving the use of simulation and technology in nursing education. Her recent publications and national and international presentations have concentrated on critical care and technology in nursing. Dr. Goldsworthy has eight texts to her credit including all four editions of *Medical-Surgical Nursing in Canada, Simulation Simplified: A Practical Guide for Nurse Educators,* and *Arrhythmia and 12-Lead EKG Interpretation.*

SECTION EDITORS FOR THE US 10TH EDITION

Jeffrey Kwong, DNP, MPH, ANP-BC, FAANP

Jeffrey Kwong is an Assistant Professor of Nursing at Columbia University School of Nursing where he also serves as Director of the Adult-Gerontology Primary Care Nurse Practitioner Program. He has worked in the area of adult primary care with a special focus on HIV for over 20 years. He received his undergraduate degree from the University of California–Berkeley, his nurse practitioner degree from the University of California–San Francisco, and completed his doctoral training at the University of Colorado–Denver. He also has a Master's Degree in Public Health with a focus on Health Education and Behavioral Sciences from the University of Califorina–Los Angeles and was appointed a Hartford Geriatric Interprofessional Scholar while completing his gerontology education at NYU. In addition to teaching, Dr. Kwong maintains a clinical practice at Gotham Medical Group in New York City. In 2015 he was inducted as a Fellow in the American Association of Nurse Practitioners.

Dottie Roberts, RN, EdD, MSN, MACI, RN, OCNS-C, CMSRN, CNE

Dottie Roberts received her Bachelor of Science in nursing from Beth-El College of Nursing, Colorado Springs, Colorado, Master of Science in adult health nursing from Beth-El College of Nursing and Health Sciences, Master of Arts in curriculum and instruction from Colorado Christian University, Colorado Springs, Colorado, and EdD in healthcare education from Nova Southeastern University, Ft. Lauderdale, Florida. She has over 25 years of experience in medical-surgical and orthopaedic nursing, and holds certifications in both specialties. She has also taught in two baccalaureate programs in the Southeast and is certified as a nurse educator. For her dissertation, Dottie completed a phenomenological study on facilitation of critical-thinking skills by clinical faculty in a baccalaureate nursing program. She has been Executive Director of the Orthopaedic Nurses Certification Board since 2005 and editor of "*MEDSURG Nursing,*" official journal of the Academy of Medical-Surgical Nurses, since 2003. Her free time is spent travelling, reading, and cross-stitching.

CANADIAN CONTRIBUTORS

Shohreh Abrouie, NP, BA Psy, MN
Clinical Nurse Specialist
Mount Sinai Hospital
Toronto, Ontario

Karen Baguley, RN, MScN
Nurse Manager
St. Joseph's Healthcare
Hamilton, Ontario

Maureen A. Barry, RN, MScN
Associate Professor, Teaching Stream
Lawrence S. Bloomberg Faculty of Nursing
University of Toronto
Toronto, Ontario

Jenifer Bennett, RN, BScN
Unit Manager
Edmonton Adult Bariatric Clinic, Surgical
    Revision Clinic, Thrombosis Clinic
Royal Alexandra Hospital
Edmonton, Alberta

Veronique M. Boscart, RN, MScN, MEd, PhD
CIHR/Schlegel Industrial Research Chair for
    Colleges in Seniors Care
School of Health & Life Sciences and
    Community Services
Conestoga College Institute of Technology
    and Advanced Learning
Kitchener, Ontario

Phil Bourget, BA (soc), BScN, MN
Professor, Nursing
Georgian College
Barrie, Ontario

Rosemary Cashman, MA, MSc(A), NP(A)
Nurse Practitioner
BC Cancer Agency
Vancouver, British Columbia

Erica Cambly, RN, MN
Assistant Professor, Teaching Stream
Lawrence S. Bloomberg Faculty of Nursing
University of Toronto
Toronto, Ontario

George Charames, PhD
Director, Molecular Diagnostics Laboratory
Pathology and Laboratory Medicine
Mount Sinai Hospital
Toronto, Ontario

Susan Chernenko, RN(EC), MN, NP
Clinical Practice Leader/Program
    Development
Toronto Lung Transplant Program, MOT
Toronto General Hospital, UHN
Toronto, Ontario

Beth Clarke, RN, MSc(A), MBA, CWOCN
Clinical Instructor, Nursing
Boston College
Boston, Massachusetts
Formerly at Bridgepoint Health
Toronto, Ontario

Debra Clendinneng, BScN, RN, MEd, PhD
Professor
Health and Community Studies
Algonquin College
Ottawa, Ontario

Shelley L. Cobbett, RN, BN, GnT, MN, EdD
Assistant Professor, Nursing
Dalhousie University
Yarmouth, Nova Scotia

Daphne Connolly, RN, MN
Nurse Educator
School of Nursing
St. Francis Xavier University
Antigonish, Nova Scotia

Kathy Danzinger, RN, BHAdmn
Program Manager
Ambulatory Care CDM
Royal Alexandra Hospital
Edmonton, Alberta

Denise Elliott, RN, BNSc, MN, CNCC(c)
Registered Nurse
Trauma and Neurosurgery Intensive Care Unit
St. Michael's Hospital
Toronto, Ontario

Mary Ann Fegan, RN, BNSc, MN
Associate Professor, Teaching Stream
Undergraduate Clinical Education
    Coordinator
Lawrence S. Bloomberg Faculty of Nursing
University of Toronto
Toronto, Ontario

Julie H. Fraser, RN, BSN, MN, GNC(c)
Clinical Nurse Specialist
Abbotsford and Mission Communities
Fraser Health
Abbotsford, British Columbia

Sandra Goldsworthy, RN, MSc, PhD, CNCC(C), CMSN(C)
Associate Dean Teaching-Learning and
    Technology;
Associate Professor
Research Professorship in Simulation
Faculty of Nursing
University of Calgary
Calgary, Alberta

Jackie Hartigan-Rogers, RN, MN
Adjunct Assistant Professor
Nursing
Dalhousie University
Yarmouth, Nova Scotia

Kimberly Hellmer, BN, MN
Clinical Nurse Educator
Safe Clinical Practice Program
Alberta Health Services
Calgary, Alberta

Shelly W. Hutchinson, RN, BSN, MN, CRE
COPD Nurse Clinician
LiveWell COPD Program
Saskatoon Health Region
Saskatoon, Saskatchewan

Lynn Jansen, RN, PhD
Associate Dean
College of Nursing, Southern Saskatchewan
    Campus
University of Saskatchewan
Regina, Saskatchewan

Sarah L. Johnston, RN, MN
Lecturer
Lawrence S. Bloomberg Faculty of Nursing
University of Toronto
Toronto, Ontario

Annemarie F. Kaan, RN, MCN, CCN(C)
Clinical Nurse Specialist—Acute and
    Chronic Heart Failure
Adjunct Professor
University of British Columbia School
    of Nursing
St Paul's Hospital
Vancouver, British Columbia

Jacqueline Klemann, RN, ACNP, MSN
Acute Care Nurse Practitioner
Alberta Health Services
Rockyview General Hospital and Peter
    Lougheed Hospital
Calgary, Alberta

Judy Knighton, RN, MScN
Clinical Nurse Specialist–Burns
Ross Tilley Burn Centre
Sunnybrook Health Sciences Centre
Toronto, Ontario

Salima Ladak, BScN, MN, PhD
Adjunct Lecturer, Lawrence S. Bloomberg
    Faculty of Nursing
University of Toronto;
Nurse Practitioner, Toronto General Hospital
    Acute Pain Service
Toronto, Ontario

Jana Lok, RN, MN, PhD, ENC(C)
Assistant Professor, Teaching Stream
Lawrence S. Bloomberg Faculty of Nursing
University of Toronto
Toronto, Ontario

Bridgette Lord, RN, MN, NP–Adult
Clinical Lead, Gattuso Rapid Diagnostic
    Centre
Princess Margaret Cancer Centre
Toronto, Ontario

**Marian Luctkar-Flude, RN, BScN,
    MScN, PhD**
Assistant Professor
School of Nursing
Queen's University
Kingston, Ontario

Lesley MacMaster, RN, BScN, MSc
Nursing Professor
York University/Georgian/Seneca
    Collaborative BScN Program
Health, Wellness and Sciences
Georgian College
Barrie, Ontario

Jane McCall, MSN, RN, PhD (c)
Nursing
University of Alberta
Edmonton, Alberta

Lynn McCleary, RN, BSc, MSc, PhD
Associate Professor, Nursing
Brock University
St. Catharines, Ontario

Susannah McGeachy, NP-PHC, MN
Nurse Practitioner
Al and Malka Green Artists' Health Centre
Toronto Western Hospital
Toronto, Ontario

Michael McGillion, BScN, RN, PhD
Associate Professor, Nursing
McMaster University
Hamilton, Ontario

Andrea Miller, MHSc, RD
Registered Dietitian
Faculty of Health Sciences
University of Ontario Institute of
    Technology
Oshawa, Ontario

**Tess Montada-Atin, BScN, MN, NP-Adult,
    CDE, CNeph(C)**
Nurse Practitioner-Adult
Nephrology, Diabetes Comprehensive Care
    Program
St. Michael's Hospital
Toronto, Ontario

Andrea Mowry, BScN, MN, CHPCN(C)
Faculty
Trent Fleming School of Nursing
Trent University
Peterborough, Ontario

**Sheila O'Keefe-McCarthy RN, BScN,
    MN, PhD**
Assistant Professor
Department of Nursing
Brock University
St. Catharine's, Ontario

Denise Ouellette, RN, MSN, CNN(C)
Clinical Nurse Specialist for the Stroke
    Network
General Internal Medicine Program
St Michael's Hospital
Toronto, Ontario

Verna C. Pangman, RN, MEd, MN
Senior Instructor
College of Nursing
University of Manitoba,
Winnipeg, Manitoba

Janet A. Piper, RN, MScN
Nursing Simulation Lab Specialist
Health and Wellness Programs
Sault College
Sault Ste. Maric, Ontario

Micki Puksa, BScN, MScN, PhD(C)
Nursing Professor
School of Health and Wellness
Georgian College
Barrie, Ontario

**Debbie Rickeard, BA, RN, BScN, MSN,
    CCRN, CNE**
Experiential Learning Specialist
Faculty of Nursing
University of Windsor
Windsor, Ontario

**Sheila Rizza, RN(EC), MN NP-Adult,
    CNCC(C), CCN(C)**
Nurse Practitioner
Heart Function Clinic
Trillium Health Partners
Mississauga, Ontario

Kathleen Rodger, RN, BSN, MN
Assistant Professor
College of Nursing
University of Saskatchewan
Regina, Saskatchewan

Ruby Sangha, BSc, BScN, MN, NP-PHC
Nurse Practitioner
Odette Cancer Centre
Sunnybrook Health Sciences Centre
Toronto, Ontario

Angela Sarro RN(EC), MN, CNN(c)
Nurse Practitioner–Adult Spine Program
Practice Leader, Krembil Neuroscience
    Program
Toronto Western Hospital
Toronto, Ontario

Kara Sealock, RN, BN, MEd, CNCC(C)
Nursing Instructor
Faculty of Nursing
University of Calgary
Calgary, Alberta

Cydnee Seneviratne, RN, PhD
Associate Dean Undergraduate Practice
    Education/Senior Instructor
Faculty of Nursing
University of Calgary
Calgary, Alberta

Rani H. Srivastava, RN, MScN, PhD
Chief of Nursing and Professional Practice
Centre for Addiction and Mental Health;
Assistant Professor
Lawrence Bloomberg Faculty of Nursing
Associate Member, School of Graduate
    Studies
University of Toronto;
Adjunct Professor
York University School of Nursing
Toronto, Ontario

**Holly Symonds-Brown, RN, MSN,
    CPMHN**
Faculty, Nursing
MacEwan University
Edmonton, Alberta

Catherine A. Thibeault, RN, PhD
Assistant Professor
Trent/Fleming School of Nursing
Trent University
Peterborough, Ontario

Jane Tyerman, RN, MScN, PhD
Nursing Professor
Trent/Fleming School of Nursing
Peterborough, Ontario

Christina Vaillancourt, MHSc, RD, CDE
Patient Care Manager Regional Nephrology
    Program
Lakeridge Health
Oshawa, Ontario

Françoise Verville, RN(NP), MN, AGD-NP
Collaborative Nurse Practitioner Program
Saskatchewan Polytechnic
Regina, Saskatchewan

Ellen Vogel, PhD, RD, FDC
Associate Professor
Faculty of Health Sciences
University of Ontario Institute of
    Technology
Oshawa, Ontario

Colina Yim, RN(EC), BScN, MN
Nurse Practitioner
Hepatology
University Health Network
Toronto, Ontario

Maysam Youssef, BSc
Consulting Dietitian
Private Practice
Whitby, Ontario

CONTRIBUTORS TO THE US 10TH EDITION

Richard B. Arbour, RN, MSN, CCRN, CNRN, CCNS, FAAN
Clinical Faculty
School of Nursing
LaSalle University
Philadelphia, Pennsylvania

Adena Bargad, RN, PhD, CNM
Assistant Professor, Columbia University
    Medical Center
Director, Sub-Specialty Program in Women's
    Health
Columbia University School of Nursing
New York, New York

Diana Taibi Buchanan, RN, PhD
Associate Professor
Biobehavioral Nursing and Health Systems
University of Washington
Seattle, Washington

Darcy Burbage, RN, MSN, AOCN, CBCN
Survivorship Nurse Navigator
Helen F. Graham Cancer Center and
    Research Institute
Newark, Delaware

Kim K. Choma, RN, DNP, WHNP
Women's Health Nurse Practitioner–Training
    Consultant
NY/NJ AIDS Education and Training
    Centers (AETC)
New York, New York

Susan Collazo, MSN, APN-CNP
Thoracic Surgery
Northwestern Memorial Hospital
Chicago, Illinois

Paula P. Cox-North, PhD, ARNP
Clinical Assistant Professor
School of Nursing
University of Washington School of Nursing
Seattle, Washington

Hazel A. Dennison, RN, DNP, APNc, CPHQ, CNE
Director of Education Services
American Nephrology Nurses Association
Anthony J. Jannetti, Pub.
Pitman, New Jersey

Jane K. Dickinson, RN, PhD, CDE
Program Coordinator/Faculty
Diabetes Education and Management
Teachers College
Columbia University
New York, New York

Rose Ann DiMaria-Ghalili, RN, PhD, CNSC
Associate Professor of Nursing
College of Nursing and Health Professions
Drexel University
Philadelphia, Pennsylvania

Mechele Fillman, RN, MSN
Nursing Practitioner
Pain Management
Stanford Healthcare
Palo Alto, California

Diana L. Gallagher, RN, MS, CWOCN, CFCN
Clinical Nursing and Education
HealthMatters Consulting
Fayetteville, Arkansas

Sherry A. Greenberg, RN, PhD, GNP-BC
Coordinator, Advanced Practice Nursing:
    Geriatrics Program
Hartford Institute for Geriatric Nursing
New York University College of Nursing
New York, New York

Angela DiSabatino Herman, RN, MS
Manager, Cardiovascular Clinical Trials
Christiana Care Health Services
Newark, Delaware

Christine R. Hoch, RN, MSN
Nursing Instructor
University of Delaware
Newark, Delaware

David M. Horner, CRNA, MS, APN
CRNA Anesthesia
Marlton Hospital
Marlton, New Jersey

Melissa L. Hutchinson, RN, MN, CCNS, CCRN
Clinical Nurse Specialist
MICU/CCU
VA Puget Sound Health Care System
Seattle, Washington

Katherine A. Kelly, RN, DNP, FNP-C, CEN
Assistant Professor of Nursing
California State University
Sacramento, California

Judy Knighton, RN, MScN
Clinical Nurse Specialist—Burns
Ross Tilley Burn Centre
Sunnybrook Health Sciences Centre
Toronto, Ontario

Nancy Kupper, RN, MSN
Associate Professor of Nursing
Tarrant County College
Fort Worth, Texas

Janet Lenart, RN, MN, MPH
Senior Lecturer and Director for Online
    Education
University of Washington School of Nursing
Seattle, Washington

Linda Littlejohns, RN, MSN, CNRN, FAAN
Neuroscience Clinical Nursing Consultant
San Juan Capistrano, California

Amy McKeever, PhD, CRNP, WHNP-BC
Assistant Professor
College of Nursing
Villanova University
Villanova, Pennsylvania

De Ann F. Mitchell, RN, PhD
Director of Nursing
Tarrant County College
Fort Worth, Texas

Carolyn Moffa, RN, MSN, FNP-C, CHFN
Clinical Leader, Heart Failure Program
Christiana Care Health System
Newark, Delaware

Eugene E. Mondor, RN, MN, CNCC(C)
Clinical Nurse Educator—Adult
   Critical Care
Royal Alexandra Hospital
Edmonton, Alberta

Janice A. Neil, RN, PhD
Associate Professor and Chair
Undergraduate Nursing Science Junior
   Division
College of Nursing
East Carolina University
Greenville, North Carolina

**Suzanne Teresa Parsell, MSN, ANP-BC,
   CUNP**
Division of Endourology
University of Michigan
Ann Arbor, Michigan

**Madona Dawn Plueger, RN, MSN,
   ACNS-BC, CNRN**
Neuroscience Clinical Nurse Specialist
Barrow Neurological Institute
St. Joseph's Hospital and Medical Center
Phoenix, Arizona

Carolee Polek, RN, PhD, AOCNS, BMTCN
Associate Professor
School of Nursing
University of Delaware
Newark, Delaware

Rosemary C. Polomano, RN, PhD, FAAN
Professor of Pain Practice
Department of Biobehavioral Health
   Sciences
University of Pennsylvania School of
   Nursing;
Professor of Anesthesiology and Critical
   Care (Secondary)
University of Pennsylvania Perelman School
   of Medicine
Philadelphia, Pennsylvania

**Matthew C. Price, RN, MS, CNP,
   ONP-C, RNFA**
Manager, Orthopedic Advanced Practice
   Providers Orthopedics
Riverside Methodist Hospital
Columbus, Ohio

**Susanne A. Quallich, RN, MSN, ANP-BC,
   NP-C, CUNP**
Andrology Nurse Practitioner
Urology
University of Michigan Health System
Ann Arbor, Michigan

**Kathleen A. Rich, RN, PhD, CCNS,
   CCRN-CSC, CNN**
Cardiovascular Clinical Specialist
Patient Care Services
IU Health La Porte Hospital
La Porte, Indiana

Sandra Irene Rome, RN, MN, AOCN, CNS
Clinical Nurse Specialist
Blood and Marrow Transplant Program
Cedars-Sinai Medical Center
Los Angeles, California

Jennifer Saylor, RN, PhD, ACNS-BC
Assistant Professor
School of Nursing
University of Delaware
Newark, Delaware

**Maureen A. Seckel, RN, MSN, APN,
   ACNS-BC, CCNS, CCRN**
Clinical Nurse Specialist
Medical Pulmonary Critical Care
Christiana Care Health System
Newark, Delaware

Rose Shaffer, RN, MSN, ACNP-CS, CCRN
Cardiology Nurse Practitioner
Thomas Jefferson University Hospital
Philadelphia, Pennsylvania

Anita Jo Shoup, RN, MSN, CNOR
Perioperative Clinical Nurse Specialist
Swedish Edmonds
Edmonds, Washington

Cindy M. Sullivan, MN, ANP-C, CNRN
Nurse Practitioner
Neurosurgery
Barrow Neurological Institute
Phoenix, Arizona

Linda A. L. Upchurch, DNP, ANP-BC
Assistant Professor
School of Nursing
Georgia Southern University
Statesboro, Georgia

Deidre D. Wipke-Tevis, RN, PhD
Associate Professor
PhD Program Director
MU Sinclair School of Nursing
University of Missouri
Columbia, Missouri

Mary K. Wollan, RN, BAN, ONC
Orthopaedic Nurse Educator
Excelen
Minneapolis, Minnesota

Kathy H. Wu, MSN, ANP-BC
Nurse Practitioner
Liver Transplant Center
New York Columbia Presbyterian Hospital
New York, New York

Meg Zomorodi, RN, PhD, CNL
Clinical Associate Professor
School of Nursing
University of North Carolina at Chapel Hill
Chapel Hill, North Carolina

**Michael E. Zychowicz, RN, DNP, ANP,
   ONP, FAAN, FAANP**
Associate Professor and Director, MSN
   Program
School of Nursing
Duke University
Durham, North Carolina

Marsha Astrop, RN, BScN, MScN
Professor
Centennial College
Toronto, Ontario

Crystal D. Avolio, RN, BScN, MSc
Professor of Nursing
St. Clair College
Windsor, Ontario

Monique Bacher, RN, BScN, MSN/Ed
Professor
Practical Nursing Program
Sally Horsfall Eaton School of Nursing
George Brown College
Toronto, Ontario

Jasmine Balakumaran, RN, BScN, MScN
Faculty
Community of Health Studies
Centennial College
Toronto, Ontario

Andrea Barron, BN, RN, MN
Nurse Educator
Centre for Nursing Studies
St. John's, Newfoundland and Labrador

Renée Berquist, RN, BScN, MN, PhD(c)
Professor
School of Baccalaureate Nursing
St. Lawrence College
Brockville, Ontario

Catherine Bock, RN, BScN, MAED
Faculty, BSN Program
Faculty of Health
Kwantlen Polytechnic University
Surrey, British Columbia

Diane Browman, RN, BScN
Nursing Instructor
Faculty of Nursing
John Abbott College
Sainte-Anne-de-Bellevue, Quebec

**Elizabeth A. Brownlee, MA,
    NP-PHC, MScN**
Professor
Health Sciences
Northern College of Applied Arts and
    Technology
Kirkland Lake, Ontario

**Mona Burrows, RN(EC), BScN, MScN,
    PHC-NP, PhD(c)**
Professor
Collaborative BScN program
St. Lawrence College/Laurentian University
Cornwall, Ontario

Patricia Connick, RegN CNCC(c)
Clinical Educator
Muskoka Algonquin Healthcare
Bracebridge, Ontario

Tracey Fallak, RN, BScN, MN
Course Leader
Nursing
Red River College
Winnipeg, Manitoba

Judith Findlay, RN, BScN, MEd
Nursing Professor
John Abbott College
Montreal, Quebec

Natasha Fontaine, RN, BN
Nurse Educator–Practical Nursing
College of the Rockies
Cranbrook, British Columbia

Laurie Freeman-Gibb, BScN, MSN, PhD
Assistant Professor
Faculty of Nursing
University of Windsor
Windsor, Ontario

Sandra Fritz, RN, BN, MN
Nursing Instructor
Division of Science and Health
Medicine Hat College
Medicine Hat, Alberta

Vernon-John Gibbins, MS, BScN, RN
Faculty Lecturer
Faculty of Nursing
University of Alberta
Edmonton, Alberta

**Odette Griscti, RN, BSc(Hons),
    MHSc, PhD**
Associate Professor
Cape Breton University
1250 Grand Lake Road
Sydney, Nova Scotia

Monica Gola RN MN CPMHN(c)
Undergraduate Program Director
School of Nursing
York University
Toronto, Ontario

Kate Hardie, RN, EdD
Associate Professor, Teaching Stream
Lawrence S. Bloomberg Faculty of Nursing
University of Toronto
Toronto, Ontario

Kerry-Anne Hogan, RN, PhD
Professor
Faculty of Health Sciences
University of Ottawa
Ottawa, Ontario

**Tania N. Killian, BScN, Bed, MEd,
    RN, CCN**
Professor
School of Health Sciences
Seneca College
Toronto, Ontario

Jutta Kurtz, RN, BScN, DE
Faculty, Nursing
Cégep Heritage College
Gatineau, Quebec

Suzanne Larochelle, RN, BScN, MEd
Teacher
Nursing Faculty
Cégep Heritage College
Gatineau, Quebec

Nicole L'Italien, RN, BScN, MN
Nursing Faculty
School of Health Sciences
College of New Caledonia
Prince George, British Columbia

Brenda Lays, RN, MScN
Nursing Instructor
Faculty of Nursing
University of Calgary
Calgary, Alberta

Jana Lok, RN, MN, PhD, ENC(C)
Assistant Professor, Teaching Stream
Lawrence S. Bloomberg Faculty of Nursing
University of Toronto
Toronto, Ontario

Tara Mackenzie-Clark, RN, MSc
Nursing Instructor
College of New Caledonia
Prince George, British Columbia

Monique Mallet-Boucher, RN, Med, MN, PhD
Senior Teaching Associate
Nursing
University of New Brunswick
Moncton, New Brunswick

April Manuel, RN, BN, MN, PhD
Assistant Professor
Faculty of Nursing
Memorial University of Newfoundland
St. John's, Newfoundland and Labrador

Karen Mason, RN, BSN, MN
Nursing Faculty
North Island College
Courtenay, British Columbia

Andrea Miller, RN, BScN, MA
Professor, Nursing
McMaster-Mohawk-Conestoga Collaborative
   BScN Program
Conestoga College
Kitchener, Ontario

Brenda Mishak, RN(NP) BSN, MN, PhD, CCHN(C)
Assistant Professor, Academic Programming
College of Nursing
University of Saskatchewan
Prince Albert, Saskatchewan

Melanic Neumeier, RN, BScN, MN
Assistant Professor, BScN Program
Faculty of Health and Community Studies
MacEwan University
Edmonton, Alberta

Tia L. Nymark, RN, BScN
Instructor, Faculty of Nursing
John Abbott College
Sainte Anne de Bellevue, Quebec

Cindy A. Olexson, RN BScN MN
Lecturer
University of Saskatchewan
Saskatoon, Saskatchewan

Brenda Orazietti, RN, BScN, CNCC(C), MEd
Lecturer, Course Director
Department of Nursing
York University
Toronto, Ontario

Beverly Pongracz, RN, MN
Faculty, Saskatchewan Bachelor of Science in
   Nursing
Saskatchewan Polytechnic
Adjunct Professor, University of Regina
Regina, Saskatchewan

Katherine Poser, RN, BScN, MNEd
Professor
School of Baccalaureate Nursing
St. Lawrence College
Kingston, Ontario

Julie Rivers, RN, BScN, MEd
Professor
Brock-Loyalist Collaborative Baccalaureate
   Nursing Program
Loyalist College
Belleville, Ontario

Margot Rykhoff, RN, BScN, MA(Ed), PhD(C)
Professor
University of New Brunswick/Humber ITAL
   Collaborative Nursing Degree Program
School of Health Sciences
Humber Institute of Technology & Advanced
   Learning
Toronto, Ontario

Karolle Saint Jean, RN, BScN, MEd
Nursing Faculty
Dawson College
Montreal, Quebec

Lynne Thibeault, NP-PHC, HBcN, MEd, DNP
Health Sciences Professor
Confederation College
Thunder Bay, Ontario

Joyce Thibodeau, RN, MSN
Faculty, Bachelor of Science in Nursing
   Program
Kwantlen Polytechnic University
Langley, British Columbia

Bonny Townsend, RN, BScN, MSN
Nursing Instructor
Faculty of Nursing and Health Studies
Grande Prairie Regional College
Grande Prairie, Alberta

Jane Tyerman, RN, MScN, PhD
Nursing Professor
Trent/Fleming School of Nursing
Trent University

Yvonne Mayne Wilkin, RN, BScN, MSc, CEFP, EdD
Faculty, Nursing
Champlain College Lennoxville
Sherbrooke, Quebec

To the Profession of Nursing and to the Important People in Our Lives

Sharon

My husband Peter and our grandchildren Malia, Halle, Aidan, Cian, Layla, Ryker, and Archer

Linda

My nieces, Stefany and Jayme, who so admirably reflect the ideals of the nursing profession and my godchild, Liz, for her love of written words.

Margaret

My husband David, our daughters Elizabeth and Ellen, and our grandsons Jaxon James and Axel

Mariann

My husband Jeff and our daughters Kate and Sarah

Maureen

My students past, present, and future.

Jana

To Shannon, who inspired me to become a nurse, and my family, colleagues and friends for your ongoing love and support.

Jane

My husband Glenn, our children Kaitlyn, Kelsey, and Aiden, my mother Jessica.

Sandra

My husband Brian and our three sons Ryan, Matthew, and Kent for always being there for me.

The Fourth Canadian Edition of *Medical-Surgical Nursing in Canada: Assessment and Management of Clinical Problems* has been thoroughly revised for the Canadian student and incorporates the most current medical-surgical nursing information presented in an easy-to-use format. More than just a textbook, this is a comprehensive resource set in the Canadian context, containing essential information that nursing students need to prepare for lectures, classroom activities, examinations, clinical assignments, and the safe, comprehensive care of patients. In addition to the readable writing style and full-colour illustrations, the text and accompanying resources include many special features to help students learn key medical-surgical nursing content, such as sections that highlight the determinants of health, patient and caregiver teaching, age-related considerations, collaborative care, cultural considerations, nutrition, home care, evidence-informed practice, patient safety, and much more.

The comprehensive content, special features, attractive layout, and student-friendly writing style combine to make this the number one medical-surgical nursing textbook, used in more nursing schools in Canada than any other medical-surgical nursing textbook.

The latest edition of *Medical-Surgical Nursing in Canada* retains the strengths of the first three editions, including the use of the nursing process as an organizational theme for nursing management. New features have been added to address some of the rapid changes in practice, and many diagrams and photos are new or improved. The content has been updated using the most recent important research and newest practice guidelines by Canadian contributors selected for their acknowledged excellence in specific content areas, ensuring a continuous thread of evidence-informed practice throughout the text. Specialists in the subject area have reviewed each chapter to ensure accuracy, and the editors have undertaken final rewriting and editing to achieve internal consistency. In other words, all efforts have been made to build on the recognized strengths of the previous Canadian editions.

ORGANIZATION

The content of this book is organized in two major divisions. The first division, Section 1 (Chapters 1 through 13), discusses concepts related to adult patients. The second division, Sections 2 through 12 (Chapters 14 through 72), presents nursing assessment and nursing management of medical-surgical problems.

The various body systems are grouped in such a way as to reflect their interrelated functions. Each section is organized around two central themes: assessment and management. Each chapter that deals with the assessment of a body system includes a discussion of the following:

1. A brief review of anatomy and physiology, focusing on information that will promote understanding of nursing care
2. Health history and noninvasive physical assessment skills to expand the knowledge base on which decisions are made
3. Common diagnostic studies, expected results, and related nursing responsibilities to provide easily accessible information
   Management chapters focus on the pathophysiology, clinical manifestations, laboratory and diagnostic study results,

collaborative care, and nursing management of various diseases and disorders. Nursing management sections are organized into assessment, nursing diagnoses, planning, implementation, and evaluation sections, following the steps of the nursing process. To emphasize the importance of patient care in various clinical settings, nursing implementation of all major health problems is organized by the following levels of care:

1. Health promotion
2. Acute intervention
3. Ambulatory and home care

CLASSIC FEATURES

- **Canadian context.** Once again, we are pleased to offer you a book that reflects the wide range of expertise of nurses from across Canada. In an effort to better reflect the nursing environments across the country, all chapters have been revised with enhanced Canadian research and statistics. SI units and metric measurements are used throughout the text, and the updated APA format, including digital object identifiers (DOIs), is used for the references.
- **Most recent research and clinical guidelines**. Every effort has been made to use the most recent research, statistics, and clinical guidelines available. References older than 5 years at the time of writing are included because they were seminal studies, or remain the most recent, authoritative source. Those references are marked "Seminal" in the References list.
- **Nursing management** is presented in a consistent and comprehensive format, with headings for Health Promotion, Acute Intervention, and Ambulatory and Home Care. In addition, over 60 customizable **Nursing Care Plans** on the Evolve website and in the text help students to understand possible nursing diagnoses, goals and nursing interventions for each condition.
- **Collaborative care** is highlighted in special Collaborative Care sections in each of the management chapters and in Collaborative Care tables throughout the text.
- **Patient and caregiver teaching** is an ongoing theme throughout the text. Chapter 4: *Patient and Caregiver Teaching* and numerous **Patient & Caregiver Teaching Guides** throughout the text emphasize the increasing importance and prevalence of patient management of chronic illnesses and conditions and the role of the caregiver in patient care.
- **Culturally competent care** is treated in Chapter 2, *Cultural Competence and Health Equity in Nursing Care,* which discusses the necessity for culturally competent nursing care; culture as a determinant of health, with particular reference to Indigenous populations; health equity and health equality issues as they relate to marginalized groups in Canada; and practical suggestions for developing cultural competence in nursing care.
- **Coverage of prioritization** includes:
  - Prioritization questions in case studies and Review Questions
  - Nursing diagnoses and interventions throughout the text listed in order of priority

- **Focused Assessment boxes** in all assessment chapters provide brief checklists that help students do a more practical "assessment on the run" or bedside approach to assessment.
- **Safety Alerts** highlight important safety issues in relation to patient care as they arise.
- **Pathophysiology Maps** outline complex concepts related to diseases in flowchart format, making them easier to understand.
- **Community-based nursing and home care** are also emphasized in this Fourth Canadian Edition. Chapter 6 contains a comprehensive discussion, which is continued throughout the text.
- **Determinants of Health boxes** focus on the determinants of health as outlined by Health Canada and the Public Health Agency of Canada, as they affect a particular disorder. The determinants are introduced and discussed in detail in Chapter 1, and then returned to throughout the text by way of Determinants of Health boxes, which have been extensively updated and revised for the new edition. Each box identifies a health issue specific to the chapter, lists the relevant determinants affecting the issue, supported by the most recent research, and includes references for further investigation.
- **Extensive drug therapy content** includes Drug Therapy tables and concise new **Drug Alerts** highlighting important safety considerations for key drugs.
- **Chronic illness,** which has become Canada's most pressing health care challenge, is discussed in depth in Chapter 5. Nurses are increasingly called on to be active and engaged partners in assisting patients with chronic conditions to live well; this chapter places chronic illness within the larger context of Canadian society.
- **Older adults** are covered in detail in Chapter 7, and are discussed throughout the text under the headings "Age-Related Considerations," and also in **Age-Related Differences in Assessment tables**.
- **Nutrition** is highlighted throughout the book, particularly in Chapter 42, *Nutritional Problems*, and in **Nutritional Therapy tables** throughout that summarize nutritional interventions and promote healthy lifestyles for patients with various health problems. Chapter 43, *Obesity*, looks in depth at this major factor contributing to so many other pathologies.
- **Complementary and alternative therapies** are discussed in Chapter 12, which addresses timely issues in today's health care settings related to these therapies, and in Complementary & Alternative Therapies boxes where relevant throughout the rest of the book that summarize what nurses need to know about therapies such as herbal remedies, acupuncture, and biofeedback, etc.
- **Sleep and sleep disorders** are explored in Chapter 9; they are key topics that impact multiple disorders and body systems, as well as nearly every aspect of daily functioning.
- **Genetics in Clinical Practice boxes** build on the foundation of Chapter 15, and highlight genetic screening and testing, as well as the clinical implications of key genetic disorders that affect adults, as rapid advances in the field of genetics continue to change the way nurses practise.
- **Ethical Dilemmas boxes** promote critical thinking with regard to timely and sensitive issues that nursing students deal with in clinical practice such as informed consent, treatment decision making, advance directives, and confidentiality.
- **Emergency Management tables** outline the emergency treatment of health problems that are most likely to require rapid intervention.

- **Assessment Abnormalities tables** in the assessment chapters alert the nursing student to abnormalities frequently encountered in practice, as well as their possible etiologies.
- **Nursing Assessment tables** summarize important subjective and objective data related to common diseases, with a sharper focus on issues most relevant to the body system under review. This focus provides for more rapid identification of salient assessment parameters and more effective use of student time.
- **Health History tables** in assessment chapters present relevant questions related to a specific disease or disorder that will be asked in patient interviews.
- **Student-friendly pedagogy:**
  - **Learning Objectives** at the beginning of each chapter help students identify the key content for a specific body system or disorder.
  - **Key Terms** lists provide a list of the chapter's most important terms and where they are discussed in the chapter. A comprehensive key terms **Glossary** with definitions may be found at the end of the book.
  - **Electronic Resources** sections at the start of each chapter draw students' attention to the wealth of supplemental content and exercises provided on the Evolve website, making it easier than ever for them to integrate the textbook content with media supplements such as animations, video and audio clips, interactive case studies, and much more.
  - **Case Studies** with photos bring patients to life. Management chapters have case studies at the end of the chapters that help students learn how to prioritize care and manage patients in the clinical setting. Unfolding case studies are included in each assessment chapter. Discussion questions that focus on prioritization and evidence-informed practice are included in most case studies. Answer guidelines are provided on the Evolve website.
  - **Review Questions** at the end of the chapter correspond to the Learning Objectives at the beginning, and thus help reinforce the important points in the chapter. Answers are provided on the same page, making the Review Questions a convenient self-study tool.
  - **Resources** at the end of each chapter contain links to nursing and health care organizations and tools that provide patient teaching and information on diseases and disorders.

NEW FEATURES

In addition to the classic strengths of this text, we are pleased to include several exciting new features:

- *New* **Unfolding assessment case** studies in every assessment chapter are an engaging tool to help students apply nursing concepts in real-life patient care. Appearing in three or four parts throughout the chapter, they introduce a patient, and then follow that patient through subjective and objective assessment to diagnostic studies and results, and include additional discussion questions to facilitate critical thinking.
- *New* **Expanded evidence-informed practice content** includes new *Translating Research into Practice* boxes that challenge students to develop critical thinking skills and apply the best available evidence to patient care scenarios; updated *Research Highlight* boxes that explore recent research in greater depth; and evidence-informed practice questions in many case studies.
- *New* **Informatics boxes** throughout the text reflect the current use and importance of technology, and touch on everything

from the proper handling of social media in the context of patient privacy, to teaching patients to manage self-care using smartphone apps, to using smart infusion pumps.

- *New* **Drug Alerts** concisely highlight important safety considerations for key drugs.
- **Safety Alerts** have been expanded throughout the book to cover surveillance for high-risk situations.
- *New* **art** enhances the book's visual appeal and lends a more contemporary look throughout.
- *Revised* **Chapter 1:** *Introduction to Medical-Surgical Nursing Practice in Canada* situates nursing practice within the unique societal contexts that continue to shape the profession of nursing in Canada. Patient-centred care, interprofessional practice and information-communication technologies are forces that have an impact on and are affected by nurses. This chapter has a new section on patient safety and quality improvement. The teamwork and interprofessional collaboration content has also been expanded to include delegation and assignment.
- *Revised* **Chapter 15:** *Genetics* has been substantially expanded to include current changes in Canadian clinical practice, such as the use of Non-Invasive Prenatal Testing (NIPT) for the detection of genetic disorders in the developing fetus; as well as promising advancements in gene therapy strategies, such as the advent of a genome editing technology, CRISPR-Cas9.

A WORD ON TERMINOLOGY

As a result of the Truth and Reconciliation Commission (TRC) recommendations, we have used the term "Indigenous peoples" when referring to First Nations, Inuit, and Métis populations in Canada as a whole. The term "Aboriginal" is no longer used as it does not recognize the inherent rights or treaty rights of the various groups.

A WORD ON LABORATORY VALUES

SI units are used for the laboratory values cited throughout the textbook. **Appendix B:** *Laboratory Values* lists SI units first, followed by U.S. conventional units in parentheses in all relevant instances. It is important to note that reference ranges for laboratory values may vary among laboratories, depending on the testing techniques used. If discrepancies should exist between the body of the text and Appendix B, the appendix should be considered the final authority.

LEARNING SUPPLEMENTS FOR THE STUDENT

- The handy **Clinical Companion** presents approximately 200 common medical–surgical conditions and procedures in a concise, alphabetical format for quick clinical reference. Designed for portability, this popular reference includes the essential, need-to-know information for treatments and procedures for which nurses play a major role. An attractive and functional four-colour design highlights key information for quick, easy reference. This edition features a strong focus on treatments and procedures in which the nurse plays a major role.
- **Evolve Student Resources** are available online at http://evolve. elsevier.com/Canada/Lewis/medsurg and include the following valuable learning aids that are organized by chapter:

- 45 Interactive **Student Case Studies** with state-of-the-art animations and a variety of learning activities that provide students with immediate feedback
- Printable **Key Points** summaries for each chapter
- 560+ **Review Questions**
- **Answer guidelines** to the case studies in the textbook
- 60+ Customizable **Nursing Care Plans**
- **Conceptual Care Map Creator** and **Conceptual Care Maps** for selected case studies in the textbook
- New **"Managing Multiple Patients"** case studies and answers for RN present scenarios with multiple patients requiring care simultaneously to develop prioritization and delegation skills
- Fluids and Electrolytes **Tutorial**
- **Audio glossary** of key terms, available as a comprehensive alphabetical glossary
- Supporting **animations** and **audio** for selected chapters
- **Virtual Clinical Excursions (VCE)** is an exciting learning tool that brings learning to life in a "virtual" hospital setting. VCE simulates a realistic, yet safe, nursing environment where the routine and rigours of the average clinical rotation abound. Students can conduct a complete assessment of a patient and set priorities for care, collect data, analyze and interpret data, prepare and administer medications, and reach conclusions about complex problems. Each lesson has a textbook reading assignment and online activities based on "visiting" patients in the hospital. Instructors receive an Implementation Manual with directions for using VCE as a teaching tool.
- More than just words on a screen, **Elsevier eBooks** come with a wealth of built-in study tools and interactive functionality to help students better connect with the course material and their instructors. Plus, with the ability to fit an entire library of books on one portable device, students can study when, where, and how they want.

TEACHING SUPPLEMENTS FOR INSTRUCTORS

- **Evolve Instructor Resources** (available online at http://evolve. elsevier.com/Canada/Lewis/medsurg) remain the most comprehensive set of instructor's materials available, containing the following:
- **TEACH for Nurses Lesson Plans** with electronic resources organized by chapter to help instructors develop and manage the course curriculum. This exciting resource includes the following:
  - Objectives
  - Teaching focus
  - Key terms
  - Student and instructor chapter resource listings
  - Detailed chapter outlines
  - Teaching strategies with learning activities and assessment methods tied to learning outcomes
  - Case studies with answer guidelines
- The **Test Bank** features over 1500 examination test questions with text page references and answers coded for nursing process and cognitive level. The ExamView software allows instructors to create new tests; edit, add, and delete test questions; sort questions by category, cognitive level, difficulty, and question type; and administer and grade online tests.

- The **Image Collection** contains more than 800 full-colour images from the text for use in lectures.
- An extensive collection of **PowerPoint Presentations** includes presentations focused on the most common diseases and disorders. The presentations have been thoroughly revised to include helpful instructor notes/ teaching tips, new illustrations and photos, and new animations.
- **Course management system**
- Access to all student resources listed above
- The **Simulation Learning System** (SLS) is an online toolkit that helps instructors and facilitators effectively incorporate medium- to high-fidelity simulation into their nursing curriculum. Detailed patient scenarios promote and enhance the clinical decision-making skills of students at all levels. The SLS provides detailed instructions for preparation and implementation of the simulation experience, debriefing questions that encourage critical thinking, and learning resources to reinforce student comprehension. Each scenario in the SLS complements the textbook content and helps bridge the gap between lecture and clinical. The SLS provides the perfect environment for students to practise what they are learning in the text for a true-to-life, hands-on learning experience.

ACKNOWLEDGEMENTS

The editors are grateful to the entire editorial team at Elsevier for their leadership and dedication in the preparation of this very comprehensive, but much needed, Canadian medical-surgical textbook. In particular, we wish to thank Acquisitions Editor, Roberta A. Spinosa-Millman, for her invaluable assistance, and Dawn Slawecki for her professionalism, sense of humour, patience, and graciousness despite pressing deadlines and for her commitment to the Canadian Lewis project from first to fourth edition. We would also like to thank Sarah Ibrahim for her help with the Lab Values appendix.

We would like to recognize the commitment and expertise of all the authors, representing diverse areas of practice and regions of Canada. It has been a genuine pleasure to work with both the first-time and returning authors on this project. We are also very grateful to the many reviewers for their valuable feedback on earlier versions of this textbook. It takes a large and coordinated team to create a textbook such as this, and we thank everyone for their individual contributions. We are proud to be able to provide a medical-surgical nursing textbook written from a Canadian perspective that provides current and accurate information to enrich the learning of our nursing students.

Concepts in Nursing Practice

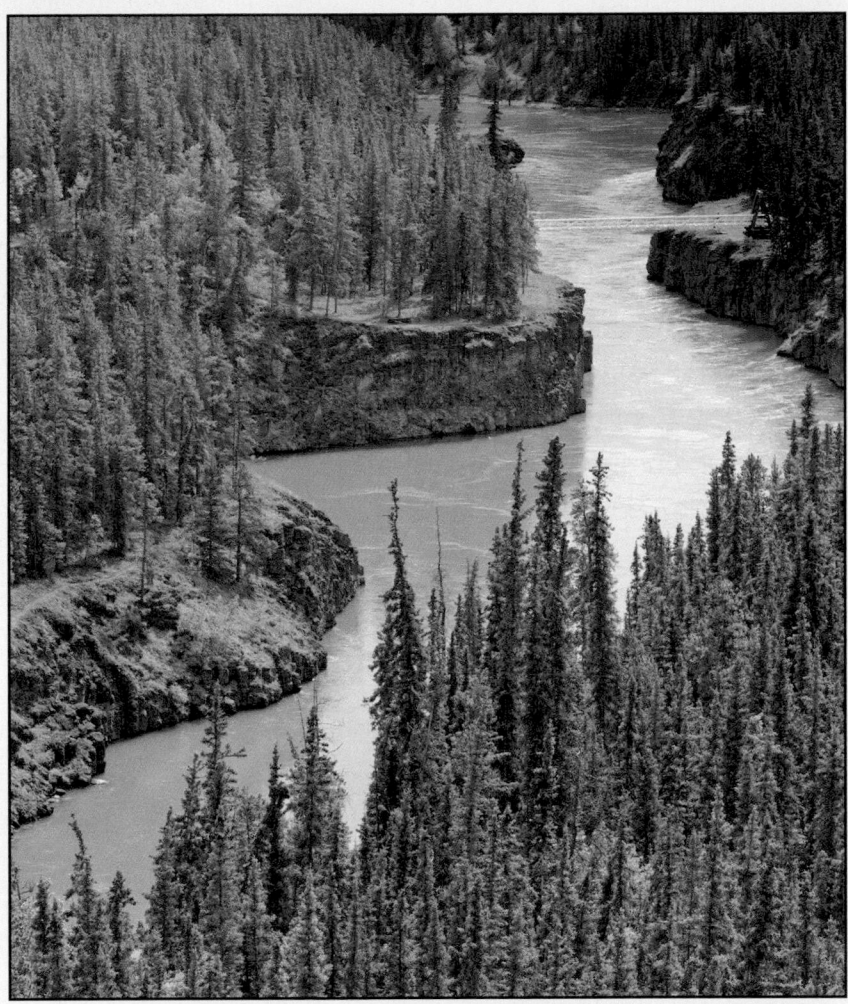

Source: Pi-Lens/Shutterstock.com.

1

Introduction to Medical-Surgical Nursing Practice in Canada

Written by: Mariann M. Harding
Adapted by: Maureen Barry

evolve WEBSITE

http://evolve.elsevier.com/Canada/Lewis/medsurg

- Review Questions (Online Only)
- Key Points
- Conceptual Care Map Creator

- Audio Glossary
- Content Updates

LEARNING OBJECTIVES

1. Describe key challenges facing the current Canadian health care system.
2. Describe the practice of professional nursing in relation to the health care team.
3. Explain how teamwork and interprofessional collaboration contribute to high-quality patient outcomes.
4. Discuss the role of integrating patient-centred care and safety and quality improvement processes into nursing practice.
5. Evaluate the role of informatics and technology in nursing practice.
6. Describe the key attributes of the practice of medical-surgical nursing.
7. Apply concepts of evidence-informed practice to nursing practice.
8. Describe the role of critical thinking and clinical reasoning skills and use of the nursing process to provide patient-centred care.

KEY TERMS

advanced nursing practice, p. 7
assessment, p. 13
clinical (critical) pathway, p. 16
collaborative problems, p. 15
continuing competence, p. 6
critical thinking, p. 10
determinants of health, p. 3
eHealth, p. 9

electronic health records (EHRs), p. 10
evaluation, p. 13
evidence-informed nursing, p. 11
expected patient outcomes, p. 15
implementation, p. 13
information and communication technologies (ICT), p. 9

medical-surgical nursing, p. 10
NurseONE, p. 13
nursing diagnosis, p. 14
nursing informatics, p. 9
nursing intervention, p. 16
nursing leadership, p. 17
nursing process, p. 13
patient-centred approach, p. 4
patient safety, p. 4
planning, p. 13

regulated health care providers, p. 5
SBAR (*situation*, *background*, *assessment*, and *recommendation*), p. 7
standard of practice, p. 6
unregulated care providers (UCPs), p. 5

THE CANADIAN HEALTH CARE CONTEXT

Health care is a subject of keen interest to the public. Repeatedly in public opinion polls, public health care has ranked as the most important public policy issue for Canadians (Canadian Federation of Nurses Unions [CFNU], 2015). In Canada, everyone has access to health care through a government-funded universal program, the costs of which are shared by the federal and the provincial/territorial governments. *The Canada Health Act* mandates that all provinces and territories provide coverage for medically necessary procedures. These include most services provided in hospitals and by family doctors. The level of health care funding from the federal government to the provinces and territories depends on the economic health of the country.

In 2003, the first ministers agreed to a 10-year Accord on Health Care Renewal. The Accord committed federal and provincial/territorial governments to work toward targeted reforms to improve access, quality, and long-term sustainability of the Canadian health care system (Health Canada, 2012). This accord expired in 2014. A new multiple-year health accord with a long-term funding agreement is in the process of being renegotiated between the federal and provincial/territorial governments with many changes expected to result in the way health care is delivered in Canada (Philpott, 2016). There is widespread agreement that the health care system has not kept pace with the changing needs of Canadians. According to the Minister of Health Mandate letter, the new accord is directed to support action in the areas of long-term funding, home care,

TABLE 1-1	PRINCIPLES TO GUIDE HEALTH CARE TRANSFORMATION IN CANADA

- *Patient-centred:* Patients must be at the centre of health care, with seamless access to the continuum of care on the basis of their needs.
- *Quality:* Canadians deserve quality services that are appropriate for patient needs, are respectful of individual choice, and are delivered in a manner that is timely, safe, effective, and according to the most currently available scientific knowledge.
- *Health promotion and illness prevention:* The health system must support Canadians in the prevention of illness and the enhancement of their well-being, with attention paid to broader social determinants of health.
- *Equitable:* The health care system has a duty to Canadians to provide and advocate for equitable access to quality care and commonly adopted policies to address the social determinants of health.
- *Sustainable:* Sustainable health care requires universal access to quality health services that are adequately resourced and delivered across the board in a timely and cost-effective manner.
- *Accountable:* The public, patients, families, providers, and funders all have a responsibility for ensuring that the system is effective and accountable.

Source: Canadian Nurses Association & Canadian Medical Association. (July, 2011). *Principles to guide health care transformation in Canada*. Retrieved from *https://www.cna-aiic.ca/~/media/cna/files/en/guiding_principles_hc_e.pdf*.

FIGURE 1-1 Nurses are frontline professionals of health care. Source: Potstock/Shutterstock.com.

innovation in digital technology, affordable access to prescription drugs, public health, and access to mental health services (Trudeau, 2015).

In September 2012, the Canadian Nurses Association (CNA) published a report titled *A Nursing Call to Action: The Health of Our Nation, the Future of Our Health System*. This report was written by an independent National Expert Commission established by CNA with leaders from disciplines such business, academia, economics, nursing, health care policy, medicine, and law. The report made recommendations to put individuals, families, and communities first in health care, with a renewed focus on quality care in both community and institutional settings. The findings of this commission, as well as other initiatives designed to re-engineer our health care system, will have a lasting effect on how nurses practise within the Canadian context.

The Canadian health care system continues to deal with major challenges, including concerns about patient safety, service delivery, fiscal constraints, age-related demographics, and the high cost of new technology and drugs. The Romanow report (Commission on the Future of Health Care in Canada, 2002), the Standing Committee on Social Affairs, Science and Technology (2002), the Mazankowski report (Premier's Advisory Council on Health for Alberta, 2001), the Commission on Medicare (Fyke, 2001), and Dagnone (2009) all emphasized the need to accelerate changes within the health care system to ensure sustainability of the system and promote the patient-centred approach desired by the public.

Together with the Canadian Medical Association, the CNA has defined a set of key principles designed to guide health care transformation in Canada. These principles are listed in Table 1-1 and are important considerations for all nurses because they will shape the re-engineered health care system of the future.

Complex Health Care Environments

Nurses practise in virtually all health care settings and communities across the country. They are the frontline providers of health care (Figure 1-1). Rapidly changing technology and dramatically expanding knowledge are adding to the complexity of health care environments. Advanced communication technologies have created a more global environment that affects the delivery of health care worldwide. The number and complexity of advances in patient care technology are transforming how care is delivered. The Human Genome Project and advances in genetics affect the prevention, diagnosis, and treatment of health problems. With advances in knowledge, ethical dilemmas and controversy arise with regard to the use of new scientific knowledge and the disparities that exist in patients' access to more technologically advanced health care. Throughout this book, expanding knowledge and technology's effect on nursing practice are highlighted in "Genetics in Clinical Practice," "Informatics in Practice," and "Ethical Dilemmas" boxes.

Diverse Populations. Patient demographics are more diverse than ever. Canadians are living longer, in part because of advances in medical science, technology, and health care delivery. As the population ages, the number of patients with chronic conditions increases. Unlike those who receive acute, episodic care, patients with chronic conditions have a multitude of needs and see a variety of health care providers in various settings over an extended period. Nurses are also caring for a more culturally and ethnically diverse population. Immigrants, particularly undocumented immigrants and refugees, often lack the resources necessary to access health care. Inability to pay for health care, as is often the case with undocumented immigrants, is associated with a tendency to delay seeking care; as a result, illnesses may become more serious.

Determinants of Health. The determinants of health are the factors that influence the health of individuals and groups. Table 1-2 displays the determinants of health recognized by the Public Health Agency of Canada (PHAC, 2013). The primary factors that shape the health of Canadians are not medical treatments or lifestyle choices but rather the living conditions (the economic, social, and political) that they experience (Mikkonen & Raphael, 2010, p. 7; Provincial Health Services Authority, 2011). These determinants can either improve a person's health status or heighten an individual's risk for disease, injury, and illness. The challenges or advantages may be specific to the individual, or they may be structural and include factors such as income and social status; social support networks; education; employment/working conditions; social environments; physical environments;

TABLE 1-2 PUBLIC HEALTH AGENCY OF CANADA: KEY DETERMINANTS OF HEALTH

Determinant of Health	Underlying Premise
Income and social status	Health status improves at each step up the income and social hierarchy. High income determines living conditions such as safe housing and ability to buy sufficient good food. The healthiest populations are those societies that are prosperous and have an equitable distribution of wealth.
Social support networks	Support from families, friends, and communities is associated with better health. Such social support networks could be very important in helping people solve problems and deal with adversity, as well as in maintaining a sense of mastery and control over life circumstances. The caring and respect that occurs in social relationships, and the resulting sense of satisfaction and well-being, seem to act as a buffer against health problems.
Education and literacy	Health status improves with level of education, which is, in turn, tied to socioeconomic status. Education contributes to health and prosperity by equipping people with knowledge and skills for problem solving and helps provide a sense of control and mastery over life circumstances. It increases opportunities for job and income security and job satisfaction. Education also improves people's ability to access and understand information to help keep them healthy.
Employment/working conditions	Unemployment, underemployment, and stressful or unsafe work are associated with poorer health. People who have more control over their work circumstances and fewer stress-related demands of the job are healthier and often live longer than those who have more stressful or riskier types of work and activities.
Social environments	The array of values and norms of a society influences in varying ways the health and well-being of individuals and populations. In addition, social stability, recognition of diversity, safety, good working relationships, and cohesive communities provide a supportive society that reduces or avoids many potential risks to good health. Social or community responses can add resources to an individual's repertoire of strategies to cope with changes and foster health.
Physical environments	The physical environment is an important determinant of health. At certain levels of exposure, contaminants in our air, water, food, and soil can cause a variety of adverse health effects, including cancer, birth defects, respiratory illness, and gastro-intestinal ailments. In the built environment, factors related to housing, indoor air quality, and the design of communities and transportation systems can significantly influence our physical and psychological well-being.
Personal health practices and coping skills	These refer to those actions by which individuals can prevent diseases and promote self-care, cope with challenges, develop self-reliance, solve problems, and make choices that enhance health. These influence lifestyle choice through at least five domains: personal life skills, stress, culture, social relationships and belonging, and a sense of control.
Healthy child development	New evidence on the effects of early experiences on brain development, school readiness, and health in later life has sparked a growing consensus about early child development as a powerful determinant of health in its own right. All of the other determinants of health, in turn, affect the physical, social, mental, emotional, and spiritual development of children and youth.
Biology and genetic endowment	The basic biology and organic makeup of the human body are a fundamental determinant of health. Genetic endowment provides an inherited predisposition to a wide range of individual responses that affect health status. Socioeconomic and environmental factors are important determinants of overall health, but in some circumstances, genetic endowment appears to predispose certain individuals to particular diseases or health problems.
Health services	Health services, particularly those designed to maintain and promote health, to prevent disease, and to restore health and function, contribute to the health of the overall population. The health services continuum of care includes treatment and secondary prevention.
Gender	Gender refers to the array of society-determined roles, personality traits, attitudes, behaviours, values, and relative power and influence that society ascribes to the two sexes on a differential basis. "Gendered" norms influence the health system's practices and priorities. Many health issues are a function of gender-based social status or roles.
Culture	Some persons or groups may face additional health risks due to a socioeconomic environment, which is largely determined by dominant cultural values that contribute to the perpetuation of conditions such as marginalization, stigmatization, loss or devaluation of language and culture, and lack of access to culturally appropriate health care and services.

Source: © All rights reserved. *What makes Canadians healthy or unhealthy?* Public Health Agency of Canada, 2013. Adapted and reproduced with permission from the Minister of Health, 2017.

personal health practices and coping skills; healthy child development; biology and genetic endowment; gender; and culture (PHAC, 2013). Table 1-2 displays the determinants of health recognized by PHAC. Because these factors or determinants intersect with each other, the overall effect can be one of multiple exclusions that are beyond individual control and that lead to compounded adverse effects on health and well-being.

Patient-Centred Care

Nurses have long demonstrated that they deliver patient-centred care that is based on each patient's unique needs and on an understanding of the patient's preferences, values, and beliefs. Patient-centred care is interrelated with both quality and safety. A patient-centred approach or a person- and family-centred care approach (Registered Nurses' Association of Ontario [RNAO], 2015) focuses on the "*whole person* as a unique individual and

not just on their illness or disease" (p. 8). In Canada, numerous provincial initiatives are under way to improve the experience of the person and their family. Many initiatives are partnering with individual users to ensure that the patient (and the patient's family) is the focus of system reform (RNAO, 2015).

Patient Safety and Quality Improvement. Patient safety is a cornerstone of nursing practice. Entry-to-practice competencies for nursing recognize the importance of the nurse's ability to assess and manage situations that may compromise patient safety (College and Association of Registered Nurses of Alberta, 2013). Although patients turn to the health care system for help with their health conditions, there is overwhelming evidence that significant numbers of patients are harmed as a result of the health care they receive, which results in permanent injury, increased lengths of hospital stay, and even death (World Health Organization, 2011). It is estimated that between 210,000 and

ETHICAL DILEMMAS

Social Networking: Confidentiality and Privacy Violation

Situation

A nursing student logs into a closed group on a social networking site and reads a posting from a fellow nursing student. The posting describes in detail the complex care the fellow student provided to an older patient in a local hospital the previous day. The fellow student comments on how stressful the day was and asks for advice on how to deal with similar patients in the future.

Ethical/Legal Points for Consideration

- Protecting and maintaining patient privacy and confidentiality are basic obligations defined in the Code of Ethics (CNA, 2017), which nurses and nursing students should uphold.
- Each province and territory has its own legislation to protect a patient's private health information. Some examples include the *Personal Information Protection Act* (PIPA) in British Columbia and the *Access to Information and Protection of Privacy Act* (ATIPPA) in Newfoundland and Labrador. Private health information is any information about the patients' past, present, or future physical or mental health. This includes not only specific details such as a patient's name or picture but also information that gives enough details that someone else may be able to identify that patient.
- A nurse may unintentionally breach privacy or confidentiality by posting patient information (diagnosis, condition, or situation) on a social networking site. Using privacy settings or being in a closed group does not guarantee the secrecy of posted information. Other users can copy and share any post without the poster's knowledge.
- Potential consequences for improperly using social networking vary according to the situation. These may include dismissal from a nursing program, termination of employment, or civil and criminal actions.
- A student nurse who experienced a stressful day and was looking for advice and support from peers could share the experience by clearly limiting the posts to the student's personal perspective (e.g., "Today my patient died. I wanted to cry") and not sharing any identifying information.

Discussion Questions

- How would you deal with the situation involving the fellow nursing student?
- How would you handle a situation in which you observed a staff member violating the provincial/territorial legislation related to a patient's private health information?

440,000 patients each year suffer some type of harm that contributes to their death because of preventable medical errors (James, 2013).

The 2004 "Canadian Adverse Events Study" confirmed that harmful incidents are a significant problem in Canadian hospitals (Baker, Norton, Flintoft, et al., 2004). A number of organizations such as the Canadian Patient Safety Institute (CPSI) are addressing patient safety issues by providing safety goals for health care organizations and identifying safety competencies for health care providers. Tools and programs in four priority areas—medication safety, surgical care safety, infection prevention and control, and home care safety—are available from the CPSI (2016).

By implementing various procedures and systems to improve health care delivery to meet safety goals, designers of health care systems are working to attain a culture of safety that minimizes the risk of harm to the patient. Because nurses have the greatest amount of interaction with patients, they are a vital part of promoting this culture of safety by providing care in a manner that reduces errors and actively promotes patient safety.

Quality and Safety Education for Nurses (QSEN). Since 2000, a number of high-profile reports have highlighted problems with the quality of health care. In one of these reports, *The Future of Nursing: Leading Change, Advancing Health,* the Institute of Medicine (2011) acknowledged the link between professional nursing practice and health care delivery. The report described how health care providers, including nurses, are not being adequately prepared to provide the highest quality care possible. Changes are recommended so that nurses will have the skills to advance health care and play leadership roles in a reformed health care system (Institute of Medicine, 2011).

One initiative to address nursing's role in solving these problems is the Quality and Safety Education for Nurses (QSEN) Institute. The QSEN Institute has made a major contribution to nursing by defining specific competencies that nurses need to have to practise safely and effectively in today's complex health care system. Table 1-3 describes each of the QSEN competencies and the knowledge, skills, and attitudes (KSAs) necessary in six key areas: (a) patient-centred care, (b) teamwork and collaboration, (c) quality improvement, (d) safety, (e) informatics and technology, and (f) evidence-based practice (QSEN, 2014). Threaded throughout the remainder of this chapter is a discussion of how professional nursing practice is focusing on acquiring the knowledge, skills, and attitudes for these competencies.

The Profession of Nursing in Canada

Health care in Canada is typically delivered by teams of workers with different responsibilities and scopes of practice. The term **regulated health care providers** refers to paid workers "covered by provincial/territorial and/or federal legislation and governed by a professional organization or regulatory authority" (Canadian Institute for Health Information [CIHI], 2013, p. 22). There are four regulated nursing groups: registered nurses (RNs), nurse practitioners, registered psychiatric nurses, or licensed practical nurses/registered practical nurses (LPN/RPNs; CNA, 2015a). In contrast, **unregulated care providers (UCPs)** or unregulated health workers are paid employees who are not licensed or registered by a regulatory body, who have no legally defined scope of practice, for whom education or practice standards may or may not be mandatory, who provide care under the direct or indirect supervision of a nurse, and who are accountable for their own actions and decisions (CIHI, 2013, p. 22; CNA, 2015a, p. 28). Some of the more common titles for UCPs include "health care aides," "personal support workers," "assistive personnel," "care team assistants," and "nursing aides."

Within Canada, nurses are granted the legal authority to use the designation "Registered Nurse" (RN) in accordance with provincial and territorial legislation and regulation. The provincial regulatory bodies set the standards for practice for RNs to protect the public in their province or territory (CNA, 2015a). RN practice is defined by the CNA (2015a) in the following way:

RNs are self-regulated health-care professionals who work autonomously and in collaboration with others to enable individuals, families, groups, communities and populations to achieve their optimal levels of health. At all stages of life, in situations of health, illness, injury and disability, RNs deliver direct health-care services, coordinate care and support clients in managing their own health. RNs contribute to the health-care system through their leadership . . . in practice, education, administration, research and policy. (p. 5)

TABLE 1-3 QUALITY AND SAFETY EDUCATION FOR NURSES (QSEN) COMPETENCIES

Competency	Knowledge, Skills, and Attitudes
Patient-Centred Care Recognize the patient or designee as the source of control and a full partner in providing compassionate and coordinated care that is based on respect for patient's preferences, values, and needs.	Provide care with sensitivity and respect, taking into consideration the patient's perspectives, beliefs, and cultural background. Assess the patient's level of comfort, and treat appropriately. Engage the patient in an active partnership that promotes health, well-being, and self-care management. Facilitate patient's informed consent for care.
Teamwork and Collaboration Function effectively within nursing and interprofessional teams, fostering open communication, mutual respect and shared decision-making to achieve quality patient care.	Value the expertise of each interprofessional member. Initiate referrals when appropriate. Follow communication practices that minimize risks associated with handoffs and transitions in care. Participate in interprofessional rounds.
Safety Minimize risk of harm to patients and providers through both system effectiveness and individual performance.	Follow recommendations from national safety campaigns. Appropriately communicate observations or concerns related to hazards and errors. Contribute to designing systems to improve safety.
Quality Improvement Use data to monitor the outcomes of care and use improvement methods to design and test changes to continuously improve the quality and safety of health care systems.	Use quality measures to understand performance. Identify gaps between local and best practices. Participate in investigating the circumstances surrounding a sentinel event or serious reportable event.
Informatics Use information and technology to communicate, manage knowledge, mitigate error, and support decision making.	Protect confidentiality of patient's protected health information. Document appropriately in electronic health records. Use communication technologies to coordinate patient care. Respond correctly to clinical decision-making alerts.
Evidence-Based or Evidence-Informed Practice Integrate best current evidence with clinical expertise and the patient/family preferences and values for delivery of optimal health care.	Read research, clinical practice guidelines, and evidence reports related to area of practice. Base individual patient care plan on patient's values, clinical expertise, and evidence. Continuously improve clinical practice on the basis of new knowledge.

Source: Reprinted from *Nursing Outlook*, 55(3), Linda Cronenwett, Gwen Sherwood, Jane Barnsteiner, Joanne Disch, Jean Johnson, Pamela Mitchell, Dori Taylor Sullivan, Judith Warren, "Quality and safety education for nurses," pages 122–131, Copyright 2007, with permission from Elsevier.

Because RNs work with other regulated providers, as well as with UCPs, they must be aware of both their own and other providers' scopes of practice. This is essential for safely enacting key nursing roles such as delegation and prioritization and for meeting the standards of practice.

Standards of Practice. A standard of practice "sets out the legal and professional basis for nursing practice: describing the desirable and achievable level of performance expected of registered nurses in their practice, against which actual performance can be measured" (College of Registered Nurses of Nova Scotia [CRNNS], 2011, p. 4). Standards are intended to promote, guide, direct, and regulate professional nursing practice (CRNNS, 2011, p. 4). Standards of practice demonstrate to the public, government, and other stakeholders that a profession is dedicated to maintaining public trust and upholding the criteria of its professional practice. Standards of practice are based on the values of the profession and articulated in the Code of Ethics for Registered Nurses (CNA, 2017). Provincial and territorial regulatory bodies for nursing are legally required to set standards for practice for RNs in order to protect the public. These standards, together with the Code of Ethics, form the foundation for nursing practice in Canada.

Because of the rapid changes in resources, expectations, and technologies that characterize health care in Canada, the practice of nursing requires a commitment to lifelong learning in order to promote the highest quality of patient outcomes. **Continuing competence** refers to "the ongoing ability of a nurse to integrate and apply the knowledge, skills, judgement and personal attributes required to practise safely and ethically in a designated role and setting" (CNA/Canadian Association of Schools of Nursing [CASN], 2004).

RNs are initially prepared at the baccalaureate level and can go on to pursue further studies at the graduate level. Many nurses also seek recognition of their clinical expertise through certification in one of the 20 specialty areas of practice through the CNA (2016). Medical-surgical nursing is one of the newer specialties to be recognized through the certification program.

Advanced Nursing Practice. As the health care system in Canada undergoes changes, advanced nursing practice (ANP) roles are also evolving to optimize patient care within the system. According to the CNA (2008, p. 2), advanced nursing practice "build[s] nursing knowledge, advanc[es] the nursing profession and contribut[es] to a sustainable and effective health care system." ANP roles focus on health assessment, diagnosis, and treatment

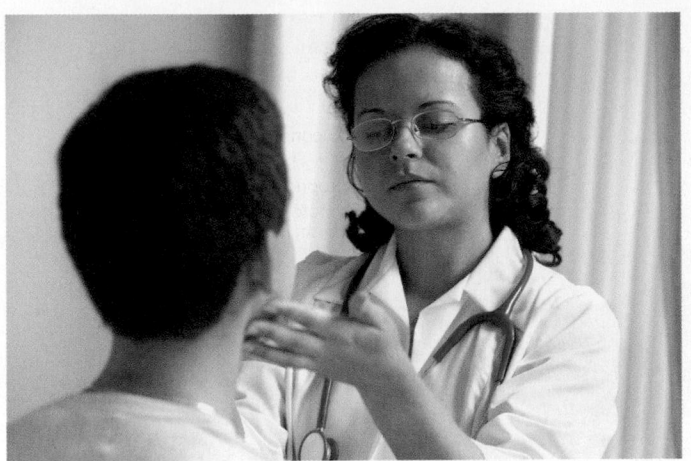

FIGURE 1-2 Advanced nursing practice (ANP) plays an important role in primary care delivery. Source: Blend Images/Shutterstock.com.

TABLE 1-4	COMPARISON OF PRIMARY GOALS FOR NURSING AND MEDICINE	
Nursing	**Medicine**	
Determines responses to health problems, level of wellness, and need for assistance	Determines etiology of illness or injury	
Provides physical care, emotional care, teaching, guidance, and counselling	Prescribes medical treatments; performs surgery	
Implements interventions aimed at promoting health, preventing illness/complications, and assisting patients to meet their own needs	Implements interventions aimed at preventing and curing injury or illness	

Source: Modified from Lewis, S. L., Dirksen, S. R., Heitkemper, M. M., et al. (2011). *Medical-surgical nursing: Assessment and management of clinical problems* (8th ed., p. 10). St. Louis: Mosby.

of conditions previously considered to be the physician's domain (Figure 1-2). According to the CNA (2008), **advanced nursing practice** is "an umbrella term describing an advanced level of clinical nursing practice that maximizes use of graduate educational preparation, in-depth nursing knowledge and expertise in meeting needs of individuals, families, groups, communities and populations. It involves analyzing and synthesizing knowledge; understanding, interpreting and applying nursing theory and research; and developing and advancing nursing knowledge and the profession as a whole" (CNA, 2008, p. 10). Examples of roles within ANP in Canada include those of the clinical nurse specialist and the nurse practitioner.

In addition to managing and delivering direct patient care, ANP nurses have significant roles in health promotion, case management, administration, and research. There is substantial variation among the provinces and territories in the framework for and specific roles of nurses working in ANP. Practice settings in which an ANP nurse may be employed include primary care, ambulatory care, long-term care, hospital care, and community care, as well as mental health care centres, physicians' offices, family health clinics, and community health facilities (CNA, 2008). In the ANP role, the nurse's focus may be, for example, the management of primary care and health promotion for a wide variety of health problems in various specialties; activities include physical examination, diagnosis, treatment of health problems, patient and family education, and counselling. In the management of complex patient care in various clinical specialty areas, the roles of ANP nurses may include direct care, consultation, research, education, case management, and administration.

Teamwork and Interprofessional Collaboration

Interprofessional Teams. Because of the increasing acuity of illnesses among patients in the health care system and the growing complexity of interventions designed to promote, restore, and maintain health, no one health discipline can work in isolation. To help patients achieve optimal health, nurses work in collaboration with a wide range of professionals, including pharmacists, physicians, occupational therapists, physiotherapists, and social workers.

Successful collaboration with other health care providers has become a cornerstone of nursing practice. In the position statement *Interprofessional Collaboration,* the CNA (2011)

recognized the growing importance of interprofessional collaboration in improving client- or patient-centred access to health care in Canada. The RNAO (2013b) described a conceptual model for developing and sustaining interprofessional health care whereby outstanding interprofessional care is a result of health care teams demonstrating expertise in six key domains: care expertise; shared power; collaborative leadership; optimizing profession, role, and scope; shared decision making; and effective group functioning (Figure 1-3).

Nurses function in independent, dependent, and collaborative roles. Each province and territory has a *Nurses' Act* that determines the scope of practice for that region. These acts allow nurses to take on delegated medical responsibilities and have a wider scope of practice when working as nurse practitioners. To function effectively in these different roles, nurses must understand how the primary goals of nursing and medicine differ (Table 1-4).

Communication Among Health Care Team Members. Effective communication is a key component of fostering teamwork and coordinating care. To provide safe, effective care, everyone involved in a patient's care should understand the patient's condition and needs. Unfortunately, many issues result from a breakdown in communication. Miscommunication often occurs during transitions of care. One structured model used to improve communication is the SBAR (situation, background, assessment, and recommendation) technique (see the inside back cover of this book). This technique provides a way for members of the health care team to talk about a patient's condition in a predictable, structured manner. Other ways to enhance communication during transitions include performing surgical time-outs, standardizing the change-of-shift process, and conducting interprofessional rounds to identify risks and develop a plan for delivering care.

Delegation and Assignment. Nurses delegate nursing care and supervise other staff members who are qualified to deliver care. *Delegation* is "a formal process through which a regulated health [care] professional (delegator) who has the authority and competence to perform a procedure under one of the controlled acts delegates the performance of that procedure to another individual (delegatee)" (CRNNS/CLPNNS, 2012, p. 2). The delegation and assignment of nursing activities is a process that, when used appropriately, can result in safe, effective, and efficient patient care.

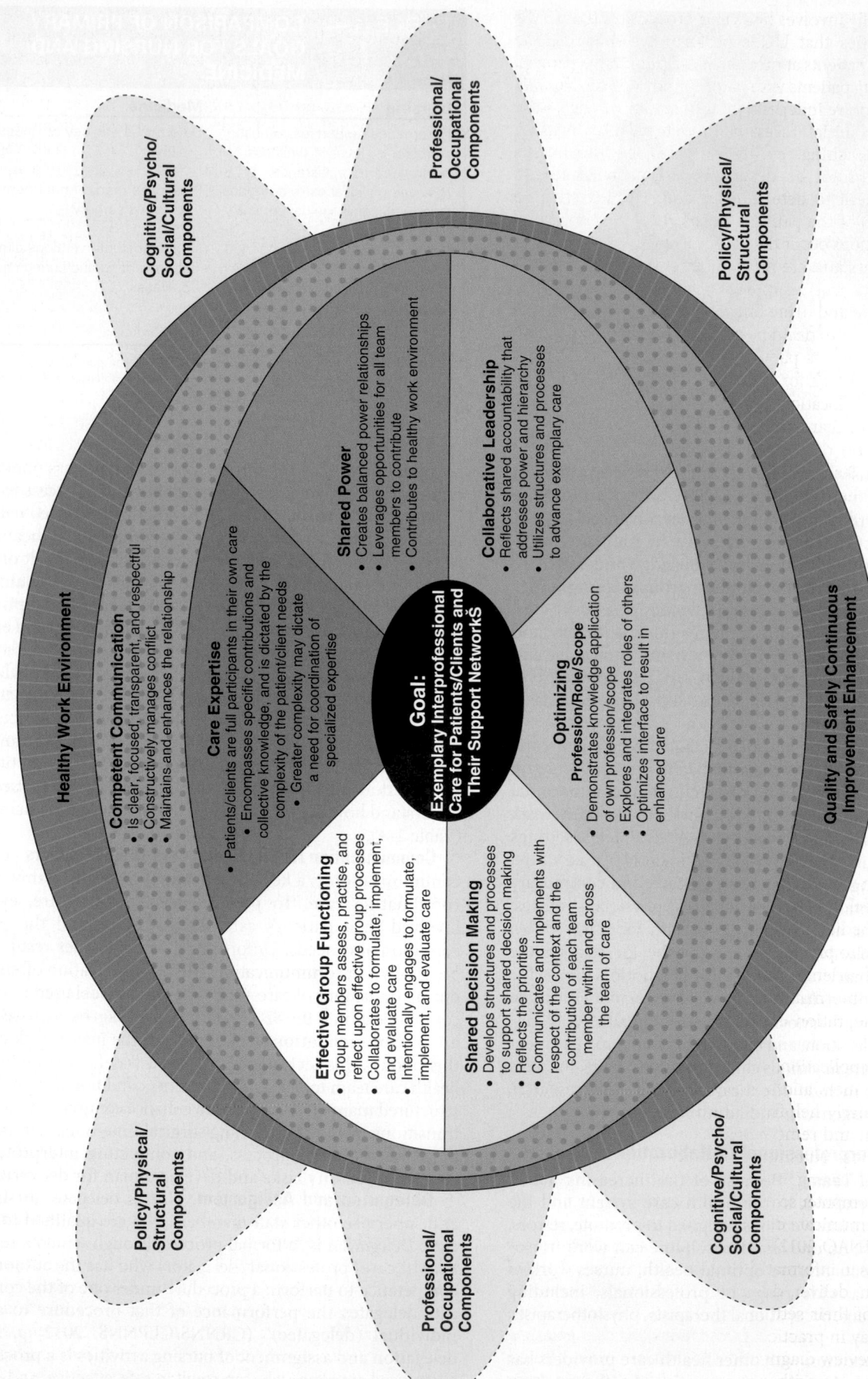

FIGURE 1-3 Conceptual model for developing and sustaining interprofessional health care. Source: Registered Nurses' Association of Ontario (2013). *Developing and sustaining interprofessional health care: Optimizing patients/clients, organizational, and system outcomes.* Toronto, Canada. Registered Nurses' Association of Ontario.

Delegation typically involves tasks and procedures that UCPs perform. The activities that UCPs perform typically include feeding and assisting patients at mealtimes, helping stable patients ambulate, and assisting patients with bathing and hygiene. Nursing interventions that require independent nursing knowledge, skill, or judgement (e.g., initial assessment, determining nursing diagnoses, patient teaching, evaluating care) are the nurse's responsibility and cannot be delegated. Nurses need to use professional judgement to determine appropriate activities to delegate on the basis of the patient's needs. The most common delegated nursing actions occur during the implementation phase of the nursing process and are for patients who are stable with predictable outcomes. For example, the nurse might delegate measuring oral intake and urine output to a UCP, but the nurse uses nursing judgement to decide whether the intake and output are adequate. Delegation is patient-specific, and the UCP can perform the delegated task for only a particular patient.

Assignment is the "allocation of nursing care among providers in order to meet patient care needs" (Nurses Association of New Brunswick/Association of New Brunswick Licensed Practical Nurses, 2015, p. 10). Staff members can be assigned only activities that are within their scope of practice. Assignment occurs at the beginning of and throughout the shift as patient care needs change.

Whether nurses delegate or are working with staff to whom they assign tasks, they are responsible for the patient's total care during their work period. Nurses are responsible for supervising the UCP who is caring for their patient. It is important to clearly communicate what tasks must be done and provide necessary guidance. Nurses are accountable for ensuring that delegated tasks are completed in a competent manner. This supervision includes evaluation and follow-up as needed by the nurse.

Delegation is a skill that is learned and must be practised to attain proficiency in managing patient care, and it requires the use of critical thinking and professional judgement.

Informatics and Technology

Rapidly changing technologies and dramatically expanding knowledge in the fields of arts and science affect all areas of health care. In telemedicine, telehealth, and telenursing, virtual technologies are used to provide professional education, consultation, and delivery of patient services. **eHealth** refers to the use of communication and information technologies in order to support the delivery and integration of clinical care within and across settings, whereas **information and communication technologies (ICT)** are tools and applications that support the management of clinical data, information, and knowledge (RNAO, 2012). These services are particularly helpful to health care providers who work or live in rural and remote areas.

Nursing Informatics. Nursing informatics is a rapidly growing specialty in nursing. **Nursing informatics** refers to the integration of nursing science, computer science, and information technology to manage and communicate data, information, and knowledge in nursing practice (RNAO, 2012). Nursing is an information-intense profession. Advances in informatics and technology have changed the way nurses plan, deliver, document, and evaluate care. All nurses, regardless of their setting or role, use informatics and technology every day in practice. Informatics has changed how nurses obtain and review diagnostic information, make clinical decisions, communicate with patients and health care team members, and document and provide care.

Technology advances have increased the efficiency of nursing care, improving the work environment and the care that nurses provide. Computers and mobile devices allow nurses to document at the time they deliver care and give them quick and easy access to information, including clinical decision-making tools, patient education materials, and references. Texting, video chat, and email enhance communication among health care team members and help them deliver the right message to the right person at the right time.

Technology plays a key role in providing safe, quality patient care. Medication administration applications improve patient safety by flagging potential errors, such as look-alike and sound-alike medications and adverse drug interactions, before they can occur. Computerized provider order entry (CPOE) systems can eliminate errors caused by misreading or misinterpreting handwritten orders. Sensor technology can decrease the number of falls by patients at high risk. Care reminder systems provide cues that decrease the amount of missed nursing care.

The ability to use technology skills to communicate and access information is now an essential component of professional nursing practice. Nurses must be able to use word processing software, communicate by email and messaging, access appropriate information, and follow security and confidentiality rules. They need to demonstrate the skills to safely use patient care technologies and navigate electronic documentation systems. The CASN (2012) outlined three entry-to-practice competencies related to nursing informatics: (a) use of relevant information and knowledge to support the delivery of evidence-informed patient care; (b) use of ICTs in accordance with professional and regulatory standards and workplace policies; and (c) use of ICTs in the delivery of patient/client care (pp. 6–10). These nursing informatics competencies are considered the minimum knowledge and skills that new graduate nurses require to practise. Throughout this book, "Informatics in Practice" boxes such as the one below offer suggestions for nurses on how to make information technology part of good nursing practice.

INFORMATICS IN PRACTICE

Responsible Use of Social Media

A nurse wants to post pictures (or videos) of himself and his nursing colleagues from the hospital.
- Before sharing anything on social media, the nurse should ensure that the posts do not reflect negatively on the nursing profession, the workplace, himself, or his colleagues as health care providers.
- The nurse should ensure that posts do not cause a breach of confidentiality and privacy for patients, colleagues, or the workplace.
- The nurse should know and follow employer policies on using social media in the workplace.

Nurses have an obligation to ensure the privacy of their patient's health information. To do so, it is necessary to understand their agency's policies regarding the use of technology. Nurses need to know the rules regarding accessing patient records and releasing personal health information, what to do if information is accidently or intentionally released, and how to protect any passwords they use. If nurses are using social media, they must be careful not to place online any personal health information that is individually identifiable and must adhere to certain principles in order to reduce risks to members of the public (Table 1-5). They must also be guided by their professional code of conduct and standards of practice.

TABLE 1-5   6 *P*S OF SOCIAL MEDIA USE
Professional: Act professionally at all times
Positive: Keep posts positive
Patient/Person-free: Keep posts patient- or person-free
Protect yourself: Protect your professionalism, your reputation, and yourself
Privacy: Keep your personal and professional life separate; respect privacy of others
Pause before you post: Consider implications; avoid posting in haste or anger

Source: International Nurse Regulator Collaborative. (2014). Social media use: Common expectations for nurses. Retrieved from *https://www.crnbc.ca/Standards/Lists/StandardResources/INRCSocialMediaUseCommonExpectforNurses.pdf.*

Electronic Health Records. Informatics is most widely used in electronic health records (EHRs), also called *electronic medical records.* An EHR is a computerized record of patient information. It is shared among all health care team members involved in a patient's care and moves with the patient: to other providers and across care settings. The ideal EHR is a single file in which team members review and update a patient's health record, document care given, and enter patient care orders, including medications, procedures, diets, and results of diagnostic and laboratory tests. The EHR should contain a patient's medical history, diagnoses, medications, treatment plans, immunization dates, allergies, and test results.

Many agencies have adopted electronic documentation. EHRs and the Canadian Health Outcomes for Better Information and Care (C-HOBIC) project are examples of electronic collection of health care data, and they are being implemented across many parts of Canada. The EHR integrates the output of a number of information systems. Several projects are under way across Canada to develop systems that form the essential building blocks of an EHR, such as digital imaging, summaries of drug prescriptions, and laboratory test results. Provinces and territories across Canada are working together with Canada Health Infoway to accelerate the development of these systems. In the C-HOBIC project, a strategy is being developed for the collection of standardized patient outcome data related to nursing care in EHRs in Saskatchewan, Manitoba, and Ontario (C-HOBIC, 2013). This project introduces a systematic, structured language for admission and discharge assessment of patients receiving acute care, complex continuing care, long-term care, or home care. Data on the following outcomes are being collected: functional status, therapeutic self-care (readiness for discharge), symptom management (e.g., pain, nausea, fatigue, dyspnea), safety (falls, pressure injuries), and patient satisfaction with nursing care (C-HOBIC, 2013). C-HOBIC will provide real-time information to nurses about how patients are benefitting from care, as well as collecting nursing-related outcomes that provide valuable information about preparing patients for discharge.

EHRs have the potential to reduce medical errors associated with traditional paper records and to improve clinical decision making, patient safety, and quality of care. Unfortunately, several obstacles remain in the way of fully implementing EHRs. Systems are expensive and technologically complex, and a number of resources are needed to implement and maintain them. In addition, communication is still lacking among computer systems and software applications in use. Finally, patients must be assured of their privacy and that information is accessed only by members of their care team with a right to know.

WHAT IS MEDICAL-SURGICAL NURSING?

Medical-surgical nursing is a challenging and dynamic type of nursing that involves caring for acutely ill adults experiencing complex variations in health (Canadian Association of Medical and Surgical Nurses [CAMSN], 2016). Because the scope of medical-surgical nursing is very broad, the nurse practising in this area is expected to acquire and maintain a great deal of knowledge and skill. This book provides the beginning nurse with much of the knowledge necessary to become a safe and competent practitioner.

The medical-surgical nurse is considered a leader and a key member of the interdisciplinary team (CNA, 2015b). Primary responsibilities of the medical-surgical nurse include prioritization, accountability, advocacy, organization, and coordination of evidence-informed care for multiple patients. Medical-surgical patients and their caregivers come from diverse backgrounds and often possess multiple, complex illnesses, and medical-surgical nurses therefore must be knowledgeable and well prepared. Because of the rapidly changing and complex health concerns that may affect multiple body systems of medical-surgical patients, safe and effective use of technology is an increasingly important competency required by these nurses. The effective medical-surgical nurse demonstrates adaptability and a strong commitment to ensuring the best possible patient outcomes.

Medical-surgical nurses practise in diverse environments, ranging from outpatient and primary care environments through the continuum of care to tertiary care hospitals (CNA, 2015a). As the largest group of nursing professionals in Canada (CAMSN, 2016), they utilize a broad range of evidence-informed knowledge and clinical skills to address the needs of acutely ill adults and their families. The CAMSN is a national organization that promotes excellence through best practice standards to provide high-quality, safe, and ethical care to patients across the continuum of care. Registered nurses may choose to seek recognition of their expertise in this specialty through postlicensure certification offered by the CNA.

Critical Thinking in Nursing

To provide high-quality care in clinical environments of increasing complexity and greater accountability, nurses need to develop higher level thinking and reasoning skills. The ability to engage in critical thinking is widely regarded as a fundamental skill in nursing education and practice. According to the Foundation for Critical Thinking, critical thinking is the art of analyzing and evaluating thinking with a view to improving it (Paul & Elder, 2014). Table 1-6 describes the characteristics of a well-cultivated critical thinker.

Alfaro-LeFevre's (2016) work suggests that "a synonym for critical thinking is reasoning because it implies careful, deliberate thought" (p. 6). *Critical thinking* is "an umbrella term that includes aspects of reasoning inside and outside of the clinical area" (p. 7). Critical thinking is not memorizing a list of facts or the steps of a procedure; instead, it is the ability to solve problems by making sense of information. Learning and using critical thinking is a continual process that occurs inside and outside of the clinical setting.

Clinical reasoning is the process used to examine and analyze patient care issues at the point of care (Alfaro-LeFevre, 2016). It involves understanding the medical and nursing implications of a patient's situation when decisions regarding patient care are made. Nurses use clinical reasoning when they identify a change

TABLE 1-6	CHARACTERISTICS OF THE WELL-CULTIVATED CRITICAL THINKER

A well-cultivated critical thinker:
- Raises vital questions and problems, formulating them clearly and precisely;
- Gathers and assesses relevant information, [and by] using abstract ideas to interpret it effectively comes to well-reasoned conclusions and solutions, testing them against relevant criteria and standards;
- Thinks open-mindedly within alternative systems of thought, recognizing and assessing, as need be, their assumptions, implications, and practical consequences; and
- Communicates effectively with others in figuring out solutions to complex problems.

Source: Paul, R., & Elder, L. (2014). *The miniature guide to critical thinking: Concepts and tools* (7th ed., p. 4). Dillon Beach, CA: Foundation for Critical Thinking.

in a patient's status, take into account the context and concerns of the patient and caregiver, and decide what to do about it.

Because of the complexity of patient care today, nurses are required to learn and implement critical thinking and clinical reasoning skills long before they obtain those skills through the experience of professional practice. Throughout this book, select boxes, case studies, and review questions promote the use of critical thinking and clinical reasoning skills.

Evidence-Informed Practice

Evidence-informed nursing is "a continuous interactive process involving the explicit, conscientious, and judicious consideration of the best available evidence to provide care" (CNA, 2010, p. 1). Basing health care decisions on evidence is essential for quality care in all domains of nursing practice. According to the CNA (2010), evidence-informed decision-making " . . . is essential to optimize outcomes for individual clients, promote healthy communities and populations, improve clinical practice, achieve cost-effective nursing care and ensure accountability and transparency in decision-making within the health-care system" (p. 1).

Four primary elements contribute to the practice of evidence-informed nursing (DiCenso, Guyatt, & Ciliska, 2005): (a) clinical state, setting, and circumstances; (b) patient preferences and actions; (c) best research evidence; and (d) health care resources (Figure 1-4). *Clinical expertise,* in which these other four components are integrated, is the nurse's "ability to use clinical skills and past experience to identify the health state of patients or populations, their risks, their preferences and actions, and the potential benefits of intervention; to communicate information to patients and their families; and to provide them with an environment they find comforting and supporting" (DiCenso et al., 2005, p. 5).

Evidence-informed practice (EIP) produces better outcomes in the most effective and efficient way. Application of EIP results in more accurate diagnoses, the most effective and efficient interventions, and the most favourable patient outcomes. The most distinguishing feature of EIP is that the new scientific base for practice is built through a summary of studies on a topic. These summaries are called *evidence syntheses, systematic reviews,* or *integrative reviews,* depending on the organization that produces them. The evidence synthesis summarizes all research results into a single conclusion about the state of the science. From this point, the clinician translates the knowledge into a clinical practice guideline, implements it through individual and

FIGURE 1-4. A model for evidence-informed clinical decisions. Source: Adapted by DiCenso, A., Guyatt, G., & Ciliska, D. (2005). In Haynes, R. B., Devereaux, P. J., & Guyatt, G. (2002). Clinical expertise in the area of evidence-based medicine and patient choice. *Evidence-Based Medicine,* 7(2), 36–38. Copyright © 2002, British Medical Journal.

FIGURE 1-5 Process of evidence-informed practice.

organizational practice changes, and evaluates it in terms of the effectiveness and efficiency of producing intended health care outcomes (Figure 1-5). Clinical practice guidelines can take the form of protocols, clinical pathways, practice guidelines, policy statements, computer-based protocols, or algorithms.

Best practice guidelines are increasingly used to guide clinical practice in health care. Such guidelines are "systematically developed statements based on best available evidence to assist

---

TABLE 1-7 STEPS OF THE EVIDENCE-INFORMED PRACTICE PROCESS

1. Ask clinical questions by using the **PICOT** format:
   Patients/population of interest
   Intervention
   Comparison or comparison group
   Outcome(s)
   Time period (as applicable)
2. Collect the most relevant and best evidence.
3. Critically appraise and synthesize the evidence.
4. Integrate all evidence with your clinical expertise and the patient's preferences and values in making a practice decision or change.
5. Evaluate the practice decision or change.
6. Share the outcomes of the decision or change.

---

practitioners' and patients' decisions about appropriate health care" (RNAO, n.d.). Examples of the current best practice guidelines include *Adult Asthma Care Guidelines for Nurses: Promoting Control of Asthma* (RNAO, 2004); *The Assessment and Management of Pain* (RNAO, 2013a); *Person- and Family-Centred Care* (RNAO, 2015); and *Caring for Persons with Delirium, Dementia & Depression* (RNAO, 2005).

Throughout this book, two different types of "Evidence-Informed Practice" (EIP) boxes are available for selected topics. "Research Highlight" boxes provide answers to specific clinical questions. These boxes contain the PICOT (**p**atients/population of interest, **i**ntervention, **c**omparison or comparative group, **o**utcome[s], and **t**ime period as applicable) question (Table 1-7); critical appraisal of the syntheses of evidence or primary studies; implications for nursing practice; and the source of the evidence. "Translating Research into Practice" boxes provide an opportunity for you to practise your critical thinking skills in applying evidence to patient scenarios. Evidence can support current practice and increase confidence that nursing care will continue to produce the desired outcome, or evidence may necessitate a change in practice.

Steps in the Evidence-Informed Practice Process. The six steps of the EIP process are provided in Table 1-7 and Figure 1-5.

Step 1. Step 1 is to ask a clinical question in the PICOT format. Developing the clinical question is the most important step in the EBP process (Echevarria & Walker, 2014). A good clinical question sets the context for integrating evidence, clinical judgement, and patient preferences. In addition, the question guides the literature search for the best evidence to influence practice.

An example of a clinical question in PICOT format is "In adult patients undergoing abdominal surgery (**p**atients/population), is splinting with an elasticized abdominal binder (**i**ntervention) or a pillow (**c**omparison) more effective in reducing pain associated with ambulation (**o**utcome) on the first postoperative day (**t**ime period)?" A properly stated clinical question may not have all components of PICOT; some include only four components. The (T) timing or (C) comparison component may not be appropriate for a particular question.

Step 2. Step 2 is to search for the best evidence in the literature. The question directs the clinician to the databases that are most appropriate. The search begins with the strongest external evidence to answer the question. Preappraised evidence tools, such as systematic reviews and evidence-informed guidelines, are appropriate time-saving resources in the EIP process. Systematic

reviews of randomized controlled trials are considered the strongest level of evidence to answer questions about interventions (i.e., cause and effect). However, a limited number of systematic reviews are available to answer the many clinical questions. In addition, systematic reviews or meta-analyses may not always provide the most appropriate answers to all clinically meaningful questions.

If the clinical question is about how a patient experiences or copes with a health problem or lifestyle change, searching for a metasynthesis of qualitative evidence may be the most appropriate approach. When research is insufficient to guide practice, evidence from opinion leaders or authorities or reports from expert committees may be all that exist. This type of evidence should not be the sole substantiation for interventions. Care based on expert opinions requires diligent, ongoing, rigorous outcome evaluation to generate stronger evidence.

Step 3. Step 3 is to critically appraise and synthesize the data from studies found in the search. A successful critical appraisal process focuses on three essential questions: (a) Are the results of the study valid? (b) What are the results? (c) Are the findings clinically relevant to the clinician's patients? The purpose of critical appraisal is to determine not only the flaws of a study but also the value of the research to practice. To conclude what the best practice is, clinicians must determine the strength of the evidence and synthesize the findings in relation to the clinical question.

Step 4. Step 4 involves implementing the evidence in practice. Recommendations that are based on sufficient, strong evidence (e.g., interventions with systematic reviews of well-designed randomized controlled trials) can be implemented in practice in combination with clinicians' expertise and patient preferences. Clinical judgement will influence how patient preferences and values are assessed, integrated, and entered into the decision-making process. For example, although evidence may support the effectiveness of morphine as an analgesic, its use in a patient with renal failure may not be appropriate.

Step 5. Step 5 is to evaluate identified outcomes in the clinical setting. Outcomes must match the clinical project that has been implemented. For example, when the effectiveness of morphine for pain control is compared with that of fentanyl, evaluating the cost of each medication will not provide the required data about clinical effectiveness. Outcomes must reflect all aspects of implementation and capture the interdisciplinary contributions elicited by the EIP process.

Step 6. Step 6 is to share the outcomes of the EIP change. If nurses performing research do not share the outcomes of EIP, then other health care providers and patients cannot benefit from what they learned from their experience. Information is shared locally through unit- or hospital-based newsletters and posters and regionally and nationally through journal publications and presentations at conferences.

Implementation of Evidence-Informed Practice. To implement EIP, nurses continuously seek scientific evidence that supports the care that they provide. The incorporation of evidence should be balanced with clinical expertise and should take into account each patient's unique circumstances and preferences. EIP closes the gap between research and practice, resulting in care that produces more reliable and predictable outcomes than does care that is based on tradition, opinion, and a trial-and-error method. EIP provides nurses with a mechanism to manage the explosion of new literature, introduction of new technologies, concern about health care costs, and increasing emphasis on quality care and patient outcomes.

In collaboration with the First Nations and Inuit Health Branch of Health Canada, the CNA launched a Web-based portal for nurses, called **NurseONE** (see the "Resources" section at the end of this chapter). The portal provides opportunities for nurses to access libraries and information related to evidence-informed practice and clinical practice issues through a dedicated Web-based portal.

Throughout this book, two different types of EIP boxes are used to show how EIP is used in nursing practice. The "Translating Research into Practice" boxes provide initial answers to specific clinical questions. These boxes contain the clinical question, critical appraisal of the supportive evidence, implications for nursing practice, and the source of the evidence. "Applying the Evidence" boxes provide an opportunity for nurses to practise their critical thinking skills in applying EIP to patient scenarios.

THE NURSING PROCESS

The nursing process is one strategy to assist nursing students in understanding the steps involved in providing effective nursing care. The **nursing process** is an assertive, problem-solving approach to the identification and treatment of patient health problems. It provides a framework to organize the knowledge, judgements, and actions that nurses supply in patient care (Wilkinson, 2011). Using the nursing process, the nurse can focus on the unique responses of patients to actual or potential health problems.

Phases of the Nursing Process

The nursing process consists of five phases: assessment, diagnosis, planning, implementation, and evaluation (Figure 1-6). **Assessment** involves collecting subjective and objective information about the patient. The nursing diagnosis phase involves analyzing the assessment data, drawing conclusions from the information, and labelling the human response. **Planning** consists of setting goals and expected outcomes with the patient and, when feasible, the patient's family and determining strategies for accomplishing the goals. **Implementation** involves the use of nursing interventions to activate the plan. The nurse also promotes self-care and family involvement when appropriate. **Evaluation** is an extremely important part of the nursing process that is too often not addressed sufficiently. In the evaluation phase, the nurse first determines whether the identified outcomes have been met. Then the overall accuracy of the assessment, diagnosis, and implementation phases is evaluated. If the outcomes have not been met, new approaches are considered and implemented as the process is repeated.

Interrelatedness of Phases

The five phases of the nursing process do not occur in isolation from one another. For example, nurses may gather data about the wound condition (assessment) as they change the soiled dressing (implementation). There is, however, a basic order to the nursing process, which begins with assessment. Assessment provides the data on which planning is based. An evaluation of the nature of the assessment data usually follows immediately, resulting in the formulation of a diagnosis. A plan based on the nursing diagnosis then directs the implementation of nursing interventions. Evaluation continues throughout the cycle and provides feedback on the effectiveness of the plan or the need for revision. Revision may be needed in the data collection method, the diagnosis, the expected outcomes or goals, the plan, or the intervention method. Once initiated, the nursing process is not only continuous but also cyclical in nature.

Assessment Phase

Data Collection. Sound data form the foundation for the entire nursing process. Collection of data is a prerequisite for diagnosis, planning, and intervention (Figure 1-7). Humans have needs and problems in biophysical, psychological, sociocultural, spiritual, and environmental domains. A nursing diagnosis made without supporting data pertaining to all of these dimensions can lead to incorrect conclusions and depersonalized care. For example, if a hospitalized patient does not sleep all night, a disturbed sleep pattern may be mistakenly diagnosed, whereas, in fact, the patient may have worked nights her entire adult life, and it is normal for her to be awake at night. Information concerning her sleeping habits is necessary to provide individualized care to her by ensuring that sleep medication is not routinely administered to her at 2200 hours. The importance of person-centred assessment in the process of clinical decision making cannot be overemphasized.

Because nursing interventions are only as sound as the data on which they are based, the database must be accurate and complete. When possible, collateral information obtained from sources such as the patient's record, other health care workers,

FIGURE 1-6 The nursing process.

Implementation
1. Nurse-initiated
2. Physician-initiated
3. Collaborative

Assessment
1. Subjective data
2. Objective data

Evaluation
1. Outcomes met?
2. If not, re-evaluate:
 • Data
 • Diagnosis
 • Etiologies
 • Outcomes
 • Interventions

Planning
1. Priorities
2. Nursing care plan:
 • Outcomes
 • Interventions

Diagnosis
1. Data analysis
2. Problem identification
3. Nursing diagnosis label—NANDA-I

FIGURE 1-7 Collection of data is a prerequisite for diagnosis, planning, and intervention. Source: bikeriderlondon/Shutterstock.

the patient's family, and the nurse's observations should be validated with the patient. If the patient's statements seem questionable, they should be validated by a knowledgeable person.

Diagnosis Phase

Data Analysis and Problem Identification. The diagnosis phase begins with clustering of information and, after analysis of the assessment data, ends with an evaluative judgement about a patient's health status. Analysis involves sorting through and organizing the information and determining unmet needs, as well as the strengths, of the patient. The findings are then compared with documented norms to determine whether anything is interfering or could interfere with the patient's needs or ability to maintain his or her usual health pattern.

After a thorough analysis of all available information, one of two possible conclusions is reached: (1) the patient has no health problems that necessitate nursing intervention or (2) the patient needs nursing assistance to solve a potential or actual health problem.

Nursing Diagnosis. The term *nursing diagnosis* has many different meanings. To some, it merely connotes the identification of a health problem. More commonly, a nursing diagnosis is viewed as the conclusion about an identified cluster of signs and symptoms. The diagnosis is generally expressed as concisely as possible according to specific guidelines.

Nursing diagnosis is the act of identifying and labelling human responses to actual or potential health problems. Throughout this book, the term *nursing diagnosis* means (1) the process of identifying actual and potential health problems and (2) the label or concise statement that describes "a clinical judgment concerning a human response to health conditions/life processes, or a susceptibility for that response, by an individual, family, group or community. . . . A nursing diagnosis provides the basis for selection of nursing interventions to achieve outcomes for which the nurse has accountability" (NANDA International [NANDA-I], 2017, p. 115). Many human responses that are identified result from a disease process. For example, a patient may have the medical diagnosis of chronic obstructive pulmonary disease (COPD). In this case, the nursing diagnosis would focus on how the COPD affects the patient's daily functioning. Examples of patient responses to COPD might be anxiety, activity intolerance, or an inability to maintain a household. Appendix A contains a comprehensive list of nursing diagnoses relevant to care of the medical-surgical patient.

Diagnostic Process. The diagnostic process involves analysis and synthesis of the data collected during assessment of the patient. Data that indicate dysfunctional or risk patterns are clustered, and a judgement about the data is made. It is important to remember that not all conclusions resulting from data analysis lead to nursing diagnoses. Nursing diagnoses refer to health states that nurses can legally diagnose and treat. Data may also point to health problems that nurses treat collaboratively with other health care providers. During this phase of the nursing process, the nurse identifies both nursing diagnoses and treatments that necessitate collaborative nursing intervention.

Nursing diagnostic statements are considered acceptable when written as two- or three-part statements. When written in three parts, the statement is in the PES (**p**roblem, **e**tiology, and **s**igns and symptoms) format (Carpenito-Moyet, 2012; Gordon, 2014). A two-part statement is deemed acceptable if the signs and symptoms data are easily available to other nurses caring for the patient through the nursing history or progress notes. "Risk" nursing diagnoses are also two-part statements because signs

and symptoms are not relevant. Use of a three-part statement is recommended during the learning process:

Problem (P): A brief statement of the patient's potential or actual health problem (e.g., pain)

Etiology (E): A brief description of the probable cause of the problem; contributing or related factors (e.g., related to surgical incision, localized pressure, edema)

Signs and symptoms (S): A list of the objective and subjective data cluster that leads the nurse to pinpoint the problem; critical, major, or minor defining characteristics (e.g., as evidenced by verbalization of pain, isolation, withdrawal)

It is important to remember that gathering the "S" comes first in the diagnostic process, even though it is last in the PES statement format.

Identifying the Problem. The NANDA International (NANDA-I; formerly known as the North American Nursing Diagnosis Association) classification system is one framework that is useful for formulating actual nursing diagnoses and at-risk diagnoses. Clinically relevant cues are clustered into functional health patterns on the basis of Gordon's (2014) 11 functional health patterns. Gordon's functional health patterns are health perception–health management pattern; nutritional–metabolic pattern; elimination pattern; activity–exercise pattern; sleep–rest pattern; cognitive–perceptual pattern; self-perception–self-concept pattern; role–relationship pattern; sexuality–reproductive pattern; coping–stress tolerance pattern; and value–belief pattern.

The process of making a nursing diagnosis from clustered cues begins with the recognition of dysfunctional patterns. Checking the definition of nursing diagnoses classified according to the functional pattern helps identify the appropriate label for the problem. Before final selection of any nursing diagnosis for the patient, the nurse verifies the diagnostic statement with the defining characteristics listed with the diagnosis (Carpenito-Moyet, 2012; Gordon, 2014; NANDA-I, 2017). The nursing diagnosis deemed most accurate is based on the individual patient's data.

Etiology. The etiology underlying a nursing diagnosis is identified in the diagnostic statement. Taking time to properly link the problem with its etiology directs the nurse to the correct interventions. Interventions to manage the problem are planned by directing nursing efforts toward the etiology. The etiology can be a pathophysiological, maturational, situational, or treatment-related factor (Carpenito-Moyet, 2012). The etiology is written after the diagnostic label. These two components are separated by the phrase "related to." For example, in Nursing Care Plan 1-1, the nursing diagnosis is *"Activity intolerance* related to *imbalance between oxygen supply/demand."* The etiology directs the nurse to select the appropriate interventions to modify the factor of fatigue. When the etiology is not included in the diagnosis, the nurse is not able to plan the correct intervention to treat the specific cause of the problem. When possible, the etiology should be validated with the patient. When the etiology is unknown, the statement reads "related to unknown etiology." When identifying "risk-for" nursing diagnoses, the specific risk factors present in the patient's situation are identified as the etiology, and the phrase "as evidenced by" is used rather than "related to".

Signs and Symptoms. Signs and symptoms are the clinical cues that, in a cluster, point to the nursing diagnosis. The signs and symptoms are often included in the diagnostic statement after the phrase "as evidenced by." The complete nursing diagnostic statement in Nursing Care Plan 1-1 is "*Activity intolerance* related to *imbalance between oxygen supply/demand* as evidenced by *abnormal heart rate response to activity, exertional dyspnea, and fatigue.*" Throughout

NURSING CARE PLAN 1-1

Heart Failure*

NURSING DIAGNOSIS	**Activity intolerance** related to *imbalance between oxygen supply/demand* as evidenced by *abnormal heart rate response to activity, exertional dyspnea, and fatigue.*

Expected Patient Outcomes	Nursing Interventions and *Rationales*
• Achieves a realistic program of activity that balances physical activity with energy-conserving activities • Vital signs, O₂ saturation, and colour are within normal limits in response to activity	**Energy Management** • Encourage alternate rest and activity periods *to reduce cardiac workload and conserve energy.* • Provide calming diversionary activities *to promote relaxation to reduce O₂ consumption and to relieve dyspnea and fatigue.* • Monitor patient's oxygen response (e.g., pulse rate, cardiac rhythm, colour, O₂ saturation, and respiratory rate) to self-care or nursing activities *to determine level of activity that can be performed.* • Teach patient and caregiver techniques of self-care *to minimize O₂ consumption (e.g., self-monitoring and pacing techniques for performance of ADLs).* **Activity Therapy** • Collaborate with occupational therapist, physiotherapist, or both *to plan and monitor activity and exercise program.* • Determine patient's commitment to increasing frequency or range of activities, or both, *to provide patient with obtainable goals.*

*The complete nursing care plan for heart failure is provided in Nursing Care Plan 37-1 in Chapter 37.
ADLs, activities of daily living.

this book, you will see nursing diagnoses listed for many diseases and patient situations. These are NANDA-I approved diagnoses and related factors, and sometimes include additional explanatory non-NANDA-I material in parentheses.

Collaborative Problems. Collaborative problems are potential or actual complications of disease or of treatment that nurses manage together with other health care providers (Carpenito-Moyet, 2012). A look at the primary goals of nursing helps in differentiating between nursing and medical diagnoses (see Table 1-3). During the diagnosis phase of the nursing process, the nurse identifies the risks for these physiological complications in addition to nursing diagnoses. Identification of collaborative problems requires knowledge of pathophysiology and possible complications of medical treatment. For example, collaborative problems with heart failure described in Nursing Care Plan 1-1 could include pulmonary edema, hypoxemia, dysrhythmias, cardiogenic shock, or a combination of these (Carpenito-Moyet, 2012). In the interdependent role, nurses use both physician-prescribed and nursing-prescribed interventions to prevent, detect, and manage collaborative problems.

Collaborative problem statements are usually written as "potential complication: _____" (e.g., "potential complication: pulmonary edema") without a "related to" statement. When potential complications are used in this textbook, "related to" statements have been added to increase understanding and link the potential complication to possible causes.

Planning Phase

Priority Setting. After the nursing diagnoses and collaborative problems are identified, the nurse must determine the urgency of the identified problems. Diagnoses of the highest priority necessitate immediate intervention. Those of lower priority can be addressed later. When setting priorities, the nurse should first intervene for life-threatening problems involving airway, breathing, or circulation issues.

Maslow's (1954) hierarchy of needs also acts as a useful guide in determining priorities. These needs include the physical needs; safety, love, and belonging; esteem; and self-actualization. Lower-level needs must be satisfied before a higher level can be addressed.

Another guideline in setting priorities is to determine the patient's perception of what is important. When the patient's priorities are not congruent with the actual situation, the nurse may have to give explanations or do some teaching to help the patient understand the need to do one thing before another. Often it is more efficient to meet the need that the patient deems a priority before moving on to other priorities.

Identifying Outcomes. After priorities are established, expected outcomes or goals for the patient are identified. *Outcomes* are simply the results of care. Expected patient outcomes are *goals* that articulate what is desired or expected as a result of care. The terms *goals* and *expected outcomes* are often used interchangeably: both terms describe the degree to which the patient's response, as identified in the nursing diagnosis, should be prevented or changed as a result of nursing care. Expected outcomes should be agreed upon with the patient, if feasible, just as priorities of interventions are considered with the patient when possible. Although the ultimate goal for the patient is to maintain or attain a state of dynamic equilibrium at the highest possible level of wellness, the setting of more specific expected outcomes, both short- and long-term, is necessary for systematic evaluation of the patient's progress. Expected patient outcomes identified in the planning stage indicate which criteria are to be used in the evaluation phase of the nursing process.

The nurse identifies both long-term and short-term goals by writing specific expected patient outcomes in terms of desired, realistic, measurable patient behaviours to be accomplished by a specific date. For example, a short-term expected outcome for the patient in Nursing Care Plan 1-1 might be "The patient will maintain normal vital signs in response to activity in 2 days," whereas a long-term expected outcome might be "The patient will identify a realistic activity level to achieve or maintain by the time of discharge." These outcomes would be evaluated in 2 days and at discharge, and the care plan would be revised as necessary if the outcomes were not met. However, these statements are less than optimal because they provide no criteria by which to evaluate the patient's degree of progress from admission to discharge.

Determining Interventions. After patient outcomes are identified, nursing interventions to accomplish the desired status of

FIGURE 1-8 Collaboration among the patient, the family, and the nurse is necessary in setting goals and coordinating high quality care. Source: privilege/Shutterstock.com.

the patient should be planned. A **nursing intervention** is any treatment based on clinical judgement and knowledge that a nurse performs to enhance patient outcomes (Bulechek, Butcher, Dochterman, et al., 2013).

Sound knowledge, good judgement, and decision-making ability are necessary to effectively choose the interventions that the nurse will use (Figure 1-8). The nurse should foster the use of a research-based approach to interventions. In the absence of a nursing research base, scientific principles from the behavioural and biological sciences should guide the selection of interventions.

Implementation Phase. Carrying out the specific, individualized plan constitutes the implementation phase of the nursing process. The nurse performs the interventions or may designate and supervise other health care workers who are qualified to intervene. Throughout the implementation phase, the nurse must evaluate the effectiveness of the methods chosen to implement the plan.

Evaluation Phase. All phases of the nursing process must be evaluated (see Figure 1-4). Evaluation occurs after implementation of the plan but also continuously throughout the process. The nurse evaluates whether sufficient assessment data have been obtained to allow a nursing diagnosis to be made. The diagnosis is, in turn, evaluated for accuracy. For example, pain might have actually been related to a wound itself or to pressure from a constricting dressing.

Next, the nurse evaluates, with the patient when possible, whether the expected patient outcomes and interventions are realistic and achievable. If not, a new plan should be formulated. This may involve revision of expected patient outcomes and interventions. Consideration must be given to whether the plan should be maintained, modified, totally revised, or discontinued in view of the patient's status.

NURSING CARE PLANS

When the nurse has determined the nursing diagnoses, the outcomes, and the interventions for a patient, the plan is recorded to ensure continuity of care by other nurses and health care providers. The plan should contain specific directions for carrying out the planned interventions, including how, when, for how long, how often, where, by whom, and with what resources the activities should be performed.

Various methods and formats are used to record the nursing care plan. One of the important factors influencing a choice of care plan format has to do with the frameworks used in a particular agency. Care plans are often written on a specific form adopted by an institution, but they may also be entered electronically to organize nursing data. Every nurse who cares for the patient must have access to the plan, whether handwritten or computer generated, to provide the planned care. The care plan is part of the patient's medical record and may be used in legal proceedings. The nurse must document the patient's nursing care requirements, changes that are made as the plan is implemented, and the outcomes of the nursing interventions. Not every activity that the nurse implements with the patient will be recorded on the care plan.

Standardized care plans are sometimes used as guides for routine nursing care and as a basis for developing individualized care plans. When standardized care plans are used, they should be personalized and specific to the unique needs and problems of each patient.

Beginning in 2009, all nurses practising in Quebec were required to develop and update therapeutic nursing plans. Such plans are a compulsory and permanent part of the patient's record.

Concept Maps

A concept map is another method of recording a nursing care plan. In a concept map care plan, the nursing process is recorded in a visual diagram of patient problems and interventions that illustrates the relationships among clinical data. Nurse educators use concept mapping to teach nursing process and care planning. There are various formats for concept maps. *Conceptual care maps* blend a concept map and a nursing care plan. On a conceptual care map, assessment data used to identify the patient's primary health concern are centrally positioned. Diagnostic testing data, treatments, and medications surround the assessment data. Positioned below are nursing diagnoses that represent the patient's responses to the health state. Listed with each nursing diagnosis are the assessment data that support the nursing diagnosis, outcomes, nursing interventions with rationales, and evaluation. After completing the map, connections can be drawn between identified relationships and concepts. A conceptual care map creator is available online on the website for this book. For selected case studies at the end of the management chapters, related concept maps are available on the website at http://evolve.elsevier.com/Canada/Lewis/medsurg.

Clinical (Critical) Pathways

Care related to common health problems experienced by many patients is delineated with the use of clinical (critical) pathways. A **clinical (critical) pathway** directs the entire health care team in the daily care goals for select health care problems. It includes a nursing care plan, specific interventions for each day of hospitalization, and a documentation tool.

The clinical pathway organizes and sequences the caregiving process at the patient level to better achieve desired quality and cost outcomes. It is a cyclical process organized for specific case types by all related health care departments. The case types selected for clinical pathways are usually those that occur in high volume and are highly predictable, such as myocardial infarction, stroke, and angina.

The clinical pathway describes the patient care required at specific times in the treatment. A multidisciplinary approach helps the patient progress toward desired outcomes within an estimated length of stay. The exact content and format of clinical pathways vary among institutions.

DOCUMENTATION

It is critical that the patient's progress be documented in a systematic way. Proper documentation enables safe and effective patient care. Patient records are also frequently used as evidence when there are legal issues related to negligence and competency. Nurses in Canada should be aware of the Canadian Nurses Protective Society. This is the agency that provides liability coverage and is a source of information and education on issues such as documentation and charting.

Many documentation methods and formats are used, depending on personal preference, agency policy, and regulatory standards. Many provinces are now moving to implement EHRs (see "Electronic Health Records" earlier in this chapter). Funding and support are available through organizations such as the Canada Health Infoway. Patient progress may be documented by nurses with the use of flow sheets; narrative notes; SOAP (subjective, objective, assessment, plan) charting (described in the next section); clinical pathways; and computer-based charting. Every method or combination of methods is designed to document the assessment of patient status, the implementation of interventions, and the outcome of interventions.

Charting

There are several methods of documentation that address the nursing process. The SOAP method is a common way of evaluating and recording patient progress. Some institutions use SOAPIER notes (subjective, objective, assessment, plan, intervention, evaluation, and revision of plan). A SOAP or SOAPIER progress note is problem specific and incorporates the elements in Table 1-8. The following is the process of SOAP documentation.

1. Additional subjective and objective data related to the area of concern are gathered.
2. On the basis of old and new data, the patient's progress toward the expected patient outcome and the effectiveness of each intervention are assessed.

TABLE 1-8   COMPONENTS OF A SOAP PROGRESS NOTE

SOAP Component	Explanation
Subjective	Information supplied by patient or knowledgeable other person
Objective	Information obtained by nurse directly by observation or measurement, from patient records, or through diagnostic studies
Assessment	Nursing diagnosis or problem according to subjective and objective data
Plan	Specific interventions related to a diagnostic or problem with consideration of diagnostic, therapeutic, and patient education needs

3. On the basis of the reassessment of the situation, the initial plan is maintained, revised, or discontinued.

The following is an example of SOAP charting for the nursing diagnosis "*Risk for infection* as evidenced by *alteration in skin integrity and invasive procedure* (surgery)":

S: Wound is more painful today
O: Temperature of 39.4°C, facial grimacing in response to movement, dressing saturated with purulent drainage
A: Risk for wound infection
P: Notify surgeon, take temperature q2h, reinforce dressing.

A second method of documentation is the PIE (**p**roblem, **i**ntervention, and **e**valuation) method, which is similar to SOAP charting and is also problem oriented. It does not include assessment data because those are recorded on flow sheets.

A third documentation format is DAR (**d**ata, both subjective and objective; **a**ction or nursing intervention; and **r**esponse of the patient) progress notes. It is also called *focus charting*, and it addresses patient concerns, not just problems.

Charting by exception is another method of documentation that focuses on documenting deviations from predefined normal findings. Assessments are standardized on flow sheets, and nurses make a narrative note only when there are exceptions to the standardized statements.

FUTURE CHALLENGES OF NURSING

Nursing roles continually evolve as society changes and health care providers learn to integrate new knowledge and technology into current practices. Although nursing is defined in different ways, past and current definitions of nursing include commonalities of health, illness, and caring. It is important that these concepts are addressed in nursing education as greater demands are placed on the profession. Future nursing practice will continue to call for the use of reasoning, analytic thinking skills, and synthesis of rapidly expanding knowledge to assist patients in maintaining or attaining optimal health.

An increasing emphasis on leadership, accountability, courage and persistence, innovation and risk taking, and decision making is essential if nursing is to move forward. Nursing leadership refers not only to people holding certain positions but also to an attitude and approach in which lifelong learning and a commitment to excellence in practice are valued. In its attempt to keep pace, nursing would do well to remember what the Red Queen in *Through the Looking Glass* said to Alice: "Now here, you see, it takes all the running you can do to keep in the same place. If you want to get somewhere else, you must run at least twice as fast as that" (Carroll, 1865/1973). This appears to be the future of nursing. Nursing leaders must ask some fundamental questions about what the contribution of nurses must be for the twenty-first century. We must increasingly challenge the status quo by relying on research and the wisdom that results from asking difficult questions. Nurse leaders must have an attitude of open-mindedness while remaining grounded in values that overcome the tendency to promote self-interest.

REVIEW QUESTIONS

The number of the question corresponds to the same-numbered learning outcome at the beginning of the chapter.

1. Which of the following is a current challenge facing the Canadian health care system?
   a. Lack of long-term funding model between provinces/territories and federal government
   b. Lack of innovation in health care
   c. Expanding knowledge and technology
   d. Health care ranking as a low-priority public health policy issue by Canadians

2. Which of the following is an example of a nursing activity that reflects the Canadian Nurses Association's definition of nursing?
   a. Establishing that the client with jaundice has hepatitis
   b. Determining the cause of hemorrhage in a postoperative client on the basis of vital signs
   c. Identifying and treating dysrhythmias that occur in a client in the coronary care unit
   d. Determining that a client with pneumonia cannot effectively cough up pulmonary secretions

3. Which of the following characteristics of health care teams are important for outstanding interprofessional care? (Select all that apply.)
   a. Care expertise
   b. Diverse mix of health care providers
   c. Collaborative leadership
   d. Effective group functioning
   e. Clear differentiation between roles

4. The nurse is caring for a client with diabetes who has just undergone debridement of an infected toe. Which of the following statements best demonstrates client-centred care?
   a. "Administer analgesics every 4 hr prn."
   b. "Keep foot elevated to promote venous return."
   c. "Elicit expectations of client and family for relief of pain, discomfort, or suffering."
   d. "Initiate the process of teaching the client and family about self-care management."

5. What are advantages of using informatics in health care delivery? (Select all that apply.)
   a. Reduced need for nurses in acute care
   b. Increased client anonymity and confidentiality
   c. The ability to achieve and maintain high standards of care
   d. Access to standard plans of care for many health problems
   e. Improved communication of the client's health status to the health care team

6. Which of the following actions best describes the work of medical-surgical nurses?
   a. Providing care only in acute care hospital settings
   b. Requiring certification by the Canadian Nurses Association in this specialty
   c. Addressing the needs of acutely ill adults and their families
   d. Caring primarily for perioperative clients

7. "In adults older than 60 with chronic obstructive pulmonary disease, is structured pulmonary rehabilitation more effective than classroom instruction in reducing the incidence of exacerbation?" In this question, what is the outcome of interest?
   a. Adults older than age 60
   b. Adults with chronic obstructive pulmonary disease
   c. Structured pulmonary rehabilitation
   d. Reduced incidence of exacerbation

8. The nurse identifies the nursing diagnosis of *constipation* related to *laxative abuse* for a client. What is the most appropriate expected client outcome related to this nursing diagnosis?
   a. The client will stop the use of laxatives.
   b. The client ingests adequate fluid and fibre.
   c. The client passes normal stools without aids.
   d. The client's stool is free of blood and mucus.

1. a; 2. d; 3. a, c, d; 4. c; 5. c, d, e; 6. c; 7. d; 8. c.

🧬 evolve

For even more review questions, visit *http://evolve.elsevier.com/Canada/Lewis/medsurg.*

REFERENCES

Alfaro-LeFevre, R. (2016). *Critical thinking, clinical reasoning and clinical judgment* (6th ed.). St. Louis: Saunders.

Baker, G. R., Norton, P. G., Flintoft, V., et al. (2004). The Canadian Adverse Events Study: The incidence of adverse events among hospital patients in Canada. *CMAJ : Canadian Medical Association Journal = Journal de l'Association Medicale Canadienne, 170*(11), 1678–1686. doi:10.1503/cmaj.1040498. (Seminal).

Bulechek, G. M., Butcher, H. K., Dochterman, J. M., et al. (2013). *Nursing interventions classification (NIC)* (6th ed.). St. Louis: Mosby.

Canadian Association of Medical and Surgical Nurses. (2016). *About us*. Retrieved from *https://medsurgnurse.ca/about-us/.*

Canadian Association of Schools of Nursing. (2012). *Nursing informatics competencies: Entry-to-practice competencies for registered nurses*. Ottawa: Author. Retrieved from *http://www.casn.ca/wp-content/uploads/2014/12/Nursing-Informatics-Entry-to-Practice-Competencies-for-RNs_updated-June-4-2015.pdf.*

Canadian Federation of Nurses Unions. (2015). *Towards a health and social accord. Issue brief*. Retrieved from *https://nursesunions.ca/sites/default/files/towards_a_health_social_accord_issue_brief.pdf.*

Canadian Health Outcomes for Better Information and Care (C-HOBIC). (2013). *C-HOBIC. FAQs*. Retrieved from *http://c-hobic.cna-aiic.ca/faq/default_e.aspx.*

Canadian Institute for Health Information. (2013). *Canada's health care providers, 1997 to 2011—A reference guide: Overview and methodological notes*. Ottawa: Author. Retrieved from *https://secure.cihi.ca/estore/productFamily.htm?pf=PFC2161&lang=en&media=0.*

Canadian Nurses Association. (2008). *Advanced nursing practice: A national framework*. Retrieved from *https://www.cna-aiic.ca/~/media/cna/page-content/pdf-en/anp_national_framework_e.pdf.* (Seminal).

Canadian Nurses Association. (2010). *Position statement: Evidence-informed decision-making and nursing practice*. Retrieved from *https://www.cna-aiic.ca/~/media/cna/page-content/pdf-en/ps113_evidence_informed_2010_e.pdf?la=en.*

Canadian Nurses Association. (2011). *Position statement: Interprofessional collaboration.* Retrieved from *http://cna-aiic.ca/~/media/cna/page-content/pdf-en/interproffessional-collaboration_position-statement.pdf.*

Canadian Nurses Association. (2012). *A nursing call to action: The health of our nation, the future of our health system.* Retrieved from *https://www.cna-aiic.ca/~/media/cna/files/en/nec_report_e.pdf?la=en.*

Canadian Nurses Association. (2015a). *Framework for the practice of registered nurses in Canada, 2015.* Retrieved from *https://www.cna-aiic.ca/~/media/cna/page-content/pdf-en/framework-for-the-pracice-of-registered-nurses-in-canada.pdf?la=en.*

Canadian Nurses Association. (2015b). *Medical-surgical nursing certification: Exam blueprint and specialty competencies.* Retrieved from *https://nurseone.ca/~/media/nurseone/files/en/ms2015_blueprint_final_e.pdf.*

Canadian Nurses Association. (2016). *Specialties.* Retrieved from *https://nurseone.ca/en/certification/what-is-certification/competencies-per-specialty-area.*

Canadian Nurses Association. (2017). *Code of ethics for registered nurses.* Retrieved from *https://www.cna-aiic.ca/html/en/Code-of-Ethics-2017-Edition/files/assets/basic-html/page-1.html#.*

Canadian Nurses Association & Canadian Association of Schools of Nursing. (2004). *Joint position statement: Promoting continuing competence for registered nurses.* Retrieved from *https://www.cna-aiic.ca/~/media/cna/page-content/pdf-en/promoting-continuing-competence-for-registered-nurses_position-statement.pdf?la=en.* (Seminal).

Canadian Patient Safety Institute. (2016). *About CPSI.* Retrieved from *http://www.patientsafetyinstitute.ca/en/About/Pages/default.aspx.*

Carpenito-Moyet, L. J. (2012). *Handbook of nursing diagnosis* (14th ed.). Philadelphia: Lippincott.

Carroll, L. (1973). *Alice's adventures in Wonderland and through the looking glass.* New York: Collier. (Original work published 1865).

College and Association of Registered Nurses of Alberta. (2013). *Entry-to-practice competencies for the registered nurses profession.* Retrieved from *http://www.nurses.ab.ca/content/dam/carna/pdfs/DocumentList/Standards/RN_EntryPracticeCompetencies_May2013.pdf.*

College of Registered Nurses of Nova Scotia. (2011). *Standards of practice for registered nurses.* Retrieved from *http://crnns.ca/wp-content/uploads/2015/02/RNStandards.pdf.*

College of Registered Nurses of Nova Scotia & College of Licensed Practical Nurses of Nova Scotia. (2012). *Assignment and delegation guidelines for registered nurses and licensed practical nurses.* Retrieved from *https://crnns.ca/wp-content/uploads/2015/02/AssignmentandDelegationGuidelines.pdf.*

Commission on the Future of Health Care in Canada. (2002). *Romanow report proposes sweeping changes to Medicare.* Retrieved from *http://publications.gc.ca/collections/Collection/CP32-85-2002E.pdf* (Seminal).

Dagnone, T. (2009). *For patient's sake: Commissioner's recommendations.* Retrieved from *https://www.saskatchewan.ca/government/health-care-administration-and-provider-resources/saskatchewan-health-initiatives/patient-first-review.* (Seminal).

DiCenso, A., Guyatt, G., & Ciliska, D. (2005). *Evidence-based nursing: A guide to clinical practice.* St. Louis: Mosby. (Seminal).

Echevarria, I. M., & Walker, S. (2014). To make your case, start with a PICOT question. *Nursing, 44*(2), 18–19. doi:10.1097/01.NURSE.0000442594.00242.f9.

Fyke, K. J. (2001). *Caring for Medicare: Sustaining a quality system. Commission on Medicare Final Report (AKA Fyke Report).*

Regina: Government of Saskatchewan. Retrieved from *http://publications.gov.sk.ca/details.cfm?p=12038.* (Seminal).

Gordon, M. (2014). *Manual of nursing diagnosis* (13th ed.). Boston: Jones & Bartlett.

Health Canada. (2012). *Canada's health care system.* Retrieved from *http://www.hc-sc.gc.ca/hcs-sss/pubs/system-regime/2011-hcs-sss/index-eng.php.*

Institute of Medicine. (2011). *The future of nursing: Leading change, advancing health.* Washington, DC: National Academies Press. Retrieved from *http://books.nap.edu/openbook.php?record_id=12956&page=R1.*

James, J. T. (2013). A new, evidence-based estimate of patient harms associated with hospital care. *Journal of Patient Safety, 9*(3), 122–128. doi:10.1097/PTS.0b013e3182948a69.

Maslow, A. (1954). *Motivation and personality.* New York: Harper & Row. (Seminal).

Mikkonen, J., & Raphael, D. (2010). *Social determinants of health: The Canadian facts.* Toronto: York University School of Health Policy and Management. Retrieved from *http://www.thecanadianfacts.org/the_canadian_facts.pdf.*

NANDA International. (2017). *Nursing Diagnoses: Definitions and Classification 2018–2020* (11th ed.). New York: Thieme.

Nurses Association of New Brunswick and Association of New Brunswick Licensed Practical Nurses. (2015). *Guidelines for intraprofessional collaboration: Registered nurses and licensed practical nurses working together.* Retrieved from *http://www.anblpn.ca/downloads/working_together.pdf.*

Paul, R., & Elder, L. (2014). *The miniature guide to critical thinking: Concepts and tools* (7th ed.). Dillon Beach, CA: Foundation for Critical Thinking.

Philpott, J. (2016). *Health Canada 2016–17. Report on plans and priorities.* Retrieved from *http://www.healthycanadians.gc.ca/publications/department-ministere/hc-report-plans-priorities-2016-2017-rapport-plans-priorites-sc/index-eng.php.*

Premier's Advisory Council on Health for Alberta. (2001). *A framework for reform.* Retrieved from *http://www.health.alberta.ca/documents/Mazankowski-Report-2001.pdf.* (Seminal).

Provincial Health Services Authority. (2011). *Towards reducing health inequities: A health system approach to chronic disease prevention. A discussion paper.* Retrieved from *http://www.phsa.ca/population-public-health-site/Documents/TowardsReducingHealthInequitiesFinalDiscussionPape.pdf.*

Public Health Agency of Canada. (2013). *What makes Canadians healthy or unhealthy?* Retrieved from *http://www.phac-aspc.gc.ca/ph-sp/determinants/determinants-eng.php#income.*

Quality and Safety Education for Nurses. (2014). *QSEN Institute: Pre-licensure KSAs.* Retrieved from *http://qsen.org/competencies/pre-licensure-ksas.*

Registered Nurses' Association of Ontario. (2004). *Adult asthma care guidelines for nurses: Promoting control of asthma.* Retrieved from *http://rnao.ca/bpg/guidelines/adult-asthma-care-guidelines-nurses-promoting-control-asthma.*

Registered Nurses' Association of Ontario. (2005). *Caring for persons with delirium, dementia & depression.* Retrieved from *http://rnao.ca/bpg/fact-sheets/caring-persons-delirium-dementia-depression.*

Registered Nurses' Association of Ontario. (2012). *Nurse educator eHealth resource.* Retrieved from *http://rnao.ca/ehealth/educator_resource.*

Registered Nurses' Association of Ontario. (2013a). *The assessment and management of pain* (3rd ed.). Retrieved from *http://rnao.ca/bpg/guidelines/assessment-and-management-pain.*

Registered Nurses' Association of Ontario. (2013b). *Developing and sustaining interprofessional health care: Optimizing patient, organizational and system outcomes*. Retrieved from *http://rnao.ca/sites/rnao-ca/files/DevelopingAndSustainingBPG.pdf*.

Registered Nurses' Association of Ontario. (2015). *Person- and family-centred care*. Retrieved from *http://rnao.ca/bpg/guidelines/person-and-family-centred-care*.

Registered Nurses' Association of Ontario. (n.d.). *Nursing best practice guidelines: Definition of terms*. Retrieved from *http://pda.rnao.ca/content/definition-terms#bpg*.

Standing Committee on Social Affairs, Science and Technology. (2002). *The health of Canadians—The federal role. Final report. Volume 6: Recommendations for reform*. Retrieved from *http://www.parl.gc.ca/Content/SEN/Committee/372/soci/rep/repoct02vol6-e.htm*. (Seminal).

Trudeau, J. (2015). *Minister of Health mandate letter*. Retrieved from *http://pm.gc.ca/eng/minister-health-mandate-letter*.

Wilkinson, J. (2011). *Nursing process and critical thinking* (4th ed.). Upper Saddle River, NJ: Prentice Hall.

World Health Organization. (2011). *What is patient safety?* In *Patient safety curriculum guide: Multi-professional edition* (pp. 92–111). Retrieved from *http://apps.who.int/iris/bitstream/10665/44641/1/9789241501958_eng.pdf*.

RESOURCES

Canadian Association of Medical and Surgical Nurses (CASMN)
http://medsurgnurse.ca/

Canadian Association of Schools of Nursing (CASN)
http://www.casn.ca

Canada Health Infoway
https://www.infoway-inforoute.ca/

Canadian Health Outcomes for Better Information and Care (C-HOBIC) Project
http://c-hobic.cna-aiic.ca/about/default_e.aspx

Canadian Nurses Association (CNA)
https://www.cna-aiic.ca/en

Canadian Nurses Protective Society
http://www.cnps.ca/

Canadian Nursing Students' Association (CNSA)
http://cnsa.ca/about-us/

Canadian Nursing Informatics Association
http://cnia.ca/

Canadian Patient Safety Institute
http://patientsafetyinstitute.ca

NurseONE
http://www.nurseone.ca

Registered Nurses' Association of Ontario (RNAO)
http://www.rnao.org/bestpractices

NANDA International (NANDA-I)
http://www.nanda.org/

Quality and Safety Education for Nurses (QSEN)
http://qsen.org/

Sigma Theta Tau International (STT)
http://www.nursingsociety.org

For additional Internet resources, see the website for this book at *http://evolve.elsevier.com/Canada/Lewis/medsurg*

Cultural Competence and Health Equity in Nursing Care

Written by: Rani H. Srivastava

ⓔvolve WEBSITE

http://evolve.elsevier.com/Canada/Lewis/medsurg

- Review Questions (Online Only)
- Key Points
- Answer Guidelines for Case Study

- Conceptual Care Map Creator
- Audio Glossary
- Content Updates

LEARNING OBJECTIVES

1. Define the terms *culture, cultural competence, cultural safety, ethnocentrism, cultural imposition, world view, health literacy,* and *health equity.*
2. Identify the determinants of health and health inequities for Indigenous populations.
3. Describe the factors that lead to health inequities in culturally diverse populations.
4. Explain the links between cultural competence, patient safety, and patient- or family-centred care.

5. Describe strategies for successfully communicating with a person with limited English proficiency.
6. Examine ways that a nurse's own cultural background may influence how that nurse delivers nursing care.
7. Describe strategies for demonstrating cultural competence and promoting health equity in care encounters.
8. Identify the benefits and challenges associated with a diverse workforce.

KEY TERMS

acculturation, p. 24
cultural competence, p. 25
cultural imposition, p. 24
cultural safety, p. 24
culture, p. 24

diversity, p. 25
ethnicity, p. 25
ethnocentrism, p. 24
explanatory model, p. 26
health literacy, p. 22

health inequality, p. 22
health inequity, p. 22
health literacy, p. 22
intersectionality, p. 25
race, p. 25

racialization, p. 25
stereotyping, p. 25
world view, p. 24

THE NEED FOR CULTURAL COMPETENCE

In today's increasingly multicultural environment, nurses come in contact with individuals from many different cultures, as patients and as colleagues, during their professional careers. This diversity can be enriching as it offers unique opportunities to learn from patients, families, and each other. At the same time, differences in culture can affect the safety and quality of care.

Because of the changes in demographic and cultural compositions of Canada and other countries, all health care providers must understand the influence of culture on health beliefs, practices, and outcomes. Culture influences individual beliefs about health, illness, care, cure, and even expectations of health care providers. Understanding these differences is crucial for providing care that is safe, meaningful, and effective for patients and families.

Canadian society is an ethnocultural mosaic characterized by immigrant population, linguistic diversity, and religious diversity.

According to data from the 2011 National Health Survey (NHS), foreign-born individuals represented approximately one-fifth (20.6%) of Canada's total population (Statistics Canada, 2013a). This is a slight increase from the 2006 census. Since the mid-1980s, Canadian immigration patterns have been undergoing a significant shift with regard to the countries from which people come. Before the 1970s, the majority of immigrants to Canada came from European countries such as the United Kingdom, Italy, Germany, and the Netherlands; however, the proportion of European-born immigrants has continued to decline steadily. By 2006, immigrants born in Asia (including the Middle East) made up 58% of all newcomers to Canada, and in 2011, the top three countries of origin were the Philippines, China, and India, followed by the United States, Pakistan, the United Kingdom, Iran, South Korea, Colombia, and Mexico. Although the majority of immigrants tend to settle in four provinces—Ontario, British Columbia, Quebec, and Alberta—changing demographics are evident across all of the provinces and cities (Statistics Canada, 2013a).

The shift in countries of origin for immigrants has led to increased linguistic and religious diversity, as well as increases in the proportion of newcomers who are also members of visible minorities. The term *visible minority*, as used by Statistics Canada, is defined as "persons, other than Aboriginal persons, who are non-Caucasian in race or non-white in colour" (Statistics Canada, 2013b). In 2011, 1 per 5 people identified themselves as a member of a visible minority. Of this number, approximately one-third were born in Canada, and approximately two-thirds (65%) were born outside the country and came to Canada as immigrants (Statistics Canada, 2013a).

Language diversity has also continued to increase in Canada; nearly 73% of Canadian immigrants have reported a first language other than English or French (Statistics Canada, 2013a). Nearly 200 languages have been reported as first languages, the most frequent being the Chinese languages, Tagalog, Spanish, and Punjabi (Statistics Canada, 2013a).

Another noteworthy trend is the relatively young age of the immigrant population. In 2011, the majority of individuals who had come to Canada since 2006 were between 25 and 54; approximately 20% were children aged 14 and younger; 15% were between the ages of 15 and 24 (Statistics Canada, 2013a). These trends provide insights into the potential health needs that will arise for this population in the coming years.

Although these changing demographics portend new challenges and opportunities in providing health care to a multi-ethnic population, it is important to remember that newcomer status is only one marker of cultural diversity. Indigenous people are the original inhabitants of Canada, but they are not part of the dominant Canadian cultural group. Instead, they are considered a minority group and experience many of the challenges faced by newcomers with regard to language and cultural beliefs in accessing health care (Statistics Canada, 2013b). In addition, the historical legacy of colonization and discrimination has led to social, psychological, and cultural crises in the Indigenous population that necessitate a deeper understanding of the unique challenges for this community, including the context of colonial policies and practices both past and present (Allan & Smylie, 2015).

Individuals with identities other than Indigenous, immigrant, or visible minority status also experience threats to patient safety and quality care. These include but are not limited to people with nondominant sexual orientation, nondominant gender identity, language disability, low socioeconomic status, and mental or physical disabilities.

The need for culturally appropriate care has been highlighted by increasing evidence of health inequities in these populations and a growing recognition that a lack of cultural competence (a concept discussed in depth later in this chapter) leads to unsafe care. Cultural competence is recognized as a critical attribute for the provision of safe, effective, quality care and an entry to practice level competency for registered nurses in Canada (Canadian Nurses Association, 2010; Douglas, Rosenkoetter, Pacquiao, et al., 2014).

In a culturally diverse nation such as Canada, it is important to recognize that those who differ from the majority are not just different with regard to their values and beliefs, and how they respond in certain situations; being different from the majority or the "norm" also puts them at a disadvantage in terms of power dynamics (Srivastava, 2014). This is discussed later in the chapter.

HEALTH EQUITY

As discussed in Chapter 1, health status of individuals and communities is influenced by many factors: social, economic, and political. Health equity is an important concept in the pursuit of quality care for all individuals, regardless of their background and socioeconomic status. **Health equity** is present when individuals have the opportunity to achieve their full health potential and is often described as the absence of unfair systems and policies that cause health inequalities (Canadian Medical Association [CMA], 2013). Health equity is concerned with creating equal opportunities for good health for everyone in two ways: (a) decreasing the negative effect of the social determinants of health and (b) by improving services to enhance access and reduce exclusion.

An understanding of health equity requires an understanding of two related but distinct concepts: health inequality and health inequity. **Health inequality** is a broad term that refers to differences in the health status of individuals and groups as a result of factors such as biological and genetic makeup, physical environments, actions of the health care system, and broad social and economic issues (CMA, 2013). **Health inequity** refers to health inequalities that are a result of factors that are generally considered to be *unfair* or *unjust and modifiable* (Public Health Agency of Canada, 2011).

For example, differences in health status that are based on genetics or developmental processes such as aging lead to inequalities in health but are not considered unfair. However, Canadians who live in remote or northern regions do not have the same access to nutritious foods, such as fruits and vegetables, as do other Canadians, and this lack of access to healthy foods results in poor nutrition, which in turn can affect health significantly; this is an example of heath inequity. As a result of inequities in health, groups of people who are already socially disadvantaged (because of socioeconomic status, sex, or membership in a minority racial, ethnic, or religious group) are at further disadvantage with regard to health.

Health Inequities Among Indigenous and Other Marginalized Populations

Indigenous populations in Canada experience many health inequities, as is evident from the significantly higher rates of illnesses such as tuberculosis, diabetes, and cardiovascular disease and by the higher rates of suicide and self-injury among these groups (Wasekeesikawa & Perley-Dutcher, 2013). Many factors contribute to these inequities. Living in remote or northern regions is one potential contributing factor; however, the health of Indigenous Canadians is also affected by the loss of culture, including language and connection to land; by racism and stigmatization; and by loss of connection with Indigenous identity and spirituality (Canadian Institute of Health Research [CIHR], 2015; Wasekeesikawa & Perley-Dutcher, 2013). These losses can be traced back to the history of colonization and policies resulting in cultural destruction and trauma (Allan & Smylie, 2015).

Table 2-1 provides additional examples of some social and health inequities experienced by marginalized populations.

Health Literacy

Another factor that can potentially compromise a person's ability to achieve health equity is health literacy. In Canada, **health literacy** is defined as the "ability to access, comprehend, evaluate and communicate information as a way to promote, maintain

TABLE 2-1 EXAMPLES OF HEALTH INEQUITIES EXPERIENCED BY MARGINALIZED POPULATIONS

- People who experience racial discrimination self-report poor or fair health more often than do those who do not experience it (Levy, Ansara, & Stover, 2013).
- People who reported experiencing racial discrimination were more likely to report depressive symptoms than did people who did not report experiencing racial discrimination (Levy, Ansara, & Stover, 2013).
- Smoking rates are more than two times higher among the three Indigenous groups than among the non-Indigenous population. Indigenous people were also twice as likely to be exposed to second-hand smoke in the home (Gionet & Roshanafshar, 2015).
- Suicide rates are five to seven times higher among Indigenous youth than among non-Indigenous youth. Suicide rates among Indigenous youth are among the highest in the world, at 11 times the national average (Health Canada, 2013).
- Transgendered people experience extremely high levels of depression and suicide. More than half of transgendered people in Ontario have levels of depressive symptoms consistent with clinical depression, and 43% had a history of attempting suicide (Bauer & Scheim, 2015).
- The health of immigrants begins to decline soon after arrival in Canada; "visible minority" status is a statistically significant factor in the decline of immigrant health (Nestel, 2012).

Sources: Gionet, L., & Roshanafshar, S. (2015). Select health indicators of First Nations people living off reserve, Métis and Inuit. Ottawa: Ministry of Industry; Health Canada. (2013). First Nations & Inuit health: Suicide prevention. Retrieved from http://www.hc-sc.gc.ca/fniah-spnia/promotion/suicide/index-eng.php; Levy, J., Ansara, D., & Stover, A. (2013). Racialization and health inequities in Toronto. Toronto: Toronto Public Health; and Nestel, S. (2012). *Colour coded health care: The impact of race and racism on Canadians' health.* Toronto: The Wellesley Institute.

and improve health in a variety of settings across the life-course" (Public Health Agency of Canada, 2014). This includes being able to access and navigate the health care system. Lack of health literacy has been identified as a significant challenge across a number of population groups, including many cultural communities, and is associated with a variety of poor health outcomes (Kalich, Heinemann, & Ghahari, 2015; Paasche-Orlow, 2011). (Health literacy is discussed further in Chapter 4.)

Equity in Nursing Care

The growing evidence of health inequities across a variety of groups is challenging previous assumptions about how to provide quality health care for everyone in the context of a diverse society. Without cultural competence, patients, families, and communities are at risk for a lack of care or for receiving care that is ineffective or unsafe. A commitment to health equity and social justice, along with a focus on determinants of health, is a key principle for primary health care as well (see Chapter 6). Nurses promote health equity by adopting a social justice approach and providing services that are accessible and devoid of discrimination and prejudice, by removing unnecessary complexity in care, and by developing cross-cultural communication competencies that empower individuals and communities to make informed, effective choices (Paasche-Orlow, 2011).

The importance of health equity has been recognized internationally, and considerable work is happening at both national and provincial levels. Pathways to Health Equity for Aboriginal Peoples is an example of national effort launched by the CIHR (2015). Another example is the development of a health equity impact assessment (HEIA) tool as a decision support tool to help identify how a program, policy, or initiative will affect population groups in different ways. When unintended potential effects are recognized, mitigating strategies can be put in place to reduce the negative and maximize the positive effects (Ontario Ministry of Health and Long Term Care, 2013).

Culture as a Determinant of Health

As discussed in Chapter 1, culture is one of the 12 determinants of health identified by the Public Health Agency of Canada (2013). It is also considered one of the *social* determinants of health, which are linked to the colonial history of Canada and ongoing inequitable social and political structures and systems.

Health and illness are inextricably linked to cultural issues. Culture influences how illness is perceived and experienced, what symptoms are reported, what remedies are sought, and who is consulted in the process (Srivastava, 2007a). The effect of culture on health is significant and pervasive and can be both positive and negative.

Fowler and Reimer-Kirkham (2012) identified several positive influences of religion and culture, including countering effects of stress and isolation, positive psychosocial and physiological effects of fellowship and community, and finding meaning in illness and suffering. As noted earlier, although loss of cultural identity and supports can produce ill health, experience from the Indigenous communities also highlights the positive relationship between supporting traditions and beliefs of a community and good health (Anderson & Olson, 2013).

Language barriers pose a major threat to patient safety and quality of care (Flores, 2014; King, Desmarais, Lindsay, et al., 2015). The resettlement process for immigrants and refugees presents inherent challenges as these individuals experience difficulties in employment, housing, and access to social support. In addition, such individuals may face health risks from a social environment in which dominant cultural values perpetuate conditions of marginalization, stigmatization, loss or devaluation of language and culture, and lack of access to culturally appropriate diet, activity, and health care services. Disruptions in traditional lifestyles can also lead to greater social exclusion and to increased use of substances such as alcohol, tobacco, and other substances. As a result of cultural differences between patients and health service providers, patients may delay seeking help, health care providers may ignore symptoms that are important to patients, and patients may not follow through with prescribed treatments.

Of importance is that although culture is regarded as a determinant of health, it should not be confused with being the *cause* of inequities; rather the inequities are rooted in the social determinants of health.

EXPLORING THE CONCEPTS: DEFINITIONS AND MEANINGS

One of the greatest difficulties associated with developing cultural competence in health care has been a lack of clarity about the meaning of terms such as *culture, cultural competence,* and *cultural safety,* as well as related terms such as *diversity, ethnicity, race,* and *minority.* For example, the term *visible minority* is often used as though it refers to a single group of people, but it actually refers to a wide range of heterogeneous groups whose experiences have been historically different and who hold different positions in the economic and political systems (Nestel, 2012). Terminology related to cultural diversity is subject to multiple interpretations and continues to evolve over time.

Cultural Safety and Cultural Competence

In Canada, both *cultural safety* and *cultural competence* are concepts used to guide the provision of safe, effective, equitable, patient-centred care. Frameworks for both concepts have different origins but have many similarities with regard to key attributes and skills needed by nurses and other health care providers.

The concept of cultural safety is based on the notion of biculturalism and was initially developed in New Zealand to draw attention to the effect of colonization on the health of the indigenous Maori people. **Cultural safety** focuses on the power imbalances that lead to a disregard for health and illness beliefs of the indigenous people and to a privileging of the dominant cultural values. In Canada, the notion of cultural safety continues to be applied largely to health care for Indigenous people. It recognizes the effects of colonization, historical trauma created by forced social assimilation, and the resulting loss of cultural cohesion (Racine, 2014). The extent to which the concept of cultural safety applies to immigrant, refugee, ethnic, and other racialized populations remains unclear.

The call for "culturally competent care" in nursing can be traced back to the 1960s, when Madeleine Leininger advocated for the use of culturally based health knowledge and care to ensure appropriate and effective care for individuals and groups with differences in values, beliefs, explanatory models of illness (discussed later in this chapter), and systems of healing (Srivastava, 2007a).

Some authors view cultural safety as an extension of cultural competence on a continuum, whereby cultural competence is a process and cultural safety is the outcome; others view it as a fundamental paradigm shift that focuses on social and political power and redefines the provider–patient relationship with emphasis on self-determination. Although cultural safety has a greater focus on race relations and on historical and current government practices and policies, both frameworks articulate the need for inclusivity; respect for unique history, traditions, and beliefs of individuals and groups; communicating in culturally appropriate ways; and a recognition of the effect of the broader social determinants of health on individuals, families, and communities.

In this chapter, the term *cultural competence* is used largely because the notion of competence implies acquisition and use of specific knowledge and skills in an intentional way to ensure the provision of quality care. The fundamental tenets underlying culturally competent care are (a) the need to uncover and address one's own assumptions about people and situations; (b) the importance of purposefully seeking out similarities and differences between individuals and groups in order to be responsive to people's varying needs; (c) the importance of addressing the dynamics of difference that lead to unequal social power and social exclusion at the levels of both the individual and the broader system; and (d) promoting inclusivity and self-determination of goals for individuals and communities. These tenets form the basis of the relational approach to cultural care (Srivastava, 2008). Throughout this text, special "Culturally Competent Care" sections highlight knowledge and skills relevant to providing culturally competent health care.

"Culture" and Other Related Terms

The term **culture** is difficult to define. Although many people equate culture with ethnicity, race, country of origin, or religion, this is an erroneous oversimplification. Culture can include many dimensions, including ethnicity, language, religion, sex,

TABLE 2-2 KEY CHARACTERISTICS OF CULTURE

Culture is...
- *Learned* through the processes of language acquisition and socialization
- *Shared* by all members of the same cultural group
- *Adapted* to specific conditions such as environmental factors
- *Dynamic* and ever-changing in relation to historical, political, and social conditions
- *Invisible* and often sensed but not seen
- *Selective*, thereby distinguishing members of one group from those of another and differentiating between groups

Source: Adapted from Srivastava, R. (2007). Culture care framework I: Overview and cultural sensitivity. In R. Srivastava (Ed.), *The healthcare professional's guide to clinical cultural competence* (pp. 53–74). Toronto: Elsevier Canada.

socioeconomic class, professional status, age, sexual orientation, group history, and life experiences (Garneau & Pepin, 2015). Culture affects ways of perceiving, behaving in, and evaluating the world, and it serves as a guide for people's values, beliefs, and practices, including those related to health and illness. Culture is not something that belongs to particular individuals; everyone has a culture. Culture exists at the levels of the individual, group, and larger society, and with regard to achieving health equity, the culture of health care providers and the health care system matters as much as the culture of the patient (Srivastava, 2008).

Cultural values are often unconsciously developed and are responsible for many inherent biases, including perceptions of acceptable and unacceptable behaviour. Cultural beliefs and ways of being are often referred to as a **world view**. A world view is a paradigm or a set of assumptions, values, concepts, and practices that influences how people perceive, interpret, and relate to the world around them.

Culture has a number of distinguishing features (Table 2-2 highlights six key characteristics). Although individuals within a cultural group have many similarities through their shared values, beliefs, and practices, there is also much diversity within groups. Individual differences continue to exist, and each person is culturally unique.

Ethnocentrism is a tendency of people to believe that their way of viewing and responding to the world is the most correct, most natural, and superior one. To some extent, this is a universal tendency; each person has the greatest familiarity with and a preference for his or her own way of doing things. However, the conscious or unconscious belief that a particular way is the only way or the best way for everyone is problematic and can cause a person to categorize others' beliefs as unusual, inferior, bizarre, and therefore inappropriate. Ethnocentrism can prevent people from considering alternative perspectives and from respecting others' world views.

Cultural imposition, a closely related concept, is the situation in which a person's own cultural beliefs and practices are, intentionally or unintentionally, imposed on another person or group of people. In health care, it can result in disregarding or trivializing a patient's health beliefs or practices.

Cultural practices change over time through processes such as acculturation. **Acculturation** is a multidimensional process in which individuals and groups undergo stages of adjustment, as well as changes in several domains such as language, socioeconomic status, values, and attitudes (Lopez-Class, Castro, & Ramirez, 2011). This process may be a gradual change that results in increased similarity between two cultures.

Ethnicity refers to characteristics of a group whose members share a common social, cultural, linguistic, or religious heritage and often implies a geographical or national affiliation (Browne & Varcoe, 2014). **Race** is controversial in that it is both a biological and social construct. The term *race* is sometimes used to highlight biological differences and physical characteristics such as skin colour, bone structure, or blood group. However, the biological basis of race is frequently challenged. Children of mixed-race couples can have varying degrees of skin pigmentation and physical characteristics, and yet all the children of a mixed-race couple share similar genetic makeup and social culture. As a social construct, race has been used to denote superiority and inferiority, whereby the assigned status limits or increases opportunities and leads to assumptions about individuals and groups; thus the social meaning of race is often more important than the biological meaning (Nestel, 2012).

Such categorization or differentiation according to race is described as a process of racialization. **Racialization** is closely linked to discrimination, in which members of a particular cultural group are treated unfairly. Ethnicity and race have an intersectional relationship in that the racial diversity occurs within ethnically defined groups and vice versa, and the effect on health is often interrelated (Nestel, 2012; Veenstra, 2011).

In a large and growing body of research, racism has been linked to poor health (see Nestel, 2012). The effect of racism is multifaceted. Individuals experiencing racism may resort to high-risk behaviours, such as substance abuse, self-harm, or simply delaying seeking health care. Racism can influence physical health by causing chronic, negative emotional states such as anxiety, depression, and diminished self-esteem or identity, which, in turn, can have direct effects on biological processes such as the cardiovascular and immune systems and can increase vulnerability to infections, diabetes, high blood pressure, heart attack, stroke, depression, and aggression (Nestel, 2012). Racism also influences health indirectly through differential exposures and opportunities related to other determinants of health such as education and employment (or affects self-worth when negative messages are internalized).

In **stereotyping**, members of a specific culture, race, or ethnic group are automatically assumed to have characteristics associated with that group, without further exploration of what the individuals—or, for that matter, what the cultural group itself—are actually like. This oversimplified approach does not take into account individual differences that exist within a culture. Stereotyping can occur with patients or health care providers. In health care, as well as in other settings, being a member of a particular ethnic group does not make the person an expert on other members of that same group. Such stereotyping can lead to false assumptions and negative attitudes that adversely affect a patient's care.

Diversity is another term that is related to culture. For some people, the term simply refers to differences or variations across individuals and social groups, whereas for others, it represents a sum of differences, usually with regard to unequal access to power, privilege, and resources. In general, in the health care context, diversity implies difference from the majority or dominant group that is assumed to be the norm (Srivastava, 2008). Diverse groups and communities, in this context, have marginalized status in society, and diversity initiatives often become synonymous with asserting human rights, freedom from discrimination, social justice, and, more recently, health equity.

Intersectionality is described as a framework for understanding how multiple social identities such as race, gender, sexual orientation, and economic status interact with each other to reflect interlocking systems of privilege and oppression. No single social identity is responsible for these systems; rather, they all interact with each other to create a new unique identity, which results in varying degrees of exclusion and disadvantage (National Collaborating Centre for Healthy Public Policy, 2015; Veenstra, 2011).

CULTURAL COMPETENCE

Cultural competence is a complex concept that has evolved from older terms such as *cultural sensitivity* and *cultural awareness*. Whereas cultural sensitivity and awareness refer to an appreciation of and respect for cultural differences, competence takes the concept one step further and refers to the ability to actually apply knowledge and skill appropriately in interactions with patients. **Cultural competence** is a process that involves the application of knowledge, attitudes, and skills that enhance cross-cultural communication; foster meaningful, respectful interactions with others; and, in so doing, address issues of exclusion that can affect health outcomes. Cultural competence includes valuing diversity, knowing about cultural norms and traditions of the populations being served, and accounting for these differences when care is provided (Douglas, Rosenkoetter, Pacquiao, et al., 2014; Srivastava, 2014).

The International Council of Nurses (2013) noted that nurses demonstrate cultural competence by developing self-awareness without letting it have undue influence on their treatment of patients from other backgrounds, by having knowledge and understanding of a patient's culture, by accepting and respecting cultural differences, and by adapting care to be congruent with a patient's culture. Cultural competence does not mean knowing everything about a particular culture; rather, it is an evolving process that is grounded in knowledge of a number of concepts, reflection, and action (Blanchet-Garneau & Pepin, 2015).

There are many definitions, frameworks, and models of cultural competence, each highlighting a different aspect of culture and attributes of cultural competence (Shen, 2015; Srivastava, 2007a). However, three key domains are evident across these frameworks: (a) an *affective* domain, which reflects an awareness of and sensitivity to cultural values, needs, and biases; (b) a *behavioural* domain, which reflects skills necessary to be effective in cross-cultural encounters; and (c) a *cognitive* domain, which involves cultural knowledge, as well as theory, research, and cross-cultural approaches to care. Together, these domains can be considered the *ABCs* of cultural competence.

To fully understand the complexities of cultural competence and its relationship to health equity, however, two other domains must also be present. The *dynamics* of difference (D) highlights the fact that the effect of difference is based on differences in world views, as well as on the stigma and racism associated with minority group status and social power imbalances. The practice *environment (E)* consists of the context of care and the supports that may or may not be available; the goal of *equity* is assumed as well (Srivastava, 2008). Understanding and actively addressing the dynamics of difference is consistent with nursing role expectations of social justice advocacy. Working towards social justice requires understanding the effect of unequal relationships, being aware of the mechanisms of oppression and systemic bias, and the ability to identify and challenge the inequities that are based on social power.

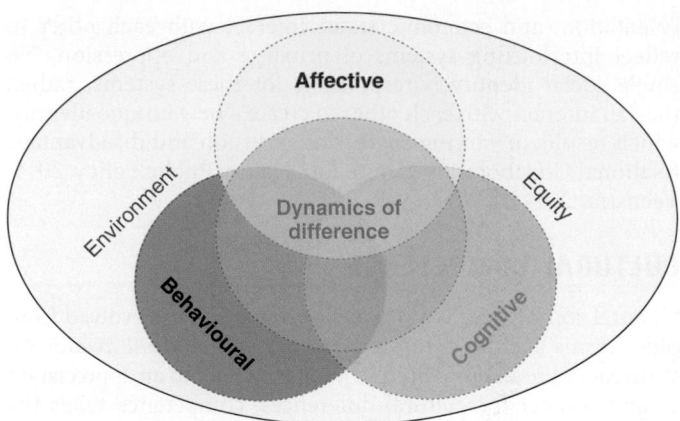

FIGURE 2-1 The ABCDEs of cultural competence. Source: Adapted from Srivastava, R. (2008). The ABC [and DE] of cultural competence in clinical care. *Ethnicity and Inequalities in Health and Social Care, 8*(11), 25–31 (p. 31).

Figure 2-1 shows the ABCDE framework for cultural competence. Table 2-3 presents examples of attributes that describe the ABC domains of cultural competence. The influence of the dynamics of difference and the environment is evident throughout the affective, behavioural, and cognitive domains and is thus not highlighted separately in the table.

Affective Domain

The affective domain of cultural competence is concerned with both attitude and awareness. This domain is often seen as the first step toward achieving cultural competence. Openness, a desire to learn, valuing differences, respect for others, and developing humility are characteristic of this domain (Douglas, Rosenkoetter, Pacquiao, et al., 2014; Srivastava, 2014). This domain is characterized by acceptance of the notion of multiple world views and norms and by the recognition that no one way is universally beneficial.

Cultural awareness is a conscious learning process in which individuals become appreciative of and sensitive to their own culture, as well as the cultures of other people. Awareness can be subcategorized into three components: self-awareness, awareness of others, and awareness of the dynamics of difference (see the "Dynamics of Difference" section later in this chapter). Every person is a cultural being; therefore, any nurse–patient interaction is affected by the cultures of both the nurse and the patient. The nurse is influenced by his or her cultural background, by the culture of the nursing profession, and by the culture of the health care setting in which the interaction occurs.

The first step in developing cultural awareness is for the nurse to examine his or her own biases toward people from different cultures. Identifying how these views may influence the care encounter is a critical step in recognizing ethnocentrism and avoiding cultural imposition. Development of self-awareness requires the nurse to engage in ongoing critical self-reflection and being amenable to feedback from other people (see the "Nurse's Self-Assessment" section later in this chapter). Awareness of other people as cultural beings is based on recognition of multiple world views and norms. Cultural differences are not issues of right or wrong; they are simply about being different.

Behavioural Domain

The behavioural domain concerns the actual application of knowledge and awareness and is also described as cultural skill.

Through the intentional use of these skills, the health care provider can determine the most appropriate goals and interventions by performing a comprehensive assessment of not only patients' complaints and symptoms but also their values, beliefs, and practices. Different cultural groups have different beliefs about the causes of illness and the appropriateness of various treatments. It is important for the nurse to try to determine the patient's explanatory model (set of beliefs regarding what causes the disease or illness and the methods that would potentially treat the condition best). It is also important to determine how experiences and beliefs affect health-seeking behaviours. Table 2-4 lists key questions that can be used to learn about the patient's explanatory model of illness and care. These questions do not have to be asked in the order they are listed, and they can be adapted to the situation. Through these questions, nurses can identify cultural values and beliefs that are important to the patient in a given situation (College of Nurses of Ontario, 2009).

The behavioural or skills domain is complex and requires competency in awareness, knowledge, and application of the generalized awareness of cultural issues to specific clinical situations.

Cross-Cultural Communication. Communication is foundational for every aspect of the clinical encounter; therefore, cross-cultural communication is a key area in which to develop cultural skill (see Table 2-3). Cultural differences are often cited as a barrier to effective communication, leading to poor adherence to regimens, dissatisfaction with care, and adverse health outcomes (Flores, 2014; King, Desmarais, Lindsay, et al., 2015). Culturally safe communication that includes communication of cultural understanding and respect is an essential tool in forming a therapeutic relationship with the client. It is critical for establishing trust, for informed consent, for decision making, for ability to partner in care, and for self-management of chronic illnesses (Canadian Nurses Association, 2010; International Council of Nurses, 2013).

Verbal and Nonverbal Communication. Cultural influences on communication are evident in both verbal and nonverbal communication. Verbal communication includes not only the language or dialect but also the voice tone, volume, timing, and a person's willingness to share thoughts and feelings. Nonverbal communication includes eye contact, use of touch, body language, style of greeting, and the spatial arrangement taken up by the participants. Culture influences the ways that feelings are expressed, as well as which verbal and nonverbal expressions are appropriate in given situations.

Nonverbal communication includes silence, touch, and eye contact, and the norms vary across cultures. For example, many Indigenous people are comfortable with silence and interpret silence as essential for thinking and carefully considering a response. In these interactions, silence shows respect for the other person and demonstrates the importance of the remarks. In traditional Japanese and Chinese cultures, the speaker may stop talking and leave a period of silence for the listener to think about what has been said before continuing. In other cultures (e.g., French, Spanish, and Russian), silence may be interpreted as meaning agreement.

Although nurses are often taught to maintain direct eye contact, patients who are Asian, Arab, or Indigenous may avoid direct eye contact and consider direct eye contact disrespectful or aggressive. Other factors to consider include the role of sex, age, status, or position on what is considered to be appropriate eye contact. For example, Muslim-Arab women avoid eye contact

TABLE 2-3 THE ABCS OF CULTURAL COMPETENCE

Component	Description
Affective (Awareness) Domain	
Attitude	• Humility and a recognition of the need for ongoing learning and *unlearning*
	• Genuine curiosity and desire to learn; valuing differences
	• Nonjudgemental stance in encountering situations and perspectives that are different from those of self or the norm
	• Commitment to the goal of social justice, inclusivity, and equity
Awareness of self, others, and dynamics of difference	• Self-awareness of values, beliefs, and biases, including unconscious bias
	• Critical reflexivity to examine and critique own beliefs
	• Awareness of own social location and privilege
	• Awareness of challenges with cross-cultural communication
	• Awareness of cultural influences on information seeking, conflict, and decision making
	• Recognition of the historical effects of racism and discrimination in society and health care
Behavioural (Skills) Domain	
Assessment	• Ask the correct questions in the correct way (knowing what and knowing how)
	• Establish trust and health care provider's credibility
	• Elicit patient's explanatory model of illness
	• Assess for the effect of social determinants on current situation
Cross-cultural communication	• Determine patient's values, strengths, and goals
	• Adapt own communication style to address cultural nuances and differences in information processing and decision making
	• Provide information in ways that are consistent with patient's linguistic and health literacy needs
	• Become familiar with different communication styles and patterns
Collaborative decision making	• Elicit patient's values, preferences, and explanatory models of health and illness
Empowering and promoting patient choice	• Recognize the need for and make use of interpreters for language support
	• Accommodate values and preferences and negotiate approaches to obtain mutually agreed-upon goals
Advocacy across differences	• Review cultural conflicts as opportunities to learn from differences
	• Reframe situations to mitigate biases that are held by the health care provider or the patient
	• Promote health literacy
	• Support informed patient choices
Development of resources (personal and organizational) to support practice	• Identify own privilege and use it appropriately to further goals of equity
	• Recognize and address the dynamics of difference at patient–clinician level and at patient–health care system level
	• Connect patients with resources within their community to promote greater autonomy and self-management
	• Explore opportunities to partner with and learn from colleagues, patients, and communities that are culturally different from self or own
	• Seek information on different cultural groups through the internet, media, movies, and visits to cultural and community centres
	• Seek out the insider cultural perspectives and meanings of events and traditions
	• Develop relationship with service agencies that support health for specific cultural groups and communities
Cognitive (Knowledge) Domain	
Generic cultural knowledge	• Understand the effect of culture on health and health seeking behaviours
	• Understand the difference between individualistic and collectivist cultures
	• Recognize dimensions of care that are likely to be influenced by culture in a particular setting (e.g., end-of-life care)
	• Identify bio-physiological determinants of health and illness in minority groups
	• Identify social determinants of health: effects of race, culture, health status, employment, and so forth
	• Understand health disparities and health equity issues
	• Identify the effect of health policy on culturally diverse groups, particularly those whose members are economically disadvantaged
	• Understand the effect of diversity on team functioning
Specific cultural knowledge	• Develop in-depth knowledge of particular communities served, including religious and cultural beliefs and traditions; cultural strengths and resources; and health inequities particular to the group or groups, such as issues of access to health care, congruence of health care with the culture, and incidence and prevalence of major illnesses
	• Learn about commonly held world views and healing traditions
	• Identify the effect of life events such as migration, settlement, and racism
	• Review the care process for own clinical specialty and identify processes and treatments that are particularly susceptible to cultural differences
	• Do not make assumptions on the basis of cultural background; instead, use knowledge as a beginning point for further assessment and inquiry

Sources: Adapted from Srivastava, R. (2008). The ABC (and DE) of cultural competence in clinical care. *Ethnicity and Inequalities in Health and Social Care, 8*(1), 25–31; and from Douglas, M. K., Rosenkoetter, M., Pacquiao, D. F., et al. (2014). Guidelines for implementing culturally competent nursing care. *Journal of Transcultural Nursing, 25*(2), 109–121. doi:10.1177/1043659614520998.

TABLE 2-4	QUESTIONS FOR DETERMINING THE PATIENT'S EXPLANATORY MODEL OF ILLNESS AND CARE

1. "What do you call the problem?"
2. "What do you think has caused the problem?"
3. "Why do you think it started when it did?"
4. "What do you think the sickness or illness does to you? How does it work?"
5. "How severe is the sickness? Will it have a long or short course?"
6. "What are the major problems or difficulties this sickness has caused in your life?"
7. "What have you done for this problem up to now?"
8. "What kind of treatment do you think you should receive?"
9. "What are the most important results you hope to achieve from the treatment?"
10. "What do you fear most about the sickness?"
11. "What do you fear most about the treatment?"
12. "Who else should be consulted or involved in your care?"

Source: From Srivastava, R. (2007). Culture care framework I: Overview and cultural sensitivity. In R. Srivastava (Ed.), *The healthcare professional's guide to clinical cultural competence* (p. 89). Toronto: Elsevier Canada. Adapted from Kleinman, A., Eisenberg, L., & Goode, B. (1978). Culture, illness, and care: Clinical lessons from anthropologic and cross cultural research. *Annals of Internal Medicine, 88,* 251–258.

with men other than their husbands and when in public situations in order to exhibit modesty.

The degree of physical contact and touch, across gender and age varies across cultures. In certain cultures (e.g., Muslim), health care providers may be prohibited from touching patients of the opposite sex (Marcus, 2016). Many Asians believe that touching a person's head is a sign of disrespect, especially because the head is believed to be the source of a person's strength. Observing how a patient interacts with others and asking permission to touch before touching are appropriate ways of respecting the patient's cultural values.

CULTURALLY COMPETENT CARE

COMMUNICATION SKILLS

It is not sufficient for nurses to simply learn about cross-cultural communication issues; they must also develop and adapt their communication skills to connect with different cultural groups (see Table 2-3). Some groups may respond effectively to direct questions, whereas others respond more comfortably in interactions that are less direct. For example, instead of telling a person what to do, a nurse may phrase the teaching in a less directive way: "Many people who experience this illness find it helpful to do. ..." Nurses must understand that when a patient says, "Yes," it can have multiple interpretations, including "Go on," "I hear you," "I understand," or "I agree." Understanding and agreement must be validated through other means.

Negotiation skills are also important in cultural competence because nurses are often required to negotiate interventions and goals that range along the gamut of mainstream and traditional ways of healing.

Providing Effective Language Support. Providing effective language support through the use of language aids, including interpreters, is essential for patient safety. Nurses and other health care providers often feel that they can get by without interpreters by using a few words in the patient's language and actions to demonstrate meaning; however, this is a fallacy and compromises

TABLE 2-5	WORKING EFFECTIVELY WITH INTERPRETERS

General Considerations
- If possible, the interpreter should meet with the patient ahead of time to establish rapport before the interpreting begins.
- Allow extra time for the session.
- Use trained bilingual–bicultural interpreters instead of the patient's family or children.
- Consider personal attributes of the interpreter such as age, gender, ethnicity, and dialect that may influence communication; use the services of an agency interpreter if possible.
- Be aware of common issues such as the following:
  - Words that cannot be translated
  - Being too rushed
  - The interpreter's answering for the patient
  - Conflict between the interpreter and the patient (if this occurs, stop the session immediately)
- Verify translations to avoid misunderstandings, mistakes, and distortions.

Before the Interpretation Session
- Get to know the interpreter.
- Provide an overview of the situation (patient, goals, and procedures).
- Ask for concerns or issues from the interpreter's perspective.
- Remind interpreter to interpret *everything*.
- Ask the interpreter to share his or her cultural insights with you but to differentiate these from the interpretation itself.
- Reinforce confidentiality.

During the Interpretation Session
- Face the patient directly.
- Speak in the first person.
- Introduce yourself, allowing the interpreter to interpret.
- Describe the role of the interpreter, the interpreter service's mandate, and the purpose of the session.
- Ask the interpreter to introduce himself or herself and his or her role in both languages.
- Address questions to the patient, not to the interpreter.
- Use simple language, and avoid jargon and technical terminology.
- Speak in one- to two-sentence bursts to allow for easier translation.
- Ensure that the interpreter understands what is to be translated.
- Allow the interpreter to ask open-ended questions if necessary to clarify what the patient says.
- Observe the patient for off-target reactions (signalling mistakes in interpretation).
- Observe and evaluate what is going on before you interrupt the interpreter.

After the Interpretation Session and Follow-Up Strategies
- Consider providing written instructions as appropriate.
- Ask the patient whether he or she has anything to ask or convey.
- Provide information on how the patient may request an interpreter's services in the future.
- Discuss the process and outcomes of the session with the interpreter.

quality care. Nurses must identify encounters where linguistic support is required through trained interpreters, seek out appropriate supports and demonstrate the abilities to effectively work with interpreters (International Council of Nurses, 2013). Table 2-5 lists strategies for working effectively with interpreters, and Table 2-6 lists strategies for communicating with patients with limited proficiency in English.

Although in-person interpretation by trained health care interpreters is considered optimal, organizations and individuals

TABLE 2-6 COMMUNICATING WITH PATIENTS WITH LIMITED ENGLISH PROFICIENCY

1. Be polite and formal.
2. Gesture to yourself and say your name, offering a handshake, nod, smile, or other greeting. If possible, greet patient in the patient's preferred language. This indicates that you are aware of and respect the patient's culture.
3. Proceed in an unhurried manner. Pay attention to any effort by the patient or family to communicate.
4. Speak in a low, moderate voice. Avoid talking loudly. Remember that there is a tendency to raise the volume and pitch of your voice when the listener appears not to understand. The listener may perceive that you are shouting or angry, or both.
5. Use simple words, such as "pain" instead of "discomfort." Avoid medical jargon, idioms, and slang. Avoid using contractions (e.g., "don't," "can't," "won't"). Use nouns repeatedly instead of pronouns. For example:
   - Do not say: "He has been taking his medicine, hasn't he?"
   - Do say: "Does Ahmad take medicine?"
6. Pantomime words and simple actions while you verbalize them.
7. Organize what you say, giving information and instructions in the proper sequence. For example:
   - Do not say: "Before you rinse the bottle, sterilize it."
   - Do say: "First, wash the bottle. Second, rinse the bottle."
8. Discuss one topic at a time. Avoid using conjunctions. For example:
   - Do not say: "Are you cold and in pain?"
   - Do say: "Are you cold [while pantomiming]? [Wait for patient's response.] Are you in pain?"
9. Validate understanding by having the patient repeat instructions, demonstrate the procedure, or act out the meaning.
10. Do not ask questions that can be answered with only "yes" or "no."
11. Summarize often, including your understanding of what the person is saying and checking whether your understanding is correct.

Source: Data from Jarvis, C., & Browne, A. J. (2014). *The interview.* In C. Jarvis, A. J. Brown, J. MacDonald-Jenkins, et al. (Eds.), *Physical examination and health assessment* (2nd Canadian ed.). Toronto: Elsevier; and from Srivastava, R. (2007). Culture care framework I: Overview and cultural sensitivity. In R. Srivastava (Ed.), *The healthcare professional's guide to clinical cultural competence* (pp. 53–74). Toronto: Elsevier Canada.

can often use technology-aided solutions such as telephone or remote interpretation. Caution is needed for using smart phones and applications such as Google Translate because they can pose risks to accuracy and thus patient safety, and such translation must be carefully validated (Flores, 2014).

Cognitive Domain

Cultural knowledge is a crucial element of cultural competence. To provide culturally competent care, nurses must identify and seek out the cultural knowledge they need (see Table 2-3). Cultural knowledge can be divided into two categories: generic cultural knowledge and specific cultural knowledge (Fung, Lo, Srivastava, et al., 2012).

Generic cultural knowledge is foundational knowledge that applies across a variety of cultural groups. The most fundamental aspect of generic cultural knowledge is understanding the effect of culture on health- and illness-related behaviours. Generic knowledge can be broken down into several broad areas that nurses should be aware of, such as variations in world views and explanatory models of illness; beliefs about care, cure, caregivers, and healing systems; family roles and relationships; migration and settlement; norms about time and personal space; and

spirituality and religion. These areas are discussed in greater detail in the following section.

Specific cultural knowledge focuses on learning about the particular cultural population that the nurse is working with. Because of the number of cultural groups in Canada, a detailed discussion of specific cultural knowledge is beyond the scope of this chapter. Nurses should educate themselves (see Table 2-3) about specific cultures they encounter frequently in their practice and always be amenable to learning more as circumstances require. For example, if the nurse is working in a community with large numbers of South Asian and Chinese people, it is important to learn more about the beliefs and issues relevant to these communities. Nurses working with the Indigenous community need to acquire deeper understanding of the legacy of residential schools and the associated trauma. Other examples of specific cultural knowledge include focusing on specific health issues faced by particular populations, such as immigrant women or the transgendered community (Srivastava, 2007a). (Table 2-3 lists other attributes of this component of cultural competence.)

In addition to determining the kind of generic and specific knowledge that is needed, nurses must critically appraise how knowledge is developed and used. Culture is concerned with shared patterns, not universal truths. Therefore, cultural knowledge should not be used to obscure individual differences. Individualized assessments are important to determine the extent to which the patient shares the beliefs and practices ascribed to the culture. Familiarity with cultural norms is helpful but should be used cautiously, inasmuch as it may lead to cultural stereotyping. It is important for nurses to reflect on how they acquired the knowledge and the extent to which the knowledge is unique to the individual, reflective of the broader cultural group, or reflective of cultural processes in general. It is also important to treat cultural knowledge as tentative hypotheses that can be verified and expanded upon by the patients and families.

Generic Cultural Knowledge

Care, Cure, Caregivers, and Healing Systems. Cultural norms have a significant influence on how illness is understood, what remedies are deemed appropriate and desirable, and who provides the care. Whereas in some cultures patients seek professional help, others rely more on family, friends, or spiritual and religious leaders. It is important to ascertain a patient's beliefs about the cause of illness, as well as perceptions of severity, expected treatment, prognosis, and effects (see Table 2-4).

Canadian health care systems and health professions also have a cultural basis in the dominant white, Eurocentric culture. The biomedical approach to health care, although regarded as the conventional treatment in North America, is one of several philosophical and scientifically based systems of healing. Other such systems include homeopathy, traditional Chinese medicine, Indigenous medicine, and Ayurvedic medicine (a form of traditional Hindu medicine). Although it is not possible for a health care provider to have expertise in all the healing systems, familiarity with the major systems and with their basic principles can be helpful. Individuals often use multiple healing systems, and a critical part of patient assessment is knowledge of what conventional treatments, as well as other folk or herbal treatments, are being used. Nurses need to understand their role in supporting and providing complementary and alternative therapy (College of Nurses of Ontario, 2014). Complementary and alternative therapies are further discussed in Chapter 12.

The Canadian approach to health care delivery is often team-based; different members of the team have different roles,

TABLE 2-7 CULTURAL AND SYSTEM FACTORS AFFECTING HELP SEEKING

Economic Factors
- Patients may not obtain health care because they cannot pay the costs associated with travel for health care, medications, or treatments.
- Patients may lack health insurance.

Health Care System
- Patients may not make or keep appointments because of the time lag between the onset of an illness and an available appointment.
- Hours of operation of health care facilities may not accommodate patients' work schedules or need to use public transportation.
- Patients may be relying on friends and family for transportation, language support, or navigation within the system.
- Lack of culturally sensitive health care programs and approaches may deter people from seeking health care.
- Patients may not have a primary care provider and thus use emergency departments for health care.
- Patients may lack knowledge about the availability of existing health care resources and may not know how to navigate the health care system.

Beliefs and Practices
- Care provided in established health care programs may not be perceived as culturally relevant.
- Patients may delay seeking care because of mistrust or because of a preference for folk medicine and herbal remedies.
- Dietary preferences may affect adherence to specific therapeutic diets.
- Patients may stop treatment or discontinue visits for health care because the symptoms are no longer present and they thus perceive that further care is not required.
- Patients may have negative associations with hospitals and extended-care facilities, such as death or abandonment.
- Patients may have prior negative experience with culturally insensitive health care providers or discriminatory practices.
- Patients may mistrust the dominant population and institutions.

and boundaries with regard to who does what are often very clear. In many cultures, people are used to having a single authoritative healer and may regard others as helpers (Srivastava, Srivastava, & Srivastava, 2012). Lack of familiarity with roles and mistrust can jeopardize patient safety because information may not be disclosed or shared appropriately with the health care team.

Help seeking is also influenced by system factors, some of which are presented in Table 2-7.

CULTURALLY COMPETENT CARE

CLOCK TIME

Patient values regarding time orientation and personal space can also affect the care delivery process. Health care providers in hospitals and clinics are often frustrated because many patients show up late for appointments and seem to have no regard for appointments and schedules. In reality, this may be a result of several factors, including issues of transportation, ability to navigate the health care system, and time orientation. The value of clock time and punctuality is different across cultures. In collectivist cultures—that is, cultures in which the relationships and interconnectedness between people are valued over the needs of the individual—it is often more important to attend to a social

role than to arrive on time for an appointment with a health care provider. Hence, the lack of adherence to the appointment time can be attributed to competing demands, and a lack of appreciation for punctuality and should not be interpreted as a blatant disregard or disrespect for the health care providers or the system.

Biology, Physiology, and Pharmacology. The racial and ethnic influences on biological and physiological processes are often viewed as controversial because these influences are considered more to be social categories than scientific categories. However, clinical realities should not be ignored. Gender differences exist in the prevalence of illness, expression of illness, and response to pharmaceutical agents. The occurrence of certain diseases in different racial and ethnic populations is also different. However, it is important to note that when an illness is prevalent in a particular culture, neither the individual nor the cultural background is the cause of illness; rather, the broader determinants of health must be assessed to understand and address disparities.

Genetic predisposition also varies across racial and ethnic lines. For example, sickle cell disease is a common genetic disorder among people of African descent. By being aware of such illness incidences, health care providers can perform a focused and thorough assessment and can avoid stereotypical assumptions (e.g., that an Indigenous patient is a "drunken Indian" when the real issue is diabetic ketoacidosis, or that a young Black man is a drug addict when really he is experiencing pain from sickle cell disease). Having knowledge of increased vulnerability can enhance clinical decision making and prevent misdiagnosis or unnecessary delays that lead to poor care.

There is increasing evidence that ethnicity influences responses to certain medications. These variations are a result of physiological and pathophysiological differences; pharmacogenetics and genetics; environmental factors such as diet, nutritional status, smoking, and alcohol use; and simultaneous use of herbal remedies (Ramamoorthy, Pacanowski, Bull, et al., 2015). Some European and African patients metabolize drugs at a slower rate, which leads to high drug levels, whereas some Japanese and Indigenous patients metabolize drugs more quickly. Differences in rates of metabolism mean that individuals from Japan, China, Thailand, and Malaysia require lower doses of drugs such as codeine than does a European person.

Differential response has also been documented for drug classifications such as antihypertensive, antipsychotic, and antianxiety agents. In general, Black persons respond better to diuretics than to beta blockers and angiotensin-converting enzyme (ACE) inhibitors; Chinese patients require lower doses of antipsychotic drugs; and Japanese patients require lower doses of antimanic agents (Lilley, Harrington, Snyder, et al., 2010). Although some drugs may have population-specific recommendations, it is important for nurses to be vigilant to variations in dosage response and side effects. For nurses working in particular specialty areas, it is important to learn about the ethnocultural variations in response to the particular classification of medications commonly taken by their clinical population.

Family Roles and Relationships. Family structures and roles differ from one culture to another (Figure 2-2). For this reason, it is important for the nurse to determine who should be involved in the communication and decision making related to health care. For example, individualistic cultures emphasize individual rights, goals, and needs, whereas collectivist cultures assign greater priority to the needs of the group (family or community), and there is an emphasis on interdependence rather than independence

FIGURE 2-2 Family roles and relationships differ from one culture to another. Source: Shutterstock.com.

(Carteret, 2011). In countries such as Canada and the United States, people hold strong beliefs related to autonomy, and each adult individual is expected to make decisions and sign consent forms when receiving health care. In contrast, in Asian cultures, the head of the household or the eldest son is expected to make health care decisions. In collectivist cultures, including Indigenous communities, affiliation is valued over confrontation, and cooperation is preferred to competition. When the nurse encounters a family that values collectivity over individualism, conflicts may arise in how decisions are made. There may be a delay in treatment while the patient waits for significant family members to arrive before giving consent for a procedure or treatment. In other instances, the patient may make a decision that is best for the family but may have negative or adverse consequences for the patient. By being aware of such values, the nurse is better prepared to advocate for and support the patient.

Expectations regarding caregiving also vary across cultures. In Asian and Latin American cultures, caregiving is seen as a duty, and it is often deemed unacceptable to place the responsibility of care in the hands of strangers (Pharr, Francis, Terry, et al., 2014). The same expectations do not hold for European families. Thus it is important for nurses to understand and support caregiver burden from a cultural perspective.

Spirituality and Religion. Spirituality and religion are aspects of culture that may affect a person's beliefs and decisions about health and illness. *Spirituality* commonly refers to a person's efforts to find purpose, meaning, and a sense of belonging (Camp, 2011; Taylor, 2012). *Religion* is a more formal and organized system of beliefs, including belief in or worship of God, and involves prayer and one or more rituals. Religion is based on beliefs about life, death, good and evil, and pain and suffering. Religious and spiritual beliefs have been shown to positively influence health outcomes, particularly in the care of patients with mental health and addiction issues (Camp, 2011). It is important for health care providers to understand the role of religion, spirituality, and culture in health and illness. For some ethnocultural groups, culture, spirituality, and religion are inseparable. For example, the Indigenous culture and way of life are entwined with the religious and spiritual beliefs, and these

extend to health and wellness. Similarly, Hinduism is as much a way of life as it is a religion and is also associated with a healing system that may influence perceptions of care and cure (Srivastava, Srivastava, & Srivastava, 2012). Many people differentiate between spirituality and religion and may identify with being spiritual but may not be religious.

Nurses can use many interventions to meet a patient's spiritual and religious needs. These interventions include use of prayer, scriptures, listening, and referral. Attention to spirituality is an important aspect of holistic care throughout the life span; however, it can take on increasing significance in end-of-life care, inasmuch as this is often a time when patients reaffirm their beliefs.

It is also important for nurses to be aware of their own assumptions about spirituality and religion and how they may differ from patients. Not all religions have the same end goals and may, in fact, vary greatly in their central theological questions and objectives (Fowler, 2012). Concepts such as "sin" and "heaven" may be central to Christian theological understanding but are not central concerns in religions such as Buddhism and Hinduism. Even the relationship between the mind, body, and spirit varies among religions (Srivastava, Srivastava, & Srivastava, 2012). It is therefore important to ascertain what religion and spirituality means to particular individuals and groups, how it may affect health and wellness, and the nurses' role in offering support.

Migration and Settlement. Understanding the influence of migration and resettlement processes on health is another area of generic cultural knowledge. Research indicates that new immigrants tend to be in better overall health than the general resident population. This finding, known as the *healthy immigrant effect,* is not surprising inasmuch as immigrants are screened before being granted admittance to Canada. However, this advantage does not last, and even after 20 years in the country, the health of immigrants, as determined by age-standardized mortality rates, is generally poorer than those of the Canadian-born population (Pottie, Greenway, Feightner, et al., 2011). In a systematic review, Vang, Sigouin, Flenon, and colleagues (2015) noted that the healthy immigrant effect is linked to immigrants' duration of residence in the country and appears to be strongest during adulthood but less so during childhood, adolescence, and late life.

Recent immigrants are at risk for health problems for many reasons. The settlement process is associated with many losses and can cause physical stress and mental distress. New immigrants often experience challenges in areas of the social determinants such as employment, housing, social support, and access to services. They are also at risk for social exclusion through underemployment, workplace stress, and unemployment. Older immigrants are especially affected by changes in role, social position, and potentially social isolation in a new country. Factors such as fatigue, stress, and racism—and, for refugees, premigratory circumstances—can result in serious physical and psychological trauma. Many newcomers face difficulties in accessing the health care system because of a lack of familiarity with the system, limited language proficiency, transportation difficulties, or inability to take time away from other responsibilities related to work and family (Kalich, Heinemann, & Ghahari, 2015). However, not all differences in access are limited by socioeconomic and language difficulties. Roberts (2012) pointed out that immigrant women access health care differently than men, on the basis of their desire to seek health care versus medical care and their use of family and community-based networks as guides.

Dynamics of Difference

In the ABCDE framework, *dynamics of difference* is not a distinctly separate domain; rather, it is evident across the ABC domains. The dynamics of difference must be understood at two levels: (a) the nurse–patient level, and (b) the patient–health care system level (Srivastava, 2014). Power differences exist in all nurse–patient relationships; however, these can be magnified, often through unconscious bias, when clinicians and clients belong to different cultural groups. To ensure that clients' rights and autonomy are respected, it is important for health care providers to be aware of their own biases and to be vigilant for processes that can be marginalizing. At the system level, understanding the dynamics of difference means understanding the effect of systematic oppression and institutional racism.

Understanding the effect of colonization and other social determinants of health (including historical trauma, racism, discrimination, and culturally destructive processes such as residential schools for Indigenous communities) helps shape awareness of how differences matter, and which differences matter more than others in particular contexts (Allan & Smylie, 2015). Demonstrating cultural competence means understanding and navigating power dynamics at both levels. Specific actions to address the dynamics of difference are outlined throughout Table 2-3.

Critical self-reflection and attention to the dynamics of difference, as well as cultural similarities and differences between the patient's culture and that of the health care provider, are essential for providing care that is truly patient centred (Douglas, Rosenkoetter, Pacquiao, et al., 2014; Srivastava, 2014).

Environment and Equity

In the ABCDE framework, *environment* and *equity* do not refer to a separate domain; rather, they refer to the importance of the context of care and the goal of equity. *Environment* highlights the importance of understanding, developing, and utilizing resources at the individual and organizational levels for ongoing learning, consultation, and referral (Fung, Lo, Srivastava, et al., 2012; Douglas et al., 2014). Examples of such resources include colleagues who can share experience and expertise in cross-cultural care; language support aids such as interpreters or telephonic services; information and education about the people and communities served; and access to spiritual and faith leaders.

Understanding the Difference Between Equity and Equality

Equity refers to the goal of health equity or quality care for all. Health care providers need to embrace the concept of health equity and understand the difference between equity and equality. The concept of equality refers to sameness in *process* (e.g., everyone gets the same treatment). That of equity, on the other hand, focuses on sameness in *outcomes*. To achieve equality in outcomes, people need to be treated differently—according to their needs.

Imagine three people of different heights trying to see over a 4-ft (122-cm) fence to watch a ball game. Kyle is an adult, 6 ft (183 cm) in height; Larry is a teenager, 4 ft (122 cm) in height; and Michael is a child who is 2.5 ft (76 cm) in height. As a way of providing support for onlookers, the park provides 12-inch crates on which people can stand on to see over the fence.

In a system in which equality is the driving principle, each person gets one crate to stand on. As a result, Kyle, who is able to see over the fence with no difficulty, is even taller; Larry, who is able to see if he stood on tip-toe, can now stand on the crate

FIGURE 2-3 Illustration of the difference between equity and equality. Source: Interaction Institute for Social Change/Artist: Angus Maguire. *interactioninstitute.org, madewithangus.com.*

and see the game more comfortably. But Michael, even with the crate, still reaches 6 inches (15 cm) below the top of the fence and therefore is still not able to see the game. The outcome is not much different than before the crates were provided, except for some benefit to Larry. The return on investment of crates is minimal, and the crate for both Kyle and Michael is a wasted resource.

In a system in which equity is the driving force, the resource of the three crates is distributed according to need. Kyle does not receive a crate to stand on, Larry gets one crate, and Michael gets two crates. The outcome is that all three individuals are able to see over the fence comfortably (Figure 2-3).

In the first scenario of resource distribution according to the principle of equality, everyone is assumed to be in the same situation and to have the same needs. This is simply not true. Differences in race, gender, income, and other factors means individuals vary in the strengths and needs they bring to every interaction. When these are recognized, interventions can be targeted on the basis of need. The result is optimal outcome with minimal waste.

NURSE'S SELF-ASSESSMENT

Developing an understanding of one's own culture through reflection and self-assessment is a crucial first step toward cultural competence in clinical care. Evidence indicates that health care providers' attitudes, whether they are conscious of them or not, have a significant influence on their interactions with other people (Browne & Varcoe, 2014; Srivastava, 2007b). Self-awareness includes being aware of one's motivation and the value that one places on cultural competence. Is the motivation purely to avoid problems for the health care provider, or is there genuine desire to learn from differences and achieve equity in health for everyone? In the interest of striving for the latter, nurses must recognize both conscious and unconscious bias that may exist at the personal, interpersonal, or organizational level. Many tools are available to assist in this process (Registered Nurses' Association of Ontario, 2007). For example, Harvard University researchers have developed the Implicit Association Test (IAT) (see the Resources at the end of this chapter), a measure of attitudes and beliefs that people may not even know exist within themselves (Banaji & Greenwald, 2013).

CULTURALLY COMPETENT PATIENT ASSESSMENT

A cultural assessment should be a fundamental part of all patient assessments. Conducting a cultural assessment means asking key questions with regard to language, diet, religion, and acculturation and eliciting the patient's explanatory model of health and illness (see Table 2-4).

A patient assessment achieves cultural competence not only through the questions that are asked but also through the use of cultural knowledge and skill to determine when and how to explore particular issues. It is critical to build trust by adopting an approach that conveys respect, a nonjudgemental attitude, and genuine curiosity to understand the patient perspective. Many health care processes require close physical contact, discussions of an intimate nature, or both; thus personal boundaries can be particularly significant with regard to a patient's disclosures and cooperation with activities. Issues concerning personal space and gender often surface during activities involving physical assessment and personal care. Health care providers must use sensitivity in talking with patients to find approaches that best fit the patients' health care needs and personal preferences.

Table 2-8 summarizes nursing actions that are part of a culturally competent health assessment.

BRIDGING CULTURAL DISTANCES: THE LEARN MODEL

Key characteristics of cultural competence are the ability to effectively apply the ABCDEs of cultural competence: cultural awareness, knowledge, and skills in clinical situations; the ability to keep in mind the dynamics of difference; supports available through the practice environment; and the goal of equity.

TABLE 2-8 CULTURALLY COMPETENT HEALTH ASSESSMENT

- Become aware of your own values, beliefs, and biases.
- Develop humility and a critical awareness that your own expertise is probably ethnocentric.
- Know that racism, heterosexism, classism, sexism, genderism, ageism, ableism, and so forth, are taught, not innate, and that the unlearning process is ongoing.
- Perceive patients/consumers as experts of their own realities.
- Work to build trust.
- Communicate in ways that are nonjudgemental and show respect for differences.
- Use open-ended questions to understand patients' priorities and perceptions.
- Pay attention to the economic and social contexts of patients' and families' lives.
- Inquire about health beliefs, practices, and help-seeking behaviours.
- Inquire about the role of religion and spirituality in health and illness.
- Identify sources of support cultural support (friends, family, community).
- Advocate with and for patients, and learn how to be an ally across diversity and oppression.
- Challenge discrimination, marginalization, and oppression.
- Assist patients in becoming informed, knowledgeable, and empowered.
- Embrace learning as an ongoing process.

Throughout this chapter, strategies that can be used to bridge gaps and differences across cultures have been discussed. One model useful for summarizing this discussion is the LEARN (listen, explain, acknowledge, recommend, and negotiate) model (Table 2-9) which offers simple but comprehensive guidelines for cross-cultural health care.

The LEARN model enables the nurse to reveal and acknowledge patients' values and perspectives and practice in a professional manner by sharing his or her expertise. By listening first, the nurse is less likely to give the impression of being hurried or too busy and will be able to tailor explanations in ways that are relevant for the patient.

WORKING IN DIVERSE TEAMS

Interactions between patients and health care providers are not the only situations in which cross-cultural issues and challenges can arise. The increasing diversity in society also affects the makeup of the health care team (Figure 2-4).

In general, workforce diversity is viewed as a positive attribute and a valuable resource to support the development of cultural competence and the provision of culturally relevant care. A diverse working team creates opportunities for cultural encounters and interactions that can result in greater cultural understanding and better delivery of care; however, diversity in the workforce has challenges. Although culturally diverse groups have more potential to generate a greater variety of ideas and other resources than do culturally homogeneous groups, racially and ethnically mixed groups actually experience more conflict and miscommunication than do homogeneous groups. When health care

TABLE 2-9 LEARN MODEL FOR CROSS-CULTURAL CARE

Listen with sympathy and understanding to the patient's perception of the problem.
Explain your perception of the problem.
Acknowledge and discuss the differences and similarities.
Recommend treatment.
Negotiate agreement.

Source: Berlin, E. A., & Fowkes, W. C., Jr. (1983). A teaching framework for cross-cultural health care—Application in family practice in cross-cultural medicine. *The Western Journal of Medicine, 12*(139), 93–98.

FIGURE 2-4 Nurses working together in a multicultural health environment.
Source: Sean Locke Photography/Shutterstock.com.

providers from different cultures and countries work together as members of the health care team, opportunities for miscommunication and conflict naturally arise (Adeniran, Bhattacharya, & Srivastava, 2015; Premji & Etowa, 2014).

The cultural origins of miscommunication and conflict in the workplace are often interconnected with cultural beliefs, values, and etiquette. Examples of such origins are the meaning, purpose, and value of work; family obligations; time orientation; gender roles and sexual orientation; and historical rivalries among groups. Cultural misunderstandings can lead to tensions within the working team, miscommunication, and wrongful assumptions, all of which result in work stress and poor outcomes for patients. These challenges can be minimized through the same principles of respect, empathy, and learning from difference that apply to nurse–patient interactions.

Even though there is a strong belief that culturally competent care necessitates a diverse workforce, workforce diversity does not necessarily result in cultural competence. Development and demonstration of cultural competence requires intentional work as discussed throughout the chapter and outlined in Table 2-3.

CONCLUSION

The need for cultural competence is a fundamental issue of health care quality and patient safety, and achieving it requires a commitment to principles of inclusiveness and equity. Developing cultural competence (see Table 2-3) is a journey in which nurses can begin with generic knowledge and, with time and experience, acquire additional knowledge specific to populations

and aspects of care. It is important for the nurse to combine the use of this information and knowledge with critical reflection and critical thinking. This approach adds both depth and breadth to the nurse's clinical competence and ability to provide patient-centred care.

CASE STUDY

Communication

Patient Profile

Source: szifei/ Shutterstock. com

Mrs. Jagwant is a 45-year-old woman who is admitted to the hospital for investigation of a tumour. She is accompanied by her husband. Dr. Stuart, the attending physician, explains to the couple that the prognosis is excellent and the treatment involves radiation. She plans to schedule the first treatment the following week.

Mr. and Mrs. Jagwant have been in Canada for approximately 3 years, and both speak English, albeit with an accent. There have been no difficulties in communicating in English with either Mr. or Mrs. Jagwant, although Mr. Jagwant tends to do most of the talking. While Dr. Stuart is explaining the diagnosis, they listen intently, nod periodically, and do not raise any questions or objections to the plan. Dr. Stuart assumes that the patient is in agreement with her plan.

Discussion Questions
1. Do you agree with Dr. Stuart's assessment?
2. What factors may be influencing the couple's silence?
3. What actions could be taken by the nurse who is present for this discussion or the doctor that reflect cultural competence?

REVIEW QUESTIONS

The number of the question corresponds to the same-numbered objective at the beginning of the chapter.

1. Which of the following is an example of forcing one's own cultural beliefs and practices on another person?
   a. Stereotyping
   b. Ethnocentrism
   c. Cultural relativity
   d. Cultural imposition
2. Which of the following is true about inequities between Indigenous health and the health of the general population? *(Select all that apply.)*
   a. They result from lifestyle choices.
   b. They result from differences in living conditions, such as housing and education.
   c. They result from conflict between systems of Indigenous medicine and Western health care concepts.
   d. They result from bias and discrimination from the mainstream system.
3. Which of the following is true about health inequity?
   a. Health inequities are caused largely by cultural factors compounded by social disadvantage.
   b. Health inequities are largely caused by different beliefs, practices, and lifestyles associated with the cultural communities.
   c. Health inequities can be reduced by improving services to enhance access and reduce exclusion.
   d. In a country in which access to health care is universal, health inequities are largely issues of health care quality.
4. Which of the following *most* accurately describes cultural factors that may affect health?
   a. Diabetes and cancer rates differ by cultural and ethnic groups.

   b. Most clients find that religious rituals help them during times of illness.
   c. There is limited ethnic variation in physiological responses to medications.
   d. Silence during a nurse–client interaction usually means that the client understands the instructions.
5. In communications with a client who speaks a language different from the nurse's, which of the following interventions is important?
   a. Have a family member translate.
   b. Use a trained medical interpreter.
   c. Use specific medical terminology so that there will be no mistakes in the information communicated.
   d. Focus on the translation rather than the nonverbal communication.
6. Why is it important for the nurse to develop cultural self-awareness? *(Select all that apply.)*
   a. This enables the nurse to clearly articulate the nurse's own values to the client.
   b. This enables the nurse to prevent ethnocentrism.
   c. This enables the nurse to prevent cultural imposition.
   d. This enables the nurse to challenge his or her own assumptions and stereotypes.
7. Which of the following strategies are appropriate for demonstrating cultural competence in clinical care? *(Select all that apply.)*
   a. Explaining to the client and family how the Canadian health care system works
   b. Exploring economic and social factors affecting the client and family
   c. Pairing the client with a provider from the client's own cultural community
   d. Exploring the client's explanatory model of illness

8. How does a diverse workforce influence a nurse's ability to provide care?
   a. It facilitates matching clients with health care providers of the same ethnicity.
   b. It exposes the nurse to different values, beliefs, and world views.
   c. It leads to greater creativity and innovation and to the development of appropriate interventions for diverse clients.

d. It meets mandated objectives of the federal and provincial governments.

1. d; 2. c, d; 3. c; 4. a; 5. b; 6. c, d; 7. b, d; 8. b.

⊜volve

For even more review questions, visit *http://evolve.elsevier.com/Canada/Lewis/medsurg.*

REFERENCES

Adeniran, R. K., Bhattacharya, A., & Srivastava, R. (2015). Facilitators and barriers to advancing in the nursing profession: Voices of U.S.- and internationally educated nurses. *Clinical Scholars Review, 8*(2), 241–248.

Allan, B., & Smylie, J. (2015). *First Peoples, second class treatment: The role of racism in the health and well-being of Indigenous peoples in Canada.* Toronto: The Wellesley Institute.

Anderson, K. A., & Olson, S. (2013). *Leveraging culture to address health inequalities: Examples from Native communities.* Washington, DC: National Academy of Sciences.

Banaji, M., & Greenwald, A. (2013). *Blindspot.* New York: Delacorte Press.

Bauer, G. R., & Scheim, A. I. (2015). *Transgender people in Ontario, Canada: Statistics to inform human rights policy.* London, ON: Trans Pulse Project.

Blanchet-Garneau, A., & Pepin, J. (2015). Cultural competence: A constructivist definition. *Journal of Transcultural Nursing, 26*(1), 9–15. doi:10.1177/1043659614541294.

Browne, A., & Varcoe, C. (2014). Cultural and social considerations in health assessment. In C. Jarvis (Ed.), *Physical examination & health assessment* (2nd Canadian ed., pp. 27–44). Toronto: Elsevier.

Camp, M. (2011). Religion and spirituality in psychiatric practice. *Current Opinion in Psychiatry, 24*, 507–513. doi:10.1097/YCO.0b013e32834bb8f4.

Canadian Institute of Health Research (2015). *Pathways to health equity for Aboriginal peoples: Overview.* Retrieved from *http://www.cihr-irsc.gc.ca/e/47003.html.*

Canadian Medical Association (2013). *Health equity and the social determinants of health: A role for the medical profession.* Retrieved from *https://www.cma.ca/Assets/assets-library/document/en/advocacy/PD13-03-e.pdf.*

Canadian Nurses Association (2010). *Promoting cultural competence in nursing.* Ottawa: Author. (Seminal).

Carteret, M. (2011). *Cultural values of Latino patients and families. Dimensions of culture.* Retrieved from *http://www.dimensionsofculture.com/2011/03/cultural-values-of-latino-patients-and-families/.*

College of Nurses of Ontario (2009). *Culturally sensitive care.* Toronto: Author. (Seminal).

College of Nurses of Ontario (2014). *Complementary therapies.* Toronto: Author.

Douglas, M. K., Rosenkoetter, M., Pacquiao, D. F., et al. (2014). Guidelines for implementing culturally competent nursing care. *Journal of Transcultural Nursing, 25*(2), 109–121. doi:10.1177/1043659614520998.

Flores, G. (2014). Families facing language barriers in healthcare: When will policy catch up with the demographics and evidence? *The Journal of Pediatrics, 164*(6), 1261–1264.

Fowler, M. (2012). Religion in nursing. In M. Fowler, S. Reimer-Kirkham, R. Sawatzky, et al. (Eds.), *Religion, religious ethics, and nursing* (pp. 1–26). New York: Springer.

Fowler, M., & Reimer-Kirkham, S. (2012). Religious ethics, religious social ethics and nursing. In M. Fowler, S. Reimer-Kirkham, R. Sawatzky, et al. (Eds.), *Religion, religious ethics, and nursing* (pp. 27–60). New York: Springer.

Fung, K., Lo, H. T., Srivastava, R., et al. (2012). Organizational cultural competence consultation to a mental health institution. *Transcultural Psychiatry, 49*, 165–184.

International Council of Nurses (2013). *Cultural and linguistic competence.* Retrieved from *http://www.icn.ch/images/stories/documents/publications/position_statements/B03_Cultural_Linguistic_Competence.pdf.*

Kalich, A., Heinemann, L., & Ghahari, S. (2015). A scoping review of immigrant experience of health care access barriers in Canada. *Journal of Immigrant and Minority Health, 18*(3), 1–13.

King, G., Desmarais, C., Lindsay, S., et al. (2015). The roles of effective communication and client engagement in delivering culturally sensitive care to immigrant parents of children with disabilities. *Disability and Rehabilitation, 37*(15), 1372–1381. doi:10.3109/09638288.2014.972580.

Lilley, L., Harrington, S., Snyder, J., et al. (2010). Ethnocultural, legal, and ethical considerations. In B. Swart (Ed.), *Pharmacology for Canadian health care practice* (2nd ed., pp. 57–72). Toronto: Elsevier.

Lopez-Class, M., Castro, F. G., & Ramirez, A. G. (2011). Conceptions of acculturation: A review and statement of critical issues. *Social Science & Medicine, 72*, 1555–1562.

Marcus, E. (2016). Muslim women's preferences in the medical setting: How might they contribute to disparities in health outcomes? *Journal of Women's Health, 25*(6), 561–562. doi:10.1089/jwh.2016.5875.

National Collaborating Centre for Healthy Public Policy (2015). *Health inequalities and intersectionality.* Retrieved from *http://www.ncchpp.ca/docs/2015_Ineg_Ineq_Intersectionnalite_En.pdf.*

Nestel, S. (2012). *Colour coded health care: The impact of race and racism on Canadians' health.* Toronto: The Wellesley Institute.

Ontario Ministry of Health and Long-Term Care (2013). *Health equity impact assessment.* Retrieved from *http://www.health.gov.on.ca/en/pro/programs/heia.*

Paasche-Orlow, M. (2011). Caring for patients with limited health literacy: A 76-year-old man with multiple medical problems. *The Journal of the American Medical Association, 306*(10), 1122–1129. doi:10.1001/jama.2011.1203.

Pharr, J., Francis, C., Terry, C., et al. (2014). Culture, caregiving, and health: Exploring the influence of culture on family caregiver experiences. *ISRN Public Health,* Article ID 689826. Retrieved from *http://dx.doi.org/10.1155/2014/689826.*

Pottie, K., Greenway, C., Feightner, J., et al. (2011). Evidence based clinical guidelines for immigrants and refugees. *Canadian Medical Association Journal, 183*(12), E824–E925. doi:10.1503/cmaj.090313.

Premji, S., & Etowa, J. B. (2014). Workforce utilization of visible and linguistic minorities in Canadian nursing. *Journal of Nursing Management, 22*(1), 80–88.

Public Health Agency of Canada (2011). *Reducing health inequalities: A challenge for our times*. Ottawa: Author.

Public Health Agency of Canada (2013). *What makes Canadians healthy or unhealthy?* Retrieved from *http://www.phac-aspc.gc.ca/ph-sp/determinants/determinants-eng.php#income*.

Public Health Agency of Canada (2014). *About health literacy*. Retrieved from *http://www.phac-aspc.gc.ca/cd-mc/hl-ls/index-eng.php#tabs-2*.

Racine, L. (2014). The enduring challenge of cultural safety in nursing. *Canadian Journal of Nursing Research, 46*(2), 6–9.

Ramamoorthy, A., Pacanowski, M. A., Bull, J., et al. (2015). Racial/ethnic differences in drug disposition and response: Review of recently approved drugs. *Clinical Pharmacology & Therapeutics, 97*(3), 263–273.

Registered Nurses' Association of Ontario (2007). *Embracing diversity: Developing cultural competence*. Toronto: Author. (Seminal).

Roberts, M. (2012). *Immigrant women access health care differently*. Retrieved from *http://healthydebate.ca/opinions/immigrant-women-access-health-care-differently*.

Shen, Z. (2015). Cultural competence models and cultural competence assessment instruments in nursing: A literature review. *Journal of Transcultural Nursing, 26*(3), 308–321.

Srivastava, R. (2007a). Culture care framework I: Overview and cultural sensitivity. In R. Srivastava (Ed.), *The healthcare professional's guide to clinical cultural competence* (pp. 53–74). Toronto: Elsevier Canada. (Seminal).

Srivastava, R. (2007b). Culture care framework II: Culture knowledge, resources, and bridging the gap. In R. Srivastava (Ed.), *The healthcare professional's guide to clinical cultural competence* (pp. 75–100). Toronto: Elsevier Canada. (Seminal).

Srivastava, R. (2008). The ABC (and DE) of cultural competence in clinical care. *Ethnicity and Inequalities in Health and Social Care, 8*(1), 25–31. (Seminal).

Srivastava, R. (2014). Culture, religion, and family-centred care. In R. Zlotnik-Shaul (Ed.), *Ethics and law in paediatric patient and family centred care* (pp. 57–77). New York: Springer.

Srivastava, R., Srivastava, B., & Srivastava, R. (2012). Hinduism and nursing. In M. Fowler, S. Reimer-Kirkham, R. Sawatzky, et al. (Eds.), *Religion, religious ethics, and nursing* (pp. 173–196). New York: Springer.

Statistics Canada (2013a). *Immigration and ethnocultural diversity in Canada*. Ottawa: Ministry of Industry. Retrieved from *http://www12.statcan.gc.ca/nhs-enm/2011/as-sa/99-010-x/99-010-x2011001-eng.cfm*.

Statistics Canada (2013b). *Aboriginal peoples in Canada: First Nations people, Métis and Inuit*. Ottawa: Ministry of Industry.

Taylor, E. J. (2012). Religion at the bedside: Why? In E. J. Taylor (Ed.), *Religion: A clinical guide for nurses* (pp. 3–14). New York: Springer.

Vang, Z., Sigouin, J., Flenon, A., et al. (2015). The healthy immigrant effect in Canada: A systematic review. *Population Change and Lifecourse Strategic Knowledge Cluster Discussion Paper Series, 3*(1). Retrieved from *http://ir.lib.uwo.ca/pclc/vol3/iss1/4/*. Article 4.

Veenstra, G. (2011). Race, gender, class, and sexual orientation: Intersecting axes of inequality and self-rated health in Canada. *International Journal for Equity in Health, 10*, 3. Retrieved from *http://equityhealthj.biomedcentral.com/articles/10.1186/1475-9276-10-3*.

Wasekeesikaw, F. J., & Perley-Dutcher, L. (2013). *Understand Aboriginal health: What all nurses need to know*. Retrieved from *https://www.cna-aiic.ca/~/media/cna/page-content/pdf-fr/aboriginal_health_june2013_e.pdf?la=en*.

RESOURCES

Canadian Indigenous Nurses Association
http://www.indigenousnurses.ca

Canadian Institute of Health Research: Pathways to Health Equity for Aboriginal Peoples: Overview
http://www.cihr-irsc.gc.ca/e/43630.html

Citizenship and Immigration Canada
http://www.cic.gc.ca/english/

Ethnicity Online
http://www.ethnicityonline.net/

Hamilton Health Sciences: Building Cultural Competency in Practice
http://www.hhsc.ca/body.cfm?id=1782

National Aboriginal Health Organization
http://www.naho.ca/

Ontario Ministry of Children and Youth Services: Achieving Cultural Competence
http://www.children.gov.on.ca/htdocs/English/topics/specialneeds/achieving_cultural_competence.aspx

Ontario Ministry of Health and Long-Term Care: Health Equity Impact Assessment (HEIA)
http://www.health.gov.on.ca/en/pro/programs/heia/

Ontario Multicultural Health Applied Research Network
http://www.ryerson.ca/omh/index.html

SickKids Cultural Competence E-Learning Modules Series
http://www.sickkids.ca/ProgramsandServices/centre-for-innovation-and-excellence/Health-Equity-Cultural-Competence/Cultural-Competence-E-Learning-Module-Series/Cultural-Competence-E-Learning.html

Dimensions of Culture: Cross Cultural Communications for Health Professionals
http://www.dimensionsofculture.com/

National Center for Cultural Competence: Georgetown University
http://nccc.georgetown.edu/

Project Implicit: Harvard University Implicit Association Test
https://implicit.harvard.edu/implicit/education.html

The Disparities Solutions Center
http://mghdisparitiessolutions.org/

Transcultural C.A.R.E. Associates
http://transculturalcare.net

Think Cultural Health
https://www.thinkculturalhealth.hhs.gov/

U.S. Department of Health & Human Services, Office of Minority Health: Cultural Competence
http://minorityhealth.hhs.gov/omh/browse.aspx?lvl=1&lvlid=6

For additional Internet resources, see the website for this book at *http://evolve.elsevier.com/Canada/Lewis/medsurg*.

Health History and Physical Examination

Written by: Jennifer Saylor
Adapted by: Mary Ann Fegan

evolve WEBSITE

http://evolve.elsevier.com/Canada/Lewis/medsurg

- Review Questions (Online Only)
- Key Points
- Conceptual Care Map Creator

- Audio Glossary
- Content Updates

LEARNING OBJECTIVES

1. Explain the purpose, components, and techniques of a patient's health history and physical examination.
2. Obtain a nursing history with the use of a common health history format.

3. Select appropriate techniques of inspection, palpation, percussion, and auscultation for physical examination of a patient.
4. Differentiate among comprehensive, focused, and emergency types of assessment in terms of indications, purposes, and components.

KEY TERMS

auscultation, p. 42
database, p. 37
general survey statement, p. 41

inspection, p. 41
nursing history, p. 37
objective data, p. 37

palpation, p. 42
percussion, p. 42

physical examination, p. 41
subjective data, p. 37

During the assessment phase of the nursing process, the nurse documents a patient's health history and performs a physical examination. The findings of this assessment (a) contribute to a database that identifies the patient's current and past health status and (b) provide a baseline against which future changes can be evaluated. The purpose of the nursing assessment is to enable the nurse to make clinical judgements or nursing diagnoses about the patient's health status (Jarvis, Browne, MacDonald-Jenkins, et al., 2014). Assessment is the first step of the nursing process, but it is performed continuously throughout the nursing process to validate nursing diagnoses, evaluate nursing interventions, and determine whether patient outcomes and goals have been met.

DATA COLLECTION

In the broadest sense, the **database** is all the health information about a patient. This includes the data from the nursing history and physical examination, the data from the medical history and physical examination, results of laboratory and diagnostic tests, and information contributed by other health care providers.

The focus of nursing care is the diagnosis and treatment of human responses to actual or potential health problems or life processes. The information obtained from the **nursing**

history and physical examination is used to determine the patient's strengths and responses to a health problem. For example, for a patient with a diagnosis of diabetes, the patient's responses may include anxiety or a lack of knowledge about self-management of the condition. The patient may also experience the physical response of fluid volume deficit because of the abnormal fluid loss caused by hyperglycemia. These human responses to the condition of diabetes are diagnosed and treated by nurses. During the nursing history interview and physical examination, the nurse obtains and records the data to support the identification of nursing diagnoses (Figure 3-1).

The purpose of the health history is to collect both subjective and objective data. **Subjective data,** also known as *symptoms,* are collected in an interview with the patient or caregiver, or both, during the nursing history. This type of data includes information that can be described or verified only by the patient or caregiver. It is what the person tells the nurse either spontaneously or in response to a direct question.

Objective data, also known as *signs,* are data that can be observed and measured. The nurse obtains this type of data by using inspection, palpation, percussion, and auscultation during the physical examination. Objective data are also acquired by diagnostic testing. Patients often provide subjective data while the nurse is performing the physical examination.

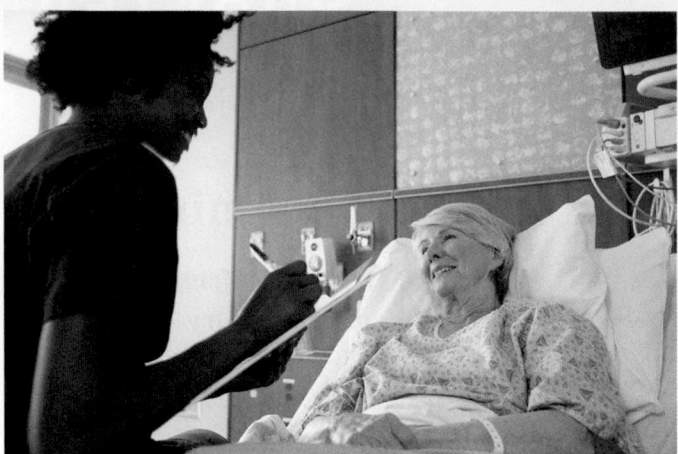

FIGURE 3-1 Obtaining a nursing history is an important role of the nurse. Source: Monkey Business Images/Shutterstock.com.

The nurse also observes objective signs while interviewing the patient. All findings related to a specific problem, whether subjective or objective, are known as *clinical manifestations* of that problem.

Interviewing Considerations

The purpose of the patient interview is to obtain a complete health history (e.g., subjective data) about the patient's past and present health status. Effective communication is a key factor in the interview process. Creating a climate of trust and respect is crucial for establishing a therapeutic relationship, as is the nurse's ability to engage in reflective practice. This ability includes the required capacities of self-awareness, self-knowledge, empathy, and awareness of boundaries and limits of the professional role (Registered Nurses' Association of Ontario, 2006). The nurse needs to communicate acceptance of the patient as an individual by using an open, responsive, nonjudgemental approach. Nurses communicate not only through language but also in their manner of dress, gestures, and body language. Modes of communication are learned through one's culture and influence: not only the words, gestures, and posture one uses but also the nature of information that is shared with others (see Chapter 2 for discussion on culture).

In addition to understanding the principles of effective communication, the nurse must develop a personal style of relating to patients. Although no single style fits all people, the wording of questions can increase the probability of eliciting the needed information. Asking questions, particularly those related to sensitive areas such as sexual functioning and economic status, becomes easier with training and experience.

The amount of time needed to complete a nursing history may vary with the format used and the experience of the nurse. The nursing history may be completed in one or several sessions, depending on the setting and the patient. For example, several short sessions might be needed for an older adult patient with a low energy level to allow time for the patient to provide the needed information. The nurse must also make a judgement about the amount of information collected on initial contact with the patient. In interviews with patients with chronic disease, patients in pain, and patients in emergency situations, the nurse should ask only questions that are pertinent to a specific problem. The nurse can complete the health history interview at a more appropriate time.

Before beginning the nursing history, the nurse should explain to the patient that the purpose of a detailed history is to collect information that will provide a health profile for comprehensive health care, including health promotion. This detailed information is collected during the patient's entry into the health care system, and subsequently, only updates are needed. The nurse should explain that personal and social data are needed to individualize the plan of care. This explanation is necessary because the patient may not be accustomed to sharing personal information and may need to know the purpose of such questioning. The nurse should assure the patient that all information will be kept confidential. The Canadian Nurses Association (CNA) requires that nurses protect the confidentiality of all information obtained in the context of the professional relationship and practise within the bounds of relevant laws governing privacy and confidentiality of personal health information. The CNA *Code of Ethics for Registered Nurses* provides helpful guidelines for ensuring confidentiality in nursing practice (CNA, 2017). To obtain factual, easily categorized information, a direct interview technique can be used. Closed-ended questions such as, "Have you had surgery before?" that require brief, specific responses are used. When asking sensitive personal and social questions, the nurse can communicate the acceptance or normality of behaviours by prefacing questions with phrases such as "most people" or "frequently." For example, stating, "Many people taking antihypertensive drugs have concerns about sexual functioning; do you have any you would like to discuss?" shows the patient that a particular situation may not be unique to that patient.

Another method of putting the patient at ease is to word the question so that an affirmative answer appears expected. An example of this technique is to ask, "What do you like to drink at a party?" instead of "Do you drink?" "How often do you drink alcohol?" is another way of obtaining information related to alcohol intake. These questions are open ended, encouraging the patient to discuss the issue in the patient's own words and at his or her own pace (Wilson & Giddens, 2013).

The nurse must judge the reliability of the patient as a historian. An older adult may give a false impression about her or his mental status because of a prolonged response time or visual and hearing impairment. The complexity and long duration of health problems may make it difficult for an older adult or a chronically ill younger patient to be an accurate historian.

It is important for the nurse to determine the patient's priority concerns and expectations because the nurse's priorities may be different from the patient's. For example, the nurse's priority may be to complete the health history, whereas the patient is interested only in relief from symptoms. Until the patient's priority need is met, the nurse will probably be unsuccessful in obtaining complete and accurate data.

Teamwork and Collaboration

Ongoing data collection is expected of all members of the health care team. In acute care settings, the initial (admission) nursing assessment must be completed by a registered nurse (RN) and within the timeframe determined by the employer. Table 3-1 shows the roles of various nursing personnel in data assessment and collection.

Data Organization

Assessment data must be systematically obtained and organized so that the nurse can readily analyze and make judgements about the patient's health status and any health problems. Information

TABLE 3-1 DATA ASSESSMENT AND COLLECTION: ROLES OF NURSING PERSONNEL

Role of Registered Nurse (RN)
- On admission, complete a comprehensive assessment (see Table 3-4).
- Document patient's health history by interviewing patient, caregiver, or both.
- Perform physical examination, using inspection, palpation, percussion, and auscultation as appropriate.
- Document findings from the health history and physical examination in the patient's record.
- Organize patient data into functional health patterns, if appropriate.
- Develop and prioritize nursing diagnoses and collaborative problems for the patient.
- Throughout patient's hospitalization, perform focused assessments that are based on patient's history or clinical manifestations (see Table 3-6).

Role of Registered Practical Nurse (RPN)
- Collect and document specific patient data as delegated by the RN (after the RN has developed the plan of care on the basis of findings of the admission assessment).
- Perform focused assessment that is based on patient's history or clinical manifestations, or as instructed by the RN (see Table 3-6).

Role of Personal Support Worker (PSW)
- Report patient's subjective complaints to RN or RPN.
- Perform activities of daily living, personal care, transferring patient in and out of bed as delegated by RN or RPN.

about the patient in various health care settings can be gathered in numerous approaches and formats. The format used in this chapter for obtaining a nursing history includes the following sequence of categories, similar to those outlined by Jarvis, Browne, MacDonald-Jenkins, and colleagues (2014). These assessment data provide a generic database for all health care practitioners:
1. Biographical data
2. Reason for seeking care
3. Current health status or history of current illness
4. Past medical history
5. Family medical history
6. Functional assessment
7. Review of systems

CULTURALLY COMPETENT CARE

ASSESSMENT

The process of obtaining a health history and performing a physical examination is an intimate experience for the nurse and the patient. As noted earlier in the chapter, a person's culture influences patterns of communication and what information is shared with others. During the interview and physical examination, the nurse must be sensitive to issues of eye contact, space, modesty, and touching, as discussed in Chapter 2. Knowing the cultural norms related to male–female relationships is especially important during the physical examination. To avoid violating any culturally based practices, the nurse can ask the patient about cultural values. The nurse should determine whether the patient would like to have someone else present during the history taking or physical examination or would prefer someone of the same gender to perform the history taking and physical examination (Jarvis, Browne, MacDonald-Jenkins, et al., 2014).

NURSING HISTORY: SUBJECTIVE DATA

Biographical Data

The nurse records the patient's name, address, contact information, age, birthdate, marital status, ethnocultural background, primary language, and current occupation. Advance care directives can be documented among these data (see Chapter 13). Also important to include here is the source of history: who is providing the information, how reliable the informant seems, and any special circumstances, such as the use of an interpreter (Jarvis, Browne, MacDonald-Jenkins, et al., 2014).

Reason for Seeking Care

The reason for seeking care is a brief statement in the patient's own words describing the reason for the visit. This statement is documented in quotation marks to indicate the patient's exact words (e.g., "My head has been aching for 3 days"; "My child has a fever and has been vomiting since last evening").

Current Health or History of Current Illness

This section is a chronological record of the reason for seeking care, beginning with the first time the symptom appeared until now. Symptoms experienced by the patient are not observed, so the symptom must be explored. Table 3-2 shows a mnemonic (PQRSTU) to help remember the areas to explore if a symptom is reported. The information that is obtained may help determine the cause of the symptom. A common symptom assessed is pain (see Chapter 10). For example, if a patient states that he has "pain in his leg at times," the nurse would assess and record the data with the use of PQRSTU:

> Has right midcalf pain that usually occurs at work when climbing stairs after lunch (P). Pain is alleviated by stopping and resting for 2 to 3 minutes. Patient thinks this pain is a "muscle cramp" and states he has been "eating a banana every day for extra potassium" but "it hasn't helped" (U, P). Pain is described as "stabbing" and is nonradiating (Q, R). Pain is so severe (rating 9 on 0–10 scale) that patient cannot continue activity (S). Onset is abrupt, occurring once or twice daily. It last occurred yesterday while he was cutting the lawn (T).

Past Health History

The past health history provides information about the patient's prior state of health. The patient is asked specifically about major childhood and adult illnesses, injuries, hospitalizations, and surgeries. This documentation should include questions about any infectious diseases such as human immunodeficiency virus (HIV) infection, hepatitis, methicillin-resistant *Staphylococcus aureus* (MRSA) infection, and vancomycin-resistant enterococcal (VRE) infection. Specific questions are more effective than simple questions of whether the patient has had any illness or health problems in the past. For example, the question "Do you have a history of diabetes?" elicits better information than does "Do you have any chronic health problems?"

Medications. The nurse obtains specific details related to past and current medications, including prescription and illicit drugs, over-the-counter drugs, vitamins, herbs, and dietary supplements. Patients frequently do not consider herbs and dietary supplements as drugs. It is important to ask specifically about their use because

TABLE 3-2	INVESTIGATION OF PATIENT-REPORTED SYMPTOM	
Factor	**Questions for Patient and Caregiver**	**Record**
Precipitating and **p**alliative	Were there any events that came before the symptom? What makes it better? Worse? What have you done for the symptom? Did this help?	Influence of physical and emotional activities Patient's attempts to alleviate (or treat) the symptom
Quality	Tell me what the symptom feels like (e.g., aching, dull, pressure, burning, stabbing).	Patient's own words (e.g., "Like a pinch or stabbing feeling")
Radiation	Where do you feel the symptom? Does it move to other areas?	Region of the body Local or radiating, superficial or deep
Severity	On a scale of 0–10, with 0 meaning no pain and 10 being the worst pain you could imagine, what number would you give your symptom?	Pain rating number (e.g., 5/10)
Timing	When did the symptom start? Any particular time of day, week, month, or year? Has the symptom changed over time? Where are you and what are you doing when the symptom occurs?	Time of onset, duration, periodicity, and frequency Course of symptoms Where patient is and what patient is doing when the symptom occurs
Understanding	Understand the patient's perception of the problem: What do you think it means?	Patient's own words about what the problem means to him or her

they can interact adversely with existing or newly prescribed medications (see Chapter 12, Table 12-7). Older adult and chronically ill patients should be questioned about medication routines; for these patients, polypharmacy, changes in absorption, distribution, metabolism, and elimination of and reaction to drugs can pose serious potential problems (Touhy, Jett, Boscart, et al., 2011).

Allergies. The patient's history of allergies to drugs, latex, contrast media, food, and the environment (e.g., pollen) should be explored. Documentation should include a detailed description of any and every allergic reaction reported by the patient.

Surgery or Other Treatments. All surgeries, along with the date of the event, the reason for the surgery, and the outcome should be recorded. Possible outcomes include complete resolution of the problem and residual effects. The nurse should ask about and record any blood products that the patient has received.

Family History

The nurse should ask about the health of family members, as well as the ages at and cause of death of blood relatives, such as parents, siblings, and grandparents. Common questions include those about any family history of heart disease, high blood pressure, stroke, diabetes, blood disorders, cancer, sickle cell disease, arthritis, allergies, obesity, alcoholism, mental health issues or illness, seizure disorder, kidney disease, and tuberculosis (Jarvis, Browne, MacDonald-Jenkins, et al., 2014). A genogram or family tree will help the nurse accurately document this information.

Functional Health Assessment

The nurse assesses the patient's functional health to identify positive, dysfunctional, and potential dysfunctional patterns. Dysfunctional health patterns result in nursing diagnoses, and potential dysfunctional patterns identify risk conditions for problems. Gordon's (2014) functional health pattern framework for assessment can assist the nurse in differentiating between areas for independent nursing intervention and areas necessitating collaboration or referral. The nurse may identify patients with effective health function who express a desire for a higher level of wellness.

It is also important to consider the social determinants of health to ensure a complete and relevant health history assessment. The nurse should explore the patient's living conditions by asking about employment; working conditions; well-being; health and social services received; and ability to obtain quality education, food, and housing, among other factors (Mikkonen & Raphael, 2010).

Health Perception–Health Management. Assessment of the patient's health perception and health management focuses on the patient's perceived level of health and well-being and on personal practices for maintaining health. The patient is asked to describe his or her personal health and any concerns about it. The patient's opinions of the effectiveness of health maintenance practices can be explored with questions about what helps and what hinders his or her well-being. The patient should be asked to rate his or her health as excellent, good, fair, or poor. When possible, this information is best recorded in the patient's own words. Asking about the type of health care providers that the patient uses is important. For example, if the patient is Indigenous Canadian, a traditional healer may be considered the primary health care provider. If the patient is of Chinese origin, a Chinese healer who practices traditional Chinese medicine may be the primary health care provider.

The purpose of questions for this pattern is also to identify risk factors with regard to family history (e.g., cardiac disease, cancer, genetic disorders), history of personal health habits (e.g., tobacco, alcohol, drug use), and history of exposure to environmental hazards (e.g., asbestos). If the patient is hospitalized, the nurse should ask about the expectations for this experience. The patient can be asked to describe his or her understanding of the current health problem, including its onset, course, and treatment. These questions elicit information about a patient's knowledge of the health problem and ability to use appropriate resources to manage the problem.

Nutrition–Metabolic. The nurse must assess the patient's processes of ingestion, digestion, absorption, and metabolism. A 24-hour dietary recall should be obtained from the patient to evaluate the quantity and quality of foods and fluids consumed. If a problem is identified, the nurse may ask the patient to keep a 3-day food diary for a more careful analysis of dietary intake. The effect of psychological factors such as depression, anxiety, stress, and self-concept on nutrition should be assessed. In addition, socioeconomic and cultural factors such as food budget, who prepares the meals, and food preferences are also determined. To determine whether the patient's present condition has interfered with eating and appetite the nurse can explore any symptoms of nausea, intestinal gas, or pain. Food allergies should be differentiated from food intolerances, such as lactose or gluten intolerance.

Elimination. To assess bowel, bladder, and skin function, the nurse should ask the patient about the frequency of bowel and bladder activity, including laxative and diuretic use. The skin is assessed again in the elimination pattern in terms of its excretory function.

Activity–Exercise. The nurse assesses the patient's usual pattern of exercise, work activity, leisure, and recreation. The patient should be questioned about his or her ability to perform activities of daily living and any specific problems noted.

Sleep–Rest. It is important for the nurse to describe the patient's perception of his or her pattern of sleep, rest, and relaxation in a 24-hour period. This information can be elicited by the question "Do you feel rested when you wake up?"

Cognitive–Perceptual. Assessment of this area involves a description of all of the senses and cognitive functions. In addition, pain is assessed as a sensory perception in this pattern. (See Chapter 10 for details on pain assessment.) The patient should be asked about any sensory deficits that affect the ability to perform activities of daily living. Ways in which the patient compensates for any sensory–perceptual problems should be recorded. To plan for patient teaching, the nurse can ask the patient how he or she communicates best and what he or she understands about the illness and treatment plan. (See Chapter 4 for details on patient teaching.)

Self-Perception–Self-Concept. The nurse should explore the patient's self-concept, which is crucial for determining the way the person interacts with others. Included are attitudes about self, perception of personal abilities, body image, and general sense of worth. The nurse should ask the patient for a self-description and about how his or her health condition affects self-concept. A patient's expressions of helplessness or loss of control frequently reflect an inability to care for himself or herself.

Role–Relationship. The nurse should explore the patient's roles and relationships, including major responsibilities. The patient should be asked to describe family, social, and work roles and relationships and to rate his or her performance of the expected behaviours related to these. The nurse should determine whether patterns in these roles and relationships are satisfactory or whether strain is evident. The nurse should note the patient's feelings about how the current condition affects his or her roles and relationships. It is important to assess whether the patient has access to family and friends who can help out when needed.

Sexuality–Reproductive. The nurse evaluates the patient's satisfaction or dissatisfaction with personal sexuality and reproductive issues. Assessing these aspects is important because many illnesses, surgical procedures, and drugs affect sexual function. A patient's sexual and reproductive concerns may be expressed and teaching needs may be identified through information obtained in this assessment.

The interview should be appropriate to the sex, age, and developmental stage of the patient. Obtaining information related to sexuality may be difficult for the nurse. However, it is important to document a health history and screen for sexual function and dysfunction in a nonjudgemental way and to provide information as appropriate or to refer the patient to a more experienced health care provider.

Coping–Stress Tolerance. The nurse should describe the patient's general coping pattern and the effectiveness of the coping mechanisms. Assessment of this pattern involves analyzing the specific stressors or problems that confront the patient, the patient's perception of the stressors, and the patient's response to the stressors. The nurse should document any major losses or stressors experienced by the patient in the previous year. Strategies used by the patient to deal with stressors and relieve tension should be noted. Individuals and groups that make up the patient's social support networks should be recorded and explored to help assess the level of support available to the patient.

Value–Belief. The nurse should describe the values, goals, and beliefs (including spiritual) that guide health-related choices. The patient's ethnic background and the effects of culture and beliefs on health practices should be documented. The patient's wishes about continuation of religious or spiritual practices and the use of religious articles should be noted and respected.

PHYSICAL EXAMINATION: OBJECTIVE DATA

General Survey

After the nursing history, the nurse makes a **general survey statement**. This reflects a general impression of a patient, including behavioural observations. This initial survey begins with the nurse's first encounter with the patient and continues during the health history interview.

Although the nurse may include other data that seem pertinent, the major areas included in the general survey statement are (a) body features, (b) mental state, (c) speech, (d) body movements, (e) obvious physical signs, (f) nutritional status, and (g) behaviour. Vital signs, height, and weight or body mass index (calculated from height and weight [kg/m^2]), or both, may be included. The following is a sample of a general survey statement:

> Mrs. H. is a 34-year-old Italian woman, BP 130/84, P 88, R 18. Alert but anxious. Speech rapid with trailing thoughts. Wringing hands and shuffling feet during interview. Skin flushed, hands clammy. Overweight relative to height (body mass index, 28.3 kg/m^2). Sits with eyes downcast and shoulders slumped and avoids eye contact.

Physical Examination

The **physical examination** is the systematic assessment of a patient's physical status. Throughout the physical examination, the nurse explores any positive findings, using the same criteria as those used during the investigation of a symptom in the nursing history (see Table 3-2). A *positive finding* indicates that the patient has or had the particular problem or sign under discussion (e.g., if the patient with jaundice has an enlarged liver, it is a positive finding). Relevant information about this problem should then be gathered.

Negative findings may also be significant. A *negative finding* is the absence of a sign or symptom usually associated with a problem. For example, peripheral edema is common with advanced liver disease. If edema is not present in a patient with advanced liver disease, this should be specifically documented as "no peripheral edema."

Techniques. Four major techniques are used in performing the physical examination: inspection, palpation, percussion, and auscultation. The techniques are usually performed in this sequence, except for the abdominal examination (inspection, auscultation, percussion, and palpation). Performing palpation and percussion of the abdomen before auscultation can alter bowel sounds and produce false findings. Not every assessment area requires the use of all four assessment techniques (e.g., for the musculo-skeletal system, only inspection and palpation are required).

Inspection. **Inspection** is the visual examination of a part or region of the body to assess normal conditions or deviations.

FIGURE 3-2 Palpation is the examination of the body using touch. Source: Jarvis, C. (2012). *Physical examination and health assessment* (6th ed.). St Louis: Saunders.

FIGURE 3-3 Percussion technique: tapping the interphalangeal joint. Only the middle finger of the nondominant hand should be in contact with the skin surface. Normal percussion sounds for lung tissue are *resonant;* for air-filled viscus (e.g., intestines), *tympany;* for dense organs (e.g., liver), *dull;* and for areas with no air present (e.g., bone, muscle), *flat.* Source: Modified from Seidel, H.M., Ball, J.W., Dains, J.E., et al. (2011). *Mosby's guide to physical examination* (7th ed.). St. Louis: Saunders.

Inspection is more than just looking. This technique is deliberate, systematic, and focused. The nurse must compare what is seen with the known, generally visible characteristics of the body part being inspected. For example, most 30-year-old men have hair on their legs. Absence of hair may indicate a vascular problem and signals the need for further investigation, or it may be normal for a patient of a particular ethnicity (e.g., First Nations men have little body hair).

Palpation. Palpation is the examination of the body through the use of touch. Using light and deep palpation can yield information about masses, pulsations, organ enlargement, tenderness or pain, swelling, muscular spasm or rigidity, elasticity, vibration of voice sounds, crepitus, moisture, and texture. Different parts of the hand are more sensitive for specific assessments. For example, the palmar surface (base of fingers) should be used to feel vibrations; the dorsa (back) of the hands and fingers, to assess skin temperature; and tips of the fingers, to palpate the abdomen (Jarvis, Browne, MacDonald-Jenkins, et al., 2014) (Figure 3-2).

Percussion. Percussion is a technique of tapping the body directly or indirectly with the fingertips to produce a sound and vibration to obtain information about the underlying area (Figure 3-3). The sounds and the vibrations are specific to the underlying structures. A change from an expected sound may indicate a problem. For example, dullness in the right lower quadrant instead of the normal tympany should be explored. (Specific percussion sounds of various body parts and regions are discussed in the appropriate assessment chapters.)

Auscultation. Auscultation is listening to sounds produced by the body to assess normal conditions and deviations from normal. This technique is particularly useful in evaluating sounds from the heart, lungs, abdomen, and vascular system. The bell of the stethoscope is more sensitive to low-pitched sounds (e.g., heart murmurs). The diaphragm of the stethoscope is more sensitive to high-pitched sounds (e.g., bowel sounds). Some stethoscopes have only a diaphragm, designed to transmit low- and high-pitched sounds. To listen for low-pitched sounds, the examiner holds the diaphragm lightly on the patient's skin. For high-pitched sounds, the examiner presses the diaphragm firmly on the skin (Jarvis, Browne, MacDonald-Jenkins, et al., 2014; Figure 3-4). (Specific auscultatory sounds and techniques are discussed in the appropriate assessment chapters.)

FIGURE 3-4 Auscultation is listening to sounds produced by the body to assess normal conditions and deviations from normal. Source: Courtesy Linda Bucher, RN, PhD, CEN, CNE, Staff Nurse, Virtua Memorial Hospital, Mt. Holly, NJ.

Equipment. The nurse should collect the equipment needed for the physical examination before beginning (Table 3-3). This saves the time and energy for the nurse and the patient. (The uses of specific equipment are discussed in the appropriate assessment chapters.)

Organization of the Examination. The physical examination should be performed systematically and efficiently. Explanations should be given to the patient as the examination proceeds, and the patient's comfort, safety, and privacy should be considered. By being confident and self-assured, considerate, and unhurried, the nurse will help reduce any anxiety the patient may be feeling about the examination (Jarvis, Browne, MacDonald-Jenkins, et al., 2014). Following the same sequence every time helps ensure that the nurse does not forget a procedure, a step in the sequence, or a portion of the body. Table 3-4 presents an outline of a comprehensive and organized physical examination. Adaptations of the physical examination often are useful for older adult patients, who may have age-related problems such as decreased mobility, limited energy, and perceptual changes.

Recording Physical Examination. At the conclusion of the examination, the nurse records the normal and abnormal findings in the patient's record. Table 3-5 provides an example of how to record the findings of a physical examination of a healthy adult. See Chapter 7, Table 7-2, and the age-related assessment findings in each assessment chapter for helpful references in recording age-related assessment differences.

TYPES OF ASSESSMENT

Various types of assessment are used to obtain information about a patient. These approaches can be divided into three types: comprehensive, focused, and emergency (Table 3-6). The nurse must decide what type of assessment to perform according to the clinical situation. Sometimes the health care employer provides guidelines, and other times it is a nursing judgement.

Comprehensive Assessment

A *comprehensive assessment* includes detailed documentation of the health history and a physical examination of all body systems. This is typically performed on the patient's admission to the hospital or at the onset of care in a primary care setting.

Focused Assessment

A *focused assessment* is an abbreviated health history and examination. It is used to evaluate the status of previously identified problems and monitor for signs and symptoms of new problems. It can be performed when a specific problem

---

TABLE 3-3 EQUIPMENT FOR PHYSICAL EXAMINATION*

- Alcohol swabs
- Blood pressure cuff
- Cotton balls
- Examining table or bed
- Eye chart (e.g., Snellen eye chart)
- Paper cup with water
- Patient gown
- Pocket flashlight
- Reflex hammer
- Stethoscope (with bell and diaphragm or a dual-purpose diaphragm; 38- to 46-cm tubing)
- Tongue blades
- Watch (with second hand or digital)

*These are examples of commonly used equipment; other equipment may be used, depending on the situation.

TABLE 3-4 OUTLINE FOR PHYSICAL EXAMINATION

1. General Survey
Observe general state of health (patient is seated):
- Body features
- Mental state and level of orientation
- Speech
- Body movements
- Physical appearance
- Nutritional status
- Behaviour

2. Vital Signs
Record vital signs:
- Blood pressure—both arms for comparison
- Apical/radial pulse
- Respiration
- Temperature
- Oxygen saturation
- Height and weight; calculation of body mass index (BMI)

3. Integument
Inspect and palpate skin for the following:
- Colour
- Integrity (e.g., lesions, breakdown, lacerations)
- Scars, tattoos, piercings
- Bruises, rash
- Edema
- Moisture
- Texture
- Temperature
- Turgor
- Vascularity
Inspect and palpate nails for the following:
- Colour
- Lesions
- Size
- Shape
- Angle
- Capillary refill time

4. Head and Neck
Inspect and palpate head for the following:
- Shape and symmetry of skull
- Masses
- Tenderness
- Condition of hair and scalp
- Temporal arteries
- Temporo-mandibular joint
- Sensory (cranial nerve V; light touch, pain)
- Motor (cranial nerve VII; showing teeth, pursing lips, raising eyebrows)
- Facial expression (cranial nerve VII; looking up, wrinkling forehead)
- Strength (cranial nerve XI; raising shoulders against resistance)
Inspect and palpate (occasionally auscultate) neck for the following:
- Skin (vascularity and visible pulsations)
- Symmetry
- Pulses and bruits (carotid)
- Midline structure (trachea, thyroid gland, cartilage)
- Lymph nodes (preauricular, postauricular, occipital, mandibular, tonsillar, submental, anterior and posterior cervical, infraclavicular, supraclavicular)
Test visual acuity. Inspect and palpate eyes/eyebrows for the following:
- Position and movement of eyelids (cranial nerve VII)
- Visual fields (cranial nerve II)
- Extraocular movements (cranial nerves III, IV, VI)
- Cornea, sclera, conjunctiva
- Pupillary response (cranial nerve III)
- Retinal (red) reflex*
Inspect and palpate nose and sinuses for the following:
- External nose: shape, blockage
- Internal nose: patency of nasal passages, shape, turbinates or polyps, discharge
- Frontal and maxillary sinuses

Continued

TABLE 3-4 OUTLINE FOR PHYSICAL EXAMINATION—cont'd

Inspect and palpate ears for the following:
- Placement
- Pinna
- Auditory acuity (whispered voice, ticking watch) (cranial nerve VIII)
- Mastoid process
- Auditory canal
- Tympanic membrane

Inspect and palpate mouth for the following:
- Lips (symmetry, lesions, colour)
- Buccal mucosa (Stensen's and Wharton's ducts)
- Teeth (absence, state of repair, colour)
- Gums (colour, receding from teeth)
- Tongue for strength (cranial nerve XII; asymmetry, ability to stick out tongue, ability to move tongue side to side, fasciculations)
- Palates
- Tonsils and pillars
- Uvular elevation (cranial nerve IX)
- Posterior pharynx
- Gag reflex (cranial nerves IX and X)
- Jaw strength (cranial nerve V)
- Moisture
- Colour
- Floor of mouth

5. Extremities
Observe size and shape, symmetry and deformity, involuntary movements. Inspect and palpate arms, fingers, wrists, elbows, and shoulders for the following:
- Strength
- Range of motion
- Joint pain
- Swelling
- Pulses (radial, brachial)
- Sensation (light tough, pain, temperature)
- Test reflexes: triceps, biceps, brachioradialis

Inspect and palpate legs for the following:
- Strength
- Range of motion
- Joint pain
- Swelling, edema
- Hair distribution
- Sensation (light touch, pain, temperature)
- Pulses (dorsalis pedis, posterior tibialis)
- Test reflexes: patellar, Achilles, plantar

6. Posterior Thorax
- Inspect for muscular development, scoliosis, respiratory movement, approximation of AP diameter.
- Palpate for symmetry of respiratory movement, tenderness of CVA, spinous processes, tumours or swelling, tactile fremitus
- Percuss for pulmonary resonance
- Auscultate for breath sounds
- Auscultate for egophony, bronchophony, and whispered pectoriloquy

7. Anterior Thorax
- Assess breasts for configuration, symmetry, dimpling of skin
- Assess nipples for rash, direction, inversion, retraction
- Inspect for apical impulse, other precordial pulsations
- Palpate the apical impulse and the precordium for thrills, lifts, heaves, tenderness
- Inspect neck for venous distension, pulsations, waves
- Palpate lymph nodes in the subclavian, axillary, and brachial areas
- Palpate breasts
- Auscultate for rate and rhythm, character of S_1 and S_2 in the aortic, pulmonic, Erb point, tricuspid, and mitral areas; bruits at carotid, epigastrium

8. Abdomen
- Inspect for scars, shape, symmetry, bulging, muscular position and condition of umbilicus, movements (respiratory, pulsations, presence of peristaltic waves)
- Auscultate for peristalsis (e.g., bowel sounds), bruits
- Percuss and then palpate to confirm positive findings: check liver (size, tenderness), spleen, kidney (size, tenderness), urinary bladder (distension)
- Palpate femoral pulses, inguinofemoral nodes, and abdominal aorta

9. Neurological
Observe motor status.
- Gait
- Toe walk
- Heel walk
- Drift

Observe coordination.
- Finger to nose
- Romberg sign
- Heel to opposite shin

Observe the following:
- Proprioception (position sense of great toe)

10. Genitalia*
Male External Genitalia
- Inspect penis, noting hair distribution, prepuce, glans, urethral meatus, scars, ulcers, eruptions, structural alterations, discharge
- Inspect epidermis of perineum, rectum
- Inspect skin of scrotum; palpate for descended testes, masses, pain

Female External Genitalia
- Inspect hair distribution; mons pubis, labia (minora and majora); urethral meatus; Bartholin's, urethral, and Skene's glands (may also be palpated, if indicated); introitus; any discharge
- Assess for presence of cystocele, prolapse
- Inspect perineum, rectum

AP, anteroposterior; *CVA,* costovertebral angle; *S_1* and *S_2,* first and second heart sounds.
*Additional techniques can be performed by qualified nurses in specialized settings. A retinal reflex (red reflex) examination would be performed with the eye examination. Speculum and bimanual examination of women and the prostate gland examination of men would be performed after inspection of genitalia. For examination of the genitalia, a second person may have to be present in the room.

(e.g., pneumonia) is identified. The patient's clinical manifestations should alert the nurse to the appropriate focused assessment. For example, abdominal pain indicates the need for a focused assessment of the abdomen. Some patients require a focused assessment of more than one body system. A complaint of headache may indicate the need to perform musculo-skeletal, neurological, and head and neck examinations. Assessment chapters throughout the text include "Focused Assessment" boxes.

Emergency Assessment

In an emergency or a critical care situation, an *emergency assessment* may be performed. This involves a rapid documentation of the history and rapid examination of a patient while vital functions are maintained.

Using Assessment Approaches

Assessment in a hospital inpatient setting, particularly in acute care, is markedly different from assessment in other settings. Focused

TABLE 3-5 HOW TO RECORD FINDINGS OF A NORMAL PHYSICAL EXAMINATION OF A HEALTHY ADULT

Example
Patient's Name _____
Age _____

General Status
Well-nourished, well-hydrated, well-developed White [woman or man] in NAD, appears stated age, speech clear and evenly paced; is alert and oriented × 3; cooperative, calm

Skin
Clear s̄ lesions, warm and dry, trunk warmer than extremities, turgor returns quickly, no ↑ vascularity, no varicose veins

Nails
Well-groomed, round 160-degree angle s̄ lesions, nail beds pink, nails flexible

Hair
Thick, brown, shiny, normal [male or female] distribution

Head
Normocephalic, sinuses nontender

Eyes
Visual fields intact on gross confrontation
VA: Right eye 20/20
Left eye 20/20
Both eyes 20/20
s̄ glasses
EOM: Intact on all gazes s̄ ptosis, nystagmus
Pupils: PERRLA, negative cover and uncover test results

Ears
Pinnae intact, in proper alignment; external canal patent; small amount of cerumen present; TMs intact; pearly-grey LMs, LR visible, not bulging; whisper heard at 90 cm (3 ft)

Nose
Patent bilaterally; turbinates pink, no swelling

Mouth
Moist and pink, soft and hard palates intact, uvula rises midline on "ahh," 24 teeth present and in good repair

Throat
Tonsils surgically removed, no redness

Tongue
Moist, pink, size appropriate for mouth

Neck
Supple, s̄ masses, s̄ bruits, lymph nodes nonpalpable and nontender
Thyroid: Palpable, smooth, not enlarged
ROM: Full, intact, strong
Trachea: Midline, nontender

Breasts
Soft, nonpendulous, s̄ venous pattern, s̄ dimpling, puckering
Nipples: s̄ inversion, point in same direction, areola dark and symmetrical, no discharge, no masses, nontender

Axilla
Hair present, shaved, no lesions, nontender

Thorax and Lungs
AP < transverse diameter, resp rate 18, reg rhythm, no ↑ in tactile fremitus, no tenderness, lungs resonant throughout, diaphragmatic excursion 4 cm bilaterally, chest expansion symmetrical, lung fields clear throughout

Heart
Rate 82, reg rate and rhythm; no lifts, heaves
Apical impulse: 5th ICS at MCL; no palpable thrills; S_1, S_2 louder, softer in appropriate locations; no S_3, S_4; no murmurs, rubs, clicks
Carotid, femoral, pedal, and radial pulses present; equal, 2+ bilaterally

Abdomen
No pulsations visible; rounded, active bowel sounds; no bruits or CVA tenderness; no palpable masses

Liver
Lower border percussed at costal margin, smooth, nontender; approx 9-cm span

Spleen
Nonpalpable, nontender

Neurological System
Cranial nerves I-XII intact
Motor (drift, toe stand) intact
Coord (FN, Romberg) intact
Reflexes: See diagram

Grading Scale
0   No response
1+ Diminished
2+ Normal
3+ Increased
4+ Hyperactive
Sensation (touch, vibration, proprioception) intact

Musculo-Skeletal System
Well developed, no muscle wasting; s̄ crepitus, nodules, swelling
ROM: Full, intact, and equal bilaterally; no scoliosis
Strength: Equal, strong bilaterally 5/5
Gait: Walks erect 60-cm steps, arms swinging at side s̄ staggering

Female Genitalia*
External genitalia: No swelling, redness, tenderness in BUS; normal hair distribution, no cysts
Vagina: No lesions, discharge, bulging; pink
Cervix: Os closed; pink, no lesions, erosions, nontender
Uterus: Small, firm, nontender
Adnexa: No enlargement; nontender
Rectovaginal: Sphincter intact; confirms above findings

Male Genitalia
Normal male hair distribution, negative inguinal hernia
Penis: Urethral opening patent; no redness, swelling, discharge; no lesions, structural alterations
Scrotum: Testes descended; no redness, masses, tenderness
Rectal*: No lesions, redness; sphincter intact; prostate small, nontender

Psychological Status
Affect appropriate
Orientation: Oriented ×3
Mood: Pleasant, appropriate
Thought content: Intelligent, coherent
Memory: Remote and recent intact
Signature _____

*These data would be obtained from an examination of the genitalia if the nurse has the appropriate training.
AP, anteroposterior; *BUS*, Bartholin's gland, urethral meatus, Skene's duct; *coord*, coordination; *CVA*, costovertebral angle; *EOM*, extraocular movements; *FN*, finger to nose; *ICS*, intercostal space; *LMs*, landmarks; *LR*, light reflex; *MCL*, midclavicular line; *NAD*, no acute distress; *PERRLA*, pupils equal, round, reactive to light and accommodation; *reg*, regular; *resp*, respiration; *oriented ×3*, oriented to person, place, and time; *ROM*, range of motion; s̄, without; S_1, S_2, S_3, and S_4, heart sounds; *TM*, tympanic membrane; *VA*, visual acuity.

TABLE 3-6 TYPES OF ASSESSMENT FOR VARIOUS SITUATIONS

The following describes types of assessment that the nurse may use in various situations.

Description	When and Where Performed	Where to Find in Book
Comprehensive • Detailed assessment of all body systems (head-to-toe assessment)	• Onset of care in primary or ambulatory care setting • On admission to hospital, rehabilitation, or long-term care setting • On initial home care visit	• Assessment chapters for each body system • Outline for physical examination (see Table 3-4) • Findings for normal physical examination (see Table 3-5)
Focused • Abbreviated assessment that focuses on one or more body systems that are the focus of care • Includes an assessment related to a specific problem (e.g., pneumonia, specific abnormal laboratory findings) • Includes monitoring for signs and symptoms of new problems	• In the emergency department for non–life-threatening situations • Throughout hospital admission: at beginning of a shift and as needed throughout shift • Revisit in ambulatory care setting or home care setting	• "Focused Assessment" boxes in each assessment chapter • Tables on nursing assessment of specific diseases throughout book
Emergency • Limited to assessing life-threatening conditions (e.g., inhalation injuries, anaphylaxis, myocardial infarction, shock, stroke) • Conducted to ensure survival. Assessment focuses on elements in the primary survey (e.g., airway, breathing, circulation disability) • After lifesaving interventions are initiated, brief systematic assessment performed to identify any and all other injuries or problems	• Performed in any setting when signs or symptoms of a life-threatening condition appear (e.g., emergency department, critical care unit, surgical setting, ambulatory care setting, home setting)	• Chapter 71, Tables 71-3 and 71-5 • Emergency management tables throughout the book and listed in Table 71-1

TABLE 3-7 CLINICAL APPLICATION FOR TYPES OF ASSESSMENT

The following is an example of how various types of assessment would be used for a patient progressing from the emergency department to a clinical unit of a hospital.

Timeline	Type of Assessment
Emergency Department Patient arrives in acute respiratory distress. Problem is identified, critical interventions are performed, and patient's condition is stabilized.	Emergency assessment (see Table 71-3) Focused assessment of the respiratory and related body systems (e.g., cardiovascular); comprehensive assessment of all body systems may begin
Clinical Unit Patient is admitted to a monitored clinical unit. At beginning of each shift, patient is reassessed per orders and more frequently as determined by the nurse.	Complete comprehensive assessment of all body systems within proper timeframe Focused assessment of respiratory system and other related body systems per agency protocol; focused assessment of one or more appropriate body systems if new symptoms are reported.

assessment of hospitalized patients is frequent and performed by many different people. Such a team approach mandates a high degree of consistency among different health care providers.

While providing ongoing care for a patient, the nurse constantly refines her or his mental image of the patient. With experience, the nurse will derive a mental image of a patient's status from a few very basic details, such as "85-year-old Black woman admitted for COPD [chronic obstructive pulmonary disease] exacerbation." The nurse's view of her becomes clearer as a more complete verbal report is received, such as length of stay, laboratory results, physical findings, and vital signs. Next, the nurse performs her or his own assessment, using a focused approach. During this assessment, the nurse confirms or revises the findings that were read in the medical record and received from other health care providers.

The process does not end once the nurse has completed her or his first assessment of a patient during rounds. The nurse will have to continue to gather information about her or his patients throughout the shift. Everything that the nurse learned previously about each patient is considered in with regard to new information. For example, while the nurse is performing a respiratory assessment on a patient with COPD, crackles are heard in the lungs. This finding should lead the nurse to perform a cardiovascular assessment because cardiac problems (e.g., heart failure) can also cause crackles. As the nurse gains experience, the importance of new findings will be more obvious.

Table 3-7 shows how the nurse can perform different types of assessments on the basis of a patient's progress through a given hospitalization. When a patient arrives at the emergency department with a life-threatening condition, the nurse performs an emergency assessment on the basis of the elements of a primary survey (e.g., airway, breathing, circulation, disability; see Chapter 71, Table 71-3). Once the patient is stabilized, the nurse can begin a focused assessment of the respiratory and related body systems. Once the patient is admitted, a comprehensive assessment of all body systems, whether they are involved in the current clinical problem or not, is performed.

PROBLEM IDENTIFICATION AND NURSING DIAGNOSES

After completing the history and physical examination, the nurse analyzes the data and develops a list of nursing diagnoses and collaborative problems. See Chapter 1 for a description of the nursing process, including the identification of nursing diagnoses and collaborative problems.

▮ REVIEW QUESTIONS

The number of the question corresponds to the same-numbered outcome at the beginning of the chapter.

1. The patient's health history and physical examination findings enable the nurse with information to primarily take which action?
   a. Diagnose a medical problem.
   b. Investigate the client's signs and symptoms.
   c. Classify subjective and objective client data.
   d. Identify nursing diagnoses and collaborative problems.

2. If a patient is concerned that his illness is threatening his job security, in which functional health pattern would the nurse place this information?
   a. Role–relationship
   b. Cognitive–perceptual
   c. Coping–stress tolerance
   d. Health perception–health management

3. The nurse is preparing to examine a client's abdomen. Number the proper order of the steps in the assessment of the abdomen, with 1 = the first technique and 4 = the last technique.
   ___ Inspection
   ___ Palpation
   ___ Percussion
   ___ Auscultation

4. Which situation would require the nurse to perform a focused assessment? *(Select all that apply.)*
   a. A client denies a current health problem.
   b. A client reports a new symptom during rounds.
   c. A previously identified problem needs reassessment.
   d. A baseline health maintenance examination is required.
   e. An emergency problem is identified during physical examination.

1. d; 2. a; 3. 1, 4, 3, 2; 4. b, c.

⊝volve

For even more review questions, visit *http://evolve.elsevier.com/Canada/ Lewis/medsurg*.

REFERENCES

Canadian Nurses Association (CNA). (2017). *Code of ethics for registered nurses.* Retrieved from *https://www.cna-aiic.ca/~/media/ cna/page-content/pdf-en/code-of-ethics-2017-edition-secure -interactive.pdf?la=en.*

Gordon, M. (2014). *Manual of nursing diagnosis* (13th ed.). Boston: Jones & Bartlett. (Seminal).

Jarvis, C., Browne, A., MacDonald-Jenkins, J., et al. (Eds.), (2014). *Physical examination and health assessment* (2nd Canadian ed.). Toronto: Elsevier/Saunders.

Mikkonen, J., & Raphael, D. (2010). *Social determinants of health: The Canadian facts.* Toronto: York University School of Health Policy and Management. Retrieved from *http:// www.thecanadianfacts.org.* (Seminal).

Registered Nurses' Association of Ontario. (2006). *Establishing therapeutic relationships. Supplement.* Retrieved from *http:// rnao.ca/sites/rnao-ca/files/storage/related/943_BPG_TR_ Supplement.pdf.* (Seminal).

Touhy, T. A., Jett, K. F., Boscart, V., et al. (2011). *Ebersole and Hess' gerontological nursing and healthy aging* (1st Canadian ed.). Toronto: Mosby.

Wilson, S., & Giddens, J. (2013). *Health assessment for nursing practice* (5th ed.). St. Louis: Mosby.

For additional Internet resources, see the website for this book at *http://evolve.elsevier.com/Canada/Lewis/medsurg*

4

Patient and Caregiver Teaching

Written by: Linda Bucher
Adapted by: Verna C. Pangman

 WEBSITE

http://evolve.elsevier.com/Canada/Lewis/medsurg

- Review Questions (Online Only)
- Key Points
- Answer Guidelines for Case Study

- Conceptual Care Map Creator
- Audio Glossary
- Content Updates

LEARNING OBJECTIVES

1. Prioritize four specific goals of patient and caregiver teaching.
2. Examine teaching implications of adult learning principles.
3. Analyze specific competencies that enhance the nurse's effectiveness as a teacher.
4. Formulate strategies to manage the challenges to the nurse's teaching effectiveness.
5. Examine the intended role of the family in patient teaching.

6. Explain the basic steps in the teaching–learning process.
7. Relate physical, psychological, and sociocultural characteristics of the patient to the teaching–learning process.
8. Describe the components of a correctly written learning outcome.
9. Appraise advantages, disadvantages, and uses of various teaching strategies.
10. Examine common methods of short- and long-term evaluation.

KEY TERMS

andragogy, p. 49
empathy, p. 51
facilitator, p. 56
family conferences, p. 48

learning, p. 49
learning needs, p. 55
learning outcomes, p. 55
learning style, p. 55

peer teaching, p. 56
self-efficacy, p. 53
stages of behavioural change, p. 50

teaching, p. 49
teaching plan, p. 49
teaching process, p. 52

ROLE OF PATIENT AND CAREGIVER TEACHING

Teaching patients and caregivers (any family member or significant other) is a dynamic and interactive process. It is one of the most major and challenging roles that nurses face in the current health care system. Constraints on staff time and resources, coupled with the shortened average length of inpatient hospitalizations, can affect the nurse's ability to engage in patient education. Inadequate patient teaching frequently results in devastating consequences for the patient and caregiver. Conversely, teaching patients about promoting, maintaining, and restoring their health is a required nursing skill that most often results in a positive outcome, enhancing the patient's quality of life.

Nurses engage in patient education to help patients and their caregivers focus on optimizing their health and to enable them to cope with acute and chronic health problems. Specifically, teaching goals include (a) maintenance of health, (b) health promotion and prevention of disease, (c) management of illness, and (d) appropriate selection and use of treatment and resources. Furthermore, these goals facilitate maintaining a high level of wellness that is meaningful and relevant for the patient throughout the lifespan. Effective teaching can assist people to make informed decisions about their lifestyle, health practices, and treatment choices. For patients who have acute health problems, quality teaching can prevent complications and promote recovery. For patients with chronic illnesses, increased knowledge can promote self-care and independence.

Patient education can occur wherever nurses practice. Teaching situations include the community, schools, industry, ambulatory care centres, hospitals, long-term care facilities, and homes.

Family conferences are held mainly in hospitals and long-term care settings. These conferences provide opportunities for patients and their caregivers, along with members of the interdisciplinary health care team, to identify needs for information and assistance with health care matters (Fineberg, Kawashima, & Asch, 2011). In fact, the involvement of the caregiver is considered one of the key variables influencing patient outcomes (Bastable, Gramet, Jacobs, et al., 2011). In family conferences, the nurse uses knowledge and skills to teach the patient and caregiver about the availability of resources and about strategies to promote health, as well as to assess additional care needs.

The teaching episodes expected from nurses are not complex. For example, teaching a patient to cough effectively and to breathe deeply after surgery can help the patient prevent atelectasis. However, when a patient has specific learning needs concerning management of a health problem or the strategies of health promotion, a teaching plan should be developed and implemented with the patient.

A teaching plan is a learner-centred approach for action to achieve the goals and learning outcomes agreed upon by the patient and nurse. The nurse, in cooperation with the patient, chooses activities and experiences to facilitate learning to improve the health of the patient. It then becomes necessary to evaluate the extent to which outcomes were attained (Billings & Halstead, 2016). This chapter describes the steps involved in providing patient and caregiver education and discusses factors that contribute to successful educational experiences.

TEACHING–LEARNING PROCESS

Teaching is much more than the simple intent of imparting information. Teaching is a process of deliberately planning experiences and sharing knowledge to meet learner outcomes in the cognitive, affective, and psychomotor domains. As well as being planned, teaching always endeavours to incorporate incidental experiences. Effective teaching can be conducted with a combination of methods such as simulation, use of printed materials, and assistive technology (computers) to influence the patient's knowledge and behaviour (Bastable, Gramet, Jacobs, et al., 2011). Learning is much more than listening to instruction. According to Kozier, Erb, Berman, and colleagues (2014), learning is a cognitive ability that is reflected by a change in behaviour (knowledge, attitudes, or skills or a combination of these) that can be observed and measured. A vital aspect of the nursing role is to understand which factors promote learning and what motivates the learner to learn (Bastable, Gramet, Jacobs, et al., 2011).

In patient education, the teaching–learning process involves the patient, the nurse, and the caregiver or social support system. The interdisciplinary team may also partake and can demonstrate accountability and responsibility for patient education on the basis of solid principles of teaching and learning.

Adult Learners

Adult Learning Principles. Through educational research and theoretical development pertaining specifically to adults, investigators have identified specific principles and characteristics that differentiate learning by adults from learning by children. These concepts provide a foundation for the effective teaching of adults. Many of the theories of adult learning have arisen from the work of Knowles (1990), who identified seven principles of andragogy (adult learning) that are deemed essential for the nurse to consider when teaching adults. These principles and their implications for patient teaching are presented in Table 4-1.

Determinants of Learning. Because of the combined effects of health care trends and population demographics, the nurse must carefully assess all of the determinants of learning for the patient for whom the nurse has teaching responsibility. The three determinants of learning that require learning assessments are identified in Table 4-2.

Motivation of Adult Learners. One important factor that is strongly associated with motivation is *emotional readiness*

TABLE 4-1   PRINCIPLES OF ADULT EDUCATION APPLIED TO PATIENT TEACHING

Principle	Teaching Implications for the Nurse
Adults are independent learners.	• The teacher is a facilitator who directs the patient to resources but is not the source of all information. • Patients expect to make decisions about their own lives and learning experiences and to take responsibility for those decisions. • Respect for the patient's independence can be reflected in statements such as "What do you think you need to learn about this topic?"
Readiness to learn arises from life's changes.	• Patients see life processes as problems to be solved. • Readiness and motivation to learn are high when new tasks are faced. • Crises in health are "teachable moments."
Past experiences are resources for learning.	• Patients have had many life experiences and have engaged in informal learning for years. • Motivation is increased when patients believe that they already know something about the subject from past experiences. • Identifying past knowledge and experiences can familiarize patients with a new situation and increase their confidence.
Adults learn best when the topic is of immediate value.	• Patients need to apply learning immediately. • Long-term goals may have little appeal. • Short-term, realistic goals should be encouraged. • Education should be focused on information that the patient views as being needed right now.
Adults approach learning as problem solving.	• Patients seek out various resources for specific learning to help them deal with a problem. • Information that is not relevant to the problem is not readily learned. • When the patient does not recognize relevancy, explanations for the need to learn something should be offered. • Teaching should target the specific problem or circumstance.
Adults see themselves as doers.	• Patients learn better by doing. • Demonstrations, computer activities, and practice of skills should be offered when appropriate.
Adults resist learning when conditions are incongruent with their self-concepts.	• Patients do not learn when they are treated as children and told what they must do. • Patients need control and self-direction to maintain their sense of self-worth.

TABLE 4-2   DETERMINANTS OF LEARNING

• The needs of the learner. Assist learner to identify, clarify, and prioritize his or her needs and interests.
• The state of readiness to learn. Seize the moment when the learner demonstrates an interest in learning the material necessary to maintain optimal health.
• The preferred learning style for processing knowledge and information. Assess the various teaching techniques and the teaching–learning conditions under which these learners are most likely to perceive, process, store, and recall health-related material.

Source: From Bastable, S. B. (2008). *Essentials of patient education.* Sudbury, MA: Jones & Bartlett.

(Bastable, 2008). When a nurse is teaching an adult, it is important to identify what that adult values so that motivation can be enhanced. If the adult perceives a need for information to enhance health or avoid illness or if the adult believes that a behaviour change has health value, motivation to learn is increased. Humans seek out experiences that stimulate their desire and effort to learn. Therefore, learning activities must be stimulating to maintain a desire to reach a goal. *Motivational interviewing* has been shown to promote behaviour change in patients in various health care settings. It is a counselling approach that serves many goals, such as increasing rapport, helping patients feel understood, reducing the likelihood of resistance to change, and allowing patients to explore their inner thoughts and motivation. This approach supports self-efficacy in patients, meaning that patients' confidence in their ability to change is acknowledged as critical to successful change efforts (Lundahl, Kunz, Brownell, et al., 2010). (See Chapter 11 for more information regarding motivational interviewing.)

When a change in health-related behaviours is recommended, patients and their families may progress through a series of steps before they are willing, or able, to accept the need for and make the change. Six stages of change have been identified in the transtheoretical model of health behaviour change developed by Prochaska and Velicer (1997). The **stages of behavioural change** and their implications for patient teaching are described in Table 4-3. It is important to note that an individual's progress through these stages occurs at his or her own pace and that progression through the stages is often nonlinear and cyclic. Therefore, it is reasonable to expect the patient to experience periods of relapse, whereby the process must be restarted—sometimes repeatedly. Accurate assessment of the patient's stage of change helps the nurse guide the patient through one stage and on to the next.

Nurse as Teacher

Required Competencies

Knowledge of Subject Matter. The scope of nursing practice is extensive, and its settings are diverse. Although it is impossible to be expert in all areas, the nurse can develop confidence as a teacher by acquiring knowledge of the matter that is to be taught. For example, if a nurse is teaching a patient about the management of hypertension, the nurse must be able to explain what hypertension is, why it is important to treat the disease, and what the patient needs to know about exercise, diet, and the effects of medication, both expected and untoward. The nurse should be able to teach the patient to use blood pressure equipment to monitor the blood pressure and to identify situations that should be reported to health care providers. In addition, the nurse should provide the patient with sources of additional information such as brochures, appropriate websites, and support organizations (e.g., Canadian Heart and Stroke Foundation).

It is not unusual for the patient to ask questions that the nurse may not be able to answer. If unsure of the response, the nurse should inform the patient of this, seek additional information to answer the question, and then return to the patient to provide the response.

Communication Skills. Patient education is an interactive and dynamic process. Through effective communication skills, a nurse can establish a valuable partnership among the nurse himself or herself, the patient, and the caregiver. In such a partnership, a nurse can provide a highly supportive environment conducive

TABLE 4-3	STAGES OF CHANGE IN THE TRANSTHEORETICAL MODEL	
Stage	**Patient Behaviour**	**Nursing Implications**
1. Precontemplation	Is not considering a change; is not ready to learn	Provide support and increase awareness of condition; describe benefits of change and risks of not changing
2. Contemplation	Thinks about a change; may verbalize recognition of need to change; says, "I know I should" but identifies barriers	Introduce what is involved in changing the behaviour; reinforce the stated need to change
3. Preparation	Starts planning the change, gathers information, sets a date to initiate change, shares decision to change with others	Reinforce the positive outcomes of change, provide information and encouragement, develop a plan, help set priorities, and identify sources of support
4. Action	Begins to change behaviour through practice; is tentative and may experience relapses	Reinforce behaviour with reward, encourage self-reward, discuss choices to help minimize relapses and regain focus, and help patient plan how to deal with potential relapses
5. Maintenance	Practises the behaviour regularly; is able to sustain the change	Continue to reinforce behaviour; provide additional education on the need to maintain change
6. Termination	Change has become part of lifestyle; behaviour is no longer considered a change	Evaluate effectiveness of the new behaviour; no further intervention is needed

Source: Adapted from Prochaska, J., & Velicer, W. (1997). The transtheoretical model of health behaviour change. *American Journal of Health Promotion, 12*(1), 38–48. Retrieved from *http://dx.doi.org/10.4278/0890-1171-12.1.38.*

to the empowerment of the patient and caregivers (Hain & Sandy, 2013).

Empowerment has become increasingly important in the education of patients and caregivers. Empowerment focuses on the individual's capacity to make decisions about his or her health and the level of control he or she has related to health (McAllister, Dunn, Payne, et al., 2012).

Specifically, nurses can help patients identify their own internal strengths and self-care abilities, both of which can be called upon to address health care issues. Nurses can address the need for caregivers to support the rights of patients and ensure that patients have access to the resources necessary to achieve optimal health.

During the teaching process, the nurse should use basic therapeutic communication skills and strategies to support, educate, and empower patients to cope effectively with health-related issues (Arnold & Boggs, 2016). These basic communication skills encompass both verbal and nonverbal

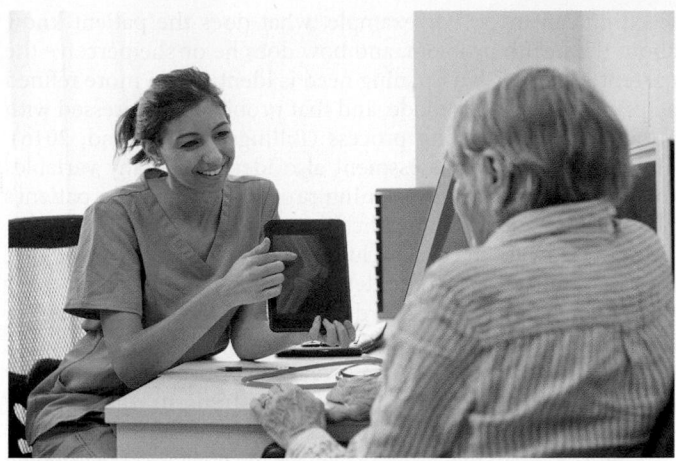

FIGURE 4-1 Open, relaxed positioning of the patient and nurse at the same eye level promotes communication in teaching and learning. Source: Monkey Business Images/Shutterstock.com.

TABLE 4-4	SUGGESTED APPROACHES TO OVERCOMING CHALLENGES TO NURSE–TEACHER EFFECTIVENESS	
Challenge	**Approaches**
Lack of time	Preplan. Set realistic goals. Use time with patient efficiently, and use all possible opportunities for teaching, such as when bathing the patient or changing a dressing. Break teaching and practice sessions into small blocks of time. Advocate for time for patient teaching. Carefully document what was taught and the time spent teaching in order to emphasize that it is a primary role of nursing and that it takes time.
Lack of knowledge	Broaden knowledge base. Read, study, and ask questions. Screen teaching materials, participate in other teaching sessions, observe more experienced nurse–teachers, and attend classes.
Incongruent goals	Establish agreed-upon, written goals. Develop a plan, and discuss it with the patient before teaching begins. Revise expectations based on patient's needs.
Diverse patient needs	Ensure teaching methods address the learner needs (i.e., challenges with communication, education level of patient).
Powerlessness, frustration	Recognize personal reaction to stress. Develop a support system. Rely on friends and family for positive encouragement. Network with other nurses, health care providers, and community leaders to change the situation. Become proactive in legislative processes affecting health care delivery.

components, and they are described in Chapter 3 in the section "Interviewing Considerations." The value of effective communication skills is to promote safe and empathic ways for patients to explore their illness experience. Terms that convey respect for culture, spiritual beliefs, and the educational level of the patient and also that of the caregiver are essential. In communication, the use of medical jargon is unnecessary and can be omitted (Arnold & Boggs, 2016). To provide positive nonverbal messages, the nurse must sit in an open, relaxed position facing the patient, with his or her eyes level with those of the patient (Figure 4-1).

It is important for the nurse to develop the art of active listening. This means paying attention to what is said, as well as observing the patient's nonverbal cues. The nurse concentrates on the patient as a communicator of vital information and does not interrupt the patient. Nodding in response to the patient's statements and rephrasing and verbally reflecting what the patient is saying help clarify communication. Allowing time for listening without appearing hurried requires thoughtful organization and planning on the part of the nurse. Listening attentively and red-flagging issues allow the nurse to obtain important information needed for the assessment phase of the teaching process.

Empathy. Empathy can be defined as the quality to enter into the world of another so as not to judge, sympathize, or correct but to establish mutual understanding. Empathy means putting aside one's own concerns for a moment and adopting the patient's viewpoint. With regard to patient teaching, empathy means assessing the patient's needs before implementing a teaching plan. For example, a nurse working in a rural outpatient clinic is asked to teach a patient with newly diagnosed diabetes the symptoms of hypoglycemia. The nurse enters the room and finds the patient sitting very still, with gaze fixed and mouth slightly ajar. The empathic approach to this situation may include sitting in a chair next to the patient and discussing the feelings that the patient is experiencing before starting the discussion on the complications of diabetes.

Challenges to Nurse–Teacher Effectiveness. The perceived lack of time is a major challenge that detracts from the effectiveness of the teaching effort. When time is limited, the nurse should inform the patient at the beginning of the interaction how much time can be devoted to the session. To make the most

of limited time, the nurse and patient must set priorities for the patient's learning so that important teaching can be accomplished during any contact with the patient or caregiver.

Disagreement between the nurse and patient with regard to the expectations of teaching may also be a challenge. The nurse must accept the fact that some patients or caregivers may not be willing to discuss the health problem or its implications. The patient or caregiver may be in denial or hold ideas and values that conflict with those of conventional health care. Although the nurse may face hostility or resentment, he or she must respect the patient's response to the health problem.

Another important challenge for the nurse who is attempting to provide patient education is the current health care system. Decreased length of hospitalization has resulted in the discharge of patients into the community with only the basic elements of educational plans established. At the same time, health care is offering increasingly complex treatment options. This situation results in greater educational needs of the patient and caregiver. Furthermore, patients and caregivers face greater difficulty using resources as the complexity of the health care system increases. Strategies that can be used to address these challenges are presented in Table 4-4.

Caregiver and Holistic Support

Support provided by the caregiver is important to a patient's sense of physical, psychological, and spiritual well-being. It is important that nurses focus on the caregiver dynamics and interactional patterns (Wright & Leahey, 2013). For example, caregivers who live with chronic disease develop expertise in managing symptoms and adjust their lifestyles and environments. When they meet with nurses, caregivers often bring a wealth of information and personal experience to the encounter. The nurse can initiate conversations about the care and support of the patient and discover that caregivers provide diagnoses, advice, remedies, and support to their family members in both sickness and health. One particularly important nursing strategy is that of commending the caregiver for being supportive to the patient (Wright & Leahey, 2013).

To develop a successful teaching plan, the nurse must view the patient's needs within the context of the caregiver's needs. For example, the nurse may teach a patient with right-sided paresis (weakness) self-feeding techniques with the use of special implements, but at a home visit, the nurse finds the patient being fed by the spouse. On questioning, the spouse reveals that it is too difficult to watch the patient struggle with feeding and that it is easier to feed the patient. This is an example of a situation in which both the patient and the spouse need additional teaching about the goals of self-care. Such situations represent opportunities for home care and community health nurses to partner with acute care nurses by evaluating the teaching that is performed in the hospital and providing ongoing patient teaching in the community.

PROCESS OF PATIENT TEACHING

Patient teaching is a distinct and definable activity that includes strategies that help patients and caregivers make informed decisions about the patient's health (Epstein, 2013). These decisions can facilitate proper care for illnesses and the implementation of health-promotion interventions to aid in recovery. In fact, participation in patient education helps patients and caregivers obtain the information and education they want and need (Canadian Partnership Against Cancer, 2012).

Many different approaches are used in the process of patient education. However, the approach used most frequently by nurses is actually a parallel of the nursing process. Both the **teaching process** and the nursing process involve development of a plan that includes assessment, diagnosis, the setting of patient outcomes or objectives, intervention, and evaluation. The teaching process, like the nursing process, may not always flow in sequential order, but the steps serve as checkpoints that the teaching–learning process has been considered.

The Situated Clinical Decision-Making framework by Gillespie and Paterson (2009) has been adapted specifically for educative nursing practice. This tool encourages the nurse to develop toward becoming an expert educator in working with patients and caregivers in nursing practice (Paterson & Young, 2015). This framework focuses on the important concepts of respect, reflection, and collaboration. Central to the framework are knowing the patient, understanding the individual's past experiences in relation to health and illness, and understanding his or her preferences, supports, and resources when making important clinical decisions (Gillespie & Paterson, 2009). Another central component is caring, which provides the interpersonal context in which educative nursing practice occurs with the patient and caregivers (Paterson & Young, 2015).

Assessment

During the general nursing assessment, the nurse gathers data that determine whether the patient has learning needs that teaching can meet. For example, what does the patient know about the health problem, and how does he or she perceive the current problem? If a learning need is identified, a more refined assessment of need is made, and that problem is addressed with an appropriate teaching process (Billings & Hallstead, 2016). The general nursing assessment also identifies many variables that affect the teaching–learning process, such as the patient's physical and mental state of health and sociocultural characteristics. Caregivers may be included in the assessment, and that information can be used to determine their abilities to care for the patient at home. According to Levine (2011), *caregiver assessment* refers to a systematic process of gathering information that not only describes a caregiver situation but identifies the particular issues, needs, resources, and strengths of the family caregiver.

The assessment that is performed for the purpose of developing a teaching plan includes particularly the physical, psychological, spiritual, and sociocultural characteristics that affect learning, as well as the patient's characteristics that influence the teaching–learning process. Key questions addressing each of these areas are included in Table 4-5.

Physical Characteristics. The age of the patient is an important factor to consider in the teaching plan. The patient's experiences, rate of learning, and ability to retain information are affected by age. Challenges to effective learning such as sensory impairments (e.g., hearing or vision loss) decrease sensory input and can alter learning. For the patient with impaired vision, magnifying glasses and bright lighting may help with reading teaching materials. Hearing loss can be compensated for with hearing aids or teaching techniques that involve more visual stimuli. Central nervous system (CNS) function may be affected by disorders of the nervous system, such as stroke and head trauma, but also by other diseases, such as renal disease, hepatic impairment, and cardiovascular failure. Patients with alterations in CNS function have difficulty learning and may require information to be presented in small amounts and with frequent repetitions. Manual dexterity is needed to perform procedures such as self-administered injections or blood pressure monitoring. Problems performing manual procedures might be resolved with the use of adaptive equipment.

Pain, fatigue, and certain medications influence the patient's ability to learn. Nobody can learn effectively when in severe pain. When the patient is experiencing pain, the nurse should provide only brief explanations and follow up with more detailed instruction when the pain has been managed. A fatigued or weakened patient cannot learn effectively because of the inability to concentrate. Such inability can be caused by sleep disruption, which is common during hospitalization, frequently resulting in patients who are exhausted at the time of discharge. Also, many chemotherapeutic drugs cause nausea, vomiting, and headaches that affect the patient's ability to assimilate new information. The nurse must adjust the teaching plan to accommodate these factors by setting high-priority goals that are based on needs and are realistic. Teaching methods should also be adjusted to accommodate for any limitations that arise in the patient's ability to learn.

Psychological Characteristics. Psychological factors have a major influence on the patient's ability to learn. Anxiety and depression are common reactions to illness. Although mild anxiety increases the learner's perceptual and learning abilities, moderate and severe anxiety limit learning. For example, the patient with newly diagnosed diabetes who is depressed about the diagnosis

TABLE 4-5	ASSESSMENT OF CHARACTERISTICS THAT AFFECT PATIENT TEACHING: CHARACTERISTICS AND KEY QUESTIONS

Physical
- What is the patient's age and sex?
- Is the patient acutely ill?
- Is the patient fatigued? In pain?
- What is the primary diagnosis?
- Are there other medical problems?
- What is the patient's hearing ability? Visual ability? Motor ability?
- What medications does the patient take? Do they affect learning?
- What is the physical environment in which the teaching will take place: the hospital classroom? The patient's room?

Psychological
- What is the patient's current mental status?
- Does the patient appear anxious, afraid, depressed, or defensive?
- Is the patient in a state of denial?
- What is the patient's level of self-efficacy?
- Is the "timing to teach" appropriate?

Sociocultural
- Is the patient employed?
- What is the patient's current or past occupation?
- How does the patient describe his or her financial status?
- What is the patient's living arrangement?
- Does the patient have family or close friends?
- What are the patient's beliefs regarding his or her illness or treatment?
- What is the patient's cultural–ethnic identity?
- Is proposed teaching consistent with the patient's cultural values?
- Has the patient's primary language been assessed for teaching purposes?

Educational
- What is the literacy level of the patient?
- What does the patient already know?
- What does the patient think is most important to learn first?
- What prior learning experiences establish a frame of reference for current learning needs?
- What is the patient's level of motivation?
- What has the patient's health care provider told the patient about the health problem?
- Is the patient ready to change behaviour or learn?
- Can the patient identify behaviours and habits that would make the problem better or worse?
- How does the patient learn best: through reading? Listening? Physical activities?
- In what kind of environment does the patient learn best: in a formal classroom? In an informal setting, such as home or office? Alone or among peers?
- In what way can the family be involved in patient education?

may not listen or respond to instructions about blood glucose testing. Engaging with the patient in a discussion about these concerns or referring the patient to an appropriate support group may enable the patient to learn that management of diabetes is possible.

Patients also respond to the stress of illness with a variety of defence mechanisms, such as denial, rationalization, and even humour. A patient who denies having cancer is not receptive to information related to treatment options. A patient using rationalization may imagine any number of reasons for avoiding change or for rejecting instruction; for example, a patient with

cardiovascular disease who does not want to change dietary habits may relate stories of persons who have eaten bacon and eggs every morning for years and lived to be 100 years of age. Humour is used by some patients to filter reality or decrease anxiety. For example, it is not uncommon for patients to assign a name or a characteristic to an intestinal stoma. The nurse must determine when a patient is using humour excessively to avoid facing reality. A nursing diagnosis for this situation could be *ineffective coping* related to *insufficent sense of control*. Humour can be important and useful in the teaching process as well but should focus only on a situation or an idea, not on personal characteristics. It is also important to note that while some patients respond well to humour, others do not.

One important psychological determinant of successful adoption of new behaviours is the patient's sense of self-efficacy. The term self-efficacy refers to an individual's sense of confidence in his or her ability to perform a set of actions. In fact, the greater a person's confidence, the more likely he or she is to initiate and persist in that particular activity. Self-efficacy is the mediator between knowledge and action (Williams, Kessler, & Williams, 2015). Appropriate teachings by the nurse will provide the patient with the knowledge and skill to cope with upcoming problems, which in turn will decrease the patient's anxiety. Self-efficacy is strongly related to outcomes of illness management.

The nurse should proceed from simple to more complex content to establish a positive experience of success. Both role play, to rehearse new behaviours, and peer learning are teaching strategies that can increase feelings of self-efficacy in patients, caregivers, and family members.

Sociocultural Characteristics. Sociocultural characteristics influence a patient's perception of health, illness, health care, life, and death. Social elements include the patient's lifestyle, status within a family, occupation, income, education, housing arrangement, and living location. Cultural elements include dietary and sleep patterns, exercise, sexuality, language, values, and beliefs. The patient and family may value the presence of an interpreter who can decrease the embarrassment of miscommunication.

Socioeconomic Factors. Knowing the patient's current or past occupation may assist the nurse in determining what vocabulary to use during teaching. For example, an auto mechanic might understand the volume overload associated with heart failure through the metaphor of an engine flooding. An engineer may bring the principles of physics associated with gravity and pressures to bear when discussing vascular problems. This technique of teaching requires creativity but can promote a patient's understanding of pathophysiological processes.

Literacy and Health Literacy. Health literacy is the individual's capacity to read, comprehend, and act on health information. A health-literate patient, therefore, has the capacity to acquire, process, and use health information (Spreos, 2011). Health literacy is critical to Canadians' capacity to manage their health (Mitic & Rootman, 2012). As the health care environment has become more complex, individuals with limited literacy have been shown to experience greater difficulty understanding and acting on health information. In essence, adults with low-level literacy scores do not possess the basic skills required to function within the twenty-first century health care system (Toronto & Weatherford, 2015). Even patients with high general health literacy can exhibit low health literacy in the presence of complicated health information (Rootman & Gordon-El-Bihbety, 2008).

Knowing whether a patient has poor health literacy skills is critical. Such knowledge enables the nurse to match verbal instructions and the readability level of materials to the health literacy skills of the patient (Spreos, 2011). Printed educational materials are used extensively for the purpose of teaching patients and caregivers. Depending on the patient's health literacy, nonprint teaching materials, such as videotapes, audiotapes, demonstrations, models, pictograms, and other visual aids, may provide patients with information concerning diagnosis, prognosis, treatment, and health-promotion strategies in terms that are understandable. The use of health informatics strategies, such as telehealth, can improve access to health teaching for patients and caregivers in rural or underserviced areas. Virtual education forums are being used extensively as they allow individuals across Canada online access to professionally led educational presentations about how to live well with a particular illness, such as osteoporosis (Osteoporosis Canada, 2017).

Nurses must structure their approach to health care education so that expectations are consistent with the needs of patients. The nurse must be a facilitator of learning by assisting patients and caregivers to access, use, and evaluate the wide range of available information. Nurses can empower their patients through the creative and efficient use of information technology. Therefore, they must remain up to date with new technology-based tools and learn how and when to use technology in their practice, while also being cognizant that each patient, family, and community is a unique entity with specific needs that are met within the context of the relationship (Cullen & Wagner, 2015). For instance, nurses can provide email consultation and clinical information available on the Internet. Through technology, patients can become enlightened and empowered to take more active roles in their own health care.

According to the Organisation for Economic Co-operation and Development (OECD; 2008) and Statistics Canada and OECD (2005), five levels of literacy have been identified. People with Level 1 literacy had very poor skills; for example, they were unable to determine the correct dose of medication from information on the package. People with Level 2 literacy required material to be simple and clearly laid out, and only tasks that were not overly complex could be included in the material. People at this level could read but had poor test results. They may have had everyday literacy-related coping skills but were unable to meet new demands, such as learning new job skills. People with Level 3 literacy had the minimum skills necessary for everyday life in a complex society, such as graduation from high school and acceptance to a postsecondary institution. People at this level were able to integrate several sources of information and solve more complex problems. People with Levels 4 and 5 literacy had higher-order skills in information processing. The majority of results are found in Table 4-6.

The two most commonly used health literacy tools in health care settings are the Rapid Estimate of Adult Literacy in Medicine (REALM) and the Test of Functional Health Literacy in Adults (TOFHLA; Altin, Finke, Kautz-Freimuth, et al., 2014). The REALM is a test of an individual's ability to recognize and pronounce words, whereas the TOFHLA is a measure of the ability to read, comprehend text, and perform computations involving health-related tasks. The two tests were modelled after general functional literacy measures and provide estimates of literacy ability when applied to health care contexts. However, recent publications suggest that neither is able to measure the full breadth of health literacy (Pleasant, McKinney, & Rikard, 2011; Kirk, Grzywacz, Arcury, et al., 2012).

TABLE 4-6	SKILL LEVELS AND DISTRIBUTION WITHIN CANADA

- Notable variations in scores exist across provinces and territories, in all three domains (literacy, numeracy, and PS-TRE).
- Literacy and numeracy scores are highest at ages 24 to 34 and are lower among older age groups.
- Individuals aged 16 to 34 are found to be most proficient in PS-TRE. Despite higher levels of proficiency in PR-TRE among youth (16 to 24), 9% display proficiency at the lowest level in PS-TRE.
- Men have higher numeracy skills than women across the entire PIAAC age spectrum while, in general, both genders display similar proficiencies in literacy and PS-TRE.
- Higher education is associated with greater literacy and PS-TRE skills.
- The employed population displays greater information-processing skills than the unemployed and not-in-the-labour-force populations.
- Literacy and numeracy skills of unemployed and not-in-the-labour-force populations are similar. However, not being in the labour force is associated with lower PS-TRE skills compared to the unemployed population.
- Information-processing skills of Indigenous populations, immigrants, and official-language minority populations vary considerably across provinces and territories.

PIAAC, Programme for the International Assessment of Adult Competencies; *PS-TRE,* problem solving in technology-rich environments.
Source: Adapted from Statistics Canada. (2013). *Skills in Canada: First results from the Programme for the International Assessment of Adult Competencies (PIAAC)* (Catalogue no. 89-555-X). Retrieved from *http://www.statcan.gc.ca.*

Newer instruments have been developed for health care providers, including the Newest Vital Sign (NVS) (Stagliano & Wallace, 2013). As a screening tool, NVS identifies patients at risk for low health literacy. The test result provides information about the patient that allows health care providers to adapt their communication practices in an effort to achieve better health outcomes. Another tool is the Brief Health Literacy Screen (BHLS), which is a brief self-report health literacy assessment tool that addresses not only written health literacy but also verbal health literacy and the ability of patients to remember health information and instructions provided by a health care provider (Sand-Jecklin & Coyle, 2014).

Housing Arrangements and Living Location. The patient should be asked about living arrangements that can affect the teaching–learning process. Whether the patient lives alone, with friends, or with caregivers is a determinant of who else is included in the teaching process. If the patient lives in another city or a rural area, at a distance from the site of teaching, the nurse might be expected to make arrangements for continued teaching in the patient's area. Similarly, the nurse may have to modify instructions if the patient does not have access to electricity, a phone, or a computer.

CULTURALLY COMPETENT CARE

Understanding how to provide culturally competent patient care is important for nurses in today's society (Douglas, Pierce, Rosenkoetter, et al., 2011). *Cultural competence* is a dynamic learning process that requires nurses to apply knowledge, skills, attitudes, or personal attributes to maximize respectful relationships with diverse populations of patients, their caregivers, and co-workers (Canadian Nurses Association [CNA], 2010).

A conflict between the patient's cultural beliefs and values and the behaviours promoted by teaching can affect the teaching–learning process. For example, a patient who views being overweight as a sign of financial success may have difficulty accepting the need for diet and exercise unless the importance of blood pressure control is understood.

As part of the assessment process, patients could be asked to describe their beliefs regarding health and illness. The nurse must determine the patient's use of cultural remedies and traditional healers and, for teaching to be effective, incorporate cultural health practices into the teaching plan. In addition, it is important to know who has authority in the patient's culture. Whether this is a community leader, a spiritual leader, or a traditional healer, the patient may defer to the authority's decision making. In this case, the nurse could, if feasible, attempt to work with the decision makers in the patient's cultural group.

Learner Characteristics. Finally, the nurse should assess patient characteristics that are directly related to the development of the teaching plan. These factors include the patient's learning needs, readiness to learn, and learning style.

Learning Needs. Learning needs are the new knowledge and skills that an individual must acquire to be able to meet an objective or a goal. The assessment of learning needs should first be used to determine what the patient already knows, whether the patient has misinformation, and whether the patient has any history of experiences with health problems. The learning needs of patients with chronic illnesses are different from those of patients with newly diagnosed health problems. The nurse then identifies the information, the behaviours, or the skills known to improve patient outcomes that should be included in the teaching plan.

What a patient should learn about managing an illness or what behaviours should be changed to promote health may seem obvious to the nurse. However, there is often a significant difference between what health care providers think is important for patients to learn and what patients want to know.

To individualize learning needs for a particular patient, the nurse may give the patient a list of the recommended topics and ask the patient to number the topics in order of importance. Another method includes writing each topic in question format on a single card and asking the patient to sort the cards in priority. For example, the questions on the cards for a patient with Parkinson's disease might include "When is the most important time to take my medications?" and "What can I do to help with the freezing when I walk?" By allowing a patient to prioritize his or her own learning needs, the nurse can address the patient's most important needs first. When life-threatening complications are a factor, the nurse can encourage the patient to prioritize learning this information by explaining why the item is a "need-to-know" topic.

Readiness to Learn. Before implementing the teaching plan, the nurse should determine which stage of change the patient is in (see Table 4-3). If the patient is only in the precontemplation stage, the nurse may just provide support and increase the patient's awareness of the problem until the patient is ready to consider a change in behaviour. When the patient leaves the hospital, continuity of care is important; that is, hospital and community nurses should be aware of a transition phase for a patient as adjustment to the community continues. They can share information about the patient's learning stage by means of nurse-to-nurse discharge summaries, continue to evaluate the patient's readiness to learn, and implement the teaching plan as the patient progresses through the stages of change.

Learning Style. Each person has a distinct style of learning, as individual as his or her personality. Learning style is the way in which each individual understands and responds to a learning situation (Billings & Hallstead, 2016). The three major learning styles are (a) visual (usually reading), (b) auditory (listening), and (c) physical or kinesthetic (doing things). People often use more than one learning style. To assess a patient's learning style, the nurse might ask how the patient learns best, whether reading or listening is the preferred method to gain information, and how the patient has learned in the past. Adult learners require a variety of approaches to learning, and nurses must be creative in their delivery of health information. However, if a patient identifies a specific learning style, the nurse should use that method whenever possible. In addition to learning styles, it is valuable to know the patient's world views and how the individual perceives his or her health and illness. Further information on world views can be found in the discussions on culture in Chapter 2 and on chronic illness in Chapter 5.

Diagnosis

From the assessment, the nurse obtains information about what the patient knows, believes, and is able to do, and then compares this information with what the patient wants to know, needs to know, and needs to be able to do. Identifying the gap between the known and unknown helps determine the nursing diagnosis. With teaching, a strength can be validated or a deficiency can be corrected. An example of a desirable outcome that could facilitate validation of a patient's strength is *developing a dietary regimen.* A common nursing diagnosis for learning needs is *deficient knowledge.*

Planning

After the assessment and identification of the nursing diagnosis, the next steps in the education process include setting goals, determining learning outcomes, and planning the learning experience. Together, the patient and nurse should prioritize the patient's learning needs and agree upon the goals and learning outcomes. If the physical or psychological condition of the patient begins to interfere with his or her participation, the patient's caregiver can then assist the nurse in the planning phase.

It is important to write attainable goals and clear learning outcomes. Goals are broad, clear, and general statements of what the patient *wants to accomplish.* Learning outcomes are the *achieved* results of what was learned (Billings & Halstead, 2016)—the competencies and the knowledge that the patient has achieved and can demonstrate successfully after the teaching–learning has occurred. For example, the patient who is diabetic will be able to demonstrate how to give an insulin injection to himself or herself safely and with precision.

Table 4-7 shows a sample teaching plan that could be adapted to address any patient's learning needs.

Selecting Teaching Strategies. Selection of a particular strategy is determined by at least three factors: (a) patient characteristics (e.g., age, educational background, degree of illness, culture, learning style); (b) subject matter; and (c) available resources. Some teaching strategies that can be employed to achieve learning objectives follow. Each has advantages and disadvantages that render it more or less suitable to a particular patient and learning situation (Figure 4-2).

Patient Workshop. In the patient workshop, the lecture format is an efficient, versatile, and economical teaching strategy that can be used when time is limited or when a group of patients

TABLE 4-7 SAMPLE TEACHING PLAN

Purpose
To provide patient with information necessary to correctly change a colostomy appliance

Goal
The patient will be able to affix accurately and independently a colostomy appliance to a stoma.

Learning Outcomes	Content Outline	Method of Instruction	Time Allotted	Resources	Method of Evaluation
After a 25-min. teaching session, the patient will be able to do the following:					
1. Demonstrate, in order, the steps required to prepare and affix correctly the colostomy appliance (cognitive)	List of the steps Description of the various items required	1:1 instruction	4 min.	Description of equipment	Post-testing • Verbal • Written • Other
2. In the presence of the nurse, accurately measure and affix the colostomy appliance to the stoma (psychomotor)	Technique as per hospital policy and procedure Procedure for measuring stoma and affixing the appliance	Demonstration and return demonstration	13 min.	All equipment required; e.g., colostomy appliance, measuring grid, adhesive paste (Stomahesive), stoma model	Observation of return demonstration
3. Express to the nurse any feelings of discomfort regarding the ostomy and its care (affective)	Discuss common concerns Explore patient's feelings	Discussion	8 min.	Video of patient vignettes Handouts	Question and answer

Source: Modified from Bastable, S. B. (2008). *Essentials of patient education.* Sudbury, MA: Jones & Bartlett. Reprinted with permission.

FIGURE 4-2 Effective teaching with a variety of materials. Source: Courtesy Linda Bucher, RN, PhD, CEN, CNE, Staff Nurse, Virtua Memorial Hospital, Mount Holly, NJ.

and family members can benefit from acquiring some core information. The nurse presents a series of related ideas or facts to one person or to a group. It is important to remember that the average adult learner can remember five to seven points at a time. Disadvantages of the lecture format are that it often has negative "school learning" connotations and that the extent of individual learning is difficult to evaluate. The lecture–discussion can overcome some of the disadvantages of the lecture alone. With this strategy, the nurse presents specific information by using the lecture technique and follows up with a discussion, during which patients and their caregivers ask questions and exchange points of view with the nurse. This strategy assists the patient

in becoming an active participant in the learning process and creates a more informal give-and-take learning environment. Some patients may be reluctant to actively engage in discussions.

Discussion. The purpose of discussion may be to exchange points of view concerning a topic or to arrive at a decision or conclusion. The nurse can discuss content with an individual or with a group, keeping the specific learning objectives in mind and clarifying information as needed. Participants' questions help the nurse identify and correct inaccurate information. This strategy is a good choice when the patient or patients have previous experience with a subject and have information to share, such as about smoking cessation or convalescence after coronary artery bypass surgery. The discussion allows the patient or caregivers to participate actively and to apply their own experiences and observations to the learning process.

Group Teaching. There are two main types of group teaching. In the first, the nurse acts as a **facilitator**, helping the group to share insights about a common problem. As facilitator, the nurse participates by keeping information moving among all group members. The nurse may introduce the patient to an existing group or may recruit a group of patients with similar problems, such as women who have multiple sclerosis.

A second kind of group teaching involves peer teaching. **Peer teaching** is teaching that is conducted within the setting of groups of peers, such as a self-help or support group. In a peer-teaching setting, the participants learn from one another without the additional input of an instructor. A support group is a self-help organization that can provide continuing information, shared experiences, acceptance, understanding, and useful suggestions about a problem or concern. Patients with health issues such as cancer, alcoholism, Parkinson's disease, compulsive overeating, diabetes, or heart disease frequently find benefit from peer-teaching situations. The nurse should actively look for opportunities to refer a patient or caregiver to a support group. This action should

FIGURE 4-3 Careful teaching using demonstration–return demonstration has been shown to increase the probability of successful learning by the patient. Source: Courtesy Linda Bucher, RN, PhD, CEN, CNE, Staff Nurse, Virtua Memorial Hospital, Mount Holly, NJ.

be taken in addition to, not instead of, the nurse's planned teaching sessions.

Demonstration–Return Demonstration. The demonstration–return demonstration is a strategy commonly used by nurses. The purpose is to show the patient how to perform a motor skill–based task, such as a dressing change, injection, or blood pressure measurement (Figure 4-3). The focus is on the correct procedure and its application. The nurse presents the demonstration in an informal manner, defines and explains unfamiliar terms, and watches the patient for signs of confusion or uncertainty. The nurse clarifies and repeats as necessary. Then the patient returns the demonstration with the nurse as observer. The entire process should require no more than 15 to 20 minutes. Achieving motor skills requires practice, so the patient must practise the procedure between teaching sessions.

Role Play. Role play is another strategy that the nurse might employ, depending on teaching objectives. This format is most often used when patients need to examine their attitudes and behaviours; understand the viewpoints and attitudes of others; or practise carrying out thoughts, ideas, or decisions. The nurse provides information and clear instructions to role players and observers and provides time for feedback and evaluation. Role-playing requires maturity, confidence, and flexibility on the part of the participants. It is important to remember that patients sometimes may feel uncomfortable and inhibited with this method; however, initial discomfort can usually be overcome with patience and support. Role-playing takes time, which must be factored into the teaching plan. An example of the use of role-playing is that of a wife who needs to rehearse how to talk with her husband about his need to quit smoking. In this case, practising the discussion with the nurse ahead of time is often a helpful strategy.

Use of Audiovisual Materials. Audiovisual materials, including DVDs, computer-based programs, charts, podcasts, or simple transparencies, are commonly used to supplement other teaching strategies. This strategy can enhance the presentation of information because it promotes learning through both visual and auditory stimulation. To use this strategy effectively, the nurse must preview and evaluate the teaching materials for accuracy, completeness, and appropriateness to the learning objectives before showing them to the patient and family. CDs are relatively easy to use and are usually inexpensive. The use of audiovisual materials can be extremely beneficial, particularly when teaching content that is largely visual, such as the steps and processes of procedures (dressing changes, injections, hemodialysis). Computer-based programs designed for interactive learning of specific health information are widely available.

Use of the Internet. The Internet is widely used by patients for self-education. Many patients use their own computers or those available at public libraries to access health information on the Internet. The Internet also offers established educational programs designed for specific learners. However, the use of the Internet as a source of information is problematic. It offers a large number of high-quality health resources and poses seemingly unlimited opportunities to inform, teach, and connect health care providers with patients; at the same time, much Internet-borne information is incomplete, misleading, or inaccurate.

The nurse is challenged by several factors when using the Internet as a teaching tool. The nurse must have adequate computer competency to review and evaluate information and programs available on the Internet. Personal computer competency is especially necessary to teach patients and caregivers who are unfamiliar with computers, especially older adults, how to access information. All patients who use the Internet must be taught how to identify reliable and accurate information. The nurse should encourage patients to use sites established by the government, universities, or reputable medical or health-related associations (e.g., the Canadian Medical Association, Canadian Diabetes Association, Canadian Heart and Stroke Foundation, and Public Health Agency of Canada). The list of resources at the end of this chapter includes select reliable patient-education websites for the nurse to review and refer for patient use.

Use of Printed Materials. Printed materials are most often used in combination with other teaching strategies presented in this section. For instance, after a lecture on the physiological effects of smoking, the nurse might distribute a pamphlet from the Canadian Cancer Society that reviews and reinforces the topic. For another patient, the nurse might select a book or magazine article written by a woman who has had a mastectomy and suggest that the patient read this material to prepare for future teaching sessions. Written materials are always recommended for patients whose preferred learning style is reading.

Written resources must be appropriate for the reading level of the patient. Before written materials are used with patients, the nurse should evaluate the readability level if it is not indicated on the materials. If patients are to understand and benefit from all offered education materials, then information must be selected, revised, or redesigned so that even those patients at the lowest literacy level can comprehend it.

Major resources for acquiring relevant printed materials include the hospital or care facility library, the pharmacy, the public library, government agencies, universities, volunteer organizations, websites, and research centres. Written materials, including computer-based programs, should be reviewed by the nurse before being used. In addition to reading level, the following criteria for review are suggested: (a) accuracy, (b) completeness, (c) suitability to meet specific learning goals, (d) inclusion of pictures and diagrams to stimulate interest, (e) focus on one main idea or concept per pamphlet or program, (f) inclusion of information the patient would like to know, and (g) gender and culture sensitivity of the material (Bastable, 2008).

Games and Simulation. A game provides a framework for inserting content to create learning activities. Frameworks are easily adaptable to a wide variety of content and learning outcomes for patients. Typically, a game requires rules for player moves and termination criteria so that winners can be determined. Simulation games have been shown to enhance educational experience so that games provide more than a mere review of content. Debriefing, an important aspect of the learning process, occurs after the game in the form of a discussion focused on concepts, generalizations, and the applications of topics covered in the game. This end process assists learners to recognize that learning has occurred within the fun experience of the game (Jaffe, 2013).

Implementation

During the implementation phase, the nurse uses the planned strategies to present information and demonstrations. Verbal and nonverbal communication skills, active listening, and empathy are incorporated into the process.

In implementing the teaching plan, the nurse should remember the principles of adult learning and the determinants of learning. Reinforcement and reward are important. Techniques to enhance the teaching process with adults are presented in Table 4-8.

Evaluation

Evaluation is the final step in the learning process. It is a measure of the degree to which the patient has mastered the learning objectives. The nurse monitors the performance level of the patient so that changes can be made as needed. The nurse might find that the patient has already achieved the goals. However, if certain goals are not reached, the nurse should reassess the patient and alter the teaching plan. If the patient has developed new needs, the nurse then plans new goals, content, and strategies accordingly.

For example, an older man with diabetes mellitus enters the hospital with a blood glucose level of 30.5 mmol/L. When the nurse observes the patient preparing his insulin injection, she notices that he incorrectly fills the syringe with 20 units of insulin and 20 units of air, instead of 40 units of insulin. After correcting the dosage and questioning the patient, the nurse concludes that

the patient could not accurately see the markings on the syringe and may have been administering insufficient insulin to himself for a long time. The patient may require special equipment and new teaching on how to use it so he can administer the insulin safely and accurately.

Evaluation techniques may be short-term or long-term. Short-term evaluation techniques are used to evaluate quickly the patient's mastery of a concept, skill, or behaviour change; short-term evaluation can be accomplished in the following ways:

1. *Observe the patient directly.* "Let me see how you administer your injection." Through observation, the nurse determines whether the patient has mastered the task, whether further instruction is needed, or whether the patient is ready for new or additional content.

2. *Observe verbal and nonverbal cues.* If the patient asks the nurse to repeat instructions, asks questions, shakes his or her head, loses eye contact, or otherwise expresses doubt about understanding, the patient may be indicating that further instruction is needed or that an alternative approach should be taken.

3. *Ask direct questions.* "What are the major food groups?" "How often must you change your dressing?" "What should you do if you develop chest pain after returning home?" Open-ended questions almost always provide more information about the patient's understanding than do questions that call for only a "yes" or "no" answer.

4. *Use a written measurement tool, graded for accuracy.* Paper-and-pencil tests can actually increase anxiety in patients. Many adults "freeze" or "go blank" when given a test or asked to write something that will be graded. Assess the patient's comfort and learning style before using a written method of evaluation.

5. *Talk with a member of the patient's family or support system.* "Is he eating regularly?" "How is he handling the walker?" "When is she taking her medications?" Because the nurse cannot observe the patient 24 hours a day, the nurse should receive information from other people who have contact with the patient.

6. *Seek the patient's self-evaluation of progress.* By seeking out a patient's opinion, the nurse is allowing the patient to provide input into the evaluation process. Long-term evaluation necessitates follow-up by the nurse, outpatient clinic, or outside health care organization. The nurse should set up a schedule of visits for the patient before the patient leaves the hospital or clinic or refer the patient to the proper agencies. The nurse keeps written documentation of follow-up telephone calls or emails to urge the patient to maintain the follow-up schedule. The patient's caregivers should be familiar with the follow-up plan so that everyone is involved in the patient's long-term progress.

Continuity of Educational Care

The nurse is responsible for communicating with the health care providers involved in the patient's long-term follow-up. To ensure continuity, the nurse should telephone, visit, or email these providers and supply them with the patient's education plan. This information needs to be charted and routinely updated in the patient's medical record.

Documentation of the Educational Process

Documentation is an essential component of the entire teaching–learning transaction. The nurse records everything,

---

TABLE 4-8	**TECHNIQUES TO ENHANCE PATIENT LEARNING**

- Keep the physical environment relaxed and nonthreatening.
- Maintain a respectful, warm, and enthusiastic attitude.
- Let the patient's expressed needs direct what information is provided.
- Focus on "must-know" information; "nice-to-know" information can be added if time allows.
- Involve the patient and family in the process; emphasize active participation.
- Be aware of and take into consideration the patient's previous experiences.
- Emphasize the relevancy of the information to the patient's lifestyle, and suggest how it may provide an immediate solution to a problem.
- Individualize the teaching plan, even if standardized plans are used.
- Emphasize helping the patient to learn, rather than simply transmitting subject matter.
- Review written materials with the patient.
- Ask frequently for feedback.
- Affirm progress with rewards valued by the patient to reinforce desired behaviours.

from the assessment through short- and long-term plans for evaluation. As mentioned, copies of the documentation should be forwarded to the organization or health care provider providing long-term follow-up. The teaching objectives, the content, the strategies, and the evaluation results should be written clearly and completely because many members of the health care team will use these records in different places and for various reasons.

The Standardized Teaching Plan

Standardized teaching plans are often included in care maps and clinical pathways, and they have become an accepted method of developing a teaching plan. Standardized teaching plans contain the widely accepted knowledge and skills that a patient and caregivers need with regard to a specific health problem or procedure. However, the nurse should always individualize these plans to meet the patient's specific needs.

CASE STUDY

Example of the Teaching Process

Source: Nadino/ Shutterstock .com.

Mrs. Emily Crowe is admitted to the hospital for preliminary testing and preparation for a hysterectomy. The nurse is aware that a patient undergoing a hysterectomy is often deeply concerned about her self-concept as a woman. The nurse also knows that such patients need to express their feelings in an atmosphere of support and understanding. Therefore, the nurse has sought to listen attentively and ask questions carefully in order to assess the patient's feelings about and knowledge of the surgical procedure she is about to undergo. The nurse has asked open-ended questions, such as, "How do you feel about having the surgery?" and "What concerns do you have about undergoing a hysterectomy?" By establishing both a climate of trust and a counselling relationship, the nurse has completed the assessment that follows.

Biophysical Dimension

Age 44, female, high school English teacher and coach of girls' high school basketball team; good general health. Height and weight proportional and average for age. Patient reports that she jogs five evenings a week. No sensory impairment; vision, hearing, and reaction time seem normal.

Psychological Dimension

Patient appears mildly anxious about surgery and seems worried about her husband's acceptance of her sexuality. She is also worried about missing work and leaving her classes to a substitute teacher. She states that she does not "let physical problems get me down" and that she dislikes "pills and hospitals." She states that she is used to "teaching" and not "being taught," and she tries to dominate any conversation or input from the nurse.

Sociocultural Dimension

Married with one child (son), age 23. Mother had a mastectomy at age 51; father healthy. Two younger sisters; both experienced difficult pregnancies but are otherwise healthy. Patient describes caregiver communication as very good. She describes her lifestyle as work oriented and says that her friends are primarily teaching colleagues. She places a high priority on work and family.

Learning Style

Responds well to formal lectures. Enjoys reading and group discussions.

Determining Learning Outcomes

After a brief period of rest and adjustment to the unfamiliar hospital environment, Mrs. Crowe states that she would like to learn more about the details of the upcoming planned surgical procedure. Together, Mrs. Crowe and the nurse identify the following objectives:

After the teaching session, I (Mrs. Crowe) will be able to do the following:

1. Describe the surgical procedure (hysterectomy) to the nurse.
2. Express to the nurse and my husband my feelings about maintaining an active and fulfilling sex life.
3. Complete arrangements with my family and school principal for convalescence and return to normal activities.
4. List the general recovery experiences that are expected, and prioritize circumstances under which to seek medical advice.
5. Discuss "old wives' tales" regarding hysterectomy and verbalize concerns regarding undergoing the hysterectomy.
6. Identify ways to avoid constipation, weight gain, and potential periods of depression during the recovery period.
7. Propose ways to return comfortably to baseline sexual activities.

Discussion Questions

1. What factors might impede Mrs. Crowe from learning?
2. What teaching strategies might be the most effective for Mrs. Crowe?
3. What observations will inform the nurse that the teaching session was effective for Mrs. Crowe? (Consider verbal and nonverbal behaviours.)
4. How can the learning be reinforced?

ℯvolve

Answers available at http://evolve.elsevier.com/Canada/Lewis/medsurg.

REVIEW QUESTIONS

The number of the question corresponds to the same-numbered objective at the beginning of the chapter.

1. A nurse in a clinic is teaching the client, a middle-aged Italian woman, about methods to relieve her symptoms of menopause. Which of the following is the best goal of this teaching episode?
   a. To prevent early onset of disease
   b. To maintain health promotion
   c. To alter the client's cultural belief regarding the use of herbs
   d. To provide information for selection and use of treatment options
2. What should the nurse do when planning experiences with consideration of adult learning principles?

   a. Present material in an efficient lecture format
   b. Recognize that adults enjoy learning regardless of the relevance to their personal lives
   c. Provide opportunities for the client to learn from other adults with similar experiences
   d. Postpone practice of new skills until the client can independently practise the skill at home
3. Which of the following skills is necessary for the nurse in the role of teacher?
   a. Determining when clients are too distressed physically or psychologically to learn

b. Assuring the client that the nurse understands what is necessary for the client to learn

c. Developing standardized teaching plans for use with all clients

d. Presenting information in medical language to increase the client's vocabulary and understanding of pathophysiology

4. When the nurse is feeling stressed about the limited time available for client teaching, which of the following strategies would be most beneficial? *(Select all that apply)*

a. Setting realistic goals that have high priority for the client

b. Referring the client to a nurse–educator in private practice for teaching

c. Observing more experienced nurse–teachers to learn how to teach faster and more efficiently

d. Providing reading materials for the client instead of discussing information the client needs to learn

e. Rescheduling the client for a later date

5. Which of the following is the best reason the nurse would choose to include family members in client teaching?

a. They provide most of the care for clients.

b. Clients have been shown to have better outcomes when caregivers are involved.

c. The client may be too ill or too stressed by the situation to understand teaching.

d. Family members might feel rejected and unimportant if they are not included in the teaching.

6. Which step of the teaching process is involved when the nurse, the client, and the client's family decide together what strategies would be best to meet the learning objectives?

a. Planning

b. Evaluation

c. Assessment

d. Implementation

7. A nurse is spending time with a client who is undergoing a diagnostic procedure. Which of the following comments by the client best indicates a teachable moment?

a. "I have to email a friend in a few moments."

b. "How long will this procedure take?"

c. "I have had this procedure before."

d. "I'm trying not to think about it."

8. Which of the following is an example of a correctly worded learning outcome?

a. The client will lose 11.5 kg in 6 weeks.

b. The client should understand the implications of the condition.

c. The client will read two pamphlets on the subject of breast self-examination.

d. The client's spouse demonstrates to the nurse how to correctly change a colostomy bag before discharge.

9. What are the benefits of role play as a teaching strategy? *(Select all that apply)*

a. Encourages self-reflection

b. Increased self-efficacy of the client

c. Rehearses new behaviours

d. Increases self-efficacy of caregivers

10. Which of these approaches would best provide short-term evaluation of teaching effectiveness?

a. Observing the client and asking direct questions

b. Monitoring the client for 3 to 6 months after the teaching

c. Monitoring for the behaviour change for up to 6 weeks after discharge

d. Asking the client what he or she found helpful about the teaching experience

1. d; 2. c; 3. a; 4. a, e; 5. b; 6. a; 7. b; 8. d; 9. a, b, c, d; 10. a.

⊜volve

For even more review questions, visit *http://evolve.elsevier.com/Canada/Lewis/medsurg.*

REFERENCES

Altin, S., Finke, I., Kautz-Freimuth, S., et al. (2014). The evolution of health literacy assessment tools: A systematic review. *BMC Public Health, 14,* 1–13. doi:10.1186/1471-2458-14-1207.

Arnold, E., & Boggs, K. (2016). *Interpersonal relationships: Professional communication skills for nurses* (7th ed.). St. Louis: Elsevier.

Bastable, S. B. (2008). *Essentials of patient education.* Sudbury, MA: Jones & Bartlett. (Seminal).

Bastable, S. B., Gramet, P., Jacobs, K., et al. (2011). *Health professional as educator.* Sudbury, MA: Jones & Bartlett.

Billings, D., & Hallstead, J. (2016). *Teaching in nursing: A guide for faculty* (5th ed.). St. Louis: Saunders.

Canadian Nurses Association. (2010). *Promoting cultural competence in nursing.* Retrieved from *https://www.cna-aiic.ca/~/media/cna/page-content/pdf-en/ps114_cultural_competence_2010_e.pdf?la=en.* (Seminal).

Canadian Partnership Against Cancer. (2012). *Knowledge management initiative—Helping to move information and evidence into action.* Retrieved from *http://www.partnershipagainstcancer.ca/impact/2012-13/knowledge-management-stories.* (Seminal).

Cullen, M., & Wagner, S. (2015). The nursing process in the 21st century. In D. Gregory, C. Raymond-Seniuk, L. Patrick, et al. (Eds.), *Fundamentals: Perspectives on the art and science of Canadian nursing* (pp. 187–188). Philadelphia: Wolters Kluwer Health.

Douglas, M., Pierce, J., Rosenkoetter, M., et al. (2011). Standards of practice for culturally competent nursing: 2011 Update. *Journal of Transcultural Nursing, 22*(4), 317–333. doi:10.1177/1043659611412965.

Epstein, R. M. (2013). Whole mind and shared mind in clinical decision-making. *Patient Education and Counseling, 90*(2), 200–206.

Fineberg, I., Kawashima, M., & Asch, S. (2011). Communication with families facing life-threatening illness: A research-based model for family conferences. *Journal of Palliative Medicine, 14*(4), 421–427. doi:10.1089/jpm.2010.0436.

Gillespie, M., & Paterson, B. (2009). Helping novice nurses make effective clinical decisions: The situated clinical decision-making framework. *Nursing Education Perspectives, 30*(3), 164–170. (Seminal).

Hain, D. J., & Sandy, D. (2013). Partners in care: Patient empowerment through shared decision-making. *Nephrology Nursing Journal, 40*(2), 153–158.

Jaffe, L. (2013). Games are multidimensional in educational situations. In M. J. Bradshaw & J. Lowenstein (Eds.), *Teaching strategies for health education and health promotion* (6th ed.), (pp. 171–179). Burlington, MA: Jones and Bartlett.

Kirk, J. K., Grzywacz, J. G., Arcury, T. A., et al. (2012). Performance of health literacy tests among older adults with diabetes. *Journal of General Internal Medicine, 27*(5), 534–540.

Knowles, M. (1990). *The adult learner: A neglected species* (4th ed.). Houston: Gulf Publishing. (Seminal).

Kozier, B., Erb, G., Berman, A., et al. (2014). *Fundamentals of Canadian nursing: Concepts, process, and practice* (3rd Canadian ed.). Toronto: Pearson Canada.

Levine, C. (2011). Supporting family caregivers: The hospital nurse's assessment of family caregiver needs. *The American Journal of Nursing, 111*(10), 47–51. doi:10.1097/01.naj.0000406420.35084.a1.

Lundahl, B., Kunz, C., Brownell, C., et al. (2010). A meta-analysis of motivational interviewing: Twenty-five years of empirical studies. *Research on Social Work Practice, 20*(2), 137–160. doi:10.1177/1049731509347850. (Seminal).

McAllister, M., Dunn, G., Payne, K., et al. (2012). Patient empowerment: The need to consider it as a measurable patient-reported outcome for chronic conditions. *BMC Health Services Research, 12*(57), 1–8. doi:10.1186/1472-6963-12-157.

Mitic, W., & Rootman, I. (2012). *An interdisciplinary approach for health literacy for Canadians.* Retrieved from *http://www.cpha.ca/uploads/portals/h-l/intersectorial_e.pdf.*

Organisation for Economic Co-operation and Development. (2008). *Adult literacy.* Retrieved from *http://www.oecd.org/document/2/0,3343,en_2649_39263294_2670850_1_1_1_1,00.html.* (Seminal).

Osteoporosis Canada. (2017). *Virtual forum.* Retrieved from *http://www.osteoporosis.ca/osteoporosis-and-you/copn/virtual-forum/.*

Paterson, B., & Young, L. (2015). D. Gregory, C. Raymond-Seniuk, L. Patrick, et al. (Eds.), *Fundamentals: Perspectives on the art and science of Canadian nursing* (p. 260). Philadelphia: Wolters Kluwer Health.

Pleasant, A., McKinney, J., & Rikard, R. (2011). Health literacy measurement: A proposed research agenda. *Journal of Health Communication, 16*(Suppl. 3), 11–21. doi:10.1080/10810730.2011.604392.

Prochaska, J. O., & Velicer, W. F. (1997). The transtheoretical model of health behaviour change. *American Journal of Health Promotion, 12*(1), 38. doi:10.4278/0890-1171-12.1.38. (Seminal).

Rootman, I., & Gordon-El-Bihbety, D. (2008). *A vision for a health literate Canada: Report of the expert panel on health literacy.* Retrieved from *http://www.cpha.ca/uploads/portals/h-l/report_e.pdf.* (Seminal).

Sand-Jecklin, K., & Coyle, S. (2014). Efficiently assessing patient health literacy: The BHLS instrument. *Clinical Nursing Research, 23*(6), 581–600. doi:10.1177/1054773813488417.

Spreos, C. (2011). Promoting health literacy: A nursing imperative. *The Nursing Clinics of North America, 46,* 321–333. doi:10.1016/j.cnur.2011.05.007.

Stagliano, V., & Wallace, L. (2013). Brief health literacy items predict newest vital sign scores. *Journal of the American Board of Family Medicine, 26,* 558–565. doi:10.3122/jabfm.2013.05.130096.

Statistics Canada & Organisation for Economic Co-operation and Development. (2005). *Learning a living: First results of the Adult Literacy and Life Skills survey.* Retrieved from *http://www.oecd.org/education/innovation-education/34867438.pdf.*

Toronto, C., & Weatherford, B. (2015). Health literacy education in health professions schools: An integrative review. *The Journal of Nursing Education, 54*(12), 669–676. doi:10.3928/01484834-20151110-02.

Williams, B. W., Kessler, H. A., & Williams, M. V. (2015). Relationship among knowledge acquisition, motivation to change, and self-efficacy in CME participants. *The Journal of Continuing Education in the Health Professions, 35*(S1), S13–S21. doi:10.1002/chp.21291.

Wright, L., & Leahey, M. (2013). *Nurses and families* (6th ed.). Philadelphia: Davis.

RESOURCES

Canada Public Health Agency, National Literacy and Health Program
http://www.cpha.ca/en/programs/portals/h-l/resources.aspx

Canadian Association for the Study of Adult Education (CASAE)
http://www.casae-aceea.ca/

Health Canada
http://www.hc-sc.gc.ca/index-eng.php

Learning Disabilities Association of Canada
http://www.ldac-acta.ca/

Learning Disabilities Resource Community
http://www.ldac-acta.ca/

Healthfinder.gov, Office of Disease Prevention and Health Promotion, U.S. Department of Health and Human Resources
http://www.healthfinder.gov

LD Online (Learning Disabilities and Attention-Deficit/Hyperactivity Disorder [ADHD])
http://www.ldonline.org/indepth/adhd

MedicineNet.com
http://www.medicinenet.com

MedlinePlus Health Information
http://www.nlm.nih.gov/medlineplus

For additional Internet resources, see the website for this book at *http://evolve.elsevier.com/Canada/Lewis/medsurg.*

Chronic Illness

Written by: Jane Tyerman

evolve WEBSITE

http://evolve.elsevier.com/Canada/Lewis/medsurg

- Review Questions (Online Only)
- Key Points
- Conceptual Care Map Creator

- Audio Glossary
- Content Updates

LEARNING OBJECTIVES

1. Describe the impact of chronic illness in Canada.
2. Define and describe acute and chronic illness and the relationships between these concepts.
3. Identify key factors contributing to the development of chronic illness.
4. Differentiate between chronic illness and disability.
5. Discuss the psychosocial implications of living with a chronic illness.

6. Describe the ways in which chronic illness may affect family members or significant others.
7. Discuss key conceptual models of chronic illness.
8. Describe the role of self-management in chronic illness.
9. Identify emerging models of providing care to individuals with chronic illness.v

KEY TERMS

acute illness, p. 64
best buys, p. 65
caregiver burden, p. 70
chronic illness, p. 62
comorbidity, p. 64
disability, p. 66
disease, p. 64
fatigue, p. 69

health, p. 64
health-related hardiness (HRH), p. 68
health-related quality of life (HRQL), p. 69
illness, p. 64
illness behaviour, p. 66
illness trajectory, p. 70

informal caregiver, p. 70
lifestyle, p. 64
modifiable risk factors, p. 65
morbidity, p. 63
mortality, p. 63
multimorbidity, p. 64
nonmodifiable risk factors, p. 65

quality of life, p. 69
self-management, p. 71
shared decision making, p. 67
signs, p. 64
stigmatization, p. 69
symptoms, p. 64

Chronic disease is a leading cause of preventable death and disability as it accounts for approximately two-thirds of deaths globally (World Health Organization [WHO], 2014b). **Chronic illness** refers to health problems that persist over extended periods and that are often (but not always) associated with participation and activity limitations (disability). Chronic illnesses demand a complex response from patients and families over an extended time period. This response also involves coordinated inputs from a wide range of health care providers, as well as access to essential treatments (Clark, Gong, & Kaciroti, 2014). Care for people with chronic illness is ideally embedded within a health care system that promotes patient empowerment.

Unfortunately, the Canadian health care system is still largely built around an acute, episodic model of care that is unable to address the needs of those with chronic health problems. The current mismatch between the episodic care orientation of the existing health care system and the needs of people living in the community with chronic illnesses has led to a

host of well-documented failures in care provision. These failures include high rates of hospital readmissions; medical errors; underdiagnosis of conditions; inconsistent monitoring of chronic conditions; lack of patient-centredness; insufficient health education; duplication of resources; inappropriate omission of resources; and preventable injuries (Bodenheimer & Berry-Millett, 2009). Innovative models of providing care for people with chronic illness, such as virtual wards, are currently being evaluated in Canada and hold promise for improving care in the future (Canadian Agency for Drugs and Technology, 2011).

Because we need to organize the vast amount of knowledge about the medical-surgical nursing care of people within a cohesive framework, most textbooks are organized along the lines of body systems and common medical diagnoses. It is critical to recognize, however, that medical diagnosis alone does not predict service needs, length of hospitalization, level of care, or functional outcomes and tells us nothing about the person experiencing the condition or how this person will

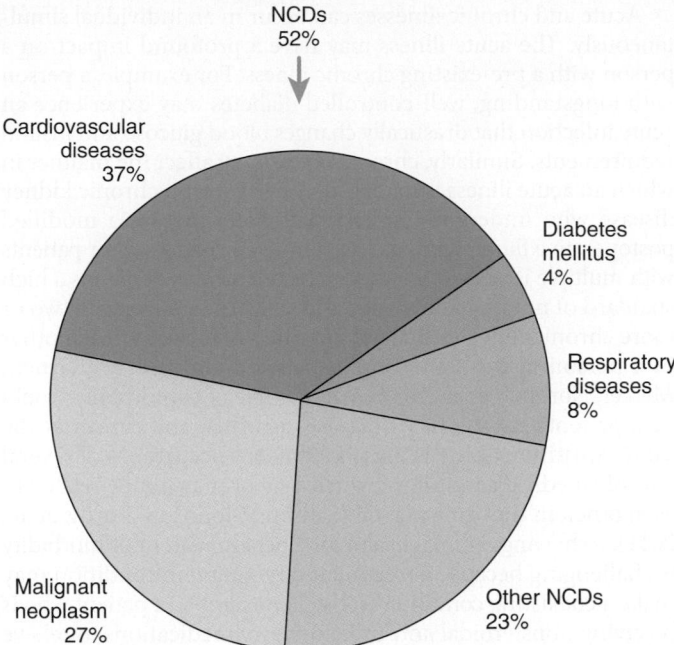

NCDs
52%

Cardiovascular
diseases
37%

Diabetes
mellitus
4%

Respiratory
diseases
8%

Other NCDs
23%

Malignant
neoplasm
27%

FIGURE 5-1 Main causes of global deaths younger than age 70 years for 2012. Source: Reprinted from *Global Status Report on Noncommunicable Diseases 2014,* WHO, Page No. 10, Copyright 2014.

TABLE 5-1 CHRONIC ILLNESS IN CANADA

Cancer
- About 2 in 5 Canadians will develop cancer in their lifetime; mortality rate is 1 in 4.
- 196 900 people are diagnosed with cancer each year.
- 78 000 Canadians die each year due to cancer.

Diabetes
- About 1 in 16 Canadians (6.2%) is living with diabetes, and it is estimated that an additional 0.9% of the population (nearly 300 000) remain undiagnosed.
- The prevalence of diabetes increased by 21% from 2002 to 2007.
- Among adults 20 years and older, mortality rates for those with diabetes (deaths usually due to a complication of diabetes, like cardiovascular disease) were twice as high as for those without diabetes.

Cardiovascular Diseases
- 1.6 million Canadians have heart disease or are living with the effects of a stroke.
- In 2007, cardiovascular diseases were responsible for about 70 000 deaths.
- Death rates have decreased since the late 1960s, probably due to lower smoking rates and improved treatment.

Chronic Respiratory Diseases
- Over 3 million Canadians live with a chronic respiratory disease.
- Tobacco remains the most important preventable risk factor for chronic respiratory diseases.

Source: Canadian Cancer Society's Advisory Committee on Cancer Statistics. (2015). *Canadian cancer statistics 2015.* Toronto: Canadian Cancer Society. Retrieved from *http://www.cancer.ca/~/media/cancer.ca/CW/cancer%20information/cancer%20101/ Canadian%20cancer%20statistics/Canadian-Cancer-Statistics-2015-EN.pdf?la=en*; and Public Health Agency of Canada. (2011). *Chronic diseases in Canada.* Reproduced with permission from the Minister of Health, 2012. Retrieved from *http://www. phac-aspc.gc.ca/media/nr-rp/2011/2011_0919-bg-di-eng.php.*

respond to nursing care. In providing truly holistic and comprehensive care, nurses assume a perspective that includes behavioural, psychosocial, and environmental factors. Understanding the illness experience allows for the implementation of effective interventions specific to the needs of the individual, family, or group (Henly, Wyman, & Findorff, 2011). This chapter seeks to situate the information contained in the remainder of this textbook within such a framework.

THE EPIDEMIOLOGY OF CHRONIC DISEASES

Noncommunicable diseases (NCDs) accounted for well over half (68%) of the world's 56 million deaths in 2012, with more than 40% resulting in the premature death of adults under the age of 70 years (WHO, 2014). Chronic heart disease, lung diseases, cancer, and diabetes ranked highest among NCDs, with cardiovascular diseases (37%) being responsible for the highest proportion of global deaths in 2012, followed by cancers (27%), chronic respiratory diseases (8%), and diabetes (4%) (WHO, 2014) (Figure 5-1).

In Canada, chronic illnesses also make a substantial contribution to morbidity and mortality. Approximately 50% of Canadians over age 20 are living with at least one chronic condition, and 14.8% of Canadians report having two or more chronic conditions (Public Health Agency of Canada [PHAC], 2015). One in four Canadian adults is obese, and approximately 1 in 10 children in Canada is obese, a condition that could lead to the development of chronic disease in adulthood (PHAC, 2015). Canada's aging population, along with the rising rates of some risk factors for chronic diseases, is driving the chronic disease challenge. About two-thirds of deaths in Canada each year result from chronic diseases. Table 5-1 illustrates how chronic illnesses affect Canadians.

Of concern is the fact that chronic diseases and related risk factors are significantly higher among Canada's Indigenous peoples when compared to the national average. For example, the prevalence of diabetes among First Nations adults living on reserves is 19.7%, compared to 5.2% among the general Canadian population, and human immunodeficiency virus (HIV) infection is 2.8 times higher in Indigenous persons (Health Canada, 2010). The most common chronic conditions in First Nations adults are asthma, diabetes, heart disease, and high blood pressure (Health Canada, 2010).

Morbidity refers to the rates of disease in a population, whereas **mortality** refers to the rates of deaths. Musculo-skeletal conditions such as arthritis and osteoporosis are the most prevalent and costly chronic conditions in Canada. In 2008, heart disease and stroke were the underlying causes of death for as many as one in three Canadians (Statistics Canada, 2011), with stroke being the leading cause of death (PHAC, 2011). In 2015, an estimated 200 000 new cases of cancer and 78 000 deaths occurred in Canada, with cancer surpassing cardiovascular disease (heart and cerebro-vascular) as the leading cause of death in Canada (Canadian Cancer Society's Advisory Committee on Cancer Statistics, 2015). Lung, prostate, breast, and colorectal cancer, the four most common cancer types in Canada, account for over 50% of all new cancer cases (Canadian Cancer Society's Advisory Committee on Cancer Statistics, 2015). Lung cancer has the highest mortality rate, causing more cancer deaths than the other three cancer types combined.

TABLE 5-2	CHARACTERISTICS OF ACUTE AND CHRONIC ILLNESSES
Description	**Characteristics**
Acute Illness	
Disease that has a rapid onset and short duration *Examples:* colds, influenza, acute gastro-enteritis	• Usually self-limiting • Responds readily to treatment • Complications infrequent • After illness, return to previous level of functioning
Chronic Illness	
Disease that is prolonged, does not resolve spontaneously, and is rarely cured completely	• Permanent impairments or deviations from normal • Irreversible pathological changes • Residual disability • Special rehabilitation required • Need for long-term medical or nursing management or both

HEALTH, ACUTE ILLNESS, AND CHRONIC ILLNESS

Health and illness may be viewed along a continuum upon which individuals journey throughout life. Health, according to the WHO (2014a), is "a state of complete physical, mental, and social well-being and not merely the absence of disease or infirmity." The state of health is dependent upon complex interactions between multiple social and economic factors, the physical environment, and individual behaviour. These factors are referred to as *determinants of health*.

Disease is a condition that a practitioner views from a pathophysiological model (Lubkin & Larsen, 2013). Illness, conversely, is the human experience of symptoms and suffering. This term refers to how the disease is perceived, lived with, and responded to by individuals and their families (Lubkin & Larsen, 2013). Nursing practice must be informed by both knowledge of disease and understanding of the illness experience.

Table 5-2 compares the characteristics of acute and chronic illness. Acute illness is typically characterized by a sudden onset, with signs and symptoms related to the disease process itself. Signs are typically objective manifestations of a condition, whereas symptoms refer to the subjective reports of the patient. Acute illness ends in a relatively short time, sometimes in recovery and sometimes in death (Lubkin & Larsen, 2013). Chronic illness often continues indefinitely. Strauss, Corbin, Fagerhaugh, and colleagues (1984) viewed chronic illness as an experience of problems that may change but do not go away. The onset of a chronic illness may be sudden, or it may develop insidiously over a long period. Some chronic illnesses are characterized by exacerbations and remissions, whereas other chronic illnesses cause persistent symptoms throughout their course.

Chronic (or noncommunicable) illnesses are typically characterized as having an uncertain etiology, multiple risk factors, long latency, prolonged duration, and a noninfectious origin and can be associated with impairments or functional disability. Cardiovascular disease, diabetes, arthritis and other musculo-skeletal diseases, cancers, chronic lung diseases, and chronic neurological disorders (including depression) are conditions recognized by the Centers for Disease Control and Prevention (2011a) as chronic illnesses.

Acute and chronic illnesses can occur in an individual simultaneously. The acute illness may have a profound impact on a person with a pre-existing chronic illness. For example, a person with longstanding, well-controlled diabetes may experience an acute infection that drastically changes blood glucose and insulin requirements. Similarly, chronic illness may affect the manner in which an acute illness is managed. A person with chronic kidney disease who undergoes surgery will likely require a modified postoperative fluid regimen. The complexity of caring for patients with multiple illnesses, whether acute or chronic, demands a high standard of nursing knowledge and skill. The presence of two or more chronic illnesses that are not directly related to each other in a person at the same time is called comorbidity (Barnett, Mercer, Norbury, et al., 2012). An example of comorbidity would be a patient's having heart disease, arthritis, and cancer at the same. Multimorbidity is the simultaneous occurrence of several chronic medical conditions, which may or may not be related to each other, in the same person (Salisbury, Johnson, Purdy, et al., 2011). Achieving optimal health for a person with multimorbidity is challenging because a treatment targeting one condition may make a coexisting condition worse. For example, a patient who is receiving nonsteroidal anti-inflammatory medications to relieve pain from arthritis finds that the medication worsens hypertension and renal disease.

Having multiple chronic medical conditions is associated with many negative outcomes: patients have decreased quality of life, more psychological distress, longer hospital stays, more postoperative complications, a higher cost of care, and higher mortality (Barnett, Mercer, Norbury, et al., 2012). In addition, multimorbidity affects the care process and may result in complex self-care needs; challenging organizational problems (accessibility, coordination, consultation time); polypharmacy; increased use of emergency facilities; difficulty in applying guidelines; and fragmented, costly, and ineffective care (Barnett, Mercer, Norbury, et al., 2012).

FACTORS CONTRIBUTING TO CHRONIC ILLNESS

The key determinants of health (see Chapter 1, Table 1-2) are also critical considerations in the development of chronic illness. Although some chronic conditions have a specific and unique etiology, there are common factors identified by large, longitudinal studies that play an important role in the development of many types of chronic illness.

Lifestyle factors such as substance use and misuse and high-risk activities can be harmful to a person's long-term health. Studies such as the Framingham Heart Study and the Nurses' Health Study have demonstrated clear associations between chronic illness and tobacco use, alcohol misuse, high blood pressure, physical inactivity, obesity, and unhealthy diet (Centers for Disease Control and Prevention, 2011a). The term *lifestyle* not only includes choices made by individuals but also recognizes the influence of social, economic, and environmental factors on the decisions people make about their health. A healthy lifestyle is determined by an individual's behaviours within his or her social environment. As a key determinant of health, the social environment involves a strong social network (e.g., family, peers, community, workplace) and the ability to connect with others (PHAC, 2013). Poverty and socioeconomic disadvantage are recognized to have a major impact on the development of chronic illness (Lubkin & Larsen, 2013). Income significantly

Chronic diseases share common risk factors and conditions

Non-modifiable risk factors

Behavioural risk factors

Cultural and environmental conditions

Intermediate conditions:

High blood pressure (or hypertension)

Elevated blood lipids (or hyperlipidemia)

Overweight/obesity

Pre-diabetes

Disease endpoints: Cardiovascular diseases Diabetes Arthritis Chronic respiratory diseases Several cancers

FIGURE 5-2 Chronic diseases share common risk factors and conditions. Source: © All rights reserved. Chronic Disease Risk Factors. Public Health Agency of Canada, 2015. Adapted and reproduced with permission from the Minister of Health, 2017.

Risk Factors for Chronic Illness

Both individuals and communities may possess risk factors for the development of chronic illness (PHAC, 2014). The recognition of these common risk factors and conditions is the conceptual basis for an integrated approach to chronic disease.

Individual risk factors can be classified as background, behavioural, or intermediate. Sex, age, level of education, and genetic characteristics are examples of background risk factors. Smoking, unhealthy diet, and physical inactivity would fall into the category of behavioural risk factors. Intermediate risk factors include comorbid conditions such as diabetes, hypertension, and obesity or being overweight. Besides risks that occur at the individual level, community-level factors can also contribute significantly to the development of chronic illnesses. Examples of community-level risk factors include social and economic conditions, such as poverty, employment, and family composition; environmental conditions, such as climate and air pollution; cultural conditions, such as practices, norms, and values; and urbanization, which influences housing and access to products and services (PHAC, 2014).

Figure 5-2 illustrates the conceptual model used by the Centre for Chronic Disease Prevention at the PHAC to examine risk factors for chronic illness. Although some risk factors, such as age, sex, and genetic makeup, cannot be changed (**nonmodifiable risk factors**), many behavioural risk factors are considered **modifiable**. Cultural and environmental risk factors, such as air pollution, may play a significant role in the development of chronic illness and may be modifiable in some cases.

PREVENTION OF CHRONIC ILLNESS

Prevention of chronic illness is the best way to deal with the chronic disease epidemic. Although not all chronic illnesses are preventable, four behavioural risk factors are considered key contributors to many of these conditions: tobacco use, unhealthy diet, insufficient physical activity, and the harmful use of alcohol

TABLE 5-3 "BEST BUYS" FOR CHRONIC ILLNESS PREVENTION

- Creating through laws completely smoke-free environments
- Warning about the dangers of tobacco use
- Enforcing bans on tobacco advertising, promotion, and sponsorship
- Raising taxes on tobacco
- Restricting access to retailed alcohol
- Enforcing bans on alcohol advertising
- Raising taxes on alcohol
- Reducing salt content of food
- Replacing *trans* fat in food with polyunsaturated fat
- Promoting public awareness about diet and physical activity, including through mass media

Source: Reprinted from *Global Status Report on Noncommunicable Disease 2014*, WHO, Page No. 10, Copyright 2014. Retrieved from *http://apps.who.int/iris/bitstream/10665/148114/1/9789241564854_eng.pdf*.

(WHO, 2014b). Decades of research have determined the most effective means, or "best buys," of preventing chronic illness. "**Best buys**," according to the WHO (2014b), are actions that should be undertaken immediately to produce accelerated results in terms of lives saved, diseases prevented, and heavy costs avoided. Table 5-3 identifies these "best buys."

The Role of Genetics

Genetics, or the study of how a specific characteristic is passed from one generation to another, has long been recognized to play an important role in the development of certain chronic illnesses. Cystic fibrosis and Huntington's disease are two chronic illnesses for which genetic testing is available. Genetic testing can also show an inherited predisposition to several different types of cancer, including breast and ovarian cancer, melanoma, and colon cancer. Research continues to explore the development of screening methods for many other chronic illnesses, such as Alzheimer's disease.

With the completion of human genome sequencing, however, the role of genetic factors will assume increasing importance in prevention, detection, and treatment of many chronic illnesses. The student is referred to Chapter 15 for an in-depth discussion of genetics in nursing practice.

The Role of Aging

Chronic illnesses are on the increase as populations age and individuals live with one or more chronic conditions for decades. The profile of diseases contributing most heavily to death, illness, and disability among Canadians has changed dramatically over the past century. Whereas infectious diseases commonly posed the greatest threat to health in the past, improved sanitation, vaccination, and public health surveillance and the advent of antibiotics have been key factors in prolonging life expectancy rates. Life expectancy for Canadians is extending. In 2010, it was 78.5 years for males and 82.7 years for females; it is projected that males born in 2031 will have an average life expectancy of 81.9 years, and females, 86.0 years (Statistics Canada, 2015).

Aging is associated with the development of many chronic illnesses. As people age, they are more likely to have at least one chronic condition, and the oldest adults (aged ≥85 years) are more likely than those aged 65 to 74 years to have at least three chronic conditions (36% versus 20%) (Canadian Institute for Health Information [CIHI], 2011). The association between obesity, hypertension, and hypercholesterolemia in middle age

Before the text "affects an individual's life expectancy, ability to obtain and provide nutritious food and good housing, and access to health care (PHAC, 2014)."

and dementia in older adulthood has been identified (Ballard, Gauthier, Corbett, et al., 2011). The most frequently reported chronic conditions among persons aged 65 and older are hypertension (47%, ≈2 million seniors), followed by arthritis (27%, ≈1.2 million seniors) (CIHI, 2011). The most common combinations of chronic conditions among seniors are hypertension and arthritis (14%) and hypertension and heart disease (12%) (CIHI, 2011).

DISABILITY IN CHRONIC ILLNESS

Chronic illness is often associated with disability, although many people are not disabled by their chronic illness. Disability is a term whose definition continues to be refined after significant global debate. It is a complex interaction between health conditions, personal factors, and the environment. As interpreted by the Supreme Court of Canada, disability "includes a wide and evolving range of permanent, temporary or intermittent impairments, both physical and mental, which can result in functional limitations as the person interacts with others and potentially with socially constructed barriers (Government of Canada, 2014, p. 9).

Two different conceptual models of disability have shaped the manner in which we think about disability (WHO, 2002): the medical model and the social model. The medical model views disability as directly caused by disease, trauma, or another health condition. From the medical model perspective, disability necessitates medical care provided in the form of individual treatment by health care providers to "correct" the problem with the individual. The social model of disability, conversely, sees disability as a socially created problem and not an inherent attribute of an individual (Barnes, 2012). The social model perspective calls for a political response, because the problem is created by an unaccommodating physical environment brought about by attitudes and other features of the social environment.

The WHO has taken the position that neither the medical nor the social model is fully adequate to define *disability*, although both models make a significant contribution to the discussion. Disability, according to the WHO (2002), is a complex phenomenon at the levels of both the body and society. Disability always comprises an interaction between features of the person and features of the overall context in which the person lives. In other words, both medical and social responses are appropriate and necessary to the problems associated with disability, but a model of disability that synthesizes both approaches is required. The integration of the medical and social approaches is contained in the biopsychosocial model, upon which the International Classification of Functioning, Disability and Health, known as the ICF (WHO, 2002), is based. Parallel to the determinants of health (see Chapter 1, Table 1-2), disability and functioning are viewed by the ICF as the outcomes of interactions between health conditions (diseases, disorders, and injuries) and contextual factors. Contextual factors are composed of external environmental factors (i.e., social attitudes, architectural characteristics, and legal and social structures, as well as climate, terrain, and so forth) as well as internal personal factors (i.e., gender, age, coping styles, social background, education, profession, past and current experience, overall behaviour pattern, character, and other factors that influence how disability is experienced by the individual).

Figure 5-3 identifies the three levels of human functioning classified by ICF: functioning at the level of the body or body

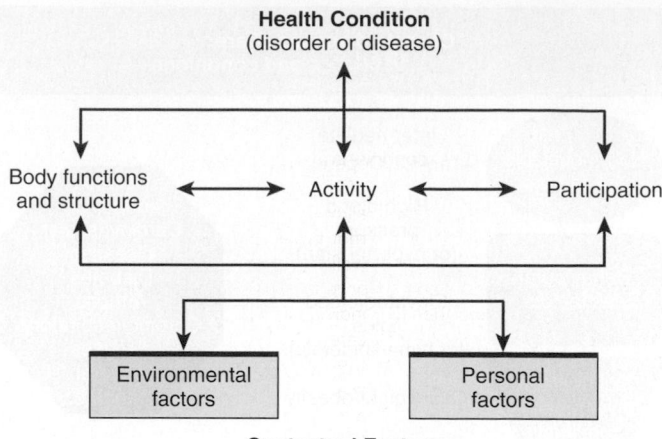

FIGURE 5-3 The International Classification of Functioning, Disability and Health (ICF) Bio–Psycho–Social Model. Source: Reprinted from *Towards a Common Language for Functioning, Disability and Health*, WHO, Page No. 9, Copyright 2002.

part, of the whole person, and of the whole person in a social context. Disability involves dysfunction at one or more of these same levels: impairments, activity limitations, and participation restrictions.

The ICF acknowledges that every human being can experience a decrement in health and thereby experience some degree of disability. Disability is a universal experience at some point in life and is not something that happens only to a minority of individuals.

PSYCHOSOCIAL DIMENSIONS OF CHRONIC ILLNESS

The interaction between mind and body has received increasing and well-deserved attention in recent years. Because chronic illness affects the whole person, and not just a particular body system, the psychosocial dimensions of chronic illness assume great significance. The relational core of nursing practice, which emphasizes nurse–patient dialogue, partnership, and conscious participation, is integral to the care of persons with chronic illness (Kramer-Kile, Osuji, Larsen, et al., 2014).

The following section will address a number of key concepts related to the psychosocial dimensions of chronic illness. Although these concepts are described individually in this section, the student should remember that a holistic perspective embraces the many facets of patients as unique individuals, and it is the interplay between these dimensions that shapes the overall experience of chronic illness.

Illness Behaviour

Illness behaviour refers to the varying ways individuals respond to physical symptoms: how they monitor internal states, define and interpret symptoms, make attributions, take remedial actions, and use various sources of informal and formal care (Mechanic, 1995). The "sick role" was first described in 1951 by Talcott Parsons. Sickness was seen by Parsons as a form of deviant behaviour that permitted the avoidance of social responsibilities (Lubkin & Larsen, 2013). A form of learned behaviour, the sick role was achieved through failure to keep well. Table 5-4 describes the characteristics of the sick role.

TABLE 5-4	CHARACTERISTICS OF THE SICK ROLE
Component of the Role	**Associated Behaviours and Expectations**
Sick person is exempt from normal social roles.	Dependent on the nature and severity of illness. More severe illness allows patients to be exempt from more roles. Requires legitimization (validation) by a physician.
Sick person is not responsible for his or her condition.	Not responsible for becoming sick, the individual therefore has a right to be cared for. Physical dependency and the right to emotional support are therefore acceptable. Will need a curative process apart from personal willpower or motivation to get well.
Obligation to want to become well.	Being ill is seen as undesirable. Because privileges and exemptions of the sick role can become secondary gains, the motivation to recover assumes primary importance.
Obligation to seek and cooperate with technically competent help.	The patient needs technical expertise that the physician and other health care providers have. Cooperation with these providers for the common goal of getting well is mandatory.

Source: Copyright 2001. From *Medical Sociology* by COCKERHAM, WILLIAM C. Reproduced by permission of Taylor and Francis Group, LLC, a division of Informa plc., via Copyright Clearance Center.

TABLE 5-5	EFFECTIVE STRATEGIES AND BARRIERS TO COMMUNICATION DURING DIFFICULT CONVERSATIONS
Effective Strategies	**Barriers to Communication**
• Open and honest communication • Ongoing and early conversations • Communicating about treatment goals • Balancing hope and reality in communicating bad news • Taking cues from the patient about how much information he or she is able to process at one time	• Provider discomfort with issues (e.g., death and dying) • Lack of experience, training, or knowledge of protocols • Lack of good mentorship • Patient factors (e.g., reluctance to talk or face an issue, language barrier, unrealistic prognosis, not ready to hear news) • Age of the patient (i.e., a younger patient can make the discussion more difficult)

Source: Adapted from Kissane, D. W., Bylund, C. L., Banerjee, S. C., et al. (2012). Communication skills training for oncology professionals. *Journal of Clinical Oncology*, *30*(11), 1242–1247.

Parsons's sick-role model, although useful for acute illnesses, has been criticized on many fronts because it does not address important issues related to the chronic illness experience. It fails to consider characteristics of chronic illness, the long-term nature of the illness, the reality that an expectation of full recovery is often not reasonable, the management role expected of the patient and family, and the adjustment to permanent change (Lubkin & Larsen, 2013). In the sick-role model, patients are seen as victims of their illness and are subordinate to physicians. This perspective differs significantly from the paradigm of the "expert patient," in which the patient knows his or her condition and its management far better than his or her health care providers (National Health Service, 2011). Unfortunately, many health care providers apply the sick-role model to patients with chronic illnesses in acute care settings (Lubkin & Larsen, 2013). The frequent readmissions often required by patients with chronic illness may create frustration for staff, who are bored by what they see as repetitive, tiresome care (Lubkin & Larsen, 2013). Patients with chronic illness who have experience with the health care system may use their knowledge to gain what they want or need from the system, demanding certain treatments, a specific schedule, or particular routines (Lubkin & Larsen, 2013). These patients may be perceived as "disruptive" to the normal routine of a hospital unit. Lack of sensitivity on the part of health care providers may lay the foundation for energy-draining power struggles with the patient (Thorne, 2006). Relationships between patients and health care providers tend to be most productive when providers are able to recognize limitations in their own expertise and to respect the expertise of patients and their families. Patients with chronic illness have been found to move from "naive trust" to "disenchantment" and on to a stage of "guarded alliance" in their relationship with health care providers. Nurses must recognize the need to establish credibility and trust with patients who have chronic illness.

More recent work by Thorne (2006) and Thorne, Oglov, Armstrong, and Hislop (2007) noted the critical importance of communication between patients with chronic illness and health care providers. Effective communication must be timely, appropriate, and compassionate (Potter, Perry, Ross-Kerr, et al., 2014). Discussions evoking heightened emotions such as breaking bad news or those requiring patients to make end-of-life decisions are also difficult and stressful experiences for the nurse. Table 5-5 provides a comparison of effective and problematic communication.

Ensuring clarity, a straightforward approach, receptiveness, and responsiveness to questions and providing written information to complement what was said are helpful characteristics of good communication. Unhelpful communications include those in which there is a mismatch between what patients feel their information needs are at a particular time and the manner in which health care providers supply this information. It is useful for nurses to reflect on the question "Am I treating this patient the way I would want to be treated?"

Given their own expertise and experience with health care, many individuals with chronic illness are demanding a new model of care in which they are truly equal partners. **Shared decision making** is a decision-making process engaged in jointly by patients and their health care providers (Barry & Edgman-Levitan, 2012). It is a central tenet of the patient-centred approach described in Chapter 1. Shared decision making exemplifies the partnership between provider and patient and is essential for ethical care as it respects autonomy (the right to make informed choices), beneficence (the balance between benefits and risk of actions), and nonmaleficence (the avoidance of harm).

Self-Efficacy

The development and maintenance of self-efficacy is critical to effective self-management of chronic illness. Self-management programs based on self-efficacy principles have been demonstrated to be highly effective in reducing symptoms and facilitating

TABLE 5-6	TEACHING TECHNIQUES FOR BEHAVIOUR CHANGE

Teaching techniques that assist patients to learn behaviour change strategies include:
- Setting goals collaboratively with the patient, using templates that can be modified based on the patient's context
- Assessing a patient's readiness for self-management, based on tools that the patient can use in the future
- Helping the patient to break down goals and tasks into small steps as part of an action plan, using specific tools and templates that can be modified based on the patient's context
- Providing personalized feedback and helping the patient learn how to ask for, receive, and use feedback
- Teaching self-monitoring, using tools and templates
- Helping the patient obtain social support and informing the patient of and linking the patient to community resources
- Helping the patient assess his or her commitment to key tasks
- Building in follow-up processes to help patients measure their progress and milestone attainment

Source: Registered Nurses' Association of Ontario. (2010). *Strategies to Support Self-Management in Chronic Conditions: Collaboration with Clients.* Toronto, Canada. Registered Nurses' Association of Ontario.

behaviour change (Lubkin & Larsen, 2013) (Table 5-6). Effective self-management relies on a patient-centred care approach in which the individual works in partnership with health care providers to develop solutions to issues related to the patient's chronic condition (Registered Nurses' Association of Ontario [RNAO], 2010). Self-efficacy may be considered a type of self-confidence; it is the belief of an individual that he or she can successfully execute the behaviour required to produce the desired outcomes (Bandura, 1977). People's beliefs about their personal efficacy constitute a major aspect of their self-knowledge, according to Bandura's social cognitive theory. Judgements about personal self-efficacy can determine which behaviours will be attempted, how much effort will be devoted to the behaviour, and how long a person will persist in continuing that behaviour. Weight loss, for example, is often recommended as a means of promoting health. The patient's self-efficacy beliefs will influence the strategies the person might use to attempt to lose weight (perhaps calorie reduction or a combined program of calorie reduction and exercise); how much effort he or she might direct toward this process (a daily walking program or a once-per-week walking program); and how long he or she continues the intended program (for a few weeks or several years).

Both outcome expectancies and efficacy expectancies have to be considered in light of self-efficacy. An *outcome expectancy* is the individual's belief that a specific behaviour will lead to certain outcomes. For example, the patient who tells the nurse that exercising helps people to lose weight is voicing an outcome expectancy. An *efficacy expectancy* is the individual's belief that she or he is able to achieve the outcome. The patient who tells the nurse that she or he is not able to exercise is voicing an efficacy expectancy. It is helpful if both outcome and efficacy expectancies are positive. A patient who believes that exercise helps other people lose weight but that it will not help her or him lose weight might benefit from some of the following influences.

Four primary influences shape an individual's self-efficacy beliefs: mastery; vicarious experience; verbal persuasion and other social influences; and physiological and affective states that help us judge our capability and our vulnerability to dysfunction (Lubkin & Larsen, 2013). *Mastery* reflects a belief about whether or not "we have what it takes to succeed" and is considered the most influential source of self-efficacy. Many chronic illnesses necessitate the mastery of certain skills—for example, monitoring heart rate and exertion level during exercise—to achieve a sense of self-efficacy. *Vicarious experience* is the observation of others' performances, from which we learn through modelling and against which we measure our own performance. These experiences inform our self-efficacy beliefs. In our weight loss example, the patient may be encouraged by the example of fellow participants in a walking program who have achieved weight loss through exercise. When people are *verbally persuaded* that they are capable of performing a certain task, their self-efficacy beliefs may be enhanced. Nurses are in a key position to provide the verbal support the patient may need to undertake the exercise program. Finally, *physiological and affective states* such as stress have an impact on our self-efficacy beliefs. A patient who has just lost his or her job and is experiencing significant financial stress may not have the energy to begin a walking program.

Health-Related Hardiness

Health-related hardiness (HRH), a concept first described by Kobasa (1979) and expanded by Pollock, Christian, and Sands (1990) to apply to people with chronic illness, is a personality resource that buffers stress and allows people to experience a high degree of stress without falling ill. Hardy people are considered to possess three general characteristics: control, commitment, and challenge. *Control* refers to the belief that the individual can influence the events in his or her experience. *Commitment* refers to an ability to feel deeply committed to the activities of life. *Challenge* is the anticipation of change. The person with HRH, when confronted with a health stressor, possesses sufficient self-mastery and confidence to appraise and modify responses appropriately (control) and cognitively reappraises the health stressor so it is viewed as stimulating and beneficial or as an opportunity for growth (challenge). This is exemplified by the perception of individuals with diabetes that they have some control over their disease. *Hardiness* has recently been replaced by the term *resilience*, which shifts the emphasis from its being an inherent trait to its being an ability one can develop (Trivedi, Bosworth, & Jackson, 2011). Motivation and competence thus develop to enhance the patient's health status and to facilitate coping with the health stressor (Pollock & Duffy, 1990). Higher levels of hardiness or resilience show better psychosocial adaptation to chronic illness; thus nurses can make use of interventions that foster a sense of control, commitment, or challenge. These interventions are discussed in the subsequent nursing management chapters.

Mood Disorders

Along with assessments of self-efficacy and health-related hardiness, assessment for the presence of a mood disorder such as depression or anxiety is a key element in the nursing assessment of patients with chronic illness since this population experiences a high burden of mood disorders (Barnett, Mercer, Norbury, et al., 2012). Illness-related anxiety and stress can trigger symptoms of depression. Prevalence rates of depression for patients with cardiac disease range from 20 to 40% while between 12 and 18% of persons with diabetes experience depression (Celano & Huffman, 2011; Katon, 2011). The burden imposed by mood disorders on persons with chronic illness, their families, and

Canadian society is significant. Major depression, in particular, may adversely affect the course of chronic illness and amplify disability (National Institute of Mental Health, 2015). The presence of a mood disorder in a person with a chronic physical illness has been found to be associated with short-term disability, the need for help with instrumental activities of daily living, and suicidal ideation.

The likelihood of depression increases with the number of chronic conditions affecting a patient. This is due in part to the fact that inflammation has been proven to be an important etiological factor in mood disorders. Individuals with inflammatory illnesses such as cardiovascular disease, cancer, Parkinson's disease, chronic obstructive pulmonary disease (COPD), and multiple sclerosis (MS) often struggle with depression (Felger & Lotrich, 2013; McNamara & Lotrich, 2012). This new understanding of the mechanism by which inflammation influences mood disorders will lead to the development of preventive and therapeutic treatments.

In spite of the evidence that mood disorders are common in persons with chronic physical illness, conditions such as depression remain both under-recognized and undertreated in this population. The nurse must be alert for the presence or the development of depressive symptoms when caring for patients with chronic illness.

Fatigue

Fatigue is often associated with chronic illness and has been described as one of the most distressing symptoms people with chronic illness experience. Fatigue may be both a symptom of an underlying condition and an outcome of that condition. It interferes with normal, customary, and desired activities and pervades every aspect of life. The invisibility of fatigue is one of the most frustrating aspects of the experience and leads to lack of understanding and misunderstanding by others. The impact of fatigue on functioning is substantial and under-recognized.

Although there is no universally accepted definition of **fatigue**, it is generally recognized to be a complex, multidimensional experience. A classic nursing definition of *fatigue* was developed by Ream and Richardson (1996, p. 527), who stated that fatigue is "a subjective, unpleasant symptom which incorporates total body feelings ranging from tiredness to exhaustion, creating an unrelenting overall condition which interferes with individuals' ability to function to their normal capacity."

There are many reasons that fatigue is common in people with chronic illness. Pain, mood disorders, sleep problems, physical deconditioning, metabolic abnormalities, infection, dietary problems, hypoxia, and medications can lead to profound fatigue. It is important for the patient to incorporate interventions to reduce fatigue such as yoga, acupuncture, and nutritional supplements.

Stigma

People with chronic illness often experience **stigmatization**, in which they are regarded others as unworthy or disgraceful. Canadian culture contributes to this stigmatization, as it places value on youth, physical fitness, and productivity. Such stigma can have a significant impact on the quality of life of those who are challenged to meet these standards due to the constraints of illness. They may be set apart and labelled by others according to the disease they have and the treatments they use. Lubkin and Larsen (2013) note that older adults and the chronically ill carry a "yoke of undesirability" in health care settings, where caring for these groups is seen as less rewarding in terms of recovery, treatment, and economics than caring for other types of patients. Stigma is an important concept in nursing because it may influence the manner in which care is provided as well as the patient's willingness to disclose information. Individuals who are concerned about being stigmatized if they disclose certain facts may feel threatened and be less likely to share this information. For instance, people with substance abuse problems may not share information with their nurse about the nature and frequency of their drug usage. Lacking this vital information, health care providers may make care decisions that inadvertently adversely affect patient outcomes.

There are several types of stigma. The stigma of physical deformity relates to situations in which there is a difference between the expected and valued norm of perfect physical condition and the actual physical condition of the person (Lubkin & Larsen, 2013). The changes or deformities in physical appearance that may occur as a result of chronic illness set the individual apart. The person with multiple sclerosis, for example, may have difficulty walking or require the use of a mobility aid, which can create stigmatization. Character blemishes, often associated with undesirable traits such as dishonesty, addiction, lack of control, or mental illness, are another type of stigma (Lubkin & Larsen, 2013). Moral judgements are made about the "unworthy" character of the individual. For example, a woman with obesity may experience the stigma of character blemish when others pass judgement about her being responsible for her illness because she is unable to control her appetite and because of her perceived laziness. This leads to the scenario of "blaming the victim" and is not uncommon among health care providers.

Quality of Life

Given the many physical and psychosocial challenges inherent in the experience of living with a chronic illness, **quality of life** is a primary outcome measure in evaluating treatment for many health conditions. *Quality of life*, in its broadest definition, refers to subjective evaluations of both the positive and the negative aspects of life (Centers for Disease Control and Prevention, 2011b). Quality of life is influenced by a host of factors, including financial status, employment, housing, spirituality, social support network, and health. The term **health-related quality of life (HRQL)** has often been used as a means of focusing on the ways health influences and is influenced by overall quality of life. At an individual level, HRQL usually includes perceptions of physical and mental health status and the key variables that are associated with health status, such as health conditions, functional ability, social support, and socioeconomic status (Centers for Disease Control and Prevention, 2011b). At a community level, HRQL includes resources, conditions, policies, and practices that influence a population's health perceptions and functional status. The concept of HRQL enables health agencies to examine broader areas of healthy public policy around a common theme (Centers for Disease Control and Prevention, 2011b).

LIVING WITH CHRONIC ILLNESS

Reduced quality of life, depression, fatigue, and stigma, together with physical symptoms, may make living with a chronic illness a daily challenge for many individuals and their families. Over time, the losses a person sustains as a result of living with a chronic illness cause a decrease in self-esteem. Loss of self is a primary source of suffering for people with chronic illness.

Experiencing social isolation, living a restricted life, and being a burden to others all contribute to this loss of self.

People with chronic conditions use various strategies to try to maintain a "normal life." Normalization is a key strategy in living with chronic illness. When individuals fail to exhibit an expected norm, they become viewed as abnormal. Individuals with chronic illness may attempt to conceal their disease from others to pass themselves off as "normal," which is an idealized notion of being the same as the rest of the presumably normal population. Although the objective of this behaviour is to fit in, this strategy may serve as a constant source of stress because of the danger of being discovered.

"Covering" a visible chronic illness is a strategy employed by some individuals. Covering involves acknowledging the condition while attempting to decrease any anxiety and stress experienced by those who do not have the same condition (Egan, Harcourt, Rumsey, et al., 2011). An example of covering may be making jokes about the condition in an effort to downplay the illness. The nurse must be sensitive to the strategies used by patients with chronic illness and explore with the person whether these strategies are adaptive and helpful or whether they are maladaptive. It is also important for the nurse to recognize that cultural expectations may limit a person's coping strategies. When a culture devalues chronic disease, such as mental illness, people often remain undiagnosed and fail to receive adequate treatment.

CHRONIC ILLNESS AND CAREGIVING

Living with a chronic illness affects not only the individual who has the condition but also those in the patient's immediate social network. Nursing assessment of a person with a chronic illness is incomplete without considering the way in which significant others are affected. Families are frequently called on—and sometimes friends and neighbours—to provide the often complex and long-term care necessitated by some chronic illnesses. In fact, more than 8 million Canadians (28% of the population) provide care to people with long-term health problems (Turcotte, 2013). The term informal caregiver is defined as anyone who provides care without pay and who usually has personal ties to the care recipient (Lubkin & Larsen, 2013).

Family caregivers in Canada are predominantly female and are most likely to be providing care to a spouse or partner or to a parent. Even though it is generally thought that older adults are the ones requiring care, it is important to know that older Canadians are often key care providers to spouses, children, grandchildren, friends, and neighbours.

The vast majority of people with chronic conditions live in the community. The shift away from institutionalization has meant that most of the responsibility for caregiving is left to families and friends. While this shift has reduced the demands on and costs of health care and social systems, it has done so often at the expense of the care provider. It has been demonstrated that the overall health of caregivers is adversely affected by the caregiving experience. One in five considers caregiving to have negatively impacted his or her own physical and emotional health (Statistics Canada, 2013). The overall physical, emotional, and financial cost of caregiving is known as caregiver burden. Issues that arise include increasing difficulty meeting the physical demands of the caregiving role; lack of time to engage in adequate self-care and health-promotion activities; the physiological sequelae of psychological distress, predisposing the individual to changes in immune function; and increased risk of hypertension and cardiovascular

disease (Capistrant, Moon, Berkman, et al., 2011). The nurse plays a critical role in assessing the level of caregiver distress present, if any, and taking appropriate action to attempt to reduce or eliminate the factors that contribute to the distress.

CONCEPTUAL MODELS OF CHRONIC ILLNESS

Conceptual models are useful in understanding the chronic illness experience, particularly because caring for a patient with a chronic illness requires a different framework for practice than may be useful in caring for a patient with an acute illness. The following section highlights several of the key models of chronic illness.

Illness Trajectory

The concept of an illness trajectory was first advanced in 1967 by Glaser and Strauss as a way of understanding the complex, dynamic path of chronic illness. An illness trajectory can be defined as an experiential pathway along which the person with an illness progresses. Some illnesses have more predictable trajectories than others, but all trajectories are subject to individual variation. There have been a number of conceptualizations of illness trajectories. Rolland (1987) identified three critical time phases within the illness trajectory:

Crisis phase: The period before and immediately after diagnosis, when learning to live with symptoms and illness-related demands takes place.

Chronic phase: The time span between initial diagnosis and the final time phase, when the key task is continuing to live as normal a life as possible in the face of the abnormality of having a chronic illness whose outcomes are uncertain.

Terminal phase: This phase is marked by issues surrounding grief and death. Depending on the illness, some patients will enter this phase only after many years.

Further important work in the area of illness trajectories was conducted by Corbin (1998). These authors defined a trajectory of the course of an illness over time, identifying nine phases: (a) pretrajectory; (b) trajectory onset; (c) stable; (d) unstable; (e) acute; (f) crisis; (g) comeback; (h) downward; and (i) dying. Table 5-7 describes the phases and the associated goals of management. Although the illness trajectory is set in motion by pathophysiology and changes in health status, there are strategies that patients, families, and health care providers can use to shape the course of the trajectory. Shaping means that the illness trajectory can be altered by actions that stabilize the disease course, minimize exacerbations, and better control symptoms (Corbin & Strauss, 1992). This model recognizes that each person's illness trajectory is unique.

These models provide a useful starting point from which to consider the concept of trajectories of chronic illness, although they have been criticized for not fully recognizing individual variation.

Shifting Perspectives Model of Chronic Illness

Models that describe living with a chronic illness as a phased process have also been criticized because they imply that an end goal exists and that this goal can be reached only if the person has lived long enough to progress through previous stages. The Shifting Perspectives Model of Chronic Illness (Figure 5-4) described by Paterson shows living with a chronic illness as an ongoing, continually shifting process. This perspective of chronic illness contains elements of both illness and wellness. As the reality of the illness experience and its context change, the person's

TABLE 5-7   ILLNESS TRAJECTORY PHASES AND GOALS OF MANAGEMENT

Phase	Definition	Goal of Management
Pretrajectory	Genetic factors or lifestyle behaviours that place an individual or community at risk for the development of a chronic condition.	Prevent onset of chronic illness
Trajectory onset	Appearance of noticeable symptoms; includes period of diagnostic workup as person begins to discover and cope with implications of diagnosis.	Form appropriate trajectory projection and scheme
Stable	Illness course and symptoms are under control. Biography and everyday life activities are being managed within limitations of illness. Illness management centres in the home.	Maintain stability of illness, biography, and everyday activities
Unstable	Period of instability to keep symptoms under control or reactivation of illness. Biographical disruption and difficulty in carrying out everyday life activities. Adjustment being made in regimen; care usually taking place at home.	Return to stable
Acute	Severe and unrelieved symptoms or the development of illness complications necessitating hospitalization or bed rest to bring illness course under control. Biographical and everyday life activities temporarily placed on hold or drastically cut back.	Bring illness under control and resume normal biographical and everyday life activities
Crisis	Critical or life-threatening situation necessitating emergency treatment or care. Biography and everyday life activities suspended until crisis passes.	Remove life threat
Comeback	A gradual return to an acceptable way of life within limits imposed by disability or illness.	Set in motion and continue the trajectory projection and scheme
Downward	Illness course characterized by rapid or gradual physical decline accompanied by increasing disability or difficulty in controlling symptoms.	Adapt to increasing disability with each major downward turn
Dying	Final days or weeks before death. Characterized by gradual or rapid shutting down of body processes, biographical disengagement, and closure and relinquishment of everyday interest and activities.	Bring closure, let go, and die peacefully

Source: Corbin, J. (2002). Introduction and overview: Chronic illness and nursing. In R. Hyman & J. Corbin (Eds.), *Chronic illness: Research and theory for nursing practice* (pp. 4–5). New York: Springer.

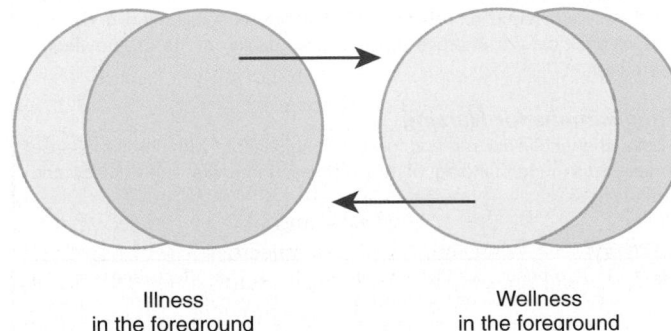

Illness in the foreground   Wellness in the foreground

FIGURE 5-4 The Shifting Perspectives Model of Chronic Illness. Source: Paterson, B. (2001). The shifting perspectives model of chronic illness. *Journal of Nursing Scholarship, 33*(1), 21–26. Copyright © 2001, John Wiley and Sons.

perspective shifts in the degree to which illness or wellness is in the foreground or background of their world. Perspectives of chronic illness are not seen as right or wrong but as reflections of people's needs and situations.

When illness is in the foreground, individuals are focused on the sickness, suffering, loss, and burden associated with living with a chronic illness. This perspective is marked by self-absorption and difficulty attending to the needs of others. This perspective often occurs in people who are newly diagnosed or overwhelmed by their illness. When wellness is in the foreground, the person attempts to create consonance between self-identity and the identity shaped by the disease and between the construction of the illness by others and by life events (Paterson, 2001). The body is objectified and placed at a distance; it is not allowed to control the person. This perspective can be gained by learning

as much as possible about the disease, creating supportive environments, developing skills such as negotiating, identifying the body's unique patterns of response, and sharing with others knowledge about living with the illness. This distance provides for a focus on social, emotional, and spiritual aspects of life, rather than a focus on the diseased body.

The perspective that is in the foreground shifts depending upon circumstances. Perceived threats to control may cause a shift in the foreground from wellness to illness, as may self-help groups that focus on sickness (Paterson, 2001). Returning to having wellness in the foreground may result from changes or interventions that resolve or accommodate the situation that has resulted in the illness focus.

SELF-MANAGEMENT

Self-management is the foundation for optimizing health outcomes for people living with chronic illness. A large body of empirical literature demonstrates that successful self-management is related to better overall physical and psychological health outcomes (Clark, Gong, & Kaciroti, 2014). **Self-management** refers to "the ability of the individual, in conjunction with family, community, and healthcare professionals, to manage symptoms, treatments, lifestyle changes, and psychosocial, cultural, and spiritual consequences of health conditions" (Richard & Shea, 2011, p. 261). This emphasizes the primary role patients have in managing their illness to achieve the best possible quality of life (Canadian Nurses Association, 2014). Every day, patients decide what they are going to eat, whether they will exercise, and to what extent they will take their prescribed medications. These activities, although usually undertaken in cooperation with a health care provider, go beyond merely adhering to a prescribed behavioural regimen. As Glasgow and Anderson (1999, p. 2090) noted:

> Patients are in control. No matter what we as health professionals do or say, patients are in control of these important self-management decisions. When patients leave the clinic or office, they can and do veto recommendations a health professional makes.

The actions people take to manage their conditions are often based on the advice given by health care providers. Sometimes, however, patients choose not to accept this advice, resulting in less than optimal outcomes (Clark, Gong, & Kaciroti, 2014).

Compliance, adherence, and self-care make up the three levels of patient response to health care recommendations on a continuum of self-care. *Compliance* reflects coercion of the patient to engage in particular recommendations, whereas *adherence* implies conformity of the patient to the recommendations. *Self-care* connotes a therapeutic alliance between the patient and the provider. *Adherence* is now the term most widely accepted because it incorporates the notion of the patient agreeing with the treatment plan presented by the health care provider.

Partnership between the nurse and the patient, which focuses on an open, caring, mutually responsive, and nondirective dialogue, is a key aspect of relational nursing practice and is essential in the promotion of self-management. The process of self-management involves empowering the patient, thereby ensuring some autonomy with respect to adjusting the regimen as necessary. Four tasks related to coping with chronic illness are as follows: (a) processing emotions, including grieving, in response to health or functioning; (b) adjusting to the changes to self and life as a result of the illness; (c) integrating illness into daily life; and (d) determining the meaning of the illness so as to help identify tasks and skills that will promote personal growth and satisfaction (Schulman-Green et al., 2012).

The nurse must be alert to potential barriers to successful self-management. People of low socioeconomic status and those who are marginalized are more difficult to attract and retain in self-management programs. Similarly, patients who have limited health literacy may be seriously compromised in their ability to self-manage their conditions successfully. In addition to health literacy, other barriers to self-management that the nurse must be sensitive to the presence of include poorer health, financial constraints, and persistent depressive symptoms (Hinder & Greenhalgh, 2012). The principles of self-management have been the foundation of numerous chronic illness management programs. Evidence-informed self-management (see, for example, the "Evidence-Informed Practice" box) starts with the premise that there is a partnership between patients and health care providers. New paradigms of self-management examine the beliefs and the problems of people with chronic illness, connecting this information with health care providers' views of what knowledge patients must have and what behaviours they must change to manage their condition.

THE EMERGING PARADIGM OF CHRONIC CARE

Our present health care system is organized around an acute, episodic model of care that fails to meet the needs of many patients, including those with chronic illnesses. Patients, families, caregivers, health care providers, and decision makers must recognize that a new model of care must be enacted that better addresses the needs of those with chronic illness. The shortcomings of the current health care system are well-known

EVIDENCE-INFORMED PRACTICE
Research Highlight

How Effective Is the Teach-Back Method on Adherence and Self-Management in Health Education For People With Chronic Disease?

Clinical Question
Adults aged 18 years and over with one or more chronic disease(s) (P), teach-back method used in a chronic disease education program (I), chronic disease education program that did not use the teach-back method (C), on health outcomes and use of health care services (O) adherence, self-management, disease-specific knowledge, readmission, knowledge retention, self-efficacy, and quality of life.

Best Available Evidence
A systematic review of randomized control trials (RTC), non-randomized control trials, cohort studies, before–after studies and case-control studies.

Critical Appraisal and Synthesis of Evidence
The reviewers assess a broad range of studies that used the teach-back method. Four studies found improved disease-specific knowledge; one study showed a statistically significant improvement in medication and diet adherence among type 2 diabetics in the intervention group compared to the control group (p < 0.001). Two studies found a statistically significant improvement in self-efficacy (p = 0.0026 and p < 0.001) in the intervention group. One study examining quality of life in heart failure patients did not improve with the intervention (p = 0.59). Although not statistically significant, five studies found lower hospitalization and readmission rates. Two studies showed improvement in daily weighing among heart failure patients, and in adherence to diet, exercise, and foot care among those with type 2 diabetes.

Conclusions
The health education teach-back method improves disease-specific knowledge, adherence, and self-efficacy. There was a positive association with self-care, reduction in hospital readmission, hospitalization, or deaths. Teach-back did not improve health-related quality of life or knowledge retention.

Implications for Nursing
Using the teach-back method for educating patients with chronic disease maximizes understanding of the disease, improves self-efficacy and self-care skills.

Reference for Evidence
Dinh, T. T., Bonner, A., Clark, R., et al. (2016). The effectiveness of the teach-back method on adherence and self-management in health education for people with chronic disease: A systematic review. *JBI Library of Systematic Reviews, 14*(1), 210–247.

P, Patient population of interest; *I*, intervention or area of interest; *C*, comparison of interest or comparison group; *O*, outcomes of interest (see Chapter 1).

to the dissatisfied patients, the frustrated families, and the weary staff who have struggled to deal with the complexities of chronic illness. In response, the Canadian government has established priorities that will support health care system innovations such as telehealth and that will enhance the integration and coordination of home care services, especially for Indigenous and northern communities (Health Canada, 2015) (see Chapter 6 for further information). There is increasing evidence that patient-centred care, a concept described in Chapter 1, produces better outcomes for patients than do traditional approaches (Battersby, Lawn, & Pols, 2010). Table 5-8 describes what patients with chronic illness want from the health care system and what they believe has been missing. These reasonable expectations are embedded within the chronic care model.

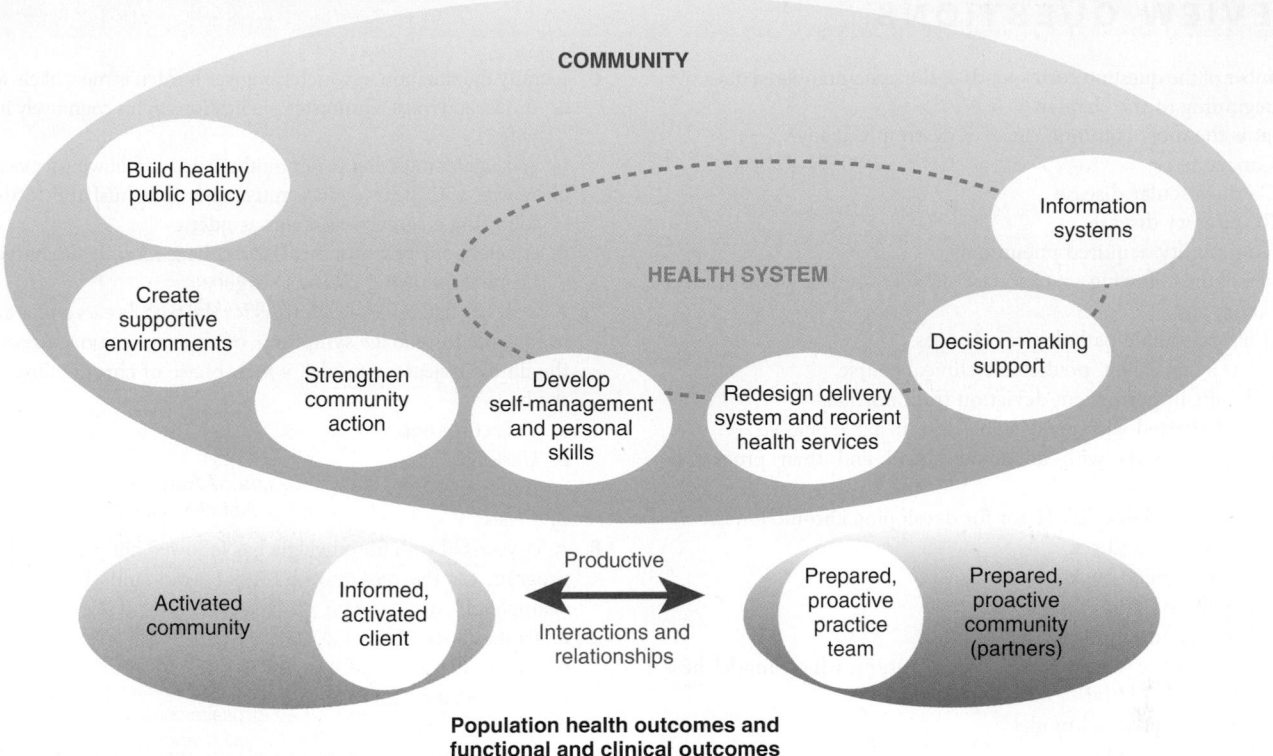

COMMUNITY

Build healthy public policy

Create supportive environments

Strengthen community action

HEALTH SYSTEM

Information systems

Decision-making support

Develop self-management and personal skills

Redesign delivery system and reorient health services

Activated community

Informed, activated client

Productive
Interactions and relationships

Prepared, proactive practice team

Prepared, proactive community (partners)

Population health outcomes and functional and clinical outcomes

FIGURE 5-5 The Expanded Chronic Care Model. Source: Barr, V., Robinson, S., Marin-Link, B., et al. (2003). The Expanded Chronic Care Model: An integration of concepts and strategies from population health promotion and the chronic care model. *Healthcare Quarterly, 7*(1), 73–82.

TABLE 5-8	**WHAT PATIENTS WITH CHRONIC ILLNESS WANT FROM THE HEALTH CARE SYSTEM**

Access to information concerning:
• Diagnosis and its implications
• Available treatments and their consequences
• Potential impact on the patient's future
• Continuity of care and ready access to it
• Coordination of care, particularly with specialists
• Infrastructure improvements (scheduling, wait times, prompt care)
• Ways to cope with symptoms such as pain, fatigue, disability, and loss of independence
• Ways to adjust to disease consequences such as uncertainty, fear and depression, anger, loneliness, sleep disorders, memory loss, exercise needs, nocturia, sexual dysfunction, and stress

Source: Holman, H., & Lorig, K. (2004). Patient self-management: A key to effectiveness and efficiency in care of chronic disease. *Public Health Reports, 119*, 239–243.

Building on the notion of self-management and the need for an integrated, patient-centred system of care, the chronic care model was first advanced by Bodenheimer, Wagner, and Grumbach (2002). This model predicted that improvements in the following six interrelated components would improve care for persons with chronic illness: (a) self-management support, (b) clinical information systems, (c) delivery system redesign, (d) decision support, (e) health care organization, and (f) community resources. The original model was expanded to include

a greater focus on prevention and health promotion by Barr, Robinson, Marin-Link, and colleagues (2003). The Expanded Chronic Care Model (ECCM) appears in Figure 5-5.

The ECCM supports the important role that the social determinants of health play in influencing individual, community, and population health. Support of self-management and the development of personal skills for health and wellness in the ECCM may be accomplished by providing information and enhancing life skills. For example, smoking cessation programs are a cost-effective means of positively affecting health.

Delivery system redesign and reorientation of health services encourage health care providers to move beyond the provision of cure-focused services to an expanded mandate that promotes a holistic perspective. Decision support encompasses the gathering of evidence not only on disease and treatment but also on staying healthy. Information systems can be used to evaluate established systems and support new ways of providing care. Healthy public policy involves working toward organizational and governmental legislation and policy that foster greater equity in society and leads to safer and healthier goods, services, and environments. The ECCM notes the significant impact of social supports on overall health and quality of life. It promotes the creation of supportive environments that are safe, stimulating, satisfying, and enjoyable. The creation of safe, affordable housing is one example in this area. Finally, strengthening community action involves working together with community groups to set priorities and achieve goals that enhance the health of the community.

Nurses have a vital role to play within the vision of the ECCM and can serve as leaders in the challenge to improve the care of Canadians living with chronic illness.

REVIEW QUESTIONS

The number of the question corresponds to the same-numbered objective at the beginning of the chapter.

1. What is the most common cause of death in Canada?
   a. Cancer
   b. Cardiovascular disease
   c. Respiratory disease
   d. Community-acquired pneumonia

2. Which of the following are characteristics of a chronic illness? *(Select all that apply)*
   a. It has reversible pathological changes.
   b. It has a consistent, predictable clinical course.
   c. It results in permanent deviation from normal.
   d. It is associated with many stable and unstable phases.
   e. It always starts with an acute illness and then progresses slowly.

3. Select the modifiable risk factor for developing chronic illness.
   a. Activity level and sex
   b. Age and genetic background
   c. Air pollution and occupation
   d. Smoking and weight

4. According to the World Health Organization, which model best accounts for disability?
   a. The biopsychosocial model
   b. The medical model
   c. The social model
   d. The shifting perspectives model

5. Which statement from a 47-year-old client with COPD reflects her efficacy expectancy?
   a. "I have this disease only because I worked in an auto body shop for years and was exposed to toxic fumes."
   b. "I know I can't quit smoking. I've tried too many times in the past 5 years."
   c. "My mother quit smoking, and she still died from lung disease."
   d. "It's too late to quit smoking now, so what's the point of trying?"

6. Identify the situation in which caregiver burden is most likely to occur.
   a. A husband must administer medications to his cognitively impaired wife.
   b. A daughter must empty her mother's drains following a mastectomy.
   c. A wife with heart failure must assist her husband to the toilet following a cerebro-vascular accident.
   d. A neighbour prepares meals for a client recently discharged from hospital following cataract surgery.

7. A client has had multiple sclerosis for the past 2 years and is admitted to hospital to manage symptoms of an exacerbation. According to the illness trajectory model, which phase of chronic illness would she be in?
   a. Trajectory onset
   b. Unstable
   c. Acute
   d. Crisis

8. A 53-year-old with fibromyalgia has followed her prescribed exercise program for the past month. What would this behaviour be an example of?
   a. Compliance
   b. Adherence
   c. Self-management
   d. Chronic care

9. A nurse is part of a citizen group initiative to start a food bank for disadvantaged people. Within the ECCM, in which domain does this work of the nurse fall?
   a. Delivery system redesign
   b. Healthy public policy
   c. Social support
   d. Strengthening community

1. a; 2, c, d; 3. d; 4. a; 5. b; 6. c; 7. c; 8. b; 9. d.

ℰvolve

For even more review questions, visit *http://evolve.elsevier.com/Canada/Lewis/medsurg.*

REFERENCES

Ballard, C., Gauthier, S., Corbett, A., et al. (2011). Alzheimer's disease. *Lancet, 377*, 1019–1031.

Bandura, A. (1977). *Social learning theory.* Orrville, OH: Prentice-Hall. (Seminal).

Barnes, C. (2012). *Understanding the social model of disability. Routledge handbook of disability studies.* Oxon and New York: Routledge.

Barnett, K., Mercer, S. W., Norbury, M., et al. (2012). Epidemiology of multimorbidity and implications for health care, research, and medical education: A cross-sectional study. *The Lancet, 380*(9836), 37–43. doi:10.1016/S0140-6736(12)60240-2.

Barr, V. J., Robinson, S., Marin-Link, B., et al. (2003). The Expanded Chronic Care Model: An integration of concepts and strategies from population health promotion and the chronic care model. *Hospital Quarterly, 7*(1), 73–82. (Seminal).

Barry, M. J., & Edgman-Levitan, S. (2012). Shared decision making—the pinnacle of patient-centered care. *New England Journal of Medicine, 366*(9), 780–781.

Battersby, M., Lawn, S., & Pols, R. (2010). Conceptualization of self-management. In D. Kralik, B. Paterson, & V. Coates (Eds.), *Translating chronic illness research into practice* (pp. 85–110). Chennai, India: Wiley Blackwell. (Seminal).

Bodenheimer, T., & Berry-Millett, R. (2009). *Care management of patients with complex health care needs. Research Synthesis Report No. 19.* The Robert Wood Johnson Foundation. Retrieved from *http://www.rwjf.org/en/library/research/2009/12/care-management-of-patients-with-complex-health-care-needs.html.* (Seminal).

Bodenheimer, T., Wagner, E. H., & Grumbach, K. (2002). Improving primary care for patients with chronic illness. *Journal of the American Medical Association, 288*, 1775–1779. doi:10.1001/jama.288.14.1775. (Seminal).

Canadian Agency for Drugs and Technology. (2011). *The use of virtual wards to reduce hospital readmissions in Canada.* Retrieved from *https://www.cadth.ca/sites/default/files/pdf/ES-27_virtual_wards_e.pdf.*

Canadian Cancer Society's Advisory Committee on Cancer Statistics. (2015). *Canadian cancer statistics 2015.* Toronto: Canadian Cancer Society. Retrieved from *http://www.cancer.ca/~/media/cancer.ca/CW/cancer%20information/cancer%20101/Canadian%20cancer%20statistics/Canadian-Cancer-Statistics-2015-EN.pdf?la=en.*

Canadian Institute for Health Information (CIHI). (2011). *Seniors and the health care system: What is the impact of multiple chronic conditions?* Retrieved from *https://www.cihi.ca/en/info_phc_chronic_seniors_en.pdf.*

Canadian Nurses Association. (2014). *Effectiveness of registered nurses and nurse practitioners in supporting chronic disease self-management.* Retrieved from *https://www.cna-aiic.ca/~/media/cna/page-content/pdf-en/effectiveness_of_rns_and_nps_in_self-care_managment_e.pdf?la=en.*

Capistrant, B. D., Moon, J. R., Berkman, L. F., et al. (2011). Current and long-term spousal caregiving and onset of cardiovascular disease. *Journal of Epidemiology and Community Health, 66*(10), 951–956.

Celano, C. M., & Huffman, J. C. (2011). Depression and cardiac disease: A review. *Cardiology in Review, 19*(3), 130–142.

Centers for Disease Control and Prevention. (2011a). *Chronic disease prevention and health promotion.* Retrieved from *https://www.cdc.gov/chronicdisease/index.htm/.*

Centers for Disease Control and Prevention. (2011b). *Health-related quality of life.* Retrieved from *http://www.cdc.gov/hrqol/concept.htm.*

Clark, N. M., Gong, M., & Kaciroti, N. (2014). A model of self-regulation for control of chronic disease. *Health Education & Behavior, 41*(5), 499–508.

Corbin, J. (1998). The Corbin and Strauss chronic illness trajectory model: An update. *Scholarly Inquiry for Nursing Practice, 12*(1), 33–41. (Seminal).

Corbin, J., & Strauss, A. (1992). A nursing model for chronic illness management based upon the trajectory framework. In P. Woong (Ed.), *The chronic illness trajectory framework.* New York: Springer. (Seminal).

Egan, K., Harcourt, D., Rumsey, N., et al. (2011). A qualitative study of the experiences of people who identify themselves as having adjusted positively to a visible difference. *Journal of Health Psychology, 16*(5), 739–749. doi:10.1177/1359105310390246.

Felger, J. C., & Lotrich, F. E. (2013). Inflammatory cytokines in depression: Neurobiological mechanisms and therapeutic implications. *Neuroscience, 246*, 99–229. doi:10.1016/j.neuroscience.2013.04.060.

Glaser, B., & Strauss, A. (1967). *The discovery of grounded theory: Strategies for qualitative research.* New York: Aldine Transaction. (Seminal).

Glasgow, R. E., & Anderson, R. M. (1999). In diabetes care, moving from compliance to adherence is not enough. *Diabetes Care, 22*(12), 2090–2092. (Seminal).

Government of Canada. (2014). *Convention on the rights of persons with disabilities: First report of Canada.* Retrieved from *http://www.ccdonline.ca/media/international/Convention%20on%20the%20Rights%20of%20Persons%20with%20Disabilities%20-%20First%20Report%20of%20Canada.pdf.*

Health Canada. (2010). *A statistical profile of the health of First Nations in Canada.* Retrieved from *http://www.hc-sc.gc.ca/fniah-spnia/pubs/aborig-autoch/2010-stats-profil-determinants/index-eng.php#a1.*

Health Canada. (2015). *Health Canada 2015-16 report on plans and priorities.* Retrieved from *http://www.hc-sc.gc.ca/ahc-asc/performance/estim-previs/plans-prior/2015-2016/report-rapport-eng.php#a2.1.*

Henly, S. J., Wyman, J. F., & Findorff, M. J. (2011). Health and illness over time: The trajectory perspective in nursing science. *Nursing Research, 60*(Suppl. 3), S5. doi:10.1097/NNR.0b013e318216dfd3.

Hinder, S., & Greenhalgh, T. (2012). "This does my head in." Ethnographic study of self-management by people with diabetes.

BMC Health Services Research, 12(1), 83. doi:10.1186/1472-6963-12-83.

Katon, W. J. (2011). Epidemiology and treatment of depression in patients with chronic medical illness. *Dialogues in Clinical Neuroscience, 13*(1), 7.

Kobasa, S. C. (1979). Stressful events, personality and health: An inquiry into hardiness. *Journal of Personality and Social Psychology, 37*(1), 1–11. (Seminal).

Kramer-Kile, M. L., Osuji, J. C., Larsen, P. D., et al. (2014). *Chronic illness in Canada: Impact and intervention.* Burlington, MA: Jones & Bartlett.

Lubkin, I. M., & Larsen, P. D. (2013). *Chronic illness: Impact and interventions* (8th ed.). Toronto: Jones & Bartlett.

McNamara, R. K., & Lotrich, F. E. (2012). Elevated immune-inflammatory signaling in mood disorders: A new therapeutic target? *Expert Review of Neurotherapeutics, 12*(9), 41–49. doi:10.1586/ern.12.98.

Mechanic, D. (1995). The concept of illness behaviour. *Journal of Chronic Diseases, 15*(2), 189–194. (Seminal).

National Health Service. (2011). *The Expert Patients Programme—What is an expert patient?* London: Author. Retrieved from *http://www.nhs.uk/Conditions/Expert-patients-programme-/Pages/Whatisanexpertpatient.aspx.*

National Institute of Mental Health. (2015). *Chronic illness and mental health.* Retrieved from *http://www.nimh.nih.gov/health/publications/chronic-illness-mental-health-2015/index.shtml.*

Paterson, B. (2001). The shifting perspectives model of chronic illness. *Journal of Nursing Scholarship, 33*(1), 21–26. doi:10.1111/j.1547-5069.2001.00021.x. (Seminal).

Pollock, S. E., Christian, B. J., & Sands, D. (1990). Responses to chronic illness: Analysis of psychological and physiological adaptation. *Nursing Research, 39*(5), 300–304. doi:10.1097/00006199-199009000-00014. (Seminal).

Pollock, S. E., & Duffy, M. E. (1990). The Health-Related Hardiness Scale: Development and psychometric analysis. *Nursing Research, 39*(4), 218–222. doi:10.1097/00006199-199007000-00008. (Seminal).

Potter, P. A., Perry, A. G., Ross-Kerr, J. C., et al. (Eds.), (2014). *Canadian fundamentals of nursing* (5th Canadian ed.). Toronto: Elsevier Canada.

Public Health Agency of Canada (PHAC). (2011). *Tracking heart disease and stroke in Canada—Stroke highlights 2011.* Retrieved from *http://www.phac-aspc.gc.ca/cd-mc/cvd-mcv/sh-fs-2011/index-eng.php.*

Public Health Agency of Canada (PHAC). (2013). *What makes Canadians healthy or unhealthy.* Retrieved from *http://www.phac-aspc.gc.ca/ph-sp/determinants/determinants-eng.php.*

Public Health Agency of Canada (PHAC). (2014). *The Chief Public Health Officer's report on the state of public health in Canada, 2014: Public health in the future.* Retrieved from *http://www.phac-aspc.gc.ca/cphorsphc-respcacsp/2014/index-eng.php.*

Public Health Agency of Canada (PHAC). (2015). *Centre for Chronic Disease Prevention: Strategic plan 2016–2019.* Retrieved from *http://www.phac-aspc.gc.ca/cd-mc/ccdp-strategic-plan-2016-2019-plan-strategique-cpmc-eng.php.*

Ream, E., & Richardson, A. (1996). Fatigue: A concept analysis. *International Journal of Nursing Studies, 33*(5), 519–529. doi:10.1016/0020-7489(96)00004-1. (Seminal).

Registered Nurses' Association of Ontario (RNAO). (2010). *Nursing best practice guideline: Strategies to support self-management in chronic conditions: Collaboration with clients.* Retrieved from *http://rnao.ca/bpg/guidelines/strategies-support-selfmanagement-chronic-conditions-collaboration-clients.*

Richard, A. A., & Shea, K. (2011). Delineation of self-care and associated concepts. *Journal of Nursing Scholarship, 43,* 255–264. doi:10.1111/j.1547-5069.2011.01404.x.

Rolland, J. S. (1987). Chronic illness and the life cycle: A conceptual framework. *Family Process, 26*(2), 203–211. (Seminal).

Salisbury, C., Johnson, L., Purdy, S., et al. (2011). Epidemiology and impact of multimorbidity in primary care: A retrospective cohort study. *British Journal of General Practice, 61*(582), e12–e21. doi:10.3399/bjgp11X548929.

Schulman-Green, D., Jaser, S., Martin, F., et al. (2012). Processes of self-management in chronic illness. *Journal of Nursing Scholarship, 44*(2), 136–144. doi:10.1111/j.1547-5069.2012 .01444.x.

Statistics Canada. (2011). *Mortality, summary list of causes 2008.* Ottawa: Author. Retrieved from *http://www.statcan.gc.ca/bsolc/ olc-cel/olc-cel?catno=84F0209X&CHROPG=1&lang=eng.*

Statistics Canada. (2013). *Portrait of caregivers, 2012.* Retrieved from *http://www.statcan.gc.ca/pub/89-652-x/89-652-x2013001-eng.pdf.*

Statistics Canada. (2015). *Life expectancy at birth (LE), healthy expectancy expected (HLE) at birth, and the proportion of life in poor health, by gender, 45 more developed countries, 2010.* Retrieved from *http://www.statcan.gc.ca/pub/82-003-x/2014012/ article/14127/tbl/tbla-eng.htm.*

Strauss, A. L., Corbin, J., Fagerhaugh, S., et al. (1984). *Chronic illness and the quality of life.* St. Louis: Mosby. (Seminal).

Thorne, S. (2006). Patient–provider communication in chronic illness: A health promotion window of opportunity. *Family and Community Health, 29*(Suppl. 1S), 4S–11S. doi:10.1097/00003727-200601001-00003. (Seminal).

Thorne, S., Oglov, V., Armstrong, E., et al. (2007). Prognosticating futures and the human experience of hope. *Palliative and Supportive Care, 5,* 227–239. doi:10.1017/S1478951507000399. (Seminal).

Trivedi, R. B., Bosworth, H. B., & Jackson, G. L. (2011). Resilience in chronic illness. In *Resilience in aging* (pp. 181–197). New York: Springer.

Turcotte, M. (2013). *Family caregiving: What are the consequences?* Retrieved from *http://www.statcan.gc.ca/pub/75-006-x/2013001/ article/11858-eng.htm.*

World Health Organization (WHO). (2002). *Towards a common language for functioning, disability and health. ICF: The International Classification of Functioning, Disability and Health.* Retrieved from *http://www.who.int/nmh/publications/ncd_ report2010/en/.* (Seminal).

World Health Organization (WHO). (2014a). *Basic documents* (48th ed.). Retrieved from *http://apps.who.int/iris/bitstream/ 10665/148114/1/9789241564854_eng.pdf.*

World Health Organization (WHO). (2014b). *Global status report on noncommunicable diseases 2014.* Geneva: Author. Retrieved from *http://apps.who.int/iris/bitstream/10665/148114/1/9789241564854 _eng.pdf.*

RESOURCES

Canada's World Health Organization (WHO) Collaborating Centre on Chronic Noncommunicable Disease
http://www.phac-aspc.gc.ca/about_apropos/whocc-ccoms/ index-eng.php

Canadian Lung Association
http://www.lung.ca

Carers Canada
http://www.carerscanada.ca

Heart and Stroke Foundation of Canada
http://www.heartandstroke.ca/

Improving Chronic Illness Care (Robert Wood Johnson Foundation)
http://www.improvingchroniccare.org/

"My Tool Box" Chronic Disease Self-Management Program
http://mytoolbox.mcgill.ca/index.php?ref=toolboxworkshopsdetails .html

National Myalgic Encephalomyelitis (Chronic Fatigue Syndrome) and Fibromyalgia Action Network
http://www.fm-cfs.ca/

Public Health Agency of Canada: Chronic Diseases
http://www.phac-aspc.gc.ca/cd-mc/index-eng.php

Public Health Agency of Canada: Determinants of Health
http://www.phac-aspc.gc.ca/ph-sp/determinants/index-eng.php

Registered Nurses' Association of Ontario Clinical Best Practice Guidelines: Strategies to Support Self-Management in Chronic Conditions: Collaboration With Clients
http://rnao.ca/sites/rnao-ca/files/Strategies_to_Support_ Self-Management_in_Chronic_Conditions_-_Collaboration_ with_Clients.pdf

Siteman Cancer Center: "Your Disease Risk" interactive questionnaire
http://www.yourdiseaserisk.wustl.edu

For additional Internet resources, see the website for this book at *http://evolve.elsevier.com/Canada/Lewis/medsurg.*

Community-Based Nursing and Home Care

Written by: Julie H. Fraser

With contributions from: Barbara L. Mildon

evolve WEBSITE

http://evolve.elsevier.com/Canada/Lewis/medsurg

- Review Questions (Online Only)
- Key Points
- Answer Guidelines for Case Study

- Conceptual Care Map Creator
- Audio Glossary
- Content Updates

LEARNING OBJECTIVES

1. Understand the history of community nursing.
2. Define *primary health care* and explain its importance to the health care system and community health nursing practice.
3. Describe the trends that are threatening the sustainability of Canada's health care system.
4. Describe the role that home care plays in promoting the sustainability of Canada's health care system.
5. Understand how home care in Canada is organized and funded.
6. Describe the practice of the home health nurse, including key clinical competencies.

KEY TERMS

chronic disease management, p. 79	home health nursing, p. 77	nurse practitioners (NPs), p. 78	primary care, p. 79
family-centred care, p. 82	hospice palliative care, p. 83	nursing-sensitive outcomes, p. 85	primary health care, p. 79
			public health nursing, p. 78

The community offers a diversity of exciting and professionally fulfilling roles in which community health nurses (CHNs) make a meaningful difference to the health of individuals, families, communities, and populations. Home and community care have increasingly been recognized as essential components of the health care system (Canadian Nurses Association [CNA], 2013, Canadian Healthcare Association, 2009; Health Council of Canada, 2008a; Nagle, 2008; Canadian Home Care Association [CHCA], 2013). This chapter is a discussion of community-based nursing, including its history, roles, and practice, with an emphasis on home health care.

In its report of the 2015 nursing workforce, the Canadian Institute for Health Information (CIHI, 2015a) reported that 14.6% of regulated nurses worked in the community health sector, which includes community health centres, home care nursing organizations, nursing stations (outpost or clinic), and public health departments or units.

THE HISTORY OF HOME HEALTH NURSING

Home health nursing (also known as *visiting nursing, district nursing,* and *home care nursing*) is a specialized area of nursing practice firmly rooted in community health nursing. "The role is characterized by the flexibility, adaptability, and creative approaches to situations and problems encountered in the context of service delivery where clients live" (Community Health Nurses of Canada [CHNC], 2010, p. 7). This specifically includes "teaching, curative interventions, end of life care, rehabilitation, support, maintenance, social adaptation and integration, and support for the family caregiver" (American Nurses Association, 2008, p. 2).

The history of home health nursing in Canada can be traced back through the centuries. Voluntary, charitable organizations were the first to address the health needs of citizens in the community. For example, the Grey Nuns, founded in Montreal in 1738, established hospitals and refuges and travelled to the homes of ill persons to provide care (Allemang, 2000). Thus the philosophy of attending to the well-being of the individual, as well as to the health of the community at large, came to uniquely characterize community health nursing (Chalmers & Kristjanson, 1992). In 1897, the Victorian Order of Nurses (VON) was established in Canada, followed in 1908 by the Saint Elizabeth Visiting Nurses Association. It has been speculated that the association of volunteerism and charity with community nursing has contributed to the continuing struggle for recognition of the formal education required by CHNs and for appropriate compensation (Chalmers & Kristjanson, 1992).

As this history demonstrates, home health nursing was already well established when public health nursing emerged. Public health nursing came into existence as a result of scientific breakthroughs, including vaccinations, pasteurization, the germ theory of disease, and antisepsis, which provided the basis for preventing infection. The movement of people from rural areas to cities fostered ideal conditions for disease transmission, necessitating new attention to sanitation (Allemang, 2000). In view of these changes, public health nursing focused on health promotion and disease prevention, and home health nurses attended to the needs of people already ill, while also incorporating health promotion and disease prevention into their care. The links between public health and home care nursing were captured by Emory (1953), who identified that the inclusion of both bedside nursing and health teaching delineates home health nursing as a branch of public health nursing.

Public health nursing is defined today as a specialized area of nursing practice in which the nurse combines knowledge from public health science, primary health care (including the determinants of health), nursing science, and the social sciences and focuses on promoting, protecting, and preserving the health of populations. Public health nursing recognizes that a community's health is closely linked to the health of its members and is often reflected first in individual and family health experiences. It recognizes, in turn, that healthy communities and systems that support health contribute to opportunities for health for individuals, families, groups, and populations. Public health nurses practise in increasingly diverse settings such as community health centres, schools, street clinics, youth centres, and nursing outposts and with diverse partners to meet the health needs of specific populations (adapted from Canadian Public Health Association, 2010, p. 8).

The shared history of visiting and public health nursing continues to unify the two groups of CHNs, who are now joined by nurses in many other community-based roles.

COMMUNITY HEALTH NURSING ROLES

CHNs "promote, protect and preserve the health of individuals, families, groups, communities and populations in the settings where they live, work, learn, worship and play in an ongoing and episodic process" (CHNC, 2011, p. 4). A variety of titles exist for nurses who work in community-based settings. These titles include *public health nurse, home health nurse, prevention nurse, faith community nurse* (also called *parish nurse*), *family practice nurse, outpost* or *rural–remote nurse, case manager, primary care nurse, outreach nurse, occupational health nurse,* and *school nurse.* More recent community health nursing roles that have been introduced include those of the forensic nurse, the sexual assault nurse examiner, the nurse entrepreneur, and the nurse practitioner (also known as a *family* or *adult nurse practitioner*).

Nurse practitioners (NPs) are "autonomous health professionals with advanced education [who] provide essential health services grounded in professional, ethical and legal standards" (CNA, 2010, p. 5). NPs "integrate their in-depth knowledge of advanced nursing practice and theory, health management, health promotion, disease/injury prevention, and other relevant biomedical and psychosocial theories to provide comprehensive health services" (CNA, 2010, p. 5). Their education and experience allow them to function both independently and collaboratively in a range of settings (CNA, 2010). Primary care clinics are an example of a setting where both NPs and other nurses are demonstrating positive impacts on individuals' health outcomes (CNA, 2014).

Although the community is the context of care for community-based nurses, they possess an understanding of the entire health system continuum. For example, a person may be hospitalized in a burn unit after suffering burns in a fire at home. When the patient's condition is no longer critical, he or she may be transferred to a general medical-surgical unit and then to a rehabilitation facility. Once the patient is back home, a home health nurse may visit to care for unhealed burn injuries, to provide care for other health needs, or both. When the individual is ready to return to work, an occupational health nurse may be involved to facilitate the reintegration to the workplace.

The continuum of care does not always include hospitalization. Health problems may be identified in a variety of outpatient settings, including physicians' offices, workplace health units, health care clinics, or community health centres. For example, a patient may be screened for diabetes mellitus at work by an occupational health nurse. Screening results may prompt a referral to a family physician or nurse practitioner, who makes the diagnosis of diabetes. Instead of hospitalization, the patient may be monitored by a chronic disease management nurse or certified diabetes educator in the family practice office or community health centre, who will collaborate with the patient to design a care plan. The care plan may include monitoring and education in a variety of settings, as well as follow-up by a home health nurse to initiate, teach, and monitor the prescribed insulin therapy. In turn, the home health nurse would communicate with the appropriate members of the health care team to promote comprehensive, timely, and appropriate patient care.

A HEALTH CARE SYSTEM UNDER PRESSURE

Several trends are putting pressure on Canada's health care system and influencing its evolution. The significance of select trends for CHNs is highlighted in the sections below.

Changing Demographics

The average age of Canadians is increasing (older adults are discussed further in Chapter 7). In 2015, for the first time, Statistics Canada reported that there were more persons aged 65 years and older (16.1%) in Canada than children aged 0 to 14 years (16%) and that the number of older adults will continue to increase to 20.1% of the population by 2024 (Statistics Canada, 2015). It has been reported that persons aged 65 and older accounted for 45.4% of health care expenditures by provincial and territorial governments in 2009 (CIHI, 2015b). In addition, community-based services for older persons, such as home nursing and personal care support, day care programs, and foot care programs, are playing important roles. In 2011, one in six Canadians aged 65 and older had received home care services (CHCA, 2013).

Health Human Resources. Nurses are the largest group of health care providers in Canada (CIHI, 2015a). Concerns about a nursing shortage continue to be raised across the country (CNA, 2012) and globally (World Health Organization, 2015a). According to CIHI (2015a), in 2014, nurses aged 40 to 59 represented 52.6% of registered nurses, 48.2% of licensed practical nurses, and 57.2% of registered practical nurses. Not only are nurses aging, but many may also retire before the traditional retirement age of 65 (CIHI, 2015a). The health of nurses is also causing concern: a national survey reported that 61% of nurses had taken time off in the previous year for health reasons and that the average number of days absent from work among all nurse respondents was 14.5 per nurse (Statistics Canada, 2006). More nurses than non-nurse health care providers reported musculo-skeletal problems, and nurses were more likely to have experienced depression in the previous year than were non-nurse health care providers (Statistics Canada, 2006).

Concern about a shortage of nurses and other health care providers in home care has also been documented (CHCA, 2013; Canadian Healthcare Association, 2009; Carter, 2009). Shortages cause concern because they lengthen waiting lists for services, impose a burden on family members who take on the care of loved ones, and may undermine quality of care due to providers' feeling rushed because of high numbers of patients.

Patient Safety. Since the release of a report entitled *To Err Is Human: Building a Safer Health System* (Institute of Medicine, 1999), the health care system has focused increasingly on enhancing patient safety. Factors influencing safety for home care patients include lack of control over a patient's home environment, lack of uniformity of procedures in private homes in comparison to hospital units, and a reliance on unpaid or untrained caregivers (Canadian Patient Safety Institute [CPSI], 2013; Lang, 2010; Lang, Edwards, & Fleiszer, 2008), as well as challenges in coordinating services from hospital to the home, the cost of equipment and supplies, and continuity of care within the home care team (CPSI, 2013). A pan-Canadian study revealed that 13% of individuals receiving home care services will experience an adverse event, 50% of which are considered preventable (CPSI, 2013). Adverse events in the home include falls, medication-related incidents, and infections resulting from such interventions as urinary catheterization or venous access or wounds (CPSI, 2013).

Sustainability of the Health Care System

Health care costs consume between 22% (Yukon) and 46% (Nova Scotia) of provincial and territorial budgets in Canada (CIHI, 2016a). Costs of over $228 billion per year (CIHI, 2016b) have raised an alarm regarding the ability to sustain Canada's health care system and have prompted calls for health care system reform or renewal. In particular, elements identified as in need of change include policies and programs that address the determinants of health, access to a consistent primary care provider, and a national strategy on chronic disease prevention and management (Morgan, Zamora, & Hindmarsh, 2007). These elements are reflected in the philosophy and principles of primary health care.

Primary Health Care. Community health nursing practice is informed and guided by nursing theory and knowledge, social sciences, public health science, and the philosophy and principles of primary health care (CHNC, 2011). According to the Declaration of Alma Ata (World Health Organization, 1978),

> Primary health care is essential health care based on practical, scientifically sound, and socially acceptable methods and technology made universally accessible to individuals and families in the community through their full participation and at a cost that the community and country can afford.

There are six key principles of primary health care:

1. Universal access to health care services on the basis of need
2. Focus on the determinants of health as part of a commitment to health equity and social justice

3. Active participation on the parts of individuals and communities in decisions that affect their health and lives
4. Partnership with other disciplines, communities, and sectors for health (intersectoral approach)
5. Appropriate use of knowledge, skills, strategies, technology, and resources
6. Focus on health promotion–illness prevention throughout the life experience from birth to death

Although the terms *primary care* and *primary health care* are often used interchangeably, there is an important difference between them. The focus of primary care is disease, and the key participants are health care providers. In contrast, primary health care is both a philosophy and an approach to the delivery of health care (Health Canada, 2012). Its focus is system-wide, and key participants are intersectoral partners in the fields of health, social services, housing, and the environment. Primary health care includes a range of activities from the health care of individuals to activity on the determinants of health. Confusion often arises between the terms *primary care* and *primary health care* because the health care provider whom an individual visits for health care is often known as the individual's primary care provider. Moreover, having access to a consistent primary care provider (e.g., a family physician or nurse practitioner) is an essential component of primary health care. Lack of access to a consistent primary care provider may result in more visits to an emergency department or more hospitalizations (Health Council of Canada, 2008b). It may also result in a delay in seeking care, fragmented care, and less effective chronic disease management.

Primary health care is increasingly being embraced as a strategy to shift the health system's emphasis from diagnosis and treatment of illness and injury to health promotion and disease prevention. This shift is also known as *reforming the system*. Decreasing the prevalence and severity of illness through effective chronic disease management has been identified as a key strategy to promote the well-being of Canadians and the sustainability of the health care system (Health Council of Canada, 2008b; Morgan, Zamora, & Hindmarsh, 2007). Chronic disease management refers to the use of elements and tools within the health care system (e.g., information systems, decision support tools, self-management promotion, and realignment of health services) and within the community (e.g., a supportive environment, health policy, and strengthened community action) to help patients living with chronic diseases (Canadian Public Health Association, 2008). Primary health care encompasses values and principles that are central to the practice of nurses: promoting health, preventing disease, and working with other members of the multidisciplinary team. Thus it is imperative that all nurses be aware of primary health care philosophy and principles and incorporate them into their practice (CNA, 2014).

HOME CARE

Definition and Importance of Home Care

Home care in Canada is defined as

> an array of services for people of all ages, provided in the home and community setting, that encompasses health promotion and teaching, curative intervention, end-of-life care, rehabilitation, support and maintenance, social adaptation, and integration and support for the informal (family) caregiver. (CHCA, 2013, p. xi)

In 2011, 1.4 million Canadians received home care services (CHCA, 2013). Home care, however, is *not* one of the insured services covered by the *Canada Health Act,* the legislation that created and protects Canada's universal, publicly funded health care system. Therefore, provinces and territories have no legal obligation federally to ensure that their citizens have access to home care services. A recent Nanos poll found that 90% of Canadians consider home care essential to aging at home (CNA, 2015). Although every province and territory now has a home care program, they offer varied access to and types of programming (CHCA, 2013). Canadian Home Care Association (2013) has established national harmonized principles of care: (a) patient- and family-centred, (b) integrated, (c) accessible, (d) evidence-informed, (e) sustainable, and (f) accountable. The Canadian Nurses Association (2015) and Canadian Medical Association (2015) have called on the federal government to adopt national home care standards.

Home Care Services

The CHCA (2013) reported that home care programs are designed to promote independence; prevent, delay, or substitute for acute or long-term care; assist with the use of community services; and supplement the care and support provided by friends and family. Recipients of home care include individuals who are frail or disabled or who have an acute or chronic medical condition. Some require only intermittent services; others need assistance 24 hours a day. Family members may also receive home care services such as respite care to support them in their caregiving efforts. Equipment for the home such as electrical beds, wheelchairs, pressure-relief mattresses, commodes, walkers, raised toilet seats, and other assistive devices may also be provided.

Home care services may be categorized as acute, chronic, palliative, or rehabilitative. In addition, coordination and management of admission to a facility may be provided when it is no longer possible for the individual to remain at home (CHCA, 2013). Services may be provided in the home (e.g., private home or residential facility) or in adult day centres, workplaces, schools, shelters, or clinics. Community clinics staffed by home care nurses have been shown to be cost-effective and are attractive to patients who are well enough to leave their homes because they can choose their own appointment time and not have to wait in their homes for the nurse's arrival (VanDeVelde-Coke, 2004). However, it is important to note that skilled nursing observation and assessment of the patient's home environment, social supports, caregiver stress, and risk for falls cannot be achieved in a clinic, and thus serious health problems may be overlooked (Pastor, 2006).

Quality and Accountability in Home Care

As a demonstration of quality and accountability, many home care provider organizations voluntarily apply for accreditation from Accreditation Canada. However, accreditation is mandatory only in Quebec, where it is obtained through the Quebec Council of Accreditation (Accreditation Canada, 2015).

Standardized home care data are collected to demonstrate the impact of nursing on safety and quality outcomes (Doran, Mildon, & Clarke, 2011). For example, CIHI has developed the Home Care Reporting System (HCRS), which is a standardized data set to support comparison of specific indicators for home care. At present, eight provinces and territories are submitting to the HCRS partial or complete data generated by their use of the Resident Assessment Instrument—Home Care (RAI-HC)

TABLE 6-1	FUNDING MECHANISMS FOR HOME CARE

1. Publicly funded, provincial–territorial health care plan
2. Private insurance (e.g., employment benefit plans)
3. Veterans Affairs Canada
4. First Nations and Inuit branch of Health Canada
5. Indigenous and Northern Affairs Canada
6. Workers' compensation boards
7. Private payment (also known as *self-payment* or *out-of-pocket payment*)
8. Associations and foundations (e.g., Canadian Red Cross)

(CIHI, 2015c). Nurses are involved in collecting such data, which is then used for several purposes. For example, data from the RAI-HC system are now being used to gain a more comprehensive understanding of the health status and demographics of specific groups of home care patients such as those with heart failure (Foebel, Hirdes, Heckman, et al., 2011). The data also support quality monitoring and comparison among health care provider organizations (Hutchinson, Draper, & Sales, 2009) and the identification of patient outcomes (Doran, Hirdes, Poss, et al., 2009).

Funding and Utilization of Home Care Services

The majority of home care is funded by provincial and territorial governments through health budgets that are administered by regional health authorities, departments of health and social services, local health integration networks, or, in Ontario, community care access centres. The federal government also funds home care services through departments such as the First Nations and Inuit Branch of Health Canada and Veterans Affairs Canada (Table 6-1).

The use of home care services in Canada has grown considerably since the 1990s. In the period 1994 to 1995, the government spent $1.6 billion on home care. By 2003/04, home care spending had risen to $3.4 billion and represented 4.2% of total government health spending (Canadian Healthcare Association, 2009). Even though in 2010/11 spending grew to $5.9 billion, the total government spending ratio remained relatively the same at 4.1% (CHCA, 2013). Factors contributing to the rising costs include not only the increased numbers of individuals using the services but also the costs associated with medical technology and equipment, access to mobile electronic records, and demand for both professional and supportive care for older adults with complex health care needs who are discharged from hospitals.

Sometimes the frequency or duration of the government-funded home care services (e.g., the number of nursing visits, the number of hours of supportive care services such as homemaking, and length of time on the program) is not deemed sufficient by the patient or the family. In those instances, they may choose to purchase additional services either through insurance or with their own financial resources. The Canadian Healthcare Association (2009) reported that between 2 and 5% of Canadians purchase home care services not funded by government. In addition, it is estimated that 70 to 80% of the care of older adults in the community is provided by family and friends, which, if paid, would amount to approximately $25 billion annually (Carers Canada, n.d.).

Home Health Care Team

Nursing Roles. The home health care team is composed of the *home health nurse* and a variety of team members who work

TABLE 6-2 MEMBERS OF THE HOME HEALTH CARE TEAM

Member	Description
Community health nurse	A registered nurse whose practice specialty promotes the health of individuals, families, communities, and populations and an environment that supports health. A CHN practices in diverse settings such as homes, schools, shelters, churches, community health centres, and on the street (CHNC, 2011).
Home care or home health nurse	A CHN who uses knowledge from primary health care (including the determinants of health), nursing science, and social sciences to focus on disease prevention, health restoration and maintenance, or palliation for patients, their caregivers, and families (CHNC, 2011) and who generally travels to the patient to provide care.
Case manager	The health care team member who leads the process of case management: "a collaborative strategy undertaken by health care professionals and clients to maximize the client's ability and autonomy through advocacy, communication, education, identification of and access to requisite resources, and service coordination" (CHCA, 2007, p. 3).
Community health worker or home support worker	An unlicensed care provider who assists individuals with ADLs such as bathing, dressing, and meal preparation, as well as IADLs such as housekeeping, shopping, and social recreational activities (Canadian Research Network for Care in the Community, 2010).
Nurse practitioner	An advanced-practice nurse who provides "direct care focusing on health promotion and the treatment and management of health conditions. [Nurse practitioners] are registered nurses with additional educational preparation and experience who possess and demonstrate the competencies to autonomously diagnosis, order and interpret diagnostic tests, prescribe pharmaceuticals and perform specific procedures within their legislated scope of practice" (CNA, 2008, p. 16).
Clinical nurse specialist	An advanced-practice nurse who provides expertise for specialized populations. Clinical nurse specialists play a leading role in the development of clinical guidelines and the use of evidence, provide expert consultation, and facilitate system change (CNA, 2008).

ADLs, activities of daily living; *CHCA*, Canadian Home Care Association; *CNA*, Canadian Nurses Association; *CHN*, community health nurse; *CHNC*, Community Health Nurses of Canada; *IADLs*, instrumental activities of daily living.

in close collaboration with the patient, the family, and medical practitioners (Table 6-2). Nurses who work on the home health care team include registered nurses and licensed practical nurses, as well as nurse practitioners and clinical nurse specialists. Home health nurses are *registered nurses* and *licensed practical nurses* who provide a variety of nursing assessments, planning and implementing of interventions, and teaching to assist individuals in optimizing their health in their home setting. *Nurse practitioners* use their in-depth nursing knowledge and their advanced scope of practice to diagnose and treat acute and chronic diseases. Nurse practitioners often provide care for homebound patients who do not have access to a primary care physician (CNA, 2008). *Clinical nurse specialists* promote the use of evidence-informed practice and system changes by providing expert consultation and leadership in guideline and policy development in the

community setting (CNA, 2008). *Unregulated care providers* make an essential contribution to quality of life for the patient by supporting the patient's activities of daily living (ADLs), including bathing, preparing meals, and performing household chores and personal errands (Canadian Research Network for Care in the Community, 2010). They provide an important social connection with patients and are often the team members who spend the most time with them. These individuals also may provide delegated or assigned nursing care for patients with long-term frequent and predictable health needs (e.g., daily routine medication). Rehabilitation specialists—including physiotherapists, occupational therapists, and speech–language pathologists—are crucial members of the home care team, as are social workers, pharmacists, dietitians, and respiratory therapists. The role of the *case manager* is to coordinate the comprehensive care plan and services for the patient, including arranging for and funding services. All members of the home health care team work collaboratively to evaluate the patient's progress, make appropriate changes to the care plan, and develop the discharge plan. The home health care team members actively include the patient's family members in all aspects of care.

Home Health Care Patients

Although home health nurses may care for newborns, young children, teenagers, and adults of all ages, in the period 2009 to 2010, 82% of individuals who received home care services were 65 years of age or older (CIHI, 2011)—a statistic that reflects Canada's aging population. The individuals served also reflect the growing cultural diversity in Canada. The most common diagnosed health conditions in home care patients relate to dementia, cardiovascular disease, musculo-skeletal and neurological diseases, and other common chronic diseases (e.g., cancer, chronic obstructive pulmonary disease, diabetes). CHNs in all roles play an important part in the prevention and management of chronic illness by (a) promoting regular health screening, (b) incorporating health promotion and disease prevention strategies into their practice, and (c) assisting individuals and families in managing chronic illness in the home.

As they face the physical and cognitive decline associated with many chronic conditions, many home care patients live alone. Nearly 40% of home care patients (CIHI, 2011) receive home support services to assist with both their ADLs and instrumental ADLs, and close to one-third receive nursing services (CIHI, 2011). The majority of patients who receive home care services require long-term supportive care or acute, short-term-focused services (e.g., postoperative care); smaller percentages receive end-of-life and rehabilitative care (CIHI, 2011). These patient characteristics have implications for home care nurses' role, competencies, and standards.

Home Health Nursing Practice

Overview. Home health nursing is a unique and diverse practice that requires specific clinical competencies. Home health nurses navigate the full spectrum of traffic and weather conditions and cope with unexpected situations ranging from power failures to uncooperative family pets. They work in isolation and use strategies to protect patient privacy and confidentiality within neighbourhoods. Home health nurses need to be extremely organized and be able to work with a high level of autonomy. They require knowledge of community resources and proficiency in time management, case management, communication, and physical, psychosocial, and environmental assessment, as well as in care planning and evaluation. They must understand and work within funding models, service limits, productivity expectations, referral processes, and employer and funder reporting requirements. Many of these competencies differ from those of nurses in other care settings and sectors. Accordingly, the CHNC (2011) developed standards of practice for community health nurses. The following seven interrelated standards of practice form the core expectations for community health nursing:

1. Health promotion
2. Prevention and health protection
3. Health maintenance, restoration, and palliation
4. Professional relationships
5. Capacity building
6. Access and equity
7. Professional responsibility and accountability

On the basis of the standards, detailed practice competencies were developed by CHNC in 2010, and these are described later in this chapter.

Home Health Nursing and Family-Centred Care. Nursing in the home occurs in a very different context than nursing in the hospital. In the hospital, the health care team has the dominant role and the environment is controlled. In the home, the patient, caregiver, or family (or a combination of these) plays the dominant role; the nurse is a guest in the house and must adapt to the home environment. Consequently, it is especially important that the home health nurse demonstrate a holistic, nonjudgemental, and family-centred philosophy and negotiate the care with the patient and family.

Family-centred care is "bringing the perspectives of patients and families directly into the planning, delivery, and evaluation of health care, and thereby improving its quality and safety" (Institute for Patient- and Family-Centered Care [IPFCC], 2011, p. 3). The core concepts of family-centred care include dignity and respect, information sharing, participation, and collaboration (IPFCC, 2011). The patient's knowledge, beliefs, values, and culture are considered in the planning and provision of care. Information sharing must be timely, accurate, unbiased, and complete to ensure patients and families can participate in decision making to the extent they choose (MacKay & Gregory, 2011). Family-centred care also involves collaboration among health care providers and patients and their families to develop, implement, and evaluate policies, programs, and professional education.

Family-centred care involves the recognition that an illness experienced by one family member will affect the entire family (Saint Elizabeth Health Care, 2011). Families often provide care for ill members and assist in decision making about all aspects of the care provided, including priority setting. Visits by community health care professionals are usually episodic, leaving the family with the burden of care. Home health nursing visits may be as frequent as several times a day or as infrequent as once a month. Visits may be lengthy, such as the initial visit, when the extensive admission assessment is completed; or they may be fairly short, such as visits to assess health status, including wound healing, pain control, or symptom management. Nursing care during a visit may be administered according to a predetermined routine such as one specified in a care pathway, or it may be directed toward newly arising symptoms or health concerns.

In some situations, an older patient may be cared for by a spouse of similar age with chronic illnesses. In other situations, an older parent needing care may live with a busy middle-aged family member with dependent children, or a person may be caring for a dying spouse at home. In these situations, it is not uncommon for caregivers to become physically, emotionally, and economically overwhelmed with the responsibilities and demands of caring for a family member (Carers Canada, n.d.; Saint Elizabeth Health Care, 2010). The home health nurse is a lifeline for the family, helping them understand their loved one's health condition and needs, cope with changing roles and responsibilities, and make decisions about ongoing care arrangements.

Assessment of the signs of caregiver burnout (e.g., sleeplessness, difficulty concentrating) is a critical role of the home care nurse (Saint Elizabeth Health Care, 2010). The focus of care is on empowering the patient and family to meet the identified health care needs while also feeling in control of their lives. The goals of care may be short- or long-term in nature. One way a nurse can help family members cope with their increased responsibilities is to provide referrals to various support groups in the community or to other resources. The nurse can also work with the case manager to advocate for additional home care services to reduce the burden of care, for example, through a personal support worker, more frequent nursing visits, short-term respite placement, or support from a social worker.

CULTURALLY COMPETENT CARE

HOME HEALTH NURSING PRACTICE

Home health care is delivered within the context of the family's and the patient's cultural values and beliefs. Strategies to overcome language barriers may be needed, and the home health nurse is more likely than other nurses to encounter the patient's use of healing practices arising from cultural beliefs and the use of home remedies and complementary and alternative therapies. The ability to apply culturally relevant care is one of the competencies expected of home health nurses (CHNC, 2010). The home health nurse demonstrates culturally sensitive care by having an understanding of how culture can affect beliefs and behaviours (College of Nurses of Ontario, 2009) and the social and spiritual needs of the individual. Exploring and recognizing the individual's cultural practices, values, and needs and including them in the plan of care are essential to home health nursing practice. (Culture is discussed in Chapter 2, and complementary and alternative therapies are discussed in Chapter 12.)

Home Health Nursing Practice Knowledge and Skills. It is generally acknowledged that the acuity of patients who require home health nursing has been rising steadily and is now very high (CNA, 2013; Lang & Edwards, 2006). As Lang and Edwards (2006) observed,

> Unlike working on a specialized unit in a hospital, home care providers must maintain a *breadth* of general and specific knowledge. This poses a significant safety challenge because of the diversity and varied frequency of health conditions and treatments. It is not unusual to come across particular conditions or treatments only once every few months, making it difficult to maintain competence. This is heightened by: the trend for earlier discharge from hospitals and the corresponding increase in the acuity of patients receiving home care services; the lack of resources for continuing education and proficiencies; and the isolated nature of the practice of home care. (p. 24)

Specific competencies for home care nurses have been established in Canada (CHNC, 2011) and in the United States (American Nurses Association, 2008). These competencies reflect the knowledge, skills, judgement, and attitudes associated with home care nursing practice. The CHNC (2011) listed three

TABLE 6-3	SPECIFIC COMPETENCIES FOR CANADIAN HOME CARE NURSES

Elements of Home Health Nursing
- Assessment, monitoring, and clinical decision making
- Care planning and care coordination
- Health maintenance, restoration, and palliation
- Teaching and education
- Communication
- Relationships
- Access and equity
- Building capacity

Foundations of Home Health Nursing
- Health promotion
- Illness prevention and health protection

Quality and Professional Responsibility
- Quality care
- Professional responsibility

Source: Community Health Nurses of Canada. (2010). Home health nursing competencies (version 1.0). Toronto: Author. Retrieved from *http://login.greatbignews. com/UserFiles/289/documents/HomeHealthNursingCompetenciesVersion1March2010. pdf*.

FIGURE 6-1 Nurse providing skilled care in the home. Source: Victorian Order of Nurses Canada.

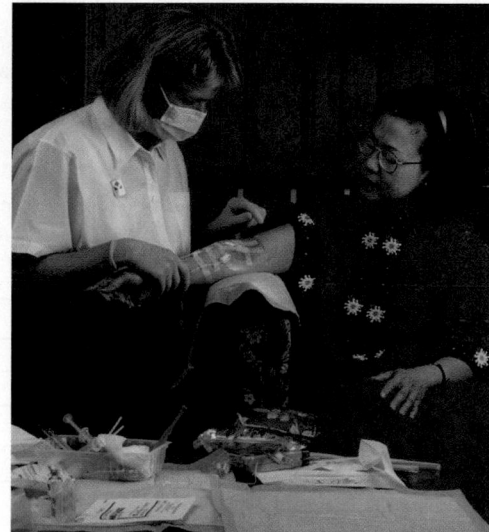

FIGURE 6-2 Nurse providing peripherally inserted central catheter (PICC) care in the home. Source: Victorian Order of Nurses Canada.

categories of competencies: (a) elements of home health nursing, (b) foundations of home health nursing, and (c) quality and professional responsibility (Table 6-3). Competencies associated with the elements of home health nursing focus on the nursing activities, functions, goals, and outcomes that are central to home care nursing practice (CHNC, 2011). Competencies associated with the foundations of home care nursing are related to the philosophy of primary health care and the core knowledge necessary in home care nursing practice (CHNC, 2011). Competencies associated with quality and professional responsibility focus on the strategies and activities that demonstrate professionalism and promote quality care (CHNC, 2011). Because many of the standards and competencies of community health nursing are unique, this branch of nursing is recognized as a specialty practice by the Canadian Nurses Association. Today, any nurse whose practice is community-based may choose to earn a national credential—CCHN (Certified in Community Health Nursing—Canada)—to indicate her or his expertise.

In addition to needing specific skills, home health nurses require general knowledge of the range of health care equipment or assistive devices used to promote independence. They must also be familiar with a wide variety of medical supplies and devices, such as chest and wound drainage tubes, intravenous therapy supplies, urinary catheters, enterostomy supplies, wound care products, enteral feeding equipment (Figure 6-1), central vascular access devices (Figure 6-2), and infusion pumps. Understanding rehabilitation techniques and terminology is helpful in collaborating with therapists, supporting the patient's progress, and evaluating the plan of care. Home care nurses also teach self-management strategies to assist individuals in managing chronic disease; the ideal result is to delay their placement in a residential home or admission to hospital. Assigning and delegating care to members of the health care team as part of the overall plan of care is a critical competency. Clinical documentation skills are also important for reflecting professional accountability and substantiating recommendations made about the patient's needs, the care provided, and the patient's response.

Establishing and maintaining a therapeutic nurse–patient relationship is fundamental for effective home care nursing practice. Therefore, effective communication strategies and techniques are crucial. Because family members are encouraged to learn how to administer treatments and manage equipment, the nurse must be able to teach certain skills to both the patient and family. Providing such care may seem overwhelming to them initially. The home health nurse assesses the readiness of the caregiver to assume the care, teaches it in a way that is most helpful for the learner, and evaluates the outcomes of care, including the coping of the caregiver.

Hospice palliative care is another important component of home health nursing practice. The Canadian Hospice Palliative Care Association defines **hospice palliative care** as

an approach that improves the quality of life of patients and their families facing the problems associated with life-threatening illness, through the prevention and relief of suffering by means of early identification and impeccable assessment and treatment of pain and other problems, physical, psychosocial and spiritual. (as cited in World Health Organization, 2015b)

Hospice palliative care is not limited to those with cancer diagnoses; it "is appropriate for any patient and/or family living

Competency Assessment Planning and Evaluation Tool (CAPE Tool)
Home Care Nurse, Fraser Health, Surrey, BC

EXCERPT

Date of first assessment   Date of second assessment   Preceptee   Preceptor   Facilitator

CRNBC Standards (College of RNs of BC)			Home Care Nurse Standards	
CRNBC	HCNs		HCNs	
1	5	Responsibility and accountability	1	Promoting health: • Health promotion • Prevention and health protection • Health maintenance restoration and palliation
2	1, 2, 3	Specialized body of knowledge	2	Building individual and community capacity
3	1, 2, 3	Competent application of knowledge	3	Building relationships
4	3, 4	Code of ethics	4	Facilitating access and equity
5	1, 4	Provision of service to the public	5	Demonstrating professional responsibility and accountability
6	5	Self-regulation		

	CRNBC Standards (College of RNs of BC)	Initial Self-Assessment	2.5-Month Self-Assessment	1-Year Self-Assessment	Learning Activities/ Resources	• Reviewed with Mentor/ Preceptor Clinical Educator/CRN Manager Peer • Planned Learning Activities	KEY: 1. Needs education and practice 2. Knowledgeable but needs practice 3. Competent: Independent practice 4. Proficient practice 5. Expert practice Achievement and Validation of Competency (include examples from clinical practice and learning plan) Date and Signature
CRNBC STD.	*COMPETENCY STATEMENTS*						
	1. RESPONSIBILITY/ACCOUNTABILITY/SELF-REGULATION						
1, 6	1. Recognizes own limitations in professional practice and seeks help from appropriate resoures when needed.						
1, 6	2. At all times practices in a safe manner, is accountable, and takes responsibility for own practice.						
	3. Maintains own mental, physical, emotional well being.						
	4. Practices safety and ethically according to: • FH standards, protocols, policies • CRNBC standards of practice/HCN community standards and phibsophy						
	5. Responsible and accountable for regular and prompt attendance at work.						

FIGURE 6-3 A sample orientation tool. Source: Fraser Health, Surrey, BC.

with, or at risk of developing, a life-threatening illness due to any diagnosis, with any prognosis, regardless of age, and at any time they have unmet expectations and/or needs, and are prepared to accept care" (Canadian Hospice Palliative Care Association, 2009, p. 8). The home health nurse is often the linchpin in achieving the highest possible quality of life for the patient and family throughout the palliative and bereavement experience.

Trends in Home Health Nursing

New Nursing Graduates and Licensed Practical Nurses in Home Health Nursing. Because of the breadth and depth of knowledge and skills required by the home health nurse, it was widely believed for many years that nurses required a minimum of 2 years of acute care hospital experience before being hired as a home health nurse. Furthermore, registered nurses generally received hiring preference over licensed practical nurses because it was believed that registered nurse preparation provided the best foundation for home care nursing. However, partly because of the growing nursing shortage, enhancements to the scope of practice and educational programs for licensed practical nurses, and the need to provide long-term interventions to a growing population with complex and unpredictable care needs, many home health employers now hire both registered nurses and licensed practical nurses right after graduation. To support these new graduates and new home health nurses, a variety of intensive orientation programs and tools have been developed to complement student placement and employment experiences (Meadows, 2009). Figure 6-3 depicts a sample orientation tool.

Technology in Home Health Nursing Practice

Surgical innovations, such as microscopic surgical techniques that have transformed many operations into day-surgery procedures, and medical interventions, such as advances in life support of premature infants, have allowed individuals to live longer and have shifted both acute and long-term care to community-based settings. An array of mechanical devices—including ventilators, infusion pumps, and peritoneal dialysis night cyclers—have been redesigned and miniaturized for portability and ease of use, making it possible for patients to remain at home while receiving intravenous antibiotics, chemotherapy, or total parenteral nutrition. Internet-based education and information programs are now common, and telemonitoring systems are enabling nurses and other health care providers to assess a patient's physical status from a remote location (Figure 6-4). As well, digital cameras are being used to take pictures of complex wounds; the pictures are then transferred via computer to a wound specialist for expert assessment and treatment recommendations (Figure 6-5).

Home care nurses are accessing clinical information and best practice evidence at the point of care through devices such as smartphones; such devices are also used to document patient health data that, in turn, is used to monitor and track clinical outcomes (Ontario Ministry of Health and Long-Term Care, 2008). Several of the nursing best practice guidelines published by the Registered Nurses' Association of Ontario are now available as applications for hand-held devices, including the iPhone and Android smartphones. Indeed, today's home health nurses are as likely to arrive at the patient's home holding a digital device, a digital camera, or a laptop or tablet as they would a stethoscope. Computerized clinical documentation systems (Figure 6-6) and electronic health records are now being used by a growing number of home health nurses. The home health nurse is able to review the patient's history and plan of care and update the electronic health record as care is given. The accessibility of electronic health records facilitates continuity of care, promotes quality, and reduces documentation time. The complexity of ensuring privacy and confidentiality, however, grows with nurses managing both technological devices and transitional paper charts.

Measurement of Nursing-Sensitive Outcomes

Nursing-sensitive outcomes are "those that are relevant, based on nurses' scope and domain of practice, and for which there is empirical evidence linking nursing inputs and interventions to

FIGURE 6-5 Home health nurse examining digital photos of a wound, using Pixalere software. Source: Fraser Health, Surrey, BC.

FIGURE 6-4 Patient at a telemonitoring station in his home. Source: Saint Elizabeth Health Care, Markham, ON.

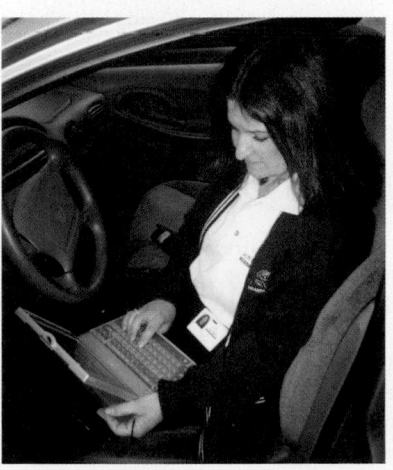

FIGURE 6-6 Home health nurse using a laptop computer in her car. Source: Saint Elizabeth Health Care, Markham, ON.

the outcomes" (Doran, 2003, pp. vii–ix). Nurses need to know the outcomes associated with their care in order to assess the effectiveness of the patient's care plan and make revisions as indicated. They may also use outcomes data to evaluate their own practice or that of their team or program. Decision makers and funders require outcomes data to support budget needs, program design and delivery, and the development of accountability mechanisms such as balanced scorecards. Research has demonstrated that it is feasible for nurses to collect electronic or manual data on nursing-sensitive outcomes in home health, acute care hospitals, and long-term care settings (Doran, Harrison, Laschinger, et al., 2004). On the basis of those results, the Canadian Health Outcomes for Better Information and Care

(C-HOBIC, 2015), a two-phase project, was launched to test the collection of patient outcome information related to nursing care in the electronic health records of Ontario, Prince Edward Island, and Saskatchewan.

SUMMARY

Nursing in the community represents a dynamic and fulfilling practice specialty for nurses. Community-based nursing is an essential component of the health care system and offers the opportunity to positively influence the health and outcomes of individuals, communities, and populations.

CASE STUDY

Home Health Care for Patient With Infected Leg Ulcer

Source: Shutterstock.com.

Patient Profile

Melody Tennant, 43 years old, has been referred to home care for care of her infected leg wound and intravenous antibiotics. She lives alone in an apartment with her cat in an area of town identified as having a high number of calls to the police. Ms. Tennant worked as a food server but is currently out of work. She is candid with the nurse completing her admission and shares the fact that she has been trying to stop her intravenous drug use for years. Her right lower leg ulcer is the result of injection drugs 6 months ago. The injection site became a "sore" and "just never healed." Ms. Tennant went to the walk-in clinic when she could no longer stand the pain and her boyfriend noticed her leg was pink and warm to touch. The walk-in clinic physician sent her to the emergency department, where a methicillin-resistant *Staphylococcus aureus* (MRSA)–infected leg wound was diagnosed.

Subjective Data
- Has a history of being hepatitis B positive (3 years)
- Has varicose veins in both legs; worries that, because of these, the home care nurses will want her to wear support stockings, which she finds "ugly"
- Complains of pain in her right lower leg and asks for "something to take the edge off"

Objective Data
Physical Examination
- Peripheral intravenous site (saline lock) in left hand
- Dressing to right lower leg: 10- × 10-cm foam dressing with adhesive edges

- Right lower leg ulcer: 10% pink base, 90% yellow base, irregular flat edges. Wound size is 0.5 cm deep, 7 cm long, 4.4 cm wide. Periwound skin is deep pink, and the diameter of the right lower leg calf is greater than that of the left.

Collaborative Care
- Methadone, 50 mg PO once daily
- Vancomycin, 1 000 mg intravenously BID
- Multivitamin, 1 tablet PO daily
- High-protein diet

Discussion Questions
1. *Priority decision:* What are the initial priorities for the home health nurse?
2. What other members of the health care team should be involved in the care of Ms. Tennant? What are their roles and responsibilities?
3. *Priority decision:* What type of patient education program should be implemented? What are the priority teaching goals to promote self-management?
4. What should the nurse consider in the nutrition assessment? How will the nurse address economic considerations related to Ms. Tennant's diet?
5. How can the nurse address Ms. Tennant's coping skills and use community resources to intervene with her mental health and substance use?
6. What types of supplies will Ms. Tennant need? What diagnostics, teaching, and community resources should accompany the use of these supplies?
7. What are the expected long-term outcomes for Ms. Tennant?

ⓔvolve

Answers are available at http://evolve.elsevier.com/Canada/Lewis/medsurg.

■ REVIEW QUESTIONS

The number of the question corresponds to the same-numbered objective at the beginning of the chapter.

1. Which of the following statements is correct about public health nursing?
   a. It predates home health nursing.
   b. It focuses on health promotion and disease prevention.
   c. It does not include health teaching.
   d. It takes place predominantly in private homes.

2. Which of the following statements best describes nurses working in community health settings?

a. They function autonomously in meeting client needs.
b. They focus only on client needs specific to the setting.
c. They use the same skills as in acute care settings.
d. They use case-management skills along the continuum of care.

3. Which of the following trends is affecting home care and threatening the sustainability of Canada's health care system?
   a. The long wait times for surgery
   b. The increased number of people hospitalized with acute illness
   c. The shortage of health care providers
   d. The high rate of health care–associated infections

4. Which of the following best describes primary health care?
   a. The first health care provider a client sees
   b. Public health nursing
   c. A philosophy that emphasizes health promotion, disease prevention, and client participation in care
   d. A theoretical model

5. Which of the following statements best reflects the reality of home care services in Canada?
   a. The use of home health services is increasing.
   b. The use of home health services is decreasing.
   c. Home health services are not yet available in all provinces and territories.
   d. Home health services are used more by families than by single clients.

6. Which of the following is a home care nurse competency? *(Select all that apply)*

a. Appreciate and understand the roles and responsibilities and the contributions of other regulated and unregulated health care workers involved in the client's care plan.
b. Assist clients and their families to recognize that their capacity for managing their own health care needs is limited by the resources available to them.
c. Limit participation in collaborative, interdisciplinary, and intersectoral partnerships to enhance the health of clients and families.
d. Keep knowledge current to ensure optimal case management.

1. b; 2. d; 3. c; 4. c; 5. a; 6. a, b.

Ⓔvolve

For even more review questions, visit *http://evolve.elsevier.com/Canada/Lewis/medsurg.*

REFERENCES

Accreditation Canada. (2015). *The value and impact of health care accreditation: A literature review.* Retrieved from *https://accreditation.ca/publications-menu.*

Allemang, M. (2000). *Community nursing: Promoting Canadians' health.* Toronto: W. B. Saunders Canada. (Seminal).

American Nurses Association. (2008). *Home health nursing: Scope and standards of practice.* Silver Spring, MD: Author. (Seminal).

Canadian Healthcare Association. (2009). *Home care in Canada: From the margins to the mainstream.* Ottawa: Author. Retrieved from *http://www.healthcarecan.ca/wp-content/themes/camyno/assets/document/PolicyDocs/2009/External/EN/HomeCareCanada_MarginsMainstream_EN.pdf.* (Seminal).

Canadian Health Outcomes for Better Information and Care (C-HOBIC). (2015). *About C-HOBIC.* Retrieved from *http://c-hobic.cna-aiic.ca/about/default_e.aspx.*

Canadian Home Care Association (CHCA). (2007). *Implementing case management as a strategy for systems integration: Experiences from the CHCA national partnership project.* Ottawa: Author. Retrieved from *http://www.cdnhomecare.ca/media.php?mid=1557.* (Seminal).

Canadian Home Care Association (CHCA). (2013). *Portraits of home care in Canada.* Ottawa: Author.

Canadian Hospice Palliative Care Association. (2009). *Canadian hospice palliative care nursing standards of practice.* Ottawa: Canadian Hospice Palliative Care Association Nursing Standards Committee. Retrieved from *http://www.chpca.net/media/7505/Canadian_Hospice_Palliative_Care_Nursing_Standards_2009.pdf.* (Seminal).

Canadian Institute for Health Information. (2011). *Health care in Canada, 2011. A focus on seniors and aging.* Retrieved from *https://secure.cihi.ca/free_products/HCIC_2011_seniors_report_en.pdf.*

Canadian Institute for Health Information. (2015a). *Regulated nurses: Canadian trends, 2014.* Ottawa: Author. Retrieved from *https://secure.cihi.ca/estore/productFamily.htm?locale=en&pf=PFC2898&lang=en.*

Canadian Institute for Health Information. (2015b). *National health expenditure trends, 1975 to 2015.* Ottawa: Author. Retrieved from *https://www.cihi.ca//en/spending-and-health-workforce/spending/national-health-expenditure-trends.*

Canadian Institute for Health Information. (2015c). *HCRS metadata.* Ottawa: Author. Retrieved from *https://www.cihi.ca/en/types-of-care/community-care/home-care/hcrs-metadata.*

Canadian Institute for Health Information. (2016a). *How does health spending differ across provinces and territories?* Retrieved from *https://www.cihi.ca/en/spending-and-health-workforce/spending/national-health-expenditure-trends/nhex2016-topic6.*

Canadian Institute for Health Information. (2016b). *How much does Canada spend on health care?* Retrieved from *https://www.cihi.ca/en/spending-and-health-workforce/spending/national-health-expenditure-trends/nhex2016-topic1.*

Canadian Medical Association. (2015). *Palliative care—Canadian Medical Association's national call to action.* Retrieved from *https://www.cma.ca/Assets/assets-library/document/en/advocacy/palliative-care-report-online-e.pdf.*

Canadian Nurses Association (CNA). (2008). *Advanced nursing practice: A national framework.* Retrieved from *https://www.cna-aiic.ca/~/media/cna/page-content/pdf-en/anp_national_framework_e.pdf.* (Seminal).

Canadian Nurses Association (CNA). (2010). *Canadian nurse practitioner core competency framework.* Ottawa: Author. Retrieved from *https://www.cna-aiic.ca/~/media/cna/files/en/competency_framework_2010_e.pdf.* (Seminal).

Canadian Nurses Association (CNA). (2012). *Registered nurses education in Canada statistics 2009–2010.* Retrieved from *http://casn.ca/wp-content/uploads/2014/10/FINALNSFS20092010sENGJanuary252012Copy.pdf.*

Canadian Nurses Association (CNA). (2013). *Optimizing the role of nursing in home health.* Ottawa: Author. Retrieved from *https://www.cna-aiic.ca/~/media/cna/page-content/pdf-en/optimizing_the_role_of_nursing_in_home_health_e.pdf?la=en.*

Canadian Nurses Association (CNA). (2014). *Optimizing the role of nurses in primary care in Canada.* Ottawa: Author. Retrieved from *https://cna-aiic.ca/~/media/cna/page-content/pdf-en/optimizing-the-role-of-nurses-in-primary-care-in-canada.pdf.*

Canadian Nurses Association (CNA). (2015). *Establish standards for home care.* Retrieved from *http://cna-aiic.ca/~/media/cna/page-content/pdf-en/establish-standards-for-home-care_e.pdf.*

Canadian Patient Safety Institute (CPSI). (2013). *Safety at home. A pan-Canadian home care study of safety.* Retrieved from *http://www.patientsafetyinstitute.ca/en/toolsResources/Research/commissionedResearch/SafetyatHome/Documents/Safety At Home Care.pdf.*

Canadian Public Health Association. (2008). *A tool for strengthening chronic disease prevention and management.* Retrieved from *https://www.cpha.ca/sites/default/files/uploads/resources/chronicdiseasetool/intro_e.pdf.* (Seminal).

Canadian Public Health Association. (2010). *Public health—Community health nursing practice in Canada: Roles and activities* (4th ed.). Ottawa: Author. Retrieved from *http://www.cpha.ca/uploads/pubs/3-1bk04214.pdf*. (Seminal).

Canadian Research Network for Care in the Community. (2010). *Home support workers in the continuum of care for older people.* Retrieved from *http://www.ryerson.ca/content/dam/crncc/knowledge/infocus/factsheets/InFocus%20Home%20Support%20Workers.pdf*.

Carers Canada. (n.d.). *Carer facts.* Retrieved from *http://www.carerscanada.ca/carer-facts/*.

Carter, A. (2009). Nursing shortage predicted to be hardest on home healthcare. *Home Healthcare Nurse, 27*(3), 198–Seminal).

Chalmers, K. I., & Kristjanson, L. J. (1992). Community health nursing practice. In A. J. Baumgart & J. Larsen (Eds.), *Canadian nursing faces the future* (2nd ed., pp. 153–179). St. Louis: Mosby. (Seminal).

College of Nurses of Ontario. (2009). *Practice guideline: Culturally sensitive care.* Retrieved from *http://www.cno.org/globalassets/docs/prac/41040_culturallysens.pdf*. (Seminal).

Community Health Nurses of Canada (CHNC). (2010). *Home health nursing competencies* (version 1.0). Toronto: Author. Retrieved from *http://login.greatbignews.com/UserFiles/289/documents/HomeHealthNursingCompetenciesVersion1March2010.pdf*. (Seminal).

Community Health Nurses of Canada (CHNC). (2011). *Canadian community health nursing: Professional practice model and standards of practice.* Toronto: Author. Retrieved from *http://www.chnc.ca/documents/CHNC-ProfessionalPracticeModel-EN/index.html#/1*. Revised March 2011.

Doran, D. M. (Ed.), (2003). *Nursing sensitive outcomes: State of the science.* Sudbury, MA: Jones and Bartlett. (Seminal).

Doran, D., Harrison, M. B., Laschinger, H., et al. (2004). *Collecting data on nursing-sensitive outcomes in different care settings: Can it be done? What are the benefits?: Report of the Nursing and Health Outcomes Feasibility Study.* Retrieved from *http://www.ontla.on.ca/library/repository/mon/15000/261600.pdf*. (Seminal).

Doran, D. M., Hirdes, J., Poss, J., et al. (2009). Identification of safety outcomes for Canadian home care clients: Evidence from the Resident Assessment Instrument—Home Care reporting system concerning emergency room visits. *Healthcare Quarterly, 12*(Special Issue), 40–48. (Seminal).

Doran, D. M., Mildon, B., & Clarke, S. (2011). Towards a national report card in nursing: A knowledge synthesis. *Canadian Journal of Nursing Leadership, 24*(2), 38–57.

Emory, F. (1953). *Public health nursing in Canada: Principles and practice* (Rev. ed.). Toronto: Macmillan. (Seminal).

Foebel, A. D., Hirdes, J. P., Heckman, G. A., et al. (2011). A profile of older community-dwelling home care clients with heart failure in Ontario. *Chronic Diseases in Canada, 31*(2), 49–57.

Health Canada. (2012). *Health system: About primary health care.* Retrieved from *http://healthycanadians.gc.ca/health-system-systeme-sante/services/primary-primaires/about-apropos-eng.php*.

Health Council of Canada. (2008a). *Fixing the foundation: An update on primary health care and home care renewal in Canada.* Toronto: Author. Retrieved from *http://www.healthcouncilcanada.ca/tree/2.26-HCC_PHC_Main_web_E.pdf*. (Seminal).

Health Council of Canada. (2008b). *Rekindling reform: Health care renewal in Canada, 2003–2008. Summary.* Retrieved from *http://www.healthcouncilcanada.ca/tree/2.46-HCC_5YRPLAN_WEB_FA.pdf*. (Seminal).

Hutchinson, A. M., Draper, K., & Sales, A. E. (2009). Public reporting of nursing home quality of care: Lessons from the United States experience for Canadian policy discussion. *Healthcare Policy, 5*(2), 87–105. (Seminal).

Institute for Patient- and Family-Centered Care. (2011). *Advancing the practice of patient- and family-centered care in hospitals: How to get started.* Retrieved from *http://www.ipfcc.org/pdf/getting_started.pdf*.

Institute of Medicine. (1999). *To err is human: Building a safer health system.* Washington, DC: Author. (Seminal).

Lang, A. (2010). There's no place like home: Research, practice and policy perspectives regarding safety in home care. *International Journal for Quality in Health Care, 22*(2), 75–76. doi:10.1093/intqhc/mzq007. (Seminal).

Lang, A., & Edwards, N. (2006). *Safety in home care: Broadening the patient safety agenda to include home care services.* Retrieved from *http://www.patientsafetyinstitute.ca/en/toolsResources/Research/commissionedResearch/SafetyinHomeCare/Pages/default.aspx*. (Seminal).

Lang, A., Edwards, N., & Fleiszer, A. (2008). Safety in home care: A broadened perspective of patient safety. *International Journal for Quality in Health Care, 20*(2), 130–135. doi:10.1093/intqhc/mzm068. (Seminal).

MacKay, L. J., & Gregory, D. J. (2011). Exploring family-centered care among pediatric oncology nurses. *Pediatric Oncology Nursing, 28*(1), 43–52. doi:10.1177/1043454210377179.

Meadows, C. (2009). Integrating new graduate nurses in home health care. *Home Healthcare Nurse, 27*(9), 561–568. doi:10.1097/01.NHH.0000361929.52668.10. (Seminal).

Morgan, M. W., Zamora, N. E., & Hindmarsh, M. F. (2007). An inconvenient truth: A sustainable healthcare system requires chronic disease prevention and management transformation. *Healthcare Papers, 7*(4), 39–42. (Seminal).

Nagle, L. M. (2008). Show me the way to stay home. *Canadian Journal of Nursing Leadership, 12*(4), 29–32. (Seminal).

Ontario Ministry of Health and Long-Term Care. (2008). *Backgrounder: PDA initiative for Ontario nurses.* Retrieved from *http://www.southeastlhin.on.ca/Page.aspx?id=198030AB9B96468187D76EB5BA720912*. (Seminal).

Pastor, D. K. (2006). Home sweet home: A concept analysis of home visiting. *Home Healthcare Nurse, 24*(6), 389–394. (Seminal).

Saint Elizabeth Health Care. (2010). *Caregiver compass.* Retrieved from *https://www.saintelizabeth.com/Caring-for-Family/Caregiver-Compass.aspx*. (Seminal).

Saint Elizabeth Health Care. (2011). *Client-centred care in the Canadian home and community sector: A review of key concepts.* Retrieved from *http://www.cdnhomecare.ca/content.php?doc=256*.

Statistics Canada. (2006). *Findings from the 2005 National Survey of the Work and Health of Nurses* (Cat. No. 83-003-XPE). Ottawa: Author. Retrieved from *https://www.cihi.ca/en/nursing_nswhn_summary2005_en.pdf*. (Seminal).

Statistics Canada. (2015). *Canada's population estimates: Age and sex.* Ottawa: Author. Retrieved from *http://www.statcan.gc.ca/daily-quotidien/150929/dq150929b-eng.htm?HPA*.

VanDeVelde-Coke, S. A. (2004). *The effectiveness and efficiency of providing home care visits in nursing clinics versus the traditional home setting.* Ottawa: Canadian Health Services Research Foundation. (Seminal).

World Health Organization. (1978). *Primary health care: Report of the International Conference on Primary Health Care, Alma-Ata, USSR, September 6–12, 1978*. Retrieved from *http://www.who.int/topics/primary_health_care/en/*. (Seminal).

World Health Organization. (2015a). *Strategic directions for nursing and midwifery development 2016–2020. The way forward. Zero draft for consultation. 3rd Version.* Geneva: Author. Retrieved from *http://www.who.int/hrh/news/2015/midwifery_nurse_SDMN_consultation/en/*.

World Health Organization. (2015b). *WHO definition of palliative care.* Retrieved from *http://www.who.int/cancer/palliative/definition/en/*.

RESOURCES

Canadian Gerontological Nursing Association
http://www.cgna.net

Canadian Home Care Association
http://www.cdnhomecare.ca/

Canadian Hospice Palliative Care Association
http://www.chpca.net/

Canadian Institute for Health Information (CIHI)
http://www.cihi.ca

Canadian Nurses Association
http://www.cna-aiic.ca/

Canadian Patient Safety Institute
http://www.patientsafetyinstitute.ca/

Canadian Research Network for Care in the Community
http://www.crncc.ca/

Chronic Disease Prevention Alliance of Canada (CDPAC)
http://www.cdpac.ca/

Community Health Nurses of British Columbia
https://www.chnc.ca/en/community-health-nurses-of-british-columbia

Community Health Nurses of Canada (CHNC)
http://www.chnc.ca

Community Health Nurses' Initiatives Group (CHNIG) of the Registered Nurses' Association of Ontario
http://www.chnig.org

Ontario Association of Community Care Access Centres
http://www.oaccac.on.ca

Saint Elizabeth Health Care
http://www.saintelizabeth.com

Victorian Order of Nurses (VON) Canada
http://www.von.ca

Home Healthcare Nurses Association
http://www.hhna.org

Institute for Healthcare Improvement
http://www.ihi.org/ihi

National Association for Home Care & Hospice
http://www.nahc.org

National Gerontological Nursing Association
http://www.ngna.org

For additional Internet resources, see the website for this book at *http://evolve.elsevier.com/Canada/Lewis/medsurg*.

Older Adults

Written by: Sherry A. Greenberg
Adapted by: Veronique M. Boscart

evolve WEBSITE

http://evolve.elsevier.com/Canada/Lewis/medsurg

- Review Questions (Online Only)
- Key Points
- Answer Guidelines for Case Study

- Conceptual Care Map Creator
- Audio Glossary
- Content Updates

LEARNING OBJECTIVES

1. Describe the effects of ageism on the care of older adults.
2. List the major biological theories about aging.
3. Describe the needs of special populations of older adults.
4. Describe nursing interventions to assist chronically ill older adults.
5. Describe common problems of older adults in relation to acute illness and the role of the nurse in assisting them.

6. Describe challenges and concerns related to the caregiving role.
7. Identify care alternatives to meet specific needs of older adults.
8. Identify the legal and ethical issues related to the care of older adults.
9. Identify the role of the nurse in health screening and promotion and in disease prevention for older adults.

KEY TERMS

ageism, p. 91
assisted-living facilities (ALFs), p. 100

elder abuse, p. 98
elder mistreatment, p. 98
elder neglect, p. 98

ethnogeriatrics, p. 97
frail older adults, p. 96
gerontological nursing, p. 90

long-term care (LTC) facilities, p. 100
polypharmacy, p. 104

Gerontological nursing is a nursing specialty that revolves around the care of older adults. The nurse delivers care from a patient-centred perspective, valuing what is important to the patient. This chapter presents specific information about older adults to assist nurses in providing medical-surgical care to such patients in a variety of settings, such as inpatient care units, clinics, ambulatory care units, community and home health care, long-term and chronic care, nursing homes, and emergency care departments. Gerontological care presents opportunities and challenges that call for highly skilled assessment and creative adaptations of interventions.

DEMOGRAPHICS OF AGING

Older adults are one of the fastest-growing populations in Canada. There is no absolute threshold chronological age at which a person becomes "old." Most Canadian statistical summaries define older adults as those aged 65 and older. Psychologists have further divided the "old" into three groups: the young-old, aged 65 to 74 years; the middle-old, aged 75 to 84 years; and the old-old, older than 85 years. Since 1980, the older population has grown about twice as fast as the overall population: 14.4% of the population were aged 65 and older in

2011 (Statistics Canada, 2011a). This rapid growth is expected to continue well into the future. The population aged 65 years and older is projected to double by 2036 (Statistics Canada, 2010a). By then, almost 10.4 million people will be older adults, representing 23.7% of the total population (Statistics Canada, 2011a).

In general, Canada's population is younger than those of most Western industrialized countries, and yet a large proportion of older adults are immigrants. By 2031, one in four Canadians will be an immigrant, and one in three will belong to a visible minority (Statistics Canada, 2011a). Approximately 5% of the Indigenous population in Canada were aged 65 years or older in 2006; this proportion is expected to increase to 6.5% by 2017 (Health Council of Canada, 2013). Furthermore, there are significant age-related differences between Canada's provinces and territories; the largest share of the older population is in Nova Scotia (16.5%) and New Brunswick (16.2%), and the smallest is in Northwest Territories (5.6%) and Nunavut (3.2%; Statistics Canada, 2011a).

The most rapidly increasing age group is those of people 85 years and older. Since 1960, this group has increased 250%. In addition, there are currently 5 852 centenarians living in Canada; this number is projected to increase to 45 000 by 2046 (Statistics Canada, 2011c).

Gender can have a significant effect on various aspects of aging. Women usually live longer than men. Female Canadians born today have a life expectancy of 83 years, and male Canadians have a life expectancy of 79 years (Statistics Canada, 2017). The majority of adults older than 65 years remain in their home; 7.9% reside in a care facility (Statistics Canada, 2011b).

Because the needs and expectations of the population are changing rapidly, nurses need to acquire and demonstrate the required knowledge levels, clinical expertise, and leadership skills, and a strong understanding of health organizations and policy to deliver the best care possible to older adults.

ATTITUDES TOWARD AGING

Today's health care system promotes the concept of aging from a holistic perspective, in which health and wellness are defined as a balance between a person's internal and external environments and the person's emotional, spiritual, social, cultural, and physical processes. According to this perspective, aging is influenced by many factors, including emotional and physical health, developmental stage, socioeconomic status, culture, and ethnicity.

As people age, they are exposed to more and different life experiences. The accumulation of these differences creates a great diversity among older adults. Nurses should acknowledge and incorporate this diversity and older adults' perceptions of aging. Research has indicated that older adults who report a high sense of subjective well-being live longer, healthier lives than do older adults with a low sense of subjective well-being (Diener & Chan, 2011). Age is important, but it may not be the most relevant factor for determining the appropriate care of an individual older adult. In approaching aging from a viewpoint of health and well-being, a person's strengths, resilience, resources, and capabilities are emphasized, rather than her or his existing pathological conditions.

Unfortunately, myths and stereotypes about aging are found throughout society and are often supported by media (Victor, 1994). These stereotypes provide the basis of commonly held misconceptions that lead to errors in nursing assessments and limitations to interventions. For example, if nurses perceive older people to be confused or disoriented, necessary assessments for delirium will be neglected, which can result in morbidity and mortality (Baker, Taggart, Nivens, et al., 2015).

This negative attitude based on age is defined as ageism. Ageism leads to discrimination and disparities in the care of older people. Research has indicated that nurses who demonstrate an ageist attitude provide lower quality care to their older patients (Skirbekk & Nortvedt, 2014). In today's aging society, it is essential for nurses to demonstrate expertise, knowledge, and practice to care for older adults. Nurses can receive a Specialty Certification in Gerontological Nursing with the Canadian Nurses Association (CNA) to demonstrate their capabilities in providing care and services to older adults and their families.

BIOLOGICAL THEORIES OF AGING

Several theories aim at describing the process of aging. From a biological view, aging is defined as the progressive loss of function. The exact cause of biological aging remains to be determined, but aging is clearly a multifactorial process involving genetics, diet, and environment (Daniel & Tollefsbol, 2015). Nurses' knowledge of biological changes is important because it allows for differentiation between the normal

TABLE 7-1	SUMMARY OF SOME BIOLOGICAL THEORIES OF AGING
Theory	**Dynamics**
Free radical	Oxidation of fats, proteins, and carbohydrates creates free electrons that attach to other molecules, altering cellular function.
Cross-link	Lipids, proteins, carbohydrates, and nucleic acid react with chemicals or radiation to form bonds that cause an increase in cell rigidity and instability.
Immunological-autoimmunological	Alteration of B and T cells leads to loss of capacity for self-regulation; normal cells or cells with age-related changes are recognized as foreign matter; system reacts by forming antibodies to destroy these cells.

aging process and health problems that necessitate specific interventions.

Several theories regarding biological aging are currently proposed. An overview of some biological theories of aging is presented in Table 7-1.

Free Radical Theory

The *free radical theory* was initially proposed in 1956 by Harman, but has become the focus of new research only more recently. A free radical is a highly reactive atom or molecule that carries an unpaired electron and thus is prone to combine with another molecules, which causes an oxidative process. This process, also called *oxidative stress,* can ultimately disrupt cell membranes and alter DNA and protein synthesis. Common diseases such as atherosclerosis and cancer are associated with oxidative stress (Shaw, Werstuck, & Chen, 2014). Free radicals are natural by-products of many normal cellular processes and are also created under the influence of noxious environmental factors such as smog, tobacco smoke, and radiation. Numerous natural protective mechanisms are in place to prevent oxidative damage. Research since 2000 has focused on the roles of various antioxidants, including vitamins C and E, in slowing down the oxidative process and, ultimately, the aging process.

Cross-Link Theory

According to the *cross-link theory,* over time and as a result of exposure to chemicals and radiation in the environment, cross-links form between lipids, proteins, and nucleic acids (Höhn & Grune, 2013). These cross-links result in decreased flexibility and elasticity, and this causes increased rigidity in tissues (e.g., blood vessels). Such changes in cell structure may explain the observable changes associated with aging, such as wrinkles and a decreased distensibility of arterial blood vessels. However, it is unlikely that such changes account for all of the physical events associated with aging.

Immunological Theory

According to the *immunological theory,* declining functional capacity of the immune system is the basis of the aging process (Fuente & Miquel, 2009). It suggests that aging is not a passive wearing-out of systems but an active self-destruction mediated by the immune system. This theory is based on observations of an age-associated decline in T cell functioning, accompanied by a decrease in resistance and an increase in autoimmune diseases with aging. The result is an autoimmune phenomenon in which normal body cells are mistaken as foreign and are attacked by the individual's own immune system.

Despite the many different theoretical views, the exact cause of aging is unknown. Nurses need to be aware that each older person exhibits an individual aging process, which will necessitate a unique approach.

AGE-RELATED PHYSIOLOGICAL CHANGES

Age-related changes affect every body system and are part of healthy aging. However, the age at which specific changes become evident differs from person to person. For instance, a person may have greying hair at age 45 but relatively unwrinkled skin at age 80. Nurses need to recognize and assess age-related changes because they form the basis to differentiate from non–age-related changes. Table 7-2 presents an overview of assessments based on age-related physiological changes and associated clinical manifestations.

OLDER POPULATIONS AT HIGH RISK

Some subgroups within the older population, such as women, adults with cognitive challenges, and individuals from minority groups, are at a higher risk for developing certain conditions or for their conditions to be misdiagnosed. Some people belong to several of these subgroups, and their care requires skilled expertise in nursing assessment, interventions, and evaluations.

Older Women

Gender is an important factor that influences the natural history of diseases and determines management and treatment in situations in which gender roles and preferences could influence care-seeking behaviour and treatment. For example, female patients tend to be older and more likely to rely on children for support, whereas male patients are more likely to have a spouse as a caregiver (Gruneir, Forrester, Camacho, et al., 2013). Home care clients and residents in long-term care facilities are predominantly female, given contemporary differences in life expectancy and caregiving patterns. With dementia, the progression of disease is faster in

TABLE 7-2 AGE-RELATED DIFFERENCES IN ASSESSMENT

Age-Related Changes and Associated Clinical Manifestations

Function	Normal Age Changes	Clinical Manifestations
Cardiovascular System		
Cardiac output	• Force of contraction decreases • Fat and collagen increase • Heart muscle weakens • Ventricular wall thickens	• Myocardial oxygen demand increases • Stroke volume and cardiac output decrease • Fatigue, shortness of breath, and tachycardia occur • Blood flow to vital organs and periphery decreases
Cardiac rate and rhythm	• Dependence of atrial contraction increases • Fibres from bundle of His are lost • Mitral valve stretching occurs • Ventricles are slower to relax • Sinus node pacemaker cells decrease in number	• HR slows to increase with stress • Maximum HR decreases (e.g., in 80-year-old, HR = 120 bpm; in 20-year-old, HR = 200 bpm) • Possible AV block • Recovery time from tachycardia is prolonged • Frequency of premature beats increases
Structural changes	• Aortic valves become sclerotic and calcify • Baroreceptor sensitivity decreases • Mild fibrosis and calcification of valves occur	• Diastolic murmur is present in 50% of older people • Heart-position landmarks change
Arterial circulation	• Elastin and smooth muscle are reduced • Vessel rigidity increases • Vascular resistance increases • Aorta becomes dilated	• Systolic BP modestly increases • Rigidity of arteries contributes to coronary artery disease and peripheral vascular disease
Venous circulation	• Vessel tortuosity increases	• Inflamed, painful, or cordlike varicosities appear
Peripheral pulses	• Arteries become more rigid	• Pulses are weaker but equal • Circulation to periphery slows • Feet and hands are cold
Respiratory System		
Structures	• Cartilage degeneration occurs • Vertebral rigidity occurs • Strength of muscles decreases • Respiratory muscles atrophy • Rigidity of thoracic wall increases • Ciliary action decreases	• Kyphosis occurs • Anterior-posterior diameter increases • Use of accessory muscles decreases • Chest becomes rigid and barrel-shaped • Respiratory excursion decreases • Ability to cough and deep breathing ability diminish
Change in ventilation and perfusion	• Pulmonary vascular bed shrinks • Alveoli decrease in number • Alveolar walls thicken • Elastic recoil decreases	• Lung compliance decreases • Total lung volume is unchanged • Vital capacity decreases • Residual lung volume increases • Mucus thickens • PaO_2 and O_2 saturation decreases • Hyperresonance
Ventilation control	• Response to hypoxia and hypercarbia diminishes	• Ability to maintain acid-base balance decreases • Respiratory rate 12–24/min

TABLE 7-2 AGE-RELATED DIFFERENCES IN ASSESSMENT

Age-Related Changes and Associated Clinical Manifestations—cont'd

Function	Normal Age Changes	Clinical Manifestations
Integumentary System		
Skin	• Amounts of collagen and subcutaneous fat decrease • Sweat glands decrease in number • Epidermal cell turnover slows • Skin tissue fluid decreases • Capillary fragility increases • Pigment cells decrease in number • Sebaceous gland activity decreases • Sensory receptors diminish • Thresholds for touch, vibration, heat, and pain increase	• Skin elasticity decreases • Wrinkles and folds increase • Extremity fat is lost; fat on trunk increases • Skin heals more slowly • Skin more dry • Skin tears and bruises easily • Skin colour uneven • Skin lesions increase in number • Ability to respond to heat and cold decreases • Ability to feel light touch decreases • Cutaneous pain sensitivity declines
Hair	• Melanin decreases • Germ centres and hair follicles decrease in size and number	• Hair turns grey or white • Hair quantity decreases and thins • Amounts of scalp, pubic, and axillary hair decrease • Amount of facial hair on men decreases • Amount of facial hair on women increases
Nails	• Blood supply to nail bed decreases • Longitudinal striations increase	• Growth slows • Nails are brittle and thicken • Nails are easily split • Potential for fungal infection increases
Urinary System		
Kidney	• Renal mass decreases • Number of functioning nephrons decreases • Glomerular filtration rate decreases • Renal plasma flow decreases	• Protein in urine increases • Potential for dehydration increases • Creatinine clearance decreases • Serum levels of creatinine and BUN increase • Excretion of toxins and drugs decreases • Nocturia increases
Bladder	• Amounts of bladder smooth muscle and elastic tissue decrease	• Capacity decreases • Control decreases; potential for stress incontinence increases
Micturition	• Sphincter control decreases	• Frequency, urgency, and nocturia increase
Reproductive System		
Male structures	• Prostate enlarges • Testicular volume decreases • Sperm count decreases • Seminal vesicles atrophy • Serum testosterone levels remain constant • Estrogen level increases	• Sexual response becomes less intense • Achieving an erection takes longer • Erection is maintained without ejaculation • Force of ejaculation decreases
Female structures	• Estradiol, prolactin, and progesterone levels diminish • Sizes of ovaries, uterus, cervix, fallopian tubes, and labia decrease • Associated glands and epithelium atrophy • Elasticity in the pelvic area decreases • Breast tissue decreases • Vaginal pH becomes alkaline	• Responses to changing hormone levels are altered • Cervical and vaginal secretions decrease • Intensity of sexual response decreases • Potential for vaginal infections increases • Potential for vaginal and uterine prolapse increases
Gastro-Intestinal System		
Oral cavity	• Dentine decreases • Gingival retraction occurs • Bone density is lost • Papillae of tongue decrease in number • Taste thresholds for salt and sugar increase • Salivary secretions decrease	• Taste perception changes • Potential for loss of teeth is increased • Gingivitis is more likely to occur • Gums may bleed, and dry mouth occurs • Oral mucosa is dry
Esophagus	• Pressure of lower esophageal sphincter decreases • Motility decreases	• Epigastric distress occurs • Dysphagia occurs • Potential for hiatal hernia and aspiration is increased
Stomach	• Gastric mucosa atrophies • Blood flow decreases	• Gastric emptying decreases
Small intestine	• Intestinal villi decrease in number • Enzyme secretions decrease • Motility decreases	• Intestinal transit slows • Absorption of fat-soluble vitamins is delayed

Continued

TABLE 7-2   AGE-RELATED DIFFERENCES IN ASSESSMENT

Age-Related Changes and Associated Clinical Manifestations—cont'd

Function	Normal Age Changes	Clinical Manifestations
Gastro-Intestinal System—cont'd		
Large intestine	• Blood flow decreases • Motility decreases • Sensation of defecation urge decreases	• Potential for constipation and fecal impaction increases
Pancreas	• Pancreatic ducts become distended • Lipase production decreases • Pancreatic reserve is impaired	• Fat absorption is impaired • Glucose tolerance decreases
Liver	• Number and size of cells decrease • Hepatic protein synthesis is impaired • Ability to regenerate liver cells decreases	• Lower border extends past costal margin • Drug metabolism decreases
Musculo-Skeletal System		
Skeleton	• Intervertebral disc space narrows • Cartilage of nose and ears increases	• Height diminishes 2.5–10 cm (1–4 inches) • Nose and ears lengthen • Kyphosis occurs • Pelvis widens
Bone	• Amounts of cortical and trabecular bone decrease	• Bone resorption exceeds bone formation • Potential for osteoporotic fractures increases
Muscles	• Number of muscle fibres decreases • Muscle fibres atrophy • Muscle regeneration slows • Contraction time and latency period are prolonged • Flexion of joints increases • Ligaments stiffen • Tendons become sclerotic • Tendon flexor reflexes decrease	• Strength decreases • Agility decreases • Rigidity in neck, shoulders, hips, and knees increases • Potential for restless legs syndrome increases
Joints	• Cartilage erosion occurs • Calcium deposits increase • Water in cartilage decreases	• Mobility decreases • ROM becomes limited • Osteoarthritis can occur
Nervous System		
Structure	• Neurons in brain and spinal cord are lost • Brain size decreases • Dendrites atrophy • Amount of major neurotransmitters decreases • Size of ventricles increases	• Conduction of nerve impulses slows • Peripheral nerve function is lost • Reaction time decreases • Response time slows • Potential for altered balance, vertigo, and syncope increases • Postural hypotension becomes more common • Proprioception diminishes • Sensory input decreases • EEG alpha waves slow down
Sleep	• Amount of deep sleep decreases • Amount of REM sleep decreases	• Falling asleep becomes more difficult • Period of wakefulness increases
Visual System		
Eye structure	• Orbital fat is lost • Eyebrows and eyelashes turn grey or white • Elasticity of eyelid muscles decreases • Tear production decreases	• Eyes become sunken • Eyes become dry • Potential for ectropion and entropion increases • Potential for conjunctivitis increases
Cornea	• Corneal sensitivity decreases • Corneal reflex decreases • Arcus senilis becomes more common	• Potential for corneal abrasion is increased
Ciliary	• Aqueous humor secretion decreases • Ciliary muscle atrophies	• Ability of lens to accommodate declines • Presbyopia occurs • Peripheral vision decreases
Lens	• Lens becomes less elastic, more dense	• Lens becomes yellow and opaque • Ability to adapt to light and dark lessens • Tolerance of glare decreases • Incidence of cataracts increases • Night vision is impaired
Iris and pupil	• Pigment is lost • Pupil size decreases • Amount of vitreous gel debris increases	• Visual acuity decreases • Pupils appear constricted • Floaters are common

TABLE 7-2 AGE-RELATED DIFFERENCES IN ASSESSMENT

Age-Related Changes and Associated Clinical Manifestations—cont'd

Function	Normal Age Changes	Clinical Manifestations
Auditory System		
Structure	• Hairs in external auditory canals of men increase • Ceruminal glands decrease in number	• Potential for conductive hearing loss increases • Cerumen is drier • Sound conduction decreases
Middle ear	• Middle-ear bone joints degenerate • Eardrum thickens	
Inner ear	• Vestibular structures decline • Hair cells are lost • Cochlea atrophies • Organ of Corti atrophies	• Sensitivity to high tones and perception of "s," "t," "f," and hard "g" sounds decrease • Understanding of speech decreases • Discrimination of background voice decreases • Equilibrium–balance deficits occur • Potential for tinnitus increases
Immune System	• Amount of secretory IgA declines • Thymus gland becomes involuted • Amount of lymphoid tissue decreases • Antibody production is impaired • Proliferative response of T and B cells decreases • Number of autoantibodies increases	• Potential for infection on mucosal surfaces increases • Cell-mediated immune response is impaired • Malignancy incidence increases • Response to acute infection is weakened • Recurrence of latent herpes zoster and tuberculosis is more likely • Susceptibility to autoimmune disease increases

AV, atrioventricular; *BP*, blood pressure; *bpm*, beats per minute; *BUN*, blood urea nitrogen; *EEG*, electroencephalographic; *HR*, heart rate; *IgA*, immunoglobulin A; *PaO₂*, arterial partial pressure of oxygen; *REM*, rapid eye movement; *ROM*, range of motion.

women, even after age is controlled in analysis (Irvine, Laws, Gale, et al., 2012). Other differences include a higher risk for inappropriate medications to be prescribed to women (Gruneir, Forrester, Camacho, et al., 2013).

In addition to having a high number of chronic health conditions, older people face challenges such as reduced financial resources, lack of informal caregiving responsibilities, or both; these challenges have a significant effect on the health of older women. As a result, older women often experience disparities in treatment in comparison with men, including unequal access to quality health care (see Chapter 2). Nurses should act as advocates for women's equity in the health care system. Advocacy organizations such as the Canadian Women's Health Network can be helpful in this undertaking. Last but of importance, older women are more likely to be victims of family violence than are older men, in part because they usually live longer (Bennett & Kingston, 2013). Several resources, organizations, and programs are in place to raise awareness of, prevent, diagnose, and address the abuse of older people in Canada. The Registered Nurses' Association of Ontario (RNAO) has partnered with the CNA for the pan-Canadian Promoting Awareness of Elder Abuse in Long-Term Care Homes (PEACE) initiative. Resources are listed at the end of this chapter.

Older Adults With Cognitive Impairments

The majority of older adults do not have any noticeable decline in mental abilities. There will be some normal age changes, such as a memory lapse or benign forgetfulness, which are significantly different from cognitive impairment. These normal age changes are often referred to as *age-associated memory impairment* (Table 7-3).

An older adult who is forgetful can benefit from using memory aids, attempting recall in a calm and quiet environment, and actively engaging in memory improvement techniques. Memory aids include clocks, calendars, notes, marked pillboxes, safety alarms on stoves, and identity necklaces or bracelets. Memory

TABLE 7-3 AGE-RELATED DIFFERENCES IN ASSESSMENT

Effects of Aging on Cognitive Functioning

Function	Manifestations of Healthy Aging
Fluid intelligence (the ability to solve new problems or use logic in new situations)	Declines
Crystallized intelligence (the ability to use learned knowledge and experience)	Improves
Vocabulary and verbal reasoning	Improves
Spatial perception	Remains constant or improves
Synthesis of new information	Declines
Mental performance speed	Declines
Short-term recall memory	Declines
Long-term recall memory	Remains constant

improvement techniques include word association, mental imaging, and mnemonics.

Declining physical health is an important factor in cognitive impairment. Older people who experience sensory losses or cerebrovascular disease may show a decline in cognitive functioning. An appropriate cognitive assessment includes hearing and vision, functional ability, memory recall, orientation, use of judgement, and appropriateness of emotional state. Standard mental status examinations and behavioural descriptions provide data for determining cognitive status. Cognitive impairment is further discussed in Chapter 62.

Older Adults Living in Rural Settings

Between 19% and 30% of older Canadians live in rural areas (Strengthening Rural Canada Initiative, 2014), and some face

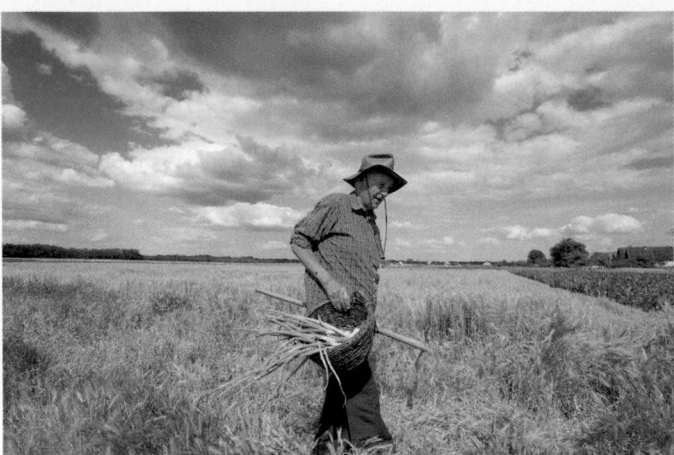

FIGURE 7-1 Transportation is a possible barrier to providing service to older adults in rural areas. Source: Budmir Jevtic/Shutterstock.com.

TABLE 7-4	NUTRITIONAL ASSESSMENT OF OLDER ADULTS

The acronym **SCALES** can remind the nurse to assess important nutritional indicators:
Sadness, or mood change
Cholesterol level: high
Albumin level: low
Loss or gain of weight
Eating problems
Shopping and food preparation problems

barriers to remaining at home and staying active and engaged in their communities. Such barriers include a lack of or limited availability of support to enable older people to remain independent, as well as very limited housing and transportation options. In addition, older adults in rural and remote areas are frequently required to travel out of their communities for health services, which creates challenges (Spina & Menec, 2015). Some research has indicated that older adults living in rural areas present with more symptoms of ill health than do older adults living in urban areas (Bacsu, Jeffery, Johnson, et al., 2012). Furthermore, rural communities offer fewer health-promoting activities, such as structured exercise programs (Spina & Menec, 2015), and are often underserved by health care providers.

Nurses working with older adults in rural communities must clearly recognize the lifestyle values and practices of rural life (Figure 7-1) and acknowledge that lack of or difficulty with transportation is a possible barrier to providing service. Alternative service approaches such as computer-based Internet sources and chat rooms, videos, radio, community centres, and church social events should be used to promote healthful practices or to conduct health screening. The development of telehealth devices for monitoring people in their home environments has enhanced the ability to provide care to isolated individuals.

Older Adults Who Are Homeless

According to careful estimates, Canada might have 6 000 homeless older people; however, older adults account for only a little more than 1.7% of shelter users (Gaetz, Donaldson, Richter, et al., 2013), which may be explained by a much higher mortality rate among chronically homeless people (Hwang, Wilkins, Tjepkema, et al., 2009). Key factors associated with homelessness include (a) a low income, (b) reduced cognitive capacity, and (c) living alone. According to Statistics Canada, 3.6% of men and 7.6% of women 65 years of age and older are living below the low-income cut-off, the point at which a family is spending 70% or more of their income on necessities (food, clothing, and shelter; Statistics Canada, 2010b). Among older Canadians, single or widowed women are at higher risk for living in poverty. Such low-income older people may become homeless because of a lack of affordable housing.

When homeless, older individuals may have increased new health problems or experience an exacerbation of existing problems because most services provided to the homeless population are not designed to reach out to older adults. Long-term care placement is often an alternative to homelessness, especially when the individual is cognitively impaired and alone. A distinct fear of such institutionalization may explain why older homeless people do not use shelter- and meal-site services. Homelessness among older people requires more research related to risk factors as well as solutions.

Frail Older Adults

Frail older adults is a term used to identify older adults who, because of declining physical health and resources, are most vulnerable to poor outcomes. *Frailty* has been defined as the presence of three or more of the following: unplanned weight loss (≥10 lb [4.5 kg] in the past year), weakness, poor endurance and energy, slowness, and low activity (Clegg, Young, Iliffe, et al., 2013). Risk factors include disability, multiple chronic illnesses, and the presence of geriatric syndromes. Frailty is not related directly to age per se, although age is a risk factor. Hardiness or psychological strength may be a significant factor in preventing frailty among older adults.

Most frail older adults have difficulty coping with declining functional abilities and decreasing daily energy. When stressful life events (e.g., the death of a loved one) occur and daily strain (e.g., caring for an ill spouse) is present, the frail individual may have difficulties with the effects of stress and may become ill. Common health problems of the frail older adult include mobility and strength limitations, sensory impairment, cognitive decline, and falls.

The frail older adult is at particular risk for malnutrition and problems with hydration (Clegg, Young, Iliffe, et al., 2013). Malnutrition and dehydration are related to sociopsychological factors such as living alone, depression, and low income. Physical factors such as loss of vision or hearing, declining cognitive status, inadequate dental care, physical fatigue, and limited mobility also add to the risks of malnutrition and dehydration. Because many frail older adults have therapeutic diets and multiple drug regimens, their nutritional state may be altered. It is important for the nurse to monitor the frail older adult for adequate calorie, protein, iron, calcium, vitamin D, and fluid intake.

Assessment tools that include a focus on physical, social, and environmental risk factors (Table 7-4) have been developed to monitor older patients for poor nutritional status. In addition, it is important to review the medications that an older adult takes because many medications affect appetite and can therefore affect nutritional status. Once an older adult's nutritional needs are identified, interventions can include home-delivered meals, dietary supplements, food stamps, dental referrals, congregate dining sites, home visits by registered dietitians, and vitamin supplements.

Older Adults With Chronic Illness

Daily living with chronic or persistent illness is a reality for many older adults. Although people of all ages have chronic health problems, illness is most common in older adults. It is estimated that 76% of older adults had one or more chronic condition in 2010 (Canadian Institute for Health Information, 2011). The most common conditions for older Canadians are high blood pressure (47%), arthritis (27%), and heart disease (19%; Canadian Institute for Health Information, 2011). Other chronic persistent conditions such as diabetes, vision or hearing problems, and dementia also have a significant effect on health-related quality of life for older adults.

Chronic illness is composed of multiple health problems that have a protracted, unpredictable course. Diagnosis and the acute phase of a chronic persistent illness are often managed in an acute care setting, and all other phases of such an illness are usually managed at home. The management of a chronic illness can profoundly affect the lives and the self-concepts of the affected older person and the family. Although health status encompasses acute and chronic illness, it also includes an individual's level of daily functioning. Functional health includes activities of daily living (ADLs), such as bathing, dressing, eating, toileting, and transferring. Instrumental activities of daily living (IADLs), such as using a telephone, shopping, preparing food, housekeeping, doing laundry, arranging transportation, taking medications, and handling finances, are also included in a functional health assessment.

As age increases, functional health declines, and disability increases. Nurses caring for older adults need to advocate for appropriate, comprehensive assessment in which health and disease states are diagnosed accurately, as well as for the utilization of health-promotion strategies.

Treatment for chronic conditions can often cause new problems. As one disease is treated, another may be affected. For example, the use of a drug with anticholinergic properties, such as a tricyclic antidepressant (e.g., amitriptyline [Elavil]), may cause urinary retention. In older adults, disease symptoms are atypical, and sometimes manifestations of disease are asymptomatic. For example, the only symptom of cardiac disease may be fatigue. Pathological entities with similar symptoms are often confused. Negative consequences of chronic illness include physical suffering, loss, worry, grief, depression, functional impairment, and increased dependence (Lundman & Jansson, 2007). Daily living with chronic illness can be very difficult for older adults. The nurse must involve the patient in any decision making related to interventions, goals planning, and quality of life and well-being (Table 7-5).

Socially Isolated Older Adults

As people age and social networks contract, they may become increasingly isolated and lonely. Although social isolation and loneliness are related factors, they are distinctly different concepts. Social isolation is defined as being separated from one's environment to the point of having few satisfying and rewarding relationships. Loneliness, conversely, is one's feeling of dissatisfaction with social contacts in terms of quantity or quality, or both (Holwerda, Deeg, Beekman, et al., 2014). Thus the feeling of loneliness can be present even if an older person is living with another person, with family, or in an institution. It is the quality of the social contacts that is critical for the maintenance of well-being and hardiness.

Both social isolation and loneliness have consistently been found to be associated with poorer physical and psychological health (Holwerda, Deeg, Beekman, et al., 2014). Although many social, personal, and health factors are involved in social isolation and loneliness, it is difficult to predict which older adults are most at risk for poor health. Older adults who are isolated and lonely should be closely monitored. Keeping these vulnerable older adults engaged in meaningful social relationships and activities is a significant health-promoting intervention, and nurses have an important role to play.

CULTURALLY COMPETENT CARE

OLDER ADULTS

The term **ethnogeriatrics** is used to describe the specialty area of providing culturally competent care to older people who are identified with a particular ethnic group (Touhy, Jett, Boscart, et al., 2011; Figure 7-2). Canada is officially a multicultural society, and culturally diverse care is essential in order to provide for the needs of a very diverse group of older adults. Vast differences or heterogeneity are found among and within various ethnic groups in relation to health beliefs and practices, access to and utilization of health care, health risks, family dynamics and caregiving, decision-making processes and priorities, and responses to interventions and changes in health care policies (Huff, Kline, & Peterson, 2014). Nurses are challenged to provide culturally competent care in all types of settings and communities: home care settings, institutionalized settings, day programs, and acute and chronic health care facilities. Although it is unrealistic to expect a health care provider to be proficient in working with every category and subgroup of minority older people, it is possible to develop levels of awareness, skill, and sensitivity that can be applied to interactions with older people of ethnic minorities and their families. The nurse must assess each older adult's ethnic orientation. Several tools or instruments can

TABLE 7-5	SUPPORTIVE INTERVENTIONS FOR OLDER ADULTS WITH CHRONIC ILLNESS

- Prevent social isolation.
- Control symptoms of the chronic illness.
- Adjust to changes in the course of the disease.
- Prevent and manage episodes of acute illness.
- Carry out prescribed therapies for the chronic illness.
- Use technology to enhance function, independence, and safety.

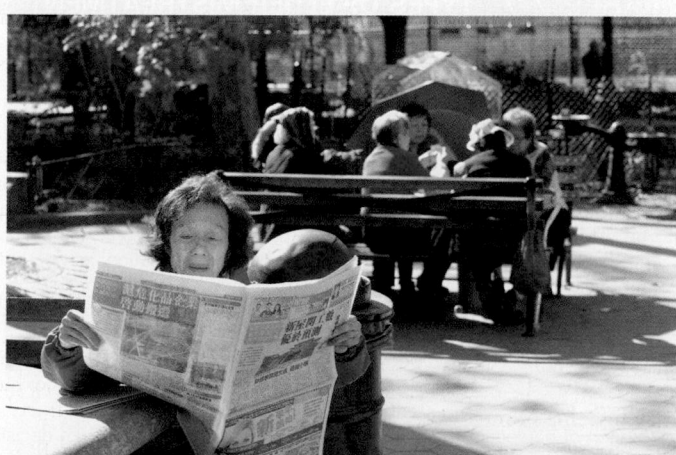

FIGURE 7-2 Culture and heritage can be important facets of many older adults' lives. Source: W8 Photography/Shutterstock.com.

assist nurses in eliciting health care beliefs and help identify a patient's perceptions of alternative beliefs (see the Resources at the end of this chapter; Kleinman, Isenberg, & Good, 1978; Touhy, Jett, Boscart, et al., 2011). Culturally competent care is discussed in Chapter 2.

SOCIAL SUPPORT AND THE OLDER ADULT

Social support is essential for all older adults to maintain their level of well-being. Social support occurs at three levels. Family and kinship relations are most often the first level of providers of social support. Second, a semiformal level of support is found in clubs, places of worship, neighbourhoods, and senior citizen centres. Third, older adults may be linked to a formal system of social welfare agencies, health facilities, and government support. In general, the nurse is part of the formal support system.

Caregivers

A caregiver is someone who provides supervision and direct care and coordinates services. In Canada, 8.1 million caregivers provide an estimated 70% to 80% of all home care, thereby supporting the public system for an estimated $24 to $31 billion (Sinha, 2013). Caregiving includes many tasks but focuses mostly on assisting older patients with ADLs and IADLs, providing emotional and social support, and managing health care.

Caregivers often experience their caregiving as rewarding, but it can also be a physically and emotionally demanding task, even leading to increased medical illnesses and a greater risk of mortality for the caregiver (Sinha, 2012; Table 7-6).

Some caregivers may develop a sense of being overwhelmed and have feelings of inadequacy, powerlessness, and depression (Kim, Chang, Rose, et al., 2011). The stress of caregiving may result in emotional problems such as depression, anger, and resentment. The burden of caregiving can be isolating, inasmuch as it limits social, emotional, and interactional opportunities. Time commitments, fatigue, and at times, socially inappropriate behaviours of the dependent older adult contribute to social isolation. The socially isolated caregiver must be identified, and plans should be designed to meet his or her needs for social support and interaction.

Many family members involved in direct caregiving activities also identify rewards associated with this role. Positive aspects of caregiving include knowing that a loved one is receiving good care (often in a home environment), learning and mastering new tasks, and finding opportunities for intimacy. At the same time, the tasks involved in caregiving often provide opportunities for family members to learn more about one another and strengthen their relationships.

The nurse should consider the caregiver as a patient and plan interventions to reduce caregiver strain if necessary. The nurse can communicate a sense of empathy to the caregiver while allowing discussion about the burdens and joys of caregiving. The caregiver can be taught about age-related changes and diseases and specific caregiving techniques. The nurse can also assist the caregiver in seeking help from the formal social support system regarding matters such as respite care, housing, health coverage, and finances. Finally, the nurse should monitor the caregiver for indications of declining health, emotional distress, and caregiver role strain.

Elder Mistreatment and Abuse

Elder abuse can be defined as "any action by someone in a relationship of trust that results in harm or distress to an older person. Neglect is a lack of action by that person in a relationship of trust with the same result" (Public Health Agency of Canada [PHAC], 2012). The term elder mistreatment is used to describe acts of commission (elder abuse) or omission (elder neglect) that harm or threaten to harm an older adult's health or welfare. Elder abuse may occur in private homes or in any type of care facilities. *Institutional abuse* refers to abuse of people living in long-term care homes and residential care facilities. An older person may experience more than one form of abuse (Table 7-7).

TABLE 7-6   CAREGIVER CHALLENGES
• Lack of respite or relief from caregiving • Conflict in the family unit related to decisions about caregiving • Lack of understanding of the time and energy needed for caregiving • Inability to meet personal self-care needs, such as socialization and rest • Inadequate information about specific tasks of caregiving • Financial depletion of resources as a result of a caregiver's inability to work and the increased cost of care

TABLE 7-7   TYPES OF ELDER MISTREATMENT

Types	Characteristics	Manifestations
Physical abuse	Slapping; restraining; incorrect positioning; oversedation	Bruises, bilateral injuries, repeated injuries in various stages of healing; use of several emergency departments
Physical neglect	Withholding of food, water, medications, clothing, hygiene; failure to provide physical aids such as dentures, eyeglasses, hearing aid; failure to ensure safety	Pressure injuries; loss of body weight; laboratory values showing dehydration (e.g., HCT; serum sodium) and malnutrition (serum protein); poor personal hygiene
Psychological or emotional abuse	Berating; harassment; intimidation, threats of punishment or deprivation; treating older person like a child; isolation	Depression, withdrawn behaviour; agitation; ambivalent attitude toward caregiver
Psychological or emotional neglect	Failure to provide social stimulation; leaving alone for long periods; failure to provide companionship	Depression, withdrawn behaviour; agitation; ambivalent attitude toward caregiver
Sexual abuse	Touching inappropriately; forcing sexual contact	Unexplained vaginal or anal bleeding; bruises; unexplained STIs or genital infections
Financial abuse	Denying access to personal resources; stealing money or possessions; coercing to sign contracts or durable power of attorney; making changes in will or trust	Living situation is below level of personal resources; sudden change in personal finances or transfer of assets
Violation of personal rights	Denying right to privacy or right to make decisions regarding health care or living environment; forcible eviction	Sudden inexplicable changes in living situation; confusion

HCT, hematocrit; *STIs,* sexually transmitted infections.

Overall, elder abuse is an underreported problem and has been difficult to quantify. According to police reports, in 2010 nearly 2 800 Canadians older than 65 were victims of family violence, and grown children were most often the perpetrators of violence against older people (Statistics Canada, 2010c). Victims often do not report it because of isolation; impaired cognitive or physical function; feelings of shame, embarrassment, guilt, or self-blame; fear of reprisal; pressure from family members; fear of losing the home and independence; and cultural norms. Health care providers may fail to report it because of lack of confidence in identifying or reporting victims; perceived inability to successfully intervene; and a desire to avoid responsibility for further action.

The primary risk factors for elder abuse are the characteristics of the abuser. Abusers tend to be adult children who are dependent on the parent for housing and financial means; have a history of violence or antisocial behaviour; are unemployed; and are disabled because of substance abuse or mental illness, or both (Department of Justice Canada, 2009). Victim characteristics, such as frailty, dementia, immobility, and social isolation also add to the risk of mistreatment. These characteristics increase the likelihood that an older person is unable to seek help or defend herself or himself.

The nursing approach to a suspected victim of elder abuse should begin with a carefully documented history and a thorough examination for mistreatment. Nurses should assess the individual for the presence of dehydration, malnutrition, pressure injuries, poor personal hygiene, and lack of compliance with the medical regimen. Of importance is that failure to follow the care plan, unauthorized use of restraints, and use of medication or isolation as punishment are also considered forms of abuse.

Key assessment findings include (a) explanations for findings (e.g., injuries) that are not consistent with objective data and (b) contradictory explanations from the patient and the caregiver. The nurse should follow the facility or employer intervention protocol for elder abuse. A screening tool for abuse by a caregiver is available as a pocket tool from the National Initiative for the Care of the Elderly (see the Resources at the end of this chapter).

In institutionalized settings, nurses should be alert to patterns of recurrent infections, poor hygiene, lack of interest in activities or eating, behavioural changes, new incontinence, sleep problems, and complaints about staff. Specific nursing interventions to reduce the risk of elder abuse include close management of the patient's plan of care and regular review of the use of restraints and psychotropic medications in addition to the interventions listed in Table 7-8.

When managing elder abuse, the nurse must be familiar with both federal and provincial laws governing reporting procedures and patient privacy. Information on mandatory reporting can be found on the Canadian Network for Prevention of Elder Abuse website.

UNIVERSAL HEALTH CARE

The older population requires specific consideration within Canada's health care system. Because of the growth in the older population and the associated increase in chronic health conditions, the health care needs of this population sector are greater than in other population segments.

The Canadian health care system is based on the *Canada Health Act* (1984) and is publicly funded. Health care is administered and delivered by the provinces and territories. The system is referred to by Canadians as "Medicare" and provides for universal

TABLE 7-8 NURSING MANAGEMENT OF ELDER MISTREATMENT

- It is mandatory to make reports to the appropriate provincial or territorial body about the suspicion of abuse or neglect.
- The nurse should screen for possible elder abuse, including domestic violence.
- A thorough history should be documented and a head-to-toe assessment conducted. It is important to document the findings, including any statements made by the patient or an accompanying adult.
- If an older adult appears to be in immediate danger, a safety plan should be developed and implemented in collaboration with the interdisciplinary team involved in the person's care.
- The nurse should identify, collect, and preserve physical evidence (e.g., dirty or bloody clothing, dressings, or sheets).
- After obtaining consent, photographs should be taken to document physical findings of suspected abuse or neglect. If possible and appropriate, this should be done before the alleged victim is treated or bathed.
- If abuse is suspected, the findings should be reported to the appropriate provincial agency or law enforcement, or both, as mandated by local laws.
- Social work, forensic nursing, and other consultations should be initiated as appropriate.

comprehensive coverage for "medically necessary" services, including primary health care, care in hospitals, and surgical–dental services. Each province and territory determines which services are publicly funded, and so there is significant variation among areas for "not urgent" services such as the provision of home care, long-term care, medications outside of hospital, physiotherapy, optometry services, and other services. As a result of the focus on Canada's health care reform, there has been increased advocacy for more realistic provision of health care for older adults, including an emphasis on health promotion and expanded community care (Health Canada, 2016; Hollander, Chappell, Prince, et al., 2007).

CARE ALTERNATIVES FOR OLDER ADULTS

Most older adults prefer to continue living at home, but they may have to move to a more restrictive environment at a time of crisis. Several living arrangements and care options for older people are described as follows.

Independent Living Options

Many older adults stay in their place of residence and do not move to a different home or geographic location as they age. The community becomes important to older adults as an environment that is safe and that supports social contacts. Older adults needs privacy and companionship, as well as a sense of belonging. The community should be accessible. Older adults may need housing assistance in the form of property tax relief and assistance with home repair and the cost of utilities (Figure 7-3). A variety of subsidized, low-income housing arrangements are available for older adults in many areas.

For an older adult who chooses to remain in the home as functional abilities decline, some home adaptations and modifications can be made to accommodate for some functional decline, including walker and wheelchair accessibility, increased lighting, and safety devices in bathrooms and kitchens. The *Safe Living Guide—A Guide to Home Safety for Seniors* (see the Resources at the end of this chapter) includes strategies for home adaptations that improve safety and accessibility.

FIGURE 7-3 Home maintenance is part of an older adult's independent lifestyle. Source: Halfpoint/Shutterstock.com.

FIGURE 7-4 Social interaction and acceptance are important for older adults. Source: belushi/Shutterstock.com.

Adult lifestyle communities or retirement communities may be an option for some older adults. These communities are age-segregated, self-contained developments and provide social activities, security, and recreational facilities. Some retirement communities offer expanded health care and social support services. An entrance fee and monthly fees for continuing care are charged. Chapter 6 discusses community-based care settings.

Assisted-living facilities (ALFs) are residential care facilities that provide housing and personal care. Because over half of community-based older adults require assistance with ADLs or IADLs, this is the most rapidly developing area of care. According to a Canadian Mortgage and Housing Corporation (2016) survey, up to 9.1% of Canadians aged 75 years and older lived in 2 812 ALFs in 2016. Services vary per facility. Nurses working in this area are challenged by questions related to regulations, use of the services of unregulated care providers, assessment to ensure safe "fit of resident to facility," and shared resident decision making. The Canadian Accreditation Council is developing standards for use in accreditation of ALFs (see the Resources at the end of this chapter).

Community-Based Care for Older Adults

Many older adults with special care needs can be aided by services in the community, such as adult day care programs or home health care.

Adult Day Care Programs. *Adult day care programs* provide daily supervision, social activities, management of chronic disease, and ADL assistance for older adults who are cognitively impaired and for people who have problems with ADLs. The services offered in the adult day care programs are based on patient needs. Restorative programs offer health monitoring, therapeutic activities, one-on-one ADL training, individualized care planning, and personal care services. Programs designed for people with cognitive impairments offer therapeutic recreation, support for family, family counselling, and social involvement. Adult day care programs provide relief to the caregiver, allow continued employment for the caregiver, and delay institutionalization for the patient. Centres are regulated and standards are set by the province. Costs are not covered by health insurance but are tax deductible as dependent care. The nurse's role consists of knowing the available adult day care services and assessing the needs of the patient.

Home Health Care. Home health care can be a cost-effective care alternative for an older person who is homebound but has health needs that are intermittent or acute. In 2011, one in every six older people received home care services; and up to 2.2 million people across this country—many of them vulnerable older people—relied on home care services to enable them to stay safely in their homes (Accreditation Canada & Canadian Home Care Association, 2015). Home health care services offer skilled nursing care and care by other regulated health care providers, nonregulated workers, volunteers, friends, and family members, all to help an older adult remain in the community. Emphasis of the care and services is often on the management of chronic disease, supporting ADLs, and promoting well-being. Home health care is discussed in more detail in Chapter 6.

Long-Term Care Facilities

Long-term care (LTC) facilities are a placement alternative for adults who can no longer live alone, who need continuous supervision, who have three or more disabilities involving ADLs, or who are frail. Three main factors precipitate placement in an LTC facility: (a) rapid deterioration of the patient's condition, (b) the caregiver's inability to continue care, and (c) an alteration in or loss of family support system. Changes in orientation (e.g., increased confusion), incontinence, or a major health event (e.g., stroke, fall) can accelerate the need for placement in LTC.

Since 2005, LTC facilities have been caring for residents with more complex health care needs (Hirdes, Mitchell, Maxwell, et al., 2011). Not only has the prevalence of chronic diseases such as diabetes, heart failure, and arthritis increased, but also conditions such as frailty and dementia necessitate high-quality care by a competent and interprofessional workforce. Nurses are instrumental in the care planning and chronic disease management to address an older person's health care needs while balancing the person's quality of life and wishes. Many LTC facilities provide an environment that truly represents the best of caring and quality of life and an extraordinary commitment and dedication of staff. Several initiatives are under way to shift from an institutional model to LTC facilities as places that nurture quality of life and well-being for older people (Figure 7-4).

LEGAL AND ETHICAL ISSUES

Legal assistance is an issue for many older adults concerned about advance directives, estate planning, taxation issues, and appeals for denied services. In Canada, legal aid is available for

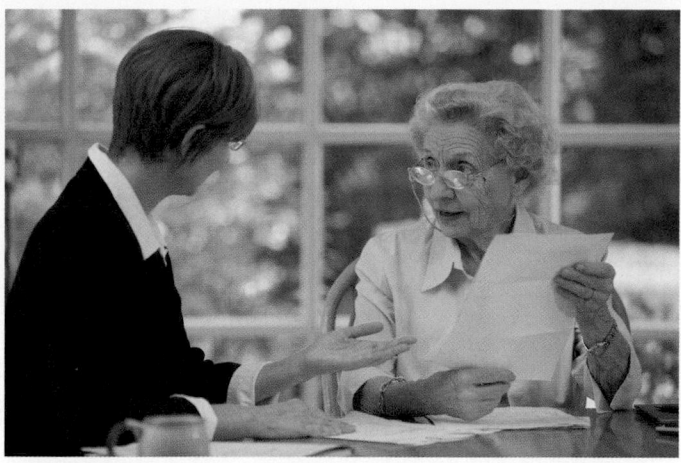

FIGURE 7-5 Some residential facilities for older adults post notices announcing when free legal help is available. Source: EdBockStock/Shutterstock.com.

all citizens (Figure 7-5). There is some variation between provinces and territories about legal matters affecting capacity, advanced directives, and consent.

Mental capacity is a person's ability to make decisions. It is a legal construct, not a clinical condition (Touhy, Jett, Boscart, et al., 2011). To be deemed capable of making a decision, the person must *understand* information that is relevant to making a decision, *evaluate* data, and *appreciate* the consequences of the decision or of not making a decision (Wahl, 2008). People are presumed to have capacity unless there is clear evidence to the contrary and the person has been legally deemed incapable. Capacity can improve, decrease, or fluctuate (Wahl, 2008).

A *power of attorney* is a legal document and legal device in which one person designates another person (e.g., family member, friend) to act on his or her behalf.

There are primarily two types of advance directives: instruction directives and those in which a substitute decision maker or proxy is named (CNA, 1998). An instruction directive (or *living will*) specifies what kinds of interventions are desirable for different health situations. In a proxy directive, the patient specifies who is to make health care decisions if he or she becomes unable to make his or her wishes known. Often, these two terms are used interchangeably; however, they serve different purposes (CNA, 1998). (Advance directives are discussed in Chapter 13.)

The nurse who works with older adults will encounter areas of ethical concern that influence practice and care. Issues may include the need to evaluate the patient's ability to make decisions, resuscitation, treatment of infections, issues of nutrition and hydration, and transfer to more intensive treatment units. These situations are often complex and emotionally charged. The nurse can assist the patient, the family, and other health care providers by acknowledging when an ethical dilemma is present, by keeping current on the ethical implications of biotechnology, and by advocating for an institutional ethics committee to help in the decision-making process. For more information, see the "Resources" section at the end of the chapter.

NURSING MANAGEMENT
OLDER ADULTS

NURSING ASSESSMENT

The assessment of an older adult provides the database and baseline information for the rest of the nursing process; however,

it is a complex undertaking. First, older people may face any health problem with fear or anxiety, and the problem may present in an atypical manner. In addition, health care providers may be perceived as helpful, but institutions may be perceived as negative, potentially harmful places. The nurse beginning an assessment needs to establish a nurse–patient relationship by communicating a sense of concern and care by use of direct and honest statements, appropriate eye contact, and direct touch when appropriate. When beginning the assessment process, the nurse should attend to primary needs first: for example, ensure that the patient is free of pain, is adequately hydrated, is wearing appropriate clothing, and does not need to go to the bathroom. All assistive devices such as glasses and hearing aids should be in place. The interview should be short so that the patient does not become fatigued. The nurse should allow adequate time to give information, as well as to respond to any questions. The medical history may be lengthy, and the nurse must determine what normal age changes are and which information is relevant. If possible, medical records and any current medications should be reviewed.

To truly assess an older adult, a comprehensive geriatric assessment is required (Ramani, Furmedge, & Reddy, 2014). The focus of a comprehensive geriatric assessment is to determine appropriate interventions to maintain and enhance the functional and cognitive abilities of the patient. This assessment is interdisciplinary and, at a minimum, includes the medical history, the physical examination, a functional abilities assessment, a cognitive assessment, and an assessment of social and financial resources. The interdisciplinary team may represent many disciplines, but at minimum it should include the nurse, the physician, and the social worker. After the assessment is complete, the interdisciplinary team meets with the patient and family to present the team's findings and recommendations.

Nursing assessment is a key component of the comprehensive geriatric assessment. Elements in a comprehensive nursing assessment include a history, documented in a functional health pattern format (see Chapter 3); physical assessment; cognitive assessment; assessment of ADLs and IADLs; and a social–environmental assessment. Evaluation of cognitive status is particularly important for older adults because results of this evaluation often determine a patient's potential for independent living. Evaluation of the results of a comprehensive nursing assessment helps determine the services needed. A good match between needs and services should be the goal of the assessment. The nurse also collects data regarding community resources that are needed to assist the patient and her or his family to maintain maximal functioning.

The comprehensive nursing assessment should be based on instruments that are reliable, valid, and specific to older adults. Several standardized assessment tools for gerontology are available and can be used in accordance with the purpose of the assessment and the status of the patient. However, difficulties often arise in the interpretation of the results of findings because of age-related changes and parameters that are not well defined for older adults. The nurse is in an important position to recognize and correct inaccurate interpretation of laboratory test results.

NURSING DIAGNOSES

With few exceptions, the same nursing diagnoses apply to an older adult as to a younger individual. However, the causes and defining characteristics are related to age and are unique to older adults. Table 7-9 lists nursing diagnoses that are seen in older

TABLE 7-9   NURSING DIAGNOSES

Associated With Age-Related Changes

Cardiovascular System
- Activity intolerance
- Decreased cardiac output
- Fatigue

Reproductive System
- Disturbed body image
- Ineffective sexuality pattern
- Sexual dysfunction

Respiratory System
- Impaired gas exchange
- Ineffective airway clearance
- Ineffective breathing pattern
- Risk for aspiration
- Risk for infection

Gastro-Intestinal System
- Constipation
- Imbalanced nutrition: less than body requirements
- Impaired oral mucous membrane
- Obesity

Integumentary System
- Impaired skin integrity

Nervous System
- Impaired memory
- Risk for acute confusion
- Hyperthermia
- Hypothermia

Urinary System
- Deficient fluid volume
- Impaired urinary elimination

Senses
- Disturbed body image
- Impaired verbal communication
- Social isolation

Musculo-Skeletal System
- Impaired physical mobility
- Chronic pain
- Risk for injury
- Self-care deficits
- Sedentary lifestyle

Immune System
- Risk for infection

FIGURE 7-6 Strength training is an example of a health promotion activity for older adults. Source: belushi/Shutterstock.com.

adults as a result of age-related changes. The identification and management of nursing diagnoses result in higher quality care and improved patient function.

PLANNING

When setting goals with an older adult, the nurse must identify the patient's strengths and abilities. Caregivers, if appropriate, should be included in goal development. Personal characteristics such as hardiness, persistence, and the ability to learn contribute to the setting of individualized goals. Priority goals for the patient may be focused on well-being, such as gaining a sense of control, feeling safe, and reducing stress.

NURSING IMPLEMENTATION

When carrying out a plan of action, the nurse may have to modify the approach and techniques used according to the physical and cognitive status of a particular older patient. Sensory changes, such as auditory and visual deficits, may interfere with communication. Small body size, common among frail older adults, may necessitate the use of pediatric equipment (e.g., blood pressure cuff). Bone and joint changes often necessitate assistance with transfers, altered positioning, and use of gait belts and lift devices. An older adult with declining energy reserves may require additional time to complete tasks. A slower pace of interaction, more limited scheduling of interventions and activities, and the availability of a bedside commode or other adaptive equipment may be necessary.

Cognitive impairment, if present, mandates careful explanations and a calm approach to avoid producing anxiety in the patient. Depression can result in apathy, malnutrition, and a decline in mobility. Several guidelines and interventions are available to enhance nursing care for people with cognitive impairment (Touhy, Jett, Boscart, et al., 2011).

HEALTH PROMOTION. Health promotion and prevention of health problems in older adults is one of the most important areas for nurses and is focused mainly on three areas: reduction in diseases, increased participation in health promotion activities, and targeted services that reduce health hazards. The Division of Aging and Seniors of the PHAC provides federal leadership on health issues affecting older adults, including fall prevention, emergency preparedness, and age-friendly communities (PHAC, 2017).

Within gerontology, nurses need to place a high value on health promotion and positive health behaviours. Several programs have been successfully developed for chronic health condition screening, smoking cessation, geriatric foot care, vision and hearing screening, stress reduction, exercise programs, drug usage, crime prevention, elder mistreatment, delirium prevention and treatment and home hazards assessment (RNAO, 2017). The nurse can carry out and teach older adults about the need for specific preventive services. The nurse interested in health promotion for older adults can reference Health Canada's "Healthy Living" web page (see the Resources at the end of this chapter).

Health promotion and prevention can be included in nursing interventions at any location where nurses and older adults interact and at any level of care delivery. The nurse can use health promotion activities to strengthen patients' self-care, increase their personal responsibility for their own health, and increase independent functioning that will enhance their well-being (Figure 7-6).

Teaching Older Adults. Throughout the continuum of care, nurses are involved in instructing and teaching older adults specific self-care practices to enhance health and well-being and modify disease processes (Table 7-10). Individual patient teaching is discussed in Chapter 4.

ACUTE CARE SETTINGS. When an emergency arises and a person cannot be cared for at home or in a residential care environment, admittance to an acute care hospital might be necessary. Some conditions that might necessitate hospitalization include exacerbations of chronic conditions, stroke, fluid and electrolyte imbalances, pneumonia, and trauma caused by falls. Unfortunately, the complexity of the acute situation often results in the loss of the whole-person perspective and focuses the care only on the diseased part. Nurses' integrated approach and emphasis on individualized care are primordial to restoring an older adult's health and well-being within this setting.

TABLE 7-10 PATIENT & CAREGIVER TEACHING GUIDE

Older Adults

Challenges for Older Adults	Specific Strategies
• Time needed to learn is increased. • New learning must relate to the patient's actual experience. • Anxiety and distractions decrease learning. • Lack of willingness to take risks and cautiousness decrease motivation to learn. • Sensory–perceptual deficits and cognitive decline necessitate modifications in teaching techniques.	• Present material at a slower rate. • Use visual aids when possible. • Use peer educators when appropriate. • Encourage participation of a spouse or family member. • Use simple phrases or sentences, and provide for repetition. • Support the belief that change in behaviour is worth the effort. • Emphasize that a person is never too old to learn new things.

Source: Adapted from Rankin, S. H., Stallings, K. D., & London, F. (2004). *Patient education: Principles and practice* (5th ed.). Philadelphia: Lippincott.

TABLE 7-11 CARE OF THE HOSPITALIZED OLDER ADULT

• Identify patients at risk for iatrogenic effects of hospitalization.
• Plan and communicate discharge goals and assess needs as soon as a person is admitted.
• Involve interdisciplinary teams and providers who focus on the special needs of older adults.
• Conduct a comprehensive geriatric assessment, and be aware of the complexity and interplay of several conditions.
• Involve appropriate community-based services (see Chapter 6).

FIGURE 7-7 The nurse assists an older person in a geriatric rehabilitation facility. Source: GWImages/Shutterstock.com.

In addition, an acute care stay often results in negative consequences for older patients, including functional decline and iatrogenic events, such as falls, pressure injuries, and delirium, (Fox, Persaud, Maimets, et al., 2012). To prevent any of these complications, care of such patients requires an interdisciplinary approach, including very succinct nursing components (Table 7-11). Involvement of the patient and the family is essential in supporting the individualized perspective and creating a support network for when the patient is discharged.

Geriatric Rehabilitation. Geriatric rehabilitation interventions are focused on adapting to a new situation or recovering from trauma. Collaborative and interdisciplinary teams focus on building up functional reserve and emotional wellness, with the use of appropriate assistive equipment and supportive personal care, and creating a supportive network in which an older adult can live as independently as possible. The patient can receive rehabilitative assistance through inpatient rehabilitation (limited days are covered), day programs, or home care programs (Figure 7-7).

Rehabilitation of older adults is influenced by several factors. First, older adults show greater initial variability in functional capacity than do adults at any other age. Pre-existing factors associated with reaction time, visual acuity, fine motor ability, physical strength, cognitive function, and motivation affect the rehabilitation potential of older adults.

Within the interdisciplinary team, nurses assess and develop interventions for existing chronic illnesses; fears and anxieties specific to falling; fatigue; sensory–perceptual deficits; malnutrition; and social and financial challenges. Many older adults lose functional ability in the acute care setting because of inactivity and immobility. This deconditioning can occur as a result of unstable acute medical conditions or environmental barriers that limit mobility. Older adults can improve flexibility, strength, and aerobic capacity even into very old age. The interdisciplinary team develops passive and active range-of-motion exercises to prevent deconditioning and subsequent functional decline.

Last, the goal of geriatric rehabilitation is to strive for maximal function and physical and cognitive capabilities with regard to the individual's current health status. For example, a woman with a history of osteoporosis receives a falls-risk appraisal and specific exercises to build stability and balance. Older adult patients with diabetes receive a geriatric foot assessment and appropriate follow-up care.

Assistive Devices. Using appropriate assistive devices such as dentures, glasses, hearing aids, walkers, wheelchairs, adaptive utensils, elevated toilet seats, and skin protective devices can greatly improve independency for older adults. The need for and use of these devices are assessed by the interdisciplinary team, and findings are included in the patient's care plan. Electronic monitoring equipment can be used to monitor heart rhythms, blood pressure, and potential falls, as well as to locate the wandering patient in the home or LTC facility. Computerized assistive devices can be used to help patients with speech difficulties following stroke, and pocket-sized devices can serve as memory aids.

Safety. Environmental safety is crucial in the maintenance of health and independence by older adults. With normal sensory age changes, slowed reaction time, decreased thermal and pain sensitivity, changes in gait and balance, and medication effects, older adults are prone to accidents. Most accidents, such as trips and falls, occur in or around the home. Older adults' impaired thermoregulating system can cause hypothermia and heat prostration (hyperthermia).

The nurse and the care team can provide valuable counsel regarding environmental safety and changes. Measures such as enhanced lighting, coloured step strips, tub and toilet grab bars, and stairway handrails can be effective in "safety-proofing" the living quarters of an older adult. The nurse can also advocate for home fire and security alarms. Uncluttered floor space, railings, increased lighting and night lights, and clearly marked stair edges are some of the easiest and most practical adaptations.

In addition, an older adult who moves to a different location needs a thorough orientation to the environment. The nurse should repeatedly reassure the patient that he or she is safe and attempt to answer all questions. The unit should foster orientation to time and place by displaying large-print clocks, avoiding complex or visually confusing wall designs, clearly designating doors, and using simple bed and nurse-call systems. Beds should be close to the floor to prevent serious injury from falls. Lighting should be adequate while avoiding glare. Environments that provide consistent caregivers and an established daily routine assist older adults.

Medication Use. Medication use in older adults necessitates thorough and regular assessment and care planning. Twenty-seven percent of older patients reported taking five or more medications on a regular basis (Reason, Terner, Moses McKeag, et al., 2012). The frequency of adverse drug reactions increases as the number of prescribed drugs increases, and as a result, hospital admissions of older adults are often for drug reactions.

Age-related changes alter the pharmacodynamics and pharmacokinetics of drugs. Drug–drug, drug–food, and drug–disease interactions all influence the absorption, distribution, metabolism, and excretion of drugs. Figure 7-8 illustrates the effects of aging on drug metabolism. The most dramatic changes with aging are related to drug metabolism and clearance. Overall, by age 75 to 80, there is a 50% decline in the renal clearance of drugs. Hepatic blood flow decreases markedly with aging, and the enzymes largely responsible for drug metabolism are decreased as well. Thus the drug half-life is increased in older patients as compared with one who is younger (Jett, 2016).

In addition to changes in the metabolism of drugs, older adults may have medication-related difficulty resulting from malnutrition and dehydration, cognitive decline, altered sensory perceptions, limited hand mobility, and the high cost of many prescriptions. Common reasons for drug errors made by older adults are listed in Table 7-12. **Polypharmacy** (the use of multiple medications by a patient who has more than one health problem), overdosage, or forgetting to take medications are recognized as major risk factors for adverse effects in older adults (Reason, Terner, Moses McKeag, et al., 2012).

TABLE 7-12   COMMON CAUSES OF MEDICATION ERRORS BY OLDER ADULTS

- Poor eyesight
- Forgetting to take drugs
- Use of nonprescription (over-the-counter) drugs
- Use of medications prescribed for someone else
- Failure to understand instructions or the importance of drug treatment
- Refusal to take medication because of undesirable adverse effects

Drug-receptor interaction
- Brain receptors become more sensitive, making psychoactive drugs very potent.

Metabolism
- Liver mass shrinks.
- Hepatic blood flow and enzyme activity decline.
- Metabolism drops to $1/2$ to $2/3$ the rate of young adults.
- Enzymes lose ability to process some drugs, thus prolonging drug half-life.

Absorption
- Gastric emptying rate and gastro-intestinal motility slow.
- Absorption capacity of cells and active transport mechanism decline.

Circulation
- Vascular nerve control is less stable.
- Antihypertensives, for example, may overshoot, dropping BP too low.
- Digoxin, for example, may slow the heart rate too much.

Excretion
- In kidneys, renal blood flow, glomerular filtration rate, renal tubular secretion and reabsorption, and number of functional nephrons decline.
- Age-related changes increase half-life for renally excreted drugs.
- Oral antidiabetic drugs, among others, stay in the body longer.

Distribution
- Lean body mass falls.
- Adipose stores increase.
- Total body water declines, raising the concentration of water-soluble drugs, such as digoxin, which can cause heart dysfunction.
- Plasma protein levels decrease, reducing sites available for protein-bound drugs and raising blood levels of free drug.

FIGURE 7-8 The effects of aging on drug metabolism. Source: Redrawn from Benzon, J. (1991). Approaching drug regimens with a therapeutic dose of suspicion. *Geriatric Nursing, 12*(4), p. 1813.

TABLE 7-13 DRUG THERAPY

Medication Use by Older Adults

1. Conduct a medication reconciliation review with the physician and the pharmacist.
2. Emphasize medications that are essential.
3. Discuss use of medication that is not essential or counterproductive.
4. Screen use of medications—including over-the-counter drugs, herbaceuticals, eyedrops and eardrops, antihistamines, and cough syrups—by using a standard assessment tool.
5. Assess medication interactions.
6. Assess patient's alcohol use.
7. Encourage the use of written or other medication-reminder systems.
8. Monitor drug dosage; normally, the dosage should be less than that for a younger person.
9. Encourage the patient to use one pharmacy.
10. Work with health care providers and pharmacists to establish routine drug profiles on all older adult patients.
11. Advocate (with drug companies) for low-income prescription support services and generic substitutions.
12. Assess financial status and discuss which medications are essential to buy for older adult patients.

To accurately assess drug use and knowledge, many nurses ask their older adult patients to bring all medications to the health care appointment (including over-the-counter medications, prescriptions, herbal remedies, and nutritional preparations) that they take regularly or occasionally. The nurse and pharmacist can then accurately assess all medications that the patient is taking, including drugs that the patient may have overlooked or thought unimportant to include. Some medications can be tapered or discontinued, especially those medications that may be causing harm or are no longer providing benefit. Specific guidelines for deprescribing of proton pump inhibitors, benzodiazepines, and antipsychotics in older adults have been developed and can be found at the website of the Ontario Pharmacy Evidence Network (see the Resources at the end of this chapter).

Additional nursing interventions to assist older adults in following a safe medication routine are listed in Table 7-13.

Several medications are considered inappropriate or dangerous for older adults and are identified on the Beers list (American Geriatrics Society 2015 Beers Criteria Update Expert Panel, 2015). This list has been recommended as a "best practice" by several Canadian regulating and professional organizations (see the Resources at the end of this chapter for the web link.)

Depression. Many older people have experienced multiple, simultaneous stressors, such as loss of loved ones, dealing with chronic illness, financial stress, and social isolation. For some older adults, the accumulation of these stressors can result in a mental health issue. The prevalence of mental illness is the same among older adults as among the general population (3%–10%), except for dementia and delirium, which is more prevalent among older adults (Inouye, Westendorp, & Saczynski, 2013). Rates of depressive symptoms in institutionalized older adults are higher than those in the community (González-Colaço Harmand, Meillon, Rullier, et al., 2014). Unfortunately, depression is an underrecognized problem for many older adults.

Depression can exacerbate medical conditions by affecting nutritional intake, mobility, or drug regimens. An older adult who is at high risk for or exhibits depressive symptoms should be encouraged to seek treatment. Because many patients feel unworthy of special attention and may withdraw and become isolated, the nurse may have to enlist the support of the family in helping the patient seek treatment. Nursing assessment consists of observation of appearance and behaviour and examination of cognitive function, functional abilities, anxiety, adjustment reactions, depression, substance abuse, and suicidal risk. A comprehensive guide to assessment and treatment of depression in older adults is available at the website of the Hartford Institute for Geriatric Nursing (see the Resources at the end of the chapter).

Specific interventions include nonpharmacological approaches and, if needed, pharmacological treatment. Depression is often reversible with prompt and appropriate treatment. Older patients experience improvement with appropriate medication, psychotherapy (Krishna, Jauhari, Lepping, et al., 2011), or psychosocial interventions (Kiosses, Leon, & Areán, 2011), or a combination of these.

Sleep. Adequacy of sleep is often a concern for older adults because of altered sleep patterns. Older people experience a marked decrease in deep sleep and are easily aroused. In individuals older than 75, the percentage of sleep time spent in the rapid eye movement (REM) stage decreases. In addition, older adults have difficulty maintaining prolonged sleep. Although the demand for sleep decreases with age, older adults may be disturbed by insomnia and complain that they spend more time in bed but still feel tired. Many older people prefer to spread sleep periods throughout 24 hours with short naps that, combined, provide adequate rest. Other factors that contribute to sleep difficulties include medical problems, such as sleep apnea and restless legs syndrome, as well as effects of medications (e.g., furosemide [Lasix]). In many cases, a later bedtime promotes a better night's sleep and a feeling of being refreshed on awakening.

Behavioural Management. Patients with cognitive impairment often are confused and anxious during specific care situations (e.g., while showering) or when left alone. These people might respond with certain behaviours, such as wandering, trying to resist care, or pushing away the care provider. In addressing these responsive behaviours, it is important for the nurses to understand that the person with cognitive impairment is responding to a "perceived threat." Ignoring this behaviour and continuing the care task will only cause the person to become more anxious or frightened and result in an exacerbation of this responsive behaviour. In caring for people with these behaviours, nurses need to understand *why* they respond in such a way, and the nurse should intervene with competent and compassionate person-centred care.

The nurse should check for changes in vital signs and urinary and bowel patterns that could account for behavioural problems. It is important to use a relational approach with a focus on empathy and nurturing and to keep care assignments consistent. When a patient is agitated by the environment, either the patient or the stimulus should be moved. Most responsive behaviours can be redirected with activities such as holding a towel during the bath or exercising or walking with staff when starting to wander. Reality orientation can be used to recall the patient to time, place, and person. A family member can be asked to stay with the patient until the person becomes calmer. The patient should be monitored frequently, and all interventions should be documented. An interdisciplinary approach is important to identify the best redirective strategies. The use of evidence-informed nursing interventions significantly reduces the use of physical and chemical (drug therapy) restraints (Enns, Rhemtulla, Ewa, et al., 2014; RNAO, 2012).

Use of Restraints. Restraints are physical, environmental, or chemical measures used to limit the activity or control the behaviour of a person or a portion of his or her body (RNAO, 2012). Devices such as seat belts, "geri-chairs," or side rails that cannot be removed by the patient are considered physical restraints, and it has been proven that these actually increase a person's risks for falls and injury (Enns, Rhemtulla, Ewa, et al., 2014). Chemical restraints are any form of psychoactive medication used not to treat illness but to intentionally inhibit a patient's particular behaviour or movement. Several researchers have indicated that antipsychotic medications have limited effectiveness and significant risks for older persons with cognitive impairment (Enns, Rhemtulla, Ewa, et al., 2014; RNAO, 2012). Despite abundant research findings, chemical and physical restraints continue to be used in the care of people with responsive behaviours. Several Best Practice Guidelines outline alternatives for care (RNAO, 2011, 2012).

EVALUATION. The evaluation phase of the nursing process is similar for all patients. Evaluation is ongoing throughout the nursing process. The results of the evaluation direct the nurse to continue the care plan or revise it as indicated.

TABLE 7-14 EVALUATING NURSING CARE FOR OLDER ADULTS

Evaluation questions may include the following:
1. Has there been an identifiable change in ADLs, IADLs, cognitive status, or disease signs and symptoms?
2. Does the patient consider his or her health and well-being state to be improved?
3. Does the patient think the treatment is helpful?
4. Do the patient and the caregiver think the care is worth the time and cost?
5. Can the nurse document positive changes that support interventions?

ADLs, activities of daily living; *IADLs*, instrumental activities of daily living.

When evaluating nursing care for an older adult, the nurse should focus on improving or maintaining the patient's functional and cognitive status and his or her quality of life and well-being, rather than a cure. Useful questions to consider when evaluating the care plan for an older adult are included in Table 7-14.

CASE STUDY

Older Adults

Source: Muellek Josef/Shutterstock.com.

Patient Profile
Lee Xiang, a 79-year-old Chinese woman, was admitted through the emergency department with shortness of breath. She was diagnosed with community-acquired pneumonia. Her history also indicates that she has chronic obstructive pulmonary disease (COPD), hypertension, diabetes, mild cognitive impairment, depression, macular degeneration, and significant hearing loss.

Subjective Data
- Had a stroke 5 years ago and has right-sided weakness.
- Has a two-pack/week history of tobacco use but quit smoking after her stroke.
- Has not seen primary care physician in 1 year.
- In past year has had an unplanned weight loss of 20 pounds.
- Spends her days either in bed or in a recliner watching television.

Psychosocial Data
- Came to the Canada 15 years ago from China.
- Speaks Mandarin with limited English proficiency.
- Lives with her unemployed adult son, who provides assistance with ADLs and IADLs.
- Has three daughters who live within a 2-hour drive.
- Has limited financial resources.
- Her son has not visited her in the hospital, but her daughters raise concerns about their mother's care and safety at home, given their brother's history of gambling addiction.
- When daughters ask their brother about how he is caring for his mother, he says, "I'm doing the best I can. She refuses help. She refuses to go to the doctor. What do you want me to do? She's old. She does what she wants."

Objective Data
- Matted hair, poor oral hygiene, overgrown toenails.
- Two stage III sacral pressure injury.
- Unstageable right heel pressure injury.
- Multiple small bruises on her forearms and shins.
- 5 × 10-cm bruise in the middle of her back.

Discussion Questions
1. Compare Mrs. Xiang's experience as an older woman to known gender differences for older adults.
2. Define *ageism*, and explain how it may be manifested in this case.
3. What risk factors does Mrs. Xiang have for development of frailty? Which of these factors are modifiable?
4. ***Priority Decision:*** On the basis of your assessment of Mrs. Xiang, what are the priority nursing diagnoses?
5. ***Priority Decision:*** What are the priority nursing interventions for Mrs. Xiang?
6. Explain ethnogeriatric considerations that affect Mrs. Xiang and how they will influence your nursing care.
7. Based on your knowledge of caregiver support and care alternatives for older adults, what support is required for the son and daughters, and what setting or settings might be appropriate for Mrs. Xiang on hospital discharge?
8. What risk factors does Mrs. Xiang have for becoming a victim of elder mistreatment?

*e*volve
Answers available at *http://evolve.elsevier.com/Canada/Lewis/medsurg*.

REVIEW QUESTIONS

The number of the question corresponds to the same-numbered objective at the beginning of the chapter.

1. What is one characteristic of ageism?
   a. Denial of negative stereotypes regarding aging.
   b. Positive attitudes towards older adults that are based on age.
   c. Negative attitudes towards older adults that are based on age.
   d. Negative attitudes towards older adults that are based on physical disability.

2. The prevalence of autoimmune diseases increases with aging. Which theory of aging accounts for this phenomenon?
   a. Immune theory of aging.
   b. Programmed theory of aging.
   c. Neuroendocrine theory of aging.
   d. Intrinsic mutation theory of aging.

3. Which of the following nursing interventions would promote a sense of self-worth for an older adult member of an ethnic minority?
   a. Informing the person about ethnic support services.
   b. Allowing the person to rely on ethnic health beliefs and practices.
   c. Using an interpreter to provide explanations and teaching.
   d. Emphasizing that a therapeutic diet does not allow ethnic foods.

4. Which of the following nursing actions would be helpful to a chronically ill older adult? *(Select all that apply.)*
   a. Discussing future lifestyle changes.
   b. Informing the patient that the condition is stable.
   c. Treating the patient as a competent manager of the disease.
   d. Encouraging the patient to "fight" the disease as long as possible.

5. When older adults become ill, which of the following are they more likely to do than younger adults?
   a. Complain about the symptoms of their problems.
   b. Refuse to carry out lifestyle changes to promote recovery.
   c. Seek medical attention because of limitations on their lifestyle.
   d. Alter their daily living activities to accommodate new symptoms.

6. What should the nurse know about a patient's caregivers?
   a. They may need the nurse to assist them in reducing caregiver strain.
   b. They are usually trained health care workers who do not live with the client.
   c. They are generally strong and healthy but need teaching to carry out care activities.
   d. They are often reluctant to share the burden of caregiving with other family members.

7. For an older adult requiring constant assistance and living with an employed daughter, what is an appropriate care choice?
   a. Adult day care.
   b. Nursing home care.
   c. A retirement centre.
   d. An assisted-living home.

8. What is a characteristic of a living will?
   a. Legally binding.
   b. Encourages the use of artificial means to prolong life.
   c. Allows a person to direct her or his health care in the event of terminal illness.
   d. Designates who can act for the patient when the patient is unable to do so for himself or herself.

9. In promotion of health for older adults, what is the primary focus of nursing interventions?
   a. Disease management.
   b. Controlling symptoms of illness.
   c. Teaching positive health behaviours.
   d. Teaching the role of nutrition in enhancing longevity.

1. c; 2. a; 3. a; 4. a, c; 5. d; 6. a; 7. a; 8. c; 9. c.

evolve

For even more review questions, visit *http://evolve.elsevier.com/Canada/Lewis/medsurg.*

REFERENCES

Accreditation Canada & Canadian Home Care Association. (2015). *Home care in Canada. Advancing quality improvement and integrated care.* Retrieved from *https://accreditation.ca/sites/default/files/home-care-in-canada-report.pdf.*

American Geriatrics Society 2015 Beers Criteria Update Expert Panel. (2015). American Geriatrics Society 2015 Updated Beers Criteria for Potentially Inappropriate Medication Use in Older Adults. *Journal of the American Geriatrics Society, 63*(11), 2227–2246. doi:10.1111/jgs.13702.

Bacsu, J. R., Jeffery, B., Johnson, S., et al. (2012). Healthy aging in place: Supporting rural seniors' health needs. *Online Journal of Rural Nursing and Health Care, 12*(2). Retrieved from *http://rnojournal.binghamton.edu/index.php/RNO/article/view/52.*

Baker, N. D., Taggart, H. M., Nivens, A., et al. (2015). Delirium: Why are nurses confused? *Medsurg Nursing, 24*(1), 15–23. PMID: 26306346.

Bennett, G., & Kingston, P. (2013). *Elder abuse: Concepts, theories and interventions.* New York: Springer.

Canadian Institute for Health Information. (2011). *Seniors and the healthcare system: What is the impact of multiple chronic conditions?* Retrieved from *https://secure.cihi.ca/free_products/air-chronic_disease_aib_en.pdf.*

Canadian Mortgage and Housing Corporation. (2016). *Seniors' housing report—Canada highlights.* Retrieved from *https://www.cmhc-schl.gc.ca/odpub/esub/65991/65991_2016_A01.pdf.*

Canadian Nurses Association. (1998). *Advance directives: The nurse's role.* Retrieved from *https://cna-aiic.ca/~/media/cna/page-content/pdf-en/ethics_pract_advance_directives_may_1998_e.pdf?la=en.* (Seminal).

Clegg, A., Young, J., Iliffe, S., et al. (2013). Frailty in elderly people. *Lancet, 381*(9868), 752–762. doi:10.1016/S0140-6736(12)62167-9.

Daniel, M., & Tollefsbol, T. O. (2015). Epigenetic linkage of aging, cancer and nutrition. *The Journal of Experimental Biology, 218,* 59–70. doi:10.1242/jeb.107110.

Department of Justice Canada. (2009). *Abuse of older adults: Department of Justice Canada overview paper.* Ottawa: Author. Retrieved from *http://publications.gc.ca/collections/collection_2009/justice/J2-354-2009E.pdf.* (Seminal).

Diener, E., & Chan, M. Y. (2011). Happy people live longer: Subjective well-being contributes to health and longevity. *Applied Psychology: Health and Well-Being, 3*(1), 1–43. doi:10.1111/j.1758-0854.2010.01045.

Enns, E., Rhemtulla, R., Ewa, V., et al. (2014). A controlled quality improvement trial to reduce the use of physical restraints in older hospitalized adults. *Journal of the American Geriatrics Society, 62*(3), 541–545. doi:10.1111/jgs.12710.

Fox, M. T., Persaud, M., Maimets, I., et al. (2012). Effectiveness of acute geriatric unit care using Acute Care for Elders components: A systematic review and meta-analysis. *Journal of the American Geriatrics Society, 60*(12), 2237–2245. doi:10.1111/jgs.12028.

Fuente, M. D., & Miquel, J. (2009). An update of the oxidation-inflammation theory of aging: The involvement of the immune system in Oxi-Inflamm-Aging. *Current Pharmaceutical Design, 15*, 3003–3026. doi:10.2174/138161209789058110. (Seminal).

Gaetz, S., Donaldson, J., Richter, T., et al. (2013). *The state of homelessness in Canada 2013*. Toronto: Canadian Homelessness Research Network Press.

González-Colaço Harmand, M., Meillon, C., Rullier, L., et al. (2014). Cognitive decline after entering a nursing home: A 22-year follow-up study of institutionalized and noninstitutionalized elderly people. *Journal of the American Medical Directors Association, 15*(7), 504–508. doi:10.1016/j.jamda.2014.02.006.

Gruneir, A., Forrester, J., Camacho, X., et al. (2013). Gender differences in home care clients and admission to long-term care in Ontario, Canada: A population-based retrospective cohort study. *BMC Geriatrics, 13*(1), 48. doi:10.1186/1471-2318-13-48.

Harman, D. (1956). Aging: A theory based on free radical and radiation chemistry. *Journal of Gerontology, 11*(3), 298–300. doi:10.1093/geronj/11.3.298. (Seminal).

Health Canada. (2016). *Canada's health care system (Medicare)*. Ottawa: Author. Retrieved from *https://www.canada.ca/en/health-canada/services/canada-health-care-system.html*.

Health Council of Canada. (2013). *Canada's most vulnerable: Improving health care for First Nations, Inuit, and Métis seniors*. Retrieved from *http://healthcouncilcanada.ca/content_ab.php?mnu=2&mnu1=48&mnu2=30&mnu3=55*.

Hirdes, J. P., Mitchell, L., Maxwell, C. J., et al. (2011). Beyond the "Iron Lungs of Gerontology": Using evidence to shape the future of nursing homes in Canada. *Canadian Journal on Aging, 30*(3), 371–390. doi:10.1017/S0714980811000304.

Höhn, A., & Grune, T. (2013). Lipofuscin: Formation, effects and role of macroautophagy. *Redox Biology, 1*(1), 140–144. doi:10.1016/j.redox.2013.01.006.

Hollander, M. J., Chappell, N. L., Prince, M. J., et al. (2007). Providing care and support for an aging population: Briefing notes on key policy issues. *Healthcare Quarterly, 10*(3), 34–45. doi:10.12927/hcq.2007.18923. (Seminal).

Holwerda, T. J., Deeg, D. J. H., Beekman, A. T. F., et al. (2014). Feelings of loneliness, but not social isolation, predict dementia onset: Results from the Amsterdam Study of the Elderly (AMSTEL). *Journal of Neurology, Neurosurgery, and Psychiatry, 85*, 135–142. doi:10.1136/jnnp-2012-302755.

Huff, R. M., Kline, M. V., & Peterson, D. V. (2014). *Health promotion in multicultural populations: A handbook for practitioners and students* (3rd ed.). Thousand Oaks, CA: Sage Publications.

Hwang, S. W., Wilkins, R., Tjepkema, M., et al. (2009). Mortality among residents of shelters, rooming houses, and hotels in Canada: 11 year follow-up study. *British Medical Journal, 339*, b4036. doi:10.1136/bmj.b4036. (Seminal).

Inouye, S. K., Westendorp, R. G. J., & Saczynski, J. S. (2013). Delirium in elderly people. *Lancet, 383*(9920), 911–922. doi:10.1016/S0140-6736(13)60688-1.

Irvine, K., Laws, K. R., Gale, T. M., et al. (2012). Greater cognitive deterioration in women than men with Alzheimer's disease: A meta analysis. *Journal of Clinical and Experimental Neuropsychology, 34*(9), 989–998. doi:10.1080/13803395.2012.712676.

Jett, K. (2016). Geropharmacology. In P. Ebersole, P. Hess, & A. Luggen (Eds.), *Toward healthy aging: Human needs and nursing response* (9th ed., pp. 101–114). St. Louis: Mosby.

Kim, H., Chang, M., Rose, K., et al. (2011). Predictors of caregiver burden in caregivers of individuals with dementia. *Journal of Advanced Nursing, 68*, 846–855. doi:10.1111/j.1365-2648.2011.05787.x.

Kiosses, D. N., Leon, A. C., & Areán, P. A. (2011). Psychosocial interventions for late-life major depression: Evidence-based treatments, predictors of treatment outcomes, and moderators of treatment effects. *The Psychiatric Clinics of North America, 34*(2), 377–401. doi:10.1013/j.psc.2011.03.011.

Kleinman, A., Eisenberg, L., & Good, B. (1978). Culture, illness, and care: Clinical lessons from anthropologic and cross-cultural research. *Annals of Internal Medicine, 88*(2), 251–258. (Seminal).

Krishna, M., Jauhari, A., Lepping, P., et al. (2011). Is group psychotherapy effective in older adults with depression? A systematic review. *International Journal of Geriatric Psychiatry, 26*(4), 331–340. doi:10.1002/gps.2546.

Lundman, B., & Jansson, L. (2007). The meaning of living with a long-term disease: To revalue and be revalued. *Journal of Clinical Nursing, 16*, 109–115. doi:10.1111/j.1365-2702.2007.01802.x. (Seminal).

Public Health Agency of Canada. (2012). *Elder abuse: It's time to face the reality*. Retrieved from *http://www.phac-aspc.gc.ca/sfv-avf/sources/age/age-abuse-broch/index-eng.php#Wha*.

Public Health Agency of Canada. (2017). *Aging and seniors*. Ottawa: Author. Retrieved from *https://www.canada.ca/en/public-health/services/health-promotion/aging-seniors.html*.

Ramani, L., Furmedge, D., & Reddy, S. P. H. (2014). Comprehensive geriatric assessment. *British Journal of Hospital Medicine, 75*(8), C122–C125.

Reason, B., Terner, M., Moses McKeag, A., et al. (2012). The impact of polypharmacy on the health of Canadian seniors. *Family Practice, 29*(4), 427–432. doi:10.1093/fampra/cmr124.

Registered Nurses' Association of Ontario. (2012). *Nursing Best Practice Guidelines. Promoting safety: Alternative approaches to the use of restraints*. Toronto: Author. Retrieved from *http://rnao.ca/bpg/guidelines/promoting-safety-alternative-approaches-use-restraints*.

Registered Nurses' Association of Ontario. (2017). *Nursing best practice guidelines*. Toronto: Author. Retrieved from *http://rnao.ca/bpg*.

Shaw, P. X., Werstuck, G., & Chen, Y. (2014). Oxidative stress and aging diseases. *Oxidative Medicine and Cellular Longevity, 2014*, 569146. doi:10.1155/2014/569146.

Sinha, S. K. (2012). *Living longer, living well*. Report submitted to the Minister of Health and long-term care and the minister responsible for seniors on recommendations to Inform a Senior Strategy for Ontario. Retrieved from *https://www.google.com/#q=%22Living+longer%2C+living+well%22+sinha*.

Sinha, S. K. (2013). *Portrait of caregivers, 2012*. Retrieved from *http://www.statcan.gc.ca/pub/89-652-x/89-652-x2013001-eng.htm*.

Skirbekk, H., & Nortvedt, P. (2014). Inadequate treatment for elderly patients: Professional norms and tight budgets could cause "ageism" in hospitals. *Health Care Analysis, 22*(2), 192–201. doi:10.1007/s10728-012-0207-2.

Spina, J., & Menec, V. H. (2015). What community characteristics help or hinder rural communities in becoming age-friendly? Perspectives from a Canadian prairie province. *Journal of Applied Gerontology, 34*(4), 444–464. doi:10.1177/0733464813496164.

Statistics Canada. (2010a). *Population projections for Canada, provinces and territories: 2009 to 2036*. Retrieved from *http://www.statcan.gc.ca/pub/91-520-x/91-520-x2010001-eng.pdf*.

Statistics Canada. (2010b). *Life expectancy at birth and at age 65 by sex and by geography*. Ottawa: Ministry of Industry. Retrieved from *http://www.statcan.gc.ca/tables-tableaux/sum-som/l01/cst01/health72a-eng.htm*.

Statistics Canada. (2010c). *Family violence against seniors*. Retrieved from *http://www.statcan.gc.ca/pub/85-002-x/2012001/article/11643/hl-fs-eng.htm#a4*.

Statistics Canada. (2011a). *Ethnic diversity and immigration*. Retrieved from *http://www.statcan.gc.ca/pub/11-402-x/2011000/chap/imm/imm-eng.htm*.

Statistics Canada. (2011b). *Living arrangements of seniors*. Retrieved from *https://www12.statcan.gc.ca/census-recensement/2011/as-sa/98-312-x/98-312-x2011003_4-eng.cfm*.

Statistics Canada. (2011c). *Generations in Canada*. Retrieved from *https://www12.statcan.gc.ca/census-recensement/2011/as-sa/98-311-x/98-311-x2011003_2-eng.cfm*.

Statistics Canada. (2017). *Aboriginal statistics at a glance*. Retrieved from *http://www.statcan.gc.ca/pub/89-645-x/2010001/life-expectancy-esperance-vie-eng.htm*.

Strengthening Rural Canada Initiative. (2014). *Strengthening rural Canada: Fewer and older: The coming demographic crisis in rural Ontario*. Retrieved from *http://strengtheningruralcanada.ca/wp-content/uploads/Executive-Summary-Fewer-and-Older-The-Coming-Demographic-Crisis-in-Rural-Ontario.pdf*.

Touhy, T., Jett, K., Boscart, V. M., et al. (2011). *Gerontological nursing and healthy aging* (1st Canadian ed.). Toronto: Elsevier Canada.

Victor, C. R. (1994). *Old age in modern society: A textbook of social gerontology* (2nd ed.). New York: Springer.

Wahl, J. (2008). *Who assesses capacity under what circumstances?* Toronto: Advocacy Centre for the Elderly. Retrieved from *http://www.advocacycentreelderly.org/appimages/file/Who%20Assesses%20Capacity%20-%20November%202008.pdf*. (Seminal).

RESOURCES

Canadian Accreditation Council
http://www.canadianaccreditation.ca/

Canadian Association on Gerontology (CAG)
http://www.cagacg.ca

Canadian Centre for Elder Law
http://www.bcli.org/ccel

Canadian Coalition for Seniors' Mental Health
http://www.ccsmh.ca

Canadian Gerontological Nursing Association
http://www.cgna.net

Canadian Network for the Prevention of Elder Abuse
http://www.cnpea.ca

Canadian Patient Safety Institute
http://www.patientsafetyinstitute.ca/en/Pages/default.aspx

Canadian Women's Health Network
http://www.cwhn.ca/

Canadian Network for the Prevention of Elder Abuse
http://cnpea.ca/en/

Government of Canada—Seniors Canada On-line
https://www.getcybersafe.gc.ca/cnt/prtct-yrslf/prtctn-fml/snrs-nln-en.aspx

Guide to Health and Social Services for Aboriginal People in Manitoba
http://www.wrha.mb.ca/aboriginalhealth/services/files/AHSGuide.pdf

Health Canada: Healthy Living: Seniors
http://www.hc-sc.gc.ca/hl-vs/seniors-aines/index_e.html

Health Canada: Just for You—Seniors
http://www.hc-sc.gc.ca/hl-vs/jfy-spv/seniors-aines_e.html

National Initiative for the Care of the Elderly
http://www.nicenet.ca

Oaknet Legal Resources by Province and Territory
http://www.oaknet.ca/node/112

Ontario Pharmacy Evidence Network
http://www.open-pharmacy-research.ca

Promoting Awareness of Elder Abuse in Long-Term Care Homes (PEACE) pan-Canadian initiative
https://www.nurseone.ca/en/knowledge-features/elder-abuse
http://rnao.ca/bpg/initiatives/promoting-awareness-elder-abuse-longterm-care

Public Health Agency of Canada—Division of Aging and Seniors
http://www.phac-aspc.gc.ca/seniors-aines/index_pages/aboutis_e.htm

Public Health Agency of Canada: Medication Matters: How You Can Help Seniors Use Medication Safely
http://publications.gc.ca/site/eng/9.695567/publication.html

Public Health Agency of Canada: Reaching Out: A Guide to Communicating With Aboriginal Seniors
http://publications.gc.ca/site/archivee-archived.html?url=http://publications.gc.ca/collections/Collection/H88-3-30-2001/pdfs/com/reach_e.pdf

Public Health Agency of Canada: *The Safe Living Guide—A Guide to Home Safety for Seniors*
http://www.phac-aspc.gc.ca/seniors-aines/publications/public/injury-blessure/safelive-securite/index-eng.php

University of Victoria: Cultural safety learning modules
http://web2.uvcs.uvic.ca/courses/csafety/mod1/index.htm
http://web2.uvcs.uvic.ca/courses/csafety/mod2/index.htm
http://web2.uvcs.uvic.ca/courses/csafety/mod3/index.htm

Hartford Institute for Geriatric Nursing
https://hign.org

For additional Internet resources, see the website for this book at *http://evolve.elsevier.com/Canada/Lewis/medsurg*

Stress and Stress Management

Written by: Sharon L. Lewis and Peter N. Bonner
Adapted by: Jane Tyerman

℮volve WEBSITE

http://evolve.elsevier.com/Canada/Lewis/medsurg

- Review Questions (Online Only)
- Key Points
- Answer Guidelines for Case Study

- Conceptual Care Map Creator
- Audio Glossary
- Content Updates

LEARNING OBJECTIVES

1. Define the terms *stressor, stress, demands, coping, adaptation,* and *allostasis.*
2. Describe the three stages of Hans Selye's general adaptation syndrome.
3. Explain the role of coping in managing stress.
4. Describe the role of the nervous and endocrine systems in the stress process.
5. Describe the effects of stress on the immune system.
6. Describe the effects of stress on health and illness.
7. Describe coping strategies that can be used by persons experiencing stress.
8. List variables that may influence an individual's response to stress.
9. Describe the nursing assessment and management of a patient experiencing stress.

KEY TERMS

alarm reaction, p. 112
allostasis, p. 112
coping, p. 116
coping resources, p. 116
emotion-focused coping, p. 116

eustress, p. 111
general adaptation syndrome, p. 112
imagery, p. 118
problem-focused coping, p. 116

psychoneuroimmunology, p. 114
resilience, p. 113
sense of coherence, p. 112
stage of exhaustion, p. 112

stage of resistance, p. 112
stress, p. 110
stressors, p. 110

Stress is a fact of daily living that can have a positive or negative effect on the mind and body. Stress, especially if it is intense or chronic, is linked to numerous psychological and physiological disorders. Anticipating potentially stressful situations, identifying stress, and implementing appropriate measures to minimize its effect is an important aspect in health promotion and disease prevention. Because high levels of stress are common among patients and their caregivers, nurses play a very important role in helping patients manage stressful events. Understanding the relationship of stress to physical and emotional health and how people cope with stress is the primary focus of this chapter.

DEFINITION OF STRESS

Stress is the inability to cope with perceived (real or imagined) demands or threats to an individual's mental, emotional, or spiritual well-being (Seward, 2014). Like pain or grief, it is a subjective condition: It is what the affected person says it is.

Stress occurs when individuals perceive that they cannot adequately cope with demands being made on them or when their well-being is threatened (Lazarus & Folkman, 1984). These stress-inducing demands are known as **stressors** (Selye, 1983). What is perceived as stressful and the response to the stressor vary greatly among individuals and are influenced by a multitude of factors such as genetic makeup, life experience, family influences, and culture. This is demonstrated in the following examples:

- A woman becomes depressed and refuses to participate in normal self-care activities after a laparoscopic hysterectomy. In this situation, the removal of her uterus is a great stressor because the woman perceives it as a loss of her womanhood and femininity.
- A patient who is told she has type 2 diabetes reacts with a smile. However, the patient is relieved because for weeks she has been worrying that her symptoms were related to terminal cancer.

Many different events, factors, or stimuli can be thought of as stressors. They can be physiological or emotional–psychological

TABLE 8-1	EXAMPLES OF STRESSORS
Physiological	**Emotional–Psychological**
• Burns	• Diagnosis of cancer
• Chronic pain	• Marital and other family problems
• Birth of a baby	• Failing an examination
• Infectious diseases	• Inadequate financial resources
• Excessive noise	• Grieving
• Inadequate nutrition	• Prolonged period of caregiving
• Running a marathon	

PATHOPHYSIOLOGY MAP

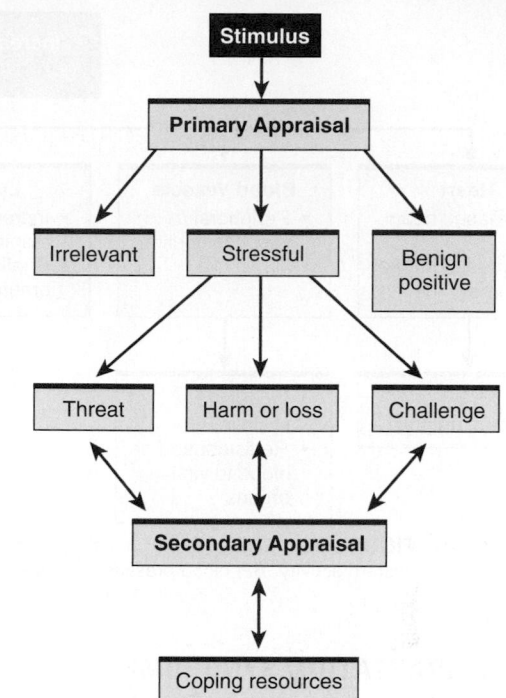

FIGURE 8-1 Cognitive appraisal process.

(Table 8-1) and positive or negative. The key aspect of stressors is that they require an individual to adapt to a situation (Lazarus & Folkman, 1984). There are differences in the behavioural and physiological adaptive responses to a stressor that are based on the duration of the stressor (acute or chronic) and intensity of the stressor (mild, moderate, or severe). For example, an individual dealing with the chronic stress of caring for a loved one may also be exposed to a multitude of acute episodic stressors (e.g., car accident, influenza).

Daily hassles are experiences and conditions of daily living that are viewed as irritating, frustrating, and distressing. The frequency and intensity of daily hassles have a stronger relationship with somatic illness than do major life events (Lazarus & Folkman, 1984). Examples of daily hassles are traffic, waiting, misplacing or losing things, deadlines, and planning meals. Not all stress is bad. Selye (1983) coined the term **eustress** to refer to stress associated with positive events such as the birth of a baby, going for a run, falling in love, or attending a much-anticipated event. A little stress can motivate and inspire an individual to achieve a goal and become more confident or stronger physically. Uplifts may modify the negative effects of daily hassles. Although studies of the effects of negative experiences (hassles or life events) are more plentiful, it is generally accepted that emotions such as humour and behaviours such as laughter are associated with healthy physiological and psychological functioning (Berk, 2015; Kuiper, 2012).

WORK-RELATED STRESS

Work-related stress occurs when there is an imbalance between work demands and a worker's ability to cope with these demands. Nursing-related work demands can include poor working conditions, work overload, shift work, and time pressures. Other demands stem from the individual's role in the organization (e.g., role conflict), career development (e.g., underpromotion), relationships at work (e.g., difficulties in delegating responsibilities), and the organizational climate (e.g., restrictions on behaviour). The extensive research on these factors and their effects validates inclusion of occupation and work experience as essential factors in patient assessment. According to 2010 General Social Survey (Statistics Canada, 2015), 37% of employed Canadians reported that they were experiencing high degrees of stress, citing work as their main source of stress. Decreasing staffing resources for managing increasing workload has been shown to be one of the most significant factors contributing to emotional exhaustion and burnout in nurses (Aiken et al., 2011; Duffield et al., 2011). This burnout is reflective of the nursing attrition rate, which peaked in 2013 at 7.1% and exceeded the number of nurses entering the workforce (Canadian Institute for Health Information, 2016).

THEORIES OF STRESS

Three different but complementary stress theories have influenced most contemporary approaches to the study of stress. The current understanding of stress began with Hans Selye, who performed his research at McGill University in Montreal in the late 1930s. He conceptualized stress as a response to a demand or stressor that elicits a series of physiological changes to which the person must adapt. This process is known as *general adaptation syndrome* and is discussed in the next section.

According to a second stress theory, stress is a stimulus that causes a response. This theory originated with Holmes and Masuda (1966) and Miller and Rahe (1997), who developed the Social Readjustment Rating Scale to assess the effects of life changes on health. The major assumption of this theory is that frequent life changes make people more vulnerable to illness. Life changes can range from minor violations of the law to the death of a loved one.

A third stress theory focuses on person–environment interactions and is referred to as the *transaction* or *interaction theory*. Proponents of this theory were Lazarus and Folkman (1984), who emphasized the role of *cognitive appraisal* (Figure 8-1) in assessing stressful situations and selecting coping options. They conceptualized cognitive appraisal as a judgement or evaluative process whereby the individual recognizes the degree of stress and its effect on well-being; as a result of this appraisal, the individual uses coping resources that respond to the demand placed upon them. Cognitive appraisal is divided into two stages: primary and secondary appraisal. Primary appraisal focuses on the influence or effect of the stressor; secondary appraisal involves positive or negative perceptions that the individual holds concerning his or her ability to overcome the stressor.

PATHOPHYSIOLOGY MAP

FIGURE 8-2 "Fight-or-flight" reaction. Alarm reaction responses resulting from increased sympathetic nervous system activity. *BP*, blood pressure; *GI*, gastro-intestinal; *SNS*, sympathetic nervous system.

GENERAL ADAPTATION SYNDROME

The **general adaptation syndrome** is composed of three stages: alarm reaction, stage of resistance, and stage of exhaustion. Once the environmental event or stressor stimulates the central nervous system, multiple responses occur because of activation of the hypothalamic–pituitary–adrenal axis and the autonomic nervous system.

The first stage of the stress response is the **alarm reaction**, in which the individual perceives a stressor physically or mentally and the fight-or-flight response is initiated (Figure 8-2). When the stressor is of sufficient intensity to threaten the steady state or homeostasis of the individual, it leads to a series of physiological changes that promote adaptation. This temporarily decreases the individual's resistance and may even result in disease or death if the stress is prolonged and severe.

Ideally, the individual quickly moves from the alarm reaction to the **stage of resistance**, in which physiological reserves are mobilized to increase the resistance to stress. At this time, adaptation may occur. The amount of resistance to the stressor varies among individuals, depending on the level of physical functioning, coping abilities, and total number and intensity of stressors experienced. For example, a person who has been exercising regularly and is physically fit has a greater ability to adapt to the stress of emergency surgery than does a person who is deconditioned and leads a sedentary lifestyle.

Although few overt physical signs and symptoms occur in the resistance stage in comparison with the alarm stage, the person is expending energy in an attempt to adapt. **Allostasis** is the process of achieving homeostasis in the presence of a challenge (Sterling, 1988). When internal and external resources are adequate, the individual may recover successfully from a stressor and return to his or her baseline state. If homeostasis is not achieved, and if these allostatic responses do not terminate, adaptation does not occur, and the person may move to the final phase of the general adaptation syndrome.

The **stage of exhaustion** is that final stage. It occurs when all of the energy for adaptation has been expended. Physical symptoms of the alarm reaction may briefly reappear in a final effort by the body to survive. A terminally ill person who becomes alert and has stronger vital signs shortly before death exemplifies this phenomenon. The individual in the stage of exhaustion usually becomes ill and may die if assistance from outside sources is not available. This stage can often be reversed by external sources of adaptive energy, such as medication or psychotherapy. Selye's research indicated that there is a predictable, uniform pattern in the physiological response to various stressors.

FACTORS AFFECTING RESPONSE TO STRESS

Why do people respond differently to stress, and why do some cope better with stress than do others? Factors that affect an individual's response to stress include internal and external influences, a fact that underscores the importance of using a holistic approach in assessing the effect of stress on an individual. See the "Determinants of Health" box for additional factors affecting people's response to stress.

In attempts to understand why some individuals do not experience negative consequences from stress, researchers have identified key personal characteristics, such as hardiness, sense of coherence, resilience, and attitude as possible factors that buffer the effect of stress. *Hardiness* is a combination of three characteristics: commitment, control, and openness to change. Together they provide protection against stress and depression (Hasel, Besharat, Abdolhoseini, et al., 2013). An *internal locus of control* is the perception that the person's life is self-determined, as opposed to being directed by outside or external events, luck, or chance (an *external locus of control*). Hardiness is discussed in more detail in Chapter 5.

Sense of coherence, first described by Antonovsky (1987), is a concept closely related to hardiness and is thought to be a key determinant of health. Sense of coherence is reflected in an optimistic view of the world and perceived ability to function optimally in that world. An individual with a strong sense of coherence has an enduring tendency to see his or her life as ordered, manageable, and meaningful.

DETERMINANTS OF HEALTH

Factors Affecting an Individual's Response to Stress

Employment and Working Conditions
- Jobs with high skill utilization, increased psychological demands, job insecurity, and low levels of social support at work are associated with increased levels of psychological distress.*
- Shift work is correlated with poor lifestyle habits such as snacking and decreased physical activity.†
- Shift work is also linked to depression, anxiety, stress-related chronic diseases, and insomnia.†

Health Practices and Coping Skills
Personal Health Practices and Coping Styles
- Individuals who are physically active have lower levels of stress.‡
- Strong support social systems enhance the capacity for an individual to cope with stress.§
- Stress predisposes an individual to emotional eating and impairs sleep hygiene.¶

References

*Marchand, A., Drapeau, A., & Beaulieu-Prévost, D. (2012). Psychological distress in Canada: the role of employment and reasons of non-employment. *International Journal of Social Psychiatry, 58*(6), 596–604.

†Johnstone, A. M., Giles, K., Maloney, N. G., et al. (2015). Effect of shift work on stress and eating behaviour (the NeuroFAST study). *Proceedings of the Nutrition Society, 74*(OCE3), E201. doi: 10.1017/S002966511500227X.

‡Lippke, S., Wienert, J., Kuhlmann, T., et al. (2015). Perceived stress, physical activity and motivation: Findings from an internet study. *Target, 5*, 8.

§Sippel, L. M., Pietrzak, R. H., Charney, D. S., et al. (2015). How does social support enhance resilience in the trauma-exposed individual? *Ecology & Society, 20*(4), Article 10.

¶Dweck, J. S., Jenkins, S. M., & Nolan, L. J. (2014). The role of emotional eating and stress in the influence of short sleep on food consumption. *Appetite, 72*, 106–113.

Resilience is another characteristic that is believed to moderate or buffer the negative effects of stress. **Resilience** is defined as the ability to be resourceful, be flexible, and recover from stressful situations and return to prior levels of functioning. Resilient individuals tend to employ more effective coping and problem-solving strategies, to possess higher self-esteem, and to be less likely to perceive an event as stressful or taxing.

Attitude can also influence the effect of stress on a person. People with positive attitudes view situations differently than do those with negative attitudes. A person's attitude also influences how he or she manages stress. To some extent, positive emotional attitudes can prevent disease and prolong life. Optimistic people tend to recover more quickly, whereas pessimistic people are likely to deny the problem, distance themselves from the stressful event, focus on stressful feelings, or allow the stressor to interfere with achieving a goal (Mayo Clinic, 2015). In addition to personal characteristics, being surrounded by a strong social support system and receiving positive support from friends and family have a significant effect on an individual's ability to cope with stressors.

PHYSIOLOGICAL RESPONSE TO STRESS

The following discussion is divided into descriptions of the nervous, endocrine, and immune systems. These systems, and thus the physiological stress responses, are interrelated (Figure 8-3). Stress activation of these systems also affects other systems,

PATHOPHYSIOLOGY MAP

FIGURE 8-3 Neurochemical links among the nervous, endocrine, and immune systems. The communication among these three systems is bidirectional.

such as the cardiovascular, respiratory, gastro-intestinal, renal, and reproductive systems.

The complex process by which an event is perceived as a stressor and the body responds is not fully understood. A person's response to a stressor determines the effect it will have on the body. In addition, the body responds physiologically to both actual (physiological) and perceived (emotional–psychological) stressors.

Nervous System

Cerebral Cortex. In the cerebral cortex, the emotional–psychological event (stressor) is evaluated with reference to past experiences and future consequences, and a course of action is planned. These functions are involved in the perception of a stressor.

Limbic System. The limbic system lies in the inner midportion of the brain near the base of the brain. The limbic system is an important mediator of emotions and behaviour. When the limbic system is stimulated, emotions, feelings, and behaviours that ensure survival and self-preservation may occur.

Reticular Formation. The reticular formation is located between the lower end of the brainstem and the thalamus. It contains the reticular activating system, which is crucial for the state of wakefulness. When stimulated, the reticular activating system sends impulses to the limbic system and the cerebral cortex, which produce arousal and emotional responses to the stressor. Stress usually increases the degree of wakefulness and can lead to sleep disturbances.

Hypothalamus. The hypothalamus, which lies at the base of the brain just above the pituitary gland, has many functions that assist in adaptation to stress. It is the central connection between the nervous and endocrine systems in the stress response. Emotional–psychological (perceived) stressors activate the limbic system, which in turn stimulates the hypothalamus. The hypothalamus sends signals via nerve fibres to stimulate the sympathetic nervous system. It also releases hormones that regulate the secretion of adrenocorticotrophic hormone (ACTH) by the anterior pituitary gland (Figure 8-4). Physiological (actual) stressors may originate in the limbic system or in portions of the brain that receive sensory information, which in turn then stimulate the hypothalamus (see Chapter 50).

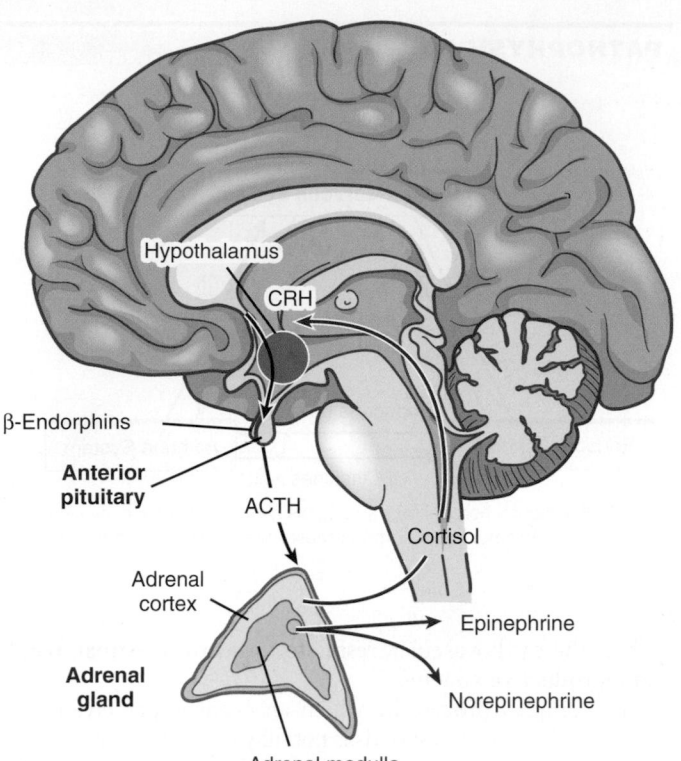

FIGURE 8-4 Hypothalamic-pituitary-adrenal axis. *ACTH,* adrenocorticotrophic hormone; *CRH,* corticotropin-releasing hormone.

Endocrine System

Once the hypothalamus is activated in response to stress, the endocrine system becomes involved. The sympathetic nervous system stimulates the adrenal medulla to release epinephrine and norepinephrine (catecholamines), which initiates a protective reflex called the *fight-or-flight response* (see Figure 8-2). This, along with the actual response of the body to the catecholamines, is referred to as the *sympatho-adrenal response.* Stress activates the hypothalamic–pituitary–adrenal axis (see Figure 8-4). In response to stress, the hypothalamus releases corticotropin-releasing hormone, which stimulates the anterior pituitary to release pro-opiomelanocortin (POMC). Both ACTH (a hormone) and β-endorphin (a neuropeptide) are derived from POMC. Endorphins have analgesic-like effects and blunt pain perception during stress situations involving pain stimuli. ACTH, in turn, stimulates the adrenal cortex to synthesize and secrete corticosteroids (e.g., cortisol) and, to a lesser degree, aldosterone. The posterior pituitary increases production of antidiuretic hormone, which leads to water retention and a decrease in urine output (Figure 8-5).

Corticosteroids are essential for the stress response. Cortisol, a primary corticosteroid, produces a number of physiological effects that potentiate or blunt aspects of the stress response, such as increasing blood glucose levels, potentiating the action of catecholamines (epinephrine, norepinephrine) on blood vessels, and inhibiting the inflammatory response. The resulting increases in cardiac output, blood glucose levels, oxygen consumption, and metabolic rate enable the fight-or-flight response (see Figure 8-2). Dilation of blood vessels supplying skeletal muscle increases blood supply to the large muscles, which provides for quick movement, and increased cerebral blood flow heightens mental

alertness. The increase in blood volume (which results from increases in extracellular fluid and shunting of blood away from the gastro-intestinal system) helps maintain adequate circulation to vital organs in case of traumatic blood loss.

By mediating the inflammatory response, cortisol plays an important role in "turning off" aspects of the stress response, which if uncontrolled can become self-destructive. This is best exemplified by the suppression of proinflammatory mediators, such as the cytokines, tumour necrosis factor, and interleukin-1. The persistent release of such mediators is believed to initiate organ dysfunction in conditions such as sepsis. Thus corticosteroids act not only to support the adaptive response of the body to a stressor but also to suppress an overzealous and potentially self-destructive response.

Summary of Neuroendocrine System Stress Response

In summary, the fight-or-flight response is a very important mechanism of the body for adapting to acute stress. This response is triggered by stressors, regardless of whether they are physiological or emotional–psychological. The acute stress response is a state of physiological and psychological arousal characterized by increased sympathetic nervous system activity that leads to increases in heart and respiratory rate, blood pressure, muscle tension, and brain activity, and to decreases in skin temperature.

Immune System

Psychoneuroimmunology is an interdisciplinary science in which investigators seek to understand the interactions among psychological, neurological, and immune responses (Pariante, 2015). It is now known that the brain is connected to the immune system by neuroanatomical and neuroendocrine pathways; thus stressors have the potential to cause alterations in immune function (Figure 8-6). The network that links the brain and immune system is bidirectional, allowing for back-and-forth communication among these systems; therefore, not only do emotions modify the immune response but also the products of immune cells send signals back to the brain and alter its activity (see Figure 8-3). Much of the communication from the immune system to the brain is mediated by cytokines, which are crucial in the coordination of the immune response. For example, interleukin-1 (a cytokine made by monocytes) acts on the temperature-regulatory centre of the hypothalamus and initiates the febrile response to infectious pathogens.

Nerve fibres extend from the nervous system and reach synapses on cells and tissues (i.e., spleen, lymph nodes) of the immune system. In turn, the cells of the immune system have receptors for many neuropeptides and hormones, which enable them to respond to nervous and neuroendocrine signals. As a result, the mediation of stress by the central nervous system leads to corresponding changes in immune cell activity.

Both acute and chronic stress can affect immune function. Acute stress stimulates increased proliferation of cellular immune components such as neutrophils and natural killer cells, which are the body's first line of defence against infection (Segerstrom, 2012). The stress response is designed to be beneficial, however, only for acute short-term stress. Chronic stress appears to have a negative effect on both the cellular and humoral (antibody) immune systems (Segerstrom, 2012). Immune responses may be either suboptimal and thus ineffective when needed or hypervigilant, leading to chronic inflammatory states that exacerbate chronic stress and predispose affected persons to cardiovascular diseases (Steptoe & Kivimäki, 2012).

Stress
(usually caused by injurious or extreme stimuli)

Stimulates **limbic system** and other parts of **cerebral cortex**

Stimulates **hypothalamus**

| ↑ CRH release | Stimulates **sympathetic centres** and **adrenal medulla** | Stimulates **posterior pituitary gland** |

| Stimulates **anterior pituitary gland** to ↑ secretion of ACTH | ↑ Catecholamine levels (norepinephrine and epinephrine) in blood | ↑ ADH secretion |

| **Stimulates Adrenal Cortex**
• Marked ↑ glucocorticoid (cortisol) secretion
• Moderate ↑ mineralocorticoid (aldosterone) secretion | **"Fight-or-Flight" Response**
↑ Heart rate, blood pressure, and blood glucose concentration | Antidiuresis (↓ urine, ↑ water retention) |

| **Cortisol Effects**
• ↑ Catabolism of tissue proteins, gluconeogenesis, producing hyperglycemia
• ↓ Lymphocytes and immune responses
• ↓ Eosinophils and allergic responses | **Aldosterone Effects**
↑ Sodium and water reabsorption (sodium and water retention) | ↑ Blood volume |

FIGURE 8-5 Current concepts of the stress syndrome. *ADH,* antidiuretic hormone; *ACTH,* adrenocorticotrophic hormone; *ADH,* antidiuretic hormone; *CRH,* corticotropin-releasing hormone.

TABLE 8-2	**EXAMPLES OF CONDITIONS ASSOCIATED WITH MALADAPTATION TO STRESS**

• Angina	• Insomnia
• Asthma	• Irritable bowel syndrome
• Depression	• Low back pain
• Dyspepsia	• Menstrual irregularities
• Eating disorders	• Peptic ulcer disease
• Headaches	• Sexual dysfunction

EFFECTS OF STRESS ON HEALTH

Acute stress leads to physiological changes that are important to human adaptation and survival. However, if stress is excessive or prolonged, these physiological responses can be maladaptive and lead to harm and disease. When stress is chronic and unrelieved, the body's defences can no longer keep up with the demands. Over time, stress takes a toll (Figure 8-7) and plays a role in the development or progression of conditions related to maladaptation (Table 8-2).

Chronic and intense stress may have profound effects on brain structure and function, especially the hippocampus. The hippocampus plays an important role in long-term memory and other cognitive functions such as spatial learning. Chronic release of corticosteroids in response to stress appears to act in concert with certain neurotransmitters to produce hippocampal damage (Marin, Lord, Andrews, et al., 2011). Studies of people who have endured traumatic events (e.g., domestic violence, childhood neglect, war) reveal decreased hippocampal volume, activation, and activity. This is thought to explain the memory impairment/fragmentation and dissociation with the traumatic event that are common in post-traumatic stress disorder (Marin, Lord, Andrews, et al., 2011).

Stress can affect cognitive function, causing deterioration in concentration, memory problems, sleep disturbances, and impairment in decision making. In addition, stress can cause a wide variety of changes in behaviour. Such changes include withdrawing from others or becoming unusually talkative, eating disorders, substance abuse, or becoming irritable (Janusek, Cooper, & Matthews, 2012) . Stress can induce fatigue, and the resulting exhaustion limits a person's ability to cope. Fatigue is discussed in more detail in Chapter 5.

Although hypertension in acute stress is thought to be transient, studies demonstrate a strong association between chronic, maladaptive stress and sustained hypertension, which is a major risk factor for cardiovascular disease (Government of Canada, 2015). Other conditions that may be either precipitated or aggravated by stress include obesity, migraine headaches, irritable

PATHOPHYSIOLOGY MAP

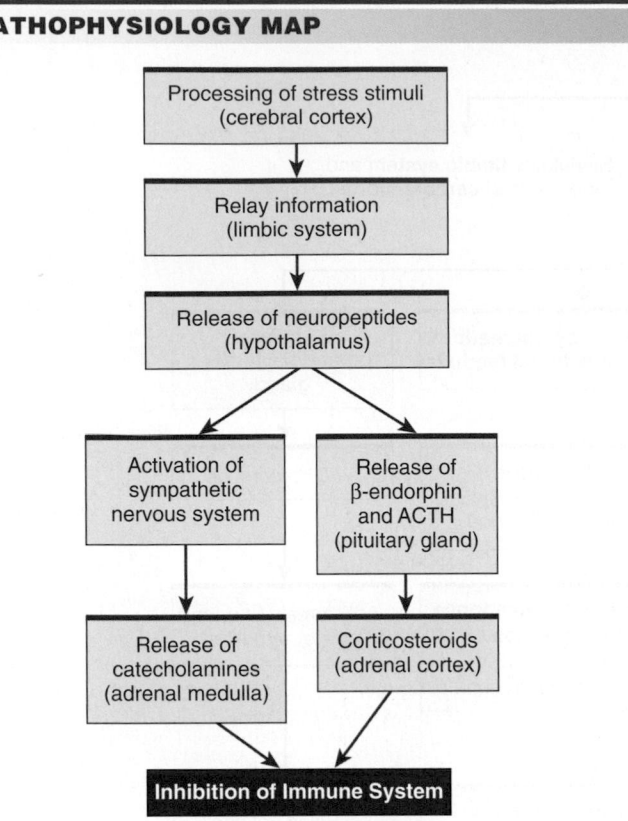

FIGURE 8-6 The psychological and neuroendocrine response to stress alters immune function. *ACTH,* adrenocorticotrophic hormone.

FIGURE 8-7 Chronic stress can take a toll on the body, resulting in poor concentration and memory problems. Source: Syda Productions/Shutterstock.com.

bowel syndrome, and peptic ulcers (Koenig, Walker, Romeo, et al., 2011). Not only can stress induce immunosuppression, making a person more vulnerable to infectious diseases, but also it may exacerbate or increase the risk of progression of immune-based diseases such as multiple sclerosis, asthma, rheumatoid arthritis, and cancer (Janusek, Cooper, & Matthews, 2012; Koenig, Walker, Romeo, et al., 2011). Many questions about stress and the immune response remain unanswered. For example, it is not known how much stress is needed to cause these changes or how much of an alteration in the immune system is necessary before an affected person becomes susceptible to disease. A current challenge for researchers in the field of psychoneuroimmunology is to study stress-induced immune changes and their relationship to health and to illness outcomes.

TABLE 8-3	EXAMPLES OF COPING RESOURCES
Internal Coping Resources	
Health, Energy, Morale	**Problem-Solving Skills**
• Robust health	• Collection of information
• High energy level	• Identification of problem
• High morale	• Generation of alternatives
• Positive beliefs	• Social skills
• Self-efficacy	• Communication skills
• Spirituality	• Compatibility
External Coping Resources	
Social Networks	**Utilitarian Resources**
• Family members	• Finances
• Co-workers	• Self-help books
• Social contacts	• Social agencies

TABLE 8-4 EXAMPLES OF EMOTION- AND PROBLEM-FOCUSED COPING		
Stressor	**Emotion-Focused Coping**	**Problem-Focused Coping**
Receiving a diagnosis of terminal cancer	Seeking spiritual guidance from one's place of worship	Preparing advanced health care directives
Exacerbation of chronic obstructive pulmonary disease (COPD)	Joining a support group	Quitting smoking
Renal failure that necessitates frequent travel for dialysis	Enjoying relaxing music and reading during travel time	Arranging for a volunteer driver
Extended hospital stay for stem cell transplantation	Communicating on Skype with family/ friends regularly while in hospital	Arranging for child/ family care before hospital admission

COPING

Coping is a person's cognitive and behavioural efforts to manage specific external or internal stressors that seem to exceed available resources (Lazarus & Folkman, 1984). Coping can be either positive or negative. Positive coping includes activities such as exercise and use of social support. Negative coping may include substance abuse and denial. Availability of coping resources affects an individual's ability to cope with stressful situations. **Coping resources** are internal or external assets, characteristics, or actions that a person draws upon to manage stress (Table 8-3).

Coping strategies function broadly in two ways: as emotion-focused or problem-focused efforts (Table 8-4). **Emotion-focused coping** involves managing the emotions that an individual feels when a stressful event occurs. Examples of emotion-focused coping include discussion of feelings with a friend or relaxing in a hot bath. **Problem-focused coping** is a cognitive approach in which the person attempts to find solutions to the problems causing the stress. For example, setting priorities, collecting information, and seeking advice would be considered problem-focused coping. Emotion- and problem-focused strategies can be employed alone or in combination to cope with the same stressor. Although it may not appear to be working toward a solution, emotion-focused coping is a valid and appropriate way to deal with various stressful situations. Two primary purposes of emotion-focused coping are to alleviate negative emotions and to create a sense of well-being. When a situation is unchangeable or uncontrollable, emotion-focused coping may dominate. If a problem can be changed or controlled, problem-focused cognitive coping may be more effective. Problem-focused coping strategies enable an individual to look at a challenge objectively, take action to address the problem, and thereby reduce the stress.

A key concept to successful coping is *coping flexibility,* which involves the ability to assess the nature of the stressor, determine what aspects can be controlled, and change and adapt coping strategies over time and across different stressful conditions. Stressful situations are best handled when an individual practises flexible coping, inasmuch as certain strategies work more effectively than others, depending on the circumstances, and overreliance on one type of coping strategy can be incapacitating. Regular exercise, especially aerobic movement, results in improved circulation, increased release of endorphins, and an enhanced sense of well-being. Numerous strategies have been shown to prevent or mitigate the effects of stress and are discussed in subsequent sections of this chapter.

RELAXATION STRATEGIES

Benson (1975) described *relaxation response* as a state of physiological and psychological deep rest. It is characterized by decreased central nervous system and sympathetic nervous system activity, which leads to decreases in heart and respiratory rates, blood pressure, muscle tension, and brain activity and an increase in skin temperature. The relaxation response can be elicited through a variety of relaxation strategies, including relaxation breathing, meditation, imagery, muscle relaxation, prayer, and physical exercise. It is an effective intervention for stress-related disorders, including chronic pain, insomnia, and hypertension. Individuals who regularly engage in relaxation strategies are able to deal better with their stressors, to increase their sense of control over stressors, and to reduce their tension (Fjorback, Arendt, Ørnbøl, et al., 2011). In addition to common strategies discussed in the following section, the relaxation response can be elicited through methods listed in Table 8-5.

Relaxation Breathing

Relaxation breathing forms the basis for most relaxation strategies, and an individual can perform it while sitting, standing, or lying down. It is especially useful in reducing stress during a stressful or anxiety-provoking experience. Techniques for relaxation breathing are presented in Table 8-6.

Before a person practises relaxation breathing, it is important to assess his or her normal breathing pattern. To do this, the person begins by placing one hand gently on the abdomen below the waistline and the other hand on the centre of the chest. Without changing the normal breathing pattern, the person takes several breaths. During inhalation, the person takes notice of which hand rises the most. When relaxation breathing is performed properly, the hand on the abdomen should rise more than the hand on the chest. Chest breathing, which involves the upper chest and shoulders, is associated with inefficient breathing, and often occurs during anxiety and distress. Relaxation breathing, which involves the diaphragm, is natural for newborns and sleeping adults and is associated with efficient breathing.

TABLE 8-5 EXAMPLES OF STRESS MANAGEMENT TECHNIQUES

Technique	Description
Thought stopping	A self-directed behavioural approach is used to gain control of self-defeating thoughts. When these thoughts occur, the individual stops the thought process and focuses on conscious relaxation.
Humour	Humour in the form of laughter, cartoons, funny movies, riddles, CDs, comic books, and joke books can be used for both the nurse and the patient.
Assertive behaviour	This behaviour entails open, honest sharing of feelings, desires, and opinions in a controlled way. The individual who has behaves assertively is less subject to stress.
Yoga	This activity incorporates exercise, postures, regulated breathing and meditation to decrease stress and to promote physical and mental well-being.
Social support	This may take the form of organized support and self-help groups, relationships with family and friends, professional help, or some combination.
Journal keeping	The individual expresses self in written form, such as personal events, thoughts, feelings, memories, and perceptions. This may allow the individual to increase self-awareness and coping.
Colouring	Colouring is a relaxation technique that lowers activity of the amygdala, a part of the brain involved in controlling negative emotions that are affected by stress. The colouring and creating of mandalas, a circular design with concentric shapes, embraces creativity and has been shown to decrease negative thoughts (Babouchkina & Robbins, 2015).
Biofeedback	This is a method of monitoring and controlling physiological responses to stressful or challenging events; these responses include skin temperature, muscle tension, heart rate, brain waves, and skin conductance (see Chapter 12).

CD, compact disc.

🌸 COMPLEMENTARY & ALTERNATIVE THERAPIES

Stress

In addition to cognitive and behavioural coping strategies, a number of complementary and alternative therapies have been shown to help people to cope with their stress. See Chapter 12 for a discussion of the role of St. John's wort and kava in coping with stress. It is important to read the "Natural Products" section to ensure patient safety when considering herbal preparations in managing any disorders. Chapter 12 also contains discussions of other complementary and alternative therapies that may be used in managing stress, such as yoga, therapeutic and healing touch, massage, and prayer.

Meditation

Meditation is an ancient relaxation strategy used to reduce stress and enhance well-being through focused mindfulness. In people who meditate regularly, the brain is reoriented from a stressful fight-or-flight mode to one of acceptance and contentment (Shonin, Van Gordon, & Griffiths, 2014). Studies have demonstrated possible links between meditation and health. Health benefits include a regeneration of pancreatic cells, which increases the metabolism of glucose in adipose tissue and the liver; a reduction in blood pressure and regression of coronary artery disease; a decline in body mass index; an increased airflow to the lungs; and improved immunity (Ankad, Herur, Patil, et al., 2011; Balaji, Varne, & Ali, 2012). Individuals typically start learning

TABLE 8-6 RELAXATION STRATEGIES

Rhythmic Breathing

1. Find a quiet, peaceful environment.
2. Assume a comfortable position, whether sitting or lying down, ensuring that arms and legs are not crossed.
3. Close your eyes, and breathe in and out slowly, saying, "Breathe in, 2, 3, 4; breathe out, 2, 3, 4." The key is a "signal breath" involving deep inhalation through the nose and forceful exhalation through the mouth. The signal breath precedes and follows each repetition of the exercise.
4. Continue to breathe in and out slowly, using abdominal breathing, feeling more relaxed with each breath. As with any breathing exercise, if you begin feeling light-headed, discontinue exercise for 30 seconds and then start again. Initially, relaxation breathing may feel unusual. With practice it becomes easier, and the relaxing benefits are soon obvious.
5. When you are ready to end a breathing relaxation exercise, count silently from 1 to 3; on 1, move your lower body; on 2, move your upper body; on 3, breathe in deeply, open your eyes, and while breathing out slowly, say silently, "I am relaxed and alert." Stretch as if just waking up.

Relaxation by Sensory Pacing

1. Follow steps 1 and 2 of rhythmic breathing.
2. Slowly repeat and finish each of the following sentences:
   "Now I am aware of seeing...."
   "Now I am aware of feeling...."
   "Now I am aware of hearing...."
   Repeat and complete each sentence four times, then three times, then twice, and finally once.
3. Allow the eyes to close when they feel heavy.

Progressive Relaxation

See the later section "Muscle Relaxation" as well as Table 8-7, for more detail.

1. Follow steps 1, 2, 3, and 4 of rhythmic breathing.
2. Once you are breathing slowly and comfortably, tighten and relax specific muscle groups in ordered succession, concentrating on the feeling of relaxing the muscle. Starting with the feet and moving upward, ending with the face, is an effective technique.
3. Lie still for a few minutes, experiencing the relaxed muscles. Continue to breathe slowly and deeply, feeling tension flow out and relaxation increasing with each breath.
4. When you are ready to get up, count backwards from 4 to 1 and slowly rise.

Modified Autogenic Relaxation

1. Follow steps 1, 2, 3, and 4 of rhythmic breathing.
2. Repeat each of the following phrases to yourself four times, saying the first part of the phrase while breathing in for 2 to 3 seconds, holding the breath for 2 to 3 seconds, and then saying the last part of the phrase while breathing out for 2 to 3 seconds:

Breathing In	Breathing Out
I am	relaxed.
My arms and legs	are heavy and warm.
My heartbeat	is calm and regular.
My breathing	is free and easy.
My abdomen	is loose and warm.
My forehead	is cool.
My mind	is quiet and still.

TABLE 8-7 BASIC GUIDE TO MEDITATION

- Find a quiet place, with no distractions.
- Sit in a comfortable position, and close your eyes.
- "Shut out the world" so that your brain can stop processing information coming from your senses.
- Pick a word or phrase that means something to you, whose sound or rhythm is soothing when repeated (e.g., "one," "peace," "shalom," "salaam," "The Lord is my shepherd").
- Breathe slowly, and practise relaxation breathing.
- Say the word or phrase again and again, or try saying it silently to yourself with every exhalation.
- The monotony will help you focus.
- Do not be concerned when other thoughts come to mind; just acknowledge them and return calmly to your word or phrase.
- Continue for 10 to 20 minutes, but even 5 minutes can leave you feeling calm and refreshed. Rise slowly.
- Practise once or twice daily.

TABLE 8-8 IMAGERY: CREATING A "SPECIAL PLACE"

- Begin by finding a comfortable position, closing your eyes, and taking several slow, deep breaths.
- Imagine a place where you feel completely comfortable and peaceful. It may be a real place or one you imagine; it may be one from your past or some place you have always wanted to go.
- Allow this image to take form, slowly. As it takes form in your imagination, look around, to your left, to your right. Enjoy the scenery: the colours, the texture, and the shapes. Engage all senses: sight, hearing, touch, smell, and taste.
- Listen carefully to the sounds of your place. What do you hear?
- Is there a gentle breeze or sunshine warming your face? Imagine picking up or touching some favourite objects from this special place. Take in a deep breath through your nose, and notice the rich smells around you. Perhaps your favourite flower is in bloom, or you smell the scents of the ocean.
- Take another deep breath and relax. Enjoy the peace, comfort, and safety of this special place.
- This is your special place. You relax and feel thankful that you are here, in your special place.
- You can return to this place any time that you wish.

the technique with only 5 to 10 minutes of meditation at a time and increase the time as the practice becomes more comfortable. Table 8-7 is a guide to meditation. It is important to note that meditation takes practice, and people are often not successful at first, and so beginners should not feel discouraged.

Imagery

Imagery is the use of the mind to generate images that have a calming effect on the body (Table 8-8; Figure 8-8). It involves the use of mental focus and incorporates all the senses to create physiological and emotional changes. It is a simple relaxation technique that requires no equipment other than an active imagination. Guided imagery is a variation of imagery in which images are suggested by another person (either live or in a recording).

Imagery can be used in many clinical settings for stress reduction and pain relief. Benefits of imagery include reduction in anxiety, decrease in muscle tension, improvement in comfort

FIGURE 8-8 Imagery. Creating a "special place" should involve the physical senses, such as a place where rustling leaves can be heard, flowers are smelled, wind is felt, and a colourful landscape is seen. Source: Muriel Lasure/Shutterstock.com.

during medical procedures, enhancement of immune function, decrease in recovery time after surgery, and improvement in sleep. Health care providers may use imagery in their own lives or may use guided imagery with their patients. Imagery is used to create a safe and special place for mental retreat.

Imagery can also be used to specifically target a disease, problem, or stressor. For example, patients with cancer may imagine sharks gobbling up their cancer cells or radiation and chemotherapy entering the body like healing rays of light that destroy cancer cells. Special images can be created to alleviate symptoms (such as pain) or to treat disorders (such as depression); for example, a person may imagine troubles attached to helium balloons and visualize releasing them into the sky. *Relaxation by colour exchange* is a technique that combines rhythmic breathing and imagery. Patients are instructed to focus on an area of pain or tension and assign a colour to it. While breathing in, they can imagine a warm white light coming into their body and surrounding this area. They then imagine the colour of discomfort leaving their body through their breath as they exhale. It should be noted that relaxation by colour exchange is a very new stress reduction technique that does not yet have an evidence base to support its efficacy.

Music for Relaxation

Music can help achieve relaxation and bring about healthy changes in emotional or physical states. Listening to relaxing music may act as a diversion from a stressful situation. In addition, healing vibrations from music can return the mind and body to better balance.

Music has been used in many clinical settings. In general, music appears to affect functions such as such as heart rate, arterial pressure, gastric and bowel secretions, muscle tone, sweat glands, and temperature regulation (Chan, Wong, & Thayala, 2011). It has been shown to decrease anxiety and pain and to evoke the relaxation response (Bauer, Cutshall, Anderson, et al., 2011). Music with low-pitch tones, without words, and that has approximately 60 to 80 beats per minute is considered to be soothing. Mozart's compositions are the most popular form of music used for relaxation. In contrast, fast-tempo music can stimulate and uplift a person.

Music can be incorporated into clinical practice. It is noninvasive, safe, inexpensive, and easy to use. First, it is important to establish the purpose and benefit of using music with the patients in a given clinical setting and to assess each individual patient's interest and preference in music. The patient should be in a comfortable position, and the possibility of interruptions should minimized: for example, by the use of headphones or earphones. For optimal benefit, music should be played for at least 20 to 30 minutes per day at least twice a day. Patients' responses to the music should be evaluated through questions about how it sounds and how it makes them feel.

Muscle Relaxation

Muscle tension is a universal reaction to stress. As the stress response sets in, muscles of the entire body tend to tighten. Muscle relaxation is therefore a common method of eliciting the relaxation response. There are two types of muscle relaxation: progressive and passive. *Progressive muscle relaxation* (PMR) involves the tensing and the relaxing of muscles. This method is intended to help patients differentiate between when a muscle is tensed and when it is relaxed. This recognition enables an individual to reduce muscle tension when it occurs during times of stress. PMR is based on the principle that when the muscles are relaxed, the mind relaxes. In a session of PMR, relaxation typically begins at the extremities and gradually moves across the whole body. An example of PMR can be found in Table 8-6. Patients with muscle or connective tissue damage and those with low back pain should not use PMR. In addition, PMR should not be used by patients with increased intracranial pressure, uncontrolled hypertension, or severe coronary artery disease.

In *passive muscle relaxation,* on the other hand, the mind focuses only on relaxation of the muscles. It is performed similarly to PMR, moving from one extremity to the rest of the body, with the exception that the muscles are never tightened. In passive muscle relaxation, the focus is simply on relaxing each muscle group separately. This form of muscle relaxation may be used more frequently by individuals who have chronic pain that may be exacerbated by the tension involved during PMR.

NURSING MANAGEMENT
STRESS

NURSING ASSESSMENT

Patients face an array of potential stressors that can have health consequences. Nurses are well positioned to assess patients and their significant others, to assist them in identifying periods in which they are at high risk for stress, and to implement stress management strategies. Three major areas are important in assessment of stress: demands, human responses to stress, and coping. The Perceived Stress Scale (Roberti, Harrington, & Storch, 2006) is a measure of how stressful a person perceives his or her life to be at that time. Although further research is needed to connect the identification of stressors with managing them, the Distress Thermometer (Snowden, White, Christie, et al., 2011) identifies areas of particular concern to patients. Caregiver stress is a well-identified phenomenon that may occur in a variety of situations, such as caring for a spouse with Alzheimer's disease, an older parent, or a child with cancer, and thus should also be considered in a stress assessment. Communication support, adequate education and resources, social support and a positive approach from nursing staff are shown to improve the quality of life of caregivers (Wittenberg-Lyles, Washington, Demiris, et al., 2014).

DEMANDS. Stressors, or demands, on the patient may include major life changes, events or situations such as disfiguring or debilitating surgery, or daily hassles. Demands may be categorized as external (e.g., job-related situations, extended hospitalization) or internal (e.g., perception of goals or commitments, physical effects of disease or injury). It is important to keep in mind the many potential stressors that predispose people to stress and take a proactive approach to address them before patients present with stress-related symptoms. The number of simultaneous demands, the duration of these demands, primary appraisal or perception of the demands (see Figure 8-1), previous experience with similar demands, and the patient's family and loved ones' responses to the demands should be considered in the health assessment. Demands may also be categorized as representing harm or loss, threat, or challenge. Eliciting the demand's personal meaning to the patient provides useful insight for planning interventions and self-management strategies with patients. Distinct groups such as immigrants and Indigenous people may have specific stressors such as language barriers and limited understanding of Western medical practices and available resources that may predispose them to stress, and these stressors should be considered when a nursing assessment is performed.

HUMAN RESPONSES TO STRESS. Physiological effects of demands that are appraised as stressful are mediated primarily by the sympathetic nervous system and the hypothalamic–pituitary–adrenal system. Examples of such effects are responses such as increased heart rate, increased blood pressure, loss of appetite, hyperventilation, sweating, and dilated pupils. Symptomatic experiences may include headache, musculo-skeletal pain, gastro-intestinal upset, skin disorders, insomnia, and chronic fatigue. In addition, the patient may exhibit some of the stress-related illnesses or diseases of adaptation (see Table 8-2).

Behavioural manifestations may include accident proneness, anxiety, crying, frustration, and shouting. Behaviour in other aspects of life may include absenteeism or tardiness at work, avoidance of conversations, or procrastination. Observable cognitive responses include self-reports of excessive demand, inability to make decisions, impaired speech, and forgetfulness or inability to concentrate. Some of these responses may also be apparent in stressed caregivers.

COPING. Secondary appraisal by the patient, or the patient's evaluation of coping resources and options, is important to assess (see Figure 8-1). Resources such as supportive family members, adequate finances, and the ability to solve problems are examples of positive resources (see Table 8-3). Knowledge of the patient's resources assists the nurse in supporting existing resources and developing strategies to expand the patient's sources of support to include family, friends, and community resources. Positive social support and possessing a large social network (relatives, friends, spiritual groups, support groups) have been shown to exert powerful effects on the negative distress associated with illness. Conversely, aversive relationships (punishing, demanding, distancing relationships) may add to life stress and intensify illness-associated pain and distress.

Coping strategies include cognitive and behavioural efforts to meet demands. The use and effectiveness of problem-focused and emotion-focused coping efforts should be addressed (see Table 8-4). These efforts may be categorized as direct action, avoidance of action, seeking information, defence mechanisms, and seeking the assistance of other people. The probability that a certain coping strategy will bring about the desired result is another important aspect to be assessed. Effective coping

skills can be taught, and nurses are in a prime position to teach these skills.

NURSING IMPLEMENTATION

The first step in managing stress is to become aware of its presence. The role of the nurse is to facilitate and enhance the processes of coping and adaptation that include identifying and expressing stressful feelings. Nursing interventions depend on the severity of the stress experience or demand. The person with multiple traumas expends energy in an attempt to physically survive. The nurse's efforts are directed to life-supporting interventions and to the inclusion of approaches aimed at the reduction of additional stressors to the patient. The individual who has endured significant trauma is much less likely to adapt or recover if faced with additional stressors such as sleep deprivation or an infection.

The importance of cognitive appraisal in the stress experience should prompt the nurse to assess whether changes in the way a person perceives and labels particular events or situations (cognitive reappraisal) are possible. Some experts also propose that the nurse consider the positive effects that result from successfully meeting stressful demands. Greater emphasis should also be placed on the part that cultural values and beliefs can play to enhance or constrain various coping options.

Because dealing with physical, social, and psychological demands is an integral part of daily experiences, the coping behaviours that are used should be adaptive and should not be a source of additional stress to the individual. Generalizing about which coping strategies are the most adaptive is not possible. However, in evaluating coping behaviours, the nurse should examine the short-term outcomes (i.e., the effect of the strategy on the reduction or mastery of the demands and the regulation of the emotional response) and the long-term outcomes that relate to health, morale, and social and psychological functioning. Nursing students often experience high levels of stress because of the demands of their educational programs; Table 8-9 provides some useful suggestions for coping.

Various factors affect an individual's response to stressors (see the "Determinants of Health" box earlier in this chapter). Resistance to stress can be increased with a lifestyle that supports optimal health regardless of sex, age, and economic status. Healthy behaviours are also cumulative; that is, the greater the number of these behaviours habitually practised by the individual, the better that person's health is. These behaviours include the following practices.

TABLE 8-9	COPING STRATEGIES FOR THE NURSING STUDENT

- Be realistic: do not try to be superhuman.
- Learn to "let go" of things that are outside your control.
- Learn to adapt and to be flexible.
- Learn acceptance of yourself.
- Share your feelings.
- Keep a sense of humour; laugh often.
- Learn and use relaxation breathing, imagery, meditation, or prayer.
- Live a healthy lifestyle (exercise, nutrition, adequate sleep, not smoking, moderate use of alcohol).
- Develop hobbies.
- Take time to relax every day.
- If it is needed, obtain professional counselling.

1. Sleeping regularly 7 to 8 hours per night
2. Eating breakfast
3. Eating regular, well-balanced meals with minimal, healthy snacking
4. Eating moderately to maintain an ideal weight
5. Exercising moderately
6. Enjoying recreational and relaxing activities with friends
7. Drinking alcohol in moderation or not at all
8. Not smoking (best outcome if the person has never smoked)
9. Learning to successfully handle life's stressors and hassles

Good mental health practices are important for good health as well. These practices result primarily in a realistic, positive self-concept and the ability to solve problems. Teaching problem-solving skills can equip individuals to better handle present and future encounters with stressful circumstances.

Stress-reducing activities can be incorporated into nursing practice (Table 8-10). The activities provide mechanisms whereby an individual is able to develop a sense of control of the situation. As stress-reducing practices are incorporated into daily activities, the individual is able to increase his or her confidence and self-reliance and limit the emotional response to the stressful circumstances. Possessing a sense of control over one's life, believing that one is able to overcome adversity, and being committed to that end are important characteristics that can avert the harmful effects inherent in the stress response.

The nurse can assume a primary role in planning stress-reducing interventions. Specific relaxation strategies are presented in Table 8-6. Specific stress-reducing activities within the scope of nursing practice (some of which may require additional training) include relaxation training, guided imagery, cognitive reappraisal, music therapy, exercise, time management, decisional control,

TABLE 8-10	IMPLEMENTING STRESS MANAGEMENT IN CLINICAL PRACTICE

- Learn relaxation–coping techniques by practising them on your own; then practise teaching them to peers before teaching them to patients. Attend seminars and workshops on stress management to learn more.
- Be aware of potential stressors that the patients face.
- Assess your patients for the demands placed on them, their response to these demands, and coping resources being used or available to them.
- Choose the language you use carefully, and be aware of your nonverbal communication. Words or gestures that express overt alarm or ambiguity may increase the stress experience for the patient.
- Pick coping strategies and stress management strategies that are appropriate for your clinical area.
- Take advantage of opportunities to teach coping and relaxation strategies to patients.
- Anticipate setbacks. They provide feedback about what you are doing wrong. Do *not* quit practising!

assertiveness training, massage, meditation, and humour (see Table 8-5). There is ample evidence of the effectiveness of stress management interventions in a variety of illnesses. Nurses are in an ideal situation to take the lead in integrating stress management into their practice. Nurses are also well equipped to develop and test the effectiveness of new approaches to manage stress and promote positive health outcomes. However, it is important for the nurse to recognize when the patient, family, or caregivers need to be referred to a professional with advanced training in counselling.

CASE STUDY

Stress Associated With Cancer Diagnosis and Treatment

Source: Chris from Paris/ Shutterstock .com.

Patient Profile

Mrs. Zyskowski, a Polish immigrant, received a diagnosis of stage 2 breast cancer at age 44. Her treatment plan included lumpectomy followed by a regimen of chemotherapy and then radiation therapy. She attributed her breast cancer to her depression, which developed while she cared for her mother, who suffered from Alzheimer's disease. Her mother passed away 6 months before the breast cancer diagnosis.

After completion of her lengthy breast cancer therapy, Mrs. Zyskowski's depression worsened. She no longer had her frequent visits to the breast cancer centre, and she missed the interaction with the nurses and other patients. In addition, Mrs. Zyskowski feared that her cancer would recur, and she worried that she would "pass it on" to her two teenage daughters. She would not discuss her fears with her husband or daughters because she did not want to burden them. She began to lose weight and constantly felt fatigued. She felt "alone" with her cancer and lost interest in other aspects of her life. She thought about joining a cancer support group but was embarrassed by her Polish accent.

Discussion Questions

1. Consider Mrs. Zyskowski's situation, and describe the physiological and psychological stressors that she is dealing with. Describe the possible effects of these stressors on her health status.
2. What are some other potential stressors that Mrs. Zyskowski may be experiencing that the nurse should anticipate and assess further for?
3. What specific nursing interventions can be included in Mrs. Zyskowski's management that will enhance her adaptability?
4. On the basis of Mrs. Zyskowski's profile, what resources are available to Mrs. Zyskowski to help her cope with her cancer diagnosis and treatment?
5. Should Mrs. Zyskowski join a cancer support group? If so, how might this benefit her?
6. **Priority decision:** On the basis of the assessment data provided, what are the priority nursing diagnoses? Are there any collaborative problems?

Answers are available at *http://evolve.elsevier.com/Canada/Lewis/medsurg*.

REVIEW QUESTIONS

The number of the question corresponds to the same-numbered objective at the beginning of the chapter.

1. How does Selye define stress?
   a. Any stimulus that causes a response in an individual
   b. A response of an individual to environmental demands
   c. A physical or psychological adaptation to internal or external demands
   d. The result of a relationship between an individual and the environment that exceeds the individual's resources

2. A client who has undergone extensive surgery for multiple injuries has a period of increasing blood pressure, heart rate, and alertness. Which stage of general adaptation syndrome are these symptoms most characteristic of?
   a. The resistance state of general adaptation syndrome
   b. The alarm reaction of the general adaptation syndrome
   c. The stage of exhaustion of general adaptation syndrome
   d. An individual response stereotype

3. Which of the following actions best demonstrates that a client is using an emotion-focused coping process? *(Select all that apply.)*
   a. Joining a support group for women with breast cancer
   b. Considering the advantages and disadvantages of the various treatment options
   c. Delaying treatment until her family can take a weekend trip together
   d. Telling the nurse that she has a good prognosis because the tumour is small
   e. Engaging in meditation

4. The nurse would expect which of the following findings in a client as a result of the physiological effect of stress on the limbic system?
   a. An episode of diarrhea while awaiting painful dressing changes
   b. Refusing to communicate with nurses while awaiting a cardiac catheterization
   c. Inability to sleep the night before beginning to self-administer insulin injections
   d. Increased blood pressure, decreased urine output, and hyperglycemia after a car accident

5. Which of the following best demonstrates that the nurse is applying knowledge of the effects of stress on the immune system?
   a. Encouraging clients to sleep for 10 to 12 hours per day
   b. Encouraging clients to receive regular immunizations when they are stressed
   c. Encouraging clients to use emotion-focused rather than problem-focused coping strategies
   d. Encouraging clients to avoid exposure to upper respiratory infections when physically stressed

6. Chronic stress or daily hassles may place a person at higher risk of developing which of the following conditions? *(Select all that apply.)*
   a. Osteoporosis
   b. Colds and flu
   c. Low blood pressure
   d. Irritable bowel syndrome
   e. Depression

7. During a stressful circumstance that is uncontrollable, which type of coping strategy is the most effective?
   a. Avoidance
   b. Coping flexibility
   c. Emotion-focused coping
   d. Problem-focused coping

8. Which of the following clients is least likely to respond to stress effectively?
   a. One who feels that the situation is directing his or her life
   b. One who sees the situation as a challenge to be addressed
   c. One who has a clear understanding of his or her values and goals
   d. One who uses more problem-focused than emotion-focused coping strategies

9. Which of the following is an appropriate nursing intervention for a client who has a nursing diagnosis of *ineffective coping* related to *inadequate resources*?
   a. Controlling the environment to prevent sensory overload and promote sleep
   b. Encouraging the client's family to offer emotional support by frequent visiting
   c. Arranging for the client to phone family and friends to maintain emotional bonds
   d. Asking the client to describe previous stressful situations and how she managed to resolve them

1. d; 2. b; 3. a, e; 4. c; 5. d; 6. b, d, e; 7. c; 8. a; 9. d.

ⓔvolve

For even more review questions, visit *http://evolve.elsevier.com/Canada/Lewis/medsurg*.

REFERENCES

Aiken, L. H., Sloane, D. M., Clarke, S., et al. (2011). Importance of work environments on hospital outcomes in nine countries. *International Journal for Quality in Health Care, 23*(4), 357–364.

Ankad, R. B., Herur, A., Patil, S., et al. (2011). Effect of short-term pranayama and meditation on cardiovascular functions in healthy individuals. *Heart Views, 12*(2), 58. doi:10.4103/1995-705X.86016.

Antonovsky, A. A. (1987). *Unraveling the mystery of health: How people manage stress and stay well.* San Francisco, CA: Jossey-Bass. (Seminal).

Babouchkina, A., & Robbins, S. J. (2015). Reducing negative mood through mandala creation: A randomized controlled trial. *Art Therapy, 32*(1), 34–39. doi:10.1080/07421656.2015.994428.

Balaji, P. A., Varne, S. R., & Ali, S. S. (2012). Physiological effects of yogic practices and transcendental meditation in health and disease. *North American Journal of Medical Sciences, 4*(10), 442. doi:10.4103/1947-2714.101980.

Bauer, B. A., Cutshall, S. M., Anderson, P. G., et al. (2011). Effect of the combination of music and nature sounds on pain and anxiety in cardiac surgical patients: A randomized study. *Alternative Therapies in Health and Medicine, 17*(4), 16–23.

Benson, H. (1975). *The relaxation response.* New York: Avon. (Seminal).

Berk, R. A. (2015). The greatest veneration: Humor as a coping strategy for the challenges of aging. *Social Work in Mental Health, 13*(1), 30–47.

Canadian Institute for Health Information. (2016). *Regulated nurses 2015.* Retrieved from *https://secure.cihi.ca/free_products/Nursing_Report_2015_en.pdf*.

Chan, M. F., Wong, Z. Y., & Thayala, N. V. (2011). The effectiveness of music listening in reducing depressive symptoms in adults: A systematic review. *Complementary Therapies in Medicine, 19*(6), 332–348. doi:10.1016/j.ctim.2011.08.003.

Duffield, C., Diers, D., O'Brien-Pallas, L., et al. (2011). Nursing staffing, nursing workload, the work environment and patient outcomes. *Applied Nursing Research, 24*(4), 244–255.

Fjorback, L. O., Arendt, M., Ørnbøl, E., et al. (2011). Mindfulness-based stress reduction and mindfulness-based cognitive therapy: A systematic review of randomized controlled trials. *Acta Psychiatrica Scandinavica, 124*(2), 102–119. doi: 10.1111/j.1600-0447.2011.01704.x.

Government of Canada. (2015). *Heart disease—Heart health.* Retrieved from *http://healthycanadians.gc.ca/diseases-conditions -maladies-affections/disease-maladie/heart-disease-eng.php.*

Hasel, K. M., Besharat, M. A., Abdolhoseini, A., et al. (2013). Relationships of personality factors to perceived stress, depression, and oral lichen planus severity. *International Journal of Behavioral Medicine, 20*(2), 286–292.

Holmes, T., & Masuda, M. (1966). Magnitude estimations of social readjustments. *Journal of Psychosomatic Research, 11*(2), 219–225. (Seminal).

Janusek, L. W., Cooper, D. T., & Matthews, H. L. (2012). Stress, immunity, and health outcomes. In V. H. Rice (Ed.), *Handbook of stress, coping, and health* (pp. 43–70). Thousand Oaks, CA: Sage.

Koenig, J. I., Walker, C. D., Romeo, R. D., et al. (2011). Effects of stress across the lifespan. *Stress (Amsterdam, Netherlands), 14*(5), 475–480. doi:10.3109/10253890.2011.604879.

Kuiper, N. A. (2012). Humor and resiliency: Towards a process model of coping and growth. *Europe's Journal of Psychology, 8*(3), 475–491.

Lazarus, R., & Folkman, S. (1984). *Stress, appraisal, and coping.* New York: Springer. (Seminal).

Marin, M. F., Lord, C., Andrews, J., et al. (2011). Chronic stress, cognitive functioning and mental health. *Neurobiology of Learning and Memory, 96*(4), 583–585. doi:10.1016/j.nlm.2011.02.016.

Mayo Clinic. (2015). *Positive thinking: Stop negative self-talk to reduce stress.* Retrieved from *http://www.mayoclinic.org/healthy-living/ stress-management/in-depth/positive-thinking/art-20043950.*

Miller, M. A., & Rahe, R. H. (1997). Life changes scaling for the 1990s. *Journal of Psychosomatic Research, 43*(3), 279–292. (Seminal).

Pariante, C. M. (2015). Psychoneuroimmunology or immunopsychiatry? *The Lancet Psychiatry, 2*(3), 197. doi:10.1016/ S2215-0366(15)00042-5.

Roberti, J. W., Harrington, L. N., & Storch, E. A. (2006). Further psychometric support for the 10-item version of the Performance Stress Scale. *Journal of College Counseling, 9*(2), 135–147. Retrieved from *http://onlinelibrary.wiley.com/ doi/10.1002/j.2161-1882.2006.tb00100.x/abstract.* (Seminal).

Segerstrom, S. (Ed.), (2012). *The Oxford handbook of psychoneuroimmunology.* New York: Oxford University Press.

Selye, H. (1983). The stress concept: Past, present, and future. In C. L. Cooper (Ed.), *Stress research: Issues for the eighties* (pp. 1–20). New York: Wiley. (Seminal).

Seward, B. L. (2014). *Managing stress: Principles and strategies for health and well-being* (8th ed.). Burlington, Mass: Jones & Bartlett.

Shonin, E., Van Gordon, W., & Griffiths, M. D. (2014). Meditation awareness training (MAT) for improved psychological well-being: A qualitative examination of participant experiences. *Journal of Religion and Health, 53*(3), 849–863. doi:10.1007/ s10943-013-9679-0.

Snowden, A., White, C. A., Christie, Z., et al. (2011). The clinical utility of the distress thermometer: A review. *British Journal of Nursing, 20*(4), 220–227.

Statistics Canada. (2015). *What's stressing the stressed? Main sources of stress among workers.* Retrieved from *http://www.statcan.gc.ca/ pub/11-008-x/2011002/article/11562-eng.htm.*

Steptoe, A., & Kivimäki, M. (2012). Stress and cardiovascular disease. *Nature Reviews. Cardiology, 9*(6), 360–370. doi:10.1038/nrcardio .2012.45.

Sterling, P. E. J. (1988). Allostasis: A new paradigm to explain arousal pathology. In S. R. Fisher (Ed.), *Handbook of life stress, cognition and health* (pp. 629–649). New York: Wiley.

Wittenberg-Lyles, E., Washington, K., Demiris, G., et al. (2014). Understanding social support burden among family caregivers. *Health Communication, 29*(9), 901–910. doi:10.1080/10410236 .2013.815111.

RESOURCES

Addiction Assessment: Centre for Addiction and Mental Health
http://www.camh.net

Canadian Centre for Occupational Health and Safety
http://www.ccohs.ca/

Canadian Institute of Stress
http://www.stresscanada.org

Canadian Mental Health Association Branches
http://www.addcoach4u.com/support/canadianmentalhealthbr.html

Centre for the Neurobiology of Stress
http://www.utsc.utoronto.ca/~cnstress

Heart and Stroke Foundation of Canada
http://www.heartandstroke.ca

NurseONE
http://www.nurseone.ca

Public Health Agency of Canada
http://www.phac-aspc.gc.ca/chn-rcs/index-eng.php

For additional Internet resources, see the website for this book at *http://evolve.elsevier.com/Canada/Lewis/medsurg*

9

Sleep and Sleep Disorders

Written by: Diana Taibi Buchanan
Adapted by: Holly Symonds-Brown

℮volve WEBSITE

http://evolve.elsevier.com/Canada/Lewis/medsurg

- Review Questions (Online Only)
- Key Points
- Answer Guidelines for Case Study
- Conceptual Care Map Creator
- Audio Glossary
- Content Updates

LEARNING OBJECTIVES

1. Define *sleep*.
2. Describe physiological sleep mechanisms and stages of sleep.
3. Explain the relationship of various diseases/disorders and sleep disorders.
4. Describe the etiology, clinical manifestations, and collaborative and nursing management of insomnia.
5. Describe the etiology, clinical manifestations, and collaborative and nursing management of narcolepsy.
6. Describe the etiology, clinical manifestations, collaborative care, and nursing management of obstructive sleep apnea.
7. Describe parasomnias, including sleepwalking, sleep terrors, and nightmares.
8. Select appropriate strategies for managing sleep problems associated with shift work.

KEY TERMS

cataplexy, p. 132
circadian rhythms, p. 125
circadian rhythm sleep–wake disorders (CRSWDs), p. 132
continuous positive airway pressure (CPAP), p. 134

delayed sleep phase disorder (DSPD), p. 132
insomnia, p. 128
narcolepsy, p. 132
obstructive sleep apnea (OSA), p. 133

parasomnias, p. 135
shift work sleep disorder, p. 136
sleep, p. 124
sleep disorders, p. 124

sleep-disordered breathing, p. 133
sleep disturbances, p. 124
sleep hygiene, p. 129
sleep terrors, p. 135
wake behaviour, p. 125

SLEEP

Sleep is a state during which an individual lacks conscious awareness of environmental surroundings and from which the individual can be easily aroused. Sleep is distinct from unconscious states such as coma, from which the individual cannot be aroused. Sleep is a basic, dynamic, highly organized, and complex behaviour that is essential for normal functioning and survival. A third of most humans' lives is spent in sleep (Gamaldo, Chung, Kang, et al., 2014). Both behavioural and physiological functions are influenced by sleep. Some of these include memory, mood, cognitive function, hormone secretion, glucose metabolism, immune function, body temperature, and renal function.

Sleep requirements vary over the lifespan and are affected by health, lifestyle, and gender (Gamaldo, Chung, Kang, et al., 2014; Hirshkowitz, Whiton, Albert, et al., 2015). Most adults require at least 7 to 9 hours of sleep within a 24-hour period

(Hirshkowitz, Whiton, Albert, et al., 2015). The term **sleep disturbances** refers broadly to situations of poor quality sleep. *Insufficient sleep* refers to obtaining less sleep than a person requires to be fully awake and alert during the day (Figure 9-1). *Fragmented sleep* is characterized by frequent arousals or actual awakenings that interrupt sleep continuity. Sleep disturbances can be related to a variety of physical, emotional, environmental, and lifestyle factors.

Sleep disorders are conditions that specifically affect the quality of sleep and wake behaviour. The classification of sleep disorders is complex; 81 different types have been identified. Table 9-1 lists the seven categories of sleep disorders with some examples based on the International Classification of Sleep Disorders—Third Edition (ICSD-3; Sateia, 2014).

More than 3 million Canadians have a sleep disorder, and many are unaware that they have a problem (Morin, LeBlanc, Bélanger, et al., 2011; Public Health Agency of Canada, 2009). On average, Canadians sleep approximately 6.5 hours on

FIGURE 9-1 Sleep disorders are common in our society. Source: Iakov Filimonov/Shutterstock.com.

TABLE 9-1   SELECTED SLEEP DISORDERS

Type of Disorder	Characteristics
Insomnia	• Chronic • Short term
Sleep-related breathing disorders	• Obstructive sleep apnea • Central sleep apnea syndromes
Central disorders of hypersomnolence	• Types 1 and 2 narcolepsy • Hypersomnia related to a medical condition • Hypersomnia related to medication or substance
Sleep-related movement disorders	• Periodic limb movement disorder • Restless legs syndrome
Circadian rhythm sleep–wake disorders	• Delayed sleep–wake phase disorder • Shift work sleep disorder
Parasomnias	• Sleepwalking • Sleep terrors • Nightmare disorder
Other sleep disorders	

workdays and 7.5 hours on non-workdays. In one survey, 40.2% of Canadians reported at least one symptom of insomnia for a minimum of 3 nights a week in the previous month, and close to 20% of the survey respondents reported being dissatisfied with the quality of their sleep (Morin, LeBlanc, Bélanger, et al., 2011). People with chronic health problems or physical disability are at greatest risk for sleep disorders (Ahn, Jiang, Smith, et al., 2014).

Untreated sleep disorders pose considerable health and economic consequences. Sleepiness during driving has become a national epidemic. An estimated 20% of fatal driving collisions involve driver fatigue (Transport Canada, 2011). Some work-related accidents have been linked to sleep problems (Uehli, Mehta, Miedinger, et al., 2014). Each year, sleep disorders, sleep loss, and excessive daytime sleepiness add billions of dollars to the cost of health care and to the economic effect of work-related accidents and lost productivity (Knauert, Naik, Gillespie, et al., 2015). Many sleep disorders go untreated because health care providers often do not ask, and patients often do not talk, about sleep problems.

PHYSIOLOGICAL SLEEP MECHANISMS

Sleep–Wake Cycle

The nervous system controls the cyclical changes between waking and sleep. No single neuronal structure regulates sleep and waking; rather, a complex arrangement of structures controls these behaviours. Key nuclei in the brain stem, hypothalamus, and thalamus are involved in the regulation of sleep and wake behaviours.

Wake Behaviour. Wake behaviour is associated with an activated cortical brain wave (electroencephalographic [EEG]) pattern. The reticular activating system in the middle of the brain stem is associated with generalized EEG activation and behavioural arousal. Various neurotransmitters (glutamate, acetylcholine, norepinephrine, dopamine, histamine, serotonin) are involved in wake behaviour. Histamine neurons in the hypothalamus stimulate cortical activation and wake behaviour. The sedating properties of many over-the-counter (OTC) medications result from inhibiting one of these arousal systems (especially acetylcholine and histamine).

Neuropeptides also influence wake behaviour. *Orexin* (also called hypocretin) is found in the lateral hypothalamus. Orexin stimulates wake behaviour through activating the reticular activating system. Decreased levels of orexin or its receptors lead to difficulties staying awake and in the syndrome called *narcolepsy* (Levenson, Kay, & Buysse, 2015). (Narcolepsy is discussed later in this chapter.)

Sleep Behaviour. *Sleep behaviour* is regulated by a variety of neurological structures and neurotransmitters. Ventral lateral and median preoptic areas of the brain interact with other areas of the brain such as the hypothalamus and the brain stem to induce sleep by inhibiting the arousal centres. Sleep-promoting neurotransmitters and peptides include melatonin, adenosine, somatostatin, growth hormone–releasing hormone, delta-sleep–inducing peptide, prostaglandins, and proinflammatory cytokines (interleukin-1, tumour necrosis factor α, interleukin-6; Levenson, Kay, & Buysse, 2015). Proinflammatory cytokines are important in mediating sleepiness and lethargy associated with infectious illness. Certain peptides, such as cholecystokinin, released by the gastrointestinal tract after food ingestion, may mediate the sleepiness that follows eating meals *(postprandial sleepiness)*.

Circadian Rhythms

Many biological rhythms of behaviour and physiology fluctuate within a 24-hour period. These circadian rhythms (from the Latin *circa dies,* "approximately a day") persist when people are placed in isolated environments free of external time cues because the rhythms are controlled by internal (endogenous) clock mechanisms. The suprachiasmatic nucleus in the hypothalamus is the master clock of the body. The 24-hour cycle is synchronized to the environmental light and dark periods through specific light detectors in the retina. Pathways from the suprachiasmatic nucleus innervate sleep-promoting cells in the anterior hypothalamus and wake-promoting cells of the lateral hypothalamus and brain stem.

Light is the strongest time cue for the sleep–wake rhythm. Because of this, light can be used as therapy to shift the timing of the sleep–wake rhythm. For example, bright light used early in the morning causes the sleep–wake rhythm to move to an earlier time; bright light used in the evening causes the sleep–wake rhythm to move to a later time. *Melatonin* is an endogenous hormone produced by the pineal gland in the brain from the amino acid tryptophan. In the central nervous system, melatonin decreases *sleep latency* (time it takes to fall asleep) and increases *sleep efficiency* (time spent asleep in comparison with time spent in bed). The secretion of melatonin is tightly linked to the environmental light–dark cycle. Under normal day–night conditions, more melatonin is released in the evening as it gets dark. Light exposure in the evening hours can suppress the secretion of melatonin (LeGates, Fernandez, & Hattar, 2014.) This can have implications for sleep quality in hospitalized patients, shift workers, and people who are exposed to computer and TV screens in the evening.

Sleep Architecture

On the basis of electrical recordings of brain activity with polysomnography (PSG), sleep can be divided into two major states: *rapid eye movement (REM)* and *non–rapid eye movement (NREM)*. Most adults transition from wake to sleep *(sleep onset latency)* in approximately 10 to 20 minutes. Once asleep, a person goes through sleep cycles. A typical sleep cycle lasts 90 minutes and is repeated throughout the duration of the person's total sleep time. *Sleep architecture* refers to the pattern of a person's sleep stage cycling.

Non–Rapid Eye Movement Sleep. In healthy adults, the largest percentage of sleep time, approximately 75% to 80%, is spent in NREM sleep. NREM sleep is subdivided into three stages (Scammell, 2015b).

Stage 1 occurs in the beginning of sleep, with slow eye movements, and is a transition phase from wakefulness to sleep. It is short in duration, lasting 1 to 7 minutes, during which the person can be easily awakened. Stage 2 is a period of sound sleep. The heart rate slows down and the body temperature drops. This stage lasts 10 to 25 minutes. Stage 3 is deep sleep, or slow-wave sleep, and is the deepest stage of sleep. During this stage, the sleeper is less responsive to environmental stimuli and unresponsive to sound. This stage lasts 20 to 40 minutes and is most common earlier in a person's total sleep time. Dreaming is more common in this stage than in other stages of NREM sleep, although not as common as in REM sleep.

Rapid Eye Movement Sleep. REM sleep accounts for 20% to 25% of sleep and occurs more in the later part of a person's total sleep time. REM sleep follows NREM sleep. In a healthy adult, REM sleep occurs four to five times during a period of 7 to 8 hours of sleep. This stage is considered paradoxical because the brain waves resemble wakefulness but movement of the skeletal muscles is inhibited. REM sleep is the period when the most vivid dreaming occurs.

EFFECTS OF SLEEP DEPRIVATION

Sleep deprivation and poor quality of sleep are associated with changes in body function (Figure 9-2) and health problems (Table 9-2). In patients with chronic illnesses, especially cardiovascular disease and stroke, sleep disorders are directly associated with increased risk for mortality and morbidity (Stopford, Ravi, & Nayar, 2013). Sleep loss is associated with decreases in immune function and body temperature and with endocrine changes, including a decrease in growth hormone levels. Cognitive function and performance on simple behavioural tasks become impaired within 24 hours of sleep loss. The effects of sleep loss are cumulative. Chronic loss of sleep places the individual at risk for a decrease in cognitive function, depression, impaired daytime functioning, social isolation, and overall reduction in quality of life (Sutton, 2014).

An insufficient amount of nighttime sleep has a harmful effect on carbohydrate metabolism and endocrine function. Individuals who report less than 6 hours of sleep a night have a higher body mass index (BMI) and are more likely to be obese. Sleep restriction and sleep fragmentation have been linked to decreased insulin

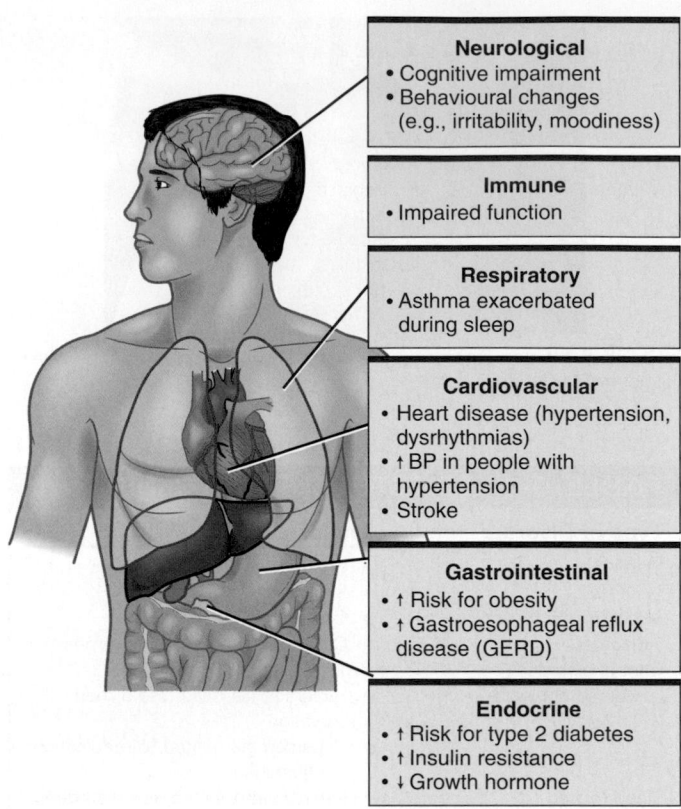

FIGURE 9-2 Effects of sleep deprivation and sleep disorders on the body. *BP,* blood pressure.

sensitivity and increased risk for diabetes (Reutrakul & Van Cauter, 2014). In women with shortened or disturbed sleep, the risk for heart disease was found to be double that of women with adequate sleep (Rod, Kumari, Lange, et al., 2014).

SLEEP DISTURBANCES IN THE HOSPITAL

Hospitalization, especially in the intensive care unit (ICU), is associated with decreases in total sleep time, sleep efficiency, and REM sleep. Pre-existing sleep disorders may be aggravated or triggered in the hospital. Environmental sleep-disruptive factors, psychoactive medications, and acute and critical illness all contribute to poor sleep. Symptoms such as pain, dyspnea, and nausea can also contribute to sleep loss in acutely ill patients.

Medications commonly used in acutely and critically ill patients can further contribute to sleep loss, by exacerbating sleep dis-ordered breathing (discussed later in this chapter) or by altering sleep architecture. Nightmares can also occur as a result of medication and are commonly reported by patients in the ICU. The longer the stay in the ICU, the more likely the patient is to have nightmares. Drug classes most likely to cause nightmares are sedative–hypnotics, β-adrenergic antagonists, dopamine agonists, and amphetamines.

Hospitalized patients are also at risk for poor sleep partly because of disruptions in circadian rhythm. The hospital or long-term care facility represents a new environment, and thus normal cues linked to sleep may be absent. Bright lights during the night can also disrupt sleep. The hospital and ICU environ-mental noise (e.g., staff paging system, respirator alarms, bedside monitors, infusion alarms, staff conversations near patients) during both the day and the night can result in sleep difficulties.

TABLE 9-2 RELATIONSHIP OF SLEEP DISTURBANCES TO SELECTED DISEASES AND DISORDERS

Disease/Disorder	Sleep Disturbance	Disease/Disorder	Sleep Disturbance
Respiratory Asthma	• Exacerbated during sleep • Reports of more insomnia	**Cardiovascular (CV)**	• With sleep apnea/sleep disorders, increased risk for CV disorders, including hypertension, dysrhythmias, and coronary artery disease
Chronic obstructive pulmonary disease (COPD)	• Associated with poor sleep quality, nocturnal O_2 desaturation, and coexisting sleep apnea	Heart failure	• Sleep d0sturbances (insomnia, PLMD, SDB) common
Obstructive sleep apnea	• Linked to heart disease (hypertension, stroke, coronary artery disease, dysrhythmias) • Impairment of glucose control similar to that occurring in type 2 diabetes • Associated with cancer		• Signs of heart failure exacerbation (Cheyne-Stokes breathing and central apnea) in relation to fluid overload • Central sleep apnea correlated with poor left ventrical function
		Central sleep	• In people with hypertension, further elevations in blood pressure as result of inadequate sleep
Renal End-stage renal disease	• Disrupted nocturnal sleep with excessive daytime sleepiness • In patients on dialysis, high incidence of SDB, PLMD, and RLS, which is a significant predictor of mortality in such patients	**Gastrointestinal** Obesity	• Association between short sleep duration and excess body weight; short sleep duration may result in metabolic changes that are linked to obesity. • Higher BMI in people who sleep <6 hr than in people who sleep >8 hr • Poor sleep associated with low levels of leptin and high levels of ghrelin
Immune Disorders Human immunodeficiency virus (HIV)	• Sleep disturbances and fatigue highly prevalent and associated with lower rates of survival	Gastro-esophageal reflux disease (GERD)	• Reflux of gastric contents into the esophagus during sleep because of incompetent lower esophageal sphincter
Endocrine Diabetes	• Insufficient sleep linked to increased risk for type 2 diabetes • Insulin resistance increased in healthy people with sleep deprivation • Sleep duration and quality predictive of Hb A1c levels, an important marker of blood glucose control	Chronic liver disease	• Associated with excessive sleepiness, nocturnal arousal, and incidence of RLS
		Bowel disorders	• Associated with increased insomnia
		Neurological Parkinson's disease	• Associated with difficulty initiating or maintaining sleep, parasomnias, and excessive daytime sleepiness
Musculoskeletal Arthritis	• Increased rates of RLS and SDB; disease activity linked to sleep complaints	Alzheimer's disease	• SDB (frequently sleep apnea) common • Circadian rhythm alterations with nocturnal wandering, daytime sleepiness, and sleep disruption and awakening
Fibromyalgia	• Dysfunctional sleep regulation in relation to altered circadian rhythms and lower concentrations of sleep-dependent hormones (growth hormone, prolactin)	Pain (acute and chronic)	• Decreased quantity and quality of sleep; poor sleep can intensify pain
Chronic fatigue syndrome	• Sleep disturbances, including decreases in total sleep time, reported	**Depression**	• Can result in insomnia or hypersomnia • Amount and quality of REM sleep often affected by anti-depressant medication
Cancer	• Higher rates of insomnia reported • Chemotherapy for cancer treatment associated with fragmented sleep		

Sources: Centers for Disease Control and Prevention (2011). *Sleep and chronic disease.* Retrieved from *http://www.cdc.gov/sleep/about_sleep/chronic_disease.html*; and from National Sleep Foundation (2016). *Sleep disorders.* Retrieved from *https://sleepfoundation.org/sleep-disorders-problems.*
BMI, Body mass index; *Hb A1c,* hemoglobin A1c; *PLMD,* periodic limb movement disorder; *RLS,* restless legs syndrome; *SDB,* sleep-disordered breathing.

In addition, patient care activities (e.g., dressing changes, blood draws, vital sign monitoring) disrupt sleep. Patients in critical care areas have been found to have poor quantity and quality of sleep, with predominantly stage 1 and 2 sleep (Tracy & Chlan, 2011). Sleep can continue being poor after the patient's hospitalization and can affect the long-term recovery and health. Staff prioritization of sleep over other competing critical care demands and the lack of research into sleep promotion within the ICU can affect use of sleep-promoting interventions (Hopper, Fried, & Pisani, 2015).

Decreased sleep duration influences pain perception. Psychological factors, such as anxiety and depression, also modify the sleep–pain relationship. Adequate pain management improves the duration and quality of sleep, but medications commonly used to relieve pain, especially opioids, also alter sleep and place the individual at risk for sleep-disordered breathing. Withdrawal of opioids is associated with rebound effects on sleep architecture.

Nurses have a critical role in creating an environment conducive to sleep. This includes the scheduling of medications and procedures during both day and night. Typical sleep architecture should be considered when interventions and care are planned. When any necessary care episodes are scheduled 90 minutes (or a multiple of that) after a patient has fallen asleep, sleep disruption has been decreased. Reducing light and noise levels or use of earplugs can promote opportunities for sleep.

SLEEP DISORDERS

INSOMNIA

The most common sleep disorder is insomnia. Insomnia is defined as difficulty falling asleep, difficulty staying asleep, waking up too early, or poor quality of sleep. Insomnia is a common problem, affecting approximately one in three adults.

Acute insomnia refers to difficulties falling asleep or remaining asleep and experiencing daytime fatigue for at least 3 nights per week over a 2-week period. *Chronic insomnia* is defined by the same symptoms and a daytime complaint (e.g., fatigue, poor concentration, interference with social or family activities) that occur at least 3 times a week and persist for 3 months or longer. Chronic insomnia occurs in 10% to 15% of Canadians and is more common in women than in men (Morin, LeBlanc, Bélanger, et al., 2011). Chronic insomnia increases in people older than 45 years, and the incidence is higher in divorced, widowed, and separated individuals, as well as in individuals with low socio-economic status and lower amounts of education (Morin, LeBlanc, Bélanger, et al., 2011).

Etiology and Pathophysiology

Behaviours, maladaptive cognitions, lifestyle, diet, and medications contribute to and perpetuate insomnia. *Inadequate sleep hygiene* refers to practices or behaviours that are inconsistent with quality sleep. Consumption of stimulants (e.g., caffeine, nicotine, methamphetamine, other drugs of abuse), especially before bedtime, results in insomnia. Insomnia is a common adverse effect of many medications (e.g., antidepressants, anti-hypertensives, corticosteroids, psychostimulants, analgesics). Insomnia can be exacerbated or perpetuated by consumption of alcohol to help induce sleep, smoking close to bedtime, taking long naps in the afternoon, sleeping in until late in the morning, nightmares, exercise near bedtime, and jet lag. *Maladaptive cognitions* concern personal beliefs and interpretations of sleep-related experiences; this is the key area addressed by cognitive–behavioural interventions for sleep (discussed later in this chapter).

Once chronic insomnia is manifested, symptoms are likely to persist over time. Individuals with insomnia may engage in behaviours that perpetuate disturbed sleep by keeping irregular sleep–wake schedules, using OTC medications or alcohol as sleep aids, and spending more time in bed trying to sleep. Increased attention to one's environment, worry or fear about not obtaining sufficient sleep, and poor sleep habits can lead to a conditioned arousal.

Clinical Manifestations

Manifestations of insomnia include (1) difficulty falling asleep *(long sleep latency)*, (2) frequent awakenings *(fragmented sleep)*, (3) prolonged nighttime awakenings or awakening too early and not being able to fall back to sleep, and (4) feeling unrefreshed on awakening (as a result of *nonrestorative sleep*). Daytime consequences of insomnia may manifest as tiredness, trouble concentrating at work or school, altered mood, and falling asleep during the day. Behavioural manifestations of poor sleep include irritability, forgetfulness, confusion, difficulty staying awake during the day, and anxiety.

Diagnostic Studies

Self-Report. The diagnosis of insomnia is based on subjective complaints and on an evaluation of a 1- or 2-week sleep diary completed by the patient. A panel of sleep experts created the Consensus Sleep Diary to standardize the type of information that clinicians collect in sleep diaries (Carney, Buysse, Ancoli-Israel, et al., 2012). In ambulatory care settings, the evaluation of insomnia requires a comprehensive sleep history to establish the type of insomnia and to screen for possible comorbid psychiatric, medical, or sleep disorder conditions that would necessitate specific treatment. Questionnaires such as the Pittsburgh Sleep Quality Index and the Consensus Sleep Diary (see the Resources at the end of this chapter) are examples of questionnaires commonly used to assess sleep quality (Buysse, Reynolds, Monk, et al, 1989; Carney, Buysse, Ancoli-Israel, et al., 2012; Johns, 1991).

Actigraphy. Actigraphy is a relatively noninvasive method of monitoring rest and activity cycles. A small actigraph watch, which can be worn on the wrist like a watch, is used to measure gross motor activity (Figure 9-3). The watch continually records the movements. After the data are collected, they are downloaded to a computer, and algorithms are used to analyze the data. Actigraphy is not required to diagnose insomnia but can be used to confirm patient's sleep self-reports and clarify sleep and activity patterns during treatment.

Polysomnography. A clinical PSG study is not necessary to establish a diagnosis of insomnia. A PSG study is performed only if there are symptoms or signs of a sleep disorder, such as sleep-disordered breathing (discussed later in this chapter). In a PSG study, electrodes simultaneously record physiological measures that define the main stages of sleep and wakefulness. These measures include (a) muscle tone, recorded with electromyography; (b) eye movements, recorded with electro-oculography; and (c) brain activity, recorded through an EEG study. To determine additional characteristics of specific sleep disorders, other measures are made during PSG. These include airflow at the nose and mouth, respiratory effort around the chest and abdomen, heart rate, noninvasive oxygen saturation, and electromyographic study of the anterior tibialis muscles (used to detect periodic leg movements). In addition, a

FIGURE 9-3 Actigraph watch worn while the patient is sleeping. Source: Courtesy Itamar Medical, Inc.

patient's gross body movements are monitored continuously by audiovisual means.

Collaborative Care

Treatments are oriented toward symptom management (Table 9-3). A key to management is to change behaviours that perpetuate insomnia. This often encompasses cognitive–behavioural strategies and education about sleep, including sleep hygiene. **Sleep hygiene** is a variety of different practices that are important for normal, quality nighttime sleep and daytime alertness (Table 9-4).

TABLE 9-3   COLLABORATIVE CARE

Insomnia

Diagnostic Measures	Collaborative Therapy

• History
• Self-report
  • Sleep assessment (see Table 9-6)
  • Pittsburgh Sleep Quality Index*
  • Epworth Sleepiness Scale*
  • Consensus Sleep Diary*
• Physical assessment
• Polysomnography
	Nondrug Therapy
	• Sleep hygiene (see Table 9-4)
	• Cognitive behavioural therapy for insomnia
	
	Drug Therapy (see Table 9-6)
	• Benzodiazepines
	• Benzodiazepine-receptor–like agents
	• Antihistamines
	
	Complementary and Alternative Therapies
	• Melatonin
	• Acupressure
	• Acupuncture
	• Tai chi

*See the Resources for this chapter.

TABLE 9-4   PATIENT & CAREGIVER TEACHING GUIDE

Sleep Hygiene

The nurse should include the following instructions when teaching a patient who has sleep disturbances/disorders:
• Try to set a bedtime that will allow you adequate sleep hours.
• Go to bed only when you are feeling sleepy.
• Keep a regular schedule of bedtime and awakening times (including weekends).
• Use bedtime routines that help you relax, such as warm baths or listening to music.
• Avoid bright light exposure in evenings (screen-time exposure from smart phones, computers, tablets, and TVs should be considered, as well as environmental lighting).
• Your bed should be used only for sleep and sex.
• Do not have beer, wine, or any other alcohol within 6 hours of your bedtime.
• Do not have a cigarette or any other source of nicotine before bedtime.
• Do not consume caffeine in late afternoon and evening.
• Do not go to bed hungry, but do not eat a big meal near bedtime, either.
• Avoid any strenuous exercise close to bedtime.
• Avoid sleeping pills, or use them cautiously.
• Make your bedroom quiet, dark, and a little bit cool.
• Maintain a healthy diet and exercise routine.

Source: Adapted from American Academy of Sleep Medicine. (2016). *Healthy sleep habits*. Retrieved from *www.sleepeducation.com/essentials-in-sleep/healthy-sleep-habits*.

Cognitive–Behavioural Therapies. Cognitive–behavioural therapy for insomnia (CBT-i) is effective in the management of insomnia and should be the first method of therapy (Williams, Roth, Vatthauer, et al., 2013). CBT-i for insomnia includes a structured treatment plan of behavioural routines, relaxation practices, and thought management strategies related to promoting sleep. Examples of strategies that can be included within CBT-i are relaxation training, guided imagery, and cognitive strategies that address dysfunctional ideas about sleep. CBT-i also includes education about good sleep hygiene practices (see Table 9-4). Often a full lifestyle behaviour plan is devised to include regular exercise (performed several hours before bedtime), regular bedtime routines, and time limits for staying in bed. CBTs require individuals to change behaviour and be able to sustain a change in routine. Supporting a patient's behaviour changes requires evaluation of his or her motivation and resources for change before treatments are initiated. Full CBT-i treatment requires providers to have training; it is often delivered by nurses working in primary care and mental health settings. Although not all nurses are trained in CBT-i, they can education people about sleep hygiene and use the principles of CBT-i to help patients set up new routines. For example, individuals with insomnia can be encouraged to avoid watching television, playing video games, or reading in bed. Time in bed should be limited to the actual time that the individual can sleep. Naps and consumption of large meals, alcohol, and stimulants need to be avoided. Naps are less likely to affect nighttime sleep if they are limited to 20 to 30 minutes.

Drug Therapy. Despite their perceived usefulness for short-term acute insomnia, medications for sleep are not without risks. Sedatives are linked with increased rates of overall mortality and are linked to adverse events such as falls, motor vehicle accidents, and poisonings. Use of sedatives in Canada has increased sharply in comparison with other prescribed medications (Vozoris & Leung, 2011). The use of sedatives in the management of chronic insomnia, particularly in older adults, is not recommended (American Geriatric Society 2012 Beers Criteria Update Expert Panel, 2012). Many individuals with insomnia become used to taking OTC or prescription medications to treat insomnia and risk becoming dependent on them, both psychologically and physically (Chapter 11 has more information on substance dependence). *Rebound insomnia* is common with abrupt withdrawal of hypnotic medications. The resulting daytime fatigue can negatively influence the patient's efforts to use nondrug approaches.

Classes of medications used to treat insomnia include benzodiazepines and benzodiazepine receptor–like drugs (Table 9-5). Although antidepressants, antihistamines, and antipsychotics are sometimes used as sleep aids, there is actually insufficient evidence to support their use for insomnia (MacFarlane, 2012).

Benzodiazepines. Benzodiazepines such as diazepam (Valium) work by activating the γ-aminobutyric acid (GABA) receptors to promote sleep. The prolonged half-life of some of these drugs (e.g., flurazepam and nitrazepam) can result in daytime sleepiness, amnesia, dizziness, and rebound insomnia so are not recommended. Temazepam and triazolam are benzodiazepines considered to be suitable for short-term treatment of insomnia because of their fast onset and short half-life, which results in less pronounced daytime effects. None of the benzodiazipines are recommended for use in people older than 65 years (Tanenbaum, 2015). Tolerance to these drugs develops and increases the risk for dependence (see Chapter 11 for more

TABLE 9-5	DRUG THERAPY

Insomnia

Drug Class	Specific Drug
Benzodiazepines	• Nitrazepam (Mogadon) • Flurazepam • Temazepam (Restoril) • Triazolam
Benzodiazepine receptor–like drugs	• Zopiclone (Rhovane, Imovane) • Zolpidem
Over-the-counter sleep aids Antihistamines	• Diphenhydramine (Benadryl, Nytol, Unisom)
Natural health products	• Melatonin • Valerian

information on benzodiazepine abuse); therefore, it is recommended that the use of benzodiazepines be limited to less than 7 days or to intermittent use of no more than 3 days a week. In addition, benzodiazepines interact with alcohol and other central nervous system depressants.

Benzodiazepine Receptor–like Agents. Because the safety profile of the so-called Z-drugs (e.g., zolpidem and zopiclone) is better than that of benzodiazepines, Z-drugs are the drug of first choice for insomnia. Adverse effects such as daytime effects, dependence, and motor impairment can still occur; thus close monitoring and short-term use for less than 7 days are recommended (MacFarlane, 2012). Because of the potential delay of activity, these drugs should not be taken with food and should be taken close to bedtime, in combination with other sleep hygiene practices, to enhance sleep.

Antidepressants. Trazodone, mirtazapine, and amitriptyline are antidepressants with sedating properties. Trazodone is one of the drugs most commonly prescribed in Canada to treat insomnia. However, there is little evidence supporting their use in nondepressed patients, and the potential for adverse effects such as anti-cholinergic effects, dizziness, orthostatic hypotension, and cardiac conduction abnormalities is significant (Davidson, 2012).

Antihistamines. Many individuals with insomnia self-medicate with OTC sleep aids. Most OTC agents include diphenhydramine (Benadryl, Nytol, Unisom). These agents are less effective than benzodiazepines, and tolerance develops quickly. In addition, they cause adverse effects, including daytime sedation, impaired cognitive function, blurred vision, urinary retention, and constipation, and they increase the risk for increased intraocular pressure. Agents that contain diphenhydramine are not intended for long-term use and should not be used by older adults.

Complementary and Alternative Therapies. Many types of complementary therapies and herbal products are used as sleep aids. Common herbal medicines used in Canada are chamomile, melatonin, and valerian root. Other therapies include the use of acupuncture, acupressure, tai chi, and music.

Herbal Supplements. Chamomile and valerian are herbs that have been used for many years as a sleep aids and to relieve anxiety. Valerian has been found to help with sleep problems related to menopausal symptoms (Taavoni, Ekbatani, & Haghani, 2015). Researchers in only a few small studies have examined chamomile to date, with inconclusive results (Taslaman, 2014). Overall, the current available evidence to support the use of valerian or chamomile to treat insomnia is lacking, and further research is warranted (Leach & Page, 2014).

As noted earlier in the chapter, melatonin is a hormone produced by the pineal gland, which plays an important role in sleep cycle regulation (Lerchl & Reiter, 2012). Melatonin can be somewhat helpful with sleep initiation and efficacy (Costello, Lentino, Boyd, et al., 2014). Although effects on insomnia have been found to be less significant than those of other prescription sleep medications, melatonin is considered much safer (Ferracioli-Oda, Qawasmi, & Bloch, 2013). Melatonin has also been used with sleep phase disorders such as jet lag and shift work disorder, although research evidence for this is weak and further study is required (Costello, Lentino, Boyd, et al., 2014).

Acupuncture. Acupuncture is an invasive technique that must be performed by a trained provider. Acupuncture has been found in several research trials to improve sleep quality, although due to inconsistent research methods it is not conclusive that it is an effective treatment for insomnia (Cheuk, Yeung, Chung, et al., 2012). Acupressure is a massage technique that can be administered by patients themselves, nursing staff, families, and caregivers. This area of Chinese medicine has been showing promising results with a variety of populations, but continued research is required to help define the optimum treatment routine and longevity of effect (Simoncini, Gatti, Quirico, et al., 2015).

Other Therapeutic Sleep Aids. Tai chi is a nonstrenuous exercise and has relaxation effects that have been found to be effective for increasing sleep quality in older adults and people with cardiac disease (Lo & Lee, 2014). Music is another complementary therapy for insomnia (see the following "Complementary & Alternative Therapies" box).

🌿 COMPLEMENTARY & ALTERNATIVE THERAPIES
Effect of Music on Sleep Quality

Scientific Evidence
Several studies, including randomized control trials, have demonstrated the effectiveness of listening to music as a method to improve sleep quality.

Nursing Implications
• Music is a well-tolerated, nonpharmacological intervention.
• Music is accessible to people in both home and hospital environments.
• Further research on the use of music for sleep may help specify who can benefit the most from the intervention and what factors support its use.

Source: Summarized from Jespersen, K. V., Koenig, J., Jennum, P., et al. (2015). Music for insomnia in adults. *Cochrane Database of Systematic Reviews*, No. 8, Article CD010459. doi:10.1002/14651858.CD010459.pub2.

NURSING MANAGEMENT
INSOMNIA

NURSING ASSESSMENT

Nurses are in a key position to assess sleep problems in patients and their family caregivers. Sleep assessment is important in helping patients to identify environmental factors that may contribute to poor sleep. Family caregivers may experience sleep disruptions because of the necessity of providing care to patients in the home. These sleep disruptions can increase the burden of caregiving.

Both subjective and objective methods are used to assess sleep duration and quality. Report of poor sleep is similar to that of pain in that it is a subjective complaint. Many patients may not tell their health care provider about their sleep problems.

TABLE 9-6 NURSING ASSESSMENT

Sleep

The following questions can serve as an initial assessment regarding sleep:
1. What time do you normally go to bed at night? What time do you normally wake up in the morning?
2. Do you often have trouble falling asleep at night?
3. About how many times do you wake up at night?
4. If you do wake up during the night, do you usually have trouble falling back asleep?
5. Does your bed partner say or are you aware that you frequently snore, gasp for air, or stop breathing?
6. Does your bed partner say or are you aware that you kick or thrash about while asleep?
7. Are you aware that you ever walk, eat, punch, kick, or scream during sleep?
8. Are you sleepy or tired during much of the day?
9. Do you usually take one or more naps during the day?
10. Do you usually doze off without planning to during the day?
11. How much sleep do you need to feel alert and function well?
12. Are you currently taking any type of medication or other preparation to help you sleep?

Source: Harrison G. Bloom, Imran Ahmed, Cathy A. Alessi, Sonia Ancoli Israel, Daniel J. Buysse, Meir H. Kryger, Barbara A. Phillips, Michael J. Thorpy, Michael V. Vitiello, Phyllis C. Zee. (2009). Evidence-based recommendations for the assessment and management of sleep disorders in older persons. *Journal of the American Geriatrics Society*, 57 (5), 761. © 2009, Copyright the Authors. Journal compilation © 2009, The American Geriatrics Society..

TABLE 9-7 CAFFEINE CONTENT OF SELECTED FOODS AND BEVERAGES

Food/Beverage	Caffeine (mg)
Coffee, brewed (237 mL)	135
Coffee, instant (237 mL)	76–106
Coffee, decaffeinated	5
Black tea, leaf or bag (237 mL)	50
Green tea	30
Herbal tea, all varieties	0
Diet cola (355 mL)	39–50
Cola (355 mL)	36–46
Dr. Pepper (237 mL)	41
Energy drinks (Red Bull, Monster, Rock Star; 237 mL)	80
Chocolate cake (1 piece)	36
Milk chocolate bar (28 g piece)	7
Dark chocolate bar (28 g piece)	19
Hot chocolate (237 mL)	5

Source: Based on Health Canada. (2012). *Caffeine in food*. Retrieved from: http://www.hc-sc.gc.ca/fn-an/securit/addit/caf/food-caf-aliments-eng.php.

Therefore, the best way to detect sleep problems is for the nurse to ask about sleep on a regular basis. A sleep history should involve characteristics of sleep, such as the duration and pattern of sleep, and of daytime alertness. Before using any questionnaire, the patient's cognitive function, reading level (if a paper form is used), and language abilities are assessed.

Examples of questions to assess sleep are presented in Table 9-6. The nurse should also assess lifestyle factors that can influence sleep, such as work schedules, diet, and use of caffeine and other stimulants. In asking about how much alcohol is consumed each week, the nurse should find out whether the patient is using alcohol or other substances as sleep aids.

The nurse should ask the patient about sleep aids, both OTC and prescription medications. It is important to note the drug dose and frequency of use, as well as any adverse effects (e.g., daytime drowsiness, dry mouth). Many individuals also consume herbal or dietary supplements to improve sleep. The exact components and concentrations of herbs and supplements often are unknown, and patients may experience adverse effects. Additional sleep aids include white noise devices or relaxation strategies.

The nurse can encourage individuals to keep a sleep diary for 2 weeks. (See the link to the Consensus Sleep Diary in the Resources at the end of this chapter.) Other standardized questionnaires such as the Epworth Sleepiness Scale (see the Resources at the end of this chapter) may be used to assess daytime sleepiness.

The patient's medical history can also provide important information about factors that contribute to poor sleep. For example, men with benign prostatic hyperplasia often report frequent awakenings during the night for voiding. Psychiatric problems such as depression, anxiety, post-traumatic stress disorder, and drug abuse are associated with sleep disturbances. Sleep disturbances often develop as a consequence or complication of a chronic or terminal condition (e.g., heart disease, dementia, cancer, renal failure). Medical conditions that cause pain such as fibromyalgia or arthritis can also disrupt sleep.

The nurse should ask the patient about work schedules, as well as cross-country and international travel. Shift work can contribute to reduced or poor-quality sleep. Work-related effects of poor sleep may include poor performance, decreased productivity, and job absenteeism.

NURSING DIAGNOSES

Specific nursing diagnoses related to sleep include *insomnia, sleep deprivation, disturbed sleep pattern,* and *readiness for enhanced sleep.*

NURSING IMPLEMENTATION

Nursing interventions depend on the severity and duration of the sleep problem, as well as on the characteristics of the individual. Occasional difficulty getting to sleep or awakening during the night is not unusual. However, prolonged sleep disruptions become problematic.

The nurse can assume a primary role in teaching about sleep hygiene (see Table 9-4). An important component of sleep hygiene is reducing dietary intake of substances containing caffeine. To reduce caffeine intake, the patient must be aware of the content of caffeine and related stimulants such as guarana and yerba mate in certain foods and beverages (Health Canada, 2012). Table 9-7 provides examples of the caffeine content of beverages and foods. Health Canada recommends no more than 400 mg of caffeine per day for the general adult population and lower amounts for children and women of child-bearing age.

Nurses are also in an ideal position to take the lead in suggesting and implementing change in patients' homes and institutional environments to enhance sleep. Reducing light and noise levels can enhance sleep. Awareness of time passing and watching the clock can add to anxieties about not falling asleep or returning to sleep.

Patients require education about sleeping medications. With the benzodiazepines and zopiclone (Imovane), the patient is taught to take the drug right before bedtime, to be prepared to get a full night's sleep of at least 6 to 8 hours, and not to plan activities the next morning that require highly skilled psychomotor coordination. The patient should also avoid high-fat foods that can alter drug absorption. To avoid oversedation, these medications should not be taken with alcohol or other central nervous system depressants. Although sleep hygiene education may be helpful, individuals with chronic insomnia require more in-depth training in cognitive–behavioural strategies so referral to a trained provider may be required.

Patient follow-up with regard to medications is important. The nurse should ask the patient about daytime sleepiness, nightmares, and any difficulties in activities of daily living. For patients who have been taking sleeping medications for a period of time, withdrawal of the drug should be tapered.

NARCOLEPSY

Narcolepsy is a chronic degenerative neurological disorder caused by the brain's inability to regulate sleep–wake cycles normally.

The onset of narcolepsy typically occurs in adolescence (Scammell, 2015a). There are two categories of narcolepsy: type 1 and type 2. With both types of narcolepsy, people experience excessive daytime sleepiness despite adequate sleep. Affected individuals fall asleep for periods lasting from a few seconds to several minutes (Cook, 2013). In significant contrast to people with other sleep disorders, people with narcolepsy awaken refreshed from sleep but become sleepy in a few hours. This excessive sleepiness interferes with sedentary activities and is accompanied by cognitive impairments in attention and working memory (Moraes, Rossini, & Reimão, 2012).

Narcolepsy type 1 is characterized by episodes of cataplexy, which is a brief and sudden loss of skeletal muscle tone or muscle weakness. Its manifestations range from a brief episode of muscle weakness to complete postural collapse and falling to the ground. Laughter, anger, or surprise often triggers episodes. Approximately 60% to 70 % of patients with narcolepsy experience cataplexy (Cook, 2013). Patients with narcolepsy, particularly those with cataplexy, have decreased quality of life because of excessive daytime sleepiness. Other common symptoms of narcolepsy are listed in Table 9-8.

Etiology and Pathophysiology

Type 1 narcolepsy is caused by a loss of hypothalamic neurons that produce orexin (discussed earlier in the chapter; Scammell,

TABLE 9-8   COMMON SYMPTOMS OF NARCOLEPSY

Sleep paralysis: a temporary (few seconds to minutes) paralysis of skeletal muscles (except respiratory and extraocular muscles) that occurs in the transition from REM sleep to waking.
Fragmented nighttime sleep
Altered REM sleep regulation (including daytime episodes of REM while awake)
Hypnagogic hallucinations (brief hallucinations that occur at the onset of sleep)
Other sleep disorders such as periodic limb movement disorders, obstructive sleep apnea, REM sleep behaviour disorder
Weight gain
Depression
Anxiety
Chronic pain
Autonomic dysregulation

Sources: Based on Cook, N. (2013). Understanding narcolepsy the wider perspective. *British Journal of Neuroscience Nursing, 9*(2), 76–82; and Scammell, T. E. (2015a). Narcolepsy. *New England Journal of Medicine, 373*(27), 2654–2662. doi:10.1056/NEJMra1500587.
REM, rapid eye movement.

2015a). The cause of type 2 narcolepsy is thought to be similar but remains unknown.

Diagnostic Studies

Narcolepsy is diagnosed on the basis of a history of sleepiness, PSG findings, and daytime *multiple sleep latency tests* (MSLTs). MSLTs are sleep studies in which the patient is encouraged to fall asleep every 2 hours during the day for approximately 20 minutes. Short sleep latencies and onset of REM sleep in more than two MSLTs are diagnostic signs of narcolepsy.

Collaborative Care

Drug Therapy. Narcolepsy cannot be cured. But excessive daytime sleepiness and cataplexy, the most disabling symptoms of the disorder, can be controlled with drug treatment in most affected patients. Drug management of narcolepsy includes amphetamine-like stimulants to relieve excessive daytime sleepiness and antidepressant drug therapy to control cataplexy (Scammell, 2015a). Sodium oxybate is sometimes used at night to produce a deep non-REM sleep that over time reduces both daytime sleepiness and cataplexy. Because of the significant risk of adverse reactions, this is used only for moderate to severe symptoms of sleepiness and cataplexy.

Behavioural Therapy. None of the current drug therapies cures narcolepsy or allows patients to consistently maintain a full, normal state of alertness. As a result, drug therapy is combined with various behavioural strategies similar to those for insomnia (discussed earlier in this chapter).

Safety precautions, especially in driving, are crucial for patients with narcolepsy. Excessive daytime sleepiness and cataplexy can result in serious injury or death if not treated. Individuals with untreated narcolepsy symptoms are involved in automobile accidents approximately five times more frequently than is the general population.

Patient support groups are also useful for many patients with narcolepsy and their family members. Social isolation can occur because of symptoms. Patients with narcolepsy can be stigmatized as being lazy and unproductive because of lack of public and professional understanding about this disorder.

CIRCADIAN RHYTHM SLEEP–WAKE DISORDERS

Circadian rhythm sleep–wake disorders (CRSWDs) are characterized by good quality sleep at the wrong time of day (Gamaldo, Chung, Kang, et al., 2014). This occurs because of lack of synchrony between the circadian time-keeping system and the environment, which disrupts the sleep–wake cycle. Delayed sleep phase disorder (DSPD) is the most common CRSWD. With this disorder, people have difficulty falling asleep (staying awake until 0100–0300 hours) and typically sleep later into the morning (waking between 1000 and 1200 hours). Because most people need to get up in the morning for school or work/care responsibilities, chronic sleep restriction and daytime sleepiness result. Typically, DSPD begins in adolescence when there is a normal shift in the sleep–wake drives that then continues into adulthood. Attentional and mood-related issues can result from the chronic sleep restriction and be overlooked as inherent traits. The altered sensitivity of the circadian system is thought to be genetic in origin (Nesbitt & Djik, 2014). People with this disorder are at risk for health sequelae of chronic sleep restriction (see the section "Effects of Sleep Deprivation" later in the chapter).

Open airway—awake
Tongue
Epiglottis
Oropharynx   Soft palate

Closed airway—asleep

Nasal CPAP

FIGURE 9-4 How sleep apnea occurs. **A,** The patient predisposed to obstructive sleep apnea (OSA) has a small pharyngeal airway. **B,** During sleep, the pharyngeal muscles relax, allowing the airway to close. Lack of airflow results in repeated apneic episodes. **C,** With continuous positive airway pressure (CPAP), the airway is splinted open, which prevents airflow obstruction. Source: Modified from LaFleur Brooks, M. (2012). *Exploring medical language: a student-directed approach* (8th ed.) St. Louis: Mosby.

Shift work disorder is another type of CRSWD and is discussed in the section "Special Sleep Needs of Nurses" later in the chapter.

SLEEP-DISORDERED BREATHING

The term **sleep-disordered breathing** indicates abnormal respiratory patterns associated with sleep. These include snoring, apnea, and hypopnea, characterized by increased respiratory effort that leads to frequent arousals. Sleep-disordered breathing results in frequent sleep disruptions and alterations in sleep architecture. Obstructive sleep apnea is the sleep-disordered breathing problem most commonly diagnosed.

Obstructive Sleep Apnea

Obstructive sleep apnea (OSA), also called *obstructive sleep apnea–hypopnea syndrome,* is characterized by partial or complete obstruction of the upper airway during sleep. *Apnea* is the cessation of spontaneous respirations that lasts longer than 10 seconds. *Hypopnea* is a condition characterized by shallow (30%–90% reduction in airflow) respirations. Airflow obstruction occurs because of narrowing of the air passages with relaxation of muscle tone during sleep, which leads to apnea and hypopnea, or when the tongue and the soft palate fall backward and partially or completely obstruct the pharynx (Figure 9-4).

Each obstruction may last from 10 to 90 seconds. During the apneic period, the patient can experience *hypoxemia* (decreased partial pressure of arterial oxygen or partial oxygen saturation) and *hypercapnia* (increased partial pressure of arterial carbon dioxide). These changes are ventilatory stimulants and cause brief arousals, but the patient may not fully awaken. The patient has a generalized startle response, snorts, and gasps, which cause the tongue and soft palate to move forward and the airway to open. Apnea and arousal cycles occur repeatedly, throughout the night.

Sleep apnea affects 5.4 million Canadians but is considered to be underreported (Public Health Agency of Canada, 2009). The risk increases with obesity (BMI > 35 kg/m²), age older than 50 years, neck circumference greater than 43 cm (17 inches), craniofacial abnormalities that affect the upper airway, and acromegaly. People who smoke are more likely to have OSA than are those who do not smoke. OSA is twice as common in men as in women until after menopause, when the prevalence is similar.

The STOP-BANG (**s**nore, **t**ired, **o**bstruction, **p**ressure–**B**MI, **a**ge, **n**eck, **g**ender) questionnaire summarizes the key risk factors

TABLE 9-9   STOP-BANG

STOP

S (Snore): Have you ever been told that you snore?	Yes	No
T (Tired): Are you often tired during the day?	Yes	No
O (Obstruction): Do you know if you stop breathing, or has anyone witnessed you stop breathing while you are asleep?	Yes	No
P (Pressure): Do you have high blood pressure, or are you on medication to control high blood pressure?	Yes	No

If the person answers "Yes" to two or more of the STOP questions, she or he is at risk for OSA and should contact her or his primary care provider. The second component of this questionnaire (BANG) provides risk assessment of moderate to severe risk of OSA.

BANG

B (BMI): Is your body mass index [BMI] greater than 28?	Yes	No
A (Age): Are you 50 years or older?	Yes	No
N (Neck): Are you a male with a neck circumference greater than 43 cm or a female with a neck circumference greater than 41 cm?	Yes	No
G (Gender): Are you a male?	Yes	No

Source: Chung, F., Yegneswaran, B., Liao, P., et al. (2008). STOP questionnaire: A tool to screen patients for obstructive sleep apnea. *Anesthesiology, 108,* 812–821. doi:10.1097/ALN.0b013e31816d83e4.
OSA, obstructive sleep apnea.

and is increasingly used as a quick and reliable screening tool for OSA (Nagappa, Liao, Wong, et al., 2015; Table 9-9). In the BANG portion, the more questions that a patient answers, "Yes," the greater is the patient's risk of having moderate to severe OSA.

Clinical Manifestations and Diagnostic Studies

Clinical manifestations of sleep apnea include frequent arousals during sleep, insomnia, excessive daytime sleepiness, and witnessed apneic episodes. The patient's bed partner may complain about the patient's loud snoring. Other symptoms include morning headaches (from hypercapnia or increased blood pressure that causes vasodilation of cerebral blood vessels), personality changes, and irritability. Women with OSA have higher rates of mortality from the disorder than do men. Hypoxemia associated with OSA is worse in patients with chronic obstructive pulmonary disease (COPD) than in those without COPD.

Complications that can result from untreated sleep apnea include hypertension, right-sided heart failure from pulmonary hypertension caused by chronic nocturnal hypoxemia, and cardiac dysrhythmias, and the risk for stroke is increased. Symptoms of sleep apnea alter many aspects of the patient's life. If problems are identified, appropriate referrals need to be made. Cessation of breathing reported by the bed partner is usually a source of great anxiety because of the fear that breathing may not resume.

Assessment of the patient with OSA includes thorough documentation of sleep and medical histories. The previously mentioned clinical manifestations of OSA should be assessed, as should less obvious symptoms, which may include cardiovascular symptoms, muscle pain, and mood changes.

A diagnosis of sleep apnea is made on the basis of PSG findings. This diagnosis requires documentation of apneic events (no airflow with respiratory effort) or hypopnea (airflow diminished 30% to 50% with respiratory effort) of at least 10 seconds' duration. OSA is defined as more than five apnea/hypopnea events per hour accompanied by a 3% to 4% decrease in oxygen saturation. In severe cases of apnea, apneic events may number more than 30 to 50 per hour of sleep. Typically, PSG studies are performed in a sleep laboratory with technicians monitoring the patient. In some instances, portable sleep studies are conducted in the home setting (see the "Informatics in Practice" box on sleep apnea diagnosis and monitoring). Overnight pulse oximetry assessment may be an alternative to determine whether nocturnal oxygen supplementation is indicated.

FIGURE 9-5 Examples of positive airwave pressure devices for sleep apnea. **A,** Patient wearing a nasal mask and headgear (positive pressure only to nose). **B,** Patient wearing nasal pillows (positive pressure only to nose). **C,** Patient wearing a full face mask (positive pressure to both nose and mouth). Source: Goldman, I., Schafer, A. I. (2012). *Goldman's Cecil medicine* (24th ed.). Philadelphia: Saunders.

INFORMATICS IN PRACTICE

Sleep Apnea Diagnosis and Monitoring

- Home respiratory monitoring is a cost-effective alternative for diagnosing sleep-related breathing disorders that allows some patients the convenience of sleeping in their own home.
- Home respiratory monitoring is used as part of a comprehensive sleep evaluation in patients likely to have moderate to severe obstructive sleep apnea but who do not have heart failure, obstructive lung disease, or neuromuscular disease.
- Home respiratory monitoring is used to monitor the effectiveness of non-CPAP therapies for patients with sleep-related breathing disorders.
- Wireless monitors can detect changes in vital signs and pulse oximetry, raising an alarm if values fall outside of set parameters.
- A patient may benefit from telehealth to diagnose and monitor for sleep apnea in the home.

CPAP, continuous positive airway pressure.

NURSING AND COLLABORATIVE MANAGEMENT SLEEP APNEA

Mild sleep apnea (5 to 10 apneic/hypopneic events per hour) may respond to simple measures. Conservative treatment at home begins with simply sleeping on the side rather than on the back. The patient is instructed to avoid sedatives and consuming alcoholic beverages for 3 to 4 hours before sleep. Sleep medications often make OSA worse. Because excessive weight worsens and weight loss reduces sleep apnea, referral to a weight loss program may be indicated. Bariatric surgery reduces OSA (Freedman, 2014). It is essential to instruct the patient on the dangers of driving or using heavy equipment (Fleetham, Ayas, Bradley, et al., 2011).

Symptoms may resolve in up to half of patients with OSA who use a special mouth guard, also called an *oral appliance,* during sleep to prevent airflow obstruction. Oral appliances bring the mandible and tongue forward to enlarge the airway space, thereby preventing airway occlusion. Some individuals find beneficial a support group in which concerns and feelings can be expressed and strategies for resolving problems can be discussed.

In patients with more severe symptoms (>15 apneic/hypopneic events per hour), continuous positive airway pressure (CPAP) by mask is the treatment of choice. With CPAP, the patient applies a nasal mask that is attached to a high-flow blower (Figure 9-5). The blower is adjusted to maintain sufficient positive pressure (5 to 25 cm H_2O) in the airway during inspiration and expiration to prevent airway collapse. Some patients cannot adjust to wearing a mask over the nose or mouth or to exhaling against the high pressure. With a technologically more sophisticated therapy, bilevel positive airway pressure (BiPAP), a higher inspiration pressure and a lower pressure during expiration can be delivered. With BiPAP, the apnea can be relieved with a lower mean pressure and may be better tolerated.

Although CPAP is highly effective in reducing apnea and hypopnea, adherence to the regimen is poor; many people discontinue its use within the first year. Approximately two-thirds of patients using CPAP report adverse effects such as nasal stuffiness. Discomfort, noise, and claustrophobia are other reasons for discontinuation of use. Patient education, including the patient's choice of mask and device and exposure to CPAP before initiation of therapy, and behavioural therapy (e.g., tracking use with a symptom diary) have been shown to be important elements associated with successful adherence to CPAP treatment (Wozniak, Lasserson, & Smith, 2014).

Surgical Interventions

Tonsillectomy (removal of tonsillar glands) is used if a patient with OSA has large tonsils. If other measures fail, surgical interventions may be attempted to help manage the airway. Patients are carefully selected for these surgeries, inasmuch as there has been no conclusive evidence that they are actually beneficial for sleep apnea. The most common procedure is uvulo-palato-pharyngoplasty, which involves excision of the tonsillar pillars, the uvula, and the posterior soft palate with the goal of removing the obstructing tissue.

Special Concerns for Hospitalization With Obstructive Sleep Apnea

CPAP treatment should be maintained throughout hospitalization stay. When patients with a history of OSA are hospitalized, health care staff must be aware that the administration of opioid analgesics and sedating medications (benzodiazepines, barbiturates, hypnotics) may worsen OSA symptoms by depressing respiration. This will necessitate that the patient wear the CPAP or BiPAP when resting or sleeping (Fleetham, Ayas, Bradley, et al., 2011).

Perioperative concerns include an increased risk for difficult endotracheal intubation and a need for increased monitoring the postoperative period. In patients with sleep-disordered breathing, OSA may be exacerbated in the postoperative period in relation to medications they receive during anaesthesia. All patients with OSA should be monitored for pulse oximetry after surgery, and those at increased risk for cardiac events should also receive cardiac monitoring postoperatively (Fleetham, Ayas, Bradley, et al., 2011).

SLEEP MOVEMENT DISORDERS

In sleep movement disorders, involuntary movement during sleep disrupts sleep and leads to daytime sleepiness. Periodic limb movement disorder (PLMD) is a type of sleep movement disorder characterized by involuntary, periodic movement of the legs, arms, or both that affects people only during sleep. Sometimes abdominal, oral, and nasal movement accompanies PLMD. Movements typically occur for 0.5 to 10 seconds, in intervals separated by 5 to 90 seconds. PLMD causes poor-quality sleep, which may lead to sleep maintenance insomnia, excessive daytime sleepiness, or both. PLMD and restless legs syndrome often occur simultaneously, but they are distinct disorders. (Restless legs syndrome is discussed in Chapter 61.)

PLMD is diagnosed on the basis of a detailed history from the patient or bed partner, or both, and PSG findings. PLMD is treated by medications aimed at reducing or eliminating the limb movements or the arousals. Dopaminergic drugs (pramipexole [Mirapex] and ropinirole [Requip]) are preferred.

Parasomnias

Parasomnias are defined as unusual and often undesirable behaviours that occur during sleep or during arousal from sleep. They can include abnormal movements and dream-related behaviours, emotions, and perceptions. They are divided into three clusters: non–rapid eye movement, rapid eye movement, and "other."

Rapid Eye Movement Parasomnias. Parasomnias that occur during REM sleep include REM sleep behaviour disorder, nightmare disorder, and recurrent isolated sleep paralysis (Sateia, 2014). Parasomnias may result in fragmented sleep and fatigue. *Nightmare disorder* is a parasomnia characterized by recurrent awakening with recall of the frightful or disturbing dream. *Nightmares* are vivid dreams that cause fear and anxiety as they unfold, and they result in a startled awakening (Nadorff, Lambdin, & Germain, 2014). These normally occur during the final third of sleep and in association with REM sleep. The startled awakening differentiates them from bad dreams (Nadorff, Lambdin, & Germain, 2014). Nightmares are more common in childhood but can persist into adulthood. Disturbed sleep, anxiety, sleep avoidance, and increased risk for suicidality are consequences of nightmare disorder. Nightmares are commonly reported by patients in the ICU and are probably adverse effects of medication because REM sleep is often absent in critically ill patients. The longer the stay in the ICU, the more likely the patient is to have nightmares. Drug classes most likely to cause nightmares are

sedative–hypnotics, β-adrenergic antagonists, dopamine agonists, and amphetamines.

Treatments for nightmare disorder include prazosin (antihypertensive) and psychological interventions such as imagery rehearsal therapy and exposure treatment (Nadorff, Lambdin, & Germain, 2014). In research studies, nabilone (a synthetic cannaboid) has shown promise in people experiencing nightmares related to post-traumatic stress disorder (Cameron, Watson, & Robinson, 2014; Jetly, Heber, Fraser, et al., 2015).

Non–Rapid Eye Movement Parasomnias. NREM parasomnias include sleepwalking, sleep terrors, sleep-related eating disorder, and confusional arousal. *Sleepwalking* behaviours can range from sitting up in bed, moving objects, and walking around the room to driving a car. During a sleepwalking event, the affected individual does not speak and may have limited or no awareness of the event. On awakening, the individual does not remember the event. In the ICU, a parasomnia may be misinterpreted as ICU psychosis. In addition, sedated ICU patients can exhibit manifestations of an NREM parasomnia.

Sleep terrors (night terrors) are characterized by a sudden awakening from sleep along with a loud cry and signs of panic. There is an intense autonomic response, including increased heart rate, increased respiration, and diaphoresis. Factors in the ICU such as sleep disruption and deprivation, fever, stress (physical or emotional), and exposure to noise and light can contribute to sleep terrors.

AGE-RELATED CONSIDERATIONS

SLEEP

Sleep, like many physiological functions, change as people age. Even with healthy aging, there are expected changes in sleep patterns, including a decrease in the amount of deep sleep, overall shorter total sleep time at night, decreased sleep efficiency, more awakenings, and increased napping (Gooneratne & Vitiello, 2014). Sleep requirements for older adults are 7 to 8 hours per 24-hour cycle (Hirshkowitz, Whiton, Albert, et al., 2015) (Figure 9-6).

FIGURE 9-6 Many older people have sleep problems. Source: Anneka/Shutterstock.com.

Despite these expected changes, the incidence of sleep disturbances and disorders is also increased in older adults. Insomnia, OSA, PLMD, and REM sleep behaviour disorder in particular are increased in prevalence among older adults (Carrier, Lafortune, & Drapeau, 2012).

A key issue is that multiple factors impair the ability of older adults to obtain quality sleep. Chronic conditions that are more common in older adults—including COPD, diabetes, dementia, chronic pain, and cancer—can affect sleep quality and increase the prevalence of insomnia (Carrier, Lafortune, & Drapeau, 2012). Prescribed and OTC medications used to treat these conditions can contribute to sleep problems. Daily stress and poor social support have also been linked to insomnia in older adults (Choi, Irwin, & Cho, 2015).

Insomnia may have detrimental effects on cognitive function in healthy older adults. Chronic disturbed sleep in an older adult can result in disorientation, delirium, impairment of intellect, disturbances in cognition, and increased risk of accidents and injury (see precipitating factors for delirium in Chapter 62).

Getting out of bed during the night to use the bathroom increases the risk for falls. Older adults may use OTC medications or alcohol as a sleep aid (see Chapter 11), which can further increase the risk of falls at night.

Because many older adults may not tell their health care providers about their sleep problems, a sleeping assessment (see Table 9-6) can be used to detect sleep disturbances. Napping during the day should not be considered problematic unless the person is complaining of insomnia or excessive daytime sleepiness. In the case of insomnia, daytime napping should be restricted (Carrier, Lafortune, & Drapeau, 2012). Screening for sleep disorders is important because of their higher prevalence among older adults. Sleep hygiene education and CBT-i are useful interventions for insomnia in older adults. Drug therapies are more challenging for older adults. Whenever possible, long-acting benzodiazepines should be avoided (Tanenbaum, 2015). Older adults receiving benzodiazepines are at increased risk of daytime sedation, falls, and cognitive and psychomotor impairment (see Table 62-1). They also have increased sensitivity to hypnotic and sedative medications. For this reason, drug therapies for sleep disturbances are started at low doses and monitored carefully. Hypnotic drugs should be used for as brief a period as possible, in most cases not exceeding 2 to 3 weeks of treatment. OTC sleep medications are not recommended for older adults because of their anticholinergic effects (American Geriatric Society, 2012; Beers Criteria Update Expert Panel, 2012).

SPECIAL SLEEP NEEDS OF NURSES

Nursing is one of several professions that necessitate night shift and rotating shift schedules. In many acute care and long-term care settings, nurses volunteer or are asked to work a variety of day and night shifts, often alternating and rotating them. Unfortunately, many nurses who do shift work report less job satisfaction and more job-related stress (Matheson, O'Brien, & Reid, 2014) than those who do not.

Nurses on permanent night or rapidly rotating shifts are at increased risk of experiencing shift work sleep disorder, characterized by insomnia, sleepiness, and fatigue. Nurses on rotating shifts get the least amount of sleep. With repeated periods of inadequate sleep, the sleep debt grows. Poor sleep is the strongest predictor of chronic fatigue in nurses doing shift work. As a result, rotating and night shift schedules pose specific challenges for the individual nurse's health and for patients' safety.

Shift work alters the synchrony between circadian rhythms and the environment, which leads to sleep disruption. Nurses working the night shift are often too sleepy to be fully alert at work and too alert to sleep soundly the next day. Sustained alterations in circadian rhythms such as that imposed by rotating shift work have been linked to negative health outcomes, including increased risk of morbidity and mortality in association with cardiovascular problems. In addition, mood disorders such as anxiety are more severe in nurses who work rotating shifts. Gastrointestinal disturbances are also more common in nurses who do shift work than in those who do not.

From a patient safety perspective, disturbed sleep and subsequent fatigue can make for a workplace hazard (errors and accidents) for nurses, as well as for their patients (Johnson, Jung, Brown, et al., 2014). Fatigue can result in diminished memory or distortions in perceptual skills, judgement, and decision-making capabilities. Lack of sleep affects the ability to cope and handle stress. Subsequently, the reduced ability to handle stress may result in physical, mental, and emotional exhaustion (Eanes, 2015).

The problem of sleep disruption is one that is critically important in nursing. Workplace policy and nursing education programs have a significant role to play in helping nurses access strategies to ensure adequate sleep. Several strategies may help reduce the distress associated with rotating shift work. These include brief scheduled periods of on-site napping, especially during the night shift, to help with the chronobiological regulation of sleep (Silva-Costa, Rotenberg, Griep, et al., 2015). Napping during shift has been found to improve recovery time from night shift and to enhance safety on the job of shift workers (Fallis, McMillan, & Edwards, 2011). On-site napping may be beneficial only if the amount of domestic work performed in the daytime hours after night shift is limited (Silva-Costa, Rotenberg, Griep, et al., 2015). Maintaining a consistent sleep–wake schedule even on days off is optimum but perhaps unrealistic. For night shift work, scheduling the sleep period for just before going to work increases alertness and vigilance, improves reaction times, and decreases accidents during night shift work. It is important that nurses self-manage the effect of sleep disruption through the use of sleep hygiene practice. Sleep hygiene skills and self-care practices could be considered as required learning for nursing students because sleep quality has been found to decrease as nurses transition from school to workplace (Ye & Smith, 2015).

CASE STUDY

Insomnia

Source: Blend Images/ Shutterstock .com.

Patient Profile

Donna Parsons, a 49-year-old woman, is seen in the preoperative clinic. She is scheduled for a right shoulder (rotator cuff) repair. She tore her rotator cuff while playing tennis 1 year ago. It is no longer painful, but her range of motion is limited. During the preoperative screening, she reports chronic fatigue. She is postmenopausal, according to self-report. In the past year since the end of her periods, she has experienced daily hot flashes and sleep problems. She denies any other health problems. On a usual workday, she drinks two cups of hot tea and one can of diet cola. Currently, she is taking OTC diphenhydramine for sleep. Her partner, who has accompanied her to the clinic, states that her snoring has gotten worse and it is interfering with his sleep.

Subjective Data
- Complains of hot flashes and nighttime sweating
- Complains of daytime tiredness and fatigue
- States that she has trouble getting to sleep and staying asleep

Objective Data
Physical Examination
- Laboratory evaluations within normal limits
- Overweight (20% over ideal body weight for height)
- Blood pressure (BP): 155/92 mm Hg
- Limited lateral and posterior rotation of right shoulder

Diagnostic Studies
- Nighttime polysomnography study reveals episodes of obstructive sleep apnea

Collaborative Care
- CPAP nightly
- Referred for weight reduction counselling

Discussion Questions
1. What are Ms. Parsons's risk factors for sleep apnea?
2. What specific sleep hygiene practices could Ms. Parsons use to improve the quality of her sleep?
3. How does CPAP work?
4. What are the potential health risks associated with sleep apnea?
5. *Priority decision:* According to the assessment data provided, what are the priority nursing diagnoses? Are there any collaborative problems?
6. *Priority decision:* For the day of surgery, what are the priority nursing interventions for Ms. Parsons?

evolve

Answers are available at *http://evolve.elsevier.com/Canada/Lewis/medsurg*

REVIEW QUESTIONS

The number of the question corresponds to the same-numbered outcome at the beginning of the chapter.

1. Sleep is *best* described as a
   a. Loosely organized state similar to coma
   b. State in which pain sensitivity decreases
   c. Quiet state in which there is little brain activity
   d. State in which an individual lacks conscious awareness of the environment

2. Which statement is true regarding rapid eye movement (REM) sleep? *(Select all that apply.)*
   a. The EEG pattern is quiescent.
   b. Muscle tone is greatly reduced.
   c. It only occurs once in the night
   d. It is separated by distinct physiological stages.
   e. The most vivid dreaming occurs during this phase.

3. Sleep loss is associated with which of the following symptoms? *(Select all that apply.)*
   a. Increased body mass index
   b. Increased insulin resistance
   c. Enhanced cognitive functioning
   d. Increased immune responsiveness

4. Which of the following points should the nurse emphasize when providing education to the client with insomnia?
   a. The importance of daytime naps
   b. The need to exercise before bedtime
   c. The need for long-term use of hypnotics
   d. Avoidance of caffeine-containing beverages before bedtime

5. A nurse is establishing a care plan for a client in whom narcolepsy has recently been diagnosed. Which of the following areas would the nurse want to address as a priority?
   a. Risk for injury
   b. Ineffective coping
   c. Risk for dehydration
   d. Ineffective family coping

6. A client with sleep apnea would like to avoid using a nasal CPAP device if possible. Which of the following suggestions should the nurse make to help him reach his goal?
   a. Lose excess weight.
   b. Take a nap during the day.
   c. Eat a high-protein snack at bedtime.
   d. Use mild sedatives or alcohol at bedtime.

7. A client on the surgical unit has a history of parasomnia (sleep-walking). Which of the following is true with regard to parasomnia?
   a. Hypnotic medications reduce the risk of sleepwalking.
   b. The client is often unaware of the activity on awakening.
   c. The client should be restrained at night to prevent personal harm.
   d. The potential for sleepwalking is reduced by exercise before sleep.

8. Which of the following strategies would reduce sleepiness during nighttime work?
   a. Exercising before work
   b. Sleeping for at least 2 hours before work time
   c. Taking melatonin before working the night shift
   d. Walking for 10 minutes every 4 hours during the night shift

1. d; 2. b, e; 3. a, b; 4. d; 5. a; 6. a; 7. b; 8. b.

evolve

For even more review questions, visit *http://evolve.elsevier.com/Canada/Lewis/medsurg*.

REFERENCES

Ahn, S., Jiang, L., Smith, M. L., et al. (2014). Improvements in sleep problems among the chronic disease self-management program participants. *Family & Community Health, 37*(4), 327–335. doi:10.1097/fch.0000000000000045.

American Academy of Sleep Medicine. (2016). *Healthy sleep habits.* Retrieved from *www.sleepeducation.com/essentials-in-sleep/healthy-sleep-habits.*

American Geriatric Society 2012 Beers Criteria Update Expert Panel. (2012). American Geriatrics Society updated Beers criteria for potentially inappropriate medication use in older adults. *Journal of the American Geriatrics Society, 60*, 616–631. doi:10.1111/j.1532-5415.2012.03923.x.

Buysse, D. J., Reynolds, C. F., III, Monk, T. H., et al. (1989). The Pittsburgh Sleep Quality Index: A new instrument for psychiatric practice and research. *Psychiatry Research, 28*, 193–213. Seminal.

Cameron, C., Watson, D., & Robinson, J. (2014). Use of a synthetic cannabinoid in a correctional population for posttraumatic stress disorder–related insomnia and nightmares, chronic pain, harm reduction, and other indications: a retrospective evaluation. *Journal of Clinical Psychopharmacology, 34*(5), 559–564. doi:10.1097/JCP.0000000000000180.

Carney, C., Buysse, D. J., Ancoli-Israel, S., et al. (2012). The Consensus Sleep Diary: Standardizing prospective sleep self-monitoring. *Sleep, 35*(2), 287–302. Retrieved from *http://dx.doi.org/10.5665/sleep.1642.*

Carrier, J., Lafortune, M., & Drapeau, C. (2012). Sleep in the elderly—When to reassure, when to intervene. *Insomnia Rounds, 1*(4). Retrieved from *https://css-scs.ca/downloadfolder/150-004_Eng.pdf.*

Cheuk, D. K. L., Yeung, W. F., Chung, K. F., et al. (2012). Acupuncture for insomnia. *The Cochrane Database of Systematic Reviews,* (9), Article CD005472, doi:10.1002/14651858.CD005472.pub3.

Choi, H., Irwin, M., & Cho, H. J. (2015). Impact of social isolation on behavioral health in elderly: Systematic review. *World Journal of Psychiatry, 5*(4), 432–438. doi:10.5498/wjp.v5.i4.432.

Cook, N. (2013). Understanding narcolepsy: The wider perspective. *British Journal of Neuroscience Nursing, 9*(2), 76–82.

Costello, R. B., Lentino, C. V., Boyd, C. C., et al. (2014). The effectiveness of melatonin for promoting healthy sleep: A rapid evidence review of the literature. *Nutrition Journal, 13*, 106. doi:10.1186/1475-2891-13-106.

Davidson, J. R. (2012). Treating chronic insomnia in primary care-Early recognition and management. *Insomnia Rounds, 1*(3), 1–6. Retrieved from *https://css-scs.ca/downloadfolder/150-003_Eng.pdf.*

Eanes, L. (2015). The potential effects of sleep loss on a nurse's health. *American Journal of Nursing, 115*(4), 34–42. doi:10.1097/01.NAJ.0000463025.42388.10.

Fallis, W. M., McMillan, D. E., & Edwards, M. P. (2011). Napping during night shift: Practices, preferences, and perceptions of critical care and emergency department nurses. *Critical Care Nurse, 31*(2), e1–e11. doi:10.4037/ccn2011710.

Ferracioli-Oda, E., Qawasmi, A., & Bloch, M. H. (2013). Meta-analysis: Melatonin for the treatment of primary sleep disorders. *PLoS ONE, 8*(5), e63773. doi:10.1371/journal.pone.0063773.

Fleetham, J., Ayas, N., Bradley, D., et al. (2011). The Canadian Thoracic Society Sleep Disordered Breathing Committee. Canadian Thoracic Society 2011 guideline update: Diagnosis and treatment of sleep disordered breathing. *Canadian Respiratory Journal, 18*(1), 25–47.

Freedman, N. (2014). Improvements in current treatments and emerging therapies for adult obstructive sleep apnea. *F1000prime Reports, 6*, 1. doi:10.12703/P6-36.

Gamaldo, C. E., Chung, Y., Kang, Y. M., et al. (2014). Tick-tock-tick-tock: The impact of circadian rhythm disorders on cardiovascular health and wellness. *Journal of the American Society of Hypertension, 8*(12), 921–929. doi:10.1016/j.jash.2014.08.011.

Gooneratne, N. S., & Vitiello, M. V. (2014). Sleep in older adults: Normative changes, sleep disorders, and treatment options. *Clinics in Geriatric Medicine, 30*(3), 591–627. doi:10.1016/j.cger.2014.04.007.

Health Canada. (2012). *Caffeine in food.* Retrieved from *http://www.hc-sc.gc.ca/fn-an/securit/addit/caf/food-caf-aliments-eng.php.*

Hirshkowitz, M., Whiton, K., Albert, S. M., et al. (2015). National Sleep Foundation's updated sleep duration recommendations: Final report. *Sleep Health, 1*, 233–243. Retrieved from *http://www.sciencedirect.com/science/article/pii/S2352721815001606.*

Hopper, K., Fried, T. R., & Pisani, M. A. (2015). Health care worker attitudes and identified barriers to patient sleep in the medical intensive care unit. *Heart and Lung: The Journal of Critical Care, 44*(2), 95–99. doi:10.1016/j.hrtlng.2015.01.011.

Jetly, R., Heber, A., Fraser, G., et al. (2015). The efficacy of nabilone, a synthetic cannabinoid, in the treatment of PTSD-associated nightmares: A preliminary randomized, double-blind, placebo-controlled cross-over design study. *Psychoneuroendocrinology, 51*, 585–588. doi:10.1016/j.psyneuen.2014.11.002.

Johns, M. W. (1991). A new method for measuring daytime sleepiness: The Epworth Sleepiness Scale. *Sleep, 14*, 540–545. Retrieved from *http://www.journalsleep.org/ViewAbstract.aspx?pid=24884.* Seminal.

Johnson, A. L., Jung, L., Brown, K. C., et al. (2014). Sleep deprivation and error in nurses who work the night shift. *Journal of Nursing Administration, 44*(1), 17–22. doi:10.1097/NNA.0000000000000016.

Knauert, M., Naik, S., Gillespie, M. B., et al. (2015). Clinical consequences and economic costs of untreated obstructive sleep apnea syndrome. *World Journal of Otorhinolaryngology—Head and Neck Surgery, 1*(1), 17–27. doi:10.1016/j.wjorl.2015.08.001.

Leach, M. J., & Page, A. T. (2014). Herbal medicine for insomnia: A systematic review and meta-analysis. *Sleep Medicine Reviews, 24*, 1–12.

LeGates, T. A., Fernandez, D. C., & Hattar, S. (2014). Light as a central modulator of circadian rhythms, sleep and affect. *Nature Reviews. Neuroscience, 15*, 443. doi:10.1038/nrn3743.

Lerchl, A., & Reiter, R. J. (2012). Treatment of sleep disorders with melatonin. *BMJ (Clinical Research Ed.), 345*, e6968. doi:10.1136/bmj.e6968. Retrieved from *http://www.bmj.com/content/345/bmj.e6968.abstract.*

Levenson, J. C., Kay, D., & Buysse, D. J. (2015). Pathophysiology of insomnia. *Chest, 147*(4), 1179–1192. doi:10.1378/chest.14-1617.

Lo, C. M., & Lee, P. H. (2014). Feasibility and Effects of TAI CHI for the Promotion of Sleep Quality and Quality of Life. *Journal of Gerontological Nursing, 40*(3), 46–52, 7p. doi:10.3928/00989134-20131028-08.

MacFarlane, J. (2012). Taking control of acute insomnia: Restoring healthy sleep patterns. *Insomnia Rounds, 1*(2), 1–6.

Matheson, A., O'Brien, L., & Reid, J. A. (2014). The impact of shiftwork on health: A literature review. *Journal of Clinical Nursing, 23*(23-24), 3309–3320.

Moraes, M., Rossini, S., & Reimão, R. (2012). Executive attention and working memory in narcoleptic outpatients. *Arquivos de Neuro-Psiquiatria, 70*(5), 335–340.

Morin, C. M., LeBlanc, M., Bélanger, L., et al. (2011). Prevalence of insomnia and its treatment in Canada. *Canadian Journal of Psychiatry, 56*, 540–548. Retrieved from *http://journals.sagepub .com/doi/pdf/10.1177/070674371105600905, http://publications .cpa-apc.org/media.php?mid=1212.*

Nagappa, M., Liao, P., Wong, J., et al. (2015). Validation of the STOP-Bang questionnaire as a screening tool for obstructive sleep apnea among different populations: A systematic review and meta-analysis. *PLoS ONE, 10*(12), e0143697. doi:10.1371/journal .pone.0143697.

Nadorff, M. R., Lambdin, K. K., & Germain, A. (2014). Pharmacological and non-pharmacological treatments for nightmare disorder. *International Review of Psychiatry, 26*(2), 225–236. Retrieved from *http://dx.doi.org/10.3109/09540261.2014.888989.*

Nesbitt, A. D., & Dijk, D. J. (2014). Out of synch with society: An update on delayed sleep phase disorder. *Current Opinion Pulmonary Medicine, 20*, 581–587. doi:10.1097/MCP.0000000000000095.

Public Health Agency of Canada (2009). *What is the impact of sleep apnea on Canadians? Fast facts from the Canadian community health survey—Sleep apnea rapid response.* Retrieved from *http:// www.phac-aspc.gc.ca/cd-mc/sleepapnea-apneesommeil/pdf/ sleep-apnea.pdf.*

Reutrakul, S., & Van Cauter, E. (2014). Interactions between sleep, circadian function, and glucose metabolism: implications for risk and severity of diabetes. *Annals of New York Academy of Sciences, 1311*, 151–173. doi:10.1111/nyas.12355.

Rod, N. H., Kumari, M., Lange, T., et al. (2014). The joint effect of sleep duration and disturbed sleep on cause-specific mortality: Results from the Whitehall II cohort study. *PLoS ONE, 9*(4), e91965. doi:10.1371/journal.pone.0091965.

Sateia, M. J. (2014). International Classification of Sleep Disorders—Third Edition: Highlights and recommendations. *Chest, 146*(5), 1387–1394. doi:10.1378/chest.14-0970.

Scammell, T. E. (2015a). Narcolepsy. *New England Journal of Medicine, 373*(27), 2654–2662. doi:10.1056/NEJMra1500587.

Scammell, T. E. (2015b). Overview of sleep: The neurologic processes of the sleep–wake cycle. *The Journal of Clinical Psychiatry, 76*(5), e13.

Silva-Costa, A., Rotenberg, L., Griep, R. H., et al. (2015). Napping on the night shift among nursing staff: Potential benefits for workers' health. *Anna Nery School Journal Of Nursing, 19*(1), 33–39. doi:10.5935/1414-8145.20150005.

Simoncini, M., Gatti, A., Quirico, P., et al. (2015). Acupressure in insomnia and other sleep disorders in elderly institutionalized patients suffering from Alzheimer's disease. *Aging Clinical & Experimental Research, 27*(1), 37–42. doi:10.1007/ s40520-014-0244-9.

Stopford, E., Ravi, K., & Nayar, V. (2013). The association of sleep disordered breathing with heart failure and other cardiovascular conditions. *Cardiology Research and Practice, 2013*, Article ID 356280. doi:10.1155/2013/356280.

Sutton, E. L. (2014). Insomnia. *Medical Clinics of North America, 98*, 566–581. doi:10.1016/j.mcna.2014.01.008.

Taavoni, S., Ekbatani, N., & Haghani, H. (2015). Effect of valerian and lemon balm combined capsules on postmenopausal sleep disorder, a triple blind randomized placebo control clinical trial. *European Psychiatry, 30*(S1), 28–31. doi:10.1016/S0924-9338 (15)31376-6.

Tanenbaum, C. (2015). Inappropriate benzodiazepine use in the elderly patients and its reduction. *Journal of Psychiatry & Neuroscience, 40*(3), E27–E28. doi:10.1503/jpn.140355.

Taslaman, M. (2014). The efficacy and safety of herbal medicine for insomnia in adults: An overview of recent research. *Australian Journal of Herbal Medicine, 26*(3), 86–93. Retrieved from *http:// search.informit.com.au/documentSummary;dn=608432227099870 ;res=IELHEA.*

Tracy, M. F., & Chlan, L. (2011). Nonpharmacological interventions to manage common symptoms in patients receiving mechanical ventilation. *Critical Care Nurse, 31*(3), 19–28. doi:10.4037/ ccn2011653.

Transport Canada. (2011). *Road safety in Canada.* Retrieved from *http://www.tc.gc.ca/eng/motorvehiclesafety/tp-tp15145-1201 .htm#s37.*

Uehli, K., Mehta, A. J., Miedinger, D., et al. (2014). Sleep problems and work injuries: A systematic review and meta-analysis. *Sleep Medicine Reviews, 18*, 61–73. Retrieved from *http://dx.doi.org/ 10.1016/j.smrv.2013.01.004.*

Vozoris, N. T., & Leung, R. S. (2011). Sedative medication use: Prevalence, risk factors, and associations with body mass index using population-level data. *Sleep, 34*(7), 869–874.

Williams, J., Roth, A., Vatthauer, K., et al. (2013). Cognitive behavioral treatment of insomnia. *Chest, 143*, 554.

Wozniak, D. R., Lasserson, T. J., & Smith, I. (2014). Educational, supportive and behavioural interventions to improve usage of continuous positive airway pressure machines in adults with obstructive sleep apnoea. *The Cochrane Database of Systematic Reviews*, (1), Article CD007736, doi:10.1002/14651858.CD007736 .pub2.

Ye, L., & Smith, A. (2015). Developing and testing a sleep education program for college nursing students. *Journal of Nursing Education, 54*(9), 532–535, 4p. doi:10.3928/01484834 -20150814-09.

RESOURCES

Canadian Lung Association, Sleep Apnea
http://www.lung.ca/diseases-maladies/apnea-apnee_e.php

Canadian Sleep Society
https://css-scs.ca

Consensus Sleep Diary
http://www.topalbertadoctors.org/download/1922/Sleep%20 Diary.pdf?_20170204003431

American Academy of Sleep Medicine
http://www.aasmnet.org

Better Sleep Council
http://www.bettersleep.org

Epworth Sleepiness Scale
http://epworthsleepinessscale.com

Narcolepsy Network
http://www.narcolepsynetwork.org

National Sleep Foundation
http://www.sleepfoundation.org

Pittsburgh Sleep Quality Index
http://uacc.arizona.edu/sites/default/files/ psqi_sleep_questionnaire_1_pg.pdf

For additional Internet resources, see the website for this book at *http://evolve.elsevier.com/canada/lewis/medsurg*

CHAPTER

10

Pain

Written by: Rosemary C. Polomano and Mechele Fillman
Adapted by: Michael McGillion, Sheila O'Keefe-McCarthy,
and Salima S. J. Ladak

℮volve WEBSITE

http://evolve.elsevier.com/Canada/Lewis/medsurg

- Review Questions (Online Only)
- Key Points
- Answer Guidelines for Case Study
- Conceptual Care Map Creator
- Student Case Study
  - Pain
- Audio Glossary
- Content Updates

LEARNING OBJECTIVES

1. Define pain.
2. Describe the neural mechanisms of pain and pain modulation.
3. Differentiate between nociceptive, neuropathic, somatic, and visceral types of pain.
4. Explain the physical and psychological effects of unrelieved pain.
5. Describe the components of a comprehensive pain assessment.
6. Describe effective pain management techniques used across many professional disciplines.
7. Describe pharmacological and nonpharmacological methods of pain relief.
8. Explain the nurse's role and responsibility in pain management.
9. Discuss ethical issues related to pain and pain management.
10. Evaluate the influence of one's own knowledge, beliefs, and attitudes about pain assessment and management.

KEY TERMS

analgesic ceiling, p. 154
breakthrough pain, p. 147
ceiling effect, p. 152
dermatomes, p. 143
equianalgesic dose, p. 151

modulation, p. 145
neuropathic pain, p. 146
nociception, p. 142
nociceptive pain, p. 146
pain, p. 141

pain perception, p. 145
patient-controlled analgesia (PCA), p. 158
physical dependence, p. 161
suffering, p. 142

titration, p. 151
transduction, p. 142
transmission, p. 143
trigger point, p. 159
windup, p. 144

PAIN

Pain is a complex experience with sensory-discriminative, motivational–affective, and cognitive–evaluative dimensions. For many people, it is a major problem that causes suffering and reduces quality of life. Pain is one of the major reasons that people seek health care, and effective pain relief is a basic human right (Canadian Pain Society [CPS], 2010). A thorough understanding of the multiple dimensions of pain is important for effective assessment and management of patients with pain. Nurses have a central role in pain assessment and management. Components of the nursing role include (a) assessing pain and documenting and communicating this information to other health care providers, (b) ensuring delivery of effective pain relief measures, (c) evaluating the effectiveness of these interventions, (d) monitoring ongoing effectiveness of pain management strategies, and (e) providing education to patients and their families regarding pain management approaches and

possible adverse effects. This chapter presents current knowledge about pain and pain management to enable the nurse to assess and manage pain successfully in collaboration with other health care providers.

MAGNITUDE OF THE PAIN PROBLEM

According to Canadian Community Health Survey data from 2007, more than 1.5 million Canadians between 12 and 44 years of age suffer chronic pain, which, for 60%, interferes with daily activities (Ramage-Morin & Gilmour, 2010). Unrelieved, persistent pain is an epidemic in Canada and the United States. More than 50 million people are affected with musculo-skeletal pain, such as back pain and arthritis, that goes unrelieved for 5 years or more (American Academy of Pain Management, n.d.). In Canada, pain is the most common cause of disability among working-age adults; up to 60% eventually lose their jobs or incur substantial loss of income (Lynch, 2011). The global prevalence of pain has a major negative economic impact, with estimated annual values of lost productivity ranging from $297.4 billion to $335.5 billion (2010 U.S. dollars). These values include days of work missed (ranging from $11.6 to $12.7 billion); hours of work lost (from $95.2 to $96.5 billion); and reduction in wages (from $190.6 billion to $226.3 billion) (Institutes of Medicine, 2011). Those with chronic pain now gainfully employed are expected to lose up to 28.5 productive working days per year (Lynch, 2011). Unfortunately, cumulative evidence indicates that, across the lifespan, people in a variety of settings continue to experience considerable acute and persistent pain despite the availability of treatment options (Choinière, Watt-Watson, Victor, et al., 2014; Lynch, 2011; McGillion & Watt-Watson, 2015; Watt-Watson & Murinson, 2013). Despite management standards and directives from nongovernmental organizations such as the Canadian Pain Society (2010) and the Registered Nurses' Association of Ontario (RNAO, 2013), more than four decades' worth of evidence documents inadequate pain management practices as the norm across health care settings and patient populations (McGillion & Watt-Watson, 2015; Watt-Watson & Murinson, 2013). For example, alarming numbers of Canadians are still left in pain after surgery, even in our top hospitals. Evidence suggests that up to 50% of patients report pain in the moderate-to-severe range following surgical procedures (Choinière, Watt-Watson, Victor, et al., 2014).

The prevalence of chronic pain increases with age, with estimates that as many as 65% of community-dwelling older adults and up to 80% of older adults in long-term care facilities experience it. Chronic pain in these populations is under-recognized and undertreated (Katz, 2014). People living with cancer—whether the disease is newly diagnosed, is being actively treated, or is in a more advanced stage—also consistently receive inadequate pain treatment (Lynch, 2011; O'Mara, 2014). The prevalence of moderate to severe pain among people with head and neck cancers, for example, has been reported to be as high as 70% (Chaturvedi, Anderson, Lortet-Tieulent, et al., 2013; O'Mara, 2014). Consequences of untreated pain include unnecessary suffering, physical dysfunction, psychosocial distress (which manifests in such forms as anxiety or depression), impairment in recovery from acute illness and surgery, immuno-suppression, and sleep disturbances (Lynch, 2011; O'Mara, 2014).

In the acutely ill patient, unrelieved pain can result in increased morbidity as a result of respiratory dysfunction, increased heart rate and cardiac workload, increased muscular contraction and spasm, decreased gastro-intestinal (GI) motility, and increased catabolism (Table 10-1). Screening for the presence of pain is recommended to be an institutional priority. In general, it is recommended that pain be assessed—in all clinical care settings for all patients—at least once per day (RNAO, 2013).

When left untreated, acute pain can also progress to persistent pain. Common surgical procedures have resulted in patients' experiencing persistent pain after surgery in 5 to 50% of cases; for some (2 to 10%), this pain is moderate to severe (Pergolizzi, Raffa, & Taylor, 2014). Rationales for the undertreatment of pain vary. Among health care providers, frequently cited reasons include a lack of knowledge and skills to adequately assess and treat pain; misconceptions about pain; and inaccurate and inadequate information regarding addiction, tolerance, respiratory depression, and other adverse effects of opioids (McMillan, Tittle, Hagan, et al., 2000; O'Keefe-McCarthy, McGillion, Clarke, et al., 2015). These reasons are indeed common among nurses, who routinely administer the lowest prescribed analgesic dose when

TABLE 10-1	CONSEQUENCES OF UNRELIEVED PAIN
System	**Responses**
Endocrine	↑ Adrenocorticotrophic hormone (ACTH), ↑ cortisol, ↑ antidiuretic hormone (ADH), ↑ epinephrine, ↑ norepinephrine, ↑ growth hormone, ↑ renin, ↑ aldosterone levels; ↓ insulin, ↓ testosterone levels
Metabolic	Gluconeogenesis, glycogenolysis, hyperglycemia, glucose intolerance, insulin resistance, muscle protein catabolism, ↑ lipolysis
Cardiovascular	↑ Heart rate, ↑ cardiac output, ↑ peripheral vascular resistance, hypertension, ↑ myocardial oxygen consumption, ↑ coagulation
Respiratory	↓ Tidal volume, atelectasis, shunting, hypoxemia, ↓ cough, sputum retention, infection
Genitourinary	↓ Urinary output, urinary retention
Gastro-intestinal	↓ Gastric and bowel motility
Musculo-skeletal	Muscle spasm, impaired muscle function, fatigue, immobility
Neurological	↓ Cognitive function; mental confusion
Immunological	↓ Immune response

Source: Adapted from McCaffery, M., & Pasero, C. (1999). *Pain: A clinical manual for nursing practice* (2nd ed.). St. Louis: Mosby.

a range of doses is prescribed (McGillion & Watt-Watson, 2015; Voshall, Dunn, & Shelestak, 2013). Such practices do little to provide relief from unremitting pain and are not consistent with current pain management guidelines (RNAO, 2013). The need to improve prelicensure pain education for health care providers in Canada is dire. One national study revealed that students in just one-third of health sciences programs (e.g., dentistry, medicine, nursing, pharmacy, rehabilitation sciences, veterinary medicine) could identify designated, mandatory curricular content dedicated to pain (Watt-Watson, McGillion, Hunter, et al., 2009).

Among patients, misconceptions about pain and opioids also play a major role in the under-reporting and undertreatment of pain (Cogan, Ouimette, Vargas-Schaffer, et al., 2014). Examples include the belief that pain is inevitable and a result of worsening disease and the desire to be a "good" patient who does not complain (Cogan, Ouimette, Vargas-Schaffer, et al., 2014; O'Keefe-McCarthy, McGillion, Nelson, et al., 2014).

Unfortunately, wait times for expert pain-related care in Canada exceed 1 year at more than one-third of publicly funded pain clinics (Lynch, 2011), and many regions have no access to appropriate care.

DEFINITIONS OF PAIN

McCaffery and Pasero's seminal definition that pain is "whatever and whenever the person says it is" changed practice by focusing health care providers' attention on the subjectivity of pain (McCaffery & Pasero, 1999). Patients' self-reports about their pain are key to effective pain management. This definition at the simplest level may cause problems because patients do not always admit to pain or use the word *pain*. The International Association for the Study of Pain (IASP) defined **pain** as "an unpleasant sensory and emotional experience associated with actual or potential tissue damage, or described in terms of such damage" (Merskey & Baranowski, 2012).

Pain is multidimensional and subjective, as the IASP definition emphasizes. The patient's self-report, therefore, is the most valid means of assessment. A person's inability to communicate verbally does not negate the possibility of that individual's experiencing pain or the need for appropriate pain-relieving treatment. In the case of patients who are nonverbal or cognitively unable to rate pain, gathering nonverbal information is critical for pain assessment.

The IASP definition of pain underlines the fact that pain can be experienced in the absence of identifiable tissue damage. It is important to differentiate pain that involves perception of a noxious (tissue-damaging) stimulus from pain involving nociception, which may not be perceived as painful. Nociception is the activation of the primary afferent nociceptors (PANs) with peripheral terminals (free nerve endings) that respond differently to noxious stimuli. Nociceptors function primarily to sense and transmit pain signals. If nociceptive stimuli are blocked, pain is not perceived.

Pain is not synonymous with *suffering*, although pain can cause substantial suffering. Suffering has been defined as "the state of severe distress associated with events that threaten the intactness (biopsychosocial integrity) of the person" (Cassell, 1982, p. 32). Suffering can occur in the presence or absence of pain, and pain can occur with or without suffering. For example, the woman awaiting breast biopsy may suffer emotionally because of anticipated loss of her breast. She may have acute pain in the breast after the biopsy (due to the procedure itself) without emotional suffering if the biopsy result is negative for malignancy. Conversely, she may have biopsy-related pain with emotional suffering if the biopsy result is positive for malignancy.

DIMENSIONS OF PAIN AND THE PAIN PROCESS

Pain is a complex experience involving several dimensions: *physiological, sensory-discriminative* (i.e., the perception of pain by the individual that addresses the pain location, intensity, pattern, and quality), *motivational–affective, behavioural, cognitive–evaluative*, and *sociocultural* (Figure 10-1). In 1965, Melzack and Wall built on prior understanding of pain mechanisms in order to develop their gate control theory of pain (Melzack & Wall, 1987). Although the gate control theory is limited to providing a basic understanding of acute pain mechanisms, it is seminal work that remains critical

FIGURE 10-1 Multidimensional nature of pain. Developed by M. McCaffery, C. Pasero, and J. A. Paice. Modified from McCaffery, M., & Pasero, C. (1999). *Pain: A clinical manual for nursing practice* (2nd ed.). St. Louis: Mosby.

to the understanding of the pain process, including transduction, transmission, perception, and modulation of pain. Pain experience and response result from complex interactions among these dimensions. In the following discussion, each dimension and the ways in which different dimensions influence pain are described.

Physiological Dimension of Pain

Understanding the physiological dimension of pain requires knowledge of neural anatomy and physiology. The neural mechanism by which pain is perceived consists of four major steps: transduction, transmission, perception, and modulation (Fields, 1987). Figure 10-2 outlines these four steps.

Transduction. Transduction is the conversion of a mechanical, thermal, or chemical stimulus to a neuronal action potential. Transduction occurs at the level of the peripheral nerves, particularly the free nerve endings, or PANs. Noxious (tissue-damaging) stimuli can include thermal damage (e.g., sunburn), mechanical damage (e.g., surgical incision, pressure from swelling), or chemical damage (e.g., from toxic substances). These stimuli cause the release of numerous chemicals into the peripheral microenvironment of the PAN. Some of these chemicals—such as histamines, bradykinin, prostaglandins, nerve growth factor, and arachidonic acid—activate or sensitize the PAN to excitation (Mogil, 2012; Mifflin & Kerr, 2014). If the PAN is activated or excited, it fires an action potential to the spinal cord.

An action potential is necessary to convert the noxious stimulus to an impulse and move the impulse from the periphery to the spinal cord. A pain action potential can result from two sources: (a) a release of the sensitizing and activating chemicals (*nociceptive pain*) or (b) abnormal processing of stimuli by the nervous system (*neuropathic pain);* both of these sources produce a change in the charge along the neuronal membrane (Kerstman, Ahn, Battu, et al., 2013; Mifflin & Kerr, 2014). In other words, when the PAN terminal is transduced, the PAN membrane becomes depolarized. Sodium enters the cell, and potassium exits the cell, thereby generating an action potential. The action potential is then transmitted along the entire length of the neuron to cells in the spinal cord.

Inflammation and the subsequent release of the chemical mediators listed above lower the excitation threshold of PANs and increase the likelihood of transduction. This increased susceptibility is called *sensitization*. Several chemicals, such as leukotrienes, prostaglandins, and substance P, are probably involved in this process of sensitization. It is known that the release of substance P, a chemical stored in the distal terminals of the PAN, sensitizes the PAN and dilates nearby blood vessels, resulting in subsequent development of edema and release of histamine from mast cells (Mogil, 2012; Pelletier, Higgins, Bourbonnais, 2015).

Therapies directed at altering either the PAN environment or the sensitivity of the PAN are used to prevent the transduction and initiation of an action potential. Decreasing the effects of chemicals released at the periphery is the basis of several pharmacological approaches to pain relief. For example, nonsteroidal anti-inflammatory drugs (NSAIDs), such as ibuprofen (Advil, Motrin) and naproxen (Naprosyn, Aleve), and corticosteroids, such as dexamethasone (Decadron), exert their analgesic effects by blocking pain-producing chemicals. NSAIDs block the action of cyclo-oxygenase, and corticosteroids block the action of phospholipase, thereby interfering with the production of prostaglandins.

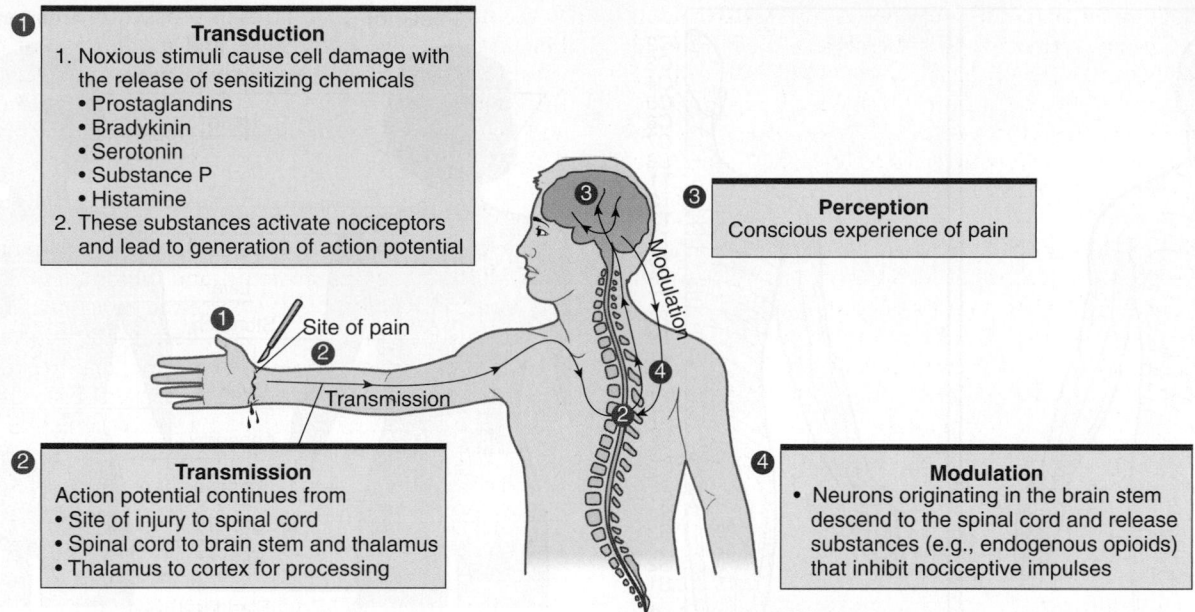

① Transduction
1. Noxious stimuli cause cell damage with the release of sensitizing chemicals
   • Prostaglandins
   • Bradykinin
   • Serotonin
   • Substance P
   • Histamine
2. These substances activate nociceptors and lead to generation of action potential

③ Perception
Conscious experience of pain

② Transmission
Action potential continues from
• Site of injury to spinal cord
• Spinal cord to brain stem and thalamus
• Thalamus to cortex for processing

④ Modulation
• Neurons originating in the brain stem descend to the spinal cord and release substances (e.g., endogenous opioids) that inhibit nociceptive impulses

Site of pain
Transmission
Modulation

FIGURE 10-2 Nociceptive pain originates when the tissue is injured. Transduction *(1)* occurs when chemical mediators are released. Transmission *(2)* involves the conduct of the action potential (short-term change in the electrical potential travelling along a cell) from the periphery (injury site) to the spinal cord and then to the brain stem, thalamus, and cerebral cortex. Perception *(3)* is the conscious awareness of pain. Modulation *(4)* involves signals from the brain going back down the spinal cord to modify incoming impulses. Source: Developed by M. McCaffery, C. Pasero, & J. A. Paice. Modified from McCaffery, M., & Pasero, C. (1999). *Pain: clinical manual* (2nd ed.). St. Louis: Mosby.

Transmission. Transmission is the movement of pain impulses from the site of transduction to the brain (see Figure 10-2) (Fields, 1987). Three segments are involved in nociceptive signal transmission: (a) transmission along the nociceptor fibres to the level of the spinal cord, (b) processing in the dorsal horn, and (c) transmission to the thalamus and the cortex. Each step in the transmission process is important in pain perception.

Transmission to the Spinal Cord. One nerve cell extends the entire distance from the periphery to the dorsal horn of the spinal cord with no synapses. For example, an afferent fibre from the great toe travels from the toe through the fifth lumbar nerve root into the spinal cord; it is one cell. Once generated, an action potential travels all the way to the spinal cord unless it is blocked by a sodium channel inhibitor or disrupted by a lesion at the central terminal of the fibre (e.g., by a dorsal root entry zone lesion) (Fields, 1987).

Two types of peripheral nerve fibres are responsible for the transmission of pain impulses from the site of transduction to the level of the spinal cord: the A fibres (A-alpha, A-beta, and A-delta) and the C fibres. Neurons that project from the periphery to the spinal cord are also referred to as *first-order neurons*. Each type of fibre has different characteristics that determine its conduction rate (Table 10-2). A-alpha and A-beta fibres are large fibres enclosed within myelin sheaths that allow them to conduct impulses at a rapid rate. A-delta fibres are smaller with thinly myelinated sheaths. Because of their smaller size, however, they conduct at a slower rate than the larger A-alpha and A-beta fibres. C fibres are the smallest fibres and are unmyelinated. They conduct at the slowest rate. The conduction rates have important implications for the modulation of noxious information from A-delta and C fibres (Fields, 1987).

Stimulation of different fibres results in different sensations. Stimulation of A-delta fibres results in pain described as pricking,

TABLE 10-2	CHARACTERISTICS OF PERIPHERAL NERVE FIBRES		
Type of Fibre	**Size**	**Myelinization**	**Conduction Velocity***
A-alpha	Large	Myelinated	Rapid
A-beta	Large	Myelinated	Rapid
A-delta	Small	Myelinated	Medium
C	Smallest	Not myelinated	Slow

*The conduction rates are important because information carried to the spinal cord by the more rapidly conducting nerve fibres reaches dorsal horn cells sooner than does information carried by the fibres that conduct more slowly.

sharp, well localized, and short in duration. C-fibre activation pain is described as a dull, aching, burning sensation and is characterized by its diffuse nature, slow onset, and relatively long duration. The A-alpha (sensory muscle) and A-beta (sensory skin) fibres typically transmit nonpainful sensations such as light pressure to deep muscles, soft touch to skin, and vibration. All of these fibres extend from the peripheral tissues through the dorsal root ganglia to the dorsal horn of the spinal cord. The manner in which nerve fibres enter the spinal cord is central to the notion of spinal dermatomes. Dermatomes are areas on the skin that are innervated primarily by a single spinal cord segment. Figure 10-3 illustrates different dermatomes and their innervations.

Dorsal Horn Processing. Once the nociceptive signal arrives in the central nervous system (CNS), it is processed within the dorsal horn of the spinal cord. This processing includes the release of neurotransmitters from the afferent fibre into the synaptic cleft. These neurotransmitters bind to receptors on nearby cell bodies and dendrites of cells that may be located elsewhere in the dorsal horn. Some of these neurotransmitters (e.g., aspartate, glutamate,

FIGURE 10-3 Spinal dermatomes representing organized sensory input carried via specific spinal nerve roots. *C,* cervical; *L,* lumbar; *S,* sacral; *T,* thoracic.

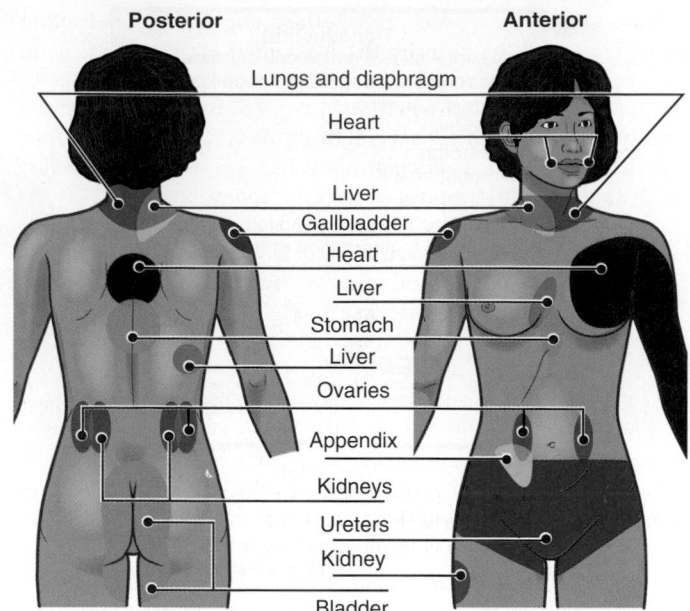

FIGURE 10-4 Typical areas of referred pain.

substance P) produce activation of nearby cells, whereas others (e.g., γ-aminobutyric acid, serotonin, norepinephrine) inhibit such activation. In turn, these nearby cells release other neurotransmitters. The effects of the complex neurochemistry can facilitate or modulate (i.e., inhibit) transmission of noxious stimuli. In this area, exogenous and endogenous opioids also play an important role by binding to opioid receptors and blocking the release of neurotransmitters, particularly substance P. Endogenous opioids, which include enkephalins and β-endorphins, are chemicals that are synthesized and secreted by the body. They are capable of producing effects that are similar to those of exogenous opioids such as morphine.

The dorsal horn of the spinal cord contains specialized cells called *wide dynamic range neurons.* These neurons receive input from noxious stimuli primarily carried by A-delta and C-fibre afferent pathways (especially from viscera) and from non-noxious stimuli from A-beta fibres; they also receive indirect input from dendritic projections (Mogil, 2012; Kerstman, Ahn, Battu, et al., 2013; Mifflin & Kerr, 2014). These stimuli come from distant areas, providing a neural explanation for referred pain. Inputs from both nociceptive fibres and A-beta fibres converge on the wide dynamic range neuron, and when the message is transmitted to the brain, pain in the originating area of the body becomes poorly localized. The concept of referred pain must be considered when a person with injury to or disease involving visceral organs

reports pain in a certain location. The location of a tumour, for instance, may be distant from the pain location reported by the patient (Figure 10-4). For example, liver disease is located in the right upper abdominal quadrant, but pain frequently is referred to the anterior and posterior neck region and to a posterior flank area. If referred pain is not considered in the evaluation of a pain location report, diagnostic tests and therapy could be misdirected.

Sensitization, or enhanced excitability, can also occur at the level of the spinal neurons, known as *central sensitization* (Mifflin & Kerr, 2014; Kerstman, Ahn, Battu, et al., 2013; Pelletier, Higgins, & Bourbonnais, 2015). Peripheral tissue damage or nerve injury can cause central sensitization, and continued nociceptive input from the periphery is necessary to maintain it (Mifflin & Kerr, 2014; Kerstman, Ahn, Battu, et al., 2013; Pelletier, Higgins, & Bourbonnais, 2015). With ongoing stimulation of the slowly conducting unmyelinated C-fibre nociceptors, firing of specialized dorsal horn neurons gradually increases. This process is known as **windup** and is dependent on the activation of *N*-methyl-D-aspartate (NMDA) receptors. NMDA receptors produce alterations in neural processing of afferent stimuli that can persist for long periods. For this reason, an important goal of therapy is to prevent persistent pain by avoiding central sensitization. Currently, the NMDA antagonist most commonly used is the anaesthetic medication ketamine (Ketalar). Unfortunately, intolerable adverse effects, such as hallucinations, limit its usefulness. Development of newer NMDA-antagonist drugs is ongoing and shows promise for potentially blocking central sensitization with fewer adverse effects.

Transmission to the Thalamus and the Cortex. From the dorsal horn, nociceptive stimuli are communicated to the *third-order neurons,* primarily in the thalamus, and several other areas of the brain. Fibres of dorsal horn projection cells enter the brain through several pathways, including the spinothalamic tract and the spinoreticular tract. Distinct thalamic nuclei receive nociceptive input from the spinal cord and have projections to several regions in the cerebral cortex, where the perception of pain is believed to occur.

Perception. Pain perception is the recognition of, definition of, and response to pain by the individual experiencing it. In the brain, nociceptive input is perceived as pain. There is no single, precise location where pain perception occurs. Instead, pain perception involves several brain structures. For example, it is believed that the reticular activating system is responsible for the autonomic response of warning the individual to attend to the pain stimulus; the somatosensory system is responsible for localization and characterization of pain; and the limbic system is responsible for the emotional and behavioural responses to pain. Cortical structures are also thought to be crucial to constructing the meaning of the pain. Therefore, behavioural strategies such as distraction, relaxation, and imagery (distraction and relaxation are discussed later in this chapter; imagery is discussed in Chapter 8) are effective pain-reducing therapies for many people. By directing attention away from the pain sensation, patients can reduce the sensory and affective components of pain. For example, blood flow to the anterior central gyrus, an area intimately involved with the perception of the unpleasantness of pain, can be altered by hypnosis.

Modulation. Modulation involves the activation of descending pathways that exert inhibitory or facilitatory effects on the transmission of pain. Depending on the type and degree of modulation, the nociceptive stimuli may or may not be perceived as pain. Modulation of pain signals can occur at the level of the periphery, the spinal cord, the brain stem, and the cerebral cortex. Centrally, modulation of nociceptive impulses occurs via descending fibres that influence dorsal horn neuronal activity. Complex neurochemistry involving excitatory and inhibitory neurotransmitters such as enkephalin, γ-aminobutyric acid, serotonin, and norepinephrine is involved in this nociceptive modulation; as a result, pain transmission is inhibited (Salter, 2014). A number of pain management medications exert their effects through the modulatory systems. For example, tricyclic antidepressants, such as amitriptyline (Elavil), are used in the management of persistent noncancer pain and cancer pain. These medications interfere with the reuptake of serotonin and norepinephrine, thereby increasing their availability to inhibit noxious stimuli and produce analgesia. Baclofen (Lioresal), an analogue of the inhibitory neurotransmitter γ-aminobutyric acid, can interfere with the transmission of nociceptive impulses and thus produce analgesia for many chronic conditions, particularly those accompanied by muscle spasms. Table 10-3 briefly summarizes how pain-relieving medications can affect pain transduction, transmission, perception, and modulation.

Sensory-Discriminative, Motivational–Affective, Behavioural, Cognitive–Evaluative, and Sociocultural Dimensions of Pain

Pain is subjective; the experience of pain and related responses vary from person to person. Because of the complex neural mechanisms of nociceptive processing, pain is a multidimensional sensory and affective experience that has cognitive, behavioural, and sociocultural aspects.

The *sensory-discriminative* component of pain is the recognition of the sensation as painful. Elements of sensory pain include pattern, area, intensity, and nature (PAIN). Information about these elements and knowledge about the pain process are indispensable to clinical decision making and appropriate pain therapy.

The *motivational–affective* component of pain encompasses the emotional responses to the pain experience. These affective

TABLE 10-3 DRUG THERAPY

Interrupting the Pain Pathway

Pain Mechanism	Mechanism of Action
Transduction	
NSAIDs	Block prostaglandin production
Local anaesthetics	Block action potential initiation
Antiseizure drugs (e.g., gabapentin [Neurontin])	Block action potential initiation
Corticosteroids	Block action potential initiation
Transmission	
Opioids	Block release of substance P
Cannabinoids	Inhibit mast cell degranulation and response of nociceptive neurons
Perception	
Opioids	Decrease conscious experience of pain
NSAIDs	Inhibit cyclo-oxygenase action
Adjuvants (e.g., antidepressants)	Dependent on specific adjuvant
Modulation	
Tricyclic antidepressants (e.g., amitriptyline [Elavil])	Interfere with reuptake of serotonin and norepinephrine

NSAIDs, nonsteroidal anti-inflammatory drugs.

responses include anger, fear, depression, and anxiety, negative emotions that impair the patient's quality of life. They become part of a vicious cycle in which pain leads to negative emotions such as depression, which in turn intensifies pain perception, leading to more depression and impairment of function. It is important for nurses to recognize this cycle and intervene appropriately (Richardson, 2014).

The *behavioural* component of pain comprises the observable actions used to express or control the pain. For example, facial expressions such as grimacing may reflect pain or discomfort. Posturing may be used to decrease pain associated with specific movements. A person often adjusts his or her daily physical and social activities in response to the pain. In this way, pain, especially persistent pain, has profound effects on functioning (RNAO, 2013).

The *cognitive–evaluative* component of pain consists of beliefs, attitudes, memories, and the meaning of the pain for the individual. The meaning of the pain stimulus can contribute to the pain experience. For example, a woman in labour may experience severe pain, but for her it is associated with a joyful event; moreover, she may feel control over her pain because of training she received in prenatal classes and the knowledge that the pain is self-limited. In contrast, a woman with persistent, nonspecific musculo-skeletal pain may be plagued by thoughts that the pain is "not real." Many people with persistent pain like this experience challenges from health care providers and others who question whether their pain is a legitimate experience (McGillion & Watt-Watson, 2015).

Such anxieties, fears, and stressors have been identified as potential intensifiers of perceived pain and related burden (O'Keefe-McCarthy, McGillion, Clarke, et al., 2015). The meaning of pain and related responses are critical aspects of nursing pain assessment. The *cognitive* dimension also includes pain-related beliefs and the cognitive coping strategies that people use. For example, some people cope with pain by distracting themselves, whereas others struggle with feelings that the pain is untreatable

TABLE 10-4   COMPARISON OF NOCICEPTIVE AND NEUROPATHIC PAIN

Nociceptive Pain	Neuropathic Pain
Definition	
Processing of noxious stimuli by an intact nervous system; usually responsive to analgesics (e.g., opioids, NSAIDs) or physical modalities	Abnormal processing of sensory input as a result of injury of the peripheral or central nervous system; treatment includes a variety of analgesics (e.g., antidepressants, opioids, antiseizure drugs)
Types	
Somatic Pain	**Centrally Generated Pain**
Arises from bone, joint, muscle, skin, or connective tissue; usually aching or throbbing in quality and well localized	• Deafferentation pain, caused by injury to either the peripheral or central nervous system (e.g., phantom pain may reflect injury to peripheral nerve)
	• Sympathetically maintained pain, associated with dysregulation of the autonomic nervous system (e.g., reflex sympathetic dystrophy)
Visceral Pain	**Peripherally Generated Pain**
Arises from organs, such as the gastro-intestinal tract and bladder. Can be further subdivided as follows:	• Painful polyneuropathies, in which pain is felt along the distribution of many peripheral nerves (e.g., diabetic neuropathy, alcohol-nutritional neuropathy, Guillain-Barré syndrome)
• Tumour involvement of the organ capsule that causes aching and fairly well-localized pain	• Painful mononeuropathies, usually associated with a known peripheral nerve injury and in which pain is felt at least partly along the distribution of the damaged nerve (e.g., nerve root compression, trigeminal neuralgia)
• Obstruction of hollow organ that causes intermittent cramping and poorly localized pain	

NSAIDs, nonsteroidal anti-inflammatory drugs.

TABLE 10-5   DIFFERENCES BETWEEN ACUTE AND PERSISTENT PAIN

Characteristic	Acute Pain	Persistent Pain
Onset	Sudden	Gradual or sudden
Duration	Usually within the normal time for healing	May start as acute injury but continues past the normal time for healing to occur
Severity	Mild to severe	Mild to severe
Cause of pain	In general, a precipitating illness or event (e.g., surgery) can be identified	May not be known; original cause of pain may differ from mechanisms that maintain the pain
Course of pain	↓ Over time and goes away as recovery occurs	Typically, pain persists and may be ongoing, episodic, or both
Typical physical and behavioural manifestations	Manifestations reflect sympathetic nervous system activation: • ↑ Heart rate • ↑ Respiratory rate • ↑ Blood pressure • Diaphoresis, pallor • Anxiety, agitation, confusion NOTE: Responses normalize quickly owing to adaptation	Predominantly behavioural manifestations: • Changes in affect • ↓ Physical movement and activity • Fatigue • Withdrawal from other people and social interaction
Usual goals of treatment	Pain control with eventual elimination	Minimizing pain to the extent possible; focusing on enhancing function and quality of life

and overwhelming. Cognitions about the pain contribute to patients' goals for and expectations of pain relief and treatment outcomes.

The *sociocultural* dimension of pain encompasses factors such as demographic features (e.g., age, sex, education, socioeconomic status), support systems, social roles, past pain experiences, and cultural aspects that contribute to the pain experience (Sturgeon & Zautra, 2013). Female sex, for example, has been found to influence nociceptive processes and the acceptability and usage of and response to analgesics such as NSAIDs and opioids (McGillion, Arthur, Cook, et al., 2012a; O'Keefe-McCarthy, McGillion, Clarke, et al., 2015).

CAUSES AND TYPES OF PAIN

Pain is generally classified as nociceptive, neuropathic, or both, according to the underlying pathological process. Nociceptive pain and neuropathic pain have different characteristics (Table

10-4). Because of its temporal nature, pain may be acute or persistent; some people may experience both, depending on the problem (Table 10-5).

Nociceptive Pain

Nociceptive pain is caused by damage to somatic or visceral tissue. *Somatic pain,* characterized as aching or throbbing that is well localized, arises from bone, joint, muscle, skin, or connective tissue. *Visceral pain,* which may result from stimuli such as tumour involvement or obstruction, arises from internal organs such as the intestines and the bladder. Examples of nociceptive pain include pain from a surgical incision or a broken bone, arthritis, or cardiac ischemia. Nociceptive pain is usually responsive to both nonopioid and opioid medications.

Neuropathic Pain

Neuropathic pain is caused by damage to nerve cells or changes in spinal cord processing. Typically described as burning, shooting, stabbing, or electrical in nature, neuropathic pain can be sudden, intense, short-lived, or lingering. Neuropathic pain is difficult to treat, and management includes opioids, antiseizure drugs, and antidepressants. Neuropathic pain can be either central or peripheral in origin.

Table 10-5 lists the classification of pain as acute or persistent. Acute pain and persistent pain have different causes, courses, manifestations, and treatment. Examples of acute pain include postoperative pain, labour pain, pain from trauma (e.g., lacerations, fractures, sprains) and infection (e.g., dysuria), and angina. For acute pain, treatment includes analgesics for symptom control treatment of the underlying cause (e.g., splinting for a fracture, antibiotic therapy for an infection). Normally, acute pain diminishes over time as healing occurs. Persistent pain continues beyond the normal time expected for healing. Persistent pain is often disabling and accompanied by anxiety and depression. Sometimes, persistent pain is further classified as cancer and noncancer pain. Persistent cancer-related pain arises from many causes, including disease progression, diagnostic procedures, anticancer therapies, and infection (von Gunten, 2011).

Cancer pain often is considered separately because its cause can be determined, its course differs from that of nonmalignant pain (cancer pain often worsens with documented disease progression), and the use of opioids in its treatment is more widely accepted than in the treatment of noncancer pain (von Gunten, 2011).

PAIN ASSESSMENT

The goals of a nursing pain assessment are (a) to describe the patient's sensory, affective, behavioural, and sociocultural pain experience for the purpose of implementing pain management techniques and (b) to identify the patient's goal for therapy and resources and strategies for effective self-management. The nurse is responsible for gathering and documenting assessment data and for making collaborative decisions with the patient and other health care providers about pain management. The following sections describe key components in pain assessment.

Sensory-Discriminative Component

Every pain assessment should include evaluation of the sensory-discriminative component: pattern, area, intensity, and nature (PAIN) of the pain. Information about these elements is essential to identifying appropriate therapy for the type and severity of the pain (RNAO, 2013).

Before beginning any assessment, the nurse must recognize that patients may use words other than *pain*. For example, older adults may deny that they have pain but respond positively when asked if they have discomfort, soreness, or aching (Tracy & Morrison, 2013). For these patients, repeatedly using open-ended questions including descriptors to understand pain may elicit more information than close-ended questions. The words that the patient uses in describing pain must be documented, and when the patient is asked about pain, the patient's words should be used consistently.

Pattern of Pain. Pain onset (when it starts) and duration (how long it lasts) are components of the pain pattern. Acute pain typically increases during wound care, ambulation, coughing, and deep breathing. Acute pain associated with surgery or injury tends to diminish over time, with recovery as tissues heal. In contrast, persistent pain may be ongoing, episodic, or both. For example, a person with persistent osteoarthritis pain may

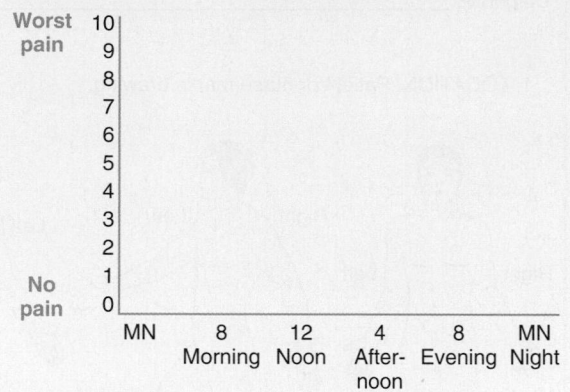

FIGURE 10-5 A method of tracking pain over time.

experience increased stiffness and pain on arising in the morning. As the joint is gently mobilized, the pain often decreases.

A patient may have constant, round-the-clock pain or discrete periods of intermittent pain. **Breakthrough pain** is moderate to severe pain that occurs despite treatment. Many patients with cancer experience breakthrough pain. It is usually rapid in onset and brief in duration, with highly variable intensity and frequency of occurrence. *Episodic, procedural,* or *incident pain* is a transient increase in pain that is caused by a specific activity or event that precipitates the pain (e.g., dressing changes, movement, eating, position changes, and certain procedures such as catheterization).

Figure 10-5 shows one method for the patient to document the pain pattern so as to report how the intensity of the pain changes with time. A similar method could be used to document the changes in the area or the nature of the pain.

Area of Pain. The area or location of pain assists in identifying possible causes of the pain and in determining treatment. Some patients may be able to specify one or more precise locations of their pain, whereas others may describe very general areas or comment that they "hurt all over." The location of the pain may also be *referred* from its origin to another site (see Figure 10-4), as described earlier in the chapter. Pain may also *radiate* from its origin to another site. For example, angina pectoris is known to radiate from the chest to the jaw, to the shoulders, or down the left arm. Sciatica is pain that originates from compression or damage to the sciatic nerve or its roots within the spinal cord. The pain is projected along the course of the peripheral nerve, causing painful shooting sensations down the back of the thigh and the inside of the leg.

Typically, information about the location of pain is elicited by asking the patient to (a) describe the site or sites of pain, (b) point to painful areas on the body, or (c) mark painful areas on a body diagram (Figure 10-6). Because many patients have more than one site of pain, it is important to make certain that the patient describes every location and identifies which one is most problematic.

Intensity of Pain. An assessment of the severity, or intensity, of pain provides a reliable measurement for determining the type of treatment as well as for evaluating the effectiveness of therapy. Pain scales are useful in helping the patient communicate the intensity of pain and in guiding treatment. Scales must be adjusted to age and level of cognitive development. Numerical

Initial Pain Assessment Tool

Date _____

Client's Name _____ Age_____ Room_____

Diagnosis_____ Physician _____

Nurse _____

1. LOCATION: Patient or nurse marks drawing.

Right   Left   Right   Left

Left   Right   Left

Right

R   L   L   R

LEFT   RIGHT

Right   Left

Left   Right

2. INTENSITY: Client rates the pain. Scale used: _____

    Present: _____

    Worst pain gets: _____

    Best pain gets: _____

    Acceptable level of pain: _____

3. QUALITY: (Use client's own words, e.g., prick, ache, burn, throb, pull, sharp) _____

_____

4. ONSET, DURATION, VARIATIONS, RHYTHMS: _____

_____

5. MANNER OF EXPRESSING PAIN: _____

_____

_____

6. WHAT RELIEVES THE PAIN? _____

_____

_____

7. WHAT CAUSES OR INCREASES THE PAIN? _____

_____

_____

8. EFFECTS OF PAIN: (Note decreased function, decreased quality of life)

    Accompanying symptoms (e.g., nausea)_____

    Sleep _____

    Appetite _____

    Physical activity _____

    Relationship with others (e.g., irritability) _____

    Emotions (e.g., anger, suicidal thoughts and behaviours, crying) _____

    Concentration _____

    Other _____

9. OTHER COMMENTS:_____

10. PLAN: _____

May be duplicated for use in clinical practice. From McCaffery M, Pasero C: Pain: Clinical manual, p. 60. Copyright © 1999, Mosby Inc.

FIGURE 10-6 Initial pain assessment tool. (May be duplicated for use in clinical practice.) Source: McCaffery, M., & Pasero, C. (1999). *Pain: Clinical manual for nursing practice* (2nd ed., p. 60). St. Louis: Mosby.

FIGURE 10-7 Simple descriptive word tool and visual analogue scale (VAS) used to assess a patient's pain. *If used as a graphic rating scale, a 10-cm baseline is recommended. †A 10-cm baseline is recommended for VAS scales. Source: McCormack, H. M., Horne, D. J., & Sheather, S. (1988). Clinical applications of visual analogue scales: A critical review. *Psychological Medicine, 18*(4), 1007–1019. Reproduced with permission.

scales (e.g., 0="no pain" and 10="the worst pain"), verbal descriptor scales (e.g., none, a little [1–3], moderate [4–6], and severe [7–10]), or visual analogue scales (a 10-cm line with one end labelled "no pain" and the other end labelled "worst possible pain") can be used by most adults to rate the intensity of their pain (Figure 10-7). For patients who are unable to respond to other pain intensity scales, a series of faces ranging from "smiling" to "crying" can be used. These scales have been investigated for use in a variety of patient populations, including young children and older adults. Results indicate that they provide valid and reliable assessment data (Craig, Prkachin, & Grunau, 2011).

Nature of Pain. The *nature* of pain refers to the quality or characteristics of the pain. Many commonly used words to describe the nature of pain are included in the McGill Pain Questionnaire (MPQ; see the Resources at the end of this chapter). The MPQ is a widely used measure of subjective pain experience with well-established reliability, validity, sensitivity, and discriminative capacity in divergent acute and chronic pain populations (Katz & Melzack, 2011). Two major strengths of the MPQ are that (a) it provides a comprehensive assessment of the nature of pain problems in a short time frame (5 to 10 minutes) and (b) it includes subsets of verbal pain descriptors associated with both nociceptive and neuropathic pain (Katz & Melzack, 2011).

For example, patients may describe neuropathic pain as burning, cold, shooting, stabbing, or itchy. Nociceptive pain may be described as sharp, aching, throbbing, or cramping.

Motivational–Affective, Behavioural, Cognitive–Evaluative, and Sociocultural Components

Comprehensive pain assessment includes evaluation of all pain dimensions and should be completed upon a patient's admission to a facility and repeated at regular intervals in order to evaluate response to treatment. In an acute care setting, time limitations may dictate an abbreviated assessment of the affective, behavioural, cognitive, and sociocultural dimensions of pain. At a bare minimum, patients' expression of pain and the effect of pain on sleep, daily activities, relationships, physical activity, and emotional

TABLE 10-6   NURSING ASSESSMENT
Pain Data

Subjective Data
Important Health Information
Past health history: Includes onset, location, intensity, quality, patterns, and expression of pain; coping strategies; past pain experiences (e.g., in childhood, in family members, other pain problems, pain relief measures used in the past and their effectiveness); pain triggers; effect of pain on emotions, relationships, sleep, work and school, family routines, leisure, and other activities; interviews with family members; meaning of pain to patient; records from any psychiatric treatment related to the pain; review of the use of health care services in relation to the pain problem (e.g., emergency department visits, treatment at pain clinics, visits to primary health care providers and specialists); influence of cultural, ethnic, or religious factors on pain intensity, interpretation of the pain, and pain management strategies
Medications: Use of any prescription, over-the-counter, or herbal products or other medications for pain relief; alcohol use

Symptoms
Fatigue; limitations in activities; pain related to muscle use; decreased libido; constipation related to opioid or tricyclic medication use (or both); depression; anxiety; mood or self-image problems

Objective Data
Complete physical examination, including evaluation of functional limitations
Psychosocial evaluation

well-being should be assessed. Strategies that the patient has used or tried to control the pain (effective or not) should also be documented.

When possible and relevant, assessment should also include examination of the psychological and social factors associated with patients' subjective experience of pain and, in particular, the meaning of the pain experience; *pain* meaning may often feature prominently in patients' treatment progress (O'Keefe-McCarthy, McGillion, Clarke, et al., 2015). Data related to meaning may be particularly useful in care planning for patients who exhibit high levels of pain-related behaviour, functional impairment, or pain-related distress. Such responses, for example, may be found in patients suffering moderate to severe persistent cardiac pain (McGillion, Arthur, Cook, et al., 2012a; O'Keefe-McCarthy, McGillion, Clarke, et al., 2015).

Measurement of beliefs related to the meaning of pain is complex. For clinical assessment purposes, key areas of inquiry with patients about the meaning of pain and related beliefs should include effective pain control in relation to current intervention strategies, pain-related disability, value placed on comfort and solace from other people, and the effect of emotions on the experience of pain.

Comprehensive assessment information is necessary to ensure effective treatment, as shown in Table 10-6.

Advances in Pain Assessment Research

Optimal ways to assess pain continue to be examined in several populations. The Postoperative Pain Assessment Skills Tool (PAST), for example, was developed by McGillion, Dubrowski, Stremler, and colleagues (2011) as a tool to develop health care providers' pain assessment skills. The PAST is divided into two components: a pain assessment checklist and a global rating scale. The assessment checklist examines pain sensory characteristics;

treatment history; impact of pain on functional status, perception of self, and relationships; and past pain experiences. The global rating scale uses a series of scales to evaluate the health care provider's interpersonal skills and empathy while conducting a pain assessment, degree of coherence during the pain assessment interview, and skillful use of verbal and nonverbal expression (McGillion, Dubrowski, Stremler, et al., 2011). The PAST has been found to be a reliable tool for providing real-time feedback to nurses and other health care providers while conducting comprehensive pain assessments under time-constrained conditions (in keeping with the realities of institutional clinical settings). Results also suggest that this tool can be used effectively by novice and experienced nurses who wish to advance their pain assessment skills (McGillion, Dubrowski, Stremler, et al., 2011).

PAIN TREATMENT

Basic Principles

All pain treatment is guided by the same underlying principles. Although treatment regimens range from short-term management to multimodal, long-term therapy for many persistent pain problems, all treatment should follow the same basic standards, as stated by the CPS (2010) and the RNAO 2013 Pain Assessment and Management Best Practice Guidelines:

- Routine assessment is essential for effective management. Pain is a subjective experience involving multiple characteristics including biological and psychosocial factors, all of which must be considered for comprehensive assessment and management.
- Unrelieved acute pain complicates recovery. Unrelieved pain after surgery or injury results in more complications, longer hospital stays, greater disability, and potentially long-term pain.
- Patients' self-report of pain should be used whenever possible. For patients unable to report pain, a nonverbal assessment method must be used.
- Health care providers have a responsibility to assess pain routinely, to accept patients' pain reports and document them, and to intervene in order to manage pain.
- The best approach to pain management involves patients, families, and health care providers. Patients and families must be informed of their right to the best pain care possible and encouraged to communicate the severity of their pain.
- Many patients—in particular, vulnerable populations; ethnic minorities including infants, children, and adolescents; older adults, adults, and children with limited ability to communicate; and patients with past or current substance use problems—are at high risk for suboptimal or inappropriate pain management. Health care providers must understand that adequate pain relief is a basic human right, must be aware of their own biases and misinformation, and must ensure that all patients are treated respectfully. Patients with a history of opioid tolerance or addiction may have higher opioid requirements following a new episode of acute pain. Care should be taken that these patients do not experience withdrawal due to undermedication.
- Treatment must be based on the patient's and family's goals for pain treatment, which should be discussed upon initial pain assessment. Sometimes these goals can be described in terms of pain intensity (e.g., the desire for pain intensity to decrease from an "8 out of 10" to a "3 out of 10"). Other patients may express a functional goal (e.g., a person may want the pain to be relieved to an extent that allows him or her to perform daily activities). Over the course of prolonged

therapy, these goals should be reassessed, and progress should be documented. If the patient has unrealistic goals for therapy, such as wanting to be completely rid of all persistent arthritis pain, the nurse should work with the patient to establish a more realistic goal.

- Treatment plans should involve a combination of pharmacological and nonpharmacological therapies. Although medications are often considered the mainstay of therapy, particularly for moderate to severe pain, nonpharmacological strategies should be incorporated to increase the overall effectiveness of the treatment plan and to allow for the reduction of medication dosages to minimize adverse effects. Examples of therapies are discussed later in the chapter.
- A multidimensional and interdisciplinary approach is necessary for optimal pain management; multiple perspectives, from all members of the interprofessional team, should be incorporated.
- All therapies must be evaluated to ensure that they are meeting the patient's goals. Therapy must be individualized for each patient, and, often, achieving an effective treatment plan requires trial and error. Medications, dosages, and routes are commonly adjusted to achieve maximal benefit while minimizing adverse effects. This trial-and-error process can become frustrating for the patient and family. They need to be reassured that pain relief is possible and that the health care team will continue to work with them to achieve adequate pain relief.
- Adverse effects of medications must be prevented or managed. Adverse effects are a major reason for treatment failure and nonadherence despite the fact that most patients' pain can be effectively managed (RNAO, 2013). Adverse effects are managed in one of several ways, described in Table 10-7. The nurse plays a key role in monitoring for and treating adverse effects, as well as in teaching the patient and family how to minimize adverse effects.
- Patient and caregiver teaching should be a cornerstone of the treatment plan. Content should include information about the cause or causes of the pain, pain assessment methods, treatment goals and options, expectations for pain management, instruction regarding the proper use of drugs, management of adverse effects, and nonpharmacological and self-help measures for pain relief (RNAO, 2013). Teaching should be documented, and the patient's and caregiver's comprehension of this teaching should be evaluated.

Drug Therapy for Pain

Although a physician or nurse practitioner prescribes the medications, it is the nurse's responsibility to evaluate the effectiveness and adverse effects of what is prescribed. It is also a nursing

---

TABLE 10-7   DRUG THERAPY

Examples of Ways to Manage Adverse Effects of Opioids

- Ensuring a schedule for the dosing regimen to maintain blood levels
- Using stool softeners and stimulant laxatives to prevent constipation
- Using an antiemetic to prevent nausea
- Changing to a different medication in the same class
- Using an administration route that minimizes drug concentrations at the site of the adverse effect (e.g., intraspinal administration of opioids is sometimes used to minimize high drug levels that produce sedation, nausea, and vomiting)

TABLE 10-8 EXAMPLES OF COMMON EQUIANALGESIC DOSES

Drug	Approximate Equianalgesic Parenteral Dosage	Approximate Equianalgesic Oral Dosage	Alert/Special Considerations
Morphine	10 mg	30 mg	
Hydromorphone (Dilaudid)	1–1.5 mg	4–7.5 mg	
Oxycodone	Not available	20 mg	
Codeine	120 mg	200 mg	
Methadone and tramadol	—	—	Methadone and tramadol conversion morphine dose equivalents have not been reliably established. Methadone conversion requires a licensed expert's assessment based on the patient's history of opioid consumption.
Meperidine (Demerol)	75 mg	300 mg	Prolonged use may increase risk of toxicity (e.g. seizures) from accumulation of the meperidine metabolite, normeperidine.

Sources: Adapted from National Opioid Use Guideline Group. (2010). Oral opioid analgesic conversion table. In *Canadian guideline for safe and effective use of opioids for chronic non-cancer pain* (p. 75). Retrieved from *http://nationalpaincentre.mcmaster.ca/documents/opioid_guideline_part_b_v5_6.pdf.*

responsibility to document and communicate the outcomes of analgesic therapy and to suggest changes when appropriate, using knowledge and skills related to several pharmacological and pain management concepts. These include calculating equianalgesic doses, scheduling analgesic doses, titrating opioids, and selecting from the prescribed analgesic drugs.

Equianalgesic Dose. The term equianalgesic dose refers to a dose of one analgesic that produces pain-relieving effects equivalent to those of another analgesic. The concept of equivalence is important when substituting one analgesic for another in the event that a particular medication is ineffective or causes intolerable adverse effects and when the administration route of opioids is changed (e.g., from parenteral to oral). In general, opioids are administered in equianalgesic doses—important to know because no upper dosage limit has been established for many of these drugs. Equianalgesic charts and conversion programs are widely available in textbooks, in clinical guidelines, in health care facility pain protocols, and on the Internet. Table 10-8 provides an example of common equianalgesic dosages compared with 10 mg of parenteral morphine, which is the standard basis for comparison. Although equianalgesic charts are useful tools, health care providers must understand their limitations: Equianalgesic dosages are approximate, and individual patient response must be routinely assessed. In addition, discrepancies exist among different published equianalgesic charts. All changes in opioid therapy must be carefully monitored and adjusted for the individual patient. When possible, health care providers should use equianalgesic conversions that have been approved for their facility or clinic and should consult a pharmacist before making changes.

Scheduling Analgesics. Appropriate analgesic scheduling should focus on prevention or ongoing control of pain rather than on providing analgesics only after the patient's pain has become moderate to severe. A patient should receive medication before procedures and activities that are expected to produce pain. Similarly, a patient with constant pain should receive analgesics around the clock rather than on an as-needed basis. These strategies control pain before it starts and usually result in lower analgesic requirements. Fast-acting drugs should be used for incident or breakthrough pain, whereas long-acting analgesics are more effective for constant pain. Examples of fast-acting and sustained-release analgesics are described later in this section.

Titration. Analgesic titration is dosage adjustment that is based on assessment of the adequacy of analgesic effect versus

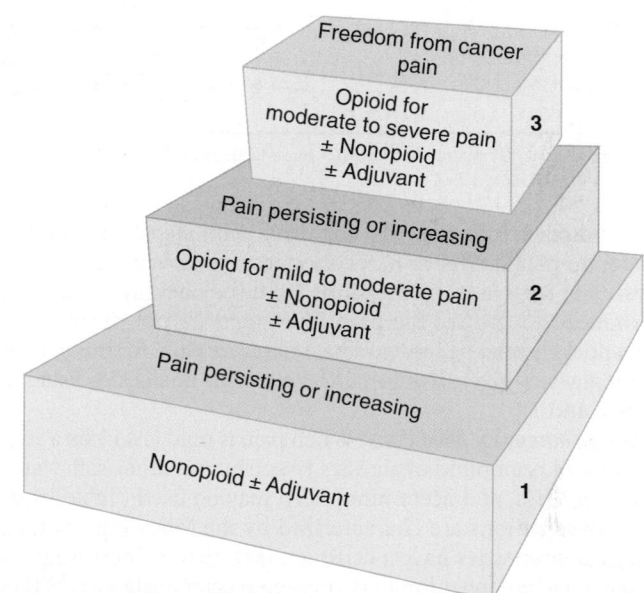

FIGURE 10-8 The analgesic ladder proposed by the World Health Organization. Source: Reprinted from *Cancer,* WHO, WHO analgesic ladder, WHO, Copyright 2018.

the adverse effects produced. The amount of analgesic needed to manage pain varies widely, and titration is an important strategy in addressing this variability. An analgesic dosage can be titrated upward or downward, depending on the situation. For example, in a postoperative patient, the dosage of analgesic generally decreases over time as the acute pain resolves. On the other hand, opioids for persistent, severe chronic noncancer pain may be titrated upward over the course of therapy to maintain adequate pain control; this titration requires expert specialty care according to Canadian guidelines for chronic opioid therapy (National Opioid Use Guideline Group [NOUGG], 2010). The goal of titration is to use the lowest dosage of opioid that provides effective pain control with the fewest adverse effects.

Analgesic Ladder. Several national and international groups have published practice guidelines recommending a systematic plan for using analgesic drugs. One widely used system is the analgesic ladder proposed by the World Health Organization (WHO) (Figure 10-8). The WHO treatment plan emphasizes that different medications are administered, depending on the severity of pain, by means of a three-step ladder approach.

TABLE 10-9 DRUG THERAPY

Comparison of Select Nonopioid Analgesics

Drug	Analgesic Efficacy in Comparison to Standards	Nursing Considerations
Acetaminophen (Tylenol)	Comparable to Aspirin	Rectal suppository available; sustained-release preparations available; maximum daily dosage of 4 g
Salicylates		
Acetylsalicylic acid (Aspirin)	Standard for comparison	Rectal suppository available; sustained-release preparations available Possibility of upper GI bleeding
Nonsteroidal Anti-Inflammatory Drugs (NSAIDs)		
Ibuprofen (Motrin, Advil)	Superior at 200–650 mg of aspirin	Usually well tolerated despite the potential for upper GI bleeding
Indomethacin	25 mg comparable with 650 mg of Aspirin	Not routinely used because of high incidence of adverse effects; rectal, intravenous, and sustained-release oral forms available
Ketorolac (Toradol)	30–60 mg equivalent to 6–12 mg of morphine	Treatment should be limited to maximum of 7 days; may precipitate renal failure in dehydrated patients
Diclofenac (Voltaren)	25–50 mg BID to TID; has a longer duration than 650 mg of aspirin	Available in oral, ophthalmic, and topical preparations
Cyclo-oxygenase-2 (COX-2) inhibitors (Celecoxib)	Similar to NSAIDs	Fewer GI complaints, including bleeding; more costly than other NSAIDs
Meloxicam (Mobicox)	Similar to other NSAIDs	May cause fewer GI adverse effects, including bleeding, than do other NSAIDs, but risk is still present; is more costly than other NSAIDs

BID, twice per day; *GI*, gastro-intestinal; *TID*, three times per day.

Step 1 medications are used for mild pain; step 2, for mild to moderate pain; and step 3, for moderate to severe pain. If pain persists or increases, medications from the next higher step are introduced to control the pain. The steps are not meant to be sequential if someone has moderate to severe pain: for this person, the analgesics given would be the stronger analgesics listed in steps 2 and 3.

Drug Therapy for Mild Pain. When pain is mild (1 to 3 on a scale of 0 to 10), nonopioid analgesics (Aspirin and other salicylates, other NSAIDs, and acetaminophen) may be used (Table 10-9). These medications are characterized by the following: (a) their analgesic properties have a **ceiling effect**: that is, increasing the dose beyond an upper limit provides no greater analgesia; (b) they do not produce tolerance or physical dependence; and (c) many are available without a prescription. It is important to monitor over-the-counter analgesic use to avoid serious problems related to medication interactions, adverse effects, and overdosage.

DRUG ALERT: NSAIDs
- NSAIDs (except Aspirin) have been linked to a higher risk for cardio-vascular events such as myocardial infarction, stroke, and heart failure.
- Patients who have just had heart surgery should not take NSAIDs.

A number of nonopioid analgesics such as acetylsalicylic acid (ASA, Aspirin) and NSAIDs inhibit the chemicals that activate the PAN (Figure 10-9). Thus when these medications are used, the PAN is transduced less often, or a larger stimulus is needed to produce transduction.

Aspirin is effective for mild pain, but its use is limited by its common adverse effects, including gastric upset and bleeding. Other salicylates such as choline magnesium trisalicylate cause fewer GI disturbances and bleeding abnormalities. Similarly to Aspirin, acetaminophen (Tylenol) has analgesic and antipyretic effects, but it has no antiplatelet or anti-inflammatory effects. Acetaminophen is well tolerated; however, dosages higher than 4 000 mg per day, acute overdosage, or use by patients with alcoholism or liver disease can result in severe hepatotoxicity.

The NSAIDs represent a broad class of medications with varying efficacy and adverse effects. Some NSAIDs possess

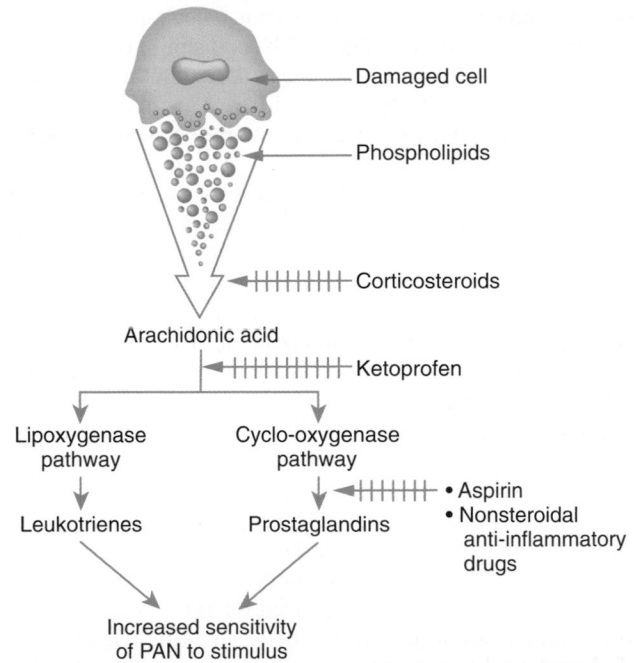

FIGURE 10-9 Schematic representation of two pathways that lead to the production of chemicals that cause the primary afferent nociceptor (PAN) to be more easily excited. Medications that block the synthesis of these chemicals are also shown.

analgesic efficacy equal to that of Aspirin, whereas others have somewhat higher efficacy. Patients vary greatly in their responses to a specific NSAID, so when one NSAID does not provide relief, another should be tried. NSAIDs inhibit the cyclo-oxygenase-1 (COX-1) and -2 (COX-2) enzymes, which produce prostaglandins involved in inflammation. Because prostaglandins also play a key role in protecting the lining of the stomach from acids, adverse

TABLE 10-10 DRUG THERAPY

Opioid Analgesics Commonly Used for Mild to Moderate Pain

Drug	Comments	Nursing Considerations
Morphine-Like Agonists		
Codeine	Weak opioid: Many preparations are combinations with nonopioid analgesics; codeine is a prodrug and metabolized to morphine; 1–30% of people metabolize too efficiently and 10–20% are unable to metabolize it	For mild to moderate pain, preparations of codeine and other opioids are limited by the dosage of nonopioid analgesic (e.g., the maximum dosage of acetaminophen is 44 g in 24 hours)
Tramadol (Ultram)	Maximum dosage: 400 mg in 24 hours	May cause seizures, although rarely
Mixed Agonist–Antagonists		
Pentazocine (Talwin)	*Not recommended*	Can precipitate withdrawal in people taking opioids on a regular basis; frequently causes psychotomimetic effects
Butorphanol	Not available orally; not scheduled under *Controlled Drugs and Substances Act*; butorphanol nasal spray is used to treat migraine headaches	May precipitate withdrawal in people taking opioids on a regular basis; may cause psychotomimetic effects; reacts with many other medications; not widely prescribed

Source: Adapted from Inturrisi, C., & Lipman, A. (2010). Opioid analgesics. In S. M. Fishman, J. C. Ballantyne, & J. P. Rathmell (Eds.), *Bonica's management of pain* (4th ed., pp. 1174–1175). London, UK: Wolters-Kluwer/Lippincott Williams & Wilkins.

TABLE 10-11 DRUG THERAPY

Opioids Commonly Used for Severe Pain

Drug	Comments	Nursing Considerations
Morphine	Standard comparison for opioid analgesics; sustained-release preparation (MS Contin) available	For all opioids: use with caution in people with impaired ventilation, bronchial asthma, increased intracranial pressure, liver failure; in some people, the metabolite M6G may cause excessive vomiting and hallucinations, necessitating a change of opioid
Morphine-Like Agonists		
Hydromorphone (Dilaudid)	—	Well tolerated; also available in elixir form for patients unable to swallow tablets
Oxycodone (slow-release formulation is OxyNeo)	May be given alone or combined with acetaminophen; immediate- and slow-release preparations are available; formulated to deter potential misuse	For moderate to severe pain; usually well tolerated
Methadone	Good oral potency; 24- to 36-hour half-life, which necessitates careful monitoring	Licence required to prescribe; accumulates with repeated doses; on days 2–5, dosage size and frequency must be reduced
Fentanyl	Available as sublingual tablet, as injection, or, for persistent pain, as transdermal preparation (Duragesic)	Immediate onset after administration by intravenous route; within 7–8 min. after intramuscular route; onset after transdermal route may take several hours; not recommended for acute pain management
Meperidine (Demerol)	Not recommended as first-line treatment for acute pain and should not be used for persistent pain management	Not well absorbed through oral route and should not be used; normeperidine (toxic metabolite with half-life of 14–21 hours) accumulates with repetitive dosing, causing CNS excitation and seizures; naloxone potentiates excitation and must not be used; avoid in patients taking monoamine oxidase inhibitors (e.g., selegiline)
Mixed Agonist–Antagonists		
Butorphanol	Not available orally; not scheduled under *Controlled Drugs and Substances Act*	May precipitate withdrawal in opioid-dependent patients

Source: Adapted from Inturrisi, C., & Lipman, A. (2010). Opioid analgesics. In S. M. Fishman, J. C. Ballantyne, & J. P. Rathmell (Eds.), *Bonica's management of pain* (4th ed., pp. 1174–1175). London, UK: Wolters-Kluwer/Lippincott Williams & Wilkins.
CNS, central nervous system.

effects of NSAIDs can be serious and include bleeding tendencies secondary to decreased platelet aggregation, GI problems ranging from dyspepsia to ulceration and hemorrhage, renal insufficiency, and, on occasion, CNS dysfunction. For certain chronic conditions, such as rheumatoid arthritis and osteoarthritis, NSAIDs that more selectively inhibit cyclo-oxygenase-2 (COX-2) only are used. The COX-2 enzyme does not play a role in protecting the stomach or intestinal tract, and therefore its selective inhibition is not associated with the same risk for injury to these organs as is the inhibition of COX-1. A common example of a COX-2 inhibitor is meloxicam (Mobicox). Cautious use of anti-inflammatory medications, long-term, has been recommended due to increased risk for cardiovascular accidents (Sanchez, Tenias, Arias, et al., 2015).

Drug Therapy for Mild to Moderate Pain. When pain is moderate in intensity (4 to 6 on a scale of 0 to 10) or mild but persistent despite nonopioid therapy, step 2 medications are indicated. Medications commonly used for mild to moderate pain are listed in Table 10-10.

One class of step 2 medications is opioids. Opioids include many drugs (Table 10-11; also see Table 10-10) that produce their effects by binding to receptors. Opioid receptors are found

FIGURE 10-10 Opioid receptor subtypes. **A,** Agonist action. **B,** Antagonist action. **C,** Agonist–antagonist action. **D,** Partial antagonist action. *M,* mu receptor; *K,* kappa receptor; *D,* delta receptor.

in the CNS, on the terminals of sensory nerves, and on the surface of immune cells. There are three major opioid receptors, traditionally referred to as *mu, kappa,* and *delta.* The receptors have been reclassified as OP1 (delta), OP2 (kappa), and OP3 (mu). Most clinically useful opioids bind to the mu receptors. Mu agonists include morphine, oxycodone, hydromorphone (Dilaudid), and methadone. Opioid *agonists* (e.g., morphine) bind to the receptors and cause analgesia. *Antagonists* (e.g., naloxone) bind to the receptors but do not produce analgesia; they also block other effects of opioid receptor activation, such as sedation and respiratory depression. Mixed *agonists naloxone,* such as pentazocine (Talwin) and butorphanol, should not be used because they bind as agonists on the kappa receptor and, as weak antagonists or partial agonists, on the mu receptor (Figure 10-10). When a mixed agonist–antagonist is given to someone taking an agonist (e.g., morphine), it will act like an agonist–antagonist, such as naloxone, and reverse any analgesic effect. These opioid agonist–antagonists also cause more dysphoria and agitation. In addition, they have an analgesic ceiling (a dosage at which no additional analgesia is produced regardless of further dosage increases) and can precipitate withdrawal in a patient who is physically dependent on agonist drugs.

At step 2, prescriptions for commonly used opioids are often for products combining an opioid with a nonopioid analgesic (e.g., oxycodone [Oxycontin] or codeine plus acetaminophen [Tylenol No. 3]), which may limit the opioid dose that can be given. Oxycodone is now administered for severe pain as well. Although propoxyphene (Darvon) is classified as a step 2 drug, it is not recommended in analgesia guidelines because its effectiveness is limited and its toxic metabolite can cause seizures. Propoxyphene is not approved for use in Canada. A third type of medication available for mild to moderate pain is tramadol (Ultram). Tramadol is a weak mu-receptor agonist and is thought to inhibit the reuptake of norepinephrine and serotonin. It has approximately the same efficacy as acetaminophen plus codeine. The most common adverse effects, which are similar to those of other opioids, include nausea, constipation, dizziness, and sedation.

Drug Therapy for Moderate to Severe Pain. Step 3 drugs are recommended for moderate to severe pain (4 to 10 on a scale of 0 to 10) or when step 2 drugs do not produce effective pain relief. Most commonly used step 3 analgesics are mu-receptor agonists, although these medications also bind with the other receptors. These medications are effective for moderate to severe pain because they are potent, have no analgesic ceiling, and can be delivered via many routes of administration. Step 3 drugs are listed in Table 10-11.

Morphine is one of the opioids most commonly prescribed for moderate to severe pain, although fentanyl (Duragesic), hydromorphone (Dilaudid), methadone (Metadol), and oxycodone also are used extensively. A long-acting morphine formulation (MS Contin) is available to treat moderate to severe persistent pain in patients who require continuous, round-the-clock therapy for an extended period. Meperidine (Demerol), a mu-receptor agonist, is no longer recommended for acute or persistent pain because of the high incidence of neurotoxicity (e.g., seizures) associated with the accumulation of its neurotoxic metabolite, normeperidine. Moreover, any adverse effect cannot be reversed by naloxone, which potentiates the effect of normeperidine. In addition, a hyperpyrexic syndrome with delirium, which can cause death, can occur if meperidine is given to patients taking monoamine oxidase inhibitors. Although step 3 opioids have no analgesic ceiling, people can experience dose-limiting adverse effects. In opioid-naive patients, adverse effects include constipation, nausea and vomiting, sedation, respiratory depression, and pruritus. With continued use, most adverse effects diminish; the exception is constipation. Less common adverse effects include urinary retention, myoclonus, dizziness, confusion, and hallucinations.

DRUG ALERT: Opioids
- Opioids may cause respiratory depression.
- If respirations are 12 or fewer breaths per minute, withhold medication and contact the health care provider.
- Methadone may cause respiratory depression.
- In increased doses, methadone can cause cardiac toxicity, specifically QT prolongation.
- Transdermal fentanyl should not be used for management of acute pain.

Constipation is the most common opioid adverse effect. Because tolerance to opioid-induced constipation does not occur, a bowel regimen should be instituted at the beginning of opioid therapy and should continue for as long as the person takes opioids. Although dietary roughage, fluids, and exercise should be encouraged to the extent possible, these measures rarely are sufficient by themselves. Thus most affected patients should immediately begin taking a gentle stimulant laxative (e.g., senna [Senokot]) plus a stool softener (e.g., docusate sodium [Colace]). Other agents (e.g., milk of magnesia, bisacodyl [Dulcolax], lactulose) can be added if necessary. Left untreated, constipation can lead to fecal impaction and paralytic ileus that can be difficult to differentiate from obstruction.

Nausea often is a problem in opioid-naive patients. The use of antiemetics such as ondansetron (Zofran), metoclopramide, hydroxyzine (Atarax), or a prochlorperazine can prevent or minimize opioid-related nausea and vomiting until tolerance develops, which usually occurs within 1 week. Metoclopramide is particularly effective when a patient complains of gastric fullness. Opioids delay gastric emptying, and this effect can be reversed by metoclopramide. If nausea and vomiting are severe and persistent, as with morphine because of the metabolite M6G, changing to a different opioid such as oxycodone or hydromorphone may be necessary.

Two of the most common concerns associated with opioids are sedation and respiratory depression. Sedation may occur initially in opioid-naive patients, although patients handling pain without relief may be sleep deprived. Respiratory depression is rare in opioid-tolerant patients when opioids are titrated to analgesic effect. Individuals at risk for respiratory depression include opioid-naive patients, older-adult patients, and patients with underlying lung disease. If respiratory depression occurs and stimulating the patient (e.g., calling and shaking patient) does not reverse the somnolence or increase the respiratory rate and depth, naloxone (0.4 mg in 10 mL saline), an opioid antagonist, can be administered intravenously or subcutaneously in 0.5 mL increments every 2 minutes. However, if the patient has been taking opioids regularly for more than a few days, naloxone should be used judiciously and titrated carefully because its use can precipitate severe, agonizing pain, profound withdrawal symptoms, and seizures. Because the half-life (60 to 90 minutes) of naloxone is shorter than that of most opioids, nurses should monitor the patient's respiratory rate because it can drop again 1 to 2 hours after naloxone administration.

Itching may occur with opioids, most frequently when they are administered via intraspinal routes. An antihistamine such as diphenhydramine (Benadryl) often is effective. If measures are ineffective, a low-dose opioid antagonist (e.g., naloxone) or a mixed agonist–antagonist can be used, but the patient must be carefully assessed for reversal of analgesia and withdrawal.

SAFETY ALERT
- The most appropriate opioid depends on the patient's clinical profile and the nature of the pain problem (e.g., mild to moderate, severe).
- Patients should be advised that opioids can cause cognitive effects, impairing their ability to drive.
- It is important to recognize that some women rapidly metabolize codeine to morphine. In the case of postoperative patients who are breastfeeding, the infant may be at risk for fatal opioid toxicity. If codeine is prescribed to breastfeeding mothers, consultation with the physician and other health care team members is crucial to ensure careful monitoring (NOUGG, 2010). The patient should be advised to monitor the infant for signs of CNS depression, including poor feeding and limpness, and to contact the health care provider immediately if any such signs are noted.

Adjuvant Analgesic Therapy. Adjuvant analgesic therapies are medications used in conjunction with opioid and nonopioid analgesics. Adjuvants are sometimes referred to as *coanalgesics.* They include medications that enhance pain therapy through one of three mechanisms: (a) enhancing the effects of opioids and nonopioids, (b) possessing analgesic properties of their own, or (c) counteracting the adverse effects of other analgesics. Commonly used analgesic adjuvants are listed in Table 10-12. Figure 10-11 shows the sites of actions of pharmacological and nonpharmacological therapies for pain. Adjuvant drugs are used at every step in the WHO ladder.

Antidepressants. Tricyclic antidepressants have analgesic properties at dosages lower than those effective for depression. They enhance the descending inhibitory system by preventing synaptic reuptake of serotonin and norepinephrine. Higher levels of serotonin and norepinephrine in the synaptic cleft inhibit the transmission of nociceptive signals in the CNS. Tricyclic antidepressants have been shown to be effective for a variety of pain syndromes, especially those involving neuropathic pain. Anticholinergic effects such as dry mouth, urinary retention, sedation, and orthostatic hypotension may lessen patients' acceptance of using the drug and adherence to the regimen.

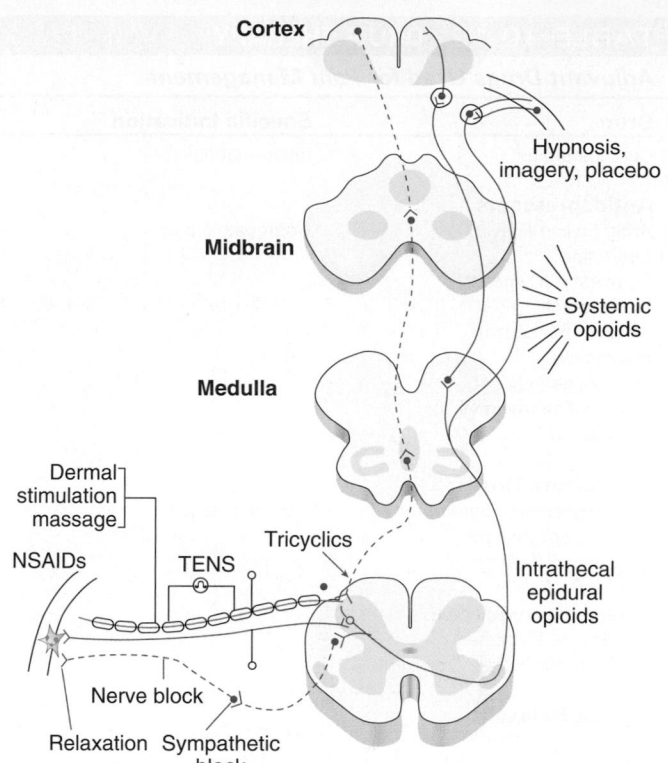

FIGURE 10-11 The sites of commonly used pharmacological and nonpharmacological analgesic therapies. *NSAIDs,* nonsteroidal anti-inflammatory drugs; *TENS,* transcutaneous electrical nerve stimulation.

DRUG ALERT: Tricyclic Antidepressants
- Tricyclic antidepressants have been implicated in prolonged QT intervals.

Antiseizure Drugs. Antiseizure drugs such as gabapentin (Neurontin), carbamazepine (Tegretol), and clonazepam (Rivotril) stabilize the membrane of the neuron and prevent transmission. These medications are effective for some neuropathic pain and for prophylactic treatment of headaches.

Corticosteroids. Corticosteroid medications, which include dexamethasone and methylprednisolone (Medrol), are used to treat several types of pain, including acute and persistent cancer pain, pain secondary to spinal cord or brain compression, and some neuropathic pain syndromes. Mechanisms of action are unknown but may involve the ability of corticosteroids to decrease edema and inflammation and, in some cases, to shrink tumours. Corticosteroids have many adverse effects, especially when used chronically in high dosages. Adverse effects include hyperglycemia, fluid retention, dyspepsia and GI bleeding, impairment in healing, muscle wasting, osteoporosis, and susceptibility to infection.

Local Anaesthetics. Oral, parenteral, and topical applications of local anaesthetics are used to interrupt transmission of pain signals to the brain. Local anaesthetics are given for acute pain resulting from surgery or trauma. Persistent neuropathic pain also may be controlled with local anaesthetics. Adverse effects can include dizziness, paresthesias, and seizures (at high dosages). Incidence and severity of adverse effects depend on dosage and route of administration. These medications also affect cardiac conductivity and may cause dysrhythmias and myocardial depression.

Administration Routes. Opioids and other analgesic medications can be delivered via many routes. This flexibility allows the health

TABLE 10-12 DRUG THERAPY

Adjuvant Drugs Used for Pain Management

Drug	Specific Indication	Nursing Considerations
Corticosteroids	Inflammation	Avoid high dosage for long-term use
Antidepressants Amitriptyline (Elavil) Bupropion Duloxetine (Cymbalta) Desipramine Doxepin (Sinequan) Imipramine Maprotiline Nortriptyline (Aventyl) Venlafaxine	Neuropathic pain	Monitor for anticholinergic adverse effects
Antiseizure Drugs Carbamazepine (Tegretol) Clonazepam (Rivotril) Gabapentin (Neurontin) Pregabalin (Lyrica) Oxcarbazepine (Trileptal) Topiramate (Topamax) Valproic acid (Epival, Depakene)	Neuropathic pain	Start with low dosages, increase slowly to appropriate level for effect Clonazepam and carbamazepine: Check liver function, renal function, electrolytes, and blood cell counts at baseline, at 2 wks. and at 6 wks. Gabapentin: Monitor for idiosyncratic adverse effects (e.g., ankle swelling, ataxia, sedation)
Muscle Relaxant Baclofen (Lioresal)	Neuropathic pain (e.g., trigeminal neuralgia, muscle spasms)	Monitor for weakness, urinary dysfunction; avoid abrupt discontinuation because of CNS irritability
Anaesthetics: Systemic or Oral Mexiletine	Diabetic neuropathy; neuropathic pain	Monitor for adverse effects, including dizziness, perioral numbness, paresthesias, tremor; can cause seizures, dysrhythmias, and myocardial depression at high dosages; avoid in patients with pre-existing cardiac disease
Anaesthetics: Local Topical EMLA: lidocaine 2.5% + prilocaine 2.5%	Local skin analgesic before venipuncture, incision; possibly effective for postherpetic neuralgia	Must be applied under an occlusive dressing (e.g., Tegaderm, DuoDerm) or on an anaesthetic disc; absorption from the genital mucosa is more rapid and onset time is shorter (5–10 min.) than after application to intact skin; common adverse effects include mild erythema, edema, skin blanching
Capsaicin	Pain associated with arthritis, postherpetic neuralgia, diabetic neuropathy	Apply sparingly, rub well into affected area; wash hands with soap and water after application; adverse effects include skin irritation (burning, stinging) at the application site and cough
Psychostimulants Dextroamphetamine (Dexedrine) Methylphenidate (Ritalin)	Managing opioid-induced sedation	Adverse effect is insomnia; avoid administering late in the day; usually well tolerated at low dosages
Cannabinoids Nabilone	Neuropathic pain	Recommended as an adjuvant for neuropathic pain in cases where therapeutic effect is not achieved via gabapentin

EMLA, eutectic mixture of local anaesthetics.

care provider to (a) target a particular anatomical source of the pain, (b) achieve therapeutic blood levels rapidly when necessary, (c) avoid certain adverse effects through localized administration, and (d) provide analgesia when patients are unable to swallow. The following discussion highlights the uses and nursing considerations for analgesics delivered through a variety of routes.

Oral. In general, oral administration is the route of choice for the patient with a functioning GI system. Oral medications are usually less expensive than those delivered by other routes. Many opioids are available in oral preparations, such as liquid and tablet formulations. To obtain analgesia equivalent to that provided by doses administered intramuscularly or intravenously,

oral doses must be higher. For example, 10 mg of parenteral morphine is equivalent to approximately 30 mg of orally administered morphine. Generally, oral administration is the route required for opioid-naive patients because of the first-pass effect of hepatic metabolism. This means that oral opioids initially are absorbed from the GI tract into the portal circulation and shunted to the liver. Partial metabolism in the liver occurs before the medication enters systemic circulation and becomes available to peripheral receptors or before it can cross the blood–brain barrier and access CNS opioid receptors, a process necessary to produce analgesia. Many opioids are available in oral preparations, such as liquid and tablet form. Oral opioids are as effective as parenteral opioids if the dose administered is large enough to compensate for the first-pass metabolism.

Oral preparations also are available in immediate-release and sustained-release preparations. For example, morphine is available in immediate-release solutions or tablets. These products are effective in providing rapid, short-term pain relief; concentration in the blood typically peaks within 30 to 60 minutes. Sustained-release oral morphine tablets are administered every 8 to 12 hours; the most common preparation is morphine ER (MS Contin). As with other sustained-release preparations, this product should not be crushed, broken, or chewed. Oxycodone also comes in a sustained-release capsule (OxyNeo). Other opioids with sustained-release formulations include hydromorphone and tramadol. The time to maximum blood plasma dose concentration typically ranges from 30 to 60 minutes and from 2 to 4 hours for immediate-release and sustained-release formulations, respectively.

Sublingual and Buccal. Opioids administered under the tongue or held in the mouth and absorbed into systemic circulation are exempt from the first-pass effect.

Intranasal. Intranasal administration allows delivery of medication to highly vascular mucosa and avoids the first-pass effect. Butorphanol is one of the few intranasal analgesics available. This medication is most commonly indicated for migraine headaches. Several intranasal opioids such as fentanyl drugs are being investigated (Dale, 2010).

Rectal. The rectal route is often overlooked but is particularly useful when the patient cannot take an analgesic by mouth. Rectal suppositories that are effective for pain relief include hydromorphone (Dilaudid) and morphine.

Transdermal. Fentanyl (Duragesic) is available as a transdermal patch system for application to nonhairy skin. This delivery system is useful for the patient who cannot tolerate oral analgesic drugs. Absorption from the patch is slow. Therefore, transdermal fentanyl is not suitable for rapid dosage titration but can be effective if the patient's pain is stable and the dosage required to control it is known. Patches may have to be changed every 48 hours rather than the recommended 72 hours, depending on individual patient responses.

Currently, creams and lotions containing 10% trolamine salicylate (e.g., Aspercreme, Myoflex) are available. These medications have been recommended by the manufacturers for joint and muscle pain. This Aspirin-like substance is absorbed locally. The topical route of administration precludes gastric irritation, but the other adverse effects of high-dosage salicylate are not necessarily prevented.

Ointments, lotions, gels, liniments, and balms (most of which are over-the-counter products) are sometimes applied topically to achieve pain relief. Common ingredients include methyl salicylate combined with camphor, menthol, or both. On application, these medications usually produce a strong hot or cold sensation and should not be used after massage or a heat treatment, when blood vessels are already dilated. Skin testing is advisable when the patient has not used the particular medication before because the strengths of the medications vary and different intensities of sensation are produced. These products are indicated for arthralgia, bursitis, myalgia, and tendinitis.

Other topical analgesic medications, such as capsaicin (e.g., Flex-ol) and prilocaine plus lidocaine (eutectic mixture of local anaesthetics [EMLA]), and anti-inflammatory medications such as Voltaren (1% diclofenac) also provide analgesia. Derived from red chili pepper, capsaicin depletes and prevents reaccumulation of substance P in the peripheral sensory neurons. It can control pain associated with postherpetic neuralgia, diabetic neuropathy, and arthritis. EMLA is useful for control of pain associated with venipunctures, ulcer debridement, and possibly postherpetic neuralgia. The area to which EMLA is applied should be covered with a plastic wrap for 30 to 60 minutes before a painful procedure begins.

Parenteral Routes. The parenteral route includes subcutaneous and intravenous administration. The only opioid that must be injected intramuscularly is meperidine, and this drug is not recommended because its toxic metabolite, normeperidine, can accumulate with repeated administration, causing CNS excitation. Single-dose administration (subcutaneous or intravenous) is possible via parenteral routes. The intramuscular route, although frequently used, is not recommended because these injections cause significant pain, result in unreliable absorption, and, with chronic use, can result in abscesses and fibrosis. Onset of analgesia after subcutaneous administration is slow, and thus the subcutaneous route is rarely used for acute pain management. However, continuous subcutaneous infusions are effective for persistent cancer pain. This route is especially helpful for people with abnormal GI function and limited venous access. Intravenous administration is the best option when immediate analgesia and rapid titration are necessary. Continuous intravenous infusions provide excellent steady-state analgesia through stable blood levels.

Intraspinal Delivery. Intraspinal (epidural or intrathecal) opioid therapy involves inserting a catheter into the subarachnoid space (for intrathecal delivery) or the epidural space (for epidural delivery) and injecting an analgesic, by either intermittent bolus doses or continuous infusion. Percutaneously placed temporary catheters are used for short-term therapy (2 to 4 days), and surgically implanted catheters are used for long-term therapy. Although the lumbar region is the most common site of placement, epidural catheters may be placed at any point along the neuroaxis (cervical, thoracic, lumbar, or caudal). Intraspinally administered analgesics are highly potent because they are delivered close to the receptors in the dorsal horn of the spinal cord. Thus much lower doses of analgesics are needed for intraspinal delivery in comparison with other routes, including intravenous. Drugs that are delivered intraspinally include morphine, fentanyl, and hydromorphone. Nausea, itching, and urinary retention are common adverse effects of intraspinal opioids.

Complications of intraspinal analgesia include catheter displacement and migration, neurotoxicity (especially of certain medications when infused intraspinally), and infection. Clinical manifestations of catheter displacement or migration depend on catheter location. Movement of a catheter out of the intrathecal or epidural space causes a decrease in pain relief with no improvement even when additional analgesic is administered. Correct placement of an intrathecal catheter can be checked by aspirating cerebrospinal fluid. Migration of a catheter into a blood vessel causes an increase in adverse effects because of systemic medication distribution. A number of medications and chemicals are highly neurotoxic when administered intraspinally. These include many substances, such as preservatives (e.g., alcohol and phenol), antibiotics, potassium, and total parenteral nutrition supplements. To avoid inadvertent injection of intravenous medications into an intraspinal catheter, the catheter should be clearly marked as an intraspinal access device, and only preservative-free medications should be injected.

Infection rarely occurs with intraspinal analgesia. However, it is a serious complication that can be difficult to detect. The skin around the exit site should be carefully assessed for inflammation, drainage, or pain. Signs and symptoms of an intraspinal infection include diffuse back pain, pain or paresthesias during bolus injection, and unexplained sensory or motor deficits. Fever may or may not be present. Acute bacterial infection (meningitis) is manifested by fever, headache, and altered mental status. Infection is avoided with regular, meticulous wound care and with the use of sterile technique in caring for the catheter and injecting drugs.

Patient-Controlled Analgesia. A specific type of subcutaneous, intravenous, or intraspinal delivery system is patient-controlled analgesia (PCA), or *demand analgesia*. PCA is an infusion system that allows the patient to self-administer a dose of opioid through a pump when needed: The patient pushes a button to receive a bolus infusion of an analgesic within preprogrammed intervals. PCA is used widely for the management of acute pain, including postoperative pain and cancer pain. Often, the patient also receives an additional continuous basal infusion (known as *PCA plus basal*) at a preset dose and rate. The addition of a continuous basal infusion to a PCA regimen improves nighttime pain relief and promotes better sleep postoperatively. Common opioids used in the PCA administration method include morphine, fentanyl, and hydromorphone (Dilaudid).

Use of PCA begins with patient teaching. The patient needs to understand the benefits and principles of PCA therapy, the mechanics of obtaining a medication dose (i.e., the operation of the pump and button), and how to titrate the medication to achieve good pain relief. The patient should be encouraged to use the PCA pump prophylactically by self-administering the analgesic before ambulation, physiotherapy, and dressing changes. The patient also needs to be reminded that apart from the involved health care providers, he or she is the only person who should press the button. The patient should also be assured—for safety reasons and to avoid excessive sedation or respiratory depression—that the pump is programmed to deliver a maximum number of doses per hour; pressing the button after the maximum dose is administered will not result in additional analgesic. If the maximum doses are inadequate to relieve pain, by order of a physician or nurse practitioner, the pump can be reprogrammed to increase the amount or frequency of administration. In addition, bolus doses can be given by the nurse if they are included in the physician's orders. The patient should also be encouraged to report adverse effects such as nausea and vomiting or pruritus so that they can be managed effectively. To make a smooth transition from infusion PCA to oral therapy, the dosage of oral medication should be increased (as ordered) as the PCA analgesic is tapered.

Surgical Therapy for Pain

Nerve Blocks. Nerve blocks are used to reduce pain by temporarily or permanently interrupting transmission of nociceptive input. This is achieved with local anaesthetics or neurolytic drugs (e.g., alcohol, phenol). Neural blockade with local anaesthetics is sometimes used for perioperative pain. For intractable persistent pain, nerve blocks are used when more conservative therapies fail. Nerve blocks have been a successful pain management technique for more localized persistent pain states, such as peripheral vascular disease, trigeminal neuralgia, causalgia, and some cancer pain. A nerve block may be considered advantageous for managing localized pain caused by malignancy and in debilitated patients who could not otherwise withstand a surgical procedure for pain relief.

Interventional Therapy

Therapeutic Nerve Blocks. Nerve blocks generally involve one-time or continuous infusion of local anaesthetics into a particular area to produce pain relief. Such relief is also referred to as *regional anaesthesia*. Nerve blocks interrupt all afferent and efferent transmission to the area and thus are not specific to nociceptive pathways. They include local infiltration of anaesthetics into a surgical area (e.g., for excision of a breast lump, inguinal hernia surgery, intra-articular infiltration after joint surgery, amputation, subcostal incisions) and injection of anaesthetics into a specific nerve (e.g., occipital or pudendal nerve) or nerve plexus (e.g., brachial or celiac plexus). Nerve blocks often are used during and after surgery to manage pain. For longer-term relief of chronic pain problems, local anaesthetics can be administered via a continuous infusion.

For intractable persistent pain, neuroablative nerve blocks (see next section) with phenol or alcohol may be used. For example, a neurolytic celiac plexus block may be induced for pain caused by pancreatic cancer, or an intercostal neurolytic block may be induced for post-thoracotomy pain. Heat and microwaves, used in many neurolytic procedures, produce nerve tissue destruction.

Neuroablative Techniques. *Neuroablative interventions* are performed for severe pain that is unresponsive to all other therapies. Neuroablative techniques destroy nerves, thereby interrupting pain transmission. Destruction is accomplished by surgical resection or thermocoagulation, including radiofrequency coagulation. Neuroablative interventions that destroy the sensory division of a peripheral or spinal nerve are classified as neurectomies, rhizotomies, and sympathectomies. Neurosurgical procedures that ablate the lateral spinothalamic tract are classified as cordotomies if the tract is interrupted in the spinal cord or as tractotomies if the interruption is in the medulla or the midbrain of the brain stem. Figure 10-12 depicts the sites of neurosurgical procedures for pain relief. Both cordotomy and tractotomy can be performed with the aid of local anaesthesia by a percutaneous technique.

Neuroaugmentation. Neuroaugmentation involves electrical stimulation of the brain and the spinal cord. Spinal cord stimulation is performed much more often than deep brain stimulation. Technological advances have enabled the use of multiple leads and multiple electrode terminals so as to stimulate large areas. In Canada and the United States, common uses of spinal cord stimulation are for chronic back pain secondary to nerve damage that is unresponsive to other therapies (van Tulder & Koes, 2013) and chronic refractory angina (McGillion, Arthur, Cook, et al., 2012b).

Potential complications include those related to the surgery (bleeding and infection), migration of the pulse generator (which usually is implanted in the subcutaneous tissues of the upper gluteal or pectoralis area), and nerve damage.

Nonpharmacological Therapy for Pain

Nonpharmacological pain management strategies can reduce the dose of an analgesic required to control pain and thereby minimize adverse effects of drug therapy. Some strategies are believed to alter ascending nociceptive input or stimulate descending pain modulation mechanisms. Nonpharmacological pain relief methods can be categorized as physical or cognitive strategies (Table 10-13).

Physical Pain Relief Strategies

Massage. Massage is a common therapy for pain, and many massage techniques exist. Examples include moving the hands or fingers over the skin slowly or briskly with long strokes or in

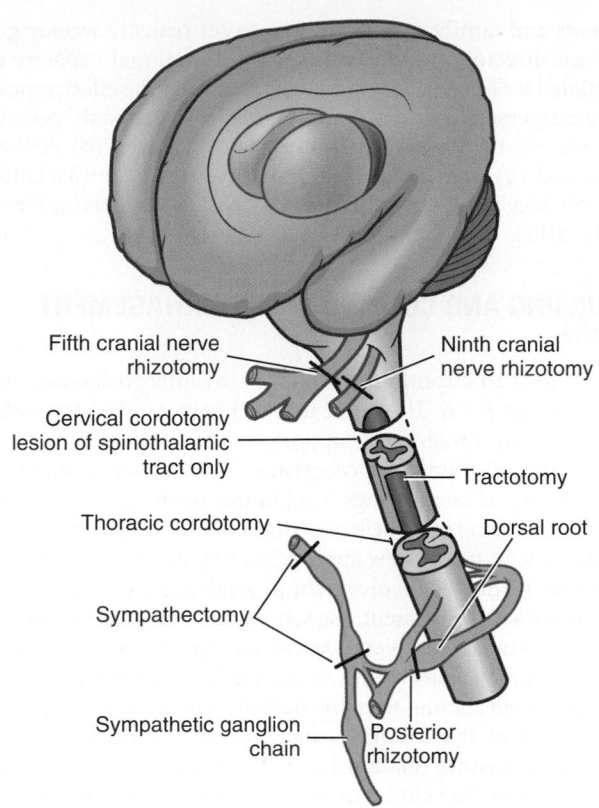

FIGURE 10-12 Sites of neurosurgical procedures for pain relief.

FIGURE 10-13 Transcutaneous electrical nerve stimulation (TENS). Source: Praisaeng/Shutterstock.com.

TABLE 10-13	NONPHARMACOLOGICAL THERAPIES FOR PAIN
Physical Therapies	**Cognitive Therapies**
• Acupuncture	• Distraction
• Application of heat and cold	• Hypnosis
• Exercise	• Imagery
• Massage	• Relaxation strategies
• Percutaneous electrical nerve stimulation (PENS)	• Self-management
• Transcutaneous electrical nerve stimulation (TENS)	

circles (superficial massage) or applying firm pressure to the skin to maintain contact while massaging the underlying tissues (deep massage). Specific massage techniques include acupressure and trigger-point massage. A **trigger point** is a circumscribed hypersensitive area within a tight band of muscle that is the result of acute or persistent muscle strain. Several common trigger points have been identified on the neck, back, and arms. Trigger-point massage is performed by either application of strong, sustained digital pressure, deep massage, or gentler massage with ice followed by muscle heating. (Massage is discussed further in Chapter 12).

Exercise. Exercise is a critical part of the treatment plan for patients with persistent pain, particularly those with musculo-skeletal pain. Many patients become physically deconditioned as a result of their pain, which in turn can exacerbate pain. Exercise acts through many mechanisms to relieve pain: it enhances circulation and cardiovascular fitness, reduces edema, increases muscle strength and flexibility, and enhances physical

and psychosocial functioning. A safe exercise program should be tailored to the physical needs and lifestyle of the patient and should include mild to moderate aerobic exercise, stretching, and strengthening exercises. The program also should be supervised by trained personnel (e.g., physiologist, physiatrist, registered nurse with specialty training, exercise physiologist, physiotherapist).

Transcutaneous Electrical Nerve Stimulation. *Transcutaneous electrical nerve stimulation* (TENS) delivers an electric current through electrodes applied to the skin surface over the painful region, at trigger points, or over a peripheral nerve. A TENS system consists of two or more electrodes connected by lead wires to a small, battery-operated stimulator (Figure 10-13). Usually, a physiotherapist is responsible for administering TENS therapy, although nurses also can be trained in the technique.

TENS may be used for acute pain, including postoperative pain, visceral pain, and pain associated with physical trauma. Although the effect of TENS on persistent pain is less clear, it may be effective in such cases (Song, Popescu, & Bell, 2014).

Application of Heat. Application of heat for pain management has been used for centuries. The premise is that applying heat to skin will increase blood flow and reduce pain-related neurotransmitter activity (RNAO, 2013). Heat therapy includes application of either moist or dry heat to the skin and can be superficial or deep. Superficial heat can be applied through an electric heating pad (dry or moist), a hot pack, hot moist compresses, or a hot water bottle. For exposure to large areas of the body, patients can immerse themselves in a hot bath, shower, or whirlpool. Physical therapy departments provide deep-heat therapy through such techniques as shortwave diathermy, microwave diathermy, and ultrasound therapy. Patient teaching regarding heat therapy is described in Table 10-14.

Application of Cold. Like heat therapy, application of cold therapy has long been used for pain relief. Cold therapy competes for nerve transmission and reduces sensation, effects that can be especially helpful for pain that resembles a burning sensation (RNAO, 2013). Cold therapy involves the application of either moist or dry cold to the skin. Dry cold can be applied by means of an ice bag, and moist cold by means of towels soaked in ice water, cold hydrocollator packs, or immersion in a cold bath or under running cold water. Icing with ice cubes or blocks of ice made to resemble popsicles is another technique used for pain relief. Cold therapy is believed to be more effective than heat

TABLE 10-14	PATIENT & CAREGIVER TEACHING GUIDE

Application of Heat and Cold

When patients use superficial heating techniques, they should be taught the following:
- Do not use heat on an area that is being treated with radiation therapy, is bleeding, has decreased sensation, or has been injured in the past 24 hours.
- Do not use any menthol-containing products (e.g., Vicks VapoRub) with heat applications because this combination may cause burns.
- Cover the heat source with a towel or cloth to prevent burns.
- Do not apply heat directly to transdermal analgesic preparations, such as fentanyl, as heat application may alter drug bioavailability.

When patients use superficial cold techniques, they should be taught the following:
- Cover the cold source with a cloth or towel.
- Do not apply cold to areas that are being treated with radiation therapy, have open wounds, or have poor circulation.
- If it is not possible to apply the cold directly to the painful site, try applying it directly above or below the painful site or on the opposite side of the body on the corresponding site (e.g., left elbow if the right elbow hurts).

for a variety of painful conditions, including acute pain from trauma or surgery, acute flares of arthritis, muscle spasms, and headache. Patient teaching regarding cold therapy is described in Table 10-14.

Cognitive Techniques. A variety of cognitive strategies and behavioural approaches can alter the affective, cognitive, and behavioural components of pain. Some of these techniques require little training and often are adopted independently by the patient. For others, a trained therapist must administer therapy.

Distraction. The redirection of attention on something other than the pain is a simple but powerful strategy to relieve pain. Distraction-induced analgesia involves introducing competition for attention between a highly salient sensation (pain) and some other information-processing activity. Distraction can be achieved by engaging the patient in any activity that can hold his or her attention (e.g., watching TV, conversing, listening to music, playing a game). Recent evidence suggests that distraction may be most effective in those who exhibit persistent pain–related catastrophizing behaviours due to great attention to pain overall (Schreiber, Campbell, Martel, et al., 2014).

Relaxation Strategies. Relaxation strategies reduce stress, decrease acute anxiety, distract from pain, alleviate muscle tension, combat fatigue, facilitate sleep, and enhance the effectiveness of other pain relief measures (Shengelia, Parker, Ballin, et al., 2013). Elicitation of the relaxation response requires a quiet environment, a comfortable position, and a mental device as a focus of concentration (e.g., a word, a sound, or the breath). Relaxation strategies include relaxation breathing, music, imagery, meditation, and progressive muscle relaxation (Crawford, Lee, & Bingham, 2014). (See Chapters 8 and 12 for additional information.)

Self-Management. Self-management training is now in widespread use in Canada as an effective, adjunctive strategy for managing the effect of chronic pain on day-to-day functioning and quality of life (McGillion, O'Keefe-McCarthy, Carroll, et al., 2014; McGillion, LeFort, Webber, et al., 2011). By structured rehearsal of various cognitive and behavioural self-management techniques (e.g., energy conservation, pacing, sleep promotion, relaxation, communication skills, safe exercise),

patients and family members learn to set realistic weekly goals that are directed at increasing overall functional capacity and emotional well-being. Strong evidence supports the effectiveness of self-management training for (a) improving participants' perceived self-efficacy or ability to achieve selected goals, (b) reducing pain, and (c) improving perceived quality of life (McGillion, O'Keefe-McCarthy, Carroll, et al., 2014; McGillion, LeFort, Webber, et al., 2011).

NURSING AND COLLABORATIVE MANAGEMENT
PAIN

The nurse is an important member of the interprofessional pain management team. The nurse acts as planner, educator, patient advocate, interpreter, and supporter of the patient in pain and of the patient's family or caregivers. Because any patient in a wide variety of care settings (e.g., home, hospital, clinic) can be in pain, the nurse must be knowledgeable about current therapies and flexible in trying new approaches to pain management. The extent of the nurse's involvement depends on the unique factors associated with the patient, the setting, and the cause of the pain. Many nursing roles were described earlier in this chapter: conducting pain assessments, administering therapies, monitoring for adverse effects, and teaching patients and caregivers. However, the success of these actions depends on the nurse's ability to establish a trusting relationship with the patient and caregivers and to address the concerns that they have regarding pain and its treatment.

EFFECTIVE COMMUNICATION

Patients need to feel confident that their reporting of pain will be believed and will not be perceived as "complaining." The patient and family also need to know that the nurse considers the pain significant and is committed to helping the patient obtain pain relief and cope with any unrelieved pain. Pharmacological and nonpharmacological interventions should be incorporated into the treatment plan, and the patient should be supported through the period of trial and error that may be necessary to implement an effective therapeutic plan. It also is important to clarify responsibilities of pain relief. The nurse should help the patient understand the roles of the interprofessional health care team members, as well as the roles and expectations of the patient.

In addition to addressing specific aspects of pain assessment and treatment, the nurse evaluates the total effect that the pain may have on the lives of the patient and family. Thus, other possible nursing diagnoses must also be considered. Table 10-15 lists possible nursing diagnoses that may be appropriate for assessing and managing pain. Table 10-16 addresses teaching needs of patients and caregivers in relation to pain management.

BARRIERS TO EFFECTIVE PAIN MANAGEMENT

Pain is a complex, multidimensional, and subjective experience, and its management is influenced greatly by psychosocial, sociocultural, and legal and ethical factors. These factors include emotions, behaviours, misconceptions, and attitudes of patients and family members about pain and the use of pain therapies. Achieving effective pain management requires careful consideration of these factors.

Concerns regarding tolerance, dependence, and addiction are common barriers to effective pain management, inasmuch as these phenomena are often misunderstood. Patients, family members, and health care providers often share these concerns.

TABLE 10-15 NURSING ASSESSMENT

Pain-Related Nursing Diagnoses

- Activity intolerance
- Acute pain
- Anxiety
- Chronic pain
- Constipation
- Disturbed sleep pattern
- Fatigue
- Fear
- Hopelessness
- Ineffective coping
- Ineffective role performance
- Interrupted family processes
- Powerlessness
- Risk for self-mutilation
- Social isolation
- Acute confusion

TABLE 10-16 PATIENT & CAREGIVER TEACHING GUIDE

Pain Management: Teaching Needs

The goals of teaching related to pain management include the expectation that the patient and the caregivers understand the following:

- The need to maintain a record of pain intensity and effectiveness of treatment
- No need to wait until pain becomes severe to take medications or use nonpharmacological therapies for pain relief
- The possibility that the dosage of medication will have to be adjusted over time to maximize long-term effectiveness
- The potential adverse effects (e.g., nausea and vomiting, constipation, sedation and drowsiness, itching, urinary retention, sweating) and complications associated with opioid therapy or other pain relief therapies
- The need to report when pain is not relieved to tolerable levels

It is important for the nurse to understand and be able to explain the differences among these various concepts (RNAO, 2013).

TOLERANCE. *Tolerance* is "a state of adaptation in which exposure to a drug induces changes that result in diminution of one or more of the drug's effects over time" (NOUGG, 2010, p. 126). In the case of opioids, steady-state dosing can lead to tolerance of unwanted opioid adverse effects (Ballantyne, 2014). However, development of tolerance to an opioid itself is characterized by the need for increasing or more frequent doses of the opioid to maintain the same degree of analgesic effect. Although tolerance is not as common as once thought, it is essential to assess for increased analgesic needs in patients receiving persistent opioid therapy (Ballantyne, 2014). The first sign of tolerance may be that the patient begins to experience regular end-of-dose failure. If manifestations of possible tolerance appear, appropriate evaluations should be made to rule out other causes of increased analgesic needs, such as disease progression or infection. Approaches to managing tolerance are (a) to increase the dosage of the analgesic, (b) to substitute another medication in the same class (e.g., changing from morphine to oxycodone), or (c) to add a medication from a different drug class that will augment pain relief without increasing adverse effects. It is important to note that there is no ceiling effect for opioid-agonist drugs and to recognize that drug tolerance is not synonymous with addiction.

PHYSICAL DEPENDENCE. Like tolerance, physical dependence is an expected physiological response to ongoing exposure to pharmacological agents. "Physical dependence is a state of adaptation manifested by a drug class–specific withdrawal syndrome that can be produced by abrupt cessation, rapid dose reduction, decreasing blood level of the drug, and/or administration of

TABLE 10-17 MANIFESTATIONS OF WITHDRAWAL FROM OPIOIDS

Type	Response
• Mood • Physical and behavioural	• Anxiety, agitation • Restlessness • Diaphoresis • Fever • Flulike symptoms (e.g., nausea, muscle aches) • Tremor • Tachycardia

an antagonist" (NOUGG, 2010, p. 124). Symptoms of opioid withdrawal are listed in Table 10-17.

When opioids are no longer needed to provide pain relief, a tapering schedule should be used in conjunction with careful monitoring. A typical tapering schedule begins with calculating the 24-hour dose used by the patient and dividing by 2. Of this decreased amount, 25% is given every 6 hours. After 2 days, the daily dose is reduced by an additional 25% every 2 days until the 24-hour oral dose is 30 mg (morphine equivalent) per day. After 2 days on this minimum dosage, the opioid is then discontinued. Despite this slow weaning schedule, the nurse should assess carefully for signs of opioid withdrawal. In addition to assessing and preventing opioid withdrawal, it is also important to recognize that other commonly prescribed medications for pain also can induce physical dependence and therefore must be slowly tapered. These include benzodiazepines and muscle relaxants.

ADDICTION. *Addiction* is defined as

a primary, chronic, neurobiological disease with genetic, psychosocial, and environmental factors influencing its development and manifestations. It is characterized by behaviours that include one or more of the following: impaired control over drug use, compulsive use, continued use despite harm, and craving. (NOUGG, 2010, p. 124)

Tolerance and physical dependence are not indicators of addiction. Rather, they are normal physiological responses to chronic exposure to certain drugs, including opioids.

Substance use disorders, including illicit drug use and misuse of prescription opioids, affect about 10% of the general population (Jovey, 2010). The available data are of limited quality and suggest that in patients being treated for persistent pain, the risk of concurrent substance use or addiction is generally the same or higher than that in patients without a substance use disorder (Jovey, 2010). For patients without a history of substance use disorder, the risk is thought to be significantly lower. For example, a 2010 Cochrane Review revealed that signs of addiction were present in 0.3% of patients without a documented history of substance use disorder who were being treated with opioids for persistent noncancer pain (Noble, Treadwell, Tregear, et al., 2010). People with a history of addiction can be managed successfully on opioids for their pain with careful monitoring; however, in this population, the risk for addiction may be higher. Expectations of the health care team and the patient must be discussed openly and documented. Signs and symptoms of possible addiction must be monitored, and interventions promptly initiated.

In addition to fears about addiction, physical dependence, and tolerance, other barriers hinder effective pain management.

TABLE 10-18   PATIENT & CAREGIVER TEACHING GUIDE

Reducing Patient-Related Barriers to Pain Management

Barrier	Nursing Considerations
Fear of addiction	• Provide accurate definition of *addiction*. • Explain that addiction is uncommon in patients taking opioids for pain relief.
Fear of tolerance	• Provide accurate definition of *tolerance*. • Teach that tolerance is a normal physiological response to long-term opioid therapy. If tolerance does develop, the medication may have to be changed (e.g., morphine in place of oxycodone). • Teach that there is no upper limit to pure opioid agonists (e.g., morphine). Dosages can be increased indefinitely, and the patient should not save medication for when the pain is worse. • Teach that tolerance to analgesic effects of opioids develops more slowly than do many adverse effects (e.g., sedation, respiratory depression). Tolerance does not ameliorate constipation; thus a regular bowel program should be started early.
Concern about adverse effects	• Teach methods to prevent and to treat common adverse effects. • Emphasize that adverse effects such as sedation and nausea decrease with time. • Explain that different medications have unique adverse effects and that other pain medications can be tried to reduce the specific adverse effect. • Teach nonpharmacological therapies to minimize the dosage of medication needed to control pain.
Fear of injections	• Explain that oral medicines are preferred. • Emphasize that even if the oral route becomes unusable, transdermal or in-dwelling parenteral routes can be used rather than injections.
Desire to be a good patient	• Explain that patients are partners in their care and that the partnership requires open communication on the parts of both patient and nurse. • Emphasize to patients that they have a responsibility to keep the nurse informed about their pain.
Desire to be stoic	• Explain that although stoicism is a valued behaviour in many cultures, failure to report pain can result in undertreatment and severe, unrelieved pain.
Forgetting to take analgesic	• Provide and teach use of pill containers. • Provide methods of record keeping for drug use. • Recruit family members as appropriate to assist with the analgesic regimen.
Fear of distracting the health care provider from treating the disease	• Explain that reporting pain is important for treating both the disease and its symptoms.
Concern that pain signifies disease progression	• Explain that increased pain or analgesic needs may reflect tolerance. • Emphasize that new pain may come from a non–life-threatening source (e.g., muscle spasm, urinary tract infection). • Institute pharmacological and nonpharmacological strategies to reduce anxiety. • Ensure that the patient and family members have current, accurate, comprehensive information about the disease and the prognosis. • Provide psychological support.
Sense of fatalism	• Explain that research has shown that pain can be managed in most patients. • Explain that with most therapies, a period of trial and error is necessary. • Emphasize that adverse effects can be managed.
Ineffectiveness of medication	• Teach that there are multiple options within each category of medication (e.g., opioids, NSAIDs) and that another medication from the same category may provide better relief. • Emphasize that finding the best treatment regimen often requires trial and error. • Incorporate nonpharmacological approaches in treatment plan.

Source: Adapted from Ersek, M. (1999). Enhancing effective pain management by addressing patient barriers to analgesic use. *Journal of Hospice & Palliative Nursing, 1,* 87–96.
NSAIDs, nonsteroidal anti-inflammatory drugs.

These include concern about adverse effects, difficulties with remembering to take medications, desire to handle pain stoically, and not wanting to distract the health care provider from treating the disease. Table 10-18 lists examples of patient-related barriers to effective pain management and includes strategies to address the barriers.

INSTITUTIONALIZING PAIN EDUCATION AND MANAGEMENT

Besides patient and family barriers, other major barriers to effective pain management arise in connection with the health care provider: inadequate education, misconceptions about pain, and lack of organizational support (McGillion & Watt-Watson, 2015). Traditionally, medical and nursing school curricula have spent little time teaching future physicians and nurses about pain and effective pain management, although this is changing.

This lack of emphasis was partially responsible for the insufficiency of health care providers' knowledge of and skills for treating pain adequately. Moreover, pain assessment and treatment were not priorities in clinical practice. Health care providers have misbeliefs about pain. Similar to patients, many clinicians confuse physical dependence, tolerance, and addiction and are more likely to assess pain by observing behaviours than by believing or eliciting a patient report (McGillion & Watt-Watson, 2015). Over the past few decades, some improvements have been made in overcoming these barriers. Some prelicensure, undergraduate health care programs are now devoting more time to addressing pain (Hunter, Watt-Watson, McGillion, et al., 2008; Watt-Watson & Murinson, 2013), and there is growing interest in interprofessional educational intervention trials for health care providers that target common pain-related misbeliefs.

The International Association for the Study of Pain has published a core curriculum on pain that was developed for the learning needs of a range of health care provider groups. Provincial organizations such as the RNAO (2013) have also developed evidence-informed practice guidelines on pain that are readily accessible (see the "Resources" section at the end of this chapter for the weblinks).

Health care institutions are also directing more, much-needed attention to their support of pain management. Researchers and health care providers have documented the central role of institutional commitment and practices in changing clinical practice; without institutional support, pain outcomes are unlikely to change. The pain management standards from the Canadian Pain Society's (2010) *Position Statement on Pain Relief* (see the "Resources" section at the end of this chapter) emphasize that patients have a right to the best pain relief possible and that measures to prevent or reduce acute pain are a priority. Many large tertiary and quaternary university-affiliated care settings now have specialized teams to manage pain. One such example is the establishment of dedicated acute pain services (APS) that include advanced-practice nurses. These services provide expert management of postsurgical pain and complex pain conditions. Advanced-practice nurses, often nurse practitioners, work collaboratively with anaesthesiologists and allied health care providers to assess and manage pain and also to serve in leadership roles to promote best practice guidelines (Ladak, McPhee, Muscat, et al., 2013).

ETHICAL ISSUES IN PAIN MANAGEMENT

Fear of Hastening Death by Administering Analgesics

It is common for the health care provider, patient, and family members to be concerned that providing sufficient medication to relieve pain will precipitate the death of a terminally ill person (Voshall, Dunn, & Shelestak, 2013). The ethical justification for administering analgesics despite the possibility of hastening death follows the bioethical principle of the *rule of double effect*: that if an unwanted consequence (e.g., hastened death) occurs as a result of an action taken to achieve a moral good (e.g., pain relief), the action is justified according to ethical theory (Voshall, Dunn, & Shelestak, 2013). Unrelieved pain has negative psychological effects, such as feelings of hopelessness and depression, with high rates of suicide (Lynch, 2011).

Use of Placebos in Pain Assessment and Treatment

Placebos have been used inappropriately in the past to determine whether patients' pain was "real." Using medication placebos for pain, such as a saline injection instead of an opioid or an oral dosage of an inappropriate medication, is unethical.

AGE-RELATED CONSIDERATIONS

PAIN

Persistent pain is a common problem in older adults and is often associated with significant physical disability and psychosocial problems. The most common sources of pain among older adults are musculo-skeletal conditions, such as osteoarthritis and low back pain, and previous fracture sites. Persistent pain often results in depression, sleep disturbance, decreased mobility, increased use of health care services, and physical and social role dysfunction. Despite its high prevalence, pain in older adults often is inadequately assessed and treated. However, there are several barriers to pain assessment in the older patient. In general, the barriers discussed earlier in the chapter are more prevalent among this population. For example, many older-adult patients believe that pain is a normal, inevitable part of aging. They may also believe that nothing can be done to relieve the pain. Older adults may not report pain for fear of being a "burden" or a "bad patient." They may have greater fears of taking opioids than patients in other age groups. Nurses must be vigilant in asking older people about their pain and its effects.

Another barrier to pain assessment in older adults is the relatively high prevalence of cognitive, sensory-perceptual, and motor problems that interfere with a person's ability to process information and to communicate (Gagliese & Melzack, 2003). Also, hearing and vision deficits may complicate assessment. Therefore, pain assessment tools may have to be adapted for older adults. For example, it may be necessary to use a large-print pain intensity scale. Although there is some concern that older adults have difficulty using pain scales, it has been documented that many older adults, even those with mild to moderate cognitive impairment, can use quantitative scales accurately and reliably (see Figure 10-7).

As for other patients with persistent pain, a thorough physical examination should be performed and the history thoroughly documented to identify causes of pain, possible therapies, and potential problems. Because depression and functional impairments are common among older adults with pain, the possibility of these also must be assessed.

Treatment of pain in older adults also is complicated by several factors. First, older adults metabolize drugs more slowly than do younger patients and thus are at greater risk for higher blood levels and adverse effects. For this reason, the adage "start low and go slow" is applied to analgesic therapy in this age group. Second, the use of NSAIDs in older adults is associated with a high frequency of serious GI bleeding. For this reason, acetaminophen should be used whenever possible. Third, many older people take multiple medications for one or more chronic conditions. The addition of analgesics can result in dangerous drug interactions and more adverse effects. Fourth, cognitive impairment and ataxia can be exacerbated when analgesics such as opioids, antidepressants, and anticonvulsant drugs are used, a possibility that again necessitates health care providers to titrate medications slowly and monitor carefully for adverse effects.

Treatment regimens for older adults must incorporate nonpharmacological modalities. Exercise and patient teaching are particularly important nonpharmacological interventions for older adults with persistent pain. The roles of family and paid caregivers also should be included in the treatment plan.

SPECIAL POPULATIONS

Cognitively Impaired Individuals

Although patient self-report is a gold standard of pain assessment in most circumstances, severe cognitive impairment often prevents patients from communicating clearly about their pain. For these individuals, behavioural and physiological changes may be the only indicators that they are in pain. Therefore, the nurse must be astute at recognizing behavioural symptoms of pain.

Several scales have been developed to assess pain in cognitively impaired older patients (Gagliese & Melzack, 2014). Typically, these scales help assess pain according to common behavioural indicators such as the following:

- Vocalization: moaning, grunting, crying, sighing
- Facial expressions: grimacing, wincing, frowning, clenching teeth

- Breathing: noisy, laboured
- Body movements: restlessness, rocking, pacing
- Body tension: clenching fist, resisting movement
- Consolability: inability to be consoled or distracted

Because it is not possible to validate the meaning of the behaviours, nurses should rely on their own knowledge of the patient's usual behaviour. If the nurse does not know the patient's baseline behaviours, she or he should obtain this information from other caregivers, including family members. When pain behaviours are present, pain therapy should be instituted on an empirical basis, and patients should be carefully reassessed to evaluate treatment effectiveness.

PATIENTS WITH SUBSTANCE USE PROBLEMS

Individuals with a past or current substance use disorder have the right to receive effective pain management. A comprehensive pain assessment is imperative, including a detailed history, physical examination, psychosocial assessment, and diagnostic workup to determine the cause of the pain. The use of screening tools to determine the possible risk for addiction has been described above. The goal of the pain assessment is to facilitate the establishment of a treatment plan that will relieve the individual's pain effectively, as well as prevent or minimize withdrawal symptoms.

Opioids may be used effectively and safely in patients with substance dependence when indicated for pain control. Opioid agonist and antagonist drugs (e.g., pentazocine [Talwin], butorphanol) should not be used in this population because they may precipitate withdrawal. The use of "potentiators" and psychoactive medications that do not have analgesic properties should also be avoided. In individuals who are tolerant to CNS depressants, larger doses of opioids or increased frequency of medication administration is necessary to achieve pain relief.

Effective pain management for people with addiction is challenging and requires expert leadership and consultation for assessment and facilitation of a planned, interprofessional team approach according to current Canadian guidelines (NOUGG, 2010). Team members must be aware of their own attitudes and misbeliefs about people with substance use problems, which have the possibility of resulting in undertreatment of pain.

CASE STUDY

Pain

Source: Samuel Borges Photography/Shutterstock.com.

Patient Profile

Mrs. Cato is a 112-kg, 43-year-old Caribbean woman admitted for an incision and drainage of a right renal abscess. Her renal function is not impaired. She has a history of low back pain and takes oxycodone, 5 to 10 mg, every 6 hours as needed.

Subjective Data

- Lives alone
- Desires 0 pain during therapy but will accept 1 to 2 on a scale of 0 to 10
- Reports incision-area pain as a 2 or 3 between dressing changes and as a 10 during dressing changes
- States sharp, throbbing pain persists 1 to 2 hours after dressing change
- Reports pain between dressing changes controlled by two oxycodone tablets

Objective Data

- Requires twice-a-day dry-to-dry dressing changes for 1 week
- Morphine, 2 to 15 mg intravenously, for every dressing change
- Oxycodone, 5 to 10 mg, for breakthrough pain between dressing changes

Discussion Questions

1. Initially, what dosage of intravenous morphine should be given?
2. Describe the assessment data that support the dosage selected in Question 1.
3. How long should the nurse wait after the intravenous morphine dose to begin the dressing change?
4. If an initial dose of 6 mg intravenous morphine reduces the pain to a 6 during the dressing change, what nursing action is indicated for the next dressing change?
5. What nursing action is indicated if Mrs. Cato has pain 5 hours after her dressing change?
6. When Mrs. Cato is discharged, needing dressing changes for 3 days at home, how would the home care nurse organize her care? (The nurse knows that Mrs. Cato has obtained adequate pain relief with 8 mg of intravenous morphine.)

ⓔvolve

Answers are available at *http://evolve.elsevier.com/Canada/Lewis/medsurg.*

■ REVIEW QUESTIONS

The number of the question corresponds to the same-numbered objective at the beginning of the chapter.

1. Pain is best described as
   a. A creation of a person's imagination
   b. An unpleasant, subjective experience
   c. A maladaptive response to a stimulus
   d. A neurological event resulting from activation of nociceptors

2. Which of the following inhibiting neurotransmitters is known for its involvement in pain modulation?
   a. Dopamine
   b. Acetylcholine
   c. Prostaglandin
   d. Norepinephrine

3. Which of the following words is most likely to be used to describe neuropathic pain? (*Select all that apply*)
   a. Dull   d. Burning
   b. Mild   e. Sickening
   c. Aching   f. Electric

4. Which of the following is true of unrelieved pain?
   a. It is to be expected after major surgery.
   b. It is to be expected in a person with cancer.
   c. It is dangerous and can lead to many physical and psychological complications.
   d. It is an annoying sensation, but it is not as important as other physical care needs.

5. Which of the following is a critical step in the pain assessment process?
   a. Assessment of critical sensory components
   b. Teaching the client about pain therapies
   c. Conducting a comprehensive pain assessment
   d. Provision of appropriate treatment and evaluation of its effect

6. Which of the following is an example of distraction to provide pain relief?
   a. TENS
   b. Music
   c. Exercise
   d. Biofeedback

7. Which of the following are appropriate nonopioid analgesics for mild pain? *(Select all that apply)*
   a. Oxycodone
   b. Ibuprofen
   c. Lorazepam
   d. Acetaminophen
   e. Acetaminophen with codeine

8. Which of the following is an important nursing responsibility related to pain?
   a. Encourage the client to stay in bed.
   b. Help the client appear not to be in pain.
   c. Believe what the client says about the pain.
   d. Assume responsibility for eliminating the client's pain.

9. A nurse is administering a prescribed dose of an intravenous opioid titrated for a person with severe pain related to a terminal illness. Which of the following actions is reflective of this practice?
   a. Euthanasia
   b. Assisted suicide
   c. Enabling the client's addiction
   d. Palliative pain management

10. A nurse believes that clients with the same type of tissue injury should have the same amount of pain. Which of the following statements best describes this belief?
    a. It will contribute to appropriate pain management.
    b. It is an accurate statement about pain mechanisms and an expected goal of pain therapy.
    c. The nurse's belief will have no effect on the type of care provided to people in pain.
    d. It is a common misconception about pain and a major contributor to ineffective pain management.

1. b, 2. d, 3. d, 4. f, 5. c, 6. b, 7. b, d, 8. c, 9. d, 10. d.

⟲volve

For even more review questions, visit *http://evolve.elsevier.com/Canada/Lewis/medsurg*.

REFERENCES

American Academy of Pain Management. (n.d.). *The cost of pain to business and society due to ineffective pain care.* Retrieved from *http://www.painmed.org/PatientCenter/Cost_of_Pain.aspx*.

Ballantyne, J. C. (2014). Adaptation to continuous opioid use: The role of tolerance, dependence, and memory. In S. N. Raja & C. L. Sommer (Eds.), *Pain 2014 refresher course: 15th World Congress on Pain* (pp. 375–380). Washington, DC: IASP Press. Retrieved from *http://ebooks.iasp-pain.org/pain_2014_refresher_courses*.

Canadian Pain Society. (2010). *Position statement on pain treatment as a human right.* Retrieved from *http://www.canadianpainsociety.ca/?page=PositionStatement*. (Seminal).

Cassell, E. J. (1982). The nature of suffering and the goals of medicine. *New England Journal of Medicine, 306,* 639. doi:10.1056/NEJM198203183061104. (Seminal).

Chaturvedi, A. K., Anderson, W. F., Lortet-Tieulent, J., et al. (2013). Worldwide trends in incidence rates for oral cavity and oropharyngeal cancers. *Journal of Clinical Oncology, 31*(36), 4550–4559. doi:10.1200/JCO.2013.50.3870.

Choinière, M., Watt-Watson, J., Victor, J. C., et al. (2014). Prevalence of and risk factors for persistent postoperative nonanginal pain after cardiac surgery: A 2-year prospective multicentre study. *Canadian Medical Association Journal, 186*(7), E213–E223. doi:10.1503/cmaj.131012.

Cogan, J., Ouimette, M. F., Vargas-Schaffer, G., et al. (2014). Patient attitudes and beliefs regarding pain medication after cardiac surgery: Barriers to adequate pain management. *Pain Management Nursing, 15*(3), 574–579. doi:10.1016/j.pmn.2013.01.003.

Craig, K. D., Prkachin, K. M., & Grunau, R. E. (2011). The facial expression of pain. In D. C. Turk & R. Melzack (Eds.), *Handbook of pain assessment* (3rd ed., pp. 117–134). New York: Guilford.

Crawford, C., Lee, C., & Bingham, J. (2014). Sensory art therapies for the self-management of chronic pain symptoms. *Pain Medicine, 15*(S1), S66–S75. doi:10.1111/pme.12409.

Dale, O. (2010). Intranasal administration of opioids/fentanyl—Physiological and pharmacological aspects. *European Journal of Pain Supplements, 4*(S3), 187–190. doi:10.1016/j.eujps.2010.06.001. (Seminal).

Fields, H. (1987). *Pain.* Toronto: McGraw-Hill. (Seminal).

Gagliese, L., & Melzack, R. (2014). Pain in older persons. In S. B. McMahon, M. Koltzenburg, I. Tracey, et al. (Eds.), *Melzack and Wall textbook of pain* (6th ed., pp. 315–320). Philadelphia, PA: Elsevier.

Gagliese, L., & Melzack, R. (2003). Age-related differences in the qualities but not the intensity of chronic pain. *Pain, 104*(3), 597–608. doi:10.1016/S0304-3959(03)00117-9. (Seminal).

Hunter, J., Watt-Watson, J., McGillion, M., et al. (2008). An interfaculty pain curriculum: Lessons learned from six years' experience. *Pain, 140*(1), 74–86. doi:10.1016/j.pain.2008.07.010. (Seminal).

Institutes of Medicine of the National Academies. (2011). *Relieving pain in America: A blueprint for transforming prevention, care, education, and research* (p. 260). Washington, DC: National Academies Press. Retrieved from *http://books.nap.edu/openbook.php?record_id=13172&page=260*.

Jovey, R. D. (2010). Pain and addiction: Prevalence, neurobiology, definitions. In J. Mogil (Ed.), *Pain 2010—An updated review: Refresher course syllabus* (pp. 315–321). Seattle: IASP Press. (Seminal).

Katz, B. (2014). Pain in older adults: Special considerations. In S. N. Raja & C. L. Sommer (Eds.), *Pain 2014 refresher course: 15th World Congress on Pain* (pp. 365–372). Washington, DC: IASP Press. Retrieved from *http://ebooks.iasp-pain.org/pain_2014_refresher_courses*.

Katz, J., & Melzack, R. (2011). The McGill Pain Questionnaire: Development, psychometric properties, and usefulness of the long form short form, and short form-2. In D. C. Turk & R. Melzack (Eds.), *Handbook of pain assessment* (3rd ed., pp. 45–66). New York: Guilford.

Kerstman, E., Ahn, S., Battu, S., et al. (2013). Neuropathic pain. *Handbook of Clinical Neurology, 110*, 175.

Ladak, S. S., McPhee, C., Muscat, M., et al. (2013). The journey of the pain resource nurse in improving pain management practices: Understanding role implementation. *Pain Management Nursing, 14*(2), 68–73. doi:10.1016/j.pmn.2011.02.002.

Lynch, M. E. (2011). The need for a Canadian pain strategy. *Pain Research and Management, 16*(2), 77–80. doi:10.1155/2011/654651.

McCaffery, M., & Pasero, C. (1999). *Pain: A clinical manual for nursing practice* (2nd ed.). St. Louis, MO: Mosby. (Seminal).

McGillion, M., Arthur, H. M., Cook, A., et al. (2012a). Nonischemic chest pain following successful PCI at a regional referral centre in southern Ontario. *The Canadian Journal of Cardiology, 28*, S60–S69. doi:10.1016/j.cjca.2011.10.017.

McGillion, M., Arthur, H. M., Cook, A., et al. (2012b). Joint Canadian Cardiovascular Society-Canadian Pain Society Guidelines for the Management of Patients with Refractory Angina. *Canadian Journal of Cardiology, 28*, S20–S41. doi:10.1016/j.cjca.2011.07.007.

McGillion, M., Dubrowski, A., Stremler, R., et al. (2011). The Postoperative Pain Assessment Skills pilot trial. *Pain Research and Management, 16*, 433–439.

McGillion, M., LeFort, S., Webber, K., et al. (2011). Pain self management—Theory and process for clinicians. In M. Lynch, K. Graig, & P. Peng (Eds.), *Clinical pain management: A practical guide* (pp. 193–199). Oxford: Blackwell Publishing.

McGillion, M., O'Keefe-McCarthy, S., Carroll, S., et al. (2014). Impact of self-management interventions on stable angina symptoms and health-related quality of life: A meta-analysis. *BMC Cardiovascular Disorders, 14*(14), doi:10.1186/1471-2261-14-14.

McGillion, M., & Watt-Watson, J. (2015). Pain assessment and management in Canada: We've come a long way but there are challenges on the road ahead. *The Canadian Journal of Nursing Research, 47*(1), 9–16.

McMillan, S. C., Tittle, M., Hagan, S., et al. (2000). Management of pain and pain-related symptoms in hospitalized veterans with cancer. *Cancer Nursing, 23*(5), 327–336. doi:10.1097/00002820-200010000-00001. (Seminal).

Melzack, R., & Wall, P. D. (1987). *The challenge of pain*. New York: Penguin Books. (Seminal).

Merskey, H., & Baranowski, A. P. (Eds.), (2012). Pain terms: A current list with definitions and notes on usage. In *Classification of chronic pain* (2nd ed., pp. 209–214). Seattle: IASP Press. Retrieved from *http://www.iasp-pain.org/PublicationsNews/Content.aspx?ItemNumber=1673.*

Mifflin, K. A., & Kerr, B. J. (2014). The transition from acute to chronic pain: Understanding how different biological systems interact. *Canadian Journal of Anaesthesia, 61*(2), 112–122.

Mogil, J. S. (2012). Pain genetics: Past, present and future. *Trends Genetic, 28*(6), 258–266. doi:10.1016/j.tig.2012.02.004.

National Opioid Use Guideline Group [NOUGG]. (2010). *Canadian guideline for safe and effective use of opioids for chronic non-cancer pain*. Retrieved from *http://nationalpaincentre.mcmaster.ca/opioid/.* (Seminal).

Noble, M., Treadwell, J. R., Tregear, S. J., et al. (2010). Long-term opioid management for chronic non-cancer pain. *The Cochrane Database of Systematic Reviews*, (1), CD006605, doi:10.1002/14651858.CD006605.pub2. (Seminal).

O'Keefe-McCarthy, S., McGillion, M., Clarke, S., et al. (2015). Pain and anxiety in rural acute coronary syndrome patients awaiting diagnostic cardiac catheterization. *Journal of Cardiovascular Nursing, 30*(6), 546–557. doi:10.1097/JCN0000000000000203.

O'Keefe-McCarthy, S., McGillion, M., Nelson, S., et al. (2014). Acute coronary syndrome pain and anxiety in a rural emergency department: Patient and nurse perspectives. *Canadian Journal of Nursing Research, 46*(2), 80–100.

O'Mara, A. (2014). The worldwide problem of cancer. In S. N. Raja & C. L. Sommer (Eds.), *Pain 2014 refresher course: 15th World Congress on Pain* (pp. 99–104). Washington, DC: IASP Press. Retrieved from *http://ebooks.iasp-pain.org/pain_2014_refresher_courses.*

Pelletier, R., Higgins, J., & Bourbonnais, D. (2015). Is neuroplasticity in the central nervous system the missing link to our understanding of chronic musculoskeletal disorders? *BMC Musculoskeletal Disorders, 16*(1), 1. doi:10.1186/s12891-015-0480-y.

Pergolizzi, J. V., Raffa, R. B., & Taylor, R. (2014). Treating acute pain in light of chronification of pain. *Pain Management Nursing, 15*(1), 380–390.

Ramage-Morin, L., & Gilmour, H. (2010). Chronic pain at ages 12 to 44 (Catalogue no. 82-003-XPE). *Health Reports, 21*(4). Retrieved from *http://www.statcan.gc.ca/pub/82-003-x/2010004/article/11389-eng.pdf.* (Seminal).

Registered Nurses' Association of Ontario (RNAO). (2013). *Assessment and management of pain*. Toronto, ON: Author. Retrieved from *http://rnao.ca/bpg/guidelines/assessment-and-management-pain.*

Richardson, P. (2014). Spirituality, religion and palliative care. *Annals of Palliative Medicine, 3*(3), 150–159.

Salter, M. W. (2014). Neurobiology of acute and persistent pain: Spinal cord mechanisms. In S. N. Raja & C. L. Sommer (Eds.), *Pain 2014 refresher course: 15th World Congress on Pain* (pp. 3–12). Washington, DC: IASP Press. Retrieved from *http://ebooks.iasp-pain.org/pain_2014_refresher_courses.*

Sanchez, S., Tenias, B., Arias, A., et al. (2015). Cardiovascular risk associated with use of non-steroidal anti-inflammatory drugs: Cohort study. *Revista Espanola de Salud Publica, 896*, 627–632.

Schreiber, K. L., Campbell, C., Martel, M. O., et al. (2014). Distraction analgesia in chronic pain patients: The impact of catastrophizing. *Anesthesiologists, 121*(6), 1292–1301. doi:10.1097/ALN.0000000000000465.

Shengelia, R., Parker, S. J., Ballin, M., et al. (2013). Complementary therapies for osteoarthritis: Are they effective? *Pain Management Nursing, 14*(4), e274–e288. doi:10.1016/j.pmn.2012.01.001.

Song, J. J., Popescu, A., & Bell, R. L. (2014). Present and potential use of spinal cord stimulation to control chronic pain. *Pain Physician, 17*(3), 235–246.

Sturgeon, J. A., & Zautra, A. J. (2013). Psychological resilience, pain catastrophizing, and positive emotions: Perspectives on comprehensive modeling of individual pain adaptation. *Current Pain Headache Report, 17*(3), 1–9. doi:10.1007/s11916-012-0317-4.

Tracy, B., & Morrison, S. (2013). Pain management in older adults. *Clinical Therapeutics, 31*(1), 1659–1668. doi:10.1016/j.clinthera.2013.09.026.

Van Tulder, M., & Koes, B. (2013). Low back pain. In S. B. McMahon, M. Koltzenburg, I. Tracey, et al. (Eds.), *Melzack and Wall textbook of pain* (6th ed., pp. 683–693). Philadelphia: Elsevier.

Von Gunten, C. F. (2011). Pathophysiology of pain in cancer. *Journal of Pediatric Hematology/Oncology, 33*, S12–S18.

Voshall, B., Dunn, K. S., & Shelestak, D. (2013). Knowledge and attitudes of pain management among faculty. *Pain Management Nursing, 14*(4), e226–e235.

Watt-Watson, J., McGillion, M., Hunter, J., et al. (2009). A survey of prelicensure pain curricula in health science faculties in Canadian Universities. *Pain Research and Management, 14*(6), 439–444. (Seminal).

Watt-Watson, J., & Murinson, B. B. (2013). Current challenges in pain education. *Pain Management, 3*(5), 351–357. doi:10.2217/pmt.13.39.

RESOURCES

Canadian Guideline for Safe and Effective Use of Opioids for Chronic Non-Cancer Pain (NOUGG)
http://nationalpaincentre.mcmaster.ca/opioid/

Canadian Pain Coalition
http://www.canadianpaincoalition.ca

Canadian Pain Society Position Statement on Pain Relief
http://www.canadianpainsociety.ca/?page=PositionStatement

McGill Pain Questionnaire
http://www.chcr.brown.edu/pcoc/MCGILLPAINQUEST.PDF

Registered Nurses' Association of Ontario Best Practice Guidelines: Assessment and Management of Pain
http://rnao.ca/bpg/guidelines/assessment-and-management-pain

Winnipeg Regional Health Authority—Pain Assessment and Management: Clinical Practice Guidelines
http://www.wrha.mb.ca/extranet/eipt/files/EIPT-017-001.pdf

Agency for Healthcare Research and Quality
http://www.ahcpr.gov

American Pain Society
http://americanpainsociety.org/

City of Hope Pain & Palliative Care Resource Center
http://prc.coh.org/res_inst.asp

Core Curriculum for Professional Education in Pain
http://issuu.com/iasp/docs/core-corecurriculum?mode=embed &layout=http%3A%2F%2Fskin.issuu.com%2Fv%2Fdarkicons %2Flayout.xml&showFlipBtn=true

International Association for the Study of Pain
http://www.iasp-pain.org

For additional Internet resources, see the website for this book at *http://evolve.elsevier.com/Canada/Lewis/medsurg*.

evolve WEBSITE

http://evolve.elsevier.com/Canada/Lewis/medsurg

- Review Questions (Online Only)
- Key Points
- Answer Guidelines for Case Study

- Conceptual Care Map Creator
- Customizable Nursing Care Plan
  - Alcohol Withdrawal

- Audio Glossary
- Content Updates

LEARNING OBJECTIVES

1. Gain a broad understanding of the prevalence of substance use in Canada.
2. Situate substance use within the continuum of use perspective.
3. Discuss the core aspects of a caring and collaborative nursing relationship with people experiencing substance use–related conditions.
4. Describe the harm-reduction model.
5. Discuss screening and assessment of people experiencing substance use–related conditions.
6. Identify common substances of abuse, their effects, and associated health consequences.
7. Discuss nursing interventions for nicotine dependence, alcohol dependence, and opioid dependence.

8. Describe how to care for patients who experience intoxication, overdose, or withdrawal from stimulants, depressants, or hallucinogens.
9. Describe nursing management of the surgical patient with substance use.
10. Discuss the nursing management of pain in the patient who is substance dependent.
11. Describe the use of motivational interviewing as an approach to helping patients who use substances explore the possibility of behaviour change.
12. Discuss substance use conditions specific to the older adult.

KEY TERMS

brain reward system, p. 169
cross-tolerance, p. 184
Korsakoff syndrome, p. 184
lapses, p. 189
motivational interviewing,
   p. 188

opiates, p. 185
opioids, p. 185
potentiation, p. 181
psychological dependence,
   p. 169
relapse, p. 170

relief craving, p. 170
reward craving, p. 170
substance use disorder, p. 170
tolerance, p. 170
transtheoretical model of
   change, p. 188

Wernicke's encephalopathy,
   p. 184
withdrawal, p. 172
withdrawal management,
   p. 184

SUBSTANCE USE IN CANADA

Substance use and abuse affect a broad spectrum of Canadians, regardless of age, gender, socioeconomic class, educational level, cultural background, or geographic region. As such, it is important for nurses to routinely assess for substance use with every individual in all practice settings and to determine whether the pattern of use is problematic. Substance use is defined as the use or misuse of substance(s) despite the associated negative personal and social consequences. The American Psychiatric Association (APA, 2013) no longer recommends the use of the term *addiction* as a diagnostic label because it has an uncertain definition and negative connotation.

According to the Canadian Alcohol and Drug Use Monitoring Survey (CADUMS) (Health Canada, 2014), in 2012, 78.4% of Canadians aged 15 years and older reported past-year consumption of alcohol; 10.2% reported cannabis use; and 10.6% reported use of either cocaine, cannabis, speed, methamphetamines, Ecstasy, or hallucinogens (Table 11-1). Since 2013, the risk for abuse of fentanyl, a powerful opioid, has risen; in Canada, between 2009 and 2014, there have been at least 655 deaths where fentanyl was found to be the cause or a contributing cause, and it is thought that this figure is an underestimate (Canadian Centre on Substance Abuse, 2015). The results of the 2012 Canadian Tobacco Use Monitoring Survey

(CTUMS) indicate that 16% (4.6 million) of Canadians aged 15 years and older are current smokers (Health Canada, 2012). This is a significant decrease from 1999, when 25% (6.1 million) of this population were reported to be current smokers (Health Canada, 2012).

The significant personal and social costs of substance use to Canadians and their families manifest as poor physical and mental health, stress, relationship strain, and increased morbidity and mortality related to substance use. Not only do nurses play a key role in screening for, assessing, and promoting healthy choices regarding the use of substances; they also need to monitor for substance misuse.

TABLE 11-1	HIGHLIGHTS FROM THE CANADIAN ALCOHOL AND DRUG USE MONITORING SURVEY (CADUMS) 2012

Alcohol
- 78.4% of Canadians reported drinking alcohol in the past year.
- 82.7% of men and 74.4% of women reported alcohol use in the past year.
- 18.6% of women drank more than 10 drinks per week, and the same percentage of men had 15 drinks per week.
- Average age of first alcohol consumption was 15.9 years.
- Youth aged 15 to 24 years had the highest rates of alcohol consumption.

Cannabis
- The prevalence of past-year use of cannabis reported by adults aged 25 years and older was 8.4%.
- The rate of cannabis use among males (13.7%) was double that among women (7%).

Other Drug Use
- The most commonly reported illicit drugs after cannabis were Ecstasy (0.6%), hallucinogens (1.1%), and cocaine or crack (1.1%).
- The rate of illicit drug use among males (3.1%) was almost triple that among females (1.1%).
- The rate of drug use by youths 15–24 years of age was five times higher than that reported by adults 25 years and older.
- The rates of psychoactive pharmaceutical use and abuse remain steady (24.1%) among adults. The prevalence was higher among females (26.7%) than males (21.3%).

Source: Health Canada. (2014). *Canadian Alcohol and Drug Use Monitoring Survey: Summary of results for 2012.* Retrieved from http://www.hc-sc.gc.ca/hc-ps/drugs-drogues/stat/_2012/summary-sommaire-eng.php#s3.

SUBSTANCE USE FROM A CONTINUUM OF USE PERSPECTIVE

People who use substances have often been categorized, especially by health care providers, as those whose use is classified as *substance abuse* and those whose use is classified as *substance dependence*. It is more helpful to situate substance use along a continuum of use, capturing a spectrum ranging from nonuse to substance dependence. A continuum allows for a broader understanding of the range and severity of substance use behaviours across populations (Figure 11-1) (Herie & Skinner, 2010). Knowing the severity of substance use allows the health care team to work with the patient, tailoring treatment according to individual needs and preferences.

This chapter focuses on the role of the medical-surgical nurse in identifying and working with patients in acute care settings who have a history of substance use. In this setting, nurses must recognize substance use, understand its effects on the patient's health, and help the patient manage withdrawal. The health care setting provides an opportunity for substance use screening and education. Vital aspects of the nursing role are determining if the patient is motivated to change substance use behaviour and making referrals to substance use treatment and rehabilitation programs. Failing to address a patient's substance use is a breach of professional responsibility.

Neurophysiology of Substances of Abuse

Substances of abuse are psychoactive in nature, meaning they affect key areas of the brain involved in pleasure and reinforcement. Caffeine is one example of a substance of abuse. Caffeine is a stimulant with reinforcing psychoactive qualities that result in mental alertness and enhanced mood. If taken regularly over a period of time, abrupt cessation of caffeine can lead to mild withdrawal symptoms. Substances with a higher index of abuse, such as cocaine or nicotine, engage the reward–pleasure system of the brain more intensely and more quickly. Substances with higher risk for dependency are those that possess fast onset and intense psychoactive characteristics (Koob, Kandel, Baler, et al., 2015; Reiss, Fiellin, Miller, et al., 2014).

Substances of abuse increase the availability of dopamine in the "pleasure area" of the mesolimbic system of the brain. This mechanism, the **brain reward system**, creates the sensation of pleasure in reaction to certain behaviours that are required for survival of the human species, such as eating and sex (Burchum & Rosenthal, 2016). **Psychological dependence**, the emotional and mental reliance on a substance because of the pleasurable

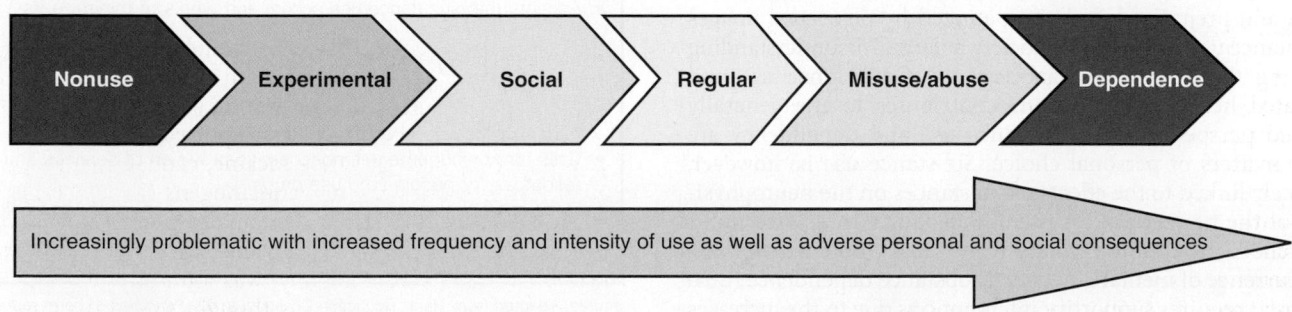

FIGURE 11-1 Continuum of use for substance use. Source: Herie, Marilyn, and Skinner, Wayne, *Substance Abuse in Canada* © 2010 Oxford University Press Canada. Reprinted by permission of the publisher.

and reinforcing effects of the substance, can result. Normally, neurons in the mesolimbic system release dopamine at a slow rate, producing normal affect or mood. Both endogenous and exogenous opiates have been found to increase the firing rate of dopaminergic neurons. Cocaine has been shown to decrease the reuptake of dopamine at the synapse, thereby decreasing its breakdown and increasing the amount of available dopamine. Nicotine, alcohol, marihuana, amphetamines, and caffeine also increase dopaminergic neuron activity at the synapse. The resulting increase in mesolimbic dopamine produces mood elevation and euphoria, factors that provide strong motivation to repeat the experience. Substances of abuse also increase the availability of other neurotransmitters, such as serotonin and γ-aminobutyric acid (GABA), but dopamine's effect on the reward system appears to be pivotal to the process of substance use and dependency (Taber, Black, Porrino, et al., 2012).

The *Diagnostic and Statistical Manual of Mental Disorders,* Fifth Edition (*DSM-5*), has replaced the terms *substance abuse* and *substance dependence* with substance use disorder (APA, 2013). Specific diagnostic criteria determine the level of severity of the disorder as mild, moderate, or severe. Substance use disorders result from the prolonged effects of psychoactive substances on the brain. Repeated long-term use of substances of abuse changes the neural circuitry involving the dopamine neurotransmitter system and reduces the responsiveness of dopamine receptors. This decreased responsiveness leads to tolerance, the need for a larger dose of a substance to obtain the original effects, and also reduces the sense of pleasure from experiences that previously resulted in positive feelings. Without the substance, the individual experiences depression, anxiety, and irritability. To feel normal, the individual must take the substance.

A key aspect of substance use is the formation of the memory of the pleasurable experience of the substance that is long-lasting even in periods of nonuse. Relief craving, the intense desire for a substance, usually experienced after decreased use, is the result of the memory aspect related to the brain reward pathway. An important type of craving experienced by people who have experienced problematic substance use or dependency is reward craving, which occurs when in the presence of people, places, or things that they have previously associated with taking the substance. Cue-induced reward craving may occur after long periods of abstinence and is a common cause of relapse, or returning to substance use after a period of abstinence (Koob, Kandel, Baler, et al., 2015).

ATTITUDES TOWARD PEOPLE EXPERIENCING SUBSTANCE-RELATED PROBLEMS

People with substance use–related conditions face significant stigma and prejudice largely perpetuated by pejorative images of substance use in media and society at large. Misunderstanding regarding the biopsychosocial aspects of substance use and associated health complications contributes to the generally accepted perspective that substance use and dependency are purely matters of personal choice. Substance use is, however, intimately linked to the effects of substances on the neurophysiology of the brain reward system. Substance use is a complex biopsychosocial condition that involves the whole person. The co-occurrence of mental illness and substance dependence (dual diagnosis) requires supportive interventions due to the increases in the severity of symptoms and poor outcomes for both disorders (Padwa, Larkins, Crevecoeur-MacPhail, et al., 2013).

Nurses must explore their own attitudes about people who use and abuse substances. It is critical to work with patients in a nonjudgemental and collaborative way. A positive nurse–patient dialogue about the impact of substance use can significantly improve health outcomes and increase the likelihood that the person will attempt to reduce harms associated with substance use.

THE HARM-REDUCTION PERSPECTIVE

Harm reduction focuses on reducing the harms associated with substance use across the continuum of use, from abstinence to high-risk use (Table 11-2). The harms targeted for reduction include the very real personal, social, and physical harms related to use of a substance from a public health perspective (Canadian Nurses Association, 2012). Laws against drinking and driving and nonsmoking bylaws are examples of harm-reduction strategies to protect people from the harms related to alcohol and smoking. Other examples include evidence-informed interventions such as needle-exchange programs and safer-sex education; these reduce the harms associated with high-risk substance use without demanding that the person stop such use.

Foundational to harm reduction are respect for patient autonomy and a nonjudgemental approach. Harm reduction is collaborative and honours the patient's inherent dignity and ability to make informed decisions. There is considerable evidence to support harm reduction (Collins, Clifasefi, Logan, et al., 2012). Nurses must support patients' healthy choices and help them avoid risks associated with substance use (Carter & MacPherson, 2013).

Health Complications of Substance Use

Health complications and harms related to substances of abuse are related to three general factors: the substance, the route, and related high-risk behaviours. First, the inherent properties of the substance itself will have specific physiological harms associated with its use such as liver damage related to alcohol use and emphysema related to smoking. Second, the route by which the substance is taken will pose specific harms. For example, harms associated with oral consumption are different in nature

TABLE 11-2	KEY ELEMENTS OF HARM REDUCTION

Harm Reduction
- Represents a value-neutral view of drug use and drug user with no moral, legal, or medical-reductionist limitations
- Accepts that at any given time some people are not ready to choose abstinence
- Promotes multiple services at one site as an alternative to traditional complex multisite service approaches
- Accepts that substance use occurs and works to minimize its harmful effects
- Promotes user participation in planning and creating programs and policies designed to serve them
- Recognizes that users are capable of making choices and taking responsibility in prevention of harm, treatment, and recovery
- Calls for nonjudgemental, noncoercive provision of services and resources for people who use drugs
- Does not attempt to minimize or ignore the many real and tragic harms and dangers associated with drug use
- Does not exclude abstinence as an option

Source: Adapted from Harm Reduction Coalition. (n.d.). *Principles of harm reduction.* Retrieved from *http://harmreduction.org/about-us/principles-of-harm-reduction/*; and Marlatt, G. A. (1996). Harm reduction: Come as you are. *Addictive Behaviours, 21*(6), 779–788. doi:10.1016/0306-4603(96)00042-1.

TABLE 11-3 COMMON HEALTH PROBLEMS RELATED TO SUBSTANCE USE

Substance	Health Problems*
Cocaine	Cardiac dysrhythmias, myocardial ischemia and infarction
	Seizures, stroke
	Psychosis
Amphetamines	Cardiac dysrhythmias, myocardial ischemia and infarction
	Liver, lung, kidney damage
	Mood disturbances, violent behaviour, psychoses
Sedative–hypnotics	Memory impairment
	Personality changes, depression
Opioids	Sexual dysfunction
	Gastric ulcers
	Glomerulonephritis
Inhalants	Cognitive and motor impairment
	Acute and chronic kidney injury
Cannabis	Bronchitis, chronic cough
	Depression, anxiety, schizophrenia
	Memory impairment
Behaviours	
Injecting drugs	Blood clots, phlebitis, skin infections
	Hepatitis B and C
	HIV/AIDS
	Other infections: endocarditis, tuberculosis, pneumonia, meningitis, tetanus, bone and joint infections, lung abscesses
Snorting drugs	Nasal sores, septal necrosis or perforation
	Chronic sinusitis
Risky sexual behaviour	HIV/AIDS
	Hepatitis B and C
	Sexually transmitted infections
Personal neglect	Malnutrition, impaired immunity
	Accidental injuries

Source: Adapted from National Institute on Drug Abuse. (2012). *Medical consequence of drug abuse*. Retrieved from *http://www.drugabuse.gov/related-topics/medical-consequences-drug-abuse*.
HIV/AIDS, human immunodeficiency virus/acquired immune deficiency syndrome.
*Throughout the text, the health problems related to substance use are discussed in the appropriate chapters where substance use–related behaviours are identified as risk factors for these problems.

TABLE 11-4 BRIEF SCREENING TOOL FOR SUBSTANCE USE

1. Single-Question Tests
Use one of the following questions to screen for the presence of alcohol, drug, or tobacco use.
- How often in the past year have you had five (men) or four (women) or more drinks in a day?
- How many times in the past year have you used illegal drugs or prescription medications for nonmedical reasons?
- In the past year, how often have you used tobacco products?

2. Two-Question Tests
Use the following two questions to screen for alcohol or drug use.
- In the past year, have you ever drunk or used drugs more than you meant to?
- Have you felt you wanted or needed to cut down on your drinking or drug use in the past year?

Source: Reprinted from *Primary Care: Clinics in Office Practice*, 41(2), Strobbe, S., "Prevention and screening, brief intervention, and referral to treatment for substance use in primary care," pages 185–213, Copyright 2014, with permission from Elsevier.

TABLE 11-5 DRUG ABUSE SCREEN TEST (DAST-10)

In the last 12 months:		
1. Have you used drugs other than those required for medical reasons?	No	Yes
2. Do you abuse more than one drug at a time?	No	Yes
3. Are you always able to stop using drugs when you want to?	No	Yes
4. Have you had "blackouts" or "flashbacks" as a result of drug use?	No	Yes
5. Do you ever feel bad or guilty about your drug use?	No	Yes
6. Does your spouse (or parents) ever complain about your involvement with drugs?	No	Yes
7. Have you neglected your family because of your use of drugs?	No	Yes
8. Have you engaged in illicit activities in order to obtain drugs?	No	Yes
9. Have you ever experienced withdrawal symptoms or felt sick when you stopped taking drugs?	No	Yes
10. Have you had medical problems as a result of your drug use?	No	Yes

Source: Skinner, H. A. (1982). Drug Abuse Screening Test. *Addictive Behaviors, 7*(4), 363–371. doi:10.1016/0306-4603(82)90005-3.

from those associated with inhalation or intravenous use. Third, high-risk sexual behaviours, exposure to violence and trauma, and placing one's personal safety at risk may occur during substance use (Table 11-3).

NURSING MANAGEMENT SUBSTANCE USE

ASSESSMENT

The nurse engages with patients to understand if they use substances in ways that place them at risk. As a baseline, the nurse asks every patient about the use of all substances, including alcohol, prescribed medications, over-the-counter (OTC) drugs, caffeine, tobacco, and recreational drugs. He or she may use a simple one- or two-question screening test for substance use (Table 11-4) or the more in-depth Drug Abuse Screening Test (DAST-10), shown in Table 11-5. If there are any indications of substance use, the nurse determines when the patient last used

the substance so that drug interactions or the onset of withdrawal can be anticipated. The nurse attempts to identify factors that influence the onset of withdrawal, including the substance used, dose taken, method of intake, and length of time the patient has been using the substance. Screening for alcohol abuse is discussed later in this chapter.

Health problems associated with substance use may be revealed through assessment of general appearance and nutritional status and through examination of the abdomen, skin, and cardiovascular, respiratory, and neurological systems. The presence of a mental health condition, such as anxiety, bipolar disorder, or depression, increases the risk for substance use disorder (Strobbe, 2014). Serum and urine drug screens can identify the types and amounts of substances present in the body. A complete blood count, serum electrolytes, blood urea nitrogen, creatinine, and liver function tests evaluate for electrolyte imbalances and cardiac, kidney, or liver dysfunction.

TABLE 11-6	MANIFESTATIONS SUGGESTIVE OF SUBSTANCE USE

- Vague physical complaints
- Insomnia, fatigue
- Headaches
- Seizure disorder
- Mood changes, anorexia, weight loss
- Overuse of mouthwash or toiletries
- Appearance of being older than stated age, unkempt appearance
- Leisure activities that involve alcohol, drugs, or both
- Sexual dysfunction, decreased libido, erectile dysfunction
- Trauma secondary to falls, auto accidents, fights, or burns
- Driving while intoxicated
- Failure of standard doses of sedatives to have a therapeutic effect
- Financial problems, including those related to spending for substances
- Defensive or evasive answers to questions about substance use and its importance in the person's life
- Problems in areas of life function (e.g., frequent job changes; marital conflict, separation, or divorce; work-related accidents, tardiness, absenteeism; legal problems; social isolation, estrangement from friends or family)

During the assessment, the nurse observes patient behaviours such as denial, avoidance, under-reporting or minimizing of substance use, or provision of inaccurate information. Possible behaviours and physical manifestations suggesting substance use are listed in Table 11-6. The list is not comprehensive.

NURSING DIAGNOSES

Nursing diagnoses for patients with substance use problems include but are not limited to the following:

- *Acute confusion* related to substance misuse (*e.g.*, as evidenced by *alteration in cognitive functioning, agitation, misperception, and hallucinations*)
- *Risk for injury* as evidenced by *alteration in cognitive function* (impaired judgement)
- *Ineffective health maintenance* related to *ineffective coping strategies, impaired decision-making*

PLANNING

The nurse and the patient should establish goals related to (a) achieving the best possible physiological functioning, (b) acknowledging substance use, (c) understanding the biopsychosocial effects of substance use, and (d) participating in treatment or harm-reduction strategies.

NURSING IMPLEMENTATION

URGENT CARE SITUATIONS. Urgent care situations precipitated by substance use involve acute intoxication, overdose, or withdrawal. The patient may also present with trauma or injuries. Intoxication responses usually last less than 24 hours and are directly related to the ingestion of psychoactive substances. Overdose occurs with the ingestion of an excessive dose of one drug or with a combination of similarly acting drugs. Overdose leads to toxic reactions that may include respiratory and circulatory arrest and other life-threatening complications. Table 11-7 lists commonly abused substances, routes, and effects.

Overdose. An overdose is an emergency situation, and management is based on the type of substance involved. If multiple substances have been ingested, a complex and potentially confusing clinical picture can result. The first priority of care in the case of overdose is always the patient's ABCs (airway, breathing, and circulation). Continuous monitoring of neurological status, including level of consciousness and respiratory and cardiovascular function, is critical until the patient is stable. Vital signs and intake and output should be monitored. Emergency management of overdose and toxicity of central nervous system (CNS) stimulants and CNS depressants is presented later in the chapter in Tables 11-13 and 11-20.

Pharmacological agents are administered as ordered to counteract toxic effects of drugs. Naloxone or flumazenil may be administered when a depressant effect is present but the ingested drug is unknown. Naloxone rapidly reverses the effects of opioids, and flumazenil reverses the effects of benzodiazepine overdose. The effects of these antagonists necessitate frequent monitoring because these drugs have a short half-life and may need to be readministered after the initial reversal of toxic effects. Specific antagonists are not available for other drugs of abuse, but a variety of other medications may be used to control symptoms.

The patient who has overdosed on sedative–hypnotics other than benzodiazepines must be treated aggressively and may require dialysis to decrease the drug level and to prevent irreversible CNS-depressant effects and death. Gastric lavage and administration of activated charcoal may be instituted if the drug was taken orally within 4 to 6 hours. CNS stimulants are not used in the treatment of depressant-drug overdose.

As soon as the patient is stable, a thorough history and physical examination must be attempted. When the patient is unwilling or unable to give a history, a collateral history should be obtained from the patient's significant others. Recent substance use, including type, amount, and time, and the presence of any chronic illnesses, are important in planning ongoing care. A patient who intentionally overdosed should not return home until seen by a psychiatric professional.

Withdrawal. The nurse must be alert to the possibility of withdrawal in any patient who has a history of substance use. Withdrawal is defined as a constellation of physiological and psychological responses that occur upon abrupt cessation or reduced intake of a substance on which an individual is dependent. In general, withdrawal signs and symptoms are opposite in nature from the direct effects of the drug (Table 11-8). Because abused substances are psychoactive, changes are consistently noted in the neurological system. These changes often manifest as acute anxiety and protracted depression. Withdrawal from CNS depressants, including alcohol, benzodiazepines, and barbiturates, can be dangerous and may be life-threatening. When caring for patients who are withdrawing from any substance, nurses should monitor physiological function, ensure safety and comfort, prevent the progression of symptoms, provide reassurance and orientation, and determine if the patient is motivated to engage in long-term treatment.

Perioperative Care. An individual who abuses substances is more likely to have accidents and injuries that necessitate surgery. Optimally, health problems such as malnutrition, dehydration, and infection should be treated before surgery is performed. All trauma victims must be carefully assessed for signs and symptoms of substance overdose and withdrawal that could lead to adverse drug interactions with analgesics or anaesthetics. For example, if an accident victim has injuries that cause CNS depression, alcohol use may be missed.

TABLE 11-7 EFFECTS OF FREQUENTLY USED SUBSTANCES

Substance	Physiological and Psychological Effects	Effects of Overdose	Withdrawal Symptoms
Stimulants			
Nicotine	Increased arousal and alertness; performance enhancement; increased heart rate, cardiac output, and blood pressure; cutaneous vasoconstriction; fine tremor, decreased appetite; antidiuretic effect; increased gastric motility	Rare: Nausea, abdominal pain, diarrhea, vomiting, dizziness, weakness, confusion, decreased respirations, seizures, death from respiratory failure	Craving, restlessness, depression, hyperirritability, headache, insomnia, decreased blood pressure and heart rate, increased appetite
Cocaine Amphetamines: amphetamine, dextroamphetamine (Dexedrine), methamphetamine, crystal methamphetamine (crystal meth), methylenedioxy-methamphetamine (MDMA, Ecstasy), methylphenidate (Ritalin)	Euphoria, grandiosity, mood swings, hyperactivity, hyperalertness, restlessness, anorexia, insomnia, hypertension, tachycardia, marked vasoconstriction, tremor, dysrhythmias, seizures, dilated pupils, diaphoresis	Agitation; increased temperature, heart rate, respiratory rate, blood pressure; cardiac dysrhythmias, myocardial infarction, hallucinations, seizures, possible death	Severe craving, severely depressed mood, exhaustion, prolonged sleep, apathy, irritability, disorientation
Caffeine	Mood elevation, increased alertness, nervousness, jitteriness, irritability, insomnia; increased respirations, heart rate, and force of myocardial contraction; relaxation of smooth muscle, diuresis	Rare: Hyperstimulation, nervousness, confusion, psychomotor agitation, anxiety, dizziness, tinnitus, muscle twitching, elevated blood pressure, tachycardia, extrasystoles, increased respiratory rate	Headache, irritability, drowsiness, fatigue
Depressants			
Alcohol Sedative–hypnotics • Barbiturates: phenobarbital (Phenobarb), pentobarbital • Benzodiazepines: diazepam (Valium), chlordiazepoxide (Librax), alprazolam (Xanax) • Nonbarbiturates–nonbenzodiazepines: chloral hydrate	Initial relaxation, emotional lability, decreased inhibitions, drowsiness, lack of coordination, impaired judgement, slurred speech, hypotension, bradycardia, bradypnea	Shallow respirations; cold, clammy skin; weak, rapid pulse; hyporeflexia, coma, possible death	Anxiety, agitation, insomnia, diaphoresis, tremors, delirium, seizures, possible death
Opioids			
Heroin Morphine Opium Codeine Fentanyl (Duragesic) Meperidine (Demerol) Hydromorphone (Dilaudid) Pentazocine (Talwin) Oxycodone hydrochloride (Percocet) Methadone	Analgesia, euphoria, drowsiness, detachment from environment, relaxation, constricted pupils, constipation, nausea, decreased respiratory rate, slurred speech, impaired judgement, decreased sexual and aggressive drives	Slow, shallow respirations; clammy skin; constricted pupils; coma; possible death	Watery eyes, dilated pupils, runny nose, yawning, tremors, pain, chills, fever, diaphoresis, nausea, vomiting, diarrhea, abdominal cramps
Cannabis			
Marihuana Hashish	Relaxation, euphoria, lack of motivation, slowed time sensation, abrupt mood changes, impaired memory and attention, impaired judgement, reddened eyes, dry mouth, lack of coordination, decreased reflexes, tachycardia, increased appetite	Fatigue, paranoia, panic reactions, hallucinogen-like psychotic states	None except for rare insomnia, hyperactivity
Hallucinogens			
Lysergic acid diethylamide (LSD) Psilocybin (mushrooms) Dimethyltryptamine (DMT) Diethyltryptamine (DET) Methylenedioxy-amphetamine (MDA) Methylenedioxy-methamphetamine (MDMA, Ecstasy) Mescaline (peyote) Phencyclidine (PCP)	Perceptual distortions, hallucinations, delusions (PCP), depersonalization, heightened sensory perception, euphoria, mood swings, suspiciousness, panic, impaired judgement, increased body temperature, hypertension, flushed face, tremor, dilated pupils, constricted pupils (PCP), nystagmus (PCP), violence (PCP)	Prolonged effects and episodes, anxiety, panic, confusion, blurred vision, increases in blood pressure and temperature, seizures, coma, death (PCP), skeletal muscle contraction, dehydration, paranoia, psychosis	None

Continued

TABLE 11-7   EFFECTS OF FREQUENTLY USED SUBSTANCES—cont'd

Substance	Physiological and Psychological Effects	Effects of Overdose	Withdrawal Symptoms
Inhalants			
Aerosol propellants Fluorinated hydrocarbons Nitrous oxide (in deodorants, hairspray, pesticide, canned whipped cream, spray paint, cookware coating products) Solvents (gasoline, kerosene, nail polish remover, typewriter correction fluid, cleaning solutions, lighter fluid, paint, paint thinner, glue) Anaesthetic agents (nitrous oxide, chloroform) Nitrites (amyl nitrite, butyl nitrite)	Euphoria, decreased inhibitions, giddiness, slurred speech, illusions, drowsiness, clouded sensorium, tinnitus, nystagmus, dysrhythmias, cough, nausea, vomiting, diarrhea; irritation to eyes, nose, mouth	Anxiety, respiratory depression, cardiac dysrhythmias, loss of consciousness, sudden death, suicide	None

TABLE 11-8   ONSET, PEAK, DURATION, AND WITHDRAWAL ONSET OF ABUSED SUBSTANCES

Substance and Route	Onset	Peak	Duration	Onset of Withdrawal Symptoms
Inhaled				
Nicotine	Immediate	5 min.	5–15 min.	3–4 hr.
Marihuana	5–20 min.	30–60 min.	3–7 hr.	—
Cocaine	Immediate	5–30 min.	60 min.	9 hr.
Inhalants	Immediate	10–15 min.	20–45 min.	—
Intravenous				
Cocaine	Immediate	10–20 min.	20–30 min.	2 hr.
Opioids	Immediate	60–90 min.	2–4 hr.	8–10 hr.
Amphetamines	Immediate	10–20 min.	20–30 min.	2 hr.
Oral				
Alcohol	15–20 min.	60–90 min.	12–14 hr.	6–12 hr.
Amphetamines	10–30 min.	60–90 min.	2–4 hr.	8–10 hr.
Sedative–hypnotics	15–30 min.	2–4 hr.	4–12 hr.	12–16 hr.
Caffeine	10–20 min.	30 min	3–7 hr.	12–24 hr.
Opioids	30 min.	2 hr.	4–8 hr.	8–10 hr.
Intranasal				
Cocaine	3–5 min.	5–30 min.	2–4 hr.	4 hr.
Amphetamines	3–5 min.	5–20 min.	45 min.	2 hr.
Buccal				
Nicotine	10–15 min.	20–30 min.	30–60 min.	1–2 hr.

TABLE 11-9   CONSIDERATIONS FOR PATIENTS WITH PROBLEMATIC SUBSTANCE USE WHO ARE UNDERGOING SURGERY

- Standard amounts of anaesthetic and analgesic drugs may not be sufficient if patient is cross-tolerant.
- Anaesthetic agents may have a prolonged sedative effect if the patient has liver dysfunction. This situation necessitates an extended observation period.
- Patients have an increased susceptibility to cardiac and respiratory depression.
- Patients have an increased risk for bleeding, postoperative complications, and infection.
- Withdrawal symptoms from substances may be delayed for up to 5 days because of effects of anaesthetics and pain medications.
- Dosage of pain medications must be reduced gradually.

Special precautions must be taken for the patient who is intoxicated or alcohol dependent and requires surgery. The patient dependent on substances is at high risk for postoperative complications and death. Acute withdrawal and delirium tremens (DTs) may be triggered by the cessation of alcohol consumption. The patient who is alcohol dependent but is not currently drinking usually requires an increased level of anaesthesia because of cross-tolerance. The intoxicated individual needs a decreased level of anaesthesia because of the synergistic effect of the alcohol. Vital signs, including body temperature, must be closely monitored to identify signs of withdrawal, possible infections, and respiratory or cardiac problems (Marley, Calabrese, & Thompson, 2014).

A patient's pattern of use may be unknown at the time of elective surgery. Preoperative assessment must include a thorough health history and assessment of substance use, including questions related to alcohol, nicotine, and caffeine use (both nicotine and caffeine are discussed later in this chapter). Respiratory changes in smokers make introduction of endotracheal and suction tubes more difficult and increase the risk for postoperative respiratory problems. During the patient's surgical recovery period, the nurse should be alert for signs and symptoms of drug interactions with pain medications or anaesthesia or for signs of withdrawal. Postoperative headaches, for example, may be caused by caffeine withdrawal in heavy users. Special nursing considerations for the substance-abusing patient undergoing surgery are presented in Table 11-9.

Acute Pain Management Considerations. Health care providers may demonstrate reluctance to treat acute pain with opioid medications in people who use substances. However, it must be noted that the effective treatment of acute pain is a key priority for all people, including those who use substances. It is appropriate, therefore, to use opioid analgesia to help all people manage acute pain.

If the patient acknowledges opioid use, it is important to determine the types and the amounts of drug used. It is best to avoid exposing the patient to the drug of abuse, and effective equianalgesic doses of other opioids may be determined if daily drug doses are known. Severe pain should be treated with opioids. The use of one opioid is preferred, but nonopioid and adjuvant analgesics and nonpharmacological pain relief measures may also be used as appropriate. Withdrawal symptoms can exacerbate pain and lead to medication-seeking behaviour. To maintain opioid blood levels and prevent withdrawal symptoms, health care providers should provide analgesics around the clock. Supplemental doses should be used to treat breakthrough pain. For patients who abuse opioids to achieve adequate pain control, the nurse should advocate for these patients to receive much higher doses than those used in drug-naive patients.

STIMULANTS AND STIMULANT WITHDRAWAL

Substances in this category of agents stimulate the CNS and generally cause increased alertness, increased heart rate, and a sense of euphoria.

Withdrawal from cocaine and amphetamines does not usually cause obvious physical symptoms, but physical and behavioural manifestations do occur. Craving for the drug is intense during the first hours to days of drug cessation and may continue for weeks. The nurse may identify withdrawal symptoms in a patient dependent on cocaine or amphetamines who is hospitalized for management of other health problems. Nursing management of withdrawal symptoms is supportive and includes measures to decrease agitation and restlessness in the early phase and to allow the patient to sleep and eat as needed in later phases. Mild symptoms of stimulant withdrawal can also be experienced by the patient dependent on caffeine when meals and fluids are withheld before diagnostic testing or during a surgical experience. A nicotine replacement system should be provided for tobacco users to control symptoms of withdrawal when they are hospitalized.

NICOTINE

Characteristics

Nurses are likely to encounter patients with tobacco use disorder (TUD). Persons with TUD are dependent on the drug nicotine due to using tobacco products. Nicotine has a rapid onset of action, making it one of the most rapidly addicting substances of abuse. A number of products contain nicotine, including smoked tobacco (cigarettes, cigars, pipes), smokeless tobacco (chew, snuff, dip), and some electronic cigarettes. Smoking tobacco is the most popular form of tobacco use in Canada (Reid, Hammond, Rynard, et al., 2015); in 2013, 19% of the population over the age of 12 smoked daily or occasionally (Statistics Canada, 2013). Considering the magnitude and severity of the risks associated with nicotine dependence, it is crucial that nurses screen for and offer interventions for nicotine dependence.

Physiological Effects of Use

When nicotine is absorbed, it produces a wide range of effects in the peripheral nervous system and CNS. Responses include increased blood pressure, heart rate, cardiac output, coronary blood flow, and cutaneous vasoconstriction. During smoking, nicotine is absorbed quickly into the bloodstream and travels to the brain in a matter of seconds. In the brain, the action of nicotine on nicotinic receptors causes general CNS stimulation with increased alertness and arousal. The effects last about 1 to 2 hours before withdrawal symptoms occur, leaving the person feeling tired, irritable, and anxious. The need to have the "high" again makes the person crave more nicotine, leading to addiction. After withdrawal from nicotine, cue-induced relief craving may cause smoking relapse. The effects of nicotine are listed in Table 11-7.

Smoking tobacco is the most harmful method of nicotine use and injures nearly every organ in the body (Figure 11-2). Although those who use smokeless tobacco are at lower risk for lung disease, it is not without complications. Holding tobacco in the mouth is associated with periodontal disease and cancer of the mouth, cheek, tongue, throat, and esophagus (Centers for Disease Control and Prevention, 2015).

Electronic cigarettes resemble and feel like traditional cigarettes. These battery-operated devices turn nicotine and other chemicals, including propylene glycol, glycerin, and flavourings, into an aerosol or vapour. These devices do not contain tobacco. Emerging information indicates e-cigarettes are not harmless. E-cigarettes containing nicotine have the potential to increase the risk for cardiovascular and respiratory problems (Hajek, Etter, Benowitz, et al., 2014), and the liquid nicotine solutions used in refillable e-cigarettes may cause poisoning or skin irritation. Although e-cigarettes are thought to be harmful to health, they are likely to be substantially less harmful than tobacco cigarettes. However, the long-term health effects of vaping have not been examined and are therefore unknown at this time.

Health Complications

The complications of nicotine abuse are related to dose and method of ingestion. Cigarette smoking is the single most preventable cause of death. Cigarette smoking also causes chronic lung disease, cardiovascular disease, stroke, and cataracts. Smoking during pregnancy can cause stillbirth, low birth weight, sudden infant death syndrome (SIDS), and other serious pregnancy complications (Cui, Shooshtari, Forget, et al., 2014). In addition, many of these substances, such as carbon monoxide, tar, arsenic, and lead, are poisonous and toxic to the human body. Together with the increased myocardial oxygen consumption that nicotine causes, carbon monoxide significantly decreases the oxygen available to the myocardium. The result is an even greater increase in heart rate and myocardial oxygen consumption that may lead to myocardial ischemia.

The chronic respiratory irritation caused by cigarette smoke is the most important risk factor in the development of lung cancer and chronic obstructive pulmonary disease (COPD). Chronic irritation from smoking also is a factor in the increased incidence of cancer of the mouth, larynx, and esophagus in those who smoke tobacco in any form. Smokeless tobacco users also experience the systemic effects of nicotine on the cardiovascular system, increasing the risk for cardiovascular disease.

Women are at greater risk than men for smoking-related diseases. Women who smoke have almost double the risk of myocardial infarction than men and may also have nearly double the risk of lung cancer as men. Smoking in women is associated with greater menstrual bleeding and duration of dysmenorrhea as well as greater variability in menstrual cycle length. In addition, there is strong evidence that breast and cervical cancer risks are increased among women who smoke (American College of Obstetricians and Gynecologists, 2010).

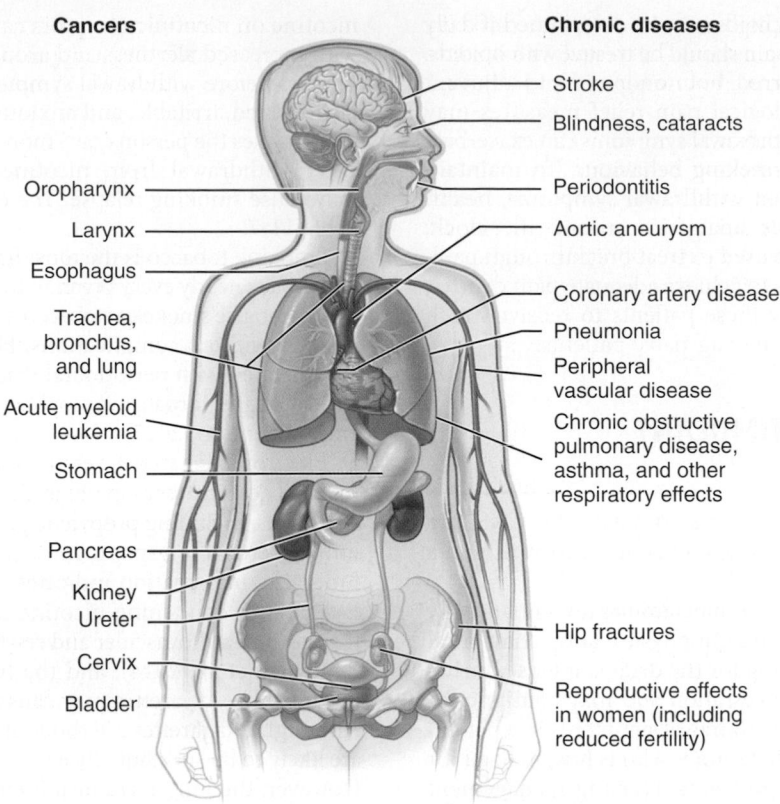

Cancers

Oropharynx
Larynx
Esophagus
Trachea, bronchus, and lung
Acute myeloid leukemia
Stomach
Pancreas
Kidney
Ureter
Cervix
Bladder

Chronic diseases

Stroke
Blindness, cataracts
Periodontitis
Aortic aneurysm
Coronary artery disease
Pneumonia
Peripheral vascular disease
Chronic obstructive pulmonary disease, asthma, and other respiratory effects
Hip fractures
Reproductive effects in women (including reduced fertility)

FIGURE 11-2 Health effects of smoking. Source: Samet, J. M. (2013). Tobacco smoking. *Thoracic Surgery Clinics, 23*(2), 103.

Collaborative Care: Nursing Interventions for Tobacco Use Disorder

A combination of medications, behavioural approaches, and support is believed to be most effective in addressing nicotine dependence and long-term tobacco cessation.

Tobacco Use Cessation. With each patient encounter, the nurse should ask about tobacco use, assess the person's level of motivation to change, and advise the person about the importance of quitting. The Registered Nurses' Association of Ontario (RNAO; 2007) algorithm "Ask, advise, assist, arrange" is an effective approach for working collaboratively with people with nicotine dependence. This approach identifies minimal and intensive clinical interventions that can be used at each patient encounter, depending on the time available (see the Resources at the end of this chapter). These interventions are designed to identify tobacco users, encourage them to quit, determine their willingness to quit, assist them in quitting, and arrange for follow-up to prevent relapse. Simply screening for and assessing for smoking has significant impact as an intervention to help people quit smoking. Smoking cessation is the single most effective intervention to increase quality of life and decrease the morbidity and mortality directly caused by smoking. The Tobacco Free RNAO website contains many resources that nurses can use to help patients quit smoking (see the Resources at the end of this chapter).

Nicotine Replacement Therapy and Pharmacotherapeutic Interventions for Nicotine Dependence. A variety of smoking cessation products are available to help support users in quitting, including prescription medicines as well as OTC products such as nicotine patches, inhalers, and gum. Nicotine replacement therapy (NRT) products are one type of smoking cessation solution. These products reduce the craving and withdrawal symptoms associated with cessation by supplying the body with smaller amounts of nicotine (Table 11-10). Because most health care facilities are tobacco-free environments, admitted patients who are addicted to nicotine may experience withdrawal symptoms since they are unable to smoke. Offering NRT to those who desire it will assist in controlling withdrawal symptoms during hospitalization and promote continued cessation after discharge.

Non-nicotine products also play a role in helping users quit. Varenicline (Champix) is a drug used to aid smoking cessation. Varenicline is unique in that it has both agonist and antagonist actions. Its agonist activity at one subtype of nicotinic receptor provides some nicotine effects to ease withdrawal symptoms. If the person does resume smoking, its antagonist action blocks the effects of nicotine at another subtype of nicotinic receptor, making smoking less enjoyable. Bupropion (Zyban), an antidepressant drug, reduces the urge to smoke, reduces some symptoms of withdrawal, and helps prevent weight gain associated with smoking cessation. Product manufacturers advise that these products should be used with counselling and that physicians and patients should consider using NRT before non-nicotine products (Government of Canada, 2013a).

Along with using a smoking cessation product, users who wish to quit are more likely to succeed if they participate in a tobacco cessation program. Nurses should be aware of community resources that assist users who are motivated to quit. Many programs teach users to avoid high-risk situations for smoking relapse and help them develop coping skills, such as cigarette refusal skills, assertiveness, alternative activities, and peer support systems.

The advice and motivation provided by health care providers can be a powerful force in smoking cessation. *Best Practice Guidelines on Smoking Cessation*, available on RNAO's website, is an excellent resource for the nurse helping patients to quit smoking: see Appendix D, "The Benefits of Quitting Smoking"; Appendix H, "Ask, Advise, Assist, Arrange Protocol"; and Appendix L, "Quit Smoking: First-Line Medications Compared." A link to this document appears in the Resources at the end of this chapter. Table 11-11 lists inpatient tobacco cessation interventions.

COCAINE AND OTHER STIMULANTS

Characteristics

In 2013, 0.9% of Canadians reported using cocaine or crack within the past year (Government of Canada, 2013b). The most common method of cocaine use is intranasal (snorting), but it may be smoked as "crack" cocaine (Figure 11-3) or in "freebase" form, injected intravenously, taken orally, or absorbed through mucous membranes. It must be manipulated either by placing it in a pipe to smoke it or by melting it down with a heat source and then adding liquid for the purpose of intravenous use.

The different types of amphetamines and related drugs such as methylphenidate are stimulant drugs that speed up the CNS. Stimulants may be prescribed for treatment of narcolepsy or attention deficit disorders and for weight control. However, methamphetamine and smokable methamphetamine crystals ("crystal meth," "ice") are in great demand on the street. These drugs act like the hormone adrenalin, which is a natural stimulant. Other drugs with similar effects include cocaine, Ecstasy, ephedrine, and caffeine. In 2013, 1% of Canadians aged 15 years and

---

TABLE 11-10 CARING FOR THE PATIENT WITH TOBACCO USE DISORDER

The Five *A*s for Users Who Desire to Quit	The Five *R*s for Users Unwilling to Quit
1. **Ask:** Identify all tobacco users at every contact. a. "Have you used any form of tobacco in the past 6 months?" b. "Do you smoke (even a puff now and again) or use tobacco products of any kind?" c. "Have you ever considered stopping?" 2. **Advise:** Strongly urge all tobacco users to quit. a. "As your nurse, the most important advice I can give you is to quit smoking." 3. **Assess:** Determine willingness to make a quit attempt. 4. **Assist:** Develop a plan with the patient to help the patient quit (e.g., counselling, medication). 5. **Arrange:** Schedule follow-up or refer patient to smoking cessation program.	1. **Relevance:** Ask the patient to indicate why quitting is personally relevant (e.g., health). 2. **Risks:** Ask the patient to identify his or her potential risks consequences of tobacco use. 3. **Rewards:** Ask the patient to identify potential benefits of stopping tobacco use. 4. **Roadblocks:** Ask patient to identify barriers or impediments to quitting. 5. **Repetition:** Repeat process every clinic visit.

Source: Agency for Healthcare Research and Quality. (2008). *AHCPR supported clinical practice guideline: Treating tobacco use and dependence: 2008 update.* Washington, DC: U.S. Public Health Service; and Registered Nurses Association of Ontario. (2007). *Best practice guideline: Integrating smoking cessation into nursing practice.* Toronto: Author. Retrieved from *http://rnao.ca/bpg/guidelines/integrating -smoking-cessation-daily-nursing-practice*.

TABLE 11-11 INPATIENT TOBACCO CESSATION INTERVENTIONS

Take the following steps for every hospitalized patient:
1. Ask each patient on admission if he or she uses tobacco, and document tobacco use status.
2. For current tobacco users, list tobacco use status on the admission problem list and as a discharge diagnosis.
3. Use counselling and medication to help all tobacco users maintain abstinence and to treat withdrawal symptoms.
4. Provide advice and assistance on how to quit during hospitalization and remain abstinent after discharge.
5. Arrange for follow-up regarding smoking status. Supportive contact should be provided for at least a month after discharge.

Source: Agency for Healthcare Research and Quality. (2008). *AHCPR supported clinical practice guideline: Treating tobacco use and dependence: 2008 update.* Washington, DC: U.S. Public Health Service.

FIGURE 11-3 A, Powder cocaine, which can be easily snorted or injected. **B,** Crack cocaine, a chalklike derivative of cocaine whereby cocaine is mixed with other substances such as baking soda. Source: A, Tatiana Popova/Shutterstock.com; B, Kevin L Chesson/Shutterstock.com.

older reported using a stimulant (including those prescribed for attention deficit disorder) in the past 12 months. Sixteen percent of people who used stimulants reported abusing them. The rate of abuse for youth aged 15 to 19 was 32% (20 000), and for young adults aged 20 to 24, 40% (14 000) (Government of Canada, 2013b).

Effects of Use

All stimulants work in part by increasing the amount of dopamine in the brain, producing euphoria and increasing energy and alertness. This action on the brain reward system magnifies pleasure and leads to rapid dependence. Cocaine and other stimulants also affect the peripheral nervous system and the cardiovascular system. Amphetamines are similar to cocaine and produce euphoria, hyperactivity, and increased heart rate and blood pressure. Initial use results in increased alertness, improved performance, relief of fatigue, and anorexia. As with cocaine use, amphetamines used over time may lead to irritability, anxiety, paranoia, and hostile and violent behaviours. Additional physical and psychological effects are presented in Table 11-12.

Smoking and intravenous (IV) methods result in the fastest absorption and the highest "rush." Effects of cocaine use are short, which is the main reason people who use cocaine are compelled to seek out and purchase more and more cocaine throughout the day to sustain the euphoric effects and why a great deal of money can be spent on cocaine over a short period of use. During periods of use, the person may not be sleeping, eating, or performing self-care. Amphetamines have a longer half-life than cocaine and, because they are usually taken orally,

have a longer effect. Patients with stimulant toxicity present with *sympathetic overdrive* (increased stimulation of the sympathetic nervous system). The patient experiences restlessness, hypervigilance, agitated delirium, impaired judgement, and paranoia with psychotic symptoms. Table 11-12 describes the effects of cocaine and amphetamine use.

Withdrawal

Cocaine withdrawal is usually accompanied by intense dysphoria, fatigue, and irritability. In the first 9 hours to 14 days, withdrawal is characterized by intense craving and cocaine-seeking behaviour. There is marked agitation, feelings of depression, exhaustion, and a need to sleep. Eventually mood is stabilized, but a desire to return to the drug, especially prompted by cue-induced craving, remains for a long period of time.

Abrupt cessation of stimulants can lead to a "crash." The patient may be depressed and experience fatigue, prolonged sleep, vivid dreams, irritability, increased appetite, and disorientation. Supportive care includes maintaining a quiet environment and allowing the patient to sleep and eat as desired. If a patient has severe depression, the nurse should initiate suicide precautions and refer for further treatment.

Complications

Routes of administration have important health complications. IV administration may result in collapse and scarring of the veins at the injection site, cellulitis, wound abscess, endocarditis, hepatitis B virus (HBV) and hepatitis C virus (HCV) infection, and human immunodeficiency virus (HIV) infection. With intranasal use, the nasal septum and mucosa may be damaged, and frequent sniffing and rhinitis are common signs of chronic intranasal use. Pulmonary damage from smoking crack may be apparent as evidenced by black or dark brown sputum and a form of pneumonia known as "crack lung." Bilateral loss of eyebrow and eyelash hair may occur during "freebasing." Dental caries and loose or broken teeth are also frequently seen as a consequence of using cocaine by any route.

A *stimulant psychosis* may occur with the chronic use of any stimulant. A cocaine psychosis usually progresses from paranoid delusions to visual hallucinations of "snow lights" (coloured lights perceived when cocaine is administered) and tactile hallucinations of bugs crawling under the skin. Skin excoriations from scratching; needle marks; and elevated blood pressure, heart rate, and temperature are findings that help differentiate a stimulant psychosis from schizophrenia.

Collaborative Care

Emergency management of cocaine intoxication will depend on the findings at the time of treating the patient and may be complicated by the possibility that the patient has combined cocaine use with that of heroin, alcohol, or phencyclidine hydrochloride (PCP). Symptoms of cocaine and stimulant toxicity and emergency management are presented in Table 11-13.

CAFFEINE

Characteristics

Caffeine is the most widely used psychoactive substance in the world and, in most people, can be safely used to promote alertness and alleviate fatigue. Although weaker than other stimulant drugs, caffeine shares their characteristics of intoxication, tolerance, and withdrawal symptoms with regular and consistent patterns.

TABLE 11-12	EFFECTS OF COCAINE AND AMPHETAMINE USE	
	Early Effects	**Long-Term Effects**
Central nervous system	Excitation, euphoria, restlessness, talkativeness	Depression, hallucinations, tremors, visual disturbances, seizures, headache, insomnia, stroke
Cardiovascular system	Tachycardia, hypertension, angina, dysrhythmias, palpitations	Dysrhythmias, hypotension, heart failure, myocardial infarction, cardiomyopathy
Respiratory system	Increased respiratory rate, dyspnea, chest pain, epistaxis	Chronic cough, inflamed throat, congestion of lungs, brown or black sputum production, pneumonia, respiratory distress and/or arrest, pulmonary edema, rhinorrhea, rhinitis, erosion and perforation of the nasal septum
Reproductive system	Heightened sexual desire, delayed orgasm and ejaculation; women may have difficulty achieving orgasm	Difficulty maintaining erection and ejaculating; loss of interest in sexual activity; women may develop aberrant sexual behaviour
Gastro-intestinal system	Decreased appetite	Dehydration, weight loss, nausea; intestinal ischemia may cause gangrenous bowel
Psychological	Behaviour changes or mood swings	Depression or suicidal thoughts

TABLE 11-13 EMERGENCY MANAGEMENT

Cocaine and Amphetamine Toxicity

Etiology	Assessment Findings	Interventions
Intranasal, inhalation, parenteral, oral, vaginal, rectal, or sublingual administration of cocaine; oral or parenteral administration of amphetamines	**Cardiovascular** • Palpitations • Tachycardia • Hypertension • Dysrhythmias • Myocardial ischemia or infarction **Central Nervous System** • Feeling of impending doom • Euphoria • Agitation • Combativeness • Seizures • Hallucinations • Confusion • Paranoia • Fever **Other** • Track marks • Consumption of bags of cocaine	**Initial** • Ensure patent airway • Anticipate need for intubation if respiratory distress evident • Establish IV access and initiate fluid replacement as appropriate • Obtain a 12-lead ECG • Treat ventricular dysrhythmias as appropriate with lidocaine, bretylium, or procainamide • Administer IV haloperidol for psychosis • Administer IV diazepam (Valium) or lorazepam (Ativan) for seizures • Naloxone IV should be given if CNS depression is present and concurrent opiate use is suspected • Anticipate the need for propranolol (Inderal) or labetalol for hypertension and tachycardia **Ongoing** • Monitor vital signs, level of consciousness, cardiac rhythm • Use restraints only if needed to protect the patient and staff

CNS, central nervous system; *ECG*, electrocardiogram; *IV*, intravenous.

The consumption of energy drinks high in caffeine content among children and youth is a growing health concern. In addition to being a component of many beverages, caffeine is found in numerous prescription and OTC analgesics, stimulants, appetite suppressants, and cold and flu preparations.

Effects of Use

Caffeine is a relatively weak CNS stimulant. It is a diuretic and a myocardial stimulant. It relaxes smooth muscles, promotes vasodilation, constricts cerebral arteries, increases gastric acid secretion, and enhances contraction of skeletal muscles. Oral doses of 200 mg (two cups of coffee) can elevate mood, produce insomnia, increase irritability, cause anxiety, and offset fatigue. Heavy intake of 500 mg or more per day is known to cause intoxication manifested by nervousness, insomnia, gastric hyperacidity, muscle twitching, confusion, tachycardia or cardiac dysrhythmias, and psychomotor agitation. The effects of caffeine are presented in Table 11-7.

Physical and psychological dependence on caffeine have been found with chronic use of more than 500 mg/day. However, dependence may occur in some individuals at lower doses, especially in children and youth who have smaller body mass. The most commonly reported withdrawal symptoms are headache, irritability, drowsiness, and fatigue that occur within 12 to 24 hours following abstinence (see Table 11-7). Caffeine withdrawal may be responsible for some cases of headache that occur after general anaesthesia.

Complications

Habitual caffeine users are reported to have slightly higher blood pressure, heart rates, and basal metabolic rates (see Table 11-7). Because symptoms of chronic use develop gradually, most people with caffeine dependence do not link sleep disruption, anxiety, and other symptoms with caffeine intake. Women with high consumption of caffeine are at particular risk for loss of bone mineral density, a risk for the development of osteoporosis later in life. In toxic doses, caffeine influences behaviour patterns and may precipitate panic states.

Collaborative Care

Management of the patient with symptoms of caffeine dependence includes assisting the patient to gradually reduce or stop the intake of caffeine. A list of caffeinated products itemizing their caffeine content may be helpful to the patient who quits coffee only to unknowingly substitute other foods and beverages containing caffeine. Substituting decaffeinated beverages may also help. Toxic reactions to caffeine and lethal doses of caffeine are managed symptomatically, with attention to maintaining respirations and controlling hypertension, dysrhythmias, and seizures.

DEPRESSANTS

Substances classified as depressants have common physiological effects and include alcohol, sedatives, hypnotics, and opioids. Depressants are also widely recognized for their abuse potential, which leads to rapid development of tolerance, dependence, and medical emergencies involving overdose and withdrawal.

ALCOHOL

Characteristics

Alcohol is the most widely consumed substance of abuse in North America. In Canada, 76% of the population aged 15 and older drink alcohol (Government of Canada, 2013b). The use of alcohol, whether by occasional drinkers or by those who are alcohol dependent, is linked to negative consequences, including automobile accidents, arrests, violence, poor job performance, trauma, and associated injuries requiring emergency intervention.

Alcohol dependence is currently viewed as a chronic, progressive, potentially fatal condition if left untreated. Numerous factors appear to be interrelated in the development of alcohol dependence and may include genetic and biological factors, psychosocial factors, and cultural–environmental background. Alcohol dependence generally occurs over a period of years and may be preceded by heavy social drinking.

Health teaching about the risks associated with consuming more than the recommended low-risk drinking guidelines (Table 11-14) is essential. Although there is evidence of the health benefits of consuming wine, it must be noted that the health benefits are associated with low consumption of one standard drink (142 mL [5 oz.] glass of 12% alcohol wine), and, in fact, consumption of more than this amount is associated with adverse health risks such as increased risk for hypertension and cardiovascular disease.

Effects of Use

Alcohol affects almost all cells of the body and has complex effects on the neurons in the CNS, leading to slowed respirations and heart rate; it also affects memory, judgement, and coordination (Mukherjee, 2013). Absorption is slower in the presence of water or food, especially proteins and fats. Faster absorption occurs when alcohol is mixed with carbonated liquids. Canada's low-risk drinking guidelines (see Table 11-14) recommend that women limit consumption to 10 standard drinks per week, with no more than two drinks per day most days and that men limit consumption to no more than 15 standard drinks per week, with no more than three drinks per day most days.

The effects of alcohol are related to the blood alcohol concentration (BAC) in the body and individual susceptibility. Alcohol is measurable in the blood within 15 to 20 minutes of ingestion, peaks in 60 to 90 minutes, and is excreted in 12 to 24 hours. BAC is affected by the amount consumed, the drinking rate, body size and composition, drink concentration, and hormones (Table 11-15). As such, children and youth who have lower body mass are more susceptible to the effects of alcohol. People who have developed high tolerance to the effects of alcohol have greater risk for complicated withdrawal from alcohol that can lead to seizures and death.

Alcohol Intoxication

Intoxication, as evidenced by increasing BAC, results in behavioural and physical changes (see Table 11-15). Behavioural effects may include relaxation, sedation, disinhibition, aggression, impaired judgement, irritability, euphoria, depression, and emotional lability. Physical signs include slurred speech, lack of motor coordination, nystagmus, and flushing resulting from dilation of peripheral blood vessels. Disturbances in memory and blackouts may occur in dependent drinkers. People are at higher risk for self-injurious behaviours while intoxicated, as a result of impaired judgement and impulsivity. People are also at risk for significant mood dysregulation and depression, and risk for suicide is an important consideration. Fatalities caused by drinking and driving, head injuries, physical trauma, and violence are closely linked to alcohol intoxication.

Acute Alcohol Intoxication. It is important to obtain as accurate a history as possible, using collateral information as necessary, and assess for injuries, trauma, diseases, and hypoglycemia. Patients with alcohol intoxication may also be hypoglycemic from a lack of food intake. Vital signs and level of consciousness should be monitored. Generally, the heart

---

TABLE 11-14   CANADA'S LOW-RISK DRINKING GUIDELINES

Drinking is a personal choice. If you choose to drink, these guidelines can help you decide when, where, why, and how much.

Guideline 1
Reduce your long-term health risks by drinking no more than:
- 10 drinks per week for women, with no more than two drinks per day most days
- 15 drinks per week for men, with no more than three drinks per day most days
Plan nondrinking days every week to avoid developing a habit.

Guideline 2
Reduce your risk for injury and harm by drinking no more than three drinks (for women) and four drinks (for men) on any single occasion.
Plan to drink in a safe environment. Stay within the weekly limits outlined in Guideline 1.

Guideline 3
Do not drink when you are:
- Driving a vehicle or using machinery and tools
- Taking medicine or other drugs that interact with alcohol
- Doing any kind of dangerous physical activity
- Living with mental or physical health problems
- Living with alcohol dependence
- Pregnant or planning to be pregnant
- Responsible for the safety of others
- Making important decisions

Guideline 4
If you are pregnant or planning to become pregnant, or if you are about to breastfeed, the safest choice is to drink no alcohol at all.

Guideline 5
If you are a child or youth, you should delay drinking until your late teens. Talk with your parents about drinking. Alcohol can harm the way your brain and body develop.
If you are drinking, plan ahead, follow local alcohol laws, and stay within the limits outlined in Guideline 1.

Defining "a Drink"
For these guidelines, "a drink" means:
- 341 mL (12 oz.) bottle of 5% alcohol beer, cider, or cooler
- 142 mL (5 oz.) glass of 12% alcohol wine
- 43 mL (1.5 oz.) serving of 40% distilled alcohol (e.g., rye, rum, gin)
Low-risk drinking helps to promote a culture of moderation.
Low-risk drinking supports healthy lifestyles.

Tips
Set limits for yourself and abide by them.
Drink slowly. Have no more than two drinks in any three hours.
For every drink of alcohol, have one nonalcoholic drink.
Eat before and while you are drinking.
Always consider your age, body weight, and health problems that might suggest lower limits.
Although drinking may provide health benefits for certain groups of people, do not start to drink, or increase your drinking, for health benefits.

Source: Butt, P., Beirness, D., Gliksman, L., et al. (2011). *Alcohol and health in Canada: A summary of evidence and guidelines for low-risk drinking.* Ottawa, ON: Canadian Centre on Substance Abuse.

---

rate is normal in uncomplicated intoxication but elevated in withdrawal.

The nurse should remain with the patient as much as possible, orienting to reality as necessary. Agitation and anxiety are common, and the patient should be assessed for increasing

TABLE 11-15 BLOOD ALCOHOL CONCENTRATION AND RELATED EFFECTS

BAC* (mmol/L)	Psychophysiological Effect
4.3	Light and moderate drinkers begin to feel some effects. Approximate BAC is reached after one drink.†
8.7	Most people begin to feel relaxed.
13.0	Judgement is mildly impaired. People are less able to make rational decisions about their capabilities (e.g., driving skills).
17.4	Definite impairment of muscle coordination and driving skills occurs. Person is legally intoxicated according to Canada's *Criminal Code*.‡
21.7	Clear deterioration of reaction time and control is observed. Person is legally intoxicated in most provinces and territories. Some provinces permit slightly higher levels than those permitted by the federal government.
26.0	Vomiting occurs unless this level is reached slowly.
32.6	Balance and movement are impaired. Equivalent of one-half pint of whisky is circulating in the bloodstream.
65.1	Many people lose consciousness.
86.8	Most people lose consciousness, and some die. For 50% of adult humans, 86.8 mmol/L is the accepted lethal dose.§
97.7	Breathing stops; person eventually dies.

BAC, blood alcohol concentration.
*BAC is generally recorded in millimoles per litre (mmol/L) of blood. BAC is dependent on how much alcohol is consumed, how fast it is consumed, and the person's weight.
†One drink is 341 mL beer, 142 mL wine, or 43 mL distilled spirits, all of which provide the same amount of alcohol.
‡Canada Safety Council. (2009). *Canada's blood alcohol laws among the strictest in the Western world.* Retrieved from http://canadasafetycouncil.org/news/canada-s-blood-alcohol-laws-among-strictest-western-world; provincial and territorial blood alcohol limits for drivers vary.
§Dalawari, P. (2014). Ethanol level. Retrieved from http://emedicine.medscape.com/article/2090019-overview#a1.

TABLE 11-16 STAGES OF ALCOHOL WITHDRAWAL

Time of Appearance After Alcohol Last Used	Symptoms
6–12 hours	Minor withdrawal symptoms: insomnia, tremors, anxiety, gastro-intestinal upset, headache, diaphoresis, palpitations, anorexia, nausea, tachycardia, hypertension
12–14 hours	Visual, auditory, or tactile hallucinations
24–48 hours	Withdrawal seizures: generalized tonic–clonic seizures
48–72 hours	Alcohol-withdrawal delirium (delirium tremens): hallucinations (predominantly visual), disorientation, agitation, diaphoresis

Source: Sachdeva, A., Choudhary, M., & Chandra, M. (2015). Alcohol withdrawal syndrome: Benzodiazepines and beyond. *Journal of Clinical and Diagnostic Research, 9*(9), VE01–VE07. doi:10.7980/JCDR/2015/13407.6538.

belligerence and a potential for violence. The patient is also at high risk for injury because of lack of coordination and impaired judgement, and protective measures should be used. It is critical to continue assessment and interventions until the BAC has decreased to at least 21.7 mmol/L and until any associated disorders or injuries have been ruled out.

Alcohol Withdrawal

If there is any indication of alcohol or other CNS-depressant use when a patient is hospitalized, the nurse should always question when the patient last used the substance. This information will help the nurse anticipate drug interactions or the time of possible onset of withdrawal symptoms. After excessive drinking, individuals may experience hangovers manifested by malaise, nausea, headache, thirst, and a general feeling of fatigue.

A patient with alcohol dependence who is hospitalized for other health conditions often develops alcohol withdrawal when the ingestion of alcohol is abruptly stopped. The signs and symptoms of alcohol withdrawal generally begin 6 to 12 hours after the patient's last drink and may last for 3 to 5 days. Characteristic symptoms include tremulousness, anxiety, increased heart rate, increased blood pressure, sweating, nausea, vomiting, hyper-reflexia, agitation, and insomnia. The most common severe manifestations are hallucinations and seizures. Seizures are most likely to occur 24 to 48 hours after the last drink in untreated alcohol withdrawal (Table 11-16). Alcohol-withdrawal delirium is a serious and potentially lethal complication that usually has its onset 48 to 72 hours after the last drink. Delirium components include disorientation, visual or auditory hallucinations, and agitation. Death may be caused by hyperthermia, peripheral vascular collapse, or cardiac failure.

Key nursing intervention and management of alcohol withdrawal is based on early and accurate assessment. Nurses should assess for tachycardia, dehydration, fever, diaphoresis, dysrhythmias, and liver impairment, in addition to cognition and level of consciousness. The Clinical Institute Withdrawal Assessment for Alcohol Scale, Revised (Table 11-17) is a standardized assessment tool that can be used to assess and monitor for withdrawal symptoms caused by alcohol withdrawal. Treatment of intermediate withdrawal usually involves the administration of a benzodiazepine (chlordiazepoxide, diazepam, lorazepam, and oxazepam are most commonly used) to prevent withdrawal-related seizure (Sachdeva, Choudhary, & Chandra, 2015). If the person has compromised liver function or is an older adult, a short-acting benzodiazepine may be preferred (Hammond, Niciu, Drew, et al., 2015). A recent report suggests that non-benzodiazepine anticonvulsant drugs may be beneficial (Hammond, Niciu, Drew, et al., 2015).

A quiet, calm environment is important to prevent exacerbation of symptoms. The use of restraints and IV lines should be avoided whenever possible. Supportive care is needed to ensure adequate rest and nutrition. Nursing care for the patient in alcohol withdrawal is presented in Nursing Care Plan 11-1.

Complications

Physical complications of chronic alcohol abuse are outlined in Table 11-18 and are frequently the reasons that alcohol-dependent individuals seek health care. Complications may also arise from the interaction of alcohol with commonly prescribed or OTC drugs. Drugs that interact with alcohol in an additive manner include antihypertensives, antihistamines, antianginals, and salicylates (Aspirin). Alcohol taken with Aspirin may cause or exacerbate gastro-intestinal (GI) bleeding. Alcohol taken with acetaminophen (Tylenol) may increase the risk for liver damage. Potentiation, a drug interaction causing a response greater than the sum of the individual responses to each drug, occurs when

TABLE 11-17 CLINICAL INSTITUTE WITHDRAWAL ASSESSMENT FOR ALCOHOL (CIWA)

Patient Name:_____ (Last Name, First Name)
Time:_____ Total Score (max score=67)_____ Temp: _____BP:____/____ Apex rate:_____ Resps:_____ Initials:____
_____ (print name and credentials) (signature)
(dd/mm/yyyy):_____ F0136-20100721 Chart Tab: Assessments/Plans Patient ID Label

Nausea & Vomiting

Ask: "Do you feel sick to your stomach? Have you vomited?" *Observation:*

0 No nausea/vomiting
1
2
3
4 Intermittent nausea with dry heaves
5
6
7 Constant nausea, frequent dry heaves and vomiting

Tremor

Arms extended and fingers spread apart.
  Observation:
0 No tremor
1 Not visible, but can be felt fingertip to fingertip
2
3
4 Moderate, with patient's arms extended
5
6
7 Severe, even with arms not extended

Paroxysmal Sweats

Observation:
0 No sweat visible
1 Barely perceptible sweating, palms moist
2
3
4 Beads of sweat obvious on forehead
5
6
7 Drenching sweats

Anxiety

Ask: "Do you feel nervous?" *Observation:*
0 No anxiety, at ease
1 Mildly anxious
2
3
4 Moderately anxious, or guarded, so anxiety is
  inferred
5
6
7 Acute panic as seen in severe delirium or acute
  schizophrenic reactions

Agitation

Observation:
0 Normal activity
1 Somewhat more than normal activity
2
3
4 Moderately fidgety and restless
5
6
7 Paces back and forth during most of interview, or
  constantly thrashes about

Tactile Disturbances

Ask: "Have you any itching, pins and needles sensations, any burning, any numbness, or do you feel bugs crawling on or under your skin?" *Observation:*

0 None
1 Very mild itching, pins and needles, burning or numbness
2 Mild itching, pins and needles, burning or numbness
3 Moderate itching, pins and needles, burning or numbness
4 Moderately severe hallucinations
5 Severe hallucinations
6 Extremely severe hallucinations
7 Continuous hallucinations

Auditory Disturbances

Ask: "Are you more aware of sounds around you? Are they harsh? Do they frighten you? Are you hearing anything that is disturbing to you? Are you hearing things you know are not there?" *Observation:*

0 Not present
1 Very mild harshness or ability to frighten
2 Mild harshness or ability to frighten
3 Moderate harshness or ability to frighten
4 Moderately severe hallucinations
5 Severe hallucinations
6 Extremely severe hallucinations
7 Continuous hallucinations

Visual Disturbances

Ask: "Does the light appear to be too bright? Is its colour different? Does it hurt your eyes? Are you seeing anything that is disturbing to you? Are you seeing things you know are not there?" *Observation:*

0 Not present
1 Very mild sensitivity
2 Mild sensitivity
3 Moderate sensitivity
4 Moderately severe hallucinations
5 Severe hallucinations
6 Extremely severe hallucinations
7 Continuous hallucinations

Headache, Fullness in Head

Ask: "Does your head feel different? Does it feel like there is a band around your head?" Do not rate for dizziness or lightheadedness. Otherwise, rate severity.

0 Not present
1 Very mild
2 Mild
3 Moderate
4 Moderately severe
5 Severe
6 Very severe
7 Extremely severe

Orientation & Clouding of Sensorium

Ask: "What day is this? Where are you? Who am I?" *Observation:*
0 Oriented and can do serial additions
1 Cannot do serial additions or is uncertain about date
2 Disoriented for date by no more than 2 calendar days
3 Disoriented for date by more than 2 calendar days
4 Disoriented for place and/or person

Source: Brands, B., Kahan, M., Selby, P., et al. (Eds.). (2000). *Management of alcohol, tobacco and other drug problems: A physician's manual* (p. 77). Toronto: Centre for Addiction and Mental Health.

NURSING CARE PLAN 11-1

Alcohol Withdrawal

NURSING DIAGNOSIS	**Risk for injury** as evidenced by *alteration in psychomotor functioning* (sensorimotor deficits)
Expected Patient Outcomes	**Nursing Interventions and *Rationales***
• Reports no falls or injuries • Experiences decrease in tremors and psychomotor activity • Reports no seizures • Verbalizes risk for injury associated with alcohol use before discharge	• Assess for risk factors such as impaired mobility (e.g., unsteady gait), sensory deficits, tremors, impaired judgement, confusion, seizure activity *to plan appropriate preventive measures.* • Assess for signs of injury such as lacerations, bruises, or burns *to treat appropriately.* • Monitor vital signs frequently, especially heart rate, *because prompt recognition of extreme autonomic nervous system response is necessary for early intervention to prevent progression of symptoms.* • Administer benzodiazepines as ordered *to control hyperactivity*, thiamine *to reduce neurological complications (e.g., Wernicke's encephalopathy)*, and antiseizure medications as ordered *to prevent seizures.* • Use seizure precautions *to prevent injury.*
NURSING DIAGNOSIS	**Acute confusion** related to *substance misuse* as evidenced by *alteration in cognitive functioning, misperception, agitation, hallucinations* related to *sensory overload* as evidenced by *impaired interpretation of environmental stimuli, disorientation, and hallucinations*
Expected Patient Outcomes	**Nursing Interventions and *Rationales***
• Reports no hallucinations • Remains oriented to person, place, and time	• Assess patient's orientation and cognition *to determine appropriate interventions.* • Provide quiet and nonstimulating environment *to reduce external stimuli and calm overactive CNS.* • Orient to nurse and environment with each contact; use calm, approach; provide consistent staff; explain procedures and what is expected *to assist in orientation and decrease anxiety.* • Administer benzodiazepines as ordered *to reduce CNS stimulation.* • Administer antipsychotic medication (e.g., haloperidol [Haldol]) if ordered *to decrease severity of hallucinations.* (Be aware that Haldol lowers the seizure threshold.)
NURSING DIAGNOSIS	**Ineffective breathing pattern** related to *hyperventilation and respiratory muscle fatigue*
Expected Patient Outcomes	**Nursing Interventions and *Rationales***
• Maintains effective breathing • Reports no indications of hypoxia	• Monitor respiratory rate, depth, and pattern *so appropriate interventions may be taken.* • Position patient on side and in semi-Fowler's position *to reduce possibility of aspiration and to enhance lung expansion by lowering diaphragm.* • Monitor effects of medications given for withdrawal *to detect respiratory depression.* • Encourage coughing and deep breathing *to prevent complications of hypoventilation.* • Administer supplemental oxygen *to treat hypoxia.*

CNS, central nervous system.

TABLE 11-18 EFFECTS OF CHRONIC ALCOHOL ABUSE

Body System	System Effects
Central nervous system	Alcoholic dementia; Wernicke's encephalopathy (confusion, nystagmus, paralysis of ocular muscles, ataxia); Korsakoff syndrome (confabulation, amnesic disorder); impairment of cognitive function, psychomotor skills, abstract thinking, and memory; depression, attention deficit, labile moods, seizures, sleep disturbances
Peripheral nervous system	Peripheral neuropathy including pain, paresthesias, weakness
Immune system	Increased risk for tuberculosis and viral infections, especially pneumonia; increased risk for cancer of oral cavity, pharynx, esophagus, liver, colon, rectum, and possibly breast
Hematological system	Bone marrow depression, anemia, leukopenia, thrombocytopenia, blood clotting abnormalities
Musculo-skeletal system	Painful or tender swelling of large muscle groups; painless progressive muscle weakness and wasting; osteoporosis
Cardiovascular system	Elevated pulse and blood pressure; decreased exercise tolerance; cardiomyopathy (irreversible); increased risk for hemorrhagic stroke, coronary artery disease, hypertension, sudden cardiac death
Hepatic system	Steatosis (reversible)—nausea, vomiting, hepatomegaly; alcoholic hepatitis (reversible)—anorexia, nausea, vomiting, fever, chills, abdominal pain, cirrhosis; cancer
Gastro-intestinal system	Gastritis, peptic ulcer, esophagitis, esophageal varices, enteritis, colitis, Mallory–Weiss tear, pancreatitis
Digestive system	Decreased appetite, indigestion, malabsorption, vitamin deficiencies
Urinary system	Diuretic effect from inhibition of antidiuretic hormone
Endocrine and reproductive system	Altered gonadal function, testicular atrophy, decreased beard growth, decreased libido, diminished sperm count, gynecomastia, glucose intolerance, early menopause, fetal alcohol spectrum disorder
Integumentary system	Palmar erythema, spider angiomas, rosacea, rhinophyma

an additional CNS depressant is taken with alcohol, increasing the effect. Heavy drinkers may be tolerant (require an increased dose for effect) to other depressant drugs such as benzodiazepines or opioids, even if they have never used these drugs. This is called **cross-tolerance**.

Complications Associated With Chronic Alcoholism. One complication of chronic alcohol abuse is **Wernicke's encephalopathy**, an inflammatory, hemorrhagic, degenerative condition of the brain. Wernicke's encephalopathy is caused by a thiamine deficiency resulting from poor diet and alcohol-induced suppression of thiamine absorption. Because Wernicke's encephalopathy is potentially reversible, IV thiamine is often administered to intoxicated patients. Untreated or progressive Wernicke's encephalopathy may lead to **Korsakoff syndrome**, an irreversible form of amnesia characterized by loss of short-term memory and an inability to learn (Xiong & Kenedi, 2016).

Collaborative Care

Cessation of drinking is the short-term goal that is accomplished through **withdrawal management**. Withdrawal management consists of interventions and processes aimed at addressing the physiological and psychological symptoms that occur in response to stopping a substance on which physiological and psychological dependence has developed. Management of alcohol withdrawal frequently includes the use of medications to decrease symptoms, increase the level of comfort, and decrease the risk of seizures and DTs. Table 11-19 presents the clinical manifestations of alcohol withdrawal and suggested drug treatment.

Patients should be referred to inpatient or intensive outpatient programs for continued support and treatment if they so desire. Treatment includes behavioural therapy and may also include drugs that block the desired effects of alcohol or agents that prevent drinking by causing aversive consequences when alcohol is consumed, such as naltrexone.

TABLE 11-19	CLINICAL MANIFESTATIONS OF ALCOHOL WITHDRAWAL AND SUGGESTED DRUG TREATMENT
Clinical Manifestations	**Drug Treatment**

• Gross tremors
• Seizures
• Hallucinations
• Minor withdrawal syndrome
  • Tremulousness, anxiety
  • Increased heart rate
  • Increased blood pressure
  • Sweating
  • Nausea
  • Hyper-reflexia
  • Insomnia
• Major withdrawal
  • DTs
  • Altered level of consciousness
  • Visual–auditory hallucinations
  • Increased hyperactivity without seizures
	• Benzodiazepines (e.g., chlordiazepoxide [Librax])
	• Thiamine (to prevent Wernicke's encephalopathy)
	• Multivitamins (folic acid, B vitamins)
	• Phenytoin (Dilantin) for seizures or past history of seizures
	• Magnesium sulphate (if serum magnesium is low)
	• Temazepam (Restoril) for sedation
	• Haloperidol (Haldol) for hallucinations

DTs, delirium tremens
NOTE: For DTs, provide intravenous fluids (do not overhydrate), cooling blanket, well-lit quiet room, consistent staff, and frequent checks of vital signs; check for hypoglycemia; assess any other health problems.

SEDATIVE–HYPNOTICS

Characteristics

Commonly abused sedative–hypnotic agents include barbiturates, benzodiazepines, and barbiturate-like drugs. Benzodiazepine-class medications are effective and important in the treatment of panic attacks and severe anxiety. However, in practice, benzodiazepine medications are widely prescribed for generalized anxiety and, at times, for sleep disturbance for long periods of time, which can contribute to the development of tolerance and risk for misuse. A person who becomes tolerant to the effects may increase the dose and frequency of use without medical advice or indication. A second and more common pattern that has the potential for misuse or dependency involves illegal sources and often begins with intermittent use by teenagers or young adults at parties.

Effects of Use

Sedative–hypnotic drugs act primarily on the CNS, causing sedation at low doses and sleep at high doses. Excessive amounts produce an initial euphoria and an intoxication that includes impaired judgement, slurred speech, and loss of inhibitions and motor coordination. Although benzodiazepines are believed to have a wide margin of safety, they are not without adverse reactions, including rebound anxiety and insomnia with short-acting drugs and confusion and memory loss with long-acting drugs. These drugs are usually taken orally, but barbiturates may be injected intravenously. The effects of sedative–hypnotics are presented in Table 11-7.

Tolerance to the sedative effects develops rapidly, necessitating higher doses to achieve euphoria. Withdrawal from sedative–hypnotics can be very serious. The patient may develop anxiety, tremors, weakness, nausea with or without vomiting, muscle cramps, and increased reflexes. After 24 hours, the patient begins craving the drug and may experience delirium, seizures, and respiratory and cardiac arrest.

Complications

An overdose of a sedative–hypnotic may cause death as a result of respiratory depression. Symptoms of overdose are listed in Table 11-20. Complications associated with IV use of the drugs (e.g., blood-borne infections) can also occur.

Withdrawal From Sedative–Hypnotics. Withdrawal from sedative–hypnotics can be highly variable, and the severity and the onset of symptoms depend on many factors, including the drug, the pattern of use, the dose and duration of use, and the presence of concurrent alcohol use. Symptoms may begin 12 hours after cessation of a short-acting drug and more than 100 hours after cessation of a long-acting drug. Withdrawal from high doses is potentially life-threatening and necessitates close monitoring in an inpatient setting. Management is symptomatic and includes a gradual reduction in drug dosage; abrupt cessation of the drug is not recommended. Long-acting agents such as diazepam (Valium), chlordiazepoxide (Librax), clonazepam, or phenobarbital may be substituted for the drug and tapered after stabilization. Mild to moderate symptoms can persist for 2 to 3 weeks after a 3- to 5-day period of acute symptoms.

Collaborative Care

Overdoses of benzodiazepines may be treated with flumazenil, a specific benzodiazepine antagonist. There are no known antagonists to counteract the effects of other sedative–hypnotic medications. Emergency life support measures must be taken

TABLE 11-20 EMERGENCY MANAGEMENT

Overdose of Depressant Drugs

Etiology	Assessment Findings	Interventions
Ingestion, inhalation, or injection of CNS depressants—accidental or intentional	• Aggressive behaviour • Agitation • Confusion • Lethargy • Stupor • Hallucinations • Depression • Slurred speech • Pinpoint pupils • Nystagmus • Seizures • Needle tracks • Cold, clammy skin • Rapid, weak pulse • Slow or rapid shallow respirations • Decreased O$_2$ saturation • Hypotension • Dysrhythmia • ECG changes • Cardiac or respiratory arrest	**Initial** • Ensure patent airway • Anticipate intubation if respiratory distress evident • Establish IV access • Obtain temperature • Obtain 12-lead ECG • Obtain information about substance (name, route, when taken, amount) • Obtain specific drug levels or comprehensive toxicology screen • Obtain a health history including drug use and allergies • Administer antidotes as appropriate • Perform gastric lavage if necessary • Administer activated charcoal and cathartics as appropriate **Ongoing** • Monitor vital signs, temperature, level of consciousness, O$_2$ saturation, cardiac rhythm

CNS, central nervous system; *ECG*, electrocardiogram; *IV*, intravenous, *O$_2$*, oxygen.

in cases of overdose. Medically supervised tapering off over an extended period of time is recommended for withdrawal management of people with benzodiazepine dependency.

OPIOIDS

Characteristics

Opiates are substances that are directly derived from the opium poppy, such as morphine and codeine. Opioids is an umbrella term that includes both opiates and the many semisynthetic and synthetic narcotic agents used as analgesics. Commonly abused opioids are identified in Table 11-7. Opioid antagonists include naloxone.

Heroin, oxycodone, and fentanyl are commonly used street drugs. Although the rates of opioid dependency are lower than those for other illegal drugs, their use is associated with high levels of crime, violence, HIV infection, and death from overdose. Heroin is emerging as a drug of choice because it is often cheaper than prescription opioids (Canadian Public Health Association, 2014).

The vast majority of people who are prescribed opioid medications for the treatment of acute and chronic pain do not develop problematic or aberrant use patterns. However, certain risk factors, including the presence of mental health disorder or physical ill-health, as well as some sociodemographic factors, will increase the risk of nonmedical use (Katz, El-Gabalawy, Keyes, et al., 2013). Individuals who have experienced trauma are at greater risk for developing a substance use disorder (Macy & Goodbourn, 2012).

Effects of Use

By acting on opiate receptors and neurotransmitter systems in the CNS, opioids cause CNS depression and a major effect on the brain reward system. As drugs of abuse, they are taken orally, sniffed, smoked, or taken intravenously. The primary effects include analgesia, drowsiness, slurred speech, detachment from the environment, hunger, decreased respiratory rate, GI peristalsis,

and decreased pupil size. Tolerance to the analgesic effects of opioids develops slowly, whereas tolerance to the euphoric psychological effects develops much more quickly; therefore, people who are misusing opioids for a sense of euphoria will require increasingly high amounts to achieve the same effect. Physiological tolerance to opioids is lost very quickly. After a few days of abstinence, lower tolerance may lead to fatal overdoses should people resume taking the same amount they had been accustomed to taking.

Opioid Overdose

Signs of overdose of opioids include pinpoint pupils, clammy skin, depressed respiration, and decreased level of consciousness that can lead to coma and death if the overdose is not treated. Unintentional overdose frequently occurs with recreational use of the drugs because of the unpredictability in potency and purity. Opioid overdose is a medical emergency and should be treated in an acute medical setting. Treatment includes administering a naloxone infusion and maintaining airways. Giving naloxone 0.4 mg to 2.0 mg intravenously puts the person into withdrawal temporarily and, as such, repeat doses may be required. Signs of overdose are presented in Table 11-7.

Opioid Withdrawal

Withdrawal from opioids occurs with decreased amounts or cessation of the drug after a period of moderate to heavy use. Symptoms may include craving, abdominal cramps, diarrhea, nausea, and vomiting. They are extremely uncomfortable and similar to a bout of stomach flu (Table 11-21). Opioid withdrawal usually peaks 2 to 3 days after the last use and resolves by days 5 to 7. Interventions to support withdrawal include comfort measures and medications for relief of symptoms.

Complications

A key consideration in people with regular chronic use of opioids is opioid-induced constipation, which can lead to bowel obstruction. An important point of health teaching for patients is to

TABLE 11-21	SYMPTOMS OF OPIOID WITHDRAWAL VERSUS OPIOID INTOXICATION
Opioid Overdose	**Opioid Withdrawal**
Early Signs • Nodding off/drowsiness • Slurred speech • Emotional lability • Myosis	• Dysphoric mood • Nausea or vomiting • Abdominal cramps • Myalgia (muscle pain) • Lacrimation (teary eyes) • Rhinorrhea (runny nose) • Mydriasis, piloerection • Sweating • Diarrhea
Late Signs • Respiratory depression • Prolonged QT interval • Ventricular arrhythmias • Coma	• Yawning • Fever • Insomnia • Anxiety • Agitation • Fatigue • Tachycardia

Source: Registered Nurses' Association of Ontario. (2009). *Supporting clients on methadone maintenance treatment: Clinical Best Practice Guidelines* (p. 107). Toronto: Author. Retrieved from *http://rnao.ca/sites/rnao-ca/files/Supporting_Clients_on_Methadone_Maintenance_Treatment.pdf.*

advise them to avoid bulk-forming laxatives, which in fact will make the constipation worse. Osmotic agents that will aid in the relief of opioid-induced constipation are recommended. As mentioned above, a lower tolerance can result in the risk of death caused by unintentional overdose. Health problems associated with opioid use are presented in Table 11-3.

Collaborative Care

Opioid dependency is a chronic and relapsing condition, and thus a long-term treatment approach is taken. Best outcomes are achieved with psychosocial interventions plus pharmacotherapy (Vancouver Coastal Health and Providence Health Care Opioid Use Disorder Treatment Committee, 2015).

Withdrawal Management. Withdrawal management alone is not recommended (Vancouver Coastal Health and Providence Health Care Opioid Use Disorder Treatment Committee, 2015). However, pharmacological treatment using methadone or buprenorphine in combination with psychosocial intervention has been found to be very effective (Amato, Davoli, Minozzi, et al., 2013).

Methadone. Methadone is a potent long-acting agonist opioid that, at the right dose, allows the person who takes it to feel comfortable and free of withdrawal symptoms for 24 hours. Methadone is dispensed as a liquid mixed with juice that is taken daily. Until a period of stability is achieved, as evidenced by improved psychosocial functioning and abstinence from substance use, the person is dosed daily at a pharmacy or specialized clinic. With stability, the patient may be provided take-home doses of methadone, as long as he or she can be responsible for ensuring safe storage and handling.

In the surgical setting, it is important to review the routine and medication history of the person who is taking methadone to ensure that no doses have been missed; it is also essential to confirm when the person last took a dose to avoid double-dosing and overdosage. Upon discharge, the health care team must coordinate care to ensure that the patient can resume dosing in the community to avoid any missed doses. Since methadone can be sedating, people on methadone maintenance therapy should be advised to avoid using other sedating substances such as alcohol and benzodiazepines.

Buprenorphine. Buprenorphine has properties of being both a partial opioid agonist and an antagonist and is less sedating than methadone. It is available as a sublingual oral tablet for substitution therapy. It is taken once daily and, like methadone, allows the person to be free of withdrawal symptoms for 24 hours at the right dose. Buprenorphine has a better safety profile than methadone, in that the risk of overdose is much lower, because buprenorphine binds to more receptors. Therefore, if additional opioids are used, they have fewer receptors to bind to, thereby reducing the risk for overdosage (Handford, Kahan, Srivastava, et al., 2011).

Maintenance. The choice of agonist treatment for long-term maintenance depends on the patient's history, the presence of other illnesses, patient preference, and response to treatment. It is critical, however, that the patient receive psychosocial support. While there is no strong evidence supporting any one particular psychotherapy approach, monitoring and supporting the patient's mental health is an essential aspect of care (Vancouver Coastal and Providence Health Care Opioid Use Disorder Treatment Committee, 2015).

HALLUCINOGENS

Hallucinogens are a variety of psychoactive substances that produce a change in level of consciousness, alter mood, and induce hallucinations. Table 11-7 identifies common hallucinogens and their effects.

Characteristics

According to the Government of Canada (2013b), about 11% of all Canadians aged 15 and older had used cannabis at least once in the past year, and about 28% of those who had used cannabis in the past 3 months reported that they used it every day or almost every day. *Cannabinoids* are chemicals found in the cannabis plant, and the chemical most responsible for the psychoactive effects is tetrahydrocannabinol (THC). At low to moderate doses, THC produces effects similar to alcohol and other CNS depressants. These include euphoria, decreased inhibition, and impaired coordination. Long-term use is associated with a wide range of effects, particularly on cardiopulmonary and mental health. Adolescents who use cannabis regularly are at higher risk for psychotic symptoms, particularly when there is coexisting or family history of psychosis (George & Vaccarino, 2015). Cannabinoids may be natural or synthetic.

The Canadian government has legalized the use of marihuana for specific medical reasons. Physicians may prescribe pharmaceutical cannabinoids, nabilone (an oral tablet containing a synthetic THC), or herbal marihuana. Illegal synthetic THC derivatives (e.g., K2, Spice), which contain varying amounts of different ingredients, have unpredictable effects and are more toxic. In some instances, death has occurred with a single use.

Effects of Use

Marihuana produces three principal effects: euphoria, sedation, and hallucinations. The most commonly affected organs are the brain and the cardiovascular and respiratory systems. Signs of intoxication are presented in Table 11-7. Problems of chronic use include impaired short-term memory, decreased motor coordination, tremors, and increased heart and respiratory rates. A condition known as *amotivational syndrome,* characterized by apathy, dullness, and disinterest, may also occur. Patients with *acute marihuana toxicity* can present with acute psychotic episodes, especially if the patient used a synthetic derivative. Cannabis can induce tachycardia and hypertension, triggering dysrhythmias and myocardial infarction.

Withdrawal can occur in a hospitalized patient who is a heavy cannabis user. The patient may experience irritability, anxiety, anorexia, chills, disturbed sleep, fever, and tremors (Hesse & Thylstrup, 2013). No specific drug therapy is effective in treating withdrawal. Supportive care includes measures such as administration of analgesics and hydration to ensure patient comfort. Panic and flashbacks are managed by providing a quiet environment and reassuring the patient, and benzodiazepines may provide symptom relief.

Collaborative Care

In acute marihuana intoxication, the nurse should perform a physical examination, a toxicology screen, and a thorough history. The main interventions are to provide a quiet environment and to support and reassure the patient by explaining what is happening. The patient should understand that the level of intoxication may fluctuate over several days as metabolites are released.

INHALANTS

Inhalation is the major route of ingestion for a number of common household and industrial volatile substances. Forms of use include sniffing, huffing, bagging, and spraying. Because inhalants are readily accessible, are inexpensive, and produce a rapid high, their use among preadolescents and adolescents is high.

There are four main classes of inhalants: volatile solvents, aerosols, anaesthetic agents, and nitrites. Inhalants are rapidly absorbed and reach the CNS quickly. Most are depressants, and their effects are similar to those of alcohol, including slurred speech, lack of coordination, euphoria, and dizziness. The effects are relatively brief, lasting only 60 to 90 minutes. Long-term use can result in neurological problems, including damage to parts of the brain that control cognition, movement, vision, and hearing. Common agents and their effects are presented in Table 11-3.

The patient with inhalant toxicity may experience dizziness, euphoria, disinhibition, nystagmus, slurred speech, and lethargy. The effects usually resolve within minutes to a few hours. Managing inhalant toxicity usually consists of providing supportive care. However, in some cases, users need emergency treatment for dysrhythmias, heart failure, or CNS hyperactivity (e.g., seizures).

NURSING MANAGEMENT ADDICTIVE BEHAVIOURS

NURSING ASSESSMENT AND SCREENING

Early recognition and identification of a patient with substance use disorder is crucial to successful treatment outcomes for any health problem. A health history should include questioning about the use of all substances, including prescribed medications, OTC drugs, herbal and homeopathic products, caffeine, tobacco, alcohol, and recreational drugs, noting pattern, amount, frequency of use, reasons for use, and reasons for nonuse. Screening tools

for drug abuse were presented in Tables 11-3 and 11-4. The nurse must be alert to signs and symptoms of the many health problems associated with substance use that may be apparent during the physical examination. Assessment of the patient's general appearance and nutritional status and examination of the abdomen, the skin, and the cardiovascular, respiratory, and neurological systems often reflect problems associated with substance use.

Although various screening tools are available, one that nurses easily use to identify alcohol dependence is the Alcohol Use Disorders Identification Test (AUDIT) (Table 11-22). A person with a score of eight points or less is considered not to have problematic use, whereas nine points or above suggests problematic use and warrants further assessment. Another instrument frequently used is the CAGE (cut down, annoy, guilt, eye-opener drinks) questionnaire (Table 11-23).

NURSING DIAGNOSES

Nursing diagnoses for the patient in alcohol withdrawal may include but are not limited to those presented in Nursing Care Plan 11-1. In addition, other nursing diagnoses for an individual with substance use may include but are not limited to the following:

- *Ineffective coping* related to *inadequate confidence in ability to deal with situation*
- *Risk for infection* as evidenced by *invasive procedure* (IV drug use)
- *Imbalanced nutrition: less than body requirements* related to *insufficient dietary intake*
- *Ineffective health maintenance* related to *impaired decision-making* (substance misuse)
- *Dysfunctional family processes* related to *substance misuse*

PLANNING

Nurses need to effectively assess for, manage, and evaluate patients experiencing intoxication, overdose, and withdrawal symptoms because these clinical situations will arise in all settings, from the emergency department to a surgical environment. But most important, positive, nonjudgemental, supportive, and therapeutic dialogue is fundamental.

NURSING IMPLEMENTATION

HEALTH PROMOTION. Prevention of substance use problems and addictive behaviours includes primary, secondary, and tertiary prevention. Primary prevention targets primarily adolescents and young adults by offering education about short- and long-term effects, negative outcomes and effects of continued use of addictive substances. Secondary prevention focuses on early detection of substance use, interventions through peer or employee assistance programs, and continuing education about substance-free alternatives and stress-management techniques. Tertiary prevention addresses dependence and includes motivating individuals to enter addiction treatment and referring to treatment and relapse-prevention programs.

MOTIVATIONAL INTERVIEWING: ENGAGING IN A SUPPORTIVE DIALOGUE WITH PEOPLE WITH PROBLEMATIC SUBSTANCE USE. The nurse is in a unique position to motivate and facilitate behaviour change while caring for patients in primary and acute care settings. When a patient seeks care for health problems related to substance use or when hospitalization interferes with the normal use of substances, the patient's awareness of problems associated with addictive behaviours is increased. Intervention by nurses

TABLE 11-22   ALCOHOL USE DISORDERS IDENTIFICATION TEST (AUDIT)

Please answer each question by checking one of the circles in the second column.

		Score				Score
1. How often do you have a drink containing alcohol?	• Never • Monthly or less • 2–4 times/mo. • 2–4 times/wk. • 4+ times/wk.	(0) (1) (2) (3) (4)	6. How often during the last year have you needed a first drink in the morning to get yourself going after a heavy drinking session?	• Never • Less than monthly • Monthly • Weekly • Daily or almost daily	(0) (1) (2) (3) (4)	
2. How many drinks containing alcohol do you have on a typical day when you are drinking?	• 1 or 2 • 3 or 4 • 5 or 6 • 7 to 9 • 10 or more	(0) (1) (2) (3) (4)	7. How often during the last year have you had a feeling of guilt or remorse about drinking?	• Never • Less than monthly • Monthly • Weekly • Daily or almost daily	(0) (1) (2) (3) (4)	
3. How often do you have six or more drinks on one occasion?	• Never • Less than monthly • Monthly • Weekly • Daily or almost daily	(0) (1) (2) (3) (4)	8. How often during the last year have you been unable to remember what happened the night before because you had been drinking?	• Never • Less than monthly • Monthly • Weekly • Daily or almost daily	(0) (1) (2) (3) (4)	
4. How often during the last year have you found that you were not able to stop drinking once you had started?	• Never • Less than monthly • Monthly • Weekly • Daily or almost daily	(0) (1) (2) (3) (4)	9. Have you or someone else been injured as a result of your drinking?	• No • Yes, but not in the last year • Yes, during the last year	(0) (2) (4)	
5. How often in the last year have you failed to do what was normally expected of you because you were drinking?	• Never • Less than monthly • Monthly • Weekly • Daily or almost daily	(0) (1) (2) (3) (4)	10. Has a relative, friend, doctor, or other health worker been concerned about your drinking or suggested that you cut down?	• No • Yes, but not in the last year • Yes, during the last year	(0) (2) (4)	

Scoring for AUDIT: Questions 1 through 8 are scored 0, 1, 2, 3, or 4. Questions 9 and 10 are scored 0, 2, or 4 only. The minimum score (nondrinkers) is 0, and the maximum possible score is 40. A score of 9 or more indicates hazardous or harmful alcohol consumption.
Source: Reprinted from *The Alcohol Use Disorders Identification Test,* 2nd edition, WHO, p. 17, Copyright 2001.

TABLE 11-23   CAGE QUESTIONNAIRE ADAPTED TO INCLUDE DRUGS (CAGE AID)

Have you felt you ought to cut down on your drinking *(or drug use)*?
_____Yes _____No

Have people annoyed you by criticizing your drinking *(or drug use)*?
_____Yes _____No

Have you felt bad or guilty about your drinking *(or drug use)*?
_____Yes _____No

Have you ever had a drink (or used drugs) first thing in the morning to steady your nerves or get rid of a hangover *(or to get the day started)*?
_____Yes _____No

Note: In the general population, two or more positive answers indicates a need for a more in-depth assessment.
Source: Fleming, M. F., & Barry, K. L. (1992). *Addictive disorders.* St. Louis: Mosby; and Ewing, J. A. (1984). Detecting alcoholism: The CAGE questionnaire. *Journal of the American Medical Association, 252,* 1905–1907. doi:10.1001/jama.1984 .03350140051025.

TABLE 11-24   KEY ASPECTS OF SUCCESSFUL MOTIVATIONAL INTERVIEWING

- Express empathy.
- Provide positive reinforcement and encouragement for gains made by the patient.
- Listen rather than tell.
- Gently persuade, with the understanding that change is up to the patient.
- Identify discrepancy between patient's goals or values and current behaviour.
- Help the patient recognize the discrepancies between where he or she is and where he or she hopes to be.
- Avoid argument and direct confrontation, which can cause defensiveness and a power struggle.
- Adjust to, rather than oppose, patient resistance.
- Focus on the patient's strengths to support the hope and optimism needed to make changes.

at this time can be a crucial factor in promoting behaviour change.

Motivational interviewing is "a directive, patient-centred counselling style for eliciting behaviour change by helping patients to explore and resolve ambivalence" (Rollnick & Miller, 1995, p. 326). Motivational interviewing uses nonconfrontational interpersonal techniques to motivate patients to change behaviour by eliciting talk about substance use. Patients are able to hear themselves speak and gain awareness of how they perceive their substance use. The role of the nurse is to listen and reflect back to the person, bring to light positive change talk, and recognize that ambivalence is normal and expected when anyone is confronted with having to make a change. The key aspects of successful motivational interviewing are presented in Table 11-24.

The stages of change identified in the **transtheoretical model of change** include precontemplation, contemplation, preparation, action, maintenance, and termination (Prochaska & Velicer, 1997), as described in Chapter 4. The stages are not viewed as linear but, rather, as a cycle through which patients move back and forth. During the process of change, relapse and small lapses (very short periods of substance use, followed by quick return to maintaining nonuse) are part of the journey and a normal aspect of behaviour change. Patients who do not change behaviours or who return to substance use after a period of cessation are often labelled "noncompliant" and "unmotivated." However, this development may reflect a normal relapse or may indicate that the interventions used do not consider the patient's stage of change. It is important for the nurse to identify the patient's current stage of readiness for change and the stage to which the patient is moving.

In the precontemplation stage, patients are not concerned about their substance use and are not considering changing their behaviour. During this stage, it is most important for the nurse to help the patient increase awareness of risks and problems related to the current behaviour. A patient in the contemplation stage of change often experiences ambivalence. The patient sees that the behaviour is a problem and that change is necessary yet feels that change is too difficult or that the pleasures of continuing the behaviour are worth the risks. During this stage of change, the nurse should help the patient thoughtfully consider the positive and negative aspects of the substance use. It is useful to summarize the patient's concerns and affirm the patient's ambivalence. As the patient moves from contemplation to preparation, a commitment to change can be strengthened by helping the patient develop self-efficacy. Self-efficacy in this case is the patient's optimism that substance use behaviours can be changed. The nurse should support even the smallest effort to change. The resolution of acute health problems or discharge from the hospital often occurs before the patient moves to the preparation and action stages of change. If the patient demonstrates a readiness to change, as evidenced by entering the contemplation stage or beyond, the nurse must support the continuation of the change process by making appropriate referrals to community resources.

ETHICAL DILEMMAS

Duty to Report

Situation

A patient who has been treated for severe alcohol-withdrawal complications discloses to the nurse that he is a long-distance truck driver and has been working for the past 10 years. As part of the substance use assessment, the nurse learns that he seems to have developed high tolerance to alcohol, with daily consumption and only short periods of abstinence since his divorce last year. He had no previous substance use history or problematic substance use before last year.

Important Points for Consideration

- Nurses have an ethical obligation to prevent harm to patients and the public.
- Nurses are responsible for communicating concerns regarding harms to the patient as well as communicating them to the patient's team of health care providers.
- Nurses must know the legal reporting obligations regarding driver licensing for their province or territory.

Clinical Decision-Making Questions

1. How should the nurse handle this situation?
2. What are the provisions of the province or territory's legal reporting obligations regarding impaired driving?

AGE-RELATED CONSIDERATIONS

Nurses and other health care providers are much less likely to recognize substance misuse and substance use in older adults than in younger adults. Older adults do not fit the image that people in today's society have of those who abuse substances. In addition, patterns of substance use in older adults are considerably different from those in younger and middle-aged adults. Because alcohol and substance use among older adults is often mistaken for other conditions associated with the aging process (e.g., neuropathy, anemia, mental status changes), the problem often goes undiagnosed and untreated.

The prescription drugs used by older adults are primarily psychoactive in nature, including sedative–hypnotic, anxiolytic, and opioid agents. Simultaneous use of OTC drugs, prescription drugs, and alcohol occurs in many older adults. This presents a pattern of drug misuse and abuse that is not commonly seen in younger populations.

The effects of alcohol and other psychoactive substances increase with aging. Age-related decreases in circulation, metabolism, and excretion slow the body's detoxification of drugs, potentiate tolerance, and accelerate physical dependence (physiological adaptation to ongoing exposure such that use and cessation cause an expected physiological response). Physiological changes that accompany aging may lead to intoxication at levels of intake that may not have been a problem earlier in life.

The adverse effects of interaction of alcohol and other drugs also increase with aging. When taken with alcohol, sedative–hypnotic drugs, minor tranquilizers, and CNS depressants have additive and synergistic effects. Misuse and abuse of psychoactive agents, either alone or in combination, by older adults may cause confusion, disorientation, delirium, memory loss, and neuro-muscular impairment. The effects of alcohol and drug use can also be mistaken for medical or psychiatric conditions common among older adults, such as insomnia, depression, poor nutrition, heart failure, and frequent falls. Withdrawal symptoms also occur in the older adult when alcohol, opioids, or sedative–hypnotics are abruptly stopped, and these symptoms may be more severe than in younger individuals. Because of the possibility of alcohol use in older adults, the nurse should always consider that behaviour changes in the older patient may be caused by alcohol use or withdrawal.

Identification of substance misuse, abuse, and dependence in the older patient presents a challenge. Evidence of addictive disorders is not always obvious in the older adult since, as mentioned above, manifestations may be similar to those caused by common health problems of old age. As with all patients, it is important for the nurse to discuss all drug and alcohol use with older patients, including use of OTC, herbal, and homeopathic medications. The nurse should also assess the patient's knowledge of the medications that he or she takes. It is important, too, to screen for warning signs such as unexplained falls, neglect of personal hygiene, and complaints of mood, sleep, or memory problems.

Patient education for the older adult includes teaching about the desired effects, possible adverse effects, and appropriate use of prescribed and OTC medications. The nurse should recommend that the patient use only one pharmacy because many pharmacies maintain a medication profile on each individual that may prevent problems with drug interactions. Patients should be advised not to drink alcohol when using prescribed and OTC medications.

Developmental, physical, and psychosocial changes that occur with aging contribute to late-onset abuse of alcohol and other drugs. The older adult may have difficulty coping with losses that occur with increasing age, such as retirement, death of family and friends, relocation, social isolation, and poor health.

The nurse should monitor people who are experiencing losses and identify those who are having difficulty coping. Home visits by a nurse provide a good opportunity for assessment of the problems and also provision of valuable support. A nurse who suspects an alcohol or substance use disorder in an older patient should refer the patient for treatment. It is a mistaken belief that older people have little to gain from alcohol and drug dependence treatment. As with younger patients, the rewards of treatment can lead to greater quality and quantity of life for older adults.

CASE STUDY

Substance Use

Source: Pavel Kriuchkov/ Shutterstock. com.

Patient Profile
Mrs. Carla Muller, a 78-year-old woman, is admitted to the emergency department after falling and injuring her right shoulder and arm. She has been widowed for 4 years and lives alone. Recently, her best friend died. Her only family is a daughter who lives out of town. When the nurse contacts the daughter by phone, the daughter tells the nurse that her mother appears to have been more disoriented and confused over the past year when they have talked on the phone.

Subjective Data
- Is complaining of severe pain in her right shoulder and upper arm.
- Admits she had some wine in the late afternoon to stimulate her appetite.
- Has experienced several falls in the past 2 months.
- Reports that she fell after taking her sleeping pill, prescribed by her physician because she does not sleep well.
- Speaks with hesitation and slurs.
- Says she smokes about half a pack of cigarettes a day.

Objective Data
Physical Examination
- Oriented to person and place, but not time.
- Blood pressure 162/94, pulse 92, respirations 24.

- Bruising and edema of right upper arm.
- Tremors of hands.

Diagnostic Tests
- Radiographic examination reveals comminuted fracture of the proximal humerus necessitating surgical repair.
- Blood alcohol concentration (BAC) 26 mmol/L.
- Complete blood count: hemoglobin 106 g/L; hematocrit 0.38 (38%).

Discussion Questions
1. What other information is needed to assess Mrs. Muller's condition?
2. How should questions regarding these areas be addressed?
3. What factors may contribute to Mrs. Muller's use of psychoactive substances?
4. *Priority decision:* What priority nursing interventions are appropriate during Mrs. Muller's preoperative period?
5. What possible complications and other health problems may become apparent during Mrs. Muller's postoperative recovery?
6. What nursing interventions are appropriate following Mrs. Muller's surgery?
7. *Priority decision:* Based on the assessment data presented, what are the priority nursing diagnoses for Mrs. Muller? Are there any collaborative problems?

℮volve
Answers are available at *http://evolve.elsevier.com/Canada/Lewis/medsurg.*

■ REVIEW QUESTIONS

The number of the question corresponds to the same-numbered objective at the beginning of the chapter.

1. Which of these statements is true?
   a. Only a small percentage of Canadians are affected by substance use issues.
   b. Tobacco use is the leading cause of preventable morbidity and mortality.
   c. The highest incidence of substance use is among youth.
   d. Substance use is more prevalent in urban areas.

2. What term best describes a pattern of compulsive, continued use of a substance despite significant personal harms and withdrawal syndromes?
   a. Abuse
   b. Substance use disorder
   c. Tolerance
   d. Addictive behaviour

3. When engaging a client experiencing substance use or dependency, which of the following is the nursing intervention based on?
   a. A comprehensive and thorough screening and assessment of substance use
   b. A holistic biopsychosocial approach to care

   c. A nonjudgemental, collaborative therapeutic relationship that honours client autonomy and choice
   d. Assessment of safety concerns and stabilization of acute illness

4. When using a harm-reduction approach with clients experiencing substance use problems, what is the key aim of the nurse?
   a. To provide harm-reduction supplies and health teaching
   b. Not to coerce or force the individual to quit his or her substance use
   c. To ensure that clients have access to health care services
   d. To reduce the harms associated with substance use

5. When screening and assessing for substance use, which of the following are some key aspects to cover?
   a. Use of substances, pattern of use, route, frequency of use, and date and time of last use
   b. Medical history and psychiatric history
   c. Social supports
   d. Legal history

6. What is a long-term effect of addictive substances on the brain?
   a. Increased availability of dopamine
   b. Destruction of the mesolimbic system

c. Loss of pleasure from experiences that previously resulted in enjoyment

d. Potentiation of effects of similar drugs taken when the individual is drug free

7. Which of the following is the most appropriate nursing intervention for a client who is seen at the clinic for increasing shortness of breath but who is not interested in quitting smoking?

a. Accept the client's decision and do not intervene until the client expresses a desire to quit.

b. Realize that some smokers will never quit and that trying to assist them only increases the client's and the nurse's frustration.

c. Increase the client's motivation to quit by explaining that continued smoking will only increase the breathing problems.

d. Ask the client at every clinic visit to identify the relevance, the risks, the benefits of quitting, and the barriers to quitting.

8. While caring for a client who is experiencing alcohol withdrawal, what actions should the nurse take? *(Select all that apply)*

a. Monitor neurological status on a routine basis.

b. Provide a quiet, nonstimulating, dimly lit environment.

c. Pad the side rails and place suction equipment at the bedside.

d. Orient the client to environment and person with each contact.

e. Administer antiseizure drugs and sedatives to relieve symptoms during withdrawal.

9. A client who is dependent on IV barbiturates is scheduled for surgery following an automobile accident. What is important for the nurse to recognize in this case?

a. The client may need less pain medication during the postoperative period.

b. The client should be provided with tapering doses of barbiturates following surgery.

c. The client may have an immediate onset of withdrawal symptoms when given anaesthetic and analgesic agents.

d. The client has a low risk for physical withdrawal symptoms but is likely to experience craving and drug-seeking behaviour during the postoperative period.

10. Which of the following is important in pain management of clients dependent on opioids or other CNS depressants?

a. Realize the goal is to treat acute pain.

b. Avoid treating the pain.

c. Understand that opioid analgesia may worsen an addictive disease.

d. Addiction treatment remains a priority while the client is in pain.

11. In which of the following behaviours should the nurse engage during motivational interviewing with a client? *(Select all that apply)*

a. Insist that the client maintain abstinence while undergoing therapy.

b. Relate motivational techniques to the client's stage of behaviour change.

c. Use any method of communication that will make the client change behaviour.

d. Identify discrepancy between the client's goals or values and current behaviour.

e. Ask a prescribed set of questions to increase the client's awareness of addiction behaviours.

12. To which factors are substance use problems in older adults most commonly related?

a. Use of drugs and alcohol as a social activity

b. Misuse of prescribed and OTC drugs and alcohol

c. Continued use of illegal drugs initiated during middle age

d. A pattern of binge drinking for weeks or months with periods of sobriety

1. b; 2. b; 3. c; 4. d; 5. a; 6. c; 7. d; 8. a, c, d, e; 9. b; 10. a; 11. b, d; 12. b.

⊝volve

For even more review questions, visit *http://evolve.elsevier.com/Canada/ Lewis/medsurg.*

REFERENCES

Amato, L., Davoli, M., Minozzi, S., et al. (2013). Methadone at tapered doses for the management of opioid withdrawal. *The Cochrane Database of Systematic Reviews*, (2), CD003409. doi:10.1002/14651858.CD003409.pub4.

American College of Obstetricians and Gynecologists. (2010). Committee opinion no. 471: Smoking cessation during pregnancy. *Obstetrics and Gynecology*, 116(5), 1241–1244. doi:10.1097/ AOG.0b013e3182004fcd. (Seminal).

American Psychiatric Association (2013). *Diagnostic and statistical manual of mental disorders* (5th ed.). Washington, DC: Author.

Burchum, J. R., & Rosenthal, L. D. (2016). *Lehne's pharmacology for nursing care* (9th ed.). St. Louis: Elsevier Saunders.

Canadian Centre on Substance Abuse. (2015). *CCENDU bulletin: Deaths involving fentanyl in Canada, 2009–2014*. Retrieved from *http://www.ccsa.ca/Resource%20Library/CCSA-CCENDU-Fentanyl -Deaths-Canada-Bulletin-2015-en.pdf*.

Canadian Nurses Association. (2012). *Joint position statement: Harm reduction*. Retrieved from *https://cna-aiic.ca/~/media/cna/ page-content/pdf-en/jps_harm_reduction_2012_e.pdf*.

Canadian Public Health Association. (2014). Heroin: A drug of choice? *CPHA-ACSP Health Digest*, 38(1), Retrieved from *http:// www.cpha.ca/en/about/digest/38-1/3.aspx*.

Carter, C., & MacPherson, D. (2013). *Getting to tomorrow: A report on Canadian drug policy*. Vancouver, BC: Canadian Drug Policy Coalition. Retrieved from *http://www.drugpolicy.ca/progress/ getting-to-tomorrow*.

Centers for Disease Control and Prevention. (2015). *Smoking & tobacco use: Health effects of cigarette smoking*. Retrieved from *http://www.cdc.gov/tobacco/data_statistics/fact_sheets/health_ effects/effects_cig_smoking/*.

Collins, S., Clifasefi, S., Logan, D., et al. (2012). Current status, historical highlights and basic principles. In G. Marlatt, M. Larimer, & K. Witkiewitz (Eds.), *Harm reduction: Pragmatic strategies for management of high-risk behaviours* (2nd ed.). New York: Guilford Press.

Cui, Y., Shooshtari, S., Forget, E., et al. (2014). Smoking during pregnancy: Findings from the 2009–2010 Canadian community health survey. *PLoS ONE*, 9(1), e84640. doi:10.1371/journal .pone.0084640.

George, T., & Vaccarino, F. (2015). (Eds.). *Substance abuse in Canada: The effects of cannabis use during adolescence*. Ottawa: Canadian Centre on Substance Abuse. Retrieved from *http:// www.ccsa.ca/Resource%20Library/CCSA-Effects-of-Cannabis-Use -during-Adolescence-Report-2015-en.pdf*.

Government of Canada. (2013a). *Champix (varenicline tartrate) and Zyban (bupropion hydrochloride)—Revision to the consumer information of non-nicotine smoking cessation aids—For the public.* Retrieved from *http://healthycanadians.gc.ca/recall-alert-rappel -avis/hc-sc/2013/33623a-eng.php.*

Government of Canada. (2013b). *Canadian tobacco, alcohol, and drug survey (CTADS): 2013 summary.* Retrieved from *http:// healthycanadians.gc.ca/science-research-sciences-recherches/ data-donnees/ctads-ectad/summary-sommaire-2013-eng.php.*

Hajek, P., Etter, J., Benowitz, N., et al. (2014). Electronic cigarettes: Review of use, content, safety, effects on smokers and potential for harm and benefit. *Addiction (Abingdon, England), 109*(11), 1801–1810. doi:10.1111/add.12659.

Hammond, C., Niciu, M., Drew, S., et al. (2015). Anticonvulsants for the treatment of alcohol withdrawal syndrome and alcohol use disorders. *CNS Drugs, 29*(4), 293–311. doi:10.1007/ s40263-015-0240-4.

Handford, C., Kahan, M., Srivastava, A., et al. (2011). *Buprenorphine/ naloxone for opioid dependence: Clinical practice guideline.* Toronto: Centre for Addiction and Mental Health.

Health Canada. (2012). *Canadian Tobacco Use Monitoring Survey (CTUMS): Annual results.* Retrieved from *http:// healthycanadians.gc.ca/publications/healthy-living-vie-saine/ tobacco-monitoring-survey-2012-enquete-surveillance-tabac/index -eng.php.*

Health Canada. (2014). *Canadian Alcohol and Drug Use Monitoring Survey: Summary of results for 2012.* Retrieved from *http:// www.hc-sc.gc.ca/hc-ps/drugs-drogues/stat/_2012/summary -sommaire-eng.php.*

Herie, M., & Skinner, W. (2010). *Substance abuse in Canada.* Toronto: Oxford University Press.

Hesse, M., & Thylstrup, B. (2013). Time-course of the *DSM-5* cannabis withdrawal symptoms in poly-substance abusers. *BMC Psychiatry, 13*(1), 258.

Katz, C., El-Gabalawy, R., Keyes, K., et al. (2013). Risk factors for incident nonmedical prescription opioid use and abuse and dependence: Results from a longitudinal nationally representative sample. *Drug and Alcohol Dependence, 132*(1-2), 107–113. doi:10.1016/j.drugalcdep.2013.01.010.

Koob, G., Kandel, D., Baler, R., et al. (2015). Pathophysiology of addiction. In A. Tasman, J. Kay, J. Lieberman, et al. (Eds.), *Psychiatry* (4th ed.). Chichester, UK: John Wiley and Sons. doi: 10.1002/9781118753378. ch22.

Macy, R., & Goodbourn, M. (2012). Promoting successful collaborations between domestic violence and substance abuse treatment service sectors: A review of the literature. *Trauma, Violence and Abuse, 13*(4), 234–251. doi:10.1177/ 1524838012455874.

Marley, R., Calabrese, T., & Thompson, K. (2014). Preoperative evaluation and preparation of the client. In J. Nagelhout & K. Plaus (Eds.), *Nurse Anesthesia* (5th ed., pp. 335–381). St. Louis: Elsevier Saunders.

Mukherjee, S. (2013). Alcoholism and its effects on the central nervous system. *Current Neurovascular Research, 10*(3), 256–262. doi:10.2174/15672026113109990004.

Padwa, H., Larkins, S., Crevecoeur-MacPhail, D. A., et al. (2013). Dual diagnosis capability in mental health and substance use disorder treatment programs. *Journal of Dual Diagnosis, 9*(2), 179–186.

Prochaska, J. O., & Velicer, W. F. (1997). The transtheoretical model of health behavior change. *American Journal of Health Promotion, 12*, 38–48. doi:10.4278/0890-1171-12.1.38. (Seminal).

Registered Nurses' Association of Ontario (2007). *Integrating smoking cessation into daily nursing practice.* Toronto: Author. Retrieved

from *http://rnao.ca/bpg/guidelines/integrating-smoking-cessation -daily-nursing-practice.* (Seminal).

Reid, J., Hammond, D., Rynard, V., et al. (2015). *Tobacco use in Canada: Patterns and trends, 2015 edition.* Waterloo, ON: Propel Centre for Population Health Impact, University of Waterloo. Retrieved from *http://tobaccoreport.ca/2015/ TobaccoUseinCanada_2015.pdf.*

Reiss, R., Fiellin, D. A., Miller, S. C., et al. (2014). (Eds.). *Principles of addiction medicine* (5th ed.). Philadelphia: Wolters Kluwer/ Lippincott Williams & Wilkins.

Rollnick, S., & Miller, W. R. (1995). What is motivational interviewing? *Behavioural and Cognitive Psychotherapy, 23*, 325–334. doi:10.1017/S135246580001643X. (Seminal).

Sachdeva, A., Choudhary, M., & Chandra, M. (2015). Alcohol withdrawal syndrome: Benzodiazepines and beyond. *Journal of Clinical and Diagnostic Research: JCDR, 9*(9), VE01–VE07. doi:10.7860/JCDR/2015/13407.6538.

Statistics Canada. (2013). *Smoking, 2013.* Retrieved from *http:// www.statcan.gc.ca/pub/82-625-x/2014001/article/14025-eng.htm.*

Strobbe, S. (2014). Prevention and screening, brief intervention and referral to treatment for substance use in primary care. *Primary Care Clinic Office Practice, 41*, 185–213. doi:10.1016/j .pop.2014.02.002.

Taber, K., Black, D., Porrino, L., et al. (2012). Neuroanatomy of dopamine: Reward and addiction. *Journal of Neuropsychiatry and Clinical Neuroscience, 24*(1), 1–4. doi:10.1176/appi .neuropsych.24.1.1.

Vancouver Coastal Health and Providence Health Care Opioid Use Disorder Treatment Committee. (2015). *A guideline for the clinical management of opioid addiction.* Retrieved from *http:// www.vch.ca/media/Opioid-Addiction-Guideline.pdf.*

Xiong, G., & Kenedi, C. (2016). *Wernicke-Korsakoff syndrome.* Retrieved from *http://emedicine.medscape.com/article/288379-overview.*

RESOURCES

CAMH and McMaster Addictions Curriculum Project
http://machealth.ca/programs/camh_and_mcmaster_addictions _curriculum_project/

Canadian Cancer Society
http://www.cancer.ca/?sc_lang=en

Canadian Centre on Substance Abuse (CCSA)
http://www.ccsa.ca

Canadian Foundation for Drug Policy
http://www.cfdp.ca

Canadian Institute for Health Information
http://www.cihi.ca

Canadian Mental Health Association
http://ontario.cmha.ca/public_policy/addressing-mental-health -and-addictions-needs-in-primary-care/#.WKVQHTvytPY

Canadian Network of Substance Abuse and Allied Professionals
http://www.cnsaap.ca

Centre for Addiction and Mental Health
http://www.camh.net

The Lung Association
http://www.lung.ca

Program Training and Consultation Centre
http://www.ptcc-cfc.on.ca

Public Health Agency of Canada: Substance Use/Addictions
http://www.phac-aspc.gc.ca/chn-rcs/saa-toxicomanie-eng.php

Registered Nurses' Association of Ontario (RNAO) Best Practice Guideline: Integrating Smoking Cessation Into Daily Nursing Practice
http://rnao.ca/sites/rnao-ca/files/Integrating_Smoking_Cessation_into_Daily_Nursing_Practice.pdf

> **Appendix D: The Benefits of Quitting Smoking**
>
> **Appendix H: Ask, Advise, Assist, Arrange Protocol**
>
> **Appendix L: Quit Smoking First-Line Medications Compared**

Tobacco Free RNAO
http://tobaccofreernao.ca

Alcoholics Anonymous
http://www.aa.org/

International Nurses Society on Addictions
http://www.intnsa.org

Narcotics Anonymous
http://www.na.org

World Health Organization: Mental Health
http://www.who.int/mental_health

ⓔvolve

For additional Internet resources, see the website for this book at *http://evolve.elsevier.com/Canada/Lewis/medsurg.*

12

Complementary and Alternative Therapies

Written by: Virginia (Jennie) Shaw
Adapted by: Jane Tyerman

ⓔvolve WEBSITE

http://evolve.elsevier.com/Canada/Lewis/medsurg

- Review Questions (Online Only)
- Key Points
- Answer Guidelines for Case Study

- Conceptual Care Map Creator
- Audio Glossary
- Content Updates

LEARNING OBJECTIVES

1. Describe commonly used complementary and alternative therapies.
2. List indications for the use of traditional Chinese medicine (TCM).
3. Describe the general types of herbal therapy and indications for their use.
4. List concepts to be included in patient teaching with regard to herbal supplements.

5. Describe the practice of holistic nursing through the use of complementary and alternative therapies.
6. Describe the process of assessing patients' use of complementary and alternative therapies.
7. Describe the roles of the nurse in integrating complementary and alternative therapies into nursing practice.

KEY TERMS

acupuncture, p. 197	healing touch, p. 201	neurofeedback, p. 196,	traditional Chinese medicine
alternative therapies, p. 194	herbal therapy, p. 197	Table 12-4	(TCM), p. 196
complementary therapies,	holistic nursing, p. 203	prayer, p. 202	
p. 194	massage therapy, p. 198	therapeutic touch, p. 201	

The general health of Canadians is steadily improving, as evidenced by lower mortality rates and increased life expectancy. Biomedical and technological advances have contributed to these improvements. However, conventional therapy has been less helpful in alleviating symptoms of chronic illnesses, and chronic health challenges are at an epidemic high. Furthermore, conventional (Western, mainstream) approaches to health care tend to be depersonalized and often fail to account for all aspects of an individual—that is, not only body but also mind and spirit. Canada's Indigenous peoples have healing traditions that attempt to balance the four parts of the person: the physical, mental, emotional, and spiritual.

Increasing access to global perspectives has resulted in greater exposure to healing philosophies from many cultures, offering both consumers and health care providers many new ideas about health and healing (Fontaine, 2014).

Various terms have been used to describe health-related approaches that are considered outside the mainstream of the system of health care dominant in Canada and other Western cultures: *alternative, complementary, integrative, nontraditional,*

unconventional, holistic, natural, and *unorthodox.* Currently, the term most frequently used to refer to such modalities and practices is *complementary and alternative therapies.* According to Health Canada (2012), **complementary therapies** are therapies that accompany traditional Western health practices, whereas **alternative therapies** are used instead of traditional health practices. Most of these practices were developed outside of conventional biomedical approaches and are generally available without medical authorization. Furthermore, many of these modalities are similar to autonomous nursing interventions such as touch, massage, stress management, and activities to facilitate wellness and enrich health.

Complementary and alternative therapies are harmonious with many of the values of nursing (Canadian Nurses Association [CNA], 2017; College & Association of Registered Nurses of Alberta, 2011; College of Nurses of Ontario, 2014a). These values include a view of humans as holistic beings, an emphasis on healing, recognition that the professional–patient relationship should be a partnership, and a focus on health promotion and illness prevention. Nursing's interest in complementary and alternative perspectives is reflected in the formation of specialty nursing groups. For example, the Canadian Holistic Nurses Association (CHNA; n.d.) was established to recognize holistic nursing as a specialty and to ensure holistic practices are considered within a health maintenance and promotion framework. Despite this, nurses may face challenges in providing alternative therapies, such as a lack of knowledge for adequate patient education and the fact that these techniques are often not supported within a biomedical health care system.

To provide direction, the College of Nurses of Ontario (CNO; 2014b) has published practice guidelines for complementary and alternative therapies, which identify the responsibilities of the nurse: (a) to ensure the appropriateness of the chosen therapy, (b) to have adequate knowledge, skill, and judgement to provide the therapy safely and effectively, and (c) to understand the potential outcomes of the therapy. Additionally, nurses need to be aware that patients often under-report or do not report their use of alternative and complementary modalities to their health care provider because of fear of being judged or of not having their health care needs met. It is important that the nurse be nonjudgemental and amenable to the patient's needs.

Health care providers have raised important questions about the effectiveness and safety of complementary and alternative approaches in view of their increased use by consumers. In response to these questions, the Canadian Interdisciplinary Network for Complementary and Alternative Medicine Research (INCAM) was established to foster excellence in complementary and alternative medicine (CAM) research. Its objectives are to build a sustainable network that facilitates and supports research, promote knowledge transfer among researchers, and thus avoid the duplication of research efforts (see the Resources at the end of this chapter). It is difficult to classify the enormous array of complementary and alternative health practices. For analytical purposes, the National Center for Complementary and Integrative Health (NCCIH, 2015) classified these therapies into specific groups: natural products, mind and body practices, and other CAM approaches. Table 12-1 offers descriptions of major categories. Tables 12-2, 12-3, and 12-4 describe select therapies within each category. The list of therapies continually changes as practices proven safe and effective become accepted as "mainstream" health care practices.

TABLE 12-1   NCCIH CATEGORIES OF COMPLEMENTARY AND ALTERNATIVE THERAPIES

Category	Description
Mind and body practices	Therapies focused on the effects of mind–body practices on the brain, mind, body, and behaviours. Science of psychoneuroimmunology demonstrates the strength of this mind–body connection (see Table 12-2).
Natural products	Substances found in nature that are used for their effect on health and wellness (see Table 12-3).
Other CAM practices	Therapies not included in the other categories of CAM therapies (see Table 12-4).

Source: National Center for Complementary and Integrative Health (NCCIH). (2015). *Complementary, alternative, or integrative health: What's in a name?* Retrieved from *https://nccih.nih.gov/health/integrative-health.*
CAM, complementary and alternative medicine.

ALTERNATIVE MEDICAL SYSTEMS

Alternative medical systems are complete methods of health-related theory and practice that were developed outside of the Western

TABLE 12-2   MIND AND BODY PRACTICES

Examples	Description
Relaxation breathing	Slow, diaphragmatic breathing and exercises, used to elicit the relaxation response. See Chapter 8 for further information.
Meditation	State of being with increased concentration and awareness. Focuses one's attention and increases self-awareness. Two branches exist: (a) inclusive/mindfulness and (b) exclusive/concentrative. Mindfulness meditation focuses on "living in the moment" without judgement. Concentrative meditation involves "moving inward," often initiated by concentrating on the breath, a mantra, or an object. Outcomes may include relaxation, spiritual growth, and personal healing.
Biofeedback	Method of learned control of physiological responses of the body (Fontaine, 2011). Information about one or more physiological functions is received, interventions are used, and a feedback loop allows for voluntary control of certain functions.
Yoga	Activity that includes mental and physical exercises, ethical principles, and guidelines for healthy living. Part of the Ayurvedic medical system. Canadians use yoga mostly for its physical benefits and for stress reduction.
Guided imagery	Use of the mind to generate images that have a calming effect on the body. Involves use of vision, sound, smell, and taste, as well as movement, position, and the sense of touch. Outcomes may include reduction of anxiety, relaxation, enhanced immunity, and changes in hormonal responses.
Hypnotherapy	Attainment of a state of attentive, focused concentration with suspension of some peripheral awareness. May be effective in promoting healing, decreasing pain, managing chronic illness, and preparing for surgery and other procedures (Fontaine, 2011).
Music therapy	Listening to music and creating music. Type of music used is individually determined. Outcomes may include relaxation, decreased anxiety, and decreased pain.
Art therapy	Creative expression through a variety of artistic mediums. May be used to facilitate expression of emotions, memories, and conscious and unconscious concerns. Outcomes may include decreased stress, as well as facilitation of healing from past distress or trauma.
Chiropractic therapy	Therapy that restores and maintains health by proper aligning the spine through a variety of adjustment and manipulation techniques. Correct spinal alignment facilitates self-healing and improves health and well-being.
Pressure point therapy	Application of finger and hand pressure to specific areas of the body (acupressure points defined by charts of energy meridians) to improve energy flow, relieve pain, and stimulate the body's innate healing abilities.
Massage therapy	Manipulation of soft tissues to improve health and promote healing. Outcomes include relaxation, reduced tension, improved immune function, increased flexibility, and pain relief.
Hand-mediated biofield energies	Therapeutic touch involves the use of the practitioner's hands to assess and balance the patient's energy field. Healing intent is incorporated. This technique is based on the belief that healing is facilitated when the human energy field is in balance.
Reiki	A Japanese therapy that involves use of the hands to affect the human energy field, with the intent to heal.

TABLE 12-3   NATURAL PRODUCTS

Examples	Description
Herbal therapy	Use of unrefined plant-based products to treat, prevent, or cure disease. Effects are slow and less dramatic than effects of pharmaceutical drugs.
Nutraceuticals	Vitamin and mineral supplements. The best source of vitamins and minerals is a well-balanced diet. Nonetheless, many Canadians take supplements regularly.
Nutritional therapy	Special diets for health promotion. Such diets must be studied for potential benefit.
Aromatherapy	Use of plants' essential oils for their beneficial effect. Canadians seek out this therapy primarily for stress reduction and use these oils via inhalation or topical application. In some other cultures, essential oils are used more comprehensively in health care.
Probiotic therapy	Use of live microorganisms that are similar to those found in the human digestive tract and that aid digestion.

biomedical model, often in other cultures. For some countries, these are their traditional systems. Traditional Chinese medicine is one of the subcategories that NCCIH has identified.

Traditional Chinese Medicine

Traditional Chinese medicine (TCM) is one of the world's oldest and most comprehensive medical systems. It has evolved over several thousand years of cultural and philosophical developments, as well as extensive clinical observation and testing. Several major concepts constitute Chinese medicine. The principle of *yin and yang* is a core tenet of Chinese art, philosophy, and science, as well as TCM. Various states are associated with yin energies (feminine energy—cold, heavy, moist, negative) and yang energies (masculine energy—hot, dry, light, positive). Yin and yang are viewed as dynamic, interacting, and interdependent energies, neither of which can exist without the other, each containing some part of the other within it (Figure 12-1). These energies are a part of everything in nature and must be maintained in a harmonious state of balance to achieve optimal health. Imbalance is associated with illness. TCM modalities are used to restore balance between yin and yang energies.

Strengths of TCM include its individualized system of diagnosis and treatment, as well as its focus on prevention. Assessment tools include a comprehensive health history, tongue examination, and pulse examination. TCM includes an array of modalities,

TABLE 12-4   OTHER COMPLEMENTARY AND ALTERNATIVE MEDICINE PRACTICES

Examples	Description
Manipulation of energy fields: bio-electromagnetics	Magnet therapy based on the principle that every animal, plant, and mineral has an electromagnetic field that allows other objects to interact with it as part of one unified energy system (Fontaine, 2011); magnets are frequently used to reduce pain, relieve swelling and inflammation, and promote healing of soft tissue and bone.
Neurofeedback (neurotherapy and EEG biofeedback)	A noninvasive drug-free technique whereby electrodes are placed on the scalp to monitory brain activity. Inappropriate waveforms are decreased and appropriate waveforms are increased through positive computer-generated visual or auditory reinforcement (Cortese, Ferrin, Brandeis, et al., 2016). This treatment is used for such conditions as epilepsy, stroke, depression, fibromyalgia, PTSD, and ADHD.
Homeopathy	Therapy based on the adage "like cures like." Remedies are specially prepared from the same substance that causes the symptom or problem. Extremely small amounts of the substance are used for the remedy. The remedies are generally safe and free from interactions with other medications. Remedies are believed to work through an energy transfer.
Naturopathy	Therapy based on promotion of health rather than on symptom management. Focus is on enhancing the body's natural healing response through a variety of individualized interventions such as nutrition, herbology, homeopathy, physical therapies, and counselling. Naturopathic physicians are graduates of accredited naturopathic medical schools, and licensing varies by province or territory.
Whole Medical Systems	
Ayurvedic medicine	A practice based on the balance of mind, body, and spirit and developed in India. Disease is viewed as an imbalance between a person's life force (*prana*) and basic metabolic condition (*dosha*). Interventions include breathing exercises, nutrition, detoxification, herbs, meditation, and yoga.
Traditional Chinese medicine (TCM)	One of the world's oldest, most holistic medical systems. Based on restoring and maintaining the balance of vital energy (*qi*). Interventions include acupressure, acupuncture, Chinese herbology, cupping, moxibustion, nutrition, meditation, tai chi, and qigong.
Spiritual Therapies	
Indigenous health care	Practices based on a domain wherein all things have a "spirit." Community is valued and plays a role in the healing process. Gratitude to and harmony with nature are central themes. Medicine men and women use herbs and natural medicines, spiritual rituals, and ceremonies. It is imperative that nurses recognize the importance of incorporating Indigenous healing traditions in the care of Indigenous patients (Beaulieu, 2012; Phillips, 2010).
Prayer	Communication with a deity or the sacred. Found in all cultures. A frequently used therapy. Nurses may incorporate prayer into their practice.

Sources: Beaulieu, T. (2012). *Exploring Indigenous and Western therapeutic integration: Perspectives and experiences of Indigenous elders* (Unpublished master's thesis). University of Toronto, Toronto; Cortese, S., Ferrin, M., Brandeis, D., et al. (2016). Neurofeedback for attention-deficit/hyperactivity disorder: Meta-analysis of clinical and neuropsychological outcomes from randomized controlled trials. *Journal of the American Academy of Child & Adolescent Psychiatry, 55*(6), 444–455; Fontaine, K. L. (2011). *Complementary and alternative therapies for nursing* (3rd ed.). Upper Saddle River, NJ: Pearson Education; Phillips, M. (2010). *Understanding resilience through revitalizing traditional ways of healing in a Kanien'kehá:ka community* (Unpublished master's thesis). Concordia University, Montreal. Retrieved from *http://spectrum.library.concordia.ca/7071*. *ADHD*, attention-deficit/hyperactivity disorder; *EEG*, electroencephalogram; *PTSD*, post-traumatic stress disorder.

FIGURE 12-1 Symbol of yin and yang. The circle representing the whole is divided into yin (black) and yang (white). The small circles of opposite colour within those regions illustrate that within the yin, there is yang, and within the yang, there is yin. The dynamic curve dividing them indicates that yin and yang are continuously shifting in balance. Thus yin and yang create each other, control each other, and transform into each other.

TABLE 12-5	CONDITIONS FOR WHICH ACUPUNCTURE MAY BE BENEFICIAL
Pain Management • Low back pain • Headache pain • Osteoarthritis • Cervical neck pain • Musculo-skeletal and myofascial pain • Fibromyalgia	**Gynecological and Obstetric Conditions** • Induction of labour • Infertility • Menopausal symptoms • Dysmenorrhea
Surgical Analgesia • Procedural analgesia • Postoperative pain • Postoperative nausea and vomiting	**Asthma** **Gastro-Intestinal Conditions** • Irritable bowel syndrome • Chronic constipation
Chemotherapy-Induced Nausea	
Neurological Disorders • Acute stroke • Stroke rehabilitation	**Substance Abuse** • Smoking cessation • Opioid dependence

the most common of which are acupuncture and Chinese herbal medicine. These modalities are used together to replenish and smooth the flow of qi (pronounced "chee") throughout the body. When yin and yang are in balance, qi, or the fundamental life force, flows evenly through the body, leading to good health. Qi is a form of energy found in all life; when it is disrupted, illness and pain can occur. Other TCM interventions include acupressure, moxibustion, cupping, Chinese massage, meditative physical exercise (e.g., tai chi and qigong), and nutrition counselling. Tai chi and qigong are slow-movement exercises that focus on breathing.

Acupuncture. Acupuncture is the primary treatment modality used by TCM practitioners. In 1983, the Chinese Medicine and Acupuncture Association of Canada was federally incorporated in order to unite practitioners of TCM and acupuncture in Canada. In acupuncture, fine needles are inserted into the circulation of qi underneath the skin's surface. The insertion points depend on the diagnosis and the nature of the complaint. With proper point selection and manipulation, acupuncture corrects disruptions in the flow of qi.

Clinical studies have indicated that acupuncture is effective in reducing pain, fighting inflammation, accelerating wound healing, and promoting nerve regeneration (Crane, Ogborn, Cupido, et al., 2012; Fontaine, 2014; Swanson, Keithley, Johnson, et al., 2015; Vickers, Cronin, Maschino, et al., 2012). Table 12-5 has a more complete listing of the uses of acupuncture. Acupuncture is considered a safe therapy when the practitioner has been appropriately trained and uses disposable needles. Patients should review the credentials of their practitioners.

Acupressure. Acupressure is a natural, hands-on healing therapy based on the same principles as acupuncture. Finger pressure is applied along the body's energy meridians. Acupressure works by accessing and releasing blocked or congested energy in the body. Acupressure can be used for many conditions, including postoperative nausea, chemotherapy-induced nausea, and headaches. Jin Shin Do and reflexology are other forms of pressure-point therapies that stimulate certain areas within the body to help balance the body's energies (Fontaine, 2014).

MIND–BODY MEDICINES

Mind–body interventions include a variety of techniques designed to facilitate the mind's capacity to affect bodily function. These include behavioural, psychological, social, and spiritual approaches

to health. Specific examples of therapies and approaches are included in Table 12-2. Within this category, the methods NCCIH considers "mainstream" include behavioural approaches such as psychotherapy, certain uses of hypnosis, biofeedback, patient education, and support groups. Nurses frequently use many of these bio-behavioural approaches.

NATURAL PRODUCTS

Biologically based therapies include herbal therapies (phytotherapy), special diet therapies, and ortho-molecular medicine (see Table 12-3).

Herbal Therapies

Herbal therapy is the use of individual herbs or combinations of herbs for therapeutic benefit. An herb is a plant or plant part (bark, roots, leaves, seeds, flowers, or fruit) that produces and contains chemical substances that act on the body. It is estimated that approximately 25 000 plant species are used medicinally throughout the world, and approximately 30% of modern prescription drugs are derived from plants. Botanical medicine is the oldest known form of medicine; archaeological evidence suggests that Neanderthals used plant-based remedies 60 000 years ago. Today, about 80% of the world's population relies extensively on plant-derived remedies (Fontaine, 2011).

Since the early 1980s, interest in herbal therapies has increased in countries whose health care practices are dominated by the biomedical model. Interest in herbal products is related to several factors, including the high cost of and the potential for severe adverse effects associated with pharmaceutical drugs. Herbal remedies are considered "natural" and therefore may be viewed as safer and more appealing. Since they are directly available to consumers, individuals can assume more autonomy with regard to their health care.

More than 73% of Canadians now consume natural health products in the form of traditional herbal products, vitamins and mineral supplements, and homeopathic preparations. To ensure that these products are safe, Health Canada established the Office of Natural Health Products in 2008. In January 2004, the Natural Health Products Regulations were implemented to ensure the safety of over-the-counter (OTC) products. In contrast, in the United States, herbal products used for medicinal value are classified as dietary supplements. As such, they lie outside the jurisdiction of many of the safety and regulatory rules covering foods and drugs.

Clinical Applications of Herbal Therapy. Medicinal plants work in much the same way as drugs; both are absorbed and trigger biological effects that can be therapeutic. Many have more than one physiological effect and thus can be used for more than one condition. A number of herbs have been determined to be safe and effective for a variety of conditions. Boxes with descriptions of herbs related to specific diseases are found throughout this book (see the accompanying "Complementary & Alternative Therapies" box).

COMPLEMENTARY & ALTERNATIVE THERAPIES

Information related to the following complementary and alternative therapies can be found throughout this text.

- Acupuncture
- Bilberry
- Biofeedback
- Echinacea
- Garlic
- Ginger
- Ginkgo biloba
- Ginseng
- Glucosamine
- Goldenseal
- Guided imagery
- Herbs and supplements that affect blood clotting
- Herbs and supplements that affect blood glucose levels
- Herbs and supplements used for menopause
- Herbs for surgical patients
- Herbs that affect healing
- Lipid-lowering agents
- Milk thistle
- Music therapy
- Saw palmetto
- Valerian
- Zinc

Although most herbal therapies can safely be used without professional assistance, adverse effects and interactions with prescription drugs can and do occur. Adverse effects resulting from the use of herbal remedies may be under-reported, which thus promotes the impression that herbal remedies are completely safe to use. Because consumers tend not to discuss their use of herbal therapies with their primary health care provider, herb–drug interactions may also be under-reported. For safety, patients who are scheduled for surgery should be advised to stop taking herbal remedies 2 to 3 weeks before surgery. Patients who are being treated with conventional drug therapy should be advised to discontinue herbal remedies that produce similar pharmacological effects because the combination may lead to an excessive reaction or to unknown interaction effects. General patient teaching guidelines related to herbal therapy use are presented in Table 12-6.

Patients who take herbal therapies should be advised to adhere to the suggested dosage. If taken in high doses, herbal preparations can be toxic. The potency of a particular herbal remedy can vary widely because of factors such as where and how it was grown, how it was harvested, and how it was processed. Herbal medicines should be purchased only from reputable manufacturers. Health Canada (2015) advises Canadians to use only herbal products that have been approved for sale under the Natural Health Products Regulations. If the product has been assessed, it will have a drug identification number (DIN) or natural products number (NPN) on its label. This certifies that the product has passed a review of formulation, labelling, and instructions for

---

TABLE 12-6   PATIENT & CAREGIVER TEACHING GUIDE

Herbal Therapies

When teaching patients and caregivers about herbal therapies the nurse should:

- Ask the patient about use of herbal therapies. Document a complete history of herbal use, including amounts, brand names, and frequency of use. Ask the patient about allergies.
- Investigate whether herbs are used instead of or in addition to traditional medical treatments. Find out whether herbal therapies are used to prevent disease or to treat an existing problem.
- Instruct the patient to inform health care providers of any intention to take herbal treatments before doing so.
- Make the patient aware of the risks and benefits associated with herbal use, including reactions when herbs are taken in combination with other drugs.
- Advise the patient using herbal therapies to be aware of any adverse effects while taking herbal treatments and to immediately report them to the health care provider.
- Make the patient aware that moisture, sunlight, and heat may alter the components of herbal products.
- Inform the patient of the need to be aware of the reputation of the manufacturers of herbal products and the safety of the product before buying herbal treatments.
- Encourage the patient to read labels of herbal therapies carefully. Advise the patient not to take more of an herb than is directed.
- Inform the patient that most herbal therapies should be discontinued at least 2 to 3 weeks before surgery.
- Inform the patient that the employees of health food stores may not have any educational background in the actions, interactions, and efficacies of the herbal therapies sold in the store they are working in. It is the responsibility of the patient to ensure that the information received comes from someone who has the appropriate background and education to be providing that information.

---

use. Because of the potential for adverse effects, pregnant women, nursing mothers, and older adults with liver or cardiovascular disease should use caution in consuming herbal products. Commonly used herbs are listed in Table 12-7, and some are pictured in Figure 12-2. Commonly used dietary supplements are found in Table 12-8.

MANIPULATIVE AND BODY-BASED PRACTICES

Manipulative and body-based practices include interventions and approaches to health care that are based on manipulation or movement of the body. Examples include chiropractic therapy, pressure-point therapies, massage, and hand-mediated biofield therapies. Massage therapy is one of the body-based practices nurses commonly use.

Massage Therapy

Massage therapy includes a range of techniques that the practitioner uses to manipulate the soft tissues and joints of the body. Involving touch and movement, massage is typically delivered with the hands, although elbows, forearms, or feet may be used. Massage techniques are used in body work, sports training, physiotherapy, nursing, chiropractic therapy, osteopathy, and naturopathy. Benefits of massage include effects on the musculo-skeletal, circulatory, lymphatic, and nervous systems. Massage also positively affects mental and emotional states. Massage therapy continues to grow in popularity; most people who use massage therapy do so as a means of reducing stress.

TABLE 12-7 COMMONLY USED HERBS*

Name	Uses Informed by Scientific Evidence	Comments
Aloe	Treat constipation	• Should be used no longer than 7 days for constipation • May cause electrolyte imbalances • May lower blood glucose level
Black cohosh	Decrease menopausal symptoms	• Generally safe when used for up to 6 months by healthy, nonpregnant women • May lower blood pressure
Echinacea	Treat upper respiratory tract infections	• Should be used with caution by patients with conditions affecting the immune system • May lead to liver inflammation • Only short-term use is recommended
Evening primrose	Treat eczema, skin irritation	• Contraindicated in individuals with seizure disorders
Feverfew	Prevent migraine headaches	• May increase risk of bleeding • Stopping long-term use may lead to withdrawal symptoms
Garlic	May decrease cholesterol and low-density lipoproteins (studies have been inconsistent)	• May increase risk of bleeding • May lower blood glucose level
Ginger	Ease nausea and vomiting during pregnancy	• May increase risk of bleeding • Should not exceed 1 g/day during pregnancy • Supervision by health care provider is recommended for pregnant women considering use of ginger
Ginkgo biloba	Treat symptoms of claudication	• Generally well tolerated in recommended dosages for up to 6 months • May increase risk of stroke • May increase risk of bleeding • May affect blood glucose levels
Ginseng (*Panax* species, including Asian and American ginseng)	May improve mental performance May enhance immune system May lower blood glucose level in type 2 diabetes mellitus	• May increase or decrease blood pressure • May increase risk of bleeding • May lower blood glucose levels • May reduce effectiveness of warfarin • Should be avoided by patients with hormone-sensitive conditions, such as breast cancer
Hawthorn	Treat mild to moderate heart failure	• May add to the effects of cardiac glycosides, antihypertensives, and cholesterol-lowering drugs
Kava	Treat anxiety	• Should be used only under the supervision of a health care provider • Should be avoided by patients with liver problems and by patients taking medications that affect the liver • May increase drowsiness • Should be used with caution with herbs or supplements that are metabolized by the kidneys • May lower blood glucose levels
Milk thistle	Treat hepatitis caused by viruses or alcohol; treat cirrhosis	• May interfere with the liver's cytochrome P450 enzyme system
St. John's wort	Treat mild to moderate depression for a short term (studies on benefits of use are contradictory)	• Well tolerated in recommended dosages for 1–3 months • May lead to serious interactions with herbs, supplements, OTC drugs, or prescription drugs • Interferes with metabolism of drugs that use cytochrome P450 enzyme system • May lead to increased adverse effects when taken with other antidepressants • Advise patients to consult a health care provider before self-medicating with St. John's wort
Zinc	Treat upper respiratory tract infections	• Relatively safe • Should not be taken with dairy products or caffeine, which will reduce its absorption

OTC, over-the-counter.
*Advise patients who are pregnant or lactating to consult a health care provider before they use any herbs. Scientific evidence for the use of most herbs during pregnancy or lactation is limited.
Source: Natural Standard. Retrieved from *http://www.naturalstandard.com*.

Clinical Applications of Massage Therapy. Until the 1970s, nurses were taught to perform "P.M. care," which consisted of a back rub and other measures to promote relaxation and sleep. After that time, P.M. care and back rubs became the exception rather than the rule. Yet today, with the increased focus on providing holistic care, nurses are again recognizing the benefits of massage. Massage promotes health and wellness and has been shown to improve quality of life (Hymel & Rich, 2014; Toth, Marcantonio, Davis, et al., 2013). The role of the nurse in massage differs from that of the registered massage therapist. Whereas massage therapists can provide more comprehensive massage therapies, nurses can use specific massage techniques as part of nursing care when indicated by findings in patient assessment. For example, a back massage can be used to help promote sleep. For a bedridden patient, gentle massage can stimulate circulation. When a nurse determines that massage may be indicated in

FIGURE 12-2 Herbs. **A,** Ginger. **B,** Echinacea. **C,** Chamomile. **D,** St. John's wort. Sources: A, COLOA Studio/Shutterstock.com; B, tazzymoto/Shutterstock.com; C, Nella/Shutterstock.com; D, Scisetti Alfio/Shutterstock.com.

TABLE 12-8 COMMONLY USED DIETARY SUPPLEMENTS*

Name	Uses Informed by Scientific Evidence	Comments
Chondroitin sulfate	Treat osteoarthritis	• Should be used with caution in patients who have bleeding disorders or are taking anticoagulants • Avoid in patients who are at risk for or diagnosed with prostate cancer
Coenzyme Q_{10}	Treat hypertension	• May decrease blood glucose levels
Fish oil/omega-3 fatty acids	Treat hypertension or hypertriglyceridemia Prevent cardiovascular disease	• May increase risk of bleeding • May increase blood glucose levels in patients with diabetes • May increase low-density lipoprotein (LDL) level
Glucosamine	Treat osteoarthritis	• May decrease effectiveness of insulin or other drugs used to control blood glucose levels • May increase risk of bleeding
Melatonin	Treat jet lag Decrease sleep latency (time to fall asleep)	• May increase risk of bleeding • Should be used with caution in patients who have bleeding disorders or are taking anticoagulants • May decrease blood pressure • Should be used with caution in patients with diabetes or hypoglycemia • Should be used with caution by patients with seizure disorder
Probiotics (live bacteria or yeast)	Re-establish gut flora, especially after prolonged antibiotic therapy	• Should be used with caution in patients with compromised immune system or gastro-intestinal disorders

*Advise patients who are pregnant or lactating to consult a health care provider before they use any supplements. Scientific evidence for use during pregnancy or lactation is limited.
Source: Natural Standard. Retrieved from http://www.naturalstandard.com.

meeting a patient goal, the nurse must first assess the patient's preference regarding touch and massage. The nurse should consider cultural and social beliefs and discuss potential benefits with the patient. The indicated plan of care (e.g., hand massage, back massage) can then be implemented, and reassessment can be performed after the massage.

Massage Techniques. Nursing use of massage typically begins with *effleurage,* or gliding strokes, to promote relaxation. Stroking is done from distal to proximal, along the long axis of the muscle

(Figure 12-3, A). After relaxing the muscles with *effleurage, pétrissage,* or a kneading stroke, may be used to gently lift and knead the muscle (see Figure 12-3, B). Gently scented lotions or diluted essential oils may be included in the massage. Forms of massage are often used for pregnant women. Essential oils should not be used for massage on a pregnant patient because they can be harmful to the fetus (Fontaine, 2014).

A simple hand massage (Figure 12-4) can be used for a calming and relaxing effect, especially for patients who are

FIGURE 12-3 Massage. **A,** Using *effleurage* to relax the back. **B,** Using *pétrissage* to relax arm muscles. Source: Lori Karhu, RMT, RN, San Antonio, TX.

FIGURE 12-4 A, Hand massage. **B,** Technique of hand massage: Bend the wrist backward and forward to relax the wrist, then massage the wrist and top of the hand, using circular movements. **C,** Massage the palm of the hand with the cushions of the thumbs, using circular movements. **D,** Massage each finger from the base to the tip. Source: Lori Karhu, RMT, RN, San Antonio, TX.

anxious or agitated. When a patient is frustrated or agitated, a hand massage can act as a distraction and return the person to a calm state.

Family members can be taught to perform massage on their loved one, providing a way for family members to participate in patient care. This can be therapeutic for both the patient and the family, even when the loved one is mentally ill or unresponsive. Massage is beneficial during all aspects of the life continuum. During the end-of-life process, hospice nurses may incorporate massage into their nursing care, inasmuch as the massaging touch can lessen pain and restlessness. Massage is contraindicated in patients who have had recent injuries, trauma, or, surgery and in patients with open wounds, deep venous thrombosis, inflammation or infections, bleeding, edema, or decreased sensation.

Hand-Mediated Biofield Energies

Energy therapies are those that involve the manipulation of energy fields. They focus on energy fields originating within the body (biofields, or human energy fields) (Gerard, 2012) or those from other sources (electromagnetic fields). Examples of biofield therapies include therapeutic touch, healing touch, and Reiki. Biofield healing therapies (see Table 12-2) are based on the theory that energy systems in the body need to be balanced and repatterned to enhance healing. Some forms of energy therapy manipulate biofields by applying pressure or manipulating the body by placing the hands in, or through, these fields.

Therapeutic Touch. Therapeutic touch is a method of detecting, balancing, and repatterning the human energy field. It is a contemporary interpretation of several ancient healing practices. It involves the conscious use of the hands to direct or modulate human energy fields. Therapeutic touch was developed in the 1970s by a nurse, Dolores Krieger, and a traditional healer, Doris Kunz. According to Krieger (1997), therapeutic touch is based on the assumptions that a human being is an open energy system, a balanced flow of energy underlies good health, and illness is a reflection of an imbalance in an individual's energy field.

Clinical Applications of Therapeutic Touch. During the actual treatment, nurses use their hands to assess the patient's energy field. Hands are positioned 5 to 15 cm from the body. The energy field is assessed for bilateral similarities or differences in the flow of energy. The next step is clearing and balancing the energy field. Nurses then work with the energy field of the patient, involving the intentionality (the conscious effort to bring about healing or to be healed) of the patient and the intentionality of the nurse. The session ends with a smoothing of the energy. Therapeutic touch is not a diagnostic tool but is used as a form of treatment in conjunction with a biomedical treatment plan.

Research has been conducted on the effectiveness of therapeutic touch for a wide range of conditions, including wound healing; sleep promotion; enhancement of immune function; and the reduction of anxiety, agitation, postoperative pain, tension headache, and stress. The research findings have been inconclusive, which indicates the need for further research. Specialized instruction is needed to perform therapeutic touch. Some individuals are able to "feel" the energy field more readily than others. However, with patience, determination, and a desire to help others, anyone (including family members) can learn to use therapeutic touch.

Healing Touch. Healing touch is a nurse-based program founded in the 1980s by a nurse, Janet Mentgen. It is a biofield therapy that encompasses a group of noninvasive techniques that use the hands to clear, energize, and balance the human and environmental energy fields. The nurse gently places his or her hands on or near the patient's clothed body. In accordance with established guidelines, the nurse assesses the patient's energy field, realigns energy flow, eliminates energy blockages, reactivates the mind–body–spirit connection, and then evaluates the process (Healing Beyond Borders, 2015; Healing Touch Canada, 2016). It is an organized system designed to assist the patient to self-heal.

Clinical Applications of Healing Touch. Research on energy therapies is in the early stages. However, research does indicate that healing touch may be effective in reducing blood pressure, improving mood, reducing stress and anxiety, and reducing pain (Thomas, Stephenson, Swanson, et al., 2013). Education for healing touch is a multilevel program leading to certification. Information on classes, resources, and practice is available at the Healing Beyond Borders website (see the Resources at the end of this chapter).

OTHER COMPLEMENTARY AND ALTERNATIVE MEDICINE PRACTICES

Spiritual Therapies

Prayer. Prayer (described in Table 12-4) is one of the mind–body interventions used most commonly by all cultures, and yet it is difficult to define. Viewed globally, prayer can be described as connecting with the sacred. An ancient healing practice, prayer has been acknowledged in health care literature. Terms such as *distant healing*, *mental healing*, and *spiritual healing* are used as researchers attempt to study the outcomes of prayer. The term *theosomatic medicine* has been developed to describe the study of health as related to an apparent connection between a deity and the human body. In exploring this connection, religious involvement has been found to be generally associated with lower levels of illness and higher levels of wellness. Prayer has been linked to the prevention of illness and to healing from disease (Fontaine, 2011).

Forms of Prayer. Forms of prayer include meditative prayer, ritualistic prayer, colloquial prayer, and intercessory (or petitionary) prayer. Meditative prayer involves openness to the divine and does not require words or thoughts. Ritualistic prayer involves repeated words and phrases and is commonly associated with formal liturgy. Colloquial prayer involves spontaneous thought and conversation with the divine. Intercessory prayer involves making a request for specific needs to be met (Fontaine, 2011).

Clinical Applications of Prayer. Nurses are committed to spiritual care as part of their holistic practice. Spiritual assessments can guide nurses in identifying patients' needs. Different formats or tools for assessment may be used.

Nurses need cross-cultural knowledge about prayer practices, awareness of patients' spiritual needs, and engagement in rigorous research that examines the effects of prayer. Nursing literature indicates that prayer is an intervention valued by many patients (Fontaine, 2011). Patients may request intercessory prayer: that is, for someone to pray with them or for them. Self-reflection is important in this situation. Knowing their own beliefs and values, nurses can decide to meet the patient's request directly. However, many nurses feel uncomfortable praying with their patients. Barriers to praying with patients include lack of time, personal discomfort, lack of experience, and lack of private space (Fontaine, 2011). If, for whatever reason, the nurse feels uncomfortable or is unable to address the patient's request directly, the nurse may consult with a spiritual director or religious leader. In most hospitals, chaplains of various faiths and denominations are available to meet with patients. Because many patients find prayer comforting, especially during times of illness, nurses must ensure that spiritual needs are met.

Nurses also report using prayer in more personal ways (Fontaine, 2011; Helming, 2011). Many nurses who are hesitant to pray with their patients say that they do pray for their patients. Some also describe using prayer before their shift or as they start their day, seeking inner guidance for effective nursing care. Nurses may use prayer for emotional support, motivation, spiritual awareness, or enhanced professional performance.

AGE-RELATED CONSIDERATIONS

COMPLEMENTARY AND ALTERNATIVE THERAPIES

Older adults with non–life-threatening, chronic conditions are most likely to use complementary and alternative therapies. For older adults, safety concerns involve herb–drug interactions or toxicity from polypharmacy and age-related changes in pharmacokinetics (Touhy, Jett, Boscart et al., 2012). Decreased renal and liver function may slow metabolism and excretion of herbs and dietary supplements. Because older patients are a more vulnerable population, the nurse must discuss the risks and benefits of using herbal products and also encourage patients to inform their health care provider of any herbal product or dietary supplement that they are taking.

NURSING MANAGEMENT
COMPLEMENTARY AND ALTERNATIVE THERAPIES

The role of the nurse with regard to complementary and alternative therapies is evolving. Roles of the nurse may include (a) assessing patients' use of complementary and alternative therapies and their risk for complications or adverse interactions with conventional therapies; (b) serving as a resource about complementary or alternative therapies, including teaching patients about these options, providing information about evidence concerning effectiveness, and making referrals to qualified practitioners; (c) serving as a provider of therapies for which the nurse obtains training and certification, such as therapeutic touch or acupuncture; and (d) conducting research about complementary and alternative approaches. The nurse must be able to perform these roles nonjudgementally. If patients believe they are being judged because of their use of complementary or alternative therapies, they will stop communicating and will withhold this information from their health care providers.

A resource for nurses and patients in Canada with regard to complementary and alternative therapies and practitioners is the Natural Health Practitioners of Canada (NHPC). "The NHPC is committed to promoting and improving the health of Canadians through information about holistic treatments" (NHPC, 2016).

ASSESSMENT

Collection of data on patients' use of complementary and alternative therapies is part of a thorough nursing assessment. It is especially important because most patients do not voluntarily tell their health care provider about their use of these therapies. However, they usually share this information with a nurse when asked. Nurses must ask general open-ended questions, while remaining nonjudgemental and respectful of the patient's response.

Examples of assessment questions to ask include the following:

1. What are you doing to maintain or improve your health and well-being?
2. How involved are you in planning and carrying out your health-related care?
3. What is your view of the ideal relationship between yourself and your primary health care provider?
4. Do you have any conditions that have not responded to conventional medicine? If so, have you tried any other approaches?
5. Are you using any vitamin, mineral, dietary, or herbal supplements or energy-based therapies?
6. Are you interested in obtaining information about alternative or complementary approaches?

Along with assessing use, the nurse needs to document the effectiveness of interventions that the patient uses.

SERVING AS A RESOURCE AND PROMOTING SAFETY

According to the Canadian Nurses Association's Code of Ethics, nurses must respect and promote people's autonomy and help them both express their health needs and obtain desired information in order to make informed decisions (CNA, 2017). A wide variety of therapies fall within the category of complementary and alternative therapies, and some of these therapies may be ineffective or even harmful. However, patients self-select these therapies, generally without consulting a health care provider. Safety concerns encompass the reliability of information, the safety and effectiveness of therapies, and the regulation of practitioners. Patients most commonly get their information about such therapies from health food stores, word of mouth, books, magazines, and the Internet. Patients need to be encouraged to seek professional assistance with these decisions. If a patient questions the nurse on how to find a registered practitioner of natural health practices in Canada, the nurse can refer the patient to the NHPC's website (see the Resources at the end of this chapter). This organization maintains a directory of registered natural health practitioners in Canada. Serving as a patient advocate, the nurse provides information on both conventional therapies and complementary and alternative therapies. Patients should be advised that complementary therapies do not replace conventional therapies but can often be used in combination with conventional therapies. By providing information for the patient, the nurse fosters informed decision making.

To serve as a resource for patients, nurses must first develop their own knowledge base. Even if specific information about complementary and alternative therapies is not provided in basic nursing programs, nurses are educated to be critical thinkers and problem solvers. Thus nurses are prepared to seek ongoing education regarding complementary and alternative therapies and to continue to read and critique research on these therapies.

As ethical practitioners, nurses need to be aware of their biases and judgements with regard to complementary and alternative therapies. Biased and judgemental attitudes do not allow the nurse to provide the best care possible for the patient.

PROVIDING HOLISTIC SELF-CARE AND HOLISTIC NURSING PRACTICE

Some individuals choose to become nurses because they want to care for others—to be a caregiver for their patients. This is a compelling reason to choose nursing. Yet many nurses fail to recognize that "caring for others" can occur only when their values and practices include "care for self" (Fontaine, 2011). Self-care (caring for one's own general level of health and well-being) is essential on both a personal and professional level. On a personal level, self-care involves commitment to maintaining one's own level of wellness. Keeping one's mind, body, and spirit healthy is required so that one has the strength to care for others. On a professional level, self-care is important because nurses are role models. They are role models for family, friends, patients, other health care providers, and the community. By demonstrating self-care practices, nurses motivate other people to achieve greater health and wellness.

Learning about complementary and alternative therapies can be one pathway to self-care. Initially, nurses are eager to learn about complementary and alternative therapies so that they can provide better patient care and be holistic in their approach. However, nurses often find that these therapies can also be used personally to enhance their own level of health and wellness. Because many different therapies are included as part of complementary and alternative therapies, each individual nurse should be able to find ways to promote personal well-being. Examples

of therapies commonly used by nurses for personal well-being include relaxation breathing, meditation, prayer, yoga, massage, and music.

Professional nursing, from the outset, included care of the whole person, which is the concept of mind–body–spirit. However, the Western biomedical model, with its focus on the physical body, transformed nursing practice into a more "medical" model. The relatively recent increase in the use of complementary and alternative therapies provides an opportunity for nursing to return to its origin and a focus on holistic nursing practice. **Holistic nursing** incorporates mind–body–spirit principles into the development of a caring–healing relationship with patients. Core concepts of holistic nursing include the following: (a) the nurse accepts patients as they are, without judgement and with compassion; (b) the nurse's care is based on holism and integrates mind–body–spirit principles; (c) the nurse serves as a facilitator, recognizing the patient's capacity for self-healing; (d) the nurse incorporates self-care and self-responsibility, recognizing the greater interconnectedness of all individuals; and (e) the nurse's practice is guided by holistic education and research (Dossey & Keegan, 2013).

Nursing interventions include therapeutic listening and empathy. The nurse also promotes a therapeutic environment and honours cultural diversity. The holistic nurse may also choose to integrate complementary and alternative therapies as part of nursing practice, recognizing the value of both conventional and complementary and alternative therapies.

SERVING AS A PROVIDER

Nursing has a long history of providing therapies that have been considered complementary and alternative. These include massage, relaxation therapy, music therapy, and therapeutic touch, as well as other strategies to promote comfort, reduce stress, improve coping, and promote symptom relief. The practice of nursing is defined in legislation throughout Canada and commonly includes promoting, maintaining, and restoring health and assessing and providing care through supportive, preventive, therapeutic, rehabilitative, and palliative means. Nurses also support a holistic approach that supports and values patient choice while promoting health and well-being (CNA, 2015; CNO, 2014b; College & Association of Registered Nurses of Alberta, 2011). The requirements for use of a specific complementary or alternative therapy are not different from those for other nursing interventions. The nurse should have specific training in the use of the therapy and should be aware of the evidence base that addresses the conditions for which the therapy is indicated, the effectiveness of the therapy, and the potential for adverse outcomes or synergistic effects. Nurses are responsible for ensuring that the patient has given consent for a given therapy. The patient must be aware of the proposed benefit and any potential risks involved. The nurse must document the effectiveness of the interventions. A mechanism must be in place to evaluate the care outcomes.

PARTICIPATING IN RESEARCH

Nurses are responsible for critiquing and applying relevant research findings to their practice, as well as participating in the identification of researchable problems. Applying research evidence on complementary and alternative therapies into practice is one strategy for developing evidence-informed approaches. Participating on teams whose focus is to develop evidence-informed protocols that address appropriate use of complementary and alternative therapies is another effective approach. Practising with a questioning mind can facilitate identification of research questions that can be investigated with research-trained health care providers. Types of research considerations that can be addressed through questions include describing the extent of patients' use of specific therapies, exploring patients' experiences of using various complementary and alternative therapies, and documenting the effectiveness of therapies commonly used by nurses.

Patient interest and participation in complementary and alternative therapies are increasing. Therefore, nurses must be knowledgeable about the multiple therapies available and must develop effective strategies to document the use of these therapies. It is also important for nurses to keep abreast of the current research in this area to provide accurate information to both patients and other health care providers. Nurses are well positioned to become the link between conventional therapy and complementary and alternative therapies.

CASE STUDY

Abdominal Distress

Patient Profile

Jane Craigo, a 21-year-old university student, was seen in the student health centre for increasing episodes of abdominal fullness and discomfort with alternating diarrhea and constipation.

Subjective Data
- Reports that irritable bowel syndrome was diagnosed several years ago
- Was told to eat more fibre, drink at least eight glasses of water per day, consume foods such as peas, prunes, and oatmeal
- States that she has tried to change her diet but due to her limited budget cannot afford fresh fruits and vegetables

Source: sematadesign/ Shutterstock. com

- Consumes mainly fast foods, due to her busy schedule
- Drinks six to eight colas per day because she does not like water
- Has not been able to effectively reduce her abdominal distress

- Is taking a heavy course load this semester
- Has to work 20 hours each week for her work–study contract

Discussion Questions
1. Assess what Ms. Craigo is currently doing to help alleviate the symptoms.
2. Explain the psychological stressors that may be contributing to Ms. Craigo's abdominal discomfort.
3. Describe how her current diet may be affecting her, both physiologically and psychologically.
4. What complementary or alternative therapy (or therapies) would be appropriate for Ms. Craigo?
5. How could the nurse recommend complementary therapies to Ms. Craigo's physician? What arguments could support their use?

Answers are available at *http://evolve.elsevier.com/Canada/Lewis/medsurg.*

REVIEW QUESTIONS

The number of the question corresponds to the same-numbered objective at the beginning of the chapter.

1. Which of the following statements best describes complementary and alternative therapies?
   a. They are used as a primary form of treatment.
   b. They contradict the values of nursing.
   c. They are based on extensive scientific research.
   d. They were developed outside the Western biomedical model.
2. Which of the following clients is most likely to benefit from treatment by a traditional Chinese medicine practitioner?
   a. A client with pneumonia
   b. A client with mental illness
   c. A client with chronic back pain
   d. A postoperative client with low blood pressure
3. Which of the following herbal treatments can cause life-threatening adverse effects when combined with antidepressants?
   a. Ginkgo biloba
   b. St. John's wort
   c. Kava
   d. Valerian
4. Which herbs can increase a client's risk of bleeding? (*Select all that apply*)
   a. Aloe
   b. Kava
   c. Garlic
   d. Ginger
   e. Feverfew

5. Which of the following statements describes holistic nursing? (*Select all that apply*)
   a. Holistic nursing focuses on physical health.
   b. Holistic nursing is practised only by experienced nurses.
   c. Holistic nursing promotes self-care and self-responsibility.
   d. Holistic nursing is based on the biomedical model of health care.
   e. Holistic nursing incorporates mind–body–spirit principles.
6. In assessing a client's use of complementary and alternative therapies, which of the following actions is a priority to include?
   a. Assess the client's compliance with all treatment modalities.
   b. Determine the client's knowledge of the therapies that he or she is using.
   c. Use the term *alternative therapies* when assessing the client's use of these therapies.
   d. Reinforce the benefits of traditional Western medicine.
7. Which of the following best describes the role of the nurse involved with complementary and alternative therapies?
   a. Caring for clients rather than caring for self
   b. Prescribing the appropriate herbal therapies for a client
   c. Serving as a resource to guide clients in the safe use of therapies
   d. Advocating for use of complementary and alternative therapies instead of conventional health care

1. d; 2. c; 3. b; 4. a, c, d, e; 5. c, e; 6. b; 7. c.

For even more review questions, visit *http://evolve.elsevier.com/Canada/ Lewis/medsurg.*

REFERENCES

Canadian Holistic Nurses Association. (n.d.). *About us*. Retrieved from *http://www.chna.ca/about-us/*.

Canadian Nurses Association (CNA). (2017). *Code of ethics for registered nurses*. Ottawa: Author. Retrieved from *https://www.cna-aiic.ca/~/media/cna/page-content/pdf-en/code-of-ethics-2017-edition-secure-interactive.pdf?la=en*.

Canadian Nurses Association (CNA). (2015). *Framework for the practice of registered nurses in Canada 2015*. Ottawa: Author. Retrieved from *https://www.cna-aiic.ca/~/media/cna/page-content/pdf-en/framework-for-the-pracice-of-registered-nurses-in-canada.pdf?la=en*.

College & Association of Registered Nurses of Alberta. (2011). *Complementary and/or alternative therapy and natural health products: Standards for registered nurses*. Edmonton: Author. Retrieved from *http://www.nurses.ab.ca/content/dam/carna/pdfs/DocumentList/Standards/RN_CompAltTherapy_Jan2011.pdf*.

College of Nurses of Ontario (CNO). (2014a). *Practice guidelines: Complementary therapies*. Toronto: Author. Retrieved from *http://www.cno.org/globalassets/docs/prac/41021_comptherapies.pdf*.

College of Nurses of Ontario (CNO). (2014b). *Competencies for entry-level registered nurse practice*. Toronto: Author. Retrieved from *https://www.cno.org/globalassets/docs/reg/41037_entrytopracitic_final.pdf*.

Crane, J. D., Ogborn, D. I., Cupido, C., et al. (2012). Massage therapy attenuates inflammatory signaling after exercise-induced muscle damage. *Science Translational Medicine, 4*(119), 119ra13.

Dossey, B., & Keegan, L. (2013). *Holistic nursing: A handbook for practice* (6th ed.). Burlington, MA: Jones & Bartlett.

Fontaine, K. L. (2011). *Complementary and alternative therapies for nursing* (3rd ed.). Upper Saddle River, NJ: Pearson Education.

Fontaine, K. L. (2014). *Complementary and alternative therapies for nursing* (4th ed.). Upper Saddle River, NJ: Pearson Education.

Gerard, B. (2012). Health care reform begins with caring for ourselves. *Beginnings (American Holistic Nurses' Association), 32*(4), 8–10.

Healing Beyond Borders. (2015). *What is healing touch?* Retrieved from *http://healingbeyondborders.org/index.php/about/what-is-healing-touch/about-healing-touch*.

Healing Touch Canada. (2016). *What is healing touch?* Retrieved from *http://www.healingtouchcanada.net/htc/newwhat.html*.

Health Canada. (2012). *About natural health products*. Ottawa: Author. Retrieved from *http://www.hc-sc.gc.ca/dhp-mps/prodnatur/about-apropos/cons-eng.php*.

Health Canada. (2015). *Information on homeopathic products*. Retrieved from *http://www.hc-sc.gc.ca/dhp-mps/prodnatur/about-apropos/info_homeo-eng.php*.

Helming, M. B. (2011). Healing through prayer: A qualitative study. *Holistic Nursing Practice, 25*(1), 33–44. doi:10.1097/HNP.0b013e3181fe2697.

Hymel, G. M., & Rich, G. J. (2014). Health psychology as a context for massage therapy: A conceptual model with CAM as mediator. *Journal of Bodywork and Movement Therapies, 18*(2), 174–182.

Krieger, D. (1997). *Therapeutic touch inner workbook: Ventures in transpersonal healing*. Santa Fe, NM: Bear. (Seminal).

National Center for Complementary and Integrative Health. (2015). *Complementary, alternative, or integrative health. What's in a name?* Retrieved from *https://nccih.nih.gov/health/integrative-health*.

Natural Health Practitioners of Canada (NHPC). (2016). *About us*. Retrieved from *http://www.nhpcanada.org/en/aboutus/index.html*.

Swanson, B., Keithley, J. K., Johnson, A., et al. (2015). Acupuncture to reduce HIV-associated inflammation. *Evidence-based Complementary and Alternative Medicine, 2015*. doi:10.1155/2015/908538.

Thomas, L. S., Stephenson, N., Swanson, M., et al. (2013). A pilot study: The effect of healing touch on anxiety, stress, pain, pain medication usage, and physiological measures in hospitalized sickle cell disease adults experiencing a vaso-occlusive pain episode. *Journal of Holistic Nursing, 31*(4), 234–247. doi:10.1177/0898010113491631.

Toth, M., Marcantonio, E. R., Davis, R. B., et al. (2013). Massage therapy for patients with metastatic cancer: A pilot randomized controlled trial. *The Journal of Alternative and Complementary Medicine, 19*(7), 650–656.

Touhy, T. A., Jett, K. F., Boscart, V., et al. (2012). *Ebersole and Hess' gerontological nursing & healthy aging* (1st Canadian ed.). Toronto: Elsevier.

Vickers, A. J., Cronin, A. M., Maschino, A. C., et al. (2012). Acupuncture for chronic pain: Individual patient data meta-analysis. *Archives of Internal Medicine, 172*(19), 1444–1453. doi:10.1001/archinternmed.2012.3654.

RESOURCES

Acupuncture Canada
https://www.acupuncturecanada.org

Acupuncture Foundation of Canada Institute (AFCI)
http://www.afcinstitute.com

Canadian Association for Parish Nursing Ministry
http://www.capnm.ca

Canadian Association of Naturopathic Doctors (CAND)
http://www.naturopathicassoc.ca

Canadian Chiropractic Association
http://www.ccachiro.org

Canadian Holistic Nurses Association
http://www.chna.ca

Canadian Interdisciplinary Network for Complementary and Alternative Medicine Research (INCAM)
http://www.incamresearch.ca

College of Traditional Chinese Medicine & Pharmacology Canada
http://www.ctcmpc.ca

Healing Beyond Borders
https://www.healingbeyondborders.org

Healing Touch Canada
http://www.healingtouchcanada.net

Massage.ca
http://massage.ca/professional_development.html

Natural Health Practitioners of Canada
http://www.nhpcanada.org

Registered Nurses' Association of Ontario (RNAO) Complementary Therapies Nurses' Interest Group (CTNIG)
http://www.rnao-ctnig.org

National Center for Complementary and Integrative Health (NCCIH)
https://nccih.nih.gov

For additional Internet resources, see the website for this book at *http://evolve.elsevier.com/Canada/Lewis/medsurg*.

13

Palliative Care at the End of Life

Written by: Linda A. L. Upchurch
Adapted by: Andrea Mowry

℮volve WEBSITE

http://evolve.elsevier.com/Canada/Lewis/medsurg

- Review Questions (Online Only)
- Key Points
- Student Case Study
  - Chronic Myelogenous Leukemia Including End-of-Life Care

- Conceptual Care Map Creator
- Audio Glossary
- Content Updates

LEARNING OBJECTIVES

1. Describe nursing management of common physical manifestations at the end of life.
2. Describe nursing management of common psychosocial manifestations at the end of life.
3. Explain the process of grief and bereavement.
4. Discuss some of the variables that affect end-of-life care.
5. Discuss key ethical and legal issues related to hospice palliative care.
6. Explore the special needs of family caregivers of a dying patient.
7. Discuss the special needs of the nurse who cares for dying patients and their families.

KEY TERMS

advance care planning, p. 211
advance directives, p. 211
bereavement, p. 209
certification of death, p. 216

Cheyne-Stokes respiration, p. 208
death, p. 208
death rattle, p. 208
end-of-life (EOL) care, p. 207

grief, p. 209
hospice, p. 206
hospice palliative care, p. 206
integrated palliative approach, p. 207

palliative, p. 206
pronouncement of death, p. 216
spirituality, p. 209

HOSPICE PALLIATIVE CARE

The term **hospice** originates from the Latin word *hospes*, a term that referred to either a travelling guest or a traveller's host (Lutz, 2011). In the 1960s, the pioneering work of Dame Cicely Saunders, a nurse, social worker, and physician, revived the hospice tradition; the first modern hospice, St. Christopher's Hospice, established in 1967 in England, provides end-of-life (EOL) services for patients with advanced malignant disease (Canadian Hospice Palliative Care Association [CHPCA], 2016).

The term **palliative** (relief of suffering to improve quality of life) also originates from a Latin word, *palliaire*, which means "to cloak." In 1974, Dr. Balfour Mount, a Canadian physician at the Royal Victoria Hospital in Montreal, first coined the term *palliative care* to refer to treatment with the goal of symptom relief (Lutz, 2011). The World Health Organization (WHO) formally described palliative care as "an approach that improves the quality of life of patients and their families facing the problems associated with a life-threatening illness, through the prevention and relief of suffering by means of early identification and impeccable assessment and treatment of pain and other problems, physical, psychosocial and spiritual"

(WHO, 2015). Specific goals of palliative care are listed in Table 13-1.

In Canada, the term **hospice palliative care**—defined in Chapter 6 as care aimed at improving the quality of life of patients with life-threatening illness and of their families through the relief of pain and suffering—is used to recognize the convergence of hospice and palliative care into one movement that has the same principles of practice and continues to evolve in an effort to reflect changes in people's experience with illness and dying (CHPCA, 2013a). Advances in medical treatments have helped people live longer, now often many years with illness. The course of an illness and timing of death is becoming harder to predict as more treatments become available to extend life. Hospice palliative care is available to individuals and families throughout the illness experience, including end of life and bereavement, playing an increasingly significant role as the illness progresses. At the beginning of the illness, the primary focus is on therapy to treat or manage the illness and a lesser focus on hospice palliative care that aims to relieve suffering and improve quality of life (Figure 13-1). Over the course of an illness, the blend of therapies will vary, depending on the

TABLE 13-1 GOALS OF PALLIATIVE CARE

- Provide relief from symptoms, including pain.
- Regard dying as a normal process.
- Affirm life and neither hasten nor postpone death.
- Support holistic patient care and enhance quality of life.
- Offer support to patients to live as actively as possible until death.
- Offer support to the family during the patient's illness and in their own bereavement.

Source: Reprinted from *Cancer*, WHO, WHO Definition of Palliative Care, Copyright 2018.

FIGURE 13-1 One goal of end-of-life care is to improve the quality of the patient's remaining life. Source: JG Photography/Alamy Stock Photo.

FIGURE 13-2 The role of hospice palliative care during illness. Source: Canadian Hospice Palliative Care Association. (2013a). *A model to guide hospice palliative care.* Retrieved from *http://www.chpca.net/media/319547/norms-of-practice-eng-web.pdf*.

patient's and family's issues, their goals of care, and treatment priorities (CHPCA, 2013a; Figure 13-2).

Integrated Hospice Palliative Care Approach

The *Canada Health Act* (1984) is the overarching legislation covering Canada's national medicare program (Library of Parliament, 2005). This publicly funded health care system is administered on a provincial or territorial basis. Developing the integrated palliative approach to care is a health priority in Canada (CHPCA, 2013b).

More than 240 000 Canadians die each year, most in advanced age (Statistics Canada, 2011a). The number of Canadians dying each year is expected to increase by 38% to 332 000 by 2030

(Statistics Canada, 2010). Interestingly, the cause of death differs by age group. Among people aged 1 to 44 years, the leading cause of death is accidents, followed by cancer. Among people aged 45 to 64 years, most deaths are attributable to cancer and a smaller proportion to heart disease. People aged 65 and older are most likely to die from cancer or heart disease, followed by stroke, chronic lower respiratory diseases, and Alzheimer's disease (Statistics Canada, 2011a). Hospice palliative care and end-of-life care are best provided as an integral part of health care and should be available in all settings of care, including acute care facilities/hospitals, long-term/continuing care facilities, community care/individual homes, free-standing/residential hospices, and shelters (Quality End of Life Care Coalition of Canada [QELCCC], 2010).

An **integrated palliative approach** to care focuses on meeting a patient's and family's full range of needs—physical, psychosocial, and spiritual—at all stages of illness, not just at the end of life. It is a shared-care model: one that shifts hospice palliative care from being a specialized service to a more generalized integrated service available to people with life-limiting conditions regardless of where they live and receive care (CHPCA, 2013b). The primary care practitioners—physicians, nurses, home care nurses, personal support workers, long-term care staff, and hospital staff—continue to provide care with support of the expert hospice palliative care team. The expert hospice palliative care team takes the lead only when a patient has complex, intensive, or tertiary EOL needs, when normal medical management has not been able to relieve symptoms (CHPCA, 2015).

Because the provision of health care is a provincial or territorial responsibility, hospice palliative care services vary across the country. In an effort to develop a national standard of palliative care, the CHPCA has produced "The Way Forward" as a national vision (CHPCA, 2013b; Table 13-2).

End-of-Life Care

End-of-life (EOL) care refers to care given during the last months, weeks, or days of a patient's life. In June 2000, the Senate of Canada issued a report, "Quality End-of Life Care: The Right of Every Canadian" (Carstairs, 2000), which contained recommendations that would ensure access to high quality EOL care for all Canadians. The Quality End of Life Care Coalition of Canada (QELCCC, 2012) supported these recommendations that would ensure that Canadians are able to die with dignity, free of pain, and surrounded by their loved ones, in a setting of their own choice. There are well-documented gaps between the EOL care that Canadians prefer and the care that they actually receive (Cook, Rocker, & Heyland, 2013).

Seriously ill individuals in hospitals and their family members have identified the following features of quality end-of-life care: trust in the treating physician, avoidance of unwanted life support, effective communication, continuity of care, and death with dignity (Cook, Rocker, & Heyland, 2013). Most people state that they would prefer to die at home (Holdsworth, Gage, Coulton, et al., 2015). However, much of the care of someone dying at home is left to the dying person's family and friends, who report feeling unprepared and lacking resources. The nature of some illnesses exceed the caregiver's ability to meet the needs of the dying individual in the home, which often results in an admission to hospital at the end of life. The freestanding/residential hospice is an alternative setting for patients who are unable to remain at home but do not require acute care (Cook, Rocker, & Heyland, 2013).

TABLE 13-2   SUCCESS FACTORS FOR AN INTEGRATED PALLIATIVE APPROACH TO CARE

Vision
- Commitment to person-centred care
- Focus on building capacity in the community
- Focus on changing organizational structure
- Senior management support

People
- Dedicated coordinators
- Interprofessional teams
- Strong role of and more support for family physicians
- Support for providers in long-term care facilities
- Key roles for nurses
- Relationships, partnerships, and networks

Delivery of Care
- Integration of primary, secondary, and tertiary care
- Cultural sensitivity
- Single access point and case management
- Round-the-clock community support and care
- Advance care planning

Supportive Tools
- Common frameworks, standards, and assessment tools
- Flexible approaches to education
- Shared records
- Research, evaluation, and quality improvement

Source: Based on Canadian Hospice Palliative Care Association (CHPCA, 2013). *Innovative models of integrated hospice palliative care. The Way Forward initiative: An integrated approach to care.* Retrieved from http://www.hpcintegration.ca/media/40546/TWF-innovative-models-report-Eng-webfinal-2.pdf.

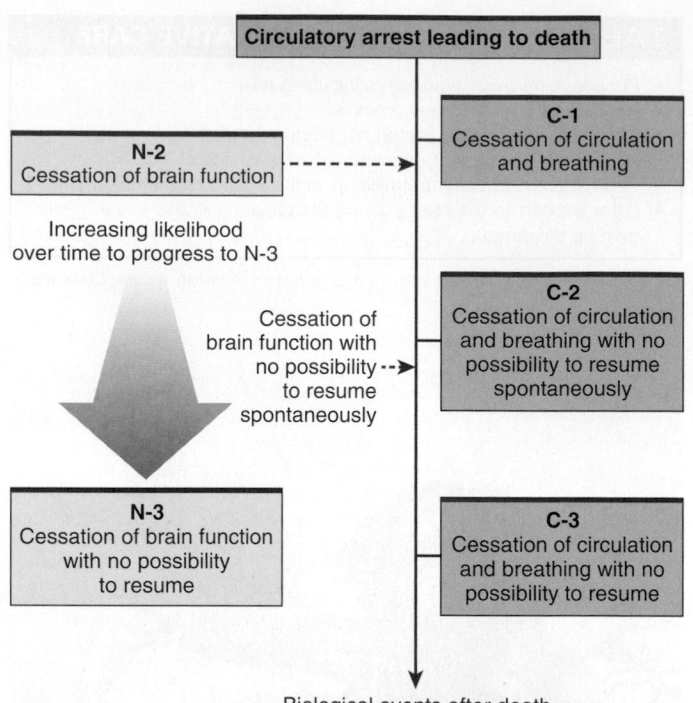

FIGURE 13-3 Physiological sequences in the dying process: integrated neurological and circulatory sequences (applies to cases of circulatory arrest). Source: Shemie, S. D., Hornby, L., Baker, A., et al. (2014). International guideline development for the determination of death. *Intensive Care Medicine, 40,* 788–797. © The Author(s) 2014. This article is published with open access at Springerlink.com. Attribution 4.0 International (CC BY 4.0) license, https://creativecommons.org/licenses/by/4.0/

Death

For many years, society has debated the criteria for death, and this is particularly of concern in the context of organ failure support, organ replacement technology, and organ transplantation. Several major sequential events occur in the dying process of terminally ill individuals who experience a circulatory arrest, when cardiopulmonary resuscitation (CPR) is not medically indicated, and whose EOL care involves limiting or withdrawing life-sustaining therapies (Figure 13-3). The individual's circulation and breathing stop. Because no attempts to restore circulation are made, after approximately 2 to 5 minutes, cessation of breathing and circulation is permanent. The individual may be determined to be dead (Shemie, Hornby, Baker, et al., 2014). There is an inseparable link between circulation and brain function, and therefore the neurological and circulatory sequences are integrated in the dying process.

Death is the permanent loss of capacity for consciousness and all brainstem functions. This may result from permanent cessation of circulation or catastrophic brain injury. In the context of death determination, *permanent* refers to loss of function that cannot resume spontaneously and will not be restored through intervention. The minimum acceptable clinical standards to test for the cessation of circulatory function are (1) absence of palpable pulse, (2) absence of breath sounds, (3) absence of heart sounds, (4) absence of respiratory effort or chest wall motion, (5) loss of pulsatile arterial blood pressure according to noninvasive measurement, and (6) coma and fixed pupils, observed continuously and confirmed after 2 to 5 minutes (Shemie, Hornby, Baker, et al., 2014). In individuals who have suffered a catastrophic brain injury, in which death follows the withdrawal of life-sustaining therapies, death entails a different sequence of events, which is beyond the scope of this discussion.

PHYSICAL MANIFESTATIONS OF THE END OF LIFE

As death approaches, metabolism is reduced and body functions gradually slow down until they all end. Respiratory changes are common at the end of life. Respirations may be rapid or slow, shallow, and irregular. Breath sounds may become wet and noisy, both audibly and on auscultation. Noisy, wet-sounding respirations, termed the **death rattle** or *terminal secretions*, are caused by mouth breathing and accumulation of mucus in the airways. **Cheyne-Stokes respiration** is a pattern of breathing characterized by alternating periods of apnea and deep, rapid breathing. When respirations cease, the heart stops beating within a few minutes. Physical manifestations of approaching death are listed in Table 13-3.

Although death in a hospice palliative care setting is anticipated, a significant minority of deaths (10%) are unexpected. A longer trajectory of illness is associated with unexpected death, and signs of impending death are observed less frequently (Bruera, Chisholm, Dos Santos, et al., 2015).

PSYCHOSOCIAL MANIFESTATIONS OF THE END OF LIFE

A variety of feelings and emotions can affect the dying patient and family at the end of life (Table 13-4). Most patients and families struggle with the news of a terminal diagnosis and the

TABLE 13-3 PHYSICAL MANIFESTATIONS OF APPROACHING DEATH

System	Manifestations	System	Manifestations
Sensory system • Hearing • Taste and smell • Sight	• Usually last sense to disappear • Decreased with disease progression • Blurring of vision • Sinking and glazing of eyes • Blink reflex absent • Eyelids may remain half open	**Gastro-intestinal (GI) system**	• Loss of appetite and thirst sensations • Slowing or cessation of GI function (may be attributed to opioid medications) • Accumulation of gas • Distension and nausea • Loss of sphincter control, which produces incontinence • Bowel movement before imminent death or at time of death
Cardiovascular system	• Increased heart rate; later slowing and weakening of pulse • Irregular rhythm • Decrease in blood pressure • Delayed absorption of drugs administered intramuscularly or subcutaneously	**Musculo-skeletal system**	• Increasing weakness • Gradual loss of ability to move • Sagging of jaw as a result of loss of facial muscle tone • Difficulty speaking • Possibly more difficulty with swallowing • Difficulty maintaining body posture and alignment • Loss of gag reflex • Jerking (myoclonus), seen in patients receiving large amounts of opioids
Respiratory system	• Increased respiratory rate • Cheyne-Stokes respiration (pattern of respiration characterized by alternating periods of apnea and deep, rapid breathing) • Inability to cough or clear secretions, which results in grunting, gurgling, or noisy congested breathing (death rattle or terminal secretions) • Irregular breathing, gradually slowing down to terminal gasps (may be described as "guppy breathing")	**Integumentary system**	• Mottling on hands, feet, arms, and legs • Cold, clammy skin • Cyanosis of nose, nail beds, and knees • "Waxlike" skin when death is very near
Urinary system	• Gradual decrease in urinary output • Incontinent of urine • Inability to urinate		

TABLE 13-4 PSYCHOSOCIAL MANIFESTATIONS OF APPROACHING DEATH

• Altered decision making • Anxiety about unfinished business • Decreased socialization • Fear of loneliness • Fear of meaninglessness of one's life • Fear of pain	• Helplessness • Life review • Peacefulness • Restlessness • Saying goodbyes • Unusual communication • Vision-like experiences • Withdrawal

realization that there is no cure. The patient and family may feel overwhelmed, fearful, powerless, and fatigued. The family's response depends in part on the type and length of the illness and their relationship with the person.

The patient's needs and wishes must be respected. Patients need time to think and express their feelings. Response time to questions may be sluggish because of fatigue, weakness, and confusion.

GRIEF AND BEREAVEMENT

Anticipatory grief is a form of grieving that takes place before the actual death; in other words, in anticipation of the death. Patients nearing the end of life may also experience anticipatory grief. As a patient approaches the end of life, it is common to begin to think of what life will be like when the person has died. The extent to which loved ones have explored and experienced anticipatory grief has an influence on their grief after the actual death (National Cancer Institute, 2014).

Grief is a normal reaction to loss and may manifest itself in both psychological and physiological ways. Psychological responses may include anger, guilt, anxiety, sadness, depression, despair, or a combination of these. Physiological reactions may include disruption in sleep, changes in appetite, physical symptoms, and illness. These experiences may be quite intense immediately after the death and diminish over time. If they persist over a significant period of time, referral to a grief counsellor or health care provider should be considered.

Elisabeth Kübler-Ross (1969) was a pioneer in the recognition and description of grief. In her model of grief, she described five stages (Table 13-5). As other theorists built on this work, they realized that the stages are not linear. Indeed, not every person experiences all the stages of grieving. It is not uncommon to reach a stage and then revert to an earlier stage.

Kübler-Ross's work was pioneering in that she was the first theorist to describe what she was observing in people who were grieving. Her "Stages of Grief" have been criticized as a model for therapy. William Worden further developed Kübler-Ross's work and began talking about "grief work." He developed a counselling model to assist people in the work of grief. Worden's (2009) model outlines "Four Tasks of Mourning" that must be accomplished in grief work (Figure 13-4).

Bereavement is the period after the death of a loved one during which grief is experienced and mourning occurs. The time spent in bereavement depends on a number of factors, including cultural norms, the nature of the relationship with the deceased person, and the degree to which the surviving person was able to prepare for the loss before death. Bereavement and grief counselling are core components of patient- and family-centred hospice palliative care.

SPIRITUAL NEEDS

Assessment of spiritual needs in EOL care is a key consideration (Table 13-6). Spirituality is defined as the beliefs, values, and

TABLE 13-5   KÜBLER-ROSS'S MODEL OF GRIEF

Stage	What a Person May Say	Characteristics
Denial	No, not me. It cannot be true.	Denying the loss has taken place and possibly withdrawing. This response may last minutes to months.
Anger	Why me?	Possibly being angry at the person who inflicted the hurt (even after death) or at the world for letting it happen. Possibly being angry with self for letting an event (e.g., car accident) take place, even if nothing could have stopped it.
Bargaining	Yes, me, but…	Making bargains with God, asking, "If I do this, will you take away the loss?"
Depression	Yes, me, and I am sad	Feeling numb, although anger and sadness may remain subconsciously.
Acceptance	Yes, me, but it is okay	Tapering off of anger, sadness, and mourning; accepting the reality of the loss.

Source: From ON DEATH AND DYING by Dr. Elisabeth Kubler-Ross. Copyright © 1969 by Elisabeth Kubler-Ross; copyright renewed © 1997 by Elisabeth Kubler-Ross. Reprinted with the permission of Scribner, a division of Simon & Schuster, Inc. All rights reserved.

Worden's tasks of mourning

Task #1 — To accept the reality of the loss

To work through the pain of grief — Task #2

Task #3 — To adjust to an environment in which the deceased is missing

To find an enduring connection with the deceased while embarking on a new life — Task #4

FIGURE 13-4 Worden's tasks of mourning. Source: Worden, J. W. (2009). *Grief counselling and grief therapy: A handbook for the mental health practitioner.* Retrieved from *http://www.whatsyourgrief.com/wordens-four-tasks-of-mourning/.*

TABLE 13-6   SPIRITUAL ASSESSMENT

1. Who or what provides you strength and hope?
2. Do you use prayer in your life?
3. How do you express spirituality?
4. How would you describe your philosophy of life?
5. What type of spiritual or religious support do you desire?
6. What is the name of your clergy, minister, chaplain, pastor, rabbi?
7. What does suffering mean to you?
8. What does dying mean to you?
9. What are your spiritual goals?
10. Is there a role of a church, synagogue, mosque, or temple in your life?
11. Has belief in God been important in your life?
12. How does your faith help you cope with illness?
13. How do you keep going day after day?
14. What helps you get through this health care experience?
15. How has illness affected you and your family?

Source: © Joint Commission Resources: Provision of Care, Treatment, and Services (PC) (Critical Access Hospitals/Critical Access Hospitals). Oakbrook Terrace, IL: Joint Commission on Accreditation of Healthcare Organizations, 2018. Reprinted with permission.

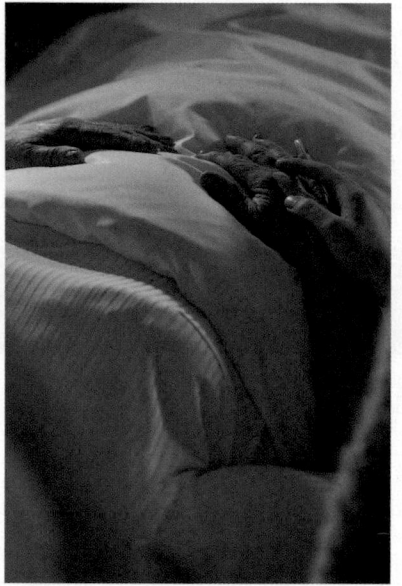

FIGURE 13-5 Spiritual needs are an important consideration in end-of-life care. Source: Photographee.eu/Shutterstock.com.

practices that relate to the search for existential meaning and purpose. It may or may not include a belief in a higher power (Skalla & Ferrell, 2015; Figure 13-5). Some patients may choose to pursue a spiritual path; others may not. Nurses, however, must respect the patient's wishes with regard to spiritual guidance or pastoral care services and make referrals as appropriate.

CULTURALLY COMPETENT CARE

AT THE END OF LIFE

Although death is universal, the ways in which people understand and experience death vary across cultures. Yet variations in rituals within cultural groups, religious faiths, and individuals remind us of the importance of not overgeneralizing culturally attributed qualities (Oyebode & Owens, 2013). Although Canada's immigrants in the sixteenth to nineteenth centuries came from Europe, today's newcomers are more likely to be from Asia, the Middle East, Africa, the Caribbean, and Central and South America (Statistics Canada, 2011b).

Some cultural and religious experiences and expressions of death are subdued and intensely private, whereas for others the experience may involve the community as a whole and be a very public affair with public expressions of grief. Some cultures shield or protect the dying from information about their illness. Effective nurses seek to understand the cultural or religious practices and attitudes toward death that are specific to their patients (LoPresti, Dement, & Gold, 2014). This understanding must not only relate to the care of dying patients but also extend to practices or rituals concerning the care of the body upon and immediately after death.

Within Canada, people of Indigenous origin are the fastest growing populace. There was a 20.1% increase (232 385 people) between 2006 and 2011, in comparison with a 5.2% increase in the non-Indigenous population. The largest numbers live in Ontario, Manitoba, Saskatchewan, and British Columbia (Statistics Canada, 2011b).

Ontario has created a health program, Aboriginal Navigators, in an effort to increase Indigenous people's access to health care services by removing barriers and increasing cultural sensitivity among health care providers. This has taken the form of increasing understandings of the role of extended family, family gatherings for support, community leaders, healers, and medicine men and women within Indigenous culture. Furthermore, an openness within the health care community to learn and understand about the connection to the spirit world, to ceremony, and to sacred and ceremonial items such as feathers, tobacco, sweet grass, cloth, and stones, as well as diet for healing, can all be respectfully incorporated into a patient's plan of care (Hampton, Baydale, Bourassa, et al., 2010). (Further considerations around culturally competent care are discussed in Chapter 2.)

LEGAL AND ETHICAL ISSUES AFFECTING END-OF-LIFE CARE

Patients and families struggle with many questions related to a terminal illness and the dying experience. It is important to create a therapeutic relationship in which patients feel safe in exploring their fears and questions. Common questions may be related to how much control the patient may have over decisions about care: "What if my heart stops?" (resuscitation/mechanical ventilation), "Who would make decisions for me if I can't?" (advance directives/power of attorney), "If it's too much for me, can I decide when I want to die?" (physician-assisted dying), and "Can I donate my body to science?" (organ/tissue donation).

Advance Care Planning and Advance Directives

Legislation pertaining to advance care planning in Canada is specific to each province or territory. However, the principles underlying advance care planning are common across the country: the intrinsic value and uniqueness of each person, the person's right to self-determination, and autonomous decision making.

Health care providers always speak with patients about their health care and treatment options. The intent of an *advance care plan* is that when the patient is no longer able to give direction or consent, the patient's substitute decision maker or advance care plan, or both, will ensure the patient's wishes are known. Each province and territory has its own legislation outlining who may be designated as a substitute decision maker.

Advance care planning is a process of a patient's thinking about and sharing his or her wishes for future health and personal care. It is a means by which an individual can tell others what

---

ETHICAL DILEMMAS

End-of-Life Care

Situation

Suzanne Simard is a terminally ill 50-year-old woman with metastatic breast cancer. She has developed severe bone pain that is not adequately controlled by her current dosage of intravenous (IV) morphine. She moans at rest and verbalizes severe pain from any movement to reposition her. Even though she appears to sleep at intervals, she requests pain medicine frequently, and her family is demanding additional pain medicine for her. At the interdisciplinary team conference, the nurses have discussed the need for more effective pain control but are concerned that additional pain medicine could hasten her death.

Important Points for Consideration

- Adequate pain relief is an important outcome for all patients, but in particular for patients who are terminally ill. The *principle of beneficence* imposes the obligation to provide the necessary care to benefit the patient.
- One goal of treatment of the terminally ill is to provide adequate pain control to alleviate suffering. This goal is based on the *principle of nonmaleficence:* preventing or reducing harm to the patient. The secondary effect of hastening the patient's death is ethically justified. This is referred to as the principle of *double effect.*
- Adequate pain relief at the end of life continues to be a major concern of health care providers and consumers.

Clinical Decision-Making Questions

1. In Ms. Simard's situation, what type of discussion needs to occur among members of the health care team, the patient, and the family as this phase of the care of the terminally ill is approached?
2. Distinguish between palliative sedation and physician-assisted death, and the promotion of comfort and relief of pain in dying patients.

would be important if he or she were ill and unable to communicate. An individual may choose a substitute decision maker and identify this person through a written document such as a power of attorney (or similar document).

An individual may express his or her wishes or directions as generally or as specifically as he or she wishes through an advance care plan (formerly known as a *living will*). When advance directives—legal documents specifying an individual's decisions regarding end-of-life care and specifying alternative decision makers as required—are written, they should be made available to the health care providers and to the substitute decision maker. The CHPCA has led a national initiative promoting and educating the general public, as well as health care providers, on the importance of advance care planning. The "Speak Up" website lists a variety of tools, workbooks, and other information (see the Resources at the end of this chapter).

In all cases, a substitute decision maker must act on a patient's prior expressed wishes, if known, and in a manner that would be consistent with what the patient would have done when capable.

Nurses play an important role in educating individuals about their health condition and in providing factual information about the probable risks and benefits of treatment options. Patients are then encouraged to consider this information in the context of the steps to the development of an advance care plan (Table 13-7).

Resuscitation

Do-not-resuscitate (DNR) decisions are unique instructions that have developed in acute care hospitals since the 1970s. Because cardiopulmonary resuscitation (CPR) is the default response to respiratory or cardiac arrest, a DNR decision requires informed consent (Jalkin & Olver, 2011). This is a very specific example

TABLE 13-7	DEVELOPING AN ADVANCE CARE PLAN
Steps	**Important Considerations**
Learn about your condition and medical treatment: Some may improve your quality of life, whereas others may only keep you alive longer. **Think about you:** What are your values, wishes, beliefs, and understanding about your care and specific medical treatments? **Talk about your wishes:** It is important to discuss your wishes with your loved ones, your family physician, and your health care team. **Choose a substitute decision maker:** Choose someone who would honour and follow your wishes if you cannot speak for yourself. **Record your wishes:** It is a good idea to write down or make a recording of your wishes. Give a copy to your health care provider and substitute decision maker.	• What makes each day worthwhile? • What makes you happy? • How do your decisions about your illness, your care, and your treatment affect your loved ones? Does this change the way you feel about treatment? • Do you have fears or worries regarding your treatment? • Do you have a preference regarding location of care (for example, at home, in a health care institution) if your condition gets worse? • Is there anything that feels "undone" about your life? • Whom can you rely on to help you through any challenges? • Do your religious, cultural, or personal beliefs affect your decisions?

Source: Based on Advance Care Planning National Task Group. (2015). *Five steps of advance care planning* (Speak Up campaign video). Retrieved from *https://www.youtube.com/watch?v=mPtu-FpY1Kw.*

of an event that can often be anticipated and addressed in an advance care directive.

A physician's DNR order is required and should be specific enough to reflect the patient's expressed wishes, whether through direct discussion with the patient, through the advance directives, or from the patient's substitute decision maker. It is now common for a physician to reflect this understanding of the patient's wishes with a written order of "comfort measures only," meaning that treatment associated with pain control and symptom management are carried out, but the natural physiological progression to death is not delayed or interrupted. The use of this type of language means that care is not withheld but rather is supportive while allowing nature to take its course. It is meant to promote comfort and dignity at the end of life. Alberta Health Services has designed "Goals of Care Designations" to facilitate conversations and documentation of an individual's values and wishes related to medical care, resuscitative care, and comfort care (see the Resources at the end of this chapter).

Physician-Assisted Dying

The issue of physician-assisted dying has been debated in Canada for decades, and several cases have been before the Supreme Court of Canada. On February 6, 2015, the Supreme Court of Canada, in its decision in *Carter v. Canada (Attorney General)*, unanimously struck down the Criminal Code prohibitions against assisted dying under certain specific circumstances (Ontario Ministry of Health and Long Term Care & Attorney General, 2015). Accordingly, the federal government, as well as provincial and territorial governments, were given 1 year to draft any necessary legislation and regulations pertinent to physician-assisted dying. As an interesting sidebar, on January 15, 2016, the Supreme Court of Canada granted a 4-month extension at the request of

Canada's newly elected government, so that April 2016 became the date for such legislation to be in place (Supreme Court of Canada, 2016).

In November 2015, a report titled "Provincial–Territorial Advisory Group on Physician-assisted Dying" (Ontario Ministry of Health and Long-Term Care & Attorney General, 2015) was published; it offered policymakers recommendations directed toward a uniquely Canadian approach to this critical social policy issue.

Palliative Sedation

Physician-assisted dying should not be confused with palliative sedation. *Palliative sedation* is an infrequent and extraordinary intervention that necessitates interprofessional expertise. Rigorous guidelines are strictly followed to intentionally produce sedation in order to relieve intractable symptoms in the last days of a patient's life (Alberta Health Services, 2015). The intent of palliative sedation is to control refractory symptoms and suffering, not to shorten life or to hasten death (Abarshi, Papavasiliou, Preston, et al., 2014), as is the case with physician-assisted death.

Promoting the relief of suffering is a nurse's ethical obligation, and it may include appropriate administration of medications (e.g., opioids) that have the potential to cause sedation. The *principle of double effect* justifies the use of medications that cause sedation as an adverse effect, an unintended harm, as its primary role is to relieve suffering and that are not intended to hasten death. Careful titration of medication, which is based on the patient's response, can improve the likelihood that the patient will receive the correct proportion of medication and minimize the potential for harm (Abarshi, Papavasiliou, Preston, et al., 2014).

The use of opioids for symptom management at the end of life is often misunderstood and feared by patients, families, and some health care providers. For this reason, many patients do not receive adequate medication, which may lead to physical and emotional suffering from uncontrolled pain and symptoms. This is an opportunity for the nurse to educate the patient and family about physical dependence on and tolerance of medications. A terminally ill patient should not be concerned with physical dependence when the goal of treatment is comfort until death. (Pain management is discussed in Chapter 10.)

Organ and Tissue Donation

In Canada, oversight and administration of health services, including organ donation, are the responsibility of provincial and territorial governments. Deceased donor services are managed by organ procurement organizations, and living donor services are managed by individual hospitals (Gill, Klarenbach, Barnieh, et al., 2014). All people who are 16 years of age or older and are competent may choose organ and tissue donation. Only patients who have sustained a nonrecoverable injury and are on life support may donate organs. However, all patients have the potential to donate tissue (e.g., eyes, bones, heart valves, and skin) after death (Ontario Trillium Gift of Life Network).

Nurses should be aware of ethical and legal issues and the patient's wishes. Advance directives and organ donor information should be located in the patient's medical record and identified on that record or in the nursing care plan. All caregivers responsible for the patient need to know the patient's wishes. In addition, nurses are responsible for becoming familiar with provincial or territorial, local, and agency procedures related to documentation of EOL care. (Altered Immune Response and Transplantation is discussed in Chapter 16.)

NURSING MANAGEMENT END OF LIFE

Nurses spend more time with patients near the end of the patient's lives than do any other health care providers. Nursing care of terminally ill and dying patients is holistic and encompasses all psychosocial and physical needs. Respect, dignity, and comfort are important for the patient and family. Although there is no cure for the person's disease, the treatment plan still consists of assessment, planning, implementation, and evaluation. The main difference is that the focus of care is on the management of the symptoms of the disease, not necessarily the disease itself. In addition, nurses who care for the dying need to recognize their own needs when dealing with grief and dying.

NURSING ASSESSMENT

Assessment of a terminally ill or dying patient varies with the patient's diagnosis, life expectancy, and rate of decline. Depending on the reason for admission, the assessment might be comprehensive or limited to essential data. Nurses must be sensitive and not impose repeated, unnecessary assessments on a dying patient. When possible, health history data that are available in the medical record should be used in the nursing assessment. The nurse documents the specific event or change in condition that caused the patient to enter the health care facility. The patient's medical diagnoses, medication profile, and allergies are recorded.

A comprehensive symptom assessment according to the acronym *OPQRSTUV* (**o**nset, **p**rovoking/**p**alliating, **q**uality, **r**egion/**r**adiation, **s**everity, **t**reatment, **u**nderstanding/effect on the examiner, and **v**alues; Fraser Health Authority, 2009) and a physical assessment should be completed so that prompt interventions can be initiated. In addition, comorbid conditions or acute episodes of problems such as diabetes mellitus or headache should be evaluated and managed. The nurse should elicit information about the patient's abilities, food and fluid intake, patterns of sleep and rest, and response to the stress of terminal illness; assess the patient's ability to cope with the diagnosis and prognosis of the illness; and determine the family's capacity to manage the needed care and to cope with the illness and its consequences. (Health history and physical assessment are discussed in Chapter 3.)

The physical assessment is abbreviated and focuses on changes that accompany terminal illness and the specific disease process (Hui, Dos Santos, Chisholm, et al., 2015). The frequency of assessment depends on the patient's stability, but a full assessment is completed at least every 8 hours in the institutional setting. For patients cared for in their homes, assessment may occur weekly. As changes occur, assessment and documentation may have to be completed more frequently. If the patient is in the final hours of life, the physical assessment may be limited to gathering essential data (e.g., level of distress).

Key elements of a social assessment include determining the relationships and patterns of communication among the family members. If multiple family members are present, the nurse should listen to varying concerns from different members. Differences in expectations and interpersonal conflict can result in family disruptions during the dying process and after the death of the loved one. Social assessment also includes evaluating the goals of the patient and family.

As the patient nears death, the nurse should monitor the patient for multiple systems that often are failing during the EOL period. This requires vigilance and attention to physical changes that are often subtle. Neurological assessment is especially important and includes evaluation of level of consciousness, presence of reflexes, and pupil responses. Evaluation of vital signs, skin colour, and temperature helps detect changes in circulation. The nurse should monitor and describe respiratory status, character and pattern of respirations, and characteristics of breath sounds. Nutritional and fluid intake, urine output, and bowel function should also be monitored because they provide assessment data for renal and gastrointestinal functioning. Skin condition should be assessed on an ongoing basis because skin becomes fragile and may easily break down.

In the last hours of life, assessments should be limited to only those that are needed to determine the patient's comfort. Assessment of pain and respiratory status may be the most important during this time. It may be more peaceful and comforting to the patient and family to refrain from overstimulation that may occur from certain types of assessments, such as measuring blood pressure or checking for pupillary response. As the patient's death approaches, the nurse's efforts may be better spent providing emotional support to the patient and family rather than performing tasks that will have no effect on the patient's physical care. (Tools for practice can be found at the Canadian Virtual Hospice and Pallium Canada websites, listed in the "Resources" section at the end of this chapter.)

NURSING DIAGNOSES

Several nursing diagnoses deal with psychosocial manifestations (Table 13-8) and physical manifestations (Table 13-9) associated with EOL care.

TABLE 13-8 NURSING DIAGNOSES

Psychosocial Manifestations of the End of Life

• Anxiety, death	• Loneliness, risk for
• Confusion, acute	• Sleep pattern, disturbed
• Confusion, chronic	• Social interaction, impaired
• Coping, ineffective	• Social isolation
• Denial, ineffective	• Sorrow, chronic
• Family processes, interrupted	• Spiritual distress
• Fear	• Spiritual well-being, readiness for enhanced
• Grieving, risk for complicated	• Verbal communication, impaired
• Grieving, complicated	
• Hopelessness	

TABLE 13-9 NURSING DIAGNOSES

Physical Manifestations of the End of Life

• Airway clearance, ineffective	• Oral mucous membrane, impaired
• Aspiration, risk for	• Pain, acute
• Bed mobility, impaired	• Pain, chronic
• Bowel incontinence	• Physical mobility, impaired
• Breathing pattern, ineffective	• Self-care deficits
• Cardiac output, decreased	• Skin integrity, impaired
• Constipation	• Swallowing, impaired
• Diarrhea	• Thermoregulation, ineffective
• Fatigue	• Tissue integrity, impaired
• Gas exchange, impaired	• Tissue perfusion, ineffective
• Infection, risk for	• Incontinence, functional urinary
• Injury, risk for	
• Nausea	
• Nutrition, imbalanced: less than body requirements	

PLANNING

The patient and family need to be involved in planning and coordinating EOL care. In some cases, a family conference may be helpful to develop a coordinated plan of care.

The nurse develops a comprehensive plan to support, teach, and evaluate patients and families. Nursing care goals during the last stages of life involve comfort and safety measures and care of the patient's emotional and physical needs. These goals may also include determining where the patient would prefer to die and whether this is possible. For example, the patient may prefer to die at home, but the family may not be in favour. Many factors contribute to the decision of the patient and family. Interprofessional EOL care should include the physician, nurse, social worker, and chaplain, as well as other members of the hospice palliative care team. The nurse should advocate for the patient so that his or her wishes are met as much as possible.

NURSING IMPLEMENTATION

Psychosocial care and physical care are interrelated for both the dying patient and the family. Support and education are important components of EOL care. Patients and families need ongoing information regarding the disease, the dying process, and any care that will be provided. They need information on how to cope with the many issues during this period of their lives. Anxiety and grief may be barriers to learning and understanding at the end of life for both the patient and the family. (Tools for practice can be found at the Canadian Virtual Hospice and Pallium Canada websites, listed in the "Resources" section at the end of this chapter.)

PSYCHOSOCIAL CARE. As the patient's death approaches, the nurse should encourage the family to respond appropriately to the psychosocial manifestations of the end of life. Table 13-10 discusses management of psychosocial manifestations near death.

Anxiety and Depression. Patients often exhibit signs of anxiety and depression during the EOL period. Anxiety is an uneasy feeling whose cause is not easily identified. Anxiety is frequently related to fear.

Causes of anxiety and depression may include uncontrolled pain and dyspnea, psychosocial factors related to the disease process or impending death, altered physiological states, and drugs used in high dosages. Encouragement, support, and teaching decrease some of the anxiety and depression. Management of anxiety and depression may include both medications and nonpharmacological interventions. Relaxation strategies such as relaxation breathing, muscle relaxation, music, and imagery may be useful. (Complementary and alternative therapies are discussed in Chapter 12.)

Anger. Anger is a common and normal response in the grief process. A grieving person cannot be forced to accept loss. The surviving family members may be angry with the dying loved one who is leaving them. The nurse should encourage the expression of feelings, but at the same time realize how difficult it is to come to terms with loss. The nurse may be the target of the anger; however, it is critical to understand the source of the expressed emotion and not to react on a personal level.

Hopelessness and Powerlessness. Feelings of hopelessness and powerlessness are common during the EOL period. The nurse should encourage realistic hope within the limits of the situation. The patient and family should be allowed to deal with what is within their control, and the nurse should help them to recognize what is beyond their control. When possible, the patient's involvement in decision making about care should be supported, to foster a sense of control and autonomy.

Fear. Fear is a common emotion associated with dying. Four specific fears associated with dying are fear of pain, fear of shortness of breath, fear of loneliness and abandonment, and fear of meaninglessness.

Fear of Pain. Many people assume that pain always accompanies dying and death. Physiologically, there is no absolute

---

TABLE 13-10   NURSING MANAGEMENT

Psychosocial Care at the End of Life

Characteristic	Nursing Management
Withdrawal Patient near death may seem withdrawn from the physical environment; however, the patient may be able to hear but unable to respond.	• Converse as though the patient were alert, using a soft voice and gentle touch.
Unusual Communication This may indicate that an unresolved issue is preventing the dying person from letting go. Patient may become restless and agitated or perform repetitive tasks (may also indicate terminal delirium).	• Encourage the family to talk with and reassure the dying person.
Vision-Like Experiences The patient may talk to people who are not there or see places and objects not visible. Vision-like experiences assist the dying person in coming to terms with meaning in life and transition from it.	• Affirm the dying person's experience as a part of transition from this life.
Saying Goodbyes It is important for the patient and family to acknowledge their sadness, mutually forgive one another, and say goodbye.	• Encourage the dying person and family to verbalize their feelings of sadness, loss, and forgiveness and to touch, hug, and cry. • Allow the patient and family privacy to express their feelings and comfort one another.
Spiritual Needs The patient or family may request spiritual support, such as the presence of a chaplain.	• Assess spiritual needs. Allow patient to express his or her spiritual needs. • Encourage visit by appropriate spiritual care service provider, chaplain, or family member.

indication that death is always painful. Psychologically, pain may result from the anxieties and separations related to dying. Terminally ill patients who do experience physical pain should have pain-relieving medications available around the clock (Pereira, 2013). Nurses must assure the patient and family that drugs will be given promptly when needed and that adverse effects of drugs can and will be managed. Reassessment of pain after medications are given is an important nursing action. Patients can participate in their own pain relief by discussing pain relief measures and their effects. Most patients want their pain relieved without the adverse effects of grogginess or sleepiness. Pain relief measures do not have to deprive the patient of the ability to interact with others.

Fear of Shortness of Breath. Respiratory distress and dyspnea occur in some patients near the end of life. The sensation of breathlessness results in anxiety for both the patient and family. Current therapies include opioids, bronchodilators, and oxygen, depending on the cause of the dyspnea. Anxiety-reducing medications (anxiolytics) may help produce relaxation.

Fear of Loneliness and Abandonment. Most terminally ill and dying people fear loneliness and do not want to be alone. Many dying patients are afraid that loved ones who are unable to cope with the patient's imminent death will abandon them. The simple presence of someone provides support and comfort (Figure 13-6). Holding hands, touching, and listening are important nursing interventions. Providing companionship allows the dying person a sense of security.

Fear of Meaninglessness. Fear of meaninglessness leads most people to review their lives. They review their intentions during life, examining actions and expressing regrets about what might have been. *Life review* helps patients recognize the value of their lives. Nurses can assist patients and their families in identifying the positive qualities of the patient's life. Practical ways of helping may include looking at photo albums or collections of important mementos. Sharing thoughts and feelings may enhance spirituality and provide comfort for the patient at this time. A patient may wish to leave a legacy through writing letters to read or making a video to be viewed at future events when they will no longer be present (Waldrop & Meeker, 2014). Nurses must respect and accept the practices and rituals associated with the patient's life review while remaining nonjudgemental.

Communication. No two conversations are the same, inasmuch as they are shaped by the unique circumstances, coping styles, and personalities of the individuals involved. Difficult discussions include any information that adversely affects one's expectations for the future. How the person experiences and processes difficult news is dependent on not only the words used but also how the message is delivered (Boles, 2015). Nurses may use several approaches to difficult conversations that share common features. Suggested approaches are "ask–tell–ask," "tell me more," responding to emotions with the NURSE protocol (naming, understanding, respecting, supporting, and exploring) and the SPIKES six-step protocol (setup, perception, invitation, knowledge, empathize, and summarize and strategize; Back, Arnold, Baile, et al., 2005).

Effective communication techniques used in conversations among the interprofessional team, patient, and family are essential at the end of the patient's life. Empathy and active listening are essential communication components in EOL care (Figure 13-7). Empathy is the identification with and understanding of another person's situation, feelings, and motives. Active listening, an active process required in the development of empathy toward another person's feeling, is paying attention to what is said, observing the patient's nonverbal cues, and not interrupting.

There may also be silence. Silence is frequently related to the overwhelming feelings experienced at the end of life. Silence can also allow time to gather thoughts. Listening to the silence sends a message of acceptance and comfort. Communication also must be respectful of the patient's ethnic, cultural, and religious backgrounds.

Patients and family members may have difficulties expressing themselves emotionally. The nurse must allow time for them to express their feelings and thoughts, making time to listen and interact in a sensitive way to enhance the relationship among the nurse, the patient, and the family. A family conference is one way to create a environment more conducive to large group conversations.

Family members must be prepared for changes in emotional and cognitive function that occur at end of the patient's life. Unusual communication by the patient may take place at the end of life. The patient's speech may become confused, disoriented,

FIGURE 13-6 Dying patients typically want someone whom they know and trust to stay with them. Source: © Can Stock Photo/jgroup.

FIGURE 13-7 Therapeutic communication is an important aspect of end-of-life nursing care. Source: © Can Stock Photo/diego_cervo.

or garbled. Patients may speak to or about family members or others who have predeceased them, give instructions to those who will survive them, or speak of projects yet to be completed. Active, careful listening allows for the identification of specific patterns in the dying person's communication and decreases the risk for inappropriate labelling of behaviours.

PHYSICAL CARE. Nursing management related to physical care at the end of life focuses on symptom management and comfort rather than treatments for curing a particular disease or disorder (Table 13-11). The priority is meeting the patient's physiological and safety needs. Physical care addresses the needs for oxygen, nutrition, pain relief, mobility, elimination, and skin care. People who are dying deserve and require the same physical care as do patients who are expected to recover. If possible, it is important to discuss with the patient and family the goals of care before treatment begins. Documentation of the discussion regarding wishes and preferences may take the form of an advance directive or simply recorded in the medical chart to clearly communicate with the interdisciplinary team.

POSTMORTEM CARE. The pronouncement of death is not a reserved act or a delegated medical function, and is within the scope of nursing practice, for an expected death related to a terminal illness (College of Registered Nurses of British Columbia, 2015, p. 10). Although the death is anticipated, the pronouncement of death should be made with certainty and compassion. Death is considered to have occurred when cardiac and respiratory functions have ceased. The pronouncement of death is verification of an absence of an apical pulse and respirations and that the pupils are fixed and dilated. A certification of death—a legal medical document stating that the patient is dead—is usually required within 24 hours of a death. This function is in the purview of a physician or medical examiner, who is required to both sign the document and indicate the cause of death (College & Association of Registered Nurses of Alberta, 2011).

After the patient is pronounced dead, prepare or delegate preparation of the body for immediate viewing by the family with consideration for cultural customs and in accord with employer policies and procedures. In some cultures, it may be important to allow the family to prepare or assist in caring for the body. In general, the nurse should close the eyes, replace dentures, wash the body as needed (placing pads under the perineum to absorb urine and feces), and remove tubes and dressings (if appropriate). The body is straightened, the pillow is positioned to support the head, and a small rolled towel is placed under the chin to hold the mouth closed.

The family should be allowed privacy and as much time as they need with the deceased person. In the case of an unexpected or unanticipated death, preparation of the patient's body for viewing or release to a funeral home depends on provincial law and employer policies and procedures. The deceased person should never be referred to as "the body." Care of and discussion related to the person should continue to be respectful even after death.

SPECIAL NEEDS OF CAREGIVERS IN END-OF-LIFE CARE

Special Needs of Family Caregivers

Family caregivers are important in meeting the patient's physical and psychosocial needs. The role of caregivers includes working and communicating with the patient and other family members, supporting the patient's concerns, and helping the patient resolve any unfinished business. Families often face emotional, physical, and economic consequences as a result of caring for a family member who is dying. The caregiver's responsibilities do not end when the person is admitted to an acute care, inpatient hospice, or long-term care facility.

An understanding of the grieving process as it affects both the patient and family is important. Being present during a family member's dying process can be highly stressful. The nurse should recognize signs and behaviours among family members who may be at risk for abnormal grief reactions, and be prepared to intervene if necessary. Warning signs may include dependency and negative feelings about the dying person, inability to express feelings, sleep disturbances, a history of depression, difficult reactions to previous losses, perceived lack of social or family support, low self-esteem, multiple previous bereavements, alcoholism, or substance abuse. Caregivers with concurrent life crises (e.g., divorce) will be especially at risk.

Family caregivers and other family members need encouragement to continue their usual activities as much as possible. They need to discuss their activities and maintain some control over their lives. The nurse should inform caregivers about appropriate resources for support, including respite care. Resources such as community counselling and local support may assist some people in working through their grief.

The nurse should encourage caregivers to build a support system of extended family, friends, faith community, and clergy. The caregivers should have people to call on at any time to express any feelings they are experiencing.

Special Needs of Nurses

Many nurses who care for dying patients do so because they are passionate about providing high-quality EOL care. Caring for patients and their families at the end of life is challenging and rewarding but also intense and emotionally charged (Sliter, Sinclair, Yuan, et al., 2014). A bond or connection may develop between the nurse and the patient or family. The nurse should be aware of how grief personally affects him or her. When the nurse provides care for terminally ill or dying patients, he or she is not immune to feelings of loss. It is common to feel helpless and powerless when dealing with death. The nurse may need to express feelings of sorrow, guilt, and frustration. It is important to recognize one's own values, attitudes, and feelings about death.

Interventions are available that may help ease the nurse's physical and emotional stress. The nurse should be aware of what he or she can and cannot control. Recognizing personal feelings allows openness in exchanging feelings with the patient and family. Realizing that it is okay to cry with the patient or family during the end of life may be important for the nurse's well-being.

To meet the nurse's personal needs, she or he should focus on interventions that will help decrease stress. The nurse can get involved in hobbies or other interests, schedule time for her- or himself, ensure time for sleep, maintain a peer support system, and develop a support system beyond the workplace (Wittenberg-Lyles, Goldsmith, & Reno, 2014). Specialized hospice palliative care teams can help the nurse cope through professionally assisted groups, informal discussion sessions, and flexible time schedules.

TABLE 13-11   NURSING MANAGEMENT

Physical Care at the End of Life

Characteristics	Nursing Management
Pain • May be a major symptom associated with terminal illness and is the one most feared • Can be acute or chronic • Possible causes of bone pain: metastases, fractures, arthritis, and immobility • Aggravated by physical and emotional stressors	• Assess pain thoroughly and regularly to determine the quality, intensity, location, and contributing and alleviating factors. • Minimize possible irritants such as wet skin, heat or cold, and pressure. • Administer medications around the clock in a timely manner and on a regular basis to provide constant relief, rather than waiting until the pain is unbearable and then trying to relieve it. • Provide complementary and alternative therapies such as guided imagery, massage, and relaxation techniques as needed (see Chapter 12). • Evaluate effectiveness of pain relief measures frequently to ensure that the patient is on a correct, adequate drug regimen. • Do not delay or deny pain relief measures to a terminally ill patient.
Delirium • A state characterized by confusion, disorientation, restlessness, clouding of consciousness, incoherence, fear, anxiety, excitement, and often hallucinations • May be misidentified as depression, psychosis, anger, or anxiety • May be caused by use of opioids or corticosteroids, as well as by their withdrawal • May be exacerbated by underlying disease process • Generally considered a reversible process	• Perform a thorough assessment for reversible causes of delirium, including pain, constipation, and urinary retention. • Provide a room that is quiet, well lit, and familiar to reduce the effects of delirium. • Reorient the dying person with delirium to person, place, and time with each encounter. • Administer ordered benzodiazepines and sedatives as needed. • Stay physically close to a frightened patient. Reassure in a calm, soft voice with touch and slow strokes of the skin. • Provide family with emotional support and encouragement in their efforts to cope with the behaviours associated with delirium.
Anxiety/Restlessness • May occur as death approaches and cerebral metabolism slows • May occur with tachypnea, dyspnea, or sweating	• Assess for previous anxiety disorder. • Assess for spiritual distress or concerns related to death as causes of restlessness and agitation. • Assess for urinary retention and stool impaction. • Do not restrain. • Use soothing music; slow, soft touch; and calm, soft voice. • Limit the number of people at the patient's bedside.
Dysphagia • May occur because of extreme weakness and changes in level of consciousness • Difficulty swallowing • Aspiration of liquids or solids, or both • Drooling/inability to swallow secretions	• Identify the least invasive alternative routes of administration for drugs needed for symptom management. • If necessary, use alternative (rectal, buccal, transdermal) medication routes. • Suction orally as needed. • Modify diet as tolerated/desired (soft, pureed, chopped meats). • Hand feed small meals. • Elevate the patient's head for meals and for at least 30 minutes after. • Discontinue nonessential medications. • Discuss risk of aspiration with patient/family.
Weakness and Fatigue • Expected at the end of life • Exacerbated by metabolic demands related to disease process	• Assess the patient's tolerance for activities. • Time nursing interventions to conserve the patient's energy. • Help the patient identify and complete valued or desired activities. • Provide support as needed to maintain patient's positions in bed or chair. • Provide frequent rest periods for the patient.
Dehydration • May occur during the last days of life • Hunger and thirst rare in the last days of life • Tendency for dying patients to take in less food and fluid	• Assess mucous membranes frequently for dryness, which can lead to discomfort. • Maintain complete, regular oral care to provide for comfort and hydration of mucous membranes. • Encourage consumption of ice chips and sips of fluids, or use moist cloths to provide moisture to the mouth. • Use moist cloths and swabs for an unconscious patient to prevent aspiration. • Apply lubricant to the lips and oral mucous membranes as needed. • Do not force the patient to eat or drink. • Teach the family that hunger and thirst are rare in the last days of life. • Reassure the family that cessation of food and fluid intake is a natural part of the process of dying.

Continued

TABLE 13-11 NURSING MANAGEMENT

Physical Care at the End of Life—cont'd

Characteristics	Nursing Management
Dyspnea • Subjective symptom • Accompanied by fear of suffocation and anxiety • Can be exacerbated by underlying disease process • Progressive difficulty with coughing and expectorating secretions	• Assess respiratory status regularly. • Elevate the patient's head, or position the patient on one side to improve chest expansion. • Use a fan or air conditioner to facilitate movement of cool air. • Teach and encourage the use of pursed-lip breathing. • Administer supplemental oxygen as ordered. • Suction as necessary to remove accumulation of mucus from the airways. Suction cautiously when a patient is in the terminal phase. • Administer expectorant as ordered.
Myoclonus • Mild to severe jerking or twitching, sometimes associated with use of high dose of opioids • Possible complaints of involuntary twitching of extremities	• Assess for initial onset, duration, and any discomfort or distress experienced by patient. • If myoclonus is distressing or becoming more severe, discuss possible drug therapy modifications with the health care provider. • Changes in opioid medication may alleviate or decrease myoclonus.
Skin Breakdown Difficulty maintaining skin integrity at the end of life Risk for development increased by immobility, urinary and bowel incontinence, dry skin, nutritional deficits, anemia, friction, and shearing forces Skin integrity possibly impaired by disease and other processes As death approaches, decrease of circulation to the extremities; become cool, mottled, and cyanotic	• Assess skin for signs of breakdown. • Implement protocols to prevent skin breakdown by controlling drainage and odour and by keeping the skin and any wound areas clean. • Perform wound assessments as needed. • Follow appropriate nursing management protocol for dressing wounds. • Follow appropriate nursing management protocol for a patient who is immobile, but consider realistic outcomes of skin integrity in relation to maintenance of comfort. • Follow appropriate nursing management to prevent skin irritations and breakdown from urinary and bowel incontinence. • Use blankets to cover for warmth. Never apply heat. • Prevent the effects of shearing forces.
Bowel Patterns • Constipation possibly caused by immobility, use of opioid medications, depression, lack of fibre in the diet, and dehydration • Diarrhea possible as muscles relax or as a result of fecal impaction related to the use of opioids and immobility	• Assess bowel function. • Assess for and remove fecal impactions. • Encourage movement and physical activities as tolerated. • Encourage fibre in the diet if appropriate. • Encourage fluid intake if appropriate. • Use suppositories, stool softeners, laxatives, or enemas if ordered. • Assess patient for confusion, agitation, restlessness, and pain, which may be signs of constipation.
Urinary Incontinence • May result from disease progression or changes in the level of consciousness • Relaxation of perineal muscles soon before death	• Assess urinary function. • Use absorbent pads for urinary incontinence. • Follow appropriate nursing protocol for the consideration and use of indwelling or external catheters. • Follow appropriate nursing management to prevent skin irritations and breakdown from urinary incontinence.
Anorexia, Nausea, and Vomiting • May be caused by complications of disease process • Nausea exacerbated by drugs • All exacerbated by constipation, impaction, and bowel obstruction	• Assess the patient for complaints of nausea or vomiting. • Assess possible contributing causes of nausea or vomiting. • Have family provide the patient's favourite foods. • Discuss modifications to the drug regimen with the health care provider. • Provide antiemetics before meals if ordered. • Offer and provide frequent meals with small portions of favourite foods. • Offer culturally appropriate foods. • Provide frequent mouth care, especially after the patient vomits. • Ensure uninterrupted mealtimes. • If ordered, administer medications (e.g., megestrol, corticosteroids) to increase appetite. • Teach family that appetite naturally decreases at the end of life.
Candidiasis • White, cottage cheese–like oral plaques • Fungal overgrowth in the mouth as a result of chemotherapy, immunosuppression, or both	• Administer oral antifungal nystatin if ordered. • Clean dentures and other dental appliances to prevent re-infection. • Provide oral hygiene, and use a soft toothbrush.

REVIEW QUESTIONS

The number of the question corresponds to the same-numbered objective at the beginning of the chapter.

1. The client is in the terminal stages of lung cancer. On assessment, it is noted that the client has alternating periods of apnea and deep, rapid breathing. Which of the following is the correct terminology to use in documenting this assessment data?
   a. Tachypnea
   b. Stertorous respirations
   c. Dyspnea
   d. Cheyne-Stokes respirations

2. The client has inoperable pancreatic cancer. Until recently, they have been very active in a book club, but no longer wants to attend. Which common end of life psychological manifestation is the client demonstrating?
   a. Decreased socialization
   b. Decreased disease progression
   c. Decreased sense of helplessness
   d. Decreased perception of pain and touch

3. A client died 2 years ago but his wife refuses to donate his belongings to charity. She often sits in the bedroom, crying and talking to her long-dead husband. What type of grief is the wife experiencing?
   a. Adaptive grief
   b. Disruptive grief
   c. Anticipatory grief
   d. Prolonged grief

4. A female client, in the terminal stages of a disease, experiences choking when she given food or fluids. The family is concerned that the client is starving. What is the most helpful response from the nurse? *(Select all that apply)*
   a. "Allow me to show you how to moisten her mouth."
   b. "If you give her food, she will choke to death."
   c. "I can order you a tray and you can try to feed her if you like."
   d. "People who are dying usually don't experience hunger or thirst."

5. The client did not have an advance directive when he suffered a serious stroke. Who is responsible for identifying end-of-life measures to be instituted when the patient cannot communicate his or her specific wishes?
   a. Adult children
   b. Notary and attorney
   c. Physician and family
   d. Physician and nursing staff

6. When a male client was diagnosed with renal failure, his new wife asked his children from a previous marriage to help with their father's care. Each of the children refused to help and his wife cared for him without help until his death. Which factors may predispose the children to an abnormal grief reaction? *(Select all that apply)*
   a. Negative feelings about the deceased person
   b. Lack of experience with other deaths in the family
   c. Difficulties with substance misuse
   d. Residing geographically far away

7. The nurse has been working full time with terminally ill clients for 3 years. The nurse has been experiencing irritability and mixed emotions when expressing sadness since four clients died on the same day. What should the nurse change to optimize the quality of her nursing care?
   a. Full-time work schedule
   b. Past feelings toward death
   c. Patterns for dealing with grief
   d. Demands for involvement in care

1. d; 2. a; 3. d; 4. a, d; 5. c; 6. a, b, c, d; 7. c.

⊜volve

For even more review questions, visit *http://evolve.elsevier.com/Canada/ Lewis/medsurg.*

REFERENCES

Abarshi, E. A., Papavasiliou, E. R., Preston, N., et al. (2014). The complexity of nurses' attitudes and practice of sedation at the end of life: A systematic review. *Journal of Pain and Symptom Management, 47*(5), 915–925. doi:10.1016/j.jpainsymman.2013.06 .011. Retrieved from *http://www.jpsmjournal.com/article/S0885 -3924(13)00396-5/pdf.*

Alberta Health Services. (2015). *Edmonton Zone Palliative Care Program: Palliative sedation guideline.* Retrieved from *http:// www.palliative.org/NewPC/_pdfs/management/Palliative%20 Sedation%20Final%20Dec%202015.pdf.*

Back, A. L., Arnold, R. M., Baile, W. F., et al. (2005). Approaching difficult communication tasks in oncology. *A Cancer Journal for Clinicians, 55,* 164–177. doi:10.3322/canjclin.55.3.164. (Seminal).

Boles, J. (2015). Bearing bad news: Supporting patients and families through difficult conversations. *Pediatric Nursing, 41*(6), 306–308.

Bruera, S., Chisholm, G., Dos Santos, R., et al. (2015). Frequency and factors associated with unexpected death in an acute palliative care unit: Expect the unexpected. *Journal of Pain and Symptom Management, 49*(5), 822–827. Retrieved from *http://dx.doi.org/ 10.1016/j.jpainsymman.2014.10.011.*

Carstairs, S. (Subcommittee Chair). (2000). *Quality end-of-life care: The right of every Canadian. Subcommittee to Update "Of Life and Death" of the Standing Senate Committee on Social Affairs, Science and Technology. Final report.* Retrieved from *https://sencanada.ca/ content/sen/committee/362/upda/rep/repfinjun00-e.htm.* (Seminal).

Canadian Hospice Palliative Care Association. (2013a). *A model to guide hospice palliative care.* Ottawa: Author. Retrieved from *http://www.chpca.net/media/319547/norms-of-practice-eng-web.pdf.*

Canadian Hospice Palliative Care Association. (2013b). *Innovative models of integrated hospice palliative care. The Way Forward initiative: an integrated approach to care.* Retrieved from *http:// www.hpcintegration.ca/media/40546/TWF-innovative-models-report -Eng-webfinal-2.pdf.*

Canadian Hospice Palliative Care Association. (2015). *The Way Forward national framework: A roadmap for an integrated palliative care approach to care.* Retrieved from *http://www .hpcintegration.ca/media/60044/TWF-framework-doc-Eng-2015 -final-April1.pdf.*

Canadian Hospice Palliative Care Association. (2016). *The Canadian Hospice Palliative Care Association … A history.* Retrieved from *http://www.chpca.net/about-us/history.aspx.*

College & Association of Registered Nurses of Alberta. (2011). *Pronouncement of death: Guidelines for regulated members.* Edmonton, AB: Author. Retrieved from *http://www.nurses.ab.ca/ content/dam/carna/pdfs/DocumentList/Guidelines/PronounceDeath _Sept2011.pdf.*

College of Registered Nurses of British Columbia. (2015). *Scope of practice for registered nurses.* Vancouver: Author. Retrieved from *https://crnbc.ca/Standards/Lists/StandardResources/433Scopefor RegisteredNurses.pdf.*

Cook, D., Rocker, G., & Heyland, D. (2013). Enhancing the quality of end-of-life care in Canada. *Canadian Medical Association Journal, 185*(16), 1383–1384.

Fraser Health Authority. (2009). *Symptom assessment acronym.* Retrieved from *http://www.fraserhealth.ca/media/Symptom AssessmentRevised_Sept09.pdf.* (Seminal).

Gill, J. S., Klarenbach, S., Barnieh, L., et al. (2014). Financial incentives to increase Canadian organ donation: Quick fix or fallacy? *American Journal of Kidney Diseases, 63*(1), 133–140. Retrieved from *http://dx.doi.org/10.1053/j.ajkd.2013.08.029.*

Hampton, M., Baydale, A., Bourassa, C., et al. (2010). Completing the circle: Elders speak about end-of-life care with Aboriginal families in Canada. *Journal of Palliative Care, 26*(1), 6–14. (Limited Publications). (Seminal).

Holdsworth, L. M., Gage, H., Coulton, S., et al. (2015). A quasi-experimental controlled evaluation of the impact of a hospice rapid response community service for end-of-life care on achievement of preferred place of death. *Palliative Medicine, 29*(9), 817–825. doi:10.1177/0269216315582124.

Hui, D., Dos Santos, R., Chisholm, G., et al. (2015). Beside clinical signs associated with impending death in patients with advanced cancer: Preliminary findings of a prospective, longitudinal cohort study. *Cancer, 121*(6), 960–967. doi:10.1002/cncr.29048.

Jalkin, J. A., & Olver, I. (2011). Dying cancer patients talk about physician and patient roles in DNR decision making. *Health Expectations, 14,* 147–158. doi:10.1111/j.1369-7625.2010.00630.x. (Seminal).

Kübler-Ross, E. (1969). *On death and dying.* New York: Macmillan. (Seminal).

Library of Parliament. (2005). *The Canada Health Act: Overview and options 94-4E.* Retrieved from *http://www.parl.gc.ca/content/lop/ researchpublications/944-e.pdf.* (Seminal).

LoPresti, M. A., Dement, F., & Gold, H. T. (2014). End-of-life care for people from ethnic minority groups: a systematic review. *American Journal of Hospice Palliative Medicine, 33*(3), 291–305. doi:10.1177/1049909114565658.

Lutz, S. (2011). The history of hospice and palliative care. *Current Problems in Cancer, 35*(6), 304–309. doi:10.1016/j .currproblcancer.2011.10.004.

National Cancer Institute. (2014). *Grief, bereavement, and coping with loss (PDQ®)—Health professional version.* Retrieved from *http://www.cancer.gov/about-cancer/advanced-cancer/caregivers/ planning/bereavement-hp-pdq.*

Ontario Ministry of Health and Long-Term Care & Attorney General. (2015). *Provincial–territorial expert advisory group on physician-assisted dying: Final report.* Retrieved from *http:// www.health.gov.on.ca/en/news/bulletin/2015/docs/eagreport _20151214_en.pdf.*

Ontario Trillium Gift of Life Network. (n.d.). *Organ and tissue donation: Frequently asked questions for health professionals.* Retrieved from *https://www.giftoflife.on.ca/resources/pdf/FAQ _for_HP_(fact_sheet)_EN.pdf.*

Oyebode, J. R., & Owens, R. G. (2013). Bereavement and the role of religious and cultural factors. *Cruse Bereavement Care, 32*(2), 60–64. doi:10.1080/02682621.2013.812828.

Pereira, J. L. (2013). *The Pallium palliative pocketbook.* Ottawa: Pallium Canada.

Quality End-of-Life Care Coalition of Canada (QELCCC). (2010). *Blueprint for Action 2010 to 2020.* Retrieved from *http://www .qelccc.ca/media/3749/eng_progress_report_20102012-07-10_2.pdf.* (Seminal).

Quality End-of-Life Care Coalition of Canada. (2012). *Executive summary.* Retrieved from *http://www.qelccc.ca/media/3806/ microsoft_word_-_3_executive_summary_2012.pdf.*

Shemie, S. D., Hornby, L., Baker, A., et al. (2014). International guideline development for the determination of death. *Intensive Care Medicine, 40,* 788–797. doi:10.1007/s00134-014-3242-7.

Skalla, K., & Ferrell, B. (2015). Challenges in assessing spiritual distress in survivors of cancer. *Clinical Journal of Oncology Nursing, 19*(1), 99–104. doi:10.1188/15.CJON.99-104.

Sliter, M. T., Sinclair, R. R., Yuan, Z., et al. (2014). Don't fear the reaper: Trait death anxiety, mortality salience, and occupational health. *The Journal of Applied Psychology, 99*(4), 759–769. doi:10.1037/a0035729.

Statistics Canada. (2010). *Population projections for Canada, provinces and territories, 2009 to 2036.* Catalogue No. 91-520-X. Ottawa: Author. Retrieved from *http://www.statcan.gc.ca/pub/ 91-520-x/91-520-x2010001-eng.pdf.*

Statistics Canada. (2011a). *The 10 leading causes of death, 2011.* Retrieved from *http://www.statcan.gc.ca/pub/82-625-x/2014001/ article/11896-eng.htm.*

Statistics Canada. (2011b). *Aboriginal peoples in Canada: First Nations People, Métis and Inuit.* Retrieved from *http://www12 .statcan.gc.ca/nhs-enm/2011/as-sa/99-011-x/99-011-x2011001 -eng.pdf.*

Supreme Court of Canada. (2016). *Carter v. Canada (Attorney General).* Supreme Court Judgments 2016 SCC 4. Retrieved from *http://scc-csc.lexum.com/scc-csc/scc-csc/en/item/15696/index.do.*

Waldrop, D. P., & Meeker, M. A. (2014). Final decisions: How hospice enrollment prompts meaningful choices about life closure. *Palliative and Supportive Care, 12,* 211–221. doi:10.1017/ S1478951512001113.

Wittenberg-Lyles, E., Goldsmith, J., & Reno, J. (2014). Perceived benefits and challenges of an oncology nurse support group. *Clinical Journal of Oncology Nursing, 18*(4), E71 E76. doi:10.1188/14.CJON.E71-E76.

Worden, J. W. (2009). *Grief counseling and grief therapy: A handbook for the mental health practitioner* (4th ed.). New York: Springer. (Seminal).

World Health Organization. (2015). *WHO definition of palliative care.* Retrieved from *http://www.who.int/cancer/palliative/ definition/en/.*

RESOURCES

Advance Care Planning: "Speak Up"
http://www.advancecareplanning.ca

Alberta Health Services: "Goals of Care Designations"
https://myhealth.alberta.ca/Alberta/Pages/advance-care-planning -goals-of-care-designations.aspx

Canadian Cancer Society
http://www.cancer.ca

Canadian Home Care Association
http://www.cdnhomecare.ca/

Canadian Hospice Palliative Care Association
http://www.chpca.net

Canadian Virtual Hospice
http://www.virtualhospice.ca

Casey House Hospice
http://www.caseyhouse.com

Pallium Canada
http://www.pallium.ca

Temmy Latner Centre for Palliative Care
http://www.tlcpc.org/

Trillium Gift of Life Network
http://www.giftoflife.on.ca

Victoria Hospice Society
http://www.victoriahospice.org

Worldwide Hospice Palliative Care Alliance
http://www.thewhpca.org

For additional Internet resources, see the website for this book at *http://evolve.elsevier.com/Canada/Lewis/medsurg*

Pathophysiological Mechanisms of Disease

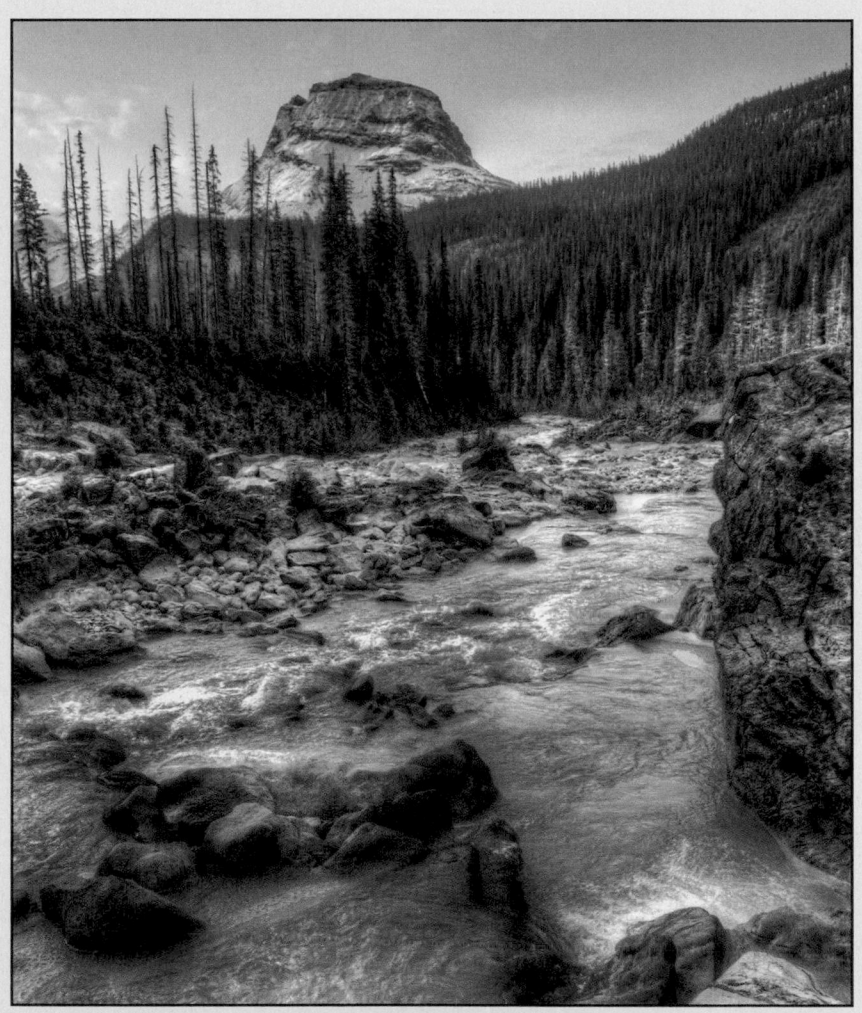

Source: BGSmith/Shutterstock.com.

Inflammation and Wound Healing

Written by: Sharon L. Lewis
Adapted by: Beth Clarke

evolve WEBSITE

http://evolve.elsevier.com/Canada/Lewis/medsurg

- Review Questions (Online Only)
- Key Points
- Answer Guidelines for Case Study
- Student Case Study
  - Pressure Injuries

- Customizable Nursing Care Plans
  - Fever
  - Pressure Injury
- Audio Glossary
- Content Updates

LEARNING OBJECTIVES

1. Explain the mechanisms that enable the cell to adapt to sublethal injury.
2. Describe the causes and mechanisms of lethal cell injury.
3. Differentiate among types of cell necrosis.
4. Describe the components and functions of the mononuclear phagocyte system.
5. Describe the inflammatory response, including vascular and cellular responses and exudate formation.
6. Explain local and systemic manifestations of inflammation and their physiological bases.
7. Describe the pharmacological, dietary, and nursing management of inflammation.

8. Differentiate between healing by primary, secondary, and tertiary intention.
9. Describe the factors that delay wound healing and common complications of wound healing.
10. Describe the risk assessment process for pressure injuries.
11. Discuss measures to prevent the development of pressure injuries.
12. Explain the causes and clinical manifestations of pressure injuries.
13. Discuss collaborative and nursing management of a patient with pressure injuries.

KEY TERMS

adhesions, p. 231
anaplasia, p. 224
apoptosis, p. 224
atrophy, p. 224
dehiscence, p. 231
dry gangrene, p. 225
dysplasia, p. 224

evisceration, p. 232
fibroblasts, p. 230
fistula, p. 232
hyperplasia, p. 224
hypertrophic scar, p. 232
hypertrophy, p. 223
inflammatory response, p. 225

integrins, p. 226
keloid, p. 232
lethal injury, p. 223
metaplasia, p. 224
necrosis, p. 224
pressure injury, p. 237
regeneration, p. 229

repair, p. 229
selectins, p. 226
shearing force, p. 237
sublethal injury, p. 223
wet gangrene, p. 225

CELL INJURY

Cell injury can be sublethal or lethal. **Sublethal injury** alters function without causing cell destruction. The changes caused by this type of injury are potentially reversible if the harmful stimulus is removed. **Lethal injury** is an irreversible process that causes cell death.

Cell Adaptation to Sublethal Injury

Cell adaptations to sublethal injuries are common and are part of many normal physiological processes, but they may also result from pathological changes. For example, prolonged exposure to sunlight stimulates melanin production, which

provides protection of deeper skin layers; increased melanin production causes tanning of the skin. Lack of muscular activity can lead to atrophy and decreased tone of muscles. Adaptive processes of the cell include hypertrophy, hyperplasia, atrophy, and metaplasia. Other responses, which are considered maladaptive, are dysplasia and anaplasia.

Hypertrophy. **Hypertrophy** is an expansion in the size of cells, which results in increased tissue mass without cell division. *Physiological hypertrophy* results from increased workload on an organ or tissue that is not caused by disease. Examples include an increase in the muscle mass that occurs during weight training, uterine expansion during pregnancy from hormonal stimulation, and enlargement of the sex organs during puberty.

Pathological hypertrophy occurs as a result of disease: for example, enlargement and thickening of the heart ventricle in a person with severe hypertension in response to increased cardiac workload. *Compensatory hypertrophy* occurs in response to increased workload caused by reduced function: for example, when a kidney is removed, the remaining kidney enlarges as a result of increased work demand.

Hyperplasia. Hyperplasia is a multiplication of cells as a result of increased cellular division. *Physiological hyperplasia* is an adaptive response to normal body changes. For example, cells of the uterus undergo hyperplasia during pregnancy, and the female breast undergoes hyperplasia during puberty and lactation. Examples of *pathological hyperplasia* are endometrial hyperplasia, caused by excessive estrogen secretion, and acromegaly, caused by excessive production of growth hormone. *Compensatory hyperplasia* is a process whereby cells of certain organs regenerate. For example, if portions of the liver are removed, the remaining cells undergo increased mitosis to compensate.

Atrophy. Atrophy is a decrease in the size of a tissue or organ as a result of a reduction in the number or size of individual cells. It is frequently caused by disease (e.g., musculo-skeletal disease), lack of blood supply (e.g., thrombus formation), the natural aging process (e.g., atrophy of ovaries after menopause), inactivity (e.g., decreased muscle size), or nutritional deficiency.

Metaplasia. Metaplasia is the transformation of one cell type into another in response to a change in physiological condition or an external irritant. An example of *physiological metaplasia* is the change of circulating monocytes to macrophages as they migrate into inflamed tissues. An example of *pathophysiological metaplasia* is the change of normal pseudostratified columnar epithelium of the bronchi to squamous epithelium in response to chronic cigarette smoking. These squamous cells can later become cancerous.

Dysplasia. Dysplasia is an abnormal differentiation of dividing cells that results in changes in their size, shape, and appearance. Minor dysplasia is found in some areas of inflammation. Dysplasia is potentially reversible if the stimulus for the change is removed. Dysplasia is frequently a precursor of malignancy, as in cervical dysplasia.

Anaplasia. Anaplasia is cell differentiation to a more immature or embryonic form. Malignant tumours are often characterized by anaplastic cell growth.

Causes of Lethal Cell Injury

Many different agents and factors can cause lethal cell injury (Table 14-1). The mechanisms of actual cell death may include deterioration of the nucleus, such as pyknosis (nuclear condensation and shrinking), karyolysis (dissolution of nucleus and contents), disruption of cell metabolism, and rupture of the cell membrane. Microbial invasion often results in cell injury and death. Infection occurs when pathogens invade and multiply in body tissue.

Cell Apoptosis and Necrosis

Apoptosis and necrosis are the two fundamental types of cell death. Programmed cell death (apoptosis) is a normal, anticipated event that occurs in some regenerating tissues to create homeostasis, such as bone marrow, skin, and gut epithelium. In contrast, necrosis is tissue death that occurs as a result of a traumatic injury, infection, or exposure to a toxic chemical that causes a local inflammatory response, which results from the release of

---

TABLE 14-1	**CAUSES OF LETHAL CELL INJURY**
Cause	**Effect on Cell**
Hypoxia or ischemic injury	Compromised cell metabolism, acute or gradual cell death
Physical agents	
• Heat	Denaturation of protein, acceleration of metabolic reactions (see Chapter 27)
• Cold	Decreased blood flow from vasoconstriction, slowed metabolic reactions, thrombosis of blood vessels, freezing of cell contents that forms crystals and can cause cell to burst (see Chapter 71)
• Radiation	Alteration of cell structure and activity, alteration of enzyme systems, mutations (see Chapter 18)
• Electrothermal injury	Interruption of neural conduction, fibrillation of cardiac muscle, coagulative necrosis of skin and skeletal muscle (see Chapter 27)
• Mechanical trauma	Transfer of excess kinetic energy to cells, causing rupture of cells, blood vessels, tissue; examples include the following: *Abrasion:* scraping of skin or mucous membrane *Laceration:* severing of vessels and tissue *Contusion (bruise):* crushing of tissue cells, causing hemorrhage into skin *Puncture:* piercing of body structure or organ *Incision:* surgical cutting
Chemical injury	Alteration of cell metabolism, interference with normal enzymatic action within cells (see Chapter 27)
Microbial injury	
• Viruses	Taking over of cell metabolism and synthesis of new particles that may cause cell rupture; cumulative effect may produce clinical disease
• Bacteria	Destruction of cell membrane or cell nucleus, production of lethal toxins
Immunological*	
• Antigen–antibody response	Release of substances (histamine, complement) that can injure and damage cells
• Autoimmune response	Activation of complement, which destroys normal cells and produces inflammation (see Chapter 16)
Neoplastic growth	Cell destruction from abnormal and uncontrolled cell growth (see Chapter 18)
Normal substances (e.g., digestive enzymes, uric acid)	Release into abdomen, causing peritonitis and crystallization of excess accumulation in joints and renal tissue

*See Chapter 16 for a more detailed discussion.

intracellular contents after the rupture of the outer membrane of the dead cells. Various types of tissue necrosis occur in different organs or tissues (Table 14-2; Figure 14-1).

Dry gangrene can result from degenerative changes that occur with certain chronic diseases, such as atherosclerosis or diabetes, when the blood supply to the lower extremities is gradually reduced (see Figure 14-1). **Wet gangrene**, which can quickly become fatal, occurs as the result of a sudden rapid elimination of blood flow, such as that seen in a severe burn or traumatic crush injury. It is malodorous because of extensive tissue liquefaction, which makes the affected area soft, and the odour is often indicative of a bacterial infection.

DEFENCE AGAINST INJURY

To protect against injury and infection, the body has various defence mechanisms: (a) the skin and mucous membranes (see Chapter 25); (b) the mononuclear phagocyte system; (c) the inflammatory response; and (d) the immune system (see Chapter 16).

Mononuclear Phagocyte System

The *mononuclear phagocyte system* consists of monocytes and macrophages and their precursor cells. In the past, the mononuclear phagocyte system was called the *reticuloendothelial system*. However, it is not a body system with distinctly defined tissues and organs. Rather, it consists of phagocytic cells located in various tissues and organs. The phagocytic cells are either fixed or free (mobile). The macrophages of the liver, spleen, bone marrow, lungs, lymph nodes, and nervous system are fixed phagocytes. The monocytes in blood and the macrophages found in connective tissue are mobile, or wandering, phagocytes.

Monocytes and macrophages originate in the bone marrow. Monocytes spend a few days in the blood and then enter tissues and change into macrophages. Tissue macrophages are larger and more phagocytic than monocytes.

The functions of the macrophage system include recognition and phagocytosis of foreign material such as microorganisms, removal of old or damaged cells from circulation, and participation in the immune response (see Chapter 16).

Inflammatory Response

The **inflammatory response** is a biological response to cell injury caused by pathogens, irritants, or chronic health conditions. Through this response, the inflammatory agent is neutralized and diluted, necrotic materials are removed, and an environment suitable for healing and repair is established. The term *inflammation* should not be confused with *infection*. Infections almost always cause inflammation, but not all inflammations are caused by infections. Furthermore, neutropenic individuals may not mount an inflammatory response to infection. An infection involves invasion of tissues or cells by microorganisms such as bacteria, fungi, and viruses. Inflammation can also be caused by heat, radiation, trauma, chemicals, allergens, or an autoimmune reaction (see Table 14-1). Under these conditions, the presence of an infection represents a superimposed invasion of microorganisms.

The mechanism of inflammation is basically the same regardless of the injuring agent. The intensity of the response depends on the extent and the severity of injury and on the reactive capacity of the injured person. The inflammatory response can be divided into a vascular response, a cellular response, formation of exudate, and healing. Figure 14-2 illustrates the vascular and cellular responses to injury.

Vascular Response. After cell injury, arterioles in the area briefly undergo transient vasoconstriction, which is stimulated by the sympathetic nervous system. Platelets adhere to vessels and aggregate to seal the injured area, forming a fibrin-platelet clot, and they release proinflammatory mediators such as histamine,

FIGURE 14-1 Gangrene of the toes. Gangrenous necrosis 6 weeks after frostbite injury. Source: Courtesy of Cameron Bangs, MD. From Auerbach, P. S. (2007). *Wilderness medicine* (6th ed., p. 201). St. Louis: Elsevier.

TABLE 14-2	TYPES OF NECROSIS
Type	**Description**
Coagulative necrosis	Caused by ischemia. Ischemia results in decreased levels of adenosine triphosphate (ATP), increased levels of cytosolic Ca^{2+}, and free radical formation, each of which eventually causes membrane damage. A myocardial infarct is an example of a localized area of coagulative necrosis.
Liquefactive necrosis	Usually caused by focal bacterial infections because they can attract polymorphonuclear leukocytes (PMNs). The enzymes in the PMNs are released to fight the bacteria but also dissolve the tissues nearby, which causes pus to accumulate and the tissue to liquefy. An abscess is an example of a liquefactive necrotic process.
Caseous necrosis	A distinct form of coagulative necrosis that occurs in mycobacterial infections (e.g., tuberculosis) or in tumour necrosis, in which the coagulated tissue no longer resembles the cells but is in chunks of unrecognizable debris.
Gangrene	Necrosis of an appendage (usually the limbs). The term may also be used to describe necrosis of an appendix or gallbladder. This form of necrosis applies to ischemic necrosis, usually with superimposed bacterial action (wet gangrene) but sometimes in toes without bacterial effects (dry gangrene or mummification).

Source: Adapted from Krafts, K. (2012). *A quick summary of six types of necrosis*. Retrieved from *http://www.pathologystudent.com/?p=5770*.

PATHOPHYSIOLOGY MAP

FIGURE 14-2 Vascular and cellular responses in inflammation.

which cause vasodilation. This results in *hyperemia* (increased blood flow in the area) in which filtration pressure increases, causing endothelial cell retraction and an increase in capillary permeability. Movement of fluid from capillaries into tissue spaces is thus facilitated. Initially composed of serous fluid, this inflammatory exudate later contains plasma proteins, primarily albumin, which exerts oncotic pressure that further draws fluid from blood vessels, and the tissue become edematous.

As the plasma protein fibrinogen leaves the blood, it is activated by the products of the injured cells to become fibrin. Fibrin strengthens the blood clot formed by platelets. In tissue, the clot functions to trap bacteria, prevent their spread, and serve as a framework for the healing process. Platelets release growth factors that begin the healing process.

Cellular Response. Phagocytes produce nitric oxide, whose role in the inflammatory response is to inhibit vascular smooth muscle contraction and growth, platelet aggregation, and leukocyte adhesion to endothelium. Cytokines are released by macrophages, which causes endothelial cells to express cellular adhesion molecules: **selectins** (cell surface carbohydrate-binding proteins that mediate cell adhesion, involved in leukocyte extravasation during the immune response) and **integrins** (cell receptors that mediate attachment between endothelial cells and surrounding tissues, also involved in leukocyte extravasation during the

immune response). The blood flow through capillaries in the area slows as fluid is lost and viscosity increases. Neutrophils and monocytes move to the inner surface of the capillaries (margination) and then, in ameboid manner, through the capillary wall *(diapedesis)* to the site of injury.

Chemotaxis is the directional migration of white blood cells (WBCs) along a concentration gradient of chemotactic factors, which are substances that attract WBCs to the site of inflammation. Chemotaxis is the mechanism for ensuring accumulation of neutrophils and monocytes at the site of injury.

Neutrophils. Neutrophils are the first leukocytes to arrive at the site of inflammation (within 6 to 12 hours). They phagocytize (engulf) bacteria, other foreign material, and damaged cells. Because of their short lifespan (24 to 48 hours), dead neutrophils soon accumulate. In time, a mixture of dead neutrophils, digested bacteria, and other cell debris collect as a creamy substance *(pus)*.

To keep up with the demand for neutrophils, the bone marrow releases more neutrophils into circulation. This results in an elevated WBC count, especially the neutrophil count. Sometimes the demand for neutrophils increases to the extent that the bone marrow releases immature forms of neutrophils (bands) into circulation. (Mature neutrophils are called *segmented neutrophils.*) The finding of increased numbers of band neutrophils in

TABLE 14-3 MEDIATORS OF INFLAMMATION

Mediator	Source	Mechanisms of Action
Histamine	Stored in granules of basophils, mast cells, platelets	Causes vasodilation and increased vascular permeability by stimulating contraction of endothelial cells and creating widened gaps between cells
Serotonin	Stored in platelets, mast cells, enterochromaffin cells of GI tract	Causes vasodilation and increased vascular permeability by stimulating contraction of endothelial cells and creating widened gaps between cells; stimulates smooth muscle contraction
Kinins (e.g., bradykinin)	Produced from precursor factor kininogen as a result of activation of Hageman factor (XII) of clotting system	Cause contraction of smooth muscle and dilation of blood vessels; result in stimulation of pain
Complement components (C3a, C4a, C5a)	Anaphylatoxic agents generated from complement pathway activation	Stimulate histamine release; stimulate chemotaxis
Fibrinopeptides	Produced from activation of the clotting system	Increase vascular permeability; stimulate chemotaxis for neutrophils and monocytes
Prostaglandins and leukotrienes	Produced from arachidonic acid	Prostaglandins E_1 and E_2 cause vasodilation; leukotriene B_4 stimulates chemotaxis
Cytokines	Secreted by white blood cells and other cells For more information on cytokines, see Table 16-3	Act as messengers between cell types; instruct cells to alter their proliferation differentiation, secretion, or activity

GI, gastrointestinal.

circulation is called *a shift to the left* and is commonly observed in patients with acute bacterial infections. (See Chapter 32 for a discussion of neutrophils.)

Monocytes. Monocytes are the second type of phagocytic cells that migrate from circulating blood. They are attracted by chemotactic factors and usually arrive at the site within 3 to 7 days after the onset of inflammation. On entering the tissue spaces, monocytes transform into macrophages. Together with the tissue macrophages, they assist in phagocytosis of the inflammatory debris. The macrophage role is important in cleaning the area before healing can occur. Macrophages have a long lifespan; they may stay in the damaged tissues for weeks and multiply, and they are important in orchestrating the healing process.

In some cases, macrophages perform tasks other than phagocytosis. They may accumulate and fuse to form a *multinucleated giant cell*. The giant cell attempts to phagocytize particles too large for macrophages and is then encapsulated by collagen, which leads to the formation of a granuloma. A classic example of this process occurs in tuberculosis of the lung. Although the *Mycobacterium* bacillus is walled off, a chronic state of inflammation exists. The granuloma formed is a cavity of necrotic tissue.

Lymphocytes. Lymphocytes arrive later at the site of injury. Their primary role is related to humoral and cell-mediated immunity (see Chapter 16).

Eosinophils and Basophils. Eosinophils and basophils have a more selective role in inflammation. Eosinophils are released in large quantities during an allergic reaction. They release chemicals that act to control the effects of histamine and serotonin. They are also involved in phagocytosis of the allergen-antibody complex. Eosinophils contain highly caustic chemicals that are capable of destroying a parasite's cell surfaces. The histamine and heparin that basophils carry in their granules are released during inflammation.

Chemical Mediators. Mediators of the inflammatory response are listed in Table 14-3.

Complement System. The complement system is an enzymatic cascade consisting of pathways to mediate inflammation and destroy invading pathogens. Major functions of the complement system are enhanced phagocytosis, increased vascular permeability, chemotaxis, and cellular lysis. All of these activities are important in the inflammatory response.

When the complement system is activated, the components are generated in the sequential order of C1, C4, C2, C3, C5, C6, C7, C8, and C9. The numbering reflects the order of their discovery. Some components have subparts designated by lowercase letters, such as C3a, C3b, and C5a. The primary pathway for activation of the complement system is through fixation of component C1 to an antigen–antibody complex. Immunoglobulins G and M are responsible for fixing complement. Each activated complex can act on the next component, which creates a cascade effect.

In an alternative pathway, C3 is activated without prior antigen–antibody fixation. Bacterial products, lipopolysaccharides, and neutrophil proteases can stimulate the complement sequence, beginning with C3 and with activation of C5 through C9.

Complement activation increases phagocytosis through opsonization and chemotaxis. *Opsonization* occurs when the antigen, in combination with complement factor C3b and immunoglobulin, sticks to the surface of phagocytic cells. This leads to more rapid phagocytosis. In addition, complement component C5a promotes chemotaxis.

The components C3a, C5a, and C4a are termed *anaphylatoxins* and bind to receptors on mast cells and basophils, thus triggering histamine release. Histamine causes smooth muscle contraction, vasodilation, and an increase in vascular permeability.

The entire complement sequence of C1 to C9 must be activated for cell lysis to occur. The final components (C8, C9) act on the cell surface, causing rupture of the cell membrane and lysis. In autoimmune disorders, healthy tissue can be damaged by complement activation and the resulting inflammatory response. Examples of this include rheumatoid arthritis and systemic lupus erythematosus.

TABLE 14-4   TYPES OF INFLAMMATORY EXUDATE

Type	Description	Examples
Serous	Results from fluid that has low cell and protein content; seen in early stages of inflammation or when injury is mild	Skin blisters, pleural effusion
Catarrhal	Found in tissues in which cells produce mucus; mucus production is accelerated by inflammatory response	Runny nose in association with upper respiratory tract infection
Fibrinous	Occurs with increasing vascular permeability and fibrinogen leakage into interstitial spaces; excessive amounts of fibrin coating of tissue surfaces may cause tissues to adhere	Adhesions
Purulent (pus)	Consists of WBCs, microorganisms (dead and alive), liquefied dead cells, and other debris	Furuncle (boil), abscess, cellulitis (diffuse inflammation in connective tissue)
Hemorrhagic	Results from rupture or necrosis of blood vessel walls; consists of RBCs that escape into tissue	Hematoma

RBCs, red blood cells; *WBCs*, white blood cells.

Prostaglandins and Leukotrienes. *Prostaglandins* are substances that can be synthesized from the phospholipids of cell membranes of most body tissues, including blood cells. On stimulation by chemotactic factors or phagocytosis or after cell injury, phospholipids can be converted to arachidonic acid, which is then oxidized by two different pathways.

The *cyclo-oxygenase metabolic pathway* leads to the production of prostaglandins of the D, E, F, and I series and of thromboxanes (formed on activation of platelets). Prostaglandins of the E and I series are potent vasodilators and inhibit platelet and neutrophil aggregation. Prostaglandin E_2 (PGE_2) can also sensitize pain receptors to arousal by stimuli that would normally be painless. PGE_2 is also a potent pyrogen, acting on the temperature-regulating area of the hypothalamus. Thromboxane A_2 is a potent vasoconstrictor and platelet-aggregating agent. Prostaglandins are generally considered proinflammatory, contributing to increased blood flow, edema, and pain. Metabolism of arachidonic acid by the lipoxygenase pathway leads to the production of leukotrienes. Leukotriene B_4 is a potent chemotactic factor. Leukotrienes C_4, D_4, and E_4 form the slow-reacting substance of anaphylaxis, which constricts smooth muscles of bronchi and increases capillary permeability.

Drugs that inhibit prostaglandin synthesis are useful clinically. Nonsteroidal anti-inflammatory drugs (NSAIDs) are used to treat many acute and chronic inflammatory conditions. Acetylsalicylic acid blocks platelet aggregation; it also has anti-inflammatory action. Prostacyclin (prostaglandin I_2) has been used to prevent platelet deposition in extracorporeal systems, such as hemodialysis and heart–lung bypass oxygenators.

Another group of drugs that inhibit prostaglandins is the corticosteroids. They are valuable in the treatment of asthma because they inhibit leukotriene production and thus prevent bronchoconstriction. (Other mediators of the inflammatory response are described in Table 14-3.)

Exudate Formation. Exudate consists of fluid and leukocytes that move from the circulation to the site of injury. The nature and quantity of exudate depend on the type and the severity of the injury and the tissues involved (Table 14-4).

Clinical Manifestations. The local manifestations of inflammation include redness, heat and swelling, and pain (Table 14-5). Systemic manifestations of inflammation include leukocytosis with a shift to the left, malaise, nausea and anorexia, increased pulse and respiratory rate, and fever. The causes of these systemic changes may be related to complement activation and the release of cytokines from stimulated WBCs. Three of these

TABLE 14-5   LOCAL MANIFESTATIONS OF INFLAMMATION

Manifestations	Cause
Redness	Hyperemia from vasodilation
Heat	Increased metabolism at inflammatory site
Pain	Change in pH; nerve stimulation by chemicals (e.g., histamine, prostaglandins); pressure from fluid exudate
Swelling	Fluid shift to interstitial spaces; fluid exudates accumulation

cytokines—interleukin-1, interleukin-6, and tumour necrosis factor—are important in causing the generalized symptoms of inflammation, such as malaise, as well as inducing fever. An increase in pulse and respiration follows the rise in metabolism as a result of a rise in body temperature. (Cytokines are discussed in Chapter 16.)

Fever. The release of cytokines initiates metabolic changes in the temperature-regulating centre of the hypothalamus, thus causing fever (Figure 14-3). The synthesis of PGE_2 is the most critical metabolic change because it acts directly to increase the thermostatic set point. The hypothalamus then activates the autonomic nervous system to stimulate increased muscle tone and shivering and decreased perspiration and blood flow to the periphery. Epinephrine released from the adrenal medulla increases the metabolic rate. The net result is fever.

With the physiological thermostat fixed at a higher-than-normal temperature, the rate of heat production is increased until the body temperature reaches the new set point. As the set point is raised, the hypothalamus signals an increase in heat production and conservation to raise the body temperature to the new level. At this point, the affected individual feels chilled and shivers. The shivering response is the body's way of raising its temperature until the new set point is reached. The body is hot, and yet the individual paradoxically piles on blankets and may go to bed to get warm. When the circulating body temperature reaches the set point of the core body temperature, the chills and warmth-seeking behaviour cease (Dinarello & Porat, 2015). The febrile response is classified into four stages, described in Table 14-6.

The released cytokines and the fever they trigger activate the body's defence mechanisms. Beneficial aspects of fever include increased killing of microorganisms, increased phagocytosis by neutrophils, and increased proliferation of T cells. Higher body

PATHOPHYSIOLOGY MAP

FEVER

FIGURE 14-3 Production of fever. When monocytes or macrophages are activated, they secrete cytokines such as interleukin-1 (IL-1), interleukin-6 (IL-6), and tumour necrosis factor (TNF), which reach the hypothalamic temperature-regulating centre. These cytokines promote the synthesis and secretion of prostaglandin E_2 (PGE_2) in the anterior hypothalamus. PGE_2 increases the thermostatic set point, and the autonomic nervous system is stimulated, which results in shivering, muscle contraction, and peripheral vasoconstriction.

TABLE 14-6 STAGES OF THE FEBRILE RESPONSE

Stage	Characteristics
Prodrome	Nonspecific complaints such as mild headache, fatigue, general malaise, muscle aches
Chill	Cutaneous vasoconstriction, "goose pimples," pale skin; feeling of being cold; generalized, shaking chill; shivering that causes body to reach new temperature set by control centre in hypothalamus
Flush	Sensation of warmth throughout body; cutaneous vasodilation; warming and flushing of skin
Defervescence	Sweating; decrease in body temperature

temperatures may also enhance the activity of interferon, the body's natural virus-fighting substance (see Chapter 16).

Types of Inflammation. The basic types of inflammation are acute, subacute, and chronic. In *acute inflammation,* the healing occurs in 2 to 3 weeks and usually leaves no residual damage. Neutrophils are the predominant cell type at the site of inflammation. A *subacute inflammation* has the features of the acute process but lasts longer. For example, infective endocarditis is a smouldering infection with acute inflammation, but it persists for weeks or months (see Chapter 39).

Chronic inflammation lasts for weeks, months, or even years. The injurious agent persists or repeatedly injures tissue. The predominant cell types present at the site of inflammation are lymphocytes and macrophages. Examples of chronic inflammation include rheumatoid arthritis, osteomyelitis, and tuberculosis. The prolongation and chronicity of any inflammation may be the

TABLE 14-7 REGENERATIVE ABILITY OF DIFFERENT TYPES OF TISSUES

Tissue Type	Regenerative Ability
Epithelial	
Skin, linings of blood vessels, mucous membranes	Cells readily divide and regenerate.
Connective Tissue	
Bone	Active tissue heals rapidly.
Cartilage	Regeneration is possible but slow.
Tendons and ligaments	Regeneration is possible but slow.
Blood	Cells actively regenerate.
Muscle	
Smooth	Regeneration is usually possible (particularly in GI tract).
Cardiac	Damaged muscle is replaced by connective tissue.
Skeletal	Connective tissue replaces severely damaged muscle; in moderately damaged muscle, some regeneration occurs.
Nerve	
Neurons	Cells of these tissues are generally nonmitotic; they do not replicate or replace themselves if irreversibly damaged.
Glial	Cells regenerate; scar tissue often forms when neurons are damaged.

GI, gastrointestinal.

result of an alteration in the immune response (e.g. autoimmune disease). C-reactive protein is an acute-phase protein whose plasma concentration increases in response to inflammation, and thus it can be a useful inflammatory marker.

Healing Process. The final phase of the inflammatory response is healing. Healing includes two major components: regeneration and repair. **Regeneration** is the replacement of lost cells and tissues with cells of the same type. **Repair** is healing as a result of lost cells being replaced by connective tissue. Repair is the more common type of healing and usually results in scar formation.

Regeneration. The ability of cells to regenerate depends on the cell type (Table 14-7). Labile cells—such as cells of the skin, lymphoid organs, bone marrow, and mucous membranes of the gastrointestinal, urinary, and reproductive tracts—divide constantly. Injury to these organs is followed by rapid regeneration.

Stable cells retain their ability to regenerate but do so only if the organ is injured. Examples of stable cells are liver, pancreas, kidney, and bone cells.

Permanent cells such as neurons of the central nervous system and cardiac muscle cells do not regenerate. Damage to these cells can lead to permanent loss. Healing occurs by repair with scar tissue.

Repair. Repair is a more complex process than is regeneration. Most injuries heal by connective tissue repair. Repair healing occurs by primary, secondary, or tertiary intention (Figure 14-4).

Primary Intention. *Primary intention* healing takes place when wound margins are neatly approximated, as in a surgical incision or a paper cut. A continuum of processes is associated with primary healing (Table 14-8). These processes include three phases: the initial (inflammatory) phase, the granulation

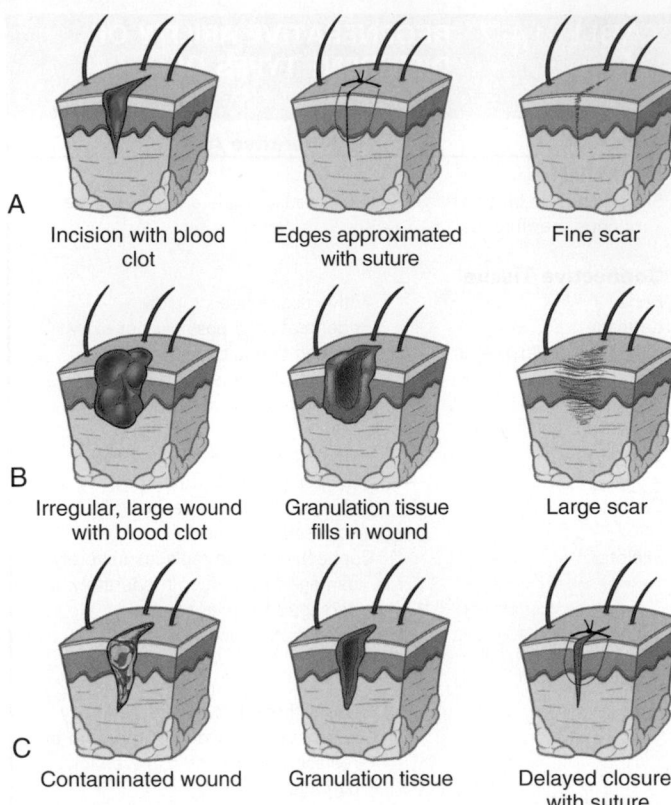

A Incision with blood clot | Edges approximated with suture | Fine scar

B Irregular, large wound with blood clot | Granulation tissue fills in wound | Large scar

C Contaminated wound | Granulation tissue | Delayed closure with suture

FIGURE 14-4 Types of wound healing. **A,** Primary intention. **B,** Secondary intention. **C,** Tertiary intention.

TABLE 14-8 PHASES IN PRIMARY INTENTION HEALING

Phase	Activity
Initial (3 to 5 days)	Approximation of incision edges; migration of epithelial cells; clot serving as meshwork for starting capillary growth
Granulation (5 days to 4 weeks)	Migration of fibroblasts; secretion of collagen; abundance of capillary buds; fragility of wound
Scar contracture (7 days to several months)	Remodelling of collagen; strengthening of scar

(proliferative/reconstructive) phase, and the maturation phase and scar contraction.

Initial (Inflammatory) Phase. *The initial phase* lasts for 3 to 5 days. The edges of the incision are aligned and sutured (or stapled) in place. The incision area fills with blood from the cut blood vessels, and blood clots form and platelets release growth factors to begin the healing process. This forms a matrix for WBC migration and an acute inflammatory reaction occurs.

The area of injury is composed of fibrin clots, erythrocytes, neutrophils (dead and dying), and other debris. Macrophages ingest and digest cellular debris, fibrin fragments, and red blood cells. Extracellular enzymes from macrophages and neutrophils help digest fibrin. As the wound debris is removed, the fibrin clot serves as a framework for future capillary growth and migration of epithelial cells.

Granulation (Proliferative/Reconstructive) Phase. *The granulation phase* is the second step and lasts from 5 days to 3 weeks.

The components of granulation tissue include proliferating fibroblasts; proliferating capillary sprouts (angioblasts); various types of WBCs; exudate; and loose, semifluid, ground substance.

Fibroblasts are immature connective tissue cells that migrate into the healing site and secrete collagen. In time, the collagen is organized and restructured to strengthen the healing site. At this stage, it is termed *fibrous* or *scar tissue.*

During the granulation phase, the wound is pink and vascular. Numerous red granules (young budding capillaries) are present. At this point, the wound is friable, at risk for dehiscence, and resistant to infection.

Surface epithelium at the wound edges begins to regenerate. In a few days, a thin layer of epithelium migrates across the wound surface in a one-cell thick layer until it contacts cells spreading from the opposite direction. The epithelium thickens and begins to mature, and the wound now closely resembles the adjacent skin. In a superficial wound, re-epithelialization may take 3 to 5 days.

Maturation Phase and Scar Contraction. The *maturation phase,* in which scar contraction occurs, overlaps with the granulation phase. It begins 7 days after the injury and continues for several months or years, during which time collagen fibres are further organized, and the remodelling process occurs. Fibroblasts disappear as the scar becomes stronger. The active movement of the myofibroblasts causes contraction of the healing area, helping to close the defect and bring the skin edges closer together to form a mature scar. In contrast to granulation tissue, a mature scar is virtually avascular and pale.

Secondary Intention. Wounds with wide or irregular wound margins that cannot be approximated will heal by *secondary intention.* Examples include chronic wounds, such as venous ulcers, and wounds caused by trauma or pressure. The inflammatory reaction that occurs is often greater than in primary healing, which creates more debris, cells, and exudate. The debris may have to be cleaned away (debrided) before healing can take place.

In some instances, a surgical incision may become infected, which creates additional inflammation. The wound may reopen (dehiscence), and healing by secondary intention must then take place.

The process of healing by secondary intention is essentially the same as that of healing by primary intention. The major differences are the larger defect and the gaping wound edges. Healing and granulation take place from the edges inward and from the bottom of the wound upward until the defect is filled. There is more granulation tissue, and the result is a much larger scar.

Tertiary Intention. *Tertiary intention* (delayed primary intention) healing occurs when a wound is intentionally left open because if the wound is closed immediately, healing could be impaired by contamination (e.g., animal bite or foreign body), infection/high risk of infection, edema, or poor circulation. The wound is later closed surgically after the problem is controlled or resolved. Healing by tertiary intention usually results in a larger and deeper scar than does healing by primary or secondary intention.

Wound Classification. Correctly classifying a wound requires identifying the underlying cause. Wounds can be categorized by cause (surgical or nonsurgical), duration (acute or chronic), level of contamination, or depth of tissue affected (superficial, partial thickness, or full thickness). A superficial wound involves only the epidermis. Partial-thickness wounds extend into the dermis.

FIGURE 14-5 Wounds classified by colour assessment. **A,** Black wound. **B,** Yellow wound. **C,** Red wound. **D,** Mixed-colour wound. Source: Courtesy Molnlyche Health Care, Eddystone, PA. In Potter, P. A., & Perry, A. G. (2009). *Fundamentals of nursing* (8th ed., p. 1285). St. Louis: Elsevier.

Full-thickness wounds cause destruction to the deepest layer of tissue because they involve the subcutaneous tissue and sometimes even extend into the fascia and underlying structures such as muscle, tendon, or bone (see Figure 27-3). Pressure injuries are the only type of wound that are staged (Wound, Ostomy and Continence Nurses Society, 2016; see Table 14-13 later in this chapter).

Another system that is sometimes used clinically to categorize open wounds is based on the colour of the wound (red, yellow, black) rather than on the depth of tissue destruction (Figure 14-5). It can be used to describe any wound allowed to heal by secondary or tertiary intention. When a wound contains two or three colours at the same time, it should be classified according to the least desirable colour present (e.g., if there is any black in the wound, the wound is deemed "black").

Delay of Healing. In a healthy person, wounds heal at a normal, predictable rate. Little can be done to accelerate this process. However, some factors delay wound healing. These are summarized in Table 14-9.

Complications of Healing. Complications of wound healing may include adhesions, contractures, dehiscence and evisceration, excess granulation tissue, fistula formation, infection, hemorrhage, and formation of hypertrophic scars and keloids.

Adhesions. Adhesions are bands of scar tissue that form between or around organs. They may develop in the abdominal cavity or between the lungs and pleura. Adhesions in the abdomen may cause an intestinal obstruction. Those between the lungs and the pleura necessitate decortication, or stripping of pleura, to enable normal ventilation.

Contractures. Wound contraction is an important part of healing. This process may become abnormal when contraction is excessive, which results in deformity, or *contracture*. Shortening

FIGURE 14-6 Dehiscence after a cholecystectomy. Source: From Bale, S., & Jones, V. (2006). *Wound care nursing: A patient-centered approach* (2nd ed., p. 20). St. Louis: Mosby.

of muscle or scar tissue, especially over joints, results from excessive fibrous tissue formation. Contractures frequently occur in burn injuries, when extensive skin and subcutaneous tissue are lost (see Chapter 27).

Dehiscence and Evisceration. Dehiscence is the separation and disruption of previously joined wound edges. It usually occurs when a primary healing site bursts open (Figure 14-6). Dehiscence has three possible contributing causes. First, an infection may cause an inflammatory process. Second, the granulation tissue may not be strong enough to withstand the forces imposed on the wound: for example, if a fluid pocket (seroma or hematoma) develops between the tissue layers. Third, obese individuals are

TABLE 14-9 FACTORS DELAYING WOUND HEALING

Factor	Effect on Wound Healing
Nutrition	
• Vitamin C deficiency	Delays formation of collagen fibres and capillary development
• Protein deficiency	Decreases supply of amino acids for tissue repair
• Zinc deficiency	Impairs epithelialization
Inadequate blood supply	Decreases supply of nutrients to injured area, decreases removal of exudative debris, inhibits inflammatory response
Smoking	Nicotine is a potent vasoconstrictor and impedes blood flow to healing areas, which results in tissue ischemia and impairs wound healing
Corticosteroid drugs	Impair phagocytosis by WBCs, inhibit fibroblast proliferation and function, depress formation of granulation tissue, inhibit wound contraction
Infection	Increases inflammatory response and tissue destruction
Anemia	Reduces supply of oxygen to tissues
Advanced age	Slows collagen synthesis by fibroblasts, impairs circulation, imposes need for longer time for epithelialization of skin, alters phagocytic and immune responses
Obesity	Decreases blood supply in fatty tissue
Diabetes mellitus	Decreases collagen synthesis, retards early capillary growth, impairs phagocytosis (result of hyperglycemia), reduces supply of O_2 and nutrients as a result of vascular disease
Poor general health	Causes generalized absence of factors necessary to promote wound healing
Mechanical friction on wound	Destroys granulation tissue, prevents apposition of wound edges
Cold temperature	Decreases cellular activity and fibroblast proliferation
Excessive moisture	Promotes formation of hypergranulation tissue, which prevents the migration of epithelial cells

WBCs, white blood cells.

at a high risk for dehiscence because adipose tissue has less blood supply, which can slow healing. **Evisceration** occurs when wound edges separate to the extent that intestines protrude through the wound.

Excess Granulation Tissue. *Excess granulation tissue* or hypergranulation tissue ("proud flesh") may protrude above the surface of the healing wound. If the granulation tissue is cauterized or cut off, healing continues in a normal manner.

Fistula Formation. A **fistula** is an abnormal passage that forms between organs or a hollow organ and the skin. For example, a connection between the bowel and the skin would be referred to as an *enterocutaneous fistula;* a connection between the bowel and the bladder would be referred to as an *enterovesical fistula.*

Infection. A wound has an increased risk of *infection* when it contains necrotic tissue, when the blood supply is decreased, when the immune function is depressed, or if a patient is malnourished, has multiple stressors, or is diabetic.

Hemorrhage. Bleeding is normal immediately after tissue injury and ceases with clot formation. *Hemorrhage* occurs as abnormal internal or external blood loss caused by suture failure, clotting abnormalities, dislodged clot, infection, or erosion of a blood vessel by a foreign object (tubing, drains) or infection process.

Formation of Hypertrophic Scars and Keloids. Hypertrophic keloid scars form when the body produces excess collagen. A **hypertrophic scar** is inappropriately large, red, raised, and hard (Figure 14-7). However, it remains confined to the wound edges and regresses in time. In contrast, a **keloid** is a protrusion of scar tissue that extends beyond the wound edges and may form tumour-like masses of scar tissue (Figure 14-8). Keloids are permanent, without any tendency to subside. A person with keloids often feels tenderness, pain, and hyperesthesia in the area of the scar, particularly in the early stages of development. Keloid formation is thought to be hereditary and occurs more often in dark-skinned people, particularly Black individuals. Neither complication is life-threatening, but both can have serious cosmetic implications.

FIGURE 14-7 Hypertrophic scarring. Source: Courtesy Dr. C. Lawrence, Wound Healing Research Unit, Cardiff, Wales, UK. In Bale, S., & Jones, V. (2006). *Wound care nursing: A patient-centered approach* (2nd ed., p. 16). St. Louis: Mosby.

NURSING MANAGEMENT
INFLAMMATION AND HEALING

NURSING IMPLEMENTATION

HEALTH PROMOTION. The best management of inflammation is the prevention of infection, trauma, surgery, and contact with potentially harmful agents. This is not always possible; for example, a simple mosquito bite causes an inflammatory response. Because occasional injury is inevitable, concerted efforts to minimize inflammation and infection are needed.

Adequate nutrition is essential so that the body has the necessary factors to promote healing when injury occurs. Individuals at risk for wound-healing complications are those with malabsorption problems (e.g., Crohn's disease, gastrointestinal surgery, liver disease), deficient intake or high energy demands (e.g., malignancy, major trauma or surgery, sepsis,

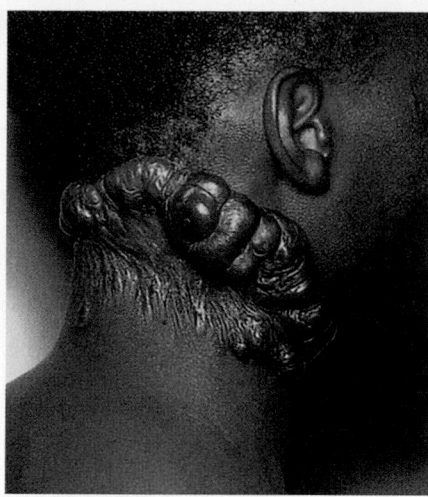

FIGURE 14-8 Keloid scarring. Source: Courtesy Dr. C. Lawrence, Wound Healing Research Unit, Cardiff, Wales, UK. In Bale, S., & Jones, V. (2006). *Wound care nursing: A patient-centered approach* (2nd ed., p. 17). St. Louis: Mosby.

fever), or diabetes. An individual should always be considered at risk for delayed wound healing if the following have occurred: (a) loss of 20% or more of total body weight in the preceding 6 months or (b) 10% loss of total body weight in the preceding 2 months.

Special nutritional measures facilitate wound healing. Fluid intake must be high to replace fluid loss from perspiration and exudate formation. An increased metabolic rate intensifies water loss. For every 1°C increase in body temperature above 37.8°C, metabolism increases by 13%. A diet high in protein, carbohydrate, and vitamins with moderate fat intake is necessary to promote healing. Protein is needed to correct the negative nitrogen balance that results from the increased metabolic rate. Protein is also necessary for synthesis of immune factors, leukocytes, fibroblasts, and collagen. Carbohydrate is needed for the increased metabolic energy required for inflammation and healing. If carbohydrate intake is deficient, the body breaks down protein for the needed energy. Fats are also a necessary component in the diet to help in the synthesis of fatty acids and triglycerides, which are part of the cellular membrane. Vitamin C is needed for capillary synthesis, capillary formation, and resistance to infection. The B-complex vitamins are necessary as coenzymes for many metabolic reactions. If a vitamin B deficiency develops, metabolism of protein, fat, and carbohydrate is disrupted. Vitamin A is also needed in healing because it aids in the process of epithelialization. It increases collagen synthesis and tensile strength of the healing wound. Patients are sometimes given vitamin A to counteract the effects of steroids on wound healing.

If the patient is unable to eat, enteral feedings and supplements should be the first choice if the gastrointestinal tract is functional. Parenteral nutrition is indicated when enteral feedings are contraindicated or not tolerated. (Enteral nutrition and parenteral nutrition are discussed in Chapter 42.)

The manifestations of inflammation and infection must be recognized early so that appropriate treatment can begin. Treatment may be rest, drug therapy, or specific care of the injured site. Immediate treatment may prevent the extension and complications of prolonged inflammation.

ACUTE INTERVENTION

Observation and Vital Signs. The ability to recognize the clinical manifestations of inflammation is important. In a patient who is immunosuppressed (e.g., taking corticosteroids or receiving chemotherapy), the classic manifestations of inflammation may be masked. In such a patient, early symptoms of inflammation may be malaise or "just not feeling well."

Observation and recording of wound characteristics are essential. The consistency, colour, and odour of any drainage should be recorded and reported if abnormal. *Staphylococcus* and *Pseudomonas* organisms commonly cause purulent drainage. Exudate from wounds colonized with *Pseudomonas* often has a distinctive bright "highlighter" yellow or green appearance.

Vital signs are important to note with any inflammation, especially when an infectious process is present. When infection is present, temperature may rise, and pulse and respiration rates may increase. If a wound infection develops in a postoperative patient, vital signs change within 3 to 5 days after surgery.

Fever. Although fever is usually regarded as harmful, an increase in body temperature is an important host defence mechanism. Steps are frequently taken to lower body temperature to relieve the anxiety of the patient and medical personnel. Because a mild fever does little harm, imposes no great discomfort, and may benefit host defence mechanisms, antipyretic drugs are rarely essential for patient welfare. Moderate fevers (up to 39.5°C) usually produce few problems in most patients. However, if the patient is very young or very old, is extremely uncomfortable, or has a significant medical problem (e.g., severe cardiopulmonary disease, brain injury), the use of antipyretics should be considered. Fever in an immunosuppressed patient should be treated rapidly and antibiotic therapy begun because infections can rapidly progress to septicemia. (Neutropenia is discussed in Chapter 33.)

Fever (especially if the temperature exceeds 40°C) can be damaging to body cells, and delirium and seizures can occur. At temperatures higher than 41°C, regulation by the hypothalamic temperature control centre becomes impaired, and many cells, including those in the brain, can be damaged.

Older adults have a blunted febrile response to infection (Dinarello & Porat, 2015). The body temperature may not rise to the level expected for a younger adult, or the onset of fever may be delayed. The blunted response can delay diagnosis and treatment. By the time fever (as defined for younger adults) is present, the illness may be severe.

Several drugs are commonly used to lower the body temperature set point in the hypothalamus (Table 14-10). Aspirin specifically blocks prostaglandin synthesis in the hypothalamus and elsewhere in the body. Acetaminophen acts on the heat-regulating centre in the hypothalamus. Some NSAIDs (e.g., ibuprofen [Motrin, Advil]) have antipyretic effects. Corticosteroids are antipyretic through the dual mechanisms of inhibiting interleukin-1 production and preventing prostaglandin synthesis. The action of these drugs results in dilation of superficial blood vessels, increased skin temperature, and sweating.

Antipyretics should be given around the clock to prevent acute swings in temperature. These agents cause a sharp decrease in temperature. When the antipyretic wears off, the body may initiate a compensatory involuntary muscular contraction (i.e., chill) to raise the body temperature back up to its previous level. To prevent this unpleasant adverse effect, these agents should be administered regularly at 2- to 4-hour intervals. Although sponge baths increase evaporative heat loss, there is no evidence that they decrease the body temperature unless antipyretic drugs

TABLE 14-10   DRUG THERAPY

Inflammation and Healing

Drug	Mechanisms of Action
Antipyretic Drugs	
Salicylates (Aspirin)	Lower temperature by action on heat-regulating centre in hypothalamus, resulting in peripheral dilation and heat loss; interfere with formation and release of prostaglandins; selectively depress CNS
Acetaminophen (Tylenol)	Lowers temperature by action on heat-regulating centre in hypothalamus
NSAIDs (e.g., ibuprofen [Motrin, Advil])	Inhibit synthesis of prostaglandins
Anti-inflammatory Drugs	
Salicylates (Aspirin)	Inhibit synthesis of prostaglandins, reduce capillary permeability
Corticosteroids (e.g. prednisone)	Interfere with tissue granulation, induce immunosuppressive effects (decreased synthesis of lymphocytes), prevent liberation of lysosomes
NSAIDs (e.g., ibuprofen [Motrin], naproxen [Naprosyn], celecoxib [Celebrex])	Inhibit synthesis of prostaglandins
Vitamins	
Vitamin A	Accelerates epithelialization
Vitamin B complex	Acts as coenzymes
Vitamin C	Assists in synthesis of collagen and new capillaries
Vitamin D	Facilitates calcium absorption

CNS, central nervous system; *NSAIDs,* nonsteroidal anti-inflammatory drugs.

have been given to lower the set point; otherwise, the body will initiate compensatory mechanisms (e.g., shivering) to restore body heat. The same principle applies to the use of cooling blankets; they are most effective in lowering body temperature when the set point has also been lowered. The nursing care of the patient with a fever is presented in Nursing Care Plan 14-1, available on the Evolve website.

RICE. Rest, ice, compression, and elevation (RICE) constitute a key concept in the treatment of soft tissue injuries and related inflammation.

Rest. Rest helps the body use its nutrients and oxygen for the healing process. The repair process is facilitated when fibrin and collagen are allowed to form across the wound edges with little disruption.

Ice and Heat. At the time of initial trauma, cold application is usually appropriate to promote vasoconstriction and decreases swelling, pain, and congestion from increased metabolism in the area of inflammation. Heat may be used later (e.g., after 24 to 48 hours) and when swelling has subsided to promote healing by increasing the circulation to the inflamed site and subsequent removal of debris. Heat is also used to localize the inflammatory agents. Warm, moist heat may help debride the wound site if necrotic material is present.

Compression and Immobilization. Compression counters vasodilation and development of edema after an injury. Compression by direct pressure over a laceration occludes blood vessels to stop bleeding. Compression bandages provide support to injured joints that have tendons and muscles unable to provide support on their own. Distal pulses and capillary refill should be assessed before and after application of compression to assess whether compression has compromised circulation (e.g., as evidenced by pale colour of skin or loss of sensation).

Immobilization of the inflamed area promotes healing by decreasing the tissues' metabolic need. Immobilization with a cast, splint, or bandage supports fractured bones and prevents further tissue injury from sharp bone fragments that could sever nerves or blood vessels (causing hemorrhage).

Elevation. Elevation of an injured extremity reduces the edema at the inflammatory site by increasing venous and lymphatic return. Elevation helps reduce pain associated with blood engorgement at the injured site. Elevation may be contraindicated in patients with significantly reduced arterial circulation.

Wound Management. The type of wound management and dressings required depend on the type, extent, and characteristics of the wound and the phase of healing (Registered Nurses' Association of Ontario [RNAO], 2016). The purposes of wound management include (a) cleaning and debriding the wound to remove debris and dead tissue from the wound bed, (b) controlling inflammation and treating infection to prepare the wound for healing, and (c) providing moisture balance for healable wounds, and moisture reduction for nonhealable and maintenance wounds (Sibbald, Elliott, Ayello, et al., 2015). Treatment of pressure injuries is discussed in more detail later in this chapter.

For wounds that heal by primary intention, it is common to cover the incision with a dry, sterile dressing that is removed as soon as the drainage stops or in 2 to 3 days. Protective sprays or wipes that form a transparent film on the skin may be used for dressings on a clean incision or injury. Sometimes a surgeon leaves a surgical wound uncovered or removes the dressing within 48 hours after surgery (Lisy, 2014).

Wound healing management by secondary intention depends on the cause of the wound and the type of tissue in the wound. The red-yellow-black concept of wound care (see Figure 14-5) can be used to describe the wound, and dressing selection depends on the characteristics of the wound. Examples of wound dressing types are presented in Table 14-11.

Red Wound. A *red wound* can be superficial or deep and is clean and red or pink in appearance. Examples include skin tears, pressure injuries, partial-thickness or second-degree burns, and wounds created surgically that are allowed to heal by secondary intention. The goal of treatment is gentle cleansing and protection of the wound (LeBlanc & Baranoski, 2014). Wounds should be cleaned with normal saline, potable or sterile water, or noncytotoxic wound cleansers (RNAO, 2016). Clean wounds that are granulating and re-epithelializing should be kept slightly moist and protected from further trauma until they heal naturally (Ayello & Baranoski, 2014). A dressing that keeps the wound surface clean and slightly moist is optimal in promoting epithelialization.

🔍 EVIDENCE-INFORMED PRACTICE

Research Highlight

What Is the Effect of Tap Water on Wound Cleansing?
Clinical Question
In patients with an infected wound (P), what is the effect of tap water (I) versus normal saline or no cleansing (C) on infection and healing rates (O)?

Best Available Evidence
Randomized controlled trials and quasi-randomized controlled trials

Critical Appraisal and Synthesis of Evidence
- Ten trials (n = 35 to 705 per trial) involving people who had acute infected wounds. In seven trials, researchers compared infection and healing rates between wounds treated with water and those treated with normal saline. In three trials, investigators compared wound cleansing (with various solutions) with no cleansing at all.
- No significant differences were found in infection rate and healing between wounds cleansed with tap water and those not cleansed at all.
- Tap water was more effective than saline in reducing wound infection rate.

Conclusion
- Using tap water to cleanse acute wounds does not increase infection rate and, in some cases, it may reduce infection.

Implications for Nursing Practice
- The option of using tap water should be carefully considered when other wound cleansing solutions are not accessible.
- Water quality, type of wound, and the patient's overall health should be evaluated before tap water is used.
- If potable tap water is not available, boiled water that is cooled or distilled water may be used in wound cleansing.

Reference for Evidence
Fernandez, R., Griffiths, R. (2012). Water for wound cleansing. *Cochrane Database Syst Rev*, (2), CD003861.

P, Patient population of interest; *I*, intervention or area of interest; *C*, comparison of interest or comparison group; *O*, outcomes of interest (see Chapter 1).

Unnecessary manipulation during dressing changes may destroy new granulation tissue and break down fibrin formation.

Yellow Wound. A *yellow wound* has nonviable necrotic tissue, which creates an ideal environment for bacterial growth. The goal of treatment is absorption of excessive drainage and removal of nonviable tissue (described in the next section). Topical antimicrobials and bactericidals (e.g., povidone-iodine, sodium hypochlorite [Dakin's solution], hydrogen peroxide, acetic acid, and chlorhexidine) may be used to cleanse wounds containing debris that are highly colonized or infected. They should never be used to treat clean granulating wounds (RNAO, 2016).

Black Wound. A *black wound* is covered with thick, dry, necrotic tissue called *eschar* that is black, brown, or grey. Examples of black wounds include third-degree burns and gangrenous ulcers. The risk of wound infection increases in proportion to the amount of necrotic tissue present. The immediate treatment is removal of the nonviable eschar. The debridement method used depends on the amount of debris and the condition of the wound tissue (Wilcox, Carter, & Covington, 2013). There are several approaches to debridement:

1. *Surgical debridement.* This fast and cost-effective method of debridement is indicated when large amounts of tissue are nonviable and the patient has sepsis. Sharp surgical debridement is selective and can be performed in the operating room or at the patient's bedside, depending on the extent of necrotic material (Woo, Keast, Parsons, et al., 2015). Only wounds that have an adequate blood supply and are considered "healable" should be debrided surgically.

2. *Mechanical debridement.* This method is used when debris is minimal. One example is wet-to-dry dressings, in which open-mesh gauze is moistened with normal saline, packed into the wound surface, and allowed to dry. Wound debris adheres to the dressing. When the dressing is removed, the debris is trapped in the gauze and is mechanically separated from the wound bed. One disadvantage to this method is that it is nonselective and destroys some healthy tissue. Mechanical debridement can be painful, and the patient should receive appropriate pain management before the removal of a wet-to-dry dressing. Another method of mechanical debridement is pressurized wound irrigation, in which water is delivered at high or low pressure to remove bacteria, foreign matter, and necrotic tissue from the wound. It is important to ensure that the pressure is not too high, as this could drive bacteria and debris deeper into the wound and damage granulation tissue. Whirlpool is another method of mechanical debridement that can be effective at loosening and removing surface wound debris, but it should be used with caution because it can cause tissue maceration and bacterial cross-contamination. Mechanical debridement should not be used for clean granulating wounds.

3. *Autolytic debridement.* Hydrogels, semiocclusive dressings, or occlusive dressings (see Table 14-11) may be used to promote softening of dry eschar by autolysis. This is a slow but selective and painless process that enables the body's own endogenous enzymes to selectively rehydrate, soften, and liquefy necrotic tissue. These types of dressings are used in noninfected wounds with necrotic tissue and adequate circulation. The use of a skin protectant around the wound helps prevent maceration.

4. *Enzymatic debridement.* In this method, a topical ointment containing proteolytic enzymes is applied to the necrotic tissue in the wound and then covered with a moist dressing such as saline-moistened gauze and changed daily. Santyl collagenase is the only product in this category currently available in Canada. The wound pH must be between 6 and 8 for optimal enzyme activity; therefore, cleansing products containing detergents or heavy metals such as mercury or silver should not be used.

5. *Biosurgical debridement.* In this debridement method, medical grade maggots are applied directly to a wound in a controlled and contained environment. The maggots clean the wound by digesting dead tissue with their proteolytic, digestive enzymes. They also kill bacteria by ingesting them and can destroy biofilm.

Negative-Pressure Wound Therapy. This therapy involves the application of negative pressure (suction) to the wound bed. The vacuum creates continuous or intermittent negative pressure at the wound base to remove fluid, exudate, and infectious material and to promote blood flow. The wound is cleansed, and the periwound area is protected with a skin protectant and transparent film. Then a foam or gauze dressing (depending on the manufacturer) is cut to the dimensions of the wound. A large occlusive dressing is applied over the top, and a small hole is made over the dressing where the tubing is attached (Figure 14-9). Wound types suitable for this therapy include chronic, acute, traumatic, and dehisced wounds; partial-thickness burns; diabetic ulcers;

TABLE 14-11   TYPES OF WOUND DRESSINGS

Type	Description	Examples
Gauze	Provides absorption of exudate. Supports debridement if applied and kept moist. Can be used to maintain moistness of wound surface. Can be used as filler dressings in sinus tracts.	Nu Gauze (numerous products available)
Nonadherent dressing	Woven or nonwoven dressings may be impregnated with petrolatum or antimicrobial drugs. Minimally absorbent. Used on minor wounds or skin tears.	Adaptic, Jelonet, Bactigras, Inadine
Transparent film	Semipermeable membrane that permits gaseous exchange between wound bed and environment. Minimally absorbent so that environment is kept moist in presence of exudate. Bacteria do not penetrate membrane. Used for dry, noninfected wounds, wounds with minimal drainage, or stage 1 pressure injuries to help prevent friction and shear.	Bioclusive, OpSite, Tegaderm, Mefilm
Acrylic clear	Used for superficial and partial-thickness wounds with light drainage.	Tegaderm Absorbent
Hydrocolloid dressing	Occlusive dressing does not allow O_2 to diffuse from atmosphere to wound bed. Occlusion does not interfere with wound healing and supports debridement. Used for superficial and partial-thickness wounds with light to moderate drainage.	Comfeel, DuoDERM, Restore, Tegasorb
Foam	Product comes in many shapes and sizes. Absorbs moderate to heavy amount of exudate. Used for partial- or full-thickness wounds or infected wounds.	Allevyn, Hydrasorb, Lyofoam, Mepilex, Biatain, Tegaderm Foam
Alginate, calcium alginate, and hydrofibre dressings	Large volume of exudate can be absorbed. Dressing forms a gel-like substance that supports autolytic debridement and maintains moistness of wound surface. Fills wound cavities and obliterates dead space. Available in rope or sheet form. For partial- or full-thickness wounds or infected wounds with heavy drainage. Dressing should not be used for lightly draining or dry wounds because it can desiccate the wound bed. A secondary dressing is required.	Aquacel, Kaltostat, Tegagen, Seasorb, Fibracol, Algisite, Algisite M, Melgisorb
Hypertonic dressing	Sheet, ribbon, or gel impregnated with sodium chloride concentrate. Should not be used on dry wounds (which should be treated with a hydrogel). May be painful on sensitive tissue.	Mesalt, Hypergel
Hydrogel	Gently eliminates necrotic tissue by autolytic debridement. Maintains moistness of wound surface. Provides limited absorption of exudate. Available as sheet, gel, and impregnated gauze. A secondary dressing is required. Used for partial- or full-thickness wounds with minimal drainage, and necrotic wounds. Has a cooling effect on the wound and thus is effective in managing pain.	IntraSite Gel, DuoDERM Hydroactive Gel, Normlgel, Nu-Gel, Tegagel, Tegaderm Hydrogel wound filler
Charcoal dressing	Dressing that contains odour-absorbent charcoal layered within the product. Some products contain silver to enhance antimicrobial capability.	Actisorb, Carbonet, CarboFlex
Antimicrobial dressing	Broad spectrum against bacteria. Silver, polyhexamethylene biguanide (PHMB), cadexomer iodine, methylene blue/crystal violet, or honey with vehicle for delivery: sheets, foams, alginates, ribbons, gels, or paste. Products are not to be used on patients with known hypersensitivity to any product components.	Acticoat, AMD Antimicrobial Foam, Iodosorb, Allevyn Ag, Mepilex Ag, Aquacel Ag, Contreet, Silvercel, SilvaSorb, Tegaderm Ag Mesh, Hydrofera Blue, Medihoney
Biological dressing	Living human fibroblasts provided in sheets at ambient or frozen temperatures. Extracellular matrix. Collagen-containing preparations. Hyaluronic acid. Not to be used on wounds with infections, sinus tracts, or excessive exudate, or on patients with hypersensitivity to any of the product components.	Apligraf, Dermagraft, Oasis Wound Matrix, Promogran, Tegaderm Matrix

Source: Information on antimicrobials and biological dressings from Sibbald, G., Orsted, H., Coutts, P., & Keast, D. (2006). Best practice recommendations for preparing the wound bed: Update 2006. *Wound Care Canada, 4*(1), 309–405.

FIGURE 14-9 Negative-pressure wound therapy. **A,** Femoral wound that is not healing. **B,** Negative-pressure wound therapy in place. **C,** Granulation tissue formation after therapy. Source: From Abai, B., Zickler, R. W., Pappas, P. J., et al. (2007). Lymphorrhea responds to negative pressure wound therapy. *Journal of Vascular Surgery, 45*(3),610–613. doi:http://dx.doi.org/10.1016/j.jvs.2006.10.043.

stage 3 and stage 4 pressure injuries; flaps; and grafts. Contraindications include malignancy, untreated osteomyelitis, fistula, eschar, and active bleeding. It is important to count and document the number of pieces of foam or gauze used in the wound. For further information on negative-pressure wound therapy, refer to the Ontario Ministry of Health and Long-Term Care document *Negative Pressure Wound Therapy* (see the Resources at the end of this chapter).

Hyperbaric Oxygen Therapy. Hyperbaric oxygen therapy is the systemic delivery of oxygen at increased atmospheric pressures. The patient is placed in an enclosed chamber in which 100% oxygen is administered at 1.5 to 3.0 times the normal atmospheric pressure. This form of therapy accelerates granulation tissue formation and wound closure by increasing blood and tissue oxygen content in hypoxic tissues, which stimulates fibroblast proliferation and collagen synthesis.

Electrical Stimulation. With this therapy, a generator connected to electrodes is attached to the periwound skin, and an electrical charge is delivered to the wound tissues to produce a physiological response. Electrical stimulation may be used as an adjunct to regular wound care to promote healing and wound closure with stalled but healable stage 2, 3, and 4 pressure injuries that have not responded to other interventions. It should not be used if a patient has osteomyelitis, cancer, an implanted electronic device, or a blood clot in the leg. It should never be applied over a pregnant uterus, dressings with metallic or ionic components, or excitable tissues.

Psychological Implications. The patient may be distressed at the thought or sight of an incision or wound because of fear of scarring or disfigurement. Drainage from a wound may also cause alarm. The patient needs to understand the healing process and the normal changes that occur as the wound heals. When a nurse is changing a dressing, inappropriate facial expressions can alert the patient to problems with the wound or the nurse's ability to care for it. Wrinkling of the nose by the nurse may convey disgust to the patient. A nurse should also be careful not to focus on the wound to the extent that the patient is not treated as a total person.

AMBULATORY AND HOME CARE. Because patients are being discharged earlier after surgery and many undergo surgery as outpatients, it is important that the patient, the family, or both know how to care for the wound and perform dressing changes. Wound healing may not be complete for 4 to 6 weeks or longer. Adequate rest and good nutrition are essential. Physical and emotional stress should be minimized. The wound should be observed for complications such as infection. The patient should be able to recognize the signs and symptoms of infection and note changes in wound colour and the amount of drainage. The health care provider should be notified of any signs of abnormal wound healing.

Medications are often taken for a period after recovery from an acute infection. Drug-specific adverse effects should be reviewed with the patient, and he or she should be instructed to contact the health care provider if any of these effects occur. The patient must be taught the necessity to continue the drugs for the specified time. For example, a person who is instructed to take an antibiotic for 10 days may stop taking the drug after 5 days because symptoms disappear. However, if a full course of antibiotic is not taken, the infection may not be entirely eliminated, and remaining organisms may also become resistant to the antibiotic.

PRESSURE INJURIES

Causes and Pathophysiological Features

A pressure injury is a localized injury to the skin or underlying soft tissue, usually over a bony prominence or related to a medical or other device as a result of pressure or pressure in combination with shear, friction, or both. Pressure injuries are generally considered an indicator of the quality of care, and most are regarded as avoidable. However, there are instances in which skin breakdown can be considered unavoidable: in the case of patients who have limited movement because of hemodynamic instability; inability to provide nutrition and fluids; or at the end of life (Edsberg, Langemo, Baharestani, et al., 2014).

According to the Canadian Institute for Health Information, pressure injuries are a financial burden to the health care system, in addition to the effect they have on mortality, morbidity, and quality of life. The prevalence of pressure injuries in Canada was reported as 0.4% in acute care, 2.4% in home care, 14.1% in complex continuing care, and 6.7% in long-term care (Canadian

TABLE 14-12	RISK FACTORS FOR PRESSURE INJURIES

- Advanced age
- Anemia
- Contractures
- Diabetes mellitus
- Elevated body temperature
- Immobility
- Impaired circulation
- Incontinence
- Low diastolic blood pressure (<60 mm Hg)
- Mental deterioration
- Neurological disorders
- Nutritional deficiencies
- Obesity
- Pain
- Prolonged surgery
- Prolonged use of steroids
- Vascular disease

Institute for Health Information, 2013). The most common sites for pressure injury development are the sacrum, ischium, trochanter, coccyx, heels, and malleolus. Factors that influence the development of pressure injuries include the intensity and duration of the pressure, as well as the ability of the patient's tissue to tolerate the externally applied stress (Doughty & McNichol, 2016). Besides pressure, shearing force (pressure exerted on the skin when it adheres to the bed and the underlying skin layers slide in the direction of body movement), *friction* (two surfaces rubbing against each other), and *excessive moisture* (incontinence or perspiration) contribute to pressure injury formation (RNAO, 2016). Factors that increase a patient's risk for the development of pressure injuries are presented in Table 14-12. A pressure injury risk assessment and comprehensive skin assessment should be conducted within 8 hours of the patient's admission and with any change in patient condition. A risk-based prevention plan should then be developed (National Pressure Ulcer Advisory Panel [NPUAP], 2014).

Clinical Manifestations

The clinical manifestations of pressure injuries depend on the extent of the tissue that is involved. They are staged according to their deepest level of tissue damage. Table 14-13 illustrates the pressure injury stages according to the NPUAP (2016) guidelines. When slough or necrotic eschar is present, it is not possible to stage the ulcer until the devitalized tissue is removed by debridement. Clinicians describe such pressure injuries as *unstageable* (RNAO, 2016).

When full-thickness pressure injuries heal, fat, muscle, and dermis are replaced with granulation tissue, and the original integrity of the tissue is lost. Reverse staging—for example, stating that a stage 3 ulcer has healed into a stage 2 ulcer—is thus not appropriate. Rather, the ulcer would be known as a "healing stage 3 ulcer." It is important to note the location of previously healed pressure injuries in an initial admission assessment because history of a pressure injury is a risk factor for recurrence.

NURSING AND COLLABORATIVE MANAGEMENT
PRESSURE INJURIES

Management of a patient with a pressure injury encompasses not only care of the wound itself but also support measures for

TABLE 14-13   STAGING OF PRESSURE INJURIES

Deep Tissue Pressure Injury

Intact or nonintact skin with localized area of persistent nonblanchable, deep red, maroon, purple discoloration or epidermal separation revealing a dark wound bed or blood filled blister. Pain and temperature change often precede skin colour changes. Discoloration may appear differently in darkly pigmented skin. This injury results from intense or prolonged pressure and shear forces at the bone–muscle interface. The wound may evolve rapidly to reveal the actual extent of tissue injury, or it may resolve without tissue loss. If necrotic tissue, subcutaneous tissue, granulation tissue, fascia, muscle, or other underlying structures are visible, the injury is a full-thickness pressure injury (unstageable, stage 3, or stage 4). The *term deep tissue pressure injury* does not describe vascular, traumatic, neuropathic, or dermatological conditions.

Diagram **Clinical Presentation***

Deep Tissue Pressure Injury

Stage 1

Intact skin with a localized area of nonblanchable erythema, which may appear differently in darkly pigmented skin. Presence of blanchable erythema or changes in sensation, temperature, or firmness may precede visible changes. Colour changes do not include purple or maroon discoloration; these may indicate deep tissue pressure injury.

Diagram **Clinical Presentation**

Stage 1 Pressure Injury – Darkly Pigmented

Stage 1 Pressure Injury – Lightly Pigmented

Note: For additional information regarding the staging of pressure injuries, refer to the Registered Nurses' Association of Ontario. (2016). *Assessment and management of pressure injuries for the interprofessional team. (3rd edition.).* Available at *http://rnao.ca/bpg/guidelines/pressure-injuries.*

Source: Descriptions, drawings, and photos (with exceptions noted as follows) of pressure injury stages copyrighted by National Pressure Ulcer Advisory Panel (NPUAP) website. (2016). *Educational and clinical resources.* Available at *http://www.npuap.org/resources/educational-and-clinical-resources.* Used with permission.

*Photograph of deep tissue injury on heel from Fleck, C. A. (2007). Deep tissue injury: What, why, and when? *Wound Care Canada, 5*(2), 10–53.

TABLE 14-13   STAGING OF PRESSURE INJURIES—cont'd

Stage 2

Partial-thickness loss of skin with exposed dermis. The wound bed is viable, pink or red, moist, and may also appear as an intact or ruptured serum-filled blister. Neither adipose (fat) nor deeper tissues are visible. Granulation tissue, slough, and eschar are not present. These injuries commonly result from adverse microclimate and shear in the skin over the pelvis and shear in the heel. This stage should not be used to describe moisture-associated skin damage, including incontinence-associated dermatitis, intertriginous dermatitis, medical adhesive–related skin injury, or traumatic wounds (skin tears, burns, abrasions).

Diagram   **Clinical Presentation**

Stage 3

Full-thickness loss of skin, in which adipose (fat) is visible in the ulcer and granulation tissue and epibole (rolled wound edges) are often present. Slough or eschar, or both, may be visible. The depth of tissue damage varies by anatomical location; deep wounds can develop in areas of significant adiposity. Undermining and tunnelling may occur. Fascia, muscle, tendon, ligament, cartilage, and bone are not exposed. If slough or eschar obscures the extent of tissue loss, the injury is considered an unstageable pressure injury.

Diagram   **Clinical Presentation**

Stage 4

Full-thickness skin and tissue loss with exposed or directly palpable fascia, muscle, tendon, ligament, cartilage, or bone in the ulcer. Slough, eschar, or both may be visible. Epibole (rolled edges), undermining, or tunnelling, or a combination of these, often occurs. Depth varies by anatomical location. If slough or eschar obscures the extent of tissue loss, the injury is considered an unstageable pressure injury.

Diagram   **Clinical Presentation**

Continued

TABLE 14-13 STAGING OF PRESSURE INJURIES—cont'd

Unstageable

Full-thickness skin and tissue loss in which the extent of tissue damage within the ulcer cannot be confirmed because it is obscured by slough or eschar. If slough or eschar is removed, a stage 3 or stage 4 pressure injury is revealed. Stable eschar (i.e., dry, adherent, intact without erythema or fluctuance) on the heel or ischemic limb should not be softened or removed.

Diagram	Clinical Presentation†‡

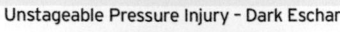
Unstageable Pressure Injury – Dark Eschar

Unstageable Pressure Injury – Slough and Eschar

Medical Device–Related Pressure Injury

Medical device–related pressure injuries result from the use of devices designed and applied for diagnostic or therapeutic purposes. The resultant pressure injury generally conforms to the pattern or shape of the device. The injury should be staged according to the staging system just described.

Example

Mucosal Membrane Pressure Injury

Mucosal membrane pressure injury is found on mucous membranes on which a medical device has been in use at the location of the injury. Because of the anatomy of the tissue, these injuries cannot be staged.

Diagram	Clinical Presentation§

Mucous Membrane

†Photograph of unstageable pressure injury (first row, middle column) courtesy Alison Anger, RN(EC), PHC-NP, BScN, MSc, ET.
‡Photograph of unstageable pressure injury to heel courtesy Beth Clarke, RN, MSc(A), MBA, CWOCN.
§Photograph of mucosal membrane pressure injury used with permission of I. Razmus and L. Lewis.

the whole person, such as adequate nutrition, pain management, control of other medical conditions, and pressure relief. Evidence-informed practice is to keep a pressure injury slightly moist, rather than dry, to enhance re-epithelialization. In addition to the nurse, other members of the health care team, such as the physician, the dietitian, the physiotherapist, and the occupational therapist, can provide valuable input into the complex treatment necessary to prevent and manage pressure injuries. Both conservative and surgical strategies are used in the treatment of pressure injuries, depending on the stage and the condition of the injury. Therapeutic and nursing management are discussed together because the activities are interrelated.

NURSING ASSESSMENT

Patients should be assessed for pressure injury risk initially on admission to the hospital and at periodic intervals thereafter on the basis of the patient's condition and the care setting. The nurse should conduct a thorough head-to-toe skin assessment on admission to identify and document pressure injuries. The skin and wounds should be reassessed on an ongoing basis and the treatment plan modified accordingly (RNAO, 2016).

SAFETY ALERT
- In acute care, the patient should be reassessed every 24 hours.
- In long-term care, a resident should be reassessed weekly for the first 4 weeks after admission and at least monthly or every 3 months thereafter.
- In home care, the patient should be reassessed at each nurse visit.

Risk assessment should be performed with a validated assessment tool such as the Braden scale (Table 14-14). To obtain a patient's pressure injury risk assessment score on the Braden scale, the nurse adds the numerical scores for the factors in each of the six subscales (sensory perception, moisture, activity, mobility, nutrition, and friction and shear). Scores can range from 6 to 23. The lower the numerical score on the Braden scale, the higher is the patient's predicted risk of developing a pressure injury. Incremental changes in the score indicate the level of risk: no risk (19 to 23), at risk (15 to 18), at moderate risk (13 to 14), at high risk (10 to 12), and at very high risk (≤9). Knowing the level of risk can help the health care provider determine how aggressive the preventive measures should be. The Braden scale has also been modified (Braden Q scale) for use with the pediatric population (Manning, Gauvreau, & Curley, 2015).

Identification of stage 1 pressure injuries may be difficult in patients with dark skin. Table 14-15 presents techniques to help assess darker skin. Subjective and objective data that should be obtained from a person with a pressure injury are presented in Table 14-16.

NURSING DIAGNOSES

Nursing diagnoses for the patient with a pressure injury may include, but are not limited to, the following:
- *Impaired skin integrity* related to *pressure over bony prominence*
- *Impaired tissue integrity* related to *inadequate nutrition*

PLANNING

The overall goals are that the patient with a pressure injury will (a) have no deterioration of the ulcer stage, (b) reduce or eliminate the factors that lead to pressure injuries, (c) have improved nutritional status, (d) have increased mobility, (e) not develop an infection in the pressure injury, (f) have healing of pressure injuries, and (g) have no recurrence.

NURSING IMPLEMENTATION

HEALTH PROMOTION. Nurses are responsible for identifying patients at risk for the development of pressure injuries (see Tables 14-12 and 14-14). Once a patient has been identified as being at risk for pressure injury development, prevention strategies should be implemented. Prevention remains the best treatment for pressure injuries (Houghton, Campbell, & Clinical Practice Guidelines Panel, 2013; Paul, McCutcheon, Tregarthen, et al., 2014; Roe & Williams, 2014).

SAFETY ALERT
- The patient should be repositioned frequently to prevent pressure injuries.
- Devices to reduce pressure and shearing force (e.g., alternating pressure mattresses, foam mattresses, lift sheets, wheelchair cushions, padded commode seats, heel boots [foam, air]) should be used, as appropriate.
- These devices are not adequate substitutes for frequent repositioning.

Acute Intervention. Once a pressure injury has developed, the nurse should initiate interventions that are based on the ulcer characteristics (e.g., stage, size, location, amount of exudate, type of wound, presence of infection or pain) and the patient's general status (e.g., nutritional state, level of mobility).

Measuring the Wound. The size of the pressure injury should be carefully documented. A wound-measuring tape can be used to note the ulcer's maximum length and width in centimetres (Figure 14-10). To find the depth of the ulcer, gently place a sterile cotton-tipped applicator into the deepest part of the ulcer.

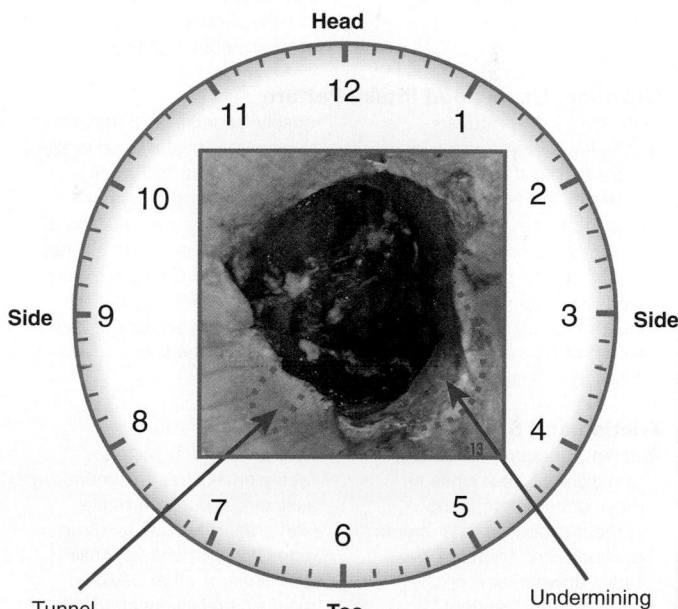

FIGURE 14-10 Wound measurements are made in centimetres. The first measurement is oriented from head to toe, the second is from side to side, and the third is the depth (if any). Any tunnelling (when a cotton-tipped applicator is placed in the wound, the applicator moves) or undermining (when a cotton-tipped applicator is placed in wound, there is a "lip" around the wound) is charted like a clock, the 12 o'clock position being toward the patient's head. This wound would be charted as a full-thickness, red wound, 7 cm × 5 cm × 3 cm, with a 3-cm tunnel at the 7 o'clock position and 2-cm undermining from the 3 o'clock to 5 o'clock positions. Source: Courtesy Robert B. Babiak, RN, BSN, CWOCN, San Antonio, TX.

TABLE 14-14   BRADEN SCALE FOR PREDICTING PRESSURE INJURY RISK

Patient's Name _____

Evaluator's Name _____

Date of Assessment _____

Point Value

1	2	3	4	Score
Sensory Perception: Ability to Respond Meaningfully to Pressure-Related Discomfort				
Completely limited: Unresponsive (does not moan, flinch, or grasp) to painful stimuli, due to diminished level of consciousness or sedation or limited ability to feel pain over most of body	Very limited: Responds only to painful stimuli; cannot communicate discomfort except by moaning or restlessness or has a sensory impairment that limits the ability to feel pain or discomfort over half of body	Slightly limited: Responds to verbal commands, but cannot always communicate discomfort or the need to be turned or has some sensory impairment that limits ability to feel pain or discomfort in one or two extremities	No impairment: Responds to verbal commands; has no sensory deficit that would limit ability to feel or to voice pain or discomfort	
Moisture: Degree to Which Skin Is Exposed to Moisture				
Constantly moist: Skin is kept moist almost constantly by perspiration, urine, and so on; dampness is detected every time patient is moved or turned	Very moist: Skin is often, but not always, moist; linen must be changed at least once per shift	Occasionally moist: Skin is occasionally moist, necessitating an extra linen change approximately once per day	Rarely moist: Skin is usually dry; linen requires changing [only] at routine intervals	
Activity: Degree of Physical Activity				
Bedfast: Confined to bed	Chairfast: Ability to walk [is] severely limited or nonexistent; cannot bear own weight or must be assisted into chair or wheelchair	Walks occasionally: Walks occasionally during day, but for very short distances, with or without assistance; spends most of each shift in bed or chair	Walks frequently: Walks outside room at least twice per day and inside room at least once every 2 hours during waking hours	
Mobility: Ability to Change and Control Body Position				
Completely immobile: Does not make even slight changes in body or extremity position without assistance	Very limited: Makes occasional slight changes in body or extremity position but unable to make frequent or significant changes independently	Slightly limited: Makes frequent though slight changes in body or extremity position independently	No limitation: Makes major and frequent changes in position without assistance	
Nutrition: Usual Food Intake Pattern				
Very poor: Never eats a complete meal; rarely eats more than half of any food offered; eats two servings or less of protein (meat or dairy products) per day; takes fluids poorly; does not take a liquid dietary supplement or is NPO and/or maintained on clear liquids or [IV supplements] for more than 5 days	Probably inadequate: Rarely eats a complete meal and generally eats only about half of any food offered; protein intake includes only three servings of meat or dairy products per day; occasionally will take a dietary supplement or receives less than optimum amount of liquid diet or tube feeding	Adequate: Eats over half of most meals; eats four servings of protein (meat or dairy products) per day; occasionally will refuse a meal, but will usually take a supplement when offered or is on a tube feeding or total parenteral nutrition regimen that probably meets most of nutritional needs	Excellent: eats most of every meal; never refuses a meal; eats four or more servings of protein (meat or dairy products); occasionally eats between meals; does not require supplementation	
Friction and Shear				
Problem: Requires moderate to maximum assistance in moving; complete lifting without sliding against sheets is impossible; frequently slides down in bed or chair, necessitating frequent repositioning with maximum assistance; spasticity, contractures, or agitation leads to almost constant friction	Potential problem: Moves feebly or requires minimum assistance; during a move, skin probably slides to some extent against sheets, chair, restraints, or other devices; maintains relatively good position in chair or bed most of the time but occasionally slides down	No apparent problem: Moves in bed and in chair independently and has sufficient muscle strength to lift up completely during move; maintains good position in bed or chair		

IVs, intravenous nutrition; *NPO,* nothing by mouth (status).

Source: From Braden, B., & Bergstrom, N. (1994). Predictive validity of the Braden scale for pressure sore risk in a nursing home population. *Research in Nursing & Health,* 17, 459. Copyright, Braden and Bergstrom, 1988. Reprinted with permission. All rights reserved.

EVIDENCE-INFORMED PRACTICE
Translating Research Into Practice

The nurse is caring for Sarjana Wali, an obese 86-year-old woman with a history of diabetes, hypertension, and chronic kidney disease. Ms. Wali spends most of her time in bed or in a wheelchair and now has a stage 1 pressure injury on her sacral area. The nurse is delivering discharge teaching to the patient's daughter, who is her primary caregiver. The nurse explains the importance of preventing further skin breakdown and that the daughter needs to reposition her mother every 2 to 4 hours during the night. Ms. Wali's daughter tells the nurse that at night, she will reposition her mother only if her mother wakes up to use the commode; otherwise, she must have uninterrupted sleep because she watches her two young grandchildren during the day.

Best Available Evidence	Clinician Expertise	Patient Preferences and Values
Repositioning remains the primary method of reducing risk for pressure injuries. Pressure-reducing devices (e.g., foam mattress, padded commode seats) can also be used but should not be a substitute for repositioning.	Patients with pressure injuries should be repositioned at least every 2 to 4 hours while in bed and should shift weight every 15 minutes when in a chair. Stage 1 pressure injuries can rapidly deteriorate to stage 2 if proper care is not taken.	Ms. Wali's caregiver expresses the need to have a certain amount of uninterrupted sleep to maintain multiple family responsibilities. The caregiver states that she will reposition her mother at least every 2–4 hours while she is in bed during the day and every 15 minutes when she is in a wheelchair. Ms. Wali's caregiver states she will purchase a foam mattress, wheelchair cushion, and padded commode seat to help prevent further skin issues.

Decision and Action
The nurse discusses the importance of repositioning as the primary method to prevent pressure injuries and decrease the progression of existing pressure injuries to more serious ones. Ms. Wali's daughter reiterates that she will not be able to reposition her mother every 2 to 4 hours during the night. The nurse can understand her decision and document this discussion in the patient's discharge teaching record.

Reference for Evidence
National Pressure Ulcer Advisory Panel, European Pressure Ulcer Advisory Panel, & Pan Pacific Pressure Injury Alliance (Haesler, E., Ed.) (2014). *Prevention and treatment of pressure ulcers: Quick reference guide*. Perth, Australia: Cambridge Media. Retrieved from *http://www.npuap.org/wp-content/uploads/2014/08/Updated-10-16-14-Quick-Reference-Guide-DIGITAL-NPUAP-EPUAP-PPPIA-16Oct2014.pdf*.

TABLE 14-15 ASSESSING PATIENTS WITH DARK SKIN

To assess patients with dark skin, the nurse should:
- Look for changes in skin colour, such as skin that is darker (purplish, brownish, bluish) than surrounding skin.
- Use natural light or a halogen light source to accurately assess the skin colour. Fluorescent light casts blue light, which can make skin assessment difficult.
- Assess the skin temperature of the area by using his or her hand. The area may feel warm initially and then cooler.
- Touch the skin to feel its consistency. Boggy or edematous observation may indicate a stage 1 pressure injury.
- Ask the patient if he or she has any pain or itchy sensation.

TABLE 14-16 NURSING ASSESSMENT
Pressure Injuries

Subjective Data
Important Health Information
Past health history: Stroke, spinal cord injury; prolonged bed rest or immobility; circulatory impairment; poor nutrition; altered level of consciousness; history of previous pressure injury; immunological abnormalities; advanced age; diabetes; anemia; trauma
Medications: Use of opioids, hypnotics, systemic corticosteroids, nicotine
Surgery or other treatments: Recent surgery

Symptoms
Incontinence of urine, feces, or both; weakness, debilitation, inability to turn and position body; pain or altered cutaneous sensation in injured area; decreased awareness of pressure on body areas; decreased fluid, calorie, or protein intake; vitamin or mineral deficiencies

Objective Data
General
Obesity; emaciation; clinically significant malnutrition as indicated by low serum albumin level, decreased total lymphocyte count, and decreased body weight (15% less than ideal body weight); contractures

Integumentary
Diaphoresis, edema, and discoloration, especially over bony areas such as sacrum, hips, elbows, heels, knees, ankles, shoulders, and ear rims, progressing to increased tissue damage characteristic of ulcer stages*

Possible Findings
Leukocytosis if infection present, positive cultures for microorganisms from pressure injury

*See Table 14-13.

The length of the portion of the applicator that probed the ulcer can then be measured.

Documentation. Healing of the wound can be documented with several available pressure injury healing tools such as the NPUAP Pressure Ulcer Scale of Healing (PUSH) tool. Some employers require that pictures of the pressure injury be taken initially and at regular intervals during the course of treatment. See the "Informatics in Practice" box for suggestions on digital imaging.

Wound Irrigation. Pressure injuries should be cleaned with 100 to 150 mL of a noncytotoxic solution, such as normal saline, that does not damage fibroblasts. It is important to

INFORMATICS IN PRACTICE
Digital Images

To monitor wound progress, use digital photography.
For the best images:
- Include a ruler with date, length, width, and depth of the wound in each photo.
- Position the patient the same way for each photo.
- Take the photo from the same angle each time. Pointing perpendicularly at the wound is best.
- Use natural light, without flash, whenever possible.
- Show the wound on a solid background, avoiding shiny underpads.

use enough irrigation pressure (4 to 15 psi) to clean the area adequately without causing trauma or damage to the wound, which can be accomplished with the use of a 100-mL saline squeeze bottle or a 30-mL syringe with an 19-gauge angiocatheter (RNAO, 2016).

Local Wound Care. After the pressure injury has been cleansed, it should be covered with an appropriate dressing. Some factors to consider in selecting a dressing are maintenance of a moist environment, prevention of wound desiccation (drying out), ability to absorb the wound drainage, location of the wound, amount of caregiver time, cost of the dressing, presence of infection, and the setting of care delivery. For further information on preparing the wound bed and localized wound care, refer to the Canadian Association of Wound Care website (see the Resources at the end of this chapter). (Dressings are discussed in Table 14-11.)

Stage 2 through stage 4 pressure injuries are considered contaminated or colonized with bacteria. For patients with chronic wounds or who are immunocompromised, the clinical signs of infection (purulent exudate, odour, erythema, induration, warmth, tenderness, edema, pain, fever, and elevated WBC count) may not be present even though the wound is infected.

The maintenance of adequate nutrition is an important nursing responsibility for the patient with a pressure injury (RNAO, 2016). Many such patients are debilitated and have a poor appetite as a result of inactivity. Clinically significant malnutrition is defined as a serum albumin level lower than 30 g/L, a total lymphocyte count lower than 1.8×10^9/L, or a body weight decrease of more than 5% over a 6- to 12-month period. Oral feedings must be adequate in calories, proteins, fluids, vitamins, and minerals to meet the patient's nutritional requirements. The intake needed to correct and maintain a nutritional balance may be 30 to 35 calories per kilogram per day and 1.25 to 1.50 g of protein per kilogram per day. Nasogastric feedings can be used to supplement the oral feedings. Parenteral nutrition consisting of amino acid and glucose solutions is administered when oral and nasogastric feedings are inadequate. (Parenteral and enteral nutrition are discussed in Chapter 42.) Nursing Care Plan 14-2 (available on the Evolve website) outlines the care for the patient with a pressure injury.

An appropriate support surface for both bed and chair or wheelchair should relieve pressure and keep the patient off of the damaged area. In some circumstances, reconstruction of the pressure injury site by operative repair, including skin grafting, skin flaps, musculo-cutaneous flaps, or free flaps, may be necessary.

Ambulatory and Home Care. Pressure injuries affect the quality of life of patients and their caregivers. Because recurrence is common, the education of both the patient and the care provider in prevention techniques is extremely important. The care provider needs to know the causes of pressure injuries, prevention techniques, early signs, nutritional support, and best practice for wound management. Because many patients with a pressure injury require extensive care for other health problems, it is important that the nurse support the caregiver in confronting the added responsibility of pressure injury treatment.

EVALUATION

Expected outcomes for the patient with a pressure injury are presented in Nursing Care Plan 14-2 on the Evolve website.

CASE STUDY

Inflammation and Infection

Source: © Kristiina Paul.

Patient Profile

Mr. Fred Roger, a 58-year-old man, is admitted to the hospital emergency department with partial-thickness burns that involved his face, neck, and upper trunk. He also has a lacerated right leg. His injuries occurred about 36 hours earlier, when he fell out of a tree onto his gas grill (which was lit) while he was trying to get his cat.

Subjective Data
• Complains of slightly hoarse voice and irritated throat
• States that he tried to treat himself because he does not regularly see the same primary care health provider
• Has been coughing up sooty sputum
• Complains of severe pain in left hip

Objective Data
Physical Examination
• Leg wound is gaping and looks infected; temperature is 38.4°C
• Radiographs reveal a fractured right tibia and a fractured left hip

Laboratory Studies
• WBC count is 26.4×10^9/L with 80% neutrophils (10% bands)

Collaborative Care
• Surgery is performed to repair the left hip

Discussion Questions
1. What clinical manifestations of inflammation did Mr. Roger exhibit, and what are their pathophysiological mechanisms?
2. What type of exudate formation developed?
3. What is the basis for the elevated temperature?
4. What is the significance of his WBC count and differential?
5. Because his wound was gaping, primary tissue healing was not possible. How might healing take place? What complications could he develop?
6. What are Mr. Roger's risk factors for developing a pressure injury?
7. **Priority Decision:** On the basis of the assessment data provided, what are the priority nursing diagnoses? Are there any collaborative problems?

🔵volve
Answers are available at *http://evolve.elsevier.com/Canada/Lewis/medsurg*

REVIEW QUESTIONS

The number of the question corresponds to the same-numbered objective at the beginning of the chapter.

1. In which context is physiological hyperplasia commonly found?
   a. A distended urinary bladder
   b. The female breast during lactation
   c. The bronchi of a chronic cigarette smoker
   d. An enlarged myocardium in heart failure

2. When radiation therapy is used in the treatment of cancer, how does it achieve the desired effect, which is death of cancer cells?
   a. Altering cellular metabolism and activity
   b. Producing mutations that interfere only with cancer cell function
   c. Accelerating metabolic reactions to reduce the normal life span of cells
   d. Stimulating synthesis of new particles that cause cell rupture and death

3. Which of the following is an example of coagulation necrosis?
   a. Autophagocytosis
   b. Myocardial infarction
   c. Malignant brain tumour
   d. Peripheral vascular disease

4. Which of the following will be experienced by a client with an impaired mononuclear phagocyte system?
   a. Increased circulation of histamine
   b. Decreased susceptibility to infection
   c. Decreased vascular response to cell injury
   d. Decreased surveillance for damaged or mutated cells

5. One day after abdominal surgery a client has incisional pain, 37.5°C temperature, slight erythema at the incision margins, and 30 mL of serosanguineous drainage in the Jackson-Pratt drain. On the basis of this assessment, what conclusion would the nurse make?
   a. The abdominal incision shows signs of an infection.
   b. The client is having a normal inflammatory response.
   c. The abdominal incision shows signs of impending dehiscence.
   d. The client's physician must be notified about her condition.

6. The nurse assessing a client with a chronic leg wound finds local signs of erythema and pain at the wound site. What would the nurse anticipate being ordered to assess the client's systemic response?
   a. Serum protein analysis
   b. WBC count and differential
   c. Punch biopsy of centre of wound
   d. Culture and sensitivity testing of the wound

7. A client in the unit has a 39.8°C temperature. Which intervention would be most effective in restoring normal body temperature?
   a. Use a cooling blanket while the client is febrile.
   b. Administer antipyretics on an around-the-clock schedule.
   c. Provide increased fluids and instruct the unlicensed assistive personnel to give sponge baths.
   d. Give prescribed antibiotics and provide warm blankets for comfort.

8. A nurse is caring for a client who has a pressure injury that is treated with debridement, irrigations, and moist gauze dressings. How should the nurse anticipate healing to occur?
   a. Tertiary intention
   b. Secondary intention
   c. Regeneration of cells
   d. Remodelling of tissues

9. A nurse is caring for a client with diabetes who is scheduled for amputation of his necrotic left great toe. The client's WBC count is 15.0×10^9/L, and he has coolness of the lower extremities, weighs 34 kg more than his ideal body weight, and smokes two packs of cigarettes per day. Which priority nursing diagnosis addresses the primary factor affecting the client's ability to heal?
   a. *Readiness for enhanced nutrition*
   b. *Impaired tissue integrity* related to *insufficient knowledge about protecting tissue integrity*
   c. *Ineffective peripheral tissue perfusion* related to *sedentary lifestyle*
   d. *Ineffective coping* related to *ineffective tension release strategies*

10. An 89-year-old client with end-stage renal disease is assessed to have a score of 16 on the Braden scale. On the basis of this information, how should the nurse plan for this client's care?
    a. Implement a 1-hour turning schedule with skin assessment
    b. Place a hydrocolloid on the client's sacrum to prevent breakdown
    c. Elevate the head of bed to 90 degrees when the client is supine
    d. Continue with weekly skin assessments with no additional special precautions

11. A 65-year-old client who has had a stroke and has limited mobility has a purple area of suspected deep tissue injury on the left greater trochanter. Which nursing diagnoses are most appropriate? *(Select all that apply)*
    a. *Acute pain* related to *physical injury agent*
    b. *Impaired skin integrity* related to *pressure over bony prominence*
    c. *Impaired tissue integrity* related to *insufficient knowledge about protecting tissue integrity*
    d. *Risk for infection* as evidenced by *malnutrition*

12. An 82-year-old man is being cared for at home by his family. A pressure injury on his right buttock measures $1 \times 2 \times 0.8$ cm in depth, and pink subcutaneous tissue is completely visible on the wound bed. Which stage would the nurse document on the wound assessment form?
    a. Stage 1
    b. Stage 2
    c. Stage 3
    d. Stage 4

13. Which one of the orders should a nurse question in the plan of care for an elderly client who is immobile as the result of a stroke and has a stage 3 pressure injury?
    a. Cover the ulcer with a foam dressing.
    b. Turn and position the client every hour.
    c. Clean the ulcer every shift with Dakin's solution.
    d. Assess for pain and medicate before dressing change.

1. b; 2. a; 3. b; 4. d; 5. b; 6. b; 7. b; 8. b; 9. b; 10. a; 11. b, c; 12. c; 13. c.

⟳ volve

For even more review questions, visit *http://evolve.elsevier.com/Canada/Lewis/medsurg.*

REFERENCES

Ayello, E. A., & Baranoski, S. (2014). Wound care prevention. *Nursing, 44*(4), 32–40. doi:10.1097/01.NURSE.0000444531.73951.ae.

Canadian Institute for Health Information (2013). *Compromised wounds in Canada.* Retrieved from *https://secure.cihi.ca/free_products/AiB_Compromised_Wounds_EN.pdf.*

Dinarello, C. A., & Porat, R. (2015). Fever and hyperthermia. In D. L. Kasper, A. S. Fauci, D. L. Longo, et al. (Eds.), *Harrison's principles of internal medicine* (19th ed.). Toronto: McGraw-Hill. doi:10.1001/jama.308.17.1813-b.

Doughty, D., & McNichol, L. (2016). *Wound Ostomy Continence Nurses Society core curriculum: Wound management.* Philadelphia: Wolters-Kluwer.

Edsberg, L. E., Langemo, D., Baharestani, M. M., et al. (2014). Unavoidable pressure injury: State of the science and consensus outcomes. *Journal of Wound, Ostomy, and Continence Nursing, 41*(4), 313–334. doi:10.1097/WON.0000000000000050.

Houghton, P. E., Campbell, K., & Clinical Practice Guidelines Panel (2013). *Canadian best practice guidelines for the prevention and management of pressure ulcers in people with Spinal Cord Injury: A resource handbook for clinicians.* Toronto: Ontario Neurotrauma Foundation.

LeBlanc, K., & Baranoski, S. (2014). Skin tears: Best practices for care and prevention. *Nursing, 44*(8), 36–46. doi:10.1097/01.NURSE.0000445744.86119.58.

Lisy, K. (2014). Early vs. delayed removal of dressings covering surgical wounds. *American Journal of Nursing, 114*(8), 23. doi:10.1097/01.NAJ.0000453038.93499.69.

Manning, M. J., Gauvreau, K., & Curley, M. A. (2015). Factors associated with occipital pressure ulcers in hospitalized infants and children. *American Journal of Critical Care, 24*(4), 342–348. doi:10.4037/ajcc2015349.

National Pressure Ulcer Advisory Panel (NPUAP) (2014). *New 2014 prevention and treatment of pressure ulcers: Clinical practice guidelines.* Retrieved from *http://www.npuap.org/resources/educational-and-clinical-resources/prevention-and-treatment-of-pressure-ulcers-clinical-practice-guideline/.*

Paul, R., McCutcheon, S. P., Tregarthen, J. P., et al. (2014). Sustaining pressure ulcer best practices in high-volume cardiac care environment. *American Journal of Nursing, 114*(8), 34–44. doi:10.1097/01.NAJ.0000453041.16371.16.

Registered Nurses' Association of Ontario (RNAO) (2016). *Assessment and management of pressure injuries for the interprofessional team* (3rd ed.). Retrieved from *http://rnao.ca/bpg/guidelines/pressure-injuries.*

Roe, E., & Williams, D. L. (2014). Using evidence-based practice to prevent hospital-acquired pressure ulcers and promote wound healing. *American Journal of Nursing, 114*(8), 61–65. doi:10.1097/01.NAJ.0000453050.31618.ec.

Sibbald, R. G., Elliott, J. A., Ayello, E. A., et al. (2015). Optimizing the moisture management tightrope with wound bed preparation 2015©. *Advances in Skin and Wound Care, 28*(10), 466–476. doi:10.1097/01.ASW.0000470851.27030.98.

Wilcox, J. R., Carter, M. J., & Covington, S. (2013). Frequency of debridement and time to heal: A retrospective cohort study of 312,744 wounds. *JAMA Dermatology, 149*(4), 1050–1058. doi:10.1001/jamadermatol.2013.4960.

Woo, K. Y., Keast, D., Parsons, N., et al. (2015). The cost of wound debridement: A Canadian perspective. *International Wound Journal, 12*(4), 402–407. doi:10.1111/iwj.12122.

Wound, Ostomy and Continence Nurses Society (2016). *Guideline for prevention and management of pressure ulcers (injuries).* Mt. Laurel, NJ: Author.

RESOURCES

Canadian Association for Enterostomal Therapists
http://www.caet.ca

Canadian Association of Wound Care
http://www.cawc.net

Canadian Institute for Health Information
http://www.cihi.ca/

Community and Hospital Infection Control Association (CHICA)—Canada
http://www.chica.org

Ontario Ministry of Health and Long-Term Care
http://www.health.gov.on.ca/en/

Ontario Ministry of Health and Long-Term Care, Medical Advisory Secretariat
Negative Pressure Wound Therapy: An Evidence-Based Analysis. *http://www.hqontario.ca/Evidence/Publications-and-OHTAC-Recommendations/Ontario-Health-Technology-Assessment-Series/Negative-Pressure-Wound-Therapy-An-Evidence-Update*

Ontario Wound Care Interest Group
http://ontwig.ca/

Public Health Agency of Canada
http://www.phac-aspc.gc.ca

Registered Nurses' Association of Ontario (RNAO)—Best Practice Guidelines
http://rnao.ca/bpg

Regroupement Québécois en Soins de Plaies
www.rqsp.ca

Toronto Medical Laboratories and Mount Sinai Hospital Department of Microbiology, MicroWeb
http://www.microbiology.mtsinai.on.ca

Agency for Health Care Policy
http://www.ahrq.gov/

Centers for Disease Control and Prevention
http://www.cdc.gov

European Pressure Ulcer Advisory Panel (EPUAP)
http://www.epuap.org

European Wound Management Association
http://www.ewma.org

International Federation of Infection Control
http://www.theific.org/

International Wound Infection Institute
http://www.woundinfection-institute.com/

National Pressure Ulcer Advisory Panel
http://www.npuap.org

Ostomy Wound Management
http://www.o-wm.com/

World Council of Enterostomal Therapists
http://www.wcetn.org

World Health Organization
http://www.who.int/en

World Wide Wounds
http://www.worldwidewounds.com

Wound, Ostomy and Continence Nurses Society
http://www.wocn.org

For additional Internet resources, see the website for this book
at *http://evolve.elsevier.com/Canada/Lewis/medsurg*

Genetics

Written by: Sharon L. Lewis
Adapted by: George S. Charames
With contributions from: Kelly Metcalfe

evolve WEBSITE

http://evolve.elsevier.com/Canada/Lewis/medsurg

- Review Questions (Online Only)
- Key Points
- Conceptual Care Map Creator

- Audio Glossary
- Content Updates

LEARNING OBJECTIVES

1. Describe the significance of the Human Genome Project for nurses and the field of health care.
2. Define common terms related to genetics and genetic disorders: *autosome, carrier, heterozygous, homozygous, mutation, recessive,* and *sex-linked*.
3. Compare and contrast the most common categories of genetic disorders.
4. Describe taking a family history or pedigree using the common nomenclature.
5. Identify the common types of genetic testing.
6. Outline the role of the nurse in working with patients and families with possible or actual genetic conditions.
7. Explore the complex ethical and social implications of genetic testing.

KEY TERMS

allele, p. 249, Table 15-1	deoxyribonucleic acid (DNA), p. 249	heterozygous, p. 249, Table 15-1	ribonucleic acid (RNA), p. 250
amniocentesis, p. 254			sex-linked gene, p. 249, Table 15-1
autosome, p. 249, Table 15-1	gene therapy, p. 256	homozygous, p. 249, Table 15-1	transcription, p. 250
carrier, p. 249, Table 15-1		mutation, p. 249, Table 15-1	translation, p. 251
chorionic villus sampling (CVS), p. 254	genetics, p. 249 genotype, p. 249	recessive allele, p. 249, Table 15-1	

Genomics (the study of genomes) is a central science for all nursing practice because essentially all diseases and conditions have a genetic or genomic component. Health care for all people will increasingly include genetic and genomic information along the pathways of prevention, screening, diagnostics, prognostics, selection of treatment, and monitoring of treatment effectiveness (Consensus Panel on Genetic/Genomic Nursing Competencies, 2009).

Genetics has a great impact on health and disease; therefore, the study of genetics has become increasingly important for health care providers. Common disorders such as heart disease and most cancers arise from a complex interplay among multiple genes and between genes and factors in the environment (World Health Organization, 2016).

The molecular basis of more than 4 600 disorders is now known (Online Mendelian Inheritance in Man [OMIM], 2017). This identification of a genetic basis for many diseases has affected the study of genetics and genomics and their relevance

to nurses and, accordingly, has directly influenced the care of patients at risk for or diagnosed with such a disease. Nurses need to know the basic principles of genetics, be familiar with the impact that genetics has on health and disease, and be prepared to assist the patient and family in dealing with genetics issues (Calzone, Jenkins, Nicol, et al., 2013; Munro, 2015). In addition, nurses must become knowledgeable regarding the application of genetic discoveries to clinical care and assume leadership in preparing to meet patients' needs for the future (Daack-Hirsch, et al., 2013). Nurses are at the interface of translating new human genome research discoveries into clinical practice and will increasingly care for individuals and families who have a genetic condition or a health issue with a genetic component.

HUMAN GENOME PROJECT

The Human Genome Project (HGP) is one of the most significant health-related advances of modern times. The HGP began in

1990 as an international effort to analyze the structure of human DNA and determine the location on chromosomes of all human genes. It involved more than 2 000 scientists from 20 institutions in six countries. The human genome was completely sequenced by 2003, with the sequence of more than 3 billion DNA bases determined. An estimated 20 000 genes exist in the human genome. The HGP has enabled the characterization of more than 15 000 genes to date (OMIM, 2017).

The contribution of the HGP has helped to improve the diagnosis of genetic-related diseases, allowed for earlier detection through improved surveillance methods, and offered improved targeted therapies, and continues to play a critical role in determining personal and familial risks. A comprehensive website covering the topic of the HGP can be found at Human Genome Project Information (see the Resources at the end of this chapter).

BASIC PRINCIPLES OF GENETICS

Genetics is the study of inheritance. Table 15-1 presents a glossary of terms commonly used in the study of genetics.

TABLE 15-1	GLOSSARY OF GENETIC TERMS
Term	**Definition**
Allele	One of two or more alternative forms of a gene that can occupy a particular chromosomal locus
Autosome	Any chromosome that is not a sex chromosome
Carrier	An individual who carries a copy of a mutated gene for a recessive disorder
Chromosome	A gene-carrying structure in the nucleus of all human cells that consists of DNA and protein
Codominance	Two dominant versions of a trait that are both expressed in the same individual
Congenital disorder	Condition present at birth
Dominant allele	Gene that is expressed in the phenotype of a heterozygous individual
Gene	Unit of hereditary information located on a specific part of a chromosome
Genome	An organism's complete set of genetic material present in a cell
Hereditary	A disease or condition being transmitted from parent to offspring
Heterozygous	Having two different alleles for one given gene
Homozygous	Having two identical alleles for one given gene
Locus	Position of a gene on a chromosome
Mutation	A change in the DNA sequence of a gene, affecting the expression of the gene (changing the original manner of expression)
Oncogene	Gene that is able to initiate and contribute to the conversion of normal cells to cancer cells
Pedigree	Family tree that contains the genetic characteristics and disorders of that particular family
Phenotype	Clinically expressed traits of an individual
Proto-oncogenes	Normal cellular genes that are important regulators of normal cellular processes; mutations can activate them to become oncogenes
Recessive allele	An allele that has no noticeable effect on the phenotype in a heterozygous individual
Sex-linked gene	A gene located on a sex chromosome
Trait	Physical characteristic that one inherits, such as hair and eye colour

Chromosomes, Genes, and DNA

An individual's heritable collection of genetic material is called the genotype. The physical and observable characteristics of an individual (e.g., eye colour, weight) are called *phenotypes*. The phenotypes may or may not be caused by the genotype. Genetic material is mostly packaged into threadlike structures called *chromosomes*, and chromosomes are located within the cell nucleus (Figure 15-1). Humans have two sets of 23 chromosomes (46 in total) in nearly every cell in the human body except the gametes (egg and sperm cells), which have only one set of 23 chromosomes. Two sets of chromosomes is termed *diploid*, while one set of chromosomes is termed *haploid*. One set is inherited from the mother, and one set is inherited from the father during conception. Twenty-two pairs of chromosomes, called *autosomes*, are the same in both men and women. The twenty-third pair is referred to as the sex chromosomes. A male has an X and a Y chromosome, and a female has two X chromosomes. The genetic material on each of the non-sex chromosome pairs is *homologous* to each other, meaning that they have the same position and order (Figure 15-2).

Chromosomes are composed of proteins and a long, thin molecule called deoxyribonucleic acid (DNA). DNA is the hereditary material (meaning it can be passed on to daughter cells and subsequent generations) in cells that contains the instructions that drive most cellular processes, typically through making functional proteins. The segments of DNA that contain these instructions are called *genes*. Although most DNA is contained within the nucleus, some DNA can be found outside the nucleus (e.g., mtDNA is in the mitochondria).

The specific structure of DNA is a double helix in which two strands (polynucleotide chains) run in opposite directions (Figure 15-3). The two strands are held together by hydrogen bonds between pairs of bases: adenine (A), thymine (T), guanine (G), and cytosine (C). DNA is composed of a sugar (deoxyribose),

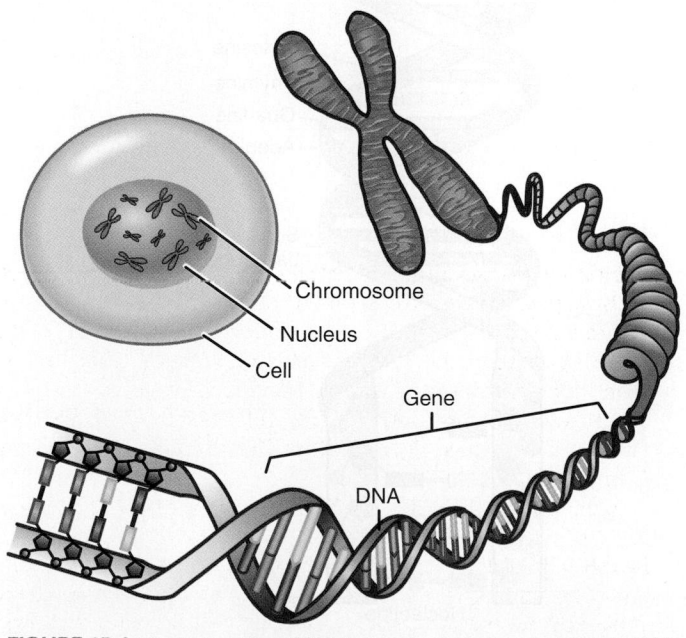

FIGURE 15-1 The long, stringy DNA that makes up genes is spooled within chromosomes inside the nucleus of a cell. (Note that a gene would actually be a much longer stretch of DNA than what is shown here.) Source: National Institute of General Medical Science. National Institutes of Health, U.S. Department of Health and Human Services (2010). *The new genetics*. Retrieved from https://publications.nigms.nih.gov/thenewgenetics/thenewgenetics.pdf.

FIGURE 15-2 Human chromosomes. Source: Turnpenny, P. D. (2007). *Emery's elements of medical genetics* (13th ed., p. 34). Edinburgh/Philadelphia: Churchill Livingstone/Elsevier.

a phosphate group, and one of the four nitrogenous bases. One unit, a sugar group combined with a phosphate group and one of the four bases, is called a *nucleotide*. The bases on each strand of DNA are paired in a specific manner. Adenine always pairs with thymine, and guanine pairs with cytosine. The specific nature of the genetic information encoded in the human genome lies in the nucleotide sequence within the DNA.

How Proteins Are Made

DNA must undergo replication, transcription, and translation before a functional protein is made. A new DNA strand must be synthesized before cell division. In order for synthesis to occur, the two DNA strands separate and unwind and become templates for new strands. DNA is formed and replicated in the cell nucleus, whereas protein synthesis takes place in the cytoplasm of the cell. Transcription and translation, the latter following the former, take place when the genetic code is transported from the cell nucleus to the cytoplasm (Figure 15-4). **Ribonucleic acid (RNA)** is the nucleic acid that is involved in these processes. RNA is similar to DNA; however, it is composed of only one strand (as opposed to two strands in DNA), and the nitrogenous base thymine (T) is replaced with uracil (U). **Transcription** takes place when RNA is synthesized from the DNA template. Genes are made up of coding (exons) and noncoding (introns) regions. In transcription, the noncoding regions (introns) are removed, or spliced out. As a result, a messenger RNA (mRNA) is created and can move across the nuclear membrane into the cytoplasm. This is where, based

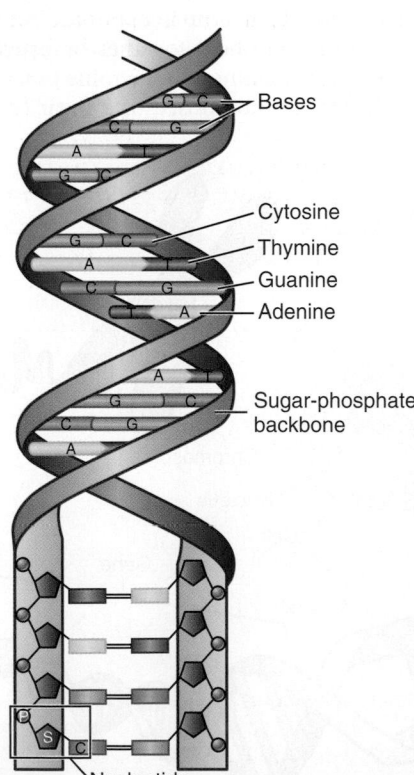

FIGURE 15-3 DNA consists of two long, twisted chains made up of nucleotides. Each nucleotide contains one base, one phosphate molecule *(P)*, and the sugar molecule deoxyribose *(S)*. The bases in DNA nucleotides are adenine *(A)*, thymine *(T)*, cytosine *(C)*, and guanine *(G)*. Source: Adapted from *The new genetics* (2010). National Institute of General Medical Science. National Institutes of Health. U.S. Department of Health and Human Services.

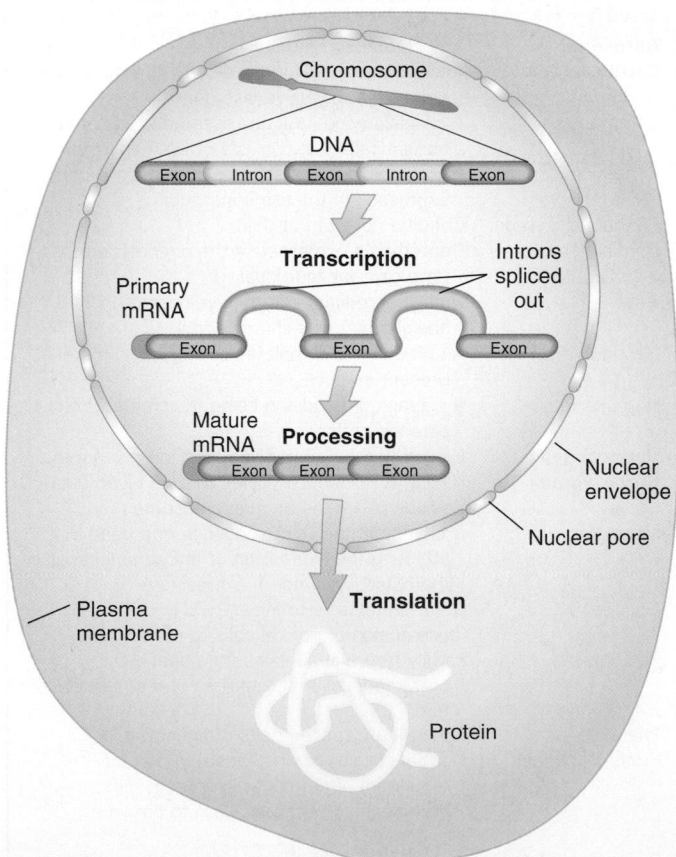

FIGURE 15-4 A summary of the steps leading from DNA to protein creation. Replication and transcription occur in the cell nucleus. The mRNA is then transported to the cytoplasm, where translation of the mRNA into amino acid sequences composing a protein occurs. Source: Jorde, L., Cary, J., & Bamshad, M. (2010). *Medical genetics* (4th ed., p. 10). St. Louis: Mosby.

on the sequence of the mRNA, the protein is manufactured in a process called **translation**. In translation, the mRNA sequence acts as a template for the formation of a chain of amino acids. Three successive nucleotides (e.g., CCG) are termed a *codon,* and one codon specifies the production of one amino acid. Proteins are made up of many amino acids. Translation is accomplished by a cytoplasmic particle called the *ribosome.*

Genes are generally stable and are passed from one generation to the next. However, sometimes a change in the gene occurs, referred to as a *variant* or *mutation*. It should be noted that, currently, the field of genetics and genomics typically prefers to describe any difference in a person's nucleotide sequence as compared to a reference sequence as a *variant*. Humans have numerous genetic variants in their DNA, which make us all unique; not all variants manifest in disease. Genetic differences that cause disease are termed *pathogenic variants,* while changes that do not cause disease are called *benign variants.* Outside of this community (and in this chapter), *mutation* is used interchangeably with *pathogenic variant*.

Mutations can occur in the germ line (sperm and eggs) or in the somatic (non-sex) cells after fertilization. Germ-line mutations are those that are passed from one generation to the next and can account for familial syndromes. Approximately 2% of the DNA is composed of sequences that code for specific proteins, and the other 98% is made up of noncoding regions. DNA sequence changes can code for different amino acids that cause structural changes to the protein, and can affect its function.

PRIMARY CATEGORIES OF GENETIC CONDITIONS

Within each human, alterations in genes or in combinations of them can cause genetic disorders. These disorders can be classified into three categories: (1) single-gene disorders; (2) chromosomal disorders; and (3) multifactorial disorders.

Single-Gene Disorders

A disorder caused by a single gene may have a mutation present on only one chromosome of a pair (matched with a normal allele on the homologous chromosome) or on both chromosomes of the pair. These disorders usually exhibit obvious and characteristic inheritance patterns in families and are also referred to as *Mendelian*. Examples of single-gene disorders include cystic fibrosis (CF), Marfan syndrome, and sickle-cell anemia. There are three primary single-gene, or Mendelian, inheritance patterns: (1) autosomal dominant, (2) autosomal recessive, and (3) X-linked. If the mutant gene is located on an autosome, the genetic disorder is called *autosomal*. If the mutant gene is on the X chromosome, the genetic disorder is called *X-linked*. In medical genetics, a family history of clinical information with respect to a hereditary condition is illustrated using a collection of symbols (Figure 15-5) and is called a *pedigree*.

Autosomal Dominant. An autosomal dominant trait is one that manifests in the heterozygous state, that is, in a person who has both an abnormal (mutated) and a normal gene. The mutated gene dominates the normal gene. Families with conditions that suggest autosomal dominant inheritance exhibit several characteristics:
1. The affected offspring has one affected parent (with each pregnancy in an affected parent, there is a 50% chance that the characteristic will be passed to the child).
2. Unaffected people do not transmit the trait to their children.
3. Males and females are equally likely to inherit the trait.
4. The trait does not skip generations.

Some examples of autosomal dominant disorders are achondroplasia, Marfan syndrome, neurofibromatosis type 1, and brachydactyly. See Figure 15-6 for an example of a pedigree of a family with an autosomal dominant trait.

Punnett squares can be used to determine inheritance possibilities. The Punnett square in Figure 15-7 illustrates the mating of a parent affected with the autosomal dominant trait and an unaffected parent. The probability that the affected parent will pass on the mutated gene to a child is 0.5. Therefore, on average, 50% of the offspring will inherit the trait.

Autosomal Recessive. In the majority of recessive conditions, an affected offspring results from a mating between two unaffected carriers of the mutated gene. The offspring inherits two copies of the mutated gene, one from each parent, which results in the offspring exhibiting the disorder. The parents of these offspring

○	Normal female	
□	Normal male	
◇	Unknown sex, normal	
●	Affected female	
■	Affected male	
◆	Affected child of unknown sex	
◫	Male heterozygote (carrier of recessive allele)	
◐	Female heterozygote (carrier of recessive allele)	
•	Spontaneous abortion or stillbirth	
⊘	Deceased	
○—□	Mating	
○=□	Consanguineous mating	
	Dizygotic twins (two eggs)	
	Monozygotic twins (one egg)	
↗	Proband or propositus/proposita	
I, II	Roman numerals designate generation number	
1, 2	Arabic numerals designate individuals within generations	

FIGURE 15-5 Conventional symbols used in pedigrees. Source: Adkison, L. (2012). *Elsevier's integrated review: Genetics* (2nd ed., p. 30). Philadelphia: Elsevier/Saunders.

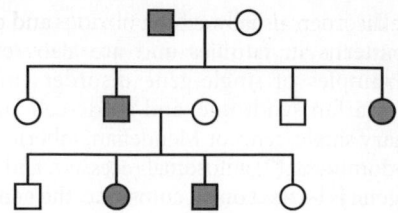

FIGURE 15-6 Pedigree of a family with an autosomal dominant trait.

FIGURE 15-8 Pedigree of a family with an autosomal recessive trait.

	Unaffected parent	
	a	a
A	Aa	Aa
a	aa	aa

(left column header: Affected parent)

FIGURE 15-7 The Punnett square illustrates the mating of an unaffected individual *(aa)* with an individual who is heterozygous for an autosomal dominant disease gene *(Aa)*. The genotypes of affected offspring are shaded.

	Carrier parent	
	A	a
A	AA	Aa
a	Aa	aa

(left column header: Carrier parent)

FIGURE 15-9 Punnett square illustrates the mating of two heterozygous carriers of an autosomal recessive gene. The genotype of the affected offspring is shaded. Source: Jorde, L., Cary, J., & Bamshad, M. (2010). *Medical genetics* (4th ed., p. 61). St. Louis: Mosby.

do not exhibit the trait associated with having the mutation because they each carry only one copy of the mutated gene (they are heterozygous carriers). Families with conditions that suggest autosomal recessive inheritance exhibit several characteristics:

1. Most affected individuals have parents that have normal phenotypes (do not exhibit the trait).
2. On average, one in four children is affected.
3. Males and females are equally likely to be affected.
4. Affected people who mate with normal people tend to have phenotypically normal children.

Some examples of autosomal recessive disorders are albinism, CF, and phenylketonuria. See Figure 15-8 for an example of a pedigree of a family with an autosomal recessive trait. The Punnett square illustrating the mating of two heterozygous parents of an autosomal recessive gene is shown in Figure 15-9.

X-Linked. An X-linked recessive trait is one determined by a gene carried on the X chromosome, and it usually manifests only in males. In males, there is only one X chromosome (the other is a Y chromosome), whereas females have two X chromosomes. A male with a mutation in a gene on the X chromosome will exhibit the disorder, because he has no corresponding normal gene to mask the mutated gene's effects. Diseases inherited in an X-linked manner are transmitted by healthy heterozygous female carriers to males, who are thus affected, as well as by affected males to their carrier daughters, with a future risk to male grandchildren. Families with conditions that suggest X-linked recessive inheritance exhibit several characteristics:

1. Unaffected males do not transmit the disorder.
2. Affected males do not transmit the disorder to their sons.
3. All daughters of an affected male are heterozygous carriers and may be unaffected or mildly affected.

4. Heterozygous women transmit the mutant allele to 50% of the sons (who are affected) and to 50% of the daughters (who are heterozygous carriers).

Some examples of X-linked recessive disorders are hemophilia A and Duchenne muscular dystrophy (DMD). See Figure 15-10 for an example of a pedigree of a family with an autosomal recessive trait. The Punnett square in Figure 15-11 illustrates the mating of a female carrier of an X-linked recessive disorder and a normal male.

X-linked dominant inheritance disorders are those in which the dominant gene is carried on the X chromosome and are typically characterized by affected females and lethal in males. X-linked dominant disorders are rarer than X-linked recessive disorders. Some examples include Rett syndrome (*MECP2* gene) and incontinentia pigmenti (*IKBKG* gene).

X-inactivation occurs in all cells in females. In brief, it is a process in which one of the two X chromosomes is randomly inactivated early in development. Skewing of X-inactivation (as well as other mechanisms) can result in the expression of disease in females for recessive conditions. For this reason, the terms *recessive* and *dominant* when referencing X-linked inheritance are less utilized.

Chromosomal Disorders

Abnormalities of chromosomes may be either numerical or structural and may involve one or more autosomes, sex chromosomes, or both together. The most common type of clinically significant chromosomal abnormality involves the number of chromosomes, called *aneuploidy*. In the case of aneuploidy, there are either extra or missing chromosomes. Aneuploidy results

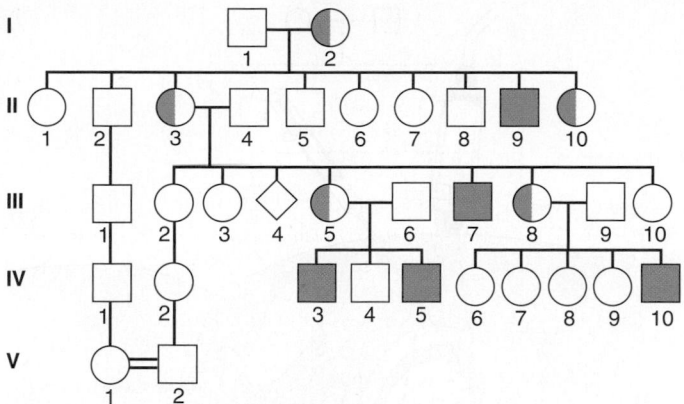

FIGURE 15-10 X-linked inheritance of hemophilia A among descendants of Queen Victoria (I-2) of England. *Roman numerals,* generation number; *Arabic numerals,* individuals within generations. Source: Adkison, L. (2012). *Elsevier's integrated review: Genetics* (2nd ed., p. 33). Philadelphia: Elsevier/ Saunders.

FIGURE 15-11 Punnett square representation of the mating of a heterozygous female who carries an X-linked recessive disease gene with a normal male. X^1, chromosome with normal allele; X^2, chromosome with disease allele. Source: Jorde, L., Cary, J., & Bamshad, M. (2010). *Medical genetics* (4th ed., p. 85). St. Louis: Mosby.

from an error during meiotic cell division, creating a sperm or an egg with too many or too few chromosomes, which is passed on to the offspring during conception. Most aneuploid offspring have either trisomy (three chromosomes) or monosomy (only one chromosome) instead of the normal pair of chromosomes. The most common trisomy that survives birth is trisomy 21 (Down syndrome). In these offspring, there are three copies of chromosome 21. Other examples of aneuploidy are trisomy 13 and trisomy 18. Monosomy for an entire chromosome is almost always lethal, with the exception of monosomy for the X chromosome, as seen in Turner's syndrome.

Abnormalities of chromosome structure result from chromosome breakage and subsequent reconstitution in an abnormal combination. These new configurations can be either balanced or unbalanced. In balanced rearrangements, the chromosome is complete, with no loss or gain of genetic material. These rearrangements are generally harmless except in rare cases in which one of the break points damages an important functional gene. When a chromosome rearrangement is unbalanced, the chromosomal complement contains an incorrect amount of chromosome material, and the clinical effects are usually serious. Chromosomal instability happens during conception and can

occur in all cells; it can also occur somatically and possibly lead to cancers (typically caused by single-gene defects) (Charames & Bapat, 2003).

Multifactorial Inheritance

Disorders that are caused by multifactorial inheritance occur as a result of an interaction between one or more genes (polygenic) or between one or more genes and environmental influences. Multifactorial inheritance is thought to be the basis for most common diseases, including cancer, heart disease, and multiple sclerosis. A primary characteristic of this type of inheritance is familial aggregation of diseases. Multifactorial conditions tend to run in families, but the pattern of inheritance is not as predictable as with single-gene disorders. The chance of recurrence of disease traits within families, although greater than the population risk, is less than that for families with single-gene disorders. The degree of risk for a multifactorial disorder occurring in relatives is related to the number of genes they share in common with the affected individual. The closer the degree of relationship, the more genes they have in common. The degree of risk also increases with the severity of the disorder. Although multifactorial conditions run in families, the risk is generally less than the 25% or 50% seen in Mendelian conditions. Identical twins, exactly alike genetically, may not always have the same condition when inheritance is multifactorial. This indicates that there are nongenetic factors that also play a role in the expression of multifactorial traits. For instance, the risk for coronary heart disease increases with smoking or obesity, and the risk for emphysema in individuals with α_1-antitrypsin deficiency increases greatly with smoking.

Characteristics of multifactorial inheritance include the following:

1. There is a similar risk for first-degree relatives (offspring, siblings, or parents).
2. Identical twins are not 100% concordant, indicating that there are nongenetic factors involved.
3. The greater the number of affected relatives, the higher the recurrence risk.
4. The severity of the disorder and occasionally the sex of the affected individual may modify the risk.

Throughout the book, genetic disorders are highlighted in "Genetics in Clinical Practice" boxes.

GENETICS IN CLINICAL PRACTICE

Boxes Throughout This Text

Genetic Disorder	Chapter
α_1-Antitrypsin	31
Alzheimer's disease	62
Ankylosing spondylitis	67
Autoimmune diseases	64
Breast cancer	54
Diabetes mellitus types 1 and 2	52
Familial adenomatous polyposis (FAP)	45
Familial hypercholesterolemia	36
Hemochromatosis	33
Hemophilia A and B	33
Hereditary nonpolyposis colorectal cancer (HNPCC)	45
Huntington's disease	61
Ovarian cancer	56
Polycystic kidney disease	48
Sickle-cell disease	33
Skin malignancies	25

GENETICS IN CLINICAL PRACTICE

Taking a Family History

A detailed three-generation family history, or *pedigree,* offers great insight into possible genetic conditions within a family. A pedigree is a symbolic representation of family members indicating specific details about each individual. General family history screening should be obtained for each family member, with details for at least three generations. Information (including age, disease status, and vital status) should be collected on the patient, his or her children, and the patient's siblings, parents, aunts, uncles, and grandparents. Standard nomenclature should be used when constructing a pedigree (see Figure 15-5). This initial pedigree can highlight certain areas, such as those pertinent to a specific condition (e.g., cancer), for further questioning. A pedigree targeting the possibility of a hereditary cancer syndrome will gather even more details about the incidence of cancer, the types of cancer, ages at diagnosis, and outcomes. Information about paternal and maternal ethnicity should also be gathered because some genetic mutations are found more commonly in certain ethnic groups.

Genetic Testing

Genetic testing is the analysis of DNA, chromosomes, proteins, or metabolites, or some combination. Testing can be done on blood or other bodily samples and involves looking for a genetic mutation that indicates the presence or absence of a genetic condition or predisposition to (i.e., increased risk for) a genetic condition. Genetic testing can be used in a multitude of ways. A genetic screening test may be useful in determining the potential risk for development of a disease in one's lifetime. Such tests may be done in a variety of settings and at any point during the lifespan, including prenatally, at birth, or throughout childhood and adulthood. Some tests screen for the possibility of a disease and are predictive of expression of disease. Other tests are done to determine whether an individual is a carrier of a mutated gene, which may be passed on to an offspring.

Prenatal Diagnosis and Screening. The main objective of prenatal diagnosis is to give parents information so they can make informed decisions during pregnancy. The potential benefits of prenatal testing include the following: (a) decreasing the anxiety of at-risk parents (when test results return as normal); (b) providing risk information to parents before conception so an informed choice can be made regarding future pregnancies; (c) allowing parents to prepare psychologically for the birth of an affected child; and (d) providing risk information to parents when pregnancy termination is an option. Prenatal diagnostic tests can be either invasive (e.g., amniocentesis, chorionic villus sampling) or noninvasive (e.g., maternal serum screening, ultrasonography). The newest noninvasive screen for chromosomal anomalies (such as trisomies 13, 18, and 21) is a blood test, done as early as 10 weeks gestation, that examines the circulating cell-free fetal DNA in the maternal blood and measures the relative abundance of markers on these chromosomes. This screen is called noninvasive prenatal testing (NIPT) and has a detection rate of >98% and a false-positive rate of <2%.

Amniocentesis. Amniocentesis is traditionally performed 15 to 17 weeks after a pregnant woman's last menstrual period. It can be used to diagnose neural tube defects, chromosome abnormalities, metabolic disorders, and molecular defects. A needle is inserted through the abdominal wall into the amniotic sac while the fetus is being monitored using ultrasound (Figure

FIGURE 15-12 A schematic illustration of an amniocentesis, in which 20 to 30 mL of amniotic fluid is withdrawn transabdominally (with ultrasound guidance), usually at 15 to 17 weeks' gestation. Source: Jorde, L., Cary, J., & Bamshad, M. (2010). *Medical genetics* (4th ed., p. 268). St. Louis: Mosby.

15-12). Between 20 and 30 mL of amniotic fluid, which contains living cells (amniocytes) shed by the fetus, is removed. Cytogenetic studies are done after culture of the amniocytes. Common indications for amniocentesis are (a) maternal age older than 35 years; (b) previous child with chromosome abnormality; (c) history of structural chromosome abnormality in one parent; (d) family history of genetic defect that is diagnosable by biochemical or DNA analysis; and (e) risk for neural tube defect. A risk of 0.1 to 1% for miscarriage is associated with this procedure (Akolekar, Beta, Picciarelli, et al., 2015).

Chorionic Villus Sampling. Chorionic villus sampling (CVS) may be done in the first trimester, usually between 11 and 12 weeks' gestation. It is performed by aspirating fetal trophoblastic tissue (chorionic villi) by either the transcervical or the transabdominal approach for prenatal evaluation of the chromosomal, enzymatic, and DNA status of the fetus (Figure 15-13).

CVS has the advantage of providing a diagnosis much earlier in a pregnancy than amniocentesis for couples who may consider termination as an option. CVS is associated with a slightly higher risk for miscarriage (0.2 to 1.5%) (Akolekar, Beta, Picciarelli, et al., 2015).

Screening for Carriers of Genetic Disease. This type of genetic screening is done on healthy individuals (i.e., those unaffected with a genetic condition) to determine whether they carry a mutation that could be passed to offspring and cause genetic diseases. Typically, this test is done for autosomal recessive and X-linked disorders. Individuals may opt for this type of genetic screening if there is a family history of a genetic disease or if they are in an ethnic group that has a greater risk of carrying a certain genetic mutation. Examples of disorders for which testing is available are Tay–Sachs disease, CF, and fragile X syndrome.

Presymptomatic and Predisposition Testing. Predictive testing includes both presymptomatic and predisposition testing. In presymptomatic testing, an individual has genetic testing to determine whether she or he carries a genetic mutation for a genetic disorder. Typically, individuals electing this testing are members of a family that exhibits a genetic disorder. An example of this would be genetic testing for Huntington's disease, an adult-onset condition characterized by progressive neurological degeneration. The gene responsible for Huntington's disease is 100% penetrant; that is, everyone who inherits this mutation will exhibit the disease and, since there is no cure, will die of the disease. For members of families in which Huntington's disease is present, the decision to undergo predictive testing may be difficult. In Canada, the uptake rate for predictive testing is approximately 18% of the estimated Canadian population at risk for the disease (Creighton, Almqvist, MacGregor, et al., 2003).

Genetic testing is also available to determine an individual's predisposition for developing a genetic condition and is now used in prenatal, pediatric, and adult populations. Many genes that, when mutated, cause an individual to be predisposed to a disease have been identified. However, not all individuals who have the genetic mutation will get the disease. An example of genetic testing that is available is for *BRCA1* and *BRCA2*. Mutations in these genes are responsible for an increased risk for breast cancer (≤80% lifetime risk) and ovarian cancer (≤40% lifetime risk) (Petrucelli, Daly, & Feldman, 2013). Typically, families that carry mutations in these genes have numerous members who have been diagnosed with breast or ovarian cancers (Figure 15-14). Other characteristics that suggest a possible *BRCA1* or *BRCA2* mutation in a family are onset of breast cancer at a young age (<50 years), male breast cancer, and bilateral breast cancer (cancer in both breasts). The advantage of testing for mutations in *BRCA1* and *BRCA2* is that women at high risk for developing breast and ovarian cancers can be identified before the development of cancer. These women can then begin vigilant breast and ovarian cancer screening at an earlier age, or they can elect for preventive options. Included in preventive options are prophylactic surgery (both bilateral mastectomy and bilateral oophorectomy) or chemopreventive drugs (e.g., tamoxifen). Each option offers varying cancer risk reduction, and there are both medical and psychological adverse effects that may result. A Canadian publication reported increasing uptake of preventive options by women with a *BRCA1* or *BRCA2* mutation: 21% of women had a prophylactic mastectomy, 54% of women had a bilateral oophorectomy (preventive removal of the ovaries), and 6% took tamoxifen (Metcalfe, Ghadirian, Rosen, et al., 2007).

Genetic Counselling

Genetic counselling is the process of helping people understand and adapt to the medical, psychological, and familial implications of genetic contributions to disease (National Society of Genetic Counselors [NSGC], n.d.). This process integrates the following:

- Interpretation of family and medical histories to assess the chance of disease occurrence or recurrence
- Education about inheritance, testing, management, prevention, resources, and research
- Counselling to promote informed choices and adaptation to the risk or condition

Andermann and Narod (2002) reported on current practices of genetic counsellors in Ontario who serve a population of over 11 million people. The cost of most genetic counselling was covered by the provincial health plan. There were no private genetic services—either testing or counselling—and there were no patient copayments. The report found that 45% of genetic consultations were for preconception or prenatal diagnosis, 22% were for breast and ovarian cancer, 5% were for other adult cancers, and 14% were for the evaluation of pediatric conditions.

FIGURE 15-13 A schematic illustration of a transcervical chorionic villus sampling procedure. With ultrasound guidance, a catheter is inserted, and several milligrams of villus tissue is aspirated. Source: Jorde, L., Cary, J., & Bamshad, M. (2010). *Medical genetics* (4th ed., p. 269). St. Louis: Mosby.

FIGURE 15-14 Pedigree for family with the *BRCA1* mutation. *Numbers without symbols* represent the current ages of family members. *Numbers with symbols* represent the age at which the diagnosis was made. *BR*, breast cancer; *d.*, age of death; *OV*, ovarian cancer; *PROS*, prostate cancer.

Although genetics can be integrated into most nurses' practices, some nurses specialize in genetics. "Genetic nurses have specialized education and training in genetics in addition to generic training in healthcare practice with the goal of caring for people's genetic and genomic health" (International Society of Nurses in Genetics, 2010, p. 1). Genetic nurses help people at risk for or affected by diseases with a genetic component to achieve and maintain health. They perform risk assessments, analyze the genetic contribution to disease risk, and discuss the impact of risk on health care management for individuals and families. They also provide genetic education, provide nursing care to patients and families, and conduct research in genetics. The International Society of Nurses in Genetics (ISONG) is an organization of nurses around the world who work in genetics (see the Resources at the end of this chapter.).

Genetic counsellors are health care providers with specialized graduate degrees and experience in the areas of medical genetics and counselling. They provide information and support to families who have members with birth defects or genetic disorders and to families who may be at risk for a variety of inherited conditions. They identify families at risk, investigate the problem that the family has, interpret information about the disorder, analyze inheritance patterns and risks for recurrence, and review available options with the family. Genetic counsellors also provide supportive counselling to families, serve as patient advocates, and refer individuals and families to community or provincial or territorial support services (NSGC, n.d.).

Gene Therapy

Gene therapy is an experimental technique that is used to replace or functionally repair defective or missing genes with normal genes. A normal gene can be inserted into a human chromosome to counteract the effects of a missing or abnormal gene. Although gene therapy is a promising treatment option for a number of diseases (including inherited disorders, some types of cancer, and certain viral infections), the technique remains risky and is still under study to make sure that it will be safe and effective. Gene therapy is currently being tested only for the treatment of diseases that have no cures (National Library of Medicine, 2017).

The first approved gene therapy trials involved children with severe combined immunodeficiency disease caused by adenosine deaminase deficiency. T lymphocytes from these children were obtained, and the missing gene was inserted into these T cells (Figure 15-15). The new T cells were then reinjected into the children's bloodstreams. The gene signalled the cells to produce the missing enzyme, and these children were capable of developing a functioning immune system.

Gene therapy shows promise for treating a wide array of problems that do not respond to conventional methods of intervention. Although gene therapy is not currently used in clinical practice, the treatment strategies closest to being incorporated into mainstream therapies are those that address immunodeficiency disease, hemophilia, and ischemic vascular disease. Before gene therapy can become a practical approach to treating disease, scientists must find improved methods of delivering the genes to directly target the affected cells and must ensure that the new genes can be controlled by the body (National Library of Medicine, 2017).

Methods of Gene Delivery. One of the major hurdles in gene therapy is finding a way to insert the gene into the body. Genes that are inserted directly into a cell usually do not function. Instead, a carrier, called a *vector*, is used to deliver the gene. The

FIGURE 15-15 Gene therapy for adenosine deaminase (ADA) deficiency attempts to correct this immunodeficiency state. The viral vector containing the therapeutic *ADA* gene is inserted into the patient's lymphocytes. These cells can then make the ADA enzyme.

most common vectors are attenuated or modified versions of viruses. The viruses are modified so they cannot cause disease when used in humans (National Library of Medicine, 2017).

Some types of viruses, such as retroviruses, integrate their genetic material (including the new gene) into a chromosome in the human cell. Other viruses, such as adenoviruses, introduce their DNA into the nucleus of the cell, but the DNA is not integrated into a chromosome.

The vector can be injected or given by the intravenous (IV) route directly into a specific tissue in the body, where it is taken up by the individual cells. Alternatively, a sample of the patient's cells can be removed and exposed to the vector in a laboratory setting. The cells containing the vector are returned to the patient. If the treatment is successful, the new gene delivered by the vector will make a functioning protein.

Examples of Gene Therapy for Cancer. One of the first gene therapy protocols used in treating cancer patients involved the addition of a gene for tumour necrosis factor (TNF). The vector with the gene for TNF was inserted into lymphocytes aimed at sites of malignant melanoma. This approach allows a high dose of TNF to be delivered to the tumour only and avoids systemic adverse effects.

The purpose of the multidrug resistance (MDR) clinical gene therapy trials is to modify the effects of high-dose chemotherapy in bone marrow cells by inserting the *MDR* gene. Bone marrow stem cells are separated and cultured with a virus carrying the genetic material for the *MDR* gene. The virus transfers the *MDR* gene into the patient's stem cells. These stem cells and their offspring become resistant to the toxic effects of chemotherapy by acquiring the ability to pump the chemotherapeutic drugs out of the cells before the drugs are able to kill the cells.

Gene Editing: Using the CRISPR-Cas9 System in Gene Therapy. One of the major challenges with gene therapy has been the efficient delivery of a corrected copy of a DNA segment to a specific site within the genome and into enough patient cells to correct the inherited gene defect (reviewed in Collins & Thrasher, 2015). Originally identified in bacterial systems, CRISPR (**c**lustered **r**egularly **i**nterspaced **s**hort **p**alindromic **r**epeats) RNA and a CRISPR-associated (Cas) protein together can use specific RNA sequences (as a guide) to direct the complex to the site of interest, cut DNA, and then attempt to repair it by introducing new DNA. This method has been used in the laboratory to inactivate integrated human immunodeficiency virus (HIV) genomes and to correct genetic defects in disorders such as CF. While the off-target effects are still being evaluated, CRISPR-Cas9 is currently the most promising advance in gene therapy.

NURSING MANAGEMENT
GENETICS

Nurses must be knowledgeable about the fundamentals of genetics. By understanding the influence that genetics has on health and disease, the nurse can assist the patient and family in making critical decisions related to genetic issues, such as genetic testing. The nurse also should collaborate with the health care team or physician to involve a genetic counsellor. The nurse should be able to give patients and their families accurate information pertaining to genetics, genetic diseases, and probabilities of genetic disorders. Inheritance patterns can be assessed by the nurse and explained to the patient and family through the use of Punnett squares (see Figures 15-7, 15-9, and 15-11) or family pedigrees (see Figures 15-6, 15-8, and 15-10). Maintaining patient confidentiality and respecting the patient's values and beliefs are critical because the information from the counsellor may have major implications for many people who are involved. Examples of applications of genetics in nursing practice include the following (Consensus Panel, 2009):

- Recognizing a newborn infant who is at risk for morbidity and mortality because of genetic metabolism errors
- Identifying an asymptomatic adolescent who is at high risk for hereditary colorectal cancer based on his or her family history
- Identifying a couple who is at risk for having a child with a genetic condition
- Assisting with the selection of a drug or dose of a drug, based on genetic markers, in the treatment of an adult with cancer
- Helping an individual or family with questions related to genetic information or services to find reliable information

Genetic testing may raise many psychological issues. Knowledge of a carrier status of a genetic disorder may influence a person's career plans and decisions about marriage and childbearing. It may also affect significant others when grappling with serious life and health care issues.

Furthermore, there are ethical concerns. At a societal level, who should know the result of a genetic test? How should society or the government protect the privacy of individuals' test results and protect individuals from discrimination? Genetic information should not be misused to stigmatize individuals or particular ethnic groups. Attention must be paid to better understand psychosocial needs of individuals, societal responses, and health care policy related to genetic testing. On a personal level, genetic test results offer individuals insight into conditions that may already exist or that may develop in the future. This type of information may cause internal ethical dilemmas. Prenatal genetic testing, for example, may raise ethics issues for parents. Parents who learn prenatally that their baby has a genetic condition must consider the future of the pregnancy. A fetus identified as having trisomy 21 (Down syndrome) will be born with physical and developmental abnormalities; however, predicting the severity of these abnormalities is difficult. This complicates the situation for parents who have to decide whether or not to terminate the pregnancy. In addition, for some individuals, cultural and religious beliefs often factor into this decision making.

Genetic testing for adult-onset conditions also may raise ethical dilemmas. With testing for adult-onset conditions (e.g., breast cancer), issues related to "duty to warn" may surface. For example, if a woman is told that she has a *BRCA1* mutation, there are significant implications for her blood relatives. Once a *BRCA1* mutation is identified in a family, all blood relatives are eligible to receive genetic testing for the specific mutation. However, if the individual does not share her genetic test results with her family, the family members may be unaware of their chance of having the *BRCA1* mutation and of their significantly increased risk of developing breast and ovarian cancers. The lack of this knowledge may result in a family member's being denied the opportunity to choose a cancer prevention option and developing cancer as a result.

Many of the ethical concerns described in this chapter can also become a legal issue depending on the jurisdiction of the parties involved. As we increase our knowledge of genetic diseases and can better predict what variants mean for the patient (i.e., survival, prognostics, etc.), discrimination based on the genetic findings in healthy individuals has become a major disadvantage. In 2008, the United States government passed a federal law called the *Genetic Information Nondiscrimination Act* (GINA), which protects individuals from genetic discrimination in health insurance and employment but not in life or disability insurance. Individual states have built on the federal law, such as California's CalGINA law (enacted in 2012), which extends the protection to other areas, such as housing, mortgage lending, education, and public accommodations. Until recently, Canada was the only G8 member without some sort of legislative protection; however, in 2017, the federal government voted in a bill to prevent genetic discrimination (Kirkup, 2017).

Ethical issues must be considered carefully when working with families undergoing genetic testing. These issues are often dealt with in genetic counselling offered by genetic counsellors or genetic nurses. The Committee on Assessing Genetic Risks, Division of Health Sciences Policy, Institute of Medicine, emphasizes autonomy, confidentiality, privacy, and equity as essential to analysis of questions related to genetic testing ("Social, Legal," 1994). Nurses must be aware of these ethical principles when providing care to individuals and families.

ETHICAL DILEMMAS

Genetic Testing

Situation

A 30-year-old woman informs the nurse that she is 3 months pregnant. She has two children with her current husband. This pregnancy was unplanned, and her youngest child has cystic fibrosis (CF). She expresses concern regarding the possibility of having another child with CF. She mentions that she would like to have genetic testing on her fetus. Her husband asks the nurse if they will have another child with CF.

Important Points for Consideration

- With complete and accurate information, the woman and her husband can make a decision on their own without coercion from others.
- With genetic testing, the patient and her family can find out whether or not their child will have CF.
- Genetic counselling is recommended before and after obtaining genetic testing because of the complexity of the information and the emotional issues involved.
- The nurse, knowing that CF is an autosomal recessive condition, can use Punnett squares (see Figures 15-7, 15-9, and 15-11) to show

the woman and her husband the probability of having another child with CF.

- Genetic testing in the fetus is most informative if the two pathogenic variants are first identified in the affected child. Without the known familial causative variants, prenatal testing cannot rule out the possibility that testing did not find the underlying cause (but may be outside of the tested regions of the gene). Therefore, a negative test result may not mean the fetus will not be born with CF.

Clinical Decision-Making Questions

1. What information should the nurse give the patient regarding genetic testing in order for her and her husband to make a decision?
2. What options are available for this couple?
3. How should the nurse assist this couple in making a decision about possibly terminating the pregnancy if the results of the genetic testing show that the fetus tested positive for the CF gene?

■ REVIEW QUESTIONS

The number of the question corresponds to the same-numbered objective at the beginning of the chapter.

1. What will the Human Genome Project accomplish? *(Select all that apply)*
   a. Help determine risk for genetic-related disease
   b. Allow for earlier detection of genetic predisposition to disease
   c. Improve the diagnosis of disease
   d. Recommend definitive treatments based on a person's genetic makeup

2. What does it mean if a person is heterozygous for a given gene?
   a. The person is a carrier for a genetic disorder.
   b. The person is affected by the genetic disorder.
   c. The person has two identical alleles for the gene.
   d. The person has two different alleles for the gene.

3. A 53-year-old male client presents with a constellation of symptoms that leads the nurse to believe that his disease is of a genetic etiology. His disease manifested when he was a teenager. The client's 29-year-old son is affected with the same disease. The client's 27-year-old daughter is healthy with an unremarkable clinical history. However, her two sons are similarly affected as their uncle. Which of the following is a mode of inheritance that most likely applies to this family?
   a. Autosomal dominant
   b. Autosomal recessive
   c. Genetic diversity
   d. Genetic drift

4. What is a family pedigree?
   a. The family ancestry traced through the father
   b. The family line of descent through the mother
   c. The depiction of an autosomal recessive gene disorder
   d. A family tree drawn in the form of a diagram

5. Which of the following would be a reason for a client or potential parents to undergo genetic testing?

   a. To determine the sex of an unborn child through amniocentesis
   b. To predict the potential for developing diabetes
   c. To help couples at risk for genetic disorders to make an informed choice before conception
   d. To screen for the possibility of undiagnosed breast cancer

6. Which of the following is the best response for the nurse who is asked by a pregnant woman about the risk associated with invasive prenatal testing?
   a. Amniocentesis is associated with a 1 to 5% risk for miscarriage.
   b. Chorionic villus sampling (CVS) is associated with a much lower risk for miscarriage than amniocentesis because it is less invasive.
   c. Both amniocentesis and CVS are associated with a low risk for miscarriage (<1.5%).
   d. CVS is the preferred method of prenatal testing because it can be done as late as 18 weeks gestation.

7. Why might prenatal genetic testing cause ethical, social, or legal dilemmas for parents? *(Select all that apply)*
   a. The sex of the child would be known.
   b. Decisions about the future of the pregnancy (including termination) would be left to the parents.
   c. Health care providers would know about the genetic conditions of the unborn child.
   d. Family members might question the couple's decision to undergo genetic testing.
   e. Genetic testing results on the fetus could identify nonpaternity situations and have subsequent legal ramifications.

1. a, b, c; 2. d; 3. a; 4. d; 5. c; 6. c; 7. b, e.

ℰvolve

For even more review questions, visit *http://evolve.elsevier.com/Canada/Lewis/medsurg*.

REFERENCES

Akolekar, R., Beta, J., Picciarelli, G., et al. (2015). Procedure-related risk of miscarriage following amniocentesis and chorionic villus sampling: A systematic review and meta-analysis. *Ultrasound in Obstetrics and Gynecology, 45*, 16–26. doi:10.1002/uog.14636.

Andermann, A., & Narod, S. A. (2002). Genetic counselling for familial breast and ovarian cancer in Ontario. *Journal of Medical Genetics, 39*, 695–696. doi:10.1136/jmg.39.9.695. (Seminal).

Calzone, K. A., Jenkins, J., Nicol, N., et al. (2013). Relevance of genomics to healthcare and nursing practice. *Journal of Nursing Scholarship, 45*(1), 1–2. doi:10.1111/j.1547-5069.2012.01464.x.

Charames, G. S., & Bapat, B. (2003). Genomic instability and cancer. *Current Molecular Medicine, 3*, 589–596. doi:10.2174/1566524033479456. (Seminal).

Collins, M., & Thrasher, A. (2015). Gene therapy: Progress and predictions. *Proceedings. Biological Sciences, 282*(1821), 20143003. doi:10.1098/rspb.2014.3003.

Consensus Panel on Genetic/Genomic Nursing Competencies (2009). *Essentials of genetic and genomic nursing: Competencies, curricula guidelines, and outcome indicators* (2nd ed.). Silver Spring, MD: American Nurses Association. Retrieved from *http://www.genome.gov/Pages/Careers/HealthProfessionalEducation/geneticscompetency.pdf*. (Seminal).

Creighton, S., Almqvist, E. W., MacGregor, D., et al. (2003). Predictive, pre-natal and diagnostic genetic testing for Huntington's disease: The experience in Canada from 1987 to 2000. *Clinical Genetics, 63*, 462–475. doi:10.1034/j.1399-0004.2003.00093.x. (Seminal).

Daack-Hirsch, S., Jackson, B., Belchez, C. A., et al. (2013). Integrating genetics and genomics into nursing curricula: You can do it too! *The Nursing Clinics of North America, 48*(4), 661–669. doi:10.1016/j.cnur.2013.08.005.

International Society of Nurses in Genetics (ISONG). (2010). *Provision of quality genetic services and care: Building a multidisciplinary, collaborative approach among genetic nurses and genetic counselors.* Retrieved from *http://www.isong.org/pdfs2013/PS_Quality_Genetic_Services_Care.pdf*. (Seminal).

Kirkup, K. (2017, March 8). *Liberal backbenchers defy Justin Trudeau on genetic-testing disclosure bill. Canadian Press.* Retrieved from *https://www.thestar.com/news/canada/2017/03/08/genetic-testing-bill-up-for-vote-is-constitutional-trudeau-says.html*.

Metcalfe, K., Ghadirian, P., Rosen, B., et al. (2007). Variation in rates of uptake of preventive options in BRCA1 and BRCA2 mutation carriers across Canada. *Open Medicine, 1*, E92–E98. Retrieved from *https://www.ncbi.nlm.nih.gov/pmc/articles/PMC2802012/*. (Seminal).

Munro, C. L. (2015). Individual genetic and genomic variation: A new opportunity for personalized nursing interventions. *Journal of Advanced Nursing, 71*(1), 35–41. doi:10.1111/jan.12552.

National Library of Medicine (2017). Gene therapy. In *Help me understand genetics.* Retrieved from *https://ghr.nlm.nih.gov/primer/therapy/genetherapy*.

National Society of Genetic Counselors (NSGC). (n.d.). *About genetic counselors: Frequently asked questions.* Retrieved from *http://www.nsgc.org/page/faqs*.

Online Mendelian Inheritance in Man (OMIM). (2017). *OMIM entry statistics.* Retrieved from *https://www.omim.org/statistics/entry*.

Petrucelli, N., Daly, M. B., & Feldman, G. L. (2013). *BRCA1 and BRCA2 hereditary breast and ovarian cancer.* Retrieved from *http://www.ncbi.nlm.nih.gov/books/NBK1247/*.

Social, legal, and ethical implications of genetic testing. (1994). In L. Andrews, J. Fullarton, & N. Holtzman, et al. (Eds.), *Assessing genetic risks: Implications for health and social policy* (pp. 247–289). Washington, DC: National Academy Press. (Seminal).

World Health Organization. (2016). *Genes and human disease.* Retrieved from *http://www.who.int/genomics/public/geneticdiseases/en/index3.html*.

RESOURCES

Canadian Directory of Genetic Support Groups
http://www.lhsc.on.ca/programs/medgenet

Genetic Resources Ontario
http://www.geneticresourcesontario.ca

Genome Canada
http://www.genomecanada.ca

Public Health Agency of Canada
http://www.phac-aspc.gc.ca/index-eng.php

American College of Medical Genetics and Genomics
http://www.acmg.net

Centers for Disease Control and Prevention, Public Health Genomics
http://www.cdc.gov/genomics

Genetic Testing Registry (GTR)
http://www.ncbi.nlm.nih.gov/gtr/

Genetic Alliance
http://www.geneticalliance.org

The Genetic Information Nondiscrimination Act of 2008 (GINA)
http://www.eeoc.gov/laws/statutes/gina.cfm

Genetics Program for Nursing Faculty
https://www.cincinnatichildrens.org/education/clinical/nursing/genetics

Human Genome Project
https://www.genome.gov/10001772/all-about-the--human-genome-project-hgp/

International Society of Nurses in Genetics (ISONG)
http://www.isong.org

National Human Genome Research Institute
http://www.nhgri.nih.gov

Online Mendelian Inheritance in Man (OMIM)
https://www.omim.org

Understanding Gene Testing
http://www.accessexcellence.org/AE/AEPC/NIH

For additional Internet resources, see the website for this book at *http://evolve.elsevier.com/Canada/Lewis/medsurg*.

16

Altered Immune Response and Transplantation

Written by: Sharon L. Lewis
Adapted by: Susan Chernenko

evolve WEBSITE

http://evolve.elsevier.com/Canada/Lewis/medsurg

- Review Questions (Online Only)
- Key Points
- Answer Guidelines for Case Study
- Conceptual Care Map Creator
- Audio Glossary

- Supporting Media
  - Function of B Cells
  - Function of T Cytotoxic Cells
- Content Updates

LEARNING OBJECTIVES

1. Describe the functions and components of the immune system.
2. Compare and contrast humoral and cell-mediated immunity regarding lymphocytes involved, types of reactions, and effects on antigens.
3. Characterize the five classes of immunoglobulins.
4. Differentiate among the four types of hypersensitivity reactions in terms of immunological mechanisms and resulting alterations.
5. Identify the clinical manifestations and emergency management of a systemic anaphylactic reaction.
6. Describe the assessment and collaborative care of a patient with chronic allergies.
7. Explain the relationship between the human leukocyte antigen system and certain diseases.
8. Describe the etiological factors, the clinical manifestations, and the treatment modalities of autoimmune diseases.
9. Describe the etiological factors and categories of immunodeficiency disorders.
10. Describe the various kinds of organ transplantation and the types of rejection that may be experienced after transplantation.
11. Identify the types of immuno-suppressive therapy and their adverse effects.
12. Describe alternative strategies that have been explored to address organ donor shortages.

KEY TERMS

anergy, p. 266
antigen, p. 260
apheresis, p. 275
autoimmunity,
 p. 274

cell-mediated immunity,
 p. 266
cytokines, p. 263
human leukocyte antigen
 (HLA) system, p. 277

humoral immunity, p. 265
hypersensitivity reaction,
 p. 266
immunity, p. 260
immuno-competence, p. 266

immunodeficiency, p. 276
immuno-suppressive therapy,
 p. 279
monoclonal antibodies, p. 283
organ transplantation, p. 277

This chapter discusses the normal immune response and the altered immune responses of hypersensitivity (including allergies), autoimmunity, and immunodeficiency. Histocompatibility, organ transplantation, and immuno-suppressive therapy are also presented.

NORMAL IMMUNE RESPONSE

Immunity is the body's ability to resist disease. Immune responses serve the following three functions (Mak, Saunders, & Jett, 2014):
1. *Defence:* The body protects against invasions by microorganisms and prevents the development of infection by attacking foreign antigens and pathogens.

2. *Homeostasis:* Damaged cellular substances are digested and removed. Through this mechanism, the body's different cell types remain uniform and unchanged.
3. *Surveillance:* Mutations continually arise in the body but are normally recognized as foreign cells and destroyed.

Antigens

An antigen is a substance that elicits an immune response. Most antigens are composed of proteins. However, other substances such as large polysaccharides, lipoproteins, and nucleic acids can act as antigens. All of the body's cells have antigens on their surface that are unique to that person and enable the body to recognize itself. The immune system normally

TABLE 16-1	TYPES OF ACQUIRED SPECIFIC IMMUNITY

Active
Natural
Natural contact with antigen through clinical infection (e.g., disease and recovery from chicken pox, measles, and mumps)

Artificial
Immunization with antigen (e.g., immunization with live or killed vaccines)

Passive
Natural
Transplacental and colostrum-mediated transfer from mother to infant (e.g., maternal immunoglobulins in neonate)

Artificial
Injection of serum from immune human (e.g., injection of human γ-globulin)

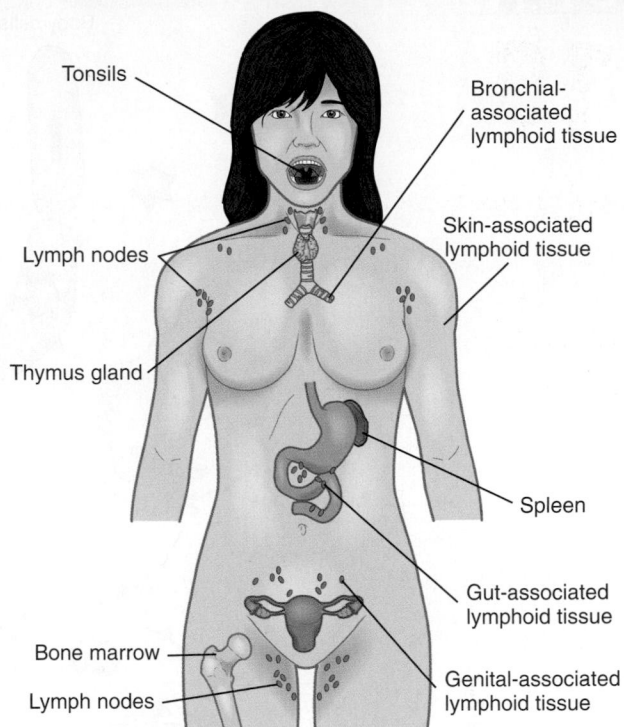

FIGURE 16-1 Organs of the immune system.

becomes "tolerant" to the body's own molecules and therefore is nonresponsive to "self" antigens.

Types of Immunity

Immunity is classified as innate or acquired.

Innate Immunity. *Innate immunity* is present at birth, and its primary role is first-line defence against pathogens. This type of immunity produces a nonspecific response, with neutrophils and monocytes being the white blood cells (WBCs) primarily involved. Innate immunity is not antigen specific, so it can respond within minutes to an invading microorganism without prior exposure to that organism (Mak, Saunders, & Jett, 2014).

Acquired Immunity. *Acquired immunity* is the development of immunity, either actively or passively (Table 16-1).

Active Acquired Immunity. *Active acquired immunity* results from the invasion of the body by foreign substances such as microorganisms, which leads to the development of antibodies and sensitized lymphocytes. With each reinvasion of the microorganisms, the body responds more rapidly and vigorously to fight off the invader. Active acquired immunity may result naturally from a disease or artificially through inoculation of a less virulent antigen (e.g., immunization). Because antibodies are synthesized, immunity takes time to develop but is long-lasting.

Passive Acquired Immunity. *Passive acquired immunity* implies that the host receives antibodies to an antigen rather than synthesizing them. This may take place naturally through the transfer of immunoglobulins across the placental membrane from mother to fetus or artificially through injection with γ-globulin (serum antibodies). The benefit of this immunity is its immediate effect. Unfortunately, passive immunity is short-lived because the person does not synthesize the antibodies and consequently does not retain memory cells for the antigen.

Lymphoid Organs

The lymphoid system is composed of central (or primary) and peripheral lymphoid organs. The central lymphoid organs are the thymus gland and bone marrow. The peripheral lymphoid organs are the lymph nodes; tonsils; spleen; and gut-, genital-, bronchial-, and skin-associated lymphoid tissues (Figure 16-1).

Lymphocytes are produced in the bone marrow and eventually migrate to the peripheral organs. The thymus is involved in the differentiation and maturation of T lymphocytes and is therefore essential for a cell-mediated immune response. During childhood, the thymus gland is large; however, it shrinks with age, thus becoming a collection of reticular fibres, lymphocytes, and connective tissue in older adults.

When antigens are introduced into the body, they may be carried by the bloodstream or lymph channels to regional lymph nodes. The antigens interact with B and T lymphocytes and macrophages in the lymph nodes. The two important functions of lymph nodes are (a) filtration of foreign material brought to the site and (b) circulation of lymphocytes.

Lymphoid tissue is found in the submucosa of the respiratory (bronchus-associated), gastro-intestinal (gut-associated), and genito-urinary (genital-associated) tracts. This tissue protects the body surface from external microorganisms. The tonsils are a typical example of lymphoid tissue.

The spleen, a peripheral lymph organ, is important as the primary site for filtering foreign antigens from the blood.

The skin-associated lymph tissue primarily consists of lymphocytes and Langerhans cells (a type of dendritic cell) found in the epidermis of skin. When Langerhans cells are depleted, the skin cannot initiate an immune response. Therefore, a delayed hypersensitivity reaction (as determined by skin testing with injected antigens) does not occur.

Cells Involved in Immune Response

Mononuclear Phagocytes. The mononuclear phagocyte system includes monocytes in the blood and macrophages throughout the body. Mononuclear phagocytes have a critical role in the immune system. They are responsible for capturing, processing, and presenting the antigen to the lymphocytes. The antigen then stimulates a humoral or cell-mediated immune response. Capturing is accomplished through phagocytosis. The macrophage-bound antigen, which is highly immunogenic, is presented to

FIGURE 16-2 The immune response to a virus. **A,** A virus invades the body through a break in the skin or another portal of entry. The virus must make its way inside a cell in order to replicate itself. **B,** A macrophage recognizes the antigens on the surface of the virus. The macrophage digests the virus and displays pieces of the virus (antigens) on its surface. **C,** T helper cells recognize the antigen displayed and bind to the macrophage. This binding stimulates the production of cytokines (interleukin-1 [IL-1] and tumour necrosis factor [TNF]) by the macrophage and interleukin-2 (IL-2) and γ-interferon (γ-IFN) by the T helper cells. These cytokines are intercellular messengers that provide communication among the cells. **D,** IL-2 instructs other T helper cells and T cytotoxic cells to proliferate (multiply). T helper cells release cytokines, causing B cells to multiply and produce antibodies. **E,** T cytotoxic cells and natural killer cells destroy infected body cells. **F,** The antibodies bind to the virus and mark it for macrophage destruction. **G,** Once the virus is gone, activated T and B cells are turned off by suppressor T cells. Memory B and T cells remain behind to respond quickly if the same virus attacks again.

circulating T or B lymphocytes and thus triggers an immune response (Figure 16-2).

Lymphocytes. Lymphocytes are produced in the bone marrow (Figure 16-3). They then differentiate into B and T lymphocytes.

B Lymphocytes. Early research on B lymphocytes (bursa-equivalent lymphocytes) in birds showed that they mature under the influence of the bursa of Fabricius; hence the name *B cells*. However, this lymphoid organ does not exist in humans. The bursa-equivalent tissue in humans is the bone marrow. B cells differentiate into *plasma cells* when activated and produce antibodies (called *immunoglobulins*) (Table 16-2).

T Lymphocytes. Cells that migrate from the bone marrow to the thymus differentiate into T lymphocytes (thymus-dependent cells). The thymus secretes hormones, including thymosin, that stimulate the maturation and differentiation of T lymphocytes. T cells make up 70 to 80% of the circulating lymphocytes and are primarily responsible for immunity to intracellular viruses,

tumour cells, and fungi. T cells live from a few months to an individual's lifespan and account for long-term immunity.

T lymphocytes can be categorized into T cytotoxic and T helper cells. Antigenic characteristics of WBCs have now been classified using monoclonal antibodies. These antigens are classified as *clusters of differentiation*, or *CD, antigens*. Many types of WBCs, especially lymphocytes, are referred to by their CD designations. All mature T cells have the CD3 antigen (Kasper, Fauci, Hauser, et al., 2015).

T Cytotoxic Cells. T cytotoxic (CD8) cells are involved in attacking antigens on the cell membrane of foreign pathogens and releasing cytolytic substances that destroy the pathogen. These cells have antigen specificity and are sensitized by exposure to the antigen (Kasper, Fauci, Hauser, et al., 2015). Much like B lymphocytes, some sensitized T cells do not attack the antigen but remain as memory T cells. As in the humoral immune response, a second exposure to the antigen

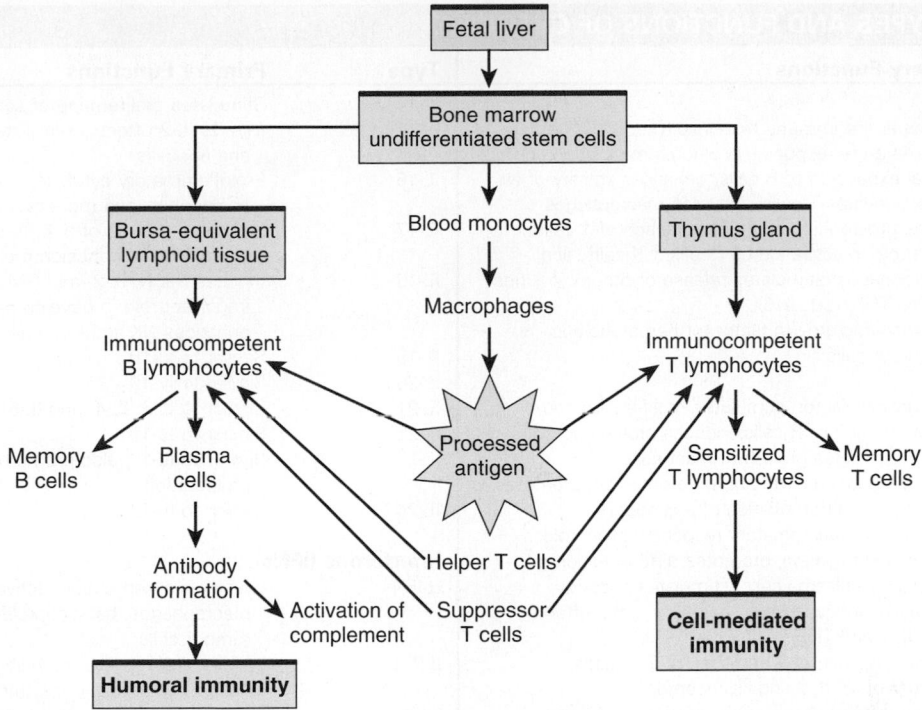

FIGURE 16-3 Relationships and functions of macrophages, B lymphocytes, and T lymphocytes in an immune response.

Class	Relative Serum Concentration (%)	Location	Characteristics
TABLE 16-2	**CHARACTERISTICS OF IMMUNOGLOBULINS**		
IgG	76	Plasma, interstitial fluid	Is only immunoglobulin that crosses placenta Is responsible for secondary immune response
IgA	15	Body secretions, including tears, saliva, breast milk, colostrum	Lines mucous membranes and protects body surfaces
IgM	8	Plasma	Is responsible for primary immune response Forms antibodies to ABO blood antigens
IgD	1	Plasma	Is present on lymphocyte surface Assists in the differentiation of B lymphocytes
IgE	0.002	Plasma, interstitial fluids	Causes symptoms of allergic reactions Fixes to mast cells and basophils Assists in defence against parasitic infections

Ig, immunoglobulin.

results in a more intense and rapid cell-mediated immune response.

T Helper Cells. T helper (CD4) cells are involved in the regulation of cell-mediated immunity and the humoral antibody response. T helper cells differentiate into subsets of cells that produce distinct types of cytokines (discussed in a later section). These subsets are called T_H1 cells and T_H2 cells. T_H1 cells stimulate phagocyte-mediated ingestion and killing of microbes, the key component of cell-mediated immunity. T_H2 cells stimulate eosinophil-mediated immunity, which is effective against parasites and is involved in allergic responses.

Natural Killer Cells. Natural killer (NK) cells are also involved in cell-mediated immunity. These cells are not T or B cells but are large lymphocytes with numerous granules in the cytoplasm. Prior sensitization is not required for the generation of NK cells. These cells are involved in the recognition and killing of virus-infected cells, tumour cells, and transplanted grafts; however, the mechanism of recognition is not fully understood. NK cells

have a significant role in immune surveillance for malignant cell changes.

Dendritic Cells. Dendritic cells are a system of cells that play a significant role in cell-mediated immune response. They are found in the skin (called *Langerhans cells*), the lining of the nose, the lungs, the stomach, and the intestines, and when in an immature state, they can be found in the blood. Their primary function is to capture antigens at sites of contact with the external environment (e.g., skin, mucous membranes) and then transport this antigen until it encounters a T cell with specificity for the antigen. Dendritic cells have an important function in activating the immune response (William, 2013).

Cytokines

The immune response involves complex interactions of T cells, B cells, monocytes, and neutrophils. These interactions depend on cytokines (soluble factors secreted by WBCs and a variety of other cells in the body), which act as messengers between the

TABLE 16-3 TYPES AND FUNCTIONS OF CYTOKINE

Type	Primary Functions	Type	Primary Functions
Interleukins (ILs)		IL-14	Stimulates proliferation of activated B cells
IL-1	Augments the immune response; mediates the inflammatory response; promotes maturation and clonal expansion of B cells; enhances activity of NK cells; activates T cells; activates macrophages	IL-15	Mimics IL-2 effects; stimulates proliferation of T cells and NK cells
IL-2	Induces proliferation and differentiation of T cells; plays role in activation of T cells, NK cells, and macrophages; stimulates release of other cytokines (α-IFN, TNF, IL-1, IL-6)	IL-16	Proinflammatory cytokine; chemoattractant of T cells, eosinophils, and monocytes
		IL-17	Promotes release of IL-6, IL-8, G-CSF; enhances expression of adhesion molecules
IL-3 (multicolony-stimulating factor)	Hematopoietic growth factor for hematopoietic precursor cells	IL-18	Induces α-IFN, IL-2, and GM-CSF production; plays important role in development of T helper cells; enhances NK activity; inhibits production of IL-10
IL-4	B-cell growth factor: stimulates proliferation and differentiation of B cells; induces proliferation of T cells; stimulates growth of mast cells	IL-19	Similar to IL-10
		IL-20	Similar to IL-10
		IL-21	Similar to IL-2, IL-4, and IL-5
IL-5	Promotes B-cell growth and differentiation; promotes growth and differentiation of eosinophils	IL-22	Similar to IL-10
		IL-23	Similar to IL-12; also promotes memory T-cell proliferation
IL-6	Enhances the inflammatory response; plays role in B-cell stimulation; promotes differentiation of B cells into plasma cells; stimulates antibody secretion; induces fever; has synergistic effects with IL-1 and TNF	IL-24	Similar to IL-10
		Interferons (IFNs)	
IL-7	Promotes growth of T and B cells; increases expression of IL-2 and its receptor	α-IFN	Inhibits viral replication; activates NK cells and macrophages; has antiproliferative effects on tumour cells
IL-8	Involved in chemotaxis of neutrophils and T cells; stimulates superoxide and granule release	β-IFN	Inhibits viral replication; inhibits certain white blood cells; is used in the treatment of multiple sclerosis
IL-9	Acts as mitogen, supporting proliferation in absence of antigen; enhances T-cell survival; plays role in mast cell activation	γ-IFN	Activates macrophages, neutrophils, and NK cells; promotes B-cell differentiation; inhibits viral replication
IL-10	Inhibits cytokine production by T and NK cells; promotes B-cell proliferation and antibody responses; is potent suppressor of macrophage function	**Tumour Necrosis Factor (TNF)**	
		TNF	Activates macrophages and granulocytes; promotes the immune and inflammatory responses; kills tumour cells; is responsible for extensive weight loss associated with chronic inflammation and cancer
IL-11	Is a multifunctional regulator of hematopoiesis and lymphopoiesis; plays role in osteoclast formation; elevates platelet count; inhibits proinflammatory cytokine production	**Colony-Stimulating Factors (CSFs)**	
		G-CSF	Stimulates proliferation and differentiation of neutrophils; enhances functional activity of mature PMNs
IL-12	Promotes α-IFN production; plays role in induction of T helper cells; activates NK cells; stimulates proliferation of activated T and NK cells	GM-CSF	Stimulates proliferation and differentiation of PMNs and monocytes
IL-13	Promotes B-cell growth and differentiation; inhibits proinflammatory cytokine production	M-CSF	Promotes the proliferation, differentiation, and activation of monocytes and macrophages

G-CSF, granulocyte colony-stimulating factor; *GM-CSF,* granulocyte-macrophage colony-stimulating factor; *M-CSF,* macrophage colony-stimulating factor; *NK,* natural killer; *PMN,* polymorphonuclear neutrophil.

cell types. Cytokines instruct cells to alter their proliferation, differentiation, secretion, or activity.

Currently more than 100 different cytokines are known, and they can be classified into distinct categories (Mak, Saunders, & Jett, 2014). Some of these cytokines are listed in Table 16-3. In general, the interleukins act as immuno-modulatory factors; colony-stimulating factors act as growth-regulating factors for hematopoietic cells; and interferons are antiviral and immuno-modulatory.

The net effect of an inflammatory response is determined by a balance between proinflammatory and anti-inflammatory mediators. Sometimes cytokines are classified as proinflammatory or anti-inflammatory. However, it is not that straightforward since many other factors (e.g., target cells, environment) influence the inflammatory response to a given injury or insult.

Cytokines serve a beneficial role in hematopoiesis and immune function but can also have detrimental effects such as those observed in chronic inflammation, autoimmune diseases, and

sepsis. Cytokines such as erythropoietin (see Chapters 18, 35, and 49), colony-stimulating factors, interferons (see Chapter 18), and interleukin-2 (see Chapter 18) are used clinically.

Three types of interferons have now been identified (Table 16-3). Interferons help the body's natural defences attack tumours and viruses (Table 16-4). Interferons are not directly antiviral but produce an antiviral effect in cells by reacting with them and inducing the formation of a second protein termed *antiviral protein* (Figure 16-4). This protein mediates the antiviral action of interferons by altering the cell's protein synthesis and prevents the virus from replicating.

Comparison of Humoral and Cell-Mediated Immunity

Humans need both humoral and cell-mediated immunity to remain healthy. Each type of immunity has unique properties and different modes of action and reactions against particular antigens. Table 16-5 compares humoral and cell-mediated immunity.

TABLE 16-4 CLINICAL USES OF CYTOKINES

Cytokine	Clinical Uses
α-Interferon (Intron A)	Hepatitis B and C Kaposi's sarcoma Hairy cell leukemia Lymphomas Melanoma Renal cell carcinoma Multiple myeloma
β-Interferon β-Interferon-1b (Betaseron) β-Interferon-1a (Avonex, Rebif)	Multiple sclerosis
Colony-Stimulating Factors: G-CSF, GM-CSF Filgrastim (Neupogen)	Neutropenia
Soluble Tumour Necrosis Factor Receptor Etanercept (Enbrel)	Rheumatoid arthritis
Interleukin-2 Aldesleukin (Proleukin)	Renal cell carcinoma Malignant melanoma Lymphoma Acute myelocytic leukemia
Erythropoietin Darbepoetin alfa (Aranesp) Epoetin alfa (Eprex)	Anemia
Interleukin-1 Receptor Antagonist Anakinra (Kineret)	Rheumatoid arthritis

G-CSF, granulocyte colony-stimulating factor; *GM-CSF,* granulocyte-macrophage colony-stimulating factor.

TABLE 16-5 COMPARISON OF HUMORAL IMMUNITY AND CELL-MEDIATED IMMUNITY

Characteristics	Humoral Immunity	Cell-Mediated Immunity
Cells involved	B lymphocytes	T lymphocytes, macrophages
Products	Antibodies	Sensitized T cells, lymphokines
Memory cells	Present	Present
Protection	Bacteria Viruses (extracellular) Respiratory and gastro-intestinal pathogens	Fungi Viruses (intracellular) Chronic infectious agents Tumour cells
Examples	Anaphylactic shock Atopic diseases Transfusion reaction Bacterial infections	Tuberculosis Fungal infections Contact dermatitis Graft rejection Destruction of cancer cells

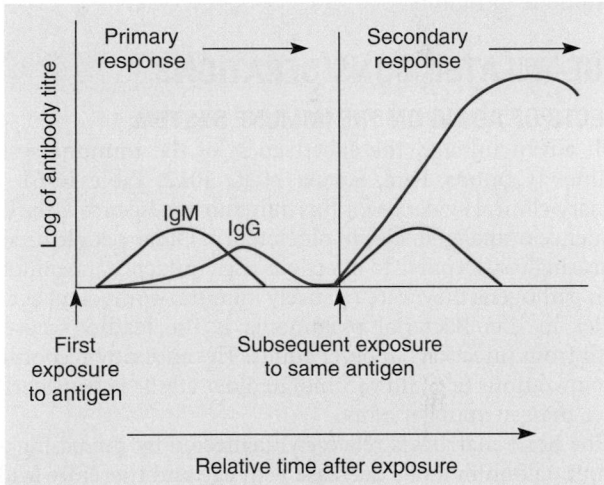

FIGURE 16-5 Primary and secondary immune responses. The introduction of antigen induces a response dominated by two classes of immunoglobulins: immunoglobulin M (IgM) and immunoglobulin G (IgG). IgM predominates in the primary response; some amount of IgG appears later. After the host's immune system is primed, another challenge with the same antigen induces the secondary response, in which some IgM and large amounts of IgG are produced.

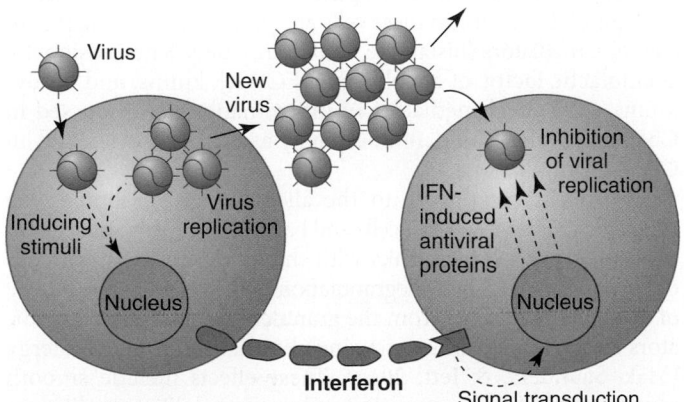

FIGURE 16-4 Mechanism of action of interferons. The virus attacks a cell. The cell begins to synthesize viral DNA and interferons. Interferons serve as intercellular messengers. Interferons induce the production of antiviral proteins. The virus is not able to replicate in the cell.

Humoral Immunity. **Humoral immunity** is antibody-mediated immunity. The term *humoral* comes from the Greek word *humor,* which means "body fluid." Since antibodies are produced by plasma cells (differentiated B cells) and found in plasma, the term *humoral immunity* is used. Production of antibodies is an essential component in a humoral immune response. Each of the five classes of immunoglobulins (Igs)—that is, IgG, IgA, IgM, IgD, and IgE—has specific characteristics (see Table 16-2).

When a pathogen (especially bacteria) enters the body, it may encounter a B lymphocyte specific for antigens located on that bacterial cell wall. In addition, a monocyte or macrophage may phagocytize the bacteria and present its antigens to a B lymphocyte. The B lymphocyte recognizes the antigen because it has receptors on its cell surface specific for that antigen. When the antigen comes in contact with the cell surface receptor, the B cell becomes activated, and most B cells differentiate into plasma cells (see Figure 16-3). The mature plasma cell secretes immunoglobulins. Some stimulated B lymphocytes remain as memory cells.

The primary immune response becomes evident 4 to 8 days after the initial exposure to the antigen (Figure 16-5). IgM is the first type of antibody formed. Because of the large size of the IgM molecule, this immunoglobulin is confined to the intravascular space. As the immune response progresses, IgG is produced and can move from intravascular to extravascular spaces.

When the individual is exposed to the antigen the second time, a secondary antibody response occurs. This response occurs faster (1 to 3 days), is stronger, and lasts for a longer time than a primary response. Memory cells account for the memory of the first exposure to the antigen and the more rapid production of antibodies. IgG is the primary antibody found in a secondary immune response.

IgG crosses the placental membrane and provides the newborn with passive acquired immunity for at least 3 months. Infants may also get some passive immunity from IgA in breast milk and colostrum.

Cell-Mediated Immunity. Immune responses that are initiated through specific antigen recognition by T cells are termed cell-mediated immunity. Several cell types and factors are involved in cell-mediated immunity, including T lymphocytes, macrophages, and NK cells. Cell-mediated immunity is of primary importance in (a) immunity against pathogens that survive inside of cells, including viruses and some bacteria (e.g., *Mycobacterium* species); (b) immunity against fungal infections; (c) rejection of transplanted tissues; (d) contact hypersensitivity reactions; and (e) tumour immunity.

AGE-RELATED CONSIDERATIONS

EFFECTS OF AGING ON THE IMMUNE SYSTEM

With advancing age, the effectiveness of the immune system declines (Camous, Pera, Solana, et al., 2012; Table 16-6). The primary clinical evidence for this immuno-senescence is the high incidence of malignancies in older adults. Older people become increasingly susceptible to infections (e.g., influenza, pneumonia) from pathogens they were relatively immuno-competent against earlier in life. Bacterial pneumonia is the leading cause of death from infections in older adults. The antibody response to immunizations (e.g., flu vaccine) in older adults is considerably lower than in younger adults.

The bone marrow is relatively unaffected by increasing age. Immunoglobulin levels decrease with age and therefore lead to a suppressed humoral immune response in older adults. Thymic involution (shrinking) occurs with aging, along with decreased numbers of T cells. These changes in the thymus gland are a primary cause of immuno-senescence. Both T and B cells show deficiencies in activation, transit time through the cell cycle, and subsequent differentiation. However, the most significant alterations involve T cells. As thymic output of T cells diminishes, the differentiation of T cells increases. Consequently, memory cells accumulate, rather than new precursor cells responsive to previously unencountered antigens.

The delayed hypersensitivity response, as determined by skin testing with injected antigens, is frequently decreased or absent in older adults. This altered response reflects anergy (an immuno-deficient condition characterized by lack of or diminished reaction to an antigen or a group of antigens).

ALTERED IMMUNE RESPONSE

Immuno-competence is the state in which the body's immune system can identify and inactivate or destroy foreign substances. When the immune system is incompetent or under-responsive, severe infections, immunodeficiency diseases, and malignancies may occur. When the immune system overreacts, hypersensitivity disorders such as allergies and autoimmune diseases may occur.

Hypersensitivity Reactions

Sometimes the immune response is overreactive against foreign antigens or reacts against its own tissue, resulting in tissue damage. This is termed a hypersensitivity reaction. Autoimmune diseases, a type of hypersensitivity response, occur when the body fails to recognize self-proteins and reacts against self-antigens.

Hypersensitivity reactions may be classified according to the source of the antigen, the time sequence (immediate or delayed), or the basic immunological mechanisms causing the injury. Four types of hypersensitivity reactions exist (Table 16-7). Types I, II, and III are immediate and are examples of humoral immunity. Type IV is a delayed hypersensitivity reaction and is related to cell-mediated immunity.

Type I: IgE-Mediated Reactions. Anaphylactic reactions are type I reactions that occur only in susceptible people who are highly sensitized to specific allergens. IgE antibodies, produced in response to the allergen, have a characteristic property of attaching to mast cells and basophils (Figure 16-6; see also Chapter 31, Figure 31-2). Within these cells are granules containing potent chemical mediators (histamine, serotonin, leukotrienes, eosinophil chemotactic factor of anaphylaxis [ECF-A], kinins, and brady-kinin). (Chemical mediators of inflammation are discussed in Chapter 14 and Table 14-3. Anaphylaxis is also discussed in Chapters 14 and 31.)

On the first exposure to the allergen, IgE antibodies are produced and bind to mast cells and basophils. On any subsequent exposures, the allergen links with the IgE bound to mast cells or basophils and triggers degranulation of the cells and the release of chemical mediators from the granules. These chemical mediators attack target tissues, causing clinical symptoms of allergy (Mak, Saunders, & Jett, 2014). These effects include smooth muscle contraction, increased vascular permeability, vasodilation, hypotension, increased secretion of mucus, and itching. Fortunately, the mediators are short-acting, and their effects are reversible. The mediators and their effects are summarized in Table 16-8.

A genetic predisposition to the development of allergic diseases exists. The capacity to become sensitized to an allergen, rather than the specific allergic disorder, appears to be an inherited trait. For example, a father with asthma may have a son who has allergic rhinitis.

The clinical manifestations of an anaphylactic reaction depend on whether the mediators remain local or become systemic or whether they affect particular organs. When the mediators remain localized, a cutaneous response termed the *wheal-and-flare*

TABLE 16-6 AGE-RELATED DIFFERENCES IN ASSESSMENT

Effects of Aging on the Immune System

- ↓ Autoantibodies
- ↓ Cell-mediated immunity
- ↓ Delayed hypersensitivity response
- ↓ Expression of IL-2 receptors
- ↓ IL-1 and IL-2 synthesis
- ↓ Primary and secondary antibody responses
- ↓ Proliferative response of T and B cells
- Thymic involution

IL-1, interleukin-1; *IL-2*, interleukin-2.

TABLE 16-7 TYPES OF HYPERSENSITIVITY REACTIONS

	Type I: Anaphylactic Reactions	Type II: Cytotoxic Reactions	Type III: Immune-Complex Reactions	Type IV: Delayed Hypersensitivity Reactions
Antigen	Exogenous pollen, food, drugs, dust	Cell surface of RBCs Basement membrane	Extracellular fungal, viral, bacterial	Intracellular or extracellular
Antibody Involved	IgE	IgG IgM	IgG IgM	None
Complement Involved	No	Yes	Yes	No
Mediators of Injury	Histamine SRS-A	Complement lysis Neutrophils	Neutrophils Complement lysis	Cytokines T cytotoxic cells Monocytes, macrophages Lysosomal enzymes
Examples	Allergic rhinitis Asthma	Transfusion reaction Goodpasture's syndrome	Serum sickness Systemic lupus erythematosus Rheumatoid arthritis	Contact dermatitis Tumour rejection Transplant rejection
Skin Test	Wheal and flare	None	Erythema and edema in 3 to 8 hours	Erythema and edema in 24 to 48 hours (e.g., tuberculin test)

IgE, immunoglobulin E; *IgG*, immunoglobulin G; *IgM*, immunoglobulin M; *RBC*, red blood cell; *SRS-A*, slow-reacting substance of anaphylaxis.

TABLE 16-8 MEDIATORS OF ALLERGIC RESPONSE

Type and Source	Biological Activity	Clinical Manifestations
Histamine Mast cell and basophil granules	Increase vascular permeability; constrict smooth muscle; stimulate irritant receptors	Edema of airways and larynx; bronchial constriction; urticaria, angioedema, pruritus; nausea, vomiting, diarrhea; shock
Leukotrienes Metabolites of arachidonic acid by lipoxygenase pathway	Constrict bronchial smooth muscle; increase vascular permeability	Bronchial constriction; enhanced effect of histamine on smooth muscle
Prostaglandins Metabolites of arachidonic acid by cyclo-oxygenase pathway	Stimulate vasodilation; constrict smooth muscle	Wheal-and-flare reaction on skin; hypotension; bronchospasm
Platelet-Activating Factor Mast cell	Aggregates platelets; stimulates vasodilation	Increase in pulmonary artery pressure; systemic hypotension
Kinins Kininogen	Stimulates slow, sustained smooth muscle contraction; increases vascular permeability; stimulates secretion of mucus; stimulates pain receptors	Angioedema with painful swelling; bronchial constriction
Serotonin Platelets	Increase vascular permeability; stimulate smooth muscle contraction	Mucosal edema; bronchial constriction
Anaphylatoxins C3a, C4a, C5a from complement activation	Stimulate histamine release	Edema of airways and larynx; bronchial constriction; urticaria, angioedema, pruritus; nausea, vomiting, diarrhea; shock

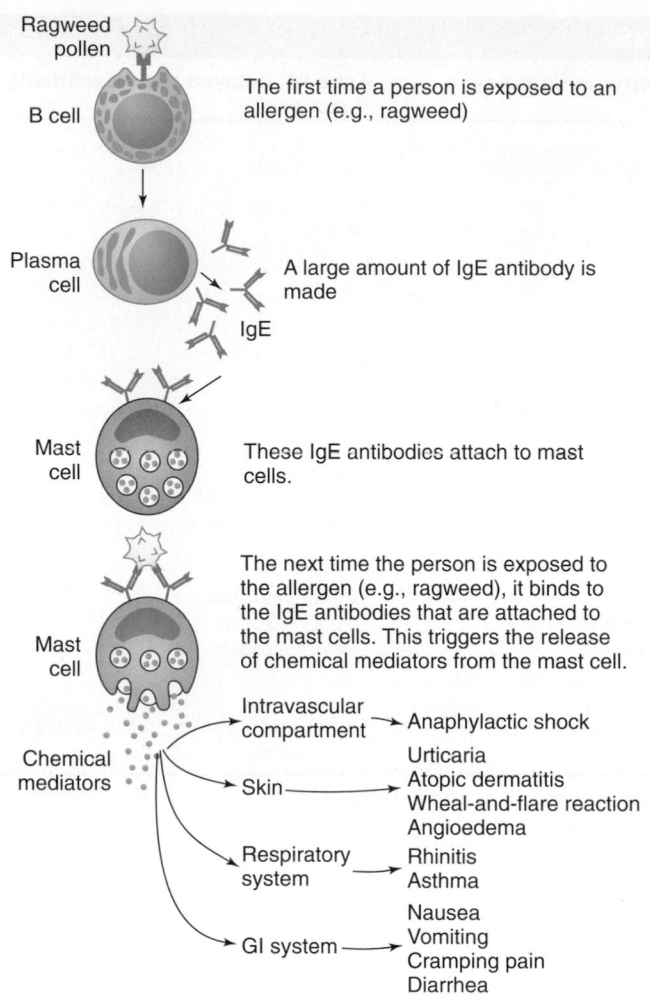

Ragweed pollen

B cell — The first time a person is exposed to an allergen (e.g., ragweed)

Plasma cell — A large amount of IgE antibody is made

IgE

Mast cell — These IgE antibodies attach to mast cells.

Mast cell — The next time the person is exposed to the allergen (e.g., ragweed), it binds to the IgE antibodies that are attached to the mast cells. This triggers the release of chemical mediators from the mast cell.

Chemical mediators

Intravascular compartment → Anaphylactic shock

Skin → Urticaria
Atopic dermatitis
Wheal-and-flare reaction
Angioedema

Respiratory system → Rhinitis
Asthma

GI system → Nausea
Vomiting
Cramping pain
Diarrhea

FIGURE 16-6 Steps in a type I allergic reaction. *GI,* gastro-intestinal; *IgE,* immunoglobulin E.

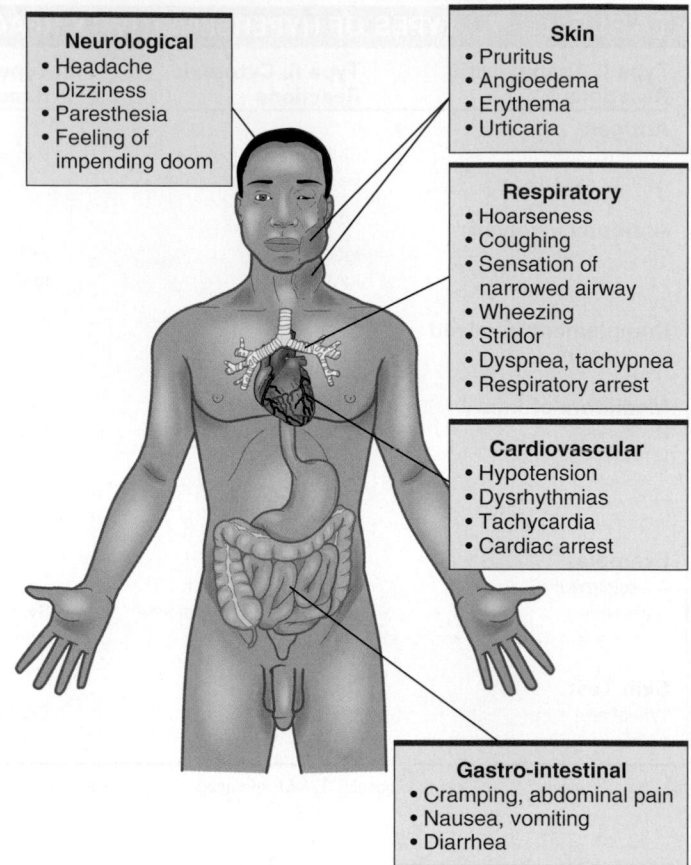

Neurological
• Headache
• Dizziness
• Paresthesia
• Feeling of impending doom

Skin
• Pruritus
• Angioedema
• Erythema
• Urticaria

Respiratory
• Hoarseness
• Coughing
• Sensation of narrowed airway
• Wheezing
• Stridor
• Dyspnea, tachypnea
• Respiratory arrest

Cardiovascular
• Hypotension
• Dysrhythmias
• Tachycardia
• Cardiac arrest

Gastro-intestinal
• Cramping, abdominal pain
• Nausea, vomiting
• Diarrhea

FIGURE 16-7 Clinical manifestations of a systemic anaphylactic reaction.

reaction occurs. This reaction is characterized by a pale wheal (pink, raised, edematous, pruritic areas) containing edematous fluid, surrounded by a red flare from the hyperemia. The reaction occurs in minutes or hours and is usually not dangerous. A classic example of a wheal-and-flare reaction is the mosquito bite. The wheal-and-flare reaction serves a diagnostic purpose as a means of demonstrating allergic reactions to specific allergens during skin tests.

Common allergic reactions include anaphylaxis and atopic reactions.

Anaphylaxis. Anaphylaxis can occur when mediators are released systemically (e.g., after injection of a drug, after an insect sting). The reaction occurs within minutes and can be life-threatening as a result of bronchial constriction and subsequent airway obstruction and vascular collapse. The target organs affected are depicted in Figure 16-7. Initial symptoms include edema and itching at the site of the exposure to the allergen. Shock can occur rapidly and is manifested by a rapid, weak pulse; hypotension; dilated pupils; dyspnea; and possibly cyanosis. This is compounded by bronchial edema and angioedema. Death occurs if emergency treatment is not initiated. Treatment can range from epinephrine administered subcutaneously for mild symptoms to full circulatory support with oxygen and vasopressor therapy (Waserman, Chad, Francoeur, et al., 2010). Some of the

important allergens leading to anaphylactic shock in hypersensitive people are listed in Table 16-9. Medications are the leading cause of anaphylaxis-related deaths (Moore, Kemp, & Kemp, 2015).

Atopic Reactions. An estimated 20% of the population are atopic, which means they have an inherited tendency to become sensitive to environmental allergens. The atopic diseases that can result are allergic rhinitis, asthma, atopic dermatitis, urticaria, and angioedema.

Allergic rhinitis, or hay fever, is the most common type I hypersensitivity reaction. It may occur year-round (perennial allergic rhinitis), or it may be seasonal (seasonal allergic rhinitis). Airborne substances such as pollens, dust, or moulds are the primary cause of allergic rhinitis. Perennial allergic rhinitis may be caused by dust, moulds, and animal dander. Seasonal allergic rhinitis is commonly caused by pollens from trees, weeds, or grasses. The target areas affected are the conjunctivas of the eyes and the mucosa of the upper respiratory tract. Symptoms include nasal discharge, sneezing, lacrimation, mucosal swelling with airway obstruction, and pruritus around the eyes, nose, throat, and mouth. (Treatment of allergic rhinitis is discussed in Chapter 29.)

Many patients with asthma have an allergic component to their disease. These patients frequently have a history of atopic disorders (e.g., infantile eczema, allergic rhinitis, food intolerances). Inflammatory mediators produce bronchial smooth muscle constriction, excessive secretion of viscous mucus, edema of the mucous membranes of the bronchi, and decreased lung compliance. Because of these physiological alterations, affected patients manifest dyspnea, wheezing, coughing, tightness in the chest,

TABLE 16-9 ALLERGENS THAT CAUSE ANAPHYLACTIC SHOCK

Drugs
- Aspirin
- Cephalosporins
- Chemotherapeutic drugs
- Insulins
- Local anaesthetics
- Nonsteroidal anti-inflammatory drugs
- Penicillins
- Sulfonamides
- Tetracycline

Insect Venoms
- Hymenoptera*

Foods
- Eggs
- Nuts
- Shellfish
- Chocolate

- Milk
- Peanuts
- Fish
- Strawberries

Animal Sera
- Tetanus antitoxin
- Diphtheria antitoxin
- Rabies antitoxin
- Snake venom antitoxin

Treatment Measures
- Blood products (whole blood and components)
- Allergenic extracts in hyposensitization therapy
- Iodine-contrast media for intravenous pyelography or angiography

*Wasps, hornets, yellow jackets, bumblebees, and ants.

FIGURE 16-8 Eczema of the lower leg. Source: Morison, M. J. (2001). *Nursing management of chronic wounds.* Edinburgh: Mosby.

and thick sputum. (Pathophysiology and management of asthma are discussed in Chapter 31.)

Atopic dermatitis is a chronic, inherited skin disorder characterized by exacerbations and remissions. It is caused by several environmental allergens that are difficult to identify. Although patients with atopic dermatitis have elevated IgE levels and positive skin tests, the histopathological features do not represent the typical, localized wheal-and-flare type I reactions. The skin lesions are more generalized and involve vasodilation of blood vessels, resulting in interstitial edema with vesicle formation (Figure 16-8). (Dermatitis is discussed in Chapter 26.)

Urticaria (hives) is a cutaneous reaction against systemic allergens that occurs in atopic people. It is characterized by transient wheals that vary in size and shape and may occur throughout the body. Urticaria develops rapidly after exposure to an allergen and may last minutes or hours. Histamine causes localized vasodilation (erythema), transudation of fluid (wheal), and flaring. Flaring is caused by dilation of blood vessels on the edge of the wheal. Histamine is responsible for the pruritus associated with the lesions. (Urticaria is discussed further in Chapter 26.)

Angioedema is a localized cutaneous lesion similar to urticaria but involving deeper layers of the skin and submucosa. The principal areas of involvement include the eyelids, lips, tongue, larynx, hands, feet, gastro-intestinal tract, and genitalia. Swelling usually begins in the face and then progresses to the airways and other parts of the body. Dilation and engorgement of the capillaries secondary to release of histamine cause the diffuse swelling. Welts are not apparent as in urticaria. The outer skin appears normal or has a reddish hue. The lesions may burn, sting, or itch and, if in the gastro-intestinal tract, can cause acute abdominal pain. The swelling may occur suddenly or over several hours and usually lasts for 24 hours.

Type II: Cytotoxic and Cytolytic Reactions. Cytotoxic and cytolytic reactions are type II hypersensitivity reactions involving the direct binding of IgG or IgM antibodies to an antigen on the cell surface. Antigen–antibody complexes activate the complement system, which mediates the reaction. Cellular tissue is destroyed in one of two ways: (a) activation of the complement cascade resulting in cytolysis or (b) enhanced phagocytosis.

Target cells frequently destroyed in type II reactions are erythrocytes, platelets, and leukocytes. The tissue damage usually occurs rapidly. Some of the antigens involved are the ABO blood group, rhesus (Rh) factor, and drugs. Pathophysiological disorders characteristic of type II reactions include ABO incompatibility transfusion reaction, Rh incompatibility transfusion reaction, autoimmune and drug-related hemolytic anemias, leukopenia, thrombocytopenia, erythroblastosis fetalis (hemolytic disease of the newborn), and Goodpasture's syndrome. Tissue damage usually occurs rapidly.

Hemolytic Transfusion Reactions. A classic type II reaction occurs when a recipient receives ABO-incompatible blood from a donor. Naturally acquired antibodies to antigens of the ABO blood group are in the recipient's serum but are not present on the erythrocyte membranes (see Chapter 32, Table 32-9). For example, a person with type A blood has anti-B antibodies, a person with type B blood has anti-A antibodies, a person with type AB blood has no antibodies, and a person with type O blood has both anti-A and anti-B antibodies.

If the recipient receives a transfusion with incompatible blood, antibodies immediately coat the foreign erythrocytes, causing agglutination (clumping). The clumping of cells blocks small blood vessels in the body, using and thus depleting existing clotting factors, which leads to bleeding. Within hours, neutrophils and macrophages phagocytize the agglutinated cells. As complement is fixed to the antigen, cell lysis occurs, which in turn causes the release of hemoglobin into the urine and plasma. In addition, a cytotoxic reaction causes vascular spasms in the kidney that further block the renal tubules. Acute kidney injury can result from hemoglobinuria. (Blood transfusions are discussed in Chapter 33.)

Goodpasture's Syndrome. Goodpasture's syndrome is a rare disorder involving the lungs and the kidneys. An antibody-mediated autoimmune reaction occurs involving the glomerular and alveolar basement membranes. The circulating antibodies combine with tissue antigen to activate the complement system, which causes deposits of IgG to form along the basement membranes of the lungs or the kidneys. This reaction may result in pulmonary hemorrhage and glomerulonephritis. (Goodpasture's syndrome is discussed further in Chapter 48.)

Type III: Immune-Complex Reactions. Tissue damage in immune-complex reactions, which are type III reactions, occurs secondary to antigen–antibody complexes. Soluble antigens combine with immunoglobulins of the IgG and IgM classes to form complexes that are too small to be effectively removed by the mononuclear phagocyte system. Therefore, the complexes deposit in tissue or small blood vessels. They cause activation of the complement system and release of chemotactic factors that lead to inflammation and destruction of the involved tissue.

Type III reactions may be local or systemic and immediate or delayed. The clinical manifestations depend on the number of complexes and their location in the body. Common sites for deposit are the kidneys, skin, joints, blood vessels, and lungs. Severe type III reactions are associated with autoimmune disorders such as systemic lupus erythematosus (SLE), acute glomerulonephritis, and rheumatoid arthritis. (SLE and rheumatoid arthritis are discussed further in Chapter 67, and acute glomerulonephritis is discussed further in Chapter 48.)

Type IV: Delayed Hypersensitivity Reactions. A delayed hypersensitivity reaction—a type IV reaction—is also called a *cell-mediated immune response*. Although cell-mediated immune responses are usually protective mechanisms, tissue damage occurs in delayed hypersensitivity reactions.

The tissue damage in a type IV reaction does not occur in the presence of antibodies or complement. Rather, sensitized T lymphocytes attack antigens or release cytokines, some of which attract macrophages into the area. These macrophages are responsible for most of the tissue destruction. A delayed hypersensitivity reaction takes 24 to 48 hours to occur.

Clinical examples of a delayed hypersensitivity reaction include contact dermatitis (Figure 16-9); hypersensitivity reactions to bacterial, fungal, and viral infections; and transplant rejection. Some drug sensitivity reactions also fit this category.

Contact Dermatitis. Allergic contact dermatitis is an example of a delayed hypersensitivity reaction involving the skin. The reaction occurs when the skin is exposed to substances that easily penetrate the skin to combine with epidermal proteins. The substance then becomes antigenic, and over a period of 7 to 14 days, memory cells for the antigen form. On subsequent exposure to the substance, a sensitized person develops eczematous skin lesions within 48 hours. The most common potentially antigenic substances encountered are metal compounds (e.g., those containing nickel, mercury); rubber compounds;

FIGURE 16-9 Contact dermatitis in reaction to rubber. Source: Morison, M. J. (2001). *Nursing management of chronic wounds*. Edinburgh: Mosby.

poison ivy, poison oak, and poison sumac; cosmetics; and some dyes.

In acute contact dermatitis, the skin lesions appear erythematous and edematous and are covered with papules, vesicles, and bullae. The involved area is very pruritic but may also burn or sting. When contact dermatitis becomes chronic, the lesions resemble atopic dermatitis because they are thickened, scaly, and lichenified. The main difference between contact dermatitis and atopic dermatitis is that contact dermatitis is localized and restricted to the area exposed to the allergens, whereas atopic dermatitis is usually widespread.

Microbial Hypersensitivity Reactions. The classic example of a microbial cell-mediated immune reaction is the body's defence against the tubercle bacillus. Tuberculosis (TB) results from invasion of lung tissue by the highly resistant tubercle bacillus. The organism itself does not directly damage the lung tissue. However, antigenic material released from the tubercle bacilli reacts with T lymphocytes, initiating a cell-mediated immune response. The resulting response causes extensive caseous necrosis of the lung.

After the initial cell-mediated immune reaction, memory cells persist; therefore, subsequent contact with the tubercle bacillus or an extract of purified protein from the organism causes a delayed hypersensitivity reaction. This is the basis for the purified protein derivative (PPD) TB skin test, which yields results 48 to 72 hours after the intradermal injection. (TB is discussed in Chapter 30.)

ALLERGIC DISORDERS

Although an alteration of the immune system may manifest in many ways, allergies or type I hypersensitivity reactions are seen most frequently.

Assessment

For a thorough assessment of a patient with allergies, a comprehensive health history, physical examination, diagnostic workup, and skin testing for allergens must be performed.

Health History. A comprehensive history that covers family allergies, past and current allergies, and social and environmental factors is essential. The information may be obtained from the patient or the family about atopic reactions in relatives in order to identify at-risk patients. Identifying past and current allergens that may have triggered a reaction is essential for controlling or preventing allergic reactions. In addition to identification of the allergen, information about the clinical manifestations and the course of allergic reaction should be obtained. The patient's use of any over-the-counter (OTC) or prescription medications used to treat the allergies should be documented.

Social factors (patient's lifestyle and stressors), environmental factors, and physical environment should be reviewed in connection with the appearance of allergic symptoms. Questions about pets, trees, plants, air pollutants, floor coverings, and cooling and heating systems in the home or workplace can yield valuable information about potential allergens. In addition, a daily or weekly food diary may be helpful. Of particular importance is a screening for any reaction to medications.

Physical Examination. A comprehensive head-to-toe physical examination should be given to a patient with allergies, with particular attention focused on the site of the allergic manifestations. A comprehensive assessment that includes subjective and objective data should be obtained from the patient (Table 16-10).

TABLE 16-10 NURSING ASSESSMENT

Allergies

Subjective Data

Important Health Information

Past health history: Recurrent respiratory problems; seasonal exacerbations; unusual reactions to insect bites or stings; past and present allergies; altered home and work environment, presence of pets; family history of allergies

Medications: Unusual reactions to any medications; use of over-the-counter drugs; use of medications for allergies

Symptoms

Food intolerances; vomiting; abdominal cramps, diarrhea; fatigue; hoarseness, cough, dyspnea; itching, burning, stinging of eyes, nose, throat, or skin; chest tightness; malaise

Objective Data

Integumentary

Rashes, including urticaria, wheal-and-flare, papules, vesicles, bullae; dryness, scaliness, scratches, irritation

Eyes, Ears, Nose, and Throat

Eyes: Conjunctivitis; lacrimation; rubbing or excessive blinking; dark circles under the eyes ("allergic shiner")

Ears: Diminished hearing; immobile or scarred tympanic membranes; recurrent ear infections

Nose: Nasal polyps; nasal voice; nose twitching; itchy nose; rhinitis; pale, boggy mucous membranes; sniffling; repeated sneezing; swollen nasal passages; recurrent, unexplained nosebleeds; crease across the bridge of nose ("allergic salute")

Throat: Continual throat clearing; swollen lips or tongue; red throat; palpable neck lymph nodes

Respiratory

Wheezing, stridor; thick sputum

Possible Findings

Eosinophilia of serum, sputum, or nasal and bronchial secretions; ↑ serum IgE levels; positive skin tests; abnormal chest and sinus radiographs

Ig, immunoglobulin.

Diagnostic Studies

Many specialized immunological techniques can be performed to detect abnormalities of lymphocytes, eosinophils, and immunoglobulins. A complete blood cell count (CBC) with WBC differential is done, including an absolute lymphocyte count and eosinophil count. Cellular immunodeficiency is diagnosed if the lymphocyte count is below 1.2×10^9/L. T-cell and B-cell quantification is used to diagnose specific immunodeficiency syndromes. The eosinophil count is elevated with type I hypersensitivity reactions involving IgE. The serum IgE level is also generally elevated in type I hypersensitivity reactions and serves as a diagnostic indicator of atopic diseases.

Sputum and nasal and bronchial secretions may also be tested for the presence of eosinophils. If asthma is suspected, pulmonary function tests (especially forced expiratory volume) are helpful.

Allergy skin testing is the preferred method for determining immediate reactions to allergens, but in some cases blood testing may be ordered. Allergy blood testing is recommended if a person (a) is using a medication that interferes with skin test results (e.g., antihistamines, corticosteroids) and cannot stop taking it for a few days, (b) cannot tolerate the many needle scratches required for skin testing, or (c) has a skin disorder (e.g., severe eczema, dermatitis, psoriasis).

Skin Tests. Skin testing is used to identify the specific allergens that are causing the allergy symptoms. With the use of empirical allergy medications as the treatment of choice for most people with allergic rhinitis, it has become common practice to omit skin testing for specific allergens in these patients. However, diagnosing an allergy to a specific antigen enables the patient to avoid an allergen and makes the patient a candidate for immunotherapy. Unfortunately, skin testing cannot be done on patients who cannot be removed from medications that suppress the histamine response or on patients with food allergies.

Procedure. Skin testing may be performed by three different methods: (a) a scratch or prick, (b) an intradermal test, or (c) a patch test. The areas of the body usually used in testing are the arms and the back. Allergen extracts are applied to the skin in rows with a corresponding control site opposite the test site. Saline or another diluent is applied to the control site. In the *scratch test*, the epidermal skin layer is scratched with a pricking device, and the allergen extract is applied at the site. In the intradermal test, the allergen extract is injected intradermally under the skin, similar to a PPD test for TB. In the patch test, an allergen is applied to a patch that is placed on the skin.

Results. In the scratch and intradermal tests, the reaction typically occurs within 5 to 10 minutes. In the patch test, the patches need to be worn for 48 to 72 hours. If the person is hypersensitive to the allergen, a positive reaction will occur within minutes after insertion in the skin and may last for 8 to 12 hours. A positive reaction is manifested by a local wheal-and-flare response.

The size of the positive reaction is not always correlated with the severity of allergy symptoms. Also, false-positive and false-negative results may occur. Negative results from skin testing do not necessarily mean the person does not have an allergic disorder, and positive results do not necessarily mean that the allergen caused the clinical manifestations. Positive results imply that the person is sensitized to that allergen. Therefore, correlating skin test results with the patient's history is important.

Precautions. A highly sensitive person is always at risk for developing an anaphylactic reaction to skin tests. Therefore, a patient should never be left alone during the testing period. Sometimes, skin testing is completely contraindicated, and blood allergy testing is used. If a severe reaction does occur with a skin test, the extract is immediately removed, and anti-inflammatory topical cream is applied to the site. For intradermal testing, the arm is used so that a tourniquet can be applied during a severe reaction. A subcutaneous injection of epinephrine may also be necessary.

Collaborative Care

After an allergic disorder is diagnosed, the therapeutic treatment is aimed at reducing exposure to the offending allergen, treating the symptoms, and, if necessary, desensitizing the person through immunotherapy.

Anaphylaxis. Anaphylactic reactions occur suddenly in hypersensitive patients after exposure to the offending allergen. They may occur after parenteral injection of drugs (especially antibiotics), administration of blood products, and after insect stings. The cardinal principle in management is speed: (a) in recognizing signs and symptoms of an anaphylactic reaction, (b) in establishing and maintaining a patent airway, (c) in preventing spread of the allergen with the use of a tourniquet,

✚ TABLE 16-11   EMERGENCY MANAGEMENT

Anaphylactic Shock

Cause
- Injection of, inhalation of, ingestion of, or topical exposure to substance that produces profound allergic response

See Table 16-9 for more complete listing.

Assessment Findings

See Figure 16-7.

Interventions
Initial
- Ensure patent airway.
- Remove insect stinger if it is present.
- Administer epinephrine 1:1000, 0.2 to 0.5 mL subcut for mild symptoms; repeat at 20-minute intervals.
- Epinephrine 1:10000, 0.5 mL IV at 5- to 10-minute intervals for severe reaction.
- Administer high-flow oxygen via nonrebreather mask.
- Place patient in recumbent position, and elevate his or her legs.
- Keep patient warm.
- Administer diphenhydramine (Benadryl) IM or IV.
- Administer histamine H_2 blockers such as cimetidine.
- Maintain patient's blood pressure with fluids, volume expanders, vasopressors (e.g., dopamine, norepinephrine bitartrate [Levophed]).

Ongoing Monitoring
- Monitor vital signs, respiratory effort, oxygen saturation, level of consciousness, and cardiac rhythm.
- Anticipate intubation in cases of severe respiratory distress.
- Anticipate cricothyrotomy or tracheostomy in cases of severe laryngeal edema.

IM, intramuscularly; *IV*, intravenously; *subcut*, subcutaneously.

(d) in administering drugs, and (e) in performing treatment for shock (Waserman, Chad, Francoeur, et al., 2010). Table 16-11 summarizes the emergency treatment of anaphylactic shock.

In severe cases of anaphylaxis, hypovolemic shock may occur because of the loss of intravascular fluid into interstitial spaces secondary to increased capillary permeability (Vacca & McMahon-Bowen, 2013). Peripheral vasoconstriction and stimulation of the sympathetic nervous system occur to compensate for the fluid shift. However, unless shock is treated early, the body will no longer be able to compensate, and irreversible tissue damage will occur, leading to death. (Hypovolemic shock is further discussed in Chapter 69.)

All health care workers must be prepared for the rare but life-threatening anaphylactic reaction, which requires immediate medical and nursing interventions. It remains extremely important to identify all of the patient's allergies and document them in all appropriate areas in the chart (Yunker & Wagner, 2014).

Chronic Allergies. Most allergic reactions are chronic and are characterized by remissions and exacerbations of symptoms. Treatment focuses on identification and control of allergens, relief of symptoms through drug therapy, and hyposensitization of a patient to an offending allergen.

Allergen Recognition and Control. The nurse plays an important role in helping the patient make lifestyle adjustments to minimize exposure to the offending allergens and offers preventive measures that will help control the allergic symptoms. The nurse must reinforce that the patient will never be desensitized or completely symptom free, even with drug therapy and immunotherapy.

Of primary importance is the need to identify the offending allergen, at times performed through skin testing. In the case of food allergies, an elimination diet is sometimes helpful. If an allergic reaction occurs, all food previously eaten should be avoided at first and then gradually reintroduced sequentially until the offending food is identified.

Many allergic reactions, especially asthma and urticaria, may be aggravated by fatigue and emotional stress. The nurse can initiate a stress-management program with the patient that includes relaxation techniques when the patient comes for repeated immunotherapy treatments.

Sometimes, control of allergic symptoms necessitates environmental control, including changing an occupation, moving to a different climate, or giving up a favourite pet. In the case of airborne allergens, sleeping in an air-conditioned room, damp-dusting daily, covering mattresses and pillows with hypoallergenic covers, and wearing a mask outdoors may be helpful.

With an identified drug allergy, the patient should be instructed not only to avoid the drug but also to notify all health care providers of drug intolerance. The patient should wear a medical alert bracelet listing the particular drug allergy and have the offending drug listed on all medical and dental records.

For a patient allergic to insect stings, commercial bee-sting kits containing injectable epinephrine and a tourniquet are available. The nurse should instruct the patient and family on the technique of applying the tourniquet and self-injecting the subcutaneous epinephrine. These patients should wear a medical alert bracelet and carry a bee-sting kit whenever they go outdoors.

Drug Therapy. The major categories of drugs used for symptomatic relief of chronic allergic disorders include antihistamines, sympathomimetic or decongestant drugs, corticosteroids, antipruritic drugs, and mast cell–stabilizing drugs. Many of these drugs may be obtained over the counter.

Antihistamines. Antihistamines are the best drugs for treatment of allergic rhinitis and urticaria; however, they are less effective for severe allergic reactions (see Chapter 29, Table 29-2). They act by competing with histamine for H_1-receptor sites and thus blocking the effect of histamine. Best results are achieved if they are taken as soon as allergy symptoms appear. Antihistamines can be used effectively to treat edema and pruritus but are relatively ineffective in preventing bronchoconstriction. With seasonal rhinitis, antihistamines should be taken during peak pollen seasons. (Antihistamines are discussed further in Chapter 29.)

Sympathomimetic or Decongestant Drugs. The major sympathomimetic drug is epinephrine (Adrenalin), which is the drug of choice to treat an anaphylactic reaction. Epinephrine is a hormone produced by the adrenal medulla that stimulates α- and β-adrenergic receptors. Stimulation of the α-adrenergic receptors causes vasoconstriction of peripheral blood vessels. Stimulation of β-adrenergic receptors causes relaxation of the bronchial smooth muscles. Epinephrine also acts directly on mast cells to stabilize them against further degranulation. The action of epinephrine lasts only a few minutes. For the treatment of anaphylaxis, the drug must be given parenterally (subcutaneously, intramuscularly, or intravenously).

Several specific, minor sympathomimetic drugs differ from epinephrine because they can be taken orally or nasally and last for several hours. Included in this category are phenylephrine (Neo-Synephrine) and pseudoephedrine (Sudafed). The minor sympathomimetic drugs are used primarily to treat allergic rhinitis.

Corticosteroids. Nasal corticosteroid sprays are very effective in relieving the symptoms of allergic rhinitis (see Chapter 29, Table 29-2). Occasional patients may experience such severe manifestations of allergies that a brief course of oral corticosteroids is required.

Antipruritic Drugs. Topically applied antipruritic drugs protect the skin and provide relief from itching. They are most effective when the skin is not broken. Common OTC drugs include calamine lotion, coal tar solutions, and camphor. Menthol and phenol may be added to lotions to produce an antipruritic effect.

Mast Cell–Stabilizing Drugs. Nedocromil (Alocril) is a mast cell–stabilizing drug that inhibits the release of histamines, leukotrienes, and other agents from the mast cell after antigen–IgE interaction. It is currently available for topical ophthalmic use only.

Leukotriene Receptor Antagonists. Leukotriene receptor antagonists (LTRAs) block leukotriene, one of the major mediators of the allergic inflammatory process. They may be used in the treatment of allergic rhinitis and asthma. These medications can be taken orally. (For more information, refer to Chapters 29 and 31.)

Immunotherapy. Immunotherapy is the recommended treatment for control of allergic symptoms when the allergen cannot be avoided and drug therapy is not effective. Relatively few patients with allergies have symptoms so intolerable that they require allergy immunotherapy. Immunotherapy is absolutely indicated only in individuals with anaphylactic reactions to insect venom. It involves administration of small titres of an allergen extract in increasing strengths until hyposensitivity to the specific allergen is achieved. For best results, the patient should continue to avoid the offending allergen whenever possible because complete desensitization is impossible. Unfortunately, not all allergy-related conditions respond to immunotherapy. Food allergies cannot be safely treated with this therapy, and eczema may worsen with immunotherapy.

Mechanism of Action. The IgE level is elevated in atopic individuals. When IgE combines with an allergen in a hypersensitive person, a reaction occurs in which histamine is released in various body tissues. Allergens more readily combine with IgG than with other immunoglobulins. Therefore, immunotherapy involves injecting allergen extracts that will stimulate increases in IgG levels. The binding of IgG to allergen-reactive sites interferes with allergen binding to mast cell–bound IgE, preventing mast cell degranulation and thus reducing the number of reactions that cause tissue damage. The goal of long-term immunotherapy is to maintain high levels of "blocking" IgG. In addition, allergen-specific T suppressor cells develop in individuals receiving immunotherapy.

Method of Administration. Allergens included in immunotherapy are chosen based on the results of skin testing with a panel of allergens.

Subcutaneous Immunotherapy. Subcutaneous immunotherapy (SCIT) involves the subcutaneous injection of titrated amounts of allergen extracts biweekly or weekly. The dose is small at first and is increased slowly until a maintenance dosage is reached. In general, it takes 1 to 2 years of immunotherapy to reach the maximal therapeutic effect. Therapy may be continued for about 5 years. After that, discontinuing therapy is considered. In many patients, a decrease in symptoms is sustained after the treatment is discontinued. For patients with severe allergies or sensitivity to insect stings, maintenance therapy is continued indefinitely. Best results are achieved when immunotherapy is administered throughout the year.

Sublingual Immunotherapy. Sublingual immunotherapy (SLIT) involves allergen extracts taken under the tongue. SLIT has been used in Europe for decades and has recently become available in Canada. Products include a five-grass pollen tablet (Oralair), a single-grass pollen tablet (Grastek), and a ragweed pollen tablet (Ragwitek) (Lee, Nolte, & Benninger, 2015).

SLIT is self-administered (usually daily) by patients at home, although the initial dose is usually given under medical supervision. Some patients experience local application-site reactions (e.g., oral pruritus, throat irritation, tongue swelling), but systemic allergic reactions are markedly fewer than with SCIT. Local reactions subside in many patients within a few days to a week.

An advantage of SLIT is the convenience of an oral therapy that is self-administered and that patients can use at home. The main disadvantage of SLIT is that it requires the patient to be consistently compliant with therapy (Compalati, Braido, & Canonica, 2013).

NURSING MANAGEMENT
IMMUNOTHERAPY

The nurse is often the professional primarily responsible for administering SCIT. Adverse reactions should always be anticipated, especially when a new strength of the dose is used, after a previous reaction occurred, or after a dose is missed. Early signs and symptoms indicative of a systemic reaction include pruritus, urticaria, sneezing, laryngeal edema, and hypotension. Emergency measures for anaphylactic shock should be initiated immediately. A local reaction should be described according to the degree of redness and swelling at the injection site. If the area is greater than the size of a quarter in an adult, the reaction should be reported to the health care provider so that the allergen dosage may be decreased.

Immunotherapy always carries the risk for a severe anaphylactic reaction. Therefore, when injections are given, a health care provider, emergency equipment, and essential medications should be available.

Accurate record keeping is invaluable because it can prevent an adverse reaction to the allergen extract. Before giving the injection, the nurse should check the patient's name against the name on the vial, check the vial strength, the amount of the previous dose, the date of the previous dose, and any reaction information previously identified.

The nurse should always administer the allergen extract in an extremity away from a joint so that a tourniquet can be applied in the event of a severe reaction. The site should be rotated for each injection. Before giving an injection, the nurse must aspirate for blood to ensure the allergen extract is not injected into a blood vessel. An injection directly into the bloodstream can potentiate an anaphylactic reaction. After the injection is given, the patient should be carefully observed for 20 minutes because systemic reactions typically occur immediately. However, the patient should be warned that a delayed reaction can occur as long as 24 hours later.

Latex Allergies

Allergies to latex products have become a problem of increasing proportion, affecting both patients and health care providers. The increase in allergic reactions has coincided with the sharp increase in glove use related to the introduction of universal precautions against infectious diseases in 1987. The more frequent and prolonged the exposure to latex, the greater the likelihood of developing a latex allergy.

In addition to gloves, many other latex-containing products are used in health care, such as blood pressure cuffs, stethoscopes, tourniquets, intravenous (IV) tubing, syringes, electrode pads, oxygen masks, tracheal tubes, colostomy and ileostomy pouches, urinary catheters, anaesthetic masks, and adhesive tape. Latex proteins can become aerosolized through powder on gloves and can result in serious reactions when inhaled by sensitized individuals. It is recommended that all health care facilities use powder-free gloves to avoid respiratory exposure to latex proteins (Canadian Centre for Occupational Health and Safety [CCOHS], 2014).

Types of Latex Allergies. Two types of latex allergies can occur: type IV allergic contact dermatitis and type I allergic reactions. Type IV contact dermatitis is caused by the chemicals used in the manufacturing process of latex gloves. It is a delayed reaction that occurs within 6 to 48 hours. Typically, the person first has dryness, pruritus, fissuring, and cracking of the skin, followed by redness, swelling, and crusting at 24 to 48 hours. The dermatitis may extend beyond the area of physical contact with the allergen. Chronic exposure can lead to lichenification, scaling, and hyperpigmentation.

A type I allergic reaction is a response to the natural rubber latex proteins and occurs within minutes of contact with the proteins. These types of allergic reactions can manifest as various reactions ranging from skin redness, urticaria, rhinitis, conjunctivitis, or asthma to full-blown anaphylactic shock. Systemic reactions to latex may result from exposure to latex protein via various routes, including the skin, mucous membranes, lungs, or blood.

Latex-Food Syndrome. Because some proteins in rubber are similar to food proteins, some foods may cause an allergic reaction in people who are allergic to latex. This is called *latex-food syndrome.* The most common of these foods are banana, avocado, chestnut, kiwi, tomato, water chestnut, guava, hazelnut, potato, peach, grape, and apricot. In people with latex allergy, most have a positive allergy test to at least one related food.

NURSING AND COLLABORATIVE MANAGEMENT LATEX ALLERGIES

The identification of patients and health care providers who are sensitive to latex is crucial to preventing adverse reactions. A thorough health history and history of any allergies should be documented, especially for patients with any complaints of latex contact symptoms. Not all latex-sensitive individuals can be identified, even with a carefully documented history. Risk factors include long-term multiple exposures to latex products (e.g., health care providers, individuals who have undergone multiple surgical procedures, rubber-industry workers). Additional risk factors include a patient history of allergic rhinitis, asthma, and allergies to certain foods (listed earlier). The Canadian Centre for Occupational Health and Safety (CCOHS) has published recommendations for preventing allergic reactions to latex in the workplace (2014) (Table 16-12).

Latex precaution protocols should be used for patients identified as having either a positive reaction to a latex allergy test or a history of signs and symptoms related to latex exposure. Many health care facilities have created latex-free product carts that can be used for patients with latex allergies.

TABLE 16-12	RECOMMENDATIONS FOR PREVENTING ALLERGIC REACTIONS TO LATEX IN THE WORKPLACE

1. Powder-free, nonlatex gloves with reduced protein content should be used.
2. Those who wear latex gloves should avoid oil-based hand creams or lotions, which can cause deterioration of latex.
3. Good work and housekeeping practices can help prevent contact with latex-containing dust in the workplace, including contact with eyes and face; hands should be washed after glove removal.
4. Education programs about latex allergies are available in some workplaces.
5. People who suspect an allergy to latex rubber products should consult an allergist to determine if the allergy is to latex (natural) rubber or to chemicals in synthetic rubbers.
6. The symptoms of latex allergy include skin rash; hives; flushing; itching; nasal, eye, or sinus symptoms; asthma; and (rarely) shock.
7. Health care providers (e.g., physicians, nurse practitioners, and dentists) should be notified of any allergy so that they can decide if alternative products should be used in any treatment that normally requires the use of rubber products.

Source: Adapted from Canadian Centre for Occupational Health and Safety. (2014). *Latex allergy.* Retrieved from *https://www.ccohs.ca/oshanswers/diseases/latex.html;* and National Institute for Occupational Safety Health. (n.d.) *NIOSH alert: Preventing allergic reactions to natural rubber latex in the workplace.* Retrieved from *http://www.cdc.gov/niosh/docs/97-135/pdfs/97-135.pdf.*

Multiple Chemical Sensitivities

Multiple chemical sensitivities (MCS) is a subjective illness marked by recurrent, nonspecific symptoms attributed to low levels of chemical, biological, or physical agents. Common causative substances include smoke, pesticides, plastics, synthetic fabrics, scented products, petroleum products, and paint fumes. Women between the ages of 30 and 50 are more likely to develop the symptoms. MCS is a controversial diagnosis and is not formally recognized as an illness by the Canadian Medical Association or other authorities (Sears, 2007).

These symptoms are usually subjective and are not found during physical examination. The patient experiences wide-ranging symptoms, but evidence of pathological processes or physiological dysfunction is lacking. Symptoms include headache, fatigue, dizziness, nausea, congestion, itching, sneezing, sore throat, chest pain, breathing problems, muscle pain or stiffness, skin rash, diarrhea, bloating, gas, confusion, difficulty concentrating, memory problems, and mood changes.

Diagnosis is usually made based on a patient's health history as there is no established test to diagnose MCS. Treatment includes minimizing or avoiding the chemicals that may trigger the symptoms and creating a chemical-free and odor-free home and workplace.

Psychotherapy is recommended as a primary option. In patients who are unwilling to undergo psychotherapy but willing to accept medications, antidepressants including selective serotonin reuptake inhibitors (SSRIs) (e.g., citalopram [Celexa]) have been used for treatment. Drugs for anxiety and sleep have also been used.

AUTOIMMUNITY

Autoimmunity is an immune reaction to self-proteins: the immune system no longer differentiates self from nonself. For unknown reasons, immune cells that are normally unresponsive (tolerant of self-antigens) are activated. In autoimmunity, autoantibodies and autosensitized T cells cause pathophysiological tissue damage (Mak, Saunders, & Jett, 2014).

The cause of autoimmune diseases remains unknown. Age is thought to play a role since the number of circulating autoantibodies increases in people over age 50. However, the principal factors in the development of autoimmunity are (a) the inheritance of susceptibility genes, which may contribute to the failure of self-tolerance, and (b) initiation of autoreactivity by triggers, such as infections, that may activate self-reactive lymphocytes.

Autoimmune diseases tend to occur in clusters, so an individual may have more than one autoimmune disease (e.g., rheumatoid arthritis and Addison's disease), or the same or related autoimmune diseases may be found in other members of the same family. This observation has led to the concept of genetic predisposition to autoimmune disease.

Most of the genetic research in this area correlates certain human leukocyte antigen (HLA) types with an autoimmune condition. (HLAs and disease association are discussed later in this chapter.) Even in a genetically predisposed person, some triggering event is necessary for the initiation of autoreactivity. This event may include infection with an agent such as a virus (Mak, Saunders, & Jett, 2014). Viral infections can alter cells or tissues that make them antigenic. There is some evidence that viruses may be involved in the development of diseases such as type 1 diabetes mellitus. Rheumatic fever and rheumatic heart disease are autoimmune responses triggered by streptococcal infection and mediated by antibodies against group A β-hemolytic streptococci that cross-react with heart muscles, heart valves, and synovial membranes.

Medications can also be precipitating factors in autoimmune diseases. For example, hemolytic anemia can result from methyldopa (Novo-Medopa) administration, and procainamide (Apo-Procainamide) can induce the formation of antinuclear antibodies and cause a lupus-like syndrome.

Gender and hormones also have a role in autoimmune diseases, with more women than men affected. During pregnancy, symptoms of many autoimmune diseases improve; however, after delivery, the disease frequently worsens.

Autoimmune Diseases

In general, autoimmune diseases are grouped according to organ-specific and systemic diseases. (Table 16-13 lists examples of autoimmune diseases.) SLE is a classic example of a systemic autoimmune disease characterized by damage to multiple organs. It occurs most frequently in women, with onset at 20 to 40 years of age. The cause is unknown, but there appears to be a loss of self-tolerance for the body's own deoxyribonucleic acid (DNA) antigens.

In SLE, tissue injury appears to be the result of the formation of antinuclear antibodies. For an unknown reason (possibly a viral infection), the cell membrane is damaged and DNA is released into the systemic circulation, where it is viewed as nonself material. This DNA is normally sequestered inside the nucleus of cells. On release into circulation, the DNA antigen reacts with an antibody. Some antibodies are involved in immune-complex formation, and others may cause damage directly. Once the complexes are deposited, complement is activated and further damages the tissue, especially the renal glomerulus. (SLE is discussed further in Chapter 67.)

TABLE 16-13	EXAMPLES OF AUTOIMMUNE DISEASES*
Systemic Diseases	**Endocrine System**
• Systemic lupus erythematosus (SLE)	• Addison's disease
• Rheumatoid arthritis	• Thyroiditis
• Progressive systemic sclerosis (scleroderma)	• Hypothyroidism
• Mixed connective tissue disease	• Type 1 diabetes mellitus
Organ-Specific Diseases	**Gastro-Intestinal System**
Blood	• Pernicious anemia
• Autoimmune hemolytic anemia	• Ulcerative colitis
• Immune thrombocytopenic purpura	**Kidney**
	• Goodpasture's syndrome
	• Glomerulonephritis
Central Nervous System	**Liver**
• Multiple sclerosis	• Primary biliary cirrhosis
• Guillain-Barré syndrome	• Autoimmune hepatitis
Muscle	**Eye**
• Myasthenia gravis	• Uveitis
Heart	
• Rheumatic fever	

*These diseases are discussed in various chapters throughout the book.

Apheresis

Apheresis has been effectively used to treat autoimmune diseases and other diseases and disorders. Apheresis is a procedure in which components of the blood are separated and then one or more of those components is removed. Compound words are often used to describe an apheresis procedure, depending on the blood components being collected. For example, platelet-pheresis is the removal of platelets, usually for collection from normal individuals to infuse into patients with low platelet counts (e.g., patients taking chemotherapy who develop thrombocytopenia). *Leukocytapheresis* is a general term indicating the removal of WBCs, a technique used in chronic myelogenous leukemia to remove high numbers of leukemic cells.

Apheresis is also used in hematopoietic stem cell transplantation to collect stem cells from peripheral blood. These stem cells can then be used to repopulate a person's bone marrow after high-dose chemotherapy (see the section "Peripheral Stem Cell Transplantation" in Chapter 18).

Plasmapheresis. Plasmapheresis is the removal of plasma-containing components that cause or are thought to cause disease. It can also be used to obtain plasma from healthy donors to administer to patients as replacement therapy.

When plasma is removed, it is replaced by substitution fluids such as saline, fresh-frozen plasma, or albumin. Therefore, the term *plasma exchange* more accurately describes this procedure.

Plasmapheresis has been used to treat autoimmune diseases such as SLE, glomerulonephritis, Goodpasture's syndrome, myasthenia gravis, thrombocytopenic purpura, rheumatoid arthritis, and Guillain-Barré syndrome. Many disorders for which plasmapheresis is being used are characterized by circulating autoantibodies (usually of the IgG class) and antigen–antibody complexes. The rationale for performing therapeutic plasmapheresis in autoimmune disorders is to remove pathological substances present in plasma. Immuno-suppressive therapy has been used to prevent recovery of IgG production, and plasmapheresis has been used to prevent antibody rebound.

In addition to removing antibodies and antigen–antibody complexes, plasmapheresis may remove inflammatory mediators (e.g., complement) that are responsible for tissue damage. In the treatment of SLE, plasmapheresis is usually reserved for patients in an acute attack who are unresponsive to conventional therapy.

Plasmapheresis involves the removal of whole blood through an IV needle and then the circulation of the blood through a cell separator. Inside the separator, the blood is divided into plasma and its cellular components by centrifugation or membrane filtration. Plasma, platelets, WBCs, or erythrocytes can be separated selectively. The undesirable component is removed, and the remainder is returned to the patient. The plasma is generally replaced with normal saline, lactated Ringer's solution, fresh-frozen plasma, plasma protein fractions, or albumin. When blood is manually removed, only 500 mL may be taken at one time. However, with the use of apheresis procedures, more than 4 L of plasma can be removed in 2 to 3 hours.

As with administration of other blood products, nurses must be aware of adverse effects associated with plasmapheresis. The most common complications are hypotension and citrate toxicity. Hypotension is usually the result of vasovagal reaction or transient volume changes. Citrate is used as an anticoagulant and may cause hypocalcemia, which may manifest as headache, paresthesias, and dizziness.

IMMUNODEFICIENCY DISORDERS

The condition in which the immune system does not adequately protect the body is **immunodeficiency**. Immunodeficiency disorders involve an impairment of one or more immune mechanisms, which include (a) phagocytosis, (b) humoral response, (c) cell-mediated immune response, (d) complement, and (e) a combined humoral and cell-mediated deficiency. Immunodeficiency disorders are primary if the immune cells are improperly developed or absent and secondary if the deficiency is caused by illnesses or treatment. Primary immunodeficiency disorders are rare and often serious, whereas secondary disorders are more common and less severe.

Primary Immunodeficiency Disorders

The basic categories of primary immunodeficiency disorders are (a) phagocytic defects, (b) B-cell deficiency, (c) T-cell deficiency, and (d) a combined B-cell and T-cell deficiency (Kasper, Fauci, Hauser, et al., 2015; Table 16-14).

Secondary Immunodeficiency Disorders

Some important factors that may cause secondary immunodeficiency disorders are listed in Table 16-15. Drug-induced immuno-suppression is the most common. Immuno-suppressive therapy is prescribed for patients to treat autoimmune disorders and to prevent transplant rejection. In addition, immuno-suppression is a serious adverse effect of drugs used in cancer chemotherapy. Generalized leukopenia often results from chemotherapeutic drugs, leading to a decreased humoral and cell-mediated immune response. Therefore, secondary infections are common in immuno-suppressed patients.

Malnutrition alters cell-mediated immune responses. When protein is deficient over a prolonged period, the thymus gland

TABLE 16-14	PRIMARY IMMUNODEFICIENCY DISORDERS	
Disorder	**Affected Cells**	**Genetic Basis**
Chronic granulomatous disease	PMNs, monocytes	Sex-linked
Job syndrome	PMNs, monocytes	—
Bruton (X-linked) agammaglobulinemia	B	Sex-linked
Common variable hypogammaglobulinemia	B	—
Selective IgA, IgM, or IgG deficiency	B	Some sex-linked
DiGeorge syndrome (thymic hypoplasia)	T	—
Severe combined immunodeficiency disease	Stem, B, T	Sex-linked or autosomal recessive
Ataxia-telangiectasia	B, T	Autosomal recessive
Wiskott–Aldrich syndrome	B, T	Sex-linked
Graft-versus-host disease	B, T	—

IgA, immunoglobulin A; *IgG,* immunoglobulin G; *IgM,* immunoglobulin M; *PMN,* polymorphonuclear neutrophil.

TABLE 16-15	CAUSES OF SECONDARY IMMUNODEFICIENCY

- Age
  - Infants
  - Older adults
- Anaesthesia
- Burns
- Cachexia
- Chemotherapeutic drugs
- Cirrhosis
- Corticosteroids
- Dietary deficiency
- Drug-induced immunodeficiency
- Malnutrition
- Predisposing factors
  - Acquired immune deficiency syndrome (AIDS)
  - Alcoholic cirrhosis
  - Chronic renal disease
  - Diabetes mellitus
  - Malignancies
  - Systemic lupus erythematosus
- Radiation
- Stress
- Surgery
- Trauma

atrophies, and lymphoid tissue decreases. In addition, an increased susceptibility to infections always exists with malnourishment.

Hodgkin's lymphoma also greatly impairs the cell-mediated immune response, and patients may die from severe viral or fungal infections. (Hodgkin's lymphoma is discussed in Chapter 18.) Viruses, especially rubella, may cause immunodeficiency by direct cytotoxic damage to lymphoid cells. Systemic infections can place such a demand on the immune system that resistance to a secondary or subsequent infection becomes impaired.

Radiation can destroy lymphocytes either directly or through depletion of stem cells. As the radiation dose is increased, more bone marrow atrophies, leading to severe pancytopenia and suppression of immune function. Splenectomy in children is especially dangerous and may lead to septicemia simply from respiratory tract infections.

The immune response involves interrelationships among the nervous, endocrine, and immune systems and can be altered by stress (see Chapter 8).

Human Leukocyte Antigen System

The antigens responsible for rejection of genetically unlike tissues are called the *major histocompatibility antigens.* These antigens are products of histocompatibility genes. In humans, they are called the human leukocyte antigen (HLA) system. The genes for the HLA antigens are linked and occur together on the sixth chromosome. HLAs are present on all nucleated cells and platelets. The HLA system plays an important part in the body's immune response to foreign substances and, therefore, is used in matching organs and tissues for transplantation.

An important characteristic of HLA genes is that they are highly polymorphic (variable). Each HLA locus can have many different possible alleles, and thus many combinations exist. Each person has two alleles for each locus, one inherited from each parent. Both alleles of a locus are expressed independently (i.e., they are codominant). The proteins encoded by certain genes are known as *antigens.*

The entire set of A, B, C, and D/DR genes (the HLA genes) is located on one chromosome and is termed a *haplotype.* The complete set is inherited as a unit. One haplotype is inherited from each parent (Figure 16-10). This means that a person has HLA genes that are one-half identical to those of each parent. The HLA genes of one person have a 25% chance of being identical to the HLA genes of a sibling.

In organ transplantation, A, B, and DR are primarily used for compatibility matching. The specific allele at each locus is identified by a number. For example, a person could have an HLA of A2, A6, B7, B27, DR4, and DR7. Currently more than 8000 HLA alleles have been identified for the various HLA genes.

Human Leukocyte Antigen and Disease Associations. The early interest in HLA was stimulated by its potential role in matching donors and recipients of organ transplants. Since that time, interest in the association between HLA and disease has grown.

A number of diseases show significant associations with specific HLA alleles. People who have these alleles are much more likely to develop the associated disease than those who do not have the allele. However, the possession of a particular HLA allele does not mean that the person will necessarily develop the associated disease—only that the relative risk is greater than in the general population.

Most of the HLA-associated diseases are classified as autoimmune disorders. Examples of associations between HLA types and diseases include (a) the presence of HLA-B27 with ankylosing spondylitis, (b) the presence of HLA-DR2 and HLA-DR3 with SLE, (c) the presence of HLA-DR3 and HLA-DR4 with diabetes mellitus, and (d) the presence of HLA-DR2 with narcolepsy.

It is now known that at least part of the genetic basis of HLA-associated diseases lies in the HLA region, but the actual mechanisms involved in these associations are still unknown. However, most individuals who inherit an HLA type associated with a disease never actually develop the disease. While the discovery of HLA associations with certain diseases is a major breakthrough in understanding the genetic basis of these diseases, this information is, at present, of little practical clinical importance. Nevertheless, there is promise for the development of clinical applications in the future. For example, in families with certain autoimmune diseases, it may be possible to identify the members who are at greatest risk for developing the same or a related autoimmune disease. These people would need close medical supervision, implementation of preventive measures (if possible), and early diagnosis and treatment to prevent chronic complications.

ORGAN TRANSPLANTATION

During the 1960s, organ and tissue transplantation was considered an experimental procedure reserved for patients with critical end-stage medical disease. However, as a result of advances in medical technology, including histocompatibility testing, surgical procedures, and improved immuno-suppressive regimens, organ transplantation has resulted in improved survival rates and quality of life. Organ transplantation is the transfer of a whole or partial organ from one individual to another for the purpose of replacing the recipient's damaged or failing organ with a working one from the donor. Commonly transplanted organs and tissues include the heart, lungs, liver, kidneys, pancreas, corneas, skin, bone marrow, heart valves, bone, and connective tissues (Figure 16-11). Corneas are transplanted to prevent or correct blindness, and skin grafts are used to assist in managing burns. Bone marrow or stem cells are transplanted to help patients with leukemias and other hematological malignancies.

Organs can be successfully transplanted together; for example, a patient may receive both a pancreas transplant for pancreatic insufficiency and a kidney transplant for renal failure.

Some organs may be transplanted in segments rather than in their entirety. Liver and lung lobes may be transplanted, or an intestine may be used in segments, thus allowing one person's organ donation to benefit multiple recipients. This technique not only enables living donors to donate part of an organ while maintaining their functioning organ but also addresses the high rate of mortality among patients on the waiting list that results from poor organ donation rates.

FIGURE 16-10 Patterns of human leukocyte antigen (HLA) inheritance. **A,** HLA genes are located on chromosome 6. **B,** The two haplotypes of the father are labelled P¹ and P², and the haplotypes of the mother are labelled M¹ and M². Each child inherits two haplotypes, one from each parent. **C,** Therefore, only four combinations—P¹M¹, P¹M², P²M¹, P²M²—are possible, and the offspring have a 25% chance of having identical HLA haplotypes.

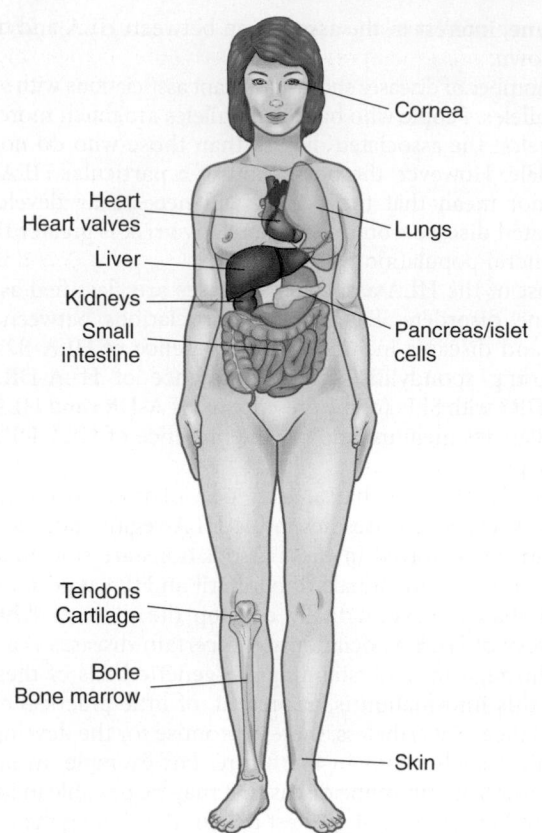

- Cornea
- Heart
- Heart valves
- Lungs
- Liver
- Kidneys
- Small intestine
- Pancreas/islet cells
- Tendons
- Cartilage
- Bone
- Bone marrow
- Skin

FIGURE 16-11 Tissues and organs that can be transplanted.

Organ donations can be taken from two sources: deceased (cadaveric) and living donors. Patients are matched to available donors through ABO blood and HLA typing, medical urgency, body size, and, for some organs, length of time on the waiting list. Currently, most donated organs originate from deceased donors. The majority of living donors are relatives of the recipient, although a number are also unrelated living donors.

In order to become an organ or tissue donor, an individual either signs an organ and tissue donor card or registers his or her consent through the provincial registry. However, despite registering as an organ or tissue donor, the individual is encouraged to discuss the decision with loved ones because doctors will not proceed with donation without the consent of family members. (Organ donation is discussed further in Chapter 71.)

Nurses caring for a patient in the intensive care unit or emergency department who has a diagnosis of brain death should discuss with the health care team the option of organ donation for the patient's family. The local organ procurement organization should then be contacted to speak with the family.

Tissue Typing

The recipient usually receives a transplant from an ABO blood group–compatible donor (see Chapter 32, Table 32-10). The donor and recipient do not need to share the same Rh factor.

HLA Typing. HLA typing is done on potential donors and recipients. Currently only the A, B, and DR antigens are thought to be clinically significant for transplantation. Because each locus has two alleles that encode for antigens, a total of six antigens are identified. In transplantation, an attempt is made to match as many antigens as possible between the HLA-A, HLA-B, and HLA-DR loci. Antigen matches of five and six antigens and

certain four-antigen matches have been found to have better clinical outcomes (i.e., the patient is less likely to reject the transplanted organ), especially in kidney and bone marrow transplants.

The degree of HLA matching required or deemed suitable for successful solid organ transplantation depends on the type of organ. Certain organ and tissue transplants require a closer histocompatibility match than other organs. For example, a cornea transplant can be accepted by nearly any individual because corneas are avascular, and therefore no antibodies reach the cornea to cause rejection. In kidney and bone marrow transplantation, HLA matching is very important, since these transplants are at high risk for graft rejection. On the other hand, for liver transplants, HLA mismatches have little impact on graft survival. Heart and lung transplants fall somewhere in between, but minimizing HLA mismatches significantly improves survival. In addition, for liver, lung, and heart transplants, fewer donors are available; therefore, it can be more difficult to obtain good HLA matches.

Transporting, storing, and then implanting donated organs take time and the "best" match may live many miles from the "ideal" recipient. The need to have the "best" matches has to be balanced against the time it takes to retrieve, transport, and transplant a donated organ.

Panel of Reactive Antibodies. A panel of reactive antibodies (PRA) indicates the recipient's sensitivity to various HLAs before receiving a transplant. To detect preformed antibodies to HLA, the recipient's serum is mixed with a randomly selected panel of donor lymphocytes to determine reactivity. The potential recipient may have been exposed to HLA antigens by means of previous blood transfusions, pregnancy, or a previous organ transplant.

PRA allows for the determination of whether a recipient is of high or low reactivity to potential donors. The results for the PRA are calculated in percentages. A high PRA indicates that the person has a large number of cytotoxic antibodies and is highly sensitized, which means there is a reduced chance of finding a crossmatch-negative donor. In patients awaiting transplantation, a PRA panel is usually done on a routine basis. In highly sensitized patients (high PRA), plasmapheresis and IV immunoglobulin (IVIG) can be used to reduce the number of circulating antibodies.

Crossmatch. A crossmatch is done to determine the existence of antibodies against the potential donor. A crossmatch uses serum from the recipient mixed with donor lymphocytes to test for any preformed anti-HLA antibodies to the potential donor organ. The crossmatch can be used as a screening test when possible living donors are being considered or once a cadaver donor is selected.

A negative crossmatch indicates that no preformed antibodies are present and it is safe to proceed with transplantation. A positive crossmatch indicates that the recipient has cytotoxic antibodies to the donor and is an absolute contraindication in living donor transplants such as in kidney transplants. Live donor transplants may be done for patients with a positive crossmatch if no other live donors (with a negative crossmatch) exist. In this situation, plasmapheresis or IVIG can be performed to remove antibodies.

It is not always possible to complete a crossmatch prior to transplantation. If a retrospective crossmatch has to be done, the results will have implications for immuno-suppression protocols after the transplantation.

Transplant Rejection

Rejection is one of the major contributing factors for organ loss after solid organ transplantation. Organ rejection can occur if the HLA profile of the donor organ does not identically match that of the recipient. Rejection can be prevented through close matching of ABO and HLA profiles of the donor and recipient. Unfortunately, because many differing HLA profiles have been found in humans, a perfect match is impossible, with the exception of tissue matching of identical twins. Three forms of rejection can develop: hyperacute, acute, or chronic. Prevention, early diagnosis, and treatment of rejection are essential for long-term graft function.

Hyperacute Rejection. Hyperacute rejection (also called *antibody-mediated* or *humoral rejection*) occurs minutes to hours after transplantation. Hyperacute rejection may result from antibody development through a number of mechanisms, some of which are not clearly understood. Recipients who have received prior blood transfusions may have antibodies to major histocompatibility complex antigens from the transfused blood that may match those in the graft (donated organ), which results in hyperacute rejection. Furthermore, multiple prior pregnancies may have exposed a woman to paternal antigens of the fetus, resulting in the development of antibodies. In the absence of these factors, antibody-mediated rejection may occur nonetheless, and the cause often remains unknown.

Acute Rejection. Acute rejection most commonly occurs days to months after transplantation. This type of rejection is mediated by the recipient's T cytotoxic lymphocytes, which attack the foreign organ (Figure 16-12). In addition to cell-mediated rejection, another type of acute rejection occurs when the recipient develops antibodies to the transplanted organ (humoral rejection). Many transplant recipients experience at least one rejection episode after transplantation. These episodes are usually reversible with alteration in or additional immuno-suppressive therapy that may include increased corticosteroid doses or polyclonal

or monoclonal antibody treatment. Unfortunately, increased doses of immuno-suppressants increase the risk for infection. To combat acute rejection, all patients with transplants require lifelong use of immuno-suppressants, putting them at a high risk for infection, especially in the first few months after transplantation, when the immuno-suppressant doses are highest.

Chronic Rejection. Chronic rejection is a process that occurs over months to years and is considered irreversible. The transplanted organ is infiltrated with large numbers of T and B cells, which is characteristic of an ongoing, low-grade, immune-mediated injury. Chronic rejection results in fibrosis and scarring. In heart transplants, it manifests as accelerated coronary artery disease. In lung transplants, it manifests as bronchiolitis obliterans, which is inflammation and fibrosis of the small airways. In liver transplants, it is characterized by loss of bile ducts. In kidney transplants, it manifests as fibrosis and glomerulopathy.

No definitive therapy is yet available for chronic rejection. Switching immuno-suppressive therapy has yielded some improvement for patients; however, treatment has largely been supportive. Ultimately, the prognosis for patients with chronic rejection remains poor, and if possible, such patients should be offered the option of retransplantation.

IMMUNO-SUPPRESSIVE THERAPY

The goal of immuno-suppressive therapy is to adequately suppress the immune response to prevent rejection of the transplanted organ and yet maintain sufficient immunity to prevent overwhelming infection. Immuno-suppressive therapy is also used to treat autoimmune diseases.

Many of the medications used to achieve immuno-suppression have adverse effects. The most common medications, routes of administration, mechanisms of action, and adverse effects are listed in Table 16-16. In a combination of medications that work in different phases of the immune response, lower doses of each drug produce effective immuno-suppression and minimize adverse effects. The major immuno-suppressive agents are (a) calcineurin inhibitors, which include cyclosporin (Sandimmune, Neoral) and tacrolimus (Prograf); (b) corticosteroids (prednisone, methylprednisolone [Solu-Medrol] by IV route); (c) mycophenolate mofetil (CellCept); and (d) sirolimus (Rapamune). Azathioprine (Imuran) and cyclophosphamide (Procytox) are also used but less frequently, because of the effectiveness of the newer generation of immuno-suppressants. Antithymocyte globulin, antilymphocyte globulin, and muromonab-CD3 (OKT 3) are medications administered intravenously for short periods to prevent early rejection (induction therapy) or to reverse acute rejection.

Immuno-suppressive protocols are highly variable among transplant centres, with different combinations of medications being used. Most patients are initially on triple therapy, which includes a calcineurin inhibitor, a corticosteroid, and either mycophenolate mofetil (CellCept) or azathioprine (Imuran). The doses of immuno-suppressant drugs are reduced over time after the transplant, with some organ groups able to wean off corticosteroids entirely.

Calcineurin Inhibitors

This group of drugs, including tacrolimus (Prograf) and cyclosporin (Sandimmune, Neoral), is the foundation of most immuno-suppression regimens. These drugs prevent a cell-mediated attack against the transplanted organ (Figure 16-13).

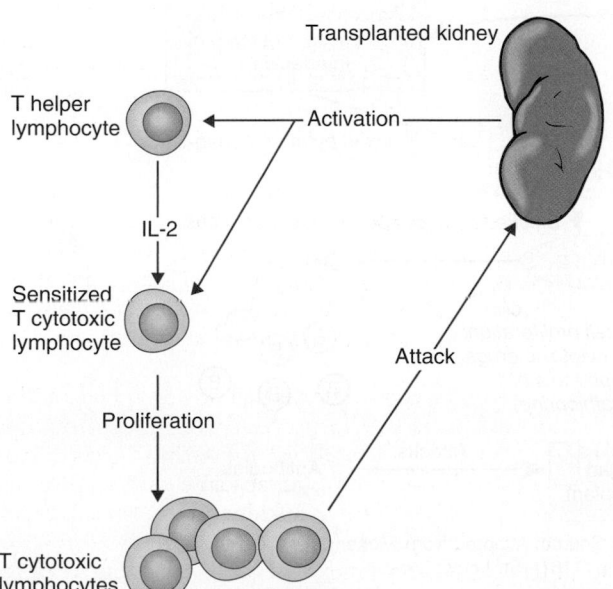

FIGURE 16-12 Mechanism of action of T cytotoxic lymphocyte activation and attack of transplanted tissue. The transplanted organ (e.g., kidney) is recognized as foreign, and the immune system is activated. T helper cells are activated to produce interleukin-2 (IL-2), and T cytotoxic lymphocytes are sensitized. After the T cytotoxic cells proliferate, they attack the transplanted organ.

TABLE 16-16 DRUG THERAPY

Immuno-Suppressive Therapy

Agent	Route	Mechanism of Action	Adverse Effects
Corticosteroids: prednisone, methylprednisolone (Solu-Medrol)	PO, IV	Suppress inflammatory response; inhibit cytokine production and T-cell activation	Peptic ulcers, hypertension, GI bleeding, osteoporosis, aseptic necrosis, Na$^+$ and H$_2$O retention, acne, muscle weakness, easy bruising, delayed healing, hyperglycemia, ↑ appetite, mood alterations, leukopenia, cataracts, dyslipidemia, ↓ resistance to infection
Tacrolimus (Prograf)	PO, IV	Inhibits calcineurin; prevents production and release of IL-2, IL-4, and α-interferon; inhibits production of T cytotoxic lymphocytes	Nephrotoxicity, neurotoxicity, seizures, tremors, nausea and vomiting, hyperglycemia, hypertension, alopecia, lymphoma, ↓ resistance to infection
Cyclosporine (Sandimmune, Neoral*)	PO, IV	Inhibits calcineurin; prevents production and release of IL-2, IL-4, and α-interferon; inhibits production of T cytotoxic lymphocytes	Nephrotoxicity, neurotoxicity, headaches, seizures, tremors, hyperglycemia, hypertension, nausea and vomiting, dyslipidemia, gingival hyperplasia, hirsutism, hepatotoxicity, lymphoma, ↓ resistance to infection
Mycophenolate mofetil (CellCept)	PO, IV	Antimetabolite that inhibits purine synthesis; suppresses proliferation of T and B cells	Diarrhea, nausea and vomiting, leukopenia, thrombocytopenia, ↓ resistance to infection, ↑ incidence of malignancies
Sirolimus (Rapamune)	PO	Suppresses lymphocyte proliferation; inhibits B cells from synthesizing antibodies	Diarrhea, dyslipidemia, hypercholesterolemia, arthralgias, delayed wound healing, thrombocytopenia, ↓ resistance to infection, ↑ incidence of malignancies
Muromonab-CD3 (OKT3)	IV push	Monoclonal antibody that binds to CD3 receptors on lymphocytes, causing cell lysis; inhibits function of cytotoxic T cells	Fever, chills, tachycardia, pulmonary edema, muscle and joint pain, diarrhea, hypertension or hypotension, aseptic meningitis, ↓ resistance to infection, ↑ incidence of malignancies
Basiliximab (Simulect)	IV	Monoclonal antibody that acts as IL-2 receptor antagonist by inhibiting the binding of IL-2; inhibits T-cell activation and proliferation	Generally no adverse effects
Polyclonal antibody serums: ATG, ALG (Thymoglobulin, ATGAM)	IV	Polyclonal antibodies directed against lymphocytes; particularly deplete T cells	Serum sickness (fever, chills, muscle and joint pain), tachycardia, back pain, shortness of breath, hypotension, anaphylaxis, leukopenia, thrombocytopenia, rash, ↓ resistance to infection, ↑ incidence of malignancies

ALG, antilymphocyte globulin; *ATG*, antithymocyte globulin; *GI*, gastro-intestinal; *IL-2*, interleukin-2; *IL-4*, interleukin-4; *IV*, intravenous (route); *PO*, by mouth.
*Neoral is a microemulsion with better absorption than Sandimmune.

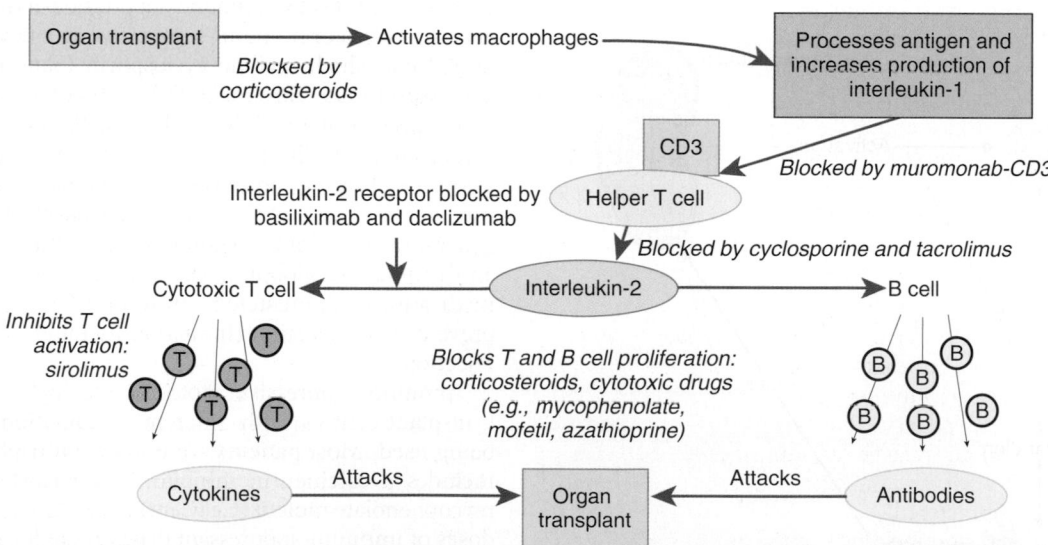

FIGURE 16-13 Sites of action for immuno-suppressive agents. Source: Adapted from McKenry, L., Tessier, E., & Hogan, M. (2006). *Mosby's pharmacology in nursing* (22nd ed., p. 1161). St. Louis: Mosby.

They do not cause bone marrow suppression or alterations of the normal inflammatory response. They are generally used in some combination with corticosteroids, mycophenolate mofetil (CellCept), and sirolimus (Rapamune). Tacrolimus (Prograf) is the most widely used calcineurin inhibitor with cyclosporin used less frequently.

Adverse effects of calcineurin inhibitors are dose related and include nephrotoxicity; therefore, drug levels are closely monitored.

> **DRUG ALERT—Tacrolimus (Prograf) and Cyclosporin (Sandimmune, Neoral)**
> - A substance in grapefruit and grapefruit juice prevents metabolism of these drugs. Consuming grapefruit or grapefruit juice while using these drugs could increase their toxicity.

Mycophenolate Mofetil (CellCept)

Mycophenolate mofetil (CellCept) inhibits purine synthesis with suppressive effects on both T and B lymphocytes. The major limitation of this drug is its gastro-intestinal toxicities, including nausea, vomiting, and diarrhea. In many cases, the adverse effects can be diminished by reduction in the dose or administration of smaller doses more frequently. Myfortic is an enteric-coated form of mycophenolate mofetil that has a similar adverse effect profile.

> **DRUG ALERT—Mycophenolate Mofetil (CellCept)**
> - When given IV, it must be reconstituted in D$_5$W and no other solution.
> - Do not give as IV bolus. Give over 2 or more hours.

Sirolimus (Rapamune)

Sirolimus (Rapamune) is an immuno-suppressive drug that suppresses T-cell activation and proliferation. At relatively low doses, it has a synergistic effect with cyclosporin (Sandimmune, Neoral), tacrolimus (Prograf), and corticosteroids.

Monoclonal Antibodies

Monoclonal antibodies are used for preventing and treating acute rejection episodes. Muromonab-CD3 (OKT 3) was the first monoclonal antibody to be used in clinical transplantation. It is a mouse monoclonal antibody that binds with the CD3 antigen found on the surface of human thymocytes and mature T cells. It interferes with the function of the T lymphocyte, the pivotal cells involved with graft rejection. It is administered via IV bolus. All T cells are affected, rather than just the subset active in graft rejection. Within minutes of the initial infusion of muromonab-CD3 (OKT 3), the number of circulating T cells decreases significantly.

A flulike syndrome occurs during the first few days of treatment, as a result of cytokine release. Adverse effects include fever, rigors, headache, myalgias, and various gastro-intestinal disturbances. To reduce the expected adverse effects of muromonab-CD3 (OKT 3), patients should receive acetaminophen (Tylenol), diphenhydramine (Benadryl), and intravenous corticosteroids before the dose is administered.

Newer generation monoclonal antibodies basiliximab (Simulect) (Ponticelli, 2014) and daclizumab (Zenapax) are a hybrid of mouse and human antibodies. They have fewer adverse effects than muromonab-CD3 (OKT 3) because large parts of the molecule have been replaced with human IgG. They target the IL-2 receptor and impair lymphocyte proliferation. Another monoclonal antibody is alemtuzumab (MabCampath), which targets the CD52 antigen found on T and B cells and the mono-cytes and macrophages. It can cause prolonged T-cell depletion.

Polyclonal Antibodies

Antilymphocyte globulin and antithymocyte globulin are used as induction therapy or to treat acute rejection. The purpose of induction therapy is to provide significant immuno-suppression to an individual immediately after transplantation to prevent early rejection. These agents are prepared by immunizing horses or rabbits with human lymphoid material (thymocytes, lymph nodes, or spleen cells) and then harvesting and purifying the resultant antibody.

Allergic reactions to the foreign proteins from the host animal, manifested by fever, arthralgias, and tachycardia, are common but usually not severe enough to preclude use. These adverse effects can be attenuated by administering the preparation slowly, over 4 to 6 hours, and administering premedication such as acetaminophen (Tylenol), diphenhydramine (Benadryl), and methylprednisolone (Solu-Medrol). The main toxic effects of polyclonal antibodies are lymphopenia and thrombocytopenia, caused by antibody contaminants that are not completely removed during preparation of the antibodies.

Graft-Versus-Host Disease

Graft-versus-host (GVH) disease occurs when an immuno-incompetent (immunodeficient) patient receives a transfusion or transplant with immuno-competent cells. A GVH response is most commonly seen in hematopoietic stem cell transplants. In most transplantation situations, the biggest concern is the patient's (host's) rejection of the organ or transplant. However, in GVH disease, the graft (donated tissue) rejects the host (recipient) tissue (Flowers & Martin, 2015).

The GVH response may begin 7 to 30 days after transplant-ation. Once the reaction is started, little can be done to modify its course. The exact mechanism involved in this reaction is not completely understood. However, it involves donor T cells' attacking and destroying vulnerable host (recipient) cells.

The target organs for the GVH phenomenon are the skin, the gastro-intestinal tract, and the liver. The skin disease may be a maculopapular rash, which may be pruritic or painful. It initially involves the palms and the soles of the feet but can progress to a generalized erythema with bullous formation and desquamation (shedding of the outer layer of skin). The liver disease may manifest as mild jaundice with elevated levels of liver enzymes and progress to hepatic coma. The GI manifestations may include mild to severe diarrhea, severe abdominal pain, gastro-intestinal bleeding, and malabsorption.

The biggest problem with GVH disease is differing types of infection at different time periods. Bacterial and fungal infections predominate immediately after transplantation, when granulo-cytopenia is occurring. Later, the development of interstitial pneumonitis is the predominant problem.

Once GVH disease is established, there is no adequate treatment. Although corticosteroids are often used, the suscept-ibility to infection then increases. The use of immuno-suppressive agents (e.g., methotrexate, cyclosporin [Sandimmune, Neoral]) has been most effective as a preventive rather than as a treatment measure. Irradiated blood products before administration is another measure to prevent T-cell replication.

ALTERNATIVE STRATEGIES

In the past decade, there has been a rapid rise in solid organ transplantation worldwide because of the increased incidence of organ failure and greater improvements in post-transplantation

ETHICAL DILEMMAS
Transplantation

Situation

A 24-year-old female patient is admitted to hospital with evidence of acute organ rejection. The patient informs the nurse in confidence that she does not take her antirejection medications regularly because she is very busy with work and school. The patient also states that she usually feels so well that she does not think she needs to take them every day. She asks the nurse not to inform the health care team that she has been missing some of her antirejection medications.

Important Points for Consideration

- Building a trusting relationship with patients is key in the health care environment; however, the larger implications for the patient's health supersede the issue of confidentiality. There are some limits to confidentiality, including potential or real harm to self or others.
- The nurse is a member of the treatment team.
- Organ rejection can cause reduced organ function and potential loss of the graft and subsequent death for the patient. With complete information, the patient can understand the importance of adherence to the medication regimen.

Critical Thinking Questions

1. How should the nurse respond to this patient's request for confidentiality? Should the nurse inform the treatment team? If so, should he or she tell the patient?
2. What information should the nurse give the patient regarding the importance of taking her antirejection medications?
3. How could the nurse work with the patient who has a busy schedule and forgets to take her medications?

outcomes. However, cadaveric organ donation rates have not met demand; thus waiting lists are long, and increasing numbers of patients die waiting for a suitable organ (Gómez, Pérez, & Manyalich, 2014). The number of patients waiting for an organ transplant in Canada in 2013 was 4 361, but only 2 367 organs were transplanted. Approximately 246 people die annually waiting for an organ transplant in Canada (Canadian Institute for Health Information, 2015). Various strategies worldwide have been implemented to offset the critical organ shortage, some with modest success, others remaining under scientific investigation and ethical debate (see the "Ethical Dilemmas" box).

Transplantation of Organs From Deceased Donor

One of the most rapid increases in organ recovery rates has been from deceased people who are declared dead on the basis of cardiopulmonary criteria (irreversible cessation of circulatory and respiratory function) rather than neurological criteria of "brain death" (irreversible loss of all functions of the entire brain, including the brain stem) (Hernandez-Alejandro, Wall, Jevnikar, et al., 2011). Such patients typically are on a ventilator because of devastating and irreversible brain injury (not complete brain death) from trauma or intracranial bleeding. Furthermore, in some of these patients, complete cessation of the heartbeat with subsequent cardiac resuscitation was followed by irreversible brain injury as the result of a long period of anoxia (lack of oxygen). Further treatment has been deemed futile, and end-of-life care management implemented. Often, family members express interest in organ donation. The potential donor must meet cardiac death criteria at onset of asystole or absence of a heartbeat. In order to avoid conflict of interest, those involved in end-of-life care or declaration of death of the potential donor are not involved in the care of the transplant recipient. Organs most commonly

recovered for donation include the kidneys, the liver, the pancreas, and the lungs (Hernandez-Alejandro, Wall, Jevnikar, et al., 2011). In 2012 in Canada, 166 organs were recovered after deceased cardiac death and successfully transplanted into recipients (Canadian Institute for Health Information, 2015).

Xenotransplantation

Xenotransplantation is the replacement of a patient's diseased and malfunctioning organ with an organ harvested from another species. Animals considered as a possible source of organs for human use include primates (because of their genetic similarities to humans) and pigs (because of their large availability). Organs from primates have been largely dismissed because of logistical difficulties. The pig is believed to be the most appropriate candidate because of comparable organ size, large litters, and rapid gestation. Difficulties in successful organ transplantation from one species to another, as in from pig to human, include multiple biological barriers. First, the significant degree of antigen disparity means that there is more for the human immune system to recognize and reject. Second, the possibility of diseases "jumping" the species barrier and infecting humans, such as porcine endogenous retroviruses, is one of the main reasons people remain sceptical and concerned regarding xenotransplantation. This possibility has decreased enthusiasm for xenotransplantation as an alternative to allogeneic organ transplantation (Health Canada, 2010). However, despite strong scepticism, much scientific research and advancement in this area continues.

Ex Vivo Transplantation

A novel strategy to help overcome donor lung shortages has been through the development of normothermic ex vivo lung perfusion (EVLP) (Figure 16-14). The injured donor lungs are reassessed and conditioned through the EVLP system by mimicking the lung's natural physiological environment and by providing oxygen and other substrates necessary for active metabolism. Through the use of EVLP, therapeutic interventions can be performed in the donor lungs that reduce the degree or negative influence of pulmonary edema, pulmonary emboli, gastric aspiration, pneumonia, and lung inflammation (Reeb & Cypel, 2016).

Stem Cell Transplantation

Stem cells are the subject of much discussion. It is believed that the use of stem cells may allow for the regeneration of lost tissue and restoration of function in many chronic diseases such as Parkinson's disease, Alzheimer's disease, heart disease, diabetes mellitus, and spinal cord injuries.

Stem cells are cells in the body that have the ability to differentiate into other cells. Stem cells can be divided into two types: embryonic and adult. Embryonic stem cells have the ability to become any one of the hundreds of types of cells in the human body. They are derived from human embryo cells that are 4 to 5 days old. These stem cells are pluripotent and can differentiate into any cell type that they are stimulated to become. Because of their versatility, embryonic stem cells are preferred for use in medical research. Donor eggs, like stem cells, can be used with existing adult tissue to produce new tissue. In a process known as *nuclear transfer* or *therapeutic cloning,* the nucleus is removed from the egg and replaced with the nucleus of the desired tissue. Then, as the egg divides, a 200-cell blastocyst of the desired tissue is created. Adult stem cells are undifferentiated cells that are found in small numbers in most adult tissues; they have been

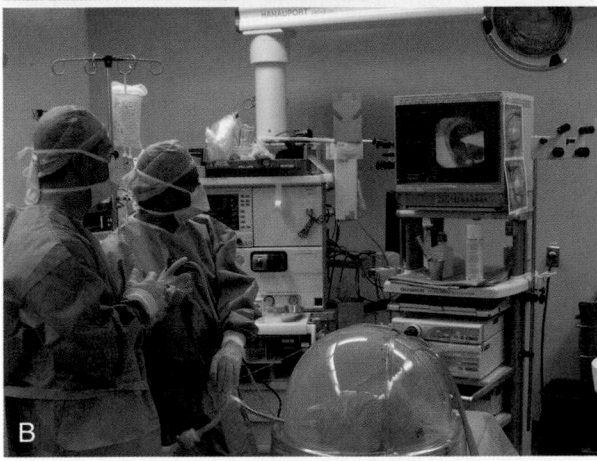

FIGURE 16-14 The Toronto EVLP System. **A,** Surgeons working on the ex vivo lung. **B,** Thoracic Surgeons at Toronto General Hospital, Dr. Marcelo Cypel and Dr. Shaf Keshavjee Director of the Toronto Lung Transplant Program, perform a bronchoscopy on the ex vivo lung for clinical evaluation. Published with the permission of Dr. Shaf Keshavjee, Director, Toronto Lung Transplant Program, University Health Network.

FIGURE 16-15 Monoclonal antibodies are identical antibodies made by clones of a single antibody-producing cell. The target antigen is injected into a mouse. Plasma cells are harvested from the spleen of the mouse and fused with myeloma cells. The fused cells, or hybridomas, are then cloned. A clone can secrete monoclonal antibodies over a long period.

discovered in the skin, the gastro-intestinal tract, and bone marrow. They are also found in newborns and can be extracted from umbilical cord blood. The primary roles of adult stem cells in the body are to maintain and repair tissues in which they are found. They are usually thought of as multipotent cells, giving rise to a closely related family of cells within the tissue. For example, hematopoietic stem cells form all the various cells in blood, whereas skin stem cells produce new skin cells. Scientists hope that adult stem cells can be coaxed into providing tissue for unrelated organs.

Stem cells found within the bone marrow are the body's site of hematopoiesis. The cells are prolific by design and are already being donated in the treatment of certain diseases, such as leukemia. Cells similar to the stem cells found in bone marrow can be found in the umbilical cord and blood from the placenta. These cells are used in situations similar to those of bone marrow. Studies are being conducted to find future uses that will allow the cells to become other tissues in the body (National Institutes of Health, 2015). With increasing waiting lists for organ transplantation, embryonic stem cell research may be the key to solving the problem of organ shortages through organ regeneration. However, conflicts exist regarding creating embryonic stem cells for therapeutic purposes such as organ development, with much debate over the definition of human life at the earliest stages

versus a potentially life-saving therapy. Much discussion continues in this area internationally.

NEW TECHNOLOGIES IN IMMUNOLOGY

Hybridoma Technology: Monoclonal Antibodies

Monoclonal antibodies are homogeneous populations of identical antibody molecules produced by specialized tissue cell culture lines. They are manufactured through cell fusion techniques and standard in vitro tissue culture systems (Figure 16-15). The two essential biological components are immunized mice or rats and myeloma tumour cell lines, which are of lymphoid origin. Single antibody-forming cells (lymphocytes) from rodents previously immunized with antigen are fused with myeloma cells to create hybrid cells with properties of both parent cell types. Like the myeloma parent cell, the hybrids have an unlimited capacity to reproduce. The hybrids produce the single type of antibody molecule that they inherited from the normal, antibody-forming parent cell. Hybrid cells derived in this way can produce unlimited quantities of specific antibodies. With appropriate selection techniques, producing monoclonal antibodies to virtually any antigen is possible. Because the monoclonal antibodies are a completely homogeneous population, their use incurs fewer problems than does that of conventional polyclonal antisera.

Monoclonal antibodies are used widely in many areas of medicine and biological science. Thousands of monoclonal antibodies have been made against many different types of antigens. Monoclonal antibodies have begun to replace conventional antibodies in blood banking and are used in the identification of organisms in bacteriology laboratories. Monoclonal antibodies have also been extensively used in radioimmunoassays to measure serum levels of various substances (e.g., parathyroid hormone). They have been useful in quantifying types of WBCs and subtypes of lymphocytes and in the diagnosis of leukemia. More recently, monoclonal antibodies have been used in the treatment of malignancies (see Chapter 18). They have been used to treat transplant rejection episodes, to purge bone marrow of tumour cells in bone marrow transplants, and to remove mature T cells that cause GVH disease in bone marrow transplant recipients.

A major limitation of monoclonal antibody use for humans is that they are mouse antibodies and therefore can elicit an antibody response by the host against the foreign agent. Human hybridomas have been produced through the use of human myelomas. These hybrids synthesize human monoclonal antibodies and are therefore advantageous for in vivo use in diagnosis and therapy.

CASE STUDY

Anaphylactic Reaction

Source: Creative Family/Shutterstock.com.

Patient Profile

Kiara Riley, a 21-year-old university student, is brought to the emergency department by ambulance from her school lunch room after a sudden change in level of consciousness and difficulty with speech.

Subjective Data

Conscious on admission but confused, disoriented, very restless, and anxious.

Objective Data

Physical Assessment

- Vital signs on admission: BP 82/58, pulse 124/minute, respirations 8/minute, temp 39.3°C, O$_2$ saturation 84% on 100% oxygen
- Skin: mild facial edema, urticaria, itchy eyes
- Respiratory: tightness of throat, shortness of breath, runny nose
- Gastro-intestinal tract: nausea, mild abdominal pain

A few of her friends arrive at the emergency department, and it is discovered that she had eaten some cookies that were thought to have peanuts in them right before the event occurred. Family could not be contacted to determine if Ms. Riley had a previous documented allergy to nuts/peanuts. Her friends were unaware of such an allergy in her history but do not remember seeing her eating nuts of any kind in the past.

Discussion Questions

1. What kind of reaction is the patient experiencing?
2. *Priority decision:* Based on the assessment data provided, what are the priority nursing diagnoses?
3. *Priority decision:* What are the priority nursing interventions for Ms. Riley?
4. What first-line medication would likely be administered, and how is it going to work to assist the patient?
5. Based on the assessment data provided and the diagnoses, what future nursing care should be provided for this patient?

evolve

Answers are available at *http://evolve.elsevier.com/Canada/Lewis/medsurg*.

REVIEW QUESTIONS

The number of the question corresponds to the same-numbered objective at the beginning of the chapter.

1. What is the function of monocytes in immunity?
   a. They stimulate the production of T and B lymphocytes.
   b. They produce antibodies on exposure to foreign substances.
   c. They bind antigens and stimulate natural killer cell activation.
   d. They capture antigens by phagocytosis and present them to lymphocytes.

2. Which of the following is a function of cell-mediated immunity?
   a. Formation of antibodies
   b. Activation of the complement system
   c. Surveillance for malignant cell changes
   d. Opsonization of antigens to allow phagocytosis by neutrophils

3. Which immunoglobulin from maternal transmission protects newborns in the first 3 to 6 months of life from bacterial infections?
   a. IgG
   b. IgA
   c. IgM
   d. IgE

4. Which primary immunological disorder typically occurs in a type I hypersensitivity reaction?
   a. Binding of IgG to an antigen on a cell surface
   b. Deposit of antigen–antibody complexes in small vessels
   c. Release of lymphokines to interact with specific antigens
   d. Release of chemical mediators from IgE-bound mast cells and basophils

5. Which response may alert the nurse that a possible anaphylactic shock reaction may be occurring immediately after a client has received an intramuscular penicillin injection?
   a. Edema and itching at the injection site
   b. Sneezing and itching of the nose and eyes
   c. A wheal-and-flare reaction at the injection site
   d. Chest tightness and production of thick sputum

6. Which is the most appropriate response when a person requests a friend who is a nurse to administer his allergy shot?
   a. It is illegal for nurses to administer injections outside of a medical setting.
   b. He or she is qualified to do it if the friend has epinephrine in an injectable syringe provided with his extract.
   c. Avoiding the allergens is a more effective way of controlling allergies, and allergy shots are not usually effective.
   d. Immunotherapy should be administered only in a setting where emergency equipment and drugs are available.

7. Association between HLA antigens and diseases is most commonly found in what disease conditions?
   a. Malignancies
   b. Infectious diseases
   c. Neurological diseases
   d. Autoimmune disorders

8. A client is undergoing plasmapheresis for treatment of SLE. What effect does plasmapheresis have?
   a. Removes T lymphocytes in the client's blood that are producing antinuclear antibodies
   b. Removes normal particles in the client's blood that are being damaged by autoantibodies
   c. Exchanges the client's plasma that contains antinuclear antibodies with a substitute fluid
   d. Replaces viral-damaged cellular components of the client's blood with replacement whole blood

9. What is the most common cause of secondary immunodeficiencies?
   a. Drugs
   b. Stress
   c. Malnutrition
   d. Human immunodeficiency virus

10. Which of the following accurately describes rejection after transplantation?
    a. Hyperacute rejection can be treated with mycophenolate mofetil.
    b. Acute rejection can be treated with sirolimus or tacrolimus.
    c. Chronic rejection can be treated with tacrolimus or cyclosporin.
    d. Hyperacute rejection can usually be avoided if crossmatching is done before transplantation.

11. Which of the following does the nurse understand regarding acute rejection of a transplanted lung? (*Select all that apply*)
    a. A new transplant should be considered immediately.
    b. Acute rejection can be treated with high-dose corticosteroids.
    c. Acute rejection always leads to chronic rejection.
    d. Acute rejection is treated with muromonab-CD3.
    e. Acute rejection is common after a transplant and is treated with augmentation of immuno-suppression.

12. Which of the following statements best describes cardiac death in a deceased donor?
    a. Severe brain damage; coma has progressed to a state of wakefulness without detectable awareness
    b. Irreversible loss of all functions of the entire brain, including the brain stem
    c. Devastating and irreversible brain injuries (not complete brain death) from trauma or intracranial bleeding; complete cessation of the heartbeat may have occurred, and after subsequent cardiac resuscitation, irreversible brain injury results from a long period of lack of oxygen
    d. Inability to be awakened; fails to respond normally to pain or light, does not have sleep–wake cycles, and does not take voluntary actions

1. d; 2. c; 3. a; 4. d; 5. a; 6. d; 7. d; 8. c; 9. a; 10. d; 11. b, e; 12. c.

⊖volve

For even more NCLEX review questions, visit *http://evolve.elsevier.com/ Canada/Lewis/medsurg.*

REFERENCES

Camous, X., Pera, A., Solana, R., et al. (2012). NK cells in healthy aging and age-associated diseases. *BioMed Research International, 2012.* doi:10.1155/2012/195956.

Canadian Centre for Occupational Health and Safety (CCOHS). (2014, February). *Latex allergy.* Retrieved from *http://www.ccohs.ca/oshanswers/diseases/latex.html.*

Canadian Institute for Health Information. (2015). *Canadian Organ Replacement Register annual report: Treatment of end-stage organ failure in Canada, 2004 to 2013.* Retrieved from *https://secure.cihi.ca/free_products/2015_CORR_AnnualReport_ENweb.pdf.*

Compalati, E., Braido, F., & Canonica, G. W. (2013). Sublingual immunotherapy: Recent advances. *Allergology International, 62*(4), 415–423. doi:10.2332/allergolint.13-RAI-0627.

Flowers, M. E., & Martin, P. J. (2015). How we treat chronic graft-versus-host disease. *Blood, 125*(4), 606–615. doi:10.1182/blood-2014-08-551994.

Gómez, M. P., Pérez, B., & Manyalich, M. (2014). International registry in organ donation and transplantation—2013. *Transplantation Proceedings, 46*(4), 1044–1048. doi:10.1016/j.transproceed.2013.11.138.

Health Canada. (2010). *Revised fact sheet on xenotransplantation.* Retrieved from *http://www.hc-sc.gc.ca/dhp-mps/brgtherap/activit/fs-fi/xeno_fact-fait-eng.php.*

Hernandez-Alejandro, R., Wall, W., Jevnikar, A., et al. (2011). Organ donation after cardiac death: Donor and recipient outcomes after the first three years of the Ontario experience. *Canadian Journal of Anesthesia/Journal canadien d'anesthésie, 58*(7), 599–605. doi:10.1007/s12630-011-9511-9.

Kasper, D., Fauci, A., Hauser, S., et al. (2015). *Harrison's principles of internal medicine* (19th ed.). New York: McGraw Hill Professional.

Lee, S., Nolte, H., & Benninger, M. S. (2015). Clinical considerations in the use of sublingual immunotherapy for allergic rhinitis. *American Journal of Rhinology & Allergy, 29*(2), 106–114. doi:10.2500/ajra.2015.29.4148.

Mak, T., Saunders, M. E., & Jett, B. D. (2014). *Primer to the immune response.* Oxford, UK: Elsevier Ltd.

Moore, L. E., Kemp, A. M., & Kemp, S. F. (2015). Recognition, treatment, and prevention of anaphylaxis. *Immunology and Allergy Clinics of North America, 35*(2), 363–374. doi:10.1016/j.iac.2015.01.006.

National Institutes of Health. (2015). *Stem cell information [home page].* Retrieved from *http://stemcells.nih.gov/info/basics/pages/basics1.aspx.*

Ponticelli, C. (2014). Basiliximab: Efficacy and safety evaluation in kidney transplantation. *Expert Opinion on Drug Safety, 13*(3), 373–381. doi:10.1517/14740338.2014.861816.

Reeb, J., & Cypel, M. (2016). Ex vivo lung perfusion. *Clinical Transplantation, 30*(3), 183–194. doi:10.1111/ctr.12680.

Sears, M. E. (2007). *The medical perspective on environmental sensitivities.* Ottawa: Canadian Human Rights Commission. (Seminal).

Vacca, V. M., & McMahon-Bowen, E. (2013). Anaphylaxis. *Nursing, 43*(11), 16–17. doi:10.1097/01.NURSE.0000435204.03647.3f.

Waserman, S., Chad, Z., Francoeur, M. J., et al. (2010). Management of anaphylaxis in primary care: Canadian expert consensus recommendations. *Allergy, 65*(9), 1082–1092. doi:10.1111/j.1398-9995.2010.02418.x. (Seminal).

William, P. E. (2013). *Fundamental immunology*. Philadelphia: Lippincott Williams & Wilkins.

Yunker, N. S., & Wagner, B. J. (2014). A pharmacologic review of anaphylaxis. *Plastic Surgical Nursing, 34*(4), 183–189. doi:10.1097/PSN.0000000000000072.

RESOURCES

Alberta Organ and Tissue Donation Registry
http://www.health.alberta.ca/services/ organ-tissue-donor-registry.html

Asthma Society of Canada
http://www.asthma.ca

B.C. Transplant
http://www.transplant.bc.ca

Canadian Association for Clinical Microbiology and Infectious Diseases
http://www.cacmid.ca

Canadian Centre for Occupational Health and Safety (CCOHS)
http://www.ccohs.ca

Canadian Society of Allergy and Clinical Immunology (CSACI)
http://www.csaci.ca

Transplant Manitoba
http://www.transplantmanitoba.ca/decide/gift-of-life

Transplant Quebec
http://www.transplantquebec.ca/en

Trillium Gift of Life Network
http://www.giftoflife.on.ca

Access Excellence: Understanding Gene Testing
http://www.accessexcellence.org/AE/AEPC/NIH

Centers for Disease Control and Prevention, Public Health Genomics
http://www.cdc.gov/genomics

National Institute of Nursing Research (NINR), Division of Intramural Research
https://www.ninr.nih.gov/researchandfunding/dir

For additional Internet resources, see the website for this book at *http://evolve.elsevier.com/Canada/Lewis/medsurg*.

Infection and Human Immunodeficiency Virus Infection

Written by: Jeffrey Kwong
Adapted by: Jane McCall

ⓔvolve WEBSITE

http://evolve.elsevier.com/Canada/Lewis/medsurg

- Review Questions (Online Only)
- Key Points
- Answer Guidelines for Case Study
- Student Case Study
- Human Immunodeficiency Virus (HIV) Infection and Acquired Immunodeficiency Syndrome (AIDS)
- Conceptual Care Map Creator
- Audio Glossary
- Content Updates

LEARNING OBJECTIVES

1. Discuss the effect of emerging and re-emerging infections on health care.
2. Review infection prevention and control strategies.
3. List the modes and variables involved in the transmission of the human immunodeficiency virus (HIV).
4. Describe the pathophysiological processes of HIV infection.
5. Outline HIV disease progression against the spectrum of untreated HIV infection.
6. List the diagnostic criteria for acquired immune deficiency syndrome (AIDS).
7. Explain the methods of testing for HIV infection.
8. Discuss the collaborative management of HIV infection.
9. Discuss the long-term consequences of HIV infection and treatment of HIV infection.
10. Explain the characteristics of opportunistic diseases associated with AIDS.
11. Describe the nursing management of HIV-infected patients and those at risk for HIV infection.
12. Compare and contrast the methods of HIV prevention that eliminate risk and those that decrease risk.

KEY TERMS

acquired immunodeficiency syndrome (AIDS), p. 293
acute retroviral syndrome, p. 297
bacteria, p. 287

emerging infectious disease, p. 289
fungi, p. 288
human immunodeficiency virus (HIV), p. 295

opportunistic diseases, p. 297
oral hairy leukoplakia, p. 297
protozoa, p. 288
retroviruses, p. 295
reverse transcriptase, p. 296

viral load, p. 294
viremia, p. 296
viruses, p. 288
window period, p. 295

▌INFECTIONS

An infection is an invasion of the body by a *pathogen* (any microorganism that causes disease) and the resulting signs and symptoms that develop in response to the invasion. Infections can be divided into two categories: localized and systemic. A localized infection is limited to a small area. Systemic infections are widespread throughout the body and are often spread via the blood.

CAUSES OF INFECTIONS

A number of microorganisms can cause infections. The most common are bacteria, viruses, fungi, and protozoa. Bacteria are one-celled microorganisms that are found virtually everywhere on earth and are involved in fermentation, putrefaction, infectious diseases, and nitrogen fixation. They were first observed by Anton Van Leeuwenhoek, who named them "animalcules." A number of bacteria are considered to be normal flora. Under normal circumstances, they live harmoniously in or on the human body without causing disease. These normal flora act protectively and prevent the overgrowth of other microorganisms. *Escherichia coli* organisms, for example, are bacteria that are normal flora in the large intestine (Huether & McCance, 2012).

Bacteria cause disease in two ways. They can enter the body and grow inside human cells (e.g., tuberculosis [TB]), or they can secrete toxins that damage cells. Bacteria are divided into

TABLE 17-1 COMMON DISEASE-CAUSING BACTERIA

Type	Diseases Caused
Clostridium organisms	
• *C. botulinum*	Food poisoning with progressive muscle paralysis
• *C. tetani*	Tetanus (lockjaw)
Corynebacterium diphtheriae	Diphtheria
Escherichia coli	Urinary tract infections, peritonitis
Haemophilus organisms	
• *H. influenzae*	Nasopharyngitis, meningitis, pneumonia
• *H. pertussis*	Pertussis (whooping cough)
Helicobacter pylori	Peptic ulcers, gastritis
Klebsiella and *Enterobacter* organisms	Urinary tract infections, peritonitis, pneumonia
Legionella pneumophila	Pneumonia (legionnaires disease)
Mycobacterium organisms	
• *M. leprae*	Hansen's disease (leprosy)
• *M. tuberculosis*	Tuberculosis
Neisseria organisms	
• *N. gonorrhoeae*	Gonorrhea, pelvic inflammatory disease
• *N. meningitidis*	Meningococcemia, meningitis
Proteus organisms	Urinary tract infections, peritonitis
Pseudomonas aeruginosa	Urinary tract infections, meningitis
Salmonella organisms	
• *S. typhi*	Typhoid fever
• Other *Salmonella* organisms	Food poisoning, gastro-enteritis
Shigella organisms	Shigellosis, diarrhea with abdominal pain and fever (dysentery)
Staphylococcus aureus	Skin infections, pneumonia, urinary tract infections, acute osteomyelitis, toxic shock syndrome
Streptococcus organisms	
• *S. faecalis*	Genito-urinary infection, infection of surgical wounds
• *S. pneumoniae*	Pneumococcal pneumonia
• *S. pyogenes* (group A β-hemolytic streptococci)	Pharyngitis, scarlet fever, rheumatic fever, acute glomerulonephritis, erysipelas, pneumonia
• *S. pyogenes* (group B β-hemolytic streptococci)	Urinary tract infections
• *S. viridans*	Bacterial endocarditis
Treponema pallidum	Syphilis

TABLE 17-2 COMMON DISEASE-CAUSING VIRUSES

Type	Diseases Caused
Adenoviruses	Upper respiratory tract infection, pneumonia
Arbovirus	Syndrome of fever, malaise, headache, myalgia; aseptic meningitis; encephalitis
Coronavirus	Upper respiratory tract infection
Coxsackieviruses A and B	Upper respiratory tract infection, gastro-enteritis, acute myocarditis, aseptic meningitis
Echoviruses	Upper respiratory tract infection, gastro-enteritis, aseptic meningitis
Hepatitis A, B, C, D, E	Viral hepatitis
Human herpesviruses	
• Cytomegalovirus (CMV)	Gastro-enteritis; pneumonia and retinal damage in immuno-suppressed individuals; infectious mononucleosis–like syndrome
• Epstein-Barr virus	Mononucleosis, Burkitt's lymphoma (possibly)
• Herpes simplex, type 1	Herpes labialis ("fever blisters"), genital herpes infection
• Herpes simplex, type 2	Genital herpes infection
• Varicella-zoster	Chickenpox; shingles
HIV	HIV infection, AIDS
Influenza A and B	Upper respiratory tract infection
Mumps	Parotitis, orchitis in postpubertal males
Papovavirus	Warts
Parainfluenza types 1–4	Upper respiratory tract infection
Parvovirus	Gastro-enteritis
Poliovirus	Poliomyelitis
Poxviruses	Smallpox
Reoviruses 1, 2, 3	Upper respiratory tract infection
Respiratory syncytial virus	Gastro-enteritis, respiratory tract infection
Rhabdovirus	Rabies
Rhinovirus	Upper respiratory tract infection, pneumonia
Rotaviruses	Gastro-enteritis
Rubella	German measles
Rubeola	Measles
West Nile virus	Flulike symptoms, meningitis, encephalitis

AIDS, acquired immune deficiency syndrome; *HIV,* human immunodeficiency virus.

categories on the basis of the shape of their cells. Cocci, including streptococci and staphylococci, are round cells. Bacilli are rod-shaped and include tetanus and TB. Bacilli that are curved rods include *Vibrio* bacteria, one of which causes cholera. Table 17-1 lists common pathogenic bacteria and the diseases that they cause (Huether & McCance, 2012).

Viruses can also cause infections. The word *virus* comes from the Latin term *virus,* meaning "poison." Unlike bacteria, viruses are not cells. They consist of either RNA or DNA and a protein envelope. Viruses can reproduce only in the cells of a living organism and are therefore obligate parasites. Examples of diseases caused by viruses are presented in Table 17-2 (Huether & McCance, 2012).

Fungi are organisms similar to plants, but they lack chlorophyll. Mycosis is any disease caused by a fungus. Pathogenic fungi cause infections that are usually localized to a small area, but in an immuno-compromised person, they can become disseminated.

Athlete's foot and ringworm are two common mycotic infections. Some fungi are normal flora in various places in the body, but when overgrowth occurs, disease can result. Overgrowth of *Candida albicans,* for example, causes oral candidiasis (thrush), esophageal candidiasis, intestinal symptoms, and vaginitis, depending on the affected site (Huether & McCance, 2012). Other fungi and their respective mycotic infections are listed in Table 17-3. Fungal infections of the lungs are presented in Chapter 30 (see Table 30-9) and fungal infections of the skin in Chapter 26 (see Table 26-8).

Protozoa are single-cell, animal-like microorganisms. Protozoa can be divided into four categories: amoebas, ciliates, flagellates, and sporozoa. Protozoa normally live in soil and bodies of water. When they are introduced into the human body, infection can result. Amoebic dysentery and giardiasis are caused by protozoan parasites. Malaria is caused by a sporozoa called *Plasmodium malariae* (Huether & McCance, 2012).

TABLE 17-3	COMMON DISEASE-CAUSING FUNGI	
Organism	**Diseases Caused**	**Organs Affected**
Aspergillus fumigatus	Aspergillosis	Lungs*
	Otomycosis	Ears
Blastomyces dermatitidis	Blastomycosis	Lungs, various organs
Candida albicans	Candidiasis	Intestines
	Vaginitis	Vagina
	Thrush	Skin,† mouth
Coccidioides immitis	Coccidioidomycosis	Lungs*
Pneumocystis jiroveci	Pneumocystis pneumonia	Lungs*
Sporothrix schenckii	Sporotrichosis	Skin, lymph vessels
Trichophyton species	Tinea pedis	Skin†
Microsporum species	Tinea capitis	Skin
Epidermophyton species	Tinea corporis	Skin†

*See Table 30-9 (Fungal Infections of the Lung).
†See Table 26-8 (Common Fungal Infections of the Skin and Mucous Membranes).

EMERGING INFECTIONS

An **emerging infectious disease** is an infectious disease whose incidence has recently increased or threatens to increase in the immediate future. Examples of emerging infections are described in Table 17-4. Emerging infectious diseases can originate from unknown sources, contact with animals, changes in known diseases, natural disasters, or even biological warfare. For example, the coronavirus that causes severe acute respiratory syndrome (SARS) and the West Nile virus come from animal sources, whereas other pathogens, such as *Staphylococcus aureus,* have emerged because a previously treatable organism developed resistance to antibiotics. Climate change has resulted in an increase of disease-carrying mosquitoes, as well as increases in rodent numbers and in hantavirus. Earthquakes, such as the large one in Haiti in 2010, are associated with the spread of waterborne diseases such as cholera. The battle against infectious disease is an age-old problem. However, modern technologies have changed how disease spreads. Global travel, population density, encroachment into new environments, and the misuse of antibiotics have all increased the risk for widespread new or untreatable infectious diseases (Public Health Agency of Canada [PHAC], 2015b).

It is interesting that, not too long ago, many people believed that science had conquered infectious disease. Unfortunately, infections remain the leading cause of death worldwide. More than 30 newly recognized infectious diseases have emerged since the 1980s, including human immunodeficiency virus (HIV) infection, Lyme disease, hepatitis C, SARS, avian flu, and Ebola virus disease. In addition, some diseases once thought to be under control, including TB and drug-resistant strains of other bacteria, have re-emerged (PHAC, 2015b).

Results of studies in zoonosis (the science of transmission of diseases from animals to humans) indicate that many known infectious diseases come from animals and insects (vectors). The SARS outbreak in China in 2003, for instance, was linked to the civet cat, a small carnivorous mammal found throughout much of Asia and Africa. (SARS is discussed in Chapters 70 and 72.) Animal-borne infections are difficult to predict and prevent.

West Nile virus is transmitted by a virus carried by mosquitoes. Mosquitoes acquire the virus as they draw blood from infected birds (PHAC, 2014). The virus does not cause illness in the mosquito but can be transferred to animals and humans as

TABLE 17-4	EXAMPLES OF EMERGING INFECTIONS
Microorganism	**Related Disease**
Bacteria	
Borrelia burgdorferi	Lyme disease
Campylobacter jejuni	Diarrhea
Escherichia coli O157:H7	Hemorrhagic colitis, hemolytic uremic syndrome
Helicobacter pylori	Peptic ulcer disease
Legionella pneumophila	Legionnaires disease
Vibrio cholerae 0139	New strain associated with epidemic cholera
Viruses	
Ebola virus	Ebola hemorrhagic fever
Hantavirus	Hantavirus pulmonary syndrome (found in North and South America)
	Hemorrhagic fever with renal syndrome (found mainly in Europe and Asia)
H1N1 virus	H1N1 (swine) flu
Hepatitis A virus	Enterically transmitted hepatitis
Hepatitis C virus	Parenterally transmitted hepatitis
Hepatitis E virus	Enterically transmitted hepatitis
HIV	HIV infection and AIDS
HHV-6	Roseola
HHV-8	Associated with Kaposi's sarcoma and Castleman's disease in immuno-suppressed patients, patients with AIDS
West Nile virus	West Nile fever
Avian influenza A (H5N1) virus	Avian flu
Zika virus	Zika fever, microcephaly
Parasites	
Cryptosporidium parvum	Acute and chronic diarrhea

AIDS, acquired immunodeficiency syndrome; *HHV,* human herpesvirus; *HIV,* human immunodeficiency virus.

the mosquito continues to feed. Bird deaths are an indicator of the spread of the West Nile virus and can serve as an early warning sign of an outbreak that can spread quickly if action is not taken in a timely manner (PHAC, 2014). (West Nile virus is discussed in Chapter 59.) Another serious disease transmitted by animals is Lyme disease, which is caused by the bite of a black-legged tick. Lyme disease is most common in the northeastern and north central United States, as well as on the west coast, including British Columbia. Lyme disease has, however, also been reported in Ontario. (See Chapter 67 for further discussion on Lyme disease.)

Sometimes, an organism alters its normal path of transmission. In the past, influenza A viruses were typically spread from birds to pigs to humans. More recently, in cases such as the avian flu outbreak, the virus has been spread directly from chickens to humans. This was first demonstrated in Hong Kong in 1997 and also in the Netherlands in 2003. Infected people generally suffer from conjunctivitis or mild influenza-like symptoms. However, 200 deaths related to avian flu have occurred worldwide (PHAC, 2015a). Upon discovery of an outbreak, all chickens in the area are typically slaughtered to remove the source of the infection.

The disease caused by Ebola virus is an emerging entity that has presented an ongoing challenge to public health since it was first observed in 1976. Ebola virus causes a severe hemorrhagic fever and is usually lethal. Therapeutic and preventive measures are extremely limited. The natural reservoir and path of transmission of the virus are unknown, which makes it impossible to effectively combat the disease (Government of Canada, 2016a). In 2014, there was a large outbreak of Ebola in West Africa that was unusually difficult to control. This outbreak was also the first time Ebola was seen outside of Africa, with cases reported in the United States and Europe (World Health Organization [WHO], 2016).

A relatively new and emerging entity is the outbreak caused by Zika virus. Originally identified in Africa and Asia in the 1950s and historically occurring in low numbers, it has occurred in a large outbreak in South and Central America, with some cases reported in the United States and Canada. Zika virus generally causes a relatively mild infection, manifested by muscle and joint pain, headache, rash, and conjunctivitis. It is spread primarily by mosquitoes, but there is some evidence of sexual transmission. Zika does not pose a risk to most people; however, women who are infected with the virus during pregnancy are more likely to have a baby with microcephaly (Government of Canada, 2016b).

Re-Emerging Infections

Vaccines and proper medications have led to the near eradication of some infections. However, infective agents can always re-emerge if conditions are right. Table 17-5 illustrates some diseases that have re-emerged in recent decades.

For example, the incidence of TB began to decrease steadily in the mid-1950s. However, by 2013, the declining trend stabilized and incidence levelled out to 4.7 cases per 100,000 people in Canada (PHAC, 2015b). One factor that has influenced the continued incidence of TB in Canada is the increase in people with HIV, whose depressed immune systems allow pathogens such as TB bacilli to cause disease. There has been an increase in drug-resistant TB, although, in Canada, the rates remain relatively low (PHAC, 2015b). International travel creates a new dilemma for the local eradication of diseases. Measles, for instance, is no longer considered endemic in Canada, but it remains a leading cause of morbidity in developing countries. Some measles cases in Canada have been found in people who have travelled to these measles-endemic countries and in people in religious nonimmunizing communities (PHAC, 2015b).

Resistant Organisms

Antibiotic-resistant organisms, also called *multidrug-resistant organisms* or *superbugs*, are bacteria whose growth and reproduction are unaffected by particular antibiotics. Microorganisms can become resistant to classic antibiotics (e.g., penicillin), as well as to newer antibiotic and antiviral agents.

Methicillin-resistant *S. aureus* (MRSA), vancomycin-resistant enterococci, health care–associated *Clostridium difficile*, and carbapenem-resistant enterobacteriaceae are four of the most troublesome resistant bacteria in North America (PHAC, 2014). Table 17-6 lists the most common antibiotic-resistant bacteria.

Bacteria are highly adaptable organisms that have evolved genetic and biochemical means of resisting antimicrobial actions. Genetic mechanisms include mutation and acquisition of new DNA. Biochemically, bacteria resist antibiotics by producing enzymes that destroy or inactivate the drugs. Drug target sites are then altered so that the antibiotic cannot bind to or enter the bacteria. If the drug cannot enter the cell, it cannot kill the bacteria (WHO, 2015a). MRSA can be acquired in a hospital setting and in the community. In health care workers exposed to MRSA, their bodies can become colonized, and they can spread the infection to other health care workers and to patients. The organism can remain viable for days on environmental surfaces and clothing. It is important to understand that many people are colonized with antibiotic-resistant organisms, but they are not infected. However, certain patients are at particular risk of becoming infected including those who are immuno-suppressed

TABLE 17-5 EXAMPLES OF RE-EMERGING INFECTIONS

Microorganism	Infection	Description
Bacteria		
Corynebacterium diphtheriae	Diphtheria	Localized infection of mucous membranes or skin
Bordetella pertussis	Pertussis	Acute, highly contagious respiratory disease that is characterized by loud whooping inspiration; also known as *whooping cough*
Mycobacterium tuberculosis	Tuberculosis	Chronic infection transmitted by inhalation of infected droplets (see Chapter 30)
Viruses		
Dengue viruses (flaviviruses)	Dengue fever	Acute infection transmitted by mosquitoes and occurring mainly in tropical and subtropical regions
Parasite		
Giardia	Giardiasis	Diarrheal illness that usually originates in fecal-contaminated water; also known as travellers' diarrhea

TABLE 17-6 COMMON ANTIBIOTIC-RESISTANT ORGANISMS AND TREATMENT

Bacteria	Resistant To	Preferred Treatment
Clostridium difficile	Associated with the overuse of certain antibiotics, including fluoroquinolones, cephalosporins, and clindamycin	Metronidazole (Flagyl) Vancomycin (Vancocin) Fidaxomicin (Dificid) Stool transplantation
Staphylococcus aureus	Methicillin*	Vancomycin (Vancocin)
Enterococcus faecalis	Vancomycin (Vancocin), streptomycin, gentamicin	Penicillin G or ampicillin
Enterococcus faecium	Vancomycin, streptomycin, gentamicin	Penicillin G or ampicillin
Carbapenem-resistant enterobacteriaceae	Carbapenem class of antibiotics	Fosfomycin (Monurol) Tigecycline (Tygacil)

*No longer used clinically.

(e.g., receiving chemotherapy), have invasive devices (e.g., indwelling catheters), or have breaks in the skin barrier (e.g., surgical wounds). Vancomycin-resistant enterococci are hardier than MRSA and can remain viable on environmental surfaces for weeks. Alcohol preparations are the most effective antimicrobial agents, followed by chlorhexidine gluconate (PHAC, 2012a). The PHAC (2012b) recommended that infection control for antibiotic-resistant organisms consist of routine practices or standard precautions (see Tables 17-8 and 17-9 later in this chapter), which should be used for all patient care.

Drug resistance is a particularly difficult problem in dealing with infectious diseases. Health care providers can contribute to the development of drug-resistant organisms by (a) administering antibiotics for viral infections, (b) succumbing to pressures from patients to prescribe unnecessary antibiotic therapy, (c) using inadequate drug regimens to treat infections, or (d) using broad-spectrum or combination agents for infections that should be treated with first-line medications. Patients who miss doses or do not take antibiotics for the full duration of the prescribed therapy also contribute to the development of resistance. In addition, limited resources or access to medications makes it difficult for some patients to get adequate treatment for infections. Patients and their families should be taught that the proper use of antibiotics (Table 17-7) is crucial to treatment success and prevention of drug-resistant pathogens.

HEALTH CARE–ASSOCIATED INFECTIONS

Health care–associated infections (HAIs; formerly called *nosocomial infections*) are infections that are acquired as a result of exposure to a microorganism in any setting in which health care is delivered (e.g., acute or long-term care facility, ambulatory clinic, home)

TABLE 17-7 PATIENT & CAREGIVER TEACHING GUIDE

Decreasing Risk for Antibiotic-Resistant Infection

1. **Do Not Take Antibiotics to Prevent Illness.** Doing this increases the risk for developing resistant infection.
   - Exceptions include taking antibiotics before certain surgical procedures and taking antibiotics before dental work if the patient has a heart valve disorder.
2. **Wash Hands Frequently.** Handwashing is the most important way to prevent an infection.
3. **Follow Directions.** Not taking antibiotic as prescribed or skipping doses can encourage the development of antibiotic-resistant bacteria.
4. **Finish the Antibiotic.** Patients must not stop taking antibiotic when they feel better. If they stop taking the antibiotic early, the hardiest bacteria survive and multiply. Eventually a patient could develop an infection resistant to many antibiotics. Patients should never have leftover antibiotics.
5. **Do Not Request an Antibiotic for Flu or Colds.** If the health care provider says that an antibiotic is not needed, chances are that this is true. Antibiotics are effective against bacterial infections but not viruses, which cause colds and flus.
6. **Do Not Take Leftover Antibiotics.** People often save unfinished antibiotics for later use or borrow leftover drugs from family or friends. This is dangerous because (a) the leftover antibiotic may not be appropriate for the patient, (b) the illness may not be a bacterial infection, (c) old antibiotics can lose their effectiveness, and in some cases, ingesting them can even be fatal, and (d) there will not be enough doses in a leftover bottle to allow for a full treatment.

and are related to receiving health care. More than 8 000 people die in Canadian hospitals each year as a result of infections acquired during their hospitalization (PHAC, 2013). More than 200 000 Canadians acquire a health care–associated infection each year (PHAC, 2013). Surgical patients are at greater risk. In addition, some bacteria that are not normally pathological can cause infections in patients who are immuno-compromised as a result of illness or treatment of illness. HAIs can be caused by any organism, but certain bacteria—including *E. coli, S. aureus, Enterobacter aerogenes, C. difficile,* and various types of streptococci—are the more common culprits. At least 30% of HAIs can be prevented by following infection prevention strategies (PHAC, 2012b). HAIs are often transmitted from patient to patient through direct contact by health care providers. Hand hygiene (handwashing or use of alcohol-based hand rub) between patient visits and procedures and the appropriate use of personal protective equipment (PPE) such as gloves remain the first lines of defence in preventing the spread of HAIs. It is important to remember that *C. difficile* is not killed by alcohol-based hand rub. Handwashing with soap and water must be followed in this instance. Isolated infections can be caused when bacteria that are normally present in one area of the body are introduced into another area. Therefore, nurses must take care to change gloves and use hand hygiene when changing tasks, even when working with one patient (PHAC, 2012a).

AGE-RELATED CONSIDERATIONS

INFECTION IN OLDER ADULTS

The rate of HAIs is significantly higher among older adults than among younger patients (PHAC, 2013). Individuals in long-term care facilities are at special risk for HAI. Age-related changes (e.g., impaired immune function, comorbid conditions such as diabetes, physical disabilities) can contribute to higher infection rates. HAIs common in older adults include pneumonia, urinary tract infections, skin infections, and TB. Urinary tract infections are more common in older adults who reside in long-term care facilities than in those who live at home. They are often found in patients who have indwelling catheters. Infections in older adults often have atypical manifestations, such as cognitive and behavioural changes, before the emergence of fever, pain, or alterations in laboratory values. Disease should typically be suspected if a patient demonstrates changes in the ability to perform daily activities or in cognitive function. In addition, underlying diseases, increased frequency of drug reactions, and institutionalization can all complicate the management of the older adult with infection.

> **SAFETY ALERT**
> Nurses should not rely on the presence of fever to indicate infection in older adults because many have lower core body temperatures and decreased immune responses.

INFECTION PREVENTION AND CONTROL

Infection Precautions

If a patient develops an infection that is considered a risk to others, infection precautions may be needed. The purpose of these precautions is to prevent the transmission of organisms from patients to health care providers, from health care providers to patients, and from one patient to another. The Centers for Disease Control and Prevention (CDC) issue isolation precaution guidelines that are used in many health care institutions in Canada and around the world. Health Canada has issued similar recommendations (PHAC, 2012b).

Both sets of guidelines contain two levels of precautions (Table 17-8): *routine practices,* or *standard precautions,* which are designed for the care of all patients in hospitals and health care facilities regardless of their diagnosis or presumed infection status, and *additional precautions,* or *transmission-based precautions,* which are used for patients known to be or suspected of being infected with epidemiologically important pathogens that can be transmitted by airborne or droplet transmission or by contact with dry skin or contaminated surfaces.

The system of routine practices or standard precautions applies to (a) blood; (b) all body fluids, secretions, and excretions regardless of whether they contain visible blood; (c) nonintact skin; and

TABLE 17-8 SUMMARY OF ROUTINE PRACTICES AND ADDITIONAL PRECAUTIONS FOR PREVENTING THE TRANSMISSION OF INFECTION IN HEALTH CARE

Routine Practices or Standard Precautions	Additional or Transmission-Based Precautions		
	Airborne*	Droplet*	Contact
When to Use			
All patients	Used in addition to routine practices or standard precautions for patients known to be or suspected of being infected with microorganisms transmitted by airborne droplet (e.g., measles, varicella, tuberculosis). Requires negative-pressure room.	Used in addition to routine practices or standard precautions for patients known to be or suspected of being infected with microorganisms transmitted by droplets (e.g., *Haemophilus influenzae, Neisseria meningitidis, Streptococcus pneumoniae, Mycoplasma pneumoniae,* febrile respiratory illness).	Used in addition to routine practices or standard precautions for specified patients known to be or suspected of being infected with epidemiologically important microorganisms that can be transmitted by direct contact with patient or environmental surfaces (e.g., enteric pathogens, multidrug-resistant bacteria, *Clostridium difficile,* herpes simplex).
Hand Hygiene			
Hand hygiene (the removal or killing of microorganisms on the hands) is done either by handwashing or by use of alcohol-based hand rubs. Using alcohol-based hand rubs is more effective than washing hands (even with antibacterial soap) when hands are not visibly soiled. Hand hygiene should be performed (a) before initial patient contact or contact with the patient's environment, (b) before aseptic procedures, (c) after body fluid exposure risk, and (d) after contact with a patient or the patient's environment.	Same as routine practices or standard precautions.	Same as routine practices or standard precautions.	Same as routine practices or standard precautions.
Gloves			
Nurses wear nonsterile gloves when touching blood, body fluids, secretions, excretions, and contaminated items; they put on clean gloves just before touching mucous membranes and nonintact skin; they remove gloves promptly after use, before touching noncontaminated items, environmental surfaces, or going to another patient.	Same as routine practices or standard precautions.	Same as routine practices or standard precautions.	In addition to glove use as described in routine practices or standard precautions, nurses wear gloves when entering the patient's room and whenever providing direct patient care or having hand contact with potentially contaminated surfaces or items in patient's environment.
Mask, Eye Protection, Face Shield			
Nurses wear mask and eye protection or face shield to protect mucous membranes of eyes, nose, and mouth during procedures and patient care activities likely to generate splashes or sprays of blood, body fluids, secretions, and excretions. These should be worn within 1 m of coughing patient.	In addition to routine practices or standard precautions, nurses wear respiratory protection when entering room of patient known to have or suspected of having tuberculosis. *Note:* Nurses should check the facility's policy for use of respirator.	In addition to routine practices or standard precautions, a mask should be worn.	Same as routine practices or standard precautions.

TABLE 17-8 SUMMARY OF ROUTINE PRACTICES AND ADDITIONAL PRECAUTIONS FOR PREVENTING THE TRANSMISSION OF INFECTION IN HEALTH CARE—cont'd

Routine Practices or Standard Precautions	Additional or Transmission-Based Precautions		
	Airborne*	Droplet*	Contact
Gown Nurses wear clean, nonsterile gown to protect skin and prevent soiling of clothing during procedures and patient care activities likely to generate splashes or sprays of blood, body fluids, secretions, or excretions or likely to cause soiling of clothing. Gown is removed promptly when tasks are completed; hands are washed.	Same as routine practices or standard precautions.	Same as routine practices or standard precautions.	Clean, nonsterile gown is worn if substantial contact is anticipated with patient, surfaces, or items in environment and if patient is incontinent or has diarrhea, an ileostomy, a colostomy, or uncontained wound drainage. Gown is removed carefully when tasks are completed; hands are washed.
Linen Handle, transport, and process used linen in manner that prevents skin and mucous membrane exposure, contamination of clothing, and environmental soiling.	Same as routine practices or standard precautions.	Same as routine practices or standard precautions.	Same as routine practices or standard precautions.
Patient Transport	Movement and transport of patient from room should be limited to instances of essential purposes only; if transport or movement is necessary, patient dispersal of droplet nuclei is minimized by placement of surgical mask on patient, if possible.	Movement and transport of patient from room should be limited to instances of essential purposes only; if transport or movement is necessary, patient dispersal of droplet nuclei is minimized by placement of surgical mask on patient, if possible.	Movement and transport of patient from room should be limited to instances of essential purposes only; if transport is necessary, precautions are maintained to minimize contamination of environmental surfaces or equipment.

Source: © All rights reserved. Routine practices and additional precautions for preventing the transmission of infection in health care settings. Public Health Agency of Canada, 2013. Adapted and reproduced with permission from the Minister of Health, 2017.
*In the case of certain infections (e.g., chicken pox and disseminated zoster), a combination of airborne and contact transmission precautions may be required. For certain other infections (e.g., influenza and invasive group A streptococci), a combination of droplet and contact precautions is required.

(d) mucous membranes. Routine practices or standard precautions are designed to reduce the risk of transmission of microorganisms from both recognized and unrecognized sources of infection in hospitals. Routine practices or standard precautions should be applied to all patients regardless of diagnosis or infection status.

Additional or transmission-based precautions are designed for patients suspected of or documented as being infected with highly transmissible or epidemiologically important pathogens for which additional precautions beyond routine practices or standard precautions are needed to interrupt transmission in hospitals. The three types of additional or transmission-based precautions are *airborne precautions, droplet precautions,* and *contact precautions.* They may be used in combination for diseases that have multiple routes of transmission. When used either by themselves or in combination, these precautions are used in addition to routine practices or standard precautions.

Preventing Occupational Infections in Health Care Workers

In 2002, Health Canada issued updated standards for preventing and controlling occupational infections in health care workers. These standards mandated that any employer whose employees are potentially exposed to blood from needles and other sharps must implement sharps safety devices wherever feasible. Many provinces have implemented mandatory use of safety-engineered needles and needle-free infusion devices. In addition, employees at risk need to be provided with appropriate PPE. Health care

workers must minimize or eliminate exposure to infectious material. When that is not possible, appropriate PPE must be selected. These include gloves, clothing, and facial protection (Table 17-9). Appropriate PPE will vary, depending on the situation (PHAC, 2012b).

In the event that a health care worker is exposed to blood or body fluids, as a result of either a needle stick or a mucous membrane splash, the worker should seek immediate medical attention to assess the level of risk for acquiring a bloodborne virus from the incident. If the risk is deemed serious enough to put the worker at risk for acquiring HIV, postexposure prophylaxis is initiated. There is no postexposure prophylaxis for hepatitis C virus. Statistics have been compiled since the early 1990s about the rates of HIV seroconversion in health care workers as a result of an accidental exposure, and in fact, the rates are extremely low; however, cases have been documented, and so it is important for nurses to use routine practices or standard precautions with every patient with whom they come into contact (PHAC, 2012b).

HUMAN IMMUNODEFICIENCY VIRUS INFECTION

The HIV epidemic in Canada and the United States began in the early 1980s. HIV had been circulating in sub-Saharan Africa since the early 1920s (Pepin, 2011), but it was not until 1981 that public health officials documented the presence of a new disease that would become known as the **acquired immunodeficiency**

TABLE 17-9   HEALTH CANADA RECOMMENDATIONS FOR THE USE OF PERSONAL PROTECTIVE EQUIPMENT FOR HEALTH CARE WORKERS

Equipment	Indications for Use
Medical gloves	Should be worn for all procedures that might involve direct skin or mucous membrane contact with blood or fluids capable of transmitting bloodborne pathogens. May also be indicated for other activities (e.g., procedures involving other infectious agents, toxins, or contaminated equipment).
Masks and protective eyewear (e.g., goggles, safety glasses) or face shields	Should be worn to protect mucous membranes, nonintact skin, and conjunctiva during procedures that are likely to generate splashes of blood or fluids capable of transmitting bloodborne pathogens.
Gowns or aprons	Should be worn during procedures that are likely to generate splashes of blood or fluids capable of transmitting bloodborne pathogens. Assessment of the specific risk will determine the type of gown required (e.g., fluid-resistant).

Source: Public Health Agency of Canada (2012). *Routine practices and additional precautions for preventing the transmission of infection in health care settings.* Ottawa: Author. Retrieved from *www.publications.gc.ca/collections/collection_2013/aspc-phac/HP40-83-2013-eng.pdf.*

syndrome (AIDS). Interestingly, people had been dying of AIDS in North America for several decades before it was identified. This first documented case in Canada was in 1959. By 1985, the causative agent, HIV, had been identified, and AIDS was determined to be the end stage of chronic HIV infection. In addition, an antibody test was developed and routes of transmission were determined. Drug therapy to treat the infection became available in 1987 with the release of zidovudine (ZDV, azidothymidine [AZT], Retrovir) and has since expanded. Since 1994, several important advances have been made, including the development of laboratory tests to assess the number of HIV particles in the blood (viral load), the production of new drugs, combination drug therapy, the ability to test for antiretroviral drug resistance, treatment to decrease the risk of transmission from mother to baby (AIDSinfo, 2016a), and the use of treatment as prevention (Montaner, 2011). In developed countries around the world, these advances have led to decreases in the number of HIV-related deaths, improved quality of life, and decreases in the number of cases of congenital HIV infection. Unfortunately, these advances are not effective or available for all those who need them. Although great progress has been made, the HIV epidemic is not over. There are signs that it is levelling off, with fewer new infections each year, but it continues to take its toll, inasmuch as approximately 7000 people are newly infected every day (United Nations AIDS [UNAIDS], 2015a). Nursing care for patients with HIV infection continues to be a critical need that must change as new findings and treatment advances emerge.

SIGNIFICANCE OF THE PROBLEM

Almost 2.4 million people were living with HIV infection in North America and Western Europe at the end of 2014, with an estimated 85 000 new infections and 26 000 HIV-related deaths that year (UNAIDS, 2015b). Of those living with the infection, 260 000 (25%) were adolescent and adult women, and 11 000 were children younger than age 15. At the end of 2014, Health Canada estimated that approximately 75 500 people in Canada were living with HIV infection (including those living with AIDS) and that approximately 21% were not aware that they were infected (PHAC, 2015d). Although the numbers are increasing, the number of new cases per year is declining. In addition, treatment has provided major advances in the ability to keep HIV-infected people healthy for longer periods, and the death rate has fallen dramatically. Globally, HIV infection has been devastating. Since the beginning of the pandemic, more than 60 million people have been infected, and more than 30 million of those have died (UNAIDS, 2015b). At the end of 2014, an estimated 36.9 million people—including 2.2 million children younger than age 15—were living with HIV infection. During that year, 2.0 million people were newly infected with HIV, and more than 1.8 million died of HIV-related causes (PHAC, 2015b).

The burden of HIV is not evenly distributed. Since the beginning of the epidemic, sub-Saharan Africa has been the most devastated, but Asia, Russia, India, Central America, and South America also have rampant epidemics. In developing countries, the major mode of transmission is through heterosexual sex, and women and children bear a large part of the burden of illness. Industrialized countries have fared better but have not been able to eliminate the infection or provide appropriate care to all HIV-infected individuals. For the most part, HIV infection remains a disease of marginalized individuals: those who are disenfranchised by virtue of sex, race, sexual orientation, poverty, drug use, or lack of access to health care.

TRANSMISSION OF HUMAN IMMUNODEFICIENCY VIRUS

HIV is a fragile virus. It can be transmitted only under specific conditions that allow contact with infected body fluids, including blood, semen, vaginal secretions, and breast milk. HIV is transmitted through sexual intercourse with an infected partner, exposure to HIV-infected blood or blood products, as a result of either contaminated transfusion or needle sharing, and perinatally at the time of delivery or through breastfeeding (CDC, 2015a).

HIV-infected individuals can transmit HIV to others within a few days after becoming infected. After that, the ability to transmit HIV is lifelong. Transmission of HIV is subject to the same requirements as other microorganisms: a large enough amount of the virus must enter the body of a susceptible host. Duration and frequency of contact, volume of fluid, virulence and concentration of the organism, and host immune status all affect whether infection actually occurs after an exposure. The viral load in the blood, the semen, the vaginal secretions, or the breast milk of the "donor" is an important variable. In HIV infection, large amounts of virus can be found in the blood during the first 2 to 6 months after infection and again during the late stages of the disease (Figure 17-1). Unprotected sexual or blood exposure to an infected individual is more risky during these periods, although HIV can be transmitted during all phases of the disease (CDC, 2015a).

HIV is not spread casually. The virus cannot be transmitted through hugging, dry kissing, shaking hands, sharing eating utensils, using toilet seats, or attending school or working with an HIV-infected person. It is not transmitted through tears, saliva,

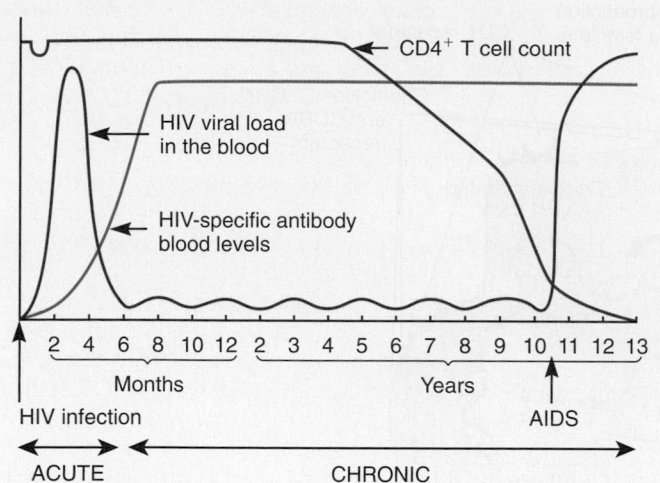

FIGURE 17-1 Viral load in the blood and CD4⁺ T cell counts across the spectrum of untreated human immunodeficiency virus (HIV) infection. *AIDS,* acquired immune deficiency syndrome.

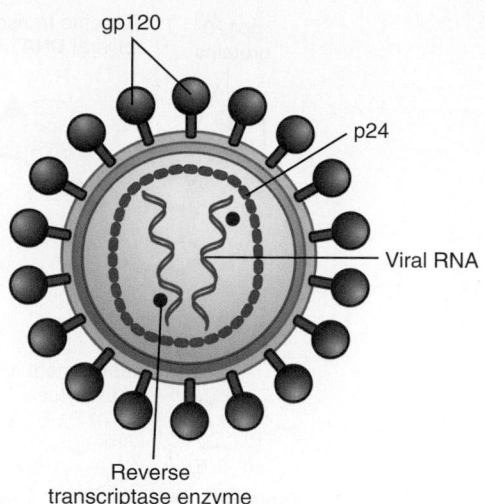

FIGURE 17-2 The human immunodeficiency virus (HIV) is surrounded by an envelope made up of proteins (including glycoprotein 120 [gp120]) and contains a core of viral RNA and proteins (including p24).

urine, emesis, sputum, feces, or sweat. Repeated studies have failed to demonstrate transmission of the virus by respiratory droplets, enteric routes, or casual encounters in any setting. Health care workers have a very low risk of acquiring HIV at work, even after a needle-stick injury (Kuhar, Henderson, Struble, et al., 2013). Should a health care worker become exposed, she or he should follow the hospital policy for reporting needle-stick incidents.

Sexual Transmission

The most common mode of HIV transmission is unprotected sexual contact with an HIV-infected partner. Sexual activity involves contact with semen, vaginal secretions, blood, or a combination of these, all of which have lymphocytes that may contain HIV. During any form of sexual intercourse (anal, vaginal, or oral), the risk of infection is greater for the partner who receives the semen, although infection can also be transmitted to the inserting partner. This occurs because the receiver has prolonged contact with infected fluids, and it helps explain why it is easier to infect women than men during heterosexual intercourse. Sexual activities that cause trauma to local tissues can increase the risk of transmission. In addition, genital lesions from other sexually transmitted infections (e.g., herpes, syphilis) significantly increase the likelihood of HIV transmission.

Contact With Blood and Blood Products

HIV is transmitted by exposure to contaminated blood through the accidental or intended sharing of injection equipment. Sharing equipment to inject illegal drugs is a major means of transmission in many large metropolitan areas and is becoming more common in smaller cities and rural areas. Once used, equipment used to inject any drug, whether prescribed or not, is contaminated, potentially with HIV, other bloodborne organisms, or both, and sharing that equipment can result in disease transmission.

In Canada, an estimated 1150 individuals were infected with HIV through blood transfusions between 1978 and 1985. In 1985, the practices of routine screening of blood donors to identify at-risk individuals and testing donated blood for the presence of HIV were implemented, which improved the safety of the blood supply. HIV infection as a result of blood transfusions is

now rare. In 2001, a new, highly sensitive nucleic acid amplification test (NAAT) was implemented by the Canadian Blood Services to detect HIV genetic material in blood of potential donors. The NAAT has a much shorter window period—the time between exposure to HIV infection and when the test yields an accurate result—than does antibody testing and is now the standard test for donated blood in Canada.

Puncture wounds are the most common means of work-related transmission. The risk of infection after a needle-stick exposure to HIV-infected blood is 0.3% to 0.4% (or 3–4 in 1000). The risk is higher if the exposure involves blood from a patient with a high viral load, from a deep puncture wound, from a needle with a hollow bore and visible blood, from a device used for venous or arterial access, or from a patient who dies within 60 days. Splash exposures of blood on skin with an open lesion present some risk, but it is much lower than from a puncture wound (HIV.gov, 2015; Kuhar, Henderson, Struble, et al., 2013; PHAC, 2016).

Perinatal Transmission

Perinatal transmission from an HIV-infected mother to her infant can occur during pregnancy, delivery, or breastfeeding (CDC, 2015b; PHAC, 2010). On average, 25% of infants born to women with untreated HIV infection are born with HIV. Fortunately, the risk of transmission can be reduced to less than 1% in settings where pregnant women are routinely tested for HIV infection and, if found to be infected, treated with antiretroviral therapy (ART) (Burdge et al., 2003).

PATHOPHYSIOLOGY

Human immunodeficiency virus (HIV) is an RNA virus. RNA viruses are called **retroviruses** because they replicate in a "backward" manner (transcribing their RNA and DNA after entering a cell). Like all viruses, HIV cannot replicate unless it is inside a living cell. HIV can enter a cell when the glycoprotein 120 (gp120) "knobs" (Figure 17-2) on the viral envelope bind to specific CD4 receptor sites and CCR5 and CXCR4 co-receptor sites on the cell's surface (Figure 17-3). Once bound, viral genetic material enters the cell. In the cell, viral RNA is transcribed into

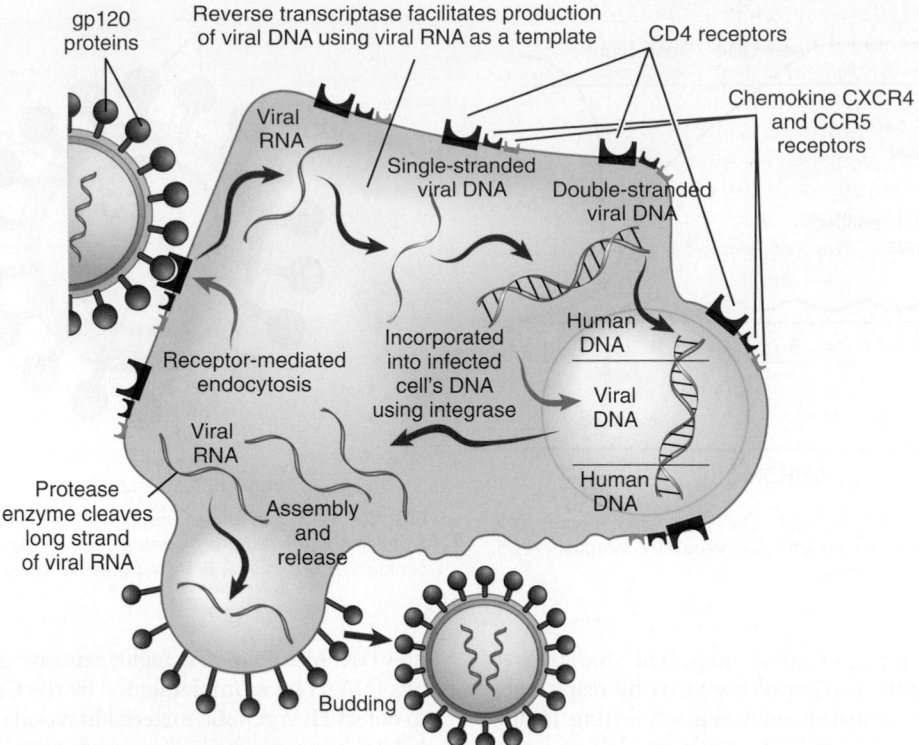

FIGURE 17-3 The human immunodeficiency virus (HIV) has glycoprotein 120 (gp120) that attaches to CD4 and chemokine CXCR4 and CCR5 receptors on the surface of CD4+ T cells. Viral RNA then enters the cell, produces viral DNA in the presence of reverse transcriptase, and incorporates itself into the cellular genome in the presence of integrase, causing permanent cellular infection and the production of new virions. New viral RNA develops initially in long strands that are cut in the presence of protease and leave the cell through a budding process that ultimately contributes to cellular destruction.

a double strand of viral DNA with the assistance of **reverse transcriptase,** an enzyme made by HIV and other retroviruses. At this point, viral DNA can enter the cell's nucleus and, using an enzyme called integrase, splice itself into the genome, becoming a permanent part of the cell's genetic structure. There are two consequences of this action: (a) because all genetic material is replicated during cellular division, all daughter cells from the infected cell will also be infected; and (b) because the genome now contains viral DNA, the cell's genetic codes can direct the cell to make HIV. Production of HIV within the cell is a complicated process that results in long strands of HIV RNA. These are cut into appropriate lengths with the assistance of the enzyme protease during the budding sequence (AIDSinfo, 2016b).

Initial infection with HIV results in **viremia** (large amounts of virus in the blood). This is followed within a few weeks by a prolonged period during which HIV levels in the blood remain low even without treatment (see Figure 17-1). During this time, which may last for 10 to 12 years, there are few clinical symptoms. It was initially thought that this phase represented a latency period during which very little viral activity occurred. It is now known that HIV replication occurs at rapid and constant rates in the blood and lymph tissues from early in the infection. A steady-state viral load can be maintained in the body of infected individuals for many years. To do this, 108 to 109 new viruses are produced each day. A major consequence of rapid replication is that errors can occur in the copying process, causing mutations that can contribute to resistance to ART and limit treatment options.

In a normal immune response, foreign antigens interact with B cells and T cells. In the initial stages of HIV infection, these cells respond and function normally. B cells make HIV-specific antibodies that are effective in reducing viral loads in the blood, and activated T cells mount a cellular immune response to viruses trapped in the lymph nodes (AIDSinfo, 2016b).

HIV infects human cells whose surfaces have CD4 receptors. These cells include lymphocytes, monocytes and macrophages, astrocytes, and oligodendrocytes. Immune dysfunction in HIV disease is caused predominantly by damage to and destruction of CD4+ T cells (also known as T helper cells or CD4+ T lymphocytes). These cells are targeted because they have more CD4 receptors on their surfaces than do other CD4 receptor–bearing cells. This is unfortunate because CD4+ T cells play a key role in the ability of the immune system to recognize and defend against pathogens.

Adults without immune dysfunction normally have 800 to 1200 CD4+ T cells per microlitre of blood. The normal life span of a CD4+ T cell is about 100 days, but HIV-infected CD4+ T cells die after an average of only 2 days. The compromise of the immune system is also caused by the chronic state of immune activation that is a result of HIV infection. This activation leads to elevated levels of inflammatory markers and destruction of T helper cells (Wasserman, Segal-Maurer, Wehbeh, et al., 2011).

Viral activity destroys about 1 billion CD4+ T cells every day. Fortunately, the bone marrow and the thymus are able to produce enough CD4+ T cells to replace the destroyed cells for many years. Eventually, however, the ability of HIV to destroy CD4+ T cells exceeds the body's ability to replace the cells. The result is a decline in the CD4+ T-cell count and a decrease in immune capability. In general, the immune system remains healthy with more than 500 CD4$^+$ T cells per microlitre. Immune problems start to occur when the count drops below this number. Severe problems develop with fewer than 200 CD4$^+$ T cells per microlitre and a CD4 fraction of less than 15%. Eventually in HIV infection, so many CD4$^+$ T cells are destroyed that not enough remain to regulate immune responses (see Figure 17-1). The major concern related to immune suppression is the development of opportunistic diseases (infections and cancers that occur in immuno-suppressed patients that can lead to disability, disease, and death).

CLINICAL MANIFESTATIONS AND COMPLICATIONS

The typical course of untreated HIV infection follows the pattern shown in Figure 17-4. However, it is important to remember that HIV is highly individualized. The information depicted in Figure 17-4 represents data from large groups of people and should not be used to predict an individual's lifespan after HIV infection.

Acute Infection

Development of HIV-specific antibodies (seroconversion) is frequently accompanied by a flulike syndrome of fever, swollen lymph glands, sore throat, headache, malaise, nausea, muscle and joint pain, diarrhea, or a diffuse rash, or a combination of these. These symptoms, called acute retroviral syndrome, generally occur 1 to 3 weeks after the initial infection and last for 1 to 2 weeks, although some of the symptoms may continue for several months. During this time, a high level of HIV in the blood is noted, and CD4$^+$ T-cell counts fall temporarily but quickly return to baseline (see Figure 17-1). In most infected people, acute retroviral symptoms are moderate and may be mistaken for a cold or flu. In some infected people, neurological complications, such as aseptic meningitis, peripheral neuropathy, facial palsy, or Guillain-Barré syndrome, have developed (Smith, Rutstein, Powers, et al., 2013).

Chronic Infection

Early Chronic Infection. The median interval between untreated HIV infection and a diagnosis of AIDS is about 10 years. During this time, CD4$^+$ T-lymphocyte counts remain above 500 cells per microlitre (normal) or slightly decreased, and the viral load in the blood remains low. This phase has been referred to as *asymptomatic disease,* but fatigue, headache, low-grade fever, night sweats, persistent generalized lymphadenopathy, and other symptoms often occur.

Because most of the symptoms during early infection are vague and nonspecific for HIV, people with HIV infection may not be aware that they are infected. According to the PHAC (2015d), approximately 21% of individuals infected with HIV are estimated to be unaware of their status. During this time, infected people continue activities that may include high-risk sexual and drug-using behaviours, which creates a public health problem because infected people can transmit HIV to others even if they have no symptoms. Personal health is also affected because people who do not know they are infected have no motivation to seek treatment or to make changes in health habits that could beneficially alter the quality and quantity of their lives.

Intermediate Chronic Infection. When the CD4$^+$ T-cell count drops below 500 cells per microlitre (as low as 200 cells per microlitre), the viral load rises, and HIV infection advances to a more active stage. Symptoms and signs that occurred in earlier phases tend to become worse, manifesting as persistent fever, frequent drenching night sweats, chronic diarrhea, recurrent headaches, and fatigue severe enough to interrupt normal routines. Other problems that may occur at this time include localized infections, lymphadenopathy, and nervous system manifestations.

The most common infection associated with this phase of HIV disease is oropharyngeal candidiasis, or thrush (Figure 17-5). *Candida* organisms rarely cause problems in healthy adults, but such problems do occur in most HIV-infected people at some time. Other infections that can occur at this time include shingles (caused by the varicella-zoster virus), persistent vaginal candidal infections, outbreaks of oral or genital herpes, bacterial infections, and Kaposi's sarcoma (Figure 17-6). Oral hairy leukoplakia, an Epstein-Barr virus infection that causes painless, white, raised lesions on the lateral aspect of the tongue, can also occur (Figure 17-7). Oral lesions may provide the earliest indication of HIV infection.

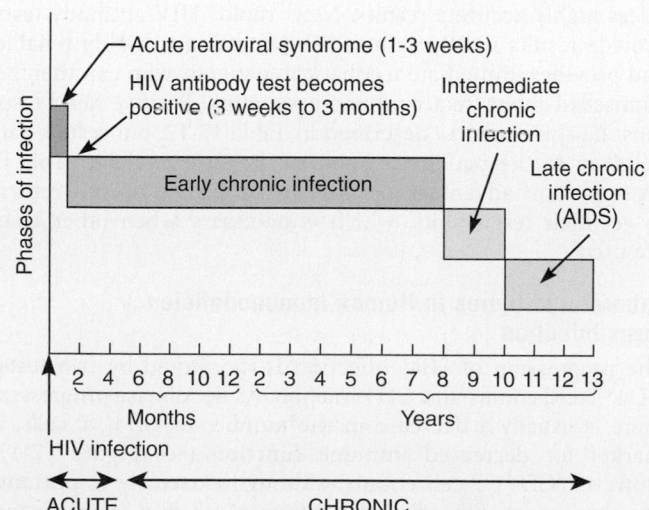

FIGURE 17-4 Timeline for the spectrum of untreated human immunodeficiency virus (HIV) infection. The timeline represents the course of the illness from the time of infection to the clinical manifestations of disease. *AIDS*, acquired immune deficiency syndrome.

FIGURE 17-5 Oral thrush involving the hard and soft palate surfaces. Source: Emond, R., Welsby, P., & Rowland, H. (2003). *Colour atlas of infectious diseases* (4th ed.). Edinburgh: Mosby.

FIGURE 17-6 Kaposi's sarcoma: malignant vascular lesion on the torso. The lesions can appear anywhere on the skin surface and on internal organs. Lesions vary in size from pinpoint to very large (several centimetres) and may appear in a variety of shades. Source: Courtesy of Jeffrey Kwong.

FIGURE 17-7 Oral hairy leukoplakia on the lateral aspect of the tongue. Source: Set of slides published in 1992 by Jon Fuller, MD, and Howard Libman, MD, at Boston University School of Medicine, Boston.

Late Chronic Infection or Acquired Immune Deficiency Syndrome. A diagnosis of AIDS cannot be made until the HIV-infected patient meets the criteria established by the WHO (2007).

These criteria (Table 17-10) are more likely to occur when the immune system becomes severely compromised. As the viral load increases, the absolute number and percentage of T cells decrease and the risk of developing opportunistic diseases increases.

Opportunistic diseases, often reactivations of a prior infection, generally do not occur in the presence of a functioning immune system. Numerous infections, a variety of malignancies, wasting, and dementia can result from HIV-related immune impairment (Table 17-11). Organisms that do not usually cause disease in people with functioning immune systems can cause severe, debilitating, disseminated, and life-threatening infections during this stage. Several opportunistic diseases are likely to occur at the same time, further compounding the difficulties of diagnosis and treatment. Advances in HIV treatment have led to significant decreases in opportunistic diseases because successful treatment helps maintain the immune system's function.

DIAGNOSTIC STUDIES

Diagnosis of Human Immunodeficiency Virus Infection

The most useful screening tests for HIV are those that detect HIV-specific antibodies. The major problem with these tests is

TABLE 17-10	DIAGNOSTIC CRITERIA FOR AIDS

AIDS is diagnosed when an individual with HIV infection develops at least one of these conditions:
- Atypical disseminated leishmaniasis
- Central nervous system toxoplasmosis
- Chronic cryptosporidiosis
- Chronic herpes simplex virus infection
- Chronic isosporiasis
- Cytomegalovirus disease (other than liver, spleen, or lymph nodes)
- Disseminated mycosis (coccidiomycosis or histoplasmosis)
- Disseminated nontuberculous mycobacterial infection
- Esophageal candidiasis
- Extrapulmonary cryptococcosis (including meningitis)
- Extrapulmonary tuberculosis
- HIV encephalopathy
- HIV wasting syndrome (*wasting* is defined as a loss of 10% or more of ideal body mass)
- Invasive cervical carcinoma
- Kaposi's sarcoma
- Lymphoma (cerebral or B-cell non-Hodgkin's)
- *Pneumocystis* pneumonia
- Progressive multifocal leukoencephalopathy
- Recurrent bacterial pneumonia
- Recurrent nontyphoid *Salmonella* bacteremia
- Symptomatic HIV-associated cardiomyopathy
- Symptomatic HIV-associated nephropathy

Source: World Health Organization. (2007). *WHO case definitions of HIV for surveillance and revised clinical staging and immunological classification of HIV-related disease in adults and children.* Geneva: Author. Retrieved from *http://www.who.int/hiv/pub/guidelines/HIVstaging150307.pdf.*
AIDS, acquired immune deficiency syndrome; HIV, human immunodeficiency virus.

that there is a median delay of 2 months after infection before antibodies can be detected (see Figure 17-1). However, there is a newer test, the fourth-generation enzyme immunoassay (EIA), which combines antibody detection with p24 antigen. This test has a shorter window period. The window period is concerning because in an infected individual, an HIV antibody test will not yield positive results during this time, even though the individual is infected. HIV-antibody screening is generally done in the sequence shown in Table 17-12. This process produces highly accurate results. New "rapid" HIV-antibody tests provide results in 20 minutes. Rapid testing is highly reliable and provides immediate feedback to patients, who can then be counselled about treatment and prevention. Positive rapid tests must be confirmed as described in Table 17-12, but results can be given to the patient as soon as they are available. This is an important advantage because many people do not return to get their test results, which is necessary when other tests are used.

Laboratory Studies in Human Immunodeficiency Virus Infection

The progression of HIV infection is monitored by two tests: CD4+ T-cell counts and CD4 fraction. As the disease progresses, there is usually a decrease in the number of CD4+ T cells, a marker for decreased immune function (see Figure 17-1). However, CD4+ T-cell counts, although extremely important, reveal only part of the clinical picture because even in uninfected people, CD4 counts vary greatly from day to day, which makes accurate assessment of immune status difficult. In contrast, CD4 fraction is a stable number for most people, with a normal range of 27% to 60%. A CD4 fraction of less than 15% is associated with immune compromise. Laboratory tests that measure viral

TABLE 17-11 DRUG THERAPY

Manifestations and Treatment of Common Opportunistic Diseases Associated With HIV Infection

Organism and Disease	Clinical Manifestations	Prophylaxis* and Treatment†
Candida albicans	Thrush, esophagitis, vaginitis; whitish yellow patches in mouth, esophagus, GI tract, vagina	Treatment: fluconazole (Diflucan), clotrimazole, nystatin, itraconazole (Sporanox); if infection is resistant to fluconazole: amphotericin B (Fungizone) Secondary prophylaxis (only if subsequent episodes are frequent or severe recurrences): fluconazole (Diflucan), itraconazole (Sporanox)
Castleman's disease (caused by HHV-8)	Generalized malaise, night sweats, rigors, fever, anorexia, weight loss Eventually lymphadenopathy, hepatosplenomegaly, ascites, edema, pulmonary and pericardial effusions	Treatment: antivirals such as IV ganciclovir (Cytovene) or oral valganciclovir (Valcyte) Chemotherapy, either single drug or combined: the CHOP protocol is most recommended
Cervical cancer	Cancerous lesions in the cervix Vaginal bleeding, pain during intercourse	Surgical excision of the cancerous lesion Chemotherapy Radiotherapy
Coccidioides immitis	Pneumonia: fever, weight loss, cough	Treatment: amphotericin B (Fungizone), fluconazole (Diflucan), itraconazole (Sporanox) Secondary prophylaxis (to prevent recurrence of documented disease): fluconazole (Diflucan), amphotericin B (Fungizone), itraconazole (Sporanox)
CNS lymphoma	Cognitive dysfunction, motor impairment, aphasia, seizures, personality changes, headache	Treatment: radiation, chemotherapy
Cryptococcus neoformans	Meningitis, cognitive impairment, motor dysfunction, fever, seizures, headache	Treatment: amphotericin B (Fungizone), fluconazole (Diflucan), itraconazole (Sporanox) Secondary prophylaxis (to prevent recurrence of documented disease): fluconazole (Diflucan), amphotericin B (Fungizone), itraconazole (Sporanox) Therapeutic lumbar punctures to reduce intracranial pressure
Cryptosporidium muris	Gastro-enteritis, watery diarrhea, abdominal pain, weight loss	Treatment: antidiarrheals, nitazoxanide (Alinia), paromomycin (Humatin)
CMV	Retinitis: retinal lesions, blurred vision, loss of vision Esophagitis, stomatitis: difficulty swallowing; colitis, gastritis: bloody diarrhea, pain, weight loss Pneumonitis: respiratory symptoms Neurological disease: CNS manifestations	Treatment: ganciclovir (Cytovene), foscarnet (Foscavir), cidofovir (Vistide), valganciclovir (Valcyte) Secondary prophylaxis (to prevent recurrence of documented disease): ganciclovir (Cytovene), foscarnet (Foscavir), cidofovir (Vistide), valganciclovir (Valcyte)
Hepatitis B virus (HBV)	Jaundice, fatigue, abdominal pain, loss of appetite, nausea, vomiting, joint pain; 30% of affected patients may have no signs or symptoms	Primary prevention: HBV vaccine series; screening and vaccination of people with no evidence of previous HBV infection; encouragement of patients to reveal injection drug use, whether they are sexually active men who have sex with men, sexual partners or household contacts of HBV-infected individuals, and those with HCV; HAV vaccine series should be given to prevent additive effects and advanced liver damage; screening and vaccination of people without evidence of previous HAV infection Treatment: adefovir dipivoxil (Hepsera), α-interferon, lamivudine (3TC), entecavir (Baraclude)
hepatitis C virus (HCV)	Jaundice, fatigue, abdominal pain, loss of appetite, nausea, vomiting, dark urine; 80% may have no signs or symptoms	Prophylaxis: none for HCV; HAV and HBV vaccines series should be given to prevent additive effects and advanced liver damage; screening and vaccination of people without evidence of previous HAV or HBV infection Treatment: α-interferon, ribavirin (Virazole), boceprevir (Victrelis)
Herpes simplex virus (HSV)	Type 1 (HSV1): orolabial and mucocutaneous vesicular and ulcerative lesions; keratitis: visual disturbances; encephalitis: CNS manifestations Type 2 (HSV2): genital and perianal vesicular and ulcerative lesions	Treatment: acyclovir (Zovirax), famciclovir (Famvir), valacyclovir (Valtrex), foscarnet (Foscavir), cidofovir (Vistide) Secondary prophylaxis (only if subsequent episodes are frequent or severe): acyclovir (Zovirax), famciclovir (Famvir), valacyclovir (Valtrex)
Histoplasma capsulatum	Pneumonia: fever, cough, weight loss Meningitis: CNS manifestations; disseminated disease	Treatment: amphotericin B (Fungizone), itraconazole (Sporanox), fluconazole (Diflucan) Secondary prophylaxis (to prevent recurrence of documented disease): itraconazole (Sporanox), amphotericin B (Fungizone)

Continued

TABLE 17-11   DRUG THERAPY

Manifestations and Treatment of Common Opportunistic Diseases Associated With HIV Infection—cont'd

Organism and Disease	Clinical Manifestations	Prophylaxis* and Treatment†
Influenza virus	Fever (usually high, 38°C–40°C), headache, extreme tiredness, dry cough, sore throat, runny or stuffy nose, muscle aches; nausea, vomiting, and diarrhea can occur	Primary prevention: inactivated trivalent influenza virus vaccine; provided annually, before influenza virus season; revaccination if initial vaccine was given when CD4+ T cell count was <200/mcL Treatment: supportive therapy
JC papovavirus	Progressive multifocal leukoencephalopathy, CNS manifestations, mental and motor declines	Treatment: supportive therapy
Kaposi's sarcoma (caused by HHV-8)	Vascular lesions on the skin, mucous membranes, and viscera, with wide range of presentation: firm, flat, raised, or nodular; pinpoint to several centimetres in size; hyperpigmented, multicentric; can cause lymphedema and disfigurement, particularly when confluent; not usually serious unless it occurs in the respiratory or GI systems	Treatment (dependent on severity of lesions): cancer chemotherapy, α-interferon, local irradiation; cryotherapy for skin lesions
Mycobacterium avium complex	Gastro-enteritis, watery diarrhea, weight loss	Primary prophylaxis (initiate when CD4+ T cell count is <50/mcL): clarithromycin (Biaxin) or azithromycin (Zithromax), rifabutin (Mycobutin). Prophylaxis may be stopped when CD4+ T cell count of >100/mcL is documented for 6–12 mo; restarted if CD4+ T cell count falls to <50/mcL. Disseminated disease or TB must be ruled out. Treatment: clarithromycin (Biaxin), ethambutol (Etibi), rifabutin (Mycobutin), azithromycin (Zithromax), ciprofloxacin (Cipro), levofloxacin (Levaquin), amikacin
Multicentric Castleman's disease (caused by HHV-8)	Fever, anemia, elevated C-reactive protein levels, widespread lymphadenopathy, weight loss, respiratory symptoms, edema, pulmonary and pericardial effusions and splenomegaly	Treatment: gancyclovir (Cytovene), systemic chemotherapy (CHOP) and rituximab (Rituxan)
Mycobacterium tuberculosis	Respiratory and disseminated disease; productive cough, fever, night sweats, weight loss	See Chapter 30 (first-line drug therapy for TB; [see Table 30.6], drug regimen options for treatment of TB [see Table 30.7])
Pneumocystis jiroveci pneumonia	Pneumonia, nonproductive cough, hypoxemia, progressive shortness of breath, fever, night sweats, fatigue	Primary prophylaxis: initiate when CD4+ T cell count is <200/mcL: TMP/SMX (Septra), dapsone, dapsone with pyrimethamine, folinic acid, aerosolized pentamidine, atovaquone (Mepron). Adverse effects of TMP/SMX and dapsone (especially rash, fever, and anemia) are common and may limit use. Treatment: TMP/SMX, pentamidine, dapsone, trimethoprim, clindamycin, primaquine, atovaquone (Mepron); with hypoxia, use corticosteroids
Toxoplasma gondii	Encephalitis, cognitive dysfunction, motor impairment, fever, altered mental status, headache, seizures, sensory abnormalities	Primary prophylaxis: (1) TMP/SMX *or* (2) dapsone + pyrimethamine + leukovorin *or* (3) atovaquone ± pyrimethamine + leukovorin Treatment: (1) sulphadiazine *or* (2) clindamycin + pyrimethamine + leukovorin *or* (3) atovaquone + pyrimethamine + leukovorin *or* (4) azithromycin + pyrimethamine + leukovorin
Varicella-zoster virus (VZV)	Shingles: erythematous maculopapular rash along dermatomal planes, pain, pruritus Ocular: progressive outer retinal necrosis	Primary prophylaxis: varicella-zoster immune globulin administered only after significant exposure to chicken pox or shingles for patients with no history of disease or negative result of VZV antibody test Treatment: acyclovir (Zovirax), famciclovir (Famvir), valacyclovir (Valtrex)

Source: Data from British Columbia Centre for Excellence in HIV/AIDS. (2009). *Therapeutic guidelines for opportunistic infections.* Vancouver: Author. Retrieved from *www.cfenet .ubc.ca/sites/default/files/uploads/docs/Opportunistic_Infection_Therapeutic_Guidelines2009.pdf.*
*If available. In most cases, effective antiretroviral therapy is the best prevention for all opportunistic diseases.
†In most cases, adequate antiretroviral therapy is the best treatment for all opportunistic diseases.
CHOP, cyclophosphamide, hydroxydaunomycin, Oncovin, prednisone; *CMV,* cytomegalovirus; *CNS,* central nervous system; *GI,* gastro-intestinal; *HAV,* hepatitis A virus; *HHV-8,* human herpesvirus 8; *HIV,* human immunodeficiency virus; *IgG,* immunoglobulin G; *IV,* intravenous; *JC,* "John Cunningham" virus; *TB,* tuberculosis; *TMP/SMX,* trimethoprim-sulphamethoxazole.

activity also allow a better assessment of clinical status and disease progression. Viral load (also referred to as *viral burden*) is the number of viral particles in a sample of blood. Viral loads can be determined with HIV RNA polymerase chain reaction (PCR) or branched-chain DNA (bDNA) tests. Viral load is reported either as less than 40 copies per millilitre, as a definitive number

between 40 and 10 million, or as more than 10 million. These tests provide information that helps determine when to initiate therapy, the efficacy of therapy, and whether clinical goals are being met.

Various abnormal results of laboratory tests of the blood are common in untreated HIV infection and may be caused by HIV,

TABLE 17-12 HIV-ANTIBODY TEST SCREENING PROCESS

All HIV testing should be accompanied by pretest and post-test counselling. The following additional steps are used in the process of testing blood for antibodies to HIV:

1. A highly sensitive EIA is performed to detect serum antibodies that bind to HIV antigens on test plates. Blood samples with negative findings on this test are reported as negative. The EIA testing can be done either with a conventional blood sample or with a rapid point-of-care test.
   - Post-test counselling should include an assessment of risk behaviours and especially seek to identify recent risks.
   - If recent risks are identified, patient should be encouraged to undergo retesting 3 weeks, 6 weeks, and 3 months later.
2. If the EIA of the blood shows positive findings, the test is repeated.
3. If the findings of the EIA of the blood are repeatedly positive, a more specific confirming test, such as the WB or IFA, is done.
   - WB testing involves the use of gel electrophoresis on purified HIV antigens. These are incubated with serum samples. If antibody in the serum is present, it can be detected.
   - IFA is used to identify HIV in infected cells. Blood is treated with a fluorescent antibody against p17 or p24 antigen and then examined under a fluorescent microscope.
4. Blood that is reactive in all of the first three steps is reported as positive for HIV antibodies.
5. If the results are inconclusive, the following steps are taken:
   - If in-depth risk assessment reveals that the individual does not have a history of high-risk activities, reassure the patient that he or she is extremely unlikely to be infected with HIV, and suggest retesting in 3 months.
   - If in-depth risk assessment reveals that the individual does have a history of high-risk activities, repeat antibody test at 1, 2, and 6 months; discuss harm reduction measures to protect partners from infection; consider tests for HIV-antigen detection such as an NAAT.

EIA, enzyme immunoassay; *HIV*, human immunodeficiency virus; *IFA*, immuno-fluorescence assay; *NAAT*, nucleic antigen amplification test; *WB*, Western blot.

opportunistic diseases, or complications of drug or radiation therapy. The white blood cell count is often decreased, especially neutrophil counts (neutropenia); low platelet counts (thrombocytopenia) may be caused by antiplatelet antibodies or drug therapy; and anemia is associated with the chronic disease process, as well as with common adverse effects of some of the antiretroviral agents. Altered results of liver function tests are common. These may be caused by disease processes or drug therapy and may be more common with newer drug therapy. Co-infection with hepatitis B virus (HBV) or hepatitis C virus must be identified early because these infections may have a more serious course in a patient with HIV infection and may ultimately limit options for ART (Gunthard, Aberg, Eron, et al., 2014).

It is now possible to test for resistance to antiretroviral drugs in people being treated for HIV infection. Two types of assays are used: genotype and phenotype. The genotype assay detects drug-resistant viral mutations that are present in the reverse transcriptase and protease genes. The phenotype assay is a measure of the growth of the virus in various concentrations of antiretroviral drugs (much like bacteria–antibiotic sensitivity tests). These assays are especially useful in making decisions about new drug combinations in patients who are not responding to their current therapies. Genotyping is usually done before the patient starts his or her first treatment regimen because it is possible to acquire resistant virus. The PHAC (2015c) estimated that approximately 9.8% of infected individuals have resistant virus at the time of infection.

Another test that is frequently done before patients begin ART is a human leukocyte antigen (HLA) B5701 antigen test. If this test result is positive, the patient will probably have a hypersensitivity to abacavir (Ziagen), one of the nucleoside reverse transcriptase inhibitors.

A test that may be performed is therapeutic drug monitoring. This test is indicated for patients who continue to have replicating virus in the presence of ART without evidence of nonadherence. It reveals whether the patient is effectively metabolizing her or his ART regimen and has a therapeutic level of drug in her or his system.

COLLABORATIVE CARE

Collaborative management of the HIV-infected patient focuses on monitoring HIV disease progression and immune function, initiating and monitoring ART, preventing the development of opportunistic diseases, detecting and treating opportunistic diseases, managing symptoms, and preventing or decreasing the complications of treatment. Ongoing assessment and health care provider–patient interactions are required to accomplish these objectives.

The initial visit provides an opportunity to gather baseline data and to establish rapport. A complete history and physical examination, including an immunization history and psychosocial and dietary evaluations, should be conducted. Findings from the history, assessment, and laboratory tests help determine the patient's needs. This is a good time to initiate patient education related to the spectrum of HIV disease, treatment, preventing transmission to others, improving health, and family planning. Patient input should be used to develop a plan of care, and necessary referrals can be made. Of importance is that a patient with newly diagnosed infection may be in a state of shock or denial and be unable to understand or retain information. The nurse should be prepared to repeat and clarify information over the course of several months. If case reports are required by the public health department, they should be completed at this time.

Drug Therapy for Human Immunodeficiency Virus Infection

The goals of drug therapy in HIV infection are to (a) decrease the viral load, (b) maintain or raise $CD4^+$ T-cell counts, (c) delay the development of HIV-related symptoms and opportunistic diseases, and (d) prevent transmission. Guidelines on the use of antiretroviral agents are updated regularly (Gunthard, Aberg, Eron, et al., 2014). HIV treatment guidelines incorporate the use of the following principles:

1. Treatment decisions should be individualized by risk for disease progression, indicated by higher viral loads and lower $CD4^+$ T-cell counts and by a patient's desires for therapy.
2. Combination ART suppresses HIV replication and limits the potential for antiretroviral resistance, which is the major factor that limits treatment effect. The most effective means to suppress HIV replication is simultaneous initiation of at least three effective antiretroviral drugs from at least two different drug classes in optimum schedules and full dosages. In general, therapy begins with two nucleoside (or nucleotide) reverse transcriptase inhibitors and a nonnucleoside reverse transcriptase inhibitor or a protease inhibitor that is boosted with ritonavir. The nucleosides and nucleotides are considered the foundation of ART.

TABLE 17-13   DRUG THERAPY

Recommendations for Initiating Antiretroviral Therapy in Treatment-Naive Adults With Established HIV-1 Infection*

Measure	Recommendation (Rating)
Symptomatic HIV disease	Treatment is recommended regardless of CD4+ T cell count. The strength of the recommendation increases as the CD4+ T cell count decreases and in the presence of certain conditions.
Asymptomatic HIV disease	
• CD4+ T cell count <500 microlitres	Antiretroviral therapy recommended
• CD4+ T cell count ≥500 microlitres†	Antiretroviral therapy recommended
Pregnant women	Treatment recommended
HIV RNA load >100,000 copies/mL	Treatment recommended
Rapid decline in CD4+ T cell count of >100 mcL/yr	Treatment recommended
Active hepatitis B or C co-infection	Treatment recommended
Active or high risk for cardiovascular disease	Treatment recommended
HIV-associated nephropathy	Treatment recommended
Symptomatic primary HIV infection	Treatment recommended
High risk for secondary transmission (e.g., serodiscordant couples)	Treatment recommended

Source: Gunthard, Aberg, Eron, et al. (2014). Antiretroviral treatment of adult HIV infection: 2014 Recommendations of the International AIDS Society—USA panel. *Journal of the American Medical Association, 304*(3), 321–333.
*In nonpregnant adults only. For all individuals, regardless of whether they are receiving treatment, intensive counselling to prevent secondary transmission is recommended.
†Considerations include high viral load (>100,000 HIV RNA copies/mL), rapid decline in CD4+ T cell count (>100/mcL/yr), high risk of cardiovascular disease, active hepatitis B or C co-infections, or presence of HIV-associated nephropathy.
ART, antiretroviral therapy; *HIV*, human immunodeficiency virus.

TABLE 17-14   DRUG THERAPY

Mechanisms of Action of Drugs Used to Treat HIV Infection

Drug Classification	Mechanism of Action
Nonnucleoside reverse transcriptase inhibitors	Combine with reverse transcriptase enzyme to block the process needed to convert HIV RNA into HIV DNA
Nucleoside reverse transcriptase inhibitors	Insert a bit of protein (a nucleoside) into the developing HIV DNA chain, blocking further development of the chain and leaving the production of the new strand of HIV DNA incomplete
Nucleotide reverse transcriptase inhibitors	Inhibit the action of reverse transcriptase
Protease inhibitors	Prevent the protease enzyme from cutting HIV proteins into the proper lengths needed to allow viable virions to assemble and bud out from the cell membrane
Integrase inhibitors	Prevents viral DNA integration into the CD4+ cell chromosome
Fusion inhibitors (entry inhibitors)	Prevent binding of HIV to cells, thus preventing entry of HIV into healthy cells

HIV, human immunodeficiency virus; *RNA*, ribonucleic acid.

that resistance develops rapidly when they are used alone or taken in inadequate doses. For that reason, combinations of three or more antiretroviral drugs, prescribed at full strength, should be used. Protease inhibitors and NNRTIs also have a number of dangerous and potentially lethal interactions with other commonly used drugs, including over-the-counter drugs and herbal therapies. For example, St. John's wort can interfere with ART by lowering the blood levels of protease inhibitors and non-nucleoside reverse transcriptase inhibitors (AIDS InfoNet, 2014). Some herbs (e.g., echinacea, astragalus) should not be used because they can enhance the replication of HIV.

Treatment protocols can reduce viral loads by 90% to 99% in most cases, but adverse effects and other problems are common (Gunthard, Aberg, Eron, et al., 2014). Antiretroviral agents used in HIV infection and their adverse effects are detailed in Table 17-15. Some patients are not able to use combination therapies because of the expense, adverse effects, or inability to adhere to required schedules.

DRUG ALERT—Efavirenz (Sustiva)
- In pregnant patients, efavirenz can be used after the first 8 weeks of pregnancy.
- Once-a-day doses should be taken at bedtime (at least initially) to help patients cope with adverse effects, including dizziness and confusion.
- Patients should be informed that many people who use the drug have reported vivid and sometimes bizarre dreams.

Preventing Transmission of Human Immunodeficiency Virus

A new and emerging use of ART is pre-exposure prophylaxis (PrEP), which is a comprehensive HIV-prevention strategy to reduce the risk of sexually acquired HIV infection in adults at high risk (Gunthard, Aberg, Eron, et al., 2014). PrEP should be used in conjunction with other proven prevention interventions such as condoms, risk reduction counselling, and regular HIV testing.

The combination of tenofovir with emtricitabine, known as *Truvada*, is used to reduce the risk of HIV infection in uninfected

3. Infected women should receive optimal ART even if pregnant.
4. HIV-infected persons, even those with viral loads below detectable limits and those receiving effective ART, should be considered infectious and should avoid behaviours associated with transmission of HIV and other infectious pathogens. There is evidence, however, that the risk of HIV transmission decreases with lower viral loads. There is an increasing acceptance of the need to start ART at a higher CD4+ T-cell count because it has become clear that a suppressed viral load leads to significantly lower infectivity (Montaner, 2011).

Recommendations for starting therapy in the chronically infected patient are summarized in Table 17-13.

Currently approved drugs include four groups that inhibit the ability of HIV to make a DNA copy early in replication, one group that inhibits the ability of the virus to reproduce in the late stages of replication, and one group that prevents entry of HIV into the cell (Table 17-14). *Nucleoside reverse transcriptase inhibitors, nonnucleoside reverse transcriptase inhibitors* (NNRTIs), and *nucleotide reverse transcriptase inhibitors* work by inhibiting the activity of reverse transcriptase; *protease inhibitors* work by interfering with the activity of the enzyme protease, and *integrase inhibitors* work by interfering with the enzyme integrase. *Fusion inhibitors* (entry inhibitors) work by inhibiting the binding of HIV to cells. A major problem with most drugs used in ART is

TABLE 17-15 DRUG THERAPY

Antiretroviral Agents Used to Treat HIV Infection*†

Drug	Adverse Effects	Drug	Adverse Effects
Nucleoside reverse transcriptase inhibitors	Common adverse effects: Lactic acidosis with hepatic steatosis, a rare but potentially life-threatening problem; lipodystrophy, especially fat atrophy and mitochondrial toxicity	• Tipranavir (Aptivus)	Nausea, diarrhea, headache, clinical hepatitis, increased serum transaminases, hepatic decompensation, symptoms of sulpha allergy, rash, or photosensitivity
• Abacavir (Ziagen)	Nausea; hypersensitivity reaction, including fever, nausea, vomiting, diarrhea, lethargy, malaise, sore throat, shortness of breath, cough, rash; may produce life-threatening event if hypersensitivity is rechallenged	• Kaletra (lopinavir + ritonavir combination)	Nausea, diarrhea, taste perversion, perioral and circumoral paresthesia, hepatitis
		Integrase inhibitors	
• Didanosine (Videx-EC)	Headache, nausea, vomiting, diarrhea, rash	• Dolutegravir (Tivicay)	Rash, increased liver enzymes, tiredness, fever, insomnia, headache
• Emtricitabine (FTC, Emtriva)	Headache, diarrhea, nausea, rash, skin discoloration	• Raltegravir (Isentress)	Diarrhea, nausea, headache, fever
		Entry inhibitors	
• Lamivudine (3TC)	Minimal toxic effects, nausea, nasal congestion	• Enfuvirtide (Fuzeon)	ISRs, fatigue, nausea, diarrhea, insomnia, peripheral neuropathy, hypersensitivity reaction, pneumonia
• Zidovudine (AZT, Retrovir)	Nausea, vomiting, anemia, leukopenia, fatigue, headache, insomnia, pancreatitis	• Maraviroc (Celsentri)	Persistent cough, URT infections, and GI upset
Nucleotide reverse transcriptase inhibitor		Combination therapy	
• Tenofovir disoproxil fumarate (Viread)	Nausea, vomiting, diarrhea	• Atripla (tenofovir + emtricitabine + efavirenz)	Nausea and vomiting, cough, increased pigmentation on soles of feet and palms of hands, diarrhea, drowsiness, indigestion, headache, strange dreams, fatigue
Nonnucleoside reverse transcriptase inhibitors	Common adverse effects: rash, erythema multiforme, increased liver enzymes, hepatotoxicity	• Combivir (lamivudine + zidovudine)	Headache, nausea, vomiting, unexpected tiredness, diarrhea, loss of appetite, insomnia, muscle pain
• Delavirdine (Rescriptor)	Headache, fatigue, GI upset, neutropenia, pruritus	• Complera (rilpivarine + emtricitabine + tenofovir disoproxil fumarate)	Dizziness, feeling sleepy during the daytime, headache, rash, nausea, stomach pain
• Efavirenz (Sustiva)	Dizziness, trouble concentrating, unusual dreams, confusion, anxiety, depression, diarrhea, encephalopathy; false-positive cannabinoid test	• Genvoya (elvitegravir + cobicistat + tenofovir alefanamide + emtricitabine)	Headache, fatigue, nausea, diarrhea
• Etravirine (Intelence)	Rash, diarrhea, nausea, flatulence, abdominal pain		
• Nevirapine (Viramune)	GI upset, headache, generalized rash	• Kivexa (abacavir + lamivudine)	Unexpected tiredness, diarrhea, nausea, headache
• Rilpivirine (Edurant)	Depression, insomnia, headache	• Prezcobix (darunavir + cobicistat)	Diarrhea, rash, headache, nausea, vomiting
Protease inhibitors	Common adverse effects: dysglycemia, hyperlipidemia, lipodystrophy	• Stribild (elvitegravir + cobicistat + truvada emtricitabine + tenofovir)	Headache, diarrhea, nausea, vomiting, vivid dreams, anxiety, rash, dizziness, insomnia, loss of appetite
• Atazanavir (Reyataz)	Nausea, diarrhea, hyperbilirubinemia	• Triumeq (dolutegravir + abacavir + lamivudine)	Nausea, vomiting, diarrhea, headache, abdominal discomfort/pain
• Darunavir (Prezista)	Diarrhea, nausea, headache		
• Fosamprenavir (Telzir)	Diarrhea, nausea, vomiting, headache	• Trizivir (lamivudine + zidovudine + abacavir)	Diarrhea, nausea, vomiting, loss of appetite, headache, insomnia, unexpected tiredness, muscle pain
• Indinavir (Crixivan)	Nausea, diarrhea, asymptomatic hyperbilirubinemia, interstitial nephritis, kidney stones (patient should drink 2–4 L of fluid a day)		
• Nelfinavir (Viracept)	Diarrhea, flatulence, nausea, rash	• Truvada (tenofovir and cmtricitabine)	Dizziness, headache, nausea, vomiting, flatulence
• Ritonavir (Norvir)—most often used in low doses with other protease inhibitors to boost effect	Nausea, diarrhea, vomiting, taste perversion, circumoral and perioral paresthesia, hepatitis		

Sources: British Columbia Centre for Excellence in HIV/AIDS. (2015). *Therapeutic guidelines for antiretroviral treatment of adult HIV infection.* Vancouver: Author. Retrieved from *http://www.cfenet.ubc.ca/our-work/initiatives/therapeutic-guidelines/adult-therapeutic-guidelines;* and Canadian AIDS Treatment Information Exchange (CATIE). Retrieved from *http://www.catie.ca/en/home.*
*Current recommendations for therapy mandate combinations of three or more of these drugs. Treatment with only one drug is rarely acceptable.
†Many of these drugs cause serious and potentially fatal interactions when used in combination with other commonly used drugs, some of which are available over the counter.
GI, gastro-intestinal; *ISRs,* injection site reactions; *URT,* upper respiratory tract.

individuals who are at significant risk of acquiring HIV. Truvada is also currently used in combination with other antiretroviral agents for the treatment of HIV-infected people.

Drug Therapy for Opportunistic Diseases

Management of HIV is complicated by the many opportunistic diseases that can develop as the immune system deteriorates. A preferred approach to opportunistic diseases is to prevent their occurrence. A number of opportunistic diseases associated with HIV can be delayed or prevented through the use of adequate ART, vaccines (including hepatitis B, influenza, and pneumococcal), and disease-specific prevention measures. Prophylaxis, used according to established criteria, contributes significantly to preventing morbidity and mortality. Although it is usually not possible to eradicate opportunistic diseases once they occur, treatments are available that can control them. Advances in the prevention, diagnosis, and treatment of opportunistic diseases have contributed significantly to increased life expectancy. Table 17-11 lists prophylaxis and treatments for some common HIV-related opportunistic diseases.

Vaccination

Despite considerable research, a vaccine for HIV still eludes scientists. The problems that impede HIV vaccine development are numerous. HIV lives inside cells, where it can "hide" from circulating immune factors. HIV also mutates rapidly, so that infected individuals develop HIV variants that may not all respond to a simple vaccine (Greenwood, Salisbury, & Hill, 2011). In addition, two strains of HIV (HIV-1 and HIV-2) cause AIDS, and at least nine clades (subtypes) of HIV-1 exist around the world. A vaccine developed for one clade may not be effective against the others.

There are also social, ethical, and economic issues related to vaccination. Vaccine efficacy will eventually have to be established in human testing: How will volunteers be recruited? How will true protection be determined? Will volunteers be exposed to HIV after immunization to test immunity? Because HIV is a global problem, with developing countries bearing the brunt of the epidemic, there is also concern about developing a vaccine that can be widely distributed in a short amount of time at an acceptable cost. Will vaccines, once developed, be accepted? Despite the overwhelming nature of these issues, considerable research is in progress. Vaccines in various stages of development are being tested. The development of a successful vaccine would be extremely helpful in controlling the epidemic but would not replace current prevention methods because no vaccine is likely to be 100% effective.

NURSING MANAGEMENT
HUMAN IMMUNODEFICIENCY VIRUS INFECTION

NURSING ASSESSMENT

Nursing assessment for an individual not known to be infected with HIV should focus on behaviours that could put the person at risk for HIV infection and other sexually transmitted and bloodborne diseases. Nurses can help individuals assess risks by asking four basic questions: (a) "Have you ever had a blood transfusion or used clotting factors? If so, was it before 1985?" (b) "Have you ever shared needles, syringes, or other injecting equipment with another person?" (c) "Have you ever had a sexual experience in which your penis, vagina, rectum, or mouth came into contact with another person's penis, vagina, rectum, or mouth?" and (d) "Have you ever had an STI?" These questions elicit the minimum data needed to initiate a risk assessment. A positive response to any of these questions necessitates an in-depth exploration of the issues specific to the identified risk.

Further assessment is needed when an HIV infection is diagnosed. Subjective and objective data that should be obtained are presented in Table 17-16. Nursing assessments should be ongoing because early recognition and treatment of problems can decrease the progression of HIV infection. A complete history and a thorough systems review can help the nurse identify problems in a timely manner.

NURSING DIAGNOSES

Nursing diagnoses related to HIV infection are dictated by several variables: the stage (e.g., is prevention of HIV infection the issue? Are there concerns related to ongoing infection? Is the patient

⟳ EVIDENCE-INFORMED PRACTICE
Translating Research Into Practice

A nurse in an HIV clinic is counselling Mr. Simms, a 25-year-old gay man, and his partner. Mr. Simms is receiving antiretroviral therapy. His viral load is very low, and his CD4[+] T cell count is normal. He tells the nurse that since the medications are working, he and his partner (who is not infected with HIV) have decided to forgo the use of condoms. They tell the nurse that they are in a committed relationship and have no other partners. The nurse spends time explaining to both of them the risks of unprotected sex: his partner may get infected with HIV even with a low viral load (although the risk is decreased).

Best Available Evidence	Clinician Expertise	Patient Preferences and Values
One of the best ways to prevent HIV transmission from an infected person to an uninfected person is by using condoms.	The nurse knows that risk-reducing sexual activities in this situation include the continued use of condoms. However, the nurse also knows that a very low viral load decreases the risk of HIV transmission.	After listening, the patient tells the nurse that he and his partner do not like using condoms. Both understand the risks and believe that while the medications are working, the risk is low and worth the risk.

Decision and Action
The nurse must respect Mr. Simm's decision. The nurse reminds him of the importance of maintaining his medication regimen and attending his appointments at the clinic. The nurse explains that this will be even more important now to keep Mr. Simms's infection under control.

Reference for Evidence
Cohen, M. S., McCauley, M., & Gamble, T. R. (2012). HIV treatment as prevention and HPTN 052. *Current opinion in HIV and AIDS, 7*(2), 99. doi:10.1097/COH.0b013e32834f5cf2.

in a terminal phase of the disease?), presence of specific etiological problems (e.g., respiratory distress, depression, wasting), and social factors (e.g., issues related to self-esteem, sexuality, family interactions, finances). Because HIV infection is a complex and individually experienced disease, a broad spectrum of nursing diagnoses may include, but not be limited to, those presented in Table 17-17.

PLANNING

Prevention of HIV infection presents a number of challenges for the patient, many of which are related to the difficulties of behaviour change. Nurses can be instrumental in this process. Nursing interventions to prevent disease transmission depend on assessment of the patient's individual risk behaviours, knowledge, and skill deficits. Nursing orders based on these assessments will encourage the patient to learn safer, healthier, and less risky behaviours. Infection with HIV affects the entire range of a person's life: not only physical health but also social, emotional, economic, and spiritual well-being. Once a person is infected, current treatment cannot eliminate HIV from the body. The overriding goals of therapy are therefore to keep the viral load as low as possible for as long as possible; to maintain or restore a functioning immune system; to improve the patient's quality of life; to reduce the potential for transmission of the virus; to reduce HIV-related disease, disability, and death; and to prevent reinfection. Nursing interventions can assist the patient to

TABLE 17-16 NURSING ASSESSMENT

HIV-Infected Patient

Subjective Data

Important health information	*Past health history:* Route of infection; hepatitis; other STIs; tuberculosis; foreign travel; frequent viral, fungal, or bacterial infections; alcohol and drug use
	Medications: Use of immuno-suppressive drugs
Symptoms	Malaise, chronic fatigue, weight loss, anorexia, nausea, vomiting; lesions, bleeding, or ulcerations of lips, mouth, gums, tongue, or throat; sensitivity to acidic, salty, or spicy foods; difficulty swallowing; abdominal cramping
	Skin rashes, lesions, or colour changes; pruritus; nonhealing wounds
	Persistent diarrhea, change in character of stools; painful urination
	Cough, shortness of breath
	Insomnia; night sweats
	Headaches, stiff neck, chest pain, rectal pain, retrosternal pain
	Blurred vision, photophobia, diplopia, loss of vision; hearing impairment; confusion, forgetfulness, attention deficit, changes in mental status, memory loss, personality changes, muscle weakness, difficulty walking; paresthesias, hypersensitivity in feet
	Lesions on genitalia (internal or external), pruritus or burning sensation in vagina, painful sexual intercourse, changes in menstruation, vaginal or penile discharge

Objective Data

General	Lethargy, persistent fever, lymphadenopathy, peripheral wasting, fat deposits in truncal areas and upper back; social withdrawal
Integumentary	Decreased skin turgor, dry skin, or diaphoresis; pallor, cyanosis; lesions, eruptions, discolorations, or bruises of skin and mucous membranes; vaginal or perianal excoriation; alopecia, delayed wound healing
Eyes	Presence of exudate; retinal lesions or hemorrhage; papilledema
Respiratory	Tachypnea, dyspnea, intercostal retractions; crackles, wheezing, productive or nonproductive cough
Cardiovascular	Pericardial friction rub, murmur, bradycardia, tachycardia
Gastro-intestinal	Mouth lesions, including blisters (HSV), white-grey patches (*Candida*), painless white lesions on lateral aspect of the tongue (hairy leukoplakia), discolorations (Kaposi's sarcoma); gingivitis, tooth decay or loosening; redness or white patchy lesions of throat; vomiting, diarrhea, incontinence; rectal lesions; hyperactive bowel sounds, abdominal masses, hepatosplenomegaly
Musculo-skeletal	Muscle wasting
Neurological	Ataxia, tremors, lack of coordination; sensory loss; slurred speech, aphasia; memory loss, apathy, agitation, depression, inappropriate behaviour; decreasing levels of consciousness, seizures, paralysis, coma
Reproductive	Genital lesions or discharge, abdominal tenderness secondary to pelvic inflammatory disease
Possible findings	Positive result of HIV antibody assay (EIA or ELISA, confirmed by WB or IFA); viral load levels detectable by bDNA or PCR, ↓ CD4$^+$ lymphocytes, reversal of CD4:CD8 ratio; ↓ WBC count, lymphopenia, anemia, thrombo-cytopenia; electrolyte imbalances; abnormal results of liver function tests; ↑ cholesterol, triglyceride, and blood glucose levels

bDNA, branched-chain deoxyribonucleic acid; *EIA,* enzyme immunoassay; *ELISA,* enzyme-linked immunosorbent assay; *HIV,* human immunodeficiency virus; *HSV,* herpes simplex virus; *IFA,* immuno-fluorescence assay; *PCR,* polymerase chain reaction; *STIs,* sexually transmitted infections; *WB,* Western blot; *WBC,* white blood cell count.

TABLE 17-17 NURSING DIAGNOSES: HIV INFECTION

- Anxiety
- Breathing pattern, ineffective
- Body image, disturbed
- Caregiver role strain
- Coping, ineffective
- Confusion, acute or chronic
- Decisional conflict
- Denial, ineffective
- Diarrhea
- Disuse syndrome, risk for
- Fatigue
- Family processes, interrupted
- Fear
- Grieving
- Headache
- Health management, ineffective
- Hyperthermia
- Nutrition, imbalanced: less than body requirements
- Oral mucous membrane integrity, impaired
- Pain, acute or chronic
- Powerlessness
- Relocation stress syndrome
- Self-care deficits
- Self-esteem, chronic low
- Self-esteem, situational low
- Sleep pattern, disturbed
- Social isolation
- Spiritual distress

(a) adhere to drug regimens; (b) promote a healthy lifestyle; (c) prevent opportunistic disease; (d) protect others from HIV; (e) maintain or develop healthy, supportive relationships; (f) maintain activities and productivity; (g) come to terms with issues related to disease, death, and spirituality; and (h) cope with the frequent symptoms caused by HIV and its treatments (Canadian Association of Nurses in AIDS Care [CANAC], 2013). Goals are individualized and change as new treatment protocols develop or as HIV disease progresses.

NURSING IMPLEMENTATION

The complexity of HIV disease is related to its chronic nature. As with most chronic and infectious diseases, primary prevention and health promotion are the most effective health care strategies. When prevention fails, however, disease results. HIV infection has no cure and continues for life. If a patient does not receive ART, it causes increasing physical disability, contributes to impaired health, and ultimately causes death.

Nursing interventions at every stage of HIV disease can be instrumental in improving the quality and quantity of the patient's life. Nurses who emphasize a holistic and individualized approach to care are well suited to and capable of providing optimal care to these patients. Table 17-18 presents a synopsis of nursing goals, assessments, and interventions at each stage of HIV infection.

HEALTH PROMOTION. A major goal of health promotion is to prevent disease. Even with recent successes in the treatment of HIV, prevention is crucial for control of the epidemic. Another goal of health promotion is to detect disease early so that if primary prevention has failed, early intervention can be implemented.

TABLE 17-18 NURSING INTERVENTIONS IN HIV DISEASE

Levels of Care; Goals	Assess	Interventions
Health Promotion 1. Prevent HIV infection 2. Detect HIV infection early	*Risk factors:* What behaviours or social, physical, emotional, pathological, and immune factors place the patient at risk? Does the patient need to be tested for HIV?	Education, including knowledge, attitudes, and behaviours, with an emphasis on risk reduction, to accomplish the following: • General population: covering general information • Pregnant women: covering general information and information specific to HIV infection and pregnancy; offering prenatal HIV testing in the first trimester Individual patient: specific to assessed need Empowering patients to take control of prevention measures Providing HIV-antibody testing with pretest and post-test counselling
Acute Intervention 1. Promote health and limit disability 2. Manage problems caused by HIV infection	*Physical health:* Is patient experiencing problems? *Mental health status:* How is the patient coping? *Resources:* Does the patient have family and social support? Is the patient accessing community services? Is money or insurance a problem? Does the patient have access to spiritual support?	Case management Education regarding HIV, the spectrum of infection, options for care, signs and symptoms to watch for, treatment options, immune enhancement, harm reduction, and ways to adhere to treatment regimens Referral to needed resources Establishing long-term, trusting relationship with patient, family, and significant others Providing emotional and spiritual support Providing care during acute exacerbations: recognition of life-threatening developments, life support, rapid intervention with treatments and drugs, patient and family emotional support during crisis, comfort, and hygiene needs Developing resources for legal needs: discrimination prevention, wills and powers of attorney, child care wishes Empowering patient to identify needs, direct care, and seek services
Ambulatory and Home Care 1. Maximize quality of life 2. Resolve life and death issues	*Physical health:* Are new symptoms developing? Is the patient experiencing drug adverse effects or interactions? *Mental health:* How is the patient coping? What adjustments have been made? *Finances:* Can the patient maintain health care and basic standards of living? *Family, social, and community supports:* Are these available? Is the patient using supports in an effective manner? Do family or significant others need education, encouragement, or stress relief? *Spirituality issues:* Does the patient desire support from a religious organization? Are spirituality issues private and personal? What assistance does the patient need?	Continuing case management Educating about changing treatment options and continued adherence Empowering patient to continue to direct care and to make desires known to family members and significant others Continuing physical care for chronic disease process: treatments, drugs, comfort, and hygiene needs Supporting patient and family and significant others in a trusting relationship Referral to resources that will assist in meeting identified needs Promoting health maintenance measures Assistance with end-of-life issues: resuscitation orders, comfort measures, funeral plans, and the like Referral to palliative care

HIV, human immunodeficiency virus.

INFORMATICS IN PRACTICE

Use of Internet and Mobile Devices to Manage Human Immunodeficiency Virus Infection

• Reputable websites such as government agencies (e.g., Health Canada) and well-known academic and medical institutions offer resources and support for patients that can assist them in coping with their illness and educate them about signs and symptoms of serious illness. (See also the Resources at the end of this chapter.)
• By monitoring their health and quickly spotting warning signs of serious illnesses, patients are able to alert their physicians and receive earlier treatment.
• These systems can help the patient manage antiretroviral therapy by sending medication reminders by text or email.

Prevention of Human Immunodeficiency Virus Infection. HIV infection is preventable. At this time, education and behaviour change are the most effective prevention tools. Educational messages should be specific to the patient's need, culturally sensitive, language appropriate, and age specific. Nurses are excellent resources for this type of education, but nurses must be comfortable with and know how to talk about sensitive topics such as sexuality and drug use (CANAC, 2013).

Prevention behaviours have been known and recommended since the mid-1980s. The nurse must remember that a range of activities can reduce the risk of HIV infection and that individuals will choose different techniques. The goal is for the person to develop safer, healthier, and less risky behaviours than are currently being used. These techniques can be divided into *safe activities* (those that eliminate risk) and *risk-reducing activities* (those that decrease risk but do not eliminate it). The more consistently and correctly prevention methods are used, the more effective they are in preventing HIV infection.

Research shows that the majority of new HIV infections were transmitted by individuals who were not aware that they were infected. An estimated 21% of HIV-infected people in Canada do not know that they are infected (PHAC, 2015c). These facts helped British Columbia develop the Seek and Treat for Optimal Prevention of HIV/AIDS (STOP) program. As a result of this program, HIV testing has been expanded to populations not historically considered to be at risk, and the program also ensures that all individuals in whom HIV is diagnosed get rapid access to treatment, which is known to prevent transmission.

Decreasing Risks Related to Sexual Intercourse. Safe sexual activities significantly decrease the risk of exposure to HIV in semen and vaginal secretions. Abstaining from all sexual activity is the most effective way to accomplish this goal, but there are safe options for those who cannot or do not wish to abstain. *Outercourse* (limiting sexual behaviour to activities in which the mouth, penis, vagina, or rectum does not come into contact with a partner's mouth, penis, vagina, or rectum) is safe because there is no contact with blood, semen, or vaginal secretions. Outercourse includes massage, masturbation, mutual masturbation, telephone sex, and other activities that meet the "no contact" requirements. *Insertive sex* between partners who are not infected with HIV or not at risk of becoming infected with HIV is considered to be safe, although it is important for a person to know his or her partner's status.

Reducing the risk of sexual activities through the use of barriers decreases the risk of contact with HIV. Barriers should be used during insertive sexual activity (oral, vaginal, or anal) with a partner who is known to be HIV infected or with a partner whose HIV status is not known. The most commonly used barrier is the male condom. Male condoms have been shown to be almost 100% effective in preventing the transmission of HIV when used correctly and consistently. Major points for the correct use of male condoms are discussed in Table 17-19. Female condoms are also available. Use can be complicated, and so careful instruction and practice are necessary (Table 17-20). In addition, squares of latex (known as dental dams) or plastic food wrap can be used to cover the external female genitalia during oral sexual activity.

Decreasing Risks Related to Substance Misuse. Misuse of substances, including alcohol and tobacco, is harmful. It can cause immune suppression and malnutrition, as well as a host of psychosocial problems. However, substance use in and of itself does not cause HIV infection. The major risk for HIV infection is related to sharing injecting equipment or having unsafe sexual experiences while under the influence of substances. The basic rules are as follows: (a) Do not inject illicit drugs; (b) If you do inject illicit drugs, do not share equipment; and (c) Do not have sexual intercourse when under the influence of any drug (including alcohol) that impairs decision-making ability (HIV.gov, 2014).

The safest mechanism is to abstain from substance misuse. Although this is the best option for people who do not currently misuse substances, it may not be a viable alternative for users who are not prepared to quit or for those who have no access to treatment services. The risk of HIV infection for individuals who misuse drugs can be eliminated if they use alternatives to injecting, such as smoking, snorting, or ingesting the drug. Risk for HIV can also be eliminated if users do not share injecting

---

TABLE 17-19 PATIENT & CAREGIVER TEACHING GUIDE

Proper Use of the Male Condom

- Use only condoms ("rubbers") that are made out of latex or polyurethane. "Natural skin" condoms have pores that are large enough for HIV to penetrate.
- Store condoms in a cool, dry place and protect them from trauma. The friction caused by carrying them in a back pocket, for instance, can wear down the latex.
- Do not use a condom if the expiration date has passed or if the package looks worn or punctured.
- Lubricants used in conjunction with condoms must be water soluble. Oil-based lubricants can weaken latex and increase the risk of tearing or breaking.
- Nonlubricated, flavoured, or unflavoured condoms can provide protection during oral intercourse.
- The condom must be placed on the erect penis before any contact is made with the partner's mouth, vagina, or rectum to prevent exposure to pre-ejaculatory secretions that may contain HIV.
- Remove the penis and condom from the partner's vagina or rectum immediately after ejaculation and before the erection is lost. Hold the condom at the base of the penis and remove both penis and condom at the same time. This keeps semen from leaking around the condom as the penis becomes flaccid.
- Remove the condom after use, wrap in tissue, and discard. Do not flush down the toilet because this can cause plumbing problems.
- Condoms are not reusable! A new condom must be used for every act of intercourse.

HIV, human immunodeficiency virus.

TABLE 17-20 PATIENT & CAREGIVER TEACHING GUIDE

Proper Use of the Female Condom

Female condoms consist of a polyurethane sheath with two spring-form rings.
- The smaller ring is inserted into the vagina and holds the condom in place internally. This ring can be removed if the condom is to be used for anal intercourse. It should not be removed if the condom is to be used for vaginal intercourse.
- The larger ring surrounds the opening to the condom. It functions to keep the condom in place while protecting the external genitalia.

Use only water-soluble lubricants with female condoms.
- Female condoms come prelubricated and with a tube of additional lubricant.
- Lubrication is needed to protect the condom from tearing during sexual intercourse and can also decrease the noise that results from friction of the penis against the condom.

Some men have reported that the female condom feels better than the male condom. Other men like male condoms better. The only way to find out which type of condom works best is to try both.

Practise inserting the female condom. Lubrication makes the condom slippery, but do not get discouraged; just keep trying.

During sexual intercourse, ensure that the penis is inserted into the female condom through the outer ring. It is possible for the penis to miss the opening, thus making contact with the vagina and defeating the purpose of the condom.

Do not use a male condom at the same time as a female condom.

After intercourse, remove the condom before standing up.
- Twist the outer ring to keep the semen inside, gently pull the condom out of the vagina, and discard.

Do not flush down the toilet because this can cause plumbing problems.

Do not reuse a female condom.

TABLE 17-21 PATIENT & CAREGIVER TEACHING GUIDE

Proper Use of Injection Equipment

- When drugs are injected, it is always preferable to use new, sterile syringes, needles, cookers, and cotton (works).
- Find out if there is a needle and syringe exchange program in your community. If there is, take used equipment in, and you will be provided with new works.
- Swab skin with an alcohol preparation before injecting.
- Use a tourniquet to assist in locating veins.
- Always inject with the bevel facing up on the needle.
- If you must share your equipment, it is very important to clean the works thoroughly with bleach before use.
- First, rinse the used needle and syringe twice with tap water.
- Then, fill the syringe with full-strength household bleach, shake for 30 seconds, and squirt the bleach out.
- Repeat the bleaching process a second time, being sure to shake the bleach-filled syringe for 30 seconds.
- Finally, rinse equipment twice with tap water.
- Do not share your bleach or rinse water.
- Do not share your cooker. If you must share your cooker, clean it with bleach and water before using it again.
- Supervised injection sites are another viable alternative for preventing the spread of infection, and there is political will to open such sites in various parts of the country.

equipment. Injecting equipment ("works") includes needles, syringes, cookers (spoons or bottle caps used to mix the drug), cotton, and rinse water. None of this equipment should be shared. Another safe tactic is for the user to have access to sterile equipment. This can be accomplished through community needle and syringe exchange programs and supervised injection sites that provide sterile equipment to users in exchange for used equipment. Opposition to these programs is supported by the fear that ready access to injecting supplies will increase drug use. However, studies have shown that in communities where exchange programs have been established, drug use does not increase, rates of HIV infection are controlled, and there are overall economic benefits (Arkin, 2011).

Cleaning equipment before use is a risk-reducing activity. It decreases the risk for those who share equipment (Table 17-21). This process takes time and may be difficult for a person who begins to suffer drug withdrawal during the process.

Decreasing Risks of Perinatal Transmission. The best way to prevent HIV infection in infants is to prevent HIV infection in women. Women who are already infected with HIV should be asked about their reproductive desires. Women who choose not to have children need to have birth control methods discussed in detail. Should they become pregnant, abortion may be desired and should be discussed in conjunction with other options.

If HIV-infected pregnant women are appropriately treated during pregnancy, the rate of perinatal transmission can be decreased from 25% to less than 1%. The current standard of care is that all women who are pregnant or contemplating pregnancy should be counselled about HIV infection, informed of their choices, routinely offered access to voluntary HIV-antibody testing, and, if infected, offered optimal ART (Burdge et al., 2003).

Decreasing Risks at Work. The risk of infection from occupational exposure to HIV is low but real. The Canadian Centre for Occupational Health and Safety requires employers to protect workers from exposure to blood and other potentially infectious materials. Precautions and safety devices decrease the risk of direct contact with blood and body fluids. Precautions for the prevention of occupational exposure to bloodborne diseases are discussed earlier in this chapter. Should significant exposure to HIV-infected fluids occur, postexposure prophylaxis with combination ART that is based on the type of exposure, the volume of the exposure, and the status of the source patient has been shown to significantly decrease the risk of infection. The possibility of treatment makes reporting of all blood exposures even more critical.

Human Immunodeficiency Virus Testing and Counselling. Testing is the only sure way to determine whether a person has HIV infection. Any individual who is at risk for HIV infection should be encouraged to be tested. When findings are negative, testing can relieve anxieties about past behaviours and provide opportunities for prevention education. When findings are positive, testing provides the needed impetus to seek treatment and to protect sexual and drug-using partners. All testing for HIV should be accompanied by pretest and post-test counselling (Table 17-22) as mandated by the World Health Organization (2015b).

ACUTE INTERVENTION

Early Intervention. Early intervention after detection of HIV infection can promote health and limit or delay disability. Because the course of HIV is variable, assessment is very important. Nursing interventions are based on and tailored to patient needs noted during assessment. The nursing assessment in HIV disease should focus on early detection of symptoms, opportunistic diseases, and psychosocial problems (see Table 17-18).

Initial Response to a Diagnosis of Human Immunodeficiency Virus Infection. Reactions to a positive result of an HIV-antibody test are similar to the reactions of people who are diagnosed with any life-threatening, debilitating, or chronic illness. They include anxiety, panic, fear, depression, denial, hopelessness, thoughts of suicide, anger, and guilt (French, Greeff, Watson, et al., 2015). Many of these reactions are also experienced by the patient's family members, friends, and caregivers. As time passes, patients and their loved ones must confront common issues associated with a life-threatening illness. These include difficult treatment decisions; feelings of loss, anger, powerlessness, depression, and grief; social isolation imposed by self or others; altered concepts of the physical, social, emotional, and creative self; thoughts of suicide; and the possibility of death. The nurse can help the patient obtain control over treatment and life decisions. Empowerment is particularly important because many individuals with HIV infection experience multiple losses, including that of control, which can be overwhelming. Empowerment is facilitated by education and honest discussions about the patient's health status and treatment options.

Antiretroviral Therapy. Multidrug therapy protocols have been shown to significantly reduce viral loads and reverse clinical progression of HIV (Gunthard, Aberg, Eron, et al., 2014). However, nurses must be aware that the protocols are complex, the drugs have adverse effects and interactions, and they do not work for everyone. These factors can contribute to problems with adherence to treatment regimens, a dangerous situation because of the high risk of developing drug resistance. Nurses are often the health care providers that work the most closely with patients who are trying to cope with these issues. Interventions include teaching about (a) advantages and disadvantages of new treatments, (b) dangers of poor adherence to therapeutic regimens, (c) how and when to take each drug, (d) drug interactions to avoid, and (e) adverse effects that must be reported to the health care provider. Table 17-23 provides guidance for patient teaching in these areas.

TABLE 17-22 PRETEST AND POST-TEST COUNSELLING ASSOCIATED WITH HIV-ANTIBODY TESTING

General Guidelines

1. Many people who are being tested for HIV are fearful about the test results:
   - The nurse should establish rapport with the patient.
   - The nurse should assess the patient's ability to understand HIV counselling.
   - The nurse must determine the patient's ability to access support systems.
2. The benefits of testing should be explained:
   - Testing provides an opportunity for education that can decrease the risk of new infections.
   - Infected individuals can be referred for early intervention and support programs.
3. Adverse aspects of testing should be discussed:
   - Confidentiality issues: breaches of confidentiality have led to discrimination.
   - A positive test result affects all aspects of the patient's life (e.g., personal, social, economic) and can raise difficult emotions (anger, anxiety, guilt, and thoughts of suicide).

Pretest Counselling

1. Determining the patient's risk factors and when the last risk factor occurred; counselling should be individualized according to these parameters.
2. Providing education to help the patient reduce future risk of exposure.
3. Providing education that will help the patient protect sexual and drug-sharing partners.
4. Discussing problems related to the delay between infection and an accurate test. Testing will have to be repeated at intervals for up to 6 months after each possible exposure. Discuss the need to use measures to decrease the risks to the patient and the patient's partners during that interval.
5. Discussing the possibility of false-negative tests, which are most likely to occur during the window period.
6. Assessing support systems. Provide telephone numbers and resources as needed.
7. Discussing the responses the patient anticipates having to the test results (positive and negative).
8. Outlining assistance that will be offered if the test result is positive.

Post-Test Counselling

1. If the test result is negative, pretest counselling and prevention education should be reinforced. The patient should be reminded that the test must be repeated at intervals for up to 6 months after the most recent high-risk exposure.
2. If the test result is positive, the nurse must understand that the patient may be in emotional shock and not hear much of what the nurse says.
3. The nurse should provide resources for medical and emotional support and help the patient get immediate assistance:
   - Evaluating suicide risk and follow-up as needed.
   - Determining need to test others who have had high-risk contact with the patient.
   - Discussing retesting to verify results. This tactic supports hope for the patient, but, of more importance, it keeps the patient in the health care system. While waiting for the second test result, the patient has time to think about and adjust to the possibility of having HIV infection.
   - Encouraging optimism.
4. The nurse should remind the patient that effective treatments are available; HIV infection is not a death sentence.
5. Health habits that can improve the immune system should be reviewed.
6. The nurse should arrange for the patient to speak to HIV-infected people who are willing to share with and assist patients with new diagnoses during the time between when the test results are available and treatment begins.
7. The nurse should emphasize that a positive HIV test result means that the patient is infected but does not necessarily mean that the patient has AIDS.
8. The patient should be educated to prevent new infections. HIV-infected people should be instructed to avoid donating blood, organs, or semen; to avoid sharing razors, toothbrushes, or other household items that may contain blood or other body fluids; and to protect sexual and needle-sharing partners from blood, semen, and vaginal secretions.

AIDS, acquired immune deficiency syndrome; *HIV,* human immunodeficiency virus.

When to Start Antiretroviral Therapy. ART has been in a state of continuous change since the first antiretroviral drug became available in 1987. When new drugs were developed, health care providers had the ability to combine and substitute drugs. However, as new treatments have improved the quality and quantity of patients' lives, problems have emerged. For a while, the preferred treatment strategy was known as "hit it early, hit it hard." This was thought to be appropriate because decreasing the viral load provides for better health outcomes. However, adverse effects and lack of regimen adherence caused many patients to question their ability to sustain ART for long periods of time. Because of this, for several years, treatment was delayed until the CD4+ T-cell count dropped below 500. However, it has become clear that when viral load is suppressed, the possibility of transmission of the virus is reduced. For this reason, current recommendations are that all people infected with HIV should receive treatment, regardless of their CD4+ T-cell count (Gunthard, Aberg, Eron, et al., 2014).

Given patient readiness, without which lack of adherence may be a problem, treatment should be initiated at the time of diagnosis because suppressing viral loads is helpful in reducing transmission rates (Montaner, 2011) and because it has become apparent that a CD4+ T-cell count of less than 500 is associated with non–AIDS-related issues such as cardiovascular disease, renal disease, and some cancers (Gunthard, Aberg, Eron, et al., 2014). Nurses can provide in-depth education and counselling for patients as they struggle to make this decision (CANAC, 2013).

Adherence. Adherence to drug regimens is a critical component of drug therapy for people with HIV infection and an area in which nurses are particularly well prepared to provide assistance (Enriquez & McKinsey, 2011). Taking drugs as ordered (right dose and time) every day is important for all drug therapy. Taking drugs as prescribed (right dose and time) is important for all drug therapy, but with HIV infection, missing even a few doses can lead to drug resistance. The difficulty of adhering consistently is clear to anyone who has tried to take a 10-day course of antibiotics. Patients with HIV infection have to take anywhere from 3 to 20 pills a day, at precise times during the day. This process must be repeated every day for the rest of their lives, even though they often suffer uncomfortable adverse effects. Patients can be helped to adhere to difficult treatment regimens

TABLE 17-23 PATIENT & CAREGIVER TEACHING GUIDE

Use of Antiretroviral Drugs

Resistance to antiretroviral drugs is a major problem in treating HIV infection. To decrease the risk of developing resistance:

1. Take at least three different antiretroviral drugs at a time; discuss other options with your health care provider.
2. Know what medications you are taking and how to take them (some have to be taken with food, some must be taken on an empty stomach, some cannot be taken together). If you do not understand, ask. Get your nurse to write the instructions clearly for you.
3. Take the full dose prescribed, and take it on schedule. If you cannot take the drug because of adverse effects or other problems, report it to your health care provider.
4. Take all of the drugs prescribed. It is important that you take them more than 95% of the time. Do not quit taking one drug while continuing the others. If you cannot tolerate one of your drugs, your health care provider will recommend a completely new set of drugs.
5. Many of the antiretroviral drugs interact with other drugs, including a number of common drugs you can buy without a prescription. Be sure your health care provider and pharmacist know all of the drugs that you are taking, and do not take any new drugs without checking for possible interactions.
6. The goal of antiretroviral therapy is to decrease the amount of virus in your blood. This is called your viral load. Viral load can be determined by tests such as the PCR or bDNA. The results are reported in absolute numbers. The goal is to get your viral load to an undetectable level. Most health care providers will check this number on a regular basis regardless of whether you are taking antiretroviral agents.
7. In 2 to 4 weeks after you start on drug therapy (or change your therapy), your health care provider will test your viral load to find out whether the drugs are working. These results are reported in absolute numbers or in "logs" (logarithms: a mathematical concept). All you have to know is that you want to see the viral load drop. If reports are in logs, you want to see a drop of at least 1 log, which means that 90% of your viral load has been eliminated. If your viral load drops by 2 logs, your viral load will have been 95% eliminated. If your viral load drops by 3 logs, your viral load will have been 99% eliminated.
8. An undetectable viral load means that the amount of virus is extremely low and viruses cannot be found in the blood through the use of the current technology. It does not mean that the virus is gone, for much of the virus will be in lymph nodes and organs where the tests cannot detect it. It also does not mean that you are no longer able to transmit HIV to others; you will need to continue protecting all of your sexual and drug-using partners.

AIDS, acquired immune deficiency syndrome; *bDNA,* branched-chain DNA; *HIV,* human immunodeficiency virus; *PCR,* polymerase chain reaction.

TABLE 17-24 PATIENT & CAREGIVER TEACHING GUIDE

Signs and Symptoms That Patients With HIV Infection Need to Report

Report the Following Signs and Symptoms Immediately to a Health Care Provider

- Any change in level of consciousness: lethargy, difficulty arousing, inability to arouse, unresponsiveness, unconsciousness
- Headache accompanied by nausea and vomiting, changes in vision, or changes in ability to perform coordinated activities, or after any head trauma
- Vision changes: blurry or black areas in vision field, new floaters
- Persistent shortness of breath related to activity and not relieved by a short rest period
- Nausea and vomiting accompanied by abdominal pain
- Dehydration: inability to eat or drink because of nausea, diarrhea, or mouth lesions; severe diarrhea or vomiting; dizziness with standing
- Yellow discoloration of the skin
- Any bleeding from the rectum that is not related to hemorrhoids
- Pain in the flank with fever and inability to urinate for more than 6 hours
- New onset of weakness in any part of the body, new onset of numbness that is not obviously related to pressure, new onset of difficulty speaking
- Chest pain not obviously related to cough
- Seizures
- New rash accompanied by fever
- New oral lesions accompanied by fever
- Severe depression, anxiety, hallucinations, delusions, or being a possible danger to self or others

Report the Following Signs and Symptoms Within 24 Hours

- New or different headache; constant headache not relieved by aspirin or acetaminophen
- Headache accompanied by fever, nasal congestion, or cough
- Burning, itching, or discharge from the eyes
- New or productive cough
- Vomiting two or three times a day
- Vomiting accompanied by fever
- New, significant, or watery diarrhea (>6 times a day)
- Painful urination, bloody urine, urethral discharge
- New, significant rash (widespread, painful, itchy, or following a path down the leg or arm, around the chest, or on the face)
- Difficulty eating because of mouth lesions
- Vaginal discharge, pain, or itching

with electronic reminders, beepers, timers on pillboxes, and calendars. Group support and individual counselling can also help, but the best approach is to learn about the patient's lifestyle and assist with problem solving related to taking medications within the confines of that life (CANAC, 2013).

Health Promotion. HIV disease progression may also be delayed by promoting a healthy immune system, regardless of whether the patient chooses to use ART. Useful interventions for HIV-infected patients include (a) nutritional support to maintain lean body mass and ensure appropriate levels of vitamins and micronutrients; (b) moderation or elimination of alcohol intake, smoking, and drug use; (c) adequate rest and exercise; (d) stress reduction; (e) avoidance of exposure to new infectious agents; (f) mental health counselling; and (g) involvement in support

groups and community activities. In the absence of ART, however, disease progression can be delayed only for a finite amount of time.

Patients should be taught to recognize symptoms that may indicate disease progression or drug adverse effects so that prompt medical care can be initiated. Table 17-24 provides an overview of symptoms that patients should report. In general, patients should have as much information as needed to make informed decisions about health care. These decisions then dictate the appropriate interventions.

Acute Exacerbations. Chronic diseases are characterized by acute exacerbations of recurring problems. This is especially true in HIV disease, in which infections, cancers, debility, and psychosocial and economic issues may interact to overwhelm the patient's ability to cope. Nursing care becomes more complex if the patient's immune system deteriorates and new problems arise to compound existing difficulties. When opportunistic diseases or difficult adverse effects of treatment develop, symptom management, education, and emotional support are necessary (CANAC, 2013).

Nursing care assumes primary importance in helping patients prevent the many opportunistic diseases associated with HIV infection. The best prevention of opportunistic disease is adequate treatment of the underlying HIV infection.

Ongoing Care. HIV-infected patients share problems experienced by all individuals with chronic diseases, but these problems are exacerbated by social constructs surrounding HIV. Chronic diseases are characterized by negative social attitudes that label the patient as weak-willed or immoral for being sick. In HIV, this stigma is compounded by several factors. HIV-infected people may be seen as lacking control over urges to have sex or use drugs. It is then easy to jump to the conclusion that they brought the disease on themselves and, therefore, somehow deserve to be sick. Behaviours associated with HIV infection may be viewed as immoral (e.g., homosexuality, having many sexual partners) and are sometimes illegal (e.g., injecting heroin, sex work). The fact that infected individuals can transmit the virus to others furthers the negative, stigmatizing social concept of HIV. Social stigmatization supports discrimination in all facets of life. According to the Canadian Human Rights Commission (1996) policy on HIV/AIDS, all Canadians have the right to equality and dignity without discrimination, regardless of HIV/AIDS status.

The chronic nature of HIV infection can cause family stress, social isolation, dependence, frustration, lowered self-image, loss of control, and economic pressures. An interesting observation is that all of these variables may have contributed to the patient's infection in the first place. Low self-esteem, searching for social contact, frustration, and economic difficulties all contribute to drug use and risky sexual behaviours.

Disease and Drug Adverse Effects. Physical problems related to HIV disease or the treatment of HIV can interrupt the patient's ability to maintain a desired lifestyle. HIV-infected patients frequently experience anxiety, fear, diarrhea, depression, peripheral neuropathy, pain, nausea and vomiting, and fatigue. These are symptoms that nurses deal with routinely, and the interventions for them do not change significantly on the basis of the primary diagnosis. Individual considerations do, of course, influence the way that the nurse approaches the patient. Nursing management of diarrhea, for instance, still includes helping patients collect specimens, recommending dietary changes, encouraging fluid and electrolyte replacement, instructing the patient about skin care, and managing skin breakdown around the perianal area. Nursing approaches for HIV-related fatigue include teaching patients to assess fatigue patterns, determine contributing factors, set activity priorities, conserve energy, schedule rest periods, exercise, and avoid substances such as caffeine, nicotine, alcohol, and other drugs that may disturb sleep.

A new set of metabolic disorders has emerged among HIV-infected patients, especially those who have been infected for a long time and who have been receiving ART. These disorders include changes in body shape (fat deposits in the abdomen, the upper back, and the breasts, along with fat loss in the arms, the legs, and the face) caused by lipodystrophy (Figure 17-8); dyslipidemia (elevated triglycerides and decreases in high-density lipoproteins); insulin resistance and hyperglycemia; bone disease (osteoporosis, osteopenia, avascular necrosis); lactic acidosis; and cardiovascular disease. It is still not clear why these disorders develop, but the reason is probably a combination of factors such as long-term infection with HIV, adverse effects of ART, genetic predisposition, and chronic stress (Leung & Glesby, 2011).

FIGURE 17-8 Manifestations of lipodystrophy. Source: James, W. D., Berger, T., & Elston, D. (2006). *Andrews' diseases of the skin: Clinical dermatology* (10th ed.) St. Louis: Saunders.

Management of metabolic disorders currently focuses on detecting problems early, dealing with the symptoms, and helping the patient cope with new problems and additional drugs. It is important to recognize and treat these problems early, especially because cardiovascular disease and lactic acidosis are potentially fatal complications. A frequent first intervention is to change ART because some drugs are more often associated with these problems than are others (see Table 17-15). Lipid abnormalities are generally treated with lipid-lowering drugs, dietary changes, and exercise. Insulin resistance is treated with hypoglycemic drugs and weight loss. Bone disease may be improved with exercise, dietary changes, and calcium and vitamin D supplements.

Body changes that combine fat accumulation and wasting are major problems for patients with this syndrome. Human growth hormone, testosterone, and anabolic steroids have been used to help resolve these changes, but the results are inconclusive. Some patients may undergo plastic surgery procedures such as liposuction or facial implants to deal with the body changes associated with fat redistribution. There is little evidence that exercise or dietary changes make any difference. Nursing interventions must focus on helping the patient make treatment decisions and on dealing with negative changes in body image (CANAC, 2013).

End-of-Life Care. Despite new developments in the treatment of HIV infection, many patients eventually experience disease progression, disability, and death. Sometimes these occur because treatments do not work for the patient. Sometimes the patient's HIV infection becomes resistant to all available drug therapies. In addition, ART is now allowing people living with HIV to live longer and to develop diseases of aging, such as cardiovascular and endocrine problems that lead to death. Nursing care during the terminal phase of any disease must focus on keeping the patient comfortable, facilitating emotional and spiritual acceptance of the finite nature of life, and helping the patient's significant others deal with grief and loss. Nurses become pivotal care providers during the terminal phase of illness, especially in HIV disease, for which patients and families often choose terminal care at home. (End-of-life care is discussed in Chapter 13.)

EVALUATION

The expected outcomes are that the patient at risk for HIV infection will do the following:

- Analyze personal risk factors
- Develop and implement a personal plan to decrease risks
- Get tested for HIV infection

The expected outcomes are that the patient with HIV infection will do the following:

- Describe basic aspects of the effects of HIV on the immune system
- Compare and contrast various treatment options for HIV disease
- Work with a team of health care providers to achieve optimal health
- Prevent transmission of HIV to others

ETHICAL DILEMMAS

Duty to Treat

Situation

A nurse in a community clinic has just discovered that Ms. Joyce Ming, a patient with respiratory problems, has human immunodeficiency virus (HIV) infection. The nurse is concerned about contact with Ms. Ming and her body fluids. She requests that she not be assigned to Ms. Ming's care. The nurse believes that she has the right to refuse to care for Ms. Ming because she has her own family to support and protect.

Important Points for Consideration

- According to the Canadian Nurses Association's *Code of Ethics*, the nurse must not discriminate in the provision of nursing care on the basis of cultural or socioeconomic background or health status.
- Health care providers have contact with patients every day who may have infectious blood or other body fluids.
- Infection precautions are instituted to protect health care workers from potentially infectious blood or other body fluids.

- There are two situations in which nurses can refuse to care for patients if employers are notified in advance: (a) when caring for a patient would conflict with a nurse's deeply held religious belief or (b) when there might be greater potential harm to the nurse than benefit to the patient (e.g., if the nurse were immuno-compromised).
- The Canadian Human Rights Commission Policy (1996) on HIV/AIDS (acquired immune deficiency syndrome) prohibits discrimination based on HIV/AIDS status.
- If a nurse's primary concern is personal safety, the nurse needs to re-examine her or his commitment to the nursing profession.

Clinical Decision-Making Questions

1. How should a nurse address this issue if a colleague refused to provide care for a patient with HIV infection?
2. If nurses could select which patients they would care for, how would that affect their ability to care for patients in general?

CASE STUDY

At Risk for Human Immunodeficiency Virus Disease

Source: Blend Images/ Shutterstock. com.

Patient Profile

Mr. Emilio Chavez, a 20-year-old university student, comes to the student health centre with pain on urination.

Subjective Data

- Describes pain as "Just like it felt when I had the clap last year"
- Provides a history of sexual activity since age 15; reports lifetime sexual partners as six women and two men
- Denies injected-drug use, tobacco use, or corticosteroid therapy
- Uses alcohol (mainly beer) at weekend parties and has smoked marijuana, but not recently
- Recent sexual activity has been on weekends during or after beer parties

Objective Data
Physical Examination
- 180 cm tall, 76 kg, temperature 38°C, purulent urethral discharge noted

Laboratory Studies
- Urine test for *Neisseria gonorrhoeae* yields positive result

Collaborative Care
- Intramuscular injection with ceftriaxone, 250 mg
- Doxycycline, 100 mg orally, twice daily for 7 days

Discussion Questions

1. Why should Mr. Chavez be encouraged to be tested for human immunodeficiency virus (HIV)?
2. How will the nurse counsel Mr. Chavez about the testing process? How can the nurse help him prepare for the test and the test results?
3. What further questions will the nurse need to ask Mr. Chavez before the nurse can determine his educational needs?
4. Ask a classmate to be "Mr. Chavez" and role-play HIV risk assessment, risk-reduction counselling, pretest and post-test counselling.
5. **Priority Decision:** What are the main considerations to cover when teaching about barrier methods of protection? Are there cultural components that may affect the nurse's approach to teaching about condoms?
6. How will the nurse discuss the issue of partner notification with Mr. Chavez?
7. **Priority Decision:** Mr. Chavez's HIV test result comes back positive. What are the priority nursing decisions? What psychosocial issues would the nurse consider? What are the most important things for Mr. Chavez to know at the first meeting with him after he gets his diagnosis? How might he react, and how should the nurse deal with it?

ⓔvolve

Answers are available at *http://evolve.elsevier.com/Canada/Lewis/medsurg*

REVIEW QUESTIONS

The number of the question corresponds to the same-numbered objective at the beginning of the chapter.

1. What are nursing responsibilities regarding emerging and re-emerging infections? *(Select all that apply)*
   a. Educating clients about risks of developing emerging and re-emerging infections
   b. Maintaining awareness of unusual disease patterns
   c. Participating in immunization programs
   d. Using infection control procedures
   e. Examining prescribing practices to ensure appropriate antibiotic use

2. Which of the following antibiotic-resistant organisms are resistant to normal hand soap?
   a. Vancomycin-resistant enterococci
   b. Methicillin-resistant *Staphylococcus aureus*
   c. Penicillin-resistant *Streptococcus pneumoniae*
   d. β-Lactamase–producing *Klebsiella pneumoniae*

3. How is human immunodeficiency virus (HIV) transmitted?
   a. Most commonly as a result of sexual contact
   b. In all infants born to women with HIV infection
   c. Only when there is a large viral load in the blood
   d. Frequently in health care workers with needle-stick exposures

4. Which is the common physiological change after HIV infection?
   a. The virus replicates mainly in B lymphocytes before spreading to CD4$^+$ T cells in lymph nodes.
   b. The immune system is impaired predominantly by infection and destruction of CD4$^+$ T cells.
   c. Infection of monocytes may occur, but these cells are destroyed by antibodies produced by oligodendrocytes.
   d. A long period develops during which the virus is not found in the blood and there is little viral replication.

5. Which of the following statements is false?
   a. "Infection with HIV results in a chronic disease with acute exacerbations."
   b. "Untreated HIV infection can remain in the early chronic stage for a decade or more."
   c. "Late-stage infection is often called *acquired immune deficiency syndrome (AIDS)*."
   d. "Opportunistic diseases occur more often when the CD4$^+$ T-cell count is high and the viral load is low."

6. When is AIDS diagnosed in an HIV-infected person?
   a. When an AIDS-defining illness develops.
   b. When the amount of HIV in the blood increases.
   c. When the CD4:CD8 ratio is reversed to less than 2:1.
   d. When the person has oral hairy leukoplakia, an infection caused by Epstein-Barr virus.

7. What does screening for HIV infection generally involve?
   a. Laboratory analysis of blood to detect HIV antigen
   b. Electrophoretic analysis of HIV antigen in plasma
   c. Laboratory analysis of blood to detect HIV antibodies
   d. Analysis of lymph tissues for the presence of HIV RNA

8. What is the indication for use of antiretroviral drugs?
   a. Cure acute HIV infection
   b. Treat opportunistic diseases
   c. Decrease viral RNA levels
   d. Supplement radiation therapy and surgery

9. Which statement about metabolic adverse effects of ART is true? *(Select all that apply)*
   a. "These are annoying symptoms that are ultimately harmless."
   b. "ART-related body changes include central fat accumulation and peripheral wasting."
   c. "Lipid abnormalities include increases in triglycerides and decreases in high-density cholesterol."
   d. "Insulin resistance and hyperlipidemia can be treated with drugs to control glucose and cholesterol."
   e. "Insulin resistance and hyperlipidemia are more difficult to treat in HIV-infected clients than in uninfected people."

10. Which of the following descriptions of opportunistic diseases in HIV infection is correct?
   a. Usually occur one at a time
   b. Generally slow to develop and progress
   c. Occur in the presence of immuno-suppression
   d. Curable with appropriate pharmacological intervention

11. Of the following, which is the most appropriate nursing intervention to help an HIV-infected client adhere to the treatment regimen?
   a. Give the client a DVD and a brochure to view and read at home.
   b. Volunteer to "set up" a drug pillbox for a week at a time.
   c. Inform the client that the adverse effects of the drugs are bad but that they go away after a while.
   d. Assess the client's lifestyle and find adherence cues that fit into the client's lifestyle.

12. Which strategy can the nurse teach the client to eliminate the risk of transmission of HIV?
   a. Using sterile equipment to inject drugs
   b. Cleaning equipment used to inject drugs
   c. Taking zidovudine (azidothymidine [AZT], ZDV, Retrovir) during pregnancy
   d. Using latex barriers to cover genitals during sexual contact

1. a, b, c, d, e; 2. a; 3. a; 4. b; 5. d; 6. a; 7. c; 8. c; 9. b, c, d; 10. c; 11. d; 12. a.

⊜volve

For even more review questions, visit *http://evolve.elsevier.com/Canada/Lewis/medsurg*.

REFERENCES

AIDS InfoNet. (2014). *Fact sheet 729: St. Johns wort (hypericin).* Retrieved from *http://www.aidsinfonet.org/fact_sheets/view/729*.

AIDSinfo. (2016a). *Preventing mother-to-child transmission of HIV.* Retrieved from *https://aidsinfo.nih.gov/education-materials/fact-sheets/20/50/preventing-mother-to-child-transmission-of-hiv*.

AIDSinfo. (2016b). *The HIV life cycle.* Retrieved from *https://www.aidsinfo.nih.gov/education-materials/fact-sheets/19/73/the-hiv-life-cycle*.

Arkin, E. (2011). Studies confirm effectiveness of harm reduction for people who inject drugs. *HIV/AIDS policy & law review/ Canadian HIV/AIDS Legal Network, 15*(3), 29.

Burdge, D. R., Money, D. M., Forbes, J. C., et al.; Canadian HIV Trials Network Working Group on Vertical HIV Transmission. (2003). Canadian consensus guidelines for the management of pregnancy, labour and delivery and for postpartum care in HIV-positive pregnant women and their offspring (summary of 2002 guidelines). *Canadian Medical Association Journal, 168*(13), 1671–1674. (Seminal).

Canadian Association of Nurses in AIDS Care. (2013). *Best practice guidelines: Caring for clients who are at risk for or living with HIV/AIDS*. Vancouver: Author. Retrieved from *http://www.canac.org/wp-content/uploads/2015/11/CANAC_BPG_v2013.pdf*.

Canadian Human Rights Commission. (1996). Canadian Human Rights Commission policy on HIV/AIDS. *Canadian HIV/AIDS Policy & Law Newsletter, 3*(1), 7–8. Retrieved from *http://www.chrc-ccdp.ca/legislation_policies/aids-en.asp*. (Seminal).

Centers for Disease Control and Prevention. (2015a). *HIV transmission*. Atlanta: Author. Retrieved from *http://www.cdc.gov/hiv/basics/transmission.html*.

Centers for Disease Control and Prevention. (2015b). *HIV among pregnant women, infants and children*. Atlanta: Author. Retrieved from *https://www.cdc.gov/hiv/group/gender/pregnantwomen/*.

Enriquez, M., & McKinsey, D. S. (2011). Strategies to improve HIV treatment adherence in developed countries: Clinical management at the individual level. *HIV/AIDS (Auckland, N.Z.), 3*, 45–51. doi:10.2147/HIV.S8993.

French, H., Greeff, M., Watson, M. J., et al. (2015). HIV stigma and disclosure experiences of people living with HIV in an urban and a rural setting. *AIDS Care, 27*(8), 1042–1046. doi:10.1080/09540121.2015.1020747.

Government of Canada. (2016a). *Ebola virus disease*. Retrieved from *http://healthycanadians.gc.ca/diseases-conditions-maladies-affections/disease-maladie/ebola/index-eng.php*.

Government of Canada. (2016b). *Zika virus*. Retrieved from *http://healthycanadians.gc.ca/diseases-conditions-maladies-affections/disease-maladie/zika-virus/index-eng.php*.

Greenwood, B., Salisbury, D., & Hill, A. V. S. (2011). Vaccines and global health. *Philosophical Transactions of the Royal Society, 366*(1579), 2733–2742. doi:10.1098/rstb.2011.0076.

Gunthard, H. F., Aberg, J. A., Eron, J. J., et al. (2014). Antiretroviral treatment of adult HIV infection: 2104 Recommendations of the International Antiviral Society—USA panel. *Journal of the American Medical Association, 312*(4), 410–425. doi:10.1001/jama.2014.8722.

HIV.gov. (2014). *How are drug use and HIV related?* Washington, DC: U.S. Department of Health and Human Services. Retrieved from *https://www.aids.gov/hiv-aids-basics/prevention/reduce-your-risk/substance-abuse-use*.

HIV.gov. (2015). *Post-exposure prophylaxis (PEP)*. Washington: Author. Retrieved from *http://www.aids.gov/hiv-aids-basics/prevention/reduce-your-risk/post-exposure-prophylaxis/*.

Huether, S. E., & McCance, K. L. (2012). *Understanding pathophysiology* (5th ed.). St. Louis: Elsevier/Mosby.

Kuhar, D. T., Henderson, D. K., Struble, K. A., et al. (2013). Updated US Public Health Service guidelines for the management of occupational exposures to human immunodeficiency virus and recommendations for post-exposure prophylaxis. *Infection Control and Hospital Epidemiology, 34*(9), 875–892. doi:10.1086/672271.

Leung, V. L., & Glesby, M. J. (2011). Pathogenesis and treatment of HIV lipohypertrophy. *Current Opinions in Infectious Diseases, 24*(1), 43–49. doi:10.1097/QCO.06013e3283420eef.

Montaner, J. S. (2011). Treatment as prevention: A double hat trick. *Lancet, 378*(9787), 208–209. doi:10.1016/50140-6736(11)60821-0.

Pepin, J. (2011). *The origin of AIDS*. Cambridge, UK: Cambridge University Press.

Public Health Agency of Canada. (2010). *Perinatal HIV transmission in Canada*. Ottawa: Author. Retrieved from *http://www.phac-aspc.gc.ca/aids-sida/publication/epi/2010/7-eng.php* (Seminal).

Public Health Agency of Canada. (2012a). *Hand hygiene practices in health care settings*. Ottawa: Author. Retrieved from *http://www.publications.gc.ca/collections/collection_2012/aspc-phac/HP40-74-2012-eng.pdf*.

Public Health Agency of Canada. (2012b). *Routine practices and additional precautions for preventing the transmission of infection in health care settings*. Ottawa: Author. Retrieved from *http://www.publications.gc.ca/collections/collection_2013/aspc-phac/HP40-83-2013-eng.pdf*.

Public Health Agency of Canada. (2013). *Healthcare associated infections: Due diligence*. Ottawa: Author. Retrieved from *http://www.phac-aspc.gc.ca/cphorsphc-respcacsp/2013/infections-eng.php*.

Public Health Agency of Canada. (2014). *Canadian Communicable Disease Report* (Vol. 40). Retrieved from *http://www.phac-aspc.gc.ca/publicat/ccdr-rmtc/15vol40/index-eng.php*.

Public Health Agency of Canada. (2015a). *Canadian Antimicrobial Resistance Surveillance System Report 2015*. Ottawa: Author. Retrieved from *http://www.healthycanadians.gc.ca/publications/drugs-products-medicaments-produits/antibiotic-resistance-antibiotique/antimicrobial-surveillance-antimicrobioresistance-eng.php#a8-2-8*.

Public Health Agency of Canada. (2015b). *Canadian Communicable Disease Report* (Vol. 41). Retrieved from *http://www.phac-aspc.gc.ca/publicat/ccdr-rmtc/15vol41/index-eng.php*.

Public Health Agency of Canada. (2015c). *Population-Specific HIV/AIDS Status Report: People Living with HIV/AIDS*. Retrieved from *http://www.phac-aspc.gc.ca/aids-sida/publication/ps-pd/people-personnes/chapter-chapitre-2-eng.php*.

Public Health Agency of Canada. (2015d). *Summary: Estimates of HIV incidence, prevalence and proportion undiagnosed in Canada, 2014*. Retrieved from *https://www.canada.ca/content/dam/canada/health-canada/migration/healthy-canadians/publications/diseases-conditions-maladies-affections/hiv-aids-estimates-2014-vih-sida-estimations/alt/hiv-aids-estimates-2014-vih-sida-estimations-eng.pdf*.

Public Health Agency of Canada. (2016). *Canadian Guidelines on Sexually Transmitted Infections*. Retrieved from *http://www.phac-aspc.gc.ca/std-mts/sti-its/cgsti-ldcits/section-5-8-eng.php*.

Smith, M. K., Rutstein, S. E., Powers, K. A., et al. (2013). The detection and management of early HIV infection: A public health emergency. *Journal of Acquired Immune Deficiency Syndromes, 63*, S187–S189.

United Nations AIDS (UNAIDS). (2015a). *AIDS by the numbers*. Geneva: Author. Retrieved from *http://www.unaids.org/en/resources/documents/2015/aids_by_the_numbers_2015*.

United Nations AIDS (UNAIDS). (2015b). *Fact sheet 2015*. Geneva: Author. Retrieved from *http://www.unaids.org/sites/default/files/media_asset/20150901_FactSheet_2015-en.pdf*.

Wasserman, P., Segal-Maurer, S., Wehbeh, W., et al. (2011). Wasting disease, chronic immune activation and inflammation in HIV infected patients. *Topics in Clinical Nutrition, 26*(1), 14–28. doi:10.1097/TIN.0b013e318209e3a0.

World Health Organization. (2007). *WHO case definitions of HIV for surveillance and revised clinical staging and immunological classification of HIV related disease in adults and children*. Geneva: Author. Retrieved from *http://www.who.int/hiv/pub/guidelines/HIVstaging150307.pdf*. (Seminal).

World Health Organization. (2015a). *Antimicrobial resistance*. Geneva: Author. Retrieved from *http://www.who.int/mediacentre/factsheets/fs194/en/*.

World Health Organization. (2015b). *HIV/AIDS*. Geneva: Author. Retrieved from *http://www.who.int/mediacentre/factsheets/fs360/en*.

World Health Organization. (2016). *Ebola virus disease: Disease outbreak news*. Retrieved from *http://www.who.int/csr/don/archive/disease/ebola/en/*.

RESOURCES

BC Centre for Excellence in HIV/AIDS
http://www.cfenet.ubc.ca

Canadian Aboriginal AIDS Network
http://www.caan.ca

Canadian AIDS Society
http://www.cdnaids.ca

Canadian AIDS Treatment Information Exchange (CATIE)
http://www.catie.ca

Canadian Association of Nurses in HIV/AIDS Care
http://www.canac.org

Canadian Blood Services
http://www.bloodservices.ca

Canadian Centre for Occupational Health and Safety
http://www.ccohs.ca

Canadian HIV/AIDS Legal Network
http://www.aidslaw.ca

Canadian Lyme Disease Foundation
https://canlyme.com

Canadian Nurses Association *Code of Ethics for Registered Nurses*
https://www.cna-aiic.ca/~/media/cna/page-content/pdf-en/code-of-ethics-2017-edition-secure-interactive.pdf?la=en

Canadian Public Health Association
http://www.cpha.ca

CTAC
http://www.ctac.ca

Canadian Working Group on HIV and Rehabilitation
http://www.hivandrehab.ca

Health Canada: HIV and AIDS
https://www.canada.ca/en/health-canada/services/health-concerns/diseases-conditions/hiv-aids-diseases-conditions.html

HIV/AIDS Epi Update
http://www.phac-aspc.gc.ca/aids-sida/publication/epi/2010/1-eng.php

Infection Prevention and Control Canada (IPAC)
https://ipac-canada.org

Positive Living Society of British Columbia
http://www.positivelivingbc.org

Positive Women's Network
http://www.pwn.bc.ca

Proceedings of the Consensus Conference on Infected Healthcare Workers: Risk for Transmission of Bloodborne Pathogens
http://www.collectionscanada.gc.ca/webarchives/20071124025757/http://www.phac-aspc.gc.ca/publicat/ccdr-rmtc/98vol24/24s4/index.html

Public Health Agency of Canada
http://www.phac-aspc.gc.ca

Public Health Agency of Canada—Surveillance
http://www.phac-aspc.gc.ca/surveillance-eng.php

Joint United Nations Programme on HIV/AIDS (UNAIDS)
http://www.unaids.org

For additional Internet resources, see the website for this book at *http://evolve.elsevier.com/Canada/Lewis/medsurg*

Cancer

Written by: Carolee Polek
Adapted by: Rosemary Cashman

⊖volve WEBSITE

http://evolve.elsevier.com/Canada/Lewis/medsurg

- Review Questions (Online Only)
- Key Points
- Customizable Nursing Care Plans
  - Radiation
  - Chemotherapy
- Conceptual Care Map Creator
- Audio Glossary
- Content Updates

LEARNING OBJECTIVES

1. Describe the prevalence, the incidence, and the death rates of cancer in Canada.
2. Describe the biological processes involved in cancer.
3. Differentiate the three phases of cancer development.
4. Describe the role of the immune system in relation to cancer.
5. Describe the use of the classification systems for cancer.
6. Explain the role of the nurse in the prevention and detection of cancer.
7. Explain the use of surgery, radiation therapy, chemotherapy, and biological therapy in the treatment of cancer.
8. Differentiate between external beam radiation and brachytherapy.
9. Identify the classifications of chemotherapeutic agents and methods of administration.
10. Describe the effects of radiation therapy and chemotherapy on normal tissues.
11. Identify the types and effects of biological therapy agents.
12. Describe the nursing management of patients receiving radiation therapy, chemotherapy, and biological therapy.
13. Describe the nutritional therapy for patients with cancer.
14. Describe the complications that can occur in advanced cancer.
15. Describe the appropriate psychosocial support of a patient with cancer and the patient's family.

KEY TERMS

benign neoplasms, p. 319
biological therapy, p. 340
bone marrow transplantation, p. 343
brachytherapy, p. 333
cancer, p. 316
carcinogens, p. 319

carcinoma, p. 324
carcinoma in situ, p. 325
extravasation, p. 329
histological grading, p. 324
immunological surveillance, p. 323
malignant neoplasms, p. 319

metastasis, p. 321
nadir, p. 332
oncogenes, p. 319
proto-oncogenes, p. 319
radiation, p. 333
sarcoma, p. 324
staging, p. 324

tumour angiogenesis, p. 321
tumour-associated antigens, p. 323
tumour suppressor genes, p. 319
vesicants, p. 329

DEFINITION AND INCIDENCE

Cancer is a group of more than 200 diseases characterized by uncontrolled and unregulated growth of cells. It can occur in persons of all ages and all ethnicities and is a major health problem. In 2016, the Canadian Cancer Society's Steering Committee on Cancer Statistics estimated that 202 400 new cancer cases (excluding 78 300 nonmelanoma skin cancers) would be diagnosed and that 78 000 people would die from cancer in Canada. As the population ages, the incidence of cancer rises. Among people with cancer, 43% of new cases and 62% of deaths caused by cancer occur in those who are at least 70 years of age. Cancer is more common among women between the age of 20 and 59, primarily because of breast and thyroid cancer. In all other age groups, cancer is more common in male patients. Cancer incidence and death rates also increase from west to east across the country. Of the 202 400 new cases of cancer predicted in 2016, it was estimated that slightly more than half (50.4%) would be lung, breast, colorectal, or prostate cancers. Because thousands of Canadians are expected to die from cancer every year, there are significant repercussions on Canadian families and the economy (Canadian Cancer Society's Steering Committee on Cancer Statistics, 2016). Estimated cancer incidences and mortality rates by site (type) and sex are presented in Tables 18-1 and 18-2.

TABLE 18-1	NEW CASES FOR CANCER BY SITE (TYPE) AND SEX, CANADA, 2016		
Male		**Female**	
Type	New Case Estimate	Type	New Case Estimate
Prostate	21 600	Breast	25 700
Lung	14 400	Lung	14 000
Colorectal	14 500	Colorectal	11 600
Non-Hodgkin's lymphoma	4 400	Non-Hodgkin's lymphoma	3 600
Bladder	6 600	Uterus	6 600
Kidney	4 100	Thyroid	5 300

Source: Canadian Cancer Society's Steering Committee on Cancer Statistics. (2016). *Canadian Cancer Statistics 2016*. Toronto: Canadian Cancer Society.

TABLE 18-2	ESTIMATED DEATHS FOR CANCER BY SITE AND SEX, CANADA, 2016		
Male		**Female**	
Type	Deaths	Type	Deaths
Lung	10 900	Lung	9 800
Prostate	4 000	Breast	4 900
Colorectal	5 000	Colorectal	4 300
Pancreas	2 400	Pancreas	2 400
Bladder	1 650	Ovary	1 750

Source: Canadian Cancer Society's Steering Committee on Cancer Statistics. (2016). *Canadian Cancer Statistics 2016*. Toronto: Canadian Cancer Society.

Prevalence is the total number of people who are living with a diagnosis of cancer. Advances in research in the areas of early detection, treatment, and supportive therapies have resulted in more people surviving cancer, especially in the pediatric population. Prevalence is, therefore, more often and more usefully defined as patients still alive 10 years after the initial diagnosis with cancer. Over a lifetime, it is estimated that two in five Canadians (45% of male Canadians and 42% of female Canadians) will develop cancer and one in four (29% of male Canadians and 24% of female Canadians) will die from it (Canadian Cancer Society's Steering Committee on Cancer Statistics, 2016). In 2012, cancer was the leading cause of death in Canada, accounting for 30% of all deaths, with cardiovascular diseases (heart and cerebro-vascular diseases) in second place (25% of deaths; Statistics Canada, 2015). Lung cancer remains the leading cause of premature death from cancer (Canadian Cancer Society's Steering Committee on Cancer Statistics, 2016), and tobacco use has long been recognized as a significant risk for the development of this and other types of cancer. Smoking prevalence and amount have declined in the Canadian population overall; however, smoking rates among Indigenous peoples are more than twice as high as those in the non-Indigenous population (39% versus 20.5%; Gionet & Roshanafshar, 2013).

Cancer incidence and mortality are tracked by province and territory through cancer registries. Statistics document the incidence and prevalence of cancer but cannot reveal the physiological and psychosocial effect of cancer on individuals, families, and society. Nurses play a critical role in shaping attitudes and promoting behaviours that prevent the development of cancer and facilitate adjustment to living with cancer.

Progress Made in Cancer Prevention: Modifiable Risk Factors

Many well-known and common cancer risk factors are preventable. For example, in addition to tobacco use, known risk factors include excessive body weight, lack of physical activity, unhealthy eating habits, alcohol consumption, and excessive exposure to the sun. Several of these factors are related to other chronic diseases such as diabetes, kidney failure, chronic obstructive lung disease, and cardiovascular disease. The Canadian Cancer Society reported a worrisome rising trend in obesity: The percentage of obese Canadians increased from 15% in 2003 to 18% in 2010 (Gotay, Katzmarzyk, Janssen, et al., 2012). In addition, as recently as 2014, 46% of Canadians were physically inactive (Statistics Canada, n.d.). All of these risk factors are within the control of each individual. If these lifestyle factors were modified, the rates of cancers and other chronic diseases would be reduced (Table 18-3). Concerted efforts in health promotion and disease prevention strategies are required in every province to alert and educate the public about what they can do to achieve improvements in health and longevity.

BIOLOGICAL PROCESSES OF CANCER

The term *cancer* encompasses many diseases of multiple causes that can arise in any cell of the body capable of evading regulatory controls over proliferation and differentiation. Two major dysfunctions present in the process of cancer are defective cellular *proliferation* (growth) and defective cellular *differentiation*.

Defects in Cellular Proliferation

Normally, most tissues of the human adult contain a population of predetermined, undifferentiated cells known as *stem cells. Predetermined* means that the stem cells of a particular tissue will ultimately differentiate and become mature, functioning cells of that tissue and only that tissue.

Cell proliferation originates in the stem cell and begins when the stem cell enters the cell cycle (Figure 18-1). The time from when a cell enters the cell cycle to when the cell divides into two identical cells is called the *generation time of the cell.* A mature cell continues to function until it degenerates and dies.

All cells of a tissue are controlled by an intracellular mechanism that determines when cellular proliferation is necessary. Under normal conditions, a state of dynamic equilibrium is constantly maintained (i.e., rate of cellular proliferation equals rate of cellular degeneration). Normally, the process of cellular division and proliferation is activated only in the event of cellular degeneration or death. Cellular proliferation also occurs if the body has a physiological need for more cells. For example, the white blood cell (WBC) count normally increases in the presence of infection.

Another mechanism for proliferation control in normal cells is *contact inhibition.* Normal cells "respect" the boundaries and territory of the cells surrounding them; they do not invade a territory that is not their own. The neighbouring cells are thought to inhibit cellular growth through the physical contact of the surrounding cell membranes. Cancer cells grown in tissue culture are characterized by loss of contact inhibition. These cells breach cellular boundaries and will grow on top of one another and also on top of or between normal cells.

The rate of normal cellular proliferation differs in each body tissue. In some tissues, such as bone marrow, hair follicles, and

TABLE 18-3 MODIFIABLE RISK FACTORS FOR SELECTED CANCER TYPES

Cancer Type	Smoking	Overweight/ Obesity	Physical Activity	Poor Diet	Sun Exposure/ Outdoor Tanning	Alcohol Consumption	Infections (Viruses and Bacteria)	Pharmaceuticals	Occupational/ Environmental Exposure (Nonsolar)
Bladder	X								X
Body of uterus		X	X					X	
Breast		X	X			X		X	X
Brain/CNS									X
Cervix	X						X	X	
Colorectal	X	X	X	X		X			X
Oesophagus	X	X		X		X			X
Hodgkin's lymphoma								X	
Kidney	X	X							X
Larynx	X					X			X
Leukemia	X							X	X
Liver	X	X				X	X	X	X
Lung	X								X
Melanoma					X				X
Multiple myeloma									
Non-Hodgkin's lymphoma							X		
Oral	X			X		X	X		X
Ovary	X	X						X	X
Pancreas	X	X							
Prostate		X							
Stomach	X			X			X		
Testis									
Thyroid									X

Source: Canadian Cancer Society's Advisory Committee on Cancer Statistics. *Canadian Cancer Statistics 2015*. Toronto, ON: Canadian Cancer Society; 2015. *CNS*, central nervous system.

FIGURE 18-1 Cell life cycle and metabolic activity. Generation time is the period from one M (mitosis) phase to the next. Cells not in the cycle but capable of division are in the resting phase (G₀). *DNA*, deoxyribonucleic acid; *GI*, gastro-intestinal; *RNA*, ribonucleic acid. Source: Adapted from Kumar, V., Abbas, A. K., Fausto, N., et al. (2010). *Robbins and Cotran pathologic basis of disease* (8th ed., p. 86). Philadelphia: W. B. Saunders.

epithelial lining of the gastro-intestinal (GI) tract, the rate of cellular proliferation is rapid. In other tissues, such as myocardium, neurons, and cartilage, cellular proliferation is slow or does not occur at all.

Cancer cells usually proliferate in the manner and at the same rate as the normal cells of the tissue from which they arise. However, cancer cells respond differently than normal cells to the intracellular signals that regulate the state of dynamic equilibrium. Whereas normal cell proliferation is regulated according to the body's needs, cell division in cancer is dysregulated and haphazard, and proliferation of cancer cells is indiscriminate and continuous. In this way, with each cell division creating two or more offspring cells, the tumour mass continuously doubles in size: 1 cell → 2 cells → 4 cells → 8 cells → 16 cells, and so on. This is termed the *pyramid effect*. The time required for a tumour mass to double in size is known as its *doubling time*.

According to the stem cell theory, the loss of intracellular control of proliferation results from a mutation of the stem cells (Tannock, Hill, Bristow, et al., 2013). The stem cells are viewed as the target or the origin of cancer development. The DNA of the stem cell is substituted or permanently rearranged. When this happens, the stem cell has mutated. Once the cell has mutated, one of three things can occur: (a) the cell can die, either from the damage resulting from the mutation or from initiation of a programmed cellular suicide called *apoptosis;* (b) the cell can recognize the damage and repair itself; or (c) the mutated cell can survive and pass along the damage to its daughter cells. Mutated cells that survive have the potential to become malignant (i.e., cells with invasive and metastatic potential), especially if the progeny cells acquire additional mutations.

Proliferating cells rely on a genetic blueprint for tissues and organs, which is found on chromosomes within the nucleus of the cell. Structures called *telomeres,* consisting of a repeated DNA code, are found at the end of chromosomes and serve to protect the genetic data within the chromosomes and facilitate normal cell division. Each time a cell divides, the telomere becomes shorter, and a small sequence of genetic material is not copied. Ultimately, the cell is unable to undergo further division, becomes inactive (senescent), and dies. Cancer cells produce an enzyme called *telomerase* that prevents telomere shortening and allows the cells to escape senescence and death. Telomerase thus promotes the immortalization of cells and has a role in the development of cancer, as well as in the process of aging.

Defects in Cellular Differentiation

Cellular differentiation is normally an orderly process in which the cell progresses from a state of immaturity to a state of maturity. Because all body cells are derived from fertilized ova, all cells have the potential to perform all body functions. As cells differentiate, this potential is narrowed, and the mature cell is capable of performing only specific functions (Figure 18-2).

In cellular differentiation, the phasing out of cellular potential is stable and orderly. Under normal conditions, the differentiated cell is stable and does not *dedifferentiate* (i.e., revert to a previous undifferentiated state).

The exact mechanism that controls cellular differentiation and proliferation is not completely understood. Two types of normal genes are important regulators of normal cellular processes: **Proto-oncogenes** promote growth, whereas **tumour**

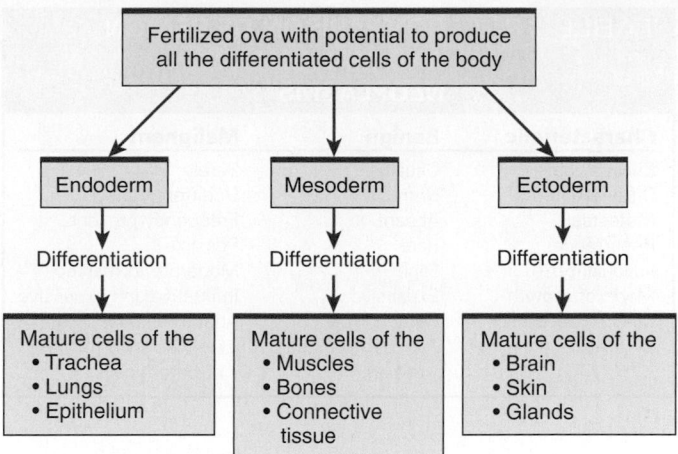

FIGURE 18-2 Normal cellular differentiation.

suppressor genes, such as tumour protein 53, suppress growth. Both can be affected by mutations. Those that alter the expression of proto-oncogenes can activate them to function as **oncogenes** (tumour-inducing genes). Mutations that alter tumour suppressor genes render them inactive, which results in a loss of their tumour suppressor ability.

The proto-oncogene has been described as the genetic lock that keeps the cell in its mature functioning state. When this lock is "unlocked," as may occur through exposure to **carcinogens** (cancer-causing agents capable of producing cellular alterations) or oncogenic viruses, genetic alterations and mutations occur. The abilities and properties that the cell had during fetal development are again expressed. Oncogenes interfere with normal cell expression under some conditions, causing the cell to become malignant. This cell regains fetal properties and function. For example, some cancer cells produce new proteins, such as those characteristic of the embryonic and fetal periods of life. These proteins, located on the cell membrane, include carcinoembryonic antigen (CEA) and alpha-fetoprotein. They can be detected in human blood by laboratory studies (see "Role of the Immune System" section). Other cancer cells, such as small cell carcinoma of the lung, produce hormones (see "Complications Resulting From Cancer" section) that are ordinarily produced by cells arising from the same embryonic cells as the tumour cells.

Tumours can be classified as benign or malignant. In general, **benign neoplasms** are well-differentiated, and **malignant neoplasms** are undifferentiated. Malignant tumour cells have the ability to invade and metastasize, unlike benign neoplasms. Other differences between benign and malignant neoplasms are listed in Table 18-4.

Development of Cancer

In this section, a theoretical model of the development of cancer is described. The cause and development of each type of cancer are likely to be multifactorial. It is not known how many tumours have a chemical, environmental, genetic, immunological, or viral origin. Cancers may arise spontaneously from causes that are thus far unclear.

It is a common misunderstanding that the development of cancer is a rapid, haphazard event. However, the natural history of cancer is an orderly process comprising several stages and occurring over a period of time. These stages are *initiation, promotion,* and *progression* (Figure 18-3).

TABLE 18-4	COMPARISON OF BENIGN AND MALIGNANT NEOPLASMS	
Characteristic	**Benign**	**Malignant**
Encapsulated	Usually	Rarely
Differentiated	Normally	Undifferentiated
Metastasis	Absent	Frequently present
Recurrence	Rare	Possible
Vascularity	Slight	Moderate to marked
Mode of growth	Expansive	Infiltrative and expansive
Cell characteristics	Fairly normal; similar to those of parent cells	Abnormal; bear little resemblance to those of parent cells

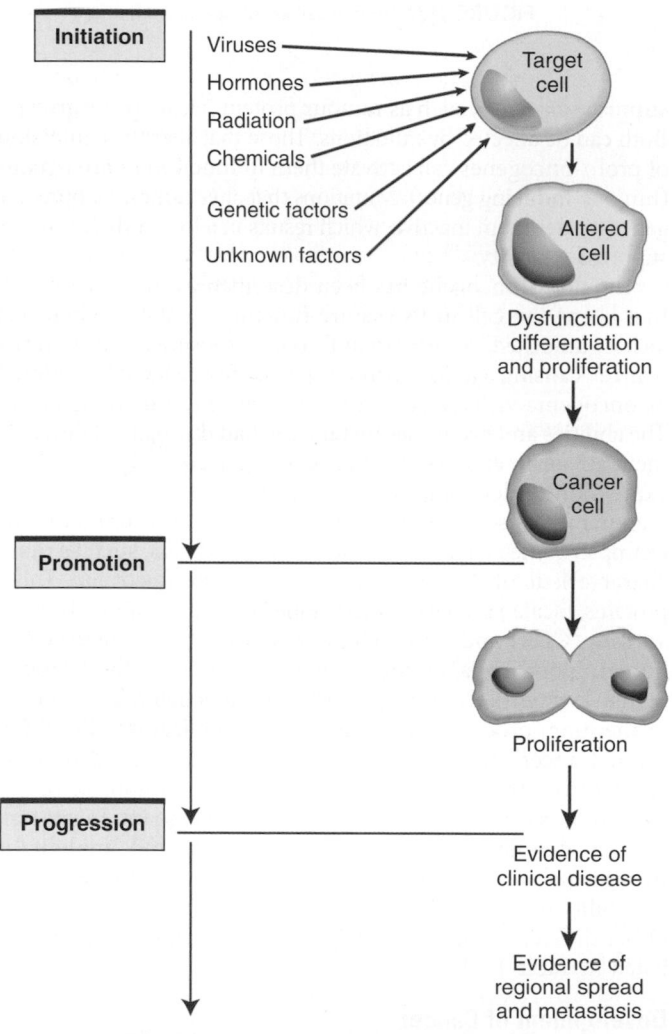

FIGURE 18-3 Process of cancer development.

Initiation. The first stage, *initiation*, is a mutation in the cell's genetic structure resulting from an inherited mutation, an error that occurs during DNA replication or after exposure to a carcinogen. This altered cell has the potential for developing into a *clone* (progeny of a single cell) of neoplastic cells.

Many carcinogens are detoxified by protective enzymes and harmlessly excreted. If this protective mechanism fails, carcinogens can enter a cell's nucleus and alter its DNA. The cell may die or

repair itself. However, if cell death or repair does not occur before cell division, the cell replicates into daughter cells, each with the same genetic alteration. Carcinogens may be chemical, radioactive, or viral in nature. In addition, some genetic anomalies increase the susceptibility of individuals to certain cancers. Common characteristics of carcinogens are that their effects in the stage of initiation are usually irreversible and additive.

Chemical Carcinogens. Chemicals were identified as cancer-causing agents in the latter part of the 18th century, when Percival Pott noted that chimney sweeps had a higher incidence of cancer of the scrotum in association with exposure to soot residues in chimneys. Over time, more chemical agents were identified as actual and potential carcinogens. Evidence indicated that individuals undergoing sustained exposure to certain chemicals had a greater incidence of certain cancers than others. Because of the long latency period from the time of exposure to the development of cancer, identifying cancer-causing chemicals is difficult. Chemicals that cause cancer in animals may or may not cause the same specific cancer in humans. Some chemicals are cancer causative in their environmental form, but others must first undergo specific changes to become carcinogenic.

Certain drugs have also been identified as carcinogens. Drugs that are capable of interacting with DNA (e.g., alkylating agents) and immuno-suppressive agents have the potential to cause neoplasms in humans. The use of alkylating agents (e.g., cyclo-phosphamide and nitrogen mustards), either alone or in combination with radiation therapy, has been associated with an increased incidence of acute myelogenous leukemia in persons treated for Hodgkin's disease, non-Hodgkin's lymphomas, and multiple myeloma. These secondary leukemias are relatively refractory to treatment. Secondary leukemia has also been observed in persons who have undergone transplantation surgery and taken immuno-suppressive drugs.

Radiation. Early in the 20th century, ionizing radiation (described later) was found to cause cancer in almost any human body tissue. The safe threshold for exposure to radiation is not known, and there is considerable debate surrounding the effect of exposure to low-dose radiation over time. Radiation damages cellular DNA. Certain malignancies have been linked to radiation:

1. Leukemia, lymphoma, thyroid cancer, and other cancers increased in incidence in the general population of Hiroshima and Nagasaki after the atomic bomb explosions.
2. A higher incidence of bone cancer occurs in persons exposed to radiation in certain occupations, such as radiologists, radiation chemists, and uranium miners.
3. Thyroid cancer has a higher incidence among persons who have received radiation to the head and neck area for treatment of a variety of disorders, such as acne, tonsillitis, sore throat, or enlarged thyroid gland.
4. The incidence of childhood cancer is higher among children exposed to radiation during fetal life.

Ultraviolet radiation has long been associated with melanoma, squamous cell carcinoma, and basal cell carcinoma of the skin. Skin cancer is by far the most common type of cancer in North America. Melanoma is a particularly aggressive skin cancer that responds poorly to treatment. Although the cause of melanoma is probably multifactorial, mounting evidence suggests that ultraviolet radiation secondary to sunlight exposure is linked to the development of melanoma.

Viral and Bacterial Carcinogens. Certain DNA and RNA viruses, termed *oncogenic viruses,* can transform the cells they infect and induce malignant transformation. Viruses have been identified as causative agents of cancer in animals and humans. For example, cells from patients with Burkitt's lymphoma have consistently shown evidence of the presence of the Epstein-Barr virus (EBV) in vitro. This virus also causes infectious mononucleosis; it is unclear which precise process results in infectious disease versus lymphoma. Persons with acquired immunodeficiency syndrome (AIDS), which is caused by a retrovirus, have a higher incidence of Kaposi's sarcoma (see Chapter 17). Other viruses that have been linked to the development of cancer include hepatitis B and C viruses, associated with hepatocellular carcinoma, and human papillomavirus, associated with squamous cell carcinomas such as cervical, anal, and head and neck cancers. *Helicobacter pylori* is a bacterium found in the stomach of two-thirds of the world's population and is implicated in the development of gastric and duodenal ulcers, as well as of some gastric cancers.

Genetic Susceptibility. Cancer-related genes have been identified that increase an individual's susceptibility to the development of certain cancers. For example, a woman with mutations in the gene *BRCA1* or *BRCA2* has a 40% to 85% risk of developing breast cancer in her lifetime. However, 95% of women who develop breast cancer do not possess these genetic mutations. On the basis of current knowledge, it is believed that only 5% to 10% of cancers have a strong genetic link (Loud & Hutson, 2011).

Promotion. A single alteration of the genetic structure of the cell is not sufficient to result in cancer. However, the odds of cancer development are increased with the presence of promoting agents. *Promotion,* the second stage in the development of cancer, is characterized by the reversible proliferation of the altered cells. Consequently, with an increase in the altered cell population, the likelihood of sustained mutagenesis is increased.

An important distinction between initiation and promotion is that the activity of promoters is reversible. This is a key concept in cancer prevention. Promoting factors include dietary fat, obesity, cigarette smoking, and alcohol consumption. The withdrawal or reduction of these factors can reduce the risk of cancer development.

Several promoting factors exert activity against specific types of body tissues or organs, and these agents tend to promote the development of specific kinds of cancer. For example, cigarette smoke is a promoting agent in bronchogenic carcinoma and, in conjunction with alcohol intake, promotes the development of esophageal and bladder cancers. Some carcinogens (*complete carcinogens*) are capable of both initiating and promoting the development of cancer. Tobacco is an example of a complete carcinogen, capable of initiating and promoting the development of cancer.

A period of time, ranging from 1 to 40 years, elapses between the initial genetic alteration and the actual clinical evidence of cancer. This period, called the *latency period,* is now theorized to comprise both the initiation and the promotion stages in the natural history of cancer (DeVita, Lawrence, & Rosenberg, 2014). The variation in the length of time that elapses before the cancer becomes clinically evident is associated with the mitotic rate of the tissue of origin and environmental factors. For most cancers, the process of developing takes years or even decades.

For the disease process to become clinically evident, the cells must reach a "critical mass." A 1-cm tumour (the size usually detectable on palpation) contains 1 billion cancer cells. A 0.5-cm tumour is the smallest that can be detected by current diagnostic measures, such as magnetic resonance imaging (MRI).

Progression. *Progression* is the final stage in the natural history of a cancer. This stage is characterized by increased growth rate of the tumour, as well as by increased invasiveness and spread of the cancer to a distant site (**metastasis**). Certain biochemical and morphological alterations take place during this stage, enabling the tumour to survive and thrive in its primary environment and throughout the process of metastasis.

Some cancers metastasize early in the process of development (e.g., premenopausal breast cancer), whereas others spread regionally and rarely metastasize (e.g., glioblastoma multiforme, basal cell carcinoma of the skin). Certain cancers seem to have an affinity for a particular tissue or organ as a site of metastasis (e.g., colon cancer spreads to the liver); other cancers are unpredictable in their pattern of metastasis (e.g., melanoma). Frequent sites of metastasis are the lungs, the brain, the bone, the liver, and the adrenal glands (Figure 18-4). Metastasis is a multistep process beginning with the rapid growth of the primary tumour (Figure 18-5). As the tumour increases in size, development of its own blood supply is crucial for its survival and growth. The process of the formation of blood vessels within the tumour itself is termed **tumour angiogenesis** and is facilitated by tumour angiogenesis factors produced by the cancer cells. As the tumour grows, it can begin to mechanically invade surrounding tissues, growing into areas of the least resistance.

Certain subpopulations of tumour cells are able to detach from the primary tumour, invade the tissue surrounding the tumour, and penetrate the walls of lymphatic or vascular vessels for metastasis to a distant site. Unique capabilities of some tumour cells facilitate this process. First, rapid proliferation of malignant

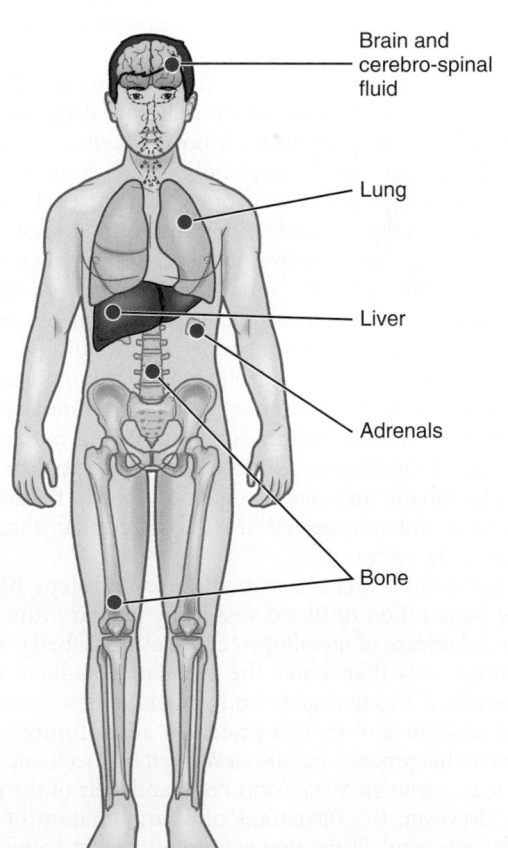

FIGURE 18-4 Main sites of bloodborne metastasis. Source: Stevens, A., & Lowe, J. (2000). *Pathology: Illustrated review in color* (2nd ed.). London: Mosby.

FIGURE 18-5 The pathogenesis of cancer metastasis. To produce metastases, tumour cells must detach from the primary tumour and enter the circulation, survive in circulation, adhere to capillary basement membrane, obtain entrance into the organ parenchyma, respond to growth factors, proliferate and induce angiogenesis, and evade host defences. Source: Reprinted by permission from Macmillan Publishers Ltd: NATURE REVIEWS CANCER, Fidler, I. T. (2003). The pathogenesis of cancer metastasis: the 'seed and soil' hypothesis revisited, 3, 453-458, copyright © 2003.

cells causes mechanical pressure that lead to penetration of surrounding tissues. Second, certain cells have decreased cell-to-cell adhesion in comparison with normal cells. This property allows these cancer cells to physically detach from their site of origin and invade vascular and organ structures. In addition, motility factors are produced by both tumour and normal cells, and changes in the tumour's cytoskeleton further facilitate movement of tumour cells. Some cancer cells produce matrix metalloproteases, a family of lytic enzymes that can erode the basement membrane (a tough barrier surrounding tissues and blood vessels) of the tumour itself, as well as lymph and blood vessels, muscles, nerves, and most epithelial boundaries, which allows for the spread of the tumour. Once free from the primary tumour, metastatic tumour cells frequently travel to distant organ sites via lymphatic and haematogenous routes. Because these two routes are interconnected, it is theorized that tumour cells metastasize via both routes.

Haematogenous metastasis involves several steps, beginning with the penetration of blood vessels by primary tumour cells through the release of metalloproteases, as described previously. The tumour cells then enter the circulation, adhere to small blood vessels of distant organs, and penetrate these vessels, again with the assistance of metalloproteases. Most tumour cells do not survive this process and are destroyed by mechanical mechanisms (e.g., turbulence of blood flow) and cells of the immune system. However, the formation of a combination of tumour cells, platelets, and fibrin deposits may protect some tumour cells from destruction in blood vessels.

In the lymphatic system, tumour cells may be "trapped" in the first lymph node confronted, or they may bypass regional lymph nodes and travel to more distant lymph nodes. This phenomenon, termed *skip metastasis,* is exhibited in certain malignancies, such as esophageal cancers, and is the basis for questions about the effectiveness of dissection of regional lymph nodes for the prevention of some distant metastases. Tumour cells that do survive the process of metastasis must create and maintain an environment in the distant organ site that is favourable to their growth and development. This is facilitated by the ability of tumour cells to evade cells of the immune system and to produce a vascular supply within the metastatic site similar to that developed in the primary tumour site. Vascularization is critical for the supply of nutrients to the metastatic tumour and for the removal of waste products. Metalloproteases contribute to vascularization through release of angiogenesis promoters such as vascular endothelial growth factor (VEGF).

Cells of the primary tumour and metastatic site may develop from a single cell or may be *clones* (cells derived from a single cell of origin). However, as the primary and metastatic sites develop, the cells quickly become more heterogeneous as they repeatedly undergo spontaneous genetic mutations. The heterogeneous nature of the cells in primary and metastatic tumours makes them difficult to treat, inasmuch as they are more likely to become resistant to chemotherapy and radiation therapy. Surgical removal may be effective for some small, circumscribed tumours.

Role of the Immune System

This section is limited to a discussion of the role of the immune system in the recognition and destruction of tumour cells. (For a detailed discussion of immune system function, see Chapter 16.)

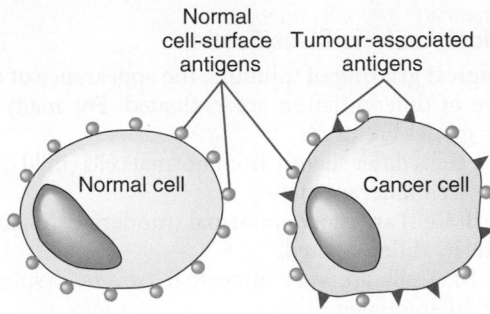

FIGURE 18-6 Tumour-associated antigens appear on the cell surface of malignant cells.

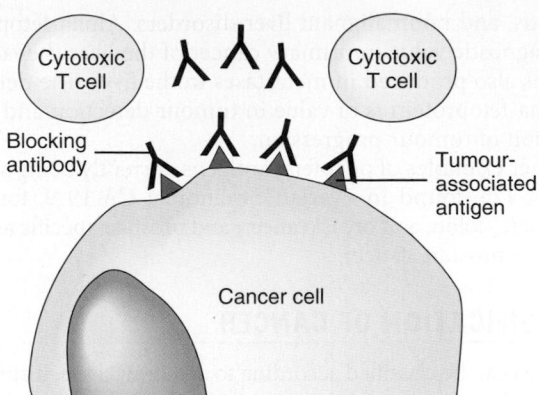

FIGURE 18-7 Blocking antibodies prevent T cells from interacting with tumour-associated antigens and from destroying the malignant cell.

The immune system has the potential to distinguish normal (self) from abnormal (nonself) cells. For example, cells of transplanted organs can be "perceived" by the immune system as nonself entities and thus elicit an immune response. This response can ultimately result in the rejection of the organ. Similarly, cancer cells can be perceived as nonself entities and elicit an immune response that results in their rejection and destruction. However, unlike transplanted cells, cancer cells arise from normal "self" cells, and although mutated and thus different, the immune response that is mounted against cancer cells may be inadequate to reject and destroy the cancer cells.

Some cancer cells have changes on their cell surface antigens as a result of malignant transformation. These altered antigens are termed **tumour-associated antigens** (Figure 18-6). It is believed that one of the functions of the immune system is to respond to tumour-associated antigens. The response of the immune system to antigens of the malignant cells is termed **immunological surveillance**. Lymphocytes continually check cell surface antigens and detect and destroy cells with abnormal or altered antigenic determinants. It has been proposed that malignant transformation occurs continuously and that the malignant cells are destroyed by the immune response. Under most circumstances, immunological surveillance prevents these transformed cells from developing into clinically detectable tumours.

Virtually every cell type involved in normal immune responses and every function used to inactivate or remove antigens have been demonstrated in immune responses to tumours. These immune responses involve cytotoxic T cells, natural killer (NK) cells, macrophages, and B lymphocytes.

Cytotoxic T cells are thought to play a dominant role in resisting tumour growth. These cells are capable of killing tumour cells. T cells are also important in the production of cytokines (e.g., interleukin-2 [IL-2] and interferon-gamma [IFN-gamma], which stimulate T cells), NK cells, B cells, and macrophages.

NK cells are able to directly lyse tumour cells spontaneously without any prior sensitization. These cells are stimulated by IFN-gamma and IL-2 (released from T cells), which results in increased cytotoxic activity.

Monocytes and macrophages have several important roles in tumour immunity. Macrophages can be activated by IFN-gamma (produced by T cells) to kill tumour cells, but they may also injure normal cells. Macrophages also secrete cytokines, including interleukin-1 (IL-1), tumour necrosis factor (TNF), and colony-stimulating factors. The release of IL-1, coupled with the presentation of the processed antigen, stimulates activation and production of T lymphocytes. Interferon-alfa augments the killing ability of NK cells. TNF causes hemorrhagic necrosis of tumours

and exerts cytocidal or cytostatic actions against tumour cells. Colony-stimulating factors regulate the production of various blood cells in the bone marrow and stimulate the function of various WBCs.

B lymphocytes produce specific antibodies that bind to and destroy tumour cells by complement fixation and lysis. These antibodies are often detectable in the serum and the saliva of an affected patient.

Mechanisms of Escape From Immunological Surveillance. The process by which cancer cells evade the immune system is termed *immunological escape.* Theorized mechanisms by which cancer cells can escape immunological surveillance include (a) suppression of factors that stimulate T cells to react to cancer cells, (b) weak surface antigens that allow cancer cells to "sneak through" immunological surveillance, (c) the development of tolerance of the immune system to some tumour antigens, (d) suppression of the immune response by products secreted by cancer cells, (e) the induction of suppressor T cells by the tumour, and (f) blocking antibodies that bind tumour-associated antigens, thus preventing their recognition by T cells (Figure 18-7).

Oncofetal Antigens. *Oncofetal antigens* are a type of tumour antigen. They are found on both the surface and the inside of cancer cells, as well as on and inside fetal cells. These antigens are an expression of the shift of cancerous cells to a more immature metabolic pathway, an expression usually associated with embryonic or fetal periods of life. The reappearance of fetal antigens in malignant disease is not well understood, but it is believed to occur as a result of the cell's regaining its embryonic capability to differentiate into many different cell types.

Examples of oncofetal antigens are CEA and alpha-fetoprotein. CEA is found on the surface of cancer cells derived from the GI tract and from normal cells from the fetal gut, liver, and pancreas. Normally, it disappears during the last 3 months of gestation. CEA was originally isolated from colon cancer cells. However, elevated CEA levels have also been found in nonmalignant conditions (e.g., cirrhosis of the liver, ulcerative colitis, and heavy smoking). At present, the major value of CEA is its use as an indicator of the success of cancer treatment. For example, the persistence of elevated preoperative CEA titres after surgery indicates that the tumour was not completely removed. A rise in CEA levels after chemotherapy or radiation therapy may indicate recurrence or spread of the cancer.

Alpha-fetoprotein is produced by malignant liver cells, as well as fetal liver cells. Alpha-fetoprotein levels have also been found to be elevated in some cases of testicular carcinoma, viral hepatitis, and nonmalignant liver disorders. Alpha-fetoprotein has diagnostic value in primary cancer of the liver (hepatoma), but it is also produced in metastases to the liver. The detection of alpha-fetoprotein is of value in tumour detection and determination of tumour progression.

Other examples of oncofetal antigens currently being studied are CA-125, found in ovarian carcinoma; CA-19-9, found in pancreatic, colon, and breast cancer; and prostate-specific antigen, found in prostate cancer.

CLASSIFICATION OF CANCER

Tumours can be classified according to anatomical site, histological analysis (grading), and extent of disease (staging). Tumour classification systems are intended to provide a standardized way to (a) communicate the cancer status of a patient to the members of the health care team, (b) assist in determining the most effective treatment plan, (c) evaluate the treatment plan, (d) help determine the prognosis, and (e) compare patients with similar conditions for statistical purposes.

Anatomical Site Classification

In the *anatomical classification* of tumours, the tumour is identified by the tissue of origin, the anatomical site, and the behaviour of the tumour (i.e., benign or malignant; Table 18-5). A **carcinoma** originates from embryonal *ectoderm* (skin and glands) and *endoderm* (mucous membrane linings of the respiratory, GI, and genito-urinary tracts). A **sarcoma** originates in the connective tissue of the body (fat, muscles, blood vessels, nerves, bones, or cartilage). Lymphomas and leukemias originate from the hematopoietic system.

Histological Analysis Classification

In **histological grading** of tumours, the appearance of cells and the degree of differentiation are evaluated. For many tumour cells, four grades are used:
- *Grade I*: Cells differ slightly from normal cells (mild dysplasia) and are well differentiated.
- *Grade II*: Cells are more abnormal (moderate dysplasia) and moderately differentiated.
- *Grade III*: Cells are very abnormal (severe dysplasia) and poorly differentiated.
- *Grade IV*: Cells are immature and primitive (anaplasia) and undifferentiated; cell of origin is difficult to determine.

Classifying Extent of Disease

Classifying the extent and spread of disease is termed **staging**. This classification system is based on a description of the extent of the disease rather than on cell appearance. The extent to which the disease has spread has important ramifications for prognosis. Although there are similarities in the staging of cancers, there are many differences between them, and thus they are based on a thorough knowledge of the natural history of each specific type of cancer.

Clinical Staging. The clinical staging classification system determines the extent of the disease process of cancer within the body by stages:
- *Stage 0*: cancer in situ
- *Stage I*: tumour limited to the tissue of origin; localized tumour growth
- *Stage II*: limited local spread
- *Stage III*: extensive local and regional spread
- *Stage IV*: metastasis

This classification system has been used as a basis for staging in cancer of the cervix (see Chapter 56, Table 56-11) and Hodgkin's disease (see Chapter 33, Figure 33-14).

TNM Classification System. The *TNM classification system* represents the standardization of the clinical staging of cancer by the Geneva-based International Union Against Cancer. This classification system (Table 18-6) is used to determine the extent of the disease process of cancer according to three parameters: tumour size (T), degree of regional spread to the lymph nodes (N), and metastasis (M).

TABLE 18-5 ANATOMICAL CLASSIFICATION OF TUMOURS

Site	Benign	Malignant
Epithelial Tissue Tumours*	Suffix: *-oma*	Suffix: *-carcinoma*
Surface epithelium	Papilloma	Carcinoma
Glandular epithelium	Adenoma	Adenocarcinoma
Connective Tissue Tumours†	Suffix: *-oma*	Suffix: *-sarcoma*
Fibrous tissue	Fibroma	Fibrosarcoma
Cartilage	Chondroma	Chondrosarcoma
Striated muscle	Rhabdomyoma	Rhabdomyosarcoma
Bone	Osteoma	Osteosarcoma
Nervous Tissue Tumours	Suffix: *-oma*	Suffix: *-oma*
Pineal region	Pineocytoma	Pineoblastoma
Nerve cells	Ganglioneuroma	Neuroblastoma
Hematopoietic Tissue Tumours		
Lymphoid tissue	—	Hodgkin's disease, non-Hodgkin's lymphoma
Plasma cells	—	Multiple myeloma
Bone marrow	—	Lymphocytic and myelogenous leukemia

*Body surfaces, lining of body cavities, and glandular structures.
†Supporting tissue, fibrotic tissue, and blood vessels.

TABLE 18-6 TNM CLASSIFICATION SYSTEM

Primary Tumour Size (T)	
T_0	No evidence of primary tumour
T_{is}	Carcinoma in situ
T_1–T_4	Ascending degrees of increase in tumour size and involvement
T_X	Primary tumour cannot be assessed
Involvement of Regional Lymph Nodes (N)	
N_0	No evidence of disease in lymph nodes
N_1–N_3	Ascending degrees of nodal involvement
N_X	Regional lymph nodes cannot be assessed
Distant Metastases (M)	
M_0	No distant metastases
M_1	Distant metastases
M_X	Distant metastases cannot be assessed

Staging of the disease may be performed initially and at repeated intervals. Clinical diagnostic staging is performed at the time of diagnosis to determine the most effective treatment plan. Examples of diagnostic studies that may be performed to assess for spread of disease include bone and liver scanning, ultrasonography, computed tomography, positron emission tomography, and MRI.

Surgical staging is used to describe the extent of the disease process after biopsy or surgical exploration. For example, a laparotomy and a splenectomy may be performed in the staging of Hodgkin's disease. During staging laparotomy, lymph node biopsy samples are obtained, and margins of any masses are marked with metal clips. These clips are used as markers when radiotherapy is used as a treatment modality.

After the extent of the disease is determined, the stage classification is not changed. The original description of the extent of the tumour remains part of the original record. If additional treatment is needed, or if treatment fails, restaging is performed to determine the extent of the disease process at the time of re-treatment.

Carcinoma in situ is a commonly used term in classification of cancer. It is defined as a lesion with all the histological features of cancer except invasion. If left untreated, carcinoma in situ eventually becomes invasive.

In addition to tumour classification systems, there are also classification systems that can be used to describe the functional status of patients with cancer. The Karnofsky Performance Status scale is an example of a functional assessment scale (see the Resources at the end of this chapter).

PREVENTION AND DETECTION OF CANCER

The nurse has a prominent role in the prevention and detection of cancer. Early detection and prompt treatment are directly responsible for increased survival rates among patients with cancer. Public education should include the following recommendations:

1. Reduce or eliminate exposure to carcinogens and cancer promoters, such as cigarette smoke and sun exposure.
2. Eat a balanced diet that includes fresh fruits, vegetables, omega-3 fatty acids, and fibre. Following *Eating Well With Canada's Food Guide* helps to ensure a healthy diet (Health Canada, 2011; see Chapter 42, Figure 42-1).
3. Participate regularly (a minimum of 30 minutes, 5 times per week) in mild to moderate physical activity such as biking, walking, or running.
4. Maintain a healthy weight for your body type.
5. Limit alcohol use to one or two drinks per day.
6. Get to know your body. Learn and practise self-examination (e.g., breast self-examination, testicular self-examination). Report any changes to your doctor or dentist.
7. Follow cancer screening guidelines (see the Resources at the end of this chapter). Early detection of cancer has a positive effect on prognosis.
8. Know the seven warning signs of cancer (Table 18-7).

When the public is educated about cancer, care should be taken to minimize the fear that surrounds the diagnosis. Teaching strategies that address the specific needs of the target audience (e.g., the needs of older adults in comparison with those of high school students or new immigrants to Canada) are most effective. Although the general public requires information that supports healthy behaviours, those at an increased risk of cancer are the target population for effective cancer control. These individuals must be motivated to learn to change negative health behaviours in order to achieve and maintain an optimal state of health. Nurses can have a definite effect in convincing people that change in lifestyle patterns will have a positive influence on health. To be successful, nurses must identify potential challenges and barriers and develop appropriate strategies to facilitate uptake of information about effective cancer control.

TABLE 18-7	SEVEN WARNING SIGNS OF CANCER
C	**C**hange in bowel or bladder habits
A	**A** sore that does not heal
U	**U**nusual bleeding or discharge from any body orifice
T	**T**hickening or a lump in the breast or elsewhere
I	**I**ndigestion or difficulty in swallowing
O	**O**bvious change in a wart or mole
N	**N**agging cough or hoarseness

DIAGNOSIS OF CANCER

The threat of a cancer diagnosis creates tremendous anxiety for an individual and his or her family. Patients typically undergo several days to weeks of diagnostic studies. During this time, fear of the unknown may be more stressful than the actual diagnosis of cancer.

While the patient is waiting for the results of the diagnostic studies, the nurse should be available to actively listen to the patient's concerns. Communication plays a pivotal role in optimal patient care. Essential elements of the establishment of a therapeutic relationship with the patient are the ability to listen, ask questions sensitively, and avoid false reassurances. During this time of high anxiety, the patient needs repetition and reinforcement of information, the opportunity to ask questions, and clarification of the diagnostic workup. Explanations should be clear and tailored to meet the specific needs of patients and families. Content that is particularly threatening or detailed may overwhelm patients, and the nurse should thus be sensitive to the individual's ability to absorb the information. Written information at the level of the patient's literacy is helpful for reinforcement of verbal information.

A diagnostic plan for the person in whom cancer is suspected includes health history, potential or actual risk factors, physical examination, and specific diagnostic studies. (The specifics of the health history and the screening physical examination are presented in Chapter 3.)

The health history includes particular emphasis on risk factors, such as family history of cancer, exposure to or ingestion of known carcinogens (e.g., cigarette smoking, exposure to occupational pollutants or chemicals), diseases characterized by chronic inflammation (e.g., ulcerative colitis), and drug ingestion (e.g., hormone therapy). Other important information is related to dietary habits, ingestion of alcohol, lifestyle, and patterns and degree of coping with perceived stressors.

The physical examination should be thorough, with particular attention to the respiratory system, the GI system (including the colon, rectum, and liver), the lymphatic system (including the spleen), the breasts, the skin, the reproductive system (testes and prostate gland in men; cervix, uterus, and ovaries in women), and the musculo-skeletal and neurological systems.

The choice of diagnostic studies depends on the suspected primary or metastatic site or sites of the cancer. (Specific procedures related to each body system are discussed in the respective assessment chapters.) Studies that may be conducted in the process of diagnosing cancer include the following:

1. Cytology studies (e.g., Papanicolaou [Pap] test)
2. Hematology and chemistry studies (e.g., complete blood cell count [CBC], liver and renal function tests)
3. Sigmoidoscopic or colonoscopic examination (including fecal occult blood test)
4. Radiological studies (e.g., chest radiography, mammography, computed tomography, MRI)
5. Radioisotope scanning (e.g., bone, lung, liver, brain)
6. Assays for the presence of oncofetal antigens (such as CEA and alpha-fetoprotein) or of genetic markers (such as *BRCA1* and *BRCA2*)
7. Bone marrow examination (if a haematolymphoid malignancy is suspected)
8. Biopsy

Biopsy. The *biopsy* procedure is the definitive means of diagnosing cancer, and the results guide treatment decisions. In a biopsy, a piece of tissue is surgically removed from the suspect area for histological examination by a pathologist. This examination helps determine whether the tissue is benign or malignant, the anatomical tissue from which the tumour arises, and the degree of cellular differentiation (i.e., how closely the specimen cells resemble the normal cells of the tissue).

The procedure may be a needle biopsy, an incisional biopsy, or an excisional biopsy. In a *needle biopsy*, cells and tissue fragments are obtained through a large-bore needle guided into the tissue of investigation (e.g., bone marrow, prostate gland, breast, liver, or kidney tissues).

Incisional biopsy performed with a scalpel or dermal punch is a common technique for obtaining a tissue sample from, for example, a skin lesion. The premise that incisional biopsy may contribute to the spread of cancer has not been proven.

Excisional biopsy involves removal of the entire tumour. It is usually used for small tumours (<2 cm in diameter), skin lesions, intestinal polyps, and breast masses. This procedure can be therapeutic in addition to diagnostic. When a tumour is not easily accessible, a major surgical procedure (laparotomy, thoracotomy, craniotomy) is necessary to obtain the tumour tissue. Biopsy specimens from the GI tract, respiratory tract, and genitourinary system can usually be obtained by endoscopic procedures, such as flexible sigmoidoscopy.

COLLABORATIVE CARE

Goals and Modalities

The goal of cancer treatment is cure, control, or palliation (Figure 18-8). Factors determining the therapeutic approach include the cell type of the cancer, the location and size of the tumour, and the extent of the disease. The patient's physiological and psychological status and personal desires are also important elements in determining the treatment plan. All factors influence the goals of care, the modalities chosen for treatment, and the length of time the treatment is administered. Evidence-informed treatment guidelines have been developed in a number of provinces and territories to guide treatment decisions. Examples include provincial guidelines in British Columbia and Ontario (see the Resources at the end of this chapter).

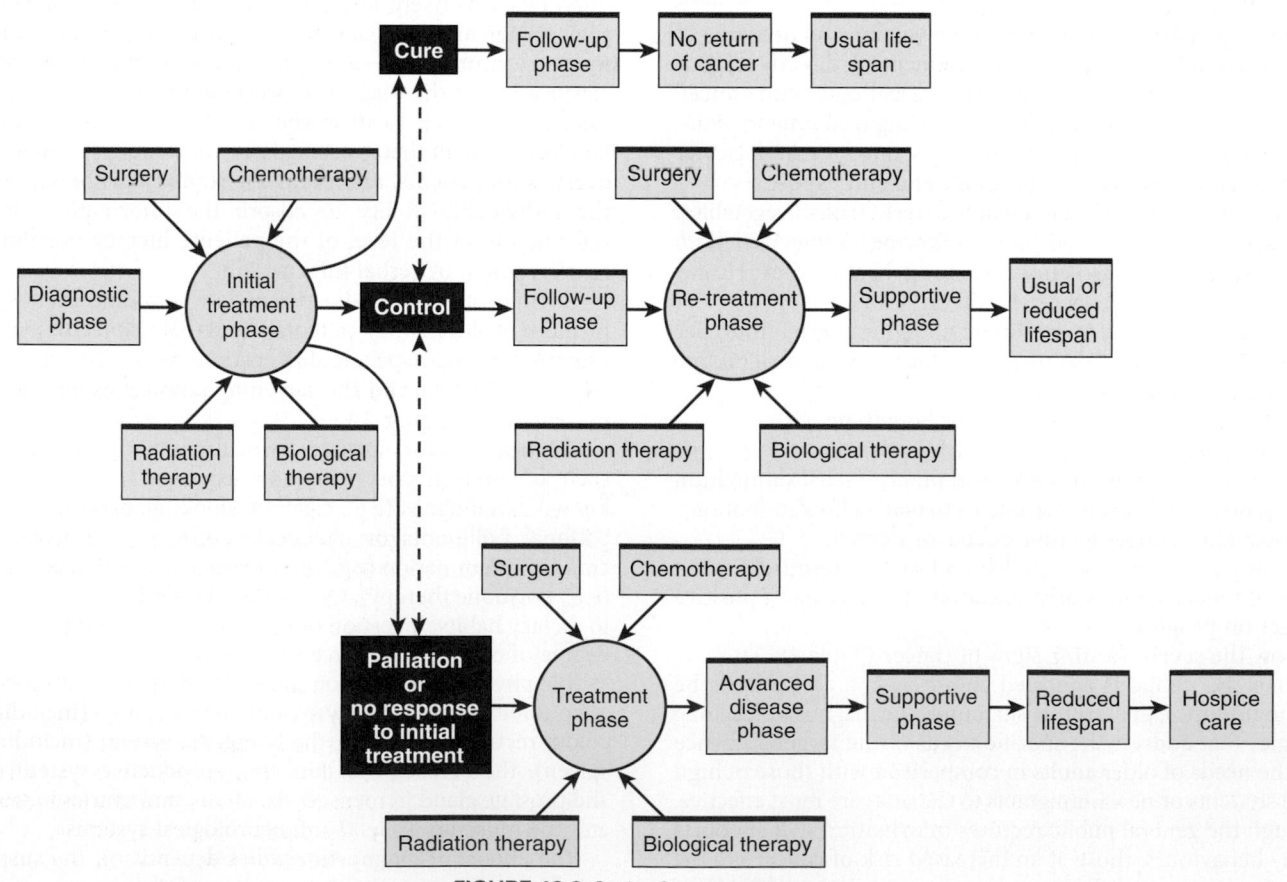

FIGURE 18-8 Goals of cancer treatment.

When caring for patients with cancer, the nurse should know the goals of the treatment plan to communicate with and support patients. When cure is the goal, treatment that has the greatest likelihood of eradicating the disease is offered. With many kinds of cancer, therapy has the potential for inducing permanent remission; therapy may be an initial course of treatment or treatment that extends for several weeks, months, or years. Basal cell carcinoma of the skin is usually cured by surgical removal of the lesion or by several weeks of radiation therapy. Acute lymphocytic leukemia in children has the potential for cure. The treatment plan for this type of cancer includes the administration of several chemotherapeutic drugs on a scheduled basis over a span of 6 months to several years. Head and neck cancers may be cured with combination therapy that includes surgery and radiation, with or without chemotherapy. The risk of disease recurrence differs according to the tumour type. In general, the risk for recurrent disease is greatest after completion of treatment and gradually decreases with the passage of time. Tumours with a rapid mitotic rate (e.g., testicular cancer) are considered to be in remission if cancer is not detected in a 2-year time span after treatment. For tumours that have a slower mitotic rate (e.g., postmenopausal breast cancer), the patient must be free of disease 20 years or longer before he or she can be considered cured of cancer.

Control is the goal of the treatment plan for many cancers that cannot be completely eradicated but are responsive to cancer therapies. Such cancers usually are not cured but are controlled by therapy for variably extended periods in a manner similar to other chronic illnesses, such as diabetes mellitus, chronic lung disease, and heart failure. An example of this type of cancer is chronic lymphocytic leukemia (see Chapter 33). The affected patient undergoes the initial course of therapy and continues maintenance therapy for a time or is monitored closely so that early signs and symptoms of disease recurrence or progression can be detected.

Palliation may also be a goal of the treatment plan. With palliation, relief or control of symptoms and the optimization of quality of life are the primary objectives, rather than cure or control of the disease process. Radiation therapy to relieve the pain of bone metastasis is an example of a palliative cancer treatment. Palliative care may be undertaken for days, weeks, months, or years.

The goals of cure, control, and palliation are achieved through the use of four treatment modalities: surgery, radiation therapy, chemotherapy, and biological therapy. These modalities can be used alone or in any combination in the initial treatment phase, as well as in the repeated treatment phases of cancer. For many cancers, two or more of the treatment modalities (referred to as *concurrent, combined-modality,* or *multimodality therapy*) are used to achieve the goal of cure or control for a long period.

INFORMATICS IN PRACTICE

Managing Symptoms of Cancer

- When patients arrive at some clinics, they are handed a tablet computer. While in the waiting room or chemotherapy infusion unit, they use the touch of a finger to select the symptoms they have been experiencing.
- Health care providers can review the information and provide care aimed at managing patients' specific symptoms.
- After the visit, the notes are stored in the patient's electronic health record. This system can assist with quality of care by determining whether standards of care were followed.

Clinical Trials

A *clinical trial* is a research study conducted on humans and designed with the intent of evaluating new treatments or supportive care interventions. The evaluation of treatments in cancer research begins in the laboratory with animal studies. From these studies, the treatments determined to be most effective, with mild or medically manageable levels of toxicity, are further evaluated in a series of studies on patients with cancer. Progress in cancer care depends on research. New drugs or treatments, evaluated for the first time in human beings, are studied in three phases:

- In *phase I trials,* researchers test a new drug or treatment in a small group of people (20 to 80) for the first time to evaluate its safety, determine a safe dosage range, and identify adverse effects.
- In *phase II trials,* the study drug or treatment is given to a larger group of people (100 to 300) to determine whether it is effective for a specific medical problem and to further evaluate its safety and adverse effects.
- In *phase III trials,* the study drug or treatment is given to large groups of people (1000 to 3000) to confirm its effectiveness, monitor adverse effects, compare it with commonly used treatments, and collect information that will allow the drug or treatment to be used safely.

Institutional review boards in each agency that conducts research closely guard the rights of the patients participating in clinical trials. These boards not only review clinical trials at their inception but also continue to review and monitor each study until its completion. Informed consent is a process in which the clinical trial physician and nurse give the patient full information regarding the nature of the treatment being evaluated and the potential risks and benefits of entering the clinical trial. The patient must understand that he or she may decide to leave a clinical trial at any time or refuse to participate in the trial without threat of compromised care or treatment.

The guidelines for the administration of a research protocol are included in the study's protocol and are monitored closely by the study investigators and clinical trial nurses to ensure safe and uniform treatment of patients.

SURGICAL THERAPY

Surgery is the oldest form of cancer treatment and was for many years the only method of cancer diagnosis and treatment. Removal of the tumour and a margin of the surrounding normal tissue may cure localized cancers, but it is ineffective if the cancer has metastasized to other locations.

Cure and Control

Several principles are applicable when surgery is used to cure or control the disease process of cancer (Figure 18-9):

1. Cancer that arises from a tissue with a slow rate of cellular proliferation or replication is the most amenable to surgical treatment.
2. A margin of normal tissue surrounding the tumour should be resected along with the tumour.
3. Only as much tissue as necessary is removed.
4. When appropriate, adjuvant therapy is used to eliminate residual micrometastases. The risk for metastatic disease is tumour dependent. The decision regarding adjuvant therapy is customized to the patient's tumour type, stage, comorbid conditions, and preferences.

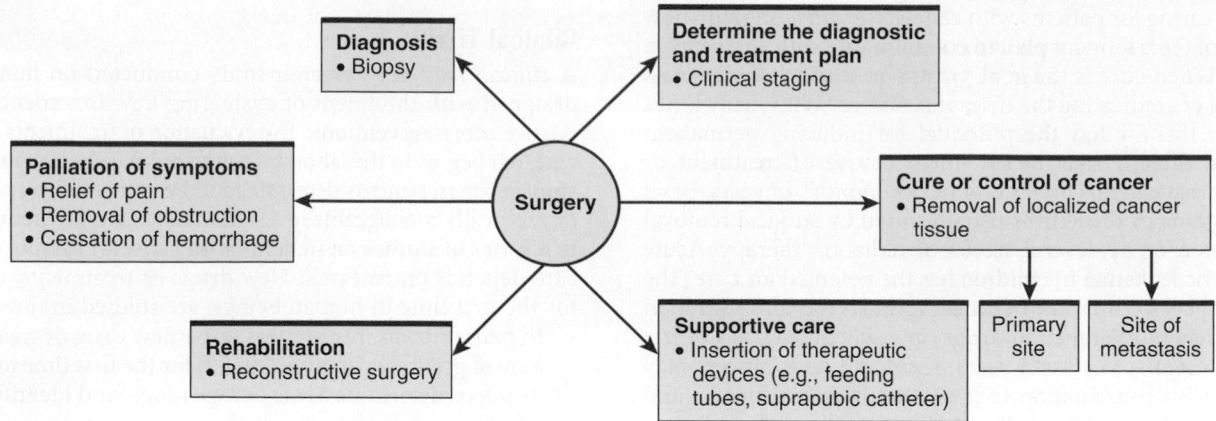

FIGURE 18-9 Role of surgery in the treatment of cancer.

5. Preventive measures are used to reduce the surgical seeding of cancer cells.

6. The usual sites of regional spread may be surgically removed for diagnostic or therapeutic purposes.

Examples of surgical procedures used for cure or control of cancer include radical neck dissection, lumpectomy, mastectomy, pneumonectomy, orchiectomy, thyroidectomy, and bowel resection.

A *debulking* or *cytoreductive* procedure may be used if the tumour cannot be completely removed (e.g., is attached to a vital organ). When this occurs, as much tumour as possible is removed, and the patient may be given chemotherapy or radiation therapy. This type of surgical procedure may increase the effectiveness of chemotherapy or radiation therapy because the target disease is reduced in volume.

Supportive and Palliative Surgical Procedures

Surgical procedures can also be used to provide supportive care and palliate symptoms throughout the disease process of cancer. Examples of supportive surgical procedures include the following:

1. Insertion of feeding tubes in the stomach for patients with head and neck cancers or cancer of the esophagus.
2. Creation of a colostomy to allow healing of rectal abscess.
3. Suprapubic cystostomy in cases of advanced prostatic cancer.

When cure or control of cancer is no longer possible, relief from distressing symptoms may be achieved through surgical procedures, including the following:

1. Debulking of tumour to relieve pain or pressure.
2. Colostomy for the relief of a bowel obstruction (see Chapter 45).
3. Laminectomy for the relief of spinal cord compression.

Rehabilitative Management

Cancer surgery may cause a change in a person's body image or function. It may be challenging for patients to cope with these changes on top of the distress of a diagnosis of cancer. As the treatment for certain cancers becomes more effective, the length of time that a patient must live with an alteration created by treatment will be increased. If quality of life is to be maintained, the body image must be one that a patient is able to adapt to and cope with on a daily basis. The rehabilitative role of surgery in cancer care has grown in prominence to improve patients' quality of life. Breast reconstruction after a mastectomy is an example of a rehabilitative surgical procedure. The use of prostheses, such as

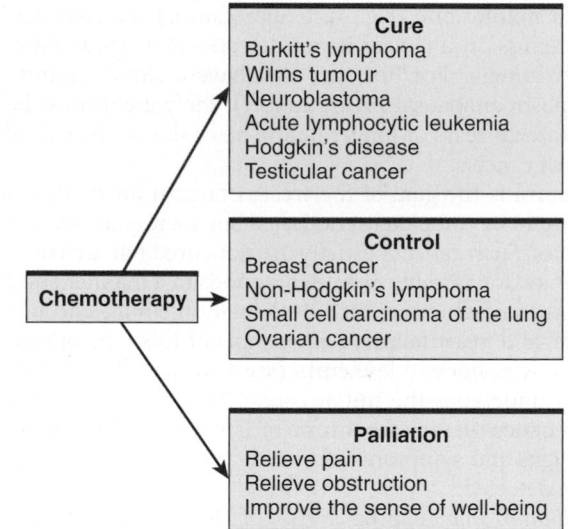

FIGURE 18-10 Goals of chemotherapy.

artificial eyes or limbs, and the care of ostomies are other major contributions to rehabilitative management.

CHEMOTHERAPY

The use of chemicals as a systemic therapy for cancer has been evolving. In the 1940s, chemotherapy was in its infancy. Nitrogen mustard, a chemical warfare agent used in World Wars I and II, was used in the treatment of lymphoma and acute leukemia, and a folic acid antimetabolite (5-fluorouracil) was found to have antitumour activity. In the 1970s, chemotherapy was established as an effective treatment modality for cancer. Chemotherapy is now used in the treatment of many solid tumours and is the primary therapy for hematological malignancies, including leukemia and lymphoma. Chemotherapy has evolved significantly to become a therapeutic option that can cure some cancers, control others, or palliate symptoms when cure or control is no longer achievable (Figure 18-10). Although practice standards in different provinces and territories vary, nurses administering chemotherapy must be specifically trained in the protocols, administration, and possible adverse effects (Canadian Association of Nurses in Oncology, 2011).

Effect on Cells

The effect of chemotherapy is at the cellular level. All cells, whether malignant or normal, enter the cell cycle for replication and proliferation (see Figure 18-1). The effects of the chemotherapeutic agents may be described in relationship to the cell cycle. The two major categories of chemotherapeutic drugs are cell cycle phase–nonspecific and cell cycle phase–specific drugs.

Cell cycle phase–nonspecific chemotherapeutic drugs have their effect on the cells that are in the process of cellular replication and proliferation, as well as those in the resting phase (G_0).

Cell cycle phase–specific chemotherapeutic drugs have their effect on cells that are in the process of cellular replication or proliferation (G_1, S_1, G_2, or M). These drugs exert their most significant effect during specific phases of the cell cycle. Cell cycle phase–specific and cell cycle phase–nonspecific agents are often administered in combination with one another. The aim of this approach is to promote a better response through the use of agents that function by differing mechanisms and at different points in the cell cycle.

The goal of chemotherapy is to reduce the number of cancer cells present in the primary and metastatic tumour site or sites. Several factors determine the response of cancer cells to chemotherapy:

1. *Mitotic rate of the tissue from which the tumour arises.* The more rapid the mitotic rate, the greater the response to chemotherapy. Chemotherapy is the treatment of choice for acute leukemia, Wilms tumour (in conjunction with surgery), and neuroblastoma. These cancer cells have a rapid rate of cellular proliferation.
2. *Size of the tumour.* The lower the tumour burden (i.e., the fewer cancer cells), the greater the response to chemotherapy.
3. *Age of the tumour.* The "younger" the tumour, the greater the response to chemotherapy. Developing tumours have a higher percentage of proliferating cells.
4. *Location of the tumour.* Certain anatomical sites provide a protected environment, or "sanctuary," from the effects of chemotherapy. For example, only a few drugs (such as nitrosoureas and temozolomide) cross the blood–brain barrier.
5. *Presence of resistant tumour cells.* Mutation of cancer cells within the tumour mass can result in variant cells that are resistant to chemotherapy. Resistance can also occur because of the biochemical inability of some cancer cells to convert the drug to its active form. This resistance is passed on to new daughter cells.

As a tumour first begins to grow, most of its cells are actively dividing. As the tumour increases in size, more cells become inactive and convert to a resting state (G_0). Because many chemotherapeutic agents are most effective against dividing cells, cells can escape death by staying in the G_0 phase. The major challenge of chemotherapy for cancer is overcoming the drug resistance of resting and noncycling cells.

Classification of Chemotherapeutic Drugs

Chemotherapeutic drugs are categorized or classified according to their structure and mechanisms of action (Table 18-8). Each drug in a particular classification has many similarities, but major differences among the drugs are also evident.

Preparation and Administration of Chemotherapeutic Agents

It is very important to know the specific guidelines for administration of chemotherapeutic drugs. These drugs may also pose occupational hazards for health care providers. A health care provider preparing or administering chemotherapeutic agents may absorb the drug through inhalation of particles and through skin contact when reconstituting a powder in an open ampule. There may also be some risk in handling the body fluids and excreta of patients receiving chemotherapy. Guidelines for the safe handling of chemotherapeutic agents have been developed by the National Institute for Occupational Safety and Health (NIOSH) and the Oncology Nursing Society (see the Resources at the end of this chapter).

Methods of Administration

Several routes are used to administer chemotherapeutic agents (Table 18-9). The oral and intravenous routes are the most commonly used. The major concerns associated with the intravenous administration of antineoplastic drugs are the potential for irritation or damage to the vessels; problems with the venous access device or catheter, including infection; and extravasation (infiltration of drugs into tissues surrounding the infusion site), which causes local tissue damage. Many chemotherapeutic drugs are irritants or vesicants, agents that cause severe local tissue breakdown and necrosis when accidentally infiltrated into the skin (Figure 18-11).

Pain is the cardinal symptom of extravasation, although extravasation has been known to occur without causing pain. Swelling, redness, and the presence of vesicles on the skin are other signs of extravasation. After a few days, the tissue may begin to ulcerate and necrose, and closure with skin grafts is often required.

To minimize these risks and to avoid physical discomfort, chemotherapeutic drugs may be administered by means of a central venous access device. Cancer care increasingly involves combination therapies that entail venous access; therefore, the use of these devices has increased. Central venous access devices are placed in large blood vessels and enable frequent, continuous, or intermittent administration of chemotherapeutic agents, biological therapeutic agents, and other products. They are indicated in instances of limited venous access, intensive chemotherapy, continuous infusion of vesicant agents, and projected long-term need for venous access. (Central venous access devices are discussed further in Chapter 19.)

The advantages of venous access devices are that they provide for rapid dilution of chemotherapeutic agents, decreased incidence of extravasation, and reduced need for venipuncture. In addition to their usefulness in administration of chemotherapeutic agents,

FIGURE 18-11 Extravasation injury from infiltration of chemotherapeutic drug. Source: Weinzweig, N. & Weinzweig, J. (2005). *The mutilated hand.* Philadelphia: Mosby.

TABLE 18-8 DRUG THERAPY

Classification of Chemotherapeutic Drugs

Mechanisms of Action	Examples
Alkylating Agents	
Cell Cycle Phase–Nonspecific Agents	
Damage DNA by causing breaks in the double-strand helix (similar to the effect of radiation therapy); if repair does not occur, cells die immediately (cytocidal) or when they attempt to divide (cytostatic)	Mechlorethamine (formerly known as *nitrogen mustard*), cyclophosphamide (Procytox), chlorambucil (Leukeran), melphalan (Alkeran), busulfan (Myleran), dacarbazine (DTIC), lomustine (CCNU, CeeNU), oxaliplatin (Eloxatin), streptozocin (Zanosar), cisplatin, carboplatin
Antimetabolites	
Cell Cycle Phase–Specific Agents (Primarily S Phase)	
Interfere with enzyme function and synthesis of DNA by mimicking naturally occurring metabolites required by the cell for synthesis of DNA and RNA (cytocidal)	Methotrexate, cytarabine (Cytosar), fluorouracil (5-FU), mercaptopurine (6-MP), thioguanine (6-TG), fludarabine (Fludara), hydroxyurea (Hydrea), gemcitabine (Gemzar), cladribine (Leustatin)
Antitumour Antibiotics	
Cell Cycle Phase–Nonspecific Agents	
Modify function of DNA and interfere with transcription of RNA (cytocidal or cytostatic)	Doxorubicin (Adriamycin), bleomycin (Blenoxane), mitomycin, daunorubicin (Daunomycin), dactinomycin (Cosmegen), idarubicin (Idamycin), epirubicin (Ellence), mitoxantrone
Plant Alkaloids (Mitotic Inhibitors)	
Cell Cycle Phase–Specific Agents (G₂ and M Phases)	
Interrupt cellular replication in mitosis at metaphase (cytocidal)	Vinblastine, vincristine, etoposide (VePesid), paclitaxel (Taxol), docetaxel (Taxotere), teniposide (Vumon)
Nitrosoureas	
Cell Cycle Phase–Nonspecific Agents	
Similar to alkylating agents; break DNA helix and interfere with DNA replication (cytocidal or cytostatic)	Carmustine (BCNU), lomustine (CCNU, CeeNU)
Corticosteroids	
Cell Cycle Phase–Nonspecific Agents	
Disrupt the cell membrane and inhibit synthesis of protein; decrease circulating lymphocytes; inhibit mitosis; depress immune system; increase feeling of well-being	Cortisone, hydrocortisone (Cortef), methylprednisolone (Medrol), prednisone, dexamethasone
Hormone Therapy	
Cell Cycle Phase–Nonspecific Agents	
Interfere with hormone receptors and proteins, inhibiting tumour growth	Androgens (testosterone), estrogens, progestins
Aromatase Inhibitors	
Inhibit the enzyme aromatase, a cytochrome P450 enzyme involved in estrogen synthesis	Anastrozole (Arimidex), letrozole (Femara), exemestane (Aromasin)
Selective Estrogen Receptor Modulator (SERM)	
Selectively modulates estrogen receptors, thus acting as an estrogen antagonist	Raloxifene (Evista)
Miscellaneous	
Destroys exogenous supply of L-asparagine, which is needed for cellular proliferation; L-asparagine can be synthesized by normal cells but not by cancer cells	L-Asparaginase (Elspar)
Antiestrogens used in breast cancer	Tamoxifen (Nolvadex), fulvestrant (Faslodex)
Suppress mitosis at interphase; appear to alter preformed DNA, RNA, and protein	Procarbazine (Matulane)

DNA, deoxyribonucleic acid; *RNA,* ribonucleic acid.
Note: Each cancer agency in Canada has a formulary of protocols and practice guidelines; strict adherence to these guidelines is critical in the clinical setting. With new clinical trial research, drug protocols change; thus, the list in this table may not remain current.

venous access devices can be used to administer additional fluids such as blood products, parenteral nutrition, or other drugs, as well as for venous blood sampling. The disadvantages are that the presence of central catheters can lead to increased incidence of blood clots, and they can be a source of systemic infection, particularly if a patient becomes immuno-suppressed during therapy. Three major types of venous access devices used in oncology care are tunnelled catheters, peripherally inserted central catheters, and implanted infusion ports. (See Chapter 19 for a detailed discussion of these venous access devices.)

TABLE 18-9 DRUG THERAPY

Methods of Administration of Chemotherapeutic Drugs

Method	Examples
Oral	Cyclophosphamide
Intramuscular	Bleomycin
Intravenous	Doxorubicin, vincristine
Intracavitary (pleural, peritoneal)	Radioisotopes, alkylating agents, methotrexate
Intrathecal	Methotrexate, cytarabine
Intra-arterial	Dacarbazine (DTIC), 5-fluorouracil (5-FU), methotrexate, floxuridine
Perfusion	Alkylating agents
Continuous infusion	5-FU, methotrexate, cytarabine
Subcutaneous	Cytarabine

FIGURE 18-12 A, Cross-section of the implantable pump displaying its two chambers: the drug chamber (inner) and the charging fluid chamber (outer). As the drug chamber is filled, the bellows expand, compressing the charging fluid in the outer chamber. The resulting increased pressure in the outer chamber forces the drug through a membrane filter and preset flow restrictor, thus ensuring a nearly constant flow. **B,** Infusaid pump. Source: Courtesy Strato/Infusaid, Inc., Norwood, MA.

Infusion Pumps. Infusion pumps are used primarily for the continuous infusion of chemotherapeutic agents by intravenous, subcutaneous, intra-arterial, and epidural routes. Infusion pumps can be worn externally or implanted surgically.

Implanted infusion pumps are used primarily for intra-arterial administration of chemotherapeutic agents (Figure 18-12). This approach enables continuous infusion of the chemotherapeutic agent directly to the area of the tumour while sparing patients the systemic effects of the drug. Some implanted pumps have two silicone septa. The second septum can be used for bolus medication administration. The most common use of this method of chemotherapeutic administration has been hepatic artery infusion in the treatment of liver metastasis, usually from primary colon cancer.

Implanted pumps also consist of a catheter that is threaded into the designated artery. The catheter is attached to a pump apparatus that consists of two chambers: an inner chamber that serves as the drug reservoir and an outer chamber that contains vapour pressure, which provides a source of power for the pump. The pump is implanted surgically in a subcutaneous pocket. Access to the pump is via a silicone septum with a Huber point needle. Flow rate of the pump can be affected by drug concentration, the length and diameter of the silicone rubber (Silastic) catheter, and the patient's body temperature. Thus dose alterations may be required if the patient experiences a change in temperature or travels to higher altitudes. Complications that have been associated with implanted infusion pumps include infection, thrombosis, clotting of the catheter, and pump malfunction.

Other access devices used in the treatment of the person with cancer include the Tenckhoff catheter, used in the administration of intraperitoneal chemotherapeutic agents, and the Ommaya reservoir, which delivers agents directly to the central nervous system (CNS).

Regional Administration of Chemotherapeutic Agents. Regional treatment with chemotherapy involves the delivery of the drug directly to the tumour site. The advantage of administering chemotherapy by this method is that higher concentrations of the drug can be delivered to the tumour with reduced systemic toxicity. Several regional delivery methods have been developed, including intra-arterial, intraperitoneal, intrathecal or intraventricular, and intravesical bladder chemotherapy.

Intra-Arterial Chemotherapy. In intra-arterial chemotherapy, the drug is delivered to the tumour via the arterial vessel supplying the tumour. This method has been used for the treatment of osteogenic sarcoma; cancers of the head and neck, the bladder, the brain, and the cervix; melanoma; primary liver cancer; and metastatic liver disease. One method of intra-arterial drug delivery involves the surgical placement of a catheter that is subsequently connected to an external infusion pump or an implanted infusion pump for infusion of the chemotherapeutic agent. In general, intra-arterial chemotherapy results in reduced systemic toxicity. The type of toxic effects experienced by patients depends on the toxicity profile of the chemotherapy agent and the site of the tumour being treated.

Intraperitoneal Chemotherapy. Intraperitoneal chemotherapy involves the delivery of chemotherapeutic agents to the peritoneal cavity for treatment of peritoneal metastases from primary colorectal and ovarian cancers and malignant ascites. Temporary Silastic catheters (e.g., Tenckhoff, Hickman, Groshong) are percutaneously or surgically placed into the peritoneal cavity for short-term administration of chemotherapeutic agents. Alternatively, an implanted port can be used to administer chemotherapeutic agents intraperitoneally. Complications of intraperitoneal chemotherapy delivery include abdominal pain; catheter occlusion, dislodgement, and migration; and infection.

Intrathecal or Intraventricular Chemotherapy. Cancers that metastasize to the CNS—most commonly breast, lung, and GI cancers; leukemia; and lymphoma—are difficult to treat because the blood–brain barrier often prevents distribution of chemotherapeutic agents to this area. One method used to treat metastasis to the CNS is intrathecal chemotherapy. This method involves a lumbar puncture and injection of chemotherapeutic drugs into the subarachnoid space. However, this method has resulted in incomplete distribution of the drug in the CNS, particularly to the cisternal and ventricular areas.

To ensure more uniform distribution of chemotherapeutic drugs to the cisternal and ventricular areas, an Ommaya reservoir is often inserted. An Ommaya reservoir is a Silastic, dome-shaped disc with an extension catheter that is surgically implanted through the cranium into a lateral ventricle. In addition to providing more consistent drug distribution, the Ommaya reservoir averts the need for repeated painful lumbar punctures.

Complications of intrathecal or intraventricular chemotherapy include meningitis and leukoencephalopathy (Beauchesne, 2010).

Intravesical Bladder Chemotherapy. Many patients with superficial transitional cell cancer of the bladder have recurrent disease after traditional surgical therapy. Instillation of chemotherapeutic agents into the bladder promotes destruction of cancer cells and reduces the incidence of recurrent disease. Additional benefits of this therapy include reduced urinary and sexual dysfunction. The chemotherapeutic agent is instilled into the bladder via a urinary catheter and retained for 1 to 3 hours. Complications of this therapy include dysuria, urinary frequency, hematuria, and bladder spasms.

Effects of Chemotherapy on Normal Tissues

Chemotherapeutic agents cannot selectively distinguish between normal cells and cancer cells. Adverse and toxic effects results from the destruction of normal cells, especially those that proliferate rapidly, such as the cells of the bone marrow, the GI lining, and the integumentary system (Table 18-10). The body's response to the products of cellular destruction in the circulation may cause fatigue, anorexia, and taste alterations.

TABLE 18-10 CELLS WITH RAPID RATE OF PROLIFERATION

Cells and Generation Time	Effect of Cell Destruction
Bone marrow stem cell: 6–24 hr	Myelosuppression; infection, bleeding, anemia
Neutrophils: 12 hr	Leukopenia, infection
Epithelial cells lining the gastro-intestinal tract: 12–24 hr	Anorexia, stomatitis, esophagitis, nausea and vomiting, diarrhea
Ova or testes: 24–36 hr	Reproductive dysfunction
Cells of the hair follicle: 24 hr	Alopecia

The adverse effects of these drugs can be classified as acute, delayed, or chronic. Acute toxic effects include vomiting, allergic reactions, and dysrhythmias. Delayed effects include mucositis, alopecia, and bone marrow suppression. Mucositis can result in mouth sores, gastritis, and diarrhea. Chronic toxicity involves damage to organs such as the heart, the liver, the kidneys, and the lungs.

Treatment Plan

When chemotherapy is used in the treatment of cancer, several drugs may be given in combination. Multidrug regimens have proved to be particularly effective in the treatment of many types of cancer. The drugs given are carefully selected to kill the cancer cells most effectively and yet allow the normal cells to repair themselves and proliferate. The dose of each drug is carefully calculated according to the body weight or the body surface area (i.e., body weight and height) of the patient being treated. The principles of combination chemotherapy include the following:

1. The drugs used in the treatment plan are effective against the cancer being treated.
2. When drugs are given in combination, a synergistic effect occurs.
3. The combination includes cell cycle phase–specific drugs, cell cycle phase–nonspecific drugs, and drugs that have different mechanisms of action.
4. The combination includes drugs that have different toxic adverse effects.
5. The combination includes drugs that cause nadirs at different time intervals. The nadir is the lowest level of the peripheral blood cell counts (particularly WBC) that occurs secondary to bone marrow depression. The nadir after administration of most chemotherapeutic drugs occurs in 7 to 28 days.

An example of a treatment regimen is the FOLFOX (**fol**inic acid, **f**luorouracil, and **ox**aliplatin) regimen (Table 18-11). The agents in this drug protocol differ in mechanisms of action, toxic adverse effects, and nadir, but the combination is synergistic in nature, and the dosage schedule includes a time of drug administration and a time of rest from drug administration. The rest period is necessary to allow the normal cells to proliferate and repair the damaged tissue. The patient is evaluated before the administration of each course of chemotherapy to determine how well he or she is tolerating the treatment and whether the normal cells have recovered sufficiently for the next dose to be given.

TABLE 18-11 DRUG THERAPY

FOLFOX Chemotherapeutic Drug Schedule

Schedule: FOLFOX + bevacizumab (Avastin) is given to treat advanced colon cancer. FOLFOX* includes 5-fluorouracil ("FOL") administered as a continuous intravenous infusion over 46 hours on days 1 and 2; leucovorin (folinic acid; "F") administered intravenously over 2 hours on days 1 and 2; and oxaliplatin (Eloxatin [OX]), administered intravenously over 2 hours on day 1. Bevacizumab is administered intravenously over 2 hours on day 1. This schedule is repeated every 2 weeks. The number of cycles depends on a patient's situation.

	Week 1		Week 3		Week 5		Week 7	
Drug	Day 1	Day 2	Day 1	Day 2	Day 1	Day 2	Day 1	Day 2
5-Fluorouracil	X	X	X	X	X	X	X	X
Leucovorin (folinic acid)	X	X	X	X	X	X	X	X
Oxaliplatin (Eloxatin)	X		X		X		X	
Bevacizumab (Avastin)	X		X		X		X	

*There are slightly different versions of the FOLFOX regimen.

RADIATION THERAPY

Radiation therapy is a local treatment modality for cancer. It is one of the oldest methods of cancer treatment. Historically, workers exposed to radiation had a higher incidence of skin desquamation and developed carcinomas of the fingers. Both Marie Curie and her daughter Irène Joliot-Curie developed leukemia as a result of radiation exposure.

The observation that radiation exposure caused tissue damage led scientists to explore the use of radiation to treat tumours. The hypothesis was that if radiation resulted in the destruction of the highly mitotic skin cells of workers, it could be used in a controlled way to prevent the continued growth of highly mitotic cancer cells. It was not until the 1960s that sophisticated equipment and treatment planning facilitated the delivery of adequate radiation doses to tumours and tolerable doses to normal tissues. Today, radiotherapy has a central role in the treatment of cancer.

Effects of Radiation

Radiation is the emission and distribution of energy through space or a material medium. The energy produced by radiation, when absorbed into tissue, produces ionization and excitation. This local energy and the resultant generation of free radicals break chemical bonds in DNA, which may lead to lethal or sublethal damage. Lethal damage causes sufficient chromosomal disruption that the cell is unable to replicate. Sublethal DNA damage may be repaired between radiation doses or, alternatively, may accumulate with repetitive doses, leading to cell death. Cancer cells are especially vulnerable to the effects of cumulative radiation doses because they are less capable of repairing sublethal damage than are normal cells. When repetitive, *fractionated* (or divided) doses of radiation are delivered to a tumour, damage to malignant cells is maximized, and normal cells are more likely to recover. The principles of radiotherapy dosing and fractionation are guided by cellular response to radiation, known as the *four Rs* of radiobiology: **r**epair of cellular damage, **r**edistribution of cells in the cell cycle, **r**epopulation with normal cells, and **r**eoxygenation of hypoxic tumour areas.

Cellular Death and Tissue Reactions. *Cellular death* related to radiation is defined as an irreversible loss of proliferative capacity. Cells may undergo several mitoses and then die. A cell that retains its proliferative capacity is a clonogenic cell because it is able to produce new clones or colonies of similar cells. After radiation, cancer is considered controlled if the cells that remain are nonclonogenic.

Cellular sensitivity to radiation varies throughout the cell cycle; cells are most sensitive in the M and G$_2$ phases and least sensitive during the S, or synthesis, phase (see Figure 18-1). Cells treated during the M and G$_2$ phases of the cell cycle are more likely to suffer lethal damage. The damage to DNA in cells that are not in the M phase is expressed when the cells divide.

The amount of time that is required for the manifestations of radiation damage is determined by the mitotic rate of the tissue. Sufficient numbers of cells within the tissue must be killed to establish a noticeable effect. This is true for both normal and cancer cells. Rapidly dividing cells in the GI tract, oral mucosa, and bone marrow die fast or exhibit other early acute responses to irradiation. Tissues with slowly proliferating cells—such as those of cartilage, bone, and kidneys—manifest late responses to irradiation.

This differential rate of cellular death explains the timing of clinical manifestations related to radiation therapy. Normal cells within the radiation field are also affected by treatment. For each normal cell type, there is a maximally tolerated radiation dose. Administration of radiation above the maximally tolerated doses results in limited ability of normal cells to recover from damage and in potentially irreversible adverse effects. Treatment planning and computerized dosimetry ensure that normal tissue tolerance is not exceeded (Behrend, 2011).

Table 18-12 lists the relative radiosensitivities of a variety of tumours. In responsive tumours, even a large tumour burden is affected by therapy. In less responsive tumours, a large tumour burden may result in a slower and perhaps incomplete response.

Simulation and Treatment

Simulation is a part of radiation treatment planning used to determine the optimal treatment method. The patient lies on a table in the treatment position. The critical normal structures to be included in the treatment field or portal are identified under fluoroscopy. An image is taken to verify the field, and marks are placed on the skin so that the field can be reproduced on a daily basis. Immobilization devices (e.g., casts, bite blocks, thermoplastic face masks) are typically used to help the patient maintain a stable position (Figure 18-13). Computerized dosimetry, accomplished with computed tomographic scanning, is used to produce a treatment plan for delivering the maximum amount of radiation to the tumour within the acceptable dosage limits for normal tissue.

External Radiation. Teletherapy (*external beam irradiation*) is the most common form of radiation treatment delivery. With this technique, the patient is exposed to radiation from a megavoltage treatment machine. The radiation source may include cobalt-60, which emits gamma rays from a radioactive source. Therapy may be delivered by a cyclotron, which produces neutrons or protons, or by a linear accelerator, which generates ionizing radiation from electricity and with which multiple levels of energy can be utilized (Figure 18-14).

Internal Radiation. Another radiation delivery system is brachytherapy ("close" treatment). In this method, radioactive materials are implanted or inserted directly into the tumour or close to the tumour. An implant may be temporary; the source is placed into a catheter or tube that is inserted into the tumour

TABLE 18-12	**TUMOUR RADIOSENSITIVITY**		
High Radiosensitivity	**Moderate Radiosensitivity**	**Mild Radiosensitivity**	**Poor Radiosensitivity**
• Hodgkin's disease	• Bladder carcinoma	• Colon adenocarcinoma	• Malignant gliomas
• Neuroblastoma	• Breast adenocarcinoma	• Gastric adenocarcinoma	• Malignant melanoma
• Non-Hodgkin's lymphoma	• Esophageal carcinoma	• Renal adenocarcinoma	• Osteosarcoma
• Ovarian dysgerminoma	• Oropharyngeal carcinoma	• Soft tissue sarcomas (e.g., chondrosarcoma)	• Testicular nonseminoma
• Testicular seminoma	• Prostate carcinoma		
• Wilms tumour	• Skin carcinoma		
	• Uterine and cervical carcinoma		

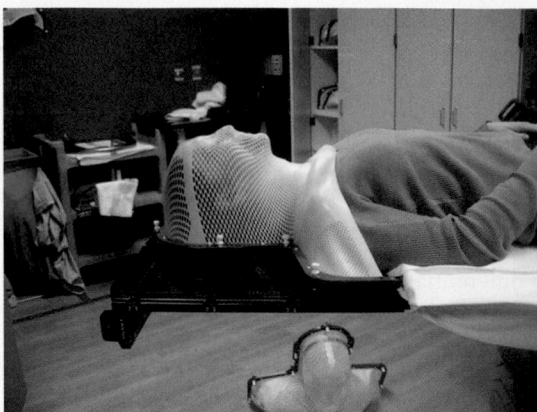

FIGURE 18-13 Immobilization device. Use of a head holder and immobilization mask may be used to ensure accurate positioning for daily treatment of head and neck cancer. Source: Courtesy Jormain Cady, Virginia Mason Medical Center, Seattle, WA.

FIGURE 18-14 Linear accelerator. Varian Clinac EX linear accelerator with multiple photon and electron energy levels available for use according to the treatment plan. Patient is positioned on radiation treatment table for treatment of head and neck cancer. Source: Courtesy Jormain Cady, Virginia Mason Medical Center, Seattle, WA.

TABLE 18-13	MEASUREMENT OF RADIATION
Unit	**Definition**
Curie (Ci)	A measure of the number of atoms of a particular radioisotope that disintegrate in 1 second
Roentgen (R)	A measure of the radiation required to produce a standard number of ions in air; a unit of exposure to radiation
Rad	Measurement of radiation dosage absorbed by the tissues
Rem	Measurement of the biological effectiveness of various forms of radiation on the human cell (1 rem = 1 rad)
Gray (Gy)	100 rads = 1 Gy
Centigray (cGy)	1 Gy = 100 cGy

procedure. The radiation safety officer determines how much time at a specific distance can be spent with the patient, according to the dose delivered by the implant. Because the source is nonpenetrating, small differences in distance are critical. Only care that must be delivered near the source, such as checking placement of the implant, is performed in close proximity. Shielding, if available, should be used, and the health care provider should not deliver care without wearing a film badge. This badge indicates any radiation exposure. The film badge should not be shared, should not be worn anywhere other than at work, and should be returned according to the employer's protocol.

Measurement of Radiation

Several different units are used to measure radiation (Table 18-13). Grays (Gy) and centigrays (cGy) are the units currently used in clinical practice.

Goals of Radiation Therapy

The goals of radiation therapy are cure, control, and palliation. To accomplish these treatment goals, radiation therapy can be used alone or as an adjuvant treatment modality with surgery, chemotherapy, biological therapy, or some combination of these.

Cure is the goal when radiation therapy is used alone for treating patients with basal cell carcinoma of the skin, tumours confined to the vocal cords, and stage I or IIA Hodgkin's disease. Radiation therapy can be combined with surgery and chemotherapy to cure certain cancers; for example, (a) stages IIB, IIIA, and IIIB Hodgkin's disease (in combination with chemotherapy); (b) Ewing's sarcoma (in combination with chemotherapy); (c) head and neck cancer (in combination with surgery and chemotherapy); and (d) stages I and II breast cancer (in combination with surgery).

Control of the disease process for a time may be a reasonable goal in some situations. Initial treatment is offered at the time of diagnosis, and additional treatment may be instituted if symptoms of disease recur. Most patients enjoy a satisfactory quality of life during the symptom-free period. Radiation therapy can be combined with surgery to further enhance the local control of cancer. It can be given preoperatively to reduce the size of the tumour so that it can be more easily resected, or it can be given postoperatively to destroy any remaining tumour cells. Intraoperative radiation therapy is now available at some research centres. In this procedure, radiation is administered directly to the site of the tumour during surgery.

area and left in place for several days. This method is commonly used for tumours of the head and neck and for prostate and gynecological malignancies. Implants may also be permanent, whereby radioactive seeds are inserted into tumours: for example, in the prostate. Brachytherapy is clinically appropriate when the radiation dose necessary to eradicate the tumour exceeds the dose tolerance of nearby normal tissues. The sources used in brachytherapy are not as energetic or penetrating as those used in the external beam machines and thus deliver most of the dose locally. External beam radiation therapy and brachytherapy may be used in combination.

To care for a patient with a radiation implant, the nurse must be aware that the patient is radioactive. Patients with temporary implants are radioactive during the time the source is in place. If the patient has a permanent implant, the radioactive exposure to the outside and to other people is low, and the patient may be discharged with precautions. The principles of time, distance, and shielding are used in caring for the patient with an implant. Nursing care should be organized so that time spent in direct contact with the patient is kept to a minimum. The patient should be informed of these restrictions before the implantation

Inoperable tumours can be treated with radiation therapy. These tumours are large and have extended regionally. An example of an inoperable cancer treated for control with radiation therapy is small (oat) cell cancer of the lung.

Palliation is often the goal of radiation therapy, with the aim of controlling symptoms resulting from the disease process. Tumours can be reduced in size to relieve symptoms such as pain and obstruction. Examples of the use of radiation therapy for palliation include relief from the following:

1. Pain associated with bone metastasis
2. Pain and neurological symptoms associated with brain metastasis
3. Spinal cord compression
4. Intestinal obstruction
5. Superior vena cava obstruction
6. Bronchial or tracheal obstruction
7. Bleeding (e.g., bladder and intrabronchial)

NURSING MANAGEMENT
RADIATION THERAPY AND CHEMOTHERAPY

The nurse has an important role in educating patients about their treatment regimens and the management of adverse effects and disease symptoms. Teaching should be tailored to the needs and abilities of patients and their families. Nurses can also assist patients to cope with the psychosocial issues associated with a cancer diagnosis. Anxiety and fear may pervade a patient's day-to-day experience and become a barrier to his or her ability to navigate through treatment. The nurse can mobilize a collaborative team of health care providers, community resources, and the patient's family to provide and reinforce information, facilitate transportation to the cancer centre, and ensure adequate physical, emotional, and spiritual support. One of the most important responsibilities of the nurse is that of differentiating between toxic effects of treatments and progression of the malignant process. The nurse must also distinguish tolerable adverse effects from acute toxic effects of chemotherapeutic agents. For example, nausea and vomiting are expected and controllable adverse effects of many drugs. However, if paresthesia occurs with the use of vincristine or if signs of heart failure appear with the use of doxorubicin (Adriamycin), these serious reactions must be reported to the physician so that drug dosages can be modified or the drug discontinued. Some toxic effects associated with chemotherapy may not be reversible. For example, ototoxicity may be an irreversible effect of cisplatin therapy, especially at high doses. Periodic testing of hearing may be necessary to monitor for this toxic effect. A nurse also advises patients about the availability of supportive therapies (e.g., antiemetics, anti-diarrheals) to optimize quality of life during treatment.

Common adverse effects and specific nursing considerations related to problems caused by cancer therapy are presented in Table 18-14. Fatigue, anorexia, bone marrow suppression, skin reactions, mucosal reactions, and pulmonary, GI, and reproductive effects are discussed in the following sections. (See NCP 18-1 and NCP 18-2 for care of the patient undergoing radiation or chemotherapy, available on the Evolve website.)

NURSING IMPLEMENTATION

FATIGUE. Fatigue is a commonly reported adverse effect of cancer therapy, affecting at least 80% of patients with cancer (Harris, Ross, & Sanchez-Reilly, 2014). The pathophysiological mechanisms that result in cancer treatment–induced fatigue are unclear. Accumulation of metabolites from the destruction of cells during treatment is one probable cause. The metabolites include lactate, hydrogen ions, and other end products of cellular destruction and result in decreased muscle strength. Energy production in patients with cancer may also be altered by cachexia, anorexia, fever, and infection. Fatigue associated with radiotherapy generally begins during the third to fourth weeks of treatment, persists after treatment ends, and then gradually subsides. Chemotherapy-related fatigue may become chronic after therapy. Factors such as weight loss, anemia, depression, nausea, and other symptoms exacerbate the sensation of fatigue.

Maintaining good nutrition and adequate hydration, alternating periods of rest and activity, relying on family members for assistance with responsibilities, and managing pain and anxiety may help reduce fatigue. The nurse can prepare patients for the expected adverse effect of fatigue, so that they do not assume that it is a sign of treatment failure. A patient may report more energy on some days than on others. Encouraging a patient to identify days or times during the day when he or she feels better may assist in understanding his or her body's responses and maximizing energy reserves. Ignoring the fatigue or overstressing the body when fatigue is tolerable may lead to an increase in symptoms. Mild physical activity programs are usually within the abilities of patients and have been found to ameliorate symptoms of fatigue, lessen anxiety, and facilitate sleep in patients with cancer (Mustian, Sprod, Janelsins, et al., 2012). Family caregivers of patients with cancer are also prone to fatigue and poor energy levels. Remaining as active as a patient is able has been shown to improve mood and avoid the debilitating cycle of fatigue-depression-fatigue that can occur.

ANOREXIA. Anorexia may develop as a general reaction to treatment. The mechanisms underlying the development of anorexia are unclear, but several theories exist. Macrophages release TNF and IL-1 in an attempt to fight the cancer. Both TNF and IL-1 have an appetite-suppressing (anorexic) effect. It is hypothesized that as tumours are destroyed by therapy, increased levels of these factors are released into the system and cross the blood–brain barrier, affecting the satiety centre. Large tumours produce more of these factors, thus resulting in the cachexia observed in patients with advanced cancer. In addition, radiation treatments to the head and neck and the GI system exacerbate eating difficulties. Anorexia peaks at about 4 weeks of treatment and seems to resolve more quickly than fatigue when treatment ends.

Patients with anorexia need to be monitored carefully during treatment to ensure that weight loss does not become excessive. Body weight should be measured at least twice weekly. Small, frequent meals of high-protein, high-calorie foods are better tolerated than large meals (see the Resources at the end of this chapter). Nutritional supplements may be required.

BONE MARROW SUPPRESSION. Myelosuppression is a common and significant effect of many chemotherapeutic modalities and may also occur with radiotherapy. Chemotherapy is a systemic treatment with the ability to affect every vulnerable cell in the body, whereas radiotherapy is delivered locally, so that only the cells within the treatment field are affected. Concurrent chemotherapy and irradiation generally increase the risk of toxic effects on the bone marrow. The onset of bone marrow suppression is related to the lifespan of the blood cell type. WBCs are affected within 1 week, platelets in 2 to 3 weeks, and red blood cells (RBCs) in 2 to 3 months. The severity of myelosuppression is related to the type and the dose of chemotherapeutic drug or

TABLE 18-14 **NURSING MANAGEMENT OF PROBLEMS CAUSED BY RADIATION THERAPY AND CHEMOTHERAPY**

Problem	Cause	Nursing Management
Gastro-intestinal System		
Stomatitis, mucositis, esophagitis	Destruction of cells in radiation treatment field Destruction of epithelial cells by chemotherapy Inflammation and ulceration, which result from rapid cell destruction	• Be aware that eating, swallowing, and talking may be difficult and necessitate changes in diet and fluid intake. • Encourage patient to use artificial saliva. • Assess oral mucosa daily. Teach the patient to do this, and encourage the patient to practise good oral hygiene. • Use evidence-informed guidelines and protocols to minimize the occurrence or reduce the severity of oral mucositis. • Discourage use of irritants such as tobacco and alcohol, spicy foods, and drinks. • Apply topical anaesthetics, such as lidocaine (Xylocaine Viscous) or oxethazaine.
Nausea and vomiting	Cellular breakdown, which stimulates vomiting centre in brain Drugs, which also stimulate vomiting centre Destruction of GI lining by radiation and chemotherapy	• Counsel the patient to eat and drink when not nauseated. • Administer antiemetics, and teach the patient and family caregiver when to use antiemetic therapy to maximize symptom control.
Anorexia	Release of TNF and IL-1 from macrophages, which has appetite-suppressant effect General reaction to therapy	• Use diversional activities (if appropriate). • Monitor the patient's weight. • Encourage the patient to eat small, frequent meals of high-protein, high-calorie foods (e.g., Ensure or other supplements). • Reassure family caregivers, and teach them to provide gentle encouragement to the patient.
Diarrhea	Denuding of epithelial lining of intestines	• Suggest low-fibre, low-residue diet. • Increase fluids. • Provide antidiarrheal agents as needed.
Constipation	Autonomic nervous system dysfunction Neurotoxic effects of plant alkaloids (vincristine, vinblastine) Use of opioids	• Encourage the patient to use a diary to monitor bowel movements and report to the health care team as needed. • Provide stool softeners and laxatives as needed. • Encourage intake of high-fibre foods.
Hepatotoxicity	Toxic effects from chemotherapeutic drugs	• Monitor liver function values.
Hematological System		
Anemia	Bone marrow depressed as a result of therapy Malignant infiltration of bone marrow by cancer	• Monitor hemoglobin and hematocrit levels. • Encourage intake of foods that promote RBC production (see Chapter 33, Table 33.5).
Leukopenia	Depression of bone marrow as a result of chemotherapy or radiation therapy Febrile neutropenia Infection resulting from immuno-suppression (most frequent cause of morbidity and death in patients with cancer) Infection in respiratory and genitourinary systems (usual sites of infection)	• Monitor WBC count, especially neutrophils. • Educate and counsel patients and family caregivers to do the following: Monitor changes in temperature, and report any elevation immediately to the health care team. Advise the patient to maintain good personal hygiene, including frequent handwashing. Recommend that the patient report any signs of infection (swelling, unusual cough, vomiting, severe headache, redness) immediately at the nearest hospital. Advise the patient to avoid large crowds and people with infections.
Thrombo-cytopenia	Bone marrow depression secondary to chemotherapy Malignant infiltration of bone marrow Spontaneous bleeding, which can occur with platelet counts at or below 20×10^9/L	• Observe for signs of bleeding (e.g., petechiae, ecchymosis). • Monitor hemoglobin, hematocrit, and platelet counts. • Recommend use of a soft-bristle toothbrush and electric razor.
Integumentary System		
Alopecia (usually temporary with chemotherapy and usually permanent in response to radiation)	Destruction of hair follicles by chemotherapy or radiation to scalp	• Suggest ways to cope with hair loss (e.g., hairpieces, scarves, wigs). • Discuss effect of hair loss on self-image. • Recommend cutting long hair before therapy. • Advise the patient to avoid excessive shampooing, brushing, and combing of hair. • Recommend avoiding use of electric hair dryers, curlers, and curling irons.

TABLE 18-14	NURSING MANAGEMENT OF PROBLEMS CAUSED BY RADIATION THERAPY AND CHEMOTHERAPY—cont'd	

Problem	Cause	Nursing Management
Skin reactions	Extravasation of vesicant chemotherapeutic drugs Radiation therapy damage to skin	• Protect the patient from extravasation through careful attention to delivery of chemotherapeutic drugs and assessment of venous access. • Recommend lubricating dry skin with nonirritating creams. • Recommend avoiding the use of harsh soaps. • Advise the patient to wear loose clothing and cotton underwear and to avoid tight garments. • Inform the patient that photosensitivity may occur.
Genitourinary System		
Cystitis	Destruction of cells lining the bladder by chemotherapy Adverse effect of radiation when located in treatment field	• Monitor manifestations such as urgency, frequency, and hematuria. • Discuss these changes with the patient.
Reproductive dysfunction	Damage of cells of testes or ova by therapy	• Provide information about effects on fertility and referral to fertility resources (e.g., sperm banking) before delivery of radiation to the pelvis, high-dose chemotherapy, or bone marrow transplantation.
Nephrotoxicity	Accumulation of drugs in the kidney and tumour lysis, which cause necrosis of proximal renal tubules	• Monitor BUN and serum creatinine levels.
Nervous System		
Increased intracranial pressure	Radiation-related edema in central nervous system	• Administer steroids and pain medication. • Monitor neurological status.
Peripheral neuropathy	Paresthesias, areflexia, skeletal muscle weakness, and smooth muscle dysfunction, which can occur as adverse effects of plant alkaloids and cisplatin	• Monitor for such manifestations in patients receiving these drugs.
Respiratory System		
Pneumonitis (develops 2–3 mo after start of treatment) Fibrosis (develops after 6–12 mo and is evident on radiographs)	Radiation Adverse effects of some chemotherapeutic drugs	• Monitor for dry, hacking cough; fever; and exertional dyspnea.
Cardiovascular System		
Pericarditis and myocarditis (complication when chest wall is irradiated; may occur up to 1 yr after treatment)	Inflammation secondary to radiation injury Adverse effect of some chemotherapeutic drugs	• Monitor for clinical manifestations of these disorders. • Monitor heart function with ECG studies and cardiac ejection fractions.
Cardiotoxicity	Some chemotherapeutic drugs (e.g., doxorubicin, daunorubicin) can cause ECG changes and rapidly progressive heart failure	• Drug therapy may have to be modified.
Biochemical		
Hyperuricemia, secondary gout, and obstructive uropathy	Cell destruction by chemotherapy	• Monitor uric acid levels. • Allopurinol (Zyloprim) may be given as a prophylactic measure. • Encourage high fluid intake.
Multidimensional Effects		
Fatigue	Increased metabolic rate Anabolic processes that result in accumulation of metabolites from cell breakdown	• Counsel the patient that fatigue is an expected adverse effect of therapy but that there are ways to manage fatigue, such as sleep hygiene, moderate exercise, and pacing activities. • Encourage the patient to rest when fatigued, to maintain usual lifestyle patterns as closely as possible, and to pace activities in accordance with energy level.
Pain	Compression or infiltration of tumour involving nerves Inflammation, ulceration, or necrosis of tissues	• Use an analgesic ladder to provide basis for pain medication administration. • Teach use of imagery, relaxation therapy, and other alternative measures (see Chapters 8 and 12).

BUN, blood urea nitrogen (serum urea [nitrogen]); *ECG*, electrocardiographic; *GI*, gastro-intestinal; *IL-1*, interleukin 1; *RBC*, red blood cell; *TNF*, tumour necrosis factor; *WBC*, white blood cell.

the specific radiation field and to the extent of bone marrow reserves. In an adult, about 40% of active marrow is in the pelvis, and 25% is in the thoracic and lumbar vertebrae.

Blood cell counts (including WBCs, neutrophils, RBCs, and platelets) must be closely monitored. Neutropenia is most common in patients receiving chemotherapy and puts them at risk for serious infections or sepsis. WBC growth factors may be used to stimulate regeneration of adequate numbers of leukocytes and prevent treatment delays. Thrombo-cytopenia may cause spontaneous bleeding or hemorrhage and may necessitate a platelet transfusion if counts fall below 20×10^9/L. If anemia occurs and the hemoglobin level drops below 6 mmol/L, the patient may require blood transfusions.

SKIN REACTIONS. Like the bone marrow, the skin cells are rapidly proliferating and are therefore vulnerable to the effects of radiation and chemotherapy. Both acute and chronic changes can occur in the skin within the radiation field. The skin-sparing property of modern radiation equipment limits the severity of these reactions. Although the skin reaction begins as early as the first treatment, it is initially transitory. Erythema may develop 1 to 24 hours after a single treatment. Erythema is an acute response followed by dry desquamation (Figure 18-15). If the rate of cellular sloughing is faster than the ability of the new epidermal cells to replace dead cells, a wet desquamation occurs, with exposure of the dermis and oozing of serum (Figure 18-16). Skin reactions are particularly evident in areas subjected to pressure, such as behind the ear and in gluteal folds, the perineum, the breast, the collar line, and bony prominences.

Although skin care protocols vary among institutions, they are founded on basic skin care principles. Dry reactions are uncomfortable and result in pruritus. Wet reactions result in discomfort and drainage. Dry skin should be lubricated with a lotion or solution that contains no metal, alcohol, perfume, or additives that irritate the skin. Wet reactions must be kept clean and protected from further damage. Prevention of infection and facilitation of wound healing are the therapeutic goals.

Irradiated skin should be protected from extremes of temperature to prevent trauma. Heating pads, ice packs, and hot water bottles cannot be used in the treatment field. Constricting garments, rubbing, harsh chemicals, and deodorants may also traumatize the skin and should be avoided. The use of corticosteroids and hydrogen peroxide is controversial because of their interference with wound healing. The guidelines presented in Table 18-15 are not intended to replace protocols or guidelines developed by the cancer agency or hospital program.

Alopecia (hair loss) is restricted to the radiation field when caused by radiotherapy but affects all body hair (including eyelashes and eyebrows) when caused by chemotherapeutic agents. For some patients, hair loss causes profound distress. Chemotherapy-induced

FIGURE 18-15 Dry desquamation.

FIGURE 18-16 Wet desquamation.

TABLE 18-15 PATIENT & CAREGIVER TEACHING GUIDE

Radiation Skin Reactions

Patient and caregiver teaching for radiation skin reactions should include the following:

1. Gently cleanse the skin in the treatment field with a mild soap (Ivory, Dove), tepid water, and a soft cloth. Rinse thoroughly and gently pat dry.
2. Apply nonmedicated, nonperfumed, moisturizing lotion or creams, such as baby lotion, oil, aloe gel or cream to alleviate dry skin. This substance must be gently cleansed from the treatment field before each treatment and reapplied after. (Note: Care differs from institution to institution.)
3. Rinse the area with saline solution. Expose the area to air as often as possible. If copious drainage is present, nonadhesive absorbent dressings are warranted, and they must be changed as soon as they become wet. Observe the area daily for signs of infection.
4. Avoid wearing tight-fitting clothing such as brassieres, girdles, and belts over the treatment field.
5. Avoid wearing harsh fabrics, such as wool and corduroy. A lightweight cotton garment is best. If possible, expose the treatment field to air.
6. Use gentle detergents such as Ivory Snow to wash clothing that will come in contact with the treatment field.
7. Avoid direct exposure to the sun. If the treatment field is in an area that is exposed to the sun, wear protective clothing such as a wide-brimmed hat during exposure to the sun. (Note: In general, people should avoid sun exposure regardless of whether they are in treatment or not; use of protective clothing and sunscreen on exposed areas should be recommended.)
8. Prevent application of heat from all sources (hot water bottles, heating pads, and sun lamps) on the treatment field.
9. Avoid exposing the treatment area to cold temperatures (ice bags or cold weather).
10. Avoid swimming in salt water or in chlorinated pools during the time of treatment.
11. Avoid the use of all medication, deodorants, perfumes, powders, or cosmetics on the skin in the treatment field. Tape, dressings, and adhesive bandages should also be avoided unless permitted by the radiation therapist. Avoid shaving the hair in the treatment field.
12. Continue to protect sensitive skin after the treatment is completed by doing the following:
    a. Continue to avoid direct exposure to the sun. A sunscreen agent and protective clothing must be worn if there is potential for exposure to the sun.
    b. If shaving is necessary in the treatment field, use an electric razor.

alopecia is temporary; hair regrowth begins 3 to 4 weeks after therapy is terminated. Radiotherapy-induced hair loss may be temporary or permanent, depending on the dose administered. Patients may be directed to the Canadian Cancer Society's "Look Good, Feel Better" program for support and advice about wigs and head coverings (see the Resources at the end of this chapter).

ORAL, OROPHARYNGEAL, AND ESOPHAGEAL REACTIONS. The mucosal lining of the GI tract is sensitive to the effects of radiation therapy and to certain antineoplastic drugs, especially 5-fluorouracil. As a result, nutritional status may be compromised by treatment. Salivary flow often decreases, with resultant xerostomia (dry mouth), during radiotherapy to the head and neck. Food must be dissolved in saliva to be tasted. Taste loss is progressive during therapy, and by the end of treatment, many patients report that all food has lost its flavour. Thick saliva is less able to perform the functions of cleansing teeth and moistening food. Difficulty swallowing, which characterizes esophageal reactions, further impedes eating. Patients report feeling that they have a "lump" as they swallow and that "foods get stuck."

Meticulous oral assessment and prompt intervention are essential to prevent infection and facilitate nutritional intake. Oral care includes pretreatment evaluation by a dentist to perform all necessary dental work before the initiation of treatment. The patient must be taught to examine the mouth and gums daily. Mucous membranes, characteristics of saliva, and ability to swallow must be assessed regularly. The patient should also be taught how to perform oral care at least before and after each meal and at bedtime. A saline solution of 1 teaspoon of salt in 1 L of water is an effective cleansing agent. One teaspoon of sodium bicarbonate may be added to the oral care solution to decrease odour, alleviate pain, and dissolve mucin. Tooth brushing and flossing are critical unless contraindicated by decreased platelet counts. Compliance with this protocol significantly reduces the risk of radiation caries, which develops as a result of loss of saliva. Saliva substitutes are available and may be offered to patients, although many patients find that drinking small amounts of water frequently has an equivalent effect.

Antacids, diphenhydramine (Benadryl), and lidocaine (Xylocaine Viscous) have been mixed in equal proportions to use as a component of oral care. The solutions may be swallowed to alleviate esophagitis. Any coating solution must be cleansed and not allowed to build up on the mucosa, where it could serve as a medium for infection. Infection, particularly with *Candida albicans,* can occur in individuals receiving head and neck radiation, and its incidence increases dramatically in protocols involving concomitant chemotherapy. Antifungal agents may be prescribed to treat the infection. Alleviation of mucositis may be achieved through the use of coating and analgesic compounds. Palifermin (Kepivance) may be effective in reducing the severity and duration of oral mucositis in patients receiving stem cell transplants, and cryotherapy involving ice chips helps prevent mucositis associated with 5-fluorouracil and melphalan therapy. The use of sucralfate, chlorhexidine, antimicrobial lozenges, and colony-stimulating factor mouthwash is not recommended (Eilers, Asakura, Blecher, et al., 2014; Lalla, Bowen, Barasch, et al., 2014).

Feedings of soft, nonirritating high-protein and high-calorie foods should be offered frequently throughout the day. Extremes of temperature, as well as tobacco and alcohol, should be avoided. Nutritional supplements (e.g., Ensure) as an adjunct to meals and fluid intake may be encouraged. The patient should be weighed at least twice each week to monitor weight loss. Families are an integral part of the health care team. As taste loss increases, the family's role in assisting the patient to eat becomes increasingly critical. If family members are not available, alternative support, such as visits by volunteers and home aides, is indicated.

PULMONARY EFFECTS. Pulmonary effects of cancer therapies may be irreversible and progressive. The effects of radiation on the lung include both acute and late reactions. Radiation doses in the lung are magnified because the dose cannot be reduced through tissue. Pneumonitis can be an acute inflammatory reaction related to radiation. This reaction is often asymptomatic, although cough, fever, and night sweats may increase. Treatment with bronchodilators, expectorants, bed rest, and oxygen is preferable to treatment with corticosteroids.

The most common pulmonary toxic effects associated with chemotherapy include pulmonary edema, interstitial fibrosis, and pneumonitis. The chemotherapeutic agents most strongly associated with these complications include bleomycin, busulfan, carmustine, cyclophosphamide, and some targeted agents (e.g., gefitinib [Iressa]). The pulmonary effects of treatments may be difficult to distinguish from those related to the disease and are frightening to patients because they may involve an exacerbation of the symptoms that precipitated the cancer diagnosis. Cough and dyspnea may increase. The cough becomes more productive because alveoli that had been blocked are opened as the tumour responds to treatment. As treatment continues, the cough can become dry as the mucosa begins to be altered by the radiation. Cough suppressants may be indicated for use at night.

Oxygen, if prescribed for symptomatic pneumonitis, must be used judiciously if a patient has chronic obstructive pulmonary disease (see Chapter 31). Oxygen therapy in such patients can cause carbon dioxide retention and respiratory acidosis and may be lethal. If a patient experiences dyspnea, anxiety may be pronounced. Lying flat on the radiation treatment table and being alone in the room may potentiate anxiety.

GASTRO-INTESTINAL EFFECTS. The mucosa of the GI tract is highly proliferative: Surface cells are replaced every 2 to 6 days, and thus they are highly vulnerable to cancer therapies. The intestinal mucosa is one of the most radiosensitive tissues. Radiation alters gastric secretion by direct injury to cells. The secretion of mucus, hydrochloric acid, and pepsin decreases with further treatment. Nausea, vomiting, and diarrhea are early responses to irradiation of the GI tissue and may occur immediately after the first treatment. The occurrence of these symptoms in response to cancer therapies may be related to the release of serotonin from the GI tract, which then stimulates the chemoreceptor trigger zone and the vomiting centre in the brain. Further GI irritation is related to direct injury to epithelial cells.

Several antiemetic drugs are available (see Chapter 44 and Table 44.1). Metoclopramide, ondansetron (Zofran), granisetron (Kytril), aprepitant (Emend), and dexamethasone have been used to decrease nausea and vomiting caused by chemotherapy. The introduction of antiemetic clinical practice guidelines and effective implementation of the guidelines in the oncology settings are essential methods for managing this treatment adverse effect. Administration of antiemetics before treatment alleviates the nausea and vomiting. Patients may find that eating a light meal of nonirritating food before treatment is also helpful. *Anticipatory nausea and vomiting* may develop in patients receiving radiation or chemotherapy when these symptoms are poorly controlled. This conditioned response results in the experience of nausea and vomiting when a patient encounters cues associated with the treatment: for example, walking through the doors of the cancer centre or merely seeing the oncologist, even outside of the treatment centre. In some individuals, this response persists after treatment ends. Aggressive emesis control, including the use of prophylactic antiemetics and antianxiety agents, is recommended.

Patients experiencing nausea and vomiting must be assessed for signs and symptoms of dehydration and alkalosis. Fluid intake is recorded to ensure that the volume consumed and retained is adequate. Diarrhea may be a reaction of the bowel mucosa to radiation. The small bowel is extremely sensitive and does not tolerate significant radiation doses. Administering treatments when a patient has a full bladder may serve to move the small bowel out of the treatment field. Nonirritating diets and low-residue diets, as well as antidiarrheal and antispasmodic drugs, are recommended. Lukewarm sitz baths may alleviate discomfort and cleanse the rectal area. The rectal area must be kept scrupulously clean and dry to maintain mucosal integrity. The nurse should inspect the perianal area. Number, volume, consistency, and character of stools per day should be recorded by patients, as should any potentially aggravating or alleviating factors related to bowel movements. Adequate food and fluid intake promote healing and mucosal integrity. Systemic analgesia is warranted for the painful skin irritations that may develop.

REPRODUCTIVE EFFECTS. The effects of radiation and chemotherapy on the ovary and testes are determined by the dose delivered and the type of chemotherapy used. The testes are highly sensitive to radiation, and the testicles are protected whenever possible. Doses of 15 to 30 cGy temporarily decrease the sperm count; aspermia results at 35 to 230 cGy. In some cases, 200 cGy may result in permanent aspermia. In patients receiving 300 to 600 cGy, the sperm count either recovers in 2 to 5 years or does not recover at all. Pretreatment status may be a significant factor because a low sperm count and loss of motility are seen in individuals with testicular cancer and Hodgkin's disease before any therapy. Combined modality treatment or prior chemotherapy with alkylating agents enhances and prolongs the effects of radiation on the testes. When radiation is used alone with conventional doses and appropriate shielding, testicular recovery often occurs. Compromised reproductive function in men may also result from erectile dysfunction after pelvic irradiation and its related vascular and neurological effects.

The radiation dose necessary to induce ovarian failure changes with age. Permanent cessation of menses occurs at 500 to 1000 cGy in 95% of women younger than 40 years, and at 375 cGy, the percentage is higher in women older than 40 years. Unlike the testes, the ovaries have no avenue for repair; therefore, the ovaries are shielded whenever possible. Other factors that influence reproductive or sexual functioning in women include reactions in the cervix and endometrium. These tissues withstand a high radiation dose with minimal sequelae, which accounts for the ability to treat endometrial and cervical cancer with high external and brachytherapeutic doses. Acute reactions such as tenderness, irritation, and loss of lubrication compromise sexual activity. Late effects of combined internal and external therapy include loss of elasticity, loss of lubrication, and vaginal shortening related to fibrosis. Supportive nursing care during brachytherapy for gynecological cancer is critical to the well-being and psychological functioning of women experiencing this treatment; the patient and the patient's partner require information about the expected effects of treatment in relation to reproductive and sexual issues. Potential infertility can be a significant consequence for the individual, and counselling is indicated. Pretreatment harvesting of sperm or ova may be considered. Specific suggestions to manage adverse effects that have an effect on sexual functioning include use of a water-soluble vaginal lubricant and a vaginal dilator after pelvic irradiation. The nurse must be competent in discussing issues related to sexuality, offering specific suggestions and making referrals for ongoing counselling when indicated.

LATE EFFECTS OF RADIATION TREATMENT AND CHEMOTHERAPY

Cancer survivors are achieving higher rates of long-term remission and survival because of advancements in treatment modalities. However, these forms of therapy (especially radiation treatment and chemotherapy) may produce long-term sequelae termed *physiological late effects* that occur months to years after cessation of therapy. Every body system can be affected to some extent by chemotherapy and radiation therapy. The effects of radiation on the body's tissues are caused by cellular hypoplasia of stem cells and alterations in the fine vasculature and fibroconnective tissues. In addition to the acute toxic effects, chemotherapy can have long-term effects related to the loss of cells' proliferative reserve capacity. The additive effects of multiagent chemotherapy before, during, or after a course of radiotherapy can significantly increase the risks of physiological late effects.

Cancer survivors may also be at risk for leukemias and other secondary malignancies resulting from therapy for the primary cancer. However, the potential risk for developing a second malignancy does not contraindicate the use of cancer treatment. The overall risk of developing neoplastic complications is low, and the latency period may be long.

The cancer treatments most frequently implicated in causing secondary malignancy are the alkylating chemotherapeutic agents and high-dose radiation, which can induce cancers at the exposure site. The exact mechanism of oncogenesis secondary to irradiation and chemotherapy remains unclear. It could be related to interactions between immuno-suppressive factors, direct cellular damage, and carcinogenic effects, along with other environmental carcinogens.

Acute leukemias occurring as secondary malignancies have been most widely reported after treatment for Hodgkin's disease, but they also occur in survivors of ovarian, lung, and breast cancers. Secondary malignancies other than leukemias include multiple myeloma after radiation therapy for breast cancer; non-Hodgkin's lymphoma after treatment for Hodgkin's disease; and cancers of the bladder, the kidney, and the ureters after the use of cyclophosphamide. Radiation therapy for breast, lung, ovarian, uterine, and thyroid cancers; for non-Hodgkin's lymphoma; and for Hodgkin's disease has been linked to secondary osteosarcoma of the rib, scapula, clavicle, humerus, sternum, ilium, and pelvis. Fibrosarcomas have been reported several years after radiation therapy for malignant glioma and pituitary adenoma. Unfortunately, secondary malignancies are usually resistant to therapy, but supportive care and palliative care are options for the patient.

BIOLOGICAL AND TARGETED THERAPY

Biological therapy is treatment involving the use of biological agents such as interferons, interleukins, monoclonal antibodies, and growth factors to modify the relationship between the host and the tumour. Biological agents are assuming a larger role in cancer treatment, either alone or in combination with surgery, radiation therapy, and chemotherapy. An understanding of the principles of cellular interaction underlies the development of agents that modify the relationship between the host and the tumour by altering the biological response of the host to the tumour cells. Biological agents may affect host–tumour response in three ways: (a) They have direct antitumour effects; (b) they restore, augment, or modulate host immune system mechanisms; and (c) they have other biological effects, such as interfering with the cancer cells' ability to metastasize or differentiate (Table 18-16; Figure 18-17).

Tumour cells express tumour antigens on their surfaces that can be recognized and destroyed by the body's immune cells. Cytokines are glycoprotein products of immune cells, such as lymphocytes and macrophages, and are capable of defence functions. Cytokines

TABLE 18-16 DRUG THERAPY

Biological and Targeted Therapy

Drug	Mechanism of Action	Indications	Adverse Effects
Cytokines and Immuno-modulators			
Interferon alfa-2b (Intron A)	Inhibits DNA and protein synthesis Suppresses cell proliferation Increases cytotoxic effects of NK cells	Hairy cell leukemia, chronic myelogenous leukemia, malignant melanoma, renal cell carcinoma, non-Hodgkin's lymphoma, ovarian cancer, multiple myeloma, Kaposi's sarcoma, pancreatic carcinoma	Flu-like syndrome (fever, chills, myalgia, headache), cognitive changes, fatigue, nausea, vomiting, anorexia, weight loss
Interleukin-2 (aldesleukin [Proleukin])	Stimulates proliferation of T and B cells Activates NK cells	Metastatic renal cell cancer, metastatic melanoma	Same as those of interferon alfa-2b; capillary leak syndrome, resulting in hypotension; bone marrow suppression
Levamisole	Potentiates monocytes and macrophage function	Stage III colon cancer (given in combination with 5-fluorouracil)	Diarrhea, metallic taste, nausea, fever, chills, mouth sores, headache
Bacille Calmette-Guérin vaccine	Induces an immune response that prevents angiogenesis of tumour	In situ bladder cancer	Flu-like syndrome, nausea, vomiting, rash, cough
Tyrosine Kinase Inhibitors			
Cetuximab (Erbitux)	Inhibits epidermal growth factor receptor, which is coupled with tyrosine kinase	Colorectal cancer, in combination with radiotherapy for head and neck carcinoma	Rash, dry skin, infusion reactions, interstitial lung disease, fatigue, fever
Erlotinib (Tarceva) and gefitinib (Iressa)	Same as for cetuximab	Non–small cell lung cancer	Rash, diarrhea, interstitial lung disease
Imatinib (Gleevec)	Inhibits *bcr-abl* tyrosine kinase	Chronic myeloid leukemia	Nausea, diarrhea, myalgia, fluid retention
Sorafenib (Nexavar)	Inhibits several tyrosine kinases, some of which are involved in angiogenesis	Advanced renal cell carcinoma	Rash, diarrhea, hypertension; redness, pain, swelling, or blisters on hands and feet
Monoclonal Antibody to CD20			
Rituximab (Rituxan)	Binds CD20 antigen, causing cytotoxicity	Non-Hodgkin's lymphoma (B cell)	Fever, chills, nausea, headache, angioedema
Ibritumomab tiuxetan–yttrium-90 (Zevalin)	Binds CD20 antigen, causing cytotoxicity and radiation injury	Non-Hodgkin's lymphoma (B cell)	Bone marrow suppression, fatigue, nausea, chills
Angiogenesis Inhibitor			
Bevacizumab (Avastin)	Binds vascular endothelial growth factor, thereby inhibiting angiogenesis	Colorectal cancer	Hypertension, colon bleeding and perforation, impaired wound healing, thrombo-embolism, diarrhea
Proteosome Inhibitor			
Bortezomib (Velcade)	Inhibits proteasome activity, which functions to regulate cell growth	Multiple myeloma	Bone marrow suppression, nausea, vomiting, diarrhea, peripheral neuropathy, fatigue
Monoclonal Antibodies			
Gemtuzumab ozogamicin (Mylotarg)	Binds CD33 antigen (expressed on leukemic cells) to deliver cytotoxic drug into the DNA	Acute myeloid leukemia	Bone marrow suppression, fever, chills, nausea
Alemtuzumab (Campath)	Binds CD52 antigen (found on T and B cells, monocytes, NK cells, neutrophils)	Chronic lymphocytic leukemia (B cell)	Bone marrow suppression, chills, fever, vomiting, diarrhea, fatigue
Trastuzumab (Herceptin)	Binds HER2	Breast cancer (HER2 positive)	Cardiotoxicity

HER2, human epidermal growth factor receptor 2; *NK*, natural killer.

FIGURE 18-17 Sites of action of targeted therapy. *EGFR*, epidermal growth factor receptor; *HER2*, human epidermal growth factor receptor 2; *VEGF*, vascular endothelial growth factor.

include interferons, interleukins, colony-stimulating factors, and TNF. Interferons were the first type of cytokine to be studied as a cancer therapy. Interferons protect cells infected by viruses from attack by other viruses and inhibit replication of viral DNA. The antiproliferative effects of interferons are not completely understood. However, they have been shown to inhibit DNA and protein synthesis in some tumour cells and to stimulate the expression of tumour antigens on tumour cell surfaces. Because the interferons have antiviral and antitumour effects, they are used to treat a number of medical conditions, including hepatitis C and Kaposi's sarcoma. The severity of adverse effects of interferons depends on the dose and the route of administration. One of the most common adverse effects is flu-like syndrome, which includes fever, chills, myalgia, and headache. Targeted therapy interferes with cancer growth by targeting specific cellular receptors and pathways that are important for tumour growth. The targeted therapies are more selective for specific molecular targets than are cancer drugs and are thus able to kill cancer cells without damaging normal cells. Targeted therapies include tyrosine kinase inhibitors, monoclonal antibodies, antiangiogenic agents such as VEGF receptor inhibitors, and interleukins.

Tyrosine kinases are important enzymes that activate the signalling pathways regulating cell proliferation and survival. For example, epidermal growth factor receptor (EGFR) is expressed in cells of epithelial origin, which rely on these receptors for repair and maintenance. EGFR is overexpressed in a wide variety of tumours, including non–small cell lung cancer, head and neck cancers, and pancreatic tumours and gliomas. Overexpression of EGFR is correlated with poor prognosis, increased recurrence rates, and resistance to chemotherapy. As such, it is an appealing target for cancer therapy. Erlotinib (Tarceva) and gefitinib (Iressa) are examples of EGFR tyrosine kinase inhibitors used in the treatment of non–small cell lung cancer.

Produced by B lymphocytes, monoclonal antibodies are antibodies (immunoglobulins) that are capable of binding to specific target cells, including tumour cells. Monoclonal antibodies can be unconjugated or conjugated. Unconjugated monoclonal antibodies are used alone to attack tumour cells directly. Conjugated monoclonal antibodies are attached to agents such as radioisotopes, toxins, chemotherapeutic agents, and other biological agents. The goal of this approach is to deliver the monoclonal antibody complex directly to the targeted cancer cells for their ultimate destruction. The antibodies also may stimulate an immune response in patients. Hybridoma technology

for the production of monoclonal antibodies is described in Chapter 16.

The first monoclonal antibody approved for use in oncological treatment was rituximab (Rituxan), an unconjugated monoclonal antibody directed against the CD20 antigen found on the surface of B lymphocytes. Human epidermal growth factor receptor 2 (HER2) is overexpressed in certain cancers (especially breast cancer) and is associated with more aggressive disease and decreased rates of survival. Trastuzumab (Herceptin) is an unconjugated monoclonal antibody that binds to HER2 and inhibits the growth of breast cancer cells that express the HER2 protein.

The most common type of conjugated monoclonal antibody is an immunotoxin, a molecule formed when a monoclonal antibody is conjugated to a plant or bacterial cell toxin. The most frequently used bacterial toxins to date have been *Pseudomonas* exotoxin and diphtheria toxin. Unfortunately, immunotoxins have shown poor clinical efficacy thus far and are associated with significant toxic effects.

Monoclonal antibodies are administered by infusion. Patients may experience infusion-related symptoms, which can include fever, chills, urticaria, mucosal congestion, nausea, diarrhea, and myalgias. There is also a risk, although rare, of anaphylaxis associated with the administration of monoclonal antibodies. This potential exists because most monoclonal antibodies are produced by mouse lymphocytes and thus represent a foreign protein to the human body. Onset of anaphylaxis can occur within 5 minutes of administration and can be a life-threatening event. (See Chapter 16 for a discussion of nursing management of anaphylaxis.) Other toxic effects of monoclonal antibodies may include hepatotoxicity, bone marrow depression, and CNS effects. Patients who receive trastuzumab may also experience cardiac dysfunction, especially when it is administered in higher doses or in combination with anthracycline antibiotics such as doxorubicin (Adriamycin).

Angiogenesis inhibitors work by preventing the mechanisms and pathways necessary for the vascularization of tumours. Bevacizumab (Avastin), a recombinant human monoclonal antibody, is active against the VEGF molecule, a crucial regulator of normal and pathological angiogenesis. Adverse effects of bevacizumab include hypertension, hemorrhage, and thromboembolic events. Its use is indicated in the treatment of colorectal cancer, and trials are being conducted to treat a number of other cancers.

Interleukins are a family of cytokines that act primarily between lymphocytes to induce activation of the immune system or alteration in the functional capacity of tumour cells. To date, 29 interleukins have been discovered, and each is designated by number, but only IL-2 has been approved as an anticancer agent. Aldesleukin (Proleukin) is a recombinant form of IL-2 used in the treatment of metastatic renal cell carcinoma, acute myelogenous leukemia, and lymphoma.

A major toxic effect of IL-2 therapy is capillary leak syndrome, which occurs as a result of changes in capillary permeability and vascular tone. As a consequence of the increase in capillary permeability, fluids shift from intravascular to extravascular compartments. This causes intravascular fluid depletion. Manifestations of capillary leak syndrome include hypotension, peripheral edema, ascites, interstitial pulmonary infiltrates, weight gain, and decreased systemic vascular resistance. Additional toxic effects of IL-2 therapy include renal, cardiovascular, pulmonary, GI, and integumentary toxic effects; bone marrow suppression; and changes in cognitive function. (Note: Provincial and territorial care programs and drug benefits programs may vary; the nurse should consult the employer's protocols and formulary.)

Hematopoietic Growth Factors

Colony-Stimulating Factors. Colony-stimulating factors are a family of glycoproteins produced by various cells. These glycoproteins stimulate production, maturation, regulation, and activation of cells of the hematological system. After release, colony-stimulating factors attach to receptors on the cell surface of peripheral blood cells and hematopoietic precursors (precursors of mature blood cells). They then stimulate production, maturation, release from the bone marrow, and functional ability of blood cells. The name of the colony-stimulating factor is based on the specific cell line it affects: granulocyte colony–stimulating factor (G-CSF), granulocyte-macrophage colony–stimulating factor (GM-CSF), macrophage colony–stimulating factor (M-CSF), and multicolony-stimulating factor, also known as *interleukin-3* (IL-3).

Colony-stimulating factors have a number of potential clinical uses. They may hasten recovery from bone marrow depression after standard and high-dose chemotherapy and bone marrow transplantation or decrease bone marrow suppression associated with administration of chemotherapeutic agents. Colony-stimulating factors may also re-establish bone marrow function in aplastic anemia, myelodysplastic syndrome, and leukemia and may be effective in the management of sepsis.

G-CSF is available as filgrastim (Neupogen) for the treatment of neutropenia. Pegfilgrastim (Neulasta) is a longer-acting form of filgrastim. G-CSF stimulates the production and function of neutrophils. It can be administered subcutaneously or by intravenous infusion. The most commonly reported adverse effect of G-CSF therapy is medullary bone pain, which occurs most often in the lower back, the pelvis, and the sternum. This pain generally develops at the time the neutrophil count begins to recover and lasts for about 24 hours. The pain associated with G-CSF therapy is usually relieved with nonopioid analgesics.

GM-CSF is available as sargramostim (Leukine, Prokine) for the treatment of (a) neutropenia associated with bone marrow transplantation, (b) bone marrow transplant failure or delay in bone marrow engraftment, and (c) acute myelogenous leukemia after chemotherapy. GM-CSF stimulates the production and function of neutrophils, eosinophils, and monocytes. In addition, GM-CSF stimulates these cells to produce cytokines. GM-CSF can be administered either subcutaneously or by intravenous infusion. The most common adverse effects associated with GM-CSF administration include medullary bone pain (similar to the bone pain associated with G-CSF administration), leukocytosis, and eosinophilia.

IL-3 is a multipotential stimulator of hematopoietic stem cells. IL-3 has been shown to stimulate the growth of neutrophils, monocytes, eosinophils, basophils, and platelet cell lines. IL-3 is being investigated for the treatment of bone marrow failure and for its ability to enhance myeloid recovery after chemotherapy, radiotherapy, and bone marrow transplantation. M-CSF is also undergoing investigation for its potential role in cancer treatment.

Erythropoietin. Erythropoietin is a colony-stimulating factor responsible for stimulating growth of the erythroid precursor cells that ultimately mature into RBCs. Erythropoietin is produced naturally by the kidneys. Erythropoietin was initially approved for the management of chronic anemia associated with end-stage renal disease. Subsequently, approval was expanded to include the use of erythropoietin (Eprex) for the management of chemotherapy-related anemia. Darbepoetin alfa (Aranesp), a long-acting form of erythropoietin, is now available.

Toxic and Adverse Effects of Biological Agents

The administration of one biological agent usually induces the endogenous release of others. The release and action of these biological agents result in systemic immune and inflammatory responses. The toxic effects and adverse effects of biological agents are related to dose and schedule. Common adverse effects, especially with interferons, include constitutional flu-like symptoms such as headache, fever, chills, myalgias, fatigue, malaise, weakness, photosensitivity, anorexia, and nausea. The severity of the flu-like symptoms associated with interferon therapy generally decreases over time. Acetaminophen administered every 4 hours, as prescribed, often reduces the severity of the flu-like syndrome. Many patients undergoing treatment with biological agents receive premedication with acetaminophen in an attempt to prevent or decrease the intensity of these symptoms. In addition, large amounts of fluids help decrease the intensity of symptoms.

Tachycardia and orthostatic hypotension are also commonly reported. IL-2 and monoclonal antibodies can cause capillary leak syndrome, with resulting pulmonary edema. Other toxic and adverse effects may involve the CNS and the renal, hepatic, and cardiovascular systems. These effects are found particularly with interferons and IL-2.

NURSING MANAGEMENT BIOLOGICAL THERAPY

Problems experienced by patients receiving biological therapy may differ in type or severity from those observed with more traditional forms of cancer therapy. For example, capillary leak syndrome and pulmonary edema are problems that necessitate expertise in critical care nursing. Bone marrow depression occurring with administration of biological agents is generally more transient and milder than that observed with chemotherapy, but fatigue associated with biological therapy can be so severe that it may constitute a dose-limiting toxic effect.

Nursing interventions for flu-like syndrome include the administration of acetaminophen before treatment and every 4 hours after treatment. Intravenous meperidine (Demerol) has been used to control the severe chills associated with some biological agents. Other nursing measures include monitoring of vital signs and temperature, planning for periods of rest for patients, and assisting with activities of daily living.

With interferon and IL-2 therapy, numerous neurological deficits have been observed. The nature and extent of these problems have not been completely elucidated. However, these problems are frightening to patients and the family, who must be taught to observe for neurological problems (e.g., confusion, memory loss, difficulty making decisions, insomnia), report their occurrence, and institute appropriate safety and support measures. (Note: Provincial care programs and drug benefits programs may vary: the nurse should consult the employer's protocols and formulary.)

BONE MARROW AND STEM CELL TRANSPLANTATION

Bone marrow transplantation (BMT) is an effective, lifesaving procedure for a number of malignant and nonmalignant diseases (Table 18-17). BMT allows for the safe use of very high doses

TABLE 18-17   USES FOR BONE MARROW TRANSPLANTATION

Malignant Diseases	Nonmalignant Diseases
• Acute and chronic myelogenous leukemia	• Aplastic anemia
• Acute lymphocytic leukemia	• Immunodeficiency diseases
• Hodgkin's lymphoma	• Severe autoimmune diseases
• Multiple myeloma	• Sickle cell disease
• Myelodysplastic syndrome	• Thalassemia
• Neuroblastoma	
• Non-Hodgkin's lymphoma	
• Ovarian cancer	
• Sarcoma	
• Testicular cancer	

of chemotherapeutic agents or radiation to patients whose tumours are resistant or unresponsive to standard doses of chemotherapeutic agents and radiation. BMT offers hope to many patients whose disease is responsive to increased doses of systemic therapy. The numbers of BMT and transplantation programs in Canada have increased dramatically since 2005.

Whether the diagnosis is a malignant or nonmalignant disease, the goal of BMT is cure. Cure rates are still low but are steadily increasing. Even if there is no cure, most transplantation procedures result in a period of remission. BMT is an intensive procedure with many risks, and some patients die from complications of BMT or from relapse of the original disease. Because it is a highly toxic therapy, patients must weigh the significant risks of treatment-related death or treatment failure (relapse) against the hope of cure.

Types of Bone Marrow Transplants

Bone marrow transplants can be allogeneic, autologous, or syngeneic. In *allogeneic marrow transplantation,* the infused bone marrow is acquired from a donor who has been matched to the recipient in terms of human leukocyte antigen (HLA) tissue typing. HLA typing involves testing WBCs to identify genetically inherited antigens common to both donor and recipient that are important in compatibility of transplanted tissue. (HLA tissue typing is discussed in Chapter 16.) The donor is often a family member, but an unrelated donor may be found through a bone marrow registry. The goal is to administer large doses of systemic therapy and then "rescue" the bone marrow through the engraftment and subsequent normal proliferation and differentiation of the donated marrow in the recipient. The most common indication for allogeneic transplantation is leukemia.

In *autologous marrow transplantation,* patients receive their own bone marrow. The aim of this approach is to enable patients to receive intensive chemotherapy or radiation while supporting them with their own bone marrow. In this type of BMT, the patient's own marrow is removed, treated, stored, and reinfused.

A third type of BMT, *syngeneic marrow transplantation,* involves obtaining stem cells from one identical twin and infusing them into the other. Identical twins have identical HLA types and are a perfect match.

Procedures

Harvest Procedures. Bone marrow can be "harvested" through a procedure conducted in the operating room with the patient under general or spinal anaesthesia in which multiple bone marrow aspirations are carried out, usually from the iliac crest but also from the sternum. The entire harvesting procedure usually takes 1 to 2 hours, and the patient can be discharged after recovery. After the procedure, the donor may experience pain at the collection site, which can be treated with mild analgesics. The donor's body replaces the bone marrow in a few weeks.

After harvesting, autologous bone marrow may be treated (*purged*) to remove cancer cells. Many different pharmacological, immunological, physical, and chemical agents have been used for this purpose. The bone marrow is then frozen (*cryopreserved*) and stored until it is used for transplantation. In allogeneic transplantation, the marrow can be harvested, processed, and infused into the recipient within a few hours of donation.

Preparative Regimens. In malignant diseases, the goal of BMT is to rescue the marrow after the patient has received high doses of chemotherapeutic agents, with or without radiation, aimed at treating the underlying disease. After harvesting of the marrow, the patient is given high-dose chemotherapy with or without radiation therapy. Total body irradiation can be used for immuno-suppression or to treat the disease.

After the therapy, the marrow that was removed is thawed and administered to the patient intravenously to replace the destroyed marrow. The stem cells reconstitute, or "rescue," the recipient's hematopoietic system. Usually 2 to 4 weeks are required for the transplanted marrow to start producing hematopoietic blood cells. During this pancytopenic period, it is critical for the patient to be in a protective isolation environment and receive supportive care. RBC and platelet transfusions are usually necessary to maintain the necessary quantity of circulating RBCs and platelets.

Complications. Bacterial, viral, and fungal infections are common after BMT. Prophylactic antibiotic therapy may reduce their incidence. A potentially serious complication of allogeneic transplant is graft-versus-host disease. This occurs when the T lymphocytes from the donated marrow (graft) respond to the recipient (host) cells as if they were foreign and begin to attack certain organs such as the skin, the liver, and the intestines. Graft-versus-host disease is discussed in Chapter 16. Another major adverse event is inadequate oral intake, which results in dehydration and malnutrition and thereby necessitates intensive nutritional support through a variety of interventions, such as oral supplementation and enteral feeding.

Peripheral Stem Cell Transplantation

An alternative to the harvest procedure is *peripheral stem cell transplantation* (PSCT). Peripheral (circulating) stem cells are capable of repopulating the bone marrow. PSCT is a type of transplantation that differs from BMT primarily in the method of stem cell collection. Because the blood contains fewer stem cells than does the bone marrow, stem cells from the bone marrow can be mobilized into the peripheral blood through chemotherapy or hematopoietic growth factors. Common growth factors that are used are GM-CSF and G-CSF. The donor's blood is collected, the peripheral stem cells are separated by means of a cell separator machine, and then the blood is returned through a venous line to the patient. This procedure is called *leukapheresis* and usually takes 2 to 4 hours to complete. In autologous transplantation, the stem cells are purged to kill any cancer cells and then frozen and stored until used for transplantation. Although many of the same steps (harvesting, intensive chemotherapy, reinfusion) of BMT are used in PSCT, the hematological recovery period in PSCT is shorter and produces fewer, less severe complications.

Cord Blood Stem Cells

Umbilical cord blood is rich in hematopoietic stem cells, and successful allogeneic transplantation has been performed with the use of this source. Cord blood can be HLA typed and cryopreserved. A disadvantage of cord blood is the possibly insufficient numbers of stem cells for transplantation into adults.

GENE THERAPY

Gene therapy involves the transfer of exogenous genes (transgenes) into the cells of patients in an effort to correct the defective gene. The effect of gene therapy for cancer can be a temporary gene transfer with the additional goal of instigating an immune response to the transgene. The use of this new therapeutic approach for cancer is currently investigational. Several clinical trials are under way to evaluate the safety, tolerability, and efficacy of gene therapy for malignancies such as melanoma, brain tumours, and mesothelioma. (Gene therapy is discussed in Chapter 15.)

COMPLICATIONS RESULTING FROM CANCER

Patients may develop complications related to the continual growth of the malignancy or the adverse effects of treatment.

Nutritional Problems

Malnutrition. Many patients with cancer experience protein and calorie malnutrition, characterized by depletion of fat and muscle. (Assessment of the degree of malnutrition is discussed in Chapter 42.) See the Resources at the end of this chapter for lists of foods suggested for increasing the protein intake to facilitate repair and regeneration of cells; high-caloric foods that provide energy and minimize weight loss; and a sample high-calorie, high-protein diet.

The nurse should suggest a referral to a dietitian as soon as a 5% weight loss is noted or if the patient has the potential for protein and caloric malnutrition. Albumin and prealbumin levels should be monitored. Once a 4.5-kg weight loss occurs, it is difficult to maintain optimal nutritional status. The patient can be taught to use nutritional supplements in place of milk when cooking or baking. Foods to which nutritional supplements can be easily added include scrambled eggs, pudding, custard, mashed potatoes, cereal, and cream sauces. Packages of instant breakfast can be used as indicated or sprinkled on cereals, desserts, and casseroles.

Malnutrition may occur as a result of the effects of cancer and cancer treatments. Patients may also radically alter their diets because of beliefs that certain foods support the growth or treatment of cancer. A discussion about the patient's dietary practices thus facilitates mutual understanding and education.

If the malnutrition cannot be treated with dietary intake, it may be necessary to use enteral or parenteral supplementation as an adjunct nutritional measure. (Enteral and parenteral nutrition are discussed in Chapter 42.)

Altered Taste Sensation. It is theorized that cancer cells release substances that resemble amino acids and stimulate the bitter taste buds. Patients may also experience an alteration in the sweet, sour, and salty taste sensations. Meat may taste bitter to patients. The physiological basis of these taste alterations is unclear. It is important to help patients (a) understand the changes that will be experienced and (b) find foods that are appealing.

Many Canadians are from different cultural and ethnic groups, and the nurse must be aware of possible differences in meal preparation and selection that are acceptable to patients. Patients can be encouraged to experiment with spices and other seasoning agents to taste in an attempt to mask the taste alterations.

Infection

Infection can cause death in a patient whose immune system is suppressed as a result of cancer treatment. The usual sites of infection include the lungs, genitourinary system, mouth, rectum, peritoneal cavity, and blood (septicemia). Infection occurs as a result of the ulceration and necrosis caused by the tumour, compression of vital organs by the tumour, and neutropenia caused by the disease process or the treatment of cancer. A critical aspect of nursing care is teaching about infection risk associated with neutropenia. A patient with a body temperature of 38°C (100.5°F) or higher should be seen at the hospital or cancer centre as soon as possible. Assessment most often includes signs and symptoms of fever, determination of possible cause, and complete blood cell count.

Many patients are neutropenic when an infection develops. In such individuals, infection causes significant morbidity and may be rapidly fatal if not treated promptly. The classical manifestations of infection are often not present in a patient with neutropenia and a depressed immune system. (Neutropenia is discussed in Chapter 33.)

Oncological Emergencies

Oncological emergencies are life-threatening events that can occur as a result of cancer or cancer treatment. These emergencies can be obstructive, metabolic, or infiltrative.

Obstructive Emergencies. Obstructive emergencies are caused primarily by tumour obstruction of an organ or a blood vessel. Obstructive emergencies include superior vena cava syndrome, spinal cord compression syndrome, third space syndrome, and intestinal obstruction.

Superior Vena Cava Syndrome. *Superior vena cava syndrome* results from obstruction of the superior vena cava by a tumour. The clinical manifestations include facial edema, periorbital edema, distension of veins of the neck and chest, headache, and seizures. A mediastinal mass is often visible on chest radiographs. The most common causes are Hodgkin's disease, non-Hodgkin's lymphoma, and lung cancer. Superior vena cava syndrome is considered a serious medical problem, and management usually involves radiation therapy to the site of obstruction and treatment of the primary tumour. Chemotherapeutic agents may be administered concurrently with the radiation therapy

Spinal Cord Compression. *Spinal cord compression* is a neurological emergency caused by the presence of a malignant tumour in the epidural space of the spinal cord. The most common primary tumours that produce this problem are melanoma and cancers of the breast, lung, prostate, GI system, and kidneys. Lymphomas also pose a risk if diseased lymph tissue invades the epidural space. The manifestations are back pain that is intense, localized, and persistent, accompanied by vertebral tenderness and aggravated by the Valsalva manoeuvre; motor weakness and dysfunction; sensory paresthesia and loss; and autonomic dysfunction. One of the clinical symptoms that reflect autonomic dysfunction is a change in bowel or bladder function. The nurse should carefully assess for potential signs or symptoms related to cord compression. Radiation therapy is used for patients with slowly progressive neurological deficits and radiosensitive tumours. Surgery is usually recommended for patients with rapidly progressive neurological signs, especially if the tumours are relatively radiologically resistant.

Third Space Syndrome. *Third space syndrome* involves a shifting of fluid from the vascular space to the interstitial space that results primarily from extensive surgical procedures, biological therapy, or septic shock. Initially, affected patients exhibit signs of hypovolemia, including hypotension, tachycardia, low central venous pressure, and decreased urine output. Treatment includes fluid, electrolyte, and plasma protein replacement. During recovery, hypervolemia can occur, resulting in hypertension, elevated central venous pressure, weight gain, and shortness of breath. Treatment generally involves reduction in fluid administration and fluid balance monitoring.

Intestinal Obstruction. Intestinal obstruction occurs when partial or complete obstruction of the intestine prevents the passage of the intestinal contents through the GI tract. This can cause nausea, vomiting, abdominal pain, or even more serious problems, such as bowel necrosis. It necessitates prompt treatment. Chapter 45 contains a complete discussion of intestinal obstruction.

Metabolic Emergencies. Metabolic emergencies are caused by the production of ectopic hormones directly from the tumour or are secondary to cancer treatment. Ectopic hormones can arise in tumours because their cells are less differentiated than normal cells, enabling re-expression of genes that are suppressed in normal development. Metabolic emergencies include syndrome of inappropriate antidiuretic hormone (SIADH), hypercalcemia, tumour lysis syndrome (TLS), septic shock, and disseminated intravascular coagulation.

Syndrome of Inappropriate Antidiuretic Hormone. SIADH results from abnormal or sustained production of antidiuretic hormone (see Chapter 51). SIADH occurs most frequently with carcinoma of the lung but can also occur with cancers of the pancreas, duodenum, brain, esophagus, colon, ovary, prostate, bronchus, and nasopharynx and with leukemia, mesothelioma, reticulum cell sarcoma, Hodgkin's disease, thymoma, and lymphosarcoma. Cancer cells in these tumours are actually able to manufacture, store, and release antidiuretic hormone. The chemotherapeutic agents vincristine and cyclophosphamide (Procytox) also stimulate the release of antidiuretic hormone from the pituitary or tumour cells. Symptoms of SIADH include weight gain, weakness, anorexia, nausea, vomiting, personality changes, seizures, and coma. Treatment of SIADH includes fluid restriction and, in severe cases, intravenous administration of 3% sodium chloride solution.

Hypercalcemia. Hypercalcemia can occur in the presence of cancer that involves the bone, as in metastatic disease of the bone or multiple myeloma, or when a parathyroid hormone–like substance is secreted by cancer cells in the absence of bone metastasis (Kurtin, 2014). Hypercalcemia resulting from malignancies that have metastasized occurs most frequently in patients with lung, breast, kidney, colon, ovarian, or thyroid cancer. Hypercalcemia resulting from secretion of parathyroid hormone–like substance occurs most frequently in patients with hypernephromas; squamous cell carcinoma of the lung; head and neck, cervical, and esophageal cancers; lymphomas; and leukemia. Immobility and dehydration can contribute to or exacerbate hypercalcemia.

The primary manifestations of hypercalcemia include apathy, depression, fatigue, muscle weakness, electrocardiographic changes, polyuria and nocturia, anorexia, nausea, and vomiting. Serum levels of calcium in excess of 3 mmol/L can be life-threatening. Chronic hypercalcemia can result in nephrocalcinosis and irreversible renal failure. The long-term treatment of hypercalcemia is aimed at the primary disease. Acute hypercalcemia is treated by hydration (3 L/day), diuretic administration (particularly loop diuretics), and a bisphosphonate, a drug that inhibits the action of osteoclasts. Infusion of a bisphosphonate is the treatment of choice.

Tumour Lysis Syndrome. Acute TLS is a metabolic complication that occurs in some patients with cancer and is frequently triggered by chemotherapy. It results from the rapid destruction of a large number of tumour cells, which can cause fatal biochemical changes. TLS is often associated with tumours that have high growth rates and are sensitive to the effects of chemotherapy. If not identified and treated quickly, TLS can result in acute renal failure.

The four hallmark signs of TLS are hyperuricemia, hyperphosphatemia, hyperkalemia, and hypocalcemia. TLS usually occurs within the first 24 to 48 hours after the initiation of chemotherapy and may persist for approximately 5 to 7 days. The primary goal of TLS management is preventing renal failure and severe electrolyte imbalances. The primary treatment includes increasing urine production through hydration therapy and decreasing uric acid concentrations through administration of allopurinol (Lydon, 2011).

Septic Shock and Disseminated Intravascular Coagulation. Septic shock is discussed in Chapter 69, and disseminated intravascular coagulation is discussed in Chapter 33.

Infiltrative Emergencies. Infiltrative emergencies occur when malignant tumours infiltrate major organs secondary to cancer therapy. The most common infiltrative emergencies are cardiac tamponade and carotid artery rupture.

Cardiac Tamponade. Cardiac tamponade results from fluid accumulation in the pericardial sac, constriction of the pericardium by tumour, or pericarditis secondary to radiation therapy for the chest. Manifestations include a heavy feeling over the chest, shortness of breath, tachycardia, cough, dysphagia, hiccups, hoarseness, nausea, vomiting, excessive perspiration, decreased level of consciousness, pulsus paradoxus, distant or muted heart sounds, and extreme anxiety. Emergency management is aimed at reduction of fluid around the heart and includes surgical establishment of a pericardial window or an indwelling pericardial catheter. Supportive therapy includes administration of oxygen therapy, intravenous hydration, and vasopressor therapy.

Carotid Artery Rupture. Rupture of the carotid artery occurs most frequently in patients with cancer of the head and neck as a result of invasion of the arterial wall by tumour or erosion after surgery or radiation therapy. Bleeding can manifest as minor oozing or, in the case of a bursting of the artery, spurting of blood. In the presence of bursting, pressure should be applied to the site with a finger. Intravenous fluid and blood products are administered in an attempt to stabilize the patient for surgery. Surgical management involves ligation of the carotid artery above and below the rupture site and reduction of local tumour.

MANAGEMENT OF CANCER PAIN

Moderate to severe pain occurs in approximately 50% of patients receiving active treatment for cancer and in 80% of those with advanced cancer. Despite progress made in cancer therapies, the incidence of cancer-related pain has not changed in decades. Cancer pain is commonly undertreated for a number of reasons, and this has a profound effect on patients' mood, functional status, and quality of life (Brant, 2011).

Inadequate pain assessment is a significant barrier to effective pain management. Data such as vital signs and patient behaviours are not reliable indicators of pain, especially longstanding, chronic pain. Therefore, it is essential that every patient with cancer be assessed for pain by the question "Do you have pain?" If the patient's self-report is affirmative, further data are obtained and documented initially and at regular intervals regarding the onset, the location, and the intensity of the pain, what it feels like, and how it is relieved. Patterns of change also should be assessed. The patient's pain report must be accepted as the primary source of assessment data. Drug therapy includes nonsteroidal anti-inflammatory medications, opioids, and adjuvant pain medications. Analgesic medications should be administered on a regular schedule, around the clock, with additional doses as needed for breakthrough pain. Oral administration of the medication is preferred. It is important to remember that with opioid drugs, such as morphine, the appropriate dose is whatever is necessary to control the pain with the least intrusive adverse effects. Principles of patient-controlled analgesia should also be followed. Fear of addiction is not warranted but must be addressed as part of patient teaching relevant to pain control because for both the patient and the nurse, it represents a significant barrier to appropriate pain management.

Nonpharmacological interventions, including relaxation therapy and imagery, can be effectively used to manage pain (see Chapter 12). (Additional strategies to relieve pain are discussed in Chapter 10.) More information on cancer pain management is available from cancer agency clinical practice guidelines, such as those on the BC Cancer Agency website (see the Resources at the end of this chapter).

PSYCHOSOCIAL CARE

Psychosocial care is an important aspect of cancer care. Supportive care includes services and strategies to help cancer patients and their families cope with the cancer experience. Because of the effectiveness of cancer treatment, cancer is cured in many patients, or the disease is controlled for long periods. In view of this trend in survival, an optimal quality of life must be maintained after the diagnosis of cancer. By understanding the effect of cancer on the patient and the family and by promoting services that can provide financial, social, and psychological counselling, the nurse can be more effective in assisting patients and families throughout their cancer experience.

A diagnosis of cancer may precipitate a crisis in the lives of the patient and his or her family, and repercussions may affect all aspects of their lives. Common fears experienced by the patient with cancer include disfigurement, dependency, unrelieved pain, financial depletion, abandonment, and death.

To cope with these fears, patients with cancer may use and experience different behavioural patterns: shock, anger, denial, bargaining, depression, helplessness, hopelessness, rationalization, acceptance, and intellectualization. These behavioural patterns may occur at any time during the process of cancer. However, some patterns appear to occur more frequently or at a greater intensity at certain specific stages of the disease process. The following factors may determine how a patient will cope with the diagnosis of cancer:

1. *Ability to cope with stressful events in the past* (e.g., loss of job, major disappointment): By simply asking how the patient has coped with stressful events, the nurse can obtain an understanding of the patient's coping patterns, the effectiveness of the usual coping patterns, and the usual coping time framework.
2. *Availability of significant others:* Patients who have effective support systems tend to cope more effectively than do patients who do not have a meaningful, available support system.
3. *Ability to express feelings and concerns:* Patients who are able to express feelings and needs and who seek and ask for help appear to cope more effectively than do patients who internalize feelings and needs.
4. *Age at the time of diagnosis:* Age determines the coping strategies to a great degree. For example, a young mother with cancer may have concerns that differ from those of a 70-year-old woman with cancer.
5. *Extent of disease:* Cure or control of the disease process is usually easier to cope with than the reality of terminal illness.
6. *Disruption of body image:* Such disruption (e.g., by radical neck dissection, alopecia, mastectomy) may intensify the psychological effect of cancer.
7. *Presence of symptoms:* Symptoms such as fatigue, nausea, diarrhea, and pain may intensify the psychological effect of cancer.
8. *Past experience with cancer:* If past experiences with cancer have been negative, the patient will probably view his or her current status as negative.
9. *Attitude associated with the cancer:* A patient who feels in control and has a positive attitude about cancer and cancer treatment is better able to cope with the diagnosis and treatment of cancer than is a patient who feels hopeless, helpless, and out of control.

To facilitate the development of a hopeful attitude about cancer and to support the patient and the family during the various stages of the process of cancer, the nurse should act on the following suggestions:

1. Be available and continue to be available for discussion with the patient and family, especially during difficult times.
2. Actively assess the patient's needs for counselling and refer him or her to appropriate services when necessary.
3. Listen actively to fears and concerns.
4. Offer strategies to enhance coping behaviours.
5. Provide essential information as the patient asks for it, and be sensitive to information overload.
6. Establish a therapeutic relationship based on trust and confidence; be open, honest, and caring in the approach.
7. Be "present" with the patient to offer comfort and assurance that the nurse cares about him or her.
8. Understand and collaborate with the patient to set realistic, reachable short- and long-term goals.
9. Encourage the patient to maintain usual lifestyle patterns.
10. Maintain hope. Hope varies, depending on the status of the patient: hope that the symptoms are not serious, hope that the treatment is curative, hope for independence, hope for relief of pain, hope for a longer life, or hope for a peaceful death. Hope provides control over what is occurring and is the basis of a positive attitude toward cancer and cancer care. The development of an advanced care plan may help to clarify patients' attitudes and provide reassurance that their wishes for future care will be respected. Consider the spiritual aspects of care; support patients in exploring their belief systems and in finding meaning that transcends cultural and religious boundaries. Nurses can assist patients

ETHICAL DILEMMAS

Medical Futility

Situation

A 65-year-old woman has breast cancer with metastasis to the liver and bone. The family asks the nurse why their mother is not receiving chemotherapy. In addition, family members want to make certain that she will be resuscitated should her heart stop. They are aware of her diagnosis and that she may have less than 1 month to live. The nurse was told in morning rounds that the woman does not want any treatment that would prolong her life.

Important Points for Consideration

- If the patient is competent, the patient is legally and ethically the decision maker with regard to his or her own care in consultation with the patient's family and the health care team as desired.
- Members of the health care team have no obligation to provide care that is medically futile. Care that is futile may be inappropriate, prolong dying, or provide little or no benefit to the patient.
- Palliative care is health care that would provide comfort, control pain, reduce symptoms, or improve the quality of her remaining life, as defined by the patient.
- Patients or families do not have a right to demand treatment that offers no clear benefit to the patient.
- The nurse should work in collaboration with other members of the health care team to have discussions with the family members, ease the acceptance of their mother's diagnosis, incorporate their mother's goals into the plan of care, discuss a do-not-resuscitate (DNR) order and a referral to hospice, and plan for her eventual death.

Clinical Decision-Making Questions

1. How can the nurse help the patient communicate her wishes to her family?
2. How can the nurse and the health care team help the family plan end-of-life care that incorporates the wishes of their mother?

modalities, nutritional supplements, and herbal therapies. The "unofficial" use of complementary and alternative medicines in oncology is widespread and has the potential to help (e.g., by relieving symptoms) or to harm (e.g., through associated toxic effects or by preventing or diminishing the effects of proven therapies). Patients may need support in understanding the difference between complementary and alternative therapies and the risks and benefits associated with complementary and alternative medicine.

Organizations and journals available as resources for the nurse are listed in the Resources section at the end of this chapter. The "Ethical Dilemmas" box is a description of considerations of nurse–family interactions when treatment is considered medically futile.

AGE-RELATED CONSIDERATIONS

CANCER

Cancer is usually a disease of aging. Most cancers occur in people older than 65 years. Cancer is the leading cause of death in people 65 to 74 years of age. Clinical manifestations of cancer in an older adult may be mistakenly attributed to age-related changes and ignored by the person.

Older adults are particularly vulnerable to the complications of both cancer and cancer therapy. This is because of their decline in physiological functioning, social and emotional resources, and cognitive function. The functional status and comorbid conditions of an older adult should be taken into consideration when a treatment plan is selected (Puts, Hardt, Monette, et al., 2012). Age alone is not a sufficient predictor of tolerance or response to treatment (Cheung, Le, Gagliese, et al., 2011).

Because of advances in the treatment of cancer, cancer therapies benefit an increasing number of older adults, including patients with suboptimal health. Some important questions to consider when cancer is diagnosed in an older person include the following: Will the treatment provide more benefit than harm? Will the patient be able to tolerate the treatment safely? What is the patient's choice of therapy?

in identifying their strengths and developing skills to cope with the emotional aspects of having cancer.

11. Encourage and facilitate patients' participation in their care. This may include considering their interest in the use of integrative therapies such as support groups, mind–body

REVIEW QUESTIONS

The number of the question corresponds to the same-numbered objective at the beginning of the chapter.

1. Which of the following is consistent with trends in the incidence and death rates of cancer?
   a. Lung cancer is the most common type of cancer in men.
   b. Breast cancer is the leading cause of cancer deaths in women.
   c. A higher percentage of women than men have lung cancer.
   d. The incidence of cancer increases as the population ages.
2. What features of cancer cells distinguish them from normal cells? *(Select all that apply.)*
   a. Cells lack contact inhibition.
   b. Cells return to a previous undifferentiated state.
   c. Oncogenes maintain normal cell expression.
   d. Proliferation occurs when there is a need for more cells.
   e. New proteins characteristic of embryonic stage emerge on cell membrane.
3. Which is a characteristic feature of the stage of progression in the development of cancer?
   a. Oncogenic viral transformation of target cells
   b. A reversible steady growth facilitated by carcinogens

   c. A period of latency before clinical detection of cancer
   d. The proliferation of cancer cells in spite of host control mechanisms
4. What is the primary protective role of the immune system in relation to malignant cells?
   a. Surveillance for cells with tumour-associated antigens
   b. The binding with free antigen released by malignant cells
   c. The production of blocking factors that immobilize cancer cells
   d. The response to a new set of antigenic determinants on cancer cells
5. What is the primary difference between benign and malignant neoplasms?
   a. The rate of cell proliferation
   b. The site of malignant tumour
   c. The requirements for cellular nutrients
   d. The characteristic of tissue invasiveness
6. Which nursing roles are important for the prevention and detection of cancer?
   a. Health promotion in relation to eating low-fibre, refined-carbohydrate diets
   b. Teaching about cancer risk factors

c. Encouraging the public to participate in regular screening tests for all detectable cancer sites

d. Using people's natural fear of cancer to motivate changes in unhealthy lifestyles

7. Which principle underpins a therapeutic approach to cancer?
   a. Surgery is the single most effective treatment for cancer.
   b. Initial treatment is always directed toward cure of the cancer.
   c. A combination of treatment modalities is effective for controlling many cancers.
   d. None of the above.

8. Which points would be part of nursing teaching for a client undergoing brachytherapy of the cervix?
   a. The client will learn that she must undergo simulation to locate the treatment area.
   b. The client will be taught about the treatment and need for staff time limitations in relation to her care.
   c. The client will be taught that she may experience desquamation of the skin on the abdomen and upper legs.
   d. The client will require shielding of the ovaries during treatment to prevent ovarian damage.

9. Which is the most effective method of administering a chemotherapeutic agent that is a vesicant?
   a. Giving it orally.
   b. Giving it intra-arterially.
   c. Using an Ommaya reservoir.
   d. Using a central venous access device.

10. Why does stomatitis, a common adverse effect of chemotherapeutic agents, occur?
    a. The site of the malignancy is near the oral cavity.
    b. The general health of the client with cancer is poor.
    c. Chemotherapeutic drugs have a local and irritating effect on epithelial cells.
    d. Rapidly dividing cells of the mucous membranes of the mouth are being destroyed.

11. In teaching the client about IL-2, which information will the nurse include?
    a. It stimulates the immune system.
    b. It inhibits DNA and protein synthesis in tumour cells.
    c. It decreases the antigenic expression of antigens on tumour cell surfaces.
    d. It prevents bone marrow suppression associated with chemotherapy.

12. Which information will the nurse provide to a client receiving radiation therapy or chemotherapy?
    a. Effective birth control methods should be used for the rest of the client's life.
    b. Notify the health care team if nausea and vomiting are experienced during treatment so that these can be managed.
    c. After successful treatment, the client returns to previous functional level.
    d. The cycle of fatigue-depression-fatigue that may occur during treatment can be reduced by restricting activity.

13. Which is an inappropriate nursing intervention to promote nutrition in the client with cancer?
    a. Providing bland, pureed food because the person's taste sensation is altered
    b. Providing increased protein for normal cell recovery and immune system function
    c. Encouraging the client to eat a high-calorie, high-protein snack every few hours to prevent weight loss
    d. Alerting the physician that nutritional supplements may be needed when the client has a 4-kg weight loss

14. What is the primary cause of syndrome of SIADH in cancer?
    a. Autoimmune reaction
    b. Gram-negative septicemia
    c. Invasiveness of cancer cells
    d. Ectopic hormonal production

15. A client has recently received a diagnosis of early-stage breast cancer. Which of the following is most appropriate for the nurse to focus on?
    a. Maintaining the client's hope
    b. Preparing a will and advance directives
    c. Discussing replacement child care for client's children
    d. Discussing the client's past experiences with her grandmother's cancer

1. d; 2. a, b, e; 3. d, 4. a; 5. d, 6. b; 7. c; 8. b; 9. d; 10. d; 11. a; 12. b; 13. a; 14. d; 15. a

ⓔvolve

For even more review questions, visit *http://evolve.elsevier.com/Canada/ Lewis/medsurg*.

REFERENCES

Beauchesne, P. (2010). Intrathecal chemotherapy for treatment of leptomeningeal dissemination of metastatic tumours. *The Lancet Oncology, 11*(9), 871–879. (Seminal).

Behrend, S. W. (2011). Radiation treatment planning. In C. H. Yarbro, D. Wujcik, & B. H. Gobel (Eds.), *Cancer nursing: Principles and practice* (7th ed., pp. 269–311). Sudbury, MA: Jones & Bartlett.

Brant, J. M. (2011). Pain and discomfort. In J. L. Lester & P. Schmitt (Eds.), *Cancer rehabilitation and survivorship: Transdisciplinary approaches to personalized care* (pp. 37–48). Pittsburgh: Oncology Nursing Society.

Canadian Association of Nurses in Oncology. (2011). *Standards of care, roles, and competencies*. Ottawa: Author.

Canadian Cancer Society's Steering Committee on Cancer Statistics. (2016). *Canadian cancer statistics 2016*. Toronto: Canadian Cancer Society.

Cheung, W. Y., Le, L. W., Gagliese, L., et al. (2011). Age and gender differences in symptom intensity and symptom clusters among patients with metastatic cancer. *Supportive Care in Cancer, 19*, 417–423. doi:10.1007/s00520-010-0865-2.

DeVita, V. T., Lawrence, T. S., & Rosenberg, S. A. (Eds.), (2014). *DeVita, Hellman, and Rosenberg's cancer: Principles and practice of oncology* (9th ed.). Philadelphia: Lippincott, Williams & Wilkins.

Eilers, J. G., Asakura, Y., Blecher, C. S., et al. (2014). *ONS PEP Resource: Mucositis*. Retrieved from *https://www.ons.org/ practice-resources/pep/mucositis*.

Gionet, L., & Roshanafshar, S. (2013). *Select health indicators of First Nations people living off reserve, Métis and Inuit*. Statistics Canada Catalogue no. 82-624-X. Retrieved from *http://www.statcan.gc.ca/ pub/82-624-x/2013001/article/11763-eng.htm*.

Gotay, C. C., Katzmarzyk, P. T., Janssen, I., et al. (2012). Updating the Canadian obesity maps: An epidemic in progress. *Canadian Journal of Public Health, 104*(1), e64–e68.

Harris, B., Ross, J., & Sanchez-Reilly, S. (2014). Sleeping in the arms of cancer: A review of sleeping disorders among patients with cancer. *The Cancer Journal*, 20(5), 299–305. doi:10.1097/PPO .0000000000000067.

Health Canada. (2011). *Eating well with Canada's Food Guide*. Retrieved from *http://www.hc-sc.gc.ca/fn-an/food-guide-aliment/ order-commander/index-eng.php#a1*.

Kurtin, S. (2014). Hypocalcemia/hypercalcemia. In D. Camp-Sorrell & R. A. Hawkins (Eds.), *Clinical manual for the oncology advanced practice nurse* (3rd ed., pp. 1275–1288). Pittsburgh: Oncology Nursing Society.

Lalla, R. V., Bowen, J., Barasch, A., et al.; Mucositis Guidelines Leadership Group of the Multinational Association of Supportive Care in Cancer and International Society of Oral Oncology (MASCC/ISOO). (2014). MASCC/ISOO clinical practice guidelines for the management of mucositis secondary to cancer therapy. *Cancer*, 120, 1453–1461.

Loud, J. T., & Hutson, S. P. (2011). Genetic risk and hereditary cancer syndromes. In C. H. Yarbro, D. Wujcik, & B. H. Gobel (Eds.), *Cancer nursing: Principles and practice* (7th ed., pp. 135–165). Sudbury, MA: Jones & Bartlett.

Lydon, J. (2011). Tumor lysis syndrome. In C. H. Yarbro, D. Wujcik, & B. H. Gobel (Eds.), *Cancer nursing: Principles and practice* (7th ed., pp. 1014–1030). Burlington, MA: Jones & Bartlett Learning.

Mustian, K. M., Sprod, L. K., Janelsins, M., et al. (2012). Exercise recommendations for cancer-related fatigue, cognitive impairment, sleep problems, depression, pain, anxiety and physical dysfunction: A review. *Oncology & Hematology Review*, 8, 81–88.

Puts, M. T. E., Hardt, J., Monette, J., et al. (2012). Use of geriatric assessment for older adults in the oncology setting: A systematic review. *Journal of the National Cancer Institute*, 104, 1133–1163. doi:10.1093/jnci/djs285.

Statistics Canada. (n.d.). *Health indicator profile, annual estimates, by age group and sex, Canada, provinces, territories, health regions (2013 boundaries) and peer groups, occasional (CANSIM Table 105-0501)*. Retrieved from *http://www5.statcan.gc.ca/cansim/a26 ?lang=eng&id=1050501*.

Statistics Canada. (2015). *Health fact sheets: The 10 leading causes of death, 2012*. Retrieved from *http://www.statcan.gc.ca/pub/82-625 -x/2015001/article/14296-eng.htm*.

Tannock, I. F., Hill, R. P., Bristow, R. G., et al. (Eds.). (2013). *The basic science of oncology* (5th ed.). New York: McGraw-Hill.

RESOURCES

Advance Care Planning
http://www.advancecareplanning.ca/

BC Cancer Agency: Cancer Management Guidelines
http://www.bccancer.bc.ca/HPI/CancerManagementGuidelines/ default.htm

BC Cancer Agency: Pain & Symptom Management
http://www.bccancer.bc.ca/HPI/CancerManagementGuidelines/ SupportiveCare/PainSymptomManagement

Canadian Association of Nurses in Oncology (CANO)
http://www.cano-acio.ca

Canadian Association of Provincial Cancer Agencies (CAPCA)
http://www.capca.ca

Canadian Association of Psychosocial Oncology (CAPO)
http://www.capo.ca

Canadian Breast Cancer Research Alliance (CBCRA)
http://www.breast.cancer.ca

Canadian Cancer Society
http://www.cancer.ca

Canadian Cancer Society: Look Good, Feel Better
http://www.cancer.ca/en/support-and-services/support-services/ look-good-feel-better-qc/?region=qc

Canadian Cancer Society: Talk to an Information Service
http://www.cancer.ca/canada-wide/support%20services/cancer%20 information%20service.aspx

Canadian Hospice Palliative Care Association
http://www.chpca.net

Canadian Institute of Health Information (CIHI)
https://www.cihi.ca/en

Canadian Oncology Nursing Journal (CONJ)
http://cano.malachite-mgmt.com/?page=CONJOnline

Canadian Virtual Hospice
http://www.virtualhospice.ca

Cancer Care Ontario: Program in Evidence-Based Care: Practice Guidelines
https://www.cancercare.on.ca/cms/One.aspx?portalId=1377 &pageId=10144

Cancer News on the Net
http://www.cancernews.com

Cancer Research Society
http://www.cancer-research-society.ca

Canadian Strategy for Cancer Control
http://www.partnershipagainstcancer.ca

Cancer Symptoms
http://www.cancer-symptoms.com

Colorectal Cancer Association of Canada
http://www.colorectal-cancer.ca/

Evidence-Informed Treatment Guidelines in British Columbia
http://www.bccancer.bc.ca

Evidence-Informed Treatment Guidelines in Ontario
https://www.cancercare.on.ca

Institute for Clinical Evaluative Studies (ICES)
http://www.ices.on.ca

Prostate Cancer Canada Network (CPCN)
http://prostatecancer.ca/

Psychosocial Oncology Research Training (PORT)
http://www.port.mcgill.ca

Screening Guidelines for Early Detection of Cancer in Asymptomatic People
http://www.cancer.ca/en/prevention-and-screening/early-detection- and-screening/screening/?region=on

American Association for Cancer Education (AACE)
http://www.aaceonline.com

International Society of Nurses in Cancer Care
http://www.isncc.org

Karnofsky Performance Status Scale
http://oncologypro.esmo.org/Guidelines-Practice/Practice-Tools/Performance-Scales

National Coalition for Cancer Survivorship (NCS)
http://www.canceradvocacy.org

National Institute for Occupational Safety and Health (NIOSH): Preventing Occupational Exposures to Antineoplastic and Other Hazardous Drugs in Health Care Settings
http://www.cdc.gov/niosh/docs/2004-165/pdf

Nutritional Therapy: High Calorie Foods
http://www.mayoclinic.org/diseases-conditions/cancer/in-depth/cancer/art-20045046?pg=2

Nutritional Therapy Protein Foods With High Biological Value
https://www.oncolink.org/support/nutrition-and-cancer/during-and-after-treatment/protein-needs-during-cancer-treatment

OncoLink (cancer information site)
http://www.oncolink.upenn.edu

Oncology Nursing Society
https://www.ons.org

Union for International Cancer Control
http://www.uicc.ch

For additional Internet resources, see the website for this book at *http://evolve.elsevier.com/Canada/Lewis/medsurg*

Fluid, Electrolyte, and Acid–Base Imbalances

Written by: Mariann M. Harding
Adapted by: Jana Lok

evolve WEBSITE

http://evolve.elsevier.com/Canada/Lewis/medsurg

- Review Questions (Online Only)
- Key Points
- Answer Guideline for Case Study
- Student Case Study
  - Hyponatremia/Fluid Volume Imbalance
- Conceptual Care Map Creator
- Fluids and Electrolytes Tutorial
- Audio Glossary
- Content Updates

LEARNING OBJECTIVES

1. Describe the composition of the major body fluid compartments.
2. Define processes involved in the regulation of the movement of water and electrolytes between the body fluid compartments.
3. Describe the etiology, laboratory diagnostic findings, clinical manifestations, and nursing and collaborative management of the following disorders:
   a. Water excess and deficit
   b. Sodium and volume imbalances: hypernatremia and hyponatremia
   c. Potassium imbalance: hyperkalemia and hypokalemia
   d. Magnesium imbalance: hypermagnesemia and hypomagnesemia

   e. Calcium imbalance: hypercalcemia and hypocalcemia
   f. Phosphate imbalance: hyperphosphatemia and hypophosphatemia
4. Identify the processes of acid–base regulation.
5. Discuss the etiology, laboratory diagnostic findings, clinical manifestations, and nursing and collaborative management of the following acid–base imbalances: metabolic acidosis, metabolic alkalosis, respiratory acidosis, and respiratory alkalosis.
6. Describe the composition and indications for use of common intravenous fluid solutions.
7. Discuss types and nursing management of commonly used central venous access devices.

KEY TERMS

acidosis, p. 370
active transport, p. 354
alkalosis, p. 370
anions, p. 353
buffers, p. 370
cations, p. 353

diffusion, p. 354
electrolytes, p. 353
facilitated diffusion, p. 354
fluid spacing, p. 357
homeostasis, p. 352
hydrostatic pressure, p. 355

hypertonic, p. 355
hypotonic, p. 355
ions, p. 353
isotonic, p. 355
oncotic pressure, p. 356
osmolality, p. 355

osmolarity, p. 355
osmosis, p. 354
osmotic pressure, p. 354
pH, p. 370
tetany, p. 367
valence, p. 353

HOMEOSTASIS

Body fluids and electrolytes play an important role in homeostasis. Homeostasis is the state of equilibrium in the internal environment of the body, naturally maintained by adaptive responses that promote healthy survival (Mosby, 2016). Maintenance of the composition and volume of body fluids within narrow normal limits is necessary to maintain homeostasis (McCance & Huether, 2014). During normal metabolism, the body produces many acids. These acids alter the internal environment of the body, including fluid and electrolyte balances, and must also be regulated to maintain homeostasis. Many diseases and their treatments have the ability to affect fluid and

electrolyte balance. For example, a patient with metastatic breast cancer may develop hypercalcemia. Chemotherapy prescribed to treat the cancer may result in nausea and vomiting and, subsequently, dehydration and acid–base imbalances. Correction of the dehydration with intravenous (IV) fluids must be monitored closely to prevent fluid overload.

It is important for the nurse to anticipate the potential for alterations in fluid and electrolyte balance associated with certain disorders and medical therapies, to recognize the signs and symptoms of imbalances, and to intervene with the appropriate actions. This chapter describes the normal control of fluids, electrolytes, and acid–base balance; etiologies that disrupt homeostasis and resultant manifestations; and actions that the health care provider can take to prevent imbalance or restore fluid, electrolyte, and acid–base balance.

WATER CONTENT OF THE BODY

Water is the primary component of the body, accounting for approximately 60% of adult body weight. Water content varies with sex, body mass, and age (Figure 19-1). Lean body mass has a higher percentage of water than does adipose tissue; therefore, the more fat present in the body, the less the total water content. Women generally have a lower percentage of body water because they tend to have less lean body mass than do men. In older adults, the body water content is lower as a result of decreased lean body mass. Thus older adults are at an increased risk for fluid-related problems.

Body Fluid Compartments

The two major fluid compartments in the body are intracellular spaces (inside the cells) and the extracellular spaces (outside the cells) (Figure 19-2). Approximately two-thirds of body water is located within cells and is called *intracellular fluid* (ICF); the ICF constitutes approximately 42% of body weight. The body of a 70-kg man would contain approximately 42 L of water, of which 30 L would be intracellular. *Extracellular fluid* (ECF) consists primarily of interstitial fluid and intravascular fluid (plasma). The ECF constitutes one-third of the body water, or approximately 17% of the total weight; this would amount to approximately 11 L in a 70-kg man. Approximately one-third of the ECF is in the plasma space (3 L in a 70-kg man), and two-thirds is in the interstitial space (8 L in a 70-kg man). Other ECF components include lymph and transcellular fluids. Transcellular fluids account for approximately 1 L and include cerebro-spinal fluid; fluid in the gastro-intestinal (GI) tract and joint spaces; and pleural, peritoneal, intraocular, and pericardial fluid.

Calculation of Fluid Gain or Loss

One litre of water weighs 1 kg. Body weight change, especially sudden change, is an excellent indicator of overall fluid volume loss or gain. For example, if a patient drinks 240 mL of fluid, weight gain will be 0.24 kg. A patient receiving diuretic therapy who loses 2 kg in 24 hours has experienced a fluid loss of approximately 2 L. An adult patient who is fasting might lose approximately 0.5 to 1 kg per day. A weight loss exceeding this is probably caused by loss of body fluid.

ELECTROLYTES

Electrolytes are substances whose molecules dissociate or split into ions when placed in solution. **Ions** are electrically charged molecules. **Cations** are positively charged ions. Examples include sodium (Na^+), potassium (K^+), calcium (Ca^{2+}), and magnesium (Mg^{2+}) ions. **Anions** are negatively charged ions. Examples include bicarbonate (HCO_3^-), chloride (Cl^-), and phosphate (PO_4^{3-}) ions. Most proteins bear a negative charge and are thus anions. The electrical charge of an ion is termed its **valence**. Cations and anions combine according to their valences.

Measurement of Electrolytes

The measurement of electrolytes is important to the nurse in evaluating electrolyte balance, as well as in determining the composition of electrolyte preparations. The concentration of electrolytes can be expressed in milligrams per decilitre (mg/dL), millimoles per litre (mmol/L), or milliequivalents per litre (mEq/L). The international standard symbol for measuring electrolytes is mmol/L. One mole (mol) of a substance is the molecular (or atomic) weight of that substance expressed in grams; hence, a millimole (mmol) of a substance is the atomic weight in milligrams. Sodium's atomic weight is 23 mg; therefore, 23 mg of sodium is 1 mmol of sodium. Sodium and chloride are monovalent elements that carry one electron and will match one to one: 1 mmol of sodium combines with 1 mmol of chloride.

An element with two electrons, such as calcium, requires two monovalent partners. To avoid keeping track of how to match millimoles, the milliequivalent is the favoured unit of measure for electrolytes. The following formula is used to convert millimoles to milliequivalents:

$$mEq = (mmol/L) \times valence$$

Electrolytes in body fluids are active chemicals that unite in varying combinations. Thus it is more practical to express

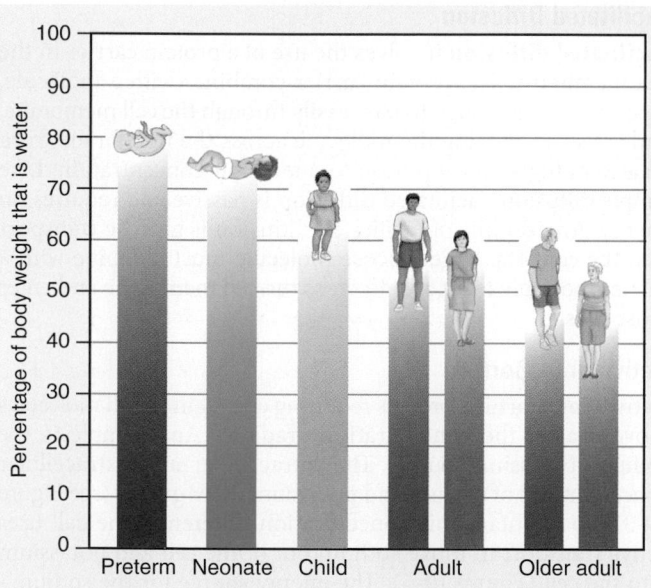

FIGURE 19-1 Levels of body water over the lifespan.

Plasma: (3 L)

Interstitial fluid (IF): (10 L)

Intracellular fluid (ICF): (28 L)

FIGURE 19-2 Relative volumes of three body fluids. Values represent fluid distribution in a young male adult. *ICF*, intercellular fluid; *IF*, interstitial fluid.

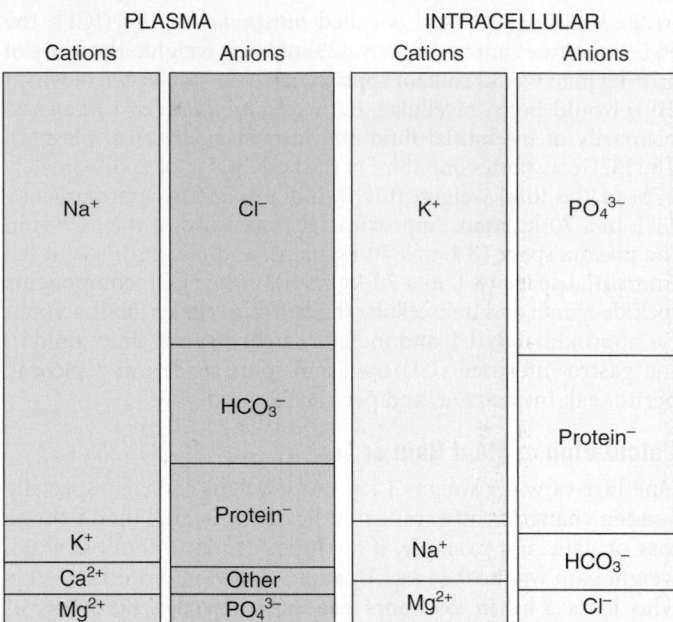

FIGURE 19-3 The relative concentrations of the major cations and anions in the intracellular space and the plasma.

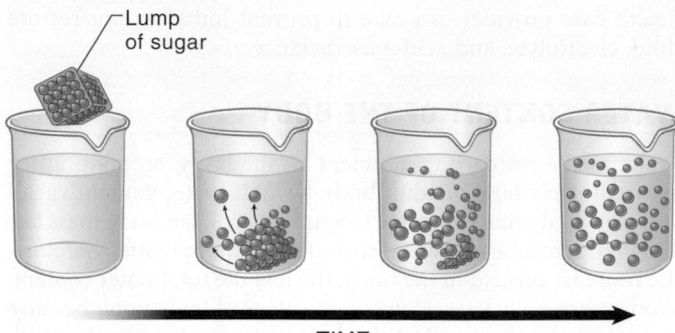

FIGURE 19-4 Diffusion is the movement of molecules from an area of high concentration to an area of low concentration. In this example, the sugar molecules eventually are evenly distributed. Source: Patton, K. T., & Thibodeau, G. A. (2016). *Anatomy and physiology* (9th ed., p. 99). St. Louis: Mosby.

their concentration as a measure of chemical activity (or milliequivalents) rather than as a measure of weight. Ions combine milliequivalent for milliequivalent: they match 1 to 1. For example, 1 mEq (1 mmol) of sodium combines with 1 mEq (1 mmol) of chloride, and 1 mEq (0.5 mmol) of calcium combines with 1 mEq (1 mmol) of chloride. This combining power of electrolytes is important for maintaining the balance of positively charged ions (cations) and negatively charged ions (anions) within body fluids.

Electrolyte Composition of Fluid Compartments

Electrolyte composition varies between the ECF and the ICF. The overall concentration of the electrolytes is approximately the same in the two compartments. However, concentrations of specific ions differ greatly (Figure 19-3). In the ECF, the main cation is sodium, with small amounts of potassium, calcium, and magnesium. The primary ECF anion is chloride, with small amounts of bicarbonate, sulfate, and phosphate anions. In the ICF, the most prevalent cation is potassium, with small amounts of magnesium and sodium. The predominant ICF anion is phosphate, with some protein and a small amount of bicarbonate.

MECHANISMS CONTROLLING FLUID AND ELECTROLYTE MOVEMENT

Different processes—such as simple diffusion, facilitated diffusion, and active transport—are involved in the movement of electrolytes and water between the ICF and the ECF. Water movement is driven by two forces: hydrostatic pressure and osmotic pressure.

Diffusion

Diffusion is the movement of molecules from an area of high concentration to one of low concentration (Figure 19-4). The membrane separating the two areas must be permeable by the diffusing substance for the process to occur. Net movement of molecules stops when the concentrations are equal in both areas.

Simple diffusion requires no external energy. Gases (e.g., oxygen, nitrogen, carbon dioxide) and substances (e.g., urea) can permeate cell membranes and are distributed throughout the body.

Facilitated Diffusion

Facilitated diffusion involves the use of a protein carrier in the cell membrane. The protein carrier combines with a molecule, especially one too large to pass easily through the cell membrane, and assists in moving the molecule across the membrane from an area of high concentration to one of low concentration. Like simple diffusion, facilitated diffusion is passive and requires no energy. An example of facilitated diffusion is glucose transport into the cell. The large glucose molecule must combine with a carrier molecule to be able to cross the cell membrane and enter most cells.

Active Transport

Active transport is a process requiring energy in which molecules move against the concentration gradient. An example is the sodium–potassium pump. The intracellular and extracellular concentrations of sodium and potassium differ greatly (see Figure 19-3). To maintain this concentration difference, the cell uses active transport to move sodium out of the cell and potassium into the cell (Figure 19-5). The energy source for the sodium–potassium pump is adenosine triphosphate (ATP).

Osmosis

Osmosis is the movement of water between two compartments separated by a semipermeable membrane, one that allows the movement of water but not solute. Water moves through the membrane from an area of low solute concentration to an area of high solute concentration (Figure 19-6). Osmosis requires no outside energy sources and stops when the concentration differences disappear or when hydrostatic pressure builds and is sufficient to oppose any further movement of water. Diffusion and osmosis are important in maintaining the fluid volume of body cells and the concentration of the solute.

Osmotic pressure is the amount of pressure necessary to stop the osmotic flow of water. Osmotic pressure can be understood by imagining a chamber in which two compartments are separated by a semipermeable membrane (see Figure 19-6). Water moves to the more concentrated side of the chamber until the pressure generated by the height of the higher column of water opposes further movement.

FIGURE 19-5 Sodium–potassium pump. As sodium (Na⁺) diffuses into the cell and potassium (K⁺) diffuses out of the cell, an active transport system supplied with energy from adenosine triphosphate (ATP) delivers Na⁺ back to the extracellular compartment and K⁺ to the intracellular compartment.

FIGURE 19-6 Osmosis is the process of water movement through a semipermeable membrane from an area of low solute concentration to an area of high solute concentration. Source: Patton, K. T., & Thibodeau, G. A. (2016). *Anatomy and physiology* (9th ed., p. 102). St. Louis: Mosby.

Osmotic pressure is determined by the concentration of solutes in solution. It is measured in milliosmoles (mOsm) and may be expressed as either fluid osmolarity or fluid osmolality. Although the terms *osmolarity* and *osmolality* are often used interchangeably, they are different measurements. Osmolarity is a measure of the total milliosmoles of solute per unit of total volume of solution: that is, the total milliosmoles per litre of solution (mOsm/L), or the concentration of molecules per volume of solution. Osmolality is a measure of the osmotic force of solute per unit of weight of solvent: that is, the number of milliosmoles per kilogram of water (mOsm/kg, or mmol/kg), or the concentration of molecules per weight of water. Osmolality is the preferred measure for evaluating the concentration of plasma, urine, and body fluids (McCance & Huether, 2014).

Measurement of Osmolality. Osmolality is approximately the same in the various body fluid spaces. Determining osmolality is important because it indicates the water balance of the body. To assess the state of the body water balance, the clinician can measure or estimate plasma osmolality. Normal plasma osmolality is between 280 and 300 mmol/kg. A value greater than 295 mmol/kg indicates that the concentration of particles is too great or that the water content is too little. This condition is termed *water*

deficit. A value less than 285 mmol/kg indicates too little solute for the amount of water or too much water for the amount of solute. This condition is termed *water excess*. Both conditions are clinically significant.

Plasma and urine osmolality can be measured in most clinical laboratories. Because the major determinants of the plasma osmolality are sodium, glucose, and urea, the effective plasma osmolality can be calculated from the concentrations of those compounds with the following equation:

$$\text{Effective osmolality} = 2 \times (Na^-)p + (glucose)p/18$$

where $(Na^-)p$ and $(glucose)p$ are the plasma concentrations of sodium and glucose in milliequivalents per litre (mEq/L) and milligrams per decilitre (mg/dL), respectively. The sodium concentration is multiplied by 2 to account for the presence of an equivalent number of anions. Glucose concentration is divided by one-tenth of its molecular weight to calculate the number of osmotically active particles per litre.

It is sometimes recommended that the measurement of blood urea nitrogen (BUN)* be included in the calculation of plasma osmolality. This is done by adding a third term to the effective osmolality equation (+ BUN/2.8), with the BUN expressed in milligrams per decilitre. However, the urea moves freely between body fluid compartments; it has no lasting effect on water movement across cell boundaries and is sometimes dubbed an "ineffective osmole." The actual osmolality is calculated more accurately if the BUN is used. However, the measure of the effective plasma osmolality without consideration of the BUN term is the more physiologically meaningful estimate. Osmolality of urine can range from 100 to 1300 mmol/kg, depending on the amount of antidiuretic hormone (ADH) and the renal response to it.

Osmotic Movement of Fluids. Cells are affected by the osmolality of the fluid that surrounds them. Fluids with the same osmolality as the cell interior are **isotonic**. Solutions in which the solutes are less concentrated than they are in cells are **hypotonic** (hypo-osmolar). Those with solutes more concentrated than they are in cells are **hypertonic** (hyperosmolar).

Normally, the ECF and the ICF are isotonic to one another; so no net movement of water occurs. In the metabolically active cell, there is a constant exchange of substances between the compartments, but no net gain or loss of water occurs.

If a cell is surrounded by hypotonic fluid, water moves into the cell, causing it to swell and possibly to burst. If a cell is surrounded by hypertonic fluid, water leaves the cell to dilute the ECF; the cell shrinks and may eventually die (Figure 19-7).

Hydrostatic Pressure

Hydrostatic pressure is the force within a fluid compartment. In the blood vessels, hydrostatic pressure is the blood pressure generated by the contraction of the heart. Hydrostatic pressure in the vascular system gradually decreases as the blood moves through the arteries until it is approximately 40 mm Hg at the arterial end of a capillary. Because of the size of the capillary bed and fluid movement into the interstitium, the pressure decreases to approximately 10 mm Hg at the venous end of the capillary. Hydrostatic pressure is the major force that pushes water out of the vascular system at the capillary level.

---

*Serum urea (nitrogen).

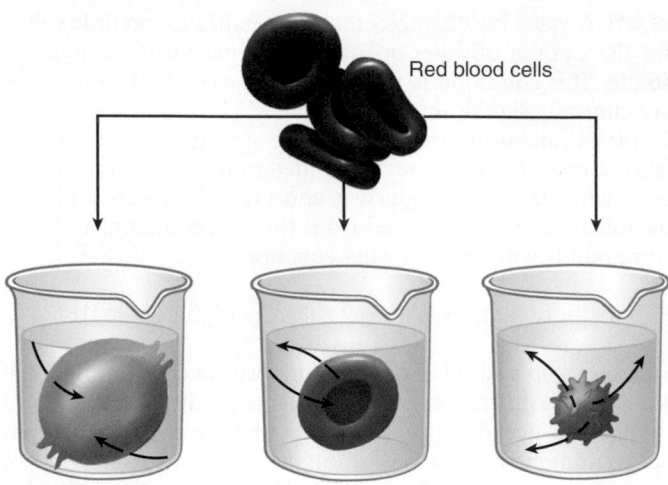

A Hypotonic solution   **B** Isotonic solution   **C** Hypertonic solution

FIGURE 19-7 Effects of water status on red blood cells. **A,** Hypotonic solution (H$_2$O excess) results in cellular swelling. **B,** Isotonic solution (normal H$_2$O balance) results in no change. **C,** Hypertonic solution (H$_2$O deficit) results in cellular shrinking. Source: Patton, K. T., & Thibodeau, G. A. (2016). *Anatomy and physiology* (9th ed., p. 102). St. Louis: Mosby.

Oncotic Pressure

Oncotic pressure (colloidal osmotic pressure) is osmotic pressure exerted by colloids in solution. The major colloid in the vascular system contributing to the total osmotic pressure is protein. Protein molecules attract water, pulling fluid from the tissue space to the vascular space (Porth, 2013). Unlike electrolytes, proteins have large molecular sizes, which prevents them from leaving the vascular space through pores in capillary walls. Plasma oncotic pressure is approximately 25 mm Hg. Some proteins are found in the interstitial space; they exert an oncotic pressure of approximately 1 mm Hg.

FLUID MOVEMENT IN CAPILLARIES

There is normal movement of fluid between the capillary and the interstitium. The amount and direction of movement are determined by the interaction of (1) capillary hydrostatic pressure, (2) plasma oncotic pressure, (3) interstitial hydrostatic pressure, and (4) interstitial oncotic pressure.

Capillary hydrostatic pressure and interstitial oncotic pressure cause the movement of water out of the capillaries. Plasma oncotic pressure and interstitial hydrostatic pressure cause the movement of fluid into the capillary. At the arterial end of the capillary (Figure 19-8), capillary hydrostatic pressure exceeds plasma oncotic pressure, and fluid is moved into the interstitium. At the venous end of the capillary, the capillary hydrostatic pressure is lower than plasma oncotic pressure, and fluid is drawn back into the capillary by the oncotic pressure created by plasma proteins.

Fluid Shifts

If capillary or interstitial pressures are altered, fluid may abnormally shift from one compartment to another, which results in edema or dehydration.

Shifts of Plasma to Interstitial Fluid. Accumulation of fluid in the interstitium (*edema*) occurs if venous hydrostatic pressure rises, plasma oncotic pressure decreases, or interstitial oncotic

FIGURE 19-8 Dynamics of fluid exchange between the capillary and the tissue. Equilibrium exists between forces filtering fluid out of the capillary and forces absorbing fluid back into the capillary. Note that the hydrostatic pressure is greater at the arterial end of the capillary than at the venous end. The net effect of pressures at the arterial end of the capillary causes a movement of fluid into the tissue. At the venous end of the capillary, there is net movement of fluid back into the capillary.

pressure rises. Edema may also develop if the lymphatic outflow is obstructed, which causes decreased removal of interstitial fluid.

Elevation of Venous Hydrostatic Pressure. Increasing the pressure at the venous end of the capillary inhibits fluid movement back into the capillary. Causes of increased venous pressure include fluid overload, heart failure, liver failure, obstruction of venous return to the heart (e.g., by tourniquets, restrictive clothing, venous thrombosis), and venous insufficiency (e.g., manifested by varicose veins).

Decrease in Plasma Oncotic Pressure. Fluid remains in the interstitium if the plasma oncotic pressure is too low to draw fluid back into the capillary. Decreased oncotic pressure is seen when the plasma protein content is low. This can result from excessive protein loss (renal disorders), deficient protein synthesis (liver disease), and deficient protein intake (malnutrition).

Elevation of Interstitial Oncotic Pressure. Trauma, burns, and inflammation can damage capillary walls and allow plasma proteins to accumulate in the interstitium. The resultant increased interstitial oncotic pressure draws fluid into the interstitium and holds it there.

Shifts of Interstitial Fluid to Plasma. Fluid is drawn into the plasma space whenever there is an increase in the plasma osmotic or oncotic pressure. This could happen with administration of colloids, dextran, mannitol, or hypertonic solutions. Fluid is drawn from the interstitium. In turn, water is drawn from cells via osmosis, which causes equilibration of the osmolality between the ICF and the ECF.

Increasing the tissue hydrostatic pressure is another way of causing a shift of fluid into plasma. The wearing of elastic compression gradient stockings or hose to decrease peripheral edema is a therapeutic application of this effect.

FLUID MOVEMENT BETWEEN EXTRACELLULAR FLUID AND INTRACELLULAR FLUID

Changes in the osmolality of the ECF alter the volume of cells. Increased ECF osmolality (water deficit) pulls water out of cells until the two compartments have a similar osmolality. Water deficit is associated with symptoms that result from cell shrinkage as water is pulled into the vascular system. For example, neurological symptoms are caused by altered central nervous system (CNS) function as brain cells shrink. Decreased ECF osmolality (water excess) develops as the result of gain or retention of excess water. In this case, cells swell. Again, the primary symptoms are neurological as a result of brain cell swelling as water shifts into the cells.

FLUID SPACING

Fluid spacing is a term sometimes used to describe the distribution of body water. *First spacing* describes the normal distribution of fluid in the ICF and ECF compartments. *Second spacing* refers to an abnormal accumulation of interstitial fluid (i.e., edema). *Third spacing* occurs when fluid accumulates in a portion of the body from which it is not easily exchanged with the rest of the ECF. Third-spaced fluid is trapped and essentially unavailable for functional use. Examples of third spacing are ascites, sequestration of fluid in the abdominal cavity with peritonitis, and edema associated with burns, trauma or sepsis.

REGULATION OF WATER BALANCE

Hypothalamic Regulation

Water balance is maintained by a balance of intake and excretion. A body fluid deficit or an increase in plasma osmolality is sensed by hypothalamic osmoreceptors, which in turn stimulate thirst and ADH release. Thirst causes the patient to drink. Hypothalamic ADH, which is stored in the posterior pituitary gland, induces water reabsorption in the renal distal and collecting tubules. Together, these factors result in increased free water in the body and decreased plasma osmolality. Once plasma osmolality is normalized, secretion of ADH is suppressed, and thus urinary excretion is restored.

An intact thirst mechanism is critical because it is the primary protection against the development of hyperosmolality. The patient who cannot recognize or act on the sensation of thirst is at risk for fluid deficit and hyperosmolality. The sensitivity of the thirst mechanism decreases in older adults.

The desire to consume fluids is also affected by social and psychological factors not related to fluid balance. A dry mouth will cause the patient to drink, even when there is no measurable body water deficit. This is normally compensated by equivalent water excretion. A patient with psychiatric issues may display psychogenic polydipsia that may lead to water intoxication.

Pituitary Regulation

Under hypothalamic control, the posterior pituitary gland releases ADH, which causes the distal tubules and collecting ducts in the kidneys to regulate water retention by becoming more permeable by water. Water is reabsorbed from the tubular filtrate into the blood and not excreted in urine. Factors that stimulate ADH release include increased plasma osmolality, stress, nausea, nicotine, and morphine. For instance, it is common for patients to have a lower serum osmolality after surgery, possibly because of the stress of surgery and opioid analgesia.

A pathological condition seen occasionally is *syndrome of inappropriate antidiuretic hormone* (SIADH; see Chapter 51). Causes of SIADH include abnormal ADH production in CNS disorders (e.g., brain tumours, brain injury) and certain malignancies (e.g., small cell lung cancer). The inappropriate secretion of ADH causes water retention, which causes plasma osmolality

FIGURE 19-9 Factors affecting aldosterone secretion. *ACTH,* adrenocorticotrophic hormone.

to decrease below the normal value and causes a relative increase in urine osmolality with a decrease in urine volume.

Reduction in the release or action of ADH produces diabetes insipidus (see Chapter 51). A copious amount of dilute urine is excreted because the renal tubules and collecting ducts do not appropriately reabsorb water. A patient with diabetes insipidus exhibits extreme polyuria and, if alert, polydipsia (excessive thirst). Symptoms of dehydration and hypernatremia develop if the water losses are not adequately replaced.

Adrenal Cortical Regulation

ECF volume is maintained by a combination of hormonal influences. ADH affects only water reabsorption. Hormones released by the adrenal cortex help regulate both water and electrolytes. Two groups of hormones secreted by the adrenal cortex are glucocorticoids and mineralocorticoids. The glucocorticoids (e.g., cortisol) have primarily an anti-inflammatory effect and increase serum glucose levels, whereas the mineralocorticoids (e.g., aldosterone) enhance sodium retention and potassium excretion (Figure 19-9). When sodium is reabsorbed, water follows as a result of osmotic changes.

Cortisol is the most common example of a naturally occurring glucocorticoid. In large doses, cortisol has both glucocorticoid (glucose level–elevating and anti-inflammatory) and mineralocorticoid (sodium-retaining) properties. The adrenocortical hormone cortisol is secreted normally and whenever stress levels are increased. Many body systems, including fluid and electrolyte balance, are affected by stress (Figure 19-10).

Aldosterone is a naturally occurring mineralocorticoid with potent sodium-retaining and potassium-excreting capability. Decreased renal perfusion or decreased sodium in the distal portion of the renal tubule activates the renin-angiotensin-aldosterone system, which results in aldosterone secretion. In addition to this system, increased serum potassium, decreased serum sodium, and adrenocorticotrophic hormone (ACTH) stimulate aldosterone secretion. Aldosterone increases sodium and water reabsorption

FIGURE 19-10 Effects of stress on fluid and electrolyte balance. *ACTH,* adrenocorticotrophic hormone; *ADH,* antidiuretic hormone; *CRH,* corticotropin-releasing hormone.

Substance	Amount
Intake	
Fluids	1200 mL
Solid food	1000 mL
Water from oxidation	300 mL
Total	2500 mL
Output	
Insensible loss (skin and lungs)	900 mL
Urine	1500 mL
In feces	100 mL
Total	2500 mL

TABLE 19-1   NORMAL FLUID BALANCE IN THE ADULT

in the renal distal tubules, which causes plasma osmolality to decrease and fluid volume to be restored (see Figure 19-9).

Renal Regulation

The primary organs for regulating fluid and electrolyte balance are the kidneys (see Chapter 47). The kidneys regulate water balance through adjustments in urine volume. Similarly, urinary excretion of most electrolytes is adjusted so that a balance is maintained between overall intake and output. The total plasma volume is filtered by the kidneys many times each day. In the average adult, the kidneys reabsorb 99% of this filtrate, producing approximately 1.5 L of urine per day. As the filtrate moves through the renal tubules, selective reabsorption of water and electrolytes and secretion of electrolytes result in the production of urine, whose composition and concentration are greatly different from those of the plasma. This process helps maintain normal plasma osmolality, electrolyte balance, blood volume, and acid–base balance. The renal tubules are the site for the actions of ADH and aldosterone.

When renal function is severely impaired, the kidneys cannot maintain fluid and electrolyte balance. This condition results in edema, potassium and phosphorus retention, acidosis, and other electrolyte imbalances (see Chapter 49). Renal function is typically decreased in older adults, which increases their risk for fluid and electrolyte imbalances. In particular, the ability to concentrate urine may be reduced in older adults.

Cardiac Regulation

Atrial natriuretic factor (ANF) is a hormone released by the cardiac atria in response to increased atrial pressure (increased volume, such as what occurs in heart failure) and high serum sodium levels. The primary actions of ANF are vasodilation and increased urinary excretion of sodium and water, which decreases blood volume (McCance & Huether, 2014).

Gastro-intestinal Regulation

Daily water intake and output are between 2 000 and 3 000 mL (Table 19-1). The GI tract accounts for most of the water intake. Water intake includes fluids, water from food metabolism, and water present in solid foods. Lean meat is approximately 70% water, whereas the water content of many fruits and vegetables approaches 100%.

Most of the body's water is excreted by the kidneys, and a small amount of water is normally eliminated by the GI tract in feces. The GI tract normally secretes approximately 8 000 mL of digestive fluids each day, of which most is reabsorbed. This is why diarrhea and vomiting, which prevent GI reabsorption of secreted fluid, can lead to significant fluid and electrolyte loss.

Insensible Water Loss

Insensible water loss, which is invisible vaporization from the lungs and the skin, assists in regulating body temperature. Normally, approximately 900 mL per day is lost. The amount of water loss is increased by accelerated body metabolism, which occurs with increased body temperature and exercise.

Water loss through the skin should not be confused with the vaporization of water excreted by sweat glands. Only water is lost by insensible perspiration. Excessive sweating *(sensible perspiration)* caused by fever or high environmental temperatures may lead to large losses of water and electrolytes.

AGE-RELATED CONSIDERATIONS

FLUID AND ELECTROLYTES

Older adults experience normal physiological changes that increase susceptibility to fluid and electrolyte imbalances. Structural changes in the kidneys and a decrease in the renal blood flow lead to a decrease in the glomerular filtration rate, decreased creatinine clearance, the loss of the ability to concentrate urine and conserve water, and narrowed limits for the excretion of water, sodium, potassium, and hydrogen ions. Hormonal changes include decreases in renin and aldosterone and increases in ADH and atrial natriuretic peptide (ANP; Touhy & Jett, 2016).

Loss of subcutaneous tissue and thinning of the dermis lead to increased loss of moisture through the skin and an inability to respond to heat or cold quickly. Older adults experience a decrease in the thirst mechanism, which results in decreased fluid intake despite increases in osmolality and serum sodium level. Frail older adults, especially if ill, are at increased risk for free-water loss and subsequent development of hypernatremia secondary to impairment of the thirst mechanism, and increased risk for adverse social and environmental conditions (Hooper, Bunn, Jimoh, et al., 2014).

Healthy older adults usually consume adequate fluids to remain well hydrated. However, functional changes may occur that affect the individual's ability to independently obtain fluids. Musculoskeletal changes, such as stiffness of the hands and fingers, can lead to a decreased ability to hold a glass or cup. Mental status changes, such as confusion or disorientation, or changes in ambulation status may lead to a decreased ability to obtain fluids. As a result of incontinent episodes, an older adult may intentionally restrict fluid intake (Hooper, Bunn, Jimoh, et al., 2014).

To help older adult patients, the health care provider must understand the homeostatic changes that occur in this population. It is important to avoid the pitfalls of ageism, wherein fluid and electrolyte problems may be inappropriately attributed to the natural processes of aging. The nurse needs to adapt assessment and nursing implementation to account for these physiological and functional changes. Suggestions for alterations in nursing care for older adults are presented throughout this chapter and in Chapter 7.

FLUID AND ELECTROLYTE IMBALANCES

Fluid and electrolyte imbalances occur to some degree in most patients with a major illness or injury because illness disrupts the normal homeostatic mechanism. Some fluid and electrolyte imbalances are directly caused by injury or disease (e.g., burns, heart failure). At other times, therapeutic measures (e.g., IV fluid replacement, diuretics) cause or contribute to fluid and electrolyte imbalances.

The imbalances are commonly classified as *deficits* or *excesses*. Each imbalance is discussed separately. Normal values are listed in Table 19-2. In actual clinical situations, more than one imbalance occurring in the same patient is common. For example, a patient undergoing prolonged nasogastric suction will lose Na^+, K^+, H^+, and Cl^-. These imbalances may result in deficiencies of both Na^+ and K^+, as well as metabolic alkalosis and fluid volume deficit.

Sodium and Extracellular Fluid Volume Imbalances

Sodium plays a major role in maintaining the concentration and the volume of the ECF. Sodium is the main cation of the ECF and the primary determinant of ECF osmolality. Sodium imbalances are typically associated with parallel changes in osmolality. Because sodium affects the water distribution between the ECF and the ICF, it affects osmolality. Sodium is also important in the generation and transmission of nerve impulses and the regulation of acid–base balance. Serum sodium is measured in milliequivalents per litre or millimoles per litre.

The GI tract absorbs sodium from foods. Typically, daily intake of sodium far exceeds the body's daily requirements. Sodium leaves the body through urine, sweat, and feces. The kidneys are the primary regulator of sodium balance. The kidneys regulate the ECF concentration of sodium by excreting or retaining water

TABLE 19-2	NORMAL SERUM ELECTROLYTE VALUES
Electrolyte	**Normal Value**
Anions	
Bicarbonate (HCO_3^-)	21–28 mmol/L
Chloride (Cl^-)	98–106 mmol/L
Phosphate (PO_4^{3-})	0.97–1.45 mmol/L
Protein	64–83 g/L
Cations	
Potassium (K^+)	3.5–5.0 mmol/L
Magnesium (Mg^{2+})	0.74–1.07 mmol/L
Sodium (Na^+)	135–145 mmol/L
Calcium (Ca^{2+}) (total)	2.25–2.75 mmol/L
Calcium (ionized)	1.05–1.30 mmol/L

under the influence of ADH. Aldosterone also plays a part in sodium regulation by promoting sodium reabsorption from the renal tubules. The serum sodium level reflects the ratio of sodium to water, not necessarily the loss or gain of sodium. Thus changes in the serum sodium level may reflect either a primary water imbalance, a primary sodium imbalance, or a combination of the two. Sodium imbalances are typically associated with imbalances in ECF volume (Figures 19-11 and 19-12).

Hypernatremia. The serum sodium level may become elevated as a result of water loss or sodium gain. Because sodium is the major determinant of the ECF osmolality, hypernatremia causes hyperosmolality. In turn, hyperosmolality causes a shift of water out of the cells, which leads to cellular dehydration.

As discussed earlier, the primary protection against the development of hyperosmolality is thirst. As the plasma osmolality increases, the thirst centre in the hypothalamus is stimulated, and the individual seeks fluids.

Hypernatremia is not a problem in an alert person who has access to water, can sense thirst, and is able to swallow. Hypernatremia secondary to water deficiency is often the result of an impaired level of consciousness or an inability to obtain fluids. Unconscious patients and certain cognitively impaired patients are at risk because of an inability to express thirst and act on it.

Several clinical states can produce water loss and hypernatremia (Table 19-3). A deficiency in the synthesis of ADH or in its release from the posterior pituitary gland (central diabetes insipidus) or a decrease in kidney responsiveness to ADH (nephrogenic diabetes insipidus) can result in profound diuresis, causing a water deficit and hypernatremia. Hyperosmolality can result from administration of concentrated hyperosmolar tube feedings and osmotic diuretics (mannitol), as well as from hyperglycemia associated with uncontrolled diabetes mellitus. These situations result in osmotic diuresis. Dilute urine is lost, leaving behind a high solute load. Other causes of hypernatremia include excessive sweating and increased sensible losses from high fever.

Sodium intake in excess of water intake can also lead to hypernatremia. Causes of sodium gain include IV administration of hypertonic saline or sodium bicarbonate, use of sodium-containing drugs, excessive oral intake of sodium (ingestion of seawater), and primary aldosteronism (hypersecretion of aldosterone), which in turn is caused by a tumour of the adrenal glands.

Symptoms are primarily the result of changes in the plasma osmolality that lead to changes in the volume of cellular water (see Table 19-3). Dehydration of neurons leads to neurological

FIGURE 19-11 Differential assessment of extracellular fluid (ECF) volume.

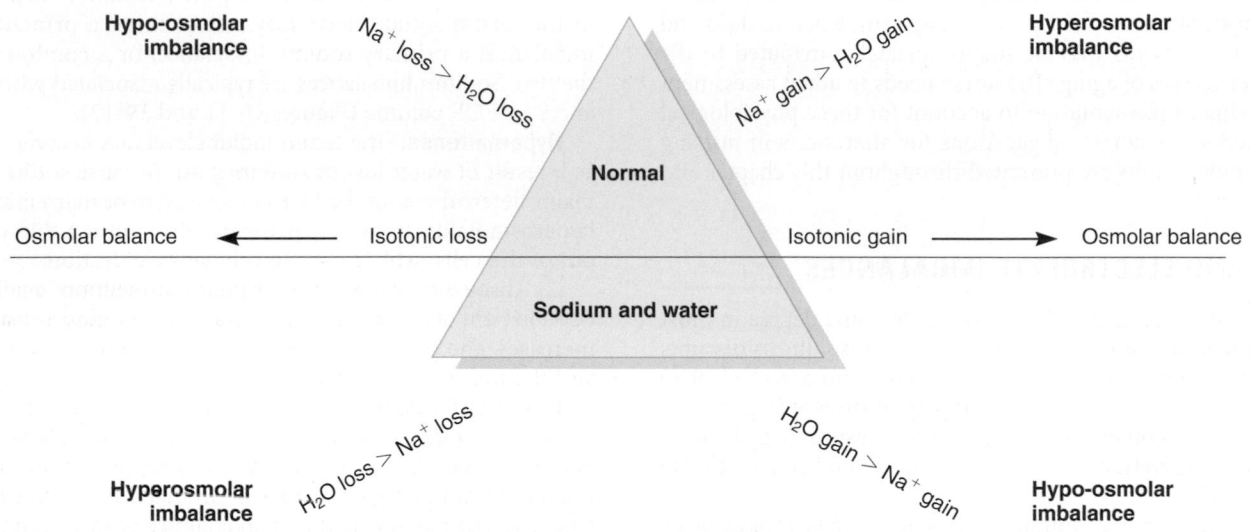

FIGURE 19-12 Isotonic gains and losses affect mainly the extracellular fluid (ECF) compartment, with little or no water movement into the cells. Hypertonic imbalances cause water to move from inside the cell into the ECF to dilute the concentrated sodium, which results in cell shrinkage. Hypotonic imbalances cause water to move into the cell, which results in cell swelling.

manifestations such as intense thirst, lethargy, agitation, seizures, and even coma. Sodium excess also has a direct effect on the irritability and conduction of neurons, causing them to be more easily excited. Patients with hypernatremia will also exhibit the symptoms of any accompanying volume imbalance.

Collaborative Care. The goal of treatment in hypernatremia that is caused by either water loss or sodium gain is to treat the underlying cause. In the treatment of primary water deficit, fluid is replaced either orally or by IV infusion with isotonic fluids, such as 0.9% sodium chloride (Harring, Deal, & Kuo, 2014). Serum sodium levels must be reduced gradually to prevent too rapid a shift of water back into the cells. Overly rapid correction of hypernatremia can result in cerebral edema. The risk is greatest in patients who have developed hypernatremia over several days or longer.

The goal of treatment for sodium excess is to dilute the sodium concentration with salt-free IV fluids, such as 5% dextrose in water, and to promote excretion of the excess sodium by administering diuretics. Dietary sodium intake is often restricted. (See Chapter 51 for specific treatment of diabetes insipidus.) To prevent hypernatremia in older adults or cognitively impaired patients, it is important to pay close attention to fluid intake and losses. Regular administration of oral fluids must be incorporated into these patients' plan of care (Hooper, Bunn, Jimoh, et al., 2014).

Hyponatremia. Hyponatremia (low serum sodium) may result from a loss of sodium-containing fluids, water excess in relation to the amount of sodium (dilutional hyponatremia), or a combination of both (see Table 19-3). Hyponatremia is usually associated with ECF hypo-osmolality that results from the excess water. To restore balance, fluid shifts out of the ECF and into the cells, leading to cellular edema. Common causes of hyponatremia caused by water excess are inappropriate use of sodium-free or hypotonic IV fluids. This may occur in patients after surgery or major trauma, during administration of fluids in patients with renal failure, or in patients with psychiatric

TABLE 19-3 WATER AND SODIUM IMBALANCES: CAUSES AND CLINICAL MANIFESTATIONS

Water Excess: Hyponatremia (Na+ Level <136 mmol/L)	Water Deficit: Hypernatremia (Na+ Level >145 mmol/L)
Causes	
Sodium loss	Water loss (sodium concentration)
• GI losses: diarrhea, vomiting, fistulas, NG suction	• ↑ Insensible water loss or perspiration (high fever, heatstroke)
• Renal losses: diuretics, adrenal insufficiency, Na+ wasting renal disease	• Diabetes insipidus
• Skin losses: burns, wound drainage	• Osmotic diuresis
Water gain (sodium dilution)	Sodium gain
• SIADH	• IV hypertonic NaCl
• Heart failure	• IV sodium bicarbonate
• Excessive hypotonic IV fluids	• IV excessive isotonic NaCl
• Primary polydipsia	• Primary hyperaldosteronism
	• Saltwater near-drowning
Clinical Manifestations	
Decreased ECF volume (sodium loss)	Decreased ECF volume (water loss)
• Irritability, apprehension, confusion	• Intense thirst; dry, swollen tongue
• Postural hypotension	• Restlessness, agitation, twitching
• Tachycardia	• Seizures, coma
• Rapid, thready pulse	• Weakness
• ↓ CVP	• Postural hypotension, ↓ CVP
• ↓ Jugular venous filling	• Weight loss
• Nausea, vomiting	
• Dry mucous membranes	
• Weight loss	
• Tremors, seizures, coma	
Normal or increased ECF volume (water gain)	Normal or increased ECF volume (sodium gain)
• Headache, lassitude, apathy	• Intense thirst
• Weakness, confusion	• Restlessness, agitation, twitching
• Nausea, vomiting	• Seizures, coma
• Weight gain	• Flushed skin
• ↑ BP, ↑ CVP	• Weight gain
• Muscle spasms, seizures, coma	• Peripheral and pulmonary edema
	• ↑ BP, ↑ CVP

BP, blood pressure; *CVP,* central venous pressure; *ECF,* extracellular fluid; *GI,* gastro-intestinal; *IV,* intravenous; *NaCl,* sodium chloride; *NG,* nasogastric; *SIADH,* syndrome of inappropriate antidiuretic hormone.

TABLE 19-4 CAUSES OF ECF VOLUME IMBALANCES

ECF Volume Deficit	ECF Volume Excess
Increased loss	Increased retention
• Vomiting	• Heart failure
• Diarrhea	• Cushing's syndrome
• Fistula drainage	• Chronic liver disease with portal hypertension
• GI tract suction	• Long-term use of corticosteroids
• Excessive sweating	• Renal failure
• Third-space fluid shifts (e.g., burns, intestinal obstruction)	
• Overuse of diuretics	
• Hemorrhage	
Decreased intake	Increased intake
• Nausea	• Rare when renal function is adequate
• Anorexia	• Excessive IV administration of fluids
• Inability to drink	
• Inability to obtain water	

ECF, extracellular fluid; *GI,* gastro-intestinal; *IV,* intravenous.

hyponatremia can cause confusion, vomiting, seizures, and even coma. If hyponatremia is severe and develops rapidly, irreversible neurological damage or death from brain herniation can occur (Verbalis, Goldsmith, Greenberg, et al., 2013).

Collaborative Care. In hyponatremia that is caused by water excess, fluid restriction is often all that is needed to treat the problem. If severe symptoms (seizures) develop, small amounts of IV hypertonic saline solution (3% sodium chloride [NaCl]) are administered to restore the serum sodium level while the body is returning to a normal water balance. Treatment of hyponatremia associated with abnormal fluid loss includes fluid replacement with sodium-containing solutions. The nurse must monitor serum sodium levels and the patient's response to therapy to avoid rapid correction or overcorrection. Rapidly increasing levels of sodium can cause osmotic demyelination syndrome with permanent damage to nerve cells in the brain. An accurate record of fluid input and output is essential. Commercially available oral rehydration fluids containing electrolytes may help prevent the development of hyponatremia in the home setting.

Extracellular Fluid Volume Imbalances. ECF volume deficit (hypovolemia) and ECF volume excess (hypervolemia) are commonly occurring clinical conditions (Table 19-4). ECF volume imbalances are typically accompanied by one or more electrolyte imbalances. As previously discussed, volume imbalances are often associated with changes in the serum sodium level. Fluid volume deficit can occur with abnormal loss of body fluids (e.g., through diarrhea, fistula drainage, hemorrhage, polyuria), decreased intake, or a plasma–to–interstitial fluid shift. Although the terms are often used interchangeably, fluid volume deficit and dehydration are not the same; *dehydration* refers to loss of pure water alone without a corresponding loss of sodium. Fluid volume excess may result from excessive intake of fluids, abnormal retention of fluids (e.g., heart failure, renal failure), or interstitial–to–plasma fluid shift. Although shifts in fluid between the plasma and the interstitium do not alter the overall volume of the ECF, these shifts do result in changes in the clinically important intravascular volume.

Collaborative Care. The goal of treatment for fluid volume deficit is to correct the underlying cause and to replace both water and electrolytes. Balanced IV solutions, such as lactated

disorders associated with excessive water intake. In SIADH, dilutional hyponatremia results from abnormal retention of water. (See Chapter 51 for a discussion of the causes of SIADH.)

Losses of sodium-rich body fluids from the GI tract, the kidneys, or the skin indirectly result in hyponatremia. Because these fluids are either isotonic or hypotonic, sodium is lost with an equal or greater proportion of water. However, hyponatremia develops as the body responds to the fluid volume deficit with activation of the thirst mechanism and by releasing ADH. The resultant retention of water lowers the sodium concentration.

The manifestations of hyponatremia are due to cellular swelling and first appear in the CNS (see Table 19-3). Mild hyponatremia has minor, nonspecific neurological symptoms, including headache, irritability, and difficulty concentrating. More severe

Ringer's solution, are usually given. Isotonic NaCl is used when rapid volume replacement is indicated. Blood is administered when volume loss is caused by blood loss.

The goal of treatment for fluid volume excess is removal of sodium and water without producing abnormal changes in the electrolyte composition or osmolality of ECF. The primary cause must be identified and treated. IV therapy is usually not indicated for this type of fluid imbalance. Diuretics and fluid restriction are the primary forms of therapy. Restriction of sodium intake may also be indicated. If the fluid excess leads to ascites or pleural effusion, an abdominal paracentesis or thoracentesis may be necessary.

NURSING MANAGEMENT
SODIUM AND VOLUME IMBALANCES

NURSING DIAGNOSES

Nursing diagnoses and collaborative problems for patients with various fluid and sodium imbalances include, but are not limited to, the following:

ECF volume excess:

- *Excess fluid volume* related to *excessive sodium intake*
- *Ineffective airway clearance* related to *retained secretions*
- *Risk for impaired skin integrity* as evidenced by *alteration in fluid volume* (edema)
- *Disturbed body image* related to *alteration in self-perception*
- Potential complications: pulmonary edema, ascites

ECF volume deficit:

- *Deficient fluid volume* related to *insufficient fluid intake*
- *Decreased cardiac output* (related to excessive ECF losses or decreased fluid intake)
- Potential complication: hypovolemic shock

Hypernatremia:

- *Risk for injury* as evidenced by *alteration in cognitive functioning* (seizures)

Hyponatremia:

- *Risk for injury* as evidenced by *alteration in cognitive functioning* (decreased level of consciousness)

NURSING IMPLEMENTATION

INTAKE AND OUTPUT. The 24-hour records of intake and output contain valuable information regarding fluid and electrolyte problems. Sources of excessive intake or fluid losses can be identified on a properly recorded intake-and-output flow sheet. Intake should include oral, IV, and tube feedings and retained irrigants. Fluid output includes urine, excess perspiration, wound or tube drainage, vomitus, and diarrhea. Fluid loss from wounds and perspiration should be estimated. Urine specific gravity can be measured. Readings higher than 1.030 indicate that the urine is concentrated, whereas those lower than 1.005 indicate that the urine is diluted.

CARDIOVASCULAR CHANGES. Monitoring patients for cardiovascular changes is necessary to prevent or detect complications from sodium and volume imbalances. Signs and symptoms of ECF volume excess and deficit are reflected in changes in blood pressure, pulse force, and jugular venous visibility. In fluid volume excess, the pulse is full and bounding. Because of the expanded intravascular volume, the pulse is not easily obliterated by the pressure cuff. Increased volume causes distension of neck veins (jugular venous distension) and increased blood pressure.

In mild to moderate fluid volume deficit, compensatory mechanisms include sympathetic nervous system stimulation of the heart and peripheral vasoconstriction. Stimulation of the heart increases heart rate and, in combination with vasoconstriction, maintains blood pressure within normal limits. A change in position from lying to sitting or standing may elicit a further increase in heart rate or a decrease in blood pressure (orthostatic hypotension). If vasoconstriction and tachycardia provide inadequate compensation, hypotension occurs when the patient is recumbent. Severe fluid volume deficit can cause a weak, thready pulse that is easily obliterated and flattened neck veins. Severe, untreated fluid deficit results in shock.

RESPIRATORY CHANGES. Both fluid excess and fluid deficit affect respiratory status. Fluid excess results in pulmonary congestion and pulmonary edema as increased hydrostatic pressure in the pulmonary vessels forces fluid into the alveoli. Affected patients exhibit shortness of breath, irritative cough, and moist crackles on auscultation. Patients with fluid deficit demonstrate an increased respiratory rate because of decreased tissue perfusion and resultant hypoxia.

NEUROLOGICAL CHANGES. Changes in neurological function may occur with sodium and water imbalances. With increased water volume and hyponatremia, water moves by osmosis into the brain cells. Alternatively, decreased water volume and hypernatremia cause water to shift out of the brain cells, with resultant shrinkage. In addition, profound volume depletion may cause an alteration in sensorium secondary to reduced cerebral tissue perfusion.

Assessment of neurological function includes evaluation of (1) the level of consciousness, which includes responses to verbal and painful stimuli and the determination of a person's orientation to time, place, and person; (2) pupillary response to light and equality of pupil size; and (3) voluntary movement of the extremities, degree of muscle strength, and reflexes. Nursing care focuses on maintaining patient safety.

DAILY WEIGHT MEASUREMENTS. Accurate daily weight measurements are the easiest way to estimate volume status. An increase of 1 kg is equal to 1000 mL (1 L) of fluid retention (provided that the person has maintained usual dietary intake or has not been on nothing-by-mouth [NPO] status). However, weight changes can be relied on only if obtained under standardized conditions. Obtaining an accurate weight depends on the patient's being weighed at the same time every day, with the same garments on, and on the same carefully calibrated scale. Excess bedding should be removed, and all drainage bags should be emptied before the weighing. If bulky dressings or tubes are present, which may not necessarily be used every day, a notation regarding these variables should be recorded on the flow sheet or nursing notes.

SKIN ASSESSMENT AND CARE. Clues to fluid volume deficit and excess can be detected by inspection of the skin. Skin should be examined for turgor and mobility. Normally, a fold of skin, when pinched, moves readily and, on release, rapidly returns to its former position. Skin areas over the sternum, the abdomen, and the anterior forearm are the usual sites for evaluation of tissue turgor (Figure 19-13). In older people, decreased skin turgor is less predictive of fluid deficit because of the loss of tissue elasticity (Hooper, Bunn, Jimoh, et al., 2014).

In ECF volume deficit, skin turgor is diminished; there is a lag in the pinched skinfold's return to its original state (referred to as *tenting*). In mild fluid deficits, the skin may appear warm,

FIGURE 19-13 Assessment of skin turgor. When normal skin is pinched, it resumes shape in seconds. If the skin remains wrinkled for 20 to 30 seconds, the patient has poor skin turgor. Source: de Vries Feyens, C., & de Jager, C. P. C. (2011, January). Images in medicine: Decreased skin turgor. Dr. P. Marazzi/Science Source.

dry, and wrinkled. These signs may be difficult to evaluate in an older adult because the patient's skin may be normally dry, wrinkled, and nonelastic. In more severe deficits, the skin may be cool and moist if there is vasoconstriction to compensate for the decreased fluid volume. Oral mucous membranes are dry, the tongue may be furrowed, and many affected individuals complain of thirst. Routine oral care is critical for the comfort of a patient who is dehydrated or has a fluid restriction order.

Edematous skin may feel cool because of fluid accumulation and a decrease in blood flow secondary to the pressure of the fluid. The fluid can stretch the skin, causing it to feel taut and hard. The nurse assesses edema by pressing with a thumb or forefinger over the edematous area. A grading scale (ranging from 1+ [slight edema; 2-mm indentation] to 4+ [pitting edema; 8-mm indentation]) is used to standardize the description if an indentation remains when pressure is released. The nurse must evaluate for edema in areas where soft tissues overlie a bone, particularly the tibia, fibula, and sacrum.

Good skin care for the person with fluid volume excess or deficit is important. Edematous tissues must be protected from extremes of heat and cold, prolonged pressure, and trauma. Frequent skin care and changes in position protect the patient from skin breakdown. Elevation of edematous extremities helps promote venous return and fluid reabsorption. Dehydrated skin needs frequent care without the use of soap. The application of moisturizing creams or oils increases moisture retention and stimulates circulation.

OTHER NURSING MEASURES. The nurse should administer IV fluids as ordered and carefully monitor the rates of infusion of IV fluid solutions, especially when large volumes of fluid are being given. This is especially true in patients with cardiac, renal, or neurological problems. Patients receiving tube feedings need supplementary water added to their enteral formula. The amount of water depends on the osmolarity of the feeding and the patient's condition.

Patients with nasogastric suction should not be allowed to drink water because it will increase the loss of electrolytes. On occasion, such patients may be given small amounts of ice chips to suck. A nasogastric tube should always be irrigated with isotonic saline solution and not with water. Water causes diffusion of electrolytes into the gastric lumen from mucosal cells; the electrolytes are then suctioned away.

Nurses in hospital and community settings should encourage and often assist older or debilitated patients in maintaining an adequate oral intake. This may be accomplished by giving patients a drink as part of the morning care, encouraging extra sips of fluid with medications, and including a drink of fluids as part of one-on-one conversations.

Potassium Imbalances

Potassium is the major ICF cation; 98% of the body potassium is intracellular. For example, potassium concentration within muscle cells is approximately 140 mmol; potassium concentration in the ECF is 3.5 to 5.0 mmol. The sodium–potassium pump in cell membranes maintains this concentration difference by pumping potassium into the cell and sodium out, a process fuelled by the breakdown of ATP. The ratio of ECF potassium to ICF potassium is the major factor in the resting neuron's membrane potential. Many of the symptoms related to potassium imbalance are caused by changes in the ratio of ECF potassium to ICF potassium (increased or decreased ECF potassium; McCance & Huether, 2014).

Potassium is critical for many cellular and metabolic functions. It is necessary for the transmission and conduction of nerve impulses, maintenance of normal cardiac rhythms, and skeletal and smooth muscle contraction. As the major intracellular cation, potassium regulates intracellular osmolality and promotes cellular growth. Potassium moves into cells during the formation of new tissues and leaves the cell during tissue breakdown (McCance & Huether, 2014). Potassium also plays a role in acid–base balance, which is discussed with acid–base regulation later in this chapter.

Diet is the source of potassium. The typical Western diet contains approximately 50 to 100 mEq of potassium daily, mainly from fruits, dried fruits, and vegetables. Many salt substitutes contain substantial potassium. Patients may receive potassium from parenteral sources, including IV fluids, stored transfused blood, and potassium–penicillin.

The kidneys are the primary route for potassium loss. Approximately 90% of the daily potassium intake is eliminated by the kidneys; the remainder is lost in the stool and sweat. If kidney function is significantly impaired, toxic levels of potassium may be retained. There is an inverse relationship between sodium and potassium reabsorption in the kidneys. Factors that cause sodium retention (e.g., low blood volume, increased aldosterone level) cause potassium loss in the urine. Large urine volumes can be associated with excess loss of potassium in the urine. The ability of the kidneys to conserve potassium is weak even when body stores are depleted (McCance & Huether, 2014).

Disruptions in the dynamic equilibrium between ICF and ECF potassium often cause clinical problems. Among the factors causing potassium to move from the ECF to the ICF are the following:

- Insulin
- Alkalosis
- β-Adrenergic stimulation (catecholamine release in stress, coronary ischemia, delirium tremens, or administration of β-adrenergic agonist drugs)

- Rapid cell building (administration of folic acid or cobalamin [vitamin B_{12}] to patients with megaloblastic anemia, which results in marked production of red blood cells [RBCs])

Factors that cause potassium to move from the ICF to the ECF include acidosis, trauma to cells (as in massive soft tissue damage or in tumour lysis), and exercise. Both digoxin-like drugs and β-adrenergic–blocking drugs (e.g., propranolol [Inderal]) can impair entry of potassium into cells, which results in the higher ECF potassium concentration. Causes of potassium imbalance are summarized in Table 19-5.

Hyperkalemia. Hyperkalemia (high serum levels of potassium) may be caused by a massive intake of potassium, impaired renal excretion, shift of potassium from the ICF to the ECF, or a combination of these factors. The most common cause of hyperkalemia is renal failure. Hyperkalemia is also common in patients with massive cell destruction (e.g., burn or crush injury, tumour lysis), rapid transfusion of aged blood, and catabolic state (e.g., severe infections). Metabolic acidosis, particularly when the chloride level is normal, is associated with a shift of potassium ions from the ICF to the ECF as hydrogen ions move into the cell. Adrenal insufficiency leads to retention of potassium ions in the serum because of aldosterone deficiency. Certain drugs, such as potassium-sparing diuretics (e.g., spironolactone [Aldactone], triamterene) and angiotensin-converting enzyme (ACE) inhibitors (e.g., enalapril [Vasotec], lisinopril [Prinivil]), may contribute to the development of hyperkalemia. Both of these types of drugs reduce the kidneys' ability to secrete and therefore excrete excess potassium (see Table 19-5).

Clinical Manifestations. Hyperkalemia causes membrane depolarization, altering cell excitability. Skeletal muscles become weak or paralyzed. The first symptom may be leg cramping. The most clinically significant problems are the disturbances in cardiac conduction. The initial finding is tall, peaked T waves. As potassium increases, cardiac depolarization decreases, leading to loss of P waves, a prolonged PR interval, ST segment depression, and a widening QRS complex (Figure 19-14). Heart block, ventricular fibrillation, or cardiac standstill may occur. Other clinical manifestations are listed in Table 19-5.

TABLE 19-5   POTASSIUM IMBALANCES: CAUSES AND CLINICAL MANIFESTATIONS

Hypokalemia (K+ Level < 3.5 mmol/L)	Hyperkalemia (K+ Level > 5.0 mmol/L)
Causes	
Potassium loss	Excess potassium intake
• GI losses: diarrhea, vomiting, fistulas, NG suction	• Excessive or rapid parenteral administration
• Renal losses: diuretics, hyperaldosteronism, magnesium depletion	• Potassium-containing drugs (e.g., potassium-penicillin)
• Skin losses: diaphoresis	• Potassium-containing salt substitute
• Dialysis	
Shift of potassium into cells	Shift of potassium out of cells
• Increased insulin (e.g., IV dextrose load)	• Acidosis
• Alkalosis	• Tissue catabolism (e.g., fever, sepsis, burns)
• Tissue repair	• Crush injury
• ↑ Epinephrine (e.g., stress)	• Tumour lysis syndrome
Lack of potassium intake	Failure to eliminate potassium
• Starvation	• Renal disease
• Diet with low potassium content	• Potassium-sparing diuretics
• Failure to include potassium in parenteral fluids if NPO status is in effect	• Adrenal insufficiency
	• ACE inhibitors
Clinical Manifestations	
Fatigue	Irritability
Muscle weakness	Anxiety
Leg cramps	Abdominal cramping, diarrhea
Nausea, vomiting, ileus	Weakness of lower extremities
Soft, flabby muscles	
Paresthesias, decreased reflexes	Paresthesias
Weak, irregular pulse	Irregular pulse
Polyuria	Cardiac standstill if hyperkalemia is sudden or severe
Hyperglycemia	
Electrocardiographic Changes	
ST segment depression	Tall, peaked T wave
Flattened T wave	Prolonged P–R interval
Presence of U wave	ST depression
Ventricular dysrhythmias (e.g., PVCs)	Loss of P wave
	Widening QRS complex
Bradycardia	Ventricular fibrillation
Enhanced digitalis effect	Ventricular standstill

ACE, angiotensin-converting enzyme; *GI*, gastro-intestinal; *IV*, intravenous; *NG*, nasogastric; *NPO*, nothing by mouth; *PVC*, premature ventricular contraction.

NURSING AND COLLABORATIVE MANAGEMENT HYPERKALEMIA

NURSING DIAGNOSES

Nursing diagnoses and collaborative problems for patients with hyperkalemia include, but are not limited to, the following:
- *Risk for injury* as evidenced by *alteration in sensation*
- Potential complication: dysrhythmias

NURSING IMPLEMENTATION

Treatment of hyperkalemia consists of the following (see Chapter 49, Table 49-4):
1. Eliminating oral and parenteral potassium intake.
2. Increasing elimination of potassium. This is accomplished through the use of diuretics, dialysis, and use of ion-exchange resins such as sodium polystyrene sulphonate (Kayexalate). Increased fluid intake can enhance renal potassium elimination.
3. Forcing potassium from the ECF to the ICF. This is accomplished by administration of IV insulin (along with glucose so that the patient does not become hypoglycemic) or by administration of IV sodium bicarbonate in the correction of acidosis. In rare cases, a β-adrenergic agonist (e.g., epinephrine) is administered.
4. Reversing the membrane effects of the elevated ECF potassium by administering calcium gluconate intravenously. Calcium ion can immediately reverse the effect of the depolarization on cell excitability.

In cases in which the elevation of potassium level is mild and the kidneys are functioning, it may be sufficient to withhold potassium from the diet and IV sources and increase renal elimination by administering fluids and possibly diuretics. Kayexalate, which is administered via the GI tract, binds potassium in exchange for sodium, and the resin is excreted in feces (see Chapter 49). All patients with clinically significant hyperkalemia should be monitored electrocardiographically

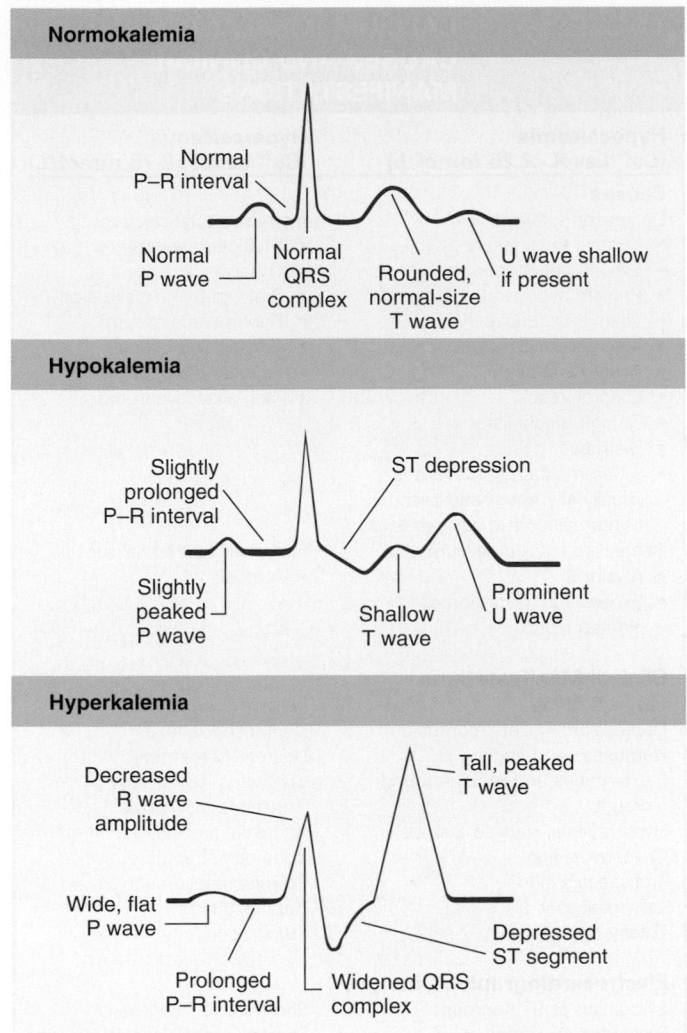

Normokalemia

Normal
P–R interval

Normal
P wave

Normal
QRS
complex

Rounded,
normal-size
T wave

U wave shallow
if present

Hypokalemia

Slightly
prolonged
P–R interval

ST depression

Slightly
peaked
P wave

Shallow
T wave

Prominent
U wave

Hyperkalemia

Decreased
R wave
amplitude

Tall, peaked
T wave

Wide, flat
P wave

Prolonged
P–R interval

Widened QRS
complex

Depressed
ST segment

FIGURE 19-14 Electrocardiographic changes associated with alterations in potassium status. Source: Redrawn from McCance, K. L., & Huether, S. E. (2014). *Pathophysiology: The biologic basis for disease in adults and children* (7th ed., p. 117). St. Louis: Mosby.

to detect dysrhythmias and to monitor the effects of therapy. Patients with moderate hyperkalemia should additionally receive one of the treatments to force potassium into cells, usually IV insulin and glucose. The patient experiencing dangerous cardiac dysrhythmias should receive IV calcium gluconate immediately; this serves to protect the patient while the potassium is being eliminated and forced into cells. Hemodialysis is an effective means of removing potassium from the body in patients with renal failure.

Hypokalemia. Hypokalemia (low serum levels of potassium) can result from abnormal losses of potassium caused by a shift of potassium from ECF to ICF or, in rare cases, by deficient dietary potassium intake. The most common causes of hypokalemia are abnormal losses, via either the kidneys or the GI tract. Abnormal losses occur in patients with diuresis, particularly in patients with an elevated aldosterone level. Aldosterone is released when the circulating blood volume is low; it causes sodium retention in the kidneys but loss of potassium in the urine. Magnesium deficiency may contribute to the development of potassium depletion. Low plasma magnesium stimulates renin

release and subsequently increases aldosterone levels, which results in potassium excretion. GI tract losses of potassium secondary to diarrhea, laxative abuse, vomiting, and ileostomy drainage can cause hypokalemia.

Metabolic alkalosis can cause a shift of potassium into cells in exchange for hydrogen, thus lowering the potassium level in the ECF and causing symptomatic hypokalemia. Hypokalemia is sometimes associated with the treatment of diabetic ketoacidosis because of a combination of factors, including an increased urinary potassium loss and a shift of potassium into cells with the administration of insulin and correction of acidosis. A less common cause of hypokalemia is the sudden initiation of cell formation; for example, the formation of RBCs as in treatment of anemia with cobalamin, folic acid, or erythropoietin.

Clinical Manifestations. Hypokalemia alters resting membrane potential. It most commonly is associated with hyperpolarization, or increased negative charge within the cell. This causes excitability problems in many types of tissue. The most serious clinical problems are cardiac. The incidence of potentially lethal ventricular dysrhythmias is increased in hypokalemia. Patients should be monitored with electrocardiography for signs of hypokalemia. These changes include impaired repolarization, which results in a flattening of the T wave and eventually in emergence of a U wave. The P wave amplitude may increase and may become peaked (see Figure 19-14). Patients taking digoxin experience increased digoxin toxicity if their serum potassium level is low. Skeletal muscle weakness and paralysis may occur with hypokalemia. As with hyperkalemia, symptoms are most often observed in the legs. Respiratory muscles and those innervated by cranial nerves are not involved. Muscle cramping and muscle cell breakdown (known as rhabdomyolysis) can be caused by hypokalemia. This can cause myoglobin to appear in the plasma and the urine, which can, in turn, lead to renal failure.

Smooth muscle function is altered by hypokalemia. Affected patients may experience decreased GI motility (e.g., paralytic ileus), altered airway responsiveness, and impaired regulation of arteriolar blood flow, all of which possibly contribute to muscle cell breakdown. Finally, hypokalemia can impair function in nonmuscle tissue. With prolonged hypokalemia, the kidneys are unable to concentrate urine, and diuresis occurs. Release of insulin is impaired, which often leads to hyperglycemia. Clinical manifestations of hypokalemia are presented in Table 19-5.

NURSING AND COLLABORATIVE MANAGEMENT HYPOKALEMIA

NURSING DIAGNOSES

Nursing diagnoses and collaborative problems for patients with hypokalemia include, but are not limited to, the following:

- *Risk for injury* as evidenced by *alteration in psychomotor functioning* (muscle weakness, hyporeflexia)
- Potential complication: dysrhythmias

NURSING IMPLEMENTATION. Hypokalemia is treated by administration of potassium chloride (KCl) supplements and increasing dietary intake of potassium. KCl supplements can be given orally or intravenously. Except in severe deficiencies, KCl is never given unless the urine output is at least 0.5 mL/kg of body weight per hour. KCl supplements added to IV solutions should never exceed 60 mmol (mEq/L). The preferred level is 40 mmol. IV KCl infusion rates should not exceed 10 mEq per hour unless the patient is in a critical care setting with continuous ECG monitoring and

TABLE 19-6	PATIENT & CAREGIVER TEACHING GUIDE

Prevention of Hypokalemia

1. Teach the patient and caregivers the signs and symptoms of hypokalemia and to report them to the health care provider.
2. For the patient taking potassium-losing diuretics:
   - Explain the importance of increasing dietary potassium intake, especially if the patient is receiving a thiazide or loop diuretic.
   - Teach the patient which foods have high potassium content (see Chapter 49, Table 49-9).
   - Explain that salt substitutes contain approximately 50-60 mEq of potassium per teaspoon and help raise potassium if the patient is taking a potassium-losing diuretic.
3. For the patient taking potassium-sparing diuretics:
   - Explain that salt substitutes and foods with high potassium content should be avoided.
4. For the patient taking oral potassium supplements:
   - Instruct the patient to take the medication as prescribed to prevent overdosage and to take the supplement with a full glass of water to help it dissolve in the GI tract.
5. For the patient taking digitalis preparations and others at risk for hypokalemia:
   - Explain the importance of having serum potassium levels monitored regularly because a low potassium level enhances the action of digitalis.

GI, gastro-intestinal.

central line access for administration (Medford-Davis & Rafique, 2014). When given intravenously, potassium may cause pain in the area of the vein where it is entering. Because KCl is irritating to the vein, assess IV sites at least hourly for phlebitis and infiltration. Infiltration can cause necrosis and sloughing of the surrounding tissue. The nurse must teach patients ways to prevent hypokalemia (Table 19-6). Patients at risk for hypokalemia should have serum potassium levels monitored regularly.

SAFETY ALERT
- KCl given intravenously must always be diluted.
- Never give KCl via IV push or in concentrated amounts.
- IV bags containing KCl should be inverted several times to ensure even distribution in the bag.
- Never add KCl to a hanging IV bag, to prevent giving a bolus dose.

Calcium Imbalances

Calcium is obtained from ingested foods. However, only approximately 30% is absorbed in the GI tract. More than 99% of the body's calcium is combined with phosphorus and concentrated in the skeletal system. Bones serve as a readily available store of calcium. Thus to avoid wide variations in serum calcium levels, the movement of calcium into or out of the bone is regulated. Usually, the amounts of calcium and phosphorus found in the serum have an inverse relationship; that is, as one increases, the other decreases (McCance & Huether, 2014). The functions of calcium include transmission of nerve impulses, myocardial contractions, blood clotting, formation of teeth and bone, and muscle contractions.

Calcium is present in the serum in three forms: free or ionized; bound to protein (primarily albumin); and complexed with phosphate, citrate, or carbonate. The ionized form is the biologically active form. Approximately half of the total serum calcium is ionized.

Calcium is typically measured in millimoles per litre (mmol/L). As usually reported, serum calcium levels reflect the total calcium

TABLE 19-7	CALCIUM IMBALANCES: CAUSES AND CLINICAL MANIFESTATIONS

Hypocalcemia (Ca^{2+} Level <2.25 mmol/L)	Hypercalcemia (Ca^{2+} Level >2.75 mmol/L)
Causes	
Decreased total calcium	Increased total calcium
• Chronic renal failure	• Multiple myeloma
• Elevated phosphorus	• Other malignancy
• Primary hypoparathyroidism	• Prolonged immobilization
• Vitamin D deficiency	• Hyperparathyroidism
• Magnesium deficiency	• Vitamin D overdose
• Acute pancreatitis	• Thiazide diuretics
• Loop diuretics	• Milk–alkali syndrome
• Chronic alcoholism	
• Diarrhea	
• ↓ Serum albumin (patient is usually asymptomatic because of normal ionized calcium level)	
Decreased ionized calcium	Increased ionized calcium
• Alkalosis	• Acidosis
• Excess administration of citrated blood	
Clinical Manifestations	
Easy fatigability	Lethargy, weakness
Depression, anxiety, confusion	Depressed reflexes
Numbness and tingling in extremities and region around mouth	Decreased memory
	Confusion, personality changes, psychosis
Hyperreflexia, muscle cramps	Anorexia, nausea, vomiting
Chvostek's sign	Bone pain, fractures
Trousseau's sign	Polyuria, dehydration
Laryngeal spasm	Nephrolithiasis
Tetany, seizures	Stupor, coma
Electrocardiographic Changes	
Elongation of ST segment	Shortened ST segment
Prolonged Q–T interval	Shortened Q–T interval
Ventricular tachycardia	Ventricular dysrhythmias
	Increased digitalis effect

level (all three forms), although ionized calcium levels are sometimes reported separately. The levels listed in Table 19-7 reflect total calcium levels. Changes in serum pH alter the level of ionized calcium without altering the total calcium level. Acidosis decreases calcium binding to albumin, which leads to more ionized calcium, and alkalosis increases calcium binding, which leads to decreased ionized calcium. Alterations in serum albumin levels affect interpretation of total calcium levels. Low albumin levels result in a drop in the total calcium level, although the level of ionized calcium does not change as much.

Calcium balance is controlled by parathyroid hormone (PTH), calcitonin, and vitamin D (McCance & Huether, 2014). PTH is produced by the parathyroid gland. Its production and release are stimulated when serum calcium levels are low. PTH increases bone resorption (movement of calcium out of bones), increases GI absorption of calcium, and increases renal tubule reabsorption of calcium.

Calcitonin is produced by the thyroid gland, and its production and release are stimulated when serum calcium levels are high. It opposes the action of PTH and thus lowers the serum calcium level by decreasing GI absorption, increasing calcium deposition into bone, and promoting renal excretion.

Vitamin D is formed through the action of ultraviolet rays on a precursor found in the skin or is ingested in the diet. Vitamin D is important for absorption of calcium from the GI tract. Causes of calcium imbalances are listed in Table 19-7.

Hypercalcemia. Approximately two-thirds of hypercalcemia cases are caused by hyperparathyroidism, and one-third are caused by malignancy, especially from breast cancer, lung cancer, and multiple myeloma (Wilson, Shannon, & Stang, 2011). Malignancies lead to hypercalcemia through bone destruction from tumour invasion or through tumour secretion of a parathyroid-related protein, which stimulates calcium release from bones. Hypercalcemia is also associated with vitamin D overdose. Prolonged immobilization results in bone mineral loss and increased calcium concentration. Hypercalcemia rarely occurs as a result of increased calcium intake (e.g., ingestion of antacids containing calcium, excessive administration during cardiac arrest).

Excess calcium blocks the effect of sodium in skeletal muscles, which leads to reduced excitability of both muscles and nerves (McCance & Huether, 2014). Manifestations of hypercalcemia include impaired memory, confusion, disorientation, fatigue, muscle weakness, constipation, cardiac dysrhythmias, and renal calculi (see Table 19-7).

NURSING AND COLLABORATIVE MANAGEMENT HYPERCALCEMIA

NURSING DIAGNOSES

Nursing diagnoses and collaborative problems for patients with hypercalcemia include, but are not limited to, the following:
- *Risk for injury* as evidenced by *alteration in sensation*
- Potential complication: dysrhythmias

NURSING IMPLEMENTATION

The basic treatment of hypercalcemia is promotion of excretion of calcium in urine by administration of a loop diuretic (e.g., furosemide [Lasix], ethacrynic acid [Edecrin]) and hydration of the patient with isotonic saline infusions. IV saline therapy necessitates careful monitoring. Fluid overload can occur in patients who cannot excrete the excess sodium because of impaired renal function.

Synthetic calcitonin can also be administered to lower serum calcium levels. A diet with low calcium content may be prescribed. Mobilization with weight-bearing activity is encouraged so as to enhance bone mineralization. In hypercalcemia associated with malignancy, the drug of choice is pamidronate (Aredia), which inhibits the activity of osteoclasts. Pamidronate is preferred because it does not have cytotoxic adverse effects and it inhibits bone resorption without inhibiting bone formation and mineralization.

Hypocalcemia. Any condition that causes a decrease in the production of PTH may result in the development of hypocalcemia. This may occur with surgical removal of a portion of or injury to the parathyroid glands during thyroid or neck surgery. Acute pancreatitis is another potential cause of hypocalcemia. Lipolysis, a consequence of pancreatitis, produces fatty acids that combine with calcium ions, which leads to a decrease in serum calcium levels. A patient who receives multiple blood transfusions can become hypocalcemic because the citrate used to anticoagulate the blood binds with the calcium. Sudden alkalosis may also result in symptomatic hypocalcemia despite a normal total serum calcium level. The high pH increases calcium binding to protein, decreasing the amount of ionized calcium.

FIGURE 19-15 Tests for hypocalcemia. **A,** Chvostek's sign is contraction of facial muscles in response to a light tap over the facial nerve in front of the ear. **B,** Trousseau's sign is a carpal spasm induced by **C,** inflating a blood pressure cuff above the systolic pressure for a few minutes.

Hypocalcemia can occur if the diet has low calcium content or if loss of calcium is increased as a result of laxative abuse and malabsorption syndromes. (See Table 19-7 for the clinical manifestations and etiologies of hypocalcemia.)

Low calcium levels allow sodium to move into excitable cells, which increases depolarization. This results in increased nerve excitability and sustained muscle contraction that is referred to as **tetany.** Clinical signs of tetany include Trousseau's and Chvostek's signs. *Trousseau's sign* refers to carpal spasms induced by inflating a blood pressure cuff on the arm (Figure 19-15). The blood pressure cuff is inflated above the systolic pressure. Carpal spasms become evident within 3 minutes if hypocalcemia is present. *Chvostek's sign* is contraction of facial muscles in response to a tap over the facial nerve in front of the ear (see Figure 19-15). Other manifestations of tetany are laryngeal stridor, dysphagia, and numbness and tingling around the mouth or in the extremities.

Because calcium is necessary for cardiac contractions, hypocalcemia results in decreased cardiac contractility and ECG changes. Clinical manifestations of hypocalcemia are listed in Table 19-7.

NURSING AND COLLABORATIVE MANAGEMENT HYPOCALCEMIA

NURSING DIAGNOSES

Nursing diagnoses and collaborative problems for patients with hypocalcemia include, but are not limited to, the following:
- *Risk for injury* as evidenced by *alteration in cognitive functioning* (tetany and seizures)
- Potential complications: fracture, respiratory arrest

NURSING IMPLEMENTATION

Treatment of hypocalcemia is aimed primarily at correcting the cause. Treating mild or asymptomatic hypocalcemia involves a diet of calcium-rich foods and calcium and vitamin D supplementation. IV preparations of calcium, such as calcium gluconate, are administered when severe symptoms of hypocalcemia are impending or present. Oral calcium supplements, such as calcium carbonate, may be used when patients are unable to consume enough calcium in the diet, such as those who do not tolerate dairy products. Pain and anxiety must be adequately treated in patients with suspected hypocalcemia because hyperventilation-induced respiratory alkalosis can precipitate hypocalcemic symptoms. Any patient who undergoes thyroid or neck surgery must be observed closely in the immediate postoperative period for manifestations of hypocalcemia because of the proximity of the surgery to the parathyroid glands.

Phosphate Imbalances

Phosphorus is a primary anion in the ICF and is essential to the function of muscle, RBCs, and the nervous system. It is deposited with calcium for bone and tooth structure. It is also involved in the acid–base buffering system, in the mitochondrial energy production of ATP, in cellular uptake and use of glucose, and as an intermediary in the metabolism of carbohydrates, proteins, and fats.

For maintenance of normal phosphate balance, renal functioning must be adequate because the kidneys are the major route of phosphate excretion. A small amount is lost in the feces. A reciprocal relationship exists between phosphorus and calcium in that a high serum phosphate level tends to cause a low calcium concentration in the serum.

Hyperphosphatemia. The major condition that can lead to hyperphosphatemia is acute or chronic renal failure that results in an altered ability of the kidneys to excrete phosphate. Other causes include chemotherapy for certain malignancies (lymphomas), excessive ingestion of milk or phosphate-containing laxatives, and large intakes of vitamin D that increase GI absorption of phosphorus (Table 19-8).

Clinical manifestations of hyperphosphatemia (presented in Table 19-8) relate primarily to metastatic calcium–phosphate precipitates. Ordinarily, calcium and phosphate are deposited only in bone. However, an increased serum phosphate concentration along with calcium precipitates readily, and calcified deposits can develop in soft tissue such as those of the joints, arteries, skin, kidneys, and corneas (see Chapter 49). Other manifestations of hyperphosphatemia are neuro-muscular irritability and tetany, which are related to the low serum calcium levels often associated with high serum phosphate levels.

Management of hyperphosphatemia is aimed at identifying and treating the underlying cause. Ingestion of foods and fluids with high phosphorus content (e.g., dairy products) should be restricted. Adequate hydration and correction of hypocalcemic conditions can enhance the renal excretion of phosphate. For patients with renal failure, measures to reduce serum phosphate levels include calcium supplements, phosphate-binding agents or gels, and dietary phosphate restrictions (see Chapter 49).

Hypophosphatemia. Hypophosphatemia (low serum phosphate) is seen in patients who are malnourished or have malabsorption syndromes. Other causes include alcohol withdrawal and use of phosphate-binding antacids. Hypophosphatemia may also occur during parenteral nutrition with inadequate phosphorus replacement. Table 19-8 lists causes of phosphorus imbalances.

Most of the clinical manifestations of hypophosphatemia (presented in Table 19-8) are related to a deficiency of ATP

TABLE 19-8	PHOSPHATE IMBALANCES: CAUSES AND CLINICAL MANIFESTATIONS	
Hypophosphatemia (PO_4^{3-} Level <0.97 mmol/L)	**Hyperphosphatemia (PO_4^{3-} Level >1.45 mmol/L)**
Causes	
Malabsorption syndrome	Renal failure
Nutritional recovery syndrome	Chemotherapeutic agents
Glucose administration	Enemas containing phosphorus (e.g., Fleet enema)
Total parenteral nutrition	Excessive ingestion (e.g., milk, phosphate-containing laxatives)
Alcohol withdrawal	
Phosphate-binding antacids	
Recovery from diabetic ketoacidosis	Large vitamin D intake
Respiratory alkalosis	Hypoparathyroidism
Clinical Manifestations	
Central nervous system dysfunction (confusion, coma)	Hypocalcemia
Rhabdomyolysis	Muscle problems; tetany
Renal tubular wasting of Mg^{2+}, Ca^{2+}, HCO_3^-	Deposition of calcium–phosphate precipitates in skin, soft tissue, corneas, viscera, blood vessels
Cardiac problems (dysrhythmias, decreased stroke volume)	
Muscle weakness, including respiratory muscle weakness	
Osteomalacia	

or 2,3-diphosphoglycerate (2,3-DPG), an enzyme in RBCs. Both conditions result in impaired cellular energy resources and oxygen delivery to tissues. Hemolytic anemia may occur because of the fragility of the RBCs. Acute manifestations include CNS depression, confusion, and other mental changes. Other manifestations include muscle weakness and pain, dysrhythmias, and cardiomyopathy.

Management of a mild phosphorus deficiency may involve oral supplementation and ingestion of foods with high phosphorus content (e.g., dairy products). Severe hypophosphatemia can be serious and may necessitate IV administration of sodium phosphate or potassium phosphate. Frequent monitoring of serum phosphate levels is necessary to guide IV therapy. Sudden symptomatic hypocalcemia, secondary to increased calcium phosphorus binding, is a potential complication of IV administration of phosphorus.

Magnesium Imbalances

Magnesium, the second most abundant intracellular cation, plays an important role in essential cellular processes. It is a cofactor in many enzyme systems, including those responsible for carbohydrate metabolism, DNA and protein synthesis, blood glucose control, and blood pressure regulation. Magnesium is required for the production and use of adenosine triphosphate (ATP), the energy source for the sodium–potassium pump. Muscle contraction and relaxation, normal neurological function, and neurotransmitter release depend on magnesium.

Approximately 50% to 60% of the body's magnesium is contained in bone. Magnesium concentration is regulated by GI absorption and renal excretion. The kidneys are able to conserve magnesium in times of need and to excrete excesses. Factors that regulate calcium balance (e.g., PTH) appear to influence magnesium balance. Manifestations of magnesium balance are

TABLE 19-9	CAUSES OF MAGNESIUM IMBALANCES
Hypomagnesemia (Mg^{2+} Level <0.74 mmol/L)	**Hypermagnesemia (Mg^{2+} Level >1.07 mmol/L)**
Diarrhea Vomiting Chronic alcoholism Impaired GI absorption Malabsorption syndrome Prolonged malnutrition Large urine output NG suction Poorly controlled diabetes mellitus Hyperaldosteronism	Renal failure (especially if patient is given magnesium products) Excessive administration of magnesium for treatment of eclampsia Adrenal insufficiency

GI, gastro-intestinal; *NG,* nasogastric.

TABLE 19-10	CAUSES OF PROTEIN IMBALANCES
Hypoproteinemia (Protein Level <64 g/L)	**Hyperproteinemia (Protein Level >83 g/L)**
Decreased food intake Starvation Diseased liver Massive burns Loss of albumin in renal disease Major infection	Dehydration Hemoconcentration

often mistaken for those of calcium imbalances. Because magnesium balance is related to calcium and potassium balance, all three cations should be assessed together. Causes of magnesium imbalances are listed in Table 19-9.

Hypermagnesemia. Hypermagnesemia usually occurs only with an increase in magnesium intake accompanied by renal insufficiency or failure. In patients with chronic renal failure, ingesting products containing magnesium (e.g., Maalox, milk of magnesia) will cause excess magnesium. Magnesium excess could develop in pregnant women who receive magnesium sulphate (MgSO$_4$) for the management of eclampsia.

Excess magnesium inhibits acetylcholine release at the myoneural junction and calcium movement into cells, impairing nerve and muscle function. Initial manifestations include hypotension, facial flushing, lethargy, urinary retention, nausea, and vomiting. As the serum magnesium level increases, deep tendon reflexes are lost, followed by muscle paralysis and coma. Respiratory and cardiac arrest can occur.

Management begins with avoiding magnesium-containing drugs and limiting diet intake of magnesium-containing foods (e.g., green vegetables, nuts, bananas, oranges, peanut butter, chocolate). If renal function is adequate, increased fluids and diuretics promote urinary excretion. In patients with impaired renal function, dialysis is required. If hypermagnesemia is symptomatic, calcium gluconate administered by IV infusion opposes the effects of the excess magnesium on cardiac muscle.

Hypomagnesemia. Magnesium deficiency occurs in patients with limited magnesium intake or increased gastro-intestinal or renal losses. Causes of hypomagnesemia from insufficient food intake include prolonged fasting or starvation and chronic alcoholism (Table 19-9). Another potential cause is prolonged parenteral nutrition without magnesium supplementation. Fluid loss from the GI tract, inflammatory bowel disease, and proton pump inhibitors interfere with magnesium absorption. Many diuretics and osmotic diuresis from high glucose levels may cause magnesium loss through increased urinary excretion (Demssie, Patel, Kumar, et al., 2014).

Clinically, hypomagnesemia resembles hypocalcemia and may contribute to the development of hypocalcemia as a result of the decreased action of PTH. Neuro-muscular manifestations are common, such as muscle cramps, tremors, hyperactive deep tendon reflexes, Chvostek's sign, and Trousseau's sign. Neurological manifestations include confusion, vertigo, and seizures.

Magnesium deficiency can lead to cardiac dysrhythmias, such as torsades de pointes and ventricular fibrillation. Hypomagnesemia

is associated with digitalis toxicity. Hypomagnesemia may also be associated with hypokalemia that does not respond well to potassium replacement. This occurs because intracellular magnesium is crucial for normal function of the sodium–potassium pump.

Mild magnesium deficiencies can be treated with oral supplements and increased dietary intake of foods with high magnesium content (e.g., green vegetables, nuts, bananas, oranges, peanut butter, chocolate). If the condition is severe, parenteral IV or intra-muscular magnesium (e.g., MgSO$_4$) should be administered. The nurse should monitor vital signs and use an infusion pump because rapid administration can lead to hypotension and cardiac or respiratory arrest.

Protein Imbalances

Plasma proteins, particularly albumin, are a significant determinant of plasma volume. Because of their large molecular size, they remain in the vascular space and contribute to the colloidal oncotic pressure. Causes of protein imbalances are listed in Table 19-10. Hypoproteinemia can occur over time. Causes related to intake are anorexia, malnutrition, starvation, fad dieting, and poorly balanced vegetarian diets. Poor absorption of protein can occur in certain GI malabsorptive diseases, such as pancreatic insufficiency and inflammatory bowel disease. Protein can shift out of the intravascular space with inflammation. Increased breakdown of proteins occurs with elevated basal metabolic rates and catabolic states, such as fever, infection, and certain malignancies. Use of protein increases with cell growth and repair after surgical wounds or burns. Hemorrhage with loss of RBCs can be a cause of protein deficit. Impaired synthesis of albumin occurs in liver failure. The kidneys can lose large amounts of protein, especially albumin, in nephrotic syndrome (see Chapter 48).

Clinical manifestations of protein deficit include edema (caused by decreased oncotic pressure), slow healing, anorexia, fatigue, anemia, and muscle loss that results from the breakdown of body tissue to meet the body's need for protein. Intravascular fluid readily accumulates in the peritoneal cavity, which leads to ascites, when the vascular oncotic pressure is decreased in hypoproteinemia.

Management of protein deficit includes providing a high-carbohydrate, high-protein diet and dietary protein supplements. If the patient cannot meet the needs for protein orally, enteral nutrition or total parenteral nutrition may be used. (Protein-calorie malnutrition is discussed in Chapter 42.)

Hyperproteinemia is rare, but it can occur with dehydration-induced hemoconcentration.

Acid–Base Imbalances

The body normally maintains a steady balance between acids produced during metabolism and bases that neutralize and

TABLE 19-11	TERMS IN ACID–BASE PHYSIOLOGY
Acid	Donor of hydrogen ion (H⁺); separation of an acid into H⁺ and its accompanying anion in solution
Acidemia	Signifying an arterial blood pH of <7.35
Acidosis	Process that adds acid or eliminates base from body fluids
Alkalemia	Signifying an arterial blood pH of >7.45
Alkalosis	Process that adds base or eliminates acid from body fluids
Anion gap	Calculation approximating normally unmeasured anions in the plasma; helpful in differential diagnosis of acidosis
Base	Acceptor of hydrogen ions; chemical combining of acid and base when hydrogen ions are added to a solution containing a base; bicarbonate (HCO₃⁻) is most abundant base in body fluids
Buffer	Substance that reacts with an acid or base to prevent a large change in pH
pH	Negative logarithm of the H⁺ concentration

FIGURE 19-16 The normal range of plasma pH is 7.35 to 7.45. A normal pH is maintained by a ratio of 1 part carbonic acid to 20 parts bicarbonate.

promote the excretion of the acids. Many health problems may lead to acid–base imbalances in addition to fluid and electrolyte imbalances. Patients with diabetes mellitus, chronic obstructive pulmonary disease, and kidney disease frequently develop acid–base imbalances. Vomiting and diarrhea may cause loss of acids and bases in addition to loss of fluids and electrolytes. The kidneys are an essential buffer system for acids, and in older adults, the kidneys are less able to compensate for an acid load. Older adults also have decreased respiratory function, which impairs compensation for acid–base imbalances. In addition, tissue hypoxia from any cause may alter acid–base balance. The nurse must always consider the possibility of acid–base imbalance in patients with serious illnesses.

pH and Hydrogen Ion Concentration. The acidity or alkalinity of a solution depends on its hydrogen ion (H⁺) concentration. An increase in H⁺ concentration leads to acidity; a decrease leads to alkalinity. (Definitions related to acid–base balance are presented in Table 19-11.)

Although acids are produced by the body daily, the H⁺ concentration of body fluids is small (0.0004 mEq/L). This tiny amount is maintained within a narrow range to ensure optimal cellular function. H⁺ concentration is usually expressed as a negative logarithm (symbolized as **pH**) rather than in milliequivalents. The use of the negative logarithm reveals an inverse relationship: the higher the pH, the lower the H⁺ concentration. In contrast to a pH of 7, a pH of 8 represents a ten-fold decrease in H⁺ concentration.

The pH of a chemical solution may range from 1 to 14. A solution with a pH of 7 is considered neutral. Acidic solutions have a pH less than 7, whereas alkaline solutions have a pH greater than 7. Blood is slightly alkaline (pH of 7.35-7.45). Medically, if a patient's blood pH drops below 7.35, the patient has **acidosis**, even though the blood may never become truly acidic. If the blood pH is greater than 7.45, the patient has **alkalosis** (Figure 19-16).

Acid–Base Regulation. The body's metabolic processes constantly produce acids. These acids must be neutralized and excreted to maintain acid–base balance. Normally, the body has three mechanisms by which it regulates acid–base balance to maintain the arterial pH between 7.35 and 7.45: the buffer systems, the respiratory system, and the renal system.

The regulatory mechanisms react at different speeds. Buffers react immediately; the respiratory system responds in minutes and reaches maximum effectiveness in hours; and the renal response takes 2 to 3 days to respond maximally, but the kidneys can maintain balance indefinitely in patients with chronic imbalances.

Buffer System. The buffer system is the fastest-acting system and the primary regulator of acid–base balance. Buffers act chemically to change strong acids into weaker acids or to bind acids to neutralize their effect. All body fluids contain buffers. The major buffer system in ECF is carbonic acid–bicarbonate. Other buffers include phosphate, protein, and hemoglobin. The cell can act as a buffer by the shifting of H⁺ in and out of the cell. When ECF levels of H⁺ are increased, H⁺ enters the cell in exchange for potassium. This may result in hyperkalemia. Conversely, with decreased H⁺ levels, H⁺ enters plasma in exchange for potassium. This is why alkalosis can cause hypokalemia.

A buffer consists of a weakly ionized acid or a base and its salt. Buffers function to minimize the effect of acids on blood pH until they can be excreted from the body. The carbonic acid (H_2CO_3)–bicarbonate (HCO_3^-) buffer system neutralizes hydrochloric acid (HCl) in the following manner:

$$HCl + NaHCO_3 \rightarrow NaCl + H_2CO_3$$
(strong acid) (weak base)   (salt)   (weak acid)

In this way, combining a strong acid with a base prevents the acid from causing a large decrease in pH. The carbonic acid is broken down to H_2O and CO_2. The lungs excrete CO_2, either combined with insensible H_2O as carbonic acid or alone as CO_2.

The phosphate, protein, and hemoglobin buffer systems act in the same way as the bicarbonate system. The main components of the phosphate system are monohydrogen phosphate (HPO_4^{2-}) and dihydrogen phosphate ($H_2PO_4^-$). A phosphate, combined with sodium, can neutralize a strong acid such as HCl by forming NaCl and sodium biphosphate (NaH_2PO_4), a weak acid. If a strong base, such as sodium hydroxide (NaOH), is present, sodium biphosphate (NaH_2PO_4) neutralizes it to a weaker base (Na_2HPO_4) and H_2O.

Intracellular and extracellular proteins constitute an effective buffering system throughout the body. The protein buffering system acts like the bicarbonate system. Some of the amino acids of proteins contain free acid radicals such as –COOH, which can dissociate into CO_2 and H^+. Other amino acids have basic radicals such as $-NH_3OH$, which can dissociate into NH^{3+} and OH^-; the OH^- can combine with an H^+ to form H_2O.

Using the "chloride shift" mechanism, hemoglobin regulates pH by shifting chloride in and out of RBCs in exchange for bicarbonate. This shift is regulated according to the level of oxygen in blood.

The cell can also act as a buffer by shifting hydrogen in and out of the cell. With an accumulation of H^+ in the ECF, the intracellular compartment can accept hydrogen in exchange for another cation (e.g., Na^+).

The body buffers an acid load better than it neutralizes base excess. Buffers cannot maintain pH without the adequate functioning of the respiratory and renal systems.

Respiratory System. The lungs help maintain a normal pH by excreting CO_2 and water, which are by-products of cellular metabolism. When released into circulation, CO_2 enters RBCs and combines with H_2O to form H_2CO_3. The carbonic acid dissociates into hydrogen ions and bicarbonate. The free hydrogen is buffered by hemoglobin molecules, and the bicarbonate diffuses into the plasma. In the pulmonary capillaries, this process is reversed, and CO_2 is formed and excreted by the lungs. The overall reversible reaction is expressed as the following:

$$CO_2 + H_2O \rightleftharpoons H_2CO_3 \rightleftharpoons H^+ + HCO_3^-$$

The amount of CO_2 in the blood directly relates to carbonic acid concentration and subsequently to H^+ concentration. With increased respirations, less CO_2 remains in the blood. This leads to less carbonic acid and fewer H^+ molecules. With decreased respirations, more CO_2 remains in the blood. This leads to increased amounts of carbonic acid and more H^+.

The rate of excretion of CO_2 is controlled by the respiratory centre in the medulla in the brainstem. If increased amounts of CO_2 or H^+ are present, the respiratory centre stimulates an increased rate and depth of breathing. Respirations are inhibited if the centre senses low H^+ or CO_2 levels.

As a compensatory mechanism, the respiratory system acts on the $CO_2 + H_2O$ side of the reaction by altering the rate and depth of breathing to "blow off" (through hyperventilation) or "retain" (through hypoventilation) CO_2. If a respiratory problem is the cause of an acid–base imbalance (e.g., respiratory failure), the respiratory system cannot play its usual role to correct a pH alteration.

Renal System. Under normal conditions, the kidneys reabsorb and conserve all of the bicarbonate they filter. The kidneys can generate additional bicarbonate and eliminate excess H^+ as compensation for acidosis. The three mechanisms of acid elimination include (1) secretion of small amounts of free hydrogen into the renal tubule, (2) combination of H^+ with ammonia (NH_3) to form ammonium (NH_4^-), and (3) excretion of weak acids.

The body depends on the kidneys to excrete a portion of the acid produced by cellular metabolism. Thus the kidneys normally excrete an acidic urine (average pH is 6). As a compensatory mechanism, the pH of the urine can decrease to 4 and increase to 8. If the renal system is the cause of an acid–base imbalance (e.g., renal failure), it loses its ability to correct a pH alteration.

Alterations in Acid–Base Balance. An acid–base imbalance is produced when the ratio of 1:20 between acid and base content is altered (Table 19-12; see also Figure 19-16). A primary disease or process may alter one side of the ratio (e.g., CO_2 retention in pulmonary disease). The compensatory process is an attempt to maintain the other side of the ratio (e.g., increased renal bicarbonate reabsorption). When the compensatory mechanism fails, an acid–base imbalance results. The compensatory process may be inadequate because either the pathophysiological process is overwhelming or there is insufficient time for the compensatory process to function.

Acid–base imbalances are classified as respiratory or metabolic. *Respiratory imbalances* affect carbonic acid concentrations; *metabolic imbalances* affect the base bicarbonate. Therefore, acidosis can be caused by an increase in carbonic acid (respiratory acidosis) or a decrease in bicarbonate (metabolic acidosis). Alkalosis can be caused by a decrease in carbonic acid (respiratory alkalosis) or an increase in bicarbonate (metabolic alkalosis). Imbalances may be further classified as acute or chronic. Chronic imbalances allow greater time for compensatory changes.

Respiratory Acidosis. *Respiratory acidosis* (carbonic acid excess) occurs with hypoventilation (see Table 19-12). Hypoventilation results in a buildup of CO_2; subsequently, carbonic acid accumulates in the blood. Carbonic acid dissociates, causing liberation of H^-, and the pH decreases. If CO_2 is not eliminated from the blood, acidosis results from the accumulation of carbonic acid (Figure 19-17, *A*).

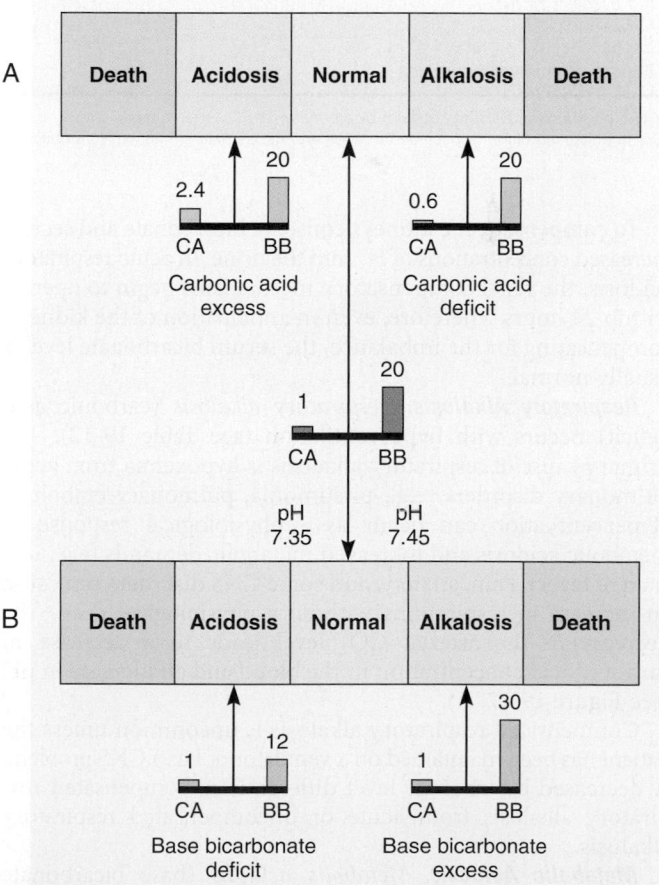

FIGURE 19-17 Kinds of acid–base imbalances. **A,** Respiratory imbalances caused by carbonic acid (CA) excess and CA deficit. *BB*, base bicarbonate. **B,** Metabolic imbalances caused by BB deficit and BB excess.

TABLE 19-12   ACID–BASE IMBALANCES

Common Causes	Pathophysiology	Laboratory Findings
Respiratory Acidosis		
Chronic obstructive pulmonary disease	CO_2 retention by lungs from hypoventilation	↓ Plasma pH
Barbiturate or sedative overdose	Compensatory response to HCO_3^- retention	↑ $PaCO_2$
Chest wall abnormality (e.g., obesity)	by kidneys	HCO_3^- normal (uncompensated)
Severe pneumonia		↑ HCO_3^- (compensated)
Atelectasis		Urine pH <6 (compensated)
Respiratory muscle weakness (e.g., Guillain-Barré syndrome)		
Mechanical hypoventilation		
Respiratory Alkalosis		
Hyperventilation (caused by hypoxia, pulmonary emboli, anxiety, fear, pain, exercise, fever)	Increased CO_2 excretion by lungs from hyperventilation	↑Plasma pH
		↓ $PaCO_2$
Stimulated respiratory centre caused by septicemia, encephalitis, brain injury, salicylate poisoning	Compensatory response of HCO_3^- excretion by kidneys	HCO_3^- normal (uncompensated)
		↓ HCO_3^- (compensated)
Mechanical hyperventilation		Urine pH > 6 (compensated)
Metabolic Acidosis		
Diabetic ketoacidosis	Gain of fixed acid, inability to excrete acid or loss of base	↓ Plasma pH
Lactic acidosis		$PaCO_2$ normal (uncompensated)
Starvation	Compensatory response of CO_2 excretion by lungs	↓ PCO_2 (compensated)
Severe diarrhea		↓ HCO_3^-
Renal tubular acidosis		Urine pH <6 (compensated)
Renal failure		
Gastro-intestinal fistulas		
Shock		
Metabolic Alkalosis		
Severe vomiting	Loss of strong acid or gain of base	↑ Plasma pH
Excess gastric suctioning		$PaCO_2$ normal (uncompensated)
Diuretic therapy*	Compensatory response of CO_2 retention by lungs	↑ PCO_2 (compensated)
Potassium deficit		↑ HCO_3^-
Excess $NaHCO_3$ intake		Urine pH >6 (compensated)
Excessive mineralocorticoids		

HCO_3^-, bicarbonate; $NaHCO_3$, sodium bicarbonate; $PaCO_2$, arterial partial pressure of CO_2; PCO_2, partial pressure of CO_2.
*Commonly used diuretics such as thiazides and furosemide are known to produce mild alkalosis by affecting tubular excretion of electrolytes and bicarbonate.

To compensate, the kidneys conserve bicarbonate and secrete increased concentrations of H^+ into the urine. In acute respiratory acidosis, the renal compensatory mechanisms begin to operate within 24 hours. Therefore, even in anticipation of the kidneys' compensating for the imbalance, the serum bicarbonate level is usually normal.

Respiratory Alkalosis. Respiratory alkalosis (carbonic acid deficit) occurs with hyperventilation (see Table 19-12). The primary cause of respiratory alkalosis is hypoxemia from acute pulmonary disorders (e.g., pneumonia, pulmonary embolus). Hyperventilation can occur as a physiological response to metabolic acidosis and increased metabolic demands (e.g., in a state of fever). Pain, anxiety, and some CNS disorders can cause an increase in respirations without a physiological need. The decrease in the arterial CO_2 level leads to a decrease in carbonic acid concentration in the blood and an increase in pH (see Figure 19-17, *A*).

Compensated respiratory alkalosis is uncommon unless the patient has been maintained on a ventilator or has a CNS problem. A decreased bicarbonate level differentiates compensated respiratory alkalosis from acute or uncompensated respiratory alkalosis.

Metabolic Acidosis. Metabolic acidosis (base bicarbonate deficit) occurs when an acid other than carbonic acid accumulates in the body or when bicarbonate is lost from body fluids (see Table 19-12 and Figure 19-17, *B*). In both cases, a bicarbonate

deficit results. Ketoacid accumulation in diabetic ketoacidosis and lactic acid accumulation with shock are examples of accumulation of acids. Severe diarrhea results in loss of bicarbonate. In renal disease, the kidneys lose their abilities to reabsorb bicarbonate and secrete H^+.

The compensatory response to metabolic acidosis is to increase CO_2 excretion by the lungs. Many affected patients develop Kussmaul's respiration (deep, rapid breathing). In addition, the kidneys attempt to excrete additional acid.

If metabolic acidosis is present, calculating the *anion gap* helps determine the source of the acidosis. The anion gap is the difference between the measured serum cations and anions in ECF. The anion gap is calculated according to the following formula:

$$\text{Anion gap (in mmol/L)} = Na^+ - (HCO_3^- + Cl^-)$$

A normal anion gap is 8 to 16 mmol/L. The anion gap increases in metabolic acidosis associated with acid gain (e.g., lactic acidosis, diabetic ketoacidosis) but is normal in metabolic acidosis caused by bicarbonate loss (e.g., diarrhea).

Metabolic Alkalosis. Metabolic alkalosis (base bicarbonate excess) occurs when acid is lost (as a result of prolonged vomiting or gastric suction) or when bicarbonate increases (from ingestion of baking soda) occurs (see Table 19-12 and Figure 19-17, *B*). The compensatory mechanism is a decreased respiratory rate to

TABLE 19-13	CLINICAL MANIFESTATIONS OF ACIDOSIS	
Respiratory ($\uparrow$ PCO$_2$)	**Metabolic ($\downarrow$ HCO$_3^-$)**
Neurological	
Drowsiness	Drowsiness
Disorientation	Confusion
Dizziness	Headache
Headache	Coma
Coma	
Cardiovascular	
$\downarrow$ Blood pressure	$\downarrow$ Blood pressure
Ventricular fibrillation (related to hyperkalemia from compensation)	Dysrhythmias (related to hyperkalemia from compensation)
Warm, flushed skin (related to peripheral vasodilation)	Warm, flushed skin (related to peripheral vasodilation)
Gastro-intestinal	
No significant findings	Nausea, vomiting, diarrhea, abdominal pain
Neuro-muscular	
Seizures	No significant findings
Respiratory	
Hypoventilation with hypoxia (lungs are unable to compensate when there is a respiratory problem)	Deep, rapid respirations (compensatory action by the lungs)

HCO$_3^-$, bicarbonate; *PCO$_2$*, partial pressure of CO$_2$.

TABLE 19-14	CLINICAL MANIFESTATIONS OF ALKALOSIS	
Respiratory ($\downarrow$ PCO$_2$)	**Metabolic ($\uparrow$ HCO$_3^-$)**
Neurological	
Lethargy	Dizziness
Light-headedness	Irritability
Confusion	Nervousness
	Confusion
Cardiovascular	
Tachycardia	Tachycardia
Dysrhythmias (related to hypokalemia from compensation)	Dysrhythmias (related to hypokalemia from compensation)
Gastro-intestinal	
Nausea	Anorexia
Vomiting	Nausea
Epigastric pain	Vomiting
Neuro-muscular*	
Tetany	Tremors
Numbness	Hypertonic muscles
Tingling of extremities	Muscle cramps
Hyperreflexia	Tetany
Seizures	Tingling of fingers and toes
Respiratory	
Hyperventilation (lungs are unable to compensate when there is a respiratory problem)	Hypoventilation (compensatory action by the lungs)

HCO$_3^-$, bicarbonate; *PCO$_2$*, partial pressure of CO$_2$.
*Alkalosis decreases calcium binding to protein.

increase plasma CO$_2$. However, once hypoxemia occurs or plasma CO$_2$ reaches a certain level, stimulation of chemoreceptors increases respirations. Renal excretion of bicarbonate also occurs.

Mixed Acid–Base Disorders. A mixed acid–base disorder occurs when two or more acid–base disturbances are present at the same time. The pH will depend on type, severity, and acuity of each of the simple disorders involved. Respiratory acidosis combined with metabolic alkalosis (e.g., chronic obstructive pulmonary disease treated with diuretic therapy) may result in a near-normal pH, whereas respiratory acidosis combined with metabolic acidosis causes a greater decrease in pH than either disorder alone. An example of a mixed acidosis appears in a patient in cardiopulmonary arrest. Hypoventilation elevates the CO$_2$ level, and anaerobic metabolism produces lactic acid. An example of a mixed alkalosis is the case of a patient who is hyperventilating because of postoperative pain and is also losing acid as a result of nasogastric suctioning.

Clinical Manifestations. Clinical manifestations of acidosis and alkalosis are summarized in Tables 19-13 and 19-14. Because a normal pH is vital for all cellular reactions, the clinical manifestations of acid–base imbalances are generalized and nonspecific. The actual compensatory mechanisms also produce some clinical manifestations. For example, the deep, rapid respirations of a patient with metabolic acidosis are an example of respiratory compensation. In alkalosis, hypocalcemia may concurrently be present and accounts for many of the clinical manifestations.

Blood Gas Values

Arterial blood gas (ABG) values provide valuable information about a patient's acid–base status, the origin of the imbalance, an idea of the body's ability to regulate pH, and a reflection of the patient's overall oxygen status. Acid–base disturbances are diagnosed and compensatory processes identified in the following six steps:

1. Determining whether the pH is acidotic or alkalotic. A value of 7.4 is the starting point. Values less than 7.4 characterize the pH as acidotic and values greater than 7.4 characterize the pH as alkalotic. If the pH is between 7.35 and 7.45, and the CO2, HCO$_3^-$, and arterial partial pressure of oxygen (PaO$_2$) are within normal limits, the ABG values are normal. If any value is abnormal, then step 2 follows.

2. Analyzing the arterial partial pressure of carbon dioxide (PaCO$_2$) to determine whether the patient has respiratory acidosis or alkalosis. Levels of CO$_2$ are controlled by the lungs, and CO$_2$ is thus considered the respiratory component of the ABG. Because carbonic acid forms when CO$_2$ is dissolved in blood, high CO$_2$ levels indicate acidosis, and low CO$_2$ levels indicate alkalosis.

3. Analyzing the HCO$_3^-$ level to determine whether the patient has metabolic acidosis or alkalosis. Levels of HCO$_3^-$, the metabolic component of the ABG value, are controlled primarily by the kidneys. Because HCO$_3^-$ is a base, high levels of HCO$_3^-$ result in alkalosis, and low levels result in acidosis.

4. Determining whether the CO$_2$ or the HCO$_3^-$ level matches the acid or base alteration of the pH. For example, if the pH is acidotic and the CO$_2$ level is high (respiratory acidosis) but the HCO$_3^-$ level is high (metabolic alkalosis), the CO$_2$ is the parameter that matches the pH derangement. The patient's acid–base imbalance would be diagnosed as respiratory acidosis.

TABLE 19-15 NORMAL ARTERIAL BLOOD GAS VALUES

Parameter	Arterial
pH	7.35–7.45
PCO_2	35–45 mm Hg
Bicarbonate (HCO_3^-) level	21–28 mmol/L
PO_2*	80–100 mm Hg
Base excess	0 ±2.0 mEq/L

PCO_2, partial pressure of carbon dioxide; PO_2, partial pressure of oxygen.
*Decreases above sea level and with increasing age.

TABLE 19-16 ARTERIAL BLOOD GAS (ABG) ANALYSIS

ABG Values
pH 7.30
$PaCO_2$ 25 mm Hg
HCO_3
16 mEq/L
PaO_2 90 mm Hg

Analysis
1. pH of <7.4 indicates acidosis.
2. $PaCO_2$ is low, indicating respiratory alkalosis.
3. HCO_3^- level is low, indicating metabolic acidosis.
4. Metabolic acidosis matches the pH.
5. The $PaCO_2$ level does not match but is in the opposite direction, which indicates the lungs are attempting to compensate for the metabolic acidosis.
6. The PaO_2 indicates adequate oxygenation of the blood.

Interpretation
This ABG value is interpreted as representing metabolic acidosis with partial compensation. If the pH returns to the normal range, the patient is said to have full compensation.

ABG, arterial blood gas; HCO_3^-, bicarbonate; $PaCO_2$, partial pressure of arterial CO_2; PaO_2, partial pressure of oxygen.

5. Deciding whether the body is attempting to compensate for the pH change. If the parameter that does not match the pH is moving in the opposite direction, the body is attempting to compensate. In step 4, the HCO_3^- is alkalotic; this is in the opposite direction of respiratory acidosis and is considered compensation. If compensatory mechanisms are functioning, the pH will return toward 7.4. When the pH is back to normal, the patient has *full compensation*. The body will not over-compensate for pH changes. If both parameters match the pH, it is possible that a combined respiratory or metabolic acidosis or alkalosis is present. For example, if the pH is acidotic, the CO_2 level is high (respiratory acidosis), and the HCO_3^- level is low (metabolic acidosis), the patient's underlying acid–base imbalance is combined respiratory-metabolic acidosis.
6. Assessing the PaO_2 and O_2 saturation. If these values are abnormal, hypoxemia is present.
   Table 19-15 lists normal ABG values, and Table 19-16 provides a sample ABG value with interpretation. (Refer to Table 19-12 for the laboratory findings of the four major acid–base disturbances.) Table 19-17 explains the ROME (respiratory, opposite, metabolic, equivalent) mnemonic to clarify acid–base imbalances. (Blood gases are discussed further in Chapter 28.)

TABLE 19-17 ROME: MNEMONIC FOR ACID–BASE IMBALANCES

For acid–base imbalances, the mnemonic ROME can be used.
In **r**espiratory conditions, the pH and the $PaCO_2$ are in **o**pposite directions.
- In respiratory alkalosis, the pH is ↑ and the $PaCO_2$ is ↓.
- In respiratory acidosis, the pH is ↓ and the $PaCO_2$ is ↑.
In **m**etabolic conditions, the pH and the HCO_3^- go in the same direction (**e**qual or **e**quivalent). The $PaCO_2$ may also go in the same direction.
- In metabolic alkalosis, pH and HCO_3^- are ↑ and the $PaCO_2$ is ↑ or normal.
- In metabolic acidosis, pH and HCO_3^- are ↓ and the $PaCO_2$ is ↓ or normal.

Type of Imbalance	Respiratory: Opposite		Metabolic: Equivalent	
	pH	$PaCO_2$	pH	HCO_3^-
Acidosis	↓	↑	↓	↓
Alkalosis	↑	↓	↑	↑

HCO_3^-, bicarbonate; $PaCO_2$, arterial partial pressure of carbon dioxide.

ASSESSMENT OF FLUID, ELECTROLYTE, AND ACID–BASE IMBALANCES

Subjective Data

Important Health Information

Past Health History. The patient should be questioned about any health history of past problems involving the kidneys, the heart, the GI system, or the lungs that could affect the current fluid, electrolyte, and acid–base balance. Medical information about specific diseases such as diabetes mellitus, diabetes insipidus, chronic obstructive pulmonary disease, ulcerative colitis, and Crohn's disease should be obtained from the patient. The patient should also be questioned about the incidence of a prior fluid, electrolyte, or acid–base disorder.

Medications. The patient's current and past use of medications must be assessed. The ingredients in many drugs, especially over-the-counter drugs, are often overlooked as sources of sodium, potassium, calcium, magnesium, and other electrolytes. Many prescription drugs, including diuretics, corticosteroids, and electrolyte supplements, can cause fluid and electrolyte problems.

Surgery or Other Treatments. The patient should be asked about previous or current renal dialysis, kidney surgery, or bowel surgery that resulted in a temporary or permanent external collecting system, such as a colostomy or nephrostomy.

Other Subjective Data. If the patient is currently experiencing a problem related to fluid, electrolyte, and acid–base balance, a careful description of the illness, including onset, course, and treatment, should be obtained.

The nurse should ask the patient about diet and any special dietary practices. Weight reduction diets, fad diets, or any eating disorders, such as anorexia or bulimia, can lead to fluid and electrolyte problems. If the patient is on a special diet, such as one of low sodium content or high potassium content, the nurse should assess the patient's ability to adhere to the dietary prescription.

The patient's usual bowel and bladder habits should be noted. Any deviations from the expected elimination pattern, such as diarrhea, nocturia, or polyuria, should be carefully documented.

The patient's exercise pattern is important to determine because excessive perspiration secondary to exercise could result in a fluid and electrolyte problem. Also, the patient's exposure to extremely high temperatures as a result of leisure or work activity should be determined. The patient should be asked what practices are followed to replace fluid and electrolytes lost through excessive perspiration.

The patient should be queried about any changes in sensations, such as numbness, tingling, fasciculations (uncoordinated twitching of a single muscle group), or muscle weakness, that could indicate a fluid and electrolyte problem. In addition, both the patient and the caregivers should be asked whether any changes in mentation or alertness have been noted, such as confusion, memory impairment, or lethargy.

Objective Data

Physical Examination. There is no specific physical examination to assess fluid, electrolyte, and acid–base balance. Common abnormal assessment findings of major body systems offer clues to possible imbalances (Table 19-18).

Laboratory Values. Assessment of serum electrolyte values is a good starting point for identifying fluid and electrolyte imbalance (see Table 19-2). However, serum electrolyte values often provide only cursory information. Each value reflects the concentration of the particular electrolyte in the ECF but does not necessarily provide information concerning the concentration of the electrolyte in the ICF. For example, the majority of the potassium in the body is intracellular. Changes in serum potassium values may be the result of a true deficit or an excess of potassium, or it may reflect the movement of potassium into or out of the cell over the course of acid–base imbalances.

An abnormal serum sodium level may reflect a sodium problem or, more possibly, a water problem. A reduced hematocrit value could indicate anemia, or it could be caused by fluid volume excess. Other laboratory tests that are helpful in evaluating the presence of or risk for fluid, electrolyte, and acid–base imbalances include serum and urine osmolality, serum glucose level, serum urea nitrogen (BUN) values, serum creatinine level, urine specific gravity, and urine electrolyte concentrations.

In addition to arterial and venous blood gas values, serum electrolyte data can provide important information concerning a patient's acid–base balance. Changes in the serum bicarbonate (often reported as total CO_2 or CO_2 content on an electrolyte panel) indicate the presence of metabolic acidosis (low bicarbonate level) or alkalosis (high bicarbonate level). Calculation of the anion gap can help determine the source of metabolic acidosis. The anion gap is increased in metabolic acidosis associated with acid gain (e.g., lactic acidosis, diabetic ketoacidosis) but remains normal in metabolic acidosis caused by bicarbonate loss (e.g., diarrhea).

ORAL FLUID AND ELECTROLYTE REPLACEMENT

In all cases of fluid, electrolyte, and acid–base imbalances, the treatment is directed toward correction of the underlying cause. The specific diseases or disorders that cause these imbalances are discussed in various chapters throughout this text. Mild fluid and electrolyte deficits can be corrected with the use of oral rehydration solutions containing water, electrolytes, and glucose. Glucose not only provides calories but also promotes sodium absorption in the small intestine. Commercial oral rehydration

TABLE 19-18 ASSESSMENT ABNORMALITIES

Fluid and Electrolyte Imbalances

Finding	Possible Cause
Skin	
Poor skin turgor	Fluid volume deficit
Cold, clammy skin	Na^+ deficit, shift of plasma to interstitial fluid
Pitting edema	Fluid volume excess
Flushed, dry skin	Na^+ excess
Pulse	
Bounding pulse	Fluid volume excess, shift of interstitial fluid to plasma
Rapid, weak, thready pulse	Shift of plasma to interstitial fluid, Na^+ deficit, fluid volume deficit
Weak, irregular, rapid pulse	Severe K^+ deficit
Weak, irregular, slow pulse	Severe K^+ excess
Blood Pressure	
Hypotension	Fluid volume deficit, shift of plasma to interstitial fluid, Na^+ deficit
Hypertension	Fluid volume excess, shift of interstitial fluid to plasma
Respirations	
Deep, rapid breathing	Compensation for metabolic acidosis
Shallow, slow, irregular breathing	Compensation for metabolic alkalosis
Shortness of breath	Fluid volume excess
Moist crackles	Fluid volume excess, shift of interstitial fluid to plasma
Skeletal Muscles	
Cramping of exercised muscle	Ca^{2+} deficit, Mg^{2+} deficit, alkalosis
Carpal spasm (Trousseau's sign)	Ca^{2+} deficit, Mg^{2+} deficit, alkalosis
Flabby muscles	K^+ deficit
Positive Chvostek's sign	Ca^{2+} deficit, Mg^{2+} deficit, alkalosis
Behaviour or Mental State	
Picking at bedclothes	K^+ deficit, Mg^{2+} deficit
Inappropriate indifference	Fluid volume deficit, Na^+ deficit
Apprehension	Shift of plasma to interstitial fluid
Extreme restlessness	K^+ excess, fluid volume deficit
Confusion and irritability	K^+ deficit, fluid volume excess, Ca^{2+} excess, Mg^{2+} excess, H_2O excess
Decreased level of consciousness	H_2O excess

solutions are now available in markets and pharmacies for home use.

INTRAVENOUS FLUID AND ELECTROLYTE REPLACEMENT

IV fluid and electrolyte therapy are commonly used to treat many different fluid and electrolyte imbalances. Many patients need maintenance IV fluid therapy only while they cannot take fluids orally (e.g., during and after surgery). Other patients need corrective or replacement therapy for losses that have already occurred. The amount and the type of solution are determined by the normal daily maintenance requirements and by imbalances

TABLE 19-19   COMPOSITION AND USE OF COMMONLY PRESCRIBED CRYSTALLOID SOLUTIONS

Solution	Tonicity	Concentration (mmol/kg)	Glucose Content (g/L)	Indications and Considerations
Dextrose in Water				
5%	Isotonic, but physiologically hypotonic	278	50	Provides free water necessary for renal excretion of solutes Used to replace water losses and treat hypernatremia Provides 170 cal/L Does not provide any electrolytes
10%	Hypertonic	556	100	Provides free water only, no electrolytes Provides 340 cal/L
Saline (Sodium Chloride [NaCl])				
0.45%	Hypotonic	154	0	Provides free water in addition to Na^+ and Cl^- Used to replace hypotonic fluid losses Used as maintenance solution, although it does not replace daily losses of other electrolytes Provides no calories
0.9%	Isotonic	308	0	Used to expand intravascular volume and replace extracellular fluid losses Only solution that may be administered with blood products Contains Na^+ and Cl^- in excess of plasma levels Does not provide free water, calories, other electrolytes May cause intravascular overload or hyperchloremic acidosis
3.0%	Hypertonic	1026	0	Used to treat symptomatic hyponatremia Must be administered slowly and with extreme caution because it may cause dangerous intravascular volume overload and pulmonary edema
Dextrose in Saline				
5% in 0.225%	Isotonic	355	50	Provides Na^+, Cl^-, and free water Used to replace hypotonic losses and treat hypernatremia Provides 170 cal/L
5% in 0.45%	Hypertonic	432	50	Same as 0.45% NaCl except provides 170 cal/L
5% in 0.9%	Hypertonic	586	50	Same as 0.9% NaCl except provides 170 cal/L
Multiple-Electrolyte Solutions				
Ringer's solution	Isotonic	309	0	Similar in composition to plasma except that it has excess Cl^-, no Mg^{2+} and no HCO_3^- Does not provide free water or calories Used to expand the intravascular volume and replace extracellular fluid losses
Lactated Ringer's (Hartmann's) solution	Isotonic	274	0	Similar in composition to normal plasma except does not contain Mg^{2+} Used to treat losses from burns and lower GI tract May be used to treat mild metabolic acidosis but should not be used to treat lactic acidosis Does not provide free water or calories

Source: Adapted from Heitz, U. E., & Horne, M. M. (2005). *Pocket guide to fluid, electrolyte, and acid–base balance* (5th ed., p. 70). St. Louis: Mosby.
GI, gastro-intestinal; *HCO_3^-*, bicarbonate.

identified by laboratory results. Table 19-19 is a list of commonly prescribed IV solutions. The available selections have remained fairly constant over the years. With IV fluid replacement therapy, local complications may occur, including phlebitis, ecchymosis, extravascular fluid infiltration, infection, thrombosis, and venous spasm. Systemic complications may also occur, such as bacteremia and sepsis, air embolism, and pulmonary edema.

Solutions

Hypotonic. A hypotonic solution provides more water than electrolytes, diluting the ECF. Osmosis then produces a movement of water from the ECF to the ICF. After osmotic equilibrium has been achieved, the ICF and the ECF have the same osmolality, and both compartments have been expanded. Examples of hypotonic fluids are listed in Table 19-19. Maintenance fluids are usually hypotonic solutions (e.g., 0.45% NaCl) because normal daily losses are hypotonic. Additional electrolytes (e.g., KCl) may be added to maintain normal levels. Hypotonic solutions have the potential to cause cellular swelling, and patients should be

monitored for changes in mentation, which may indicate cerebral edema (Porth, 2013).

Although 5% dextrose in water is considered an isotonic solution, the dextrose is quickly metabolized, and the net result is the administration of free water (hypotonic) with proportionately equal expansion of the ECF and ICF. One litre of a 5% dextrose solution provides 50 g of dextrose, or 170 calories. Although this amount of dextrose is not enough to meet caloric requirements, it helps prevent ketosis associated with starvation. Pure water must not be administered intravenously because it would cause hemolysis of RBCs.

Isotonic. Administration of an isotonic solution expands only the ECF. There is no net loss or gain from the ICF. An isotonic solution is the ideal fluid replacement for a patient with an ECF volume deficit. Examples of isotonic solutions include lactated Ringer's solution and 0.9% NaCl. Lactated Ringer's solution contains sodium, potassium, chloride, calcium, and lactate (the precursor of bicarbonate) in approximately the same concentrations as those of the ECF. Its use is contraindicated in the presence of lactic acidosis because of the body's decreased ability to convert lactate to bicarbonate.

Isotonic saline (0.9% NaCl) has a sodium concentration (154 mmol/L) somewhat higher than that of plasma (135–145 mmol/L) and a chloride concentration (154 mmol/L) significantly higher than the plasma chloride level (98–106 mmol/L or mEq/L). Therefore, excessive administration of isotonic NaCl can cause elevation of sodium and chloride levels. Isotonic saline may be used when a patient has sustained both fluid and sodium losses or as vascular fluid replacement in hypovolemic shock.

Hypertonic. A hypertonic solution initially raises the osmolality of ECF and expands it. It is useful in treatment of hypovolemia and hyponatremia. Examples are listed in Table 19-19. In addition, the higher osmotic pressure causes water to shift out of the cells and into the ECF. Hypertonic solutions (e.g., 3% NaCl) necessitate frequent monitoring of blood pressure, lung sounds, and serum sodium levels and should be used with caution because of the risk for intravascular fluid volume excess, as well as for intracellular dehydration (Porth, 2013).

Although concentrated dextrose and water solutions (≥10% dextrose) are hypertonic solutions, once the dextrose is metabolized, the net result is the administration of water. The free water provided by these solutions ultimately causes both the ECF and the ICF to expand. The primary use of these solutions is in the provision of calories. Concentrated dextrose solutions may be combined with amino acid solutions, electrolytes, vitamins, and trace elements to provide total parenteral nutrition (see Chapter 42). Solutions containing 10% dextrose or less may be administered through a peripheral IV catheter. Solutions with greater concentrations of dextrose must be administered through a central catheter so that dilution is adequate to prevent shrinkage of RBCs.

Intravenous Additives. Additives in basic IV solutions replace specific losses. KCl, calcium chloride (CaCl), MgSO$_4$, and HCO$_3^-$ are common additives. The use of each was described earlier in the discussion of the specific electrolyte deficiencies. Many premixed IV solutions containing specific additives are available. Use of these solutions reduces error inasmuch as they contain the correct amount of the electrolytes in the proper volumes and types of IV solution. Recommendations for administering potassium vary, but in general, no more than 10 to 20 mEq per hour is considered safe for routine administration. Potassium can be safely diluted as 40 mEq/L of solution, with a maximum of 60 mEq/L. It must never be administered undiluted or by IV push because it can cause fatal cardiac reactions.

Plasma Expanders. Plasma expanders stay in the vascular space and increase the osmotic pressure. Plasma expanders include colloids, dextran, and hetastarch. Colloids are protein solutions such as plasma, albumin, and commercial plasmas. Albumin is available in 5% and 25% solutions. The 5% solution has an albumin concentration similar to that of plasma and expands the intravascular fluid millilitre for millilitre. In contrast, the 25% albumin solution is hypertonic and causes additional fluid to move from the interstitium. Dextran is a complex synthetic sugar. Because dextran is metabolized slowly, it remains in the vascular system for a prolonged period but not as long as the colloids. It causes additional fluid to move into the intravascular space. (Indications for plasma volume expanders are discussed in Chapter 69.)

If the patient has lost blood, whole blood or packed RBCs are necessary. Packed RBCs have the advantage of giving the patient primarily RBCs; the blood bank can use the plasma for blood components. Whole blood, with its additional fluid volume,

may cause circulatory overload. Although packed cells have a decreased plasma volume, they will increase the oncotic pressure and pull fluid into the intravascular space. Loop diuretics may be administered with blood to prevent symptoms of fluid volume excess in anemic patients who are not volume depleted. (Administration of blood is discussed in Chapter 33.)

CENTRAL VENOUS ACCESS DEVICES

Central venous access devices (CVADs) are catheters that are placed in large blood vessels (e.g., subclavian vein, jugular vein) when access to the vascular system is needed frequently. In contrast to CVADs, the basic IV catheter is inserted into a peripheral vein in the hand, inside of the arm, or antecubital fossa and is used for short-term IV access. Central venous access can be achieved by three different methods: centrally inserted catheters, peripherally inserted central catheters (PICCs), or implanted ports. Centrally inserted catheters and implanted ports must be placed by a physician, whereas PICCs can be inserted by a nurse with specialized training.

CVADs enable frequent, continuous, rapid, or intermittent administration of fluids and medications. They allow for the administration of drugs that are potential vesicants, blood and

---

🔍 EVIDENCE-INFORMED PRACTICE

Research Highlight

Do Heparin Flushes Decrease Occlusions in Central Venous Catheters?

Clinical Question

For patients with intermittently used central venous catheters (P), do heparin solution flushes (I) versus normal saline flushes (C) decrease catheter occlusions (O)?

Best Available Evidence

Cochrane systematic review of six studies with a total of 1433 participants.

Critical Appraisal and Synthesis of Evidence

- Study participants were adult patients with a central venous catheter (CVC) or a peripherally inserted central catheter (PICC).
- Primary outcomes included occlusion of CVCs and duration (in days) of catheter patency.
- There were wide variations in guideline recommendations and practice surrounding the effectiveness of heparin flushing of CVCs.
- Potential harms were associated with heparin use, especially in critically ill patients.

Conclusions

- No conclusive evidence favours intermittent flushing with heparin over flushing with 0.9% normal saline with regard to safety or efficacy.
- More studies of central venous access maintenance are needed to guide evidence-informed practice.

Implications for Nursing Practice

- Maintenance of catheter patency is critical.
- Flushing devices with saline solution may be a safe and effective alternative to heparin flushes for catheter maintenance.

Reference for Evidence

López-Briz, E., Ruiz Garcia, V., Cabello, J. B., et al. (2013). Heparin versus saline solution flushing for prevention of occlusion in central venous catheters in adults. Health. *The Cochrane Database of Systematic Reviews*, (10), CD008462, doi:10.1002/14651858.CD008462.pub2.

P, patient population of interest; *I*, intervention or area of interest; *C*, comparison of interest or comparison group; *O*, outcome(s) of interest (see Chapter 1 of this textbook).

TABLE 19-20	INDICATIONS FOR USE OF CENTRAL VENOUS ACCESS DEVICE*
Medical Condition	**Indications for Use**
Medication administration	
• Cancer	Chemotherapy, infusion of irritating or vesicant medications
• Infection	Long-term administration of antibiotics
• Pain	Long-term administration of pain medication
• Drugs and other substances that increase risk for phlebitis	Epoprostenol (Flolan), calcium chloride, potassium chloride, amiodarone (Cordarone)
Nutritional replacement	Infusion of parenteral nutrition
	Solutions with higher dextrose content can be infused through CVAD (versus peripheral line)
Blood samples	Multiple diagnostic blood tests over a period of time
Blood transfusions	Infusion of blood or blood products in acute situations, as well as over a period of time
Renal failure	Performing hemodialysis (especially on an acute basis) or continuous renal replacement therapy
Shock, burns	Infusion of high volumes of fluid and electrolyte replacement
Hemodynamic monitoring	Measuring CVP to assess fluid balance
Heart failure	Performing ultrafiltration
Autoimmune disorders	Performing plasmapheresis

CVAD, central venous access device; *CVP*, central venous pressure.
*This list is not all-inclusive, and these are examples only.

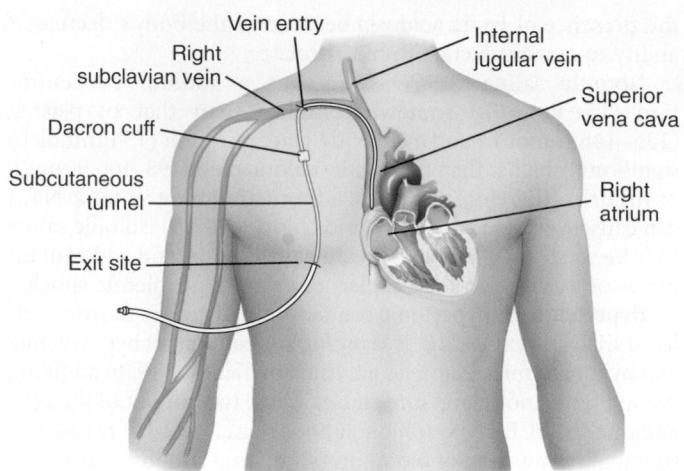

FIGURE 19-18 Tunnelled central venous catheter. Note tip of the catheter in the superior vena cava.

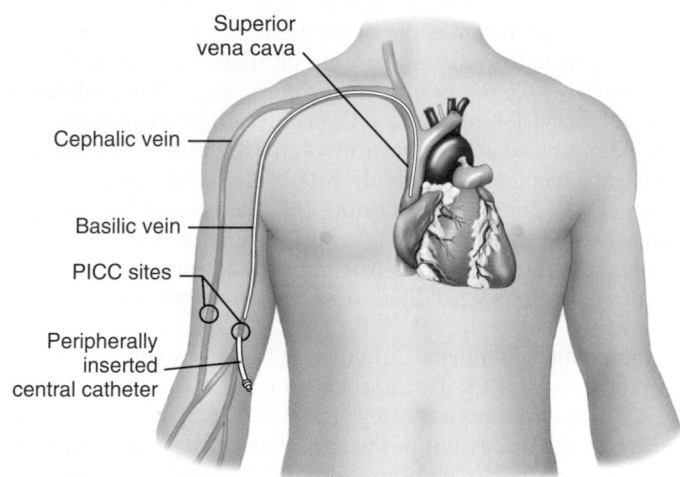

FIGURE 19-19 Peripherally inserted central catheter (PICC) can be inserted into the basilic or cephalic vein.

blood products, and parenteral nutrition. They may also be used for hemodynamic monitoring and venous blood sampling. These devices are indicated for patients who have limited peripheral vascular access or who have a projected need for long-term vascular access. Table 19-20 provides examples of medical conditions in which CVADs are used.

Advantages of CVADs include a reduced need for multiple venipunctures, decreased risk of extravasation injury, and immediate access to the central venous system. Although the incidence is decreased, extravasation can nonetheless occur if the device being used is displaced or damaged. The major disadvantages of CVADs are an increased risk of systemic infection and the invasiveness of the insertion procedure.

Centrally Inserted Catheters

The tip of centrally inserted catheters (also called central venous catheters [CVCs]) rests in the distal end of the superior vena cava near its junction with the right atrium (Figure 19-18). The other end of the catheter exits through a separate incision on the chest or abdominal wall. Nontunnelled catheters are placed usually in the subclavian or internal jugular vein and more rarely in the femoral vein. They are best for patients with short-term needs in an acute care setting. Surgically placed tunnelled catheters (e.g., Hickman catheters) are suitable for long-term needs. Tunnelling of the catheter through subcutaneous tissue and the synthetic cuff used to anchor the catheter provide stability and decrease infection risk. Accurate placement must be verified by chest radiography before the catheter can be used. After the site heals, the catheter does not require a dressing, which makes it easier for the patient to maintain the site at home. Care requirements

include injection cap change, cleansing, flushing, and dressing change.

CVCs are available as single-, double-, triple-, or quadruple-lumen catheters. Multilumen catheters are useful in critically ill patients because each lumen can be simultaneously used to provide a different therapy. For example, incompatible drugs can be infused in separate lumens without mixing, and a third lumen can provide access for blood sampling. Specific types of long-term central catheters are Hickman catheters, for which clamps are needed to make sure the valve is closed, and Groshong catheters, which have a valve that opens as fluid is withdrawn or infused and remains closed when not in use.

Peripherally Inserted Central Catheters

PICCs are central venous catheters inserted into a vein in the arm. The basilic vein is preferred because of its large diameter. PICC lines are inserted at or just above the antecubital fossa and advanced to a position with the tip ending in the distal one third of the superior vena cava (Figure 19-19). Single-, double-, or triple-lumen PICCs are available; those with double lumens are preferred because they allow for simultaneous uses. PICCs are used with patients who need vascular access for 1 week to 6 months, but they can be in place for longer periods.

The technique for placement of a PICC line involves insertion of the catheter through a needle with the use of a guide wire or forceps to advance the line. Advantages of the PICC over a CVC are lower infection rate, fewer insertion-related complications, decreased cost, and ability to be inserted at the patient's bedside or in the outpatient area.

Complications of PICC lines include catheter occlusion and phlebitis (Table 19-21). If phlebitis occurs, it usually happens within 7 to 10 days after insertion. The nurse must not use the arm with the PICC to obtain a blood pressure reading or draw blood. When the blood pressure cuff is inflated, the PICC can touch the vein wall, which increases the risk of vein damage and thrombosis.

Implanted Infusion Ports

An implanted infusion port is a CVC connected to a single or double implanted subcutaneous injection port (Figure 19-20, *A*). The catheter is placed into the desired vein, and the other end is connected to a port that is surgically implanted in a subcutaneous pocket on the chest wall. The port consists of a metal sheath with a self-sealing silicone septum. Drugs are injected through the skin into the port. After being filled, the reservoir slowly releases the medicine into the bloodstream.

The port is accessed via the septum by means of a special noncoring needle that has a deflected tip, which prevents damage to the septum that could render the port useless (see Figure 19-20, *B*). Implanted ports are convenient for long-term therapy and can remain in the body for years. Because the port is hidden, it offers cosmetic advantages (Zaghal, Khalife, Mukherji, et al., 2012). Care requirements include regular flushing. Formation of "sludge" (accumulation of clotted blood and drug precipitate) may also occur within the port septum.

Complications

The potential for complications associated with CVADs is always present. Astute monitoring and assessment may assist in early identification of potential complications. Table 19-21 lists potential complications of CVADs.

TABLE 19-21	POTENTIAL COMPLICATIONS OF CENTRAL VENOUS ACCESS DEVICES	
Possible Cause	**Clinical Manifestations**	**Nursing and Collaborative Management**
Catheter Occlusion		
Clamped or kinked catheter	Sluggish infusion or aspiration	Instructing patient to change position, raise arm, and cough
Tip against wall of vessel	Inability to infuse or aspirate	and cough
Thrombosis		Assessing for and alleviating clamping or kinking
Precipitate buildup in lumen		Flushing with normal saline with a 10-mL syringe; do not force flush
		Fluoroscopy to determine cause and site
		Anticoagulant or thrombolytic agents
Embolism		
Catheter breakage	Chest pain	Administering oxygen
Dislodgement of thrombus	Respiratory distress (dyspnea, tachypnea, hypoxia, cyanosis)	Clamping catheter
Entry of air into circulation		Placing patient on left side with head down (air emboli)
	Hypotension	
	Tachycardia	Notifying physician
Catheter-Related Infection (Local or Systemic)		
Contamination during insertion or use	Local: redness, tenderness, purulent drainage, warmth, edema	Local
Migration of organisms along catheter		• Culture of drainage from site
Immuno-suppression of patient	Systemic: fever, chills, malaise	• Warm, moist compresses
		• Catheter removal if indicated
		Systemic
		• Blood cultures
		• Antibiotic therapy
		• Antipyretic therapy
		• Catheter removal if indicated
Pneumothorax		
Perforation of visceral pleura during insertion	Decrease in or absence of breath sounds	Administering oxygen
	Respiratory distress (cyanosis, dyspnea, tachypnea)	Positioning in semi-Fowler's position
	Chest pain	Preparing for chest tube insertion
	Unilateral distension of chest	
Catheter Migration		
Improper suturing	Sluggish infusion or aspiration	Fluoroscopy to verify position
Insertion site trauma	Edema of chest or neck during infusion	Assistance with removal and new CVAD placement
Changes in intrathoracic pressure	Patient complaint of gurgling sound in ear	
Forceful catheter flushing	Dysrhythmias	
Spontaneous movement	Increased external catheter length	

CVAD, central venous access device.

FIGURE 19-20 A, Cross-section of implantable port displaying access of the port with the Huber-point needle. Note the deflected point of the Huber-point needle, which prevents coring of the port's septum. **B,** Two Huber-point needles used to enter the implanted port. The 90-degree needle is used for top-entry ports for continuous infusion. Source: **A,** Courtesy Pharmaceia Deltec, Inc., St. Paul, MN.

NURSING MANAGEMENT
CENTRAL VENOUS ACCESS DEVICES

Nursing management of CVADs includes assessment, dressing change and cleansing, injection cap changes, and flushing. Although institution policies and procedures may differ for specific types of CVADs, there are some general guidelines to be followed.

Catheter and insertion site assessment includes inspecting the site for redness, edema, warmth, drainage, and tenderness or pain. Observing the catheter for misplacement or slippage is important. The nurse should perform a comprehensive pain assessment, particularly noting any complaints of chest or neck discomfort, arm pain, or pain at the insertion site. Newly placed CVADs should not be used until the tip position is verified with a chest radiograph.

Dressing change and cleansing of the catheter insertion site should be performed according to institution policies and procedures with strict sterile technique. Transparent semipermeable dressings or gauze and tape can be used. If the site is bleeding, a gauze dressing may be preferable; otherwise, transparent dressings are preferred because they allow observation of the site without having to be removed. Transparent dressings may be left in place for up to 1 week. The dressing should be changed immediately if it becomes damp, loose, or soiled.

The skin around the catheter insertion suite should be cleansed according to institution policy. A chlorhexidine-based preparation is the cleansing agent of choice. Its effects last longer than either povidone-iodine or isopropyl alcohol, offering improved killing of bacteria (Marschall, Mermel, Fakih, et al., 2014). When chlorhexidine is used, cleansing the skin with friction is critical for preventing infection (Weinstein & Hagle, 2014). When applying a new dressing, the nurse should allow the area to air-dry completely. The lumen ports are secured to the skin above the dressing site. The nurse should document the date and time of the dressing change and initial the dressing.

Injection caps must be changed at regular intervals with the use of strict sterile technique according to institution policy or when they are damaged from excessive punctures. The patient should be taught to turn the head to the opposite side of the CVAD insertion site during cap change. If the catheter cannot be clamped and is open to air, the patient should be asked to lie flat in bed and perform the Valsalva manoeuvre to prevent an air embolism.

Flushing is one of the most effective ways to maintain lumen patency and to prevent occlusion of the CVAD. It also keeps incompatible drugs or fluids from mixing. The lumen is flushed with a normal saline solution in a syringe that has a barrel capacity of 10 mL or more to avoid excess pressure on the catheter. If resistance is felt, force should not be applied; this could result in rupture of the catheter or in the creation of an embolism if a thrombus is present. Because of the risk of contamination and infection, prefilled syringes or single-dose vials are preferred over multiple-dose vials. During flushing, the push–pause method is preferred over a continual even push of saline into the catheter. The push–pause technique creates turbulence within the catheter lumen, promoting the removal of debris that adheres to the catheter lumen. This technique involves injecting the saline with a rapid alternating push–pause motion, instilling 1 to 2 mL with each push on the syringe plunger.

REMOVAL OF CENTRAL VENOUS ACCESS DEVICES

CVADs should be removed according to institution policy and the nurse's scope of practice. In many agencies, nurses with demonstrated competency can remove PICCs and nontunnelled CVCs. The procedure involves removing any sutures and then gently withdrawing the catheter. The patient is instructed to perform the Valsalva manoeuvre as the last 5 to 10 cm of the catheter is withdrawn. The nurse immediately applies pressure to the site with sterile gauze to prevent air from entering and to control bleeding. The catheter tip is inspected to ensure that it is intact. After bleeding has stopped, an antiseptic ointment and sterile dressing are applied to the site.

CASE STUDY

Fluid and Electrolyte Imbalance

Patient Profile

Sarah Stern, a 73-year-old woman with lung cancer, has been receiving chemotherapy on an outpatient basis. She completed her third treatment 5 days ago and has been experiencing nausea and vomiting for 2 days even though she has been taking prochlorperazine as directed. Ms. Stern's daughter brings her to the hospital, where she is admitted to the medical unit. The admitting nurse performs a thorough assessment.

Source: elbud/
Shutterstock
.com.

Subjective Data

- Complains of lethargy, weakness, and a dry mouth
- States she has been too nauseated to eat or drink anything for 2 days

Objective Data

- Heart rate, 110; pulse, thready
- Blood pressure, 100/65 mm Hg
- Weight loss of 2.2 kg since she received her chemotherapy treatment 5 days ago
- Dry oral mucous membranes

Discussion Questions

1. According to her clinical manifestations, what fluid imbalance does Ms. Stern have?
2. What additional assessment data should the nurse obtain?

3. What are the patient's risk factors for fluid and electrolyte imbalances?
4. The nurse draws blood for a serum chemistry evaluation. What electrolyte imbalances are likely to be found and why?
5. Ms. Stern is at risk for which acid–base imbalance? Describe the changes that would occur in Ms. Stern's ABG values with this acid–base imbalance. How would her body compensate?
6. What is the interprofessional team's priority at this time for Ms. Stern?
7. The physician orders dextrose 5% in 0.45% saline to infuse at 100 mL per hour. What type of solution is this, and how will it help Ms. Stern's fluid imbalance?
8. **Priority Decision:** What are the priority nursing interventions for Ms. Stern?
9. **Evidence-Informed Practice:** Ms. Stern has a double-lumen PICC in her left arm. One lumen is connected to the IV infusion; the other is unused. What is the recommended practice for maintaining the patency of the unused lumen?

evolve

Answers available at *http://evolve.elsevier.com/Canada/Lewis/medsurg*.

REVIEW QUESTIONS

The number of the question corresponds to the same-numbered objective at the beginning of the chapter.

1. In which of the following fluid compartments is the majority of the body's water contained?
   a. Interstitial
   b. Intracellular
   c. Extracellular
   d. Intravascular

2. Which mechanism is involved with equalizing the fluid concentration when the blood plasma has a higher osmolality than the intracellular fluid in blood cells?
   a. Osmosis
   b. Diffusion
   c. Active transport
   d. Facilitated diffusion

3a. An older woman was admitted to the medical unit with GI bleeding and fluid volume deficit. What are the clinical manifestations of the latter problem? *(Select all that apply)*
   a. Weight loss
   b. Dry oral mucosa
   c. Full bounding pulse
   d. Engorged neck veins
   e. Decreased central venous pressure

3b. Which of the following nursing actions is required for clients with hyponatremia?
   a. Fluid restriction
   b. Administration of hypotonic intravenous fluids
   c. Administration of a cation exchange resin
   d. Increased water intake for clients on nasogastric suction

3c. Which of the following should the nurse monitor for when a client is receiving a loop diuretic?
   a. Restlessness and agitation
   b. Paresthesias and irritability
   c. Weak, irregular pulse and poor muscle tone
   d. Increased blood pressure and muscle spasms

3d. Which of the following clients would be at greatest risk for the potential development of hypermagnesemia?
   a. An 83-year-old man with lung cancer and hypertension
   b. A 65-year-old woman with hypertension taking β-adrenergic blockers
   c. A 42-year-old woman with systemic lupus erythematosus and renal failure
   d. A 50-year-old man with benign prostatic hyperplasia and a urinary tract infection

3e. In a client who has just undergone a total thyroidectomy, it is especially important for the nurse to assess which of the following?
   a. Weight gain
   b. Depressed reflexes
   c. Positive Chvostek's sign
   d. Confusion and personality changes

3f. Care of the client experiencing hyperphosphatemia secondary to renal failure includes which of the following?
   a. Calcium supplements
   b. Potassium supplements
   c. Magnesium supplements
   d. Fluid replacement therapy

4. How do the lungs act as an acid–base buffer?
   a. By increasing respiratory rate and depth when CO_2 levels in the blood are high, thereby reducing acid load
   b. By increasing respiratory rate and depth when CO_2 levels in the blood are low, thereby reducing base load
   c. By decreasing respiratory rate and depth when CO_2 levels in the blood are high, thereby reducing acid load
   d. By decreasing respiratory rate and depth when CO_2 levels in the blood are low, thereby increasing acid load

5. A client has the following arterial blood gas results: pH, 7.52; partial pressure of carbon dioxide in the arterial blood ($PaCO_2$), 30 mm Hg; HCO_3^- level, 24 mmol/L. These results indicate the presence of which acid–base disturbance?
   a. Metabolic acidosis
   b. Metabolic alkalosis
   c. Respiratory acidosis
   d. Respiratory alkalosis

6. What is the typical fluid replacement for the client with a fluid volume deficit?
   a. Dextran
   b. 0.45% Saline
   c. Lactated Ringer's solution
   d. 5% Dextrose in 0.45% saline

7. The nurse is unable to flush a central venous access device and suspects occlusion. Which of the following would be the best nursing intervention?
   a. Apply warm moist compresses to the insertion site.
   b. Attempt to force 10 mL of normal saline into the device.
   c. Place the client on the left side with head-down position.
   d. Instruct the client to change positions, raise arm, and cough.

1. b; 2. a; 3a. a, b, e; 3b. a; 3c. c; 3d. c; 3e. c; 3f. a; 4. a; 5. d; 6. c; 7. d.

⊖volve

For even more review questions, visit *http://evolve.elsevier.com/Canada/Lewis/medsurg*.

REFERENCES

Demssie, Y. N., Patel, L., Kumar, M., et al. (2014). Hypomagnesaemia: Clinical relevance and management. *British Journal of Hospital Medicine, 75*(1), 39.

Harring, T. R., Deal, N. S., & Kuo, D. C. (2014). Disorders of sodium and water balance. *Emergency Medicine Clinics of North America, 32*(2), 379–401. doi:10.1016/j.emc.2014.01.001.

Hooper, L., Bunn, D., Jimoh, F. O., et al. (2014). Water-loss dehydration and aging. *Mechanisms of Ageing and Development, 136–137*(Complete), 50–58. doi:10.1016/j.mad.2013.11.009.

Marschall, J., Mermel, L. A., Fakih, M., et al. (2014). Strategies to prevent central line–associated bloodstream infections in acute care hospitals: 2014 update. *Infection Control, 35*(07), 753–771. doi:10.1086/591059.

McCance, K. L., & Huether, S. E. (2014). *Pathophysiology: The biologic basis for disease in adults and children* (7th ed.). St. Louis: Mosby.

Medford-Davis, L., & Rafique, Z. (2014). Derangements of potassium. *Emergency Medicine Clinics of North America, 32*(2), 329–347. doi:10.1016/j.emc.2013.12.005.

Mosby (2016). *Mosby's dictionary of medicine, nursing, and health professions* (10th ed.). St. Louis: Mosby.

Porth, C. M. (2013). *Pathophysiology: Concepts of altered health states* (9th ed.). Philadelphia: Lippincott.

Touhy, T. A., & Jett, K. F. (2016). *Ebersole and Hess' toward healthy aging* (9th ed.). St. Louis: Mosby.

Verbalis, J. G., Goldsmith, S. R., Greenberg, A., et al. (2013). Diagnosis, evaluation, and treatment of hyponatremia: Expert panel recommendations. *The American Journal of Medicine, 126*(10), S1–S42. doi:10.1016/j.amjmed.2013.07.006.

Weinstein, S. M., & Hagle, M. E. (2014). *Plumer's principles and practice of infusion therapy* (9th ed.). Philadelphia: Lippincott Williams & Wilkins.

Wilson, B. A., Shannon, M. A., & Stang, C. L. (2011). *Pearson intravenous drug guide* (2nd ed., pp. 2011–2012). Upper Saddle River, NJ: Prentice Hall.

Zaghal, A., Khalife, M., Mukherji, D., et al. (2012). Update on totally implantable venous access devices. *Surgical Oncology, 21*(3), 207–215. doi:10.1016/j.suronc.2012.02.003.

RESOURCES

Acid–Base Physiology @ The Anaesthesia Education Web site
http://www.anaesthesiamcq.com/AcidBaseBook/ABindex.php

Acid–Base Tutorial
http://www.acid-base.com/

Body Fluid Volumes Calculator
http://www.globalrph.com/body_fluid_volumes.htm

For additional Internet resources, see the website for this book at *http://evolve.elsevier.com/Canada/Lewis/medsurg*

Perioperative Care

Source: Pi-Lens/Shutterstock.com.

CHAPTER
20

Nursing Management
Preoperative Care

Written by: Janice A. Neil
Adapted by: Debra Clendinneng

evolve WEBSITE

http://evolve.elsevier.com/Canada/Lewis/medsurg

- Review Questions (Online Only)
- Key Points
- Answer Guidelines for Case Study
- Conceptual Care Map Creator
- Audio Glossary
- Content Updates

LEARNING OBJECTIVES

1. Identify the common purposes and settings of surgery.
2. Describe the scope of practice for the perianesthesia nurse.
3. Describe the purpose and components of a preoperative nursing assessment.
4. Explain the purpose and components of informed consent for surgery.
5. Examine the nursing role in the physical, psychological, and educational preparation of the patient undergoing surgery.
6. Prioritize nursing responsibilities related to day-of-surgery preparation for the surgical patient.
7. Identify the purposes and types of preoperative medications.
8. Apply knowledge of special considerations in the preoperative preparation for the older-adult surgical patient.

KEY TERMS

ambulatory surgery, p. 385
elective surgery, p. 384

emergency surgery, p. 384
informed consent, p. 394

same-day admission,
p. 385

The Canadian health care system focuses on the health and well-being of all Canadians and has a renewed commitment to support innovation in and improve health care delivery to First Nations communities (Health Canada, 2015). Despite Canadians' commitment to health promotion and illness prevention, there are patients with diseases or conditions that require surgical interventions (Health Quality Ontario, 2012). Surgery may be performed for any of the following purposes:

1. *Diagnosis:* Determination of the presence or extent of pathological abnormality (e.g., lymph node biopsy or bronchoscopy).
2. *Cure or repair:* Elimination or repair of a pathological condition (e.g., removal of a ruptured appendix or benign ovarian cyst) or repair of anatomy (e.g., fracture fixation).
3. *Palliation:* Alleviation of symptoms without cure (e.g., cutting a nerve root [rhizotomy] to remove symptoms of pain or creating a colostomy to bypass an inoperable bowel obstruction).
4. *Prevention:* For example, removal of a premalignant or partial colectomy in a patient with familial adenomatous polyposis to prevent cancer.

5. *Exploration:* Surgical examination to determine the nature or extent of a disease (e.g., laparotomy).
6. *Cosmetic improvement:* For example, repair of a burn scar or changing breast shape.

Terminology used in surgical procedures combines anatomical vocabulary with prefixes and suffixes derived primarily from Latin and Greek. The use of this language pattern allows us to determine what operation or procedure is being done. Table 20-1 provides a sampling of suffixes that are commonly combined with an anatomical part or organ in naming surgical procedures.

SURGICAL SETTINGS

Surgery may be urgent (emergency surgery) or carefully planned (elective surgery). Regardless of where the surgery is performed or whether it is emergency or elective surgery, nurses are vital in preoperative patient preparation, caring for the patient during surgery, and facilitating the patient's recovery postoperatively.

Suffix	**Meaning**	**General Surgery**	**Orthopedic Surgery**	**Urological Surgery**
-ectomy	Excision/removal	Appendectomy	Discectomy	Nephrectomy
-oscopy	Looking into	Gastroscopy	Knee arthroscopy	Cystoscopy
-ostomy	Creation of opening into	Colostomy		Ureterostomy
-otomy	Cutting into/incision	Tracheotomy	Arthrotomy	Cystotomy
-plasty	Repair/reconstruction	Mammoplasty	Total hip arthroplasty	Ureteroplasty

TABLE 20-1   SUFFIXES DESCRIBING COMMON SURGICAL PROCEDURES

Surgical Wait Times

Currently, all provinces in Canada collect and report on surgical wait times for cancer, heart, joint replacement, and sight-restoration surgery. Provincial wait times are compared using a pan-Canadian benchmark for the various categories (Canadian Institute for Health Information [CIHI], 2016). Efforts to reduce wait times for elective surgery in Canada had mixed results from 2011 to 2016. For instance, the wait time for cataract surgery increased, while the wait time for joint surgery remained stable despite the increased number of procedures performed. Wait times for urgent repair of hip fractures, which is associated with a high mortality risk in seniors, decreased significantly in those five years. Despite all the contextual variables, Canada remains committed to reducing surgical and diagnostic wait times and continues to perform well when compared internationally (CIHI, 2016).

Elective Inpatient Surgery

The most common inpatient surgeries in Canada are Caesarean section, knee replacement, fractures, coronary artery angioplasty, and hip replacement surgery (CIHI, 2015). Patients requiring hospitalization for surgery are usually admitted the day of their surgery (**same-day admission**).

Ambulatory Surgery. In Canada, for the majority of surgeries, the patient is discharged on the same day. **Ambulatory surgery**, also called *same-day surgery,* can be conducted in emergency departments, endoscopy clinics, doctors' offices, and outpatient surgery units in hospitals. These procedures can be performed using general, regional, or local anaesthetic, usually take less than 2 hours, necessitate less than a 3- to 4-hour stay in the postanaesthesia care unit (PACU), and do not require overnight hospitalization. Sometimes patients are admitted to hospital postoperatively if they experience difficulty with pain control, nausea, or vomiting.

Several nurses are involved in the surgical patient's continuum of care through the preoperative, intraoperative, and postoperative phases. The following information gathered by the perianesthesia nurse before surgery assists these nurses in planning care:

- The disorder necessitating surgery
- Awareness of comorbidities
- Identification of the patient's response to the stress of surgery
- Assessment of results of preoperative diagnostic tests
- Consideration of bodily alterations, impact of comorbidities, risks, and potential complications associated with surgery

This preoperative assessment is communicated and documented to ensure continuity of care.

The preoperative nursing measures included in this chapter are applicable to the preparation of any patient undergoing surgery. Measures to prepare for specific surgical procedures (e.g., abdominal, thoracic, or orthopedic surgery) are covered in appropriate chapters of this text.

PREOPERATIVE ADMISSION ASSESSMENT

The patient's initial contact for preoperative evaluation is done at the preoperative admission clinic (PAC), where the patient is interviewed by a perianesthesia nurse. The interview is done well in advance of surgery in order to ensure time to (Andrews & Cartwright, 2016):

- Obtain consults or diagnostic testing
- Ensure that the patient's emotional status and medical regimen (e.g., glycemic control) are satisfactory
- Make arrangements for family care and transportation

The purposes of the preoperative assessment are (1) to decrease surgical delays or cancellations by obtaining patient health information (e.g., physical assessment and American Society of Anesthesiologists physical status); (2) to evaluate and reduce patient anxiety by providing clear explanations, correcting misconceptions, and supporting physiological, cognitive, and psychosocial perspectives (Andrews & Cartwright, 2016); and (3) to educate and allow questions from the patient and family or caregiver regarding the preparation for surgery and anaesthetic protocols. The information provided includes:

- Protocol for taking routine medication on day of surgery
- Which medications (e.g., anticoagulants) or herbal remedies to stop prior to surgery and when to stop them
- Nothing-by-mouth (NPO) instructions
- Pain management options
- Infection prevention and wound care
- Postoperative discharge and care (see Chapter 22)

DAY-OF-SURGERY ASSESSMENT

All surgical patients have a physical assessment completed and documented by a physician. The extent of the exam is dependent on the type of surgery and anaesthesia required.

On the day of surgery, the nurse does a focused preoperative assessment that reviews existing information, reinforces teaching, and reviews discharge plans (Odom Forren, 2013). Each hospital or facility has a concise preoperative checklist that helps the nurse meet the following goals:

- Confirm and identify changes to patient's physical status by reviewing the physical exam, confirming preoperative consultations are complete (e.g., by a cardiology, internal medicine, physiotherapy, or wound care nurse) and communicate mobility or sensory deficits to the perioperative team.
- Determine the patient's psychological status and reinforce coping strategies.
- Establish baseline data (i.e., vital signs) for comparison in the intraoperative and postoperative period.
- Review prescription medications, over-the-counter drugs, and herbal medications that may affect the surgical outcome.
- Ensure that preoperative laboratory and diagnostic test results are documented and communicated to appropriate personnel.

- Support the patient's language, family, culture, and spiritual or religious needs that may affect the surgical experience.
- Determine whether the patient has adequate information from the surgeon to make an informed decision to have surgery, and ensure that the consent form is signed by the patient and physician.
- Ensure the patient understands the discharge plan and has postoperative support. This may involve consulting with and setting up postoperative care with rehabilitative facilities or community nursing agencies.

Subjective Data

Psychosocial Assessment. The meaning of surgery should be explored with the patient as each person has a different perception and anxiety level regarding the procedure, anaesthesia, and postoperative pain (Odom-Forren, 2013). Stress can negatively impact surgical outcomes, such as causing a longer, more painful postoperative recovery (Pereira, Figueiredo-Braga, & Carvalho, 2015). Many factors influence the patient's susceptibility to stress, including the use of positive coping strategies, such as taking an active role, relaxation training, using distraction, and practising other pain control techniques. Past experiences, current health, socioeconomic status, and age also impact stress. Calm, confident nursing communication can help allay patients' fears (Odom-Forren, 2013). (See Chapter 8 for a discussion of stress.)

Older adults may perceive hospitalization for surgery as a physical decline or loss of mobility and independence. They may fear being placed in a long-term care facility, which some view as a place to die. The nurse is instrumental in alleviating anxieties and restoring the self-esteem of these surgical patients (see "Age-Related Considerations" at the end of the chapter), by identifying stressors that can negatively affect them (Table 20-2). Children and their caregivers also experience anxiety related to surgery despite increased knowledge of perioperative events (Tourigny, Clendinneng, Chartrand, et al., 2011). Nurses reassure anxious parents and reduce children's emotional distress by correcting erroneous ideas and providing timely information in the perioperative period. The nurse uses language that is familiar to the child or youth and caregivers in order to increase their understanding of surgical consent and of perioperative processes. If the patient and caregivers do not speak English, it is ideal to have an interpreter to disseminate information. Not all hospitals can provide an interpreter, so families may bring an English-speaking representative with them to the preoperative interview. (The use of interpreters is discussed in Chapter 2.)

Anxiety. Patients may be anxious when facing surgery because of lack of knowledge, for example, not knowing what to expect during the surgical experience or having uncertainty about the outcome of surgery and the potential findings of diagnostic procedures. Some may worry about allowing strangers to take control of their life or even have concerns about not waking from anaesthesia. Studies have shown that preoperative education that includes information about perianesthesia helps decrease anxiety and allay fears (Campbell, 2015). Further, Pereira, Figueiredo-Braga, and Carvalho (2015) demonstrated that nurses' using an empathic, patient-centred approach during the preoperative interview results in improved patient satisfaction, lower pain levels, and faster wound healing.

Patients may be concerned when surgical or anaesthetic interventions, for example, blood transfusions, are in conflict with religious or cultural beliefs. The requesting physician should discuss the need for blood replacement with the patient and

---

TABLE 20-2 PSYCHOSOCIAL ASSESSMENT OF THE PATIENT BEFORE SURGERY

Situational Changes
- Determine support systems, including family, other caregivers, significant others, and religious or spiritual orientation.
- Define degree of personal control, decision making, and independence.
- Consider the impact of surgery and hospitalization on family and dependents and financial impacts related to recovery time and medical expenses.
- Identify the presence of hope and anticipation of positive results.

Concerns With the Unknown
- Identify specific areas and depth of anxiety and fears.
- Identify expectations of surgery, changes in current health status, and effects on daily living.

Concerns With Body Image
- Identify current roles or relationships and view of self.
- Determine perceived or potential changes in role or relationships and their impact on body image.

Past Experiences
- Review previous surgical experiences, hospitalizations, and treatments.
- Determine responses to those experiences (positive and negative).
- Identify current perceptions of surgical procedure in relation to the above and information from others (e.g., a neighbour's view of a personal surgical experience).

Knowledge Deficit
- Identify what preoperative information this specific patient wants to receive.
- Assess understanding of the surgical procedure, including preparation, care, interventions, preoperative activities, restrictions, and expected outcomes.
- Identify the accuracy of information the patient has received from others, including the health care team, family, friends, and the media.

---

obtain an informed consent, noting patient consent or refusal for transfusion on the patient's chart. This discussion presents an opportunity to provide information to patients about autologous blood donation if they are undergoing surgeries with a higher likelihood of requiring a transfusion (Ontario Regional Blood Coordinating Network, 2013).

Common Fears. The primary reasons patients fear surgery are the fear of dying under anaesthesia, permanent disability resulting from the operation, pain, change in body image, or receiving a poor prognosis during a diagnostic procedure (e.g., breast biopsy). Patients can become fearful after independently hearing or reading about the risks of surgery and during the informed consent process when the surgeon explains all aspects of the operation to the patient.

Fear of death can be extremely stressful for the patient. If the nurse identifies that a patient has a fear of death, this information must be communicated to the surgeon immediately. It is important that the surgeon talk with the patient in order to understand where the fear originates and to assuage anxiety. *Fear of pain and discomfort* during and after surgery is common. If the fear appears extreme, the nurse should notify the anaesthesiologist so that appropriate preoperative medication (such as an antianxiety medication) can be ordered. The patient should be reassured that medications are available to minimize or eliminate pain during and after surgery. Drugs can be given that provide an amnesic effect so that the patient will not remember what occurs during the surgical episode. These medications can cause temporary cognitive deficits following surgery that the patient must be informed of. The nurse should stress that the patient should ask for pain medications as needed following surgery and that taking these medications will not contribute to an addiction but may assist with postoperative recovery. (Pain is discussed in Chapter 10.)

Fear of mutilation or alteration in body image can occur whether the surgery is minor or radical, such as amputation. Even the presence of just a small scar on the body can be bothersome to some patients. The nurse assesses these concerns with an open, nonjudgemental attitude.

Fear of anaesthesia may arise from fear of the unknown, from tales of others' bad experiences, or from previous personal experience. Some patients are concerned about information provided about hazards or complications (e.g., brain damage, paralysis, family history of malignant hyperthermia). Other patients have a fear of losing control while under the influence of anaesthesia. If these fears or questions are identified, the nurse should inform the anaesthesiologist immediately so that he or she can reassure the patient and confirm that a nurse and the anaesthesiologist will be present at all times during surgery.

Fear of disruption of life functioning or patterns can present in varying degrees. A patient may fear permanent disability or loss of life or have concerns about physical limitations after surgery. Also common are concerns about separation from family and worry about how a spouse or children will manage. Financial concerns may surface as a result of an anticipated loss of income because of missed work. If the nurse identifies any of these fears, consultation with a social worker, a spiritual or cultural advisor, a psychologist, or family members may provide valuable assistance to the patient.

Coping With Surgery. The way patients transition through the perioperative period can impact their postoperative recovery. Many draw on their spirituality, seeking inner peace and sources of hope. As patients, especially outpatients, move through the surgical experience in an accelerated fashion, the perioperative team must be responsive to the patient's health goals, hopes, and fears in order to provide the necessary support. Perioperative caregivers who listen to the patient's story may be perceived as a "person who offers spiritual care during a point of vulnerability and need" (Griffin, 2013, p. 251). Griffin also advises health care providers to engage in meaningful relationships with the perioperative patient before surgery and to mitigate feelings of vulnerability in the intimidating operating room (OR) environment.

Health History. During the preoperative interview, the nurse should ask about the patient's diagnosed medical conditions and current health issues. An organized approach using hospital guidelines and subjective questioning elicits good information regarding the patient's health history. Initially, the nurse should determine whether the patient understands the reason for surgery. For example, the patient scheduled for a total knee replacement may indicate that the reason for surgery is increasing pain and mobility problems. Detailed information on past hospitalizations, previous surgeries, dates of the surgeries, and any adverse reactions or problems with surgery or anaesthetics is documented. As an example, the patient may have experienced a bad wound infection or a reaction to an analgesic following a prior surgery.

Women should be asked about their menstrual and obstetrical history, including the date of their last menstrual period and the number of pregnancies and deliveries they have had. If the patient states that she might be pregnant, this information should be immediately communicated to the surgeon to avoid maternal and subsequent fetal exposure to anaesthetics during the first trimester. Questioning an adolescent regarding her reproductive functioning may be embarrassing for her and should be done in privacy with parents or guardians out of the room.

The nurse may identify inherited conditions by asking about the patient's family health history. A family history of cardiac and endocrine disease should be recorded. If a patient reports a mother or father with hypertension, sudden cardiac death, myocardial infarction, or coronary artery disease, the nurse should be alerted to the possibility that the patient may have a similar predisposition or condition. A family history of diabetes should be investigated because of the familial predisposition to both type 1 and type 2 diabetes mellitus. Tendencies toward these conditions may be exacerbated during surgery and affect physiological function during and after surgery. Since inherited traits, such as sickle cell trait, contribute to the choice of anaesthesia and impact surgical outcomes, they must be considered in family histories (Odom-Forren, 2013). Anaesthesia care providers obtain the patient's and family's anaesthetic history, particularly adverse reactions to or problems with anaesthesia, such as malignant hyperthermia. This rare metabolic disease is characterized by hyperthermia with rigidity of skeletal muscles and can result in death. The genetic predisposition for malignant hyperthermia susceptibility is well documented, and anaesthetic care plans are preventive (Rothrock, 2015). (Malignant hyperthermia is discussed in Chapter 21.)

Medications. As part of the preoperative interview, the nurse documents the patient's current medication use, including the use of over-the-counter (OTC) drugs and herbal products. Patients may be asked to bring their medication bottles when attending the PAC so that the nurse can accurately chart the names and dosages because patients who use a variety of medications may not remember specific details. At this time, it is important also to investigate whether the patient is taking the medication as ordered or has stopped taking it because of cost, adverse effects, or the belief that ongoing therapy is no longer needed.

Medications and herbal products may interact with anaesthetics, often increasing or decreasing potency and effectiveness, or they may be needed during surgery to maintain physiological function. It is important to consider the effects of medications used for heart disease, hypertension, immuno-suppression, seizure control, anticoagulation, and endocrine replacement. Insulin or oral hypoglycemic agents may require dosage or agent adjustments during the perioperative period because of increased body metabolism, decreased caloric intake, stress, and anaesthesia. Many patients use OTC acetylsalicylic acid (Aspirin) or are on anticoagulant therapy such as warfarin sodium (Coumadin), heparin, clopidogrel (Plavix), or others that inhibit platelet aggregation and may contribute to postoperative bleeding complications. Surgeons often require that patients stop taking acetylsalicylic acid (Aspirin) for at least 2 weeks before surgery. It is also important to stress that stopping some medications abruptly can cause complications. The preoperative nurse should check with an anaesthesiologist to ensure which medications should be stopped and which should be taken the day of surgery.

The use of herbal therapy and dietary supplements is common, but many patients do not disclose to health care providers that they take these supplements unless specifically asked (Larner, 2015). Therefore, it is essential for the nurse to ask about the use of vitamins, herbal supplements, and other alternative substances (see Chapter 12, Table 12-7). These products may interfere with anaesthesia and potentially cause complications during surgery, such as effects on blood pressure, increased sedation, cardiac effects, electrolyte alterations, and inhibition of platelet aggregation. In patients taking anticoagulants or platelet aggregation inhibitors, the use of specific herbal products can cause excessive postoperative bleeding that may necessitate a return to the OR. These types of supplements must be discontinued before surgery, as ordered by the physician (Larner, 2015). Some effects of specific herbs that can be of concern during the perioperative period are identified in the "Complementary & Alternative Therapy" box.

In the preoperative interview, the nurse should ask the patient about recreational drug use and any substance use disorder.

🌸 COMPLEMENTARY & ALTERNATIVE THERAPIES

Effects of Herbs and Supplements During the Perioperative Period

Herb	Perioperative Considerations
Echinacea	May cause immune suppression if taken over long term. Use to be discontinued as far in advance of surgery as possible.
Ephedra	Stimulant, decongestant, bronchodilator, taken for weight loss. Multiple cardiovascular and GI adverse effects. Use to be discontinued at least 24 hours preoperatively.
Feverfew	May increase clotting time. Preoperative use to be avoided.
Garlic	May increase clotting time and potentiate effects of anticoagulants. Use to be discontinued at least 7 days preoperatively.
Ginger	May increase bleeding, especially in patients taking anticoagulants. To be avoided preoperatively.
Ginkgo biloba	May increase bleeding, especially in patients taking anticoagulants. Use to be discontinued at least 36 hours preoperatively.
Ginseng	May falsely elevate digoxin levels and potentiate MAOIs. Contraindicated for cardiac disorders, hypertension, and hypoglycemia. Use to be discontinued 7 days preoperatively.
Goldenseal	May cause hypotension; may increase edema and potentiate effect of insulin. Preoperative use to be avoided.
Kava	May prolong the effects of certain anaesthetics and have adverse effect on motor reflexes. Use to be discontinued at least 24 hours preoperatively.
Licorice	Certain preparations may cause elevated BP or electrolyte imbalance. Not to be used for more than 7 days preoperatively.
Saw palmetto	May have additive effects with other hormone therapies.
St. John's wort	May prolong the effects of anaesthetic agents, potentiate opioids, and cause electrolyte imbalance.
Valerian	Potentiates sedative–hypnotics; may prolong anaesthesia recovery time. Dose to be tapered for 1–2 weeks preoperatively.
Vitamin E	May increase bleeding and may increase heart rate.

BP, blood pressure; *GI*, gastro-intestinal; *MAOI*, monoamine oxidase inhibitor.
Sources: American Society of Anesthesiologists. (2003). *What you should know about herbal and dietary supplement use and anesthesia.* Park Ridge, IL: Author; Rothrock, J. C. (Ed.). (2015). *Alexander's care of the patient in surgery* (15th ed., pp. 1171–1172). St. Louis: Elsevier.

Substances most likely to be abused include tobacco, alcohol, opioids, marihuana, and cocaine. Questions should be asked matter-of-factly and information given that recreational drug use may affect the type and amount of anaesthesia required. When patients are aware of the potential interactions of these drugs with anaesthetics, most will respond honestly about their drug use. Chronic alcohol use may place the patient undergoing surgery at risk because of lung, gastro-intestinal, or liver damage. When liver function is decreased, metabolism of anaesthetic agents is prolonged, nutritional status is altered, and the potential for postoperative complications is increased. Alcohol withdrawal can also occur during lengthy surgery or in the postoperative period but can be avoided with appropriate planning and management (see Chapter 11).

When assessing medication use, drug intolerance and drug allergies should be considered. Drug intolerance usually results in adverse effects that are uncomfortable or unpleasant for the patient but not life-threatening. These effects can include nausea, constipation, diarrhea, or *idiosyncratic* (opposite from expected) reactions. A true drug allergy produces hives, an anaphylactic reaction, or both, causing cardiopulmonary compromise, including hypotension, tachycardia, bronchospasm, and possibly pulmonary edema. Awareness of drug intolerance and drug allergies, however, makes it possible to maintain patient comfort, safety, and stability. For example, some anaesthetic drugs contain sulphur, so the anaesthesiologist should be notified of a history of allergy to sulphur. Any drug intolerance or drug allergy identified must be documented and flagged on the patient's chart, and, on the day of surgery, an allergy wristband is put on the patient. Depending on institutional protocol, the nurse may be responsible for entering the identified allergy in the electronic medical record so that all health care providers and the pharmacy have knowledge of any medication or related allergy.

All findings of the medication history are documented and communicated to the intraoperative and postoperative teams. Although the anaesthesiologist will determine the appropriate schedule and dose of the patient's routine medications before and after surgery based on the medication history, the nurse must ensure that all of the patient's medications are identified, administer the medications as ordered, and monitor the patient for potential interactions and complications.

Allergies. The nurse should inquire about nonpharmaceutical allergies to foods, metals, chemicals, tape, and pollen. The patient with a history of any allergic response has a greater potential for demonstrating hypersensitivity reactions to drugs administered during anaesthesia. Patients should also be screened for possible latex allergies (Operating Room Nurses Association of Canada, 2015) (see Chapters 16 and 21). Centimole (2013) recommends that patients who report the following be considered at risk for latex allergy:

- History of contact dermatitis and atopic immunological reactions
- Allergies to nuts, bananas, avocados, figs, chestnuts, papayas
- Neural tube defects
- Multiple operations
- Repeated bladder catheterizations

High-risk groups for latex allergy also include health care providers. Latex allergies produce reactions ranging from mild skin redness to anaphylaxis (Centimole, 2013).

Review of Systems. A thorough body systems review is performed and documented before surgery by members of the perioperative team. This review of systems is described in detail in Chapter 3. The surgeon does a preoperative physical examination (PE) and patient history and orders appropriate preoperative laboratory tests and consultations before the day of surgery. In the immediate preoperative period, there is seldom time for the nurse to do a full physical assessment, so nurses rely on the chart documentation. The following are important points for the nurse to assess immediately before surgery to ensure a seamless, safe experience for the patient.

Nervous System. Preoperative evaluation of neurological functioning includes assessing the patient's ability to respond to questions, follow commands, and maintain orderly thought patterns. Alterations in the patient's hearing (e.g., requiring hearing aids) and vision (e.g., requiring glasses, development of glaucoma) may affect responses and ability to follow directions. A person's ability to pay attention, concentrate, and respond appropriately is documented to use as the baseline for postoperative comparison.

Impaired cognitive function may affect the patient's ability to prepare for surgery, and the nurse must determine whether all preoperative procedures were carried out—for example, bowel preparations. If confusion is noted and persistent, it is important to determine whether there are appropriate resources and support to assist the patient after surgery.

Cognitive function is of major importance in the assessment of older-adult patients. Although major surgery is a predisposing factor for delirium, other predictive conditions for delirium are dehydration, malnutrition, immobility, urinary catheters, medications, and infection (Rothrock, 2015). Nonverbal older patients and those with chronic conditions such as Alzheimer's disease must be assessed for their interpretation of pain before surgery so that postoperative pain scales can be used effectively. It has been demonstrated that older adults are at risk for undetected pain due to beliefs that pain must be endured and that they should not disturb nurses with complaints of pain (Rothrock, 2015). These preoperative findings are extremely important for postoperative comparison.

Cardiovascular System. The purpose of evaluating cardiovascular function is to determine the presence of pre-existing disease or existing problems so that the patient's condition can be effectively monitored during the surgical and recovery periods. If there is a history of cardiac problems, including hypertension, angina, dysrhythmias, heart failure, or myocardial infarction, or use of pacemakers or implanted cardiac devices, the patient may need a cardiology and anaesthesia consult before surgery.

If pertinent, clotting and bleeding times and other relevant laboratory results must also be on the chart before surgery. For example, for the patient who receives digitalis therapy, serum potassium levels must be documented. If the patient has a history of congenital, rheumatic, or valvular heart disease, antibiotic prophylaxis before surgery may be given to decrease the risk for bacterial endocarditis. Further, the nurse should confirm that the patient has not taken anticoagulants, as an international normalized ratio (INR) may need to be drawn before surgery.

Respiratory System. The patient should be asked about any recent or chronic upper respiratory infections. The presence of an upper airway infection may result in the cancellation or postponement of elective surgery because the patient has an increased anaesthetic risk. If the patient has a history of respiratory problems, he or she will have an anaesthetic consult before surgery and an appropriate workup.

If a patient has asthma, the nurse should inquire about the patient's recent use of inhaled or oral corticosteroids and bronchodilators. The patient with a severe active airway infection, chronic obstructive pulmonary disease, or asthma is at risk for pulmonary complications, including bronchospasm, laryngospasm, hypoxemia, and atelectasis.

The patient who smokes should be encouraged to stop at least 6 weeks before surgery to decrease the risk for intraoperative and postoperative respiratory complications. Many patients may find this difficult given the added stress of impending surgery (Registered Nurses' Association of Ontario, 2015). The greater the patient's pack-years of smoking, the greater the patient's risk for pulmonary complications.

Obesity; spinal, chest, or airway deformities; and sleep apnea can compromise respiratory function. Depending on the patient's history and PE findings, baseline pulmonary function tests and arterial blood gas tests may be ordered before surgery.

Urinary System. Before surgery, the patient's urinary system status should be documented. Results of any renal function tests, such as serum creatinine and blood urea nitrogen (serum urea [nitrogen]), ordered before surgery should be available on the patient's chart.

Male patients who have problems voiding may have an enlarged prostate, which would hinder the insertion of a urinary catheter during surgery and also impair voiding in the postoperative period. This information is documented for the perioperative team. The nurse should inform patients if they will have a catheter after surgery.

Integumentary System. Any skin rashes, boils, ulcers, or other dermatological conditions should be noted. A history of pressure injuries may necessitate extra padding during surgery, and skin problems may affect postoperative healing.

Musculo-Skeletal System. The nurse should note mobility problems in any affected joints, as these restrictions influence intraoperative and postoperative positioning and can affect ambulation. Spinal anaesthesia may be difficult if the patient cannot flex her or his lumbar spine adequately to allow easy needle insertion. If the neck is affected, intubation and airway management may be difficult.

Endocrine System. Diabetes mellitus is a risk factor for both anaesthesia and surgery. The patient with diabetes is at risk for the development of hypoglycemia, hyperglycemia, ketosis, cardiovascular alterations, delayed wound healing, and infection. Preoperative capillary blood glucose tests should be done to determine baseline levels. It is important to clarify with the patient's surgeon or anaesthesiologist whether the patient should take the usual dose of insulin on the day of surgery. Some practitioners prefer that the patient take only half of the usual dose; others ask that the patient take either the usual dose or no insulin at all. Regardless of the preoperative insulin orders, the patient's capillary blood glucose will be determined periodically and managed, if necessary, with regular (short-acting, rapid-onset) insulin.

It should also be determined whether the patient has a history of thyroid dysfunction. Either hyperthyroidism or hypothyroidism can place the patient at surgical risk because of alterations in metabolic rate. If the patient takes a thyroid replacement drug, the nurse should check with the anaesthesiologist about administration of the drug the day of surgery. If the patient has a history of thyroid dysfunction, laboratory tests may be ordered to determine current levels of thyroid function.

Immune System. Patients with active chronic infections, such as hepatitis, acquired immune deficiency syndrome, or tuberculosis, may be suitable for surgery; however, if the patient has a history of immuno-suppression or takes immuno-suppressive drugs, this will be noted in the patient chart. Impairment of the immune system can lead to delayed wound healing and postoperative infections. If the patient has an acute infection (e.g., active skin rash, acute sinusitis, flu, etc.), elective surgery is frequently cancelled. (Infection control guidelines are discussed in Chapter 17.)

Fluid and Electrolyte Status. The patient should be questioned about vomiting, diarrhea, or difficulty swallowing. Drugs that the patient takes that alter fluid and electrolyte status, such as diuretics, should also be identified because serum electrolyte levels may need to be evaluated before surgery. Most patients have restricted fluids because of NPO status before surgery; it is the responsibility of the anaesthesiologist to administer intravenous (IV) fluids and electrolyte therapy to maintain proper hydration.

Nutritional Status. Nutritional extremes in patients require consideration in the perioperative period. For example, if the patient is extremely obese, having notification before surgery allows the perioperative nurse time to prepare the necessary equipment and instrumentation. Obesity stresses the cardiac and pulmonary systems and predisposes the patient to obstructive sleep apnea, which in turn can indicate difficult intubation and post-extubation complications. Ventricular arrhythmias and hypertension are other potential complications (Clifford, 2013).

Malnutrition is a result of inadequate intake of protein or calories. It can cause poor tolerance for anaesthetic drugs, altered wound healing, and susceptibility to infections and cause an increased risk for morbidity and mortality (Jackson, 2015). Many older adults are at risk for malnutrition and fluid volume deficits. If the patient is very thin, the perioperative team should be notified so as to have adequate pressure-reducing positioning devices (pressure points on all patients are protected routinely) on the operating bed. Pressure reduction helps prevent pressure injuries, especially during lengthy procedures. Nutritional deficiencies impair the ability to recover from surgery, so if the nutritional problem is severe, surgery may be postponed until the patient's weight and nutritional deficiencies are corrected.

Impaired nutritional status may affect postoperative recovery and should be identified if the patient will remain in the hospital after surgery. This is particularly true of the undernourished geriatric patient who is at high risk for postoperative morbidity and mortality (Papanier Wells & Flanagan, 2015).

Nursing Assessment: Patient About to Undergo Surgery. The review of the patient's health provides valuable data about the patient's physical and psychological status as well as cultural values and beliefs related to his or her health care. Questions to ask a patient about to undergo surgery are listed in Table 20-3.

Objective Data

Physical Examination. In Canada, the health authority in each province or territory may have its own policies on preoperative health assessments, but it is important to have a PE documented on the chart in case surgical complications arise. This examination may be done in advance of surgery or on the day of surgery.

Findings from the patient's history and PE will enable the anaesthesiologist to assign the patient a physical status rating for anaesthesia administration reference. The classification system

TABLE 20-3 **HEALTH HISTORY**
Patient About to Undergo Surgery

Subjective Data
Past Health History
- Have you had surgeries in the past?* Which ones?* Did you have any complications?*
- Have you or any family members ever experienced any problems with anaesthesia?*
- Do you have any past hospitalizations?*
- Do you have any chronic health conditions?
- Do you have a history of high blood pressure or cardiac disease?*
- Do you have any history of dyspnea, coughing, hemoptysis, COPD, or asthma?*

Current Health History
- What is your usual or present height and weight? Have you had a recent weight gain or loss?*
- Do you at present have an upper respiratory infection?*
- Do you wear glasses, contact lenses, or a hearing aid?*
- Do you smoke?* If yes, how many packs daily? For how many years?
- What is your usual use of alcohol?
- Do you have any problems healing?*
- Do you have any musculo-skeletal problems that might affect positioning during surgery or activity level after surgery?*
- Do you have any limitation in mobility of your neck?* (Might affect intubation for surgery)
- Do you require any special equipment for ambulation?*
- How would you describe your pain tolerance? What methods have you found effective for pain relief?
- Do you have anxiety related to the surgery?
- Will you have the support you feel you need following discharge?

Medications
- Are you currently taking any prescribed medications, over-the-counter medications, or herbal or vitamin supplements?*
- Do you have any allergies or sensitivities to any foods or medications?*

COPD, chronic obstructive pulmonary disease.
*If yes, describe.

commonly used was developed by the American Society of Anesthesiologists as a way to provide a standardized way to assess the expected anaesthesia outcome for the surgical patient and provide health care providers consistent communication about the patient's physical status and fitness for surgery (Marley, Calabrese, & Thompson, 2014) (Table 20-4). Many physiological stressors may put the patient at risk for surgical complications, whether the surgery is an elective or an emergency procedure. A physiological assessment of the patient who is about to undergo surgery is presented in Table 20-5. If the PE is done immediately before surgery, it will be a more focused assessment because of the impending procedures that must be completed before surgery. The nurse should review the documentation already present on the patient's chart, including the review of systems and the physician's PE report. All findings must be documented, with any relevant findings immediately communicated to members of the perioperative team.

Laboratory and Diagnostic Testing. Preoperative laboratory and electrocardiogram testing is obtained based on the patient's history in order to determine their surgical and anaesthetic risk. Diagnostic tests must be ordered judiciously according to hospital protocol in order to reduce unnecessary testing (Marley, Calabrese, & Thompson, 2014). For example, if the patient is taking an anticoagulant (including Aspirin), a coagulation profile may be

TABLE 20-4 ASA PHYSICAL STATUS CLASSIFICATION SYSTEM

Rating	Examples
ASA I: Healthy normal patient	Healthy, nonsmoking, no or minimal alcohol intake
ASA II: Patient with mild systemic disease	Mild disease, minimal functional limitations (e.g., currently smoking, social alcohol intake, pregnancy, obesity, controlled diabetes, controlled hypertension, mild lung disease)
ASA III: Patient with severe systemic disease	Substantial functional limitations with one or more moderate to severe diseases (e.g., poorly controlled diabetes, hypertension, COPD, active hepatitis, premature infant, myocardial ischemia, CVA)
ASA IV: Patient with severe systemic disease that is a constant threat to life	*Examples:* Recent (<3 months) myocardial infarction, CVA, ongoing cardiac ischemia, sepsis, acute respiratory disease, DIC
ASA V: Moribund patient not expected to survive without surgery	*Examples:* Ruptured abdominal/thoracic aneurysm, massive trauma, massive intracranial bleed, ischemic bowel plus cardiac or multiple organ failure
ASA VI: Brain-dead patient	Organs being removed for donation

COPD, chronic obstructive pulmonary disease; *CVA,* cerebro-vascular accident; *DIC,* disseminated intravascular coagulation.
Source: Based on ASA physical status classification system, 2014, of the American Society of Anesthesiologists. A copy of the full text can be obtained from ASA, 1061 American Lane, Schaumburg, Illinois 60173-4973 or online at *www.asahq.org.*

TABLE 20-5 PHYSIOLOGICAL ASSESSMENT OF THE PATIENT BEFORE SURGERY*

Neurological System
- Determine orientation to time, place, and person.
- Identify presence of confusion, disorderly thinking, or inability to follow commands.
- Identify past history of strokes, TIAs, or diseases of the central nervous system such as Parkinson's disease or multiple sclerosis.
- Identify history of headaches or issues with vision or hearing.

Cardiovascular System
- Identify acute or chronic problems; focus on the presence of angina, hypertension, heart failure, and recent history of myocardial infarction.
- Palpate baseline radial pulse for rate and characteristics.
- Inspect for edema, noting location and severity.
- Take baseline blood pressure.
- Identify any medication or herbal product that may affect coagulation (e.g., acetylsalicylic acid, ginkgo biloba, ginger).
- Review laboratory and diagnostic tests for cardiovascular function when indicated.

Respiratory System
- Identify acute or chronic problems; note the presence of infection or COPD.
- Assess history of smoking and encourage the patient to stop before surgery by educating him or her about the increased risk for complications.
- Determine baseline respiratory rate and rhythm, regularity of pattern, and pulse oximetry.
- Observe for cough, dyspnea, use of accessory muscles of respiration, and cyanosis.

Urinary System
- Identify any pre-existing disease and ability of the patient to void. Prostate enlargement may affect catheterization during surgery and ability to void after surgery.
- Review laboratory and diagnostic tests for renal function when indicated.

Hepatic System
- Review any history of substance abuse, especially alcohol and intravenous drug use.
- Review laboratory and diagnostic tests for liver when indicated.

Endocrine and Hematological Systems
- Identify pre-existing problems with bleeding or hematological and endocrine disorders.

Integumentary System
- Assess mucous membranes for dryness and intactness.
- Determine skin status; note drying, bruising, or breaks in integrity of surface.
- Inspect skin for rashes, boils, or infection, especially around the planned surgical site.
- Assess skin moisture and temperature.
- Inspect the mucous membranes and skin turgor for presence of dehydration.
- Identify any history of problems with wound healing.

Musculo-Skeletal System
- Examine skin–bone pressure points and pressure injuries.
- Assess for limitations in joint pain, range of motion, and muscle weakness.
- Assess mobility, gait, and balance.

Gastro-Intestinal–Nutritional System
- Identify history of gastro-intestinal disorders or problems with elimination.
- Determine food and fluid intake patterns and any recent weight loss.
- Weigh patient.
- Assess for the presence of dentures and bridges (loose dentures or teeth may be dislodged during intubation).

COPD, chronic obstructive pulmonary disease; *TIA,* transient ischemic attack.
*See related body system chapters for more specific assessments and related laboratory studies.

done; a patient on diuretic or digoxin therapy may need to have a potassium level obtained; a patient taking medications for dysrhythmias will have a preoperative electrocardiogram. Blood glucose monitoring should be done for patients with diabetes. Findings may necessitate dosage or drug adjustments during the perioperative period because of increased body metabolism, decreased caloric intake, stress, and anaesthesia. Regulation of

the stability of the blood glucose levels during surgery will promote a more positive outcome. Commonly ordered preoperative laboratory tests can be found in Table 20-6.

Offices and PACs may do the preoperative tests days before surgery. Thus, the nurse must ensure that all laboratory reports are on the chart. Lack of these reports may result in a delay or cancellation of the surgery.

TABLE 20-6 COMMON PREOPERATIVE LABORATORY TESTS

Test	Area Assessed
ABGs, oximetry	Pulmonary and metabolic function
Blood glucose	Metabolic status, diabetes mellitus
Blood studies: RBC, Hb, Hct, platelets, WBC, WBC differential	Anemia, immune status, infection
Blood type, screen, and crossmatch	Blood availability for replacement (elective surgery patients may have own blood available—autologous)
Blood urea nitrogen*	Renal function
Chest radiograph	Pulmonary disorders, cardiac enlargement
Creatinine	Renal function
Electrocardiogram	Cardiac disease, electrolyte abnormalities
Electrolytes	Metabolic status, renal function, diuretic adverse effects
Liver function tests	Liver function
Pregnancy	Reproductive status
Prothrombin (INR) or partial thromboplastin time	Bleeding tendencies
Pulmonary function studies	Pulmonary status
Urinalysis	Renal status, hydration, urinary tract infection and disease

ABGs, arterial blood gases; *Hct,* hematocrit; *Hb,* hemoglobin; *INR,* international normalized ratio; *RBC,* red blood cell; *WBC,* white blood cell.
*Serum urea (nitrogen).

NURSING MANAGEMENT
PATIENT ABOUT TO UNDERGO SURGERY

Preoperative nursing interventions are derived from the nursing assessment and must reflect each individual patient's specific needs. Physical preparations will be determined by the pending surgery and the routines of the surgery setting. Psychological preparations should be tailored to each patient's needs. Preoperative teaching may be minimal or extensive. General information for surgery should be given.

PREOPERATIVE EDUCATION

Preoperative education empowers the patient to make informed health decisions and to participate effectively during the surgical experience. Preoperative teaching increases patient compliance with instructions and satisfaction and may reduce fear, anxiety, stress, the duration of hospitalization, and recovery time following discharge. In our multicultural Canadian society, challenges nurses may encounter in perianesthesia teaching include language barriers; cultural perceptions of health, hospitals, and surgery; and the individualized time required to allay the patient's concerns and anxiety level.

In most surgical settings, patients attend the PAC within a month of their scheduled surgery. However, even in unplanned surgery, there is time for the nurse to present information to the patient about the surgery and the postoperative period. The only time patients may not receive any information about their surgery is in an emergency situation where there is no time for teaching. In the PAC, information is presented to the patient in verbal, video, and written forms, which patients and caregivers can review at their leisure.

In preparing the patient for surgery, the nurse identifies the patient's educational needs by determining age, language, reading level, emotional status, and motivation to understand surgery and the perianesthesia process. Preoperative teaching concerns three types of information: sensory, process, and procedural. Different patients, with varying cultures, backgrounds, and experience, may want different types of information. Patients wanting *sensory information* want to know what they will see, hear, smell, and feel during the surgery. The nurse may tell them that the OR will be cold, but they can ask the perioperative nurse for a warm blanket; the lights in the OR are very bright; or there will be lots of sounds that are unfamiliar and specific smells. Patients wanting *process information* may not want specific details but desire the general flow of what is going to happen. Patients can be advised that a nurse and anaesthesiologist will speak with them in the preoperative unit; then they will go to the OR, and, when they wake up, they will be in the PACU. After this, they will be transferred back to their postoperative room or home. With *procedural information,* desired details are more specific: for example, an IV line will be started while patients are in the holding area, and, in the OR, patients will be asked to move onto the narrow bed, and a safety strap will be put over their thighs.

Preoperative patient teaching is a perianesthesia nursing team effort; PAC nurses initiate teaching, perioperative nurses continue it, and the postoperative and discharge nurses reinforce and supplement it. Community nurses who visit the patient at home, in the community, or in extended-care facilities after surgery must also be cognizant of the surgical teaching plan. All teaching should be documented in the patient's medical record. A patient and caregiver teaching guide for preoperative preparation is presented in Table 20-7. Additional information related to patient teaching may be found in Chapter 4.

GENERAL SURGERY INFORMATION. The nurse also provides information specific to the operation being performed and the educational needs of the patient (Table 20-8). All patients should receive instruction about deep breathing, incentive spirometry, coughing, and mobilizing after surgery. This education is essential because patients may not want to do these activities after surgery unless they are taught the rationale for them and practise them before surgery. Patients and caregivers should be told whether there will be tubes, drains, monitoring devices, or special equipment after surgery and that these devices enable the nurse to safely care for the patient.

Examples of individualized teaching may include how to use incentive spirometers or postoperative, patient-controlled analgesia pumps. Examples of surgery-specific information include having an immobilizer (for a patient undergoing a total joint replacement), having an epidural catheter for postoperative pain control, or waking up in the intensive care unit (for a patient requiring extensive surgery).

AMBULATORY SURGERY INFORMATION. The ambulatory surgery patient or the patient admitted to hospital the day of surgery will need to receive information before admission. The teaching is generally done in the surgeon's office or PAC and reinforced on the day of surgery. Some ambulatory surgical centres have the staff telephone the patient the evening before surgery to answer last-minute questions and to reinforce teaching.

Information provided includes the need for preoperative shower, bowel prep, or medication; arrival time at the hospital; and the time of surgery. Arrival time is usually a minimum of 2 hours before the scheduled time of surgery to allow for the

TABLE 20-7 PATIENT & CAREGIVER TEACHING GUIDE

Preoperative Preparation

Sensory Information
- Holding area is often noisy.
- Drugs and cleaning solutions may cause chemical odours.
- Operating room can be cold; warming blankets are available.
- Talking may be heard in the OR but will be distorted because of masks. Questions should be asked if something is not understood.
- OR bed will be narrow. A safety strap will be applied over the thighs.
- Lights in the OR can be very bright.
- Machines (making ticking and pinging noises) may be heard when awake. Their purpose is to monitor and ensure safety.

Procedural Information
- What to bring and what type of clothing to wear on the day of surgery.
- Any changes in time of surgery.
- Fluid and food restrictions—fasting guidelines.
- Physical preparation required (e.g., bowel or skin preparation with antibacterial cleanser).
- Purpose of frequent vital signs assessment.
- Pain control and other comfort measures (including any pain scales that a specific hospital might use to assess pain).
- Coughing and deep-breathing practice (possibly using incentive spirometry).
- How to use a pillow to assist with splinting after surgery.
- Insertion of intravenous lines.
- Procedure for anaesthesia administration.
- Importance of transferring, turning, mobilizing pain management, and postoperative exercises.
- Expected procedure for discharge and postoperative support.

Process Information
Information About General Flow of Surgery
- Admission area.
- Preoperative holding area, OR, and PACU (recovery area).
- Families can usually stay in holding area until surgery.
- Families may be able to enter recovery area as soon as patient is awake.
- Identification of any technology that may be present on awakening, such as monitors and central lines.

Where Families Can Wait During Surgery and Postoperative Roles
- Patient and family members need to be encouraged to verbalize concerns.
- OR staff will notify family when surgery is completed.
- Surgeon will usually talk with family following surgery.
- A competent adult must accompany the patient upon discharge and continue monitoring the patient at home as per the discharge instructions.
- Caregivers have requisite information to contact a health care provider with concerns and questions after discharge.

OR, operating room.

EVIDENCE-INFORMED PRACTICE

Translating Research Into Practice

Gurden Kaur is a 57-year-old woman scheduled for a knee replacement. She has been NPO since midnight and was scheduled to be the third surgical case of the day. Unfortunately, several emergency surgeries have resulted in delays, and she is not expected to leave for surgery for another 4 hours. She tells the nurse that she has a "headache" from missing her "morning coffee." She says she is hungry and thirsty, and, since surgery has been delayed, she would like a cup of coffee.

Best Available Evidence	Clinician Expertise	Patient Preferences and Values
For healthy adults, the minimum fasting period for clear liquids before surgery is 2 hours.	NPO restrictions are meant to prevent aspiration and vomiting during surgery. Patients who are NPO from midnight frequently complain of hunger and thirst while waiting for surgery. Patients who regularly drink caffeine in the morning often experience a "caffeine withdrawal" headache when fasting. Clear liquids consist of water, fruit juices without pulp, carbonated beverages, clear tea, and black coffee.	Patient is requesting something to drink given the extended period of fast due to the delay in surgery.

Decision and Action
The nurse knows that the current protocol of keeping all patients NPO after midnight for surgery does not reflect the best available evidence and that a multidisciplinary task force is working to review and revise the protocol. The nurse decides to call the anaesthesia care provider to discuss Ms. Kaur's situation and request that clear liquids be ordered for her.

References for Evidence

Crenshaw, J. T. (2011). Preoperative fasting: Will the evidence ever be put into practice? *American Journal of Nursing, 111*(10), 38–43. doi:10.1097/01 .NAJ.0000406412.57062.24.
Merchant, R., Chartrand, D., Dain, S., et al. (2016). Guidelines to the practice of anaesthesia—Revised edition 2016. *Canadian Journal of Anaesthesia, 63*(1), 86–112. doi:10.1007/s12630-015-0470.

NPO, nothing by mouth.

completion of the preoperative assessment and paperwork. Information given can also include the day-of-surgery events such as patient registration, parking, what to wear, what to bring, and the need to have a responsible adult present for transportation home after surgery.

Restriction of fluids and food is necessary preoperatively to minimize the risk for aspiration when administering general anaesthesia and to decrease the risk for postoperative nausea and vomiting. Fasting, however, is associated with dehydration, hypoglycemia, electrolyte imbalance, and patient discomfort; therefore, the patient must follow guidelines accurately (Falconer, Skouras, Carter, et al., 2014). Dobson, Chong, Chow, and colleagues (2017) recommend instituting guidelines that vary according to patient age and pre-existing medical conditions. Guidelines apply to all forms of anaesthesia, including local and monitored anaesthesia care. Patients undergoing emergency surgery must be assessed to determine the risk of delaying surgery versus the risk for gastric content aspiration. The type and amount of food ingested is considered when determining the duration of fasting, and adults and children should be encouraged to drink clear fluids up to 2 hours before surgery (see Table 20-9). Educating the patient regarding the rationale for adhering to NPO orders improves patient compliance and leads to a decrease in surgical delays and cancellations.

TABLE 20-8   SUMMARY OF PREOPERATIVE TEACHING

Topic	What to Teach the Patient	Rationale
Nutrition	• NPO guidelines • Diet increased slowly • Nausea is common—there are medications to help with this	• NPO guidelines help keep the stomach empty, reducing the potential for aspiration during anaesthesia induction. • Diet is increased slowly to prevent gastric overfilling and prevent nausea.
Ambulation	• Ambulate early • May have immobilizers, have to use assistive devices • Leg exercises • May have to wear antiembolism stockings after surgery	• Early ambulation increases circulation, ventilation, muscle tone, and vital capacity; improves gastro-intestinal and urinary function; reduces pain; and supports healing. • Antiembolic stockings reduce the incidence of postoperative formation of deep vein thrombosis.
Breathing	• To perform deep breathing and coughing exercises • Splinting • Use of incentive spirometer	• Postoperative patients are at risk for pulmonary complications (e.g., pneumonia) due to increased respiratory secretions, decreased lung expansion, and depression of the respiratory centre that occurs during general anaesthesia.
Grooming	• Take a bath or shower morning of surgery—may be required to bathe using chlorhexidine • Remove nail polish, artificial fingernails, hair clips, and jewellery (including from piercings) before surgery • Remove dentures and eyeglasses (stored during surgery) • Remove external prosthetics • Remove contact lenses	• Showers remove soil and reduce the number of transient bacteria on the skin. • Nail polish prevents accurate assessment of nail beds and interferes with pulse oximetry. • Jewellery can interfere with patient positioning, cause pressure points, and get caught on equipment. • Dentures and glasses interfere with administering general anaesthesia. • External prosthetics may impair patient transfer and positioning and interfere with intraoperative equipment. • Contact lenses can cause corneal abrasions if left in during surgery.
Medications	• Take preoperative medication as ordered • Consult physician, anaesthesiologist, or surgeon regarding when and what prescribed medications, OTC medications, and herbal remedies should be stopped preoperatively	• Medication is used preoperatively to: Assist with reducing anxiety and sedating the patient Reduce oral secretions Reduce risk of aspiration of gastric contents Reduce nausea and vomiting • Prescribed and OTC medications and herbal remedies may cause surgical complications (e.g., increased bleeding, hypertension, arrhythmias) and may need to be discontinued prior to surgery
Pain control	• Ask for pain medication as needed • Types of pain control (epidural, PCA)	• Early and effective analgesia reduces postoperative problems such as: Decreased lung compliance; risk of atelectasis Decreased mobility; risk of thrombo-embolism Increased risk of myocardial ischemia Impaired immune system Delayed return of bowel and gastric function
Drains, dressings, and tubings	• Drains (e.g., Jackson-Pratt, Hemovac) • Dressings (staples, sutures) to be expected • Tubing: IV, NG, or epidural tubing	• Preoperative patient and family teaching prepares them for the presence of postoperative drains and tubes. • Patient instruction and postoperative follow-up regarding routine practices for infection control and wound management can reduce the incidence of SSI.
Safety	• Patient identification and allergy wrist band (if appropriate) in place • Instructed to call for assistance to get out of bed • Use of call bell • Instructed not to climb over the side rails	• Identification and allergy wrist bands are important so that all health care providers can identify the patient and immediately be alerted to any allergies. • Patient injury such as rail entrapment and falls can occur if patients try to climb over bed rails.
Preoperative information	• Parking • Time to be at hospital and time of surgery • Waiting areas for family • Length of expected stay	• Preoperative information provides patients and family with guidelines and can mitigate stress on the day of surgery.

IV, intravenous; *NG,* nasogastric; *NPO,* nothing by mouth; *OTC,* over-the-counter; *PCA,* patient-controlled analgesia; *SSI,* surgical site infection.

LEGAL PREPARATION FOR SURGERY

Legal preparation for surgery consists of checking that all required forms have been correctly signed and are present in the chart and that the patient and family clearly understand what is going to happen. The most important of these forms are the signed consent form for the surgical procedure on the correct side (right or left), with no abbreviations, and specific consents for anaesthesia interventions and for blood transfusion. Other forms can include those that have been completed for advance directives and powers of attorney (see Chapter 13).

CONSENT FOR SURGERY. It is critical that nurses, as patient advocates, understand the ethical and legal tenets of informed consent. From an ethical perspective, the patient, at all times, has the right to autonomously make his or her own health decisions regarding medical, surgical, or diagnostic treatment.

Before nonemergency surgery can be legally performed, the patient must voluntarily sign an **informed consent** in the presence of a witness. Informed surgical consent is an active process between the surgeon and the patient that allows the patient to assess information and make an informed decision. Legally, a

TABLE 20-9	PREOPERATIVE FASTING RECOMMENDATIONS OF THE CANADIAN ANESTHESIOLOGISTS' SOCIETY

Liquid and Food Intake	Minimum Fasting Period (hr)
After drinking clear liquids (e.g., water, clear tea, black coffee, carbonated beverages, and fruit juice without pulp)	2
After ingesting breast milk	4
After light meal (e.g., toast and clear liquids) or after drinking infant formula or nonhuman milk	6
After meal including meat, fried or fatty food	8

Source: Merchant, R., Chartrand, D., Dain, S., et al. (2016). Guidelines to the practice of anaesthesia—Revised edition 2016. *Canadian Journal of Anesthesia, 63*(1), 86–112. doi:10.1007/s12630-015-0470

written, signed, and witnessed surgical consent helps protect the patient, surgeon, hospital, and health care team. Surgical consent forms may vary among facilities; nurses must be familiar with the form and process of obtaining consent in their institution.

According to the Canadian Medical Protective Association (CMPA; 2016), three key elements are required for a consent to be considered valid:

1. It must be voluntary.
2. The patient must have the mental capacity to consent.
3. The patient must be properly informed.

Voluntary Consent. Patients must be free either to consent to or to refuse treatment without duress, fraud, or coercion. It is considered prudent to have the surgical consent signed by the patient before giving any preoperative drugs that may interfere with patient comprehension. It is the physician's legal responsibility to obtain consent; however, in most institutions, the nurse may witness the patient's signature on the consent form. Preoperatively, the nurse can be a patient advocate, by verifying that the patient voluntarily signed the consent and understands the consent and its implications. If the patient is unclear about operative plans, the nurse may need to contact the surgeon to offer additional information. The patient must be informed that permission for treatment may be withdrawn at any time, even after the consent has been signed.

Documentation of the consent discussion should be made in the patient chart, and, in many Canadian jurisdictions, a signed consent form is a legal requirement before surgery (CMPA, 2016).

Capacity to Consent. Patient understanding is complex. However, the physician must ensure the patient comprehends the consent discussion, taking into consideration such things as emotional state and language difficulties. A patient has the capacity to consent if he or she understands the nature and effects of the proposed treatment, the consequences of refusing the treatment, and any alternatives to the treatment. Capable patients have a right to refuse to consent.

In all provinces and territories except Quebec, there is no chronological age of consent; capacity to consent is determined by maturity. This means children and youth are considered capable of consenting to or of refusing treatment if their physical, mental, and emotional development allow them to fully appreciate the consequences of their decisions. Additionally, capable minors

must give permission (consent) to the physician to have their parents involved in health care decisions. In Quebec, people 14 years and older can give consent (CMPA, 2016).

The patient who is unconscious or who has diminished capacity may have the consent form signed by a responsible family member or legally appointed representative. Hospital policies should be consulted for clarification.

Life-Threatening Situations. If the patient's life or limb is at risk, the patient is unable to consent, and the substitute decision maker is not available, the doctor does what is immediately necessary based on any known wishes of the patient and then obtains consent as soon as possible.

Properly Informing the Patient. The physician relates the diagnosis, also explaining any uncertainty about the diagnosis, the proposed treatment, the risks and consequences, the probability of a successful outcome, and the consequences of leaving the medical condition untreated. The patient must know the availability, benefits, and risks of alternative treatments (see the "Ethical Dilemmas" box). Depending on the patient's unique condition, the physician may need to discuss uncommon risks, such as permanent disability or death.

ETHICAL DILEMMAS
Informed Consent

Situation
The nurse discusses with a patient his impending surgery in the preoperative holding area. It becomes obvious that this competent adult patient was not fully informed of the alternatives to this surgery, although he has signed the consent form.

Important Points for Consideration
- Informed consent requires that patients have complete information about the proposed treatment and its possible consequences as well as alternative treatments and possible consequences.
- Risks and benefits of each treatment option must also be explained in order for patients to weigh treatment options.
- It is the surgeon's responsibility to provide this information.
- An important element of informed consent is the opportunity to have questions answered about the various treatment options and their possible outcomes.
- Health care providers must not decide what is best for patients.
- As patient advocate, the nurse must ensure that the patient is not rushed into making an informed decision.

Clinical Decision-Making Questions
1. What should the nurse do?
2. What is the nurse's role as patient advocate in the informed-consent process?

DAY-OF-SURGERY PREPARATION

NURSING ROLE

Communication is a major consideration in the patient's surgical experience. Nurses can help patients understand the questions posed preoperatively by taking a "teach-back" approach to verify that patients understand the information they are given and that, if necessary, culturally appropriate translators are available (Health Quality Ontario, 2012).

Surgery preparation will vary depending on whether the patient is an inpatient or an outpatient. The nurse prepares inpatients for surgery, but in the case of outpatient procedures, the patient or a family member may have the responsibility of preoperative preparation.

Nurses, however, must ensure the following are complete before surgery: final preoperative teaching, readiness assessment, and communication of pertinent findings from diagnostic procedures and consults to appropriate health care providers. This can be challenging for investigations done outside the hospital, as in many provinces there is poor data sharing. For instance, in Ontario, only 21% of hospitals, health care organizations, and health care providers can send electronic referrals (Health Quality Ontario, 2012). The chart should include a patient history, physical examination, lab results, baseline vitals, informed consent, and nurses' notes. All critical documentation must accompany the patient or be accessible electronically in the OR.

Most institutions require that a patient has showered or bathed before surgery and is dressed in a hospital gown; underclothes may or may not be permitted. The patient should not wear cosmetics because observation of skin colour will be important. Nail polish is removed because it may skew the results of the pulse oximeter placed on the patient's fingertip and used to monitor oxygenation. An identification band, and, if applicable, an allergy band, is put on the patient. The band(s) must remain on the patient as a means of communicating important information to health care providers (Figure 20-1). If the patient has been typed and screened for possible blood transfusion, a blood band also may be applied to the patient's wrist. All patient valuables are returned to a family member or locked up according to institutional protocol. If the patient prefers not to remove a wedding ring, in most circumstances, the ring can be taped securely to the finger to prevent loss. All other jewellery (including body piercings) and prostheses such as dentures, contact lenses, and glasses, are generally removed to prevent loss or damage. Hearing aids are usually left in place to allow the patient to better follow instructions. Glasses and hearing aids, if removed, must be returned to the patient as soon as possible following surgery.

The patient must void shortly before surgery to prevent involuntary elimination under anaesthesia and reduce the possibility of urinary retention during early postoperative recovery. The patient should void before administration of any preoperative

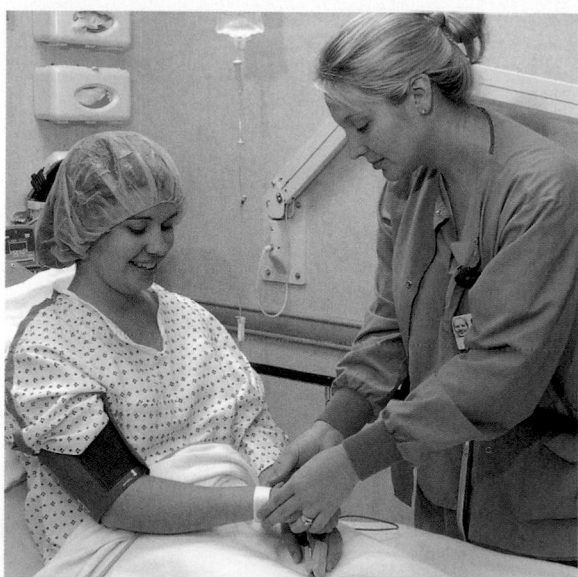

FIGURE 20-1 As part of the preoperative preparations, the nurse performs a safety check by verifying that the patient has an identification band (wristband) before going to surgery. Source: Courtesy Susan R. Volk, MSN, RN, CCRN, CPAN, Staff Development Specialist, Christiana Care Health System, Newark, DE.

medication since many preoperative medications can interfere with balance and possibly lead to a fall when the patient is in the bathroom. Voiding should be documented on the patient record. The nurse should determine that all preoperative preparations have been completed and that the signed consent for surgery is present before giving any preoperative medications.

SAFETY ALERT

Use a preoperative checklist (Figure 20-2) to ensure that all preoperative preparations have been completed before the patient is given any sedating medications.

PREOPERATIVE MEDICATIONS. Preoperative medications are used for a variety of reasons, and patients may receive a single drug or a combination of drugs. The following are examples of preoperative medications:

- *Benzodiazepines* such as midazolam, diazepam (Valium), and lorazepam (Ativan) and *barbiturates* reduce anxiety and are used for their sedative and amnesic properties.
- *Anticholinergics* such as atropine and glycopyrrolate may be given to reduce respiratory and oral secretions.
- *Opioids* such as morphine, meperidine (Demerol), and fentanyl may be given to decrease intraoperative anaesthetic requirements and to decrease pain.
- *Antiemetics* such as metoclopramide may be given to decrease nausea and vomiting after surgery.
- *Antacids* such as sodium citrate increase gastric pH, as do the following histamine H_2-receptor antagonists, in addition to decreasing gastric volume: cimetidine, famotidine (Pepcid), and ranitidine (Zantac).
- *Antibiotics* are routinely given intravenously before surgery or in the OR, with optimal initiation 30 minutes before the incision time. (Some provinces require reporting of prophylactic antibiotic use rates for specific surgical interventions to monitor surgical site infections.)
- *Eye drops* are commonly ordered and administered for the patient undergoing cataract and other eye surgery. The patient may require multiple sets of eye drops to be administered at 5-minute intervals to adequately prepare the eye for surgery.

There is no standard protocol for routine preoperative medications. In order to facilitate patient teaching and eliminate confusion, written preoperative orders clarify which medications should and should not be taken on the day of surgery. If there is any question, the nurse should clarify the orders with the anaesthesiologist. Most patients will be advised to take routine cardiac, antihypertensive, and asthma medications on the day of surgery. In the case of insulin, it is important to clarify the time and amount of the last dose before surgery.

Premedications may be administered by oral, IV, subcutaneous, or intramuscular routes. Oral medications should be given 60 to 90 minutes before the patient goes to the OR. Because patients are fluid restricted before surgery, the patient should swallow these medications with a minimal amount of water. Intramuscular and subcutaneous injections should be given 30 to 60 minutes before arrival at the OR (minimally 20 minutes). IV medications are usually administered to the patient after arrival in the preoperative holding area or OR. The medication administration must be charted immediately. The patient should be told the effects of the medications, such as relaxation, drowsiness, and dry mouth.

TRANSPORTATION TO THE OPERATING ROOM

If the patient is an inpatient, transport personnel go to the patient's room with a stretcher to transport the patient to surgery. The

Preoperative requirements	Initials
Height _____ Weight _____	
Isolation? _____ Type _____	
Allergies noted on chart	
Vital signs (Initial) T_____ P_____ R_____ BP_____	
Chart Review	
H&P on chart	
H&P within 30 days? Y N	
Signed and witnessed informed consent form on chart	
Signed consent for blood administration Y NA	
Blood type and crossmatch Y NA	
Name plate on chart	
Old chart requested and sent Y NA	
Diagnostic Results	
Hb/Hct_____/_____ NA	
PT/INR/PTT_____/_____/_____ NA	
CXR_____ NA	
ECG_____ NA	
Other labs	
Final chart review: New forms added	
Signed off	
Time to OR _____ Date _____	
Transported to OR by _____	
Final check by _____ RN	

Day of surgery	Initials
Surgical site marked Y N NA	
ID band on patient	
Allergy band on patient Y NA	
Vital signs Time _____ T_____ P_____ R_____ BP_____	
Procedures	
NPO since _____	
Capillary blood glucose Y N	
Preoperative skin prep Y N Shower Scrub Shave	
Makeup, nail polish, false fingernails, and false eyelashes removed Y NA	
Hospital gown applied Y NA	
Valuables Y N	
Dentures _____	
Wig or hairpiece _____	
Eyeglasses _____	
Contact lenses_____	
Hearing aid _____	
Prosthesis _____	
Jewellery_____	
Clothing_____	
Disposition of valuables Family Rings taped Safe	
Voided/catheter Time_____	
Preoperative medications given Time_____ NA	
Preoperative antibiotics given Time_____ NA	

FIGURE 20-2 Preoperative checklist. *BP*, blood pressure; *CXR*, chest radiograph (X-ray); *ECG*, electrocardiogram; *H&P*, history and physical examination; *Hb*, hemoglobin; *Hct*, hematocrit; *ID*, identification; *INR*, international normalized ratio; *N*, no; *NA*, not applicable; *NPO*, nothing by mouth; *OR*, operating room; *P*, pulse; *PT*, prothrombin time; *PTT*, partial thromboplastin time; *R*, respiration; *T*, temperature; *Y*, yes.

INFORMATICS IN PRACTICE

Bar-Coding in Medication Administration

- According to Institute for Safe Medication Practices (ISMP) Canada (2013), 38% of medication misadventures occur in the dose administration.
- A surgical patient who receives the appropriate preoperative antibiotic within 60 minutes of the incision being made has a decreased risk of developing a surgical site infection (Canadian Patient Safety Institute, 2014).
- Software systems that bar-code patients and medications can be used to monitor accurate dosage and time of medication administration.
- Data are tracked on a computer-based system.
- Retrospective chart reviews allow health care providers to review the data, see the time patients received antibiotics, and compare the rate of wound infections for those who did and did not receive timely treatment.

nurse assists the patient in transferring from the hospital bed to the OR stretcher, and the side rails of the stretcher are raised and secured. The nurse should ensure that the completed chart goes with the patient.

If the patient is an outpatient, the patient may be transported to the OR by stretcher or wheelchair, or, in the absence of premedication, the patient may walk, accompanied, to the OR. The method of transportation must be safe and documented by the nurse responsible for the transfer.

The family or caregivers are instructed where to wait for the patient during surgery. Many hospitals have a surgical waiting room where OR personnel communicate the status of the patient to the family. It is in this waiting room that the surgeon can locate the family after surgery and where families can be notified when surgery is complete. Some hospitals provide pagers to waiting family members so that they may eat or run errands during the surgery.

While the patient is in surgery, the patient's room is prepared to accommodate the patient's needs after surgery, the bed is made and raised to stretcher height, and, if necessary, disposable pads are placed for any anticipated drainage. There should be a basin, soap, towels, and clean gown available in the patient's room. Necessary equipment, including those for vital signs, IV administration, oxygen, suction, kidney basin, and additional pillows for positioning, should also be placed in the room and organized to facilitate entry of the stretcher or hospital bed. Having the room ready and equipped makes the patient transfer from the PACU smooth.

CULTURALLY COMPETENT CARE

PATIENT ABOUT TO UNDERGO SURGERY

In Canada, health care providers must be aware and supportive of cultural perceptions and beliefs of patients when preparing them for surgery. Decisions made because of cultural variations must be respected and valued. For example, Makokis and Makokis (2015) detail the experience of one of the authors, a 51-year-old Cree woman faced with undergoing a total hysterectomy in the Western medical system. Makokis felt the need to respect and give thanks to her uterus and ovaries, which had given her the gift of two children. She wanted to bring her body parts home from the hospital, wrapped in sage and broadcloth (both have spiritual significance), provide a ceremony for them, and commit them to Mother Earth. Makokis's preparation involved planning ahead with her gynecologist and a First Nations liaison worker. After the surgery, which was uneventful, Makokis was able to carry out her burial ceremony and felt that she had been treated with respect by the health care team.

AGE-RELATED CONSIDERATIONS

OLDER-ADULT PATIENT ABOUT TO UNDERGO SURGERY

Many surgical procedures are performed on patients older than 65 years of age, and surgery can be safely performed even on those in their 90s. Frequently performed procedures in older adults include cataract extraction, coronary and vascular procedures, prostate surgery, herniorrhaphy, cholecystectomy, total knee and hip replacements, and repair of fractured hips.

The nurse must be particularly alert when assessing and caring for the older-adult patient undergoing surgery. An event that has little effect on a younger patient may be overwhelming to the older patient. As well, the risks associated with anaesthesia and surgery increase in the older patient. As a whole, the older the patient, the greater the risk for complications after surgery (Rothrock, 2015). However, assessment and consideration of the physiological status of older adults, and not simply their chronological age, are essential when planning surgery and assessing risks. A 75-year-old woman may be biologically healthy and more like a 60-year-old in physiological responses. Conversely, a 55-year-old with multiple chronic health problems may biologically resemble a 75-year-old. The risk for surgical complications in the older adult relates to physiological aging (frailty can be predictive of postoperative outcomes) and changes that compromise organ function, reduce reserve capacity, and limit the body's ability to adapt to stress.

When preparing patients for surgery, a detailed history and complete physical examination are obtained. Preoperative laboratory tests and results, an electrocardiogram, and chest radiograph help plan the choice of and technique for anaesthesia. More than one physician may be involved in geriatric care, so the nurse coordinates the care and the physicians' orders for the patient.

Knowledge of family support is important when considering the continuity of care for the older adult, especially for same-day surgical patients who may be discharged to a family caregiver.

The nurse must remember that many older adults have sensory deficits. Vision and hearing may be diminished, and bright lights may bother those with eye problems. Physical reactions are often slowed as a result of mobility and balance problems, so more time should be allowed for the older adult to complete preoperative testing. Since thought processes and cognitive abilities also may be slowed or impaired, these patients may need extra time to understand preoperative instructions. Remember, however, that not every older person has cognitive deficits. Sensory function and cognition must be assessed and documented (Rothrock, 2015). If, for any reason, the patient cannot sign the consent form for himself or herself, a legal representative of the patient must be present to provide consent for surgery.

Some older adults live in long-term care facilities. Transportation from these agencies must be coordinated so that the arrival time allows for surgery preparation. If a long-term care patient is cognitively impaired, a falls-risk assessment should be completed.

Adding to the stress of the surgical procedure, even a minimally invasive one, the perceived situational change and loss may be overwhelming to the older adult. The threat to independence, lifestyle, and self-esteem may result in ineffective coping. The nurse must be particularly supportive and help the older adult cope with the surgical experience.

CASE STUDY

Patient About to Undergo Surgery

Source: Sergei Bachlakov/ Shutterstock .com.

Patient Profile

Mrs. Mary Goodswimmer, an 82-year-old First Nations retired librarian, is admitted to the hospital with compromised circulation of the right lower leg and a necrotic right foot. She was diagnosed with diabetes 40 years ago and takes insulin to maintain appropriate blood glucose levels. She is scheduled for surgery today for a below-knee amputation under spinal anaesthesia. She had a light breakfast at 0600 hours and a glass of apple juice at 1000 hours but has not had anything since. It is now 1300 hours on the day of surgery.

Subjective Data

- History of type 2 diabetes mellitus for 40 years
- History of renal problems
- History of vision problems
- Surgical history that includes a Caesarean section at age 30 and a cholecystectomy at age 65; did not heal well following the last surgery
- Blood glucose has not been well controlled
- Pension cheques barely cover the cost of living and medications
- Lives alone but has family who want her to move in with them following surgery
- Uses herbs to control diabetes and frequently refuses to take insulin

CASE STUDY

Patient About to Undergo Surgery—cont'd

Objective Data

Physical Examination

- Alert, cognitively intact, anxious, older woman with complaints of numbness and lack of feeling in right leg
- Weight, 65 kg; height, 160 cm
- Wears glasses
- Has macular degeneration in her right eye

Diagnostic Studies

- Admission laboratory blood glucose level was 29.8 mmol/L
- Morning finger-stick blood glucose level was 5.3 mmol/L
- Doppler pulses for lower right leg very weak; absent in right foot
- Doppler pulses in left leg present, weak in left foot
- Serum creatinine 221 mmol/L

Collaborative Care

- Scheduled for a below-the-knee amputation of the right leg as the last case of the day

Discussion Questions

1. What factors may influence Mrs. Goodswimmer's response to hospitalization and surgery?
2. **Priority decision:** Given Mrs. Goodswimmer's history, what preoperative nursing assessments should be completed and why?
3. What potential perioperative complications might be expected for Mrs. Goodswimmer?
4. **Priority decision:** What priority topics should be included in Mrs. Goodswimmer's preoperative teaching plan?
5. **Priority decision:** Based on the assessment data presented, identify the priority nursing diagnoses and related interventions. Are there any collaborative problems?
6. **Evidence-informed practice:** Mrs. Goodswimmer asks why she received insulin this morning when she has not eaten anything since midnight. How should the nurse respond to her?

ⓔvolve

Answers are available at *http://evolve.elsevier.com/Canada/Lewis/medsurg*.

REVIEW QUESTIONS

The number of the question corresponds to the same-numbered objective at the beginning of the chapter.

1. Which of the following surgical procedures involves removal of a body organ?
   a. Colostomy
   b. Laparotomy
   c. Mammoplasty
   d. Cholecystectomy

2. Which of the following is one of the most important goals of the preoperative assessment by the nurse?
   a. Determine whether the client's psychological stress is too high to undergo surgery.
   b. Identify what information the client needs to understand before surgery.
   c. Establish baseline data for comparison of the client's status in the intraoperative and postoperative periods.
   d. Determine whether the client's surgery should be done on an inpatient, an outpatient, or a same-day admission basis.

3. A client who is scheduled for a hysterectomy reports using ginkgo biloba to improve her memory. Which of the following questions is the most important for the perioperative nurse to ask the client?
   a. "How long have you used ginkgo biloba?"
   b. "How have you been able to tell if this herb is effective?"
   c. "Have you been taking this herb during the last several weeks?"
   d. "Have you experienced any adverse effects of taking this herbal product?"

4. What is the nurse's role when assisting a client with informed consent before an operative procedure?
   a. Obtains the consent when a surgeon cannot
   b. Asks the client to explain what surgical procedure she or he is having and ensures that the client understands the operation to be performed
   c. Explains all the risks of the surgical procedure
   d. Ensures that the client signs the consent form before preoperative sedation is given

5. What is a *priority* nursing intervention that will assist a client about to undergo surgery to cope with fear of pain?
   a. Describe the degree of pain expected.
   b. Explain the availability of pain medication.
   c. Divert the client when talking about pain.
   d. Inform the client of the frequency of pain medication.

6. What is important for the nurse to ensure the client does right before being transported to the operating room?
   a. The client must void before surgery.
   b. The client must sign the consent form.
   c. The client must take any oral preanaesthetic medications.
   d. The client must remove all jewellery, which is secured by the nurse.

7. What should the nurse administering preoperative medications recognize before administering the medication?
   a. Preoperative medications are used only to decrease client anxiety.
   b. Intravenous medications can be administered only by an anaesthesiologist on the day of surgery.
   c. A preoperative diazepam (Valium) tablet should be administered within 15 minutes of scheduled surgery.
   d. Preoperative opioids given to decrease pain may help reduce intraoperative anaesthetic requirements.

8. Preoperative considerations for older adults include which of the following? (*Select all that apply*)
   a. Using only large-print educational materials
   b. Speaking louder for clients with hearing aids
   c. Recognizing that sensory deficits may be present
   d. Providing warm blankets to prevent hypothermia
   e. Teaching important information early in the morning

1. d; 2. c; 3. c; 4. b; 5. a; 6. a; 7. d; 8. c, d.

ⓔvolve

For even more review questions, visit *http://evolve.elsevier.com/Canada/Lewis/medsurg*.

REFERENCES

Andrews, S., & Cartwright, S. (2016). Preoperative evaluation. In L. Schick & P. Windle (Eds.), *Perianesthesia nursing core curriculum* (3rd ed.). St. Louis: Elsevier.

Campbell, B. (2015). Anesthesia. In J. Rothrock (Ed.), *Alexander's care of the patient in surgery* (15th ed., pp. 124–152). St. Louis: Elsevier Mosby.

Canadian Institute for Health Information. (2015). *Inpatient hospitalizations, surgeries and childbirth indicators in 2013–2014*. Retrieved from *https://secure.cihi.ca/free_products/CAD _Hospitalization%20and%20Childbirth_Infosheet_ENrev-web.pdf*.

Canadian Institute for Health Information. (2016). *Wait times for priority procedures in Canada, 2016*. Retrieved from *https:// secure.cihi.ca/free_products/wait_time_report2016_en.pdf*.

Canadian Medical Protective Association (CMPA). (2016). *Informed consent*. Retrieved from *https://www.cmpa-acpm.ca/serve/docs/ ela/goodpracticesguide/pages/communication/Informed_Consent/ medical_students-e.html*.

Canadian Patient Safety Institute. (2014). *Prevent surgical site infections*. Retrieved from *http://www.patientsafetyinstitute.ca/en/ toolsResources/Pages/SSI-resources-Getting-Started-Kit.aspx*.

Centimole, Z. (2013). The immune system. In J. Odom-Forren (Ed.), *Drain's perianesthesia nursing: A critical care approach* (6th ed., pp. 227–235). St. Louis: Elsevier.

Clifford, T. (2013). Care of the obese patient undergoing bariatric surgery. In J. Odom-Forren (Ed.), *Drain's perianesthesia nursing: A critical care approach* (6th ed., pp. 639–645). St. Louis: Elsevier.

Dobson, G., Chong, M., Chow, L., et al. (2017). Guidelines to the practice of anesthesia. *Canadian Journal of Anesthesia, 64*(1), 65–91. doi:10.1007/s12630-016-0749-0.

Falconer, R., Skouras, C., Carter, T., et al. (2014). Preoperative fasting: Current practice and areas for improvement. *Updates in Surgery, 66*(1), 31–39. doi:10.1007/s13304-013-0242-z.

Griffin, A. (2013). The lived spiritual experiences of patients transitioning through major outpatient surgery. *American Operating Room Journal, 97*(2), 243–252. doi:10.1016/j.aorn .2012.11.019.

Health Canada. (2015). *Health Canada 2015–16 report on plans and priorities*. Retrieved from *https://www.canada.ca/en/ health-canada/corporate/about-health-canada/accountability -performance-financial-reporting/estimates/report-plans-priorities/ 2015-2016/health-canada-2015-2016-report-plans-priorities.html*.

Health Quality Ontario. (2012). *Quality Monitor: 2012 report on Ontario's health system*. Retrieved from *http://www.hqontario.ca/ portals/0/documents/pr/qmonitor-full-report-2012-en.pdf*.

Institute for Safe Medication Practices Canada. (2013). *Medication bar code system implementation planning: A resource guide*. Retrieved from *https://www.ismp-canada.org/barcoding/download/ ResourceGuide/BarCodingResourceGuideFINAL.pdf*.

Jackson, D. (2015). Gastrointestinal surgery. In J. Rothrock (Ed.), *Alexander's care of the patient in surgery* (15th ed., pp. 295–349). St. Louis: Elsevier Mosby.

Larner, R. (2015). Integrative health practices: Complementary and alternative therapies. In J. Rothrock (Ed.), *Alexander's care of the patient in surgery* (15th ed., pp. 1161–1174). St. Louis: Elsevier Mosby.

Makokis, P., & Makokis, J. (2015). Practising "the good way of life" from the hospital bed to mother earth. In M. Greenwood, S. de Leeuw, N. Lindsay, et al. (Eds.), *Determinants of Indigenous people's health in Canada: Beyond the social* (pp. 205–218). Toronto: Canadian Scholars' Press.

Marley, R., Calabrese, T., & Thompson, K. (2014). Preoperative evaluation and preparation of the patient. In J. Nagelhout & K. Plaus (Eds.), *Nurse anesthesia* (5th ed., pp. 336–381). St. Louis: Elsevier Saunders.

Odom-Forren, J. (2013). *Drain's perianesthesia nursing: A critical care approach* (6th ed.). St. Louis: Saunders.

Ontario Regional Blood Coordinating Network. (2013). *Informed consent and refusal of consent. Resource manual for medical directors of transfusion medicine*. Retrieved from *http:// transfusionontario.org/en*.

Operating Room Nurses Association of Canada (2015). *Standards, guidelines, and position statements for perioperative registered nursing practice* (12th ed.). Kingston, ON: Author.

Papanier Wells, M., & Flanagan, A. (2015). Geriatric surgery. In J. Rothrock (Ed.), *Alexander's care of the patient in surgery* (15th ed., pp. 1081–1103). St. Louis: Elsevier Mosby.

Pereira, L., Figueiredo-Braga, M., & Carvalho, I. (2015). Perioperative anxiety in ambulatory surgery: The impact of an empathic patient-centered approach on psychological and clinical outcomes. *Patient Education and Counseling, 99*(5), 733–738. doi:10.1016/j.pec.2015.11.016.

Registered Nurses' Association of Ontario. (2015). *Nurses and other health care professionals helping clients quit smoking*. Toronto: Author. Retrieved from *http://rnao.ca/bpg/courses/ nurses-and-other-health-care-professionals-helping-clients-quit -smoking*.

Rothrock, J. C. (2015). *Alexander's care of the patient in surgery* (15th ed.). St. Louis: Mosby.

Tourigny, J., Clendinneng, D., Chartrand, J., et al. (2011). Evaluation of a virtual tour for children undergoing same-day surgery and their parents. *Pediatric Nursing, 37*(4), 117–183.

RESOURCES

Resources for this chapter are listed in Chapter 22.

For additional Internet resources, see the website for this book at *http://evolve.elsevier.com/Canada/Lewis/medsurg*.

Nursing Management
Intraoperative Care

Written by: Anita Jo Shoup and David M. Horner*
Adapted by: Debra Clendinneng

℮volve WEBSITE

http://evolve.elsevier.com/Canada/Lewis/medsurg

- Review Questions (Online Only)
- Key Points
- Conceptual Care Map Creator
- Audio Glossary
- Content Updates

LEARNING OBJECTIVES

1. Describe the roles and responsibilities of the perioperative nurse in the management of patients undergoing surgery.
2. Differentiate the purposes of the three different areas of the surgical suite and the proper attire for each area.
3. Identify characteristics of the OR environment that contribute to patient safety and infection prevention.
4. Describe the activities and responsibilities of the members of the surgical team.
5. Prioritize the needs of patients undergoing surgery.
6. Describe basic principles of aseptic technique used in the operating room.
7. Discuss the importance of safety in the positioning of patients related to surgical procedure, equipment, and anaesthesia.
8. Differentiate between general and regional or local anaesthesia, including advantages, disadvantages, and rationale for choice of the anaesthetic technique.
9. Identify the basic techniques used to induce and maintain general anaesthesia.
10. Discuss techniques for administering local and regional anaesthesia.

KEY TERMS

anaesthesia care team, p. 405
anaesthesiologist, p. 404
circulating nurse, p. 403
epidural block, p. 413
general anaesthesia, p. 409
holding area, p. 402

laryngeal mask airway (LMA), p. 407
local anaesthesia, p. 409
malignant hyperthermia (MH), p. 415
neuraxial blocks, p. 413
operating room (OR), p. 402
procedural sedation, p. 410

regional anaesthesia, p. 410
scrub nurse, p. 404
spinal anaesthesia, p. 413
surgeon, p. 404
surgical suite, p. 401

Traditionally, surgery has been performed in hospital operating rooms (ORs). However, the advent of advanced surgical technologies, improvements in the administration of anaesthesia, and changes in the Canadian health care system have altered where and how surgery is delivered. Depending on the acuity of the surgical procedure, it can be performed on an outpatient basis in diverse environments like surgi-centres, ambulatory care settings, and clinics. Today, the majority of surgeries are minimally invasive (MIS) and offer the benefits of shorter hospital stays, decreased postoperative pain and incidence of surgical site infection, and, consequently, a faster return to a normal lifestyle (Rothrock, 2015). The impact of MIS for the surgical team is shorter procedures requiring quicker turnovers and less time available for perioperative teaching of patient and caregivers. Conversely, complex procedures and use of advanced technologies such as robotics may require longer setups and surgical time.

Despite the variety of settings and range of surgical complexity, the principles of intraoperative patient care remain the same and are discussed in detail in this chapter.

PHYSICAL ENVIRONMENT

Department Layout

The **surgical suite** is a controlled environment designed to maximize infection control and provide a seamless flow of patients, personnel, and operative instruments, equipment, and

---

*Contributed anaesthesia content.

supplies. The suite is divided into three distinct areas: unrestricted, semirestricted, and restricted. The *unrestricted* area provides access to all people in street clothes, who can interact with those in scrub uniforms. These areas typically include the patient admissions area, a staff locker room, the communication or control centre, and offices. The *semirestricted* area includes the peripheral support areas, such as work and storage areas for clean and sterile supplies. Authorized personnel can access semirestricted areas but must wear surgical attire and cover all head and facial hair. *Restricted* areas include the ORs and all areas where sterile supplies are opened. Personnel wear surgical attire and masks (Operating Room Nurses Association of Canada [ORNAC], 2017). Since the restricted area is designed to reduce cross-contamination, personnel may not bring in personal belongings, food, or beverages (ORNAC, 2017), and clean and sterile items must be separated from contaminated supplies and waste by space, time, and traffic patterns. For example, sterile surgical supplies move from the medical device reprocessing department (MDRD) through the clean core and into the restricted OR. Supplies contaminated after surgery are covered or otherwise contained and transported through the peripheral or semirestricted areas to the MDRD decontamination area (ORNAC, 2017).

Preoperative Holding Area

The preoperative **holding area** is an admission and waiting area inside or adjacent to the surgical suite. This preoperative unit may be a centralized area that accommodates numerous patients or a single-patient area immediately outside the OR designated for the surgical procedure. In the holding area, the perioperative nurse identifies and assesses the patient, gives preoperative medications, and, in some institutions, initiates intravenous (IV) infusions before the patient is transferred into the OR or to an anaesthesia block room. Hospitals that have instituted anaesthesia block rooms have the ability to do neuraxial (spinal and epidural) and peripheral nerve blocks. The presence of these holding rooms reduces anaesthesia prep time in the OR, thus increasing anaesthesia and surgical efficiency (Chazapis, Kaur, & Kamming, 2014). Family or caregivers are often permitted to wait in the holding area with the patient until it is time to be transferred to the OR. This helps relieve patient anxiety.

Operating Room

The **operating room (OR)** is a unique acute care setting specially designed for surgery (Figure 21-1) that, in a hospital, is usually adjacent to the *postanaesthesia care unit* (PACU) and the surgical intensive care unit (ICU). This positioning allows for quick patient transport and proximity to anaesthesia and surgical personnel if complications arise.

ORs are designed using infection-control and safety principles. Airborne transmission of microorganisms and dust is controlled by high-efficiency particulate air (HEPA) filters in the ventilating systems, and controlled positive pressure airflow helps remove anaesthetic gas and toxic fumes. Proper air exchange, temperature, and humidity control provide physical comfort and inhibit bacterial proliferation (ORNAC, 2017). OR furniture and equipment are manufactured from materials that resist the corroding effects of disinfectants, are adjustable, and can be moved. Equipment is checked frequently to ensure proper functioning and electrical safety. Lighting provides a low- to high-intensity range for a precise view of the surgical site (Figure 21-2). Effective integrated voice-over Wi-Fi aids communication

FIGURE 21-1 A hybrid operating room. Hybrid ORs are advanced, flexible operating rooms that combine traditional surgical capabilities with the latest imaging modalities such as radiography, computed tomographic (CT) scan, and magnetic resonance imaging (MRI) to improve operating efficiencies. Source: Courtesy of Healthcare Purchasing News. imageBROKER/Alamy Stock Photo.

FIGURE 21-2 The lighting system in an operating room must provide a range of lighting intensity for a clear view of the surgical site. Source: surassawadee/Shutterstock.com.

workflows in the OR: hands-free communication allows sterile team members to converse without touching anything and provides seamless connectivity between the OR and other support areas. Further, medical devices such as IV infusion pumps, monitors, and radiology machines can connect wirelessly to a network, providing a cord-free environment (Extreme Marketing Team, 2014).

SURGICAL TEAM

Registered Nurse

The **registered nurse (RN)** provides individualized nursing to patients throughout the surgical continuum. In order to address the patient's complex physiological, psychological, sociocultural, and spiritual responses to the surgical event, perioperative nurses require basic and expanded knowledge, skills, and abilities. The Operating Room Nurses Association of Canada (ORNAC) Standards for Perioperative Registered Nursing Practice present the evidence-informed rationale for the structure and resources required in the perioperative environment to promote safe, effective patient care through collaboration with the multidisciplinary team (ORNAC, 2017). Since 1995, perioperative nurses have been able to attain national certification through the Canadian Nurses Association (n.d.) and the designation Certified Perioperative Nurse (Canada). This certification reinforces ORNAC's mission to promote and advance excellence in perioperative patient care (ORNAC, 2017). Expanded roles of the perioperative nurse include registered nurse first assistant (RNFA) and nurse anaesthesiologist.

In the perioperative role, nurses perform either sterile activities (scrub nurse) or unsterile activities (circulating nurse). Canadian ORs have a mixture of registered and practical nurses. The scope of practice for practical nurses allows them to assume the scrub role; however, RNs may perform all aspects of perioperative practice.

Circulating Role. The scope of perioperative registered nursing practice is a continuum of nursing activities that identify and meet the patient's unique needs throughout the perioperative experience (ORNAC, 2017). Competencies include practising professionally, providing physical and supportive care, promoting a safe environment, responding to urgent situations, and managing resources (ORNAC, 2017). The perioperative nurse orchestrates the preparation of the OR with other members of the surgical team. The nurse is usually the first member of the surgical team to greet the patient on arrival to the surgical suite and advocates for the patient throughout the intraoperative experience by:

- Maintaining privacy, confidentiality, and dignity
- Providing physical care and comfort
- Ensuring safety
- Promoting communication—for example, explaining steps prior to induction and ensuring they can hear (e.g., hearing aids left in) (ORNAC, 2017)

Some specific intraoperative activities of the circulating nurse are outlined in Table 21-1.

The perioperative nurse knows that all surgical procedures have a potential for adverse outcomes, so they implement evidence-informed guidelines for surgical care by establishing and maintaining infection-control measures, keeping current on new technologies, and carrying out the Surgical Safety Checklist—an interprofessional time out before the surgical incision to verify patient information (Canadian Patient Safety Institute [CPSI], 2015).

Since the implementation of this checklist in 2009, there have been mixed reports on its efficacy. In a Canadian research study, Urbach, Govindarajan, Saskin, and colleagues (2014) reported no significant reductions in operative mortality or complications after the implementation of surgical checklists in Ontario. Conversely, Haugen, Søfteland, Almeland, and colleagues (2015) promote the use of the checklist, as their research demonstrated a robust reduction in postoperative morbidity and hospital length of stay. Institutions that perform surgery should consider the implementation of safe-surgery checklists and ensure they are applied judiciously (Stock & Sundt, 2015). (See the Resources at the end of this chapter for the Canadian adaptation of the Surgical Safety Checklist.)

Perioperative nurses use critical thinking in assessing patients on an ongoing basis and in responding to changing patient conditions. Examples of nursing activities that characterize each phase of the surgical experience are presented in Table 21-2.

The **circulating nurse** is not scrubbed, gloved, or gowned and remains in the unsterile field. This nurse documents nursing

TABLE 21-1	ACTIVITIES OF THE CIRCULATING NURSE

Circulating Role

The perioperative Registered Nurse shall practice in a manner that:

2.1.1 Assesses the health status of the patient

2.1.2 Develops, modifies, and documents the individualized plan of care, or a clinical pathway to meet the specific needs of the patient

2.1.3 Provides resources for the health care team to function efficiently

2.1.4 Provides physical comfort measures specific to each surgical patient

2.1.5 Provides appropriate care during the admission to the operating room, pre-induction, induction, intraoperative, and emergence phases

2.1.6 Performs the surgical count procedure concurrently with the scrub nurse and documents accurately

2.1.7 Uses a surgical conscience to maintain and monitor the integrity of the sterile field

2.1.8 Reduces risk by providing continuous, astute, and vigilant observation of the surgical team throughout the surgical phase, meeting the health care team and patient's needs

2.1.9 Acts as the patient's advocate throughout the perioperative period

2.1.10 Responds to complications and unexpected events during the perioperative period

2.1.11 Demonstrates leadership capabilities and skills to provide a safe and therapeutic environment for the patient

2.1.12 Organizes and coordinates appropriate resources in a timely manner in preparation for the subsequent patient

2.1.13 Provides and assists with procedures/devices required to complete patient care following the surgical procedure

2.1.14 Assists in the patient transfer and postoperative positioning

2.1.15 Accurately and appropriately documents nursing, surgical, and other health care team activities during the perioperative period

2.1.16 Promotes appropriate communication techniques to keep noise levels at a minimum

2.1.17 Assists with patient transport to a receiving unit and communicates pertinent patient information

2.1.18 Organizes and coordinates appropriate resources to ensure an efficient operating room turnover

2.1.19 Has knowledge and awareness of their organization's policies and procedures and implements appropriately

Source: Operating Room Nurses Association of Canada (ORNAC). (2017). *The ORNAC standards, guidelines, and position statements for perioperative registered nurses* (13th ed.). Kingston, ON: Author.

and medical activities throughout the perioperative period. Intraoperative documentation includes but is not limited to (ORNAC, 2017):

- Naming all personnel involved in patient care in the OR
- Recording event times, additional interventions such as fluoroscopy, and the surgical procedure performed
- Documenting the patient's positioning, surgical skin preparation, and placement of dispersive pad
- Documenting patient monitoring devices and type of anaesthesia
- Recording all equipment used on the patient including settings and serial numbers
- Noting information for prosthetic implants and other devices left in the patient such as catheters and drains
- Logging of specimens and documenting blood loss and the surgical count
- Making note of any untoward events

TABLE 21-2 EXAMPLES OF NURSING ACTIVITIES SURROUNDING THE SURGICAL EXPERIENCE

Before Assessment
Home, Clinic, Preoperative Holding Area
- Performs preoperative assessment
- Provides appropriate education to meet patient's needs
- Involves family and other caregivers in interview and education

Surgical Unit
- Coordinates patient teaching with other nursing staff
- Develops a nursing care plan

Surgical Suite
- Identifies patient
- Verifies surgical site
- Assesses patient's level of consciousness, skin integrity, mobility, emotional status, and functional limitations
- Reviews chart

Planning
- Determines a plan of care that incorporates and respects patient's value system, lifestyle, ethnicity, and culture
- Ensures all supplies and equipment needed for surgery are available, functioning properly, and sterile if appropriate

During Implementation
Maintenance of Safety
- Ensures integrity of sterile field
- Ensures that sponge, needle, and instrument counts are correct
- Positions patient to ensure correct alignment, exposure of surgical site, and prevention of injury
- Prevents chemical injury from preparation solutions, pharmaceuticals
- Ensures safe use of electrical equipment, lasers, and radiation (energy forms)
- Safely labels and administers appropriate medications
- Handles, labels, documents, and establishes chain of custody for specimens

Monitoring of Physical Status
- Monitors and reports changes in patient's vital signs
- Monitors blood loss
- Monitors urine output as applicable

Monitoring of Psychological Status
- Provides emotional support by using a patient-centric approach
- Stands near or touches patient during procedures and induction
- Ensures patient's right to privacy is maintained
- Communicates patient's emotional status to other appropriate members of health care team

After Evaluation
Postanaesthesia, Discharge Area
- Determines patient's immediate response to surgical intervention
- Monitors vital signs
- Safely administers appropriate medications
- Discharges according to protocols

Surgical Unit
- Evaluates effectiveness of nursing care in OR using patient outcome criteria
- Determines patient's level of satisfaction with care given during perioperative period
- Evaluates products used in care of patient in OR
- Determines patient's psychological status
- Assists with discharge planning

Home, Community Clinic
- Seeks patient's understanding of effects of anaesthetic drugs, surgery's impact on body image, effects of immobilization, and efficacy of pain control—including chronic pain postoperatively
- Determines family's perceptions of surgery and ability to cope and function during surgical recuperation

OR, operating room.

Practical Nurse

The scrub role is often performed by a practical nurse who has a perioperative certificate. Practical nurses may assume broader responsibilities depending on patient acuity and hospital policy.

Scrub Role. The scrub nurse is often a practical nurse who performs surgical hand asepsis, is gowned and gloved in sterile attire, and remains in the sterile field assisting the surgical team by preparing and handling instruments. The scrub nurse's duties include setting priorities and ensuring an efficient aseptic setup for the surgical procedure. The nurse monitors aseptic technique throughout the procedure, performs the surgical count concurrently with the circulating nurse, and acts as the patient's advocate during the surgical procedure (ORNAC, 2017). Additionally, the scrub nurse implements patient safety protocols through accurate administration of medication, proper handling and counting of surgical instruments and supplies, management and labelling of specimens, and completion of postoperative documentation.

Surgeon and Assistant

The surgeon performs the surgical procedure and is primarily responsible for the following:
- Preoperative medical history and physical assessment, including need for surgical intervention, choice of surgical procedure, and management of preoperative workup

- Informed consent—explaining surgical risks, complications, and alternative treatment options and obtaining written consent
- Patient safety and surgical management in the OR
- Postoperative patient management

The surgeon's assistant holds retractors to expose surgical areas and assists with hemostasis and suturing. The surgeon's assistant is usually a physician but, in educational settings, may be a surgical resident who can perform some portions of the operation under the surgeon's direct supervision. Some institutions employ RNFAs to assist in surgery under the direct supervision of the surgeon.

Registered Nurse First Assistant

The RNFA is a registered perioperative nurse with formal surgical education, skills, and knowledge who facilitates and supports the health care needs of the patient through the perioperative continuum. The scope of practice allows the RNFA to collaborate with the surgeon in planning preoperative, intraoperative, and postoperative patient care. Intraoperatively, RNFAs handle instruments, provide exposure, manipulate tissue, assist with hemostasis, and suture under direct supervision of the surgeon (ORNAC, 2017).

Anaesthesiologist

According to the Canadian Anesthesiologists' Society (2015), an anaesthesiologist is a physician responsible for a patient's comfort and safety during and after surgery. As vital members of the surgical team, anaesthesiologists are experts in administering potent drugs used to deliver general and regional anaesthesia and in ensuring absence of pain during surgery. Anaesthesiologists medically manage the unconscious or insensible patient during interventions requiring anaesthesia. This duty includes protecting vital functions, managing pulmonary and cardiac complications including cardiopulmonary resuscitation (CPR), and caring for critically ill patients.

In larger ORs and teaching hospitals, respiratory therapists or RNs can take advanced education and training in order to work with the anaesthesia care team as anaesthesia assistants. An anaesthesia care team is an anaesthesiologist-led care model in which anaesthesiologists practise among a team of other professionals such as nurse practitioners in anaesthesia care, anaesthesia assistants, RNs, and respiratory therapists.

Advanced Nursing Practice Roles

Registered Nurse Anaesthesia Assistant. A registered nurse anaesthesia assistant (RNAA) is an RN with advanced education, knowledge, and skills in anaesthesia who works in collaboration with and under the supervision of an anaesthesiologist throughout the perioperative period (ORNAC, 2017).

An additional Canadian category of anaesthesia provider is the nurse practitioner in anaesthesia care (NP-A), which requires master's level preparation. These nurse practitioners with specialist education in anaesthesia care work as part of the anaesthesia care team, providing a range of services in preoperative, intraoperative, postoperative, and ambulatory care settings (Bloomberg Faculty of Nursing, 2015).

As the scope of anaesthesia increases, more practitioners are pursuing subspecialties in anaesthesia such as those in critical care, pain medicine and pediatric care, and cardiothoracic care. Nurses in advanced practice anaesthesia roles will have more opportunity to become involved in these areas (Butterworth, Mackey, & Wasnick, 2013).

NURSING MANAGEMENT
PATIENT BEFORE SURGERY

Preoperative assessment data and health information provided by the patient and family ensure their active involvement in the care plan and establish baseline data for the perioperative team (Rothrock, 2015).

PSYCHOSOCIAL ASSESSMENT

The perioperative nurse must be knowledgeable about the patient's surgery and about its psychological ramifications in order to support the patient. For instance, many patients fear death as a complication of surgery. However, perioperative mortality rates in developed countries are very low, 1 176 per 1 million operations (Bainbridge, Martin, Arango, et al., 2012). Perioperative nurses use this type of current evidence to inform and reassure anxious patients. General questions regarding surgery or anaesthesia can be answered by the perioperative nurse: for example, "When will I go to sleep?" "Who will be in the room?" "How much of my body will be exposed and to whom?" "When will I wake up?" Specific questions relating to the surgical procedure are referred to the surgeon, who is legally responsible for informing the patient about all aspects of the operation (Rothrock, 2015).

PHYSICAL ASSESSMENT

The surgical patient receives a thorough physical preoperative assessment (see Chapter 20). *Vital signs* provide baseline data used to evaluate the effects of intraoperative medications and body positioning. *Height* and *weight* help the perioperative nurse choose the size of equipment and attachments required for the operating bed. An accurate weight helps calculate fluid requirements and medication dosage, which are determined per kilogram. *Thermoregulation* and the use of warming strategies are indicated by the patient's age, metabolic needs, and type and length of the planned surgical procedure. *Allergic reactions* may be avoided with effective preoperative screening. *Skin condition* alerts the team to the presence of open or closed lesions that may predispose infections, and noting *skeletal and muscle impairments* helps prevent injury during positioning. Knowledge of perceptual difficulty, such as a *vision or hearing impairment*, allows the nurse to adapt communication techniques to the individual. An *altered level of consciousness* indicates the need for increasing safety measures and vigilance. Identifying sources of patient *pain* and communicating this to perioperative team members ensures patient comfort throughout this period.

CHART REVIEW

Charting requirements vary with hospital policy, patient condition, and specific surgical procedures; for instance, ambulatory surgery facilities have healthier patients, so fewer preoperative tests may be required. Nursing review of the health record includes validating important findings and verifying that appropriate documentation is present, including (Steelman, 2015):

- Consents for:
  - Surgery and anaesthesia
  - Blood transfusion with notation of predeposit autologous donation or contraindications for transfusion (e.g., Jehovah's Witness)
  - Bone harvesting or allograft (receiving bone from another person)
- Preoperative checklist
- History and physical examination

ADMITTING THE PATIENT

The nurse follows hospital protocol for patient admission to the preoperative holding area and OR. The perioperative nurse greets the patient using a respectful, caring communication style and institutes comfort measures to keep the patient warm and relaxed. The identification process includes asking the patient to state his or her name, the surgeon's name, the operative procedure, and the site of surgery. This active communication process reduces the risk for error. The nurse compares the patient's unique identification number with the patient's identification band and chart (ORNAC, 2017). The admission procedure verifies items on the preoperative checklist such as NPO status, allergies, presence of dentures or prostheses, and so on. The nurse confirms informed consent, secures personal belongings, and confirms whether preoperative medication was administered (ORNAC, 2017). The patient must have time to get responses to last-minute questions. The nurse completes the chart review, documenting any abnormalities or changes. The patient is seen and assessed by the surgeon and anaesthesiologist before anaesthesia induction.

Once the admission process is complete, the patient may be offered complementary or alternative therapies to decrease anxiety and promote relaxation. Therapeutic touch, guided imagery, aromatherapy, music, and movies are modalities used for surgical patients (Jiménez-Jiménez, García-Escalona, Martín-López, et al., 2013).

NURSING MANAGEMENT INTRAOPERATIVE CARE

ROOM PREPARATION

Before the patient enters the OR, nurses start implementing the intraoperative care plan by ensuring all case-specific surgical instrumentation and supplies are available, have been properly sterilized, and are aseptically opened onto the sterile field. The scrub nurse sets up the instrument table, placing instruments and supplies in a predesignated spot so they can be handled systematically and accurately during the surgical procedure. The perioperative nurse determines the type of surgical count: full or partial, depending on the probability of leaving an instrument, sponge, or other item in the incision. Counts are conducted and documented in accordance with ORNAC guidelines and hospital policy (ORNAC, 2017).

Nurses verify the proper functioning and safe operation of electrical and mechanical equipment, ensure patient privacy by limiting personnel in the OR, and are infection-control stewards. The circulating nurse ensures that all people entering the OR are wearing surgical attire. Dress protocols include scrub pants and shirt, mask, protective eyewear, a cap or hood that covers all hair, and absence of jewellery or false nails (Figure 21-3).

Once gowned and gloved, nurses create a sterile environment by disinfecting the incision site and placing sterile sheets (drapes) over the patient to expose only the incision area. Sterile team members can touch only items in the sterile field and must keep their hands at the level of the patient.

The circulating nurse remains outside the sterile field (at least 30 cm [1 foot] away from sterile items) and supports the patient by assisting the anaesthesiologist and surgical team, monitoring aseptic practice, providing ongoing supplies and communication, and documenting care.

TRANSFERRING THE PATIENT. Once the change-over in the OR is done, the patient is identified for the final time and transported into the room for surgery. There, a sufficient number of health care providers must be available to monitor and lift the patient from the stretcher to the OR table, and the wheels of both must be locked to prevent accidents. Once the patient is on the operating table, a safety strap is placed across the patient's thighs; the electrocardiogram monitor leads, oxygen saturation monitor, and blood pressure cuff are applied; and an IV catheter is inserted if it was not started before surgery.

SCRUBBING, GOWNING, AND GLOVING. Although all personnel entering the OR must perform hand hygiene, the surgeon, scrub nurse, and surgical assistant must disinfect their hands and arms using a surgical hand antiseptic or scrub agent. The surgical hand antiseptic or scrub is a broad-spectrum agent that kills microorganisms on contact and supplies persistent protection because it inhibits microbial reproduction. There are different procedures for water-based and waterless hand preparation, and personnel must follow the manufacturer's written instructions and hospital policy (ORNAC, 2017).

After completing the scrub procedure, the team members enter the room and don sterile surgical gowns and gloves, which allow them then to manipulate and organize all sterile items for use during the procedure (Figure 21-4).

BASIC ASEPTIC TECHNIQUE

The surgical team adheres to surgical aseptic principles with the intention of eliminating patient exposure to exogenous pathogenic microorganisms and thus preventing surgical site infection (Rothrock, 2015). Members of the surgical team share responsibility for monitoring aseptic practice and initiating corrective action when the sterile field is compromised (Rothrock, 2015).

In addition to protecting the surgical patient, the safety of perioperative health care providers must also be considered. Bloodborne pathogens spread via airborne, droplet, or contact transmission, so appropriate infection-control precautions addressing specific methods of transmission are implemented to protect the surgical team (ORNAC, 2017). These guidelines emphasize routine and transmission-based precautions (see Table 17-8), engineering and work practice controls, and the use of personal protective equipment such as gloves, gowns, caps, face shields, masks, and protective eyewear (see Table 17-9 and Table 21-3).

FIGURE 21-3 Surgical attire is worn by all persons entering the operating room suite.

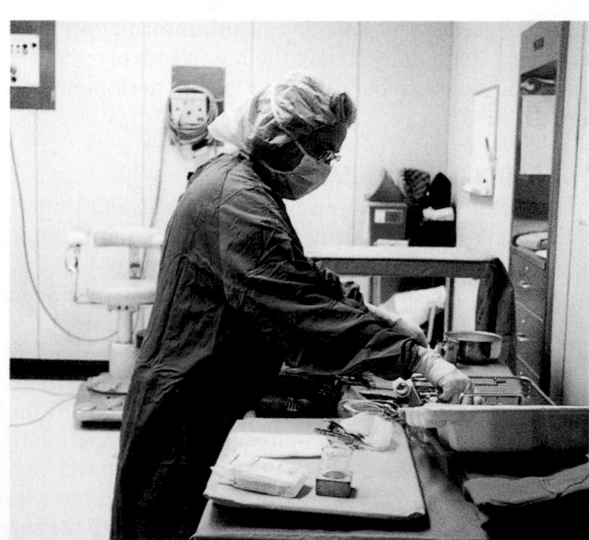

FIGURE 21-4 A sterile field is created before surgery. Source: Courtesy the Methodist Hospital, Houston, TX. Photograph by Donna Dahms, RN, CNOR.

TABLE 21-3 MAINTAINING A STERILE FIELD IN THE OPERATING ROOM

Practice

2.16.1 Opened sterile supplies/setup shall not be left unattended. They shall be continuously monitored for possible contamination.

2.16.2 Unsterile persons shall not reach over the sterile field. Movement is from unsterile to unsterile areas. They should not pass between sterile fields.

2.16.3 Unsterile health care team members shall remain at a safe distance, at least 30 cm (1 ft.), from the sterile field. When approaching the sterile field, unsterile personnel should face the sterile field. Personnel should not pass between sterile fields.

2.16.4 Sterile persons shall not reach over unsterile areas.

2.16.5 Sterile personnel shall stay within the sterile field. Sterile persons shall not walk around or go outside the operating room.

2.16.6 The scrub team should remain close to and face the sterile field. Movement shall be between sterile areas only. If position changes are necessary, scrubbed personnel shall pass face to face or back to back. When changing positions, the scrub personnel should avoid changing levels; personnel either sit or stand. Hands shall be kept above waist level.

2.16.7 Talking should be kept to a minimum.

2.16.8 The sterile setup shall not be covered.

2.16.9 Cover unsterile equipment with sterile barriers before placing them over or in the sterile field. For example, C-arms, laparoscopic cameras, certain positioning devices should be draped for use.

2.16.10 Breaks in aseptic technique shall be recognized, monitored, documented (as per health care facility policy/procedure/protocol) and corrective action taken as soon as safely possible.

Source: Operating Room Nurses Association of Canada (ORNAC). (2017). *The ORNAC standards, guidelines, and position statements for perioperative registered nurses* (13th ed.). Kingston, ON: Author.

ASSISTING THE ANAESTHESIOLOGIST

In many ORs, it is the perioperative circulating nurse who assists the anaesthesiologist. The nurse is familiar with anaesthetic modalities and effects of anaesthetic drugs and can respond to complications and emergency situations with appropriate medication and equipment (ORNAC, 2017).

Before anaesthetic induction, the circulating nurse may help establish the following monitoring:

- Temperature, pulse, and respiration
- Blood pressure
- Electrocardiogram
- Oxygen saturation
- Arterial, central venous pressure, and pulmonary artery lines
- Input and output (urine, blood loss)

During induction of general anaesthesia through an IV, the nurse remains at the patient's side to ensure safety and to assist the anaesthesiologist by ensuring all necessary equipment is available and functional (e.g., suction is on, laryngoscope is fully lighted, monitoring is initiated) (Figure 21-5). After the patient loses consciousness, the anaesthesiologist can insert a **laryngeal mask airway (LMA)**—a supraglottic airway device that is easily placed and used as a method of elective ventilation—or administer a neuro-muscular blocking drug intravenously, causing skeletal muscle relaxation and enabling the anaesthesiologist to perform a direct laryngoscopy and tracheal intubation. Under direct supervision of the anaesthesiologist, the circulating nurse may assist intubation by applying cricoid pressure, supporting head positioning, administering oxygen, and inflating the endotracheal (ET) tube (ORNAC, 2017).

When the patient is receiving regional anaesthesia (spinal, epidural, nerve block, etc.), the circulating nurse assists the anaesthesiologist by placing appropriate monitors on the patient and assisting and supporting patient positioning for the insertion (ORNAC, 2017).

FIGURE 21-5 Commonly used anaesthesia equipment. *A,* Scissors. *B,* Supplemental oxygen mask. *C,* Nasal trumpet airway. *D,* Guedel oral airway. *E,* Supraglottic airway i-gel; laryngeal mask airway (LMA) "Unique." *F,* Cook intubating LMA. *G,* Endotracheal tube. *H,* Long- and short-handled laryngoscopes with curved Macintosh and straight Miller blades. *I,* Nasogastric/orogastric tube. *J,* Peripheral nerve stimulator. *K,* Elastic bougie endotracheal tube (ETT) introducer. *L,* ETT malleable stylet. *M,* Skin temperature probe. Source: Rothrock, J. C. (2015). *Alexander's care of the patient in surgery* (15th ed., p. 141). St. Louis: Elsevier.

POSITIONING THE PATIENT

Proper patient positioning is a critical part of every procedure. The perioperative team must have in-depth knowledge about the surgical procedure in order to determine the patient's position and optimize surgical exposure. The time the patient will spend on the OR bed and any patient limitations such as arthritis or joint replacements require special consideration (Hiezenroth, 2015). Anaesthesia blocks sensory nerve impulses, so the patient will not feel pain, discomfort, or stress being placed on nerves, muscles, bones, or skin. Improper positioning, however, may result in muscle strain, joint damage, pressure injuries, and untoward effects like hypotension and oxygen desaturation.

Proper positioning is a team effort that follows administration of the anaesthetic. The anaesthesiologist indicates when to position the patient and assists the surgeon, nurses, and auxiliary staff to comply with recommended safe positioning practices (Hiezenroth, 2015).

The patient's position ensures proper anatomical alignment and functioning while allowing access to the operative site, access for anaesthesia medication administration, patient monitoring, and patent airway maintenance. Principles for positioning include (1) ensuring correct skeletal alignment; (2) preventing pressure on nerves, skin over bony prominences, and eyes; (3) providing for adequate thoracic excursion; (4) preventing occlusion of arteries and veins; (5) providing modesty in exposure; and (6) recognizing and respecting individual needs such as previously assessed aches, pains, or deformities. The perioperative nurse collaborates with the surgical team to plan, implement, and monitor the patient's position throughout the surgical procedure.

As part of the intraoperative nursing care plan, extremities are secured and appropriate padding and support for at-risk areas (e.g., eyes during prone positioning) are provided. Obtaining sufficient physical or mechanical help in positioning avoids unnecessary strain on either the patient or perioperative team (ORNAC, 2017).

Patient positions include supine, prone, Trendelenburg, lateral decubitus, and lithotomy (Figure 21-6). Supine is the most common position and is suited for abdominal, cardiac, and breast surgeries. A variation of the supine is the Trendelenburg position, used in lower abdominal or pelvic surgery, for which it is necessary to see the pelvic organs. The prone position allows easy access for back surgeries (e.g., laminectomies). The lithotomy position is used for genito-urinary procedures such as vaginal hysterectomy and transurethral resection of the prostate.

FIGURE 21-6 Common intraoperative patient positioning. **A,** Supine position: abdominal surgery. **B,** Trendelenburg position: pelvic surgery. **C,** Lithotomy position: abdominal perineal resection. **D,** Lateral decubitus position: thoracic surgery. **E,** Prone position with a Wilson frame: spinal surgery. Source: Miller, R. D. (Ed.). (2010). *Miller's anesthesia* (7th ed., pp. 1153, 1155, 1157, 1158, & 1160). Philadelphia: Churchill-Livingstone.

FIGURE 21-7 When an electrosurgical unit is used, well-vascularized muscle mass is an optimal site. Safety can be compromised by excessive hair, adipose tissue, bony prominences, fluid (edema), adhesive failure, and scar tissue. Source: Courtesy Covidien, Mansfield, MA.

Once the patient is positioned, the circulating nurse applies an adhesive, flexible gel pad called a *dispersive electrode* on a well-muscled, dry, clean area as close to the operative site as possible, avoiding any bony areas, implanted prostheses, or scar tissue (Figure 21-7). The dispersive pad is connected to the electrosurgical unit (ESU) or electrocautery, which is used by the surgeon to cauterize blood vessels and cut tissue. The dispersive electrode is a safety device that acts as a ground. If for any reason the current from the ESU is interrupted in its return through the dispersive electrode, thermal injury can occur (ORNAC, 2017). An alternative method for grounding the patient is to use a specifically designed gel mattress on the OR bed that connects to the ESU. Patient contact with the mattress provides adequate protection against tissue injury (ORNAC, 2017).

PREPARING THE SURGICAL SITE

The purpose of skin preparation, or "prepping," is to reduce the number of transient and resident skin microorganisms at and surrounding the surgical incision site. Skin prep is usually the responsibility of the circulating nurse.

Before surgical skin preparation, body-piercing jewellery is removed. Hair is not removed unless it interferes with access to the surgical incision site. The rationale is that hair removal can traumatize skin by causing minor abrasions and increase the incidence of surgical site infections (ORNAC, 2017). In light of this evidence-informed information, surgical units must form their own policies and procedures for determining when hair removal is necessary, while considering the following:

- Hair removal is done after assessment of the patient's skin.
- Hair is clipped, not shaved.
- Clipping is performed close to the time of surgery and in an area outside the OR.
- A depilatory agent may be used for hair removal.

- Hair removal should be done with single-use clippers. Clippers with reusable heads must be disinfected between uses (ORNAC, 2017).

Before prepping the skin, the nurse verifies that the surgeon has marked the incision site with an indelible ink marker. Any lesions, irritation, or abrasions on or near the incision site are documented. The incision site is cleansed using a nontoxic agent that has a fast-acting, broad-spectrum, persistent antimicrobial action and that the patient has no allergies to (Spry, 2015). The area is scrubbed in a circular motion from the clean area (site of the incision) to the dirty area (periphery), with the exception of the umbilicus. If the incision is proximal to the umbilicus, the umbilical area is prepped first to prevent contaminants splashing onto a previously prepped area (ORNAC, 2017). Prep solution must not be allowed to pool, as it may cause chemical skin burns, and it must be allowed to dry thoroughly before draping and using electrocautery or laser due to the risk for fire (alcohol and heat source) (ORNAC, 2017). After preparation of the skin, the sterile members of the surgical team drape the area leaving the incision exposed.

SAFETY CONSIDERATIONS

All surgical procedures can put the patient at risk for injury. Injuries include infections and physical injury related to positioning, anaesthesia, or equipment such as lasers and ESUs. The perioperative nurse follows safety protocols to prevent fires and burns. Airborne contaminants and surgical smoke from some equipment produce toxins and carcinogens that irritate the respiratory system and can aerosolize viruses, so smoke evacuators are used during these cases.

SAFETY ALERT

Surgery is the service with the highest percentage of adverse events in Canadian hospitals (CPSI, 2015). Due to the serious repercussions of errors made during surgery, the Canadian Patient Safety Institute recommends using the safe-surgery checklist for all cases. Before administration of anaesthesia, the surgeon, anaesthesiologist, and nursing personnel do a briefing to ensure each item on the checklist has been addressed:

- Patient identity
- Site, side, and level of surgery
- Procedure being performed
- Antibiotic prophylaxis: was initial dose given, and is repeat dose necessary?
- Final surgical positioning of patient
- Any questions or concerns from surgical team members before proceeding

Once the patient is anaesthetized, positioned, prepped, and draped, the team members take a "time out" to reconfirm patient, procedure, site or side, antibiotic dose, and positioning. The operation can then be conducted.

Before the surgeon leaves the OR, the team has a postoperative debriefing that reviews intraoperative patient care and identifies any concerns for patient recovery. These data become part of the hand-off information to the PACU or ICU nursing staff in the transfer of accountability (ORNAC, 2017).

CLASSIFICATION OF ANAESTHESIA

Anaesthesia is classified according to the effect that it has on the patient's central nervous system and pain perception. **General anaesthesia** is an altered physiological state characterized by reversible loss of consciousness, skeletal muscle relaxation, amnesia, and analgesia. **Local anaesthesia** is the loss of sensation without loss of consciousness and can be induced topically or via intracutaneous or subcutaneous infiltration. Regional anaesthesia causes a reversible loss of sensation to a region of the body by blocking nerve fibres with the administration of a local anaesthetic. Examples include spinal, epidural, or peripheral nerve blocks. An advantage of this technique is that the patient remains conscious throughout the procedure.

Procedural (formerly *conscious*) sedation is a mild depression of consciousness that results from administration of IV sedatives, analgesics, or both so patients can tolerate minor procedures yet still maintain airway control and protective airway reflexes (Campbell, 2015).

The anaesthesiologist selects the anaesthetic technique and drugs in collaboration with the patient and surgeon. Considerations for choice of anaesthesia include the patient's physical and mental status, age, and allergy and pain history; the length of the surgery; the operative procedure; and discharge plans.

General Anaesthesia

General anaesthesia is the technique of choice for lengthy surgical procedures that require skeletal muscle relaxation and for surgery that requires the patient to be in uncomfortable positions for the duration. General anaesthesia is appropriate for anxious patients and for those who refuse or have contraindications for local or regional anaesthetics.

General anaesthesia can be produced by many different drugs but is primarily administered intravenously or by inhalation. Balanced anaesthetic technique refers to the use of nitrous oxide, neuro-muscular blocking drugs, and opioids during the maintenance phase of general anaesthesia. Table 21-4 presents common anaesthetic drugs with advantages and disadvantages and the nursing interventions indicated for patients receiving them.

Intravenous Induction Agents. Routine induction of general anaesthesia in adults usually includes intravenous drug administration, such as midazolam or propofol (Diprivan). These drugs induce a pleasant sleep, with a rapid onset of action that patients find desirable. A single dose lasts only a few minutes, which is long enough for an ET to be placed and an inhalation drug to be started.

In today's clinical anaesthesia, one or two inhalation drugs, in conjunction with a variety of IV medications, are given to produce an anaesthetic state. Inhalation drugs come as a liquid, are vaporized in an anaesthetic machine, and are then delivered to the brain and body tissues via the lungs (Nagelhout, 2014). These drugs are noted for ease of administration and the ability to monitor their alveolar concentration and thus the level of anaesthesia. When the inhalation gas is discontinued at the end of surgery, the drug leaves the tissues via the bloodstream and is excreted through the lungs with ventilation, allowing for rapid reversal of anaesthesia. It is routine practice to administer 100% oxygen (O_2) during emergence to assist with recovery (Nagelhout, 2014). Inhalation drugs are most commonly administered through a mask, an LMA, or an ET tube once the patient has been induced with an IV agent. The ET tube permits control of ventilation and airway protection, both to ensure patency and to prevent aspiration. Complications of ET intubation are associated with insertion and removal and include damage to teeth and lips, laryngospasm, laryngeal edema, postoperative sore throat, and hoarseness caused by injury to or irritation of the vocal cords or surrounding tissues.

IV Drugs and General Anaesthesia. The administration of general anaesthesia is rarely limited to one agent. For instance, IV opioids, benzodiazepines, and neuro-muscular blocking drugs (muscle relaxants) result in analgesia, amnesia, and muscle relaxation. Maintenance of general anaesthesia can be achieved with total intravenous anaesthesia (TIVA) (Butterworth, Mackey, & Wasnick, 2013). On occasion, reversal agents may be required to speed up the reversal of muscle relaxants and opioids at the end of surgery. See Table 21-4 for nondepolarizing muscle relaxants.

Antiemetic drugs may be given preoperatively, intraoperatively, and postoperatively to prevent the nausea and vomiting that result from anaesthesia. (See Table 21-5 for IV drugs used in general anaesthesia.)

Opioids. Opioids are used before surgery for sedation and analgesia, intraoperatively for induction and maintenance of anaesthesia, and after surgery for pain management. Opioids alter the perception and response to painful stimuli. When administered before the end of surgery, the residual analgesia often carries over into the PACU, allowing the patient to awaken relatively pain free.

All opioids produce dose-related respiratory depression. Respiratory depression may be difficult to detect in the OR and, therefore, necessitates close observation and pulse oximetry monitoring. Respiratory depression can be reversed with naloxone.

Benzodiazepines. Benzodiazepines are commonly used before surgery for their sedative and amnestic effects, and less commonly used as induction and maintenance agents. They are used for procedural sedation, as supplemental IV sedation during local and regional anaesthesia, and for postoperative anxiety and agitation. Midazolam is an excellent amnestic drug, has a short

TABLE 21-4 DRUG THERAPY

General Anaesthesia

Drug	Advantage	Disadvantage	Nursing Implications
Preoperative Agents			
Lorazepam (Ativan)	Excellent for patients with anxiety	Must be administered cautiously to patients with hepatic or renal disease and to pediatric or geriatric patients	Ensure patients have signed consent before administering any premedication Ensure side rails on stretcher or bed are up
Midazolam	Short acting; excellent for inducing retrograde amnesia	Has a slower induction than thiopental	Used for premedication and as anaesthetic induction and maintenance agent; no pain on injection; often used in conjunction with regional anaesthetic

TABLE 21-4 DRUG THERAPY

General Anaesthesia—cont'd

Drug	Advantage	Disadvantage	Nursing Implications
Induction Agents			
Propofol (Diprivan)	Ideal for short outpatient procedures because of rapid onset of action and elimination; may be used for induction and maintenance of anaesthesia	May cause bradycardia and other dysrhythmias, hypotension, apnea, phlebitis, nausea and vomiting, hiccups	Short action leads to minimal postoperative effects; monitor injection site for phlebitis; ensure cardiac monitoring if patient condition is unstable
Ketamine (Ketalar)	Can be administered by IV or IM route; potent analgesic and amnestic	May cause hallucinations and nightmares, increased intracranial and intraocular pressure, increased heart rate, hypertension	—
Inhalation Gases *Volatile Liquids*			
Isoflurane (Forane) Desflurane (Suprane) Sevoflurane	All volatile liquids: muscle relaxation, low incidence of nausea and vomiting *Isoflurane:* less cardiac depression, devoid of toxicity to body organs *Desflurane:* rapid induction and emergence, most widely used volatile agent *Sevoflurane:* predictable effects on cardiovascular and respiratory systems, smooth, rapid induction, nonirritating to respiratory system	All volatile liquids: myocardial depression, early onset of postoperative pain because of rapid elimination	Assess and treat pain during early anaesthesia recovery; assess for adverse effects such as cardiopulmonary depression with hypotension and prolonged respiratory depression, confusion, and nausea and vomiting
Gaseous Agents			
Nitrous oxide (N_2O)	Potentiates volatile agents, allowing a reduction in both their dosage and their adverse effects, and accelerates induction	Weak anaesthetic, rarely used alone; must be administered with oxygen to prevent hypoxemia	Produces little or no toxicity; monitor for effects of volatile liquids when N_2O used as an adjunct
Induction: Depolarizing Muscle Relaxants			
Succinylcholine (Quelicin)	Used with intubation or short cases; rapid onset	Can trigger MH crisis	Requires refrigeration; may cause fasciculation
Induction: Nondepolarizing Muscle Relaxants *Intermediate Onset and Duration*			
Atracurium	Used with intubation; maintains relaxation	May have slight histamine release	Requires refrigeration
Rocuronium (Zemuron)	Rapid onset; maintains relaxation	Can increase heart rate (vagolytic)	Eliminated via the kidneys and the liver
Longer Onset and Duration			
Pancuronium	Onset 1–3 min; maintains relaxation	May increase heart rate and blood pressure	Eliminated via the kidneys
Reversal: Cholinergic Agent			
Neostigmine bromide (Prostigmin)	Reverses nondepolarizing neuromuscular blocker in 3–15 min	Cardiac arrhythmias	Given with atropine sulphate or glycopyrrolate; prevents breakdown of acetylcholine
Anticholinergics			
Atropine sulphate (Atropine)	Blocks effect of acetylcholine; can decrease vagal tone; increases heart rate, suppresses salivary, gastric, and bronchial secretions	May cause dry mouth, CNS symptoms (dizziness)	Used to treat bradycardia
Glycopyrrolate	Blocks effect of acetylcholine; can decrease vagal tone; increases heart rate; suppresses salivary, gastric, and bronchial secretions	Can have prolonged duration of effects	Does not cross blood–brain barrier; has lower incidence of dysrhythmias than atropine sulphate

CNS, central nervous system; *IM,* intramuscular; *IV,* intravenous; *MH,* malignant hyperthermia.

TABLE 21-5 DRUG THERAPY

IV Drugs Used in General Anaesthesia

Drugs	Uses During Anaesthesia	Adverse Effects	Nursing Interventions
Opioids Fentanyl Morphine sulphate Sufentanil Alfentanil	Induce and maintain anaesthesia, reduce stimuli from sensory nerve endings, provide analgesia during surgery	Respiratory depression, stimulation of vomiting centre, possible bradycardia and peripheral vasodilation (when combined with anaesthetics), high incidence of pruritus with both regional and IV administration	Assess respiratory status, monitor pulse oximetry findings, protect airway in anticipation of vomiting, use standing orders for antipruritics such as diphenhydramine (Benadryl) and low-dose naloxone
Benzodiazepines Midazolam Diazepam (Valium) Lorazepam (Ativan)	Induce and maintain anaesthesia	Potentiation of the effects of opioids, increasing the potential for respiratory depression; hypotension and tachycardia	Monitor cardiopulmonary status, level of consciousness
Antiemetics Ondansetron (Zofran) Metoclopramide Dimenhydrinate (Gravol) Promethazine (Histantil) Droperidol	Prevention of vomiting with aspiration during surgery, counteract the emetic effects of inhalation agents and opioids; droperidol often used during surgery; others more often used after surgery	*Droperidol:* dysrhythmias, laryngospasm, bronchospasm, tachycardia, hypotension, CNS alterations, extrapyramidal reactions; contraindicated for use in patients with Parkinson's disease or hypomagnesemia *Other antiemetics:* headache, dizziness, sedation, malaise, fatigue, musculo-skeletal pain, shivers, diarrhea, acute dystonic reactions, cardiovascular alterations; contraindicated for use with patients with hypomagnesemia	Monitor cardiopulmonary status, level of consciousness, and ability to move limbs *Droperidol:* administer with caution in patients with heart disease

CNS, central nervous system; *IV*, intravenous.

duration of action, and causes no pain on injection, so it is frequently used intramuscularly (IM) or intravenously for ambulatory surgery and procedural sedation. Flumazenil is a benzodiazepine antagonist that may be used to reverse marked benzodiazepine-induced respiratory depression.

Neuro-Muscular Blocking Drugs. Neuro-muscular blocking drugs (muscle relaxants) are used during general anaesthesia to facilitate airway control and to optimize surgical working conditions by providing relaxation (paralysis) of skeletal muscles. These drugs interrupt the transmission of nerve impulses at the neuro-muscular junction. Based on their mechanisms of action, neuro-muscular blocking drugs are classified as either depolarizing or nondepolarizing muscle relaxants. The effects of nondepolarizing muscle relaxants are frequently reversed toward the end of the surgery by the administration of anticholinesterase drugs (e.g., neostigmine [Prostigmin], pyridostigmine [Mestinon]).

A disadvantage of muscle relaxants of special concern to the anaesthesiologist and postanaesthesia nurse is that their duration of action may outlast the surgical procedure, and reversal agents may not be effective in completely eliminating the residual effects. Patients receiving these drugs must be carefully observed for airway patency and adequacy of respiratory muscle movement. Lack of movement or poor return of reflexes and strength may indicate the need for an artificial airway and ventilator. If the patient is intubated, the ET should not be removed without careful assessment of return of muscular strength, level of consciousness, and the minute volume (respiratory rate times tidal volume [amount of air inhaled and exhaled during a normal ventilation]).

Antiemetics. Antiemetics, as previously described, are used before, during, and after surgery to prevent and treat nausea and vomiting associated with the administration of anaesthesia. The antiemetics listed in Table 21-5 are most frequently used before and after surgery.

Local Anaesthesia

Local anaesthetics block the initiation and transmission of electrical impulses along nerve fibres. With progressive increases in local anaesthetic concentration, the transmission of autonomic, then somatic sensory, and finally somatic motor impulses is blocked. This produces autonomic nervous system blockade, anaesthesia, and skeletal muscle paralysis in the area of the affected nerve.

Local anaesthesia allows an operative procedure to be performed on a particular part of the body without loss of consciousness or sedation. Because there is little systemic absorption of the drug, recovery is rapid, and the duration of action of the local anaesthetic frequently carries over into the postoperative period, providing continued analgesia. In addition, the use of a local anaesthetic in a regional technique provides an alternative to a general anaesthetic in a physiologically compromised patient.

The disadvantages of local anaesthetics include the technical challenges of performing the block, discomfort that may be associated with injections, inadvertent IV administration producing hypotension and potential seizures, and the inability to precisely match the duration of action of the drugs administered to the duration of the surgical procedure.

Methods of Administration. There are a variety of methods for administering local anaesthetics (Table 21-6). *Topical application* is application of the agent directly to the skin, mucous membranes, or open surface. A mixture of local anaesthetics (lidocaine and prilocaine) in a skin cream form can be applied to the skin to produce localized dermal anaesthesia (see Chapter 10). Anaesthetic cream should be applied to the site 30 to 60 minutes before painful procedures. *Local infiltration* is the injection of the agent into the tissues through which the surgical incision will pass.

TABLE 21-6	METHODS FOR ADMINISTERING LOCAL ANAESTHESIA

- Topical application
- Local infiltration
- Regional injection
- Peripheral nerve block
- Intravenous regional block (Bier block)
- Spinal anaesthesia (block)
- Epidural anaesthesia (block)

Regional (peripheral) nerve block is achieved by the injection of a local anaesthetic into or around a specific nerve or group of nerves. Nerve blocks may be used to provide intraoperative anaesthesia and postoperative analgesia and for the diagnosis and treatment of chronic pain. Examples of common regional nerve blocks include brachial plexus, intercostal, and retrobulbar blocks. IV regional nerve block (e.g., Bier block) is the IV injection of a local anaesthetic into an extremity following mechanical exsanguination using a compression bandage and a tourniquet. This type of block provides not only analgesia but also the ability to work in a bloodless field.

Spinal and Epidural Anaesthesia (Neuraxial Blocks). Spinal and epidural anaesthesia are types of regional anaesthesia referred to as **neuraxial blocks.** Neuraxial anaesthesia blocks pain transmission during surgery and may be used in combination with other techniques (e.g., inhalation or IV anaesthesia) to balance anaesthetic options, thus maximizing benefits and reducing adverse effects of any particular anaesthetic modality (Olson, Pellegrini, & Movinsky, 2014).

Spinal anaesthesia involves the injection of a local anaesthetic into the cerebro-spinal fluid found in the subarachnoid space, usually below the level of L2. The local anaesthetic mixes with cerebro-spinal fluid, and depending on the extent of its spread, various levels of anaesthesia are achieved. Because the local anaesthetic is administered directly into the cerebro-spinal fluid, a spinal anaesthetic produces an autonomic, sensory, and motor blockade. Patients experience vasodilation and may become hypotensive as a result of the autonomic block, will feel no pain as a result of the sensory block, and will be unable to move as a result of the motor block. The duration of action of the spinal anaesthetic depends on the agent selected and the dose administered. A spinal anaesthetic may be used for intra-abdominal surgery; procedures involving the lower extremities, pelvis, or groin (hernia); and back and spinal surgery.

An **epidural block** involves injection of a local anaesthetic into the epidural (extradural) space via either a thoracic or a lumbar approach. The anaesthetic agent does not enter the cerebro-spinal fluid but works by binding to nerve roots as they enter and exit the spinal cord. This allows the anaesthesiologist to titrate the dosage of medication and better control the extent of sensory or motor block (Olson, Pellegrini, & Movinsky, 2014). A low concentration of local anaesthetic ensures sensory pathways are blocked but allows motor fibres to remain intact. In higher doses, both sensory and motor fibres are blocked (Figure 21-8). Epidural anaesthesia may be the sole anaesthetic for a surgical procedure, or a catheter may be placed to allow for intraoperative use and postoperative analgesia, using lower doses of epidural local anaesthetic, usually combined with an opioid. Epidural anaesthesia is commonly used during labour, as it has minimal impact on maternal and fetal physiology yet offers a comfortable

Sagittal section

FIGURE 21-8 Location of needle point and injected anaesthetic relative to dura. *A,* Epidural catheter. *B,* Single-injection epidural. *C,* Spinal anaesthesia. (Interspaces most commonly used are L4–L5, L3–L4, and L2–L3.)

delivery while allowing for immediate maternal–infant bonding. Furthermore, it provides flexibility for surgical options if the patient must convert to Caesarean section (Olson, Pellegrini, & Movinsky, 2014). Epidurals are also used for lower extremity vascular procedures and hip and knee replacements. (Table 21-7 lists some differences between epidural and spinal anaesthetics.)

During the surgical procedure that uses either spinal or epidural anaesthesia, the patient can remain fully conscious, or sedation can be achieved intravenously. The onset of spinal anaesthesia is faster than that of an epidural, but the results are similar. The patient must be closely observed for signs of autonomic nervous system blockade, including hypotension, bradycardia, nausea, and vomiting. As well, inadvertent high blocks or excessive drug dosages can lead to cardiac and respiratory depression (ORNAC, 2017).

One advantage of epidural (extradural) over spinal (subarachnoid) anaesthesia is a decreased incidence of post–spinal anaesthesia headache due to leakage of spinal fluid at the site of injection. The incidence of headache decreases with the use of smaller-gauge (25- to 27-gauge) and noncutting spinal needles.

Because there are varying perceptions of relative and absolute contraindications for administering neuraxial anaesthesia, it is preferable to formulate an anaesthetic plan specific to the patient's unique health status. The following situations and conditions must be considered when determining whether or not to use spinal or epidural anaesthesia or both (Olson, Pellegrini, & Movinsky, 2014):

- Patient refusal or inability to cooperate
- Increased intracranial pressure
- Coagulopathies
- Skin infection at injection site
- Musculo-skeletal deformities
- Hypovolemia and shock
- Diabetic neuropathies
- Cardiac fixed-volume states
- Extreme inebriation or opioid sedation

Procedural (Conscious) Sedation

Procedural sedation is achieved through administration of sedatives, with or without analgesics. It reduces the patient's

TABLE 21-7 DIFFERENCES BETWEEN EPIDURAL AND SPINAL ANAESTHETICS

Drugs	Injection Space	Potential Complications	Postoperative Monitoring
Spinal Anaesthetic (Local)			
Bupivacaine (Marcaine) Lidocaine Tetracaine (Ametop)	Most commonly used interspaces: L4–L5, L3–L4, and L2–L3	Hypotension, total spinal anaesthesia, post–dural puncture headache	Vital signs Motor and sensory block Urinary output and bladder distension Headache assessment
Spinal Anaesthetic (Analgesia)			
Fentanyl Morphine sulphate (preservative-free)	Most commonly used interspaces: L4–L5, L3–L4, and L2–L3	Hypotension; pruritus; urinary retention; nausea, vomiting; infection; epidural hematoma; oversedation *Contraindications:* Septicemia, ↑ ICP, hypovolemia, neurological disease, anticoagulation therapy, spinal fracture	Vital signs Motor and sensory block Urinary output and bladder distension Headache assessment
Epidural Anaesthetic (Local)			
Ropivacaine (Naropin) Lidocaine Bupivacaine	Between the ligamentum flavum and the dura	Bupivacaine can be associated with cardiac toxicity if injected intravascularly	Respiratory assessment Vital signs Sedation score
Epidural Anaesthetic (Analgesia)			
Morphine sulphate (preservative-free) Fentanyl Sufentanil	The dura	Hypotension; pruritus; urinary retention; nausea, vomiting; infection; epidural hematoma; oversedation *Contraindications:* Septicemia, ↑ ICP, hypovolemia, neurological disease, anticoagulation therapy, spinal fracture	Urinary output and bladder distension Assessment for pruritus, nausea, or vomiting Pain assessment Assessment for catheter migration (numbness or tingling) Assessment of dressing and insertion site Headache assessment

ICP, intracranial pressure.

anxiety and discomfort when undergoing a noninvasive or minimally invasive procedure (Orlewicz, Coleman, Dudley, et al., 2016). Examples of interventions done under procedural sedation include (a) interventional radiology, (b) endoscopy, (c) wound debridement, (d) central line and chest tube placement, (e) dental surgery, and (f) more extensive surgery such as breast biopsy and some cosmetic and reconstructive procedures. Traditionally, this monitored anaesthetic care (MAC) has been provided by and supervised by anaesthesiologists. Practice is changing, however, with many of these surgical and diagnostic procedures being done outside the OR. Patients may be monitored by other health care team members, such as nurses or anaesthesia assistants, with an anaesthesiologist close by in case of a need to convert to a general anaesthetic or in case of complications.

The Canadian Anesthesiologists' Society (2015) advises using the modified Ramsay sedation scale to determine the patient's level of consciousness. There are six levels in total, with the extremes of (1) the patient is awake, anxious, and agitated and (6) the patient is asleep and does not respond to pain.

Nurses receive education and training in procedural sedation, which is an advanced skill (ORNAC, 2017), before taking on the monitoring role. They should not perform circulating duties at the same time because complications can occur quickly.

Patient After Surgery

The anaesthesiologist anticipates the end of the surgical procedure and titrates doses of anaesthetic drugs so there will be minimal effects at the end of the surgical procedure, allowing the patient greater physiological control during the transfer to the PACU or designated recovery area.

The anaesthesiologist and the perioperative nurse or another member of the surgical team accompany the patient to the PACU. A report of the patient's status and of the procedure is communicated to staff there. The OR nurse evaluates the patient's response to nursing care based on outcome criteria established when the plan of care was developed and transfers nursing care accountability to the health care providers in the PACU using a written and verbal report. The verbal report of nursing care provides continuity of care from one health care provider to another, decreases the risk for error, and provides an opportunity for family-centred care. For instance, the perioperative nurse may have information on where the family is waiting for news of the surgical outcome. Although, traditionally, the surgeon, keeping confidentiality issues in mind, is responsible for providing postoperative information to family or significant others, some hospital policies allow a family member or significant other to visit in the PACU once the patient is stable. Hand-off communication should include the patient's situation, background, assessment, and recommendations (SBAR). Examples of information included are (Murray, 2015):

- Name and age of patient
- Preoperative diagnosis and comorbid medical problems
- Allergies
- Time of next antibiotic dose, surgical medication administration (e.g., local anaesthesia)
- Operative procedure performed
- Intake/output, vital signs
- Drains, dressing/packing
- Foley catheter, nasogastric tube, and intraoperative drainage
- Intraoperative positioning and postoperative skin assessment
- Physical issues such as loose teeth, deafness, blindness, arthritis
- Psychological disorders and language barriers
- Existence of advance directives
- Intraoperative complications if any

AGE-RELATED CONSIDERATIONS

PATIENT DURING SURGERY

Anaesthetic drugs are safe and predictable but must be administered to older adults judiciously. Currently, the majority of patients over 65 have one or more chronic problems that may be a risk factor during surgery. In conjunction with physiological deficits due to aging, these may cause varying and unique responses to anaesthetics, blood and fluid management, hypothermia, pain, and the tolerance for the surgical procedure and positioning (Papanier Wells & Flanagan, 2015).

OR nurses must understand the geriatric assessment data required to formulate an intraoperative plan of care—for example, risk for impaired skin integrity (Papanier Wells & Flanagan, 2015):

Risk is related to the patient's current skin condition, such as less elasticity due to decreased collagen, decreased turgor due to dehydration, and decreased peripheral circulation and sensation.

Outcome is that skin integrity remains intact throughout surgery.

Interventions to accomplish this outcome may include assessing the likelihood for pressure injuries, avoiding friction and shearing when moving the patient, ensuring the patient's pressure points are adequately padded when positioned, minimizing tape used to secure devices, and preventing moisture on the linens.

Evaluation takes place immediately postoperatively, when the nurse assesses and documents the patient's skin condition.

EXCEPTIONAL CLINICAL EVENTS IN THE OPERATING ROOM

Unanticipated intraoperative events demand immediate interventions by all perioperative team members. Such events include anaphylactic reactions, malignant hyperthermia, hemorrhage due to trauma or disseminated intravascular coagulation (DIC), cardiac arrest, and intraoperative death (ORNAC, 2017).

Anaphylactic Reactions

Anaphylaxis is a severe form of allergic reaction, manifesting with life-threatening pulmonary and circulatory complications. Initial clinical manifestations of anaphylaxis may be masked by anaesthesia. Anaesthesiologists administer an array of drugs to patients, such as anaesthetics, antibiotics, blood products, and plasma expanders, and because they are parenterally administered, they can stimulate an allergic response, so vigilance and rapid intervention are essential. An anaphylactic reaction causes hypotension, tachycardia, bronchospasm, and, possibly, pulmonary edema. Anaesthetics, antibiotics, and latex are responsible for many perioperative allergic reactions. (Anaphylaxis is discussed in Chapter 16.)

Latex allergy remains a concern in the perioperative setting, despite fewer surgical products being manufactured from natural rubber latex. Reactions to natural rubber latex range from urticaria to anaphylaxis, with symptoms appearing immediately or at some time during the surgical procedure.

Policies and procedures must ensure that the health care team can provide a latex-safe environment for patients and staff with potential or actual latex allergy (ORNAC, 2017). (Latex allergies are discussed in Chapter 16.)

Malignant Hyperthermia

Malignant hyperthermia (MH) is a rare, potentially fatal metabolic disease characterized by hyperthermia with rigidity of skeletal muscles that can affect genetically susceptible patients. It is triggered by commonly administered anaesthetic drugs, particularly succinylcholine (Anectine), which is given during general anaesthesia. MH susceptibility has an inherited autosomal dominant pattern, and thus children of a susceptible parent have a 50% chance of having the genetic defect (Malignant Hyperthermia Association of the United States [MHAUS], 2015). (Autosomal dominant disorders are discussed in Chapter 15.) The MH defect is hypermetabolism of skeletal muscle resulting from altered control of intracellular calcium, leading to muscle contracture, hyperthermia, hypoxemia, lactic acidosis, and hemodynamic and cardiac alterations that can result in cardiac arrest and death. The first sign of MH is often severe masseter muscle rigidity (MMR) that occurs after the administration of succinylcholine and is noted by the anaesthesiologist when trying to establish an airway. MMR should be considered an indication of MH, and treatment should be initiated right away. Other physiological changes, such as a rise in end-tidal carbon dioxide (CO_2) and body temperature, are delayed signs of MH (MHAUS, 2015).

The definitive treatment of MH is prompt administration of dantrolene (Dantrium), which slows metabolism and provides symptomatic support to correct hemodynamic instability, acidosis, hypoxemia, and elevated temperature. A treatment protocol in the form of an interactive MH-emergency smartphone application or a hardcopy poster is available from the Malignant Hyperthermia Association of the United States (MHAUS; see the Resources section at the end of this chapter).

To prevent an MH episode, the nurse must obtain a careful family history and be alert to MH susceptibility preoperatively. The patient known or suspected to be at risk for MH can be anaesthetized with minimal risk if appropriate precautions are taken. Patients with MH susceptibility should inform family members so they are aware of the health care risks and can wear a health alert bracelet or choose to be genetically tested by having a muscle biopsy (ORNAC, 2017).

Major Blood Loss

Surgery can pose a risk for blood loss. If major blood loss occurs during surgery, the circulating nurse assists the anaesthesiologist with fluid replacement. Initially, crystalloids and colloid solutions are given to maintain fluid volume, but when hemorrhage is significant, blood or blood components may be administered (Lynn & Winner, 2014). Estimating intraoperative blood loss is difficult and requires the circulating nurse to monitor and record all blood accumulation in the suction container (fluid total minus irrigation solution) and to weigh surgical sponges to account for blood from the operative site. Anaesthesiologists may perform serial hemoglobin, hematocrit, and blood gas monitoring using point-of-use monitors in the OR; however, these do not measure blood loss, so, ultimately, it is the anaesthesiologist's calculations and knowledge of the patient's condition that determine the need for blood transfusion therapy (Lynn & Winner, 2014).

NEW AND FUTURE CONSIDERATIONS

Dramatic and rapid changes in perioperative health care are occurring through disruptive technology—ideas and devices that revolutionize how surgery is conceptualized and performed.

Holomers are holographic medical electronic representations of people based on CT scans with physiological processes and vital signs. The computer-generated virtual reality image of organs allows for surgical training and practice on the "virtual patient" before surgery. Add the use of robotics, combined with computer-assisted surgery, and surgeons can achieve surgical precision and enhanced patient outcomes (Rothrock, 2015).

Research is being conducted on high-intensity focused ultrasound (HIFU), which generates heat that can either coagulate tissue and blood or vaporize tissue. By combining HIFU with diagnostic ultrasonography, it will be possible to diagnose a source of internal bleeding, focus the HIFU, and stop the bleeding externally without surgical intervention.

Miniaturization in conjunction with tissue engineering of synthetic organs (Souriau, Herrera Morales, Castagné, et al.,

2015) and intelligent prostheses will soon allow replacement of most body parts.

There is also ongoing research data leading to better treatment for patients undergoing surgery—for example, revised fasting guidelines for healthy patients undergoing elective surgery (Rothrock, 2015). (Chapter 20 discusses preoperative fasting guidelines used by the Canadian Anesthesiologists' Society.)

Another example of the surgery of the future is "bloodless surgery," which uses advanced techniques to minimize patient blood loss (Ashley, 2015).

Exciting innovations like these hold much promise for the future of surgery and of health care in general.

REVIEW QUESTIONS

The number of the question corresponds to the same-numbered objective at the beginning of the chapter.

1. What is the perioperative nurse's primary responsibility for the care of the client undergoing surgery?
   a. Developing an individualized plan of nursing care for the client
   b. Carrying out specific tasks related to surgical policies and procedures
   c. Ensuring that the client has been assessed for safe administration of anaesthesia
   d. Performing a preoperative history and physical assessment to identify client needs
2. What is the proper attire for the semirestricted area of the surgery department?
   a. Street clothing
   b. Surgical attire and head cover
   c. Surgical attire, head cover, and mask
   d. Street clothing with the addition of shoe covers
3. What is one characteristic of the OR environment that facilitates the prevention of infection in the surgical client?
   a. Adjustable lighting
   b. Conductive furniture
   c. Filters in the ventilating system
   d. Explosion-proof electrical plugs
4. Which of the following activities might a nurse perform in the role of a scrub nurse during surgery? (Select all that apply)
   a. Checking electrical equipment
   b. Preparing the instrument table
   c. Passing instruments to the surgeon and assistants
   d. Coordinating activities occurring in the operating room
   e. Maintaining accurate counts of sponges, needles, and instruments
5. What is the most important intervention to perform when a client arrives to the OR with musculo-skeletal impairments?
   a. Ensure proper preparation of the skin.
   b. Ensure the anaesthesiologist uses muscle relaxants.
   c. Ensure positioning on the OR bed to prevent injury.
   d. Provide detailed explanations about the surgical activities.
6. The practical nurse in the OR knows that which of the following is not acceptable for ensuring a sterile field?
   a. Unsterile personnel remaining at least 30 cm from the sterile field

   b. Reaching over the sterile field to place sterile items on the sterile back table
   c. Covering unsterile items such as laparoscopic cameras with sterile barriers before placing them on the sterile field
   d. Flipping a sterile item from a paper peel pack onto the sterile field
7. Which of the following is not a consideration when positioning the surgical client?
   a. Providing modesty for the client
   b. Avoiding compression of nerve tissue
   c. Providing correct skeletal alignment
   d. Ensuring that students in the room can see the operative site
8. A client is scheduled for an abdominal hysterectomy. She is extremely anxious and has a tendency to hyperventilate when upset. What is the most appropriate type of anaesthetic for this client?
   a. A spinal block
   b. An epidural block
   c. A general anaesthetic
   d. A local anaesthetic
9. Why is IV induction for general anaesthesia the method of choice for most clients?
   a. The client is not intubated.
   b. The drugs are nonexplosive.
   c. Induction is rapid and pleasant.
   d. The odour of the drug is not offensive.
10. What is the name for the injection of the local anaesthetic into the tissues through the surgical incision?
    a. Nerve block
    b. Local infiltration
    c. Topical application
    d. Regional application

1. a; 2. b; 3. c; 4. b, c, e; 5. c; 6. d; 7. d; 8. c; 9. c; 10. b.

⊖volve

For even more review questions, visit *http://evolve.elsevier.com/Canada/Lewis/medsurg.*

REFERENCES

Ashley, A. (2015, June 8). *Medicine without blood. The Atlantic.* Retrieved from *http://www.theatlantic.com/health/archive/2015/06/blood-management-bloodless-medicine-transfusions/395054/.*

Bainbridge, D., Martin, J., Arango, M., et al. (2012). Perioperative and anaesthetic-related mortality in developed and developing countries: A systematic review and meta-analysis. *Lancet, 380,* 1075–1081. doi:10.1016/S0140-6736(12)60990-8.

Bloomberg Faculty of Nursing. (2015). *Canada's first nurse practitioner in anesthesia care program celebrates recent graduates*. Retrieved from *https://bloomberg.nursing.utoronto.ca/news/canadas-first-nurse-practitioner-in-anesthesia-care-program-celebrates-recent-graduates*.

Butterworth, J., Mackey, D., & Wasnick, J. (2013). *Morgan and Mikhail's clinical anesthesiology* (5th ed.). New York: McGraw-Hill Education.

Campbell, B. (2015). Anesthesia. In J. C. Rothrock (Ed.), *Alexander's care of the patient in surgery* (15th ed., pp. 124–154). St. Louis: Elsevier.

Canadian Anesthesiologists' Society. (2015). Guidelines to the practice of anesthesia—Revised edition 2015. *Canadian Journal of Anesthesia, 62*(1), 54–79. doi:10.1007/s12630-014-0232-8.

Canadian Nurses Association. (n.d.). *Certification nursing practice specialties*. Retrieved from *https://nurseone.ca/en/certification/get-certified/certification-nursing-practice-specialties*.

Canadian Patient Safety Institute (CPSI). (2015). *Surgical care safety*. Retrieved from *http://www.patientsafetyinstitute.ca/en/Topic/Pages/Surgical-Care-Safety.aspx*.

Chazapis, M., Kaur, N., & Kamming, D. (2014). Improving the peri-operative care of patients by instituting a "block room" for regional anaesthesia. *BMJ Quality Improvement Reports, 3*(1), doi:10.1136/bmjquality.u204061.w1769.

Extreme Marketing Team. (2014). *Top 5 Wi-Fi technologies in operating rooms*. Retrieved from *http://www.extremenetworks.com/top-5-o-r-technologies-that-wi-fi-provides-operating-theaters*.

Haugen, A. S., Søfteland, E., Almeland, S. K., et al. (2015). Effect of the World Health Organization checklist on patient outcomes: A stepped wedge cluster randomized controlled trial. *Annals of Surgery, 261*(5), 821–828. doi:10.1097/SLA.0000000000000716.

Hiezenroth, P. (2015). Positioning the patient for surgery. In J. C. Rothrock (Ed.), *Alexander's care of the patient in surgery* (15th ed., pp. 382–402). St. Louis: Elsevier.

Jiménez-Jiménez, M., García-Escalona, A., Martín-López, A., et al. (2013). Intraoperative stress and anxiety reduction with music therapy: A controlled randomized clinical trial of efficacy and safety. *Journal of Vascular Nursing, 31*(3), 101–106. doi:10.1016/j.jvn.2012.10.002.

Lynn, R., & Winner, L. (2014). Fluids, electrolytes and blood component therapy. In J. Nagelhout & K. Plaus (Eds.), *Nurse anesthesia* (5th ed., pp. 382–402). St. Louis: Saunders/Elsevier.

Malignant Hyperthermia Association of the United States. (2015). *MH susceptibility and operating room personnel: Defining the risks*. Retrieved from *http://www.mhaus.org/healthcare-professionals/mhaus-recommendations/malignant-hyperthermia-susceptible-operating-room-personnel*.

Murray, E. (2015). Patient safety and risk management. In J. C. Rothrock (Ed.), *Alexander's care of the patient in surgery* (15th ed., pp. 16–46). St. Louis: Elsevier.

Nagelhout, J. J. (2014). Pharmacokinetics of inhalation anesthetics. In J. J. Nagelhout & K. L. Plaus (Eds.), *Nurse anesthesia* (5th ed., pp. 78–84). St. Louis: Elsevier/Saunders.

Olson, R., Pellegrini, J., & Movinsky, B. (2014). Regional anesthesia: Spinal and epidural anesthesia. In J. Nagelhout & K. Plaus (Eds.), *Nurse anesthesia* (5th ed., pp. 1070–1101). St. Louis: Saunders/Elsevier.

Operating Room Nurses Association of Canada (ORNAC). (2017). *The ORNAC standards, guidelines, and position statements for perioperative registered nurses* (13th ed.). Kingston, ON: Author.

Orlewicz, M. S., Coleman, A. E., Dudley, R. M., et al. (2016, November 14). *Procedural sedation. Medscape, 20*. Retrieved from *http://emedicine.medscape.com/article/109695-overview#a1*.

Papanier Wells, M., & Flanagan, A. (2015). Geriatric surgery. In J. C. Rothrock (Ed.), *Alexander's care of the patient in surgery* (15th ed., pp. 1081–1103). St. Louis: Elsevier.

Rothrock, J. C. (2015). *Alexander's care of the patient in surgery* (15th ed.). St. Louis: Elsevier.

Souriau, J., Herrera Morales, J., Castagné, L., et al. (2015). *Miniaturization and biocompatible encapsulation for implantable biomedical silicon devices. The Electrochemical Society*. doi: 10.1149/2.0221512jss.

Spry, C. (2015). Infection prevention and control. In J. C. Rothrock (Ed.), *Alexander's care of the patient in surgery* (15th ed., pp. 69–123). St. Louis: Elsevier.

Steelman, V. (2015). Concepts basic to perioperative nursing. In J. C. Rothrock (Ed.), *Alexander's care of the patient in surgery* (15th ed., pp. 1–15). St. Louis: Elsevier.

Stock, C., & Sundt, T. (2015). Timeout for checklists? *Annals of Surgery, 261*(5), 841–842.

Urbach, D. R., Govindarajan, A., Saskin, R., et al. (2014). Introduction of surgical safety checklists in Ontario, Canada. *New England Journal of Medicine, 370*, 1029–1038. doi:10.1056/NEJMsa1308261.

RESOURCES

Association of Nova Scotia PeriAnesthesia Nurses
http://anspan.weebly.com

Canadian Anesthesiologists' Society
http://www.cas.ca

Canadian Patient Safety Institute's Surgical Safety Checklist
http://www.patientsafetyinstitute.ca/en/toolsResources/Pages/SurgicalSafety-Checklist-Resources.aspx

Malignant Hyperthermia Unit, Ottawa Hospital
http://www.ottawahospital.on.ca/wps/portal/Base/TheHospital/ClinicalServices/DeptPgrmCS/Departments/Anesthesiology/MalignantHyperthermiaUnit

National Association of PeriAnesthesia Nurses of Canada
http://www.napanc.org

Ontario PeriAnesthesia Nurses Association
http://www.opana.org

Operating Room Nurses Association of Canada
http://www.ornac.ca

PeriAnesthesia Nurses Professional Practice Group of Saskatchewan
http://www.srna.org

PeriAnesthesia Nursing Association of British Columbia
https://panbc.ca

Quebec PeriAnesthesia Nurses Association
http://www.aipaq.org/en

Malignant Hyperthermia Association of the United States
http://www.mhaus.org

For additional Internet resources, see the website for this book at *http://evolve.elsevier.com/Canada/Lewis/medsurg*.

Nursing Management

Postoperative Care

Written by: Christine R. Hoch
Adapted by: Debra Clendinneng

⊖volve WEBSITE

http://evolve.elsevier.com/Canada/Lewis/medsurg

- Review Questions (Online Only)
- Key Points
- Answer Guidelines for Case Study
- Student Case Study
  - Patient Undergoing Surgery

- Customizable Nursing Care Plan
  - Postoperative Patient
- Conceptual Care Map Creator

- Audio Glossary
- Content Updates

LEARNING OBJECTIVES

1. Identify the components of an initial postanaesthesia assessment.
2. Identify the nursing responsibilities in admitting patients to the postanaesthesia care unit (PACU).
3. Explain the etiology and nursing assessment and management of potential problems of patients in the PACU.

4. Describe the initial nursing assessment and management after transfer from the PACU to the general care unit.
5. Explain the etiology and nursing assessment and management of potential problems during the postoperative period.
6. Differentiate discharge criteria from phase I and phase II postanaesthesia care.

KEY TERMS

airway obstruction, p. 420
atelectasis, p. 420
bronchospasm, p. 421, Table 22-5
delayed awakening, p. 426

emergence delirium, p. 425
epidural analgesia, p. 427
hypothermia, p. 427
hypoventilation, p. 421, Table 22-5

hypoxemia, p. 421, Table 22-5
paralytic ileus, p. 429
syncope, p. 424

The postoperative period begins immediately after surgery and continues until the patient is discharged from medical care. This chapter focuses on the postoperative nursing care required for patients undergoing surgery. After surgery, the primary focus is on protecting the patient, who has been put in physiological risk during surgery, and preventing complications while the body heals. The problems and nursing care related to specific surgical procedures are discussed in the appropriate chapters of this text.

POSTOPERATIVE CARE IN THE POSTANAESTHESIA CARE UNIT

The patient's immediate recovery period occurs in a *postanaesthesia care unit* (PACU). It is located adjacent to the operating room (OR) to minimize the transport distance of the patient after surgery and to provide ready access to surgical and anaesthesia personnel. There are three levels of postanaesthesia

care, depending on the patient's surgical procedure, anaesthesia, and individualized needs (Table 22-1).

POSTANAESTHESIA CARE UNIT ADMISSION

Admission of the patient to the PACU is a transfer of care from the anaesthesiologist and perioperative nurse to the PACU or perianesthesia nurse. These team members determine what phase of care the patient is assigned.

Postanaesthesia Care Unit Progression

The rate at which patients move through the phases of care in the PACU depends on their condition. An inpatient or outpatient who is stable and recovering well is admitted to phase I care but may rapidly be discharged to either phase II care or an inpatient unit. An accelerated system of care, *fast-tracking*, involves admitting ambulatory surgery patients who have received general, regional, or local anaesthesia directly to phase

TABLE 22-1 PHASES OF POSTANAESTHESIA CARE

Phase I
- Care during the immediate postanaesthesia period
- Focused on the patient's basic life-sustaining needs
- Constant, vigilant monitoring
Goal: Prepare patient for safe transfer to phase II or inpatient unit

Phase II
- Surgery patient is ambulatory
Goal: Prepare patient for transfer to extended-care environment or home with discharge teaching

Extended Observation
- Ongoing care for patients who will be admitted to the unit and those who require observation or interventions
Goal: Prepare patient for self-care

Source: American Society of PeriAnesthesia Nurses. (2016). *Perianesthesia nursing core curriculum* (3rd ed.). St. Louis: Elsevier.

TABLE 22-2 POSTANAESTHESIA ADMISSION REPORT

General Information
- Patient name
- Age
- Anaesthesiologist name
- Surgeon name
- Surgical procedure

Patient History
- Indication for surgery
- Medical history, medications, allergies

Intraoperative Management
- Anaesthetic medications received
- Other medications received before surgery or intraoperatively
- Blood loss
- Fluid replacement totals, including blood transfusions
- Urine output

Intraoperative Course
- Unexpected anaesthetic events or reactions
- Unexpected surgical events
- Vital signs and monitoring trends
- Results of intraoperative laboratory tests

TABLE 22-3 INITIAL POSTANAESTHESIA CARE UNIT ASSESSMENT

Airway
- Patency
- Oral or nasal airway
- Endotracheal tube

Breathing
- Respiratory rate and quality
- Auscultated breath sounds
- Pulse oximetry
- Supplemental oxygen

Circulation
- ECG monitoring—rate and rhythm
- Blood pressure
- Temperature and colour of skin
- Peripheral pulses

Neurological
- Level of consciousness
- Orientation
- Sensory and motor status

Gastro-Intestinal–Genito-Urinary
- Intake (fluids, irrigations)
- Output (emesis, urine, drains)

Surgical Site
- Dressings and drainage

Pain
- Incision
- Other

ECG, electrocardiogram.

TABLE 22-4 CLINICAL MANIFESTATIONS OF INADEQUATE OXYGENATION

Central Nervous System
- Restlessness
- Agitation
- Muscle twitching
- Seizures
- Coma

Cardiovascular System
- Hypertension
- Hypotension
- Tachycardia
- Bradycardia
- Dysrhythmias

Integumentary System
- Cyanosis
- Prolonged capillary refill
- Flushed and moist skin

Respiratory System
- Alterations ranging from increased to absent respiratory effort
- Use of accessory muscles
- Abnormal breath sounds
- Abnormal arterial blood gases

Renal System
- Urine output 30 mL/hour

II care. Patients' safety is the primary consideration when determining what level of postoperative care is provided.

Initial Assessment

On patient admission to the PACU, the anaesthesiologist and perioperative nurse give a verbal report to the admitting perianesthesia nurse. Table 22-2 summarizes the components of a complete anaesthesia report. While the patient is in the PACU, priority care includes the monitoring and management of respiratory and circulatory functions, pain, temperature, and surgical site and the assessment of the patient's response to the reversal of anaesthetic, such as sedation score and level of spinal block.

Assessment should begin with an evaluation of the patient's airway, breathing, and circulation (ABCs) (Table 22-3). The first priority is to establish a patent airway. In order to breathe adequately, the patient may need stimulation, repositioning to the right side, or a chin tilt. If these measures do not work, an oral or nasal airway may be used.

Pulse oximetry monitoring is initiated on admission because it provides a noninvasive means of assessing the adequacy of oxygenation and alerts nurses to any respiratory compromise.

Oxygen therapy is used if the patient had general anaesthesia or if ordered by the anaesthesiologist. Oxygen therapy, given via nasal cannula or face mask, aids in eliminating anaesthetic gases and meets the increased oxygen demand due to decreased blood volume or increased cellular metabolism. If the patient requires postoperative ventilation, a ventilator is provided. During the initial assessment, signs of inadequate oxygenation and ventilation should be identified (Table 22-4).

Electrocardiographic (ECG) monitoring may be initiated to determine cardiac rate and rhythm. Deviations from preoperative findings must be noted and evaluated. Blood pressure (BP) should be measured and compared with baseline readings. Invasive monitoring (e.g., arterial BP monitoring) initiated in the OR will be monitored in the PACU. Body temperature, skin colour and condition, and capillary refill should also be assessed. Any evidence of inadequate circulatory status requires prompt intervention.

The *initial neurological assessment* focuses on level of consciousness; orientation; sensory and motor status; and size, equality, and reactivity of the pupils. Hearing is the first sense to return in the unconscious patient, so the nurse should explain all activities to the patient from the moment of PACU admission, including that the surgery is completed, that the patient is in the recovery room, and that the family or significant other has been notified.

A patient who has had a regional anaesthetic (e.g., spinal or epidural) should be assessed for residual sensory and motor blockade by testing for sensation and movement.

Urinary system assessment focuses on intake, output, and fluid balance. Intraoperative fluid totals are communicated during the anaesthesia report. The PACU nurse should note the presence of all intravenous (IV) lines, irrigation solutions and infusions, and output devices such as catheters. IV infusions are regulated according to postoperative orders. If the patient is nauseated or vomiting, the nurse should administer antiemetic medications as ordered. The colour and amount of emesis should be charted.

The surgical site is assessed by noting the condition of dressings, and the colour and amount of drainage from the incision site or wound drains should be documented. All data obtained in the admission assessment are documented on a specific PACU record.

The goal of PACU care is to identify actual and potential patient problems that may occur as a result of anaesthetic administration and surgical intervention, so the perianesthesia nurse is continually assessing, adjusting diagnoses, and intervening appropriately. Common postoperative problems that require nursing interventions are airway compromise (obstruction), respiratory insufficiency (hypoxemia and hypercarbia), cardiac compromise (hypotension, hypertension, and dysrhythmias), neurological compromise (emergence delirium and delayed awakening), hypothermia, pain, and nausea and vomiting (Figure 22-1). Each of these problems and appropriate nursing interventions are discussed in this chapter.

POTENTIAL ALTERATIONS IN RESPIRATORY FUNCTION

Etiology

Postanaesthesia Care Unit. In the immediate postanaesthetic period, the most common causes of airway compromise include obstruction, hypoxemia, and hypoventilation (Table 22-5). Patients at particular risk include those who had general anaesthesia; are older; have a smoking history or lung disease; are obese; or have undergone airway, thoracic, or abdominal surgery. However, respiratory complications may occur in any patient who was anaesthetized.

Airway obstruction is a blockage of the airway, most commonly caused by the patient's tongue (Figure 22-2).

Atelectasis is a complete or partial collapse of a lung or segment of a lung that occurs when the alveoli become deflated (Figure 22-3).

Clinical Unit. Common causes of respiratory problems for postoperative patients in the clinical unit are atelectasis and

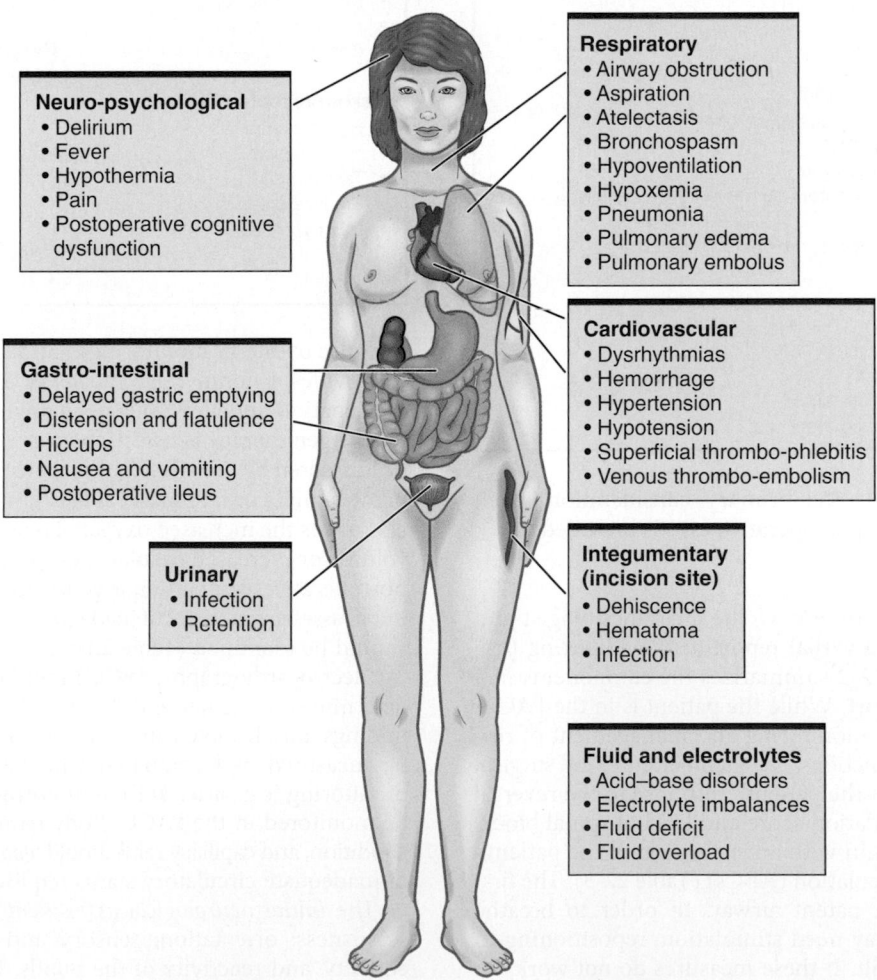

Neuro-psychological
- Delirium
- Fever
- Hypothermia
- Pain
- Postoperative cognitive dysfunction

Gastro-intestinal
- Delayed gastric emptying
- Distension and flatulence
- Hiccups
- Nausea and vomiting
- Postoperative ileus

Urinary
- Infection
- Retention

Respiratory
- Airway obstruction
- Aspiration
- Atelectasis
- Bronchospasm
- Hypoventilation
- Hypoxemia
- Pneumonia
- Pulmonary edema
- Pulmonary embolus

Cardiovascular
- Dysrhythmias
- Hemorrhage
- Hypertension
- Hypotension
- Superficial thrombo-phlebitis
- Venous thrombo-embolism

Integumentary (incision site)
- Dehiscence
- Hematoma
- Infection

Fluid and electrolytes
- Acid–base disorders
- Electrolyte imbalances
- Fluid deficit
- Fluid overload

FIGURE 22-1 Potential problems in the postoperative period.

TABLE 22-5 COMMON IMMEDIATE POSTOPERATIVE RESPIRATORY COMPLICATIONS

Complications and Causes	Mechanisms	Manifestations	Interventions
Airway Obstruction			
Tongue falling back	Muscular flaccidity associated with decreased consciousness and muscle relaxants Most pronounced in supine position Occurrence immediately after surgery but also postoperatively if patient is heavily sedated	Use of accessory muscles Snoring respirations Decreased air movement	Patient stimulation Jaw thrust Chin lift Artificial airway Side positioning
Retained thick secretions	Secretion stimulation by anaesthetic agents Dehydration of secretions	Noisy respirations Wheezing	Suctioning Deep breathing and coughing IV hydration IPPB with mucolytic agent Chest physical therapy
Laryngospasm *Cause:* Most likely to occur after removal of endotracheal tube	Irritation from endotracheal tube or anaesthetic gases	Inspiratory stridor (crowing respiration) Sternal retraction Acute respiratory distress	O₂ therapy Positive pressure ventilation IV muscle relaxant Lidocaine Corticosteroids
Laryngeal edema	Allergic reaction to medication Mechanical irritation from intubation Fluid overload	Similar to laryngospasm	O₂ therapy Antihistamines Corticosteroids Sedatives Possible intubation
Atelectasis *Cause:* Secretions or decreased lung volumes	Mucus blockage of bronchioles Reduced alveolar surfactant (the substance that holds alveoli open)	↓ Breath sounds ↓ O₂ saturation (Figure 22-3) May affect a portion or entire lobe of lungs May occur immediately or in early postoperative period	O₂ therapy Deep breathing Incentive spirometry Early mobilization
Pulmonary edema *Cause:* Accumulation of fluid in alveoli from fluid overload, left ventricular failure, prolonged airway obstruction, sepsis, or aspiration	↑ Hydrostatic pressure ↓ Interstitial pressure ↑ Capillary permeability	Crackles on auscultation Infiltrates seen on chest radiograph Fluid overload ↓ O₂ saturation Productive cough with clear to pink sputum	O₂ therapy Diuretics Fluid restriction
Pulmonary embolism *Cause:* Peripheral venous thrombus	Thrombus dislodged from peripheral venous system and lodged in pulmonary arterial system	Acute tachypnea Dyspnea Tachycardia Hypotension ↓ O₂ saturation	O₂ therapy Cardiopulmonary support Anticoagulant therapy
Aspiration *Cause:* Gastric contents (acidic) in respiratory system *Risk factors:* Obesity, pregnancy, history of hiatal hernia, GERD, peptic ulcer, or trauma	Inhalation of regurgitated gastric contents	Potentially serious airway emergency Symptoms: broncho-/laryngospasm, hypoxemia, atelectasis, interstitial edema, alveolar hemorrhage, and respiratory failure. Crackles ↓ O₂ saturation	Prevention is optimal: Premedicate with histamine H₂-receptor antagonist (e.g., famotidine [Pepcid]) before anaesthesia induction Protect airway during induction and emergence from anaesthesia when aspiration occurs O₂ therapy Cardiac support Antibiotics
Bronchospasm *Causes:* History of asthma or COPD; irritation during intubation or extubation; aspiration; suctioning; or chemical mediator release as a result of an allergic response	Increased bronchial smooth muscle tone with resultant closure of small airways Airway edema develops; secretions build up in airway	Wheezing Dyspnea Tachypnea ↓ O₂ saturation Use of accessory muscles	O₂ therapy Bronchodilators
Hypoventilation	Depression of central respiratory drive secondary to anaesthesia or pain medication Neuro-muscular blockade, neuro-muscular disease, or combination of both	↓ Respiratory rate or effort **Hypoxemia** (low oxygen tension in the blood, characterized by a variety of nonspecific clinical signs and symptoms) ↑ Arterial partial pressure of carbon dioxide—hypercapnia (PaCO₂)	O₂ therapy Ventilator assistance, manual or mechanical Reversal agent

Continued

TABLE 22-5	COMMON IMMEDIATE POSTOPERATIVE RESPIRATORY COMPLICATIONS—cont'd		
Complications and Causes	**Mechanisms**	**Manifestations**	**Interventions**
Depression of central respiratory drive	Medullary depression from anaesthetics, opioids, or sedatives	Shallow respirations ↓ Respiratory rate, apnea ↓ PaO_2 ↑ $PaCO_2$	Stimulation Reversal of opioids or benzodiazepines Mechanical ventilation Deep breathing
Poor respiratory muscle tone	Neuro-muscular blockade Neuro-muscular disease	As above	Reversal of paralysis Mechanical ventilation
Mechanical restriction	Tight casts, dressings, positioning, and obesity prevent lung expansion	As above	Elevated head of bed Repositioning Loosening of dressings
Pain	Shallow breathing to prevent incisional pain	As above Complaints of pain Guarding behaviour	Opioid analgesic therapy in reduced dosage
Hypoxemia *Causes:* Atelectasis, aspiration, broncho-/laryngospasm, pulmonary edema, pulmonary embolism	PaO_2 <60 mm Hg O_2Sat <90–92% (common cause is atelectasis)	Nonspecific clinical signs and symptoms: agitation to somnolence, hypertension to hypotension, tachycardia to bradycardia	Deep breathing Coughing Increasing oxygen delivery

COPD, chronic obstructive pulmonary disease; *GERD,* gastro-esophageal reflux disease; *IPPB,* intermittent positive pressure breathing; *IV,* intravenous; *O₂,* oxygen; *PaCO₂,* arterial partial pressure of carbon dioxide; *PaO₂,* arterial partial pressure of oxygen.

Tongue

Tongue occluding airway

Manually elevate the jaw while tilting the head back

Tongue

Airway cleared

FIGURE 22-2 Causes and relief of airway obstruction caused by the patient's tongue.

FIGURE 22-3 Postoperative atelectasis. **A,** Normal bronchiole and alveoli. **B,** Mucous plugs in bronchioles. **C,** Collapse of alveoli caused by atelectasis following absorption of air.

pneumonia, especially after abdominal or thoracic surgery. Postoperatively, bronchial secretions increase when the respiratory passages have been irritated by heavy smoking, acute or chronic pulmonary infection or disease, and the drying of mucous membranes that occurs with intubation, inhalation anaesthesia, and dehydration. Subsequent postoperative development of mucous plugs that block small bronchi and decreased surfactant production are directly related to hypoventilation, constant recumbent position, ineffective coughing, and history of smoking. Without intervention, the affected lung segment can collapse, become infected, and progress to pneumonia within 2 to 3 days postoperatively.

NURSING MANAGEMENT RESPIRATORY COMPLICATIONS

NURSING ASSESSMENT

For an adequate respiratory assessment, nurses in the PACU and clinical unit settings must evaluate airway patency; chest symmetry; and the depth, rate, and character of respirations. The chest wall should be observed for symmetry of movement with a hand placed lightly over the xiphoid process. Slow breathing or diminished chest and abdominal movement during the respiratory cycle may indicate impaired ventilation. The nurse should determine whether abdominal or accessory muscles are being used for breathing, as their use may indicate respiratory distress. Breath sounds should be auscultated anteriorly, laterally, and posteriorly. Decreased or absent breath sounds are detected when airflow is diminished or obstructed. The presence of crackles or wheezes necessitates notifying the physician.

Regular monitoring of vital signs and use of pulse oximetry in conjunction with thorough respiratory assessment permit the nurse to recognize early signs of respiratory complications. Hypoxemia from any cause may be reflected by rapid breathing, gasping, apprehension, restlessness, and a rapid or thready pulse.

The characteristics of sputum or mucus should be noted and recorded. Mucus from the trachea and throat is colourless and thin in consistency. Sputum from the lungs and bronchi can be thick with a slight yellow or pink tinge.

NURSING DIAGNOSES

Nursing diagnoses and collaborative problems related to potential postoperative respiratory complications for the patient in the PACU or clinical unit include but are not limited to the following:

- *Ineffective airway clearance* related to *excessive mucus, retained secretions*
- *Ineffective breathing pattern* related to *pain, respiratory muscle fatigue*
- *Impaired gas exchange* (related to *hypoventilation*)
- *Risk for aspiration* as evidenced by *decrease in level of consciousness, depressed gag reflex*
- Potential complications: pneumonia, atelectasis

NURSING IMPLEMENTATION

POSTANAESTHESIA CARE UNIT. Nursing interventions in the PACU are designed to prevent and treat respiratory problems. Proper patient positioning facilitates respirations and protects the airway. Unless contraindicated by the surgical procedure, the unconscious patient is positioned in a lateral "recovery" position that keeps the airway open and reduces risk for aspiration if vomiting occurs (Figure 22-4). Once conscious, the patient is usually returned to a supine position with the head of the bed elevated. This position maximizes thoracic expansion by decreasing the pressure of the abdominal contents on the diaphragm.

SAFETY ALERT

Position the unconscious patient in a lateral "recovery" position (see Figure 22-4) to keep the airway open and reduce the risk for aspiration if vomiting occurs.

CLINICAL UNIT. Deep breathing is encouraged to facilitate gas exchange and promote the return to consciousness. The patient should be taught to take in slow, deep breaths, ideally through the nose; to hold the breath; and then to exhale slowly. This type of breathing is also useful as a relaxation strategy when the patient is anxious or in pain. Other nursing interventions appropriate for specific respiratory complications are detailed in Table 22-5.

Deep breathing and coughing techniques in the postoperative phase help the patient prevent alveolar collapse and move respiratory secretions to larger airway passages for expectoration. The patient should be stimulated to take three to four deep breaths every 5 to 10 minutes. As well, the sustained maximal inspiratory (SMI) manoeuvre can be used to increase lung volumes postoperatively. The patient inhales to the limit of his or her lung capacity and holds air in the lungs for 3 to 5 seconds before exhaling. Using an incentive spirometer is helpful in providing visual feedback of respiratory effort. The patient is taught to use an incentive spirometer preoperatively by inhaling into the mechanism, holding the ball for about 3 seconds, and then exhaling. This is done 10 to 15 times, and then the patient is encouraged to cough. This technique is used to improve oxygenation and prevent or reverse atelectasis (Odom-Forren, 2013). Diaphragmatic or abdominal breathing is accomplished by inhaling slowly and deeply through the nose, holding the breath for a few seconds, and then exhaling slowly and completely through the mouth. Placing the patient's hands lightly over the lower ribs and upper abdomen allows the patient to feel the abdomen rise during inspiration and fall during expiration.

Effective coughing is essential in mobilizing secretions (see Chapter 30). If secretions are present in the respiratory passages, deep breathing often will move them up to stimulate the cough reflex, and then they can be expectorated. Splinting an abdominal incision with a pillow or a rolled blanket provides support to the incision and aids in coughing and expectoration of secretions (Figure 22-5).

The patient's position should be changed every 1 to 2 hours to allow full chest expansion and increase perfusion of both lungs. Ambulation, not just sitting in a chair, should be aggressively carried out unless contraindicated by the surgical procedure performed or other concurrent diagnoses. Adequate

FIGURE 22-4 Position of patient during recovery from general anaesthesia.

FIGURE 22-5 Techniques for splinting wound when coughing.

and regular analgesic medication should be provided because incisional pain often deters patient participation in effective ventilation and ambulation. The patient should be reassured that these activities will not cause the incision to separate. Adequate parenteral or oral hydration is essential to maintain the integrity of mucous membranes and keep secretions thin and loose for easy expectoration.

POTENTIAL ALTERATIONS IN CARDIOVASCULAR FUNCTION

Etiology

Postanaesthesia Care Unit. In the immediate postanaesthetic period, common cardiovascular complications include hypotension, hypertension, and dysrhythmias. Patients at greatest risk for alterations in cardiovascular function include those with altered respiratory function or a cardiac history, older adults, and debilitated or critically ill patients.

Hypotension is evidenced by signs of hypoperfusion to the vital organs, especially the brain, heart, and kidneys. Clinical signs of disorientation, loss of consciousness, chest pain, oliguria, and anuria reflect hypoxemia and the loss of physiological compensation. Timely intervention may prevent the devastating complications of cardiac ischemia or infarction, cerebral ischemia, renal ischemia, and bowel infarction.

A common cause of hypotension in the PACU is unreplaced intraoperative fluid and blood loss, or postsurgical internal hemorrhage. If changes in level of consciousness and vital signs are detected, treatment is directed toward restoring circulating volume. If there is no response to fluid administration, cardiac dysfunction should be presumed to be the cause of hypotension.

Primary cardiac dysfunction, as in myocardial infarction, cardiac tamponade, or pulmonary embolism, results in an acute fall in cardiac output. Secondary myocardial dysfunction occurs as a result of the negative chronotropic (rate-derived) and negative inotropic (force-derived) effects of drugs, such as β-adrenergic blockers, digoxin, or opioids. Other causes of hypotension include decreased or low systemic vascular resistance and dysrhythmias.

Hypertension, a common finding in the PACU, is most frequently the result of sympathetic nervous stimulation resulting from pain, anxiety, bladder distension, or respiratory compromise. Hypertension may result from hypothermia or pre-existing hypertension and be seen after revascularization in vascular and cardiac surgery.

Dysrhythmias are often the result of an identifiable cause other than myocardial injury. The leading causes include hypokalemia, hypoxemia, hypercarbia, alterations in acid–base status, circulatory instability, and pre-existing heart disease. Hypothermia, pain, surgical stress, and many anaesthetic agents are also capable of causing dysrhythmias.

Clinical Unit. Postoperative fluid and electrolyte imbalances contribute to alterations in cardiovascular function. Imbalances develop as a result of a combination of the body's normal response to the stress of surgery, excessive fluid losses, and improper IV fluid replacement, which directly affects cardiac output. Fluid retention during the first 2 to 5 postoperative days can be the result of the stress response (see Chapter 8). This body response maintains both blood volume and BP (see Chapter 8, Figure 8-5). Fluid retention results from the secretion and release of two hormones by the pituitary gland—antidiuretic hormone (ADH) and adrenocorticotrophic hormone (ACTH)—and activation of the renin–angiotensin–aldosterone system. ADH release leads to increased H_2O reabsorption and decreased urinary output, increasing blood volume. ACTH stimulates the adrenal cortex to secrete aldosterone. Fluid losses resulting from surgery decrease kidney perfusion, stimulating the renin–angiotensin–aldosterone system and causing marked release of aldosterone (see Chapter 19). Both of the mechanisms that increase aldosterone lead to significant sodium and fluid retention, which also increases blood volume.

Fluid overload may occur during this period of fluid retention when IV fluids are administered too rapidly, when chronic disease (e.g., cardiac or renal) exists, or with older-adult patients. Conversely, fluid deficit may be related to slow or inadequate fluid replacement, which leads to decreases in cardiac output and tissue perfusion. Untreated preoperative dehydration or intraoperative or postoperative losses from vomiting, bleeding, wound drainage, or suctioning may contribute to fluid deficits.

Hypokalemia results when potassium is lost through the urinary and gastro-intestinal (GI) tracts and not replaced by IV fluids. Low serum potassium levels directly affect the contractility of the heart, thus contributing to decreased cardiac output and overall body tissue perfusion. Adequate replacement of potassium usually entails administration of 40 mmol/day. However, it should not be given until adequate renal function has been established. A urine output of at least 30 mL/hr is generally considered indicative of adequate renal function.

Cardiovascular status is affected by the state of tissue perfusion or blood flow. The stress response contributes to an increase in clotting tendencies in the postoperative patient by increasing platelet production. Deep-vein thrombosis (DVT) may form in leg veins as a result of inactivity, body position, and pressure, all of which lead to venous stasis and decreased perfusion. DVT, common in older adults and obese or immobilized individuals, is a potentially life-threatening complication because it may lead to pulmonary embolism. Patients with a history of DVT have a greater risk for pulmonary embolism. Pulmonary embolism should be suspected in any patient complaining of tachypnea, dyspnea, and tachycardia, particularly when the patient is already receiving oxygen therapy. Manifestations may include chest pain, hypotension, hemoptysis, dysrhythmias, or heart failure. Definitive diagnosis requires pulmonary angiography. Superficial thrombo-phlebitis is an uncomfortable but less ominous complication that may develop in a leg vein as a result of venous stasis or in the arm veins as a result of irritation from IV catheters or solutions. If a piece of a clot becomes dislodged and travels to the lung, it can cause a pulmonary infarction of a size proportionate to the vessel in which it lodges.

Syncope (fainting) is another factor that reflects the cardiovascular status. It may indicate decreased cardiac output, fluid deficits, defects in cerebral perfusion, or orthostatic hypotension, a fall in BP when the patient sits or stands. This results from peripheral dilation when blood leaves the central body organs, most notably the brain, and moves to the periphery, causing the person to feel faint.

NURSING MANAGEMENT
CARDIOVASCULAR PROBLEMS

NURSING ASSESSMENT

Cardiovascular assessment involves frequent monitoring of vital signs, usually every 15 minutes or more often until they stabilize, and then less frequently. Postoperative vital signs are compared with preoperative and intraoperative readings to determine when the signs are stabilized at the patient's normal level. The anaesthesiologist or surgeon should be notified if any of the following occur:

1. Systolic BP is less than 90 mm Hg or greater than 160 mm Hg.
2. Pulse rate is less than 60 beats per minute (bpm) or greater than 120 bpm.
3. Pulse pressure (difference between systolic and diastolic pressures) narrows.
4. BP gradually decreases during several consecutive readings.
5. An irregular cardiac rhythm develops.
6. There is a significant variation from preoperative readings.

Cardiac monitoring is recommended for patients who have a history of cardiac disease and for all older-adult patients who have undergone major surgery, regardless of whether they have cardiac problems. The apical–radial pulse should be assessed, and irregularities should be reported.

Assessment of skin colour, temperature, and moisture provides valuable information for detecting cardiovascular problems. Hypotension accompanied by a normal pulse and warm, dry, pink skin usually represents the residual vasodilating effects of anaesthesia and suggests a need for continued observation. Hypotension accompanied by a rapid pulse and cold, clammy, pale skin may be caused by impending hypovolemic shock and necessitates immediate treatment.

Assessment of cardiovascular function includes regular monitoring of the patient's BP, heart rate, pulse, and skin temperature and colour. Peripheral circulation, dressing, and drains should also be assessed. Results should be compared with the preoperative status and the immediate postoperative and intraoperative findings.

NURSING DIAGNOSES

Nursing diagnoses and collaborative problems related to potential cardiovascular complications in the PACU and the clinical unit include but are not limited to:

- *Decreased cardiac output* (related to hypovolemia, dysrhythmias)
- *Ineffective peripheral tissue perfusion* related to *sedentary lifestyle* (prolonged immobility)
- *Risk for imbalanced fluid volume*
- Potential complications: hypovolemic shock, venous thromboembolism

NURSING IMPLEMENTATION

POSTANAESTHESIA CARE UNIT. Nursing interventions in the PACU are designed to prevent and treat cardiovascular complications. Treatment of hypotension should begin with oxygen therapy to promote oxygenation of hypo-perfused organs. Volume status should be assessed, and errors of BP measurement should be ruled out. Because the most common cause of hypotension is fluid loss, IV fluid boluses should be given to normalize BP. Primary cardiac dysfunction may necessitate drug intervention. Peripheral vasodilation and hypotension may necessitate administration of vasoconstrictive agents to normalize systemic vascular resistance.

Hypertension treatment addresses the cause of sympathetic nervous system stimulation. Treatment may include use of analgesics and assistance in voiding. Rewarming corrects hypothermia-induced hypertension. If the patient has pre-existing hypertension or has undergone cardiac or vascular surgery, drug therapy designed to reduce BP may be required.

Most dysrhythmias seen in the PACU have identifiable causes, so treatment is directed toward eliminating the cause. Correcting physiological alterations often corrects the dysrhythmias. In the event of life-threatening dysrhythmias, protocols of advanced cardiac life support are applied (see Chapter 38).

CLINICAL UNIT. An accurate intake and output record should be kept during the postoperative period, and laboratory findings (e.g., electrolytes, hematocrit) should be monitored. Nursing responsibilities relating to IV management are critical during this period. In particular, the nurse should be alert for symptoms of too slow or too rapid a rate of fluid replacement. The infusion site should also be assessed for discomfort and the hazards associated with the IV administration of potassium, such as cardiac arrhythmias. Thirst is one of the most annoying discomforts of postoperative patients. This may be related to the drying effects of anticholinergic drugs, anaesthetic gases, and fluid deficits. Adequate and regular mouth care is helpful while the patient cannot ingest food or drink by mouth.

When confined to bed, patients should alternately flex and extend all joints 10 to 12 times every 1 to 2 hours while awake. The muscular contraction produced by these exercises and by ambulation facilitates venous return from the lower extremities. The ambulating patient should pick up the feet rather than shuffling them so as to maximize muscular contraction. When the patient is sitting in a chair or lying in bed, there should be no pressure to impede venous flow through the popliteal space. Crossed legs, pillows behind the knees, and extreme elevation of the knee gatch must be avoided.

The use of unfractionated heparin or low-molecular-weight heparin is a prophylactic measure for venous thrombosis and pulmonary embolism (Rieker, 2014); however, a systematic review by Beitland, Sanden, Kjærvik, and colleagues (2015) revealed a beneficial effect of low-molecular-weight heparin over unfractionated heparin. Some surgeons routinely prescribe use of elastic stockings or mechanical aids such as sequential compressive devices to stimulate the massaging and milking actions that are transmitted to the veins when leg muscles contract. These devices may actually impair circulation if the legs remain inactive or if the devices are sized or applied improperly. Elastic stockings must be removed and reapplied at least twice daily for skin care and inspection.

Before the patient may ambulate, the nurse should first raise the head of the patient's bed for 1 to 2 minutes and then assist the patient to sit on the side of the bed while monitoring the radial pulse for rate and quality. If no changes or complaints are noted, ambulation can be started. Nurses should use transfer belts or have adequate personnel to assist ambulation if the patient is unsteady or unable to transfer herself or himself. If the patient complains of feeling faint during ambulation, the nurse should provide assistance to ease the patient to a supine position until recovery is evidenced by BP stability. While faintness is often frightening for the patient, it poses no real physiological danger, although injury can result from a fall.

POTENTIAL ALTERATIONS IN NEUROLOGICAL FUNCTION

Etiology

Postanaesthesia Care Unit. Occasionally, patients may wake up from anaesthesia in an agitated state referred to as *emergence delirium* (Figure 22-6). This is a reversible neurological alteration in which patients may be disoriented and exhibit bizarre behaviour (Rothrock, 2015). Emergence delirium can include restlessness;

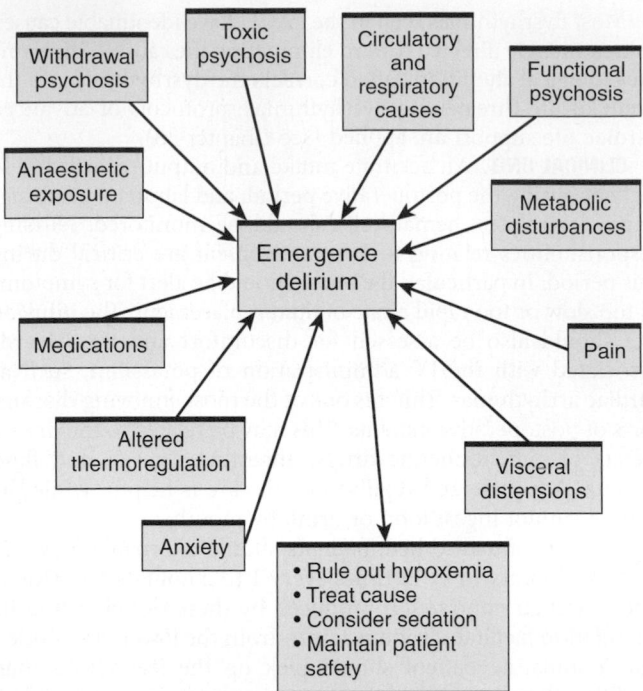

FIGURE 22-6 Emergence delirium in the postanaesthesia care unit: contributing factors and treatment. Source: Redrawn from Rothrock, J. C. (2015). *Alexander's care of the patient in surgery* (15th ed., p. 277). St. Louis: Mosby.

agitation; disorientation to place, time, and person; thrashing; and shouting. Primarily pediatric and older-adult patients are affected, and it is usually noted about half an hour after surgery but may manifest in up to 24 hours in older adults. Contributing factors include:

- Hypoxia
- Anaesthetic agents
- Bladder distension
- Immobility
- Sensory and cognitive impairments
- Inadequate pain control
- Electrolyte abnormalities
- Presence of an endotracheal tube
- Polypharmacy
- Dehydration and malnutrition
- State of anxiety before surgery

If delirium occurs, the nurse should first rule out hypoxia. Once the cause is determined, the patient can receive appropriate treatment. Nurses may also be able to positively affect the patient's recovery by using interventions that decrease anxiety (Rothrock, 2015).

Delayed awakening is another possible problem after surgery. Fortunately, the most common cause of delayed awakening is prolonged drug action, particularly of opioids, sedatives, and inhalational anaesthetics, as opposed to neurological injury. Normally, the anaesthesiologist can predict awakening based on the drugs used in surgery.

NURSING MANAGEMENT
NEUROLOGICAL COMPLICATIONS

NURSING ASSESSMENT

After surgery, the nursing assessment should include the patient's level of consciousness, orientation, and ability to follow commands; the size, reactivity, and equality of the pupils; and the patient's sensory and motor status. If the patient had a regional anaesthetic, the level of anaesthetic effect should also be determined by assessing the level of numbness and number of dermatomes blocked. If the neurological status is altered, possible causes should be determined.

NURSING DIAGNOSES

Nursing diagnoses related to potential neurological complications for the patient in the PACU and the clinical unit include but are not limited to the following:

- *Risk for acute confusion* as evidenced by *sensory deprivation, pharmaceutical agent*
- *Risk for injury* as evidenced by *alteration in cognitive functioning, alteration in sensation*
- *Impaired verbal communication* related to *central nervous system impairment, emotional disturbance*

NURSING IMPLEMENTATION

POSTANAESTHESIA CARE UNIT. The most common cause of postoperative agitation is hypoxemia, so the nurse needs to evaluate respiratory function. Once hypoxemia has been ruled out and all potentially known causes have been addressed, sedation may prove beneficial in controlling the agitation and provide patient and staff safety. Emergence delirium and delays in awakening are time limited and will resolve before the patient is discharged from the PACU. If necessary, benzodiazepines and opioids may be pharmacologically reversed with antagonists.

Until the patient is awake and able to communicate effectively, it is the responsibility of the PACU nurse to act as a patient advocate and to maintain patient safety at all times. Measures to accomplish this include having the side rails up, securing IV lines and artificial airways, verifying the presence of identification and allergy bands, and monitoring physiological status.

CLINICAL UNIT. On the postoperative unit, the nurse prevents or manages postoperative delirium by maintaining fluid and electrolyte balance, ensuring adequate nutrition and sleep, providing pain management, ensuring proper bowel and bladder function, and aiding early mobilization. Specific aids, such as clocks, calendars, and photographs, help orient the patient.

Psychological problems in the postoperative period can be limited by providing adequate support for the patient, for example, by listening to and talking with the patient, explaining, reassuring, and encouraging caregiver presence.

Some common alterations in neurological function seen on the clinical unit may be related to medications for pain management, sleep deprivation, or sensory overload. It is important that the nurse complete a central nervous system assessment for all patients who have undergone surgery. In the case of patients who are receiving pain medication, the nurse must ensure that they are responsive and oriented to person, place, and time. For patients who have received a spinal or epidural anaesthetic, the nurse must assess sensation and motor function. An ice pack may be used to check a patient's motor block as the effects of the spinal anaesthetic are resolving.

PAIN AND DISCOMFORT

Etiology

Postanaesthesia Care Unit. Despite the availability of analgesic drugs and pain-relieving techniques, pain remains a common problem and a significant fear for the patient in the PACU and during the postoperative period. Pain may be the result of surgical manipulation, positioning, or the presence of internal devices such as an endotracheal tube or a catheter, or it may occur as the patient begins to mobilize after surgery.

Clinical Unit. On the surgical unit, postoperative pain is caused by the interaction of a number of physiological and psychological factors. Skin and underlying tissues have been traumatized during surgery, and there may be reflex muscle spasms around the incision. Anxiety and fear, sometimes related to the anticipation of pain, create tension and further increase muscle tone and spasm. The effort and movement associated with deep breathing, coughing, and changing position may aggravate pain by creating tension or pull on the incisional area.

When the internal viscera are cut, no pain is felt. However, pressure in the internal viscera elicits pain. Therefore, deep visceral pain may signal the presence of a complication such as intestinal distension or bleeding that can occur in the immediate postoperative phase or abscess formation, which can be apparent within 3 to 5 days postoperatively.

NURSING MANAGEMENT
PAIN

NURSING ASSESSMENT

POSTANAESTHESIA CARE UNIT. Pain assessment may be difficult in the PACU and in the early postoperative period on the clinical unit. The patient's self-report is the most important means of measuring pain intensity. Physiological indicators such as vital signs are not good indicators of pain, as research has demonstrated no significant correlation between the patient's self-reported intensity of pain and elevated heart rate and BP (Odom-Forren, 2015). When caring for patients who cannot self-report, the nurse should observe for behavioural clues of pain such as crying, restlessness, a wrinkling face or brow, or moaning.

CLINICAL UNIT. Postoperative pain is usually most severe within the first 48 hours and subsides thereafter. Variation is considerable, however, and is affected by the procedure performed and the patient's individual pain tolerance or perception. A comprehensive pain assessment includes the following:

- Location
- Intensity, assessed using a reliable, valid pain assessment tool (e.g., verbal descriptor, numeric rating, or visual analogue)
- Quality (e.g., neuropathic pain may be described as "burning" or "shooting")
- Factors that relieve and aggravate
- Effect of pain on function
- Comfort–function goal (e.g., for the postoperative patient, link pain control to the ability to deep-breathe, turn, or ambulate)

The nurse assesses the effectiveness of all pain control measures (e.g., epidural catheters, patient-controlled analgesia [PCA]) (Odom-Forren, 2014). (See Chapter 10 for a more detailed discussion of pain assessment.)

NURSING DIAGNOSES

Nursing diagnoses for the patient experiencing pain and discomfort in the PACU and clinical unit include but are not limited to the following:

- *Acute pain* related to *physical injury agent* (surgical procedure)
- *Chronic pain* related to *injury agent, emotional distress*

NURSING IMPLEMENTATION

POSTANAESTHESIA CARE UNIT. IV opioids provide the most rapid relief. Medications are administered slowly and titrated to allow for optimal pain management with minimal to no adverse drug effects. More sustained relief may be obtained through the use of epidural catheters, PCA, or regional anaesthetic blockade. Nonpharmacological interventions are used to supplement pain medications and include such measures as touch, application of heat or cold, massage, imagery, music, biofeedback, and reuniting the patient and family (Odom-Forren, 2015).

Pain management is most successful when the treatment plan is developed by the patient, anaesthesiologists, and PACU nurse. The goals should be to determine the most effective therapy, drug, and dose and the best response to therapy. Once the patient is discharged from the PACU to an inpatient unit, the nurse replaces the PACU nurse as a member of the pain management team. (For more information on nursing assessment and management of patients in pain, see Chapter 10.)

CLINICAL UNIT. On the surgical unit, postoperative pain relief is a nursing responsibility because the surgeon's orders for analgesic medication and other comfort measures are usually written on an as-needed basis. Pain should be reassessed, as per the assessment protocol previously mentioned, when the patient complains of pain and before and after analgesic administration. When pain is stabilized, pain should be assessed at least every 4 to 8 hours during the first 1 to 2 days postoperatively (Odom-Forren, 2013). Patient complaints of either chest or leg pain should be reported, as it may indicate a complication. If it is gas pain, opioid medication may aggravate it. The nurse should notify the physician and request a change in the order if the analgesic either fails to relieve pain or makes the patient excessively lethargic or somnolent.

During the first 48 hours or longer, opioid analgesics (e.g., morphine) are required to relieve moderate to severe pain. After that, nonopioid analgesics, such as nonsteroidal anti-inflammatory drugs (NSAIDs), may be sufficient as pain intensity decreases.

Effective pain management will reduce harmful complications, promote optimal healing, and allow patients to participate in necessary activities such as ambulating (Rothrock, 2015). Although opioid analgesics are often essential for the postoperative patient's comfort, adverse effects such as constipation, nausea and vomiting, respiratory depression, and hypotension are common. Patient-controlled analgesia (PCA) is one of the most common ways to deliver opioid analgesia. PCA provides immediate analgesia and maintains a constant, steady blood level of the analgesic agent. PCA allows for self-administration of a preset bolus dose of analgesia by the patient (Odom-Forren, 2013). (PCA is discussed in Chapter 10.)

Epidural analgesia is the infusion of pain-relieving medications through a catheter placed into the epidural space surrounding the spinal cord. The goal of epidural analgesia is delivery of medication directly to opiate receptors in the spinal cord. The administration is through a bolus, continuous infusion, or patient-controlled epidural analgesia and is monitored by the nurse (Odom-Forren, 2013).

POTENTIAL ALTERATIONS IN TEMPERATURE

Etiology

Postanaesthesia Care Unit. Hypothermia sets in when a person's core temperature is less than 35°C. The perianesthesia nurse should monitor the patient's temperature with an electronic oral temperature device (Odom-Forren, 2015). Postoperative hypothermia may be the result of heat loss during long, open surgical procedures due to the low ambient temperature in the OR, the use of cold irrigation fluids, or both.

Patients predisposed to hypothermia include older adults, children under 2 years—especially neonates—burn patients, females, and patients under general or neuraxial anaesthesia (Odom-Forren, 2015). Complications from hypothermia may include prolonged emergence from anaesthesia, increased likelihood of impaired wound healing and surgical site infection, bleeding, and cardiac incidences (Odom-Forren, 2015).

Active rewarming of hypothermic patients is achieved by applying external warming devices to the body and head. Although the application of warm blankets is traditionally done in the PACU, the use of forced-air warmers is an evidence-informed initiative that also effectively rewarms patients (Odom-Forren, 2015). When using any external warming device, the nurse should monitor the patient's body temperature at 15-minute intervals and use care to prevent thermal skin injuries. Oxygen therapy via nasal prongs or mask is used to treat the increased demand for oxygen that accompanies the increase in body temperature. Shivering is usually quickly suppressed by opioids.

Clinical Unit. Temperature variation in the postoperative period provides valuable information about the patient's status. Fever may occur at any time during the postoperative period (Table 22-6). A mild elevation (≤38°C) during the first 48 hours usually reflects the surgical stress response. A moderate elevation (>38°C) is caused more frequently by respiratory congestion or atelectasis and less frequently by dehydration. After the first 48 hours, a moderate to marked elevation (>37.7°C) is usually caused by infection.

NURSING MANAGEMENT
POTENTIAL TEMPERATURE COMPLICATIONS

NURSING ASSESSMENT

Frequent assessment of the patient's temperature in the days after surgery helps detect patterns of hypothermia or fever that may be present postoperatively. The nurse should observe the patient for early signs of inflammation and infection so that any complications that arise may be treated in a timely manner. Infections may include:

- Wound infection
- Respiratory tract infection
- Urinary tract infection (secondary to catheterization)
- IV site superficial thrombo-phlebitis (temperature elevation 7 to 10 days after surgery)
- Hospital-associated diarrhea caused by *Clostridium difficile*
- Septicemia (microorganisms enter bloodstream during surgery, especially in GI or genito-urinary procedures)

NURSING DIAGNOSES

Nursing diagnoses related to potential postoperative temperature complications may include but are not limited to the following:

- *Hypothermia* related to *decrease in metabolic rate, inactivity*
- *Hyperthermia* related to *increase in metabolic activity, dehydration*
- *Risk for hypothermia* as evidenced by *inefficient nonshivering thermogenesis* (general anaesthesia, surgical procedure)

NURSING IMPLEMENTATION

POSTANAESTHESIA CARE UNIT. Passive rewarming (i.e., shivering) raises basal heat metabolism, so active rewarming using forced-air warmers or other devices, such as radiant warmers or heated water mattresses, is preferable. During rewarming, the nurse should also monitor a patient who has an increase in temperature, specifically for symptoms of malignant hyperthermia, because symptoms may not be evident until the postoperative phase. (See the discussion of malignant hyperthermia in Chapter 21). Oxygen therapy via nasal prongs or mask is used to address the increased demand for oxygen that accompanies the increased body temperature. (See Chapter 71 for more on the management of hypothermia.)

CLINICAL UNIT. The nurse's role with respect to postoperative fever may be preventive, diagnostic, therapeutic, or a combination of these. The patient's temperature is usually measured every 4 hours for the first 48 hours after surgery and then less frequently if no problems develop. As well, the nurse maintains meticulous care of the wound and the IV site and encourages airway clearance. If fever develops, chest radiographs may be done, and, depending on the suspected cause, cultures of the wound, urine, or blood may be obtained. If infection is determined to be the source of the fever, antibiotics are started right away. If the fever rises above 39.4°C, antipyretic drugs and body-cooling measures may be employed.

POTENTIAL GASTRO-INTESTINAL PROBLEMS

Etiology

Postanaesthesia Care Unit. Nausea and vomiting are significant problems in the immediate postoperative period and are often the reason for unanticipated hospital admission of day-surgery patients, increased patient discomfort, delays in discharge, and patient dissatisfaction with the surgical experience.

Clinical Unit. Slowed GI motility and altered patterns of food intake may lead to the development of several distressing postoperative symptoms that are most pronounced after abdominal surgery. Nausea and vomiting may be caused by the action of anaesthetics or opioids, delayed gastric emptying, slowed peristalsis resulting from the handling of the bowel during surgery, or resumption of oral intake too soon after surgery (Table 22-7).

TABLE 22-6	**SIGNIFICANCE OF POSTOPERATIVE TEMPERATURE CHANGES**	
Time After Surgery	**Temperature**	**Possible Causes**
≤12 hours	Hypothermia to 35°C	Effects of anaesthesia Body heat loss in surgical exposure
First 24–48 hours	Elevation to 38°C	Inflammatory response to surgical stress
	>38°C	Lung congestion, atelectasis
Third day and later	Elevation above 37.7°C	Wound infection Urinary infection Respiratory infection Phlebitis

TABLE 22-7 POSTOPERATIVE DIETS

Clear Fluids
Broth, gelatin, water, tea, black coffee

Fluids
Milk, coffee with cream, cream soups

Soft Diet
Fish, cottage cheese, pasta, eggs, mousse, pudding

Full Diet
Regular diet
Patients can also be placed on special diets, such as diabetic or low sodium.

NURSING MANAGEMENT GASTRO-INTESTINAL PROBLEMS

NURSING ASSESSMENT

NAUSEA AND VOMITING. Postoperative nausea and vomiting (PONV) is a complex physiological interaction between the following: the vomiting centre in the brain stem, the chemo-receptor trigger zone, the internal ear, the vagus nerve, the limbic system, and the cerebral cortex. PONV occurs in approximately 30% of all surgical patients and 80% of high-risk patients. PONV leads to delayed PACU or hospital discharge and, sometimes, subsequent readmission. As well as being a major cause of distress for patients, it can lead to more severe postoperative complications such as (Peterson, 2013):

- Aspiration
- Wound dehiscence
- Increased intracranial pressure
- Increased cardiovascular demand, predisposing compromised patients to myocardial infarctions

Primary risk factors for PONV include the following (Odom-Forren, 2014):

Patient-specific
- Age <50 years old
- Female gender
- History of motion sickness or PONV
- Nonsmoker

Anaesthesia-related
- Use of volatile anaesthetics
- Use of nitrous oxide
- High doses of opioids intra- and postoperatively

Surgery-related
- Duration of surgery >1 hour
- Type of surgery, specifically laparoscopy

These risk factors can be determined in the preoperative assessment so that prophylaxis can be planned using either one medication such as ondansetron (Zofran) or a combination of medications that minimize PONV.

Nonpharmacological interventions that may be used in combination for PONV or for postdischarge nausea and vomiting (PDNV) include transcutaneous electrical nerve stimulation, acupuncture, acupressure, acupoint stimulation, and aromatherapy (isopropyl alcohol and peppermint) (Odom-Forren, 2014). Nurses should document the quantity and characteristics (including colour) of the emesis.

ILEUS

Postoperative Ileus. Postoperative ileus (POI) is a delay in the return of the GI system's normal peristalsis, specifically after GI surgery. It is characterized by abdominal distension and tenderness or pain. Stomach motility returns in 1 to 2 days, and bowel motility in 3 to 5 days. Laparoscopic colon surgery is associated with a shorter period of ileus than open surgery. Abdominal distension during this time may require insertion of a nasogastric tube for symptomatic relief and the lowering of opioid doses or provision of pain relief with NSAIDs to reduce inflammation (Cagir, 2016).

Paralytic Ileus. Paralytic ileus is impairment of intestinal motility (ileus that persists for more than 2 to 3 days) postoperatively. It can be associated with the large and small intestine and resolves with treatment; it is not a mechanical obstruction. Peristalsis stops, and the patient complains of abdominal pain, distension, nausea, vomiting, and poor appetite. Nursing care on the postoperative unit consists of measuring the patient's abdominal girth for distension and auscultating the abdomen in all four quadrants to determine presence, frequency, and characteristics of bowel sounds. Bowel sounds are frequently absent or diminished, and the abdomen will sound tympanic to percussion. Early bowel sounds may signal return of small intestine motility; however, full return of bowel function is indicated by the passage of flatus or stool (Jackson, 2015). When paralytic ileus does not resolve spontaneously, the patient may require diagnostic tests to rule out mechanical blockage that would require surgical intervention.

NURSING DIAGNOSES

Nursing diagnoses and collaborative problems related to potential GI complications in the PACU and clinical unit may include but are not limited to the following:

- *Nausea* related to *noxious environmental stimuli*
- *Risk for aspiration* as evidenced by *delayed gastric emptying, depressed gag reflex, increase in intragastric pressure*
- *Risk for deficient fluid volume* as evidenced by *active fluid volume loss*
- *Imbalanced nutrition: less than body requirements* related to *inability to ingest food, inability to absorb nutrients*
- Potential complications: fluid and electrolyte imbalance

NURSING IMPLEMENTATION

POSTANAESTHESIA CARE UNIT. Intervention for *nausea and vomiting* is primarily the use of antiemetic or prokinetic drugs (see Chapter 44). In the PACU, oral fluids should be given only as indicated and tolerated. IV fluids will provide hydration until the patient is able to tolerate oral fluids. Care should also be taken to prevent aspiration in case the patient vomits while still sleepy from anaesthesia. Having suction equipment readily available at the bedside and positioning the patient in the lateral recovery position will help protect the patient from aspiration (see Figure 22-4). Other interventions that may be effective include placing the patient in the upright position; encouraging slow, deep breathing; doing mouth care; using distraction; and providing emotional support.

CLINICAL UNIT. Depending on the nature of the surgery, the patient may resume oral intake as soon as the gag reflex returns. While the patient is on nothing-by-mouth status, IV infusions are given to maintain fluid and electrolyte balance. Once oral intake is allowed, clear liquids are started and the IV infusion is continued, usually at a reduced rate. If oral intake is well tolerated by the patient, the IV is discontinued and the diet is advanced progressively until a regular diet is tolerated.

The nurse should assess the patient regularly to detect the resumption of normal intestinal peristalsis, as evidenced by the return of bowel sounds and the passage of flatus. The patient may need to be encouraged to expel flatus and be reassured that expulsion is necessary and desirable. Gas pains, which tend to become pronounced on the second or third postoperative day, may be relieved by ambulation and frequent repositioning. Positioning the patient on the right side permits gas to rise along the transverse colon and facilitates its release. Resumption of a normal diet after bowel sounds have returned will also enhance the return of normal peristalsis. A patient who does not improve with conservative measures will need to be reassessed and may require additional surgery.

POTENTIAL ALTERATIONS IN URINARY FUNCTION

Etiology

Low Urine Output. In patients with normal renal function, a urinary output of ≈30 mL/hr is expected in the PACU. This lower output is caused by increased aldosterone and antidiuretic hormone secretion resulting from the stress of surgery, fluid restriction before surgery, loss of fluids during surgery, drainage, and diaphoresis. By the second or third day, the patient's urinary output should return to the normal level of 0.5 to 1 mL/kg/hr (≈60 mL/hr). Persistent low urinary output, or oliguria, can indicate inadequate renal perfusion and pending renal failure. Restoring renal blood flow and urine production can prevent renal failure.

Acute urinary retention can occur in the postoperative period for a variety of reasons. Surgical genito-urinary trauma can cause swelling and bleeding. Anaesthesia depresses the nervous system, allowing the bladder to fill more completely than normal before the urge to void is felt. Neuraxial anaesthesia can cause autonomic blockade of sacral nerves, resulting in a hypotonic bladder. After lower abdominal or pelvic surgery, spasms or guarding of the abdominal and pelvic muscles interferes with their normal function, resulting in urinary retention. Pain may alter perception, interfering with the patient's awareness of the sensation arising as the bladder fills. Voiding may be impaired by lack of skeletal muscle activity (decreased smooth bladder muscle tone). As well, the supine position reduces the ability to relax the perineal muscles and the external sphincter.

Anticholinergic, antispasmodic, and opioid drugs are some medications that prevent the complete emptying of the bladder.

NURSING MANAGEMENT
POTENTIAL URINARY PROBLEMS

NURSING ASSESSMENT

The urine of the patient after surgery should be examined for both quantity and quality. The colour, amount, consistency, and odour of the urine should be noted. In-dwelling catheters should be assessed for patency, and urine output should be approximately 60 mL/hr. Most people urinate approximately 200 mL of urine within 6 to 8 hours after surgery. If no voiding occurs, the abdominal contour should be inspected and the bladder palpated and percussed for distension or a bladder scanner used to detect bladder volumes.

NURSING DIAGNOSES

Nursing diagnoses and collaborative problems related to potential urinary complications for the patient after surgery include but are not limited to the following:

- *Urinary retention* related to *anaesthetic drugs, pain*
- Potential complication: acute kidney injury, catheter-associated urinary tract infections (CAUTIs)

NURSING IMPLEMENTATION

There may be a postoperative order to catheterize the patient in 8 to 12 hours if voiding has not occurred; however, there are ways for the nurse to facilitate voiding. Some measures known to help include positioning the patient—sitting for women and standing for men—ambulating, putting a commode in place, providing reassurance, running water, providing water to drink, or pouring warm water over the perineum.

In assessing the need for catheterization, the nurse considers fluid intake during and after surgery and determines bladder fullness (e.g., palpable fullness above the symphysis pubis, discomfort when pressure is applied over the bladder, the presence of the urge to void). Urinary tract infections are the most common complication associated with urinary catheterization and commonly occur in the first postoperative week. Patients should be catheterized only when absolutely necessary, using aseptic protocol, and the catheter should be removed as soon as it is no longer required.

POTENTIAL ALTERATIONS IN THE INTEGUMENT

Etiology

Despite advances in surgical technologies and techniques, environmental conditions, antibiotic regimens, and sterilization methods, surgery remains an invasive procedure that can predispose patients to surgical site infections (SSIs). An SSI is an infection that occurs within 30 days of surgery or up to 1 year after implant surgery. It has at least one of the following signs or symptoms (Keast & Swanson, 2014):

- Purulent discharge
- Isolation of organisms from wound fluid or tissue
- Pain, tenderness, local edema, warmth
- Physician or health care team member diagnosis

According to the Centers for Disease Control and Prevention (CDC; 2017) in the United States, SSIs account for 31% of all health care–associated infections (HAIs) and have a mortality rate of 3%. In Canada, Keast and Swanson (2014) report that because 75% of all surgery is done on an outpatient basis, detecting and caring for SSIs in the community are the most common reasons for community nursing visits. Having community nurses provide leading-edge wound care practice is decreasing the need for patient readmission to hospital and thus saving health care costs (Canadian Nurses Association [CNA], 2013).

Wounds are a significant, costly, and preventable barrier to successful recovery from routine surgical interventions, so reducing the incidence of SSIs is essential, and much evidence is now available to support prevention practices, for example, the Wound Care Instrument developed collaboratively by the Canadian Association of Wound Care and the Canadian Association for Enterostomal Therapy (Canadian Association of Wound Care and Canadian Association for Enterostomal Therapy, 2011). (Wound healing and complications are discussed in Chapter 14.)

SSIs are caused by (Keast & Swanson, 2014):

- Introduction of endogenous bacteria (from the patient) into the wound
- Introduction of exogenous contamination (from the surgical environment) into the wound

TABLE 22-8 RECOMMENDATIONS FOR PREVENTION OF SURGICAL SITE INFECTIONS

Intervention	Guidelines for SSI Prevention
Perform holistic preoperative assessment and manage preoperative risk	Document patient's age, weight, general health, medications, coexisting health conditions, glycemic control, recent weight loss or gain, state of being overweight or obese, physical activity levels, present and past smoking history, and previous experiences with anaesthetic. *Example:* Advanced age relates to decreased healing potential and diminished immune factors. Complete a nutritional assessment or lab analysis for serum albumin and total protein or both. Improve diet preoperatively.
Manage intraoperative risk	Maintain patient homeostasis (e.g., temperature, glucose levels, O_2 saturation >95%). Ensure strict adherence to aseptic practice by surgical personnel. Minimize tissue trauma through gentle handling and limited use of electrocautery, and when closing incision, eliminate dead space below the skin. Use antibiotics prophylactically.
Manage postoperative risk	Maintain body temperature. Ensure adequate oxygenation. Use clean, intact wound dressing (e.g., waterproof dressing for 48 hours or aseptic technique for dressing change). Control pain.
Educate patients and families on signs and symptoms of SSIs	Provide information in easy-to-understand verbal and written form, including: • How to recognize an SSI (i.e., a little redness around wound edge is normal and can be expected for the first few days after surgery; redness spreading out more than 2 cm from incision, pain, swelling, or pus are SSI danger signs that must be reported to doctor) • Who to contact if infection is suspected • How to care for wound at home • Antibiotic regimen
Identify and treat SSIs	Ensure early diagnosis. Open incision to remove sutures and infected tissue and to drain. Use dressings to promote secondary healing. Follow evidence-informed recommendations for antibiotics.
Debride necrotic tissue	*(Necrotic tissue prolongs inflammation and may harbour aerobic and anaerobic bacteria and toxins.)* Choose debridement technique based on wound condition, resources, and patient condition.
Choose dressing or device to manage exudate and bacterial burden	Choose a dressing based on: • Depth of wound • Exudate and odour control • Conformability • Antimicrobial efficacy • Ease of removal • Patient safety and comfort
Consider adjunctive therapies	Use topical NPWT (e.g., for sternal and abdominal dehiscence, use growth factors, antibacterial honey, larva therapy [maggots], anti-scarring agents, and antiseptic-impregnated sutures).
Implement a surgical site surveillance program	*(Collating infection rates for individual surgeons and surgical procedures reduces infection rates and identifies trends and causative agents. Surveillance programs must be in the community and extend a minimum of 30 days postoperatively and up to 1 year for implants.)* Help evaluate effectiveness of preventive strategies. Determine compliance to guidelines (e.g., teamwork, collaboration, and effective communication).

NPWT, negative-pressure wound therapy; *SSI,* surgical site infection.
Adapted from Keast, D., & Swanson, T. (2014). Ten top tips: Managing surgical site infections. *Wounds International, 5*(3), 15–16. Retrieved from *http://www.woundinfection-institute.com/wp-content/uploads/2014/11/SSI_11422.pdf.*

• Inability of the individual to resist infection due to reduced immune capacity (disease, malnutrition, medication) or other factors

Table 22-8 provides guidelines for the prevention of SSIs.

NURSING MANAGEMENT
SURGICAL WOUNDS

NURSING ASSESSMENT

Wound assessment requires gathering information through questioning, observation, physical examination, and clinical investigation and using this information to formulate a wound care plan. It is recommended that the physical assessment be done in three zones: wound bed, wound edge, and periwound skin (Dowsett, Protz, Drouard, et al., 2015). Assessment includes:

• *Appearance:* Note the colour of wound, bruising, redness, and approximation of the incision.

• *Size:* Note the length, width, depth and shape of the wound and any signs of the wound opening (i.e., dehiscence or evisceration).

• *Exudate:* Check the wound for exudate type (e.g., watery, purulent), odour, and amount. A small amount of serous drainage is common, and it changes from sanguineous (red) to serosanguineous (pink) to serous (clear yellow). Draining will decrease over time.

• *Edema:* Excessive swelling may indicate wound complications.

• *Pain:* Sudden onset or persistent severe incisional pain may indicate infection, hemorrhage, or hematoma.

• *Drains:* Note the placement and security of drain or tube. Check the collection device; empty as required and document.

Wound dehiscence (separation and disruption of previously joined wound edges) may be preceded by a sudden discharge of brown, pink, or clear drainage. Wound evisceration (protrusion of the visceral organs though a wound opening) can occur after

TABLE 22-9   EXPECTED DRAINAGE FROM TUBES AND CATHETERS

Substance	Daily Amount	Colour	Odour	Consistency
In-Dwelling Catheter				
Urine*	500–700 mL, 1–2 days postoperative; 1 500–2 500 mL thereafter (output = 0.5–1 mL/kg/hr)	Clear, yellow	Ammonia	Watery
Nasogastric Tube, Gastrostomy Tube				
Gastric contents	≤1 500 mL/day	Pale, yellow–green, brown Bloody following gastro-intestinal surgery	Sour	Watery
Hemovac, Jackson-Pratt				
Wound drainage	Variable with procedure	Variable with procedure Usually serosanguineous	Same as wound dressing	Variable
T Tube				
Bile	500 mL	Bright yellow to dark green	Acid	Thick

*See Chapter 47.

surgery and is considered a medical emergency. If evisceration occurs, place sterile, saline-soaked towels over any extruding tissue, keep the patient on nothing-by-mouth status, observe the patient for signs and symptoms of shock, and call the surgeon immediately.

NURSING DIAGNOSES

Nursing diagnoses related to surgical wounds of the patient after surgery include but are not limited to the following:

- *Impaired skin integrity* related to *chemical injury agent*
- *Risk for surgical site infection* as evidenced by *invasive procedure, type of surgical procedure, comorbidity*

NURSING IMPLEMENTATION

When drainage occurs on the dressing, the type, amount, colour, consistency, and odour of drainage should be noted and recorded. Expected drainage from tubes is outlined in Table 22-9. The effect of position changes on drainage should also be assessed. The surgeon should be notified of any excessive or abnormal drainage and significant changes in vital signs.

Immediately after surgery, the incision is usually covered with a dressing. Surgical wound dressings are left dry and untouched for a minimum of 48 hours after surgery. This permits re-establishment of the protective, natural bacteria-proof barrier. The nurse changes the dressing according to employer policy. Wound healing and care are discussed in Chapter 14.

POTENTIAL ALTERATIONS IN PSYCHOLOGICAL FUNCTION

Etiology

Anxiety and depression may occur in the postoperative patient. These states may be more pronounced in the patient who has had radical surgery (e.g., colostomy, amputation), or who has received a poor prognosis (e.g., inoperable tumour). A history of a neurotic or psychotic disorder should alert the nurse to the possibility of postoperative anxiety and depression. However, these responses may develop in any patient as part of the grief response to loss of a body organ or disturbance in body image (e.g., mastectomy or hysterectomy) and may be exacerbated by a lowered response to stress.

The patient who lives alone or requires rehabilitation after surgery may also develop anxiety and depression when faced with the need for assistance after surgery until strength and independence can be regained. The discharge nurse may refer a patient to community service and arrange home care nursing visits before discharge if the patient needs assistance, wound therapy, or monitoring after returning home (CNA, 2013).

In caring for the older adult, nurses in Canada must be cognizant of the increasing incidence of delirium, dementia, and depression in that segment of the population. Nurses must possess the knowledge and skills to screen for and differentiate between these conditions, which can have overlapping clinical features (Registered Nurses' Association of Ontario, 2016).

After surgery, confusion or delirium may arise from physiological sources, including fluid and electrolyte imbalances; hypoxemia; medication effects; sleep deprivation; and sensory alteration, deprivation, or overload.

Delirium tremens may also occur in some patients after surgery as a result of alcohol withdrawal. Delirium tremens is a reaction characterized by restlessness, insomnia, nightmares, tachycardia, apprehension, confusion and disorientation, irritability, and auditory or visual hallucinations. (Management of delirium tremens is discussed in Chapter 11.)

NURSING MANAGEMENT PSYCHOLOGICAL FUNCTION

NURSING DIAGNOSES

Nursing diagnoses related to potential postoperative alterations in psychological function include but are not limited to the following:

- *Anxiety* related to *threat to current status*
- *Disturbed body image* related to *alteration in self-perception*
- *Disturbed sleep pattern* related to *environmental barrier* (unfamiliar setting, insufficient privacy)

NURSING IMPLEMENTATION

Nurses must observe and evaluate the patient's behaviour and plan appropriate interventions to ensure proper treatment of symptoms, prevent adverse outcomes, and improve the patient's quality of life on discharge. Supportive measures include taking time to listen to and talk with the patient, offering explanations and reassurance, and working collaboratively with family or significant others for discharge planning.

The nurse should discuss the patient's expectations for activity and the assistance that will be needed following discharge. The older patient may be particularly distressed if an immediate

TABLE 22-10	POSTANAESTHESIA AND AMBULATORY SURGERY DISCHARGE CRITERIA

Postanaesthesia Discharge Criteria
- Patient awake (or baseline)
- Vital signs stable
- No excess bleeding or drainage
- No respiratory depression
- Oxygen saturation >90%
- Report given

Ambulatory Surgery Discharge Criteria
- All PACU discharge criteria met
- No IV opioids for last 30 minutes
- Minimal nausea and vomiting
- Voided (if appropriate to surgical procedure or orders)
- Able to ambulate if age appropriate and not contraindicated
- Responsible adult present to accompany patient
- Written discharge instructions given and understood

PACU, postanaesthesia care unit; *IV*, intravenous.

return to home is not feasible. The patient must be included in discharge planning and provided with the information and support to make informed decisions about continuing care.

Recognition of alcohol withdrawal syndrome in a patient not previously known to abuse alcohol presents a particular challenge. Any unusual or disturbed behaviour should be reported immediately so that diagnosis can be made and treatment instituted.

DISCHARGE FROM THE POSTANAESTHESIA CARE UNIT

The patient leaving the PACU may be discharged to an intensive care unit, an inpatient unit, an ambulatory care unit, or home. The choice of discharge site is based on patient acuity, access to follow-up care, and the potential for postoperative complications. The decision to discharge the patient from the PACU is based on written discharge criteria, which can take the form of a standardized scoring system used to determine the patient's general condition and readiness for discharge. Examples of discharge criteria are provided in Table 22-10.

CARE OF THE POSTOPERATIVE PATIENT ON THE CLINICAL UNIT

Before discharging the patient from the PACU to the clinical unit, the PACU nurse should provide a verbal report about the patient to the receiving nurse. The report summarizes the operative and postanaesthetic period.

The nurse receiving the patient on the clinical unit assists PACU transport personnel in transferring the patient from the PACU stretcher onto the bed. Care must be taken to protect IV lines, wound drains, dressings, and traction devices. The use of a draw sheet or transfer board and sufficient personnel facilitates transfer of the patient.

On the clinical unit, vital signs should be obtained, and patient status should be compared with the report provided by the PACU. Documentation of the transfer is then completed, followed by a more in-depth assessment (Table 22-11). Postoperative orders and appropriate nursing care are then initiated.

Although many of the problems that may occur in the PACU are time limited to the immediate postoperative period, complications may occur during the extended postoperative recovery period on the clinical unit. Nursing assessment and management are based on awareness of the potential complications of surgery in general as well as complications specific to the surgical procedure. (A comprehensive nursing care plan for the postoperative patient is available on the Evolve website.)

PLANNING FOR DISCHARGE AND FOLLOW-UP CARE

Ambulatory and Inpatient Surgery Discharge

Ambulatory Surgery Discharge. Ambulatory surgery accounts for 75% to 80% of all surgical procedures in Canada (Keast & Swanson, 2014). Despite the obvious advantages of ambulatory surgery (e.g., patient convenience, lower health care costs), because these patients are in the health care setting for such a short time, it is difficult to complete all the required teaching. Optimally, the patient and any caregivers should be contacted 1 or more days before surgery to collect assessment data and to provide teaching that will be needed after surgery. The patient's lower anxiety level at this time may enhance learning.

The patient leaving an ambulatory surgery setting must be mobile and alert so as to be able to provide self-care when discharged to home. Postoperative pain must be controlled. Overall, the patient must be stable and near the level of preoperative functioning for discharge from the unit. On discharge, instructions specific to the type of anaesthesia received and the surgery are given to the patient and caregiver verbally and reinforced with written directions. The patient may not drive and must be accompanied by a responsible adult at the time of discharge. A follow-up evaluation of the patient's status is made by telephone, and any specific questions and concerns are addressed.

As more complex surgical procedures are being done on an ambulatory basis, the nurse should carefully determine not only readiness for discharge but also the home care needs of the individual, including availability of assistive personnel (e.g., family, friends), access to a pharmacy for prescriptions, access to a phone in the event of an emergency, and access to follow-up care.

Discharge From the Clinical Unit. Preparation for the patient's discharge should be an ongoing process throughout the surgical experience, beginning during the preoperative period. During the preoperative assessment, the nurse must determine if the patient will need additional health care support upon returning home. Arrangements for home care nurses and community resources are initiated so that they are in place when the patient is discharged. The patient is educated about what he or she will have to do postoperatively and, as events unfold, gradually assumes greater responsibility for self-care. As discharge approaches, the nurse should be certain that the patient and any caregivers have the following information:
- Care requirements for wound site and any dressings, including bathing recommendations
- Action and possible adverse effects of any medications and when and how to take them
- Activities allowed and prohibited; when various physical activities can be resumed safely (e.g., driving a car, returning to work, sexual intercourse, leisure activities)
- Dietary restrictions or modifications

TABLE 22-11 NURSING ASSESSMENT AND CARE OF PATIENT ON ADMISSION TO CLINICAL UNIT

General Anaesthetic Versus Spinal or Epidural Anaesthetic

General Anaesthetic

1. Verify patient identification using name band and medical record number.
2. Note any allergies and ensure presence of an allergy bracelet if applicable.
3. Record time of patient's return to unit.
4. Take baseline vital signs.
5. Assess airway and breath sounds.
6. Assess neurological status, including level of consciousness and movement of extremities.
7. Assess wound, wound closure and dressing, and drainage and nasogastric tubes.
   - Note length of tubing where applicable.
   - Ensure all drains and tubings are secured in place (minimizes risk of accidental discontinuation and resulting tissue trauma).
   - Note type and amount of drainage.
   - Note any packing to an open wound.
   - Connect tubing to gravity or suction drainage.
8. Assess colour and appearance of skin.
9. Assess urinary status.
   - Note time of voiding.
   - Note presence of catheter, if any, and total output.
   - Check for bladder distension or urge to void.
   - Note catheter patency; check integrity of insertion site and size of Foley catheter.
10. Assess pain and discomfort.
    - Note last dose and type of pain control.
    - Note current pain intensity.
11. Position for comfort and safety (bed in low position, side rails up).
12. Check IV infusion.
    - Note type of solution.
    - Note amount of fluid remaining.
    - Note flow rate.
13. Attach call light within patient's reach, and orient patient to its use.
14. Ensure that emesis basin and tissues are available.
15. Determine emotional condition and support needed.
16. Check for presence of family member or significant other.
17. Orient patient and family to immediate environment.
18. Check and carry out postoperative orders.

Spinal or Epidural Anaesthetic

1. Record time of patient's return to unit.
2. Take baseline vital signs.
3. Assess airway and breath sounds.
4. Assess neurological status, including level of consciousness and movement of extremities.
   - Assess spinal insertion or epidural insertion site; ensure that there is a continuous epidural infusion in place and that the dressing and catheter are secure.
   - Assess motor and sensory blockade from spinal anaesthetic.
5. Assess wound, wound closure, dressing, and drainage tubes.
   - Note type and amount of drainage.
   - Note any packing to an open wound.
   - Connect tubing to gravity or suction drainage.
6. Assess colour and appearance of skin.
7. Assess urinary status.
   - Note time of voiding.
   - Note presence of catheter, if any, and total output.
   - Check for bladder distension or urge to void.
   - Note catheter patency; check integrity of insertion site and size of Foley catheter.
8. Assess pain and discomfort.
   - Note last dose and type of pain control.
   - Note current pain intensity.
9. Position for comfort and safety (bed in low position, side rails up).
10. Check IV infusion.
    - Note type of solution.
    - Note amount of fluid remaining.
    - Note flow rate.
11. Attach call light within patient's reach, and orient patient to its use.
12. Ensure that emesis basin and tissues are available.
13. Determine emotional condition and support.
14. Check for presence of family member or significant other.
15. Orient patient and family to immediate environment.
16. Check and carry out postoperative orders.

IV, intravenous.

- Symptoms to be reported (e.g., development of incisional tenderness or increased drainage, discomfort in other parts of the body)
- Where and when to return for follow-up care
- Answers to any individual questions or concerns

The nurse should specifically document in the record the discharge instructions provided to the patient and family. For the patient, the postoperative phase of care continues and extends into the recuperative period. Assessment and evaluation of the patient after discharge may be accomplished by a follow-up call or by a visit from a nurse (e.g., home health nurse).

Increasingly, patients with many medical or surgical needs are being discharged from hospital. They may be transferred to transitional care facilities, to long-term care facilities, or directly to their homes (see Chapter 6). When discharged directly to home, it is expected that the patient, with assistance from family, friends, or home health care services, will continue self-care in the home. This may include dressing changes, wound care, catheter or drain care, home antibiotics, or continued physical therapy. Working through the discharge planner for the hospital unit or

through the case manager, the nurse can facilitate the transition of care from hospital-based to community-based without jeopardizing the quality of care.

INFORMATICS IN PRACTICE

Discharge Teaching

If the nurse is discharging a patient who requires a complex dressing change and thinks that written instructions are not adequate, the nurse should consider using a video either on the hospital's television system or from the Internet (e.g., YouTube). If using a video from the Internet, the nurse should check it first to ensure that the procedure is properly done. The nurse could also take a series of pictures that demonstrate how to perform the procedure. The patient and caregiver can view the video or pictures at home as a reference when performing the procedure.

AGE-RELATED CONSIDERATIONS

PATIENT AFTER SURGERY

Aging is a chronological, functional, and physiological process, and all these factors must be considered when determining the postoperative needs of the older patient. The nurse should understand that normal aging and chronic disease can impact surgical outcomes (Papanier Wells & Flanagan, 2015). The older adult has decreased respiratory function and ability to cough, due to reduced thoracic compliance. These alterations in pulmonary status increase the work of ventilation and decrease the ability to eliminate some pharmacological agents. Reactions to anaesthetic agents must be carefully monitored and their postoperative elimination assessed before the patient is left without close supervision. Pneumonia is a common postoperative complication in older adults.

Vascular function in the older adult is altered because of atherosclerosis and decreased elasticity in the blood vessels. Cardiac function is often compromised, and compensatory responses to changes in BP and fluid volume are limited. Circulating blood volume is decreased, and hypertension is common. Cardiovascular parameters must be closely monitored throughout surgery and the postoperative period.

Drug toxicity is a potential problem in the older adult as renal perfusion decreases, thus reducing elimination of drugs excreted by the kidney. Decreased liver function also leads to decreased drug metabolism and thus increased drug activity. Renal and liver function must be carefully assessed in the postoperative phase of the patient's care to prevent drug overdose and toxicity.

Observing for changes in mental status is an important part of postoperative care in older adults. Predisposing factors for postoperative delirium in this population include such things as >80 years old, alcohol abuse, lower education level, polypharmacy, sensory impairments, low mobility, and major surgery. Anaesthetics, notably anticholinergic drugs and benzodiazepines, increase the risk for delirium. One way for the nurse to lessen delirium is to ensure adequate postoperative pain control (Papanier Wells & Flanagan, 2015). An acute change in mental status can have a potentially reversible cause, such as an infection or an adverse effect of analgesic medication. (Dementia and delirium are discussed in Chapter 62.)

Pain is a multidimensional experience, and assessment should include how pain affects function, mood, activities, and quality of life. Older patients are at great risk for undertreated pain. They may be hesitant to request pain medication, believing that pain is an inevitable consequence of surgery and that acknowledging it is a sign of weakness. Nurses must be alert to nonverbal indications of pain and should also assess pain using a standardized scale that is explained to the patient each time it is used. The presence of postoperative pain should always be assumed in the cognitively impaired patient who cannot reliably respond (Papanier Wells & Flanagan, 2015). Surgery will usually result in pain, and, if untreated, pain could have a negative effect on recovery. (Pain is discussed in Chapter 10.)

A comprehensive, multidisciplinary approach is recommended when caring for older adults, and all health care personnel delivering geriatric care must be educated in it and competent. When older adults undergo surgery, nurses have the opportunity to enhance outcomes and improve the patient's quality of life (Papanier Wells & Flanagan, 2015)

CASE STUDY

Patient After Surgery

Source: Blend Images/Shutterstock.com.

Patient Profile

Edward Lee, a 74-year-old retired university professor, has just undergone surgery for a fractured hip. He fell off a ladder while painting his house. Mr. Lee's medical history includes type 2 diabetes and COPD. The surgery, performed while the patient was under general anaesthesia, lasted 3 hours.

Subjective Data

- Walks 30 to 50 km/wk
- Smokes one pack of cigarettes per day × 58 years
- Has always had problems sleeping
- Has difficulty hearing; wears hearing aid
- Is upset with injury and its impact on his life
- Is a widower and has no relatives or friends nearby who are able to assist with care
- Reports pain is 8 on a 0-to-10 scale on arrival to PACU

Objective Data

- Admitted to PACU with abduction pillow between his legs, one peripheral IV catheter, a self-suction drain from the hip dressing, an in-dwelling urinary catheter
- Oxygen (O₂) saturation 91% on 40% O₂ face mask

Interprofessional Care
Postoperative Orders

- Vital signs per PACU routine
- Capillary blood glucose level on arrival and every 4 hours: Call for blood glucose level <3.9 mmol/L to >13.9 mmol/L; follow employer guidelines for management of hypoglycemia
- 0.45% normal saline at 100 mL/hr
- Morphine via patient-controlled analgesia 1 mg q10min (20 mg max in 4 hr) for pain
- Advance diet as tolerated
- Incentive spirometry q1hr × 10 while awake
- O₂ therapy to keep O₂ saturation >90%
- Respiratory: Ventolin 2.5 mg via nebulizer every 4 hours PRN for wheezing
- Neuro-vascular checks q1hr × 4 hours
- Empty and measure self-suction drain every shift
- Strict intake and output

Discussion Questions

1. What are the potential postanaesthesia problems with Mr. Lee?
2. **Priority decision:** What priority nursing interventions would be appropriate to prevent these problems from occurring?
3. What factors may predispose Mr. Lee to the following problems: atelectasis, infection, pulmonary embolism, and nausea and vomiting?
4. What criteria would determine when Mr. Lee is sufficiently recovered from general anaesthesia to be discharged to the clinical unit?
5. What potential postoperative problems on the clinical unit might be expected?
6. **Priority decision:** Based on the assessment data presented, what are two priority nursing diagnoses? Are there any collaborative problems?

ⓔvolve

Answers are available at *http://evolve.elsevier.com/Canada/Lewis/medsurg/*.

REVIEW QUESTIONS

The number of the question corresponds to the same-numbered objective at the beginning of the chapter.

1. When a client is admitted to the PACU, what are the *priority* interventions the nurse performs?
   a. Assess the surgical site, noting presence and character of drainage.
   b. Assess the amount of urine output and the presence of bladder distension.
   c. Assess for airway patency and quality of respirations and obtain vital signs.
   d. Review results of intraoperative laboratory values and medications received.

2. A client is admitted to the PACU after major abdominal surgery. During the initial assessment, the client tells the nurse he thinks he is "going to throw up." What would be the *priority* nursing intervention?
   a. Increase the rate of the IV fluids.
   b. Obtain vital signs, including O_2 saturation.
   c. Position client in lateral recovery position.
   d. Administer antiemetic medication as ordered.

3. After admission of the postoperative client to the clinical unit, which assessment data require the *most* immediate attention?
   a. O_2 saturation of 85%
   b. Respiratory rate of 13/min
   c. Temperature of 38°C
   d. Blood pressure of 90/60 mm Hg

4. A 70-kg postoperative client has an average urine output of 25 mL/hr during the first 8 hours. Given this assessment, what would the *priority* nursing intervention(s) be?
   a. Perform a straight catheterization to measure the amount of urine in the bladder.

   b. Notify the physician and anticipate obtaining blood work to evaluate renal function.
   c. Continue to monitor the client because this is a normal finding during this time period.
   d. Evaluate the client's fluid volume status since surgery and obtain a bladder ultrasound.

5. The nurse on the postoperative unit is caring for a client who had a laparoscopic partial colectomy. On postoperative day 2, the client is complaining of abdominal distension and discomfort. Which of the following interventions may be appropriate for this client? (*Select all that apply*)
   a. Increase the dose of opioids for pain relief.
   b. Insert a nasogastric tube.
   c. Reassure the client that this complication should subside in a day or two.
   d. Monitor the client's abdominal girth by measuring for distension and auscultate the abdomen in all four quadrants.

6. Discharge criteria for the Phase II client include which of the following? (*Select all that apply*)
   a. No nausea or vomiting
   b. Ability to drive himself or herself home
   c. No respiratory depression
   d. Written discharge instructions understood
   e. Opioid pain medication given 45 minutes ago

1. c; 2. c; 3. a; 4. d; 5. b, c, d; 6. c, d, e.

⊖volve

For even more review questions, see the website for this book at *http://evolve.elsevier.com/Canada/Lewis/medsurg.*

REFERENCES

Beitland, S., Sandven, I., Kjærvik, L. K., et al. (2015). Thromboprophylaxis with low molecular weight heparin versus unfractionated heparin in intensive care patients: A systematic review with meta-analysis and trial sequential analysis. *Intensive Care Medicine, 41*(7), 1209–2119. doi:10.1007/s00134-015-3840-z.

Cagir, B. (2016). Postoperative ileus. *Medscape.* Retrieved from *http://emedicine.medscape.com/article/2242141-overview.*

Canadian Association of Wound Care and Canadian Association for Enterostomal Therapy. (2011). *The wound care instrument: Collaborative appraisal and recommendations for education.* Retrieved from *https://caet.ca/wp-content/uploads/2015/02/caet-wound-care-instrument.pdf.*

Canadian Nurses Association (CNA). (2013). *Optimizing the role of nursing in home health.* Retrieved from *http://cna-aiic.ca/~/media/cna/page-content/pdf-en/optimizing_the_role_of_nursing_in_home_health_e.pdf.*

Centers for Disease Control and Prevention. (2017). *Surgical site infection (SSI) event.* Retrieved from *https://www.cdc.gov/nhsn/pdfs/pscmanual/9pscssicurrent.pdf.*

Dowsett, C., Protz, K., Drouard, M., et al. (2015). Triangle of wound assessment. *Wounds International.* Retrieved from *http://www.woundsinternational.com/media/other-resources/_/1189/files/twa-made-easy_web.pdf.*

Jackson, D. (2015). Gastrointestinal surgery. In J. Rothrock (Ed.), *Alexander's care of the patient in surgery* (15th ed., pp. 295–349). St. Louis: Elsevier.

Keast, D., & Swanson, T. (2014). Ten top tips: Managing surgical site infections. *Wounds International, 5*(3), 13–18. Retrieved from *http://www.woundinfection-institute.com/wp-content/uploads/2014/11/SSI_11422.pdf.*

Odom-Forren, J. (2013). *Drain's perianesthesia nursing: A critical care approach* (6th ed.). St. Louis: Elsevier.

Odom-Forren, J. (2014). Postanesthesia recovery. In J. Nagelhout & K. Plaus (Eds.), *Nurse anesthesia* (5th ed., pp. 1224–1243). St. Louis: Elsevier.

Odom-Forren, J. (2015). Postoperative pain care and pain management. In J. Rothrock (Ed.), *Alexander's care of the patient in surgery* (15th ed., pp. 280–281). St. Louis: Elsevier.

Papanier Wells, M., & Flanagan, A. (2015). Geriatric surgery. In J. Rothrock (Ed.), *Alexander's care of the patient in surgery* (15th ed., pp. 1081–1103). St. Louis: Elsevier.

Peterson, C. (2013). The hepatobiliary and gastrointestinal system. In J. Odom-Forren (Ed.), *Drain's perianesthesia nursing: A critical care approach* (6th ed., pp. 214–221). St. Louis: Elsevier.

Registered Nurses' Association of Ontario. (2016). *Delirium, dementia and depression in older adults: Assessment and care* (2nd ed.). Retrieved from *http://rnao.ca/bpg/guidelines/screening-delirium-dementia-and-depression-older-adult.*

Rieker, M. (2014). Respiratory anatomy, physiology, pathophysiology and anesthetic management. In J. Nagelhout & K. Plaus (Eds.), *Nurse anesthesia* (pp. 590–661). St. Louis: Elsevier.

Rothrock, J. (2015). *Alexander's care of the patient in surgery* (15th ed.). St. Louis: Elsevier.

RESOURCES

Allergy and Asthma Information Association
http://www.aaia.ca

Canadian Allergy, Asthma, and Immunology Foundation
http://www.allergyfoundation.ca

Canadian Anesthesiologists' Society
http://www.cas.ca

Canadian Pain Society
http://www.canadianpainsociety.ca

National Association of PeriAnesthesia Nurses of Canada
http://www.napanc.org

Operating Room Nurses Association of Canada
http://www.ornac.ca

Registered Nurses' Association of Ontario
http://rnao.ca

Wounds Canada
https://www.woundscanada.ca/index.php

American College of Surgeons
http://www.facs.org

American Latex Allergy Association
http://latexallergyresources.org

American Society of Anesthesiologists
http://www.asahq.org

American Society of PeriAnesthesia Nurses (ASPAN)
http://www.aspan.org

Association of PeriOperative Registered Nurses (AORN)
http://www.aorn.org

For additional Internet resources, see the website for this book at *http://evolve.elsevier.com/Canada/Lewis/medsurg.*

Problems Related to Altered Sensory Input

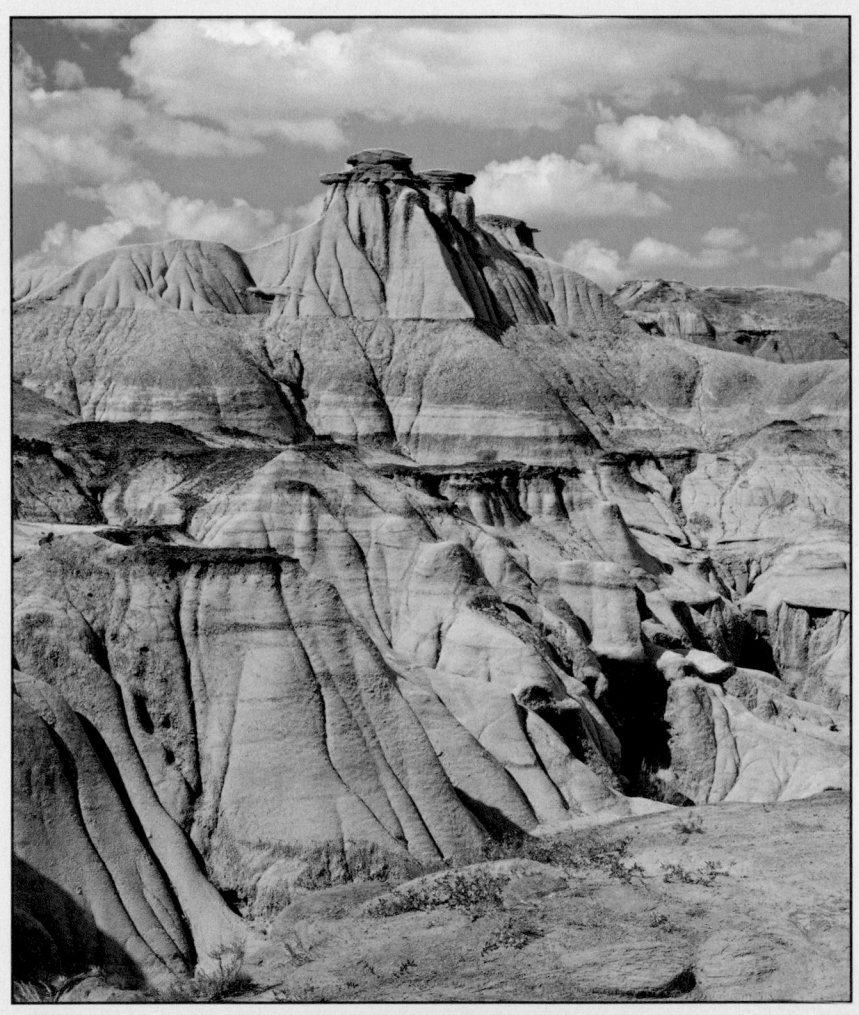

Source: Elena Elisseeva/Shutterstock.com.

23

Nursing Assessment
Visual and Auditory Systems

Written by: Sharon L. Lewis
Adapted by: Marian Luctkar-Flude

℮volve WEBSITE

http://evolve.elsevier.com/Canada/Lewis/medsurg

- Review Questions (Online Only)
- Key Points
- Answer Guidelines for Case Study
- Conceptual Care Map Creator

- Audio Glossary
- Supporting Media—Animation
  - Weber Test
- Content Updates

LEARNING OBJECTIVES

1. Describe the structures and functions of the visual and auditory systems.
2. Describe the physiological processes involved in normal vision and hearing.
3. Identify the significant subjective and objective assessment data related to the visual and auditory systems that should be obtained from the patient.
4. Describe the appropriate techniques used in the physical assessment of the visual and auditory systems.

5. Differentiate normal from common abnormal findings of a physical assessment of the visual and auditory systems.
6. Explain how age-related changes in the visual and auditory systems correspond to differences in assessment findings.
7. Describe the purpose, the significance of results, and the nursing responsibilities related to diagnostic studies of the visual and auditory systems.

KEY TERMS

accommodation, p. 441	hyperopia, p. 440	PERRLA, p. 448	sclera, p. 441
aqueous humor, p. 440	lens, p. 440	presbycusis, p. 452	tinnitus, p. 452
astigmatism, p. 440	myopia, p. 440	presbyopia, p. 440	vertigo, p. 452
conjunctiva, p. 441	nystagmus, p. 452	retina, p. 441	

THE VISUAL SYSTEM

STRUCTURES AND FUNCTIONS

The visual system consists of the external tissues and structures surrounding the eye, the external and internal structures of the eye, the refractive media, and the visual pathway. The external structures are the eyebrows, eyelids, eyelashes, lacrimal system, conjunctiva, cornea, sclera, and extraocular muscles. The internal structures are the iris, lens, ciliary body, choroid, and retina. The entire visual system is important for visual function. Light reflected from an object in the field of vision passes through the transparent structures of the eye and, in doing so, is *refracted* (bent) so that a clear image can fall on the retina. From the retina, the visual stimuli travel through the visual pathway to the occipital cortex, where they are perceived as an image.

Structures and Functions of Vision

Eyeball. The eyeball, or globe, is composed of three layers (Figure 23-1). The tough outer layer is composed of the sclera and the transparent cornea. The middle layer consists of the uveal tract (iris, choroid, and ciliary body), and the innermost layer is the retina. The anterior chamber lies between the iris and the posterior surface of the cornea, whereas the posterior chamber lies between the anterior surface of the lens and the posterior surface of the iris. These chambers are filled with aqueous humor secreted by the ciliary body. The anatomic space *(vitreous cavity)* between the posterior lens and the retina is filled with a gel substance *(vitreous humor,* or *vitreous).*

Refractive Media. For light to reach the retina, it must pass through a number of structures: the cornea, the aqueous humor, the lens, and the vitreous humor. All of these structures must remain clear for light to reach the retina and stimulate the

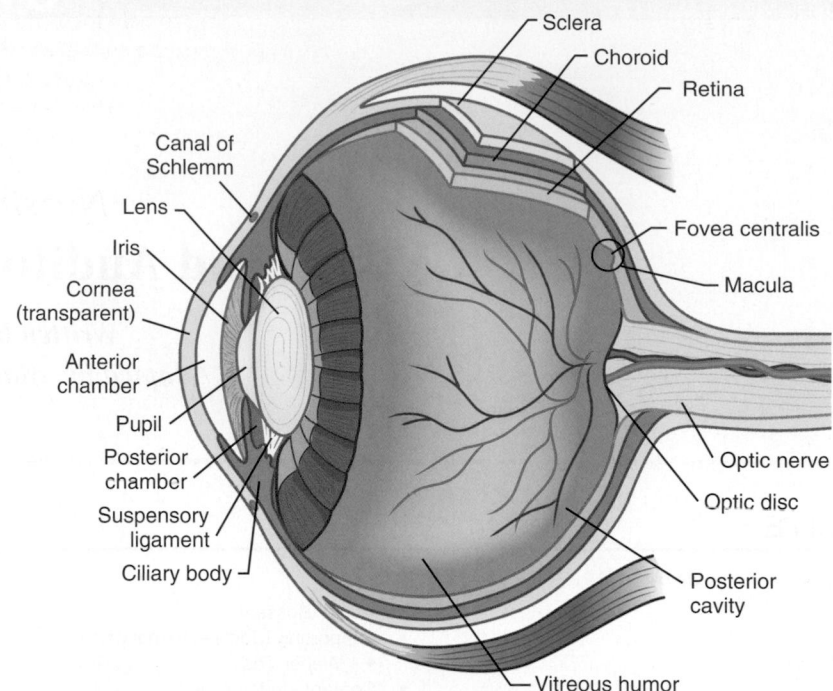

FIGURE 23-1 The human eye. Source: Adapted from Patton, K. T., & Thibodeau, G. A. (2013). *Anatomy and physiology* (8th ed., p. 527). St. Louis: Mosby.

photoreceptor cells. The cornea, which is normally transparent, is the first structure through which light passes. It is responsible for the majority of light refraction necessary for clear vision.

Aqueous humor, produced by the ciliary process, is a clear, watery fluid that fills the anterior and posterior chambers of the anterior cavity of the eye. It bathes and nourishes the lens and the endothelium of the cornea. It drains through the trabecular meshwork located in the angle. This circular canal conveys fluid into scleral veins, which enter the circulation of the body. Normal intraocular pressure is between 10 and 21 mm Hg; excess production or decreased outflow of the aqueous humor can cause an elevation in this pressure, a condition termed *glaucoma.*

The lens is a biconvex structure located behind the iris and supported in place by small fibres collectively called the *suspensory ligament* (also called the *zonule*) that connect the lens to the ciliary body. The primary function of the lens is to bend light rays, which enables them to fall onto the retina. Anything altering the clarity of the lens affects light transmission.

Vitreous humor is located in the vitreous cavity, the large area behind the lens and in front of the retina (see Figure 23-1). Light passing through the vitreous humor may be blocked by any nontransparent substance within, such as the cellular debris (often called *floaters*). The effect on vision varies, depending on the amount, type, and location of the substance blocking the light.

Refractive Errors. *Refraction* is the ability of the eye to bend light rays so that they fall on the retina. In the normal eye, parallel light rays are focused through the lens into a sharp image on the retina. The state that enables this process is termed *emmetropia,* which means that light is focused exactly on the retina, not in front of it or behind it. The condition in which the light does not focus properly is called a *refractive error.*

The individual with myopia can see near objects clearly (nearsightedness), but objects in the distance appear blurred. The individual with hyperopia can see distant objects clearly (farsightedness), but near objects appear blurred. Astigmatism is an imperfection in the curvature of the cornea or in the shape of the eye's lens that causes blurred or distorted vision for both near and far objects. Presbyopia is a normal aging change in which the lens of the eye loses its elasticity and flexibility, which results in an inability to focus on close objects, usually beginning at approximately age 40.

Visual Pathways. Once the image travels through the refractive media, it is focused on the retina, inverted, and reversed left to right. For example, if the visualized object is in the upper part of the left temporal visual field, it is focused in the lower part of the nasal retina, upside down, and as a mirror image. From the retina, the impulses travel through the optic nerve to the optic chiasm, where the nasal fibres of each eye cross over to the other side. The optic chiasm is the X-shaped space just in front of the pituitary gland where the optic nerve fibres partially cross. Fibres from the left field of both eyes form the left optic tract and travel to the left occipital cortex. The fibres from the right field of both eyes form the right optic tract and travel to the right occipital cortex. Because of this arrangement of the nerve fibres in the visual pathways, it is possible to determine the anatomical location of abnormalities in those nerve fibres from the specific visual field defect (Figure 23-2).

External Structures and Functions

Eyebrows, Eyelids, and Eyelashes. Eyebrows, eyelids, and eyelashes serve an important role in protecting the eye. They provide a physical barrier to dust and foreign particles. The eye is further protected by the surrounding bony orbit and by fat pads located below and behind the *globe,* or eyeball.

The upper and lower eyelids join at the medial and lateral canthi. The upper eyelid blinks spontaneously approximately 15 times a minute. Blinking distributes tears over the anterior surface of the eyeball and helps control the amount of light entering the visual pathway (Figure 23-3).

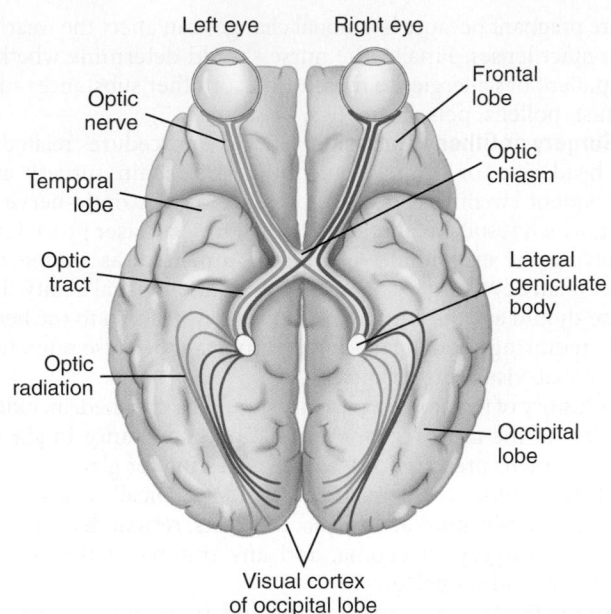

FIGURE 23-2 The visual pathway. Fibres from the nasal portion of each retina cross over to the opposite side of the optic chiasm, terminating in the lateral geniculate body of the opposite side. The location of a lesion in the visual pathway determines the resulting visual defect.

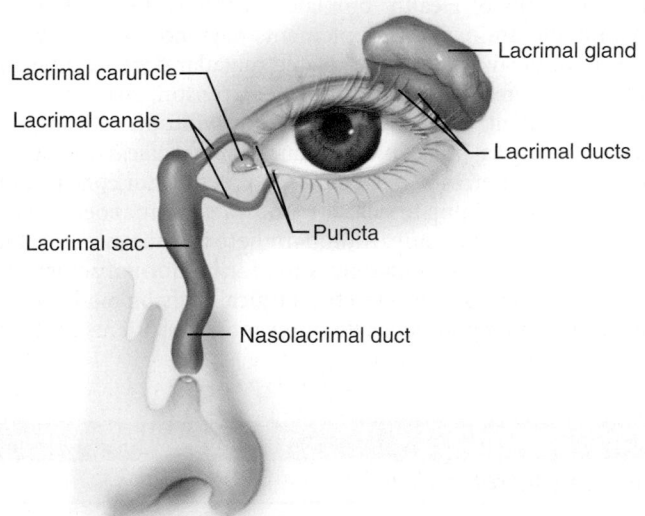

FIGURE 23-3 External eye and lacrimal apparatus. Tears produced in the lacrimal gland pass over the surface of the eye and enter the lacrimal canal. From there, the tears are carried through the nasolacrimal duct to the nasal cavity.

The eyelids open and close through the action of muscles innervated by cranial nerve (CN) VII, which is the facial nerve. Muscular action also helps hold the eyelids against the eyeball.

The **conjunctiva** is a transparent mucous membrane that covers the inner surfaces of the eyelids (the palpebral conjunctiva) and extends over the **sclera** (the bulbar conjunctiva), forming a "pocket" under each eyelid. Glands in the conjunctiva secrete mucus and tears. The sclera, an opaque structure commonly referred to as the "white" of the eye, is formed by collagen fibres meshed together. The sclera forms a tough shell that helps protect the intraocular structures.

The transparent and avascular cornea allows light to enter the eye (see Figure 23-1). The curved cornea refracts (bends) incoming light rays to help focus them on the retina. The cornea consists of six layers: the epithelium, Bowman's layer, the stroma, Dua's layer, Descemet's membrane, and the endothelium (Dua, Faraj, Said, et al., 2013). The epithelium consists of a layer of cells that helps protect the eye. Epithelial cells regenerate when damaged. The stroma consists of collagen fibrils. The cornea is maintained by the lacrimal system, which consists of the lacrimal gland and ducts, the lacrimal canals and puncta, the lacrimal sac, and the nasolacrimal duct (Figure 23-3). In addition to the lacrimal gland, other glands provide secretions to make up the mucous, aqueous, and lipid layers of the tear film. The tear film moistens the eye and provides oxygen to the cornea.

Each eye is moved by three pairs of extraocular muscles and controlled by three cranial nerves: (a) superior and inferior rectus muscles (CN III), (b) medial (CN III) and lateral rectus muscles (CN VI), and (c) superior (CN IV) and inferior oblique muscles (CN III). Neuro-muscular coordination enables simultaneous movement of the eyes in the same direction (conjugate movement).

Internal Structures and Functions

The iris (plural: irides) is the colourful part of the eye. This structure has a small, round opening in its centre, the pupil, which allows light to enter the eye. The pupil constricts through action of the iris sphincter muscle (innervated by CN III [oculomotor nerve]) and dilates through action of the iris dilator muscle (innervated by CN V [trigeminal nerve]) to control the amount of light that enters the eye.

The lens, as described previously, is a structure behind the iris whose function is to bend light rays so that they fall onto the retina. The shape of the lens is modified by action of the ciliary body as part of **accommodation,** the convergence of the eyes and the constriction of the pupils that occurs when the eyes refocus from a far object to a near object. This enables a person to focus on near objects, as in reading a book. The choroid is a highly vascular structure that nourishes the ciliary body, the iris, and the outer portion of the retina. It lies inside and parallel to the sclera and extends from the area where the optic nerve enters the eye to the ciliary body (see Figure 23-1). The ciliary body consists of the ciliary muscles, which surround the lens and lie parallel to the sclera; the ciliary zonules, which attach to the lens capsule; and the ciliary processes, which constitute the terminal portion of the ciliary body. The ciliary processes lie behind the peripheral part of the iris and secrete aqueous humor.

The **retina** is the innermost layer of the eye that extends and gives rise to the optic nerve. Neurons make up the major portion of the retina. Therefore, retinal cells cannot regenerate if destroyed. The retina lines the inside the eyeball, extending from the area of the optic nerve to the ciliary body (see Figure 23-1). It is responsible for converting images into a form that the brain can understand and process as vision. The retina is composed of two types of photoreceptor cells: rods and cones. Rods are stimulated in dim or darkened environments, and cones are receptive to colours in bright environments. The centre of the retina is the *fovea centralis*, a pinpoint depression composed only of densely packed cones (Thibodeau & Patton, 2012). This area of the retina provides the sharpest visual acuity. Surrounding the fovea is the *macula,* an area smaller than 1 square millimetre, which has a high concentration of cones and is relatively free of blood vessels. With the exception of the macula, the retina is nourished by retinal arterioles and veins. This blood supply enters the eye through the optic disc, located nasally from the macula. The optic disc is the area where the optic nerve (CN II) exits the eyeball. Within the disc is the physiological cup, a depression that can be visualized through the pupil with the ophthalmoscope. The retinal veins and arteries can also be visualized in this way and can provide information about the condition of the vascular system in general.

AGE-RELATED CONSIDERATIONS

THE VISUAL SYSTEM

Every structure of the visual system is subject to changes as the individual ages. Whereas many of these changes are relatively benign, others may compromise visual acuity severely in the older adult. The psychosocial effect of poor vision or blindness can be highly significant. Visual impairment increases with age; the number of people with vision loss doubles every decade after age 40 and triples after age 75 (National Coalition for Vision Health, 2011). Age-related changes in the visual system and differences in assessment findings are presented in Table 23-1.

ASSESSMENT

Assessment of the visual system may be as simple as determining a patient's visual acuity or as complex as collecting complete subjective and objective data pertinent to the visual system. To perform an appropriate ophthalmic evaluation, the nurse must determine which parts of the data collection are important for each patient. Table 23-2 lists suggested questions to ask while the health history is documented, to obtain subjective data related to the visual system.

Subjective Data

Past Health History. Information about the patient's health history should include both ocular and nonocular history. The nurse should ask specifically about systemic diseases—such as diabetes, hypertension, cancer, rheumatoid arthritis, sexually transmitted infections, acquired immune deficiency syndrome, muscular dystrophy, myasthenia gravis, multiple sclerosis, inflammatory bowel disease, and hypothyroidism or hyperthyroidism—because many of these diseases have ocular manifestations. It is particularly important to determine whether the patient has any history of cardiac or pulmonary disease because the eye drops often used to treat glaucoma (β-adrenergic blockers) may have serious adverse effects, including bradycardia, orthostatic hypotension, bronchospasm, and heart failure (Skidmore-Roth, 2012).

Medications. If the patient takes any medications, the nurse should obtain a complete list, including over-the-counter medicines, eye drops, herbal therapies, or dietary supplements. Many patients do not think that over-the-counter drugs, eye drops, or herbal therapies are "real" medications and may not mention their use unless specifically questioned. However, many of these drugs have ocular effects. For example, many preparations for colds contain a form of epinephrine (e.g., pseudoephedrine) that can dilate the pupil. The nurse should also note the use of any antihistamines or decongestants because these drugs can cause ocular dryness. The nurse should specifically ask whether the patient uses any prescription drugs such as corticosteroids, thyroid medications, oral hypoglycemic agents, or insulin. Long-term use of corticosteroids can contribute to development of glaucoma or cataracts. It is especially important to note whether the patient is taking any β-adrenergic blocker eye drops because they may potentiate the effects of corticosteroids. The nurse should also ask female patients whether they are taking birth control pills or are pregnant because hormonal changes can affect the wearing of contact lenses. Finally, the nurse should determine whether the patient has allergies to medications or other substances such as dust, pollens, pets, cosmetics, or scents.

Surgery or Other Treatments. Surgical procedures related to the head, eye, or brain should be noted. Brain surgery and subsequent swelling can cause pressure on the optic nerve or tract, which results in alterations in vision. Any laser procedures involving the eye should also be documented, as should the effect of any eye surgery or laser treatment on visual acuity. The nurse should ask the patient about previous trauma to the head. Also, inquiring about headaches is important because migraines may create visual disturbances.

A history of tests for visual acuity should be obtained, including the date of the most recent examination and change in glasses or contact lens prescriptions, as well as testing for glaucoma and what the results were. The nurse should specifically ask about a history of strabismus, amblyopia, cataracts, retinal detachment, refractive surgery, glaucoma, and any trauma to the eye, its treatment, and sequelae.

The patient's intake of vitamins and trace minerals can be important to ocular health. Supplementation with vitamins C and E, minerals copper and zinc, and the phytochemicals lutein and zeaxanthin may help delay the progression of eye diseases such as age-related macular degeneration (Age-Related Eye Disease Study 2 [AREDS2] Research Group, 2013). (See the "Determinants of Health" box later in this section.) However, vitamin and antioxidant supplements have not been shown to prevent or delay onset of age-related macular degeneration and may have harmful effects (Evans & Lawrenson, 2012).

For a patient who has undergone or will undergo ophthalmological surgical procedures, the nurse should assess the patient's elimination pattern and determine the potential for constipation, inasmuch as straining to defecate (the Valsalva manoeuvre) can raise intraocular pressure. Although there is some evidence that elevation of the intraocular pressure during normal activities is not detrimental in relation to the surgical incision made during eye surgery, many surgeons do not want such patients to strain.

CASE STUDY

Patient Introduction

Source: Zurijeta/
Shutterstock
.com.

Fatimah Abdullah is an 81-year-old woman who comes to the emergency department with the complaint that her vision "looks like everything is covered with spider webs."

Critical Thinking

Throughout this assessment chapter, think about Ms. Abdullah with the following questions in mind:

1. What are possible causes of Ms. Abdullah's visual disturbances?
2. What type of assessment should be most appropriate: comprehensive, focused, or emergency?
3. What questions should the nurse ask Ms. Abdullah?
4. What should be included in the physical assessment? What would the nurse be looking for?
5. What diagnostic studies might be ordered?

See pp. 445 and 448 for more information on Ms. Abdullah.

evolve
Answers available at *http://evolve.elsevier.com/Canada/Lewis/medsurg*.

TABLE 23-1 AGE-RELATED DIFFERENCES IN ASSESSMENT

Visual System

Changes	Differences in Assessment Findings
Eyebrows and Eyelashes	
Loss of pigment in the hair	Greying of eyebrows, eyelashes
Eyelids	
Loss of orbital fat, decreased muscle tone	Entropion, ectropion, mild ptosis
Tissue atrophy, prolapse of fat into eyelid tissue	Blepharodermachalasis (excessive upper eyelid skin)
Plaques	Xanthelasma
Conjunctiva	
Tissue damage related to chronic exposure to ultraviolet light or to other chronic environmental exposure	Pinguecula (small, yellowish spot seen usually on the medial aspect of the conjunctiva)
Sclera	
Lipid deposition	Yellowish (as opposed to bluish) scleral colour
Cornea	
Cholesterol deposits in peripheral cornea	Arcus senilis (milky or yellow ring encircling periphery of cornea; see Figure 23-1)
Tissue damage related to chronic exposure	Pterygium (thickened, triangular bit of pale tissue that extends from the inner canthus of the eye to the nasal border of the cornea)
Decrease in water content, atrophy of nerve fibres	Decreased corneal sensitivity and corneal reflex
Epithelial changes	Loss of corneal lustre
Accumulation of lipid deposits	Blurring of vision
Lacrimal Apparatus	
Decreased tear secretion	Dryness
Malposition of the eyelid that results in tears overflowing the eyelid margins instead of draining through the puncta	Tearing, irritated eyes
Iris	
Increased rigidity of iris	Decreased pupil size
Dilator muscle atrophy or weakness	Slower recovery of pupil size after light stimulation
Loss of pigment	Change of iris colour
Shrinking and stiffening of ciliary muscle	Decrease in near vision and accommodation
Lens	
Biochemical changes in lens proteins, oxidative damage, chronic exposure to ultraviolet light	Cataracts
Increased rigidity of lens	Presbyopia
Opacities in the lens (may also be related to opacities in the cornea and the vitreous humor)	Complaints of glare, impairment of night vision
Accumulation of yellow substances	Yellow colouring of lens
Retina	
Retinal vascular changes related to atherosclerosis and hypertension	Narrowed, pale, straighter arterioles; acute branching
Decrease in cones	Changes in colour perception, especially blue and violet
Loss of photoreceptor cells, retinal pigment, epithelial cells, and melanin	Decreased visual acuity
Age-related macular degeneration as a result of vascular changes	Loss of central vision
Vitreous Humor	
Liquefaction and detachment of the vitreous humor	Increased complaints of "floaters" or light flashes

Self-Care History. The nurse should assess the patient's ocular health care activities, including regular eye examinations and awareness of the importance of eye safety practices, such as wearing protective eyewear during potentially hazardous activities or while playing sports and avoiding noxious fumes and other eye irritants. Information about the use of sunglasses in bright light should be obtained as prolonged exposure to ultraviolet light can affect the retina and may contribute to cataract formation. Nighttime driving habits and any problems encountered in nighttime driving should be noted. For a patient who wears contact lenses, the nurse should assess the patient's use and care

habits, which may indicate a need for teaching, inasmuch as many contact lens wearers do not care for them properly (Wu, Willcox, & Stapleton, 2015). The nurse should ask about time spent working on computers or handheld devices because eye strain is a common problem. The 20/20 rule can be promoted: Every 20 minutes, patients should look away from their computer screen for 20 seconds (American Optometric Association, 2015).

Environmental exposures at home or work can cause trauma or irritation to the eyes; eye protection should be discussed. Patients should be asked whether they smoke or are regularly exposed to second-hand smoke. Smokers are at greater risk for

TABLE 23-2 HEALTH HISTORY

Visual System: Questions for Obtaining Subjective Data

Vision Difficulty
- Do you have any visual difficulties or change in your visual acuity?* Describe the change in your vision. Describe how this affects your daily life.
- Did it come on slowly or progress slowly? Does it affect one or both eyes? Is it constant or intermittent? Do you see spots or floaters move in front of your eyes?* Do you see light flashes?*
- Do you have a blind spot?* Do you have any night blindness?*
- For older adults: Are you experiencing any visual difficulties when you climb stairs or drive at night?
- Do you use any visual aids such as glasses or contact lenses?

Eye Pain
- Do you have any eye pain?*

Strabismus or Diplopia
- Have you ever had a history of crossed eyes, or do you have double vision?*

Redness or Swelling
- Do you have redness or swelling in your eyes?*
- Do you have any discharge or watering from your eyes?*

Family History
- Do you have a family or personal history of diseases such as atherosclerosis, diabetes, thyroid disease, hypertension, arthritis, or cancer that might affect your eyes?*
- Do you have a family or personal history of ocular problems such as cataracts, tumours, glaucoma, refractive errors (especially myopia and hyperopia), or retinal degenerative conditions (e.g., macular degeneration, retinal detachment, retinitis pigmentosa)?*

Nutrition and Elimination
- Do you take any nutritional supplements?*
- Does your visual problem affect your ability to obtain and prepare food?*
- Do you have to strain to void or defecate?*

Sleep
- Is your vision affected by the amount of sleep you get?*
- Is your sleep affected by your eye problem?*

Reproduction–Sexuality
- Has your eye problem caused a change in your sex life?*
- For women: Are you pregnant? Do you use birth control pills?

Self-Care History
- Do you have regular eye examinations? When was your last test?
- Do you wear glasses or contact lenses? When was the last time your eye prescription was checked? Was it changed?
- Have you ever been tested for colour vision?*
- Do you wear protective eyewear (sunglasses, safety goggles, or hats)?*
- Do you wear contact lenses? If so, how do you take care of them?
- If you use eye drops, how do you instill them?
- Do you spend long periods of time in the sun?* Do you wear sunglasses?
- Do you smoke, or are you regularly exposed to second-hand smoke?
- Have you ever been tested for glaucoma?* Results?

Social and Occupational History
- Do you have any problems at work or home because of your eyes?*
- Does your eye problem affect your ability to read?*
- Have you made any changes in your social activities because of your eyes?*
- Are your activities limited in any way by your eye problem?*
- Are there any environmental conditions at home or work that may have an effect on your eyes (e.g., smoke, dust, chemicals, flying sparks)?* If so, do you use goggles for eye protection?
- Do you participate in any leisure activities that have the potential for eye injury?*
- Do you work for long hours at the computer?*

Coping Abilities
- How does your eye problem make you feel about yourself? Has it created stress for you?*
- If you have a vision loss, how do you cope?* Are you able to maintain your same living environment?* Do you use large-print books or Braille?*

Source: Adapted from Jarvis, C., Browne, A. J., MacDonald-Jenkins, J., & Luctkar-Flude, M. (2014). *Physical examination & health assessment* (2nd Canadian ed., pp. 303–305). Toronto: Elsevier Canada.
*If yes, describe.

developing age-related macular degeneration (see the "Determinants of Health" box). If patients use eye drops, the nurse should ascertain whether they are aware of correct methods for instilling drops to avoid contamination of the container.

Social and Occupational Health History. The patient's ability to maintain necessary or desired roles and responsibilities in home, work, and social environments can be negatively affected by ocular problems. For example, macular degeneration may decrease the patient's visual acuity to a level inadequate for functioning at work. In many occupations, employees work in conditions in which eye injury may occur. For example, factory workers may be at risk from flying debris. Information should be obtained about eye safety practices, such as use of goggles or safety glasses. Workers can also be exposed to eyestrain in the office from video display terminals, poor lighting, and glare. An ergonomic consultation may be beneficial.

A patient with diabetes may not be able to see well enough to self-administer insulin. This patient may resent dependence on a family member who takes over this function. The patient with *exophthalmos* (marked protrusion of eyeballs) may be embarrassed by his or her appearance and avoid usual social activities. The nurse should sensitively inquire whether the patient's preferred roles and responsibilities have been affected by the ocular problem.

The nurse should also inquire about leisure activities during which the patient may incur an ocular injury. For example, during gardening, woodworking, and other craft activities, foreign bodies can scratch or enter the cornea or conjunctiva or even penetrate the globe. Injuries to the globe or the bony orbit can also occur after blows to the head or eye during sports activities such as racquetball, baseball, and tennis. Other leisure activities such as needlepoint, fly tying, or birdwatching may have high-level visual demands and produce eye strain.

Coping Abilities. Patients with temporary or permanent visual problems may experience emotional stress. The nurse should assess the patient's coping strategies and availability of support

DETERMINANTS OF HEALTH

Macular Degeneration

Gender
- The incidence of macular degeneration is higher among women than among men. Early-onset menopause can also increase the risk for developing macular degeneration.*

Biology and Genetic Endowment
- The risk of developing macular degeneration increases with a family history (first generation).†
- White individuals are more likely to develop macular degeneration than any other ethnic group.†
- Vision problems are more common among new immigrants and refugees than in the general Canadian population.‡

Personal Health Practices and Coping Skills
- Smoking increases the risk of developing macular degeneration four-fold. Smokers also develop the disease approximately 10 years earlier than nonsmokers. Twenty percent of vision loss may be avoided by staying smoke-free.†
- Adequate exercise and a healthy diet (leafy vegetables, omega-3 fatty acids) reduces the risk of macular degeneration. Antioxidants and zinc can slow the progression of intermediate and advanced macular degeneration and thereby minimize vision loss.†
- Ultraviolet radiation damages the retina, which leads to macular degeneration.†

References
*Jarvis, C., Browne, A. J., MacDonald-Jenkins, J., et al. (Eds.), (2014). *Physical examination and health assessment* (2nd Canadian ed.). Toronto: Elsevier.

†Canadian National Institute for the Blind (CNIB). (2015). Age-related macular degeneration. Retrieved from *http://www.cnib.ca/en/your-eyes/eye-conditions/eye-connect/AMD/Prevention/Pages/RiskFactors.aspx*

‡Pottie, K., Greenaway, C., Feightner, J., et al. (2011). Evidence-based clinical guidelines for immigrants and refugees: Vision health. *Canadian Medical Association Journal, 183*(12), E898–E900. doi:10.1503/cmaj.090313.

CASE STUDY

Subjective Data

Source: Zurijeta/ Shutterstock .com.

A focused subjective assessment of Fatimah Abdullah revealed the following information.

Vision Difficulty: Had no vision problems until today. Wears eyeglasses for seeing distances and reading. Now having difficulty reading. Reports seeing periodic light flashes and small white spots "floating" in the air. Denies eye pain, itching, or tearing.

Past Health History: Extraocular extraction of cataract on right eye with implantation of intraocular lens 2 mo ago. Type 2 diabetes mellitus and hypertension.

Medications: Glyburide (DiaBeta), 5 mg/day; metoprolol (Lopressor), 50 mg PO daily.

Self-Care History: States she was compliant with postoperative regimen of antibiotic and corticosteroid eyedrops and with office follow-up with eye surgeon. Recovery from surgery was uneventful, and eyedrops were discontinued 2 wk ago. Does not have allergies. Walks in the mall at least 1 km three times a week. No resistance or isotonic exercises. Has had difficulty moving bowels with increased straining. Trying prune juice to help.

Coping Abilities: Afraid she is having a stroke.

See pp. 442 and 448 for more information on Ms. Abdullah.

TABLE 23-3	NORMAL FINDINGS IN PHYSICAL ASSESSMENT OF THE VISUAL SYSTEM

- Visual acuity: 20/20 in both eyes; no diplopia
- External eye structures: symmetrical and without lesions or deformities
- Lacrimal apparatus: nontender and without drainage
- Conjunctiva: clear; sclera: white
- Pupils: equal, round, and reactive to light and accommodation (PERRLA)
- Lens: clear
- Extraocular movements: intact
- Optic disc margins: sharp
- Retinal vessels: normal, with no hemorrhages or spots

---

systems, and perform a more comprehensive psychosocial assessment if it is indicated.

Objective Data

Physical Examination. Physical examination of the visual system includes inspecting ocular structures and determining their functional status. Assessment of ocular structures should include examining the ocular adnexa, the external eye, and internal structures. Some structures, such as the retina and blood vessels, must be visualized with the aid of equipment, such as the ophthalmoscope. Physiological functional assessment includes determining the patient's visual acuity and ability to judge closeness and distance; assessing extraocular muscle function; evaluating visual fields; observing pupil function; and measuring intraocular pressure.

Assessment of the visual system may include all of the components described in the following material, or it may be as brief as measuring the patient's visual acuity. The nurse assesses what is appropriate and necessary for the specific patient. All of the following assessments are in the nurse's scope of practice, but some necessitate special training. Normal findings of a physical assessment of the visual system are outlined in Table 23-3. Age-related visual changes and differences in assessment findings are listed in Table 23-1. Assessment techniques related to vision are summarized in Table 23-4. Common abnormalities found during assessment are listed in Table 23-5.

The initial observation of the patient can provide information that will help the nurse focus the assessment. A patient with impaired colour vision may dress in clothing with unusual colour combinations. A patient with diplopia may hold the head in a skewed position in an attempt to see a single image. A patient with a corneal abrasion or photophobia may cover the eyes with the hands or wear dark glasses to try to block out room light. The nurse can make a crude estimate of depth perception by extending a hand for the patient to shake.

During the initial observation, the nurse should also observe the overall facial and ophthalmic appearance of the patient. The eyes should be symmetrical and normally positioned on the face. The globes should not have a bulging or sunken appearance.

Assessing Functional Status

Visual Acuity. Before the patient receives any care, the nurse should record the patient's visual acuity for medical and legal reasons. To assess distance visual acuity, the patient sits or stands 6 metres (20 feet) from the Snellen chart with the usual correction

TABLE 23-4 NURSING ASSESSMENT

Visual System

Technique	Description	Purpose
Basic Techniques		
Visual acuity testing	Patient reads from Snellen chart at a distance of 6 m (distance vision test) and from Jaeger test type at a distance of 35 cm (near vision test); examiner notes smallest print that patient can read on each chart.	To determine patient's distance and near visual acuity
Confrontation visual field test	Patient faces examiner, covers one eye, fixates on examiner's face, and counts number of fingers that the examiner brings into patient's field of vision.	To determine whether patient has a full field of vision, without obvious scotomas
Pupil function testing	Examiner shines light into patient's pupil and observes pupillary response; each pupil is examined independently; examiner also checks for consensual and accommodative response.	To determine whether patient has normal pupillary response
Extraocular muscle functioning	Patient faces examiner, holds head still, and follows (with eyes only) object that examiner moves through six cardinal positions of gaze. Examiner also tests corneal light reflex.	To determine whether muscles and cranial nerves III, IV, and VI are functioning normally
Colour vision testing	Patient identifies numbers or paths formed by pattern of dots in a series of colour plates.	To determine patient's ability to distinguish colours
Advanced Techniques*		
Tono-Pen tonometry	Covered end of probe gently touches the anaesthetized corneal surface several times; examiner records several readings to obtain a mean intraocular pressure (see Figure 23-6).	To measure intraocular pressure (normal pressure is 10–22 mm Hg)
Ophthalmoscopy	Examiner holds ophthalmoscope close to patient's eye, shining light into back of eye and looking through aperture on ophthalmoscope; examiner adjusts dial to select one of the lenses in ophthalmoscope that produces the desired amount of magnification to inspect ocular fundus.	To observe retina and optic nerve head
Keratometry	Examiner aligns the projection and notes the readings of corneal curvature.	To measure the corneal curvature; often performed before fitting of contact lenses, before refractive surgery, or after corneal transplantation

*Performed by qualified health care provider.

TABLE 23-5 ASSESSMENT ABNORMALITIES

Visual System

Finding	Description	Possible Etiology and Significance
Subjective Data		
Pain	Foreign body sensation	Superficial corneal erosion or abrasion; can result from contact lens wear or trauma or from foreign body in the conjunctiva or cornea
	Severe, deep, throbbing	Anterior uveitis, acute glaucoma, infection; acute glaucoma also associated with nausea, vomiting
Photophobia	Persistent abnormal intolerance to light	Inflammation or infection of cornea or anterior uveal tract (iris and ciliary body), conjunctivitis
Blurred vision	Gradual or sudden inability to see clearly	Refractive errors, corneal opacities, cataracts, migraine aura, retinal changes (detachment, macular degeneration)
Appearance of spots, floaters, or light flashes (photopsias)	Seeing spots, "spider webs," "a curtain," or floaters within the field of vision, or flashes or flickers of light	Most common: liquefaction of the vitreous humor (benign phenomenon); other possible causes include hemorrhage into the vitreous humor, retinal holes, or retinal tears
		Light flashes may occur as the retina is being tugged, torn, or detached
Dryness	Discomfort, sandy or gritty sensation, irritation, or burning	Decreased tear formation or changes in tear composition because of aging or various systemic diseases
Diplopia	Double vision	Abnormalities of extraocular muscle action related to muscle or cranial nerve abnormality
Glare	Headache, ocular discomfort, reduced visual acuity	Related to corneal inflammation or to opacities in cornea, lens, or vitreous humor that scatter the incoming light; can also result from light scatter around edges of an intraocular lens; worse at night, when pupil is dilated

TABLE 23-5 ASSESSMENT ABNORMALITIES

Visual System—cont'd

Finding	Description	Possible Etiology and Significance
Objective Data		
Eyelids		
Allergic reactions	Redness, excessive tearing, and itching of eyelid margins	Many possible allergens; associated eye trauma can occur from rubbing itchy eyelids
Hordeolum (stye)	Small, superficial white nodule along eyelid margin	Infection of a sebaceous gland of eyelid; causative organism is usually bacterial (most commonly *Staphylococcus aureus*)
Blepharitis	Redness, swelling, and crusting along eyelid margins	Bacterial invasion of eyelid margins; often chronic
Ptosis	Drooping of upper eyelid margin; unilateral or bilateral	Mechanical causes as a result of eyelid tumours or excess skin; myogenic causes such as myasthenia gravis or neurogenic causes
Entropion	Inward turning of upper or lower eyelid margin, unilateral or bilateral	Congenital causes resulting in development abnormalities
Ectropion	Outward turning of lower eyelid margin	Mechanical causes as a result of eyelid tumours, herniated orbital fat, or extravasation of fluid
Conjunctiva		
Conjunctivitis	Redness, swelling of conjunctiva; possibly itching	Bacterial or viral infection; may be allergic response or inflammatory response to chemical exposure
Subconjunctival hemorrhage	Appearance of blood spot on sclera; may be small or can affect entire sclera	Conjunctival blood vessels rupture, leaking blood into the subconjunctival space
Cornea and Sclera		
Corneal abrasion	Localized painful disruption of the epithelial layer of cornea; can be visualized with fluorescein dye	Trauma; overwear or improper fit of contact lenses
Jaundice	Yellow discoloration* of the entire sclera	Related to liver dysfunction or hemolytic disease
Globe		
Exophthalmos	Protrusion of globe beyond its normal position within bony orbit; sclera often visible above iris when eyelids are open	Intraocular or periorbital tumours; hyperthyroidism; Crouzon's syndrome
Pupil		
Anisocoria	Pupils are unequal (constricted)	Central nervous system disorders; in a small percentage of the population, slight difference in pupil size is normal
Abnormal response to light or accommodation	Pupils respond asymmetrically or abnormally to light stimulus or accommodation	Central nervous system disorders, general anaesthesia
Iris		
Heterochromia	Irides are different colours†	Congenital causes (Horner's syndrome); acquired causes (chronic iritis, metastatic carcinoma, diffuse iris nevus or melanoma)
Extraocular Muscles		
Strabismus	Deviation of eye position in one or more directions	Overaction or underaction of one or more extraocular muscles
Lens		
Cataract	Opacification of lens; pupil can appear cloudy or white when opacity is visible behind pupil opening	Aging, trauma, diabetes, long-term systemic corticosteroid therapy
Visual Field Defect		
Peripheral	Partial or complete loss of peripheral vision	Glaucoma; interruption of visual pathway (e.g., tumour); migraine headache
Central	Loss of central vision	Macular disease

*Yellow colour is normal after a diagnostic study necessitating intravenous fluorescein injection.
†Most cases of heterochromia occur by chance and are not associated with any other symptoms or problems.

(glasses or contact lenses) left in place unless they are used solely for reading. The nurse asks the patient to cover the left eye with an eye spoon and to read through the chart to the smallest line of letters that the patient can possibly discern. The nurse notes the smallest line the patient can read with 50% or fewer errors. The nurse then asks the patient to cover the right eye, and the process is repeated. At the left of most rows of the Snellen chart is a fraction (e.g., "20/30") in which the numerator represents the distance the patient is from the chart and the denominator represents the distance at which a normal eye could see the letters in the row. For example, a patient with a visual acuity of 20/30 sees at 20 feet what the patient with no vision problems would see at 30 feet. The larger the denominator, the worse the visual acuity. If vision is poorer than 20/30, the patient should be referred to an ophthalmologist or optometrist (Jarvis, Browne, MacDonald-Jenkins, et al., 2014). *Legal blindness* is defined as the best corrected vision in the better eye of 20/200 or worse. If a patient cannot read letters, the nurse can use an eye chart with pictures, numbers, or symbols, such as the STYCAR graded-balls test, the Sheridan-Gardiner letter-matching test, or the Snellen E chart.

To evaluate visual acuity when the patient is unable to see even the largest letters, the nurse holds up a number of fingers in front of the patient at successively closer distances and asks the patient to count them. If the patient cannot count the fingers, the nurse asks the patient to indicate whether he or she can see hand motion or light from a penlight in front of the face.

If the patient has a complaint of near vision problems, and for all patients 40 years of age or older, the nurse tests near visual acuity. The patient is instructed to hold a Jaeger chart 35 cm (14 inches) from the eyes. The nurse covers the patient's left eye with an eye spoon, asks the patient to read successively smaller lines of print from the chart, and records the visual acuity corresponding to the smallest line of print that the patient can read comfortably. The procedure is repeated with the right eye covered. A normal result is 14/14. A result of 14/20 means the person can read at 14 inches what someone with normal vision reads at 20 inches. If a screening card is not available, the nurse can assess near vision acuity by asking the patient to read from a newspaper.

Extraocular Muscle Functions. The nurse observes the corneal light reflex to evaluate for weakness or imbalance of the extraocular muscles. In a darkened room, the nurse asks the patient to look straight ahead while a penlight is shone directly on the cornea. The light reflection should be located in the centre of both corneas as the patient faces the light source.

To assess eye movement, the nurse should hold a finger or object 25 to 30 cm from the patient's nose. The patient is asked to follow the movement of the object or finger with only his or her eyes through the six cardinal positions of gaze (Figure 23-4). This test can indicate weakness or paralysis in the extraocular muscles or dysfunction in a cranial nerve (oculomotor nerve [CN III], trochlear nerve [CN IV], and abducens nerve [CN VI]).

Pupil Function. To determine pupil function, the nurse inspects the pupils and their reactions to light. Pupil size is noted before reaction to light is checked. Pupils should be equal in

size and round and should react briskly to light. With age, pupil size decreases (Jarvis, Browne, MacDonald-Jenkins, et al., 2014). In a small percentage of the population, pupils are unequal in size (anisocoria). Pupils should react to light directly (pupil constricts when a light shines into the eye) and consensually (pupil of one eye constricts when a light shines into opposite eye). Accommodation should also be present: when the patient looks at a distant object 0.6 to 0.9 metres away and then is asked to focus on an object 7 to 8 cm from the nose, the nurse should observe convergence of the patient's eyes and constriction of the pupils. Normal pupil function may be documented as PERRLA (**p**upils **e**qual, **r**ound, **r**eactive to **l**ight and **a**ccommodation).

CASE STUDY

Objective Data: Physical Examination

Physical examination findings of Fatimah Abdullah are as follows: PERRLA. No abnormalities noted on visual examination of external eye structures. EOM [extraocular movement] intact and symmetrical.

Diagnostic Studies

Ophthalmoscopic examination on Ms. Abdullah identifies a partial retinal detachment, which is confirmed via ultrasonography.

See pp. 442 and 445 for more information on Ms. Abdullah.

Source: Zurijeta/ Shutterstock .com.

Assessing Structures. The visual system is unique because the nurse can directly inspect not only the external structures but also many of the internal structures by using special equipment such as the ophthalmoscope and the slit-lamp microscope, which enables examination of conjunctiva, sclera, cornea, anterior chamber, iris, lens, vitreous humor, and retina under magnification. The *ophthalmoscope,* a hand-held instrument with a light source and magnifying lenses, is held close to the patient's eye to visualize the posterior part of the eye. Little pain or discomfort is associated with these examinations.

Eyebrows, Eyelashes, and Eyelids. All structures should be present, symmetrical, and without deformities, redness, or swelling. Eyelashes extend outward from the eyelid margins. In normal closing, the upper and lower eyelid margins just touch. The lacrimal puncta should be open and positioned properly against the globe. If the sac is inflamed, pressure over the lacrimal sac may cause purulent material to ooze from the puncta.

Conjunctiva and Sclera. The nurse can examine the conjunctiva and sclera at the same time, evaluating colour, smoothness, and presence of any lesions or foreign bodies. The conjunctiva covering the sclera is normally clear, with fine blood vessels visible, more commonly in the periphery.

The sclera is normally white, but its colour may become yellowish in older individuals because of lipid deposition in the sclera. A pale blue cast caused by scleral thinning can also be normal in older adults and infants (who have naturally thinner sclerae). A slightly yellow cast may also be normal finding in some dark-skinned people.

Cornea. The cornea should be clear, transparent, and shiny. The iris should appear flat and not bulge toward the cornea. The area between the cornea and iris should be clear, with no blood or purulent material visible in the anterior chamber.

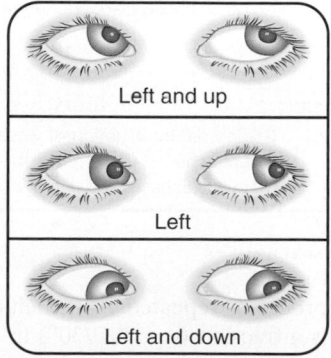

FIGURE 23-4 Six cardinal positions of gaze. Source: Adapted from Bowling, Brad. (2015). *Kanski's clinical ophthalmology: A systematic approach* (8th ed, p. 731). New York: Saunders.

Optic disc   Fovea centralis

Retinal blood vessels   Macula

FIGURE 23-5 Illustration of magnified view of retina through the ophthalmoscope. Source: Adapted from Patton, K. T., & Thibodeau, G. (2013). *Anatomy and physiology* (8th ed., p. 528). St Louis: Mosby.

FOCUSED ASSESSMENT

Visual System

Use this checklist to make sure the key assessment steps have been performed.

Subjective
Ask the patient about any of the following, and note responses.

Changes in vision (e.g., acuity, blurred)	Y	N
Eye redness, itching, discomfort	Y	N
Drainage from eyes	Y	N

Objective: Physical Examination
Inspect

Eyes for any discoloration or drainage	✓
Conjunctiva and sclera for colour and vascularity	✓
Lens for clarity	✓
Eyelid for ptosis	✓

Assess

Vision based on patient's looking at nurse or Snellen chart	✓
Extraocular movements	✓
Peripheral vision	✓
Pupil function: PERRLA	✓

PERRLA, Pupils equal, round, reactive to light and accommodation.

Iris. Both irides should be of similar colour and shape. However, a colour difference between the irides is normal in a small proportion of individuals. Round or notched areas of missing iris tissue are often the result of cataract or glaucoma surgery. The nurse should determine the cause of these round, notched, or triangular areas and document the findings.

Retina and Optic Nerve. To assess these structures, the nurse uses an ophthalmoscope to magnify the ocular structures and bring them into crisp focus (Figure 23-5). This enables the examiner to directly view arteries, veins, and the optic nerve. The nurse directs the beam of light from the ophthalmoscope obliquely into the patient's pupils and should note the appearance of a *red reflex.* This reflex is a result of light's reflecting off the retina. Any dense area in the lens or nontransparent material in the vitreous humor decreases the red reflex. The optic nerve or disc is examined for size, colour, and abnormalities. The optic disc is creamy yellow with distinct margins. A slight blurring of the nasal margin is common.

A central depression in the disc, called the *physiologic cup,* is the exit site for the optic nerve. The cup should be less than half the diameter of the disc. Normally, no hemorrhages or exudates are present in the fundus (retinal background). Careful inspection of the fundus can reveal the presence of retinal holes, tears, detachments, or lesions. Small hemorrhages can be associated with diabetes or hypertension and can appear in various shapes, such as dots or flames. Finally, the nurse examines the macula for shape and appearance. This area of high reflectivity is devoid of any blood vessels.

The nurse can obtain important information about the vascular system and the central nervous system through direct visualization with an ophthalmoscope. Skilled use of this instrument requires practice.

Focused Assessment. A focused assessment (see the following "Focused Assessment" box) may be performed by a general nurse when a patient is admitted to a medical-surgical unit or an outpatient clinic. Inspection of the eyes may be performed routinely as part

of the assessment of a hospitalized patient. In addition, the nurse should assess for and document use of glasses or contact lenses. Assessment for PERRLA may be performed routinely as part of neurological assessment of a hospitalized patient (see Chapter 58).

Special Assessment Techniques

Colour Vision. Testing the patient's ability to distinguish colours can be an important part of the overall assessment because some occupations may require accurate colour discrimination. The Ishihara colour test determines the patient's ability to distinguish a pattern of colour in a series of colour plates. Older adults have a loss of colour discrimination at the blue end of the colour spectrum and loss of sensitivity throughout the entire spectrum, especially when cataracts are present.

Stereopsis. Stereoscopic vision allows a patient to see objects in three dimensions. Any event causing a patient to have monocular vision (e.g., enucleation, patching) results in loss of stereoscopic vision, which impairs the individual's depth perception. This condition can have serious consequences: for example, if the patient trips over a step when walking or follows too closely behind another vehicle when driving.

Intraocular Pressure. Testing intraocular pressure is important because high intraocular pressure is a major risk factor for glaucoma. Intraocular pressure can be measured by a variety of methods, including the Tono-Pen (Figure 23-6). Use of the Tono-Pen is common because it is simple and results are very accurate. The surface of the anaesthetized cornea is touched lightly several times with the covered end of the probe. The instrument records several readings and provides a mean measurement on a digital light-emitting diode (LED) screen located on the front surface. Normal intraocular pressure ranges from 10 to 22 mm Hg.

DIAGNOSTIC STUDIES

Diagnostic studies provide important objective data to the nurse monitoring the patient's condition and planning appropriate interventions. Table 23-6 presents the most common basic diagnostic studies of the visual system.

SAFETY ALERT

Nurses should avoid using the abbreviations *OS* for left eye, *OD* for right eye, and *OU* for both eyes when documenting in patients' charts or transcribing medication orders because they can be easily confused with each other and with the abbreviations *AD, AS,* and *AU* for the ear. Use of these abbreviations can contribute to communication errors and potentially serious medication errors (Institute for Safe Medication Practices Canada, 2016).

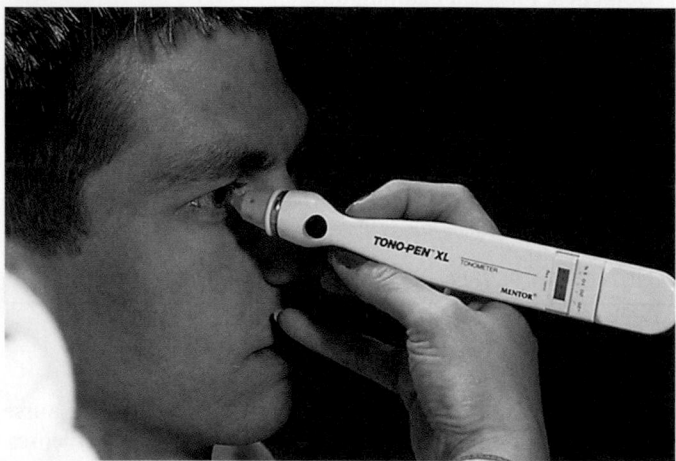

FIGURE 23-6 Tono-Pen tonometry. Source: Courtesy the Eye Institute, Department of Ophthalmology and Visual Services, University of Iowa Health Care, Iowa City, Iowa.

THE AUDITORY SYSTEM

STRUCTURES AND FUNCTIONS

The auditory system is composed of the peripheral and central auditory systems. The peripheral auditory system includes the structures of the ear itself: external, middle, and inner ear (Figure 23-7). This system is concerned with the reception and perception of sound. The external and middle portions of the ear function to conduct and amplify sound waves from the environment. The inner ear serves functions of hearing and balance. The central auditory system (the brain and its pathways) integrates and assigns meaning to what is heard.

External Ear

The external ear consists of the auricle (pinna) and the external auditory canal. The *auricle* is composed of cartilage and connective tissue covered with epithelium, which also lines the external auditory canal (see Figure 23-7). The *external auditory canal* is a slightly S-shaped tube about 2.5 cm in length in the adult. The skin that lines the canal contains fine hairs and sebaceous (oil) glands and ceruminous (wax) glands. The hairs and wax help prevent dust and other foreign objects from entering the ear canal (Herlihy, 2014).

Hair is present in the outer half of the canal. The inner half of the ear canal is highly sensitive. The function of the external ear and canal is to collect and transmit sound waves to the *tympanic membrane* (eardrum). This shiny, translucent, pearl-grey membrane is composed of epithelial cells, connective tissue, and mucous membrane. It serves as a partition and instrument of

TABLE 23-6 DIAGNOSTIC STUDIES

Visual System

Study	Description and Purpose	Patient Education*
Refractometry	Subjective measure of refractive error; multiple lenses are mounted on rotating wheels. While patient sits looking through apertures at Snellen acuity chart, lenses are changed; patient chooses lenses that make acuity sharpest. Cycloplegic drugs are used to paralyze accommodation during refraction process.	Procedure is painless; patient may need help holding the head still. Pupil dilation makes it difficult for the patient to focus on near objects; dilation may last 3–4 hr.
Ultrasonography	A-scan probe is placed on patient's anaesthetized cornea; used primarily for axial length measurement for calculating power of intraocular lens implanted after cataract extraction. B-scan probe is applied to patient's closed eyelid; used more often than A-scan for diagnosis of ocular disorders such as intraocular foreign bodies or tumours, opacities in the vitreous humor, and retinal detachments.	Procedure is painless (cornea is anaesthetized).
Fluorescein angiography	Fluorescein (a nonradioactive, non-iodine dye) is intravenously injected into antecubital or other peripheral vein, followed by serial photographs (over 10-min period) of the retina through dilated pupils. Provides diagnostic information about flow of blood through pigment epithelial and retinal vessels; often used in patients with diabetes to accurately locate areas of diabetic retinopathy before laser destruction of neovascularized area.	Fluorescein is toxic to tissue if extravasation occurs; systemic allergic reactions are rare, but the nurse should be familiar with emergency equipment and procedures. The patient should be informed that dye can sometimes cause transient nausea or vomiting and transient yellow discoloration of urine and skin.
Amsler grid test	Test is self-administered with a hand-held card printed with a grid of lines (similar to graph paper); patient fixates on centre dot and records any perceived abnormalities of the grid lines, such as wavy, missing, or distorted areas. Test is used to monitor macular problems.	Regular testing is necessary to identify any changes in macular function.

*Patient education regarding the purpose and method of testing is a nursing responsibility for all diagnostic procedures.

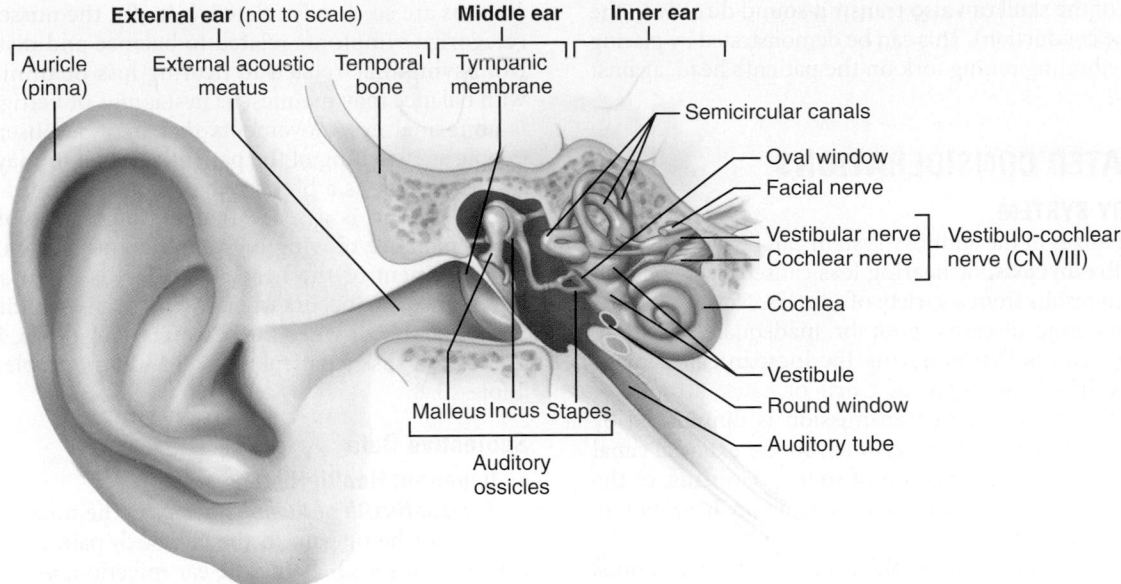

FIGURE 23-7 External, middle, and inner ear. *CN,* cranial nerve. Source: Adapted from Patton, K. T., & Thibodeau, G. A. (2013). *Anatomy and physiology* (8th ed., p. 518). St. Louis: Mosby.

sound transmission between the external auditory canal and middle ear.

Middle Ear

The middle ear cavity is an air space located in the temporal bone. Mucosa lines the middle ear and is continuous from the nasal pharynx via the Eustachian (auditory) tube. The *Eustachian tube* functions to equalize atmospheric air pressure between the middle ear and throat and allows the tympanic membrane to move freely. It opens during yawning and swallowing. Blockage of this tube can occur with allergies, nasopharyngeal infections, or enlarged adenoids.

The middle ear contains three tiny bones or *(ossicles): malleus, incus,* and *stapes.* Vibrations of the tympanic membrane cause the ossicles to move and transmit sound waves to the oval window. The resulting vibration in the oval window causes fluid in the inner ear to move and stimulate hearing receptors. The round window sits below the oval window and is covered with a thin membrane called the *fenestra cochlea;* it also opens into the inner ear and acts as a pressure valve that moves outward as fluid pressure builds in the inner ear. The superior part of the middle ear is called the *epitympanum* (attic). It also communicates with air cells within the mastoid bone. The facial nerve (CN VII) passes above the oval window of the middle ear. The thin, bony covering of the facial nerve can become damaged by chronic ear infection, skull fracture, or trauma during ear surgery. Such damage can cause problems with voluntary facial movements, eyelid closure, and taste discrimination. Permanent damage to the facial nerve can also result.

Inner Ear

The inner ear is composed of a bony labyrinth (maze) surrounding a membrane. This complex contains the functional organs for hearing and balance. The receptor organ for hearing is the *cochlea,* a coiled structure. It contains the *organ of Corti,* whose tiny hair cells respond to stimulation of selected portions of the basilar membrane according to pitch. This stimulus is converted into an electrochemical impulse and then transmitted by the cochlear branch of the vestibulo-cochlear nerve (CN VIII; formerly called the *acoustic nerve*) to the temporal lobe of the brain to process and interpret the sound.

Three semicircular canals and the vestibule make up the membranous labyrinth, which is housed in the bony labyrinth and enables the sense of balance. The membranous labyrinth is filled with endolymphatic fluid, and the bony labyrinth is filled with perilymphatic fluid. The fluid cushions these two sensitive organs and communicates with the brain and the subarachnoid spaces of the brain. The nervous stimuli are communicated by the vestibular portion of CN VIII. Debris or excessive pressure within the lymphatic fluid can cause disorders such as vertigo.

Transmission of Sound and Implications for Hearing Loss

Sound waves are conducted by air (air conduction) and picked up by the auricles and the auditory canal. The sound waves strike the tympanic membrane, causing it to vibrate. The central area of the tympanic membrane is connected to the malleus, which also starts to vibrate, transmitting the vibration to the incus and then the stapes. As the stapes moves back and forth, it pushes the membrane of the oval window in and out. Movement of the oval window produces waves in the perilymph. Pathological disturbances in the external ear canal or the middle ear may cause a conductive hearing loss, resulting in an alteration in the patient's perception of or sensitivity to sounds.

Once sound has been transmitted to the liquid medium of the inner ear, the vibration is picked up by the tiny sensory hair cells of the cochlea, which initiate nerve impulses. These impulses are carried by nerve fibres to the main branch of the acoustic portion of CN VIII and then to the brain. Disruptions of the inner ear or along the nerve pathway from the inner ear to the brain can result in sensorineural hearing loss. This may result in an alteration of the patient's perception of or sensitivity to specific tones. Impairment within the central auditory system causes *central hearing loss.* This type of hearing loss causes difficulty in understanding the meaning of words that are heard. (Types of hearing loss are discussed further in Chapter 24.)

The bones of the skull can also transmit sound directly to the inner ear (bone conduction). This can be demonstrated by placing the stem of a vibrating tuning fork on the patient's head, against the skull.

AGE-RELATED CONSIDERATIONS

THE AUDITORY SYSTEM

Age-related changes of the auditory system can result in hearing impairment. Presbycusis, or hearing loss caused by aging, can also result from insults from a variety of sources. Noise exposure, vascular or systemic diseases, poor or inadequate nutrition, ototoxic drugs, and pollution during the lifespan can damage delicate hair cells of the organ of Corti or cause atrophy of lymph-producing cells. Sound transmission is diminished by calcification of the ossicles. Dry cerumen in the external canal can also interfere with transmission of sound. Tinnitus, or the perception of ringing in the ears, may accompany hearing loss that results from the aging process.

Hearing loss, especially in an older adult, can have serious implications for the quality of life, including progressive physical and psychosocial dysfunction (Seidel, Ball, Dains, et al., 2011). As the average lifespan increases, the number of people with hearing loss will also increase. Early identification of hearing problems will ensure that patients are more active and healthy as they age.

Age-related changes in the auditory system and differences in assessment findings are presented in Table 23-7.

ASSESSMENT

Assessment of the auditory system includes assessment of the *vestibular* (balance) system because the auditory and vestibular systems are so closely related. Initially, the nurse should try to categorize symptoms related to balance and distinguish them from symptoms related to hearing loss or tinnitus. Problems with balance may manifest as nystagmus or vertigo. Nystagmus is abnormal eye movements that may be observed by other people as twitching of the patient's eyeball or may be described by the patient as a blurring of vision with head or eye movement. Vertigo is a sense that the person or objects around the person are moving or spinning and is usually stimulated by movement of the head. Dizziness is a sensation of being off-balance that occurs when the person is standing or walking. It does not occur when the person is lying down. Health history questions to ask a patient with an auditory problem are listed in Table 23-8.

Subjective Data

Important Health History

Current Health of Auditory System. The nurse should inquire about earache or pain in the ear. Such pain may be caused by ear problems such as middle ear infection, or may be referred pain originating in the teeth or temporo-mandibular joint. If pain is present, the patient should be asked to describe the pain and the treatments used for relief. If the patient has experienced any ear infections or has a history of chronic ear infections, this may contribute to increased hearing loss. Pus or bloody discharge may indicate an ear infection, whereas clear discharge may consist of cerebro-spinal fluid, particularly if the patient has received any head trauma. The nurse should note the time of onset of the hearing loss, whether it was sudden or gradual, and the person who noted the onset. Gradual hearing losses are most often noted by people who communicate regularly with the patient. Sudden losses and those exacerbated by some other condition are most often reported by the patient. If a hearing loss is identified in an older adult patient, the nurse can use the questions from the Hearing Handicap Inventory for Older Persons (Table 23-9). Referral is recommended for individuals scoring 10 or higher on the inventory.

If the patient has experienced any ringing, crackling, or buzzing sensation, the nurse should note time of onset and whether the patient is taking any medications that might cause tinnitus. Symptoms such as dizziness, tinnitus, and hearing loss are recorded in detail in the patient's own words. This careful description could help differentiate the cause.

Past Health History. Many problems related to the ear are sequelae of childhood illnesses or result from problems of adjacent organs. Consequently, a careful assessment of past health problems is important.

The patient should be questioned about previous problems regarding the ears, especially problems experienced during childhood. The frequency of acute middle ear infections (otitis media), perforations of the eardrum, drainage, and history of mumps, measles, or scarlet fever should be recorded. Congenital hearing loss can result from infectious diseases (e.g., rubella, influenza, or syphilis), teratogenic medications, or hypoxia in the first trimester of pregnancy. Information regarding family members with hearing loss and type of hearing loss is important. Some congenital hearing loss is hereditary. The age at onset of presbycusis also follows a familial pattern. Head injury should be documented because it can result in hearing loss. Information about food and environmental allergies is important because they can cause the Eustachian tube to become edematous and prevent aeration of the middle ear.

TABLE 23-7   AGE-RELATED DIFFERENCES IN ASSESSMENT

Auditory System

Changes	Differences in Assessment Findings
External Ear	
Increased production of and drier cerumen	Impacted cerumen; potential hearing loss
Increased hair growth	Visible hair, especially in men
Loss of elasticity in cartilage	Collapsed ear canal
Middle Ear	
Atrophic changes of tympanic membrane	Conductive hearing loss
Inner Ear	
Hair cell degeneration, neuron degeneration in auditory nerve and central pathways, reduced blood supply to cochlea, calcification of ossicles	Presbycusis, diminished sensitivity to high-pitched sounds, impairment in speech reception, tinnitus
Less effective vestibular apparatus in semicircular canals	Alterations in balance and body orientation
Brain	
Decline in ability to filter out unwanted and unnecessary sound	Difficulty hearing in a noisy environment, heightened sensitivity to loud sounds

TABLE 23-8   HEALTH HISTORY

Auditory System: Questions for Obtaining Subjective Data

Earache
- Do you have earache or another kind of pain in your ear?*
- Where is it located? Can you describe the pain?
- Do you have any symptoms of a cold or a sore throat?*
- What measures have you used to relieve the pain?* Were they effective?

Discharge
- Have you experienced discharge from your ears? How much and what colour?
- Have you had ear infections? How frequent? How were they treated?

Hearing Loss
- Was the hearing loss sudden or gradual?*
- Is it all your hearing or just hearing of certain sounds that has decreased?
- Where do you notice the hearing loss (e.g., conversations in a crowd, telephone conversations, watching television)?
- Have you travelled by airplane recently?
- Do you have any allergies that result in ear problems?*
- How does your hearing loss affect your daily life at home and at work?

Environmental Noise
- Do you have loud noise in your home or work environment?*
- Do you work near loud noises such as heavy machinery or drums in a band?

Tinnitus
- Have you ever experienced ringing, crackling, or buzzing in your ears?*
- Does the noise seem louder at certain times?*
- When does it bother you the most?
- What things have you tried that help?

Vertigo
- Have you felt vertigo—a spinning sensation?*
- Have you felt dizzy, as if you were falling or losing your balance?*
- Do you ever experience lightheadedness or giddiness?*
- Have you ever fallen because of the dizziness?*
- How does your dizziness affect your daily life?*

Nutrition and Elimination
- Do you have any food allergies that affect your ears?*
- Do you notice any differences in symptoms with changes in your diet?*
- Does your ear problem cause nausea that interferes with your food intake?*
- Does chewing or swallowing cause you any ear discomfort?
- Does straining during a bowel movement cause you ear pain?*

Activities of Daily Living and Exercise
- Does your ear problem cause you to change your usual activity or exercise?*
- Do you need help with certain activities (e.g., lifting, bending, climbing stairs, driving, speaking) because of symptoms?*
- Do you have any limitations in activities of daily living because of your symptoms?*
- Is your sleep disturbed by symptoms of pain, tinnitus, or dizziness?*

Self-Care History
- When did you last have your ears checked?
- How do you clean your ears?
- Do you use any devices to improve your hearing (e.g., hearing aid, special volume control, headphones for television or audio devices)?*
- How long have you used a hearing aid? Do you have any problems using or maintaining your hearing aid?*
- Do you use any means to protect your ears such as headphones or earplugs?* When?
- Do you use personal sound systems such as iPhones or MP3 players?*

Coping Abilities
- Is your ability to communicate and understand affected by your symptoms?*
- What effect has your ear problem had on your work, family, or social life?
- How does your ear problem make you feel about yourself?
- Do you consider your ear problem a stressor?*
- How do you cope with your ear problem?

Source: Adapted from Jarvis, C., Browne, A. J., MacDonald-Jenkins, J., et al. (Eds.). (2014). *Physical examination and health assessment* (2nd Canadian ed., pp. 346–348). Toronto: Elsevier Canada.
*If yes, describe.

Medications. The nurse should obtain information about current or past medications that are ototoxic (cause damage to CN VIII) and can produce hearing loss, tinnitus, and vertigo. The amount and frequency of acetylsalicylic acid (ASA; Aspirin) use is important because tinnitus can result from high ASA (Aspirin) intake. Aminoglycosides, any other antibiotics, salicylates, antimalarial agents, chemotherapeutic drugs, diuretics, and nonsteroidal anti-inflammatory drugs are groups of drugs that are potentially ototoxic (Lehne, 2012). Careful monitoring for hearing and balance problems is essential. Many drugs produce hearing loss that may be reversible if treatment is stopped. The nurse should also inquire about the use of herbal or alternative therapies, including ear candling. Health Canada (2011) does not recommend ear candling because patients have experienced burns and hearing loss as a result.

Surgery or Other Treatments. The nurse should obtain information about previous hospitalizations for ear surgery (e.g., myringotomy, tympanoplasty), tonsillectomy, and adenoidectomy.

Use of and satisfaction with a hearing aid should be documented. Problems with impacted cerumen should also be noted.

Nutrition and Elimination. Both alcohol and sodium affect the amount of endolymph in the inner ear system. Patients with Ménière's disease generally notice some improvement in their symptoms with alcohol restriction and a low-sodium diet. Improvements and exacerbations associated with food intake should be noted. The patient should also be questioned about any ear pain or discomfort that occurs with chewing or swallowing, which might decrease nutritional intake. This situation is often associated with a problem in the middle ear.

Assessment of clenching or grinding of the teeth helps differentiate problems of the ear from referred pain of the temporo-mandibular joint. The nurse should ask about dental problems and dentures.

Elimination patterns and their association with ear problems are of interest mainly in patients with perilymph fistula or in patients immediately after surgery. Frequent constipation or

TABLE 23-9	THE HEARING HANDICAP INVENTORY FOR OLDER PERSONS*

Does a hearing problem cause you

1. (E) To feel embarrassed when meeting new people?
2. (E) To feel frustrated when talking to members of your family?
3. (S) To have difficulty understanding when someone speaks in a whisper?
4. (E) To feel handicapped?
5. (S) To have difficulty when visiting friends, relatives, or neighbours?
6. (S) To attend religious services less often than you would like?
7. (E) To have arguments with family members?
8. (S) To have difficulty when listening to television or radio?
9. (E) To feel that your hearing limits or hampers your personal or social life?
10. (S) To have difficulty when in a restaurant with relatives and friends?

Source: Adapted from Bance, M. (2007). Hearing and aging. *Canadian Medical Association Journal*, 176(7), 925–927. By permission of the publisher. © 1982 Canadian Medical Association. Copied under licence from Access Copyright. Further reproduction, distribution or transmission is prohibited except as otherwise permitted by law.
*Overall scoring: *yes* = 4 points; *sometimes* = 2 points; *no* = 0 points.
(E), question referring to emotional handicap; *(S)*, question referring to social handicap.

straining with bowel or bladder elimination may interfere with healing of a perilymph fistula or its repair. A patient who has just undergone stapedectomy especially needs to prevent the increase in intracranial (and consequent inner ear) pressure associated with straining during bowel movements. Stool softeners may be ordered postoperatively for a patient who reports chronic problems with constipation.

Activities of Daily Living and Exercise. Activity and exercise review is most important in assessing a patient with vestibular problems. If vertigo is a problem, the patient should be questioned about the onset, duration, and frequency of this symptom. Patients who have Ménière's disease demonstrate increasing inability to compensate for environmental input as the day progresses. Symptoms are experienced particularly in the evening. In contrast, patients with chronic vertigo syndrome (benign paroxysmal positional vertigo) note that the symptoms improve throughout the day as adjustment to the visual and positional input from the environment occurs. The nurse and the patient should identify a list of activities and exercises that aggravate and relieve dizziness and vertigo or cause nausea or vomiting. Frequent repetition of an activity that causes symptoms (habituation) may help the body adjust so that the activity is no longer a problem.

A patient with chronic tinnitus should be questioned about sleep problems. Tinnitus can disturb sleep and activities conducted in a quiet environment. Affected patients should be asked whether they have used or tried any masking devices or techniques to drown out the tinnitus. The nurse should also assess for snoring because it can be caused by swelling or hypertrophy of tissue in the nasopharynx. This excessive tissue can impair the functioning of the Eustachian tube and cause the sensation of ear fullness or pain.

Self-Care History. Patients should be questioned about personal practices such as the most recent ear examination, use of cotton ear swabs, use of earphones for personal listening devices, and measures used to preserve hearing. Patients should be questioned about contact with environments that have excessive noise levels, such as work with jet engines and machinery, firing of firearms, and electronically amplified music. The use of protective ear covers or earplugs is good practice for people in high-noise environments and is important to document.

If the patient is a swimmer, the frequency and duration of swimming and use of ear protection should be documented. It is also important to note the type of water (pool, lake, or ocean) in which the swimming takes place to help identify contact with contaminated water. Placement of any item in the ear, including hearing aids, that can cause trauma to the skin increases risk of infection.

Coping Abilities. Patients should be questioned about the effect the ear problem has had on family life, work responsibilities, and social relationships. Hearing loss can strain family relations and create misunderstandings. Failure to acknowledge hearing loss and failure to seek treatment can further hinder family relationships. Many jobs rely on the ability to hear accurately and respond appropriately. If a hearing loss is present, the nurse should gather detailed information of its effect on the patient's job. The patient should be assisted to realistically evaluate the job situation.

The unpredictability of vertigo attacks can have devastating effects on all aspects of a patient's life. Ordinary activities such as driving, child care, housework, climbing stairs, and cooking all acquire an element of danger. The patient should be asked to describe the effect of the vertigo on the many roles and responsibilities of life. Compensatory practices to avoid the development of dangerous situations should also be noted.

Hearing loss often leaves the patient feeling isolated from valued social relationships. The nurse should historically document social activities such as playing cards, going to movies, and attending religious functions from before and since the hearing loss occurred. Comparison of the frequency and enjoyment of the events can indicate whether a problem is present. The nurse should determine whether hearing loss or deafness has interfered with the patient's establishment of a satisfactory sex life. Although intimacy does not depend on the ability to hear, it could interfere with establishing or maintaining a relationship.

Objective Data

Physical Examination. During the health history interview, the nurse can collect valuable objective data regarding the patient's ability to hear. Clues such as posturing of the head and appropriateness of responses should be noted. Does the patient ask to have certain words repeated? Does the patient intently watch the examiner but miss comments when not looking at the examiner? Such observations are significant and should be recorded. This is also important because many patients are unaware of hearing loss or do not admit to changes in hearing until moderate losses have occurred. A normal assessment of the ear is described in Table 23-10.

Age-related changes of the auditory system and differences in assessment findings are listed in Table 23-7.

External Ear. The external ear is inspected and palpated before examination of the external canal and tympanum. The auricle, preauricular area, and mastoid area are observed for symmetry of the ears, colour of skin, temperature, nodules, swelling, redness, and lesions. The auricle and mastoid areas are then palpated for tenderness and nodules. Grasping the auricle may elicit a pain response, especially if inflammation of the external ear or canal is present.

TABLE 23-10	NORMAL FINDINGS IN PHYSICAL ASSESSMENT OF THE AUDITORY SYSTEM

- Ears: symmetrical in location and shape
- Auricles and tragus: nontender, without lesions
- Canal: clear; tympanic membrane: intact; landmarks and light reflex: intact
- Ability to hear low whisper at 30 cm; Rinne's test results: air conduction is better than bone conduction; Weber's test results: no lateralization

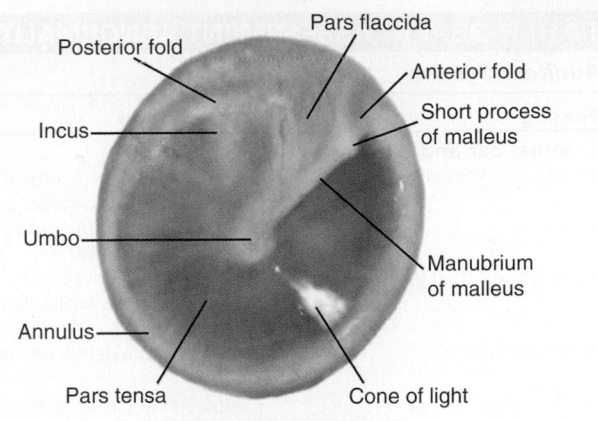

FIGURE 23-9 Illustration of normal landmarks of the right tympanic membrane, as seen through an otoscope. Source: Jarvis, C. (2015). *Physical examination and health assessment* (7th ed.). St. Louis: Elsevier.

FIGURE 23-8 Otoscopic examination of the adult ear. The auricle is pulled up and back. The examiner's hand holding the otoscope is braced against the patient's face for stabilization. Source: Courtesy Maureen Barry.

External Auditory Canal and Tympanum. Before inserting an otoscope, the nurse should inspect the canal opening for patency, palpate the tragus, and gently move the auricle to check for discomfort. A speculum only slightly smaller than the size of the ear canal is selected. The patient's head is tipped to the opposite shoulder. The top of the auricle is grasped and gently pulled up and backward in adults and slightly down and backward in children to straighten the canal. The otoscope, held in one of the examiner's hands and stabilized on the patient's head by the fingers of the other hand, is inserted slowly (Figure 23-8). A tight seal of the speculum is essential during this step of the examination. The canal is observed for size and shape and for the colour, amount, and type of cerumen. The tympanic membrane separates the external ear from the middle ear. If a large amount of cerumen is present, the tympanic membrane may not be visible. The tympanic membrane is observed for colour, landmarks, contour, and intactness (Figure 23-9). It is pearl-grey, white, or pink; shiny; and translucent.

The handle *(manubrium)* of the malleus and the end *(umbo)* are formed from the short process of the malleus and should be visible through the membrane. The somewhat anterior position and concave shape of the tympanic membrane causes the light from the otoscope to reflect back as a cone of light with crisp edges. If the tympanic membrane is bulging or retracted, the edges of the light reflex do not have the cone shape; instead, the

reflected light spreads out or moves and has irregular edges (diffuse). The circumference of the tympanum is thickened into a dense, whitish, fibrous ring, or *annulus,* except in the superior area. The tympanum within the annulus *(pars tensa)* is taut. Above the short process of the malleus is the *pars flaccida,* the flaccid part of the tympanum. The malleolar folds are anterior and posterior to the short process of the malleus. The middle and inner ear cannot be examined with the otoscope because of the tympanic membrane. Table 23-11 summarizes common abnormalities of the auditory system that are found in the assessment.

Focused Assessment. A focused assessment (see the following "Focused Assessment" box) may be performed by a general nurse when a patient is admitted to a medical-surgical unit or an outpatient clinic. The ears may be inspected routinely as part of the assessment of a hospitalized patient. In addition, the nurse should assess for the presence of a hearing aid and document whether the patient has been using it.

FOCUSED ASSESSMENT
Auditory System

Use this checklist to make sure the key assessment steps have been performed.

Subjective
Ask the patient about any of the following, and note responses.

Changes in hearing	Y	N
Ear pain	Y	N
Ear drainage	Y	N

Objective: Physical Examination
Inspect

Alignment and position of ears on head	✓
Size, shape, symmetry, colour, and skin intactness	✓
External auditory meatus for discharge or lesions	✓

Assess

Hearing, according to ability to respond to conversation, respond to a whisper, or hear a ticking watch	✓

TABLE 23-11   ASSESSMENT ABNORMALITIES

Auditory System

Finding	Description	Possible Cause and Significance
External Ear and Canal		
Sebaceous cyst behind ear	Usually within skin, possible presence of black dot (opening to sebaceous gland)	Removal or incision and drainage if painful
Tophi	Hard nodules in the helix or antihelix, consisting of uric acid crystals	Associated with gout, metabolic disorder; further diagnosis needed
Impacted cerumen	Wax that has not been excreted from the ear normally; no visualization of eardrum	Decreased hearing possible, sensation of fullness in auditory canal; removal necessary before otoscopic examination can be conducted
Discharge in canal	Infection of external ear, usually painful	Swimmer's ear, infection of external ear; possibly caused by ruptured eardrum and otitis media
Swelling of auricle, pain	Infection of glands of skin, hematoma caused by trauma	Aspiration (for hematoma)
Scaling or lesions	Change in usual appearance of skin	Seborrheic dermatitis, squamous cell carcinoma, atrophic dermatitis
Exostosis	Bony growth extending into canal, causing narrowing of canal	Possible interference with visualization of tympanum; usually asymptomatic
Tympanum		
Retracted eardrum	Appearance of shorter, more horizontal malleus; cone of light is absent or bent	Vacuum in middle ear, blockage of Eustachian tube, negative pressure in middle ear
Hairline fluid level, yellow-amber bubbles above fluid level	Caused by transudate of blood and serum; meniscus of fluid produces hairline appearance	Serous otitis media
Bulging red or blue eardrum, lack of landmarks	Middle ear filled with fluid (pus, blood)	Acute otitis media; perforation possible
Perforation of eardrum (central or marginal)	Previous perforations of the eardrum that have failed to heal; thin, transparent layer of epithelium surrounding eardrum	Chronic otitis media, mastoiditis
Recruitment	Disproportionate loudness of sound; difficulty in using hearing aid	Malfunction of inner ear

DIAGNOSTIC STUDIES

Table 23-12 describes diagnostic studies commonly used to assess the auditory system.

Tests for Hearing Acuity

Tests involving the whispered and the spoken voice can provide gross screening information about the patient's ability to hear. Audiometric testing provides more detailed information that can be used for diagnosis and treatment. In the *whispered voice test,* the examiner stands 30 to 60 cm behind the patient and, after exhaling, speaks in a low whisper. A louder whisper is used if the patient does not respond correctly. Spoken voice, increasing in loudness, is similarly used. The patient is asked to repeat numbers or words or answer questions. One ear at a time is tested while hearing in the other ear is masked to prevent sound transmission around the head. During testing, the nontest ear is masked by the patient, who occludes the ear, or by the examiner, who gently occludes the auditory canal with a finger and rubs the tragus in a circular motion.

Tuning-Fork Tests. Tuning-fork tests aid in differentiating between conductive and sensorineural hearing loss. For this examination, 512-Hz tuning forks are generally used. Both skill and experience are necessary to ensure accurate results. If a problem is suspected, further evaluation by pure-tone audiometry is essential. The most common tuning-fork tests are Rinne's test and Weber's test.

In Rinne's test, the base of an activated tuning fork is held first against the patient's mastoid bone to evaluate bone conduction and then 1 to 5 cm in front of the patient's ear canal to evaluate air conduction. The patient reports whether the sound is louder behind the ear (on the mastoid bone) or next to the ear canal. When the sound is no longer perceived behind the ear, the fork is moved next to the ear canal until the patient indicates that the sound is no longer heard. The test result is positive when the patient reports that air conduction is heard longer than bone conduction. This can indicate normal hearing or a sensorineural loss. If the patient hears the tuning fork better by bone conduction, the test result is negative, indicating that conductive hearing loss is present.

In Weber's test, an activated tuning fork is placed on the midline of the patient's skull, on the forehead, or on the teeth. The patient is asked to indicate where the sound is heard best. In conditions of normal auditory function, the patient perceives a midline tone best. If a patient has a conductive hearing loss in one ear, sound is heard louder (lateralizes) in that ear. If a sensorineural loss is present, sound is louder (lateralizes) in the unaffected ear.

Results of tuning-fork tests are subjective. A patient with inconsistent test results or questionable results should be referred for more objective audiometric evaluation.

Audiometry. *Audiometry* is beneficial as a screening test for hearing acuity and as a diagnostic test for determining the degree and type of hearing loss. The audiometer produces pure tones at varying intensities to which the patient can respond. Sound is characterized by the number of vibrations or cycles that occur each second. *Hertz* (Hz) is the unit of measurement used to classify the frequency of a tone; the higher the frequency, the higher the pitch. Hearing loss can affect certain sound frequencies. The specific pattern produced on the audiogram by these losses

TABLE 23-12   DIAGNOSTIC STUDIES

Auditory System

Study	Description and Purpose	Nursing Responsibility
Auditory		
Pure tone audiometry	Sounds are presented through earphones in soundproof room. Patient responds nonverbally when sound is heard. Response is recorded on an audiogram. Purpose is to determine patient's hearing range in terms of decibels (dB) and hertz (Hz) for diagnosing conductive and sensorineural hearing loss. Tinnitus can cause inconsistent results.	Nurse does not usually participate in examination.
Bone conduction	Tuning fork is placed on mastoid process, and hearing by bone conduction is recorded. Helps diagnose conductive hearing loss.	Nurse may perform test.
One- and two-syllable word lists	Words are presented and recorded at comfortable level of hearing to determine percentage correct and word understanding.	Nurse may perform test.
Auditory evoked potential	Procedure is similar to electroencephalography (see Chapter 58, Table 58-8). Electrodes are attached to patient in darkened room. Electrodes are placed typically at vertex, mastoid process, or earlobes and forehead. A computer is used to record auditory activity in isolation from other electrical activity of the brain.	Nurse should explain procedure to patient. Nurse should not leave patient alone in the darkened room.
Electrocochleography	Test is useful for uncooperative patient or for patient who cannot volunteer useful information. Test records electrical activity in the cochlea and auditory nerve.	Nurse does not usually participate in examination.
Auditory brainstem response	Electrical peaks along auditory pathway of inner ear to brain are measured, and diagnostic information is related to acoustical neuromas, brainstem problems, and stroke.	Nurse does not usually participate in examination.
Tympanometry (impedance audiometry)	Useful in diagnosis of middle ear effusions. A probe is placed snugly in the external ear canal, and positive and negative pressures are then applied. Compliance of the middle ear is then noted in response to the pressures.	Nurse does not usually participate in examination.
Vestibular		
Caloric test stimulus	Endolymph of the semicircular canals is stimulated by irrigation of cold (20°C) or warm (36°C) solution into ear. Patient is seated or in supine position. Observation of type of nystagmus, nausea and vomiting, falling, or vertigo is helpful in diagnosing disease of labyrinth. Decreased response indicates decreased function and thus disease of vestibular system. Other ear is tested similarly, and results from both are compared.	Nurse instructs patient to eat no more than a light meal before test, to prevent nausea. Nurse observes patient for vomiting and assists patient if necessary. Nurse ensures patient safety.
Electronystagmography	Electrodes are placed near patient's eyes, and movement of eyes (nystagmus) is recorded on graph during specific eye movements and when ear is irrigated. Study aids in diagnosing diseases of vestibular system.	Nurse instructs patient to eat no more than a light meal before test, to prevent nausea. Nurse observes patient for vomiting and assists patient if necessary. Nurse ensures patient safety.
Posturography	A balance test in which one semicircular canal can be isolated from others to determine site of lesion.	Nurse informs patient that test is time consuming and uncomfortable but that the test can be discontinued any time at patient's request.
Rotary chair testing	The patient is seated in a chair driven by a motor under computer control. Test is an evaluation of peripheral vestibular system.	Nurse instructs patient to eat no more than a light meal before test, to prevent nausea. Nurse observes patient for vomiting and assists patient if necessary. Nurse ensures patient safety.

can assist in the diagnosis of the type of hearing loss. The intensity or strength of a sound wave is expressed in terms of decibels (dB), ranging from 0 to 110 dB. The intensity of a sound required to make any frequency barely audible to the average normal ear is 0 dB. *Threshold* refers to the signal level at which pure tones are detected (pure tone thresholds) or the signal level at which the patient correctly hears 50% of the signals (speech detection thresholds).

Normal speech is approximately 40 to 65 dB; a soft whisper is 20 dB. Normally, a child and a young adult can hear frequencies from about 16 to 20,000 Hz, but hearing is most sensitive between 500 and 4000 Hz. This range is similar to that of the frequencies contained in speech. A 40- to 45-dB loss in these frequencies causes moderate difficulty in hearing normal speech. A hearing aid may be helpful because it makes sound information louder, although not clearer. A hearing aid may not be helpful to a patient who has problems with discrimination of sounds or sound information because the consonants are still not heard well enough to make speech understandable.

Screening Audiometry. Screening audiometry is the testing of large numbers of people with a fast, simple test to detect possible hearing problems. A pass–fail criterion is used to identify people who will need additional diagnostic testing. People who fail the screening should be referred to an audiologist for pure-tone (threshold) audiometry.

Pure-Tone Audiometry. A pure-tone audiometer produces tones at specific frequencies and intensities and is used by an audiologist to determine the hearing range of the patient in terms of decibels and hertz. Tinnitus can cause inconsistent results.

Specialized Tests

Specialized tests of the auditory system are most often performed in an outpatient setting by an audiologist. An audiologist can perform many additional tests with the use of audiometers and computers that record electrical activity from the middle ear, the inner ear, and the brain (see Table 23-12). The test most commonly performed by audiologists is pure-tone audiometry. More sophisticated tests are available to determine the origin of certain hearing losses. These include evoked potential studies (also called *auditory brainstem response*) and electrocochleography. Computed tomography and magnetic resonance imaging are used to diagnose the site of a lesion, such as a tumour of the auditory nerve.

Test for Vestibular Function

Table 23-12 describes diagnostic studies commonly used to assess vestibular function. Results of these tests can be altered by use of caffeine, other stimulants, sedatives, and antivertigo agents.

REVIEW QUESTIONS

The number of the question corresponds to the same-numbered objective at the beginning of the chapter.

1. In a client who has a hemorrhage in the vitreous cavity of the eye, where is the blood accumulating?
   a. In the aqueous humor
   b. Between the lens and the retina
   c. Between the cornea and the lens
   d. In the space between the iris and the lens
2. Why might intraocular pressure increase?
   a. Edema of the corneal stroma
   b. Dilation of the retinal arterioles
   c. Blockage of the lacrimal canals and ducts
   d. Increased production of aqueous humor by the ciliary process
3. Which of the following should the nurse question clients about if they are using eye drops to treat glaucoma?
   a. Use of corrective lenses
   b. Their usual sleep pattern
   c. A history of heart or lung disease
   d. Sensitivity to opioids or depressants
4. For a client with an ophthalmic problem, the nurse should always assess for which of the following?
   a. Visual acuity
   b. Pupillary reactions
   c. Intraocular pressure
   d. Confrontation visual fields

5. Which of the following normal findings would the nurse expect during assessment of the auditory system?
   a. Absence of the cone of light
   b. Pearl-grey tympanic membrane
   c. Lateralization with Weber's test
   d. Bone conduction greater than air conduction
6. Which of the following are common age-related changes in the auditory system? *(Select all that apply)*
   a. Drier cerumen
   b. Tinnitus in both ears
   c. Auditory nerve degeneration
   d. Atrophy of the tympanic membrane
   e. Greater ability to hear high-pitched sounds
7. Before fluorescein is injected for angiography, what should the nurse do? *(Select all that apply)*
   a. Obtain an emesis basin.
   b. Ask whether the client is fatigued.
   c. Administer a topical anaesthetic.
   d. Inform client that skin may turn yellow.
   e. Assess for allergies to iodine-based contrast media.

1. b; 2. d; 3. c; 4. a; 5. b; 6. a, c, d; 7. a, d.

Ⓔvolve

For even more review questions, visit *http://evolve.elsevier.com/Canada/Lewis/medsurg.*

REFERENCES

Age-Related Eye Disease Study 2 (AREDS2) Research Group. (2013). Lutein + zeaxanthin and omega-3 fatty acids for age-related macular degeneration: The Age-Related Eye Disease Study 2 (AREDS2) randomized clinical trial. *JAMA: The Journal of the American Medical Association, 309*(19), 2005–2015. doi:10.1001/jama.2013.4997.

American Optometric Association. (2015). *Computer vision syndrome.* Retrieved from *http://www.aoa.org/patients-and-public/caring-for-your-vision/protecting-your-vision/computer-vision-syndrome?sso=y.*

Dua, H. S., Faraj, L. A., Said, D. G., et al. (2013). Human corneal anatomy redefined: A novel pre-Descemet's layer (Dua's layer). *Ophthalmology, 120*(9), 1778–1785.

Evans, J. R., & Lawrenson, J. G. (2012). Antioxidant vitamin and mineral supplements for preventing age-related macular degeneration. *The Cochrane Database of Systematic Reviews*, (6), article CD000253. doi:10.1002/14651858.CD000253.pub3.

Health Canada. (2011). *It's your health: Ear candling.* Retrieved from *http://www.hearingclinic.ca/docs/cerumen-ear-wax-goc-canada.pdf.*

Herlihy, B. (2014). *The human body in health and illness* (5th ed.). St. Louis: Elsevier Saunders.

Institute for Safe Medication Practices Canada. (2016). *Do not use: List of dangerous abbreviations, symbols, and dose designations.* Retrieved from *https://www.ismp-canada.org/dangerous abbreviations.htm.*

Jarvis, C., Browne, A. J., MacDonald-Jenkins, J., et al. (2014). *Physical examination & health assessment* (2nd Canadian ed.). Toronto: Saunders Elsevier.

Lehne, R. A. (2012). *Pharmacology for nursing care* (8th ed.). Philadelphia: Saunders.

National Coalition for Vision Health. (2011). *Vision loss in Canada 2011*. Retrieved from *http://www.cos-sco.ca/wp-content/uploads/2012/09/VisionLossinCanada_e.pdf*.

Seidel, H., Ball, J. W., Dains, J. E., et al. (2011). *Mosby's guide to physical examination* (7th ed.). St. Louis: Mosby.

Skidmore-Roth, L. (2012). *Mosby's 2013 nursing drug reference* (26th ed.). St. Louis: Mosby.

Thibodeau, G., & Patton, K. (2012). *Structure and function of the body* (14th ed.). St Louis: Mosby.

Wu, Y. T., Willcox, M. D. P., & Stapleton, F. (2015). The effect of contact lens hygiene behavior on lens case contamination. *Optometry and Vision Science, 92*(2), 167–174.

RESOURCES

Resources for this chapter are listed after Chapter 24.
For additional Internet resources, see the website for this book at *http://evolve.elsevier.com/Canada/Lewis/medsurg*

CHAPTER

24

Nursing Management
Visual and Auditory Problems

Written by: Sharon L. Lewis
Adapted by: Ruby Sangha

⊖volve WEBSITE

http://evolve.elsevier.com/Canada/Lewis/medsurg

- Review Questions (Online Only)
- Key Points
- Answer Guidelines for Case Study
- Student Case Study
  - Patient Undergoing Cataract Surgery
- Customizable Nursing Care Plan
  - After Eye Surgery
- Conceptual Care Map Creator
- Audio Glossary
- Content Updates

LEARNING OBJECTIVES

1. Compare and contrast the types of refractive errors and appropriate corrections.
2. Describe the etiology of and collaborative care for extraocular disorders.
3. Review the pathophysiological features and clinical manifestations of selected intraocular disorders and the nursing management and collaborative care of affected patients.
4. Discuss the nursing measures that promote the health of the eyes and ears.
5. Explain the general preoperative and postoperative care of the patient undergoing ophthalmological or otological surgery.
6. Summarize the action and uses of drug therapy for treating problems of the eyes and ears.
7. Explain the pathophysiological features and clinical manifestations of common ear problems and the nursing management and collaborative care of affected patients.
8. Compare the causes, management, and rehabilitative potential of conductive and sensorineural hearing loss.
9. Explain the use of, care of, and patient teaching related to assistive devices for eye and ear problems.
10. Describe the common causes and assistive measures for uncorrectable visual impairment and deafness.
11. Describe the measures used to assist the patient in adapting psychologically to decreased vision and hearing.

KEY TERMS

acoustic neuroma, p. 484	cataract, p. 468	keratitis, p. 466	refractive error, p. 461
age-related macular degeneration (AMD), p. 474	conjunctivitis, p. 465	Ménière's disease, p. 483	retinal detachment, p. 472
amblyopia, p. 461	enucleation, p. 479	myopia, p. 461	retinopathy, p. 472
astigmatism, p. 461	external otitis, p. 480	otosclerosis, p. 482	strabismus, p.468
benign paroxysmal positional vertigo (BPPV), p. 484	glaucoma, p. 475	presbycusis, p. 488	
	hordeolum, p. 464	presbyopia, p. 461	
	hyperopia, p. 461		

This chapter describes visual and auditory problems, with an emphasis on their pathophysiological features and clinical manifestations and on the collaborative care and nursing management of affected patients. Assistive devices for visual and hearing impairment are also discussed.

VISUAL PROBLEMS

The eye contains numerous structures, all of which are critical for proper functioning of the visual system. These components include, most anteriorly, the tear film and cornea; the anterior segment structures, including the iris and lens; and posterior structures, including the vitreous, retina, and optic nerve. The optic nerves of both eyes meet and cross at the optic chiasm. At this point, the information from both eyes is combined and then splits according to the visual field. Information from the visual fields travels via the right or left optic tract, which terminates in the posterior part of the brain in the occipital cortex.

Loss of some or all vision doubles the difficulties associated with activities of daily living, halves the ease of social functioning, doubles the incidence of falls and mortality rates, triples the risk of depression, and quadruples the risk of hip fractures (National Coalition for Vision Health, 2011).

CORRECTABLE REFRACTIVE ERRORS

The most common visual problem is refractive error. In this defect, light rays focus either in front of or behind the retina. The cornea is responsible for two-thirds of the refractive power of the eye, and the lens is responsible for one-third of refractive power. In addition to their combined refractive power, the length of the eye is an important determinant of potential refractive error. When light rays are out of focus, the patient may experience blurry vision, eye strain (asthenopia), headaches, or generalized eye discomfort. The principal refractive errors of the eye can be corrected by the use of lenses in the form of eyeglasses or contact lenses, by refractive surgery, or by surgical implantation of an artificial lens. Refractive errors in young children should be corrected because such children may develop amblyopia (reduced or no vision in affected eye) also known as "lazy eye," which may result in permanent vision loss if not treated in early childhood, ideally before the age of 5 (Canadian Ophthalmological Society, 2007). Undetected and untreated refractive errors and cataracts in persons older than 65 can lead to falls and unintentional injuries. Falls and fractures are of particular concern because of the effect on the individual's independence and long-term health (Bell, Hawranik, & McCormac, 2011).

SAFETY ALERT
Upon admission to hospital, older adult patients should undergo vision screening and, when it is warranted, be referred to an appropriate eye care specialist.

Myopia (nearsightedness) is an inability to accommodate for objects at a distance. It causes light rays to be focused in front of the retina. Myopia may occur because of excessive light refraction by the cornea or lens or because of an abnormally long eye.

Hyperopia (farsightedness) is an inability to accommodate for near objects. The light rays focus behind the retina, and so the patient must use accommodation to focus the light rays on the retina for near objects. This type of refractive error occurs when the cornea or lens does not have adequate focusing power or when the eyeball is too short.

Presbyopia is the loss of accommodation associated with age. This condition generally appears at approximately age 40. As the eye ages, the lens becomes larger, firmer, and less elastic. These changes, which progress with aging, result in an inability to focus on near objects. The first sign of presbyopia is often the need to hold reading material farther away.

Astigmatism is caused by an irregular corneal curvature. This irregularity causes the incoming light rays to be bent unequally. Consequently, the light rays do not converge in a single point of focus on the retina. Astigmatism can occur in conjunction with any of the other refractive errors.

Aphakia is the absence of the lens, which results in significant refractive error. Without the focusing ability of the lens, images are projected behind the retina. In rare cases, the lens may be absent congenitally, or it may be removed during cataract surgery. A lens that is traumatically injured is removed and replaced with an intraocular lens (IOL) implant. The lens accounts for approximately 30% of ocular refractive power.

Nonsurgical Corrections

Corrective Glasses. Myopia, hyperopia, presbyopia, and astigmatism can be modified by the appropriate corrective lenses. Myopia necessitates a "minus" (concave) corrective lens, whereas hyperopia and presbyopia necessitate a "plus" (convex) corrective lens. Glasses for presbyopia are often called reading glasses because they are usually worn only for close work. The presbyopic correction may also be combined with a correction for another refractive error, such as myopia or astigmatism. In these combined glasses, the presbyopic correction is in the lower portion of the spectacle lens. A traditional bifocal or trifocal has visible lines. A newer type of corrective glasses for presbyopia, the progressive lens, is actually a multifocal lens in which the transition from near to far correction is graduated seamlessly over a range in the middle area of the lens. This eliminates the visible lines between the different corrective lenses. The lower lens in multifocal glasses may predispose older people to falls because viewing the environment through their lower lenses impairs important visual capabilities (contrast sensitivity and depth perception) for detecting environmental hazards, particularly in unfamiliar environments (Tareef, 2011).

Contact Lenses. Use of contact lenses is another way to correct refractive errors; they are available in rigid and soft types. The rigid types are available in standard and gas-permeable forms. Their care requires separate solutions for cleaning, storing, and wetting. The soft types are available in many forms. The most commonly used soft contact lenses are the standard and disposable forms, which are less durable and more expensive than rigid forms. Contact lenses generally provide better vision than do glasses because the patient has more normal peripheral vision without the distortion and obstruction of glasses and their frames. This is especially true with high refractive errors. Contact lenses are made from various plastic and silicone substances, which are very permeable by oxygen, have a high water content, and thus enable longer wearing time with greater comfort. If the oxygen supply to the cornea is decreased, the cornea becomes swollen, visual acuity decreases, and the patient experiences severe discomfort.

Altered or decreased tear formation can make wearing contact lenses difficult. Tear production can be decreased by medications such as antihistamines, decongestants, diuretics, hormone medications such as oral contraceptives, and the hormones produced during pregnancy. Environmental factors such as wind, fans, and dust may also decrease the tear film. Allergic conjunctivitis with itching, tearing, and redness can also affect contact lens wear.

In general, the nurse must know whether the patient wears contact lenses, the pattern of wear (daily versus extended), and care practices. Shining a light obliquely on the eyeball can help the nurse visualize a contact lens. The patient should know the signs and symptoms of contact lens problems that must be managed by the eye care professional. These symptoms are remembered better with the mnemonic device RSVP: redness, sensitivity, vision problems, and pain.

SAFETY ALERT
The nurse should stress the importance of removing contact lenses immediately when the patient experiences RSVP symptoms.

Surgical Therapy

Surgical procedures are designed to eliminate or reduce the need for eyeglasses or contact lenses and correct refractive errors by changing the focus of the eye. Surgical management for refractive errors includes laser surgery and IOL implantation.

Laser Surgery. *Laser-assisted in situ keratomileusis* (LASIK) may be considered for patients with low to moderately high degrees of myopia, hyperopia, and astigmatism. It has revolutionized refractive surgery, and millions of LASIK procedures have been performed worldwide. The procedure first involves using a laser or surgical blade to create a thin flap in the cornea. Through new "wave-front" technology, the laser is then programmed to use a map of the patient's cornea to sculpt the cornea and correct the refractive error. The flap is then repositioned and adheres on its own without sutures in a few minutes (Sutton, Lawless, & Hodge, 2014). Perceptions of glare, halos, and starbursts and poor night vision are negative consequences for some patients despite uncomplicated and successful surgery (Government of Canada, 2012).

Photorefractive keratectomy is indicated for low to moderate degrees of myopia, hyperopia, and astigmatism and is a good option for a patient with insufficient corneal thickness for a LASIK flap. In this procedure, only the epithelium is removed, and the laser is used to sculpt the cornea to correct the refractive error. *Laser-assisted epithelial keratomileusis* (LASEK) is similar to photorefractive keratectomy except that the epithelium is replaced after surgery.

Implantation. *Intracorneal ring segments* are two semicircular pieces of plastic that are implanted between the layers of the cornea to treat mild forms of myopia. They are designed to change the shape of the cornea by adjusting the focusing power. Intracorneal ring segments can be removed, and the cornea usually returns to its original shape within a few weeks.

Refractive IOL implantation is an option for patients with severe myopia or hyperopia. Like cataract surgery, it involves the removal of the patient's natural lens and implantation of an IOL, which is a small plastic lens to correct a patient's refractive error. Because this requires entering the eye, the risk of complications is higher. New accommodating IOLs correct both myopia and presbyopia.

Phakic IOLs are sometimes referred to as *implantable contact lenses*. They are implanted into the eye without removal of the eye's natural lens. They are used for patients with severe myopia and hyperopia. Unlike the refractive IOL, the phakic IOL is placed in front of the eye's natural lens. Leaving the natural lens in the eye preserves the ability of the eye to focus for reading vision. The Artisan IOL is one type of phakic IOL used for moderate to severe myopia.

UNCORRECTABLE VISUAL IMPAIRMENT

In 2012, approximately 750 000 Canadians were identified as having a *seeing disability,* defined as either difficulty seeing ordinary newsprint with corrective lenses if those are usually worn or difficulty seeing the face of someone 4 m across a room with corrective lenses if those are usually worn (Statistics Canada, 2016). The partially sighted individual may actually have significant vision. It is important in working with a visually impaired patient to understand that a person classified as blind may have useful vision. Appropriate responses and interventions depend on the nurse's understanding of an individual patient's visual abilities.

Levels of Visual Impairment
Total blindness is defined as no light perception and no usable vision. *Functional blindness* is the condition in which the patient has some light perception but no usable vision. A patient with

TABLE 24-1	DEFINITION OF BLINDNESS IN CANADA

Legal blindness is defined as follows:
- Central visual acuity for distance: 20/200 or worse in the better eye (with correction)
- Visual field: no more than 20 degrees in its widest diameter or in the better eye.

either total or functional blindness may use vision substitutes such as guide dogs and canes for ambulation. Vision enhancement techniques are not helpful.

There are approximately 108 000 legally blind Canadians (visual acuity less than 20/200) and another 278 000 with visual impairment (visual acuity between 20/50 and 20/200) (Health Professions Regulatory Advisory Council, 2010, p. 7). More than 5.5 million Canadians have a major eye disease that could cause vision loss (Canadian National Institute for the Blind [CNIB], 2015a). Most cases of vision impairment and blindness are caused by conditions such as age-related macular degeneration, glaucoma, diabetic retinopathy, and cataracts. These conditions are preventable, treatable, or both. The prevalence of vision loss in Canada is expected to increase nearly 30% by 2025 (CNIB, 2015a).

A *legally blind individual* meets the criteria developed by the federal government to determine eligibility for government programs and income tax benefits (Table 24-1). A legally blind individual may have some usable vision. The *partially sighted individual* who is not legally blind has a corrected visual acuity greater than 20/200 in the better eye and more than 20 degrees of visual field, but the visual acuity is 20/50 or worse in the better eye. The patient who is partially sighted but also legally blind can benefit greatly from vision enhancement techniques.

NURSING MANAGEMENT
VISUAL IMPAIRMENT

NURSING ASSESSMENT
It is important to determine how long a patient has had a visual impairment because recent loss of vision has particular implications for nursing care. To determine how the patient's visual impairment affects normal functioning, the nurse should question the patient about the level of difficulty encountered when he or she performs certain tasks. For example, the nurse may ask how much difficulty the patient has when reading a newspaper, writing a cheque, moving from one room to the next, or viewing television. Other questions can help the nurse determine the personal meaning that the patient attaches to the visual impairment. The nurse can ask how the vision loss has affected specific aspects of the patient's life, whether the patient has lost a job, or in what activities the patient no longer engages because of the visual impairment. Techniques such as describing where personal items are located, warning the patient when the nurse will be providing direct care, and informing the patient where food items are located on the tray are helpful strategies (Jensen, 2012). In older adult patients in all health care settings, vision can be assessed with the evidence-informed Focus on Falls Prevention Program Vision Screening Tool (Figure 24-1). This tool was specifically adapted and designed to screen vision in older patients and has proved to be successful in effectively identifying such patients who require a referral to an eye specialist. Improving vision in older patients can prevent falls and associated fractures (Bell, Hawranik, & McCormac, 2011).

FIGURE 24-1 **A,** An older patient undergoing vision screening with the Focus on Falls Prevention Program Vision Screening Tool. **B,** Focus on Falls Prevention Program Vision Screening Tool. Source: Courtesy Focus on Falls Prevention Vision Screening Program, Winnipeg, Manitoba.

Patients may attach many negative meanings to the impairment because of societal opinions about blindness. For example, patients may view the impairment as punishment or view themselves as useless and burdensome. It is also important to determine a patient's primary coping strategies, the patient's emotional reactions, and the availability and strength of the patient's support systems.

NURSING DIAGNOSES

Nursing diagnoses depend on the degree of visual impairment and how long it has been present. Nursing diagnoses for a visually impaired patient include, but are not limited to, the following:

- *Risk for injury* as evidenced by *alteration in sensation* (visual impairment)
- *Self-care deficits* related to *perceptual disorders* (visual impairment)
- *Readiness for enhanced self-care*
- *Grieving* (related to loss of vision)

PLANNING

For a patient with recently impaired vision or a patient with impaired adjustment to longstanding visual impairment, the overall goals are that the patient will (a) make a successful adjustment to the impairment, (b) verbalize feelings related to the loss, (c) identify personal strengths and external support systems, and (d) use appropriate coping strategies. If the patient has been functioning at an appropriate or acceptable level, the goal is to maintain the current level of function.

NURSING IMPLEMENTATION

HEALTH PROMOTION. When a partially sighted patient is at risk for preventable further visual impairment, the nurse should encourage the patient to seek appropriate health care. For example, the patient with vision loss from glaucoma may prevent further visual impairment by complying with prescribed therapies and suggested ophthalmological evaluations.

ACUTE INTERVENTION. The nurse provides emotional support and direct care to patients with visual impairment of recent onset. Active listening and facilitating are important components of nursing care for such a patient. The nurse should allow the patient to express anger and grief and should help the patient identify fears and successful coping strategies. The patient's family is intimately involved in the experiences that follow vision loss. With the patient's knowledge and permission, the nurse should include family members in discussions and encourage members to express their concerns.

Many people are uncomfortable around a blind or partially sighted individual because they are not sure what behaviours are appropriate. Sensitivity to the person's feelings without being overly solicitous or stifling the person's independence is vital in creating a therapeutic nursing presence.

The nurse should always communicate in a normal conversational tone and manner with the patient and address the patient directly, not the caregiver or friend who may accompany the patient. Common courtesy dictates introducing oneself and any other persons who approach a blind or partially sighted patient and saying goodbye on leaving. Making eye contact with the partially sighted patient accomplishes several objectives. It ensures that the nurse speaks while facing the patient so that the patient has no difficulty hearing the nurse. The nurse's head position confirms that the nurse is attentive to the patient. Also, establishing eye contact ensures that the nurse can observe the patient's facial expressions and reactions.

Orientation to the environment lessens patients' anxiety or discomfort and facilitates independence. In orienting a partially sighted or blind patient to a new area, the nurse should identify one object as the focal point and describe the location of other objects in relation to it. For example, the nurse may say, "The bed is straight ahead, approximately 10 steps. The chair is to the left of the bed, and the nightstand is to the right, near the head of the bed. The bathroom is to the left of the foot of the bed." The nurse should explain any activities or noises occurring in the patient's immediate surroundings.

The nurse should assist the patient in ambulating to each major object in the area, using the *sighted-guide technique.* When using this technique, the nurse stands slightly in front and to one side of the patient and offers an elbow for the patient to hold. The nurse serves as the sighted guide, walking slightly ahead of the patient with the patient holding the back of the nurse's arm. When using this technique in any situation, the nurse describes the environment to help orient the patient. For example, the nurse may say, "We're going through an open doorway and approaching two steps down. There is an obstacle on the left." To assist the patient to sit, place one of his or her hands on the back of the chair.

The nurse should be familiar with common vision deficits such as cataracts, refractive errors, macular degeneration, glaucoma, and diabetic retinopathy and their associated nursing strategies for care. For example, age-related macular degeneration entails loss of central vision, and the patient is best cared for by being approached from the side. This condition affects a person's ability to see detail required for reading, writing, preparing meals, and recognizing faces. Caring for the patient with glaucoma, which entails loss of peripheral vision, is better when the nurse directly faces the patient. Vision loss from glaucoma primarily affects a person's mobility, especially in a dynamic moving environment (Popescu, Boisjoly, Schmaltz, et al., 2011).

AMBULATORY AND HOME CARE. Rehabilitation after partial or total loss of vision can foster independence, self-esteem, and productivity. The nurse should know what services and devices are available for a partially sighted or blind patient and should be prepared to make appropriate referrals for those services and devices. For patients who are legally blind and those with low-degree vision, the primary resource for services is the Canadian National Institute for the Blind (CNIB). A list of agencies that serve the partially sighted or blind patient is available from this institute (see the Canadian Resources at the end of this chapter).

Braille or audio books for reading and a cane or guide dog for ambulation are examples of vision substitution techniques. These are usually most appropriate for patients with no functional vision. For most patients who have some remaining vision, vision enhancement techniques can provide enough help for them to learn to ambulate, read printed material, and accomplish activities of daily living.

Optical Devices for Vision Enhancement. A wide range of technological advances have become available to assist people with low-degree vision. These devices include desktop video magnification/closed-circuit units, electronic hand-held magnifiers, text-to-speech scanners, e-readers, and computer tablets (material read aloud, magnification, image zooming, brighter screen, voice recognition). Many of these devices require some training and practice for successful use. The nurse should encourage patients to practise with the device so that they can use it successfully.

Nonoptical Methods for Vision Enhancement. Approach magnification is a simple but sometimes overlooked technique for enhancing the patient's residual vision. The nurse can recommend that the patient sit closer to the television or hold books closer to the eyes, which the patient may be reluctant to do unless encouraged. Contrast enhancement techniques include watching television in black and white, placing dark objects against a light background (e.g., a white plate on a black placemat), using a black felt-tip marker to write, and using contrasting colours (e.g., a red stripe at the edge of steps or curbs). Increased lighting can be provided by halogen lamps, direct sunlight, or gooseneck lamps that can be aimed directly at the reading material or other near objects. Large type is often helpful, especially in conjunction with other optical or nonoptical vision enhancements.

EVALUATION

The overall expected outcomes are that the patient with severe visual impairment will

- Have no further loss of vision
- Be able to use adaptive coping strategies
- Not experience a decrease in self-esteem or social interactions
- Function safely within her or his own environment

AGE-RELATED CONSIDERATIONS

VISUAL IMPAIRMENT

Older adults are at an increased risk for vision loss caused by eye disease (Akpek & Smith, 2013). Older adults may have other deficits, such as cognitive impairment or limited mobility, that further affect the ability to function in usual ways. Financial resources may meet normal needs but can be inadequate in meeting increased demands of vision services or devices.

Older adult patients may become confused or disoriented when visually compromised. The combination of decreased vision and confusion increases the risk of falls, which have potentially serious consequences for older adults. Decreased vision may compromise an older adult's ability to function, which raises concerns about maintaining independence and damaging the patient's self-image. Because of decreased manual dexterity, some older adults may have difficulty instilling prescribed eye drops. It is important to provide proper instruction and demonstration. Having the patient demonstrate the technique is an important aspect of nursing education and reassurance for patients. Eye drop assistive devices are available for purchase at pharmacies in Canada, and their use can be suggested.

EYE TRAUMA

Although the eyes are well protected by the bony orbit and by fat pads, everyday activities can result in ocular trauma. Ocular injuries can involve the ocular adnexa, the superficial structures, or the deeper ocular structures. Eye trauma is one of the leading causes of vision impairment in Canada; an estimated 720 000 Canadians sustain eye injuries that necessitate medical attention every year (CNIB, 2012). Of all Canadian workers, 40% do not get needed visual aids, and approximately 200 per day suffer eye injuries. Furthermore, many of these injuries are serious enough to cause workers to lose work time, and some can lead to permanent eye damage or blindness. A Canadian online eye injury registry has been developed to gather data about the pattern and types of eye injuries that occur. Table 24-2 outlines emergency management of an eye injury. Types of ocular trauma include blunt injuries, penetrating injuries, and chemical exposure injuries. Causes of ocular injuries include automobile accidents, falls, injuries from sports and leisure activity, assaults, and work-related situations. Trauma is often a preventable cause of visual impairment. Almost 90% of all eye injuries could be prevented by the wearing of protective eyewear during potentially hazardous work, hobbies, or sports activities. The nurse's role in individual and community education is extremely important in reducing the incidence of ocular trauma.

EXTRAOCULAR DISORDERS

Inflammation and Infection

One of the most common conditions encountered by ophthalmologists is inflammation or infection of the external eye. Many external irritants or microorganisms can affect the eyelids and conjunctiva and can involve the avascular cornea. The nurse is responsible for teaching the patient appropriate interventions related to the specific disorder.

Hordeolum. An external hordeolum (commonly called a *stye*) is an infection of the sebaceous glands in the eyelid margin (Figure 24-2). The most common bacterial infective pathogen is *Staphylococcus aureus*. The affected area rapidly becomes red, swollen, circumscribed, and acutely tender. The nurse should instruct the patient to apply warm, moist compresses at least four times a day until it improves. This may be the only treatment necessary. If it tends to recur, the patient should be taught to perform eyelid scrubs daily. In addition, use of appropriate antibiotic ointments or drops may be indicated.

✚ TABLE 24-2   EMERGENCY MANAGEMENT

Eye Injury

Cause	Interventions
Trauma	**Initial**
Blunt: Fist; other blunt objects	• Determine mechanism of injury.
Penetrating: Fragments such as glass, metal, wood; knife, stick, or other large object	• Ensure airway, breathing, and circulation.
	• Assess for other injuries.
Chemical Burn	• Assess for chemical exposure.
• Alkaline	• In case of chemical exposure, begin ocular irrigation *immediately;* do not stop until emergency personnel arrive to continue irrigation. Use sterile saline or water if saline is unavailable.
• Acid	
	• Do not attempt to treat the injury (except as noted above for chemical exposure).
Thermal Burn	• Assess visual acuity.
• Direct burn from curling iron or other hot surface	• Do not put pressure on the eye.
• Indirect burn from ultraviolet light (e.g., welding torch, sun lamp)	• Instruct patient not to blow nose.
	• Stabilize foreign objects.
Foreign Bodies	• Cover injured eye or eyes with dry, sterile patches, and a protective shield.
• Glass	
• Metal	• Do not give the patient food or fluids.
• Wood	• Elevate head of bed to 45 degrees.
• Plastic	• Do not put medication or solutions in the eye unless ordered by physician.
• Ceramic	
	• Administer analgesic drugs as appropriate.
Possible Assessment Findings Depending on Cause	
• Pain	**Ongoing Monitoring**
• Photophobia	• Reassure the patient.
• Redness: diffuse or localized	• Monitor pain.
• Swelling	• Anticipate surgical repair for penetrating injury, globe rupture, or globe avulsion.
• Ecchymosis	
• Tearing	
• Blood in the anterior chamber	
• Absence of eye movements	
• Fluid drainage from eye (e.g., blood, CSF, aqueous humor)	
• Abnormal or decreased vision	
• Visible foreign body	
• Prolapsed globe	
• Abnormal intraocular pressure	
• Visual field defect	

CSF, cerebro-spinal fluid.

FIGURE 24-2 External hordeolum (stye) on the upper eyelid caused by staphylococcal infection. Source: Courtesy Cory J. Bosanko, OD, FAAO, Eye Centers of Tennessee, Crossville, Tennessee.

Chalazion. A *chalazion* is a chronic inflammatory granuloma of the meibomian (sebaceous) glands in the eyelid. A hordeolum may evolve into a chalazion. A chalazion may also occur as a response to the material released into the eyelid when a blocked gland ruptures. The chalazion usually appears on the upper eyelid as a swollen, tender, reddened area that may be painful. Initial treatment is similar to that for a hordeolum. If warm, moist

compresses are ineffective in causing spontaneous drainage, the ophthalmologist may surgically remove the lesion (this is normally an office procedure), or the ophthalmologist may inject the lesion with corticosteroids.

Blepharitis. *Blepharitis* is a chronic inflammatory process of the eyelid margin. It is a common eye disorder throughout the world and can affect any age group. The cause is unknown and probably multifactorial. Bacteria have been implicated in playing a significant role. It may be associated with several systemic diseases such as rosacea or seborrheic dermatitis. It is related to other ocular conditions such as dry eye, chalazion, conjunctivitis, and keratitis. Symptoms include a burning sensation, irritation, tearing, photophobia, blurred vision, and redness of the conjunctiva. These symptoms are usually worse in the morning because the inflamed eyelids are in close contact with the ocular surface and tear production is decreased overnight as a result of less blinking. Basic treatment includes a long-term commitment to eyelid hygiene. Warm compresses and washing the eyelid margins with baby shampoo diluted in water and applied gently with a cotton-tipped swab are recommended. An antibiotic-corticosteroid ointment can be used for short periods only.

Conjunctivitis. Conjunctivitis is an infection or inflammation of the conjunctiva, the mucous membrane that lines the eyelids and covers the conjunctiva. These infections may be caused by bacteria or viruses (Durning, 2013). Conjunctival inflammation may result from exposure to allergens or chemical irritants. Symptoms include ocular redness, discharge, burning, and sometimes itching and light sensitivity. It can occur in one or both eyes and is contagious. Careful hand hygiene and the use of individual or disposable towels help prevent the spread of the condition (Callahan, 2012).

Bacterial Infections. Acute bacterial conjunctivitis *(pinkeye)* is a common infection. Although it occurs in every age group, epidemics commonly occur among children because of their poor personal hygiene habits. In adults and children, the most common causative microorganism is *S. aureus. Streptococcus pneumoniae* and *Haemophilus influenzae* are other common causative pathogens, but they are seen more often in children than in adults. A patient with bacterial conjunctivitis may complain of discomfort, pruritus, tearing, redness, and a muco-purulent drainage. Although this initially occurs in one eye, it generally spreads within 48 hours to the unaffected eye. The infection is usually self-limiting, but treatment with antibiotic drops shortens the course of the disorder.

Viral Infections. Conjunctival infections may be caused by many different viruses. A patient with viral conjunctivitis may complain of tearing, foreign body sensation, redness, and mild photophobia. This condition is usually mild and self-limiting. However, it can be severe, with considerable discomfort and subconjunctival hemorrhaging. Adenovirus conjunctivitis may be contracted in contaminated swimming pools and through direct contact with an infected patient. Treatment is usually palliative. If the patient's symptoms are severe, topical cortico-steroids provide temporary relief but do not cure the infection. Antiviral drops are ineffective and therefore not indicated.

Chlamydial Infections. Trachoma is a chronic conjunctivitis caused by *Chlamydia trachomatis* (serotypes A through C). It is a major cause of blindness worldwide. It is responsible for visual impairment in approximately 1.8 million people, and 0.5 million of those people are irreversibly blind (World Health Organization, 2016). This preventable eye disease is transmitted mainly via contact with the hands and by flies. Adult inclusion conjunctivitis (AIC) is caused by *C. trachomatis* (serotypes D through K). Manifestations of both trachoma and AIC are mucopurulent ocular discharge, irritation, redness, and eyelid swelling. For unknown reasons, AIC does not carry the long-term consequences of trachoma. AIC also differs from trachoma in that it is common in economically developed countries, whereas trachoma is most common in underdeveloped countries. Antibiotic therapy is usually effective for trachoma and AIC.

Although antibiotic treatment may be successful in adults with AIC, these patients have a high risk of concurrent chlamydial genital infection, as well as other sexually transmitted infections. The nurse's teaching plan for this patient should include the implications of AIC for sexual activity and reproductive health.

Allergic Conjunctivitis. Conjunctivitis caused by exposure to an allergen can be mild and transitory, or it can be severe enough to cause significant swelling, sometimes causing the conjunctiva to balloon beyond the eyelids. The defining symptom of allergic conjunctivitis is itching. The patient may also complain of burning, redness, and tearing. In the acute stage, the patient may also have white or clear exudate. If the condition is chronic, the exudate is thicker and becomes mucopurulent. The patient may develop allergic conjunctivitis in response to pollens, in addition to animal dander, ocular solutions and medications, or even contact lenses. The nurse should instruct the patient to avoid the allergen if it

is known. Artificial tears can be effective in diluting the allergen and washing it from the eye. Effective topical medications include antihistamines and corticosteroids.

Keratitis. Keratitis is an inflammation or infection of the cornea that can be caused by a variety of microorganisms or by other factors. The condition may involve the conjunctiva, the cornea, or both. When it involves both, the disorder is termed *keratoconjunctivitis.*

Bacterial Infections. When the epithelial layer is disrupted, the cornea can become infected by a variety of bacteria. Topical antibiotics are generally effective, but eradicating the infection may require subconjunctival antibiotic injection or, in severe cases, intravenous antibiotics. Risk factors include mechanical or chemical corneal epithelial damage, contact lens wear, debilitation, nutritional deficiencies, immuno-suppressed states, and use of contaminated products (e.g., lens care solutions and cases, topical medications, cosmetics).

Viral Infections. Herpes simplex virus (HSV) keratitis is the most frequently occurring infectious cause of corneal blindness in the Western hemisphere. It is a growing problem, especially among immuno-suppressed patients. It may be caused by HSV-1 or HSV-2 (genital herpes), although HSV-2 ocular infection is much less common. The resulting corneal ulcer has a characteristic dendritic (tree-branching) appearance (Farooq & Shukla, 2012). Pain and photophobia are common. In up to 40% of patients, herpetic keratitis heals spontaneously. The spontaneous healing rate increases to 70% if the cornea is debrided to remove infected cells. Collaborative therapy includes corneal debridement, followed by topical therapy with trifluridine (Viroptic) for 2 to 3 weeks. Topical corticosteroids are usually contraindicated because they contribute to a longer course and possible deeper ulceration of the cornea. Drug therapy may also include oral acyclovir (Zovirax).

The varicella-zoster virus causes both chicken pox and herpes zoster ophthalmicus (HZO). HZO may occur by reactivation of an endogenous infection that has persisted in latent form after an earlier attack of varicella or by contact with a patient with chicken pox or herpes zoster. It occurs most frequently in older adults and in immuno-suppressed patients. Collaborative care of a patient with acute HZO may include analgesics for the pain, topical corticosteroids to reduce inflammation, antiviral drugs such as acyclovir (Zovirax) to reduce viral replication, mydriatic drugs to dilate the pupil and relieve pain, and topical antibiotics to combat secondary infection. The patient may apply warm compresses and povidone-iodine gel to the affected skin (gel should not be applied too near the eye).

Epidemic keratoconjunctivitis is the most serious ocular adenoviral disease. This condition is spread by direct contact, including sexual activity. In the medical setting, contaminated hands and instruments can be the source of spread. The patient may complain of tearing, redness, photophobia, and sensation of a foreign body in the eye. In most patients, the disease involves only one eye. Treatment is primarily palliative and includes ice packs and dark glasses. In severe cases, therapy can include mild topical corticosteroids to temporarily relieve symptoms and topical antibiotic ointment. The nurse's most important role is to teach the patient and caregivers the importance of good hygienic practices to avoid spreading the disease.

Other Causes of Keratitis. Keratitis may also be caused by fungi (most commonly *Aspergillus, Candida,* and *Fusarium* species), especially in the case of ocular trauma in an outdoor setting in which fungi are prevalent in the soil and moist organic matter. *Acanthamoeba* keratitis is caused by a parasite that is

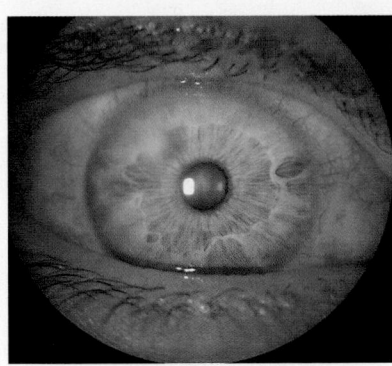

FIGURE 24-3 Corneal ulcer. Infection associated with poor contact lens care. Source: Courtesy Cory J. Bosanko, OD, FAAO, Eye Centers of Tennessee, Crossville, Tennessee.

associated with contact lens wear, probably as a result of using contaminated lens care solutions or cases. Homemade saline solution is particularly susceptible to *Acanthamoeba* contamination. The nurse should instruct all patients who wear contact lenses about good lens care practices. Medical treatment of fungal and *Acanthamoeba* keratitis is difficult. The *Acanthamoeba* organism is resistant to most drugs. If antimicrobial therapy fails, the patient may require corneal transplantation.

Exposure keratitis occurs when the patient cannot adequately close the eyelids. The patient with exophthalmos (protruding eyeball) caused by thyroid eye disease or masses posterior to the globe is susceptible to exposure keratitis.

Corneal Ulcer. Tissue loss caused by infection of the cornea produces a *corneal ulcer* (infectious keratitis) (Figure 24-3). The infection can be caused by bacteria, viruses, or fungi. Corneal ulcers are often very painful, and patients may feel as if a foreign body is in the eye. Other symptoms can include tearing, purulent or watery discharge, redness, and photophobia. Treatment is generally aggressive to prevent permanent loss of vision. Antibiotic, antiviral, or antifungal eye drops may be prescribed as frequently as every hour, night and day, for the first 24 hours. An untreated corneal ulcer can result in corneal scarring and perforation (hole in the cornea). Corneal transplantation may be indicated.

NURSING MANAGEMENT
INFLAMMATION AND INFECTION

NURSING ASSESSMENT

The nurse should assess ocular changes—such as edema, redness, decreasing visual acuity, the sensation that a foreign body is present, or discomfort—and document the findings in the patient's record. In the assessment, the nurse should also consider the psychosocial aspects of the patient's condition, especially when the patient's vision is also impaired.

NURSING DIAGNOSES

Nursing diagnoses for the patient with inflammation or infection of the external eye include, but are not limited to, the following:
- *Acute pain* related to *biological injury agent* (infection)
- *Anxiety* related to *threat to current status* (major change in health status)

PLANNING

The overall goals are that the patient with inflammation or infection of the external eye will (a) avoid spread of infection,

(b) maintain an acceptable level of comfort and functioning during the course of the specific ocular problem, (c) maintain or improve visual acuity, (d) comply with the prescribed therapy, and (e) engage in appropriate health-seeking behaviours.

NURSING IMPLEMENTATION

HEALTH PROMOTION. Careful asepsis and frequent, thorough hand hygiene are essential to prevent spreading organisms from one eye to the other, to other patients, to family members, and to the nurse. The patient and family require information about avoiding sources of ocular irritation or infection and responding appropriately if an ocular problem occurs. Patients with infective disorders that may be transmitted sexually or who have an associated sexually transmitted infection need specific information about those disorders. The nurse should inform the patient about the appropriate use and care of lenses and lens care products.

ACUTE INTERVENTION. Apply warm or cool compresses if indicated for the patient's condition. Darkening the room and providing an appropriate analgesic are other comfort measures. If the patient's visual acuity is decreased, the nurse may need to modify the patient's environment or activities for safety.

The patient may require eye drops as frequently as every hour. If the patient receives two or more different types of drops, the nurse should stagger the eye drop dosing to promote maximum absorption. For example, if two different eye drops are ordered hourly, the nurse should administer one kind of drop on the hour and the other kind of drop on the half-hour unless otherwise prescribed. This staggered schedule promotes maximum absorption. The patient who needs frequent eye drop administration may experience sleep deprivation.

AMBULATORY AND HOME CARE. The patient's primary need in the home environment is for information about required care and how to accomplish that care. The patient and family also need information about proper techniques for medication administration. If the patient's vision is compromised, the nurse should provide suggestions for alternative ways to accomplish necessary daily activities and self-care. A patient who wears contact lenses and develops infections should discard all opened or used lens care products and cosmetics to decrease the risk of reinfection from contaminated products (a common problem and a probable source of infection for many patients).

EVALUATION

The overall expected outcomes are that the patient with inflammation or infection of the external eye will
- Cooperate with the treatment plan
- Experience relief from ocular discomfort
- Effectively cope with functional changes if visual acuity is decreased
- Obtain specific information to prevent recurrent disease

DRY EYE DISORDERS

Keratoconjunctivitis sicca (dry eyes) is a common complaint, particularly of older adults and individuals with certain systemic diseases such as scleroderma and systemic lupus erythematosus. Patients with dry eyes complain of irritation or the sensation of sand in the eye and that the sensation typically worsens throughout the day. This condition is caused by a decrease in the quality or quantity of the tear film, and treatment is directed at the underlying cause. If it is caused by lacrimal duct dysfunction, the condition may respond to hot compresses and eyelid massage.

FIGURE 24-4 Strabismus with right exotropia and fixation of the left eye. Source: Courtesy Cory J. Bosanko, OD, FAAO, Eye Centers of Tennessee, Crossville, Tennessee.

FIGURE 24-5 Sutures on a donated cornea after penetrating keratoplasty (corneal transplantation). Source: Courtesy Cory J. Bosanko, OD, FAAO, Eye Centers of Tennessee, Crossville, Tennessee.

With decreased tear secretion, the patient may use artificial tears or ointments. They should be used sparingly because preservatives in the drops or overuse can cause further ocular irritation. In severe cases, closure of the lacrimal puncta may be necessary. Patients with dry eyes in association with dry mouth may have Sjögren's syndrome (see Chapter 67).

STRABISMUS

Strabismus is a condition in which the patient cannot consistently focus both eyes simultaneously on the same object (Figure 24-4). One eye may deviate inward *(esotropia)*, outward *(exotropia)*, upward *(hypertropia)*, or downward *(hypotropia)*. Strabismus in adults may be caused by thyroid disease, neuro-muscular problems of the eye muscles, retinal detachment repair, or cerebral lesions. The primary complaint with strabismus is double vision.

CORNEAL DISORDERS

Corneal Scars and Opacities

The cornea is a transparent tissue that allows light rays to enter the eye and focus on the retina, thus producing a visual image. Any wound causes the cornea to become abnormally hydrated and decreases the normal transparency. A rigid contact lens can be effective in correcting the irregular astigmatism that results from corneal scars. In other situations, the treatment for corneal scars or opacities is *penetrating keratoplasty* (corneal transplantation). In this surgical procedure, the ophthalmological surgeon removes the full thickness of the patient's cornea and replaces it with a donor cornea that is sutured into place (Figure 24-5). Vision may not be restored for up to 12 months. Corneal problems leading to blindness are uncommon, but if they occur, corneal transplantation can preserve vision that otherwise would be lost.

Corneal transplantation surgery is one of the fastest and safest of all tissue or organ transplantation procedures (Güell, El Husseiny, Manero, et al., 2014). The time between the donor's death and the removal of the tissue should be as short as possible. Most surgeons prefer this interval to be 4 hours or less. The eye banks test donors for human immunodeficiency virus (HIV) and hepatitis B and C viruses. The tissue is preserved in a special nutritive solution, and it can be kept for up to 5 days in the storage medium, if used for transplantation. Improved methods of tissue procurement and preservation, refined surgical techniques, postoperative topical corticosteroids, and careful follow-up have decreased the incidence of graft rejection. Matching the blood type of the donor and the recipient may also improve the success rate (National Eye Institute, 2013).

Keratoconus

Keratoconus is a noninflammatory, usually bilateral disease that has a familial tendency. It can be associated with Down syndrome, atopic dermatitis, Marfan syndrome, aniridia (congenital absence of the iris), and retinitis pigmentosa (hereditary disease characterized by bilateral primary degeneration of the retina beginning in childhood and progression to blindness by middle age).

The anterior cornea thins and protrudes forward, taking on a cone shape. Keratoconus usually appears during adolescence and slowly progresses between the ages of 20 and 60 years. The only symptom is blurred vision. The astigmatism may be corrected with glasses or rigid contact lenses. Intacs inserts, for example, are two clear plastic lenses surgically inserted on the cornea's perimeter to reduce astigmatism and myopia. Intacs inserts are generally used to delay the need for corneal transplantation when contact lenses or glasses no longer help a patient achieve adequate vision. The cornea can perforate as central corneal thinning progresses. In advanced cases, a penetrating keratoplasty is indicated before perforation.

INTRAOCULAR DISORDERS

Cataract

A cataract is an area of opacity within the lens. The patient may have a cataract in one or both eyes. If cataracts are present in both eyes, one cataract may affect the patient's vision more than the other. Cataracts are one of the leading causes of vision loss in Canada. Nearly 2.5 million Canadians have some form of cataract, and this number is expected to double by 2031 (CNIB, 2015c). Cataract removal is the most common surgical procedure for Canadians older than 65 years (Hatch, Campbell, Bell, et al., 2012).

Causes and Pathophysiological Processes. Although most cataracts are age related *(senile cataracts)*, they can be associated with other factors. These include blunt or penetrating trauma, congenital factors such as maternal rubella, exposure to radiation or ultraviolet light, certain drugs such as systemic corticosteroids or long-term topical corticosteroids, and ocular inflammation. Patients with diabetes mellitus tend to develop cataracts at a younger age than average.

Cataract development is mediated by a number of factors. In senile cataract formation, it appears that altered metabolic processes within the lens cause an accumulation of water and alterations in the lens fibre structure. These changes affect lens transparency, causing vision changes.

Clinical Manifestations. Patients with cataracts may complain of a decrease in vision, abnormal colour perception, and glare.

TABLE 24-3 COLLABORATIVE CARE

Cataract

Diagnostic Studies	During Surgery
• History and physical examination	• Removal of lens:
• Visual acuity measurement	• Phacoemulsification (see Figure 24-6)
• Ophthalmoscopy (direct and indirect)	• Extracapsular extraction
• Slit-lamp microscopy	• Correction of surgical aphakia
• Glare testing, potential acuity testing in selected patients	• Intraocular lens implantation (most frequent type of correction)
• Keratometry and A-scan ultrasonography (if surgery is planned)	• Contact lens
• Other tests (e.g., visual field perimetry) may be indicated to determine cause of visual loss	*Postoperative*
	• Topical antibiotic
Collaborative Therapy	• Topical corticosteroid or other anti-inflammatory drug
Nonsurgical	• Mild analgesic drug if necessary
• Prescription change for glasses	• Eye shield and activity as preferred by patient's surgeon
• Strong reading glasses or magnifiers	
• Increased lighting	
• Lifestyle adjustment	
Acute Care: Surgical Therapy	
Preoperative	
• Mydriatic, cycloplegic drugs (see Table 24-4)	
• Nonsteroidal anti-inflammatory drugs	
• Topical antibiotics	
• Antianxiety medications	

Glare results from light scatter caused by the lens opacities, and it may be significantly worse at night when the pupil dilates. The visual decline is gradual, but the rate of cataract development varies from patient to patient. Secondary glaucoma can also occur if the enlarging lens causes an increase in intraocular pressure (IOP).

Diagnostic Studies. Diagnosis is based on decreased visual acuity or other complaints of visual dysfunction. The opacity is directly observable by ophthalmoscopic or slit-lamp microscopic examination. A totally opaque lens creates the appearance of a white pupil. Table 24-3 outlines other diagnostic studies that may be helpful in evaluating the visual effect of a cataract.

Collaborative Care. The presence of a cataract does not necessarily indicate a need for surgery. For many patients, the diagnosis is made long before they actually decide to have surgery. Nonsurgical therapy may postpone the need for surgery. Collaborative care for cataracts is described in Table 24-3.

Nonsurgical Therapy. Currently, the only way to "cure" cataracts is through surgical removal. If the cataract is not removed, the patient's vision will continue to deteriorate. However, specific strategies may help the patient. In many cases, changing the patient's eyewear prescription can improve the level of visual acuity, at least temporarily. Other visual aids, such as strong reading glasses or magnifiers of some type, may help the patient with close vision. Increasing the amount of light to read or accomplish other near-vision tasks is another useful measure. The patient may be willing to adjust his or her lifestyle to accommodate for visual decline. For example, if glare makes it difficult to drive at night, a patient may elect to drive only during daylight hours and to have a family member drive at night. Sometimes, informing and reassuring the patient about the disease process makes the patient comfortable about choosing nonsurgical measures, at least temporarily.

Surgical Therapy. When palliative measures no longer provide an acceptable level of visual function, the patient is an appropriate candidate for surgery. The patient's occupational needs and lifestyle changes are also factors affecting the decision to undergo surgery. In some instances, factors other than the patient's visual needs may influence the need for surgery. Lens-induced problems such as increased IOP may necessitate lens removal. Opacities may prevent the ophthalmologist from obtaining a clear view of the retina in a patient with diabetic retinopathy or other sight-threatening pathological conditions. In those cases, the cataract may be removed to allow the surgeon to visualize the retina and adequately manage the problem.

Preoperative Phase. The patient's preoperative preparation should include an appropriate documentation of the history and a physical examination. Because almost all patients undergo the procedure under local anaesthesia, many physicians and surgical facilities do not require an extensive preoperative physical assessment. However, most patients with cataracts are older adults and may have several medical problems that should be evaluated and controlled before surgery. The surgeon may order preoperative antibiotic eye drops. The patient should not have food or fluids for approximately 6 to 8 hours before surgery. Almost all patients with cataracts are admitted to a surgical facility on an outpatient basis (see the "Evidence-Informed Practice" box). The patient is normally admitted several hours before surgery to allow adequate time for necessary preoperative procedures.

The instillation of dilating and nonsteroidal anti-inflammatory eye drops helps maintain pupil dilation and reduce inflammation, respectively. One type of drug used for dilation is a mydriatic, an α-adrenergic agonist that produces pupillary dilation by causing contraction of the iris dilator muscle. Another type of drug is a cycloplegic, an anticholinergic drug that produces paralysis of accommodation (cycloplegia) and thus pupillary dilation (mydriasis) by blocking the effect of acetylcholine on the ciliary body muscles. Examples of mydriatic and cycloplegic drugs are listed in Table 24-4, and nursing considerations are discussed in the "Nursing Management: Cataracts" section. Many patients receive preoperative antianxiety medication before the injection of local anaesthetic.

DRUG ALERT—Cycloplegics and Mydriatics
- Instruct patient to wear dark glasses to minimize photophobia.
- Monitor for signs of systemic toxicity (e.g., tachycardia, central nervous system effects).

Intraoperative Phase. Cataract extraction is an intraocular procedure. The anterior capsule is opened and the lens nucleus and cortex are removed, leaving the remaining capsular bag intact. In extracapsular extraction, the surgeon can remove the lens nucleus by "scooping" it out with a lens loop or by *phacoemulsification,* in which the nucleus is fragmented by ultrasonic vibration and aspirated from inside the capsular bag (Mayo Clinic, 2013; Figure 24-6). In either case, the remaining cortex is aspirated with an irrigation and aspiration instrument. The choice of placement and type of incision varies among surgeons. Corneoscleral incisions necessitate closure with sutures, whereas scleral tunnel incisions are self-sealing and necessitate no closing suture. The incision required for phacoemulsification is considerably

TABLE 24-4   DRUG THERAPY

Topical Medications for Pupil Dilation

Examples	Onset	Duration	Comments
Mydriatic Drugs			
Phenylephrine hydrochloric acid (Mydfrin)	45–60 min	4–6 hr	May cause tachycardia and elevation in blood pressure, especially in older adult patient; can cause a reflexive decrease in heart rate when blood pressure rises Punctal occlusion should be used to limit systemic absorption
Cycloplegic Drugs			
Tropicamide (Mydriacyl)	20–40 min	4–6 hr	1% Solution used in cycloplegic refraction; 0.5% solution used in fundus examination
Cyclopentolate HCl acid (Cyclogyl)	30–75 min	6–24 hr	Has been associated with psychotic reactions and behavioural disturbances Used in cycloplegic refraction, fundus examination, and uveitis
Homatropine hydrobromide (Isopto Homatropine)	30–60 min	1–3 days	Used in cycloplegic refraction, uveitis; may be used for pupil dilation to allow patient to see around a central lens opacity
Atropine sulphate (Isopto Atropine)	30–180 min	6–12 days	Used in cycloplegic refraction, uveitis

EVIDENCE-INFORMED PRACTICE

Research Highlight

What Surgical Location Has Better Outcomes for Cataract Surgery?

Clinical Question

In adults with cataracts (P), does day surgery (I) or inpatient surgery (C) result in better visual acuity 4 months postoperatively, and which surgical location is safer and more cost effective (O)?

Best Available Evidence

Systematic review of randomized controlled trials

Critical Appraisal and Synthesis of Evidence

- Meta-analysis of two randomized controlled trials (*n* = 1 284). Only one study with 1 034 subjects was methodologically sound, and evidence is based primarily on this study.
- No significant differences in visual acuity were found between patients who underwent day surgery and those who underwent inpatient surgery, as measured with the Snellen chart 4 months after surgery.
- Significantly more early complications (e.g., increased intraocular pressure) were reported in the patients who underwent day surgery, with no relevance to vision acuity at 4 months.
- Costs for inpatient surgery were 20% higher than those for day surgery.
- Quality-of-life scores, patient satisfaction, and cataract symptom scores were similar for both patient groups.

Conclusions

- Day surgery is safe and, subjectively, preferred by patients.
- Day surgery provides the same visual outcome as inpatient surgery.

Implications for Nursing Practice

- Provide information that day-surgery outcomes are comparable to those of inpatient surgery and less costly.
- Quality of life may be improved if day surgery allows the patient to begin home recuperation sooner.

Reference for Evidence

Fedorowicz, Z., Lawrence, D., Gutierrez, P., et al. (2011). Day care versus in-patient surgery for age-related cataract. *Cochrane Database of Systematic Reviews*, (7), CD004242. doi:10.1002/14651858.CD004242.pub4.

P, patient population of interest; I, intervention or area of interest; C, comparison of interest or comparison group; O, outcome or outcomes of interest (see Chapter 1).

FIGURE 24-6 Intraocular lens implant after cataract surgery. Source: Courtesy Cory J. Bosanko, OD, FAAO, Eye Centers of Tennessee, Crossville, Tennessee.

lens that is implanted in the capsular bag behind the iris. At the end of the procedure, additional medications such as antibiotics and corticosteroids may be administered. Depending on the type of anaesthetic, the patient's eye is covered with a patch or protective shield. If used, a patch or protective shield is usually worn overnight and removed during the first postoperative visit.

Postoperative Phase. Unless complications occur, most patients are ready to go home as soon as the effects of sedative drugs have worn off. Postoperative medications usually include antibiotic drops to prevent infection and corticosteroid drops to decrease the postoperative inflammatory response. There is some evidence that postoperative activity restrictions and nighttime eye shielding are unnecessary. However, many ophthalmologists still prefer that the patient avoid activities that increase the IOP, such as bending or stooping, coughing, or lifting.

During each postoperative examination, the ophthalmologist measures the patient's visual acuity, checks anterior chamber depth, assesses corneal clarity, and measures IOP. A flat anterior chamber may cause adhesions of the iris and cornea. The cornea may become hazy or cloudy from intraoperative trauma to the endothelium. Even on the day of surgery, the patient's uncorrected visual acuity in the operative eye may be good. However, it is not unusual or indicative of any problem if the patient's visual acuity is reduced immediately after surgery.

The postoperative eye drops are gradually reduced in frequency and finally discontinued when the eye has healed. When the eye is fully recovered, the patient receives a final prescription for glasses. The newest innovation is a multifocal IOL that corrects for both

smaller than that required with intracapsular or standard extracapsular surgery.

In almost all cases today, an IOL is implanted at the time of cataract extraction surgery. Because most patients undergo an extracapsular procedure, the lens of choice is a posterior chamber near and distance vision. Regardless of the type of IOL used, patients may still need glasses to achieve their best visual acuity.

NURSING MANAGEMENT
CATARACTS

NURSING ASSESSMENT

The nurse should assess the patient's distance and near visual acuity. If the patient is to undergo surgery, the nurse should especially note the visual acuity in the patient's nonoperative eye. With this information, the nurse can determine how visually compromised the patient may be while the operative eye is healing. In addition, the nurse should assess the psychosocial effect of the patient's visual disability and the patient's level of knowledge regarding the disease process and therapeutic options. Postoperatively, it is important to assess the patient's level of comfort and ability to follow the postoperative regimen.

NURSING DIAGNOSES

Nursing diagnoses for the patient with a cataract include, but are not limited to, the following:

- *Self-care deficits* related to *perceptual disorders* (visual impairment)
- *Anxiety* related to *unmet needs* (knowledge about surgical and postoperative experience)

PLANNING

Preoperatively, the overall goals are that the patient with a cataract will (a) make informed decisions regarding therapeutic options and (b) experience minimal anxiety. Postoperatively, the overall goals are that the patient with a cataract will (a) understand and comply with postoperative therapy, (b) maintain an acceptable level of physical and emotional comfort, and (c) remain free of infection and other complications.

NURSING IMPLEMENTATION

HEALTH PROMOTION. There are no proven measures to prevent cataract development. However, it is wise (and certainly does no harm) to suggest that the patient wear sunglasses, avoid extraneous or unnecessary radiation, and maintain good nutrition and appropriate intake of antioxidant vitamins (e.g., vitamins C and E). Also, information about vision enhancement techniques should be provided to the patient who chooses not to undergo surgery.

ACUTE INTERVENTION. Preoperatively, patients with cataracts need accurate information about the disease process and the treatment options, especially because cataract surgery is considered an elective procedure. Although cataracts are not a life-threatening condition, patients need to know that without surgery, some degree of visual disability will develop. The nurse should be available to give each patient and the family or caregivers information to help them make an informed decision about appropriate treatment.

For a patient who elects to have surgery, the nurse is able to provide information, support, and reassurance about the surgical and postoperative experience that can reduce or alleviate the patient's anxiety.

When administering topical medications for pupil dilation before surgery (see Table 24-4 for examples), the nurse should note that patients with dark irides may need a larger dose. Photophobia is common; therefore, decreasing the room lighting is helpful. These medications produce transient stinging and burning and are

TABLE 24-5	**PATIENT & CAREGIVER TEACHING GUIDE**

After Eye Surgery

Include the following information when teaching the patient and the caregiver after eye surgery.
1. Proper hygiene and eye care techniques to ensure that medications, dressings, and surgical wound are not contaminated during eye care
2. Signs and symptoms of infection and when and how to report those to allow early recognition and treatment of possible infection
3. Importance of complying with postoperative restrictions on head positioning, bending, coughing, and the Valsalva manoeuvre to optimize visual outcomes and prevent increased intraocular pressure
4. How to instill eye medications with the use of aseptic techniques and to comply with prescribed eye medication regimen to prevent infection
5. How to monitor pain, take pain medication, and report pain not relieved by medication
6. Importance of continued follow-up as recommended to maximize potential visual outcomes

Source: Adapted from Lamb, P., & Simms-Eaton, S. (2008), *Core curriculum for ophthalmic nursing* (3rd ed.). Dubuque, IA: Kendall-Hunt.

contraindicated for use in patients with narrow-angle glaucoma because angle-closure glaucoma may be produced. Mydriatic drugs can produce significant cardiovascular effects.

Table 24-5 outlines patient and caregiver teaching after eye surgery. Patients with a patch should be informed that they will not have depth perception until the patch is removed (usually within 24 hours). This necessitates special considerations to avoid possible falls or other injuries. The patient with significant visual impairment in the nonoperative eye requires more assistance while the operated eye is patched. Once the patch is removed (usually within 24 hours), most patients with visual impairment in the nonoperative eye have adequate vision for necessary activities because the implanted IOL provides immediate visual rehabilitation in the operated eye. On occasion, a patient may require 1 or 2 weeks for the visual acuity in the operated eye to reach an adequate level for most visual needs. Such a patient also needs some special assistance until the vision improves.

After cataract surgery, most patients experience little or no pain. There may be some scratchy sensation in the operative eye. Mild analgesics are usually sufficient to relieve any pain. If the pain is intense, the patient should notify the surgeon because this may indicate hemorrhage, infection, or increased IOP. The nurse should also instruct the patient to notify the surgeon of increased or purulent drainage, increased redness, or any decrease in visual acuity. (A nursing care plan for the patient after eye surgery is available on the Evolve website.)

AMBULATORY AND HOME CARE. For a patient with cataracts who has not undergone surgery, the nurse can suggest ways in which the patient may modify activities or lifestyle to accommodate the visual deficit caused by the cataract. The nurse should also provide the patient with accurate information about appropriate long-term eye care.

Patients with cataracts who undergo surgery remain in the surgical facility for only a few hours. The patient and the family are responsible for almost all postoperative care. The nurse must give them written and verbal instructions before discharge. These instructions should include information about postoperative eye care, activity restrictions, medications, follow-up visit scheduling, and signs and symptoms of possible complications. The patient's family should be included in the instruction because some patients may have difficulty with self-care activities, especially if the vision in the nonoperative eye is poor. The nurse should provide an opportunity for the patient and family to demonstrate any necessary self-care activities. Most patients experience little visual impairment after surgery.

IOL implants provide immediate visual rehabilitation, and many patients achieve a usable level of visual acuity within a few days after surgery. Also, the patient's eye may remain patched for only 24 hours, and many patients have good vision in the nonoperative eye. A few patients may experience significant visual impairment postoperatively: those who do not have an IOL implanted at the time of surgery, those who require several weeks to achieve a usable level of visual acuity after surgery, or those with poor vision in the nonoperative eye. For such patients, the time between surgery and receiving glasses or contacts can be a period of significant visual disability. The nurse can suggest ways in which the patient and the family can modify activities and the environment to maintain an adequate level of safe functioning. Suggestions may include getting assistance with going up stairs, removing area rugs and other potential obstacles, preparing meals for freezing before surgery, and obtaining audio books for diversion until visual acuity improves.

EVALUATION

The overall expected outcomes are that after cataract surgery, the patient will
- Have improved vision
- Be better able to take care of self
- Have minimal to no pain
- Be optimistic about expected outcomes

AGE-RELATED CONSIDERATIONS

Most patients with cataracts are older adults. When an older patient is visually impaired, even temporarily, she or he may experience a loss of independence, lack of control over her or his life, and a significant change in self-perception. Many older patients need emotional support and encouragement, as well as specific suggestions to allow a maximum level of independent function. The nurse should assure older patients that cataract surgery can be accomplished safely and comfortably with minimal sedation. A study in which nonagenarians (individuals aged 90 to 99) who underwent cataract surgery were compared with octogenarian patients (aged 80 to 89) revealed that nonagenarians are not at increased risk of ocular complications from cataract surgery (Tseng, Greenberg, Wu, et al., 2011).

RETINOPATHY

Retinopathy is a process of microvascular damage to the retina. It can develop slowly or rapidly and lead to blurred vision and progressive vision loss. In adults, retinopathy is most often associated with diabetes mellitus or hypertension.

Diabetic retinopathy is a common complication of diabetes mellitus, especially in patients with longstanding uncontrolled diabetes (Nentwich & Ulbig, 2015). It is the leading cause of visual disability and blindness in Canadians with longstanding uncontrolled diabetes (diabetes is discussed in Chapter 52). Because diabetes has been diagnosed in increasing numbers of Canadians, the incidence of diabetic retinopathy will continue to

FIGURE 24-7 Diabetic retinopathy. Intraretinal clot or blot hemorrhages. Source: Courtesy Cory J. Bosanko, OD, FAAO, Eye Centers of Tennessee, Crossville, Tennessee.

increase. In a Canadian study of diabetic retinopathy in Indigenous and non-Indigenous Canadians, the data indicated that ethnicity does play a significant role in the development and severity of diabetic retinopathy, but potential risk factors are not significantly different (Canadian Diabetes Association, 2013). *Nonproliferative retinopathy* is the most common form of diabetic retinopathy and is characterized by capillary microaneurysms, retinal swelling, and hard exudates. Macular edema represents a worsening of the retinopathy, inasmuch as plasma leaks from macular blood vessels. As capillary walls weaken, they can rupture, which leads to intraretinal "dot or blot" hemorrhaging (Figure 24-7). This can lead to a severe loss of central vision. As the disease advances, *proliferative retinopathy* may occur where new blood vessels grow. However, these blood vessels are abnormal, fragile, and predisposed to leak and thus predispose the patient to severe vision loss. Fluorescein angiography is used to detect diabetic macular edema, which may be treated with laser photocoagulation (Bressler, Beck, & Ferris, 2011).

Hypertensive retinopathy is caused by blockages in retinal blood vessels that result from hypertension. (Hypertension is discussed in Chapter 35.) These changes may not initially affect a person's vision. On a routine eye examination, retinal hemorrhages and macular swelling can be noted. Sustained, severe hypertension can cause swelling of the optic disc and nerve (*papilledema*) and lead to sudden visual loss. Treatment, which may be required on an emergency basis, focuses on lowering the blood pressure. Normal vision is restored in patients with treatment of the underlying cause of the hypertension.

RETINAL DETACHMENT

A **retinal detachment** is a separation of the retina and the underlying pigment epithelium, with fluid accumulation between the two layers. The incidence of nontraumatic retinal detachment is approximately 1 per 15 000 individuals each year. This number is higher when aphakic individuals are included because retinal detachment is more likely to occur in aphakic patients. In a patient with no other risk factors who has had a retinal detachment in one eye, the risk of detachment in the second eye is as high as 25% (Steel, 2014). Almost all patients with an untreated, symptomatic retinal detachment become blind in the involved eye.

Etiology and Pathophysiology

Retinal detachment has many causes, the most common of which is a retinal break. A *retinal break* is an interruption in the full

TABLE 24-6	RISK FACTORS FOR RETINAL DETACHMENT

- Increasing age
- Severe myopia
- Infection or eye trauma
- Retinopathy (diabetic)
- Eye diseases or tumours
- Cataract or glaucoma surgery
- Family or personal history of retinal detachment

Source: Adapted from Canadian National Institute for the Blind. (2015). *Retinal detachment.* Retrieved from *http://www.cnib.ca/en/your-eyes/eye-conditions/retinal-detachment/Pages/default.aspx.*

thickness of the retinal tissue, and such breaks can be classified as tears or holes. *Retinal holes* are atrophic retinal breaks that occur spontaneously. *Retinal tears* can occur as the vitreous humor shrinks during aging and pulls on the retina. The retina tears when the traction force exceeds the strength of the retina. Once the retina has a break, liquid vitreous can enter the subretinal space between the sensory layer and the retinal pigment epithelium layer, causing a *rhegmatogenous* retinal detachment. Retinal detachment can also occur when abnormal membranes mechanically pull on the retina. Such detachments are called *tractional* detachments and are less common. A third type of retinal detachment is the *secondary* or *exudative* detachment, which occurs in conditions that allow fluid to accumulate in the subretinal space (e.g., choroidal tumours, intraocular inflammation). Risk factors for retinal detachment are listed in Table 24-6.

Clinical Manifestations

Patients with a detaching retina describe symptoms that include *photopsia* (light flashes), floaters, and a "cobweb," "hairnet," or ring in the field of vision. Once the retina has detached, the patient describes a painless loss of peripheral or central vision, "like a curtain" coming across the field of vision. The area of visual loss corresponds to the area of detachment. If the detachment is in the superior nasal retina, the visual field loss is in the inferior temporal area. If the detachment is small or develops slowly in the periphery, the patient may not be aware of a visual problem. The effects of a retinal detachment can be viewed online at VisionSimulations.com (see the Resources at the end of this chapter).

Diagnostic Studies

Visual acuity measurements should be the first diagnostic procedure with any complaint of vision loss (Table 24-7). The retinal detachment can be directly visualized through direct and indirect ophthalmoscopy or slit-lamp microscopy in conjunction with a special lens to view the far periphery of the retina. Ultrasonography may be useful for identifying a retinal detachment if the retina cannot be directly visualized (e.g., when the cornea, the lens, or the vitreous humor is hazy or opaque).

Collaborative Care

Some retinal breaks are not likely to progress to detachment. The ophthalmologist simply monitors the patient, giving precise information about the warning signs and symptoms of impending detachment and instructing the patient to seek immediate evaluation if any of those signs or symptoms occurs. The ophthalmologist usually refers the patient with a detachment to a retinal specialist. Treatment objectives are to seal any retinal

TABLE 24-7	COLLABORATIVE CARE

Retinal Detachment

Diagnostic Studies
- History and physical examination
- Visual acuity measurement
- Ophthalmoscopy (direct and indirect)
- Slit-lamp microscopy
- Ultrasonography if cornea, lens, or vitreous humor is hazy or opaque

Collaborative Therapy
Preoperative
- Mydriatic, cycloplegic eye drops (see Table 24-4)
- Photocoagulation of retinal break that has not progressed to detachment

Surgery
- Laser photocoagulation
- Cryotherapy (cryopexy)
- Scleral buckling procedure
- Draining of subretinal fluid
- Vitrectomy
- Intravitreal bubble

Postoperative
- Topical antibiotic
- Topical corticosteroid
- Analgesia
- Mydriatics
- Positioning and activity as preferred by patient's surgeon

breaks and to relieve inward traction on the retina. Several techniques are used to accomplish these objectives (Schaal, Sherman, Barr, et al., 2011).

Surgical Therapy

Laser Photocoagulation and Cryopexy. These techniques seal retinal breaks by creating an inflammatory reaction that causes a chorioretinal adhesion or scar. In *laser photocoagulation,* an intense, precisely focused light beam is used to create an inflammatory reaction. The light is directed at the area of the retinal break. For retinal breaks accompanied by significant detachment, the retinal specialist may use photocoagulation intraoperatively in conjunction with scleral buckling. Tears or holes without accompanying retinal detachment may be treated prophylactically with laser photocoagulation if there is a high risk of progression to retinal detachment. When used alone, laser therapy is an outpatient procedure for which most patients require only topical anaesthesia. Patients may experience minimal adverse symptoms during or after the procedure.

Another method used to seal retinal breaks is *cryopexy.* This procedure involves the use of extreme cold to create the inflammatory reaction that produces the sealing scar. The ophthalmologist applies the cryoprobe instrument to the external globe in the area over the tear. This is usually done on an outpatient basis and with the use of a local anaesthetic. As with photocoagulation, cryotherapy may be used alone or during scleral buckling surgery. The patient may experience significant discomfort and eye pain after cryopexy. The nurse should encourage the patient to take the prescribed pain medication after the procedure.

Scleral Buckling. *Scleral buckling* is an extraocular surgical procedure that involves compressing the globe so that the pigment epithelium, the choroid, and the sclera move toward the detached retina. The retinal surgeon sutures a silicone implant against the sclera, causing the sclera to buckle inward. The surgeon may place an encircling band over the implant if there are multiple retinal breaks, if suspected breaks cannot be located, or if there is widespread inward traction on the retina (Figure 24-8). To drain any subretinal fluid, a small-gauge needle is inserted to facilitate contact between the retina and the buckled sclera. Scleral buckling is usually done as an outpatient procedure with the patient under local anaesthesia.

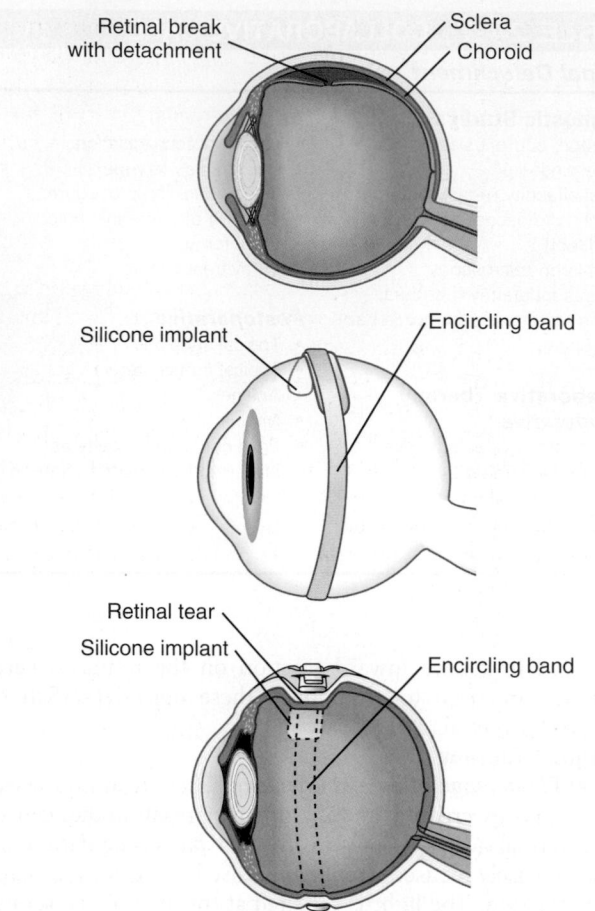

FIGURE 24-8 Retinal break with detachment *(top)*; surgical repair by scleral buckling technique *(middle* and *bottom)*.

Intraocular Procedures. In addition to the extraocular procedures described, retinal surgeons may use one or more intraocular procedures in treating some retinal detachments. *Pneumatic retinopexy* is the intravitreal injection of a gas to form a temporary bubble in the vitreous that closes retinal breaks and provides apposition of the separated retinal layers. Because the intravitreal bubble is temporary, this technique is combined with laser photocoagulation or cryotherapy (cryopexy). A patient with an intravitreal bubble must position the head so that the bubble is in contact with the retinal break. It may be necessary for the patient to maintain this position as much as possible for up to several weeks.

Vitrectomy (surgical removal of the vitreous) may be used to relieve traction on the retina, especially when the traction results from proliferative diabetic retinopathy. Vitrectomy may be combined with scleral buckling to provide a dual effect in relieving traction.

Postoperative Considerations in Scleral Buckling and Intraocular Procedures. Reattachment procedures are successful in 90% of retinal detachments (Schaal, Sherman, Barr, et al., 2011). Visual prognosis varies, depending on the extent, length, and area of detachment. Postoperatively, the patient may be on bed rest and may require special positioning to maintain proper position of an intravitreal bubble. The patient may need multiple topical medications, including antibiotics, anti-inflammatory drugs, or dilating drugs. The level of activity restriction after retinal detachment surgery varies greatly. The nurse should verify the

prescribed level of activity with the patient's surgeon and help the patient plan for any necessary assistance in relation to activity restrictions.

In most cases, retinal detachment is an urgent situation, and the patient is confronted suddenly with the need for surgery. The patient needs emotional support, especially during the immediate preoperative period when preparations for surgery can lead to additional anxiety. When the patient experiences postoperative pain, the nurse should administer prescribed pain medications and teach the patient to take the medication as necessary after discharge. The patient may go home within a few hours of surgery or may remain in the hospital for several days, depending on the surgeon and the type of repair.

Discharge planning and teaching are important, and the nurse should begin these processes as early as possible because the patient does not remain hospitalized long. Patient and caregiver teaching after eye surgery is discussed in Table 24-5. The patient is at risk for retinal detachment in the other eye. Therefore, the nurse should teach the patient the signs and symptoms of retinal detachment. The nurse can also promote use of proper protective eyewear to help avoid retinal detachments related to trauma.

AGE-RELATED MACULAR DEGENERATION

Age-related macular degeneration (AMD) is an eye disease that begins after age 60 that progressively destroys the macula (the central portion of the retina), causing irreversible central vision loss. It is the leading cause of blindness and vision loss in Canada (CNIB, 2015b). AMD is a common eye condition, affecting 1.4 million people in Canada. Canadians who have AMD outnumber those who have breast cancer, prostate cancer, Parkinson's disease, or Alzheimer's disease combined (CNIB, 2015b).

AMD is divided into two forms: dry (nonexudative) and wet (exudative). People with *dry AMD*, which is the more common form (90% of all cases), often notice close vision tasks become more difficult. In this form, the macular cells start to atrophy, leading to a slowly progressive and painless vision loss.

Wet AMD is the more severe form. Wet AMD accounts for 90% of the cases of AMD-related blindness. Wet AMD has a more rapid onset and is characterized by the development of abnormal blood vessels in or near the macula.

Etiology and Pathophysiology

AMD is related to retinal aging. Genetic factors also appear to play a major role, and family history is a major risk factor for AMD (Mackey & Hewitt, 2014). A gene responsible for some cases of AMD has been identified. People who smoke cigarettes are twice as likely to develop late AMD as are nonsmokers (National Eye Institute, 2015). Other risk factors include long-term exposure to ultraviolet light, hyperopia, and light-coloured irides. Nutritional factors may play a role in the progression of AMD. A dietary supplement of vitamin C, vitamin E, beta-carotene, and zinc decreases the progression of advanced AMD but has no effect on people with minimal AMD or those with no evidence of AMD (Chew, Clemons, Agron, et al., 2013). Mechanisms of protection are also being discovered among non-antioxidant nutrients such as omega-3 fatty acids and the B vitamins. A proper nutritious diet is thought to be more protective than nutritional supplements. The nutrients with the strongest evidence of a protective effect include zinc, lutein, zeaxanthin, docosahexaenoic acid (DHA) and eicosapentaenoic acid (EPA). Older patients are at higher risk for zinc deficiency, which may increase their risk of vision loss from AMD (Olson, Erie, & Bakri, 2011).

The dry form of AMD starts with the abnormal accumulation of yellowish extracellular deposits called *drusen* in the retinal pigment epithelium. The macular cells then undergo atrophy and degeneration. Wet AMD is characterized by the growth of new, fragile blood vessels from their normal location in the choroid to an abnormal location in the retinal epithelium. As the new blood vessels leak, scar tissue gradually forms. Acute vision loss may occur in some cases, with bleeding from subretinal neovascular membranes.

Clinical Manifestations

The patient may complain of blurred and darkened vision, the presence of *scotomas* (blind spots in the visual field), and *metamorphopsia* (distortion of vision). Many people may not notice unilateral early changes in their vision if the other eye is not affected.

Diagnostic Studies

In addition to visual acuity measurement, the primary diagnostic procedure is ophthalmoscopy. The examiner looks for drusen and other fundus changes associated with AMD. The Amsler grid test may help define the involved area, and the result provides a baseline for future comparison. Fundus photography and intravenous angiography with fluorescein or indocyanine green dyes, or both, may help to further define the extent and type of AMD.

Collaborative Care

Vision often does not improve for most people with AMD. Limited treatment options for patients with wet AMD include several medications that are injected directly into the vitreous cavity. Ranibizumab (Lucentis), and bevacizumab (Avastin) are selective inhibitors of endothelial growth factor that helps to slow vision loss in wet AMD. Adverse effects can include blurred vision, eye irritation, eye pain, and photosensitivity. The injections are given at 4- to 6-week intervals, depending on which drug is used. Retinal stability is determined by ocular coherence tomography, which allows the physician to identify fluid in the central retina to determine the need for continued intravitreal injections.

Photodynamic therapy entails the use of verteporfin (Visudyne) intravenously and a "cold" laser to excite the dye. This procedure is used for cases of wet AMD and destroys the abnormal blood vessels without permanent damage to the retinal pigment epithelium and photoreceptor cells. Verteporfin is a photosensitizing drug that becomes active when exposed to the low-level laser light wave. Until the drug is completely excreted by the body, it can be activated by exposure to sunlight or other high-intensity light such as halogen; therefore, patients are cautioned to avoid direct exposure to sunlight and other intense forms of light for 5 days after treatment. After receiving therapy, patients must be completely covered because any exposure to skin by sunlight could activate the drug in that area, which would result in a thermal burn.

People at risk for developing advanced AMD should consider supplements of vitamins and minerals (in consultation with their health care provider). The cessation of smoking may also help in halting the progression of dry AMD to a more advanced stage.

Many patients with assistive devices for low-degree vision can continue reading and retain a licence to drive during the daytime and at lowered speeds. The permanent loss of central vision has significant psychosocial implications for nursing care. Nursing

management of patients with uncorrectable visual impairment is discussed earlier in the chapter and is appropriate for patients with AMD. The nurse should avoid giving the impression that "nothing can be done" about the problem when caring for a patient with AMD. Although therapy will not recover lost vision, much can be done to augment the remaining vision.

GLAUCOMA

Glaucoma is a group of disorders characterized by elevated IOP and its consequences: optic nerve atrophy and peripheral visual field loss. Glaucoma is the second most common reason for vision loss in Canadians. It affects more than 400 000 Canadians and 67 million people worldwide (Glaucoma Research Society of Canada, 2016). Risk factors for glaucoma include family history, age, nearsightedness, diabetes, and ethnicity (e.g., individuals of African descent are more likely to develop the disease). The incidence of glaucoma increases with age. Blindness from glaucoma is largely preventable with early detection and appropriate treatment.

Etiology and Pathophysiology

A proper balance between the rate of aqueous production (referred to as *inflow*) and the rate of aqueous reabsorption (referred to as *outflow*) is essential to maintain the IOP within normal limits. The place where the outflow occurs is the *angle* where the iris meets the cornea. When the rate of inflow is greater than the rate of outflow, IOP can rise above the normal limits. If IOP remains elevated, vision loss may be permanent.

Primary open-angle glaucoma (POAG) is the most common type of glaucoma. In POAG, the outflow of aqueous humor is decreased in the trabecular meshwork. The drainage channels become clogged, and damage to the optic nerve can then result.

Primary angle-closure glaucoma is due to a reduction in the outflow of aqueous humor that results from angle closure. Usually this is caused by the lens's bulging forward as a result of the aging process. Angle closure may also occur as a result of pupil dilation in the patient with anatomically narrow angles. An acute attack may be precipitated by situations in which the pupil remains in a partially dilated state long enough to cause an acute and significant rise in the IOP. This may occur because of drug-induced mydriasis, emotional excitement, or darkness. Drug-induced mydriasis may occur not only from topical ophthalmic preparations but also from many systemic medications (both prescription and over-the-counter drugs). The nurse should check drug records and documentation before administering medications to the patient with angle-closure glaucoma and instruct the patient not to take any mydriatic medications.

Clinical Manifestations

POAG develops slowly and without symptoms of pain or pressure. The patient usually does not notice the gradual visual field loss until peripheral vision has been severely compromised. Eventually, patients with untreated glaucoma have "tunnel vision," in which only a small centre field can be seen and all peripheral vision is absent.

Acute angle-closure glaucoma causes definite symptoms, including sudden, excruciating pain in or around the eye. This is often accompanied by nausea and vomiting. Visual symptoms include blurred vision, ocular redness, and seeing coloured halos around lights. The acute rise in IOP may also cause corneal edema, which gives the cornea a frosted appearance.

FIGURE 24-9 The optic disc. **A,** In the normal eye, the optic disc is pink with little cupping. **B,** In glaucoma, the optic disc is pale, and optic cupping is present. (Note the appearance of the retinal vessels, which travel over the edge of the optic cup and appear to dip into it.)

Manifestations of subacute or chronic angle-closure glaucoma appear more gradually. The patient who has had a previous, unrecognized episode of subacute angle-closure glaucoma may report a history of blurred vision, ocular redness, eye or brow pain, or seeing coloured halos around lights. The effects of glaucoma can be viewed online at VisionSimulations.com (see the Resources at the end of this chapter).

Diagnostic Studies

IOP is usually elevated in glaucoma (normal IOP is 10–21 mm Hg). In cases of elevated pressures, the ophthalmologist usually repeats the measurements over time to verify the elevation. In open-angle glaucoma, IOP is usually between 22 and 32 mm Hg. In acute angle-closure glaucoma, IOP may exceed 50 mm Hg.

In open-angle glaucoma, slit-lamp microscopy reveals a normal angle. In angle-closure glaucoma, the examiner may note a markedly narrow or flat anterior chamber angle, an edematous cornea, a fixed and moderately dilated pupil, and ciliary injection (hyperemia of the ciliary blood vessels produces redness).

Measures of peripheral and central vision provide other diagnostic information. Whereas central acuity may remain 20/20 even in the presence of severe peripheral visual field loss, visual field perimetry may reveal subtle changes in the peripheral area of the retina early in the disease process, long before actual scotomas develop. In acute angle-closure glaucoma, central visual acuity is reduced if corneal edema is present, and the visual fields may be markedly decreased.

As glaucoma progresses, *optic disc cupping* may be one of the first signs of chronic open-angle glaucoma. The optic disc becomes wider, deeper, and paler (light grey or white); these characteristics are visible with direct or indirect ophthalmoscopy (Figure 24-9).

Collaborative Care

The primary focus of glaucoma therapy is to keep the IOP low enough to prevent optic nerve damage. Therapy varies with the type of glaucoma. The diagnostic studies and collaborative care of glaucoma are summarized in Table 24-8.

TABLE 24-8 COLLABORATIVE CARE

Glaucoma

Diagnostic Studies	**Surgical Therapy**
• History and physical examination	• Argon laser trabeculoplasty (ALT)
• Visual acuity measurement	• Trabeculectomy with or without filtering implant
• Tonometry	
• Ophthalmoscopy (direct and indirect)	***Acute Angle-Closure Glaucoma***
• Slit-lamp microscopy	• Topical cholinergic drug
• Gonioscopy	• Hyperosmotic drug
• Visual field perimetry	• Laser peripheral iridotomy
	• Surgical iridectomy
Collaborative Therapy	
Chronic Open-Angle Glaucoma	
Drug Therapy*	
• β-Adrenergic blockers	
• α-Adrenergic agonists	
• Cholinergic drugs (miotics)	
• Carbonic anhydrase inhibitors	

*See Table 24-9.

Chronic Open-Angle Glaucoma. Initial treatment in chronic open-angle glaucoma is with drugs (Table 24-9). The patient must understand that continued treatment and supervision are necessary because the drugs control, but do not cure, glaucoma.

Argon laser trabeculoplasty (ALT) is a noninvasive option to lower IOP when medications are not successful or when the patient either cannot or will not use the drug therapy as recommended. ALT is an outpatient procedure that necessitates only topical anaesthesia. The laser stimulates scarring and contraction of the trabecular meshwork, which opens the outflow channels. ALT reduces IOP approximately 75% of the time. The patient uses topical corticosteroids for approximately 3 to 5 days after the procedure. The most common postoperative complication is an acute rise in IOP. The ophthalmologist examines the patient 1 week and again 4 to 6 weeks after surgery.

Filtration surgery, also called a *trabeculectomy,* may be indicated if medical management and laser therapy are not successful. The success rate of this surgery is 75% to 85%.

Acute Angle-Closure Glaucoma. Acute angle-closure glaucoma is an ocular emergency that necessitates immediate intervention. Miotics and oral or intravenous hyperosmotic drugs are usually successful in immediately lowering the IOP (see Table 24-8). A laser peripheral iridotomy or surgical iridectomy is necessary for long-term treatment and prevention of subsequent episodes. These procedures allow the aqueous humor to flow through a newly created opening in the iris and into normal outflow channels. One of these procedures may also be performed on the other eye as a precaution because many patients often experience an acute attack in the other eye.

SAFETY ALERT

Patients who take miotic drugs must be warned that they may experience decreased visual acuity, especially in dim light.

NURSING MANAGEMENT GLAUCOMA

NURSING ASSESSMENT

Because glaucoma is a chronic condition that necessitates long-term management, the nurse must assess the patient's ability

TABLE 24-9 DRUG THERAPY

Acute and Chronic Glaucoma

Drug	Action	Adverse Effects	Nursing Considerations
β-Adrenergic Blockers			
Betaxolol (Betoptic)	Cardioselective β₁-adrenergic blocker; probably decreases aqueous humor production	Transient discomfort; systemic reactions (rarely reported) include bradycardia, heart block, pulmonary distress, headache, depression	Topical drugs; minimal effect on pulmonary and cardiovascular parameters Contraindicated for use in patients with bradycardia, cardiogenic shock, or overt cardiac failure. Systemic absorption can have additive effect with systemic β₁-adrenergic blocking drugs.
Levobunolol (Betagan) Timolol maleate (Timoptic)	Noncardioselective β₁- and β₂-blockers; probably decrease aqueous humor production	Transient ocular discomfort, blurred vision, photophobia, blepharoconjunctivitis, bradycardia, decreased blood pressure, bronchospasm, headache, depression	Topical drops; same effects and contraindications as for betaxolol; also contraindicated for use in patients with asthma or severe COPD
α-Adrenergic Agonists			
Apraclonidine (Iopidine) Brimonidine tartrate (Alphagan)	α-Adrenergic agonists; probably decrease aqueous humor production	Ocular redness; irregular heart rate	Topical drops; used to control or prevent acute rise in IOP after laser procedure (used before and immediately after ALT and iridotomy, Nd:YAG laser capsulotomy) For patient at risk for systemic reactions, teaching includes instructions to occlude puncta
Latanoprost (Xalatan)	Prostaglandin-F analogue	Increased brown iris pigmentation, ocular discomfort and redness, dryness, itching, and sensation of foreign body	Topical drops Teach patient not to take more than 1 drop per evening and to remove contact lens 15 min before instilling
Cholinergic Drugs (Miotics)			
Carbachol (Isopto Carbachol)	Parasympathomimetic; stimulates iris sphincter contraction, causing miosis and opening of trabecular meshwork, facilitating outflow of aqueous humor; also partially inhibits activity of cholinesterase	Transient ocular discomfort, headache, ache in brow area, blurred vision, decreased adaptation to darkness, syncope, excessive salivation, dysrhythmias, vomiting, diarrhea, hypotension, retinal detachment in susceptible individual (rare)	Topical drops Caution patient about decreased visual acuity caused by miosis, particularly in dim light
Pilocarpine (Isopto Carpine)	Parasympathomimetic; stimulates iris sphincter contraction, causing miosis and opening of trabecular meshwork, facilitating outflow of aqueous humor	Same as those of carbachol	Topical drops Same cautions as for carbachol
Carbonic Anhydrase Inhibitors *Systemic*			
Acetazolamide Methazolamide	Decreases production of aqueous humor	Paresthesias, especially "tingling" sensation in extremities; hearing dysfunction or tinnitus; loss of appetite; taste alteration; GI disturbances; drowsiness; confusion	Oral nonbacteriostatic sulphonamides Anaphylaxis and other sulpha type of allergic reactions may occur in patient allergic to sulpha drugs Diuretic effect can lower electrolyte levels Ask patient about acetylsalicylic acid (ASA; Aspirin) use; drug should not be given to patient receiving high-dose ASA (Aspirin) therapy
Topical			
Brinzolamide (Azopt) Dorzolamide (Trusopt)	Decreases production of aqueous humor	Transient stinging, blurred vision, redness	Same as for systemic drugs

Continued

TABLE 24-9   DRUG THERAPY

Acute and Chronic Glaucoma—cont'd

Drug	Action	Adverse Effects	Nursing Considerations
Combination Therapy			
Timolol maleate and dorzolamide (Cosopt)	Combination of two drugs (β-adrenergic blocker and topical carbonic anhydrase inhibitors)	Same as those for timolol maleate and dorzolamide (described previously)	—
Hyperosmolar Drugs			
Mannitol solution (Osmitrol)	Increases extracellular osmolarity so that intracellular water moves to the extracellular and vascular spaces, reducing IOP	Nausea, vomiting, diarrhea, thrombophlebitis, hypertension, hypotension, tachycardia	Intravenous solution; used in acute glaucoma attacks or preoperatively when decreased IOP is desired Nurse must assess patient for susceptibility to pulmonary edema and HF before administering hyperosmolar drugs

ALT, argon laser trabeculoplasty; *COPD,* chronic obstructive pulmonary disease; *GI,* gastro-intestinal; *HF,* heart failure; *IOP,* intraocular pressure; *Nd:YAG,* neodymium:yttrium–aluminum–garnet (laser).

to understand and adhere to the rationale and regimen of the prescribed therapy. In addition, the nurse should assess the patient's psychological reaction to the diagnosis of a potentially sight-threatening chronic disorder. The nurse must include the patient's caregiver in the assessment process because the chronic nature of this disorder affects the family in many ways. Some families may become the primary providers of necessary care, such as eye drop administration, if the patient is unwilling or unable to accomplish these self-care activities. The nurse also assesses visual acuity, visual fields, IOP, and fundus changes when appropriate.

NURSING DIAGNOSES

Nursing diagnoses for the patient with glaucoma include, but are not limited to, the following:

- *Risk for injury* as evidenced by *sensory integration dysfunction* (visual acuity deficits)
- *Self-care deficits* related to *perceptual disorders* (visual impairment)
- *Readiness for enhanced self-care*
- *Acute pain* related to *physical injury agent* (surgical process)

PLANNING

The overall goals are that the patient with glaucoma will (a) have no progression of visual impairment, (b) understand the disease process and the rationale for therapy, (c) comply with all aspects of therapy (including medication administration and follow-up care), and (d) have no postoperative complications.

NURSING IMPLEMENTATION

HEALTH PROMOTION. Loss of vision from glaucoma is a preventable problem. It is important to teach the patient and caregiver about the risk of vision loss from glaucoma and that this risk increases with age. The nurse should stress the importance of early detection and treatment in preventing visual impairment. A comprehensive ophthalmic examination is invaluable in identifying persons with glaucoma or those at risk of developing glaucoma. The Canadian Ophthalmological Society (2007) recommended an eye examination every 3 to 5 years until the age of 40 and then every 2 to 4 years until the age of 65. Patients with risk factors such as family history of glaucoma and those of African descent should have annual eye examinations. Because so many eye diseases tend to occur in older adults,

those older than 65 should have an examination every 2 years (annually if they have any risk factors; Canadian Ophthalmological Society, 2007).

ACUTE INTERVENTION. Acute nursing interventions are directed primarily toward patients with acute angle-closure glaucoma and patients undergoing surgery for glaucoma. A patient with acute angle-closure glaucoma requires immediate IOP-lowering medication, which the nurse must administer in a timely and appropriate manner according to the ophthalmologist's prescription. Most surgical procedures for glaucoma are outpatient procedures. In the acute situation, the patient needs postoperative instructions and may require nursing comfort measures to relieve discomfort related to the procedure. Patient and caregiver teaching after eye surgery is discussed in Table 24-5.

AMBULATORY AND HOME CARE. Because of the chronic nature of glaucoma, the patient needs encouragement to follow the therapeutic regimen and follow-up recommendations prescribed by the ophthalmologist. The patient needs accurate information about the disease process and treatment options, including the rationale underlying each option. In addition, the patient needs information about the purpose, the frequency, and the technique of administering prescribed antiglaucoma drugs. In addition to verbal instructions, all patients should receive written instructions that contain the same information. The nurse may encourage adherence by helping the patient identify the most convenient and appropriate times for medication administration or by advocating a change in therapy if the patient reports unacceptable adverse effects.

EVALUATION

The overall expected outcomes are that the patient with glaucoma will

- Have no further loss of vision
- Adhere to the recommended therapy
- Safely function within own environment
- Obtain relief from pain associated with the disease and surgery

AGE-RELATED CONSIDERATIONS

Many older patients with glaucoma have systemic illnesses or take systemic medications that may affect their glaucoma therapy. In particular, patients who take a β-adrenergic blocking drug for glaucoma may experience an additive effect if they are also taking a systemic β-adrenergic blocking drug. All β-adrenergic blocking glaucoma drugs are contraindicated for use in patients that have bradycardia, a greater than first-degree heart block, cardiogenic shock, and overt cardiac failure. The non–cardioselective β-adrenergic blocking glaucoma drugs are also contraindicated in patients with severe chronic obstructive pulmonary disease (COPD) or asthma. The hyperosmolar drugs may precipitate heart failure or pulmonary edema in susceptible patients. Older patients receiving high-dose acetylsalicylic acid (ASA; Aspirin) therapy for rheumatoid arthritis should not take carbonic anhydrase inhibitors. The α-adrenergic agonists can cause tachycardia or hypertension, which may have serious consequences in older patients. The nurse must teach older patients to occlude the puncta to limit the systemic absorption of glaucoma medications.

INTRAOCULAR INFLAMMATION AND INFECTION

The term *uveitis* is used to describe inflammation of the uveal tract, the retina, the vitreous cavity, or the optic nerve. This inflammation may be caused by bacteria, viruses, fungi, or parasites. *Cytomegalovirus retinitis* is an opportunistic infection that occurs in patients with acquired immune deficiency syndrome (AIDS) and in other immuno-suppressed patients. The causes of sterile intraocular inflammation include autoimmune disorders, AIDS, malignancies, or disorders associated with systemic diseases such as inflammatory bowel disease. Pain and photophobia are common symptoms.

Endophthalmitis is an extensive intraocular inflammation of the vitreous cavity. Bacteria, viruses, fungi, or parasites can all induce this serious inflammatory response. The mechanism of infection may be endogenous, in which the infecting pathogen arrives at the eye through the bloodstream, or exogenous, in which the infecting pathogen is introduced through a surgical wound or a penetrating injury. Although rare, endophthalmitis is a devastating complication of intraocular surgery or penetrating ocular injury and can lead to irreversible blindness within hours or days. Manifestations include ocular pain, photophobia, decreased visual acuity, headaches, reddened and swollen conjunctiva, and corneal edema.

When all the layers of the eye (vitreous humor, retina, choroid, and sclera) are involved in the inflammatory response, the patient has *panophthalmitis*. In the final stages of extensive cases, the scleral coat may undergo bacterial or inflammatory dissolution. Subsequent rupture of the globe spreads the infection into the orbit or eyelids.

Treatment of intraocular inflammation depends on the underlying cause. Intraocular infections must be treated with antimicrobial drugs, which may be delivered topically, subconjunctivally, intravitreally, systemically, or in some combination. Sterile inflammatory responses necessitate anti-inflammatory drugs such as corticosteroids. The patient with intraocular inflammation is usually uncomfortable and may be noticeably anxious and frightened. The nurse must provide accurate information and emotional support to the patient and the family. In severe cases, enucleation may be necessary. When patients lose visual function or even the entire eye, they grieve over the loss. The nurse's role includes helping patients through the grieving process.

ENUCLEATION

Enucleation is the removal of the eye. The primary indication for enucleation is the combination of blindness and pain in the eye. These may result from glaucoma, infection, or trauma. Enucleation may also be indicated in ocular malignancies, although many malignancies can be managed with cryotherapy, radiation, and chemotherapy. The surgical procedure includes severing the extraocular muscles close to their insertion on the globe, inserting an implant to maintain the intraorbital anatomy, and suturing the ends of the extraocular muscles over the implant. The conjunctiva covers the joined muscles, and a clear conformer is placed over the conjunctiva until the permanent prosthesis is fitted. A pressure dressing helps prevent postoperative bleeding.

Postoperatively, the nurse observes the patient for signs of complications, including excessive bleeding or swelling, increased pain, displacement of the implant, or temperature elevation. Patient teaching should include instructions about the instillation of topical ointments or drops and wound cleansing. The nurse should also instruct the patient how to insert the conformer into the socket in case it falls out. The patient is often devastated by the loss of an eye, even when enucleation occurs after a lengthy period of painful blindness. The nurse should recognize and validate the patient's emotional response and provide support to the patient and the family.

Approximately 6 weeks after surgery, the wound is sufficiently healed for the permanent prosthesis. The prosthesis is fitted by an ocular specialist and designed to match the remaining eye. The nurse should teach the patient how to remove, cleanse, and insert the prosthesis. Special polishing is required periodically to remove dried protein secretions.

OCULAR TUMOURS

Benign and malignant tumours can occur in many areas of the eye, including the conjunctiva, retina, and orbit. Malignancies of the eyelid include basal cell and squamous cell carcinomas (see Chapter 26).

Uveal melanoma is a cancerous neoplasm of the iris, choroid, or ciliary body. It is the most common primary intraocular malignancy in adults, but it is much rarer than skin melanoma. Approximately 200 cases are diagnosed in Canada each year (Melanoma Network of Canada, 2015). It is more frequently found in light-skinned people older than 60 with chronic exposure to ultraviolet light. Genetic factors such as a mutated gene may also increase a person's risk (Nielsen, Dogrusöz, Bleeker, et al., 2015). Uveal melanoma can arise from pre-existing nevi in the eye. Tumours may be asymptomatic or associated with vision loss depending on their size and location and presence of hemorrhage and retinal detachment. As with other cancers, cancer stage and cell type are important variables in the patient's prognosis. Diagnostic testing may include ultrasonography, magnetic resonance imaging (MRI), and fine-needle aspiration biopsy. Uveal melanoma commonly appears as a dome-shaped, well-circumscribed, solid brown to golden pigment in the iris, choroid, or ciliary body (Figure 24-10). Many patients do not lose the affected eye, and some may experience good vision after treatment in that eye.

Depending on the status of the involved eye, treatment options can include enucleation, plaque radiation therapy (brachytherapy), external beam radiation, transpupillary photocoagulation, eye wall resection, and exenteration. Within 15 years, approximately 50% of all patients with uveal melanoma will develop metastases, most commonly in the liver.

FIGURE 24-10 Uveal melanoma. A large tumour in the choroid, the most common location in the eye for melanoma. Source: Courtesy Cory J. Bosanko, OD, FAAO, Eye Centers of Tennessee, Crossville, Tennessee.

OCULAR MANIFESTATIONS OF SYSTEMIC DISEASES

Many systemic diseases are accompanied by significant ocular manifestations. Ocular signs and symptoms may be the first finding or complaint in a patient with a systemic disease. One example is the patient with undiagnosed diabetes who seeks ophthalmic care for blurred vision. A thorough history and careful examination of the patient can reveal that the underlying cause of the blurred vision is lens swelling resulting from hyperglycemia. Another example is the patient who seeks care for a conjunctival lesion. The ophthalmologist may be the first health care provider to make the diagnosis of AIDS on the basis of the presence of a conjunctival Kaposi's sarcoma.

AUDITORY PROBLEMS

EXTERNAL EAR AND CANAL

Trauma

Trauma to the external ear can cause injury to the subcutaneous tissue that may result in a hematoma. If the hematoma is not aspirated, inflammation of the membranes of the ear cartilage (perichondritis) can result. Blows to the ear can also cause a conductive hearing loss if the ossicles in the middle ear are damaged or the tympanic membrane (TM) is perforated. Head trauma that injures the temporal lobe of the cerebral cortex can impair the ability to understand the meaning of sounds.

External Otitis

The skin of the external ear and the ear canal is subject to the same problems as skin anywhere on the body. **External otitis** involves inflammation or infection of the epithelium of the auricle and ear canal. Swimming may alter the flora of the external canal as a result of chemicals and contaminated water. This can result in an infection often referred to as "swimmer's ear." Trauma from picking the ear or using sharp objects (e.g., hairpins) to clean the ear frequently causes the initial break in the skin. Piercing of auricular cartilage carries a greater risk of infection than does soft-tissue piercing (Lee & Gold, 2011).

Causes. Infections and skin conditions may cause external otitis. Bacteria or fungi may be the cause. *Pseudomonas aeruginosa* is the most common bacterial cause. Fungi, including *Candida albicans* and *Aspergillus* species, especially thrive in warm, moist climates. The warm, dark environment of the ear canal provides a good medium for the growth of microorganisms.

Malignant external otitis is a serious infection caused by *P. aeruginosa*. It occurs mainly in older patients with diabetes. The infection, which can spread from the external ear to the parotid gland and temporal bone (osteomyelitis), is usually treated with antibiotics.

Clinical Manifestations and Complications. Ear pain *(otalgia)* is one of the first signs of external otitis. Even in mild cases, a patient may experience significant discomfort with chewing, moving the auricle, or pressing on the tragus. Swelling of the ear canal can muffle hearing. Drainage from the ear may be serosanguineous (blood-tinged fluid) or purulent (white to green thick fluid). Fever occurs when the infection spreads to surrounding tissue. Facial nerve paralysis may occur with malignant external otitis.

NURSING AND COLLABORATIVE MANAGEMENT EXTERNAL OTITIS

Diagnosis of external otitis is made by otoscopic examination of the ear canal. The nurse must be careful to avoid pain when pulling on the patient's auricle to straighten out the canal or when inserting the otoscope speculum. The eardrum may be difficult to see because of swelling in the canal. Culture and sensitivity studies of the drainage may be done. Moist heat, mild analgesics, and topical anaesthetic drops usually control the pain. Topical antibiotics include polymyxin B (Polysporin), neomycin (Neosporin), and chloramphenicol (Pentamycetin). Nystatin (Nyaderm) is used for fungal infections. Corticosteroids may also be used to decrease inflammation unless the infection is fungal, in which case their use is contraindicated. If the surrounding tissue is involved, systemic antibiotics are prescribed. Improvement should occur in 48 hours, but the patient must adhere to the prescribed therapy for 7 to 14 days for complete resolution.

Hands should be washed before and after otic drops (eardrops) are administered. The drops should be administered at room temperature; cold drops can cause vertigo by stimulating the semicircular canals, and heated drops can burn the tympanum. The tip of the dropper should not touch the ear during administration, so as to prevent contamination of the entire bottle. The ear is positioned so that the drops can run down into the canal. The patient should maintain this position for 2 minutes to allow the drops to spread. Sometimes drops are placed onto a wick of cotton that is placed in the canal. The nurse should instruct the patient not to push the cotton farther into the ear. Careful handling and disposal of material saturated with drainage is important. The nurse should also instruct the patient on methods to reduce the risk of external otitis (Table 24-10).

Cerumen and Foreign Bodies in the External Ear Canal

Impacted cerumen can cause discomfort and decreased hearing. In older adults, the earwax becomes dense and drier. Hair becomes thicker and coarser, entrapping the hard, dry cerumen in the canal. Symptoms of cerumen impaction are outlined in Table 24-11. Management involves irrigation of the canal with body-temperature solutions to soften the cerumen. Special syringes, varying from a simple bulb syringe to special irrigating equipment, can be used. The patient is placed in a sitting position with an emesis basin under the ear. The auricle is pulled up and back, and the flow of solution is directed above or below the impaction. It is important that the ear canal not be completely

TABLE 24-10 PATIENT & CAREGIVER TEACHING GUIDE

Prevention of External Otitis

Include the following instructions when teaching the patient and caregiver how to prevent external otitis.
1. Do not put anything in your ear canal unless requested by your health care provider.
2. Report itching if it becomes a problem.
3. Cerumen (earwax) is normal.
   - It lubricates and protects the canal.
   - Report chronic excessive cerumen if it impairs your hearing.
4. Keep your ears as dry as possible.
   - Use earplugs if you are prone to swimmer's ear.
   - Turn your head to each side for 30 sec at a time to help water run out of the ears.
   - Do not dry with cotton-tipped applicators.
   - A hair dryer set to low and held at least 6 in from the ear can speed water evaporation.

TABLE 24-11 MANIFESTATIONS OF CERUMEN IMPACTION

- Hearing loss
- Otalgia
- Tinnitus
- Vertigo
- Cough
- Cardiac depression (vagal stimulation)

occluded with the syringe tip. If irrigation does not remove the cerumen, mild lubricant drops may be used to soften it. Severe impaction may need to be removed by the health care provider.

Attempts to remove a foreign object from the ear canal may result in pushing it farther into the canal. Vegetable matter in the ear tends to swell and may create a secondary inflammation, which makes removal more difficult. Mineral oil or lidocaine drops can be used to kill an insect before removal under microscope guidance. Removal of impacted objects should be performed by the health care provider.

Ears should be cleaned with a washcloth and finger. Cotton-tipped applicators should be avoided: Penetration of the middle ear by a cotton-tipped applicator can cause serious injury to the TM and ossicles. The use of cotton-tipped applicators can also cause cerumen to become impacted against the TM and impair hearing.

Malignancy of the External Ear

Skin cancers are the only common malignancies of the ear. Rough sandpaper-like changes to the upper border of the auricle are premalignant lesions (actinic keratoses) associated with chronic sun exposure. They are often removed with liquid nitrogen. Malignancies in the external ear canal include basal cell carcinoma in the auricle and squamous cell carcinoma in the ear canal. If left untreated, they can invade underlying tissue. The nurse should teach the patient about the dangers of sun exposure and the importance of using hats and sunscreen when outdoors.

MIDDLE EAR AND MASTOID

Acute Otitis Media

Acute otitis media (AOM) is an infection of the tympanum, ossicles, and space of the middle ear. Swelling of the auditory tube as a result of colds or allergies can trap bacteria, causing a middle ear infection. Pressure from the inflammation pushes on the TM, causing it to become red, bulging, and painful. AOM is usually a childhood disease because in children the auditory tube that drains fluids and mucus from the middle ear is shorter and narrower, and its position is flatter, than that in adults (Le Saux & Robinson, 2016). Pain, fever, malaise, and reduced hearing are signs and symptoms of infections. Referred pain from the temporomandibular joint, teeth, gums, sinuses, or throat may also cause ear pain. Clinical practice guidelines include strategies such as observation, antibiotics, and pain control (Thornton, Parrish, & Swords, 2011).

Collaborative care involves the use of antibiotics to eradicate the causative organism. Amoxicillin (Amoxil) is the current therapy of choice in North America. Surgical intervention is generally reserved for patients who do not respond to medical treatment. A *myringotomy* involves an incision in the tympanum to release the increased pressure and exudate from the middle ear. A tympanostomy tube may be placed for short- or long-term drainage. Prompt treatment of an episode of AOM generally prevents spontaneous perforation of the TM. In the adult patient for whom allergy may be a causative factor, antihistamines may also be prescribed.

Otitis Media With Effusion

Otitis media with effusion is an inflammation of the middle ear with a collection of fluid in the middle ear space. The fluid may be thin, mucoid, or purulent. If the Eustachian tube does not open and allow equalization of atmospheric pressure, negative pressure within the middle ear pulls fluid from surrounding tissues. This problem commonly follows upper respiratory tract or chronic sinus infections, barotrauma (caused by pressure change), or otitis media.

Complaints include a feeling of fullness of the ear, a "plugged" feeling or popping sensation, and decreased hearing. The patient does not experience pain, fever, or discharge from the ear. It is normal to have otitis media with effusion for weeks to months after an episode of AOM. It usually resolves in 75% to 90% of cases without treatment but may recur.

Chronic Otitis Media and Mastoiditis

Etiology and Pathophysiology. Repeated attacks of AOM may lead to chronic otitis media, especially in adults who have a history of recurrent otitis in childhood. Organisms involved in chronic otitis media include *S. aureus, Proteus mirabilis,* and *P. aeruginosa.* Because the mucous membrane is continuous, both the middle ear and the air cells of the mastoid bone can be involved in the chronic infectious process.

Clinical Manifestations. *Chronic otitis media* is characterized by a purulent exudate and inflammation that can involve the ossicles, Eustachian tube, and mastoid bone. It is often painless and may be accompanied by hearing loss, nausea, and episodes of dizziness. Hearing loss is a complication from inflammatory destruction of the ossicles, a TM perforation, or accumulation of fluid in the middle ear space.

Complications. Untreated conditions can result in TM perforation and the formation of a *cholesteatoma* (a mass of epithelial cells and cholesterol in the middle ear). The cholesteatoma enlarges and can destroy the adjacent bones. Unless removed surgically, it can cause extensive damage to the ossicles and impair hearing.

Diagnostic Studies. Otoscopic examination of the TM may reveal colour changes and mobility or a perforation (Figure 24-11).

FIGURE 24-11 Perforation of the tympanic membrane (TM). Source: Flint, P., Haughey, Lund, V., et al. (Eds.). (2010). *Cummings otolaryngology: Head and neck surgery* (5th ed.). St Louis: Mosby.

TABLE 24-12 COLLABORATIVE CARE

Chronic Otitis Media

Diagnostic Studies	Collaborative Therapy
• History and physical examination	• Ear irrigations
• Otoscopic examination	• Otic, oral, or parenteral antibiotics
• Culture and sensitivity tests of middle ear drainage	• Analgesics
• Mastoid radiography	• Antiemetics
	• Surgery
	• Tympanoplasty*
	• Mastoidectomy

*See Table 24-13.

Culture and sensitivity tests of the drainage are necessary to identify the organisms involved so that the appropriate antibiotic therapy can be prescribed. Audiography may demonstrate a hearing loss as great as 50 to 60 dB if the ossicles have been damaged or separated. Sinus radiographic studies, MRI, or computed tomography of the temporal bone may demonstrate bone destruction, absence of ossicles, or the presence of a mass.

Collaborative Care. The aims of treatment are to clear the middle ear of infection, repair the perforation, and preserve hearing (Table 24-12). Systemic antibiotic therapy is initiated on the basis of results of the culture and sensitivity tests. In addition, the patient may need to undergo frequent evacuation of drainage and debris in an outpatient setting. Otic and oral antibiotics are used to reduce infection. In many cases of chronic otitis media, the causative pathogen is resistant to antibiotics.

Surgical Therapy. Chronic TM perforations often do not heal with conservative treatment, and surgery is necessary. *Tympanoplasty (myringoplasty)* involves reconstruction of the TM, the ossicles, or both. A *mastoidectomy* is often performed with a tympanoplasty to remove infected portions of the mastoid bone. Removal of tissue stops at the middle ear structures that appear capable of conducting sound. Sudden pressure changes in the ear and postoperative infections can disrupt the surgical repair during the healing phase or cause facial nerve paralysis.

NURSING MANAGEMENT
CHRONIC OTITIS MEDIA

AFTER TYMPANOPLASTY

Routine preoperative care is provided before tympanoplasty and includes teaching postoperative expectations (Table 24-13).

TABLE 24-13 PATIENT & CAREGIVER TEACHING GUIDE

After Ear Surgery

Include the following instructions when teaching the patient and caregiver after ear surgery.
1. Avoid sudden head movements.
2. Do not try to get out of bed without assistance.
3. Take drugs to reduce dizziness if prescribed.
4. Change positions slowly.
5. Avoid getting the head wet (including showering) until directed by surgeon.
6. Report fever, pain, an increase in hearing loss, or drainage from the ear.
7. Do not cough or blow the nose because this causes increased pressure in the Eustachian tube and middle ear cavity and disrupts healing.
8. If you need to cough or sneeze, leave the mouth open to help reduce the pressure.
9. Avoid crowds because respiratory infections may be contracted.
10. Avoid situations in which pressure or popping in the ears is normally experienced, such as high elevations or airplane travel.

After surgery, the patient is positioned flat and side-lying with the operated side up. It is normal for hearing to be impaired during the postoperative period if there is packing in the ear. A cotton-ball dressing is used for the incision made through the external auditory canal (endaural incision). The patient should be instructed to change the cotton packing and dressing daily. If a postauricular incision is used and a drain is in place, a mastoid dressing is used. A small gauze pad is cut to fit behind the ear, and fluffs are applied over the ear to prevent the outer circular head dressing from placing pressure on the auricle. The nurse should monitor the amount and type of drainage postoperatively, as well as the tightness of the dressing, to prevent tissue necrosis.

Otosclerosis

Otosclerosis is a hereditary autosomal dominant disease and the most common cause of hearing loss in young adults (Ferri, 2012). Spongy bone develops from the bony labyrinth, causing immobilization of the footplate of the stapes in the oval window. This reduces the transmission of vibrations to the inner ear fluids and results in conductive hearing loss. Although otosclerosis is typically bilateral, hearing loss may progress more rapidly in one ear. The patient is often unaware of the problem until the loss becomes so severe that communication is difficult.

Otoscopic examination may reveal a reddish blush of the tympanum (Schwartz's sign) caused by the vascular and bony changes within the middle ear. Tuning fork tests help identify the conductive component of the hearing loss. On Rinne's test, sound is heard longer when the stem of the tuning fork is touching the mastoid bone (bone conduction) than when placed next to the ear (air conduction). In Weber's test, the sound is heard better through the skull bone in the ear than through air when conductive hearing loss is greater. Audiography demonstrates good hearing by bone conduction but poorer hearing by air conduction (air–bone gap). The difference between air and bone conduction levels of hearing is usually at least 20 to 25 dB in otosclerosis.

Collaborative Care. The hearing loss associated with otosclerosis may be stabilized by the use of sodium fluoride with

TABLE 24-14   COLLABORATIVE CARE

Otosclerosis

Diagnostic Studies	Collaborative Therapy

• History and physical examination
• Otoscopic examination
• Rinne's test
• Weber's test
• Audiometry
• Tympanometry
	• Hearing aid
	• Surgery (stapedectomy or fenestration)
	• Drug therapy
	  • Sodium fluoride with vitamin D
	  • Calcium carbonate

TABLE 24-15   COLLABORATIVE CARE

Ménière's Disease

Diagnostic Studies	Surgical Therapy
• History and physical examination • Audiometric studies (including speech discrimination, tone decay) • Vestibular tests (including caloric test, positional test) • Electronystagmography • Neurological examination • Glycerol test	**Conservative Surgical Intervention** • Endolymphatic shunt • Vestibular nerve section **Destructive Surgical Intervention** • Labyrinthotomy • Labyrinthectomy
Collaborative Therapy **Acute Care** **Drug Therapy (One or More)** • Sedatives • Benzodiazepines • Anticholinergics • Antiemetics • Antihistamines	**Ambulatory or Home Care** • Diuretics • Antihistamines • Calcium channel blockers • Sedatives • Hydrops diet: restriction of sodium, caffeine, nicotine, alcohol, and foods with monosodium glutamate (MSG)

vitamin D and calcium carbonate to retard bone resorption and encourage calcification of bony lesions. Amplification of sound by a hearing aid can be effective because the inner ear function is normal. Surgical treatment involves partial removal of the stapes *(stapedectomy)* or complete removal with prosthesis insertion *(fenestration)*. Collaborative care of otosclerosis is described in Table 24-14.

These procedures are usually performed with the patient under conscious sedation. The ear with poorer hearing is repaired first, and the other ear may be operated on within a year. An endaural incision is made under visualization through the operating microscope. Gelfoam is used on the incision flap to limit bleeding. A cotton ball is placed in the ear canal, and a small dressing is used to cover the ear.

During surgery, patients often report an immediate improvement in hearing in the operated ear. Because of the accumulation of blood and fluid in the middle ear, the hearing level decreases postoperatively but improves with healing. After stapedectomy, 90% of patients experience an improvement in hearing, in many instances to near normal.

NURSING MANAGEMENT
OTOSCLEROSIS

Nursing management of patients undergoing stapedectomy or fenestration is similar to that for patients who have undergone tympanoplasty. Postoperatively, patients may experience dizziness, nausea, and vomiting as a result of intraoperative stimulation of the labyrinth. Some patients demonstrate nystagmus because of disturbance of the perilymph fluid. The patient should take care to avoid sudden movements that may induce or exacerbate dizziness. The patient should avoid actions that increase inner ear pressure, such as coughing, sneezing, lifting, bending, and straining during bowel movements.

INNER EAR PROBLEMS

Three symptoms that indicate disease of the inner ear are vertigo, sensorineural hearing loss, and tinnitus. Symptoms of vertigo arise from the vestibular labyrinth, whereas hearing loss and tinnitus arise from the auditory labyrinth. Manifestations of inner ear problems overlap with some manifestations of central nervous system disorders.

Ménière's Disease

Ménière's disease (endolymphatic hydrops) is characterized by symptoms caused by inner ear disease, including episodic vertigo, tinnitus, fluctuating sensorineural hearing loss, and a sense of aural fullness. The patient experiences significant disability because of sudden, severe attacks of vertigo with nausea, vomiting, sweating, and pallor. Symptoms usually begin between the ages of 30 and 60 years (Tassinari, Mandrioli, Gaggioli, et al., 2015).

The cause of the disease is unknown, but it results in an excessive accumulation of endolymph in the membranous labyrinth. The volume of endolymph increases until the membranous labyrinth ruptures. Attacks may be preceded by a sense of fullness in the ear, increasing tinnitus, and muffled hearing. Patients with Ménière's disease may experience the feeling of being pulled to the ground ("drop attacks"). Some patients report that they feel as if they are whirling in space. Attacks may last hours or days and may occur several times a year. The clinical course of the disease is highly variable.

NURSING AND COLLABORATIVE MANAGEMENT
MÉNIÈRE'S DISEASE

Collaborative care of Ménière's disease (Table 24-15) includes diagnostic tests to rule out other causes of symptoms, including central nervous system disease. Audiography demonstrates a mild, low-frequency sensorineural hearing loss. Vestibular tests indicate decreased function.

A glycerol test may aid in the diagnosis. An oral dose of glycerol is given, followed by serial audiography over 3 hours. Improvement in hearing or speech discrimination supports a diagnosis of Ménière's disease. The improvement is attributed to the osmotic effect of glycerol that pulls fluid from the inner ear. Although a positive test result is diagnostic of Ménière's disease, a negative test result does not rule out the condition.

During the acute attack, antihistamines, anticholinergic drugs, and benzodiazepines can be used to decrease the abnormal sensation and lessen symptoms such as nausea and vomiting. Acute vertigo is treated symptomatically with bed rest, sedation, and antiemetics or antivertigo drugs for motion sickness. The patient requires reassurance and counselling that the condition is not life-threatening. Management between attacks may include diuretics, antihistamines, calcium channel blockers, and a low-sodium diet. Diazepam (Valium) may be used to reduce the vertigo. Over time, most patients respond to the prescribed medications, but the attacks and hearing loss remain unpredictable.

Frequent and incapacitating attacks are indications for surgical intervention. Decompression of the endolymphatic sac and shunting are performed to reduce the pressure on the cochlear hair cells and to prevent further damage and hearing loss. If relief is not achieved, the vestibular nerve may be resected. When involvement is unilateral, surgical ablation of the labyrinth, resulting in loss of the vestibular and hearing cochlear function, is performed. Careful management can decrease the possibility of progressive sensorineural loss in many patients.

Nursing interventions are planned to minimize vertigo and provide for patient safety. During an acute attack, the patient is kept in a quiet, darkened room in a comfortable position. The patient needs to be taught to avoid sudden head movements or position changes. Fluorescent or flickering lights or television may exacerbate symptoms and should be avoided. An emesis basin should be available because vomiting is common. To minimize the patient's risk of falling, the nurse should keep the side rails up and the bed low in position when the patient is in bed. The patient should be instructed to call for assistance when getting out of bed. Medications and fluids are administered parenterally, and intake and output are monitored. When the attack subsides, the patient should be assisted with ambulation because unsteadiness may remain.

Benign Paroxysmal Positional Vertigo

Benign paroxysmal positional vertigo (BPPV) is a common cause of vertigo. Approximately 50% of cases of vertigo may be due to BPPV. In BPPV, free-floating debris in the semicircular canal causes vertigo with specific head movements, such as those involved with getting out of bed, rolling over in bed, and sitting up from lying down (HealthLinkBC, 2014). The debris ("ear rocks") is composed of small crystals of calcium carbonate derived from the utricle in the inner ear. The utricle may be injured by head trauma, infection, or degeneration as a result of the aging process. However, for many patients, a cause cannot be found.

Symptoms include dizziness, vertigo, light-headedness, loss of balance, and nausea. Hearing loss is not characteristic, and symptoms tend to be intermittent. The symptoms of BPPV may be confused with those of Ménière's disease. Diagnosis is based on the results of auditory and vestibular tests.

Although BPPV is bothersome, it is rarely a serious problem unless an affected person falls. The Epley manoeuvre (canalith repositioning procedure) is effective in providing symptom relief for many patients (Balatsouras & Korres, 2012). In this manoeuvre, the ear debris is moved from areas in the inner ear that cause symptoms and repositioned into areas where they do not cause these problems. The Epley manoeuvre does not address the actual presence of debris; rather, it changes their location. A trained health care provider can instruct the patient in how to perform the Epley manoeuvre.

Acoustic Neuroma

An **acoustic neuroma** is a unilateral benign tumour that occurs where the vestibulo-cochlear nerve (cranial nerve VIII) enters the internal auditory canal. Early diagnosis is important because the tumour can compress the trigeminal and facial nerves and arteries within the internal auditory canal. Symptoms usually begin at 40 to 60 years of age.

Early symptoms are associated with compression and destruction of cranial nerve VIII. They include unilateral, progressive,

sensorineural hearing loss; reduced touch sensation in the posterior ear canal; unilateral tinnitus; and mild, intermittent vertigo. Diagnostic tests include neurological, audiometric, and vestibular tests; computed tomographic scans; and MRI.

Surgery to remove small tumours generally preserves hearing and vestibular function. Large tumours (>3 cm) and the surgery required to remove them can leave the patient with permanent hearing loss and facial paralysis. The nurse should instruct the patient to report any clear, colourless discharge from the nose. This may be cerebro-spinal fluid, and such leaks increase the risk of infection.

Hearing Loss and Deafness

Hearing loss is the fastest growing and one of the most prevalent, chronic conditions facing Canadians today (Hearing Foundation of Canada, 2014). Hearing loss has many causes; age-related presbycusis and noise-induced hearing loss are two of the most common. Nearly half the persons who need assistance with hearing disorders are 65 years of age or older. With the aging of the population, the prevalence of hearing loss is increasing. At age 50, one of every eight persons is hearing impaired. A disturbing trend is the number of young adults showing signs of hearing loss. The tiny hair cells located inside the ear pick up sound waves and convert them into electrical signals that the brain can interpret. When loud sounds are listened to constantly, the vibrations destroy the tiny hair cells, which contributes to hearing loss. Unlike other cells in the body, hair cells never grow back once they are damaged (Health Canada, 2012). Earbuds are of particular concern because volumes must be high in order to block out environmental distractions (Portnuff, Fligor, & Arehart, 2011). Causes of hearing loss are listed in Figure 24-12.

Types of Hearing Loss

Conductive Hearing Loss. *Conductive hearing loss* occurs when conditions in the outer or middle ear impair the transmission of sound through air to the inner ear. A common cause is otitis media with effusion. Other causes are impacted cerumen, TM

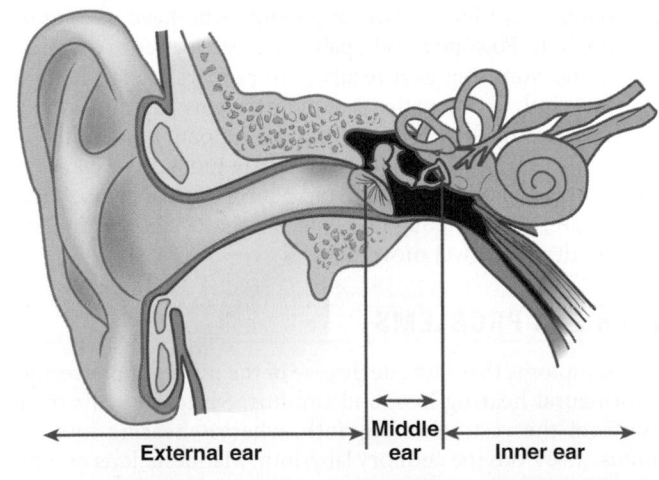

External ear	Middle ear	Inner ear
• Impacted cerumen	• Otitis media	• Ménière's disease
• Foreign bodies	• Serous otitis	• Noise-induced
• External otitis	• Otosclerosis	hearing loss
	• Tympanic	• Presbycusis
	membrane	• Ototoxicity
	trauma	
	• Cholesteatoma	
	• Acoustic neuroma	

FIGURE 24-12 Causes of hearing loss, by location.

perforation, otosclerosis, and narrowing of the external auditory canal (Harkin & Kelleher, 2011).

Audiography demonstrates an air–bone gap of at least 15 decibel (dB). The term *air–bone gap* represents the situation in which hearing sensitivity is better by bone conduction than by air conduction. Patients may speak softly because they hear their own voices, which are conducted by bone, as being loud. Such patients hear better in a noisy environment. If correction of the cause is not possible, a hearing aid may help if the loss is greater than 40 to 50 dB.

Sensorineural Hearing Loss. *Sensorineural hearing loss* is caused by impairment of function of the inner ear or the vestibulo-cochlear nerve (cranial nerve VIII). Congenital and hereditary factors, noise trauma over time, aging (presbycusis), Ménière's disease, and ototoxicity can cause sensorineural hearing loss.

Ototoxic drugs include ASA (Aspirin), nonsteroidal anti-inflammatory drugs (NSAIDs), antibiotics (aminoglycosides, erythromycin, vancomycin), loop diuretics, and chemotherapy drugs.

Systemic infections, such as Paget's disease of the bone, immune diseases, diabetes mellitus, bacterial meningitis, and trauma, are associated with this type of hearing loss. The two main problems associated with sensorineural loss are (a) the inability to understand speech despite the ability to hear sound and (b) the lack of understanding of the problem by other people. The ability to hear high-pitched sounds, including consonants, diminishes. Sounds become muffled and difficult to understand. An audiogram demonstrates a loss in decibel levels at the 4 000-Hz range and eventually the 2 000-Hz range. A hearing aid may help some patients, but it only makes sounds and speech louder, not clearer.

Mixed Hearing Loss. Mixed hearing loss results from a combination of conductive and sensorineural causes. Careful evaluation is needed if corrective surgery for conductive loss is planned because the sensorineural component of the hearing loss will still remain.

Central and Functional Hearing Loss. Central hearing loss involves the inability to interpret sound, including speech, because of a problem in the brain (central nervous system). Careful documentation of the history is helpful because there is usually a reference to deafness within the family. The patient should be referred to a qualified hearing and speech service if it is indicated.

Functional hearing loss may be caused by an emotional or a psychological factor. The patient does not seem to hear or respond to pure-tone subjective hearing tests, but no physical cause can be identified. Psychological counselling may help.

Classification of Hearing Loss. Hearing loss can also be classified by the decibel (dB) level or loss as recorded on the audiogram. Normal hearing is in the 0- to 15-dB range. Table 24-16 describes the levels hearing loss.

Clinical Manifestations. Common early signs of hearing loss are answering questions inappropriately, not responding when not looking at the speaker, asking others to speak up, and showing irritability with others who do not speak up. Other behaviours that suggest hearing loss include straining to hear, cupping the hand around the ear, reading lips, and an increased sensitivity to slight increases in noise level. Often, the patient is unaware of minimal hearing loss or may compensate by using these mannerisms. Family and friends who get tired of repeating or talking loudly are often first to notice hearing loss.

Deafness is often called the "unseen handicap" because it is not until conversation is initiated with a deaf adult that the difficulty in communication is realized. It is important that the health care provider be aware of the need for thorough validation of the deaf person's understanding of health teaching. Descriptive visual aids can be helpful.

Interference in communication and interaction with others can be the source of many problems for the patient and caregiver. Often the patient refuses to admit or may be unaware of impaired hearing. Irritability is common because the patient must concentrate very hard to understand speech. The loss of clarity of speech is most frustrating to a patient with sensorineural hearing loss. The patient may hear what is said but not understand it. Withdrawal, suspicion, loss of self-esteem, and insecurity are commonly associated with advancing hearing loss.

NURSING AND COLLABORATIVE MANAGEMENT HEARING LOSS AND DEAFNESS

HEALTH PROMOTION

ENVIRONMENTAL NOISE CONTROL. Noise is the most preventable cause of hearing loss. Figure 24-13 lists the levels of environmental noise generated by common indoor and outdoor sounds. Sudden severe loud noise (acoustic trauma) and chronic exposure to loud noise (noise-induced hearing loss) can damage hearing. Acoustic trauma causes hearing loss by destroying the hair cells of the organ of Corti. Sensorineural hearing loss as a result of increased and prolonged environmental noise, such as amplified sound, is occurring in young adults at an increasing rate. Amplified music (e.g., on iPods or MP3 players) should not exceed 50% of maximum volume. Health teaching must emphasize avoidance of continued exposure to noise levels greater than 70 dB.

In work environments known to have high noise levels (>85 dB), ear protection should be worn. Canadian Occupational Health and Safety regulations Part VII, Sections 7.1 to 7.8, deal with workplace noise (Department of Justice Canada, 2011). A variety of protectors that are worn over the ears or in the ears to prevent hearing loss are available. Periodic audiometric screening should be part of the health maintenance policies of industry. This provides baseline data on hearing to measure subsequent hearing loss.

Employees should participate in hearing conservation programs in work environments. Such programs should include noise exposure analysis, provision for control of noise exposure (hearing protectors), measurements of hearing, and employee–employer notification and education. Young adults should be encouraged to keep amplified music at a reasonable level and limit their exposure time. Hearing loss caused by noise is irreversible.

IMMUNIZATIONS. Various viruses in utero can cause deafness as a result of damage and malformations affecting the ear. The

TABLE 24-16	CLASSIFICATION OF HEARING LOSS	
Decibel (dB) Loss	**Meaning**
0–15	Normal hearing
16–25	Slight hearing loss
26–40	Mild impairment
41–55	Moderate impairment
56–70	Moderately severe impairment
71–90	Severe impairment
>90	Profound deafness*

*Most people in this category have been deaf since birth (congenitally deaf).

Outdoor sounds	NOISE LEVEL (dB)	Indoor sounds
	110	Rock concert
B-747-200 takeoff	100	Indoor subway
Gas lawnmower at 1 metre	90	Blender at 1 metre
Noisy urban daytime	80	Shouting at 1 metre
	70	Vacuum cleaner at 3 metres Normal speech at 1 metre
Commercial area	60	
Quiet urban daytime	50	Large business office
		Small theatre
Quiet suburban nighttime	40	Library
	30	
Quiet rural nighttime	20	Broadcast and recording studio
	10	

Hearing threshold

FIGURE 24-13 Levels of common environmental sounds.

nurse should promote childhood and adult immunizations, including the measles-mumps-rubella (MMR) vaccine. Rubella infection during the first 8 weeks of gestation is associated with an 85% incidence of congenital rubella syndrome, which causes sensorineural deafness. Women of child-bearing age should be tested for antibodies to these viral diseases. Women should avoid pregnancy for at least 3 months after being immunized. Immunization must be delayed if the woman is pregnant. Women who are susceptible to rubella can be vaccinated safely during the postpartum period.

OTOTOXIC SUBSTANCES. Drugs commonly associated with ototoxicity include salicylates, loop diuretics, chemotherapy drugs, and antibiotics. Chemicals used in industry (e.g. toluene, carbon disulphide, mercury) may damage the inner ear. Patients who are receiving ototoxic drugs or are exposed to ototoxic chemicals should be monitored for signs and symptoms associated with ototoxicity, including tinnitus, diminished hearing, and changes in equilibrium. If these symptoms develop, immediate withdrawal of the drug may prevent further damage and may cause the symptoms to disappear.

ASSISTIVE DEVICES AND TECHNIQUES

HEARING AIDS. The patient with a suspected hearing loss should have a hearing assessment by a qualified audiologist. If a hearing aid is indicated, it should be fitted by an audiologist or by a speech and hearing specialist. Many types of hearing aids are available, each with advantages and disadvantages (see Table 24-17). The conventional hearing aid serves as a simple amplifier.

For patients with bilateral hearing impairment, binaural hearing aids provide the best sound lateralization and speech discrimination. The nurse must give careful instruction on its use and maintenance and must assist the patient during the period of adjustment. The goal of hearing aid therapy is improved hearing with consistent use. Patients who are motivated and optimistic about using a hearing aid are more successful users. The nurse should determine the patient's readiness for hearing aid therapy, including acknowledgement of a hearing problem, the patient's feelings about wearing a hearing aid, the degree to which hearing loss affects life, and any difficulties the patient has manipulating small objects such as putting a battery in a hearing aid.

Initially, use of the hearing aid should be restricted to quiet situations in the home. The patient must first adjust to voices (including the patient's own) and household sounds. The patient should also experiment by increasing and decreasing the volume, as situations require. As the patient adjusts to the increase in sounds and background noise, he or she can progress to situations in which several people are talking simultaneously. Next, the environment can be expanded to the outdoors and then to such environments as a shopping mall or grocery store. Adjustment to different environments occurs gradually, depending on the individual patient.

When the hearing aid is not being worn, it should be placed in a dry, cool area where it will not be inadvertently damaged or lost. The battery should be disconnected or removed when not in use. Battery life averages 1 week, and patients should be

TABLE 24-17 TYPES OF HEARING AIDS

Type	Advantages	Disadvantages
Completely in the canal (mild to moderate hearing loss)	Smallest and least visible aid Protected from sounds such as wind noise	Costly No space for add-ons such as directional microphones or volume controls Small, short-lived batteries
In the canal (mild to severe hearing loss)	More powerful than aids completely in the canal Has adjustable features such as noise reduction	Small size of aid with its additional features may be difficult to operate for patients with visual loss or arthritis
In the ear (mild to severe hearing loss)	Powerful amplification Inserts and adjusts easily Longer-lasting batteries	Visible May pick up wind noise readily
Behind the ear (all types of hearing loss)	Most powerful aid Adjusts easily Longest battery life	Largest, most visible aid Newer models may be smaller and less obvious

TABLE 24-18 COMMUNICATION WITH PATIENTS WHO HAVE HEARING IMPAIRMENTS

Nonverbal Aids	Verbal Aids
• Draw attention with hand movements. • Have speaker's face in good light. • Avoid covering mouth or face with hands. • Avoid chewing, eating, and smoking while talking. • Maintain eye contact. • Avoid distracting environments. • Avoid careless expression that the patient may misinterpret. • Use touch. • Move close to better ear. • Avoid light behind speaker.	• Speak normally and slowly. • Do not overexaggerate facial expressions. • Do not overenunciate. • Use simple sentences. • Rephrase sentence; use different words. • Write name or difficult words. • Do not shout. • Speak in normal voice directly into better ear.

advised to purchase only a month's supply at a time. Ear moulds should be cleaned weekly or as needed. Toothpicks or pipe cleaners may be used to clear a clogged ear tip.

SPEECH READING. *Speech reading*, commonly called *lip reading*, can be helpful in increasing communication. It enables patients to achieve approximately 40% understanding of the spoken word. Patients are able to use visual cues associated with speech, such as gestures and facial expression, to help clarify the spoken message. In speech reading, many words look alike to the patient (e.g., "rabbit" and "woman"). If a patient wears glasses, the glasses should be used to facilitate speech reading. The nurse can help the patient by using and teaching verbal and nonverbal communication techniques as described in Table 24-18.

SIGN LANGUAGE. *Sign language* is used as a form of communication for people with profound hearing impairment. It involves gestures and facial features such as eyebrow motion and lip-mouth movements.

There is no one universal sign language. American Sign Language is used in the United States and the English-speaking parts of Canada. Quebec Sign Language, known in French as *Langue des signes québécoise* or *Langue des signes du Québec (LSQ)*, is the sign language of deaf communities in francophone Canada, primarily in Quebec.

COCHLEAR IMPLANT. The *cochlear implant* is used as a hearing device for people with severe to profound sensorineural hearing loss in one or both ears. The system consists of an external microphone placed behind the ear, a speech processor and a transmitter implanted under the skin that change sounds into electrical impulses, and a group of electrodes placed within the cochlea that stimulate the auditory nerves in the ear (Figure 24-14). Cochlear implants send information that covers the entire range of sound frequencies. The cochlear implant electrodes are inserted as far as possible into the cochlea to send both high- and low-frequency information. For patients with conductive and mixed hearing loss, the cochlear Baha system may be surgically implanted. The system works through direct bone conduction and becomes integrated with the skull bone over time.

Extensive training and rehabilitation are essential in order to receive maximum benefit from these implants. The positive aspects of a cochlear implant include providing sound to the person who heard none, improving lip-reading ability, monitoring

FIGURE 24-14 Cochlear implant.

TABLE 24-19	CLASSIFICATION OF PRESBYCUSIS	
Type	**Hearing Change**	**Prognosis**
Sensory Atrophy of auditory nerve; loss of sensory hair cells	Loss of high-pitched sounds	Little effect on speech understanding; good response to sound amplification
Neural Degenerative changes in cochlea and spinal ganglion	Loss of speech discrimination	Amplification alone not sufficient
Metabolic Degenerative changes in cochlea and spinal ganglion	Uniform loss for all frequencies accompanied by recruitment*	Good response to hearing aid
Cochlear Stiffening of basilar membrane, which interferes with sound transmission in the cochlea	Range of hearing loss increases from low to high frequencies; speech discrimination affected with higher frequency losses	Ameliorated by appropriate forms of amplification

*Abnormally rapid increase in loudness as sound intensity increases.

the loudness of the person's own speech, improving the sense of security, and decreasing feelings of isolation. With continued research, the cochlear implant may offer the possibility of aural rehabilitation for a wider range of hearing-impaired individuals.

The U.S. Food and Drug Administration has created an informational website on cochlear implants (see the Resources at the end of this chapter). The site includes an animated movie to help visualize the implants and how they work.

ASSISTED LISTENING DEVICES. Numerous devices are now available to assist hearing-impaired persons. Direct amplification devices, amplified telephone receivers, alerting systems that flash when activated by sound, an infrared system for amplifying the sound of the television, and a combination FM receiver and hearing aid are all devices that the nurse can explore on the basis of the patient's needs. People with profound deafness may be assisted by text-telephone alerting systems that flash when activated by sound, by closed captioning on television, and by specially trained dogs. Such dogs are trained to alert their owners to specific sounds within the environment, which thus increases the person's safety and independence.

AGE-RELATED CONSIDERATIONS

HEARING LOSS

Presbycusis, hearing loss associated with aging, includes the loss of peripheral auditory sensitivity, a decline in word recognition ability, and associated psychological and communication issues. Because consonants (high-frequency sounds) are the letters by which spoken words are recognized, an older adult with presbycusis has a diminished ability to understand the spoken word. Vowels are heard, but some consonants fall into the high-frequency range and cannot be differentiated. This may lead to confusion and embarrassment because of the difference in what was said and what was heard (Öberg, 2015).

The cause of presbycusis is related to degenerative changes in the inner ear. Noise exposure is thought to be a common factor. Table 24-19 describes the classification of specific causes and associated hearing changes of presbycusis. Many patients have more than one type of presbycusis. The prognosis for hearing depends on the cause of the loss. Sound amplification with the appropriate device is often helpful in improving the understanding of speech. In other situations, an audiological rehabilitation program can be valuable.

Many older adults are reluctant to use a hearing aid for sound amplification. Reasons cited most often include cost, appearance, insufficient knowledge about hearing aids, amplification of competing noise, and unrealistic expectations. Most hearing aids and batteries are small, and neuro-muscular changes such as stiff fingers, enlarged joints, and decreased sensory perception often make the care and handling of a hearing aid a difficult and frustrating experience for an older person. Some older persons may also tend to accept their losses as part of aging and believe there is no need for improvement.

CASE STUDY

Glaucoma and Diabetic Retinopathy

Patient Profile

Lena Andrews is a 68-year-old woman who has osteo-arthritis and type 2 diabetes mellitus, diagnosed 15 years earlier. She now has diabetic retinopathy. She returns to the eye clinic for continued evaluation and care of the primary open-angle glaucoma (POAG) and re-examination for changes in diabetic retinopathy. Her current medical regimen for POAG includes topical timolol maleate, 0.5% extended (Timoptic XE), once daily in each eye, and latanoprost (Xalatan), 0.005%, in each eye, at bedtime. At her last examination it was noted that she had microaneurysms and hard exudates of the retina.

Source: Blend Images/ Shutterstock .com.

Subjective Data

- She can no longer read the newspaper and reports that medication labels are difficult to read.
- States that she is not always successful in getting the eye drops instilled because her hands are gnarled and painful from osteoarthritis.

Objective Data

- Distant and near visual acuity are stable at 20/60 in the right eye and 20/50 in the left eye. This is a reduction from 20/40 in both eyes at her last visit.
- Intraocular pressures are stable at 20 mm Hg in both eyes. Visual field testing in the left eye reveals a new scotoma.
- Fluorescein angiography reveals diabetic macular edema in both eyes.

Collaborative Care

- Brimonidine (Alphagan), 0.15%, in left eye 15 min before and immediately after argon laser trabeculoplasty (ALT)

- Argon laser treatment in left eye to seal leaking microaneurysym from macular edema
- Checking intraocular pressure (IOP) after ALT
- Continuing previous glaucoma drop regimen
- Follow-up examination for glaucoma in 2 weeks for possible ALT in right eye
- Follow-up examination for diabetic macular edema in 8 weeks

Discussion Questions

1. What is the cause of Ms. Andrews's new nonproliferative retinopathy?
2. Why might laser photocoagulation be an appropriate therapy for macular edema?
3. What is the purpose of the fluorescein angiography?
4. **Priority decision:** What priority topics should be discussed in discharge teaching?
5. In what way could glaucoma cause vision loss if Ms. Andrews's eye pressures are not properly monitored?
6. **Priority decision:** What are the priority nursing interventions for Ms. Andrews?
7. **Priority decision:** On the basis of the assessment data, what are the priority nursing diagnoses? Are there any collaborative problems?
8. **Evidence-informed practice:** Ms. Andrews wants to know if her glaucoma is related to her diabetes. How should the nurse respond to her question?

⊖volve

Answers are available at *http://evolve.elsevier.com/Canada/Lewis/medsurg.*

REVIEW QUESTIONS

The number of the question corresponds to the same-numbered objective at the beginning of the chapter.

1. Why does presbyopia occur in older individuals?
   a. The retina degenerates.
   b. The lens becomes inflexible.
   c. The corneal curvature becomes irregular.
   d. It is associated with cataract development.
2. What is the most important nursing intervention for clients with epidemic keratoconjunctivitis?
   a. Applying patches to the affected eyes.
   b. Accurately measuring intraocular pressure.
   c. Monitoring near visual acuity every 4 hours.
   d. Teaching client and family members good hygiene techniques.
3. What should clients with eye inflammation or an eye infection be taught?
   a. Wear dark glasses to prevent irritation from ultraviolet light.
   b. Acute conditions commonly lead to chronic problems.
   c. Apply a cold compress with pressure to the inflamed area frequently.
   d. Regular, careful hand hygiene may prevent the infection from spreading.
4. Which of the following client behaviours would the nurse promote for healthy eyes and ears? (*Select all that apply*)

a. Wearing protective sunglasses when bicycling.
b. Supplemental intake of B vitamins and magnesium
c. Playing amplified music at 75% of maximum volume.
d. Notifying the health care provider if tinnitus occurs during antibiotic therapy.
e. For women, avoiding pregnancy for 4 weeks after receiving measles-mumps-rubella (MMR) immunization.

5. What should the nurse do to prepare clients for retinal detachment surgery?
   a. Explain how to care for an ocular prosthesis.
   b. Assure clients that they can expect 20/20 vision after surgery.
   c. Teach the family how to recognize when the client is hallucinating.
   d. Assess the client's level of knowledge about retinal detachment and provide information appropriate to the situation.
6. What should be included in the nursing plan for a client who needs to administer antibiotic eardrops?
   a. Cool the drops so that they decrease swelling in the canal.
   b. Be careful to avoid touching the tip of the dropper bottle to the ear.
   c. Placement of a cotton wick to assist in administering the drops is not recommended.
   d. Keep the head tilted for 5 to 7 minutes after administering the drops to prevent them from running out of the ear canal.

7. The nurse would suspect otosclerosis from assessment findings of hearing loss in which of the following clients?
   a. A 26-year-old woman with three biological children younger than 5 years of age.
   b. A 52-year-old man whose hearing loss is accompanied by vertigo and tinnitus.
   c. A 42-year-old woman who has a history of serous otitis media.
   d. A 63-year-old man who can hear high-pitched sounds more effectively than low-pitched sounds.

8. Which of the following statements best describes a client who has a sensorineural hearing loss?
   a. The client has difficulty understanding speech.
   b. The client experiences clearer sounds with the use of a hearing aid.
   c. The client may have a reversal of damage caused by ototoxic drugs.
   d. The client hears low-pitched sounds better than high-pitched sounds.

9. Which of the following would the nurse tell the client who is newly fitted with bilateral hearing aids? *(Select all that apply)*
   a. Replace the batteries monthly.
   b. Clean the ear moulds weekly or as needed.
   c. Clean ears with cotton-tipped applicators daily.
   d. Disconnect or remove the batteries when not in use.
   e. Initially restrict usage to quiet listening in the home.

10. Which strategies would best assist the nurse in communicating with a client who has a hearing loss? *(Select all that apply)*
    a. Overenunciate speech.
    b. Exaggerate facial expression.
    c. Raise the voice to a higher pitch.
    d. Write out names or difficult words.
    e. Speak normally and slowly.

11. Which of the following statements best describes clients with permanent visual impairment?
    a. They feel most comfortable with other visually impaired persons.
    b. They may feel threatened when others make eye contact during a conversation.
    c. They usually need others to speak louder so they can communicate appropriately.
    d. They may experience the same grieving process that is associated with other losses.

1. b; 2. d; 3. d; 4. a; 5. d; 6. b; 7. a; 8. a; 9. b, d; 10. d, e; 11. d.

ⓔvolve

For even more review questions, visit *http://evolve.elsevier.com/Canada/Lewis/medsurg.*

REFERENCES

Akpek, E. K., & Smith, R. A. (2013). Overview of age-related ocular conditions. *American Journal of Managed Care, 19*(5 Suppl.), S67–S75.

Balatsouras, D. G., & Korres, S. G. (2012). Subjective benign paroxysmal positional vertigo. *Otolaryngology–Head and Neck Surgery: Official Journal of American Academy of Otolaryngology-Head and Neck Surgery, 146*(1), 98–103. doi:10.1177/0194599811425158.

Bell, S., Hawranik, P. G., & McCormac, K. (2011). Focus on falls prevention: A quality improvement initiative. *AER Journal: Research and Practice in Visual Impairment and Blindness, 4*(3), 133.

Bressler, N., Beck, R., & Ferris, F. (2011). Panretinal photocoagulation for proliferative diabetic retinopathy. *New England Journal of Medicine, 365*, 1520–1526. doi:10.1056/NEJMct0908432.

Callahan, D. (2012). Conjunctivitis. *Digital Journal of Ophthalmology.* Retrieved from *http://www.djo.harvard.edu/site.php?url=/patients/pi/410.*

Canadian Diabetes Association. (2013). *Clinical practice guidelines: Retinopathy.* Retrieved from *http://guidelines.diabetes.ca/browse/Chapter30.*

Canadian National Institute for the Blind. (2012). *Eye safety—Take it personally.* Retrieved from *http://www.cnib.ca/en/your-eyes/safety/Pages/default.aspx.*

Canadian National Institute for the Blind. (2015a). *Fast facts about vision loss.* Retrieved from *http://www.cnib.ca/en/about/media/vision-loss/pages/default.aspx.*

Canadian National Institute for the Blind. (2015b). *About AMD.* Retrieved from *http://www.cnib.ca/en/your-eyes/eye-conditions/eye-connect/AMD/About/Pages/default.aspx.*

Canadian National Institute for the Blind. (2015c). *Cataracts.* Retrieved from *www.cnib.ca/en/your-eyes/eye-conditions/Cataracts/Pages/default.aspx.*

Canadian Ophthalmological Society evidence-based clinical practice guidelines for the periodic eye examinations in adults in Canada. (2007). *Canadian Journal of Ophthalmology, 42*(1), 39–45. doi:10.3129/canjophthalmol.06-126e. (Seminal).

Chew, E. Y., Clemons, T. E., Agron, E., et al. (2013). Long-term effects of vitamins C and E, β-carotene, and zinc on age-related macular degeneration. *Ophthalmology, 120*(8), 1604–1611. doi:10.1016/j.ophtha.2013.01.021.

Department of Justice Canada. (2011). *Canada occupational health and safety regulations (SOR/86-304).* Retrieved from *http://laws.justice.gc.ca/eng/regulations/SOR-86-304/index.html.*

Durning, M. V. (2013). Patient education series: Conjunctivitis. *Nursing, 43*(7), 39. doi:10.1097/01.NURSE.0000431137.97779.b1.

Farooq, A. V., & Shukla, D. (2012). Herpes simplex epithelial and stromal keratitis: An epidemiologic update. *Survey of Ophthalmology, 57*(5), 448–462. doi:10.1016/j.survophthal.2012.01.005.

Ferri, F. (2012). *Ferri's clinical advisor 2012.* St. Louis: Mosby.

Glaucoma Research Society of Canada. (2016). *Learning about glaucoma.* Retrieved from *http://www.glaucomaresearch.ca/en/about/about_glaucoma.shtml.*

Government of Canada. (2012). *Laser eye surgery.* Retrieved from *https://www.canada.ca/en/health-canada/services/medical-procedures/laser-eye-surgery.html?_ga=1.120126344.1853370565.1458502526.*

Güell, J. L., El Husseiny, M. A., Manero, F., et al. (2014). Historical review and update of surgical treatment for corneal endothelial diseases. *Ophthalmology and Therapy, 3*(1-2), 1–15. doi:10.1007/s40123-014-0022-y.

Harkin, H., & Kelleher, C. (2011). Caring for older adults with hearing loss. *Nursing Older People, 23*(9), 22–28.

Hatch, W. V., Campbell, E. L., Bell, C. M., et al. (2012). Projecting the growth of cataract surgery during the next 25 years. *Archives of Ophthalmology, 130*(11), 1479–1481. doi:10.1001/archopthalmol.2012.838.

Health Canada. (2012). *Noise-induced hearing loss.* Retrieved from *http://www.hc-sc.gc.ca/hl-vs/iyh-vsv/environ/hearing_loss-perte _audition-eng.php.*

Health Professions Regulatory Advisory Council. (2010). *Report to the Minister of Health and Long-Term Care on interprofessional collaboration among eye care health professionals.* Retrieved from *http://www.coptont.org/docs/hprac_eyes_report-March2010.pdf.* (Seminal).

HealthLinkBC. (2014). *Benign paroxysmal positional vertigo (BPPV).* Retrieved from *http://www.healthlinkbc.ca/healthtopics/content .asp?hwid=hw263714.*

Hearing Foundation of Canada. (2014). *Statistics.* Retrieved from *www.hearingfoundation.ca//?s=statistics.*

Jensen, L. (2012). Focusing your care: Working with clients with vision loss. *Canadian Nurse, 108*(3), 28–33.

Lee, T. C., & Gold, W. L. (2011). Necrotizing pseudomonas chondritis after piercing of the upper ear. *Canadian Medical Association Journal, 183*(7), 819–821. doi:10.1503/cmaj.100018.

Le Saux, N., & Robinson, J. L. (2016). Management of acute otitis media in children six months of age and older. *Paediatrics & Child Health, 21*(1), 39–50. Retrieved from *www.cps.ca/ documents/position/acute-otitis-media.*

Mackey, D. A., & Hewitt, A. W. (2014). Genome-wide association study success in ophthalmology. *Current Opinion in Ophthalmology, 25*(5), 386–393. doi:10.1097/ ICU.0000000000000090.

Mayo Clinic. (2013). *Cataract surgery: What you can expect.* Retrieved from *http://www.mayoclinic.org/tests-procedures/ cataract-surgery/basics/what-you-can-expect/prc-20012917.*

Melanoma Network of Canada. (2015). *A guide to uveal melanoma.* Retrieved from *https://www.melanomanetwork.ca/wp-content/ uploads/2015/04/140622-MNC_UvealGuideBooklet_FIN2_lr1.pdf.*

National Coalition for Vision Health. (2011). *Vision loss in Canada.* Retrieved from *http://www.cos-sco-ca/wp-content/uploads/2012/ 09/VisionLossinCanada_e.pdf.*

National Eye Institute. (2013). *Facts about the cornea and corneal disease [NEI health information].* Retrieved from *http://www .nei.nih.gov/health/cornealdisease/.*

National Eye Institute. (2015). *Facts about age-related macular degeneration.* Retrieved from *https://nei.nih.gov/health/ maculardegen/armd_facts.*

Nentwich, M. M., & Ulbig, M. W. (2015). Diabetic retinopathy— ocular complications of diabetes mellitus. *World Journal of Diabetes, 6*(3), 489–499. doi:10.4239/wjd.v6.i3.489.

Nielsen, M., Dogrusöz, M., Bleeker, J. C., et al. (2015). The genetic basis of uveal melanoma. *Journal Français d'Ophthalmologie, 38*(6), 516–521. doi:10.1016/j.jfo.2015.04.003.

Öberg, M. (2015). Hearing care for older adults: Beyond the audiology clinic. *American Journal of Audiology,* doi:10.1044/2015_AJA-14-0077. [Epub ahead of print].

Olson, J. H., Erie, J. C., & Bakri, S. J. (2011). Nutritional supplementation and age-related macular degeneration. *Seminars in Ophthalmology, 26*(3), 131–136. doi:10.3109/08820538.2011 .577131.

Popescu, M. L., Boisjoly, H., Schmaltz, H., et al. (2011). Age-related eye disease and mobility limitations in older adults. *Investigative Ophthalmology & Visual Science, 52*(10), 7168–7174. doi:10.1167/ iovs.11-7564.

Portnuff, C. D. F., Fligor, B. J., & Arehart, K. H. (2011). Teenage use of portable listening devices: A hazard to hearing? *Journal of American Academy of Audiology, 22*(10), 663–677. doi:10.3766/ jaaa.22.10.5.

Schaal, S., Sherman, M. P., Barr, C. C., et al. (2011). Primary retinal detachment repair: Comparison of 1-year outcomes of four surgical techniques. *Retina (Philadelphia, Pa.), 31*(8), 1500–1504. doi:10.1097/IAE/0b013e31820d3f55.

Statistics Canada. (2016). *Canadian survey on disability: Seeing and hearing disabilities, 2012.* Retrieved from *http://www.statcan.gc.ca/ daily-quotidien/160229/dq160229c-eng.htm.*

Steel, D. (2014). Retinal detachment. *BMJ Clinical Evidence,* pii: 0710.

Sutton, G., Lawless, M., & Hodge, C. (2014). Laser in situ keratomileusis in 2012: A review. *Clinical & Experimental Optometry, 97*(1), 18–29. doi:10.1111/cxo.12075.

Tareef, A. A. (2011). Falls in the elderly, spectrum and prevention. *Canadian Family Physician, 57*(7), 771–776. Retrieved from *https://www.ncbi.nlm.nih.gov/pmc/articles/PMC3135440/.*

Tassinari, M., Mandrioli, D., Gaggioli, N., et al. (2015). Ménière's disease treatment: A patient-centered systematic review. *Audiology & Neurotology, 20*(3), 153–165. doi:10.1159/000375393.

Thornton, K., Parrish, F., & Swords, C. (2011). Topical vs. systemic treatments for acute otitis media. *Pediatric Nursing, 37*(5), 263–267, 242. Retrieved from *http://www.pediatricnursing.net/ issues/11sepoct/abstr5.html.*

Tseng, V. L., Greenberg, P. B., Wu, W.-C., et al. (2011). Cataract surgery complications in nonagenarians. *Ophthalmology, 118*(7), 1229–1235. doi:10.1016/j.ophtha.2010.11.023.

World Health Organization. (2016). *Prevention of blindness and visual impairment: Trachoma.* Retrieved from *http://www.who.int/ blindness/causes/trachoma.*

RESOURCES

Alberta Association of the Deaf
http://www.aadnews.ca/

Alliance for Equality of Blind Canadians
http://www.blindcanadians.ca/

BC and Alberta Guide Dog Services
http://www.bcguidedog.com/

Canadian Association of the Deaf
http://www.cad.ca/

Canadian Association of Optometrists
http://opto.ca/

Canadian Council of the Blind (CCB)
http://ccbnational.net

Canadian Glaucoma Society
http://www.cgs-scg.org/

Canadian Hard of Hearing Association
http://www.chha.ca/chha/

Canadian Hearing Society
http://www.chs.ca/

Canadian Helen Keller Centre
http://www.chkc.org/

Canadian National Institute for the Blind (CNIB)
http://www.cnib.ca

Canadian Ophthalmological Society
http://www.cos-sco.ca

Foundation Fighting Blindness
http://www.blindness.org/

Hearing Foundation of Canada
http://hearingfoundation.ca

Misericordia Health Centre: Buhler Eye Care Centre
http://www.misericordia.mb.ca/Programs/EyeCare.html

Misericordia Health Centre: Focus on Falls Prevention Vision Screening Program
http://www.misericordia.mb.ca/AboutUs/VisionScreening.html

Montreal Association for the Blind: MAB-Mackay Rehabilitation Centre
http://www.mabmackay.ca/

Society of Deaf and Hard of Hearing Nova Scotians
http://sdhhns.org/

The Ottawa Hospital Eye Institute
http://www.ottawahospital.on.ca/wps/portal/Base/TheHospital/ClinicalServices/DeptPgrmCS/Programs/EyeInstitute

American Academy of Audiology
http://www.audiology.org/Pages/default.aspx

American Academy of Ophthalmology
http://www.aao.org/

American Society of Cataract and Refractive Surgery
http://ascrs.org/

American Society of Ophthalmic Registered Nurses
http://www.asorn.org/

Glaucoma Research Foundation
http://www.glaucoma.org/

International Hearing Society
http://ihsinfo.org/IhsV2/Home/Index.cfm

Macula Foundation, The
http://maculafoundation.org/

National Eye Institute of the National Institutes of Health
http://www.nei.nih.gov/

National Center on Deaf-Blindness
http://www.nationaldb.org/

University of Michigan Kellogg Eye Center
http://www.kellogg.umich.edu/

U.S. Food and Drug Administration: Cochlear Implants
http://www.fda.gov/MedicalDevices/ProductsandMedicalProcedures/ImplantsandProsthetics/CochlearImplants/default.htm

VisionSimulations.com
http://visionsimulations.com/

For additional Internet resources, see the website for this book at *http://evolve.elsevier.com/Canada/Lewis/medsurg*

Nursing Assessment

Integumentary System

Written by: Diana L. Gallagher
Adapted by: Susannah McGeachy

evolve WEBSITE

http://evolve.elsevier.com/Canada/Lewis/medsurg

- Review Questions (Online Only)
- Key Points
- Answer Guidelines for Case Study
- Conceptual Care Map Creator
- Audio Glossary
- Content Updates

LEARNING OBJECTIVES

1. Describe the structures and the functions of the integumentary system.
2. Link the age-related changes in the integumentary system to differences in assessment findings.
3. Identify the significant subjective and objective data related to the integumentary system that should be obtained from a patient.
4. Describe specific assessments to be made during the physical examination of the skin and the appendages.
5. Compare the critical components for describing primary and secondary lesions.
6. Identify appropriate techniques used in the physical assessment of the integumentary system.
7. Differentiate normal from common abnormal findings of a physical assessment of the integumentary system.
8. Summarize the structural and assessment differences in lighter- and darker-skinned individuals.
9. Describe the purpose, significance of results, and nursing responsibilities related to diagnostic studies of the integumentary system.

KEY TERMS

alopecia, p. 494	erythema, p. 501, Table 25-7	keratinocytes, p. 493	pruritus, p. 498
dermis, p. 494	hirsutism, p. 501, Table 25-7	melanocytes, p. 494	sebaceous glands, p. 495
epidermis, p. 493	intertriginous, p. 500	mole (nevus), p. 501, Table 25-7	vitiligo, p. 501, Table 25-7

The integumentary system is the largest body organ and comprises skin, hair, nails, and glands. The skin is further divided into two layers: the epidermis and the dermis. The subcutaneous tissue is immediately under the dermis (Figure 25-1).

STRUCTURES AND FUNCTIONS OF THE SKIN AND APPENDAGES

Structures

The epidermis is the outermost layer of the skin. The dermis, the second skin layer, contains collagen bundles and supports the nerve and vascular network. Subcutaneous tissue lies below the dermis and is composed primarily of fat and loose connective tissue.

Epidermis. The epidermis, the thin avascular superficial layer of the skin, is made up of an outer dead portion that serves as a protective barrier and a deeper, living portion that folds into the dermis. Together these layers measure 0.05 to 0.1 mm in thickness. The epidermis is nourished by blood vessels in the dermis. The epidermis regenerates with new cells every 28 days and is composed of two main types of cells: keratinocytes and melanocytes (Woodford & Yao, 2013).

Keratinocytes are synthesized from epidermal cells in the basal layer and outnumber melanocytes ten to one (Woodford & Yao, 2013). Initially, these cells are undifferentiated. As they mature *(keratinize),* they move to the surface, where they flatten and die to form the outer skin layer *(stratum corneum).* Keratinocytes produce a fibrous protein, called *keratin,* which is vital to the skin's protective barrier function. The upward movement of keratinocytes from the basement membrane to the stratum corneum takes approximately 4 weeks. If dead cells slough off too rapidly, the skin will appear thin and eroded. If

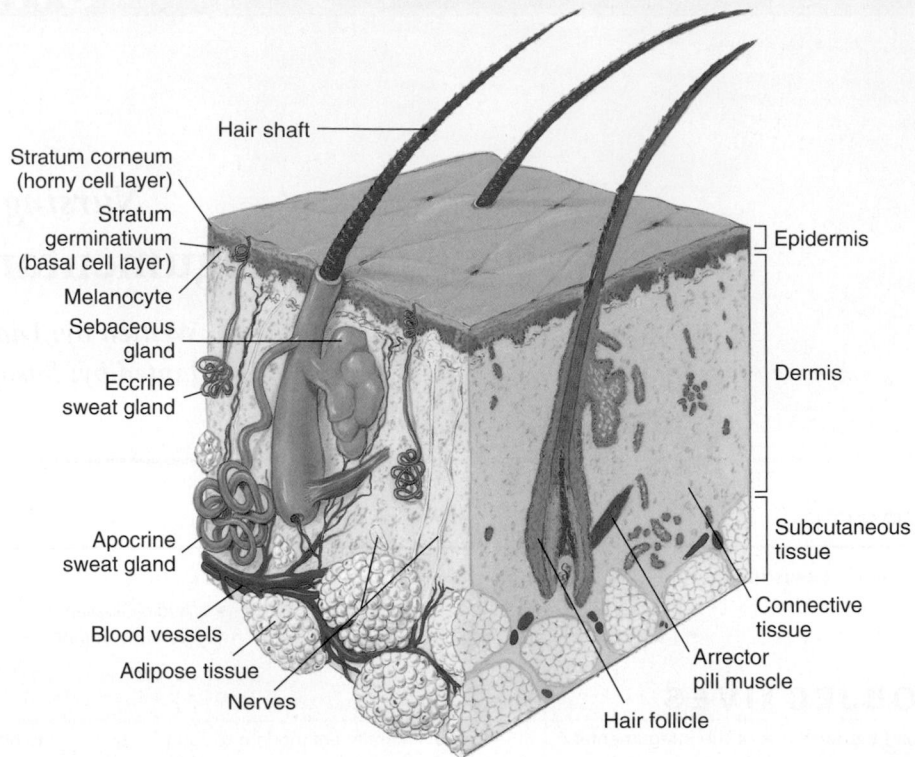

Hair shaft

Stratum corneum
(horny cell layer)

Stratum
germinativum
(basal cell layer)

Melanocyte

Sebaceous
gland

Eccrine
sweat gland

Apocrine
sweat gland

Blood vessels

Adipose tissue

Nerves

Epidermis

Dermis

Subcutaneous
tissue

Connective
tissue

Arrector
pili muscle

Hair follicle

FIGURE 25-1 Microscopic view of the skin in longitudinal section. Source: Jarvis, C., Browne, A. J., MacDonald-Jenkins, J. et al. (2014). *Physical examination and health assessment* (2nd Canadian ed., p. 220). Toronto: Elsevier.

new cells form faster than old cells are shed, the skin becomes scaly and thickened. Changes in this cell cycle account for many skin problems, such as psoriasis.

Melanocytes are contained in the deep, basal layer *(stratum germinativum)* of the epidermis. They contain melanin, a pigment that gives colour to the skin and hair and protects the body from damaging ultraviolet (UV) sunlight. Sunlight and hormones stimulate these cells to produce melanin. The wide range of skin and hair colours are a result of varying amounts of melanin produced; more melanin results in darker skin colour (Marks & Miller, 2013).

Dermis. The **dermis** is the connective tissue below the epidermis. The dermis is highly vascular, with a thickness varying from 1 to 4 mm. The dermis is divided into two layers: an upper, thin papillary layer and a deeper, thicker reticular layer (Woodford & Yao, 2013). The papillary layer is folded into ridges, which form congenital patterns called *fingerprints* and *footprints*. The reticular layer contains collagen, elastic, and reticular fibres.

Collagen forms the greatest part of the dermis and is responsible for the mechanical strength of the skin. The primary cell type in the dermis is the fibroblast. Fibroblasts produce collagen and elastin and are important in wound healing. Nerves, lymphatic vessels, hair follicles, and sebaceous and sweat glands are also found in the dermis.

Subcutaneous Tissue. While not part of the skin, the subcutaneous tissue is often discussed with the integument because it attaches the skin to underlying tissues such as the muscle and bone. The subcutaneous tissue contains loose connective tissue and fat cells, which store lipids, regulate temperature, and provide shock absorption. The anatomical distribution of subcutaneous tissue varies according to gender, heredity, age, and nutritional status.

Skin Appendages. Appendages of the skin include the hair, the nails, and glands (sebaceous, apocrine, and eccrine). These structures develop from the epidermal layer and receive nutrients, electrolytes, and fluids from the dermis. Hair and nails form from specialized keratin that becomes hardened.

Hair grows on most of the body except for the lips, the palms of the hands, and the soles of the feet (Patton & Thibodeau, 2013). The colour of the hair is a result of heredity and is determined by the type and the amount of melanin in the hair shaft. Hair grows approximately 1 cm per month. People lose an average of 25 to 100 hairs each day (Marks & Miller, 2013). When hair is not replaced, for example, due to normal aging, an endocrine disorder, a medication reaction, anticancer medication, or a skin disease, baldness, or **alopecia** (partial or complete lack of hair), results.

Fingernails and toenails are made of heavily keratinized cells. The part of the nail that you can see is the nail body. The rest is the nail root. A fold of skin hides most of the nail root. The cuticle borders this skin fold. Nail growth begins in the nail root. The portion of the nail root you can see is called the *lunula*. This white, crescent-shaped area is the site of mitosis and nail growth (Figure 25-2). Under the nail is an area of epidermis called the *nail bed*. The nail bed contains many blood vessels. Fingernails grow at a rate of 0.7 to 0.84 mm per week, with toenail growth 30% to 50% slower (Patton & Thibodeau, 2013). A lost fingernail usually regenerates in 3 to 6 months, while a lost toenail may require 12 months or longer to regenerate. Nail growth varies based on a person's age and health. Nails grow faster in men and in warm weather. Nail colour ranges from pink to yellow or brown depending on skin colour. Colour and texture variations in the nails may represent normal or abnormal conditions. Pigmented longitudinal bands *(melanonychia*

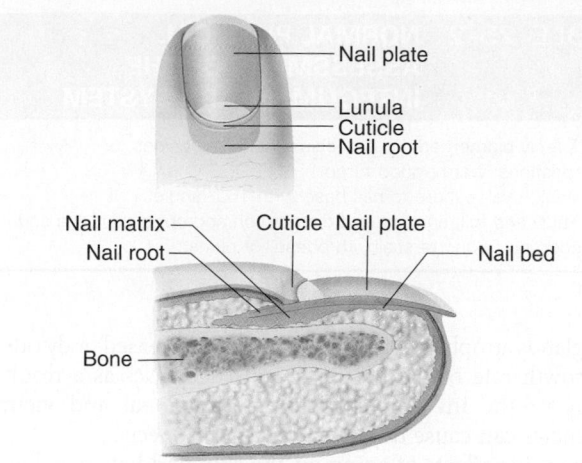

FIGURE 25-2 Structure of a nail. Source: Patton, K. T., & Thibodeau, G. A. (2016). *Essentials of anatomy and physiology* (9th ed., p. 196). St. Louis: Mosby.

FIGURE 25-3 Pigmented nail bed normally seen with dark skin colour. Source: Habif, T. P. (2016). *Clinical dermatology: A color guide to diagnosis and therapy* (6th ed., p. 766). St. Louis: Mosby.

striata) occur in the nail bed of most people with dark skin (Figure 25-3).

Two major types of glands are associated with the skin: sebaceous and sweat glands. The sebaceous glands secrete *sebum,* a lipid-rich substance that waterproofs and lubricates the skin and hair and inhibits bacterial and fungal growth. These glands depend on sex hormones, particularly testosterone, to regulate sebum secretion and production. Sebum production varies depending on age, sex, and hormone levels. Sebaceous glands are present on all areas of the skin except the palms and soles and are most abundant on the face, the scalp, the upper chest, and the back.

There are two varieties of sweat glands: apocrine and eccrine. The apocrine sweat glands are located mainly in the axillae, breast areolae, umbilical and anogenital areas, external auditory canals, and eyelids. These glands become active at puberty due to reproductive hormones. They secrete a milky, odourless substance, which interacts with skin surface bacteria to produce adult body odour (Jarvis, Browne, MacDonald-Jenkins, et al., 2014). In contrast, eccrine sweat glands are widely distributed over the body. Two square centimetres of skin contains about 1 000 of these sweat glands. Sweat is a transparent watery solution composed of salts, ammonia, urea, and other wastes. The main function of these glands is to cool the body by evaporation,

FIGURE 25-4 Photoaging. Irregular pigmentation and keratoses occur on sun-damaged skin on the forehead. Source: Gawkrodger, D., & Ardern-Jones, M. R. (2012). *Dermatology* (5th ed.). Edinburgh: Churchill Livingstone.

excrete waste products through the pores of the skin, and moisturize surface cells.

Functions of the Integumentary System

The skin's primary function is to protect the underlying tissues of the body from the external environment. The skin acts as a barrier against invasion by bacteria and viruses and prevents excessive water loss. The fat in the subcutaneous layer insulates the body and provides protection from trauma. Melanin screens and absorbs ultraviolet radiation. Nerve endings and receptors located within the skin provide sensory information on environmental stimuli to the brain related to pain, heat and cold, touch, pressure, and vibration. In addition, the skin regulates heat loss by responding to changes in internal and external temperature with vasoconstriction, vasodilation, and excretion of sweat. Evaporation of water from the lungs and skin results in the loss of 600 to 900 mL of water daily. Sebum and sweat lubricate the skin surface. Furthermore, endogenous synthesis of vitamin D, which is critical to calcium and phosphorus balance, occurs in the epidermis.

The skin is also a delivery system for drugs. An increasing number of systemic drugs are effectively delivered via patches or creams applied directly to the skin.

AGE-RELATED CONSIDERATIONS

EFFECTS OF AGING ON THE INTEGUMENTARY SYSTEM

Skin changes related to aging include decreased turgor, thinning, dryness, wrinkling, vascular lesions, increased skin fragility, and benign neoplasms. Although many changes are only of cosmetic concern, others can be serious and need careful evaluation. Age-related changes of the integumentary system and differences in assessment findings are listed in Table 25-1.

With advancing age, the junction between the dermis and the epidermis becomes flattened, and the epidermis contains fewer melanocytes. In addition, the dermis loses volume and has fewer blood vessels. Scalp, pubic, and axillary hair becomes depigmented and thinner. A loss of melanin results in grey or white hair. The nail plate thins, and nails become brittle, thicker, and more prone to splitting and yellowing.

Chronic UV exposure is the major contributor to photoaging and wrinkling of the skin (Canadian Dermatology Association [CDA], 2015a). Sun damage to the skin is cumulative (Figure 25-4). The wrinkling of sun-exposed areas such as the face and hands is more marked than in sun-shielded areas such as the buttocks. Poor nutrition, with decreased intake of protein, calories, and vitamins, further contributes to aging of the skin. With

TABLE 25-1 AGE-RELATED DIFFERENCES IN ASSESSMENT

Integumentary System

Changes	Differences in Assessment Findings
Skin	
• Decreased subcutaneous fat, muscle laxity, degeneration of elastic fibres, collagen stiffening	Increased wrinkling, sagging breasts and abdomen, redundant flesh around eyes, slowness of skin to flatten when pinched (tenting)
• Decreased extracellular water, surface lipids, and sebaceous gland activity	Dry, flaking skin with possible signs of excoriation caused by scratching
• Decreased activity of apocrine and sebaceous glands	Dry skin with minimal to no perspiration, uneven skin coloration
• Increased capillary fragility and permeability	Bruising
• Increased focal melanocytes in basal layer with pigment accumulation	Solar lentigines on face and backs of hands
• Diminished blood supply	Decrease in rosy appearance of skin and mucous membranes; skin cool to touch; diminished awareness of pain, touch, temperature, and peripheral vibration
• Decreased proliferative capacity	Diminished rate of wound healing
• Decreased immuno-competence	Increase in neoplasms
Hair	
• Decreased melanin and melanocytes	Grey or white hair
• Decreased oil	Dry, coarse hair; scaly scalp
• Decreased density of hair	Thinning and loss of hair
• Cumulative androgen effect; decreasing estrogen levels	Facial hirsutism, baldness
Nails	
• Decreased peripheral blood supply	Thick, brittle nails with diminished growth
• Increased keratin	Longitudinal ridging
• Decreased circulation	Prolonged return of blood to nails on blanching

TABLE 25-2 NORMAL PHYSICAL ASSESSMENT OF THE INTEGUMENTARY SYSTEM

Skin: Evenly pigmented; no petechiae, purpura, lesions, or excoriations; warm; good turgor.
Nails: Pink; oval; adhere to nail base with 160° angle.
Hair: Shiny and full; amount and distribution appropriate for age and gender; no flaking of scalp, forehead, or pinna.

sweat glands atrophy, causing dry skin and decreased body odour. The growth rate of the hair and nails decreases as a result of atrophy of the involved structures. Hormonal and vitamin deficiencies can cause dry, thin hair and alopecia.

The visible effects of aging on the skin and hair may have a profound psychological effect on many people. Although fine wrinkling of the skin, thinning hair, and brittle nails are normal changes with aging, they may result in an altered self-image (Jarvis, Browne, MacDonald-Jenkins, et al., 2014).

ASSESSMENT OF THE INTEGUMENTARY SYSTEM

A general assessment of the skin begins at the initial contact with the patient and continues throughout the examination. Specific areas are examined during examination of other body sites unless the reason for seeking care is a dermatological problem. Record a general statement about the physical condition of the patient's skin (Table 25-2). When a skin problem is noted, investigate by gathering further subjective data. Health history questions are presented in Table 25-3.

CASE STUDY

Patient Introduction

Source: DGLimages/ Shutterstock .com.

Ms. Danielle Arquette is a 74-year-old woman who comes to her primary care clinic with concerns related to various "spots" on her face. She says they have been there for a while, and she thought they were just "age spots" but got concerned after her friend was diagnosed with a malignant melanoma.

Critical Thinking

The following questions should be kept in mind while studying this assessment chapter:
1. What are the possible causes of Ms. Arquette's facial lesions?
2. What questions should the patient be asked to determine the possible causes?
3. What should be included in the physical assessment? What specific characteristics of the skin lesions should the nurse look for?
4. What diagnostic studies might be ordered?

See pp. 498 and 503 for more information on Ms. Arquette.

⊖volve
Answers available at *http://evolve.elsevier.com/Canada/Lewis/medsurg.*

aging, collagen fibres stiffen, elastic fibres degenerate, and the amount of subcutaneous tissue decreases. These changes, with the added effects of gravity, lead to wrinkling.

Benign neoplasms related to the aging process can occur. These growths include seborrheic keratoses, vascular lesions such as cherry angiomas, and skin tags. Actinic keratoses appear on areas of chronic sun exposure, especially in people with a fair complexion. These premalignant cutaneous lesions place an individual at increased risk for squamous cell and basal cell carcinomas. The photoaged person is more susceptible to skin cancers because of decline in the capacity to repair cellular deoxyribonucleic acid (DNA) damage caused by UV exposure (CDA, 2015b). Chronic UV exposure from tanning beds causes the same damage as UV from the sun.

Subcutaneous fat decreases with age, leading to increased risk of traumatic injury, hypothermia, and skin shearing, which may lead to pressure injuries. With aging, the apocrine and eccrine

Subjective Data

Past Medical History. Past medical history (PMH) reveals previous trauma, surgery, or disease that involves the skin. Many diseases have dermatological manifestations. The nurse needs to determine if the patient has noticed any problems such as jaundice, delayed wound healing, cyanosis, or pallor. It is

TABLE 25-3 HEALTH HISTORY

Integumentary System: Questions for Obtaining Subjective Data

Past History

- Do you have any history of previous trauma, surgery, or prior disease that involves the skin?*
- Do you have any dermatological manifestations of systemic problems such as jaundice (liver disease), delayed wound healing (diabetes mellitus), cyanosis (respiratory disorder), or pallor (anemia)?*
- Do you have a history of chronic or unprotected exposure to UV light such as use of tanning beds or history of radiation treatments?*
- Have you had any skin-related problems that occurred as a result of taking prescription or OTC medications?*
- Have you ever taken vitamins, hormones, antibiotics, corticosteroids, or antimetabolites?
- Are you taking any complementary or alternative medicines?*
- Are you using any medications to treat hair loss?*
- Have you used prescription or OTC medications to treat a primary skin problem, such as acne, or a secondary skin problem, such as itching? If so, please state the name, length of use, method of application, and effectiveness of the medication.
- Have you ever had surgery on your skin, including cosmetic surgery?*
- Do you have any body art, piercings, or tattoos?* Did you experience any complications such as skin infections, allergic reactions, dental problems, or MRI burns?
- Have you ever had a skin biopsy?* If so, what were the results?
- Have you had any treatments specifically for a skin problem (e.g., phototherapy, radiation therapy, cosmetic "peels")?

Family History

- Do you have a family history of any skin diseases, including congenital and familial diseases (e.g., alopecia and psoriasis) and systemic diseases with dermatological manifestations (e.g., diabetes, thyroid disease, cardiovascular diseases, immune disorders)?
- Do you have any family or personal history of skin cancer, particularly melanoma?

Self-Care History

- Describe your daily hygiene practices.
- What skin products are you currently using?
- Do you do anything to protect yourself from the sun?* How frequently do you use sun protection, and what is the SPF number of your sunscreen products?
- Has your birth control method, if used, caused a skin problem?*

Nutritional History

- Are there any changes in the condition of your skin, hair, nails, and mucous membranes that might be related to dietary changes?*
- Do you have food allergies that cause a skin reaction?

Social, Environment, or Occupational History

- Do you have any pets?
- Do you have any food, pet, or drug allergies?*
- Do you have any unusual skin reactions to insect bites and stings?*
- Are there any environmental skin irritants at your current or previous workplace or home?*
- Do your leisure activities involve the use of any chemicals that are potentially toxic to the skin?*

Cognitive–Perceptual

- Do you have any unusual sensations of heat, cold, or touch?*
- Do you have any pain associated with your skin condition?*
- Do you have any joint pain?*

Coping Abilities

- Does stress play a role in the onset of your skin condition, or does stress exacerbate the condition?
- What strategies have you used to manage your skin condition?

General

- Describe any current skin condition, including onset, course, and treatment (if any).
- Describe any changes in the condition of your skin, hair, nails, and mucous membranes.
- Have you noticed any changes in skin pigmentation? Any changes in the size or shape or colour of a mole? Any excessive bruising? Any unusual hair loss? Any change in the strength, colour, or nature of your nails? Any itching?
- Have you noticed any changes in the way sores or lesions heal?*
- Have you noticed changes in your skin related to excessive sweating, dryness, or swelling?*
- Does your skin condition keep you awake or awaken you after you have fallen asleep?*

MRI, magnetic resonance imaging; *OTC*, over-the-counter; *SPF*, sun protection factor; *UV*, ultraviolet.
*If yes, describe.
Source: Based on Jarvis, C., Browne, A., MacDonald-Jenkins, J., et al. (2014). *Physical examination and health assessment* (2nd Canadian ed.). Toronto: Elsevier.

important to obtain specific information related to sensitivities, allergies, and skin reactions to insect bites and stings. Any history of chronic or unprotected exposure to UV light should be noted.

Medications. Many vitamins, hormones, antibiotics, corticosteroids, and antimetabolites have adverse effects that are manifested in the skin, so the patient should be asked about any skin-related changes that occurred after taking medications. Additionally, it is important to document the use of medications (i.e., drug's name, length of use, method of application, and effectiveness) to treat a primary or secondary skin problem.

Surgery or Other Treatments. The nurse should determine if any surgical procedures, including cosmetic surgery, were done on the skin. Any previous biopsy results should be recorded, as should any treatments done specifically for a skin problem or for another health problem. Any treatments undergone for cosmetic purposes should also be documented.

Family History. The nurse should obtain information about any family history of skin diseases or systemic diseases with dermatological manifestations. Any family or personal history of skin cancer, particularly melanoma, must also be noted.

Self-Care History. The patient should be questioned about health and hygiene practices related to the integumentary system, including the brand name, quantity, and frequency of use of personal care products (e.g., shampoos, moisturizing agents, cosmetics). Any current skin problems, including onset, symptoms, course, and treatment, should be recorded, as well as the frequency of use and the sun protection factor (SPF) of sunscreen products.

Nutritional History. A diet history reveals the adequacy of nutrients essential to healthy skin such as vitamins A, D, E, and C; dietary fat; and protein. The nurse should question the patient regarding recent dietary changes; any food allergies that cause a skin reaction; and conditions of the skin such as dehydration, edema, and **pruritus** (itching), which can indicate alterations in fluid balance. If urinary or fecal incontinence is a problem, the nurse should determine the condition of the skin in the anal and perineal areas.

Social, Environmental, and Occupational Health History. The patient should be questioned about environmental factors that affect the skin such as occupational exposure to chemicals, irritants, sun, and unusually cold or unhygienic conditions. Contact dermatitis caused by allergies and irritants is a common problem associated with occupation, as well as with some hobbies. The patient's participation in any recreational activities involving significant sun exposure should be determined and documented, as should any changes in the skin during exercise or other activities.

Cognitive–Perceptual. The patient's perception of the sensations of health, cold, pain, and touch should be determined. The nurse should note any discomfort associated with a skin condition, especially when observed in intact skin. As well, joint pain and the mobility of joints should be assessed and recorded, since a skin condition may cause alterations in mobility.

Coping Abilities. The patient should be asked about the role that stress may play in creating or exacerbating the skin condition. The nurse should determine what coping strategies the patient uses to manage the skin condition. For example, pruritus can be distressing and cause major alterations in normal sleep patterns, while acne can be disfiguring and lead to significant threat to self-image.

Objective Data

Physical Examination. A physical examination of the skin begins with a systematic, general inspection and then a more specific assessment of problem areas. The nursing assessment should note changes in the colour, turgor, temperature, dryness,

⌛ GENETICS IN CLINICAL PRACTICE

Skin Malignancies

- The primary risk factor leading to skin cancers, including melanoma, is environmental exposure to UV radiation. UV radiation damages DNA, causing an error in the genetic code and resulting in abnormal skin cells (Han, Chien, & Kang, 2014).
- However, inherited genetic factors can increase the risk for skin cancer. A person who has a first-degree relative (e.g., parent, full sibling) who had a melanoma has an increased risk for developing melanoma (CDA, 2015b).
- The risk for skin cancer is also increased in people who have a fair complexion (light-coloured skin that easily freckles, red or blond hair, and blue or light-coloured eyes).

thickness, and vascularity of the skin. The findings may be normal, relative to age, genetic factors, and environmental exposures, or may represent primary or secondary skin lesions (Tables 25-3 and 25-4). General principles when conducting an assessment of the skin are as follows:

1. Use a private examination room of moderate temperature with good lighting; a room with exposure to daylight is preferred.
2. Ensure that the patient is comfortable and in a gown that allows easy access to all skin areas.
3. Be systematic and proceed from head to toe.
4. Compare symmetrical parts.
5. Perform a general inspection followed by a lesion-specific examination.
6. Use the metric system when taking measurements.
7. Use appropriate terminology and nomenclature when reporting or documenting.

Photographs are useful to accurately capture findings and to monitor skin lesions over time. Follow clinical agency protocol regarding obtaining a patient's consent to photograph skin lesions for inclusion in the medical record.

Inspection. The skin should be inspected for general colour and pigmentation, vascularity, bruising, and the presence of lesions or discolorations. The critical factor in assessment of skin colour is change. A skin colour that is normal for a particular patient can be a sign of a pathological condition in another patient. The most reliable areas in which to assess erythema, cyanosis, pallor, and jaundice are the areas of least pigmentation, such as sclerae, conjunctivae, nail beds, lips, and buccal mucosa. The true skin colour is best observed in photoprotected areas, such as the buttocks. Activity, sun (UV) exposure, emotions, cigarette smoking, and edema, as well as respiratory, renal, cardiovascular, and hepatic disorders, can all directly affect the colour of the skin.

In the general inspection, the nurse should note the presence of body art such as piercings and tattoos. The nose, ears, eyebrows, lips, navel, and nipples are common sites of piercing. Tattoos and needle track marks should be identified, and their location and the characteristics of the surrounding skin area noted. Tattoo pigments deposited in the skin may cause itching, pain, and sensitivity for several weeks after the tattoo is placed.

The skin should be examined for possible problems related to vascularity, such as areas of bruising, and vascular and purpuric lesions, such as *angiomas* (benign tumours of blood or lymph vessels), *petechiae* (tiny purple-red macules on skin), ecchymoses (bruises, larger than petechiae), or *purpuras* (purple patches characterized by ecchymoses or other small hemorrhages) (Figure 25-5). Placing direct pressure on a lesion can provide important

CASE STUDY

Subjective Data

Source: DGLimages/ Shutterstock .com.

A focused subjective assessment of Danielle Arquette reveals the following:
- *PMH:* Negative except for an appendectomy at age 16.
- *Medications:* None at present. No known allergies.
- *Self-care:* Currently washes her face with a skin cleanser in the morning and at nighttime. After cleansing, she applies a moisturizer with SPF 15. She has used these facial products for the past 3 years, since she first started noticing small age spots appearing. Before that, she used just soap and water.
- *Nutritional:* Ms. Arquette reports that her skin seems to be drier as she ages but otherwise no changes besides the "age spots or whatever they are."

Denies any changes in the way cuts or sores heal. No weight loss. Takes 400 IU of vitamin D daily; does not take any other supplemental vitamins or minerals.
- *Elimination:* Although skin is a little dry, she does not perceive it to be excessively dry. Denies excessive sweating or any swelling.
- *Social, environmental, and occupational:* Loves to garden and go for walks outdoors. Reports a history of frequent, sometimes severe, sunburns as a child. No use of sunscreen growing up but does remember her mother making her wear T-shirts over her bathing suits to help prevent sunburn. Has used sunscreen for the past 20 years when outdoors. Reapplies as needed.
- *Coping abilities:* Denies any pain or discomfort associated with skin lesions. Fearful that she might have skin cancer.

See p. 503 for more information on Ms. Arquette.

TABLE 25-4 PRIMARY SKIN LESIONS

Lesion	Description
Macule	Circumscribed, flat area with a change in skin colour; <0.5 cm in diameter; if lesion >0.5 cm, it is a *patch* *Examples:* freckles, petechiae, measles, flat mole (nevus), café-au-lait spots, vitiligo (complete depigmentation)
Papule	Elevated, solid lesion; <0.5 cm in diameter; if lesion is >0.5 cm in diameter, it is a *nodule* *Examples:* wart (verruca), elevated moles, lipoma, basal cell carcinoma
Vesicle	Circumscribed, superficial collection of serous fluid; <0.5 cm in diameter *Examples:* varicella (chicken pox), herpes zoster (shingles) (Figure 25-6), second-degree burn
Plaque	Circumscribed, elevated, superficial, solid lesion; >0.5 cm in diameter *Examples:* psoriasis, seborrheic and actinic keratoses
Wheal	Firm, edematous, irregularly shaped area; diameter variable *Examples:* insect bite, urticaria
Pustule	Elevated, superficial lesion filled with purulent fluid *Examples:* acne, impetigo

FIGURE 25-5 Purpura as seen in acute meningococcemia. Source: Dr. François Bricaire/ScienceSource.

FIGURE 25-6 Herpes zoster (shingles) on the anterior chest, classic dermatomal distribution. Source: James, W. D., Berger, T. G., & Elston, D. M. (2011). *Andrews' diseases of the skin* (11th ed.). Philadelphia: Saunders.

information. If the lesion blanches on direct pressure and then refills, the redness is caused by dilated blood vessels. If the discoloration remains, it is the result of subcutaneous or intradermal bleeding or the presence of a nonvascular lesion. Bruising that has a pattern—for example, in the shape of a hand or fingers—should be documented, as should bruises at different stages of resolution. These may be indications of other health problems or abuse and require further investigation.

If lesions are found on the skin, their colour, size, height, distribution, location, and shape should be recorded. Lesions may be primary or secondary. Primary skin lesions develop on previously unaltered skin. The common characteristics of primary skin lesions are shown in Table 25-4. Secondary skin lesions are lesions that change with time or occur because of factors such as scratching or infection. Secondary skin lesions are shown in Table 25-5.

Skin lesions are usually described in terms of their configuration (shape, whether solitary or forming a pattern in relation to other lesions) and distribution (arrangement of lesions over an area of skin) (Table 25-6). For example, herpes zoster (shingles) lesions are characteristically vesicular and have a linear distribution clustered along one or more dermatomes (Figure 25-6). Any unusual odours should also be noted. Skin sites with lesions,

TABLE 25-5   SECONDARY SKIN LESIONS

Lesion	Description
Fissure	Linear crack or break from the epidermis to the dermis; dry or moist *Examples:* athlete's foot, cracks at corner of the mouth
Scale	Excess, dead epidermal cells produced by abnormal keratinization and shedding *Examples:* flaking of skin after a drug reaction or sunburn
Scar	Abnormal formation of connective tissue that replaces normal skin *Examples:* surgical incision, healed wound
Ulcer	Loss of the epidermis, extending into the dermis; crater-like, irregular shape *Examples:* pressure injury, chancre
Atrophy	Depression in skin resulting from thinning of the epidermis or dermis *Examples:* aged skin, striae
Excoriation	Area in which epidermis is missing, exposing the dermis *Examples:* abrasion, scratch

TABLE 25-6   LESION DISTRIBUTION TERMINOLOGY

Term	Description
Asymmetric	Unilateral distribution
Confluent	Merging together
Diffuse	Wide distribution
Discrete	Separate from other lesions
Generalized	Diffuse distribution over large area of body surface
Grouped	Cluster of lesions
Localized	Limited areas of involvement that are clearly defined
Satellite	Single lesion in proximity to a large grouping
Solitary	A single lesion
Symmetrical	Bilateral distribution
Zosteriform	Bandlike distribution along a dermatome area

FIGURE 25-7 Intertrigo. Candidal rash in body folds. Source: Graham-Brown, R., Bourke, J., & Cunliffe, T. (2008). *Dermatology: Fundamentals of practice.* Edinburgh: Mosby.

such as rashes, may be colonized with yeast or bacteria, which can be associated with distinctive odours in intertriginous areas (Figure 25-7). **Intertriginous** areas are where skin surfaces overlap and rub on each other (e.g., below the breasts, axillae, and groin).

The nurse's inspection should include all body hair, noting the distribution, texture, and quantity of hair. Changes in the normal distribution of body hair and growth may indicate an endocrine or vascular disorder. The nails should be observed for shape, thickness, curvature, and surface, and any grooves, pitting, ridges, or detachment from nail bed should be noted. Changes in nail smoothness or thickness can occur with anemia, psoriasis, thyroid problems, decreased vascular circulation, and some infections.

Palpation. Palpating the skin provides information about temperature, turgor and mobility, moisture, and texture. The nurse should use the back of her or his own hand to gauge skin temperature, since the skin on the back of the examiner's hand is thinner than on the palm and therefore more sensitive to temperature changes. The patient's skin should be warm, not hot. Skin temperature increases with increased blood flow to the dermis. Localized temperature increase occurs with burns and local inflammation. A generalized increase will result from fever. A decreased skin temperature may occur when shock or other circulatory problems, chilling, or infection is present.

Turgor refers to the elasticity of the skin. The nurse should assess turgor by gently pinching an area of skin under the clavicle or on the back of the hand. Skin with good turgor should move easily when lifted and should immediately return to its original position when released (see Figure 19-13). Dehydration and aging may cause loss of turgor, leading to skin tenting (Table 25-7).

TABLE 25-7 ASSESSMENT ABNORMALITIES

Integumentary System

Finding	Description	Possible Etiology and Significance
Alopecia	Loss of hair (localized or general; especially the head, but there can be hair loss on other parts of the body as well, from patches to total body hair loss) (see Figure 25-8)	Heredity, friction, rubbing, traction, trauma, stress, infection, inflammation, chemotherapy, pregnancy, emotional shock, tinea capitis, immunological factors or unknown causation
Angioma	Tumour consisting of blood or lymph vessels	Increased incidence normal with aging, liver disease, pregnancy, varicose veins
Carotenemia (carotenosis)	Yellow discoloration of skin, no yellowing of sclerae, most noticeable on palms and soles	Excessive ingestion of vegetables containing carotene (e.g., carrots, squash), hypothyroidism
Comedone (acne lesion)	Enlarged hair follicle plugged with sebum, bacteria, and skin cells; can be open (blackhead) or closed (whitehead)	Heredity, certain drugs, hormonal changes with puberty and pregnancy
Cyanosis	Slightly bluish-grey or dark purple discoloration of the skin and mucous membranes caused by presence of excessive amounts of reduced hemoglobin in capillaries	Cardiorespiratory problems; vasoconstriction, asphyxiation, anemia, leukemia, and malignancies
Cyst	Sac containing fluid or semisolid material	Obstruction of a duct or gland, parasitic infection
Ecchymosis	Large, bruiselike lesion caused by collection of extravascular blood in dermis and subcutaneous tissue	Trauma, bleeding disorders
Erythema	Redness occurring in patches of variable size and shape	Heat, certain drugs, alcohol, ultraviolet rays, any problem that causes dilation of blood vessels to the skin
Hematoma	Extravasation of blood of sufficient size to cause visible swelling	Trauma, bleeding disorders
Hirsutism	Male-pattern distribution of hair in women	Abnormality of ovaries or adrenal glands, decrease in estrogen level, heredity
Hypopigmentation	Congenital or acquired loss of melanin resulting in lighter depigmented areas	Heredity, chemical or pharmacological agents, nutritional factors, burns, inflammation and infection, vitiligo (patchy loss of skin pigment common on hands, face, and genital region) (Figure 25-9)
Intertrigo	Dermatitis of overlying surfaces of the skin	Moisture, irritation, obesity; may be complicated by *Candida* infection (see Figure 25-7)
Jaundice	Yellow (in White people) or yellowish-brown (in Black people) discoloration of the skin, best observed in the sclera; secondary to increased bilirubin in the blood	Liver disease, red blood cell hemolysis, pancreatic cancer, common bile duct obstruction
Keloid	Hypertrophied scar beyond margin of incision or trauma (see Figure 14-8)	Predisposition more common in dark-skinned individuals
Lichenification	Thickening of the skin with accentuated skin markings	Repeated scratching, rubbing, and irritation usually due to pruritus or neurosis
Mole (nevus)	Benign overgrowth of melanocytes	Defects of development; excessive numbers of large, irregular moles; sometimes hereditary
Petechiae	Pinpoint, discrete deposit of blood <1–2 mm in the extravascular tissues; visible through the skin or mucous membrane	Inflammation, marked dilation, blood vessel trauma, blood dyscrasia that results in bleeding tendencies (e.g., thrombo-cytopenia)
Telangiectasia	Visibly dilated, superficial, cutaneous small blood vessels, commonly found on face and thighs	Aging, acne, sun exposure, alcohol use, liver failure, corticosteroids, radiation, certain systemic diseases, skin tumours
Tenting	Failure of skin to return immediately to normal position after gentle pinching	Aging, dehydration, cachexia
Varicosity	Increased prominence of superficial veins	Interruption of venous return (e.g., from tumour, incompetent valves, inflammation), commonly found on lower legs with aging
Vitiligo	Complete absence of melanin (pigment) resulting in chalky white patch (see Figure 25-9)	Autoimmune, heredity, thyroid disease

Skin moisture (level of dampness or dryness of the skin) increases in intertriginous areas and with high humidity. Skin moisture varies with environmental temperature, muscular activity, body weight, and body temperature. The skin should be intact with no flaking, scaling, or cracking. Skin generally becomes drier with increasing age. *Texture* refers to the fineness or coarseness of the skin. The skin should feel smooth and firm, with the surface evenly thin in most areas. Thickened callous areas are normal on the soles and palms and relate to weight bearing. Increased thickness is often work related and a result of excessive pressure. Excessive calluses on the soles of patients with neuropathy or diabetes predispose them to developing lesions. Common assessment abnormalities of the skin are described in Table 25-7.

Risk assessment to predict a patient's pressure injury risk should be done using a validated assessment tool such as the Braden Scale. (See Chapter 14, Table 14-14, for the Braden Scale for Predicting Pressure Sore Risk.)

A focused assessment is used to evaluate the status of previously identified integumentary problems and to monitor for signs of new problems. A focused assessment of the integumentary system is presented in the box on the following page.

Assessment of Dark Skin Colour

The structures of dark skin are no different than those of lighter skin, but they are often more difficult to assess (Table 25-8). Colour variation is easiest to assess in parts of the body where the epidermis is thin and pigmentation is not influenced by sun exposure, such as the lips, mucous membranes, nail beds, and protected areas such as the buttocks. As well, palmar and plantar surfaces are lighter than other skin areas.

FOCUSED ASSESSMENT
Integumentary System

This checklist can be used to make sure the key assessment steps have been done.

Subjective
The patient should be asked about any of the following and responses noted:

Hair loss (unusual or rapid)	Y	N
Changes in the skin (e.g., lesions, bruising)	Y	N
Nail discoloration	Y	N

Objective: Diagnostic
The following should be checked for results and critical values:

Biopsy results	✓
Albumin	✓

Objective: Physical Examination
The following should be inspected:

Skin for colour, integrity, scars, lesions, signs of breakdown	✓
Facial and body hair for distribution, colour, quantity, and hygiene	✓
Nails for shape, contour, colour, thickness, and cleanliness	✓
Dressings if present	✓
Palpation is used to determine the following:	
Skin for temperature, texture, moisture, thickness, turgor, and mobility	✓

FIGURE 25-8 Traction alopecia. Hair loss in scalp because of prolonged tension from hair roller, braiding, or straightening combs. Source: Hurwitz, S. (1993). *Clinical pediatric dermatology: A textbook of skin disorders of childhood and adolescence* (2nd ed.). Philadelphia: Saunders.

TABLE 25-8   ASSESSMENT VARIATIONS IN LIGHTER- AND DARKER-SKINNED INDIVIDUALS

Lighter Skin	Darker Skin
Cyanosis	
Greyish-blue tone, especially in nail beds, earlobes, lips, mucous membranes, and palms and soles of feet	Ashen or greyish colour most easily seen in the conjunctiva of the eye, mucous membranes, and nail beds
Ecchymosis	
Dark red, purple, yellow, or green colour, depending on age of bruise	Purple to brownish-black; difficult to see unless occurring in an area of light pigmentation
Erythema	
Reddish tone, possibly accompanied by increased skin temperature secondary to localized inflammation	Deeper brown or purple skin tone with evidence of increased skin temperature secondary to inflammation
Jaundice	
Yellowish colour of skin, sclera, fingernails, palms of hands, and oral mucosa	Yellowish-green colour most obviously seen in sclera of eye (do not confuse with yellow eye pigmentation, which may be evident in darker-skinned individuals), palms, and soles
Pallor	
Pale skin colour that may appear white or ashen; also evident on lips, nail beds, and mucous membranes	Underlying red tone in brown or black skin is absent, causing the skin to appear yellowish, ashen, or grey
Petechiae	
Lesions appear as small, reddish purple pinpoints, best observed on abdomen and buttocks	Difficult to see; may be evident in the buccal mucosa of the mouth or the conjunctiva of the eye
Rash	
May be visualized as well as felt with light palpation	Not easily visualized, but may be felt with light palpation
Scar	
Generally heals, showing narrow scar line	Higher incidence of keloid development, resulting in a thickened, raised scar (see Chapter 14, Figure 14-8)

FIGURE 25-9 Vitiligo. Total loss of pigment in the affected area. Source: Graham-Brown, R., Bourke, J., & Cunliffe, T. (2008). *Dermatology: Fundamentals of practice.* Edinburgh: Mosby.

Rashes are often difficult to observe in darker-skinned individuals and may need to be palpated (Jarvis, Browne, MacDonald-Jenkins, et al., 2014). Wrinkling also is less apparent among this population.

People with dark skin are predisposed to certain skin and hair conditions. *Keloid* is a protrusion of scar tissue that extends beyond the wound edges and may form tumour-like masses (e.g., ear piercing) (see Chapter 14, Figure 14-8). Vitiligo is total loss of pigment in the affected area (Figure 25-9). In *dermatosis papulosa nigra*, the person has small, pigmented wartlike papules, commonly on the face. *Nevus of Ota* is a slate-grey or blue-grey birthmark located on the forehead and face around the eye area. It may also involve the sclera (Figure 25-10). *Traction alopecia* may be the result of trauma from hair rollers or from tight braiding

FIGURE 25-10 Nevus of Ota. Flat grey to blue pigmentation in the upper trigeminal area, which is more common in darker-skinned individuals. Source: Gawkrodger, D., & Ardern-Jones, M. R. (2012). *Dermatology* (5th ed.). Edinburgh: Churchill Livingstone.

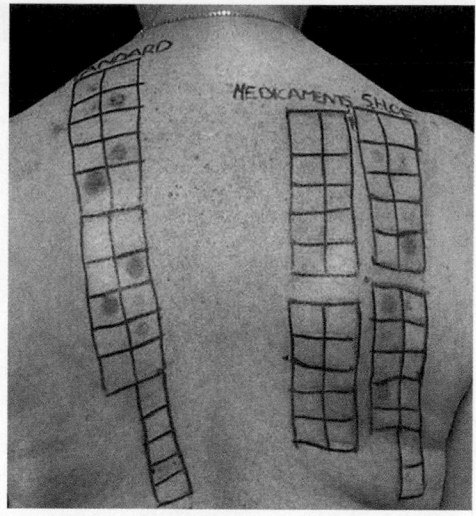

FIGURE 25-11 Patch test. Results from an application of possible allergens to the skin show positive reactions in the sites labelled "standard" and "shoe." Source: Graham-Brown, R., Bourke, J., & Cunliffe, T. (2008). *Dermatology: Fundamentals of practice.* Edinburgh: Mosby.

of the hair (see Figure 25-8). The hair loss may be temporary or permanent. *Pseudofolliculitis* is an inflammatory response to ingrown hairs that may occur after shaving, which results in pustules and papules.

In patients with darker skin, colour may not be a reliable indicator of systemic conditions (e.g., flushed skin with fever). Cyanosis may be difficult to determine because a normal bluish hue occurs in dark-skinned people. Dark skin rarely shows a blanch response, making it more difficult to identify pressure injuries.

DIAGNOSTIC STUDIES OF THE INTEGUMENTARY SYSTEM

Diagnostic studies provide the nurse important information for monitoring the patient's condition and planning appropriate interventions. These studies are considered to be objective data. Table 25-9 presents diagnostic studies common to the integumentary system.

The main diagnostic techniques related to skin problems are inspection of an individual lesion and the taking of a careful history related to the problem. If a definitive diagnosis cannot be made through these techniques, additional tests may be indicated such as dermatoscopy (examination of the skin through a lighted instrument with optical magnification) (Marchetti & Marghoob, 2014).

Biopsy is one of the most common diagnostic tests used in the evaluation of a skin lesion. A biopsy is indicated in all conditions in which a malignancy is suspected or a specific diagnosis is questionable. Techniques include punch, incisional, excisional, and shave biopsies. The method used is related to factors such as the site of the biopsy, the cosmetic result desired, and the type of tissue to be obtained.

Other diagnostic procedures used include stains and cultures for fungal, bacterial, and viral infections. *Direct immuno-fluorescence* is a technique used on skin biopsy specimens and may be indicated in certain conditions such as bullous diseases and systemic lupus erythematosus. In contrast, *indirect immuno-fluorescence* is performed on a blood sample. Patch testing (Figure 25-11) and photopatch testing may be used in the evaluation of allergic contact dermatitis and photoallergic reactions (Goldsmith, Katz, Gilchrest, et al., 2012).

CASE STUDY

Objective Data

Source: DGLimages/Shutterstock.com.

Physical Examination

Physical examination findings of Danielle Arquette's skin are as follows:

- Complexion fair. Wrinkles around eyes, above upper lip, and on sides of cheeks bilaterally. Normal skin temperature and turgor.
- Lesions on upper right forehead measuring 2 × 3 mm; on left forehead near hairline measuring 1 × 2 mm; and on left lower cheek measuring 2 × 2.5 mm.
- All lesions are slightly erythematous but do not blanch when direct pressure is applied. Borders distinct. Minimal elevation noted on palpation.
- No skin lesions noted on rest of body.

Throughout this chapter, consider which diagnostic studies would likely be performed for Ms. Arquette and also identify patient problems and the appropriate nursing interventions for her while she is in the clinic.

Diagnostic Studies

Ms. Arquette's primary care provider examines the lesions via dermatoscopy and also uses a Wood's lamp to rule out a fungal infection. She suspects basal cell carcinoma, which is confirmed by a shave biopsy.

See pp. 496 and 498 for more information on Ms. Arquette.

TABLE 25-9   DIAGNOSTIC STUDIES

Integumentary System

Study	Description and Purpose	Nursing Responsibility
Biopsy		
Punch	Special punch biopsy instrument of appropriate size is used. Instrument is rotated to appropriate level to include dermis and some fat. Suturing may or may not be done. Provides full-thickness skin for diagnostic purposes.	Verify that consent form is signed (if needed). Assist with preparation of site, anaesthesia, procedure, and hemostasis. Apply dressing, and give postprocedure instructions to patient. Properly identify specimen.
Excisional	Useful when good cosmetic results or entire removal or both are desired. Skin closed with subcutaneous and skin sutures.	Same as above.
Incisional	Wedge-shaped incision made in lesion too large for excisional biopsy. Useful when larger specimen than shave biopsy is needed.	Same as above.
Shave	Single-edged razor blade used to shave off superficial lesions or small sample of a large lesion. Provides thin specimen for diagnostic purposes.	Same as above.
Microscopic Tests		
Potassium hydroxide (KOH)	Hair, scales, or nails are examined for superficial fungal infection. Specimen is put on a glass slide, and potassium hydroxide solution of 10%–20% concentration added.	Instruct patient regarding purpose of test. Prepare slide.
Culture	The test identifies fungal, bacterial, and viral organisms. For *fungi*, scraping or swab of skin is performed. For *bacteria*, material is obtained from intact pustules, bullae, or abscesses. For *viruses*, vesicle or bulla is scraped and exudate taken from base of lesion.	Instruct patient regarding purpose and procedure. Properly identify specimen. Follow instructions for storage of specimen if not immediately sent to laboratory.
Mineral oil slides	The test checks for infestations. Scrapings are placed on slide with mineral oil and viewed microscopically.	Instruct patient about purpose of test. Prepare slide.
Immuno-fluorescent studies	Some cutaneous diseases have specific, abnormal antibody proteins that can be identified by fluorescent studies. Both skin and serum can be examined.	Inform patient about purpose of test. Assist in obtaining specimen. For punch biopsy of tissue, place specimen in special fixative (e.g., Michel's), and not formalin.
Miscellaneous		
Wood's lamp (black light)	Examination of skin with long-wave ultraviolet light causes specific substances to fluoresce (e.g., *Pseudomonas* organisms, fungal infections, vitiligo).	Explain purpose of examination and that it is not painful. Room is darkened for examination.
Patch test	Used to determine whether patient is allergic to specific testing material. Small amount of potentially allergenic material is applied, usually to skin on back.	Explain purpose and procedure to patient. Instruct patient to return in 48–72 hr for removal of allergens and evaluation. Inform patient if re-evaluation is needed at 96 hr (see Figure 25-11).

REVIEW QUESTIONS

The number of the question corresponds to the same-numbered objective at the beginning of the chapter.

1. What is the primary function of the skin?
   a. Insulation
   b. Protection
   c. Sensation
   d. Absorption

2. Which of the following are age-related changes in the hair and nails? (*Select all that apply*)
   a. Oily scalp
   b. Scaly scalp
   c. Thinner nails
   d. Thicker, brittle nails
   e. Longitudinal nail ridging

3. When assessing self-care habits in relation to the skin, what does the nurse question the client about?
   a. Joint pain
   b. Use of sunscreen products
   c. Recent changes in exercise tolerance
   d. Family history of melanoma

4. During the physical examination of a client's skin, which of the following would the nurse do?
   a. Use a flashlight if the room is poorly lit.
   b. Note cool, moist skin as a normal finding.
   c. Pinch up a fold of skin to assess for turgor.
   d. Perform a lesion-specific examination first and then a general inspection.

5. The nurse assessed the client's skin lesions as firm, edematous, and irregularly shaped with variable diameter. What would these lesions be called?
   a. Wheals
   b. Papules
   c. Pustules
   d. Plaques

6. What is the *most* appropriate technique for the nurse to use in assessing the skin for temperature and moisture?
   a. Palpation
   b. Inspection
   c. Percussion
   d. Auscultation

7. On inspection of the client's skin, the nurse notes the complete absence of melanin pigment in patchy areas on the client's hands. What is this assessment finding called?
   a. Vitiligo
   b. Nevus of Ota
   c. Telangiectasia
   d. Lichenification

8. Individuals with dark skin are more likely to develop which of the following?
   a. Keloids
   b. Wrinkles
   c. Rashes
   d. Skin cancer

9. Under what circumstance is diagnostic testing recommended for skin lesions?
   a. When a health history cannot be obtained
   b. When a more definitive diagnosis is needed
   c. When percussion reveals an abnormal finding
   d. When treatment with prescribed medication has failed

1. b; 2. b, d, e; 3. b; 4. c; 5. a; 6. a; 7. a; 8. a; 9. b

⊖volve

For even more review questions, visit *http://evolve.elsevier.com/Canada/Lewis/medsurg*.

REFERENCES

Canadian Dermatology Association (CDA). (2015a). *Photoaging.* Retrieved from *http://www.dermatology.ca/skin-hair-nails/skin/photoaging/#!/skin-hair-nails/skin/photoaging/what-is-photoaging/*.

Canadian Dermatology Association (CDA). (2015b). *Skin cancer.* Retrieved from *http://www.dermatology.ca/skin-hair-nails/skin/skin-cancer/#!/skin-hair-nails/skin/skin-cancer/malignant-melanoma/*.

Goldsmith, L., Katz, S., Gilchrest, B., et al. (2012). *Fitzpatrick's dermatology in general medicine* (8th ed.). New York: McGraw-Hill.

Han, A., Chien, A., & Kang, S. (2014). Photoaging. *Dermatologic Clinics, 32,* 291–299.

Jarvis, C., Browne, A., MacDonald-Jenkins, J., et al. (2014). *Physical examination and health assessment* (2nd Canadian ed.). Toronto: Elsevier.

Marchetti, M., & Marghoob, A. (2014). Dermoscopy. *Canadian Medical Association Journal, 186*(15), 1167. doi:10.1503/cmaj.140008.

Marks, J., & Miller, J. (2013). *Principles of dermatology* (5th ed.). St Louis: Mosby.

Patton, K. T., & Thibodeau, G. A. (2013). *Anatomy and physiology* (8th ed.). St. Louis: Mosby.

Woodford, C., & Yao, C. (Eds.). (2013). *Toronto notes 2013: Comprehensive medical reference and review* (29th ed.). Toronto: Toronto Notes for Medical Students, Inc.

For additional Internet resources, see Chapter 26 and the website for this book at *http://evolve.elsevier.com/Canada/Lewis/medsurg*.

WEBSITE

http://evolve.elsevier.com/Canada/Lewis/medsurg

- Review Questions (Online Only)
- Key Points
- Answer Guidelines for Case Study
- Customizable Nursing Care Plan
  - Chronic Skin Lesions
- Conceptual Care Map Creator
- Audio Glossary
- Content Updates

LEARNING OBJECTIVES

1. Specify health-promotion practices related to the integumentary system.
2. Explain the etiology, clinical manifestations, and nursing and collaborative management of common acute dermatological problems.
3. Explain the etiology, clinical manifestations, and collaborative management of malignant dermatological disorders.
4. Explain the etiology, clinical manifestations, and collaborative management of bacterial, viral, and fungal infections of the integument.
5. Explain the etiology, clinical manifestations, and collaborative management of infestations and insect bites.
6. Explain the etiology, clinical manifestations, and collaborative management of allergic dermatological disorders.
7. Explain the etiology, clinical manifestations, and collaborative management care related to benign dermatological disorders.
8. Summarize the psychological and physiological effects of chronic dermatological conditions.
9. Explain the indications and nursing management related to common cosmetic procedures and skin grafts.

KEY TERMS

acne vulgaris, p. 519,
  Table 26-11
actinic keratosis, p. 510
basal cell carcinoma (BCC), p. 510
cellulitis, p. 514, Table 26-6

cryosurgery, p. 522
curettage, p. 522
dysplastic nevi (DNs), p. 513
herpes zoster, p. 515,
  Table 26-7

impetigo, p. 514, Table 26-6
lichenification, p. 524
malignant melanoma,
  p. 511
psoriasis, p. 517

squamous cell carcinoma
  (SCC), p. 510
sun protection factor (SPF),
  p. 507
urticaria, p. 518, Table 26-10

HEALTH PROMOTION

Health-promotion practices related to the skin often parallel practices appropriate for general good health. The skin reflects both physical and psychological well-being. Specific health-promotion activities appropriate to good skin health include avoidance of environmental hazards; adequate rest, hygiene, and nutrition; and skin self-examination.

Environmental Hazards

Sun Exposure. Years of exposure to the sun cause cumulative skin damage. The ultraviolet (UV) rays of the sun cause degenerative changes in the dermis, resulting in premature aging (e.g., loss of elasticity, thinning, wrinkling, and drying of the skin). Prolonged and repeated sun exposure is a major factor in precancerous and cancerous lesions (Health Canada, 2013). Actinic keratoses, basal cell carcinoma (BCC), squamous cell carcinoma (SCC), and malignant melanoma are dermatological problems associated directly or indirectly with sun exposure. The earth's ozone layer, which protects the world's creatures from excessive exposure to UV radiation, continues to thin because of environmental pollutants, leading to increased risk for sun damage and skin cancer.

It is important for the nurse to emphasize safe sun practices to patients. Specific wavelengths of the sun (Table 26-1) have different effects on the skin. Sunlight is composed of visible light and UV light; UV light may be further divided into UVA and UVB. Both types can damage the skin and increase the risk for skin cancer. When sun exposure is excessive, the turnover time of the skin is shortened and results in peeling. Individuals

TABLE 26-1	WAVELENGTHS OF THE SUN AND EFFECTS ON SKIN
Wavelength	**Effect**
Long (UVA)	• Causes elastic tissue damage and actinic skin damage
	• Is responsible for tanning due to increased melanin production
	• Contributes to formation of skin cancer
Middle (UVB)	• Is responsible for sunburn
	• Is a major factor in development of skin cancer
Short (UVC)	• Does not reach earth; is blocked by atmosphere

UVA, ultraviolet A light; *UVB,* ultraviolet B light; *UVC,* ultraviolet C light.

TABLE 26-2	SUNSCREEN INGREDIENTS AND ULTRAVIOLET LIGHT PROTECTION	
Sunscreen Ingredients		**Ultraviolet Light Protection**
Chemical		
Benzophenones		UVA and UVB
PABA and PABA esters		UVB
(Removed from many sunscreen products because of clothing staining and allergic reactions, including contact dermatitis)		
Cinnamates		UVB
Salicylates		UVB
Miscellaneous		
Methyl anthranilate		UVB
Parsol (Avobenzone)		UVA
Physical Sunscreens		
Titanium dioxide		UVA and UVB
Zinc oxide		UVA and UVB

PABA, para-aminobenzoic acid; *UVA,* long wavelength of ultraviolet light; *UVB,* middle wavelength of ultraviolet light.

with fair skin should be especially cautious about excessive sun exposure because they have less melanin and, thus, less natural protection.

Nurses play an important role in educating patients on sun-safety strategies including sun avoidance, protective clothing, and sunscreen. The greatest risk of damaging sun exposure is between the hours of 10:00 a.m. and 4:00 p.m., so avoiding the sun or using protection is paramount during these hours (Health Canada, 2014). Even on overcast days, serious sunburn can occur, because up to 80% of UV rays can penetrate the clouds. Other factors that increase sunburn risk include being at high altitudes, where atmospheric protection from UV rays is decreased, being in snow, and being in or near water, as water and snow reflect a significant portion of the sun's rays back toward the skin. The UV index is a scale used by Environment Canada to communicate the risk for harmful UV exposure; it is regularly included in local weather forecasts and is available online. At an index of 3 (moderate) or higher, Health Canada (2014) recommends using sun-protective measures.

Eye protection is important to consider when spending time in the sun, as UV rays can potentially cause retinal damage and may be a contributing factor in cataract development. The nurse should advise patients to use sunglasses with UVA and UVB protection, particularly when the UV index is 3 or above (Government of Canada [GOC], 2012a).

Sun-protective measures for the skin include carrying an umbrella, wearing a large-brimmed hat and long-sleeved clothing, and applying sunscreen to exposed skin. Two types of sunscreens filter both UVA and UVB wavelengths: chemical and physical. Chemical sunscreens are light creams, lotions, or sprays that absorb or filter UV light, resulting in diminished UV light penetration. In contrast, physical sunscreens (e.g., titanium dioxide, zinc oxide) are thick, opaque, heavy creams that reflect UV radiation, blocking all UVA and UVB radiation. Sunscreen products are rated according to their **sun protection factor (SPF)** (GOC, 2012b). SPF measures the effectiveness of a sunscreen in filtering and absorbing UVB radiation. "Broad-spectrum" products offer protection against UVA radiation as well (GOC, 2012b) (Table 26-2).

In general, a sunscreen with a minimum SPF of 15 should be used daily (GOC, 2012b). Sunscreens with an SPF of 15 or more filter 92% of the UVB responsible for erythema and make sunburn unlikely in most individuals when applied appropriately. The Canadian Dermatology Association (CDA, 2017a) recommends a broad-spectrum sunscreen with an SPF of 30 or higher to prevent premature aging of the skin and skin cancer, particularly for outdoor workers, athletes, and spectators. Sunscreen should

be applied 20 to 30 minutes before going outside. It must be reapplied after swimming or profusely sweating to maintain good sun protection even if the product is "waterproof." Sunscreens with physical filters such as zinc oxide or titanium dioxide that scatter and reflect both UVA and UVB rays are recommended for prominent parts like the nose, cheeks, shoulders, and ears (GOC, 2012b). Tanning booths and sun lamps are still commonly used to artificially tan skin, despite well-known associated risks including photoaging (premature aging of the skin due to UV exposure) and skin cancers. Indoor tanning increases a person's risk of developing melanoma by 75% if used before the age of 35 and increases the risk of developing other skin malignancies such as SCC and BCC (GOC, 2012c). Indoor tanning especially increases cancer risk for individuals who are younger than 18 years of age, have fair or freckled skin, burn easily, have lots of moles, have had previous skin cancer or a family history of skin cancer, or use medication that increases sensitivity to UV (CDA, 2017b). Sunless tanning creams are cosmetic creams absorbed by the epidermis only to give the appearance of tan (GOC, 2012d). In 2000, the CDA published a position statement that self-tanning products are safe. However, it is important to note that these products provide *no* sun protection and must be used in conjunction with appropriate SPF products and sun-avoidance strategies.

Certain topical and systemic medications potentiate the effect of the sun, even with brief exposure. Categories of drug therapy that may contain common photosensitizing medications are listed in Table 26-3. Many drugs are included in these categories, and the photosensitivity of each individual drug should be examined. The chemicals in these medications absorb light and release energy that harms cells and tissues. The clinical manifestations of drug-induced photosensitivity (Figure 26-1) are similar to those of exaggerated sunburn. These include swelling, erythema, vesicles, and papular, plaquelike lesions. Skin that is at risk for photosensitivity reactions can be protected by the use of sunscreen products. Educating patients about photosensitizing effects of their medications is an important nursing role.

EVIDENCE-INFORMED PRACTICE
Research Highlight

Is Sun-Protective Counselling Effective?
Clinical Question
In adults (P) does sun-protective counselling (I) improve safe sun behaviours (O)?

Best Available Evidence
Systematic review of randomized controlled trials (RCTs)

Critical Appraisal and Synthesis of Evidence
- Five RCTs (*n* = 6949) of middle-aged white men and women and three RCTs (*n* = 897) of young adults examined the effect of counselling on sun-protective behaviours. Trials ranged from one to several sessions of in-person counselling, phone counselling, or tailored written feedback according to risk.
- Counselling with tailored feedback influenced sun-protective behaviours in older adults.
- Appearance-focused counselling reduced indoor tanning use among young women.

Conclusion
- Relevant counselling by primary health care providers can increase sun-protective behaviours and decrease indoor tanning.

Implications for Nursing Practice
- Promote safe sun behaviours for patients to decrease ultraviolet exposure, including sunscreen use, sun-avoidance hours, and protective clothing.
- Emphasize the dangers of tanning booth use among college students.
- Tailor sun-safety interventions to the target population.

Reference for Evidence
Lin, J., Eder, M., & Weinmann, S. (2011). Behavioral counseling to prevent skin cancer: A systematic review for the U.S. Preventive Services Task Force. *Annals of Internal Medicine, 154*(3), 190–201. doi:10.7326/0003-4819-154-3-201102010-00009.

P, Patient population of interest; *I,* intervention or area of interest; *O,* outcomes of interest (see Chapter 1).

EVIDENCE-INFORMED PRACTICE
Translating Research Into Practice

A nurse is helping in a skin cancer screening clinic. Sara Walters, a 24-year-old woman with a fair skin type (blond hair and blue eyes), is completing her health history before her screening examination. She indicates that she visits an indoor tanning salon every other week because being tan makes her feel "more attractive." The nurse spends time explaining the increased risk for skin cancer associated with the use of tanning booths.

Best Available Evidence	Clinician Expertise	Patient Preferences and Values
Canadian Dermatology Association and International Agency for Cancer Research report a strong link between exposure to indoor tanning devices and development of skin cancer and melanoma.	The nurse notes that Ms. Walters has the following skin cancer risk factors: fair skin, blond hair, blue eyes, frequent use of tanning booths.	After listening, the patient tells the nurse that she will consider reducing the frequency of her visits—going only when she has an important event to attend.

Decision and Action
The nurse accepts Ms. Walters's decision, tells her that this is a step in the right direction, and encourages her to consider completely stopping her use of the tanning booth.

References for Evidence
Canadian Dermatology Association (2016). *Indoor tanning.* Retrieved from *http://www.dermatology.ca/programs-resources/programs/sap/indoor-tanning.*
Government of Canada (2012). *Tanning beds and lamps.* Retrieved from *http://www.healthycanadians.gc.ca/healthy-living-vie-saine/environment-environnement/sun-soleil/bed_lamps-lits_lampes-eng.php.*

TABLE 26-3   DRUG THERAPY
Categories of Drugs That May Cause Photosensitivity

Categories	Examples
Anticancer drugs	Methotrexate (Metoject), vinorelbine
Antidepressants	Amitriptyline (Elavil), clomipramine (Anafranil), doxepin (Silenor)
Antidysrhythmics	Quinidine, amiodarone
Antifungals	Ketoconazole (Ketoderm, Nizoral)
Antihistamines	Diphenhydramine (Benadryl), chlorpheniramine (Chlor-Tripolon)
Antimicrobials	Tetracycline, sulfamethoxazole-trimethoprim (Septra), azithromycin (Zithromax), ciprofloxacin (Cipro)
Antipsychotics	Chlorpromazine, haloperidol
Diuretics	Furosemide (Lasix), hydrochlorothiazide
Hypoglycemics	Tolbutamide, chlorpropamide
Nonsteroidal anti-inflammatory drugs	Diclofenac (Arthrotec, Voltaren), piroxicam, sulindac (Apo-Sulin)

FIGURE 26-1 Intense eruption in areas exposed to sunlight after patient started on hydrochlorothiazide. Source: Habif, T. P. (2016). *Clinical dermatology: A color guide to diagnosis and therapy* (6th ed., p. 454). St. Louis: Mosby.

Cold Exposure. Excessive or prolonged exposure to cold can cause damage to the skin and underlying tissue, or frostbite. Assessment and management of frostbite are discussed further in Chapter 71.

Irritants and Allergens. Patients may seek treatment for irritant or allergic dermatitis, which are two types of contact dermatitis. *Irritant contact dermatitis* is produced by direct chemical injury to the skin. *Allergic contact dermatitis* is an antigen-specific, type IV delayed hypersensitivity response. This response requires sensitization and occurs only in individuals who are predisposed to react to a particular antigen (see Chapter 16).

The nurse should counsel patients to avoid known irritants (e.g., ammonia, harsh detergents). Skin patch testing (application of allergens) can sometimes be helpful in determining the most likely sensitizing agent. Sometimes the health care provider is the first to detect a contact allergy to various metals, gloves (latex), and adhesives. The nurse must also be aware that pre-scribed and over-the-counter (OTC) topical and systemic drugs used to treat a variety of conditions may contain fragrances and preservatives that cause dermatological reactions. Health Canada (2016) maintains a database (called MedEffect) of suspected adverse reactions, including dermatological problems, to Canadian-marketed health products. Consumers and health care providers may report suspected reactions online, by phone, or by mail.

Radiation. Although most radiology departments are extremely cautious in protecting both themselves and their patients from the effects of excessive radiation, the nurse should support the patient in making informed decisions by ensuring the patient understands the benefits and risks of proposed radiological procedures. Discussing the purpose of the procedure, common adverse effects, and rare adverse effects can assist patients in their decision and increase patient engagement in the plan of care. Radiographic studies are invaluable in both diagnosis and therapy, but they can cause serious adverse effects to the skin, including erythema, dry and moist desquamation, edema, and changes in pigmentation.

Rest and Sleep

Sleep is restorative to the skin. Pruritic skin diseases often interfere with sleep. Helping patients obtain high-quality sleep is an important health-promotion consideration. Adequate rest increases the patient's ability to tolerate itching, thereby decreasing skin damage from scratching.

Exercise

Exercise has numerous psychological and physiological benefits, including dilation of the blood vessels and improved perfusion of the dermis. However, caution must be used to avoid or protect from overexposure to heat, cold, and sun during outdoor exercise.

Hygiene

The patient's skin type, lifestyle, culture, age, and gender influence hygiene practices. The normal acidity of the skin and perspiration protect against bacterial overgrowth. Most soaps are alkaline and neutralize the skin surface, leading to loss of protection. Using mild, moisturizing soaps or "nonsoap" lipid-free cleansers, and avoiding hot water and vigorous scrubbing can noticeably decrease local skin irritation. Skin piercings where jewellery has been inserted can be cared for with antibacterial soaps that do not contain sulfites.

In general, the skin and hair should be washed often enough to remove excess oil and excretions and to prevent odour. Older people should avoid the use of harsh, heavily scented soaps and shampoos (such as Dial or Irish Spring) because of the increasing dryness of their skin and scalp; unscented products marketed "for sensitive skin" are generally preferable. Cold weather and indoor heating systems further contribute to dry and pruritic skin conditions, particularly during winter months. Patients should be advised that applying moisturizers immediately after bathing while the skin is still damp helps seal in moisture.

Nutrition

A well-balanced diet adequate in all food groups can produce healthy skin, hair, and nails (see *Canada's Food Guide* in Chapter 42). Important elements of skin nutrition appear in Table 26-4.

Obesity has an adverse effect on the skin. The increase in subcutaneous fat can lead to stretching and overheating. Over-heating secondary to the greater insulation provided by fat causes an increase in sweating, which inflames and dries the skin. Obesity is a risk factor for poor wound healing and type 2 diabetes mellitus. Increased skin folds contribute to skin problems. Skin in these intertriginous (skin on skin) areas is predisposed to skin tags *(acrochordons),* candidiasis (yeast), intertrigo (bacteria, fungi, yeast), and erythrasma (bacteria) infections.

Self-Treatment

Self-diagnosis and treatment of skin problems can be dangerous; and the wide variety of OTC skin preparations, confusing.

In general, the nurse should stress the duration of the treatment and the need to follow package directions closely. Skin problems may be slow to produce symptoms and slow to resolve. If the

TABLE 26-4 NUTRITIONAL THERAPY

Nutrients Essential for Healthy Skin, Hair, and Nails

Nutrient	Supportive Function	Impact of Nutrient Deficiency
Vitamin A	• Maintenance of normal epithelial cell structure • Wound healing	• Conjunctival dryness • Poor wound healing
Vitamin B complex (niacin, pyroxidine, biotin)	• Complex metabolic functions	• Erythema/rashes • Bullae • Seborrhea-like lesions • Alopecia

Vitamin C (ascorbic acid)	• Connective tissue formation
	• Wound healing
		• Symptoms of scurvy (severe deficiency):
		  • Petechiae
		  • Bleeding gums
		  • Purpura

Vitamin D3 (cholecalciferol)	• Bone health • Produced in skin cells after UVB exposure	• Decreased bone mineral density • Muscle weakness and pain
Vitamin K	• Blood clotting cascade	• Decreased prothrombin synthesis • Easy bruising
Protein	• Cell growth and maintenance • Wound healing	• Poor wound healing • Dry, flaky skin • Brittle nails and hair
Unsaturated fatty acids (e.g., linoleic acid, arachidonic acid)	• Integrity of cellular and subcellular membranes	• Decreased tissue metabolism

package insert of an OTC drug says its use should not exceed 7 days, patients should heed this warning. If any systemic signs of inflammation or extension of the skin problem (e.g., an increased number of lesions or increased erythema or swelling) develop, self-care should be stopped and the patient should seek the help of a health care provider.

MALIGNANT SKIN NEOPLASMS

Skin cancer is the most common cancer diagnosed in Canada and worldwide, with incidence in Canada steadily increasing since the early 1980s (GOC, 2015). Skin cancers are either nonmelanoma or melanoma. The fact that skin lesions are so visible increases the likelihood of early detection and diagnosis; a marked majority of cancerous skin lesions are first detected by patients or their family members (CDA, 2017c).

Teach patients to self-examine their skin at least monthly. The cornerstone of the skin self-examination is the "ABCDE rule." Examine skin lesions for **a**symmetry, **b**order irregularity, **c**olour change or variation, **d**iameter of 6 mm or more, and an **e**volving appearance (Figure 26-2). The nurse should emphasize to patients that persistent skin lesions that do not heal, lesions once flat and now raised, or lesions once small and recently growing or changing in appearance are warning signs. These should be examined by a health care provider. Skin malignancies generally grow slowly, and early detection and treatment often leads to a highly favourable prognosis.

RISK FACTORS

Risk factors for skin malignancies include having fair skin, blond or red hair, light eye colour, history of chronic sun exposure, family or personal history of skin cancer, outdoor occupations, frequent outdoor recreational activities, indoor tanning, and smoking (Canadian Cancer Society, 2015). Patients treated with photochemotherapy, which is called *PUVA* and is a combination of oral methoxsalen (**p**soralen) and **UVA** radiation, may be at greater risk for melanoma. Individuals with darker skin are less susceptible to skin cancer because of naturally occurring increased melanin, an effective sunscreen. Melanoma may still occur in

these patients, however, most often on the palms, the soles, and the mucous membranes.

NONMELANOMA SKIN CANCERS

Nonmelanoma skin cancers (basal cell and squamous cell carcinomas) are the most common forms of skin cancer, with a projected 78 000 diagnoses in Canada in 2015 alone (GOC, 2015). Nonmelanoma skin cancers do not develop from melanocytes. They develop in the basement membrane of the skin. Although there are few deaths from nonmelanoma skin cancers, they have the potential for severe local destruction, permanent disfigurement, and disability.

Nonmelanoma skin cancers usually develop in sun-exposed areas, such as the face, head, neck, back of the hands, and arms, and are more common in patients over age 50. The most common causative factor is sun exposure. There are some differences between basal and squamous cell cancers. SCCs usually occur on the head and neck, where there is the highest degree of UV radiation. BCCs do not follow that pattern and may occur in sun-protected areas.

Actinic Keratosis

Actinic keratosis, also known as *solar keratosis,* consists of hyperkeratotic papules and plaques occurring on sun-exposed areas. Actinic keratoses are premalignant skin lesions that affect nearly all older individuals with light skin. They are the most common precancerous skin lesion. The clinical appearance of actinic keratoses can be highly varied. The typical lesion is an irregularly shaped, flat, slightly erythematous papule with indistinct borders and an overlying hard keratotic scale or horn (Table 26-5). Because actinic keratosis is impossible to differentiate from squamous cell carcinoma, treatment should be aggressive. Nonsurgical procedures are the first-line treatment (see Table 26-5). Any lesion that persists should be evaluated for a possible biopsy.

Basal Cell Carcinoma

Basal cell carcinoma (BCC) is a locally invasive malignancy arising from epidermal basal cells. It is the most common type of skin cancer but the least deadly. BCC usually occurs in middle-aged to older adults. It commonly develops at the site of earlier trauma, such as scarring, thermal burns, and injuries (Habif, 2011).

Clinical manifestations are described in Table 26-5. Some BCCs are pigmented, with curled borders and an opaque appearance. They may be hard to distinguish from melanoma. A tissue biopsy is needed to confirm the diagnosis. BCCs rarely metastasize (Figure 26-3). However, if BCC is left untreated, massive tissue destruction may result.

Treatment depends on the tumour location and histological type, history of recurrence, and patient characteristics (see Table 26-5). Location and size are important factors in determining the best treatment.

Squamous Cell Carcinoma

Squamous cell carcinoma (SCC) is a malignant neoplasm of keratinizing epidermal cells. It frequently occurs on sun-exposed skin. While less common than BCC, SCC can be aggressive, has the potential to metastasize, and may lead to death if not treated early and correctly. Pipe, cigar, or cigarette smoking contributes to the formation of SCC on the mouth and lips. Immuno-suppression leads to a dramatic increase in the incidence of SCC.

FIGURE 26-2 The ABCDEs of melanoma. **A,** Asymmetry: one half is unlike the other half. **B,** Border irregularity: edges are ragged, notched, or blurred. **C,** Colour: varied pigmentation; shades of tan, brown, and black. **D,** Diameter: greater than 6 mm (diameter of a pencil eraser). **E,** Evolving; changing appearance (not pictured; change in shape, size, colour, or other characteristic is noted over a length of time). Source: The Skin Cancer Foundation, New York, NY.

TABLE 26-5   PREMALIGNANT AND MALIGNANT CONDITIONS OF THE SKIN

Etiology and Pathophysiology	Clinical Manifestations	Treatment and Prognosis
Actinic Keratosis Actinic (sun) damage. Premalignant skin lesion, precursor of squamous cell carcinoma.	Flat or elevated, dry, hyperkeratotic scaly papule; felt more than seen. Adherent rough scale on red base, which returns when removed. Often multiple. Often on erythematous sun-exposed areas; increase in number with age.	Cryosurgery, chemical caustics, topical application of 5-FU over entire area for 14–28 days or topical application of imiquimod (Aldara) over ≥16 wk. Photodynamic or later therapies. Recurrence possible even with adequate treatment.
Dysplastic Nevi Morphologically between common acquired nevi and melanoma. May be precursor of cutaneous malignant melanoma.	Often >5 mm; irregular border, possibly notched. Variegated colour of tan, brown, black, red, or pink with single mole. Presence of at least one flat portion, often at edge of mole. Frequently multiple. Most common site is the back, but possible in uncommon mole sites such as scalp or buttocks.	Increased risk for melanoma. Careful monitoring of people suspected of familial tendency to melanoma or dysplastic nevi. Excisional biopsy for suspicious lesions.
Basal Cell Carcinoma Change in basal cells. No maturation or normal keratinization. Continuing division of basal cells and formation of enlarging mass. Related to excessive sun exposure, genetic skin type, radiographic radiation, scars, and some types of nevi.	*Nodular and ulcerative:* Small, slowly enlarging papule. Borders semitranslucent or "pearly," with overlying telangiectasia. Erosion, ulceration, and depression of centre. Normal skin markings lost (see Figure 26-3). *Superficial:* Erythematous, pearly, sharply defined, barely elevated multinodular plaques; similar to eczema but nonpruritic.	Excisional surgery, chemosurgery, electrosurgery, Mohs (microscopically controlled) surgery, cryosurgery; 90% cure rate; slow-growing tumour that invades local tissue; metastasis rare; 5-FU and imiquimod (Aldara) for superficial lesions.
Squamous Cell Carcinoma Frequent occurrence on previously damaged skin (e.g., from sun, radiation, scar). Malignant tumour of squamous cell of epidermis. Invasion of dermis, surrounding skin.	*Superficial:* Thin, scaly, erythematous plaque without invasion into the dermis. *Early:* Firm nodules with indistinct borders, scaling, and ulceration. *Late:* Covering of lesion with scale or horn from keratinization. Most common on sun-exposed areas such as face and hands.	Surgical excision, cryosurgery, radiation therapy, chemotherapy, Mohs surgery, or electrodessication and curettage. Untreated lesion may metastasize to regional lymph nodes. High cure rate with early detection and treatment.
Cutaneous T-Cell Lymphoma (Mycosis Fungoides) Origination in skin. Localized, chronic, slowly progressing disease. Possible etiologies of environmental toxins and chemical exposure.	Classic presentation involving three stages—patch (early), plaque, and tumour (advanced). History of persistent macular eruption followed by gradual appearance of indurated erythematous plaques on the trunk that appear similar to psoriasis. Pruritus, lymphadenopathy.	Treatment usually controls symptoms, not curative. UVB, PUVA, corticosteroids, topical nitrogen mustard, radiation therapy, systemic chemotherapy, extracorporeal photopheresis. Disease course is unpredictable; 10% will have progressive disease.
Malignant Melanoma Neoplastic growth of melanocytes anywhere on skin, eyes, or mucous membranes. Classification according to major histological mode of spread. Potential invasion and widespread metastases.	Irregular colour, surface, and border. Varying colour including red, white, blue, black, grey, and brown. Flat or elevated. Eroded or ulcerated. Often <1 cm in size. Most common sites are back, chest, and legs.	Wide surgical excision and possible sentinel lymph node evaluation depending on depth. Correlation of survival rate with depth of invasion. Poor prognosis unless diagnosis and treatment early. Spreading by local extension, regional lymphatic vessels, and bloodstream. Adjuvant therapy after surgery may be indicated if lesion >1.5 mm in depth.

5-FU, 5-fluorouracil; *PUVA,* psoralen plus ultraviolet A light (phototherapy); *UVB,* ultraviolet B light.

Manifestations and treatment of SCC are described in Table 26-5. A biopsy should always be performed when a lesion is suspected to be SCC. There is a high cure rate with early detection and treatment.

MALIGNANT MELANOMA

Malignant melanoma is a tumour arising in melanocytes, the cells producing melanin. Melanoma causes the majority of skin cancer deaths. Estimates in 2016 were that nearly 6 800 new cases would be diagnosed in Canada in that calendar year, and over 1 200 Canadians would die from the disease (Canadian Cancer Society's Advisory Committee on Cancer Statistics, 2016). Since 2001, the incidence of Canadians diagnosed with melanoma has risen steadily at 2% to 3% per year. Melanoma can occur in the eyes, ears, gastro-intestinal tract, leptomeninges, and oral and genital mucous membranes. When it begins in the skin, it is called *cutaneous melanoma*. Melanoma has the ability to metastasize to any organ, including the brain and heart.

FIGURE 26-3 Basal cell carcinoma. Note rolled border and central erosion. Pearly papule with slight erythema. Source: Swartz, M. H. (2010). *Textbook of physical diagnosis: History and examination* (6th ed., p. 159). Philadelphia: Saunders.

DETERMINANTS OF HEALTH

Melanoma

Biology and Genetic Endowment
- There are genetic links associated with the development of melanoma (e.g., xeroderma pigmentosum, Werner syndrome).
- There is an increased risk if a first-degree relative has been diagnosed with melanoma.

Personal Health Practices and Coping Skills
- Individuals who have had more than one blister sunburn in youth have a higher risk of developing melanoma, a risk that increases with each successive sunburn.
- Radiation exposure (i.e., environmental or occupational) increases an individual's risk for developing melanoma.

Gender
- Melanoma is more common in men than in women.

Source: Canadian Cancer Society. (2016). *Risk factors for melanoma.* Retrieved from *http://www.cancer.ca/en/cancer-information/cancer-type/skin-melanoma/risks/?region=on#possible.*

Although the exact cause of melanoma is unknown, a combination of environmental and genetic factors is involved. Excessive exposure to UV radiation from the sun plays a leading role in the development of melanomas, but artificial sources of UV radiation, such as sun lamps and tanning booths, also play a role. UV radiation damages the deoxyribonucleic acid (DNA) in skin cells, causing mutations in their genetic code and altering the cells. Although anyone can develop melanoma, the risk is greatest for people who have red or blond hair, blue or light-coloured eyes, and light-coloured skin that freckles easily. These individuals have less melanin and thus less protection from UV radiation. The use of immuno-suppressive drugs and a history of dysplastic nevi also increase a person's risk.

Additionally, a person may have a genetic predisposition toward getting melanoma. Between 5% and 10% of people with melanoma have a first-degree relative (e.g., parent, full sibling) who had melanoma. This risk increases significantly if multiple relatives have a history of melanoma. Mutated genes have been identified in some families who have a high familial incidence of melanoma. Furthermore, having multiple and atypical moles, particularly atypical dysplastic nevi, increases individual risk for melanoma (CDA, 2017c). Other factors that affect a person's likelihood for developing melanoma are listed in the "Determinants of Health" box.

Clinical Manifestations

About 25% of melanomas occur in existing nevi or moles; about 20% occur in dysplastic nevi (see Table 26-5). Melanomas frequently occur on the lower legs and on the back in women and on the trunk, the head, and the neck in men. Because most melanoma cells continue to produce melanin, melanoma tumours are often dark brown or black. Individuals should consult their health care provider immediately if their moles or lesions show any of the clinical signs (ABCDEs) of melanoma (see Figure 26-2). Any sudden or progressive increase in the size, the colour, or the shape of a mole should be evaluated.

Collaborative Care

One of the initial steps in correctly diagnosing a suspicious lesion is dermoscopic examination. Dermatoscopes use magnification to see patterns and structures not visible with the naked eye and can assist the health care provider in determining if a lesion

FIGURE 26-4 Breslow measurement of tumour thickness. **A,** Thin (0.08-mm) superficial spreading melanoma, good prognosis. **B,** Thick nodular melanoma with lymph node involvement, poor prognosis. Source: Gawkrodger, D., & Ardern-Jones, M. R. (2012). *Dermatology* (5th ed.). Edinburgh: Churchill Livingstone.

without the obvious ABCDE signs should be biopsied. Biopsy is a critical tool for identifying a lesion. All suspicious lesions should be biopsied using an excisional biopsy technique. They should not be shave-biopsied, shave-excised, or electrocauterized. These techniques fail to provide an accurate measurement of depth.

The most important prognostic factor is tumour thickness at the time of the diagnosis. Two methods to determine thickness are currently being used. The *Breslow measurement* indicates tumour depth in millimetres (Figure 26-4), and the *Clark level* indicates the number of skin layers involved (one to five); the higher the number, the deeper the melanoma.

Treatment depends on the site of the original tumour, stage of the cancer, and the patient's age and general health. The staging of melanoma (stages 0–4) is based on tumour size, nodal involvement, and presence of metastasis. In stage 0, the melanoma is confined to one place (in situ) in the epidermis. Melanoma is nearly 100% curable by excision if diagnosed at stage 0. The 5-year survival rate depends on the sentinel node biopsy results, which indicate whether metastasis has occurred. If spread to regional lymph nodes has occurred (stage 3), the patient has a 61.7% chance of 5-year survival (Howlader, Noone, Krapcho, et al., 2015). If metastasis to other organs occurs (stage 4), treatment then is palliative.

The initial treatment of malignant melanoma is wide surgical excision. Melanoma that has spread to the lymph nodes or nearby sites usually requires additional (adjuvant) therapy such as chemotherapy, immunotherapy, targeted therapy, radiation therapy, or a combination of therapies. Examples of chemotherapeutic drugs that are used include dacarbazine and temozolomide. These may be given alone or in combination with other drugs, such as cisplatin, carmustine, carboplatin, or vincristine, to improve the response rate.

Immunotherapy can include cytokines (interferon alfa, interleukin-2), programmed cell death protein 1 (PD-1) inhibitors, or cytotoxic T-lymphocyte antigen 4 (CTLA-4) inhibitors. PD-1 inhibitors include nivolumab (Opdivo) and pembrolizumab (Keytruda). These drugs block PD-1, a protein on T cells that normally keeps these cells from attacking other cells in the body. By blocking PD-1, these drugs boost the immune response against melanoma cells. Ipilimumab (Yervoy), a CTLA-4 inhibitor, also boosts the immune system, but it has a different target. It blocks CTLA-4, a protein that normally helps keep T cells in check. By blocking the action of CTLA-4, ipilimumab boosts the immune response against melanoma cells (Kim, Trinh, & Hwu, 2014).

Targeted therapy for melanoma includes BRAF and MEK inhibitors. About half of all melanomas have mutations in the *BRAF* gene, which makes an altered BRAF protein that signals melanoma cells to proliferate. Vemurafenib (Zelboraf) and dabrafenib (Tafinlar) are BRAF-inhibitor drugs that attack the BRAF protein directly. The *MEK* gene is involved in the activation of the BRAF pathway. Therefore, a MEK-inhibitor drug, trametinib (Mekinist), can be used to treat melanomas with *BRAF* gene changes.

Atypical/Dysplastic Nevus

An abnormal nevus pattern called *dysplastic nevus syndrome* places a person at increased risk for melanoma. Approximately 2% to 8% of the white population has moles classified as **dysplastic nevi (DNs)**. DNs, or atypical moles, are moles that are larger than usual (>5 mm across) and have irregular borders and various shades of colour. These nevi may have the same ABCDE characteristics as melanoma, but they are less pronounced. The earliest clinically detectable abnormality associated with DNs is an increase in the number of morphologically normal-looking nevi that occur in children between 2 and 6 years of age. Another proliferation occurs around adolescence, and new nevi continue to appear throughout the person's life. The average number of normal nevi in adults is about 40; individuals with DNs may have over 100 normal-appearing nevi. The nurse should obtain a detailed family history related to melanoma and DNs. The risk of developing melanoma doubles with the presence of one DN, and having multiple DNs increases the risk up to twelve-fold.

FIGURE 26-5 Impetigo. Superficial pustules covered by a thick, honey-coloured crust. Source: Habif, T. P. (2016). *Clinical dermatology: A color guide to diagnosis and therapy* (6th ed., p. 329). St. Louis: Mosby.

FIGURE 26-6 Cellulitis with characteristic erythema, tenderness, and edema. Source: Habif, T. P. (2011). *Clinical dermatology: A color guide to diagnosis and therapy* (5th ed., p. 274). St. Louis: Mosby.

SKIN INFECTIONS AND INFESTATIONS

Bacterial Infections

The skin provides an ideal environment for bacteria growth because of its abundant supply of nutrients and water and its warm temperature; it is home to numerous microorganisms, including bacteria. Bacterial infection occurs when the balance between the host and the microorganisms is altered. Infection can be primary, following a break in the skin, or it can be secondary, appearing in already damaged skin or as a sign of a systemic disease. *Staphylococcus aureus* and group A β-hemolytic streptococci are the major types of bacteria responsible for primary and secondary skin infections, including impetigo (Figure 26-5), erysipelas, cellulitis (Figure 26-6), lymphangitis, and furuncles (Table 26-6).

Healthy people can develop bacterial skin infections. Predisposing factors such as moisture, obesity, atopic dermatitis, systemic corticosteroids and antibiotics, and chronic disease such as diabetes mellitus all increase the likelihood of infection. Good hygiene practices and general good health inhibit bacterial infections. If an infection is present, the resulting drainage is infectious. Good skin hygiene and infection-control practices are necessary to prevent the spread of infection.

TABLE 26-6 COMMON BACTERIAL INFECTIONS OF THE SKIN

Etiology and Pathophysiology	Clinical Manifestations	Treatment and Prognosis
Impetigo Group A β-hemolytic streptococci, staphylococci, or combination of both. Associated with poor hygiene. Primary or secondary infection. Contagious.	Vesiculo-pustular lesions that develop a thick, honey-coloured crust surrounded by erythema. Pruritic. Most common on face as primary infection (Figure 26-5).	**Systemic Antibiotics** Oral penicillin, benzathine penicillin G by IM route, erythromycin. **Local Treatment** Warm saline or aluminum acetate soaks followed by soap-and-water removal of crusts. Topical antibiotic cream or ointment (mupirocin [Bactroban], fusidic acid [Fucidin]). Meticulous hygiene essential. With no treatment, glomerulonephritis is possible when streptococcal strain is nephritogenic.
Folliculitis Usually staphylococci; present in areas subjected to friction, moisture, oiliness, or shaving. Increased incidence in patients with diabetes mellitus.	Small pustule at hair follicle opening with minimal erythema. Development of crusting; most common on scalp, beard, extremities in men. Tender to touch.	Warm compresses of water or aluminum acetate solution. Antistaphylococcal soap (e.g., Hibiclens, Lever 2000, Dial) and water cleansing. Topical antibiotics (e.g., mupirocin [Bactroban], fusidic acid [Fucidin]). Heals usually without scarring. If lesions are extensive and deep, with possible scarring and loss of involved hair follicles, treatment with systemic antibiotics is necessary.
Furuncle Deep infection with staphylococci around hair follicle, often associated with severe acne or seborrheic dermatitis.	Tender erythematous area around hair follicle. Draining pus and core of necrotic debris on rupture. Most common on face, back of neck, axillae, breasts, buttocks, perineum, thighs. Painful.	Incision and drainage, possibly with packing. Antibiotics. Meticulous care of involved skin including frequent application of warm, moist compresses.
Furunculosis Increased incidence in patients with obesity, diabetes, chronic illness, or those regularly exposed to moisture or pressure.	Lesions as above. Malaise, regional adenopathy, fever.	Incision and drainage of painful nodules. Warm, moist compresses. Systemic antibiotic after culture and sensitivity study of drainage (usually semisynthetic, penicillinase-resistant oral penicillin such as cloxacillin. Measures to reduce surface staphylococci include antimicrobial cream to nares, armpits, and groin and antiseptic to entire skin. Often recurrent with scarring. Prevention or correction of predisposing factors. Meticulous personal hygiene.
Carbuncle Multiple, interconnecting furuncles.	Many pustules appearing in erythematous area, most commonly at nape of neck.	Treatment same as for furuncles. Often recurrent despite production of antibodies. Slow healing with scar formation.
Cellulitis Inflammation of subcutaneous tissues; possibly secondary complication or primary infection. Often following break in skin. *Staphylococcus aureus* and streptococci usual causative agents. Deep inflammation of subcutaneous tissue from enzymes produced by bacteria.	Hot, tender, erythematous, and edematous area with diffuse borders (Figure 26-6). Chills, malaise, and fever.	Moist heat, immobilization and elevation, systemic antibiotic therapy, hospitalization if severe. Progression to gangrene possible if untreated.
Erysipelas Superficial cellulitis primarily involving the dermis. Group A β-hemolytic streptococci.	Red, hot, sharply demarcated plaque that is indurated and painful. Bacteremia possible. Most common on face and extremities. Toxic signs, such as fever, ↑ WBC count, headache, malaise.	Systemic antibiotics, usually penicillin. Hospitalization often required.

IM, intramuscular; *WBC,* white blood cell.

Viral Infections

Similar to viral infections elsewhere in the body, viral infections of the skin are difficult to treat. When a virus infects a cell, a skin lesion may develop. Lesions can also result from an inflammatory response to the viral infections. Herpes simplex (Figure 26-7), herpes zoster (see Chapter 25, Figure 25-6), and warts (Figure 26-8) are the most common viral infections affecting the skin (Table 26-7).

Fungal Infections

Because of the large number of identified fungi, it is almost impossible to avoid exposure to some pathological varieties. However, some fungi, including candidiasis and tinea unguium (Figure 26-9), can cause infections of the skin, hair, and nails. Common fungal infections of the skin are presented in Table 26-8. Most infections are relatively harmless in healthy adults, but they can be embarrassing and distressing to the patient.

Microscopic examination of the scraping of suspicious skin lesions in 10% to 20% potassium hydroxide (KOH) is an easy, inexpensive diagnostic measure to determine the presence of fungus. The appearance of hyphae (threadlike structures) is indicative of a fungal infection.

FIGURE 26-7 Herpes viral infection on the lips. Typical presentation with vesicles on the lips and extending onto the skin. Source: Habif, T. P. (1996). *Clinical dermatology: A color guide to diagnosis and therapy* (3rd ed.). St. Louis: Mosby.

TABLE 26-7 COMMON VIRAL INFECTIONS OF THE SKIN

Etiology and Pathophysiology	Clinical Manifestations	Treatment and Prognosis
Herpes Simplex Virus (HSV) Types 1 and 2		
Oral or genital HSV infections can be serotyped as either HSV-1 or HSV-2; both are recurrent, lifelong viral infections. Exacerbated by sunlight, trauma, menses, stress, and systemic infection. Contagious to those not previously infected. Transmission by respiratory droplets or virus-containing fluid (e.g., saliva, cervical secretions). Infection in one area readily transmitted to another area by contact.	***First Episode*** Symptoms occurring 3–7 days or more after contact. Painful local reaction. Single or grouped vesicles on erythematous base. Systemic symptoms (e.g., fever, malaise) possible or asymptomatic presentation possible (see Figure 26-7). ***Recurrent Episodes*** Typically milder and shorter; recur in similar spot; characteristic grouped vesicles on erythematous base.	Soothing, moist compresses; petroleum jelly to lesions. Usually not scarring. Antiviral agents (e.g., acyclovir [Zovirax], famciclovir [Famvir], and valacyclovir [Valtrex]) depending on location, frequency of outbreaks.
Herpes Zoster (Shingles)		
Activation of the varicella-zoster virus. Incidence increases with age and in immuno-suppressed patients. Potentially contagious to anyone who has not had varicella.	Linear distribution along dermatome of grouped vesicles on erythematous base. Usually unilateral on trunk, face, and lumbosacral areas. Burning, pain, and neuralgia preceding outbreak. Mild to severe pain during outbreak (see Chapter 25, Figure 25-6).	Symptomatic. Antiviral agents (e.g., acyclovir [Zovirax], famciclovir [Famvir], and valacyclovir [Valtrex]) effective for prevention of postherpetic neuralgia (PHN) if given within 72 hours of lesion appearance. Wet compresses, silver sulfadiazine (Flamazine) to ruptured vesicles. Analgesia. Gabapentin (Neurontin) to treat PHN. Usually heals without complications, but scarring and PHN possible. Vaccine (Zostavax II) to reduce risk for shingles and PHN is available for adults 60 years or older who previously had chicken pox.
Verruca Vulgaris		
Caused by human papilloma virus (HPV). Spontaneous disappearance in 1–2 yr possible. Mildly contagious by autoinoculation. Specific response dependent on body part affected. Prevalence greater in youth and immuno-suppressed.	Circumscribed, hypertrophic, flesh-coloured papule limited to epidermis. Painful on lateral compression.	Multiple treatments, including surgery: blunt dissection with scissors or curette, liquid nitrogen therapy keratolytic agents (e.g., cantharidin/salicylic acid [Cantharone Plus]), podophyllin (Podofilm), CO₂ laser destruction. Possibility of scarring.
Plantar Warts		
Caused by human papilloma virus (HPV).	Wart on bottom surface of foot, growing inward because of pressure of walking or standing. Painful when pressure applied. Interrupted skin markings. Cone-shaped with black dots (thrombosed vessels) when wart removed (Figure 26-8).	Topical immunotherapy (imiquimod [Vyloma]), cryotherapy, salicylic acid, duct tape.

Infestations and Insect Bites

The possibilities for exposure to infestations (harbouring insects or worms) and insect bites are numerous (Table 26-9). In many instances, an allergy to the venom plays a major role in the reaction. In other cases, the clinical manifestations are a reaction to eggs, feces, or body parts of the invading organism. Some individuals react with a severe hypersensitivity (anaphylaxis), which can be life-threatening. (Anaphylaxis is discussed in Chapter 16).

Prevention of insect bites by avoidance or by the use of repellents is somewhat effective. Meticulous hygiene related to personal articles, clothing, bedding, and examination and care of pets, as well as careful selection of sexual partners, can reduce the incidence of infestations. Routine inspection is necessary in geographical areas where there is a risk of tick bites and Lyme disease.

FIGURE 26-9 Tinea unguium (onychomycosis). Fungal infection of toenails. Crumbly, discoloured, and thickened nails. Source: Gawkrodger, D., & Ardern-Jones, M. R. (2012). *Dermatology: An illustrated colour text* (5th ed.). Edinburgh: Churchill Livingstone.

FIGURE 26-8 Plantar wart. **A,** Keratotic lesion. **B,** After excision. Source: Swartz, M. H. (2010). *Textbook of physical diagnosis: History and examination* (6th ed.). Philadelphia: Saunders.

TABLE 26-8 COMMON FUNGAL INFECTIONS OF THE SKIN AND THE MUCOUS MEMBRANES

Etiology and Pathophysiology	Clinical Manifestations	Treatment and Prognosis
Candidiasis Caused by *Candida albicans*; also known as *moniliasis*. 50% of adults are symptom-free carriers. Appears in warm, moist areas such as groin area, oral mucosa, and submammary folds. HIV infection, chemotherapy, radiation, and organ transplantation related to depression of cell-mediated immunity that allows yeast to become pathogenic.	**Mouth:** White, cheesy plaque, resembles milk curds. **Vagina:** Vaginitis, with red, edematous, painful vaginal wall, white patches, vaginal discharge, pruritus, and/or pain on urination and intercourse. **Skin:** Diffuse papular erythematous rash with pinpoint satellite lesions around edges of affected area.	Microscopic examination and culture. Azole antifungals (e.g., fluconazole [Canesoral, Diflucan], ketoconazole [Ketoderm, Nizoral]) or other specific medication, such as vaginal suppository or oral mouthwash. Abstinence from intercourse or use of condom. Skin hygiene to keep area clean and dry. Powder effective on nonmucosal skin surfaces to prevent reinfection.
Tinea Corporis Various dermatophytes, commonly referred to as *ringworm*.	Typical annular (ringlike), scaly appearance; well-defined margins. Erythematous.	Cool compresses. Topical antifungals for isolated patches (e.g., miconazole [Monistat], clotrimazole [Canasten], ketoconazole [Ketoderm, Nizoral]).
Tinea Cruris Various dermatophytes, commonly referred to as *jock itch*.	Well-defined, scaly plaques in groin area. Does not affect mucous membranes.	Topical antifungal cream or solution.
Tinea Pedis Various dermatophytes, commonly referred to as *athlete's foot*.	Interdigital scaling and maceration. Scaly plantar surfaces sometimes with erythema and blistering. May be pruritic. Less commonly painful.	Topical antifungal cream, gel, solution, spray, or powder (e.g., tolnaftate [Tinactin], clotrimazole [Canasten]).
Tinea Unguium (Onychomycosis) Various dermatophytes. Incidence increases with age.	Toenails more commonly affected than fingernails. Scaliness under distal nail plate. Brittle, thickened, broken, or crumbling nails with yellowish discoloration (see Figure 26-9).	Oral antifungal (terbinafine [Lamisil], itraconazole [Sporanox]). Topical antifungals (e.g., ciclopirox [Penlac], efinaconazole [Jublia]) minimally effective but an option if unable to tolerate system drug. Thinning of toenails if needed. Nail avulsion (removal) is an option.

HIV, human immunodeficiency virus.

TABLE 26-9 COMMON INFESTATIONS AND INSECT BITES

Etiology and Pathophysiology	Clinical Manifestations	Treatment and Prognosis
Bees and Wasps *Hymenoptera* species.	Intense, burning, local pain. Swelling and itching. Severe hypersensitivity, possibly leading to anaphylaxis.	Cool compresses. Local application of antipruritic lotion. Antihistamines if indicated. Usually uneventful recovery.
Bedbugs *Cimicidae* species. Usually feed at night. Present in furniture, clothing, walls during day.	Wheal surrounded by vivid flare. Firm urticaria transforming into persistent lesion. Severe pruritus. Often grouped in threes appearing on noncovered parts of body.	Bedbug controlled by chlorocyclohexane. Lesions usually requiring no treatment. Severe itching possibly necessitating use of antihistamines or topical corticosteroids.
Pediculosis (Head Lice, Body Lice, Pubic Lice) *Pediculus humanus*, var. *capitis*; *Pediculus humanus*, var. *corporis*; *Phthirus pubis*. Obligate parasites that suck blood, leave excrement and eggs on skin, live in seams of clothing (if body lice) and in hair as nits. Transmission of pubic lice often by sexual contact.	Minute, red, noninflammatory. Points flush with skin. Progression to papular wheal-like lesions. Pruritus with secondary excoriation, especially parallel linear excoriations in intrascapular region. Firmly attached to hair shaft in head and body lice.	Pyrethrins (R&C Shampoo), permethrin 1% (Nix Crème Rinse), isopropyl myristate/cyclomethicone (Resultz) to treat various parts of body. Apply as directed. Screen and treat all possible close contacts: bed partners, playmates. Do not share head gear.
Scabies *Sarcoptes scabiei*. Mite penetrates stratum corneum, deposits eggs. Allergic reaction resulting from presence of eggs, feces, mite parts. Transmission by direct physical contact, only occasionally by shared personal items. Rarely seen in dark-skinned people.	Severe itching, especially at night, usually not on face. Presence of burrows, especially in interdigital webs, flexor surface of wrists, genitalia, and anterior axillary folds. Erythematous papules (may be crusted), possible vesiculation, interdigital web crusting.	5% permethrin topical lotion, one overnight application with second application 1 wk later, may yield 95% eradication. Treat all cohabitants and sexual partners. Treat environment with plastic covering for 5 days, launder all clothes and linen with bleach. Antibiotics if secondary infections present. Residual pruritus possible up to 4 weeks after treatment. Recurrence possible if inadequately treated.
Ticks *Borrelia burgdorferi* (spirochete transmitted by ticks in certain areas) causes Lyme disease. Distribution shifts yearly, but generally endemic in Nova Scotia, southern and eastern Ontario, southeast Manitoba, and southern British Columbia, with isolated occurrences in the southern part of the provinces bordering the United States.	Spreading, ringlike rash 3–4 wk after bite. Rash commonly in groin, buttocks, axillae, trunk, and upper arms and legs. May be warm, itchy, or painful. Flulike symptoms. Cardiac, arthritic, and neurological manifestations possible. Unreliable laboratory test. No acquired immunity.	Oral antibiotics such as doxycycline or tetracycline. Intravenous antibiotics for arthritic, neurological, and cardiac symptoms. Rest and healthy diet. Most patients recover (see discussion of Lyme disease in Chapter 67).

ALLERGIC DERMATOLOGICAL PROBLEMS

Dermatological problems associated with allergies and hypersensitivity reactions may present a challenge to the clinician (Table 26-10). The pathophysiology related to allergic and contact dermatitis is discussed in Chapter 16. A careful family history and discussion of exposure to possible offending agents can provide valuable data. Patch testing involves the application of allergens to the patient's skin (usually on the back) for 48 hours and evaluation of the test sites for signs of reaction; this is useful in determining possible causative agents. The best treatment of allergic dermatitis is avoidance of the causative agent. The extreme pruritus of contact dermatitis and its potential for chronicity make it a frustrating problem for clinicians and patients, especially if the offending agent cannot be identified.

BENIGN DERMATOLOGICAL PROBLEMS

The list of benign dermatoses is extensive; nonetheless, some of the most commonly seen and distressing problems include psoriasis, acne vulgaris, and seborrheic keratoses. Benign problems are summarized in Table 26-11.

Psoriasis is a common inherited benign disorder that is characterized by the eruption of reddish, silver-scaled maculopapules, predominantly on the elbows, knees, scalp, and trunk. It currently affects 1 million people in Canada (CDA, 2017d) and usually develops in individuals between 15 and 35 years old. One-third of people with psoriasis have at least one relative with the disease. Diagnosis is often based on the skin's appearance (Figure 26-10). Lesions merge to form plaques. The affected area is normally rounded, with adherent silver scales that bleed easily when removed.

While most people with psoriasis have mild disease, many with severe disease often have a weakened immune system, diabetes mellitus, depression, and cardiovascular disease. Psoriatic arthritis affects 10% to 30% of all people with psoriasis (CDA, 2017d). (Psoriatic arthritis is discussed in Chapter 67.) The chronicity of psoriasis can be severe and disabling. People withdraw from social contacts because of visible lesions, and quality of life can diminish.

TABLE 26-10   COMMON ALLERGIC CONDITIONS OF THE SKIN

Etiology and Pathophysiology	Clinical Manifestations	Treatment and Prognosis
Allergic Contact Dermatitis Manifestation of delayed hypersensitivity, absorbed agent acting as antigen, sensitization after one or more exposures, appearance of lesions 2–7 days after contact with allergen.	Red papules and plaques, sharply circumscribed with occasional vesicles. Usually pruritic. Area of dermatitis frequently takes shape of causative agent (e.g., metal allergy and bandlike dermatitis on ring finger).	Elimination of contact allergen. Topical or systemic corticosteroids. Antihistamines. Skin lubrication.
Urticaria Usually allergic phenomenon. Erythema and edema in upper dermis resulting from a local increase in permeability of capillaries (histamine response).	Spontaneously occurring, raised or irregularly shaped wheals. Varying size; usually multiple. May occur anywhere on the body.	Removal of triggering agent, if known. Oral antihistamine. Cool compresses. Systemic corticosteroids if severe.
Drug Reaction May be caused by any drug that acts as antigen and causes hypersensitivity reaction. Certain drugs (e.g., penicillin) more prone to reactions. Not all reactions are allergic; some are intolerance (e.g., gastric upset).	Rash of any morphology. Often red, macular and papular, semiconfluent, generalized rash with abrupt onset. Appearance as late as 14 days after cessation of drug. Possibly pruritic. Some reactions may be life-threatening, requiring immediate and intensive care.	Withdrawal of drug if possible. Antihistamines, topical or systemic corticosteroids may be necessary depending on severity of symptoms.
Atopic Dermatitis Exaggerated cutaneous response to environmental allergens. Genetically influenced, chronic, relapsing disease associated with immunological irregularity involving inflammatory mediators. Associated with allergic rhinitis and asthma. Most severe in childhood.	Multiple presentations include acute, subacute, and chronic stages. All are pruritic. Common in an antecubital and popliteal space in adults. Acute stage with bright erythema, oozing vesicles, with extreme pruritus. Subacute stage with scaly, light red to red-brown plaques. Chronic stage with thickened skin and accentuation of skin markings (lichenification), possible hypopigmentation or hyperpigmentation. Dry skin.	Lubrication of dry (xerotic) skin; restoration of skin barrier function. Topical immuno-modulators (pimecrolimus [Elidel], tacrolimus [Protopic]). Corticosteroids. Phototherapy for severe inflammation and pruritus. Reduction of stress reduces flares. Antibiotics for secondary infection as needed.

FIGURE 26-10 Psoriasis. Characteristic inflammation and scaling. Source: Habif, T. P. (2010). *Clinical dermatology. A color guide to diagnosis and therapy* (5th ed.). St Louis: Mosby.

DRUG ALERT—Isotretinoin (Accutane)
- Used to treat acne
- Can cause serious damage to fetus
- Contraindicated in women who are pregnant or want to become pregnant while on the drug
- Blood donation prohibited for those taking the drug and for 1 month after treatment ends
- Linked to liver function test abnormalities

COLLABORATIVE CARE: DERMATOLOGICAL PROBLEMS

Diagnostic Studies

A careful history is of prime importance in the diagnosis of skin problems. The health care provider must be skilled at detecting evidence that could reveal the cause of a large number of skin diseases and conditions. Individual lesions must be inspected as part of the physical examination. Thorough history, physical examination, and appropriate diagnostic tests guide therapy.

Collaborative Care

Many different treatment methods are used in dermatology. Advances in this field have brought relief to patients with previously chronic, untreatable conditions. Many therapies require specialized equipment and are usually reserved for use by a dermatologist.

Phototherapy. Ultraviolet light (UVL) of different wavelengths may be used to treat many dermatological conditions, including psoriasis, cutaneous T-cell lymphoma, atopic dermatitis, vitiligo, and pruritus. Light sources available include broadband UVB, narrowband UVB, and long-wave UV (UVA). One form of phototherapy involves the use of psoralen plus UVA light (PUVA). Psoralen is a photosensitizing drug given to patients for a prescribed amount of time before exposure to UVA.

Treatments are generally given two to four times a week. Adverse effects of oral psoralen include nausea and vomiting,

TABLE 26-11   COMMON BENIGN CONDITIONS OF THE SKIN

Etiology and Pathophysiology	Clinical Manifestations	Treatment and Prognosis
Acne Vulgaris Inflammatory disorder of sebaceous glands. More common in teenagers but possible development and persistence in adulthood. Flare can occur before menses, with use of corticosteroids, or with use of androgen-dominant oral contraceptives.	Noninflammatory lesions, including open comedones (blackheads) and closed comedones (whiteheads). Inflammatory lesions, including papules, pustules, and cysts. Most common on face, neck, and upper back. Nodular or inflammatory acne produces deeper lesions and can lead to significant scarring (see Figure 26-11).	Mechanical removal of multiple lesions with comedo extractor. Topical benzoyl peroxide or other antimicrobial. Topical retinoids. Systemic antibiotics if severe. Aim of treatment is to suppress new lesions and minimize scarring. Spontaneous remission possible. Use of isotretinoin (Accutane) for severe nodulocystic acne to possibly provide lasting remission (see "Drug Alert" box for contraindications). Pregnancy testing and monitoring of liver function, lipids, and depression essential.
Nevi (Moles) Grouping of normal cells derived from melanocyte-like precursor cells.	Hyperpigmented areas that vary in form and colour. Flat, slightly elevated, verrucoid, dome-shaped, sessile, or papillomatous. Preservation of normal skin markings. Hair growth possible.	No treatment necessary except for cosmetic reasons. Skin biopsy for suspicious or changing nevi.
Psoriasis Autoimmune chronic dermatitis, which involves excessively rapid turnover of epidermal cells. Genetic predisposition. Usually develops before age 40.	Sharply demarcated, silvery, scaling plaques on the scalp, elbows, knees, palms, soles, and fingernails. Itching, burning pain. Localized or general, intermittent or continuous. Symptoms vary from mild to severe (see Figure 26-10).	Goal is to reduce inflammation and suppress rapid turnover of epidermal cells. No cure, but control is possible. Topical treatments including corticosteroids, tar, anthralin, intralesional injection of corticosteroids for chronic plaques, sunlight, natural or artificial UVB, PUVA, UVA (alone or with topical or systematic potentiation [psoralen]) and clobetasol propionate 0.05% spray (Clobex). Systemic treatments include antimetabolites (e.g., methotrexate), immuno-suppressants (e.g., cyclosporin [Apo-Cyclosporine]), and biological therapies (e.g. adalimumab [Humira], etanercept [Enbrel], infliximab [Remicade], ustekinumab [Stelara]) for moderate to severe plaque form of disease.
Seborrheic Keratoses Benign growths. Exact etiology unknown. Increasing number with age; no association with sun exposure.	Irregularly round or oval, often verrucous, flat-topped papules or plaques. Well-defined shape, appearance of being "stuck on." Increase in pigmentation with time. Usually multiple and possibly itchy (Figure 26-12).	Removal by curettage or cryosurgery for cosmetic reasons or to eliminate source of irritation. Biopsy if unable to differentiate from melanoma.
Acrochordons (Skin Tags) Common after midlife. Appearance on neck, axillae, and upper trunk secondary to mechanical friction or redundant skin (correlated with obesity).	Small, skin-coloured, soft, pedunculated papules, irregularly round or oval. May become irritated.	Surgical removal for cosmetic reasons or to eliminate source of irritation only. Usually just "clipping off" without anaesthesia.
Lipoma Benign tumour of adipose tissue, often encapsulated. Most common in 40- to 60-yr-old age group.	Rubbery, compressible, round mass of adipose tissue. Single or multiple. Variable in size, possibly extremely large. Most common on trunk, back of neck, and forearms.	Usually no treatment; biopsy to differentiate from liposarcoma; excision only when indicated.
Vitiligo Unknown cause; genetically influenced, often precipitated by an event such as illness or a crisis. Most noticeable in dark-skinned people and those with a tan; complete absence of melanocytes. Noncontagious.	Focal amelanosis (complete loss of pigment). Macular. Wide variation in size and location. Usually symmetrical and may be permanent.	Topical steroids often successful in small areas. Attempts at repigmentation of larger areas with exposure to PUVA. Depigmentation of pigmented skin with extensive disease (>50% of body involved). Cosmetics and stains to conceal vitiliginous areas.
Lentigo Increased number of normal melanocytes in basal layer of epidermis related to sun exposure and aging. Also called *liver spots* or *age spots*.	Hyperpigmented, brown to black, flat macule or patch. Single or multiple. Typically on sun-exposed areas.	Evaluate carefully for progression. Treatment (only for cosmetic purposes) is liquid nitrogen or laser resurfacing. May recur. Biopsy if suspicious of melanoma.

PUVA, psoralen plus ultraviolet A light; *UVA,* ultraviolet A light; *UVB,* ultraviolet B light.

FIGURE 26-11 Acne vulgaris. Papules and pustules. Source: James, W. D., Berger, T., & Elston, D. (2011). *Andrews' diseases of the skin: Clinical dermatology* (11th ed.). Philadelphia: Saunders.

FIGURE 26-12 Seborrheic keratoses. Deeply pigmented, rough, and warty surface. Source: Callen, J. P., & Greer, K. E. (1993). *Color atlas of dermatology*. Philadelphia: Saunders.

TABLE 26-12	SKIN CONDITIONS TREATED BY LASER
• Acne scars	• Port wine stain
• Skin lesions	• Vascular lesions
• Hemangiomas	• Tattoos
• Spider veins or telangiectasias	• Rough or scarred skin
• Rosacea	• Psoriasis
• Pigmented nevi	• Wrinkles
• Hair removal	• Pigment discoloration in epidermis

sunburn, and persistent pruritus. Nurses should perform frequent skin assessments on all patients receiving phototherapy since erythema is an adverse effect of treatment. Topical corticosteroids may reduce painful erythema. Psoralen is used with extreme caution in patients with liver or renal disease because slower metabolism and excretion can lead to prolonged photosensitivity.

Prior to initiating phototherapy, the patient should understand the risks and benefits associated with UV exposure. Patients should be cautioned about the potential hazards of using photosensitizing chemicals and of further exposure to UV rays from sunlight or artificial UVL during therapy. Because the lens of the eye absorbs psoralen, patients receiving PUVA need prescription protective eyewear that blocks 100% of UVL to prevent cataract formation. Patients should be instructed to use the eyewear for 24 hours after taking the medication when outdoors or even when near a bright window because UVA penetrates glass. Ongoing monitoring is essential because of the immuno-suppressive effects of PUVA, including an increased risk of SCC, BCC, and melanoma.

Photodynamic therapy is a special type of phototherapy used to treat actinic keratosis and some malignant skin tumours. This therapy uses a photosensitizing agent in a different way than other phototherapy treatments. The patient receives the photosensitizing agent intravenously or topically, depending on the area being treated. Time is allowed for the drug to be absorbed by the target cells, and light is then applied to the area, causing the drug to react with oxygen. This starts a reaction that kills the cells (Rkein & Ozog, 2014).

Radiation Therapy. The use of radiation for the treatment of cutaneous malignancies varies greatly according to local practice and availability. Even if radiation therapy is planned, a biopsy must first be performed to obtain a pathological diagnosis. One of the advantages of radiation treatment is that it produces minimal damage to surrounding tissue, which is a prime consideration for such areas as the nose, eyelids, and canthal areas. It is a useful treatment for the older adult or the debilitated patient who cannot tolerate minor surgical procedures.

Radiation therapy usually requires multiple visits to a radiology department. It can produce permanent hair loss (*alopecia*) in the irradiated areas. Other adverse effects, depending on anatomical location and dose of radiation delivered, include telangiectasia, atrophy, hyperpigmentation, depigmentation, ulceration, hearing loss, ocular damage, atrophy, and mucositis. Careful shielding is necessary to prevent ocular lens damage if the irradiated area is around the eyes. (Radiation therapy is discussed in Chapter 18.)

Total-body skin irradiation (in which the body is bombarded with high-energy electrons) is one treatment for cutaneous T-cell lymphoma. Treatment follows a lengthy course. Patients experience varying degrees of hair loss and radiation dermatitis with transient loss of sweat gland function. This treatment causes premature aging of the skin.

Laser Technology. Laser treatment is an efficient surgical tool for many types of dermatological problems (Table 26-12). Lasers are able to produce measurable, repeatable, consistent zones of tissue damage. They can cut, coagulate, and vaporize tissue to some degree. The wavelength determines the type of delivery system used and the intensity of the energy delivered.

The surgical use of laser energy requires a focusing device to produce a small, high-density spot of energy. Several types of lasers are available. The CO_2 laser, the most common, has numerous applications as a vaporizing and cutting tool for most tissues. The argon laser emits light that is primarily absorbed by hemoglobin. It helps in the treatment of vascular and other pigmented lesions. Other, less common lasers include copper and gold vapours and neodymium: yttrium–aluminum–garnet (Nd:YAG). Written policies and procedures should cover laser safety and be reviewed by all personnel working with laser equipment.

Laser technology is increasingly being used for cosmetic treatments. The effectiveness of the treatment depends on a variety of factors, including choice of the correct laser equipment, training and skills of the laser operator, beam wavelength, power settings, duration of the energy pulse, and colour of the skin or hair. The patient must be informed about the risks of laser treatments, which include pain; reddened, bruised, and swollen skin; burns;

infection; and temporary scarring and discoloration if the wrong equipment or technique is used (CDA, 2017e).

Drug Therapy.

Antibiotics. Antibiotics are used both topically and systemically to treat dermatological problems, and they are often used in combination. If used, topical antibiotics should be applied lightly in a thin film to clean skin. Examples of common OTC topical antibiotics are polymyxin B sulphate–neomycin sulphate and bacitracin zinc (Polysporin). Prescription topical antibiotics include mupirocin (Bactroban; used for superficial *Staphylococcus* such as impetigo), gentamicin (used for *Staphylococcus* and most Gram-negative organisms), and erythromycin (used for Gram-positive cocci [staphylococci and streptococci] and Gram-negative cocci and bacilli). Topical erythromycin (e.g., erythromycin–benzoyl peroxide [Benzamycin]) and clindamycin (e.g., clindamycin phosphate–benzoyl peroxide [Clindoxyl, BenzaClin]) are used in combination with other agents for the treatment of acne vulgaris. Topical metronidazole (Metrogel) is used to treat rosacea and bacterial vaginosis.

If there are manifestations of systemic infection, a systemic antibiotic should be used. Systemic antibiotics are useful in the treatment of bacterial infections and acne vulgaris. The most frequently used are synthetic sulphur, penicillin, erythromycin (Eryc), minocycline, tetracycline, or doxycycline. These drugs are particularly useful for erysipelas, cellulitis, carbuncles, and severe, infected eczema. Culture and sensitivity of the lesion can guide the choice of antibiotic. Patients require drug-specific instructions on the proper technique of taking or applying antibiotics.

Corticosteroids. Corticosteroids are particularly effective in treating a wide variety of dermatological conditions and can be used topically, intralesionally, or systemically. Topical corticosteroids are used for their local anti-inflammatory action as well as for their antipruritic effects. Attempts to diagnose a lesion should be made before a corticosteroid preparation is applied because corticosteroids may alter the clinical manifestations. Once a sufficient amount of medication is dispensed, limits should be set on the duration and the frequency of application.

The potency of a particular preparation is related to the concentration of active drug in the preparation. With prolonged use, the more potent corticosteroid formulations can cause adrenal suppression, especially if a large surface area is covered and occlusive dressings are used. High-potency corticosteroids may produce adverse effects when their use is prolonged, including atrophy of the skin resulting from impaired cell mitosis and capillary fragility and susceptibility to bruising. In general, dermal and epidermal atrophy does not occur until a corticosteroid has been used for 2 to 3 weeks. If drug use is discontinued at the first sign of atrophy, recovery usually occurs in several weeks. Rosacea eruptions, severe exacerbations of acne vulgaris, and dermatophyte infections may also occur. Rebound dermatitis is not uncommon when therapy is stopped; this can be reduced by tapering the use of high-potency topical corticosteroids when the patient improves.

Low-potency corticosteroids such as hydrocortisone act more slowly but can be used for a longer period without producing serious adverse effects. Low-potency corticosteroids are safe to use on the face and intertriginous areas, such as the axillae and groin. The ointment form represents the most efficient delivery system. Creams and ointments should be applied in thin layers and slowly massaged into the site one to three times a day as prescribed. Accurate and adequate topical therapy is often the key to a successful outcome.

Intralesional corticosteroids are injected directly into or just beneath the lesion. This method provides a reservoir of medication with an effect lasting several weeks to months. Intralesional injection is commonly used in the treatment of psoriasis, alopecia areata (patchy hair loss), hypertrophic scars, and keloids. Triamcinolone acetonide (Kenalog) is the most common drug used for intralesional injection.

Systemic corticosteroids can have remarkable results in the treatment of dermatological conditions. However, they often have undesirable systemic effects (see Chapter 51). Corticosteroids can be administered as short-term therapy for acute conditions such as contact dermatitis caused by poison ivy. Long-term corticosteroid therapy for dermatological conditions is reserved for chronic bullous (blistering) disorders.

Antihistamines. Oral antihistamines are helpful in treating urticaria, angioedema, and pruritus that can occur with problems such as atopic dermatitis, contact dermatitis, and other allergic cutaneous reactions. Antihistamines compete with histamine for the receptor site, thus preventing its effects. Antihistamines may have anticholinergic or sedative effects or both. Several different antihistamines may have to be tried before the satisfactory therapeutic effect is achieved. Sedating antihistamines such as hydroxyzine (Atarax) and diphenhydramine (Benadryl) are often preferred for pruritus because the tranquilizing and sedative effects offer symptomatic relief. The patient should be warned about sedative effects, a particular problem when driving or operating heavy machinery. Antihistamines such as fexofenadine (Allegra), cetirizine (Reactine), and loratadine (Claritin) bind to peripheral histamine receptors, providing antihistamine action without sedation. These nonsedating antihistamines are generally not effective for controlling pruritus. Antihistamines should be used with caution in older adults because of their long half-life and their anticholinergic effects.

Topical Fluorouracil. Fluorouracil (5-FU) is a topical cytotoxic agent with selective toxicity for sun-damaged cells. It is used for the treatment of premalignant (especially actinic keratosis) and some malignant skin diseases. Because systemic absorption of the drug is minimal, systemic adverse effects are virtually nonexistent. Patient compliance can be a problem because 5-FU causes erythema and pruritus within 3 to 5 days and painful, eroded areas over the damaged skin within 1 to 3 weeks, depending on skin thickness of site. Treatment must continue with applications one to two times a day for 2 to 4 weeks. Healing may take up to 4 weeks after medication is stopped (Micali, Lacarrubba, Nasca, et al., 2014). Low-potency topical steroids are often prescribed and increase patient compliance with therapy. Because 5-FU is a photosensitizing drug, the patient must be educated to avoid sunlight during treatment. Patients should also be educated about the effect of the medication, including a warning that they will look worse before they look better. Adherence depends on thoroughness of the instruction, which should include a written handout. After effective treatment, treated skin is smooth and free of actinic keratosis. Recurrence in treated areas is possible and multiple courses of chemotherapy may be necessary over the years for individuals with severely sun-damaged skin.

Immuno-Modulators. Topical immuno-modulators, such as pimecrolimus (Elidel) and tacrolimus (Protopic), are used to treat atopic dermatitis. They work by suppressing an overreactive immune system. The adverse effects are minimal and may include a transient burning or feeling of heat at the application site. An increased risk of skin cancer and precancerous lesions may be associated with long-term use of these drugs. Another topical immuno-modulator, imiquimod (Aldara), acts to stimulate the production of interferon alfa and other cytokines to enhance cell-mediated immunity. It boosts the immune response only where applied and is safe for transplant patients. This medication is used for external genital warts, actinic keratoses, and superficial BCC. Most patients using this cream experience skin reactions including redness, swelling, blistering, excoriations, peeling, itching, and burning. Dosing varies depending on the type of lesion treated and the strength of medication prescribed (Micali, Lacarrubba, Nasca, et al., 2014).

Diagnostic and Surgical Therapy

Skin Scraping. Scraping is done with a scalpel blade to obtain a sample of surface cells (stratum corneum) for microscopic inspection and diagnosis. The most common tests of skin scrapings are potassium hydroxide (KOH) for fungus and mineral oil examination for scabies.

Electrodesiccation and Electrocoagulation. Electrical energy can be converted to heat by the tip of an electrode. This results in tissue being destroyed by burning. The major uses of this type of therapy are point coagulation of bleeding vessels to obtain hemostasis and destruction of small *telangiectasias* (dilation of groups of superficial capillaries and venules). *Electrodesiccation* uses a monopolar electrode and usually involves more superficial destruction. *Electrocoagulation* uses a dipolar electrode and has a deeper effect, with better hemostasis but an increased possibility of scarring. While minor electrosurgery on patients with a pacemaker poses minimal risk, both pacemakers and internal defibrillators can be affected by the electrical energy being used.

Curettage. Curettage is the removal and scooping away of tissue using an instrument with a circular cutting edge attached to a handle. Although the curette is not usually strong enough to cut normal skin, it is useful for scooping many types of small skin tumours and superficial lesions, such as warts, actinic keratoses, and small BCCs and SCCs. The area to be curetted is anaesthetized before the procedure. Hemostasis is obtained by use of one of several methods: electrocoagulation, ferric subsulphate (Monsel's solution), gelatin foam, aluminum chloride, or a gauze pressure dressing. Specimens are usually sent for biopsy. A small scar and hypopigmentation may form.

Punch Biopsy. Punch biopsy is a common dermatological procedure used to obtain a tissue sample for histological study or to remove small lesions. Its use is generally reserved for lesions smaller than 0.5 cm. Before local anaesthesia is used, the biopsy area is outlined so that landmarks will not be obscured by the anaesthetizing agent. The biopsy punch instrument cores out a small cylinder of skin when its sharp edge is twirled between the fingers (Figure 26-13). The core of skin is snipped from the subcutaneous fat and appropriately preserved for examination in a fixative solution. Hemostasis is achieved by using methods as used with curettage, but sites of 4 mm or larger are often closed with sutures.

Cryosurgery. Cryosurgery is the use of subfreezing temperatures to destroy epidermal lesions. Cryosurgery is a useful treatment for common benign, precancerous conditions including common and genital warts, cutaneous tags, thin seborrheic keratoses, lentigines, actinic keratoses, BCC, and SCC. Topical liquid nitrogen is the agent most commonly used for cryosurgery (Marks & Miller, 2013). The mechanism of injury involves direct cellular freezing as well as vascular stasis (stoppage or slowdown in the flow of blood), which develops after thawing. Intracellular

FIGURE 26-13 Punch biopsy. **A,** Removal of skin for diagnostic purposes. **B,** Specimen obtained. Source: Graham-Brown, R., Bourke, J., & Cunliffe, T. (2008). *Dermatology: Fundamentals of practice.* Edinburgh: Mosby.

ice formation causes the cell to rupture during thaw, leading to cell death and necrosis of the treated tissue.

Liquid nitrogen can be applied topically (directly onto the lesion) with a direct spray or cotton-tipped applicator. Patients usually feel a stinging cold sensation. The lesion will first become swollen and red, and it may blister. A scab forms and falls off in 1 to 3 weeks. The skin lesion is sloughed off along with the scab. Growth of new skin follows. The low temperature of the liquid nitrogen easily destroys melanocytes, leaving an area of hyperpigmentation resembling a scar. The size of the area to be treated may limit the use of cryotherapy. The major disadvantages of this treatment are lack of a tissue specimen for histological confirmation of cell type before destruction and potential for destruction of adjacent healthy tissue.

Excision. Excision is an option if the lesion involves the dermis. Complete closure of the excised area usually results in a good cosmetic outcome. One type of excision is *Mohs surgery* (Figure 26-14), which is a microscopically controlled removal of a cutaneous malignancy. In this procedure, the health care provider removes tissue sections in thin horizontal layers. All of the specimen's margins are examined to determine whether any malignant cells remain. Any residual tumour not removed by the first surgical excision is removed in serial excisions performed the same day. Benefits of Mohs surgery are preserving normal tissue, producing the smallest possible wound, and completely removing the cancer before surgical closure. Although this can become a lengthy procedure, it is done in an outpatient setting using local anaesthesia.

NURSING MANAGEMENT DERMATOLOGICAL PROBLEMS

AMBULATORY AND HOME CARE

Dermatological conditions are not usually a primary reason for hospitalization. Nevertheless, many hospitalized patients will

FIGURE 26-14 A, Removal of melanoma by Mohs surgery. **B,** Following plastic surgery using a skin flap to repair defect. Source: Courtesy Peter Bonner.

TABLE 26-13 DRUG THERAPY
Common Bases for Topical Medications

Agent	Therapeutic Considerations
Powder	Promotion of dryness. Lubrication of skin fold areas to prevent irritation. Increase in evaporation, absorbing of moisture possible. Common base for antifungal preparations. Patient must be protected from inhalation.
Lotion	Oil and water emulsions. Cooling and drying effect, with residual powder film after evaporation of water. Useful in subacute pruritic eruptions.
Cream	Oil and water emulsions. Most common base for topical medications. Affords lubrication and protection.
Ointment	Oil with differing amounts of water added in suspension. Lubrication and prevention of dehydration. Petrolatum most common.
Paste	Mixture of powder and ointment. Useful when drying effect necessary because moisture is absorbed.
Gel	Nongreasy combination of propylene glycol and water. May contain alcohol. Used for acute exudative inflammation (e.g., poison ivy contact dermatitis).

exhibit concurrent skin problems that warrant nursing intervention and patient education. Nursing interventions related to dermatological conditions fall into broad categories. They are applicable to many skin problems in both inpatient and outpatient settings. A nursing care plan for the patient with chronic skin lesions is available on the Evolve website.

WET DRESSINGS. For superficial skin problems that involve inflammation, itching, and infection, wet compresses (dressings) are commonly used. They are appropriate for damaged, oozing skin. Wet compresses are an excellent way to remove crusts and scabs that are adhering to the wound surface. Wet compresses provide comfort and treatment of conditions such as poison ivy, insect bites, and skin infections.

It is important to understand how to do a wet dressing correctly. Unless there is a concern about water quality, tap water at room temperature is the best choice. If drinkable water is not available, filtered, bottled, or sterile water may be used. Depending on the skin problem, additives may be used. Antibacterial solutions may contain aluminum acetate (Domeboro powder), silver nitrate, or acetic acid. Close attention to appropriate concentrations is critical when additives are used. Wet compresses should generally be tepid. However, when an anti-inflammatory effect is desired, the wet dressing should be cool.

The material for wet compresses should be four to eight layers thick and slightly larger than the area being treated. Gauze or any clean material (e.g., thin cotton sheeting, thermal underwear, tube socks) may be used. Ingenuity is sometimes required when covering odd-shaped body parts. Gauze sponges with fillers (abdominal pads) should be avoided for this purpose, because they will retain too much solution, and fibres can be left in the wound if the skin is open. Compress material is placed into fresh solution and excess liquid squeezed out. The goal is a *wet* compress—not simply damp and not dripping.

Wet compresses are applied continuously or intermittently. When used continuously, new solution should be used as needed but no additional solution added since doing so can alter the concentration and damage the skin. Depending on the desired effect, intermittent compresses are placed for 10 to 30 minutes two to four times a day, always using clean materials. Careful monitoring of the skin is important. If the skin appears *macerated* (softens and turns white), the dressings should be discontinued for 2 to 3 days. The patient should be protected from discomfort and chilling. A water-resistant pad will help protect the mattress, linens, and furniture.

BATHS. Baths are appropriate when large body areas need to be treated. They also have sedative and antipruritic effects. Some medications, such as oilated oatmeal (Aveeno) and sodium bicarbonate, can be added directly to the bath water. The tub should be filled enough to cover affected areas. Both the bath water and the prescribed solution should be at a lukewarm (tepid) temperature. The patient can soak for 15 to 20 minutes three or four times a day, depending on the severity of the dermatitis and the patient's discomfort. It is important to stress to the patient that the skin must not be rubbed dry with a towel but gently patted to prevent increasing irritation and inflammation. The addition of oils makes a bathtub extremely slippery and should be avoided. If oils *are* used in the tub, the utmost caution must be used in transferring patients to prevent accidents. Applying scent-free cream or emollients (moisturizer) or topical agents to the skin directly after the bath helps sustain the hydrating effect by helping to seal moisture into hydrated cells.

TOPICAL MEDICATIONS. Topical medications are commonly used to treat cutaneous problems. The effectiveness of topical therapy depends on which base the medication is prepared in. Table 26-13 summarizes the common agents used as bases for topical preparations and their therapeutic considerations. The base selected depends on the properties needed.

Creams are very versatile and most commonly prescribed. They are a mix of organic oils, water, and usually a preservative. Ointments are primarily organic oils with little or no water. Many are preservative free. They are more lubricating than creams and offer enhanced potency of the active ingredient. They may be too occlusive for conditions with high levels of exudate or in body creases. Gels work well on the scalp, where other compounds may mat the hair, and for acute exudative conditions such as poison ivy. Lotions can be a mix of water, alcohols, and oils. They are also appropriate for the scalp but may cause stinging and drying when used in skin folds. Pastes are a compound of 50% or more powder in an ointment base. They are good for protecting the skin but are messy. A limited number of foams are available.

Some of these medications are very costly. Proper administration, as directed, will yield best results, maintain consistency, and avoid waste. As a general rule, topical medication should be applied in a thin film to clean skin and spread evenly in a downward motion in the direction of hair growth, using a gloved hand. Thick creams will spread more easily if the skin is still damp. If a secondary dressing is going to be used, the medication may be applied directly onto a dressing. The patient and caregiver will need to be taught proper dosing, application technique, anticipated results, and common reactions. Patients and caregivers should be reminded to wash hands with soap and water after applying topical medications at home.

Occlusion with a plastic wrap is an effective way of increasing the absorption of topical corticosteroids or simple emollients. The plastic wrap traps perspiration against the outer layer of the epidermis. Applying preparations to moist skin increases absorption ten-fold. Tape or stretch wraps can keep the plastic wrap in place. For conditions on the feet or lower legs, socks can be worn over the plastic wrap. Wraps applied multiple times daily are kept in place for 2 to 8 hours. Some patients choose to use the occlusion technique at bedtime. Occlusion is recommended with discretion because it is not appropriate in areas prone to infection, such as skin creases, or when high-potency corticosteroids or antibiotics are used.

CONTROL OF PRURITUS. Pruritus (itching) can be caused by almost any physical or chemical stimulus to the skin (e.g., drugs, insects), dry skin, or any scaling skin disorder. The itch sensation is carried by the same nonmyelinated nerve fibres as pain. If the epidermis is damaged or absent, the sensation will be felt as pain rather than itch.

The itch/scratch cycle must be broken to prevent excoriation and lichenification. Control of pruritus is also important because it is difficult to diagnose a lesion that is excoriated and inflamed. Certain circumstances make itching worse. Anything that causes vasodilation, such as heat or rubbing, should be avoided. Dryness of the skin lowers the itch threshold and increases the itch sensation.

There are several approaches to help break the itch/scratch cycle. A cool environment may cause vasoconstriction and decrease itching. Hydration, wet compresses, and moisturizers (including antipruritic lotions) are normally helpful. Topical and injectable corticosteroids are occasionally ordered. Topically applied menthol, camphor, or phenol can be used to numb the itch receptors. Systemic antihistamines may provide relief while the underlying cause of the pruritus is diagnosed and treated. The principal adverse effect of most antihistamines is sedation. This may be desirable because pruritus is often worse at night and can interfere with sleep.

Lichenification is a thickening of epidermis with exaggerated markings resembling a washboard. It is caused by chronic scratching or rubbing of the skin. Lichenification is often associated with atopic dermatoses and other pruritic conditions. Although any area of the body may be affected, the hands, forearms, shins, and nape of the neck are common sites. Itching

may become habitual. The persistent scratching can cause excoriations. Treating the cause of the itching is the key to preventing lichenification.

PREVENTION OF SPREAD. Although most skin problems are not contagious, infection-control precautions indicate wearing gloves when working with any open wounds or lesions with drainage. Procedures should be explained to avoid demoralizing patients who may be sensitive about skin lesions. Careful handwashing and proper disposal of soiled dressings are the best means of preventing the spread of infections or infestations. The most common contagious lesions include impetigo, streptococcal infections, staphylococcal infections (e.g., methicillin-resistant *S. aureus* [MRSA]), fungal infections, primary chancre, scabies, and pediculosis.

PREVENTION OF SECONDARY INFECTIONS. Open skin lesions are susceptible to invasion by other viral, bacterial, or fungal organisms. Meticulous hygiene, handwashing, and dressing changes are important to minimize potential for secondary infections. Patients should be warned against scratching lesions, which can cause excoriations and create a portal of entry for pathogens. The patient's nails should be kept short to minimize trauma from scratching.

SPECIFIC SKIN CARE. Nurses are often in a position to advise patients regarding care of the skin following simple dermatological surgical procedures, such as skin biopsy, excision, and cryosurgery. Patient follow-up should be individualized. In general, instructions include dressing changes, use of topical antibiotics, and the signs and symptoms of infection. After a dermatological procedure, any oozing wound should be cleansed twice a day with a saline solution or as ordered by the health care provider. Soap and water can be used to clean a non-oozing wound. An antibiotic ointment or plain petroleum jelly may then be applied with a dressing that is both absorbent and nonadherent.

Wounds that are kept moist and covered heal more rapidly and with less scarring. The initial crust that forms should be left undisturbed as a protective coating for the damaged skin beneath. Healing crusts that have been moisturized and protected will separate naturally from healed epidermis.

A sutured wound may be covered with a variety of dressings. Sutures are generally removed within 4 to 14 days depending on the site. Sometimes alternating sutures are removed after the third day. Incision lines may require daily cleansing, usually with plain tap water. If necessary, a topical antibiotic is applied and the wound either covered with a dry sterile dressing or left open to air. The patient may experience some swelling and discomfort in the first 24 hours during the first phase of wound healing. Intermittent application of cold (ice packs) over the surgical dressing may reduce edema and promote comfort. Mild analgesics such as acetaminophen or a nonsteroidal anti-inflammatory medication should control discomfort. The patient should learn to differentiate normal inflammation from an infection. A slight red border during the first few days after a procedure is normal inflammation. Redness that persists longer than a week or extends beyond a 1 cm border, a fever above 38°C, increased pain, pronounced swelling, and purulent drainage are all signs and symptoms of a possible infection. If these occur, they should be promptly reported to the health care provider.

PSYCHOLOGICAL EFFECTS OF CHRONIC DERMATOLOGICAL PROBLEMS

Emotional stress can occur for people who suffer from chronic skin problems such as psoriasis, atopic dermatitis, or acne. The sequelae of chronic skin problems can include social and employment problems with subsequent financial implications, a poor self-image, problems with sexuality, and increasing and progressive frustration. The usual lack of overt systemic illness coupled with the visibility of the skin lesions often presents a real problem to the patient.

Nurses are positioned to help the patient remain optimistic and adhere to the prescribed regimen. The patient must be allowed to verbalize the "Why me?" question, even though there is no ready answer. Dermatology patient support groups are listed on the CDA website (see the Resources at the end of this chapter). These groups are extremely helpful in providing patient support and accurate educational materials.

The location of lesions and scars is the determining factor with respect to cosmetic implications. Facial scars are the most damaging psychologically because they are so visible. Creative use of cosmetics can do much to mask lesions and scarring. Individual sensitivity to product ingredients must be considered when selecting cosmetics. Oil-free, hypoallergenic cosmetics are available and may be beneficial for the allergic patient. Rehabilitative cosmetics are available to help camouflage and de-emphasize such lesions as *vitiligo* (loss of pigmentation), *melasma* (tan to brown patches on the face), or healed postoperative wound sites. These commercially available products are opaque, smudge resistant, and water resistant.

PHYSIOLOGICAL EFFECTS OF CHRONIC DERMATOLOGICAL PROBLEMS

Scarring and lichenification are the result of chronic dermatological problems. Scars occur when ulceration takes place and reflect the pattern of healing in the area. Scars are pink and vascular at first. With time, in lighter-skinned people, they become avascular and white, and in individuals with darker skin, they may become hyperpigmented. Different regions of the body scar differently, such as the face and neck, which heal fairly well because they are well vascularized. Scar formation is described in Chapter 14.

COSMETIC PROCEDURES

A vast array of cosmetic procedures is available, including chemical peels, toxin injections, collagen fillers, laser surgery, breast augmentation and reduction (see Chapter 54), laser surgery, facelift, eyelid lift, and liposuction. Common cosmetic topical procedures are presented in Table 26-14. Other types of common cosmetic injection procedures include the injection of botulinum toxins (Botox) and collagen (Xiaflex, Santyl). Transitory adverse effects such as mild redness, pain, swelling, and bruising may occur.

The reasons for undergoing these procedures are as varied as the techniques. The most common reason that people suffer the discomfort and financial expense (most are not covered by insurance) of a cosmetic procedure is to improve their body image. If patients feel better about themselves after having cosmetic procedures, they will often act more confident and self-assured. Often social position and economic considerations are part of the decision. Increased longevity provides a larger population to whom cosmetic procedures are especially appealing.

Regardless of the patient's reasons, the nurse should maintain a supportive, nonjudgemental attitude about these cosmetic procedures. If the patient wishes to change or enhance a body feature perceived as unattractive and has realistic expectations about the outcome, it is reasonable to support this decision.

Body Art and Tattoos

Body art through tattoos and skin piercings are popular means of self-expression. A tattoo is a permanent design that is made by injecting dyes into the skin's epidermal layer via a machine that creates tiny skin pricks. Patients should ensure tattoo and

TABLE 26-14	COMMON COSMETIC TOPICAL PROCEDURES			
Procedure	**Indications**	**Description**	**Adverse Effects**	**Patient Teaching**
Tretinoin (Retin-A)	Improves appearance of photodamaged skin, especially fine wrinkling. Reduces actinic keratosis.	Applied initially every other day, nightly as tolerated. Treatment stopped if inflammation is severe. Maximum response in 8–12 mo.	Erythema, swelling, flaking, photosensitivity, hypopigmentation. Teratogenic. Increases phototoxicity if also taking other photosensitive drugs (see Table 26-3).	Apply emollients, use sunscreen (SPF 15 or higher), use sun-avoidance measures, avoid use of abrasive or drying facial cleanser if severe sensitivity.
Chemical peels	Improves appearance of aged and photodamaged skin, acne scarring, freckles, actinic and seborrheic keratoses.	Solution applied (e.g., trichloracetic acid, phenol) in varying amounts to the skin, causing a controlled burn. Loss of melanin occurs.	Moderate swelling and crusting for 1 wk. Redness persisting 6–8 wk. Pink tone possible for several months. Photosensitivity.	Use sunscreen; avoid sun for 6 mo to prevent hyperpigmentation.
Microdermabrasion	Smoothes appearance of photodamaged and wrinkled skin, acne scarring.	Removal of the epidermis and top dermal layer by application of aluminum oxide or baking soda crystals. Re-epithelialization of abraded surface then occurs.	Light pink tone that resolves within 24 hr. Photosensitivity.	Generous application of emollients and sunscreen.
Alpha-hydroxy acids (e.g., glycolic acid, lactic acid)	Similar indications as for microdermabrasion. Also called a *minipeel* or *light chemical peel*.	Low concentrations (<10%) found in many skin care products that patients can self-administer. Higher concentrations (50%–70%) given only by a health care provider.	Photosensitivity, irritation at lower concentrations. Severe redness, oozing, and flaking skin possible for 1–4 wk with higher concentrations.	Sunscreen and sun avoidance.

SPF, sun protection factor.

piercing establishments are certified through the local public health unit and that artists use new, sterile equipment and good hand hygiene and gloves. These measures minimize the risk of contracting a bloodborne disease (e.g., human immunodeficiency virus, hepatitis C) or skin infection. Tattoo dye contains metal, so a magnetic resonance imaging scan may not be able to be done over a tattooed site. Patients should be educated on how to care for tattoos and piercings at home in order to minimize infection risk. Important points include washing hands thoroughly before applying lotions or ointments to the tattooed or pierced area and before rotating jewellery and observing for signs of infection (pain, swelling, redness, or high temperature) and allergic reactions. Oral piercings require specific care: careful mouth hygiene (ideal bacterial breeding ground), plastic jewellery because metal chips the teeth, checking for loose pieces that could be a choking risk, and a mouth guard when playing sports (Simcoe Muskoka District Health Unit, n.d.).

Elective Surgery

Laser Surgery. When a laser beam enters the skin, the light can affect skin structures by scattering, being absorbed, or passing through different layers. The spectrum of clinical application for each laser depends on the depth of the wavelength emitted and the operator technique. Laser surgery is used to treat congenital and acquired vascular lesions (cherry angiomas, spider leg veins, hemangiomas, port wine stains, and tattoo removal) and for skin resurfacing and hair removal. Lasers can reduce scarring and fine wrinkles around the lips or eyes and remove facial lesions (see Table 26-12). Swelling, redness, and bruising are common after treatment. The treated areas usually are kept moist with ointment or occlusive dressings for the first few days. The patient must protect treated skin from the sun.

Facelift. A facelift *(rhytidectomy)* is the lifting and repositioning of the lower two-thirds of the face and neck to improve appearance (Figure 26-15). Indications for this procedure include the following:

1. Redundant soft tissue resulting from disease (e.g., acne scarring).
2. Asymmetrical redundancy of soft tissues (e.g., facial palsy).
3. Redundant soft tissue resulting from trauma.
4. Preauricular lesions.

FIGURE 26-15 Facelift. **A,** Before surgery. **B,** After surgery. Source: Reprinted from *Facial Plastic Surgery Clinics of North America*, 13(3), Pastorek, N., & Bustillo, A. Deep Plane Face-Lift, Pages 433–449, Copyright 2005, with permission from Elsevier.

5. Redundant soft tissues resulting from solar elastosis (sagging of the skin as a result of sun damage), changes in body weight, and the effects of gravity.
6. Restoration of body image.

The surgical approach and the lines of incisions vary according to the nature of the deformity and the position of the hairline. Eyelid lifts *(blepharoplasty)* with similar indications are performed to remove redundant tissue and possibly improve the field of vision. Preventing hematoma formation is the most important postoperative consideration. Ice packs are usually applied during the first 24 to 48 hours to reduce swelling and decrease the possibility of hematoma formation. Usually pain is minimal. Antibiotics are used at the surgeon's discretion. Infection is not a common problem. Complications can occur if the person smokes or is involved in vigorous exercise.

Liposuction. Liposuction is a technique for removing subcutaneous fat to improve facial and body contours. Although not a substitute for diet and exercise, it can be successful in removing areas of fat from virtually any body area that is resistant to other techniques.

Liposuction is relatively free of complications. Possible contraindications include use of anticoagulants, uncontrolled hypertension, diabetes mellitus, and poor cardiovascular status. People younger than 40 years of age with good skin elasticity are the best candidates, but those over 40 can be treated successfully.

The procedure is usually performed on an outpatient basis under local anaesthesia. One or more sessions may be necessary, depending on the size of the area to be treated. A blunt-tipped cannula is inserted through a 1.3-cm incision and pushed into the fat to break it loose from the fibrous stroma. Multiple repeated thrusts disrupt the fat and create tunnels. The loosened fat is removed with a powerful suction. Afterwards, firm pressure is applied to the wounds, and compression garments are worn for 3 to 4 weeks (Afrooz, Pozner, & DiBernardo, 2014). Bandaging also helps to contour the skin. It may take several months for the results to be evident.

NURSING MANAGEMENT
COSMETIC SURGERY

Many cosmetic surgical procedures are performed in well-equipped day-surgery units or in office surgery suites. Nursing interventions are important, regardless of where the surgery was done.

PREOPERATIVE MANAGEMENT

A major preoperative management consideration relates to informed consent and realistic expectations of what cosmetic surgery can accomplish. Although this information is usually provided by the surgeon, the nurse should reinforce this information and answer questions and concerns. For instance, a facelift has little or no effect on deep wrinkling of the forehead and temples, deep nasolabial grooves, or vertical lip wrinkles. Before- and after-treatment photographs of similar cases are often useful in helping the patient to set realistic expectations.

The nurse's teaching plan should include the time frame for healing. The oozing, crusting stage of the abrasive procedure must be explained so the patient can plan time off from work if necessary. Since the third phase of wound healing does not become complete for 1 year, the patient should not anticipate complete results immediately. The final results of the cosmetic procedure are affected by the patient's age, general state of health, extent of procedure, and skin type. Efforts should be made to correct or control any existing health problem before the procedure.

POSTOPERATIVE MANAGEMENT

Most cosmetic procedures are not extremely painful. Usually, mild analgesics are sufficient to keep the patient comfortable. Although infection is not a common problem after cosmetic surgery, the nurse should assess surgical sites for signs of infection. The patient should be educated on signs of infection and know to report any such signs and symptoms immediately so that appropriate antibiotic intervention can be started.

If the surgery involved alteration to the skin's circulation, such as in a facelift, careful monitoring for adequate circulation is necessary. In light-skinned individuals, warm pink skin that blanches with pressure indicates that adequate circulation is present in the surgical area. Blanching does not occur in dark-skinned patients, so it is necessary to check for areas that are darker than surrounding skin and to check for local changes in skin texture and skin temperature. Supportive compression dressings and ice packs may be necessary early in the postoperative period.

SKIN GRAFTS

Uses

Skin grafts may be necessary to provide protection to underlying structures or to reconstruct areas for functional or cosmetic purposes. They may be used to facilitate rapid closure and minimize complications. Ideally, wounds heal by primary intention. However, large wounds, surgically created wounds, trauma, and chronic wounds can result in extensive tissue destruction, making primary intention healing impossible. In these cases, skin grafting may be necessary to close the defect. Improved surgical techniques make it possible to graft skin, bone, cartilage, fat, fascia, muscles, and nerves. For cosmetically pleasing results, the colour, thickness, texture, and hair-growing nature of skin used for grafting should match the recipient site. (See Chapter 27 for further discussion of skin grafting.)

Types

The two types of skin grafts are free grafts and skin flaps. Free grafts are further classified according to the method of providing a blood supply to the grafted skin. One method is to transfer the graft (epidermis and part or all of the dermis) to the recipient site from the donor site. If the graft is an *autograft* (from the patient's own body) or an *isograft* (from an identical twin), it will revascularize and become fixed to the new site. Chapter 27 discusses full- and split-thickness skin grafts in detail. Another method of free skin grafting is by *reconstructive microsurgery.* An operating microscope is used to immediately establish circulation in the graft by anastomosis of the blood vessels from the skin flap to the vessels in the recipient site.

Skin flaps involve moving a section of skin and subcutaneous tissue from one part of the body to another without terminating the vascular attachment *(pedicle).* Skin flaps are used to cover wounds with a poor vascular bed, to provide padding when needed, and to cover wounds over cartilage and bone. The patient may need intermediate flap placement if the recipient site is far removed from the donor site. For instance, a skin flap from the thigh to the head would require an intermediate graft. The flap is advanced to the recipient site when circulation is well established at the intermediate site. The patient's needs and the type of defect to be repaired determine the type of flap and the route of transfer. Soft tissue expansion is a technique for providing skin (1) for resurfacing a defect, such as a burn scar; (2) for removing a disfiguring mark (e.g., a tattoo); or (3) as a preliminary step in breast reconstruction. A subcutaneous tissue expander of an appropriate size and shape is placed under the skin, usually as an outpatient procedure. Weekly expansion with saline solution can be done in a health care setting or by the patient at home. This expansion procedure is repeated until the skin reaches the size needed for the repair. This may take from several weeks to 4 months. Once sufficient skin is available, the old incision is opened, the expander is removed, and the soft tissue is ready to be used as an advancement flap. The tissue expander next to a defect retains the primary tissue characteristics such as colour and texture.

Newer engineered skin substitutes (e.g., Dermagraft, Alloderm) are gaining popularity. There are a number available, and each offers its own benefits. Some are two-layered membranes with both dermal and epidermal components. Others are only one layer. The skin is engineered from neonatal foreskins and cadavers. Because the tissue is engineered, Langerhans cells are removed, reducing the risk for rejection (Nathoo, Howe, & Cohen, 2014). Engineered skin grafts have an extended shelf life. Some are cryopreserved; others, shipped overnight as they are needed. Advantages include ready availability, the avoidance of a donor site, application in outpatient settings, minimal scarring, and less pain.

CASE STUDY

Malignant Melanoma and Dysplastic Nevi

Source: tmcphotos/ Shutterstock .com.

Patient Profile
Gordon Lindquist is a 46-year-old fair-skinned man who is a contract safety officer supervising large industrial construction sites. In his leisure time, he enjoys fishing and kayaking. He comes to the clinic for evaluation of a changing lesion on his left arm.

Subjective Data
• History of a basal cell carcinoma (BCC) on his left ear in the past 4 years
• Father treated for metastatic malignant melanoma in the past 2 years
• First noted the lesion 5 months ago, when it started changing size

• Anxious the lesion might have spread and require extensive, disfiguring surgery

Objective Data
Physical Examination
• Has a 4-mm lesion, dark brown/black, scalloped with vaguely defined borders to dorsum of left forearm just distal to the elbow
• Has a large number of small nevi (>50) on back, legs, and arms
• Has four dysplastic nevi on back

Diagnostic Studies
• Excisional biopsy confirmed malignant melanoma.
• Sentinel node biopsy results were negative.
• Diagnostic tests indicate melanoma stage 1.

Continued

CASE STUDY

Malignant Melanoma and Dysplastic Nevi—cont'd

Discussion Questions

1. What risk factors for malignant melanoma does Mr. Lindquist have?
2. What are the usual clinical manifestations associated with malignant melanoma?
3. What is the prognosis for a patient with this stage of malignant melanoma?
4. What treatment options are available for him?
5. *Priority decision:* What is the priority of care for Mr. Lindquist?
6. How would the nurse address Mr. Lindquist's anxiety over the treatment outcomes?

7. What should the nurse include in the patient teaching plan to address future sun exposure?
8. *Priority decision:* Based on the assessment data presented, what are the priority nursing diagnoses? Are there any collaborative problems?
9. *Evidence-informed practice:* Mr. Lindquist wants to know whether regularly applying sunscreen will reduce his risk for developing a second melanoma. How should the nurse reply?

ⓔvolve

Answers available at *http://evolve.elsevier.com/Canada/Lewis/medsurg.*

REVIEW QUESTIONS

The number of the question corresponds to the same-numbered objective at the beginning of the chapter.

1. Which sun-safety practices would the nurse include in the teaching plan for a client who has photosensitivity? *(Select all that apply)*
   a. Wear protective clothing.
   b. Apply sunscreen liberally and often.
   c. Use tanning booths only for short durations.
   d. Avoid exposure to the sun, especially during midday.
   e. Wear any sunscreen as long as it is purchased at a drugstore.

2. In teaching a client who is using topical corticosteroids to treat acute dermatitis, what information should the nurse include? *(Select all that apply)*
   a. The cream form is the most efficient system of delivery.
   b. Short-term use of topical corticosteroids usually does not cause systemic adverse effects.
   c. Apply creams and ointments with a glove in small amounts to prevent further infection.
   d. Abruptly discontinuing the use of topical corticosteroids may cause a reappearance of the dermatitis.
   e. Malnourishment is a risk factor for systemic adverse effects from topical corticosteroids.

3. What measurement is the prognosis of a client with malignant melanoma most dependent on?
   a. The thickness of the lesion
   b. The degree of asymmetry in the lesion
   c. How much the lesion has spread superficially
   d. The amount of ulceration in the lesion

4. The nurse determines that a client with a diagnosis of which disorder is most at risk for spreading the disease?
   a. Tinea pedis
   b. Impetigo on the face
   c. Candidiasis of the nails
   d. Psoriasis on the palms and soles

5. A mother and her two children have been diagnosed with pediculosis corporis at a health centre. Which of the following is an appropriate measure in treating this condition?
   a. Application of pyrethrins to the body
   b. Topical application of an antifungal ointment
   c. Moist compresses applied frequently
   d. Administration of systemic antibiotics

6. What is a common site for the lesions associated with atopic dermatitis?
   a. Buttocks
   b. Temporal area
   c. Antecubital space
   d. Plantar surface of the feet

7. During assessment of a client, the nurse notes on the client's knee and elbow red, sharply defined plaques covered with silvery scales that the client reports as mildly itchy. What should the nurse recognize this finding to be?
   a. Lentigo
   b. Psoriasis
   c. Actinic keratosis
   d. Seborrheic keratosis

8. A patient with acne vulgaris tells the nurse that she has quit her job as a receptionist because she feels her appearance is disgusting to customers. Which of the following nursing diagnoses best describes this patient's response?
   a. *Ineffective coping* related to *insufficient social support*
   b. *Impaired skin integrity* related to *inadequate nutrition*
   c. *Anxiety* related to *unmet needs* (lack of knowledge about the disease process)
   d. *Social isolation* related to *alteration in physical appearance*

9. What important point should client teaching after a chemical peel include?
   a. Avoidance of sun exposure
   b. Application of firm bandages
   c. Limitation of vigorous exercise
   d. Use of moist heat to prevent discomfort

1. a, b, d; 2. b, d; 3. a; 4. b; 5. a; 6. c; 7. b; 8. d; 9. a.

ⓔvolve

For even more review questions, visit *http://evolve.elsevier.com/Canada/Lewis/medsurg.*

REFERENCES

Afrooz, P. N., Pozner, J. N., & DiBernardo, B. E. (2014). Noninvasive and minimally invasive techniques in body contouring. *Clinics in Plastic Surgery, 41*(4), 789–804. doi:10.1016/j.cps.2014.07.006.

Canadian Cancer Society. (2015). *Indoor tanning.* Retrieved from *http://www.cancer.ca/en/get-involved/take-action/what-we-are-doing/indoor-tanning/?region=on.*

Canadian Cancer Society's Advisory Committee on Cancer Statistics. (2016). *Canadian cancer statistics 2016.* Toronto: Canadian Cancer Society. Retrieved from *https://www.cancer.ca/~/media/cancer.ca/CW/publications/Canadian%20Cancer%20Statistics/Canadian-Cancer-Statistics-2016-EN.pdf.*

Canadian Dermatology Association (CDA). (2000). *Position statement: Use of self-tanning creams.* Retrieved from *http://www.dermatology.ca/wp-content/uploads/2013/09/Use-of-Self-Tanning-Creams-Feb-2013.pdf.*

Canadian Dermatology Association (CDA). (2017a). *Sunscreen FAQ.* Retrieved from *http://dermatology.ca/public-patients/sun-protection/sunscreen-faq.*

Canadian Dermatology Association (CDA). (2017b). *Indoor tanning information.* Retrieved from *http://dermatology.ca/public-patients/sun-protection/indoor-tanning-information.*

Canadian Dermatology Association (CDA). (2017c). *Melanoma.* Retrieved from *http://dermatology.ca/public-patients/skin/melanoma.*

Canadian Dermatology Association (CDA). (2017d). *Psoriasis.* Retrieved from *http://dermatology.ca/public-patients/skin/psoriasis/#!/skin-hair-nails/skin/psoriasis/living-with-psoriasis.*

Canadian Dermatology Association (CDA). (2017e). *Hair removal.* Retrieved from *http://www.dermatology.ca/skin-hair-nails/hair/hair-removal/#!/skin-hair-nails/hair/hair-removal/lasering.*

Government of Canada (GOC). (2012a). *Sunglasses.* Retrieved from *https://www.canada.ca/en/health-canada/services/sun-safety/sunglasses.html.*

Government of Canada (GOC). (2012b). *Sunscreens.* Retrieved from *https://www.canada.ca/en/health-canada/services/sun-safety/sunscreens.html.*

Government of Canada (GOC). (2012c). *Tanning beds and lamps.* Retrieved from *https://www.canada.ca/en/health-canada/services/sun-safety/tanning-beds-lamps.html.*

Government of Canada (GOC). (2012d). *Tanning products.* Retrieved from *https://www.canada.ca/en/health-canada/services/cosmetics/tanning-products.html.*

Government of Canada (GOC). (2015). *Canadian cancer statistics.* Retrieved from *https://www.cancer.ca/~/media/cancer.ca/CW/cancer%20information/cancer%20101/Canadian%20cancer%20statistics/Canadian-Cancer-Statistics 2015 EN.pdf?la=en.*

Habif, T. (2011). *Clinical dermatology* (5th ed.). St. Louis: Elsevier.

Health Canada. (2013). *Sun safety.* Retrieved from *http://www.hc-sc.gc.ca/hl-vs/sun-sol/index-eng.php.*

Health Canada. (2014). *The ultraviolet index and your local forecast.* Retrieved from *http://www.healthycanadians.gc.ca/healthy-living-vie-saine/environment-environnement/sun-soleil/index-uv-indice-eng.php.*

Health Canada. (2016). *Adverse reaction and medical device problem reporting.* Retrieved from *http://hc-sc.gc.ca/dhp-mps/medeff/report-declaration/index-eng.php.*

Howlader, N., Noone, A., Krapcho, M., et al. (Eds.), (2015). *SEER cancer statistics review, 1975–2012.* Bethesda, MD: National Cancer Institute. Retrieved from *http://seer.cancer.gov/csr/1975_2012.*

Kim, D. W., Trinh, V. A., & Hwu, W. J. (2014). Ipilimumab in the treatment of advanced melanoma: A clinical update. *Expert Opinion on Biological Therapy, 14*(11), 1709–1718. doi:10.1517/14712598.2014.963053.

Marks, J., & Miller, J. (2013). *Principles of dermatology* (5th ed.). St. Louis: Elsevier.

Micali, G., Lacarrubba, F., Nasca, M., et al. (2014). Topical pharmacotherapy for skin cancer: Part II. Clinical applications. *Journal of the American Academy of Dermatology, 70,* 979–991. doi:10.1016/j.jaad.2013.12.037.

Nathoo, R., Howe, N., & Cohen, G. (2014). Skin substitutes: An overview of the key players in wound management. *Journal of Clinical and Aesthetic Dermatology, 7*(10), 44–48.

Rkein, A. M., & Ozog, D. M. (2014). Photodynamic therapy. *Dermatologic Clinics, 32*(3), 415–425. doi:10.1016/j.det.2014.03.009.

Simcoe Muskoka District Health Unit. (n.d.). *Tattooing and piercing introduction.* Retrieved from *http://www.simcoemuskokahealth.org/Topics/InfectiousDiseases/BeautyAndBodyArt/TattooPiercingIntroduction.aspx.*

RESOURCES

Canadian Cancer Society
http://www.cancer.ca

Canadian Dermatology Association
http://www.dermatology.ca

Canadian Dermatology Foundation
http://www.cdf.ca

Canadian Society of Aesthetic Specialty Nurses
http://www.csasn.org/

Canadian Society of Plastic Surgeons
http://www.plasticsurgery.ca

Eczema Society of Canada
http://www.eczemahelp.ca

Melanoma Network of Canada
https://www.melanomanetwork.ca

Psoriasis Society of Canada
http://www.psoriasissociety.org

Rosaceafacts.ca
http://www.rosaceafacts.ca

Save Your Skin Foundation
http://www.saveyourskin.ca

Scleroderma Canada
http://www.scleroderma.ca

University of British Columbia, Department of Dermatology and Skin Science
http://www.derm.ubc.ca

American Academy of Dermatology
http://www.aad.org

For additional Internet resources, see the website for this book at *http://evolve.elsevier.com/Canada/Lewis/medsurg.*

Nursing Management

Burns

Written by: Judy Knighton

evolve WEBSITE

http://evolve.elsevier.com/Canada/Lewis/medsurg

- Review Questions (Online Only)
- Key Points
- Answer Guidelines for Case Study

- Student Case Study
  - Burns
- Customizable Nursing Care Plan
  - Thermal Burn Injury

- Conceptual Care Map Creator
- Audio Glossary
- Content Updates

LEARNING OBJECTIVES

1. Explain the causes of burn injuries and prevention strategies.
2. Differentiate between partial- and full-thickness burns.
3. Apply the parameters used to determine the severity of burns.
4. Compare the pathophysiological processes, clinical manifestations, complications, and collaborative management throughout the three burn phases.
5. Compare the fluid and electrolyte shifts during the emergent and the acute burn phases.
6. Differentiate the nutritional needs of the patient with a burn injury throughout the three burn phases.

7. Compare the various burn wound care techniques and surgical options for partial-thickness versus full-thickness burn wounds.
8. Prioritize nursing interventions in the management of the physiological and psychosocial needs of the patient throughout the three burn phases.
9. Examine the various physiological and psychosocial aspects of burn rehabilitation.
10. Design a plan of care to prepare the burn patient and family for discharge.

KEY TERMS

burn, p. 530
chemical burns, p. 531
contracture, p. 550
cultured epithelial autograft, p. 548

debridement, p. 543
electrical burns, p. 532
escharotomy, p. 538
excision and grafting, p. 547

full-thickness burn, p. 534
partial-thickness burn, p. 534
smoke and inhalation injuries, p. 531
thermal burns, p. 531

A **burn** is an injury to the tissues of the body caused by heat, chemicals, electric current, or radiation. The resulting effects are influenced by the temperature of the burning agent, the duration of contact time, and the type of tissue that is injured.

While there is a lack of precise data on the number of Canadians burned each year, there is some consistency between two existing data sources. The Institute for Clinical Evaluative Sciences (ICES, 2005) found that, in one year in Ontario, there were 157 emergency department visits for hot object/scald (115) and fire/flame (42) per 100 000 people. Based on a population of 35 million people in Canada, it could then be estimated that approximately 54 950 Canadians are burned each year, severely enough to require a visit to an emergency department. According to Statistics Canada (2011), 44 450 Canadians over the age of 12 years stated that they had an activity-limiting injury due to a burn, scald, or chemical burn in the previous 12 months. The highest incidence occurred within the 20–64 years age

group, and treatment predominantly occurred in the emergency department.

An estimated 486 000 Americans seek medical care each year for burns (American Burn Association [ABA], 2016). Accounting for the 2016 population difference between the United States and Canada (324 million versus 36 million), the burn incidence data appear similar. Around the world, nearly 11 million people need medical attention annually for burn injuries, and about 265 000 die as a result of burns (World Health Organization, 2016).

Although burn incidence has decreased over the past 20 years, burn injuries still occur too frequently, mainly to those in a lower socioeconomic level and with histories of substance abuse or mental illness. Most burn incidents are preventable (Taira, Cassara, Meng, et al., 2011). The focus of burn prevention has shifted from blaming individuals and changing behaviours to making legislative changes and collecting global burn data

TABLE 27-1	COMMON LOCATIONS AND SOURCES OF BURN INJURY*

Home Hazards
Kitchen and Bathroom
- Microwaved food
- Steam, hot grease, or liquids from cooking
- Hot water heaters set at 60°C or higher

General Household
- Heat lamps
- Fireplaces (e.g., gas, wood)
- Open space heaters
- Radiators (e.g., home, automobile)
- Outdoor grills (e.g., propane, charcoal)
- Frayed or defective wiring
- Multiple extension cords per outlet

- Flammables (e.g., starter fluid, gasoline, kerosene)
- Carelessness with cigarettes, matches, candles

Occupational Hazards
- Tar
- Cement
- Chemicals
- Hot metals
- Steam pipes
- Combustible fuels
- Fertilizers, pesticides
- Electricity from power lines
- Sparks from live electric sources

*List is not all-inclusive.

to address the unique prevention needs of low- and middle-income countries (Peck, 2012).

Coordinated national programs in developed countries have focused on child-resistant lighters, nonflammable children's clothing, tap water anti-scald devices, stricter building codes, hard-wired smoke detectors and alarms, and fire sprinklers. Nurses can advocate for and teach about burn risk–reduction strategies in the home and at work (Tables 27-1 and 27-2).

TYPES OF BURN INJURY

Thermal Burns

Thermal burns are caused by flame, flash fire, scald, or contact with hot objects. They are the most common type of burn injury (Figure 27-1; see Table 27-2). The severity depends on the temperature of the burning agent and duration of contact time. Scald injuries can occur in the bathroom or while cooking. Flash, flame, or contact burns can occur while cooking, smoking, burning leaves in the backyard, or using gasoline or hot oil.

Chemical Burns

Chemical burns are the result of contact with acids, alkalis, and organic compounds. Acids are found in the home and at work and include hydrochloric, oxalic, and hydrofluoric acid. Alkali burns can be more difficult to manage than acid burns since alkalis adhere to tissue, causing protein hydrolysis and liquefaction. Alkalis are found in cement, oven and drain cleaners, and heavy industrial cleansers (Summers, 2013). Organic compounds, including phenols (chemical disinfectants) and petroleum products (creosote and gasoline), produce contact burns and systemic toxicity.

Smoke and Inhalation Injury

Smoke and inhalation injuries from breathing noxious chemicals or hot air can cause damage to the tissues of the respiratory tract. Fortunately, gases are cooled to body temperature before

TABLE 27-2	TYPES OF BURN INJURY AND BURN RISK–REDUCTION STRATEGIES

Flame or Contact
- Never smoke in bed.
- Use child-resistant lighters.
- Hold regular fire exit drills in the home.
- Never leave hot oil unattended while cooking.
- Never use gasoline or other flammable liquids to start a fire.
- Never leave candles unattended or near open windows or curtains.
- Consider a flame-retardant smoking apron for older or at-risk people.
- Exercise caution when microwaving food and beverages as they can get very hot.

Scald
- Lower hot water temperature to the "lowest point" or 40°C.
- Use "anti-scald" devices with showerhead or faucet fixtures.
- Supervise bathing of small children, older adults, or anyone with impaired physical movement, physical sensation, or judgement.
- After running bath water, check temperature with back of hand or bath thermometer.

Inhalation
- Install smoke and carbon monoxide detectors and change batteries annually (if appropriate).

Chemical
- Store chemicals safely in approved containers, and label clearly.
- Ensure safety of workers and students handling chemicals (e.g., provide education, protective eyewear, gloves, masks, clothing).

Electrical
- Avoid or repair frayed wiring.
- Avoid outdoor activities during electrical (i.e., lightning) storms.
- Ensure electrical power source is shut off before beginning repairs.
- Wear protective eyewear and gloves when making electrical repairs.

TABLE 27-3	MANIFESTATIONS OF RESPIRATORY INJURY ASSOCIATED WITH BURNS

Upper Airway Injury
Edema, hoarseness, difficulty swallowing, copious secretions, stridor, substernal and intercostal retractions, total airway obstruction

Lower Airway Injury
Strongly assumed if patient was trapped in a fire in an enclosed space or clothing caught fire and if patient has facial burns or singed nasal or facial hair; symptoms include dyspnea, carbonaceous sputum, wheezing, hoarseness, altered mental status

they reach the lung tissue. The vocal cords and glottis close as a protective mechanism, so damage to the respiratory mucosa occurs less often. Smoke inhalation injuries are a major predictor of mortality in burn patients. Rapid initial and ongoing assessment are critical (Table 27-3). Assess for signs and symptoms of airway compromise and pulmonary edema that can develop over the first 12 to 48 hours (Jeschke, 2013).

There are three types of smoke and inhalation injuries:
1. *Carbon monoxide poisoning.* Carbon monoxide poisoning and asphyxiation account for the majority of deaths at a fire scene. Carbon monoxide is produced by the incomplete combustion of burning materials. It is subsequently inhaled and displaces oxygen (O_2) on the hemoglobin molecule,

FIGURE 27-1 Types of burn injury. **A,** Superficial, partial-thickness scald burn to thigh. **B,** Deep partial-thickness flame burn to hand. **C,** Full-thickness flame burn secondary to posterior chest and arm. Source: Courtesy Judy A. Knighton, RN, MScN, Toronto.

FIGURE 27-2 Electrical injury produces heat coagulation of the blood supply and contact area as electric current passes through the skin. **A,** Back and buttock *(arrows)*. **B,** Leg *(arrow)*. Source: Courtesy Judy A. Knighton, RN, MScN, Toronto.

causing carboxyhemoglobinemia, hypoxia, and, when the carbon monoxide levels exceed 20%, death. With severe carbon monoxide poisoning, skin colour is often described as "cherry red" in appearance. Carbon monoxide poisoning may occur in the absence of burn injury to the skin (e.g., smoke inhalation during a fire).

2. *Inhalation injury above the glottis.* In general, an inhalation injury above the glottis *(upper airway injury)* is thermally produced and may be caused by the inhalation of hot air, steam, or smoke. Mucosal burns of the oropharynx and larynx are manifested by redness, blistering, and edema. Mechanical obstruction can occur quickly, which represents a true medical emergency. Clues to the occurrence of this injury include the presence of facial burns, singed nasal hair, hoarseness, painful swallowing, darkened oral and nasal membranes, carbonaceous sputum, history of being burned in an enclosed space, and clothing burns around the chest and neck.

3. *Inhalation injury below the glottis.* An inhalation injury below the glottis *(lower airway injury)* is usually chemically produced. Tissue damage is related to the duration of exposure to smoke or toxic fumes. Clinical manifestations such as pulmonary edema may not appear until 12 to 24 hours after the burn, and then they may manifest as acute respiratory distress syndrome (see Chapter 70).

Electrical Burns

Electrical burns result from intense heat generated from an electric current. Direct damage to nerves and vessels, causing tissue anoxia and death, can also occur. The severity of the electrical injury depends on the amount of voltage, tissue resistance, current pathways, surface area in contact with the current, and length of time that the current flow was sustained (Figure 27-2). Tissue density affects the amount of resistance to electric current. For example, fat and bone offer the most resistance, whereas nerves and blood vessels offer the least resistance. Current that passes through vital organs (e.g., brain, heart, kidneys) produces more life-threatening sequelae than that which passes through other tissues. In addition, electric sparks may ignite the patient's clothing, causing a flame injury.

As with inhalation injury, a rapid assessment of the patient with an electrical injury should be performed. Transfer to a burn centre is indicated. The severity of an electrical injury can be difficult to determine since most of the damage is below the skin (known as the *iceberg effect*). Determination of electric current contact points and history of the injury may help reveal the likely path of the current and potential areas of injury. Contact with electric current can cause muscle contractions strong enough to fracture the long bones and vertebrae. Another reason to suspect long bone or spinal fractures is a fall resulting from the electrical injury. For this reason, consider all patients with electrical burns at risk for a cervical spine injury. Use cervical spine immobilization during transport and subsequent diagnostic testing until injury is ruled out.

Electrical injury puts the patient at risk for dysrhythmias or cardiac arrest, severe metabolic acidosis, and myoglobinuria (Saracogli, Kuzucuoglu, Yakupoglu, et al., 2014). Electric shock can cause immediate asystole or ventricular fibrillation. Delayed dysrhythmias or arrest can also occur without warning during the first 24 hours after injury. Myoglobin from injured muscle and hemoglobin from damaged red blood cells (RBCs) are released into the circulation whenever massive muscle and blood vessel damage occurs. The released myoglobin travels to the kidneys and can block the renal tubules. This can result in acute tubular necrosis (ATN) and acute kidney injury (see Chapter 49).

Cold Thermal Injury

Cold thermal injury, or frostbite, is discussed in Chapter 71.

CLASSIFICATION OF BURN INJURY

Treatment of burns is related to the severity of the injury. Severity is determined by (a) depth of burn, (b) extent of burn calculated in percentage of total body surface area (TBSA), (c) location of burn, and (d) patient risk factors (e.g., age, past medical history). Health Canada uses referral criteria to determine which burn injuries should be treated in burn centres (Table 27-4). Critical Care Services Ontario (CCSO) has adapted American Burn Association (ABA) "Burn Center Referral Criteria" to develop "Burns Centre Consultation Guidelines" (see Table 27-4). A list of provincial burn units and centres across Canada is found in

Table 27-5. The majority of patients with minor burn injuries can be managed in community hospitals or on an outpatient basis (Payne & Cole, 2012).

Goals of care include wound healing, prevention of infection, pain management, prevention of complications, and return to preinjury function.

Depth of Burn

Burn injury involves the destruction of the integumentary system. The skin is divided into three layers: epidermis, dermis, and subcutaneous tissue (Figure 27-3). The *epidermis*, or nonvascular outer layer of the skin, is approximately as thick as a sheet of

---

TABLE 27-4 CRITERIA FOR TRANSFER OF THE PATIENT WITH BURN INJURIES*

Consider transfer to a major burn centre:
- ≥20% TBSA partial- and/or full-thickness at any age
- ≥10% TBSA partial- and/or full-thickness for ages ≤10 and ≥50
- Full-thickness burns ≥5% TBSA at any age
- Burns to face, hands, feet, joints, genitalia, perineum
- Electrical burns [including lightning injury]
- Chemical burns
- Inhalation injury
- Burns with comorbidity
- Burns with patients who require special social, emotional, or rehabilitation care

Consider transfer to a minor burn centre:
- Burns >10% but <20% TBSA in adults

Remain at base site:
- Burns <10% TBSA in adults who do not require transfer but seek medical advice or an ambulatory burns clinic referral for assessment

Special considerations:
High-risk considerations which may warrant transfer at a lower clinical threshold. These considerations include:
- ≥50 years of age
- Anticoagulation
- Immuno-suppression
- Pregnancy
- Diabetes
- Other significant medical problems

TBSA, total body surface area.
Source: Critical Care Services Ontario. (n.d.). Burns centre consultation guidelines. Retrieved from *http://www.oninjuryresources.ca/downloads/news/CCSO_ BurnsCentreGuidelines_11x14-EN.PDF.*
*See also: Health Canada. (2010). Dermatological emergencies: Burns. *Clinical Practice Guidelines for Nurses in Primary Care: Adult Care.* Retrieved from *http:// www.hc-sc.gc.ca/fniah-spnia/alt_formats/pdf/services/nurs-infirm/clini/adult/ skin-peau-eng.pdf*; and American Burn Association. (2006). *Guidelines for the operation of burn centers.* Retrieved from *http://www.ameriburn.org/Chapter14.pdf.*

TABLE 27-5 CANADIAN BURN UNITS OR CENTRES BY PROVINCE,* 2015

Province	City	Hospital
Alberta	Calgary	Alberta Children's Hospital Burn Treatment Services
	Calgary	Calgary Firefighters' Burn Treatment Centre
	Edmonton	Edmonton Firefighters' Burn Treatment Unit
British Columbia	Vancouver	B.C. Professional Fire Fighters' Burn, Trauma, and High Acuity Unit
	Vancouver	B.C. Children's Hospital Burn Unit
	Victoria	Complex Wound and Burn Clinic, Royal Jubilee Hospital
Manitoba	Winnipeg	Manitoba Firefighters' Burn Unit
	Winnipeg	Winnipeg Children's Hospital Burn Unit
New Brunswick	Saint John	Saint John Regional Hospital Plastic and Burns Unit
Newfoundland and Labrador	St. John's	General Hospital Health Sciences Centre
Nova Scotia	Halifax	Queen Elizabeth II Health Sciences Centre
	Halifax	IWK Health Centre
Ontario	Hamilton	Hamilton Health Sciences Centre Burn Unit
	London	London Health Sciences Centre Burn Unit
	Ottawa	Children's Hospital of Eastern Ontario
	Toronto	Hospital for Sick Children (Sick Kids) Burn Unit
	Toronto	Sunnybrook Health Sciences Centre Ross Tilley Burn Centre
Quebec	Montreal	Hôtel-Dieu du CHUM Montreal Burn Unit
	Montreal	CHU Sainte-Justine Burn Clinic
	Montreal	McGill University Health Centre
	Quebec City	Centre d'expertise pour victimes de brulures graves de l'Est du Québec
	Quebec City	Hôpital de L'Enfant-Jésus du CHU de Québec Unité des grands brûlés
Saskatchewan	Regina	South Saskatchewan Firefighters' Burn Unit
	Saskatoon	Royal University Hospital

Source: Developed by Judy Knighton, RN, MScN, clinical nurse specialist—burns. (2015, April). Data collected for Canadian Special Interest Group Meeting, American Burn Association Meeting, Chicago.
*There are no known burn centres in Yukon, Northwest Territories, or Nunavut.

paper. It is composed of many layers of nonliving epithelial cells that provide a protective barrier to the skin, hold in fluids and electrolytes, help regulate body temperature, and keep harmful agents in the external environment from injuring or invading the body. The *dermis,* which lies below the epidermis, is approximately 30 to 45 times thicker than the epidermis. The dermis contains connective tissues with blood vessels and highly specialized structures consisting of hair follicles, nerve endings, sweat glands, and sebaceous glands. Under the dermis lies *subcutaneous tissue,* which contains major vascular networks, fat, nerves, and lymphatic vessels. The subcutaneous tissue acts as a heat insulator for underlying structures, which include the muscles, tendons, bones, and internal organs.

Burns continue to be defined by degrees: first-, second-, third-, and fourth-degree. The ABA recommends a more precise definition, classifying them according to depth of skin destruction: partial-thickness burn and full-thickness burn (see Figure 27-3).

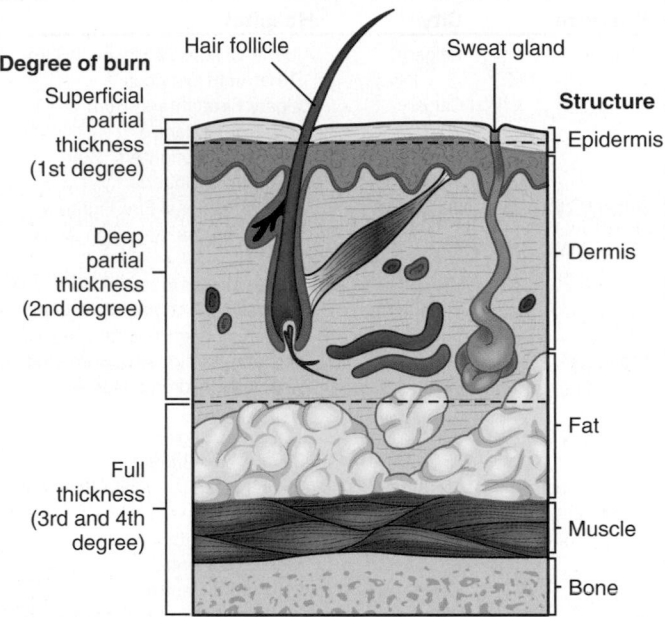

FIGURE 27-3 Cross-section of skin indicating the depth of burn and structures involved.

Partial-thickness burns have varying degrees of epidermal and dermal skin injury, with some skin elements remaining viable for regeneration. Full-thickness burns involve the destruction of all skin elements and subcutaneous tissues, with the possible involvement of muscles, tendons, and bones. Skin-reproducing (re-epithelializing) cells are located along the shafts of the hair follicles, sweat glands, and sebaceous glands. If there is significant damage to the dermis (e.g., a full-thickness burn), not enough skin cells remain to regenerate new skin. A permanent, alternative source of skin is then needed. In Table 27-6, the various burn classifications are compared according to depth of injury.

Extent of Burn

Two commonly used guides for determining the TBSA affected or the extent of a burn wound are the adult Lund–Browder chart (Figure 27-4, A) and the adult rule of nines chart (Figure 27-4, B). (First-degree burns, equivalent to a sunburn, are not included when TBSA burned is calculated.) The Lund–Browder chart is considered more accurate because the patient's age, in proportion to relative body-area size, is taken into account. The rule of nines, which is easy to remember, is considered adequate for initial assessment of an adult patient with burn injury. For irregular or odd-shaped burns, the size of the patient's hand (including the fingers) is approximately 1% TBSA.

An additional tool is the Sage Burn Diagram, a free, Internet-based tool available for estimating TBSA burned (see the Resources at the end of this chapter). There are also mobile applications (e.g., uBurn, Mersey Burns) available to estimate the percentage of burn and fluid resuscitation needs (Faraklas, Ghanem, Brown, et al., 2013). The extent of a burn is often revised after edema has subsided and demarcation of the zones of injury has occurred.

Location of Burn

The severity of the burn injury is related to the location of the burn wound. Burns to the face and neck and circumferential burns to the trunk or back can result in mechanical obstruction, secondary to edema, and leathery, devitalized tissue formation *(eschar),* both of which may inhibit respiratory function. These injuries may also include possible inhalation injury and respiratory mucosal damage.

TABLE 27-6	CLASSIFICATION OF BURN INJURY DEPTH		
Classification	**Clinical Appearance**	**Possible Cause**	**Structures Involved**
Partial-Thickness Skin Destruction			
Superficial: first-degree burn	Erythema, blanching on pressure, pain and mild swelling, no vesicles or blisters (although after 24 hr, skin may blister and peel)	Superficial sunburn Quick heat flash	Superficial epidermal damage with hyperemia; tactile and pain sensation intact
Deep: second-degree burn	Fluid-filled vesicles that are red, shiny, wet (if vesicles have ruptured); severe pain caused by nerve injury; mild to moderate edema	Flame Flash Scald Contact Chemical Tar Electrical current	Epidermis and dermis involved to varying depth; skin elements, from which epithelial regeneration occurs, remain viable
Full-Thickness Skin Destruction			
Third- and fourth-degree burns	Dry, waxy-white, leathery, or hard skin; visible thrombosed vessels; insensitivity to pain because of nerve destruction; possible involvement of muscles, tendons, and bones	Flame Scald Chemical Tar Electrical current	All skin elements and local nerve endings destroyed; coagulation necrosis present; surgical intervention advisable for healing

FIGURE 27-4 A, Adult Lund–Browder chart. By convention, areas of partial-thickness injury are coloured in blue, and areas of full-thickness in red. Superficial partial-thickness burns are not calculated. **B,** Adult rule of nines chart.

Burns to the hands, feet, joints, and eyes are of concern because they make self-care very difficult and may jeopardize future function. Burns to the hands and feet are challenging to manage because of superficial vascular and nerve supply systems that must be protected and because of the need to maintain hand function during healing.

Burns to the ears and nose are susceptible to infection because the skin is very thin and the underlying skeleton frequently exposed. Burns to the buttocks or perineum are at high risk for infection from urine or feces contamination. Circumferential burns to the extremities can cause circulatory compromise distal to the burn and, subsequently, neurological impairment of the affected extremity. Patients may also develop compartment syndrome (see Chapter 65) from direct heat damage to muscles; edema may result, and preburn vascular problems can be exacerbated.

Patient Risk Factors

The older adult heals more slowly and usually experiences more difficulty with rehabilitation than a younger adult. Any patient with pre-existing cardiovascular, respiratory, or renal disease has a poorer prognosis for recovery because of the tremendous demands placed on the body by a burn injury. The patient with diabetes mellitus or peripheral vascular disease is at high risk for poor healing especially with leg and foot burns (Somerset, Coffey, Jones, et al., 2014) General physical debilitation from any chronic disease—including alcoholism, drug abuse, or malnutrition—renders the patient less physiologically able to recover from a burn injury. In addition, the patient with a burn injury who has concurrently sustained other injuries—fractures, head injuries, or other trauma—has a poorer prognosis for recovery.

PHASES OF BURN MANAGEMENT

Historically, burn management has been organized chronologically into three phases that correspond to the key priority of each particular phase: emergent (resuscitative), acute (wound healing), and rehabilitative (restorative). Care overlaps from one phase to another. For example, although the emergent phase is seen as

beginning in the emergency department, care often begins in the prehospital phase, depending on the skill level of paramedics at the scene. Planning for rehabilitation begins on the day of the burn injury or admission to the burn unit. Formal rehabilitation begins as soon as functional assessment can be performed. Wound care is the primary focus of the acute phase, but it also takes place in both the emergent and rehabilitative phases.

PREHOSPITAL CARE

At the injury scene, priority is given to removing the person from the source of the burn and stopping the burning process. Rescuers must also protect themselves from being injured. In the case of electrical and chemical injuries, initial management involves removal of the patient from the electrical or chemical source.

Small thermal burns (<10% of TBSA) should be covered with a clean, cool, tap water–dampened towel for the patient's comfort and protection until definitive medical care is instituted. Cooling of the injured area (if small) within 1 minute helps minimize the depth of the injury. If the burn area is large (>10% TBSA) or an electrical or inhalation burn is suspected and the patient is unresponsive, attention needs to be focused first on CAB (**c**irculation, **a**irway, **b**reathing):

- *Circulation:* Check for presence of pulses and elevate the burned limb(s) above the heart to decrease pain and swelling.
- *Airway:* Check for patency, soot around nares and on the tongue, singed nasal hair, darkened oral or nasal membranes.
- *Breathing:* Check for adequacy of ventilation.

If the patient is responsive, the nurse's priorities would follow the order of the ABCs: **a**irway, **b**reathing, and **c**irculation.

To prevent hypothermia, large burns should be cooled for no more than 10 minutes. Do not immerse the burned body part in cold water because doing so might lead to extensive heat loss. Never cover a burn with ice because this can cause hypothermia and vasoconstriction of blood vessels, further reducing blood flow to the injury. Gently remove as much burned clothing as possible to prevent further tissue damage. Adherent clothing should be left in place until the patient is transferred to a hospital. The patient should be wrapped in a dry, clean sheet or blanket to prevent further contamination of the wound and to provide warmth.

Chemical burns are best treated by quickly removing the solid particles and powder from the skin. (For information on handling specific agents, refer to a hazardous materials text.)

Watch patients with inhalation injuries closely for signs of respiratory distress or compromise. Patients who have both body burns and inhalation injury must be transferred to the nearest burn unit.

Patients with burns may also have sustained other injuries that take priority over the burn wound. It is important for individuals involved in the prehospital phase of burn care to adequately communicate the circumstances of the injury to hospital-based health care providers. This is especially important when the patient's injury involves entrapment in a closed space, hazardous chemicals, electricity, or possible trauma (e.g., fall).

Prehospital management and emergency management are described for chemical burns in Table 27-7, for inhalation injury in Table 27-8, for electrical burns in Table 27-9, and for thermal burns in Table 27-10.

EMERGENT PHASE

The *emergent (resuscitative) phase* is the period of time required to resolve the immediate, life-threatening problems resulting from the burn injury (Hampson, Piantadosi, Thom, et al., 2012). This phase usually lasts up to 72 hours from the time of the burn. Primary concerns are the onset of hypovolemic shock and formation of edema. The phase ends when fluid mobilization and diuresis begin.

Pathophysiological Changes

Fluid and Electrolyte Shifts. The greatest initial threat to a patient with a major burn is hypovolemic shock. It is caused by a massive shift of fluids out of the blood vessels as a result of increased capillary permeability and can begin as early as 20 minutes after the burn injury. As the capillary walls become more permeable, water, sodium, and, later, plasma proteins (especially albumin) move into interstitial spaces and other surrounding tissue (Figure 27-5). The colloidal osmotic pressure decreases with progressive loss of protein from the vascular space. This results in the shifting of more fluid out of the vascular space into the interstitial spaces (Figure 27-6). (Fluid accumulation in the interstitium is termed *second spacing*.) Fluid also moves to areas that normally have minimal to no fluid, a phenomenon termed *third spacing*. Examples of third spacing in burn injury are exudate and blister formation, as well as edema in nonburned areas.

Other sources of fluid loss during this period are insensible losses by evaporation from large, denuded body surfaces and the respiratory system. The normal insensible loss of 30 to 50 mL per hour is increased in severely burned patients. The net result

---

✚ TABLE 27-7 EMERGENCY MANAGEMENT

Chemical Burns

Cause	Assessment Findings	Interventions
• Acids • Alkalis • Organic compounds	• Burning • Redness, swelling of injured tissue • Degeneration of exposed tissue • Discoloration of injured skin • Localized pain • Edema of surrounding tissue • Degeneration of exposed tissue (tissue destruction continuing for up to 72 hr) • Respiratory distress if chemical inhaled • Decreased muscle coordination (if organophosphate is involved) • Paralysis	**Initial** 1. If unresponsive, assess circulation, airway, and breathing before decontamination procedures are done. 2. If responsive, monitor airway, breathing, and circulation before decontamination procedures are done. 3. Stabilize cervical spine. 4. Provide supplemental oxygen as needed. 5. Anticipate intubation with significant inhalation injury, circumferential full-thickness burns to the neck and trunk, or large TBSA burn. 6. Brush dry chemical from skin before irrigation. 7. Remove nonadherent clothing, shoes, watches, jewellery, and, if face was exposed, glasses or contact lenses. 8. Flush chemical from wound and surrounding area with copious amounts of saline solution or water. 9. For chemical burn of the eye, flush from inner to outer corner of eye with water unless lactated Ringer's solution is available. 10. Cover burned areas with dry dressings or clean sheet. 11. Establish IV access with two large-bore catheters if burn >15% TBSA. 12. Begin fluid replacement. 13. Insert urinary catheter if adult burn >15% TBSA. 14. Elevate burned limb above level of heart to decrease edema. 15. Administer IV analgesic drug and assess effectiveness frequently. 16. Contact poison control centre for assistance. **Ongoing Monitoring** • Monitor airway if patient was exposed to chemicals. • Monitor urine output. • Consider possibility of systemic effect of identified chemical, and monitor and treat accordingly. • Monitor pH of eye if eye was exposed to chemicals. • Monitor pain level.

IV, intravenous; *TBSA*, total body surface area.

✚ TABLE 27-8 EMERGENCY MANAGEMENT

Inhalation Injury

Cause	Assessment Findings	Interventions
• Exposure of respiratory tract to intense heat or flames • Inhalation of noxious chemicals, smoke, or carbon monoxide	• History of being trapped in an enclosed space, of being in an explosion, or of clothing catching fire • Rapid, shallow respirations • Increasing hoarseness • Coughing • Singed nasal or facial hair • Darkened oral or nasal membranes • Smoky breath • Carbonaceous sputum • Productive cough with black, grey, or bloody sputum • Irritation of upper airways or burning pain in throat or trunk • Difficulty swallowing • Cherry-red skin colour (carbon monoxide levels >20%) • Restlessness, anxiety • Altered mental status, including confusion, coma • Decreased oxygen saturation • Dysrhythmias	**Initial** 1. If unresponsive, assess circulation, airway, and breathing. 2. If responsive, monitor airway, breathing, and circulation. 3. Stabilize cervical spine. 4. Assess for inhalation injury. 5. Assess for concurrent thermal burn. 6. Provide 100% humidified oxygen. 7. Monitor vital signs, level of consciousness, oxygen saturation, and cardiac rhythm. 8. Remove nonadherent clothing, jewellery, and, if face was exposed, glasses or contact lenses. 9. Establish IV access with two large-bore catheters if burn >15% TBSA. 10. Begin fluid replacement. 11. Insert urinary catheter if burn >15% TBSA. 12. Elevate burned limb(s) above level of heart to decrease edema. 13. Measure arterial blood gas and carboxyhemoglobin levels, and obtain chest radiograph. 14. Administer IV analgesic drug and assess effectiveness frequently. 15. Identify and treat other associated injuries (e.g., fractures, pneumothorax, head injury). 16. Cover burned areas with dry dressings or clean sheet if TBSA is large or patient is hypothermic; can cover with normal saline–moistened gauze and clean sheet if TBSA is small. 17. Anticipate need for fibre-optic bronchoscopy or intubation. **Ongoing Monitoring** • Monitor airway, breathing, and circulation. • Monitor urine output. • Monitor vital signs, level of consciousness, respiratory status, oxygen saturation, and cardiac rhythm. • Monitor pain level.

IV, intravenous; *TBSA*, total body surface area.

of the fluid shifts and losses is intravascular volume depletion. Decreased blood pressure (BP), increased heart rate, and other manifestations of hypovolemic shock are clinically detectable signs of intravascular volume depletion (see Chapter 69). If it is not corrected, irreversible shock and death may result. The circulatory status is also impaired because of hemolysis of RBCs. The RBCs are hemolyzed by circulating factors (e.g., oxygen free radicals) released at the time of the burn, as well as by the direct insult of the burn injury. Thrombosis in the capillaries of burned tissue causes an additional loss of circulating RBCs. Elevation of the hematocrit is commonly caused by hemoconcentration, which results from fluid loss. After fluid balance has been restored, hematocrit levels lower as a result of dilution.

Major shifts in sodium and potassium also occur during this phase. Sodium rapidly shifts to the interstitial spaces and remains there until edema formation ceases (Figure 27-7). A potassium shift develops initially because injured cells and hemolyzed RBCs release potassium into the circulation. (Fluid and electrolyte shifts are discussed in Chapter 19.)

Toward the end of the emergent phase, capillary membrane permeability is restored if fluid replacement is adequate. Fluid loss and edema formation cease. Interstitial fluid gradually returns to the vascular space (see Figure 27-7). Clinically, diuresis is noted with low urine specific gravities.

Inflammation and Healing. Burn injury causes coagulation necrosis, in which tissues and vessels are damaged or destroyed. Neutrophils and monocytes accumulate at the site of injury. Fibroblasts and newly formed collagen fibrils appear and begin wound repair within the first 6 to 12 hours after injury. (The inflammatory response is discussed in Chapter 14.)

Immunological Changes. Burn injury causes widespread impairment of the immune system. The skin barrier to invading organisms is destroyed, bone marrow depression occurs, and circulating levels of immunoglobulins decrease. The function of white blood cells (WBCs) becomes defective. The inflammatory cytokine cascade triggered by tissue damage impairs the function of lymphocytes, monocytes, and neutrophils. This impaired function increases the patient's risk for infection.

Clinical Manifestations

Patients with burns are likely to be in shock from hypovolemia. In many cases, areas of full-thickness and deep partial-thickness burns are initially anaesthetic because nerve endings have been destroyed. Superficial to moderate partial-thickness burns are painful. Blisters, filled with fluid and protein, may develop in partial-thickness burns. Fluid is not actually lost from the body as much as it is sequestered in the interstitium and third spaces. Patients with a larger burn area may have signs of adynamic

TABLE 27-9   EMERGENCY MANAGEMENT

Electrical Burns

Cause	Assessment Findings	Interventions
Alternating Current • Electrical wires • Utility wires **Direct Current** • Lightning • Defibrillator	• Leathery, white, or charred skin • Burn odour • Loss of consciousness • Impaired touch sensation • Minimal or no pain • Dysrhythmias • Cardiac arrest • Location of contact points • Diminished peripheral circulation in injured extremity • Thermal burns if clothing ignited • Fractures or dislocations from force of current • Head or neck injury if fall occurred • Depth and extent of wound difficult to visualize (injury should be presumed more severe than what is seen)	**Initial** 1. Remove patient from electric source while protecting rescuer. 2. If unresponsive, assess circulation, airway, and breathing. 3. If responsive, monitor airway, breathing, and circulation. 4. Stabilize cervical spine. 5. Provide supplemental oxygen as needed. 6. Monitor vital signs, level of consciousness, respiratory status, oxygen saturation, and cardiac rhythm. 7. Check pulses distal to burns. 8. Remove nonadherent clothing, shoes, watches, jewellery, and, if face was exposed, glasses or contact lenses. 9. Cover burned areas with dry dressing or clean sheet if TBSA is large or patient is hypothermic; can cover with normal saline–moistened gauze and dry sheet if TBSA is small. 10. Establish IV access with two large-bore catheters if burn >15% TBSA. 11. Begin fluid replacement. 12. Measure arterial blood gas to assess acid–base balance. 13. Insert urinary catheter if burn >15% TBSA. 14. Elevate burned limb(s) above level of heart to decrease edema. 15. Administer IV analgesic drug and assess effectiveness frequently. 16. Identify and treat other associated injuries (e.g., fractures, pneumothorax, head injury). **Ongoing Monitoring** • Monitor airway, breathing, and circulation. • Monitor vital signs, cardiac rhythm, level of consciousness, respiratory status, oxygen saturation, and neuro-vascular status of injured limbs. • Monitor urine output. • Monitor serum creatine kinase for development of myoglobinuria secondary to muscle breakdown and urine for hemoglobinuria secondary to RBC breakdown. • Anticipate possible administration of NaHCO₃ to alkalinize the urine and maintain serum pH >6.0. • Monitor pain level.

IV, intravenous; *NaHCO₃,* sodium bicarbonate; *RBC,* red blood cell; *TBSA,* total body surface area.

ileus, such as absent or decreased bowel sounds, as a result of the body's response to massive trauma and potassium shifts. Shivering may occur as a result of chilling caused by heat loss, anxiety, or pain. Ongoing nursing assessment of the ABCs, vital signs, cardiac rhythm, oxygenation, and level of consciousness are priorities during the emergent phase of burn care.

Most patients with burn injuries are quite alert and can provide answers to questions shortly after the injury or until they are intubated. They are often frightened and benefit from calm reassurance and simple explanations by all health care providers. Unconsciousness or altered mental status in a patient with burn injury is usually not a result of the burn. The most common reason for unconsciousness or altered mental status is hypoxia associated with smoke inhalation. Other possibilities include head trauma, history of substance abuse, or excessive amounts of sedation or pain medication.

Complications

The three major organ systems most susceptible to complications during the emergent phase of burn injury are the cardiovascular, respiratory, and urinary systems.

Cardiovascular System. Cardiovascular system complications include dysrhythmias and hypovolemic shock, which may progress to irreversible shock. Circulation to the extremities can be severely impaired by deep, circumferential burns and subsequent edema formation. These processes occlude the blood supply by acting like a tourniquet. If they are untreated, ischemia, paresthesias, and necrosis can occur. To restore circulation to compromised extremities, an escharotomy (a scalpel or electrocautery incision into necrotic tissue) is frequently performed after the patient's transfer to a burn unit (Figure 27-8).

Initially, blood viscosity increases with burn injuries because of fluid loss occurring in the emergent period. Microcirculation is impaired because of damage to skin structures containing small capillary systems. These two events result in a phenomenon termed *sludging.* Sludging can be corrected by adequate fluid replacement.

Respiratory System. The respiratory system is especially vulnerable to two types of injury: (a) upper airway burns, which cause edema formation and obstruction of the airway, and (b) lower airway injury (see Table 27-3). Upper airway distress may occur with or without smoke inhalation, and airway injury at either level may occur in the absence of burn injury to the skin.

Upper Airway Injury. Upper airway injury results from an inhalation injury to the mouth, oropharynx, or larynx. The injury may be caused by thermal burns or the inhalation of hot air, steam, or smoke. Mucosal burns of the oropharynx and larynx are manifested by redness, blistering, and edema. The swelling

TABLE 27-10   EMERGENCY MANAGEMENT

Thermal Burns

Cause	Assessment Findings	Interventions
• Hot liquids or solids • Flash flame • Open flame • Steam • Hot surface • UV rays	**Partial-Thickness Burn** ***Superficial; First-Degree Burn*** • Redness • Pain • Moderate to severe tenderness • Minimal edema • Blanching with pressure ***Deep; Second-Degree Burn*** • Moist blebs, blisters • Mottled white, pink to cherry red • Hypersensitive to touch or air • Moderate to severe pain • Blanching with pressure **Full-Thickness; Third- or Fourth-Degree Burn** • Dry, leathery eschar • White, waxy, dark brown, or charred appearance • Strong burn odour • Impaired sensation when touched • Absence of pain with severe pain in surrounding tissues • Lack of blanching with pressure	**Initial** 1. If unresponsive, assess circulation, airway, and breathing. If responsive, monitor airway, breathing, and circulation. 2. Stabilize cervical spine. 3. Assess for inhalation injury. 4. Provide supplemental oxygen as needed. 5. Anticipate endotracheal intubation and mechanical ventilation with circumferential, full-thickness burns to the neck, trunk, or both or with large TBSA. 6. Monitor vital signs, level of consciousness, respiratory status, oxygen saturation, and cardiac rhythm. 7. Remove nonadherent clothing, shoes, watches, jewellery, and, if face was exposed, glasses or contact lenses. 8. Cover burned areas with dry dressings or clean sheet if TBSA is large or patient is hypothermic; cover with normal saline–moistened gauze and dry sheet if TBSA is small. 9. Establish IV access with two large-bore catheters if burn >15% TBSA. 10. Begin fluid replacement. 11. Insert urinary catheter if burn >15% TBSA. 12. Elevate burned limb(s) above level of heart to decrease edema. 13. Administer IV analgesic drug and assess effectiveness frequently. 14. Identify and treat other associated injuries (e.g., fractures, pneumothorax, head injury). **Ongoing Monitoring** • Monitor airway, breathing, and circulation. • Monitor vital signs, cardiac rhythm, level of consciousness, respiratory status, and oxygen saturation. • Monitor urine output. • Monitor pain level.

IV, intravenous; *TBSA*, total body surface area; *UV*, ultraviolet.

can be massive, and the onset rapid. Flame burns to the neck and chest may make breathing more difficult because of burn eschar, which becomes tight and constricting from underlying edema. Swelling from scald burns to the face and neck can also be lethal, as can external pressure from edema pressing on the airway. Mechanical obstruction can occur quickly, presenting a true airway emergency.

Carefully assess the patient for facial burns, singed nasal hair, hoarseness, painful swallowing, darkened oral and nasal membranes, carbonaceous sputum, history of being burned in an enclosed space, and clothing burns around the neck and trunk.

Lower Airway Injury. An inhalation injury to the trachea, bronchioles, and alveoli is usually caused by breathing in toxic chemicals or smoke. Tissue damage is related to the duration of exposure to toxic fumes or smoke. Clinical manifestations of lower airway lung injury are presented in Table 27-3. Pulmonary edema may not appear until 12 to 48 hours after the burn and may manifest as acute respiratory distress syndrome (ARDS) (see Chapter 70).

Other Cardiopulmonary Problems. Burn-injured patients with pre-existing heart disease (e.g., myocardial infarction) or lung disease (e.g., chronic obstructive pulmonary disease) are at risk for complications. If fluid replacement is too vigorous, these patients can develop heart failure or pulmonary edema. Invasive measures (e.g., hemodynamic monitoring) may be necessary to monitor fluid resuscitation.

Burn-injured patients with pre-existing respiratory problems are more likely to develop a respiratory infection. Pneumonia is a common complication of major burns and the leading cause of death in patients with inhalation injury. Debilitation, abundant microbial flora, and relative immobility predispose such patients to the development of pneumonia.

Urinary System. The most common complication of the urinary system in the emergent phase is ATN. If the patient becomes hypovolemic, blood flow to the kidneys decreases, causing renal ischemia. If the decreased flow rate continues, acute kidney injury may develop.

With full-thickness and electrical burns, myoglobin (from muscle cell breakdown) and hemoglobin (from RBC breakdown) are released into the bloodstream and occlude renal tubules. Adequate fluid replacement and diuretics can counteract myoglobin and hemoglobin obstruction of the tubules.

NURSING AND COLLABORATIVE MANAGEMENT EMERGENT PHASE

In the emergent phase, patient survival depends on rapid and thorough assessment and intervention (Fahlstrom, Boyle, & Makic, 2013). The nurse and physician make the initial assessment of depth and extent of the burn and coordinate the actions of the health care team. In a community hospital, decisions must be made as to whether the patient requires inpatient or outpatient

PATHOPHYSIOLOGY MAP

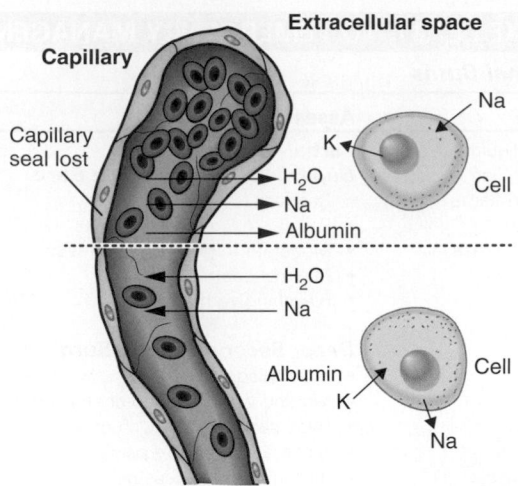

FIGURE 27-7 The effects of burn shock are shown above the dotted line. As the capillary seal is lost, interstitial edema develops. The cellular integrity is also altered, with sodium *(Na)* moving into the cell in abnormal amounts and potassium *(K)* leaving the cell. The shifts after the resolution of burn shock are shown below the dotted line. The water and sodium move back into the circulating volume through the capillary. The albumin remains in the interstitium. Potassium is transported into the cell, and sodium is transported out as the cellular integrity returns.

FIGURE 27-5 At the time of a major burn injury, there is increased capillary permeability. All fluid components of the blood begin to leak into the interstitium, causing edema and a decrease in blood volume. Hematocrit increases, and the blood becomes more viscous. The combination of decreased blood volume and increased viscosity produces increased peripheral resistance. Burn shock, a type of hypovolemic shock, rapidly ensues, and, if it is not corrected, death can result.

FIGURE 27-8 Escharotomies of the anterior chest and arm (indicated by *arrows*). Source: Courtesy Judy A. Knighton, RN, MScN, Toronto.

FIGURE 27-6 A, Facial edema before fluid resuscitation. **B,** Facial edema after 24 hours. Source: Courtesy Judy Knighton, Toronto, Canada.

care and, in the case of inpatient care, whether the patient remains in that hospital or is transferred to the closest regional burn unit (see Table 27-5). From the onset of the burn event until the patient is stabilized, nursing and collaborative management consist predominantly of airway management, fluid therapy, and wound care (Table 27-11).

Although burn management can be chronologically categorized as emergent, acute, and rehabilitative, overall care requirements are not so easily classified. Depending on the severity of the patient's condition, the duration of time spent in each phase varies greatly, and conditions improve and worsen unpredictably on a daily basis. Care changes accordingly. Whereas physiotherapy and occupational therapy are a focus of the acute and rehabilitative phases, proper positioning and splinting begin at the time of admission. Support and teaching of patients and caregivers begin on admission and intensify in the rehabilitative phase. See the accompanying nursing care plan NCP 27-1 (Patient With a Thermal Burn Injury) on the Evolve website.

TABLE 27-11 COLLABORATIVE CARE

Patient With Burn Injury

Emergent Phase	Acute Phase	Rehabilitation Phase
Fluid Therapy • Assess fluid needs.* • Begin IV fluid replacement. • Insert urinary catheter. • Monitor intake and output. **Wound Care** • Start daily shower/cleansing and wound care. • Debride as necessary. • Assess extent and depth of burns. • Administer tetanus toxoid or tetanus antitoxin. **Pain and Anxiety** • Assess and manage pain and anxiety. **Psychosocial Care** • Provide support to patient and family during initial crisis phase. **Respiratory Therapy** • Assess oxygenation needs. • Provide supplemental oxygen as needed. • Intubate if necessary. • Monitor respiratory status. **Physiotherapy and Occupational Therapy** • Place patient in position that prevents contracture formation and reduces edema. • Assess need for splints or devices such as pressure relief/reduction mattresses to decrease tissue ischemia and potential for skin breakdown. • Turn and reposition patient frequently to allow for appropriate circulation to tissues. **Nutritional Therapy** • Assess nutritional needs and begin feeding patient by most appropriate route as soon as possible.	**Fluid Therapy** • Continue to monitor intake and output. • Continue to replace fluids, depending on patient's clinical response. **Wound Care** • Continue daily shower and wound care. • Assess wound daily and adjust dressing protocols as necessary. • Observe for complications (e.g., infection). • Continue debridement (if necessary). **Pain and Anxiety** • Continue to assess for and treat pain and anxiety. **Psychosocial Care** • Continue to provide ongoing support, counselling, and education to patient and family about physical and emotional aspects of care and recovery. • Begin to anticipate discharge needs. **Respiratory Therapy** • Continue to assess oxygenation needs. • Continue to monitor respiratory status. • Monitor for signs of complications (e.g., pneumonia). **Physiotherapy and Occupational Therapy** • Have patient begin daily therapy program for maintenance of range of motion. • Assess need for splints and anticontracture positioning. • Encourage and assist patient with self-care as possible. **Nutritional Therapy** • Continue to assess diet to support wound healing. **Other Therapy** ***Early Excision and Grafting*** • Provide temporary homografts. • Provide permanent autografts. • Care for donor sites. ***Drug Therapy*** • Assess need for medications. • Continue to monitor effectiveness of and necessity for medications. • Titrate medications and discontinue as appropriate.	• Continue to counsel and teach patient and caregiver about wound care. • Discuss possible need for home care to continue wound care in the community. • Continue to counsel and teach patient and family. • Continue to encourage and assist patient in resuming self-care. • Continue to prevent or minimize contractures (surgery, physiotherapy and occupational therapy, splinting, or pressure garments), and assess likelihood for scarring. • Discuss possible reconstructive surgery. Prepare for discharge home or transfer to rehabilitation unit or hospital.

IV, intravenous.
*See Tables 27-12, 27-13, and 27-14.

AIRWAY MANAGEMENT

Airway management frequently involves early endotracheal (preferably orotracheal) intubation. Early intubation eliminates the necessity for emergency tracheostomy after respiratory problems have become apparent. In general, patients with major injuries that include burns to the face and neck require intubation within 1 to 2 hours after burn injury. (Intubation is discussed in Chapter 68.) After intubation, such patients are placed on ventilatory assistance, and the delivered oxygen concentration is determined from an assessment of arterial blood gas (ABG) values. Extubation may be indicated when the edema resolves, usually 3 to 6 days after burn injury, unless severe inhalation injury is involved. Escharotomies of the trunk may be needed to relieve respiratory distress secondary to circumferential, full-thickness burns to the neck and trunk (see Figure 27-8).

Within 6 to 12 hours after injury in which smoke inhalation is suspected, a fibre-optic bronchoscopy should be performed to assess the lower airway. Significant findings include the appearance of carbonaceous material, mucosal edema, vesicles, erythema, hemorrhage, and ulceration.

When intubation is not performed, treatment of inhalation injury includes administration of 100% humidified oxygen as needed. Patients should be placed in a high Fowler's position unless it is contraindicated (e.g., because of spinal injury), and coughing and deep breathing every hour should be encouraged. Patients should be repositioned every 1 to 2 hours, and chest physiotherapy and suctioning performed as necessary. If respiratory failure develops, intubation and mechanical ventilation are initiated. Positive end-expiratory pressure may be used to prevent collapse of the alveoli and progressive respiratory failure (see Chapter 68). Bronchodilators may be administered to treat severe bronchospasm. Carbon monoxide poisoning is treated by administering 100% oxygen until carboxyhemoglobin levels return to normal. The use of hyperbaric oxygen therapy to treat carbon monoxide poisoning is contraindicated in the presence of a body burn as it delays important burn care.

FLUID THERAPY

Establishing IV access that can accommodate large volumes of fluid is critical for fluid resuscitation and medication administration. At least two large-bore IV access routes must be obtained for patients with burns over more than 15% TBSA. For patients with burns over more than 30% TBSA, a central line for fluid and medication administration, as well as a line for blood sampling, should be considered if frequent ABGs or invasive BP monitoring is needed.

A standardized chart is used to assess the extent of the burn wound (see Figure 27-4), allowing for accurate estimation of fluid resuscitation requirements.

The type of fluid replacement is determined by size and depth of burn, age of the patient, and individual considerations, such as pre-existing chronic illness. Fluid replacement is accomplished with crystalloid solutions (usually lactated Ringer's solution), colloids (albumin), or a combination of the two. Paramedics generally administer IV saline until the patient's arrival at the hospital.

The Parkland (Baxter) formula for fluid replacement is the formula most commonly used to estimate fluid replacement (Table 27-12; see also the Parkland Formula for Burns calculator in the Resources for this chapter). It is important to remember that all formulas yield estimates, which must be titrated on the basis of the patient's physiological response. For example, in

| TABLE 27-12 | FLUID RESUSCITATION WITH THE PARKLAND (BAXTER) FORMULA* |

Formula
4 mL of lactated Ringer's solution per kilogram of body weight per percentage of TBSA burned = Total fluid requirements for first 24 hr after burn

Application
50% of total in first 8 hr
25% of total in second 8 hr
25% of total in third 8 hr

Example
For a 70-kg patient with a burn on 50% of TBSA:

4 mL × 70 kg × 50% of TBSA burned	= 14 000 mL, or 14 L, in 24 hr
50% of total in first 8 hr	= 7 000 mL (875 mL/hr)
25% of total in second 8 hr	= 3 500 mL (438 mL/hr)
25% of total in third 8 hr	= 3 500 mL (438 mL/hr)

TBSA, total body surface area.
*Formulas are guidelines. Fluid is administered at a rate to produce 0.5–1.0 mL/kg/hr of urine output.

patients with an electrical injury or inhalation injury, fluid requirements may be greater than normal and include an osmotic diuretic (mannitol) and sodium bicarbonate to alkalize the urine. Too much fluid and overestimation of TBSA contribute to the development of fluid over-resuscitation or "fluid creep" (Fahlstrom, Boyle, & Makic, 2013).

Colloidal solutions (e.g., albumin) may be given. However, administration is recommended in the first 12 to 24 hours after the burn injury, when capillary permeability returns to normal or near normal. After this time, the plasma remains in the vascular space and expands the circulating volume. The replacement volume is calculated on the basis of the patient's body weight and TBSA burned (e.g., 0.3 to 0.5 mL/kg per percentage of TBSA burned).

The adequacy of fluid replacement is best assessed according to clinical parameters. Urine output, the most commonly used parameter, and cardiac parameters are defined as follows:
1. *Urine output:* The goal is generally 0.5 to 1 mL/kg/hour for most patients with burn injuries but increases to 75 to 100 mL/ hour for patients with an electrical burn and evidence of hemoglobinuria or myoglobinuria.
2. *Cardiac factors:* Mean arterial pressure is greater than 65 mm Hg, systolic BP is greater than 90 mm Hg, and heart rate is less than 120 beats/minute. Mean arterial pressure and BP are most appropriately measured by means of an arterial line. Peripheral measurement is often invalid because of vasoconstriction and edema.

WOUND CARE

Once a patent airway, adequate circulation, and adequate fluid replacement have been established, the priority is care of the burn wound. Full-thickness burn wounds are dry and waxy white to dark brown or black and have only minor, localized sensation because nerve endings have largely been destroyed. Partial-thickness burn wounds appear pink to cherry red and are wet and shiny with serous exudate. These wounds may or may not have intact blisters and are painful when touched or open to air due to exposed nerve endings.

FIGURE 27-9 Cart shower. Showering presents an opportunity for wound care and physiotherapy. Source: Courtesy Judy A. Knighton, RN, MScN, Toronto.

FIGURE 27-10 Surgical debridement of full-thickness burns is necessary to prepare the wound for grafting. Source: Courtesy Judy Knighton, Toronto, Canada.

Cleansing and gentle debridement, with the use of scissors and forceps, can occur on a cart shower (Figure 27-9), a regular shower, or the patient's bed or stretcher. Extensive, surgical debridement is performed in the operating room (Figure 27-10). During **debridement**, necrotic skin is removed from the wound to prevent infection and promote healing. Releasing escharotomies and fasciotomies can be carried out in the emergent phase, usually in burn units by burn physicians.

Patients find the initial wound care to be both physically and psychologically demanding. Patients are showered with tap water not exceeding 40°C. A once-daily shower and dressing change in the morning, followed by a dressing change in the patient's room in the evening, are part of a common routine in many burn units. Some of the newer antimicrobial dressings can be left in place from 3 to 14 days, thereby decreasing the frequency of dressing changes.

Infection is the most serious risk, leading to further tissue injury and possible sepsis (Shahrokhi, 2014). The source of infection in burn wounds is the patient's own flora, predominantly from the skin (burned and unburned), respiratory tract, and gastro-intestinal tract. The prevention of cross-contamination between one patient and another is a priority for all members of the health care team.

Two approaches to burn wound treatment are the open method and the closed method, using multiple dressing changes. In the *open method*, the patient's burn is covered with a topical anti-microbial and has no dressing over the wound. In the *multiple-dressing change* or *closed method*, sterile gauze dressings are impregnated with or laid over a topical antimicrobial. These dressings are changed at various intervals, from every 12 to 24 hours to once every 14 days, depending on the product. Most burn units support the concept of moist wound healing and use dressings to cover the burned areas, except for the burned face.

When the patient's open burn wounds are exposed, staff must wear personal protective equipment (e.g., disposable hats, masks, gowns, gloves). When removing contaminated dressings and washing the dirty wound, the nurse may use nonsterile, disposable gloves. Sterile gloves, however, are used when applying ointments and sterile dressings. In addition, the room must be kept warm (approximately 30°C) to prevent the patient from using up valuable calories through shivering. When finished treating one patient, the nurse removes all personal protective equipment and dons new personal protective equipment before treating another patient to avoid transmitting organisms from one patient to another. Careful handwashing and the use of alcohol-based hand rub, both inside and outside each patient room, is also necessary to prevent cross-contamination. After the dressing change is completed, the equipment and immediate environment are thoroughly cleaned and disinfected. The use of plastic liners on equipment is helpful in reducing the potential contamination of the equipment and facilitates cleaning.

Coverage is the primary goal for burn wounds. In the major burn wound (>50% TBSA), there is rarely enough unburned skin for immediate grafting. This necessitates the use of other temporary wound closure methods. *Allograft (homograft) skin* (from a cadaver skin bank) is used, along with newer biosynthetic options, with varying frequency among burn units (Table 27-13).

OTHER CARE MEASURES

For certain parts of the body (e.g., face, eyes, hands, arms, ears, perineum), nursing care must be particularly meticulous. The face is highly vascular and subject to a great amount of edema. It is often covered with ointments and gauze but not wrapped, to limit pressure on delicate facial structures. Eye care for corneal burns or edema includes antibiotic ointments. All patients with facial burns should undergo an ophthalmological examination soon after admission. Periorbital edema can prevent opening of the eyes and be frightening to the patient. The nurse should provide assurance that the swelling is not permanent. Instillation of methyl cellulose drops or artificial tears into the eyes for moisture provides additional comfort for patients.

Burned hands and arms should be extended and elevated on pillows to minimize edema. Splints may need to be applied to maintain them in positions of function. Ears should be kept free of pressure because of their poor vascularization and predisposition to infection. A patient with ear burns should not rest the head on pillows because pressure on the cartilage may cause chondritis and the ear may stick to the pillowcase, causing pain and bleeding. The patient's head can be elevated with a rolled towel placed under the shoulders, with care to avoid pressure necrosis. The same holds true for a patient with neck burns. Pillows are removed and a rolled towel is placed under the shoulders to hyperextend the neck and prevent neck wound contracture.

TABLE 27-13 SOURCES OF GRAFTS

Source	Graft Name	Coverage
Porcine skin	Heterograft or xenograft (different species)	Temporary (3 days to 2 wk)
Cadaveric skin	Homograft or allograft (same species)	Temporary (3 days to 2 wk)
Patient's own skin	Autograft	Permanent
Patient's own skin and cell cultures	Cultured epithelial autograft (CEA)	Permanent
Porcine collagen bonded to silicone membrane	Biobrane	Temporary (10–21 days)
Bovine collagen and glycosaminoglycan bonded to silicone membrane	Integra	Permanent
Acellular dermal matrix derived from donated human skin	AlloDerm	Permanent
Donated neonatal foreskin fibroblasts and keratinocytes in bovine collagen sponge	OrCel	Permanent
Donated neonatal foreskin fibroblasts and keratinocytes in bovine collagen gel	Apligraf	Permanent
Bovine collagen and elastin matrix	MatriDerm	Permanent

TABLE 27-14 DRUG THERAPY

Drugs Commonly Used in Burn Treatment

Types and Names of Drugs	Purpose
Nutritional Support	
Vitamins A, C, E, and multivitamins	Promote wound healing
Minerals: zinc, iron (ferrous sulphate)	Promote cell integrity and hemoglobin formation
Analgesia	
Morphine (Statex)	Promote pain control
Sustained-release morphine (MS Contin)	
Hydromorphone (Dilaudid)	
Sustained-release hydromorphone (Dilaudid)	
Fentanyl	
Acetaminophen (Tylenol)	
Ibuprofen (Advil)	
Adjuvant analgesics (e.g., gabapentin [Neurontin], pregabalin [Lyrica])	
Sedation–Hypnosis	
Quetiapine (Seroquel)	Produce antipsychotic and sedative effects
Haloperidol (Haldol)	
Lorazepam (Ativan)	Diminish anxiety
Midazolam	Provide short-acting amnestic effects
Ketamine (Ketalar)	
Antidepressant Therapy	
Venlafaxine (Effexor XR)	Reduce depression; improve mood
Citalopram (Celexa)	
Anticoagulation Therapy	
Enoxaparin (Lovenox)	Prevent venous thromboembolism
Heparin	
Gastro-Intestinal Support	
Ranitidine (Zantac)	Decrease stomach acid and risk for Curling's ulcer
Esomeprazole (Nexium)	
Aluminum/magnesium hydroxide (Diovol)	Neutralize stomach acid

The perineum must be kept as clean and dry as possible. In addition to providing hourly urine outputs, an in-dwelling catheter prevents urine contamination of the perineal area.

Routine laboratory tests are performed to monitor fluid and electrolyte balance. ABGs are measured to determine adequacy of ventilation and perfusion in all patients with suspected or confirmed inhalation or electrical injury.

Physiotherapy is begun immediately, sometimes during showering and dressing changes and before new dressings are applied. Early range-of-motion exercises are necessary to facilitate mobilization of the extravasated fluid back into the vascular bed. Exercise also maintains function, prevents contracture, and reassures the patient that movement is still possible.

DRUG THERAPY

ANALGESICS AND SEDATIVES. Analgesics are ordered to promote patient comfort. Early in the postburn period, pain medications should be given intravenously because (a) onset of action is fastest with this route; (b) gastro-intestinal function is slowed or impaired as a result of shock or paralytic ileus; and (c) medications injected intramuscularly are not absorbed adequately in burned or edematous areas, and so medications pool in the tissues. When fluid mobilization begins, interstitial accumulation of previous intramuscular medications could cause inadvertent overdose.

Opioids commonly used for pain control are listed in Table 27-14. The need for analgesia must be re-evaluated frequently because patients' needs may change and tolerance to medications may develop over time. Initially, opioids are the drugs of choice for pain control. Sedative–hypnotics and antidepressant drugs can also be given with analgesics to control the anxiety, insomnia, or depression that patients may experience (see Table 27-14).

Analgesic requirements can vary tremendously from one patient to another. The extent and depth of burn may not be correlated with pain intensity. Hospital pharmacists, psychiatrists, and multidisciplinary pain services are valuable resources for the more complex patient situations. Effective pain control depends on assessment, prompt analgesia with dosages titrated to achieve effect, and regular evaluation.

TETANUS IMMUNIZATION. Tetanus toxoid is given routinely to all patients with burn injuries because of the likelihood of anaerobic contamination of the burn wound. If the patient has not received an active immunization in the 10 years before the burn injury, tetanus immunoglobulin should be considered.

ANTIMICROBIAL AGENTS. After the wound is cleansed, topical agents are applied and covered with a light dressing. Systemic antibiotics are not routinely used to control burn wound flora because there is little or no blood supply to the burn eschar and, consequently, little delivery of the antibiotic to the wound. In addition, the routine use of systemic antibiotics increases the chance of developing multidrug-resistant organisms. Some topical burn agents penetrate the eschar, thereby inhibiting bacterial invasion of the wound. Silver-impregnated dressings (e.g., Acticoat Flex, Aquacel Ag Burn, Exsalt T7) can be left in place anywhere from 3 to 14 days and are effective against many organisms. Silver sulphadiazine (Flamazine) and mafenide acetate (Sulfamylon) creams are also used (Sheckter, Van Vliet, Krishnan, et al., 2014). Sepsis remains a leading cause of death in patients with major burns because it may lead to multiple organ dysfunction syndrome (see Chapter 69). Systemic antibiotic therapy is initiated when invasive burn wound sepsis is clinically diagnosed or when some other source of infection (e.g., pneumonia) is identified.

Fungal infections may develop in the patient's mucous membranes (mouth and genitalia) as a result of systemic antibiotic therapy and low resistance in the host. The offending organism is usually *Candida albicans*. Oral infection is treated with nystatin mouthwash. When a normal diet is resumed, yogourt or *Lactobacillus* may be given by mouth to reintroduce the normal intestinal flora that have been destroyed by antibiotic therapy.

VENOUS THROMBO-EMBOLISM PROPHYLAXIS. For burn-injured patients at risk for venous thrombo-embolism (e.g., those with lower extremity burns, obese patients), if there are no contra-indications, it is recommended that low-molecular-weight heparin (enoxaparin [Lovenox]) or low-dose unfractionated heparin be started as soon as it is considered safe to do so (see Table 27-14). For burn-injured patients who are at high risk for bleeding, it is recommended that mechanical prophylaxis against venous thrombo-embolism, with sequential compression devices or graduated compression stockings, or both, be used until the bleeding risk decreases and heparin can be started (Faraklas, Ghanem, Brown, et al., 2013) (see Table 27-14).

NUTRITIONAL THERAPY

Early and aggressive nutritional support within several hours of the burn injury can decrease mortality risks and complications, optimize healing of the burn wound, and minimize the negative effects of hypermetabolism and catabolism (Jeschke, 2014). Nonintubated patients with a burn over less than 20% TBSA are generally able to eat enough to meet their nutritional requirements. Intubated patients and those with larger burns require additional support. Enteral feedings (gastric or intestinal) have almost entirely replaced parenteral feeding. Early enteral feeding, usually with smaller-bore tubes, preserves gastro-intestinal function, increases intestinal blood flow, promotes optimal conditions for wound healing, and prevents complications (e.g., Curling's ulcer). The patient with a large burn (>20% TBSA) can develop paralytic ileus within a few hours as a result of the body's response to major trauma. If a large nasogastric tube is inserted on admission, gastric residuals should be checked frequently to detect delayed gastric emptying. Bowel sounds should be assessed every 8 hours. In general, feedings can begin slowly at 20 to 40 mL/hour and be increased to the goal rate within 24 to 48 hours.

A *hypermetabolic state* proportional to the size of the wound occurs after a major burn injury. Resting metabolic expenditure may increase by 50% to 100% above normal in patients with major burns. Core temperature is elevated. Catecholamines, which stimulate catabolism and heat production, increase. Massive catabolism can occur and is characterized by protein breakdown and increased gluconeogenesis. Failure to supply adequate calories and protein leads to malnutrition and delayed healing. Calorie-containing nutritional supplements and milkshakes are often administered because of the great need for calories. Protein powder can also be added to food and liquids. Supplemental vitamins may be given as early as the emergent phase, with iron supplements often started in the acute phase (Nordlund, Pham, & Gibran, 2014; see Table 27-14).

ACUTE PHASE

The *acute phase* begins with mobilization of extracellular fluid and subsequent diuresis. This phase concludes when the burned area is completely covered by skin grafts or when the wounds are healed. This may take weeks or many months.

Pathophysiological Changes

Burn injury involves pathophysiological changes in many body systems. Diuresis from fluid mobilization occurs, and the patient becomes less edematous. Areas that are full- or partial-thickness burns are more evident than in the emergent phase. Bowel sounds return. The patient may now become aware of the enormity of the situation and benefit from additional psychosocial support. Some healing begins as WBCs surround the burn wound and phagocytosis occurs. Necrotic tissue begins to slough. Fibroblasts lay down matrices of the collagen precursors that eventually form granulation tissue. A partial-thickness burn wound heals from the edges and the dermal bed below if kept free from infection and *desiccation* (dryness). However, full-thickness burn wounds, unless extremely small, must be covered by skin grafts. In some cases, healing time and length of hospitalization are decreased by early excision and grafting.

Clinical Manifestations

Partial-thickness wounds form eschar, which begins separating fairly soon after injury. Once the eschar is removed, re-epithelialization begins at the wound margins and appears as red or pink scar tissue. Epithelial buds from the dermal bed eventually close in the wound, which then heals spontaneously without surgical intervention, usually within 10 to 21 days.

Margins of full-thickness eschar take longer to separate. As a result, full-thickness wounds necessitate surgical debridement and skin grafting for healing.

Laboratory Values

Because the body is attempting to re-establish fluid and electrolyte homeostasis in the initial acute phase, it is important to monitor serum electrolyte levels closely.

Sodium. *Hyponatremia* can develop from excessive gastro-intestinal suction, diarrhea, and excessive water intake. Manifestations of hyponatremia include weakness, dizziness, muscle cramps, fatigue, headache, tachycardia, and confusion. The patient with burn injuries may also develop *water intoxication*, a dilutional form of hyponatremia. To avoid this condition, the patient should drink fluids other than water, such as juice or nutritional supplements.

Hypernatremia may occur after successful fluid replacement if copious amounts of hypertonic solutions were required. Other causes may be related to tube-feeding therapy or inappropriate fluid administration. Manifestations of hypernatremia include thirst; dry, coated tongue; lethargy; confusion; and possibly seizures.

Potassium. *Hyperkalemia* is noted if the patient has renal failure, adrenocortical insufficiency, or massive deep muscle injury (e.g., electrical burn) and if large amounts of potassium are being released from damaged cells. Cardiac dysrhythmias and ventricular failure can occur with elevated potassium levels. Muscle weakness and electrocardiographic changes are observed clinically (see Chapter 19).

Hypokalemia occurs with vomiting, diarrhea, prolonged gastro-intestinal suction, and prolonged IV therapy without potassium supplementation. Constant potassium loss occurs through the burn wound.

Manifestations of hypokalemia include fatigue, muscle weakness, leg cramps, paresthesias, and decreased reflexes (see Chapter 19).

Complications

Infection. The body's first line of defence, the skin, is destroyed by burn injury. Pathogens often proliferate before phagocytosis has adequately begun. The burn wound becomes colonized with organisms. If the bacterial density at the junction of the eschar with underlying viable tissue rises to greater than 10^5/g of tissue, the burn wound is considered infected. In the presence of an infection, localized inflammation, induration, and sometimes suppuration can occur at the burn wound margins. Partial-thickness burns can convert to full-thickness wounds when the infecting organisms invade viable, adjacent, unburned tissue. Invasive wound infections may be treated with systemic antibiotics on the basis of culture results.

Burn wound infection may progress to transient bacteremia and sepsis as a result of burn wound manipulation (e.g., after showering and debridement). Manifestations of sepsis include hypothermia or hyperthermia, increased heart and respiratory rates, decreased BP, and decreased urine output. Patients may exhibit mild confusion, chills, malaise, and loss of appetite. The WBC count is usually between 10 and 20 $\times 10^9$/L.

There are functional deficits in the WBCs, and the patient remains immuno-suppressed for a time after the burn injury. The causative organisms of sepsis are usually Gram-negative bacteria (e.g., *Pseudomonas, Proteus* organisms), which increase the risk for septic shock.

When sepsis is suspected, cultures are immediately obtained from all possible sources, including the burn wound, blood, urine, sputum, oropharynx, perineal regions, and any invasive line or tube sites. However, treatment should not be delayed pending results of the culture and sensitivity studies. Therapy begins with antibiotics appropriate for the usual residual flora of the particular burn unit. The topical antibiotic in use may be continued or changed to another medication. At this stage, the patient's condition is critical, and vital signs must be monitored closely. Collaboration with infectious disease specialists is important to ensure appropriate antibiotic coverage.

Cardiovascular and Respiratory Systems. The same cardiovascular and respiratory system complications present in the emergent phase may continue into the acute phase of care. In addition, new problems might arise, necessitating timely intervention.

Neurological System. Neurologically, the patient usually has no physical symptoms, unless severe hypoxia from respiratory injuries or complications from electrical injuries occur. However, some patients may demonstrate certain behaviours that are not completely understood. A patient can become extremely disoriented, become withdrawn or combative, or have hallucinations and nightmare-like episodes. Delirium is more acute at night and occurs more often in older patients. Consultation with psychiatric or geriatric services is helpful in quickly diagnosing and treating delirium or similar behaviours. The nurse can then focus on strategies to orient and reassure a confused or agitated patient. Delirium is a transient state, lasting from a day or two to several weeks. Various causes have been considered, including electrolyte imbalance, stress, cerebral edema, sepsis, sleep disturbances, and the use of analgesics and antianxiety drugs.

Musculo-Skeletal System. The musculo-skeletal system is prone to complications during the acute phase. As the burns begin to heal and scar tissue forms, the skin is less supple and pliant. Range of motion may be limited, and contractures can occur. The muscles in the body tend to shorten in a flexed position. The patient should be encouraged to stretch and move the burned body parts as much as possible. Splinting can be beneficial in preventing or reducing contracture formation. Attention to repositioning and the use of devices such as pressure-redistribution mattresses may also be necessary to decrease the potential for tissue ischemia and skin breakdown.

Gastro-Intestinal System. The gastro-intestinal system may also exhibit complications during this phase. Paralytic ileus results from sepsis. Diarrhea may be caused by the use of enteral feedings or antibiotics. Constipation can occur as an adverse effect of opioid analgesics, decreased mobility, and a low-fibre diet. *Curling's ulcer* is a type of gastro-duodenal ulcer characterized by diffuse superficial lesions (including mucosal erosion). It is caused by a generalized stress response to decreased blood flow to the gastro-intestinal tract during the emergent phase; this response results in decreased production of mucus and increased secretion of gastric acid. The best measure for preventing Curling's ulcer is feeding the patient soon after the injury. Antacids, H_2-histamine blockers (e.g., ranitidine [Zantac]), and proton pump inhibitors (e.g., esomeprazole [Nexium]) are used prophylactically to neutralize stomach acids and inhibit the secretion of histamine and hydrochloric acid (see Table 27-14).

Endocrine System. A transient increase in blood glucose levels may occur because of stress-mediated cortisol and catecholamine release, which results in increased mobilization of glycogen stores, gluconeogenesis, and subsequent production of glucose. Insulin production and release also increase. However, insulin's effectiveness decreases because of relative insulin insensitivity; consequently, the blood glucose level becomes elevated. Later, hyperglycemia can be caused by the increased caloric intake necessary to meet metabolic requirements. When hyperglycemia occurs, the treatment is supplemental intravenous insulin, not decreased feeding. Serum glucose levels are checked frequently, and an appropriate amount of insulin is given if hyperglycemia is present. Glucometers may be used to assess blood glucose at the patient's bedside; however, serum glucose samples yield more accurate results. As the patient's metabolic demands are met and less stress is placed on the entire system, this stress-induced condition may be reversed before or at time of discharge.

NURSING AND COLLABORATIVE MANAGEMENT ACUTE PHASE

The predominant therapeutic interventions in the acute phase are (a) wound care, (b) excision and grafting, (c) pain management, (d) physiotherapy and occupational therapy, (e) nutritional therapy, and (f) psychosocial care.

WOUND CARE

The goals of wound care are to (a) prevent infection by cleansing and debriding the area of necrotic tissue that would promote bacterial growth and (b) promote wound re-epithelialization, successful skin grafting, or both.

Wound care consists of daily observation, assessment, cleansing, debridement, and dressing reapplication. Nonsurgical debridement, dressing changes, topical antimicrobial therapy, graft care, and donor site care are performed as necessary, depending on the topical cream or dressing ordered. Wounds are cleansed with soap and water or with normal saline–moistened gauze to gently remove the old antimicrobial agent and any loose necrotic tissue, scabs, or dried blood. During the debridement phase, the wound is covered with topical antimicrobial agents (e.g., silver sulphadiazine, silver-impregnated dressings). When partial-thickness burn wounds have been fully debrided, a protective greasy (paraffin or petroleum) gauze dressing is applied to protect the re-epithelializing cells as they resurface and close the open wound bed. If grafting is necessary, the meshed, split-thickness skin graft may be protected with the same greasy gauze dressings, followed by middle and outer dressings. With facial grafts, the unmeshed sheet graft is left open, so it is possible for *blebs* (serosanguinous exudate) to form between the graft and the recipient bed. Blebs prevent the graft from permanently attaching to the wound itself. The evacuation of blebs is best performed by aspiration with a tuberculin syringe and only by professionals who have received instruction in this specialized skill. (Dressings are discussed in Chapter 14 and Table 14-11.)

EXCISION AND GRAFTING

Current management of full-thickness burn wounds involves early removal of the necrotic tissue, followed by application of split-thickness autograft skin (Kamolz, 2014). In the past, patients with major burns had low rates of survival because healing and wound coverage took so long that patients usually died of sepsis or malnutrition. Currently, as a result of earlier intervention, mortality and morbidity rates have been greatly reduced. Many patients, especially those with major burns, are taken to the operating room for wound excision on day 1 or 2 (resuscitation phase). The wounds are covered with a biological dressing or allograft for temporary coverage until permanent grafting can be accomplished (see Table 27-13).

During the procedure of **excision and grafting**, devitalized tissue (eschar) is removed down to the subcutaneous tissue or the

fascia, depending on the degree of injury. Surgical excision can result in massive blood loss. Topical application of epinephrine or thrombin, application of extremity tourniquets, or application of a fibrin sealant (ARTISS) all work to decrease surgical blood loss.

Once hemostasis has been achieved, a graft is then placed on clean, viable tissue to achieve good adherence. Whenever possible, the freshly excised wound is covered with *autograft* (the person's own) skin (see Table 27-13). Fibrin sealant has been used to attach skin grafts to the wound bed. Grafts can also be stapled or sutured into place (Figure 27-11, A). Negative pressure wound therapy dressings are often placed on top of skin grafts to optimize adherence to the excised bed (Waltzman & Bell, 2014). A temporary allograft (from a cadaver skin bank) can be used to test how the recipient site will accept a graft. The allograft is then removed several days later in the operating room, and an autograft applied.

With early excision, function is restored, and scar tissue formation is minimized. Frequent observation for bleeding and circulation problems and appropriate nursing interventions can help identify and manage complications that would interfere with graft survival. Facial, neck, and hand burns require skillful nursing care to identify and manage clots quickly for the best functional and aesthetic outcomes.

Donor skin from another area of the patient's body is harvested for grafting by means of a dermatome, which removes a thin (14/1000 to 16/1000) split-thickness layer of skin from an unburned site (see Figure 27-11, B). This sample of skin can be meshed (usually a ratio of 1.5:1) to allow for greater wound coverage, or it may be applied as an unmeshed sheet graft for a better cosmetic result when grafting the face, neck, and hands. The site from which this skin was taken now becomes a new open wound.

The goals of donor site care are to promote rapid moist wound healing, decrease pain at the site, and prevent infection. The choices of dressings vary among burn centres and include greasy

FIGURE 27-11 Split-thickness skin grafting. **A,** Freshly applied split-thickness sheet skin graft to the hand. **B,** Split-thickness skin graft is harvested from a patient's thigh using a dermatome. **C,** Donor site is covered with a hydrophilic foam dressing after harvesting. **D,** Healed donor site. Source: Courtesy Judy A. Knighton, RN, MScN, Toronto.

gauze dressings, silver-impregnated dressings, and hydrophilic foam dressings (see Figure 27-11, C). Nursing care of the donor site is specific to the dressing selected. Several of the newer dressing materials offer decreased healing time, which facilitates earlier reharvesting of skin at the same site. The average healing time for a donor site is 10 to 14 days (see Figure 27-11, D).

CULTURED EPITHELIAL AUTOGRAFTS. In the patient with large body surface area burns, only a limited amount of unburned skin may be available as donor sites for grafting, and some of that available skin may be unsuitable for harvesting. Cultured epithelial autograft (CEA) is a method of obtaining permanent skin from a person with limited available skin for harvesting. CEA is grown from biopsy specimens obtained from the patient's own unburned skin. The specimens are sent to a commercial laboratory, where the keratinocytes from the biopsy sample are grown in a culture medium containing epidermal growth factor. After approximately 18 to 25 days, the keratinocytes have expanded up to 10 000 times and form confluent sheets that can be used as skin grafts. The cultured skin is returned to the burn unit, where it is placed on the patient's excised burn wounds. Because CEA tissue is made only of epidermal cells, meticulous care is required to prevent shearing injury or infection (Figure 27-12). Problems related to CEA include infection, contracture development, and poor graft take as a result of loss of thin epidermal skin during healing.

ARTIFICIAL SKIN. To be successful, artificial skin must perform all functions of natural skin and consist of both dermal and epidermal elements (Jeschke, Finerty, Shahrokhi, et al., 2013). The Integra dermal regeneration template is an example of a successful skin replacement system available in burn care today. As with CEA, it is indicated for use in the treatment of life-threatening full-thickness or deep partial-thickness burn wounds when conventional autograft is not available or advisable, as in older-adult patients or those at high risk for complications from anaesthesia. It has also been successfully used in surgical burn reconstructive procedures. As with CEA, it needs to be applied within a few days of admission for greatest success.

Integra artificial skin has a bilayer membrane composed of acellular dermis and silicone. The wound is debrided, the bilayer membrane is placed dermal layer down, and the wound is wrapped with dressings in the operating room. The dermal layer functions as a biodegradable template that induces organized regeneration of new dermis by the body. The silicone layer remains intact for 3 weeks as the dermal layer degrades and epidermal autografts become available. At this point, the silicone is removed during

a second surgical procedure and replaced by the patient's own epidermal autografts. In some situations, burn units use CEA as the source of epidermis.

Another currently available dermal replacement is AlloDerm, a cryopreserved allogenic dermis. Human allograft dermis, harvested from cadavers, is decellularized to render it immunogenic, and then it is freeze-dried. Once thawed, AlloDerm is rehydrated with ultrathin epidermal autografts immediately before placement on a newly excised wound.

PAIN MANAGEMENT

One of the most critical functions a nurse performs on behalf of a patient with burn injuries is individualized and ongoing pain assessment and management. Many aspects of burn care cause pain. However, patients experience moments of relative comfort if they receive adequate analgesia. A coordinated understanding of both physiological and psychological aspects of pain is essential if the nurse is to intervene with actions that are beneficial. (General pain management is discussed in Chapter 10.) Patients with burn injuries experience two kinds of pain: (a) continuous, background pain that might be present throughout the day and night and (b) treatment-induced pain associated with dressing changes, ambulation, and rehabilitation activities. Initial treatment is pharmacological (see Table 27-14). With background pain, a continuous intravenous infusion of an opioid allows for a steady, therapeutic level of medication. If an intravenous infusion is not present, slow-release twice-a-day opioid medications (e.g., MS Contin, sustained-release hydromorphone [Dilaudid]) are indicated. Around-the-clock oral analgesics can also be used (ibuprofen, acetaminophen). Breakthrough doses of pain medication need to be available regardless of the regimen selected. Anxiolytics (e.g., lorazepam [Ativan]), which frequently potentiate analgesics, are also indicated.

For treatment-induced pain, premedication with an analgesic and perhaps an anxiolytic via the IV or oral route, is required. For patients with an IV infusion, a potent, short-acting analgesic, such as fentanyl, is useful. During treatment or activity, doses should be low but high enough to keep the patient as comfortable as possible. Elimination of all pain is difficult to achieve, and most patients indicate satisfaction with "tolerable" levels of discomfort.

Pain can also be managed through nonpharmacological strategies. Mind–body interventions such as relaxation, hypnosis, guided imagery, biofeedback, and music therapy are considered adjuncts to traditional pharmacological treatment of pain. They

FIGURE 27-12 Cultured epithelial autograft (CEA). **A,** Intraoperative application of CEA. **B,** Appearance of healed CEA. Source: Courtesy of Epicel.

are not meant to be used exclusively to control pain but may help some patients cope with the painful aspects of care, both in the hospital and after discharge (see Chapter 8).

An important point to remember is that the more control the patient has in managing the pain, the more successful the chosen strategies are. Patient-controlled analgesia (PCA) is used in some burn units, with varying degrees of success. (PCA is discussed in Chapters 10 and 22.) Active patient participation has been found to be effective also for some patients in anticipating and coping with treatment-induced pain.

PHYSIOTHERAPY AND OCCUPATIONAL THERAPY

Rigorous physiotherapy throughout burn recovery is imperative to maintain muscle strength and optimal joint function. A good time for exercise is during and after wound cleansing, when the skin is softer and bulky dressings are removed. Passive and active range-of-motion exercises should be performed on all joints. The patient with neck burns must sleep without pillows or with the head hanging slightly over the top of the mattress to encourage hyperextension. Custom-fitted splints are designed to keep joints in a functional position. These must be re-examined frequently to ensure an optimal fit with no undue pressure that might lead to skin breakdown or nerve damage.

NUTRITIONAL THERAPY

The goal of nutritional therapy during the acute burn phase is to provide adequate calories and protein to promote healing. The patient with burn injury is in a hypermetabolic and highly catabolic state. Decreasing catecholamine release by minimizing pain, fear, anxiety, and cold can maximize the patient's comfort and conserve energy. Infection also increases the metabolic rate.

Meeting daily caloric requirements is crucial and should begin within the first 1 to 2 days after the burn injury. The daily estimated caloric needs must be regularly calculated by a dietitian and readjusted as the patient's condition changes (e.g., wound healing, sepsis).

If the patient is on a mechanical ventilator or unable to consume adequate calories by mouth, a small-bore feeding tube is placed and enteral feedings are initiated. When the patient is extubated, a swallowing assessment should be performed by a speech–language pathologist before oral feeding is commenced. The alert patient should be encouraged to eat high-protein, high-carbohydrate foods to meet increased caloric needs. Family members should be encouraged to bring in favourite foods from home. Ideally, weight loss should not be more than 10% of preburn weight. Daily calorie counts and weekly weights are monitored by the dietitian to evaluate progress.

PSYCHOSOCIAL CARE

The patient and family have many needs for psychosocial support during the often lengthy, unpredictable, and complex course of care. The social worker and nursing staff have important support and counselling roles to play. (Patient and family emotional needs are discussed later in this chapter and in Chapter 6.)

REHABILITATION PHASE

The formal *rehabilitation phase* begins when the patient's burn wounds have healed and the patient is able to resume a level of self-care activity. This can occur as early as 2 weeks or as long as 7 to 8 months after the burn injury. Goals for this period are (a) to assist the patient in resuming a functional role in

🔁 EVIDENCE-INFORMED PRACTICE

Research Highlight

Does the Type of Enteral Feeding Affect Outcomes in Burn Patients?

Clinical Question
In patients with burns (P), what is the effect of high-carbohydrate enteral feeding (I) versus high-fat enteral feeding (C) in reducing mortality, days on ventilator, and incidence of pneumonia (O)?

Best Available Evidence
Systematic review of randomized controlled trials (RCTs)

Critical Appraisal and Synthesis of Evidence
- Two RCTs (n=93) were done in the immediate postburn period involving hospitalized patients with burns covering ≥10% of the total body surface area (TBSA).
- Two types of enteral feeding were compared: high-carbohydrate, high-protein, low-fat feeding (high-carbohydrate formula) and low-carbohydrate, high-protein, high-fat feeding (high-fat formula).
- High-carbohydrate enteral feeding resulted in a reduced incidence of pneumonia compared with high-fat enteral feeding.
- Results on type of enteral feeding as it related to patient outcomes of mortality and days on ventilator were inconclusive.

Conclusion
- High-carbohydrate enteral feedings may be of benefit in reducing the risk for pneumonia.

Implications for Nursing Practice
- Further research is needed to determine if type of enteral feeding produces significantly different patient outcomes.

Reference for Evidence
Masters, B., Aarabi, S., Sidhwa, F., et al. (2012). High-carbohydrate, high-protein, low-fat versus low-carbohydrate, high-protein, high-fat enteral feeds for burns. *The Cochrane Database of Systematic Reviews*, (1), CD006122, doi:10.1002/14651858.CD006122.pub3.

P, Patient population of interest; *I*, intervention or area of interest; *C*, comparison of interest or comparison group; *O*, outcomes of interest (see Chapter 1).

society and (b) rehabilitation after functional and cosmetic reconstructive surgery (Stergiou-Kita, Grigorovich, & Gomez, 2014). Rehabilitation-focused activities that were taking place during the earlier emergent and acute phases begin in earnest once the patient's wounds have healed.

Pathophysiological Changes and Clinical Manifestations

Burn wounds can heal on their own or through skin grafting. Through epithelialization, the tissue structure destroyed by the burn injury begins to rebuild. Collagen fibres, present in the new scar tissue, assist with healing and add strength to weakened areas. The new skin appears flat and pink. In approximately 4 to 6 weeks, the area may become raised and hyperemic. If adequate range of motion is not instituted, the new tissue shortens, which causes a contracture. Mature healing is reached in about 12 months, by which time suppleness has returned and, in lighter-skinned people, the pink or red colour has faded to a slightly lighter hue than the surrounding unburned tissue. More heavily pigmented skin takes longer to regain its dark colour because many of the melanocytes have been destroyed. In many cases, the skin does not regain its original colour. Paramedical cosmetic camouflage—the topical application of pigment onto the skin—can help even out unequal skin tones and improve the patient's overall appearance and self-image.

Scarring has two components: discoloration and contour. The discoloration of scars fades somewhat with time. However, scar tissue tends to develop altered contours; that is, it is no longer flat or slightly raised but becomes elevated and enlarged above the original burned area. It is believed that pressure can help keep a scar flat. Gentle pressure can be maintained on the healed burn with custom-fitted pressure garments, worn up to 24 hours a day for as long as 12 to 18 months. They should never be worn over unhealed wounds and are removed for bathing.

Patients typically experience discomfort from itching where healing is occurring. Application of water-based moisturizers and use of oral antihistamines (e.g., diphenhydramine [Benadryl]) help reduce the itching. Massage, silicone gel sheeting (e.g., Cica-Care), gabapentin (Neurontin)/pregabalin (Lyrica), and injectable steroids may also be helpful (Carrougher, Martinez, McMullen, et al., 2013). As "old" epithelium is replaced by new cells, flaking occurs. Newly formed skin is extremely sensitive to trauma. Blisters and skin tears are likely to develop from slight pressure or friction. In addition, newly healed areas can be hypersensitive or hyposensitive to cold, heat, and touch. Grafted areas are more likely to be hyposensitive until peripheral nerve regeneration occurs. Healed burn areas must be protected from direct sunlight for 3 to 6 months to prevent hyperpigmentation and sunburn.

Complications

The most common complications during the rehabilitative phase are skin and joint contractures and hypertrophic scarring (Godleski, Oeffling, Bruflat, et al., 2013). A contracture (an abnormal, usually permanent condition of a joint, characterized by flexion and fixation) develops as a result of the shortening of scar tissue in the flexor tissues of a joint. Areas most susceptible to contracture formation include anterior and lateral neck areas, axillae, antecubital fossae, fingers, groin areas, popliteal fossae, knees, and ankles (Figure 27-13). Not only does the skin over these areas develop contractures, but also the underlying tissues, such as the ligaments and tendons, have a tendency to shorten in the healing process.

Because of pain, patients with burn injuries prefer to assume a flexed position for comfort. This position predisposes wounds to contracture formation. Proper positioning, splinting, and exercise should be instituted to minimize this complication while the skin matures. Burned legs may be wrapped with elastic (e.g., tensor [ACE]) bandages to assist with circulation to leg graft and donor sites before ambulation. This additional pressure prevents blister formation, promotes venous return, and decreases pain and itchiness. Once the skin is completely healed and less fragile, interim tubular gauze (Tubigrip, Coban) and then custom-fitted pressure garments can replace the elastic bandages.

NURSING AND COLLABORATIVE MANAGEMENT REHABILITATION PHASE

During the rehabilitation phase, both the patient and the family are actively encouraged to participate in care. Because the patient may go home with small, unhealed wounds, education and "hands-on" instruction in dressing changes and wound care are needed. If necessary, home care nursing services may be arranged to assist with wound care for the first few weeks after discharge. An emollient, water-based cream (e.g., Vaseline Intensive Care Extra Strength) that penetrates into the dermis should be used routinely on healed areas to keep the skin supple and well moisturized, thereby decreasing itching and flaking. Reconstructive surgery is frequently required after a major burn. It is important for the patient to understand the need for or possibility of further surgery before leaving the hospital.

The continuous role of exercise and physiotherapy or occupational therapy cannot be overemphasized. Computerized gaming devices can provide patients with a break from exercise routines (Parry, Carbullido, Kawada, et al., 2014). Constant encouragement and reassurance are necessary to maintain morale, particularly once the patient realizes that recovery can be slow and rehabilitation may need to be a primary focus for at least the next 12 months.

Because of the tremendous psychological effect of burn injury, health care providers should be particularly sensitive and attuned to the patient's emotions and concerns. It is essential that patients be encouraged to discuss their fears regarding loss of their lifestyle as they once knew it, loss of function, temporary or permanent deformity and disfigurement, return to work and home life, and financial burdens resulting from a long and potentially costly hospitalization and rehabilitation. Patients may benefit from being assisted toward a realistic and positive appraisal of their

FIGURE 27-13 Contractures. **A,** Foot. **B,** Neck. Source: Courtesy Judy A. Knighton, RN, MScN, Toronto, and Linda Bucher, RN, PhD.

particular situation, emphasizing what they can do instead of what they cannot do.

A person's self-esteem may be impacted by a burn injury. In some individuals, an overwhelming fear may be the loss of relationships because of perceived or actual physical disfigurement. In a society in which physical beauty is valued, alterations in body image may result in psychological distress. Encouraging appropriate independence, an eventual return to preburn activities, and interactions with other burn survivors will involve the patient in familiar activities that may bring comfort and help restore self-esteem. Counselling, which may have started in the acute phase of care, can be offered after discharge. Patients appreciate reassurance that their emotions during this period of adjustment are normal and that frustration is to be expected as they attempt to resume a normal lifestyle.

AGE-RELATED CONSIDERATIONS

BURNS

Older-adult patients with burns present many challenges for the burn team. The normal aging process puts such patients at risk for injury because of the possibility of an unsteady gait, limited eyesight, and diminished hearing. As people age, skin becomes drier, more wrinkled, and looser. The dermal layer thins, there is a loss of elastic fibres, the amount of subcutaneous adipose tissue lessens, and vascularity decreases. As a result, the thinner dermis, with reduced blood flow, sustains deeper burns with poorer rates of healing.

Once injured, older adults have more complications in the emergent and acute phases of burn resuscitation because of pre-existing medical conditions. For example, among older patients with diabetes, heart failure, or chronic obstructive pulmonary disease, morbidity and mortality rates exceed those of healthy, younger patients. Pneumonia is a frequent complication, burn wounds and donor sites take longer to heal, and surgical procedures are not as well tolerated. Weaning from a ventilator can be a challenge, and delirium from medication and anaesthesia may be a distressing, although usually self-limiting, outcome. It usually takes longer for older patients to become rehabilitated to the point at which they can safely return home. For some, a return home to independent living may not be possible. As the population ages, developing strategies to prevent burn injuries in this age group is a priority.

EMOTIONAL NEEDS OF THE PATIENT AND CAREGIVERS

For the nurse to adequately manage the enormous range of emotional responses that the patient with burn injury may exhibit, it is important to have an understanding of the circumstances of the burn, family relationships, and previous coping experiences with stressful stimuli (Kornhaber, Wilson, Abu-Kumar, et al., 2014). At any time, emotions of fear, anxiety, anger, guilt, and depression may be experienced (Table 27-15).

A common emotional response is regression. The patient may revert to behaviour that helped with stressful situations in the past. This response can be healthy and is usually short-lived. As more and more independence is expected from the patient, new fears must be confronted: "Can I do it?" "Am I a desirable partner or parent?" Open and frequent communication among the patient, family members, close friends, and burn team members is essential.

TABLE 27-15	EMOTIONAL RESPONSES OF PATIENTS WITH BURN INJURY*	
Emotion	**Possible Verbal Expression**
Fear	"Will I die?"
	"What will happen next?"
	"Will I be disfigured?"
	"Will my family and friends still love me?"
Anxiety	"I feel out of control."
	"What's going to happen to me?"
	"When will I look normal again?"
Anger	"Why did this happen to me?"
	"The nurses enjoy hurting me."
	"I hope the person who did this to me dies."
Guilt	"If only I'd been more careful."
	"I'm being punished because I did something wrong."
Depression	"It's no use going on like this."
	"I don't care what happens to me."
	"I wish people would leave me alone."

*List is not all-inclusive.

Burn survivors frequently experience thoughts and feelings that are frightening and disturbing, such as guilt about the burn accident, reliving the experience, fear of death, concern about future therapy and surgery, frustrations with ongoing discomfort and wound breakdown, and, perhaps, hopelessness about the future. Families may share some or all of these feelings. At times, family members may feel helpless to assist their loved one. Continued support from trusted and familiar burn team members is essential. Assisting with aspects of care helps family members reconnect with their loved one and assists with the transition home. Many burn survivors and their families remark on the powerful learning experience of the burn and a renewed appreciation for life, despite the ongoing challenges of a prolonged and challenging recovery (Stavrou, Weissman, Tessone, et al., 2014). Acknowledgement that such feelings are normal and valid can be therapeutic for patients and their families.

The stress of the burn injury occasionally precipitates a time-limited psychiatric or psychological crisis. Many patients realize that coping with this experience is beyond their ability. Assessment by a psychiatrist who can prescribe appropriate medication, if needed, and begin short-term counselling is frequently helpful. Early psychiatric intervention is essential if the patient has been previously treated for a psychiatric illness or if the injury resulted from a suicide attempt. The diagnosis of post-traumatic stress disorder is made in a number of patients with burn injuries. However, it has been noted that distress and trauma symptoms can act as a catalyst for positive post-traumatic growth. Coping styles and social support appear to assist in these positive changes postburn (Baillie, Sellwood, & Wisely, 2014). Treatment typically begins in the hospital, but links to community resources must be made before discharge to ensure continuity of psychological care. Once the patient is discharged, referral to a psychiatrist, psychologist, mental health counsellor, social worker, or psychiatric clinical nurse specialist may be helpful if concerns are raised at burn clinic follow-up.

Patients with burn injuries benefit from information about sexuality and intimacy (Gonçalves, Melo, Caltran, et al., 2014). Physical appearance is altered in patients who have sustained a major burn, and acceptance of any changes is difficult at first for both the patient and the significant other. The nature of skin injury causes modifications in processing sexual stimuli. Touch is an important part of sexuality, and immature scar tissue may make the sensation of touch unpleasant or may dull it. This effect is usually transient, but the patient and partner need to know that it is normal, so they will benefit from anticipatory guidance from the health care team to avoid undue emotional strain.

Patient and family support groups may assist patients and families with their emotional needs at any phase of the recovery process. Speaking with other people who have experienced burn trauma can be beneficial, both in terms of reaffirming that their feelings are normal and allowing for sharing of helpful advice (Tolley & Foroushani, 2014). The Phoenix Society (see the Resources at the end of this chapter) is an international and highly respected burn survivors' support group that has been offering invaluable support and resources to burn survivors, family members, and burn team personnel for many years.

SPECIAL NEEDS OF THE NURSING STAFF

Warm, trusting, mutually satisfying relationships frequently develop between patients with burn injuries and nursing staff, not only during hospitalization but also during the long-term rehabilitation period. The frequency and intensity of family contact can also be rewarding, as well as draining, for the nurse. Those

new to burn nursing often find it difficult at first to cope with not only the deformities caused by burn injury but also the odours, the unpleasant sight of wounds, and the reality of the pain that accompanies the burn and its treatment. With time and positive experiences, those reactions diminish.

Many nurses come to know that the care they provide makes a critical difference in helping patients not only to survive but also to cope with and triumph over a challenging and multifaceted injury. It is this belief that allows and inspires nurses to provide meaningful care to patients with burn injury and their families.

Ongoing support services for the burn nurse or critical incident stress debriefings led by a psychiatrist, psychologist, psychiatric clinical nurse specialist, or social worker may be helpful. Professional burn nursing groups (e.g., American Burn Association, Canadian Association of Burn Nurses, International Society for Burn Injuries) can serve a similar purpose by helping nursing staff cope with difficult feelings they may experience when caring for patients with burn injuries. Burn nursing is physically, psychologically, and intellectually demanding and immensely rewarding (Leggett, Wasson, Sinacore, et al., 2013). Attention to self-care helps to maintain a positive attitude and healthy work–life balance. Time with family and friends and rest and relaxation at home are essential parts of self-care and living a life with purpose and fulfillment.

CASE STUDY

Burn Injury

Source: Billion Photos/ Shutterstock .com.

Patient Profile
Elliott Curtis, a 65-year-old married man, is brought to the emergency department with burns to his face, neck, torso, right arm and hand, and right foot from a kitchen grease fire. He arrives with an 18-gauge IV line with lactated Ringer's solution infusing at 100 mL/hour, and he is receiving 100% humidified oxygen by mask.

Subjective Data
- Complains of impaired vision and swallowing difficulties
- States his burns are painful and that he is scared
- States he has "diabetes and high blood pressure"

Objective Data
Physical Examination
- Patient is awake, alert, and oriented but in some distress
- Eyes are red and irritated
- Voice is hoarse; nasal hair is singed
- Face is reddened, with blisters noted on the nose and forehead
- Right arm, right hand, anterior torso, neck, and right foot have shiny, bright red, wet wounds
- Patient is shivering

Discussion Questions
1. ***Priority decision:*** What are the priorities of care in the prehospital setting and emergency department? How should Mr. Curtis's airway, breathing, and circulation be managed?
2. ***Priority decision:*** What signs and symptoms indicate that Mr. Curtis likely has an inhalation injury? What priority interventions can be anticipated?
3. What pain medications might be considered to relieve his pain?
4. Which of the criteria for admission to the hospital burn unit does Mr. Curtis meet?
5. What metabolic disturbances would be expected soon after Mr. Curtis's admission? Explain the physiological basis for these changes.
6. How might Mr. Curtis's comorbidities affect his burn care and rehabilitation?
7. What measures should be taken to support Mr. Curtis's family?
8. ***Priority decision:*** What three priority nursing diagnoses and any collaborative problems can be identified based on the assessment data presented?
9. ***Evidence-informed practice:*** What are the most effective wound care strategies to manage Mr. Curtis's burn wounds?

evolve

Answers are available at *http://evolve.elsevier.com/Canada/Lewis/medsurg.*

REVIEW QUESTIONS

The number of the question corresponds to the same-numbered objective at the beginning of the chapter.

1. Knowing the most common causes of household fires, which prevention strategy would the nurse focus on when teaching about fire safety?
   a. Set hot water temperature at 60°C.
   b. Use only hard-wired smoke detectors.
   c. Encourage regular home fire exit drills.
   d. Never permit older adults to cook unattended.

2. Which of the following injuries is least likely to result in a full-thickness burn?
   a. Sunburn
   b. Scald injury
   c. Chemical burn
   d. Electrical injury

3. When assessing a client with a partial-thickness burn, what would the nurse expect to find? *(Select all that apply)*
   a. Blisters
   b. Exposed fascia
   c. Exposed muscles
   d. Intact nerve endings
   e. Red, shiny, wet appearance

4. A client is admitted to the burn centre with burns on his head and neck, chest, and back after an explosion in his garage. On assessment, the nurse auscultates the lung fields and hears wheezes throughout. On reassessment, the wheezes are gone and the breath sounds are greatly diminished. Which action is the most appropriate for the nurse to take next?
   a. Obtain vital signs and an immediate arterial blood gas
   b. Encourage the client to cough and auscultate the lungs again
   c. Document the findings and continue to monitor the client's breathing
   d. Anticipate the need for endotracheal intubation and notify the physician

5. Which of the following fluid and electrolyte shifts occurs during the early emergent phase?
   a. Adherence of albumin to vascular walls
   b. Movement of potassium into the vascular space
   c. Sequestering of sodium and water in interstitial fluid
   d. Hemolysis of RBCs from large volumes of rapidly administered fluid

6. Which of the following must the client with a major burn do in order to maintain a positive nitrogen balance?
   a. Eat a high-protein, low-fat, high-carbohydrate diet
   b. Increase normal adult caloric intake by about three times
   c. Eat at least 1 500 calories per day in small, frequent meals
   d. Eat rice and whole wheat for their chemical effect on nitrogen balance

7. A client has 25% of TBSA burned in a car fire. His wounds have been debrided and covered with a silver-impregnated dressing. What should the nurse's priority intervention for wound care be?
   a. To reapply a new dressing without disturbing the wound bed
   b. To observe the wound for signs of infection during dressing changes
   c. To apply cool compresses for pain relief in between dressing changes
   d. To wash the wound aggressively with soap and water three times a day

8. Which of the following is most effective in terms of pain management for the client with burn injuries? *(Select all that apply)*
   a. A pain rating tool is used to monitor the client's level of pain.
   b. Painful dressing changes are delayed until the client's pain is completely relieved.
   c. The client is educated about pain management and has some control over its management.
   d. A multimodal approach is used (e.g., sustained-release and short-acting opioids, nonsteroidal anti-inflammatory drugs, adjuvant analgesics).
   e. Nonpharmacological therapies (e.g., music therapy, distraction) replace opioids in the rehabilitation phase of a burn injury.

9. Which of the following therapeutic measures is used to prevent hypertrophic scarring during the rehabilitative phase of burn recovery?
   a. Applying pressure garments
   b. Repositioning the patient every 2 hours
   c. Performing active range of motion at least every 4 hours
   d. Massaging the new tissue with water-based moisturizers

10. A client is recovering from second- and third-degree burns over 30% of his body and is now ready for discharge. What is the first action that the nurse should take when meeting with the client?
   a. Arrange a return-to-clinic appointment and prescription for pain medications
   b. Teach the client and the caregiver proper wound care to be performed at home
   c. Review the client's current health care status and readiness for discharge to home
   d. Give the client written discharge information and websites for additional information for burn survivors

1. c, 2, a, 3, a, d, e, 4, d, 5, c, 6, a, 7, b, 8, a, c, d, 9, a, 10. c.

Ⓔvolve

For even more review questions, visit *http://evolve.elsevier.com/Canada/Lewis/medsurg.*

REFERENCES

American Burn Association (ABA). (2016). *Burn incidence and treatment in the United States: 2016.* Retrieved from *http://www.ameriburn.org/resources_factsheet.php.*

Baillie, S. E., Sellwood, W., & Wisely, J. A. (2014). Post-traumatic growth in adults following a burn. *Burns: Journal of the International Society for Burn Injuries, 40*(6), 1089–1096. doi:10.1016/j.burns.2014.04.007.

Carrougher, G. J., Martinez, E. M., McMullen, K. S., et al. (2013). Pruritus in adult burn survivors: Postburn prevalence and risk factors associated with increased intensity. *Journal of Burn Care and Research, 34*(1), 94–101. doi:10.1097/BCR.0b013e3182644c25.

Fahlstrom, K., Boyle, C., & Makic, M. B. (2013). Implementation of a nurse-driven burn resuscitation protocol: A quality improvement project. *Critical Care Nurse, 33*(1), 25–35. doi:10.4037/ccn2013385.

Faraklas, I., Ghanem, M., Brown, A., et al. (2013). Evaluation of an enoxaparin dosing calculator using burn size and weight. *Journal of Burn Care and Research, 34*(6), 621–627. doi:10.1097/BCR.0b013e3182a2a855.

Godleski, M., Oeffling, A., Bruflat, A. K., et al. (2013). Treating burn-associated joint contracture: Results of an inpatient rehabilitation stretching protocol. *Journal of Burn Care and Research, 34*(4), 420–426. doi:10.1097/BCR.0b013e3182700178.

Gonçalves, N., Melo, A., Caltran, M. P., et al. (2014). Sexuality in burn victims: An integrative literature review. *Burns: Journal of the International Society for Burn Injuries, 40*(4), 552–561. doi:10.1016/j.burns.2013.11.007.

Hampson, N. B., Piantadosi, C. A., Thom, S. R., et al. (2012). Practice recommendations in the diagnosis, management, and prevention of carbon monoxide poisoning. *American Journal of Respiratory and Critical Care Medicine, 186*(11), 1095–1101. doi:10.1164/rccm.201207-1284CI.

Institute for Clinical and Evaluative Sciences (ICES). (2005). *Injuries in Ontario: ICES atlas.* Retrieved from *http://www.ices.on.ca/ Publications/Atlases-and-Reports/2005/Injuries-in-Ontario.*

Jeschke, M. G. (2013). Critical care of burn victims including inhalation injury. In M. G. Jeschke, L.-P. Kamolz, & S. Shahrokhi (Eds.), *Burn care and treatment: A practical guide* (pp. 67–90). Germany: Springer Wien.

Jeschke, M. G. (2014). Nutrition of the burn patient and treatment of the hypermetabolic response. In M. G. Jeschke, L.-P. Kamolz, & S. Shahrokhi (Eds.), *Burn care and treatment: A practical guide* (pp. 91–110). Germany: Springer Wien.

Jeschke, M. G., Finerty, C. C., Shahrokhi, S., et al. (2013). Wound coverage technologies in burn care: Novel technologies. *Journal of Burn Care & Research, 34*(6), 612–620. doi:10.1097/BCR .0b013e31829b0075.

Kamolz, L.-P. (2014). Acute burn surgery. In M. G. Jeschke, L.-P. Kamolz, & S. Shahrokhi (Eds.), *Burn care and treatment: A practical guide* (pp. 57–66). Germany: Springer Wien.

Kornhaber, R., Wilson, A., Abu-Kumar, M. Z., et al. (2014). Coming to terms with it all: Adult burn survivors' "lived experience" of acknowledgement and acceptance. *Burns: Journal of the International Society for Burn Injuries, 40*(4), 589–597. doi:10.1016/j.burns.2013.08.038.

Leggett, J. M., Wasson, K., Sinacore, J. M., et al. (2013). A pilot study examining moral distress in nurses working in one United States burn center. *Journal of Burn Care & Research, 34*(5), 521–528. doi:10.1097/BRC.0b013e31828c7397.

Nordlund, M. J., Pham, T. N., & Gibran, N. S. (2014). Micronutrients after burn injury: A review. *Journal of Burn Care & Research, 35*(2), 121–133. doi:10.1097/BCR.0b013e318290110b.

Parry, I. S., Carbullido, C., Kawada, J., et al. (2014). Keeping up with video game technology: Objective analysis of XBox Kinect™ and PlayStation 3 Move™ for use in burn rehabilitation. *Burns: Journal of the International Society for Burn Injuries, 40*(5), 852–859. doi:10.1016/j.burns.2013.11.005.

Payne, S., & Cole, E. (2012). Treatment of acute burn blisters in unscheduled care settings. *Emergency Nurse, 20*(5), 32–37. doi:10.7748/en2012.09.20.5.32.c9291.

Peck, M. (2012). Epidemiology and prevention of burns throughout the world. In M. G. Jeschke, L.-P. Kamolz, F. Sjöberg, et al. (Eds.), *Handbook of burns: Acute burn care* (Vol. 1, pp. 19–60). Austria: Springer-Verlag/Wien.

Saracogli, A., Kuzucuoglu, T., Yakupoglu, S., et al. (2014). Prognostic factors in electrical burns: A review of 101 patients. *Burns: Journal of the International Society for Burn Injuries, 40*(4), 702–707. doi:10.1016/j.burns.2013.08.023.

Shahrokhi, S. (2014). Infections in burns. In M. G. Jeschke, L.-P. Kamolz, & S. Shahrokhi (Eds.), *Burn care and treatment: A practical guide* (pp. 43–56). Germany: Springer Wien.

Sheckter, C. C., Van Vliet, M. M., Krishnan, N. M., et al. (2014). Cost-effectiveness comparison between topical silver sulfadiazine and enclosed silver dressings for partial-thickness burn treatment. *Journal of Burn Care & Research, 35*(4), 284–290. doi:10.1097/ BCR.0b013e3182a36916.

Somerset, A., Coffey, R., Jones, L., et al. (2014). The impact of prediabetes on glycemic control and clinical outcomes postburn injury. *Journal of Burn Care & Research, 35*(1), 5–10. doi:10.1097/ BCR.0b013e3182a2adea.

Statistics Canada. (2011). *Injuries in Canada: Insights from the Canadian Community Health Survey.* Retrieved from *http:// www.statcan.gc.ca/pub/82-624-x/2011001/article/11506-eng.htm.*

Stavrou, D., Weissman, O., Tessone, A., et al. (2014). Health-related quality of life in burn patients: A review of the literature. *Burns: Journal of the International Society for Burn Injuries, 40*(5), 788–796. doi:10.1016/j.burns.2013.11.014.

Stergiou-Kita, M., Grigorovich, A., & Gomez, M. (2014). Development of an inter-professional clinical practice guideline for vocational evaluation following severe burn. *Burns: Journal of the International Society for Burn Injuries, 40*(6), 1149–1163. doi:10.1016/j.burns.2014.01.001.

Summers, A. (2013). Treating cement burns in the emergency department. *Emergency Nurse, 20*(10), 30–31. doi:10.7748/ en2013.03.20.10.30.e1112.

Taira, B. R., Cassara, G., Meng, H., et al. (2011). Predictors of sustaining burn injury: Does the use of common prevention strategies matter? *Journal of Burn Care & Research, 32*(1), 20–25. doi:10.1097/BCR/0b013e318204b2eb.

Tolley, J. S., & Foroushani, P. S. (2014). What do we know about one-to-one peer support for adults with a burn injury? A scoping review. *Journal of Burn Care & Research, 35*(3), 233–242. doi:10.1097/BCR.0b013e3182957749.

Waltzman, J. T., & Bell, D. E. (2014). Vacuum-assisted closure device as a split-thickness skin graft bolster in the burn population. *Journal of Burn Care & Research, 35*(5), e338–e342. doi:10.1097/ BCR.0000000000000009.

World Health Organization. (2016). *Burns.* Retrieved from *http:// www.who.int/mediacentre/factsheets/fs365/en.*

RESOURCES

Canadian Association of Burn Nurses
http://www.cabn.ca

Canadian Burn Survivors Community
http://canadianburnsurvivors.ca/

American Burn Association
http://www.ameriburn.org

Burn Foundation
http://www.burnfoundation.org

Burn Survivors Throughout the World
http://www.burnsurvivorsttw.org

Changing Faces
http://www.changingfaces.org.uk

International Society for Burn Injuries
http://www.worldburn.org

Parkland Formula for Burns Calculator
www.mdcalc.com/parkland-formula-for-burns

Phoenix Society for Burn Injuries
http://www.phoenix-society.org

Sage Burn Diagram
http://www.sagediagram.com

For additional Internet resources, see the website for this book at *http://evolve.elsevier.com/Canada/Lewis/medsurg.*

Problems of Oxygenation: Ventilation

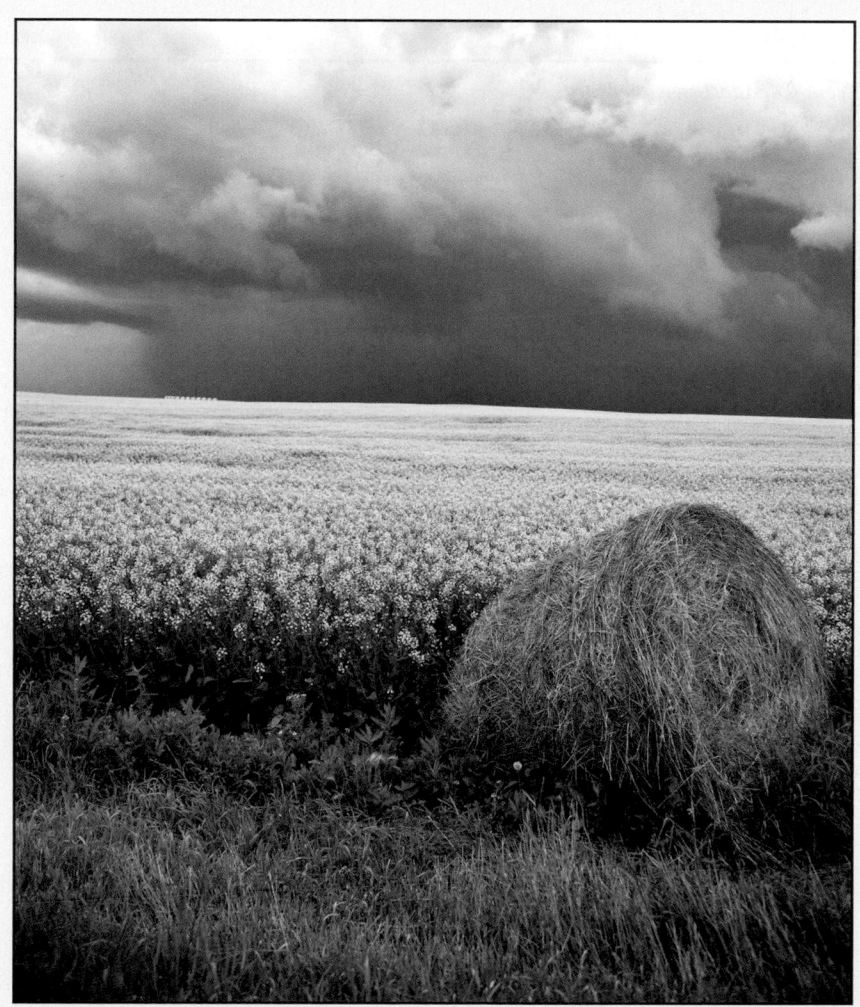

Source: Pictureguy/Shutterstock.com.

Nursing Assessment
Respiratory System

Written by: Eugene E. Mondor
Adapted by: Lesley MacMaster and Micki Puksa

⊖volve WEBSITE

http://evolve.elsevier.com/Canada/Lewis/medsurg

- Review Questions (Online Only)
- Key Points
- Answer Guidelines for Case Study
- Conceptual Care Map Creator
- Audio Glossary
- Supporting Media—Animations
  - Patterns of Respiration

- Percussion Tones Throughout the Chest
- Pulmonary Circulation
- Supporting Media—Audio
  - Bronchial Breath Sounds
  - Bronchovesicular Breath Sounds
  - High-Pitched Crackles
  - High-Pitched Wheeze

- Low-Pitched Crackles
- Low-Pitched Wheeze
- Pleural Friction Rub
- Stridor
- Vesicular Breath Sounds
- Content Updates

LEARNING OBJECTIVES

1. Describe the structures and functions of the upper respiratory tract, the lower respiratory tract, and the chest wall.
2. Describe the process that initiates and controls inspiration and expiration.
3. Describe the process of gas diffusion within the lungs.
4. Identify the respiratory defence mechanisms.
5. Describe the significance of arterial blood gas values and the oxygen–hemoglobin dissociation curve in relation to respiratory function.
6. Identify the signs and symptoms of inadequate oxygenation and the implications of these findings.
7. Describe age-related changes in the respiratory system and differences in assessment findings.
8. Identify the significant subjective and objective data related to the respiratory system that should be obtained from a patient.
9. Describe the techniques used in physical assessment of the respiratory system.
10. Differentiate normal from common abnormal findings in a physical assessment of the respiratory system.
11. Describe the purpose, significance of results, and nursing responsibilities related to diagnostic studies of the respiratory system.

KEY TERMS

adventitious sounds, p. 569
chemoreceptor, p. 562
compliance, p. 559
crackles, p. 569

dyspnea, p. 564
elastic recoil, p. 559
fremitus, p. 567
mechanical receptors, p. 562

pleural friction rub,
  p. 569
surfactant, p. 558
tidal volume, p. 558

ventilation, p. 559
wheezes, p. 569

STRUCTURES AND FUNCTIONS OF THE RESPIRATORY SYSTEM

The primary purpose of the respiratory system is gas exchange, which involves the transfer of oxygen and carbon dioxide from the atmosphere to the blood. The respiratory system is divided into two parts: the upper respiratory tract and the lower respiratory tract (Figure 28-1). The upper respiratory tract includes the nasal cavity, the pharynx, the adenoids, the tonsils, the epiglottis, the larynx, and the trachea. The major structures of the lower respiratory tract are the bronchi, the bronchioles,

the alveolar ducts, and the alveoli. With the exception of the right and left mainstem bronchi, all lower airway structures are contained within the lungs. The right lung is divided into three lobes (upper, middle, and lower) and the left lung into two lobes (upper and lower; Figure 28-2). The structures of the chest wall (ribs, pleura, muscles of respiration) are also essential for respiration.

Upper Respiratory Tract

The nose, made of bone and cartilage, is divided into two nares by the nasal septum. The interior of the nose is shaped into

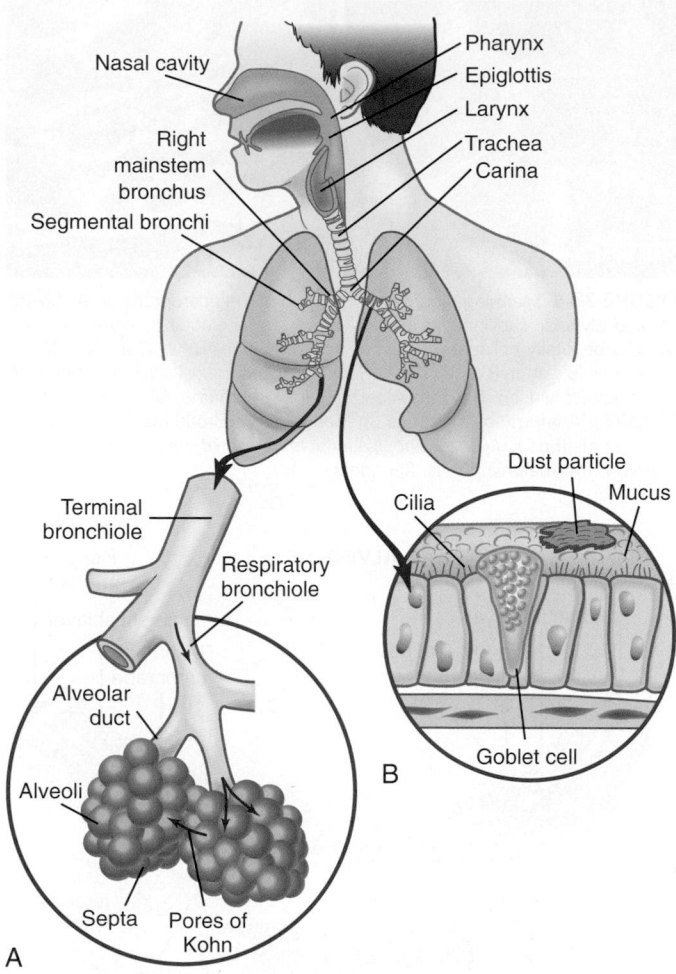

FIGURE 28-1 Structures of the respiratory tract. **A,** Pulmonary functional unit. **B,** Ciliated mucous membrane. Source: Redrawn from Price, S. A., & Wilson, L. M. (2003). *Pathophysiology: Clinical concepts of disease processes* (6th ed.). St. Louis: Mosby.

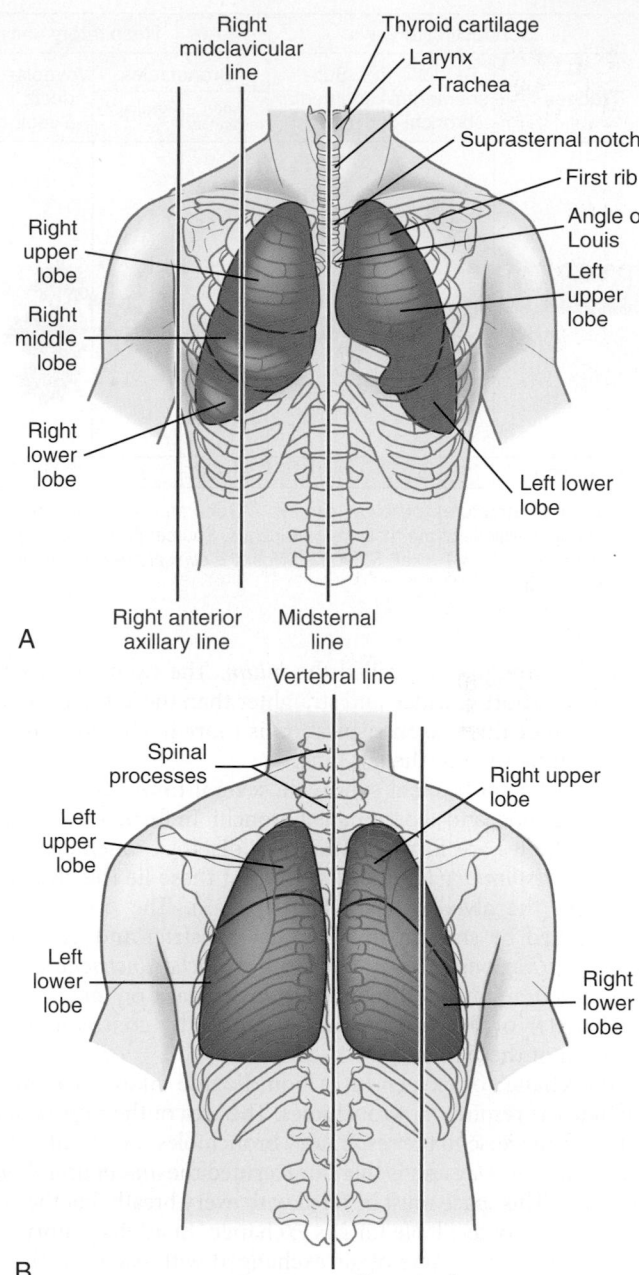

FIGURE 28-2 Landmarks and structures of the chest wall. **A,** Anterior view. **B,** Posterior view. Source: Thompson, J. M., McFarland, G., & Tucker, S. (2002). *Mosby's clinical nursing* (5th ed.). St. Louis: Mosby.

rolling projections called *turbinates* that increase the surface area for warming and moistening air. The internal portion of the nose opens directly into the sinuses. The nasal cavity is connected to the pharynx, a tubular passageway that is subdivided into three parts: in descending order, they are the nasopharynx, the oropharynx, and the laryngopharynx.

Breathing through the narrow nasal passages (rather than mouth breathing) provides protection for the lower airway. The nose is lined with mucous membrane and small hairs. Air entering the nose is warmed to near body temperature, humidified to nearly 100% water saturation, and filtered to remove particles larger than 10 mcm (e.g., dust, bacteria).

The olfactory nerve endings (receptors for the sense of smell) are located in the roof of the nose. The adenoids and the tonsils, which are small masses of lymphatic tissue, are found in the nasopharynx and the oropharynx, respectively.

The epiglottis is a small flap of tissue at the base of the tongue. During swallowing, the epiglottis covers the larynx, preventing solids and liquids from entering the lungs. A condition such as a stroke that alters swallowing ability may impair the function of the epiglottis, thus predisposing the affected person to aspiration.

After passing through the oropharynx, air moves through the laryngopharynx and the larynx, where the vocal cords are located, and then down into the trachea. The trachea is a cylindrical tube about 10 to 12 cm long and 1.5 to 2.5 cm in diameter. The support of U-shaped cartilages keeps the trachea open but allows the adjacent esophagus to expand for swallowing. The trachea bifurcates into the right and left mainstem bronchi at a point called the *carina*. The carina is located at the level of the manubriosternal junction, also called the *angle of Louis*. The carina is highly sensitive, and touching it during suctioning causes vigorous coughing (Patton & Thibodeau, 2016).

Lower Respiratory Tract

Once air passes the carina, it is in the lower respiratory tract. The mainstem bronchi, the pulmonary vessels, and nerves enter

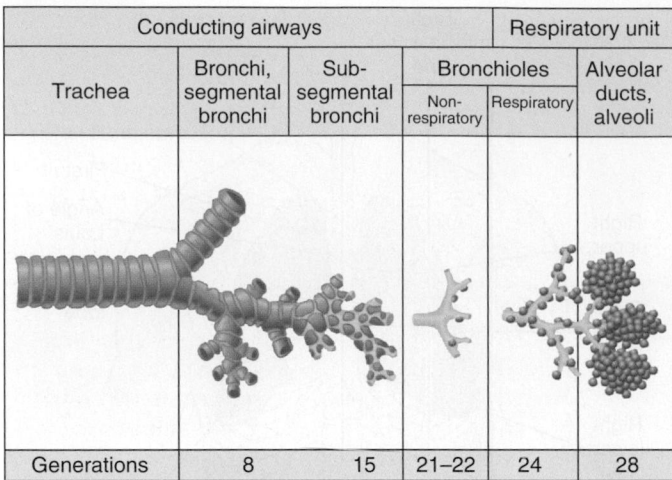

Conducting airways					Respiratory unit
Trachea	Bronchi, segmental bronchi	Sub-segmental bronchi	Bronchioles		Alveolar ducts, alveoli
			Non-respiratory	Respiratory	
Generations	8	15	21–22	24	28

FIGURE 28-3 Structures of lower airways. "Generations" refers to the number of subdivisions of the mainstem bronchus. Source: From Thompson, J. M., McFarland, G., & Tucker, S. (2002). *Mosby's clinical nursing* (5th ed.). St. Louis: Mosby.

FIGURE 28-4 Scanning electron micrograph of lung parenchyma. **A,** Alveoli *(A)* and alveolar capillary *(arrow).* **B,** Effects of atelectasis. Alveoli *(A)* are partially or totally collapsed. Source: **A,** From Bone, R. C., Dantzker, D. R., George, R. B., et al. (Eds.). (1993). *Pulmonary and critical care medicine* (Vol. 1). St. Louis: Mosby. **B,** From Albertine, K. H., Williams, M. C., & Hyde, D. M. (2005). Anatomy of the lungs. In Mason, R. J., Broaddus, V. C., Murray, J. F., et al. (Eds.), *Murray and Nadel's textbook of respiratory medicine* (4th ed.). Philadelphia: W. B. Saunders.

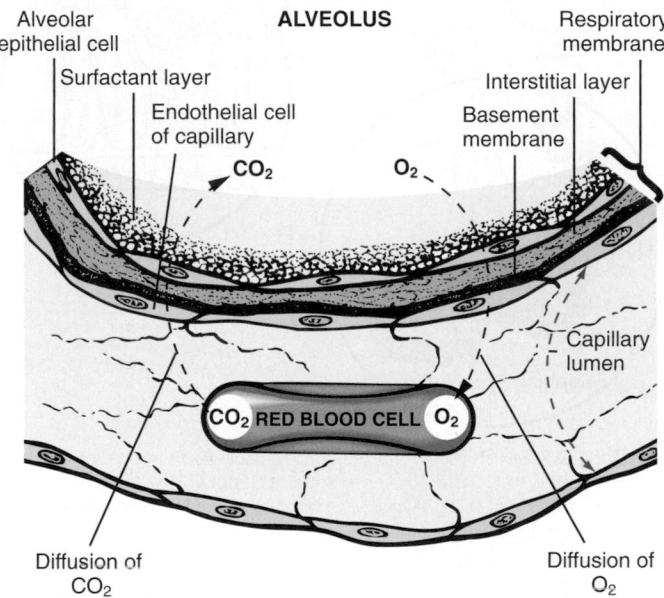

FIGURE 28-5 Illustration of a small portion of the respiratory membrane, greatly magnified. An extremely thin interstitial layer of tissue separates the endothelial cell and basement membrane on the capillary side from the epithelial cell and surfactant layer on the alveolar side of the respiratory membrane. The total thickness of the respiratory membrane is less than 5 mcm.

the lungs through a slit called the *hilum.* The right mainstem bronchus is shorter, wider, and straighter than the left mainstem bronchus. For this reason, aspiration is more likely to occur in the right lung than in the left lung.

The mainstem bronchi subdivide several times to form the lobar, segmental, and subsegmental bronchi. In further divisions, the bronchioles are formed. The most distant bronchioles are called the *respiratory bronchioles.* Beyond these lie the alveolar ducts and the alveolar sacs (Figure 28-3). The bronchioles are encircled by smooth muscles that constrict and dilate in response to various stimuli. The terms *bronchoconstriction* and *bronchodilation* are used to refer to a decrease or increase in the diameter of the airways that is caused by contraction or relaxation of these muscles.

No exchange of oxygen or carbon dioxide takes place until air enters the respiratory bronchioles. The area of the respiratory tract from the nose to the respiratory bronchioles serves only as a conducting pathway and is therefore termed the *anatomical dead space* (V_D). This space must be filled with every breath, but the air that fills it is not available for gas exchange. In adults, a normal **tidal volume,** or volume of air exchanged with each breath, is about 500 mL. Of each 500 mL inhaled, about 150 mL is V_D.

After moving through the conducting zone, air reaches the respiratory bronchioles and the alveoli (Figure 28-4). *Alveoli* are small sacs that form the functional unit of the lungs. The alveoli are interconnected by pores of Kohn, which allow movement of air from alveolus to alveolus (see Figure 28-1). Bacteria can also move through these pores; as a result, a respiratory infection can extend to previously noninfected areas. The 300 million alveoli in the adult have a total volume of about 2500 mL and a surface area for gas exchange that is about the size of a tennis court. The alveolar–capillary membrane (Figure 28-5) is very thin—less than 5 mcm thick—and is the site of gas exchange. In conditions such as pulmonary edema, excess fluid fills the interstitial space and the alveoli, markedly impairing gas exchange (Patton & Thibodeau, 2016; Weinberger, Cockrill, & Mandel, 2014).

Surfactant. The lung can be conceptualized as a collection of 300 million bubbles (alveoli), each 0.3 mm in diameter. Such a structure is inherently unstable and, as a consequence, the alveoli have a natural tendency to collapse. The alveolar surface

is composed of cells that provide structure and cells that secrete surfactant (see Figure 28-5). **Surfactant,** a lipoprotein that lowers the surface tension in the alveoli, reduces the amount of pressure needed to inflate the alveoli and decreases the tendency of the alveoli to collapse. Normally, each person takes a slightly larger breath, termed a *sigh,* after every five to six breaths. This sigh stretches the alveoli and promotes surfactant secretion.

When the amount of surfactant is insufficient, the alveoli collapse. The term *atelectasis* refers to collapsed, airless alveoli (see Figure 28-4). The patient who has just undergone surgery is at risk for postoperative atelectasis because of the effects of anaesthesia and restricted breathing with pain (see Chapter 22). In acute respiratory distress syndrome, lack of surfactant contributes to widespread atelectasis (Huether & McCance, 2017). (Acute respiratory distress syndrome is discussed further in Chapter 70.)

Blood Supply. The lungs have two different types of circulation: pulmonary and bronchial. The pulmonary circulation provides the lungs with blood for gas exchange. The pulmonary artery receives deoxygenated blood from the right ventricle of the heart and branches so that each pulmonary capillary is directly connected with many alveoli. Oxygen–carbon dioxide exchange occurs at this point. The pulmonary veins return oxygenated blood to the left atrium of the heart.

The bronchial circulation starts with the bronchial arteries, which arise from the thoracic aorta. The bronchial circulation provides oxygen to the bronchi and other pulmonary tissues. Deoxygenated blood returns from the bronchial circulation through the azygos vein into the left atrium.

Chest Wall

The chest wall is shaped, supported, and protected by 24 ribs (12 on each side). The ribs and the sternum protect the lungs and the heart from injury and, collectively, are sometimes called the *thoracic cage*. The structures of the chest wall include the thoracic cage, the pleura, and the respiratory muscles.

The chest cavity is lined with a membrane called the *parietal pleura*, and the lungs are lined with a membrane called the *visceral pleura*. The parietal and visceral pleurae are joined and form a closed, double-walled sac. The visceral pleura does not have any afferent pain fibres or nerve endings. The parietal pleura, however, does have afferent pain fibres. Therefore, irritation of the parietal pleura causes severe pain with each breath.

The space between the pleural layers is termed the *intrapleural space*. In a normal adult, this space is filled with a thin film of fluid, which serves two purposes: it provides lubrication, allowing the layers of pleura to slide over each other during breathing, and it increases cohesion between the pleural layers, thereby facilitating expansion of the pleura and lung during inspiration.

Normally, the pleural space contains 20 to 25 mL of fluid. Fluid is drained from the pleural space by the lymphatic circulation. Several pathological conditions may cause the accumulation of greater amounts of fluid; such accumulations are termed *pleural effusions*. Pleural fluid may accumulate because malignant cells block lymphatic drainage or because there is an imbalance between intravascular and oncotic fluid pressures, as occurs in heart failure. The presence of purulent pleural fluid with bacterial infection is called *empyema*.

The diaphragm is the major muscle of respiration. During inspiration, the diaphragm contracts, pushing the abdominal contents downward. At the same time, the external intercostal muscles and scalene muscles contract, increasing the lateral and anteroposterior dimension of the chest. This causes the size of the thoracic cavity to increase and intrathoracic pressure to decrease, so that air can enter the lungs.

The diaphragm is made up of two hemidiaphragms, each innervated by the right and left phrenic nerves. The phrenic nerves arise from the spinal cord between the third and fifth cervical vertebrae (C3 and C5). Injury to the phrenic nerve results in hemidiaphragmatic paralysis on the side of the injury. Complete spinal cord injuries above the level of C3 result in total diaphragmatic paralysis, and affected patients are dependent on mechanical ventilation (Herlihy, 2014).

Physiology of Respiration

Ventilation. Ventilation involves *inspiration* (movement of air into the lungs) and *expiration* (movement of air out of the lungs). Air moves in and out of the lungs because intrathoracic pressure changes in relation to pressure at the airway opening. Contraction of the diaphragm and of the intercostal and scalene muscles increases chest dimensions, thereby decreasing intrathoracic pressure. Gas flows from an area of higher pressure (atmospheric) to one of lower pressure (intrathoracic). When inspiration is difficult, neck and shoulder muscles can assist the effort. Some conditions (e.g., phrenic nerve paralysis, rib fractures, neuro-muscular disease) may limit diaphragm or chest wall movement and cause the patient to breathe with smaller tidal volumes. As a result, the lungs do not fully inflate, and gas exchange is impaired.

In contrast to inspiration, expiration is passive. The elastic recoil of the chest wall and lungs allows the chest to passively return to its normal position. Intrathoracic pressure rises, causing air to move out of the lungs. Exacerbations of asthma or emphysema cause expiration to become an active, laboured process (see Chapter 31). Abdominal and intercostal muscles assist in expelling air during laboured breathing.

Elastic Recoil and Compliance. Elastic recoil is the tendency for the lungs to recoil after being stretched or expanded. The elasticity of lung tissue is attributable to the elastin fibres that are found in the alveolar walls and that surround the bronchioles and capillaries.

Compliance (distensibility) is a measure of the elasticity of the lungs and the thorax. When compliance is decreased, inflation of the lungs is more difficult. Examples of conditions in which compliance is decreased include those that increase fluid in the lungs (e.g., pulmonary edema, acute respiratory distress syndrome); diseases that make lung tissue less elastic (e.g., pulmonary fibrosis, sarcoidosis); and conditions that restrict lung movement (e.g., pleural effusion). Compliance is decreased as a result of aging and when there is destruction of alveolar walls and loss of tissue elasticity, as in emphysema.

Diffusion. Oxygen and carbon dioxide move back and forth across the alveolar capillary membrane by diffusion. The overall direction of movement is from the area of higher concentration to the area of lower concentration. Thus oxygen moves from alveolar gas (atmospheric air) into the arterial blood, and carbon dioxide from the arterial blood into the alveolar gas. Diffusion continues until equilibrium is reached (see Figure 28-5).

The ability of the lungs to oxygenate arterial blood adequately is determined by examination of the arterial oxygen tension (PaO_2; also referred to as the *partial pressure of oxygen in arterial blood*) and arterial oxygen saturation (SaO_2). Oxygen is carried in the blood in two forms: dissolved oxygen and hemoglobin-bound oxygen. The PaO_2 represents the amount of oxygen dissolved in the plasma and is expressed in millimetres of mercury. The SaO_2 is the amount of oxygen actually bound to hemoglobin, as opposed to the amount of oxygen that the hemoglobin can carry. The SaO_2 is expressed as a percentage. For example, if the SaO_2 is 90%, this means that 90% of the hemoglobin attachments for oxygen have oxygen bound to them.

Oxygen–Hemoglobin Dissociation Curve. The affinity of hemoglobin for oxygen is described by the *oxygen–hemoglobin (oxyhemoglobin) dissociation curve* (Figure 28-6). Oxygen delivery to the tissues depends on the amount of oxygen transported to the tissues and the ease with which hemoglobin gives up oxygen once it reaches the tissues. In the upper flat portion of the curve, fairly large changes in the PaO_2 cause small changes in hemoglobin saturation. For this reason, if the PaO_2 drops from 100 to 60 mm Hg, the saturation of hemoglobin changes only 7% (from the normal 97% to 90%). In other words, the hemoglobin remains

90% saturated despite a 40–mm Hg drop in the PaO_2. This portion of the curve also explains why a patient is considered adequately oxygenated when the PaO_2 is higher than 60 mm Hg. Increasing the PaO_2 above this level does little to improve hemoglobin saturation.

The lower portion of the oxygen–hemoglobin dissociation curve indicates a different type of phenomenon. As hemoglobin is desaturated, larger amounts of oxygen are released for tissue use. This is an important method of maintaining the pressure gradient between the blood and the tissues. It also ensures an adequate oxygen supply to peripheral tissues, even if oxygen delivery is compromised.

Many factors alter the affinity of hemoglobin for oxygen. A shift to the left in the oxygen–hemoglobin dissociation curve indicates that blood picks up oxygen more readily in the lungs but delivers oxygen less readily to the tissues. This occurs in alkalosis, in hypothermia, and with a decrease in arterial carbon dioxide tension ($PaCO_2$; also referred to as the *partial pressure of carbon dioxide in the arterial blood;* see Figure 28-6). A patient

FIGURE 28-6 Oxygen–hemoglobin dissociation curve. A shift to the left indicates the hemoglobin's increased affinity for oxygen. A shift to the right indicates the hemoglobin's decreased affinity for oxygen. *2,3-DPG,* 2,3-diphosphoglycerate; *PaO₂,* partial pressure of oxygen in arterial blood; *PCO₂,* partial pressure of carbon dioxide.

with a condition that causes a leftward shift of the curve, such as hypothermia that follows open heart surgery, may be given higher concentrations of oxygen until the body temperature normalizes. This helps compensate for decreased oxygen unloading in the tissues. A shift in the curve to the right indicates the opposite: blood picks up oxygen less rapidly in the lungs but delivers oxygen more readily to the tissues. This occurs in acidosis, in hyperthermia, and when the $PaCO_2$ is increased.

Two methods are used to assess the efficiency of gas transfer in the lung: analysis of arterial blood gas (ABG) values and oximetry. These measures are usually adequate if the patient is stable and not critically ill. Many critically ill patients have a condition that impairs tissue oxygen delivery. In such patients, cardiac output, tissue oxygen consumption, mixed venous oxygen tension (PvO_2), and venous oxygen saturation (SvO_2) may also be assessed (Urden, Stacy, & Lough, 2014; see Chapter 68).

Arterial Blood Gases. ABGs are measured to determine oxygenation status and acid–base balance. ABG analysis includes measurement of the PaO_2, the $PaCO_2$, the pH, and the amount of bicarbonate (HCO_3^-) in arterial blood. The SaO_2 is either calculated or measured during this analysis. Blood for ABG analysis can be obtained by arterial puncture or from an arterial catheter in the radial or the femoral artery. Both techniques are invasive and allow only intermittent analysis. Continuous intra-arterial blood gas monitoring is also possible via a fibre-optic sensor or an oxygen electrode inserted into an arterial catheter. An arterial catheter enables ABG sampling without repeated arterial punctures.

Normal ABG values are given in Table 28-1, and ABG analysis and interpretation are further discussed in Chapter 19. The normal PaO_2 decreases with advancing age. The normal PaO_2 also varies in relation to the distance above sea level. At higher altitudes, the barometric pressure is lower, and thus the amount of inspired oxygen pressure and the PaO_2 are lower (see Table 28-1). Most airplanes are pressurized to approximate an altitude of 2400 m above sea level. A normal person can expect a 16– to 32–mm Hg fall in PaO_2 at this altitude (McCance & Huether, 2014). A patient who is already receiving oxygen therapy or whose PaO_2 is lower than 72 mm Hg while he or she is breathing room air needs a careful evaluation before air travel. Supplemental oxygen or a change in litre flow may be required during the flight.

Mixed Venous Blood Gases. For patients with normal or near-normal cardiac status, an assessment of PaO_2 or SaO_2 is usually sufficient to determine adequate oxygenation. Patients with impaired cardiac output or hemodynamic instability may have inadequate tissue oxygen delivery or abnormal oxygen

Laboratory Value	Arterial Blood Gases		Mixed Venous Blood Gases
	BP at Sea Level: 760 mm Hg	BP at 1609 m Above Sea Level: 629 mm Hg	
pH	7.35–7.45	7.35–7.45	7.31–7.41
Partial pressure of oxygen	80–100 mm Hg	65–75 mm Hg	40–50 mm Hg
Oxygen saturation	≥95%†	≥95%†	60–80%†
Partial pressure of carbon dioxide	35–45 mm Hg	35–45 mm Hg	SvO_2 is a better indicator for change in acid–base balance
HCO_3^-	21–28 mmol/L	21–28 mmol/L	21–28 mmol/L

TABLE 28-1   NORMAL ARTERIAL AND VENOUS BLOOD GAS VALUES*

*Assumes patient is 60 years of age or younger and breathing room air.
†The same normal values apply to both the venous oxygen saturation value (obtained through mixed venous blood gas sampling or oximetry via catheter) and the oxygen saturation value (obtained through pulse oximetry).
BP, barometric pressure; *HCO₃⁻,* bicarbonate.

FIGURE 28-7 A, Portable pulse oximeter displays oxygen saturation (SpO_2) and pulse rate. **B,** A pulse oximeter displays the oxygen saturation and pulse rate as a digital reading. Sources: *A,* © Can Stock Photo/praisaeng. *B,* © Can Stock Photo/masuti.

TABLE 28-2 SIGNS AND SYMPTOMS OF INADEQUATE OXYGENATION	
Signs and Symptoms	**Onset**
Central Nervous System	
Unexplained apprehension	Early
Unexplained restlessness or irritability	Early
Unexplained confusion or lethargy	Early or late
Combativeness	Late
Coma	Late
Respiratory System	
Tachypnea	Early
Dyspnea on exertion	Early
Dyspnea at rest	Late
Use of accessory muscles	Late
Retraction of interspaces on inspiration	Late
Pause for breath between sentences, words	Late
Cardiovascular System	
Tachycardia	Early
Mild hypertension	Early
Dysrhythmias (e.g., premature ventricular contractions)	Early or late
Hypotension	Late
Cyanosis	Late
Cool, clammy skin	Late
Other Body Systems	
Diaphoresis	Early or late
Decreased urinary output	Early or late
Unexplained fatigue	Early or late

consumption. The amount of oxygen delivered to the tissues or consumed can be calculated.

A catheter positioned in the pulmonary artery, termed a *pulmonary artery catheter,* is used for mixed venous sampling (see Chapter 68). Blood drawn from a pulmonary artery catheter is termed a *mixed venous blood gas sample* because it consists of venous blood that has returned to the heart from all tissue beds and "mixed" in the right ventricle. Normal mixed venous values are listed in Table 28-1. When tissue oxygen delivery is inadequate or when amount of oxygen transported to the tissues by the hemoglobin is inadequate, the PvO_2 and SvO_2 fall.

Oximetry. ABG values provide accurate information about oxygenation and acid–base balance. However, the tests are invasive, necessitate laboratory analysis, and create the risk of bleeding from an arterial puncture. Arterial oxygen saturation can be monitored continuously by means of a *pulse oximetry* probe on a finger, a toe, an ear, the forehead, or the bridge of the nose (Figure 28-7).

A pulse oximeter emits two wavelengths of light, one red and one infrared, which pass from a light-emitting diode (positioned on one side of the probe) to a photodetector (positioned on the opposite side). Well-oxygenated blood absorbs light differently than does deoxygenated blood. The oximeter determines the amount of light absorbed by the vascular bed and calculates the saturation. The oxygen saturation value obtained by pulse oximetry (SpO_2) and heart rate are displayed on the monitor

as digital readings (see Figure 28-7, *B*). The normal SpO_2 is higher than 95%.

Pulse oximetry is particularly valuable in intensive care and perioperative areas, in which sedation or decreased consciousness might mask hypoxia (Table 28-2). SpO_2 is assessed during each routine check of vital signs in many inpatient areas. Changes in SpO_2 can be detected quickly and treated (Table 28-3). Oximetry is also used during exercise testing and when flow rates are adjusted during long-term oxygen therapy. Pulse oximetry alone does not provide information about ventilation status and acid–base balance. Therefore, ABG measurements are also needed periodically.

Values obtained by pulse oximetry are less reliable if the SpO_2 is lower than 70%. At this level, the oximeter tends to underestimate saturation and may display an artificially low value. Pulse oximetry is also inaccurate if hemoglobin variants (e.g., carboxyhemoglobin, methemoglobin) are present. Other factors that can alter the accuracy of pulse oximetry include motion, low perfusion, anemia, bright fluorescent lights, intravascular dyes, thick acrylic nails, and dark skin colour. If there is doubt about the accuracy of the SpO_2 reading, ABGs should be measured to verify accuracy.

Oximetry can also be used to monitor SvO_2 via a pulmonary artery catheter. A decrease in SvO_2 suggests that less oxygen is being delivered to the tissues or that more oxygen is being consumed. Changes in SvO_2 provide an early warning of a change in cardiac output or tissue oxygen delivery. Normal SvO_2 is 60% to 80%.

Oxygen Delivery. Information from ABG values or oximetry is used to assess adequacy of oxygenation. Several questions must be asked to determine whether oxygenation is adequate:

1. What is the patient's SpO_2 or PaO_2 in comparison with expected normal values (see Table 28-1)?

TABLE 28-3   CRITICAL VALUES FOR PAO₂ AND SPO₂*

PaO₂	SpO₂	Considerations
≥70%	≥95%	Adequate unless patient is hemodynamically unstable or has O₂ unloading problem. With a low cardiac output, dysrhythmias, a leftward shift of the oxygen–hemoglobin dissociation curve, or carbon monoxide inhalation, higher values may be desirable. Benefits of a higher arterial O₂ level must be balanced against the risk of O₂ toxicity.
60%	90%	Adequate in almost all patients. Values are at steep part of oxygen–hemoglobin dissociation curve. Oxygenation is adequate, but margin of error is less than for higher values.
55%	88%	Adequate for patients with chronic hypoxemia if no cardiac problems occur. These values are also used as criteria for prescription of continuous O₂ therapy.
40%	75%	Inadequate but may be acceptable on a short-term basis if the patient also has CO₂ retention. In this situation, respirations may be stimulated by a low PaO₂. Thus, the PaO₂ cannot be raised rapidly. O₂ therapy at a low concentration (24%–28%) will gradually increase the PaO₂. Monitoring for dysrhythmias is necessary.
<40%	<75%	Inadequate. Tissue hypoxia and cardiac dysrhythmias can be expected.

*The same critical values apply for SpO₂ and arterial oxygen saturation (SaO₂). Values pertain to rest or exertion.
PaO₂, partial pressure of oxygen in arterial blood; SpO₂, the oxygen saturation value obtained by pulse oximetry.

2. What is the degree of hypoxemia, and what is the trend? Has SpO₂ or PaO₂ declined rapidly? A sudden drop in blood oxygen level can be life-threatening. A gradual decline is tolerated with fewer symptoms. Critical values for SpO₂ and PaO₂ are given in Table 28-3.
3. Is the patient exhibiting signs or symptoms of inadequate oxygenation? Changes in central nervous system, respiratory, cardiovascular, and renal function occur when tissue oxygen delivery is inadequate (see Table 28-2). Because the brain is highly sensitive to a decrease in tissue oxygen delivery, the first evidence of hypoxemia may be apprehension, restlessness, or irritability. If these signs or symptoms are observed, a change in the management plan is needed.
4. What is the oxygenation status with activity or exercise? To assess for desaturation with activity, pulse oximetry is used to monitor SpO₂ levels during a standardized 6-minute walk distance test or during activities of daily living. An SpO₂ value of 88% or less during exertion indicates the need for supplemental oxygen (McCance & Huether, 2014).

Control of Respiration

In the brain stem, the respiratory centre in the medulla responds to chemical and mechanical signals from the body. Impulses are sent from the medulla to the respiratory muscles through the spinal cord and phrenic nerves.

Chemoreceptors. A chemoreceptor is a receptor that responds to a change in the chemical composition (PaCO₂ and pH) of the fluid around it. Central chemoreceptors are located in the medulla and respond to changes in the hydrogen ion (H⁺) concentration. An increase in the H⁺ concentration (acidosis) causes the medulla to increase the respiratory rate and tidal volume. A decrease in H⁺ concentration (alkalosis) has the opposite effect. Changes in PaCO₂ regulate ventilation primarily by their effect on the pH of the cerebro-spinal fluid. When the PaCO₂ level is increased, more CO₂ is available to combine with H₂O and form carbonic acid (H₂CO₃). This lowers the pH of the cerebro-spinal fluid and stimulates an increase in respiratory rate. The opposite process occurs with a decrease in PaCO₂ level.

Peripheral chemoreceptors are located in the carotid bodies at the bifurcation of the common carotid arteries and in the aortic bodies above and below the aortic arch. The peripheral chemoreceptors respond to decreases in PaO₂ and pH and to increases in PaCO₂. These changes also cause stimulation of the respiratory centre.

In a healthy person, an increase in PaCO₂ or a decrease in pH causes an immediate increase in the respiratory rate. The process is extremely precise. The PaCO₂ does not vary more than about 3 mm Hg if lung function is normal. Conditions such as chronic obstructive pulmonary disease (COPD) alter lung function and may result in chronic elevation of PaCO₂ levels. In these circumstances, patients are relatively insensitive to further increases in PaCO₂ as a stimulus to breathe and may be maintaining ventilation largely because of a hypoxic drive from the peripheral chemoreceptors (carbon dioxide narcosis is discussed in Chapter 31).

Mechanical Receptors. Mechanical receptors (juxtacapillary and irritant) are located in lungs, upper airways, chest wall, and diaphragm. They are stimulated by a variety of physiological factors, such as irritants, muscle stretching, and alveolar wall distortion. Signals from the stretch receptors aid in the control of respiration. As the lungs inflate, pulmonary stretch receptors activate the inspiratory centre to inhibit further lung expansion. This is termed the *Hering–Breuer reflex* and prevents overdistension of the lungs. Impulses from the mechanical sensors are sent through the vagus nerve to the brain. Juxtacapillary (J) receptors are believed to cause the rapid respiration (tachypnea) observed in patients with pulmonary edema. These receptors are stimulated by the entry of fluid into the pulmonary interstitial space.

Respiratory Defence Mechanisms

Respiratory defence mechanisms are efficient in protecting the lungs from inhaled particles, microorganisms, and toxic gases. The defence mechanisms include filtration of air, the mucociliary clearance system, the cough reflex, reflex bronchoconstriction, and alveolar macrophages.

Filtration of Air. Nasal hairs filter the inspired air. In addition, the abrupt changes in direction of airflow that occur as air moves through the nasopharynx and larynx increase air turbulence. This causes particles and bacteria to contact the mucosa lining these structures. Most large particles (>5 mcm in diameter) are removed in this manner.

The velocity of airflow slows greatly after it passes the larynx, facilitating the deposition of smaller particles (1–5 mcm in size). They settle like sand in a river, a process termed *sedimentation*. Particles less than 1 mcm in size are too small to settle in this manner and are deposited in the alveoli. One example of small particles that can build up is coal dust, which can lead to pneumoconiosis (see Chapter 30). Particle size is important. Particles larger than 5 mcm are less dangerous because they are removed in the nasopharynx or bronchi and do not reach the alveoli.

Mucociliary Clearance System. Below the larynx, movement of mucus is accomplished by the mucociliary clearance system, commonly referred to as the *mucociliary escalator*. This term is used to indicate the interrelationship between the secretion of mucus and the ciliary activity. Mucus is continually secreted at a rate of about 100 mL per day by goblet cells and submucosal glands. It forms a mucous blanket that contains the impacted particles and debris from distal lung areas (see Figure 28-1). The small amount of mucus normally secreted is swallowed without being noticed. Collectins (glycoproteins which are part of the innate immune system) are secreted and produced by the lungs and contribute to protection against bacteria and viruses (McCance & Huether, 2014).

Cilia cover the airways from the level of the trachea to the respiratory bronchioles (see Figure 28-1). Each ciliated cell contains approximately 200 cilia, which beat rhythmically about 1 000 times per minute in the large airways, moving mucus toward the mouth. The ciliary beat is slower farther down the tracheo-bronchial tree. As a consequence, particles that penetrate more deeply into the airways are removed less rapidly. Ciliary action is impaired by dehydration, smoking, inhalation of high oxygen concentrations, infection, and ingestion of drugs such as atropine, anaesthetics, alcohol, and cocaine. Cilia are often destroyed by chronic bronchitis and cystic fibrosis, which results in impaired secretion clearance, a chronic productive cough, and frequent upper respiratory infections.

Cough Reflex. The cough is a protective reflex action that clears the airway by a high-pressure, high-velocity flow of air. It is a backup for mucociliary clearance, especially when this clearance mechanism is overwhelmed or ineffective. Coughing is effective in removing secretions only above the subsegmental level (large or main airways). Secretions below this level must be moved upward by the mucociliary mechanism or by interventions such as postural drainage before they can be removed by coughing.

Reflex Bronchoconstriction. Another defence mechanism is reflex bronchoconstriction. In response to the inhalation of large amounts of irritating substances (e.g., dusts, aerosols), the bronchi constrict in an effort to prevent entry of the irritants. In conditions of hyperreactive airways, such as asthma, bronchoconstriction occurs after inhalation of cold air, perfume, or other strong odours.

Alveolar Macrophages. Because ciliated cells are not found below the level of the respiratory bronchioles, the primary defence mechanism at the alveolar level is performed by alveolar macrophages. *Alveolar macrophages* rapidly phagocytize inhaled foreign particles such as bacteria. The debris is moved to the level of the bronchioles for removal by the cilia or is removed from the lungs by the lymphatic system. Particles (e.g., coal dust, silica) that cannot be adequately phagocytized tend to remain in the lungs for indefinite periods and can stimulate inflammatory responses (see Chapter 30). Because alveolar macrophage activity is impaired by cigarette smoke, people who are employed in an occupation with heavy dust exposure (e.g., mining, foundries) and smoke are at an especially high risk for lung disease.

AGE-RELATED CONSIDERATIONS

EFFECTS OF AGING ON THE RESPIRATORY SYSTEM

Age-related changes in the respiratory system and related assessment findings can be divided into alterations in structure, defence mechanisms, and respiratory control (Table 28-4).

TABLE 28-4 AGE-RELATED DIFFERENCES IN ASSESSMENT

Respiratory System

Changes	Differences in Assessment Findings
Structure	
↓ Elastic recoil	Barrel shape of chest
↓ Chest wall compliance	↓ Chest wall movement
↑ Anteroposterior diameter	↓ Respiratory excursion
↓ Functioning alveoli	↓ Vital capacity*
	↑ Functional residual capacity*
	Diminished breath sounds, particularly at lung bases
	↓ PaO₂ and SaO₂; normal pH and PaCO₂
Defence Mechanisms	
↓ Cell-mediated immunity	↓ Cough effectiveness
↓ Specific antibodies	↓ Secretion clearance
↓ Cilia function	↑ Risk of upper respiratory infection,
↓ Cough force	influenza, and pneumonia; respiratory
↓ Alveolar macrophage function	infections may be more severe and last longer
Respiratory Control	
↓ Response to hypoxemia	Greater ↓ in PaO₂ and ↑ in PaCO₂
↓ Response to hypercapnia	before respiratory rate changes
	Significant hypoxemia or hypercapnia may develop as a result of relatively minor incidents
	Retained secretions, excessive sedation, or positioning that impairs chest expansion may substantially alter PaO₂ or SpO₂ values

*See Table 28-14 for definitions of terms related to lung volumes and capacities.
PaCO₂, arterial carbon dioxide tension; *PaO₂*, arterial oxygen tension; *SaO₂*, arterial oxygen saturation; *SpO₂*, oxygen saturation value obtained by pulse oximetry.

Within the aging lung, the number of functional alveoli decreases and small airways in the lung bases close earlier in expiration. As a consequence, more inspired air is distributed to the lung apices, and ventilation is less matched to perfusion, which causes a lowering of the PaO_2. The PaO_2 associated with a given age can be calculated by means of the following equation:

$$PaO_2 \text{ (mm Hg)} = 103.5 - (0.42 \times \text{age in years})$$

For example, the normal PaO_2 for a patient 80 years of age is 70 mm Hg (103.5 − [0.42 × 80]); in comparison, the normal PaO_2 for a 25-year-old person is 93 mm Hg (103.5 − [0.42 × 25]).

The extent of these changes varies among persons of the same age. Older adults—who have experienced many years of exposure to smoking, air pollutants, and other environmental toxins—are at risk for a host of other conditions (Hoffman Wold, 2012; Jarvis, Browne, MacDonald-Jenkins, et al., 2014).

ASSESSMENT OF THE RESPIRATORY SYSTEM

Correct diagnosis depends on an accurate health history and a thorough physical examination (Table 28-5). A respiratory assessment can be performed as part of a comprehensive physical examination or as a focused evaluation. Whether all or part of the history and physical examination is completed is

TABLE 28-5 HEALTH HISTORY

Respiratory System: Questions for Obtaining Subjective Data

Cough
- Do you have a cough, and if so, when did it start? How often do you cough? Does it wake you up at night? Does activity affect your cough?* What relieves your cough?
- Do you cough up sputum?* How much do you expectorate? What colour is your sputum?
- Are you coughing up blood?*

Shortness of Breath
- Are you ever short of breath?* What brings it on?
- Do you get too short of breath to do the things you want to do?* (Note: To determine the intensity of dyspnea, the Medical Research Council Dyspnea Scale [see Chapter 31, Figure 31-12] or a visual analogue scale may be helpful [Registered Nurses' Association of Ontario, 2010, p. 93])
- Do breathing problems cause you to awaken during the night?*
- Can you lie flat at night? If not, how many pillows do you use? Do you need to sleep upright in a chair?
- What do you do when you get short of breath?

Chest Pain With Breathing
- Do you experience chest pain with breathing?* Where exactly is the pain located? What brings on the pain? What relieves the pain?

History of Respiratory Infections or Illness
- Do you have any history of breathing trouble or lung disease (e.g. shortness of breath, coughing, blood in your sputum, COPD, bronchitis, emphysema, asthma, pneumonia, sleep apnea)?*
- Have you ever been hospitalized or treated for a respiratory illness?*
- Do you have frequent colds or very severe colds, or both?*
- Do you have any allergies or sensitivities (food, environmental, medications)?*
- Do you have a family history of allergies, tuberculosis, or asthma?*

Self-Care History
- Do you use any equipment or take any medications to manage respiratory symptoms (e.g., home oxygen therapy equipment, metered-dose inhaler with spacer or nebulizer for medication administration, positive airway pressure device for relief of sleep apnea)?*
- Do you smoke?* If yes, how many packs daily? For how many years? Do you smoke cigarettes or cigars? Have you ever tried to quit? Are you living with someone who smokes?
- Are there any environmental conditions at home or work that may have an effect on your respiratory health (e.g., smoke, dust, chemicals)?* If so, do you do anything to protect your lungs or monitor your exposure?
- Have you received immunization for influenza (flu), pneumococcal pneumonia (Pneumovax), tuberculosis skin test, and/or chest radiograph? When?

Source: Based on Jarvis, C., Browne, A. J., MacDonald-Jenkins, J., et al. (Eds.). (2014). *Physical examination & health assessment* (2nd Canadian ed., pp. 441–443). Toronto: Elsevier Canada.
*If the answer is "yes," the patient should describe further.
COPD, chronic obstructive pulmonary disease.

CASE STUDY

Patient Introduction

Source: Monkey Business Images/ Shutterstock .com.

Fred Thompson is a 70-year-old man who comes to the emergency department complaining of increased shortness of breath. He states that he started using his salbutamol (Ventolin) inhaler every 4 hours a few days ago, but it does not seem to be helping. He has been having trouble sleeping or doing any activity because of the shortness of breath.

Critical Thinking

As you read through this assessment chapter, think about Mr. Thompson's symptoms with the following questions in mind:
1. What are the possible causes of Mr. Thompson's shortness of breath?
2. What type of assessment would be most appropriate for Mr. Thompson: comprehensive, focused, or emergency?
3. What questions would the nurse ask Mr. Thompson?
4. What should be included in the physical assessment? What would the nurse be looking for?
5. What diagnostic studies might be ordered?
   See pp. 567, 570, and 572 for more information on Mr. Thompson.

ⓔvolve
Answers available at. *http://evolve.elsevier.com/Canada/Lewis/medsurg*

based on problems presented by the patient and the degree of respiratory distress. If respiratory distress is severe, only pertinent information should be obtained; a thorough assessment should be deferred until the patient's condition stabilizes. Table 28-6 outlines subjective and objective data that may emerge during

the assessment that provide clues to the presence of respiratory problems.

Subjective Data

Important Health Information

Past Health History. The nurse should discuss with the patient the types of respiratory illnesses that the patient experienced during childhood (e.g., croup, respiratory syncytial virus, asthma, pneumonia, frequent colds).

The nurse should determine the frequency of upper respiratory problems (e.g., colds, sore throats, sinus problems, allergies) and whether weather changes exacerbate these problems. Patients with allergies should be questioned about possible precipitating factors such as medications or exposure to pollen, smoke, or animal dander. Characteristics of the allergic reaction—such as runny nose, wheezing, scratchy throat, or sensation of tightness in the chest—and the severity of the reaction should be documented. The frequency of asthma exacerbations and cause, if known, should also be determined. Prior use of a peak expiratory flowmeter and personal best values can be helpful information in determining the patient's current asthma status.

A history of lower respiratory tract problems, such as asthma, COPD, pneumonia, and tuberculosis, should also be documented (see the "Determinants of Health: Tuberculosis in Canada" box, Chapter 30). Respiratory symptoms are often manifestations of problems that involve other body systems. Therefore, the patient should be asked whether he or she has a history of other health problems in addition to those involving the respiratory system. For example, patients with cardiac dysfunction may experience **dyspnea** (shortness of breath) as a consequence of heart failure. Patients with human immunodeficiency virus (HIV) infection

TABLE 28-6 CLUES TO RESPIRATORY PROBLEMS

Manifestation	Description
Shortness of breath (dyspnea)	Distressing sensation of uncomfortable breathing. Most common complaint of people with respiratory problems. Person may become accustomed to the sensation and not recognize its presence. Difficult to evaluate because it is a subjective experience.
Wheezing	May or may not be heard by patient. May be described as "chest tightness."
Pleuritic chest pain	Described on a continuum from discomfort during inspiration to intense, sharp pain at the end of inspiration. Pain is usually aggravated by deep breathing and coughing.
Cough	Characteristics and timing of cough are important diagnostic clues.
Sputum production	Material coughed up from lungs. Contains mucus, cellular debris, or microorganisms and may contain blood or pus. Amount, colour, and constituents of sputum constitute important diagnostic information.
Hemoptysis	Coughing up of blood; sputum may be grossly bloody, frankly bloody, or blood-tinged. Precipitating events should be investigated.
Audible changes	Voice changes such as hoarseness and muffling, stridor (whistling sound during inspiration), or a barking cough may indicate abnormalities of upper airway, vocal cord dysfunction, or gastro-esophageal reflux disease.
Fatigue	Sense of overwhelming tiredness, not completely relieved by sleep or rest.

may experience frequent respiratory infections because immune function is compromised.

Medications. Patients should be questioned carefully about prescription and over-the-counter (OTC) drugs used to manage respiratory problems, such as antihistamines, bronchodilators, corticosteroids, cough suppressants, and antibiotics. The nurse should obtain information about the reason for taking the medication, its name, the dose and frequency, length of time taken, its effect, and any adverse effects.

If a patient is using supplemental oxygen to ease a breathing problem, the amount, the method of administration, and effectiveness of the therapy should be documented. Safety practices related to using supplemental oxygen should also be assessed.

Patients should be questioned with regard to OTC and herbal remedies used to treat respiratory illnesses such as the common cold, sore throat, and laryngitis.

Surgery or Other Treatments. The nurse should determine whether a patient has been hospitalized for a respiratory problem. If so, the dates, therapy (including surgery), and current status of the problem should be recorded. The nurse should ask about the use and results of respiratory treatments such as nebulizer, humidifier, airway clearance modalities, high-frequency chest oscillation, postural drainage, and percussion.

Current Health History. If a patient has a cough, the nurse should evaluate the quality of the cough. For example, a productive cough indicates the presence of secretions; a dry, hacking cough indicates airway irritation or obstruction; a harsh, barking cough is suggestive of upper airway obstruction from inhibited vocal cord movement related to subglottic edema. The nurse should assess whether the cough is weak or strong and whether it is productive or nonproductive of secretions. Determining the onset and chronicity of a cough is helpful in the differential diagnosis process. The pattern of the cough is determined from answers to questions such as the following: What has been the pattern of coughing? Has it been regular or irregular, and has it been related to a time of day or weather, certain activities, talking, or deep breaths? Has the cough changed over time? What efforts have been tried to alleviate the coughing? Were any prescription or OTC drugs tried?

If a patient has a productive cough, the following characteristics of sputum should be evaluated: amount, colour, consistency, and odour. The amount should be quantified in teaspoons, tablespoons, or cups per day. The nurse should note any recent increases or decreases in the amount. The normal colour is clear or slightly

whitish. If a patient smokes cigarettes, the sputum is usually clear to grey with occasional specks of brown. Patients with COPD may exhibit clear, whitish, or slightly yellow sputum, especially in the morning on rising. If a patient reports any change in sputum from baseline colour to yellow, pink, red, brown, or green, pulmonary complications should be suspected. Changes in consistency of sputum to thick, thin, or frothy should be noted. These changes may indicate dehydration, postnasal drip or sinus drainage, or possible pulmonary edema. Normally sputum should be odourless. A foul odour is suggestive of an infectious process. The patient should be asked whether the sputum was produced along with a position change (e.g., increased with lying down) or a change in activity.

Patients should be questioned about a family history of respiratory problems that may be genetic or familial tendencies, such as asthma, emphysema resulting from α_1-antitrypsin deficiency, or cystic fibrosis. A history of family exposure to tubercle bacilli should be noted.

Risk factors for tuberculosis (TB) include prior residence in Asia, Africa, Latin America, or any developing nation. People who are homeless, those who use injection drugs, Indigenous people, health care workers, residents of long-term care facilities and correctional facilities are also at increased risk of TB infection. People with certain comorbid conditions such as HIV infection and diabetes and those receiving dialysis have an increased risk of TB reactivation (Public Health Agency of Canada, The Lung Association, & Canadian Thoracic Society, 2014). Risk factors for avian influenza A (H7N9) include recent trips to China (Public Health Ontario, 2015a). It is important for the nurse to take droplet or airborne precautions with patients being assessed for new respiratory illness (Public Health Ontario, 2013; 2015b).

The nurse should also ask about current and past smoking habits and quantify exposure in pack-years by multiplying the number of packs smoked per day by the number of years smoked. For example, a person who smoked one pack per day for 15 years has a 15 pack-year history. The risk of lung cancer rises in direct proportion to the number of pack-years smoked. Smoking increases the risk of COPD and exacerbates symptoms of asthma and chronic bronchitis. In addition to asking about cigarette use, it is important to find out the use of any other tobacco products, including cigars, pipes, chewing tobacco, and smokeless tobacco products. Information about exposure to second-hand smoke is also important. The nurse should also ask whether the patient has made efforts—including the use of

CASE STUDY

Subjective Data

Source: Monkey Business Images/ Shutterstock .com.

A focused subjective assessment of Fred Thompson revealed the following information:

History of Current Illness: Has been experiencing increasing difficulty breathing since catching a cold from his granddaughter last week, even with the use of salbutamol (Ventolin). Has had increased shortness of breath on exertion and worsening paroxysmal nocturnal dyspnea. Denies any pain or confusion associated with the shortness of breath.

Past Health: COPD, hypertension, and benign prostatic hyperplasia. No history of environmental allergies. Denies history of coronary artery disease or heart failure.

Medications: Metoprolol, 50 mg/day orally; finasteride (Propecia), 5 mg/day orally; fluticasone and salmeterol (Advair) inhaler, 2 puffs per day; and salbutamol (Ventolin) inhaler, 2 puffs every 4 hours as needed. Does not use O_2 at home.

Functional Assessment: Mr. Thompson states that he usually manages his COPD well with just the fluticasone and salmeterol (Advair) inhaler and occasional use of the salbutamol (Ventolin) inhaler as needed. Has a history of 30 pack-years of smoking, having quit 5 years ago. Had a Pneumovax vaccination 5 years ago and receives the flu vaccine on an annual basis. States that he can typically walk at least 2 blocks and up and down stairs without getting short of breath. However, at this point, he cannot walk 30 metres without feeling short of breath, nor can he walk up one flight of stairs without stopping to catch his breath. Has been having difficulty sleeping with this most recent episode of shortness of breath. Typically uses just one pillow to sleep with but needed three pillows this week, and last night he slept upright in his recliner. Denies any stress or emotional disturbance that could be having an impact on his breathing. Feels slightly irritable because of lack of sleep.

See pp. 565, 570, and 572 for more information on Mr. Thompson.

prescription, OTC, and herbal remedies—to quit the use of these tobacco products.

The nurse should ask whether the patient received immunization for influenza (flu) and pneumococcal pneumonia (Pneumovax). Influenza vaccine should be administered yearly in the fall (Public Health Agency of Canada, 2015a). Pneumococcal vaccine is recommended for persons 65 years of age or older and for individuals with chronic cardiovascular disease, chronic pulmonary disease, or diabetes mellitus. The current recommendation is one dose of Pneumovax vaccine for adults aged 65 or older. This vaccine is also recommended in immunocompromised persons, such as organ transplant recipients (Public Health Agency of Canada, 2014).

Patients should be asked whether they use equipment to manage respiratory symptoms, such as home oxygen therapy equipment, metered-dose inhaler (MDI) with spacer or nebulizer for medication administration, and positive airway pressure device for relief of sleep apnea. Patients should be questioned about the type of equipment used, frequency of use, its therapeutic effect, and any adverse effects. Patients who use an MDI should be asked to demonstrate its use. Many patients do not know how to use MDI devices correctly (see Chapter 31).

Objective Data

Physical Examination. Vital signs, including temperature, pulse, respirations, and blood pressure, are important data to collect before examination of the respiratory system.

Nose. The nose is inspected for patency, inflammation, deformities, symmetry, and discharge. Each naris (nostril) is checked for air patency with respiration while the other naris is briefly occluded. The nurse tilts the patient's head backward and pushes the tip of the nose upward gently. With a nasal speculum and a good light, the nurse inspects the interior of the nose. The mucous membrane should be pink and moist, with no evidence of edema (bogginess), exudate, or bleeding. The nasal septum should be observed for deviation, perforations, and bleeding. Some nasal deviation is normal in an adult. The turbinates should be observed for polyps, which are abnormal, finger-like projections of swollen nasal mucosa. Polyps may result from long-term irritation of the mucosa, as from allergies. Any discharge should be assessed for colour and consistency. The presence of purulent and malodorous discharge could indicate the presence of a foreign body. Watery discharge could be secondary to allergies or could represent cerebro-spinal fluid. Bloody discharge could be secondary to trauma. Thick mucosal discharge could indicate the presence of infection.

Mouth and Pharynx. Using a good light source, the nurse inspects the interior of the mouth for colour, lesions, masses, gum retraction, bleeding, and poor dentition. The tongue is inspected for symmetry and presence of lesions. The nurse observes the pharynx by pressing a tongue blade against the middle of the back of the tongue. The pharynx should be smooth and moist, with no evidence of exudate, ulcerations, swelling, or postnasal drip. The colour, symmetry, and any enlargement of the tonsils are noted. The nurse stimulates the gag reflex by placing a tongue blade along the side of the pharynx behind the tonsil. A normal response (gagging) indicates that cranial nerves IX (glossopharyngeal nerve) and X (vagus nerve) are intact and that the airway is protected. Each side of the pharynx should be checked for the gag reflex.

Neck. The nurse inspects the neck for symmetry and presence of tender or swollen areas. The lymph nodes are palpated while the patient is sitting erect with the neck slightly flexed. Palpation progresses from the nodes around the ears to the nodes at the base of the skull and then to those located under the angles of the mandible to the midline. The nodes may be small, mobile, and nontender (shotty nodes), which is not a sign of a pathological condition. Nodes that are tender, hard, or fixed indicate disease. The location and characteristics of any palpable nodes are described.

Thorax and Lungs. Imaginary lines can be pictured on the chest to help in identifying abnormalities (see Figure 28-2). The locations of abnormalities can be described in relation to these lines (e.g., 2 cm from the right midclavicular line).

Chest examination is best performed in a well-lit, warm room, with measures taken to ensure the patient's privacy. Either the anterior or the posterior aspect of the chest may be examined first.

Inspection. The anterior aspect of the chest should be exposed while the patient is sitting upright or with the head of the bed upright. The patient may need to lean forward on the bedside table for support in order to facilitate breathing. First, the nurse observes the patient's appearance and notes any evidence of respiratory distress, such as tachypnea or use of accessory muscles. Next, the nurse determines the shape and symmetry of the chest. Chest movement should be equal on both sides, and the anteroposterior diameter should be less than the transverse diameter. Normal anteroposterior diameter is less than the transverse diameter by a ratio of 1:2. An increase in anteroposterior diameter (e.g., in the case of barrel-shaped chest) may be a normal age-related change or a result of lung hyperinflation, as occurs with emphysema. The nurse observes for abnormalities in the sternum, such as *pectus carinatum* (a prominent protrusion of the sternum) and *pectus excavatum* (an indentation of the lower sternum above the xiphoid process).

Next, the nurse should observe the respiratory rate, depth, and rhythm. The normal rate is 12 to 20 breaths per minute; in older persons, it is 16 to 25 breaths per minute. Inspiration should take half as long as expiration (ratio of inspiration to expiration is 1:2). The nurse should observe for abnormal breathing patterns, such as Kussmaul's (rapid, deep breathing), Cheyne–Stokes (abnormal pattern of respiration characterized by alternating periods of apnea and deep, rapid breathing), or Biot's respiration (a sequence with an irregular pattern of three to four respirations varying in depth, followed by a period of apnea) (Jarvis, Browne, MacDonald-Jenkins, et al., 2014). Skin colour provides clues to respiratory status. In dark-skinned patients, cyanosis is best observed in the conjunctivae, lips, palms, and soles of the feet. Causes of cyanosis include hypoxemia and decreased cardiac output. The fingers should be inspected for evidence of *clubbing* (an increase in the angle between the base of the nail and the fingernail to 180 degrees or more, usually accompanied by an increase in depth, bulk, and sponginess of the end of the finger). Nail beds should also be inspected for cyanosis.

When the nurse is inspecting the posterior aspect of the chest, the patient should lean forward with arms folded. This position moves the scapula away from the spine, so there is more exposure of the area to be examined. The observations that were made on the anterior part of the chest are made in the same sequence on the posterior part. In addition, any spinal curvature is noted. Spinal curvatures that affect breathing include kyphosis, scoliosis, and kyphoscoliosis.

Palpation. The nurse determines tracheal position by gently placing the index fingers on either side of the patient's trachea just above the suprasternal notch and gently pressing backward. Normal tracheal position is midline; deviation to the left or right is abnormal. Tracheal deviation occurs away from the side of a tension pneumothorax or a neck mass but toward the side of a pneumonectomy or lobar atelectasis (Wilson & Giddens, 2013). The nurse determines symmetry of chest expansion and extent of movement at the level of the diaphragm. The nurse places the hands over the lower anterior aspect of the patient's chest wall along the costal margin and moves them inward until the thumbs meet at midline. The patient is asked to breathe deeply, and the nurse observes the movement of the thumbs away from each other. Normal expansion is 2.5 cm. On the posterior side of the chest, the nurse places the hands at the level of the patient's tenth rib and moves the thumbs until they meet over the patient's spine (Figure 28-8).

Normal chest movement is symmetrical. Expansion is asymmetrical when air entry is limited by conditions involving the lung (e.g., atelectasis, pneumothorax) or the chest wall (e.g., incisional pain). Expansion is symmetrical but diminished in conditions that cause the chest to become hyperinflated or barrel-shaped and in neuro-muscular conditions (e.g., amyotrophic lateral sclerosis, spinal cord lesions). Movement may be absent or asymmetrical over a pleural effusion, an atelectasis, or a pneumothorax.

Fremitus is an abnormal, palpable vibration in the chest wall that is produced during vocalization and caused by the passage of air past thick bronchial mucus. The nurse can feel it with the hand on the chest while the patient takes a deep inspiration, and it may change or clear with coughing. It is produced by

FIGURE 28-8 Estimation of thoracic expansion. **A,** Exhalation. **B,** Maximal inhalation.

vocalization. To elicit tactile fremitus, the nurse places the palms of the hands against the patient's chest and asks the patient to repeat a phrase such as "ninety-nine." The nurse moves the hands from side to side and from top to bottom on the patient's chest (Figure 28-9). All areas of the chest should be palpated, and vibrations from an area on one side should be compared with those from the corresponding area on the other side. Tactile fremitus is most intense in the first and second interspaces lateral to the sternum and between the scapulae because these areas are closest to the major bronchi. Fremitus is less intense farther away from these areas.

Increase in, decrease in, or absence of fremitus should be noted. Fremitus is increased when the lung becomes filled with fluid or denser. This is noted with pneumonia, with lung tumours, and above a pleural effusion (the lung is compressed upward). Fremitus is decreased if the hand is farther from the lung (e.g., pleural effusion) or if the lung is hyperinflated (e.g., as in barrel-shaped chest). Absence of fremitus may be noted with pneumothorax or atelectasis. The anterior aspect of the chest is more difficult to palpate for fremitus because of the presence of large muscles and breast tissue.

Percussion. Percussion is performed to assess density or aeration of the lungs. Percussion sounds are described in Table 28-7. (The technique for percussion is described in Chapter 3.)

The anterior aspect of the chest is usually percussed with the patient in a semisitting or supine position. Starting above the clavicles, the nurse percusses downward, interspace by interspace (see Figure 28-9). The area over lung tissue should be resonant, with the exception of the area of cardiac dullness (Figure 28-10). For percussion of the posterior chest, the patient should sit leaning forward with arms folded. The posterior chest should be resonant over lung tissue to the level of the diaphragm (Figure 28-11).

Auscultation. During chest auscultation, the patient is instructed to breathe slowly and deeply in through the nose and out through the mouth. The nurse should proceed by comparing opposite areas of the chest, from the lung apices to the bases (see Figure 28-9). The stethoscope should be placed over lung tissue, not over bony prominences. At each placement of the stethoscope, the nurse should listen to at least one cycle of inspiration and expiration. Note the pitch (e.g., high, low), the duration of sound, and presence of any adventitious or abnormal sounds. The location of normal auscultatory sounds is more easily understood through visualization of a lung model (Figure 28-12).

FIGURE 28-9 Sequence for examination of the chest. **A,** Anterior sequence. **B,** Lateral sequence. **C,** Posterior sequence. For palpation, the nurse places the palms of the hands in the position designated as *1* on the right and left sides of the chest. The nurse compares the intensity of vibrations. Then the nurse repeats for all positions in each sequence. For percussion, the nurse taps the chest at each designated position, moving downward from side to side, while comparing percussion notes. For auscultation, the nurse places the stethoscope at each position and listens to at least one complete inspiratory and expiratory cycle.

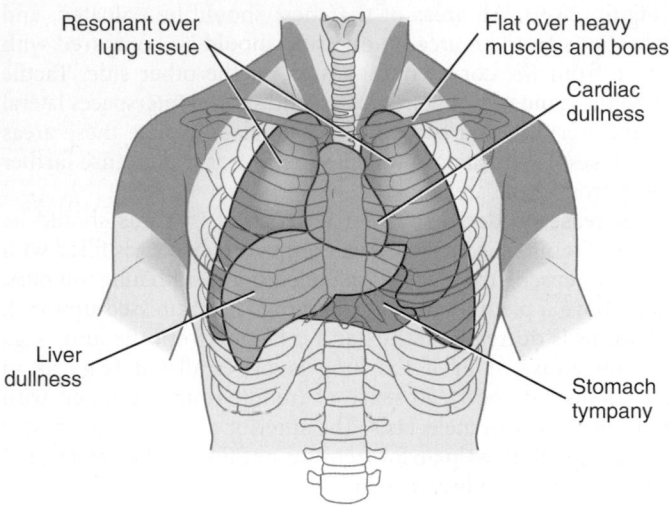

FIGURE 28-10 Diagram of percussion areas and sounds in the anterior aspect of the chest. Source: Redrawn from Thompson, J. M., McFarland, G., & Tucker, S. (2002). *Mosby's clinical nursing* (5th ed.). St. Louis: Mosby.

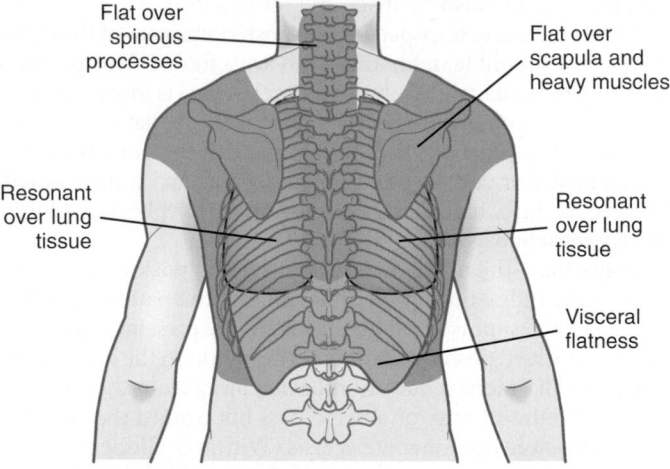

FIGURE 28-11 Diagram of percussion areas and sounds in the posterior aspect of the chest. Percussion proceeds from the lung apices to the lung bases, and sounds from opposite areas of the chest are compared. Source: Redrawn from Thompson, J. M., McFarland, G., & Tucker, S. (2002). *Mosby's clinical nursing* (5th ed.). St. Louis: Mosby.

TABLE 28-7   PERCUSSION SOUNDS

Sound	Description
Resonance	Low-pitched sound heard over normal lungs
Hyperresonance	Loud, lower-pitched sound than normal resonance heard over hyperinflated lungs, as in chronic obstructive lung disease and acute asthma
Tympany	Drumlike, loud, empty quality heard over gas-filled stomach or intestine or over pneumothorax
Dull	Medium-intensity pitch and duration heard over areas of "mixed" solid and lung tissue, such as over the top area of the liver, partially consolidated lung tissue (pneumonia), or fluid-filled pleural space
Flat	Soft, high-pitched sound of short duration heard over very dense tissue in which air is not present

The lung sounds should be heard down to the sixth rib anteriorly at the midclavicular line, the eighth rib at the midaxillary line, and the tenth rib at the scapular line in the back. In addition, during a deep breath, the lungs expand to the twelfth rib posteriorly. There are three normal breath sounds: vesicular, bronchovesicular, and bronchial. *Vesicular sounds* are relatively soft, low-pitched, gentle, rustling sounds. They are heard over all lung areas except the major bronchi. Vesicular sounds are heard longer on inspiration than on expiration, in a 3:1 ratio. *Bronchovesicular sounds* have a medium pitch and intensity and are heard anteriorly over the mainstem bronchi on either side of the sternum and posteriorly between the scapulae. Bronchovesicular sounds are heard for the same length of time on inspiration as on expiration (1:1). *Bronchial sounds* last for a shorter time on inspiration than on expiration by a ratio of 2:3, with a gap between inspiration and expiration that reflects the

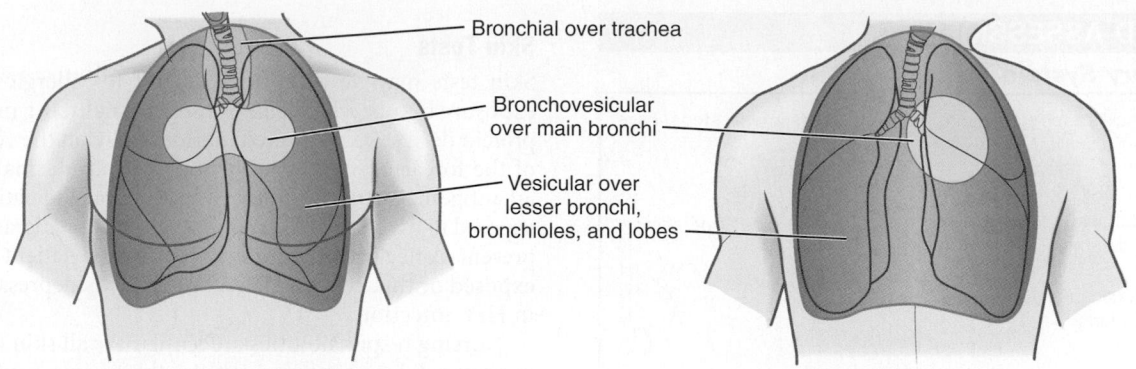

FIGURE 28-12 Normal auscultatory sounds. Source: From Beare, P. G., & Myers, J. L. (1998). *Adult health nursing* (3rd ed.). St. Louis: Mosby.

TABLE 28-8	**NORMAL PHYSICAL ASSESSMENT OF THE RESPIRATORY SYSTEM**

- Nose is symmetrical with no deformities. Nasal mucosa is pink and moist with no edema, exudate, blood, or polyps. Nasal septum is straight, without perforations.
- Oral mucosa is light pink and moist, with no exudate or ulcerations.
- Tonsils are not inflamed or enlarged.
- Pharynx is smooth, moist, and pink.
- Trachea is midline. No nodes are palpable.
- Chest is elliptical in shape, and chest expansion is symmetrical. Respirations are regular and nonlaboured, at the rate of 14/min. Breath sounds noted throughout both lung fields, without crackles or wheezes. No axillary nodes are palpable.

CASE STUDY

Objective Data: Physical Examination

Source: Monkey Business Images/ Shutterstock .com.

Physical examination findings of Fred Thompson are as follows:

BP 170/90, apical pulse 110, respiratory rate 30, temp 37°C, O_2 saturation 87% on room air. Patient sitting on edge of bed with arms resting on bedside table. Slight use of accessory muscles in neck and shoulders noted. Chest expansion equal. Respirations regular but slightly laboured with prolonged expiration. Skin colour pale with no cyanosis. No clubbing noted. Trachea midline. Bibasilar crackles, scattered rhonchi, and expiratory wheezing heard on auscultation. Moist, productive cough with yellow-tinged sputum.

Throughout this chapter, consider diagnostic studies that may be ordered for Mr. Thompson.

See pp. 565, 567, and 572 for more information on Mr. Thompson.

short pause between respiratory cycles. Bronchial sounds are louder and higher pitched and resemble air blowing through a hollow pipe. Bronchial sounds can be heard if the stethoscope is placed alongside the trachea in the neck.

The term *abnormal breath sounds* is used to describe bronchial or bronchovesicular sounds heard in the peripheral lung fields. Adventitious sounds are extra breath sounds that are abnormal. Adventitious breath sounds, described more fully in Table 28-8, include crackles (short, low-pitched sounds caused by the passage of air through an airway intermittently occluded by mucus, unstable bronchial wall, or fold of mucosa), wheezes (continuous high-pitched squeaking sound caused by rapid vibration of bronchial walls), and pleural friction rub (a creaking or grating sound that occurs when roughened, inflamed surfaces of the pleura rub together; it is evident during inspiration, expiration, or both; and does not change with coughing).

A record of normal findings in the physical assessment of the respiratory system is shown in Table 28-8. Assessment abnormalities of the thorax and lungs are listed in Table 28-9. Chest examination findings in common pulmonary problems are listed in Table 28-10. Age-related changes in the respiratory system and assessment findings are listed in Table 28-4.

A focused assessment is performed to evaluate the status of previously identified respiratory problems and to monitor for signs of new problems (see Chapter 3, Table 3-6). A focused assessment of the respiratory system is presented in the following "Focused Assessment" box.

DIAGNOSTIC STUDIES OF THE RESPIRATORY SYSTEM

Blood Studies

Common blood studies used to assess the respiratory system are the determinations of hemoglobin, hematocrit, and ABGs. Table 28-11 lists nursing responsibilities associated with these tests.

Oximetry

Oximetry is used to noninvasively monitor SpO_2 and SvO_2 (see Tables 28-1 and 28-3). Nursing care associated with oximetry is discussed in Table 28-11.

Sputum Studies

Sputum samples can be obtained by expectoration, tracheal suction, or bronchoscopy, a technique in which a flexible bronchoscope is inserted into the airways. The specimens may be examined for culture and sensitivity to identify an infecting organism (e.g., *Mycobacterium* species, *Pneumocystis jiroveci*) or to confirm a diagnosis (e.g., malignant cells). Nursing responsibilities for specimen collection are described in Table 28-11. Regardless of whether specimen tests are ordered, it is important to observe the sputum for colour, blood, volume, and viscosity.

FOCUSED ASSESSMENT

Respiratory System

Use this checklist to make sure the key assessment steps have been done.

Subjective
Ask the patient about any of the following and note the responses:

Shortness of breath	Y	N
Wheezing	Y	N
Sputum production (colour, quantity)	Y	N
Pain with breathing	Y	N
Cough	Y	N

Objective: Diagnostic
Check the following laboratory results for critical values:

Arterial blood gas measurements	✓
Chest radiographic examination	✓
Hematocrit, hemoglobin measurements	✓

Objective: Physical Examination
Observe

Respirations for rate, quality, and pattern	✓
Facial expression, level of consciousness, position patient takes to breath	

Inspect

Skin and nails for integrity and colour	✓
Accessory muscle use and position of trachea	✓
Shape, symmetry, and movement of chest wall	✓

Palpate

Chest and back for masses	✓
Tactile fremitus	

Auscultate

Lung (breath) sounds	✓

Skin Tests

Skin tests may be performed to test for allergic reactions or exposure to tubercle bacilli or fungi. Usually, 0.1 mL of purified protein derivative is injected intradermally on the ventral surface of the forearm. Skin tests involve the intradermal injection of an antigen. A positive result indicates that the patient has been exposed to the antigen. It does not indicate that disease is currently present. A negative result indicates that the patient has not been exposed or that cell-mediated immunity is depressed, as occurs in HIV infection.

Nursing responsibilities are similar for all skin tests. First, to prevent a false-negative reaction, the nurse should be certain that the injection is intradermal and not subcutaneous. After the injection, the sites should be circled and the patient instructed not to remove the marks. When charting administration of the antigen, the nurse should draw a diagram of the forearm and hand and label the injection sites. The diagram is especially helpful when more than one test is administered.

Tuberculin Skin Testing. When reading test results, the nurse should use a good light. The reading should be performed within 48 to 72 hours after the purified protein derivative is administered. It can take up to 48 hours for induration to become maximal. However, it is difficult to interpret a reaction after 72 hours (Public Health Agency of Canada, The Lung Association, & Canadian Thoracic Society, 2014). If an induration is present, a marking pen should be used to indicate the periphery (on all four sides) of the induration. As the pen touches the raised area, a mark should be made. The nurse then determines the diameter of the induration in millimetres. Reddened, flat areas are not measured. Reactions that indicate a positive and potential negative tuberculin skin test (TST) are described in Tables 28-12 and 28-13. Canadian health care settings use tuberculin purified protein (Tubersol) for skin tests. If any patient has had a previous bacille Calmette-Guérin vaccination, it will affect results. This

---

TABLE 28-9   ASSESSMENT ABNORMALITIES

Respiratory System

Finding	Description	Possible Etiology and Significance*
Inspection		
Pursed-lip breathing	Exhalation through mouth with lips pursed together to slow exhalation	COPD, asthma; suggests ↑ breathlessness; strategy taught to slow expiration, reduce dyspnea
Tripod position; inability to lie flat	Learning forward with arms and elbows supported on overbed table	COPD, asthma in exacerbation, pulmonary edema; indicates moderate to severe respiratory distress
Accessory muscle use; intercostal retractions	Neck and shoulder muscles used to assist breathing; muscles between ribs pull in during inspiration	COPD, asthma in exacerbation, secretion retention; indicates severe respiratory distress, hypoxemia
Splinting	↓ Inspiratory effort (or ↓ in tidal volume) as a result of sharp pain upon inspiration	Thoracic or abdominal incision; chest trauma, pleurisy
↑ Anteroposterior diameter	Anteroposterior chest diameter equal to transverse diameter; slope of ribs more horizontal (90 degrees) to spine	COPD, asthma, cystic fibrosis; lung hyperinflation; advanced age
Tachypnea	Rate >20 breaths/min; >25 breaths/min in older adults	Fever, anxiety, hypoxemia, restrictive lung disease; ↑ above normal respiratory rate reflects increased work of breathing
Kussmaul's respirations	Regular, rapid, and deep respirations	Metabolic acidosis; ↑ in rate aids body in ↑ CO_2 excretion
Cyanosis	Bluish coloration of skin, best seen in earlobes, under the eyelids, or in nail beds	↓ Oxygen transfer in lungs, ↓ cardiac output; nonspecific, unreliable indicator
Clubbing of fingers	↑ Depth, bulk, sponginess of distal digit of finger	Chronic hypoxemia; cystic fibrosis, lung cancer, bronchiectasis
Abdominal paradox	Inward (rather than normal outward) movement of abdomen during inspiration	Inefficient and ineffective breathing pattern; nonspecific indicator of severe respiratory distress

TABLE 28-9 ASSESSMENT ABNORMALITIES

Respiratory System—cont'd

Finding	Description	Possible Etiology and Significance*
Palpation		
Tracheal deviation	Leftward or rightward movement of trachea from normal midline position	Nonspecific indicator of change in position of mediastinal structures; medical emergency if caused by tension pneumothorax
Altered tactile fremitus	Increase or decrease in vibrations	↑ In pneumonia, pulmonary edema; ↓ in pleural effusion, lung hyperinflation; absent in pneumothorax, atelectasis
Altered chest movement	Diminished movement (can be asymmetrical or symmetrical) of two sides of chest with inspiration	Asymmetrical movement caused by atelectasis, pneumothorax, pleural effusion, splinting; symmetrical but diminished movement caused by barrel shape of chest, restrictive disease, neuro-muscular disease
Percussion		
Hyper-resonance	Loud, lower-pitched sound over areas that normally produce a resonant sound	Lung hyperinflation (COPD), lung collapse (pneumothorax), air trapping (asthma)
Dullness	Medium-pitched sound over areas that normally produce a resonant sound	↑ Density (pneumonia, widespread atelectasis), ↑ fluid pleural space (pleural effusion)
Auscultation		
Fine crackles	Series of short, explosive, high-pitched sounds heard just before the end of inspiration; rapid equalization of gas pressure when collapsed alveoli or terminal bronchioles suddenly snap open; sounds similar to rolling hair between fingers just behind ear	Interstitial fibrosis (asbestosis), interstitial edema (early pulmonary edema), alveolar filling (pneumonia), loss of lung volume (atelectasis), early phase of heart failure
Coarse crackles	Series of short, low-pitched sounds on inspiration and sometimes expiration; air passing through airway intermittently occluded by mucus, unstable bronchial wall, or fold of mucosa; sounds similar to blowing through straw under water (increase in bubbling quality with more fluid)	Heart failure, pulmonary edema, pneumonia with severe congestion, COPD
Wheezes	Continuous high-pitched squeaking sound caused by rapid vibration of bronchial walls; first evident on expiration; possibly evident on inspiration as obstruction of airway increases; possibly audible without stethoscope	Bronchospasm (caused by asthma), airway obstruction (caused by foreign body; tumour; viscous, thick increased secretions), COPD, pneumonia, bronchiectasis
Stridor	Continuous musical sound of constant pitch; result of partial obstruction of larynx or trachea	Croup, epiglottitis, vocal cord edema after extubation, foreign body
Absence of breath sounds	No sound evident over entire lung or area of lung	Pleural effusion, mainstem bronchi obstruction, widespread atelectasis, pneumonectomy, lobectomy, severe acute asthma (i.e., silent chest)
Pleural friction rub	Creaking or grating sound occurs when roughened, inflamed surfaces of pleura rub together; evident on inspiration, expiration, or both; no change with coughing; usually painful, especially on deep inspiration	Pleurisy, pneumonia, pulmonary infarct

*Only common causes are listed. (These conditions are discussed further in Chapters 29 through 31.)
COPD, chronic obstructive pulmonary disease.

CASE STUDY

Diagnostic Studies

The health care provider orders the following diagnostic studies for Fred Thompson:
- Complete blood cell count, basic metabolic panel (electrolytes, blood urea nitrogen, creatinine)
- ABGs
- Chest radiograph
- Sputum for culture and sensitivity

The ABGs demonstrate a compensated respiratory acidosis (pH, 7.37; PaCO₂, 58 mm Hg; HCO₃⁻, 29 mEq/L) with hypoxemia (PaO₂ 58 mm Hg; SaO₂, 87%). The white blood cell count is 14.3×10^9/L, and the chest radiograph shows lower lobe pneumonia. Mr. Thompson is admitted to the cardiopulmonary medical-surgical nursing unit.

See pp. 565, 567, and 570 for more information on Mr. Thompson.

Source: Monkey Business Images/Shutterstock.com.

is significant especially for people from Quebec, Newfoundland, and Indigenous populations, who regularly received this vaccine from 1940 through the 1970s (Public Health Agency of Canada, 2015b).

Radiological Studies

Chest Radiography. Chest radiographic examination is the most common method of assessing the respiratory system. It is also used to assess progression of disease and response to treatment. The views most commonly used are posteroanterior and lateral. (See Table 28-11 for nursing responsibilities related to chest radiographic examinations.)

Computed Tomography. Computed tomography (CT) may be used to examine cross-sections of the entire body. CT is used to evaluate areas that are difficult to assess by conventional radiographic study, such as the mediastinum, the hilum, and the pleura. With enhancement by a contrast medium, with a

TABLE 28-10   CHEST EXAMINATION FINDINGS IN COMMON PULMONARY PROBLEMS

Problem	Inspection	Palpation	Percussion	Auscultation
Chronic bronchitis	Barrel shape of chest; cyanosis; possible clubbing of fingers	—	Resonant	Crackles over deflated areas; wheeze may be present
Emphysema	Barrel shape of chest; tripod position; use of accessory muscles	↓ Chest expansion	Hyper-resonant or dull if consolidation is present	Crackles diminished if no exacerbation is present
Asthma (during an exacerbation)	Prolonged expiration; tripod position; pursed lips	↓ Chest expansion ↓ Fremitus if hyperinflation is present	Hyper-resonance	Wheezes; ↓ breath sounds are ominous sign if no improvement occurs (represent severely diminished air movement)
Pneumonia	Tachypnea; use of accessory muscles; cyanosis	Unequal movement with lobar involvement; ↑ fremitus over affected area	Dull over affected areas	Early: bronchial sounds Later: crackles; wheezes
Atelectasis	No change unless entire segment or lobe is involved	If area affected is small, no change If area affected is large, ↓ movement on affected side; ↑ fremitus	Dull over affected areas	Crackles (may disappear with deep breaths); absence of sounds if large area is affected
Pulmonary edema	Tachypnea; laboured respirations; cyanosis	↓ Chest expansion or normal movement	Dull or normal, depending on amount of fluid	Fine or coarse crackles
Pleural effusion	Tachypnea; use of accessory muscles	↓ Chest expansion ↑ Fremitus above effusion; absence of fremitus over effusion	Dull	Diminished or absent over effusion; egophony over effusion
Pulmonary fibrosis	Tachypnea	↓ Chest expansion	Normal	Crackles

TABLE 28-11   DIAGNOSTIC STUDIES

Respiratory System

Study	Description and Purpose	Nursing Responsibility
Blood Studies		
Hemoglobin (Hb) measurement	Value reflects amount of hemoglobin available for combination with oxygen. Venous blood is sampled. Normal level for men is 140–180 mmol/L; normal level for women is 120–160 mmol/L.	Explain procedure and its purpose.
Hematocrit (Hct) measurement	Value reflects ratio of red blood cells to plasma cells. Hematocrit is increased (polycythemia) in chronic hypoxemia. Venous blood is sampled. Normal value for men is 0.42–0.52; normal value for women is 0.37–0.47.	Explain procedure and its purpose.
ABG measurements	Values reflect acid–base balance, ventilation status, need for oxygen therapy, change in oxygen therapy, or change in ventilator settings.* Arterial blood is obtained through puncture of radial or femoral artery or through arterial catheter. Continuous ABG monitoring is also possible via a sensor or electrode inserted into the arterial catheter.	Indicate whether patient is using supplemental oxygen (percentage, amount per minute). Avoid change in oxygen therapy or interventions (e.g., suctioning, position change) for 20 min before obtaining sample. Assist with positioning (e.g., palm up, wrist slightly hyperextended if radial artery is used). Collect blood into heparinized syringe. To ensure accurate results, expel all air bubbles, and place sample on ice, unless it will be analyzed in <1 min. Apply pressure to artery for 5 min after specimen is obtained to prevent hematoma at the arterial puncture site.
Oximetry	Test monitors arterial or venous oxygen saturation. Oximetry is used for intermittent or continuous monitoring and exercise testing.†‡ Device attaches to finger, forehead, earlobe, or nose for SpO_2 monitoring or is contained in a pulmonary artery catheter for SvO_2 monitoring.	Apply probe to finger, forehead, earlobe, or bridge of nose. Before interpreting SpO_2 and SvO_2 values, first assess patient status and presence of factors that can alter accuracy of pulse oximeter reading. For SpO_2, these include motion, low perfusion, bright lights, use of intravascular dyes, acrylic nails, dark skin colour. For SvO_2, these include change in oxygen delivery or consumption. For SpO_2, notify health care provider of ±4% change from baseline or ↓ to <90%. For SvO_2, notify health care provider of ±10% change from baseline or ↓ to <60%.
Sputum Studies		
Culture and sensitivity	Purpose is to diagnose bacterial infection, select antibiotic, and evaluate treatment. Single sputum specimen is collected in a sterile container.	Instruct patient on how to produce a good specimen (see nursing responsibilities for Gram stain). If patient cannot produce specimen, bronchoscopy may be used (see Figure 28-13).
Gram stain	Staining of sputum enables classification of bacteria into gram-negative and gram-positive types. Results guide therapy until culture and sensitivity results are obtained.	Instruct patient to expectorate sputum into the container after coughing deeply. Obtain sputum (mucoid-like), not saliva. Obtain specimen in early morning because secretions accumulate during night. If sputum production is unsuccessful, try increasing oral fluid intake unless fluids are restricted. Collect sputum in sterile container (sputum trap) during suctioning or by aspirating secretions from the trachea. Send specimen to laboratory promptly.

TABLE 28-11   DIAGNOSTIC STUDIES

Respiratory System—cont'd

Study	Description and Purpose	Nursing Responsibility
Sputum Studies—cont'd		
Acid-fast smear and culture	Test is performed to collect sputum for acid-fast bacilli (tuberculosis). A series of three early morning specimens is used.	Instruct patient on how to produce a good specimen (see nursing responsibilities for Gram stain). Cover specimen and send to laboratory for analysis.
Cytology study	Purpose is to determine presence of abnormal cells that may indicate malignant condition. Single sputum specimen is collected in special container with fixative solution.	Send specimen to laboratory promptly. Instruct patient on how to produce a satisfactory specimen (see nursing responsibilities for Gram stain). If patient cannot produce specimen, bronchoscopy may be used (Figure 28-13).
Radiology		
Chest radiograph	Test is used to screen, diagnose, and evaluate change. Most common views are posteroanterior and lateral.	Instruct patient to undress to waist, put on gown, and remove any metal objects (e.g., jewellery, watch) between neck and waist.
Computed tomography (CT)	Test is performed for diagnosis of lesions difficult to assess by conventional radiographic studies, such as those in the hilum, the mediastinum, and the pleura. Images show structures in cross-section.	Same as for chest radiograph.
Magnetic resonance imaging (MRI)	Test is used for diagnosis of lesions difficult to assess by CT (e.g., lung apex near the spine).	Same as for chest radiograph. Instruct the patient to remove all metal objects (e.g., jewellery, watch) before test.
Ventilation–perfusion (VQ) scan	Test is used to identify areas of the lung not receiving airflow (ventilation) or blood flow (perfusion). It involves injection of radioisotope and inhalation of small amount of radioactive gas (xenon). A gamma ray–detecting device records radioactivity. Ventilation without perfusion is suggestive of pulmonary embolus.	Same as for chest radiograph. No precautions needed afterward because the gas and isotope transmit radioactivity for only a brief interval.
Pulmonary angiography	Study is used to visualize pulmonary vasculature and locate obstruction or pathological conditions such as pulmonary embolus. Contrast medium is injected through a catheter into the pulmonary artery or right side of the heart.	Same as for chest radiograph. Know that contrast injection may cause flushing, warm sensation, and coughing. Check pressure dressing site after procedure. Monitor blood pressure, pulse, and circulation distal to injection site. Report and record significant changes.
Positron emission tomography (PET)	Test is used to distinguish benign and malignant lung nodules. It involves IV injection of a radioisotope with short half-life.	Same as for chest radiograph. No precautions needed afterward because isotope transmits radioactivity for only a brief interval.
Endoscopic Examinations		
Bronchoscopy	Flexible fibre optic endoscope is used for diagnosis, biopsy, specimen collection, or assessment of changes. It may also be used to suction mucous plugs or to remove foreign objects. Study is typically performed in outpatient procedure room.	Instruct patient to be on NPO status for 6–12 hr. Obtain informed consent. Give sedative if it is ordered. After procedure, keep patient on NPO status until gag reflex returns, and monitor for laryngeal edema; monitor for recovery from sedatives. If biopsy was performed, monitor for hemorrhage and pneumothorax.
Mediastinoscopy	Test is used for inspection and biopsy of lymph nodes in mediastinal area.	Prepare patient for surgical intervention. Obtain informed consent. Afterward, monitor as for bronchoscopy.
Biopsy		
Lung biopsy	Specimens may be obtained by transbronchial or open lung biopsy. This test is used to obtain specimens for laboratory analysis.	Same as for bronchoscopy if procedure is performed with bronchoscope, and same as for thoracotomy (see Chapter 30) if open-lung biopsy is performed. Obtain informed consent.
Other Studies		
Thoracentesis	Test is used to obtain specimen of pleural fluid for diagnosis, to remove pleural fluid, or to instill medication. The physician inserts a large-bore needle through the chest wall into pleural space. A chest radiograph is always obtained after procedure to check for pneumothorax.	Explain procedure to patient, and obtain informed consent before procedure. Position patient sitting upright with elbows on an overbed table and feet supported. Instruct patient not to talk or cough, and assist during procedure. Observe for signs of hypoxia and verify breath sounds in all fields after procedure. Send labelled specimens to laboratory.
Pulmonary function test	Test is used to evaluate lung function. It involves use of a spirometer to diagram air movement as patient performs prescribed respiratory manoeuvres.†	Avoid scheduling test immediately after mealtime. Avoid administration of inhaled bronchodilator for 6 hr before procedure. Explain procedure to patient. Allow patient to rest after procedure.

*For normal values, see Tables 28-1.
†For normal values, see Table 28-15.
‡For critical values, see Table 28-3.
ABG, arterial blood gas; *IV,* intravenous; *NPO,* nothing by mouth; *SpO₂,* the oxygen saturation value obtained by pulse oximetry; *SvO₂,* venous oxygen saturation.

TABLE 28-12	SITUATION IN WHICH TUBERCULIN SKIN TEST REACTION IS CONSIDERED POSITIVE

Test Result	Situation in Which Reaction Is Considered Positive*
0–4 mm†	In a child younger than 5 years of age and at high risk of TB infection
≥5 mm	HIV infection
	Contact with person with infectious TB case within the past 2 years
	Presence of fibronodular disease on chest radiograph (healed TB, and not previously treated)
	Organ transplantation (related to immuno-suppressive therapy)
	Tumour necrosis factor alpha inhibitors
	Other immuno-suppressive drugs, such as corticosteroids (equivalent of ≥15 mg/day of prednisone for 1 month or more; risk of TB disease increases with higher dosage and longer duration)
	End-stage renal disease
≥10 mm	All others, including the following specific situations:
	• Test result conversion (within 2 years)
	• Diabetes, malnutrition, alcohol abuse (3 drinks/day)
	• Silicosis
	• Hematological malignancies (leukemia, lymphoma) and certain carcinomas (e.g., head and neck)

Source: © All rights reserved. *Canadian Tuberculosis Standards,* 7th Edition. Public Health Agency of Canada and Canadian Thoracic Society, 2014. Adapted and reproduced with permission from the Minister of Health, 2017.
*The goal of testing for latent tuberculosis is to identify individuals who are at increased risk for the development of tuberculosis and therefore would benefit from treatment of latent tuberculosis. Only those who would benefit from treatment should be tested; thus a decision to test presupposes a decision to treat if the test result is positive.
†In general, this level is considered negative, and no treatment is indicated.
HIV, human immunodeficiency virus; *TB,* tuberculosis.

TABLE 28-13	POTENTIAL CAUSES OF FALSE-NEGATIVE RESULT OF TUBERCULIN TEST

Category	Specific Cause
Technical (Potentially Correctable)	
Tuberculin material:	• Improper storage (exposure to light or heat)
	• Contamination, improper dilution, or chemical denaturation
Administration:	• Injection of too little tuberculin or injection made too deeply (should be intradermal)
	• Administration more than 20 minutes after tuberculin material is drawn up into the syringe
Reading:	• Inexperienced or biased reader
	• Error in recording
Biological (Not Correctable)	
Infections:	• Active TB (especially if advanced)
	• Other bacterial infection (typhoid fever, brucellosis, typhus, leprosy, pertussis)
	• HIV infection (especially if CD4 count <200)
	• Other viral infection (measles, mumps, varicella)
	• Fungal infection (South American blastomycosis)
Live virus vaccination:	• Measles
	• Mumps
	• Polio
Immuno-suppressive drugs:	• Corticosteroids
	• Tumour necrosis factor inhibitors
	• Others
Metabolic disease:	• Chronic renal failure
	• Severe malnutrition
	• Stress (surgery, burns)
Diseases of lymphoid organs:	• Lymphoma
	• Chronic lymphocytic leukemia
	• Sarcoidosis
Age:	• Infants <6 months
	• Older adults

Source: © All rights reserved. *Canadian Tuberculosis Standards,* 7th Edition. Public Health Agency of Canada and Canadian Thoracic Society, 2014. Adapted and reproduced with permission from the Minister of Health, 2017.

high-resolution technique, or with newer spiral CT, even pulmonary arteries can be inspected for emboli.

Magnetic Resonance Imaging. While in a strong magnetic field, the alignment of spinning nuclei can be changed with a superimposed radiofrequency, and the rate at which they return to alignment with the field can be measured. In magnetic resonance imaging (MRI), this technique is used to produce images of body structures. MRI has limited indications. It is most useful for evaluating images near the lung apex or the spine and for distinguishing vascular from nonvascular structures.

Ventilation–Perfusion Scan. A ventilation–perfusion scan is used primarily to check for the presence of a pulmonary embolus. There is no specific preparation or aftercare. A radioisotope is administered intravenously for the perfusion portion of the test; it outlines the pulmonary vasculature, which is then photographed. For the ventilation portion, the patient inhales a radioactive gas, which outlines the alveoli, and another photograph is taken. Normal scans show homogeneous radioactivity. Diminished appearance or absence of radioactivity is suggestive of lack of perfusion or airflow.

Pulmonary Angiography. Pulmonary angiography is used to confirm the diagnosis of an embolus if findings of the lung scan are inconclusive. A series of radiographs is taken after radiopaque dye is injected into the pulmonary artery. This test also detects congenital and acquired lesions of the pulmonary vessels.

Positron Emission Tomography. Positron emission tomography (PET) scans involve the use of radionuclides with short half-lives. PET scans are used to distinguish benign and malignant solitary pulmonary nodules. Because uptake of glucose is increased in malignant lung cells, the PET scan, in which an intravenous glucose preparation is used, can demonstrate the presence of malignant lung cells.

Endoscopic Examinations

Bronchoscopy. *Bronchoscopy* is a procedure in which the bronchi are visualized through a fibre-optic tube. Bronchoscopy may be used to obtain biopsy specimens, assess changes resulting from treatment, and remove mucous plugs or foreign bodies. Small amounts (30 mL) of sterile saline may be injected through the bronchoscope, then withdrawn, and examined for cells. This technique, termed *bronchoalveolar lavage,* is used to diagnose *Pneumocystis jiroveci* pneumonia (PCP; see Figure 28-13).

Bronchoscopy can be performed in an outpatient procedure room, in a surgical suite, or at the patient's bedside in the critical

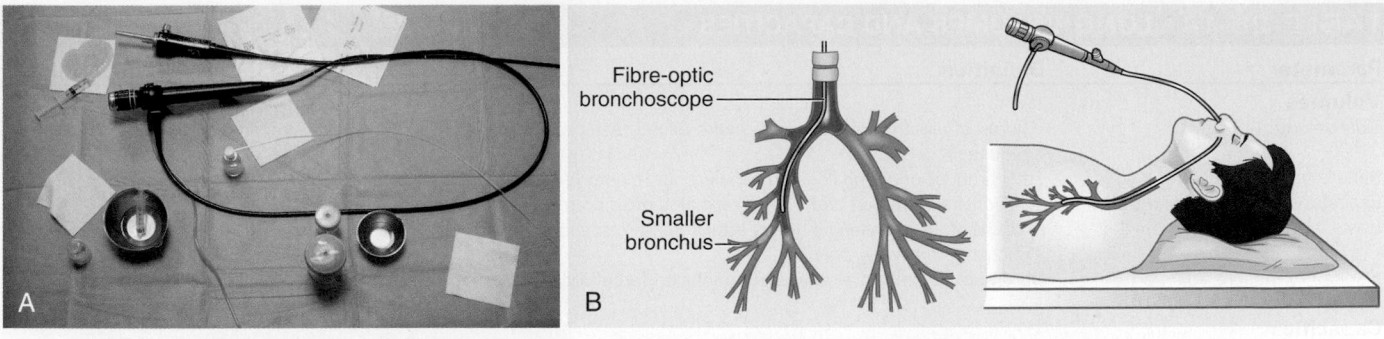

FIGURE 28-13 Fibre-optic bronchoscopy. **A,** The transbronchoscopic balloon-tipped catheter and the flexible fibre-optic bronchoscope. **B,** Procedure. The catheter is introduced into a small airway, and the balloon is inflated with 1.5 to 2 mL of air to occlude the airway. To perform bronchoalveolar lavage, 30 mL aliquots of sterile saline solution are injected and withdrawn, with gentle aspiration after each injection. Specimens are sent to the laboratory for analysis. Source: *A,* BSIP SA/Alamy Stock Photo.

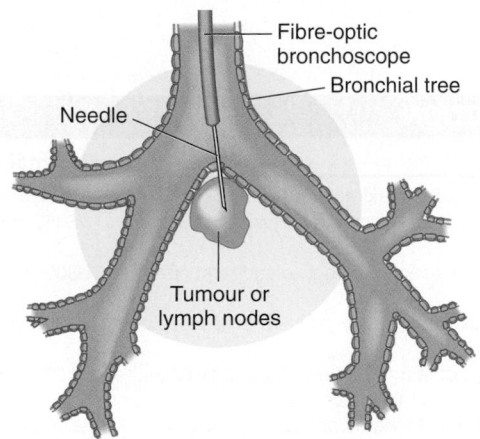

FIGURE 28-14 Transbronchial needle biopsy. In this diagram, a transbronchial biopsy needle penetrates the bronchial wall and enters a mass of subcarinal lymph nodes or tumour. Source: Redrawn from Du Bois, R. M., & Clarke, S. W. (1987). *Fiberoptic bronchoscopy in diagnosis and management.* Orlando, FL: Grune & Stratton.

FIGURE 28-15 Thoracentesis. A catheter is positioned in the pleural space to remove accumulated fluid.

care unit or on a medical-surgical floor, with the patient lying down or seated. After local anaesthetic is applied to the nasal pharynx and oral pharynx, the bronchoscope is coated with lidocaine (Xylocaine) and inserted, usually through the nose, and threaded down into the airways. A bronchoscopy can be performed on mechanically ventilated patients through the endotracheal tube. The nursing care for patients undergoing this procedure is described in Table 28-11.

Mediastinoscopy. For mediastinoscopy, an endoscope is inserted through a small incision in the suprasternal notch and advanced into the mediastinum to inspect lymph nodes and sample them for biopsy. The test is used to diagnose carcinoma, granulomatous infections, and sarcoidosis. The procedure is performed in the operating room, and the patient is given a general anaesthetic.

Lung Biopsy

Lung biopsy may be performed transbronchially or as an open lung procedure. The purpose is to obtain tissue, cells, or secretions for evaluation. Transbronchial lung biopsy involves passing a forceps or needle through the bronchoscope for a specimen (Figure 28-14). Specimens can be cultured or examined for malignant cells. A combination of transbronchial lung biopsy

and bronchoalveolar lavage is used to differentiate infection and rejection in lung transplant recipients. Nursing care is the same as for fibre optic bronchoscopy. Open lung biopsy is used when pulmonary disease cannot be diagnosed by other procedures. The patient receives a general anaesthetic, the chest is opened with a thoracotomy incision, and a biopsy specimen is obtained. Nursing care after the procedure is the same as after thoracotomy (see Chapter 30 and NCP 30-2, available on the Evolve website).

Thoracentesis

Thoracentesis is the insertion of a needle through the chest wall into the pleural space to obtain specimens for diagnostic evaluation, remove pleural fluid, or instill medication into the pleural space (Figure 28-15). The patient is positioned sitting upright with elbows on an overbed table and feet supported. The skin is cleansed, and a local anaesthetic (lidocaine [Xylocaine]) is instilled subcutaneously. A chest tube may be inserted to enable further drainage of fluid. Nursing care is described in Table 28-11.

Pulmonary Function Tests

Pulmonary function tests (PFTs) are conducted to measure lung volumes and airflow. The results of PFTs are used to diagnose pulmonary disease, monitor disease progression, evaluate

TABLE 28-14   LUNG VOLUMES AND CAPACITIES

Parameter	Definition	Normal Value
Volumes		
Tidal volume (V$_T$)	Volume of air inhaled and exhaled with each breath; only a small proportion of total capacity of lungs	0.5 L
Minute volume (MV)	Total amount of air inhaled and exhaled per minute (V$_T$ X respiratory rate).	5–8 L/min
Expiratory reserve volume (ERV)	Additional air that can be forcefully exhaled after normal exhalation is complete	1.0 L
Residual volume (RV)	Amount of air remaining in lungs after forced expiration; air available in lungs for gas exchange between breaths	1.5 L
Inspiratory reserve volume (IRV)	Maximum volume of air that can be inhaled forcefully after normal inhalation	3.0 L
Capacities		
Total lung capacity (TLC)	Maximum volume of air that lungs can contain (TLC = IRV + V$_T$ + ERV + RV)	6.0 L
Functional residual capacity (FRC)	Volume of air remaining in lungs at end of normal exhalation (FRC = ERV + RV); increase or decrease possible with lung disease	2.5 L
Vital capacity (VC)	Maximum volume of air that can be exhaled after maximum inspiration (VC = IRV + V$_T$ + ERV); generally higher in men	4.5 L
Inspiratory capacity (IC)	Maximum volume of air that can be inhaled after normal expiration (IC = V$_T$ + IRV)	3.5 L

TABLE 28-15   COMMON MEASURES OF PULMONARY FUNCTION

Measure	Description	Normal Value*
Forced vital capacity (FVC)	Amount of air that can be quickly and forcefully exhaled after maximum inspiration	>80% of predicted
Forced expiratory volume in first second of expiration (FEV$_1$)	Amount of air exhaled in first second of FVC; valuable clue to severity of airway obstruction	>80% of predicted
FEV$_1$/FVC	Ratio of value for FEV$_1$ to value for FVC; useful in differentiating obstructive and restrictive pulmonary dysfunction	>80% of predicted
Maximal midexpiratory flow rate (MMEF)	Measurement of airflow rate in middle half of forced expiration; early indicator of disease of small airways	>80% of predicted
Maximal voluntary ventilation (MVV)	Deep breathing as rapidly as possible for specified period; test for airflow, muscle strength, coordination, airway resistance; important factor in exercise tolerance	≈170 L/min
Peak expiratory flow rate (PEFR)	Maximum airflow rate during forced expiration; aids in monitoring bronchoconstriction in asthma	≤600 L/min
Maximum inspiratory pressure (MIP) or negative inspiratory force (NIF)	Amount of negative pressure generated on inspiration; indication of ability to breathe deeply and cough	≤80 cm H$_2$O

*Normal values vary with height, weight, age, and sex of patient.

disability, and evaluate response to bronchodilators. In PFTs, a spirometer is used. The patient's age, sex, height, and weight are entered into the PFT computer to calculate predicted values. The patient inserts a mouthpiece, takes as deep a breath as possible, and exhales as hard, fast, and long as possible. Verbal coaching is given to ensure that the patient continues blowing out until exhalation is complete. The computer determines the actual value achieved, predicted (normal) value, and percentage of the predicted value for each test. A normal actual value is 80% to 120% of the predicted value. Normal values for PFTs are shown in Tables 28-14 and 28-15, and the relationships between lung volumes and capacities are described in Figure 28-16.

Home spirometry may be used to monitor lung function in persons with asthma or cystic fibrosis, as well as before and after lung transplantation. Changes in spirometry values at home can warn of early lung transplant rejection or infection. Feedback from a peak expiratory flowmeter can increase the sense of control achieved when persons with asthma learn to modify activities and medications in response to changes in rates of peak expiratory flow.

Pulmonary function parameters can also be used to determine the need for mechanical ventilation or the readiness to be weaned

FIGURE 28-16 Relationship of lung volumes and capacities. *ERV*, expiratory reserve volume; *FRC*, functional residual capacity; *IC*, inspiratory capacity; *IRV*, inspiratory reserve volume; *RV*, residual volume; *TLC*, total lung capacity; *V$_T$*, tidal volume; *VC*, vital capacity.

from ventilatory support. Vital capacity, maximum inspiratory pressure, and minute ventilation are measured to make this determination (see Table 28-14).

Exercise Testing

Exercise testing is used in diagnosis, in determining exercise capacity, and for disability evaluation. A complete exercise test involves walking on a treadmill while expired oxygen and carbon dioxide, respiratory rate, heart rate, and rhythm are monitored. A modified test (desaturation test) may also be used. In that case, only SpO_2 is monitored. A desaturation test can also be used to determine the oxygen flow needed to maintain the SpO_2 at a safe level during activity or exercise in patients who use home oxygen therapy.

A timed walk can also be used to measure exercise capacity. The patient is instructed to walk as far as possible during a timed period (6 or 12 minutes), to stop when short of breath, and to continue when able. The distance walked is measured, and the data are used to monitor progression of disease or improvement after rehabilitation.

REVIEW QUESTIONS

The number of the question corresponds to the same-numbered objective at the beginning of the chapter.

1. Which of the following is the mechanism that stimulates the release of surfactant?
   a. Fluid accumulation in the alveoli
   b. Alveolar collapse from atelectasis
   c. Alveolar stretch from deep breathing
   d. Air movement through the alveolar pores of Kohn

2. Which of the following causes air to enter the thoracic cavity during inspiration?
   a. Contraction of the accessory abdominal muscles
   b. Increased carbon dioxide and decreased oxygen in the blood
   c. Stimulation of the respiratory muscles by the chemoreceptors
   d. Decreased intrathoracic pressure relative to pressure at the airway

3. Which of the following measures the lungs' ability to adequately oxygenate the arterial blood?
   a. Arterial oxygen tension
   b. Carboxyhemoglobin level
   c. Arterial carbon dioxide tension
   d. Venous carbon dioxide tension

4. Which of the following is the most important respiratory defence mechanism distal to the respiratory bronchioles?
   a. Alveolar macrophage
   b. Impaction of particles
   c. Reflex bronchoconstriction
   d. Mucociliary clearance mechanism

5. Which of the following is caused by a rightward shift of the oxygen–hemoglobin dissociation curve?
   a. Metabolic alkalosis
   b. Postoperative hypothermia
   c. Release of oxygen at the tissue level
   d. Greater affinity of oxygen for hemoglobin

6. Which of the following are very early signs or symptoms of inadequate oxygenation?
   a. Dyspnea and hypotension
   b. Apprehension and restlessness
   c. Cyanosis and cool, clammy skin
   d. Increased urine output and diaphoresis

7. During the respiratory assessment of an older adult, the nurse would expect to find which of the following? *(Select all that apply)*
   a. A vigorous cough
   b. Increased chest expansion
   c. Increased residual volume
   d. Increased breath sounds in the lung apices
   e. Increased anteroposterior (AP) chest diameter

8. Which of the following should the nurse inquire about when assessing activity and exercise related to respiratory health?
   a. Dyspnea during rest or exercise
   b. Recent weight loss or weight gain
   c. Willingness to wear oxygen equipment in public
   d. Ability to sleep through the entire night

9. Which of the following is the best tool to assess for the vibration of tactile fremitus?
   a. Palms
   b. Fingertips
   c. Stethoscope
   d. Index fingers

10. Which of the following is an abnormal finding in the assessment of the respiratory system?
    a. Presence of fremitus
    b. Inspiratory chest expansion of 2.5 cm
    c. Percussion resonance over the lung bases
    d. Symmetrical chest expansion and contraction

11. Which of the following is performed to remove pleural fluid for analysis?
    a. Thoracentesis
    b. Bronchoscopy
    c. Pulmonary angiography
    d. Sputum culture and sensitivity

1. c; 2. d; 3. a; 4. a; 5. c; 6. b; 7. c, e; 8. a; 9. a; 10. a; 11. a.

evolve

For even more review questions, visit *http://evolve.elsevier.com/Canada/Lewis/medsurg*.

REFERENCES

Herlihy, B. (2014). *The human body in health and illness* (5th ed.). St. Louis: Elsevier Saunders.

Hoffman Wold, G. (2012). *Basic geriatric nursing* (5th ed.). St. Louis: Elsevier Mosby.

Huether, S. E., & McCance, K. L. (2017). *Understanding pathophysiology* (6th ed.). St. Louis: Elsevier Mosby.

Jarvis, C., Browne, A., MacDonald-Jenkins, J., et al. (2014). *Physical examination & health assessment* (2nd Canadian ed.). Toronto: Elsevier Canada.

McCance, K. L., & Huether, S. E. (2014). *Pathophysiology: The biologic basis for disease in adults and children* (7th ed.). St. Louis: Mosby.

Patton, K. T., & Thibodeau, G. A. (2016). *Anatomy and physiology* (9th ed.). St. Louis: Mosby.

Public Health Agency of Canada. (2014). *Canadian immunization guide: Part 4—Active vaccines.* Retrieved from *http:// www.phac-aspc.gc.ca/publicat/cig-gci/p04-pneu-eng.php.*

Public Health Agency of Canada. (2015a). *An Advisory Committee Statement (ACS) National Advisory Committee on Immunization (NACI): Canadian immunization guide chapter on influenza and statement on seasonal influenza vaccine for 2015–2016* (pp. 6, 12–13). Retrieved from *http://www.phac-aspc.gc.ca/naci-ccni/ assets/pdf/flu-2015-grippe-eng.pdf.*

Public Health Agency of Canada. (2015b). *Canadian immunization guide: Bacille Calmette-Guérin (BCG) vaccine.* Retrieved from *https://www.canada.ca/en/public-health/services/publications/ healthy-living/canadian-immunization-guide-part- 4-active-vaccines/page-2-bacille-calmette-guerin-vaccine.html.*

Public Health Agency of Canada, The Lung Association, & Canadian Thoracic Society. (2014). *Canadian tuberculosis standards* (7th ed.).
Retrieved from *http://strauss.ca/OEMAC/wp-content/uploads/ 2013/11/Canadian_TB_Standards_7th-edition_English.pdf.*

Public Health Ontario. (2013). *Annex B: Best practices for prevention of acute respiratory infection in all health care settings.* Retrieved from *https://www.publichealthontario.ca/en/eRepository/PIDAC -IPC_Annex_B_Prevention_Transmission_ARI_2013.pdf.*

Public Health Ontario. (2015a). *Emergency planning and preparedness: Avian influenza A(H7N9) virus guidance for health workers and health sector employers.* Retrieved from *http:// www.health.gov.on.ca/en/pro/programs/emb/avian/workers.aspx.*

Public Health Ontario. (2015b). *Best practices for prevention, surveillance and infection control management of novel respiratory infections in all health care settings.* Retrieved from *http:// www.publichealthontario.ca/en/eRepository/Best_Practices_Novel _Respiratory_Infections.pdf.*

Urden, L. D., Stacy, K. M., & Lough, M. E. (2014). *Critical care nursing: Diagnosis and management* (7th ed.). St. Louis: Elsevier Mosby.

Weinberger, S. E., Cockrill, B. A., & Mandel, J. (2014). *Principles of pulmonary medicine* (6th ed.). Philadelphia: Elsevier Saunders.

Wilson, S. F., & Giddens, J. F. (2013). *Health assessment for nursing practice* (5th ed.). St. Louis: Mosby.

RESOURCES

Resources for this chapter are listed in Chapters 30 and 31.

For additional Internet resources, see the website for this book at *http://evolve.elsevier.com/Canada/Lewis/medsurg*

Nursing Management

Upper Respiratory Problems

Written by: Eugene E. Mondor
Adapted by: Micki Puksa and Lesley MacMaster

⊝volve WEBSITE

http://evolve.elsevier.com/Canada/lewis/medsurg

- Review Questions (Online Only)
- Key Points
- Answer Guidelines for Case Study
- Student Case Study
  - Head and Neck Cancer: Laryngectomy With Tracheostomy

- Customizable Nursing Care Plans
  - Tracheostomy
  - Total Laryngectomy and/or Radical Neck Surgery
- Conceptual Care Map Creator

- Audio Glossary
- Supporting Media—Animation
  - Anatomical Location of Sinuses
- Content Updates

LEARNING OBJECTIVES

1. Describe the clinical manifestations and nursing management of problems of the nose.
2. Describe the clinical manifestations and nursing management of problems of the paranasal sinuses.
3. Describe the clinical manifestations and nursing management of problems of the pharynx and the larynx.
4. Discuss the nursing management of the patient who requires a tracheostomy.

5. Identify the steps involved in performing tracheostomy care and suctioning an airway.
6. Describe the risk factors and warning symptoms associated with head and neck cancer.
7. Discuss the nursing management of the patient with a laryngectomy.
8. Describe the methods used in voice restoration for the patient with temporary or permanent loss of speech.

KEY TERMS

allergic rhinitis, p. 581	epistaxis, p. 580	nasal polyps, p. 587	tracheostomy, p. 587
deviated septum, p. 579	esophageal speech, p. 597	rhinoplasty, p. 580	tracheotomy, p. 587

STRUCTURAL AND TRAUMATIC DISORDERS OF THE NOSE

DEVIATED SEPTUM

Deviated septum is a deflection of the normally straight nasal septum. Most commonly, it is caused by trauma to the nose or arises from a congenital disproportion in which the size of the septum is not proportional to the size of the nose. On inspection, the septum is bent to one side, altering the air passage. Symptoms are variable. The patient may experience obstruction to nasal breathing, nasal edema, or dryness of the nasal mucosa with crusting and bleeding (epistaxis). A severely deviated septum may block drainage of mucus from the sinus cavities, resulting in infection (sinusitis; Patton & Thibodeau, 2016).

Medical management of deviated septum includes nasal allergy control, as in allergic rhinitis (discussed later in this chapter). For patients with severe symptoms, a nasal septoplasty (surgical realignment of the septum) is performed to reconstruct and properly align the deviated septum.

NASAL FRACTURE

Nasal fracture is most often caused by trauma of substantial force to the middle of the face. Some cases of facial trauma can be prevented by using protective sports equipment and protecting against falls. Complications of a nasal fracture include airway obstruction, epistaxis, meningeal tears, and cosmetic deformity.

Nasal fractures are classified as unilateral, bilateral, or complex. A *unilateral fracture* typically produces little or no displacement. *Bilateral fractures,* the most common type, give the nose a flattened look. Powerful frontal blows cause *complex fractures*, which may also shatter the frontal bones. Diagnosis is based on the health history, direct observation, and radiographic findings.

On inspection, the nurse should assess the patient's ability to breathe through each nostril and note the presence of edema, bleeding, or hematoma (Emergency Nurses Association, 2013). There may be ecchymosis under one or both eyes. Ecchymosis involving both eyes is often termed *raccoon eyes*. The nose is inspected internally for evidence of deviated septum, hemorrhage, or clear drainage. Clear, pink-tinged, or persistent drainage (i.e., rhinorrhea) after control of epistaxis suggests a cerebro-spinal (CSF) leak. A positive glucose screen can confirm the presence of CSF. Injury of sufficient force to fracture nasal bones results in considerable swelling of soft tissues. With extensive swelling, it may be difficult to verify the extent of deformity or to repair the fracture until several days later, when the edema subsides (Emergency Nurses Association, 2013).

The goals of nursing management are to reduce edema, prevent complications, and provide emotional support. Ice may be applied to the face and nose to reduce edema and bleeding. When a fracture is confirmed, the goal of management is to realign the fracture using closed or open reduction (septoplasty, rhinoplasty). These procedures re-establish cosmetic appearance and proper function of the nose and provide an adequate airway. After the patient undergoes nasal surgery, the patient should be assessed for the ability to mouth-breathe. Nasal intubation or nasogastric tube should be avoided in any patient suspected of a nasal fracture (Rothrock, 2015).

RHINOPLASTY

Rhinoplasty, the surgical reconstruction of the nose, is performed for cosmetic reasons or to improve airway function when trauma or congenital deformities result in nasal obstruction. Assessment of the patient's expectations is a critical aspect in preparation for a rhinoplasty. Expected results of surgery should be explained frankly and truthfully to prevent disappointment (Rothrock, 2015).

Collaborative Care

Rhinoplasty is performed as an outpatient procedure, using regional anaesthesia. Nasal tissue may be added or removed, and the nose may be lengthened or shortened. Plastic implants are sometimes used to reshape the nose. After surgery, nasal packing may be inserted to apply pressure and prevent bleeding or septal hematoma formation. Nasal septal splints (small pieces of plastic or Silastic) may be inserted to help prevent scar tissue formation between the surgical site and the lateral nasal wall. Adhesive-strip skin closures are placed to hold the skin against the septal cartilage. Typically, nasal packing is removed the day after surgery, and the splint is removed in 3 to 5 days. A small dressing under the nostrils is changed as often as every 2 hours during the first 24 hours. The patient is instructed to prevent pressure on the surgical site by sneezing through the mouth (Rothrock, 2015).

NURSING MANAGEMENT
NASAL SURGERY

Examples of nasal surgery include rhinoplasty, septoplasty, and nasal fracture reductions. Before surgery, the patient should be instructed to not take drugs containing acetylsalicylic acid (ASA;

Aspirin) or nonsteroidal anti-inflammatory drugs (NSAIDs) for 2 weeks to reduce the risk for bleeding. Nursing interventions during the immediate postoperative period include assessment of respiratory status, pain management, and observation of the surgical site for hemorrhage and edema. Teaching is important because the patient must be able to detect complications at home (Rothrock, 2015). There is an interim period while edema and ecchymosis resolve, before the final cosmetic effect can be achieved.

EPISTAXIS

Epistaxis (nosebleed) occurs in all age groups, especially in children and older-adult patients. Epistaxis may be caused by trauma, foreign bodies, nasal spray abuse, street drug use, anatomical malformation, allergic rhinitis, or tumours. Any condition that prolongs bleeding time or alters platelet counts will predispose the patient to epistaxis. Bleeding time may also be prolonged if the patient takes ASA (Aspirin) or NSAIDs. Conditions such as hypertension do not increase the risk for epistaxis (Bamimore & Silverberg, 2015; Emergency Nurses Association, 2013). Elevated blood pressure, however, makes bleeding more difficult to control.

Children and young adults have a tendency to develop anterior nasal bleeding, whereas older adults more commonly have posterior nasal bleeding. Anterior bleeding usually stops spontaneously or can be self-treated; posterior bleeding may require medical treatment (Bamimore & Silverberg, 2015).

NURSING AND COLLABORATIVE MANAGEMENT
EPISTAXIS

Simple first-aid measures should be attempted first to control epistaxis. The nurse should (1) keep the patient quiet; (2) place the patient in a sitting position, leaning forward, or if not possible, in a reclining position with head and shoulders elevated; (3) apply direct pressure by pinching the entire soft lower portion of the nose for 10 to 15 minutes; (4) apply ice compresses to the forehead and have the patient suck on ice; (5) apply digital pressure if bleeding continues; and (6) obtain medical assistance if bleeding does not stop (Emergency Nurses Association, 2013; Nguyen, 2015).

If first aid is not effective, management involves localization of the bleeding site and application of a vasoconstrictive agent, cauterization, or anterior packing by a health care provider. Anterior packing may consist of ribbon gauze impregnated with antibiotic ointment that is wedged firmly in the desired location and remains in place for 48 to 72 hours. If posterior packing is required, the patient should be hospitalized. Inflatable balloons may be used as a nasal pack, or gauze rolls may be inserted (Figure 29-1). Strings attached to the packing are brought to the outside and taped to the cheek for ease of removal. A nasal sling (a folded 2×2–inch gauze pad) should be taped over the nares to absorb drainage (Cooper & Gosnell, 2015).

Posterior packing may alter respiratory status, especially in older-adult patients. Some patients experience *hypoventilation* causing *hypercapnia* (increase in the partial pressure of carbon dioxide in arterial blood [$PaCO_2$]) and *hypoxemia* (decrease in the partial pressure of oxygen in arterial blood [PaO_2]) sufficient to lead to cardiac dysrhythmias or respiratory arrest. The nurse should closely monitor respiratory rate, heart rate and rhythm,

FIGURE 29-1 Method for placing posterior nasal pack. **A,** Catheter is passed through the bleeding side of the nose and pulled out through the mouth with a hemostat. Strings are tied to the catheter, and the pack is pulled up behind the soft palate and into the nasopharynx. **B,** Nasal pack in position in the posterior nasopharynx. Dental roll at the nose helps maintain correct position.

oxygen saturation using pulse oximetry (SpO_2), and level of consciousness and observe for signs of aspiration (Aghababian, Bird, Braen, et al., 2011).

Packing is painful because sufficient pressure must be applied to stop the bleeding. Nasal packing predisposes to infection from bacteria (e.g., *Staphylococcus aureus*) present in the nasal cavity. The patient should receive a mild opioid analgesic for pain (e.g., acetaminophen with codeine) and an antibiotic effective against staphylococci to protect against infection.

Posterior packs are left in place for no longer than 48 hours because of the incidence of toxic shock syndrome and are usually removed by the surgeon. Before removal, the patient should be medicated for pain because this procedure is very uncomfortable. After removal, the nares may be gently cleaned and then lubricated with petroleum jelly.

Failure of posterior packing to control epistaxis indicates the need for surgery or radiological embolization of the affected artery (Aghababian et al., 2011). The most common surgical procedure of this nature involves ligation of the internal maxillary artery, performed through a Caldwell–Luc incision under the upper lip to gain access to the artery.

The patient can be discharged after being taught about home care. The patient should be instructed to avoid vigorous nose blowing, strenuous activity, lifting, and straining for 4 to 6 weeks. The patient should be taught to sneeze with the mouth open and to avoid the use of ASA (Aspirin)–containing products or NSAIDs (Rothrock, 2015).

INFLAMMATION AND INFECTION OF THE NOSE AND PARANASAL SINUSES

ALLERGIC RHINITIS

Allergic rhinitis is the reaction of the nasal mucosa to a specific allergen. Attacks of seasonal rhinitis usually occur in the spring and fall and are caused by allergy to pollens from trees, flowers, or grasses. The typical attack lasts for several weeks during times

when pollen counts are high, then disappears, and recurs at the same time the following year. Perennial rhinitis is present intermittently or constantly. Symptoms are usually caused by specific environmental triggers such as pet dander, dust mites, moulds, or cockroaches (deSchazo & Kemp, 2016). Because symptoms of perennial rhinitis resemble the common cold, the patient may believe the condition is a continuous or repeated cold.

Clinical Manifestations

Manifestations of allergic rhinitis are nasal congestion; sneezing; watery, itchy eyes and nose; altered sense of smell; and thin, watery nasal discharge. The nasal turbinates appear pale, boggy, and swollen. With chronic exposure to allergens, the patient's responses include headache, congestion, pressure, postnasal drip, and nasal polyps (deSchazo & Kemp, 2016). The patient may complain of cough, hoarseness, snoring, or the recurrent need to clear the throat.

NURSING AND COLLABORATIVE MANAGEMENT ALLERGIC RHINITIS

Several steps are used in managing allergic rhinitis. The most important step involves identifying and avoiding triggers of allergic reactions (Table 29-1). The patient should be instructed to keep a diary of times when the allergic reaction occurs and the activities that precipitate the reaction. Steps can then be taken to avoid these triggers.

Drug therapy involves using nasal sprays, leukotriene receptor antagonists (LTRAs; deSchazo & Kemp, 2016), antihistamines, and decongestants to manage symptoms (Table 29-2). Intranasal corticosteroid and cromolyn sprays are effective for seasonal and perennial rhinitis. Nasal corticosteroid sprays are used to decrease inflammation locally; there is little absorption in the systemic circulation, and therefore, systemic adverse drug events are rare. Relief may require combining a nasal corticosteroid spray and an antihistamine. The patient using nasal inhalers needs careful instructions about proper use. Nasal decongestant sprays can be used only for up to 5 days because they can cause a rebound effect from prolonged use (deSchazo & Kemp, 2016).

Immunotherapy ("allergy injections") may be used if drugs are not tolerated, or ineffective, when a specific, unavoidable allergen is identified. Immunotherapy involves controlled exposure to small amounts of a known allergen through frequent (at least weekly) injections, with the goal to decrease sensitivity. (The mechanisms involved in the allergic response and immunotherapy are discussed in Chapter 16.)

DRUG ALERT—Antihistamines
- First-generation antihistamines (e.g., chlorpheniramine) can cause drowsiness and sedation.
- Warn patients that operating machinery and driving may be dangerous because of the sedative effect.

DRUG ALERT—Pseudoephedrine
- Large doses may produce tachycardia and palpitations, especially in patients with cardiac disease.
- Overdose in people over 60 years of age may result in central nervous system depression, seizures, and hallucinations.

ACUTE VIRAL RHINITIS

Acute viral rhinitis (common cold or acute coryza) is caused by viruses that invade the upper respiratory tract. It is the most prevalent infectious disease and is spread by airborne droplet sprays emitted by the infected person while breathing, talking,

TABLE 29-1 PATIENT & CAREGIVER TEACHING GUIDE

How to Reduce Symptoms of Allergic Rhinitis

Include the following information when teaching the patient and caregiver how to reduce symptoms of allergic rhinitis.

1. Avoidance of allergens is the best treatment.
2. Avoid house dust. Use the approach, "less is best." Focus on the bedroom. Remove carpeting. Limit furniture. Enclose pillows, mattress, and springs in airtight, vinyl encasements. Limit clothing in the bedroom to items used frequently. Place clothing in airtight, zipper-sealed, vinyl clothes bags. Install an air filter. Close the air-conditioning vent into the room.
3. Avoid house dust mites. Wash bedding in hot water (55°C), weekly. Wear a mask when vacuuming. Double-bag the vacuum cleaner. Install a filter on the outlet port of the vacuum cleaner. Avoid sleeping or lying on upholstered furniture. Remove carpets that are laid on concrete. If possible, have someone else clean the house.
4. Avoid mould spores. The three Ds that promote growth of mould spores are **d**arkness, **d**ampness, and **d**rafts. Avoid places where humidity is high (e.g., basements, camps on the lake, clothes hampers, greenhouses, stables, barns). Dehumidifiers may be helpful in humid weather and in damp spaces. Ventilate closed rooms, open doors, and install fans. HEPA (high-efficiency particulate air) filters may be beneficial. Consider adding windows to dark rooms. Consider keeping a small light on in closets. A basement light with a timer that provides light several hours a day may decrease mould growth.
5. Avoid pollens. Stay inside, with doors and windows closed, during high-pollen season. Avoid the use of fans. Install an air conditioner with a good air filter. Wash filters weekly during high pollen season. Put the car air conditioner on "recirculate" when driving. Get someone else to tend to your yard.
6. Avoid pet allergens. Remove pets from the interior of the home. Clean the living area thoroughly. Do not expect instant relief. Symptoms usually do not improve significantly for 2 months following pet removal.
7. Avoid smoke. The presence of a smoker will sabotage the best of all possible symptom-reduction programs.

TABLE 29-2 DRUG THERAPY

Allergic Rhinitis and Sinusitis

Preparation	Mechanism of Action	Adverse Effects	Nursing Actions
Corticosteroids **Nasal Spray** Beclomethasone (Apo-Beclomethasone) Budesonide (Rhinocort) Flunisolide (Apo-Flunisolide) Fluticasone (Flonase) Triamcinolone (Nasacort) Ciclesonide (Omnaris)	Inhibits inflammatory response At recommended dosage, systemic adverse effects are unlikely because of low systemic absorption Systemic effects may occur with greater-than-recommended dosages	Mild transient nasal burning and stinging; in rare instances, localized fungal infection with *Candida albicans*	• Teach patient correct use • Instruct patient to use on regular basis and not PRN • Explain to patient that the spray acts to decrease inflammation over time and does not have an immediate effect • Discontinue use if nasal infection develops
Mast Cell Stabilizer **Nasal Spray** Cromolyn spray (Apo-Cromolyn)	Inhibits degranulation of sensitized mast cells that occurs after exposure to specific antigens	Minimal adverse effects; occasional burning or nasal irritation	• Teach patient correct use • Reinforce that spray prevents symptoms • Begin 2 wk before pollen season starts and use throughout pollen season • If isolated allergy, such as to cats, use prophylactically (i.e., 10–15 min before exposure to allergen)
Leukotriene Receptor Antagonists (LTRAs) **Antagonists** Zafirlukast (Accolate) Montelukast (Singulair)	Antagonize or inhibit leukotriene activity, thereby inhibiting airway edema and bronchoconstriction through decreasing inflammatory process	Headaches, dizziness, rash, altered liver function tests, abdominal pain *Zafirlukast:* Monitor PT levels and theophylline levels if patient is taking coumadin or theophylline	• Monitor liver function tests periodically while on therapy; discontinue if values elevate • Administer on empty stomach • Do not discontinue therapy without consulting health care provider • Not to be used for acute attacks
Anticholinergic **Nasal Spray** Ipratropium bromide (Atrovent)	Blocks hypersecretory effects by competing for binding sites on the cell. Reduces rhinorrhea in the common cold and allergic and nonallergic rhinitis	Dryness of the mouth and nose may occur Does not cause systemic adverse effects	• Teach patient correct use • Reinforce that spray prevents symptoms, with onset of action within 1 hr of use • May reduce need for other rhinitis medications

TABLE 29-2   DRUG THERAPY

Allergic Rhinitis and Sinusitis—cont'd

Preparation	Mechanism of Action	Adverse Effects	Nursing Actions
Antihistamines			
First-Generation Agents			
Ethanolamines	Bind with H_1 receptors on target cells, blocking histamine binding	First-generation agents cross blood–brain barrier, bind to H_1 receptors in brain, cause sedation (diminished alertness, slow reaction time, somnolence) and stimulation (restless, nervous, insomnia)	• Warn patient that operating machinery and driving may be dangerous because of sedative effect Drowsiness usually passes after 2 wk of treatment
Diphenhydramine (Benadryl)			
Ethylenediamines			
Tripelennamine (Vagin-X)	Relieve acute symptoms of allergic response itching, sneezing, excessive secretions, mild congestion)		• Teach patient to report palpitations, change in heart rate, change in bowel, bladder habits
Alkylamines			• Instruct patient not to use alcohol with antihistamines because of additive depressant effect
Brompheniramine (Dimetane)		Some drugs (e.g., ethanolamines) are more likely to cause sedation	
Chlorpheniramine (Chlor-Tripolon)		Patients vary in their sensitivity to these adverse effects. The next most common adverse effects involve the GI system and include loss of appetite, epigastric distress, constipation, or diarrhea	• Rapid onset of action, no drug tolerance with prolonged use
			• Limited use with sinusitis
		May cause palpitations, tachycardia, urinary retention or frequency	
Second-Generation Agents			
Loratadine (Claritin)	—	Second-generation agents have limited affinity for brain H_1 receptors; cause minimal sedation; few effects on psychomotor activities, bladder function	• Teach patient to expect few, if any, adverse effects
Cetirizine (Reactine)			• More expensive than classical antihistamines
Fexofenadine (Allegra)			• Rapid onset of action, no drug tolerance with prolonged use
Desloratadine (Aerius)			• General interactions:
			• Do not take with alcohol or any form of tranquilizer or sedative
			• Do not take with any monoamine oxidase inhibitor
Decongestants			
Oral			
Pseudoephedrine (Sudafed)	Stimulate adrenergic receptors on blood vessels, promote vasoconstriction and reduce nasal edema and rhinorrhea	CNS stimulation, causing insomnia, excitation, headache, irritability, increased blood and ocular pressure, dysuria, palpitations, tachycardia	• Advise patient of adverse reactions
			• Advise that use of some preparations is contraindicated for patients with cardiovascular disease, hypertension, diabetes, glaucoma, prostate hyperplasia, hepatic and renal disease
			• Teach patient that these drugs should not be used for more than 3 days or more than three or four times a day; longer use increases risk for rebound vasodilation, which can increase congestion
Topical (Nasal Spray)			
Oxymetazoline (Dristan)	Same as above	Same as above, plus rhinitis medicamentosa (rebound nasal congestion),	—
Phenylephrine (Dimetapp)	Blocks action of histamine	headache, bitter taste, somnolence, nasal irritation	

CNS, central nervous system; *GI,* gastro-intestinal; *H_1,* histamine 1; *PRN,* as needed; *PT,* prothrombin time.

sneezing, or coughing or by direct hand contact. Frequency increases in the winter months, when people stay indoors and overcrowding is more common. Other factors, such as chilling, fatigue, physical and emotional stress, and compromised immune status, may increase susceptibility. The patient with acute viral rhinitis typically first experiences tickling, irritation, sneezing, or dryness of the nose or nasopharynx, followed by copious nasal secretions, some nasal obstruction, watery eyes, elevated temperature, general malaise, and headache. After the early profuse secretions, the nose becomes more obstructed, and the discharge is thicker. Within a few days, the general symptoms improve, nasal passages reopen, and normal breathing is re-established (Goldman & Schafer, 2012; National Institute of Allergy and Infectious Diseases [NIAID], 2016).

NURSING AND COLLABORATIVE MANAGEMENT
ACUTE VIRAL RHINITIS

Supportive therapy such as rest, fluids, proper diet, antipyretics, and analgesics is the recommended treatment. Complications

🌿 COMPLEMENTARY & ALTERNATIVE THERAPIES

Echinacea

Clinical Uses

Common cold, upper respiratory tract infection, wound healing, urinary tract infections.

Effects

Stimulates immune system; has antibacterial and anti-inflammatory activity.

Nursing Implications

Because Echinacea has immuno-modulating actions, individuals with systemic lupus erythematosus, tuberculosis, multiple sclerosis, leukemia, or acquired immune deficiency syndrome (AIDS) should not use it. Long-term use may suppress the immune system. Should not be used in conjunction with corticosteroids or immuno-suppression therapy. May be used in conjunction with antibiotics. Is considered safe when used in recommended dosages. Therapy for 10 to 14 days is usually long enough. Should not be taken for more than 8 weeks.

of acute viral rhinitis include pharyngitis, sinusitis, otitis media, tonsillitis, and lung infections. Antibiotics do not have a role in the treatment of viral rhinitis during the cold season; the patient with a chronic illness or a compromised immune status should be advised to avoid crowded, close situations and other persons who have obvious cold symptoms. Frequent hand hygiene and avoiding hand-to-face contact may help prevent direct spread.

Interventions are directed toward relieving annoying and uncomfortable symptoms. The patient should be encouraged to drink increased amounts of fluids to liquefy secretions. Antihistamine or decongestant therapy reduces postnasal drip and significantly decreases severity of cough, nasal obstruction, and nasal discharge. The patient should also be taught to recognize the symptoms of secondary bacterial infection, such as a temperature higher than 38°C (100.4°F); purulent nasal exudate; tender, swollen glands; and a sore, red throat. In the patient with pulmonary disease, signs of infection include a change in consistency, colour, or volume of the sputum. Because infection can progress rapidly, the patient with chronic respiratory disease may be taught to begin antibiotics in response to sputum changes (Goldman & Schafer, 2012; NIAID, 2016).

INFLUENZA

Approximately 10% to 20% of Canadians become infected with seasonal influenza each year, which runs from November to April. Although the majority recover completely, an estimated 4000 to 8000, mostly older adults, die every year from flu-related pneumonia. Many others die from other complications of flu (Immunize Canada, 2015). Much of the influenza-related morbidity and mortality could be prevented by vaccination of high-risk groups (Table 29-3). There are three groups of influenza viruses—A, B, and C; note that influenza C has little pathogenic potential. Influenza viruses have a remarkable ability to change over time. This ability accounts for widespread disease and the need for annual vaccination against new strains. Fewer cases of influenza result when a minor change in the virus occurs because most persons have partial immunity (Public Health Agency of Canada [PHAC], 2015a). Birds are natural carriers of influenza A viruses. Avian influenza H5N1 is circulating in some countries, especially in Asia and northeast Africa, and infecting many

🔍 EVIDENCE-INFORMED PRACTICE

Research Highlight

Do Probiotics Prevent Upper Respiratory Tract Infections?

Clinical Question

In healthy patients (P), what is the effect of probiotics (I) versus placebo (C) in preventing acute upper respiratory tract infections (URIs) (O)?

Best Available Evidence

Systematic review of randomized controlled trials (RCTs)

Critical Appraisal and Synthesis of Evidence

- Ten RCTs ($n=3451$) including healthy children and adults up to age 40.
- Intervention was ingestion of any probiotic (single or mixture of strains, any dosage regimen or route of administration) for more than 7 days, compared with placebo or no treatment.
- Most common probiotics were lactic acid bacteria and bifidobacteria, often consumed in fermented foods (e.g., yogourt) or as dietary supplements.
- Probiotics were better than placebo in reducing the occurrence of acute URIs.
- The number of URIs requiring antibiotics was lower in patients using probiotics compared with those using placebo.

Conclusion

- Probiotics are effective in reducing the incidence of URIs.

Implications for Nursing Practice

- Encourage continued probiotic use to prevent acute URIs.
- Yogourt is an excellent food source for probiotics.
- Probiotics are also available as a dietary supplement.
- Advise patients with frequent URIs of potential benefit from probiotic ingestion.
- Probiotics are typically well tolerated but can cause gastro-intestinal (GI) adverse effects
- Counsel patients of minor probiotic adverse effects, including flatulence and increased GI irritability.

Reference for Evidence

Hao, Q., Lu, Z., Dong, B., et al. (2011). Probiotics for preventing acute upper respiratory tract infections. *The Cochrane Database of Systematic Reviews, (9),* CD006895.

P, Patient population of interest; *I,* intervention or area of interest; *C,* comparison of interest or comparison group; *O,* outcomes of interest (see Chapter 1).

poultry populations and some humans (PHAC, 2013). This strain is highly pathogenic to birds and has infected a limited number of people. There is no evidence that this virus is transmitted from person to person. Although seasonal influenza immunization will not prevent avian influenza infection, immunization is recommended for those in direct contact with poultry infected with avian influenza during the culling operation. The rationale is that preventing infection with human influenza strains may reduce the theoretical potential for human–avian reassortment of genes should workers become co-infected with both influenza viruses (PHAC, 2015b).

The Canadian Pandemic Influenza Preparedness: Planning Guidance for the Health Sector document, updated in 2015, provides strategic guidance and a framework for pan-Canadian preparedness and response. It is not a response plan (PHAC, 2015a).

Clinical Manifestations

The onset of flu is typically abrupt, with systemic symptoms of cough, fever, and myalgia often accompanied by a headache and

TABLE 29-3 TARGET GROUPS FOR INFLUENZA IMMUNIZATION

Groups at High Risk

- Adults and children with cardiac or pulmonary disease
- Adults ≥65 yr old
- Healthy children between 6 and 23 mo
- Pregnant females, in the third trimester, if their delivery date is in influenza season
- Residents of nursing homes or long-term care facilities
- People with chronic conditions such as diabetes, anemia, cancer, immunodeficiency, immuno-suppression, neurological conditions, renal disease, or conditions that compromise management of respiratory secretions
- Children or adolescents on long-term acetylsalicylic acid therapy
- Health care workers, and those who provide essential community services, and other caregivers and household contacts capable of transmitting influenza to the above at-risk groups
- People at high risk for influenza complications
- People who are also travelling to areas where the flu virus is likely to be circulating

Public Health Agency of Canada. (2015). *Canadian communicable disease report: Summary of the National Advisory Committee on Immunization (NACI)*. Retrieved from *http://www.phac-aspc.gc.ca/publicat/ccdr-rmtc/15vol41/dr-rm41-10/ar-02-eng.php*.

COMPLEMENTARY & ALTERNATIVE THERAPIES

Goldenseal

Clinical Uses
Common cold, respiratory and gastro-intestinal infections, wound healing, cirrhosis of the liver, gallbladder inflammation, peptic ulcers.

Effects
Has a wide variety of effects such as anti-inflammatory properties, antimicrobial, and immuno-stimulating actions. Goldenseal can stimulate the flow of bile.

Nursing Implications
Because of the anticoagulant effects, goldenseal should not be used for longer than 2 weeks. Large doses may cause gastro-intestinal distress (e.g., diarrhea, vomiting) and possible nervous system effects. Commonly combined with Echinacea in preparations. May be used in conjunction with antibiotics. Should not be used concurrently with anticoagulants, antihypertensives, β-adrenergic blockers, or calcium channel blockers. Should not be used if person has heart or vascular disease, especially hypertension, heart failure, or dysrhythmias.

Source: Rothrock, J. (2015). *Alexander's care of the patient in surgery* (15th ed.). St. Louis: Mosby.

---

sore throat. Milder symptoms, similar to those of the common cold, may also occur. Physical findings are usually minimal, with normal assessment on chest auscultation. Dyspnea and diffuse crackles are signs of pulmonary complications. In uncomplicated cases, symptoms subside within 7 days. Some patients, particularly older adults, experience weakness or lassitude that persists for weeks. The convalescent phase may be marked by hyperactive airways and a chronic cough. Important diagnostic factors include the patient's health history and clinical findings and the presence of other cases of influenza in the community.

The most common complication of influenza is pneumonia. The patient who develops secondary bacterial pneumonia experiences gradual improvement of influenza symptoms and then worsening cough and purulent sputum. Treatment with antibiotics is usually effective if started early.

NURSING AND COLLABORATIVE MANAGEMENT INFLUENZA

The nurse should advocate regular handwashing as an effective strategy to reduce the risk for influenza. The nurse should also advocate influenza vaccination for patients at high risk, during routine office visits or, if hospitalized, at the time of discharge (see Table 29-3). The vaccine is 70% to 90% effective in preventing influenza in adults. To be effective, the vaccine must be given in the fall (mid-October), before exposure occurs. Although all healthy people between 2 and 65 years old should be encouraged to receive the vaccination, high priority should also be given to groups that can transmit influenza to high-risk persons, such as health care workers. By being vaccinated, the nurse can decrease the risk of transmitting influenza to those who have less ability to cope with the effects of this illness. Despite obvious benefits, many persons are reluctant to be vaccinated. Current vaccines are highly purified, and reactions are extremely uncommon. Soreness at the injection site is usually the only adverse effect. The only contraindications are for children younger than 6 months, people who have a hypersensitivity to eggs, or those who had a reaction to a previous immunization. People with a

---

COMPLEMENTARY & ALTERNATIVE THERAPIES

Zinc

Clinical Uses
Common cold, upper respiratory tract infections, wound healing, dermatitis, acne, herpes simplex.

Effects
Prevents replication of viruses and stimulates the immune system. Severe zinc deficiency results in severely depressed immune function and frequent infections.

Nursing Implications
Zinc supplements are available as oral tablets and lozenges. Oral zinc should not be taken with foods that will reduce its absorption, such as coffee, bran, protein, or calcium. Long-term use of zinc supplements over 15 mg/day is not recommended without medical supervision.

---

previous history of Guillain-Barré syndrome following a vaccination should avoid future vaccinations.

The primary goals in nursing management are supportive measures directed toward relief of symptoms and prevention of secondary infection. The patient should drink plenty of fluids and get plenty of rest. Older adults and those with a chronic illness may require hospitalization. Drug therapy with oral oseltamivir (Tamiflu) and inhaled zanamivir (Relenza) may be given to prevent or decrease symptoms of influenza in high-risk patients. Amantadine is effective only against influenza A. These drugs prevent the virus from budding and spreading to other cells. For maximum benefit, they should be initiated as soon as possible and ideally within 2 days of the onset of symptoms. They shorten the duration and severity of influenza and can be used prophylactically for control of outbreaks.

SINUSITIS

Sinusitis develops when the ostia (exit) from the sinuses is narrowed or blocked by inflammation or hypertrophy (swelling)

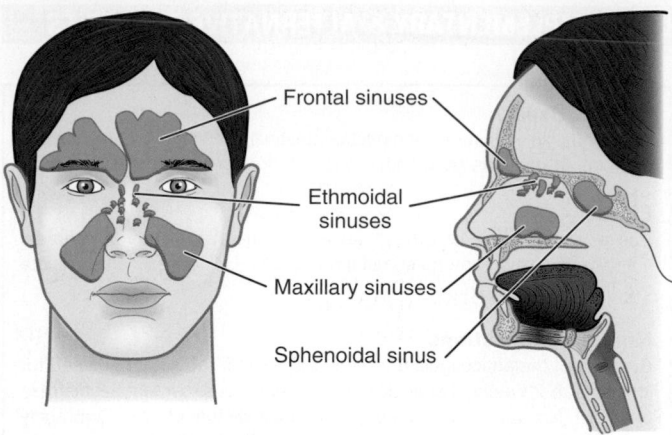

FIGURE 29-2 Location of the sinuses.

TABLE 29-4	**PATIENT & CAREGIVER TEACHING GUIDE**

Acute or Chronic Sinusitis

The following information should be included when teaching the patient and caregiver about sinusitis.

1. Keep well hydrated by drinking six to eight glasses of water daily to liquefy secretions.
2. Take hot showers twice daily; use a steam inhaler (15-min vaporization of boiled water), bedside humidifier, or nasal saline spray to promote secretion drainage.
3. Report temperature of ≥38°C, which may indicate infection.
4. Follow prescribed medication regimen:
   - Take analgesics to relieve pain.
   - Take decongestants or expectorants, or both, to relieve swelling and to thin mucus.
   - Take antibiotics, as prescribed, for infection. Be sure to take entire prescription and report continued symptoms or a change in symptoms.
   - Administer nasal sprays correctly.
5. Do not smoke, and avoid exposure to smoke—smoke is an irritant and may worsen symptoms.
6. If allergies predispose to sinusitis, follow instructions regarding environmental control, drug therapy, and immunotherapy to reduce the inflammation and prevent sinus infection.
7. Avoid use of nasogastric tube inserted via the nares.

of the mucosa (Figure 29-2). The secretions that accumulate behind the obstruction provide a rich medium for growth of bacteria, viruses, and fungi, all of which may cause infection (Tung, Landers, Li, et al., 2016). Bacterial sinusitis is most commonly caused by *Streptococcus pneumoniae, Haemophilus influenzae,* or *Moraxella catarrhalis* (Kaplan, 2014). Viral sinusitis follows an upper respiratory infection in which the virus penetrates the mucous membrane and decreases ciliary transport. Fungal sinusitis is uncommon and is usually found in patients who are debilitated or immuno-compromised.

Acute sinusitis usually results from an upper respiratory infection, allergic rhinitis, swimming, or dental manipulation, all of which can cause inflammatory changes and retention of secretions. When acute sinusitis follows viral rhinitis, symptoms worsen after 5 to 7 days and are worse than the original rhinitis. *Chronic sinusitis* is a persistent infection usually associated with allergies and nasal polyps. Chronic sinusitis generally results from repeated episodes of acute sinusitis that result in irreversible loss of the normal ciliated epithelium lining the sinus cavity.

Clinical Manifestations

Acute sinusitis causes significant pain over the affected sinus(es), purulent nasal drainage, nasal obstruction, congestion, fever, and malaise. The patient looks and feels sick. Assessment involves inspection of the nasal mucosa and palpation of the sinus points for pain. Findings that indicate acute sinusitis include a hyperemic and edematous mucosa, enlarged turbinates, and tenderness over the involved sinus(es). The patient may have recurrent headaches that change in intensity with position changes or when secretions drain (Kaplan, 2014).

Chronic sinusitis is difficult to diagnose because symptoms may be nonspecific. The patient is rarely febrile. Although there may be facial pain, nasal congestion, and increased drainage, often, severe pain and purulent drainage are absent. Symptoms may mimic those seen with allergies. Radiographic studies of the sinuses or a sinus computed tomographic (CT) scan may be performed to confirm the diagnosis. CT scans may show the sinuses to be filled with fluid or the mucous membrane to be thickened. Nasal endoscopy with a flexible scope may be used to examine the sinuses, obtain drainage for culture, and restore normal drainage.

Many patients with asthma have sinusitis. The link between these conditions is unclear. Sinusitis may trigger asthma by stimulating reflex bronchospasm. Appropriate treatment of sinusitis often causes a reduction in asthma symptoms (Calhoun, Omachi, Reddy, et al., 2016).

NURSING AND COLLABORATIVE MANAGEMENT SINUSITIS

If allergies are the precipitating cause of sinusitis, the patient needs to be instructed in ways to reduce sinus inflammation and infection, including environmental control of allergies and appropriate drug therapy (see section on allergic rhinitis earlier in this chapter). Treatment of acute sinusitis includes antibiotics to treat the infection, decongestants to promote drainage, nasal corticosteroids to decrease inflammation, and mucolytics to promote mucus flow (Table 29-4). Classical (first-generation) antihistamines increase the viscosity of mucus and promote continued symptoms, so they should be avoided. Nonsedating (second-generation) antihistamines do not cause this problem. For acute sinusitis, antibiotic therapy is usually continued for 10 to 14 days.

If symptoms do not resolve, the antibiotic should be changed to a broader-spectrum agent. With chronic sinusitis, mixed bacterial florae are often present, and infections are difficult to eliminate. Broad-spectrum antibiotics may be used for 4 to 6 weeks.

The patient should be encouraged to increase fluid intake (six to eight glasses daily) and use nasal cleaning techniques. This may include taking a hot shower in the morning and the evening, followed by blowing the nose thoroughly each time. Other interventions to cleanse the nasal passages and promote drainage include irrigating the nose with salt water (Cooper & Gosnell, 2015).

The patient with persistent or recurrent sinus complaints that are not alleviated by medical therapy may require nasal endoscopic surgery to relieve blockage caused by hypertrophy or deviated septum. This is an outpatient procedure usually performed under local anaesthesia (Cooper & Gosnell, 2015).

OBSTRUCTION OF THE NOSE AND PARANASAL SINUSES

POLYPS

Nasal polyps are benign mucous membrane masses that form slowly in response to repeated inflammation of the sinus or the nasal mucosa. Polyps, which appear as bluish, glossy projections in the naris (nostril), can exceed the size of a grape. The patient may be anxious, fearing the polyps are malignant. Clinical manifestations include nasal obstruction, nasal discharge (usually clear mucus), and speech distortion. Nasal polyps can be removed with endoscopic or laser surgery, but recurrence is common. Topical or systemic corticosteroids may slow polyp growth (Cooper & Gosnell, 2015).

FOREIGN BODIES

A variety of foreign bodies may lodge in the upper respiratory tract. Inorganic foreign bodies such as buttons and beads may cause no symptoms, lie undetected, and be accidentally discovered on routine examination. Organic foreign bodies such as wood, cotton, beans, peas, and paper produce a local inflammatory reaction and nasal discharge, which may become purulent and foul smelling. Foreign bodies should be removed from the nose through the route of entry. Sneezing with the opposite nostril closed may be effective in assisting the removal of foreign bodies. Irrigation of the nose or pushing the object backward should not be done because either could cause aspiration and airway obstruction. If sneezing or blowing the nose does not remove the object, the patient should see a health care provider.

PROBLEMS RELATED TO THE PHARYNX

ACUTE PHARYNGITIS

Acute pharyngitis is an acute inflammation of the pharyngeal walls. It may include the tonsils, palate, and uvula. It can be caused by a viral, bacterial, or fungal infection. Viral pharyngitis accounts for approximately 70% of cases. Acute follicular pharyngitis ("strep throat") results from β-hemolytic streptococcal invasion and accounts for an additional 5% to 15% of episodes (Chow & Doron, 2016; Cooper & Gosnell, 2015). Fungal pharyngitis, especially candidiasis, can develop with prolonged use of antibiotics or inhaled corticosteroids or in immuno-suppressed patients, especially those with human immunodeficiency virus (HIV).

Clinical Manifestations

Symptoms of acute pharyngitis range in severity from complaints of a "scratchy throat" to pain so severe that swallowing is difficult. Both viral and strep infections appear as a red and edematous pharynx, with or without patchy yellow exudates. Appearance is not always diagnostic. Cultures or a rapid strep antigen test is done to establish the cause and direct appropriate management. Inadequate treatment of acute streptococcal pharyngitis can result in rheumatic heart disease or glomerulonephritis.

White, irregular patches suggest fungal infection with Candida albicans. In diphtheria, a grey-white false membrane, termed a

pseudomembrane, is seen covering the oropharynx, nasopharynx, and laryngopharynx and sometimes extending to the trachea.

NURSING AND COLLABORATIVE MANAGEMENT ACUTE PHARYNGITIS

The goals of nursing management are infection control, symptomatic relief, and prevention of secondary complications. The patient with documented strep throat is treated with antibiotics. Antibiotics do not alter the course of viral infections and should not be used to treat this type of infection (Nathan & Cars, 2014). Candida infections are treated with nystatin, an antifungal antibiotic. The preparation should be swished in the mouth for as long as possible before it is swallowed, and treatment should continue until symptoms are gone. The patient should be encouraged to increase fluid intake. Cool, bland liquids and gelatin will not irritate the pharynx; the patient should avoid citrus juices, which can be irritating to the throat.

PERITONSILLAR ABSCESS

Peritonsillar abscess is a complication of acute pharyngitis or acute tonsillitis, when bacterial infection invades one or both tonsils. The tonsils may enlarge sufficiently to threaten airway patency. The patient experiences a high fever, leukocytosis, and chills. Intravenous antibiotic therapy is given along with needle aspiration or incision and drainage of the abscess. An emergency tonsillectomy may be performed, or an elective tonsillectomy may be scheduled after the infection has subsided.

PROBLEMS RELATED TO THE TRACHEA AND LARYNX

AIRWAY OBSTRUCTION

Airway obstruction may be complete or partial. Complete airway obstruction is a medical emergency. Partial airway obstruction may occur as a result of aspiration of food or a foreign body. In addition, partial airway obstruction may result from laryngeal edema following extubation, laryngeal or tracheal stenosis, central nervous system (CNS) depression, and allergic reactions. Symptoms include stridor, use of accessory muscles, suprasternal and intercostal retractions, wheezing, restlessness, tachycardia, and cyanosis. Prompt assessment and treatment are essential because partial obstruction may quickly progress to complete obstruction. Interventions to re-establish a patent airway include the obstructed airway (Heimlich) manoeuvre, cricothyroidotomy, endotracheal intubation, and tracheostomy. Unexplained or recurrent symptoms indicate the need for additional tests, such as a chest radiography, pulmonary function tests, and bronchoscopy.

TRACHEOSTOMY

A tracheotomy is a surgical incision into the trachea for the purpose of establishing an airway. A tracheostomy is the stoma (opening) that results from the tracheotomy. A tracheostomy tube is an artificial airway that is inserted into the trachea during a tracheotomy. Indications for a tracheostomy are to (1) bypass an upper airway obstruction, (2) facilitate removal of secretions, (3) permit long-term mechanical ventilation, and (4) permit oral intake and speech in the patient who requires long-term mechanical ventilation. Most patients who require mechanical ventilation are initially managed with an endotracheal tube (ETT), which can be quickly inserted in an emergency (see Chapter 68). A tracheotomy may be performed for patients requiring intubation longer than 7 to 10 days or when an airway is obstructed due to trauma, tumours, or swelling. A tracheostomy may also be required to facilitate airway clearance when spinal cord injury, neuro-muscular disease, or severe debilitation is present (Stacy, 2014). A tracheostomy tube is usually inserted by an open procedure in the operating room but can also be inserted emergently in a percutaneous procedure at the bedside (Stacy, 2014).

Several advantages make a tracheostomy a better option than an ETT for long-term nursing management and weaning from the ventilator. Without a tube in the mouth, patient comfort and mobility can be increased, and risk for long-term damage to the vocal cords is decreased. The patient is able to eat and talk with a tracheostomy because the tube enters lower in the airway (Stacy, 2014; Figure 29-3).

NURSING MANAGEMENT
TRACHEOSTOMY

PROVIDING TRACHEOSTOMY CARE

Before the tracheotomy procedure, the nurse should explain to the patient and caregivers the purpose of the procedure and inform them that the patient will not be able to speak while an inflated cuff is used. A number of complications can occur with tracheostomies (see Table 29-5).

A variety of tubes are available to meet individual patient needs (Table 29-6). All tracheostomy tubes contain a faceplate or flange, which rests on the neck between the clavicle and an outer cannula. In addition, all tubes have an obturator, which is used when inserting the tube (see Figure 29-3, A). In the event of accidental decannulation, a spare tracheostomy set, obturator and tracheal dilator, should be kept at the bedside, preferably taped at the head of the bed (Stacy, 2014).

Some tracheostomy tubes also have an inner cannula, which can be removed for cleaning (see Figure 29-3, C). The cleaning procedure removes mucus from the inside of the tube. If humidification is adequate, mucus may not accumulate and a tube without an inner cannula can be used. Care of the patient with a tracheostomy involves suctioning the airway to remove secretions (Figure 29-4 and Table 29-7) and cleaning around the stoma. In addition, tracheostomy care includes changing tracheostomy ties (Figure 29-5 and Table 29-8). If an inner cannula is used, whether disposable or nondisposable, tracheostomy care also involves inner cannula care (Stacey, 2014; see Table 29-8).

Both cuffed and uncuffed tracheostomy tubes are available. A tracheostomy tube with an inflated cuff is used if the patient is at risk for aspiration or needs mechanical ventilation. Because an inflated cuff exerts pressure on tracheal mucosa, it is important to inflate the cuff with the minimum volume of air required to obtain an airway seal. Cuff inflation pressure should not exceed 20 mm Hg or 25 cm H_2O because higher pressures may compress tracheal capillaries, limit blood flow, and predispose to tracheal necrosis. An alternative approach, termed the *minimal leak technique (MLT)*, involves inflating the cuff with the minimum

FIGURE 29-3 Types of tracheostomy tubes. **A,** Parts of a tracheostomy tube. **B,** Tracheostomy tube inserted in the airway with an inflated cuff. **C,** Fenestrated tracheostomy tube with cuff, inner cannula, decannulation plug, and pilot balloon. **D,** Tracheostomy tube with a foam cuff and obturator (one cuff is deflated on tracheostomy tube). (See Table 29-6 and NCP 29-1 for related nursing management.)

TABLE 29-5 COMPLICATIONS OF TRACHEOSTOMIES

Complication	Causes	Nursing Management
Abnormal bleeding	Surgical intervention Erosion or rupture of blood vessel, or both	• Monitor bleeding • Notify physician if it continues or is excessive
Tube dislodgement	Excessive manipulation or suctioning	• Ensure ties are secure • Keep obturator, hemostat, and new tracheostomy tube at bedside
Obstructed tube	Dried or excessive secretions	• Assess patient's respiratory status • Suction as necessary • Maintain humidification • Perform tracheostomy care • Ensure adequate hydration
Subcutaneous emphysema	Air escapes from the incision to the subcutaneous tissue	• Monitor subcutaneous emphysema • Reassure patient and family
Tracheo-esophageal fistula	Tracheal wall necrosis, leading to fistula formation	• Monitor cuff pressure • Monitor patient for coughing and choking while eating or drinking
Tracheal stenosis	Narrowing of tracheal lumen owing to scarring caused by tracheal irritation	• Monitor cuff pressure • Ensure prompt treatment of infections • Ensure ties are secure

FIGURE 29-5 Changing tracheostomy ties. **A,** A slit is cut about 2.5 cm (1 in) from the end. The slit end is put into the opening of the faceplate. **B,** A loop is made with the other end of the tape. **C,** The tapes are tied together with a double knot on the side of the neck, avoiding any blood vessels. **D,** A tracheostomy tube holder can be used in place of twill ties to make tracheostomy tube stabilization more secure. Source: **D,** Dale Medical Products, Inc.

FIGURE 29-4 Suctioning tracheostomy with closed system suction catheter. Source: Potter, P. A., Perry, A. G., Stockert, P. A., et al. (2011). *Basic nursing: Essentials for practice* (7th ed., p. 826). St. Louis: Mosby.

amount of air to obtain a seal and then withdrawing 0.1 mL of air. Disadvantages of MLT are the risk for aspiration from secretions leaking around the cuff and difficulty maintaining positive end-expiratory pressure (Stacy, 2014).

In some patients, cuff deflation is performed to remove secretions that accumulate above the cuff. Before deflation, the patient should cough up secretions, if possible, and the tracheostomy tube and mouth should be suctioned (see Figure 29-4 and Table 29-7). This step is important to prevent secretions from being aspirated during deflation. The cuff is deflated during exhalation because the exhaled gas helps propel secretions into the mouth. The patient should also cough or be suctioned after cuff deflation. The cuff should be reinflated during inspiration. The volume of air required to inflate the cuff should be monitored daily because this volume may increase if there is tracheal dilation from cuff pressure. The nurse should assess the patient's ability to protect the airway from aspiration and remain with the patient when the cuff is initially deflated, unless the patient can protect the airway from aspiration and breathe without respiratory distress.

When the patient can protect the airway from aspiration and does not require mechanical ventilation, a cuffless tracheostomy tube should be used.

Retention sutures are often placed in the tracheal cartilage when the tracheotomy is performed. The free ends should be taped to the skin in a place and manner that leaves them accessible if the tube becomes dislodged. Care should be taken not to dislodge the tracheostomy tube during the first few days when the stoma is not mature (healed). Because tube replacement can be difficult, several precautions are required: (1) a replacement tube of equal or smaller size is kept at the bedside, readily available for emergency reinsertion; (2) tracheostomy tapes are not changed for at least 24 hours after the insertion procedure; and (3) the first tube change is performed by a physician, usually no sooner than 7 days after the tracheotomy.

If accidental decannulation occurs, the retention sutures (if present) are grasped and the opening is spread with a tracheal dilator or hemostat, and the replacement tube is guided in, using

TABLE 29-6 CHARACTERISTICS AND NURSING MANAGEMENT OF TRACHEOSTOMIES

Tube	Characteristics	Nursing Management
Tracheostomy tube with cuff and pilot balloon (see Figure 29-3, A and B)	When properly inflated, low-pressure, high-volume cuff distributes cuff pressure over large area, minimizing pressure on tracheal wall	**Procedure for Cuff Inflation** • *Spontaneously breathing patient:* Inflate cuff to minimal occlusion pressure by slowly injecting air into the cuff until no sound is heard after deep breath or during inhalation with manual resuscitation bag. If using MLT, remove 0.1 mL of air while maintaining seal. MLT should not be used if there is risk for aspiration. • *Immediately after cuff inflation:* Verify that pressure is within accepted range (≤20 mm Hg or ≤25 cm H_2O) with a manometer. Record cuff pressure and volume of air used for cuff inflation in chart. **Care of Patients With an Inflated Cuff** • Monitor and record cuff pressure q8h. Cuff pressure should be ≤20 mm Hg or ≤25 cm H_2O to allow adequate tracheal capillary perfusion. If necessary, remove or add air to the pilot tubing using a syringe and stopcock. Afterward, verify that cuff pressure is within accepted range with manometer. • Report inability to keep the cuff inflated or need to use progressively larger volumes of air to keep cuff inflated. Potential causes of these problems include tracheal dilation at the cuff site or a crack or slow leak in the housing of the one-way inflation valve. If the leak is caused by tracheal dilation, the physician may intubate the patient with a larger tube. Cracks in the inflation valve may be temporarily managed by clamping the small-bore tubing with a hemostat. The tube should be changed within 24 hr.
Fenestrated tracheostomy tube (Shiley, Portex) with cuff, inner cannula, and decannulation plug (see Figures 29-3, B and 29-6, A)	When inner cannula is removed, cuff deflated, and decannulation plug inserted, air flows around tube, through fenestration in outer cannula, and up over vocal cords. Patient can then use voice.	• Signs or symptoms of aspiration need further evaluation by a speech pathologist or radiologist. • *Never* insert decannulation plug in tracheostomy tube until cuff is deflated and inner cannula removed. Prior insertion will prevent patient from breathing (no air inflow). This may precipitate a respiratory arrest. • Assess for signs of respiratory distress when a fenestrated cannula is first used. If this occurs, the cap should be removed, the inner cannula replaced, and the cuff reinflated. • Cuff management as described above.
Speaking tracheostomy tube (Portex, National) with cuff, two external tubings (see Figure 29-6, B)	Has two tubings, one leading to cuff and one to opening above the cuff. When port is connected to air source, air flows out of opening and up over the vocal cords, allowing voicing with cuff inflated.	• Once tube is inserted, wait 2 days before use so that the stoma can close around the tube and prevent leaks. • When patient desires to speak, connect port to compressed air (or oxygen). Be certain to identify correct tubing. If gas enters the cuff, it will overinflate and rupture, necessitating an emergency tube change. Use lowest flow (typically 4–6 L/min) that permits use of the voice. High flows dehydrate mucosa. • Cover port adaptor. This will cause the air to flow upward. Instruct patient to speak in short sentences because voice becomes a whisper with long sentences. • Disconnect flow when patient does not want to speak to prevent mucosal dehydration. • Cuff management as described above.
Tracheostomy tube (Bivona Fome-Cuf) foam-filled cuff (see Figure 29-3, D)	Cuff is filled with plastic foam. Before insertion, cuff is deflated. After insertion, cuff is allowed to fill passively with air. Pilot tubing is not capped, and no cuff pressure monitoring is required.	• Before insertion, withdraw all air from the cuff, using a 20-mL syringe. Cap pilot balloon tubing to prevent re-entry of air. After tracheostomy is inserted, remove cap from pilot tubing, allowing cuff to passively reinflate. • Do not inject air into tubing or cap pilot balloon tubing while in patient. Air will flow in and out in response to pressure changes (e.g., with head turning). Place tag on tubing, alerting staff not to cap or inflate cuff. • Deflate cuff daily via pilot balloon to evaluate integrity of cuff. Also assess ability to easily deflate cuff. Difficulty deflating cuff indicates a need for tube change. If aspirate returns with air, the cuff is no longer intact. • Tube can be used for up to 1 mo in patients on home mechanical ventilation. Good choice for patients who require inflated cuff at home because teaching about cuff pressure is simplified.

MLT, minimal leak technique.

the obturator. To permit airflow, the obturator is immediately removed once the tube is inserted. Another method is to insert a suction catheter to allow passage of air. The new tube is threaded over the catheter, followed by removal of the suction catheter. If the tube cannot be replaced, the level of respiratory distress is assessed. Minor dyspnea may be alleviated by use of semi-Fowler's position until assistance arrives. Severe dyspnea may progress to respiratory arrest; if this situation occurs, the stoma should be covered with a sterile dressing, and the patient should be ventilated with bag–mask ventilation until help arrives.

After the first tube change, the tube should be changed approximately once a month. When a tracheostomy has been in place for several months, the healed tract will be well formed. The patient can then be taught to change the tube using clean technique at home. Teaching will vary depending on how ill the patient is and what device has been selected.

SWALLOWING DYSFUNCTION

The patient who cannot protect the airway from aspiration requires an inflated cuff. However, an inflated cuff may promote

TABLE 29-7 PROCEDURE FOR SUCTIONING A TRACHEOSTOMY TUBE

1. The nurse should assess the need for suctioning q2h. Indications include coarse crackles or wheezes over large airways, moist cough, and restlessness or agitation if accompanied by decrease in SpO_2 or PaO_2. The patient should not be suctioned routinely or if able to clear secretions with cough.
2. If suctioning is indicated, the nurse should explain procedure to patient.
3. The necessary sterile equipment should be collected: suction catheter (no larger than half the lumen of the tracheostomy tube), gloves, water, cup, and drape. If a closed tracheal suction system is used, the catheter is enclosed in a plastic sleeve and reused. No additional equipment is needed.
4. The next step is to adjust suction pressure until the dial reads between 100 and 150 mm Hg pressure (for adults) with tubing occluded. For infants and children, the pressure should read between 50 and 100 mm Hg, depending upon the size of the child. (NOTE: The nurse should check the institution or agency's policy and procedure manuals for specific guidelines.)
5. The nurse should wash hands and put on goggles and gloves.
6. Sterile technique should be used to open package, fill cup with water, put on gloves, and connect catheter to suction. One hand should be designated as contaminated for disconnecting, bagging, and operating the suction control, and water should be suctioned through the catheter to test the system.
7. The nurse must assess SpO_2 and heart rate and rhythm to provide baseline for detecting change during suctioning.
8. Preoxygenation should be provided by using a reservoir-equipped MRB connected to 100% oxygen or by asking the patient to take three to four deep breaths while administering oxygen. The method chosen will depend on the patient's underlying disease and acuity of illness. The patient who has had a tracheostomy for an extended period and is not acutely ill may be able to tolerate suctioning without use of an MRB.
9. The nurse should gently insert catheter *without suction* to minimize the amount of oxygen removed from the lungs and then insert the catheter approximately 13 to 15 cm. Suctioning should be stopped if an obstruction is met.
10. Then the catheter should be withdrawn 1 to 2 cm and suction applied intermittently while withdrawing catheter in a rotating manner. If secretion volume is large, suctioning should be applied continuously.
11. *Suctioning time should be limited to 10 seconds.* Suctioning should be discontinued if heart rate decreases from baseline by 20 beats per minute, increases from baseline by 40 beats per minute, a dysrhythmia occurs, or SpO_2 decreases to less than 90%.
12. After each suction pass, the nurse should oxygenate with three to four breaths by MRB or deep breaths with oxygen.
13. Single-use catheters should not be reintroduced into the tracheostomy tube. (The nurse should check the institution's policy and procedure manuals.)
14. The procedure should be repeated until airway is clear, and insertions of suction catheter should be limited to as few as needed.
15. Oxygen concentration should be returned to prior setting.
16. The nurse should suction the oropharynx or use mouth suction.
17. The catheter should be disposed of by wrapping it around fingers of gloved hand and pulling glove over catheter. Then equipment should be discarded in proper waste container.
18. The nurse should auscultate to assess changes in lung sounds and then record time, amount, and character of secretions and response to suctioning.

MRB, manual resuscitation bag.

TABLE 29-8 TRACHEOSTOMY CARE

1. The nurse should explain procedure to patient.
2. A tracheostomy care kit should be used or necessary sterile equipment should be collected (e.g., suction catheter, gloves, water, basin, drape, tracheostomy ties, tube brush or pipe cleaners, 4×4–inch gauze pads, normal saline or sterile water, and tracheostomy dressing [optional]). NOTE: Clean rather than sterile technique is used at home.
3. The patient should be positioned in a semi-Fowler's position.
4. The needed materials should be assembled on bedside table next to patient.
5. The nurse should wash hands and put on goggles and clean gloves.
6. The next step is to auscultate chest sounds. If wheezes or coarse crackles are present, the patient should be suctioned if unable to cough up secretions (see Table 29-7) and then the nurse should remove soiled dressing and clean gloves.
7. The nurse should open sterile equipment, pour sterile normal saline into basins, and put on sterile gloves.
8. The inner cannula, if present, should be unlocked and removed. Many tracheostomy tubes do not have inner cannulas. Care for these tubes includes all steps except for inner cannula care.
9. If disposable inner cannula is used, it should be replaced with new cannula. If a nondisposable cannula is used, the following applies:
   a. Inner cannula should be immersed in sterile normal saline and the inside and outside of cannula cleaned using tube brush or pipe cleaners.
   b. Inner cannula should be rinsed in normal saline and shaken to dry.
   c. Inner cannula should be inserted into outer cannula with the curved part downward and then locked in place.
10. Dried secretions should be removed from stoma, outer cannula, and neck plate, using 4×4–inch gauze pad soaked in normal saline. Then the area around the stoma should be gently pat dry.
11. The nurse should maintain position of tracheal retention sutures, if present, by taping above and below the stoma.
12. Tracheostomy ties should be changed as follows: secure new ties to flanges before removing the old ones. Tie tracheostomy ties securely with room for one finger between ties and skin (see Figure 29-5). To prevent accidental tube removal, secure the tracheostomy tube by gently applying pressure to the flange of the tube during the tie changes. *Tracheostomy ties should not be changed for first 72 hours after the tracheotomy procedure.*
13. As an alternative, some patients prefer tracheostomy ties made of Velcro, which are easier to adjust.
14. If drainage is excessive, dressings should be placed around tube (see Figure 29-5). A tracheostomy dressing or unlined gauze should be used. The gauze should not be cut because threads may be inhaled or wrap around the tracheostomy tube. Dressing should be changed frequently—wet dressings promote infection and stoma irritation.
15. The nurse should repeat care three times a day and as needed.

swallowing dysfunction (dysphagia) because the cuff interferes with the normal function of the muscles used to swallow. For this reason, it is important to evaluate the risk for aspiration with the cuff deflated. The patient may be able to swallow without aspirating when the cuff is deflated but not when it is inflated. The cuff may then be left deflated or a cuffless tube substituted (Figure 29-6).

USE OF THE VOICE WITH A TRACHEOSTOMY TUBE

A number of techniques promote use of the voice in the patient with a tracheostomy. The patient who can breathe spontaneously may be able to talk by deflating the cuff, which allows exhaled

FIGURE 29-6 Speaking tracheostomy tubes. **A,** Fenestrated tracheostomy tube with cuff deflated, inner cannula removed, and tracheostomy tube capped to allow air to pass over the vocal cords. **B,** Speaking tracheostomy tube. One tube is used for cuff inflation. The second tube is connected to a source of compressed air or oxygen. When the port on the second tube is occluded, air flows up over the vocal cords, allowing use of the voice with an inflated cuff. (See Table 29-6 and NCP 29-1 for related nursing management.)

FIGURE 29-7 Passy–Muir speaking tracheostomy valve. The valve is placed over the hub of the tracheostomy tube after the cuff is deflated. Multiple options are available and can be used for ventilated and nonventilated patients. The valve contains a one-way valve that allows air to enter the lungs during inspiration and redirects air upward over the vocal cords into the mouth during expiration. Source: Image courtesy of Passy Muir, Inc. Irvine, CA.

air to flow upward over the vocal cords. This can be enhanced by the patient occluding the tube with a finger or plug. Frequently, a small cuffless tube is inserted so exhaled air can pass freely around the tube. These tracheostomy tubes and valves have been designed to facilitate use of the voice. The nurse can be an advocate in promoting use of these specialized devices. Their use can provide great psychological benefit and facilitate self-care for the patient with a tracheostomy.

A fenestrated tube has openings on the surface of the outer cannula that permit air from the lungs to flow over the vocal cords (see Figures 29-3, *C* and 29-6, *A*). A fenestrated tube allows the patient to breathe spontaneously through the larynx, speak, and cough up secretions with the tracheostomy tube in place. It can be used by the patient who can swallow without risk for aspiration but requires suctioning for secretion removal. It may also be used by the patient who requires mechanical ventilation for less than 24 hours a day (e.g., during sleep).

Before the fenestrated tube is used, the patient's ability to swallow without aspiration is determined (see Table 29-5 and Nursing Care Plan [NCP] 29-1, available on the Evolve website). If there is no aspiration, (1) the inner cannula is removed, (2) the cuff is deflated, and (3) the decannulation cap is placed in the tube (see Figure 29-6, *A*). It is important to perform the steps in order because severe respiratory distress may result if the tube is capped before the inner cannula is removed and the cuff deflated. When a fenestrated cannula is first used, the nurse should frequently assess the patient for signs of respiratory distress.

If the patient is not able to tolerate the procedure, the cap should be removed, the inner cannula replaced, and the cuff reinflated. A disadvantage of fenestrated tubes is the potential for development of tracheal polyps from tracheal tissue granulating into the fenestrated openings.

A speaking tracheostomy tube has two pigtail tubings. One tubing connects to the cuff and is used for cuff inflation, and the second connects to an opening just above the cuff (see Figure 29-6, *B*). When the second tubing is connected to a low-flow (4–6 L/min) air source, sufficient air moves up over the vocal cords to produce the voice. The patient can then use the voice, even though the cuff is inflated.

When a speaking tracheostomy valve is used, a cuffless tube must be in place, or the cuff must be deflated, to allow exhalation (Figure 29-7). Ability to tolerate cuff deflation without aspiration or respiratory distress must also be evaluated in patients using this device. If there is no aspiration, the cuff is deflated and the valve is placed over the tracheostomy tube opening. The speaking valve contains a thin plastic diaphragm that opens on inspiration and closes on expiration. During inspiration, air flows in through the valve. During expiration, the diaphragm prevents exhalation and air flows upward over the vocal cords and into the mouth.

If speaking devices are not used, the patient should be provided with a paper and pencil, a whiteboard with marker, or a computer tablet (e.g., iPad). A word (communication) board can usually be obtained from speech therapy, or one can be devised with pictures of common needs and an alphabet for spelling words.

INFORMATICS IN PRACTICE

Communication Devices for Patient With Laryngectomy

- Assisting with communication will improve a patient's quality of life after a laryngectomy.
- A tablet (e.g., iPad) or smartphone can be used with a downloaded text-to-speech application. These applications allow the patient to type in text, and then a computer voice says the text aloud.
- The nurse can also teach the patient how to use a keyboard-based communication program. The patient types on a traditional keyboard and generates speech that is transmitted through hand-held speakers.

DECANNULATION

When the patient can adequately exchange air and expectorate secretions, the tracheostomy tube can be removed. The stoma is closed with tape strips and covered with an occlusive dressing. The dressing must be changed if it gets soiled or wet. The patient should be instructed to splint the stoma with the fingers when coughing, swallowing, or speaking. Epithelial tissue begins to form in 24 to 48 hours, and the opening will close in several days. Surgical intervention to close the tracheostomy is not required.

LARYNGEAL POLYPS

Laryngeal polyps may develop on the vocal cords from vocal abuse (e.g., excessive talking, singing) or irritation (e.g., intubation, cigarette smoking). The most common symptom is hoarseness. Polyps may be treated conservatively with voice rest. Surgical removal may be indicated for large polyps, which may cause dyspnea and stridor. Polyps are usually benign but may be removed because they may later become malignant.

HEAD AND NECK CANCER

Head and neck cancer arises from mucosal surfaces and is typically squamous cell in origin. This category of tumours includes those of the paranasal sinuses, the oral cavity, and the nasopharynx, oropharynx, and larynx. (Cancer of the oral cavity is discussed in Chapter 44.) Although this type of cancer is not common, disability is great because of the potential loss of voice, disfigurement, and social consequences.

Clinical Manifestations

Early signs and symptoms of head and neck cancer vary with the tumour location (Carr, 2016). Cancer of the oral cavity may first be signalled by a painless growth in the mouth, an ulcer that does not heal, or a change in fit of dentures. Pain is a late symptom that may be aggravated by acidic food. Cancers of the oropharynx, hypopharynx, and supraglottic larynx rarely produce early symptoms and are usually diagnosed in late stages. The patient may complain of persistent unilateral sore throat or otalgia (ear pain). Hoarseness may be a symptom of early laryngeal cancer. If a lump in the neck or hoarseness lasts longer than 2 weeks, a medical evaluation is indicated. Some patients experience what feels like a lump in the throat or a change in voice quality.

Late stages of head and neck cancers have easily detectable signs and symptoms, including pain, dysphagia, decreased tongue mobility, airway obstruction, and cranial nerve neuropathies. The nurse should thoroughly examine the oral cavity, including the areas under the tongue and the dentures. The floor of the mouth, the tongue, and the lymph nodes in the neck should be bimanually palpated. There may be thickening of the normally soft and pliable oral mucosa. *Leukoplakia* (white patch) or *erythroplakia* (red patch) may be seen and should be noted for later biopsy. Both leukoplakia and carcinoma in situ (localized to a defined area) may precede invasive carcinoma by many years.

Diagnostic Studies

If lesions are suspected, the upper airways may be examined using indirect laryngoscopy—using a laryngeal mirror to visualize the laryngeal area—or a flexible nasopharyngoscope. The larynx and vocal cords are visually inspected for lesions and tissue mobility. A CT scan, magnetic resonance imaging (MRI), or positron emission tomography (PET) scan may be performed to detect local and regional spread. Neoplastic tissue is identifiable because it contains tissue of greater density or because it distorts, displaces, or destroys normal anatomical structures. Typically, multiple biopsy specimens are obtained to determine the extent of the disease (Goldman & Schafer, 2012).

Collaborative Care

The stage of the disease will be determined based on tumour size (T), number and location of involved nodes (N), and extent of metastasis (M). TNM staging classifies disease over the range between stage I through stage IV and guides treatment. Choice of treatment is based on medical history, extent of disease, cosmetic considerations, urgency of treatment, and patient choice. Approximately one-third of patients with head and neck cancers have highly confined lesions that are stage I or II at diagnosis. Such patients can undergo radiation therapy or surgery with the goal of cure.

Radiation therapy may be effective in curing early vocal cord lesions. This therapy is usually successful in eliminating the tumour while preserving the quality of the voice. If radiation therapy is not successful or the lesion is too advanced for this therapy, surgery may be performed. A *cordectomy* (partial removal of one vocal cord) is used when there is a superficial tumour involving one cord (Figure 29-8). A *hemilaryngectomy* involves removal of thyroid cartilage, a portion of the larynx and one vocal cord or part of a cord and necessitates a temporary tracheostomy. A *supraglottic laryngectomy* involves removing structures above the true cords—the false vocal cords and epiglottis. The patient is left at high risk for aspiration following surgery and requires a temporary tracheostomy. Both a hemilaryngectomy and a supraglottic laryngectomy allow the voice to be preserved, but quality is breathy and hoarse.

Advanced lesions are treated by a total laryngectomy in which the entire larynx and pre-epiglottic region is removed and a permanent tracheostomy performed. Airflow patterns before and after total laryngectomy are shown in Figure 29-9. *Radical neck dissection* frequently accompanies total laryngectomy to decrease the risk for lymphatic spread. Depending on the extent of involvement, extensive dissection and reconstruction may be performed. This procedure involves wide excision of the lymph nodes and their lymphatic channels (Figure 29-10). The following structures may also be removed or transected: sternocleidomastoid

FIGURE 29-8 Excision of laryngeal cancer. This cancer of the right vocal cord meets criteria for resection by transoral cordectomy. The cord is fully mobile and the lesion can be fully exposed. It does not approach or cross the anterior commissure.

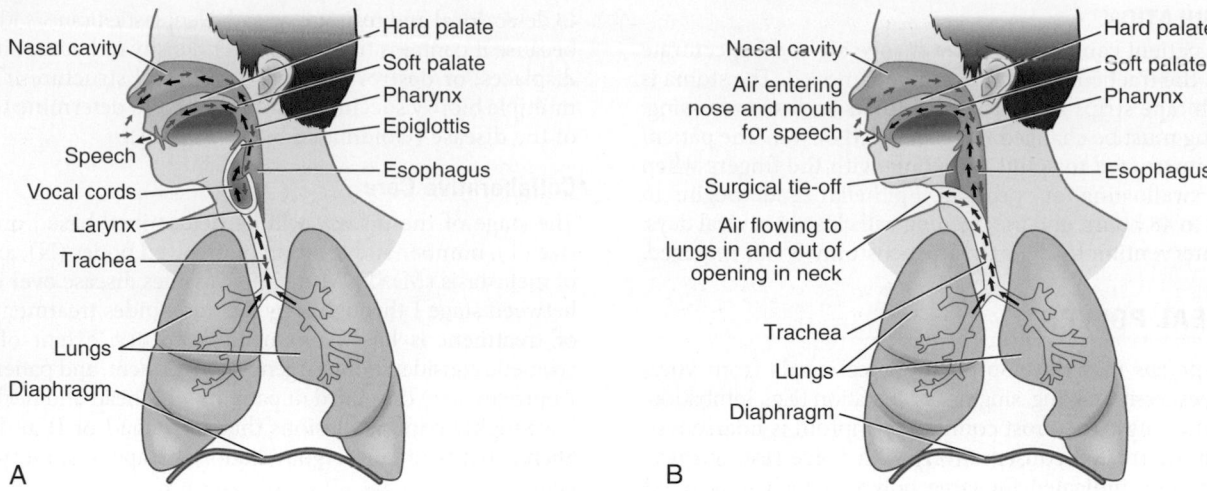

FIGURE 29-9 A, Normal airflow in and out of the lungs. **B,** Airflow in and out of the lungs after total laryngectomy. Patients using esophageal speech by trapping air in the esophagus and releasing it to create sound. Source: The American Cancer Society.

FIGURE 29-10 Radical neck incision with drains in place.

muscle and other closely associated muscles, internal jugular vein, mandible, submaxillary gland, part of the thyroid and parathyroid glands, and the spinal accessory nerve.

A *modified neck dissection* is performed whenever possible as an alternative to a radical neck dissection. The dissection is modified by sparing as many structures as possible to limit disfigurement and functional loss. A modified neck dissection usually involves dissection of the major cervical lymphatic vessels and lateral cervical space, with preservation of nerves and vessels, including the sympathetic and vagus nerves, spinal accessory nerves, and internal jugular vein. Neck dissection with vocal cord cancer usually involves one side of the neck. However, if the lesion is midline, a bilateral neck dissection may be performed. In this case, it is always modified on at least one side to minimize structural and functional deficits (Rothrock, 2015).

The patient may refuse surgical intervention for advanced lesions because of the extent of the procedure, or the patient may be judged to be at too great a medical risk to undergo the procedure. In these situations, external radiation therapy may be used as the sole treatment or in combination with chemotherapy (Rothrock, 2015).

In addition, brachytherapy, a concentrated and localized method of delivering radiation that involves placing a radioactive source into or near the tumour, may be used to treat head and neck cancer. The goal of brachytherapy is to deliver high doses of radiation to the target area while limiting exposure of surrounding tissues. Thin, hollow, plastic needles are inserted into the tumour area, and radioactive iridium seeds are placed in the needles. The seeds emit continuous radiation. Brachytherapy can be used alone or combined with external radiation or surgical intervention. (Radiation therapy and brachytherapy are discussed in Chapter 18.)

Nutritional Therapy. The patient's nutritional status should be assessed before surgery as 60% of patients with head and neck cancer initially present with malnutrition (Carr, 2016). After radical neck surgery, the patient may be unable to take in nutrients through the normal route of ingestion because of swelling, the location of sutures, or difficulty swallowing. Parenteral fluids will be given for the first 24 to 48 hours. Tube feedings are usually given via a nasogastric, nasointestinal, or gastrostomy tube that was placed during surgery. (Nasogastric and gastrostomy feedings are described in Chapter 42.) The nurse must observe for tolerance of the feedings and adjust amount, time, and formula if nausea, vomiting, diarrhea, or distension occurs. The patient is instructed about the tube feedings. When the patient can swallow, small amounts of water are given. Close observation for difficulty swallowing is essential. Suctioning may be necessary to prevent aspiration.

Swallowing problems should be anticipated when the patient resumes eating. All patients should be referred to a speech pathologist for a dysphagia/swallowing assessment and recommendations during treatment. The type and degree of difficulty vary, depending on the surgical procedure. When a supraglottic laryngectomy is performed, the surgeon excises the upper portion of the larynx, including the epiglottis and the false vocal cords. The patient can speak because the true vocal cords remain intact. However, a new technique, the supraglottic swallow, must be learned to compensate for removal of the epiglottis and minimize risk for aspiration (Table 29-9). When the patient is learning this technique, it may be helpful to start with carbonated beverages because the effervescence provides cues about the liquid's position. With this exception, thin, watery fluids should be avoided because they are difficult to swallow and increase the risk for aspiration. A better choice is nonpourable puréed foods, which are thicker and allow more control during swallowing. Swallowing can be enhanced by thickening liquids using a commercially available thickening agent. Consultation with a dietitian will assist with appropriate diet texture, while ensuring nutritional and caloric needs are maintained.

Good nutrition is important during radiation therapy because calories and protein are needed for tissue repair. Antiemetics or analgesics may be given before meals to reduce nausea and mouth pain. Bland foods may be better tolerated than more highly flavoured foods. Caloric intake may be increased by adding dry milk to foods during preparation, selecting foods high in calories, and using oral supplements. It is helpful to add sauces and gravies to food, which adds calories and moistens food so it is more easily swallowed. If an adequate intake cannot be maintained, enteral feedings may be used. When eating, the patient should always be positioned with the head elevated.

NURSING MANAGEMENT
HEAD AND NECK CANCER

NURSING ASSESSMENT

Subjective and objective data that should be obtained from a person with head and neck cancer are presented in Table 29-10.

NURSING DIAGNOSES

Nursing diagnoses for the patient with head and neck cancer include, but are not limited to, the following:

TABLE 29-9 PATIENT & CAREGIVER TEACHING GUIDE

Steps for Performing the Supraglottic Swallow

The following information should be included when teaching the patient and caregiver how to perform the supraglottic swallow.

1. Take a deep breath to aerate lungs.
2. Perform the Valsalva manoeuvre to approximate the vocal cords.
3. Place food in the mouth and swallow. Some food will enter airway and remain on top of the closed vocal cords.
4. Cough to remove food from top of vocal cords.
5. Swallow so food is moved from top of vocal cords.
6. Breathe after cough–swallow sequence to prevent aspiration of food collected on top of vocal cords.

- *Ineffective airway clearance* related to *presence of artificial airway and excessive mucus*
- *Risk for aspiration* related to *presence of oral/nasal tube and impaired ability to swallow*
- *Anxiety* related to *unmet needs* (lack of knowledge about surgical procedure and pain management)
- *Acute pain* related to *physical injury agent* (surgery)
- *Impaired verbal communication* related to *physiological condition* (removal of vocal chords)

Additional information on nursing diagnoses for the patient with head and neck cancer is presented in NCP 29-2, available on the Evolve website.

PLANNING

The overall goals are that the patient will have (1) a patent airway, (2) no spread of cancer, (3) no complications related to therapy, (4) adequate nutritional intake, (5) minimal to no pain, (6) the ability to communicate, and (7) an acceptable body image.

NURSING IMPLEMENTATION

HEALTH PROMOTION. Development of head and neck cancer is closely related to personal habits, primarily tobacco use, including the use of cigarettes, cigars, chewing tobacco, and snuff. Prolonged alcohol use has been implicated as a potentiating factor in head and neck cancer. Excessive sun exposure to the lips also increases the risk for oral cancer.

The nurse should include information about risk factors in health teaching (Carr, 2016). If cancer has been diagnosed, tobacco cessation is still important. The patient with head and neck cancer who continues to smoke during radiation therapy has a lower rate of response and survival than the patient who does not smoke during radiation therapy. In addition, risk for a second primary cancer is significantly increased in patients who continue to smoke.

ACUTE INTERVENTION. The patient and the family must be taught about the type of therapy to be performed and care required. Assessment of concerns is integral to the plan of care. The patient and family must deal with the psychological impact of the diagnosis of cancer, alteration of physical appearance, and possible need for alternative methods of communication (Carr, 2016). The care plan should include assessment of the patient's support system. The patient may not have someone to provide assistance after discharge, may not be employed, or may be employed in a job that cannot be continued.

TABLE 29-10 NURSING ASSESSMENT

Head and Neck Cancer

Subjective Data	Objective Data
Important Health Information	**Respiratory**
Past health history: Positive family history; prolonged tobacco use (cigarettes, pipes, cigars, chewing tobacco, smokeless tobacco); prolonged, heavy alcohol use	Hoarseness, chronic laryngitis, nasal voice, palpable neck mass and lymph nodes (tender, hard, fixed), tracheal deviation; dyspnea, stridor (late sign)
Medications: Prolonged use of over-the-counter medication for sore throat, decongestants	**Gastro-Intestinal**
	White (leukoplakia) or red (erythroplakia) patches inside mouth, ulceration of mucosa, asymmetrical tongue, exudate in mouth or pharynx, mass or thickening of mucosa
Symptoms	
Mouth ulcer that does not heal, change in fit of dentures, change in appetite, weight loss, swallowing difficulty (e.g., sensation of lump in throat, pain with swallowing, aspiration when swallowing)	**Possible Findings**
Fatigue with minimal exertion	Mass on direct or indirect laryngoscopy; tumour on soft tissue radiographic study, computed tomographic scan, magnetic resonance imaging, or positron emission tomography; positive biopsy
Sore throat, hoarseness, change in voice quality, referred ear pain	

Radiation Therapy. The nurse can suggest interventions to reduce adverse effects of radiation therapy. (Radiation is discussed in Chapter 18.) Fatigue is common. Patients should be encouraged to take frequent rest periods. Light, regular exercise, such as walking, may be helpful.

Dry mouth (xerostomia), the most frequent and annoying problem, typically begins within a few weeks of treatment. The patient's saliva decreases in volume and becomes thick. The change may be temporary or permanent. Pilocarpine hydrochloride (Salagen) can be effective in increasing saliva production and should be started before the initiation of radiation therapy and continued for 90 days. Symptom relief can also be obtained by increasing fluid intake, chewing sugarless gum or eating sugarless candy, using nonalcoholic mouth rinses (baking soda or glycerin solutions), and using artificial saliva.

The patient may also complain of stomatitis, especially if the oral cavity is in the field of therapy. Irritation, ulceration, and pain are common complaints. Normal saline mouth rinses after meals and at bedtime can be used to clean and soothe irritated tissues. Commercial mouthwashes and hot or spicy foods should be avoided because they are irritating. If the problem is severe, a mouthwash mixture of equal parts of antacid, diphenhydramine (Benadryl), and topical lidocaine can be used.

Skin over the irradiated area often becomes reddened and sensitive to touch. It is common for patients to require a break from their scheduled radiation program because of altered skin integrity. Only prescribed lotions and products should be used during radiation therapy. All exposure to the sun should be avoided to reduce discomfort.

Surgical Therapy. Preoperative care for the patient who is to have a radical neck dissection involves consideration of the patient's physical and psychosocial needs. Physical preparation is the same as for any major surgery, with special emphasis on oral hygiene. Explanations and emotional support are of special significance and should include postoperative measures relating to communication and feeding. The surgical procedure should be explained to the patient and family or caregivers, and the nurse should make sure that the information is understood.

Teaching must be tailored to the planned surgical procedure. For surgeries that involve a laryngectomy, teaching should include information about expected changes in speech. The nurse or speech pathologist should demonstrate means of communicating other than speaking that can be used temporarily or permanently. This may include some type of communication board.

After surgery, maintenance of a patent airway is essential. The inflammation in the surgical area may compress the trachea. A tracheostomy tube will be in place. The patient will be placed in a semi-Fowler's position to decrease edema and limit tension on the suture lines. Vital signs should be monitored frequently because of the risk for hemorrhage and respiratory compromise. Pressure dressings, packing, or drainage tubes (Hemovac, Jackson Pratt) may be used for wound management, depending on the type of surgical procedure. When a radical neck dissection is performed, wound suction using a portable system, such as a Hemovac, is generally used. If skin flaps are employed, dressings are typically not used. This allows better visualization of the incision and helps prevent excessive pressure on tissue (see Figure 29-10). The drainage should be serosanguineous and gradually decrease in volume over 24 hours. Patency of drainage tubes should be monitored every 4 hours to ensure that they are properly removing serous drainage and for the amount and character of drainage. If the tubing becomes obstructed, fluid will accumulate under the skin flap and predispose to impaired wound healing and infection. After drainage tubes are removed, the area should be closely monitored for any swelling. If fluid continues to accumulate, aspiration may be necessary.

Immediately after surgery, the patient with a laryngectomy requires frequent suctioning via the laryngectomy tube. Secretions typically change in amount and consistency over time. The patient may initially have copious blood-tinged secretions that diminish and thicken. Standard administration of saline boluses via the tracheostomy tube to loosen secretions is no longer recommended as it may increase risk for infection (Astobelli, 2013).

The patient will benefit from the use of a humidifier while hospitalized and at home.

Following a neck dissection, an exercise program should be instituted to maintain strength and movement in the affected shoulder and the neck. This is especially important when the spinal accessory nerve and the sternocleidomastoid muscles are removed or damaged. Without exercise, the patient will be left with a "frozen" shoulder and limited range of motion in the neck. This exercise program should be continued following discharge to prevent future functional disabilities. The patient may need the neck supported to be able to move the head after surgery.

Voice Rehabilitation. A speech pathologist should meet with the patient preoperatively and following a total laryngectomy to discuss voice restoration options. The International Association of Laryngectomees, an association of patients who have had laryngectomies, focuses on assisting patients to re-establish speech. Local groups, called Lost Cord Clubs, often provide member volunteers to visit the patient, preferably before surgery. Several options are available to restore speech. These include use of a voice prosthesis, esophageal speech, and an electrolarynx.

The most commonly used voice prosthesis is the Blom–Singer (Figure 29-11). This soft plastic device is inserted into a fistula made between the esophagus and the trachea. The puncture may be created at the time of surgery or afterward, depending on the preference of the surgeon. A red rubber catheter is placed in the tracheo-esophageal puncture and must remain in place until a tract is formed. Once the tract is formed, the voice prosthesis is inserted. This prosthesis allows air from the lungs to enter the esophagus by way of the tracheal stoma. A one-way valve prevents aspiration of food or saliva from the esophagus into the tracheostomy. To produce the voice, the patient manually blocks the stoma with the finger. Air moves from the lungs, through the prosthesis, into the esophagus, and out the mouth. The voice is produced by the air vibrating against the esophagus, and speech sounds are formed into words by moving the tongue, jaw, and lips. A valve may also be used with this device. When the valve is in place, the stoma does not need to be closed with the finger to speak. The prosthesis must be cleaned regularly and replaced when it becomes blocked with mucus.

An electrolarynx is a handheld, battery-powered device that creates speech with the use of sound waves. There are two main types: the intra-oral type and the neck type. One intra-oral device, the Cooper-Rand, uses a plastic tube placed in the corner of the roof of the mouth to create vibrations. To create the most normal sound when using this device, the patient should (1) avoid trying to use the tongue to hold the tube in place; (2) compress the tone generator for short intervals and speak in phrases, rather than full sentences; (3) speak using large movements of the lips, tongue, and jaw, rather than keeping the mouth partially closed;

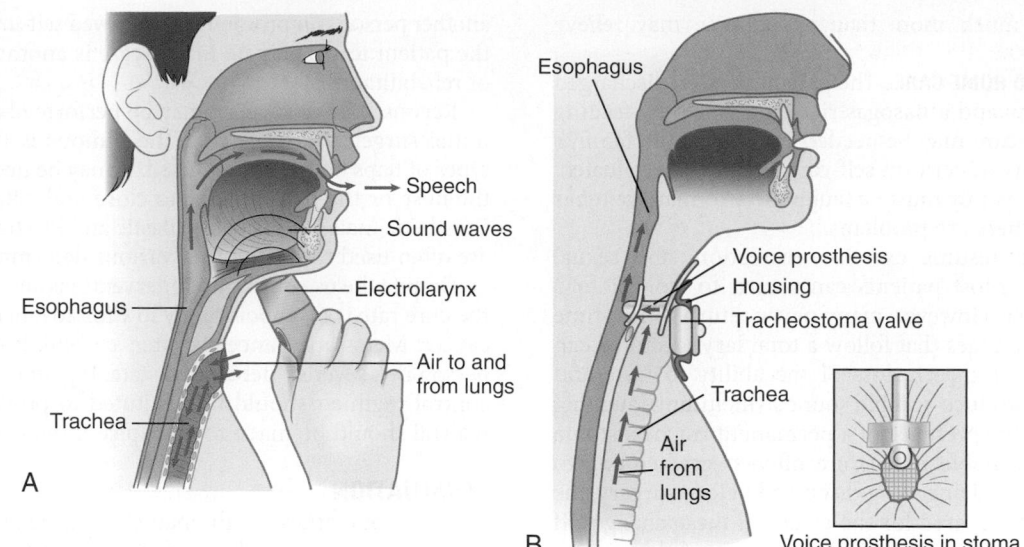

FIGURE 29-11 **A,** The sound waves created by the electrolarynx allow the person to speak. **B,** The Blom–Singer voice prosthesis and valve.

FIGURE 29-12 Artificial larynx. Battery-powered electronic artificial larynx for a patient who has had a total laryngectomy. Source: Courtesy CLG Photographics, Inc. St. Louis.

(4) talk face-to-face with the listener; and (5) practise because it takes time to develop this skill.

With the neck type of artificial larynx, the device is placed against the neck rather than in the mouth. This device is used after surgical healing is complete and no edema remains (Figure 29-12). With experience, the patient can learn to move the lips in ways that create somewhat normal-sounding speech. With both devices, voice pitch is low, and the sound is mechanical.

Esophageal speech is a method of swallowing air, trapping it in the esophagus, and releasing it to create sound. The air causes vibration of the pharyngoesophageal segment to create sound (which initially is similar to a belch). With practice, 50% of patients develop some speech skills, but only 10% develop fluent speech.

Stoma Care. Before discharge, the patient should be instructed in the care of the laryngectomy stoma. The area around the stoma should be washed daily with a moist cloth. If a laryngectomy tube is in place, the entire tube must be removed at least daily and cleaned in the same manner as a tracheostomy tube. The inner cannula may have to be removed and cleaned more frequently. A scarf, a loose shirt, or a crocheted shield can be used to shield the stoma.

The patient should cover the stoma when coughing (because mucus may be expectorated) and during any activity (e.g., shaving,

applying makeup) that might lead to inhalation of foreign materials. Because water can easily enter the stoma, the patient should wear a plastic collar when taking a shower. Swimming is contraindicated. Initially, humidification will be administered via a tracheostomy mask. After discharge, a bedside humidifier can be used. A high oral fluid intake must be maintained, especially in dry weather.

The patient should be told the importance of wearing a medical alert bracelet or other identification that alerts others in an emergency situation of the need for neck breathing. Because the patient no longer breathes through the nose, the ability to smell smoke and food may be lost. Advise the patient to install smoke and carbon monoxide detectors in the home. It is important for food to be colourful, attractively prepared, and nutritious because taste may also be diminished secondary to the loss of smell as well as to radiation therapy.

Depression. Depression is common in the patient who has had a radical neck dissection. The patient may not be able to speak because of the laryngectomy and cannot control saliva. The neck and shoulders may be numb because of the transected nerves. The facial appearance may be significantly altered, with swelling, edema, and deformities. The patient must understand that many of the physical changes are reversible as the edema subsides and the tracheostomy tube is removed. Depression may also be related to concern about the prognosis. The nurse can help the patient through the depression by allowing verbalization of feelings, conveying acceptance, and helping the patient regain an acceptable self-concept. The nurse should obtain a psychiatric referral for the patient who is experiencing prolonged or severe depression.

Sexuality. Surgery and the presence of foreign attachments such as tracheostomy and gastrostomy tubes may affect body image dramatically. The patient may feel less desirable sexually. The nurse can assist the patient by allowing discussions regarding sexuality and encouraging the patient to discuss this problem with the sexual partner. It may be difficult for the patient to discuss sexual problems verbally because of the alteration in communication. The nurse can help the patient to plan how to communicate with the sexual partner and offer support and guidance to the sexual partner. Helping the patient see that sexuality involves much more than appearance may relieve some anxiety.

AMBULATORY AND HOME CARE. The patient is often discharged with a tracheostomy and a nasogastric or gastrostomy feeding tube. Home health care may be needed initially as the family's or the patient's ability to perform self-care activities is evaluated. The patient and the family must be taught how to manage tubes and who to call if there are problems.

The patient can resume exercise, recreation, and sexual activity when able. Most patients can return to work 1 to 2 months after surgery. However, many never return to full-time employment. The changes that follow a total laryngectomy can be upsetting. Loss of speech, loss of the ability to taste and smell, inability to produce audible sounds (including laughing and weeping), and the presence of a permanent tracheal stoma that produces undesirable mucus are often overwhelming to the patient. Although changes are discussed before surgery, the patient may not be prepared for the extent of these changes. If the patient has a significant other, the reaction of this person to the patient's altered appearance is important. Acceptance by another person can promote an improved self-image. Encouraging the patient to participate in self-care is another important part of rehabilitation.

Reconstructive surgery may be performed at the time of the initial surgery or soon after the tumour is removed. Various types of flaps and grafts are used. It may be necessary to rebuild the nose or the mandible or to close oral cutaneous openings. Prosthetic materials, such as Silastic and Plastigel (which is soft), are often used to reconstruct various deformities.

Despite the use of surgical interventions and radiation therapy, the cure rate is disappointingly low for advanced head and neck cancer. Metastatic cancer is often painful, leaving the affected person in a severely debilitated state. If pain is a problem, a pain control regimen should be instituted to provide comfort, and referral should be made to a hospice if indicated.

EVALUATION

Expected outcomes for the patient with head and neck cancer who is treated surgically are addressed in NCP 29-2, available on the Evolve website.

CASE STUDY

Laryngeal Cancer

Source: goodluz/Shutterstock.com.

Patient Profile
Tomas Pereira, a 60-year-old man, was admitted for evaluation of mild pain on swallowing and a persistent sore throat over the past year. He has a history of type 2 diabetes mellitus.

Subjective Data
- States that his symptoms worsened in the past 2 mo
- Has used various cold remedies to relieve symptoms, without relief
- Has lost weight because of decrease in appetite and difficulty swallowing
- Has smoked three packs of cigarettes a day for 40 yr
- Consumes four to six cans of beer a day

Objective Data
Laryngoscopy
- Subglottic mass

Physical Examination
- Enlarged cervical nodes

Computed Tomographic Scan
- Subglottic lesion with lymph node involvement

Collaborative Care
- Percutaneous gastrostomy tube inserted preoperatively for enteral tube feeding

- Total laryngectomy with tracheostomy with inflated cuff
- Nasogastric tube postoperatively

Discussion Questions
1. What information in the assessment suggests that Mr. Pereira is at risk for cancer of the larynx?
2. What diagnostic tests are typically performed to evaluate the extent of this problem?
3. **Priority decision:** What are the priority teaching strategies for Mr. Pereira before and after laryngectomy?
4. Discuss methods used to restore speech after laryngectomy.
5. Is there anything in his history that may affect wound healing after surgery?
6. **Priority decision:** While in the recovery room, Mr. Pereira develops shortness of breath. What are the priority nursing interventions?
7. What teaching is required to help this patient assume self-care after his surgery? What precautions should the patient take because of his stoma?
8. While on the medical-surgical unit, Mr. Pereira is tearful and is staring at the wall. What should the nurse do?
9. **Priority decision:** Based on the assessment data presented, what are the priority nursing diagnoses? Are there any collaborative problems?
10. **Evidence-informed practice:** How could the nurse best meet Mr. Pereira's communication needs during the first few postoperative days?

evolve

Answers are available at *http://evolve.elsevier.com/Canada/Lewis/medsurg*

REVIEW QUESTIONS

The number of the question corresponds to the same-numbered objective at the beginning of the chapter.

1. A client is seen in the clinic for an episode of epistaxis, which is controlled by placement of anterior nasal packing. During discharge teaching, what should the nurse instruct the client to do?
   a. Use ASA (Aspirin) for pain relief.
   b. Remove the packing later that day.
   c. Skip the next dose of antihypertensive medication.
   d. Avoid vigorous nose blowing and strenuous activity.

2. A client with allergic rhinitis reports severe nasal congestion, sneezing, and watery, itchy eyes and nose, at various times of the year. What should the nurse advise the client to do?
   a. Avoid all intranasal sprays and oral antihistamines.
   b. Limit the duration of use of nasal decongestant spray to 10 days.
   c. Use oral decongestants at bedtime to prevent symptoms during the night.
   d. Keep a diary of when the allergic reaction occurs and what precipitates it.

3. A client is seen at the clinic with fever, muscle aches, sore throat with yellowish exudate, and headache. Which of the following does the nurse anticipate that the collaborative management will include? *(Select all that apply)*
   a. Antiviral agents to treat influenza
   b. Treatment with antibiotics starting ASAP
   c. A throat culture or rapid strep antigen test
   d. Supportive care, including cool, bland liquids
   e. Comprehensive history to determine possible etiology

4. What type of tracheostomy tube prevents the use of the voice?
   a. Cuffless tracheostomy tube
   b. Fenestrated tracheostomy tube
   c. Tube with an inflated foam cuff
   d. Cuffed tube with the cuff deflated

5. Which nursing action related to the tracheostomy tube cuff pressure would prevent excessive pressure on tracheal capillaries?
   a. Monitor pressure every 2 to 3 days.
   b. Ensure pressure is less than 20 mm Hg or 25 cm H_2O.
   c. Ensure pressure is less than 30 mm Hg or 35 cm H_2O.
   d. Ensure pressure is sufficient to fill the pilot balloon until it is tense.

6. Which of the following is not an early symptom of head and neck cancer?
   a. Hoarseness
   b. Change in fit of dentures
   c. Mouth ulcers that do not heal
   d. Decreased mobility of the tongue

7. While in the recovery room, a client with a total laryngectomy is suctioned and has bloody mucus with some clots. Which of the following nursing interventions would apply?
   a. Notify the physician immediately.
   b. Place the client in the prone position to facilitate drainage.
   c. Instill 3 mL of normal saline into the tracheostomy tube to loosen secretions.
   d. Continue the assessment of the client, including oxygen saturation, respiratory rate, and breath sounds.

8. How should the client use a voice prosthesis?
   a. Place a vibrating device in the mouth.
   b. Place a speaking valve over the stoma.
   c. Block the stoma entrance with a finger.
   d. Swallow air using the Valsalva manoeuvre.

1. d; 2. d; 3. c, d, e; 4. c; 5. b; 6. d; 7. d; 8. c.

⊝volve

For even more review questions, visit *http://evolve.elsevier.com/Canada/Lewis/medsurg*.

REFERENCES

Aghababian, R., Bird, S., Braen, G., et al. (2011). *The essentials of emergency medicine*. Burlington, MA: Jones & Bartlett Learning.

Astobelli, N. (2013). Chapter 33: Airway management. In R. M. Kacmarek, J. K. Stoller, & A. J. Heuer (Eds.), *Egan's fundamentals of respiratory care* (10th ed., pp. 732–786). St. Louis: Mosby Elsevier.

Bamimore, O., & Silverberg, M. A. (2015). *Acute epistaxis: Treatment and management*. Retrieved from http://emedicine.medscape.com/article/764719-overview#a4.

Calhoun, W. J., Omachi, T. A., Reddy, S. R., et al. (2016). *Allergic status is associated with increased number of asthma exacerbations*. C38, New Developments in Asthma Care, Methods, and Outcomes (A4970–A4970). American Thoracic Society. doi:10.1164/ajrccm-conference.2016.193.1_MeetingAbstracts.A4970.

Carr, E. (2016). Head and neck cancers. In J. K. Itano, J. M. Brant, F. A. Conde, et al. (Eds.), *Core curriculum for oncology* (5th ed., pp. 139–157). St. Louis: Elsevier Mosby.

Chow, A. W., & Doron, S. (2016). *Evaluation of acute pharyngitis in adults*. Retrieved from www.uptodate.com/contents/evaluation-of-acute-pharyngitis-in-adults#H1.

Cooper, K., & Gosnell, K. (2015). *Adult health nursing* (7th ed.). St. Louis: Mosby.

deSchazo, R. D., & Kemp, S. F. (2016). *Patient information: Allergic rhinitis (seasonal allergies)*. Retrieved from www.uptodate.com/contents/allergic-rhinitis-seasonal-allergies-beyond-the-basics.

Emergency Nurses Association (2013). *Sheehy's manual of emergency care* (7th ed.). St. Louis: Mosby.

Goldman, L., & Schafer, A. I. (2012). *Goldman's Cecil medicine* (24th ed.). Philadelphia: Saunders.

Immunize Canada. (2015). *Diseases and vaccines: Influenza*. Retrieved from http://www.immunize.ca/en/diseases-vaccines/influenza.aspx.

Kaplan, A. (2014). Canadian guidelines for acute bacterial rhinosinusitis. *Canadian Family Physician, 60*(227), 227–234.

Nathan, C., & Cars, O. (2014). Antibiotic resistance—problems, progress, and prospects. *New England Journal of Medicine, 371*(19), 1761–1763.

National Institute of Allergy and Infectious Diseases [NIAID]. (2016). *Common cold*. Retrieved from http://www.niaid.nih.gov/topics/commoncold/Pages/default.aspx.

Nguyen, Q. A. (2015). *Epistaxis: Patient education*. Retrieved from http://emedicine.medscape.com/article/863220-overview#a8.

Patton, K., & Thibodeau, G. (2016). *Anatomy and physiology* (9th ed.). St. Louis: Mosby.

Public Health Agency of Canada. (2013). *Canada communicable disease report CCDR: Statement on seasonal influenza vaccine for 2013–2014*. Retrieved from http://www.phac-aspc.gc.ca/publicat/ccdr-rmtc/13vol39/acs-dcc-4/index-eng.php.

Public Health Agency of Canada. (2015a). *Canadian pandemic influenza preparedness: Planning guidance for the health sector*. Retrieved from http://www.phac-aspc.gc.ca/cpip-pclcpi/report-rapport-2015-eng.php#pre.

Public Health Agency of Canada. (2015b). *An Advisory Committee Statement (ACS)-National Advisory Committee on Immunization (NACI): Canadian immunization guide chapter on influenza and statement on seasonal influenza vaccine for 2015–2016*. Retrieved from http://www.phac-aspc.gc.ca/naci-ccni/assets/pdf/flu-2015-grippe-eng.pdf.

Rothrock, J. (2015). *Alexander's care of the patient in surgery* (15th ed.). St. Louis: Mosby.

Stacy, K. M. (2014). Pulmonary therapeutic management. In L. D. Urden, K. M. Stacy, & M. E. Lough (Eds.), *Critical care nursing: Diagnosis and management* (7th ed., pp. 549–586). St. Louis: Elsevier Mosby.

Tung, H. Y., Landers, C., Li, E., et al. (2016). Allergen-encoded signals that control allergic responses. *Current Opinion in Allergy and Clinical Immunology, 16*(1), 51.

RESOURCES

Resources for this chapter are listed in Chapters 30 and 31.

For additional Internet resources, see the website for this book at *http://evolve.elsevier.com/Canada/Lewis/medsurg*

CHAPTER
30

Nursing Management

Lower Respiratory Problems

Written by: Eugene E. Mondor
Adapted by: Cydnee Seneviratne

evolve WEBSITE

http://evolve.elsevier.com/Canada/Lewis/medsurg

- Review Questions (Online Only)
- Key Points
- Answer Guidelines to Case Study
- Student Case Studies
  - Lung Cancer
  - Pulmonary Embolism and Respiratory Failure
- Customizable Nursing Care Plans
  - Pneumonia
  - Thoracotomy
- Conceptual Care Map Creator
- Audio Glossary
- Content Updates

LEARNING OBJECTIVES

1. Describe the pathophysiology, types, clinical manifestations, and collaborative care of pneumonia.
2. Explain the nursing management of the patient with pneumonia.
3. Describe the pathogenesis, classification, clinical manifestations, complications, diagnostic abnormalities, and nursing and collaborative management of tuberculosis.
4. Identify the causes, clinical manifestations, and nursing and collaborative management of pulmonary fungal infections.
5. Explain the pathophysiology, clinical manifestations, and nursing and collaborative management of bronchiectasis and lung abscess.
6. Identify the causative factors, clinical features, and management of environmental lung diseases.
7. Describe the causes, risk factors, pathogenesis, clinical manifestations, and nursing and collaborative management of lung cancer.
8. Identify the mechanisms involved and the clinical manifestations of pneumothorax, fractured ribs, and flail chest.
9. Describe the purpose, methods, and nursing responsibilities related to chest tubes.
10. Explain the types of chest surgery and appropriate preoperative and postoperative care.
11. Compare and contrast extrapulmonary and intrapulmonary restrictive lung disorders in terms of causes, clinical manifestations, and collaborative management.
12. Describe the pathophysiology, clinical manifestations, and management of pulmonary hypertension and cor pulmonale.
13. Discuss the use of lung transplantation as a treatment for pulmonary disorders.

KEY TERMS

acute bronchitis, p. 601
atelectasis, p. 633
blebs, p. 624
bronchiectasis, p. 612
chylothorax, p. 625
community-acquired pneumonia (CAP), p. 601
cor pulmonale, p. 638

empirical therapy, p. 604
empyema, p. 631
flail chest, p. 625
hemothorax, p. 625
hospital-acquired pneumonia (HAP), p. 602
lung abscess, p. 614
pleural effusion, p. 631

pleurisy (pleuritis), p. 633
pneumoconiosis, p. 615
pneumonia, p. 601
pneumothorax, p. 623
pulmonary edema, p. 634
pulmonary embolism (PE), p. 634

pulmonary hypertension, p. 636
tension pneumothorax, p. 624
thoracentesis, p. 631
thoracotomy, p. 630
tuberculosis (TB), p. 607

A wide variety of problems affect the lower respiratory system. Lung diseases that are characterized primarily by an obstructive disorder, such as asthma, emphysema, chronic bronchitis, and cystic fibrosis, are discussed in Chapter 31. All other lower respiratory problems are discussed in this chapter.

Respiratory tract infections are a common cause of morbidity and mortality worldwide. Respiratory diseases account for some of the most common reasons for hospitalization in Canada (Canadian Institute for Health Information, 2015). During the 2014/2015 influenza ("flu") season, there were 43 510 cases of influenza leading to 7 719 hospitalizations and 591 deaths in Canada (Public Health Agency of Canada [PHAC], 2016). Tuberculosis (TB), although potentially curable and preventable, is a worldwide public health threat of epidemic proportion.

ACUTE BRONCHITIS

Acute bronchitis is an inflammation of the bronchi in the lower respiratory tract that is usually caused by infection. It is one of the most common conditions seen in primary care. It usually occurs as a sequel to an upper respiratory tract infection. A type of acute bronchitis is acute exacerbation of chronic bronchitis (AECB). AECB represents acute infection superimposed on chronic bronchitis. AECB is a potentially serious condition that may lead to respiratory failure. (Chronic bronchitis is discussed in Chapter 31.)

The cause of most cases of acute bronchitis is viral (rhinovirus, influenza). However, bacterial causes are also common both in smokers (e.g., *Streptococcus pneumoniae, Haemophilus influenzae*) and nonsmokers (e.g., *Mycoplasma pneumoniae, Chlamydia pneumoniae*).

In acute bronchitis, persistent cough following an acute upper airway infection (e.g., rhinitis, pharyngitis) is the most common symptom. Cough is often accompanied by production of clear, mucoid sputum, although some patients produce purulent sputum. Associated symptoms include fever, headache, malaise, and shortness of breath on exertion. Physical examination may reveal mildly elevated temperature, pulse, and respiratory rate with either normal breath sounds or expiratory wheezing. Chest radiographic studies can differentiate acute bronchitis from pneumonia because there is no radiographic evidence of consolidation or infiltrates with bronchitis.

Acute bronchitis is usually self-limiting, and the treatment is generally supportive, including fluids, rest, and anti-inflammatory agents. Cough suppressants or bronchodilators may be prescribed for symptomatic treatment of nocturnal cough or wheezing. Antibiotics are generally not prescribed unless the person has a prolonged infection associated with constitutional symptoms (which indicate systemic disease effects) including mild to moderate pain, the person is a smoker, or the person has chronic obstructive pulmonary disease (COPD).

The patient with AECB is usually treated empirically with broad-spectrum antibiotics. Often, the patient with COPD is taught to recognize symptoms of acute bronchitis and to begin a course of antibiotics when symptoms occur. Many health care providers believe that a more severe infection often results if the patient delays taking antibiotics until after a clinical examination. Early initiation of antibiotic treatment in patients with COPD has resulted in a decrease in relapses and a decrease in hospital admissions.

PNEUMONIA

Pneumonia is an acute inflammation of the lung parenchyma caused by a microbial agent. The discovery of sulpha drugs and penicillin was pivotal in the treatment of pneumonia. Since that time, there has been remarkable progress in the development of antibiotics to treat pneumonia. However, despite the new antimicrobial agents, pneumonia is still common and is associated with significant morbidity and mortality rates.

Etiology

Normally, the airway distal to the larynx is sterile because of protective defence mechanisms. These mechanisms include the following: filtration of air, warming and humidification of inspired air, epiglottis closure over the trachea, cough reflex, mucociliary escalator mechanism, secretion of immunoglobulin A, and alveolar macrophages (see Chapter 28).

Factors Predisposing to Pneumonia. Pneumonia is more likely to result when defence mechanisms become incompetent or are overwhelmed by the virulence or quantity of infectious agents. Decreased consciousness depresses the cough and epiglottal reflexes, which may allow aspiration of oropharyngeal contents into the lungs. Tracheal intubation interferes with the normal cough reflex and the mucociliary escalator mechanism. It also bypasses the upper airways, in which filtration and humidification of air normally take place. The mucociliary escalator mechanism is impaired by air pollution, cigarette smoking, viral upper respiratory infections (URIs), and normal changes of aging. In the presence of malnutrition, the functions of lymphocytes and polymorphonuclear leukocytes are altered. Certain diseases, such as leukemia, alcoholism, and diabetes mellitus, are associated with an increased frequency of Gram-negative bacilli in the oropharynx. (Gram-negative bacilli are not normal flora in the respiratory tract.) Altered oropharyngeal flora can also occur secondary to antibiotic therapy given for an infection elsewhere in the body. The factors predisposing to pneumonia are listed in Table 30-1.

Acquisition of Organisms. Organisms that cause pneumonia reach the lung by three methods:

1. *Aspiration* from the nasopharynx or oropharynx. Many of the organisms that cause pneumonia are normal inhabitants of the pharynx in healthy adults.
2. *Inhalation* of microbes present in the air (e.g., *M. pneumoniae*, fungal pneumonias).
3. *Hematogenous spread* from a primary infection elsewhere in the body. An example is *Staphylococcus aureus*.

Types of Pneumonia

Pneumonia can be caused by bacteria, viruses, *Mycoplasma*, fungi, parasites, and chemicals. Although pneumonia can be classified according to the causative organism, a clinically effective way to classify pneumonia is as *community-acquired* or *hospital-acquired*. Classifying pneumonia is important because of differences in the likely causative organisms and the selection of appropriate antibiotics.

Community-Acquired Pneumonia. Community-acquired pneumonia (CAP) is defined as a lower respiratory tract infection of the lung parenchyma with onset in the community or during

---

TABLE 30-1 FACTORS PREDISPOSING TO PNEUMONIA

- Aging
- Air pollution
- Altered consciousness: alcohol use disorder, head injury, seizures, anaesthesia, drug overdose, stroke
- Altered oropharyngeal flora
- Bed rest and prolonged immobility
- Chronic diseases: chronic lung disease, diabetes mellitus, heart disease, cancer, end-stage renal disease
- Debilitating illness
- Human immunodeficiency virus infection
- Immuno-suppressive drugs (corticosteroids, cancer chemotherapy, immuno-suppressive therapy after organ transplant)
- Inhalation or aspiration of noxious substances
- Intestinal and gastric feedings
- Malnutrition
- Smoking
- Tracheal intubation (endotracheal intubation, tracheostomy)
- Upper respiratory tract infection

the first 2 days of hospitalization. The incidence of CAP is highest in the winter months. Smoking is an important risk factor. The causative organism in CAP is identified only 50% of the time. Organisms that are commonly implicated in CAP include *S. pneumoniae* and atypical organisms (e.g., *Legionella, Mycoplasma, Chlamydia,* viral). Modifying risk factors include the presence of COPD, recent use of antibiotics, and conditions incurring risk of aspiration.

In 2000, the Canadian Infectious Disease Society and the Canadian Thoracic Society conducted an evidence-informed update of the Canadian guidelines for initial management of CAP (Mandell, Marrie, Grossman, et al., 2000). Considering that there are over 100 microorganisms that cause pneumonia, Mandel, Marrie, Grossman, and colleagues stressed that, in addition to chest radiography and clinical evaluation, assessment and diagnosis be based on serology results as well as sputum culture, pleural fluid culture, or both, and blood cultures. Pharmacological intervention should include specific antimicrobial selection based on type of pneumonia, including where acquired, and modifying factors such as pathogens (Table 30-2).

Hospital-Acquired Pneumonia. Hospital-acquired pneumonia (HAP) is pneumonia occurring 48 hours or longer after hospital admission and not incubating at the time of hospitalization. HAP accounts for 25% of all intensive care unit infections. It is the second most common hospital-associated infection in Canada and has high mortality and morbidity rates (Rotstein, Evans, Born, et al., 2008). The microorganisms responsible for HAP are different from those organisms implicated in CAP. Bacteria are responsible for the majority of HAP infections, including *Pseudomonas, Enterobacter, S. aureus,* methicillin-resistant *Staphylococcus aureus* (MRSA), and *S. pneumoniae.* Many of the organisms causing HAP enter the lungs after aspiration of particles from the patient's own pharynx. Immuno-suppressive therapy, general debility, and endotracheal intubation may be predisposing factors. Contaminated respiratory therapy equipment is another source of infection.

Fungal Pneumonia. Fungi may also be a cause of pneumonia (see "Pulmonary Fungal Infections" later in this chapter).

Aspiration Pneumonia. *Aspiration pneumonia* refers to the sequelae of abnormal entry of secretions or substances into the lower airway. It usually follows aspiration of material from the mouth or the stomach into the trachea and subsequently the lungs. The person who has aspiration pneumonia usually has a history of loss of consciousness (e.g., as a result of seizure, anaesthesia, head injury, stroke, alcohol intake). With loss of consciousness, the gag and cough reflexes are depressed, and aspiration is more likely to occur. Another risk factor is tube feedings. The dependent portions of the lung are most often affected, primarily the superior segments of the lower lobes and the posterior segments of the upper lobes, which are dependent in the supine position.

The aspirated material—food, water, vomitus, or toxic fluids—is the pathological triggering mechanism for the development of this type of pneumonia. There are three distinct forms of aspiration

TABLE 30-2 EMPIRICAL ANTIMICROBIAL SELECTION FOR ADULT PATIENTS WITH COMMUNITY-ACQUIRED PNEUMONIA

Type of Pneumonia	Modifying Factors and/or Pathogens	First Choice	Second Choice
Outpatient without modifying factors		Macrolide*	Doxycycline
Outpatient with modifying factors	COPD (no recent antibiotics or oral steroids within past 3 months)	Newer macrolides†	Doxycycline
	COPD (antibiotics or oral steroids within past 3 months)—*Haemophilus influenzae* and enteric Gram-negative rods	"Respiratory" fluoroquinolone‡	Amoxicillin–clavulanate + macrolide or second-generation cephalosporin + macrolide
	Suspected macroaspiration—oral anaerobes	Amoxicillin–clavulanate ± macrolide, or fourth-generation fluoroquinolone‡ (e.g., moxifloxacin)	Third-generation fluoroquinolones‡ (e.g., levofloxacin) + clindamycin or metronidazole
Nursing home resident in nursing home	*Streptococcus pneumoniae,* enteric Gram-negative rods, *H. influenzae*	"Respiratory" fluoroquinolone‡ alone or amoxicillin–clavulanate + macrolide	Second-generation cephalosporin + macrolide
Nursing home resident in hospital		Identical to treatment for other hospitalized patients (see below)	
Hospitalized patient on medical ward	*S. pneumoniae, Legionella pneumophila, Chlamydia pneumoniae*	"Respiratory" fluoroquinolone‡	Second-, third-, or fourth-generation cephalosporin + macrolide
Hospitalized patient in intensive care unit	*Pseudomonas aeruginosa* not suspected (*S. pneumoniae, L. pneumophila, C. pneumoniae,* enteric Gram-negative rods implicated)	IV "respiratory" fluoroquinolone + cefotaxime, ceftriaxone, or β-lactam–β-lactamase inhibitor	IV macrolide + cefotaxime, ceftriaxone, or β-lactam–β-lactamase inhibitor
	P. aeruginosa suspected	Antipseudomonal fluoroquinolone (e.g., ciprofloxacin) + antipseudomonal β-lactam (e.g., ceftazidime, carbapenem, piperacillin–tazobactam) or aminoglycoside (e.g., gentamicin, tobramycin, amikacin)	Triple therapy with antipseudomonal β-lactam + aminoglycoside + macrolide

*Macrolide—erythromycin, azithromycin, clarithromycin.
†Newer macrolide—azithromycin, clarithromycin.
‡Respiratory fluoroquinolone—levofloxacin (third generation), gatifloxacin, and moxifloxacin (fourth generation); trovafloxacin (fourth generation) is restricted because of potential severe hepatoxicity.
COPD, chronic obstructive pulmonary disease; *IV,* intravenous.
Source: Mandell, Lionel A., Marrie, Thomas J., "Canadian Guidelines for the Initial Management of Community-Acquired Pneumonia: An Evidence-Based Update by the Canadian Infectious Diseases Society and the Canadian Thoracic Society," *Clinical Infectious Diseases,* 2000, Volume 31, Issue 2, Pages 383–421, by permission of Oxford University Press.

pneumonia. If the aspirated material is an inert substance (e.g., barium), the initial manifestation is usually caused by mechanical obstruction of airways. When the aspirated materials contain toxic fluids, such as gastric juices, there is chemical injury to the lung with infection as a secondary event, usually 48 to 72 hours later; this is identified as *chemical (noninfectious) pneumonitis.* The most important form of aspiration pneumonia is bacterial infection. The infecting organism is usually one of the normal oropharyngeal flora, and multiple organisms, including both aerobes and anaerobes, are isolated from the sputum of the patient with aspiration pneumonia. Antibiotic therapy is based on an assessment of the severity of illness, where the infection was acquired (community or hospital), and the type of organisms present.

Opportunistic Pneumonia. Patients with altered immune response are highly susceptible to respiratory infections. Specific individuals considered at risk include those who have severe protein–calorie malnutrition; those who have immune deficiencies; those who have received transplants and been treated with immuno-suppressive drugs; and patients who are being treated with radiation therapy, chemotherapeutic drugs, or corticosteroids (especially for a prolonged period). These individuals have a variety of altered conditions, including altered B- and T-lymphocyte function, depressed bone marrow function, and decreased levels or function of neutrophils and macrophages. In addition to the risk for bacterial and viral pneumonia, immuno-compromised patients may develop an infection from microorganisms that do not normally cause disease, such as *Pneumocystis jiroveci* (formerly *P. carinii*) and cytomegalovirus (CMV).

P. jiroveci is an opportunistic pathogen whose natural habitat is the lung. This organism rarely causes pneumonia in healthy individuals. *P. jiroveci* pneumonia (PJP) affects 70% of human immunodeficiency virus (HIV)–infected individuals and is the most common opportunistic infection in patients with acquired immune deficiency syndrome (AIDS). In this type of pneumonia, the chest radiograph usually shows a diffuse bilateral alveolar pattern of infiltration. In widespread disease, the lungs are massively consolidated.

Clinical manifestations are insidious and include fever, tachypnea, tachycardia, dyspnea, nonproductive cough, and hypoxemia. Pulmonary physical findings are minimal in proportion to the serious nature of the disease. Treatment consists of antibiotics. In populations at risk for development of *P. jiroveci* pneumonitis (e.g., patients with hematological malignancies or AIDS), antibiotic prophylaxis may be advocated. (PJP is discussed in Chapter 17.)

Cytomegalovirus (CMV) is a cause of viral pneumonia in the immuno-compromised patient, particularly in transplant recipients. CMV, a type of herpesvirus, gives rise to latent infections and reactivation with shedding of infectious virus. This type of interstitial pneumonia can be a mild disease, or it can be fulminant and produce pulmonary insufficiency and death. Often, CMV coexists with other opportunistic bacterial or fungal agents in causing pneumonia. Ganciclovir (Cytovene) is recommended for treatment of CMV pneumonia.

Pathophysiology

Pneumococcal pneumonia is the most common cause of bacterial pneumonia. However, regardless of causative factors, pneumonia is characterized by four stages of the disease process:
1. *Congestion.* After the pneumococcus organisms reach the alveoli via droplets or saliva, there is an outpouring of fluid

PATHOPHYSIOLOGY MAP

```
      Aspiration of S. pneumoniae
                 │
                 ▼
      Release of bacterial endotoxin
                 │
                 ▼
        Inflammatory response
      Attraction of neutrophils;
   release of inflammatory mediators;
    accumulation of fibrinous exudate,
       red blood cells, and bacteria
          │                      │
          ▼      Leukocyte       ▼
  Red hepatization  infiltration   Gray hepatization and
  and consolidation              deposition of fibrin
  of lung parenchyma (neutrophils and  on pleural surfaces;
                     macrophages)  phagocytosis in alveoli
                 │                      │
                 ▼                      │
        Resolution of infection  ◄──────┘
      Macrophages in alveoli ingest
          and remove degenerated
      neutrophils, fibrin, and bacteria
```

FIGURE 30-1 Pathophysiological course of pneumococcal pneumonia.

into the alveoli. The organisms multiply in the serous fluid, and the infection is spread. The pneumococci damage the host by their overwhelming growth and interference with lung function.
2. *Red hepatization.* There is massive dilation of the capillaries, and alveoli are filled with organisms, neutrophils, red blood cells, and fibrin (Figure 30-1). The lung appears red and granular, similar to the liver, which is why the process is called *hepatization.*
3. *Grey hepatization.* Blood flow decreases, and leukocytes and fibrin consolidate in the affected part of the lung.
4. *Resolution.* Complete resolution and healing occur if there are no complications.

The exudate becomes lysed and is processed by the macrophages. The normal lung tissue is restored, and the person's gas-exchange ability returns to normal.

Clinical Manifestations

Patients with pneumonia usually have a constellation of symptoms including sudden onset of fever, chills, a cough producing purulent sputum, and pleuritic chest pain (in some cases). In the older adult or debilitated patient, confusion or stupor (possibly related to hypoxia) may be the predominant finding. On physical examination, signs of pulmonary consolidation, such as dullness to percussion, increased fremitus, bronchial breath sounds, and crackles, may be found. The typical pneumonia syndrome is usually caused by the most common pathogen in CAP, which is *S. pneumoniae,* but can also be caused by other bacterial pathogens, such as *H. influenzae.*

Pneumonia may also manifest atypically with a more gradual onset, a dry cough, and extrapulmonary manifestations such as headache, myalgias, fatigue, sore throat, nausea, vomiting, and diarrhea. On physical examination, crackles are often heard. This presentation of symptoms is classically produced by *M. pneumoniae* but can also be caused by *Legionella* and *C. pneumoniae*. Patients with hematogenous *S. aureus* pneumonia may have only dyspnea and fever. This necrotizing infection causes destruction of lung tissue, and these patients are usually very sick.

Manifestations of viral pneumonia are highly variable but may be characterized by chills, fever, dry, nonproductive cough, and extrapulmonary symptoms. Viral pneumonia may be found in association with systemic viral diseases such as measles, varicella-zoster, herpes simplex, or influenza virus infection.

Complications

Most cases of pneumonia run an uncomplicated course. Complications generally develop more frequently in individuals with underlying chronic diseases and may include the following:

1. *Pleurisy* (inflammation of the pleura) is a relatively common accompanying problem of pneumonia.
2. *Pleural effusion* can occur. Usually, the effusion is sterile and is reabsorbed in 1 to 2 weeks. Occasionally, it necessitates aspiration by means of thoracentesis.
3. *Atelectasis* (collapsed, airless alveoli) of one or part of one lobe may occur. These areas usually clear with effective coughing and deep breathing.
4. *Delayed resolution* results from persistent infection and is seen on radiograph as residual consolidation. Usually, the physical findings return to normal within 2 to 4 weeks. Delayed resolution occurs most frequently in patients who are older or malnourished or have alcohol use disorder or COPD.
5. *Lung abscess* is not a common complication of pneumonia. It may be seen with pneumonia caused by *S. aureus* and Gram-negative pneumonias (see Lung Abscess later in this chapter).
6. *Empyema* (accumulation of purulent exudate in the pleural cavity) is relatively infrequent but necessitates antibiotic therapy and drainage of the exudate by a chest tube or by open surgery.
7. *Pericarditis* results from spread of the infecting organism from an infected pleura or via a hematogenous route to the pericardium (the fibroserous sac around the heart).
8. *Bacteremia* can occur with pneumococcal pneumonia, more so in older-adult patients.
9. *Meningitis* can be caused by *S. pneumoniae*. The patient with pneumonia who is disoriented, confused, or somnolent should have a lumbar puncture to evaluate the possibility of meningitis.
10. *Endocarditis* can develop when the organisms attack the endocardium and the valves of the heart. The clinical manifestations are similar to those of acute infective endocarditis (see Chapter 39).

Diagnostic Studies. The common diagnostic measures for pneumonia are presented in Table 30-3. History, physical examination, and chest radiographic study often provide enough information to make management decisions without costly laboratory tests.

The chest radiograph often shows a typical pattern characteristic of the infecting organism and is an invaluable adjunct in the diagnosis of pneumonia. Lobar or segmental consolidation suggests a bacterial cause, usually *S. pneumoniae* or *Klebsiella*. Diffuse pulmonary infiltrates are most commonly caused by infection with viruses, *Legionella,* or pathogenic fungi. Cavitary shadows suggest the presence of a necrotizing infection with

---

TABLE 30-3 COLLABORATIVE CARE

Pneumonia

Diagnostic	Collaborative Therapy
• History and physical examination	• Appropriate antibiotic therapy
• Chest radiograph	• Increased fluid intake (at least 3 L/day)
• Gram stain examination of sputum	• Limited activity and rest
• Sputum culture and sensitivity test (if drug-resistant pathogen or organism not covered by empirical therapy)	• Antipyretics
	• Analgesics
	• Oxygen therapy (if indicated)
• Pulse oximetry or ABGs (if indicated)	
• Complete blood cell count, differential, and routine blood chemistries (if indicated)	
• Blood cultures (if indicated)	

ABGs, arterial blood gases.

---

destruction of lung tissue commonly caused by *S. aureus,* Gram-negative bacteria, or *Mycobacterium tuberculosis.* Pleural effusions, which can occur in up to 30% of patients with CAP, can also be seen on radiographic study.

Sputum cultures are recommended in the case of the suspected presence of a drug-resistant pathogen or an organism that is not covered by the usual **empirical therapy** (therapy based on observation and experience, implemented when the condition's exact cause is not known). A Gram stain examination of the sputum provides information on the predominant causative organism. A sputum culture should be collected before initiating antibiotic therapy as a means to intervene with patients with community- or hospital-acquired pneumonia (Health Quality Ontario and Ministry of Health and Long-Term Care, 2013; Mandell, Marrie, Grossman, et al., 2000). Because of the poor sensitivity and specificity of sputum cultures, any sputum culture results should be correlated with the predominant organisms found on Gram stain examination results. Before treatment, two blood cultures may be done for patients who are seriously ill. Although microbial studies are expected before treatment, initiation of antibiotics should not be delayed.

Arterial blood gases (ABGs), if obtained, usually reveal hypoxemia. Leukocytosis is found in the majority of patients with bacterial pneumonia, usually with a white blood cell (WBC) count greater than 15×10^9/L with the presence of bands (immature neutrophils).

Collaborative Care

Prompt treatment with the appropriate antibiotic almost always cures bacterial and mycoplasma pneumonia. In uncomplicated cases, the patient responds to drug therapy within 48 to 72 hours. Indications of improvement include decreased temperature, improved breathing, and reduced chest pain. Abnormal physical findings can last for more than 7 days.

In addition to antibiotic therapy, supportive measures may be used, including oxygen therapy to treat hypoxemia, analgesics to relieve the chest pain for patient comfort, and antipyretics such as acetylsalicylic acid (ASA; Aspirin) or acetaminophen (Tylenol) for significantly elevated temperature. During the acute febrile phase, the patient's activity should be restricted, and rest should be encouraged and planned. The Health Quality Ontario and Ministry of Health and Long-Term Care CAP guidelines (2013) recommend airway clearance, supportive therapy, antiviral therapy during flu season, smoking cessation, and vaccinations for CAP in addition to antibiotic therapy.

Most individuals with mild to moderate illness who have no other underlying disease process can be treated on an outpatient basis. If there is a serious underlying disease or if the pneumonia is accompanied by severe dyspnea, hypoxemia, or other complications, the patient should be hospitalized.

Currently, there is no definitive treatment for viral pneumonia. An antiviral drug, amantadine, is approved for oral use in the treatment of influenza A virus. The neuraminidase inhibitors zanamivir (Relenza) and oseltamivir (Tamiflu) are active against both influenza A and B (see Chapter 29). An influenza vaccine is available. It is modified annually to reflect the anticipated strains in the upcoming season. The flu vaccine is considered a mainstay of prevention and is recommended annually for individuals considered to be at risk for influenza, including older adults, long-term care residents, patients with COPD or diabetes mellitus, and health care workers. For older adults with signs and symptoms of influenza, including those who have received the influenza vaccine, treatment with amantadine or a neuraminidase inhibitor is recommended. During epidemics of influenza A, especially in long-term care facilities, chemoprophylaxis with these agents is recommended for unvaccinated patients, immunodeficient patients, or those who have received the vaccine within the past 2 weeks.

Pneumococcal Vaccine. Pneumococcal vaccine is indicated primarily for the individual considered at risk who (1) has a chronic illness such as lung or heart disease or diabetes mellitus, (2) is recovering from a severe illness, (3) is 65 years of age or older, or (4) resides in a long-term care facility. Vaccination is particularly important because the rate of drug-resistant *S. pneumoniae* infections is increasing. Pneumococcal vaccine can be given simultaneously with other vaccines such as the flu vaccine, but each should be administered in a separate site (PHAC, 2015).

The current recommendation is that pneumococcal vaccine is good for a person's lifetime (PHAC, 2015). However, in the immuno-suppressed individual at risk for development of fatal pneumococcal infection (e.g., asplenic patient; patient with nephrotic syndrome, renal failure, or AIDS; or transplant recipient), revaccination is recommended every 5 years.

Drug Therapy. The main problems with the use of antibiotics to treat pneumonia are the development of resistant strains of organisms and the patient's hypersensitivity or allergic reaction to certain antibiotics.

Most cases of CAP in otherwise healthy adults do not necessitate hospitalization. The Canadian Infectious Diseases Society and Canadian Thoracic Society have guidelines aimed at classifying patients to determine therapy options (see Table 30-2).

The oral antibiotic therapy administered is frequently empirical treatment with broad-spectrum antibiotics. Once the patient is assigned a treatment classification, therapy can be based on the likely infecting organism.

For HAP, empirical antibiotic therapy should be based on the likely pathogens in the various patient groups. Even with extensive diagnostic testing, an etiological organism is often not identified. It is important to recognize when a patient is not responding to treatment. Therapy may require modification based on the patient's culture results or clinical response. Clinical response is evaluated by factors such as a change in fever, sputum purulence, leukocytosis, oxygenation, or radiographic study patterns. Improvement is often not apparent for the first 48 to 72 hours, and therapy need not be altered during this period unless deterioration is noted or culture results dictate that a different antibiotic should be used. Common antibiotics for HAP include cephalosporins (third-generation antipseudomonal [ceftazidime]), β-lactam or β-lactamase inhibitor, vancomycin (for MRSA), aminoglycosides (gentamicin), and antipseudomonal quinolones (ciprofloxacin) (Rotstein, Evans, Born, et al., 2008).

Patients with ventilator-associated pneumonia may experience rapid deterioration. Patients who deteriorate or fail to respond to therapy will require aggressive evaluation to assess non-infectious etiologies, complications, other coexisting infectious processes, or pneumonia caused by a resistant pathogen (Rotstein, Evans, Born, et al., 2008). It may be necessary to broaden antimicrobial coverage while awaiting results of cultures and other studies, such as computed tomographic (CT) scan, ultrasound, or lung scans.

Nutritional Therapy. Fluid intake of at least 3 L/day is important in the supportive treatment of pneumonia. If the patient has heart failure, fluid intake must be individualized. If oral intake cannot be maintained, intravenous (IV) administration of fluids and electrolytes may be necessary for the acutely ill patient. An intake of at least 1 500 calories per day should be maintained to provide energy for the increased metabolic processes in the patient. Small, frequent meals are better tolerated by the patient with dyspnea.

NURSING MANAGEMENT PNEUMONIA

NURSING ASSESSMENT

Subjective and objective data that should be obtained from a patient with pneumonia are presented in Table 30-4.

NURSING DIAGNOSES

Nursing diagnoses for the patient with pneumonia may include but are not limited to the following:
- *Impaired gas exchange* (related to fluid and exudate accumulation with the alveoli and surrounding lung tissue)
- *Ineffective breathing pattern* related to *pain*
- *Acute pain* related to *biological injury agent* (infection)
- *Activity intolerance* related to *respiratory condition, physical deconditioning*

Additional information on nursing diagnoses for the patient with pneumonia is presented in Nursing Care Plan (NCP) 30-1, available on the Evolve website.

PLANNING

The overall goals are that the patient with pneumonia will have (a) clear breath sounds, (b) normal breathing patterns, (c) no signs of hypoxia, (d) a normal chest radiograph, and (e) no complications related to pneumonia.

NURSING IMPLEMENTATION

HEALTH PROMOTION. Many nursing interventions are available to help prevent the occurrence of pneumonia as well as the morbidity associated with it. Teaching a patient to practise good health habits, such as proper diet and hygiene, adequate rest, and regular exercise, can help the patient maintain the natural resistance to infecting organisms. If possible, exposure to people with URIs should be avoided. If a URI occurs, it should be treated

TABLE 30-4 NURSING ASSESSMENT

Pneumonia

Subjective Data

Important Health Information

Past health history: Lung cancer, COPD, diabetes mellitus; cigarette smoking; alcohol use disorder; recent upper respiratory tract infection; chronic debilitating disease; malnutrition; altered consciousness; AIDS; exposure to chemical toxins, dust, or allergens; immobility or prolonged bed rest

Medications: Use of antibiotics, corticosteroids, chemotherapy, or any other immuno-suppressants

Surgery or other treatments: Recent abdominal or thoracic surgery, splenectomy, endotracheal intubation, general anaesthesia; tube feedings

Symptoms
- Fatigue, weakness, malaise
- Anorexia, nausea, vomiting
- Fever, chills
- Dyspnea, cough (productive or nonproductive), nasal congestion, pain with breathing
- Chest pain, sore throat, headache, abdominal pain, muscle aches

Objective Data

General

Fever, restlessness, or lethargy; splinting of affected area

Respiratory

Tachypnea; dyspnea, nasal congestion, pharyngitis; asymmetrical chest movements or retraction; decreased excursion; nasal flaring; use of accessory muscles (neck, abdomen); grunting; crackles, friction rub on auscultation; dullness on percussion over consolidated areas, increased tactile fremitus on palpation; pink, rusty, purulent, green, yellow, or white sputum (amount may be scant to copious)

Cardiovascular

Tachycardia

Neurological

Changes in mental status, ranging from confusion to delirium

Possible Findings

Leukocytosis; abnormal ABGs with ↓ or normal PaO_2, ↓ $PaCO_2$, and ↑ pH initially, and later ↓ PaO_2, ↑ $PaCO_2$, and ↓ pH; positive sputum Gram stain examination and culture; patchy or diffuse infiltrates, abscesses, pleural effusion, or pneumothorax on chest radiographic study

ABGs, arterial blood gases; *AIDS,* acquired immune deficiency syndrome; *COPD,* chronic obstructive pulmonary disease; *PaO₂,* partial pressure of oxygen in arterial blood; *PaCO₂,* partial pressure of carbon dioxide in arterial blood.

promptly with supportive measures (e.g., rest, fluids). If symptoms persist for more than 7 days, the person should obtain medical care. Individuals at risk for pneumonia (e.g., people who are chronically ill, older adults) should be encouraged to obtain both influenza and pneumococcal vaccines.

In the hospital, the nursing role involves identifying the patient at risk (see Table 30-1) and taking measures to prevent the development of pneumonia. The patient with altered consciousness should be placed in positions (e.g., side-lying, upright) that will prevent or minimize the risk for aspiration. The patient should be turned and repositioned at least every 2 hours to facilitate adequate lung expansion and to discourage pooling of secretions.

The patient who has a feeding tube generally requires that measures be taken to prevent aspiration (see Chapter 42).

Although feeding tubes are small, an interruption in the integrity of the lower esophageal sphincter still exists and can allow reflux of gastric and intestinal contents. The patient who has difficulty swallowing (e.g., a patient who has had a stroke) needs assistance in eating, drinking, and taking medication to prevent aspiration. The patient who has recently had surgery and others who are immobile need assistance with turning and measures to facilitate deep breathing at frequent intervals (see Chapter 22). The nurse must be careful to avoid overmedication with opioids or sedatives, which can cause a depressed cough reflex and accumulation of fluid in the lungs. Presence of the gag reflex should be ascertained before the administration of fluids or food to the individual who has had local anaesthesia to the throat.

To reduce the incidence of hospital-associated infections, the nurse should practise strict medical asepsis and adherence to infection-control guidelines. Poor handwashing practices allow spread of pathogens via the hands of the health care worker. Staff members should wash their hands or, if hands are not visibly soiled, use hand rubs with 60% alcohol (Infection Prevention and Control Canada, n.d.) before providing care to a patient. Respiratory devices can harbour microorganisms and have been associated with outbreaks of pneumonia. Strict sterile aseptic technique should be used when suctioning the trachea of a patient.

ACUTE INTERVENTION. Although many patients with pneumonia are treated on an outpatient basis, the NCP for a patient with pneumonia (see NCP 30-1, available on the Evolve website) is applicable to outpatients and inpatients. It is important for the nurse to remember that pneumonia is an acute, infectious disease. Although most cases of pneumonia are potentially completely curable, complications can result. The nurse must be aware of these complications and their manifestations. The infection-control nurse can be a valuable resource in assisting with the care of patients with pneumonia.

Therapeutic positioning for patients with pneumonia ensures stable oxygenation status. The "good lung down" position is used for patients with unilateral lung disease, in whom better oxygenation is achieved when the unaffected lung (good lung) is placed in the down (lateral) position to achieve maximum lung expansion. Incentive spirometry, turning, coughing, and deep breathing all increase lung volume, mobilize secretions, and prevent atelectasis. Exercise and early ambulation augment bronchial hygiene and are encouraged as tolerated.

AMBULATORY AND HOME CARE. The patient needs to be reassured that complete recovery from pneumonia is possible. It is extremely important to emphasize the need to take all of any drugs prescribed and to return for follow-up medical care and evaluation. The patient needs to be taught about the drug–drug and the food–drug interactions for the prescribed antibiotic. Adequate rest is needed to maintain progress toward recovery and to prevent a relapse. The patient should be told that it may take weeks to feel the usual vigour and sense of well-being. A prolonged period of convalescence may be necessary for the older-adult or chronically ill patient.

The patient considered to be at risk for pneumonia should be told about available vaccines and should discuss them with the health care provider. Deep-breathing exercises should be practised for 6 to 8 weeks after the patient is discharged from the hospital.

EVALUATION. The expected outcomes for the patient with pneumonia are presented in NCP 30-1, available on the Evolve website.

TUBERCULOSIS

Tuberculosis (TB) is an infectious disease caused by *M. tuberculosis*. It usually involves the lungs, but it also occurs in the larynx, the kidneys, the bones, the adrenal glands, the lymph nodes, and the meninges and can be disseminated throughout the body. TB is a reportable communicable disease; it kills more people worldwide than any other infectious disease, with an estimated 8.8 million of the world's population having been infected. In Canada, the number of reported cases of active TB has remained relatively stable, averaging 1 623 cases per year and showing some indication of decline. In 2010, the Public Health Agency of Canada (PHAC) determined that since 1970, Canadian-born people diagnosed with TB significantly declined from 67.8% to 11.8%. However, during the same period, immigrants with TB increased from 17.7% to 67.0%, and reported cases of TB in Canadian-born Indigenous peoples increased from 14.7% to 21.1% (PHAC & Canadian Lung Association, 2014). The pulmonary system continues to be the main diagnostic site of disease, representing 68% of all reported TB cases (PHAC, 2014).

The populations most at risk in Canada are the Indigenous and immigrant populations. TB among Canadian-born Indigenous peoples is 31 times higher than the national average (Assembly of First Nations, 2011). Factors or challenges the Canadian-born Indigenous peoples face that influence the transmission of TB are poor nutrition, overcrowding, poorly ventilated homes, comorbidities (diabetes, HIV) as well as limited or remote access to health care facilities (PHAC, 2014). Immigrant populations are challenged with poverty and stress related to living in a new country and are more susceptible to latent TB infection with subsequent progression to active TB (PHAC, 2014).

DETERMINANTS OF HEALTH

Tuberculosis

Income and Social Status
- Low socioeconomic groups have higher rates of TB.*

Physical Environments
- Residing in overcrowded institutions (e.g., long-term care facilities, correctional facilities), and urban homelessness increase the risk for acquiring TB.*

Personal Health Practices and Coping Skills
- Smoking and air pollution increase the risk for TB

Culture
- TB is most prevalent in immigrants and Indigenous peoples.†

Gender
- TB is more prevalent in males than in females.‡

References

*Public Health Agency of Canada. (2012). *Tuberculosis fact sheets*. Retrieved from *http://www.phac-aspc.gc.ca/tbpc-latb/fa-fi/index-eng.php*.
†Public Health Agency of Canada. (2015). *Tuberculosis in Canada 2013*. Retrieved from *http://www.phac-aspc.gc.ca/tbpc-latb/pubs/tbcan13pre/assets/pdf/tbcan13pre-eng.pdf*.
‡Öztürk, A. B., Kiliçaslan, Z., & Işsever, H. (2014). Effect of smoking and indoor air pollution on the risk of tuberculosis: Smoking, indoor air pollution and tuberculosis. *Tuberkuloz ve Toraks, 62*(1), 1–6. doi:10.5578/tt.7013.

TB, tuberculosis.

Etiology and Pathophysiology

M. tuberculosis, a Gram-positive, acid-fast bacillus, is usually spread from person to person via airborne droplets, which are produced when the infected individual with pulmonary or laryngeal TB coughs, sneezes, speaks, or sings. Once released into a room, the organisms are dispersed and can be inhaled. TB is not highly infectious, and transmission usually requires close, frequent, or prolonged exposure. Brief exposure to a few tubercle bacilli rarely causes an infection. The disease cannot be spread by hands, books, glasses, dishes, or other fomites.

The very small droplets, 1 to 5 mcm in size, contain *M. tuberculosis*. Because they are so small, the particles remain airborne indoors for minutes to hours. Once inhaled, these small particles lodge in the bronchiole and alveolus. Factors that influence the likelihood of transmission include the (a) number of organisms expelled into the air, (b) concentration of organisms (small spaces with limited ventilation would mean higher concentration), (c) length of time of exposure, and (d) immune system of the exposed person. *M. tuberculosis* replicates slowly and spreads via the lymphatic system. The organisms find favourable environments for growth primarily in the upper lobes of the lungs, kidneys, epiphyses of the bone, cerebral cortex, and adrenal glands.

Healing of the primary lesion usually takes place by resolution, fibrosis, and calcification. The granulation tissue surrounding the lesion may become more fibrous and form a collagenous scar around the tubercle. A *Ghon complex* is formed, consisting of the Ghon tubercle and regional lymph nodes. Calcified Ghon complexes may be seen on chest radiographic studies.

When a TB lesion regresses and heals, the infection enters a latent period in which it may persist without producing clinical symptoms of illness. The infection may develop into clinical disease if the persisting organisms begin to multiply rapidly, or it may remain dormant.

People who are infected with *M. tuberculosis* but do not have TB disease cannot spread the infection to other people. TB infection occurs when the bacteria are inhaled but there is an ineffective immune response and the bacteria become inactive. The majority of people mount effective immune responses to encapsulate these organisms for the rest of their lives, preventing primary infection from progressing to disease. TB infection in a person who does not have the active TB disease is not considered a case of TB and is often referred to as *latent tuberculosis infection* (LTBI). If the initial immune response is not adequate, control of the organisms is not maintained, and clinical disease results. Dormant but viable organisms persist for years. Reactivation of TB can occur if the host's defence mechanisms become impaired. The reasons for reactivation are not well understood, but they are related to decreased resistance found in older adults, individuals with concomitant diseases, and those who receive immuno-suppressive therapy.

Clinical Manifestations

In the early stages of TB, the person is usually free of symptoms. Many cases are found incidentally when routine chest radiographic studies are done, especially in older adults.

Systemic manifestations may initially consist of fatigue, malaise, anorexia, weight loss, low-grade fevers, and night sweats. The weight loss may not be excessive until late in the disease and is often attributed to overwork or other factors.

A characteristic pulmonary manifestation is a cough that becomes frequent and produces mucoid or mucopurulent sputum. Dyspnea is unusual. Chest pain characterized as dull or tight may be present. Hemoptysis is not a common finding and is usually associated with more advanced cases. Sometimes TB has more acute, sudden manifestations: the patient has high fever, chills, generalized flulike symptoms, pleuritic pain, and a productive cough.

The HIV-infected patient with TB often has atypical physical examination and chest radiographic examination findings. Classical signs such as fever, cough, and weight loss may be attributed to PCP or other HIV-associated opportunistic diseases. Clinical manifestations of respiratory problems in patients with HIV must be carefully investigated to determine the cause.

Complications

Miliary Tuberculosis. If a necrotic Ghon complex erodes through a blood vessel, large numbers of organisms invade the bloodstream and spread to all body organs. This is called *miliary* or *hematogenous* TB. The patient may be either acutely ill with fever, dyspnea, and cyanosis or chronically ill with systemic manifestations of weight loss, fever, and gastro-intestinal (GI) disturbance. Hepatomegaly, splenomegaly, and generalized lymphadenopathy may be present.

Pleural Effusion and Empyema. A pleural effusion is caused by the release of caseous material into the pleural space. The bacteria-containing material triggers an inflammatory reaction and a pleural exudate of protein-rich fluid. A form of pleurisy called *dry pleurisy* may result from a superficial tubercular lesion involving the pleura. It appears as localized pleuritic pain on deep inspiration. Empyema is less common than effusion but may occur from large numbers of organisms spilling into the pleural space, usually from rupture of a cavity.

Tuberculosis Pneumonia. Acute pneumonia may result when large amounts of tubercle bacilli are discharged from the liquefied necrotic lesion into the lung or lymph nodes. The clinical manifestations are similar to those of bacterial pneumonia, including chills, fever, productive cough, pleuritic pain, and leukocytosis.

Other Organ Involvement. Although the lungs are the primary site of TB, other body organs may also be involved. The meninges may become infected. Bone and joint tissue may be involved in the infectious disease process. The kidneys, the adrenal glands, the lymph nodes, and the genital tract (in both females and males) may also be infected.

Diagnostic Studies

Tuberculin Skin Testing. The body's immune response can be demonstrated by hypersensitivity to a tuberculin skin test. A positive reaction occurs 2 to 12 weeks after the initial infection, corresponding to the time needed to mount an immune response.

Purified protein derivative (PPD) of tuberculin is used primarily to detect the delayed hypersensitivity response. (The procedure for performing the tuberculin skin test is described in Chapter 28.) Once acquired, sensitivity to tuberculin tends to persist throughout life. A positive reaction indicates the presence of a TB infection, but it does not show whether the infection is latent or active, that is, causing a clinical illness. Because the response to TB skin testing may be decreased in the immuno-compromised patient, induration reactions equal to or greater than 5 mm are considered positive. Sometimes, a repeat PPD can cause an accelerated response (the "booster"

effect). Thus, two-step testing is recommended for initial screening of health care workers who will be getting regularly retested in the future and for those who have a decreased response to allergens. This procedure helps identify individuals with past disease and prevent a later positive PPD test from being misinterpreted as a new, infection-related PPD conversion. See Chapter 28, Tables 28-12 and 28-13, for guidelines in interpreting TB skin tests. Recent guidelines for targeted tuberculin testing emphasize targeting only high-risk groups and discourage testing low-risk individuals (PHAC & Canadian Lung Association, 2014).

Chest Radiographic Study. Although the findings on chest radiographic examination are important, it is not possible to make a diagnosis of TB solely on the basis of this examination. This is because other diseases can mimic the radiographic appearance of TB. The abnormality most commonly found in TB is multinodular lymph node involvement with cavitation in the upper lobes of the lungs. Calcification of the lung lesions generally occurs within several years of the infection.

Bacteriological Studies. The demonstration of tubercle bacilli bacteriologically is essential for establishing a diagnosis. Microscopic examination of stained sputum smears for acid-fast bacilli (AFB) is usually the first bacteriological evidence of the presence of tubercle bacilli. Three consecutive sputum specimens are collected on different days and sent for smear and culture. In addition to sputum, material for examination can be obtained from gastric washings, cerebro-spinal fluid (CSF), or pus from an abscess.

The most accurate means of diagnosis is the culture technique. The major disadvantage of this method is that it may take 6 to 8 weeks for the mycobacteria to grow. The advantage is that it can detect small quantities (as few as 10 bacteria/mL of specimen).

Nucleic acid amplification (NAA) is a rapid diagnostic test for TB. Test results are available in a few hours. They are more sensitive than AFB smears but less sensitive than TB cultures. NAA does not replace routine sputum smears and cultures, but it offers a health care provider increased confidence in the diagnosis (PHAC & Canadian Lung Association, 2014).

Since 2007, Canada has been testing using QuantiFERON-TB Gold In-Tube. The patient's blood is mixed with mycobacterial antigens and is then measured using an enzyme-linked immunosorbent assay (ELISA). If the patient is infected with TB organisms, the lymphocytes in the blood will recognize the antigens. Guidelines for when to use this rapid diagnostic tool are outlined in the Canadian Tuberculosis Standards (PHAC & Canadian Lung Association, 2014).

Collaborative Care

Hospitalization for initial treatment of TB is not necessary in most patients. Most patients are treated on an outpatient basis (Table 30-5), and many can continue to work and maintain their lifestyles with few changes. Hospitalization may be used for diagnostic evaluation, for the severely ill or debilitated, and for those who experience adverse drug reactions or treatment failures.

The mainstay of TB treatment is drug therapy. Drug therapy is used to treat an individual with clinical disease and to prevent disease in an infected person.

Drug Therapy

Active Disease. Standard therapy for active TB has been revised because of the global increase in prevalence of multidrug-resistant TB (MDR TB) (World Health Organization [WHO], 2014). MDR

TB occurs when resistance develops to two or more anti-TB drugs. In Canada, MDR TB risk factors include previous TB treatment, birth outside of Canada, and exposure to an individual or individuals diagnosed with infectious drug-resistant TB. The PHAC and Canadian Lung Association (2014) guidelines recommend prevention over management of MDR TB in order to prevent resistance. It is important to ensure proper drug and dosage regimens and management as well as not to prescribe a new single drug when a regimen is failing. It is also important that prescribed regimens are adhered to through direct observed therapy (DOT) and that nonadherent individuals are identified. As such, treatment is individualized, and an initial phase of treatment for a minimum of 8 months is recommended (PHAC & Canadian Lung Association, 2014).

The patient with active TB should be managed aggressively; treatment usually consists of a combination of at least four drugs. The reason for combination therapy is to increase the therapeutic effectiveness and decrease the development of resistant strains of *M. tuberculosis*. It has been shown that single-drug therapy can result in rapid development of resistant strains.

Drugs are divided into first-line and second-line drugs. The four first-line drugs used in Canada are isoniazid (INH), rifampin (RMP), pyrazinamide (PZA), and ethambutol (EMB) (Table 30-6). The most commonly used second-line drugs include fluoroquinolones (e.g., moxifloxacin, levofloxacin) and injectables (e.g., streptomycin, amikacin). Second-line drugs are used in special situations such as drug-resistant tuberculosis (PHAC & Canadian Lung Association, 2014).

Various drug and dosing regimens are available (Table 30-7). Fixed-dose combination anti-TB drugs may enhance adherence to treatment recommendations. Patients on antiretroviral drugs for HIV cannot take RMP because it can impair the effectiveness of the antiretroviral drugs. Other drugs are primarily used for treatment of resistant strains or in the case of the patient's developing adverse effects to the primary drugs. Many second-line drugs carry a greater risk for adverse effects and necessitate closer monitoring.

In follow-up care for patients on long-term therapy, it is important to monitor the effectiveness of drugs and the development of adverse effects. Usually, sputum specimens are initially obtained weekly and then monthly to assess the effectiveness of the medication. The regimen is considered to be effective if the patient converts to a negative TB sputum status.

Although TB tends to have a rapidly progressive course in the patient co-infected with HIV, it responds well to standard medication. The co-infected patient should receive treatment for TB for at least 6 months beyond the conversion of sputum cultures to negative status.

An important reason for follow-up care in the patient with TB is to ensure adherence to the treatment regimen. Nonadherence is a major factor in the emergence of multidrug resistance and treatment failures. Many individuals do not adhere to the treatment program in spite of understanding the disease process and the value of treatment. DOT is recommended for patients known to be at risk for nonadherence with therapy. DOT is an expensive but essential public health issue. DOT involves observing the ingestion of every dose of medication for the TB

TABLE 30-5 COLLABORATIVE CARE

Tuberculosis

Diagnostic	Collaborative Therapy

• History and physical examination
• Tuberculin skin test
• Chest radiographic study
• Bacteriological studies
  • Sputum smear
  • Sputum culture
	• Long-term treatment with antimicrobial drugs (see Tables 30-6 and 30-7)
	• Follow-up bacteriological studies and chest radiographic examinations

TABLE 30-6 DRUG THERAPY

First-Line Drug Therapy for Tuberculosis

Drug	Mechanisms of Action	Adverse Effects	Comments
First-Line Drugs			
Isoniazid (INH)	Bacteriocidal; interferes with DNA metabolism of tubercle bacillus	Peripheral neuritis, hepatotoxicity, hypersensitivity (skin rash, arthralgia, fever), optic neuritis	Metabolism primarily by liver and excretion by kidneys; pyridoxine (vitamin B₆) administration during high-dose therapy as prophylactic measure; use as single prophylactic agent for active TB in individuals whose PPD converts to positive; ability to cross blood–brain barrier; safe in pregnancy*
Rifampin (RMP)	Bacteriocidal; has broad-spectrum effects, inhibits RNA polymerase of tubercle bacillus	Drug interactions, rash, hepatitis, febrile reaction, GI disturbance, peripheral neuropathy, hypersensitivity	Most commonly used with INH; low incidence of adverse effects; suppression of effect of birth control pills; possibility of orange urine and bodily fluids; safe in pregnancy
Pyrazinamide (PZA)	Bacteriocidal; exact mechanism unknown	Hepatitis, arthralgia, fever, skin rash, hyperuricemia, GI symptoms, jaundice (rare)	High rate of effectiveness when used with streptomycin or capreomycin
Ethambutol (EMB)	Bacteriostatic; inhibits RNA synthesis	Skin rash, GI disturbance, malaise, peripheral neuritis, optic neuritis	Adverse effects uncommon and reversible with discontinuation of drug; most commonly used as substitute drug when adverse effects occur with INH or RMP; safe in pregnancy*

DNA, deoxyribonucleic acid; *GI*, gastro-intestinal; *PPD*, purified protein derivative; *RNA*, ribonucleic acid.

*Pyridoxine (vitamin B₆) supplements should be prescribed for patients who may be or are pregnant or who are breastfeeding or are diagnosed with renal failure, diabetes, seizures, malnutrition, or substance use disorder, as these patients are at risk for symptoms of pyridoxine deficiency. Canadian tuberculosis standards suggest pyridoxine dose of 25 mg.

Source: © All rights reserved. *Canadian Tuberculosis Standards*, 7th Edition. Public Health Agency of Canada, Canadian Thoracic Society and the Canadian Lung Association, 2014. Adapted and reproduced with permission from the Minister of Health, 2017.

TABLE 30-7 DRUG THERAPY

Drug Regimen Options for Treatment of Tuberculosis

Standard	Initial Phase (First 2 Months)	Continuation Phase
Regimen 1	INH + RMP + PZA +/– EMB* daily or 5 days/week	INH + RMP for 4 months daily or 3 times/week
Regimen 2	INH + RMP +/– EMB daily or 5 days/week	INH + RMP for 7 months daily or 3 times/week

*EMB can be stopped as soon as drug susceptibility testing results are available and the strain is pan-sensitive. PZA is continued for the full 2 months.
EMB, ethambutol; *INH*, isoniazid; *PZA*, pyrazinamide; *RMP*, rifampin.
Source: © All rights reserved. *Canadian Tuberculosis Standards*, 7th Edition. Public Health Agency of Canada, Canadian Thoracic Society and the Canadian Lung Association, 2014. Adapted and reproduced with permission from the Minister of Health, 2017.

TABLE 30-8 INDICATIONS FOR TREATMENT OF LATENT TUBERCULOSIS INFECTION

Treatment is indicated with positive tuberculin skin tests in people with the following:
- Known or suspected HIV infection
- Recent contact with infectious TB
- Presence of lung scar

Treatment is indicated with significant tuberculin skin test reaction in the following situations:
- Special clinical situations (immuno-suppression therapy, use of corticosteroids, diabetes mellitus, silicosis, chronic renal failure, organ transplant, hematological malignancies)
- If the person was born in a high-prevalence country, is a resident of a communal setting, is a health care worker, or is Indigenous

HIV, human immunodeficiency virus; *TB*, tuberculosis.
Source: Adapted from Public Health Agency of Canada & Canadian Lung Association. (2014). *Canadian tuberculosis standards* (7th ed.). Retrieved from https://cts.lung.ca/sites/default/files/documents/cts/Canadian%20Tuberculosis%20Standards_7th%20edition_Complete.pdf.

patient's entire course of treatment. Completing therapy is important because of the danger of reactivation of TB and the development of MDR TB seen in patients who do not complete the full course of therapy. In many regions, the public health nurse administers DOT at a clinic site. The patient needs to have follow-up visits for 12 months after completion of therapy to check for the presence of resistant strains. DOT protocols and options in remote or rural areas and in Indigenous communities remain problematic.

Teaching patients about the adverse effects of these drugs and when to seek medical attention is critical. The major adverse effect of INH, RMP, and PZA is hepatitis. Liver function tests should be monitored. Baseline liver function tests are done at the start of treatment, and routine monitoring of liver function is done if baseline tests are abnormal.

Latent Tuberculosis Infection. *Latent TB infection* (LTBI) occurs when an individual becomes infected with *M. tuberculosis* but does not become acutely ill. Drug therapy can be used to prevent a TB infection from developing into a clinical disease. Previously used terms such as *preventive therapy* and *chemoprophylaxis* were confusing. Therefore, LTBI is the preferred term. The indications for treatment of LTBI are presented in Table 30-8.

The drug generally used in treatment of LTBI is INH. It is effective and inexpensive and can be administered orally.

Vaccine. Immunization with bacille Calmette–Guérin (BCG) vaccine to prevent TB is currently in use in many parts of the world. Although millions of people have been vaccinated with BCG, the efficacy of the vaccine is not clear. BCG vaccination can result in a positive PPD reaction. The BCG vaccine reaction will wane over time, and the mean PPD reaction size among people who received BCG is less than 10 mm. Because it may be difficult to determine the relevance of increases in individuals who have undergone BCG vaccination, the PHAC and Canadian Lung Association (2014) recommend that a conversion to "positive" be defined as a reaction of 10 mm or greater. People who receive BCG are from high-prevalence areas of the world, and it is important that a positive skin reaction be evaluated for TB.

NURSING MANAGEMENT
TUBERCULOSIS

NURSING ASSESSMENT

It is important to determine whether the patient was ever exposed to a person with TB. The patient should be assessed for productive cough, night sweats, afternoon temperature elevation, weight loss, pleuritic chest pain, and crackles over the apices of the lungs. If the patient has a productive cough, an early-morning sputum specimen will be required for an AFB smear to detect the presence of mycobacteria.

NURSING DIAGNOSES

Nursing diagnoses for the patient with TB may include but are not limited to the following:
- *Ineffective airway clearance* related to *excessive mucus, retained secretions*
- *Risk for infection* (of others) as evidenced by *insufficient knowledge to avoid exposure to pathogens*
- *Ineffective health management* related to *insufficient knowledge of therapeutic regimen, insufficient social support*

PLANNING

The overall goals are that the patient with TB will (a) comply with the therapeutic regimen, (b) have no recurrence of disease, (c) have normal pulmonary function, and (d) take appropriate measures to prevent the spread of the disease.

NURSING IMPLEMENTATION

HEALTH PROMOTION. The ultimate goal related to TB in Canada is eradication. Selective screening programs in known risk groups are of value in detecting individuals with TB. The person with a positive tuberculin skin test should have a chest radiographic examination to assess for the presence of TB. Another important measure is to identify the contacts of the individual who has TB. These contacts should be assessed for the possibility of infection and the need for prophylactic drug therapy.

When an individual has respiratory symptoms such as cough, dyspnea, or sputum production, especially if accompanied by a history of night sweats or unexplained weight loss, the nurse should assess for exposure to people with TB. Even if the suspected respiratory problem is something else, such as emphysema, pneumonia, or lung cancer, it is possible that the patient may have TB as well.

ACUTE INTERVENTION. Acute in-hospital care is seldom required for the patient with TB. If hospitalization is needed, it is usually for a brief period. Patients strongly suspected of having TB should

(a) be placed in respiratory isolation; (b) receive four-drug therapy; and (c) receive an immediate medical workup, including chest radiographic examination, sputum smear, and culture. Respiratory isolation is indicated for the patient with pulmonary or laryngeal TB until the patient is considered to be noninfectious (effective drug therapy, clinical improvement, three negative AFB smears). A negative-pressure isolation room that offers six or more exchanges per hour may be used. Ultraviolet radiation of the air in the upper part of the room is another approach for reducing airborne TB organisms. Therefore, ultraviolet lights are commonly seen in clinics and homeless shelters. Masks are needed to filter out droplet nuclei. Use of institution-approved high-efficiency particulate air (HEPA) masks is indicated. The mask must be moulded to fit tightly around the nose and mouth.

The patient should be taught to cover the nose and mouth with paper tissue every time he or she coughs, sneezes, or produces sputum. The tissues should be thrown into a paper bag and disposed of with the trash, burned, or flushed down the toilet. The patient should also be taught careful handwashing techniques to be used after handling sputum and soiled tissues. Special precautions should be taken during high-risk procedures such as sputum induction, aerosolized pentamidine treatments, intubation, bronchoscopy, or endoscopy.

AMBULATORY AND HOME CARE. Patients who have responded clinically are discharged home despite positive smears if their household contacts have already been exposed and the patient is not posing a risk to susceptible people. Determination of absolute noninfectiousness requires negative cultures. Most treatment failures occur because the patient neglects to take the drug, discontinues it prematurely, or takes it irregularly. On discharge, the physician may order a combination of drugs to increase the likelihood of adherence, ensure that all drugs are taken, and reduce the risk of developing drug resistance.

It is important for the nurse to develop a therapeutic, consistent relationship with each patient. The nurse must understand the patient's lifestyle and be flexible in planning a program that facilitates the patient's participation in and completion of therapy. The nurse should teach the patient so that the patient fully understands the need for dedication to the prescribed regimen. Ongoing reassurance helps the patient understand that adherence can mean cure. If the patient cannot or will not adhere to a self-administered medication regimen, medication may have to be given by a responsible person on a daily or intermittent basis (see the "Ethical Dilemmas" box). The public health department must be notified if patient adherence to the drug regimen is questionable so that follow-up of close contacts can be accomplished. In some cases, the public health nurse will be responsible for DOT. In other situations, a spouse, grown child, other relative living with the patient, or co-worker may be asked to supervise drug taking.

Some patients may feel that there is a social stigma attached to TB. Many people still remember when TB patients were sent away to TB sanatoriums and isolated from society. These feelings should be discussed, and the patient should be reassured that an individual with TB can be cured if the prescribed regimen is followed. The Canadian Lung Association provides excellent literature for teaching about the disease as well as providing emotional support to the patient and family (Canadian Lung Association, 2015).

When the chemotherapy regimen has been completed, there is evidence of negative cultures, the patient is improving clinically, and there is radiological evidence of improvement, most

---

ETHICAL DILEMMAS

Patient Adherence

Situation

The health clinic for the homeless discovers that a man with tuberculosis has not been adhering to instructions for taking his medication. He tells the nurse that it is hard for him to get to the clinic to obtain the medication, much less to keep on a schedule. The nurse is concerned not only about this patient but also about the risks for the other people at the shelter, in the park, and at the meal sites.

Important Points for Consideration

- Adherence is a complex issue involving a person's culture and values, perceived risk for disease, availability of resources, access to treatment, and perceived consequences of available choices.
- Nurses in the community are concerned not only with providing benefits and supporting decision making for individual patients but also with the health and well-being of the entire community.
- Greater harm may result for the community when more virulent drug-resistant strains of microorganisms develop as a consequence of partial treatment or inability of the patient to complete a course of therapy.
- Advocacy for the patient and the community obliges the nurse to involve other members of the health care team, such as those in social services, to assist in obtaining the necessary resources or support to facilitate the patient's completion of the course of treatment.
- If the patient is unable to comply with the treatment program, even with necessary supports in place, concern for the public's health would take priority and necessitate placing him in a supervised living situation until his treatment is completed.

Clinical Decision-Making Questions

1. Under what circumstances are health care providers justified in overriding a patient's autonomy or decision making?
2. How would the nurse determine whether there were cultural beliefs interfering with this man's ability to understand the importance of completing the treatment? What would the nurse do about it?

---

individuals can be considered adequately treated. Follow-up care may be indicated during the subsequent 12 months, including bacteriological studies and chest radiographic examinations. Because approximately 5% of individuals experience relapses, the patient should be taught to recognize the symptoms that indicate recurrence of TB. If these symptoms occur, immediate medical attention should be sought.

The patient needs to be instructed about certain factors that could reactivate TB, such as immuno-suppressive therapy, malignancy, and prolonged debilitating illness. If the patient experiences any of these events, the health care provider must be told so that reactivation of TB can be closely monitored. In some situations, it may be necessary to put the patient on anti-TB therapy.

EVALUATION

The following are the expected outcomes for the patient with TB:

- Patient will have complete resolution of the disease.
- Patient will have normal pulmonary function.
- Patient will have absence of any complications.
- Patient will have no transmission of TB.

ATYPICAL MYCOBACTERIA

Pulmonary disease that closely resembles TB may be caused by atypical acid-fast mycobacteria. This type of pulmonary disease is indistinguishable from TB clinically and radiologically but can be differentiated by bacteriological culture. These organisms are not believed to be airborne and, thus, are not transmitted by droplet nuclei.

Atypical mycobacteria may also invade the cervical lymph nodes, causing lymphadenitis. This type of pulmonary disease typically occurs in White men with a history of COPD, cystic fibrosis, or silicosis. *Mycobacterium avium-intracellulare (MAI)* is a common cause of opportunistic infections in the patient with HIV infection (see Chapter 17).

Treatment depends on identification of the causative agent and determination of drug sensitivity. Many of the drugs used in treating TB are used in combating infections from atypical mycobacteria.

PULMONARY FUNGAL INFECTIONS

Pulmonary fungal infections are increasing in incidence. They appear most frequently in seriously ill patients being treated with corticosteroids, antineoplastic immuno-suppressive drugs, or multiple antibiotics. They are also more common in patients with AIDS or cystic fibrosis. Types of fungal infections are presented in Table 30-9. These infections are not transmitted from person to person, and the patient does not have to be placed in isolation. The clinical manifestations are similar to those of bacterial pneumonia. Skin and serology tests are available to assist in identifying the infecting organism. However, identification of the organism in a sputum specimen or in other body fluids is the best diagnostic indicator.

Collaborative Care

Amphotericin B (Fungizone) is the drug most widely used in treating serious systemic fungal infections. It must be given intravenously to achieve adequate blood and tissue levels because it is poorly absorbed from the GI tract. Amphotericin B is considered a toxic drug with many possible adverse effects, including hypersensitivity reactions, fever, chills, malaise, nausea and vomiting, thrombo-phlebitis at the injection site, and abnormal renal function. Many of the adverse effects during infusion can be avoided by premedicating with an anti-inflammatory or with diphenhydramine (Benadryl) 1 hour before the infusion. Monitoring renal function and ensuring adequate hydration are essential while a person is receiving this drug. Renal changes are at least partially reversible. Amphotericin infusions are incompatible with most other drugs. Amphotericin is frequently administered every other day after daily therapy for an initial period of several weeks. Total treatment with the drug may range from 4 to 12 weeks.

Oral antifungal drugs such as ketoconazole (Nizoral), fluconazole (Diflucan), and itraconazole (Sporanox) have also been successful in the treatment of fungal infections. Their effectiveness in treatment allows an alternative to the use of amphotericin B in many cases. Effectiveness of therapy can be monitored with fungal serology titres.

BRONCHIECTASIS

Etiology and Pathophysiology

Bronchiectasis is characterized by permanent, abnormal dilation of one or more large bronchi. The pathophysiological change that results in dilation is destruction of the elastic and muscular structures of the bronchial wall. There are two pathological types

TABLE 30-9	FUNGAL INFECTIONS OF THE LUNG
Organism	**Characteristics**
Histoplasmosis	
Histoplasma capsulatum	Indigenous to soil of the St. Lawrence River valleys; inhalation of mycelia into lungs; infected individual often free of symptoms; generally self-limiting, chronic disease similar to TB
Coccidioidomycosis	
Coccidioides immitis	Indigenous to semi-arid regions of southwestern United States (not normally found in Canada); inhalation of arthrospores into lungs; suppurative (pus-forming) and granulomatous reaction in lungs; symptomatic infection in one-third of individuals
Blastomycosis	
Blastomyces dermatitidis	Indigenous to southern Canada; inhalation of fungus into lungs; progression of disease often insidious; possible involvement of skin
Cryptococcosis	
Cryptococcus neoformans	True yeast; indigenous worldwide in soil and pigeon excreta; inhalation of fungus into lungs; possible meningitis
Aspergillosis	
Aspergillus niger or *A. fumigatus*	True mould inhabiting mouth; widely distributed; invasion of lung tissue resulting in possible necrotizing pneumonia; in individual with asthma, allergic bronchopulmonary aspergillosis may necessitate corticosteroid therapy
Candidiasis	
Candida albicans	Leading cause of mycotic infections in hospitalized and immuno-compromised hosts; ubiquitous and frequent colonization of upper respiratory and gastro-intestinal tracts; infections often following broad-spectrum antibiotic therapy (systemic or inhaled); possible development of localized pulmonary infiltrate to widespread bilateral consolidation with hypoxemia
Actinomycosis	
Actinomyces israelii	Not a true fungus; anaerobic; Gram-positive bacteria with branching hyphae; presence of necrotizing pneumonia after aspiration; pneumonitis; commonly in lower lobes with abscess or empyema formation
Nocardiosis	
Nocardia asteroides	Not a true fungus; aerobic; soil saprophyte widely distributed in nature; acquisition of infection from nature; rarely present in sputum without accompanying disease
Pneumocystis Pneumonia (PCP)	
Pneumocystis jiroveci	Rarely causes pneumonia in healthy individuals; fungus present in the environment; common opportunistic pneumonia in people with impaired immune systems, HIV infection, or both

HIV, human immunodeficiency virus; *TB*, tuberculosis.

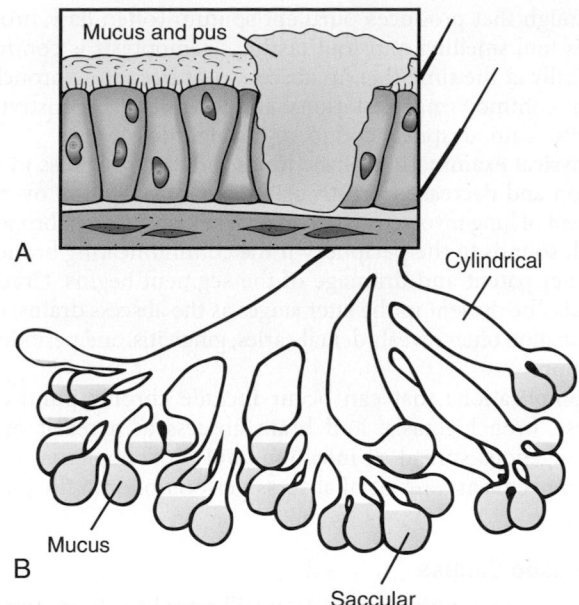

FIGURE 30-2 Pathological changes in bronchiectasis. **A,** Longitudinal section of bronchial wall where chronic infection has caused damage. **B,** Collection of purulent material in dilated bronchioles, leading to persistent infection.

of bronchiectasis: saccular and cylindrical (Figure 30-2). *Saccular bronchiectasis* occurs mainly in large bronchi and is characterized by cavity-like dilations. The affected bronchi end in large sacs. *Cylindrical bronchiectasis* involves medium-sized bronchi that are mildly to moderately dilated.

Almost all forms of bronchiectasis are associated with bacterial infections. A wide variety of infectious agents can initiate bronchiectasis, including adenovirus, influenza virus, *S. aureus, Klebsiella,* and anaerobes. Infections cause the bronchial walls to weaken, and pockets of infection begin to form. When the walls of the bronchial system are injured, the mucociliary mechanism is damaged, allowing bacteria and mucus to accumulate within the pockets. The infection becomes worse and results in bronchiectasis.

The incidence of bronchiectasis has shown a decline in recent years. The emergence of atypical mycobacteria, especially MAI, presents a new threat because MAI can progress to bronchiectasis. MAI is an opportunistic infection found in patients with HIV.

Clinical Manifestations

The hallmark of bronchiectasis is persistent or recurrent cough with production of greater than 20 mL of purulent sputum per day. The cough is paroxysmal and is often stimulated by position changes. Other manifestations include exertional dyspnea, fatigue, weight loss, anorexia, and fetid breath. On auscultation of the lungs, crackle and wheezing may be heard. Sinusitis frequently accompanies diffuse bronchiectasis. The manifestations of advanced, widespread bronchiectasis are generalized wheezing, digital clubbing, and cor pulmonale.

Diagnostic Studies

An individual with a chronic productive cough with copious purulent sputum (which may be blood streaked) should be suspected of having bronchiectasis. Chest radiographic studies are usually done and may show streaky infiltrates or may be normal. The availability of high-resolution CT scans of the chest, which have excellent sensitivity for detecting bronchiectasis, has

made diagnosis easier. Bronchoscopy can also be useful in identifying the source of secretions, in identifying sites of hemoptysis, or for collecting microbiological samples.

Sputum may provide additional information regarding the severity of impairment and the presence of active infection. Pulmonary function studies may be abnormal in advanced bronchiectasis, showing a decrease in vital capacity, expiratory flow, and maximum voluntary ventilation. Complete blood cell count may be normal or show evidence of leukocytosis or anemia from chronic infection.

Collaborative Care

Bronchiectasis is difficult to treat. Therapy is aimed at treating acute flare-ups and preventing decline in lung function. Antibiotics are the mainstay of treatment and are given on the basis of sputum culture results. Long-term suppressive therapy with antibiotics is occasionally used but is fraught with risks for antibiotic resistance. A form of treatment gaining popularity is the use of nebulized antibiotics. Studies indicate that they are safe and may reduce the number of flare-ups and hospitalizations in bronchiectatic patients (Rubin & Williams, 2014). Antipseudomonal antibiotics, such as tobramycin, are commonly used. Concurrent bronchodilator therapy is given to prevent bronchospasm. Other forms of drug therapy may include mucolytic agents and expectorants. Maintaining good hydration is important to liquefy secretions. Chest physiotherapy and other airway clearance techniques are important to facilitate expectoration of sputum. (These techniques are discussed in Chapter 31.) The individual should reduce exposure to excessive air pollutants and irritants, avoid cigarette smoking, and obtain pneumococcal and influenza vaccinations.

Surgical resection of parts of the lungs, although not used as often as in the past, may be done if more conservative treatment is not effective. Surgical resection of an affected lobe or segment may be indicated for the patient with repeated bouts of pneumonia, hemoptysis, and disabling complications. Surgery is not advisable when there is diffuse or widespread involvement. For select patients who are disabled in spite of maximal therapy, lung transplantation is an option. (Lung transplantation is discussed later in this chapter.)

NURSING MANAGEMENT BRONCHIECTASIS

The early detection and treatment of lower respiratory tract infections will help prevent complications such as bronchiectasis. Any obstructing lesion or foreign body should be removed promptly. Other measures to decrease the occurrence or progression of bronchiectasis include avoiding cigarette smoking and decreasing exposure to pollution and irritants.

An important nursing goal is to promote drainage and removal of bronchial mucus. Various airway clearance techniques can be effectively used to facilitate secretion removal. The patient should be taught effective deep-breathing exercises and effective ways to cough (see Chapter 31, Table 31-18). Chest physiotherapy with postural drainage should be done on affected parts of the lung (see Chapter 31, Figure 31-17). Some individuals require elevation of the foot of the bed by 10 to 15 cm to facilitate drainage. Pillows may be used in the hospital and at home to help the patient assume postural drainage positions. A Flutter mucus clearance device is a hand-held device that provides airway vibration during the respiratory phase of breathing (see Chapter 31, Figure 31-18). Two to four 15-minute sessions daily by a patient who has been properly trained can provide satisfactory mucus clearance. Positive expiratory pressure therapy is a breathing manoeuvre against an expiratory resistance often used in conjunction with nebulized medications. (Respiratory therapy procedures are explained in Chapter 31.)

Administration of the prescribed antibiotics, bronchodilators, or expectorants is important. The patient needs to understand the importance of taking the prescribed regimen of drugs to obtain maximum effectiveness. The patient should be aware of possible adverse effects and of adverse effects that must be reported to the physician.

Health teaching must include information regarding the importance of getting adequate rest, avoiding overexertion, consuming adequate nutrients, ensuring hydration, and performing oral care. Unless there are contraindications such as concomitant heart failure or renal disease, the patient should be instructed to drink at least 3 L of fluid daily. Generally, the patient should be counselled to use low-sodium fluids to avoid systemic fluid retention.

Direct hydration of the respiratory system may also prove beneficial in the expectoration of secretions. Usually, a bland aerosol with normal saline solution delivered by a jet-type nebulizer is used. The patient with bronchiectasis should avoid ultrasonic nebulizers because they often induce bronchospasm. At home, a steamy shower can prove effective; expensive equipment that requires frequent cleaning is usually unnecessary. It is important that the patient medicate with an inhaled bronchodilator 10 to 15 minutes before using a bland aerosol to prevent bronchoconstriction.

The patient and caregivers should be taught to recognize significant clinical manifestations to be reported to the health care provider. These manifestations include increased sputum production, grossly bloody sputum, increasing dyspnea, fever, chills, and chest pain.

LUNG ABSCESS

Etiology and Pathophysiology

A lung abscess is a pus-containing lesion of the lung parenchyma that gives rise to a cavity. The cavity is formed by necrosis of the lung tissue. In many cases, the causes and pathogenesis of lung abscesses are similar to those of pneumonia. Most lung abscesses are caused by aspiration of material from the oral cavity (the gingival crevices) into the lungs. In general, infectious agents including enteric Gram-negative organisms (e.g., *Klebsiella*), *S. aureus*, and anaerobic bacilli (e.g., *Bacteroides*) are responsible for lung abscesses and the associated infection and necrosis of the lung tissue. A lung abscess can also result from a lung infarct secondary to pulmonary embolus, malignant growth, TB, and various parasitic and fungal diseases of the lung.

The areas of the lung most commonly affected are the superior segments of the lower lobes and the posterior segments of the upper lobes. Fibrous tissue usually forms around the abscess in an attempt to wall it off. The abscess may erode into the bronchial system, causing the production of foul-smelling sputum. It may grow toward the pleura and cause pleuritic pain. Multiple small abscesses can occur within the lung.

Clinical Manifestations and Complications

The onset of a lung abscess is usually insidious, especially if anaerobic organisms are the primary cause. A more acute onset occurs with aerobic organisms. The most common manifestation

is a cough that produces purulent sputum (often dark brown) that is foul smelling and foul tasting. Hemoptysis is common, especially at the time that an abscess ruptures into a bronchus. Other common manifestations are fever, chills, prostration, pleuritic pain, dyspnea, cough, and weight loss.

Physical examination of the lungs indicates dullness to percussion and decreased breath sounds on auscultation over the segment of lung involved. There may be transmission of bronchial breath sounds to the periphery if the communicating bronchus becomes patent and drainage of the segment begins. Crackles may also be present in the later stages as the abscess drains. Oral examination often reveals dental caries, gingivitis, and periodontal infection.

Complications that can occur include chronic pulmonary abscess, bronchiectasis, and brain abscess as a result of the hematogenous spread of infection, and bronchopleural fistula and empyema as a result of abscess perforation into the pleural cavity.

Diagnostic Studies

A chest radiographic examination will reveal a solitary cavitary lesion with fluid. CT scanning is used if there is suspicion of cavitation not clearly seen. A lung abscess, in contrast to other types of abscesses, does not require assisted drainage, as long as there is drainage via the bronchus. Routine sputum cultures can be collected, but contaminants can confuse the results and it is difficult to isolate anaerobic bacteria. Pleural fluid and blood cultures may be obtained. Bronchoscopy may be used in cases of abscess in which drainage is delayed or in which there are factors that suggest an underlying malignancy.

NURSING AND COLLABORATIVE MANAGEMENT LUNG ABSCESS

Antibiotics given for a prolonged period (up to 2 to 4 months) are usually the primary method of treatment. Penicillin has historically been the drug of choice because of the frequent presence of anaerobic organisms. However, recent studies suggest that the anaerobic bacteria involved in abscesses of the lung produce β-lactamase, which is resistant to penicillin. Clindamycin has been shown to be superior to penicillin and is the standard treatment for an anaerobic lung infection. Patients with putrid lung abscesses usually show clinical improvement with decreased fever within 3 to 4 days of beginning antibiotics.

Because of the need for prolonged antibiotic therapy, the patient must be aware of the importance of continuing the medication for the prescribed period. As well, the patient needs to know about adverse effects to be reported to the health care provider. Sometimes, the patient is asked to return periodically during the course of antibiotic therapy for repeat cultures and sensitivity tests to ensure that the infecting organism is not becoming resistant to the antibiotic. When antibiotic therapy is completed, the patient is re-evaluated.

The patient should be taught how to cough effectively (see Chapter 31, Table 31-18). Chest physiotherapy and postural drainage are sometimes used to drain abscesses located in the lower or posterior portions of the lung. Postural drainage according to the lung area involved will aid the removal of secretions (see Chapter 31, Figure 31-17). Frequent (every 2 to 3 hours) mouth care is needed to relieve the foul-smelling odour and taste from the sputum. Diluted hydrogen peroxide and mouthwash are often effective.

Rest, good nutrition, and adequate fluid intake are all supportive measures to facilitate recovery. If dentition is poor and dental hygiene is not adequate, the patient should be encouraged to obtain dental care.

Surgery is rarely indicated but occasionally may be necessary when reinfection of a large cavitary lesion occurs or to establish a diagnosis when there is evidence of an underlying neoplasm or chronic associated disease. The usual procedure in such cases is a lobectomy or pneumonectomy. An alternative to surgery is percutaneous drainage, but this has a high risk for contamination of the pleural space.

ENVIRONMENTAL LUNG DISEASES

Environmental or occupational lung diseases result from inhaled dust or chemicals. The duration of exposure and the amount of inhalant have a major influence on whether the exposed individual will have lung damage, as does the susceptibility of the host.

Pneumoconiosis is a general term for lung diseases caused by the inhalation and retention of dust particles. The literal meaning of *pneumoconiosis* is "dust in the lungs." Examples of this condition are silicosis, asbestosis, berylliosis, and hantavirus, a potentially fatal disease transmitted by inhalation of aerosolized rodent excreta particles, which has had outbreaks reported in Canada and the United States. The classical response to the inhaled substance is diffuse parenchymal infiltration with phagocytic cells. This eventually results in diffuse pulmonary fibrosis (excess connective tissue). Fibrosis is the result of tissue repair after inflammation. Pneumoconiosis and other environmental lung diseases are presented in Table 30-10.

Chemical pneumonitis results from exposure to toxic chemical fumes. Acutely, there is diffuse lung injury characterized as pulmonary edema. Chronically, the clinical picture is that of bronchiolitis obliterans, which is usually associated with a normal chest radiograph or one that shows hyperinflation. An example is silo filler's disease. *Hypersensitivity pneumonitis* or extrinsic allergic alveolitis is the response seen when antigens to which an individual is allergic are inhaled. Examples include bird fancier's lung and farmer's lung.

Although many occupational respiratory diseases have declined, occupational asthma is the most common occupational lung disease (Canadian Centre for Occupational Health and Safety, 2013). *Occupational asthma* refers to the development of symptoms of shortness of breath, wheezing, cough, and chest tightness as a result of exposure to dust or fumes that trigger an allergic response. The obstruction may initially be reversible or intermittent, but continued exposure results in permanent obstructive changes. The best-known causative agent in occupational asthma is toluene di-isocyanate (TDI), which is used in the production of rigid polyurethane foam.

Lung cancer, either squamous cell carcinoma or adenocarcinoma, is the most frequent cancer associated with asbestos exposure. People who have experienced more exposure are at a greater risk for disease. There is a minimum lapse of 15 to 19 years between first exposure and development of lung cancer. Mesotheliomas, both pleural and peritoneal, are also associated with asbestos exposure.

Clinical Manifestations

Acute symptoms of pulmonary edema may be seen following early exposure to chemical fumes. However, symptoms of many environmental lung diseases may not occur until at least 10 to 15 years after the initial exposure to the inhaled irritant. Dyspnea and cough are often the earliest manifestations. Chest pain and cough with sputum production usually occur later. Complications that often result are pneumonia, chronic bronchitis, emphysema, and lung cancer. Manifestations of these complications can be the reason the patient seeks health care. Cor pulmonale is a late complication, especially in conditions characterized by diffuse pulmonary fibrosis.

Pulmonary function studies often show reduced vital capacity. A chest radiograph will often reveal lung involvement specific to the primary problem. CT scans have been shown to be useful in detecting early lung involvement.

Collaborative Care

The best approach to management is to try to prevent or decrease environmental and occupational risks. Well-designed, effective ventilation systems can reduce exposure to irritants. Wearing a mask is appropriate in some occupations. Periodic inspections and monitoring of workplaces by agencies such as the Canadian Centre for Occupational Health and Safety (CCOHS) reinforce the obligations of employers to provide a safe work environment (CCOHS, 2013). In addition, the Canada Labour Code requires that an occupational health and safety committee be established in all workplaces with 20 or more regular employees (Human Resources and Skills Development Canada, 2012).

Cigarette smoking adds increased insult to the lungs, so the person at risk for occupational lung disease should not smoke. In addition, second-hand smoke is an important source of exposure that increases risk for development of lung cancer. This risk has led to regulations requiring a smoke-free workspace for all employees.

Early diagnosis is essential if the disease process is to be halted. Places of employment in which there is a known risk for lung disease may require periodic chest radiographic examinations and pulmonary function studies for exposed employees. This measure can detect pulmonary changes before symptoms develop.

There is no specific treatment for most environmental lung diseases. The best treatment is to decrease or stop exposure to the harmful agent. Strategies are directed toward providing symptomatic relief. If there are coexisting problems, such as pneumonia, chronic bronchitis, emphysema, or asthma, they are treated.

LUNG CANCER

Lung cancer, the most preventable cancer, is the leading cause of cancer-related deaths in men and women in Canada. In 2012, lung cancer accounted for 1.59 million deaths worldwide, making it the most deadly of all cancers (WHO, 2017). It was estimated that in 2017 there would be 28 600 new cases of lung cancer in Canada and 20 100 deaths (Canadian Cancer Society's Advisory Committee on Cancer Statistics, 2017).

Lung cancer most commonly occurs in people who have a long history of cigarette smoking and who are 40 to 75 years of age, with peak incidence between 55 and 65.

Etiology

Cigarette smoking is the most important risk factor in the development of lung cancer. Smoking is responsible for approximately 85% of all lung cancers in Canada (Canadian Cancer Society, 2017a). Tobacco smoke contains 60 carcinogens

TABLE 30-10 ENVIRONMENTAL LUNG DISEASES

Agents and Industries	Description	Complications
Asbestosis		
Asbestos fibres present in insulation, construction material (roof tiling, cement products), shipyards, textiles (for fireproofing), automobile clutch and brake linings	Disease appears 15–35 yrs after first exposure. Interstitial fibrosis develops. Pleural plaques, which are calcified lesions, develop on pleura. Dyspnea, basal crackles, and decreased vital capacity are early manifestations.	Diffuse interstitial pulmonary fibrosis; lung cancer, especially in cigarette smokers; mesothelioma (rare type of cancer affecting pleura and peritoneal membrane)
Berylliosis		
Beryllium dust present in aircraft manufacturing, metallurgy, rocket fuels	Formation of noncaseating granulomas is seen. Acute pneumonitis occurs after heavy exposure. Interstitial fibrosis can also occur.	Progress of disease possible even after removal of stimulating inhalant
Bird Fancier's, Breeder's, or Handler's Lung		
Bird droppings or feathers	Hypersensitivity pneumonitis is present.	Progressive fibrosis of lung
Byssinosis		
Cotton, flax, and hemp dust (textile industry)	Airway obstruction is caused by contraction of smooth muscles. Chronic disease results from severe airway obstruction and decreased elastic recoil.	Progression of chronic disease after cessation of dust exposure
Coal Worker's Pneumoconiosis (Black Lung)		
Coal dust	Incidence is high (20%–30%) in coal workers. Deposits of carbon dust cause lesions to develop along respiratory bronchioles. Bronchioles dilate because of loss of wall structure. Chronic airway obstruction and bronchitis develop. Dyspnea and cough are common early symptoms.	Progressive, massive lung fibrosis; increased risk for chronic bronchitis and emphysema in smokers
Farmer's Lung		
Inhalation of airborne material from mouldy hay or similar matter	Hypersensitivity pneumonitis occurs. Acute form is similar to pneumonia, with manifestations of chills, fever, and malaise. Chronic, insidious form is type of pulmonary fibrosis.	Progressive fibrosis of lung
Hantavirus Pulmonary Syndrome (HPS)		
Rodent droppings inhaled while in rodent-infested areas	Acute hemorrhagic fever associated with severe pulmonary and cardiovascular collapse and death. Incubation period is 1–4 wks with prodrome (3–5 days) of flulike symptoms. No cure or specific treatment exists.	Intensive care unit with careful monitoring of fluid and electrolyte balance and blood pressure; supportive therapy and early intervention vital; research on this virus is done in high-level biocontainment facilities
Siderosis		
Iron oxide present in welding materials, foundries, iron ore mining	Dust deposits are found in lung.	—
Silicosis		
Silica dust present in quartz rock in mining of gold, copper, tin, coal, lead; also present in sandblasting, foundries, quarries, pottery making, masonry	In chronic disease, dust is engulfed by macrophages and may be destroyed, resulting in fibrotic nodules. Acute disease results from intense exposure in short period. Within 5 yrs, it progresses to severe disability from lung fibrosis.	Increased susceptibility to tuberculosis; progressive, massive fibrosis; high incidence of chronic bronchitis
Silo Filler's Disease		
Nitrogen oxides from fermentation of vegetation in freshly filled silo	Chemical pneumonitis occurs.	Progressive bronchiolitis obliterans

in addition to substances (e.g., carbon monoxide, nicotine) that interfere with normal cell development. Cigarette smoking, a lower airway irritant, causes a change in the bronchial epithelium, which usually returns to normal when smoking is discontinued. The risk for lung cancer is gradually lowered when smoking ceases, and it continues to decline with time. After 10 years following cessation of smoking, the risk for lung cancer is cut in half (Canadian Lung Association, 2016a). In 2013, 11% of Canadian youth between the ages of 15 and 19 were smokers. This number has been gradually decreasing (Canadian Tobacco, Alcohol and Drugs Survey [CTADS], 2013).

The risk of developing lung cancer is directly related to total exposure to cigarette smoke measured by total number of cigarettes smoked in a lifetime; age of smoking onset; depth of inhalation; tar and nicotine content; and the use of unfiltered cigarettes. Sidestream smoke (smoke from burning cigarettes and cigars) contains the same carcinogens found in mainstream smoke (smoke inhaled by smoker). This environmental tobacco smoke (ETS) inhaled by nonsmokers poses a 35% increased risk for the development of lung cancer in nonsmokers (Registered Nurses' Association of Ontario [RNAO], 2007). In 2013, 3.9% of Canadian children between the ages of 0 and 17 years were exposed to second-hand smoke at home every day or almost every day (CTADS, 2013). Children are more vulnerable to ETS than adults because their respiratory and immune systems are not fully developed.

Compared with nonsmokers, those who smoke pipes and cigars have also been shown to have an increased risk of developing lung cancer. Cigar smokers are at higher risk for lung cancer than pipe smokers. In fact, rates of lung cancer caused by heavy smoking of cigars and inhalation of smoke from small cigars have been shown to correlate with the rates of lung cancer caused by cigarette smoking.

Another major risk factor for lung cancer is inhaled carcinogens. These include asbestos, radon, nickel, iron and iron oxides, uranium, polycyclic aromatic hydrocarbons, chromates, arsenic, and air pollution. Exposure to these substances is common for employees of industries such as mining, smelting, or chemical or petroleum manufacturing. The cigarette smoker who is also exposed to one or more of these chemicals or to high amounts of air pollution is at significantly higher risk for lung cancer.

There are marked variations in a person's propensity to develop lung cancer. To date, no genetic abnormality has conclusively been defined for lung cancer. It is known that the carcinogens in cigarette smoke directly damage deoxyribonucleic acid (DNA). One theory is that people have different genetic carcinogen-metabolizing pathways.

Pathophysiology

The pathogenesis of primary lung cancer is not well understood. More than 90% of cancers originate from the epithelium of the bronchus (bronchogenic). They grow slowly, and it takes 8 to 10 years for a tumour to reach 1 cm in size, which is the smallest detectable lesion on a radiographic study. Lung cancers occur primarily in the segmental bronchi or beyond and have a preference for the upper lobes of the lungs (Figures 30-3 and 30-4). Pathological changes in the bronchial system show nonspecific inflammatory changes with hypersecretion of mucus, desquamation of cells, reactive hyperplasia of the basal cells, and metaplasia of normal respiratory epithelium into stratified squamous cells.

Primary lung cancers are often categorized into two broad subtypes (Table 30-11): non–small cell lung cancer (NSCLC; 85% to 90%) and small cell lung cancer (SCLC; 10% to 15%) (Canadian Cancer Society, 2017b). Lung cancers metastasize primarily by direct extension and via the blood circulation and the lymph system. The common sites for metastatic growth are liver, brain, bones, scalene lymph nodes, and adrenal glands.

Paraneoplastic Syndrome. Certain lung cancers cause *paraneoplastic syndrome*, which is characterized by various systemic manifestations caused by factors (e.g., hormones, enzymes, antigens) produced by the tumour cells. SCLCs are most commonly associated with paraneoplastic syndrome. The systemic manifestations seen are hormonal, dermatological, neuro-muscular, vascular, hematological, and connective tissue syndromes. Examples of paraneoplastic syndromes include hypercalcemia, syndrome of inappropriate antidiuretic hormone (SIADH) secretion, anemia, leukocytosis, hypercoagulable disorders, and neurological syndromes. These syndromes can respond temporarily to symptomatic treatment, but they are impossible to control without successful treatment of the underlying lung cancer.

Clinical Manifestations

Lung cancer is clinically silent for most individuals for the majority of its course. The clinical manifestations of lung cancer are usually

FIGURE 30-3 Lung cancer. Peripheral adenocarcinoma. The tumour shows prominent black pigmentation, suggestive of having evolved in an anthracotic scar. Source: Damjanov, I., & Linder, J. (1996). *Anderson's pathology* (10th ed.). St. Louis: Mosby.

FIGURE 30-4 Lung carcinoma. The grey-white tumour tissue is infiltrating the lung. Histologically, this tumour is identified as a squamous cell carcinoma. Source: Kumar, V., Abbas, A. K., Aster, J. C., et al. (2010). *Robbins and Cotran pathologic basis of disease* (8th ed.). Philadelphia: Saunders.

nonspecific and appear late in the disease process. Manifestations depend on the type of primary lung cancer, its location, and metastatic spread. Often, there is extensive metastasis before symptoms become apparent. Persistent pneumonitis that is a result of obstructed bronchi may be one of the earliest manifestations, causing fever, chills, and cough.

One of the most significant symptoms, and often the one reported first, is a persistent cough that may produce sputum. Sputum may be blood-tinged because of bleeding caused by malignancy, but hemoptysis is not a common early symptom. Chest pain may be present and localized or unilateral, ranging from mild to severe. Dyspnea and an auscultatory wheeze may be present if there is bronchial obstruction.

Later manifestations may include nonspecific systemic symptoms such as anorexia, fatigue, weight loss, and nausea and vomiting. Hoarseness may be present as a result of involvement of the recurrent laryngeal nerve. Unilateral paralysis of the

TABLE 30-11   COMPARISON OF THE TYPES OF PRIMARY LUNG CANCER

Cell Type	Risk Factors	Characteristics	Response to Therapy
Non–Small Cell Lung Cancer (NSCLC)			
Squamous cell (epidermoid) carcinoma	Almost always associated with cigarette smoking; is associated with exposure to environmental carcinogens (e.g., uranium, asbestos)	Accounts for 30% of lung cancers; is more common in men; arises from the bronchial epithelium; produces earlier symptoms because of bronchial obstructive characteristics; does not have a strong tendency to metastasize; metastasizes locally by direct extension; causes cavitating pulmonary lesions	Surgical resection is often attempted; life expectancy is better than for small cell lung cancer.
Adenocarcinoma	Has been associated with lung scarring and chronic interstitial fibrosis; is not related to cigarette smoking	Accounts for approximately 40% of lung cancers; is more common in women; often has no clinical manifestations until widespread metastasis is present; metastasizes via bloodstream; is most commonly located in peripheral portions of lungs*	Surgical resection is often attempted; cancer does not respond well to chemotherapy.
Large cell undifferentiated carcinoma	High correlation with cigarette smoking and exposure to environmental carcinogens	Accounts for 10% of lung cancers; commonly causes cavitation; is highly metastatic via lymphatics and blood; commonly peripheral rather than central	Surgery is not usually attempted because of high rate of metastases; tumour may be radiosensitive but often recurs.
Small Cell Lung Cancer (SCLC)			
Small cell anaplastic undifferentiated (includes oat cell)	Associated with cigarette smoking, exposure to environmental carcinogens	Accounts for 20%–25% of lung cancers; is most malignant form; tends to spread early via lymphatics and bloodstream; is frequently associated with endocrine disturbances; predominantly central and can cause bronchial obstruction and pneumonia	This cancer has the poorest prognosis; however, chemotherapy advances have been substantial; radiation is used as adjuvant therapy as well as palliative measure. Average median survival is 12–18 months.

*See Figure 30-3.

diaphragm, dysphagia, and superior vena cava obstruction may occur because of intrathoracic spread of the malignancy. There may be palpable lymph nodes in the neck or the axilla. Mediastinal involvement may lead to pericardial effusion, cardiac tamponade, and dysrhythmias.

Diagnostic Studies

Chest radiographic studies are widely used in the diagnosis of lung cancer. The findings may show the presence of the tumour or abnormalities related to the obstructive features of the tumour such as atelectasis and pneumonitis. The radiograph can also show evidence of metastasis to the ribs or vertebrae and the presence of pleural effusion.

CT scanning is the single most effective noninvasive technique for evaluating lung cancer. CT scans of the brain and bone scans complete the evaluation for metastatic disease. With CT scans, the location and extent of masses in the chest can be identified, as well as any mediastinal involvement or lymph node enlargement. Magnetic resonance imaging (MRI) may be used in combination with or instead of CT scans. Positron emission tomography (PET) can be a useful diagnostic tool in early clinical staging. PET allows measurement of differential metabolic activity in normal and diseased tissues.

A definitive diagnosis of lung cancer is made by identifying malignant cells. Sputum specimens are usually obtained for cytological studies. An early-morning specimen that has been obtained by having the patient cough deeply provides the most accurate results. However, malignant cells may not be obtained even in the presence of a lung cancer.

The use of the fibre-optic bronchoscope is important in the diagnosis of lung cancer, particularly when the lesions are endobronchial or close to an airway. It provides direct visualization and allows biopsy specimens to be obtained. A biopsy is usually the best method for establishing the presence of a malignant tumour.

Mediastinoscopy—the insertion of a scope via a small anterior chest incision into the mediastinum—is done to examine for metastasis in the anterior mediastinum or in the hilum or in the chest extrapleurally. It is also used to determine the stage of the lung cancer, an important step toward preparing a treatment plan. Video-assisted thoracoscopy (VAT), which involves the insertion of a scope into a small thoracic incision, may be used to explore areas inaccessible by mediastinoscopy.

Pulmonary angiography and lung scans may be performed to assess overall pulmonary status. Fine-needle aspiration (FNA) may be used to obtain a tissue sample to determine tumour histology. FNA is most useful in cases involving a peripheral lesion near the chest wall, and it is usually attempted in an effort to avoid a thoracotomy. If a thoracentesis is performed to relieve a pleural effusion, the fluid should be analyzed for malignant cells. (Table 30-12 summarizes the diagnostic management of lung cancer.)

Staging. Staging of NSCLC is performed according to the tumour–node–metastasis (TNM) staging system in a manner similar to that for other tumours (Tables 30-13 and 30-14). Assessment criteria are *T*, which denotes tumour size, location, and degree of invasion; *N*, which indicates regional lymph node involvement; and *M*, which represents the presence or absence of distant metastases. Depending on the TNM designation, the tumour is then staged, which assists in estimating prognosis and determining the appropriate therapy.

Staging of SCLC has not been useful because the cancer has usually metastasized by the time a diagnosis is made. Instead, SCLC is determined to be *limited* (confined to one hemothorax and to regional lymph nodes) or *extensive* (any disease exceeding those boundaries).

TABLE 30-12 COLLABORATIVE CARE

Lung Cancer

Diagnostic	Collaborative Therapy
• History and physical examination	• Surgery
• Chest radiographic examination	• Radiation therapy
• Sputum for cytological study	• Chemotherapy
• Bronchoscopy	• Biological therapy
• CT scan	• Bronchoscopic laser therapy
• MRI	• Phototherapy
• PET	• Airway stenting
• Spirometry (preoperative)	• Cryotherapy
• Mediastinoscopy	• Respiratory therapy
• VAT	• Nutritional therapy
• Pulmonary angiography	
• Lung scan	
• Fine-needle aspiration	

CT, computed tomography; *MRI*, magnetic resonance imaging; *PET*, positron emission tomography; *VAT*, video-assisted thoracoscopy.

Screening for Lung Cancer. In 2016, new guidelines were published recommending the screening of asymptomatic adults aged 55 to 74 with at least a 30 pack-year smoking history (who currently smoke or quit smoking less than 15 years ago). Screening is done using a low-dose CT scan every year for 3 consecutive years (Canadian Task Force on Preventive Health Care, 2016).

Collaborative Care

Cancer Care Ontario has published evidence-informed clinical guidelines for treating lung cancer. The guidelines can be accessed at its website in the Cancer Care Ontario Toolbox, under Evidence-Based Guidelines. (See the Resources at the end of the chapter.)

Surgical Therapy. Surgical resection is considered the treatment of choice in NSCLC Stages I and II because the disease is potentially curable with resection. For other NSCLC stages, surgery may be indicated in conjunction with radiation therapy, chemotherapy, or both. In limited-stage SCLC, which is rare, surgical resection, chemotherapy, and radiation therapy may be recommended.

TABLE 30-13 LUNG CANCER TUMOUR–NODE–METASTASIS CLASSIFICATIONS

T		Primary Tumour
TX		Primary tumour cannot be assessed, or tumour proven by the presence of malignant cells in sputum or bronchial washings but not visualized by imaging or bronchoscopy.
T0		No evidence of primary tumour.
Tis		Carcinoma in situ.
T1		Tumour 3 cm or less in greatest dimension, surrounded by lung or visceral pleura, without bronchoscopic evidence of invasion, more proximal than the lobar bronchus (i.e., not in the main bronchus); the uncommon superficial spreading tumour of any size with its invasive component limited to the bronchial wall, which may extend proximal to the main bronchus, is also classified as T1a.
	T1mi	Minimally invasive adenocarcinoma
	T1a	Tumour 1 cm or less in greatest dimension
	T1b	Tumour more than 1 cm but not more than 2 cm in greatest dimension
	T1c	Tumour more than 2 cm but not more than 3 cm in greatest dimension
T2		Tumour more than 3 cm but not more than 5 cm; or tumour with any of the following features (T2 tumours with these features are classified T2a if 4 cm or less or if size cannot be determined and as T2b if greater than 4 cm but not larger than 5 cm): • Involves main bronchus, regardless of distance to the carina, but without involving the carina • Invades visceral pleura • Associated with atelectasis or obstructive pneumonitis that extends to the hilar region, involving either part of the lung or the entire lung
	T2a	Tumour more than 3 cm but not more than 4 cm in greatest dimension
	T2b	Tumour more than 4 cm but not more than 5 cm in greatest dimension
T3		Tumour more than 5 cm but not more than 7 cm in greatest dimension or one that directly invades any of the following: parietal pleura (PL3), chest wall (including superior sulcus tumours), phrenic nerve, parietal pericardium; or associated separate tumour nodule(s) in the same lobe as the primary.
T4		Tumours more than 7 cm or one that invades any of the following: diaphragm, mediastinum, heart, great vessels, trachea, recurrent laryngeal nerve, esophagus, vertebral body, carina; separate tumour nodule(s) in a different ipsilateral lobe to that of the primary.
N		**Regional Lymph Nodes**
NX		Regional lymph nodes cannot be assessed.
N0		No regional lymph node metastasis.
N1		Metastasis in ipsilateral peribronchial and/or ipsilateral hilar lymph nodes and intrapulmonary nodes, including involvement by direct extension.
N2		Metastasis in ipsilateral mediastinal and/or subcarinal lymph node(s).
N3		Metastasis in contralateral mediastinal, contralateral hilar, ipsilateral or contralateral scalene, or supraclavicular lymph node(s).
M		**Distant Metastasis**
M0		No distant metastasis.
M1		Distant metastasis.
	M1a	Separate tumour nodule(s) in a contralateral lobe; tumour with pleural nodules or malignant pleural or pericardial effusion; most pleural (pericardial) effusions with lung cancer are due to tumour; in a few patients, however, multiple microscopic examinations of pleural (pericardial) fluid are negative for tumour, and the fluid is nonbloody and is not an exudate; where these elements and clinical judgement dictate that the effusion is not related to the tumour, the effusion should be excluded as a staging descriptor.
	M1b	Single extrathoracic metastasis in a single organ and involvement of a single distant (nonregional) node.
	M1c	Multiple extrathoracic metastases in one or several organs.

Used with the permission of the American College of Surgeons. The original source for this material is the *AJCC Cancer Staging Manual*, Eighth Edition (2017) published by Springer Science and Business Media LLC, www.springer.com.

TABLE 30-14	LUNG CANCER STAGING		
	Grouping		
Stage	**Tumour**	**Node**	**Metastasis**
Occult carcinoma	TX	N0	M0
Stage 0	Tis	N0	M0
Stage IA1	T1a	N0	M0
Stage 1A2	T1b	N0	M0
Stage 1A3	T1c	N0	M0
Stage IB	T2a	N0	M0
Stage IIA	T2b	N0	M0
Stage IIB	T1a–T2b	N1	M0
	T3	N0	M0
Stage IIIA	T1a–T2b	N2	M0
	T3	N1	M0
	T4	N0/N1	M0
Stage IIIB	T1a–T2b	N3	M0
	T3/T4	N2	M0
Stage IIIC	T3/T4	N3	M0
Stage IVA	Any T	Any N	M1a/M1b
Stage IVB	Any T	Any N	M1c

Used with the permission of the American College of Surgeons. The original source for this material is the *AJCC Cancer Staging Manual*, Eighth Edition (2017) published by Springer Science and Business Media LLC, www.springer.com.

When the tumour is considered operable with a potential for cure, the patient's cardiopulmonary status must be evaluated to determine the ability to withstand surgery. This is done by clinical studies of pulmonary function, ABGs, and others, as indicated by the individual's status. Contraindications for thoracotomy include hypercapnia, pulmonary hypertension, cor pulmonale, and markedly reduced lung function. Coexisting conditions such as cardiac, renal, and liver disease may also be contraindications for surgery.

A tumour may be considered inoperable. If operable, the type of surgery performed is usually a lobectomy (removal of one or more lobes of the lung) and, less often, a *pneumonectomy* (removal of one entire lung).

Radiation Therapy. Radiation therapy is used as a curative approach in the individual who has a resectable tumour but who is considered a poor surgical risk. There has been improved survival when radiation therapy is used in combination with surgery and chemotherapy. Adenocarcinomas are the most radioresistant type of cancer cell. Although SCLCs are radiosensitive, radiation (even when used in combination with chemotherapy) does not significantly improve the mortality rate because of the early metastases of this type of cancer.

Radiation therapy is also done as a palliative procedure to reduce distressing symptoms such as cough, hemoptysis, bronchial obstruction, and superior vena cava syndrome. It can be used to treat pain that is caused by metastatic bone lesions or cerebral metastasis. Radiation used as a preoperative or postoperative adjuvant measure has not been found to significantly increase survival in the patient with lung cancer.

Stereotactic Radiotherapy. Stereotactic radiotherapy (SRT), also called *stereotactic surgery* or *radiosurgery,* is a new lung cancer treatment. It is a type of radiation therapy that uses high doses of radiation delivered very accurately to the tumour. SRT provides an option to older-adult patients, patients with severe lung or heart disease, and other patients in poor health who are not good candidates for surgery. SRT is an outpatient procedure that uses special positioning procedures and radiology techniques so that a higher dose of radiation can be delivered to the tumour and a smaller part of the healthy lung is exposed.

Chemotherapy. Chemotherapy may be used in the treatment of nonresectable tumours or as adjuvant therapy to surgery in NSCLC with distant metastases. A variety of chemotherapy drugs and multidrug regimens (i.e., protocols) including combination chemotherapy have been used. These drugs include etoposide (VePesid), carboplatin, cisplatin, paclitaxel, vinorelbine, cyclophosphamide (Procytox), ifosfamide (Ifex), docetaxel (Taxotere), gemcitabine, topotecan (Hycamtin), and irinotecan (Camptosar). Chemotherapy has improved survival in patients with advanced NSCLC and is now considered standard treatment.

Biological Therapy. Biological (targeted) therapy as adjuvant therapy has been used in individuals with cancer, including malignant lung tumours. (Biological therapy is discussed in Chapter 18.)

Other Therapies

Prophylactic Cranial Radiation. Brain metastasis is a common complication of SCLC. Most chemotherapy drugs do not adequately penetrate the blood–brain barrier. Prophylactic cranial radiation may be used as a potential way to improve the prognosis of patients, especially those who have a complete response to chemotherapy. Toxicity of this therapy may include scalp erythema, fatigue, and alopecia.

Bronchoscopic Laser Therapy. Bronchoscopic laser therapy makes it possible to remove obstructing bronchial lesions. The thermal energy of the laser is transmitted to the target tissue. It is a complicated procedure that often requires general anaesthesia to control the patient's cough reflex. Relief of the symptoms from airway obstruction as a result of thermal necrosis and shrinkage of the tumour can be dramatic. However, it is not a curative therapy for cancer.

Phototherapy. Photodynamic therapy is a safe, nonsurgical therapy for lung cancer. Porfimer (Photofrin) is injected intravenously and selectively concentrates in tumour cells. After a set time (usually 48 hours), the tumour is exposed to laser light, producing a toxic form of oxygen that destroys tumour cells. Necrotic tissue is removed through a bronchoscope.

Airway Stenting. Stents can be used alone or in combination with other techniques for palliation of dyspnea, cough, or respiratory insufficiency. The advantage of an airway stent is that it supports the airway wall against collapse or external compression and can impede extension of the tumour into the airway lumen.

Cryotherapy. Cryotherapy is a technique in which tissue is destroyed as a result of freezing. Bronchoscopic cryotherapy is used to ablate (destroy) bronchogenic carcinomas, especially polypoid lesions. A repeat bronchoscopy is performed 8 to 10 days after the first session. The second examination enables assessment of cryodestruction, removal of any slough, and repeat cryotherapy if required for the treatment of large lesions.

NURSING MANAGEMENT LUNG CANCER

NURSING ASSESSMENT

It is important to determine the understanding of the patient and the family concerning the diagnostic tests (those completed as well as those planned), the diagnosis or potential diagnosis, the treatment options, and the prognosis. At the same time, the nurse can assess the level of anxiety experienced by the patient and the support provided and needed by the patient's significant others. Subjective and objective data that should be obtained from a patient with lung cancer are presented in Table 30-15.

TABLE 30-15 NURSING ASSESSMENT

Lung Cancer

Subjective Data
Important Health Information
Past health history: Exposure to second-hand smoke; airborne carcinogens (e.g., asbestos, uranium, chromates, hydrocarbons, arsenic) or other pollutants; urban living environment; chronic lung disease, including TB, COPD, bronchiectasis; smoking history; frequent respiratory infections; family history of lung cancer
Medications: Use of cough medicines or other respiratory medications

Symptoms
- Anorexia, nausea, vomiting, dysphagia (late symptom), weight loss
- Persistent cough (productive or nonproductive), dyspnea, hemoptysis (late symptom)
- Fatigue, fever, chills
- Chest pain or tightness, shoulder and arm pain; headache; bone pain (late symptom)

Objective Data
General
Fever, neck and axillary lymphadenopathy, paraneoplastic syndromes (e.g., SIADH secretion)

Integumentary
Jaundice (liver metastasis); edema of neck and face (superior vena cava syndrome), digital clubbing

Respiratory
Wheezing, hoarseness, stridor, unilateral diaphragm paralysis, pleural effusions (late signs)

Cardiovascular
Pericardial effusion, cardiac tamponade, dysrhythmias (late signs)

Neurological
Unsteady gait (brain metastasis)

Musculo-skeletal
Pathological fractures, muscle wasting (late sign)

Possible Findings
Observance of lesion on chest radiographic examination, CT scan, lung scan, or PET scan; MRI findings of mediastinal invasion, positive sputum or bronchial washings for cytological studies; positive fibre-optic bronchoscopy and biopsy findings; low serum sodium and hypercalcemia (paraneoplastic syndrome)

COPD, chronic obstructive pulmonary disease; *CT,* computed tomography; *MRI,* magnetic resonance imaging; *PET,* positron emission tomography; *SIADH,* syndrome of inappropriate antidiuretic hormone; *TB,* tuberculosis.

NURSING DIAGNOSES

Nursing diagnoses for the patient with lung cancer may include but are not limited to the following:

- *Ineffective airway clearance* related to *excessive mucus, retained secretions, foreign body in airway* (tumour)
- *Ineffective breathing pattern* related to *body position that inhibits lung expansion* (space occupying lesion)
- *Impaired gas exchange* (related to tumour obstructing airflow)
- *Anxiety* related to *unmet needs* (lack of knowledge of the disease process)
- *Grieving* (related to new cancer diagnosis and therapeutic regimen)

PLANNING

The overall goals are that the patient with lung cancer will have (a) effective breathing patterns, (b) adequate airway clearance, (c) adequate oxygenation of tissues, (d) minimal to no pain, and (e) a realistic attitude toward treatment and prognosis.

NURSING IMPLEMENTATION

HEALTH PROMOTION. The best way to halt the epidemic of lung cancer is for people to stop smoking. Important nursing activities to assist in the progress toward this goal include promoting smoking cessation programs and actively supporting education and policy changes related to smoking. Important changes have occurred as a result of the recognition that sidestream smoke is a health hazard. There are now laws that (a) require designation of nonsmoking areas in most public places, (b) prohibit smoking, and (c) ban smoking on airline flights. Other actions aimed at controlling tobacco use include restrictions on tobacco advertising on television and warning label requirements for cigarette packaging. These are examples of beginning steps toward the goal of a smokeless society. Despite the small advances being made, tobacco-producer organizations such as marketing boards and tobacco companies still have strong political influences.

The nurse should make an effort to assist patients who smoke to stop smoking. There are many resources available to help. The Registered Nurses' Association of Ontario's Best Practice Guideline *Integrating Smoking Cessation Into Daily Nursing Practice* recommends nurses use the "ask, advise, assist, arrange" protocol to motivate smokers and other tobacco users to quit (RNAO, 2007). The six stages of change identified in smokers attempting to quit include precontemplation, contemplation, preparation, action, maintenance, and termination. (The stages of change in relationship to patient teaching [Transtheoretical Model] are discussed in Chapter 4, Table 4-3.) Each stage requires specific actions to progress to the next stage. Nurses working with patients at their individual stage of change will help them progress to the next stage. For patients unwilling to quit, motivational interviewing is recommended (discussed in Chapter 11). The Canadian Lung Association (2016b) provides information on access to counselling, medications, and supports to help Canadians quit smoking. The Canadian Cancer Society (2012) launched the "Break It Off" campaign, funded by Health Canada (2014a/b), which developed smoking cessation guides for both adults and young adults. Tobacco use and dependence and strategies to assist patients to stop smoking are discussed in Chapter 11.

The evidence-informed guideline also offers the five *R*s strategy for motivating smokers to quit: **r**elevance, **r**isk, **r**eward, **r**oadblocks, and **r**epetition. Because some patients relapse months or years after having stopped smoking, nurses must continually provide interactions to prevent relapse.

Nicotine's addictive properties make quitting a difficult task that requires much support. Nicotine replacement significantly lessens the urge to smoke and increases the percentage of smokers who successfully quit smoking. There is no evidence that one product has better results than another, so the choice of agent is dependent on the health care provider and patient preferences.

The advice and motivation of health care providers can be a powerful force in smoking cessation. Nurses are in a unique position to promote smoking cessation because they see large numbers of smokers who may be reluctant to seek help. Support for the smoker includes education that smoking a few cigarettes during a cessation attempt (a slip) is much different from resuming the full smoking habit (a relapse). Despite the slip, smokers should be encouraged to continue the attempt at cessation without viewing the effort as a failure. Measures to assist an individual in quitting should be directed toward the meaning that smoking has to that individual. The nurse must be aware of resources in the community to assist the individual who is interested in quitting.

ACUTE INTERVENTION. Care of the patient with lung cancer will initially involve support and reassurance during the diagnostic evaluation. (Specific nursing measures related to the diagnostic studies are outlined in Chapter 28.)

Another major responsibility of the nurse is to help the patient and the family deal with the diagnosis of lung cancer. The patient may feel guilty about cigarette smoking having caused the cancer and need to discuss this feeling with someone who has a nonjudgemental attitude. Questions regarding the patient's condition should be answered honestly. Additional counselling from a social worker, psychologist, or member of the clergy may be needed. Specific care of the patient will depend on the treatment plan. Postoperative care for the patient having surgery is discussed later in this chapter. Care of the patient undergoing radiation therapy and chemotherapy is discussed in Chapter 18 and in NCPs 18-1 and 18-2, on the Evolve website. The nurse has a major role in providing patient comfort, teaching methods to reduce pain, assessing for signs and symptoms of progressive or recurrent disease, and assessing indications for hospitalization.

AMBULATORY AND HOME CARE. Patient teaching needs to include signs and symptoms to report, such as hemoptysis, dysphagia, chest pain, and hoarseness. The patient and caregivers should be encouraged to provide a smoke-free environment, which may include smoking cessation for multiple family members.

If the treatment plan includes the use of home oxygen, teaching must include the safe use of oxygen. The patient who has had a surgical resection with intent to cure should be followed up with carefully to watch for manifestations of metastasis. The patient and family should be told to contact the physician if symptoms such as hemoptysis, dysphagia, chest pain, and hoarseness develop. For many individuals who have lung cancer, little can be done to significantly prolong their lives. Radiation therapy and chemotherapy can be used to provide palliative relief from distressing symptoms. Constant pain becomes a major problem. (Measures used to relieve pain are discussed in Chapter 10. Care of the patient with cancer is discussed in Chapter 18.) The patient and family or caregivers may need information about palliative care options in the community.

EVALUATION

The following are the expected outcomes for the patient with lung cancer:
- Patient will have adequate breathing patterns.
- Patient will have adequate airway clearance.
- Patient will have adequate tissue oxygenation.
- Patient will have minimal to no pain.
- Patient will have realistic attitude about prognosis.

OTHER TYPES OF LUNG TUMOURS

Other types of primary lung tumours include sarcomas, lymphomas, and bronchial adenomas. Bronchial adenomas are small tumours that arise from the lower trachea or major bronchi and are considered malignant because they are locally invasive and frequently metastasize. Clinical manifestations of bronchial adenomas include hemoptysis, persistent cough, localized obstructive wheezing, and pneumonia. Bronchial adenomas can usually be treated successfully with surgical resection.

The lungs are a common site for secondary metastases and are more often affected by metastatic growth than by primary

🔍 EVIDENCE-INFORMED PRACTICE
Research Highlight

Do Noninvasive Interventions Improve Quality of Life in Patients With Lung Cancer?
Clinical Question
In lung cancer patients (P), does receiving noninvasive interventions (I) compared with receiving no additional treatment (C) improve symptoms, psychological functioning, and quality of life (O)?

Best Available Evidence
Systematic review of RCTs or quasi-RCTs

Critical Appraisal and Synthesis of Evidence
- Meta-analysis of 15 clinical trials.
- Interventions studied included nursing interventions to manage breathlessness, nursing care programs, nutritional interventions, psychotherapeutic interventions, exercise, and reflexology.

Conclusions
- Nursing interventions to manage breathlessness showed improved symptom control, performance status, and emotional functioning.
- Nursing programs were effective in delaying clinical deterioration, dependency, and symptom distress as well as improving emotional functioning and satisfaction with care.
- Exercise and nutritional interventions had no significant or lasting effects on quality of life.
- Psychological interventions and reflexology had some short-lasting positive effects on quality of life.

Implications for Nursing Practice
- It is important to develop and maintain a supportive and empathic relationship with the patient with lung cancer.
- Nurses should offer patients supportive multidisciplinary interventions that may benefit their emotional, psychological, and physical well-being.
- These interventions may also help patients with other types of cancers.
- Further research is needed to accurately assess the effectiveness of noninvasive nursing interventions on the well-being and quality of life of patients with cancer.

Reference for Evidence
Rueda, J. R., Solà, I., Pascual, A., et al. (2011). Non-invasive interventions for improving well-being and quality of life in patients with lung cancer. *Cochrane Database of Systematic Review, (9),* CD004282. doi:10.1002/14651858.CD004282.pub3.

P, Patient population of interest; *I,* intervention or area of interest; *C,* comparison of interest or comparison group; *O,* outcome(s) of interest (see Chapter 1). *RCTs,* randomized controlled trials.

lung tumours. The pulmonary capillaries, with their extensive network, are ideal sites for tumour emboli. In addition, the lungs have an extensive lymphatic network. The primary malignancies that spread to the lungs often originate in the GI or genito-urinary tracts and in the breast. General symptoms of lung metastases are chest pain and nonproductive cough.

Benign tumours of the lung are generally classified as *mesenchymal.* Their occurrence is rare, and they have the potential to become malignant. The most common mesenchymal tumours are *chondromas,* which arise in the bronchial cartilage, and *leiomyomas,* which are myomas of smooth, nonstriated muscle fibres. Mesotheliomas may be malignant or benign and originate from the visceral pleura. Benign mesotheliomas are localized lesions.

Hamartomas of the lung are the most common benign tumour. These tumours, composed of fibrous tissue, fat, and blood vessels, are congenital malformations of the connective tissue of the bronchiolar walls. Hamartomas are slow-growing tumours.

CHEST TRAUMA AND THORACIC INJURIES

Traumatic injuries fall into two major categories: (1) blunt trauma and (2) penetrating trauma. *Blunt trauma* occurs when the body is struck by a blunt object, such as a steering wheel. The external injury may appear minor, but the impact may cause severe, life-threatening internal injuries, such as a ruptured spleen.

TABLE 30-16	COMMON TRAUMATIC CHEST INJURIES AND MECHANISMS OF INJURY
Mechanism of Injury	**Common Related Injury**
Blunt Trauma	
Blunt steering-wheel injury to chest	Rib fractures, flail chest, pneumothorax, hemo-pneumothorax, cardiac contusion, pulmonary contusion, cardiac tamponade, great vessel tears
Shoulder-harness seat belt injury	Fractured clavicle, dislocated shoulder, rib fractures, pulmonary contusion, pericardial contusion, cardiac tamponade
Crush injury (e.g., heavy equipment, crushing thorax)	Pneumothorax and hemo-pneumothorax, flail chest, great vessel tears and rupture, decreased blood return to heart with decreased cardiac output
Penetrating Trauma	
Gunshot or stab wound to chest	Open pneumothorax, tension pneumothorax, hemo-pneumothorax, cardiac tamponade, esophageal damage, tracheal tear, great vessel tears

Contrecoup trauma, a type of blunt trauma, is caused by the impact of parts of the body against other objects. This type of injury differs from blunt trauma primarily in the velocity of the impact. Internal organs are rapidly forced back and forth within the bony structures that surround them so that internal injury is sustained not only on the side of the impact but also on the opposite side, where the organ or organs hit bony structures. If the velocity of impact is great enough, organs and blood vessels can literally be torn from their points of origin. This is the shearing injury that can cause transection of the aorta, hemothorax, and diaphragmatic rupture injuries. Compression injury occurs when the body cannot handle the degree of external pressure during blunt trauma, resulting in contusions, crush injuries, and organ rupture.

Penetrating trauma occurs when a foreign body impales or passes through the body tissues (e.g., gunshot wounds, stabbings). Table 30-16 describes selective traumatic injuries as they relate to the categories of trauma and the mechanism of injury. Emergency care of the patient with a chest injury is presented in Table 30-17.

Thoracic injuries range from simple rib fractures to life-threatening tears of the aorta, vena cava, and other major vessels. The most common thoracic emergencies and their management are described in Table 30-18.

PNEUMOTHORAX

A **pneumothorax** is the presence of air in the pleural space. A complete or partial collapse of a lung results from this accumulation of air. This condition should be suspected after any blunt trauma to the chest wall. Pneumothorax may be closed or open.

TABLE 30-17	EMERGENCY MANAGEMENT

Chest Trauma

Etiology	Assessment Findings	Interventions
Blunt	**Respiratory**	**Initial**
• Motor vehicle collision	• Dyspnea, respiratory distress	• Ensure patent airway.
• Pedestrian accident	• Cough with or without hemoptysis	• Administer high-flow O_2 with nonrebreather mask.
• Fall	• Cyanosis of mouth, face, nail beds, mucous membranes	• Establish IV access with two large-bore catheters. Begin fluid resuscitation as appropriate.
• Assault with blunt object	• Tracheal deviation	• Remove clothing to assess injury.
• Crush injury	• Audible air escaping from chest wound	• Cover sucking chest wound with nonporous dressing taped on three sides.
• Explosion	• Decreased breath sounds on side of injury	• Stabilize impaling objects with bulky dressings. Do not remove.
	• Decreased O_2 saturation	• Assess for other significant injuries and treat appropriately.
Penetrating	• Frothy secretions	• Stabilize flail rib segment first with hand and then by application of large pieces of tape horizontal across the flail segment.
• Knife		• After cervical spine injury has been ruled out, place patient in a semi-Fowler's position or position patient on the injured side if breathing is easier.
• Gunshot	**Cardiovascular**	
• Stick	• Rapid, thready pulse	
• Arrow	• Decreased blood pressure	**Ongoing Monitoring**
• Other missiles	• Narrowed pulse pressure	• Monitor vital signs, level of consciousness, O_2 saturation, cardiac rhythm, respiratory status, and urinary output.
	• Asymmetrical blood pressure values in arms	• Anticipate intubation for respiratory distress.
	• Distended neck veins	• Release dressing if tension pneumothorax develops after sucking chest wound is covered.
	• Muffled heart sounds	
	• Chest pain	
	• Crunching sound synchronous with heart sounds	
	• Dysrhythmias	
	Surface Findings	
	• Bruising	
	• Abrasions	
	• Open chest wound	
	• Asymmetrical chest movement	
	• Subcutaneous emphysema	

IV, intravenous; *O_2,* oxygen.

TABLE 30-18   EMERGENCY MANAGEMENT

Thoracic Injuries

Definition	Clinical Manifestations	Emergency Management
Pneumothorax Air in pleural space (see Figure 30-5)	Dyspnea, decreased movement of involved chest wall, diminished or absent breath sounds on the affected side, hyper-resonance to percussion	Chest tube insertion with chest drainage system; Heimlich (flutter) valve
Hemothorax Blood in the pleural space, usually occurs in conjunction with pneumothorax	Dyspnea, diminished or absent breath sounds, dullness to percussion, shock	Chest tube insertion with chest drainage system; autotransfusion of collected blood, treatment of hypovolemia as necessary
Tension Pneumothorax Air in pleural space that does not escape Continued increase in amount of air shifts intrathoracic organs and increases intrathoracic pressure (see Figure 30-6)	Cyanosis, air hunger, violent agitation, tracheal deviation away from affected side, subcutaneous emphysema, neck vein distension, hyper-resonance to percussion	Medical emergency: needle decompression followed by chest tube insertion with chest drainage system
Flail Chest Fracture of two or more adjacent ribs in two or more places with loss of chest-wall stability (see Figure 30-7)	Paradoxical movement of chest wall, respiratory distress, associated hemothorax, pneumothorax, pulmonary contusion	Stabilization of flail segment with intubation in some patients and taping in others; oxygen therapy; treatment of associated injuries; analgesia
Cardiac Tamponade Blood rapidly collects in pericardial sac, compresses myocardium because the pericardium does not stretch, and prevents heart from pumping effectively	Muffled, distant heart sounds, hypotension, neck vein distension, increased central venous pressure	Medical emergency: pericardiocentesis with surgical repair as appropriate

Pneumothorax associated with trauma may be accompanied by hemothorax, a condition called *hemo-pneumothorax*.

Types of Pneumothorax

Closed Pneumothorax. *Closed pneumothorax* has no associated external wound. The most common form is a spontaneous pneumothorax, which is accumulation of air in the pleural space without an apparent antecedent event. It is caused by the rupture of small blebs (air-filled alveolar dilations <1 cm in diameter on the edge of the lung at the apex of the upper lobe or superior segment of the lower lobe) on the visceral pleural space. The cause of the blebs is unknown. This condition occurs most commonly in underweight male cigarette smokers between 20 and 40 years of age. There is a tendency for this condition to recur.

Other causes of closed pneumothorax include the following:
- Injury to the lungs from mechanical ventilation
- Injury to the lungs from insertion of a subclavian catheter
- Perforation of the esophagus
- Injury to the lungs from broken ribs
- Ruptured blebs or bullae in a patient with COPD

Open Pneumothorax. *Open pneumothorax* occurs when air enters the pleural space through an opening in the chest wall (Figure 30-5, *B*). Examples include stab or gunshot wounds and surgical thoracotomies. A penetrating chest wound is often referred to as a *sucking chest wound*.

An open pneumothorax should be covered with a vented dressing. (A vented dressing is one secured on three sides with the fourth side left untaped.) This allows air to escape from the vent and decreases the likelihood of tension pneumothorax developing. If the object that caused the open chest wound is still

FIGURE 30-5 Disorders of the pleura. **A,** Fibrothorax resulting from an organization of inflammatory exudate and pleural effusion. **B,** Open pneumothorax resulting from collapse of the lung caused by disruption of the chest wall and outside air entering.

in place, it should not be removed until a physician is present. The impaling object should be stabilized with a bulky dressing.

Tension Pneumothorax. Tension pneumothorax is a pneumothorax with rapid accumulation of air in the pleural space, causing severely high intrapleural pressures with resultant tension on the heart and great vessels. It may result from either an open or a closed pneumothorax (Figure 30-6). In an open chest wound, a flap may act as a one-way valve; thus, air can enter on inspiration but cannot escape. The intrathoracic pressure increases, the lung collapses, and the mediastinum shifts toward the unaffected side, which is subsequently compressed. As the pressure increases, cardiac output is altered because of decreased venous return and compression of the vena cava and aorta. Tension pneumothorax can occur with mechanical ventilation and resuscitative efforts. It can also occur if chest tubes are clamped or become blocked in a patient with a pneumothorax. Unclamping the tube or relieving the obstruction will remedy this situation.

Tension pneumothorax is a medical emergency with both the respiratory and the circulatory systems affected. If the tension

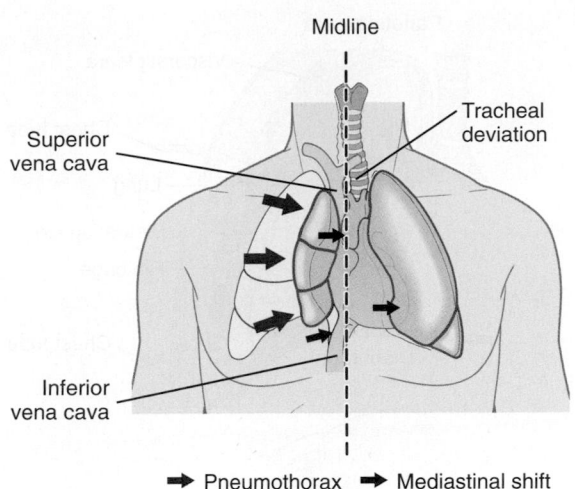

Midline

Superior
vena cava

Tracheal
deviation

Inferior
vena cava

➡ Pneumothorax   ➡ Mediastinal shift

FIGURE 30-6 Tension pneumothorax. As pleural pressure on the affected side increases, mediastinal displacement ensues with resultant respiratory and cardiovascular compromise.

in the pleural space is not relieved, the patient is likely to die from inadequate cardiac output or marked hypoxemia. Nurses and paramedics are now being trained to insert large-bore needles and chest tubes into the chest wall to release the trapped air.

Hemothorax. Hemothorax is an accumulation of blood in the intrapleural space. It is frequently found in association with open pneumothorax and is then called a *hemo-pneumothorax*. Causes of hemothorax include chest trauma, lung malignancy, complications of anticoagulant therapy, pulmonary embolus, and tearing of pleural adhesions.

Chylothorax. Chylothorax is the presence of lymphatic fluid in the pleural space because of a leak in the thoracic duct. Causes include trauma, surgical procedures, and malignancy. The thoracic duct is disrupted, and the chylous fluid, milky white with high lipid content, fills the pleural space. Total lymphatic flow through the thoracic duct is 1 500 to 2 400 mL/day. Fifty percent of those affected will heal with conservative treatment (chest drainage, bowel rest, and total parenteral nutrition). Surgery and pleurodesis are options if conservative therapy fails. *Pleurodesis* is the artificial production of adhesions between the parietal and the visceral pleurae, usually done with a chemical sclerosing agent.

Clinical Manifestations

If the pneumothorax is small, mild tachycardia and dyspnea may be the only manifestations. If the pneumothorax is large, respiratory distress may be present, including shallow, rapid respirations; dyspnea; air hunger; and decreased oxygen saturation. Chest pain and a cough with or without hemoptysis may be present. On auscultation, there are no breath sounds over the affected area, and hyper-resonance may be present. A chest radiograph shows the presence of air or fluid in the pleural space. If a tension pneumothorax develops, the patient experiences severe respiratory distress, tachycardia, and hypotension. Mediastinal displacement occurs, and the trachea shifts to the unaffected side. The patient is hemodynamically unstable.

Collaborative Care

Treatment depends on the severity of the pneumothorax and the nature of the underlying disease. If the patient is stable and the amount of air and fluid accumulated in the intrapleural space is minimal, no treatment may be needed as the pneumothorax

resolves spontaneously. If the amount of air or fluid is minimal, the pleural space can be aspirated with a large-bore needle. As a life-saving measure, needle venting (using a large-bore needle) of the pleural space may be used. A Heimlich valve may also be used to evacuate air from the pleural space. The most definitive and common form of treatment of pneumothorax and hemothorax is the insertion of a chest tube that is connected to water-seal drainage. Repeated spontaneous pneumothorax may have to be treated surgically by a partial pleurectomy, stapling, or pleurodesis to promote adherence of the pleurae to one another.

FRACTURED RIBS

Rib fractures are the most common type of chest injury resulting from trauma. Ribs 5 through 10 are most commonly fractured because they are least protected by chest muscles. If the fractured rib is splintered or displaced, it may damage the pleura and the lungs.

Clinical manifestations of fractured ribs include pain (especially on inspiration) at the site of injury. The individual splints the affected area and takes shallow breaths to try to decrease the pain. The individual is reluctant to take deep breaths, and the decreased ventilation may cause atelectasis to develop.

The main goal of treatment is to decrease pain so that the patient can breathe adequately to promote good chest expansion. Intercostal nerve blocks with local anaesthesia may be used to provide pain relief. The effect of the anaesthesia lasts for a period of hours to days. It must be repeated as necessary to provide pain relief. Opioid drug therapy must be individualized and used with caution because these drugs can depress respirations. Nonsteroidal anti-inflammatory drugs are used to reduce pain and aid with deep breathing and coughing. Patient teaching should emphasize deep breathing, coughing, use of incentive spirometry, and use of pain medications. Strapping the chest with tape or using a binder is not common practice. Most physicians believe that these measures should be avoided because they reduce lung expansion and predispose the individual to atelectasis.

FLAIL CHEST

Flail chest results from multiple rib fractures, causing instability of the chest wall (Figure 30-7). The chest wall cannot provide the bony structure necessary to maintain bellows action and ventilation. The affected (flail) area will move paradoxically to the intact portion of the chest during respiration. During inspiration, the affected portion is sucked in, and during expiration, it bulges out. This paradoxical chest movement prevents adequate ventilation of the lung in the injured area. The underlying lung may or may not have a serious injury. Associated pain and any lung injury giving rise to loss of compliance will contribute to an alteration in breathing patterns and lead to hypoxemia.

A flail chest is usually apparent on visual examination of the unconscious patient. The patient manifests rapid, shallow respirations and tachycardia. A flail chest may not be initially apparent in the conscious patient as a result of splinting of the chest wall. The patient moves air poorly, and movement of the thorax is asymmetrical and uncoordinated. Palpation of abnormal respiratory movements, crepitus of the rib, chest radiography, and ABG assessment assist in diagnosis.

Initial therapy consists of adequate ventilation, administration of humidified oxygen (O_2), careful administration of crystalloid

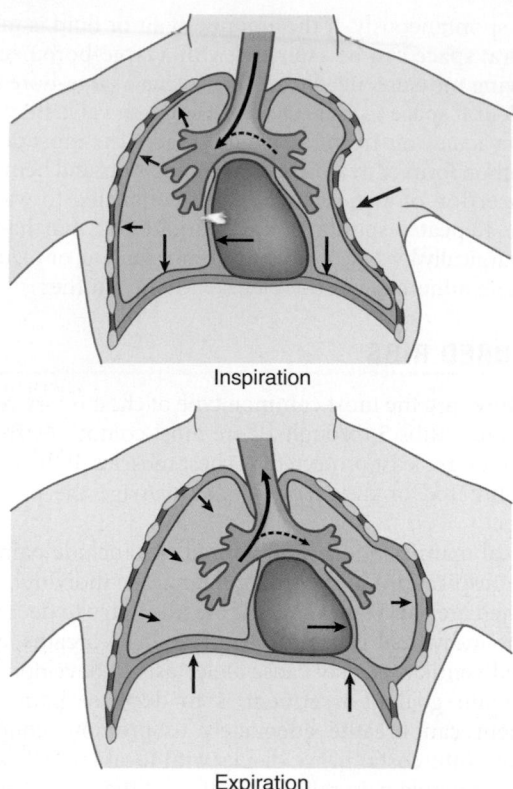

FIGURE 30-7 Flail chest produces paradoxical respiration. On inspiration, the flail section sinks in with the mediastinal shift to the uninjured side. On expiration, the flail section bulges outward with the mediastinal shift to the injured side.

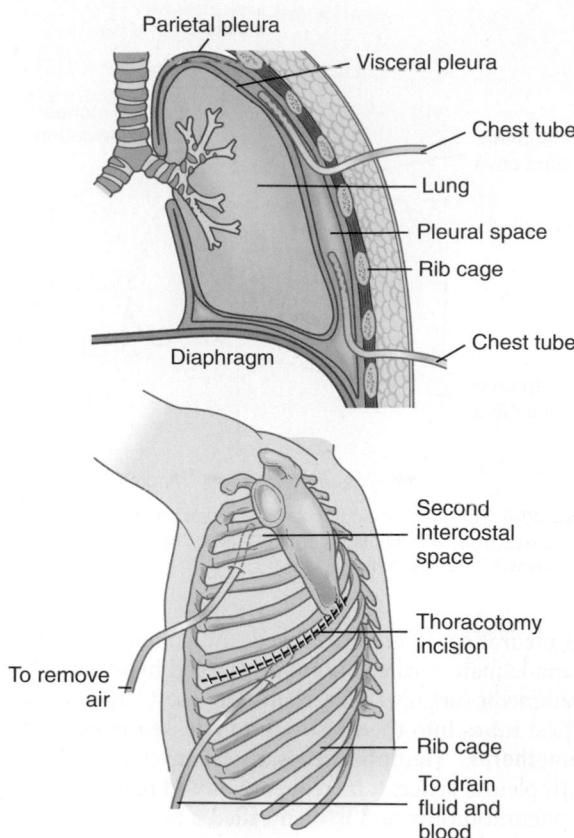

FIGURE 30-8 Placement of chest tubes.

IV solutions, and pain control. The definitive therapy is to re-expand the lung and ensure adequate oxygenation. Although many patients can be managed without the use of mechanical ventilation, a short period of intubation and ventilation may be necessary until the diagnosis of the lung injury is complete. The lung parenchyma and fractured ribs will heal with time. Some patients continue to experience intercostal pain after the flail chest has resolved.

CHEST TUBES AND PLEURAL DRAINAGE

The purpose of chest tubes and pleural drainage is to remove the air and fluid from the pleural space and to restore normal intrapleural pressure so that the lungs can re-expand. (Intrapleural pressure, also known as intrathoracic pressure, and the intrapleural space are described in Chapter 28.) Small accumulations of air or fluid in the pleural space may not require removal by thoracentesis or chest tube insertion. Instead, the air and fluid may be reabsorbed over time.

Chest Tube Insertion

Chest tubes can be inserted in the emergency department, at the patient's bedside, or in the operating room, depending on the situation. In the operating room, the chest tube is inserted via the thoracotomy incision. In the emergency department or at the bedside, the patient is placed in a sitting position or is lying down with the affected side elevated. The area is prepared with antiseptic solution, and the site is infiltrated with a local anaesthetic agent. After a small incision is made, one or two chest tubes are inserted into the pleural space. One catheter is placed

anteriorly through the second intercostal space to remove air (Figure 30-8). The other is placed posteriorly through the eighth or ninth intercostal space to drain fluid and blood. The tubes are sutured to the chest wall, and the puncture wound is covered with an airtight dressing. During insertion, the tubes are kept clamped. After the tubes are in place in the pleural space, they are connected to drainage tubing and pleural drainage, and the clamp is removed. Each tube may be connected to a separate drainage system and suction. More commonly, a Y-connector is used to attach both chest tubes to the same drainage system.

Pleural Drainage

Most pleural drainage systems have three basic compartments, each with its own separate function.

The first compartment, the *collection chamber,* receives fluid and air from the chest cavity. The fluid stays in this chamber while the air vents to the second compartment (Figure 30-9). The second compartment, called the *water-seal chamber,* contains 2 cm of water, which acts as a one-way valve. The incoming air enters from the collection chamber and bubbles up through the water. (The water acts as a one-way valve to prevent backflow of air into the patient from the system.) Initial bubbling of air is seen in this chamber when a pneumothorax is evacuated. Intermittent bubbling can also be seen during exhalation, coughing, or sneezing because of an increase in the patient's intrathoracic pressure. In this chamber, fluctuations, or "tidalling," will be seen and reflect the pressures in the pleural space. If tidalling is not seen, either the lungs have re-expanded or there is a kink or obstruction in the tubing. The air then exits the water seal and enters the suction chamber.

Water-seal chamber

Suction control chamber

Collection chamber

Air leak monitor

A

Dry suction regulator

Water-seal chamber

Suction monitor bellows

Collection chamber

Air leak monitor

B

FIGURE 30-9 Chest drainage unit. Both units have three chambers: (1) collection chamber; (2) water-seal chamber; and (3) suction control chamber. The suction control chamber requires a connection to a wall suction source that is dialed up higher than prescribed so that the suction will work. **A,** Water suction. This unit uses water in the suction control chamber to control the wall suction pressure. **B,** Dry suction. This unit controls wall suction by using a regulator control dial. Source: Getinge Group, Merrimack, NH.

A

Chest tube

Heimlich valve

Drainage bag

B

FIGURE 30-10 A, The Heimlich chest drain valve is a specially designed flutter valve that is used in place of a chest drainage unit for small, uncomplicated pneumothorax with little or no drainage and no need for suction. The valve allows for escape of air but prevents the re-entry of air into the pleural space. **B,** The valve is placed between the chest tube and the drainage bag, which can be worn under a person's clothes.

A third compartment, the *suction control chamber*, applies controlled suction to the chest drainage system. The classic suction control chamber uses tubing with one end submerged in a column of water and the other end vented to the atmosphere. It is typically filled with 20 cm of water. When the negative pressure generated by the suction source exceeds 20 cm, the air from the atmosphere enters the chamber through a vent and begins bubbling up through the water. As a result, excess pressure is relieved. The amount of suction applied is regulated by the depth of the suction control tube in the water and not by the amount of suction applied to the system. An increase in suction does not result in an increase in negative pressure to the system because any excess suction merely draws in air through the vented tubing. The suction pressure is usually ordered to be −20 cm H_2O.

Two types of suction control chambers are available on the market: wet and dry. The wet suction control chamber system is the classic system outlined previously. Bubbling is one way to tell that suction is functioning. Suction is started by turning up

the vacuum source until gentle bubbling appears. Turning the vacuum source higher just makes the bubbling more vigorous and makes the water evaporate faster. Even with gentle bubbling, water evaporates in this chamber, and water must be added periodically. The dry suction control chamber system, on the other hand, contains no water. It uses either a restrictive device or a regulator, internal to the chest drainage system, to dial the desired negative pressure. The dry system has a visual alert that indicates if the suction is working, so bubbling is not seen in a third chamber. The suction pressures are increased by turning the dial on the drainage system. Increasing the vacuum suction source will not increase the pressure (see Figure 30-9).

A variety of commercial disposable plastic chest drainage systems are available. The manufacturer's suggestions for use are included with the equipment. The plastic units allow the patient mobility and decrease the risk of breaking or spilling the drainage system.

INFORMATICS IN PRACTICE
Chest Drainage System

- A nurse needs to set up a chest drainage system but has not done so since simulation lab in nursing school.
- On the Internet, find a procedure manual, watch a video, or listen to a podcast of the procedure that would aid the nurse in this situation.

Heimlich Valves. Another device that may be used to evacuate air from the pleural space is the Heimlich valve (Figure 30-10). This device consists of a rubber flutter one-way valve within a rigid plastic tube. It is attached to the external end of the chest tube. The valve opens whenever the pressure is greater than the atmospheric pressure and closes when the reverse occurs. The

Heimlich valve functions like a water seal and is usually used for emergency transport or in special home care situations.

Small Chest Tubes. Small chest tubes ("pigtail catheters") are used in selected patients because they are less traumatic. The drains may be straight catheters or "pigtail" catheters (curled at the distal end, resembling a pig's tail). Curled catheters are considered to be less traumatic than straight catheters. These catheters, if occluded, can be irrigated by the physician using sterile water. Chemical pleurodesis can also be performed through this catheter. This system is not suitable for trauma or for drainage of blood. Owing to the smaller size, the tube can become kinked, occluded, or dislodged more easily. Small-bore chest tubes and Heimlich valves should be used with caution in patients on mechanical ventilators because there is a potential for rapid accumulation of air and a tension pneumothorax (Light, 2011).

NURSING MANAGEMENT CHEST DRAINAGE

Some general guidelines for nursing care of the patient with chest tubes and water-seal drainage systems are presented in Table 30-19. The traditional practice of routine milking or stripping of chest tubes to maintain patency is no longer recommended because it can cause dangerously high intrapleural pressure and damage to pleural tissue. Drainage and blood are not likely to clot inside chest tubes because the newer chest tubes are made with a coating that makes them nonthrombogenic. The nurse should remember that insertion of the chest tube, as well as its continued presence, can be painful to the patient. Dislodgement of the tube may occur if the tube is not stabilized.

Clamping of chest tubes during transport or when the tube is accidentally disconnected is no longer advocated. The danger of rapid accumulation of air in the pleural space causing tension pneumothorax is far greater than that of a small amount of atmospheric air entering the pleural space. Chest tubes may be momentarily clamped to change the drainage apparatus or to check for air leaks. Clamping for more than a few moments is indicated only for assessing how the patient will tolerate chest tube removal. It is done to simulate chest tube removal and identify if there will be negative clinical repercussions with tube removal. Generally, this is done 4 to 6 hours before the tube is removed, and the patient is monitored closely. If a chest tube becomes disconnected, the most important intervention is immediate re-establishment of the water-seal system and attachment of a new drainage system as soon as possible. In some hospitals, when disconnection occurs, the chest tube is immersed in sterile water ($\approx$2 cm) until the system can be re-established. It is important for the nurse to know the unit protocol, individual clinical situation (e.g., whether an air leak exists), and physician preference before resorting to prolonged chest tube clamping.

As with many procedures, the hospital may have policies and procedures referring to the care of chest tubes. Ensure that these are reviewed and followed.

COMPLICATIONS

Chest tube malposition is the most common complication. The nurse does routine monitoring to evaluate whether the chest drainage is successful by observing for tidalling in the water-seal chamber, listening for breath sounds over the lung fields, and measuring the amount of fluid drainage. Re-expansion pulmonary edema can occur after rapid expansion of a collapsed lung

in patients with a pneumothorax or with evacuation of large volumes of pleural fluid (>1 to 1.5 L). A vasovagal response with symptomatic hypotension can occur from too rapid removal of fluid.

Infection at the skin site is also a concern. Meticulous sterile technique during dressing changes can reduce the incidence of infected sites. Other complications include (a) pneumonia from not taking deep breaths, from not using an incentive spirometer, and from splinting on the affected side and (b) shoulder disuse ("frozen shoulder") from lack of range-of-motion exercises. Poor patient adherence or lack of patient teaching can contribute to these complications. Nurses can make a tremendous impact on preventing these complications.

CHEST TUBE REMOVAL

The patient with chest tubes may have chest radiographic studies to follow the course of lung expansion. The chest tubes are removed when the lungs are re-expanded and fluid drainage has ceased. Generally, suction is discontinued, and the patient is placed on gravity drainage for a period of time before the tubes are removed. The tube is removed by cutting the sutures; applying a sterile petroleum jelly gauze dressing; having the patient take a deep breath, exhale, and bear down (Valsalva manoeuvre); and then removing the tube. Pain medication is generally given before chest tube removal. The site is covered with an airtight dressing, the pleura seals itself off, and the wound heals in several days. A chest radiograph is obtained after chest tube removal to evaluate for pneumothorax, reaccumulation of fluid, or both. The wound should be observed for drainage and should be reinforced if necessary. The patient should be observed for respiratory distress, which may signify a recurrent or new pneumothorax.

CHEST SURGERY

Chest surgery is performed for a variety of reasons, some of which are unrelated to primary lung problems. For example, a thoracotomy may be performed for heart and esophageal surgery. The types of chest surgery are compared in Table 30-20.

Preoperative Care

Before chest surgery, baseline data are obtained on the respiratory and cardiovascular systems. Diagnostic studies performed are pulmonary function, chest radiography, electrocardiogram (ECG), ABGs, blood urea nitrogen (serum urea [nitrogen]), serum creatinine, blood glucose, serum electrolytes, and complete blood cell count. Additional studies of cardiac function such as cardiac catheterization may be done for the patient who is to undergo a pneumonectomy. A careful physical assessment of the lungs, including percussion and auscultation, should be done. This will allow the nurse to compare preoperative and postoperative findings.

The patient should be encouraged to stop smoking before surgery to decrease secretions and increase O_2 saturation. In the anxious period before surgery, refraining from smoking is not easy for the habitual smoker to do. Chest physiotherapy may be indicated to help drain the lungs of accumulated secretions. This is especially indicated for the patient with a lung abscess or bronchiectasis.

Preoperative teaching should include exercises for effective deep breathing and incentive spirometry. If the patient practices these techniques before surgery, the techniques will be easier to perform after surgery. The patient should be told that adequate

TABLE 30-19 CLINICAL GUIDELINES FOR CARE OF PATIENT WITH CHEST TUBES AND WATER-SEAL DRAINAGE SYSTEM

1. Keep all tubing loosely coiled below chest level. Tubing should drop straight from bed or chair to drainage unit. Do not let it be compressed.
2. Keep all connections between chest tubes, drainage tubing, and drainage collector tight, and tape at connections.
3. Observe for air fluctuations (tidalling) and bubbling in the water-seal chamber.
   - If no tidalling is observed (rising with inspiration and falling with expiration in the spontaneously breathing patient), the drainage system is blocked, the lungs are re-expanded, or the system is attached to suction.
   - If bubbling increases, there may be an air leak in the drainage system or a leak from the patient (bronchopleural leak).
4. If the chest tube is connected to suction, disconnect from wall suction to check for tidalling.
5. Suspect a system leak when bubbling is continuous.
   - To determine the source of the air leak, momentarily clamp the tubing successively from the chest tube insertion site to the drainage set, observing for the bubbling to cease. When bubbling ceases, the leak is above the clamp.
   - Retape tubing connections.
   - If leak continues, notify physician. It may be necessary to replace the drainage apparatus or to secure the chest tube with an air-occlusive dressing.
6. High fluid levels in the water seal indicate residual negative pressure.
   - The chest system may need to be vented by using the high negativity release valve available on the drainage system to release residual pressure from the system.
   - Do not lower water-seal column when wall suction is not operating or when patient is on gravity drainage.

Patient's Clinical Status

1. Monitor the patient's clinical status. Assess vital signs, lung sounds, pain.
2. Assess for manifestations of reaccumulation of air and fluid in the chest (↓ or absent breath sounds), significant bleeding (>100 mL/hr), chest drainage site infection (drainage, erythema, fever, ↑ white blood cell count), or poor wound healing. Notify physician for management plan. Evaluate for subcutaneous emphysema at chest tube site.
3. Encourage the patient to breathe deeply periodically to facilitate lung expansion, and encourage range-of-motion exercises to the shoulder on the affected side. Incentive spirometry every hour while awake may be necessary to prevent atelectasis or pneumonia.
4. Chest tubes are *not routinely clamped*. A physician order is required. A physician may order clamping for 24 hours to evaluate for reaccumulation of fluid or air before discontinuing the chest tube.

Chest Drainage

1. Never elevate the drainage system to the level of the patient's chest because doing so will cause fluid to drain back into the lungs. Secure the unit to the drainage stand. If the drainage chambers are full, notify the physician and anticipate changing the system. Do not try to empty it.
2. Mark the time of measurement and the fluid level on the drainage unit according to the unit standards. Report any change in the quantity or characteristics of drainage (e.g., clear yellow to bloody) to the physician and record the change. Notify physician if >100 mL/hr drainage.

3. Check the position of the chest drainage container. If the drainage system is overturned and the water seal is disrupted, return it to an upright position and encourage the patient to take a few deep breaths, followed by forced exhalations and cough manoeuvres.
4. If the drainage system breaks, place the distal end of the chest tubing connection in a sterile water container at a 2-cm level as an emergency water seal.
5. Do not strip chest tubes. Doing so dangerously increases intrapleural pressures. Drainage tubes may be milked (alternately folded or squeezed and then released) on physician order. Milk only if drainage has evidence of clots or obstruction. Take 15-cm strips of the chest tube and squeeze and release starting close to the chest and repeating down the tube distally.

Monitoring Wet Versus Dry Suction Chest Drainage Systems
Suction Control Chamber in Wet Suction System

1. Keep the suction control chamber at the appropriate water level by adding sterile water as needed to replace water lost to evaporation.
2. Keep the muffler covering the suction control chamber in place to prevent more rapid evaporation of water and to decrease the noise of the bubbling.
3. After filling the suction control chamber to the ordered suction amount (generally −20 cm water suction), connect the suction tubing to the wall suction.
4. Dial the wall suction regulator until continuous gentle bubbling is seen in the suction control chamber (generally 80–120 mm Hg). Vigorous bubbling is not necessary and will increase the rate of evaporation.
5. If no bubbling is seen in the suction control chamber, (a) there is no suction, (b) the suction is not set high enough, or (c) the pleural air leak is so large that suction is not high enough to evacuate it.

Suction Control Chamber in Dry Suction System (See Manufacturer's Directions)

- After connecting patient to system, turn the dial on the chest drainage system to amount ordered (generally −20 cm pressure), connect suction tubing to wall suction source, and increase the suction until the correct amount of negative pressure is indicated. There will be a high negative-pressure release valve in the system.

Chest Tube Dressings

1. Dressings are not routinely changed. If there is visible drainage, notify physician for instructions.
2. If ordered to change dressings, remove old dressing carefully to avoid removing unsecured chest tube. Assess the site, and culture site as indicated.
3. Cleanse the site with sterile normal saline. Apply sterile gauze and tape to secure the dressing. Some physicians may prefer use of petroleum gauze dressing around the tube to prevent air leak. Date the dressing and document dressing change.

Obtaining a Sample From the Chest Tube

1. Form a loop in the tubing in an area to get the most recently drained fluid.
2. Swab the sampling site of the tubing with antiseptic and allow to air-dry.
3. Aspirate from the sampling site with syringe; cap syringe; label with patient name, date, time, and source of specimen.
4. Send to laboratory.

medication will be given to reduce the pain and should be helped to splint the incision with a pillow to facilitate deep breathing.

For most types of chest surgery, chest tubes are inserted and connected to water-sealed drainage systems. The purpose of these tubes should be explained to the patient. In addition, O₂ is frequently given the first 24 hours after surgery. Range-of-motion exercises on the surgical side, similar to those for the mastectomy patient, should be taught (see Chapter 54).

The thought of losing part of a vital organ is frequently frightening. The patient should be reassured that the lungs have a large degree of functional reserve. Even after the removal of one lung, there is enough lung tissue to maintain adequate oxygenation.

TABLE 30-20 CHEST SURGERIES

Type and Description	Indication	Comments
Lobectomy Removal of one lobe of lung	Lung cancer, bronchiectasis, TB, emphysematous bullae, benign lung tumours, fungal infections	Most common lung surgery; postoperative insertion of chest tubes; expansion of remaining lung tissue to fill up space
Pneumonectomy Removal of entire lung	Lung cancer (most common), extensive TB, bronchiectasis, lung abscess	Done only when lobectomy or segmental resection will not remove all diseased lung; no drainage tubes (generally), fluid gradually fills space where lung was; patient positioned on operative side to facilitate expansion of remaining lung
Segmental Resection Removal of one or more lung segments	Lung cancer, bronchiectasis, TB	Technically difficult; done to remove lung segment; insertion of chest tubes; expansion of remaining lung tissue to fill space
Wedge Resection Removal of small, localized lesion that occupies only part of a segment	Lung biopsy, excision of small nodules	Need for chest tubes after surgery
Decortication Removal of thick, fibrous membrane from visceral pleura	Empyema	Use of chest tubes and drainage after surgery
Exploratory Thoracotomy Incision into thorax to look for injured or bleeding tissues	Chest trauma	Use of chest tubes and drainage after surgery
Thoracotomy Not Involving Lungs* Incision into thorax for surgery on other organs	Hiatal hernia repair, open-heart surgery, esophageal surgery, tracheal resection, aortic aneurysm repair	
Video-Assisted Thorascopic Surgery (VATS) VATS under general anaesthesia in OR	Procedures performed using VATS include lung biopsy, lobectomy, resection of nodules, repair of fistulas	Video-assisted technique involving insertion of a rigid scope with a distal lens into the pleura with image shown on a monitor screen, allowing surgeon to manipulate instruments passed into the pleural space through separate small intercostal incisions
Lung Volume Reduction Surgery (LVRS)	Advanced bullous emphysema, α_1-antitrypsin emphysema	Involves reducing lung volume by multiple wedge excisions or VATS (see Video-Assisted Thorascopic Surgery)

OR, operating room; *TB*, tuberculosis.
*For comments on thoracotomy not involving the lungs, see discussion of individual diseases in text.

The nurse should be available to deal with the questions asked by the patient and the family, and questions should be answered honestly. The nurse should try to facilitate the expression of concerns, feelings, and questions. (General preoperative care and teaching are discussed in Chapter 20.)

Surgical Therapy

Thoracotomy (surgical opening into the thoracic cavity) surgery is considered major surgery because the incision is large and cuts into bone, muscle, and cartilage. The two types of thoracic incisions are median sternotomy, performed by splitting the sternum, and lateral thoracotomy. The median sternotomy is primarily used for surgery involving the heart. The two types of lateral thoracotomy are posterolateral and anterolateral. The posterolateral thoracotomy is used for most surgeries involving the lung. The incision is made from the anterior axillary line below the nipple level posteriorly at the fourth, fifth, or sixth intercostal space. It is rarely necessary to remove the ribs. Strong mechanical retractors are used to gain access to the lung. The anterolateral incision is made in the fourth or fifth intercostal space from the sternal border to the midaxillary line. This procedure is commonly used for surgery or trauma victims, mediastinal operations, and wedge resections of the upper and middle lobes of the lung.

The extensiveness of the thoracotomy incision often results in severe pain for the patient after surgery. Because muscles have been severed, the patient is reluctant to move the shoulder and arm on the surgical side. Chest tubes are placed in the pleural space except in pneumonectomy surgery. In a pneumonectomy, the space from which the lung was removed gradually fills with serosanguinous fluid.

Video-Assisted Thorascopic Surgery. Video-assisted thorascopic surgery (VATS) is a thorascopic surgical procedure that, in many cases, can enable the avoidance of a full thoracotomy. The procedure involves three or four 2.5-cm incisions made on the chest that allow the thorascope (a special fibre-optic camera) and instruments to be inserted and manipulated. Video-assisted thorascopes improve visualization because the surgeon can view the thoracic cavity from the video monitor. The thorascope is equipped with a camera that magnifies the image on the monitor. Thorascopy can be used to diagnose and treat a variety of conditions of the lung, the pleura, and the mediastinum.

The candidate for this type of procedure should not have a prior history of conventional thoracic surgery because of the probability of adhesion formation, which would make access more difficult. The patient whose lesions are in the lung periphery or the mediastinum is a better candidate because of better accessibility. The patient considered for thorascopic surgery should have sufficient pulmonary function before surgery to allow the surgeon to perform conventional thoracotomy if complications occur. Complications that may occur are bleeding, diaphragmatic perforation, air emboli, persistent pleural air leaks, and tension pneumothorax.

There are many benefits of thorascopic surgery when compared with a conventional thoracotomy procedure. These include less adhesion formation, minimal blood loss, less time under anaesthesia, shorter hospitalization, faster recovery, less pain, and no need for postoperative rehabilitation therapy because of minimal disruption of thoracic structures.

Chest tubes are placed at the end of the procedure through one of the incisions. The incisions are closed with sutures or a wound-approximating adhesive bandage. Nursing assessment and care after surgery include monitoring respiratory status and lung re-expansion with the chest tubes and checking the incisions for drainage or dehiscence. The most common complication is prolonged air leak. A return to prior activities should be encouraged as quickly as possible. The hospital stay averages from 1 to 5 days, depending on the type of surgery.

Postoperative Care

Specific measures related to the care after a thoracotomy are presented in NCP 30-2, available on the Evolve website. The specific follow-up care depends on the type of surgical procedure. General postoperative care is discussed in Chapter 22.

RESTRICTIVE RESPIRATORY DISORDERS

Restrictive respiratory disorders are characterized by a restriction in lung volume (caused by decreased compliance of the lungs or chest wall). This is in contrast to obstructive disorders, which are characterized by increased resistance to airflow (see Chapter 31). Pulmonary function tests are the best means of differentiating between restrictive and obstructive respiratory disorders (Table 30-21). Mixed obstructive and restrictive disorders are often manifested. For example, a patient may have both chronic bronchitis (an obstructive problem) and pulmonary fibrosis (a restrictive problem).

Restrictive problems are generally categorized into extrapulmonary and intrapulmonary disorders. Extrapulmonary causes of restrictive lung disease include disorders involving the central nervous system, neuro-muscular system, and chest wall (Table 30-22). In these disorders, the lung tissue is normal. Intrapulmonary causes of restrictive lung disease involve the pleura or the lung tissue (Table 30-23).

PLEURAL EFFUSION

Types

The pleural space lies between the lung and the chest wall and normally contains a very thin layer of fluid. **Pleural effusion** is a

TABLE 30-21	**RELATIONSHIP OF LUNG VOLUMES TO TYPE OF VENTILATORY DISORDER**		
Lung Volumes	**Restrictive**	**Obstructive**	**Restrictive and Obstructive**
Vital capacity (VC)	↓	Normal or ↓	↓
Total lung capacity (TLC)	↓	↑	Variable
Residual volume (RV)	Normal or ↓	↑	Variable
Forced expiratory volume in 1 sec (FEV₁)	Normal or ↓	↓	↓
FEV₁/Functional vital capacity (FVC)	Normal or ↑	↓	↓

collection of fluid in the pleural space (see Figure 30-5, *A*). It is not a disease but rather a sign of a serious disease. Pleural effusion is frequently classified as *transudative* or *exudative* according to whether the protein content of the effusion is low or high, respectively. A transudate occurs primarily in noninflammatory conditions and is an accumulation of protein- and cell-poor fluid. Transudative pleural effusions (also called *hydrothorax*) are caused by (1) increased hydrostatic pressure found in heart failure, which is the most common cause of pleural effusion, or (2) decreased oncotic pressure (from hypoalbuminemia) found in chronic liver or renal disease. In these situations, fluid movement is facilitated out of the capillaries and into the pleural space.

An exudative effusion is an accumulation of fluid and cells in an area of inflammation. An exudative pleural effusion results from the increased capillary permeability characteristic of the inflammatory reaction. This type of effusion occurs secondary to conditions such as pulmonary malignancies, pulmonary infections, pulmonary embolization, and GI disease (e.g., pancreatic disease, esophageal perforation).

The type of pleural effusion can be determined from a sample of pleural fluid obtained via **thoracentesis** (a procedure to remove fluid from the pleural space). Exudates have a high protein content, and the fluid is generally dark yellow or amber. Transudates have a low protein content or contain no protein, and the fluid is clear or pale yellow. The fluid can also be analyzed for red and white blood cells, malignant cells, bacteria, and glucose.

An **empyema** is a pleural effusion that contains pus. It is caused by conditions such as pneumonia, TB, lung abscess, and infection of surgical wounds of the chest. Treatment of empyema is generally chest tube drainage. Appropriate antibiotic therapy is also needed to eradicate the causative organism. A complication of empyema is fibrothorax, in which there is fibrous fusion of the visceral and parietal pleurae (see Figure 30-5, *A*). A condition called *trapped lung* can occur with effusions and empyema. It occurs when the visceral pleura becomes encased with a fibrous peel or rind. The fibrous peel causes severe pulmonary restriction. The pathological process affecting the visceral pleura prevents the lung from expanding and from filling the thoracic cavity. A decortication surgical procedure to remove the pleural peel may be needed.

Clinical Manifestations

Common clinical manifestations of pleural effusion are progressive dyspnea and decreased movement of the chest wall on the affected

TABLE 30-22 EXTRAPULMONARY CAUSES OF RESTRICTIVE LUNG DISEASE

Disease or Alteration	Description	Comments
Central Nervous System		
Head injury, CNS lesion (e.g., tumour, stroke)	Injury to or impingement on respiratory centre, causing hypoventilation or hyperventilation; relationship of manifestations to increased intracranial pressure (see Chapters 59 and 60)	Management is directed toward treating the underlying cause, maintaining the airway, using mechanical ventilation for supportive care, and assessing for manifestations of increased intracranial pressure.
Opioid and barbiturate use	Depression of respiratory centre, respiratory rate of <12 breaths/min	Respiratory depression is caused by drug overdose or inadvertent administration of drugs to a person with respiratory difficulty. These drugs should not be administered to a person with a respiratory rate of <12 breaths/min.
Neuro-Muscular System		
Spinal cord injury	Complete cervical- and complete upper thoracic–level injuries have restrictive ventilation. The lung volumes are reduced owing to inspiratory muscle weakness	Patient with a cervical injury may need mechanical ventilator support initially.
Guillain-Barré syndrome	Acute inflammation of peripheral nerves and ganglia; paralysis of intercostal nerves leading to diaphragmatic breathing; paralysis of vagal preganglionic and postganglionic fibres leading to reduced ability of bronchioles to constrict, dilate, and respond to irritants	Patient often has to be put on mechanical ventilation for supportive care (see Chapter 63).
Amyotrophic lateral sclerosis	Progressive degenerative disorder of the motor neurons in the spinal cord, brain stem, and motor cortex; respiratory system involvement as a result of interruption of nerve transmission to respiratory muscles, especially diaphragm	See Chapter 61 for clinical manifestations and management.
Myasthenia gravis	Defect in neuro-muscular junction; respiratory system involvement as a result of interruption of nerve transmission to respiratory muscles	See Chapter 61 for clinical manifestations and management.
Muscular dystrophy	Hereditary disease; eventual involvement of all skeletal muscles; paralysis of respiratory muscles, including intercostals, diaphragm, and accessory muscles	Pulmonary problems develop late in disease process.
Chest Wall		
Chest-wall trauma (e.g., flail chest, fractured rib)	Rib fracture causing inspiratory pain; voluntary splinting of chest, resulting in shallow, rapid breathing; impaired ventilatory ability caused by paradoxical breathing	Strapping the chest wall to stabilize the fractures is not recommended because this increases the restrictive defect.
Pickwickian syndrome (extreme obesity)	Excess adipose tissue interfering with chest-wall and diaphragmatic excursion, somnolence from hypoxemia and CO_2 retention, polycythemia from chronic hypoxia	Weight loss generally causes reversal of symptoms. Prevention and prompt treatment of respiratory infections is important. Condition is worsened in supine position.
Kyphoscoliosis	Posterior and lateral angulation of the spine; restriction of ventilation as a result of alteration in thoracic excursion; increase in work of breathing; pattern of rapid, shallow breathing; reduction of lung volume; compression of alveoli and blood vessels	Only a small number of people with condition develop severe respiratory problems. Atelectasis and pneumonia are common complications.

CNS, central nervous system; *CO₂,* carbon dioxide.

side. There may be pleuritic pain from the underlying disease. Physical examination of the chest will indicate dullness to percussion and absent or decreased breath sounds over the affected area. The chest radiograph will indicate an abnormality if the effusion is greater than 250 mL. Manifestations of empyema include the manifestations of pleural effusion as well as fever, night sweats, cough, and weight loss. A thoracentesis reveals an exudate containing thick, purulent material.

Thoracentesis

If the cause of the pleural effusion is not known, a diagnostic thoracentesis is needed to obtain pleural fluid for analysis (see Chapter 28, Figure 28-15). If the degree of pleural effusion is severe enough to impair breathing, a therapeutic thoracentesis is done to remove fluid as well as to obtain fluid for analysis.

A thoracentesis is performed by having the patient sit on the edge of a bed and lean forward over a bedside table. The puncture site is determined by chest radiograph, and percussion of the chest is used to assess the maximum degree of dullness. The skin is cleaned with an antiseptic solution and anaesthetized locally. The thoracentesis needle is inserted into the intercostal space. Fluid can be aspirated with a syringe, or tubing can be connected to allow fluid to drain into a sterile collection bag. After the fluid is removed, the needle is withdrawn, and a bandage is applied over the insertion site.

Usually, only 1 000 to 1 200 mL of pleural fluid is removed at one time. Because high volumes are removed, rapid removal can result in hypotension, hypoxemia, or pulmonary edema. A follow-up chest radiograph should be obtained to detect a possible pneumothorax that could have been induced by perforation of the visceral pleura. During and after the procedure, the patient should be observed for any manifestations of respiratory distress.

Collaborative Care

The main goal of management of pleural effusions is to treat the underlying cause. For example, adequate treatment of heart failure

TABLE 30-23 INTRAPULMONARY CAUSES OF RESTRICTIVE LUNG DISEASE

Disease or Alteration	Description
Pleural disorders	Inflammation, scarring, or fluid in the pleural space causing restriction
Pleural effusion	Accumulation of fluid in pleural space secondary to altered hydrostatic or oncotic pressure; fluid collection >250 mL, showing up on chest radiograph
Pleurisy (pleuritis)	Inflammation of pleura; classification as fibrinous (dry) or serofibrinous (wet); wet pleurisy accompanied by an increase in pleural fluid and possibly resulting in pleural effusion
Pneumothorax	Accumulation of air in pleural space with accompanying lung collapse
Parenchymal disorders	Inflammation, collapse, or scarring of the lung tissue
Atelectasis	Condition of lung characterized by collapsed, airless alveoli; possibly acute (e.g., in postoperative patient) or chronic (e.g., in patient with malignant tumour)
Pneumonia	Acute inflammation of lung tissue caused by bacteria, viruses, fungi, chemicals, dusts, and other factors
Interstitial lung diseases (ILDs)	General term that includes a variety of chronic lung disorders characterized by some type of injury, inflammation, and scarring (or fibrosis); this process occurs in the interstitium (tissue between the alveoli), and the lung becomes stiff (fibrotic); can be caused by occupational and environmental exposures (see Table 30-10), infections (e.g., TB), and connective tissue disorders (e.g., rheumatoid arthritis); when all known causes of ILDs are ruled out, the condition is termed *idiopathic pulmonary fibrosis* (IPF)
Acute respiratory distress syndrome (ARDS)*	Atelectasis, pulmonary edema, congestion, and hyaline membrane lining the alveolar wall; result of variety of conditions, including shock lung, O_2 toxicity, Gram-negative sepsis, cardiopulmonary bypass, and aspiration pneumonia

*O_2, oxygen; *TB*, tuberculosis.*
*See Chapter 70 for clinical manifestations and management.

with diuretics and sodium restriction will result in decreased pleural effusions. The treatment of pleural effusions secondary to malignant disease represents a more difficult problem. These types of pleural effusions are frequently recurrent and accumulate quickly after thoracentesis. Chemical pleurodesis may be used to sclerose the pleural space and prevent reaccumulation of effusion fluid. Although doxycycline and bleomycin have been used for sclerosing with good results, talc appears to be the most effective agent for pleurodesis. Thoracoscopy can be used to perform talc pleurodesis after inspection of the pleural space. After instillation of the sclerosing agent, patients are usually instructed to rotate their positions to spread the agent uniformly throughout the pleural space. Chest tubes are left in place after pleurodesis until fluid drainage is less than 150 mL/day and no air leaks are noted.

PLEURISY

Pleurisy (pleuritis) is an inflammation of the pleura. The most common causes are pneumonia, TB, chest trauma, pulmonary infarctions, and neoplasms. The inflammation usually subsides with adequate treatment of the primary disease. Pleurisy can be classified as fibrinous (dry), with fibrinous deposits on the pleural surface, or serofibrinous (wet), with increased production of pleural fluid that may result in pleural effusion.

The pain of pleurisy is typically abrupt and sharp in onset and is aggravated by inspiration. The patient's breathing is shallow and rapid to avoid unnecessary movement of the pleura and chest wall. A pleural friction rub may occur, which is the sound over areas where inflamed visceral and parietal pleurae rub over one another during inspiration. This sound is usually loudest at peak inspiration but can be heard during exhalation as well.

Treatment of pleurisy is aimed at treating the underlying disease and providing pain relief. Taking analgesics and lying on or splinting the affected side may provide some relief. The patient should be taught to splint the rib cage when coughing. Intercostal nerve blocks may be done if the pain is severe.

ATELECTASIS

Atelectasis is a complete or partial collapse of a lung or segment of a lung that occurs when the alveoli become deflated. The most common cause of atelectasis is airway obstruction that results from retained exudates and secretions, which is frequently observed in the postoperative patient. Normally, the pores of Kohn (see Chapter 28, Figure 28-1) provide for collateral passage of air from one alveolus to another. Deep inspiration is necessary to open the pores effectively. For this reason, deep-breathing exercises are important in preventing atelectasis in the high-risk patient (e.g., postoperative, immobilized patient). (The prevention and treatment of atelectasis are discussed in Chapter 22.)

INTERSTITIAL LUNG DISEASE

Many acute and chronic lung disorders with variable degrees of pulmonary inflammation and fibrosis are collectively referred to as *interstitial lung diseases* (ILDs) or *diffuse parenchymal lung diseases*. ILDs have been difficult to classify because more than 200 known diseases have diffuse lung involvement, either as the primary condition or as a significant part of a multiorgan process, as may occur in connective tissue disorders (e.g., systemic lupus erythematosus, rheumatoid arthritis).

Among the ILDs of known cause, the largest group comprises occupational and environmental exposures, especially the inhalation of dusts and various fumes or gases. The most common ILDs of unknown etiology are idiopathic pulmonary fibrosis and sarcoidosis.

IDIOPATHIC PULMONARY FIBROSIS

Idiopathic pulmonary fibrosis (IPF) is characterized by scar tissue in the connective tissue of the lungs as a sequel to inflammation or irritation. A common risk factor for IPF is environmental or occupational inhalation of organic and inorganic substances (see discussion earlier in this chapter). Other risk factors include cigarette smoking and history of chronic aspiration. There also may be genetic risk factors.

Clinical manifestations of IPF include exertional dyspnea, nonproductive cough, and inspirational crackles with or without clubbing. High-resolution CT scan is the most definitive diagnostic study. Chest radiographic studies show changes characteristic of IPF. Pulmonary function tests show a typical pattern characteristic of restrictive lung disease (see Table 30-21). Open lung biopsy using VATS may help to differentiate the specific pathology.

The clinical course is variable, with a 5-year survival rate of 30% to 50% after diagnosis. Treatment includes corticosteroids, cytotoxic agents (azathioprine [Imuran], cyclophosphamide [Procytox]), and antifibrotic agents (colchicine). However, there is no good evidence that any of these treatments improves survival or quality of life. Lung transplantation is an option that should be considered for those who meet the criteria. (Lung transplant-ation is discussed later in this chapter.)

SARCOIDOSIS

Sarcoidosis is a chronic, multisystem granulomatous disease of unknown cause that primarily affects the lungs. The disease may also involve skin, eyes, liver, kidney, heart, and lymph nodes. The disease is often acute or subacute and self-limiting, but in many individuals, it is chronic with remissions and exacerbations. Marked pulmonary fibrosis can be present with severe restrictive lung disease. Cor pulmonale and bronchiectasis can develop in the advanced stages.

Corticosteroids are the most commonly used drugs for the treatment of pulmonary sarcoidosis. A trial of methotrexate may be considered if the patient does not respond to or cannot tolerate corticosteroid therapy. If methotrexate is ineffective or not tol-erated, cyclophosphamide (Procytox) or azathioprine (Imuran) may be initiated (King, 2017). Nonsteroidal anti-inflammatory agents, such as ibuprofen (Motrin), may help decrease acute inflammation or relieve symptoms but are not a treatment of sarcoidosis. Disease progression is monitored by pulmonary function tests, chest radiographic studies, and CT scan.

VASCULAR LUNG DISORDERS

PULMONARY EDEMA

Pulmonary edema is an abnormal, life-threatening accumulation of fluid in the alveoli and the interstitial spaces of the lungs. It is a complication of various heart and lung diseases (Table 30-24) and is considered a medical emergency.

Normally, there is a balance between the hydrostatic and the oncotic pressures in the pulmonary capillaries. If the hydrostatic pressure increases or the colloid oncotic pressure decreases, the net effect will be fluid leaving the pulmonary capillaries and entering the interstitial space, an event referred to as *interstitial edema*. At this stage, the lymphatic system can usually drain away the excess fluid. If fluid continues to leak from the pulmonary capillaries, it will enter the alveoli, an event referred to as *alveolar edema*.

TABLE 30-24	**CAUSES OF PULMONARY EDEMA**

- Heart failure
- Overhydration with intravenous fluids
- Hypoalbuminemia: nephrotic syndrome, hepatic disease, nutritional disorders
- Altered capillary permeability of lungs: inhaled toxins, inflammation (e.g., pneumonia), severe hypoxia, near-drowning
- Malignancies of the lymph system
- Respiratory distress syndrome (e.g., oxygen toxicity)
- Unknown causes: neurogenic condition, opioid overdose, high altitude

Pulmonary edema interferes with gas exchange by causing an alteration in the diffusing pathway between the alveoli and the pulmonary capillaries. The most common cause of pulmonary edema is left-sided heart failure. (The clinical manifestations and management of pulmonary edema are described in Chapter 37.)

PULMONARY EMBOLISM

Etiology and Pathophysiology

Pulmonary embolism (PE) is the blockage of pulmonary arteries by a thrombus, fat or air embolus, or tumour tissue. The word *embolus* derives from a Greek word meaning "plug" or "stopper." Emboli are mobile clots that generally do not stop moving until they lodge at a narrowed part of the circulatory system. A PE consists of material that gains access to the venous system and then to the pulmonary circulation. The embolus travels with the blood flow through ever-smaller blood vessels until it lodges and obstructs perfusion of the alveoli (Figure 30-11). Because of higher blood flow, the lower lobes of the lung are commonly affected. PE is associated with a mortality rate of up to 30% in patients who are not treated. With diagnosis and anticoagulant therapy, the mortality rate is reduced to 6% to 8% (Hogg, Thomas, Mackway-Jones, et al., 2011). Most PEs arise from deep-vein thromboses (DVT) in the deep veins of the legs. *Venous thrombo-embolism* (VTE) is the preferred term to describe the spectrum of pathology from DVT to PE (see Table 40-7). Lethal PEs most commonly originate in the femoral or iliac veins. Generally, the VTEs that are below the knee have not been considered a risk factor for PE because they rarely migrate to the pulmonary circulation without first extending above the knee.

Other sites of origin of PE include the right side of the heart (especially with atrial fibrillation), the upper extremities (rare), and the pelvic veins (especially after surgery or childbirth). Upper-extremity VTE occasionally occurs in the presence of a central venous catheters or cardiac pacing wires. These cases may resolve with removal of the catheter. Thrombi in the deep veins can dislodge spontaneously. However, it is more common for mechanical forces (e.g., sudden standing) or changes in the rate of blood flow (e.g., those that occur with Valsalva manoeuvre) to dislodge the thrombus. The majority of patients with PE caused by VTE have no leg symptoms at the time of diagnosis (Thrombosis Canada, 2015). Less common causes of

FIGURE 30-11 Large embolus from the femoral vein lying in the main left and right pulmonary arteries. Source: From the teaching collection of the Department of Pathology, University of Texas Southwestern Medical School, Dallas.

PE include fat emboli (from fractured long bones), air emboli (from improperly administered IV therapy), bacterial vegetations, amniotic fluid, and tumours. Tumour emboli may originate from primary or metastatic malignancies. Risk factors for PE include immobility or reduced mobility, surgery within the past 3 months (especially pelvic and lower-extremity surgery, including hip and knee joint replacement), history of DVT, malignancy, obesity, oral contraceptives, hormone therapy, cigarette smoking, prolonged air travel, heart failure, pregnancy, and clotting disorders.

Clinical Manifestations

The signs and symptoms in PE are varied and nonspecific, making diagnosis difficult. The classic triad—dyspnea, chest pain, and hemoptysis—occurs in only about 20% of patients. Symptoms may begin slowly or suddenly. A mild to moderate hypoxemia with a low partial pressure of carbon dioxide in arterial blood ($PaCO_2$) is a common finding. Other manifestations are cough, pleuritic chest pain, hemoptysis, crackles, fever, accentuation of the pulmonic heart sound, and sudden change in mental status as a result of hypoxemia. Massive emboli may produce abrupt hypotension, pallor, severe dyspnea, and hypoxemia. Chest pain may or may not be present. ECG may indicate tachycardia and right ventricular strain. The mortality rate of people with symptomatic PEs is approximately 10% (Thrombosis Canada, 2015). Medium-sized emboli often cause pleuritic chest pain, dyspnea, slight fever, and a productive cough with blood-streaked sputum. A physical examination may reveal tachycardia and a pleural friction rub. Small emboli frequently are undetected or produce vague, transient symptoms. The exception to this is the patient with underlying cardiopulmonary disease. In these patients, even small or medium-sized emboli may result in severe cardiopulmonary compromise. However, repeated small emboli gradually cause a reduction in the capillary bed and eventual pulmonary hypertension. An ECG and chest radiograph may indicate right ventricular hypertrophy secondary to pulmonary hypertension.

Complications

Pulmonary infarction (death of lung tissue) is most likely when the following factors are present: (a) occlusion of a large or medium-sized pulmonary vessel (>2 mm in diameter), (b) insufficient collateral blood flow from the bronchial circulation, or (c) pre-existing lung disease. Infarction results in alveolar necrosis and hemorrhage. Occasionally, the necrotic tissue becomes infected, and an abscess may develop. Concomitant pleural effusion is frequent. *Pulmonary hypertension* results from hypoxemia or from involvement of more than 50% of the area of the normal pulmonary bed. As a single event, an embolus does not cause pulmonary hypertension unless it is massive. Recurrent emboli may result in chronic pulmonary hypertension.

Diagnostic Studies

A spiral (helical) CT scan is the most frequently used test to diagnose PE (see Table 30-25). An IV injection of contrast media is required to view the blood vessels. The scanner continuously rotates while obtaining slices and does not start and stop between each slice. This allows visualization of all anatomical regions of the lungs. The computer reconstructs the data to provide a three-dimensional picture and assist in emboli visualization. If a patient cannot have contrast media, a ventilation–perfusion (VQ) scan is done.

TABLE 30-25 COLLABORATIVE CARE

Acute Pulmonary Embolism

Diagnostic	Collaborative Therapy
• History and physical examination	• Supplemental oxygen, intubation may be necessary
• Chest radiographic study	• Fibrinolytic agent
• Continuous ECG monitoring	• Unfractionated heparin IV infusion
• ABGs	• Low-molecular-weight heparin (e.g., enoxaparin [Lovenox])
• Venous ultrasound	• Warfarin (Coumadin) for long-term therapy
• CBC count with WBC differential	• Monitoring of aPTT and INR levels
• Spiral (helical) CT scan	• Limited activity
• Ventilation–perfusion (VQ) scan	• Opioids for pain relief
• Lung scan	• Inferior vena cava filter
• D-dimer level	• Pulmonary embolectomy in life-threatening situation
• Troponin level, BNP level	
• Pulmonary angiography	

ABGs, arterial blood gases; *aPTT,* activated partial thromboplastin time; *BNP,* B-type natriuretic peptide; *CBC,* complete blood cell; *CT,* computed tomography; *ECG,* electrocardiogram; *INR,* international normalized ratio; *IV,* intravenous; *WBC,* white blood cell.

The VQ scan has two components and is most accurate when both are performed:

1. Perfusion scanning involves IV injection of a radioisotope. A scanning device images the pulmonary circulation.
2. Ventilation scanning involves inhalation of a radioactive gas such as xenon. Scanning reflects the distribution of gas through the lung. The ventilation component requires the cooperation of the patient and may be impossible to perform in a critically ill patient, particularly if the patient is intubated.

D-dimer is a laboratory test that measures the amount of cross-linked fibrin fragments. These fragments are found in the circulation after clotting events such as VTE, acute myocardial infarction, unstable angina, and acute stroke. This degradation product is rarely found in healthy individuals. The disadvantage of D-dimer is that it is neither specific (other conditions cause elevation) nor sensitive because up to 50% of patients with small PEs have normal results. Patients with suspected PE and an elevated D-dimer level but normal venous ultrasound may need a lung scan or spiral CT.

Pulmonary angiography is a sensitive and specific test for PE. However, it is an invasive procedure that involves the insertion of a catheter through the antecubital or femoral vein, advancement to the pulmonary artery, and injection of contrast medium. It allows visualization of the pulmonary vascular system and location of the embolus. However, with spiral CT, pulmonary angiography is now used less frequently.

ABG analysis is important, but not diagnostic. The partial pressure of oxygen in arterial blood (PaO_2) is low because of inadequate oxygenation secondary to an occluded pulmonary vasculature preventing matching of perfusion to ventilation. The pH remains normal unless respiratory alkalosis develops as a result of prolonged hyperventilation or to compensate for lactic acidosis caused by shock. Abnormal findings are usually reported on the chest radiograph (atelectasis, pleural effusion) and on the ECG (ST-segment and T-wave changes), but they are not diagnostic for PE. Serum troponin levels are elevated in 30% to 50% of patients with PE, and, although not diagnostic, they are predictive of an adverse prognosis. Serum B-type natriuretic peptide levels, although not diagnostic, may be helpful in identifying the severity of the clinical course.

Collaborative Care

Prevention of PE begins with prevention of VTE. VTE prophylaxis includes the use of sequential compression devices, early ambulation, and prophylactic use of anticoagulant medications. To reduce mortality risk, treatment is begun as soon as PE is suspected (see Table 30-25). The objectives are to (a) prevent further growth or multiplication of thrombi in the lower extremities, (b) prevent embolization from the upper or lower extremities to the pulmonary vascular system, and (c) provide cardiopulmonary support if indicated.

Supportive therapy for the patient's cardiopulmonary status varies according to the severity of the PE. The administration of supplemental O_2 by mask or cannula is adequate for some patients. Oxygen is given in a concentration determined by ABG analysis. In some situations, endotracheal intubation and mechanical ventilation are necessary to maintain adequate oxygenation. Respiratory measures such as turning, coughing, deep breathing, and incentive spirometry are important to help prevent or treat atelectasis. If symptoms of shock are present, IV fluids are administered followed by vasopressor agents as needed to support perfusion (see Chapter 69). If heart failure is present, diuretics are used. (Heart failure is discussed in Chapter 37.) Pain resulting from pleural irritation or reduced coronary blood flow is treated with opioids, usually morphine.

Drug Therapy. Fibrinolytic drugs, such as tissue plasminogen activator (tPA) or alteplase (Activase), dissolve the PE and the source of the thrombus in the pelvis or deep leg veins, thereby decreasing the likelihood of recurrent emboli. Indications for thrombolytic therapy in PE include hemodynamic instability and right ventricular dysfunction. (Thrombolytic therapy is discussed in Chapter 40; see Table 40-10.) Because most deaths are caused by recurrent PEs, treatment should begin immediately. Properly managed anticoagulant therapy is effective in the prevention of further emboli. Heparin works to prevent future clots but does not dissolve existing clots. Although unfractionated heparin IV has traditionally been used, low-molecular-weight heparin (e.g., enoxaparin [Lovenox]) is becoming more common. Warfarin (Coumadin) should be initiated within the first 24 hours and is typically administered for 3 to 6 months. Some health care providers use Factor Xa inhibitors and direct thrombin inhibitors in the treatment of PEs. The dosage of heparin is adjusted according to the activated partial thromboplastin time (aPTT), and the dosage of warfarin is determined by the international normalized ratio (INR).

Frequent changes and titrations of heparin doses are needed initially in order to obtain a therapeutic aPTT level. Anticoagulant therapy may be contraindicated if the patient has complicating factors such as blood dyscrasias, hepatic dysfunction causing alteration in the clotting mechanism, injury to the intestine, overt bleeding, a history of hemorrhagic stroke, or neurological conditions.

Surgical Therapy. If the degree of pulmonary arterial obstruction is severe and the patient does not respond to conservative therapy, an immediate embolectomy may be indicated. Pulmonary embolectomy, a rare procedure, has a 50% mortality rate. Preoperative pulmonary angiography is necessary to identify and locate the site of the embolus. When a pulmonary embolectomy is performed, the patient also has placement of a vena cava filter. To prevent further emboli, an inferior vena cava filter may be the treatment of choice in patients who remain at high risk and for patients for whom anticoagulation is contraindicated. This device is placed at the level of the diaphragm in the inferior vena cava via the femoral vein. It prevents migration of large clots into the pulmonary system. Research has shown complications associated with this device include recurrent VTEs and post-thrombotic syndrome, in addition to misplacement, migration, and perforation (Sheares, 2011).

NURSING MANAGEMENT PULMONARY EMBOLISM

NURSING IMPLEMENTATION

HEALTH PROMOTION. Nursing measures aimed at prevention of PEs are similar to those for prophylaxis of VTEs (Association of Perioperative Registered Nurses, 2007; see the discussion of venous thrombosis in Chapter 40).

ACUTE INTERVENTION. The prognosis of a patient with PE is good if therapy is promptly instituted. The patient should be kept on bed rest in a semi-Fowler's position to facilitate breathing. An IV line should be maintained for medications and fluid therapy. The nurse should know the adverse effects of medications and observe for them. Oxygen therapy should be administered as ordered. Careful monitoring of vital signs, cardiac dysrhythmia, pulse oximetry, ABGs, and lung sounds is critical to assess the patient's status. Laboratory results should be monitored to ensure normal ranges of aPTT and INR. Nursing care includes assessing for the complications of anticoagulant therapy (e.g., bleeding, hematomas, bruising) and for PEs (e.g., hypoxia, hypotension). The nurse should perform appropriate interventions related to immobility and fall precautions. Patients are usually anxious because of pain, a sense of doom, inability to breathe, and fear of death. Explaining the situation and providing emotional support and reassurance can help relieve this anxiety.

AMBULATORY AND HOME CARE. The patient affected by thromboembolic processes may require emotional support. In addition, some patients may have an underlying chronic illness requiring long-term treatment. To provide supportive therapy, the nurse must understand and differentiate between the various problems caused by the underlying disease and those related to thrombo-embolic disease. Patient teaching regarding long-term anticoagulant therapy is critical.

Anticoagulant therapy continues for at least 3 to 6 months; patients with recurrent emboli are treated indefinitely. INR levels are drawn at intervals and warfarin dosage is adjusted. Some patients are monitored by nurses in an anticoagulation clinic. Long-term management is similar to that for the patient with VTE (see the discussion of VTE in Chapter 40). Discharge planning is aimed at limiting progression of the condition and preventing complications and recurrence. The need for the patient to return to the health care provider for regular follow-up examinations should be reinforced.

EVALUATION

The expected outcomes are that the patient who has a PE will have:

- Adequate tissue perfusion and respiratory function
- Adequate cardiac output
- Increased level of comfort
- No recurrence of PE

PULMONARY HYPERTENSION

Pulmonary hypertension comprises a variety of disorders occurring as a primary disease (primary pulmonary hypertension) or as a complication of a large number of respiratory and cardiac disorders (secondary pulmonary hypertension). Pulmonary hypertension is elevated pulmonary pressure resulting from an increase in pulmonary vascular resistance to blood flow through small arteries and arterioles.

PRIMARY PULMONARY HYPERTENSION

Primary pulmonary hypertension (PPH) is a rare, severe, and progressive disease. PPH is characterized by mean pulmonary arterial pressure greater than 25 mm Hg at rest or greater than 30 mm Hg with exercise, in the absence of a demonstrable cause. PPH is associated with a poor prognosis because there is no definitive therapy.

Etiology and Pathophysiology

The exact etiology of PPH is unknown. PPH has been linked to the use of fenfluramine in the drug Fen-Phen, which was used as an appetite suppressant to treat obesity. The drug was withdrawn from the market in 1996. PPH affects more women than men. It may have a genetic component because the incidence is higher in families. It is a rare and potentially fatal disease; the mean age at diagnosis is 36 years.

Normally, the pulmonary circulation is characterized by low resistance and low pressure. In pulmonary hypertension, the pulmonary pressures are elevated. Until recently, the pathophysiology of PPH was poorly understood. Recently, it was discovered that a key mechanism involved in PPH is a deficient release of vasodilator mediators from the pulmonary epithelium with a resultant cascade of injury (Figure 30-12).

Clinical Manifestations

Classic symptoms of pulmonary hypertension are dyspnea on exertion and fatigue. Exertional chest pain, dizziness, and exertional syncope are other symptoms. These symptoms are related to the inability of cardiac output to increase in response to increased oxygen demand. Eventually, as the disease progresses, dyspnea occurs at rest. Pulmonary hypertension increases the workload of the right ventricle and causes right ventricular hypertrophy (a condition called *cor pulmonale*) and eventually heart failure. A chest radiograph generally shows enlarged central pulmonary arteries and clear lung fields. A heart enlarged on the right may be seen. Echocardiogram usually reveals right ventricular hypertrophy.

Collaborative Care

Diagnostic evaluation includes ECG, chest radiographic study, and echocardiogram. CT and cardiac catheterization to measure pulmonary artery pressures can be used. Additional tests may be done to exclude secondary factors. Early recognition of pulmonary hypertension is essential to interrupt the self-perpetuation cycle responsible for the progression of this problem (see Figure 30-12). The mean time between onset of symptoms and diagnosis is 2 years. By the time patients become symptomatic, the disease is already in the advanced stages and the size of pulmonary artery pressure is two to three times normal.

Although there is no cure for PPH, treatment can relieve symptoms, improve quality of life, and prolong life. Diuretic therapy relieves dyspnea and peripheral edema and may be useful in reducing right ventricular volume overload. Anticoagulation therapy is recommended for patients with severe pulmonary hypertension to prevent in situ thrombus formation and venous thrombosis.

PATHOPHYSIOLOGY MAP

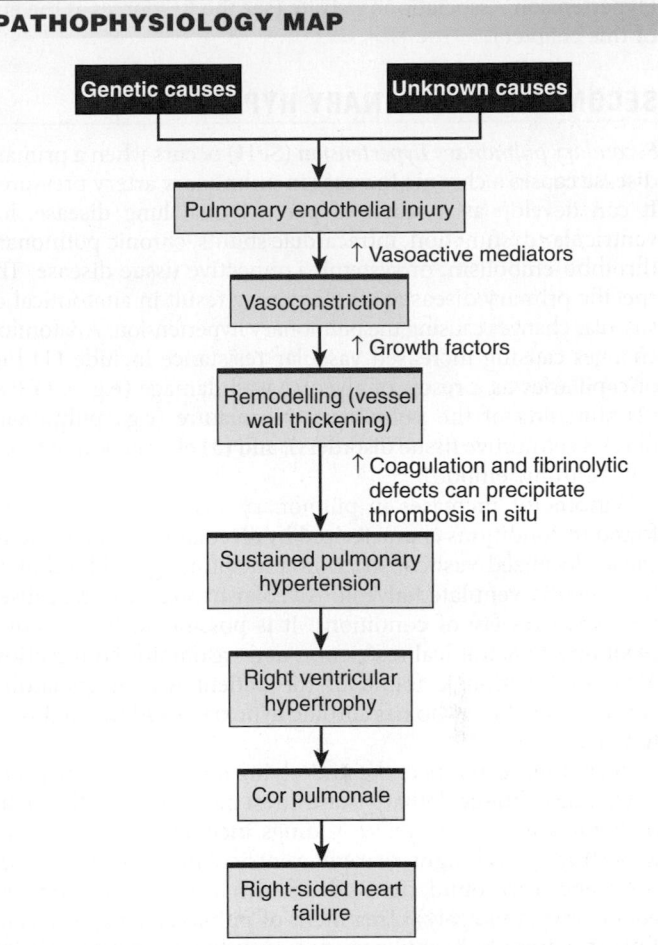

FIGURE 30-12 Pathogenesis of pulmonary hypertension and cor pulmonale.

Vasodilator therapy is used to reduce right ventricular overload by dilating pulmonary vessels and reversing remodelling. Many patients with pulmonary hypertension can be effectively managed with calcium channel blocker therapy, such as nifedipine (Adalat) and diltiazem (Cardizem).

Synthetic prostacyclins promote pulmonary vasodilation and reduce pulmonary vascular resistance and have revolutionized the management of PPH. They are now the treatment of choice for select patients unresponsive to calcium channel blockers. They can be administered orally (e.g., bosentan), subcutaneously (e.g., treprostinil), or intravenously (e.g., epoprostenol). Aerosolized forms are not yet available in Canada.

Bosentan (Tracleer) is an oral form of prostacyclin used to treat PPH. It is an active endothelin receptor antagonist. This medication works by blocking the hormone endothelin, which causes blood vessels to constrict. Treprostinil (Remodulin), a prostacyclin, is used as a continuous subcutaneous injection. It causes vasodilation of the pulmonary arterial system and inhibits platelet aggregation.

Surgical interventions include atrial septostomy, pulmonary thromboendarterectomy, and lung transplantation (Stamm, Risbano, & Mathier, 2011). Lung transplantation is the mainstay of treatment for those patients who do not respond to prostacyclins and progress to severe right-sided heart failure. Recurrence of the disease has not been reported in individuals who have undergone transplantation. A patient education and support site for pulmonary hypertension is located on the Pulmonary

Hypertension Association's website (see the Resources at the end of this chapter).

SECONDARY PULMONARY HYPERTENSION

Secondary pulmonary hypertension (SPH) occurs when a primary disease causes a chronic increase in pulmonary artery pressures. It can develop as a result of parenchymal lung disease, left ventricular dysfunction, intracardiac shunts, chronic pulmonary thrombo-embolism, or systemic connective tissue disease. The specific primary disease pathology may result in anatomical or vascular changes causing the pulmonary hypertension. Anatomical changes causing increased vascular resistance include (1) loss of capillaries as a result of alveolar wall damage (e.g., COPD), (2) stiffening of the pulmonary vasculature (e.g., pulmonary fibrosis connective tissue disorders), and (3) obstruction of blood flow (chronic emboli).

Vasomotor increases in pulmonary vascular resistance are found in conditions characterized by alveolar hypoxia. Hypoxia causes localized vasoconstriction and shunting of blood away from poorly ventilated alveoli. Alveolar hypoxia can be caused by a wide variety of conditions. It is possible to have a combination of anatomical restriction and vasomotor constriction. This combination is found in the patient with longstanding chronic bronchitis who has chronic hypoxia in addition to loss of lung tissue.

Symptoms can reflect the underlying disease, but some, such as dyspnea, fatigue, lethargy, and chest pain, are directly attributable to the SPH. Physical findings include right ventricular hypertrophy and signs of right ventricular failure (increased pulmonic heart sound, right-sided fourth heart sound, peripheral edema, hepatomegaly). Treatment of pulmonary hypertension caused primarily by pulmonary or cardiac disorders consists mainly of treating the underlying disorder. Treatment of SPH is similar to treatment of PPH.

COR PULMONALE

Cor pulmonale is a hypertrophy of the right side of the heart, with or without heart failure, resulting from pulmonary hypertension. Diseases of the lung or thorax or changes in pulmonary circulation can lead to pulmonary hypertension. Pulmonary hypertension is usually a pre-existing condition in the individual with cor pulmonale. Cor pulmonale may be present with or without overt cardiac failure. The most common cause of cor pulmonale is COPD; however, almost any disorder that affects the respiratory system can cause cor pulmonale. The etiology and pathogenesis of pulmonary hypertension and cor pulmonale are outlined in Figure 30-12.

Clinical Manifestations

Clinical manifestations of cor pulmonale include dyspnea, chronic productive cough, wheezing respirations, retrosternal or substernal pain, and fatigue. Chronic hypoxemia leads to polycythemia and increased total blood volume and viscosity of the blood. (Polycythemia is often present in cor pulmonale secondary to COPD.) Compensatory mechanisms that are secondary to hypoxemia can aggravate the pulmonary hypertension. Episodes of cor pulmonale in a person with underlying chronic respiratory problems are frequently triggered by an acute respiratory tract infection.

If heart failure accompanies cor pulmonale, additional manifestations such as peripheral edema; weight gain; distended neck

TABLE 30-26 COLLABORATIVE CARE

Cor Pulmonale

Diagnostic	Collaborative Therapy
• History and physical examination	• O₂ therapy
• ABGs	• Bronchodilators
• Serum and urine electrolytes	• Diuretics
• Monitoring with ECG	• Low-sodium diet
• Chest radiographic study	• Fluid restriction
	• Antibiotics (if indicated)
	• Digitalis (if left-sided heart failure)
	• Vasodilators (if indicated)
	• Calcium channel blockers (if indicated)

ABGs, arterial blood gases; *ECG,* electrocardiogram; *O₂,* oxygen.

TABLE 30-27 INDICATIONS FOR LUNG TRANSPLANTATION

- α₁-Antitrypsin deficiency
- Bronchiectasis
- Cystic fibrosis
- Emphysema
- Idiopathic pulmonary fibrosis
- Interstitial lung disease
- Pulmonary fibrosis secondary to other diseases (e.g., sarcoidosis)
- Pulmonary hypertension

veins; full, bounding pulse; and enlarged liver will also be found. (Heart failure is discussed in Chapter 37.) A chest radiograph will show an enlarged right ventricle and pulmonary artery.

Collaborative Care

The primary management of cor pulmonale is directed at treating the underlying pulmonary problem that precipitated the heart problem (Table 30-26). Long-term low-flow O₂ therapy is used to correct the hypoxemia and reduce vasoconstriction in chronic states of respiratory disorders. If fluid, electrolyte, and acid–base imbalances are present, they must be corrected. Diuretics and a low-sodium diet will help decrease the plasma volume and the load on the heart. Bronchodilator therapy is indicated if the underlying respiratory problem is caused by an obstructive disorder. Digitalis may be used if there is left-sided heart failure. Other treatments include those for pulmonary hypertension and comprise vasodilator therapy, calcium channel blockers, and anticoagulants. Theophylline may help because of its weak inotropic effect on the heart. When medical treatment fails, lung transplantation is an option for some patients.

Management of cor pulmonale resulting from COPD is similar to that described for COPD (see Chapter 31). Continuous low-flow O₂ during sleep; exercise; and small, frequent meals may allow the patient to feel better and be more active.

LUNG TRANSPLANTATION

Lung transplantation has evolved as a viable therapy for patients with end-stage lung disease. A variety of pulmonary disorders are potentially treatable with some type of lung transplantation (Table 30-27). Improved selection criteria, technical advances, and better methods of immuno-suppression have resulted in improved survival rates. Various transplant options are available, including single-lung transplant, bilateral-lung transplant, heart–lung transplant, and transplantation of lobes from a living related donor.

Patients being considered for a lung transplant need to undergo extensive evaluation. The candidate for lung transplantation should not have a malignancy or recent history of malignancy (within the past 2 years), renal or liver insufficiency, or HIV. The typical wait for a lung transplant is longer than 1 year. The candidate and the family undergo psychological screening to determine the ability to cope with a postoperative regimen that requires strict adherence to immuno-suppressive therapy, continuous monitoring for early signs of infection, and prompt reporting of manifestations of infection for medical evaluation.

Postoperative care includes ventilatory support, pulmonary clearance measures (bronchodilators, chest physiotherapy, and deep breathing and coughing), fluid and hemodynamic management, immuno-suppression, detection of early rejection, and prevention or treatment of infection. Infection is the leading cause of morbidity and mortality. Gram-negative bacterial pneumonia is common. Viral infection with CMV and herpes simplex occur frequently. CMV is a leading cause of mortality, which, if it is going to occur, usually happens 4 to 8 weeks after surgery. Fungal infections are also seen. Empirical antibiotic regimen is routine perioperatively for potential pathogens isolated from donor or recipient.

Immuno-suppressive therapy usually includes a triple-drug regimen of cyclosporine, azathioprine (Imuran), and prednisone. Immuno-suppressive drugs are discussed in Chapter 16 and Table 16-16.

Acute rejection can be seen as soon as 5 to 7 days after surgery. It is characterized by low-grade fever, fatigue, and oxygen desaturation with exercise. Accurate diagnosis is by transtracheal biopsy. Treatment with bolus corticosteroids results in remission of symptoms.

Bronchiolitis obliterans (an obstructive airway disease causing progressive occlusion) is considered to represent chronic rejection in lung transplant patients. The onset is often subacute, with gradual, progressive obstructive airflow defect, including cough, dyspnea, and recurrent lower respiratory tract infection. Treatment involves optimum maintenance immuno-suppression.

Discharge planning begins in the preoperative phase. Patients are placed in an outpatient rehabilitation program to improve physical endurance. The use of home spirometry has been useful in monitoring trends in lung function. Patients are taught to keep logs of medications, laboratory results, and spirometry. Patients need to be able to perform self-care activities, including medication management and ability to identify when to call the physician. Over the past decade, lung transplantation has become an increasingly important mode of therapy for patients with a variety of end-stage lung diseases.

CASE STUDY

Pneumonia and Lung Cancer

Source: Shutterstock.com.

Patient Profile
Jacob Hillen is a 52-year-old man who comes to the emergency department complaining of shortness of breath. He has not seen a health care provider for many years.

Subjective Data
- Has a 38 pack-year history of cigarette smoking
- States he has always been slender but has had 11 kg weight loss despite a normal appetite in the past few months
- Admits to a "smoker's cough" for the past 2 to 3 years; recently coughing up blood
- Is married and the father of three adult children

Objective Data
Physical Examination
- Thin, pale man, looking older than stated age
- Height 182 cm; weight 61.2 kg
- Intermittently confused and anxious with rapid shallow respirations
- Vital signs: temperature 39.2°C, heart rate 120, respiratory rate 36
- Chest wall has limited excursion on right side; auscultation of left side reveals coarse crackles but clear with cough; right side has diminished breath sounds

Diagnostic Studies
- Arterial blood gases: pH 7.51, PaO$_2$ 58 mm Hg, PaCO$_2$ 30 mm Hg, HCO$_3^-$ 22 mmol/L, O$_2$ saturation 84% (room air)
- Chest radiograph: consolidation of the right lung, especially in the base with possible mass in the area of right bronchus; pleural effusion on the right side
- Bronchoscopy with biopsy of mass: small cell lung carcinoma

Collaborative Care
- Diagnosis: pneumonia with small cell lung cancer
- Follow-up with patient and family to consider treatment options

Discussion Questions
1. How would Mr. Hillen's pneumonia be classified? Why is classification important?
2. What would the nurse's analysis of Mr. Hillen's arterial blood gas results be?
3. *Priority decision:* Based on the assessment data presented, what are the priority nursing diagnoses? Are there any collaborative problems?
4. *Priority decision:* What are the priority nursing interventions for Mr. Hillen?
5. The nurse is planning a meeting with Mr. Hillen and his family to discuss their needs. The physician tells the nurse that Mr. Hillen is terminally ill. Who should be included in this meeting?
6. *Evidence-informed practice:* Mr. Hillen's children tell the nurse that they are worried they will get lung cancer because their father has it and they grew up around his second-hand smoke. They want to know what kind of screening is available for them. How should the nurse respond?
7. What is the goal if radiation therapy is used for Mr. Hillen?
8. What issues should be addressed in the nurse's teaching of Mr. Hillen and his wife as he is prepared for discharge and care at home?

⊝volve
Answers are available at *http://evolve.elsevier.com/Canada/Lewis/medsurg*

REVIEW QUESTIONS

The number of the question corresponds to the same-numbered objective at the beginning of the chapter.

1. What clinical manifestations should the nurse expect when assessing a client with pneumococcal pneumonia?
   a. Fever, chills, and a productive cough with purulent sputum
   b. Nonproductive cough and night sweats that are usually self-limiting
   c. Gradual onset of nasal stuffiness, sore throat, and purulent productive cough
   d. Abrupt onset of fever, nonproductive cough, and formation of lung abscesses

2. A client with pneumonia has the nursing diagnosis of *ineffective airway clearance* related to *excessive mucus and retained secretions*. What would be an appropriate nursing intervention?
   a. Promote fluid hydration, as appropriate, to help liquefy secretions.
   b. Provide analgesics as ordered to promote client comfort.
   c. Administer oxygen as prescribed to maintain optimal oxygen levels.
   d. Teach the client how to cough effectively to bring secretions to the mouth.

3. A client with tuberculosis (TB) has a history of nonadherence to the medication regimen. What is the most common cause of this behaviour in clients with TB?
   a. Fatigue and lack of energy to manage self-care
   b. Lack of knowledge about how the disease is transmitted
   c. Lack of social support systems for the client and family
   d. Feelings of shame and the response to the social stigma associated with TB

4. A client has been receiving high-dose corticosteroids and broad-spectrum antibiotics for treatment of serious trauma and infection. Which of the following infections is the client most susceptible to?
   a. Aspergillosis
   b. Candidiasis
   c. Coccidioidomycosis
   d. Histoplasmosis

5. Which of the following statements best describes the treatment of lung abscess?
   a. It is best treated with surgical excision and drainage.
   b. Antibiotics for a prolonged period is the treatment of choice.
   c. Abscesses are difficult to treat and usually result in pulmonary fibrosis.
   d. Penicillin can effectively eradicate anaerobic organisms.

6. What is a common complication of many types of environmental lung diseases?
   a. Benign tumour growth
   b. Diffuse airway obstruction
   c. Liquefactive necrosis
   d. Pulmonary fibrosis

7. What type of lung cancer is generally associated with the best prognosis because it is potentially surgically resectable?
   a. Adenocarcinoma
   b. Small cell carcinoma
   c. Squamous cell carcinoma
   d. Undifferentiated large cell carcinoma

8. How does the nurse identify in a client a flail chest caused by trauma?
   a. Multiple rib fractures are determined by radiographic study.
   b. Tracheal deviation to the unaffected side is present.
   c. Paradoxical chest movement occurs during respiration.
   d. Decreased movement of the involved chest wall is apparent.

9. The nurse notes tidalling of the water level in the tube submerged in the water-seal chamber in a client with closed chest tube drainage. What should the nurse do?
   a. Continue to monitor this normal finding.
   b. Check all connections for a leak in the system.
   c. Lower the drainage collector further from the chest.
   d. Clamp the tubing at progressively more distal points from the client until the tidalling stops.

10. Which nursing measure should be instituted after a pneumonectomy?
    a. Monitor chest tube drainage and functioning.
    b. Position the client on the operative side or the back.
    c. Perform range-of-motion exercises on the affected upper extremity.
    d. Auscultate frequently for lung sounds on the affected side.

11. What is the cause of respiratory problems in clients with Guillain-Barré syndrome?
    a. Central nervous system depression
    b. Deformed chest-wall muscles
    c. Paralysis of the diaphragm secondary to trauma
    d. Interruption of nerve transmission to respiratory muscles

12. A client with chronic obstructive pulmonary disease asks why the heart is affected by the respiratory disease. Which of the following statements regarding cor pulmonale is the basis for the nurse's response to the client?
    a. Pulmonary congestion secondary to left ventricular failure
    b. Excess serous fluid collection in the alveoli caused by retained respiratory secretions
    c. Right ventricular hypertrophy secondary to increased pulmonary vascular resistance
    d. Right ventricular failure secondary to compression of the heart by hyperinflated lungs

13. Which statement(s) describe(s) the management of a client following lung transplantation? *(Select all that apply)*
    a. High doses of oxygen are administered around the clock.
    b. The use of a home spirometer will help to monitor lung function.
    c. Immuno-suppressant therapy usually involves a three-drug regimen.
    d. Most clients experience an acute rejection episode in the first 2 days.
    e. The lung is biopsied using a transtracheal method if rejection is suspected.

1. a; 2. a; 3. d; 4. b; 5. b; 6. d; 7. c; 8. c; 9. a; 10. b; 11. d; 12. c; 13. b, c, e.

ⓔvolve

For even more review questions, visit *http://evolve.elsevier.com/Canada/Lewis/medsurg*.

REFERENCES

Assembly of First Nations. (2011). *Fact sheet: Quality of life of First Nations*. Retrieved from *http://www.afn.ca/uploads/files/factsheets/ quality_of_life_final_fe.pdf*.

Association of Perioperative Registered Nurses. (2007). Guideline for prevention of venous stasis. *AORN Journal, 85*(3), 607–614, 616–624. doi:10.1016/S0001-2092(07)60131-8. (Seminal).

Canadian Cancer Society. (2012). *Canadian Cancer Society announces new Health Canada–funded smoking cessation campaign aimed at young adults*. Retrieved from *http://www .cancer.ca/en/about-us/for-media/media-releases/ontario/2012/ canadian-cancer-society-announces-new-health-canada-funded -smoking-cessation-campaign/?region=on*.

Canadian Cancer Society. (2017a). *Risk factors for lung cancer*. Retrieved from *http://www.cancer.ca/en/cancer-information/cancer -type/lung/risks/?region=on*.

Canadian Cancer Society. (2017b). *Lung cancer: Malignant tumours of the lung*. Retrieved from *http://www.cancer.ca/en/cancer -information/cancer-type/lung/lung-cancer/non-small-cell-lung -cancer/?region=ab*.

Canadian Cancer Society's Advisory Committee on Cancer Statistics. (2017). *Canadian cancer statistics 2017*. Toronto: Canadian Cancer Society. Retrieved from *http://www.cancer.ca/~/media/cancer.ca/ CW/cancer%20information/cancer%20101/Canadian%20cancer %20statistics/Canadian-Cancer-Statistics-2017-EN.pdf?la=en*.

Canadian Centre for Occupational Health and Safety. (2013). *OSH Answers fact sheets: Asthma, work related*. Retrieved from *http:// www.ccohs.ca/oshanswers/diseases/asthma.html*.

Canadian Institute for Health Information. (2015). *Reasons for inpatient hospitalization and surgery vary across Canada*. Retrieved from *https://www.cihi.ca/en/summ_inpatient_hosp _en.pdf*.

Canadian Lung Association. (2015). *Tuberculosis*. Retrieved from *https://www.lung.ca/lung-health/lung-disease/tuberculosis*.

Canadian Lung Association. (2016a). *Smoking & tobacco: Benefits of quitting smoking*. Retrieved from *https://www.lung.ca/lung-health/ smoking-and-tobacco/benefits-quitting*.

Canadian Lung Association. (2016b). *Smoking and tobacco*. Retrieved from *https://www.lung.ca/lung-health/smoking-and-tobacco*.

Canadian Task Force on Preventive Health Care. (2016). Recommendations on screening for lung cancer. *Canadian Medical Association Journal, 188*(6), 425–432. doi:10.1503/cmaj.151421.

Canadian Tobacco, Alcohol and Drugs Survey (CTADS). (2013). *Summary of results for 2013*. Retrieved from *http:// healthycanadians.gc.ca/science-research-sciences-recherches/ data-donnees/ctads-ectad/summary-sommaire-2013-eng.php*.

Health Canada. (2014a). *On the road to quitting: Guide to becoming a non-smoker*. Retrieved from *http://healthycanadians.gc.ca/ publications/healthy-living-vie-saine/non-smoker-adult-non-fumeur -adulte/alt/non-smoker-adult-non-fumeur-adulte-eng.pdf*.

Health Canada. (2014b). *On the road to quitting: Guide to becoming a non-smoker for young adults*. Retrieved from *http:// healthycanadians.gc.ca/publications/healthy-living-vie-saine/ becoming-non-smoker-youth-guide-jeunes-devenir-non-fumeur/ index-eng.php*.

Health Quality Ontario and Ministry of Health and Long-Term Care. (2013). *Quality-based procedures clinical handbook for community-acquired pneumonia*. Retrieved from *http://www .health.gov.on.ca/en/pro/programs/ecfa/docs/qbp_pneumonia.pdf*.

Hogg, K., Thomas, D., Mackway-Jones, K., et al. (2011). Diagnosing pulmonary embolism: A comparison of clinical probability scores. *British Journal of Haematology, 153*(2), 253–258. doi:10.1111/j .1365-2141.2011.08575.x.

Human Resources and Skills Development Canada. (2012). *Information on occupational health and safety*. Retrieved from *http://www12.esdc.gc.ca/sgpe-pmps/servlet/sgpp-pmps-pub?lang=en g&curjsp=p.5bd.2t.1.3ls@-eng.jsp&curactn=dwnld&pid=4769&did=3*.

Infection Prevention and Control Canada. (n.d.). *Information about hand hygiene: Position statement*. Retrieved from *http://www.ipac -canada.org/links_handhygiene.php*.

King, T. E. (2017). *Treatment of pulmonary sarcoidosis with glucocorticoids*. Retrieved from *http://www.uptodate.com/contents/ treatment-of-pulmonary-sarcoidosis-with-glucocorticoids*.

Light, R. W. (2011). Pleural controversy: Optimal chest tube size for drainage. *Respirology (Carlton, Vic.), 16*(2), 244–248. doi:10.1111/ j.1440-1843.2010.01913.

Mandell, L. A., Marrie, T. J., Grossman, R. F., et al. (2000). Summary of the Canadian guidelines for the initial management of community-acquired pneumonia: An evidence-based update by the Canadian Infectious Disease Society and the Canadian Thoracic Society. *Canadian Respiratory Journal, 7*(5), 371–382. doi:10.1086/313959. (Seminal).

Public Health Agency of Canada (PHAC). (2014). *Tuberculosis Prevention and Control in Canada: A Federal framework for action*. Retrieved from *http://www.phac-aspc.gc.ca/tbpc-latb/pubs/ tpc-pct/index-eng.php*.

Public Health Agency of Canada (PHAC). (2015). *Part 4—Active vaccines: Pneumococcal vaccines. Canadian immunization guide*. Retrieved from *http://www.phac-aspc.gc.ca/publicat/cig-gci/p04 -pneu-eng.php#approve*.

Public Health Agency of Canada (PHAC). (2016). *Reported influenza hospitalizations and deaths in Canada: 2011–12 to 2015–16 (data to April 30, 2016)*. Retrieved from *http://www.phac-aspc.gc.ca/ influenza/flu-stat-eng.php*.

Public Health Agency of Canada (PHAC) & Canadian Lung Association. (2014). *Canadian tuberculosis standards (7th ed.)*. Retrieved from *https://cts.lung.ca/sites/default/files/documents/ cts/Canadian%20Tuberculosis%20Standards_7th%20edition _Complete.pdf*.

Registered Nurses' Association of Ontario (RNAO) (2007). Integrating smoking cessation into daily nursing practice. In *Nursing best practice guidelines* (p. 32). Toronto: Author. Retrieved from *http://rnao.ca/bpg/guidelines/integrating-smoking-cessation -daily-nursing-practice*. (Seminal).

Rotstein, C., Evans, G., Born, A., et al. (2008). Clinical practice guidelines for hospital-acquired pneumonia and ventilator-associated pneumonia in adults. *The Canadian Journal of Infectious Diseases & Medical Microbiology, 19*(1), 19–53. doi:10.1155/2008/593289. (Seminal).

Rubin, B. K., & Williams, R. W. (2014). Aerosolized antibiotics for non-cystic fibrosis bronchiectasis. *Respiration; International Review of Thoracic Diseases, 88*, 177–184. doi:10.1159/000366000.

Sheares, K. K. (2011). How do I manage a patient with suspected acute pulmonary embolism? *Clinical Medicine, 11*(2), 156–159. doi:10.7861/clinmedicine.11-2-156.

Stamm, J., Risbano, M. G., & Mathier, M. A. (2011). Overview of current therapeutic approaches for pulmonary hypertension. *Pulmonary Circulation, 1*(2), 138–159. doi:10.4103/2045-8932 .83444.

Thrombosis Canada. (2015). *Pulmonary embolism (PE): Diagnosis*. Retrieved from *http://thrombosiscanada.ca/wp-content/uploads/ 2015/11/4A_Pulmonary-Embolism-Diagnosis-2015Oct26 -FINAL2.pdf*.

World Health Organization (WHO). (2014). *Companion handbook to the WHO guidelines for the programmatic management of drug-resistant tuberculosis.* Retrieved from *http://apps.who.int/iris/bitstream/10665/130918/1/9789241548809_eng.pdf?ua=1&ua=1.*

World Health Organization (WHO). (2017). *Cancer (Fact sheet No. 297).* Retrieved from *http://www.who.int/mediacentre/factsheets/fs297/en.*

RESOURCES

B.C. Cancer Agency
http://www.bccancer.bc.ca

Canadian Cancer Society
http://www.cancer.ca

Canadian Cancer Society Quit Smoking Guidelines
http://www.cancer.ca/en/support-and-services/support-services/quit-smoking/?region=on

Canadian Lung Association
http://www.lung.ca

Canadian Tuberculosis Standards (7th ed.)
http://www.phac-aspc.gc.ca/tbpc-latb/pubs/tb-canada-7/index-eng.php

Cancer Care Ontario
http://www.cancercare.on.ca

Cancer Care Ontario—Lung Cancer Evidence-Based Guidelines (PEBC)
https://www.cancercare.on.ca/toolbox/qualityguidelines

CancerControl Alberta
http://www.albertahealthservices.ca/cancer/cancer.aspx

Health Canada
http://www.hc-sc.gc.ca

Public Health Agency of Canada
http://www.phac-aspc.gc.ca

Statistics Canada
http://www.statcan.ca

Centers for Disease Control and Prevention, National Center for Health Statistics
http://www.cdc.gov/nchs/fastats

Centers for Disease Control and Prevention, Smoking & Tobacco Use
http://www.cdc.gov/tobacco

International Standards for Tuberculosis Care (ISTC)
http://www.who.int/tb/publications/2006/istc/en

National Cancer Institute
http://www.nci.nih.gov

Pulmonary Hypertension Association (PHA)
http://www.phassociation.org

For additional Internet resources, see the website for this book at *http://evolve.elsevier.com/Canada/Lewis/medsurg.*

Nursing Management
Obstructive Pulmonary Diseases

Written by: Susan Collazo
Adapted by: Kimberly Hellmer

⊝volve WEBSITE

http://evolve.elsevier.com/Canada/Lewis/medsurg

- Review Questions (Online Only)
- Key Points
- Answer Guidelines for Case Study
- Student Case Studies
  - Asthma
  - Cystic Fibrosis

- Customizable Nursing Care Plans
  - Asthma
  - Chronic Obstructive Pulmonary Disease
- Conceptual Care Map Creator
  - Conceptual Care Map for Textbook Case Study
- Audio Glossary
- Content Updates

LEARNING OBJECTIVES

1. Describe the etiology, pathophysiology, and clinical manifestations of asthma, and describe the collaborative care of patients with asthma.
2. Explain the nursing management of patients with asthma.
3. Describe the etiology, pathophysiology, and clinical manifestations of chronic obstructive pulmonary disease (COPD), and describe the collaborative care of patients with COPD.
4. Explain the effects of cigarette smoking on the lungs.
5. Explain the nursing management of patients with COPD.
6. Identify the indications for oxygen therapy, the methods of delivery, and the complications of oxygen administration.
7. Describe the etiology, pathophysiology, and clinical manifestations of cystic fibrosis, and explain the collaborative care of patients with cystic fibrosis.

KEY TERMS

absorption atelectasis, p. 676
α1-antitrypsin (AAT) deficiency, p. 665
asthma, p. 643

chest physiotherapy, p. 687
chronic bronchitis, p. 664
chronic obstructive pulmonary disease (COPD), p. 664

cor pulmonale, p. 668
cough variant asthma, p. 647
cystic fibrosis, p. 685
emphysema, p. 664

oxygen toxicity, p. 676
postural drainage, p. 687
pursed-lip breathing, p. 678

The prevalence of chronic lung disorders in Canada is an important population health concern. Current population health data indicate that the prevalence of asthma among children and youth aged 1 to 19 years is 15.7%; the prevalence of asthma among the population aged 20 years or older is 9.5%; and the prevalence of chronic obstructive pulmonary disease among the population aged 35 years or older is 9.7% (Public Health Agency of Canada [PHAC], 2015a). Among the total population, the rate of mortality due to chronic respiratory diseases is 43.8 per 100 000 (PHAC, 2015a).

Obstructive pulmonary diseases are the most common chronic lung diseases, which include conditions characterized by increased airflow resistance as a result of airway obstruction or narrowing. Airway obstruction may result from accumulated secretions, edema, inflammation of the airways, bronchospasm of smooth muscle, or destruction of lung tissue, or some combination. Asthma, chronic obstructive pulmonary disease (COPD), and cystic fibrosis are obstructive pulmonary diseases and are discussed in further depth in this chapter.

ASTHMA

Asthma is a chronic inflammatory disorder of the airways. Inflammation causes varying degrees of obstruction in the airways, which leads to recurrent episodes of wheezing, breathlessness, sensation of chest tightness, and cough, particularly at night and in the early morning. The hyper-responsiveness, or "twitchiness," of the airways is directly related to the degree of airway inflammation, in that the more airway inflammation present, the more hyper-responsive the airways are to endogenous or exogenous stimuli or triggers. Asthma occurs as a result of environmental (endogenous or exogenous) effects on the airways that trigger a series of events in the immune system of a genetically predisposed individual. These events lead to airway inflammation and bronchoconstriction (airway narrowing). A key characteristic of asthma is the episodic and reversible nature of the airway obstruction and its associated symptoms (cough, wheeze, sensation of chest tightness, dyspnea), so that an episode may resolve spontaneously or with treatment.

According to Statistics Canada (2015), more than 2.4 million (8.1%) of Canadians older than 12 years were living with asthma (9.2% of all female Canadians and 7.0% of all male Canadians). The morbidity associated with asthma is dramatic. The 2011 *Survey on Living with Chronic Diseases in Canada* identified 11.1% of Canadians with active asthma who reported a minimum of one visit to a hospital emergency room in the previous 12 months because of asthma symptoms (PHAC, 2011). Only one in three (34.4%) of Canadians with active asthma symptoms reported that their asthma was well-controlled (PHAC, 2011). In further investigation, 65.6% of respondents with active asthma were found to have at least one indicator of poorly controlled asthma (PHAC, 2011). The high rate of morbidity related to asthma may be attributed to practice that is inconsistent with the Canadian asthma consensus guidelines, inaccurate assessment of disease severity, a delay in seeking help, inadequate medical treatment, nonadherence to prescribed therapy, an increase in allergens in the environment, limited access to health care, and a lack of knowledge on the part of patients and health care providers.

Triggers of Asthma Attacks

Although the exact mechanisms that cause airway hyper-responsiveness and inflammation remain unknown, multiple stimuli or triggers are involved (Table 31-1, Figure 31-1). Numerous allergens, chemicals, and infectious pathogens can trigger airway inflammation, which leads to airway narrowing and appearance of symptoms. These triggers are discussed in the following sections.

Allergens. Some people with asthma have an exaggerated immunoglobulin E (IgE) response to certain allergens (e.g., dust, pollen, grasses, mites, roaches, moulds, animal dander, latex). These allergens attach to IgE receptors on mast cells (Figure 31-2). The IgE–mast cell complexes remain for a long time; thus a second exposure to the allergen triggers mast cell degranulation even years after the initial exposure to the allergen. Patients with allergic rhinitis or atopic dermatitis should be asked specifically about any incidence of respiratory symptoms (Global Initiative for Asthma [GINA], 2015). Allergic reactions are discussed further in Chapter 16.

Exercise. Acute airway narrowing that is induced or exacerbated during physical exertion is referred to as *exercise-induced*

PATHOPHYSIOLOGY MAP

FIGURE 31-1 Early- and late-phase responses of asthma. *IgE,* immunoglobulin E; *IL-4,* interleukin-4.

TABLE 31-1 TRIGGERS OF ASTHMA ATTACKS

Allergens
- Animal dander (e.g., from cats, dogs, horses, mice, guinea pigs)
- Household dust mites
- Cockroaches
- Pollens
- Moulds
- Air pollutants
- Diesel particulates
- Exhaust fumes
- Perfumes
- Ozone
- Sulphur dioxides
- Cigarette smoke
- Aerosol sprays

Viral upper respiratory infection
Sinusitis
Exercise
Cold, dry air
Stress

Hormones or menses
Gastro-esophageal reflux disease (GERD)

Drugs
- Acetylsalicylic acid (ASA; Aspirin)
- Nonsteroidal anti-inflammatory medications
- β-Adrenergic blockers

Occupational exposure
- Agriculture
- Metal salts
- Wood and vegetable dusts
- Industrial chemicals and plastics (isocyanates)
- Pharmaceutical drugs

Food additives
- Sulphites (bisulphites and metabisulphites) found in beer, wine, dried fruit, shrimp
- Monosodium glutamate
- Tartrazine

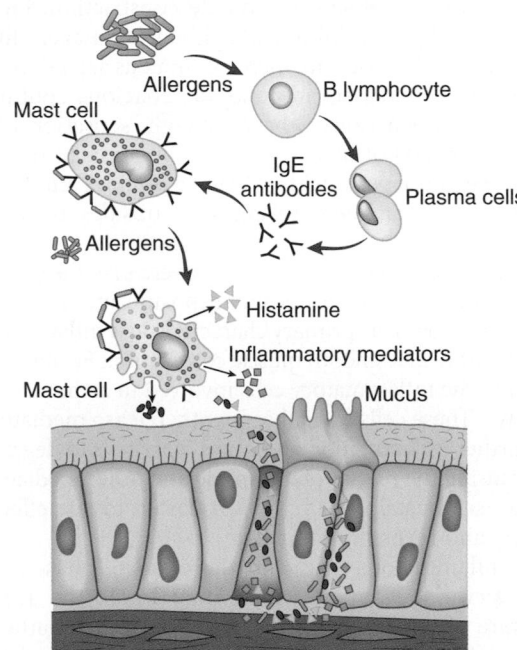

FIGURE 31-2 The early-phase response in asthma is triggered when an allergen or irritant attaches to immunoglobulin E (IgE) receptors on mast cells, which are then activated to release histamine and other inflammatory mediators.

asthma or *exercise-induced bronchospasm* (EIB). Although a substantial proportion of patients with an asthma diagnosis experience EIB, other people experience these symptoms but do not have a known diagnosis of asthma (Parsons et al., 2013). Typically, EIB occurs after, not during, vigorous exercise and is characterized by bronchospasm (airway smooth muscle contraction) that causes shortness of breath, cough, wheeze, sensation of chest tightness, or a combination of these. EIB is pronounced during activities

in cold, dry air. Airway hyper-responsiveness may result from changes in the airway mucosa caused by the hyperventilation that occurs during exercise with either the cooling or rewarming of air and capillary leakage in the airway wall.

Several strategies can be incorporated to prevent EIB: an adequate warm-up period before the activity begins; breathing through a scarf or mask during exercise in a cold or dry climate; and using inhaled short-acting β₂-adrenergic agonists either to relieve the symptoms or, 10 to 20 minutes before exercising, to ward off symptoms. Too frequent use of β₂-adrenergic agonists indicates poor asthma control, may mask asthma severity, and may cause a reduction in drug effectiveness. In such cases, patients may need escalation of therapy. (Control criteria and controller therapy are discussed further later in this chapter.) In the American Thoracic Society's clinical practice guideline for EIB, suggestions for the dietary modification are outlined for control of symptoms; these suggestions include low salt intake and dietary supplementation with fish oils and ascorbic acid (Parsons et al., 2013).

Respiratory Infections. Respiratory infections (particularly viral) are among the most common triggers of worsening asthma. Infections cause increased inflammation in the tracheo-bronchial system, resulting in increased airway hyper-responsiveness, which can last from 2 to 8 weeks after infection both in individuals with asthma and in those without asthma. Patients with asthma should take steps to reduce the possibility of infections by using proper handwashing techniques and receiving an annual influenza vaccination. Influenza vaccines are recommended for patients with asthma aged 6 months and older, especially because of the prevalence of high-risk influenza-related complications in patients with asthma (PHAC, 2015b).

Nose and Sinus Problems. Some patients with asthma have chronic sinus and nasal problems. Nasal problems include allergic rhinitis, either seasonal or perennial, and nasal polyps. Sinus problems are usually related to inflammation of the mucous membranes, most commonly from noninfectious causes such as allergies. However, bacterial sinusitis may also occur. It is important to treat these comorbid conditions because they often contribute to poor asthma control (Ducharme, Dell, Radhakrishnan, et al., 2015). (Sinusitis is discussed further in Chapter 29.)

Drugs and Food Additives. Some patients with asthma, especially those with nasal polyps, may have sensitivity to specific drugs. Some people with asthma have what is termed the *asthma triad*: nasal polyps, asthma, and sensitivity to acetylsalicylic acid (ASA; Aspirin) and nonsteroidal anti-inflammatory drugs (NSAIDs). Salicylic acid can be found in many over-the-counter drugs and some foods, beverages, and flavourings. In some asthmatic patients, wheezing develops within 2 hours after they take ASA (Aspirin) or NSAIDs (e.g., ibuprofen [Motrin]). In addition, most affected patients have profound rhinorrhea, congestion, and tearing. Facial flushing, gastro-intestinal symptoms, and angioedema can also occur. Although sensitivity to salicylates persists for many years, the nature and severity of the reaction can change over time. Such patients should avoid ASA (Aspirin) and NSAIDs. However, patients with ASA (Aspirin) sensitivity can, under the care of an allergist, be desensitized by daily administration of the drug (Simon, Dazy, & Waldram, 2015). Such patients may be more likely to benefit from antileukotriene drugs.

β-Adrenergic blockers in oral form (e.g., metoprolol) or topical eye drops (e.g., timolol [Timoptic]) may trigger asthma episodes because they induce bronchospasm. Angiotensin-converting enzyme inhibitors (e.g., lisinopril) may induce cough in susceptible individuals, thus worsening asthma symptoms. Other irritants that may precipitate asthma symptoms in susceptible patients are tartrazine (yellow dye no. 5, found in many foods) and sulphites (e.g., sodium metabisulphite), widely used in the food and pharmaceutical industries as preservatives and sanitizing agents. Sulphites are commonly found in fruits, beer, and wine and are used extensively in salad bars to protect vegetables from oxidation.

These drugs and food additives are thought to interfere with metabolic pathways, which results in enhanced production of leukotrienes, some of which are potent bronchoconstrictors. The onset of a typical reaction occurs 15 minutes to 3 hours after ingestion and is marked by profuse rhinorrhea, often accompanied by nausea, vomiting, intestinal cramps, and diarrhea. An acute episode of asthma typically begins after the nasal symptoms appear. Pretreatment with corticosteroids does not prevent the reaction. Epinephrine and antihistamines given shortly after the onset of the asthma symptoms usually control the symptoms.

Gastro-esophageal Reflux Disease. The exact mechanism by which gastro-esophageal reflux disease (GERD) triggers asthma is unknown. It is postulated that reflux of stomach acid into the esophagus can be aspirated into the lungs, which causes reflex vagal stimulation and bronchoconstriction. Although GERD is involved primarily in nocturnal asthma, it can trigger daytime asthma as well. By monitoring esophageal pH and peak expiratory flow rate (PEFR) simultaneously, the examiner can determine whether GERD is the cause of the asthma symptoms. H_2-histamine blockers or proton pump inhibitors are given to ameliorate symptoms. (GERD is discussed further in Chapter 44.)

Air Pollutants. Various air pollutants, cigarette or wood smoke, vehicle exhaust, diesel particulate, elevated ozone levels, sulphur dioxide, and nitrogen dioxide can trigger asthma attacks. Ongoing studies are being done to better understand how chronic exposure to urban air pollution and "hotspots" of air pollution within Canadian cities affect people who work and live in these areas (Government of Canada, 2013). The Air Quality Health Index (AQHI) was developed by the Government of Canada (2015) as a tool to help alert the public of health risks posed by air pollution (Figure 31-3).

Emotional Stress. Asthma is not a psychosomatic disease. However, physiological stress that elicits emotional responses such as crying, laughing, anger, and fear can lead to hyperventilation and hypocapnia, which can cause airway narrowing (GINA, 2015). An asthma exacerbation can produce panic and anxiety, which are not unexpected emotions during this experience. Panic is a normal response to not being able to breathe. The extent to which psychological factors contribute to the induction and continuation of any given acute exacerbation is unknown, but it probably varies from patient to patient and in the same patient from episode to episode.

Pathophysiology

The hallmarks of asthma are airway inflammation and airway hyper-responsiveness. The degree of bronchoconstriction is related to the degrees of airway inflammation, airway hyper-responsiveness, and exposure to endogenous and exogenous triggers (e.g., infections, allergens, histamine, and other cell mediators). Exposure to allergens or irritants initiates an inflammatory cascade involving multiple cell types, mediators, and chemokines. Typically, there are two possible types of asthmatic responses to stimuli: an early-phase response and a late-phase response.

The early-phase response in asthma is characterized by bronchospasm (see Figure 31-1). This response is triggered when an allergen or irritant attaches to IgE receptors on mast cells found beneath the basement membrane of the bronchial wall (see Figure 31-2). The mast cells become activated, and, subsequently, granules are released and the phospholipids' cell membranes are disrupted. Both processes result in the release of inflammatory mediators, including histamine, bradykinin, leukotrienes, prostaglandins, platelet-activating factor, chemotactic factors, and cytokines (e.g., interleukin-4 and interleukin-5; GINA, 2015). A similar early-phase response process can occur with exercise. These mediators cause intense inflammation in association with bronchial smooth muscle constriction, increased vasodilation and permeability, and epithelial damage. Clinically, the effects are bronchospasm, increased mucus secretion, edema formation, and increased amounts of tenacious sputum (see Figure 31-1), which cause wheeze, cough, sensation of chest tightness, shortness of breath, or a combination of these. This immediate response peaks within 30 to 60 minutes after exposure to the trigger (e.g., allergen, irritant) and subsides in another 30 to 90 minutes.

The late-phase response can be more severe than the early-phase response. It peaks 5 to 12 hours after exposure and may last from several hours to days. Its primary characteristic is inflammation, as opposed to bronchial smooth muscle contraction. Eosinophils and neutrophils, the inflammatory cells involved in asthma, infiltrate the airways. These cells can subsequently release mediators that induce further inflammation and cause mast cells to degranulate, thereby causing the release of histamine and other mediators and initiating a self-sustaining cycle. Corticosteroids are effective in preventing and reversing this cycle.

These inflammatory characteristics of a late-phase response increase airway reactivity, which may lower the threshold of exposure necessary to induce a future asthma attack and cause its symptoms to worsen. The affected person becomes hyper-responsive to allergens and nonspecific stimuli such as air pollution, cold air, and dust. In summary, prominent pathophysiological features of asthma are a reduction in airway

| 1 | 2 | 3 | 4 | 5 | 6 | 7 | 8 | 9 | 10 | ✚ |

| Low (1–3) | | Moderate (4–6) | | | High (7–10) | | | Very high (Above 10) |

FIGURE 31-3 The Air Quality Health Index (AQHI) is measured on a scale ranging from 1 to 10+. The AQHI index values are also grouped into health risk categories: 1 to 3 indicates low risk; 4 to 6, moderate risk; 7 to 10, high risk; and 10+, very high risk. These categories help patients easily and quickly identify their level of risk. Source: © All rights reserved. *The Air Quality Health Index.* Health Canada, 2015. Adapted and reproduced with permission from the Minister of Health, 2017.

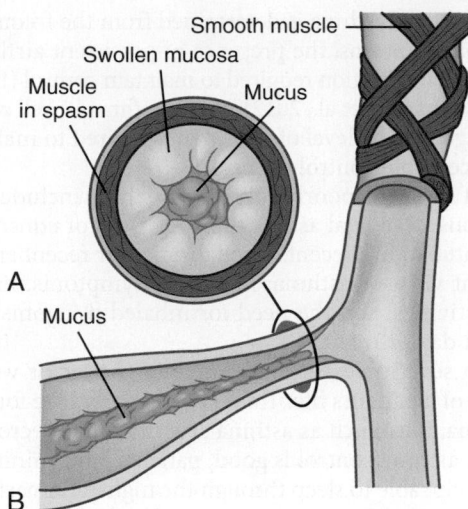

FIGURE 31-4 Factors causing obstruction (especially expiratory obstruction) in asthma. **A,** Cross section of a bronchiole occluded by muscle spasm, swollen mucosa, and mucus in the lumen. **B,** Longitudinal section of a bronchiole. Source: Asthma Society of Canada. (2016). *About asthma.* Retrieved from *http://www.asthma.ca/adults/about/whatIsAsthma.php.*

diameter and an increase in airway resistance that are related to mucosal inflammation, constriction of bronchial smooth muscle, and excess production of mucus (Figure 31-4). Accompanying these changes are hypertrophy of bronchial smooth muscle, thickening of basement membrane, hypertrophy of mucous glands, secretion of thick and tenacious sputum, hyperinflation, and air trapping in the alveoli, all of which increase the work of breathing. As a consequence of these events, respiratory muscle function may be altered, distribution of both ventilation and perfusion may be abnormal, and arterial blood gas (ABG) values may be altered, depending on severity of the disease. Asthma is considered a disease of the airways, but during an asthma attack, eventually all aspects of pulmonary function are compromised. If airway inflammation is not treated or does not resolve, progressive and irreversible lung damage may eventually occur. This irreversible airway obstruction is thought to be the result of inflammation-induced structural changes called *airway remodelling* (GINA, 2015).

Clinical Manifestations

Asthma has an unpredictable, episodic, and variable course. Recurrent episodes of wheezing, breathlessness, sensation of chest tightness, coughing, or a combination of these, particularly at night and in the early morning (typically between 0200 and 0500 hours), are common features. The onset of an attack or episode of asthma may be abrupt (minutes) or more gradual (1 hour to days). Between attacks, the patient may have no symptoms, with normal or near-normal pulmonary function, depending on the severity of disease. However, in some people, prolonged and uncontrolled asthma may result in compromised pulmonary function and chronic debilitation, resulting in irreversible or fixed airway disease.

The characteristic clinical manifestations of asthma are wheezing, cough, dyspnea, and sensation of chest tightness after exposure to a precipitating factor or trigger. Expiration is often prolonged. The inspiratory–expiratory ratio, instead of being the normal 1:2, may be prolonged to 1:3 or 1:4. As a result of bronchospasm, edema, and mucus in the bronchioles, the airways become narrower; thus it takes longer for the air to move out

of the bronchioles. This produces the characteristic wheezing, air trapping, and hyperinflation.

Wheezing is an unreliable sign for gauging the severity of an attack. Many patients with minor attacks wheeze loudly, whereas others with severe attacks do not wheeze. A patient with a severe asthma attack may have no audible wheezing because of the marked reduction in airflow. For wheezing to occur, the patient must be able to move enough air to produce the sound. Wheezing usually occurs first on exhalation. As an asthma attack progresses, the patient may wheeze during inspiration and expiration. Severely diminished breath sounds or their absence, often referred to as a "silent chest," is an ominous sign of severe obstruction and impending respiratory failure. During an acute attack, the person with asthma usually sits upright or slightly bent forward and uses the accessory muscles of respiration in an attempt to make breathing easier. The more difficult the breathing becomes, the more anxious the patient feels.

SAFETY ALERT

If a patient has been wheezing but the wheeze abruptly disappears (i.e., silent chest) and the patient is obviously in distress, the situation has become life-threatening and may necessitate mechanical ventilation.

In some patients with asthma, cough is the only symptom, which is termed cough variant asthma. The bronchospasm may not be severe enough to cause airflow obstruction, but it can increase bronchial tone and cause irritation and stimulation of the cough receptors. The cough may be nonproductive. Mobilizing secretions may be difficult as a result of their thick, tenacious, gelatinous quality.

In patients experiencing an acute attack of moderate or severe asthma, examination usually reveals signs of hypoxemia, which may include restlessness, increased anxiety, inappropriate behaviour, increased pulse and blood pressure, and *pulsus paradoxus* (a drop in systolic pressure during the inspiratory cycle of more than 10 mm Hg). The respiratory rate is significantly increased (usually >30 breaths/minute), and the use of accessory muscles is evident. The patient also has difficulty speaking in complete sentences; typically he or she is able to complete only two to five words without requiring another breath. Percussion of the lungs indicates hyper-resonance, and auscultation indicates the presence of inspiratory or expiratory wheezing.

Asthma Control and Severity

A dynamic continuum of treatment is used to manage asthma. This approach enables drug therapy to be adapted to the severity of the underlying illness and the current level of asthma control. The concepts of asthma "control" and "severity" are related to each other but not correlated (GINA, 2015). For example, even severe asthma may be well controlled, whereas mild disease may remain out of control. *Optimal asthma control* is defined by the absence of both asthma symptoms and the need for rescue bronchodilator, as well as by normal pulmonary function; however, this is difficult to achieve in all patients with asthma. As a result, according to the Canadian Asthma Consensus 2012 guidelines update, treatment needs should be based on achieving acceptable asthma control, determined through clinical and physiological criteria (Lougheed, Lemiere, Ducharme, et al., 2012; Table 31-2). Asthma control is obtained through the use of environmental control measures (reduced exposure to triggers), self-management education, written action plans, and pharmacotherapy tailored to the individual (Lougheed, Lemiere, Ducharme, et al., 2012). Asthma control must be assessed regularly and treatment adjusted accordingly.

TABLE 31-2 ASTHMA CONTROL CRITERIA

Characteristic	Frequency or Value
Daytime symptoms	<4 days/week
Nighttime symptoms	<1 night/week
Physical activity	Normal
Exacerbations	Mild, infrequent
Absence from work or school because of asthma	None
Need for a fast-acting β_2 agonist	<4 doses/week
FEV_1 or PEF	≥90% personal best
PEF diurnal variation*	<10%–15%
Sputum eosinophils†	<2%–3%

Source: Lougheed, M. D., Lemiere, C, Ducharme, F.M., et al. (2012). Canadian Thoracic Society 2012 guideline update: Diagnosis and management of asthma in preschoolers, children and adults. *Canadian Respiratory Journal, 19*(2), 127–164, Table 16.
Diurnal variation is calculated as the highest peak expiratory flow (PEF) minus the lowest peak expiratory flow rate (PEFR), divided by the highest PEFR, multiplied by 100 for morning and night (determined over a 2-week period).
†Considered in adults with uncontrolled moderate to severe asthma who are assessed in specialist centres.
FEV_1, forced expiratory volume in 1 second.

The severity of asthma is determined from the frequency and duration of symptoms, the presence of persistent airflow limitation, and the medication required to maintain control (Lougheed, Lemiere, Ducharme, et al., 2012). When asthma is well controlled, severity is gauged by level of treatment required to maintain the state of acceptable control (Figure 31-5).

Signs of severe or poorly controlled asthma include a history of a previous near-fatal asthma episode (loss of consciousness, need for intubation); recent hospitalization or recent emergency department visit for asthma; nighttime symptoms; limitations in daily activities; and the need for inhaled β_2 agonists several times each day or night.

Asthma severity levels can change for better or worse over the course of a patient's life. This is particularly true for children with asthma, inasmuch as asthma severity often decreases with age. When asthma control is good, patients have minimal to no symptoms, are able to sleep through the night, and participate in sports, exercise, and strenuous activity. Once asthma control has been maintained for at least a few weeks to months, an attempt should be made to reduce medication dosages and yet maintain

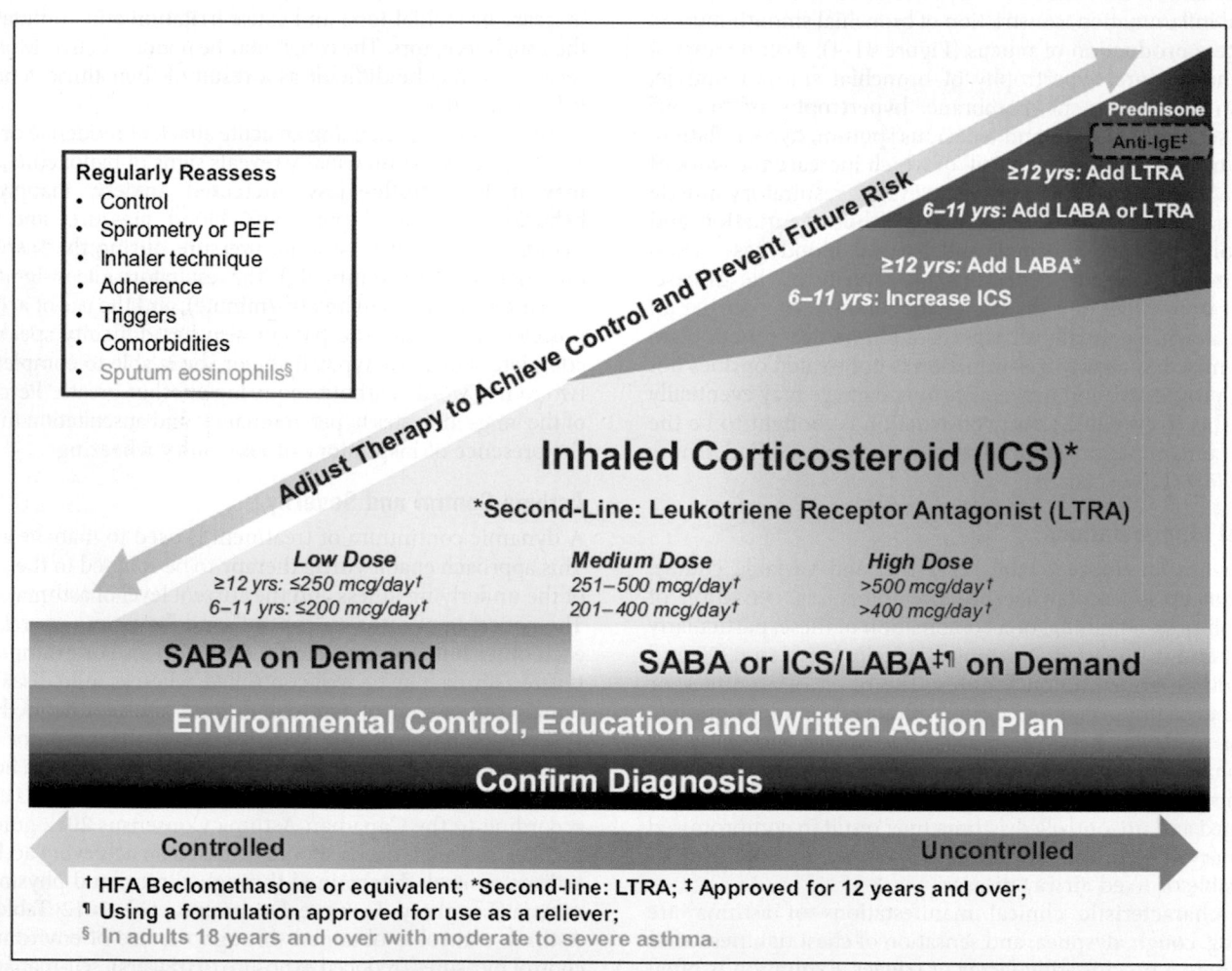

FIGURE 31-5 The 2012 Asthma Management Continuum (for children aged 6 years and older and for adults). *HFA,* hydrofluoroalkane; *IgE,* immunoglobulin E; *LABA,* long-acting β_2 agonist; *PEF,* peak expiratory flow; *SABA,* short-acting β_2 agonist. Source: Lougheed, M. D., Lemiere, C., Ducharme, F. M., et al. (2012). Canadian Thoracic Society 2012 guideline update: Diagnosis and management of asthma in preschoolers, children and adults. *Canadian Respiratory Journal, 19*(2), p. 162. Retrieved from *http://www.respiratoryguidelines.ca/guideline/asthma.*

acceptable asthma control (Lougheed, Lemiere, Ducharme, et al., 2010).

Severe Acute Asthma and Life-Threatening Asthma. Patients who present with a severe acute asthma attack, or one that is life-threatening, often report a history of progressively worsening of asthma control over days or weeks. Of the people with asthma admitted to the hospital, approximately 10% require monitoring or ventilatory assistance in the critical care unit for severe uncontrolled asthma. Common causes of severe acute attacks include viral illnesses, ingestion of ASA (Aspirin) or other NSAIDs, increases in environmental pollutants or other allergen exposure, and discontinuation of drug therapy (especially corticosteroids). The clinical manifestations of a severe attack are a consequence of increased airway resistance that results from edema, mucous plugging, and bronchospasm with subsequent air trapping and hyperinflation. The clinical manifestations are similar to those of nonsevere asthma but are more serious and prolonged. Extreme anxiety, fear of suffocation, severely increased work of breathing, and diaphoresis are common. Absence of diaphoresis may indicate significant dehydration. Sternocleidomastoid, intercostal, and supraclavicular muscle retractions reflect increased work of breathing.

Although wheezing is often audible even without a stethoscope, auscultation may not always be reliable: airflow obstruction may be so severe and airflow so insufficient that audible wheezing or other abnormal lung sounds may not be produced. Absence of a wheeze (i.e., silent chest) represents a life-threatening situation that may necessitate mechanical ventilation. The chest appears fixed in a hyperinflated position and is often described as "tight," indicating severely decreased movement of air through the constricted bronchial airways.

Forced exhalation with the use of the abdominal musculature can result in increased intrathoracic pressure transmitted to the great vessels and heart. Neck vein distension and pulsus paradoxus with a pressure of 40 mm Hg or higher may result. (Pulsus paradoxus is described in Chapter 39 and Table 39-8.) Hypertension, sinus tachycardia, and ventricular dysrhythmias may occur. These three conditions are related to hypoxemia, to the catecholamines present as a result of an endogenous response to hypoxia, and, in older patients, to underlying coronary artery disease. On the right side of the heart, an electrocardiogram may show sinus tachycardia or signs of strain secondary to pulmonary vasoconstriction, which may appear as cor pulmonale and a right axis deviation.

Hypoxemia with hypocapnia usually occurs initially as the patient attempts to hyperventilate and maintain adequate oxygenation and ventilation. As the severity of the attack increases, the work of breathing increases, which makes it more difficult for the patient to overcome the increased resistance to breathing. The patient becomes fatigued, which causes more carbon dioxide retention. ABG measurements initially reveal hypocapnia due to increased respiratory rate. Ultimately, these measurements deteriorate to manifest hypercapnia and hypoxemia. The patient must move amounts greater than 150 mL of air for air to participate in gas exchange. A moderate elevation in partial pressure of arterial carbon dioxide ($PaCO_2$) may be tolerated without intubation, and mechanical ventilation may be necessary because of respiratory arrest, altered level of consciousness, or extreme exhaustion (Leatherman, 2015).

Possible complications of a severe asthma attack include pneumothorax, pneumomediastinum, acute cor pulmonale with right ventricular failure, and severe respiratory muscle

TABLE 31-3 **COLLABORATIVE CARE**	
Asthma	
Diagnostic	**Collaborative Therapy**
• History and physical examination	• Establishing partnerships between health care providers and patients and their families
• Pulmonary function studies (spirometry; methacholine, histamine, exercise challenge test; PEFR)	• Identification and avoidance or elimination of triggers
• Chest radiograph	• Patient and family teaching
• Allergy skin testing	• Continuous assessment of asthma control and severity
• Oximetry and measurement of ABGs during acute episodes when patient is in emergency department or hospital	• Appropriate pharmacotherapy (see Tables 31-5 and 31-6)
	• Asthma action plan (see Figure 31-8)
	• Regular follow-up

ABG, arterial blood gases; *PEFR*, peak expiratory flow rate.

fatigue that leads to respiratory arrest. Respiratory arrest can be fatal.

Diagnostic Studies for Asthma

"A diagnosis of asthma should be considered in individuals of all age groups with recurrent symptoms" (Lougheed, Lemiere, Dell, et al., 2010, p. 16). Two main features must be considered in the diagnosis of asthma: symptoms and variable airflow obstruction. Several sources of information assist with confirming the diagnosis of asthma along with monitoring severity and control (Table 31-3). A detailed history is important in determining whether a person has had previous attacks of a similar nature, often precipitated by a known cause or trigger, as discussed previously in this chapter. Because asthma and allergies commonly coexist, it is also important to determine whether the patient has a history of nonpulmonary symptoms. Rhinitis, eczema, and conjunctivitis are common but not specific to asthma and indicate a predisposition to allergy.

Of further value is to determine whether the patient has a family history of asthma, allergies, and eczema because such a history increases the likelihood that the patient has asthma. Recurrent symptoms of wheeze, sensation of chest tightness, cough, or breathlessness that improve with treatment are suggestive of asthma. However, wheezing and cough occur with a variety of disorders—COPD, pulmonary embolism, GERD, obesity, vocal cord dysfunction, and heart failure—and their presence can therefore complicate the diagnosis. According to both GINA and the Global Initiative for Chronic Obstructive Lung Disease, differentiating between asthma and COPD can be challenging in a small proportion of patients, and the term *asthma–COPD overlap syndrome* (ACOS) is utilized to clinically describe disease features (GINA, 2015). This is discussed further in the section on COPD later in this chapter.

In all patients who are able to perform pulmonary testing, clinically suspected asthma should be confirmed with objective lung measurements that demonstrate post–bronchodilator therapy reversible obstruction, variable airflow limitation over time, or airway hyper-responsiveness (Lougheed, Lemiere, Dell, et al., 2010). Spirometry is the preferred test for diagnosing asthma; alternative lung testing includes variations in PEFR and bronchoprovocative challenge testing (Lougheed, Lemiere, Dell, et al., 2010; Table 31-4).

TABLE 31-4	DIAGNOSIS OF ASTHMA: PULMONARY FUNCTION CRITERIA	
Pulmonary Function Measurement	Children (6 Years of Age and Older)	Adults
Preferred: Spirometry Showing Reversible Airway Obstruction		
Reduced FEV₁/FVC	Less than lower limit of normal based on age, sex, height, and ethnicity (<0.8–0.9)*	Less than lower limit of normal based on age, sex, height, and ethnicity (<0.75–0.8)*
	and	*and*
Increase in FEV_1 after a bronchodilator or after a course of controller therapy	≥12%	≥12% (and a minimum ≥200 mL)
Alternative: Peak Expiratory Flow Variability		
Increase after a bronchodilator or after course of controller therapy	≥20%	60 L/min (minimum ≥20%)
	or	*or*
Diurnal variation†	Not recommended	>8% based on twice daily readings; >20% based on multiple daily readings
Alternative: Positive Challenge Test		
Methacholine challenge	PC₂₀ < 4 mg/mL (4–16 mg/mL is borderline; >16 mg/mL is negative)	
	or	*or*
Exercise challenge	≥10%–15% decrease in FEV_1 post-exercise	

Source: Lougheed, M. D., Lemiere, C., Ducharme, F. M., et al. (2012). Canadian Thoracic Society 2012 guideline update: Diagnosis and management of asthma in preschoolers, children and adults. *Canadian Respiratory Journal, 19*(2), 127–164.
*Approximate lower limits of normal ratios for children and adults;
†Difference between minimum morning pre–bronchodilator therapy value in 1 wk and maximum nighttime value as percentage of recent maximum.
FEV₁, forced expiratory volume in 1 second; *FVC*, forced vital capacity; *PC₂₀*, provocative concentration of methacholine producing a 20% fall in FEV_1.

Spirometry performed before and after bronchodilator treatment can best reveal whether airway obstruction is reversible. The ratio of forced expiratory volume in 1 second to the forced vital capacity (FEV_1 to FVC; see Chapter 28, Table 28-15) is a measure of airflow obstruction. For spirometry, the patient is asked to refrain from using bronchodilator medication for 6 to 12 hours before the test. The test is then completed both before and after administration of a bronchodilator to determine the degree of response. Most children 6 years of age and older should be able to perform spirometry, but a standardized clinical score such as the Pediatric Respiratory Assessment Measure (PRAM) can reduce subjectivity of assessment (Ducharme, Dell, Radhakrishnan, et al., 2015). (The normal values for pulmonary function tests are discussed in Chapter 28.)

An alternative objective pulmonary measurement is peak expiratory flow rate (PEFR), in which variable airflow limitation

overtime is measured (see Chapter 28, Table 28-15). The PEFR is a home measurement, which is not as reliable as spirometry but can be used when spirometry or challenge testing is unavailable. To determine an asthma diagnosis through this method, the patient must measure the PEFR four times per day—in the morning and evening both before and after bronchodilator treatment—for several weeks. To determine the PEFR variability, the lowest reading is subtracted from the highest reading, the result is divided by the highest reading, and this answer is then multiplied by 100. Variability in peak expiratory flow of 20% or higher is indicative of asthma.

Determining airway hyper-responsiveness with the use of methacholine, histamine, or exercise challenge testing can be useful in patients with persistent symptoms despite normal spirometry findings and to evaluate work-related asthma (Lougheed, Lemiere, Dell, et al., 2010). Challenge testing must be performed in a controlled environment by trained staff.

Chest radiographs are not necessary to diagnose asthma; however, they may be used to exclude other diagnoses, such as congenital malformations in children and heart failure in adults (Lougheed, Lemiere, Dell, et al., 2010). A chest radiograph in a patient with asthma with no clinical manifestations is usually normal; however, this radiograph should be used as a baseline on initial diagnosis. A chest radiograph obtained during an acute attack usually shows hyperinflation and may reveal other complications of asthma such as mucoid impaction, pneumothorax, atelectasis, or pneumomediastinum.

Allergy assessment is warranted in a patient with asthma and must be interpreted in view of the patient's history of exposure and symptom experience. Allergy skin testing can be helpful in determining sensitivity to specific allergens (antigens). (Allergy testing is discussed further in Chapter 16.)

If a patient is in acute distress, it is not feasible to obtain a detailed health history (although a family member may supply some pertinent information). During an acute asthma attack, bedside spirometry (FEV_1 and FVC are preferred, but usually PEFR is measured) may be used to monitor obstruction. Serial spirometric parameters, oximetry, and measurement of ABGs help provide information about the severity of the attack and the response to therapy. A complete blood cell count and serum electrolyte measurements are obtained to help monitor the course of therapy because high dosages of inhaled β_2 agonists can cause hypokalemia.

In addition to standard measures of asthma control, monitoring changes in sputum eosinophil counts is a method of measuring airway inflammation, indicating whether treatment for asthma is working (Lougheed, Lemiere, Ducharme, et al., 2012). Sputum eosinophils are not normally present in a healthy individual, but their levels are increased in individuals with known asthma who are exposed to allergens. These measurements have been used in adults and children and are becoming more easily available and reliable. However, they continue to be used most frequently in major research centres.

Collaborative Care

In 1990, Canada became the first country to produce asthma practice guidelines. These guidelines provide a medical approach to diagnosing and managing asthma informed by the best available evidence. The Registered Nurses' Association of Ontario (RNAO) also developed asthma best practice guidelines for adults (RNAO, 2017) and children (Olajos-Clow, Cicutto, Duff Cloutier, et al.,

2008) to provide nurses working in diverse settings with an evidence-informed summary of basic asthma care. The RNAO's *Best Practice Guidelines* build on and complement the Canadian Asthma Consensus Report and remain pertinent with the current Canadian Thoracic Society Asthma Management Guidelines Update (Lougheed, Lemiere, Dell, et al., 2012). The focus of the nursing guidelines is on promoting asthma control for adults and children affected by asthma. The overall goal of the guidelines is to achieve asthma control with the minimum level of pharmacotherapy while enhancing the quality of life of individuals living with asthma and reducing the personal and social burdens inflicted by the condition.

Education that builds an active partnership with patients remains the cornerstone of asthma management (see the following "Evidence-Informed Practice" box). Education should start at the time of asthma diagnosis and be integrated into every aspect of clinical asthma care. Asthma self-management should be tailored to the needs of each patient; patients' cultural beliefs and practices should be accounted for. Emphasis should be placed on evaluating outcomes in terms of a patient's level of asthma control and perceptions of improvement, especially quality of life and the ability to engage in activities of normal living such as physical activity. A listing of centres that provide asthma education to patients can be accessed through the Canadian Network for Respiratory Care (see the Canadian Resources at the end of this chapter).

General Management Approach. Several components enable successful management of asthma: (a) establishment of a confirmed diagnosis through the use of objective measures; (b) development of a partnership between health care providers and the patients and families affected by asthma; (c) limited exposure to triggers; (d) education of patients; (e) appropriate pharmacotherapy; (f) continuous assessment and monitoring of asthma control and severity; (g) implementation of a written action plan; and (h) ensuring regular follow-up.

In Canada, asthma treatment is based on the Asthma Management Continuum (see Figure 31-5), which reflects the key concepts pertaining to asthma diagnosis and management for children 6 years of age and older and for adults. Controlling the disease in order to prevent complications, morbidity, and mortality is the primary goal of asthma management (Lougheed, Lemiere, Dell, et al., 2010; Lougheed, Lemiere, Ducharme, et al., 2012). The continuum accounts for the fact that the level of control and severity of asthma change over time and that constant assessment and adjustment of therapy is necessary to achieve and maintain control. The general management approach to asthma includes confirming the diagnosis, monitoring the level of asthma control (see Table 31-3), reducing exposure to environmental triggers, providing appropriate medications, providing asthma education, and providing a written action plan.

All individuals with asthma need to have access to "a rescue medication," sometimes referred to as a *fast-acting β₂ agonist (FABA);* such medications most commonly consist of an inhaled short-acting β₂ agonist (SABA), specifically salbutamol. In rare cases, a select subgroup of individuals 12 years of age and older with moderately severe asthma but poor control and prone to exacerbations are already receiving a fixed maintenance of a FABA; this may consist of a combination of an inhaled corticosteroid (ICS) and a long-acting β₂ agonist (LABA), specifically budesonide/formoterol, for quick relief of symptoms (Lougheed, Lemiere, Ducharme, et al., 2012).

If symptoms are infrequent and lung function measurements are normal, a SABA used on an as-needed basis to relieve symptoms is all that is required. However, an ICS is also required if one or more indicators of poor control are identified in a child 6 years of age or older or in an adult (see Table 31-2; Lougheed, Lemiere, Ducharme, et al., 2012). The guidelines emphasize that most patients with asthma, unless it is very mild and manifests infrequently, require daily use of ICS in addition to a SABA as necessary (Lougheed, Lemiere, Dell, et al., 2010). If symptoms persist and are outside the limits of acceptable asthma control, the next step recommended on the Asthma Management Continuum in children 6 to 11 years old is advancement to a moderate-dosage ICS. In children 12 years of age and older and in adults, however, the appropriate second-line therapy is the addition of a LABA in the form of a combination inhaler; the third-line therapy is an increase to a moderate-dosage ICS or addition of leukotriene receptor antagonists (LTRAs). For children 6 to 11 years old in whom asthma is not controlled on a moderate-dosage ICS, the addition of a LABA or LTRA, or both, is recommended. A fourth-line therapy—addition of theophylline—may be considered for adults.

In a minority of patients, symptoms persist despite the use of these therapies. If the FEV_1 is below 60% of predicted levels or of their best value, treatment with an oral corticosteroid (prednisone) should be initiated (GINA, 2015). Long-term prednisone use may be indicated and effective for asthma that is difficult to control, but it should be avoided, if at all possible, because of its adverse effects. An anti-IgE antagonist, omalizumab (Xolair), may be considered in patients 12 years of age and older with atopic asthma that is poorly controlled despite high-dosage ICS and additional therapies, either with or without prednisone. The Asthma Management Continuum also stresses the importance of assessing symptom control, lung function, inhaler technique, adherence to therapy, avoidance of exposure to asthma triggers, the presence of comorbid conditions, and examination of sputum eosinophils (where available) on a regular basis and before therapy is advanced (Lougheed, Lemiere, Ducharme, et al., 2012).

Acute Asthma Episode. Many patients with an acute asthma episode come to the emergency department. The choice of treatment of acute asthma depends on the severity of a patient's condition and the response to initial therapy. The examiner can assess the degree of severity by measuring FEV_1 or PEFR, by identifying the degree of change in objective measurements, and by evaluating the baseline pulse oximetry value. Inhaled SABA (e.g., salbutamol) should be administered immediately and supplemental oxygen provided to keep arterial oxygen saturation (SaO_2) above 92%. In more severe cases, ABG measurements may be used to monitor SaO_2.

Inhaled β₂-adrenergic agonists are preferably administered through a metered-dose inhaler (MDI) with a spacer (a holding chamber that holds the medication for a few seconds after it has been released from the inhaler) at a frequency of four to eight puffs every 15 to 20 minutes, usually repeated three times. If the FEV_1 or PEFR is below 40% of predicted, one puff every 30 to 60 seconds (up to 20 puffs) may be administered, depending on the patient's response to and tolerance of treatment (Hodder, Lougheed, Rowe, et al., 2010). Ipratropium bromide (four to eight puffs inhaled every 15 to 20 minutes, repeated three times) may be added to salbutamol during moderate and severe acute asthma episodes. In some emergency departments, bronchodilators are

Research Highlight

Adult Asthma Care Guidelines: Promoting Control of Asthma

Clinical Questions

1. What are the appropriate nursing assessment strategies to use with adults living with asthma to achieve optimal asthma control?
2. What are the appropriate nursing management strategies to use with adults living with asthma to achieve optimal asthma control?
3. What education and training do nurses require to assist people living with asthma to achieve optimal asthma control?
4. What organization or health system–level supports are needed to enable health care providers to assist people living with asthma to achieve optimal asthma control?

Best Available Evidence

Multiple systematic reviews of asthma management practices

Synthesis of Best Available Evidence
Recommendations of Clinical Practice Guideline

Assessment

Recommendation 1.0: All individuals identified as having asthma, or suspected of having asthma, will have their level of asthma control assessed by the nurse.

Recommendation 1.1: At initial encounter, the nurse should identify adults with an asthma diagnosis by reviewing the health record for an established asthma diagnosis, supported by the use of objective lung function measurements, and by asking the following two questions:

1. Have you ever been told by a health care provider that you have asthma?
2. Have you ever used a puffer or inhaler or asthma medication for breathing problems?

Recommendation 1.2a: At every encounter, the nurse should assess the person's current level of asthma control according to the following criteria:

- Need for a fast-acting β_2 agonist <4 doses/week (including for exercise)
- Daytime symptoms <4 days/week
- Nighttime symptoms <1 night/week
- Normal physical activity levels
- Mild, infrequent exacerbations
- No absences from work or school
- Forced expiratory volume in first second (FEV_1) or peak expiratory flow (PEF) ≥ 90% of personal best*†
- Diurnal PEF variation < 10%–15%*†
- Sputum eosinophil [counts] <2%–3%*

Recommendation 1.2b: For adults with uncontrolled asthma, the nurse should determine whether the person is currently experiencing an asthma exacerbation and, if so, the severity and need for urgent medical attention.

Recommendation 1.3: At every encounter, the nurse should assess the person's risk of future asthma exacerbations according to the following criteria:

- Current control of asthma
- Severe exacerbations experienced
- Exacerbations necessitating systemic corticosteroids
- Use of emergency care or hospitalizations for asthma

Recommendation 1.4: At every encounter, the nurse should identify factors affecting the complexity of asthma management for the person, including age, sex, smoking habits, social determinants of health, triggers, and comorbid conditions.

Asthma Planning

Recommendation 2.0: The nurse should develop an individualized, person-centred asthma education plan that addresses the following:

- Learning needs
- Culture
- Health literacy
- Empowerment

Implementation

Recommendation 3.1a: The nurse should provide asthma education as an essential component of care.

Recommendation 3.1b: The nurse should educate the person on the essential skills and self-management of asthma based on the person's learning needs, including the following:

- Pathophysiology of asthma
- Medications and device technique
- Self-monitoring
- Action plans
- Trigger identification and management
- Smoking cessation (if applicable)

Recommendation 3.2: The nurse should evaluate nonpharmacological interventions for effectiveness and for potential interactions with pharmacological interventions

Recommendation 3.3a: At every encounter, the nurse should actively educate on correct inhaler device technique through observation, feedback, physical demonstration, and written instructions.

Recommendation 3.3b: The nurse should engage the person with asthma in shared decision making with regard to the selection of an inhaler device.

Recommendation 3.3c: The nurse should educate the person with asthma on the difference between controller and reliever medications, their indications, and their potential adverse effects.

Recommendation 3.4: When appropriate, the nurse should assist and educate persons with asthma to measure their peak expiratory flow.

Recommendation 3.5: To support self-management, the nurse should collaborate with the person with asthma to develop and review a documented asthma action plan, in one or a combination of the following formats:

- In writing, on paper
- Electronically
- Pictorially

Recommendation 3.6: The nurse should provide integrated asthma self-management support to adults with uncontrolled asthma who are at risk for severe exacerbations through multiple modalities/formats, such as one of the following:

- Home-care visits
- Telehealthcare

Recommendation 3.7: The nurse should refer and connect persons with asthma to one of the following:

- Primary care provider
- Certified asthma educator or certified respiratory educator

Evaluation

Recommendation 4.1: At every encounter, the nurse should evaluate the effectiveness of the overall plan of care in achieving asthma control.

Education

Recommendation 5.1a: At every encounter, the nurse should evaluate the effectiveness of the overall plan of care in achieving asthma control.

- Health care providers
- Students entering health care professions

Recommendation 5.1b: At every encounter, the nurse should evaluate the effectiveness of the overall plan of care in achieving asthma control.

Recommendation 5.3: The nurse should provide a quality assurance program and standardized training for health care providers who perform spirometry.

Organization and Policy

Recommendation 6.1: Organizations establish a corporate priority focused on the integration and evaluation of best practice asthma care across all care settings.

Recommendation 6.2: Organizations provide the resources and professional training necessary to integrate best practices for the assessment and management of adult asthma across all care settings.

Reference for Evidence

Registered Nurses' Association of Ontario (2017). *Adult asthma care: Promoting control of asthma* (2nd ed.). Toronto, ON: Registered Nurses' Association of Ontario. Retrieved from *http://rnao.ca/sites/rnao-ca/files/bpg/Adult_Asthma_FINAL_WEB.pdf*.

---

*Indicates important objective information for a complete assessment of asthma control, but may not be available.
†Performed and interpreted within health care provider's scope of practice (including appropriate knowledge and skills) and in alignment with organizational policies and procedures.
PEFR, peak expiratory flow rate.

administered via a nebulizer, but a meta-analysis of study results revealed that the MDI with a spacer works faster, is less costly, and is more effective in reducing hospitalization and improving clinical scores (GINA, 2015).

Oral corticosteroids are indicated for treatment of an acute exacerbation that necessitates a visit to the emergency department. Intravenous corticosteroids are generally administered to patients who have difficulty with swallowing. Therapy should be continued until the patient is breathing comfortably, wheezing has disappeared, and pulmonary function measurements are near baseline values.

On occasion, an asthma attack is so severe and unresponsive to treatment that the patient requires mechanical ventilation. Indications for mechanical ventilation are persistent or progressive carbon dioxide retention and respiratory acidosis, clinical deterioration (indicated by fatigue, hypersomnolence), metabolic acidosis, and cardiopulmonary arrest. In life-threatening asthma exacerbation, the goals of initiating mechanical ventilation are to achieve a partial pressure of arterial oxygen (PaO_2) of 60 mm Hg or higher, an SaO_2 of 90% or higher, and a normal pH.

Audible wheezing may occur in the airways, which indicates a response to therapy as airflow increases. As the patient begins to respond to therapy and symptoms begin to subside, it is important to remember that despite the reversibility of most of the bronchospasm, the edema and cellular infiltration of the airway mucosa and the viscous mucous plugs are still present, and improvement may take several days. Thus intensive therapy includes corticosteroids and must be continued even after clinical improvement has occurred. Patients with moderate or severe acute asthma are typically discharged home with an inhaled SABA, an added LABA or LRTA, high-dosage ICS, and an oral corticosteroid, and the addition of an anti-IgE drug should be considered as well (Lougheed, Lemiere, Dell, et al., 2010). In addition, discharge instructions should include an action plan detailing the use of the medications and the criteria for returning to the emergency department for immediate medical assistance. It is important that patients follow up with their primary asthma care provider after an emergency department visit.

Drug Therapy

Medications used to treat asthma are divided into two categories: (a) relievers and (b) controllers (Table 31-5). They are available in several forms, and various delivery devices are used to administer them. The inhaled route is preferred because the drug is delivered directly to the lungs, which minimizes systemic absorption and thus the number and intensity of adverse events. Relievers, used to ease asthma symptoms, are also known as "rescue medication" and are used intermittently as required. Controllers are maintenance therapy used on a daily basis, typically twice a day. Because inflammation is considered an early and persistent component of asthma, drug therapy is directed toward long-term suppression of inflammation (Table 31-6).

Anti-Inflammatory Drugs

Corticosteroids. Chronic inflammation is a primary component of asthma. Corticosteroids are anti-inflammatory medications that reduce bronchial hyper-responsiveness by blocking the late-phase reaction and that inhibit migration of inflammatory cells. Corticosteroids are more effective than any other long-term drug in improving asthma control. ICSs are the mainstay therapy for the long-term control of asthma (GINA, 2015). Usually,

TABLE 31-5	CATEGORIES OF ASTHMA MEDICATIONS: RELIEVERS VERSUS CONTROLLERS

Reliever Medications
Bronchodilators
- Short-acting inhaled β_2-adrenergic agonists (e.g., salbutamol)

Anticholinergics
- Ipratropium, for example*

Controller Medications
Anti-Inflammatory Drugs
- Corticosteroids
  - Inhaled (e.g., fluticasone)
  - Oral (e.g., prednisone)
- Leukotriene modifiers (e.g., montelukast)
- Anti-IgE (e.g., omalizumab)

Bronchodilators
- Long-acting inhaled β_2-adrenergic agonists (e.g., salmeterol inhalation)
- Long-acting oral β_2-adrenergic agonists (e.g., oral salmeterol)
- Methylxanthines (e.g., theophylline)

*Not considered a rescue medication if used alone; commonly used in combination with salbutamol in the emergency department for severe exacerbations.

ICSs must be administered for 1 to 2 weeks before maximum therapeutic effects can be observed. However, some ICSs (e.g., fluticasone and budesonide) begin to have a therapeutic effect in 24 hours. These drugs must be administered on a fixed schedule.

For children 6 years of age and older and adults with newly diagnosed asthma, low-dosage ICS is recommended (see Figure 31-5) and for ICS-naive patients with mild loss of control (see Table 31-2). In children 6 years of age and older and adults presenting with an asthma exacerbation necessitating a short-term regimen of systemic corticosteroids, a daily low- to moderate-dosage ICS should be initiated as maintenance therapy. In children 6 years of age and older, if low-dosage ICS is not adequate in achieving or maintaining control, then increasing to moderate-dosage ICS (see Figure 31-5) is the preferred approach. To minimize the intensity of adverse effects, however, add-on therapy should be considered in patients 12 years of age and older before ICS therapy is increased to moderate dosages and certainly before high dosages are prescribed (GINA, 2015).

When ICSs are administered, asthma can usually be controlled without significant systemic adverse events because only minimal amounts of drugs are absorbed systemically. However, ICSs administered at the highest dosage levels have been associated with adverse events such as easy bruising and accelerated bone loss (GINA, 2015). Oropharyngeal candidiasis, hoarseness, and dry cough are local adverse effects caused by ICS (GINA, 2015). Occurrence of these oropharyngeal adverse events can be reduced by mouth rinsing and gargling after every inhalation treatment. If an MDI is used, absorption can be improved, and the intensity of adverse events is reduced with the use of a spacer (Figure 31-6). However, newer drugs (e.g., ciclesonide) that are activated in the lungs (not in the pharynx) appear to minimize the intensity of these adverse events without the need for a spacer or mouth rinsing (Lougheed, Lemiere, Dell, et al., 2010).

In acute asthma exacerbations, short courses of orally administered corticosteroids are indicated for gaining prompt control (Lougheed, Lemiere, Dell, et al., 2010). In a minority of cases, maintenance dosages of oral corticosteroids are necessary to control severe chronic asthma. However, long-term use should be avoided in all age groups if possible, especially children, because of adverse effects (Lougheed, Lemiere, Dell, et al., 2010). If long-term use is indicated, a single dose in the morning, to coincide with endogenous cortisol production, and alternate-day dosing should be considered; these schedules are associated with fewer adverse effects. Long-term corticosteroid therapy is discussed further in Chapter 51.

Adults using maintenance oral corticosteroids or high dosages of ICS (>500 mcg of fluticasone and beclomethasone; >800 mcg of budesonide), or both, should be monitored for osteoporosis with bone densitometry. Patients should take adequate amounts

TABLE 31-6 DRUG THERAPY

Asthma and Chronic Obstructive Pulmonary Disease

Drug	Route of Administration	Mechanisms of Action	Adverse Effects	Comments
Bronchodilators				
Short-Acting β_2-Adrenergic Agonists				
Salbutamol (Airomir, Apo-Salvent, Ventolin)	Diskus DPI, MDI, nebules	Selectively stimulates β_2 receptors on airway smooth muscle, causing relaxation and producing bronchodilation	Tremor, tachycardia, headache, nervousness, palpitations, insomnia; excessive use can cause hypokalemia	Asthma "rescue medication" (FABA) Rapid onset of action: 1–3 min Duration of action: up to 6 hr Peak effect: 60–90 min
Terbutaline (Bricanyl)	Turbuhaler DPI	Same as for salbutamol	Same as for salbutamol	Rapid onset of action: within minutes Duration of action: 4–7 hr Peak effect: 15–60 min
Long-Acting β_2-Adrenergic Agonists				
Formoterol (Foradil, Oxeze)	Aerolizer DPI, Turbuhaler DPI	Selectively stimulates β_2 receptors on airway smooth muscle, causing relaxation and producing bronchodilation	Tremor, tachycardia, headache, nervousness, palpitations, insomnia	Rapid onset of action: 1–3 min Duration of protection: 8–12 hr Peak effect: 15 min Typically taken twice daily Oxeze has approval to be used as an asthma reliever (FABA) in asthma only in specified patients, and only when used in combination with inhaled steroid (specifically budesonide)
Salmeterol (Serevent)	Diskus DPI	Same as above	Same as above	Onset of action: 10–20 min Duration of action: 8–12 hr Typically taken twice daily; not to exceed 50 mcg q12h Not used for relief of acute exacerbations
Anticholinergics				
Ipratropium bromide (Apo-Ipravent, Atrovent HFA)	MDI, nebulizer	Blocks action of acetylcholine, resulting in bronchodilation; competitive inhibitor of muscarinic receptors	Dry mouth, cough, bad taste in mouth, nausea, headache, flushed skin; blurred vision if sprayed in eyes	Onset: 5–15 min Duration: 4–6 hr Peak effect: 1–2 hr Should be used with caution by individuals with narrow-angle glaucoma, prostatic hyperplasia, or bladder neck obstruction
Ipratropium and salbutamol (Combivent) Ipratropium and fenoterol (Duovent)	Nebulizer	Combination of anticholinergic and β_2 agonist preparations produces bronchodilation	Same as for ipratropium and short-acting β_2 agonists	Same as for ipratropium and short-acting β_2 agonists
Tiotropium bromide (Spiriva)	HandiHaler DPI	Blocks action of acetylcholine, resulting in bronchodilation; competitive inhibitor of muscarinic receptors on bronchial smooth muscle	Dry mouth, cough, bad taste in mouth, nausea, headache, constipation, urinary retention	Onset: 30 min Peak: 1–4 hr Duration: 24 hr Should be used only once per day Should be used same time each day Contact with eyes should be avoided Powder capsules sensitive to light and moisture

TABLE 31-6 DRUG THERAPY

Asthma and Chronic Obstructive Pulmonary Disease—cont'd

Drug	Route of Administration	Mechanisms of Action	Adverse Effects	Comments
Anti-Inflammatory Drugs				
Steroidal Anti-Inflammatory Drugs				
Hydrocortisone (Cortef Tab, Solu-Cortef)	Oral, intravenous	Potent anti-inflammatory and immuno-suppressive effects; interferes with inflammatory cascade; decreases edema in bronchial airways; increases number and affinity of β_2 receptors; abolishes and prevents tolerance induced with chronic use of inhaled β_2 agonists; decreases mucus secretion; effective in late-phase reaction of asthma	Short-term use (<2 wk): weight gain, increased appetite, Cushingoid appearance, menstrual changes, mood changes, skin changes (acne, striae, bruising) Longer term use (>2 wk): adrenal suppression, immuno-suppression, osteoporosis, hyperglycemia, obesity, peptic ulcers, hypertension, hypokalemia, cataracts, glaucoma, muscle weakness, catabolism, growth retardation, avascular necrosis, dysphonia	Onset: Some effects within 2–4 hr In acute severe asthma, 4–12 hr may be required before clinical response noted Reversal of bronchial hyper-responsiveness requires approximately 1 wk Alternate-day or morning therapy may minimize the intensity of adverse drug events Should be taken with food When drug is given in high doses, patient should be assessed for epigastric pain Histamine (H₂) blockers and antacids may minimize the intensity of GI effects Patient should be counselled about how to prevent osteoporosis If taken for <2 wk or <2 bursts in 1 year, no tapering of dosage required; otherwise dosage should be tapered gradually If symptoms recur during tapering, asthma care provider should be notified
Methylprednisolone (Medrol, Solu-Medrol)	Oral, intravenous			
Prednisone (Winpred)	Oral			
Prednisolone (Pediapred)				
Dexamethasone				
Beclomethasone (QVAR, Rivanase AQ)	MDI, nasal spray	Same as for hydrocortisone and others Acts locally in respiratory tract with relatively little systemic absorption at low to medium dosages	Oral candidiasis infection, hoarseness, irritated throat, dry mouth, cough	Mouth should be rinsed after use to reduce the risk for oral fungal infections, hoarseness, and dry mouth If an MDI is used, a spacer should also be used to reduce the intensity of adverse effects Nasal spray form used for allergic rhinitis Typically taken twice daily
Budesonide (Pulmicort, Rhinocort NS)	Turbuhaler DPI, nasal spray, nebulizer	Same as for beclomethasone	Same as for beclomethasone	Mouth should be rinsed after use Nasal spray form used for allergic rhinitis Typically taken twice daily
Ciclesonide (Alvesco, Omnaris NS)	MDI, nasal spray	Same as for beclomethasone	Same as for beclomethasone	Same as for budesonide
Fluticasone (Avamys NS, Flonase NS, Flovent DPI, MDI)	Diskus DPI, MDI, nasal spray	Same as for beclomethasone but with higher potency (approximately double); as a result, dosages tend to be lower	Same as for beclomethasone; bruising with higher dosages	Mouth should be rinsed after use If an MDI is used, a spacer also needed to reduce the intensity of adverse effects Nasal spray form used for allergic rhinitis Typically taken twice daily
Mometasone (Nasonex NS)	Metered-dose manual pump spray	Exact mechanism of action unknown	Headache, viral infection, pharyngitis	Treatment may be required for 2 wk before improvement noted
Combination Inhalers: Inhaled Corticosteroid and Inhaled Long-Acting β_2 Agonist (LABA)				
Budesonide and formoterol (Symbicort)	Turbuhaler DPI, diskus DPI, MDI	See text sections pertaining to inhaled corticosteroid and inhaled LABAs	See text sections pertaining to inhaled corticosteroid and inhaled LABAs	Commonly used for moderate and severe asthma Combination therapy products may simplify treatment regimen In COPD, ICS is recommended only in combination with LABA and is initiated when a person has had >1 acute exacerbation in a year
Fluticasone and salmeterol (Advair)				
Mometasone and formoterol (Zenhale)				

Continued

TABLE 31-6   DRUG THERAPY

Asthma and Chronic Obstructive Pulmonary Disease—cont'd

Drug	Route of Administration	Mechanisms of Action	Adverse Effects	Comments
Antileukotrienes				
Montelukast (Singulair)	Oral tablets, chewable tablets for children, granules	Blocks the action of leukotrienes released by inflammatory cell membranes; has bronchodilator and anti-inflammatory effects	Headache, indigestion, nausea, vomiting, diarrhea, fatigue, abdominal pain, respiratory infections	Prevents exercise-induced asthma Affects metabolism of erythromycin and theophylline Not used to relieve acute asthma episodes
Zafirlukast (Accolate)	Oral tablets	Same as for montelukast	Same as for montelukast	Same as for montelukast Bioavailability is reduced when it is taken with food
Anti–IgE Antagonist				
Omalizumab (Xolair)	Subcutaneous injection	Binds free IgE and therefore prevents IgE from binding to receptors on its effector cells, primarily mast cells and basophils, which, in turn, prevents allergens from triggering acute allergic reactions	Reaction at injection site (pain, bruising, redness, warmth)	Only for moderate to severe persistent allergic asthma with symptoms not inadequately controlled by ICS Not for acute bronchospasm Administered under direct medical supervision; patient is observed for a minimum of 2 hr after administration because anaphylaxis has been reported with use
Methylxanthines				
Theophylline (Uniphyl, Theolair) Aminophylline	Oral, intravenous	Relieves bronchoconstriction and its accompanying symptoms by dilating the muscles around the bronchi	Tachycardia, blood pressure changes, dysrhythmias, anorexia, nausea, vomiting, nervousness, irritability, headache, muscle twitching, flushing, epigastric pain, diarrhea, insomnia, palpitations	Wide variety of responses to drug metabolism Half-life: ↓ by smoking and ↑ by heart failure and liver disease Cimetidine, ciprofloxacin, erythromycin, and other drugs may rapidly ↑ theophylline levels The effect of these medications is proportionate to their concentration in the blood To be effective, they must be taken regularly, and blood concentrations should be monitored
Phosphodiesterase 4 Inhibitor				
Roflumilast (Daxas)	Oral	Selective phosphodiesterase 4 inhibitor Nonsteroidal anti-inflammatory drug that targets systemic and pulmonary inflammation associated with COPD	Diarrhea, nausea, anorexia, weight loss, headache, insomnia, anxiety; may resolve after 4 wk of continuous treatment	Indicated for use in severe COPD as a therapeutic addition to long-acting bronchodilators for patients with chronic cough, chronic sputum findings, and history of frequent exacerbations Not currently indicated for asthma Not indicated for acute bronchospasm

COPD, chronic obstructive pulmonary disease; *DPI,* dry powder inhaler; *FABA,* fast-acting β_2 agonist; *GI,* gastro-intestinal; *ICS,* inhaled corticosteroids; *IgE,* immunoglobulin E; *MDI,* metered-dose inhaler.

of calcium and vitamin D and participate in regular weight-bearing exercise. (Osteoporosis is discussed in Chapter 66.)

Antileukotrienes. In Canada, two leukotriene receptor antagonists (zafirlukast, montelukast), which block the action of leukotrienes (Lougheed, Lemiere, Dell, et al., 2010), are available. Leukotrienes are produced as a result of arachidonic acid metabolism (see Chapter 14, Table 14-3). Some leukotrienes are potent bronchoconstrictors, causing airway edema and inflammation, and thus contribute to the symptoms of asthma. The anti-inflammatory action of antileukotrienes is not as potent as that of ICS, and thus they are not recommended as a single drug in the treatment of persistent asthma (Lougheed, Lemiere, Dell, et al., 2010). These drugs are used as adjuvant or add-on therapy for individuals experiencing symptoms (uncontrolled asthma) or significant adverse events while using higher dosage ICS. Antileukotrienes may be considered as an alternative to

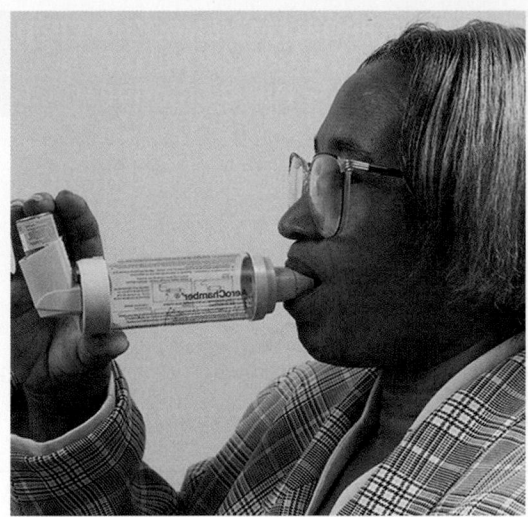

FIGURE 31-6 Example of an AeroChamber spacer used with a metered-dose inhaler. Source: Potter, P. A., Perry, A. G., Stockert, P., et al. (2011). *Basic nursing: Essentials for practice* (7th ed.). St. Louis: Mosby.

increasing dosages of ICS. They are not used to reverse bronchospasm in acute asthma attacks. An advantage of these drugs is that they are administered orally.

Anti–Immunoglobulin E Antagonists. Omalizumab (Xolair) is a monoclonal antibody to IgE that decreases circulating free IgE levels (Kuhl & Hanania, 2012). Omalizumab prevents IgE from attaching to mast cells, which thus prevents the release of chemical mediators. Health Canada has approved this drug for use by patients who have moderate to severe persistent allergic asthma and are 12 years of age and older. This medication is expensive and therefore should be reserved for specific patients: those with asthma that is difficult to control despite adherence to a regimen of high-dosage ICS and at least one additional controller therapy; those who have objectively confirmed asthma; those who have documented allergic perennial asthma; and those whose serum IgE level is 30 to 700 IU/mL. The medication is administered subcutaneously every 2 to 4 weeks and should be part of a well-controlled therapeutic trial supervised by an asthma specialist (Lougheed, Lemiere, Dell, et al., 2010).

Bronchodilators. Three classes of bronchodilator drugs are currently used in asthma therapy: β_2-adrenergic agonists, anticholinergic drugs, and methylxanthines.

β_2-Adrenergic Agonists. These drugs may be SABAs or LABAs. These medications work by binding to β_2 receptors located on airway smooth muscle, causing relaxation of the bronchial smooth muscle and thus bronchodilation. Fast-acting β_2-adrenergic agonists are the drug of choice for relief of acute symptoms of asthma (Lougheed, Lemiere, Dell, et al., 2010) and are used as rescue or reliever medication for quick relief of symptoms; therefore, they should be carried by the patient at all times. They are also used to prevent bronchospasm precipitated by exercise, with administration 10 to 15 minutes before exercise. In Canada, several SABAs are approved for this indication, including salbutamol and terbutaline (Lougheed, Lemiere, Dell, et al., 2010). These drugs begin to work within a few minutes and cause maximum dilation within 10 to 15 minutes. The duration of effect varies according to the drug, but airflow rates remain significantly elevated for 2 to 6 hours after inhalation. Adverse events from SABAs are few; they include mild tremor and

tachycardia, which diminish with repeated use without loss of bronchodilator effect. However, frequent daily use of inhaled SABAs may be associated with decreased control of asthma and provides the rationale for as-needed dosage. The frequency of use of reliever medications is a good indicator of a patient's level of asthma control (Lougheed, Lemiere, Dell, et al., 2010).

LABAs provide sustained bronchodilation (approximately 12 hr) and include formoterol and salmeterol. LABAs should be considered as add-on therapy in adults who have persistent symptoms despite low-dosage ICS and in children 6 to 11 years of age who have persistent symptoms despite use of moderate-dosage ICS (Lougheed, Lemiere, Dell, et al., 2010). Both formoterol and salmeterol can help patients reduce the amount of ICS necessary to control asthma and are useful in controlling nocturnal asthma symptoms. However, LABAs are to be used not as monotherapy but rather in combination with an ICS (Lougheed, Lemiere, Dell, et al., 2010). Neither salmeterol nor formoterol causes major adverse events when used in conjunction with ICS. Immediate adverse events are similar to those of SABAs. Salmeterol and formoterol cannot be considered interchangeable. Formoterol has a greater bronchopulmonary protective effect and is rapid acting; thus it can be used as rescue therapy for prompt relief of symptoms when taken in combination with only an ICS (Lougheed, Lemiere, Ducharme, et al., 2012). Salmeterol has a narrower therapeutic window, and dosage should stay within the recommended range.

Combination therapy inhalers that contain both a LABA and an ICS are available and commonly used. The three products available in Canada are Advair, which is a combination of salmeterol and fluticasone; Symbicort, which is a combination of formoterol and budesonide; and Zenhale, which is a combination of formoterol and mometasone. Evidence suggests that combination therapy inhalers can replace the two separate inhalers, thus simplifying therapy and probably increasing adherence to the medication regimen. There is no superior effect over using the two inhalers separately; however, using the two medications in a combination inhaler is preferred for asthma, inasmuch as it the LABA is always used with the ICS (GINA, 2015).

Anticholinergic Drugs. The parasympathetic division of the autonomic nervous system controls airway diameter. The effects of acetylcholine on the airways are increased smooth muscle contraction and mucus secretion, which result in bronchoconstriction. Anticholinergic drugs inhibit bronchoconstriction that is related to the parasympathetic nervous system. Anticholinergic bronchodilators are not recommended as first-line therapy in asthma, primarily because their action does not peak until 30 minutes to 1 hour after ingestion; therefore, they are inferior to SABAs as rescue or reliever inhalers. Anticholinergic drugs, as rescue inhalers, may be useful only in patients who are unable to tolerate SABAs (Lougheed, Lemiere, Dell, et al., 2010). The combination of ipratropium bromide with salbutamol (Combivent; a nebulized preparation) is commonly used for the emergency management of acute asthma. This combination appears to produce greater bronchodilation than does either drug used alone. The most common adverse effect of anticholinergic drugs is dry mouth. Systemic adverse events are uncommon because it is poorly absorbed.

Methylxanthines. Sustained-release methylxanthine (theophylline) preparations should be used only as controller medication for asthma that is difficult to control, after ICS, LABA, and LTRAs. Methylxanthines are bronchodilators with mild anti-inflammatory effects. Theophylline should be prescribed only by an asthma specialist because of its narrow toxic/therapeutic ratio and frequent adverse events (Lougheed, Lemiere, Dell, et al., 2010), which include nausea, headache, insomnia, gastro-intestinal distress, tachycardia, dysrhythmias, and seizures. Blood levels must be monitored regularly to determine whether the drug levels are in the therapeutic range.

Patient Education Related to Drug Therapy. Education about asthma medication is an essential component of asthma care (GINA, 2015). Information about medications with which the patient should be familiar includes name, dosage, method of administration, frequency of use, indications, adverse effects, consequences of improper use, and the importance of adherence. Specifically, with regard to asthma, patients need to be taught about the different roles and indications for using relievers and controllers. In addition to providing information, it is essential that the nurse assess a patient's ability to use inhaler devices accurately and provide coaching in the proper use of the device. Thus all nurses should know the correct use of the various devices and feel confident in their ability to assess and coach patients and their families about their proper use.

Most asthma drugs are administered by inhalation. Inhalation of drugs is preferred to oral administration because a lower dosage is required and systemic adverse events are fewer and less intense. The onset of action of bronchodilators is faster when they are delivered via inhalation. Inhalation devices include MDIs with or without spacers, dry powder inhalers (DPIs), and wet nebulizers (see Table 31-6).

Wet nebulizers are used primarily to deliver large bronchodilator doses during acute asthma attacks in emergency department and other hospital settings. In the home, they are used as a last resort for patients unable to use other inhalation devices. A trial of wet nebulization in infants and young children at home may be appropriate if an MDI with a spacer is ineffective. In response to the outbreak of severe acute respiratory syndrome (SARS), the use of wet nebulization has decreased in emergency departments and hospitals because when wet nebulization is used, aerosol is released into the environment, not just to a patient's airways; thus everyone in the room is breathing in the aerosol. MDIs with spacers are as effective as nebulizers in delivering large doses of bronchodilators during acute asthma attacks because the amount of drug delivered to the lungs is enhanced with the spacer.

Inadequate technique in the use of MDIs is widespread, and many patients demonstrate common errors (Table 31-7). If an inhaler technique can be improved and sustained, clinical benefits are likely to result (Table 31-8). Some patients need to add a spacer to the MDI or switch to a DPI to acquire a good technique. Spacers (e.g., AeroChamber, OptiChamber; see Figure 31-6) are used when patients do not have the coordination necessary to use a MDI. In addition, spacers enhance the delivery of medication to the airways and decrease the intensity of adverse events from ICS because less medication is delivered to the mouth. MDIs with spacers can be considered for all age groups and should be used when ICSs are delivered via MDI. A spacer with a face mask is recommended for young children and older adults. When spacers with face masks are used in children, however, a conversion to a spacer with a mouthpiece is encouraged as soon as the child is old enough and able to cooperate.

The DPI contains dry, powdered medication and is breath-activated (Figure 31-7). No propellant is used; instead, an aerosol is created when the patient inhales quickly and forcefully through a reservoir containing a dose of powder. Patients find DPIs easier to use than MDIs with no spacer. There are several advantages

TABLE 31-7	PROBLEMS ENCOUNTERED WITH USE OF METERED-DOSE INHALER (MDI)

1. Failing to coordinate activation with inspiration
2. Activating MDI in the mouth while breathing through nose
3. Inspiring too rapidly
4. Not holding the breath for 10 sec (or as close to 10 sec as possible)
5. Holding MDI upside down or sideways
6. Inhaling more than one puff with each inspiration
7. Not shaking MDI before use
8. Not waiting a sufficient amount of time between each puff
9. Not opening mouth wide enough, which causes medication to bounce off teeth, tongue, or palate
10. Not having adequate strength to activate MDI
11. Being unable to perform all the necessary steps

FIGURE 31-7 Example of a dry powder inhaler (DPI). Source: From Potter, P. A., Perry, A. G., Stockert, P., et al. (2011). *Basic nursing: Essentials for practice* (7th ed.). St. Louis: Mosby.

to using DPIs: (a) less manual dexterity is required; (b) the patient does not need to coordinate depressing the canister with inhaling; (c) an easily visible colour or number system indicates the number of doses left in the device; and (d) no spacer is necessary. The biggest problem with DPIs is that the medication may clump if exposed to humidity, and so they should be stored in a dry place. The care of DPIs involves wiping off the mouthpiece with a dry tissue. Water or other liquids should never be used to clean the device, which could cause clumping of the medication and cause the device to work improperly.

Various inhalation devices are used to deliver medications to the airways. It is important to work with patients individually to identify the inhalation device that best fits their needs.

Poor adherence to asthma therapy regimens is a major challenge in the long-term management of asthma. Patients commonly rely too heavily on their reliever inhalers because they provide immediate relief of symptoms and gratification, whereas no immediate benefit is felt with anti-inflammatory therapy, which must be sustained on a daily basis. It is important to explain to patients the importance and purpose of taking controller therapy

TABLE 31-8   PATIENT & CAREGIVER TEACHING GUIDE

How to Use a Metered-Dose Inhaler (MDI) Correctly

The nurse must teach the patient that the key to using all inhaled medications is proper technique. Patients should receive the following instructions to ensure that every puff of the MDI delivers the most medication possible into the lungs, rather than to the back of the throat.

1. Firmly place the metal container into the mouthpiece. Remove the cap, and shake the inhaler vigorously.
2. Breathe out only to the end of a normal breath (not a forced breath).
3. Position the mouthpiece end of the inhaler approximately 4 cm (1.5 inches) from your mouth.
4. Open your mouth widely, and tilt your head back slightly. (Another way of doing this is to close your lips around the mouthpiece, keeping teeth apart and tongue flat so the medication can flow freely into the lungs.)
5. At the same time that you start to breathe in slowly, depress the metal container into the mouthpiece to release one puff of medication.
6. Continue breathing in slowly until your lungs are full (approximately 5 seconds).
   - Once you have breathed in fully, hold your breath for 10 seconds (or as long as comfortable).
   - If you need a second puff, wait 30–60 seconds before repeating the preceding steps.

Is the Inhaler Full?

The patient needs to know the correct way to determine whether the MDI must be replaced. Shaking the canister is not a reliable method because the patient may be hearing only the propellant move in the canister when the MDI is nearly empty. The only reliable method, if the MDI does not have a counter, is to count each puff. Alternatively, the patient can plan the length of use on the basis of prescribed puffs per day: for example, if the patient uses two puffs, twice-a-day use means that the inhaler must be replaced in 50 days. Most canisters contain 200 doses. It is a good practice to keep a spare inhaler on hand.

Special Instructions for Children

Most children younger than 9 years cannot use an MDI properly. For these children, a spacer should be used with the MDI. Regardless of the child's age, spacers are recommended when a steroid inhaler is used, to reduce the risk of developing a yeast infection in the mouth or the throat and to enhance the distribution of the medication to the small airways.

How to Use a Metered-Dose Inhaler With a Spacer

Some people, no matter how hard they try, still have trouble coordinating an MDI. Fortunately, spacers (holding chambers), which hold the medication for a few seconds after it has been released from the inhaler, are available. The patient's physician or Certified Respiratory Educator may recommend one if the patient has trouble with an MDI or is using an ICS.

Spacers may also reduce occurrence of adverse drug events such as hoarseness or sore throat if the patient is taking higher dosages of ICS. Spacers can be used with most aerosol inhalers and are very easy to use. Following are instructions for using a spacer with an MDI:

1. Remove the plastic cap from the inhaler mouthpiece and the spacer mouthpiece.
2. Insert the inhaler mouthpiece into the large opening of the spacer.
3. Hold the spacer and inhaler together and shake well.
4. Forcibly exhale.
5. Put the mouthpiece of the spacer into your mouth, close your lips around it; do not cover the small slots.
6. Press the metal canister down into the inhaler to spray the medication into the spacer. Then, breathe in slowly and deeply through your mouth (for approximately 5 seconds).
7. Hold your breath for as long as you comfortably can (approximately 10 seconds).
8. Breathe out slowly through your mouth or nose.
9. If more puffs are prescribed, wait 1 minute and then repeat these steps, starting from step 3.

Caring for the Spacer

Spacers must be cleaned weekly because powder collects on the walls of a spacer with repeated use. To clean, agitate the spacer device carefully in warm tap water mixed with dish soap. Shake off excess water, do not rinse, and allow it to air dry overnight; do not dry with a towel. The soap residue left on the chamber, as well as not using a towel to dry, will prevent static cling and therefore prevent medication from clinging to the inside of the chamber.

ICS, inhaled corticosteroids; *MDI,* metered dose inhaler.
Source: Adapted from Asthma Society of Canada. (2016). *How to use your inhaler: Cleaning your spacer.* Retrieved from *http://www.asthma.ca/adults/treatment/spacers.php.*

regularly, emphasizing that maximum improvement may take more than 1 week. It is also important to emphasize that without regular use, the inflammation in the airways may progress and the asthma is likely to worsen over time.

NURSING MANAGEMENT ASTHMA

NURSING ASSESSMENT

If a patient can speak and is not in acute distress, a detailed health history, including identification of any precipitating factors and what has helped alleviate attacks in the past, should be documented. If a patient is in acute distress, some of the information may be obtained from the person accompanying the patient. Subjective and objective data to obtain from a patient with asthma are presented in Table 31-9.

NURSING DIAGNOSES

Nursing diagnoses for the patient with asthma may include, but are not limited to, the following:

- *Ineffective airway clearance* related to *excessive mucus, retained secretions*
- *Anxiety* related to *threat to current status, threat of death* (difficulty breathing)
- *Deficient knowledge* related to *insufficient information, insufficient knowledge of resources* (asthma education)

Additional information on nursing diagnoses is presented in Nursing Care Plan 31-1.

TABLE 31-9 NURSING ASSESSMENT

Asthma

Subjective Data
Important Health Information
Current health: Assess the level of asthma control (see Table 31-2); frequency and severity of asthma symptoms (wheeze, cough, sensation of chest tightness, dyspnea) in the past week, both during the day and in early morning hours and night; need for reliever medication during the past week; and usual pattern of asthma symptoms. Determine whether the patient experienced a recent worsening of asthma and how it was handled. Identify recent exposure to triggers (e.g., upper respiratory tract infection, pollen, animals, mould, dust, inhaled irritants, weather changes, exercise, smoke).
Past health history: One or more previous asthma attacks and response to treatment; previous visits to the emergency department or hospitalizations for asthma and the need for ICU admission and intubation; recent exposure to pollen, dander, feathers, mould, dust, inhaled irritants, weather changes, exercise, smoke; allergic rhinitis and eczema; sinus infections; gastroesophageal reflux; family history of asthma and allergies
Medications: Last time the reliever medication was used, what level of relief was provided, duration of relief, and frequency of the reliever use in the past week; pattern of use for controller medications; recent use of antibiotics; use of medications that may precipitate asthma, such as ASA (Aspirin), NSAIDs, β-adrenergic blockers; allergies to medications

Symptoms
• Wheezing, cough, sensation of chest tightness, dyspnea
• Decreased level of activity or exercise because of symptoms
• Interrupted sleep, fatigue; fear, anxiety, panic, depression, emotional distress

Objective Data
General
Restlessness or exhaustion, confusion, upright or forward-leaning body position

Integumentary
Eczema, diaphoresis, cyanosis (circumoral, nail beds)

Respiratory
Wheezing, crackles, diminishment or absence of breath sounds on auscultation; hyper-resonance on percussion; sputum character and quantity; increased work of breathing, demonstrated by use of accessory muscle, intercostal and supraclavicular retractions; tachypnea; prolonged expiration

Cardiovascular
Tachycardia, pulsus paradoxus, jugular venous distension, hypertension or hypotension, premature ventricular contractions

Possible Diagnostic Findings
Abnormal results of pulmonary function tests: decreased flow rates; FVC, FEV_1, PEFR, and FEV_1/FVC ratio that improve with bronchodilators and between exacerbations
↓ O_2 saturation and abnormal ABG values during moderately severe to life-threatening attacks
Serum and sputum eosinophilia
Positive results of skin tests for allergens and allergies to medication

ABG, arterial blood gas; *FEV_1,* forced expiratory volume in 1 second; *FVC,* forced vital capacity; *ICU,* intensive care unit; *NSAIDs,* nonsteroidal anti-inflammatory drugs; *PEFR,* peak expiratory flow rate.

PLANNING

The overall goals are that patients with asthma will (a) be able to participate in activities of normal life (including exercise and other physical activity) with little to no interference; (b) have normal or near-normal pulmonary function; (c) have the asthma under control; (d) experience as few adverse effects from asthma medication as possible while taking the lowest dosage of medication necessary to keep the asthma under control; and (e) possess the knowledge and skills necessary to participate in the management of the asthma.

NURSING IMPLEMENTATION

ASTHMA EDUCATION. Nurses play an essential role in preventing and controlling asthma symptoms by developing a partnership with the patient and family, providing information and education, and helping the patient and family develop the necessary skills for controlling asthma. Education is an essential component of asthma care and should occur at every encounter with patients, families, and caregivers. In order to be effective, asthma education must provide information, help develop and refine asthma-related skills, assist with problem solving, and cause behaviour change. In addition, findings of meta-analyses suggest that self-management asthma education programs can reduce the number of emergency department visits, hospitalizations, urgent care visits, nocturnal awakenings related to asthma, and days of interrupted activity and can improve quality of life (PHAC, 2011). Asthma education programs can also be cost effective. Table 31-10 details basic asthma education to be provided.

ENVIRONMENTAL CONTROL. Environmental control strategies focus on reducing exposure to asthma triggers specific to the individual. Triggers can be divided into two groups: allergens and irritants. Patients should be taught to identify known personal triggers for asthma and to reduce exposure to them (see Table 31-1). Sensitization to environmental allergens is clearly linked to asthma in children and adults (PHAC, 2011). However, before patients and families are advised to use environmental control strategies to reduce or manage exposure to allergens, it is important to understand the allergen to which they are sensitized.

House dust mites produce a common allergen that can trigger asthma. House dust mites are sightless, eight-legged microorganisms. They excrete food and digestive enzymes as a fecal particle, which is the major form of mite allergen. House dust mites require dead skin and water to survive, and thus the bed provides a perfect environment because when humans sleep, they slough off dead skin and provide humidity. As a result, control strategies focus on the bedroom and include keeping the relative humidity below 50%; encasing the mattress, box springs, and pillows in covers that are impermeable to mites and mite allergens; laundering bed linen in hot water and hot (55°C) air to dry it; and possibly removing carpets (PHAC, 2011).

Pet dander is another common allergen, and strategies to reduce exposure have been evaluated. The removal of the pet is the most effective means to reduce exposure. However, this is often not a realistic option for patients and families. As a result, numerous alternative strategies have been evaluated to minimize or reduce exposure. These strategies include excluding the pet and its dander from the bedroom by keeping the door and heating register closed; frequent vacuuming (including furniture) with a high-efficiency particulate air (HEPA)–filtered vacuum; removing carpets; and washing the pet at least twice a

◎ NURSING CARE PLAN 31-1

Asthma

NURSING DIAGNOSIS	***Ineffective airway clearance*** related to *excessive mucus, retained secretions* as evidenced by *ineffective cough, adventitious breath sounds*

Expected Patient Outcomes

- Maintains open airways
- Has normal breath sounds and respiratory rate
- Has normal or personal best objective lung function measurements (PEFR, FEV₁, FEV₁/FVC)
- Participates in normal life activities, including exercise and physical activity (identifying activity that is meaningful to the patient is helpful)

Nursing Interventions and *Rationales*

- Position patient to maximize ventilation potential *allowing for adequate chest expansion.*
- Monitor respiratory (including spirometry) and oxygenation status *to determine need for intervention or to note improvement.*
- Administer medications (e.g., bronchodilators, corticosteroids), as appropriate, *to improve respiratory function.*
- Teach patient proper use of prescribed inhalers (see Table 31-8) *to deliver adequate medication to the lungs.*
- Auscultate lung sounds after treatments *to note improvement.*
- Regulate fluid intake to optimize fluid balance and liquefy secretions *to facilitate removal.*
- Provide asthma education *to help patient understand condition and avoid triggers, when possible.*
- Establish a written asthma action plan with patient to manage exacerbations., and educating the patient about it *to ensure that patient is prepared for emergency situations.*

NURSING DIAGNOSIS	***Anxiety*** related to *threat to current status* (difficulty breathing, perceived or actual loss of control, fear of suffocation) as evidenced by *restlessness, increase in heart rate, respiratory rate, and blood pressure*

Expected Patient Outcomes

- Reports reduced anxiety or no anxiety

Nursing Interventions and *Rationales*

- Explore patterns of anxiety and feelings, perceptions, and fears *to identify precipitating factors and problem areas so that planning can be concentrated.*
- Use a calm, supportive approach *to provide reassurance.*
- Stay with patient *to promote safety and reduce fear.*
- Provide factual information concerning diagnosis, treatment, and prognosis *to help patient know what to expect.*
- Instruct patient on the use of relaxation techniques *to relieve muscle tension and slow respirations.*

NURSING DIAGNOSIS	***Deficient knowledge*** related to *insufficient information, insufficient knowledge of resources* (asthma and treatment) as evidenced by *inaccurate follow-through of instruction*

Expected Patient Outcomes

- Demonstrates appropriate use of inhalers, peak flow-meters, spacers, and nebulizers (if used)
- Maintains good asthma control
- Manages personal triggers
- Recognizes worsening asthma and initiates early treatment
- Actively participates in management decisions with the asthma care team

Nursing Interventions and *Rationales**

- Appraise patient's current level of knowledge and skills related to asthma management *to identify learning needs.*
- Teach patient to identify and manage triggers *to prevent asthma attacks.*
- Encourage patient to verbalize feelings about diagnosis, treatment, and effect on lifestyle *to offer support and increase adherence to medication regimen to improve asthma control.*
- Ensure that patient has an asthma action plan and understands its use *to enhance patient's ability to identify worsening asthma and respond appropriately.*
- Instruct the patient about the proper administration of each medication* (e.g., inhalers, spacers) *to ensure proper use.*
- Evaluate the patient's inhaler techniques *to assess correct technique and ensure maximum benefit.*
- Instruct the patient on purpose, action, dosage, indication, and duration of each medication *to promote understanding of effects and use.*
- Instruct patient about strategies to decrease the intensity of adverse drug events *to prevent or minimize the intensity of adverse drug events and enhance adherence.*
- Assist patient to identify strategies that incorporate taking medications into daily life, such as taking inhaled steroids before brushing teeth in the morning and at night, *to enhance adherence.*
- Include the family and significant others as appropriate *to ensure that a knowledgeable person is available to help when the patient needs it*

*Refer to Figures 31-6 and 31-7 and to Patient & Caregiver Teaching Guides (see Tables 31-8, 31-10, and 31-11).
FEV₁, forced expiratory volume; *FVC,* forced vital capacity; *PEFR,* peak expiratory flow rate.

TABLE 31-10	PATIENT & CAREGIVER TEACHING GUIDE

Basic Asthma Education

Basic asthma education for patients and caregivers should include:

Basic Facts About Asthma
- Basic anatomical and physiological characteristics of the lungs
- Pathophysiological changes of asthma
- Relationship of pathophysiological changes to signs and symptoms
- Asthma control criteria (signs and symptoms)

Trigger Control
- Identification of possible triggers and management strategies
- Avoidance of allergens and other triggers

Medications
- Differences between relievers and controllers
- Indications for using reliever as opposed to controller medication
- Establishing medication schedule
- Adverse effects and strategies to reduce their frequency and intensity

Device Technique
- Good inhaler technique
- Good peak flowmeter and monitoring technique (if applicable)

Self-Monitoring and Action Plan
- Development of an individualized asthma action plan
- Early recognition of worsening asthma
- Actions to take in response to worsening asthma

Follow-Up Care
- Understanding and accepting the need for regular follow-up care

week (none of these actions to be performed by the person with the allergies).

Environmental tobacco smoke is the most harmful indoor air irritant and should be avoided. Environmental tobacco smoke is a risk factor for the development of childhood asthma and frequently causes the worsening of asthma in children and adults. Among children with asthma, those whose parents smoke have more severe disease than do those whose parents do not smoke. When parents of a child with asthma stop smoking, the child's asthma improves. Nurses must encourage patients and their family members to stop smoking and assist them with identifying smoking cessation strategies.

Exercise and cold air are very common asthma triggers. Strategies to prevent exposure to cold air include the use of scarves and face masks. Exercise is just as important for individuals with asthma as those without it because it provides multiple health benefits. Asthma is not an excuse for avoiding exercise. If a form of exercise provokes asthma symptoms, the nurse can advise the patient to use a warm-up period and an inhaled SABA 10 to 15 minutes before the activity to prevent bronchospasm.

Occupational asthma, defined as asthma symptoms induced by exposure to a specific irritant in the workplace, is the most common occupational lung disease. Exposure to irritants in the occupational environment resulting in occupational asthma has been reported in 10% or less among current workers in cross-sectional studies (Tarlo & Lemiere, 2014). Objective lung function tests, along with a detailed occupational exposure history, are necessary to confirm the diagnosis of occupational asthma. If occupational asthma is suspected, the patient should

be referred to his or her primary care provider, a specialist, or an occupational hygienist.

SELF-MONITORING AND ACTION PLANS. According to the Canadian Asthma Consensus Guidelines (Lougheed, Lemiere, Dell, et al., 2010), every person with asthma should have an asthma action plan (Figure 31-8). An action plan is a written plan developed to provide the patient with a framework for monitoring and determining his or her level of asthma control and making treatment changes to achieve and maintain control. Often, action plans are designed according to a traffic-light analogy: green, yellow, and red "zones." The green zone represents good asthma control and signals "go" with current therapy. The yellow zone is a time of worsening or uncontrolled asthma and signals "caution" and the need for enhanced anti-inflammatory therapy. The red zone represents a time of danger during which the asthma is severe enough to necessitate urgent medical attention; it signals "stop" current activities in order to address this need.

Nurses must develop a partnership with patients and their families, their primary asthma care provider, and the rest of the asthma care team in order to help patients attain and effectively use an individualized asthma action plan. Systematic reviews concluded that self-management programs that included self-monitoring, either by symptoms or peak flow, combined with a written action plan and regular medical review, resulted in reduced need for health care services, fewer days lost from work, and fewer episodes of nocturnal asthma (GINA, 2015). Self-monitoring based on symptom experience alone was compared with self-monitoring based on both symptom experience and peak expiratory flow monitoring; comparable outcomes were reported (GINA, 2015). PEFR provides an objective measurement of lung function (Table 31-11). As a result, it has been advocated for detecting asthma exacerbations; however, for most people, asthma symptoms are a more sensitive measure and change earlier in the course of an exacerbation than does PEFR. The choice of whether an action plan is based on PEFR or symptom monitoring may be made according to a patient's ability to perceive symptoms and airflow limitation, the availability of peak flowmeters, and, of most importance, the patient's preferences.

The level of detail in the plan depends on the patient's understanding of asthma and preferences for monitoring (PEFR or symptoms). Key components for teaching patients and their families how to use an action plan include the signs and symptoms of worsening asthma, knowing the level of asthma control and how to adjust medications, and when to seek medical attention. The green zone represents a time when a patient's asthma is under good control (see Table 31-2); peak flow rates are usually 80% or more of predicted or of the patient's personal best (see Table 31-11). When asthma status is in the green zone, the patient should continue with the current therapeutic plan. If asthma status has been in the green zone for a couple of months, an attempt to reduce medication dosages may be warranted. The potential risk of a medication reduction is worsening asthma that necessitates an increase in medications to regain control.

The yellow zone represents a time of uncontrolled asthma, as demonstrated by symptom occurrence, the need for an inhaled short-acting bronchodilator (reliever), and, if measured, PEFR between 50% (some authorities use 60%) and 79% of predicted or personal best (see Table 31-2). In response to worsening asthma, some patients are advised to see their primary asthma care providers, whereas others are advised to increase dosages of

THE ✚ LUNG ASSOCIATION®

MY ASTHMA ACTION PLAN

Name _____   Doctor _____

Date _____   Doctor's Phone Number _____

GREEN LEVEL   My asthma is under control.

SYMPTOMS

- My breathing is normal.
- I have no trouble sleeping.
- I'm not coughing or wheezing.
- I can do all my normal activities.

PEAK FLOW

_____ to _____ (80 to 100% of your personal best)

WHAT SHOULD I DO?

I should continue using my normal medications as directed by my doctor, and re-measure my peak flow every _____ weeks/months.

Medication	Dose	Take it when?

YELLOW LEVEL   My asthma is getting worse.

SYMPTOMS

- I have symptoms, like wheezing or coughing, with activity or at night. They go away when I use my reliever.
- I'm using my reliever more than ___ times a week/day.
- I can't do many of my usual activities.

PEAK FLOW

_____ to _____ (60 to 80% of your personal best)

WHAT SHOULD I DO?

A problem is beginning. I should increase my medication as specified below until I am in the green level for _____ days or more. **If my symptoms do not improve within 4 days, I will call my doctor.**

Medication	Dose	Take it when?

RED LEVEL   I am having an asthma emergency.

SYMPTOMS

- My breathing is difficult.
- I'm wheezing often when resting.
- I'm having difficulty walking and/or talking.
- My lips and/or fingernails are blue or grey.
- My reliever does not help in 10 minutes OR is needed every 4 hours or more.

PEAK FLOW

_____ to _____ (less than 60% of your personal best)

WHAT SHOULD I DO?

I NEED TO GO TO THE HOSPITAL EMERGENCY RIGHT AWAY.

I SHOULD USE MY RELIEVER AS MUCH AS I NEED TO ON THE WAY THERE.

FIGURE 31-8 Example of an asthma action plan. Source: Modified from the Canadian Lung Association (n.d.). *Asthma action plan*. Retrieved from *https://www.lung.ca/sites/default/files/media/asthma_action_plan.pdf*.

anti-inflammatory medication. Typically, this involves initiating the use of an inhaled corticosteroid, doubling, tripling, or quadrupling the dosage of inhaled corticosteroid, or initiating a short burst of oral corticosteroids. Not all patients feel comfortable adjusting medications without seeing their asthma care provider, which highlights the importance of tailoring the type of action plan to meet the individual's needs and preferences.

The red zone represents a time of severe asthma and the need for immediate medical assistance. Indications of the red zone are difficulty completing a sentence without needing another breath; incomplete relief from reliever inhaler or use more frequently than every 2 hours; or, if the patient is using a peak flowmeter, a PEFR between less than 50% and 60% of predicted or personal best value. Affected patients are advised to use their

TABLE 31-11   PATIENT & CAREGIVER TEACHING GUIDE

How to Use a Peak Flowmeter

Follow these five steps to use a peak flowmeter:
1. Move the indicator to the bottom of the numbered scale.
2. Stand up, or sit upright.
3. Take a deep breath in, and fill your lungs completely.
4. Place the mouthpiece in your mouth and close your lips around it.
5. Blow out as hard and fast as possible in a single blow.
6. Write down the value. If coughing occurred, the value is inaccurate; do not record that value. Repeat the test.
7. Repeat steps 1 through 5 twice more.
8. Record the highest result of the three.

Finding the Personal Best Peak Flow Number

- The patient's personal best peak flow number is the highest peak flow number achieved over a 2- to 3-week period when asthma is under good control.
- Each patient's manifestations of asthma are different, and the "best" peak flow value may be higher or lower than that of another person of the same height, weight, and sex. The action plan must be based on the patient's personal best peak flow value.
- To identify the patient's personal best peak flow number, the patient should record peak flow readings
  - At least twice a day for 2 to 3 weeks
  - Upon awakening and before bed
  - Before and 15 minutes after taking a short-acting inhaled bronchodilator (reliever)

Source: Registered Nurses' Association of Ontario. (2004). Appendix I: How to use a peak flow meter. In *Adult asthma care guidelines for nurses: Promoting control of asthma* (p. 94). Toronto: Author. Retrieved from *http://rnao.ca/sites/rnao-ca/files/Adult_Asthma_Care_Guidelines_for_Nurses_-_Promoting_Control_of_Asthma.pdf.* Reprinted with permission of the Registered Nurses' Association of Ontario.

short-acting inhaled β_2 agonists on their way to the emergency department.

In developing a management plan, it is important to involve the patient's family. Family members and friends should be taught how to help the patient during an asthma exacerbation. They should know where the patient's inhalers and emergency phone numbers are located. Family members can help patients identify deteriorating levels of asthma control, inasmuch as they may notice an increase in symptoms or avoidance of certain activities before the patient notices.

It is particularly important to provide asthma education, which should occur at every encounter with the patient and family, during emergency department visits, and during hospitalization because this is a time when patients are highly motivated to learn and do not have to schedule an additional visit. The Canadian Lung Association develops and distributes several excellent resources for individuals affected by asthma. (See the Resources at the end of this chapter.)

EVALUATION. The expected outcomes for the patient with asthma are presented in Nursing Care Plan 31-1.

CHRONIC OBSTRUCTIVE PULMONARY DISEASE

Chronic obstructive pulmonary disease (COPD) is a preventable disease, characterized by persistent airflow limitation that is usually progressive. It is associated with an enhanced chronic inflammatory response in the airways and lungs, caused primarily by cigarette smoking and other noxious particles and gases. COPD exacerbations and other coexisting illnesses or comorbid conditions contribute to the overall severity of the disease (Global Initiative for Chronic Obstructive Lung Disease [GOLD], 2017).

Cardinal symptoms experienced by patients with COPD are dyspnea, difficulty breathing, or shortness of breath and limitations in activity. Symptoms are usually insidious in onset and progressive. Dyspnea is the subjective experience of shortness of breath and is the most disabling symptom in COPD (GOLD, 2017). Initially, COPD is confined to the lungs, but when disease is advanced, skeletal muscle dysfunction, right-sided heart failure, secondary polycythemia, depression, and altered nutrition are commonly observed. Past definitions of COPD included the terms *emphysema* and *chronic bronchitis*. Emphysema describes only one pathological change present in COPD: destruction of the alveoli. Chronic bronchitis, which is the presence of chronic productive cough for 3 months in 2 successive years, remains a useful epidemiological term but it, too, does not convey how airway limitation so severely affects morbidity and mortality in patients with COPD (GOLD, 2017). People with COPD often display characteristics of both chronic bronchitis and emphysema (GOLD, 2017).

The PHAC (2015a) reported that the prevalence of COPD among the population aged 35 years and older was 9.7%. The prevalence among men (9.8%) and women (9.6%) are currently comparable, although rates of COPD and of subsequent hospitalization and death are rising more rapidly among women. Hospitalization may be required in the treatment of COPD, particularly when symptoms worsen from infection. The *Survey on Living with Chronic Diseases in Canada* (SLCDC) revealed that 20% of respondents reported one or more visits to the emergency department in the previous 12 months and 8% reported one or more nights in the hospital in the previous 12 months because of COPD (PHAC, 2011). Overall, 21% of respondents to the SLCDC reported that breathing problems affect their daily life activities "quite a bit or extremely" (PHAC, 2011). COPD accounts for approximately 4.4% of all deaths in Canada, which is probably an underestimation because the primary cause of death may be listed as pneumonia or heart failure (Bryan & Navaneelan, 2015).

Causes

Cigarette Smoking. Exposure to tobacco smoke is the primary cause of 80% to 90% of COPD cases in Canada (Bryan & Navaneelan, 2015). In 2012, 16% of Canadians older than 15 years were smoking (Health Canada, 2012). Although the prevalence of cigarette smoking has decreased, it is still a major public health concern.

Clinically significant airway obstruction develops in 15% to 20% of smokers. For most Canadians who die of lung diseases related to cigarette smoking, death is preceded by a long period of debilitation characterized by frequent hospitalizations and loss of many years of productivity. Cigarette smoking remains the most preventable cause of premature death in Canada.

When cigarettes are smoked, approximately 4 000 chemicals and gases are inhaled into the lungs. Over 60 carcinogens have been isolated from cigarette smoke, including cyanide, formaldehyde, and ammonia. Nicotine is probably not a carcinogen, but it has deleterious effects. It acts by stimulating the sympathetic nervous system, resulting in increases in heart rate, peripheral vasoconstriction, blood pressure, and cardiac workload. These effects of nicotine compound the problems in a person with coronary artery disease. (The effects of nicotine are discussed further in Chapter 11.)

Cigarette smoke has several direct effects on the respiratory tract. It simulates an inflammatory response in the lung, which is most evident late in the course of COPD. The irritating effect of the smoke causes hyperplasia of goblet cells, which subsequently results in increased production of mucus and is the basis of chronic cough and sputum accumulation. In airways smaller than 2 mm in diameter, injury leads to narrowing and obstruction of the airways. Smoking reduces ciliary activity and accelerates loss of ciliated cells. Smoking also produces abnormal dilation of the distal air space with destruction of alveolar walls. Many cells develop large, atypical nuclei, which is considered a precancerous condition. Removal of the inciting stimulus is of greatest benefit early in the process but may be less effective in late disease. However, smoking cessation can prevent or delay the development of airflow limitation or slow its progression.

Carbon monoxide is a component of tobacco smoke. Carbon monoxide has a high affinity for hemoglobin and combines with it more readily than does oxygen, thereby reducing the smoker's oxygen-carrying capacity. Smokers inhale a lower percentage of oxygen than normal; as a result, less oxygen is available at the alveolar level. The heart's need for oxygen is increased because of the stimulatory effect of nicotine on the sympathetic nervous system. Because the blood's oxygen-carrying capacity is reduced, the heart must pump more rapidly to adequately supply tissues with oxygen. Carbon monoxide also seems to impair psychomotor performance and judgement.

Passive smoking (also known as *environmental tobacco smoke* or *second-hand smoke*) is the exposure of nonsmokers to cigarette smoke. In adults, involuntary smoke exposure is associated with decreased pulmonary function, increased risk for lung cancer, and increased rates of mortality from ischemic heart disease.

Occupational Chemicals and Dusts. High levels of urban air pollution are harmful to people with existing lung disease. However, the effect of outdoor air pollution as a risk factor for the development of COPD is unclear. In a person who has intense or prolonged exposure to various dusts, vapours, irritants, or fumes in the workplace, COPD can develop independently of cigarette smoking (PHAC, 2011). If the person also smokes, the risk of COPD increases (GOLD, 2017).

Infection. Recurring respiratory tract infection is a major factor contributing to the aggravation and progression of COPD (GOLD, 2017). The pathological destruction of lung tissue and the ensuing progression of COPD results from the recurring infections, which impair normal defence mechanisms, making the bronchioles and alveoli more susceptible to injury, and increase inflammation (GOLD, 2017). The most common causative organisms are *Haemophilus influenzae, Streptococcus pneumoniae,* and *Moraxella catarrhalis,* and in patients with severe to very severe COPD, *Pseudomonas aeruginosa* is probably a causative organism (GOLD, 2017). Retained secretions constitute a good medium for their proliferation.

Severe recurring respiratory tract infections in childhood have been associated with reduced lung function and increased respiratory symptoms in adulthood. It is unclear whether the development of COPD can be related to recurrent infections in adults. People who smoke and also have human immunodeficiency virus (HIV) infection have an accelerated development of COPD. Tuberculosis is also a risk factor for COPD development.

Heredity. α_1-Antitrypsin (AAT) deficiency is currently the only known genetic abnormality that leads to COPD; however, research is ongoing to identify other genes that predispose a person to developing this disease (GOLD, 2017). AAT (also termed α_1-*protease inhibitor*) is the major antiprotease in plasma, and its primary function is to inhibit neutrophil elastase. It is produced by the liver and is normally found in the lungs, where it inhibits the action of proteolytic enzymes from neutrophils (neutrophil elastase) and macrophages. Lower levels of AAT result in insufficient inactivation of neutrophil elastase, and the subsequent lysis of lung tissue causes destruction of the alveoli. Severe AAT deficiency leads to early-onset COPD. Smoking greatly exacerbates the disease process in affected patients (GOLD, 2017).

Intravenous or nebulizer-administered AAT (Prolastin) replacement therapy is available for people with AAT deficiency (GOLD, 2017). Infusions are administered weekly. Such therapy should be restricted to AAT-deficient patients who do not smoke and whose postbronchodilator FEV_1 is between 35% and 50% of predicted. Its effectiveness in slowing the progression of the disease continues to be evaluated.

Aging. Aging results in changes in the lung structure and respiratory muscles that cause a gradual loss of the elastic recoil of the lung. As a result, the lungs become smaller and stiffer. The number of functional alveoli decreases as a result of the loss of the alveolar supporting structures. Thoracic cage changes result

---

GENETICS IN CLINICAL PRACTICE

α_1-Antitrypsin (AAT) Deficiency

Genetic Basis
- Described as an autosomal recessive and codominant genetic disorder; >120 alleles.
- Gene for AAT located on chromosome 14.
- Several allelic variants of AAT gene.

Incidence and Prevalence
- Severe AAT deficiency occurs in 1 in 5 000 to 1 in 5 500 of Canadian and North American population.
- Exact prevalence of AAT deficiency in patients with diagnosed COPD: unknown, but estimated prevalence is 1%–5%.
- Severe AAT deficiency occurs in approximately 1 in 1 600 of the Scandinavian population.
- AAT deficiency is found in equal numbers of male and female patients.

Genetic Testing
- Targeted testing for AAT deficiency is recommended for individuals with COPD diagnosed before the age of 65 yr or with a smoking history of <20 pack-years.
- DNA testing is available.
- Screening of siblings is useful.
- Serum assay is available to test for AAT deficiency.

Clinical Implications
- Genetic disorder is linked to COPD.
- AAT deficiency is associated with cirrhosis, hepatitis, panniculitis, and anti–proteinase 3 antibody vasculitis.
- Treatment may include AAT replacement (Prolastin).
- Predisposes patients to early-onset COPD (in the third or fourth decade of life)
- Participation in AAT Canadian Registry is encouraged.

Source: Based on Marciniuk, D.D., Hernandez, P., Balter, M., et al. (2012). Alpha-1 antitrypsin deficiency targeted testing and augmentation therapy: A Canadian Thoracic Society clinical practice guideline. *Canadian Respiratory Journal, 19*(2), 109–116.

PATHOPHYSIOLOGY MAP

FIGURE 31-9 Pathophysiological changes of chronic obstructive pulmonary disease (COPD).

from osteoporosis and calcification of the costal cartilages. The thoracic cage becomes stiff and rigid, and the ribs are less mobile. These changes result in a decreased compliance of the chest wall and an increase in the work of breathing. These changes are similar to those in patients with emphysema. With fewer capillaries available for gas exchange, arterial oxygen levels decrease. Clinically significant emphysema is usually not caused by aging alone.

Pathophysiology

COPD is characterized by chronic inflammation found in the airways, lung parenchyma (respiratory bronchioles and alveoli), and pulmonary blood vessels (Figure 31-9). The pathogenesis of COPD is complex and involves many mechanisms. The defining features of COPD are (a) airflow limitations during forced exhalation that are caused by loss of elastic recoil and are not fully reversible and (b) airflow obstruction caused by mucus hypersecretion, mucosal edema, and bronchospasm.

In COPD, airflow limitation, air trapping, gas exchange abnormalities, mucus hypersecretion, and, in severe disease, pulmonary hypertension and systemic abnormalities are among the various disease processes that occur (see Figure 31-9). The inflammatory process starts with inhalation of noxious particles and gases (e.g., cigarette smoke) but is magnified in people with COPD. The abnormal inflammatory process causes tissue destruction and disrupts the normal defence mechanisms and repair processes of the lungs.

The predominant inflammatory cells in COPD are neutrophils, macrophages, and lymphocytes. This pattern of inflammatory cells is different from that in asthma. The inflammatory cells in COPD attract other inflammatory mediators (e.g., leukotrienes, interleukins). This cascading inflammatory process results in the activation of proinflammatory cytokines such as tumour necrosis factor. In addition, growth factors are recruited into the area and activated, which results in structural changes in the lungs.

The inflammatory process may also be magnified by oxidative stress. Oxidants are produced by cigarette smoke and other inhaled particles and are released from the inflammatory cells, such as macrophages and neutrophils, during inflammation. The oxidative stress adversely affects the lungs as it inactivates antiproteases (which prevent the natural destruction of the lungs), stimulates mucus secretion, and increases fluid in the lungs (GOLD, 2017).

After the inhalation of oxidants in tobacco or air pollution, the activity of proteases (which break down the connective tissue of the lungs) increases, and the antiproteases (which protect against the breakdown) are inhibited. Therefore, the natural balance of protease/antiprotease is tipped in favour of destruction of the alveoli and loss of the elastic recoil of the lung (GOLD, 2017).

Inability to expire air is a main characteristic of COPD. The airflow limitation occurs primarily in the smaller airways and is caused by remodelling. As the peripheral airways become obstructed, air is progressively trapped during expiration. The residual air becomes significant in severe disease as alveolar attachments to small airways (similar to rubber bands) are destroyed. The residual air, combined with the loss of elastic

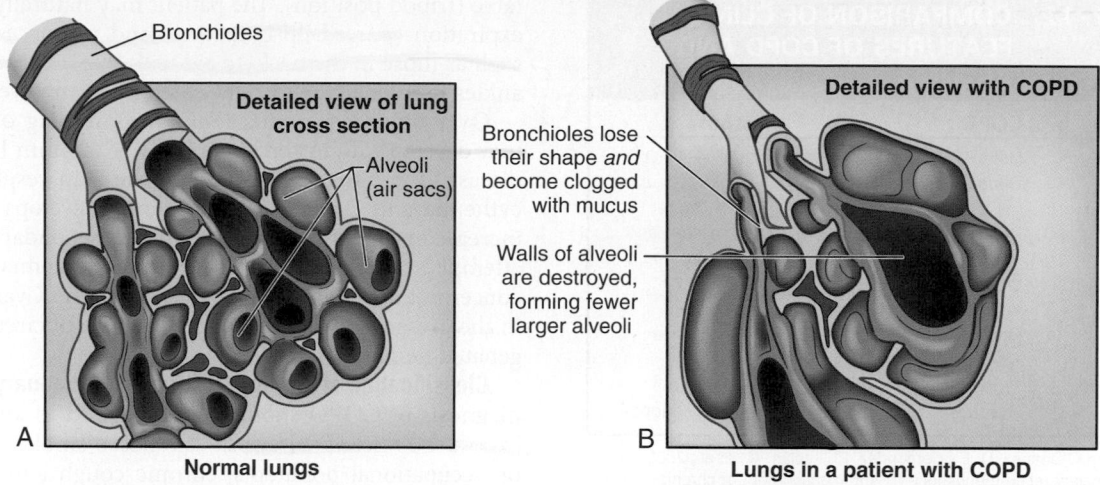

FIGURE 31-10 Illustrations of bronchioles and alveoli in the lungs. **A,** Appearance in normal lungs. **B,** Appearance as a result of changes in the lungs of a patient with chronic obstructive pulmonary disease (COPD).

recoil, makes passive expiration of air difficult, and air is trapped in the lungs. The chest hyperexpands and becomes barrel-shaped because the respiratory muscles cannot function effectively. The functional residual capacity is increased, and at this stage, the patient is trying to breathe in when the lungs are in an "over-inflated" state; thus the patient appears dyspneic, and exercise capacity is limited (GOLD, 2017).

As the disease progresses, abnormal gas exchange may occur and results in hypoxemia (decreased oxygen in the blood) and hypercapnia (increased carbon dioxide). As the air trapping worsens and alveoli are destroyed, bullae (large air spaces in the parenchyma) and blebs (air spaces adjacent to pleurae) can form (Figure 31-10). Bullae and blebs are not effective in gas exchange because the capillary bed that normally surrounds each alveolus does not exist in the bullae and bleb. Therefore, there is a significant ventilation–perfusion (VQ) mismatch, and hypoxemia results. Peripheral airway obstruction also results in VQ imbalance and, in combination with the respiratory muscle impairment, can lead to carbon dioxide retention, particularly in severe disease (GOLD, 2017).

Excess mucus production, resulting in a chronic productive cough, is a feature of predominant chronic bronchitis and is not necessarily associated with limitation in airflow. However, not all patients with COPD produce sputum. Excess mucus production is a result of an increased number of mucus-secreting goblet cells and enlarged submucosal glands, which respond to the chronic irritation of smoke or other inhalants. In addition, dysfunction of cilia leads to chronic cough and sputum production. Some of the inflammatory mediators also stimulate mucus production.

Pulmonary vasculature changes that result in mild to moderate pulmonary hypertension may occur late in the course of COPD. The small pulmonary arteries undergo vasoconstriction as a consequence of hypoxemia, and their structure changes, which results in thickening of the vascular smooth muscle as the disease advances. Because of the loss of alveolar walls and the capillaries surrounding them, the pressure in the pulmonary circulation increases. Affected patients typically do not have difficulty with hypoxemia at rest until late in the disease. However, hypoxemia may develop during exercise, and such patients may benefit from supplemental oxygen.

Pulmonary hypertension may progress and lead to hypertrophy of the right ventricle of the heart or to cor pulmonale, with or without right-sided heart failure. COPD has been shown to have effects on other body systems, especially in severe disease. These extrapulmonary changes contribute greatly to the clinical findings in affected patients and affect their survival and management. The mechanisms that cause the changes are unclear and are probably multifaceted, but systemic inflammation and inactivity of the patients are probably key factors (GOLD, 2017). Cachexia is common with a loss of skeletal muscle mass (sarcopenia), and weakness probably results from increased apoptosis (programmed cell death), muscle disuse, or a combination of both (GOLD, 2017). Patients may have weakness in all muscles of the upper and lower extremities, and the progression of muscle wasting may be gradual or accelerated, depending on the underlying disease state, and it may be accelerated at times of acute exacerbation or during recovery from illness and a time of deconditioning (GOLD, 2017). Consideration must also be given to the presence of exercise intolerance, deconditioning, and osteoporosis. Patients with severe COPD also may develop chronic anemia, anxiety, and depression. The incidence of cardiovascular disease is increased among such patients, probably as a result of an increase in C-reactive protein (another inflammatory marker linked to cardiovascular disease; GOLD, 2017).

Clinical Manifestations

Several common aspects of asthma and COPD cause diagnostic confusion. However, there are clinically important differences between COPD and asthma (Table 31-12). In addition, some patients have a mixture of asthma and COPD (e.g., those with asthma who have a significant smoking history), and it is important to identify such patients because they may benefit from combination therapy of ICS/LABA and anticholinergic medications. In addition, earlier introduction of ICS may be justified if the asthma component is prominent.

A diagnosis of COPD should be considered when a person experiences symptoms of cough, sputum production, or dyspnea; has a history of smoking or exposure to risk factors for the disease; or demonstrates both. An intermittent cough, often the earliest symptom, usually occurs in the morning with the expectoration of small amounts of mucus. A productive cough (coughing that

TABLE 31-12	COMPARISON OF CLINICAL FEATURES OF COPD AND ASTHMA	
Feature	COPD	Asthma
Age at onset	Usually >40 yr	Usually <40 yr
Smoking history	Usually >10 pack-years	Not causal but can be a trigger
Clinical symptoms	Persistent	Intermittent and variable
Sputum production	Often	Infrequent
Allergies	Infrequent	Often
Spirometry	Findings may improve but never normalize	Findings often normalize
Disease course	Progressive worsening with exacerbations	Stable with exacerbations

Source: Adapted from O'Donnell, D. E., Hernandez, P., Kaplan, A., et al. (2008). Canadian Thoracic Society recommendations for the management of chronic obstructive pulmonary disease—2008 Update—Highlights for primary care. *Canadian Respiratory Journal, 15*(Suppl. A), 1–8A.
COPD, chronic obstructive pulmonary disease.

brings up mucus) during winter months is also a common early symptom that is often exacerbated by respiratory irritants; by cold, damp air; and by respiratory infections. Patients usually seek medical help when they have an acute respiratory infection, dyspnea being the main concern. Dyspnea on exertion may also be one of the earliest symptoms. Dyspnea becomes progressively more severe to the point that it occurs at rest. Patients may dismiss the importance of dyspnea, rationalizing that "I'm just getting older." They change behaviours to avoid dyspnea and adapt, such as by using the elevator instead of stairs. The dyspnea gradually interferes with daily activities, such as carrying grocery bags, bathing, and cooking. People with COPD have described acute dyspnea as an experience inextricably related to anxiety and emotional functioning. Patients may describe dyspnea in various terms: "My breath does not go out all the way"; "It's hard work to breathe"; or that breathing feels like "heaviness" or "gasping."

Progressive dyspnea occurs as more alveoli become overdistended, trapping increasing amounts of air. This causes the diaphragm to flatten and the anteroposterior diameter of the chest to increase; as a result, the chest assumes the typical barrel shape. Effective abdominal breathing is decreased because of the flattening of diaphragm, which forces the person to rely on intercostal and accessory muscles. This type of breathing, however, is not very effective because the ribs become fixed in an inspiratory position.

Many people with advanced COPD experience weight loss and anorexia. The exact cause of these developments is not well understood. One possibility is that such patients are in a hypermetabolic state with increased energy requirements, partly because of the increased work of breathing. Even when caloric intake is adequate, weight loss still occurs. Many patients with COPD have protein-calorie malnutrition, with loss of lean muscle mass and subcutaneous fat (Langen, Gosker, Remels, et al., 2013). (Malnutrition is discussed in Chapter 42.) Fatigue is a highly prevalent symptom that affects the patient's activities of daily living (ADLs).

During physical examination, a prolonged expiratory phase of respiration, wheezes, or decreased breath sounds, or some combination is noted in some or all lung fields. The patient may sit upright with arms supported on a fixed surface such as a table (tripod position). The patient may naturally purse lips on expiration (pursed-lip breathing) and use accessory muscles, such as those in the neck, to aid with inspiration. Edema in the ankles may be a clue to right-sided heart involvement.

Over time, hypoxemia (PaO_2 <60 mm Hg or SaO_2 <88%) may develop with hypercapnia ($PaCO_2$ >45 mm Hg) later in the disease. The bluish-red colour of the skin results from polycythemia and cyanosis. Polycythemia develops as a result of increased production of red blood cells secondary to the body's attempt to compensate for chronic hypoxemia. Hemoglobin concentrations may reach 200 g/L or more. Cyanosis develops in the presence of at least 50 g/L or more of circulating unoxygenated hemoglobin.

Classification of Chronic Obstructive Pulmonary Disease. The diagnosis of COPD should be considered in any person with exposure to risk factors such as tobacco smoke, environmental or occupational pollutants, chronic cough and dyspnea, or a combination of these. The diagnosis of COPD is confirmed by spirometry, regardless of whether the patient has chronic symptoms. The FEV_1/FVC ratio of less than 70% establishes the diagnosis of COPD. COPD can be classified as mild, moderate, severe, and very severe (Table 31-13), and this classification is based on the severity of obstruction (as indicated by FEV_1). The management of COPD is based primarily on a patient's symptoms, but the staging provides a general guideline for the type of interventions.

Complications

Cor Pulmonale. Cor pulmonale is hypertrophy of the right side of the heart, with or without heart failure, that results from pulmonary hypertension. In COPD, pulmonary hypertension is caused primarily by constriction of the pulmonary vessels in response to alveolar hypoxia; acidosis further potentiates the vasoconstriction (Figure 31-11). Chronic alveolar hypoxia causes pulmonary arteriolar muscle hypertrophy. Chronic hypoxia also stimulates erythropoiesis, which causes polycythemia and increases the viscosity of the blood. Cor pulmonale is a late manifestation of COPD with a poor prognosis.

Normally, the right ventricle and the pulmonary circulatory system are low-pressure systems in comparison with the left ventricle and the systemic circulation. When pulmonary hypertension develops, the pressures on the right side of the heart must increase to push blood into the lungs. Eventually, right-sided heart failure develops.

The clinical manifestations of cor pulmonale are related to dilation and failure of the right ventricle with subsequent intravascular volume expansion and systemic venous congestion. Lung sounds are normal, or crackles may be heard in the bases of the lungs. Heart sound changes include accentuation of the pulmonic component of the second heart sound, presence of a right-sided third heart sound (right ventricular gallop), and early systolic ejection click along the left sternal border. Overt manifestations of right-sided heart failure may develop, which include distension of neck veins (jugular venous distension), hepatomegaly with right upper quadrant tenderness, ascites, epigastric distress, peripheral edema, and weight gain.

Management of cor pulmonale includes continuous administration of low-flow oxygen. Long-term oxygen therapy can slow but not reverse the progression of pulmonary hypertension in patients with COPD. Diuretics are generally used, but serum creatinine level, blood urea nitrogen level, and electrolytes must be monitored because diuretics can cause volume depletion and

TABLE 31-13 CANADIAN THORACIC SOCIETY CHRONIC OBSTRUCTIVE PULMONARY DISEASE (COPD) CLASSIFICATION OF SEVERITY BY SYMPTOMS, DISABILITY,* AND IMPAIRMENT OF LUNG FUNCTION

COPD Stage	Classification of Function	
	Symptoms	Spirometry (After Bronchodilator Treatment)
Mild	Shortness of breath from COPD† when hurrying on the level or walking up a slight hill (MRC grade 2)	$FEV_1 \geq 80\%$, $FEV_1/FVC < 0.7$
Moderate	Shortness of breath from COPD† causing the patient to stop after walking approximately 100 m (or after a few minutes) on the level (MRC grades 3 to 4)	$50\% \leq FEV_1 < 80\%$ predicted, $FEV_1/FVC < 0.7$
Severe	Shortness of breath from COPD† resulting in the patient being too breathless to leave the house, breathless when dressing or undressing (MRC grade 5), or the presence of chronic respiratory failure or clinical signs of right heart failure	$30\% \leq FEV_1 < 50\%$ predicted, $FEV_1/FVC < 0.7$
Very severe		$FEV_1 < 30\%$ predicted, $FEV_1/FVC < 0.7$

Source: O'Donnell, D. E., Aaron, S., Bourbeau, J., et al. (2007). Canadian Thoracic Society recommendations for management of chronic obstructive pulmonary disease—2007 Update. *Canadian Respiratory Journal, 14*(Suppl. B), 5B–32B, Table 3.
*Postbronchodilator FEV_1/FVC ratio of less than 0.7 is required for the diagnosis of COPD to be established.
†In the presence of non-COPD conditions that may cause shortness of breath (e.g., cardiac dysfunction, anemia, muscle weakness, metabolic disorders), symptoms may not appropriately reflect COPD disease severity. Classification of COPD severity should be undertaken with care in patients with comorbid disease or other possible contributors to shortness of breath.
FEV₁, forced expiratory volume in one second; *FVC*, forced vital capacity; *MRC*, Medical Research Council Dyspnea Scale.

PATHOPHYSIOLOGY MAP

FIGURE 31-11 Mechanisms involved in the pathophysiological process of cor pulmonale secondary to chronic obstructive pulmonary disease.

electrolyte imbalance. (Cor pulmonale is discussed further in Chapter 30.)

Acute Exacerbations of Chronic Obstructive Pulmonary Disease. Acute exacerbations are the most frequent cause of medical visits, hospitalizations, and death among people with

COPD (Abascal-Bolado, Novotny, Sloan, et al., 2015). Frequent exacerbations contribute to decreases in lung function and deterioration in quality of life. An acute exacerbation of COPD (AECOPD) is defined as a sustained worsening of respiratory symptoms, such as dyspnea, cough, or sputum production that leads to an increased use of maintenance medications or supplementation with additional medications (Beghé, Verduri, Roca, et al., 2013). The term *sustained* implies a change from baseline that lasts 48 hours or longer. Exacerbations should be characterized as purulent or nonpurulent to assist with determining the need for antibiotic therapy; purulent exacerbations necessitate antibiotic therapy. The frequency of AECOPD is, in part, related to the underlying severity of airflow obstruction, and patients with a history of frequent exacerbations are more likely to continue experiencing frequent exacerbations. The cause of AECOPD is often difficult to determine. Noninfectious triggers for exacerbations include exposure to allergens, irritants, cold air, and air pollution.

At least half of all exacerbations are thought to be infectious in nature; many of these are viral in origin, whereas the remainder are caused by bacterial infection. The most common organisms causing AECOPD are *H. influenzae, M. catarrhalis,* and *S. pneumoniae.* As COPD becomes more severe, *Pseudomonas* organisms, *Klebsiella pneumoniae,* and *Escherichia coli* are frequent causes of infection (GOLD, 2017). The antibiotics most commonly given are amoxicillin, cefuroxime, cefixime, azithromycin, clarithromycin, trimethoprim-sulphamethoxazole, doxycycline, moxifloxacin, levofloxacin, and amoxicillin with clavulanic acid. Some patients are provided with a written action plan and instructed to self-manage exacerbations by beginning antibiotics at the first signs of change in sputum production and colour. In concept, the COPD action plan is similar to the action plan used for patients with asthma (see Figure 31-8); however, the COPD action plan is specific to COPD and AECOPD. Many action plans are available. An example of an action plan can be downloaded from the website of the Canadian Lung Association (see the Resources at the end of this chapter).

Pneumonia is a frequent complication of COPD. The most common causative pathogens are *S. pneumoniae, H. influenzae,* and viruses. The most common manifestation is purulent sputum. Systemic manifestations such as fever, chills, and leukocytosis may not be present. (Treatment of pneumonia is discussed in Chapter 30.)

No diagnostic tests currently define AECOPD. A complete history and physical examination are needed to rule out other causes of increased symptoms. In patients who are very dyspneic, SaO_2 and ABGs should be measured (if oxygen saturation as measured by oximetry is low). Chest radiography should be performed for patients in the emergency department or who are admitted to the hospital because they may have pneumonia, heart failure, or pneumothorax. Increased inhaled bronchodilator dosages (β_2 agonists and anticholinergics) are administered to all patients with AECOPD; oral or systemic corticosteroids, to patients with moderate to severe airflow obstruction ($FEV_1 < 50\%$ of predicted); and antibiotics, to those with purulent sputum. Annual influenza vaccination and pneumococcal vaccination should be encouraged unless the patient has a contraindication.

Acute Respiratory Failure. An acute exacerbation leads to increased decline in overall lung function, deterioration in health status, and risk of death (GOLD, 2017). Frequently, patients with COPD wait too long to contact their health care provider when they develop fever, increased cough and dyspnea, or other symptoms suggestive of AECOPD. An exacerbation of cor pulmonale may lead to acute respiratory failure. Discontinuing bronchodilator or corticosteroid medication may also precipitate respiratory failure. The use of β-adrenergic blockers (e.g.,

propranolol [Inderal]) may exacerbate acute respiratory failure. However, cardioselective β-adrenergic blockers (e.g., atenolol, metoprolol) should not be withheld from patients with mild to moderate diseases because they do not produce clinically significant problems with respiration (Etminan, Jafari, Carleton, et al., 2012).

Indiscriminate use of sedatives and opioids, especially before or after surgery in a patient who retains carbon dioxide, may suppress ventilatory drive and lead to respiratory failure. The patient with COPD who retains carbon dioxide should be treated with low-flow rates of oxygen, and ABG values should be monitored carefully. Surgery or severe, painful illness involving the chest or abdomen may lead to splinting, ineffective ventilation, and respiratory failure. Careful preoperative screening, which includes pulmonary function tests and ABG monitoring, is important in patients with a history of heavy smoking and COPD to prevent postoperative pulmonary complications. (Respiratory failure is defined and discussed in Chapter 70.)

Depression, Anxiety, and Panic. People with COPD experience higher rates of depression, anxiety, and panic (Yohannes & Alexopoulos, 2014). Of the respondents to the SLCDC, 15% rated their mental health as "fair or poor" (PHAC, 2011). Approximately 40% of patients with COPD report clinically significant anxiety or depression (Long, Bekelman, & Make, 2014). Depression may be related to feelings of loss and grief that accompany the progressive course of the disease, as well as an overall decrease in quality of life (Long, Bekelman, & Make, 2014). A heightened experience of dyspnea is probably related to both anxiety and depression (Long, Bekelman, & Make, 2014). When a person is exceptionally dyspneic, particularly if the condition occurs suddenly, the person becomes anxious and tries to breathe faster, which affects oxygenation status. Proper screening for anxiety and depression and assessment of coping strategies and supports by health care providers are needed to reduce the intensity of these symptoms and improve quality of life.

Clinical Assessment

Goals of the clinical assessment are to determine the severity of the disease and the effect of disease on a patient's quality of life. Identification of these and other factors enable the health care provider to design an individualized treatment plan (GOLD, 2017).

Clinical assessment begins with a thorough history. Tobacco consumption should be quantified and is typically expressed in pack-years. Pack-years are calculated by multiplying the number of cigarette packs smoked daily by the number of years smoked. Nurses should ask each patient about the experience of symptoms and their effect on the individual's life. A series of probing questions is often necessary to uncover the extent of the patient's breathing difficulty and exercise curtailment. The severity of breathlessness is determined by identifying the magnitude of the task (often an ADL) necessary to cause discomfort in breathing. The Medical Research Council (MRC) Dyspnea Scale is used to assess the level of shortness of breath and disability in COPD (Figure 31-12). The history also should include an assessment of the frequency and severity of exacerbations because the findings may guide treatment choices. In addition, nurses should include an assessment of symptoms associated with comorbid conditions or complications of COPD (ankle swelling, weight loss, anxiety, depression) and the current medical treatment.

Physical examination is important for patients with COPD but is not diagnostic. Pulmonary function studies are needed to determine airflow obstruction and therefore to determine a

None

Grade 1 Breathlessness with strenuous exercise

Grade 2 Short of breath when hurrying on the level or walking up a slight hill

Grade 3 Walks slower than people of the same age on the level or stops for breath while walking at own pace on the level

Grade 4 Stops for breath after walking 100 yards

Grade 5 Too breathless to leave the house or breathless when dressing

Severe

FIGURE 31-12 Medical Research Council (MRC) Dyspnea Scale. This scale can be used to assess shortness of breath and disability in chronic obstructive pulmonary disease. Source: O'Donnell, D. E., Aaron, S., Bourbeau, J., et al. (2004). State of the art compendium: Canadian Thoracic Society recommendations for the management of chronic obstructive pulmonary disease. *Canadian Respiratory Journal, 11*(Suppl. B), 1B–59B, Table 1. Reprinted with permission of D. E. O'Donnell.

TABLE 31-14 COLLABORATIVE CARE
Chronic Obstructive Pulmonary Disease

Diagnostic
- History and physical examination
- Pulmonary function tests
- Serum α_1-antitrypsin levels
- Chest radiography (if indicated)
- Sputum specimen for Gram stain and culture (if indicated)
- ABG measurements (if indicated)
- Exercise testing with oximetry (if indicated)
- Electrocardiography (if indicated)
- Echocardiography or cardiac nuclear scans (if indicated)

Collaborative Therapy
- Smoking cessation
- Bronchodilator therapy (see Table 31-8)
- β_2-Adrenergic agonists
- Anticholinergic drugs
- Long-acting theophylline preparations (rarely used)
- Prompt treatment of exacerbations
- Corticosteroids (oral for exacerbations)
- Nonsteroidal anti-inflammatory drugs (roflumilast)
- Antibiotics for exacerbations with purulent sputum
- Influenza immunization (yearly)
- Pneumovax immunization (every 5–10 years)
- Pulmonary rehabilitation program
- Progressive plan of exercise, especially walking and upper body strengthening
- Breathing exercises
- Airway clearance techniques
- Hydration of 3 L/day (if not contraindicated)
- Relaxation techniques
- Appropriate pacing and planning of activities
- Patient and family teaching
- Long-term oxygen (if indicated)
- Nutritional supplementation if BMI is low
- Surgery in severe and advanced COPD
  - Lung volume reduction
  - Lung transplantation

ABG, arterial blood gas; *BMI*, body mass index; *COPD*, chronic obstructive pulmonary disease.

diagnosis of COPD and to assess the severity of lung impairment (GOLD, 2017). Spirometry is ordered before and after bronchodilator therapy; when the post-therapy FEV_1/FVC ratio is less than 70% of the predicted value, it confirms the presence of airway obstruction (GOLD, 2017).

Chest radiographic studies are not diagnostic of COPD but are often necessary to confirm or rule out comorbid conditions. This also applies to high-resolution computed tomography, which is not routinely required. Pulse oximetry should be used to assess all patients with an FEV_1 of less than 35% of predicted, and ABGs should be monitored in patients who have a low SaO_2 (<92%) on oximetry, especially in patients in whom respiratory failure is suspected (GOLD, 2017). In the later stages of COPD, typical findings are low PaO_2, elevated $PaCO_2$, decreased pH, and increased bicarbonate levels. The 6-minute walking test is a useful test of functional disability and provides prognostic information. It includes determination of changes in the SaO_2 with exercise.

Collaborative Care

Primary COPD management goals are the following (O'Donnell, Aaron, Bourbeau, et al., 2007; O'Donnell, Hernandez, Kaplan, et al., 2008):
1. Prevent disease progression (smoking cessation)
2. Reduce the frequency and severity of exacerbations
3. Alleviate breathlessness and other respiratory symptoms
4. Improve exercise tolerance and daily activity
5. Treat exacerbations and complications of the disease
6. Improve health status and quality of life
7. Reduce the risk of mortality

AECOPD and complications such as respiratory failure, pneumonia, and heart failure necessitate hospitalization, but otherwise patients are treated on an outpatient basis and manage their condition at home. Therapy is expected to escalate in intensity as a patient's disability progresses from MRC Dyspnea Scale grade 2 to grade 5; those with grade of 3 or higher require more intensive management, including pharmacological and

nonpharmacological interventions (O'Donnell, Aaron, Bourbeau, et al., 2007). Collaborative care guidelines are presented in Table 31-14.

Environmental and occupational irritants and triggers should be assessed for a possible negative effect, and ways to control or avoid them should be determined. Patients with COPD should receive an annual influenza vaccination and a pneumococcal vaccine (pneumococcal revaccination is recommended every 5–10 years; O'Donnell, Hernandez, Kaplan, et al., 2008). (See the "Evidence-Informed Practice: Translating Research Into Practice" box.)

Smoking Cessation. Cessation of cigarette smoking is the most significant factor in slowing the progression of COPD. After a patient stops smoking, not only does the accelerated decline in pulmonary function slow but also pulmonary function usually improves. Thus the sooner the patient stops smoking, the less pulmonary function is lost and the sooner the symptoms decrease, particularly cough and sputum production. (See the RNAO's Best Practice Guideline: *Integrating Smoking Cessation Into Daily Practice* in the Resources at the end of this chapter.)

Drug Therapy. Medications for COPD can reduce the intensity of symptoms or abolish them altogether, increase the capacity for exercise, improve overall health, and reduce the number and severity of exacerbations. Bronchodilators are the mainstay of pharmacological therapy for COPD (GOLD, 2017). Bronchodilator drug therapy relaxes smooth muscles in the airway, reduces airway resistance and dynamic hyperinflation of the lungs, and improves the ventilation of the lungs, thus reducing the degree of breathlessness. Although patients with COPD do not

◆ EVIDENCE-INFORMED PRACTICE

Translating Research Into Practice

Physical Activity and Chronic Obstructive Pulmonary Disease

A nurse in the pulmonary clinic is working with a 65-year-old man who has been recently discharged from the hospital after receiving a new diagnosis of COPD. He tells the nurse that he has been mostly inactive for the past few months because his breathing seems to worsen with activity.

Best Available Evidence	Clinician Expertise	Patient Preference and Values
Patients with COPD who participate in regular moderate physical activity (e.g., brisk walking) have fewer severe flare-ups and are less likely to be readmitted to the hospital.	Physical inactivity is common in patients with COPD. Persistent inactivity may place a patient at greater risk for hospital readmissions.	The patient tells the nurse that he misses taking walks every day with his wife and is wondering whether he would be able to resume this activity at a slow pace.

Decisions and Actions

1. What important factors should be discussed with the patient about physical activity and COPD?
2. How would the nurse assess the patient's willingness and motivation to engage in physical activity?
3. How would the nurse involve the interprofessional team members to assist the patient in regular physical activity?

Reference for Evidence

Nguyen, H., Chu, L., Liu, I., et al. (2014). Associations between physical activity and 30-day readmission risk in chronic obstructive pulmonary disease. *Annals of the American Thoracic Society, 11,* 695.

respond to bronchodilator therapy as dramatically as do those with asthma, a reduction in dyspnea and an increase in FEV_1 are usually achieved. As with asthma, the preferred route of administration is inhalation because it targets the lungs directly.

Bronchodilator medications commonly used are β_2-adrenergic agonists, anticholinergic drugs, and methylxanthines (see Table 31-6). Short-acting bronchodilators, both β_2-adrenergic agonists and anticholinergic drugs, improve pulmonary function, symptoms, and exercise function (O'Donnell, Hernandez, Kaplan, et al., 2008). SABAs and anticholinergic drugs can be used separately, but together they produce superior bronchodilation than does either drug alone. These medications are also available in nebulized combination (salbutamol and ipratropium [Combivent]). For most patients with COPD, bronchodilator therapy is best used as maintenance therapy (three or four times per day) with extra puffs on an as-needed basis for breakthrough symptoms.

Long-acting bronchodilators also play a role in COPD and are typically indicated for patients with more severe COPD who experience persistent symptoms. Like short-acting bronchodilators, long-acting bronchodilators include both β_2-adrenergic agonists (formoterol [Oxeze; Foradil], salmeterol [Serevent]), and anticholinergic drugs (tiotropium [Spiriva]). The long-acting anticholinergic drugs and LABAs produce more sustained improvements in pulmonary function, activity-related dyspnea, and quality of life than do the short-acting bronchodilators.

Tiotropium reduces the frequency of hospitalization and exacerbation, improves health status and hyperinflation, and is taken only once daily. In comparison with LABAs, tiotropium provides greater improvements in dyspnea and health status (GOLD, 2017). These two classes of long-acting bronchodilators can be used separately or in combination.

The use of theophylline in the treatment of COPD is controversial. Although it has some weak bronchodilator effects, its main value may be to improve contractility of the diaphragm and decrease diaphragmatic fatigue. The addition of theophylline to inhaled bronchodilator therapy may provide some benefit in some patients. However, the benefits and the risks need to be weighed because theophylline produces serious cardiovascular and neurological adverse effects. (Bronchodilator drugs are described in Table 31-6.)

The role of ICS in stable COPD has not been found to modify the long-term decline of FEV_1 or overall patient mortality (GOLD, 2017). ICS monotherapy does not have consistent effects on important outcomes (e.g., pulmonary function, symptoms, exacerbations). However, ICS in combination with a LABA has been found to reduce the frequency of exacerbations and to improve lung function and health status (GOLD, 2017). In Canada, two ICS and LABA combination products are currently used in the management of COPD: budesonide-formoterol (Symbicort) and fluticasone-salmeterol (Advair). The Canadian Thoracic Society Guidelines (O'Donnell, Aaron, Bourbeau, et al., 2007) suggest the addition of an ICS in combination with a LABA when the patient has moderate to severe lung impairment and has frequent AECOPD (defined as one or more per year).

A new medication, approved for the treatment of COPD in 2011, is a phosphodiesterase 4 inhibitor, roflumilast (Daxas). This drug is indicated as add-on therapy with bronchodilators for the maintenance of COPD in patients with chronic cough and sputum and frequent exacerbations.

Oral or parenteral corticosteroids are used for the treatment of AECOPD. They speed recovery time, reduce relapse rates, reduce the need for hospitalization, and improve FEV_1 and partial pressure of oxygen. The dosage and duration should be individualized, but treatment periods between 7 and 14 days are recommended for people with moderate to severe COPD (O'Donnell, Hernandez, Kaplan, et al., 2008). Continuous use of oral corticosteroids is not recommended for routine use in managing COPD because it can produce deleterious effects.

Oxygen Therapy. Oxygen therapy is frequently used in the treatment of COPD and other problems associated with hypoxemia. Oxygen is a colourless, odourless, tasteless gas that constitutes 20.95% of the atmosphere. Administering supplemental oxygen raises the partial pressure of oxygen in inspired air.

Indications for Use. Oxygen is usually administered to treat hypoxemia caused by respiratory disorders such as COPD, acute exacerbations of COPD, cor pulmonale, pneumonia, atelectasis, and lung cancer. Long-term oxygen therapy (15 hours/day or more to achieve an oxygen saturation of 90% or greater) prolongs life in patients with hypoxemia. Hypoxemia is defined as a PaO_2 lower than 55 mm Hg or lower than 60 mm Hg in the presence of cor pulmonale with a hematocrit higher than 56%. Patients with COPD are at risk of developing hypoxemia during an exacerbation.

Methods of Administration. The goal of oxygen administration is to supply the patient with adequate oxygen to maximize the oxygen-carrying ability of the blood. There are various methods of oxygen administration (Table 31-15, Figures 31-13 through

TABLE 31-15 METHODS OF OXYGEN ADMINISTRATION

Advantages	Disadvantages	Nursing Interventions
Nasal Cannula		
May be used by a mobile or restless patient Safe and simple method that is relatively comfortable and acceptable Used for patients requiring low O_2 concentrations Can be used while patient eats, talks, or coughs (see Figure 31-13, E)	Difficult to maintain in position and can be easily dislodged Patient alertness necessary to keep cannula in proper place Dryness of nasal membranes and possible pain in frontal sinuses with high flow rates (>5 L/min) Can cause pressure necrosis or excoriation of nares	Stabilize cannula during care for a restless patient. Flow rate of 2 L/min produces an O_2 concentration of approximately 28%. Amount of O_2 inhaled depends on room air and patient's breathing pattern. Most patients with COPD can tolerate 2 L/min via cannula.
Simple Face Mask		
Delivers O_2 quickly for short periods O_2 concentrations of 35%–50% achievable with flow rates of 6–12 L/min Provides adequate humidification of inspired air (see Figure 31-13, A)	Not as well tolerated as nasal cannula; lack of patient tolerance results in inadequate therapy. May be uncomfortable because a tight seal must be maintained between face and mask May produce pressure necrosis of the skin and confines heat radiating from the face to the area around the nose and mouth Must be removed to eat or drink	Wash and dry under mask q2h. Mask must fit snugly. Nasal cannula may be provided while patient is eating. Watch for pressure necrosis at the top of ears from elastic straps. (Gauze or other padding may be used to alleviate this problem.) Method requires at least 5-L/min flow to prevent accumulation of expired air in the mask.
Nasal Catheter		
Allows continuous, uninterrupted O_2 therapy Delivers O_2 even if patient is a mouth breather Does not interfere with patient care Rarely used except for short-term procedures (e.g., bronchoscopy)	Inserted into nasopharynx through a nostril and can produce excoriation of the nostril Dryness of nasal membranes with high flow rates (>6 L/min). Stomach distension with inadvertent gas flow High degree of humidification not delivered easily; catheter must be taped to patient's face	Catheter should be changed q8h, alternating the nostrils. Distance that catheter is to be inserted is measured from distance between tip of nose and earlobe. A flow rate of 5–6 L/min produces O_2 concentration of ≈30%. This method is best for short-term therapy.
Partial Rebreathing Mask		
Lightweight and easy to use. O_2 conserved by reservoir bag. Concentrations of 40%–60% achievable with flow rates of 6–10 L/min	Cannot be used when patient requires a high degree of humidity	This method is useful when blood O_2 concentrations must be raised. It is not recommended for patients with COPD and should never be used with a nebulizer. Bag should not be allowed to deflate during inspiration.
Nonrebreathing Mask		
Accurate delivery of high concentrations of O_2 O_2 flow into bag and mask during inhalation. Valve in place to prevent expired air from flowing back into bag Concentrations of 60%–90% achievable	Cannot be used when patient requires a high degree of humidity	Mask should fit snugly. Flow rate must be sufficient to keep bag from collapsing during inspiration. Bag should not be allowed to deflate during inspiration.
Oxygen-Conserving Cannula		
Has a built-in reservoir that increases O_2 concentration delivered and allows patient to use lower flow rates, usually 30%–50%, which increases comfort and lowers cost Reported to be more comfortable than standard nasal cannulas (see Figure 31-15)	Cannot be cleaned: changing cannula weekly recommended More expensive than standard cannulas and requires evaluation with measurement of ABGs and oximetry to determine correct flow Highly visible and heavy on ears	This method is generally indicated when long-term O_2 therapy is used at home rather than during hospitalization. It may be "moustache" or "pendant" type. Cannula may cause necrosis over the tops of the ears; can be padded.
Transtracheal Catheter		
Less visible than cannula. Flow requirement possibly reduced 60%–80%, which greatly increases amount of time available from portable source of O_2 Less nasal irritation occurs (see Figure 31-14)	Necessary for patient and family to learn entire program of care for tracheostoma and how to replace catheter Procedure invasive Equipment more costly	Method may not be appropriate for patient with excessive mucus production from mucous plugging.

Continued

TABLE 31-15   METHODS OF OXYGEN ADMINISTRATION—cont'd

Advantages	Disadvantages	Nursing Interventions
Tracheostomy Collar		
Can deliver high humidity and O$_2$	Possible for condensed fluid in tubing to drain into tracheostomy Water traps usually inserted Collection of secretions inside collar and around tracheostomy O$_2$ concentration lost into atmosphere because collar does not fit tightly	Collar attaches to neck with elastic strap and should be removed and cleaned at least q4h to prevent aspiration of fluid and infection.
Tracheostomy T Bar		
Better O$_2$ and humidity delivery than by tracheostomy collar because of tight fit	Possible for condensed fluid in tubing to drain into tracheostomy Water traps usually inserted	T bar must be removed for suctioning. T bar may pull on patient's tracheostomy tube, causing irritation and potential tissue damage. The nurse should monitor this closely.
Tent or Incubator		
Has ability to control temperature and humidity	Limited usefulness Difficult to maintain adequate concentrations of O$_2$ Isolates patient from environment	Tent should be flushed with O$_2$ every time it is opened. Nurse should assess for leaks around canopy.
Venturi Mask		
Delivers precise, high flow rates of O$_2$ Lightweight, cone-shaped plastic device fitted to face Available for delivery of 24%, 28%, 31%, 35%, 40%, and 50% O$_2$ Possible to apply adaptors to increase humidification (see Figure 31-13, *C*)	Uncomfortable and must be removed when patient eats Possible to talk while wearing mask, but voice may be muffled Other disadvantages: same as those for the simple face mask	Entrainment device on mask must be changed to deliver higher concentrations of O$_2$. Method is especially helpful for administering low, constant O$_2$ concentrations to patients with COPD. Air entrainment ports must not be occluded.

ABGs, arterial blood gases; *COPD*, chronic obstructive pulmonary disease.

31-16). The method selected depends on factors such as the fraction of inspired oxygen, mobility of the patient, humidification requirement, patient cooperation, comfort, cost, and available financial resources.

Oxygen delivery systems are classified as low- or high-flow systems. Because room air is mixed with oxygen, the percentage of oxygen delivered to the patient is not as precise in low-flow systems as in high-flow systems. Most methods of oxygen administration are low-flow devices that deliver oxygen in concentrations that vary in accordance with the patient's respiratory pattern. In contrast, the Venturi mask is a high-flow device that delivers fixed concentrations of oxygen independent of a patient's respiratory pattern. With the Venturi mask, oxygen is delivered to a small jet (Venturi device) in the centre of a wide-based cone (see Figure 31-13, *C*). Air is entrained (pulled) through openings in the cone as oxygen flows through the small jet. The mask has large vents through which exhaled air can escape. The degree of restriction, or narrowness, of the jet determines the amount of entrainment and the dilution of pure oxygen with room air and thus the concentration of oxygen.

Humidification. Oxygen obtained from cylinders or wall systems is dry. Dry oxygen has an irritating effect on mucous membranes and dries secretions. Therefore, it is important that oxygen be humidified when administered, either by humidification or by nebulization. A device commonly used for humidification when the patient has a catheter, cannula, or low-flow mask is a bubble-through humidifier. It is a small plastic jar filled with sterile distilled water that is attached to the oxygen source by means of a flowmeter. Oxygen passes into the jar, bubbles through

the water, and then goes through tubing to a patient's catheter, cannula, or mask. The purpose of the bubble-through humidifier is to restore the humidity conditions of room air. However, the need for bubble-through humidifiers at flow rates between 1 and 4 L/min is debatable when humidity in the environment is adequate.

Complications

Combustion. Oxygen supports combustion and increases the rate of burning; thus it is important that smoking be prohibited in an area where supplemental oxygen is being used. A "No Smoking" sign should be prominently displayed on patients' doors and in their homes and cars. Patients should also be cautioned against smoking cigarettes when using oxygen.

Carbon Dioxide Narcosis. The drive to breathe is guided by arterial and central chemoreceptors in the respiratory centre that respond to changes in carbon dioxide and oxygen levels. Normally, accumulation of carbon dioxide is the major stimulant of the respiratory centre. Over time in COPD, the respiratory centre loses its sensitivity to the elevated carbon dioxide levels, and some patients with COPD develop a tolerance for high carbon dioxide levels. In theory, for these individuals, the "drive" to breathe is hypoxemia. Thus administering oxygen to patients with COPD has been thought to weaken their drive to breathe. This has been a pervasive myth but is not a serious threat. In fact, not providing adequate oxygen to these patients is much more detrimental. Although oxygen administration should be titrated to the lowest effective dosage, many patients who have end-stage COPD require high-flow rates. They may, in fact, exhibit higher than normal levels of carbon dioxide in their blood, but this is of little concern. What is important is careful, ongoing

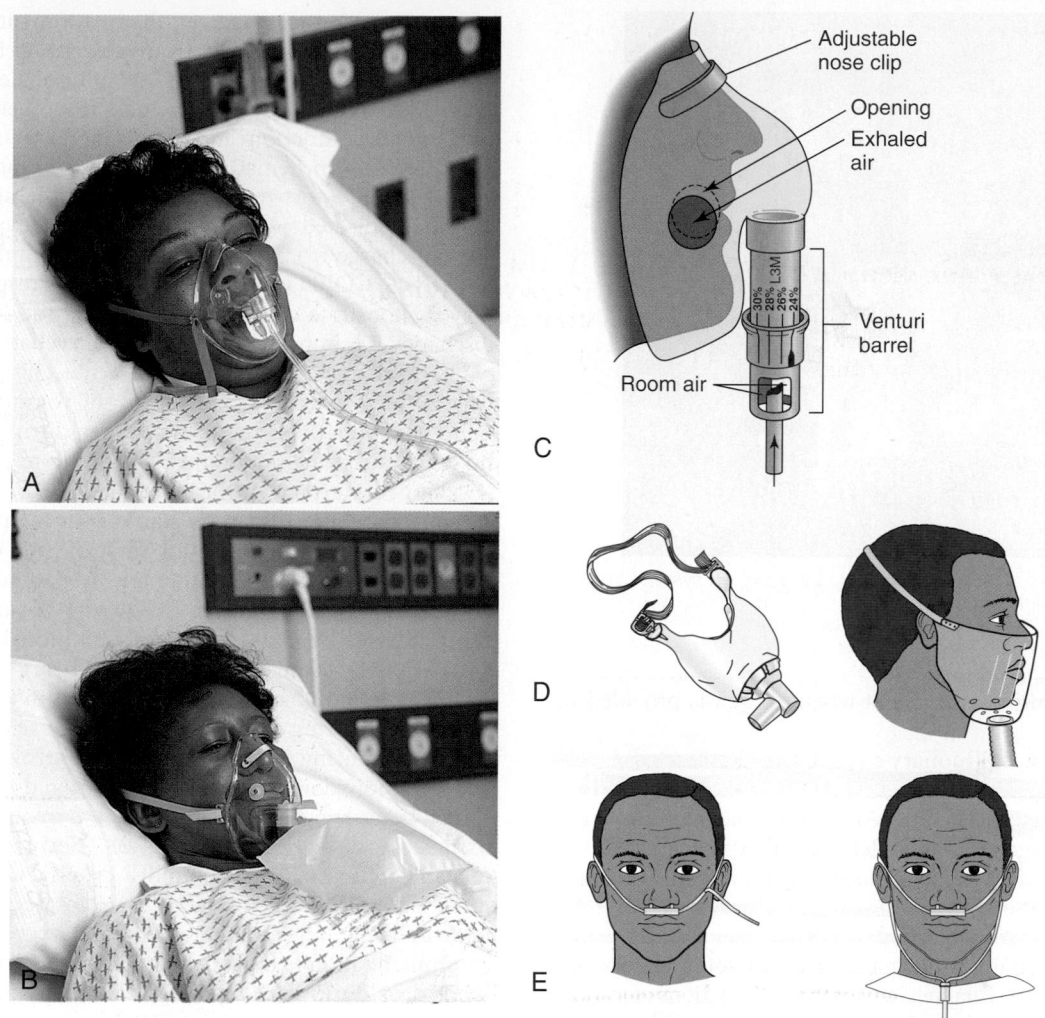

FIGURE 31-13 Methods of oxygen administration. **A,** Simple face mask. **B,** Plastic face mask with reservoir bag. **C,** Venturi mask. **D,** Tracheostomy mask. **E,** Standard nasal cannulas. Source: Adapted from Potter, P. A., & Perry, A. G. (2009). *Fundamentals of nursing* (7th ed., pp. 958–959, Figures 40-15, 40-16, and 40-17). St. Louis: Mosby.

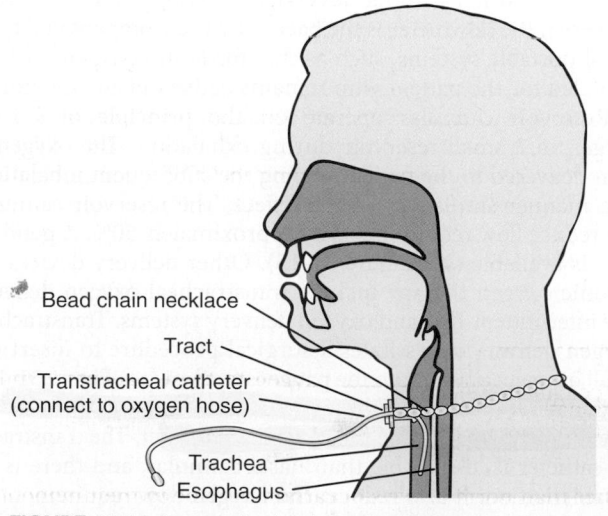

FIGURE 31-14 Transtracheal catheter for oxygen administration.

FIGURE 31-15 Pendant type of oxygen-conserving cannula.

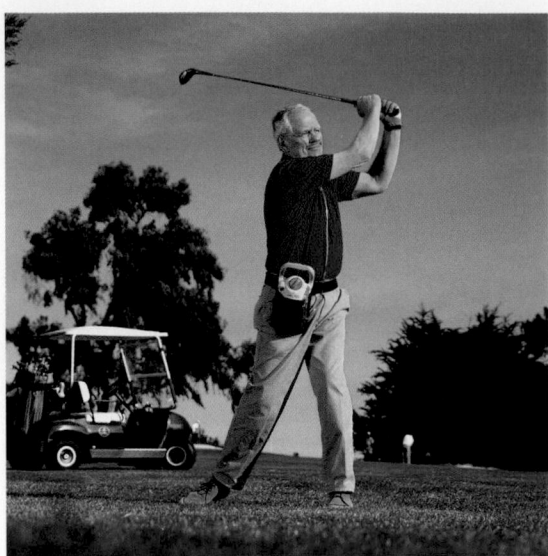

FIGURE 31-16 Golfer using Helios liquid portable oxygen system. Source: © 2017 CAIRE Inc. All Rights Reserved.

physical and cognitive assessment when oxygen is provided to these patients.

Oxygen Toxicity. Pulmonary oxygen toxicity, a condition of oxygen overdosage, may result from prolonged exposure to a high level of oxygen (PaO$_2$). Although relatively rare, the development of oxygen toxicity is determined by patient tolerance, exposure time, and dosage. High concentrations of oxygen damage alveolar–capillary membranes, inactivate pulmonary surfactant, cause interstitial and alveolar edema, and decrease lung compliance; all these changes ultimately lead to acute respiratory distress syndrome (see Chapter 70). Early manifestations of oxygen toxicity are reduced vital capacity, cough, substernal chest pain, nausea, and vomiting, paresthesia, nasal stuffiness, sore throat, and malaise. Prevention of oxygen toxicity is important in patients who are receiving oxygen. The amount of oxygen administered should be just enough to maintain the PaO$_2$ within a normal or acceptable range for each patient. A safe limit of oxygen concentrations has not yet been established. All levels above 50% and supplemental oxygen used for longer than 24 hours should be considered potentially toxic. Levels of 40% and below may be regarded as relatively nontoxic if the exposure period is short.

Absorption Atelectasis. Normally, nitrogen constitutes 79% of the air that is breathed, but it is not absorbed into the bloodstream. Its presence in the alveoli prevents alveolar collapse. When high concentrations of oxygen are given, nitrogen is washed out of the alveoli and replaced with oxygen. If airway obstruction occurs, the oxygen is absorbed into the bloodstream and the alveoli collapse. This process is called absorption atelectasis.

Infection. Infection can be a major hazard of oxygen administration. Heated nebulizers present the highest risk. The constant use of humidity supports bacterial growth, the most common infecting organism being *P. aeruginosa*. Disposable equipment that operates as a closed system should be used. The hospital should have a policy about the required frequency of equipment changes, based on the type of equipment used, and about the use of Gram staining and culturing of both equipment and respiratory secretions.

Long-Term Oxygen Therapy at Home. Improved survival and enhanced quality of life are observed in patients with COPD who receive long-term oxygen therapy to treat hypoxemia. The improved prognosis results from preventing both progression of the disease and subsequent cor pulmonale. The benefits of long-term oxygen therapy include improvements in neuropsychological function and sleep, increase in exercise tolerance, decrease in hematocrit, and reduced rates of pulmonary hypertension. Short-term home oxygen therapy (1 to 30 days) may be indicated for patients in whom hypoxemia persists after discharge from the hospital. For example, a patient with underlying COPD who develops a serious respiratory infection may demonstrate continued hypoxemia for 4 to 6 weeks after discharge. It is important to measure oxygenation status by pulse oximetry 2 to 3 months after an acute episode to determine whether long-term oxygen therapy is still warranted: At that point, up to 50% of patients requiring oxygen during an exacerbation no longer meet the requirements for long-term oxygen therapy (O'Donnell, Aaron, Bourbeau, et al., 2007).

Patients whose disease is stable with a PaO$_2$ of 55 mm Hg or lower (corresponding to an SaO$_2$ of 88% or lower) should receive long-term oxygen therapy. A patient whose PaO$_2$ is between 55 and 59 mm Hg (SaO$_2$ of 89%) and who exhibits signs of tissue hypoxia, such as cor pulmonale, erythrocytosis, and peripheral edema from right-sided heart failure, should also receive long-term oxygen therapy. In cases in which desaturation occurs only during exercise or sleep, the use of oxygen therapy specifically during exercise or sleep is controversial and must be assessed individually. The need for oxygen during these periods should be evaluated with oximetry or a 6-minute walk test. (Pulse oximetry is discussed in Chapter 28.) Several issues in Canada related to funding and eligibility criteria vary greatly across jurisdictions. Periodic re-evaluations are necessary for patients who are using long-term supplemental oxygen. In general, the recommendation is that such patients be re-evaluated every 30 to 90 days during the first year of therapy and annually after that, as long as patients remain stable.

Nasal cannulas, either regular or the oxygen-conserving type (see Figures 31-13, *E* and 31-15 and Table 31-15) are usually used to deliver oxygen from a central source in the home. The source may be a liquid oxygen storage system, compressed oxygen in tanks, or an oxygen concentrator or extractor, depending on home environment, insurance coverage, activity level, and proximity to an oxygen supply company (Table 31-16). To increase mobility in the home, the patient can use extension tubing (up to 15 m [≈50 ft]) without adversely affecting the oxygen flow delivery if the flowmeter is the back pressure–compensated type. Small portable systems, such as that for liquid oxygen, may be provided for the patient who remains active outside the home.

Reservoir cannulas operate on the principle of storing oxygen in a small reservoir during exhalation. The oxygen is then delivered to the patient during the subsequent inhalation, in a manner similar to a bolus effect. The reservoir cannulas can reduce flow requirements by approximately 50%. A pendant type is available (see Figure 31-15). Other delivery devices for chronic oxygen therapy include transtracheal oxygen delivery and intermittent-demand oxygen delivery systems. Transtracheal oxygen delivery necessitates a surgical procedure to insert the small oxygen catheter into the patient's trachea (see Figure 31-14). Nursing care involves teaching the patient and caregivers how to care for the stoma and the transtracheal catheter. The transtracheal catheter is less visible than nasal cannulas, and there is no nasal irritation. It also reduces the oxygen flow requirement by 30% to 50%.

TABLE 31-16 HOME OXYGEN DELIVERY SYSTEMS

Advantages	Disadvantages	Comments
Liquid Oxygen		
Portable unit* can be refilled by patient from reservoir. Portable unit holds 6- to 8-hr supply at 2 L/min; reservoir will last approximately 7–10 days when 2 L/min is used continuously.	Liquid system is slightly more expensive, depending on location and is not available everywhere; its use is generally limited to urban areas.	As liquid warms to gas, some is vented from the system. In summer, evaporation is accelerated and may decrease reservoir duration to <1 wk.
Compressed Oxygen Tanks or Cylinders		
Availability is good in most areas. Portability is possible with a cart. Aluminum cylinders available in varying sizes (e.g., D, E, M, H, J) are markedly lighter than steel and easier to manoeuvre.	Duration of large (H or J) tank at 2 L/min flow is approximately 50 hr; storage of four or five large cylinders in the home is necessary to have 7- to 10-day supply; portable cylinder on cart is cumbersome and heavy. Duration of E cylinder when 2 L/min is used is approximately 4–5 hr.	Some smaller tanks (D or M) may be used; these can be refilled from large cylinders and weigh approximately 4.5 kg (10 lb). Tank can be carried on shoulder strap, backpack, or fanny pack or placed on portable cart.
Concentrator or Extractor		
Because the O_2 supply is made from room air, these devices never need to be "filled." These devices are on wheels, movable from room to room. They provide compact, excellent systems for rural or homebound patients. They are convenient, safe, and reliable (assuming electricity source is reliable).	—	Concentrator should be kept in room other than bedroom if noise disturbs sleep.
Portable Oxygen Concentrator		
These are light-weight devices (3.9–17.7 kg [8.5–17 lb]) that are portable via carts or shoulder straps. Batteries last up to 8 hr with recharging in either AC or DC (e.g., car) outlets. These devices provide patient with exceptional freedom and are beneficial to an active patient who may use more than the allotted requirement of O_2 cylinders each month.	These devices can be costly. Patient must meet qualifications of O_2 company to use.	—
Pulse or Demand Delivery System (Oxygen-Conserving Device)		
These devices deliver a pulse of O_2 only during inhalation to conserve O_2. They attach to cylinders. Their use increases duration of O_2 supply. There is less drying or irritation to nasal mucosa. These devices save O_2.	These devices may not be able to provide sufficient oxygen during exertion; are costly; are less efficient at higher O_2 flow rates; are best for low activity levels. Audible pulses may be annoying. Patient must be a nose-breather to trigger the flow of O_2.	Monitor O_2 saturation during rest and exercise to determine whether oxygenation is acceptable. Consult with vendor or respiratory therapist if O_2 saturation is below desired level.

Portable usually refers to units weighing more than 4.5 kg (10 lb); ambulatory units weigh less than 4.5 kg (10 lb).

Intermittent-demand delivery systems or conserver devices are mechanically complex devices that most commonly attach to the oxygen cylinders. They deliver "pulses" of oxygen to the patient, usually during inspiration, and thus eliminate waste of oxygen during exhalation, as is experienced during continuous flow.

Home oxygen systems are usually rented from a company that sends a respiratory therapist or respiratory nurse specialist to the patient's home to teach how to use and care for the oxygen system and how to recognize when the supply is running low and must be reordered. A patient and caregiver teaching guide for the use of oxygen at home is presented in Table 31-17.

A patient who uses home oxygen should be encouraged to remain active and to travel. If long-distance travel is by automobile, arrangements can be made for oxygen to be available at the destination point. Oxygen-supply companies can often assist with these arrangements. If a patient wishes to travel by bus, train, or airplane, the patient must notify the transportation company of the need for oxygen during travel when reservations are made. A high-altitude simulation test may be performed or a mathematical formula calculated in a hospital pulmonary function laboratory to determine the oxygen prescription required. Because airplane cabins are pressurized to an elevation of 2 100 or 2 400 m (7 000 or 8 000 ft), a passenger who uses supplemental oxygen should have oxygen provided during flight. The plane's oxygen system must be used. Passengers may not use their own oxygen system during flight because it is not properly pressurized. Airlines allow patients to bring their oxygen system to be carried in the baggage compartment for use at the point of destination, but the reservoirs (liquid or tank) must be empty and the valves left open. Some patients may need to avoid prolonged exposure to high elevations during travel unless they are instructed by their health care provider how to adjust their oxygen flow to attempt to compensate for altitude.

Surgical Therapy. Two different surgical procedures have been used in management of severe COPD. One type of surgery is *lung volume reduction surgery* (GOLD, 2017). The rationale

TABLE 31-17 PATIENT & CAREGIVER TEACHING GUIDE

Home Oxygen Use

Mask or Cannula
- Ensure that the straps are not too tight.
- Remove two or three times per day to wash and dry skin where straps are placed.
- Pad any pressure points.
- Observe tops of ears for skin breakdown from pressure points.

Oral and Nasal Mucous Membranes
- Assess oral and nasal mucous membranes two or three times per day.
- Use water-based gel on lips and nasal mucosa.
- Practise frequent oral hygiene.
- Avoid dry ambient air; humidity is required whenever oxygen is used.

Decreasing Risk for Infection
- Remove mask or collar, and clean with water two or three times per day.
- Clean skin carefully and observe for cuts, scratches, and bruises.
- Change disposable equipment frequently.
- Remove secretions that are expectorated.

Decreasing Risk of Fire Injuries
- Post "No Smoking" signs in home where they can be seen.
- Do not use electric razors, portable radios, open flames, wool blankets, or mineral oils in the area where oxygen is in use.
- Do not allow smoking in the home or car.

Note: The Canadian Lung Association has good resources for patients using oxygen at home. See the Resources at the end of this chapter.

for the surgery is that by reducing the size of the hyperinflated emphysematous lungs, airway obstruction is decreased and room for the remaining normal alveoli to function is increased. The procedure reduces volume by approximately 20% to 35% of the most emphysematous lungs and improves lung and chest wall mechanics. The most common postoperative complication is pneumonia. For a subgroup of patients with severe COPD, however, lung volume reduction surgery may offer improvements in lung function, exercise capacity, quality of life, and possibly length of survival.

The second surgical procedure is *lung transplantation* for selected patients with advanced, severe COPD. In Canada between 2004 and 2013, 445 lung transplantations (double-lung, single-lung, or heart-lung) were performed in patients with COPD (Canadian Institute for Health Information [CIHI], 2015). Recipients of lung transplants who have COPD tend to have better outcomes than do those with other conditions (O'Donnell, Aaron, Bourbeau, et al., 2007). The major complications affecting long-term morbidity and mortality are (a) chronic graft dysfunction associated with obliterative bronchiolitis and (b) opportunistic infection (GOLD, 2017). Patients with COPD who receive lung transplants can achieve substantial improvements in exercise capacity and improved quality of life, and most no longer need supplemental oxygen. (Lung transplantation is discussed in Chapter 30.)

Pulmonary Rehabilitation Programs. All patients with COPD should be encouraged to maintain an active lifestyle. Pulmonary rehabilitation programs (PRPs) are used to optimize the functional status of patients with COPD—as well as their quality of life, experience of dyspnea, exercise endurance, psychosocial

INFORMATICS IN PRACTICE

Texting for Patients With Chronic Obstructive Pulmonary Disease (COPD)

- Sometimes patients with COPD or those requiring O_2 therapy experience difficulty speaking because of shortness of breath.
- Patients should be encouraged to use typed messages displayed on a monitor to communicate.
- Texting and instant messaging family and friends are good alternatives to having phone conversations.

functioning, and overall autonomy—and to reduce health care costs (Camp, Hernandez, Bourbeau, et al., 2015). The benefits observed with PRPs are often superior to the benefits of pharmacological therapy. These benefits are largely attributable to exercise. In addition, patients who attend a PRP within 1 month of an exacerbation are shown to have improved outcomes (Marciniuk, Goodridge, Hernandez, et al., 2011).

Specific components of a PRP can include exercise conditioning (aerobic conditioning and upper and lower body conditioning), breathing exercises, energy conservation, nutrition, smoking cessation, environmental factors, health promotion, patient education and self-management, psychological support, psychological counselling, and vocational rehabilitation. PRPs can be provided as inpatient, outpatient, or in-home programs. The duration of the program is typically 4 to 12 weeks or longer.

Exercise training involves both lower and upper extremity training and improves dyspnea and exercise performance. Lower extremity training focuses on aerobic training and includes walking, treadmill walking, bicycling, and cycling ergometry. Upper extremity training focuses on improving arm strength and endurance. Peripheral muscle wasting and weakness affects approximately 25% of patients with COPD. Exercise training should be performed more than three times per week. Health care providers working in PRPs assess the individual's limitations and conditioning status and develop a customized exercise program that is monitored over the length of the rehabilitation program.

Breathing Exercises. In patients with COPD, the respiratory rate increases and expiration is prolonged, to compensate for airflow obstruction and dyspnea. The accessory muscles of breathing, located in the neck and the upper part of the chest, are used excessively to promote chest wall movement. These muscles are not adapted to long-term use for breathing and, as a result, become fatigued. Breathing exercises can assist the patient during rest and activity (e.g., lifting, walking, stair climbing). The main types of breathing exercises are (a) pursed-lip breathing and (b) diaphragmatic breathing.

Pursed-lip breathing is used to prolong exhalation, prevent bronchiolar collapse and air trapping, and assist with dyspnea. Exhalation should be at least three times longer than inhalation. It is important to demonstrate and teach patients how to use this technique and for them to practise until it works for them and they feel comfortable using it. Patients should be instructed to follow this sequence:

1. Relax neck and shoulder muscles.
2. Inhale slowly through the nose to the count of 2.
3. Pucker lips as if whistling.
4. Exhale slowly and gently through the lips while mentally counting to 6.
5. Always exhale longer than inhaling.

TABLE 31-18	PATIENT & CAREGIVER TEACHING GUIDE

Huff Coughing

1. Patient assumes a sitting position with neck slightly flexed, shoulders relaxed, knees flexed, and forearms supported by pillow and, if possible, with feet on the floor.
2. Patient then drops head and bends forward while using slow, pursed-lip breathing to exhale.
3. Sitting up again, patient uses diaphragmatic breathing to inhale slowly and deeply.
4. Patient repeats steps 2 and 3 another three or four times to facilitate mobilization of secretions.
5. Before initiating a cough, patient should take a deep abdominal breath, bend slightly forward, and then cough three or four times on exhalation (huff coughing). Patient may need to support or splint the thorax or the abdomen to achieve a cough of maximum effectiveness.

Diaphragmatic (abdominal) breathing focuses on using the diaphragm instead of accessory muscles to achieve maximum inhalation and to slow the respiratory rate. There has been an overall lack of evidence in controlled studies to either support or refute the use of diaphragmatic breathing in pulmonary rehabilitation programs.

Effective Coughing. Many patients with COPD have developed ineffective coughing patterns that do not adequately clear their airways of sputum. In addition, they fear they may develop spastic coughing, which would increase dyspnea. *Huff coughing* is an effective technique that the patient can be taught easily; guidelines are presented in Table 31-18. The main goals of effective coughing are to conserve energy, reduce fatigue, and facilitate removal of secretions.

Nutritional Therapy. Weight loss and malnutrition are common among people with severe COPD and are a result of multiple factors. In these patients, energy expenditure is increased as a result of increased work of breathing (they spend 30%–50% more energy on breathing than does the average person); oxygen consumption is increased; gas exchange is inefficient; and dead space ventilation is increased. Other factors contributing to weight loss and malnutrition are decreased food intake, the effects of certain drugs, and a high systemic inflammatory response (Remels, Gosker, Langen, et al., 2013). Other factors further affecting patients' nutritional status may be dyspnea, dysphagia, dyspepsia, depression, anxiety, physical limitations, social or financial considerations, decreased sense of smell and taste, and drug and alcohol consumption. Eating becomes an effort as a result of dyspnea, especially in the later stages of COPD. In addition, a full stomach presses up on the flattened diaphragm, further increasing dyspnea and causing discomfort. It is difficult for some patients to eat and breathe at the same time; therefore, they eat inadequate amounts of food. The role of a registered dietitian is critical for nutritional screening and intervention.

Patients with COPD should try to keep body mass index (BMI) between 21 and 25 kg/m². Being either overweight or underweight can cause further problems in conjunction with COPD. However, a reduced BMI or weight loss is especially associated with poor outcomes in acute exacerbations and with increased rates of morbidity and mortality among patients with COPD. To decrease dyspnea and conserve energy, patients may need to rest (30 minutes) before eating, use a bronchodilator before meals, and select foods that can be prepared in advance. Eating five to six small meals per day helps avoid feelings of bloating and early satiety. Patients may want to avoid foods that form intestinal gas, such as cabbage, Brussels sprouts, and beans. Cold foods produce less of a sense of fullness than do hot foods. Foods that require a great deal of chewing can be served in another manner (e.g., grated, pureed). The use of frozen foods and a microwave oven may help conserve a patient's energy in food preparation. Exercises should be avoided for at least 1 hour before and after eating. In patients with late-stage or severe COPD, nutritional requirements for protein and calories may be greater than normal. They may need 1.2 to 1.3 times the normal kilocalorie requirement to even maintain their weight. A high-calorie, high-protein diet is recommended. High-protein, high-calorie nutritional supplements can be offered between meals. (Nutritional supplements are discussed in Chapter 42.)

Fluid intake should be at least 2 to 3 L per day unless contraindicated for other medical conditions, such as heart failure. Fluids should be taken between meals (rather than with them) to prevent excess stomach distension and to decrease pressure on the diaphragm. Sodium restriction may be indicated if a patient also has heart failure. In older patients, corticosteroid use increases the risk of or leads to osteoporosis. As a result, it is important to stress the necessity for adequate calcium and vitamin D intake.

AGE-RELATED CONSIDERATIONS

CHRONIC OBSTRUCTIVE PULMONARY DISEASE

Older adults have physiological changes, including reduced lean body mass and decreased respiratory muscle strength that may increase the burden of disease from COPD, including more dyspnea and less tolerance of exercise (Kobayashi, Yanai, Hanagama, et al., 2014). This causes a poorer ADL status and a higher incidence of acute exacerbations, which necessitate hospitalization. Smoking cessation is a key intervention but can be difficult to achieve.

COPD is frequently complicated by the presence of comorbid conditions such as cardiovascular disease, serious infections, osteoporosis, psychological problems (depression, anxiety), impaired cognition, and lung cancer (Areias, Carreira, & Anciães, 2014). The presence of comorbid conditions can make it difficult for patients to cope with the stress of an exacerbation. Thus assessment of comorbid conditions can assist in ensuring comprehensive and safe management, especially during an exacerbation.

Older patients may have difficulty in handling the increased secretions during an acute COPD exacerbation. The use of additional medications to manage the acute exacerbation can complicate disease management and increase the likelihood of adverse events. The nurse should assess for potential drug–drug interactions, especially in patients being treated for comorbidities. Some medications used to treat common disorders in older adults, such as hypertension, can worsen COPD symptoms. Nonspecific beta blockers should be avoided because they can also block the α₂ receptors in the airway and cause bronchoconstriction. Angiotensin-converting enzyme inhibitors may cause a dry cough or worsen a current cough.

Older adults may not adhere to drug therapies because of cognitive impairment and complexity of the polypharmacy prescribed. Arthritis in the hands can hinder the patient from using proper technique for MDIs. It is important to review MDI technique during clinic visits and have DPI or spacers prescribed (if possible) because they are easier to use. For patients with poor memory and visual impairment, an attempt should be made to simplify the medication regimen with written large-font action plans. Long-term use of ICSs has the potential of causing local and systemic side effects, including cataracts, glaucoma, and osteoporosis. Monitoring of ocular pressures, bone densitometry, and using the lowest possible ICS dose should be recommended (Battaglia, Cardillo, Lavorini, et al., 2014).

Older adult patients with COPD generally have impaired quality of life (Rinaudo, Ferrer, Terraneo, et al., 2015). An important role for the nurse is to focus on things that will improve these patients' quality of life. Psychological and emotional support becomes imperative to help them achieve successful outcomes. In the later stages of COPD, the nurse should get palliative and hospice care involved to help manage symptoms and improve the quality of the remainder of the patients' lives (Batzlaff, Karpman, Afessa, et al., 2014).

NURSING MANAGEMENT
CHRONIC OBSTRUCTIVE PULMONARY DISEASE

NURSING ASSESSMENT

Subjective and objective data that should be obtained from a patient with COPD are listed in Table 31-19.

NURSING DIAGNOSES

Nursing diagnoses for patients with COPD may include, but are not limited to, the following:

Ineffective breathing pattern related to *hyperventilation, body position that inhibits lung expansion*

Ineffective airway clearance related to *excessive mucus, retained secretions* (expiratory airflow obstruction)

Impaired gas exchange (related to alveolar hypoventilation)

Additional information on nursing diagnoses is presented in Nursing Care Plan 31-2.

PLANNING

Overall goals for patients with COPD include (a) the prevention of disease progression, (b) the ability to perform ADLs, (c) relief from breathlessness and other respiratory symptoms, (d) improvement in exercise tolerance, (e) the prevention and treatment of exacerbations, (f) improved overall quality of life, and (g) reduction in premature mortality.

NURSING IMPLEMENTATION

HEALTH PROMOTION. The best way to prevent COPD is never to smoke, and the next best step is to stop smoking immediately. (See the "Nursing Management: Lung Cancer" section in Chapter 30.) Avoiding or controlling exposure to occupational

---

TABLE 31-19   NURSING ASSESSMENT

Chronic Obstructive Pulmonary Disease (COPD)

Subjective Data	Objective Data
Important Health Information	**General**
Current health: The nurse should assess patient's experience of dyspnea (with activity and at rest) and cough. If cough is productive, the nurse should determine colour, consistency, and quantity of secretions. Current dyspnea should be measured on a quantitative scale such as a visual analogue or a numeric rating scale. (See Chapter 28 with regard to dyspnea.) The usual level of dyspnea that a patient experiences should be measured against the Medical Research Council Dyspnea Scale (see Figure 31-12).	Height, weight, BMI Distress, increased work of breathing, use of compensatory mechanisms for breathing (upright position, pursed-lip breathing), anxiety, depression, restlessness
	Integumentary
	Cyanosis (bronchitis), pallor or ruddy colour, poor skin turgor, thin skin, easy bruising, peripheral edema (cor pulmonale)
Past health history: The nurse should note whether the patient has had long-term exposure to chemical pollution, respiratory irritants, occupational fumes, and dust; the history and frequency of respiratory infections; previous hospitalizations and emergency department visits related to breathing and cardiac problems; smoking exposure (pack-years, exposure to secondary smoke, previous attempts at cessation); and personal and family history of respiratory and cardiac conditions.	**Respiratory** Rapid, shallow breathing; accessory muscle use; inability to speak at all; prolonged expiratory phase; pursed-lip breathing; wheezing, crackles, diminished breath sounds; ↓ chest excursion and diaphragmatic movement; use of accessory muscles; hyper-resonant or dull chest sounds on percussion
Medications: The nurse should record the use and duration of supplemental O_2, bronchodilators, anticholinergics, corticosteroids, antibiotics, OTC drugs, complementary therapies; effectiveness of bronchodilators and experience of adverse effects	**Cardiovascular** Tachycardia, dysrhythmias, jugular vein distension, right-sided third heart sound (cor pulmonale), edema (especially in feet)
	Gastro-intestinal Ascites, hepatomegaly (cor pulmonale)
Symptoms	**Musculo-skeletal**
• Anorexia, weight loss or gain, early satiety, difficulty eating	Muscle atrophy, ↑ anteroposterior diameter (barrel chest)
• Decreased level of activity and ability to perform ADLs or exercise. Dyspnea, palpitations, recurrent cough, use of sitting-up position for sleeping, paroxysmal nocturnal dyspnea, orthopnea, swelling of feet	**Possible Diagnostic Findings** Pulmonary function test results demonstrating airflow obstruction (e.g., ↓ FEV_1, FEV_1/FVC ratio, and PEFR; ↑ RV), ↓ SaO_2 as measured by pulse oximetry, abnormal arterial blood gas values, polycythemia
• Constipation, gas, bloating	Chest radiograph showing flattened diaphragm and hyperinflation or infiltrates
• Headache, loss of memory, inability to concentrate	ECG showing dysrhythmias
• Fatigue, insomnia, depression, anxiety, panic	

ADLs, activities of daily living; *BMI,* body mass index; *ECG,* electrocardiogram; *FEV₁,* forced expiratory volume in one second; *FVC,* forced vital capacity; *OTC,* over-the-counter; *PEFR,* peak expiratory flow rate; *RV,* residual volume; *SaO₂,* arterial oxygen saturation.

⊚ NURSING CARE PLAN 31-2

Chronic Obstructive Pulmonary Disease (COPD)

NURSING DIAGNOSIS	**Ineffective breathing pattern** related to *body position that inhibits lung expansion, fatigue, respiratory muscle fatigue* as evidenced by *use of three-point position, pursed-lip breathing, use of accessory muscles to breathe*

Expected Patient Outcomes

- Returns to baseline respiratory function
- Demonstrates an effective rate, rhythm, and depth of respirations

Nursing Interventions and *Rationales*

Ventilation Assistance

- Monitor respiratory and oxygenation status *to assess need for intervention.*
- Auscultate breath sounds, noting areas of decreased or absent ventilation and presence of adventitious sounds, *to obtain ongoing data on patient's response to therapy.*
- Encourage slow, deep breathing; turning; and coughing *to promote effective breathing techniques and secretion mobilization.*
- Administer medications (e.g., bronchodilators, inhalers) *that promote airway patency and gas exchange.*
- Position to minimize respiratory efforts (i.e., elevate head of the bed and provide overbed table for patient to lean on) *to save energy for breathing and promote chest expansion.*
- Monitor for respiratory muscle fatigue *to detect a need for ventilatory assistance.*
- Initiate a program of respiratory muscle strength and/or endurance training *to establish effective breathing patterns and techniques.*

NURSING DIAGNOSIS	**Ineffective airway clearance** related to *excessive mucus, retained secretions* as evidenced by *ineffective cough, absence of cough, diminished breath sounds*

Expected Patient Outcomes

- Has normal breath sounds for patient
- Demonstrates effective coughing
- Reports decreased dyspnea
- Maintains clear airway

Nursing Interventions and *Rationales*

- Facilitate deep breathing by sitting patient up *to maximize use of diaphragm and prolong expiratory phase.*
- Ensure adequate hydration (oral intake approximately 2–3 L/day, humidified ambient air) *to liquefy secretions for easier expectoration.*
- Teach effective cough techniques *to minimize the extent of airway collapse and to enhance airway clearance.*
- Assist with inhaled bronchodilator administration *to facilitate clearance of retained secretions.*

NURSING DIAGNOSIS	**Impaired gas exchange** (related to alveolar hypoventilation as evidenced by headache on awakening, $PaCO_2$ of ≥ 45 mm Hg and abnormal for patient's baseline, PaO_2 of <60 mm Hg, or SaO_2 of <90% at rest)

Expected Patient Outcomes

- Has $PaCO_2$ of 35–45 mm Hg or usual compensated baseline value
- Experiences return of PaO_2 to normal range for patient
- Reports improved mental status
- Reports decreased dyspnea
- Performs ADLs

Nursing Interventions and *Rationales*

- Monitor respiratory and oxygenation status *to assess need for intervention.*
- Teach pursed-lip breathing *to prolong expiratory phase and slow respiratory rate.*
- Assist patient to assume position of comfort (e.g., tripod position, elevated back rest, support of upper extremities to fix shoulder girdle) *to maximize respiratory excursion.*
- Administer and teach appropriate use of bronchodilators *to open the airways.*
- Teach signs, symptoms, and consequences of hypercapnia (e.g., confusion, somnolence, headache, irritability, decrease in mental acuity, increase in respiration, facial flush, diaphoresis) *to recognize problem early and initiate treatment.*
- Teach avoidance of central nervous system depressants *because they further depress respirations.*
- Administer O_2 if appropriate *to increase SaO_2 saturation.*
- Select O_2 supply systems and devices (e.g., nasal cannula, mask) that are appropriate for patient's ADLs (rest, sleep, exercise) *to minimize effect on preferred lifestyle.*

NURSING DIAGNOSIS	**Imbalanced nutrition: less than body requirements** related to *insufficient dietary intake, inability to ingest food* (decreased energy level, shortness of breath, gastric distention) as evidenced by *food intake less than recommended daily allowance*

Expected Patient Outcomes

- Maintains body weight within normal range for sex, height, and age
- Has normal serum protein and albumin levels

Nursing Interventions and *Rationales*

- Monitor caloric intake, weight, and serum albumin and protein levels *to determine adequacy of intake.*
- Provide menu suggestions for high-protein, high-calorie foods *to ensure maintenance of weight.*
- Give patient high-protein, high-calorie liquid supplements if necessary *to provide adequate calories and protein to prevent weight loss and muscle wasting.*
- Plan periods of rest before and after food intake *to assist with controlling fatigue and to compensate for blood flow diversion to the gastro-intestinal tract for digestion.*
- Refer to agency for financial or nutritional assistance as necessary (e.g., Meals-On-Wheels, home care) *to ensure nutritional adequacy after discharge.*
- Discuss benefit of five to six small meals throughout the day *because this reduces bloating.*

Continued

⊚ **NURSING CARE PLAN 31-2**

Chronic Obstructive Pulmonary Disease (COPD)—cont'd

NURSING DIAGNOSIS	***Disturbed sleep pattern*** related to *nonrestorative sleep pattern* (dyspnea, orthopnea, paroxysmal nocturnal dyspnea) as evidenced by *unintentional awakening, feeling unrested*
Expected Patient Outcomes	**Nursing Interventions and *Rationales***
• Sleeps at least 5 hr over a 24-hr period • Reports improved sleep pattern • Reports feeling rejuvenated on awakening	• Identify usual sleep habits and elicit reasons for difficulty sleeping *to provide baseline data.* • Monitor patient's sleep pattern, and note physical circumstances (e.g., pain or discomfort and urinary frequency) and psychological circumstances (e.g., fear or anxiety) that interrupt sleep *to initiate appropriate interventions.* • Observe for signs and symptoms of sleep apnea such as frequent awakenings at night or excessive daytime sleepiness, or noting a partner who complains of the patient's snoring or gasping for air *to initiate appropriate diagnostic tests and interventions.* • Identify patient-specific methods of relaxation, and teach patient relaxation methods *to foster sleep.* • Encourage exercise and activity during daylight hours *to ensure improved sleep at night.* • Provide patient with activity that promotes wakefulness *to limit daytime sleep.* • Instruct patient in arranging surroundings (e.g., clothing, temperature, position, noise level) *to produce an environment conducive to sleep.* • Teach patient to avoid alcoholic beverages, caffeine products, or other stimulants before bedtime *to reduce interference with sleep.*
NURSING DIAGNOSIS	***Risk for infection*** as evidenced by *insufficient knowledge to avoid exposure to pathogens, smoking, malnutrition, stasis of body fluid* (increased secretions)
Expected Patient Outcomes	**Nursing Interventions and *Rationales***
• Uses behaviours that minimize risk of infection • Experiences fewer or no respiratory infections	• Monitor for systemic and localized signs and symptoms of infection *to determine whether an infection is present.* • Teach patient to assess indicators of infection: change in sputum colour, quantity, odour, and viscosity; increase in cough and dyspnea; experience of fever, chills, diaphoresis, excessive fatigue; increase in respiratory rate; and abnormal breath sounds (gurgles, wheezing) *to determine whether an infection is present.* • Teach patient to use good handwashing and hygiene techniques and to avoid contact (when possible) with people with respiratory infections *to minimize sources of infection.* • Encourage patient to obtain vaccination for influenza and pneumococcal pneumonia *to decrease occurrence or severity of influenza or pneumonia.* • Teach proper care and cleaning of home respiratory equipment *to eliminate this source of infection.* • Instruct patient to seek medical attention for manifestations of early infection *to initiate treatment promptly.* • Teach patient to follow plan of care for managing exacerbations (e.g., increase fluid intake, initiate antibiotics and oral corticosteroid) *to initiate appropriate self-care promptly.*

ADLs, activities of daily living; *PaCO₂,* partial pressure of arterial carbon dioxide; *PaO₂,* partial pressure of arterial oxygen; *SaO₂,* arterial oxygen saturation.

and environmental pollutants and irritants is another preventive measure to maintain healthy lungs. (These factors are discussed in the section on environmental lung diseases in Chapter 30.) Early detection of airway disease is important and is the rationale for the use of spirometry or pulmonary function tests. Early identification and treatment of respiratory tract infections is important for improving the long-term prognosis of COPD. Avoiding exposure to large crowds in the peak influenza periods may be necessary, especially for older adults and patients with a history of respiratory problems. Patients should also be taught good handwashing technique, to avoid sharing food and drinks, and to keep their hands away from their nose, mouth, and ears. Influenza and pneumococcal pneumonia vaccinations are recommended.

Families with a history of both COPD and AAT deficiency should be aware of the genetic nature of the disease. Genetic counselling may be appropriate for such patients and their families.

EDUCATION. An important aspect in the long-term care of the patient with COPD is education (Table 31-20). (Patient teaching is discussed in Chapter 4.) One component of education may involve preparation of an advance care plan (see the "Ethical Dilemmas: Advance Directives" box).

EXERCISE. Walking is by far the best physical exercise for patients with COPD. Coordinated walking with slow, pursed-lip breathing without breath holding is a difficult task that requires conscious effort and frequent reinforcement. During coordinated walking and breathing, the patient is taught to breathe in through the nose while taking one step, then to breathe out through pursed lips while taking two to four steps (the number depends on a patient's tolerance). Walking should occur at a slow pace with rest periods when necessary. If supplemental oxygen has been prescribed, the patient needs to use oxygen while walking or exercising. By walking with the patient, the nurse helps decrease anxiety and helps maintain an appropriate pace. Walking also enables the nurse to observe the patient's actions and physiological responses to the activity. Many patients with moderate or severe COPD are anxious and fearful of walking or performing exercise. These patients and their families require much support while they build the confidence they need to walk or to perform daily exercises (GOLD, 2017).

Patients should be encouraged to walk 15 to 20 minutes a day and gradually increase this time. Patients can begin at a slower pace by walking for 2 to 5 minutes three times a day and slowly building up to 20 minutes a day, if possible. Adequate rest periods should be allowed. Some patients benefit from using a SABA (see Table 31-6) approximately 10 minutes before exercise. Parameters to monitor with exercise include resting pulse and pulse rate after activity. Pulse rate after exercise should not exceed 75% to 80% of the maximum heart rate (maximum heart rate = 220 − age in years). Dyspnea is usually the limiting factor, rather than increased heart rate, for exercise; therefore, the patient's

---

TABLE 31-20 PATIENT & CAREGIVER TEACHING GUIDE

Chronic Obstructive Pulmonary Disease

Goal: To assist patient and caregivers in improving quality of life through education and to promote lifestyle practices that support successful living with chronic obstructive pulmonary disease (COPD).

Teaching Topic	Strategies and Resources
• Overall guide to COPD, including topics listed below	Global Initiative for Chronic Obstructive Lung Disease (GOLD): *Patient guide: What you can do about a lung disease called COPD*, available at http://goldcopd.org/wp-content/uploads/2016/04/GOLD_PatientGuide_2012.pdf Canadian Lung Association: *COPD BreathWorks Plan*, available at http://www.lung.ca/lung-health/lung-disease/chronic-obstructive-pulmonary-disease-copd/resources or toll-free helpline at 1-866-717-COPD (2673) Living Well With COPD program: available online (see the Resources at the end of this chapter)

What Is COPD?

• Basic anatomy and physiology of lung	Models and posters of the lungs
• Basic pathophysiological changes of COPD	
• Signs and symptoms of COPD, exacerbations, cold, flu, pneumonia	
• Tests to assess breathing	

Nonpharmacological Therapy

• Breathing exercises	Demonstration and return demonstration
• Combating breathlessness and shortness of breath with "rescue breathing" techniques	RNAO dyspnea guidelines
• Pursed-lip breathing	Developing and using a schedule of daily and weekly activities
• Relaxation techniques	Pulmonary rehabilitation program
• Energy conservation techniques	
• Pacing and planning throughout the day for ADLs (pacing activity and using pursed-lip breathing with activities)	
• Regular exercise (upper and lower extremity)	
• Smoking cessation	See Chapter 11 Smoking cessation guidelines for nurses (e.g., the RNAO's Best Practice Guideline *Integrating Smoking Cessation into Daily Practice*); Quit Smoking helplines

Medications

Types (include mechanism of action)	Written medication list and schedule
• β₂-Adrenergic agonists	Having patients explain purpose of the medication and show the medication they are referring to
• Anticholinergics	
• Corticosteroids	Knowing the various colours of the inhalers because patients typically refer to them by colour
• Methylxanthines	
• Phosphodiesterase 4 inhibitor	
• Antibiotics	
Reviewing medication schedule and indications for use	
Adverse drug events	

Correct Use of Inhalation Devices

• Metered-dose inhalers with and without spacers	See Figures 31-6 and 31-7 Canadian Lung Association
• Dry powder inhalers	• Handouts
	• Inhalation device videos
	Placebo and demonstration units (provided by pharmaceutical companies) to assist with hands-on training
	Having patients demonstrate inhaler technique, and providing feedback about technique
	Checking periodically to ensure maintenance of proper technique
	Repeating process until accurate technique is demonstrated
	Exploring alternative delivery devices for patients who cannot demonstrate accurate technique

Home Oxygen

• Explaining need for O₂	Canadian Lung Association website (see the Resources at the end of this chapter)
• Explaining equipment and rationale for use	
• Guidance for home O₂ and ambulatory use	See Tables 31-16 and 31-17
• Care of oxygen equipment	

Psychosocial/Emotional Issues

Concerns about interpersonal relationships	Canadian Lung Association website (see the Resources at the end of this chapter)
• Dependency	
• Intimacy	Open discussion (sharing with patient, significant other, and family)
Emotional difficulties	
• Depression	
• Anxiety and panic	Exploring idea of attending social support groups or speaking to another person with COPD
Treatment decisions	
• Support and rehabilitation groups	

Continued

TABLE 31-20 **PATIENT & CAREGIVER TEACHING GUIDE**

Chronic Obstructive Pulmonary Disease—cont'd

COPD Management Plan		Healthy Nutrition	
• Focusing on self-management • A written action plan • Monitoring signs and symptoms • Reporting changes in symptoms • Understand causes of flares or exacerbations • Recognizing signs and symptoms of respiration infection, heart failure • Reducing the number of risk factors, especially smoking • Pulmonary rehabilitation program • Yearly follow-up	COPD management plan, developed and agreed upon by nurse and patient, that meets individual needs Assessment of patient's confidence level in managing COPD, and enhancement of skill development and confidence as necessary	• Strategies to lose weight (if patient is overweight) • Strategies to gain weight (if patient is underweight)	Consultation with dietitian
		End-of-Life and Advance Planning	
		• Identifying concerns and preferences for end-of-life care • Support of problem solving, decision making, and planning	End-of-life planning module in the Living Well With COPD program (see the Resources at the end of this chapter) Open discussion (health care team, patient, and family)

ADLs, activities of daily living; *RNAO*, Registered Nurses Association of Ontario.

perceived sense of dyspnea should be used as an indication of exercise tolerance. The patient can use the MRC Dyspnea Scale (see Figure 31-12) to determine the intensity of dyspnea.

Patients should be informed that shortness of breath often increases during exercise (as it does for a healthy individual). The activity is not being overdone unless the increased dyspnea does not return to baseline within 5 minutes after the cessation of exercise. Patients should wait approximately 5 minutes after completion of exercise, and if the dyspnea has not returned to baseline levels, then a SABA should be used. During the recovery time, the patient should use pursed-lip breathing. If dyspnea takes longer than 5 minutes to return to baseline levels, the patient has probably overdone the exercise and should proceed at a slower pace during the next exercise period. Keeping a diary or log of the exercise program may be beneficial. Diaries provide a realistic evaluation of progress, help motivate, and add to a sense of accomplishment. Stationary bicycles and treadmills can also be used and are particularly valuable when weather prevents walking outside.

Energy-Conserving Strategies. Energy conservation is another important component in COPD rehabilitation. Exercise training of the upper extremities improves function and reduces dyspnea. Many patients have already adapted alternative energy-saving practices for ADLs. Alternative or modified methods of hair care, shaving, showering, and other activities that necessitate over-the-head reaching must be explored. Assuming a tripod posture (elbows supported on a table, chest in fixed position) and placing a mirror on the table while using an electric razor or hair dryer conserves energy in comparison with standing in front of a mirror to perform these activities. If the patient uses home oxygen therapy, it must be used during activities of hygiene because these activities consume energy. Another energy-saving tip is to exhale when pushing, pulling, or exerting effort during an activity and to inhale during rest. Patients should also try to sit as much as possible when performing activities.

Sexual Activity. Modifying but not abstaining from sexual activity can contribute to a feeling of well-being. Using a SABA before sexual activity can help control dyspnea. Patients with COPD also need less energy if these guidelines are followed: (a) have sexual activity during the part of the day when breathing is best, (b) use slow pursed-lip breathing, (c) refrain from sexual activity after eating or other strenuous activity, (d) do not assume a dominant position, and (e) do not prolong foreplay. These aspects of sexual activity require open communication between partners regarding their needs and expectations and the changes that may be necessary as the result of a chronic disease (e.g., changes in body image, role reversal).

Sleep. Adequate sleep is extremely important. Getting adequate amounts of sleep can be difficult for patients with COPD. Medications may cause restlessness and insomnia. If patients experience cough during the night, the use of long-acting bronchodilators may help. Postnasal drip may cause coughing at night and can be treated with nasal saline sprays or rinses, nasal steroids, or both before sleep and in the morning. If a patient snores, stops breathing, or makes gasping breaths while sleeping and has a tendency to fall asleep during the day, the patient may need to be tested for sleep apnea (see Chapter 9).

Psychosocial Considerations. Healthy coping is often challenging for patients with COPD. Such patients frequently have to deal with many lifestyle changes that may involve a decreased ability to care for themselves and their condition, decreased energy for performing day-to-day activities and social activities, and the loss of a job. These lifestyle changes can put the patient at risk for social isolation.

When a patient first receives a diagnosis of COPD or experiences complications, the nurse should expect a variety of emotional responses. Emotions frequently encountered include guilt, depression, anxiety, social isolation, denial, and dependence. Among patients who still or used to smoke, guilt may result from the knowledge that the disease was caused largely by tobacco smoking. The patient may experience depression as he or she realizes the severity and chronicity of the disease. The nurse should convey a sense of understanding and caring to the patient. Relaxation techniques may provide benefit in terms of relief of dyspnea for some patients, but the evidence for this is unclear. Relaxation techniques include progressive muscular relaxation, positive thinking and visualization, use of music, yoga, massage, and humour (see Chapters 8 and 12). Progressive relaxation techniques are performed by having the patient listen to music, or to his or her own or another voice, and then gradually begin

ETHICAL DILEMMAS

Advance Directives

Situation

A 79-year-old man with chronic obstructive pulmonary disease is admitted to the hospital with respiratory failure. He is placed on a mechanical ventilator and responds to stimuli occasionally by opening his eyes. His living will was written 5 years ago, and a copy was given to his wife and health care provider at that time. The wife brings the document to the critical care unit and tells the nurse that the hospital must stop treating her husband and allow him to die as he requested. However, the oldest son is threatening the hospital with a lawsuit if the staff does not provide full care to his father.

Important Points for Consideration

- A living will is one type of an advance directive.
- A living will is prepared by the person in advance, indicating the person's treatment wishes should he or she become terminally ill or in a situation in which there is no hope of recovery.
- Health care providers must determine whether this respiratory crisis is reversible.
- Power of attorney for health care is another form of advance directive in which one person names another person to make health care decisions in the event that the first person is no longer able to do so.
- An advance directive respects the patient's autonomy: that is, the right to self-determination regarding health care at the end of life.
- A legally written living will is legally binding.
- Health care providers are obligated to follow the patient's advance directive when the patient is no longer able to speak for himself or herself.
- Health care providers are protected from liability when they adhere to advance directives.

Clinical Decision-Making Questions

1. What should the nurse do next with the information provided by the wife?
2. How should the nurse address the needs of each member of this family in the patient's plan of care?
3. What resources can the nurse use to facilitate decision making in this situation?

to slowly tense and relax muscle groups. Support groups at local chapters of the Canadian Lung Association, at hospitals, and at clinics can also be helpful.

End-of-Life Issues. Nurses have a responsibility to discuss with and plan for end-of-life care with patients and their families or caregivers to make sure that the necessary supports are in place to assist them through this critical terminal phase. Patients, their families, and health care providers should be involved in writing advance directives. Nurses must explore and understand the issues facing patients and their families through empathic, honest, and informative conversations. Discussions that highlight the importance of palliative care services and alleviation of terminal dyspnea lessen anticipatory fear and anxiety. The following "Ethical Dilemmas" box discusses advance directives.

EVALUATION

The expected outcomes for the patient with COPD are presented in Nursing Care Plan 31-2.

CYSTIC FIBROSIS

Cystic fibrosis (CF) is an autosomal recessive, multisystem disease characterized by altered function of the exocrine glands involving primarily the lungs, the pancreas, and the sweat glands.

(Autosomal recessive disorders are discussed in Chapter 15.) Abnormally thick, abundant secretions from mucous glands leads to a chronic, diffuse, obstructive pulmonary disorder in almost all affected patients. Exocrine pancreatic insufficiency is associated with most cases of CF. Sweat glands excrete increased amounts of sodium and chloride.

CF is a chronic fatal respiratory disease. According to the Canadian Cystic Fibrosis Registry, nearly 4 200 Canadians have cystic fibrosis (representing about 1 in 3 600 live births); the numbers of male and female patients are approximately equal, and the majority (92.7%) of CF patients are White (Cystic Fibrosis Canada, 2017). This autosomal recessive disease has a carrier rate of 1 per 25. If both parents carry the gene, the chance that their offspring will have the disease is 25%. The first signs and symptoms typically occur in early childhood, and in most patients, the disease is diagnosed by the age of 5 years. However, some patients tend to have less severe disease, and their cases are not diagnosed until they are adults.

The severity and the progression of the disease vary from person to person. Since the 1990s, the prognosis of this disease has improved dramatically as a result of early diagnosis and improvements in therapy. CF survival has improved at a rate of 1.8% per year with a median survival age of 39 years in 2010 (MacKenzie, Gifford, Sabadosa, et al., 2014). Of the 47 patients with CF who died in Canada in 2015, the median age at death was 29.7 years of age (Cystic Fibrosis Canada, 2017) and the median age of survival for Canadians with CF is currently estimated to be 52.1 years of age (Cystic Fibrosis Canada, 2017).

Etiology and Pathophysiology

CF results from mutations in a gene located on chromosome 7. The most common genetic mutation in CF occurs in what is known as the cystic fibrosis transmembrane regulator (CFTR) gene. The CFTR protein localizes to the lining of the exocrine portion of particular organs such as airways, pancreatic duct, sweat gland duct, and reproductive tract. The CFTR gene regulates sodium and chloride channels. Mutations in the CFTR gene alter this protein in such a way that the channels are blocked. As a result, cells that line the passages of the lungs, the pancreas, and other organs produce abnormally thick, sticky mucus. This mucus obstructs the airways and glands. The glands distal to the duct eventually undergo fibrosis. The high concentrations of sodium and chloride in the sweat of the patient with CF result from decreased chloride resorption in the sweat duct.

In the respiratory system, both upper and lower respiratory tracts can be affected. Upper respiratory tract manifestations include chronic sinusitis and nasal polyposis. The hallmark of respiratory involvement in CF is its effect on the airways. From being a disease of the small airways (chronic bronchiolitis), CF progresses to an entity that eventually involves the larger airways and finally causes destruction of lung tissue. Thick secretions obstruct bronchioles and lead to air trapping and hyperinflation of the lungs. The stasis of mucus provides an excellent growth medium for bacteria, which makes the airways more susceptible to serious lower respiratory tract infections. CF is thus characterized by chronic airway infection. The organisms most commonly cultured from the sputum of a patient with CF are *Staphylococcus aureus*, *H. influenzae*, and *P. aeruginosa* (Esther, Lin, Kerr, Miller, & Gilligan, 2014). These infections increase the rate of lung destruction through inflammatory mediators such as interleukins, tumour necrosis factor, and leukotrienes.

Lung disorders that can result from this pathological process include pneumonia, bronchiolitis, bronchitis, bronchiectasis, atelectasis, and emphysema. Lung tissue is progressively destroyed by inflammation and scarring, and the resultant chronic hypoxia leads to pulmonary hypertension and cor pulmonale. Blebs and large cysts in the lung are further severe manifestations of lung destruction. Other pulmonary complications include hemoptysis, which can sometimes be fatal, and pneumothorax. The degree of hemoptysis may range from scant streaking to major bleeding.

Initially, CF is an obstructive lung disease caused by the overall obstruction of the airways with mucus. Later, CF also progresses to a restrictive lung disease because of the fibrosis, lung destruction, and thoracic wall changes. Death usually results from loss of pulmonary function. Cor pulmonale is a common late complication caused by extensive loss of lung tissue and chronic hypoxia.

Pancreatic insufficiency is caused primarily by mucous plugging of the pancreatic duct and its branches, which results in fibrosis of the acinar glands of the pancreas and leads to the loss of exocrine function. Pancreatic enzymes such as trypsinogen, lipase, and amylase do not reach the intestine to digest ingested nutrients. Fat, protein, and fat-soluble vitamins (vitamins A, D, E, and K) are malabsorbed. Fat malabsorption results in steatorrhea, and protein malabsorption results in malnutrition, failure to grow, and failure to gain weight.

Diabetes mellitus may occur if the islets of Langerhans become fibrotic. CF-related diabetes mellitus affects approximately 15% of all patients with CF. It differs from type 1 diabetes in that some insulin is secreted, the disease is nonketotic, and it is slow in onset. It differs from type 2 diabetes in that affected individuals are underweight (as opposed to being obese), the onset is in a younger age population, and affected individuals are hypoinsulinemic. Routine screening of serum glucose levels is recommended. Insulin may be required for treatment of CF-related diabetes.

The sweat glands of the patient with CF secrete normal volumes of sweat but are unable to absorb sodium and chloride from sweat as it moves through the sweat duct. Therefore, these patients excrete four times the normal amount of sodium and chloride in sweat. This abnormality does not seem to affect the general health of the person, but it is useful as a diagnostic indicator.

Individuals with CF often have gastrointestinal problems. Intestinal obstruction resulting in meconium ileus is present in 10% to 15% of newborns with CF. GERD, distal intestinal obstructive syndrome (DIOS), and constipation are common. GERD is a major problem in individuals with CF. The relationship between reflux and exacerbation of respiratory disease is not known, but it is known that these two entities worsen each other.

DIOS is a syndrome that results from intermittent obstruction in the ileocecal area in patients with pancreatic insufficiency. The degree to which the bowel is obstructed may vary with each episode, and a partial obstruction may progress to a complete obstruction. Complete obstruction necessitates gastric decompression and a surgical consultation; partial and uncomplicated episodes of DIOS are treated with ingestion of a balanced polyethylene glycol electrolyte solution. Constipation develops in the sigmoid colon and progresses proximally, whereas DIOS develops in the ileocecal area and progresses distally. Careful monitoring of bowel habits and patterns is essential.

The liver may become involved. Biliary cirrhosis may not be recognized until late in the disease. Hepatobiliary disease is common in adult patients with CF. Chronic cholestasis, inflammation, fibrosis, and portal hypertension can occur.

Clinical Manifestations

The clinical manifestations of CF vary in accordance with the severity of the disease. As mentioned, meconium ileus is present in 10% to 15% of newborns with CF. Early childhood manifestations are failure to grow, digital clubbing, persistent cough with mucus production, tachypnea, and large, frequent bowel movements. The abdomen may become large and protuberant, and the extremities may develop an emaciated appearance.

The first symptom of CF in adults is frequently cough. With time, the cough becomes persistent and produces viscous, purulent, and often greenish sputum. Other respiratory problems that may be indicative of CF are recurring lung infections such as bronchiolitis, bronchitis, and pneumonia. As the disease progresses, periods of clinical stability are interrupted by exacerbations characterized by increased cough and sputum production, weight loss, and decreases in pulmonary function. Over time, the exacerbations become more frequent and lost lung function is less completely recovered, which ultimately leads to respiratory failure.

DIOS causes pain in the right lower quadrant, loss of appetite, and emesis, and a mass is often palpable. Insufficient pancreatic enzyme release causes the typical pattern of protein and fat malabsorption with frequent, bulky, foul-smelling stools.

The function of the reproductive system is altered. This finding is important because increasing numbers of people with CF are living to adulthood. Nearly all men with CF have reproductive issues because the vas deferens, which transports the sperm from the storage in the testes to the penile urethra, is congenitally absent. However, men with CF make sperm normally and thus, with assisted reproductive technology, have the capability of fathering children. In women with CF, menarche is usually delayed. During exacerbations, menstrual irregularities and secondary amenorrhea are fairly common. Affected women may be unable to become pregnant because of the increased viscosity of the cervical mucus. Many women with CF do have children, but the fertility rate is lower than among healthy women (Ahmad, Ahmed, & Patrizio, 2015). The baby of such a patient is heterozygous for CF (and hence a carrier of the CFTR gene) if the father is not a carrier. If the father is a carrier, the baby has a 50% chance of having CF. Genetic counselling can assist couples in deciding whether they want to have children and whether they want to use assisted reproductive technology to have a baby without the risk of CF. Screening of newborns can identify who will develop CF. Debate about the usefulness of this technology continues. (See Chapter 15, Figures 15-7, 15-9, and 15-11, for an explanation of genetic transmission of CF.)

Complications

Pneumothorax is a relatively uncommon but serious complication that is caused by the formation of bullae and blebs. A small amount of blood in the sputum is common in patients with CF because of chronic infection. Massive hemoptysis is life-threatening. With advanced lung disease, digital clubbing becomes evident. Respiratory failure and cor pulmonale are late complications of CF.

Diagnostic Studies

Diagnostic criteria for CF are evidence of CFTR protein malfunction on the sweat chloride test and characteristic respiratory or gastrointestinal symptoms. The sweat chloride test is performed with the pilocarpine iontophoresis method, which yields abnormal results in more than 90% of adults with CF. Pilocarpine carried by a small electric current is used to stimulate sweat production. The sweat is collected on filter paper or gauze and then analyzed for sodium and chloride concentrations. The test takes approximately 40 to 60 minutes. Values higher than 65 mEq/L for both sodium and chloride are suggestive of CF, especially in a person who has other clinical features of the disease. A second sweat chloride test is recommended to confirm the diagnosis unless two CF mutations have been identified by genetic testing (Ooi, Castellani, Keenan, et al., 2015). The degree of sodium and chloride elevation is not necessarily correlated with the severity of the disease. Secondary diagnostic studies include chest radiography, pulmonary function tests, fecal analysis for fat, and duodenoscopy for quantitative determination of pancreatic enzymes.

Because of the large number of CF mutations, DNA analysis is not used for the primary diagnostic test. A positive result of DNA analysis does, however, corroborate the diagnosis. Fetal diagnosis can be performed from specimens obtained by amniocentesis or chorionic villus sampling.

Collaborative Care

A multidisciplinary team should be involved in patients' care and should include nurses, physicians, respiratory and physical therapists, dietitians, pharmacists, and social workers. The major objectives of therapy in CF are to (a) promote clearance of secretions, (b) control infection in the lungs, and (c) provide adequate nutrition. Management of pulmonary problems in CF is directed at relieving airway obstruction and controlling infection. Drainage of thick bronchial mucus is assisted by aerosol and nebulized forms of medications to liquefy mucus and to facilitate coughing. The abnormal viscosity of secretions in CF results primarily from mucus glycoproteins and DNA from degenerated neutrophils. Drugs that degrade the high concentrations of DNA in CF sputum (e.g., DNase [Pulmozyme]) decrease sputum viscosity and increase airflow. Bronchodilators (e.g., β_2-adrenergic agonists, theophylline) may be used.

Airway clearance techniques are critical in reducing mucus. These techniques include chest physiotherapy, postural drainage, and positive expiratory pressure breathing. **Chest physiotherapy** (CPT) consists of percussion, vibration, and postural drainage. Percussion and vibration are manual or mechanical techniques used to augment postural drainage. In **postural drainage**, the principle of gravity is used to assist in bronchial clearance (Figure 31-17). Percussion and vibration are used after the patient has assumed a postural drainage position to assist in loosening the mobilized secretions. Percussion, vibration, and postural drainage may assist in bringing secretions into larger, more central airways. Effective coughing is then necessary to help raise these secretions. After each drainage position change, the patient should be given time to cough and breathe deeply. These techniques are individualized on the basis of the patient's pulmonary condition and response to the initial treatment. Sometimes it takes several hours after CPT for secretions to be expectorated. It is important to evaluate the effectiveness of CPT and its relief of symptoms; a physiotherapist who is trained in the proper technique often performs CPT. Complications associated with improperly performed CPT include fractured ribs, bruising, hypoxemia, and discomfort. CPT may not be beneficial and can be stressful

Anterior upper

Posterior upper

Apical upper

Lingula

Right middle

Superior lower

Lateral basal lower

Anterior basal

Posterior basal lower

FIGURE 31-17 Representative positions for postural drainage. *Shaded areas* in each illustration indicate the segment of the lung in which drainage is promoted.

for some patients. Some patients may develop hypoxemia and bronchospasm with CPT.

Various *airway clearance devices* are available to mobilize secretions, are easier to tolerate than CPT, and take less time than conventional CPT sessions. These devices include the Flutter device, Acapella device, and TheraPEP Therapy System. These devices involve the use of the principle of positive expiratory pressure (PEP) and may provide greater benefit to patients with COPD than other airway clearance techniques.

The Flutter mucus clearance device is also effective in promoting mucus removal (Figure 31-18). It is a handheld device that provides positive expiratory pressure. The flutter valve works by (a) causing the airways to vibrate, which loosens mucus from airway walls; (b) intermittently increasing the endobronchial pressure, which helps maintain the patency of the airway; and (c) accelerating expiratory airflow. It helps move mucus up through the airways to the mouth, where the mucus can be expectorated.

The Acapella device is another small hand-held tool that combines the benefits of both PEP therapy and airway vibrations to mobilize pulmonary secretions. It can be used in virtually any setting, inasmuch as patients are free to sit, stand, or recline while using it.

TheraPEP Therapy System can also provide sustained PEP and can simultaneously deliver aerosols so that the patient can inhale and exhale through it. TheraPEP has a mouthpiece attached to tubing connected to a small cylindrical resistor and a pressure indicator. The pressure indicator provides visual feedback about the pressure that the patient needs to hold in an exhalation to receive the PEP. (See the Resources section at the end of this chapter for a description and photo of this system.)

It is important to work collaboratively with families and patients because individuals with CF may have a preference for a certain technique that works well for them. Aerobic exercise seems to be effective in clearing the airways. Important needs to consider in planning an aerobic exercise program for a patient with CF are (a) frequent rest periods interspersed throughout the exercise regimen, (b) meeting increased nutritional demands of exercise, (c) being alert for manifestations of

hyperthermia, and (d) drinking large amounts of fluid and replacing salt losses.

Most CF patients die of complications resulting from lung infection. According to current data, antimicrobial treatment used for prophylaxis of *P. aeruginosa* has not been found beneficial and therefore is not a recommended prevention strategy (Doring, Flume, Heijerman, et al., 2012). Rigorous, early treatment of early *P. aeruginosa* colonization/infection is of great benefit to CF patients because of high eradication rates of the pathogen (Doring, Flume, Heijerman, et al., 2012). Prolonged high-dosage therapy may be necessary because many drugs are abnormally metabolized and rapidly excreted by patients with CF. Results of pharmacokinetic and kidney function studies should be monitored closely.

Although combination oral and aerosolized antimicrobial therapy is usually adequate, some patients require a 2- to 4-week course of intravenous antimicrobial therapy. If home care supports are adequate, the patient and family may choose parenteral therapy at home. The usual treatment for an acute infectious exacerbation is either an aminoglycoside combined with penicillin or a third-generation cephalosporin. Aerosolized bronchodilators may be used in selected patients, particularly before CPT. Patients with cor pulmonale or hypoxemia may require oxygen therapy. (Oxygen therapy is discussed earlier in this chapter.) Sclerosing of the pleural space or partial pleural stripping and pleural abrasion performed surgically are usually indicated for recurrent episodes of pneumothorax. (See the section on collaborative care of pleural effusions in Chapter 30.)

CF has become a leading indication for bilateral lung transplantation, accounting for 24.5% of these operations from 2004 to 2013 (CIHI, 2015). Also during this period, 356 people with cystic fibrosis received bilateral lung transplants (CIHI, 2015). (Lung transplantation is discussed in Chapter 30.) Lung transplantation for people with CF has resulted in significant improvements in pulmonary function and quality of life, as well as longer life expectancy. The survival rate among lung transplant recipients, including all primary diagnoses, is 86.8% at 1 year and 65.9% at 5 years (CIHI, 2015). The rate of survival after lung

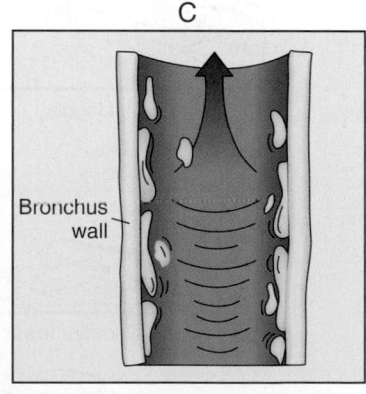

FIGURE 31-18 The Flutter mucus clearance device is a small, handheld tool that provides positive expiratory pressure therapy. It is used to facilitate removal of mucus from the lungs. **A,** It consists of a hard plastic mouthpiece, a plastic perforated cover, and a high-density stainless steel ball resting in a circular cone. **B,** The flutter effect occurs during expiration. Before exhalation, the steel ball blocks the conical canal of the Flutter device. During exhalation, the position the steel ball occupies is the result of equilibrium between the pressure of the exhaled air, the force of gravity on the ball, and the angle of the cone where the contact with the ball occurs. As the steel ball rolls and moves up and down, it creates an opening-and-closing cycle that repeats itself many times throughout each exhalation. The net result is that vibrations occur in the airways, resulting in the "fluttering" sensation. **C,** These vibrations loosen mucus from the airway walls and facilitate its movement up the airways. Source: Axcan Scandipharm, Inc., Birmingham, Alabama.

transplantation is higher among people with CF than among those with other pulmonary diseases such as COPD.

The management of pancreatic insufficiency includes pancreatic enzyme replacement of lipase, protease, and amylase (e.g., pancrelipase [Cotazym, Creon, Ultrase, Viokase] and zymase, an enzyme complex) administered before each meal and snack. A high-calorie, high-protein diet and multivitamin supplementation are recommended. Fat restriction usually is not necessary. Fat-soluble vitamin supplementation (vitamins A, D, E, and K) is necessary. Use of caloric supplements improves nutritional status. Added dietary salt is indicated whenever sweating is excessive, such as during hot weather, in the presence of fever, or from intense physical activity.

Gene therapy has been used as an experimental therapy for treating CF, but more research is still required (Mitomo, Griesenbach, Inoue, et al., 2010). (Gene therapy is discussed in Chapter 15.)

NURSING MANAGEMENT
CYSTIC FIBROSIS

NURSING ASSESSMENT

Subjective and objective data that should be obtained from a patient with cystic fibrosis are listed in Table 31-21.

NURSING DIAGNOSES

Nursing diagnoses for a patient with CF may include, but are not limited to, the following:

- *Ineffective airway clearance* related to *excessive mucus, retained secretions*
- *Ineffective breathing pattern* related to *fatigue, respiratory muscle fatigue*

- *Impaired gas exchange* (related to recurring lung infection)
- *Imbalanced nutrition: less than body requirements* related to insufficient dietary intake, inability to digest food
- *Ineffective coping* related to *high degree of threat* (decreased life expectancy, cost of treatment, limitation of career choices)

PLANNING

Overall goals for patients with CF include (a) adequate airway clearance, (b) reduction in number of risk factors associated with respiratory infections, (c) ability to perform ADLs, (d) minimizing complications related to CF, (e) adequate nutritional support to maintain appropriate BMI, and (f) active participation in planning and implementing a therapeutic regimen.

NURSING IMPLEMENTATION

Nurses and other health care providers can help young adults with CF obtain independence by helping them assume responsibility for their care. An important issue that should be discussed is sexuality. Delayed or irregular menstruation is not uncommon. There may be delayed development of secondary sex characteristics such as breasts in girls. A patient may use CF as a reason to avoid certain events or relationships. In contrast, healthy individuals may hesitate to make friends with someone who is sick, which can present a challenge for individuals with CF. Normal life transitions can present larger challenges to young adults with CF, such as building confidence and self-respect on the basis of achievements, persevering with employment goals and opportunities, developing motivation to set and achieve goals, learning to cope with the intensity and chronicity of the treatment program, and adjusting to losing independence when health fails. Disclosing the CF diagnosis to friends, potential spouses, or employers may pose challenges emotionally and financially.

TABLE 31-21 NURSING ASSESSMENT

Cystic Fibrosis (CF)

Subjective Data	Objective Data
Important Health Information	**General**
Current health: Experience of cough and mucus production (quantity, colour, consistency), dyspnea, and wheeze	Restlessness, failure to thrive
Past health history: Past respiratory and sinus infections: typical pattern, how treated, how responded to treatment; past hospitalizations and emergency department visits; when CF was diagnosed; family history of CF	**Integumentary System** Cyanosis (circumoral, nail beds), digital clubbing, salty skin
Medications: Use of bronchodilators, antibiotics, enzymes, herbs, and complementary therapies; adverse effects experienced; and adherence to treatment regimen	**Eyes** Scleral icterus
Nonpharmacological therapies: Use of postural drainage, percussion, and vibration	**Respiratory System** Runny nose, diminished breath sounds, sputum (amount, colour, tenacious), hemoptysis, increased work of breathing evidenced by use of accessory muscles of respiration, barrel chest
Symptoms	**Cardiovascular System** Tachycardia
• Runny nose; increased work of breathing; thick, tenacious sputum	**Gastro-intestinal System** Possibility of protuberant abdomen and abdominal distension and of foul, fatty stools
• Dietary intolerances, voracious appetite, weight loss, intestinal gas, bulky and foul-smelling stools, abdominal pain	
• Fatigue, restlessness, decreased exercise tolerance	**Possible Diagnostic Findings** Abnormal results of the following: pulmonary function tests, sweat chloride test, chest radiography, fecal fat analysis for fatty stools
• Anxiety, depression	
• Delayed menarche, menstrual irregularities, and secondary amenorrhea; fertility issues	

For patients with CF, respiratory intervention targets relief of bronchoconstriction, airway obstruction, and airflow limitation through the use of aggressive CPT, antibiotics, and bronchodilators. Good nutrition, nutritional supplements, and pancreatic enzymes are also important. Advances in long-term vascular access (e.g., implanted ports) have made intravenous access and administration of medication much easier and has eased the transition for intravenous treatment from hospital to home.

CPT is the mainstay of intervention for airway clearance. Home management of CF includes an aggressive plan of postural drainage with percussion and vibration, aerosol nebulization therapy, and breathing retraining. The patient is taught controlled coughing techniques and deep-breathing exercises and is encouraged to perform progressive exercise conditioning, such as a bicycling program.

Individuals and families affected by CF need significant support to cope with the many stresses imposed by the condition. Education and assistance can help them maintain a normal family life while coping with the huge physical demands associated with the condition. It is not uncommon for a person with CF to spend 2 hours a day performing CPT and 1 hour receiving nebulized medication (often antibiotics).

The family and the person with CF have a great financial and emotional burden. The cost of drugs, special equipment, and health care is often a financial hardship. Financial support for medications varies considerably across provinces. Some provinces provide complete support, whereas others have much lower levels of subsidy. In addition, some provinces cover only the cost of medications in childhood but stop coverage when the patient becomes an adult. The Canadian Cystic Fibrosis Foundation has established cystic fibrosis centres across the country to provide a comprehensive range of services to patients and families. A major advantage of the centres is the multidisciplinary team of nurses, physiotherapists, respiratory therapists, nutritionists, and doctors who work very closely with the family to tailor care to meet the family's needs.

As the person continues toward and into adulthood, the nurse and other skilled health professionals should be available to help the patient and family cope with complications resulting from the disease.

CASE STUDY

Chronic Obstructive Pulmonary Disease

Source: Jeroen van den Broek/ Shutterstock .com.

Patient Profile

Hazel Merrick is a 68-year-old married, female, retired police officer. She has been in the hospital for 3 days with an acute COPD exacerbation and will be discharged tomorrow.

Subjective Data

- Before admission, had 7 days of exceptional shortness of breath and increased volume of sputum, which turned greenish
- Had increased salbutamol use at home to five or six times a day for dyspnea
- Had jitters and racing heart
- Had three or four bouts of exacerbations of COPD in the past year that she treated at home
- Thirty pack-year history of smoking; smokes half a pack per day now to "clear out lungs" in the morning
- Eats a regular diet but "gets full fast"
- Cannot climb one flight of stairs without stopping; walks down the flat driveway 10 yards without difficulty
- Awakens two or three times per night coughing and short of breath

Objective Data
Physical Examination
- Weight, 58.5 kg (129 lb); height, 1.73 m (5 ft 8 in.); BMI, 20 kg/m²
- Blood pressure, 136/76 mm Hg; pulse, 86; respiratory rate, 28
- Increased anteroposterior diameter of chest (barrel-shaped)
- Slight use of accessory (neck) muscles with breathing
- Diminished breath sounds with occasional wheezes
- No peripheral edema

Diagnostic Studies
- Last spirometry: decreased FEV$_1$ (48%) and FEV$_1$/FVC ratio (62%)
- ABG measurements on admission: pH, 7.34; PaCO$_2$, 49 mm Hg; HCO$_3^-$, 27 mmol/L; PaO$_2$, 70 mm Hg

- WBC count: 14×10^9/L, on admission
- Chest radiograph: hyperinflation, flat diaphragm, no sign of pneumonia
- Sputum: negative for *P. aeruginosa*

Collaborative Care
- COPD stage: severe COPD with acute exacerbation
- O$_2$, 2 L via nasal catheter while in hospital
- Prednisone, 40 mg daily PO for 5 days
- Levofloxacin, 750 mg PO
- Ipratropium HFA MDI, 2 puffs four times a day
- At discharge: fluticasone, 250 mcg, and salmeterol, 50 mcg (Advair) Diskus 250/50, one inhalation q12hr

Discussion Questions
1. What classic manifestations indicate the patient had a COPD exacerbation?
2. What are some likely causes of her COPD?
3. What symptoms indicate the overuse of inhalers, and which drug would cause the symptoms described?
4. What is the only way Ms. Merrick can halt the progression of her lung disease?
5. Why would Ms. Merrick "feel full fast" when eating? What could the nurse do to minimize this issue?
6. Interpret the ABG values. What pattern can be seen?
7. ***Priority decision:*** What are nursing priorities for discharge planning and teaching?
8. ***Priority decision:*** In view of the assessment data presented, what are the priority nursing diagnoses? Are there any collaborative problems?
9. ***Evidence-informed practice:*** Ms. Merrick's son has been trying to persuade his mother to quit smoking for many years without success. He asks the nurse to tell his mother the results of her spirometry to convince her it is time to quit. Will this approach work?

ⓔvolve

Answers are available at *http://evolve.elsevier.com/Canada/Lewis/medsurg*

REVIEW QUESTIONS

The number of the question corresponds to the same-numbered objective at the beginning of the chapter.

1. A client is concerned that he may have asthma. Of the following symptoms that he relates to the nurse, which ones suggest asthma or risk factors for asthma? *(Select all that apply)*
   a. Allergic rhinitis
   b. Prolonged inhalation
   c. History of skin allergies
   d. Cough, especially at night
   e. Gastric reflux or heartburn

2. In evaluating an asthmatic client's knowledge of self-care, the nurse recognizes that additional instruction is needed when the client says which of the following?
   a. "I use my corticosteroid inhaler when I feel short of breath."
   b. "I get a flu shot every year and see my health care provider if I have an upper respiratory tract infection."
   c. "I use my inhaler before I visit my aunt who has a cat, but I visit for only a few minutes because of my allergies."
   d. "I walk 30 minutes every day but sometimes I have to use my bronchodilator inhaler before walking to prevent me from getting short of breath."

3. Which of the following clinical manifestations would the nurse recognize as a key feature of COPD?
   a. Age at onset of younger than 40 years
   b. Smoking history of more than 10 pack-years
   c. History of atopic dermatitis
   d. Infrequent sputum production

4. When teaching clients about the common adverse effects of cigarette smoke on the respiratory system, the nurse would include which of the following?
   a. Increased proliferation of ciliated cells
   b. Hypertrophy of the alveolar membrane
   c. Destruction of all alveolar macrophages
   d. Hyperplasia of goblet cells and increased production of mucus

5. A plan of care for the client with COPD could include which of the following? *(Select all that apply)*
   a. Exercise, such as walking
   b. High flow rate of O_2 administration
   c. Low-dose long-term oral corticosteroid therapy
   d. Use of peak flowmeter to monitor the progression of COPD
   e. Breathing exercises such as pursed-lip breathing that focus on exhalation

6. The nurse is preparing a client for transport for a diagnostic test and selects a Venturi mask for oxygen delivery. What is the rationale for choosing a Venturi mask?
   a. It can deliver up to 80% oxygen.
   b. It can provide continuous 100% humidity.
   c. It can deliver a precise concentration of oxygen.
   d. It can be used while a patient eats and sleeps.

7. Which studies would the nurse anticipate that the health care provider would order to diagnose cystic fibrosis?
   a. Pulmonary function test and sweat test
   b. Insulin tolerance and blood glucose
   c. Pancreatic enzymes and hormones
   d. Sweat test and vitamin B tolerance test

1. a, c, d, e; 2. d; 3. b; 4. d; 5. a, e; 6. c; 7. a.

⊖volve

For even more review questions, visit *http://evolve.elsevier.com/Canada/Lewis/medsurg.*

REFERENCES

Abascal-Bolado, B., Novotny, P. J., Sloan, J. A., et al. (2015). Forecasting COPD hospitalization in the clinic: Optimizing the chronic respiratory questionnaire. *International Journal of Chronic Obstructive Pulmonary Disease, 10,* 2295–2301. doi:10.2147/COPD.S87469.

Ahmad, A., Ahmed, A., & Patrizio, P. (2015). Cystic fibrosis and fertility. *Current Opinion in Obstetrics and Gynecology, 25*(3), 167–172. doi:10.1097/GC.0b013e32835f1745.

Areias, V., Carreira, S., Anciães, M., et al. (2014). Co-morbidities in patients with GOLD stage 4 chronic obstructive pulmonary disease. *Revista Portuguesa de Pneumologia (English Edition), 20*(1), 5–11. doi:10.1016/j.rppnen.2013.09.001.

Battaglia, S., Cardillo, I., Lavorini, F., et al. (2014). Safety considerations of inhaled corticosteroids in the elderly. *Drugs and Aging, 31*(11), 787–796. doi:10.1007/s40266-014-0213-1.

Batzlaff, C. M., Karpman, C., Afessa, B., et al. (2014). Predicting 1-year mortality rate for patients admitted with an acute exacerbation of chronic obstructive pulmonary disease to an intensive care unit: An opportunity for palliative care. *Mayo Clinic Proceedings, 89*(5), 638–643. doi:10.1016/j.mayocp.2013.12.004.

Beghé, B., Verduri, A., Roca, M., et al. (2013). Exacerbation of respiratory symptoms in COPD patients may not be exacerbations of COPD. *European Respiratory Journal, 41*(4), 993–995. doi:10.1183/09031936.00180812.

Bryan, S., & Navaneelan, T. (2015, November). *Study: Deaths from chronic obstructive pulmonary disease in Canada, 1950 to 2011. Health at a Glance* [Catalogue no. 82-624-X, Statistics Canada]. Retrieved from *http://www.statcan.gc.ca/pub/82-624-x/2015001/article/14246-eng.pdf.*

Camp, P. G., Hernandez, P., Bourbeau, J., et al. (2015). Pulmonary rehabilitation in Canada: A report from the Canadian Thoracic Society COPD Clinical Assembly. *Canadian Respiratory Journal, 22*(3), 147–152. Retrieved from *https://www.ncbi.nlm.nih.gov/pmc/articles/PMC4470547/.*

Canadian Institute for Health Information. (2015). *Canadian Organ Replacement Register update.* Retrieved from *https://www.cihi.ca/en/corr_update_winter15_en.pdf.*

Cystic Fibrosis Canada. (2017). *The Canadian Cystic Fibrosis Registry: 2015 annual report.* Retrieved from *http://www.cysticfibrosis.ca/uploads/Registry%20Report%202015/2015%20Registry%20Annual%20Report%20EN.pdf.*

Doring, G., Flume, P., Heijerman, H., et al. (2012). Treatment of lung infection in patients with cystic fibrosis: Current and future strategies. *Journal of Cystic Fibrosis, 11*(6), 461–479. doi:10.1016/j.jcf.2012.10.004.

Ducharme, F. M., Dell, S. D., Radhakrishnan, D., et al. (2015). Diagnosis and management of asthma in preschoolers: A Canadian Thoracic Society and Canadian Paediatric Society position paper. *Canadian Respiratory Journal, 20*(7), 353–371.

Esther, C. R., Lin, F. C., Kerr, A., et al. (2014). Respiratory viruses are associated with common respiratory pathogens in cystic fibrosis. *Pediatric Pulmonology, 49*(9), 926–931. doi:10.1002/ppul.22917.

Etminan, M., Jafari, S., Carleton, B., et al. (2012). Beta-blocker use and COPD mortality: A systematic review and meta-analysis. *BMC Pulmonary Medicine, 12*(48), 1–6. doi:10.1186/1471-2466-12-48.

Global Initiative for Asthma (GINA). (2015). *Global strategy for asthma management and prevention.* Retrieved from *http://ginasthma.org/wp-content/uploads/2016/01/GINA_Report_2015_Aug11-1.pdf.*

Global Initiative for Chronic Obstructive Lung Disease (GOLD). (2017). *Global strategy for the diagnosis, management and prevention of chronic obstructive pulmonary disease.* Retrieved from *http://goldcopd.org/gold-2017-global-strategy-diagnosis-management-prevention-copd/.*

Government of Canada. (2013). *Air pollution and health.* Retrieved from *http://www.hc-sc.gc.ca/ewh-semt/air/out-ext/health-sante/index-eng.php.*

Government of Canada. (2015). *Air Quality Health Index.* Retrieved from *http://www.healthycanadians.gc.ca/healthy-living-vie-saine/environment-environnement/air/quality-air-qualite-eng.php.*

Health Canada. (2012). *Canadian Tobacco Use Monitoring Survey (CTUMS) 2012.* Retrieved from *http://www.hc-sc.gc.ca/hc-ps/tobac-tabac/research-recherche/stat/ctums-esutc_2012-eng.php.*

Hodder, R., Lougheed, D. M., Rowe, B. H., et al. (2010). Management of acute asthma in adults in the emergency department: Non-ventilatory management. *Canadian Medical Association Journal, 182*(2), E55–E67. doi:10.1503/cmaj.080072. (Seminal).

Kobayashi, S., Yanai, M., Hanagama, M., et al. (2014). The burden of chronic obstructive pulmonary disease in the elderly population. *Respiratory Investigation, 52*(5), 296–301. doi:10.1016/j.resinv.2014.04.05.

Kuhl, K., & Hanania, N. A. (2012). Targeting IgE in asthma. *Current Opinion in Pulmonary Medicine, 18*(1), 1–5. doi:10.1097/MCP.0b013e32834deebb.

Langen, R. C. J., Gosker, H. R., Remels, A. H. V., et al. (2013). Triggers and mechanisms of skeletal muscle wasting in chronic obstructive pulmonary disease. *The International Journal of Biochemistry & Cell Biology, 45*(10), 2245–2256. doi:10.1016/j.biocel.2013.06.015.

Leatherman, J. (2015). Mechanical ventilation for severe asthma. *Chest, 147*(6), 1671–1680. doi:10.1378/chest.14-1733.

Long, M. B., Bekelman, D. B., & Make, B. (2014). Improving quality of life in chronic obstructive pulmonary disease by integrating palliative approaches to dyspnea, anxiety, and depression. *Journal of Hospice & Palliative Nursing, 16*(8), 514–520. doi:10.1097/NJH.0000000000000111.

Lougheed, M. D., Lemiere, C., Dell, S. D., et al. (2010). Canadian Thoracic Society Asthma Management Continuum—2010 Consensus summary for children six years of age and over, and adults. *Canadian Respiratory Journal, 17*(1), 15–24. (Seminal).

Lougheed, M. D., Lemiere, C., Ducharme, F. M., et al. (2012). Canadian Thoracic Society 2012 guideline update: Diagnosis and management of asthma in preschoolers, children and adults. *Canadian Respiratory Journal, 19*(2), 127–164.

MacKenzie, T., Gifford, A. H., Sabadosa, K. A., et al. (2014). Longevity of patients with cystic fibrosis in 2000 to 2010 and beyond: Survival analysis of the Cystic Fibrosis Foundation patient registry. *Annals of Internal Medicine, 161*(4), 233–241.

Marciniuk, D. D., Goodridge, D., Hernandez, P., et al. (2011). Managing dyspnea in patients with advanced chronic obstructive pulmonary disease: A Canadian Thoracic Society clinical practice guideline. *Canadian Respiratory Journal, 18*(2), 1–10.

Mitomo, K., Griesenbach, U., Inoue, M., et al. (2010). Toward gene therapy for cystic fibrosis using a lentivirus pseudotyped with Sendai virus envelopes. *Molecular Therapy, 18*(6), 1173–1182. doi:10.1038/mt.2010.13. (Seminal).

O'Donnell, D. E., Aaron, S., Bourbeau, J., et al. (2007). Canadian Thoracic Society recommendations for management of chronic obstructive pulmonary disease—2007 update. *Canadian Respiratory Journal, 14*(Suppl.B), 5B–32B. (Seminal).

O'Donnell, D. E., Hernandez, P., Kaplan, A., et al. (2008). Canadian Thoracic Society recommendations for management of chronic obstructive pulmonary disease—2008 update—Highlights for primary care. *Canadian Respiratory Journal, 15*(Suppl.A), 1A–8A. (Seminal).

Olajos-Clow, J., Cicutto, L., Duff Cloutier, J., et al. (2008). *Promoting asthma control in children.* Toronto: Registered Nurses' Association of Ontario. Retrieved from *http://rnao.ca/bpg/guidelines/promoting-asthma-control-children.* (Seminal).

Ooi, C. Y., Castellani, C., Keenan, K., et al. (2015). Inconclusive diagnosis of cystic fibrosis after newborn screening. *Pediatrics, 135*(6), e1377–e1385. doi:10.1542/peds.2014-2081.

Parsons, J. P., Hallstrand, T. S., Mastronarde, J. G., et al. (2013). An official American Thoracic Society clinical practice guideline: Exercise-induced bronchoconstriction. *American Journal of Respiratory and Critical Care Medicine, 187*(9), 1016–1027.

Public Health Agency of Canada (2011). *Fast facts about asthma: Data compiled from 2011 Survey on Living With Chronic Disease in Canada.* Ottawa: Author. Retrieved from *http://www.phac-aspc.gc.ca/cd-mc/crd-mrc/assets/pdf/asthma_fs_asthme-eng.pdf.*

Public Health Agency of Canada. (2015a). Chronic disease and injury indicator framework. Quick Stats, 2015 edition. *Health Promotion and Chronic Disease Prevention in Canada, 35*(10), Retrieved from *http://www.phac-aspc.gc.ca/publicat/hpcdp-pspmc/35-10/assets/pdf/ar-03-eng.pdf.*

Public Health Agency of Canada (2015b). *An Advisory Committee Statement (ACS) National Advisory Committee on Immunization (NACI): Canadian immunization guide chapter on influenza and statement on seasonal influenza for 2015–2016.* Ottawa: Author. Retrieved from *http://www.phac-aspc.gc.ca/naci-ccni/assets/pdf/flu-2015-grippe-eng.pdf.*

Registered Nurses' Association of Ontario (2017). *Adult asthma care: Promoting control of asthma* (2nd ed.). Toronto, ON: Registered Nurses' Association of Ontario.

Remels, A. H. V., Gosker, H. R., Langen, R. C. J., et al. (2013). The mechanism of cachexia underlying muscle dysfunction in COPD. *Journal of Applied Physiology, 114*(9), 1253–1262. doi:10.1152/japplphysiol.00790.2012.

Rinaudo, M., Ferrer, M., Terraneo, S., et al. (2015). Impact of COPD in the outcome of ICU-acquired pneumonia with and without previous intubation. *Chest, 147*(6), 1530–1538. doi:10.1378/chest.14-2005.

Simon, R. A., Dazy, K. M., & Waldram, J. D. (2015). Update on aspirin desensitization for chronic rhinosinusitis with polyps in aspirin-exacerbated respiratory disease (AERD). *Current Allergy and Asthma Reports, 15*(3), 1–8.

Statistics Canada. (2015). *Asthma, 2014.* Retrieved from *http://www.statcan.gc.ca/pub/82-625-x/2015001/article/14179-eng.htm.*

Tarlo, S. M., & Lemiere, C. (2014). Occupational asthma. *New England Journal of Medicine, 370*(7), 640–649. doi:10.105/NEJMra1301758.

Yohannes, A. M., & Alexopoulos, G. S. (2014). Depression and anxiety in patients with COPD. *European Respiratory Review, 23*(133), 345–349. doi:10.1183/09059180.00007813.

RESOURCES

Allergy/Asthma Information Association (AAIA)
www.aaia.ca/

Alpha 1 Canadian Registry
http://www.alpha1canadianregistry.com

Asthma Society of Canada
http://www.asthma.ca

Canadian Cancer Society
http://www.cancer.ca

Canadian Network for Respiratory Care
http://cnrchome.net/

Canadian Respiratory Health Professionals, Canadian Thoracic Society
https://crhp.lung.ca/

Canadian Thoracic Society Asthma Management Continuum—2010 Consensus Summary for Children Six Years of Age and Over, and Adults
https://www.ncbi.nlm.nih.gov/pmc/articles/PMC2866209/

Canadian Thoracic Society Guidelines
The Canadian Respiratory Guidelines (CRGC) Site
http://www.respiratoryguidelines.ca/

Cystic Fibrosis Canada
http://www.cysticfibrosis.ca

Living Well With COPD Program
http://www.livingwellwithcopd.com/

Lung Association*
http://www.lung.ca
Asthma Action Plan
https://www.lung.ca/lung-health/lung-disease/asthma/asthma
  -action-plan
Fact Sheet: Oxygen and COPD
https://www.lung.ca/sites/default/files/media/Oxygen_COPD
  _LungAssoc.pdf

---

*Most provinces have their own Lung Association.

Public Health Agency of Canada
Includes Canadian Communicable Disease Reports
http://www.phac-aspc.gc.ca/

Registered Nurses' Association of Ontario
Best Practice Guideline: Adult Asthma Care: Promoting Control
  of Asthma
http://rnao.ca/bpg/guidelines/adult-asthma-care-guidelines-nurses
  -promoting-control-asthma
Best Practice Guideline: Integrating Smoking Cessation Into Daily
  Nursing Practice
http://rnao.ca/bpg/guidelines/integrating-smoking-cessation-daily
  -nursing-practice

Alpha-1 Foundation
http://www.alpha1.org/

Cystic Fibrosis Foundation
http://www.cff.org

Global Initiative for Asthma (GINA)
http://www.ginasthma.com

Global Initiative for Chronic Obstructive Lung Disease (GOLD)
http://www.goldcopd.com

TheraPEP PEP Therapy System
https://www.smiths-medical.com/catalog/bronchial-hygiene/
  therapep/therapep-system.html

For additional Internet resources, see the website for this book at *http://evolve.elsevier.com/Canada/Lewis/medsurg*

SECTION 6

Problems of Oxygenation: Transport

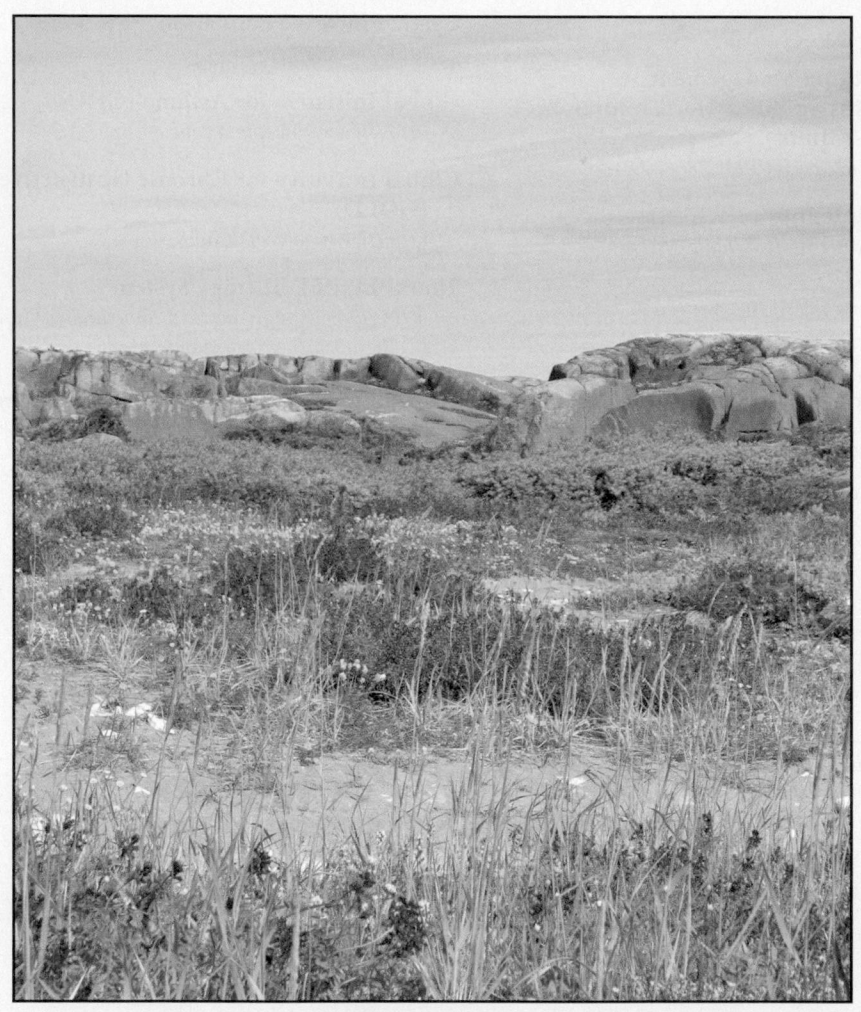

Source: wlkellar/Shutterstock.com.

Nursing Assessment
Hematological System

Written by: Sandra Irene Rome
Adapted by: Bridgette Lord

evolve WEBSITE

http://evolve.elsevier.com/Canada/Lewis/medsurg

- Review Questions (Online Only)
- Key Points
- Answer Guidelines for Case Study
- Conceptual Care Map Creator
- Audio Glossary
- Content Updates

LEARNING OBJECTIVES

1. Describe the structures and functions of the hematological system.
2. Differentiate among the different types of blood cells and their functions.
3. Explain the process of hemostasis.
4. Understand how age-related changes in the hematological system may result in differences in findings of hematological studies.
5. Describe the significant subjective and objective assessment data related to the hematological system that should be obtained from a patient.
6. Describe how to conduct a physical assessment of the hematological system.
7. Differentiate normal from abnormal physical findings of the hematological system.
8. Describe the purpose, the significance of results, and the nursing responsibilities related to diagnostic studies of the hematological system.
9. Differentiate between common normal and abnormal blood laboratory studies.

KEY TERMS

ecchymosis, p. 703	hemoglobin, p. 697	pancytopenia, p. 707	purpura, p. 705
erythropoiesis, p. 697	hemolysis, p. 697	petechiae, p. 703	stem cell, p. 695
fibrinolysis, p. 699	leukopenia, p. 708	phagocytosis, p. 698	thrombo-cytopenia, p. 708
hematopoiesis, p. 695	neutropenia, p. 708	polycythemia, p. 707	thrombo-cytosis, p. 708

Hematology is the study of blood and blood-forming tissues. The hematological system includes the bone marrow, blood, spleen, and lymph system. A basic knowledge of hematology is useful in clinical settings to evaluate a patient's ability to transport oxygen (O_2) and carbon dioxide (CO_2), coagulate blood, and combat infections. Assessment of the hematological system is based on the patient's health history, physical examination, and results of diagnostic studies.

STRUCTURES AND FUNCTIONS OF THE HEMATOLOGICAL SYSTEM

Bone Marrow

Blood cell production (hematopoiesis) occurs within the bone marrow. *Bone marrow* is the soft material that fills the central core of bones. There are two types of bone marrow (yellow [adipose] and red [hematopoietic]). The red marrow actively produces blood cells. In adults, the red marrow is located primarily in the flat and the irregular bones, such as the ends of long bones, pelvic bones, vertebrae, sacrum, sternum, ribs, flat cranial bones, and scapulae.

All three types of blood cells (red blood cells, white blood cells, and platelets) develop from a common hematopoietic stem cell within the bone marrow. This hematopoietic stem cell is best described as an immature blood cell that is able to self-renew and to differentiate into hematopoietic progenitor cells. As blood cells mature and differentiate, several different types of cells are formed (Figure 32-1). The marrow responds to increased demands for various types of blood cells by increasing production by means of a negative feedback system. The bone marrow is stimulated by various factors (e.g., erythropoietin, granulocyte colony–stimulating factor, thrombopoietin) that cause differentiation of the stem cells into one type of the committed hematopoietic cells. For example, when tissue

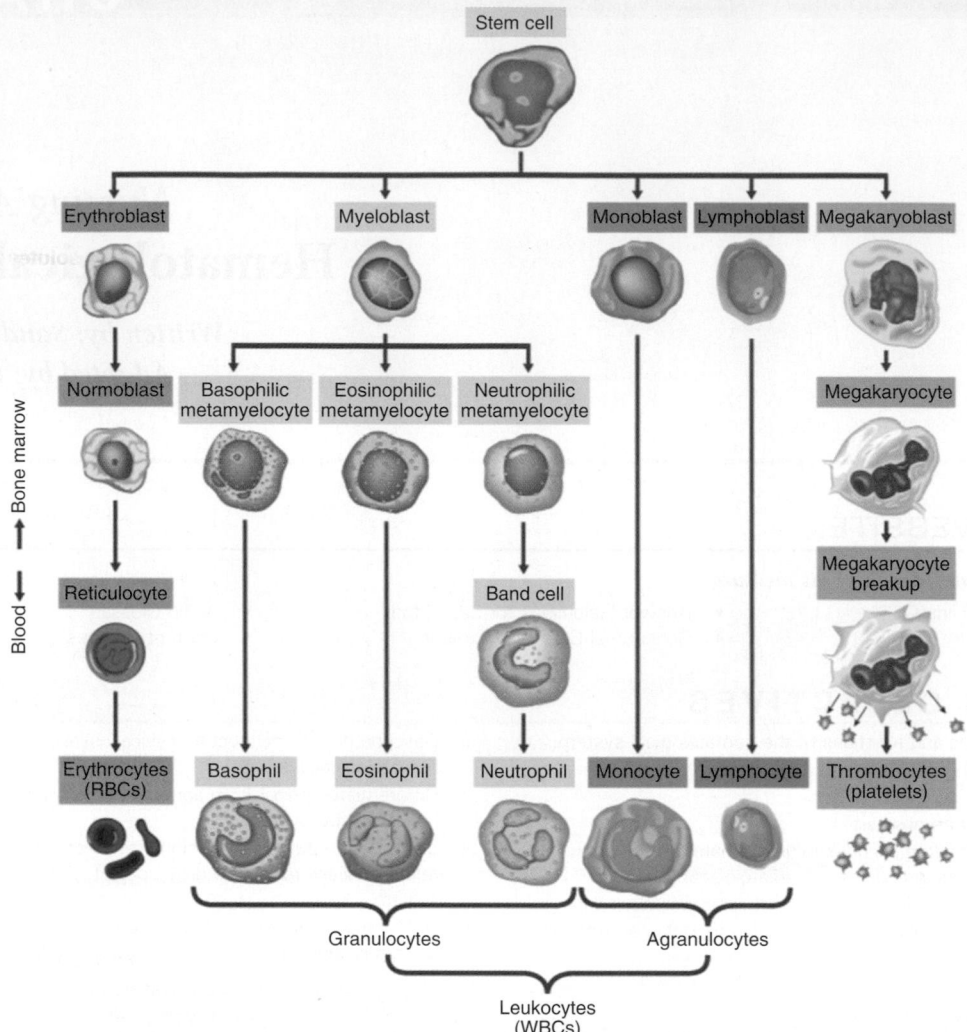

FIGURE 32-1 Development of blood cells. *RBCs,* red blood cells; *WBCs,* white blood cells.

hypoxia occurs, erythropoietin is secreted primarily by the kidney. It circulates to the bone marrow and causes differentiation of proerythroblasts in the bone marrow (Zhang, Wang, Dey, et al., 2014).

Blood

Blood is a type of connective tissue that performs three major functions: transportation, regulation, and protection (Table 32-1). Blood is responsible for the *transportation* of oxygen, nutrients, hormones, and waste products around the body. Blood also plays a role in the *regulation* of temperature, fluid and electrolyte balance, and acid–base balance. Finally, blood plays a *protective* role in its ability to coagulate (or clot) and combat infections. Blood has two major components: plasma and blood cells.

Plasma. Approximately 55% of blood is plasma (Figure 32-2). Plasma is composed primarily of water, but it also contains proteins, electrolytes, gases, nutrients, and waste. Plasma proteins include albumin, globulin, and clotting factors, mostly fibrinogen (McCance & Huether, 2015). The term *serum* refers to plasma without its clotting factors.

Blood Cells. About 45% of the blood (see Figure 32-2) is composed of formed elements, or blood cells. There are three types of blood cells: *erythrocytes,* or red blood cells (RBCs);

TABLE 32-1	FUNCTIONS OF BLOOD
Function	**Examples**
Transportation	• Oxygen from lungs to cells • Nutrients from gastro-intestinal tract to cells • Hormones from endocrine glands to tissues and cells • Metabolic waste products (e.g., CO_2, ammonia, urea) from cells to lungs, liver, and kidneys
Regulation	• Fluid and electrolyte balance • Acid–base balance • Body temperature
Protection	• Combating invasion of pathogens and other foreign substances • Maintaining homeostasis of blood coagulation

leukocytes, or white blood cells (WBCs); and *thrombocytes,* or platelets. The primary function of erythrocytes is oxygen transportation, whereas the leukocytes are involved in protection of the body from infection. Platelets mainly function to promote blood coagulation.

Erythrocytes. The primary functions of erythrocytes (RBCs) include transport of gases (both O_2 and CO_2) and assistance in

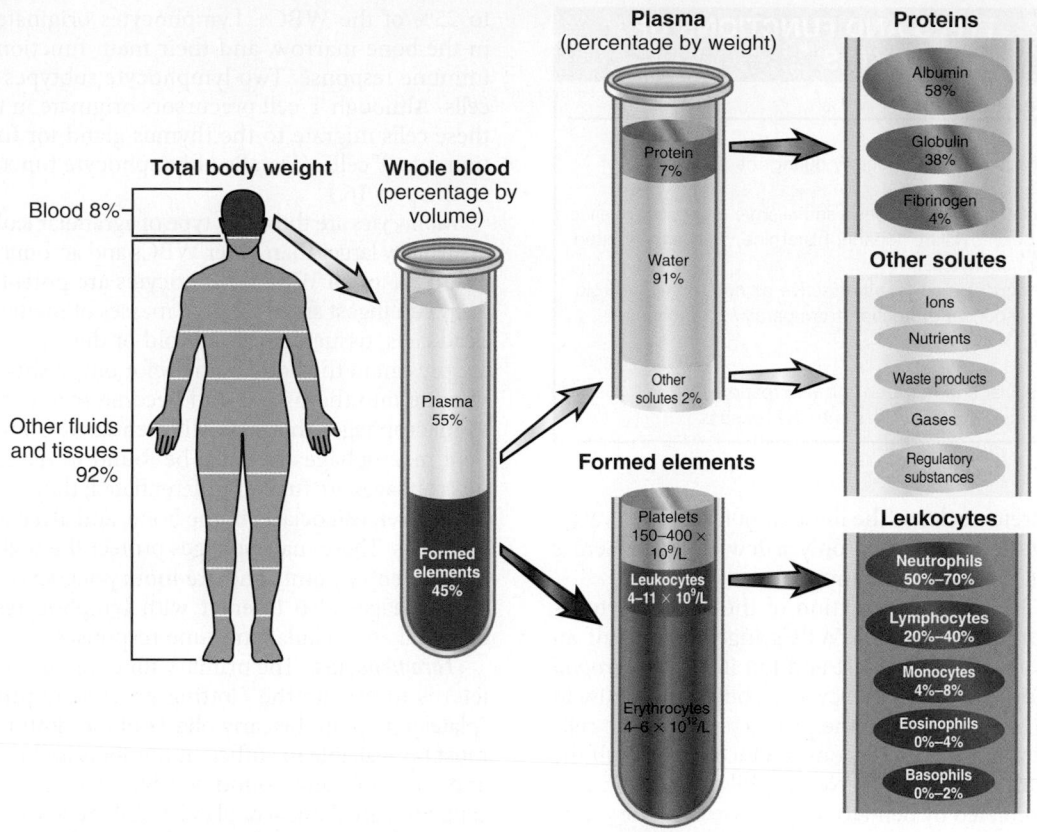

FIGURE 32-2 Approximate values for the components of blood in the adult. Normally, 45% of the blood is composed of blood cells, and 55% is composed of plasma.

maintaining acid–base balance. The composition and features of an erythrocyte are ideal for its role in gas transportation. It is a flexible cell with a unique biconcave shape. Flexibility enables the cell to alter its shape so that it can easily pass through tiny capillaries. The cell membrane is also very thin, which facilitates the diffusion of gases. Erythrocytes are composed primarily of a large molecule called **hemoglobin,** a complex compound composed of heme (an iron compound) and globin (a simple protein) that binds with O_2 and CO_2. As erythrocytes circulate through the capillaries surrounding the alveoli within the lungs, O_2 attaches to the iron on the hemoglobin. The O_2-bound hemoglobin is referred to as *oxyhemoglobin* and is responsible for the bright-red appearance of arterial blood. As erythrocytes flow to body tissues, O_2 detaches from the hemoglobin and diffuses from the capillary into tissue cells. CO_2 diffuses from tissue cells into the capillary, attaches to the globin portion of hemoglobin, and is transported to the lungs for removal. Hemoglobin also acts as a buffer and plays a role in maintaining acid–base balance. This buffering function is described further in Chapter 19.

Erythropoiesis (the process of RBC production) is regulated by cellular O_2 requirements and general metabolic activity. Erythropoiesis is stimulated by hypoxia and controlled by *erythropoietin,* a glycoprotein growth factor synthesized and released primarily by the kidneys. Erythropoietin stimulates the bone marrow to increase erythrocyte production. Approximately 2.5 million erythrocytes are produced per second, and the normal lifespan of an erythrocyte is about 120 days. Erythropoiesis is also influenced by the availability of nutrients. Many essential nutrients are necessary for erythropoiesis, including protein,

iron, copper, folate (folic acid), cobalamin (vitamin B_{12}), riboflavin (vitamin B_2), pyridoxine (vitamin B_6), pantothenic acid (vitamin B_5), niacin (vitamin B_3), ascorbic acid (vitamin C), and vitamin E. Erythrocyte production is also affected by endocrine hormones, such as thyroxine, corticosteroids, and testosterone.

Several distinct cell types evolve during erythrocyte maturation (see Figure 32-1). The *reticulocyte* is an immature erythrocyte. The reticulocyte count is a measure of the rate at which new RBCs appear in the circulation. Reticulocytes can develop into mature erythrocytes within 48 hours of their release into circulation. Therefore, assessing the number of reticulocytes is a useful means of evaluating the rate and adequacy of erythrocyte production.

Hemolysis (destruction of RBCs) by monocytes and macrophages removes abnormal, defective, damaged, and old RBCs from circulation. Hemolysis occurs in the bone marrow, liver, and spleen and results in increased levels of bilirubin that must be processed by the body. When hemolysis occurs under normal conditions, the liver is able to conjugate and excrete the bilirubin produced.

Leukocytes. Leukocytes (WBCs) appear white when separated from blood. Like erythrocytes, leukocytes originate from stem cells within the bone marrow (see Figure 32-1). There are five different types of leukocytes, each of which has a different function. Leukocytes that contain granules within the cytoplasm are called *granulocytes* (also known as *polymorphonuclear leukocytes*). Granulocytes include three types: neutrophils, basophils, and eosinophils. Leukocytes that do not have granules within the cytoplasm are called *agranulocytes* and include lymphocytes and monocytes (Table 32-2). Lymphocytes and monocytes are also referred to as *mononuclear cells* because they

TABLE 32-2   TYPES AND FUNCTIONS OF LEUKOCYTES

Type	Cell Function
Granulocytes	
Neutrophil	Phagocytosis, especially during the early phase of inflammation
Basophil	Inflammatory response and allergic response; release of bradykinin, heparin, histamine, serotonin; limited phagocytosis
Eosinophil	Phagocytosis (not as effective as neutrophil); allergic response; protection from parasitic infections
Agranulocytes	
Lymphocyte	Cellular and humoral immune response
Monocyte	Phagocytosis; cellular immune response

have only one discrete nucleus. The lifespan of leukocytes varies widely: granulocytes may live for only a few hours, whereas some lymphocytes may live for many years.

Granulocytes. The primary function of the granulocytes is phagocytosis, a process by which WBCs ingest or engulf an unwanted organism and then digest and kill it. The *neutrophil* is the most common type of granulocyte, accounting for 50% to 70% of all WBCs. Neutrophils are the primary phagocytic cells involved in acute inflammatory responses. Once they engulf the pathogen, they die in 1 to 2 days. Neutrophil production and maturation are stimulated by hematopoietic growth factors (e.g., granulocyte colony–stimulating factor [G-CSF] and granulocyte-macrophage colony–stimulating factor [GM-CSF]) (Hamilton & Achuthan, 2013).

A mature neutrophil is called a *segmented neutrophil* ("seg") because the nucleus is segmented into two to five lobes connected by strands. An immature neutrophil is called a *band* (for the bandlike or rodlike appearance of the nucleus). Although band cells are sometimes found in the peripheral circulation of normal people and are capable of phagocytosis, the mature neutrophils are more effective. An increase in neutrophils in the blood is a common diagnostic indicator of infection or tissue injury. The existence of many immature cells is termed a *shift to the left* and may be indicative of active infection or inflammation. (Shift to the left is explained further in the "White Blood Cells" section later in this chapter.)

Eosinophils account for only 2% to 4% of all WBCs. They have a similar but reduced ability for phagocytosis. One of their primary functions is to engulf antigen–antibody complexes formed during an allergic response. Elevated levels of eosinophils are also seen in some neoplastic disorders, such as lymphoma, as well as in various skin and connective tissue disorders (Lebeaux & Sene, 2012). Eosinophils are able to defend against parasitic infections.

Basophils constitute less than 2% of all leukocytes. These cells have cytoplasmic granules that contain chemical mediators such as heparin, serotonin, and histamine. If a basophil is stimulated by an antigen or by tissue injury, it responds by releasing substances from the granules. This is part of the response in allergic and inflammatory reactions. *Mast cells* are similar to basophils, but they reside in connective tissue and play a central role in inflammation, permeability of blood vessels, and smooth muscle contraction.

Agranulocytes. Agranulocytes differ from granulocytes in that their cytoplasm does not contain lysosomal granules. *Lymphocytes*, one type of agranular leukocyte, constitute 20%

to 25% of the WBCs. Lymphocytes originate from stem cells in the bone marrow, and their main function is related to the immune response. Two lymphocyte subtypes are B cells and T cells. Although T-cell precursors originate in the bone marrow, these cells migrate to the thymus gland for further differentiation into T cells. (Details of lymphocyte function are presented in Chapter 16.)

Monocytes are the other type of agranular leukocyte. These cells are usually larger than other WBCs and account for approximately 3% to 8% of all WBCs. Monocytes are potent phagocytic cells. They can ingest small or large masses of matter, such as bacteria, dead cells, tissue debris, and old or defective RBCs. These cells are present in the bone marrow for only a short time before they migrate into the tissues and become macrophages. In addition to macrophages that have differentiated from monocytes, resident macrophages can also be found in tissues. These resident macrophages are further differentiated; they include Kupffer cells in the liver, osteoclasts in the bone, and alveolar macrophages in the lungs. These macrophages protect the body from pathogens at these entry points and are more phagocytic than monocytes. Macrophages also interact with lymphocytes to facilitate the humoral and cellular immune responses.

Thrombocytes. The primary function of thrombocytes (platelets) is to initiate the clotting process by producing an initial "platelet plug" in the early phases of the clotting process. Platelets must be available in sufficient numbers and must be structurally and metabolically sound for blood clotting to occur. When capillaries are damaged, platelets adhere to the damaged capillary wall, and platelet activation is initiated. Increasing numbers of platelets accumulate to form the platelet plug, which is stabilized with clotting factors. Platelets are also important in the process of clot shrinkage and retraction.

Platelets, like other blood cells, originate from stem cells within the bone marrow (see Figure 32-1). The stem cell undergoes differentiation by transforming into a *megakaryocyte*, which fragments into platelets. Platelet production is partly regulated by *thrombopoietin*, a growth factor that acts on bone marrow to stimulate platelet production (Kaushansky, 2015).

Thrombopoietin is produced in the liver, kidneys, smooth muscle, and bone marrow. Typically, platelets have a lifespan of 8 to 10 days.

Iron Metabolism

Iron is obtained from foods and dietary supplements. On average, only 5% to 10% of the dietary iron that is consumed is absorbed by the body. Absorption primarily takes place in the duodenum and the upper jejunum. Approximately two-thirds of the body's iron is found as the heme part of the hemoglobin molecule in RBCs. The other third of iron is stored as ferritin and hemosiderin in the bone marrow, spleen, liver, and macrophages (Figure 32-3). When stored iron is not replaced, hemoglobin production is reduced.

Transferrin, which is synthesized in the liver, serves as a carrier plasma protein for iron. The degree to which transferrin is saturated with iron is a reliable indicator of the iron supply for developing RBCs.

Iron is recycled in the body after old and damaged RBCs are *phagocytized* (i.e., ingested and destroyed) by macrophages in the liver and spleen. Iron is released into the plasma and transported by transferrin to the bone marrow for RBC production. Alternatively, iron may be stored as ferritin or hemosiderin (see Figure 32-3). Only about 3% of iron is lost daily in urine, sweat,

FIGURE 32-3 Iron metabolism. Iron is ingested in the diet or from supplements. Macrophages break down ingested red blood cells. Iron is returned to the blood bound to transferrin or stored as ferritin or hemosiderin. *RBC,* red blood cell.

TABLE 32-3	**COAGULATION FACTORS**
Coagulation Factor	**Action**
I Fibrinogen	Source of fibrin to form a clot. Made in liver.
II Prothrombin	Converted to thrombin, which then activates fibrinogen into fibrin, as well as activating factors V, VII, VIII, XI, XIII; protein C; and platelets.
III Tissue factor, tissue thromboplastin	Released from damaged endothelial cells; activates the extrinsic pathway by reacting with factor VII.
IV Calcium	Required cofactor at several points in the coagulation cascade.
V Labile factor	Binds with factor X to activate prothrombin.
VI	Not in use (now obsolete).
VII Stable factor, proconvertin	Forms a complex with factor III and activates factors IX and X.
VIII Antihemophilic factor	Works with factor IX and calcium to activate factor X.
IX Christmas factor	Together with factor VIII, activates factor X.
X Stuart–Prower factor	Activates conversion of factor II (prothrombin) into thrombin.
XI Plasma thromboplastin antecedent	Activates factor IX when calcium is present.
XII Hageman factor	Activates factor XI, which starts the intrinsic pathway.
XIII Fibrin-stabilizing factor	Cross-links fibrin strands and stabilizes fibrin clot.

bile, and epithelial cells in the gastro-intestinal tract. Therefore, there is normally very little iron loss except with blood loss.

Clotting Mechanisms

Hemostasis is a term used to describe the blood clotting process. This process is important in minimizing blood loss when body structures are injured. The sequence of events is as follows: (1) vascular injury and subendothelial exposure; (2) platelet plug formation involving adhesion, aggregation, and activation; (3) fibrin clot development; and (4) clot retraction and dissolution.

Vascular Injury and Subendothelial Exposure. When a blood vessel is injured, an immediate local vasoconstrictive response occurs. Vasoconstriction reduces the leakage of blood from the vessel not only by restricting the vessel size but also by pressing the endothelial surfaces together. The latter reaction enhances vessel wall stickiness and maintains closure of the vessel even after the vasoconstriction subsides. Vascular spasm may last for 20 to 30 minutes, allowing time for the platelet response and plasma clotting factors to be activated.

Platelet Plug Formation (Adhesion, Aggregation, Activation). Damage to the endothelial lining of blood vessels exposes glycoproteins such as collagen and von Willebrand factor (vWF), to which platelets adhere. The stickiness is termed *adhesiveness,* and the formation of clumps is termed *aggregation.* As platelets adhere to the collagen fibres of a wound, platelets become spiked and much stickier. They stick to one another because of fibrin linking their glycoprotein IIb/IIIa receptors. The adhesion process causes platelets to undergo an *activation* process whereby they release their stored granules that contain adenosine diphosphate (ADP), prostaglandin, thromboxane A$_2$ (TXA$_2$), and other factors that enhance platelet plug formation and limit bleeding (Porteus & Mantanona, 2012).

In addition to their contribution in forming a platelet plug, platelets also facilitate the reactions of the plasma clotting factors

within the coagulation cascade. Platelet lipoproteins stimulate necessary conversions in the clotting process (Figure 32-4).

Fibrin Clot Development. The formation of a fibrin clot interlaced with the platelet plug is the conclusion of a complex series of reactions involving different clotting factors. The plasma clotting factors are labelled with both names and Roman numerals (Table 32-3). Plasma proteins circulate in inactive forms until stimulated to initiate clotting through one of two pathways: intrinsic or extrinsic. The *intrinsic pathway* is activated by collagen exposure from endothelial injury when the blood vessel is damaged. The *extrinsic pathway* is initiated when tissue thromboplastin is released extravascularly from injured tissues.

Regardless of whether clotting is initiated by substances inside or outside the blood vessel, coagulation ultimately follows the same final common pathway of the clotting cascade. Thrombin, in the common pathway, is the most powerful enzyme in the coagulation process (Figure 32-5). It converts fibrinogen to fibrin, which is an essential component of a blood clot.

Clot Retraction and Dissolution. Just as some blood elements foster coagulation (*procoagulants*), others interfere with clotting (*anticoagulants*). This counter-mechanism to blood clotting serves to keep blood in its fluid state. Anticoagulation may be achieved by several means: antithrombin activity, fibrinolysis, and vessel and platelet activity. As the name implies, antithrombins keep blood fluid by antagonizing thrombin, a powerful coagulant. Endogenous heparin, protein C, and protein S are examples of anticoagulants.

Another method of maintaining blood in its fluid form is fibrinolysis, a continual process resulting in the dissolution of fibrin and thus clots. The fibrinolytic system is initiated when plasminogen is converted to plasmin (see Figure 32-5). Thrombin

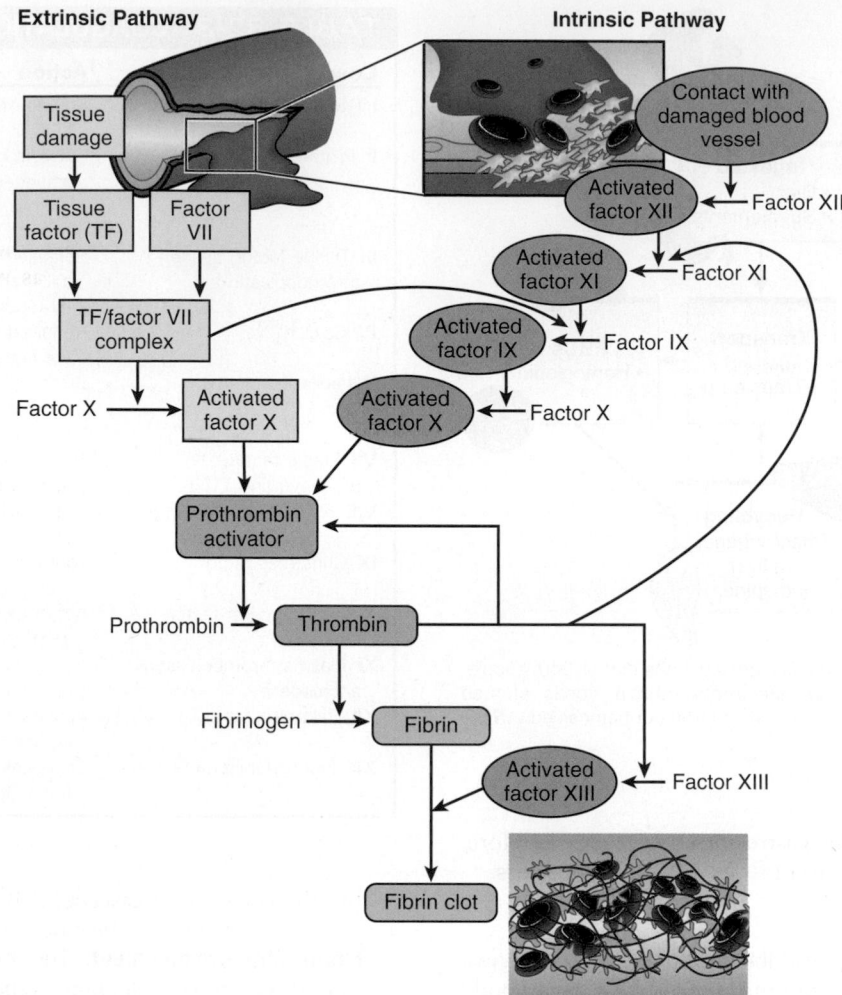

FIGURE 32-4 Coagulation mechanism showing steps in the intrinsic and the extrinsic pathways as they would occur in the test tube.

FIGURE 32-5 Fibrinolytic system. *RBC,* red blood cell.

is one of the substances that can activate the conversion of plasminogen to plasmin, thereby promoting fibrinolysis. The plasmin attacks either fibrin or fibrinogen by splitting the molecules into smaller elements known as *fibrin split products* (FSPs) or *fibrin degradation products* (FDPs). (More information about FSPs can be found in Table 32-8 later in this chapter and in the discussion of disseminated intravascular coagulation in Chapter 33.)

If fibrinolysis is excessive, the patient is predisposed to bleeding. In such a situation, bleeding results from the destruction of fibrin in platelet plugs or from the anticoagulation effects of

increased amounts of FSPs. Increased FSPs lead to impairment in platelet aggregation, reduction in prothrombin, and an inability to stabilize fibrin.

Spleen

Another component of the hematological system is the spleen, which is located in the upper left quadrant of the abdomen. The role of the spleen can be classified into the following four general functions:

1. *Hematopoietic function:* The spleen produces RBCs during fetal development.
2. *Filter function:* The spleen filters the blood. It removes old and defective RBCs from circulation by means of the mononuclear phagocyte system. Filtration also involves the reuse of iron—the spleen is able to catabolize hemoglobin released by hemolysis and return the iron component of the hemoglobin to the bone marrow for reuse. The spleen also plays an important role in filtering circulating bacteria, especially encapsulated organisms such as Gram-positive cocci.
3. *Immune function:* The spleen contains a rich supply of lymphocytes, monocytes, and stored immunoglobulins.
4. *Storage function:* The spleen serves as a storage site for platelets and RBCs. More than 300 mL of blood and one-third of platelets can be stored in the spleen.

Lymph System

The lymph system—consisting of lymph fluid, lymphatic capillaries, lymphatic ducts, and lymph nodes—carries fluid from the interstitial spaces to the blood. It is by means of the lymph system that proteins and fat from the gastro-intestinal (GI) tract and certain hormones are able to return to the circulatory system. The lymph system also returns excess interstitial fluid to the blood, which is important in preventing the development of edema.

Lymph fluid is a pale-yellow fluid that has diffused through lymphatic capillary walls. It circulates through a special vasculature, much as blood moves through blood vessels. The formation of lymph fluid increases when interstitial fluid increases, thereby forcing fluid into the lymph system. When too much interstitial fluid forms or when something interferes with the reabsorption of lymph, *lymphedema* develops. Lymphedema may occur as a complication following surgery (for example, when axillary lymph nodes are removed as part of a radical mastectomy) or if lymph drainage is disrupted following radiation to an area. The lymphatic capillaries are thin-walled vessels that have an irregular diameter. They are somewhat larger than blood capillaries and do not contain valves. Lymphatic capillaries unite to form lymphatic vessels that carry all lymph fluid to either the right lymphatic duct or to the thoracic duct. These large lymphatic ducts drain into the subclavian veins of the neck.

The *lymph nodes* are round, oval, or bean-shaped and vary in size according to their location. Structurally, lymph nodes are small clumps of lymphatic tissue and are found in groups along lymph vessels at various sites in the body. The body contains more than 200 lymph nodes, with the greatest number in the abdomen surrounding the GI tract. Lymph nodes are situated both superficially and deep. The superficial nodes can be palpated, but evaluation of the deep nodes requires radiological examination. A primary function of lymph nodes is the filtration of pathogens and foreign particles that are carried by lymph fluid to the nodes.

Liver

The liver functions as a filter. It also produces procoagulants that are essential for hemostasis and blood coagulation. In addition, when the amount of iron exceeds tissue needs (which can occur with frequent blood transfusions or with diseases that cause iron overload), the excess is stored in the liver. *Hepcidin*, a protein produced by the liver, is a key regulator of iron balance. The synthesis of hepcidin is regulated by a variety of stimuli, including existent iron stores in the body, inflammation, hypoxia, and RBC requirements (Kautz & Nemeth, 2014). Hepcidin reduces the release of stored iron from enterocytes (in the intestines) and macrophages. Thus, when iron is deficient, hepatocytes produce less hepcidin, releasing stored iron and increasing dietary absorption. Other functions of the liver are described in Chapter 46.

AGE-RELATED CONSIDERATIONS

HEMATOLOGICAL SYSTEM

Physiological aging is a gradual process that involves cell loss and organ atrophy. Aging leads to a decrease in bone marrow mass and cellularity and an increase in bone marrow fat (Ershler, Artz, & Kanapuru, 2015). Although older adults are still capable of maintaining adequate blood cell levels, the lower reserve capacity leaves them more vulnerable to possible problems with clotting, transporting O_2, and fighting infection. The result is a diminished ability to compensate for an acute or chronic illness. In addition, age-related changes result in an increased risk for clonal myeloid cancers.

Hemoglobin levels begin to decrease in both men and women after middle age. Although iron deficiency is often responsible for the low hemoglobin levels, the cause of anemia in approximately one-third of older patients is unknown. Inadequate nutritional intake of iron may be a factor, as may occult inflammation, low testosterone levels, impaired renal function, or incipient myelodysplasia (Ershler, Artz, & Kanapuru, 2015). Older adults are also not as able as younger adults to produce reticulocytes in response to hemorrhage or hypoxemia. Also, the RBC plasma membranes are more fragile in the older person. This fragility may account for a slight increase in mean corpuscular volume (MCV) and a slight decrease in mean corpuscular hemoglobin concentration (MCHC) of RBCs in some older individuals.

The total WBC count and differential are generally not affected by aging (Ershler, Artz, & Kanapuru, 2015). However, humoral antibody response and T-cell function may decrease (Bueno, Sant'Anna, & Lord, 2014). During an infection, an older adult may have only a minimal elevation in the total WBC count. This laboratory finding suggests that the bone marrow reserve of granulocytes is diminished in older adults and reflects the possible impairment in stimulation of hematopoiesis.

The number of platelets is unaffected by the aging process, but functionally the platelets may have increased adhesiveness. More important, the levels of proteins critical to coagulation change with age. There is an age-related activation of coagulation and fibrinolytic pathways that favours clot formation. The effects of aging on hematological studies are presented in Table 32-4. Immune changes related to aging are described in Chapter 16.

TABLE 32-4	AGE-RELATED DIFFERENCES IN ASSESSMENT
Effects of Aging on Hematological Studies	
Study	**Changes**
CBC Studies	
Hemoglobin	Normal; possibly slightly decreased
MCV	May be slightly increased
MCHC	May be slightly decreased
WBC count	Diminished response to infection
Platelets	Unchanged
Clotting Studies	
Partial thromboplastin time	Decreased
Fibrinogen	May be elevated
Factors V, VII, VIII, IX	May be elevated
ESR	Increased significantly
D-dimers	Increased
Iron Studies	
Serum iron	Decreased
Total iron-binding capacity	Decreased
Ferritin	Increased
Erythropoietin	May be decreased

CBC, complete blood cell count; *ESR*, erythrocyte sedimentation rate; *MCHC*, mean corpuscular hemoglobin concentration; *MCV*, mean corpuscular volume; *WBC*, white blood cell.

TABLE 32-5 HEALTH HISTORY

Hematological System: Subjective Data

Past History
- Have you had any previous problems with anemia, bleeding disorders, and blood diseases such as leukemia?*
- Have you ever received a blood transfusion?*
- Have you undergone any surgical procedures?

Family History
- Has anyone in your family had anemia, cancer, bleeding, or clotting problems?*

Social and Occupational History
- Does your occupation bring you into contact with hazardous substances?*
- Have you had any past or current occupational or household exposures to radiation or chemicals?*
- Have you had any past exposure to radiation as a medical treatment?
- Do you have a support system to assist you when needed?
- What coping strategies do you use when your symptoms get worse?

Self-Care History
- Do you smoke or drink alcohol?*
- Do you take any prescribed or over-the-counter medications?*
- Are you having or have you ever had chemotherapy?*
- Do you take any herbal products?* Home remedies?*
- Have you in the past or are you currently consuming illegal drugs? What agents? What route? How frequently? When did you last use them?
- Do you exercise regularly? What type of exercise do you do, and how frequently?*

Activities of Daily Living
- Do you have any difficulty performing daily activities because of a lack of energy?*
- Have you experienced excessive fatigue recently?*
- Do you have any shortness of breath at rest? With activity?*

Nutrition–Metabolic History
- Do you have any difficulties with eating, chewing, or swallowing?*
- Have you had a sore tongue or any mouth sores, swollen or sore gums, or excessive oral bleeding?
- How has your appetite been?
- What kind of diet do you follow? If vegetarian, do you eat eggs, milk products, fish, or chicken? Do you follow a vegan diet?
- Do you take any vitamins, nutritional supplements, or iron?*
- Have you had any changes in your weight in the past year?*
- Are nausea and vomiting a problem for you?*
- Have you ever experienced any unusual bleeding or bruising?*
- Have there been recent changes in the condition of your skin?*
- Have you noticed any swelling in your armpits, neck, or groin?*
- Have you experienced night sweats or cold intolerance?*

Elimination
- Have you had black or tarry stools?* Have you had light- or clay-coloured stools?
- Do you ever have diarrhea or a change in your bowel habits?*
- Have you noticed any blood or a dark tea colour in your urine?*
- Have you been urinating less?*
- Has your urine had a foul odour or cloudiness?

Neurological History
- Do you have any pain, such as bone, joint, or abdominal pain, or abdominal fullness?*
- Do you have pain when moving your joints?*
- Have your muscles been sore or achy recently?*
- Do you have any limitations in joint motion?*
- Do you have a problem with unsteady gait?* Have you fallen recently?*
- Have you experienced any numbness or tingling?*
- Have you had any problems with your vision, hearing, or taste?*
- Have you noticed any changes in your mental functions?*

Sleep History
- Do you feel fatigued? Are you more fatigued than usual?*
- Do you feel rested on awakening? If no, explain.

Sexual–Reproductive History
- Has your hematological problem caused any sexual or intimacy problems that concern you?*
- *Women:* When was your last menses? Is your cycle regular? How long does your bleeding usually last? How heavy is the flow? Have you had any increase in cramping or clotting?* Have there been any changes in the amount of flow?
- *Men:* Do you experience erectile dysfunction?*
- Have you had unprotected sex in the past 6 months?* Was your partner someone new or a person with whom you have had a long-term sexual relationship?

Other
- Has your current illness caused a change in your roles and relationships?*
- Does your health problem make you feel differently about yourself?*
- Do you have any other physical changes that cause you distress?*
- Do you have any personal or religious objection to receiving blood or blood products?*
- Do you have any conflicts between your planned therapy and your value–belief system?*

*If yes, describe.

ASSESSMENT OF THE HEMATOLOGICAL SYSTEM

Much of the evaluation of the hematological system is based on a thorough health history. Key questions to ask a patient with a hematological problem are presented in Table 32-5.

Subjective Data

Important Health Information

Past Medical History. It is important to learn whether the patient has had prior hematological problems or whether the patient's family has any hereditary disorders. Hematological disorders that have a strong genetic link include sickle cell anemia, hemophilia, thalassemia, and hemochromatosis. The nurse should also document other related medical conditions such as mononucleosis, malabsorption, and liver disorders (e.g., hepatitis, cirrhosis), as well as kidney or spleen disorders. A patient may have received a kidney transplant, may have lost a spleen to traumatic injury, or may have a history of intravenous drug use that may affect the risk for hematological disorders. A history of recurrent infection or problems with blood clotting should also be noted. In addition, it is important to determine how many, if any, blood transfusions a patient has had, as well as any complications experienced during administration, since the risk for transfusion reactions and iron overload increase with the number of blood transfusions.

CASE STUDY

Patient Introduction

Allison Jobena is a 73-year-old woman who is brought to the emergency department by her husband. He found his wife at home, weak and lying in bed after she had returned from work. She says she has been slowly getting more "cold and tired" but "that is what happens when you continue to work at this age." Her husband states that she has become more tired over the past couple of weeks and gets short of breath when doing simple errands. She recently developed a "bad cold and sinus infection" that improved only after two courses of antibiotics. Ms. Jobena also states, "I've noticed I've had a lot of bruising lately."

Source: Image Point Fr/ Shutterstock .com

Discussion Questions

Throughout this assessment chapter, think about Ms. Jobena with the following questions in mind:

1. What are the possible causes of Ms. Jobena's weakness, pallor, and shortness of breath?
2. What would be the nurse's priority assessment?
3. What questions should the nurse ask Ms. Jobena?
4. What should be included in the physical assessment? What would the nurse be looking for?
5. What diagnostic studies might be ordered?
   Ms. Jobena and her condition will be followed throughout this assessment chapter. See pp. 704, 705, and 711 for more information on Ms. Jobena.

ℯvolve

Answers are available at http://evolve.elsevier.com/Canada/Lewis/medsurg.

Medications. A complete medication history that includes both prescription and over-the-counter drugs taken is an important component of a hematological assessment. The use of vitamins, herbal products, or dietary supplements should specifically be addressed because many patients may not consider these to be drugs. Many drugs and supplements interfere with normal hematological functions. For example, herbal therapies such as *Panax* ginseng can alter clotting times (Li, Wang, & Xu, 2013). Chemotherapeutic drugs used to treat cancer and anti-retroviral agents used to treat human immunodeficiency virus (HIV) infection may cause bone marrow depression (see Chapters 17 and 18). A patient previously treated with chemotherapeutic drugs, particularly alkylating agents, is at a higher risk of developing a secondary malignancy such as leukemia or lymphoma. A patient receiving long-term anticoagulation therapy (e.g., warfarin [Coumadin]) may be at increased risk for bleeding.

Surgery or Other Treatments. The patient should be asked about specific past surgical procedures, specifically, splenectomy, tumour removal, prosthetic heart valve placement, surgical excision of the duodenum (in which iron absorption occurs), partial or total gastrectomy (in which parietal cells are removed, thus reducing intrinsic factor needed for the absorption of cobalamin [vitamin B_{12}]), gastric bypass (in which the duodenum may be bypassed and parietal cell surface area decreased), and ileal resection (in which cobalamin absorption takes place). The nurse should also ascertain how wound healing progressed postoperatively and if and when any bleeding problems occurred related to the surgery. Wound healing and bleeding as responses to past injuries (including minor trauma) and to dental extractions should be documented.

Approach to Obtaining a Hematological History

Social and Occupational History. The patient should be questioned about any past or current occupational or household exposures to radiation or chemicals. If such exposure has occurred, the type, amount, and duration of exposure should be determined. A person who has been exposed to radiation, as a treatment modality or by accident, has a higher incidence of certain hematological problems (see Chapter 18). The same is true of a person who has been exposed to chemicals (e.g., benzene, lead, naphthalene, phenylbutazone). These chemicals are commonly used by potters, dry cleaners, and individuals in occupations involving the use of adhesives. The nurse should assess the effect of the current illness on a patient's usual roles and responsibilities. The patient's support systems and coping skills should also be assessed.

Self-Care History. Risk factors that might disrupt the hematological system, such as alcohol and cigarette use, must be assessed. Alcohol is a caustic agent, and damage to the GI tract secondary to alcohol use can cause bleeding. *Hematemesis* (bright-red, brown, or black vomit) can be a symptom of this problem and should be investigated. Alcohol also exerts a damaging effect on platelet function and the liver, in which clotting factors are produced. Consequently, bleeding problems can develop and should be anticipated in patients with a known history of alcohol use disorder. Cigarette smoking increases low-density lipoprotein cholesterol and levels of CO_2, leading to hypoxia and altering the anticoagulant properties of the endothelium. Smoking also increases platelet reactivity, plasma fibrinogen, hematocrit, and blood viscosity, which increases the risk of developing blood clots. Illegal drug use should also be documented because many illegal drugs may affect hematopoiesis.

Activities of Daily Living. Because fatigue is a prominent symptom in many hematological disorders, the patient should be asked about feelings of tiredness. The nurse should also ask whether the patient experiences weakness and complains of heavy extremities. Symptoms of apathy, malaise, dyspnea, or palpitations should be documented. Any change in a patient's ability to perform activities of daily living (ADLs) should be noted. Whether or not the patient exercises should also be determined.

Nutritional–Metabolic History. During the patient interview and assessment, the nurse should measure the patient's weight and determine whether the patient has experienced any anorexia, nausea, vomiting, or oral discomfort. A dietary history may provide clues about the cause of anemia. Iron, cobalamin, and folic acid are necessary for the development of RBCs. Iron and folic acid deficiencies are associated with inadequate dietary intake; foods containing these substances include liver, meat (duck, chicken, beef), tofu, eggs, seafood (sardines, oysters), whole-grain and enriched breads, potatoes, leafy green vegetables (kale, spinach, bok choy), dried fruits, lentils, soybeans, and molasses. Folic acid deficiencies may be offset by a diet that includes foods that are also high in iron.

Any changes in the skin's texture or colour should be explored. The patient should be asked about any bleeding of gum tissue. Any **petechiae** (small, purplish-red lesions) or **ecchymosis** (bruising) on the skin should be noted; if they are present, the frequency, size, and cause should be documented. The location of petechiae can indicate an accumulation of blood in the skin or mucous membranes. Small vessels leak under pressure, and if platelet numbers are insufficient to stop the bleeding, petechiae may result. Petechiae may also occur in areas where clothing constricts the circulation.

The patient should also be questioned about any lumps or swelling in the neck, the armpits, or the groin. Specifically, the patient must be asked what the lumps feel like (i.e., hard or soft, tender or nontender) and if they are mobile or fixed. Primary lymph tumours are usually not painful. A nontender swollen lymph node may be a sign of Hodgkin's disease or non-Hodgkin's lymphoma. Lymph nodes that are enlarged and tender are usually associated with an acute infection. Any incidents of fever should be explored thoroughly. It should be determined whether the patient currently has a fever, recurring fevers, chills, or night sweats.

Elimination Pattern. The patient should be asked whether blood has been noted in the urine or stool or whether stools have been black and tarry. The patient should indicate whether he or she has had a recent stool Hemoccult (blood) test or colonoscopy. Also, any decrease in urinary output or diarrhea should be documented.

Neurological History. *Arthralgia* (joint pain) may be caused by a hematological problem and should be assessed. Pain in the joint may be indicative of an autoimmune disorder or may be caused by gout secondary to increased uric acid production, which in turn may be secondary to a hematological malignancy or hemolytic anemia. Aching bones may result from pressure of expanding bone marrow with diseases such as leukemia. *Hemarthrosis* (blood in a joint) can occur in patients with bleeding disorders and can be painful.

Paresthesias, numbness, and tingling may be related to a hematological disorder and should be noted. Any changes in vision, hearing, taste, or mental status should also be assessed carefully.

Sleep History. The patient's feeling of being rested after a night's sleep should be determined. Fatigue secondary to a hematological problem often does not resolve after sleep.

Sexual–Reproductive History. A careful gynecological history should be obtained from women, including the ages at menarche and menopause, duration and amount of bleeding, incidence of clotting and cramping, and any associated problems. Any intrapartum or postpartum bleeding problems should also be documented. Men should be asked whether they have any problems related to erectile dysfunction, a common occurrence in men with hematological problems. Patients should also be questioned about sexual behaviour because HIV infection is potentially a concern, particularly among populations at high risk for acquiring this disease.

Values and Beliefs. Some hematological problems are treated with blood transfusions or bone marrow transplantation. Determine whether any treatment plans may conflict with a patient's values or beliefs.

Objective Data

Physical Examination. A complete and thorough physical examination is necessary to assess all the body systems that affect or are affected by the hematological system (see Chapter 3). Disorders of the hematological system can manifest in various ways; thus a patient's presenting symptoms may not immediately point to a hematological problem. For example, paresthesias of the lower extremities may not appear to reflect a hematological problem, but when they are accompanied by other clinical findings or risk factors, cobalamin deficiency and resulting pernicious anemia may be suspected. Although a full examination should be performed on patients suspected of a hematological disorder, certain aspects of the physical examination are specifically relevant

CASE STUDY

Subjective Data

Source: Image Point Fr/ Shutterstock .com.

A focused subjective assessment of Allison Jobena revealed the following information:

Past History: History of mild osteoarthritis. Denies any personal history of anemia, cancer, or bleeding. No surgical history. Prefers to take care of self with "natural therapy" and has not seen a health care provider for 5 years, except for a recent sinus infection.

Medications: Metamucil 1 tbsp. PO daily; vitamins C, E, and D with calcium.

Family History: Ms. Jobena denies any family history of anemia, cancer, or bleeding disorders. She believes she comes from a family with great genes for longevity because they "eat organic foods."

Self-Care History: Ms. Jobena admits to drinking one glass of red wine with her evening meal. She is a nonsmoker and just cannot understand her gradual increase in shortness of breath with exertion. She states she cannot do anything anymore without having to stop and catch her breath. She says, "It's tough getting old."

Activities of Daily Living: Ms. Jobena is having difficulty performing ADLs without having to stop and catch her breath. Denies dyspnea at rest.

Nutritional–Metabolic History: Ms. Jobena and her husband eat a lot of pasta "because it is cheap." She uses a lot of garlic for flavouring and the "health benefit of it." Although not a vegetarian, she states that she eats little meat.

Elimination: Denies black or tarry stool. Occasional constipation. No problems with urination. Urine without odour.

Neurological History: Ms. Jobena states her joints are stiff on arising in the morning and after sitting, but she is able to get around okay and work at her secretarial job. States her walking is steady but weak. No history of falling. Denies any numbness or tingling. Admits to being a little hard of hearing but can still see "pretty good."

Sleep History: Typically sleeps 8 to 9 hr/night with no difficulty falling asleep. However, she still feels tired and needs to nap during her lunch break and on her days off.

Other: Prefers natural therapies over traditional medication.

See pp. 703, 705, 711 for more information on Ms. Jobena.

in hematological disorders; these include the skin, the lymph nodes, the spleen, and the liver. Examination of the skin is discussed in Chapter 25; spleen and liver examinations are described in Chapter 41.

Lymph Node Assessment. Lymph nodes are distributed throughout the body. Superficial lymph nodes can be evaluated by light palpation (Figure 32-6). Deep lymph nodes cannot be palpated and are best evaluated with radiological examination. Lymph nodes should be assessed with regard to symmetry in location, size, degree of fixation (i.e., movable, fixed), tenderness, and texture. To assess superficial lymph nodes, lightly palpate the nodes with the pads of the fingers and then gently roll the skin over the area and concentrate on feeling for possible lymph node enlargement. To be considered normal, a palpable node should be small (0.5 to 1 cm), mobile, firm, and nontender. A node that is tender, hard, fixed, or enlarged (regardless of whether it is tender or not) is abnormal and warrants further investigation. Tender nodes are usually a result of inflammation, whereas hard or fixed nodes are suggestive of malignancy (Ball, Dains, Flynn, et al., 2014).

It is important to develop a sequence for examining the lymph nodes. A convenient sequence for examination is to start at the head and neck. First, preauricular, posterior auricular, occipital, tonsillar, submandibular, submental, superficial cervical, posterior

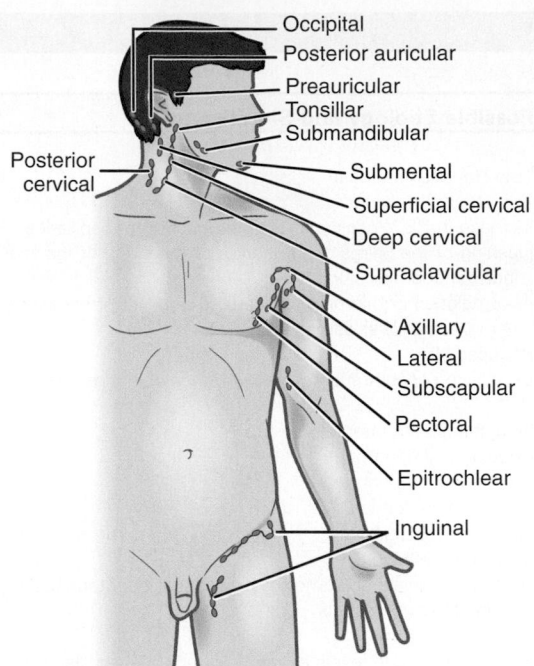

Occipital
Posterior auricular
Preauricular
Tonsillar
Submandibular
Submental
Superficial cervical
Deep cervical
Supraclavicular
Axillary
Lateral
Subscapular
Pectoral
Epitrochlear
Inguinal
Posterior cervical

FIGURE 32-6 Palpable, superficial lymph nodes.

cervical chain, deep cervical chain, and supraclavicular nodes are palpated. Next, the axillary lymph nodes and pectoral, subscapular, and lateral groups of nodes are palpated. The epitrochlear nodes, located in the antecubital fossa between the biceps and triceps muscles, are then examined. The inguinal lymph nodes, found in the groin, are palpated last.

A focused assessment of the hematological system is used to evaluate previously identified hematological problems and to monitor for signs of new problems. An example of such an assessment is presented in the "Focused Assessment" box below.

Palpation of the Liver or the Spleen. The liver and the spleen are normally not detectable through palpation of the abdomen. When they are enlarged, however, they may be detectable through percussion or palpation. The degree of enlargement of the liver is measured by the number of centimetres it extends below the rib border. The spleen may be more difficult to palpate because of its deep location in the abdomen.

Skin Assessment. In hematological disorders, assessment of the skin may yield valuable information about the hematological system. The skin should be examined over the entire body in a systematic manner (e.g., starting with the face and oral cavity and moving downward over the body). In patients with RBC disorders, the skin may be pale or, in the case of severe anemia, have a cyanotic or grayish tinge. Erythrocytosis often produces small vessel occlusions, causing a purple, mottled appearance of the face, the nose, the fingers, or the toes. Digital clubbing can occur with conditions of chronic anemia, such as sickle cell disease. Leukocyte disorders may cause infectious skin lesions or malignant nodular lesions. These lesions may occur anywhere and have a variable distribution pattern. During the physical assessment of the skin, the nurse must look carefully for petechiae (small purplish-red lesions), **purpura** (purplish-red rash), ecchymosis (bruising), and spider nevus (a form of *telangiectasia*) because these can indicate bleeding disorders (Table 32-6).

FOCUSED ASSESSMENT

Hematological System

Use this checklist to make sure the key assessment steps have been performed.

Subjective
Ask the patient about any of the following and note the responses:

Unusual bleeding (e.g., gums) or bruising	Y	N
Black, tarry stool	Y	N
Blood in vomit	Y	N
Swelling in neck, armpits, groin	Y	N
Dark-coloured urine	Y	N
Fatigue	Y	N
Heart palpitations	Y	N

Objective: Diagnostic
Check the following laboratory results for critical values:

CBC	✓
Clotting: PT, INR, aPTT, platelets	✓
Hematocrit and hemoglobin	✓

Objective: Physical Examination
Inspect

Skin for lesions or colour changes	✓

Auscultate

Blood pressure for alteration or orthostasis	✓

Palpate

Pulse for tachycardia	✓
Liver and spleen for enlargement	✓
Lymph nodes for lymphadenopathy	✓

aPTT, activated partial thromboplastin time; *CBC*, complete blood cell count; *INR*, international normalized ratio; *PT*, prothrombin time.

CASE STUDY

Objective Data: Physical Examination

Source: Image Point Fr/ Shutterstock .com.

Physical examination findings for Allison Jobena are as follows:

BP 100/70 (lying), 88/60 (standing); apical pulse 110 (lying), 124 (standing), but regular in rhythm. Respiratory rate 26, temperature 36°C (96.8°F), O₂ saturation 90% on room air. No jugular venous distension. Weight: 48 kg. Height: 155 cm. Skin pale with two ecchymoses on her arms and one on her left lower leg. A few scattered petechiae on both ankles. No jaundice noted. Conjunctivas pale. Tongue smooth and shiny. Lungs clear but diminished breath sounds in the bases bilaterally. No visible bleeding. No enlarged lymph nodes, spleen, or liver noted. General weakness with dyspnea on exertion. No numbness or tingling or peripheral edema.

Throughout this chapter, consider diagnostic studies that the nurse may order for Ms. Jobena.

See pp. 703, 704, and 711 for more information on Ms. Jobena.

DIAGNOSTIC STUDIES OF THE HEMATOLOGICAL SYSTEM

The most direct means of evaluating the hematological system is through laboratory analysis and other diagnostic studies. Diagnostic tests of the hematological system are presented in Tables 32-7 through 32-9 and Table 32-11.

TABLE 32-6 ASSESSMENT ABNORMALITIES

Hematological System

Finding	Description	Possible Etiology and Significance
Skin		
Pallor of skin or nail beds	Paleness; decrease in or absence of skin coloration (varies with patient's natural skin colour)	Low Hb level (anemia)
Flushing	Transient, episodic redness of skin (usually around face and neck)	Increase in RBC (polycythemia), congestion of capillaries Flushing of the palms of the hands or the soles of the feet may indicate anemia
Jaundice	Yellow appearance of skin and mucous membranes	Accumulation of bile pigment caused by rapid or excessive hemolysis or liver damage
Cyanosis	Bluish discoloration of skin and mucous membranes in lighter-skinned people; greyish/whitish discoloration of skin and mucous membranes in darker-skinned people	Reduced Hb Excessive concentration of deoxyhemoglobin in blood
Excoriation	Scratch or abrasion of skin	Scratching from intense pruritus
Pruritus	Unpleasant cutaneous sensation that provokes the desire to rub or scratch the skin	Hodgkin's lymphoma Cutaneous lymphomas Infiltrative leukemias Increased bilirubin level
Leg ulcers	Prominent on the malleoli on the ankles	Sickle cell disease
Angioma	Benign tumour consisting of blood or lymph vessels	Most are congenital; some may disappear spontaneously
Telangiectasia	Small angioma with tendency to bleed; focal red lesions, coarse or fine red lines	Dilation of small vessels
Spider nevus	Form of telangiectasia characterized by a round red central portion and branching radiations resembling the profile of a spider; usually develop on face, neck, or chest	Elevated estrogen levels as in pregnancy or liver disease
Petechiae	Pinpoint, nonraised, perfectly round area <2 mm; purple, dark-red, or brown in colour	Decreased numbers of platelets or clotting factors, resulting in hemorrhage into the skin Vascular abnormalities Break in blood vessel walls as a result of trauma
Purpura	Small hemorrhages in the surface of the skin or mucous membranes resulting in a rash of purple, red, or brown spots measuring 2–10 mm in diameter	Same as for petechiae
Ecchymosis (bruise)	Small hemorrhagic spot, larger than purpura; nonelevated; round or irregular	Same as for petechiae
Hematoma	A localized collection of blood, usually clotted	Same as for petechiae
Chloroma	A tumour arising from myeloid tissue and containing a pale-green pigment	Acute myelogenous leukemia that has infiltrated the skin
Plasmacytoma	A tumour arising from abnormal plasma cells	Multiple myeloma that has infiltrated tissue
Eyes		
Jaundiced sclera	Yellow appearance of the sclera	Accumulation of bile pigment resulting from rapid or excessive hemolysis or liver disease or infiltration
Conjunctival pallor	Paleness; decreased or absence of coloration in the conjunctiva	Low Hb level (anemia)
Blurred vision, diplopia, visual field cuts	Decreased visual acuity or areas of blindness (field cuts)	Anemia, extreme leukocytosis, and polycythemia may cause visual abnormalities Thrombo-cytopenia may cause intraocular hemorrhage with visual abnormalities Excessive clotting may cause thromboses in the circulation to the brain that cause visual field cuts
Nose		
Epistaxis	Spontaneous bleeding from the nares	May occur with low platelet counts, especially if the patient bends down for a long period, tries to lift a heavy item, or attempts an intense Valsalva manoeuvre
Mouth		
Gingival and mucous membrane changes	Pallor Gingival or mucosal ulceration, swelling, or bleeding	Low Hb level (anemia) Neutropenia; inability of impaired leukocytes to combat oral infections; thrombo-cytopenia Gingival hyperplasia may be present with some types of leukemia
Smooth tongue	Tongue surface is smooth and shiny; mucosa is thin and red from decreased papillae	Pernicious anemia, iron-deficiency anemia
Lymph Nodes		
Lymphadenopathy	Lymph nodes are enlarged (>1 cm diameter)	Infection, foreign infiltrations, or systemic disease such as leukemia, lymphoma, Hodgkin's lymphoma, or metastatic cancer

TABLE 32-6 ASSESSMENT ABNORMALITIES

Hematological System—cont'd

Finding	Description	Possible Etiology and Significance
Heart and Chest		
Tachycardia	Heart rate >100 beats/min	Compensatory mechanism in anemia to increase cardiac output
Palpitations	Sensation of feeling the heart beat, flutter, or pound in the chest	Anemia, fluid volume overload, hypotension with impending syncope, hypertension, or dysrhythmias may cause palpitations
Altered blood pressure	Orthostasis: >20/min increase in heart rate or >20 mm Hg decrease in blood pressure from baseline value when moving from a lying position to either sitting or standing Hypotension: <90 mm Hg systolic or >40 mm Hg drop in systolic reading from baseline BP Hypertension: >130/90 mm Hg	Orthostasis is a common manifestation in anemia, especially if accompanied by low blood volume Hypotension may indicate an infectious process, blood loss, or compromised cardiovascular compensatory mechanisms Hypertension may occur initially as a compensatory mechanism for anemia
Sternal tenderness	Abnormal sensitivity to touch or pressure on sternum	Leukemia, as a result of increased bone marrow cellularity, which causes an increase in pressure and bone erosion; multiple myeloma, as a result of stretching of periosteum
Low oxygen saturation	Oxygen-carrying capacity is reflected by the oxygen saturation as measured with pulse oximetry	Oxygen saturation may be decreased in cases of severe anemia
Abdomen		
Hepatomegaly	Palpable liver	Leukemia, cirrhosis, or fibrosis secondary to iron overload from sickle cell disease or thalassemia
Splenomegaly	Palpable spleen	Anemia, thrombo-cytopenia, leukemia, lymphomas, leukopenia, mononucleosis, malaria, cirrhosis, trauma, portal hypertension
Distended abdomen	Distended abdomen is an abdominal profile that is larger than normal; it may be soft or firm, tender or nontender, and accompanied by other symptoms such as nausea, vomiting, or rebound tenderness	Lymphoma may manifest as abdominal adenopathy, mass(es), or bowel obstruction
Nervous System		
Paresthesias of feet and hands; ataxia	Numbness sensation and extreme sensitivity experienced in central and peripheral nerves; impaired muscle movement	Cobalamin (vitamin B_{12}) deficiency or folate deficiency
Weakness	Lacking physical strength or energy	Low Hb level (anemia)
Headache, nuchal rigidity	Pain in the cranium, potentially involving one area or extending from the frontal area to the back of the neck	Generalized headache is a common manifestation of mild to moderate anemia Severe headache with or without visual disturbances may signal intracranial hemorrhage caused by thrombo-cytopenia
Musculo-Skeletal System		
Bone pain	Pain in pelvis, ribs, spine, sternum	Multiple myeloma, in relation to enlarged tumours that stretch periosteum Bone invasion by leukemia cells Bone demineralization that results from various malignancies Sickle cell disease
Joint swelling	Fluid-filled spaces surrounding the joints	Occurs with sickle cell anemia as bleeding into the joint (hemarthrosis) causes inflammation
Arthralgia	Joint pain	Sickle cell disease, as a result of hemarthrosis

Hb, hemoglobin.

Laboratory Studies

Complete Blood Cell Count. The complete blood cell count (CBC) involves several laboratory tests (Table 32-7), each of which serves to assess the three major blood cells formed in the bone marrow. In addition to the CBC, a *peripheral blood smear* may be ordered. The smear is used to look at the morphological features (shape and appearance) of the blood cells and may assist with diagnosis. For example, a large number of immature *blast* WBCs may indicate acute leukemia.

Although the status of each cell type is important, the entire system may be disrupted by diseases, as well as by the treatment of diseases. Suppression of the entire CBC is termed pancytopenia (marked decrease in the number of RBCs, WBCs, and platelets). In such cases, care is directed toward the management of anemia, infection, and hemorrhage (see Chapter 33).

Red Blood Cells. Normal values of some RBC tests are reported separately for men and for women because normal values are based on body mass and men usually have a larger body mass than do women.

The *hemoglobin* value is reduced in cases of anemia, hemorrhage, and states of hemodilution, such as those that occur when the fluid volume is excessive. RBCs are increased in polycythemia or in states of hemoconcentration, which can develop from volume depletion (dehydration).

The *hematocrit* value is determined by spinning blood in a centrifuge, which causes erythrocytes (RBCs) and plasma to separate. The RBCs, being the heavier elements, settle to the bottom. The hematocrit value represents the percentage of RBCs in comparison with the total blood volume. The hematocrit value is reduced and elevated in the same conditions that raise and lower the hemoglobin value.

The total RBC count is reported as $RBC \times 10^{12}/L$. However, the total RBC count is not always reliable in determining the adequacy of RBC function. Consequently, other data, such as

TABLE 32-7	COMPLETE BLOOD CELL COUNT STUDIES	
Study	**Description and Purpose**	**Normal Values**
Hb	Measurement of gas-carrying capacity of RBCs	Women: 117–160 g/L Men: 132–173 g/L
Hct	Measurement of packed cell volume of RBCs, expressed as a percentage of the total blood volume	Women: 0.35–0.47 Men: 0.39–0.50
Total RBC count	Count of number of circulating RBCs	Women: $3.8–5.1 \times 10^{12}$/L Men: $4.3–5.7 \times 10^{12}$/L
RBC indices		
• MCV (Hct/RBC)	Determination of relative size of RBC; low MCV reflection of microcytosis, high MCV reflection of macrocytosis	fL
• MCH (Hb/RBC)	Measurement of average weight of Hb/RBCs; low MCH is indication of microcytosis or hypochromia, high MCH is indication of macrocytosis	pg
• MCHC	Evaluation of RBC saturation with Hb; low MCHC is indication of hypochromia, high MCHC is evident in spherocytosis	g/L
• RBC morphology	Examination of the shape and size of RBCs	No variation in RBC structure
• WBC count	Measurement of total number of leukocytes	$\times 10^9$/L
• WBC differential	Determination of whether each kind of WBC is present in proper proportion; absolute value is determined by multiplying percentage of cell type by total WBC count and dividing by 100	Neutrophils: $5.0–7.0 \times 10^9$/L Eosinophils: $0.00–0.04 \times 10^9$/L Basophils: $0–0.02 \times 10^9$/L Lymphocytes: $0.2–0.4 \times 10^9$/L Monocytes: $0.04–0.08 \times 10^9$/L
• Platelet count	Measurement of number of platelets available to maintain platelet clotting functions (not measurement of quality of platelet function)	$150–400 \times 10^9$/L

Hb, hemoglobin; *Hct*, hematocrit; *MCH*, mean corpuscular hemoglobin; *MCHC*, mean corpuscular hemoglobin concentration; *MCV*, mean corpuscular volume; *RBC*, red blood cell; *WBC*, white blood cell.

hemoglobin, hematocrit, and RBC indices, must also be evaluated. The RBC count is altered by the same conditions that raise and lower the hemoglobin and hematocrit values.

RBC indices are special indicators that reflect RBC volume, colour, and hemoglobin saturation (see Table 32-7). These parameters may provide insight into the cause of anemia. (The significance of these parameters is discussed further in Chapter 33.)

White Blood Cells. The WBC count provides two different sets of information. The first is a total count of WBCs per litre of peripheral blood. Elevations in WBC count to more than 11×10^9/L are associated with infection, inflammation, tissue injury or death, and malignancies (e.g., leukemia, lymphoma). Although the degree of WBC elevation is not necessarily predictive of the severity of illness, it can provide clues to the cause. Certain types of leukemias are more likely to produce extremely high WBC counts (e.g., $>25 \times 10^9$/L). A total WBC count lower than 4×10^9/L (**leukopenia**) is associated with bone marrow depression, severe or chronic illness, and some types of leukemia.

The second aspect of the WBC count, the *differential count*, is the percentage of each type of leukocyte. The information from the WBC differential count provides valuable clues to the cause of illness. When infections are severe, more granulocytes are released from the bone marrow as a compensatory mechanism. To meet the increased demand, many young, immature polymorphonuclear neutrophils (bands) are released into circulation. More mature neutrophils are called *polymorphonuclear segmented neutrophils* ("segs"). The usual laboratory procedure is to report WBCs in order of maturity, with the less mature forms (i.e., band neutrophils) on the left side of the written report; hence, the existence of many immature cells is termed a *shift to the left*. A shift to the left may be indicative of active infection or inflammation (e.g., postsurgically). The WBC differential count is of considerable significance because it is possible for the total WBC count to remain essentially normal despite a marked change in one type of leukocyte. For example, a patient may have a normal

WBC count of 8.8×10^9/L, but the differential count may reveal a relative proportion of lymphocytes to be reduced to 10%—an abnormal finding that warrants further investigation.

When the bone marrow does not produce enough neutrophils, neutropenia occurs. **Neutropenia** is a condition associated with an absolute neutrophil count (ANC) lower than 1×10^9/L to 1.5×10^9/L; severe neutropenia is associated with an ANC lower than 0.5×10^9/L. The ANC is determined as the total WBCs multiplied by the percentage of neutrophils. Neutropenia results from a number of disease processes, such as leukemia, or from bone marrow depression (see Chapter 33) and is associated with an increased risk for infection and death from sepsis.

Platelet Count. The platelet count is the number of platelets per microlitre of blood. Normal platelet counts are between 150×10^9/L and 400×10^9/L; counts lower than 150×10^9/L signify a condition termed **thrombo-cytopenia**. Bleeding may occur with thrombo-cytopenia. Spontaneous hemorrhage is probable once platelet counts fall below 10×10^9/L. A more extensive description of clotting studies is presented in Table 32-8. **Thrombo-cytosis**, in contrast, is an excess of platelets, a disorder that occurs with inflammation and some malignant diseases. The complication related to thrombo-cytosis that is most likely to occur is excessive clotting.

Blood Typing and Rh Factor. Blood group antigens (A and B) are found only on RBC membranes and form the basis for the ABO blood typing system. The presence or absence of one or both of the two inherited antigens is the basis for the four blood groups: *A, B, AB,* and *O.* People with blood group A have A antigens, those with group B have B antigens, those with group AB have both A and B antigens, and those with group O have neither A nor B antigens. People with blood types A, B, or O have antibodies in the serum, termed *anti-A* and *anti-B,* that react with A or B antigens. These antibodies are found when the corresponding antigen is absent from the RBC membrane. For example, anti-B antibodies are found in the plasma of people with blood group A (Table 32-9).

TABLE 32-8 CLOTTING STUDIES

Study	Description and Purpose	Normal Values
Activated clotting time (ACT)	Evaluation of intrinsic coagulation status; more accurate than aPTT; used during dialysis, coronary artery bypass procedure, arteriography	70–120 sec
Activated partial thromboplastin time (aPTT)	Assessment of intrinsic coagulation by measuring factors I, II, V, VIII, IX, X, XI, and XII; longer with the use of heparin	25–35 sec
Antithrombin	Naturally occurring protein synthesized by the liver that inhibits coagulation through inactivation of thrombin and other factors; is depleted in DIC	210–300 mg/L or 0.80–1.2 of standard
Capillary fragility test (tourniquet test, Rumpel–Leede test)	Reflection of capillary integrity when positive or negative pressure is applied to various areas of the body; positive result is indication of thrombo-cytopenia, toxic vascular reactions	No petechiae, or negative
D-dimer	Assay to measure a fragment of fibrin that is formed as a result of fibrin degradation and clot lysis; used in diagnosis of hypercoagulable conditions (e.g., DIC, pulmonary embolism)	<250 mcg/L
Fibrin split products (FSP) or fibrin degradation products (FDPs)	Reflection of degree of fibrinolysis and predisposition to bleeding (if present); screening test for DIC; elevated levels associated with DIC, advanced malignancy, severe inflammation	<10 mg/L
Fibrinogen (factor I)	Reflection of level of fibrinogen; increase in fibrinogen may indicate enhancement of fibrin formation, which renders patient hypercoagulable; decrease in fibrinogen indicates that patient may be predisposed to bleeding	2–4 g/L
International normalized ratio (INR)	Standardized system of reporting PT that is based on a reference calibration model and calculated by comparison of the patient's PT with a control value	0.8–1.2
Plasminogen	Assessment of adequacy of plasminogen in patients who have multiple thrombo-embolic episodes	2.4–4.4 units/mL
Platelet count	Count of number of circulating platelets	150×10^9/L to 400×10^9/L
Prothrombin time (PT)	Assessment of extrinsic coagulation by measurement of factors I, II, V, VII, and X	11–16 sec
Thrombin time	Reflection of adequacy of thrombin; prolonged thrombin time indicates that coagulation is inadequate secondary to decreased thrombin activity	17–23 sec

DIC, disseminated intravascular coagulation.

TABLE 32-9 ABO BLOOD GROUP NAMES AND PATIENT/DONOR COMPATIBILITIES*

Recipient's Blood Group	RBC Antigen	Plasma/Serum Antibody	Compatible Donor for RBC Transfusions	Compatible Donor for Plasma Transfusions
A	A	Anti-B	A and O	A and AB
B	B	Anti-A	B and O	B and AB
AB (universal recipient)	Both A and B	Neither anti-A nor anti-B	A, B, AB, and O	AB
O	Neither A nor B	Both anti-A and anti-B	O (universal donor)	A, B, AB, and O

RBC, red blood cell.
*ABO blood groups are named for the antigen found on the RBCs. Donor compatibility is based on the antibodies present in the serum.

Blood reactions caused by ABO incompatibilities result in intravascular hemolysis of the RBCs. RBCs *agglutinate* (or clump) when a serum antibody that reacts with the antigens on the RBC membrane is present. For example, agglutination would occur in the blood of a person with type A blood if he or she received blood from a donor with B antigens (i.e., type B or AB). The anti-B antibodies in the serum of the person with type A blood would react with the B antigens on the donor RBCs, thus initiating the process that results in RBC hemolysis.

The Rhesus (Rh) system is based on a third antigen, D, which is also found on the RBC membrane. Rh-positive people have the D antigen, whereas Rh-negative people do not. Rh-positive blood is indicated with a plus sign after the ABO group name (e.g., "AB+"). A Coombs test is used to evaluate the person's Rh status (Table 32-10).

As a result of transfusion therapy or during childbirth, an Rh-negative person may be exposed to Rh-positive blood. If an Rh-negative mother gives birth to an Rh-positive infant, the mother forms an antibody, anti-D, which acts against Rh antigens. (Rh-positive people normally have no anti-D antibody.) In subsequent pregnancies, the mother's anti-D antibodies can cross the placenta and attack the RBCs of a fetus who is Rh-positive, thus causing hemolysis of the RBCs. A pregnant Rh-negative woman should receive Rho(D) immune globulin (WinRho) injections during pregnancy to prevent anti-D antibodies from forming.

Iron Metabolism. The laboratory tests used in evaluating iron metabolism include serum iron, total iron-binding capacity (TIBC), serum ferritin, and transferrin saturation. Additional tests for nutritional deficiencies leading to defective RBC production may also be performed (see Table 32-10).

Serum iron is a measurement of the amount of protein-bound iron circulating in the serum. TIBC provides a measurement of all proteins that bind or transport iron between the tissues and the bone marrow. Although this indirect measurement is a general reflection of the amount of transferrin present in the circulation, it overestimates transferrin levels by 16% to 20% because it also measures other proteins that can bind iron. These alternative proteins bind iron only when transferrin is more than half saturated. Also, TIBC varies inversely with tissue iron stores; it is higher when iron stores are low and lower when iron stores are high.

Transferrin saturation is a better indicator of the availability of iron for erythropoiesis than is serum iron because, unlike serum iron, the iron bound to transferrin is readily available for

TABLE 32-10   MISCELLANEOUS LABORATORY BLOOD STUDIES

Study/Substance Studied	Description and Purpose	Normal Values
Bilirubin	Measurement of degree of RBC hemolysis or liver's inability to excrete normal quantities of bilirubin Increase in indirect bilirubin with hemolytic problems; increase in direct bilirubin with obstructive problems (e.g., gallstones, tumour)	Total: 3.0–21 mcmol/L Direct: 1.7–5.1 mcmol/L Indirect: 1.7–17 mcmol/L
Blood smear (peripheral blood smear)	Reviews colour, size, shape, and quantity of cells in peripheral blood; can provide significant information regarding disorders affecting RBCs, WBCs, or platelets	Normal quantity of each cell type; normal size, shape, and colour of RBCs; normal WBC differential
Coombs test	Differentiation among types of hemolytic anemias; detection of immune antibodies; detection of Rh factor	Negative finding (no agglutination)
• Direct	Detection of antibodies that are attached to RBCs	Negative finding
• Indirect	Detection of antibodies in serum	Negative finding
Cobalamin (vitamin B_{12})	Level of vitamin B_{12} available for production of new RBCs	148–616 pmol/L
Erythrocyte sedimentation rate (ESR)	Measurement of sedimentation, or settling, of RBCs in 1 hr Inflammatory process causes an alteration in plasma proteins, resulting in aggregation of RBCs and making them heavier; the faster the RBCs settle, the higher the ESR is	Female • <50 yr: <20 mm/hr • >50 yr: <30 mm/hr Male • <50 yr: <15 mm/hr • >50 yr: <20 mm/hr
Erythropoietin	Measurement of degree of hormonal stimulation of the bone marrow to release RBCs	5–35 mU/mL
Ferritin	Major iron storage protein; is normally present in blood in concentrations directly related to iron storage	Female: 10–150 mcg/L Male: 12–300 mcg/L
Folic acid (folate)	Amount of folic acid or folate available for RBC production	7–36 nmol/L
Hemoglobin (Hb) electrophoresis	Proteins involved in development of the hemoglobin molecule have a definitive pattern of separation on electrophoresis; this pattern is altered with abnormal Hb synthesis, as occurs in thalassemia or in sickle cell anemia, in which sickle Hb (HbS) is increased	Normal HbA_1: 95%–98% HbA_2: 2%–3% HbF: 0.8%–2% HbS: 0% HbC: 0%
Homocysteine	Amino acid formed from methionine Rapidly metabolized through pathways that require cobalamin (vitamin B_{12}) and folic acid; increased in deficiencies of cobalamin and folic acid	3.7–12.9 mcmol/L (some variation with gender)
Iron		
• Serum iron	Reflection of amount of iron combined with proteins in serum; accurate indication of status of iron storage and use	mcmol/L
• Total iron-binding capacity (TIBC)	Measurement of all proteins available for binding iron Transferrin represents the largest quantity of iron-binding proteins; therefore, TIBC is an indirect measure of transferrin	45–76 mcmol/L
Lactic dehydrogenase (LDH)	Intracellular enzyme that is present in almost all body tissues Levels rise in response to cell damage; increased levels confirm diagnosis of injury or disease May be used as a nonspecific marker of hematological malignancy growth and response to treatment	0.83–2.5 mckat/L
Methylmalonic acid (MMA)	Indirect test for cobalamin: MMA metabolism requires cobalamin; test helps differentiate cobalamin deficiency from folic acid deficiency	<2.4 mcg/dL
Microglobulin (β_2 microglobulin)	Protein that is found on the surface of all cells Increased in patients with malignancies such as lymphoma, leukemia, or multiple myeloma; may be used as a tumour marker	Blood: 0.7–1.8 mcg/mL Urine: ≤300 mcg/L Spinal fluid: ≤2.4 mg/L
Reticulocyte count	Measurement of immature RBCs; reflection of bone marrow activity in producing RBCs	0.5%–1.5% of RBC count (0.005–0.015 of RBC count)
Serum protein electrophoresis (SPEP)	Separates proteins in the blood on basis of electrical charge; helps detect hyperglobulinemic states, as in multiple myeloma or some lymphomas	Normal banding pattern of albumin and globulins; an increase in any protein ("protein spike") is abnormal
Transferrin	The largest of proteins that bind to iron; increased in majority of people with iron-deficiency anemia	1.9–3.8 g/L
Transferrin saturation (%)	Decreased in iron-deficiency anemia and increased in hemolytic and megaloblastic anemia	15%–50%

HbA, hemoglobin alpha; *HbC*, abnormal hemoglobin that shows reduced plasticity of the erythrocyte causing hemoglobinopathy; *HbF*, fetal hemoglobin; *HbS*, sickle hemoglobin; *RBC*, red blood cell.

the body to use. To calculate transferrin saturation, the serum iron value is divided by TIBC, and the result is multiplied by 100. For example, a patient with a serum iron level of 18 mcmol/L and a TIBC of 57 mcmol/L would have a transferrin saturation of about 31.6%. Under normal conditions, the serum ferritin concentration is correlated closely with body iron stores.

Radiological Studies

Radiological studies for the hematological system involve primarily the use of computed tomography (CT) or magnetic resonance imaging (MRI) for evaluating the spleen, the liver, and the lymph nodes. Nursing responsibilities related to these studies are presented in Table 32-11.

Biopsy

Biopsy procedures specific to hematological assessment are bone marrow examination and lymph node biopsy. In general, these procedures are performed because a peripheral blood smear is nonspecific and a diagnosis cannot usually be established from a peripheral blood smear. Furthermore, a biopsy provides additional information about a hematological problem; such information is needed for diagnostic purposes, as well as for planning treatment options.

Bone Marrow Examination. Bone marrow examination is important in the evaluation of many hematological disorders. The examination of the marrow may involve aspiration alone or aspiration with biopsy. The benefits of bone marrow examination include the ability to (a) fully evaluate hematopoiesis and (b) obtain specimens for cytopathological study and evaluation for chromosomal abnormalities.

The preferred site for both aspiration and biopsy of bone marrow is the posterior superior iliac crest (Pagana & Pagana, 2014). In adults, the anterior superior iliac crest is an alternative site. Bone marrow aspiration and biopsy are performed by a physician or by a nurse with special credentials. Local anaesthesia and sedation may be used to minimize anxiety and pain.

For bone marrow aspiration, the skin over the puncture site is cleansed with a bactericidal agent. The skin, subcutaneous tissue, and periosteum are infiltrated with a local anaesthetic drug (Figure 32-7). The patient may be uncomfortable when the

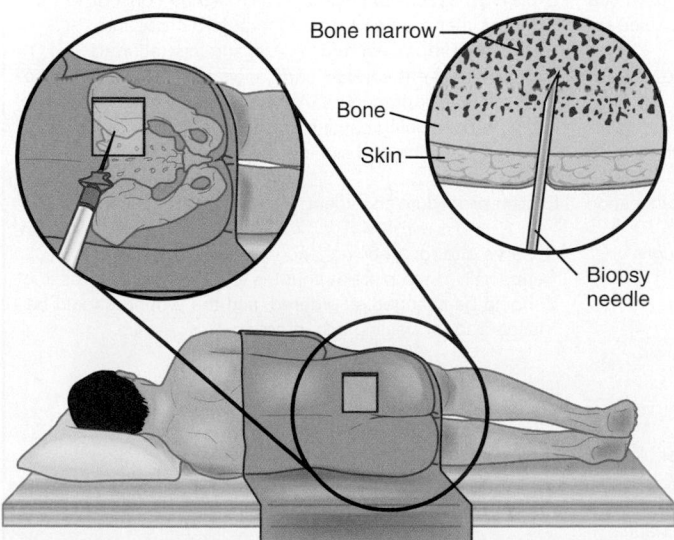

FIGURE 32-7 Bone marrow aspiration from the posterior superior iliac crest.

periosteum is penetrated. Once the area is anaesthetized, a bone marrow needle is inserted through the cortex of the bone. The stylet of the needle is then removed, the hub is attached to a 10-mL syringe, and 0.2 to 0.5 mL of the marrow fluid is aspirated. The patient may experience pain with aspiration. Although it generally lasts for only a few seconds, the pain may be quite uncomfortable. After the marrow aspiration, the needle is removed. Pressure is applied over the aspiration site to ensure hemostasis. If the patient is thrombo-cytopenic, pressure may be required for 5 to 10 minutes or longer. With severe thrombo-cytopenia, platelets may be infused before the procedure. If a bone biopsy is required, the preparatory procedure remains the same, but a different needle is used. The needle has a cutting blade that allows a specimen of the bone to be removed.

Although complications of bone marrow aspiration are minimal, there is a possibility of penetrating the bone and damaging underlying structures. Other complications include hemorrhage (particularly if the patient is thrombo-cytopenic) and infection (particularly if the patient is leukopenic).

Lymph Node Biopsy. Lymph node biopsy involves obtaining lymph tissue for histological examination to determine the diagnosis and to help plan therapy. Lymph tissue may be obtained through either an open biopsy or a closed (needle) biopsy. Negative results from a needle biopsy may indicate only that the cancer cells were not part of the tissue specimen obtained. A repeated needle biopsy or a larger tissue specimen (open biopsy) may be subsequently required.

CASE STUDY

Objective Data: Diagnostic Studies

The health care provider orders the following initial diagnostic studies for Allison Jobena:
- CBC, basic metabolic panel (electrolytes, BUN, creatinine), PT/PTT
- Arterial blood gases
- Chest radiograph

Ms. Jobena's CBC reveals an Hgb of 59 g/L, Hct of 0.18, WBC of 2.6×10^9/L, platelet count of 72×10^9/L, PT = 18 sec, aPTT = 37. Her arterial blood gases are normal, as is her chest radiograph. The health care provider orders more blood work, including a WBC differential and RBC indices, and admits Ms. Jobena to the hospital for further evaluation.

Source: Image Point Fr/ Shutterstock .com.

See pp. 703, 704, and 705 for more information on Ms. Jobena.

Molecular Cytogenetics and Gene Analysis

Testing for specific genetic or chromosomal variations in hematological conditions is often helpful in diagnosis, in determining the treatment options, and in determining prognosis. If a large number of abnormal cells are circulating in the blood, as in acute leukemia, these tests may be performed with peripheral blood samples. However, testing is usually performed on samples from bone marrow and from lymph node biopsies. For example, fluorescent in situ hybridization (FISH) can identify specific genes or portions of genes that are abnormal by attaching a probe to a targeted region of deoxyribonucleic acid (DNA). It may be used to reveal an abnormal extra chromosome 8 that is common in certain leukemias. Spectral karyotyping (SKY) allows for each set of chromosomes to be coloured individually. It can be used to identify the 9;22 translocation in the Philadelphia chromosome of chronic myelogenous leukemia. More information on genetics is available in Chapter 15.

TABLE 32-11   DIAGNOSTIC STUDIES

Hematological System

Study/Substance Studied	Description and Purpose	Nursing Responsibility
Urine Studies		
Bence Jones protein	An electrophoretic measurement is used to detect the presence of the Bence Jones protein, which is found in most cases of multiple myeloma. Negative finding is considered normal.	Acquire random urine specimen early in the morning. If a 24-hour urine collection is ordered, discard first specimen and collect all urine voided during the 24 hr, keeping on ice or refrigerated.
Radioisotope Studies		
Bone scan	Radioactive isotope is injected by IV. Used for evaluating the structure of the bones. Patient is not a source of radioactivity.	IV access is required. Patient needs to lie still during imaging.
SPECT (**s**ingle-**p**hoton **e**mission **c**omputed **t**omography) scan	Radioactive isotope is injected by IV. Images from the radioactive emissions are used to evaluate the structure of the spleen, liver, bone, and possible tumours. Patient is not a source of radioactivity.	IV access is required. Patient needs to lie still during imaging.
Radiological Studies		
Skeletal radiograph	Radiographic studies performed as a bone survey to detect lytic lesions associated with multiple myeloma. Bone scans do not identify lytic lesions very well in this condition: Because of lack of blood supply, there is no uptake of radioactive isotopes.	No specific nursing responsibilities.
Liver, spleen, or abdominal ultrasonography	Noninvasive probe is lubricated and slid across the abdomen to detect the density and borders of the abdominal organs. Irregular borders, masses, vascular structure, and biliary tree can be detected.	Patients must be comfortable lying flat, and the probe must compress the abdomen.
Positron emission tomography (PET) scan	A nuclear tracer substance is injected and is taken up by metabolically active cells. The follow-up scan shows tissues in different colours based on the metabolic rate. "Hot spots" reflect increased glucose consumption that may reflect tumours.	IV access is required for injection of the tracer substance. Patients should ingest nothing by mouth except water and medications for at least 4 hr before the test. IV solutions containing glucose may be held. Patients who are glucose intolerant or diabetic may need adjustments to their medications. Bowel preparation may also be needed, depending on the area being studied.
Computed tomographic (CT) scan	Noninvasive examination in which computer-assisted radiography is used to evaluate the lymph nodes. Contrast medium often is used in abdominal studies of the liver or the spleen. Spiral CT is used to evaluate lymph nodes.	If contrast medium is used, investigate whether patient has iodine sensitivity. IV, oral contrast, or both may be given prior to the procedure, depending on the area being studied. Patient may need to be NPO.
Magnetic resonance imaging (MRI)	Noninvasive procedure that produces sensitive images of soft tissue without the use of contrast medium. No ionizing radiation is required.	Instruct patient to remove all metal objects and ask about any history of surgical insertion of staples, plates, or other metal appliances. Patient may need to lie still in small chamber.
Biopsies/Procedures		
Bone marrow aspirate	Removal of bone marrow through a locally anaesthetized site to evaluate the status of the blood-forming tissue. Used to diagnose multiple myeloma, leukemia, and some lymphomas and to stage some solid tumours. Also performed to assess efficacy of leukemia therapy.	Explain procedure to patient. Obtain signed consent form. Ensure that a *time out** is done before procedure. Consider preprocedure analgesic administration to enhance patient comfort and cooperation. Apply pressure dressing after procedure. Assess biopsy site for bleeding.
Lumbar puncture (LP)	Purpose is to obtain cerebro-spinal fluid for testing for malignancy or infection. It may also be used to administer chemotherapy to central nervous system.	Assist in positioning patient and provide support. Observe site for bleeding and signs of infection.
Lymph node biopsy	Purpose is to obtain lymph tissue for histological examination to determine diagnosis and therapy.	Explain procedure to patient. Obtain signed consent form.
• Open	Excision of lymph node and surrounding tissue through an incision. Performed in the operating room or procedure area; either local or general anaesthesia is administered.	Observe site for bleeding, and monitor vital signs, especially if the platelet count is low. The sterile dressing should be changed as ordered, and the wound should be inspected for healing and infection.
• Closed (needle) or fine needle	Performed at patient's bedside or in an outpatient area.	
Molecular, Cytogenic, and Gene Analysis Studies		
Fluorescent in situ hybridization (FISH) Comparative genomic hybridization (CGH) Spectral karyotyping (SKY)	Tests performed on malignant cells, either peripheral blood (e.g., leukemia) or biopsy specimen (bone marrow, lymph node), to assess genetic or chromosomal abnormalities of cancer cells. May be useful in confirming diagnosis and determining treatment modalities and prognosis.	Explain purpose of testing to patient.

IV, intravenous; *NPO,* nothing by mouth.
*A time out is done just before a surgical procedure starts to verify patient identification, surgical procedure, and surgical site.

REVIEW QUESTIONS

The number of the question corresponds to the same-numbered objective at the beginning of the chapter.

1. Why might a client who lives at a high altitude normally have an increased RBC count?
   a. High altitudes cause vascular fluid loss, leading to hemoconcentration.
   b. Hypoxia caused by decreased atmospheric oxygen stimulates erythropoiesis.
   c. The function of the spleen in removing old erythrocytes is impaired at high altitudes.
   d. Impaired production of leukocytes and platelets leads to proportionally higher RBC counts.

2. What is the primary effect of malignant disorders that arise from granulocytic cells in the bone marrow?
   a. Risk for hemorrhage
   b. Altered oxygenation
   c. Decreased production of antibodies
   d. Decreased phagocytosis of bacteria

3. An anticoagulant such as warfarin that interferes with prothrombin production will alter the clotting mechanism during what process?
   a. Platelet aggregation
   b. Activation of thrombin
   c. Release of tissue thromboplastin
   d. Stimulation of factor activation complex

4. When reviewing laboratory results of an 83-year-old client with an infection, what should the nurse expect to find?
   a. Minimal leukocytosis
   b. Decreased platelet count
   c. Increased hemoglobin and hematocrit levels
   d. Decreased erythrocyte sedimentation rate (ESR)

5. What significant information related to the hematological system should be obtained from a client's health history?
   a. Jaundice
   b. Bladder surgery
   c. Early menopause
   d. Multiple pregnancies

6. What technique should the nurse use when assessing the lymph nodes?
   a. Applying gentle, firm pressure to deep lymph nodes
   b. Palpating the deep cervical and supraclavicular nodes last
   c. Lightly palpating superficial lymph nodes with the pads of the fingers
   d. Using the tips of the second, third, and fourth fingers to apply deep palpation

7. When a lymph node is palpated, which of the following is a normal finding?
   a. Hard, fixed nodes
   b. Firm, mobile nodes
   c. Enlarged, tender nodes
   d. Hard, nontender nodes

8. Nursing care for a client immediately after a bone marrow biopsy and aspiration includes which of the following? (*Select all that apply*)
   a. Administering analgesics as necessary
   b. Preparing to administer a blood transfusion
   c. Instructing on need to lie still with a sterile pressure dressing intact
   d. Monitoring vital signs and assessing the site for excess drainage or bleeding
   e. Instructing on the need for preprocedure and postprocedure antibiotics

9. A nurse is taking care of a male client who has the following laboratory values from his CBC: WBC 6.5×10^9/L, Hb 134 g/L, Hct 40%, platelets 50×10^9/L. What should the nurse be most concerned about?
   a. The client is neutropenic.
   b. The client has an infection.
   c. The client is at risk for bleeding.
   d. The client is at risk of falling due to his anemia.

1. b; 2. d; 3. b; 4. a; 5. a; 6. c; 7. b; 8. a, c, d; 9. c

ⓔvolve

For even more review questions, visit *http://evolve.elsevier.com/Canada/Lewis/medsurg*.

REFERENCES

Ball, J. W., Dains, J. E., Flynn, J. A., et al. (2014). *Seidel's guide to physical examination* (8th ed.). St. Louis: Mosby.

Bueno, V., Sant'Anna, O. A., & Lord, J. M. (2014). Ageing and myeloid-derived suppressor cells: Possible involvement in immunosenescence and age-related disease. *Age, 36*(6), 9729–9741. doi:10.1007/s11357-014-9729-x.

Ershler, W. B., Artz, A. S., & Kanapuru, B. (2015). Hematology in older persons. In K. Kaushansky, M. A. Lichtman, J. T. Prchal, et al. (Eds.), *Williams hematology* (9th ed.). New York: McGraw-Hill.

Hamilton, J. A., & Achuthan, A. (2013). Colony stimulating factors and myeloid cell biology in health and disease. *Trends in Immunology, 34*, 81–89. doi:10.1016/j.it.2012.08.006.

Kaushansky, K. (2015). Thrombopoiesis. *Seminars in Hematology, 52*(1), 4–11. doi:10.1053/j.seminhematol.2014.10.003.

Kautz, L., & Nemeth, E. (2014). Molecular liaisons between erythropoiesis and iron metabolism. *Blood, 24*(124), 479–482. doi:10.1182/blood-2014-05-516252.

Lebeaux, D., & Sene, D. (2012). Eosinophilic fasciitis (Shulman disease). *Best Practice & Research in Clinical Rheumatology, 26*(4), 449–458. doi:10.1016/j.berh.2012.08.001.

Li, C. T., Wang, H. B., & Xu, B. J. (2013). A comparative study on anticoagulant activities of three Chinese herbal medicines from the genus Panax and anticoagulant activities of ginsenosides Rg1 and Rg2. *Pharmaceutical Biology, 51*(8), 1077–1080. doi:10.3109/13880209.2013.775164.

McCance, K. L., & Huether, S. E. (Eds.), (2015). *Pathophysiology: The biologic basis for disease in adults and children* (7th ed.). St. Louis: Mosby.

Pagana, K. D., & Pagana, T. J. (2014). *Mosby's manual of diagnostic and laboratory tests* (5th ed.). St. Louis: Mosby.

Porteus, M., & Mantanona, T. (2012). Blood. In L. W. Janson & M. E. Tischler (Eds.), *The big picture: Medical biochemistry*. New York: McGraw-Hill.

Zhang, Y., Wang, L., Dey, S., et al. (2014). Erythropoietin action in stress response, tissue maintenance and metabolism. *International Journal of Molecular Sciences, 15*(6), 10296–10333. doi:10.3390/ijms150610296.

RESOURCES

Resources for this chapter are listed in Chapter 33.

Nursing Management

Hematological Problems

Written by: Sandra Irene Rome
Adapted by: Bridgette Lord

⊖volve WEBSITE

http://evolve.elsevier.com/Canada/Lewis/medsurg

- Review Questions (Online Only)
- Key Points
- Answer Guidelines for Case Study
- Student Case Studies
  - Chronic Myelogenous Leukemia, Including End-of-Life Care
  - Endometrial Cancer and Blood Transfusion

- Customizable Nursing Care Plans
  - Neutropenia
  - Thrombo-Cytopenia
- Conceptual Care Map Creator
  - Conceptual Care Map for Case Study
- Audio Glossary
- Content Updates

LEARNING OBJECTIVES

1. Describe the general clinical manifestations and complications of anemia.
2. Describe the etiologies, clinical manifestations, diagnostic findings, and nursing and collaborative management of iron-deficiency, megaloblastic, and aplastic anemias and anemia of chronic disease.
3. Explain the nursing and collaborative management of anemia secondary to blood loss.
4. Describe the pathophysiology, clinical manifestations, and nursing and collaborative management of anemia caused by increased erythrocyte destruction, including sickle cell disease and acquired hemolytic anemias.
5. Describe the pathophysiology and nursing and collaborative management of polycythemia.
6. Explain the pathophysiology, clinical manifestations, and nursing and collaborative management of various types of thrombo-cytopenia.
7. Describe the types, clinical manifestations, diagnostic findings, and nursing and collaborative management of hemophilia and von Willebrand disease.

8. Explain the pathophysiology, diagnostic findings, and nursing and collaborative management of disseminated intravascular coagulation.
9. Describe the etiology, clinical manifestations, and nursing and collaborative management of neutropenia.
10. Describe the pathophysiology, clinical manifestations, and nursing and collaborative management of myelodysplastic syndrome.
11. Compare and contrast the major types of leukemia in terms of age of onset, clinical manifestations, and diagnostic findings.
12. Explain the nursing and collaborative management of acute and chronic leukemias.
13. Compare Hodgkin's lymphoma and non-Hodgkin's lymphoma in terms of clinical manifestations, staging, and nursing and collaborative management.
14. Describe the pathophysiology, clinical manifestations, and nursing and collaborative management of multiple myeloma.
15. Describe spleen disorders and related collaborative care.
16. Describe the nursing management of transfusing blood and blood products.

KEY TERMS

ANEMIA

DEFINITION AND CLASSIFICATION

Anemia is a deficiency in the number of erythrocytes (red blood cells [RBCs]), the quantity or quality of hemoglobin (Hb), the volume of packed RBCs (hematocrit [Hct]), or a combination of these. It is a prevalent condition with many diverse causes such as blood loss, impaired production of erythrocytes, or increased destruction of erythrocytes. Because RBCs transport oxygen (O_2), erythrocyte disorders can lead to tissue hypoxia; this accounts for many of the signs and symptoms of anemia. Anemia is not a specific disease: it is a manifestation of a pathological process.

Anemia is diagnosed based on a complete blood count (CBC), reticulocyte count, and peripheral blood smear. Once anemia is identified, further investigation is done to determine its specific cause (Marks, 2013).

Anemia can result from primary hematological problems or can develop as a secondary consequence of defects in other body systems. There are also biological and genetic factors (see the "Determinants of Health" box). The various types of anemia can be grouped according to either a morphological classification (by cellular characteristics) or an etiological one (by underlying cause). Morphological classification is based on descriptive, objective laboratory information about erythrocyte size and colour (Table 33-1). Etiological classification is related to the clinical conditions causing the anemia (Table 33-2). Although the morphological system is the most accurate means of classifying anemias, it is easier to discuss patient care by focusing on the cause or etiology of the anemia.

CLINICAL MANIFESTATIONS

The clinical manifestations of anemia are caused by the body's response to tissue hypoxia. Specific manifestations vary depending on the rate at which anemia evolved, its severity, and the presence of coexisting disease. Hb levels are often used to determine the severity of anemia. Mild states of anemia (Hb 100–120 g/L) may exist without causing symptoms. If symptoms develop, it is because the patient has an underlying disease or is experiencing a compensatory response to heavy exercise. Symptoms include palpitations, dyspnea, and diaphoresis. In cases of moderate anemia (Hb 60–100 g/L), the cardiopulmonary symptoms are increased and the patient may experience them while resting as well as with activity. The patient with severe anemia (Hb <60 g/L) displays many clinical manifestations involving multiple body systems (Table 33-3).

Integumentary Changes

Integumentary changes include pallor, jaundice, and pruritus. Pallor results from reduced amounts of Hb and reduced blood flow to the skin. Jaundice occurs when hemolysis of RBCs results in an increased concentration of serum bilirubin. Pruritus occurs because of increased serum and bile salt concentrations in the skin. In addition to the skin, the sclera of the eyes and the mucous membranes should be evaluated for jaundice because they reflect the integumentary changes more accurately, especially in dark-skinned individuals.

Cardiopulmonary Manifestations

Cardiopulmonary manifestations of severe anemia result from additional attempts by the heart and lungs to provide adequate

---

TABLE 33-1 RELATIONSHIP OF MORPHOLOGICAL CLASSIFICATION AND ETIOLOGIES OF ANEMIA

Morphology	Etiology
Normocytic, normochromic (normal size and colour) MCV 80–100 fL, MCH 27–34 pg	Acute blood loss, hemolysis, chronic renal disease, chronic disease, cancers, sideroblastic anemia, refractory anemia, diseases of endocrine dysfunction, aplastic anemia, pregnancy
Macrocytic (megaloblastic), normochromic (large size, normal colour) MCV >100 fL, MCH >34 pg	Vitamin B_{12} deficiency, folate deficiency, liver disease (including effects of alcohol use disorder), medications that impair DNA synthesis, hypothyroidism
Microcytic, hypochromic (small size, pale colour) MCV <80 fL, MCH <27 pg	Iron-deficiency anemia, thalassemia, anemia of chronic disease, sideroblastic anemia, lead poisoning

DNA, deoxyribonucleic acid; *MCH*, mean corpuscular hemoglobin; *MCV*, mean corpuscular volume.

TABLE 33-2 ETIOLOGICAL CLASSIFICATION OF ANEMIA

Decreased Red Blood Cell Production
Decreased Hemoglobin Synthesis
- Iron deficiency
- Thalassemias (decreased globin synthesis)
- Sideroblastic anemia (decreased porphyrin)

Defective DNA Synthesis
- Cobalamin (vitamin B_{12}) deficiency
- Folic acid deficiency

Decreased Number of Erythrocyte Precursors
- Aplastic anemia
- Anemia of myeloproliferative disorders and myelodysplasia
- Chronic diseases or disorders
- Medications (e.g., chemotherapy)

Blood Loss
Acute
- Trauma
- Blood vessel rupture

Chronic
- Gastritis
- Menstrual flow
- Hemorrhoids

Increased Red Blood Cell Destruction
Intrinsic
- Abnormal hemoglobin (hemoglobin S—sickle cell anemia)
- Enzyme deficiency (G6PD)
- Membrane abnormalities (paroxysmal nocturnal hemoglobinuria, hereditary spherocytosis)

Extrinsic
- Physical trauma (prosthetic heart valves, extracorporeal circulation)
- Antibodies (isoimmune and autoimmune)
- Infectious agents, medications, and toxins (malaria)

DNA, deoxyribonucleic acid; *G6PD*, glucose-6-phosphate dehydrogenase.

TABLE 33-3   CLINICAL MANIFESTATIONS OF ANEMIA

Body System	Severity of Anemia		
	Mild (Hb 100–120 g/L*)	Moderate (Hb 60–100 g/L*)	Severe (Hb <60 g/L*)
Integument	None	None	Pallor, jaundice,† pruritus†
Eyes	None	None	Icteric conjunctiva and sclera, retinal hemorrhage, blurred vision
Mouth	None	None	Glossitis, smooth tongue
Cardiovascular	Palpitations	Increased palpitations, "bounding pulse"	Tachycardia, increased pulse pressure, systolic murmurs, intermittent claudication, angina, HF, MI
Pulmonary	Exertional dyspnea	Dyspnea	Tachypnea, orthopnea, dyspnea at rest
Neurological	None	"Roaring in the ears"	Headache, vertigo, irritability, depression, impaired thought processes
Gastro-intestinal	None	None	Anorexia, hepatomegaly, splenomegaly, difficulty swallowing, sore mouth
Musculo-skeletal	None	None	Bone pain
General	None	Fatigue	Sensitivity to cold, weight loss, lethargy

Hb, hemoglobin; *HF*, heart failure; *MI*, myocardial infarction.
*Applies to female values; will be slightly higher in males.
†Caused by hemolysis.

DETERMINANTS OF HEALTH

Anemia

Biology and Genetic Endowment
- Sickle cell disease has a high incidence among people of African descent but may also affect people of Latin, Caribbean, Arabian, Indian, and Mediterranean descent.
- Thalassemia has a higher incidence among people of North African, East Asian, and Mediterranean origin.
- There is a high incidence of pernicious anemia among people of African and Scandinavian descent.
- Indigenous people have a higher incidence of iron-deficiency anemia, primarily caused by inadequate diet, poor living conditions, and high infection rates.*

Reference
*Khambalia, A. Z., Aimone, A. M., & Zlotkin, S. H. (2011). Burden of anemia among indigenous populations. *Nutrition Reviews, 69*(12), 693–719. doi:10.1111/j.1753-4887.2011.00437.x.

amounts of O_2 to the tissues. Cardiac output is maintained by increasing the heart rate and the stroke volume. The low viscosity of the blood contributes to the development of systolic murmurs and bruits. In extreme cases or when concomitant heart disease is present, angina pectoris and myocardial infarction (MI) may occur if myocardial O_2 needs cannot be met. Heart failure (HF), cardiomegaly, pulmonary and systemic congestion, ascites, and peripheral edema may develop if the heart is overworked for an extended period.

NURSING MANAGEMENT
ANEMIA

This section discusses general nursing management of anemia. Specific care related to various types of anemia is discussed later in this chapter.

NURSING ASSESSMENT

Subjective and objective data that should be obtained from a patient with anemia are presented in Table 33-4.

NURSING DIAGNOSES

Nursing diagnoses for the patient with anemia include but are not limited to those presented in Nursing Care Plan (NCP) 33-1.

PLANNING

The overall goals are that the patient with anemia will (a) assume normal activities of daily living, (b) maintain adequate nutrition, and (c) develop no complications related to anemia.

NURSING IMPLEMENTATION

The numerous causes of anemia necessitate different nursing interventions specific to the needs of the patient. Nevertheless, there are certain general components of care for all patients with anemia; these are presented in NCP 33-1.

Correcting the cause of anemia is ultimately the goal of therapy. Acute interventions may include blood or blood product transfusions, drug therapy, volume replacement, and O_2 therapy to stabilize the patient. Dietary and lifestyle changes can reverse some types of anemias. The plan of care should include an ongoing assessment of the patient's knowledge regarding adequate nutritional intake and drug therapies and of the patient's compliance with safety precautions to prevent falls and injury.

AGE-RELATED CONSIDERATIONS

ANEMIA

Modest changes in RBC mass occur in older adults. In healthy older men, a decline in Hb of about 10 g/L between ages 70 and 88 years is common, in part because of the decreased production of androgens. Only a minimal decrease in Hb occurs between these ages in healthy women (≈2 g/L) (Marks, 2013).

Anemia is not a normal finding in older adults. However, its prevalence increases starting from the seventh decade of life. For the majority of older adults, anemia is related to an underlying cause such as iron or folate deficiency, bleeding, cancer, chronic disease or inflammation, or renal insufficiency. In many older patients with anemia, there is no identifiable cause (Artz & Ershler, 2013). Signs and symptoms of anemia in the

TABLE 33-4 NURSING ASSESSMENT

Anemia

Subjective Data
Important Health Information

Past health history: Recent blood loss or trauma; chronic liver, endocrine, or renal disease (including dialysis); GI disease (e.g., malabsorption syndrome, ulcers, gastritis, or hemorrhoids); inflammatory disorders (especially Crohn's disease); smoking, exposure to radiation or chemical toxins (arsenic, lead, benzenes, copper); infectious disease (e.g., HIV) or recent travel suggesting exposure to infection; angina, myocardial infarction; history of falling

Medications: Use of vitamin and iron supplements, acetylsalicylic acid (ASA) (Aspirin), anticoagulants, oral contraceptives, phenobarbital, penicillins, nonsteroidal anti-inflammatory drugs, phenacetin, omeprazole, phenytoin (Dilantin), methyldopa, sulphonamides, herbal products

Surgery or other treatments: Recent surgery, small bowel resection, gastrectomy, prosthetic heart valves, chemotherapy, radiation therapy

Dietary history: General dietary patterns, consumption of alcohol

Symptoms

- Nausea, vomiting, anorexia, dysphagia, dyspepsia, heartburn, painful tongue
- Night sweats, cold intolerance, weight loss, pruritus, pain
- Hematuria, decreased urinary output, diarrhea, constipation, flatulence, tarry stools, bloody stools
- Fatigue, muscle weakness, and decreased strength
- Dyspnea, orthopnea, cough, hemoptysis, palpitations, shortness of breath with activity
- Headache; paresthesias of feet and hands; disturbances in vision, taste, or hearing; vertigo
- Menorrhagia, metrorrhagia; recent or current pregnancy in women; male impotence

Objective Data
General

Lethargy, apathy, general lymphadenopathy, fever

Integumentary

Pale skin and mucous membranes; blue sclera, yellowing of the whites of the eyes, or icteric sclera; cheilitis; poor skin turgor; brittle, spoon-shaped fingernails; jaundice; petechiae; ecchymoses; nose or gingival bleeding; poor healing; dry, brittle, thinning hair

Respiratory

Tachypnea

Cardiovascular

Tachycardia, systolic murmur, dysrhythmias; postural hypotension, widened pulse pressure, bruits (especially carotid); intermittent claudication, ankle edema

Gastro-Intestinal

Hepato-splenomegaly; glossitis; beefy, red tongue; stomatitis; abdominal distension; anorexia

Neurological

Headache, roaring in the ears, confusion, impaired judgement, irritability, ataxia, unsteady gait, paralysis, loss of vibration sense

Possible Diagnostic Findings

↓ RBCs; ↓ Hb; ↓ Hct; ↓ or ↑ reticulocytes, MCV; ↓ serum iron, ferritin, folate, or cobalamin (vitamin B_{12}); heme (guaiac)-positive stools; ↓ serum erythropoietin level; ↓ or ↑ LDH, bilirubin, transferrin (see Table 33-6)

GI, gastro-intestinal; *Hb,* hemoglobin; *Hct,* hematocrit; *HIV,* human immunodeficiency virus; *LDH,* lactate dehydrogenase; *MCV,* mean corpuscular volume; *RBCs,* red blood cells.

older adult may include pallor, confusion, ataxia, fatigue, and worsening cardiovascular and respiratory problems. Unfortunately, anemia may go unrecognized in the older adult because manifestations of anemia may be mistaken as normal aging changes or be overlooked because of another health problem. By recognizing signs of anemia, the nurse can play a pivotal role in appropriate health assessment and related interventions for older adults.

ANEMIA CAUSED BY DECREASED ERYTHROCYTE PRODUCTION

Normally, RBC production (termed *erythropoiesis*) is in equilibrium with RBC destruction and loss. This balance ensures that an adequate number of erythrocytes are available at all times. The normal lifespan of an RBC is 120 days. Three alterations in erythropoiesis may occur that decrease RBC production: (a) decreased Hb synthesis may lead to iron-deficiency anemia, thalassemia, and sideroblastic anemia; (b) defective deoxyribonucleic acid (DNA) synthesis in RBCs (e.g., cobalamin or folic acid deficiency) may lead to megaloblastic anemias; and (c) diminished availability of erythrocyte precursors may result in aplastic anemia and anemia of chronic disease (see Table 33-2).

IRON-DEFICIENCY ANEMIA

Iron-deficiency anemia is the most common nutritional disorder in the world. It is a microcytic hypochromic anemia caused by inadequate supplies of the iron needed to synthesize hemoglobin. The people most susceptible to iron-deficiency anemia are the very young, those with poor diets, and women in their reproductive years (World Health Organization, 2016). Normally, 1 mg of iron is lost daily in urine, bile, sweat, sloughing of epithelial cells, and minor bleeding (Rote & McCance, 2014).

Etiology

Iron deficiency may develop from inadequate dietary intake, malabsorption, blood loss, or hemolysis. Iron is obtained from food and dietary supplements. Dietary iron is usually adequate to meet the needs of men and older women, but it may be inadequate for individuals with higher iron needs (e.g., menstruating or pregnant women). Table 33-5 lists nutrients needed for erythropoiesis. Malabsorption of iron may occur after certain types of gastro-intestinal (GI) surgery and in malabsorption syndromes. Surgical procedures may involve removal or bypass of the duodenum. Because iron absorption occurs primarily in the duodenum, malabsorption syndromes may involve disease of the duodenum in which the absorptive surface is altered or destroyed.

Blood loss is a major cause of iron deficiency in adults. Two millilitres of whole blood contains 1 mg of iron. The major sources of chronic blood loss are from the GI and genito-urinary (GU) systems. GI bleeding is often not apparent and, therefore, may be present for a considerable time before the problem is identified. Loss of 50 to 75 mL of blood from the upper GI tract is required for stools to appear black *(melena)*. The black colour results from the iron in the RBCs. Common causes of GI blood loss are peptic ulcer, gastritis, esophagitis, diverticuli, hemorrhoids, and neoplasia. GU blood loss occurs primarily from menstrual bleeding. The average monthly menstrual blood loss is about 45 mL and

◎ NURSING CARE PLAN 33-1

Anemia

NURSING DIAGNOSIS	**Fatigue** related to *anemia* (inadequate oxygenation of the blood) as evidenced by insufficient energy, *increase in physical symptoms* (pulse rate and blood pressure)

Expected Patient Outcomes	**Nursing Interventions and *Rationales***
• Participates in activities of daily living (e.g., bathing, dressing, grooming, feeding) without abnormal increases in pulse and blood pressure • Reports increased endurance of activity	• Correct physiological status deficits (e.g., chemotherapy-induced anemia) *to help mitigate the underlying cause of anemia.* • Encourage alternate periods of rest and activity *to provide activity without tiring the patient.* • Monitor cardiorespiratory response to activity (e.g., tachycardia, dysrhythmias, dyspnea, diaphoresis, pallor, respiratory rate) *to evaluate activity intolerance.* • Limit environmental stimuli *to reduce demands placed on patient.* • Assist the patient in assigning priority to activities *to accommodate energy levels for important activities.* • Arrange physical activities (e.g., avoid activity immediately after meals) *to reduce competition for O$_2$ supply to vital body functions.* • Assist with regular physical activities (e.g., ambulation, transfers, turning, personal care) *to minimize fatigue and risk for injury from falls.* • Instruct patient, caregiver(s), and family member(s) to recognize signs and symptoms of fatigue that require reduction in activity *to promote self-care.* • Instruct patient, caregiver(s), and family member(s) to notify health care provider if signs and symptoms of fatigue persist *to review treatment plan.*

NURSING DIAGNOSIS	**Imbalanced nutrition: less than body requirements** related to insufficient dietary intake as evidenced by *insufficient interest in food, inability to absorb nutrients*

Expected Patient Outcomes	**Nursing Interventions and *Rationales***
• Maintains dietary intake that provides minimum daily requirements of nutrients. • Experiences normal blood values of nutrients necessary to prevent anemia.	• Determine, in collaboration with dietitian, number of calories and type of nutrients needed to meet nutritional requirements *to plan interventions.* • Teach patient how to use a food diary *to help evaluate nutritional intake.* • Monitor recorded intake for nutritional content and calories *to evaluate nutritional status.* • Instruct patient about nutritional needs (i.e., encourage increased intake of protein, iron, vitamin C) *to help ensure patient gets nutrients needed for maximum iron absorption and hemoglobin production.* • Adjust diet, as necessary, *to adapt to changes in nutritional requirements.*

NURSING DIAGNOSIS	**Ineffective health management** related to *insufficient knowledge of therapeutic regimen* as evidenced by *difficulty with prescribed regimen*

Expected Patient Outcomes	**Nursing Interventions and *Rationales***
Verbalizes knowledge necessary to maintain adequate nutrition and management of medication regimen	*Nutritional Counselling* • Facilitate identification of eating behaviours to be changed. • Use accepted nutritional standards *to assist patient in evaluating adequacy of dietary intake.* • Discuss nutritional requirements and patient's perceptions of prescribed or recommended diet. • Provide referral or consultation with other members of the health care team *to help patient achieve goals and make adjustments throughout recovery.* • Review with patient measurements of hemoglobin values *to evaluate response to therapeutic plan.* *Teaching: Prescribed Medication* • Instruct the patient on the purpose and action of each medication. • Instruct the patient on dosage, route, and duration of each medication *to improve adherence.* • Instruct the patient on possible adverse effects of each medication *to ensure early detection of adverse responses to medication.*

causes the loss of about 22 mg of iron. Postmenopausal bleeding can contribute to anemia in a susceptible older woman. Pregnancy also contributes to iron deficiency because of the diversion of iron to the fetus for erythropoiesis, blood loss at delivery, and lactation (Cantor, Bougatsos, Dana, et al., 2015). In addition to anemia of chronic kidney disease, dialysis treatment may induce iron-deficiency anemia because of the blood lost in the dialysis equipment and frequent blood sampling.

Clinical Manifestations

In the early course of iron-deficiency anemia, the patient may be symptom free. As the disease becomes chronic, any of the general manifestations of anemia may develop (see Table 33-3). In addition, specific clinical symptoms may occur related to iron-deficiency anemia. Pallor is the most common finding, and *glossitis* (inflammation of the tongue) is the second most common; another finding is *cheilitis* (inflammation of the lips). In addition, the patient may report headache, paresthesias, and a burning sensation of the tongue, all of which are caused by a lack of iron in the tissues.

Diagnostic Studies

Iron-deficiency anemia will lead to a number of characteristic laboratory abnormalities (Table 33-6). Other diagnostic studies

TABLE 33-5 NUTRITIONAL THERAPY

Nutrients Needed for Erythropoiesis

Nutrient	Role in Erythropoiesis	Food Sources
Cobalamin (vitamin B$_{12}$)	RBC maturation	Red meats (especially liver), eggs, enriched grain products, dairy, fish, fortified rice and soy beverages
Copper	Mobilization of iron from tissues to plasma	Shellfish, whole grains, beans, nuts, potatoes, organ meats, sesame seeds, kale, fermented soy foods
Folic acid	RBC maturation	Leafy green vegetables, okra, liver, meat, fish, legumes, whole grains, orange juice, peanuts, avocado, lentils
Iron	Hemoglobin synthesis	Liver and muscle meats, eggs, dried fruits, legumes, leafy dark-green vegetables, whole-grain and enriched bread and cereals, beans, tofu
Niacin (vitamin B$_3$)	RBC maturation	Peanut butter, beans, meats, avocado, enriched and fortified grains, yeast extract
Pantothenic acid (vitamin B$_5$)	Hemoglobin synthesis	Meats, leafy green vegetables, cereal grains, legumes, eggs, milk, mushrooms
Pyridoxine (vitamin B$_6$)	Hemoglobin synthesis	Meats, wheat germ, legumes, potatoes, cornmeal, bananas, nuts, fish (salmon, sardines)
Riboflavin (vitamin B$_2$)	Oxidative reactions	Dairy, enriched bread, salmon, chicken, eggs, leafy green vegetables
Vitamin E	Hemoglobin synthesis, protection against oxidative damage to RBCs	Vegetable oils, meat, eggs, wheat germ, whole-grain products, seeds, nuts (pine nuts, almond butter), fish (salmon, eel)
Amino acids	Synthesis of nucleoproteins	Eggs, meat, milk and milk products, poultry, fish, legumes, nuts, tofu
Ascorbic acid (vitamin C)	Conversion of folic acid to its active forms; contribution to iron absorption	Citrus fruits, leafy green vegetables, strawberries, cantaloupe, kiwi, chili peppers

RBC, red blood cell.

are done to determine the cause of the iron deficiency (e.g., stool occult blood test). Endoscopy and colonoscopy may be used to detect GI bleeding. A bone marrow biopsy may be done if other tests are inconclusive.

Collaborative Care

The main goal of the collaborative care of iron-deficiency anemia is to treat the underlying disease that is causing reduced intake or absorption of iron. In addition, efforts are directed toward replacing iron (Table 33-7). The patient should be taught which foods are good sources of iron (see Table 33-5). If nutrition is already adequate, increasing iron intake by dietary means may not be practical. Consequently, oral or, occasionally, parenteral iron supplements are used. If the iron deficiency is from acute blood loss, the patient may require a transfusion of packed RBCs.

Drug Therapy. Oral iron should be used whenever possible because it is inexpensive and convenient. Many iron preparations are available. The following five factors should be considered in the administration of iron:

1. Iron is absorbed best from the duodenum and the proximal jejunum. Therefore, enteric-coated or sustained-release capsules, which release iron farther down in the GI tract, are counterproductive.
2. The daily dosage should provide 150 to 200 mg of elemental iron. This can be ingested in three or four daily doses, with each tablet or capsule of the iron preparation containing between 50 and 100 mg of iron. Common iron preparations and amounts of elemental iron are provided in Table 33-8.
3. Iron is best absorbed as ferrous sulphate (Fe2$^+$) in an acidic environment. For this reason and to avoid binding the iron with food, iron should be taken about an hour before meals, when the duodenal mucosa is most acidic. Taking iron with vitamin C (ascorbic acid) or orange juice, which contains ascorbic acid, also enhances iron absorption. Gastric effects, however, may necessitate ingesting iron with meals.
4. Undiluted liquid iron may stain the patient's teeth; therefore, it should be diluted and ingested through a straw.
5. GI adverse effects of iron administration may occur, including heartburn, constipation, and diarrhea. If adverse effects develop, the dosage and type of iron supplement may be adjusted. For example, many individuals who need supplemental iron cannot tolerate ferrous sulphate because of the

TABLE 33-6 LABORATORY RESULTS IN ANEMIA

Etiology of Anemia	Hb/Hct	MCV	Reticulocytes	Serum Iron	TIBC	Transferrin	Ferritin	Bilirubin	Serum B$_{12}$	Folate
Iron deficiency	↓	↓	N or slight ↓ or ↑	↓	↑	N or ↓	↓	N or ↓	N	N
Thalassemia major	↓	N or ↓	↑	↑	↓	↓	N or ↑	↑	N	↓
Cobalamin deficiency	↓	↑	N or ↓	N or ↑	N	Slight ↑	↑	N or slight ↑	↓	N
Folic acid deficiency	↓	↑	N or ↓	N or ↑	N	Slight ↑	↑	N or slight ↑	N	↓
Aplastic anemia	↓	N or slight ↑	↓	N or ↑	N or ↑	N	N	N	N	N
Chronic disease	↓	N or ↓	N or ↓	N or ↓	↓	N or ↓	N or ↑	N	N	N
Acute blood loss	↓	N or ↓	N or ↑	N	N	N	N	N	N	N
Chronic blood loss	↓	↓	N or ↑	↓	↓	N or ↓	N	N or ↓	N	N
Sickle cell anemia	↓	N	↓	N or ↑	N or ↓	N or ↓	N	↑	N	↓
Hemolytic anemia	↓	N or ↑	↑	N or ↑	N or ↓	N	N or ↑	↑	N	N

Hb, hemoglobin; *Hct,* hematocrit; *MCV,* mean corpuscular volume; *N,* normal; *TIBC,* total iron-binding capacity.

TABLE 33-7 COLLABORATIVE CARE

Iron-Deficiency Anemia

Diagnostic	Collaborative Therapy
• History and physical examination	• Identification and treatment of underlying cause
• Hct and Hb levels	• Drug therapy
• RBC count, including morphology	• Oral: ferrous sulphate or ferrous gluconate
• Reticulocyte count	
• Serum iron	• IM or IV: iron dextran, iron sucrose, sodium ferric gluconate (Ferrlecit)
• Serum ferritin	
• Serum transferrin	
• TIBC	• Nutritional therapy (see Table 33-5)
• Stool examination for occult blood	• Transfusion of packed RBCs
• Bone marrow aspirate (rarely)	

Hb, hemoglobin; *Hct,* hematocrit; *IM,* intramuscular; *IV,* intravenous; *RBC,* red blood cell; *TIBC,* total iron-building capacity.

TABLE 33-8 COMMON IRON PREPARATIONS AND ELEMENTAL IRON PROVIDED

Iron Preparation	Amount of Elemental Iron (mg)
Ferrous sulphate (300-mg tablet)	60
Ferrous gluconate (300-mg tablet)	35
Ferrous fumarate (300-mg tablet)	99
Polysaccharide iron complex	150

Source: Adapted from Canadian Pharmacists Association. (2011). *Iron preparations: Oral.* Retrieved from *https://www.e-therapeutics.ca/cps.showMonograph.action?newSearch=true&simpleIndex=BrandGeneric&simpleQuery=Iron+Preparations%3A+Oral&=#m267400n00027.*

effects of the sulphate base. However, ferrous gluconate may be an acceptable substitute. All patients should know that the use of iron preparations will cause their stools to become black because the GI tract excretes excess iron. Constipation is common, so patients should be started on stool softeners and laxatives if needed when taking iron.

DRUG ALERT—Iron
- Some preparations of IV iron have a risk of allergic reaction; the patient should be monitored accordingly.
- Oral iron should be taken about 1 hour before meals.
- Vitamin C (ascorbic acid) enhances iron absorption.

In some situations, it may be necessary to administer iron parenterally. Parenteral use of iron is indicated for malabsorption, intolerance of oral iron, a need for iron beyond oral-intake limits, or poor patient compliance in taking the oral preparations of iron. Parenteral iron may be given intramuscularly (IM) or intravenously (IV). Because IM iron solutions may stain the skin, separate needles should be used for drawing up the solution and for injecting the medication. The Z-track method should be used for injection to prevent leakage of the iron solution to the subcutaneous tissue. Some preparations of IV iron have a high risk for an allergic reaction, so the patient should be monitored accordingly.

NURSING MANAGEMENT
IRON-DEFICIENCY ANEMIA

Certain groups of individuals are at an increased risk for the development of iron-deficiency anemia. These include premenopausal and pregnant women, persons from low socio-economic backgrounds, older adults, and individuals experiencing blood loss. Nutritional education, with an emphasis on foods high in iron and on ways to maximize absorption, is important for these groups, as is adherence to both dietary and drug therapy. The patient should be informed of the need for diagnostic studies to identify the underlying cause, and the Hb and RBC counts should be reassessed periodically to evaluate the response to therapy. To replenish the body's iron stores, the patient needs to continue to take iron therapy for 2 to 3 months after the Hb level returns to normal. Patients who require lifelong iron supplementation should be monitored for potential liver problems related to the iron storage. Appropriate nursing measures are presented in NCP 33-1.

THALASSEMIA

Etiology

Thalassemia is a group of diseases involving inadequate production of normal Hb, and therefore decreased erythrocyte production. Thalassemia is caused by an absent or reduced globulin protein. Alpha-globulin chains are absent or reduced in alpha thalassemia, and beta-globin chains are absent or reduced in beta thalassemia. Hemolysis also occurs in thalassemia, but insufficient production of normal Hb is the predominant problem. Thalassemia is commonly found in members of ethnic groups whose origins are near the Mediterranean Sea, South East Asia, the Middle East, China, or Africa.

Thalassemia has an autosomal recessive genetic basis. An individual with thalassemia may have a heterozygous or homozygous form of the disease. A person who is heterozygous has one thalassemic gene and one normal gene and is said to have *thalassemia minor* (or *thalassemic trait*), a mild form of the disease. A homozygous person has two thalassemic genes, causing a severe condition known as *thalassemia major* (Porteus & Mantanona, 2012).

Clinical Manifestations

Thalassemia minor is frequently asymptomatic. A patient with thalassemia minor may exhibit mild to moderate anemia with *microcytosis* (small RBCs) and *hypochromia* (pale cells).

Thalassemia major is a life-threatening disease in which growth, both physical and mental, is often affected. The person who has thalassemia major is pale and displays other general symptoms of anemia (see Table 33-3). The symptoms develop by 2 years of age and can cause growth and development deficits. In addition, the person has pronounced splenomegaly as the spleen continuously tries to remove the damaged RBCs. Jaundice from RBC hemolysis is prominent. Hepatomegaly and cardiomyopathy may occur from iron deposition. As the bone marrow responds to the reduced O$_2$-carrying capacity of the blood, RBC production is stimulated and the marrow becomes packed with immature erythroid precursors that die. The death of these erythroid precursors stimulates further erythropoiesis, leading to chronic bone marrow hyperplasia and expansion of the marrow space. This expansion may cause thickening of the cranium and the maxillary cavity. Other complications of the disease include endocrinopathies and thromboses.

Collaborative Care

The laboratory abnormalities of thalassemia major are summarized in Table 33-6. No specific drug or diet therapies are effective in treating thalassemia. Thalassemia minor requires no treatment because the body adapts to the reduction of normal Hb; however, genetic counselling is advised.

Thalassemia major is managed with blood transfusions in conjunction with chelating agents that bind to iron: oral deferasirox (Exjade) or deferiprone (Ferriprox) or IV or subcutaneous deferoxamine (Desferal). These agents reduce the iron overloading that occurs with chronic transfusion therapy (Carson & Martin, 2014). Transfusions are administered to keep the Hb level at approximately 100 g/L in order to foster the patient's own erythropoiesis without enlarging the spleen. Zinc supplementation may be needed with transfusion therapy, though supplement amounts are reduced with chelation therapy. During chelation therapy, ascorbic acid supplementation increases urine excretion of iron; ascorbic acid should not otherwise be taken because it increases the absorption of dietary iron. Regular folic acid may be given if the patient's diet is poor. Iron supplements should not be given.

Although hematopoietic stem cell transplantation (HSCT) remains the only cure for thalassemia, issues such as the risk of the procedure, donor availability, access, and cost make HSCT a reasonable option for only a small number of patients. Regular transfusions and proper iron chelation therapy remain the mainstay of therapy for thalassemia major (Goss, Giardina, Degtyaryova, et al., 2014).

MEGALOBLASTIC ANEMIAS

Megaloblastic anemias are a group of disorders caused by impaired DNA synthesis and characterized by the presence of large RBCs. When DNA synthesis is impaired, defective RBC maturation results. These abnormal, large RBCs (macrocytic) are referred to as *megaloblasts*. Macrocytic RBCs are easily destroyed because they have fragile cell membranes. Although the overwhelming majority of megaloblastic anemias result from cobalamin (vitamin B$_{12}$) and folic acid deficiencies, this type of RBC deformity can also occur from suppression of DNA synthesis by drugs, inborn errors of cobalamin and folic acid metabolism, and *erythroleukemia* (a malignant blood disorder characterized by a proliferation of erythropoietic cells in bone marrow) (Table 33-9).

Normally, a protein termed *intrinsic factor* (IF) is secreted by the parietal cells of the gastric mucosa. IF is required for cobalamin (vitamin B$_{12}$) absorption. Cobalamin is normally absorbed in the distal ileum and if IF is not secreted, cobalamin will not be absorbed.

Etiology

Pernicious Anemia. The most common cause of cobalamin deficiency is pernicious anemia, which is caused by an absence of IF. In pernicious anemia, the gastric mucosa does not secrete IF because of either gastric mucosal atrophy or autoimmune destruction of parietal cells and possibly also because of IF itself. Pernicious anemia is a disease of insidious onset that begins in middle age or later (usually after age 40), with 60 years being the most common age at diagnosis. Pernicious anemia occurs frequently in people of African or Northern European ancestry (particularly Scandinavians). In people of African descent, the disease tends to begin early, occurs with higher frequency in women, and is often severe.

Other Causes of Cobalamin Deficiency. Cobalamin deficiency can also occur in patients who have had GI surgery such as

TABLE 33-9 CLASSIFICATION OF MEGALOBLASTIC ANEMIA

Cobalamin (Vitamin B$_{12}$) Deficiency
- Dietary deficiency
- Deficiency of gastric intrinsic factor
  - Pernicious anemia
  - Gastrectomy
  - Gastric bypass
  - Celiac disease
  - *Helicobacter pylori*
- Intestinal malabsorption
- Increased requirement (pregnancy)
- Chronic alcoholism

Folic Acid Deficiency
- Dietary deficiency (e.g., leafy green vegetables, citrus fruits)
- Malabsorption syndromes
  - Celiac disease
  - Crohn's disease
  - Small bowel resection
- Drugs interfering with absorption or use of folic acid
  - Methotrexate
  - Antiseizure drugs (e.g., phenobarbital, phenytoin [Dilantin])

- Increased requirement (pregnancy)
- Chronic alcoholism
- Chronic hemodialysis (folic acid lost during dialysis)

Drug-Induced Suppression of DNA Synthesis
- Folate antagonists
- Metabolic inhibitors
- Alkylating agents

Inborn Errors
- Defective folate metabolism
- Defective transport of cobalamin

Erythroleukemia
- Alkylating agents
- Ionizing radiation
- Familial erythroleukemia
- Myelodysplastic syndrome (MDS)

gastrectomy or gastric bypass; patients who have had a small bowel resection involving the ileum; and patients with Crohn's disease, ileitis, celiac disease, diverticulitis of the small intestine, chronic atrophic gastritis, or a combination of these. In these cases, cobalamin deficiency results from the loss of IF-secreting gastric mucosal cells or impaired absorption of cobalamin in the distal ileum. Cobalamin deficiency is also found in long-term users of histamine (H$_2$)-receptor blockers and proton pump inhibitors and in strict vegetarians (Townsley & Rodgers, 2013).

Clinical Manifestations

General symptoms of anemia related to cobalamin deficiency develop because of tissue hypoxia (see Table 33-3). GI manifestations include a sore, red, shiny tongue; anorexia; nausea; vomiting; and abdominal pain. Typical neuro-muscular manifestations include weakness, paresthesias of the feet and hands, reduced vibratory and position senses, ataxia, muscle weakness, and impaired thought processes ranging from confusion to dementia. Because cobalamin deficiency–related anemia has an insidious onset, it may take several months for these manifestations to develop.

Diagnostic Studies

Laboratory data reflective of cobalamin-deficiency anemia are presented in Table 33-6. The RBCs appear large (macrocytic) and have abnormal shapes. This structure contributes to erythrocyte destruction because the cell membrane is fragile. Serum cobalamin levels are reduced. It is important also to know serum folate levels because, if they are normal and cobalamin levels are low, it suggests that megaloblastic anemia is caused by a cobalamin deficiency. A serum test for anti-IF antibodies may be done that is specific for pernicious anemia. Because the potential for gastric cancer is increased in patients with pernicious anemia, a gastroscopy and biopsy of the gastric mucosa may also be done. Testing of serum methylmalonic acid (MMA) (elevated mainly in cobalamin deficiency) and serum homocysteine (elevated in both cobalamin and folic acid deficiencies) helps determine the cause of the anemia.

Collaborative Care

Regardless of how much is ingested, the patient is not able to absorb cobalamin if IF is lacking or if absorption in the ileum is impaired. For this reason, increasing dietary cobalamin does not correct this anemia. However, the patient should be instructed on adequate dietary intake to maintain good nutrition (see Table 33-5). Parenteral or intranasal administration of cobalamin (cyanocobalamin or hydroxocobalamin) is the treatment of choice. Without cobalamin administration, these individuals will die in 1 to 3 years. A typical treatment schedule consists of 1 000 mcg of cobalamin IM daily for 2 weeks and then weekly until the Hct is normal and then monthly for life. High-dose oral cobalamin and sublingual cobalamin are also available for those whose GI absorption is intact. As long as supplemental cobalamin is used, the anemia can be reversed. However, any longstanding neuro-muscular complications a patient has experienced may not be reversible.

Folic Acid Deficiency

Folic acid (folate) deficiency also causes megaloblastic anemia. Folic acid is required for DNA synthesis leading to RBC formation and maturation. Common causes of folic acid deficiency are listed in Table 33-9.

The clinical manifestations of folic acid deficiency are similar to those of cobalamin deficiency. The disease develops insidiously, and the patient's symptoms may be attributed to other, coexisting problems such as cirrhosis or esophageal varices. GI disturbances include dyspepsia and a smooth, swollen, beefy red or shiny tongue. The absence of neurological problems is an important diagnostic finding and differentiates folic acid deficiency from cobalamin deficiency (Stabler, 2013).

The diagnostic findings for folic acid deficiency are presented in Table 33-6. In addition, the serum folate level is low (normal is 11–57 mmol/L), and the serum cobalamin level is normal. Folic acid deficiency is treated by replacement therapy. The usual dose is 1 mg/day by mouth. In malabsorption states, up to 5 mg/day may be required. The duration of treatment depends on the reason for the deficiency. In addition to supplements, the patient should be encouraged to eat foods containing large amounts of folic acid (see Table 33-5).

NURSING MANAGEMENT
MEGALOBLASTIC ANEMIA

Because there is a familial predisposition for pernicious anemia (the most common type of cobalamin deficiency), patients who have a positive family history of pernicious anemia should be evaluated for symptoms. Although disease development cannot be prevented, early detection and treatment can help reverse symptoms more easily. Signs and symptoms of other possible causes of megaloblastic anemia should be brought to the attention of the primary health care provider.

The nursing measures presented in NCP 33-1 for the patient with anemia are appropriate for the patient with cobalamin-deficiency anemia. In addition to these measures, the nurse should ensure protection against injuries such as falls, burns, and trauma because the patient will have diminished sensations to heat and pain resulting from the neurological impairment. If heat therapy is required, the patient's skin must be evaluated at frequent intervals to detect redness.

Ongoing care is focused on ensuring good patient compliance with treatment. There must also be careful follow-up to assess for neurological difficulties that were not fully corrected by adequate cobalamin replacement therapy. Because the potential for gastric cancer may be increased in patients with atrophic gastritis–related pernicious anemia, the patient should have frequent and appropriate screening.

ANEMIA OF CHRONIC DISEASE

Chronic inflammation, autoimmune, infectious, or malignant diseases can lead to anemia of chronic disease. *Anemia of chronic disease* is associated with an underproduction of RBCs and mild shortening of RBC survival. The RBCs are usually normocytic, normochromic, and hypoproliferative. The anemia is usually mild, but it can be more severe if the underlying disorder is not treated. This type of anemia is primarily immune driven. Cytokines released with inflammatory, autoimmune, infectious, or malignant disease cause an increased uptake and retention of iron within macrophages. This leads to a diversion of iron from the circulation into storage sites and subsequent limitation of the availability of iron for erythropoiesis.

In the case of any chronic disease, additional factors may contribute to the anemia. For example, with renal disease, the primary factor causing anemia is decreased erythropoietin, a hormone made in the kidneys that is necessary for erythropoiesis. With impaired renal function, erythropoietin production is decreased (see Chapter 49).

Anemia of chronic disease must first be recognized and differentiated from anemias of other etiologies. Findings of elevated serum ferritin and increased iron stores distinguish it from iron-deficiency anemia. Normal folate and cobalamin blood levels distinguish it from megaloblastic anemias secondary to folate and cobalamin deficiencies.

The best treatment of anemia of chronic disease is correction of the underlying disorder. Unless the anemia is severe, blood transfusions are rarely indicated. Erythropoietin therapy may be used for anemia related to renal disease (see Chapter 49) or anemia related to cancer therapies. However, erythropoietin therapy is used conservatively because of the increased risk for thrombo-embolism and mortality in some patients (Bejjani, 2015).

APLASTIC ANEMIA

Aplastic anemia is a disease in which the patient has peripheral blood *pancytopenia* (decrease of all blood cell types—RBCs, white blood cells [WBCs], and platelets) and hypocellular bone marrow. The spectrum of the anemia can range from a chronic condition managed with erythropoietin or blood transfusions to a critical condition with hemorrhage and sepsis.

Etiology

The incidence of aplastic anemia is low, affecting approximately four of every 1 million people every year. There are various etiological classifications for aplastic anemia, but they can be divided into two major groups: *congenital* and *acquired*

TABLE 33-10	CAUSES OF APLASTIC ANEMIA

Congenital (Chromosomal Alterations)	Acquired
• Fanconi's syndrome • Congenital dyskeratosis • Amegakaryocytic thrombo-cytopenia • Schwachman-Diamond syndrome	• Chemical agents and toxins (e.g., benzene, arsenic) • Drugs (e.g., gold, antimicrobials) • Idiopathic/autoimmune • Radiation • Viral and bacterial infections

TABLE 33-11	MANIFESTATION OF ACUTE BLOOD LOSS	

Volume Lost*		
%	mL	Manifestations
10	500	None or rare vasovagal syncope
20	1000	No detectable signs or symptoms at rest; tachycardia with exercise and slight postural hypotension
30	1500	Normal supine blood pressure and pulse at rest; postural hypotension and tachycardia with exercise
40	2000	Blood pressure, central venous pressure, and cardiac output below normal at rest; air hunger; rapid, thready pulse and cold, clammy skin
50	2500	Shock, lactic acidosis, and potential death

*Based on an adult with a total blood volume of 5 L.

(Table 33-10). Most of the acquired aplastic anemias are idiopathic and thought to have an autoimmune basis (Scheinberg, Young, & Liu, 2013).

Clinical Manifestations

Aplastic anemia can manifest acutely (over days) or insidiously over weeks to months and can vary from mild to severe. Clinically, the patient may have symptoms caused by suppression of any or all bone marrow elements. General manifestations of anemia, such as fatigue and dyspnea, as well as cardiovascular and cerebral responses may be seen (see Table 33-3). Patients with neutropenia (low neutrophil counts) are susceptible to infection and are at risk for septic shock. Even a low-grade fever should be considered a medical emergency. Thrombo-cytopenia manifests as a predisposition to bleeding (e.g., petechiae, ecchymosis, epistaxis).

Diagnostic Studies

The diagnosis is confirmed by laboratory studies. Because all marrow elements are affected, Hb, WBC, and platelet values are often decreased in aplastic anemia. Other RBC indices are generally normal (see Table 33-6). The condition is, therefore, classified as a normocytic, normochromic anemia. The reticulocyte count is low.

Aplastic anemia can be further evaluated by assessing various iron studies. The serum iron and total iron-binding capacity (TIBC) may be elevated as initial signs of erythropoiesis suppression. Bone marrow biopsy, aspiration, and pathological examination may be done for any anemic state. However, the findings are especially important in aplastic anemia because the marrow is hypocellular, with increased yellow marrow (fat content).

NURSING AND COLLABORATIVE MANAGEMENT APLASTIC ANEMIA

Management of aplastic anemia is based on identifying and removing the causative agent (when possible) and providing supportive care until the pancytopenia reverses. Nursing interventions appropriate for the patient with pancytopenia from aplastic anemia are presented in NCP 33-1, earlier in this chapter. (See also NCP 33-2 for thrombo-cytopenia and NCP 33-3 for neutropenia, both available on the Evolve website.) Nursing actions are directed at preventing complications from infection and hemorrhage.

The prognosis for severe untreated aplastic anemia is poor. However, advances in medical management, including HSCT and immuno-suppressive therapy with antithymocyte globulin (ATG) and cyclosporin (Neoral), have improved outcomes significantly. ATG is a horse or rabbit serum that contains polyclonal antibodies against human T cells. The rationale for this therapy is that aplastic anemia is an immune-mediated disease resulting from the upregulation of T cells actively targeting and destroying the patient's own hematopoietic stem cells. ATG can cause anaphylaxis, but with premedications and careful infusion, most patients can complete the prescribed course of treatment.

The treatment of choice for younger adults who have a human leukocyte antigen (HLA)–matched donor is bone marrow transplantation. (Bone marrow transplants are discussed in Chapter 18.) The best results occur in younger patients (Bacigalupo, 2014). Prior transfusions increase the risk of graft rejection.

For the older adult or the patient without an HLA-matched donor, the treatment of choice is immuno-suppression with ATG or cyclosporine. High-dose corticosteroids may also be used. However, this therapy may be only partially beneficial.

ANEMIA CAUSED BY BLOOD LOSS

Anemia resulting from blood loss may be caused by either acute or chronic problems.

ACUTE BLOOD LOSS

Acute blood loss occurs as a result of sudden hemorrhage. Causes of acute blood loss include trauma, complications of surgery, and conditions or diseases that disrupt vascular integrity. There are two clinical concerns in such situations. First, there is a sudden reduction in the total blood volume that can lead to hypovolemic shock. Second, if the acute loss is more gradual, the body maintains its blood volume by slowly increasing the plasma volume. Although the circulating fluid volume is preserved, the number of RBCs available to carry O_2 is significantly diminished.

Clinical Manifestations

The clinical manifestations of anemia from acute blood loss are caused by the body's attempts to maintain an adequate blood volume and meet O_2 requirements. Table 33-11 summarizes the clinical manifestations of patients with varying degrees of blood volume loss. It is essential to understand that the clinical signs and symptoms the patient is experiencing are more important than the laboratory values. For example, an adult with a bleeding peptic ulcer who had a 750-mL hematemesis (15% of a normal total blood volume) within the past 30 minutes may have postural hypotension but have normal values for Hb and Hct. Over the ensuing 36 to 48 hours, most of the volume deficit will be repaired by the movement of fluid from the extravascular into the intravascular space. Only at these later times will the Hb and Hct reflect the blood loss.

The nurse should be alert to the patient's expression of pain when assessing for blood loss. Internal hemorrhage may cause pain because of tissue distension, organ displacement, and nerve compression. Pain may be localized or referred. In the case of retroperitoneal bleeding, for example, the patient may not experience abdominal pain. Instead, the patient may have numbness and pain in a lower extremity secondary to compression of the lateral cutaneous nerve, which is located in the region of the first to third lumbar vertebrae.

The major complication of acute blood loss is shock. (Shock and its management are discussed in Chapter 69.)

Diagnostic Studies

When blood volume loss is sudden, plasma volume has not yet had a chance to increase, the loss of RBCs is not reflected in laboratory data, and values may seem normal or high for 2 to 3 days. However, once the plasma is replaced, the RBC mass is less concentrated. At this time, RBC, Hb, and Hct levels are low, reflecting the blood loss.

Collaborative Care

Collaborative care is initially concerned with (a) replacing blood volume to prevent shock and (b) identifying the source of the hemorrhage and stopping the blood loss. IV fluids used in emergencies include dextran, hetastarch, albumin, and crystalloid electrolyte solutions such as lactated Ringer's. The amount of infusion varies with the solution used. (Management of shock is discussed in Chapter 69.)

Once volume replacement is established, attention can be directed to correcting the RBC loss. The body needs 2 to 5 days to manufacture more RBCs in response to increased erythropoietin. Consequently, blood transfusions (packed RBCs) may be needed if the blood loss is significant. In addition, if the bleeding is related to a platelet or clotting disorder, replacement of that deficiency must be addressed. If a large volume of blood is lost, platelets, plasma, and possibly cryoprecipitate will also be infused, because large volumes of RBCs would dilute the patient's own coagulation system.

The patient may also need supplemental iron because the availability of iron affects the marrow production of erythrocytes. When anemia exists after acute blood loss, dietary sources of iron will probably not be adequate to maintain iron stores. Therefore, oral or parenteral iron preparations are administered.

❚ NURSING MANAGEMENT ACUTE BLOOD LOSS

In the case of trauma, it may be impossible to prevent loss of blood. For the postoperative patient, carefully monitor the blood loss from various drainage tubes and dressings and implement appropriate actions. The NCP for the patient with anemia resulting from acute blood loss will most likely include administration of blood products (described at the end of this chapter).

Once the source of hemorrhage is identified, blood loss is controlled, and fluid and blood volumes are replaced, the anemia should begin to correct itself. There should be no need for long-term treatment of this type of anemia.

CHRONIC BLOOD LOSS

The sources of chronic blood loss are similar to those of iron-deficiency anemia (e.g., bleeding ulcer, hemorrhoids, menstrual and postmenopausal blood loss). The effects of chronic blood loss are usually related to the depletion of iron stores and are usually considered as iron-deficiency anemia. Management of chronic blood loss anemia involves identifying the source and stopping the bleeding. Supplemental iron may be required. The nursing measures presented in NCP 33-1 are relevant to anemia of chronic blood loss.

❚ ANEMIA CAUSED BY INCREASED ERYTHROCYTE DESTRUCTION

The third major cause of anemia is termed **hemolytic anemia**, a condition caused by the destruction or hemolysis of RBCs at a rate that exceeds production. Hemolysis can occur because of problems intrinsic or extrinsic to the RBCs. Intrinsic hemolytic anemias result from defects in the RBCs themselves caused by abnormal Hb (e.g., sickle cells), enzyme deficiencies that alter glycolysis (glucose-6-phosphate dehydrogenase [G6PD] deficiency), or RBC membrane abnormalities. Intrinsic hemolytic anemias are usually hereditary. More common are the extrinsic hemolytic anemias, which are acquired. In this type of anemia, the patient's RBCs are normal; damage is caused by external factors (see Table 33-2). The spleen is the primary site of the destruction of RBCs that are old, defective, or moderately damaged. Figure 33-1 indicates the sequence of events involved in extravascular hemolysis.

The patient with hemolytic anemia manifests the general symptoms of anemia and clinical manifestations specific to this type of anemia (see Table 33-3). Jaundice is likely because the increased destruction of RBCs causes an elevation in bilirubin

FIGURE 33-1 Sequence of events in extravascular hemolysis. *Fe,* iron; *Hb,* hemoglobin; *RBC,* red blood cell.

levels. The spleen and the liver may enlarge because of their hyperactivity, which is related to macrophage phagocytosis of the defective erythrocytes.

A major focus of treatment of hemolysis, no matter its cause, is to maintain renal function. When an RBC is hemolyzed, the Hb molecule is released and filtered by the kidneys. The accumulation of Hb molecules can obstruct the renal tubules and lead to acute tubular necrosis (see Chapter 49).

SICKLE CELL DISEASE

Sickle cell disease (SCD) is a group of inherited, autosomal recessive disorders characterized by the presence of an abnormal form of Hb in the RBC. (Autosomal recessive genetic disorders are discussed in Chapter 15.) This abnormal Hb, *hemoglobin S* (HbS), causes the erythrocyte to stiffen and elongate and take on a sickle shape in response to low levels of O_2 in the blood. HbS results from substitution of valine for glutamic acid on the beta-globin chain of Hb. Because it is a genetic disorder, SCD is usually identified during infancy or early childhood. It is an incurable disease that is often fatal by the time the affected individual reaches middle age. Death usually results from renal and pulmonary failure, infection, or stroke (Kline, 2014).

SCD is common in the African-descended population of Canada. It affects millions of people around the world, mainly those whose ancestors come from sub-Saharan Africa, Spanish-speaking regions (South America, Cuba, Central America), Saudi Arabia, India, and Mediterranean countries.

Etiology and Pathophysiology

Types of Sickle Cell Disease. Types of SCD disorders include sickle cell anemia, sickle cell–thalassemia, sickle cell–HbC disease, and sickle cell trait. *Sickle cell anemia,* the most severe of the SCD syndromes, occurs when a person is homozygous for HbS (HbSS), meaning the person has inherited HbS from both parents. *Sickle cell–thalassemia* and *sickle cell–HbC* occur when a person inherits HbS from one parent and another type of abnormal Hb (such as thalassemia or HbC) from the other parent. Both of these forms of SCD are less common and less severe than sickle cell anemia. *Sickle cell trait* occurs when a person is heterozygous for hemoglobin S (HbAS), meaning the person has inherited HbS from one parent and normal Hb (HbA) from the other parent. Sickle cell trait is typically a very mild or even asymptomatic condition.

Sickling Episodes. The major pathophysiological event of SCD is the sickling of RBCs. Sickling episodes are most commonly triggered by low O_2 tension in the blood. Hypoxia or deoxygenation of the RBCs can be caused by viral or bacterial infection, high altitude, emotional or physical stress, surgery, or blood loss. Infection is the most common precipitating factor. Other events that can trigger or sustain a sickling episode include dehydration, increased hydrogen ion concentration (acidosis), increased plasma osmolality, decreased plasma volume, and low body temperature. A sickling episode can also occur without an obvious cause.

Sickled RBCs become rigid and take on an elongated, crescent shape (Figure 33-2). Sickled cells cannot easily pass through capillaries or other small vessels and can cause vascular occlusion, leading to acute or chronic tissue injury. The resulting hemostasis promotes a self-perpetuating cycle of local hypoxia, deoxygenation of more erythrocytes, and more sickling. Circulating sickled cells are hemolyzed by the spleen, leading to anemia. Initially, the sickling of cells is reversible with reoxygenation, but it eventually

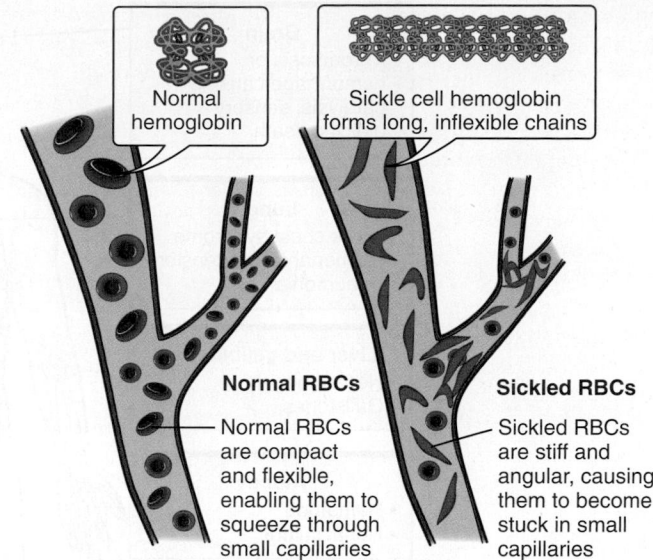

FIGURE 33-2 Sickle cell hemoglobin aggregates into long chains and alters the shape of the red blood cell.

becomes irreversible owing to cell membrane damage from recurrent sickling.

Sickle cell crisis is a severe, painful, acute exacerbation of RBC sickling causing a vaso-occlusive crisis. As blood flow is impaired by sickled cells, vasospasm occurs, further restricting blood flow. Severe capillary hypoxia causes changes in membrane permeability, leading to plasma loss, hemoconcentration, the development of thrombi, and further circulatory stagnation. Tissue ischemia, infarction, and necrosis eventually occur from lack of O_2. Shock is a possible life-threatening consequence of sickle cell crisis owing to severe O_2 depletion of the tissues and a reduction of the circulating fluid volume. Sickle cell crisis can begin suddenly and persist for days to weeks.

The frequency, extent, and severity of sickling episodes are highly variable and unpredictable but are largely dependent on the percentage of HbS present. Individuals with sickle cell anemia have the most severe form because the erythrocytes contain a high percentage of HbS.

Clinical Manifestations

The effects of SCD vary greatly from person to person, with their severity believed to result from genetic polymorphisms. Many people with sickle cell anemia are in reasonably good health the majority of the time. However, they may have chronic health problems and pain because of organ tissue hypoxia and damage (e.g., involving the kidneys or liver). The typical patient is anemic but asymptomatic except during sickling episodes. Because most individuals with sickle cell anemia have dark skin, pallor is more readily detected by examining the mucous membranes. The skin may have a greyish cast. Because of the hemolysis, jaundice is common and patients are prone to gallstones (cholelithiasis).

The primary symptom associated with sickling is pain. The pain can range from mild to excruciating. The episodes can affect any area of the body or several sites simultaneously, with the back, chest, extremities, and abdomen most commonly affected. Pain episodes are often accompanied by objective clinical signs such as fever, swelling, tenderness, tachypnea, hypertension, nausea, and vomiting.

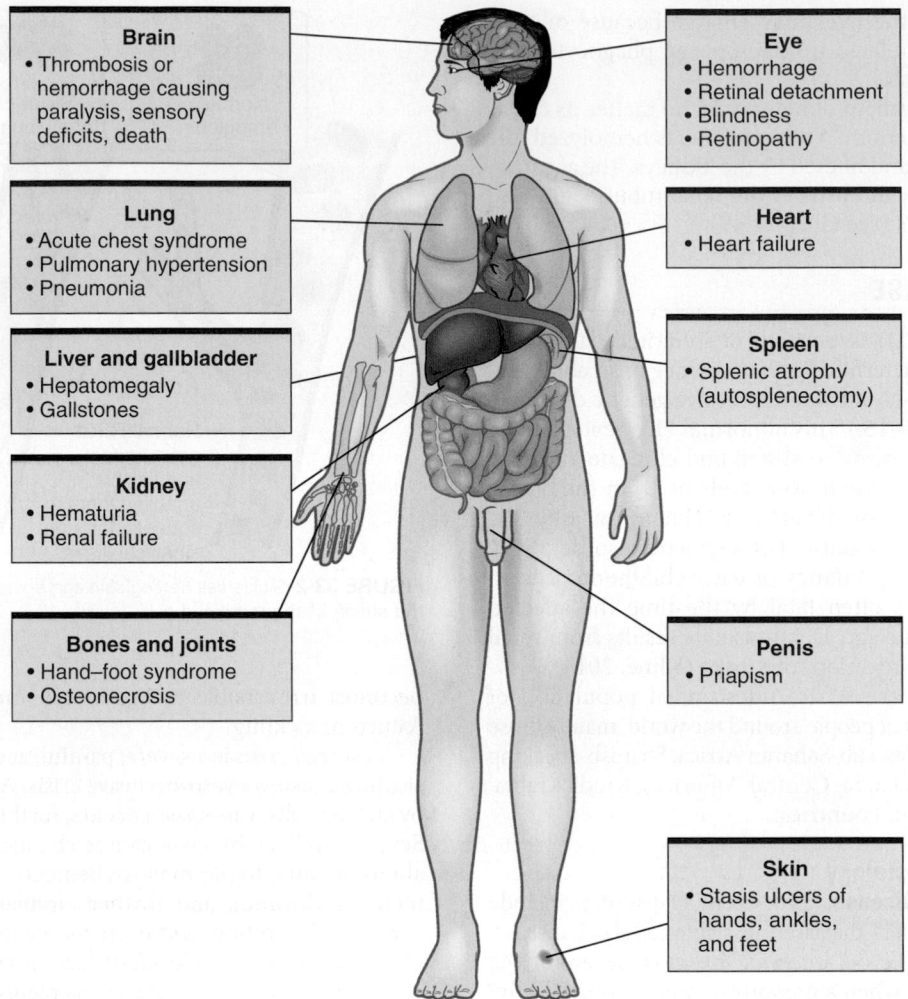

FIGURE 33-3 Clinical manifestations and complications of sickle cell disease. Source: Modified from McCance, K.L., & Huether, S. E. (2014). *Pathophysiology: The biologic basis for disease in adults and children* (7th ed.). St Louis: Mosby.

Complications

With repeated episodes of sickling, there is gradual involvement of all body systems, especially the spleen, lungs, kidneys, and brain. Organs that have a high need for O_2 are most often affected, and their involvement forms the basis for many of the complications of SCD (Figure 33-3). Infection is a major cause of morbidity and mortality in patients with SCD. One reason for this is the failure of the spleen to phagocytize foreign substances as it becomes infarcted and dysfunctional (usually by 2 to 4 years of age) from the sickled RBCs. The spleen becomes small because of repeated scarring, a phenomenon termed *autosplenectomy*.

Pneumonia is the most common infection and often is of pneumococcal origin. Infections can be severe enough to cause an aplastic and hemolytic crisis and gallstones. In turn, an *aplastic crisis* can be so severe as to cause a temporary shutdown of RBC production in the bone marrow.

Acute chest syndrome is a term used to describe acute pulmonary complications that include pneumonia, tissue infarction, and fat embolism. It affects 30% of patients with SCD; is characterized by fever, chest pain, cough, pulmonary infiltrates, and dyspnea; and may be life-threatening. Pulmonary infarctions may cause pulmonary hypertension, MI, HF, and ultimately cor

pulmonale. The heart may become ischemic and enlarged, leading to HF. Retinal vessel obstruction may result in hemorrhage, scarring, retinal detachment, and blindness. The kidneys may be injured from the increased blood viscosity and the lack of O_2, which can lead to renal failure. Pulmonary embolism or stroke can result from thrombosis and infarction of blood vessels. Bone changes may include osteoporosis and osteosclerosis after infarction. Chronic leg ulcers can result from hypoxia and are especially prevalent around the ankles. *Priapism* (persistent penile erection) may occur if penile veins become occluded.

Diagnostic Studies

A peripheral blood smear may reveal sickled cells and abnormal reticulocytes. The presence of HbS can be diagnosed by the sickling test, which uses RBCs (in vitro) and exposes them to a deoxygenation agent. As a result of the accelerated RBC breakdown, the patient has characteristic clinical findings of hemolysis (jaundice, elevated serum bilirubin levels) and abnormal laboratory test results. Hb electrophoresis may be done to determine the proportion of HbS and other variants. Skeletal radiographs demonstrate bone and joint deformities and flattening. Magnetic resonance imaging (MRI) may be used to diagnose a stroke caused by blocked cerebral vessels from sickled cells. Doppler studies may be used to assess for deep venous thromboses. Other tests may be indicated, such as a chest radiograph, to diagnose infection or organ malfunction.

NURSING AND COLLABORATIVE MANAGEMENT SICKLE CELL DISEASE

Collaborative care for a patient with SCD is directed toward (a) preventing sequelae from the disease, (b) alleviating the symptoms of the disease, (c) minimizing end–target organ damage, and (d) promptly treating serious sequelae, such as acute chest syndrome. Patients with SCD should be taught to minimize triggers of the disease by avoiding high altitudes, avoiding extreme temperatures, minimizing stress, maintaining adequate fluid intake, and treating infections promptly. Ongoing screening is also pertinent to patients with SCD. Screening for retinopathy should begin at age 10. In addition, brain scans (transcranial Doppler examinations) may be recommended. Pneumococcal, *Haemophilus influenzae,* influenza, and hepatitis immunizations should be administered.

Sickle cell crises may require hospitalization. O_2 may be administered to treat hypoxia and control sickling. Because respiratory failure is the most common cause of death, the nurse should be vigilant in assessing for any changes in respiratory status. Rest may be encouraged to reduce metabolic requirements, and deep-vein thrombosis prophylaxis (using anticoagulants) should be prescribed. Fluids and electrolytes are administered to reduce blood viscosity and maintain renal function. Priapism is managed with pain medication, fluids, and nifedipine. If it does not resolve within a few hours, a urologist may inject the corpus cavernosum with a dilute solution of epinephrine to preserve penile function.

Transfusion therapy is indicated when an aplastic crisis occurs; aggressive total RBC exchange transfusion programs may be implemented for patients who have frequent crises, serious complications such as acute chest syndrome or a brain stroke, or both. These patients, like those with thalassemia major, may require chelation therapy to reduce transfusion-produced iron overload.

Undertreatment of sickle cell pain is a major problem. Lack of understanding can lead health care providers to underestimate how much pain these patients suffer. Because of their prior opioid treatment, patients with SCD may be tolerant, and thus large doses may be needed to reduce pain to an acceptable level. During an acute crisis, optimal pain management usually includes large doses of continuous opioid analgesics along with breakthrough analgesia, often in the form of patient-controlled analgesia (PCA). (PCA is discussed in Chapter 10.)

Because patients may experience different types and sites of pain, a multimodal and multidisciplinary approach to pain management is often needed. Adjunctive measures, such as nonsteroidal anti-inflammatory agents, antineuropathic pain medications (e.g., tricyclic antidepressants, antiseizure medications), local anaesthetics, nerve blocks, transelectrodermal nerve stimulator (transcutaneous electrical nerve stimulation [TENS]), acupuncture, or some combination of these strategies may be used.

Although pain is the most common symptom in patients with SCD seeking medical care, infection is a frequent complication and must be treated. Infections, such as chronic leg ulcers, may be treated with rest, antibiotics, warm saline soaks, debridement, or grafting if necessary. Patients with acute chest syndrome are treated with broad-spectrum antibiotics, O_2 therapy, fluid

therapy, and possibly exchange transfusion. Blood transfusions have little, if any, role in the treatment between crises because patients develop antibodies to RBCs and iron overload. However, because chronic hemolysis results in increased utilization of folic acid stores, routine folic acid supplements should be taken.

Although many antisickling drugs have been tried, hydroxyurea (Hydrea) is the only one that has been shown to be clinically beneficial. This drug increases the production of fetal hemoglobin (HbF), decreases the reactive neutrophil count, increases erythrocyte volume and hydration, and alters the adhesion of sickle erythrocytes to the endothelium. The increase in HbF is accompanied by a reduction in hemolysis, an increase in Hb concentration, and a decrease in sickled cells and painful crises (Yawn, Buchanan, Afenyi-Annan, et al., 2014).

Bone marrow transplantation is the only available treatment that can cure some patients with SCD; however, it is very rarely done in Canada. The selection of appropriate recipients, the scarcity of appropriate donors, the risks involved, and the high cost/benefit ratio limit the use of bone marrow transplantation for SCD. (Bone marrow transplants are discussed in Chapter 18.) Patient teaching and support are important in the long-term care of the patient with SCD. The patient and family must understand the basis of the disease and the reasons for supportive care and ongoing screening pertinent to SCD patients, such as eye examinations. The patient must be taught ways to avoid crises, which include taking steps to avoid dehydration and reducing the chance of developing hypoxia (for example, by avoiding high altitudes and seeking medical attention quickly to counteract problems such as upper respiratory tract infections). Education on pain control is also needed because the pain during a crisis may be severe and often requires considerable analgesia. There are several smartphone applications that may help patients and support self-care. For example, a free iPhone app called sickleWell helps with maintaining medication adherence and provides information about symptoms and interventions.

Recurrent episodes of severe acute pain and unrelenting chronic pain can be profoundly disabling and depressing. Occupational therapists and physiotherapists can help the patient achieve optimum physical functioning and independence; a psychologist may be able to use cognitive–behavioural therapy to help patients with SCD cope with anxiety and depression; support groups may also be helpful. Because there are often such additional quality-of-life issues, the nurse can play an important role in ensuring that the patient's needs are met through appropriate referrals.

ACQUIRED HEMOLYTIC ANEMIA

Acquired hemolytic anemia results from hemolysis of RBCs from extrinsic factors. These factors can be separated into three categories: (a) physical destruction, (b) immune reactions, and (c) infectious agents and toxins (see Table 33-2).

Physical destruction of RBCs results from the exertion of extreme force on the cells. Traumatic events causing disruption of the RBC membrane include hemodialysis, extracorporeal circulation used in cardiopulmonary bypass, and prosthetic heart valves. In addition, the force needed to push blood through abnormal vessels, such as those that have been burned, radiated, or affected by vascular disease (e.g., diabetes mellitus) may also physically damage RBCs. RBCs can also be fragmented and destroyed as they try to pass through abnormal arterial or venous microcirculation. The RBCs are sheared as they try to pass by

🧬 **GENETICS IN CLINICAL PRACTICE**

Sickle Cell Disease

Genetic Basis
- Autosomal recessive disorder (see Chapter 15, Figure 15-8)
- Mutation in beta-globin gene *(HBB)*; sickle hemoglobin (HbS) on chromosome 11
- Various versions of beta globin result in different mutations in the *HBB* gene
- HbS variant involves substitution of valine for glutamic acid in the beta-globin gene

Incidence
- Most common inherited blood disorder in Canada
- More commonly affects people of African descent
- Also affects people of Mediterranean, Caribbean, South and Central American, Arabian, and Middle Eastern descent
- Affects 8 of every 100 000 people

Genetic Testing
- DNA testing is available.
- Electrophoresis of hemoglobin and sickling screening test are more commonly used.

Clinical Implications
- SCD requires ongoing continuity of care and extensive patient education.
- Sickle cell trait is the carrier state for SCD and represents a mild type of sickle cell disease.
- If both parents have the trait, there is a one in four chance that their child will have SCD.
- Management of SCD should focus on the prevention of sickle cell crisis.
- Genetic counselling is recommended for individuals with a family history of SCD; individuals should understand the risks of transmitting the genetic mutation.

SCD, sickle cell disease.

ETHICAL DILEMMAS

Pain Management

Situation

A 21-year-old man is admitted to the emergency department in sickle cell crisis with complaints of excruciating pain. He is known to several of the nurses and health care providers in the department. One of the nurses remarks that it must be time for his "fix" of pain medications.

Important Points for Consideration
- The experience of pain is subjective, and experts in pain management agree that "pain is what the patient says it is." The single most reliable indicator of pain is self-report.
- Pain can have serious and debilitating physical and psychological effects. The best possible pain relief should be provided in all circumstances.
- Previous episodes of acute pain or a history of chronic pain can alter physiological and psychological responses to pain and to pain medication. Care should be provided in consultation with the patient and should take into account the patient's history.
- People with pain are often stigmatized because of health care providers' lack of knowledge about pain and about long-term use of opioids or other pain medications. Competent and compassionate care should be provided to all patients.

Clinical Decision-Making Questions
1. How can the nurse educate peers regarding pain assessment and management?
2. What important factors would need to be included in the nurse's assessment and management in consultation with the patient?

excessive platelet aggregation or fibrin polymer formation, such as seen in thrombotic thrombo-cytopenic purpura (TTP) and disseminated intravascular coagulation (DIC).

Antibodies may destroy RBCs by the mechanisms involved in antigen–antibody reactions. The reactions may be of an isoimmune or autoimmune type. *Isoimmune reactions* occur when antibodies develop against antigens from another individual of the same species—in the case of humans, that is, from another person. Blood transfusion reactions typify this response, when the recipient's antibodies hemolyze donor cells.

Autoimmune reactions result when individuals develop antibodies against their own RBCs. Autoimmune hemolytic reactions may be idiopathic, developing with no prior hemolytic history as a result of the immunoglobulin G (IgG) covering the RBCs, or secondary to other autoimmune diseases (e.g., systemic lupus erythematosus), leukemia, or lymphoma, or reactions to drugs (penicillin, ibuprofen, metformin).

Infectious agents and toxins constitute the third category of acquired hemolytic disorders. Infectious agents foster hemolysis in three ways: (a) by invading the RBC and destroying its contents (e.g., parasites such as in malaria); (b) by releasing hemolytic substances (e.g., *Clostridium perfringens*); and (c) by generating an antigen–antibody reaction (e.g., *Mycoplasma pneumonia*). Various agents may be toxic to RBCs and cause hemolysis. These hemolytic toxins involve chemicals such as oxidative drugs, arsenic, lead, copper, bee stings, and snake venom.

Laboratory findings in hemolytic anemia are presented in Table 33-6. Treatment and management of acquired hemolytic anemias involve general supportive care until the causative agent can be eliminated or at least rendered less injurious to the RBCs. Because a hemolytic crisis is a potential consequence, the nurse must be ready to institute appropriate emergent therapy. This includes aggressive hydration and electrolyte replacement to reduce the risk for kidney injury caused by hemoglobin's clogging the kidney tubules and, subsequently, shock. Additional supportive care may include administering corticosteroids and blood products or removing the spleen. For chronic hemolytic anemia, folate may have to be replaced. To suppress the RBC destruction, immuno-suppressive drugs such as rituximab (Rituxan) may be used.

HEMOCHROMATOSIS

Hemochromatosis is an iron overload disorder. Although it is primarily caused by a genetic defect, hemochromatosis occurs secondary to diseases such as sideroblastic anemia. It may also be caused by liver disease and the multiple blood transfusions that are used to treat thalassemia and SCD.

The genetic disorder *(hereditary hemochromatosis)* is autosomal recessive and characterized by increased intestinal iron absorption and, as a result, increased tissue iron deposition (see the "Genetics in Clinical Practice" box). In Canada, it is one of the most common genetic disorders (Canadian Hemochromatosis Society, 2013). It most affects Canadians of Northern European descent, with an incidence of 1 in 300. One in 250 to 300 Canadians is at risk of developing the full-blown disease (homozygous with two recessive genes), and approximately one in nine is a potential carrier with one recessive gene (Canadian Hemochromatosis Society, 2013).

The normal range for total body iron is 2 to 6 g. Individuals with hemochromatosis accumulate iron at a rate of 0.5 to 1.0 g each year and may accumulate total iron concentrations exceeding

50 g. Symptoms of hemochromatosis usually develop between 40 and 60 years of age. Early symptoms are nonspecific and include fatigue, arthralgia, erectile dysfunction, abdominal pain, and weight loss. Later, the excess iron accumulates in the liver and causes liver enlargement and eventually cirrhosis. Patients with hemochromatosis are at increased risk for hepato-cellular carcinoma. Other organs also become affected, resulting in

GENETICS IN CLINICAL PRACTICE

Hemochromatosis

Genetic Basis
- Autosomal recessive disorder
- Caused by mutations in *HAMP, HFE, HFE2, SLC40A1,* and *TFR2* genes
- These genes play an important role in regulating the absorption, transport, and storage of iron
- Mutations in these genes impair the control of the iron absorption during digestion and alter the distribution of iron to other parts of the body; as a result, iron accumulates in tissues and organs

Incidence
- Most common genetic disease in people of European ancestry
- Affects approximately 1 in 300 Canadians of Northern European ancestry
- Very low prevalence in other ethnic populations

Genetic Testing
- Genetic testing is recommended for all first-degree relatives of people with the disease.
- Useful diagnostic tests include serum iron concentration, total iron-binding capacity, and transferrin saturation.
- Liver biopsy, once considered the gold standard diagnostic test, is primarily used to quantify iron deposition and estimate the prognosis and extent of the disease.

Clinical Implications
- Early treatment can prevent serious complications.
- Clinical expression is variable depending on dietary iron, blood loss, and other modifying factors.
- If untreated, progressive iron deposits can lead to multiple organ failure.

diabetes mellitus, skin pigment changes (bronzing), cardiac changes (e.g., cardiomyopathy), arthritis, and testicular atrophy. Physical examination reveals an enlarged liver and spleen and pigmentation changes in the skin. Laboratory values demonstrate an elevated serum iron, TIBC, and serum ferritin. Testing for known genetic mutations confirms the diagnosis. A liver biopsy can quantify the amount of iron and is the definitive way to establish the diagnosis.

The goal of treatment is to remove excess iron from the body and minimize any symptoms the patient may have. Iron removal is achieved by removing 500 mL of blood each week for 2 to 3 years until the iron stores in the body are depleted. Then, less frequent removal of blood is needed to maintain iron levels within normal limits. Iron chelating agents, which form a complex with iron and promote its excretion from the body, may also be used to remove excess iron.

Management of organ involvement (e.g., diabetes mellitus, HF) is the same as conventional treatment for these problems. Dietary modifications, such as avoidance of vitamin C and iron supplements, uncooked seafood, and iron-rich foods, may also assist in the reduction of iron accumulation.

The most common causes of death in people with hemochromatosis are cirrhosis, liver failure, hepatic carcinoma, and cardiac failure. With early diagnosis and treatment, life expectancy is normal. However, many cases go undetected and untreated.

POLYCYTHEMIA

Polycythemia is an abnormal condition characterized by increased RBCs. This increase in RBCs can be so great that blood circulation is impaired as a result of the increased blood viscosity (*hyperviscosity*) and volume (*hypervolemia*).

Etiology and Pathophysiology

The two types of polycythemia are primary polycythemia (or *polycythemia vera*) and secondary polycythemia (Figure 33-4). Their etiologies and pathogenesis differ, although their complications and clinical manifestations are similar. Polycythemia vera is considered a myeloproliferative disorder arising from a chromosomal mutation (e.g., Janus kinase 2 [JAK2]) in a single

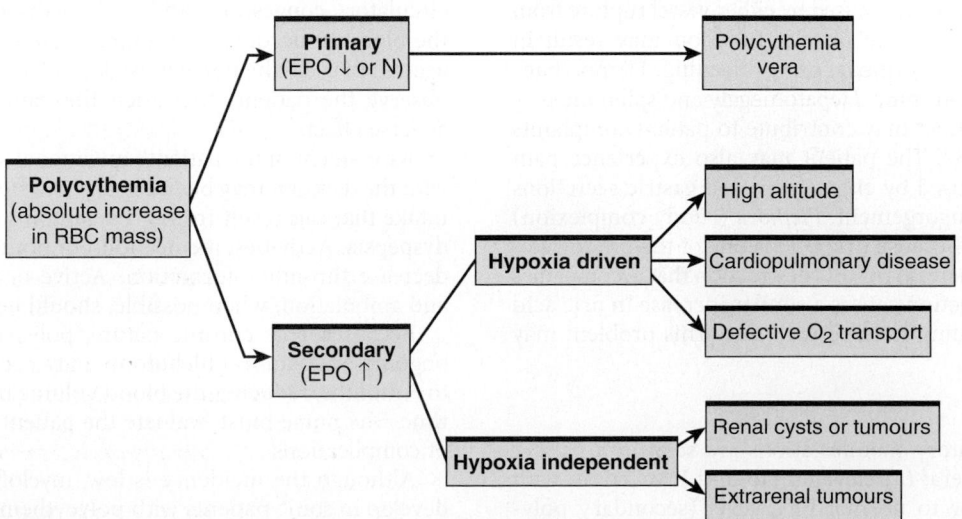

FIGURE 33-4 Differentiating between primary and secondary polycythemia. *EPO,* erythropoietin; *N,* normal; *O₂,* oxygen; *RBC,* red blood cell.

pluripotent stem cell. Therefore, not only are RBCs involved but also granulocytes and platelets, leading to increased production of each of these blood cells. The disease develops insidiously and follows a chronic, vacillating course. The median age at diagnosis is 60 years old, and it has a slight male predominance. With polycythemia vera, the patient has enhanced blood viscosity and blood volume and congestion of organs and tissues with blood. These patients have hypercoagulopathies, which predispose them to clotting. Splenomegaly and hepatomegaly are common.

Secondary polycythemia can be either hypoxia driven or hypoxia independent. In the former, hypoxia stimulates erythropoietin (EPO) production in the kidney, which in turn stimulates RBC production. The need for O_2 may be because of high altitude, pulmonary disease, cardiovascular disease, alveolar hypoventilation, defective O_2 transport, or tissue hypoxia. EPO levels may return to normal once the Hb is stabilized at a higher level. In this situation, secondary polycythemia is a physiological response in which the body tries to compensate for a problem rather than a pathological response. (Hypoxia-driven polycythemia is discussed in the section on chronic obstructive pulmonary disease in Chapter 31.) In hypoxia-independent secondary polycythemia, EPO is produced by malignant or benign tumour tissue. Serum EPO levels often remain elevated in these situations. Splenomegaly does not accompany secondary polycythemia.

Clinical Manifestations and Complications

Circulatory manifestations of polycythemia vera occur because of the hypertension caused by hypervolemia and hyperviscosity. They are often the first symptoms and include subjective complaints of headache, vertigo, dizziness, tinnitus, and visual disturbances. Generalized pruritus (often exacerbated by a hot bath) may be a striking symptom and is related to histamine release from an increased number of basophils. Paresthesias and *erythromelalgia* (painful burning and redness of the hands and feet caused by paroxysmal peripheral dilation of peripheral blood vessels) may also be present. In addition, the patient may experience angina, HF, intermittent claudication, and thrombo-phlebitis, which may be complicated by embolization. These manifestations are caused by blood vessel distension, impaired blood flow, circulatory stasis, thrombosis, and tissue hypoxia caused by the hypervolemia and hyperviscosity. The most common serious complication is stroke secondary to thrombosis.

Hemorrhagic phenomena caused by either vessel rupture from overdistension or inadequate platelet function may result in petechiae, ecchymoses, epistaxis, or GI bleeding. Hemorrhage can be acute and catastrophic. Hepatomegaly and splenomegaly from organ engorgement may contribute to patient complaints of satiety and fullness. The patient may also experience pain from peptic ulcer caused by either increased gastric secretions or liver and spleen engorgement. *Plethora* (ruddy complexion) may also be present. Because uric acid is one of the products of cell destruction, the increase in RBC destruction that accompanies excessive RBC production causes a similar increase in uric acid production, thus leading to hyperuricemia. This problem may cause a form of gout.

Diagnostic Studies

The following laboratory manifestations are seen in a patient with polycythemia vera: (a) elevated Hb and RBC count with microcytosis; (b) low to normal EPO level (secondary polycythemia will have a high level); (c) elevated WBC count with basophilia; (d) elevated platelets (thrombo-cytosis) and platelet dysfunction; (e) elevated leukocyte alkaline phosphatase, uric acid, and cobalamin levels; and (f) elevated histamine levels. Bone marrow examination in polycythemia vera shows hypercellularity of RBCs, WBCs, and platelets. Splenomegaly is found in 90% of patients with primary polycythemia but does not accompany secondary polycythemia.

Collaborative Care

Treatment is directed toward reducing blood volume and viscosity and bone marrow activity. Phlebotomy is the mainstay of treatment. The aim of phlebotomy is to reduce the Hct and keep it less than 45% to 48%. Generally, from the time of diagnosis, 300 to 500 mL of blood may be removed every other day until the Hct is reduced to normal levels. An individual managed with repeated phlebotomies eventually becomes deficient in iron, although this effect is rarely symptomatic. Iron supplementation should be avoided. Hydration therapy is used to reduce the blood's viscosity. Myelosuppressive agents such as busulphan (Myleran) and hydroxyurea (Hydrea) may be given to inhibit bone marrow activity. Interferon alfa may be used in high-risk patients. Targeted therapies such as ruxolitinib (Jakavi), which targets the JAK2 mutation, may be used (Griesshammer, Gisslinger, & Mesa, 2015). Antiplatelet agents, such as acetylsalicylic acid (ASA; Aspirin), may also be used for erythromelalgia or antithrombotic primary prophylaxis. Allopurinol may reduce the number of acute gout attacks, and antihistamines may be used to alleviate pruritus. Anagrelide (Agrylin) may be used to reduce the platelet count and inhibit platelet aggregation.

NURSING MANAGEMENT POLYCYTHEMIA VERA

Primary polycythemia vera is not preventable. However, because secondary polycythemia is generated by any source of hypoxia, maintaining adequate oxygenation may prevent problems. Therefore, controlling chronic pulmonary disease, stopping smoking, and avoiding high altitudes may be important.

When acute exacerbations of polycythemia vera develop, the nurse has several responsibilities. Depending on the institution's policies, the nurse may assist with or perform the phlebotomy. Fluid intake and output must be evaluated during hydration therapy to avoid fluid overload (which further complicates the circulatory congestion) and underhydration (which can cause the blood to become even more viscous). If myelosuppressive agents are used, the nurse must administer the drugs as ordered, observe the patient, and teach the patient about medication adverse effects.

Assessment of the patient's nutritional status in collaboration with the dietitian may be necessary to offset the inadequate food intake that can result from GI symptoms of fullness, pain, and dyspepsia. Activities, medications, or both must be instituted to decrease thrombus formation. Active or passive leg exercises and ambulation, when possible, should be initiated.

Because of its chronic nature, polycythemia vera requires ongoing evaluation. Phlebotomy may need to be done every 2 to 3 months, reducing the blood volume by about 500 mL each time. The nurse must evaluate the patient for the development of complications.

Although the incidence is low, myelofibrosis and leukemia develop in some patients with polycythemia vera (10% and 5%, respectively). These occurrences may be caused by the chemotherapeutic drugs used to treat the disease, or they may be secondary to a disorder in the stem cells that progresses to erythroleukemia.

PROBLEMS OF HEMOSTASIS

Hemostasis involves the vascular endothelium, platelets, and coagulation factors, which normally function together to stop hemorrhage and repair vascular injury. (These mechanisms are described in Chapter 32.) Disruption in any of these components may result in bleeding or thrombotic disorders.

Three major disorders of hemostasis discussed in this section are (a) thrombo-cytopenia (low platelet count), (b) hemophilia and von Willebrand disease (inherited disorders of specific clotting factors), and (c) disseminated intravascular coagulation (DIC).

THROMBO-CYTOPENIA

Etiology and Pathophysiology

Thrombo-cytopenia is a reduction of platelets to an amount below 150×10^9/L or 150 000/mcL. Acute, severe, or prolonged decreases from this normal range can result in abnormal hemostasis that manifests as prolonged bleeding from minor trauma to spontaneous bleeding without injury.

Platelet disorders can be inherited (e.g., Wiskott–Aldrich syndrome), but the vast majority are acquired (Table 33-12). A common cause of acquired abnormalities is the ingestion of certain foods, herbs, or drugs. Although some drugs are directly myelosuppressive (e.g., chemotherapeutic drugs, ganciclovir

---

TABLE 33-12 CAUSES OF THROMBO-CYTOPENIA

Inherited
- Fanconi's syndrome (pancytopenia)
- Hereditary thrombo-cytopenia

Acquired
Immune
- Immune thrombo-cytopenic purpura (ITP)
- Neonatal alloimmune thrombo-cytopenia

Nonimmune
- Shortened circulation
  - Thrombotic thrombo-cytopenic purpura (TTP)
  - Disseminated intravascular coagulation (DIC)
  - Heparin-induced thrombo-cytopenia (HIT)
  - Splenomegaly, splenic sequestration
- Turbulent blood flow (hemangiomas, abnormal cardiac valves, intra-aortic balloon pumps)
- Decreased production
  - Drug-induced marrow suppression
  - Chemotherapy
  - Viral infections (hepatitis C virus, HIV, cytomegalovirus)
  - Bacterial infection (sepsis)
  - Alcohol use disorder
  - Bone marrow suppression
  - Myelodysplastic syndrome (MDS)
  - Myelofibrosis
  - Aplastic anemia
  - Hematological malignancy (leukemias, lymphomas, myeloma)
  - Solid tumour infiltrating bone marrow
  - Radiation to the bone

HIV, human immunodeficiency virus.

[Cytovene]), the usual mechanism of acquired thrombo-cytopenia is accelerated platelet destruction caused by drug-dependent antibodies. Antibodies attack the platelets when the offending agent binds to a platelet surface glycoprotein.

A careful review of the patient's history can help to identify the causes of thrombo-cytopenia. For example, quinine may cause thrombo-cytopenia and is found in tonic water and in many herbal preparations. In addition, some drugs can affect platelet aggregation. ASA doses as low as 81 mg (a baby Aspirin) can alter the function of circulating platelets. Normal function is restored with the generation of newly formed platelets.

Immune Thrombo-Cytopenic Purpura. The most common acquired thrombo-cytopenia is a syndrome of abnormal destruction of circulating platelets termed *immune thrombo-cytopenic purpura* (ITP). It was originally termed *idiopathic thrombo-cytopenic purpura* because its cause was unknown. However, it is now known that ITP is an autoimmune disease. In ITP, platelets are coated with antibodies. Although these platelets function normally, when they reach the spleen, the antibody-coated platelets are recognized as foreign and are destroyed by macrophages.

Platelets normally survive 8 to 10 days. However, in ITP, survival of platelets is only 1 to 3 days. Generally, the clinical syndrome manifests as an acute condition in children and a chronic condition in adults.

Thrombotic Thrombo-Cytopenic Purpura. *Thrombotic thrombo-cytopenic purpura* (TTP) is an uncommon syndrome characterized by hemolytic anemia, thrombo-cytopenia, neurological abnormalities, fever (in the absence of infection), and renal abnormalities. Not all features are present in all patients. Because it is almost always associated with hemolytic–uremic syndrome (HUS), it is often referred to as TTP–HUS. The disease is associated with enhanced agglutination of platelets, which form microthrombi that deposit in arterioles and capillaries. In most cases, the syndrome is due to the deficiency of a plasma enzyme (ADAMTS-13) that usually breaks down the von Willebrand clotting factor (vWF) into normal size. (vWF is the most important protein that mediates platelet adhesion to damaged endothelial cells.) Without the enzyme, unusually large amounts of vWF attach to activated platelets, thereby promoting platelet aggregation.

TTP is seen primarily in adults between 20 and 50 years of age and has a slight female predominance. The syndrome may be idiopathic (thought to be due to an autoimmune disorder against ADAMTS-13); may be caused by certain drug toxicities, pregnancy, or infection; or may be the result of a known autoimmune disorder such as systemic lupus erythematosus or scleroderma (McCrae, Sadler, & Cines, 2013). TTP is a medical emergency because bleeding and clotting occur simultaneously.

Heparin-Induced Thrombo-Cytopenia and Thrombosis Syndrome. One of the risks associated with the broad and increasing use of heparin is the development of the life-threatening condition called *heparin-induced thrombo-cytopenia* (HIT), also called *heparin-induced thrombo-cytopenia and thrombosis syndrome* (HITTS). Typically, patients develop thrombo-cytopenia 5 to 10 days after the onset of heparin therapy. HIT should be suspected if the platelet count falls by more than 50% or falls below 150×10^9/L. As many as 3% of patients on heparin therapy develop HIT (Warkentin, 2013).

The major clinical problem of HITTS is venous thrombosis; arterial thrombosis can also develop. Deep venous thromboses and pulmonary emboli most commonly result as a complication

FIGURE 33-5 Acute idiopathic thrombo-cytopenic purpura commonly manifests with purpuric lesions of this kind, although they may often be widespread by the time medical attention is sought. Source: Forbes, C. D., & Jackson, W. F. (2003). *Color atlas and text of clinical medicine* (3rd ed., p. 437). London: Mosby.

FIGURE 33-6 Severe ecchymosis of the left hand.

of the thromboses. Additional complications may include arterial vascular infarcts resulting in skin necrosis, stroke, and end-organ damage.

In HIT, platelet destruction and vascular endothelial injury are the two major responses to what is believed to be an immune-mediated response to heparin. Platelet factor 4 (PF4) binds to heparin. This complex then binds to the platelet surface, leading to further platelet activation and release of more PF4, thus creating a positive feedback loop. Antibodies are created against this complex, and they are removed prematurely from circulation, leading to thrombo-cytopenia and platelet-fibrin thrombi. Platelet aggregation also induces heparin to be neutralized. Thus, more heparin is required to maintain therapeutic activated partial thromboplastin times (aPTTs).

Clinical Manifestations. Many patients with thrombo-cytopenia are asymptomatic. The most common symptom is bleeding, usually mucosal or cutaneous. Mucosal bleeding may manifest as epistaxis and gingival bleeding, and large bullous hemorrhages may appear on the buccal mucosa owing to the lack of vessel protection afforded by the submucosal tissue. Bleeding into the skin is manifested as petechiae or superficial ecchymoses (Figure 33-5).

Petechiae are small, flat, pinpoint, red or reddish-brown microhemorrhages. When the platelet count is low, RBCs may leak out of the blood vessels and into the skin to cause petechiae. When petechiae are numerous, the resulting reddish skin bruise is called *purpura* (see Figure 33-5). Larger purplish lesions caused by hemorrhage are termed *ecchymoses* (Figure 33-6). Ecchymoses may be flat or raised; pain and tenderness sometimes are present.

Prolonged bleeding after routine procedures such as venipuncture or IM injection may also indicate thrombo-cytopenia. Because the bleeding may be internal, the nurse must be aware of manifestations that reflect this type of blood loss, including weakness, fainting, dizziness, tachycardia, abdominal pain, and hypotension.

The major complication of thrombo-cytopenia is hemorrhage. The hemorrhage may be insidious or acute and internal or external. It may occur in any area of the body, including the joints, retina, and brain. Cerebral hemorrhage may be fatal in people with ITP. Insidious hemorrhage may first be detected by discovering the anemia that accompanies blood loss.

Diagnostic Studies

The platelet count is decreased in cases of thrombo-cytopenia. Any reduction below 150×10^9/L or 150000/mcL may be termed *thrombo-cytopenia*. However, prolonged bleeding from trauma or injury does not usually occur until platelet counts are less than 50×10^9/L or 50000/mcL. When the count drops below 10×10^9/L or 10000/mcL, spontaneous, life-threatening hemorrhages (e.g., intracranial bleeding) can occur. Platelet transfusions are generally not recommended until the count is below 10×10^9/L unless the patient is actively bleeding or critically ill with fever or sepsis.

The patient's medical history and clinical examination, along with comparisons of laboratory parameters, help to determine the etiology of the thrombo-cytopenia. Table 33-13 compares the types of thrombo-cytopenia.

Laboratory tests that assess secondary hemostasis or coagulation, such as the prothrombin time (PT) and aPTT, can yield normal results even in severe thrombo-cytopenia. Elevated values may point toward DIC. Specific assays, such as the ITP antigen-specific assay, platelet activation/function assay, or PF4–heparin complex for HIT, can be done to assist with the diagnosis. In TTP, testing for deficiency of ADAMTS-13 is not always diagnostic, so an increase of lactic dehydrogenase (LDH) is used to help establish the diagnosis. When thrombo-cytopenia occurs with anemia characterized by altered RBC morphology, including *spherocytes* (small, globular, completely hemoglobinated erythrocytes), fragmented cells *(schistocytes)*, and pronounced reticulocytosis, a diagnosis of TTP should be suspected. These findings are partially a result of intravascular fibrin deposition causing a "slicing" of RBCs. In TTP, thrombo-cytopenia may be severe, but coagulation studies are normal.

Examination of the peripheral blood smear may help distinguish acquired disorders such as ITP and TTP from congenital disorders, which may be indicated by abnormally sized platelets. Bone marrow examination is done to rule out production problems as the cause of thrombo-cytopenia (e.g., leukemia, aplastic anemia, other myeloproliferative disorders). It is performed if the other tests are inconclusive, especially in older patients suspected of having an underlying bone marrow disorder. When destruction of circulating platelets is the cause, bone marrow analysis shows *megakaryocytes* (precursors of platelets) to be normal or increased, even though circulating platelets are reduced. The absence or decreased numbers of megakaryocytes on bone marrow biopsy is consistent with thrombo-cytopenia caused by decreased bone marrow production (e.g., aplastic anemia).

TABLE 33-13 COMPARISON OF DISORDERS CAUSING THROMBO-CYTOPENIA

Laboratory Test	ITP	TTP	HIT	DIC
Platelets	↓↓↓	↓↓↓	↓↓	↓↓↓
Hemolysis				
Hb	N	↓↓	N	N, ↓
LDH	N	↑↑↑	N	↑
Reticulocytes	N	↑	N	N, ↑
Haptoglobin	N	↓	N	↓
Indirect bilirubin	N	↑	N	N, ↑
Schistocytes	N	↑↑↑	N, ↑	N, ↑
Coagulopathy				
PT	N	N	N	↑
aPTT	N	N	N	↑
D-dimer	N	N, ↑	↑	↑↑
Other Tests	ITP platelet antigen-specific assay; platelet activation/function assay, *Helicobacter pylori*, bone marrow biopsy	ADAMTS-13	Platelet activation/function assay PF4–heparin complex	

aPTT, activated partial thromboplastin time; *DIC*, disseminated intravascular coagulation; *Hb*, hemoglobin; *HIT*, heparin-induced thrombo-cytopenia; *ITP*, idiopathic thrombo-cytopenic purpura; *LDH*, lactic dehydrogenase; *N*, normal; *PF4*, platelet factor 4; ↑, increased; ↓, decreased; *PT*, prothrombin time; *TTP*, thrombotic thrombo-cytopenic purpura.

TABLE 33-14 COLLABORATIVE CARE

Thrombo-Cytopenia

Diagnostic
- History and physical examination
- Bone marrow aspiration and biopsy
- CBC including platelet count
- Specific laboratory studies

Collaborative Therapy
Immune Thrombo-Cytopenic Purpura
- Corticosteroids
- Intravenous immunoglobulin (IVIG)
- Anti-Rho(D)
- Romiplostim (Nplate)
- Eltrombopag (Revolade)
- Tranexamic acid
- Platelet transfusions (if life-threatening)
- Vaccination (pneumococcal, meningococcal, *Haemophilus influenzae* B)
- Danazol (Cyclomen)
- Immuno-suppressives (e.g., rituximab [Rituxan], cyclosporin)
- High-dose cyclophosphamide (Procytox) or combination chemotherapy
- Splenectomy

Thrombotic Thrombo-Cytopenic Purpura
- Identification and treatment of cause
- Plasmapheresis (plasma exchange)
- High-dose corticosteroids
- Splenectomy
- Chemotherapy (e.g., vincristine, vinblastine)
- Immuno-suppressives (e.g., cyclophosphamide [Procytox], rituximab [Rituxan])

Heparin-Induced Thrombo-Cytopenia
- Discontinuation of heparin
- Direct thrombin inhibitor (e.g., dabigatran [Pradaxa])
- Indirect thrombin inhibitor (e.g., fondaparinux [Arixtra])
- Plasmapheresis (plasma exchange)
- Warfarin (Coumadin)
- Thrombolytic agents

Decreased Platelet Production
- Identification and treatment of cause
- Corticosteroids
- Platelet transfusions

CBC, complete blood count.

Collaborative Care

Collaborative care of thrombo-cytopenia differs according to the etiology of the thrombo-cytopenia. Discussion of management strategies for these different etiologies appears in Table 33-14.

Immune Thrombo-Cytopenic Purpura. Multiple therapies are used to manage the patient with ITP. If the patient is asymptomatic, therapy may not be used unless the patient's platelet count is less than 10×10^9/L or 10 000/mcL. Corticosteroids (e.g., prednisone) are used to treat ITP because of their ability to suppress the phagocytic response of splenic macrophages. This suppression alters the spleen's recognition of platelets and increases the lifespan of the platelets. In addition, corticosteroids depress antibody formation and reduce capillary leakage.

Splenectomy is indicated if the patient does not respond to prednisone initially or requires unacceptably high doses to maintain an adequate platelet count. A splenectomy results in a complete or partial remission in approximately 60% to 70% of patients. The effectiveness of splenectomy is based on four factors. First, the spleen contains an abundance of the macrophages that sequester and destroy platelets. Second, structural features of the spleen enhance the interaction between antibody-coated platelets and macrophages. Third, some antibody synthesis occurs in the spleen; thus, antiplatelet antibodies decrease after splenectomy. Fourth, the spleen normally sequesters approximately one-third of the platelets, so its removal increases the number of platelets in circulation.

High doses of IV immunoglobulin (IVIG) and a component of IVIG, anti-Rho(D) (anti-D, WinRho), may be used to treat the patient who is unresponsive to corticosteroids or splenectomy. These agents work by competing with the antiplatelet antibodies for macrophage receptors. They effectively raise the platelet count, but the beneficial effects are temporary. Rituximab (Rituxan) may be used for its ability to lyse activated B cells, thereby reducing the immune recognition of platelets.

Romiplostim (Nplate) is used for patients with chronic ITP who have had an insufficient response to the other treatments or who have a contraindication to splenectomy. As a thrombopoietin receptor agonist, this medication increases platelet production. Danazol (Cyclomen), an androgen, may be used along with steroids in some patients. Although the mechanism is not totally understood, danazol reduces the ability of the body to remove antibody-coated platelets from the blood. Immuno-suppressive therapy may be used in refractory cases (see Table 33-14).

Platelet transfusions may be used to increase platelet counts in cases of life-threatening hemorrhage. Platelets should not be given prophylactically because of the possibility of antibody formation. The usual indication for administering platelets is a platelet count less than 10×10^9/L or 10 000/mcL or the presence of bleeding before a procedure.

Thrombotic Thrombo-Cytopenic Purpura. TTP may be treated in a variety of ways. The first step is to treat the underlying disorder (e.g., infection) or to remove the causative agent, if identified. If untreated, TTP usually results in irreversible renal failure and death. Plasma exchange (plasmapheresis) (see Chapter 16) is used to aggressively reverse platelet consumption by supplying the appropriate vWF and enzyme (ADAMTS-13) and removing the large vWF molecules binding with the platelets. Treatment should be continued daily until the patient's counts normalize and hemolysis has ceased. Corticosteroids may be added to this treatment. Monoclonal antibody therapy (e.g., rituximab), immuno-suppressants (e.g., cyclosporine or cyclophosphamide), and splenectomy have also been used with success. The administration of platelets is generally contraindicated because it may lead to new vWF-platelet complexes and increased clotting.

Heparin-Induced Thrombo-Cytopenia and Thrombosis Syndrome. Heparin must be discontinued when HITTS is first recognized, and heparin flushes for vascular catheters should be stopped.

To maintain anticoagulation, the patient should be started on a direct thrombin inhibitor, such as dabigatran (Pradaxa). Warfarin (Coumadin) should be started only when the platelet count has reached 150×10^9/L. If clotting is severe, the most commonly used treatment modalities are plasmapheresis to clear the platelet-aggregating IgG from the blood, protamine sulphate to interrupt the circulating heparin, thrombolytic agents to treat the thrombo-embolic events, and surgery to remove clots. Platelet transfusions are not effective because they may enhance thrombo-embolic events. Patients who have had HITTS should never be given heparin or low-molecular-weight heparin.

Acquired Thrombo-Cytopenia From Decreased Platelet Production. The management of acquired thrombo-cytopenia is based on identifying the cause and treating the disease or removing the causative agent. If the precipitating factor is unknown, the patient may receive corticosteroids. Platelet transfusions are given if life-threatening hemorrhage develops. Splenectomy is not used because the spleen does not contribute to this type of thrombo-cytopenia.

Often, acquired thrombo-cytopenia is caused by another underlying condition (e.g., aplastic anemia, leukemia) or therapy used to treat another problem. For example, in acute leukemia, all blood cell types may be depressed. In addition, the patient may receive chemotherapeutic drugs that cause bone marrow suppression. If the patient can be adequately supported throughout the course of chemotherapy-induced thrombo-cytopenia, the thrombo-cytopenia will also resolve.

NURSING MANAGEMENT
THROMBO-CYTOPENIA

NURSING ASSESSMENT

Subjective and objective data that should be obtained from a patient with thrombo-cytopenia are presented in Table 33-15.

NURSING DIAGNOSES

Nursing diagnoses for the patient with thrombo-cytopenia may include but are not limited to the following:

- *Risk for impaired oral mucous membrane integrity* as evidenced by *decrease in platelets and treatment regimen*
- *Risk for bleeding* as evidenced by *inherent coagulopathy*

TABLE 33-15 NURSING ASSESSMENT
Thrombo-Cytopenia

Subjective Data
Important Health Information
Past health history: Recent hemorrhage, excessive bleeding, or viral illness; HIV infection; cancer (especially leukemia or lymphoma); aplastic anemia; systemic lupus erythematosus; cirrhosis; exposure to radiation or toxic chemicals; disseminated intravascular coagulation; family history of bleeding problems
Medications: e.g., chemotherapeutic drugs, furosemide, gold, penicillin
Surgeries or other treatments: Recent surgery, splenectomy

Symptoms
- Bleeding gingiva; coffee-ground or bloody vomitus; epistaxis; hemoptysis; easy bruising, hematuria; dark or bloody stools; menorrhagia, metrorrhagia
- Headache; fatigue, weakness, general malaise; fainting
- Dyspnea
- Fever

Objective Data
General
Fever, lethargy

Integumentary
Petechiae, ecchymoses, purpura

Gastro-Intestinal
Splenomegaly, abdominal distension, guaiac-positive stools

Possible Findings
Platelet count $<150 \times 10^9$/L (150 000/mcL) or prolonged bleeding time, decreased hemoglobin and hematocrit; normal or increased megakaryocytes in bone marrow examination

HIV, human immunodeficiency virus.

- *Deficient knowledge* related to *insufficient information, insufficient knowledge of resources*

Additional information on nursing diagnoses is presented in NCP 33-2, available on the Evolve website.

PLANNING

The overall goals are that the patient with thrombo-cytopenia will (a) have no gross or occult bleeding, (b) maintain vascular integrity, and (c) manage home care to prevent any complications related to an increased risk for bleeding.

NURSING IMPLEMENTATION

HEALTH PROMOTION. It is important for the nurse to discourage excessive use of over-the-counter medications known to be possible causes of acquired thrombo-cytopenia. Many medications contain ASA (Aspirin) as an ingredient. ASA reduces platelet adhesiveness, thus contributing to bleeding. It is also important for the nurse to encourage people to have a complete medical evaluation if manifestations of bleeding tendencies (e.g., prolonged epistaxis, petechiae) develop. In addition, the nurse must observe for early signs of thrombo-cytopenia in the patient receiving chemotherapeutic drugs.

ACUTE INTERVENTION. The goal during acute episodes of thrombo-cytopenia is to prevent or control hemorrhage (see NCP 33-2 on the Evolve website). In the patient with thrombo-cytopenia, bleeding is usually from superficial sites; deep bleeding (into muscles, joints, and abdomen) usually occurs

TABLE 33-16 PATIENT & CAREGIVER TEACHING GUIDE

Thrombo-Cytopenia

This instruction sheet explains precautions you should take to protect yourself when your platelet count is low. Please make sure to ask your health care provider about specific precautions you should take that relate to your bleeding risk factors.

- Notify your health care provider of any manifestations of bleeding. These include the following:
  - Black, tarry, or bloody bowel movements
  - Black or bloody vomit, sputum, or urine
  - Bruising or small red or purple spots on the skin
  - Bleeding from the mouth or anywhere in the body
  - Headache or changes in how well you can see
  - Difficulty talking, sudden weakness of an arm or leg, confusion
- Ask your health care provider about restrictions in your normal activities, such as vigorous exercise, lifting weights, and so on. Generally, walking can be done safely and should be done while wearing sturdy shoes or slippers. If you are weak and at risk for falling, get help or supervision when getting out of bed.
- Do not blow your nose forcefully; gently pat it with a tissue if needed. For a nosebleed, keep your head up and apply firm pressure to the nostrils and the bridge of your nose. If bleeding continues, place an ice bag over the bridge of your nose and the nape of your neck. If you are unable to stop a nosebleed after 10 minutes, call your health care provider.
- Do not bend down with your head lower than your waist.
- Prevent constipation by drinking plenty of fluids, and do not strain when having a bowel movement. Your health care provider may prescribe a stool softener. Do not use a suppository, an enema, or a rectal thermometer without the permission of your health care provider.
- Shave only with an electric razor; do not use blades.
- Do not pluck your eyebrows or other body hair.
- Do not puncture your skin, such as by getting tattoos or body piercing.
- Avoid using any medication (e.g., ASA [Aspirin]) or herbal product that can prolong clotting time. If you are unsure about a connection between any medication or herbal product and your thrombo-cytopenia, check with your health care provider or pharmacist.
- Use a soft-bristle toothbrush to prevent injuring the gums. Flossing is also usually safe if it is done gently using the thin tape floss. Do not use alcohol-based mouthwashes because they can dry your gums and increase bleeding.
- Women: If you are menstruating, keep track of the number of pads that you use per day. When you start using more pads per day than usual or bleed more days, notify your health care provider. Do not use tampons; use sanitary pads only.
- Ask your health care provider before you have any invasive procedures done, such as a dental cleaning, manicure, or pedicure.

ASA, acetylsalicylic acid.

only when clotting factors are diminished. It is important to emphasize to the patient that a seemingly minor nosebleed or new petechiae may indicate potential hemorrhage and that the health care provider should be notified. Bleeding from the posterior nasopharynx may be difficult to detect because the blood may be swallowed. If a subcutaneous injection is unavoidable, a small-gauge needle should be used and direct pressure applied for at least 5 to 10 minutes after injection; application of an ice pack may also be helpful; IM injections should be avoided. The patient needs to understand the importance of adherence to self-care measures that reduce the risk of bleeding (Table 33-16).

In a woman with thrombo-cytopenia, the amount and duration of menstrual blood loss may exceed the usual. Counting sanitary napkins used during menses is another important intervention to detect excess blood loss. Fifty millilitres of blood will completely soak a sanitary napkin. Suppression of menses with hormonal agents may be indicated during predictable periods of thrombo-cytopenia to reduce blood loss from menses (e.g., during chemotherapy and bone marrow transplantation).

Closely monitor the platelet count, coagulation studies, hemoglobin, and hematocrit. Together these provide important information regarding potential or actual bleeding.

The proper administration of platelet transfusions is an important nursing responsibility. This is discussed under Blood Component Therapy later in this chapter.

AMBULATORY AND HOME CARE. The patient with ITP who is receiving treatment should be monitored for response to therapy. The person with acquired thrombo-cytopenia must be taught to avoid causative agents when possible (see Table 33-12). If the causative agents cannot be avoided (e.g., chemotherapy), the patient should learn to avoid injury or trauma during these periods and to detect the clinical signs and symptoms of bleeding caused by thrombo-cytopenia (see Table 33-16). Patients with either ITP or acquired thrombo-cytopenia should have periodic medical evaluations so the health care provider can assess the patient's status and intercede in situations in which exacerbations and bleeding are likely to occur. The impact of either an acute or a chronic condition on the patient's quality of life should also be addressed appropriately.

EVALUATION. The expected outcomes for the patient with thrombo-cytopenia are presented in NCP 33-2, available on the Evolve website.

HEMOPHILIA AND VON WILLEBRAND DISEASE

Hemophilia is an X-linked recessive genetic disorder caused by defective or deficient coagulation factor (see the "Genetics in Clinical Practice" box later in this chapter, and Figure 15-10). (X-linked genetic disorders are discussed in Chapter 15.) The two major forms of hemophilia, which can occur in mild to severe forms, are hemophilia A (classic hemophilia, factor VIII deficiency) and hemophilia B (Christmas disease, factor IX deficiency); von Willebrand disease is a related disorder involving a deficiency of the von Willebrand coagulation protein. Factor VIII is synthesized in the liver and circulates as a complex with vWF.

Hemophilia A is the most common form of hemophilia, accounting for approximately 80% of all cases. In Canada, both hemophilia A and hemophilia B are rare disorders. About 2 500 Canadians are known to be affected by hemophilia A and about 500 Canadians by hemophilia B. von Willebrand disease is considered the most common congenital bleeding disorder and is estimated to affect as many as 1 in 1 000 Canadians (Canadian Hemophilia Society, 2016). This disease can exist in mild to severe forms; however, life-threatening hemorrhage is rare. The deficiency and inheritance patterns of these three forms of inherited coagulopathies are compared in Table 33-17.

Clinical Manifestations and Complications

Clinical manifestations and complications related to hemophilia include (a) slow, persistent, prolonged bleeding from minor trauma and small cuts; (b) delayed bleeding after minor injuries (the delay may be several hours or days); (c) uncontrollable hemorrhage after dental extractions or irritation of the gingiva with a hard-bristle toothbrush; (d) epistaxis, especially after a

GENETICS IN CLINICAL PRACTICE

Hemophilia A and B

Genetic Basis
- X-linked recessive disorder
- *Hemophilia A:* Caused by mutations in the *F8* gene that provide instructions for making coagulation factor VIII
- *Hemophilia B:* Caused by mutations in the *F9* gene that provides instructions for making coagulation factor IX
- Mutations in the *F8* or *F9* gene lead to the production of an abnormal version of or reduced amounts of these coagulation factors.

Incidence
- *Hemophilia A:* 1 in 5000 to 10 000 male births
- *Hemophilia B:* 1 in 30 000 to 50 000 male births

Genetic Testing
- Possible with DNA technology

Clinical Implications
- Female carriers will transmit the genetic defect to 50% of their sons, and 50% of their daughters will be carriers.
- Men with hemophilia will not transmit the genetic defect to their sons, but all of their daughters will be carriers.
- Female hemophilia can occur if a man with hemophilia mates with a female carrier. However, it is a rare occurrence.
- Clinical manifestations of hemophilias A and B are very similar.
- Replacement therapy is available for factors VIII and IX (see Table 33-19).

FIGURE 33-7 Severe ecchymoses in a person with hemophilia following a fall. Source: Courtesy Peter Bonner.

FIGURE 33-8 Acute hemarthrosis of the knee is a common complication of hemophilia. Source: Forbes, C. D., & Jackson, W. F. (2003). *Color atlas and text of clinical medicine* (3rd ed., p. 441). London: Mosby.

TABLE 33-17   COMPARISON OF TYPES OF HEMOPHILIA

Disorder	Deficiency	Inheritance Pattern
Hemophilia A	Factor VIII	Recessive X-linked (transmitted by female carriers, displayed almost exclusively in men)
Homophilia R	Factor IX	Recessive X-linked (transmitted by female carriers, displayed almost exclusively in men)
von Willebrand disease	vWF; variable factor VIII deficiencies and platelet dysfunction	Autosomal dominant, seen in both genders; Recessive (in severe forms of the disease)

vWF, von Willebrand's factor.

blow to the face; (e) GI bleeding from ulcers and gastritis; (f) hematuria from GU trauma and splenic rupture resulting from falls or abdominal trauma; (g) ecchymoses and subcutaneous hematomas (Figure 33-7); (h) neurological signs, such as pain, anaesthesia, and paralysis, that may develop from nerve compression caused by hematoma formation; and (i) hemarthrosis (bleeding into the joints) (Figure 33-8), which may lead to joint deformity severe enough to cause crippling (most commonly in knees, elbows, shoulders, hips, and ankles).

These symptoms in children may lead to diagnosis during childhood. In adults, these developments may be the first sign of a mild form of the disease that escaped detection because of a childhood free of major injuries, dental procedures, or surgeries. All clinical manifestations relate to bleeding, and any bleeding episode in people with hemophilia may lead to a life-threatening hemorrhage.

Treatment rationales will depend on the severity of the hemophilia and the amount of the respective factor that is missing. About 80% of people with hemophilia have severe disease whereby they will have excessive bleeding after injuries or surgery and can also have spontaneous bleeding episodes. About 10% of people with hemophilia have moderate disease. Another 10% of people with hemophilia have mild disease, which may not even be detected until excessive bleeding is noted after surgery or a severe injury.

Diagnostic Studies

Laboratory studies are used to determine the type of hemophilia present. Any factor deficiency within the intrinsic system (factors VIII, IX, XI, or XII or vWF) will yield the laboratory results presented in Table 33-18.

Collaborative Care

The goals of collaborative care are to prevent and treat bleeding. Collaborative care for people with hemophilia or von Willebrand disease requires (a) preventive care, (b) the use of replacement

TABLE 33-18 LABORATORY RESULTS IN HEMOPHILIA

Test	Comments
Prothrombin time	Normal. No involvement of extrinsic system.
Thrombin time	Normal. No impairment of thrombin–fibrinogen reaction.
Platelet count	Normal. Adequate platelet production.
Partial thromboplastin time	Prolonged because of deficiency in any intrinsic clotting system factor.
Bleeding time	Prolonged in von Willebrand disease because of structurally defective platelets; normal in hemophilias A and B because platelets not affected.
Factor assays	Reduction of factor VIII in hemophilia A; vWF in von Willebrand disease; factor IX in hemophilia B.

vWF, von Willebrand factor.

TABLE 33-19 DRUG THERAPY

Replacement Factors Used in Treating Hemophilia

Factor VIII	Factor IX
Advate	Alprolix
Eloctate	BeneFIX
Humate P	Immunine
Kogenate FS	
Wilate	
Xyntha	

Source: Adapted from Canadian Hemophilia Society. (2016). *Clotting factor concentrates.* Retrieved from *http://www.hemophilia.ca/en/bleeding-disorders/clotting-factor-concentrates.*

therapy during acute bleeding episodes and as prophylaxis, and (c) the treatment of the complications of the disease and its therapy.

Replacement of deficient clotting factors is the primary means of supporting a patient with hemophilia. In addition to treating acute crises, replacement therapy may be given before surgery and dental care as a prophylactic measure (Oldenburg & Brackmann, 2014). Examples of replacement therapy are listed in Table 33-19. Fresh-frozen plasma, once commonly used for replacement therapy, is rarely used today.

For mild hemophilia A and certain subtypes of von Willebrand disease, desmopressin acetate (also known as DDAVP), a synthetic analogue of vasopressin, may be used to stimulate an increase in factor VIII and vWF. This medication acts on platelets and endothelial cells to cause the release of vWF, which subsequently binds with factor VIII, thus increasing their concentration. It can be administered intravenously, subcutaneously, or intranasally. Beneficial effects (e.g., decreased bleeding time) of DDAVP, when administered by IV, are seen within 30 minutes and can last for more than 12 hours. Because the effect of DDAVP is relatively short-lived, the patient must be closely monitored, and repeated doses may be necessary. It is an appropriate therapy for minor bleeding episodes and dental procedures. The intranasal form may be indicated for home therapy for some patients with mild to moderate forms of the disease.

Antifibrinolytic therapy (e.g., tranexamic acid [Cyklokapron]) inhibits fibrinolysis by inhibiting plasminogen activation in the fibrin clot, thereby enhancing clot stability. These agents are used to stabilize clots in areas of increased fibrinolysis, such as the oral cavity, and in patients with difficult-to-manage episodes of epistaxis and menorrhagia. Topical thrombin and fibrin sealants may also be used for mucosal bleeding.

Complications of treatment of hemophilia include development of inhibitors to factors VIII or IX, transfusion-transmitted infectious disorders, allergic reactions, and, with the use of factor IX, thrombotic complications, because it contains activated coagulation factors. Patients with vWF may also develop alloantibodies against vWF, the infusion of which could cause life-threatening anaphylaxis; thus, replacement factors for these patients should be devoid of vWF. The most common difficulties with acute management are starting factor replacement therapy too late and stopping it too soon. Generally, minor bleeding episodes should be treated for at least 72 hours. Surgery and traumatic injuries may need more prolonged therapy. Chronically, development of inhibitors to the factor products has occurred and necessitates individualized expert patient management.

Designated treatment centres have been established in Canada as well as in many other countries to provide multidisciplinary care of hemophilia and related disorders. Gene therapy has been used on an experimental basis to treat hemophilia. (Gene therapy is discussed in Chapter 15.)

NURSING MANAGEMENT HEMOPHILIA

NURSING IMPLEMENTATION

HEALTH PROMOTION. Genetic counselling referral is especially important now that many people with hemophilia live into adulthood. Reproductive concerns and long-term effects are issues that the nurse should include in the patient's care plan.

ACUTE INTERVENTION. Interventions are related primarily to controlling bleeding and include the following:

1. Stop the topical bleeding as quickly as possible by applying direct pressure or ice, packing the area with fibrin foam or Gelfoam, and applying a topical hemostatic medication such as thrombin.

2. Administer the specific coagulation factor to raise the patient's level of the deficient coagulation factor. Monitor the patient for signs and symptoms, such as hypersensitivity.

3. When joint bleeding occurs, in addition to administering replacement factors, it is important to totally rest the involved joint to prevent crippling deformities from hemarthrosis. Pack the joint in ice. Analgesics (e.g., acetaminophen [Tylenol], codeine) are given to reduce severe pain. However, ASA (Aspirin) and ASA-containing compounds should never be used. As soon as bleeding ceases, it is important to encourage mobilization of the affected area through range-of-motion exercises and physical therapy. Weight bearing is avoided until all swelling has resolved and muscle strength has returned.

4. Manage any life-threatening complication that may develop as a result of hemorrhage or adverse effects from coagulation factors or other medications, such as hyponatremia from use of desmopressin. For example, nursing interventions may include preventing or treating airway obstruction from hemorrhage into the neck and pharynx or assessing and treating intracranial bleeding.

AMBULATORY AND HOME CARE. Home management is a primary consideration for the patient with hemophilia because the disease follows a progressive, chronic course. The quality and the length of life may be significantly affected by the patient's knowledge of the illness and how to live with it. The patient and family can be referred to a local treatment centre or the provincial chapter of the Canadian Hemophilia Society to encourage associations with other individuals who are dealing with the problems of hemophilia. The nurse must provide ongoing assessment of the patient's adaptation to the illness. Psychosocial support and assistance should be readily available as needed.

Most of the needed long-term care measures are related to patient teaching. The patient with hemophilia must be taught to recognize disease-related problems and to know which problems can be resolved at home and which necessitate hospitalization. Immediate medical attention is required for severe pain or swelling of a muscle or joint that restricts movement or inhibits sleep and for a head injury, a swelling in the neck or the mouth, abdominal pain, hematuria, melena, and skin wounds in need of suturing.

Daily oral hygiene must be performed without causing trauma. Understanding how to prevent injuries is another consideration. The patient can learn to participate in noncontact sports (e.g., golf) and wear gloves when doing household chores to prevent cuts or abrasions from knives, hammers, and other tools. The patient should wear medical alert identification to ensure that health care providers know about the hemophilia in case of an accident. Patients or their caregivers may also be taught to self-administer the factor replacement therapies at home.

EVALUATION

The overall expected outcomes are similar to those for the patient with thrombo-cytopenia and are presented in NCP 33-2 (see the Evolve website).

DISSEMINATED INTRAVASCULAR COAGULATION

Disseminated intravascular coagulation (DIC) is a serious bleeding and thrombotic disorder. It results from the abnormally initiated and accelerated clotting and anticlotting processes that occur in response to disease or injury. The term *disseminated intravascular coagulation* can be misleading because it suggests that blood is clotting. In fact, the paradox of this condition is that it is characterized by the profuse bleeding resulting from the depletion of platelets and clotting factors. An underlying disease or condition always causes DIC. The underlying disease must be treated for the DIC to resolve.

Etiology and Pathophysiology

DIC is not a disease; it is an abnormal response of the normal clotting cascade stimulated by a disease process or disorder. The diseases and disorders known to predispose a patient to DIC are listed in Table 33-20. DIC can occur as an acute, catastrophic condition, or it may exist at a subacute or chronic level. Each condition may have one or multiple triggering mechanisms to start the clotting cascade. For example, tumours and traumatized or necrotic tissue release tissue factors into circulation. Endotoxin from Gram-negative bacteria activates several steps in the coagulation cascade.

Tissue factor is released at the site of tissue injury and by some malignancies, such as leukemia, and enhances normal coagulation mechanisms. Abundant intravascular thrombin, the most powerful coagulant, is produced (Figure 33-9). It catalyzes the conversion of fibrinogen to fibrin and enhances platelet aggregation. With widespread fibrin and platelet deposition in capillaries and arterioles, thrombosis results and can lead to

TABLE 33-20	PREDISPOSING CONDITIONS TO DEVELOPMENT OF DISSEMINATED INTRAVASCULAR COAGULATION

Acute Disseminated Intravascular Coagulation
- Shock
  - Hemorrhagic
  - Cardiogenic
  - Anaphylactic
- Septicemia
- Hemolytic processes
  - Transfusion of mismatched blood
  - Acute hemolysis from infection or immunological disorders
- Obstetric conditions
  - Abruptio placentae
  - Amniotic fluid embolism
  - Septic abortion
  - HELLP syndrome
- Malignancies
  - Acute leukemia
  - Lymphoma
  - Metastatic solid tumours

- Tissue damage
  - Extensive burns and trauma
  - Heatstroke
  - Severe head injury
  - Transplant rejections
  - Postoperative damage, especially after extracorporeal membrane oxygenation
  - Fat and pulmonary emboli
  - Snakebites
  - Glomerulonephritis
  - Acute anoxia (e.g., after cardiac arrest)
  - Prosthetic devices
  - Fulminant hepatitis

Subacute Disseminated Intravascular Coagulation
- Malignant disease
  - Myeloproliferative and lymphoproliferative malignancies
  - Metastatic cancer
- Obstetric: retained dead fetus

Chronic Disseminated Intravascular Coagulation
- Liver disease
- Systemic lupus erythematosus
- Localized malignancy

HELLP, **h**emolysis, **e**levated **l**iver enzymes, **l**ow **p**latelet count.

multiorgan failure. In addition, clotting inhibitory mechanisms, such as antithrombin III (AT III) and protein C, are depressed. This excessive clotting activates the fibrinolytic system, which in turn breaks down the newly formed clot, creating *fibrin split products* (FSPs; also called *fibrin degradation products* [FDPs]). These products have anticoagulant properties and inhibit normal blood clotting. Ultimately, with FSPs accumulating and clotting factors being depleted, the blood loses its ability to clot. Therefore, a stable clot cannot be formed at injury sites, which predisposes the patient to hemorrhage.

Chronic and subacute DIC are most commonly seen in patients with longstanding illnesses such as malignant disorders or autoimmune diseases. Occasionally, these patients have subclinical disease manifested only by laboratory abnormalities. However, the clinical spectrum ranges from easy bruising to hemorrhage and from hypercoagulability to thrombosis.

Clinical Manifestations

There are both bleeding and thrombotic manifestations in DIC. Bleeding manifestations of DIC are multifactorial (see Figure 33-9) and result from consumption and depletion of platelets and coagulation factors as well as from clot lysis and formation of FSPs that have anticoagulant properties. Bleeding manifestations include (a) integumentary manifestations, such as pallor, petechiae, purpura (Figure 33-10), oozing blood, venipuncture site bleeding, hematomas, and occult hemorrhage; (b) respiratory

Signs of microvascular thrombosis
Neurological: Multifocal, delirium, coma
Integumentary: Focal ischemia, superficial gangrene
Renal: Oliguria, azotemia, cortical necrosis
Pulmonary: Acute respiratory distress syndrome
Gastro-intestinal: Paralytic ileus

Signs of hemorrhage
Neurological: Intracerebral bleeding
Integumentary: Petechiae, ecchymoses, venipuncture oozing
Renal: Hematuria
Pulmonary: Respiratory congestion, dyspnea, hemoptysis
Mucous membranes: Epistaxis, gingival oozing
Gastro-intestinal: Massive bleeding

FIGURE 33-9 The sequence of events that occur during disseminated intravascular coagulation.

FIGURE 33-10 Disseminated intravascular coagulation resulting from staphylococcal septicemia. Note the characteristic skin hemorrhage ranging from small purpuric lesions to larger ecchymoses. Source: Forbes, D. D., & Jackson, W. F. (2003). *Color atlas and text of clinical medicine* (3rd ed., p. 443). London: Mosby.

manifestations, such as tachypnea, hemoptysis, and orthopnea; (c) cardiovascular manifestations, such as tachycardia and hypotension; (d) GI manifestations, such as upper and lower GI bleeding, abdominal distension, and bloody stools; (e) urinary manifestations, such as hematuria; (f) neurological manifestations, such as vision changes, dizziness, headache, changes in mental status, and irritability; and (g) musculo-skeletal complaints, such as bone and joint pain.

Thrombotic manifestations are a result of fibrin or platelet deposition in the microvasculature (see Figure 33-9). They include (a) integumentary changes, such as cyanosis, ischemic tissue necrosis (e.g., gangrene), and hemorrhagic necrosis; (b) respiratory changes, such as tachypnea, dyspnea, pulmonary emboli, and acute respiratory distress syndrome (ARDS); (c) cardiovascular changes, such as electrocardiogram (ECG) changes and venous distension; (d) GI changes, such as abdominal pain and paralytic ileus; and (e) urinary changes, such as oliguria, leading to renal failure.

TABLE 33-21	LABORATORY ABNORMALITIES OF ACUTE DISSEMINATED INTRAVASCULAR COAGULATION
Test	**Finding**
Screening Tests	
Prothrombin time (PT)	Prolonged
Partial thromboplastin time (PTT)	Prolonged
Activated partial thromboplastin time (aPTT)	Prolonged
Thrombin time	Prolonged
Fibrinogen	Reduced
Platelets	Reduced
Special Tests	
Fibrin split products (FSPs)	Elevated
Factor assays (for factors V, VIII, X, XIII)	Reduced but may give misleading results, as V and VIII rise with inflammation
D-dimers (cross-linked fibrin fragments)	Elevated
Antithrombin III (AT III)	Reduced
Protein C and S	Reduced
Plasminogen, tissue activator	Reduced
Peripheral blood smear	Schistocytes present

Diagnostic Studies

Tests used to diagnose acute DIC and their findings are listed in Table 33-21. As more clots are made in the body, more breakdown products from fibrinogen and fibrin are also formed. These FSPs, or FDPs, interfere with blood coagulation by (a) coating the platelets and interfering with platelet function; (b) interfering with thrombin and thus disrupting coagulation; and (c) attaching to fibrinogen, interfering with the polymerization process necessary to form a stable clot. D-dimer, a polymer

Therapy

Treat the cause

FIGURE 33-11 Intended sites of action for therapies in disseminated intravascular coagulation (DIC). *AT III*, antithrombin III; *CPR*, cardiopulmonary resuscitation; *FSPs*, fibrin split products; *RBC*, red blood cell.

resulting from the breakdown of fibrin (and not fibrinogen), is a specific marker for the degree of fibrinolysis. In general, tests that measure raw materials needed for coagulation (e.g., platelets, fibrinogen) are reduced and tests that measure clotting times are prolonged. Fragmented erythrocytes *(schistocytes)*, indicative of partial occlusion of small vessels by fibrin thrombi, may be found on blood smears.

Collaborative Care

It is important to diagnose DIC quickly, stabilize the patient (e.g., oxygenation, volume replacement), treat the underlying causative disease or problem, and provide supportive care for the manifestations resulting from the pathology of DIC itself. Depending on its severity, a variety of different methods are used to manage DIC (Figure 33-11). First, if chronic DIC is diagnosed in a patient who is not bleeding, no therapy for DIC is necessary. Treatment of the underlying disease may be sufficient to reverse the DIC (e.g., chemotherapy when DIC is caused by malignancy). Second, when the patient with DIC is bleeding, therapy is directed toward providing support with necessary blood products while treating the primary disorder.

Blood products are administered cautiously based on specific component deficiencies. Blood product support with platelets, cryoprecipitate, and fresh-frozen plasma is usually reserved for a patient with life-threatening hemorrhage. The concern is that one is adding "fuel to the fire" of already activated coagulation. However, it may be the only method to prevent death in some patients with severe hemorrhage. Therapy will stabilize a patient, prevent exsanguination or massive thrombosis, and permit institution of definitive therapy to treat the underlying cause.

A patient with manifestations of thrombosis is often treated by anticoagulation with heparin or low-molecular-weight heparin. However, these medications are used in the treatment of DIC only when the benefit (e.g., reduce clotting) outweighs the risk (e.g., further bleeding). Antithrombin III is sometimes used in fulminant DIC, although it increases the risk of bleeding. Chronic DIC does not respond to oral anticoagulants, but it can be controlled with long-term use of heparin.

▌ NURSING MANAGEMENT
▌ DISSEMINATED INTRAVASCULAR COAGULATION

▌ NURSING DIAGNOSES

Nursing diagnoses for the patient with DIC may include but are not limited to the following:

- *Risk for impaired tissue integrity* as evidenced by *insufficient fluid volume* (bleeding)
- *Acute pain* related to *physical injury agent* (bleeding)
- *Decreased cardiac output* (related to fluid volume deficit)
- *Anxiety* related to *unmet needs* (fear of the unknown)

▌ NURSING IMPLEMENTATION

Nurses must be alert to the possible development of DIC and especially to the precipitating factors listed in Table 33-20. The nurse must also remember that, because DIC is secondary to an underlying disease, appropriate care for managing the causative problem must be provided while also providing supportive care related to the manifestations of DIC.

Appropriate nursing interventions are essential to the survival of a patient with acute DIC. Astute, ongoing assessment, active attention to manifestations of DIC, and prompt administration of prescribed therapies are crucial. Table 33-14 and NCP 33-2 (see the Evolve website) provide assessments and interventions appropriate for the patient with DIC. Early detection of bleeding, both occult and overt, must be a primary goal. Assess for signs of external bleeding (e.g., petechiae, oozing at IV or injection sites) and signs of internal bleeding (e.g., increased heart rate, changes in mental status, increasing abdominal girth, pain) as well as indications that microthrombi may be causing significant organ damage (e.g., decreased urinary output). Tissue damage should be minimized and the patient protected from additional sources of bleeding.

An additional nursing responsibility is to administer blood products and medications correctly. (Blood product transfusion is discussed later in this chapter.)

NEUTROPENIA

Leukopenia refers to a decrease in the total WBC count (granulocytes, monocytes, and lymphocytes). *Granulo-cytopenia* is a deficiency of granulocytes, which include neutrophils, eosinophils, and basophils. The neutrophilic granulocytes, which play a major role in phagocytizing pathogenic microbes, are closely monitored in clinical practice as an indicator of a patient's risk for infection. A reduction in neutrophils is termed *neutropenia*. (Some clinicians use the terms *granulo-cytopenia* and *neutropenia* interchangeably because neutrophils constitute the largest proportion of granulocytes.) The *absolute neutrophil count* (ANC) is determined by multiplying the total WBC count by the percentage of neutrophils. Neutropenia is defined as a neutrophil count of less than 1 to 1.5×10^9/L, or 1 000 to 1 500/mcL. Normally, neutrophils range from 2.2 to 7.7×10^9/L. *Severe neutropenia* is defined as an ANC less than 0.5×10^9/L.

However, in considering the clinical significance of neutropenia, it is important to know whether the decrease in the neutrophil count was gradual or rapid, as well as the degree and the duration of neutropenia. The faster the drop and the longer the duration, the greater the likelihood is of developing life-threatening infection, sepsis, and death. Other factors and comorbid conditions—such as being older than 60 years of age, having an existing infection, being in a hospital, having diabetes, and other factors—can increase the risk of a serious infection.

Neutropenia is not a disease; it is a clinical consequence that occurs with a variety of conditions or diseases (Table 33-22). It can also be a predictable or an unanticipated adverse effect of taking certain drugs. The most common cause of neutropenia is iatrogenic, resulting from widespread use of chemotherapeutic and immuno-suppressive therapy in the treatment of malignancies and autoimmune diseases.

Clinical Manifestations

The patient with neutropenia is predisposed to infection with nonpathogenic organisms that constitute normal body flora as well as opportunistic pathogens. When the WBC count is depressed or immature WBCs are present, normal phagocytic mechanisms are impaired. Also, because of the diminished phagocytic response, the classic signs of inflammation—redness, heat, and swelling—may not occur. WBCs are the major component of pus. Therefore, in the patient with neutropenia, pus formation (e.g., as a visible skin

TABLE 33-22 CAUSES OF NEUTROPENIA

Drug Therapy
- Antitumour antibiotics (daunorubicin [Cerubidine], doxorubicin [Adriamycin])
- Alkylating agents (nitrogen mustards, busulfan [Myleran])
- Antimetabolites (methotrexate, 6-mercaptopurine, cytarabine)
- Anti-inflammatory drugs (phenylbutazone)
- Cardiovascular drugs (captopril, procainamide)
- Diuretics (furosemide [Lasix])
- Psychotropics and antidepressants (clozapine, imipramine)
- Miscellaneous (gold, penicillamine)
- Antimicrobial agents (ganciclovir, penicillin G, trimethoprim–sulphamethoxazole)

Hematological Disorders
- Idiopathic neutropenia
- Fanconi's anemia
- Congenital (cyclic neutropenia)
- Aplastic anemia
- Leukemia
- Myelodysplastic syndrome

Autoimmune Disorders
- Systemic lupus erythematosus
- Felty syndrome
- Rheumatoid arthritis

Infections
- Viral (e.g., hepatitis, influenza, HIV, measles)
- Fulminant bacterial infection (e.g., typhoid fever, miliary tuberculosis)
- Parasitic
- Rickettsial

Miscellaneous
- Severe sepsis
- Bone marrow infiltration (e.g., carcinoma, tuberculosis, lymphoma)
- Hypersplenism (e.g., portal hypertension, storage diseases [e.g., Gaucher's disease])
- Nutritional deficiencies (cobalamin, folic acid)
- Transfusion reaction
- Hemodialysis

HIV, human immunodeficiency virus.

lesion or as pulmonary infiltrates on a chest radiograph) is also absent.

> **SAFETY ALERT**
> - Presence of a low-grade fever in neutropenic patients is of great significance because it may indicate infection and quickly lead to septic shock and death.
> - A fever greater than 38°C and a neutrophil count less than 0.5×10^9/L is a medical emergency.

When fever occurs in a neutropenic patient, it is assumed to be caused by infection and calls for immediate attention. The immuno-compromised, neutropenic patient has little or no ability to fight infection. Thus, minor infections can lead rapidly to sepsis. The mucous membranes of the throat and mouth, skin, perianal area, and pulmonary system are common entry points for pathogenic organisms in susceptible hosts. Clinical manifestations related to infection at these sites include complaints of sore throat and dysphagia, appearance of ulcerative lesions of the pharyngeal and the buccal mucosa, diarrhea, rectal tenderness, vaginal itching or discharge, shortness of breath, and a nonproductive cough. Any minor complaint by the patient of pain or any other symptom should be taken seriously. These seemingly minor complaints can progress to fever, chills, sepsis, and septic shock if not recognized and treated in the early stages.

Systemic infections caused by bacterial, fungal, and viral organisms are common in patients with neutropenia. The patient's own flora (normally nonpathogenic) contributes significantly to life-threatening infections such as pneumonia. Organisms that are known to be common sources of infection include Gram-positive coagulase-negative staphylococci and *Staphylococcus aureus* and Gram-negative organisms such as *Escherichia coli* and *Pseudomonas aeruginosa* (Baden, Bensinger, Angarone, et al., 2014). Fungi involved include *Candida* (usually *C. albicans*) and *Aspergillus.* Viral infections caused by reactivation of herpes simplex and herpes zoster are common following prolonged periods of neutropenia, such as in HSCT patients.

Diagnostic Studies

The primary diagnostic tests for assessing neutropenia are the peripheral WBC count and bone marrow aspiration and biopsy (Table 33-23). A total WBC count of 4×10^9/L or 4000/mcL reflects leukopenia. However, only a differential count can confirm the presence of neutropenia (ANC of $1-1.5 \times 10^9$/L or 1000-1500/mcL). If the differential WBC count reflects an ANC of 0.5 to 1×10^9/L or 500 to 1000/mcL, the patient is at moderate risk for a bacterial infection. An ANC less than 0.5 to 1×10^9/L or 500 to 1000/mcL places the patient at severe risk. Note that patients with acute leukemia who present with a high WBC may in fact have neutropenia, because the majority of the WBCs are ineffective leukemia blast cells.

A peripheral blood smear is used to assess for immature forms of WBCs (e.g., bands). The Hct level, the reticulocyte count, and the platelet count are performed to evaluate bone marrow function. A review of the patient's recent past and current drug history should also be done. If the cause of neutropenia is unknown, bone marrow aspirations and biopsies are performed to examine cellularity and cell morphology. Additional studies may be done as indicated to assess spleen and liver function.

TABLE 33-23   COLLABORATIVE CARE

Neutropenia

Diagnostic	Collaborative Management
• History and physical examination	• Identification and removal of cause of neutropenia (if possible)
• Risk assessment for severity and duration of neutropenia	• Identification of site of infection (if present) and causative organism
• WBC count with differential	
• WBC morphology	• Antimicrobial therapy
• Hct and Hb values	• Blood cultures (prior to administration of antimicrobials)
• Reticulocyte and platelet count	
• Bone marrow aspiration or biopsy	• Hematopoietic growth factors (G-CSF, and GM-CSF)
• Cultures of nose, throat, sputum, urine, stool, obvious lesions, blood (as indicated)	• Strict adherence to handwashing and patient hygiene protocols
• Chest radiograph or other diagnostic tests	• Single-patient room and positive-pressure or HEPA filtration, depending on risk
	• Community isolation and home precautions if outpatient

G-CSF, granulocyte colony–stimulating factor; *GM-CSF,* granulocyte-macrophage colony–stimulating factor; *Hb,* hemoglobin; *Hct,* hematocrit; *HEPA,* **h**igh-**e**fficiency **p**articulate **a**ir; *WBC,* white blood cell.

NURSING AND COLLABORATIVE MANAGEMENT NEUTROPENIA

The factors involved in the nursing and collaborative care of neutropenia include (a) determining the cause of the neutropenia; (b) identifying the offending organisms if an infection has developed; (c) instituting prophylactic, empirical, or therapeutic antibiotic therapy; (d) administering hematopoietic growth factors (e.g., granulocyte colony–stimulating factor [G-CSF] and granulocyte-macrophage colony–stimulating factor [GM-CSF]); and (e) instituting protective practices (e.g., strict handwashing, skin and oral hygiene) (see Table 33-23).

Occasionally, the cause of the neutropenia can be easily treated (e.g., nutritional deficiencies). However, neutropenia can also be an adverse effect that must be tolerated as a necessary step in therapy (e.g., chemotherapy, radiation therapy). In some situations, the neutropenia resolves when the primary disease is treated (e.g., tuberculosis).

The nurse must monitor the neutropenic patient for signs and symptoms of infection (any fever ≥38°C) and early septic shock. Early identification of a potentially infective organism depends on acquiring cultures from various sites. Serial blood cultures (at least two) or one from a peripheral site and one from a venous access device should be done promptly and antibiotics started immediately. In addition, cultures of sputum, throat, lesions, wounds, urine, and feces may be required. It may also be necessary to do a computed tomographic (CT) scan, tracheal aspiration, bronchoscopy with bronchial brushings, or lung biopsy to diagnose the cause of pneumonic infiltrates. Despite these many tests, the causative organism is identified in only approximately half of patients with neutropenia.

When a febrile episode occurs in a patient with neutropenia, antibiotic therapy must be initiated immediately (within 1 hour), even before the determination by culture of a specific causative organism. Broad-spectrum antibiotics are usually ordered by the IV route because of the potential lethal effects of infection. However, some oral antibiotics are highly effective and routinely used for prophylaxis against infection in some patients with neutropenia. Antibiotics are often used in combinations because of their synergistic effects and in the event that multiple organisms are responsible for the infectious symptoms. Regardless of the combination, the nurse must initiate therapy promptly and observe for adverse effects of antimicrobial agents. Adverse effects common to aminoglycosides include nephrotoxicity and ototoxicity; adverse effects common to cephalosporins include rashes, fever, and pruritus.

The extended duration of neutropenia increases the infection risk of the patient. The longer the neutropenia lasts, the greater the risk of a fungal infection. Antifungal therapy is initiated in patients who produce a positive culture or in patients who do not become afebrile with broad-spectrum antibiotic coverage.

G-CSF (filgrastim [Neupogen]) and GM-CSF can be used to prevent neutropenia or to reduce its severity, its duration, or both. They should be considered for patients receiving chemotherapy based on their risk factors for neutropenia. G-CSF stimulates the production and function of neutrophils. GM-CSF stimulates the production and function of neutrophils and monocytes. These agents can be given by IV or subcutaneously. Keratinocyte growth factor may also be used to reduce the duration and severity of mucositis, which may contribute to infection. An important consideration in the care of a patient with neutropenia is the determination of the best means to protect the patient, whose own defences against infection are compromised. To accomplish this goal, the following principles must be kept in mind: (a) the patient's normal flora is the most common source of microbial colonization and infection; (b) transmission of organisms from humans most commonly occurs by direct contact with the hands; (c) air, food, water, and equipment provide additional opportunities for infection transmission; and (d) health care providers with transmissible illnesses and other patients with infections can also be sources of infection under certain conditions.

Handwashing is the single most important preventive measure in minimizing the risk of infection in the patient with neutropenia. Strict adherence to handwashing protocol by all people coming in contact with the compromised patient is the major method to prevent transmission of harmful pathogens.

Immuno-compromised patients should be separated from those who are infected or who have conditions that increase the probability of transmitting infections. A patient who is hospitalized, therefore, should be in a private room. Often, patients can be managed on an outpatient basis if the patient and caregivers can astutely monitor for fevers and other signs of infection and then report promptly to a nearby health care facility (Table 33-24). Although it is expensive to install, high-efficiency particulate air (HEPA) filtration, an air-handling method with a high-flow filtering system, can reduce or eliminate the number of aerosolized pathogens in the environment. It is often used for a patient with severe, prolonged neutropenia (e.g., patients who have undergone bone marrow transplant). Care routines in a HEPA environment are essentially the same as care in any other private room. Prophylactic antibiotics and antifungals may also be used for severely immuno-compromised patients. The patient and caregiver should be instructed on a diet that restricts potentially hazardous foods, such as raw and undercooked meats and eggs and soft cheeses with moulds.

Quality-of-life issues for the patient with neutropenia should not be overlooked. Potential patient experiences of fatigue, malaise, decrease in functioning, social isolation, depression, and perceived lack of support require appropriate interventions.

AGE-RELATED CONSIDERATIONS

THROMBO-CYTOPENIA AND NEUTROPENIA

About 55% to 60% of cancer diagnoses are currently made in individuals older than 65 years. This proportion is expected to further increase in the next 2 decades as the baby boomers move into this age group. Age-related changes of bone marrow function are rather subtle and probably not significant for the hematopoietic function of normal older individuals. These changes, however, may become clinically evident under conditions of severe hematopoietic stress, such as the administration of repeated courses of chemotherapy, radiation therapy, or both and the resultant sequelae of myelosuppression. The use of supportive therapies, such as hematopoietic growth factors, increases the likelihood that older individuals will be treated with standard and even aggressive therapies, leading to neutropenia and thrombo-cytopenia. The nurse also needs to be aware that older individuals may have signs and symptoms different from those of a younger individual. For example, the older adult may have delirium as compared with cough as a clinical manifestation of pneumonia.

MYELODYSPLASTIC SYNDROME

Myelodysplastic syndrome (MDS) is a group of related hematological disorders characterized by a change in the quantity and quality of bone marrow elements. Peripheral blood cytopenias in combination with a hypercellular bone marrow exhibiting dysplastic changes is the hallmark of MDS. In MDS, hematopoiesis is disorderly and ineffective. In Canada, it is estimated that the incidence is 75 to 162 per 100 000 adults aged 65 and older (Leukemia & Lymphoma Society, 2016). Although it can occur in all age groups, the highest prevalence is in people over 80 years of age (Shead, Hanisch, Marlow, et al., 2016).

Etiology and Pathophysiology

The exact etiology of MDS is unknown. Its manifestations result from neoplastic transformation of the pluripotent hematopoietic stem cells within the bone marrow. People who have received radiation or chemotherapy or who have been exposed to industrial solvents are at higher risk for developing MDS. Rarely, genetic disorders are responsible for the disease. Nevertheless, in 85% of MDS patients, no specific cause can be identified (Klotz, Parikh, & Battiwalla, 2013).

MDS is referred to as a *clonal disorder* because some bone marrow stem cells continue to function normally whereas others (a specific clone) do not. The abnormal clone of the stem cells is usually found in the bone marrow but eventually may be found in circulation. Occasionally, one type of MDS transforms into

---

TABLE 33-24 PATIENT & CAREGIVER TEACHING GUIDE

Neutropenia

This instruction sheet for patients explains protective precautions they should take when their neutrophil count is low. Patients should ask their health care provider about specific precautions to follow related to their particular risk factors for infection.

- *Wash your hands* frequently and make sure those around you wash their hands frequently, particularly if they help with your care. An antibacterial hand gel may also be used.
- Notify your nurse or health care provider if you have any of the following:
  - A fever greater than 38°C
  - Chills or feeling hot
  - Redness, swelling, discharge, or new painful area either on the skin or deeper in your body
  - Changes in urination or bowel movements
  - A cough, sore throat, mouth sores, or blisters
- If you are at home, take your temperature as directed and follow instructions on what to do if you have a fever.
- Avoid crowds and people with colds, flu, or infections. If you are in a public area, wear a mask and use hand-sanitizing gel frequently.
- Avoid uncooked meats, seafood, eggs, and unwashed fruits and vegetables. Ask your health care provider about specific dietary guidelines for you.
- Bathe or shower daily. A moisturizer may be used to prevent skin from drying and cracking.
- Maintain some daily activity as instructed by your health care team. This may include walking and moderate exercise while avoiding crowds.
- Brush your teeth with a soft toothbrush four times daily. You may floss once daily if it does not cause excessive pain or bleeding. Avoid alcohol-based mouthwashes.
- Do not perform gardening or clean up after pets. Feeding and petting your dog or cat is fine as long as you wash your hands well after handling.

another. Depending on the subtype, MDS may progress to acute myelogenous leukemia (AML) (Meers, 2015). In contrast to AML, in which the leukemic cells show little normal maturation, the clonal cells in MDS always display some degree of maturity. Disease progression is slower than in AML. However, eventually, the abnormal cells replace the bone marrow. Typically, life-threatening anemia, thrombo-cytopenia, and neutropenia occur during the advanced stage of MDS.

Clinical Manifestations

MDS commonly manifests as infection and bleeding caused by inadequate numbers of ineffectively functioning circulating granulocytes or platelets. MDS is often discovered in the older adult in the course of investigating symptoms of anemia, thrombo-cytopenia, or neutropenia. It may also be diagnosed incidentally from a routine CBC.

Diagnostic Studies

Bone marrow biopsy with aspirate analysis is essential for both the diagnosis and the classification of the specific types of myelodysplasia. In MDS, the bone marrow is normocellular, hypocellular, or hypercellular, and the patient has peripheral cytopenia. Laboratory data and bone marrow studies will help rule out other causes of the dysplasia, such as nonmalignant disorders, cobalamin and folate deficiencies, and infectious causes.

INFORMATICS IN PRACTICE

Use of Internet to Access Information on Unfamiliar Diseases

- Nurses assigned the care of a patient with a disease or disorder that they are not familiar with, such as thalassemia, can access the Internet and perform a quick search.
- Within minutes, nurses can learn the pathophysiology of thalassemia, treatment options, possible complications that will need monitoring, and recommended medical and nursing interventions.
- Using this readily available information helps nurses deliver high-quality, evidence-informed care.

NURSING AND COLLABORATIVE MANAGEMENT MYELODYSPLASTIC SYNDROME

Treatment of MDS is based on the premise that the aggressiveness of the treatment should match the aggressiveness of the disease. The recommended treatment depends on the amount and type of dysplasia in the bone marrow as well as genetic mutations and patient's age. Low-intensity treatments consist of hematological monitoring (serial bone marrow and peripheral blood examinations) and transfusions with blood products, including iron chelators to prevent iron overload if required. Growth factors may also be used (e.g., G-CSF, erythropoietin). Low-intensity chemotherapeutic drugs may be used, such as azacitidine (Vidaza) or lenalidomide (Revlimid). High-intensity treatments include the use of chemotherapeutic drugs similar to those used to treat and cure myeloid leukemia. High-intensity treatments are not recommended for all patients, and only about one-third of high-risk patients are treated with intensive chemotherapy, HSCT, or both.

Nursing care of a patient with MDS is similar to that of a patient with manifestations of anemia (see NCP 33-1, earlier in this chapter, for patients with anemia; see NCP 33-2 for thrombo-cytopenia and NCP 33-3 for neutropenia, both available on the Evolve website).

LEUKEMIA

Leukemia is a broad term given to a group of malignant diseases that affect the blood and blood-forming tissues of the bone marrow, lymph system, and spleen. Leukemia occurs in all age groups. It is characterized by diffuse replacement of bone marrow with proliferating leukocyte precursors. This loss of regulation in cell division results in an accumulation of dysfunctional cells. Leukemia follows a progressive course that is eventually fatal if untreated. It was estimated that, in 2017, there would be 6200 new cases and 2900 deaths in Canada due to leukemia and that males would account for more than 58% of new cases (Canadian Cancer Society, 2017a).

Etiology and Pathophysiology

Regardless of the specific type of leukemia, there is generally no single causative agent in the disease's development. Most leukemias result from a combination of factors, including genetic and environmental influences. Chromosomal changes, first recognized in chronic myelogenous leukemia, have led to discoveries of how normal genes, once transformed, can result in abnormal genes (*oncogenes*) capable of causing many types of cancers, including leukemias (see Chapter 18). Chemical agents (e.g., benzene), chemotherapeutic drugs (e.g., alkylating agents), viruses, radiation, and immunological deficiencies have all been associated with the development of leukemia in susceptible hosts. The incidence of leukemia is increased in radiologists, people who have lived near nuclear bomb test sites or nuclear reactor accidents (e.g., Chernobyl), and people previously treated with radiation therapy or chemotherapy.

Although ribonucleic acid (RNA) retroviruses cause a number of leukemias in animals, a viral cause for a human leukemia has been established only for some patients with adult T-cell leukemia. This form of leukemia is endemic in southwestern Japan and parts of the Caribbean and central Africa and is caused by the human T-cell leukemia virus type 1 (HTLV-1).

Classification

Leukemia can be classified as either acute or chronic. The terms *acute* and *chronic* refer to cell maturity and the nature of the disease's onset. *Acute leukemia* is characterized by the clonal proliferation of immature hematopoietic cells. The leukemia develops following malignant transformation of a single type of immature hematopoietic cell, followed by cellular replication and expansion of that malignant clone. *Chronic leukemias* involve more mature forms of WBCs, and the disease onset is more gradual.

Leukemia can also be classified by identifying the type of leukocyte involved, that is, whether it is of myelogenous origin or of lymphocytic origin. By combining the acute and chronic categories with the cell type involved, specific types of leukemia can be identified. Four major types of leukemia are acute lymphocytic leukemia (ALL), acute myelogenous leukemia (AML), chronic myelogenous (granulocytic) leukemia (CML), and chronic lymphocytic leukemia (CLL). The defining features of these leukemic subtypes are presented in Table 33-25.

Acute Myelogenous Leukemia. AML represents only one-fourth of all leukemias, but it makes up approximately 80% of the acute leukemias in adults. Its onset is often abrupt and dramatic.

TABLE 33-25 TYPES OF LEUKEMIA

Type	Age of Onset	Clinical Manifestations	Diagnostic Findings
Acute myelogenous leukemia (AML)	Increase in incidence with advancing age; peak incidence between 60 and 70 yr of age; accounts for 15%–20% of acute leukemia in children and 80% in adults	Fatigue and weakness, headache, mouth sores, anemia, bleeding, fever, infection, sternal tenderness, gingival hyperplasia, mild hepato-splenomegaly and lymphadenopathy	Low RBC count, Hb, Hct; low platelet count; low to high WBC count with myeloblasts; high LDH; greatly hypercellular bone marrow with myeloblasts
Acute lymphocytic leukemia (ALL)	Peak prevalence between ages 2 and 5 and after age 50	Fever; pallor; bleeding; anorexia; fatigue and weakness; bone, joint, and abdominal pain; generalized lymphadenopathy; infections; weight loss; hepato-splenomegaly; headache; mouth sores; neurological manifestations, CNS involvement, increased intracranial pressure secondary to meningeal infiltration	Low RBC count, Hb, Hct; low platelet count; low, normal, or high WBC count; high LDH; transverse lines of rarefaction at ends of metaphysis of long bones on radiograph; hypercellular bone marrow with lymphoblasts; lymphoblasts also possible in cerebro-spinal fluid; presence of Philadelphia chromosome (20%–25% of patients)
Chronic myelogenous leukemia (CML)	25–60 yr of age; peak incidence around 45 yr of age	No symptoms early in disease; then fatigue and weakness, fever, sternal tenderness, weight loss, joint pain, bone pain, massive splenomegaly, increase in sweating	Low RBC count, Hb, Hct; high platelet count early, lower count later; increase in polymorphonuclear neutrophils, normal number of lymphocytes, and normal or low number of monocytes in WBC differential; low leukocyte alkaline phosphatase; presence of Philadelphia chromosome (90% of patients)
Chronic lymphocytic leukemia (CLL)	50–70 yr of age; rare below 30 yr of age; predominance in men	No symptoms frequently; detection of disease often during examination for unrelated condition; chronic fatigue, anorexia, splenomegaly and lymphadenopathy and hepatomegaly; may progress to fever, night sweats, weight loss, fatigue, and frequent infections	Mild anemia and thrombo-cytopenia with disease progression; total WBC count >100 × 10^9/L; increase in peripheral lymphocytes; increase in presence of lymphocytes in bone marrow; hypo-gammaglobulinemia; may have autoimmune hemolytic anemia (4%–11%), idiopathic thrombo-cytopenia purpura (2%–4%)

CNS, central nervous system; *Hb,* hemoglobin; *Hct,* hematocrit; *LDH,* lactic dehydrogenase; *RBC,* red blood cell; *WBC,* white blood cell.

A patient may have serious infections and abnormal bleeding from the onset of the disease (Figure 33-12).

AML is characterized by uncontrolled proliferation of myeloblasts, the precursors of granulocytes. There is hyperplasia of the bone marrow and the spleen. The clinical manifestations are usually related to replacement of normal hematopoietic cells in the marrow by leukemic myeloblasts and, to a lesser extent, to infiltration of other organs (see Table 33-25.)

Acute Lymphocytic Leukemia. ALL is the most common type of leukemia in children and accounts for about 20% of acute leukemia in adults. In ALL, immature, small lymphocytes proliferate in the bone marrow; most are of B-cell origin. Fever is present in the majority of patients at the time of diagnosis. Signs and symptoms may appear abruptly with bleeding or fever, or they may be insidious with progressive weakness, fatigue, and bleeding tendencies.

Central nervous system (CNS) manifestations are especially common in ALL and represent a serious problem. Leukemic meningitis caused by arachnoid infiltration occurs in many patients with ALL (Cooper & Brown, 2015).

Chronic Myelogenous Leukemia. CML is caused by excessive development of mature neoplastic granulocytes in the bone marrow. The excess neoplastic granulocytes move into the peripheral blood in massive numbers and ultimately infiltrate the liver and the spleen. These cells contain a distinctive cytogenetic abnormality, the *Philadelphia chromosome*, which serves

FIGURE 33-12 Complications of acute leukemia. Spreading cellulitis of the neck and chin in this woman with acute myelogenous leukemia results from streptococcal and candidal infection. She is at risk because of previous chemotherapy and prolonged neutropenia. Source: Skarin, A. T. (1996). *Atlas of diagnostic oncology* (2nd ed.). London: Mosby-Wolfe.

as a disease marker and results from translocation of genetic material between the *BCR* gene on chromosome 22 and the *ABL* gene on chromosome 9. The protein that is encoded by the newly created *BCR–ABL* gene on the Philadelphia chromosome interferes with normal cell cycle events, such as the regulation of cell proliferation.

The natural history of CML is a chronic stable phase followed by the development of a more acute, aggressive phase referred to as the *blastic phase*. The chronic phase of CML can last for several years and can usually be well controlled with treatment. Even with treatment, the chronic phase of the disease will eventually progress to the accelerated phase, ending in a blastic phase. Once CML transforms to an acute or blastic phase, it must be treated aggressively, similar to an acute leukemia.

Chronic Lymphocytic Leukemia. CLL is the most common leukemia in adults. CLL is characterized by the production and accumulation of functionally inactive but long-lived, mature-appearing lymphocytes. The type of lymphocyte involved is usually the B cell. The lymphocytes infiltrate the bone marrow, spleen, and liver. Lymph node enlargement (lymphadenopathy) is present throughout the body, and there is an increased incidence of infection because of T-cell deficiencies or hypo-gammaglobulinemia. Complications from early-stage CLL are rare but may develop as the disease advances. Pressure on nerves from enlarged lymph nodes causes pain and even paralysis. Mediastinal node enlargement leads to pulmonary symptoms. Because CLL is usually a disease of older adults, treatment decisions must be made by considering the progression of the disease and the adverse effects of treatment. Many individuals in the early stages of CLL require no treatment. Others may be followed closely and receive treatment only when the disease progresses.

Other Leukemias. Occasionally, the subtype of leukemia cannot be identified. The malignant leukemic cells may have lymphoid, myeloid, or mixed characteristics. Frequently, these patients do not respond to treatment and have a poor prognosis. Other rare types include hairy cell and biphenotypic leukemias.

Clinical Manifestations

The clinical manifestations of leukemia are varied (see Table 33-25). Essentially, they relate to problems caused by bone marrow failure and the formation of leukemic infiltrates. Bone marrow failure results from (a) bone marrow overcrowding by abnormal cells and (b) inadequate production of normal marrow elements. The patient is predisposed to anemia, thrombo-cytopenia, and decreased number and function of WBCs.

As leukemia progresses, fewer normal blood cells are produced. The abnormal WBCs continue to accumulate because they do not go through the normal cell life cycle to death *(apoptosis)*. The leukemic cells infiltrate the patient's organs, leading to problems such as splenomegaly, hepatomegaly, lymphadenopathy, bone pain, meningeal irritation, and oral lesions. Solid masses called *chloromas* can result from collections of leukemic cells. A high leukemia WBC count in the peripheral blood can cause the blood to thicken and potentially block circulatory pathways. This is called *leukostasis* and can be life-threatening.

Diagnostic Studies

Peripheral blood evaluation and bone marrow examination are the primary methods of diagnosing and classifying the subtypes of leukemia. Morphological, histochemical, immunological, and cytogenetic methods are all used to identify cell subtypes and the stage of development of leukemic cell populations. This is important because different subtypes have different natural histories, prognoses, and chemotherapeutic regimens. Other studies such as lumbar puncture and CT scan can determine the presence of leukemic cells outside of the blood and the bone marrow.

The malignant cells in most patients with leukemia have specific cytogenetic abnormalities that are associated with distinct subsets of the disease. These cytogenetic abnormalities have diagnostic, prognostic, and therapeutic importance. For example, in CML, the finding of the Philadelphia chromosome has a good prognostic significance, but not so in ALL.

Collaborative Care

Once a diagnosis of leukemia has been made, collaborative care is focused on the initial goal of attaining remission. Age and cytogenetic analysis often help form the basis of important treatment decisions. Because chemotherapy is the mainstay of the treatment, the nurse must understand the principles of cancer chemotherapy, including cellular kinetics, the use of multiple medications rather than single drugs, and the cell cycle. (See the section on chemotherapy in Chapter 18.)

In some cases, such as with asymptomatic patients who have CLL, watchful waiting with active supportive care may be appropriate. Although a patient may not be cured, attaining remission or disease control is a realistic option for the majority of patients. In *complete remission*, there is no evidence of overt disease on physical examination, and the bone marrow and peripheral blood appear normal. A lesser state of control is known as *partial remission*. It is characterized by a lack of symptoms and a normal peripheral blood smear, but there is still evidence of disease in the bone marrow. *Minimal residual disease* is defined as tumour cells that cannot be detected by morphological examination but can be detected by molecular testing. *Molecular remission* indicates that all molecular studies are negative for residual leukemia. The patient's prognosis is directly related to the ability to maintain a remission and becomes more unfavourable with each relapse. Each time there is a relapse, the succeeding remission may be more difficult to achieve and shorter in duration.

Sometimes patients have such a high WBC count that initial emergent treatment may include the use of leukapheresis and hydroxyurea administration. The purpose of these treatments is to reduce the WBC count and the risk of leukemia-induced thrombosis.

The chemotherapeutic treatment of acute leukemia is divided into stages. The first stage, *induction therapy,* is the attempt to induce or bring about a remission. Induction is aggressive treatment that seeks to destroy leukemic cells in the tissues, peripheral blood, and bone marrow in order to eventually restore normal hematopoiesis on bone marrow recovery. During induction therapy, a patient may become critically ill because the bone marrow is severely depressed by the chemotherapeutic drugs. Throughout the induction phase, nursing interventions focus on neutropenia, thrombo-cytopenia, and anemia as well as on providing psychosocial support to the patient and family. Common chemotherapeutic drugs for induction of AML include cytarabine (Cytosar) and antitumour antibiotics (anthracyclines) such as daunorubicin (Cerubidine), idarubicin (Idamycin), or mitoxantrone. After one course of induction therapy, approximately 70% of newly diagnosed patients achieve complete remission. There is one subtype of AML, called *promyelocytic leukemia* (M3), for which tretinoin (Vesanoid) and arsenic trioxide (Trisenox) may also be used to induce a remission. It is generally assumed that leukemia cells persist undetected after induction therapy. As a result, relapse is possible within a few months if no further therapy is administered.

Terms used to describe postinduction or postremission chemotherapy include *intensification, consolidation,* and *maintenance. Intensification therapy,* or high-dose therapy, may be given immediately after induction therapy for several months. This therapy may use the same drugs as those used in induction, but at higher dosages. Other drugs that target the cell in a different way than those administered during induction may also be added.

Consolidation therapy is started after a remission is achieved. It may consist of one or two additional courses of the same drugs given during induction or involve high-dose therapy *(intensive consolidation).* The purpose of consolidation therapy is to eliminate remaining leukemic cells that may not be clinically or pathologically evident.

Maintenance therapy is treatment with lower doses of the same drugs used in induction or other drugs given every 3 to 4 weeks for a prolonged period of time. Like consolidation or intensification, the goal is to keep the body free of leukemic cells. Each leukemia calls for different maintenance therapy. In AML, maintenance therapy is rarely effective and, therefore, rarely administered.

In addition to chemotherapy, corticosteroids and radiation therapy can also have a role in the complex therapeutic plans for the patient with leukemia. Total body radiation may be used to prepare a patient for bone marrow transplantation, or radiation may be restricted to certain areas (fields) such as the liver and spleen or other organs affected by infiltrates. In ALL, prophylactic intrathecal methotrexate is given to decrease the chance of CNS involvement, which is common in this particular type of leukemia. When CNS leukemia does occur, cranial radiation may be given. Biological therapy may be indicated for specific leukemias. (Biological therapy is discussed in Chapter 18.)

Drug Therapy Regimens. Therapeutic drugs used to treat leukemia vary. Table 33-26 gives examples of treatment regimens used in various types of leukemia.

Combination chemotherapy is the mainstay of treatment for leukemia. The three purposes for using multiple drugs are to (a) decrease drug resistance, (b) minimize the drug toxicity to the patient by using multiple drugs with varying toxicities, and (c) interrupt cell growth at multiple points in the cell cycle.

Some therapeutic drugs are aimed at affecting small molecules that promote the growth and differentiation of leukemic cells. For example, arsenic trioxide (Trisenox), which is used to treat acute promyelocytic leukemia (a type of AML), causes DNA fragmentation and cell death. In addition, it inhibits cell proliferation and angiogenesis. Imatinib mesylate (Gleevec) and other tyrosine-kinase inhibitors target *BCR–ABL* protein that is present in nearly all patients with CML. Thus, this drug kills only cancer cells, leaving healthy cells alone.

The use of specific targeted therapy in the form of monoclonal antibodies is an exciting new treatment modality in hematopoietic malignancies, but cures with these therapies alone are rare. Rituximab (Rituxan) binds to the B-cell antigen (CD20) and has been used with CLL. Alemtuzumab (MabCampath) binds to CD52, a panlymphocyte antigen present on both T and B cells, and is used to treat CLL.

Hematopoietic Stem Cell Transplantation. HSCT is another type of therapy used for patients with different forms of leukemia.

TABLE 33-26 DRUG THERAPY

Treatments Used in Leukemia*

Drug Therapy	Other Therapy
Acute Myelogenous Leukemia	
Cytarabine (Cytosar), daunorubicin (Cerubidine),† idarubicin (Idamycin),† mitoxantrone, tretinoin (Vesanoid),† etoposide (Vepesid),† clofarabine (Clolar), arsenic trioxide (Trisenox), fludarabine (Fludara), azacitidine (Vidaza)	Autologous or allogeneic hematopoietic stem cell transplant (see Chapter 18)
Combination chemotherapy of cytarabine and antitumour antibiotic (most common)	
Acute Lymphocytic Leukemia	
Doxorubicin (Adriamycin), vincristine sulphate, prednisone, dexamethasone, L-asparaginase (Kidrolase) ponatinib (Iclusig), dasatinib (Sprycel), cyclophosphamide (Procytox), methotrexate, 6-mercaptopurine (Purinethol), cytarabine, imatinib (Gleevec), rituximab (Rituxan), clofarabine (Clolar)	Cranial radiation therapy, intrathecal methotrexate or cytarabine, allogeneic hematopoietic stem cell transplant (see Chapter 18)
Combination chemotherapy of several agents is common	
Chronic Myelogenous Leukemia	
Imatinib (Gleevec), dasatinib (Sprycel), ponatinib (Iclusig), nilotinib (Tasigna), bosutinib (Bosulif), hydroxyurea (Hydrea)	Radiation, hematopoietic stem cell transplant, interferon alfa, leukapheresis
Combination chemotherapy including any of the following: cytarabine, daunorubicin, methotrexate, prednisone, vincristine, L-asparaginase, 6-mercaptopurine, busulfan (Myleran)	
Chronic Lymphocytic Leukemia	
Chlorambucil (Leukeran), cyclophosphamide (Procytox), prednisone, vincristine, fludarabine (Fludara), rituximab (Rituxan), alemtuzumab (MabCampath), bendamustine (Treanda), oxaliplatin (Eloxatin), methotrexate, ofatumumab (Arzerra), idelalisib (Zydelig), obinutuzumab (Gazyva), ibrutinib (Imbruvica), lenalidomide (Revlimid)	Radiation, splenectomy, colony-stimulating factors, allogeneic hematopoietic stem cell transplant

*The classification and mechanism of action of these drugs are presented in Table 18-8 (Drug Therapy Classification of Chemotherapeutic Drugs).
†Used for acute promyelocytic leukemia.

The goal of HSCT is to totally eliminate leukemic cells from the body using combinations of chemotherapy with or without total body irradiation. This treatment also eradicates the patient's hematopoietic stem cells, which are then replaced with those of an HLA-matched sibling or volunteer donor (allogeneic), with those of an identical twin (syngeneic), or with the patient's own (autologous) stem cells that were removed (harvested) before the intensive therapy. (Hematopoietic stem cell transplantation is discussed in Chapter 18.)

The primary complications of patients who undergo allogeneic HSCT are graft-versus-host (GVH) disease, relapse of leukemia (especially ALL), and infection (especially interstitial pneumonia). GVH disease is discussed in Chapter 16. Because HSCT has serious associated risks, the patient must weigh the significant risks of treatment-related death or treatment failure (relapse) with the hope of cure.

NURSING MANAGEMENT LEUKEMIA

NURSING ASSESSMENT

Subjective and objective data that should be obtained from a patient with leukemia are presented in Table 33-27.

NURSING DIAGNOSES

Nursing diagnoses for the patient with leukemia include those appropriate for anemia, thrombo-cytopenia, and neutropenia (see NCP 33-1 in this chapter and NCPs 33-2 and 33-3 on the Evolve website).

PLANNING

The overall goals are that the patient with leukemia will (a) understand and follow the treatment plan, (b) experience minimal adverse effects and complications associated with both the disease and its treatment, and (c) establish realistic hopes and goals, and feel supported during the periods of treatment, relapse, or remission.

NURSING IMPLEMENTATION

ACUTE INTERVENTION. The nursing role during acute phases of leukemia is extremely challenging because the patient has many physical and psychosocial needs. As with other forms of cancer, the diagnosis of leukemia can evoke great fear and be equated with death. It may be viewed as a hopeless, horrible disease with many painful and undesirable consequences. The treatment and prognosis of each patient with leukemia are driven by many factors, such as age and type of leukemia. For each patient, it is important that the nurse has an understanding of the patient's type of leukemia, prognosis, treatment plan, and goals. With this information, the nurse can help the patient realize that, although the future may be uncertain, one can have a meaningful quality of life while in remission or with disease control and that, in some cases, there is reasonable hope for cure. The family also needs help adjusting to the stress of this abrupt onset of serious illness (e.g., with the patient's dependence, withdrawal, changes in role responsibilities, and alterations in body image) and the losses imposed by the sick role. The diagnosis of leukemia often brings with it the need to make difficult decisions at a time of profound stress for the patient and family.

Patients may have comorbid conditions that affect treatment decisions. Important nursing interventions include (a) maximizing the patient's physical functioning, (b) teaching patients that acute adverse effects of treatment are usually temporary, and (c) encouraging patients to discuss their quality-of-life issues. The nurse is an important advocate in helping the patient and family understand the complexities of treatment decisions and manage the adverse effects and toxicities. A patient may require long hospitalization or may need to temporarily relocate to an appropriate treatment centre. These situations can lead a patient to feel deserted and isolated at a time when support is most needed. The nurse has contact with the patient many hours a

TABLE 33-27 NURSING ASSESSMENT

Leukemia

Subjective Data
Important Health Information
Past health history: Exposure to chemical toxins (e.g., benzene, arsenic), radiation, or viruses (Epstein-Barr, HTLV-1); chromosome abnormalities (Down, Klinefelter's, and Fanconi's syndromes); immunological deficiencies; organ transplantation; frequent infections; bleeding tendencies; family history of leukemia
Medications: Chemotherapy
Surgery or other treatments: Radiation exposure; prior radiation and chemotherapy for cancer

Symptoms
- Weight loss, chills, night sweats
- Fatigue with progressive weakness; bone pain, joint pain; muscle cramps
- Dyspnea, cough
- Nausea, vomiting, anorexia, dysphagia, early satiety; mouth sores, sore throat
- Hematuria, decreased urine output
- Diarrhea, dark or bloody stools
- Headaches, confusion, numbness, tingling, visual disturbances
- Easy bruising; epistaxis; prolonged menses; menorrhagia; erectile dysfunction

Objective Data
General
Fever, generalized lymphadenopathy, lethargy

Integumentary
Pallor or jaundice; petechiae, ecchymoses, purpura, reddish-brown to purple cutaneous infiltrates, macules, and papules

Cardiovascular
Tachycardia, systolic murmurs

Gastro-Intestinal
Gingival bleeding and hyperplasia; oral ulcerations, herpes and *Candida* infections; perirectal irritation and infection; hepatomegaly, splenomegaly

Neurological
Seizures, disorientation, confusion, decreased coordination, cranial nerve palsies, papilledema

Musculo-Skeletal
Muscle wasting, bone pain, joint pain

Possible Findings
Low, normal, or high WBC count with shift to the left (blast cells); anemia, ↓ hematocrit and hemoglobin, thrombo-cytopenia, Philadelphia chromosome; hypercellular bone marrow aspirate or biopsy with myeloblasts, lymphoblasts, and markedly ↓ normal cells

HTLV-1, human T-cell leukemia virus, type 1; *WBC,* white blood cell.

day and can help reverse feelings of abandonment and loneliness by balancing the demanding technical needs with a humanistic, caring approach. The needs of the patient with leukemia are best met by a multidisciplinary team (e.g., psychiatric and oncology clinical nurse specialists, case managers, dietitians, chaplains, and social workers).

From a physical care perspective, the challenge is to make astute assessments and plan care to help the patient manage the severe adverse effects of chemotherapy. The life-threatening results of bone marrow suppression (neutropenia, thrombo-cytopenia, and anemia) require aggressive nursing interventions (see NCP

33-1, earlier in this chapter, and NCPs 33-2 and 33-3 on the Evolve website). These patients may be at risk for oncological emergencies such as tumour lysis syndrome, DIC, and leukostasis. Additional complications of chemotherapy may affect the patient's GI tract, nutritional status, skin and mucosa, cardiopulmonary status, liver, kidneys, and neurological system. (Nursing interventions related to chemotherapy are discussed in Chapter 18 and NCP 18-2 on the Evolve website.)

The nurse must be knowledgeable about all medications being administered. This knowledge must include mechanism of action, purpose, routes of administration, usual doses, potential adverse effects, safe-handling considerations, and toxic effects of the medications. In addition, the nurse must know how to assess laboratory data reflecting the effects of the medications. Patient survival and comfort during aggressive chemotherapy are significantly affected by the quality of nursing care.

AMBULATORY AND HOME CARE. Ongoing care for the patient with leukemia is necessary to monitor for signs and symptoms of disease control or relapse. For a patient requiring long-term or maintenance chemotherapy, long-term chronic disease management can become discouraging. Therefore, the patient and the family must be taught to understand the importance of the continued diligence in disease management and the need for follow-up care. Teachings must also include information about the medications and self-care measures and when to seek medical attention.

The goals of rehabilitation for long-term survivors of leukemia are to manage the physical, psychological, social, and spiritual consequences and delayed effects from the disease and its treatment. (Delayed effects from treatment are discussed in Chapter 18.) The patient may need assistance re-establishing some relationships, and friends and family may need help learning how to interact with the patient. The patient and the family must learn to regain attitudes of health and life while facing the real fear of relapse of disease. Involving the patient in survivor networks and support groups may help the patient adapt to living after a life-threatening illness. Exploring community resources (e.g., Canadian Cancer Society) may reduce the financial burden and the feelings of dependence. Spiritual support may give the patient inner strength and peace.

Vigilant follow-up care helps to ensure that the cancer survivor's unique needs are recognized and treated. Often, these needs require referral or consultation. For example, physiotherapists may be asked to develop an exercise program to prevent post-treatment deficits caused by drug-induced peripheral neuropathy. Some patients' needs may include, for instance, growth and development concerns for childhood survivors, vocational retraining, and reproductive concerns for a patient of child-bearing age. The long-term recovery following treatment for leukemia affects the quality of the patient's life.

EVALUATION

The expected outcomes are that the patient with leukemia will (a) cope effectively with diagnosis, treatment regimen, and prognosis; (b) experience no complications related to the disease or its treatment; and (c) feel comfortable and supported throughout treatment.

Lymphomas

Lymphomas are malignant neoplasms originating in the bone marrow and lymphatic structures resulting in the proliferation

TABLE 33-28	COMPARISON OF HODGKIN'S DISEASE AND NON-HODGKIN'S LYMPHOMA	
	Hodgkin's Disease	**Non-Hodgkin's Lymphoma**
Cellular origin	B lymphocytes	B lymphocytes (88%) T or natural killer lymphocytes (12%)
Extent of disease	Localized to regional, but may be more widespread	Disseminated
B symptoms*	Common	Uncommon
Extranodal involvement	Rare	Common

*B symptoms include fever, night sweats, and weight loss.

of lymphocytes. Two major types of lymphoma—Hodgkin's disease and non-Hodgkin's lymphoma (NHL)—are discussed in this chapter. NHL is the fourth most common type of cancer in Canada (Leukemia and Lymphoma Society of Canada, 2016). A comparison of these two types of lymphoma is presented in Table 33-28.

HODGKIN'S LYMPHOMA

Hodgkin's lymphoma, also called *Hodgkin's disease,* makes up about 11% of all lymphomas (Ansell, 2015). It is a malignant condition characterized by proliferation of abnormal, giant, multinucleated cells, called *Reed–Sternberg cells,* which are located in lymph nodes. The disease has a bimodal age-specific incidence, occurring most frequently in people from 15 to 30 years of age and older than 55 years (Hoppe, Advani, Ai, et al., 2015). In adults, it is twice as prevalent in men than in women. It was estimated that, in 2017, 990 people would be diagnosed with Hodgkin's lymphoma in Canada (Canadian Cancer Society, 2017b).

Etiology and Pathophysiology

Although the cause of Hodgkin's lymphoma remains unknown, several key factors are thought to play a role in its development. The main interacting factors include infection with Epstein-Barr virus (EBV), genetic predisposition, and exposure to occupational toxins. The incidence of Hodgkin's lymphoma is increased in patients with HIV.

Normally, the lymph nodes are composed of connective tissues that surround a fine mesh of reticular fibres and cells. In Hodgkin's lymphoma, the normal structure of lymph nodes is destroyed by hyperplasia of monocytes and macrophages. The main diagnostic feature of Hodgkin's disease is the presence of Reed–Sternberg cells in lymph node biopsy specimens. The disease is believed to arise in a single location (it originates in cervical lymph nodes in 80% of patients) and then spread along adjacent lymphatics. However, in recurrent disease, it may be more diffuse, and not necessarily contiguous. It eventually infiltrates other organs, especially the lungs, spleen, and liver. When the disease begins above the diaphragm, it remains confined to lymph nodes for a variable time. Disease originating below the diaphragm frequently spreads to extralymphoid sites such as the liver.

FIGURE 33-13 Enlarged cervical lymph node in the neck of a man with Hodgkin's lymphoma. Source: Howard, M. R., & Hamilton, P. J. (2013). *Haematology: An illustrated colour atlas* (4th ed.). London: Churchill Livingston.

Clinical Manifestations

The onset of symptoms in Hodgkin's lymphoma is usually insidious. The initial development is most often enlargement of cervical, axillary, or inguinal lymph nodes (Figure 33-13); a mediastinal node is the second most common location. This lymphadenopathy affects discrete nodes that remain movable and nontender. The enlarged nodes are not painful unless they exert pressure on adjacent nerves.

The patient may notice weight loss, fatigue, weakness, fever, chills, tachycardia, or night sweats. A group of initial findings including fever, night sweats, and weight loss (termed *B symptoms*) correlates with a worse prognosis. After the ingestion of even small amounts of alcohol, individuals with Hodgkin's disease may complain of a rapid onset of pain at the site of disease. The cause for the alcohol-induced pain is unknown. Generalized pruritus without skin lesions may develop. Cough, dyspnea, stridor, and dysphagia may all reflect mediastinal node involvement.

In more advanced disease, there is hepatomegaly and splenomegaly. Anemia results from increased destruction and decreased production of erythrocytes. Other physical signs vary depending on where the disease is located; for example, (a) intrathoracic involvement may lead to superior vena cava syndrome, (b) enlarged retroperitoneal nodes may cause palpable abdominal masses or interfere with renal function, (c) jaundice may occur from liver involvement, (d) spinal cord compression leading to paraplegia may occur with extradural involvement, and (e) bone pain may occur as a result of bone involvement.

Diagnostic and Staging Studies

Peripheral blood analysis, excisional lymph node biopsy, bone marrow examination, and radiological evaluation are important means of evaluating Hodgkin's lymphoma. Peripheral blood analysis often reveals a microcytic hypochromic anemia; neutrophilic leukocytosis ($15–28 \times 10^9/L$), which may be associated with lymphopenia; and an increased platelet count. Leukopenia and thrombo-cytopenia may develop, but they are usually a consequence of treatment, advanced disease, or superimposed hypersplenism. Other blood studies may show an elevated erythrocyte sedimentation rate, hypoferremia caused by excessive iron uptake by the liver and spleen, elevated leukocyte alkaline phosphatase from liver and bone involvement, hypercalcemia from bone involvement, and hypoalbuminemia from liver involvement.

Excisional lymph node biopsy offers a definitive means of diagnosis. The removed peripheral lymph node is examined for the presence of the diagnostic Reed–Sternberg cells. Bone marrow biopsy is performed as an important aspect of staging. Reed–Sternberg cells may also be found in the patient's bone marrow.

Radiological evaluation can help define all sites and determine the clinical stage of the disease. CT or MRI scans are used as initial staging tools. These scans may show mediastinal lymphadenopathy; renal displacement caused by retroperitoneal node enlargement; abdominal lymph node enlargement; and liver, spleen, bone, and brain infiltration. Gallium scans may also be used to monitor response to treatment.

NURSING AND COLLABORATIVE MANAGEMENT HODGKIN'S LYMPHOMA

The information from the various diagnostic studies is used to determine the stage of the disease (Figure 33-14). The nomenclature used in staging includes a Roman numeral (I to IV) that reflects the location and extent of the disease, followed by an *A* or *B* classification (meaning B symptoms are absent or present, respectively). Treatment depends on the nature and the extent of the disease.

Once the stage of Hodgkin's lymphoma is established, management focuses on selecting a treatment plan. The standard for chemotherapy is the ABVD regimen: doxorubicin (**A**driamycin), **b**leomycin, **v**inblastine, and **d**acarbazine. Patients with early-stage disease with favourable characteristics will receive two to four cycles of chemotherapy. Patients with early-stage but unfavourable prognostic features (e.g., the presence of B symptoms) or intermediate-stage disease will be treated with four to six cycles of chemotherapy. Advanced-stage Hodgkin's lymphoma is treated more aggressively using six to, potentially, eight cycles of chemotherapy. A more aggressive chemotherapy regimen is BEACOPP (**b**leomycin, **e**toposide, doxorubicin [**A**driamycin], **c**yclophosphamide, vincristine (former trade name **O**ncovin), **p**rocarbazine, and **p**rednisone) (Hoppe, Advani, Ai, et al., 2015). The role of radiation as a supplement to chemotherapy varies depending on sites of disease and the presence of resistant disease after chemotherapy.

A variety of chemotherapy regimes and newer drugs, such as brentuximab vedotin (Adcetris), are used to treat patients with relapsed or refractory disease. Ideally, once remission is achieved, a curative option may be intensive chemotherapy with the use of autologous or allogeneic HSCT. HSCT has allowed patients to receive higher, potentially curative doses of chemotherapy while reducing life-threatening leukopenia. Combination chemotherapy works well because, as with leukemia, drugs are used that have an additive antitumour effect without increased adverse effects. As with leukemia, therapy must be aggressive. Thus, potentially life-threatening problems are risked for the sake of attempting to achieve a remission.

Maintenance chemotherapy does not contribute to increased survival once a complete remission is achieved. Occasionally, single medications may be administered palliatively to patients who cannot tolerate intensive combination therapy. A serious consequence of the treatment for Hodgkin's lymphoma is the later development of secondary malignancies (see Chapter 18) as well as potential long-term toxicities from the treatment, such as endocrine, cardiac, and pulmonary dysfunction (Kanate, Craig, Abraham, et al., 2013). Secondary cancers often occur 10 years after treatment for Hodgkin's lymphoma, the most common of

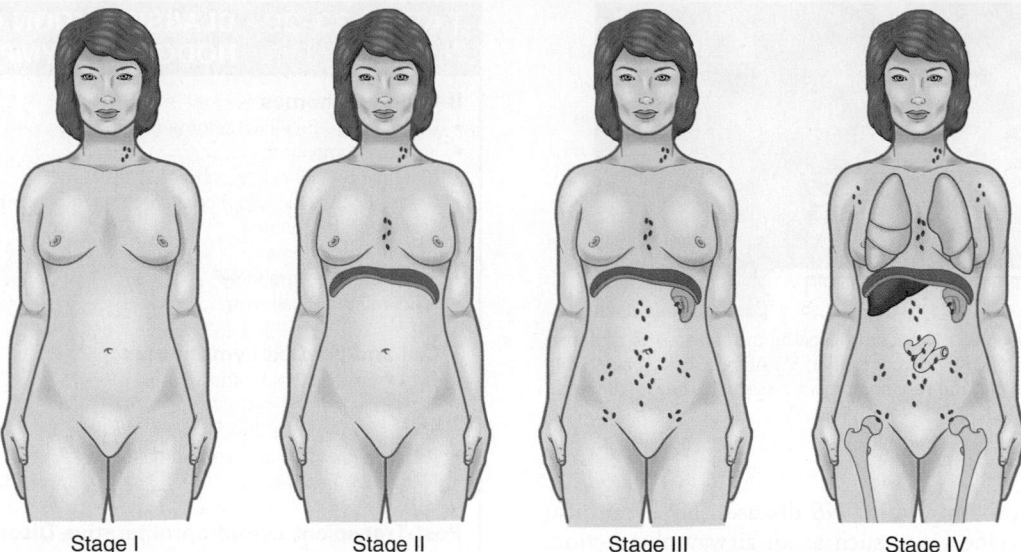

| Stage I | Stage II | Stage III | Stage IV |

FIGURE 33-14 Staging system for Hodgkin's lymphoma and non-Hodgkin's lymphoma. **Stage I,** involvement of single lymph node (e.g., cervical node). **Stage II,** involvement of two or more lymph nodes on one side of diaphragm. **Stage III,** lymph node involvement above and below the diaphragm. **Stage IV,** involvement outside the lymph nodes (e.g., liver, bone marrow). The stage is followed by the letter A (absence) or B (presence) to indicate significant systemic symptoms (e.g., fever, night sweats, weight loss).

which are breast cancer and lung cancer. Patients should have screening for early detection of these problems.

The nursing care for patients with Hodgkin's lymphoma is largely focused on managing problems related to the disease (e.g., pain caused by the tumour), pancytopenia, and other adverse effects of therapy. Because the survival of patients with Hodgkin's lymphoma depends on their response to treatment, supporting the patient through the immuno-suppressive state is extremely important.

Psychosocial considerations are just as important as they are with leukemia. However, the prognosis for Hodgkin's lymphoma is better than that for many other forms of cancer. The physical, psychological, social, and spiritual consequences of the patient's disease must be addressed. Fertility issues may be of particular concern because this disease is frequently seen in adolescents and young adults. The nurse must help ensure that these issues are addressed soon after diagnosis. Evaluation of patients for long-term effects of therapy is important because delayed consequences of disease and treatment may not be apparent for many years. (Secondary malignancies and delayed effects of treatment are discussed in Chapter 18.)

NON-HODGKIN'S LYMPHOMA

Non-Hodgkin's lymphomas (NHLs) are a heterogeneous group of malignant neoplasms of primarily B-, T-, or natural killer (NK)–cell origin that can affect people of all ages. B-cell lymphomas constitute about 88% of all NHLs. They are classified by the level of differentiation, cell of origin, and rate of proliferation. A variety of clinical presentations and courses are recognized, from indolent (slowly developing) to rapidly progressive disease. NHL is the most commonly occurring hematological cancer. It was estimated that, in 2017, there would be 8 300 new cases of NHL diagnosed in Canada and approximately 2 700 deaths due to NHL (Canadian Cancer Society, 2017c).

Etiology and Pathophysiology

As with Hodgkin's lymphoma, the cause of NHL is usually unknown. It may result from chromosomal translocations, infections, environmental factors, or immunodeficiency states. Chromosomal translocations have an important role in the pathogenesis of many NHLs. Some viruses and bacteria are implicated in the pathogenesis of NHL, including HTLV-1, EBV, human herpesvirus 8, hepatitis B and C, *Helicobacter pylori, Chlamydophila psittaci, Campylobacter jejuni,* and *Borrelia burgdorferi.* Environmental factors linked to the development of NHL include chemicals such as pesticides, herbicides, solvents, organic chemicals, and wood preservatives. NHL is also more common in individuals who have inherited immunodeficiency syndromes and who have used immuno-suppressive medications or received chemotherapy or radiation.

There is no hallmark feature in NHL that parallels the Reed–Sternberg cell of Hodgkin's lymphoma. However, all NHLs involve lymphocytes arrested in various stages of development. For example, lymphoblastic lymphoma and lymphoblastic leukemia (which has a majority of disease within the bone marrow rather than in the lymph nodes) result from malignant proliferation of small, immature B lymphocytes. Diffuse large B-cell lymphoma, the most common aggressive lymphoma in adults, is a neoplasm that originates in the lymph nodes. Burkitt's lymphoma is a highly aggressive disease thought to originate from B-cell blast cells in the lymph nodes.

Clinical Manifestations

NHLs can originate outside the lymph nodes, the method of spread can be unpredictable, and the majority of patients have widely disseminated disease at the time of diagnosis (Figure 33-15). The primary clinical manifestation is painless lymph node enlargement. Because the disease is usually disseminated when it is diagnosed, other symptoms will be present depending on where the disease has spread (e.g., hepatomegaly with liver involvement

FIGURE 33-15 Non-Hodgkin's lymphoma involving the spleen. The presence of an isolated mass is typical. Source: Kumar, V., Abbas, A. K., Fausto, N., et al. (2010). *Robbins and Cotran pathologic basis of disease* (8th ed., p. 607). Philadelphia: Saunders.

TABLE 33-29   CLASSIFICATION OF NON-HODGKIN'S LYMPHOMA*
B-Cell Lymphomas • Diffuse large B-cell lymphoma (DLBCL) • Follicular lymphoma • Marginal zone B-cell lymphoma (MALT) • Small lymphocytic lymphoma/chronic lymphocytic leukemia • Mantle cell lymphoma • Burkitt's lymphoma • Plasmablastic lymphoma • AIDS-related B-cell lymphomas **T-Cell and NK-Cell Lymphomas** • Lymphoblastic lymphoma • T-cell lymphoma • Mycosis fungoides and Sézary syndrome • Anaplastic large T-cell lymphoma • NK-cell lymphomas **Post-Transplant Lymphoproliferative Disorders (PTLD)**

AIDS, acquired immune deficiency syndrome; *MALT,* mucosa-associated lymphoid tissue; *NK,* natural killer.
*This is only a partial list.

or neurological symptoms with CNS disease). NHL can also manifest in nonspecific ways, such as an airway obstruction, hyperuricemia, renal failure or acute kidney injury from tumour lysis syndrome, pericardial tamponade, or GI complaints.

Patients with high-grade lymphomas may have lymphadenopathy and constitutional symptoms (B symptoms) such as fever, night sweats, and weight loss. The peripheral blood is usually normal, but some lymphomas manifest in a "leukemic" phase.

Diagnostic and Staging Studies

Diagnostic studies used for NHL resemble those used for Hodgkin's disease. However, because NHL is more often in extranodal sites, more diagnostic studies may be done, such as an MRI to rule out CNS or bone marrow infiltration or a barium enema or CT to visualize suspected GI involvement. Clinical staging, as described for Hodgkin's lymphoma, is used to help guide therapy (see Figure 33-14), but establishment of the precise histological subtype is extremely important. Lymph node biopsy establishes the cell type and the pattern. NHL is classified based on morphological, genetic, immunophenotypic (i.e., cell surface antigens, CD20, CD52), and clinical features.

The World Health Organization has categorized more than 30 unique types of NHL. A simple modification of the classification system is presented in Table 33-29.

Treatment is guided by cell type, cytogenetic studies, and clinical behaviour: *indolent* (low grade), *aggressive* (high grade), or *highly aggressive* (very high grade). Additional factors, known as the International Prognostic Index (IPI), may be considered for each subtype to help select the appropriate treatment for each patient. Factors considered may include the clinical stage, number of extranodal sites, age, serum LDH level, WBC count, Hb, and performance status. Immunological, cytogenetic, and molecular studies are also useful for making therapeutic decisions and assessing prognoses.

NURSING AND COLLABORATIVE MANAGEMENT NON-HODGKIN'S LYMPHOMA

Treatment for NHL involves chemotherapy and sometimes radiation (Table 33-30). Ironically, more aggressive lymphomas are more responsive to treatment and more likely to be cured. In contrast, indolent lymphomas have a naturally long course but are difficult to treat effectively.

Patients with low-grade (indolent) lymphoma may live 10 years or more without treatment. However, some initial therapies

can be well tolerated and have been shown to extend the time to progression of the disease. Therapy would be indicated if the patient has local symptoms from progressive, bulky, or painful disease or a compromise of normal organ function. Lymphomas that have an infectious basis, such as *H. pylori* gastric lymphomas, may be treated with antibiotic or antiviral therapy. HSCT may have some benefit in certain subtypes of aggressive or refractory lymphomas.

Rituximab, a genetically engineered monoclonal antibody against the CD20 antigen on the surface of normal and malignant B lymphocytes, is also used to treat NHL. Once bound to the cells, rituximab causes lysis and cell death. Numerous chemotherapy combinations have been used to try to overcome the resistant nature of this disease. Complete remissions are uncommon, but the majority of patients will respond with improvement in adenopathy and symptoms.

> **DRUG ALERT—rituximab (Rituxin)**
> • Patients must be monitored for signs of severe hypersensitivity or reaction to rituximab (Rituxan), especially with the first infusion.
> • Manifestations may include hypotension, bronchospasm, dysrhythmias, angioedema, and cardiogenic shock.
> • Patients should be screened for history of hepatitis because rituximab may reactivate the disease.

Another therapy for NHL is the monoclonal antibody ibritumomab tiuxetan (Zevalin). This antibody is linked to a radioactive isotope (yttrium-90) (see Chapter 18, Table 18-16). The monoclonal antibody targets the CD20 antigen, which is on the surface of mature B cells and B-cell tumours. This targeting allows for the delivery of radiation directly to the malignant cells. Adverse effects of these medications include pancytopenia. Nurses must be aware of the precautions to take in caring for these patients and must educate patients about safety issues to minimize the risk of radiation exposure to staff and others.

In general, T-cell lymphomas are more difficult to treat and are often treated aggressively up front followed by an HSCT. Cutaneous T-cell lymphomas may be treated with topical corticosteroids or topical chemotherapy for limited-stage disease. For more diffuse disease, treatment may include phototherapy, interferon alfa, vorinostat (Zolinza), or others.

TABLE 33-30 TREATMENT OF NON-HODGKIN'S LYMPHOMA*

Recommended Therapies	Common Chemotherapy Combinations
Indolent (Low Grade) (e.g., follicular lymphoma, marginal zone B-cell lymphoma [MALT])	
• Observation until disease progression for asymptomatic patients with low-volume tumours and normal blood counts • External beam irradiation for local, limited disease • Single-agent rituximab (Rituxan) • Single-agent chemotherapy (chlorambucil, cyclophosphamide, bendamustine, or idelalisib) • Rituximab with another agent (bendamustine, cyclophosphamide, fludarabine, cladribine, lenalidomide, chlorambucil) • Combination chemotherapy (R-CHOP or other) • Radioimmunotherapy • Hematopoietic stem cell transplant (HSCT)	• **R-CHOP: r**ituximab, **c**yclophosphamide, doxorubicin **h**ydrochloride, vincristine (former trade name **O**ncovin), **p**rednisone • **FCMR: f**ludarabine, **c**yclophosphamide **m**itoxantrone, **r**ituximab • **R-CVP: r**ituximab, **c**yclophosphamide, **v**incristine, **p**rednisone • **RFND: r**ituximab, **f**ludarabine, mitoxantrone (former trade name **N**ovantrone), **d**examethasone ± rituximab • **FC: f**ludarabine, **c**yclophosphamide
Aggressive (Intermediate or High Grade) (e.g., mantle cell, diffuse large B-cell, peripheral T-cell, natural killer–cell lymphomas)	
• Combination chemotherapy with localized radiation if needed • Aggressive combination chemotherapy for 3–8 cycles with rituximab with local radiation if needed • Intrathecal chemotherapy if needed • Single agent or other combination treatment, depending on subtype and response (e.g., bendamustine, bortezomib, cladribine, ibrutinib, lenalidomide, gemcitabine, alemtuzumab, oxaliplatin, romidepsin) • HSCT	• **R-CHOP** (see above) • **ICE** (or "RICE" with **r**ituximab): **i**fosfamide, **c**yclophosphamide, **e**toposide • **R-EPOCH: r**ituximab, **e**toposide, **p**rednisone, vincristine (former trade name **O**ncovin), **c**yclophosphamide, doxorubicin **h**ydrochloride • **ESHAP ± R: e**toposide, methylprednisolone (**S**olu-Medrol), **h**igh-dose cytarabine (former trade name **A**ra-C), cisplatin (former trade name **P**latinol), with or without **r**ituximab • **Hyper-CVAD ± R:** hyperfractionated **c**yclophosphamide, **v**incristine, doxorubicin hydrochloride (**A**driamycin), **d**examethasone alternating with high-dose methotrexate and cytarabine with or without rituximab • **DHAP ± R: d**examethasone, **h**igh-dose cytarabine (former trade name **A**ra-C), cisplatin (former trade name **P**latinol), with or without **r**ituximab • **SMILE: s**teroids, **m**ethotrexate, **i**fosfamide, L-asparaginase, **e**toposide • High-dose cytarabine and high-dose methotrexate with leucovorin rescue
Highly Aggressive (e.g., Burkitt's lymphoma, AIDS-related B-cell lymphomas)	
• Aggressive combination chemotherapy for 3–8 cycles • HSCT	• Hyper-CVAD ± R (see above) • CODOX-M: **c**yclophosphamide, vincristine (former trade name **O**ncovin), **dox**orubicin, high-dose **m**ethotrexate, with or without **r**ituximab (includes intrathecal methotrexate)

MALT, mucosa-associated lymphoid tissue.
*Not all-inclusive.

The nursing care for NHL is similar to that for Hodgkin's lymphoma. Nursing care is largely focused on managing problems related to the disease (e.g., pain caused by the tumour, spinal cord compression, tumour lysis syndrome), pancytopenia, and other adverse effects of therapy. However, because NHL can be more extensive and involve specific organs (e.g., CNS, spleen, liver, GI tract, bone marrow), it is important that the nurse have an understanding of the subtype and the extent of the disease. For example, a patient with known involvement of the colon may complain of acute abdominal pain. The patient most likely would have abdominal guarding and an enlarged and tympanic abdomen. This could indicate a bowel perforation and be considered a medical emergency. A patient with Burkitt's NHL starting chemotherapy would be at high risk for tumour lysis syndrome and would require frequent laboratory studies and monitoring, as well as strict documentation of intake and output. (For oncological problems, refer to Chapter 18.) Because most of these patients receive therapy that is potentially myelosuppressive, NCP 33-1, NCP 33-2, and NCP 33-3 would apply to these patients as well.

A patient undergoing radiation therapy has special nursing needs. The skin in the radiation field requires attention. In addition, the nurse must understand the concepts related to administration of and safety issues regarding radiation therapy (see Chapter 18 and NCP 18-1 on the Evolve website).

Psychosocial considerations are very important. Helping the patient and the family understand the disease, the treatment, and expected and potential adverse effects is paramount in enlisting their help in ensuring the patient's well-being and safety. Some aggressive treatments require close follow-up and even inpatient admission. In young patients, fertility concerns may need to be addressed. As with Hodgkin's lymphoma, evaluation of patients with NHL for long-term effects of therapy is important because delayed consequences of disease and treatment may not be apparent for many years. (Secondary malignancies and delayed effects of treatment are discussed in Chapter 18.)

MULTIPLE MYELOMA

Multiple myeloma, or *plasma cell myeloma,* is a condition in which neoplastic plasma cells infiltrate the bone marrow and destroy bone. The disease is more common in men than in women and usually develops after 40 years of age, with an average age at onset of 69 years (Röllig, Knop, & Bornhäuser, 2015). Myeloma has a higher incidence in Black ethnic groups than in White people. It was estimated that, in 2017, 2 900 new cases of multiple myeloma would be diagnosed in Canada (Canadian Cancer Society, 2017d).

Etiology and Pathophysiology

The cause of multiple myeloma is unknown. Exposure to radiation, organic chemicals (such as benzene), herbicides, and insecticides may play a role. Genetic factors, viral infection,

EVIDENCE-INFORMED PRACTICE

Translating Research Into Practice

A nurse is caring for Gerard Robineault, a 59-year-old male with non-Hodgkin's lymphoma who is receiving chemotherapy. Due to a decrease in red blood cells and platelets, he was advised to rest and avoid the high level of physical exercise he once enjoyed. He misses his active lifestyle and now admits to the nurse that he is "somewhat depressed."

Best Available Evidence	Clinician Expertise	Patient Preferences and Values
Aerobic exercise, especially walking and stretching, to maintain mobility may improve physical functioning, fatigue, and depression in patients with hematological cancers.	The nurse knows that recommendations to decrease intensive physical exercise may result in a diminished quality of life for many patients, especially for individuals who are used to being physically active.	Gerard is considering joining a neighbourhood bicycling club so that he can "feel better."

Decision and Action

1. Why is intensive or extreme exercise contraindicated in someone who is receiving chemotherapy or who is acutely ill?
2. What precautions should the nurse suggest Gerard take before he increases his exercise level?
3. How should the nurse involve Gerard in monitoring his fatigue?
4. As Gerard seeks ways to improve his quality of life, how should the nurse support him?

Reference for Evidence

Bergenthal, N., Will, A., Streckmann, F., et al. (2014). Aerobic physical exercise for adult patients with haematological malignancies. *The Cochrane Database of Systematic Reviews, 11*, doi:10.1002/14651858.CD009075.pub2.

FIGURE 33-16 Multiple myeloma. This segment of the lower thoracic spine has been sectioned to show the extensive replacement of the bone and the marrow with red gelatinous tissue. Source: Skarin, A. T. (1996). *Atlas of diagnostic oncology* (2nd ed.). London: Mosby-Wolfe.

and obesity may also influence the risk of developing multiple myeloma.

The disease process involves excessive production of plasma cells. Plasma cells are activated B cells, which produce immunoglobulins (antibodies) that normally protect the body. However, in multiple myeloma, instead of a variety of plasma cells producing antibodies to fight different infections, myeloma tumours produce monoclonal antibodies. *Monoclonal* means they are all of one kind, making them ineffective and even harmful. Not only do they not fight infections, but they also infiltrate the bone marrow. *Bence Jones proteins* are the light chain part of these monoclonal antibodies. They show up in the urine in many patients with multiple myeloma.

Furthermore, plasma-cell production of excessive amounts of cytokines (interleukins [ILs]; IL-4, IL-5, and IL-6) also plays an important role in the pathological process of bone destruction. As myeloma protein increases, normal plasma cells are reduced, a decrease that further compromises the body's normal immune response. Proliferation of malignant plasma cells and the overproduction of immunoglobulin and proteins result in the end-organ effects of myeloma to the bone marrow, bone, and kidneys and possibly the spleen, lymph nodes, liver, and even heart muscle.

Clinical Manifestations

Multiple myeloma develops slowly and insidiously. The patient often does not manifest symptoms until the disease is advanced, at which time skeletal pain is the major manifestation. Pain in the pelvis, spine, and ribs is particularly common and is triggered by movement. Diffuse osteoporosis develops as the myeloma protein destroys bone. Osteolytic lesions are seen in the skull, vertebrae, and ribs (Figure 33-16). Vertebral destruction can lead to collapse of vertebrae with ensuing compression of the spinal cord. Loss of bone integrity can lead to the development of pathological fractures.

Bony degeneration also causes calcium to be lost from bones, eventually causing hypercalcemia. Hypercalcemia may cause renal, GI, or neurological manifestations such as polyuria, anorexia, confusion, and ultimately seizures, coma, and cardiac problems. A serum *hyperviscosity syndrome* can occur in some patients, leading to cerebral, pulmonary, renal, and other organ dysfunction. Even without hyperviscosity, high protein levels caused by the presence of the myeloma protein can result in renal tubular obstruction, interstitial nephritis, and renal failure. The patient may also display manifestations of anemia, thrombo-cytopenia, and granulo-cytopenia (recurrent infections), all of which are related to the replacement of normal bone marrow with plasma cells. Neurological abnormalities may be caused by regional myeloma cell growth that compresses the spinal cord or cranial nerves or by perineuronal or perivascular deposition.

Diagnostic Studies

Evaluating multiple myeloma involves laboratory, radiological, and bone marrow examination. M protein can be found in the blood and urine. Pancytopenia, hypercalcemia, the presence of Bence Jones protein in the urine, and an elevated serum creatinine are possible findings.

Skeletal bone surveys; MRI, PET scan, or both; and CT scan show distinct lytic areas of bone erosions, generalized thinning of the bones, or fractures, especially in vertebrae, ribs, pelvis, and bones of the thigh and the upper arms. Bone marrow analysis shows significantly increased numbers of plasma cells in the bone marrow. The simplest criteria for prognosis in multiple myeloma are the blood levels of two markers: β_2-microglobulin and albumin. In general, higher levels of β_2-microglobulin and lower levels of albumin are associated with a poorer prognosis.

Collaborative Care

Collaborative care involves managing both the disease and its symptoms. The current treatment options include corticosteroids, chemotherapy, immunotherapy, targeted therapy, and HSCT (Röllig, Knop, & Bornhäuser, 2015). Multiple myeloma is seldom cured, but treatment can relieve symptoms, produce remission, and prolong life. Ambulation and adequate hydration are used to treat hypercalcemia, dehydration, and potential renal damage. Weight bearing helps the bones reabsorb some calcium, and fluids dilute calcium and prevent protein precipitates from causing renal tubular obstruction. Control of pain and prevention of pathological fractures are other goals of management. Analgesics, orthopedic supports, and localized radiation help reduce the skeletal pain.

Kyphoplasty is sometimes used to control spinal vertebral disease. *Kyphoplasty* is a minimally invasive procedure that injects cement to stabilize the vertebral compression (Terpos, Berenson, Raje, et al., 2014).

Bisphosphonates, such as pamidronate and zoledronic acid (Zometa), inhibit bone breakdown and are used for the treatment of skeletal pain and hypercalcemia. They inhibit bone resorption without inhibiting bone formation and mineralization. They are given monthly by IV infusion and are recommended for all patients with symptomatic multiple myeloma.

> **DRUG ALERT—zoledronic acid (Zometa)**
> - Patients must be adequately hydrated prior to administering zoledronic acid (Zometa).
> - Renal toxicity may occur if IV zoledronic acid is infused in less than 15 minutes.

Chemotherapy with corticosteroids is often recommended for multiple myeloma. It is used to reduce the number of plasma cells. Initial treatment depends on whether the patient is a future bone marrow transplant candidate and on anticipated tolerance of therapy. The treatment usually includes a corticosteroid plus one or two chemotherapy agents, such as melphalan (Alkeran), cyclophosphamide, doxorubicin (Adriamycin), and bendamustine (Treanda). High-dose chemotherapy followed by autologous HSCT has evolved as the standard of care in eligible patients.

Immunotherapy and targeted therapy are also used to treat multiple myeloma. Immuno-modulator drugs include thalidomide (Thalomid), lenalidomide (Revlimid), and pomalidomide (Pomalyst). Proteasome inhibitors include bortezomib (Velcade).

Drugs may be used to treat complications of multiple myeloma. For example, allopurinol (Zyloprim) may be given to reduce hyperuricemia, and IV furosemide (Lasix) promotes renal excretion of calcium. In some patients, the levels of plasma proteins are so high that it causes a hyperviscosity syndrome leading to neurological changes, renal insufficiency, and other problems related to the lack of blood flow. In this instance, plasmapheresis is used.

NURSING MANAGEMENT
MULTIPLE MYELOMA

A major focus of care relates to the bone involvement and the sequelae from bone breakdown. Maintaining adequate hydration is a primary nursing consideration to minimize problems from hypercalcemia. Fluids are administered to attain a urinary output of 1.5 to 2 L/day if the patient does not have renal compromise. In addition, weight bearing helps bones reabsorb some of the circulating calcium, and corticosteroids may augment the excretion of calcium. Once chemotherapy is initiated, the uric acid levels may rise because of the increased cell destruction. Hyperuricemia is treated by ensuring adequate hydration and using allopurinol to prevent any renal damage. Because of the myeloma proteins, the patient is at additional risk for renal dysfunction. The nurse must monitor electrolytes and fluid balance.

Because of the potential for pathological fractures, the nurse must be careful when moving and ambulating the patient. A slight twist or strain in the wrong area (e.g., a weak area in the patient's bones) may be sufficient to cause a fracture. In addition, the development of peripheral neuropathy is common with several therapies for multiple myeloma and can contribute to discomfort, the inability to perform basic activities of daily living, and the risk for injury from falling.

Pain management requires innovative and knowledgeable nursing interventions. Analgesics, such as nonsteroidal anti-inflammatory drugs, acetaminophen, or an acetaminophen–opioid combination, may be more effective than opioids alone in diminishing bone pain. Braces, especially for the spine, may also help control pain. As in any situation necessitating pain management, the nurse is responsible for assessing the patient and for implementing necessary measures to alleviate the pain. (Pain management is discussed in Chapter 10.) Patients may also be at risk for deep-vein thrombosis related to chemotherapy and immobility and should have preventive measures employed.

Assessment and prompt treatment of infection are important in the care of patients with multiple myeloma. Recurrent infections may be caused by a decrease in the production of normal immunoglobulins, the ineffectiveness of the overproduced and abnormal immunoglobulins, neutropenia that results from the bone marrow infiltration or as an adverse effect of treatment, or a combination of these. NCP 33-1 for anemia, NCP 33-2 for thrombo-cytopenia, and NCP 33-3 for neutropenia apply to the patient with multiple myeloma. (NCPs 33-2 and 33-3 are available on the Evolve website.)

The patient's psychosocial needs require sensitive, skilled management. It is important to help the patient and significant others adapt to changes fostered by chronic sickness and adjust to the losses related to the disease process while helping to maximize functioning and quality of life. The symptoms of multiple myeloma go through remission and exacerbation periods. Consequently, acute care is needed at various times during the course of the illness. The final acute phase is unresponsive to treatment and usually short. The way in which patients and families deal with confronting death may be affected by the manner in which they learned to accept and live with the chronic nature of the disease.

DISORDERS OF THE SPLEEN

The spleen can be affected by many illnesses, most of which cause some degree of *splenomegaly* (enlarged spleen) (Table 33-31). The term *hypersplenism* refers to the occurrence of splenomegaly and peripheral cytopenias (anemia, leukopenia, and thrombo-cytopenia). The degree of splenic enlargement varies with the disease. For example, massive splenic enlargement occurs with chronic myelogenous leukemia, hairy cell leukemia, and thalassemia major. Mild splenic enlargement occurs with HF and systemic lupus erythematosus.

TABLE 33-31 CAUSES OF SPLENOMEGALY

Infections and Inflammations
- Bacterial infections: endocarditis, salmonella
- Mycobacterial infections: tuberculosis
- Spirochetes: syphilis, Lyme disease
- Viral infections: hepatitis, human immunodeficiency virus, cytomegalovirus, mononucleosis
- Parasitic infections: malaria, trypanosomiasis, schistosomiasis, leishmaniasis, toxoplasmosis
- Rickettsial infections: Rocky Mountain spotted fever, typhoid fever
- Fungal infections: histoplasmosis
- Autoimmune diseases: systemic lupus erythematosus, rheumatoid arthritis

Infiltrative Diseases and Tumours or Cysts
- Acute and chronic leukemia
- Lymphomas
- Polycythemia vera
- Multiple myeloma, amyloidosis
- Other primary or secondary neoplasms and cysts
- Sarcoidosis
- Gaucher's disease

Congestion
- Cirrhosis of the liver
- Heart failure (portal hypertension)
- Portal or splenic vein thrombosis
- Sickle cell disease
- Thalassemia
- Acquired hemolytic anemia
- Immune thrombo-cytopenia

When the spleen enlarges, its normal filtering and sequestering capacity increases. Consequently, there is often a reduction in the number of circulating blood cells. In addition, there are unusual findings in the peripheral smear, such as pitted or pocked erythrocytes or Howell–Jolly bodies. These findings assist with diagnosing a malfunctioning spleen. A slight to moderate enlargement of the spleen is usually asymptomatic and found during a routine examination of the abdomen. Even massive splenomegaly can be well tolerated, but the patient may complain of abdominal discomfort and early satiety. In addition to physical examination, other techniques to assess the size of the spleen include radionuclide colloid liver–spleen scan, CT scan, MRI, and ultrasound scan.

Occasionally, laparotomy and splenectomy are indicated in the evaluation or treatment of splenomegaly. Splenectomy can have a dramatic effect in increasing peripheral RBC, WBC, and platelet counts. Another major indication for splenectomy is splenic rupture. The spleen may rupture from trauma, inadvertent tearing during other surgical procedures, and diseases such as mononucleosis, malaria, and lymphoid neoplasms.

Nursing responsibilities for the patient with spleen disorders vary depending on the nature of the problem. Splenomegaly may be painful and may necessitate analgesic administration; care in moving, turning, and positioning; and evaluation of lung expansion because spleen enlargement may impair diaphragmatic excursion. If anemia, thrombo-cytopenia, or leukopenia develops from splenic enlargement, nursing measures must be instituted to support the patient and prevent life-threatening complications. If splenectomy is performed, observation for hemorrhage and shock is required.

After splenectomy, immunological deficiencies may develop. Patients who have had splenectomy have a lifelong risk for infection, especially from encapsulated organisms such as pneumococcus (Weledji, 2014). This risk is reduced by immunization with pneumococcal vaccine (e.g., Pneumovax).

BLOOD COMPONENT THERAPY

Blood component therapy is frequently used in managing hematological diseases. Many therapeutic and surgical procedures depend on blood product support. However, blood component therapy supports the patient only temporarily so is used in the interim until the underlying problem is resolved. Because transfusions are not free from hazards, they should be used only if necessary.

Nurses must be careful to avoid developing a complacent attitude about this common but potentially dangerous therapy. Nurses also must make sure that the physician has discussed the risks, benefits, and alternatives with the patient and that this conversation is documented in the patient's medical record.

Traditionally, the term *blood transfusion* meant the administration of whole blood. Blood transfusion now has a broader meaning because of the ability to administer specific components of blood such as platelets, packed red blood cells (PRBCs), or plasma. Usually, a specific component is ordered, although whole blood may be used rarely with massive hemorrhage or for an exchange transfusion (Table 33-32).

After the Canadian blood supply was found to be tainted with viruses in the 1980s, a government inquiry known as the Krever Commission (1997) led to a new federally mandated and regulated system (Ministry of Health, 1997). For example, in Canada, all blood is tested for viruses such as HIV and hepatitis as well as other infectious organisms. Strict donor screening now takes place to reduce the risk for transfusion-transmitted infection. Although the blood supply in Canada is very safe, the Krever Commission recommended recipients be informed of the benefits, risks, and alternatives to receiving donor blood products. The new federal standards on blood and blood components are relevant to nursing policy and practice because they highlight critical areas such as proper patient and product identification as well as careful monitoring of patients receiving blood products.

Administration Procedure

Blood components may be administered with a 22-gauge IV needle, cannula, or catheter. However, larger needles (e.g., 18- or 16-gauge) may be preferred if rapid transfusions are given or if the infusion is sluggish. Smaller needles can be used for platelets, albumin, and clotting factor replacement. Whatever type of venous access used, it is important to assess patency prior to requesting the blood component from the blood bank. Most blood product administration tubing is of a "Y type" with a microaggregate filter (which filters out particulate) with one branch of the Y for the isotonic saline solution and the other branch for the blood product. Infusion pumps may be used if approved for blood administration and according to institutional policy.

SAFETY ALERT
- Dextrose solutions or lactated Ringer's solution must not be used for administering blood because they will cause RBC hemolysis.
- Additives (including medications) must not be given via the same tubing as the blood unless the tubing is first cleared with saline solution.

When the blood or blood components have been obtained from the blood bank, positive identification of the blood donor

TABLE 33-32 BLOOD PRODUCTS*

Description	Special Considerations	Indications for Use
Packed Red Blood Cells Packed RBCs are prepared from whole blood by sedimentation or centrifugation. One unit contains 250–350 mL. They can be stored up to 35 days depending on processing.	Use of RBCs for treatment allows remaining components of blood (e.g., platelets, albumin, plasma) to be used for other purposes. There is less danger of fluid overload. • Leukocyte depletion (by the blood bank or with a filter) may be used to reduce hemolytic febrile reactions in patients who receive frequent transfusions.	Severe or symptomatic anemia; acute blood loss. In general, one unit of packed red blood cells can be expected to increase a patient's Hb level by 10 g/L or Hct by 3%. One unit of RBCs can replace a blood loss of 500 ml.
Frozen Red Blood Cells Frozen RBCs are prepared using glycerol for protection. They can be stored for 10 years.	They must be used within 24 hr of thawing. Successive washings with saline solution remove the majority of WBCs and plasma proteins.	Autotransfusion; stockpiling; or rare donors for patients with allobodies. Infrequently used because filters remove most WBCs.
Platelets Platelets are prepared from fresh whole blood. Platelets may be pooled from multiple donors. A single donation by apheresis is usually 200–400 ml in volume.	Multiple units of platelets can be obtained from one donor by platelet pheresis. They can be kept at room temperature for 1–5 days depending on type of collection and storage. For patients who receive frequent transfusions or who have not responded to previous platelet transfusions, platelets that are leukocyte-reduced or HLA- or type-specific may be given to prevent alloimmunization to HLA antigens.	Bleeding caused by thrombo-cytopenia or platelet levels <10–20 × 10^9/L; use may be contraindicated in the presence of thrombo-cytopenic purpura, thrombotic thrombo-cytopenic purpura, and heparin-induced thrombo-cytopenia except for life-threatening hemorrhage. Expected increase is 10 000 mcL per unit. Failure to obtain a rise may be caused by fever, sepsis, splenomegaly, or DIC.
Fresh-Frozen Plasma Liquid portion of whole blood is separated from cells and frozen. One unit contains 200–250 mL. Plasma is rich in clotting factors but contains no platelets. It may be stored for >1 year, depending on storage, but must be used within 24 hr after thawing.	Use of plasma in treating hypovolemic shock is being replaced by use of pure preparations such as albumin plasma expanders.	Bleeding caused by deficiency in clotting factors (e.g., DIC, hemorrhage, massive transfusion, liver disease, vitamin K deficiency, excess warfarin).
Albumin Albumin is prepared from plasma. It is available in 5% or 25% solution. It can be stored for 5 years.	Albumin 25 g/100 mL is osmotically equal to 500 mL of plasma. Hyperosmolar solution acts by moving water from extravascular to intravascular space. It is heat treated and does not transmit viruses.	Hypovolemic shock, hypoalbuminemia.
Cryoprecipitates and Commercial Concentrates Cryoprecipitate is prepared from fresh-frozen plasma, with 10–20 mL/ bag. Once thawed, it must be used.	See Table 33-19.	Replacement of clotting factors, especially factor VIII, von Willebrand factor, and fibrinogen.

DIC, disseminated intravascular coagulation; *Hb,* hemoglobin; *Hct,* hematocrit; *HLA,* human leukocyte antigen; *RBCs,* red blood cells; *WBCs,* white blood cells.
*Component therapy has replaced the use of whole blood, which accounts for <10% of all transfusions. Granulocyte transfusions are not included here because they are rarely used.

and the recipient must be made. Improper product-to-patient identification causes 90% of hemolytic transfusion reactions, thus placing a great responsibility on nursing personnel to carry out the identification procedure appropriately. The nurse must follow the policy and procedures of the institution where care is being provided; many institutions have implemented a dual-checking system with two licensed individuals checking patient identification with the labelled blood component. The blood bank is responsible for typing and crossmatching the donor's blood with the recipient's blood; the result of the compatibility testing should be noted on the product bag or tag, if pertinent.

ABO compatibility is not a prerequisite for platelet transfusions. However, after multiple platelet transfusions, a patient may develop anti-HLA antibodies to the transfused platelets. With the use of lymphocyte typing to match HLA types of the donor and the recipient, multiple platelet transfusions can be given with fewer complications to those who develop antibodies to platelets. Patients with a history of reactions to platelet transfusions may be premedicated with an antihistamine and hydrocortisone to decrease the possibility of reaction.

The nurse takes the patient's vital signs before the beginning of the transfusion to obtain a baseline measure; if the patient has abnormal vital signs, such as an elevated temperature, the health care provider is called to clarify when the blood component may be administered. The blood should be administered as soon as it is brought to the patient. No blood products are to be refrigerated on the nursing unit in food or drug refrigerators because the temperature does not meet the temperature-range requirements for safe storage. Products that are not used right away (i.e., within 30 minutes of being issued) should be returned to the blood bank. During the first 15 minutes or 50 mL of blood infusion, the nurse should remain with the patient. If there are any untoward reactions, they are most likely to occur at this time. The rate of infusion during this period should be no more than 2 mL/min. PRBCs should not be infused quickly unless an emergency exists. Rapid infusion of cold blood may cause the patient to become chilled. If rapid replacement of large amounts of blood is necessary, a blood-warming device may be used. Other blood components, such as fresh-frozen plasma and platelets, may be infused over 15 to 30 minutes. Refer to your institution's policy and procedure.

After the first 15 minutes, vital signs are usually retaken, and the rate of infusion is governed by the clinical condition of the patient and the product being infused. The nurse should observe the patient periodically throughout the transfusion (e.g., every 30 minutes) and up to 1 hour after the transfusion. Most patients not in danger of fluid overload can tolerate the infusion of 1 unit of PRBCs over 2 hours. The transfusion should not take more than 4 hours to administer because of the increased risk for bacterial growth in the product once it is out of refrigeration.

Blood Transfusion Reactions

A *blood transfusion reaction* is an adverse reaction to blood transfusion therapy that can range in severity from mild symptoms to a life-threatening condition. Because complications of transfusion therapy may be significant, judicious evaluation of the patient is required. Blood transfusion reactions can be classified as acute or delayed (Tables 33-33 and 33-34).

If an *acute transfusion reaction* occurs, the following steps should be taken: (a) stop the transfusion; (b) maintain a patent IV line with saline solution; (c) notify the blood bank and the health care provider immediately; (d) recheck identifying tags and numbers; (e) monitor vital signs and urine output; (f) treat symptoms as per physician order; (g) save and return the blood bag and tubing to the blood bank for examination; (h) collect blood and urine samples at intervals as stipulated by hospital policy to evaluate for hemolysis; and (i) document the incident (and steps a–h) on a transfusion reaction form and the patient's chart. The blood bank and laboratory are responsible for identifying the type of reaction.

TABLE 33-33 ACUTE TRANSFUSION REACTIONS

Cause	Clinical Manifestations	Management	Prevention
Acute Hemolytic Reaction			
Infusion of ABO-incompatible whole blood, RBCs, or components containing 10 mL or more of RBCs. Antibodies in the recipient's plasma attach to antigens on transfused RBCs causing RBC destruction.	Reaction usually occurs in first 15 minutes. Fever with or without chills; low back, abdominal, chest or flank pain; flushing, tachycardia, dyspnea, tachypnea, hypotension, vascular collapse, hemoglobinuria, acute jaundice, dark urine, bleeding, acute kidney injury, shock, cardiac arrest, DIC, death.	Treat shock and DIC if present. Draw blood samples—slowly to avoid hemolysis—for serological testing. Send urine specimen to the laboratory. Maintain BP with IV colloid solutions. Give diuretics as prescribed to maintain urine flow. Insert in-dwelling urinary catheter or measure voided amounts to monitor hourly urine output. Dialysis may be required if renal failure occurs. Do not transfuse additional RBC-containing components until blood bank has provided newly crossmatched units.	Meticulously verify and document patient identification at each step from sample collection to component infusion.
Febrile, Nonhemolytic Reaction (Most Common)			
Sensitization to donor WBCs, platelets, or plasma proteins.	Sudden chills and fever (rise in temperature of >1°C), headache, flushing, anxiety, vomiting, muscle pain.	Give antipyretics as prescribed—avoid ASA in patients with thrombo-cytopenia. *Do not restart transfusion* unless physician orders it.	Consider leukocyte-poor blood products (filtered, washed, or frozen) for patients with a history of two or more such reactions. Give acetaminophen or diphenhydramine 30 min before transfusion.
Mild Allergic Reaction			
Sensitivity to foreign plasma proteins. More common in people with history of allergies.	Flushing, itching, pruritus, urticaria (hives).	Give antihistamine, corticosteroid, epinephrine as directed. If symptoms are mild and transient, transfusion may be restarted slowly with health care provider's order. Do not restart transfusion if fever or pulmonary symptoms develop.	Treat prophylactically with antihistamines and steroids. Consider using washed RBCs and platelets.
Anaphylactic and Severe Allergic Reaction			
Sensitivity to donor plasma proteins. Infusion of IgA proteins to IgA-deficient recipient who has developed IgA antibody.	Anxiety; urticaria; dyspnea, wheezing, progressing to cyanosis; bronchospasm; hypotension, shock, and possible cardiac arrest.	Initiate CPR if indicated. Administer O$_2$. Have epinephrine ready for injection. Antihistamines, corticosteroids, β$_2$ agonists may also be prescribed. *Do not restart transfusion.*	Transfuse extensively washed RBC products, from which all plasma has been removed. Use blood from IgA-deficient donor. Use autologous components.

TABLE 33-33 ACUTE TRANSFUSION REACTIONS—cont'd

Cause	Clinical Manifestations	Management	Prevention
Circulatory Overload Reaction			
Fluid administered faster than the circulation can accommodate. People with cardiac or renal disease at risk.	Cough, dyspnea, pulmonary congestion, adventitious breath, headache, hypertension, tachycardia, distended neck veins.	Place patient upright with feet in dependent position. Obtain chest radiograph stat if ordered. Administer prescribed diuretics, O$_2$, and/or morphine. Phlebotomy may be indicated.	Adjust transfusion volume and flow rate based on patient size and clinical status. Have blood bank divide unit into smaller aliquots for better spacing of fluid input.
Sepsis Reaction			
Transfusion of bacterially infected blood components.	Rapid onset of chills, high fever, vomiting, diarrhea, marked hypotension, or shock.	Obtain culture of patient's blood and send bag with remaining blood and tubing to blood bank for further study. Treat septicemia as directed—administration of antibiotics, IV fluids, and/or vasopressors.	Collect, process, store, and transfuse blood products according to blood banking standards, and infuse within 4 hr of starting time.
Transfusion-Related Acute Lung Injury (TRALI) Reaction			
Reaction between transfused antileukocyte antibodies and recipient's leukocytes, causing pulmonary inflammation and capillary leak.	Fever, chills, hypotension, tachypnea, frothy sputum, dyspnea, hypoxemia, respiratory failure. Noncardiogenic pulmonary edema. Leading cause of transfusion-related deaths. Arises within 1–6 hours of transfusion.	Send bag with remaining blood and tubing to blood bank for further study; draw blood to analyze ABGs and HLA or antileukocyte antibodies; obtain chest radiograph stat. Provide O$_2$ and administer corticosteroids (diuretics of no value). Initiate CPR if needed, and provide ventilatory and blood pressure support if needed.	Provide leukocyte-reduced products. Identify donors who are implicated in TRALI reactions, and do not allow them to donate.
Massive Blood Transfusion Reaction			
Can occur with replacement of 10 or more RBC units within 24 hours. RBC transfusions do not contain clotting factors, albumin, and platelets.	Hypothermia and cardiac dysrhythmias (from massive infusion of large quantities of cold blood). Citrate toxicity and hypocalcemia (from the use of citrate as a storage solution). Hyperkalemia (from potassium leaking from stored RBCs).	When patients receive massive transfusions of blood products, monitor clotting status and electrolyte levels.	Use blood-warming equipment. Infusion of 10% calcium gluconate. Because of dilution effect on coagulation due to massive RBC transfusion, platelets and plasma will also be administered.

ABGs, arterial blood gases; *ASA,* acetylsalicylic acid (Aspirin); *BP,* blood pressure; *CPR,* cardiopulmonary resuscitation; *DIC,* disseminated intravascular coagulation; *HLA,* human leukocyte antigen; *IgA,* immunoglobulin A; *IV,* intravenous; *O₂,* oxygen; *RBC,* red blood cell; *WBC,* white blood cell.

Acute Transfusion Reactions

Acute Hemolytic Reactions. The most common cause of hemolytic reactions is transfusion of ABO-incompatible blood (see Table 33-33). This is an example of a type II cytotoxic hypersensitivity reaction (see Chapter 16). Severe hemolytic reactions are rare. Mislabelling specimens and administering blood to the wrong individual cause most acute hemolytic reactions. This again points to the importance of using proper patient identifiers when drawing blood samples and when administering medications and blood products.

When an acute hemolytic reaction occurs, antibodies in the recipient's serum react with antigens on the donor's RBCs. This reaction results in agglutination of cells, which can obstruct capillaries and block blood flow. Hemolysis of the RBCs releases free Hb into the plasma. The Hb is filtered by the kidney and may be found in the urine (hemoglobinuria). Hb may obstruct the renal tubules, leading to acute kidney injury, DIC, and death (see Chapter 49).

The clinical manifestations of an acute hemolytic reaction may be mild or severe and usually develop within 15 minutes of transfusion. Free Hb in blood and urine specimens obtained at the onset of the reaction will provide evidence of an acute hemolytic reaction. Delayed transfusion reactions are defined as those occurring 24 hours to 14 days after the administration of blood.

Febrile Reactions. Febrile reactions are most commonly caused by leukocyte incompatibility. Many individuals who receive five or more transfusions develop circulating antibodies to the small amount of WBCs in the blood product. Febrile reactions can often be prevented by using additional filters in the tubing to leukocyte-deplete RBCs and platelets. Donated blood in Canada is processed to reduce the number of circulating WBCs (i.e., leuko-depleted), a process that has helped decrease the incidence of the febrile nonhemolytic and minor allergic reactions. Medications such as acetaminophen (Tylenol) and diphenhydramine (Benadryl) may be ordered and given 30 minutes before blood administration to reduce these reactions.

Allergic Reactions. Allergic reactions result from the recipient's sensitivity to plasma proteins of the donor's blood. These reactions are more common in an individual with a history of allergies. Administration of antihistamines may help prevent allergic reactions. Epinephrine or corticosteroids may be used to treat a severe reaction.

Circulatory Overload. An individual with cardiac or renal insufficiency is at risk for developing circulatory overload,

TABLE 33-34   DELAYED TRANSFUSION REACTIONS

Manifestations	Prevention and Management
Delayed Hemolytic	
Fever, mild jaundice, decreased hemoglobin. Occurs as early as 3 days or as late as several months post-transfusion as the result of destruction of transfused RBCs by alloantibodies not detected during crossmatch.	Generally, no acute treatment is required. Hemolysis may be severe enough to warrant further transfusions.
Hepatitis B*	
Elevated liver enzymes (AST and ALT), anorexia, malaise, nausea and vomiting, fever, dark urine, jaundice. Usually resolves spontaneously within 4–6 wk. Chronic carrier state can develop and result in permanent damage to the liver.	Hepatitis B virus can be detected in donated blood by the presence of hepatitis B surface antigen (HBsAg). Treat symptomatically (see Chapter 46).
Hepatitis C*	
Similar to hepatitis B, but symptoms are usually less severe. Chronic liver disease and cirrhosis may develop.	Before anti-HCV testing of donated blood began, this accounted for 90%–95% of all post-transfusion hepatitis. Treat symptomatically (see Chapter 46).
Iron Overload	
Excess iron is deposited in heart, liver, pancreas, and joints, causing dysfunction. Heart failure, dysrhythmias, impaired thyroid and gonadal function, diabetes, arthritis, cirrhosis. Occurs in patients receiving >100 units for chronic anemia (e.g., sickle cell anemia, beta thalassemia) over time.	Treat symptomatically. Deferoxamine (Desferal), which chelates and removes accumulated iron via the kidneys, administered IV or subcutaneously. Deferasirox (Exjade) and deferiprone (Ferriprox) are oral agents that chelate iron and should be started before more than 50 units of red cells are transfused.
Other	
CMV, HIV, HSV-6, Epstein-Barr virus, HTLV-1, and malaria. Most recent threats have been agents that primarily affect animals but have been transmitted to the blood supply through the food supply, or vectors such as mosquitoes or ticks. These include *Plasmodium* species (malaria), dengue fever virus, West Nile virus, *Trypanosoma cruzi* (Chagas's disease), *Babesia* species (babesiosis), human herpesvirus 8 (KS virus), and variant Creutzfeldt-Jakob disease ("mad cow disease").	Treatment is based on the cause. Ways of detecting some of these agents are now available and required, such as the nucleic acid test for West Nile virus, HIV, and *T. cruzi*. Donor screening has been the only available method to reduce the risk for donor-contaminated blood for others.

ALT, alanine aminotransferase; *AST,* aspartate aminotransferase; *CMV,* cytomegalovirus; *HCV,* hepatitis C virus; *HIV,* human immunodeficiency virus; *HSV-6,* human herpesvirus, type 6; *HTLV-1,* human T-cell leukemia virus, type 1; *KS,* Kaposi sarcoma.
*New cases of transfusion-related hepatitis B and C are not common.

especially if a large quantity of blood is infused in a short period, particularly in an older adult. PRBCs can be split by the blood bank, allowing for one-half of a unit to be given over a time frame of up to 4 hours. A fluid balance assessment, including baseline auscultation of the patient's lungs, is performed. Complaints of shortness of breath and the presence of adventitious breath sounds may indicate fluid overload in a patient.

Sepsis. Blood products can become infected from improper handling and storage. Bacterial contamination of blood products can result in bacteremia, sepsis, or septic shock.

Transfusion-Related Acute Lung Injury. Transfusion-related acute lung injury (TRALI) is characterized by the sudden development of noncardiogenic pulmonary edema (acute lung injury). It usually occurs within hours of the transfusion of blood products. With the reduction of clerical errors, leukocyte-reduced products, more effective screening, and the prevention of the transmission of infectious agents, TRALI has surpassed hemolytic reactions as the leading cause of transfusion-related death. It is thought to be caused by an antibody-mediated reaction between the recipient's leukocytes and antileukocyte antibodies from donors who were sensitized during pregnancy or by previous transfusions. TRALI causes pulmonary capillary inflammation and increased permeability, leading to respiratory distress and potentially death.

Massive Blood Transfusion Reaction. An acute complication of transfusing large volumes of blood products is termed *massive blood transfusion reaction.* Massive blood transfusion reactions can occur when replacement of RBCs or blood exceeds the total blood volume within 24 hours. In this situation, an imbalance of normal blood elements results because clotting factors, albumin, and platelets are not found in RBC transfusions. Thus, appropriate monitoring of hemostatic laboratory parameters must be done concurrently.

Additional problems such as hypothermia, citrate toxicity, hypocalcemia, and hyperkalemia may occur when massive blood transfusions are given. Hypothermia and cardiac dysrhythmias can result from rapid infusion of large quantities of cold blood. Blood-warming equipment prevents this problem. Citrate toxicity can occur when large quantities of blood products are used because citrate is part of the storage solution; calcium binds to the citrate. Citrate toxicity is likely to develop when blood is transfused at a rate of 1 unit in 10 minutes (or 8–10 units of RBCs within a few hours). Manifestations such as muscle tremors and ECG changes may be observed with hypocalcemia but can be prevented or reversed by the infusion of 10% calcium gluconate (10 mL with every litre of citrated blood). Hyperkalemia results when potassium leaks from RBCs in stored blood. Mild to severe signs and symptoms can occur, including nausea, muscle weakness, diarrhea, paresthesias, flaccid paralysis of the cardiac or respiratory muscles, and cardiac arrest. Electrolyte monitoring is an important aspect of the care of the patient receiving massive transfusions of blood products.

Delayed Transfusion Reactions. Delayed transfusion reactions include delayed hemolytic reactions (discussed previously), infections, and iron overload (see Table 33-34).

Infection. Infectious agents transmitted by blood transfusion include hepatitis B and C viruses, HIV, human herpesvirus type 6 (HSV-6), EBV, HTLV-1, cytomegalovirus (CMV), and malaria. Hepatitis is still the most common viral infection transmitted, although its incidence is decreasing. Hepatitis B virus can be detected in the blood by the presence of hepatitis B surface antigen (HBsAg). A test for hepatitis C antibodies in donor blood is used to exclude the use of any donated blood testing positive for hepatitis C. Therefore, the risk for transmission of hepatitis C has been reduced. Leukocyte-reduced blood products drastically decrease the risk for blood transfusion–associated viral infections, including CMV.

In the past, transmittal of HIV by contaminated blood and blood products posed a serious problem for individuals who received infected transfusions. Patients with hemophilia who received antihemophilic factors that had been prepared from pooled plasma of a large number of donors, some of whom were HIV-infected, have a high rate of HIV infection from transfusion sources. At present, the use of recombinant antihemophilic factors, donor education, donor screening, and HIV-antibody testing have greatly reduced the transmission of HIV by blood transfusion or factor replacement therapy.

Autotransfusion

Autotransfusion, or autologous transfusion, involves removing whole blood from a person and transfusing that blood back into the same person. Through this method, the problems of incompatibility, allergic reactions, and transmission of disease can be avoided. Methods of autotransfusion include the following:

- *Autologous donation* or *elective phlebotomy* (predeposit transfusion). A person donates blood before a planned surgical procedure. The blood can be frozen and stored for up to 10 years. Usually, the blood is stored without being frozen and is given to the person within a few weeks of donation. This technique is especially beneficial to the patient with a rare blood type or for any patient who might be expected to require limited blood product support during a major surgical procedure (e.g., elective orthopedic surgery).
- *Autotransfusion.* A newer method for replacing blood volume involves safely and aseptically collecting, filtering, and returning the patient's own blood that is lost during a major surgical procedure or from a traumatic injury. This system was originally developed in response to patients' concerns about the safety of blood from blood products. However, today it provides an important way to safely replace volume and stabilize the condition of bleeding patients. Collection devices are most often used during surgeries. Some systems allow blood to be automatically and continuously reinfused; others require collection for some period (usually no longer than 4 hours), after which the blood is reinfused. Hospitals in Canada are now required to have a blood conservation program in place.

CASE STUDY

Leukemia

Source:
Shutterstock
.com

Patient Profile
Andeep Singh, a 35-year-old man, went to the emergency department because of severe bruising caused by a fall while hiking.

Subjective Data
- Complains of oral pain and white patches covering his tongue
- Has had a 2-month history of fatigue, malaise, and flu symptoms
- Complains of shortness of breath while doing activities that previously required no exertion
- Has taken numerous prescribed antibiotics and increased rest and sleep in the past 2 months without relief of symptoms

Objective Data
Physical Examination
- Has bruises and ecchymoses from fall
- Gingiva has petechiae and patchy white spots
- Temperature 39°C, respiratory rate 26/min, pulse 110
- Has splenomegaly

Laboratory Results
- Hematocrit 0.2
- White blood cell (WBC) count 120 × 10⁹/L

- Hemoglobin (Hb) 69 g/L
- Platelet count 25 × 10⁹/L

Bone Marrow Biopsy
- Multiple myeloblasts (>50%)

Discussion Questions
1. What components of the laboratory test results suggest acute leukemia?
2. How is acute myelogenous leukemia treated?
3. What is the prognosis for Mr. Singh?
4. What are the life-threatening problems that can occur as a result of this disease and treatment? How can the nurse anticipate and assess for these problems?
5. *Priority decision:* What are the priority nursing interventions?
6. *Priority decision:* What are the priorities for patient teaching of a newly diagnosed young adult with leukemia?
7. *Priority decision:* Based on the assessment data presented, what are the priority nursing diagnoses? Are there any collaborative problems?
8. *Evidence-informed practice:* Mr. Singh becomes very fatigued after starting chemotherapy. He wants to know if he can still exercise even if he is so fatigued. What should the nurse tell him?

ⓔvolve
Answers are available at *http://evolve.elsevier.com/Canada/Lewis/medsurg.*

■ REVIEW QUESTIONS

The number of the question corresponds to the same-numbered objective at the beginning of the chapter.

1. In a severely anemic client, what would the nurse expect to find?
   a. Dyspnea and tachycardia
   b. Cyanosis and pulmonary edema
   c. Cardiomegaly and pulmonary fibrosis
   d. Ventricular dysrhythmias and wheezing

2. When obtaining assessment data from a client with a microcytic, hypochromic anemia, what would the nurse question the client about?
   a. Folic acid intake
   b. Dietary intake of iron
   c. History of gastric surgery
   d. History of sickle cell anemia

3. Nursing interventions for a client with severe anemia related to peptic ulcer disease include which of the following? (*Select all that apply*)
   a. Giving instructions in high-iron diet
   b. Taking vital signs every 8 hours
   c. Monitoring stools for occult blood
   d. Teaching self-injection of erythropoietin
   e. Administering cobalamin (vitamin B$_{12}$) injections

4. Which nursing management actions apply for a client in sickle cell crisis? (*Select all that apply*)
   a. Monitoring CBC
   b. Providing optimal pain management and O$_2$ therapy
   c. Doing blood transfusions if required and iron chelation
   d. Recommending rest as needed and deep-vein thrombosis prophylaxis
   e. Administering IV iron and a diet high in iron content

5. Which is a complication of the hyperviscosity of polycythemia?
   a. Thrombosis
   b. Cardiomyopathy
   c. Pulmonary edema
   d. Disseminated intravascular coagulation (DIC)

6. When caring for a client with thrombo-cytopenia, the patient teaching should include which instruction?
   a. To wipe her or his nose gently instead of blowing
   b. To be careful when shaving with a safety razor
   c. To continue with physical activities to stimulate thrombopoiesis
   d. To avoid acetylsalicylic acid because it may mask the fever that occurs with thrombo-cytopenia

7. The nurse would anticipate that a client with von Willebrand disease who is undergoing surgery would be treated with administration of von Willebrand factor (vWF) and which of the following?
   a. Thrombin
   b. Factor VI
   c. Factor VII
   d. Factor VIII

8. What physiological process occurs in a person with DIC?
   a. The coagulation pathway is genetically altered, leading to thrombus formation in all major blood vessels.
   b. An underlying disease depletes hemolytic factors in the blood, leading to diffuse thrombotic episodes and infarcts.
   c. A disease process stimulates coagulation processes with resultant thrombosis, as well as depletion of clotting factors, leading to diffuse clotting and hemorrhage.
   d. An inherited predisposition causes a deficiency of clotting factors that leads to overstimulation of coagulation processes in the vasculature.

9. Which of the following is (are) a priority nursing action when caring for a hospitalized client with a new-onset temperature of 39°C and severe neutropenia? (*Select all that apply*)
   a. Administering the prescribed antibiotic immediately
   b. Drawing peripheral and central line blood cultures
   c. Ensuring ongoing monitoring of the client's vital signs for septic shock

   d. Taking a full set of vital signs and notifying the physician immediately
   e. Administering transfusions of WBCs to decrease immunogenicity

10. Because myelodysplastic syndrome arises from the pluripotent hematopoietic stem cell in the bone marrow, which laboratory results would the nurse expect to find?
    a. An excess of T cells
    b. An excess of platelets
    c. A deficiency of granulocytes
    d. A deficiency of all cellular blood components

11. Which is the most common type of leukemia in older adults?
    a. Acute myelocytic leukemia
    b. Acute lymphocytic leukemia
    c. Chronic myelocytic leukemia
    d. Chronic lymphocytic leukemia

12. Why are multiple drugs often used in combinations to treat leukemia and lymphoma?
    a. There are fewer toxic and adverse effects.
    b. The chance that one drug will be effective is increased.
    c. The drugs are more effective and cause fewer adverse effects.
    d. The drugs work by different mechanisms to maximize killing of malignant cells.

13. What is the major difference between Hodgkin's lymphoma and non-Hodgkin's lymphoma?
    a. Hodgkin's lymphoma occurs only in young adults.
    b. Hodgkin's lymphoma is considered potentially curable.
    c. Non-Hodgkin's lymphoma can manifest in multiple organs.
    d. Non-Hodgkin's lymphoma is treated only with radiation therapy.

14. A client with multiple myeloma becomes confused and lethargic. What indications would the nurse expect from the diagnostic results?
    a. Indications of hyperkalemia
    b. Indications of hyperuricemia
    c. Indications of hypercalcemia
    d. Indications of central nervous system myeloma

15. What would the nurse expect to find when reviewing a client's hematological laboratory values after a splenectomy?
    a. Leukopenia
    b. Red blood cell abnormalities
    c. Decreased hemoglobin
    d. Increased platelet count

16. Which complications of transfusions can be decreased by the use of leukocyte depletion or reduction of red blood cell transfusion?
    a. Chills and hemolysis
    b. Leukostasis and neutrophilia
    c. Fluid overload and pulmonary edema
    d. Transmission of cytomegalovirus and fever

1. a; 2. b; 3. a, c; 4. a, b, c, d; 5. a; 6. a; 7. d; 8. c; 9. a, b, c, d; 10. d; 11. d; 12. d; 13. c; 14. c; 15. d; 16. d.

🔵volve

For even more review questions, visit *http://evolve.elsevier.com/Canada/Lewis/medsurg*.

REFERENCES

Ansell, S. M. (2015). Hodgkin lymphoma: Diagnosis and treatment. *Mayo Clinic Proceedings, 90*(11), 1574–1583. doi:10.1016/j.mayocp.2015.07.005.

Artz, A. S., & Ershler, W. B. (2013). Hematology in aging. In R. Hoffman, E. J. Ben, L. E. Silberstein, et al. (Eds.), *Hematology: Basic principles and practice* (6th ed.). Philadelphia: Saunders.

Bacigalupo, A. (2014). Bone marrow transplantation for acquired severe aplastic anemia. *Hematology/Oncology Clinics of North America, 28*(6), 1145–1155. doi:10.1016/j.hoc.2014.08.004.

Baden, L. R., Bensinger, W., Angarone, M., et al. (2014). Prevention and treatment of cancer-related infections. *NCCN Clinical Practice Guidelines, Version 2*. Retrieved from *http://file.trsgo.org/userfiles/file/NCCN%20Cancer-Related%20Infections%20Guideline%202015.pdf*.

Bejjani, R. (2015). Anemic control in patients with chronic kidney disease: A controversial issue. *Medsurg Nursing, 24*(1), 23–26.

Canadian Cancer Society. (2017a). *Leukemia statistics.* Retrieved from *http://www.cancer.ca/en/cancer-information/cancer-type/leukemia/statistics/?region=on.*

Canadian Cancer Society. (2017b). *Hodgkin lymphoma statistics.* Retrieved from *http://www.cancer.ca/en/cancer-information/cancer-type/hodgkin-lymphoma/statistics/?region=on.*

Canadian Cancer Society. (2017c). *Non-Hodgkin lymphoma statistics.* Retrieved from *http://www.cancer.ca/en/cancer-information/cancer-type/non-hodgkin-lymphoma/statistics/?region=on.*

Canadian Cancer Society. (2017d). *Multiple myeloma statistics.* Retrieved from *http://www.cancer.ca/en/cancer-information/cancer-type/multiple-myeloma/statistics/?region=on.*

Canadian Hemochromatosis Society. (2013). *Hemochromatosis—How common is it?* Retrieved from *http://www.toomuchiron.ca/wp-content/uploads/2013/02/hemochromatosis_how_common.pdf.*

Canadian Hemophilia Society. (2016). *An introduction to hemophilia.* Retrieved from *http://www.hemophilia.ca/en/about-the-chs/case-for-support/facts-and-figures/.*

Cantor, A. G., Bougatsos, C., Dana, T., et al. (2015). Routine iron supplementation and screening for iron deficiency anemia in pregnancy: A systematic review for the U.S. Preventive Services Task Force. *Annals of Internal Medicine, 162*(8), 566–576. doi:10.7326/M14-2932.

Carson, S. M., & Martin, M. B. (2014). Effective iron chelation practice for patients with β-thalassemia major. *Clinical Journal of Oncology Nursing, 18*(1), 102–111. doi:10.1188/14.CJON.102-111.

Cooper, S. L., & Brown, P. A. (2015). Treatment of pediatric acute lymphoblastic leukemia. *Pediatric Clinics of North America, 62*(1), 61–73. doi:10.1016/j.pcl.2014.09.006.

Goss, C., Giardina, P., Degtyaryova, D., et al. (2014). Red blood cell transfusions for thalassemia: Results of a survey assessing current practice and proposal of evidence-based guidelines. *Transfusion, 54*(7), 1773–1781. doi:10.1111/trf.12571.

Green, R. (2015). Folate, cobalamin, and megaloblastic anemias. In K. Kaushansky, M. A. Lichtman, J. T. Prchal, et al. (Eds.), *Williams hematology* (9th ed.). New York: McGraw-Hill.

Griesshammer, M., Gisslinger, H., & Mesa, R. (2015). Current and future treatment options for polycythemia vera. *Annals of Hematology, 94*(6), 901–910. doi:10.1007/s00277-015-2357-4.

Hoppe, R. T., Advani, R. H., Ai, W. Z., et al. (2015). Hodgkin lymphoma, version 2.2015. *Journal of the National Comprehensive Cancer Network, 13*(5), 554–586. Retrieved from *https://www.ncbi.nlm.nih.gov/pmc/articles/PMC4898052/.*

Kanate, A. S., Craig, M., Abraham, J., et al. (2013). Hodgkin's lymphoma. In G. P. Rodgers & N. S. Young (Eds.), *The Bethesda handbook of clinical hematology* (3rd ed.). Philadelphia: Lippincott.

Kline, N. E. (2014). Alterations of hematologic function in children. In K. L. McCance & S. E. Huether (Eds.), *Pathophysiology: The biologic basis for disease in adults and children* (7th ed.). St. Louis: Mosby.

Klotz, J., Parikh, A. R., & Battiwalla, M. (2013). The myelodysplastic syndromes. In G. P. Rodgers & N. S. Young (Eds.), *The Bethesda handbook of clinical hematology* (3rd ed.). Philadelphia: Lippincott.

Leukemia and Lymphoma Society of Canada. (2016). *Facts and statistics.* Retrieved from *http://www.llscanada.org/disease-information/facts-and-statistics.*

Marks, P. W. (2013). Approach to anemia in the adult and child. In R. Hoffman, E. J. Benz, L. E. Silberstein, et al. (Eds.), *Hematology: Basic principles and practice* (6th ed.). Philadelphia: Saunders.

McCrae, K. R., Sadler, J. E., & Cines, D. B. (2013). Thrombotic thrombocytopenic purpura and the hemolytic uremic syndrome. In R. Hoffman, E. J. Benz, L. E. Silberstein, et al. (Eds.), *Hematology: Basic principles and practice* (6th ed.). Philadelphia: Saunders.

Meers, S. (2015). The myelodysplastic syndromes: The era of understanding. *European Journal of Haematology, 94*(5), 379–390. doi:10.1111/ejh.12443.

Ministry of Health. (1997). *Commission of inquiry on the blood system in Canada.* Ottawa: Canadian Government Publishing. (Seminal).

Oldenburg, J., & Brackmann, H. (2014). Prophylaxis in adult patients with severe haemophilia A. *Thrombosis Research, 134*(1), S33–S37. doi:10.1016/j.thromres.2013.10.019.

Porteus, M., & Mantanona, T. (2012). Blood. In L. W. Janson & M. E. Tischler (Eds.), *The big picture: Medical biochemistry.* New York: McGraw-Hill.

Röllig, C., Knop, S., & Bornhäuser, M. (2015). Multiple myeloma. *Lancet, 385*(9983), 2197–2208. doi:10.1016/S0140-6736(14)60493-1.

Rote, N. S., & McCance, K. L. (2014). Structure and function of the hematologic system. In K. L. McCance & S. E. Huether (Eds.), *Pathophysiology: The biologic basis for disease in adults and children* (7th ed.). St. Louis: Mosby.

Scheinberg, P., Young, N. S., & Liu, J. M. (2013). Bone marrow failure syndromes: Aplastic anemia, acquired and constitutional; paroxysmal nocturnal hemoglobinuria; pure red blood cell aplasia; and agranulocytosis. In G. P. Rodgers & N. S. Young (Eds.), *The Bethesda handbook of clinical hematology* (3rd ed.). Philadelphia: Lippincott.

Shead, D. A., Hanisch, L. J., Marlow, L., et al. (2016). *NCCN guidelines for patients: Myelodysplastic syndromes.* National Comprehensive Cancer Network. Retrieved from *https://www.nccn.org/patients/guidelines/mds/files/assets/basic-html/page-1.html.*

Stabler, S. P. (2013). Vitamin B$_{12}$ deficiency. *The New England Journal of Medicine, 368*, 149–160. doi:10.1056/NEJMcp1113996.

Terpos, E., Berenson, J., Raje, N., et al. (2014). Management of bone disease in multiple myeloma. *Expert Review of Hematology, 7*(1), 113–125. doi:10.1586/17474086.2013.874943.

Townsley, D. M., & Rodgers, G. P. (2013). Deficiencies of vitamin B$_{12}$ and folate. In G. P. Rodgers & N. S. Young (Eds.), *The Bethesda handbook of clinical hematology* (3rd ed.). Philadelphia: Lippincott.

Warkentin, T. E. (2013). Heparin-induced thrombocytopenia. In R. Hoffman, E. J. Benz, L. E. Silberstein, et al. (Eds.), *Hematology: Basic principles and practice* (6th ed.). Philadelphia: Saunders.

Weledji, E. P. (2014). Benefits and risks of splenectomy. *International Journal of Surgery, 12*(2), 113–119. doi:10.1016/j.ijsu.2013.11.017.

World Health Organization. (2016). *Micronutrient deficiencies: Iron deficiency anaemia.* Retrieved from *http://www.who.int/nutrition/topics/ida/en/index.html.*

Yawn, B. P., Buchanan, G. R., Afenyi-Annan, A. N., et al. (2014). Management of sickle cell disease: Summary of the 2014 evidence-based report by expert panel members. *Journal of the American Medical Association, 312*(10), 1033–1048. doi:10.1001/jama.2014.10517.

RESOURCES

B.C. Cancer Agency
http://www.bccancer.bc.ca

Canadian Blood Services
http://www.bloodservices.ca

Canadian Cancer Society
http://www.cancer.ca

Canadian Hemochromatosis Society
http://www.cdnhemochromatosis.ca

Canadian Hemophilia Society
http://www.hemophilia.ca

Cancer Care Ontario
http://www.cancercare.on.ca

Childhood Cancer Foundation Canada
http://www.childhoodcancer.ca

Fanconi Canada
http://www.fanconicanada.org

Leukemia and Lymphoma Society of Canada
http://www.llscanada.org

Lymphoma Canada
http://www.lymphoma.ca

Myeloma Canada
http://www.myelomacanada.ca

Sickle Cell Association of Ontario
http://sicklecellontario.ca

Sickle Cell Association of Canada
http://www.sicklecelldisease.ca/

Thalassemia Foundation of Canada
http://www.thalassemia.ca

Global Sickle Cell Disease Network
http://www.globalsicklecelldisease.org/

National Cancer Institute
http://www.cancer.gov

National Heart, Lung, and Blood Institute
http://www.nhlbi.nih.gov

National Hemophilia Foundation
http://www.hemophilia.org

For additional Internet resources, see the website for this book at *http://evolve.elsevier.com/Canada/Lewis/medsurg.*

Problems of Oxygenation: Perfusion

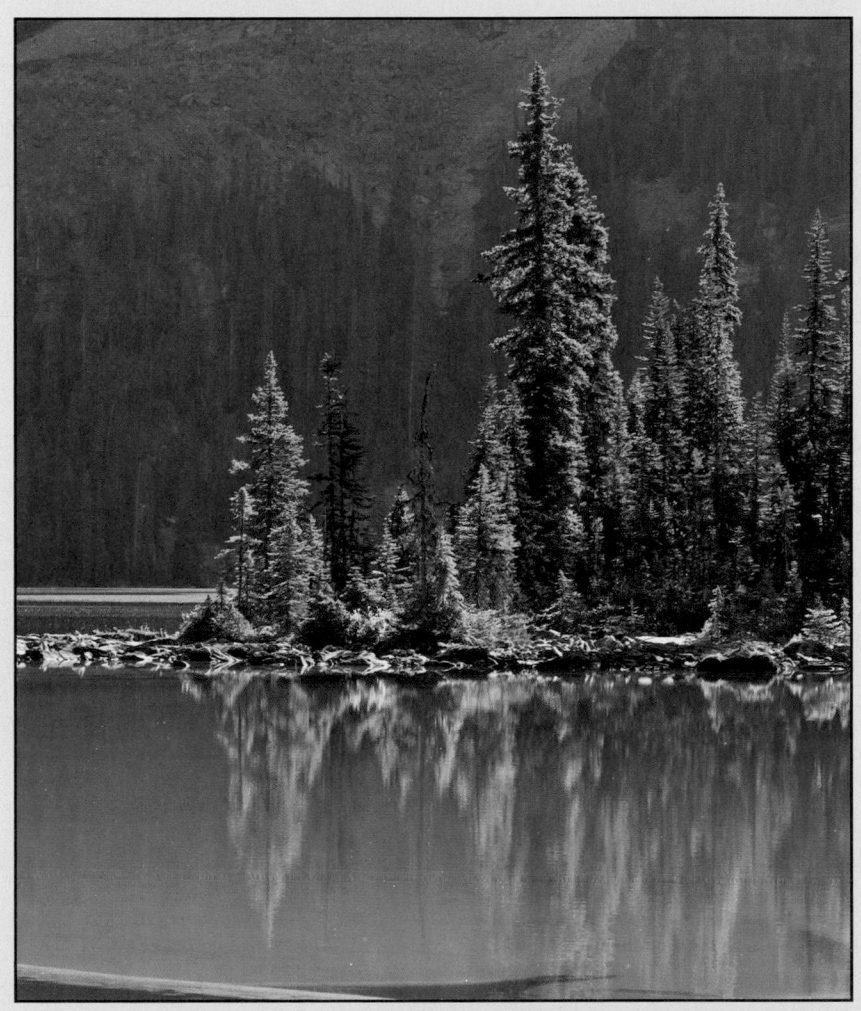

Source: Christopher Gardiner/Shutterstock.com.

Nursing Assessment

Cardiovascular System

Written by: Angela DiSabatino Herman and Linda Bucher
Adapted by: Sandra Goldsworthy

evolve WEBSITE

http://evolve.elsevier.com/Canada/Lewis/medsurg

- Review Questions (Online Only)
- Key Points
- Answers Guidelines for Case Study
- Conceptual Care Map Creator
- Audio Glossary
- Supporting Media—Animations
  - Auscultation of Heart Valves
  - Blood Flow: Circulatory System
  - Cardiac Cycle During Systole and Diastole
  - Pulse Variations

- Supporting Media—Audio
- Diastolic Murmur
- Fourth Heart Sound (S$_4$)
- Murmurs: Blowing, Harsh or Rough, and Rumble
- Murmurs: High, Medium, and Low
- First Heart Sound (S$_1$) at Various Locations
- Second Heart Sound (S$_2$) at Various Locations
- Single S$_1$

- Single S$_2$
- Systolic Murmur
- Third Heart Sound (S$_3$)
- Content Updates

LEARNING OBJECTIVES

1. Differentiate the anatomical locations and functions of the following cardiac structures: pericardial layers, atria, ventricles, semilunar valves, and atrioventricular valves.
2. Explain the relation between the coronary circulation and the areas of heart muscle supplied by each blood vessel.
3. Explain the normal sequence of events involved in the conduction pathway of the heart.
4. Differentiate the structures and functions of arteries, capillaries, and veins.
5. Describe the mechanisms involved in blood pressure regulation.
6. Select essential assessment data related to the cardiovascular system that should be obtained from a patient or caregiver.

7. Select the appropriate techniques used in the physical assessment of the cardiovascular system.
8. Discuss the differences between normal and common abnormal findings of a physical assessment of the cardiovascular system.
9. Explain the links between age-related changes of the cardiovascular system and differences in assessment findings.
10. Describe the purpose of, significance of, and nursing responsibility related to diagnostic studies of the cardiovascular system.
11. Explain the relationship of the various waveforms on an electrocardiogram with the associated cardiac event.

KEY TERMS

action potential, p. 767
afterload, p. 769
arterial blood pressure (BP), p. 770
cardiac index, p. 769
cardiac output (CO), p. 769

cardiac reserve, p. 769
coronary angiography, p. 786
diastole, p. 769
diastolic blood pressure (DBP), p. 770
ejection fraction, p. 783

heaves, p. 776
Korotkoff sounds, p. 770
mean arterial pressure, p. 770
murmurs, p. 776
point of maximal impulse (PMI), p. 776

preload, p. 769
pulse pressure, p. 770
systole, p. 769
systolic blood pressure (SBP), p. 770

STRUCTURES AND FUNCTIONS OF THE CARDIOVASCULAR SYSTEM

Heart

Structure. The heart is a four-chambered, hollow, muscular organ normally about the size of a fist. It lies within the thorax in the mediastinal space that separates the right and left pleural cavities. The heart is composed of three layers: a thin inner lining, the *endocardium*; a layer of muscle, the *myocardium*; and an outer layer, the *epicardium*. The heart is covered by a fibroserous sac called the *pericardium*. This sac consists of two layers: the inside *(visceral)* layer of the pericardium (part of

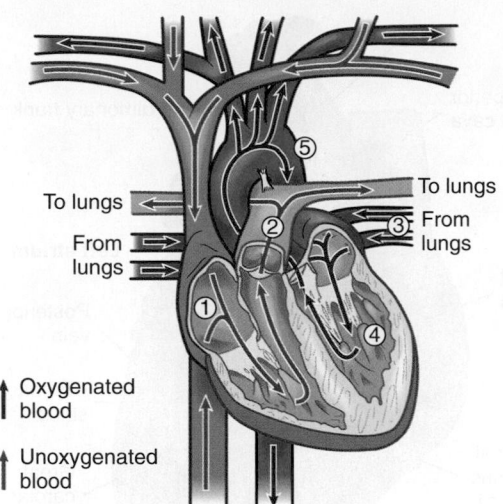

FIGURE 34-1 Schematic representation of blood flow through the heart. *Arrows* indicate direction of flow. *1,* The right atrium receives venous blood from the inferior and superior venae cavae and the coronary sinus. The blood then passes through the tricuspid valve into the right ventricle. *2,* With each contraction, the right ventricle pumps blood through the pulmonic valve into the pulmonary artery and to the lungs. *3,* Oxygenated blood flows from the lungs to the left atrium by way of the pulmonary veins. *4,* It then passes through the mitral valve and into the left ventricle. *5,* As the heart contracts, blood is ejected through the aortic valve into the aorta and thus enters the systemic circulation.

FIGURE 34-2 Anatomical structures of the atrioventricular valves.

the epicardium) and the outer *(parietal)* layer. A small amount of pericardial fluid (approximately 10–15 mL) lubricates the space between the pericardial layers *(pericardial space)* and prevents friction between the surfaces as the heart contracts (Patton & Thibodeau, 2016).

The heart is divided vertically by the septum. The interatrial septum divides the right and left atria, and the interventricular septum divides the right and left ventricles. The thickness of the wall of each chamber is different. The atrial myocardium is thinner than that of the ventricles, and the left ventricular wall is two or three times thicker than the right ventricular wall (Patton & Thibodeau, 2016). The left ventricle must be thick in order to produce the force needed to pump the blood into the systemic circulation.

Blood Flow Through the Heart. The blood flow through the heart is illustrated in Figure 34-1.

Cardiac Valves. The four valves of the heart serve to keep blood flowing in a forward direction. The cusps of the mitral and tricuspid valves are attached to thin strands of fibrous tissue termed *chordae tendineae* (Figure 34-2). Chordae are anchored in the papillary muscles of the ventricles. This support system prevents the eversion of the leaflets into the atria during ventricular contraction. The pulmonic and aortic valves (also known as *semilunar valves*) prevent blood from regurgitating into the ventricles at the end of each ventricular contraction.

Blood Supply to the Myocardium. The myocardium has its own blood supply, the *coronary circulation* (Figure 34-3). Blood flow into the coronary arteries occurs primarily during diastole. The right coronary artery and its branches usually supply the right atrium, the right ventricle, and a portion of the posterior wall of the left ventricle. The left coronary artery and its branches (left anterior descending artery and left circumflex artery) supply the left atrium and the left ventricle. In 90% of people, the atrioventricular node and the bundle of His (part of the cardiac

conduction system) receive blood supply from the right coronary artery. For this reason, obstruction of this artery often causes serious defects in cardiac conduction.

The divisions of coronary veins parallel the coronary arteries. Most of the blood from the coronary system drains into the coronary sinus, which empties into the right atrium near the entrance to the inferior vena cava (see Figure 34-3).

Conduction System. The conduction system is specialized nerve tissue responsible for creating and transporting the electrical impulse; this impulse is called the **action potential.** This impulse initiates depolarization and, subsequently, cardiac contraction. The electrical impulse is initiated by the sinoatrial node (the pacemaker of the heart; Figure 34-4). Each impulse generated at the sinoatrial node travels swiftly through the muscle fibres of the atria by internodal pathways and cell-to-cell conduction. Mechanical contraction of the atria follows the depolarization of the cells.

The electrical impulse travels from the atria to the atrioventricular node. The excitation then moves through the bundle of His and the left and right bundle branches. The left bundle branch has an anterior and a posterior fascicle. The action potential diffuses widely through the walls of both ventricles by means of *Purkinje fibres*. The efficient ventricular conduction system delivers the impulse within 0.12 second. This triggers a uniform ventricular contraction.

The cardiac cycle starts with depolarization of the sinoatrial node. The cycle's climax is ejection of blood into the pulmonary and systemic circulations. It ends with repolarization, when the contractile fibre cells and the conduction pathway cells regain their resting polarized condition. Cardiac muscle cells have a compensatory mechanism that makes them unresponsive or refractory to re-stimulation during the action potential. During systole, there is an absolute refractory period during which cardiac muscle does not respond to any stimuli. After this period, cardiac muscle gradually recovers its excitability and a relative refractory period occurs by early diastole.

Electrocardiography. The electrical activity of the heart can be detected on the body surface and recorded on an electrocardiogram (ECG). The letters *P, QRS, T,* and *U* are used to

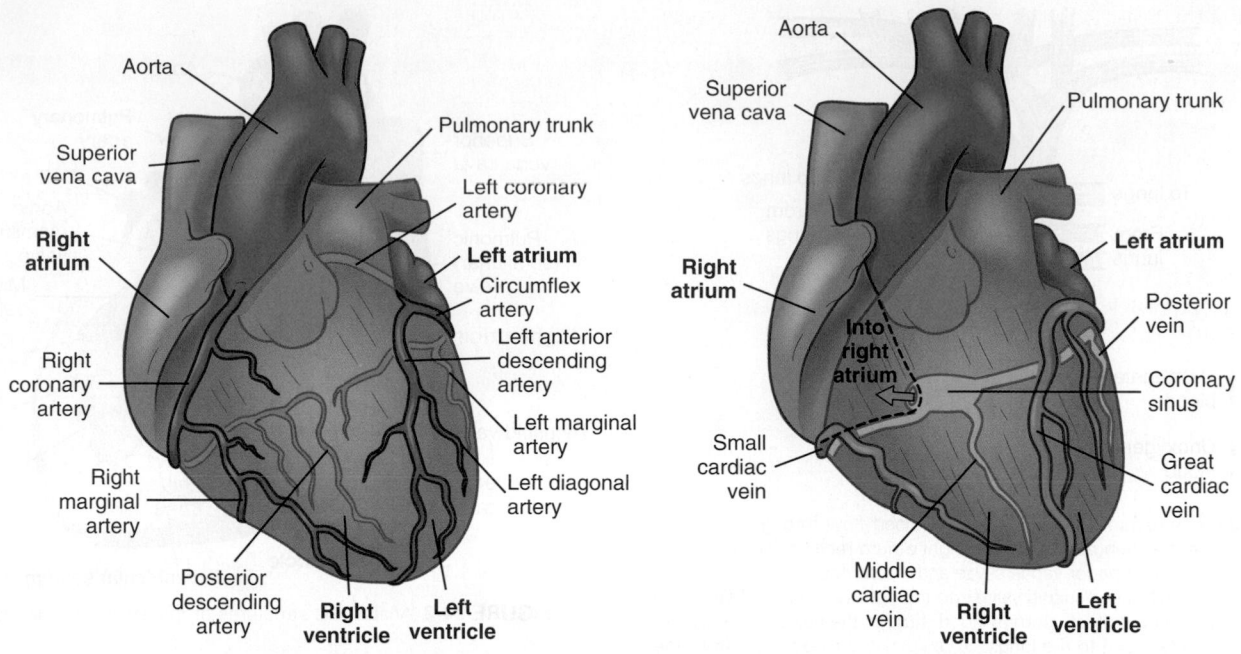

FIGURE 34-3 Coronary arteries and veins.

FIGURE 34-4 A, Conduction system of the heart. *AV,* atrioventricular; *SA,* sinoatrial. **B,** The normal electrocardiogram pattern. The P wave represents depolarization of the atria. The QRS complex indicates depolarization of the ventricles. The T wave represents repolarization of the ventricles. The U wave, if present, may represent repolarization of the Purkinje fibres or may be associated with hypokalemia. The PR, QRS, and QT intervals reflect the length of time it takes for the impulse to travel from one area of the heart to another.

identify the separate waveforms (see Figure 34-4, *B*). The first wave, P, begins with the firing of the sinoatrial node and represents depolarization of the fibres of the atria. The QRS wave represents depolarization from the atrioventricular node throughout the ventricles. There is a delay of impulse transmission through the atrioventricular node that accounts for the time sequence between the end of the P wave and the beginning of the QRS wave. The

T wave represents repolarization of the ventricles. The U wave, if present, represents delayed ventricular repolarization and may be associated with electrolyte imbalance (i.e., hypokalemia, hypomagnesemia, hypercalcemia) and is most typically observed in different types of bradycardia.

Intervals between these waves (PR, QRS, and QT intervals) reflect the length of time it takes for the impulse to travel from one area of the heart to another. These time intervals have been referenced, and deviations from these time references often indicate the presence of pathological conditions (Aehlert, 2013).

Mechanical System. Depolarization triggers mechanical activity. **Systole,** contraction of the myocardium, results in ejection of blood from the cardiac chamber. Relaxation of the myocardium, **diastole,** allows for filling of the chamber. **Cardiac output (CO)** is the measurement of the heart's mechanical efficiency. CO is the amount of blood pumped by each ventricle in 1 minute. To calculate CO, the amount of blood ejected from the ventricle with the heartbeat—the stroke volume (SV)—is multiplied by the heart rate (HR) per minute:

$$CO = SV \times HR$$

For a normal adult at rest, CO is maintained in the range of 4 to 8 L/minute. **Cardiac index** is the CO divided by the body mass index (BMI). A measure of the CO of a patient per square metre of body surface area, the cardiac index adjusts the CO to the body size. The normal cardiac index is 2.8 to 4.2 L/minute/m^2.

Factors Affecting Cardiac Output. Numerous factors can affect either the HR or the SV and thus the CO. The HR is regulated primarily by the autonomic nervous system. The factors affecting the SV are preload, contractility, and afterload (Huether & McCance, 2012). Increases in preload, contractility, and afterload increase the workload of the myocardium, which results in increased oxygen demand.

The volume of blood in the ventricles at the end of diastole, before the next contraction, is called **preload.** Preload determines the amount of stretch placed on myocardial fibres. According to Starling's law, to a point, the more the fibres are stretched (i.e., the greater the preload), the greater is their force of contraction, or contractility.

Contractility can be increased by norepinephrine, released by the sympathetic nervous system, as well as by epinephrine. Increasing contractility raises the SV by increasing ventricular emptying.

Afterload is the peripheral resistance against which the left ventricle must pump. Afterload is affected by the size of the ventricle, the wall tension, and the arterial blood pressure. If the arterial blood pressure is elevated, the ventricles meet increased resistance to ejection of blood, which increases the work demand. Eventually, this results in ventricular hypertrophy (enlargement of the cardiac muscle tissue without an increase in the size of cavities).

Cardiac Reserve. The cardiovascular system must respond to numerous situations in health and illness (e.g., exercise, stress, hypovolemia). The ability of the heart to respond to these demands by increasing CO as much as three-fold or four-fold is termed **cardiac reserve.**

The increase in CO results from an increase in HR or SV. The HR can increase to as high as 180 beats per minute for short periods without deleterious effects. The SV can be increased by an increase in either preload or contractility.

Vascular System

Blood Vessels. The three major types of blood vessels in the vascular system are the arteries, the veins, and the capillaries. Arteries carry blood away from the heart and, except for the pulmonary artery, carry oxygenated blood. Veins carry blood toward the heart and, except for the pulmonary veins, carry

FIGURE 34-5 Comparative thicknesses of layers of an artery, a vein, and a capillary.

deoxygenated blood. Small branches of arteries and veins are arterioles and venules, respectively. Blood circulates from the heart into arteries, arterioles, capillaries, venules, and veins and back to the heart.

Arteries and Arterioles. The arterial system differs from the venous system by the amount and type of tissue that makes up arterial walls (Figure 34-5). The large arteries have thick walls that are composed mainly of elastic tissue. This elastic property cushions the vessels against the impact of the pressure created by ventricular contraction, and it provides recoil that propels blood forward into the circulation. Large arteries also contain some smooth muscle. Examples of large arteries are the aorta and the pulmonary artery.

Arterioles have relatively little elastic tissue and more smooth muscle. Arterioles serve as the major control of arterial blood pressure and distribution of blood flow. They respond readily to local conditions, such as low O_2 and increasing levels of CO_2, by dilating or constricting.

Capillaries. The thin capillary wall is made up of endothelial cells, with no elastic or muscle tissue (see Figure 34-5). There are many kilometres of capillaries in an adult. The exchange of cellular nutrients and metabolic end products takes place through these thin-walled vessels.

Veins and Venules. Veins are large diameter, thin-walled vessels that return blood to the right atrium (see Figure 34-5). The venous system is a low-pressure, high-volume system. The larger veins contain semilunar valves at intervals to maintain the blood flow toward the heart and to prevent backward flow. The amount of blood in the venous system is affected by a number of factors, including arterial flow, compression of veins by skeletal muscles, alterations in thoracic and abdominal pressures, and right atrial pressure.

The largest veins are the superior vena cava, which returns blood to the heart from the head, neck, and arms, and the inferior vena cava, which returns blood to the heart from the lower part of the body. These large-diameter vessels are affected by the pressure in the right side of the heart. Elevated right atrial pressure can cause neck veins to become distended or the liver to become engorged as a result of resistance to blood flow.

Venules are relatively small vessels made up of a small amount of muscle and connective tissue. Venules collect blood from various capillary beds and channel it to the larger veins.

Regulation of the Cardiovascular System
Autonomic Nervous System. The autonomic nervous system consists of the sympathetic nervous system and the parasympathetic nervous system.

Effect on the Heart. Stimulation of the sympathetic nervous system increases the HR, the speed of impulse conduction through the atrioventricular node, and the force of atrial and ventricular contractions. This effect is mediated by specific sites in the heart called *β-adrenergic receptors* that are receptors for norepinephrine and epinephrine.

In contrast, stimulation of the parasympathetic system (mediated by the vagus nerve) causes a decrease in HR by the action on the sinoatrial node and slows conduction through the atrioventricular node.

Effect on the Blood Vessels. The source of neural control of blood vessels is the sympathetic nervous system. The α-adrenergic receptors are located in vascular smooth muscles. Stimulation of the α-adrenergic receptors results in vasoconstriction. Decreased stimulation to the α-adrenergic receptors causes vasodilation. (Sympathetic nervous system receptors that influence blood pressure are presented in Chapter 35, Table 35-1.)

The parasympathetic nerves have selective distribution in the blood vessels. Blood vessels in skeletal muscle do not receive parasympathetic input.

Baroreceptors. *Baroreceptors* in the aortic arch and the carotid sinus (at the origin of the internal carotid artery) are sensitive to stretch or pressure within the arterial system. Stimulation of these receptors sends information to the vasomotor centre in the brainstem. This results in temporary inhibition of the sympathetic nervous system and enhancement of the parasympathetic influence, which cause a decrease in HR and peripheral vasodilation. Decreased arterial pressure causes the opposite effect.

Chemoreceptors. *Chemoreceptors* are located in the aortic arch and the carotid bodies. They are capable of initiating changes in HR and arterial pressure in response to decreased arterial O_2 pressure, increased arterial CO_2 pressure, and decreased plasma pH. When the chemoreceptor reflexes in the medulla are triggered, they stimulate the vasomotor centre to increase blood pressure and, in turn, to increase cardiac activity (Huether & McCance, 2012).

Blood Pressure
The **arterial blood pressure (BP)** is a measure of the pressure exerted by blood against the walls of the arterial system. The **systolic blood pressure (SBP)** is the peak pressure exerted against the arteries when the heart contracts. The **diastolic blood pressure (DBP)** is the residual pressure of the arterial system during ventricular relaxation. BP is usually expressed as the ratio of SBP to DBP.

The two main factors influencing BP are CO and systemic vascular resistance (SVR):

$$BP = CO \times SVR$$

SVR is the force opposing the movement of blood. This force is created primarily in small arteries and arterioles.

Measurement of Arterial Blood Pressure. BP can be measured by invasive and noninvasive techniques. The invasive technique consists of catheter insertion into an artery. The catheter is attached to a recording device, and the pressure is measured directly (see Chapter 68).

Noninvasive, indirect measurement of BP can be done with a sphygmomanometer and a stethoscope. The sphygmomanometer consists of an inflatable cuff and a pressure gauge or an electronic cuff. The examiner measures BP externally by listening for sounds of turbulent blood flow through a compressed artery (termed Korotkoff sounds). The brachial artery is the usual site for measuring BP (Jarvis, Browne, MacDonald-Jenkins, et al., 2014).

After the appropriate-size cuff is placed on the extremity, the cuff is inflated to a pressure in excess of the SBP. This causes blood flow in the artery to cease. As the pressure in the cuff is lowered, the artery is auscultated for Korotkoff sounds. There are five phases of Korotkoff sounds. The first phase is a tapping sound caused by the spurt of blood into the constricted artery as the pressure in the cuff is gradually deflated. The pressure when this sound is heard is considered the SBP. The fifth phase occurs when the sound disappears, and this pressure is known as the DBP (Jarvis, Browne, MacDonald-Jenkins, et al., 2014). Clinically, the BP is recorded as SBP/DBP (e.g., 120/80 mm Hg). On occasion, an auscultatory gap is heard. An auscultatory gap is a loss of sound between the SBP and the DBP. The BP could be measured incorrectly if the cuff is not inflated to exceed the true SBP.

In addition to the manual technique, another noninvasive way to measure BP indirectly is to use automatic BP monitors (see Chapter 35). The monitor consists of a BP cuff and a lightweight microprocessing unit. This system, which records a patient's BP at preset intervals during routine activities over 24 to 48 hours, enables ambulatory BP monitoring and may help clinicians diagnose hypertension more accurately in some patients.

Pulse Pressure and Mean Arterial Pressure. Pulse pressure is the difference between the SBP and the DBP. Normally it is approximately one-third of the SBP. If the BP is 120/80 mm Hg, the normal pulse pressure is 40 mm Hg. The pulse pressure may be elevated during exercise or in individuals with atherosclerosis of the larger arteries because of increased SBP. The pulse pressure may be decreased in cardiac failure or hypovolemia.

Another measurement related to BP is mean arterial pressure. It is not the average of the DBP and SBP because the duration of diastole exceeds that of systole at normal HRs. To calculate mean arterial pressure, the DBP is added to one-third of the pulse pressure:

$$\text{Mean arterial pressure} = DBP + \tfrac{1}{3}\text{Pulse pressure}$$

A person with a BP of 120/60 mm Hg has a mean arterial pressure of 80 mm Hg.

AGE-RELATED CONSIDERATIONS

EFFECTS OF AGING ON THE CARDIOVASCULAR SYSTEM
One of the greatest risk factors for cardiovascular disease is age. Cardiovascular disease remains the leading cause of death in adults older than 85 years. It is the most common cause of hospitalization and the second leading cause of death in adults younger than age 85. The most common cardiovascular problem is coronary artery disease (CAD) secondary to atherosclerosis.

TABLE 34-1 AGE-RELATED DIFFERENCES IN ASSESSMENT

Cardiovascular System

Changes	Differences in Assessment Findings
Chest Wall	
Kyphosis	Altered chest landmarks for palpation, percussion, and auscultation; distant heart sounds
Heart	
Myocardial hypertrophy, ↑ collagen and scarring, ↓ elastin	↓ Cardiac reserve, slight ↓ HR
Downward displacement	Difficulty in isolating apical pulse
↓ CO, HR, and SV in response to exercise or stress	Slowed, ↓ response to stress; slowed recovery from activity
Cellular aging changes and fibrosis of conduction system	↓ Amplitude of QRS complex and lengthening of PR, QRS, and QT intervals; left axis deviation; irregular cardiac rhythms
Valvular rigidity from calcification, sclerosis, or fibrosis, impeding complete closure of valves	Systolic murmur (aortic or mitral) possible without being indication of cardiovascular disease
Blood Vessels	
Arterial stiffening caused by loss of elastin in arterial walls, thickening of intima of arteries, and progressive fibrosis of media	Elevation in systolic and possibly diastolic BP (e.g., 160/90 mm Hg); possibly, widened pulse pressures; more pronounced arterial pulses; diminished pedal pulses

BP, blood pressure; *CO*, cardiac output; *HR*, heart rate; *SV*, stroke volume.

It is difficult to distinguish normal aging changes from the pathophysiological changes of atherosclerosis. Many of the physiological changes in the cardiovascular system of older adults are a result of the combined effects of the aging process, disease, environmental factors, and lifetime health behaviours, rather than just age alone (North & Sinclair, 2012).

Age-related changes in the cardiovascular system and differences in assessment findings are presented in Table 34-1. With increased age, the amount of collagen in the heart increases and that of elastin decreases. These changes affect the myocardium's ability to stretch and contract. One of the major changes in the cardiovascular system is the response to physical or emotional stress. In times of increased stress, CO and SV decrease because of reduced contractility and HR response. The resting supine HR is not markedly affected by aging. When an older adult changes positions (e.g., sits upright), the sympathetic nerve pathway may be affected by fibrous tissue and fatty deposits, manifested as a blunted HR response (North & Sinclair, 2012).

Cardiac valves become thicker and stiffer from lipid accumulation, degeneration of collagen, and fibrosis. The aortic and mitral valves are most frequently affected. These changes result in either regurgitation of blood when the valve should be closed or narrowing of the orifice of the valve (stenosis) when the valve should be open. The turbulent blood flow across the affected valve results in a murmur.

The number of pacemaker cells in the sinoatrial node decreases with age. By age 75, a person may have only 10% of the normal number of pacemaker cells. Although this is compatible with adequate sinoatrial node function, it may account for the frequency of some sinus dysrhythmias in older adults. Similar decreases also occur in the number of conduction cells in the internodal tracts, bundle of His, and bundle branches. These changes contribute to the development of atrial dysrhythmias and heart blocks. The autonomic nervous system control of the cardiovascular system changes with aging. The number and function of β-adrenergic receptors in the heart decrease with age. So the older adult not only has a decreased response to physical and emotional stress, but also is less sensitive to β-adrenergic agonist drugs. The lower maximum HR during exercise results in only a two-fold increase in CO, in contrast to the three- or four-fold increase observed in younger adults.

Arterial and venous blood vessels thicken and become less elastic with age. Arteries increase their sensitivity to vasopressin (antidiuretic hormone). With aging, both of these changes contribute to a progressive increase in SBP and a decrease or no change in DBP. Thus an increase in the pulse pressure is found. Hypertension is not a normal consequence of aging and should be treated. Valves in the large veins in the lower extremities have a reduced ability to return the blood to the heart, which often results in dependent edema.

Orthostatic hypotension, which is estimated to be present in more than 30% of patients older than 70 years with systolic hypertension, may be related to medications, decreased baroreceptor function, or both. *Postprandial hypotension* (decrease in BP of at least 20 mm Hg that occurs within 75 minutes after eating) may also occur in about a third of otherwise healthy older adults. Both orthostatic and postprandial hypotension may be related to falls in older adults. Despite the changes associated with aging, the heart is able to function adequately under most circumstances.

Age-related changes in the cardiovascular system and differences in assessment findings are presented in Table 34-1.

ASSESSMENT OF THE CARDIOVASCULAR SYSTEM

Subjective Data

A careful health history and physical examination (Table 34-2) should aid the nurse in distinguishing symptoms that reflect a cardiovascular problem from those that reflect problems of other body systems. For instance, it is important to determine whether weight gain results from overeating or is a manifestation of fluid retention.

Important Health Information

History of Current Illness. The nurse should ask the patient what problem has brought him or her to the health care facility or provider and should fully explore all symptoms the patient is experiencing.

Past Health History. Many illnesses affect the cardiovascular system directly or indirectly. The patient should be questioned about a history of chest pain, shortness of breath, alcoholism or excessive drinking, anemia, rheumatic fever, streptococcal sore throat, congenital heart disease, stroke, syncope, hypertension, thrombo-phlebitis, intermittent claudication, varicosities, obesity, and edema.

Medications. An assessment of the patient's current and past use of medications should be made. This includes both over-the-counter drugs and prescription drugs. For example, acetylsalicylic

CASE STUDY

Patient Introduction

Source: ESB
Professional/
Shutterstock
.com.

Lawrence Tan, a 63-year-old man, is brought to the emergency department by ambulance at 0600 hours after calling 911 with complaints of chest pain, shortness of breath, palpitations, and dizziness. The paramedics have started an intravenous infusion and administered oxygen at 2 L/min via nasal cannula. They also administered four chewable baby acetylsalicylic acid (ASA) and a nitroglycerin tablet, and they obtained a 12-lead ECG. Mr. Tan is pain free on arrival but still complains of palpitations and dizziness.

Critical Thinking

Throughout this assessment chapter, think about Mr. Tan's symptoms with the following questions in mind:

1. What are the possible causes of Mr. Tan's chest pain, shortness of breath, palpitations, and dizziness?
2. What would be the nurse's priority assessment of Mr. Tan?
3. What questions would the nurse ask Mr. Tan?
4. What should be included in the physical assessment? What would the nurse be looking for?
5. What diagnostic studies would the nurse expect to be ordered?
See pp. 777 and 786 for more information on Mr. Tan.

evolve

Answers available at *http://evolve.elsevier.com/Canada/Lewis/medsurg.*

CASE STUDY

Subjective Data

Source: ESB
Professional/
Shutterstock
.com.

A focused subjective assessment of Lawrence Tan revealed the following information:

- *Past Medical History:* History of hypertension, mitral valve prolapse with mild regurgitation, heart failure, and type 2 diabetes mellitus.
- *Medications:* Lisinopril (Prinivil), 10 mg/day PO; metoprolol (Lopresor), 50 mg PO bid; ASA, 325 mg/day PO; furosemide (Lasix), 40 mg/day PO; and metformin (Glucophage), 500 mg PO qid.
- *Current History:* Mr. Tan denies any previous history of chest pain or CAD. He was feeling fine until this morning, when he awoke and experienced shortness of breath, chest pain, palpitations, and dizziness while walking to the bathroom. He became frightened that he was having a heart attack, so he called 911. Denies smoking or alcohol intake. Shortness of breath and chest pain are now gone, but he continues to feel palpitations and dizziness when he sits up.
- Denies any edema. States he takes Lasix in the morning and typically "pees until lunchtime." Denies nocturia.
See pp. 777 and 786 for more information on Mr. Tan.

---

acid (ASA; Aspirin), which prolongs the blood clotting time, is contained in many drugs used to alleviate cold symptoms.

A medication assessment should list the name of the drug and the patient's understanding of its purpose and adverse effects. Drugs that may adversely affect the cardiovascular system should also be assessed. Some of these and examples of their effects on the cardiovascular system are listed in Table 34-3.

Surgery or Other Treatments. The patient should also be asked about specific treatments, past surgical procedures, and hospital admissions related to cardiovascular problems. Any hospitalizations for diagnostic workups or cardiovascular symptoms should be explored. It should be noted whether an ECG or a chest radiograph was obtained for baseline data.

Objective Data
Physical Examination

Vital Signs. After the patient's general appearance has been observed, vital signs—including BP, heart and respiratory rate, and temperature—are measured. The BP should be measured while the patient is sitting, lying, and standing. An appropriate cuff size should be used for accurate readings. Normally, there is a reduction of up to 15 mm Hg in the SBP and 3 to 5 mm Hg in the DBP in the standing position. BP measurements should be taken in both arms. These readings may vary by 5 to 15 mm Hg. BP in the lower extremities is expected to be about 10 mm Hg higher than in the upper extremities.

Peripheral Vascular System

Inspection. The skin colour, hair distribution, and venous blood flow provide information about arterial blood flow and venous return. The extremities should be inspected for conditions such as edema, thrombo-phlebitis, varicose veins, and lesions such as stasis ulcers. Edema in the extremities can be caused by gravity, interruption of venous return, or elevation of right atrial pressure.

A measure used for assessing arterial flow to the extremities is the *capillary filling time.* The patient's nail beds are squeezed to produce blanching and are observed for the return of colour. When arterial capillary perfusion is normal, the colour returns within 3 seconds.

The large veins in the neck (internal and external jugular) should be inspected while the patient is gradually elevated to an upright position. Distension and prominent pulsations of these neck veins can be caused by right atrial pressure elevation.

Palpation. Palpation of the pulses in the neck and extremities also provides information on arterial blood flow. The pulses should be palpated to assess the volume and pressure within each vessel. Characteristics of the arteries on the right and left sides of the body should be compared. It is important to palpate each carotid pulse separately to avoid vagal stimulation and subsequent dysrhythmias.

When palpating the arteries identified in Figure 34-6, the assessor should note the pressure of the pulse wave, or how far the vessel wall distends when the pulse occurs. This judgement of the pulsation volume is recorded as normal, bounding, thready, or absent. A scale may be used to document pulse volume or amplitude (Jarvis, Browne, MacDonald-Jenkins, et al., 2014):
0: Absent
1+: Weak, thready
2+: Normal
3+: Full, bounding

The *rigidity* (hardness) of the vessel should also be noted. The normal pulse feels as if it is tapping, whereas a vessel wall that is narrowed or bulging vibrates. A term for a palpable vibration is *thrill.*

Auscultation. An artery that has a narrowed or bulging wall may cause blood flow to be turbulent. This abnormal flow can sound like a buzzing or humming, termed a *bruit.* It can be heard with a stethoscope placed over the vessel. Auscultation of major arteries such as the carotid arteries, the abdominal aorta, and the femoral arteries should be part of the initial cardiovascular

TABLE 34-2 HEALTH HISTORY

Cardiovascular System—Questions for Obtaining Subjective Data

Chest Pain
- Do you have any chest pain or discomfort? Please show me where it is.
- Is the pain in one spot, or does it move around?
- How long have you had this pain?
- Does it come and go, or is it constant? Does it get worse before or after meals? When is the pain worst (e.g., with a certain position or activity, with stress)?
- Can you describe how it feels (e.g., burning, stabbing, aching, heaviness, squeezing)?
- What brings the pain on (e.g., activity, stress)?
- Do any other symptoms occur when you get the pain (e.g., shortness of breath, weakness, nausea, vomiting)?*
- What works to relieve the pain (e.g., rest, change of position, medication)?*

Dyspnea
- Have you experienced any shortness of breath? If yes, what kind of activity precipitates your shortness of breath?
- Is your shortness of breath dependent on your position (e.g., lying down)?*
- How does the shortness of breath affect your daily activities?*

Orthopnea
- How many pillows do you sleep on at night? Has this number changed recently?*

Cough
- Do you have a cough? If yes, describe the duration, the frequency, and the kind of cough (e.g., dry, hoarse, congested).
- Do you cough up mucus? If yes, describe the colour and the amount.
- Is coughing associated with any activity such as talking, lying down, stress, and so on?*
- Is the coughing relieved by anything (e.g., walking, exercise, rest, medication)?*

Fatigue
- Do you tire easily?* If yes, when did you notice a change in your level of fatigue?
- Is your energy level related to the time of the day?*

Cyanosis or Pallor
- Have you ever noticed a bluish or ashen colour to your face?*

Edema
- Have you ever noticed any swelling in your feet and legs?*
- When did you first experience swelling, and have there been any recent changes?*
- Are both feet swollen to the same degree?*

Nocturia
- How many times a night do you awaken to urinate?*

Cardiac History
- Do you have any past history of hypertension, elevated cholesterol or triglycerides, heart murmur, congenital heart diseases, rheumatic fever or unexplained joint pains in your youth, recurrent tonsillitis, or anemia?
- Do you have any history of heart disease?*
- When was your last ECG, serum cholesterol blood work, or other heart-related tests?*

Family History
- Do you have any family history of heart disease, high blood pressure, obesity, diabetes, or sudden death at a young age?*

Self-Care History
- Describe your usual daily diet, including sodium and fluid intake. What is your current weight? What was your weight 1 year ago?
- Have you ever used tobacco? If yes, in what form, how much, and for how long? Have you ever tried to quit? If yes, what methods have you tried?
- How often do you drink alcohol, and how much? Have you ever been told that you have a problem with alcohol?*
- What is your usual amount of exercise per week?
- Do you take any cardiac medications (e.g., antihypertensives, diuretics, aspirin, anticoagulants), over-the-counter medications, herbal products, or street drugs?*

Source: Adapted from Jarvis, C., Browne, A. J., MacDonald-Jenkins, J., & Luctkar-Flude, M. (2014). *Physical examination & health assessment* (2nd Canadian ed., pp. 303–305). Toronto: Elsevier Canada.
ECG, electrocardiogram.
*If yes, describe.

TABLE 34-3 CARDIOVASCULAR EFFECTS OF NONCARDIAC DRUGS*

Drug Classification	Examples	Cardiovascular Effects
Anticancer agents	Daunorubicin (Cerubadine) Doxorubicin (Caelyx)	Dysrhythmias, cardiomyopathy
Antipsychotics	Chlorpromazine Haloperidol	Dysrhythmias, orthostatic hypotension
Corticosteroids	Cortisone Prednisone	Hypotension, edema, potassium depletion
Hormone therapy, oral contraceptives	Estrogen + progestin (Climara Pro)	Myocardial infarction, thrombo-embolism, stroke, hypertension
Nonsteroidal anti-inflammatory drugs (NSAIDs)†	Ibuprofen (Motrin) Celecoxib (Celebrex)	Hypertension, myocardial infarction, stroke
Psychostimulants	Cocaine Amphetamines	Tachycardia, angina, myocardial infarction, hypertension, dysrhythmias
Tricyclic antidepressants	Amitriptyline (Elavil) Doxepin (Sinequan, Silenor)	Dysrhythmias, orthostatic hypotension

*List is not all-inclusive.
†Second-generation NSAIDs, known as cyclo-oxygenase 2 (COX-2) inhibitors, have been linked to an increased risk of serious adverse cardiovascular events.

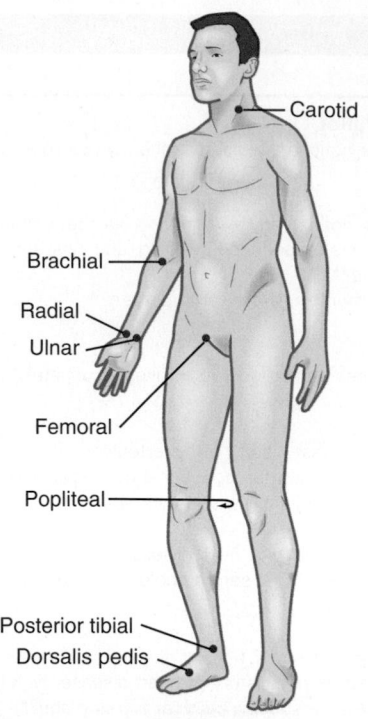

- Carotid
- Brachial
- Radial
- Ulnar
- Femoral
- Popliteal
- Posterior tibial
- Dorsalis pedis

FIGURE 34-6 Common sites for palpating arteries.

assessment. Abnormalities of the cardiovascular system are described in Table 34-4.

Thorax

Inspection and Palpation. An overall inspection and palpation of the bony structures of the thorax is the initial step in the examination.

Next, the areas where the cardiac valves project their sounds are inspected and palpated by identifying the intercostal spaces (ICSs). The raised notch, the angle of Louis, where the manubrium and the body of the sternum are joined, is readily palpable in the midline of the sternum. The angle of Louis is at the level of the second rib and can therefore be used to count ICSs and locate specific auscultatory areas.

The following auscultatory areas can be located (Figure 34-7): The aortic area, in the second ICS to the right of the sternum; the pulmonic area, in the second ICS to the left of the sternum; the tricuspid area, in the fifth left ICS close to the sternum; and the mitral area, in the left midclavicular line (MCL) at the level of the fifth ICS. A fifth auscultatory area is Erb point, located at the third left ICS near the sternum. Normally, no pulsations are felt in these areas unless the patient has a thin chest wall.

A valvular disorder may be suspected if abnormal pulsations or thrills are felt. Next, the epigastric area, which lies on either side of the midline just below the xiphoid process, is inspected and palpated. In a thin person, the pulsation of the abdominal

TABLE 34-4 ASSESSMENT ABNORMALITIES

Cardiovascular System

Finding	Description	Possible Etiology and Significance*
Inspection		
Distended neck veins	Vertical distance between intersection of angle of Louis and level of jugular distension >3 cm with patient sitting at 30- to 45-degree angle	Elevated right atrial pressure; right-sided heart failure
Central cyanosis	Bluish or purplish tinge in central areas such as tongue, conjunctivae, inner surface of lips	Inadequate O_2 saturation of arterial blood as result of pulmonary or cardiac disorders (e.g., congenital defects)
Peripheral cyanosis	Bluish or purplish tinge in extremities or nose and ears	Reduced blood flow because of heart failure, vasoconstriction, cold environment
Splinter hemorrhages	Small red to black streaks under fingernails	Infective endocarditis (infection of endocardium, usually in area of cardiac valves)
Clubbing of nail beds	Obliteration of normal angle between base of nail and skin	Endocarditis, congenital defects, prolonged O_2 deficiency
Colour changes in extremities with postural change	Pallor, cyanosis, mottling of skin after limb elevation; glossy skin	Chronic decreased arterial perfusion
Ulcers	*Venous:* necrotic crater-like lesions usually found on lower leg at medial malleolus; characterized by slow wound healing *Arterial:* lesions with pale ischemic base and well-defined edges; usually found on toes, heels, lateral malleoli	Poor venous return, varicose veins, incompetent venous valves; arteriosclerosis, diabetes
Varicose veins	Visible dilated, tortuous vessels in lower extremities	Incompetent valves in vein
Palpation		
Pulse		
Bounding	Sharp, brisk, pounding pulse	Hyperkinetic states (anxiety, fever), anemia, hyperthyroidism
Thready	Weak, slowly rising pulse; easily obliterated by pressure	Blood loss, decreased cardiac output, aortic valve disease, peripheral arterial disease
Irregular	Regularly irregular or irregularly irregular; skipped beats	Cardiac dysrhythmias
Pulsus alternans	Regular rhythm, but strength of pulse varies with each beat	Heart failure
Absent	Lack of pulse	Atherosclerosis, thrombus, trauma, embolus
Thrill	Vibration of vessel or chest wall	Aneurysm, aortic regurgitation, arteriovenous fistula
Rigidity	Stiffness or inflexibility of vessel wall	Atherosclerosis
>100 bpm	Tachycardia	May be exercise-induced; may reflect anxiety or shock; may indicate need for increased cardiac output, hyperthyroidism

TABLE 34-4 ASSESSMENT ABNORMALITIES

Cardiovascular System—cont'd

Finding	Description	Possible Etiology and Significance*
<60 bpm	Bradycardia	May be rest-induced; SA or AV node damage, athletic conditioning, adverse effect of drugs (e.g., β-adrenergic blockers), hypothyroidism
Displaced point of maximal impulse (apical pulse)	Point of maximal impulse is palpated (or auscultated) below the fifth ICS and to the left of the MCL	Left ventricular dilation
Extremities		
Unusually warm extremities	Hands and feet warmer than normal	Possible thyrotoxicosis
Cold extremities	Hands or feet, or both, cold to touch; external covering necessary for comfort	Intermittent claudication, peripheral arterial obstruction, low cardiac output, severe anemia
Pitting edema of lower extremities or sacral area	Visible finger indentation after application of firm pressure	Interruption of venous return to heart, fluid in tissues
Positive Homans sign	Presence of calf pain during sharp dorsiflexion of foot	Thrombo-phlebitis
Abnormal capillary filling time	Blanching of nail bed for >3 sec after release of pressure	Reduced arterial capillary perfusion, anemia
Asymmetry in limb circumference	Measurable swelling of involved limb	Thrombo-phlebitis, varicose veins, lymphedema
Percussion		
Abnormal cardiac borders	Left border of cardiac dullness extends beyond MCL in fifth ICS; right border of cardiac dullness extends beyond sternal border	Cardiac enlargement due to coronary heart disease, heart failure, cardiomyopathy
Auscultation		
Pulse deficit	Apical heart rate exceeds the peripheral pulse rate	Cardiac dysrhythmias
Arterial bruit	Turbulent flow sound in peripheral artery	Arterial obstruction or aneurysm
Third heart sound (S_3)	Extra heart sound, low-pitched, heard in early diastole, similar to sound of a gallop	Left ventricular failure; volume overload; mitral, aortic, or tricuspid regurgitation; hypertension (possible)
Fourth heart sound (S_4)	Extra heart sound, low-pitched, heard in late diastole, similar to sound of a gallop	Forceful atrial contraction from resistance to ventricular filling (e.g., in left ventricular hypertrophy, aortic stenosis, hypertension, coronary artery disease)
Cardiac murmurs	Turbulent sounds occurring between normal heart sounds; characterized by loudness, pitch, shape, quality, duration, timing	Cardiac valve disorder, abnormal blood flow patterns
Pericardial friction rub	High-pitched, scratchy sound heard during S_1 or S_2 or both at the apex; heard best with patient sitting and leaning forward, and at the end of expiration	Pericarditis

AV, atrioventricular; *bpm,* beats per minute; *ICS,* intercostal space; *MCL,* midclavicular line; *SA,* sinoatrial.
*Limited to common etiological factors. (Further discussion of conditions listed may be found in Chapters 35 through 40 and 68.)

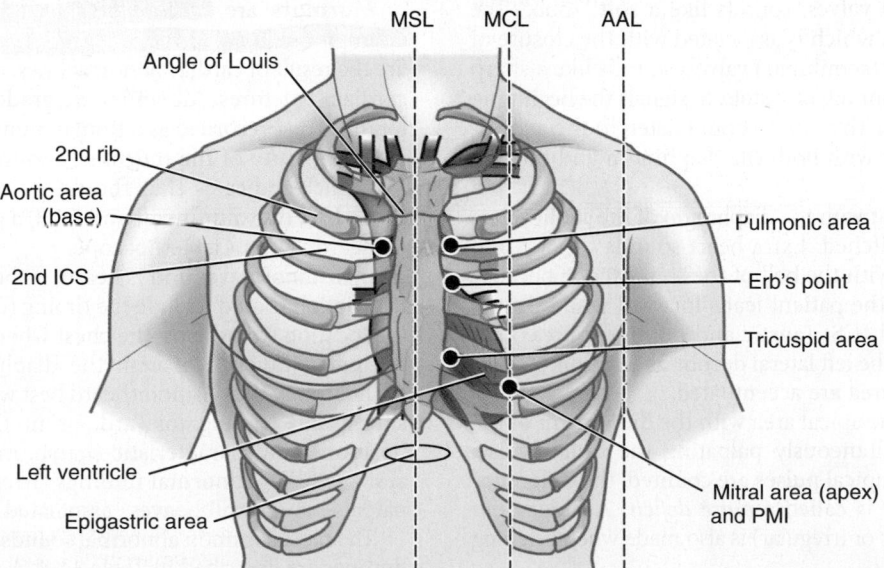

FIGURE 34-7 Orientation of the heart within the thorax and cardiac auscultatory areas. *Red lines* indicate the midsternal line (*MSL*), midclavicular line (*MCL*), and anterior axillary line (*AAL*). *ICS,* intercostal space; *PMI,* point of maximal impulse.

FIGURE 34-8 Relationship of electrocardiogram, cardiac cycle, and heart sounds (S_1, S_2).

TABLE 34-5	**NORMAL FINDINGS IN THE PHYSICAL ASSESSMENT OF THE CARDIOVASCULAR SYSTEM**
Inspection	Normal skin colour with capillary refill <3 sec; thorax symmetrical with no visible PMI; no JVD with patient at 45-degree angle
Palpation	PMI palpable in fifth ICS at MCL; no forceful pulsations, thrills, or heaves; slight palpable pulsations of abdominal aorta in epigastric area; carotid and extremity pulses 2+ and equal bilaterally; no evidence of impaired arterial flow or venous return in lower extremities
Percussion	Inability to distinguish right-sided heart border
Auscultation	S_1 and S_2 heard; HR, 72 and regular; no murmurs or extra heart sounds

HR, heart rate; *ICS,* intercostal space; *JVD,* jugular venous distension; *MCL,* midclavicular line; *PMI,* point of maximal impulse.

aorta may be visible and can normally be palpated here. Next, the precordium, which is located between the apex and the sternum, is inspected for heaves. Heaves are sustained lifts of the chest wall in the precordial area that can be seen or palpated. They may be caused by left ventricular enlargement. Normally, no pulsations are seen or felt in the precordial area.

When the patient is recumbent, the mitral valve area at the apex of the heart is inspected and palpated for the **point of maximal impulse** (PMI), the site of strongest pulsation. This pulsation or ventricular thrust lies within the MCL in the fifth ICS. If the PMI is palpable, its position is recorded in relation to the MCL and ICSs. When the PMI is to the left of the MCL, the heart may be enlarged.

Percussion. The borders of the right and left sides of the heart can be estimated by percussion. The nurse stands to the right of the recumbent patient and percusses along the curve of the rib in the fourth and fifth ICSs, starting at the midaxillary line. The percussion note over the heart is dull in comparison with the resonance over the lung and is recorded in relation to the MCL.

Auscultation. The movement of the cardiac valves creates some turbulence in the blood flow; the resulting heart sounds are normal (Figure 34-8). These sounds can be heard through a stethoscope placed on the chest wall. The first heart sound (S_1), which is associated with the closure of the tricuspid and mitral (atrioventricular) valves, sounds like a soft "lubb." The second heart sound (S_2), which is associated with the closure of the aortic and pulmonic (semilunar) valves, sounds like a sharp "dupp." S_1 signals the beginning of systole. S_2 signals the beginning of diastole (Figure 34-8). The nurse should listen to the auscultatory areas in sequence with both the diaphragm and the bell of the stethoscope.

S_1 and S_2 are heard best with the diaphragm of the stethoscope because they are high pitched. Extra heart sounds (S_3 or S_4), if present, are heard best with the bell of the stethoscope because they are low pitched. If the patient leans forward while sitting, sounds from the second ICSs (aortic and pulmonic areas) are accentuated, whereas in the left lateral decubitus position, sounds produced at the mitral area are accentuated.

The nurse listens at the apical area with the diaphragm of the stethoscope while simultaneously palpating the radial pulse. When fewer radial than apical pulses are counted, the difference between those numbers is called a *pulse deficit*. A judgement about the rhythm (regular or irregular) is also made when listening at the apex.

Palpating one carotid artery while auscultating it allows the examiner to distinguish between S_1 and S_2 and between systole and diastole. Because S_1 ("lubb") occurs almost simultaneously

with ventricular ejection, it is heard when the carotid pulse is felt.

Normally, no sound is heard between S_1 and S_2 during the periods of systole and diastole. Sounds that are heard during these periods may represent abnormalities and should be described in the assessment. An exception to this is a normal splitting of S_2, which is best heard at the pulmonic area during inspiration. Splitting of this heart sound can be abnormal if it is heard during expiration or if it is constant (fixed) during the respiratory cycle.

S_3 is a low-intensity vibration of the ventricular walls usually associated with ventricular filling. S_3 may occur in patients with left ventricular failure or mitral valve regurgitation. It is heard closely after S_2 and is known as a *ventricular gallop*. S_4 is a low-frequency vibration caused by atrial contraction. It precedes S_1 of the next cycle and is known as an *atrial gallop*. S_4 may occur in patients with CAD, left ventricular hypertrophy, or aortic stenosis.

Murmurs are sounds produced by turbulent blood flow through the heart or the walls of large arteries. Most murmurs are the result of cardiac abnormalities, but some occur in normal cardiac structures. Murmurs are graded on a six-point scale of loudness and recorded as a Roman numeral ratio: The numerator is the intensity of the murmur, and the denominator is always VI, which indicates that the six-point scale is being used. A grade I/VI murmur is soft and faint; a grade VI/VI murmur can be heard without a stethoscope.

If an abnormal sound is heard, it should be documented. The description should include the timing (during systole or diastole), the location (the site on the chest where it is heard the loudest), the pitch (heard best with the diaphragm or the bell of the stethoscope), the position (heard best when patient is recumbent, sitting and leaning forward, or in the left lateral decubitus position), the characteristic (harsh, musical, soft, short, long), and any other abnormal findings (irregular cardiac rhythms or palpable chest wall heaves) associated with the sound.

The most common abnormal sounds and abnormal assessment findings are described in Table 34-4. A method of recording data from the cardiovascular assessment is presented in Table 34-5.

A focused assessment is used to evaluate the status of previously identified cardiovascular problems and to monitor for signs of

CASE STUDY

Objective Data: Physical Examination

Physical examination findings of Lawrence Tan are as follows:
- BP, 98/70; apical pulse rate, 164; pulse irregular; respiratory rate, 20; temperature, 36.8°C; O₂ saturation, 93% on room air
- Awake, alert, and oriented ×3
- Lungs clear on auscultation; systolic murmur present
- Cardiac monitor shows atrial fibrillation with a rapid ventricular response
- +1 pedal pulses bilaterally
- No peripheral edema, jugular venous distention, or heaves noted

Throughout this chapter, consider diagnostic studies the nurse would anticipate being ordered for Mr. Tan. See pp. 772 and 786 for more information on Mr. Tan.

Source: ESB Professional/ Shutterstock .com.

FOCUSED ASSESSMENT

Cardiovascular System

Use this checklist to make sure the key assessment steps have been done.

Subjective
Ask the patient about any of the following, and note responses:

Chest pain or discomfort	Y	N
Shortness of breath (especially when lying down)	Y	N
Edema in legs or any part of body	Y	N
Leg pain during exercise	Y	N
Excess urination at night	Y	N
Palpitations	Y	N

Objective: Diagnostic
Check the following laboratory test results for critical values:

Hematocrit and hemoglobin	✓
Cardiac biomarkers (CK-MB, troponin)	✓
Electrocardiogram	✓

Objective: Physical Examination
Inspect and Palpate

Anterior chest wall for contour, lifts, and heaves	✓
Check pulses for symmetry, quality, and rhythm	✓

Auscultate

Blood pressure	✓
Heart for rate, rhythm, and sounds	✓

CK-MB, MB isoenzyme of creatine kinase.

new problems (see Table 3-6). A focused assessment of the cardiovascular system is presented in the "Focused Assessment" box afterwards.

DIAGNOSTIC STUDIES OF THE CARDIOVASCULAR SYSTEM

Numerous diagnostic procedures add to the information obtained from the history and physical examination of the cardiovascular system. These procedures are usually classified as noninvasive or invasive. Procedures in which only a needle is inserted to

FIGURE 34-9 Chest radiograph: standard posteroanterior view. Source: Drake, R. L., Vogl, A. W., & Mitchell, A. W. M. (2010). *Gray's anatomy for students* (2nd ed.). Philadelphia: Churchill Livingstone.

withdraw blood or inject contrast media are usually considered noninvasive. Catheter insertion for angiography is considered an invasive procedure. The most common studies used to assess the cardiovascular system are presented in Table 34-6.

Noninvasive Studies

Chest Radiography. A radiograph can depict cardiac contours, heart size and configuration, and anatomical changes in individual chambers (see Figure 34-9). The radiographic image records any displacement or enlargement of the heart, the presence of extra fluid around the heart (pericardial effusion), and pulmonary congestion.

Electrocardiography. The basic P, QRS, and T waveforms (see Figure 34-4) are used to assess cardiac function. Deviations from the normal sinus rhythm can indicate abnormalities in heart function. There are many types of electrocardiographic monitoring, including resting ECG, ambulatory ECG monitoring, and exercise or stress testing.

A resting ECG helps identify at one point in time primary conduction abnormalities, cardiac dysrhythmias, cardiac hypertrophy, pericarditis, myocardial ischemia, site and extent of myocardial infarction (MI), pacemaker performance, and effectiveness of drug therapy. It is also used to monitor recovery from an MI. (See Chapter 38 for a complete discussion of ECG monitoring.)

Ambulatory Electrocardiographic Monitoring. Continuous ambulatory ECG (Holter monitoring) can provide diagnostic information over a longer period than can a standard resting ECG. In Holter monitoring, a recorder is worn by the patient for 24 to 48 hours, and the resulting ECG information is then stored until it is played back for printing and evaluation. Holter monitoring gives the patient freedom to perform usual activities of daily living and those that may be associated with cardiovascular symptoms. The patient maintains a record of activities, symptoms,

Text continued on p. 783

TABLE 34-6   DIAGNOSTIC STUDIES

Cardiovascular System

Study	Description and Purpose	Nursing Responsibility
Blood Studies*		
MB isoenzyme of creatine kinase (CK-MB)	Cardiospecific isoenzyme that is released in the presence of myocardial tissue injury. Concentrations >4%–6% of total CK are highly indicative of MI. Serum levels increase within 4–6 hr after MI.	Explain to patient the purpose of serial sampling (e.g., q6–8h tid) in conjunction with serial ECGs.
Troponin (cardiac-specific)	Contractile proteins that are released after an MI. Both troponin T and troponin I are highly specific to cardiac tissue. *Reference intervals:* **Troponin I (cTnI)** Negative: <0.5 mcg/L Indeterminate or suspicious for injury to myocardium: 0.5–2.3 mcg/L Positive for myocardial injury: >2.3 mcg/L (2.3 mcg/L) **Troponin T (cTnT)** <0.1 mcg/L	Rapid point-of-care (bedside) assays are available. Serial sampling is often done in conjunction with CK-MB measurements and ECGs.
Myoglobin	Low-molecular-weight protein that is 99%–100% sensitive for myocardial injury. Serum concentrations rise 30–60 min after MI. *Reference intervals:* Male: 15.2–91.2 mcg/L Female: 11.1–57.5 mcg/L	Myoglobin is cleared from the circulation rapidly, and the test is most diagnostic if measurements are made within first 12 hr of onset of chest pain.
C-reactive protein (CRP)	Marker of inflammation that can predict risk of cardiac disease and cardiac events, even in patients with normal lipid values. CRP assay is highly sensitive. Lowest risk: <1 mg/L Moderate risk: 1–3 mg/L High risk: >3 mg/L	CRP levels are stable and can be measured nonfasting and any time during the day. In women, CRP levels may be more predictive risk factor of cardiac disease than LDLs.
Homocysteine	Amino acid produced during protein catabolism that has been identified as a risk factor for cardiovascular disease. Homocysteine may cause damage to the endothelium or have a role in formation of thrombi. *Reference intervals:* Male: 5.2–12.9 micromoles/L Female: 3.7–10.4 micromoles/L	Hyperhomocysteinemia resulting from dietary deficiencies is treated with folic acid, vitamin B_6, and vitamin B_{12} supplements.
B-type natriuretic peptide (BNP)	Peptide that causes natriuresis. Elevation indicates presence of heart failure and may help distinguish cardiac vs. respiratory cause of dyspnea. *Reference intervals:* Levels <100 ng/L are diagnostic for heart failure	Continue to monitor for signs and symptoms of heart failure.
N-terminal–pro B-type natriuretic peptide (NT–pro-BNP)	Aids in assessing the severity of heart failure in symptomatic and asymptomatic patients. In patients with renal insufficiency, concentrations may increase and may not correlate with New York Heart Association functional classification of heart failure. *Reference intervals:* ≤74 yr: 124 pg/mL >75 yr: 449 pg/mL	
Serum Lipids		
Cholesterol	A blood lipid. Elevated levels are considered a risk factor for atherosclerotic heart disease. *Reference interval:* <5 mmol/L (varies with age and gender)	Cholesterol levels can be measured in a nonfasting state.
Triglycerides	Mixtures of fatty acids. Elevations are associated with cardiovascular disease and diabetes. *Reference interval:* <1.7 mmol/L (varies with age and sex)	Triglyceride levels and lipoproteins must be measured in a fasting state (at least 12 hr, except for water); alcohol should be withheld for 24 hr before testing.

TABLE 34-6   DIAGNOSTIC STUDIES

Cardiovascular System—cont'd

Study	Description and Purpose	Nursing Responsibility
Lipoproteins† (HDL, LDL)	Soluble proteins that combine with and transport lipids in the plasma. Electrophoresis is performed to distinguish HDL from LDL. Serum lipid levels may fluctuate markedly from day to day. More than one determination is needed for accurate diagnosis and treatment. *Reference intervals* (vary with age): **HDL** • Recommended Male: >1.04 mmol/L Female: >1.3 mmol/L • Low risk for CAD: >1.55 mmol/L • High risk for CAD: <1.04 mmol/L **LDL** • Recommended: <2.59 mmol/L • Near optimal: 2.6–3.34 mmol/L • Moderate risk for CAD: 3.37–4.12 mmol/L • High risk for CAD: >4.14 mmol/L	After test is completed, risk for cardiac disease is assessed by dividing the total cholesterol level by the HDL level and obtaining a ratio. *Low risk:* Ratio <3 *Average risk:* Ratio 3–5 *Increased risk:* Ratio >5
Lipoprotein (a) (Lp[a])	Lipoprotein that contains one molecule of apolipoprotein B. Increased levels are associated with an increased risk of premature CAD and stroke. *Reference interval:* <0.3 g/L	Lp(a) levels can be obtained in a nonfasting state.
Lipoprotein-associated phospholipase A_2 (Lp-PLA_2)	Enzyme that catalyzes release of arachidonic acid. Elevated levels are associated with vascular inflammation and increased risk for CAD. Serum levels of Lp-PLA_2 are measured by the PLAC test. *Reference intervals:* *Low risk:* ≤151 nmol/min/mL *Moderate risk:* 152–194 nmol/min/mL *High risk:* ≥ 195 nmol/min/mL	Lp-PLA_2 levels can be obtained during a nonfasting state.
Chest Radiograph	X-ray imaging. Patient is placed in two upright positions to examine the lung fields and size of the heart. The two common positions are posteroanterior and lateral. Normal heart size and contour for the individual's age, sex, and size are noted.	The nurse should inquire about frequency of recent radiographic studies and possibility of pregnancy. Lead shielding is applied to areas not being viewed. Any jewellery or metal objects that may obstruct the view of the heart and lungs must be removed.
Electrocardiography (ECG)	Electronic graphing of cardiac activity. Electrodes are placed on the chest and extremities, allowing the ECG machine to record cardiac electrical activity from different views. This study can reveal rhythm of heart, activity of pacemaker, conduction abnormalities, position of heart, size of atria and ventricles, presence of injury, and history of MI.	The patient's skin is prepared, and electrodes and leads are applied. The nurse should inform patient that no discomfort is involved. Patient should be instructed to avoid moving, to decrease motion artifact.
Signal-averaged electrocardiography (SAECG)	High-resolution ECG that can identify electrical activity called *late potentials* that indicate a patient is at risk for developing ventricular dysrhythmias (e.g., ventricular tachycardia).	Same as for ECG.
Ambulatory ECG Monitoring		
Holter monitoring	Recording of ECG rhythm for 24–48 hr; rhythm changes are then correlated with symptoms recorded in patient's diary. Normal patient activity is encouraged to simulate conditions that produce symptoms. Electrodes are placed on chest, and a recorder is used to store information until it is recalled, printed, and analyzed for any rhythm disturbance. It can be performed on an inpatient or outpatient basis.	The patient's skin is prepared, and electrodes and leads are applied. The nurse should explain importance of keeping an accurate diary of activities and symptoms. The patient should take no bath or shower during monitoring. Electrodes may cause skin irritation.
Event monitor or loop recorder	Recording of rhythm disturbances that are not frequent enough to be recorded in one 24-hr period. It allows more freedom than does a regular Holter monitor. Some units have electrodes that are attached to the chest and have a loop of memory that captures the onset and end of an event. Other types are placed directly on patient's wrist, chest, or fingers and have no loop of memory but record the patient's ECG in real time. Recordings may be transmitted over the phone to a receiving unit.	The patient needs instruction in the use of equipment for recording and transmitting (if appropriate) of transient events. The nurse should teach patient about skin preparation for lead placement or steady skin contact for units not requiring electrodes. This will ensure the reception of optimal ECG tracings for analysis. The nurse should instruct patient to initiate recording as soon as symptoms begin or as soon thereafter as possible.

Continued

TABLE 34-6	**DIAGNOSTIC STUDIES**

Cardiovascular System—cont'd

Study	Description and Purpose	Nursing Responsibility
Exercise or stress testing	Study of the effect of exercise tolerance on cardiovascular function. Various protocols are used. A common protocol is to use 3-min stages at set speeds and with elevation of the treadmill belt. The patient can exercise to either predicted peak heart rate (calculated as the patient's age subtracted from 220) or to peak exercise tolerance, at which time the test is terminated. The test is also terminated for chest discomfort, significant increase or decrease in vital signs from baseline, or significant ECG changes indicating cardiac ischemia. Vital signs and ECG are monitored. The ECG is monitored after exercise for rhythm disturbances or, if ECG changes occurred with exercise, for return to baseline. Continual monitoring of vital signs and ECG rhythms for ischemic changes is important in the diagnosis of CAD. An exercise bike may be used if the patient is unable to walk on the treadmill.	The nurse should instruct patient (a) to wear comfortable clothes and shoes that can be used for walking and running and (b) about procedure and importance of reporting any symptoms that may occur. The nurse monitors vital signs and obtains 12-lead ECG before patient's exercise, during each stage of exercise, and after exercise until all vital signs and ECG changes have returned to normal. The nurse monitors patient's response throughout procedure. Contraindications include any reasons patient is unable to reach peak exercise. β-Adrenergic blockers may be withheld 24 hr before the test because they will blunt the heart rate and limit the patient's ability to achieve maximal heart rate. Caffeine-containing food and fluids are also withheld for 24 hr. Patients must refrain from smoking and strenuous exercise for 3 hr before test.
6-Minute walk test	Measurement of distance patient is able to walk on a flat surface in 6 min. Used to measure response to treatments and determine functional capacity for activities of daily living. Useful for patients who are unable to perform treadmill or exercise bike testing.	The nurse instructs patient to wear comfortable shoes and informs patient to carry or pull oxygen if it is used routinely. Patient should be encouraged to walk as quickly as possible.
Echocardiography • Contrast • M-mode • Two-dimensional • Colour-flow imaging (duplex) • Real-time three-dimensional	Ultrasound imaging of cardiac activity. Transducer that emits and receives ultrasound waves is placed in four positions on the chest above the heart. Transducer records sound waves that are bounced off the heart. Also records direction and flow of blood through the heart and transforms it to audio and graphic data that reflect valvular abnormalities, congenital cardiac defects, wall motion, ejection fraction, and cardiac function. IV contrast medium may be used to enhance images.	The patient is placed in a supine position on left side, facing equipment. The nurse instructs patient about procedure and expected sensations (pressure and mechanical movement from head of transducer). No contraindications to procedure exist.
Stress echocardiography	Combination of exercise testing and echocardiography. Resting images of the heart are taken with ultrasonography, and then the patient exercises. Postexercise images are taken immediately after exercise (within 1 min of stopping exercise). Differences in left ventricular wall motion and thickening before and after exercise are evaluated.	The nurse instructs and prepares patient for treadmill or exercise bicycle. The nurse also informs patient of importance of timely return to examination table for imaging after exercise. Contraindications include any reasons patient is unable to reach peak exercise.
Pharmacological echocardiography	Echocardiography with the use of pharmacological agent. Used as a substitute for the exercise stress test for patients unable to exercise. While echocardiography is performed, dobutamine or dipyridamole is infused intravenously, and dosage is increased in 5-min intervals to detect wall motion abnormalities at each stage.	The nurse starts IV infusion. Medication is administered per protocol. The nurse monitors vital signs before, during, and after test until baseline achieved. The nurse also monitors patient for signs and symptoms of distress during procedure. The patient is observed for adverse effects (e.g., shortness of breath, dizziness, nausea). Aminophylline may be given to prevent or reverse adverse effects of dipyridamole. Contraindications include any known allergies to medications.
Transesophageal echocardiography (TEE)	Echocardiography with an internal probe. A probe with an ultrasound transducer at the tip is swallowed while the physician controls angle and depth. As the probe passes down the esophagus, it sends back clear images of heart size, wall motion, valvular abnormalities, endocarditis vegetation, and possible source of thrombi without interference from lungs or chest ribs. Contrast medium may be injected intravenously for evaluating direction of blood flow if an atrial or ventricular septal defect is suspected. Doppler ultrasonography and colour-flow imaging can also be used concurrently.	The nurse instructs patient to avoid eating for at least 6 hr before test. Removable dentures are taken out of patient's mouth, and a bite block is placed in the mouth. IV sedative is administered, and local anaesthetic is applied to throat. The nurse monitors vital signs and oxygen saturation levels and performs suctioning as needed during procedure. The nurse also assists patient to relax. Patient may not eat or drink until gag reflex returns. Sore throat is temporary. A designated driver is needed for patient if test is done in outpatient department.
Nuclear cardiology	Radiological study with radioactive isotope (technetium-99m sestamibi). Isotope is injected intravenously. Radioactive uptake is counted over the heart by scintillation camera. Study supplies information about myocardial contractility, myocardial perfusion, and acute cell injury.	The nurse explains procedure to patient. IV line is established for injection of isotopes. The nurse must explain that radioactive isotope is used in a small, diagnostic amount and will lose most of its radioactivity in a few hours. Patient is informed that he or she will be lying still on back with arms extended overhead for 20 min. Repeat scans are performed within a few minutes to hours after the injection.

TABLE 34-6   DIAGNOSTIC STUDIES

Cardiovascular System—cont'd

Study	Description and Purpose	Nursing Responsibility
Multigated acquisition (MUGA) (cardiac blood pool) scan	Imaging with a radioactive isotope. A small amount of the patient's blood is removed, mixed with isotope (e.g., technetium-99m sestamibi with Cardiolite kit), and reinjected intravenously. The ECG is used for timing, and images are acquired during the cardiac cycle. Indicated for patients with MI, heart failure, or valvular heart disease. It also can be used to evaluate the effect of various cardiac or cardiotoxic medications on the heart.	Procedure is explained to patient. The nurse establishes IV line for removal of blood sample and reinjection of isotope and then establishes ECG monitoring. Patient is informed that procedure involves little risk.
Single-photon emission computed tomography (SPECT)	Computed tomography with radioactive isotope. Used to evaluate myocardium at risk of infarction and to determine infarction size. Small amounts of isotope (e.g., technetium-99m tetrofosmin [Myoview] or thallium-201) are injected intravenously, and recordings are made of the radioactivity emitted over a specific area of the body. Circulation of the isotope can be used to detect coronary artery blood flow, intracardiac shunts, motion of ventricles, ejection fraction, and size of the heart chambers.	The nurse explains procedure to patient, establishes IV line for injection of isotope, and establishes ECG monitoring. Patient must be informed that procedure involves little risk.
Exercise (stress) nuclear imaging	Nuclear imaging performed while patient is at rest and after exercise. The injection is given when patient reaches maximum heart rate on bicycle or treadmill. Patient is then required to continue exercise for 1 min to circulate the radioactive isotope. Scanning is done 15–60 min after exercise. A resting scan is performed 60–90 min after initial infusion or 24 hr later.	Explain procedure to patient. Instruct patient to eat only a light meal between scans. Certain medications may need to be held for 1–2 days before the scan.
Pharmacological nuclear imaging	Nuclear imaging performed with vasodilating drugs. Dipyridamole or adenosine is used to produce vasodilation when patients are unable to tolerate exercise. Vasodilation will increase blood flow to well-perfused coronary arteries. Scanning procedure is same as for exercise nuclear imaging. Aminophylline may be given to prevent or reverse adverse effects of dipyridamole (e.g., shortness of breath, dizziness, nausea). Dobutamine is used if vasodilators are contraindicated.	The nurse explains procedure to patient and instructs patient to avoid all caffeine products for 12 hr before procedure. Calcium channel blockers and β-adrenergic blockers should be avoided 24 hr before the test. The nurse observes patient for adverse effects (e.g., shortness of breath, dizziness, nausea).
Positron emission tomography (PET)	Tomographic imaging with two radionuclides. Highly sensitive in distinguishing viable and nonviable myocardial tissue. Nitrogen-13 ammonia is injected intravenously first, and scanning is performed to evaluate myocardial perfusion. A second radioactive isotope, fluorine-18 fludeoxyglucose, is then injected, and scanning is performed to show myocardial metabolic function. If the heart is normal, the two scans will match, but if the heart is ischemic or damaged, they will differ. The patient may undergo this test with or without conditions of stress. A baseline resting scan is usually obtained for comparison.	The nurse instructs patient on procedure, explaining that patient will be scanned by a machine and will need to stay still for a period of time. Patient's glucose level must be between 3.3 and 7.8 mcmol/L for accurate glucose metabolic activity. If exercise is included as part of testing, patient will need to fast and refrain from tobacco and caffeine for 24 hr before test.
Cardiovascular magnetic resonance imaging (CMRI)	Noninvasive imaging technique that obtains information about cardiac tissue integrity, aneurysms, ejection fractions, cardiac output, and patency of proximal coronary arteries. It does not involve ionizing radiation and is an extremely safe procedure. It provides images in multiple planes with uniformly good resolution.	The nurse explains procedure to patient, informing patient that the small diameter of the cylinder, along with loud noise of the procedure, may cause panic or anxiety. Antianxiety drugs and distraction strategies (e.g., music) may be recommended. Patient must lie still during MRI. Contraindicated for patients with implanted metallic devices or other metal fragments. The nurse must discern the presence of any implants before scan.
Magnetic resonance angiography (MRA)	Imaging of vascular occlusive disease and abdominal aortic aneurysms. Same as MRI but with use of gadolinium as IV contrast medium.	Contraindications include any known allergies to contrast medium and the presence of implanted metallic devices or other metal fragments.
Cardiac computed tomography (CT)	Heart-specific CT imaging technology with or without IV contrast media. It is used to visualize heart anatomy, coronary circulation, and blood vessels.	The nurse explains procedure to patient.
Computed tomographic angiography (CTA)	Use of CT with injected IV contrast medium to obtain images of blood vessels and diagnose CAD.	The nurse explains procedure to patient. Metal objects should be removed before examination. The patient may be asked not to eat or drink for several hours before the procedure.

Continued

TABLE 34-6   DIAGNOSTIC STUDIES

Cardiovascular System—cont'd

Study	Description and Purpose	Nursing Responsibility
Calcium-scoring CT scan • Electron beam computed tomography (EBCT)	Also known as *ultrafast CT;* a scanning electron beam is used to quantify calcification in coronary arteries and heart valves (see Figure 34-12). Used primarily for risk assessment in asymptomatic patients and to assess for heart disease in patients with atypical symptoms potentially resulting from cardiac causes.	The nurse explains procedure to patient and informs patient that procedure is quick and involves little or no risk.
Cardiac catheterization	Insertion of catheter into heart, via artery, to obtain information about O_2 levels and pressure readings within heart chambers. Contrast medium is injected to assist in examining structure and motion of heart.	The nurse checks patient for iodine sensitivity. Food and fluids are withheld for 6–18 hr before procedure. The nurse administers sedative and other drugs, if ordered, and informs patient about use of local anaesthesia, insertion of catheter, feeling of warmth when dye is injected, and possible fluttering sensation of heart as catheter is passed. Patient may be instructed to cough or take a deep breath when dye is injected and then is monitored by ECG throughout procedure. After procedure, the nurse assesses circulation to extremity used for catheter insertion. The nurse checks peripheral pulses, colour, and sensation of extremity every 15 min for 1 hr and then with decreasing frequency. The puncture site is observed for hematoma and bleeding. A compression device is placed over arterial site to achieve hemostasis, if indicated. The nurse monitors vital signs and ECG and assesses for hypotension or hypertension, abnormal heart rate, dysrhythmias, and signs of pulmonary emboli (e.g., respiratory difficulty).
Coronary angiography	Imaging during a cardiac catheterization in which contrast medium is injected directly into coronary arteries. Used to evaluate patency of coronary arteries and collateral circulation.	Same as for cardiac catheterization.
Noninvasive coronary computed tomographic angiography (CCTA)	A noninvasive imaging modality that can be used to evaluate the anatomy of the coronary arteries. Unlike coronary artery calcium scoring, in which noncontrast CT is used to assess atherosclerotic disease burden, CCTA allows direct visualization of the coronary artery wall and lumen with the administration of IV contrast medium.	Same as for cardiac catheterization.
Intracoronary ultrasonography	Ultrasound imaging in which a small ultrasound probe is introduced into coronary arteries during cardiac catheterization. Data are used to assess size and consistency of plaque, arterial walls, and effectiveness of intracoronary artery treatment.	Same as for cardiac catheterization.
Fractional flow reserve	Measurement of blood pressure and flow. During cardiac catheterization, a special wire is inserted into the coronary arteries to gather these measurements. Information is used to determine need for angioplasty or stent placement on nonsignificant blockages.	Same as for cardiac catheterization.
Electrophysiology study (EPS)	Invasive study used to record intracardiac electrical activity. Catheters (with multiple electrodes) are inserted via the femoral and jugular veins into the right side of the heart. The catheter electrodes record the electrical activity in different cardiac structures. In addition, dysrhythmias can be induced and terminated.	Antidysrhythmic medications may be discontinued several days before study. Patient should be on NPO status 6–8 hr before test. The nurse administers premedication to promote relaxation, if ordered. IV sedative is often used during procedure. Patient must have frequent monitoring of vital signs and continuous ECG monitoring after the procedure.
Peripheral arteriography and venography‡	Radiographic study involving injection of radiopaque contrast medium into either arteries or veins. Serial radiographs are taken to detect and visualize any atherosclerotic plaques, occlusion, aneurysms, or traumatic injury.	The nurse checks for iodine allergy and administers mild sedative, if ordered. The nurse checks extremity with puncture site for pulsation, warmth, colour, and motion after procedure. Insertion site is inspected for bleeding or swelling. The nurse observes patient for allergic reactions to dye.
Hemodynamic monitoring	Hemodynamic monitoring of arterial blood pressures, pulmonary artery pressure, pulmonary artery wedge pressure, and cardiac output to evaluate cardiovascular status and response to treatment.	Patients requiring hemodynamic monitoring are critically ill and are monitored in critical care units. See Chapter 68 for complete information on hemodynamic monitoring.

*Reference ranges for the laboratory tests vary by institution because of differences in equipment and reagents used.
†Source: American Heart Association. (2011). *What your cholesterol levels mean.* Retrieved from *http://www.heart.org/HEARTORG/Conditions/What-Your-Cholesterol-Levels-Mean_UCM_305562_Article.jsp*
‡Additional peripheral vascular diagnostic studies are found in Table 40-9.
CAD, coronary artery disease; *CK,* creatine kinase; *CK-MB,* MB isoenzyme of creatine kinase; *CT,* computed tomography; *ECGs,* electrocardiograms; *HDL,* high-density lipoprotein; *IV,* intravenous; *LDLs,* low-density lipoproteins; *MI,* myocardial infarction; *NPO,* nothing by mouth; *O₂,* oxygen.

and sleep and this record is correlated with the ECG events recorded by the device (see Table 34-6).

Transtelephonic Event Recorders. This type of recorder is helpful for monitoring less frequent ECG events. The monitor is a portable unit with which electrodes are used to transmit a limited ECG over the phone to a receiving device. A disadvantage of this type of monitoring is that if the event is of short duration, the symptoms may end before the patient puts on the device and calls the assigned number. Likewise, if patients are extremely symptomatic (e.g., syncopal), they may not be physically able to transmit the ECG.

Exercise or Stress Testing. Cardiac symptoms frequently occur only with activity because of the demand on the coronary arteries to provide more oxygen. Exercise testing is used to evaluate the heart's response to physical stress. This helps to assess cardiovascular disease and set limits for exercise programs. Exercise testing is used for individuals who do not have restrictions related to walking or using a bicycle. It is also helpful for patients with normal ECGs that limit diagnostic interpretation (e.g., those with pacemakers; see Table 34-6).

Echocardiography. In echocardiography, ultrasound waves are used to record the movement of the structures of the heart. In the normal heart, ultrasonic sound waves directed at the heart are reflected back in typical configurations. The echocardiogram provides information about abnormalities of (a) valvular structure and motion, (b) cardiac chamber size and contents, (c) ventricular muscle and septal motion and thickness, (d) the pericardial sac, and (e) the ascending aorta. The **ejection fraction**, or the percentage of end-diastolic blood volume that is ejected during systole, can also be measured. The ejection fraction provides information about the function of the left ventricle during systole.

Two commonly used types are M-mode (motion mode) and two-dimensional echocardiography. In the M-mode type, a single ultrasound beam is directed toward the heart, and the motion of the intracardiac structures is recorded, as are wall thickness and chamber size. In two-dimensional echocardiography, the ultrasound beam sweeps through an arc, producing a cross-sectional view, and shows correct spatial relationships among the structures.

Doppler technology allows for sound evaluation of the flow or motion of the scanned object (heart valves, ventricular walls, blood flow). Colour-flow (duplex) imaging is the combination of two-dimensional echocardiography and Doppler technology (Figure 34-10). Colour changes demonstrate the velocity and direction of blood flow. Pathological conditions, such as valvular leaks and congenital defects, can be diagnosed more effectively. Stress echocardiography, a combination of treadmill test and ultrasound images, is used to evaluate segmental wall motion abnormalities (Pagana, Pagana, & Pagana, 2014). A digital computer system is used to compare images before and after exercise, and wall motion and segmental function can be clearly seen. This diagnostic test provides the information of an exercise stress test combined with that obtained from an

FIGURE 34-10 Long-axis images of the aortic and mitral valve with the depth adjusted to optimize evaluation of valve anatomy and motion. The two-dimensional images *(left)* in diastole *(top)* and systole *(bottom)* show normal aortic and mitral opening and closure. The colour flow images *(right)* show normal left ventricular inflow with no aortic regurgitation in diastole *(top)* and normal antegrade flow in the left ventricular outflow tract and no mitral regurgitation in systole *(bottom)*. Source: From Otto, C. (2004). *Textbook of clinical echocardiography* (3rd ed.). St. Louis: Saunders.

echocardiogram. For patients unable to exercise, infusion of a pharmacological agent—usually dobutamine (Dobutrex) or dipyridamole (Persantine)—induces stress on the heart while the patient is resting. The same ultrasound technology is used.

In comparison with surface two-dimensional echocardiography, transesophageal echocardiography (TEE) is used to provide more precise images of the heart by eliminating interference from the chest wall and the lungs. TEE involves the use of a modified, flexible endoscope probe with an ultrasound transducer in the tip for imaging of the heart and great vessels. The probe is introduced into the esophagus to the level of the heart, and M-mode, two-dimensional, pulsed Doppler, and colour-flow images can be obtained.

TEE is used frequently in an outpatient setting primarily for evaluation of mitral regurgitation, of the presence of thrombus before cardioversion is performed, or of the source of cardiac emboli. In addition, TEE has applications in the operating room to assess presurgical and postsurgical cardiac function and in the emergency department for suspicion of aortic dissection.

The risks with TEE are minimal. However, complications may include perforation of the esophagus, hemorrhage, dysrhythmias, vasovagal reactions, and transient hypoxemia. TEE is contra-indicated if the patient has a history of esophageal disorders, dysphagia, or radiation therapy involving the chest wall. Patients must be sedated during TEE.

In contrast echocardiography, intravenous contrast agents (e.g., albumin microbubbles, agitated saline) are used to assist in delineation of the images, especially in cases of technical difficulties (Pagana, Pagana, & Pagana, 2014). When these agents are injected into the cardiac blood pool, they greatly enhance reflectivity for the ultrasound procedure.

Nuclear Cardiology. One of the most common nuclear imaging tests is the multigated acquisition (MUGA), or cardiac blood pool, scanning. This test provides information on wall motion during systole and diastole, cardiac valves, and ejection fraction (see Table 34-6).

Perfusion imaging is also used with exercise testing to determine whether the coronary blood flow changes with increased activity. Stress perfusion imaging may show an abnormality even when a resting image is normal. This procedure is used to diagnose CAD, establish a prognosis for patients with existing CAD, differentiate viable myocardium from scar tissue, and determine the potential for success of various interventions, such as coronary artery bypass surgery and percutaneous coronary intervention (Zaret & Beller, 2010; see Chapter 36).

Exercise stress perfusion imaging is always preferred but, if a patient cannot exercise, intravenous dipyridamole or adenosine (Adenocard) can be administered to dilate the coronary arteries and simulate the effect of exercise. After the drug takes effect, the isotope is injected and the imaging is performed.

Cardiovascular Magnetic Resonance Imaging. Cardiovascular magnetic resonance imaging (CMRI) can reveal areas of MI in a three-dimensional view. It is sensitive enough to find even small MIs that are not apparent with single-photon emission computed tomography imaging. CMRI aids in the final diagnosis of MI and the assessment of ejection fraction. It also plays a role in prediction of recovery from MI and in the diagnosis of congenital heart and aortic disorders and CAD (Hundley, Bluemke, & Finn, 2010).

One major advantage of CMRI is that it does not require any irradiation of the patient. In general, the use of CMRI in patients with pacemakers and ICDs is discouraged because the magnets can alter the function of the devices. When clinical need is strong and the benefits outweigh the risks, CMRI should be performed only at experienced centres (Hundley, Bluemke, & Finn, 2010). Some newer models of these devices are approved for use with MRI.

Cardiac Computed Tomography. Cardiac computed tomography (CT) is a heart-imaging test in which CT technology, with or without intravenous contrast medium (dye), is used to see the heart anatomy, coronary circulation, and great blood vessels (e.g., aorta, pulmonary veins, artery). This technology is often called *multidetector CT scanning*. Types of CT scans used to diagnosis heart disease include coronary CT angiography (CTA) and calcium-scoring CT scan (see Table 34-6).

Coronary CTA is a noninvasive test. It can be performed faster than cardiac catheterization with less risk and discomfort to the patient (Mark, Berman, & Budoff, 2010). Although the use of coronary CTA is increasing, cardiac catheterization (discussed in the next section) remains the gold standard for diagnosing coronary artery stenosis. Furthermore, when a cardiac catheterization is done, interventions (e.g., angioplasty, stent placement) can be performed if coronary blockages are found.

The calcium-scoring CT scan is used to find calcium deposits in plaque in the coronary arteries. The most common method used is electron beam CT (Figure 34-11). It can detect early coronary calcification before symptoms develop. The amount of coronary calcium is a predictor of future cardiac events.

Blood Studies. Many blood studies provide information about the cardiovascular system. For example, some reflect the O_2-carrying capacity (red blood cell count and hemoglobin) and coagulation properties (clotting times) of the blood. (See Chapter 32 and Tables 32-7 and 32-8 for hematology studies.) The studies most commonly used to assess the cardiovascular system are listed in Table 34-6.

Cardiac Biomarkers. When cells are injured, they release their contents, including enzymes and other proteins, into the circulation. These *biomarkers* are useful in the diagnosis of myocardial injury and infarction.

Cardiac-specific troponin is a myocardial muscle protein released into circulation after injury or infarction. Two subtypes,

FIGURE 34-11 Examples of coronary calcification of the left anterior descending coronary artery *(large arrow)* and left circumflex artery *(small arrow)* as seen on electron beam computed tomography. Source: From Libby, P., Bonow, R., Zipes, D., et al. (Eds.). (2008). *Braunwald's heart disease: A textbook of cardiovascular medicine* (8th ed.). St. Louis: Saunders.

cardiac-specific troponin T (cTnT) and cardiac-specific troponin I (cTnI), are specific to myocardial tissue. Normally the level in the blood is very low, and so a rise in level is diagnostic of myocardial injury. Rising levels of cTnT and cTnI are detectable within hours (on average 4 to 6 hours) of myocardial injury; these levels peak at 10 to 24 hours and can be detected for up to 10 to 14 days (see Figure 36-11). Troponin is the biomarker of choice in the diagnosis of MI. The development of high-sensitivity troponin (hs-cTnT, hs-cTnI) assays may provide even earlier detection of a cardiac event (Lee, Browne, Guest, et al., 2016).

Creatine kinase (CK) enzymes are found in a variety of organs and tissues and occur as three isozymes. These isozymes are specific to skeletal muscle (CK-MM), brain and nervous tissue (CK-BB), and the heart (CK-MB). CK-MB elevation is specific for myocardial injury or infarction. CK-MB levels begin to rise 3 to 6 hours after symptom onset, peak in 12 to 24 hours, and return to baseline within 12 to 48 hours after MI (Pagana, Pagana, & Pagana, 2014). The peak level and return to normal can be delayed in cases of large MI. Levels drop more rapidly in patients who are quickly and successfully treated for an MI. (Figure 36-11 depicts the changes in cardiac markers related to an MI.)

Myoglobin is a low-molecular-weight heme protein found in cardiac and skeletal muscle. Elevation in myoglobin levels is a sensitive indicator of very early myocardial injury but lacks specificity for MI. Its usefulness in diagnosing MI is limited (Pagana and Pagana, 2014).

To interpret diagnostic test results correctly, the time of onset of symptoms and the time of the expected presence and elevation of the biomarkers must be considered. Additional data (patient symptoms, history, and ECG changes) complete the diagnostic picture for the patient with suspected myocardial injury or MI.

C-Reactive Protein. C-reactive protein (CRP) is a protein produced by the liver during periods of acute inflammation. CRP can be measured with a high-sensitivity test (hs-CRP). An increased level of CRP is an independent risk factor for CAD. The level of CRP may also be predictive of the risk for future cardiac events in patients with unstable angina and MI, but studies have produced conflicting results.

Homocysteine. Homocysteine is an amino acid that is produced during protein catabolism. Elevated homocysteine levels can be either hereditary or acquired from dietary deficiencies of vitamin B_6, vitamin B_{12}, or folate. Elevated levels of homocysteine have been linked to a higher risk of CAD, peripheral vascular disease, and stroke. It is recommended that homocysteine testing be performed in patients with a familial predisposition for early cardiovascular disease or a history of cardiovascular disease in the absence of other common risk factors (American Heart Association, 2012).

Cardiac Natriuretic Peptide Markers. There are three natriuretic peptides: (a) atrial natriuretic peptide (ANP) from the atrium, (b) b-type natriuretic peptide (BNP) from the ventricles, and (c) c-type natriuretic peptide from endothelial and renal epithelial cells. BNP is the marker of choice for distinguishing a cardiac or respiratory cause of dyspnea. N-terminal pro–b-type natriuretic peptide (NT–pro-BNP) is also secreted in the ventricles and is more sensitive but less specific than BNP as a diagnostic marker of heart failure (Pagana, Pagana, & Pagana, 2014). When diastolic blood pressure increases (e.g., heart failure), BNP and NT–pro-BNP are released and increase natriuresis (excretion of sodium in the urine). (ANP and BNP are also discussed in Chapter 37.)

Serum Lipids. Serum lipids consist of triglycerides, cholesterol, and phospholipids. They circulate in the blood bound to protein. Thus they are often referred to as *lipoproteins*.

Triglycerides are the main storage form of lipids and make up about 95% of fatty tissue. Cholesterol, a structural component of cell membranes and plasma lipoproteins, is a precursor of corticosteroids, sex hormones, and bile salts. In addition to being absorbed from food in the gastro-intestinal tract, cholesterol can also be synthesized in the liver. Phospholipids contain glycerol, fatty acids, phosphates, and a nitrogenous compound. Although formed in most cells, phospholipids usually enter the circulation as lipoproteins synthesized by the liver. Apoproteins are water-soluble proteins that combine with most lipids to form lipoproteins.

Different classes of lipoproteins contain varying amounts of the naturally occurring lipids. These include the following:
1. *Chylomicrons:* primarily exogenous triglycerides from dietary fat
2. *Low-density lipoproteins (LDLs):* mostly cholesterol with moderate amounts of phospholipids
3. *High-density lipoproteins (HDLs):* approximately 50% protein and 50% phospholipids and cholesterol
4. *Very-low-density lipoproteins (VLDLs):* primarily endogenous triglycerides with moderate amounts of phospholipids and cholesterol

A lipid panel usually includes measurements of cholesterol, triglyceride, LDL, and HDL. Elevations in triglyceride and LDL levels are strongly associated with CAD. An increased HDL level is associated with a decreased risk of CAD (Huether & McCance, 2012). High levels of HDLs serve a protective role by mobilizing cholesterol from tissues.

Although an association exists between elevated serum cholesterol levels and CAD, a measure of total cholesterol alone is not sufficient for an assessment of CAD. To calculate a risk assessment, the ratios of total cholesterol to HDL ratio are compared over time. An increase in the ratio indicates increased risk. This provides more information than either value alone. The patient must fast before blood is drawn for a lipid panel so that food intake does not affect the results.

Plasma levels of apolipoprotein A-I (the major HDL protein) and the ratio of apolipoprotein A-I to apolipoprotein B (the major LDL protein) are stronger predictors of CAD than is the HDL cholesterol level alone. Measurements of these lipoproteins can be useful in identifying patients at risk for CAD (Pagana, Pagana, & Pagana, 2014).

Lipoprotein (a) has been studied for its role as a risk factor for CAD. Increased levels of lipoprotein (a), especially with increased levels of lactate dehydrogenase, have been linked with the progression of atherosclerosis, especially in women (Huether & McCance, 2012).

Lipoprotein-Associated Phospholipase A₂. Lipoprotein-associated phospholipase A_2 (Lp-PLA$_2$) is an inflammatory enzyme expressed in atherosclerotic plaques. Elevated levels of Lp-PLA$_2$ are related to an increased risk of CAD (Lp-PLA$_2$ Studies Collaboration, 2010).

Invasive Studies

Invasive studies are performed if definitive information is required. These studies include cardiac catheterization, coronary angiography, electrophysiology (see Table 34-6), intracoronary ultrasonography, and hemodynamic monitoring.

Cardiac Catheterization and Coronary Angiography. Cardiac catheterization is a common outpatient procedure. It provides information about CAD, coronary spasm, congenital and valvular heart disease, and ventricular function. Cardiac catheterization is also used to measure intracardiac pressures and O_2 levels, as well as CO and ejection fraction. With injection of contrast media and fluoroscopy, the coronary arteries can be seen, chambers of the heart can be outlined, and wall motion can be observed.

In cardiac catheterization, a radiopaque catheter is inserted into the right or left side of the heart, or both sides. For the right side of the heart, a catheter is inserted through an arm vein (basilic or cephalic) or a leg vein (femoral). Pressures are recorded as the catheter is moved into the vena cava, the right atrium, the right ventricle, and the pulmonary artery. The catheter is then moved until it is wedged or lodged in position. This blocks the blood flow and pressure from the right side of the heart and looks ahead through the pulmonary capillary bed to the pressure in the left side of the heart *(pulmonary artery wedge pressure)*. This pressure is used to assess the function of the left side of the heart.

In left-sided cardiac catheterization, a catheter is inserted into a femoral, brachial, or radial artery. The catheter is passed in a retrograde manner up to the aorta, across the aortic valve, and into the left ventricle.

Coronary angiography is performed with a left-sided heart catheterization. The catheter is positioned at the origin of the coronary arteries (see Figure 34-3), and contrast medium is injected into the arteries. Patients often feel a temporary flushed sensation with dye injection. The images identify the location and severity of any coronary blockages (Figure 34-12; see also Figure 36-7). Complications of cardiac catheterization include bleeding or hematoma at the puncture site; allergic reactions to the contrast media; looping or kinking of the catheter; infection; thrombus formation; aortic dissection; dysrhythmias; MI; stroke; and puncture of the ventricles, cardiac septum, or lung tissue.

Intracoronary Ultrasonography. Intracoronary ultrasonography (ICUS), also known as *intravascular ultrasonography* (IVUS), is an invasive procedure performed in the catheterization laboratory with coronary angiography. The two- or three-dimensional ultrasound images provide a cross-sectional view of the arterial walls of the coronary arteries. In this procedure, a miniature transducer attached to a small catheter is moved to the artery to be studied. Once it is in the artery, ultrasound images are obtained. The health of the arterial layers is assessed, including the composition, location, and thickness of any plaque. ICUS can help evaluate vessel response to treatments such as stent placement and atherectomy, as well as any complications that may have occurred during the procedure. Patients most often undergo ICUS in addition to angiography or a coronary intervention. Thus nursing care is similar to that after cardiac catheterization (see Table 34-6).

Fractional Flow Reserve. Fractional flow reserve is a procedure that is performed during a cardiac catheterization. It involves using a special wire that can measure pressure and flow in the coronary artery. Fractional flow reserve helps to determine the need to perform angioplasty or stent placement on nonsignificant blockages.

Hemodynamic Monitoring. Bedside hemodynamic monitoring of pressures of the cardiovascular system is frequently used to assess cardiovascular status. Invasive hemodynamic monitoring with the use of intra-arterial and pulmonary artery catheters can be performed to monitor arterial blood pressure, intracardiac pressures, and CO (see Chapter 68). The central venous pressure (CVP) is a measurement of preload and can be used to monitor the pressure in the right atrium and right ventricle. The CVP reading is influenced by the function of the left side of the heart, pressures in the pulmonary vessels, venous return to the heart, and the position of the patient when the reading is taken. The last factor must be kept in mind to obtain an accurate reading. The CVP can be used as a guide in fluid volume management of overhydration or dehydration.

CVP can be measured with a pulmonary artery catheter (see Chapter 68) or a central venous line threaded through the jugular or the subclavian vein into the superior vena cava. The normal CVP is 2 to 9 mm Hg.

FIGURE 34-12 Normal left coronary artery angiogram. Source: From Drake, R. L., Vogl, A. W., & Mitchell, A. W. M. (2010) *Gray's anatomy for students* (2nd ed.). Philadelphia: Churchill Livingstone.

CASE STUDY

Objective Data: Diagnostic Studies

The health care provider orders the following initial diagnostic studies for Lawrence Tan:

- 12-lead ECG
- Complete blood cell count, basic metabolic panel (glucose, electrolytes, blood urea nitrogen, creatinine)
- Partial thromboplastin time, prothrombin time, international normalized ratio
- Pro-BNP measurement
- Troponin, CK-MB measurement
- Thyroid-stimulating hormone, free thyroxine
- Chest radiograph

Source: ESB Professional/ Shutterstock .com.

Mr. Tan's initial troponin and CK-MB levels are within normal limits. The ECG demonstrates atrial fibrillation with a rapid ventricular response. Results of the chest radiograph, complete blood cell count, basic metabolic panel, pro-BNP measurement, and coagulation studies are all within normal limits. The health care provider orders intravenous diltiazem (Cardizem) and heparin to be started in the emergency department. Mr. Tan will be admitted to the progressive care unit and will have a consult with a cardiologist.
See pp. 772 and 777 for more information on Mr. Tan.

REVIEW QUESTIONS

The number of the question corresponds to the same-numbered objective at the beginning of the chapter.

1. A patient has a tricuspid valve disorder. Between which of the following will the blood flow be impaired?
   a. Vena cava and right atrium
   b. Left atrium and left ventricle
   c. Right atrium and right ventricle
   d. Right ventricle and pulmonary artery

2. A patient has a severe blockage in his right coronary artery. Which cardiac structures are most likely to be affected by this blockage? *(Select all that apply)*
   a. Atrioventricular node
   b. Left ventricle
   c. Coronary sinus
   d. Right ventricle
   e. Pulmonic valve

3. Where is the conduction impairment when the Purkinje system is damaged?
   a. Atria
   b. Atrioventricular node
   c. Ventricles
   d. Bundle of His

4. Why does prolonged pressure on the skin cause areas at the point of contact to redden?
   a. Arterial vasodilation from smooth muscle relaxation
   b. Compression of veins, which results in venous engorgement
   c. Occlusion of major arteries causing infarction of the tissue
   d. Tissue damage and inflammation resulting from impaired capillary blood flow

5. When a person's blood pressure rises, which compensatory homeostatic mechanism is stimulated?
   a. Chemoreceptors that inhibit the sympathetic nervous system, causing vasodilation
   b. Baroreceptors that inhibit the parasympathetic nervous system, causing vasodilation
   c. Baroreceptors that inhibit the sympathetic nervous system, causing a decrease in heart rate
   d. Chemoreceptors that stimulate the sympathetic nervous system, causing an increase in heart rate

6. If a patient's capillary refill assessment shows that the colour returns in 10 seconds, what does this indicate?
   a. A normal response
   b. Thrombus formation in the veins
   c. Lymphatic obstruction of venous return
   d. Impaired arterial flow to the extremities

7. Which auscultatory area is found at the left midclavicular line at the level of the fifth intercostal space?
   a. Aortic area
   b. Mitral area
   c. Tricuspid area
   d. Pulmonic area

8. When a palpable precordial thrill is found upon assessment, what could this indicate?
   a. Heart murmurs
   b. Gallop rhythms
   c. Pulmonary edema
   d. Right ventricular hypertrophy

9. Which of the following may be found on assessment of a 79-year-old patient?
   a. A narrowed pulse pressure
   b. Diminished carotid artery pulses
   c. Difficulty in isolating the apical pulse
   d. An increased heart rate in response to stress

10. Which of the following is an important nursing responsibility for a patient undergoing an invasive cardiovascular diagnostic study?
    a. Checking the peripheral pulses and percutaneous insertion site
    b. Instructing the patient about radioactive isotope injection
    c. Informing the patient that general anaesthesia will be given
    d. Assisting the patient to do a surgical scrub of the insertion site

11. Which of the following statements best describe the P-wave impulse?
    a. Arising at the sinoatrial node and repolarizing the atria
    b. Arising at the sinoatrial node and depolarizing the atria
    c. Arising at the atrioventricular node and depolarizing the atria
    d. Arising at the atrioventricular node and spreading to the bundle of His

1. c; 2. a, b, d; 3. c; 4. d; 5. c; 6. d; 7. b; 8. a; 9. c; 10. a; 11. b.

evolve

For even more review questions, visit *http://evolve.elsevier.com/Canada/Lewis/medsurg.*

REFERENCES

Aehlert, B. (2013). *ECGs made easy* (5th ed.). St. Louis: Mosby.

American College of Cardiology Foundation Task Force on Expert Consensus Documents, Mark, D., Berman, D., et al. (2010). ACCF/ACR/AHA/NASCI/SAIP/SCAI/SCCT 2010 Expert consensus document on coronary computed tomographic angiography: A report of the American College of Cardiology Foundation Task Force on Expert Consensus Documents. *Circulation, 121,* 2509–2543.

American Heart Association. (2012). *Homocysteine, folic acid and cardiovascular disease.* Retrieved from *http://www.heart.org/ HEARTORG/GettingHealthy/NutritionCenter/Homocysteine-Folic -Acid-and-Cardiovascular-Disease_UCM_305997_Article.jsp.*

Huether, S., & McCance, K. (2012). *Understanding pathophysiology* (5th ed.). St. Louis: Mosby.

Hundley, G., Bluemke, D., & Finn, J. (2010). ACCF/ACR/AHA/ NASCI/SCMR 2010 Expert consensus document on cardiovascular magnetic resonance: A report of the American College of Cardiology Foundation Task Force on Expert Consensus Documents. *Circulation, 121,* 2462–2508.

Jarvis, C., Browne, A., MacDonald-Jenkins, J., et al. (2014). *Physical examination and health assessment* (2nd ed.). Toronto: Elsevier.

Lee, G. R., Browne, T., Guest, B., et al. (2016). Transitioning high sensitivity cardiac troponin I (hs-cTnI) into routine diagnostic use: More than just a sensitivity issue. *Pracitcal Laboratory Medicine, 4,* 62–75. doi:10.1016/j.plabm.2016.01.001.

Lp-PLA$_2$ Studies Collaboration. (2010). Lipoprotein-associated phospholipase A$_2$ and risk of coronary disease, stroke, and mortality: Collaborative analysis of 32 prospective studies. *Lancet, 375,* 1536–1544. (Seminal).

North, B. J., & Sinclair, D. A. (2012). The intersection between aging and cardiovascular disease. *Circulation Research, 110*(8), 1097–1108.

Pagana, K., Pagana, T., & Pagana, T. (2014). *Mosby's diagnostic and laboratory test reference* (12th ed.). St. Louis: Elsevier.

Pagana, K. D., & Pagana, T. J. (2014). *Mosby's manual of diagnostic and laboratory tests* (5th ed.). St. Louis: Elsevier.

Patton, K. T., & Thibodeau, G. A. (2016). *Anatomy & physiology* (9th ed.). St. Louis: Elsevier.

Zaret, B., & Beller, G. (2010). *Clinical nuclear cardiology* (4th ed.). St. Louis: Mosby.

RESOURCES

Resources for this chapter are listed in Chapter 36.

Nursing Management
Hypertension

Written by: Melissa L. Hutchinson
Adapted by: Kara Sealock

ℯvolve WEBSITE

http://evolve.elsevier.com/Canada/Lewis/medsurg

- Review Questions (Online Only)
- Key Points
- Answer Guidelines for Case Study

- Conceptual Care Map Creator
- Audio Glossary
- Content Updates

LEARNING OBJECTIVES

1. Relate the pathophysiological mechanisms associated with primary hypertension to the clinical manifestations and complications.
2. Select appropriate strategies for the prevention of primary hypertension.
3. Describe the collaborative care for primary hypertension, including drug therapy and lifestyle modifications.

4. Explain the collaborative care of the older adult with primary hypertension.
5. Prioritize the nursing management of the patient with primary hypertension.
6. Describe the collaborative care of a patient with hypertensive crisis.

KEY TERMS

baroreceptors, p. 790
blood pressure (BP), p. 789
cardiac output (CO), p. 789
hypertension, p. 791

hypertensive crisis,
   p. 809
isolated systolic hypertension
   (ISH), p. 792

orthostatic hypotension,
   p. 806
primary (essential)
   hypertension, p. 793

secondary hypertension,
   p. 793
systemic vascular resistance
   (SVR), p. 789

Hypertension, or high blood pressure (BP), is one of the most important modifiable risk factors that can lead to the development of cardiovascular disease (CVD). As BP increases, so does the risk for myocardial infarction (MI), heart failure, stroke, and renal disease. This chapter discusses the nursing and interprofessional care of patients who are at risk for or who have hypertension.

NORMAL REGULATION OF BLOOD PRESSURE

Blood pressure (BP) is the force exerted by the blood against the walls of the blood vessel and must be adequate for tissue perfusion to be maintained during activity and rest. The maintenance of normal BP and tissue perfusion requires the integration of both systemic factors and local peripheral vascular effects. Arterial BP is primarily a function of cardiac output (CO) and systemic vascular resistance (SVR). The relationship between the two is summarized by the following equation: Arterial blood pressure = cardiac output multiplied by systemic vascular resistance (arterial BP = CO × SVR).

Cardiac output (CO) is the volume of blood ejected from the heart per minute. CO can be described as the stroke volume (SV, or the amount of blood pumped out of the left ventricle per beat [~70 mL]) multiplied by the heart rate (HR) for 1 minute. **Systemic vascular resistance (SVR)** is the force opposing the movement of blood within the blood vessels. The radius of the small arteries and arterioles is the principal factor determining vascular resistance. A small change in the radius of the arterioles creates a major change in the SVR. If SVR is increased and CO remains constant or increases, arterial BP will increase.

The mechanisms that regulate BP can affect either CO or SVR, or both. Regulation of BP is a complex process involving nervous, cardiovascular, renal, and endocrine functions (Figure 35-1). BP is regulated by both short-term (over seconds to hours) and long-term (over days to weeks) mechanisms. Short-term mechanisms, including the effects exerted by the sympathetic nervous system (SNS) and the vascular endothelium, are active within a few seconds. Long-term mechanisms include renal and hormonal processes that regulate arteriolar resistance and blood volume.

FIGURE 35-1 Factors influencing blood pressure (BP). Hypertension develops when one or more of the BP-regulating mechanisms are defective.

Sympathetic Nervous System

The nervous system, which reacts within seconds after a decrease in arterial pressure, increases BP primarily by activation of the SNS. Increased SNS activity increases HR and cardiac contractility, produces widespread vasoconstriction in the peripheral arterioles, and promotes the release of renin from the kidneys. The net effect of SNS activation is to increase arterial pressure by increasing both CO and SVR.

Changes in BP are sensed by specialized nerve cells called *baroreceptors* and transmitted to the vasomotor centres in the brain stem. Information received in the brain stem is relayed throughout the brain by complex networks of interneurons that excite or inhibit efferent nerves, thereby influencing cardiovascular function. Sympathetic efferent nerves innervate cardiac and vascular smooth muscle cells. Under normal conditions, a low level of continuous sympathetic activity maintains tonic vasoconstriction. BP may be reduced by withdrawal of SNS activity or by stimulation of the parasympathetic nervous system, which decreases the HR (via the vagus nerve) and thereby decreases CO.

The neurotransmitter norepinephrine (NE) is released from sympathetic nerve endings. NE activates receptors located in the sinoatrial node, the myocardium, and vascular smooth muscle. The response to NE depends on the type and the density of receptors present. SNS receptors are classified as α_1, α_2, β_1, and β_2 (Table 35-1). α-Adrenergic receptors located in peripheral vasculature cause vasoconstriction when stimulated by NE. β_1-Adrenergic receptors in the heart respond to NE with increased HR (chronotropic effect), increased force of contraction (inotropic effect), and increased speed of conduction (dromotropic effect). Diminished responsiveness of cardiovascular cells to sympathetic stimulation is one of the most significant cardiovascular effects of aging. The smooth muscle of the blood vessels has β_1-adrenergic and β_2-adrenergic receptors. β_2-Adrenergic receptors are activated primarily by epinephrine released from the adrenal medulla and cause vasodilation.

The sympathetic vasomotor centre, located in the medulla, interacts with many areas of the brain to maintain normal BP under various conditions. During exercise, the motor area of the cortex is stimulated, activating the vasomotor centre and the SNS through neuronal connections. This causes an appropriate increase in BP to accommodate the increased oxygen demand of the exercising muscles. During postural change from lying to standing, there is a transient decrease in BP. The vasomotor centre is stimulated and activates the SNS, causing peripheral vasoconstriction and increased venous return to the heart. If this response did not occur, there would be inadequate blood flow to the brain, resulting in dizziness. Cerebral cortical perceptions such as pain and stress activate the vasomotor centres through the neuronal connections.

Baroreceptors. Baroreceptors (pressoreceptors) are specialized nerve cells located in the carotid sinus at the bifurcation of the external and internal carotid arteries and the arch of the aorta. They are sensitive to stretching and, when stimulated by an increase in BP, send inhibitory impulses to the sympathetic vasomotor centre in the brain stem. Inhibition of sympathetic activity results in decreased HR, decreased force of contraction, and vasodilation in peripheral arterioles. Increased parasympathetic activity (vagus nerve) also reduces HR.

A fall in BP, sensed by the baroreceptors, leads to activation of the SNS. The result is constriction of the peripheral arterioles, increased HR, and increased contractility of the heart. The baroreceptors have an important role in the maintenance of BP stability during normal activities. In the presence of longstanding hypertension, the baroreceptors become adjusted to elevated levels of BP and recognize this level as "normal." Consequently, the long-term regulation of arterial pressure requires activation of other mechanisms (primarily hormonal and renal) to maintain normal BP. The baroreceptor reflex is less responsive in some older adults.

Vascular Endothelium

The vascular endothelium is a single cell layer that lines the blood vessels. Previously considered inert, it is now known to have the ability to produce vasoactive substances and growth factors. Nitric oxide, an endothelium-derived relaxing factor (EDRF), helps maintain low arterial tone at rest, inhibits growth of the smooth muscle layer, and inhibits platelet aggregation. Other substances released by the vascular endothelium with local vasodilator effects include prostacyclin and endothelium-derived hyperpolarizing factor.

Endothelin (ET), produced by the endothelial cells, is an extremely potent vasoconstrictor. There are three subclasses of ETs: ET-1, ET-2, and ET-3. ET-1 is the most potent ET in producing vasoconstriction. ET-1 also causes adhesion and aggregation of

TABLE 35-1	SYMPATHETIC NERVOUS SYSTEM RECEPTORS INFLUENCING BLOOD PRESSURE	
Adrenergic Receptor	**Location**	**Response When Activated**
α_1	Vascular smooth muscle	Vasoconstriction
	Heart	Increased contractility
α_2	Presynaptic membrane	Inhibition of norepinephrine release
	Vascular smooth muscle	Vasoconstriction
β_1	Heart	Increased contractility (positive inotropic effect)
		Increased heart rate (positive chronotropic effect)
		Increased conduction (positive dromotropic effect)
	Juxtaglomerular cells	Increased renin secretion
β_2	Smooth muscle of peripheral blood vessels in skeletal muscle, coronary arteries, lungs, kidneys, liver, islet cells, bladder, liver	Vasodilation
		Relaxation
		Gluconeogenesis
		Increase in secretion
Dopaminergic receptors	Primarily kidney and mesenteric blood vessels	Vasodilation

neutrophils and stimulates smooth muscle growth. Endothelial function and dysfunction is an area of ongoing investigation. There is some evidence that vascular endothelial dysfunction may contribute to atherosclerosis and primary hypertension. The prevention or reversal of endothelial dysfunction may become important for therapeutic interventions in the future.

Renal System

The kidneys contribute to BP regulation by controlling sodium excretion and extracellular fluid (ECF) volume (see Chapter 47). Sodium retention results in water retention, which causes an increased ECF volume. This increases the venous return to the heart, increasing the stroke volume, which elevates the BP through an increase in CO.

The renin–angiotensin–aldosterone system (RAAS) also plays an important role in BP regulation. In response to sympathetic stimulation, decreased blood flow through the kidneys, or decreased serum sodium concentration, renin is secreted from the juxtaglomerular apparatus in the kidney. Renin is an enzyme that converts angiotensinogen to angiotensin I. Angiotensin-converting enzyme (ACE) converts angiotensin I into angiotensin II (A-II), which can increase BP by two different mechanisms (see Chapter 47, Figure 47-6). First, A-II is a potent vasoconstrictor and increases vascular resistance, resulting in an immediate increase in BP. Second, over a period of hours or days, A-II increases BP indirectly by stimulating the adrenal cortex to secrete aldosterone, which causes sodium and water retention by the kidneys, resulting in increased blood volume and increased CO.

A-II also functions at a local level within the heart and the blood vessels. The local vasoactive effects of A-II (vasoconstriction

and growth promotion) may contribute to atherosclerosis and primary hypertension.

Prostaglandins (PGs) E_2 (PGE$_2$) and I_2 (PGI$_2$), secreted by the renal medulla, have a vasodilator effect on the systemic circulation. This results in decreased SVR and lowering of BP. (PGs are discussed in Chapter 14.)

Endocrine System

Stimulation of the SNS results in release of epinephrine along with a small fraction of NE by the adrenal medulla. Epinephrine increases CO by increasing HR and myocardial contractility. Epinephrine activates β_2-adrenergic receptors in peripheral arterioles of skeletal muscle, causing vasodilation. In peripheral arterioles with only α_1-adrenergic receptors (skin and kidneys), epinephrine causes vasoconstriction.

The adrenal cortex is stimulated by A-II to release aldosterone. (Release of aldosterone is also regulated by other factors, such as low sodium levels [see Chapters 50 and 51].) Aldosterone stimulates the kidneys to retain sodium and, therefore, water. This increases BP by increasing CO.

An increased blood sodium osmolarity level stimulates the release of antidiuretic hormone (ADH) from the posterior pituitary gland. ADH increases the ECF volume by promoting the reabsorption of water in the distal and the collecting tubules of the kidneys. The resulting increase in blood volume can cause an elevation in BP.

In the healthy person, these regulatory mechanisms function in response to the demands of the body. When hypertension develops, one or more of the BP-regulating mechanisms are defective.

HYPERTENSION

Hypertension is sustained elevation of systemic arterial BP and is the leading cause for visits to primary care physicians (Hypertension Canada, 2014). High BP is the most significant modifiable risk factor for cardiovascular disease and mortality in Canada (McAlister, Wilkins, Joffres, et al., 2011). High blood pressure remains a significant cardiovascular risk factor affecting 40% of the global adult population ≥25 years (World Health Organization, 2013) and is predicted to become the leading cause of death and disability worldwide by 2020 (Sliwa, Stewart, & Gersh, 2011). As indicated by Padwal, Bienek, McAlister, et al. (2015), even small incremental changes in systolic and diastolic pressures have a direct effect on mortality—for every 20-mm Hg increase in systolic BP to >115 mm Hg (or a 10-mm Hg increase in diastolic BP to >75 mm Hg), the risk for cardiovascular mortality doubles. The prevalence of diagnosed high BP has steadily increased among the Canadian population, from 12.9% in 1998–1999 (Dai, Robitaille, Bancej, et al., 2010) to 22.6% in 2012–2013 (Padwal et al., 2015). Consequently, new recommendations have appeared in the 2017 Hypertension Canada guidelines (formerly the Canadian Hypertension Education Program [CHEP] guidelines). CHEP is Hypertension Canada's "knowledge translation program that targets various healthcare professionals in clinical and community settings, provides regularly updated standardized recommendations and clinical practice guidelines to detect, treat and control hypertension" (Hypertension Canada, 2017).

Hypertension is defined as a systolic blood pressure (SBP) equal to or greater than 140 mm Hg or a diastolic blood pressure (DBP) equal to or greater than 90 mm Hg. According to the Canadian Diabetes Association (CDA) and Hypertension Canada

TABLE 35-2   TARGET VALUES FOR BLOOD PRESSURE*

Setting	Target (mm Hg)
Out-of-Office Assessments (Home or Pharmacy)	
Home blood pressure and daytime ambulatory blood pressure measurement (ABPM)*	≤135/85
24-hour ambulatory blood pressure measurement	<130/80
Office	
Diastolic and/or systolic hypertension	<140/90
Isolated systolic hypertension	<140/90 (age <80)
	<150/90 (age >80)
Diabetes (with microalbuminuria, renal disease, cardiovascular disease, or additional cardiovascular risk factors)	<130/80
Non-diabetic chronic kidney disease	<140/90
Automated office oscillometric device	<130/80
Awake	<135/85
24-hr	<130/80

*Automated blood pressure method (preferred)
Source: Adapted from Canadian Hypertension Education Program (CHEP). (2015). *2015 Canadian Recommendations for the Management of Hypertension. What's new?* (Summary document.) Markham, ON: Hypertension Canada. Retrieved from *https://drive.google.com/file/d/0B_aFVG-E49pmc1BwTFFHbHczaWlRYTR4aHNzOVQwZV9WQTd3/view*.

DETERMINANTS OF HEALTH
Hypertension

Ethnicity: Education and Literacy
- 50% of all Canadians are not aware of the impact of hypertension on kidneys, of the need to adhere to antihypertensive medication, and that hypertension is a chronic condition.
- Chinese Canadians are less aware than other Canadians of the relationship between hypertension and heart attacks; Indian Canadians are less knowledgeable than other Canadians of the association between hypertension and weight.
- Hypertension education needs to be promoted in populations of people from all ethnic backgrounds and should target individuals of lower socioeconomic status.
- Educational materials need to be available in multiple languages and use multi-modal delivery (e.g., television, radio, brochures).

Source: Cunningham, C. T., Sykes, L. L., Metcalfe, A., et al. (2014). Ethnicity and health literacy: A survey on hypertension knowledge among Canadian ethnic populations. *Ethnicity & disease, 24*(3), 276–282.

target blood pressures for persons diagnosed with hypertension and diabetes mellitus, SBP should be less than or equal to 130 mm Hg and DBP should be less than or equal to 80 mm Hg (Gilbert, Rabi, LaRochelle, et al., 2013). This is the established level at which antihypertensive therapy is effective at decreasing cardiovascular morbidity and mortality. Canadian targets for blood pressure are shown in Table 35-2. The American Joint National Committee 7 (JNC-7) defines normal BP as an SBP less than 120 mm Hg and a DBP less than 80 mm Hg. Based on JNC-7, patients with sustained hypertension are further divided into stage 1 hypertension (SBP 140–159 or DBP 90–99 mm Hg), and stage 2 hypertension (SBP =160 or DBP =100 mm Hg).

According to the Canadian Health Measures Survey (CHMS), approximately 19% of adults ages 20 to 79 years have hypertension, with the rates increasing with age. Older women have higher rates of hypertension than older men. Women with high BP have three and one-half times greater risk of developing cardiovascular disease than women with normal BP do (Heart and Stroke Foundation, 2015). See the Determinants of Health box for statistics on hypertension in selected ethnic groups.

Canada has increased awareness and treatment of hypertension compared to other developed countries (Campbell & Chen, 2010). The World Health Organization (WHO) (2013) identified hypertension as a silent killer requiring increased global public awareness necessary for early detection (WHO, 2013). According to McAlister and colleagues (2011), the status of hypertension control improved considerably between 1992 and 2009; however, the prevalence of hypertension still increased by 3% between 2012 and 2013 (Padwal et al., 2015). Large-scale education programs, such as the CHEP and Heart and Stroke Foundation, have increased people's awareness of hypertension. McAlister and colleagues (2011) found that 83% of those with hypertension are aware of their condition and 17% remain unaware. Padwal et al. (2015) found no changes in this statistical data between the years of 2012 and 2013. Despite these statistics, hypertension remains on the rise in Canada (Padwal et al., 2015) and globally

(Campbell & Niebylski, 2014). In addition, the mortality rate for individuals aged 20 to 49 years is two to four times higher for people with hypertension than those without it (Robitaille, Dai, Waters, et al., 2012).

One in five adult Canadians is affected by hypertension, which is also a major risk factor for cardiovascular disease, chronic kidney disease, and death (Daskalopoulou, Rabi, Zarnke, et al., 2015). Adults with high-normal BP (also called *prehypertension*) require annual BP assessment. Health care providers who have been specifically trained to measure BP accurately should assess BP in all adult patients, at all appropriate visits, to determine cardiovascular risk and monitor antihypertensive treatment. Home measurement of BP has been recommended since the 2008 CHEP guidelines to encourage patient self-efficacy and is consistent with the 2017 Hypertension Canada guidelines (Leung, Daskalopoulou, Dasgupta, et al., 2017). Out-of-office BP readings, including ambulatory and home readings, are recommended by Hypertension Canada to identify higher BP readings, prompting patients to seek treatment and earlier diagnosis (Leung, Daskalopoulou, Dasgupta, et al., 2017). Patient instructions for purchasing and using home BP measurement devices are available at both the Hypertension Canada and the Heart and Stroke Foundation of Canada websites. A comprehensive instructional video on home measurement of BP was developed in 2009 and can be viewed at the Hypertension Canada website (see the Resources at the end of this chapter).

The recommendations for diagnosis of hypertension and follow-up are shown in Figure 35-2. It should be emphasized that, when using BPs recorded during office visits to diagnose hypertension, the thresholds given refer to readings averaged over a specified range of visits and are not one-time measurements from the last visit.

Subtypes of Hypertension

Isolated systolic hypertension (ISH) is defined as a sustained elevation in SBP equal to or greater than 140 mm Hg with a DBP less than 90 mm Hg. (A one-time isolated reading of increased SBP is not classified as ISH.) Arterial BP increases with advancing age.

An increase of the SBP without an increase of the DBP, as occurs in ISH, increases the pulse pressure. The *pulse pressure* is the difference between the SBP and the DBP. Loss of elasticity of the large arteries contributes to this widening of the pulse

FIGURE 35-2 Criteria for the diagnosis of hypertension and recommendations for follow-up. The thresholds shown here are blood pressure *(BP)* values that are averaged across the corresponding number of visits and are not one-time measurements taken at the most recent office visit. All BP measurements are in millimetres of mercury. *ABPM,* ambulatory blood pressure monitoring; *BPM,* blood pressure monitoring; *DBP,* diastolic blood pressure; *HBPM,* home blood pressure monitoring; *SBP,* systolic blood pressure. Source: Leung, A. A., Daskalopoulou, S. S., Dasgupta, K., et al. (2017). Hypertension Canada's 2017 guidelines for diagnosis, risk assessment, prevention, and treatment of hypertension in adults. *Canadian Journal of Cardiology, 33*(5), 557-576. doi: http://dx.doi.org/10.1016/j.cjca.2017.03.005

pressure. Once considered to be harmless, a high pulse pressure is now considered an independent risk factor for cardiovascular disease and end-organ damage. ISH is associated with a two- to four-fold increased future risk for cardiomegaly, MI, or stroke. There is compelling evidence that treatment of ISH with a reduction in the SBP of 20 to 30 mm Hg results in significant cardiovascular benefits. Figure 35-3 presents the treatment algorithm for ISH.

Etiology

Hypertension can be classified etiologically as either primary or secondary.

Primary Hypertension. Primary (essential) hypertension is elevated BP and accounts for 90% to 95% of all cases of hypertension (Riaz, Dreisbach, Madhur, et al., 2012). Although the exact cause of primary hypertension has not been identified, it is considered to be a complex interaction between genes and the environment (Geller, 2015). Several contributing factors, including increased SNS activity, overproduction of sodium-retaining hormones and vasoconstrictors, increased sodium intake, greater-than-ideal body weight, diabetes mellitus, and excessive alcohol intake, have been identified. Primary

hypertension is the focus of this chapter because of its prevalence in clinical practice.

Secondary Hypertension. Secondary hypertension is elevated BP with a specific cause that often can be identified and corrected. This type of hypertension accounts for 5% to 10% of hypertension in adults and more than 80% of hypertension in children. If a person younger than age 20 or older than age 50 suddenly develops hypertension, especially if it is severe, a secondary cause should be suspected. Clinical findings that suggest secondary hypertension include unprovoked hypokalemia; abdominal bruit; variable pressures with history of tachycardia, sweating, and tremor; or a family history of renal disease.

Causes of secondary hypertension include the following: (1) coarctation or congenital narrowing of the aorta; (2) renal disease such as renal artery stenosis and parenchymal disease (see Chapter 48); (3) endocrine disorders such as pheochromocytoma, Cushing's syndrome, and hyperaldosteronism (see Chapter 51); (4) neurological disorders such as brain tumours, quadriplegia, and head injury; (5) sleep apnea; (6) medications such as sympathetic stimulants (including cocaine), monoamine oxidase inhibitors taken with tyramine-containing foods, estrogen replacement therapy, oral contraceptive pills, and nonsteroidal

* Beta-blockers are not indicated as first-line therapy for age 60 and above.

**Recommended SPC choices are those in which an ACE-I is combined with a CCB, an ARB with a CCB, or an ACE-I or ARB with a diuretic

Renin angiotensin system (RAS) inhibitors are contraindicated in pregnancy and caution is required in prescribing to women of child-bearing potential

FIGURE 35-3 Treatment of systolic/diastolic hypertension *(HTN)* without other compelling indications. *ACE,* angiotensin-converting enzyme; *ARB,* angiotensin II receptor blocker; *CCB,* calcium channel blocker; *SPC,* single pill combination. Source: Hypertension Canada. (2017). What's new? 2017 *Hypertension Canada guidelines for the management of hypertension.* Retrieved from *https://www.hypertension.ca/images/CHEP_2017/ HTN_Whats_New_2017_EN.pdf.*

anti-inflammatory drugs (NSAIDs); and (7) pregnancy-induced hypertension. Treatment of secondary hypertension is directed at eliminating the underlying cause. Secondary hypertension is a contributing factor to hypertensive urgency (see section at end of this chapter).

Pathophysiology of Primary Hypertension

For arterial pressure to rise, there must be an increase in either CO or SVR. Increased CO is sometimes found in people with early and borderline hypertension. Later in the course of hypertension, SVR rises and the CO returns to normal. The hemodynamic hallmark of hypertension is persistently increased SVR. This persistent elevation in SVR may come about in various ways. Factors that are known to be related to the development of primary hypertension or contribute to its consequences are presented in Table 35-3.

Genes. Genetic observations to date suggest that primary hypertension is polygenic and also involves numerous environmental influences. Genetic factors are thought to account for a 30% to 60% variability in BP in individuals (Singh, Mensah, & Bakris, 2010) and vary depending on the study population, from 15% to 20% or from 65% to 70%. Familial heritability is a significant factor. A child with both parents and a sibling with hypertension has a 40% to 60% chance of developing hypertension. This risk increases to 80% if the child is a monozygotic twin. It is unlikely that this risk is from a single genetic locus but, rather, from multiple genes. Similarities across populations have not been established; ongoing research is needed in the area of genetic susceptibility to hypertension.

Sodium and Water Retention. Excessive dietary intake of sodium is the most studied environmental factor and is strongly linked to the initiation of hypertension in some people. Studies of populations with a low sodium intake (usually primitive hunter–gatherer societies) show little or no hypertension and no progressive increase in BP with age as is found in industrialized societies. In addition, the prevalence of hypertension increases when people from these societies adopt industrialized lifestyles.

In many people with hypertension, when sodium is restricted, their BP falls. A high sodium intake may alter the pressure–natriuresis relationship and cause water retention. Although almost everyone in Western countries consumes a high-sodium diet, only about 20% develop hypertension. This indicates that some degree of sodium sensitivity must be present for high sodium intake to trigger the development of hypertension.

Altered Renin–Angiotensin–Aldosterone Mechanism. The RAAS is a significant mechanism in the regulation of blood volume and pressure. Its role in hypertension is complex. High plasma renin activity (PRA) results in the increased conversion of angiotensinogen to angiotensin I (see Chapter 47, Figure 47-6). A-II causes direct arteriolar constriction, promotes vascular hypertrophy, and induces aldosterone secretion. Thus, altered renin–angiotensin mechanisms may contribute to the development and maintenance of hypertension. However, only about 20% of patients with primary hypertension have high PRA.

Stress and Increased Sympathetic Nervous System Activity. The SNS also has a critical role in BP control. It has long been recognized that arterial pressure is influenced by factors such as anger, fear, and pain. Physiological responses to stress, which are normally protective, may persist to a pathological degree, resulting in prolonged increase in SNS activity. Increased sympathetic stimulation produces increased vasoconstriction, increased HR, and increased renin release. Increased renin activates the angiotensin mechanism and increases aldosterone secretion, both leading to elevated BP. People exposed to high levels of repeated psychological stress develop hypertension to a greater extent than those who do not experience as much stress.

Insulin Resistance and Hyperinsulinemia. Abnormalities of glucose, insulin, and lipoprotein metabolism are common in primary hypertension. Insulin resistance is present in 50% of patients with primary hypertension; a strong genetic component is associated with hyperinsulinemia-associated hypertension. Insulin resistance is associated with endothelial dysfunction. High insulin concentration in the blood stimulates SNS and RAAS activity and impairs nitric oxide–mediated vasodilation.

TABLE 35-3 RISK FACTORS FOR PRIMARY HYPERTENSION

Advancing age	• BP rises progressively with increasing age. • Elevated BP is present in approximately 50% of people >65 yr, with 90% of the remainder developing hypertension during their lifespan.
Heavy alcohol consumption	• Excessive alcohol intake is strongly linked to hypertension. • Canadians with hypertension should limit their daily intake to 30 mL of alcohol.
Cigarette smoking	• The incidence of hypertension is increased among those who smoke ≥15 cigarettes/day. • Canadians with hypertension and who smoke have a greater risk for secondary cardiovascular disease.
Glucose intolerance (diabetes mellitus)	• Hypertension is diagnosed three times more often in individuals diagnosed with diabetes. • When hypertension and diabetes coexist, hypertension augments the already raised risk for cardiovascular diseases and worsens outcomes.
Elevated serum lipids	• Elevated levels of cholesterol and triglycerides are primary risk factors in atherosclerosis. • Hyperlipidemia is more common in Canadians with hypertension.
High dietary sodium intake	• High sodium intake can contribute to hypertension in some patients and can decrease the efficacy of certain antihypertensive medications. • For prevention of hypertension, the daily recommended dietary sodium intake is 1 500 mg for adults ages 14–50 yr of age; 1 300 mg for adults ages 50–70 yr; and 1 200 mg for adults >70 yr.
Gender	• In young adulthood and early middle age, hypertension is more prevalent in men. • After age 55, hypertension is more prevalent in women.
Family history	• Level of BP is strongly familial. • Risk for hypertension increases for those with a close relative having hypertension.
Obesity	• Weight gain is associated with increased risk for hypertension. • According to Statistics Canada, 59% of Canadian adults are at a weight that increases their risk for hypertension. • Risk is greatest with central abdominal obesity. Waist circumference recommendations are <102 cm for men and <88 cm for women.* • Maintenance of a healthy weight and BMI of 18.5–24.9 kg/m² is recommended.*
Ethnicity	• Black people or people of South Asian descent are three times more likely to have hypertension than the general population. • Almost 50% of Black people have already developed hypertension in their 40s and 50s.
Sedentary lifestyle	• Physical activity may decrease BP. • Regular physical activity can help control weight and reduce cardiovascular risk. • Daily accumulation of 30–60 min of moderate-intensity dynamic exercise (walking, jogging, cycling, or noncompetitive swimming), 4–7 days/wk is recommended. • Higher intensities of exercise are no more effective.
Socioeconomic status	• Canadians living in low-income neighbourhoods have higher rates of hypertension.
Psychosocial stress	• Canadians exposed to repeated stress may develop hypertension more frequently than others. • Canadians who develop hypertension may respond differently to stress from those who do not.

BP, blood pressure; *BMI*, body mass index.

*Leung, A. A., Daskalopoulou, S. S., Dasgupta, K., et al. (2017). Hypertension Canada's 2017 Guidelines for diagnosis, risk assessment, prevention, and treatment of hypertension in adults. *Canadian Journal of Cardiology, 33*(5), 557-576. doi: http://dx.doi.org/10.1016/j.cjca.2017.03.005.

Additional pressor effects of insulin include vascular hypertrophy and increased renal sodium reabsorption.

Endothelial Cell Dysfunction. Vascular endothelial cells are known to be a source of multiple vasoactive substances such as nitric oxide and ET. Some people with hypertension have a reduced vasodilator response to nitric oxide. ET produces pronounced and prolonged vasoconstriction. The role of endothelial dysfunction in the pathogenesis and treatment of hypertension is an area of ongoing investigation.

Obesity. Obesity is a well-known risk factor for hypertension. Hypertension and central (visceral) obesity are major components of cardiometabolic syndrome. The relationship between hypertension and obesity is multifaceted; the etiology is complex, and it is not well elucidated. Several hormone abnormalities that are associated with obesity are linked to the development of hypertension. Enlarged adipocytes or fat cells secrete leptin, proinflammatory cytokines, and reactive oxygen species. This dysfunctional adipose tissue may induce activation of the SNS and RAAS.

Clinical Manifestations

Hypertension is a lanthanic, or silent, disease because it is frequently asymptomatic until it becomes severe and target-organ disease has occurred. A patient with severe hypertension may experience a variety of symptoms secondary to effects on blood vessels in the various organs and tissues or to the increased workload of the heart. These secondary symptoms include fatigue, reduced activity tolerance, dizziness, palpitations, angina, and dyspnea. In the past, symptoms of hypertension were thought to include headache, nosebleeds, and dizziness. However, unless BP is extremely high or low, these symptoms are not more frequent in people with hypertension than in the general population.

Complications

The most common complications of hypertension are *target-organ diseases* (Table 35-4) occurring in the heart (hypertensive heart disease), the brain (cerebro-vascular disease), the peripheral vasculature (peripheral arterial disease), the kidneys (nephrosclerosis), and the eyes (retinal damage).

Hypertensive Heart Disease

Coronary Artery Disease. Hypertension is an established major risk factor for coronary artery disease, almost doubling the risk. The mechanisms by which hypertension contributes to the development of atherosclerosis are multifactorial. The shear stress (response-to-injury hypothesis of atherogenesis) results in endothelial dysfunction, causing impairment in the synthesis and release of the potent vasodilator, nitric oxide. A decreased nitric oxide level promotes the development and acceleration of atherosclerosis and plaque formation.

TABLE 35-4	PATHOLOGICAL EFFECTS OF SUSTAINED, COMPLICATED PRIMARY HYPERTENSION	
Site of Injury	**Mechanism of Injury**	**Potential Pathological Effect**
Heart		
• Myocardium	Increased workload combined with diminished blood flow through coronary arteries	Left ventricular hypertrophy, myocardial ischemia, left heart failure
• Coronary arteries	Accelerated atherosclerosis (coronary artery disease)	Myocardial ischemia, myocardial infarction, sudden death
Aorta	Weakened vessel wall	Aneurysms, acute aortic syndromes
Kidneys	Renin and aldosterone secretion stimulated by reduced blood flow	Retention of sodium and water, leading to increased blood volume and perpetuation of hypertension
	Inflammation and ischemia	Tissue damage that compromises filtration
	High pressures in renal arterioles	Nephrosclerosis leading to renal failure
Brain	Reduced blood flow and oxygen supply; weakened vessel walls, accelerated atherosclerosis	Transient ischemic attack, cerebral thrombosis, aneurysm, hemorrhage, acute brain infarction
Eyes (retinas)	Reduced blood flow	Retinal vascular sclerosis
	High arteriolar pressure	Exudation, hemorrhage
Arterial vessels of lower extremities	Reduced blood flow and high pressures in arterioles, accelerated atherosclerosis	Intermittent claudication, arterial thrombosis, gangrene

Source: McCance, K. L., & Huether, S. E. (2014). *Pathophysiology: The biologic basis for disease in adults and children.* 7th ed. (p. 1138). St. Louis: Mosby.

FIGURE 35-4 A, Massively enlarged heart caused by hypertrophy of the muscle in the left ventricle. **B,** Compare with the thickness of the normal left ventricle. The patient suffered from severe hypertension. Source: Kumar, V., Cotran, R. S., & Robbins, S.L. (2007). *Robbins basic pathology*, 8th ed. Philadelphia: Saunders.

The intimal layer is exposed to activated white blood cells and platelets. Growth factors released by the vascular endothelium and platelets may induce smooth muscle proliferation within the lesion. These arteriolar changes may account for a high incidence of coronary artery disease and the resulting problems of angina and MI.

Left Ventricular Hypertrophy. Sustained high BP increases the cardiac workload and produces left ventricular hypertrophy (LVH) (Figure 35-4). The risk for LVH doubles with associated obesity. Initially, LVH is an adaptive or compensatory mechanism that strengthens cardiac contraction and increases CO. However, increased contractility increases myocardial work and oxygen consumption. When the heart can no longer meet the demands for myocardial oxygen, heart failure develops. Progressive LVH, especially in association with coronary artery disease, is associated with the development of heart failure.

Heart Failure. Heart failure is a common complication of a chronically elevated BP and occurs when the heart's compensatory adaptations are overwhelmed and the heart can no longer pump enough blood to meet the metabolic needs of the body (see Chapter 37). Contractility is depressed, and SV and CO are decreased. The patient may complain of shortness of breath on exertion, paroxysmal nocturnal dyspnea, and fatigue. Signs of an enlarged heart may be present on radiograph, and an electrocardiogram (ECG) may show electrical changes indicative of LVH.

Cerebro-vascular Disease. Atherosclerosis is the most common cause of cerebro-vascular disease. Hypertension is a major risk factor for cerebral atherosclerosis and stroke. Even in people with mild hypertension, the risk for stroke is four times higher than in people with normal BP. Adequate control of BP effectively diminishes the risk for stroke.

Atherosclerotic plaques are commonly distributed at the bifurcation of the common carotid artery into the internal and external carotid arteries. Portions of the atherosclerotic plaque, or the blood clot that forms on the plaque, may break off and travel to intracerebral vessels, producing a thrombo-embolism. The patient may experience transient ischemic attacks or a stroke. (These conditions are discussed in Chapter 60.)

Hypertensive encephalopathy may occur after a marked rise in BP if the cerebral blood flow is not decreased by autoregulation. *Autoregulation* is a physiological process that maintains constant cerebral blood flow despite fluctuations in arterial BP. Normally, as pressure in the cerebral blood vessels rises, the vessels constrict to maintain constant flow. When arterial BP exceeds the body's ability to autoregulate, the cerebral vessels suddenly dilate and cerebral edema develops, producing a rise in intracranial pressure. If left untreated, patients die quickly from brain damage. (Cerebral blood flow and autoregulation are discussed in Chapter 59.)

Peripheral Arterial Disease. As it does with other vessels, hypertension speeds up the process of atherosclerosis in the peripheral arterial blood vessels, leading to the development of aortic aneurysm, aortic dissection, and peripheral arterial disease (see Chapter 40). *Intermittent claudication* (ischemic muscle pain precipitated by activity and relieved with rest) is a classical symptom of peripheral arterial disease.

Nephrosclerosis. Hypertension is one of the leading causes of end-stage renal disease (ESRD). Some degree of kidney dysfunction is usually present in the patient with hypertension, even one with a minimally elevated BP. One of the earliest markers of nephropathy is microalbuminuria, the presence of protein in the urine. Kidney dysfunction is the direct result of ischemia caused by the narrowed lumen of the intrarenal blood vessels. Gradual narrowing of the arteries and arterioles leads to atrophy of the tubules, destruction of the glomeruli, and eventual death of nephrons. Initially intact nephrons can compensate, but these changes may eventually lead to renal failure. Common laboratory indications of kidney dysfunction are microalbuminuria, macroalbuminuria, elevated blood urea nitrogen (BUN), serum creatinine levels, and microscopic hematuria.

Retinal Damage. The appearance of the retina provides important information about how severe and longstanding the hypertensive process has been. The retina is the only place in the body where the blood vessels can be directly visualized. Damage seen to have occurred to retinal vessels thus provides an indication of vessel damage in the heart, the brain, and the kidneys. An ophthalmoscope is used to visualize the blood vessels of the eye. Manifestations of severe retinal damage include blurring of vision, retinal hemorrhage, and loss of vision.

Diagnostic Studies

The diagnosis of hypertension is not based on a single elevated reading (if <80/110 mm Hg) but requires several elevated readings over several weeks (see Figure 35-1). (Measurement of BP is discussed in Chapter 34.)

Table 35-5 is a list of basic laboratory studies that are performed in a person with sustained hypertension. Routine urinalysis and serum creatinine levels are used to screen for kidney involvement and to provide baseline information about kidney function. (Serum creatinine is discussed in Chapters 47 and 49.)

Measurement of serum electrolytes, especially potassium levels, is important to detect hyperaldosteronism, a cause of secondary hypertension. Blood glucose levels should be assessed to assist in the diagnosis of diabetes mellitus. Serum cholesterol and triglyceride levels provide information about additional risk factors that predispose to atherosclerosis. An ECG provides baseline information about the cardiac status. It is helpful in identifying the presence of LVH and myocardial ischemia. If the patient's age, history, physical examination findings, or severity of hypertension points to a secondary cause, further diagnostic tests may be indicated.

Ambulatory Blood Pressure Monitoring. Twenty-four–hour ambulatory BP readings are useful in the diagnosis of uncomplicated mild-to-moderate hypertension and are more accurate in predicting cardiovascular risk than office BP. This method of measuring BP is incorporated into the Hypertension Canada diagnostic algorithm to facilitate more rapid diagnosis of hypertension and reduce the risk of patients being left untreated for long periods of time while a diagnosis is being made over numerous office visits.

A fully automated system that measures BP at preset intervals over a 24-hour period is used. The equipment includes a BP cuff and a small microprocessing unit that fits into a pouch worn on a shoulder strap or belt. Patients are asked to maintain a diary of activities that may affect BP. This procedure may be helpful in patients with suspected white coat hypertension, masked hypertension, apparent drug resistance, hypotensive symptoms with hypertensive medications, episodic hypertension, or autonomic nervous system dysfunction.

TABLE 35-5   COLLABORATIVE CARE

Hypertension

Diagnosis
- History and physical examination
- Routine laboratory tests should be performed for the investigation of all patients with hypertension, including the following:
  - Urinalysis
  - Blood chemistry (potassium, sodium, creatinine, blood urea and nitrogen)
  - Fasting blood glucose
  - Fasting total cholesterol and high-density lipoprotein cholesterol, low-density lipoprotein cholesterol, and triglycerides
  - Standard 12-lead electrocardiography
- Assess urinary albumin excretion in patients with diabetes
- All patients with treated hypertension need to be monitored for the appearance of diabetes, according to the Canadian Diabetes Association (CDA) guidelines (available at *http://www. canadianjournalofdiabetes.com/article/S1499-2671%2813 %2900034-8/pdf*).

Collaborative Therapy
- Periodic monitoring of BP
  - Home BP monitoring
  - Ambulatory BP monitoring
  - Every 3–6 mo once BP is stabilized
- Nutritional therapy (see Tables 35-7 and 35-8)
  - Restricted sodium intake (reduce to 2 000 mg per day)*
  - Restricted intake of cholesterol and saturated fats
  - Maintenance of adequate intake of potassium
  - Maintenance of adequate intake of calcium and magnesium
- Weight management
- Regular, moderate physical activity
- Tobacco cessation
- Moderation in alcohol consumption
- Antihypertensive drugs (see Table 35-8)
- Patient and caregiver teaching

NOTE: During the maintenance phase of hypertension management, tests (including those for electrolytes, creatinine, and fasting lipids) should be repeated with a frequency reflecting the clinical situation.
BP, blood pressure.
*Leung, A. A., Daskalopoulou, S. S., Dasgupta, K., et al. (2017). Hypertension Canada's 2017 Guidelines for diagnosis, risk assessment, prevention, and treatment of hypertension in adults. *Canadian Journal of Cardiology, 33*(5), 557-576. doi: http:// dx.doi.org/10.1016/j.cjca.2017.03.005.

Some patients have elevated BP readings in a clinical setting and normal readings when BP is measured elsewhere. This phenomenon is referred to as *white coat hypertension*. Other patients have normal BP in the office and elevated BP at home. This condition is called *masked hypertension.*

As with most physiological phenomena, BP demonstrates diurnal variability, expressed as sleep–wakefulness difference. For day-active people, BP is highest in the early morning, decreases during the day, and is lowest at night. Some patients with hypertension do not show a normal, nocturnal fall in BP—they are called "nondippers." A decrease in nocturnal BP of less than 10% is associated with increased risk for cardiovascular events. The presence or absence of diurnal variability can be determined by continuous ambulatory BP monitoring.

Canadians with hypertension should be encouraged to use an approved BP-measuring device and use proper technique to assess BP at home. BP measured at home is a stronger predictor of cardiovascular events than office-based readings. Home measurement can help to confirm the diagnosis of hypertension, improve BP control, reduce the need for medications, help to identify white coat and masked hypertension, and improve medication adherence in nonadherent patients. An Internet-based toolbox to assist patient self-management for home BP measurement and lifestyle change can be found at the Heart and Stroke Foundation of Canada's website.

Canadian adults with high-normal BP require annual BP assessment. All Canadian adults need to have BP assessed at all appropriate clinical visits. One in five adult Canadians has hypertension, and for those age 55 with normal BP, 90% will develop hypertension if they live to an average age. All adults require ongoing assessment of BP throughout their lives.

Collaborative Care

Since the establishment of CHEP in 1999, evidence-informed recommendations for the management of hypertension have been updated annually. In 2011, CHEP joined with Hypertension Canada and Blood Pressure Canada with the goal of providing a stronger, united approach to the prevention and control of hypertension. Each year, new evidence is reviewed and integrated into previous evidence-informed guidelines to develop new guidelines (now known as Hypertension Canada guidelines), where appropriate. In order for health care providers to remain informed of updates, the guidelines and other hypertension resources are available at the Hypertension Canada website.

Risk Stratification. The risk for cardiovascular disease in people with hypertension is determined by the level of BP; the presence of target-organ damage; risk factors such as diabetes, dyslipidemia, smoking, and obesity; and other exogenous, potentially modifiable factors that can induce or aggravate hypertension (Table 35-6). Over 90% of Canadians with hypertension have other cardiovascular risks. Hypertension Canada guidelines recommend that global cardiovascular risk should be assessed in all patients. Simply counting risk factors may lead to underestimating risk.

Follow-up monitoring of BP is important. The frequency of monitoring varies initially with the level of BP. After the BP has stabilized, follow-up visits should be scheduled every 3 to 6 months to ensure continued control of BP, provide support for lifestyle changes, assess for target-organ damage, and detect adverse effects of medications.

Lifestyle Modifications. All patients with hypertension should use lifestyle modifications as either definitive or adjunctive therapy. Lifestyle modifications are directed toward reducing BP and overall cardiovascular risk factors. Modifications include (1) dietary changes, including reduced sodium intake, (2) limitation of alcohol intake, (3) regular physical activity, (4) avoidance of tobacco use (smoking and chewing), (5) stress management, and (6) weight reduction (see Figure 35-3).

Nutritional Therapy. Hypertension Canada and the Heart and Stroke Foundation of Canada recommend consumption of the Dietary Approaches to Stop Hypertension (DASH) diet, which emphasizes fruits, vegetables, and low-fat dairy products; dietary and soluble fibre; whole grains; and protein from plant sources and that is reduced in saturated fat and cholesterol. The DASH diet is recommended for both patients with hypertension and individuals with normal BP who are at increased risk of developing hypertension. Dietary management of hypertension consists of restriction of sodium; maintenance of dietary potassium, calcium, and magnesium intake; and calorie restriction if the patient is overweight (Table 35-7). (See the Government of Canada's recommended intake for sodium, and the DASH diet to lower high blood pressure, in the Resources at the end of this chapter.)

The Hypertension Canada 2017 recommendations included the reduction in salt intake for the prevention and treatment of

TABLE 35-6 ASSESSMENT OF THE OVERALL CARDIOVASCULAR RISK

Search for Target-Organ Damage
- Cerebrovascular disease
  - Stroke
    - Ischemic stroke and transient ischemic attack
    - Intracerebral hemorrhage
    - Aneurysmal subarachnoid hemorrhage
  - Dementia
    - Vascular dementia
    - Mixed vascular dementia and dementia of the Alzheimer's type
- Hypertensive retinopathy
- Left ventricular dysfunction
- Left ventricular hypertrophy
- Coronary artery disease
  - Myocardial infarction
  - Angina pectoris
- Heart failure
- Renal disease
  - Chronic kidney disease (GFR <60 mL/min/1.73 m^2)
  - Albuminuria
- Peripheral artery disease
  - Intermittent claudication

Search for Key Cardiovascular Risk Factors for Atherosclerosis
Non-Modifiable
- Age ≥55 yr
- Male
- Family history of premature cardiovascular disease (<55 yr in men and <65 yr in women)

Modifiable
- Sedentary lifestyle
- Poor dietary habits
- Abdominal obesity
- Diabetes mellitus
- Smoking
- Dyslipidemia
- Stress
- Nonadherence

Search for Exogenous, Potentially Modifiable Factors That Can Induce or Aggravate Hypertension
- Prescription drugs
  - NSAIDs, including "coxibs"
  - Corticosteroids and anabolic steroids
  - Oral contraceptives and sex hormones
  - Vasoconstricting/ sympathomimetic decongestants
  - Calcineurin inhibitors (cyclosporin, tacrolimus)
  - Erythropoietin and analogues
  - Antidepressants: MAOIs, SNRIs, SSRIs
  - Midodrine
- Other
  - Licorice root
  - Stimulants, including cocaine
  - Salt
  - Excessive alcohol use

GFR, glomerular filtration rate; *MAOIs,* monoamine oxidase inhibitors; *NSAIDs,* nonsteroidal anti-inflammatory drugs; *SNRIs,* serotonin–norepinephrine reuptake inhibitors; *SSRIs,* selective serotonin reuptake inhibitors.
Source: Adapted from Leung, A. A., Daskalopoulou, S. S., Dasgupta, K., et al. (2017). Hypertension Canada's 2017 Guidelines for diagnosis, risk assessment, prevention, and treatment of hypertension in adults. *Canadian Journal of Cardiology, 33*(5), 557-576. (Supplemental tables.) doi: http://dx.doi.org/10.1016/j.cjca.2017.03.005. Reprinted with permission.

hypertension in accordance with the recommendations of Health Canada. According to the World Health Organization (WHO), reducing salt intake is the most cost-effective measure to improve population health outcomes for all individuals, with or without hypertension (2014).

"High dietary salt causes an estimated 30% of hypertension and increases blood pressure in people with or without hypertension" (Campbell, Lackland, & Niebylski, 2014, p. 7). The daily adequate intake (AI) for sodium is 1 200 mg (52 mmol) to 1 500 mg (65 mmol) for healthy adults, decreasing with age. The upper tolerable intake level (UL) for sodium is 2 300 mg/day. There is a large discrepancy between recommended levels of sodium intake and actual sodium intake levels by Canadians. The average sodium consumption in Canada is 3 500 mg/day. Eighty percent of sodium intake comes from processed and restaurant foods, whereas only 10% is added at the table or in cooking. See "Sodium 101" and Government of Canada's "Recommended intake of sodium" in the Resources at the end of this

TABLE 35-7   NUTRITIONAL THERAPY

Hypertension

Food Group	Daily Servings	Examples	Significance to DASH Eating Pattern
Whole grains	7–8	Whole wheat breads, cereals; oatmeal; brown rice; pasta; quinoa; barley; low-fat, low-sodium crackers	Major sources of energy and fibre
Vegetables	4–5	Dark green and orange fresh or frozen vegetables, tomatoes, leafy greens, carrots, peas, squash, spinach, peppers, broccoli, sweet potatoes	Rich sources of potassium, magnesium, and fibre
Fruits	4–5	Have fruit more often than juice: apples, apricots, bananas, dates, grapes, oranges, grapefruit, melons, peaches, berries, pineapple	Important sources of potassium, magnesium, and fibre
Low-fat or fat-free dairy foods or alternatives	2–3	Skim milk, 1% milk, fortified soy beverage or yogourt, 6%–18% modified-fat cheese	Major sources of calcium and protein
Lean meats, poultry, and fish	≤170 g	Lean meats; choose fish such as char, herring, mackerel, salmon, sardines, and trout; trim fat; broil, roast, or boil; no frying; remove skin from poultry; low-sodium, low-fat deli meats	Rich sources of protein and magnesium
Nuts, seeds, and dry beans	4–5/wk	—	Rich sources of energy, magnesium, potassium, protein, and fibre
Fats and oils*	2–3 tsp	Soft margarine, mayonnaise, vegetable oil (olive, corn, canola, or safflower), salad dressing	Added fat and high-fat sources should be minimal. DASH has 27% of calories as fat, including fat in or added to foods.
Sweets	≤5/wk	Sugar, jelly, jam, hard candy, syrups, sorbet, chocolate	Sweets should be low in fat.

*Fat content changes serving counts for fats and oils: For example, 1 tablespoon of regular salad dressing equals 1 serving, 1 tablespoon of low-fat salad dressing equals ½ serving, and 1 tablespoon of fat-free salad dressing equals 0 servings.

DASH, Dietary Approaches to Stop Hypertension. The DASH eating plan is based on approximately 2 000 calories/day. The number of daily servings in a food group may vary from those listed, depending on specific caloric needs.

Source: National Heart, Lung, and Blood Institute. (2006). The DASH diet. NIH Publication No. 06-4082. Washington, DC: National Institutes of Health. Retrieved from http://www.nhlbi.nih.gov/files/docs/public/heart/hbp_low.pdf.

chapter for more educational resources about salt. (See also Chapter 37, Tables 37-6 through 37-9.)

The patient and caregivers, especially those who prepare the meals, should be taught about sodium-restricted diets. Instruction should include reading labels of over-the-counter drugs, packaged foods, and health products (e.g., baking soda–containing toothpaste) to identify hidden sources of sodium. It is helpful to review the patient's normal diet and to identify foods high in sodium. Analysis of a 3-day diet history will help identify foods high in sodium in the patient's usual diet.

Sodium restriction may be enough to control BP in some patients with stage 1 hypertension. If drug therapy is needed, a lower dose may be effective if the patient also restricts sodium intake. Furthermore, moderate sodium restriction lessens the risk for hypokalemia associated with diuretic therapy. However, people with hypertension respond differently to salt restriction. This heterogeneity of response has led to attempts to define subgroups of people with hypertension as "salt sensitive" or "salt resistant." Patients with low renin activity are more likely to respond to salt restriction with a reduction in BP.

The significance of other dietary elements for the control of hypertension is not certain. There is evidence that greater levels of dietary potassium, calcium, magnesium, and vitamin D are associated with lower BP in the general population and in those with hypertension. Based on available evidence, the Hypertension Canada 2017 guidelines advise the maintenance of adequate potassium, magnesium, and calcium intake from food sources (Leung, Daskalopoulou, Dasgupta, et al., 2017). Supplementation of potassium, calcium, and magnesium is not recommended for the prevention or treatment of hypertension. Caffeine may raise BP acutely, but there is no long-term relationship between caffeine intake and elevated BP.

Weight Reduction. Overweight individuals have an increased incidence of hypertension and increased cardiovascular disease risk. Height, weight, and waist circumference should be measured and body mass index (BMI) calculated for all adults. Maintenance of a healthy body weight (BMI 18.5–24.9 kg/m² and waist circumference <102 cm for men and <88 cm for women) is recommended for individuals who are normotensive to prevent hypertension and for Canadians with hypertension to reduce BP. All individuals with hypertension who are overweight should be advised to lose weight. Weight reduction has a significant effect on lowering BP, and the effect is seen with even moderate weight loss. When a person decreases caloric intake, sodium and fat intake may also be reduced. Although reducing the fat content of the diet has not been shown to produce sustained benefits in BP control, it may slow the progress of atherosclerosis and reduce overall cardiovascular disease risk (see Chapter 36). Weight-loss strategies should employ a multidisciplinary approach that includes dietary education, increased physical activity, and behavioural intervention.

Modification in Alcohol Consumption. Excessive alcohol consumption is strongly associated with hypertension. To reduce BP, alcohol consumption should be in accordance with Canadian low-risk drinking guidelines for both adults with hypertension and those with normal BP. Healthy adults should limit alcohol consumption to 2 drinks or fewer per day, and consumption should not exceed 14 standard drinks per week for men and 9 standard drinks per week for women. (One standard drink is considered 13.6 g or 17.2 mL of ethanol, or approximately 44 mL of 80-proof [40%] spirits, 148 mL of 12% wine, or 355 mL of 5% beer [Leung, Daskalopoulou, Dasgupta, et al., 2017].)

Physical Activity. Recommendations for individuals with normal BP (to reduce the possibility of developing hypertension) and for patients with hypertension (to reduce their BP) include the accumulation of 30 to 60 minutes of moderate-intensity dynamic exercise (such as walking, jogging, cycling, or swimming), 4 to 7 days per week, in addition to the routine activities of daily living (Leung, Daskalopoulou, Dasgupta, et al., 2017). Higher intensities of exercise are no more effective.

Moderately intense activity can lower BP, promote relaxation, and decrease or control body weight. Regular activity of this type can reduce SBP in the patient with hypertension by approximately 10 mm Hg. Sedentary people should be advised to increase activity levels gradually. People with heart disease or other serious health problems need a thorough examination, possibly including a stress test, before beginning an exercise program.

Avoidance of Tobacco Products. Nicotine contained in tobacco causes vasoconstriction and increases BP in people with hypertension. In addition, smoking tobacco is a major risk factor for cardiovascular disease. The cardiovascular benefits of discontinuing tobacco use can be seen within 1 year in all age groups. Everyone, especially people with hypertension, should be strongly advised to avoid tobacco use. The lower amounts of nicotine contained in smoking cessation aids usually will not raise BP and may be used as indicated. People who continue to use tobacco

products should be advised to monitor their BP during use. (See Chapter 11 and the Resources at the end of this chapter for links to smoking cessation materials.)

Stress Management. In patients with hypertension in whom stress may be contributing to BP elevation, stress management should be considered as an intervention. Individualized cognitive–behavioural interventions are more likely to be effective when relaxation techniques are used.

Drug Therapy. The implementation of the CHEP and Hypertension Canada recommendations has resulted in an increased use of antihypertensive medications, increased use of multiple antihypertensive medications, and improved persistence with medication use. The general goal of drug therapy is to achieve a BP of less than 140/90 mm Hg. For patients with chronic kidney disease or diabetes, target BP is less than 130/80 mm Hg. The drugs currently available for treating hypertension have two main actions: (1) to reduce SVR and (2) to decrease the volume of circulating blood (Table 35-8). The drugs used in the treatment of hypertension include diuretics, adrenergic (sympathetic) inhibitors, direct vasodilators, angiotensin inhibitors, and calcium channel blockers. The sites where the drugs exert their action and the methods of action are shown in Figure 35-5.

TABLE 35-8 DRUG THERAPY

Hypertension

Drug	Mechanism of Action	Adverse Effects	Nursing Considerations
Diuretics			
Thiazide and Related Diuretics			
Indapamide (Lozide) Metolazone (Zaroxolyn)	Inhibit NaCl reabsorption in the distal convoluted tubule; increase excretion of Na$^+$ and Cl$^-$. Initial decrease in ECF; sustained decrease in SVR. Lower BP moderately in 2–4 wk.	Fluid and electrolyte imbalances (volume depletion, hypokalemia, hyponatremia, hypochloremia, hypomagnesemia, hypercalcemia, hyperuricemia, metabolic alkalosis); CNS effects (vertigo, headache, weakness); GI effects (anorexia, nausea, vomiting, diarrhea, constipation, pancreatitis); sexual problems (impotence and decreased libido); blood dyscrasias; dermatological effects (photosensitivity, skin rash); decreased glucose tolerance	Monitor for orthostatic hypotension, hypokalemia, and alkalosis. Thiazides may potentiate cardiotoxicity of digoxin by producing hypokalemia. Dietary sodium restriction reduces the risk for hypokalemia. NSAIDs can decrease diuretic and antihypertensive effect of thiazide diuretics. Advise patient to supplement with potassium-rich foods. Current doses are lower than previously recommended. Indapamide should be administered with caution to patients with renal failure.
Loop Diuretics			
Bumetanide (Burinex) Ethacrynic acid (Edecrin) Furosemide (Lasix)	Inhibit NaCl reabsorption in the thick ascending limb of the loop of Henle. Increase excretion of Na$^+$ and Cl$^-$. More potent diuretic effect than thiazides, but shorter duration of action; less effective for hypertension.	Fluid electrolyte imbalance as with thiazides, except no hypercalcemia; ototoxicity (hearing impairment, deafness, vertigo) that is usually reversible; metabolic effects, including hyperuricemia, hyperglycemia, increased LDL cholesterol and triglycerides with decreased HDL cholesterol	Monitor for orthostatic hypotension and electrolyte abnormalities. Loop diuretics remain effective despite renal insufficiency. Diuretic effect of drug increases at higher doses.
Potassium-Sparing Diuretics			
Amiloride hydrochloride (Midamor, Novamilor)	Reduce K$^+$ and Na$^+$ exchange in the distal and collecting tubules. Reduce excretion of K$^+$, H$^+$, Ca^{2+}, and Mg^{2+}.	Hyperkalemia, nausea, vomiting, diarrhea, headache, leg cramps, and dizziness	Monitor for orthostatic hypotension and hyperkalemia. Potassium-sparing diuretics are contraindicated for use in patients with renal failure and used with caution in patients on ACE inhibitors or angiotensin II blockers. Avoid potassium supplements.
Spironolactone (Aldactone)	Inhibit the Na$^+$-retaining and K$^+$-excreting effects of aldosterone in the distal and collecting tubules.	Same as amiloride; may cause gynecomastia, impotence, decreased libido, and menstrual irregularities	

TABLE 35-8 DRUG THERAPY

Hypertension—cont'd

Drug	Mechanism of Action	Adverse Effects	Nursing Considerations
Adrenergic Inhibitors			
Central-Acting Adrenergic Antagonists			
Clonidine hydrochloride (Catapres)	Reduce sympathetic outflow from CNS. Reduce peripheral sympathetic tone, produces vasodilation; decrease SVR and BP.	Dry mouth, sedation, impotence, nausea, dizziness, sleep disturbance, nightmares, restlessness, and depression; symptomatic bradycardia in patients with conduction disorder	Sudden discontinuation may cause withdrawal syndrome, including rebound hypertension, tachycardia, headache, tremors, apprehension, and sweating. Chewing gum or hard candy may relieve dry mouth. Alcohol and sedatives increase sedation. May be given transdermally with fewer adverse effects and better patient adherence.
Methyldopa	Same as clonidine.	Sedation, fatigue, orthostatic hypotension, decreased libido, impotence, dry mouth, hemolytic anemia, hepatotoxicity, sodium and water retention, psychological depression	Instruct patient about daytime sedation and avoidance of hazardous activities. Administration of a single daily dose at bedtime minimizes sedative effect.
α₁-Adrenergic Blockers			
Doxazosin mesylate (Cardura) Prazosin hydrochloride (Minipress) Terazosin hydrochloride (Hytrin)	Block α_1-adrenergic effects, producing peripheral vasodilation (decrease SVR and BP).	Variable amount of orthostatic hypotension, depending on the plasma volume; may see profound orthostatic hypotension with syncope within 90 min after initial dose; retention of salt and water	Reduced resistance to the outflow of urine in benign prostatic hyperplasia. Taking drug at bedtime reduces risks associated with orthostatic hypotension. Has beneficial effects on lipid profile.
Phentolamine mesylate (Rogitine)	Block α_1-adrenergic receptors, resulting in peripheral vasodilation (decrease SVR and BP).	Acute, prolonged hypotension, cardiac dysrhythmias, tachycardia, weakness, flushing; abdominal pain, nausea, and exacerbation of peptic ulcer	Used in short-term management of pheochromocytoma. Also used locally to prevent necrosis of skin and subcutaneous tissue after extravasation of an α-adrenergic drug. No oral formulation.
β-Adrenergic Blockers			
Acebutolol hydrochloride (Sectral) Atenolol (Tenormin) Betaxolol hydrochloride Bisoprolol fumarate Carvedilol Metoprolol tartrate Nadolol Propranolol hydrochloride Timolol maleate	Reduce BP by antagonizing β_1-adrenergic effects. Decrease CO and reduce sympathetic vasoconstrictor tone. Decrease renin secretion by kidney.	Bronchospasm, atrioventricular conduction block, impaired peripheral circulation; nightmares, depression, weakness, reduced exercise capacity; may induce or exacerbate heart failure in susceptible patients; sudden withdrawal of β-adrenergic blockers may cause rebound hypertension and exacerbate symptoms of ischemic heart disease	β-Adrenergic blockers vary in lipid solubility, selectivity, and presence of partial sympathomimetic effect, which explains different therapeutic and adverse effect profiles of specific agents. Monitor pulse regularly. Use with caution in patients with diabetes mellitus because drug may mask signs of hypoglycemia.
Esmolol hydrochloride (Brevibloc)	Reduce BP by antagonizing β_1-adrenergic effects.	—	IV administration; has rapid onset and brief duration of action.
Combined α- and β-adrenergic blocker			
Labetalol hydrochloride (Trandate)	α_1, β_1-, and β_2-Adrenergic blocking properties, producing peripheral vasodilation and decreased heart rate. Reduce CO, SVR, and BP.	Dizziness, fatigue, nausea, vomiting, dyspepsia, paresthesia, nasal stuffiness, impotence, edema; hepatic toxicity	Same as β-adrenergic blockers. IV form available for hypertensive crisis in hospitalized patients. Patients must be kept supine during IV administration. Assess patient tolerance of upright position (severe orthostatic hypotension) before allowing upright activities (e.g., use of commode).
Direct Vasodilators			
Diazoxide (Proglycem)	Reduce SVR and BP by direct arterial vasodilation.	Reflex sympathetic activation, producing increased HR, CO, and salt and water retention; hyperglycemia, especially in patients with type 2 diabetes	IV use only for hypertensive crisis in hospitalized patients. Administer only into peripheral vein.

Continued

TABLE 35-8   DRUG THERAPY
Hypertension—cont'd

Drug	Mechanism of Action	Adverse Effects	Nursing Considerations
Hydralazine hydrochloride (Apresoline)	Reduce SVR and BP by direct arterial vasodilation.	Headache, nausea, flushing, palpitation, tachycardia, dizziness, and angina; hemolytic anemia, vasculitis, and rapidly progressive glomerulonephritis	IV use for hypertensive crisis in hospitalized patients. Twice-daily oral dosage. Not used as monotherapy because of adverse effects. Contraindicated for use in patients with coronary artery disease; used with caution in patients >40 yr of age.
Minoxidil (Loniten)	Reduce SVR and BP by direct arterial vasodilation.	Reflex tachycardia, marked sodium and fluid retention (may require loop diuretics for control), and hirsutism; may cause ECG changes (flattened and inverted T waves) not related to ischemia	Reserved for treatment of severe hypertension associated with renal failure and resistant to other therapy. Once- or twice-daily dosage.
Nitroglycerin	Relax arterial and venous smooth muscle reducing preload and SVR. At low dose, venous dilation predominates; at higher dose, arterial dilation is present.	Hypotension, headache, vomiting, flushing IV use for hypertensive crisis in hospitalized patients with myocardial ischemia	Administered by continuous IV infusion with pump or control device.
Sodium nitroprusside (Nipride)	Direct arterial vasodilation reduce SVR and BP.	Acute hypotension, nausea, vomiting, muscle twitching; signs of thiocyanate toxicity include anorexia, nausea, fatigue, disorientation	IV use for hypertensive crisis in hospitalized patients. Administered by continuous IV infusion with pump or control device. Use intra-arterial monitoring of BP. Light-resistant bags, bottles, and administration sets must be used; stable for 24 hr. Monitor thiocyanate levels with prolonged (>24–48 hr) use.

Angiotensin Inhibitors
Angiotensin-Converting Enzyme (ACE) Inhibitors

Benazepril hydrochloride (Lotensin)	Inhibit ACE; reduce conversion of angiotensin I to angiotensin II (A-II); prevent A-II–mediated vasoconstriction. Inhibit ACE when oral drugs not appropriate.	Hypotension, loss of taste, cough, hyperkalemia, acute kidney injury, skin rash, angioneurotic edema; same as oral forms	ASA and NSAIDs may reduce drug effectiveness. Addition of diuretic enhances drug effect. Should not be used with potassium-sparing diuretics. Can cause fetal morbidity or mortality. Captopril may be given orally for hypertensive crisis.
Captopril			
Enalapril sodium (Vasotec)			Given by IV route over 5 min; may be given every 6 hr.
Fosinopril sodium			
Lisinopril (Prinivil, Zestril)			
Perindopril erbumine (Coversyl)			
Quinapril hydrochloride (Accupril)			
Ramipril (Altace)			
Trandolapril (Mavik, Tarka)			
Enalaprilat injection (Vasotec IV)			

Angiotensin II Receptor Blockers

Candesartan cilexetil (Atacand)	Prevent action of angiotensin II and produce vasodilation and increased salt and water excretion.	Hyperkalemia, decreased kidney function	Full effect on BP may not be seen for 3–6 wk.
Eprosartan mesylate (Teveten)			
Irbesartan (Avapro)			
Losartan potassium (Cozaar)			
Telmisartan (Micardis)			
Valsartan (Diovan)			

Calcium Channel Blockers

Amlodipine besylate (Caduet, Norvasc)	Block movement of extracellular calcium into cells, causing vasodilation and decreased SVR.	Nausea, headache, dizziness, peripheral edema; reflex tachycardia (with dihydropyridines); reflex decrease HR (with diltiazem); constipation (with verapamil)	Use with caution in patients with heart failure. Contraindicated for use in patients with second- or third-degree heart block. Sustained-release formulations for some drugs. Avoid grapefruit consumption when on nifedipine.
Diltiazem hydrochloride (Tiazac)			
Felodipine (Plendil)			
Nifedipine (Adalat)			
Verapamil hydrochloride (Isoptin)			

ACE, angiotensin-converting inhibitor; *ASA,* acetylsalicylic acid (Aspirin); *BP,* blood pressure; *CNS,* central nervous system; *CO,* cardiac output; *ECF,* extracellular fluid; *ECG,* electrocardiogram; *GI,* gastro-intestinal; *HDL,* high-density lipoprotein; *HR,* heart rate; *IV,* intravenous; *LDL,* low-density lipoprotein; *NSAIDs,* nonsteroidal anti-inflammatory drugs; *SVR,* systemic vascular resistance.

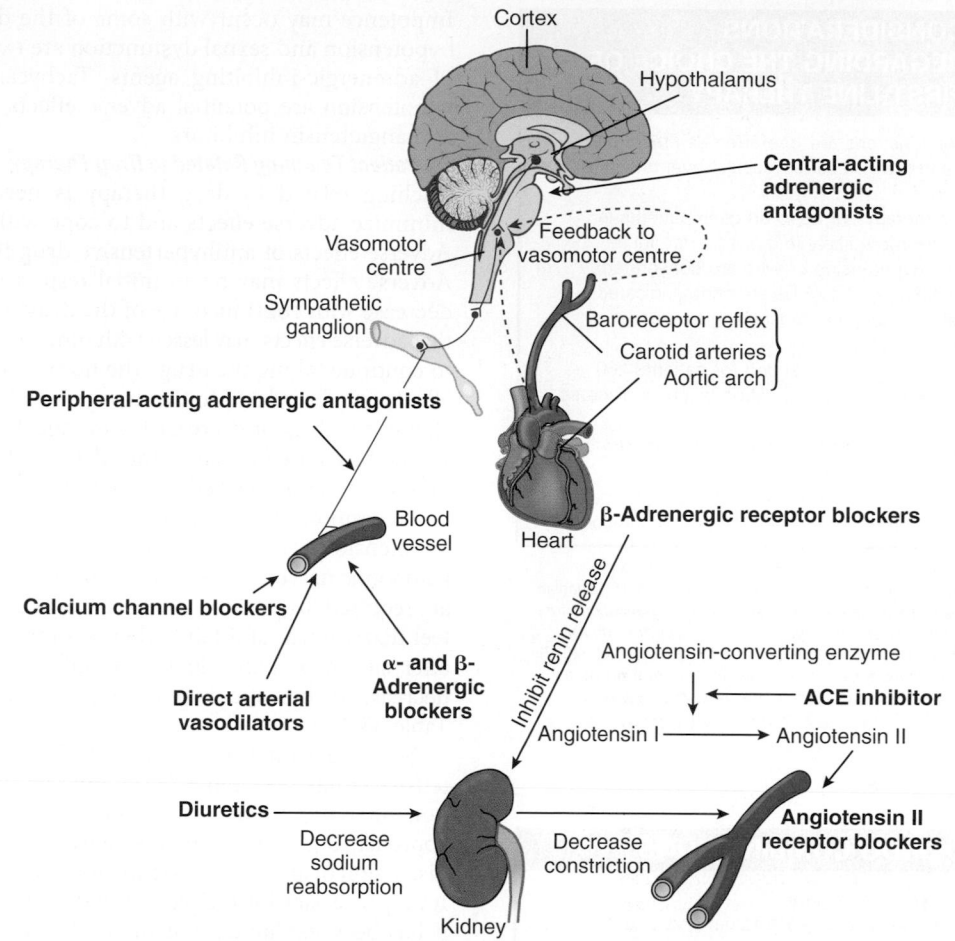

FIGURE 35-5 Site and method of action of various antihypertensive drugs. *ACE*, angiotensin-converting enzyme.
Source: U.S. Department of Health and Human Services. (2003). *The seventh report of the Joint National Committee on Detection, Evaluation, and Treatment of High Blood Pressure (JNC-7).* Washington, DC: National Institutes of Health.

Although the precise action of diuretics in the reduction of BP is unclear, it is known that they promote sodium and water excretion, reduce plasma volume, decrease sodium in the arteriolar walls, and reduce the vascular response to catecholamines. Adrenergic-inhibiting drugs act by diminishing the sympathetic effects that increase BP. Adrenergic inhibitors include drugs that act centrally on the vasomotor centre and peripherally to inhibit NE release or to block the adrenergic receptors on blood vessels. Direct vasodilators decrease the BP by relaxing vascular smooth muscle and reducing SVR. Calcium channel blockers increase sodium excretion and cause arteriolar vasodilation by preventing the movement of extracellular calcium into cells.

There are two types of angiotensin inhibitors. The first type is angiotensin-converting enzyme (ACE) inhibitors, which prevent the conversion of angiotensin I to A-II and thus reduce A-II–mediated vasoconstriction and sodium and water retention. The second type is A-II receptor blockers (ARBs), which prevent A-II from binding to its receptors in the walls of the blood vessels.

Drug therapy is recommended for all patients at low risk with stage 1 hypertension (140–159/90–99 mm Hg), although lifestyle management may be the sole therapy. For patients with diabetes or chronic kidney disease, target blood pressure is <130/80 mm Hg. Many younger Canadians with hypertension have multiple cardiovascular risks and are not treated with antihypertensive drugs. Currently, this is a gap in treatment. See the treatment algorithm of systolic–diastolic hypertension without other compelling indications, in Figure 35-3 and Tables 35-9 and 35-10.

The initial drug may be started at a low dosage for several weeks. The full effects of antihypertensive medication may not be apparent for up to 6 weeks. If the BP is not controlled, the dosage of the first-line drug can be increased. A second drug from a different class can be substituted or added if the initial drug was ineffective or there were adverse effects to the initial drug. For most patients, at least two medications (probably taken in a single tablet) will be necessary in addition to lifestyle changes. Before proceeding with the addition or substitution of medication, consideration should be given to possible reasons for the lack of response to drug therapy.

A new drug therapy has been marketed recently in Canada. Although long-term mortality and morbidity studies have yet to be published, it has been authorized for use in Canada. Aliskiren fumarate (Rasilez) is an oral direct renin inhibitor (DRI). Renin inhibition acts on the conversion of angiotensinogen to angiotensin I. This is the rate-limiting step in the production of A-II, which is a key mediator of BP, body fluid volume, and vascular remodelling. DRIs may be more effective in inhibiting RAAS when compared with ACE inhibitors or ARBs.

The addition of a third or fourth drug may be necessary, but only after the maximum doses of the first and second drugs have been achieved.

TABLE 35-9 CONSIDERATIONS REGARDING THE CHOICE OF FIRST-LINE THERAPY

- Low-dose single pill combinations are preferred as first line therapy to reduce BP and prevent cardiovascular events and reduce the risk of adverse events.
- Use caution in initiating therapy with two drugs in patients in whom adverse events are more likely (e.g., frail older adult, patients with orthostatic hypotension or who are dehydrated).
- ACE inhibitors, renin inhibitors, and ARBs are contraindicated in pregnancy, and caution is required in prescribing to women of child-bearing potential.
- β-Adrenergic blockers are not recommended for patients ≥60 yr without another compelling comorbid condition (such as diabetes mellitus or heart disease).
- Diuretic-induced hypokalemia should be avoided through the use of potassium-sparing agents, if required.
- ACE inhibitors are not recommended (as monotherapy) for patients who are Black, without another compelling comorbid condition.

ACE, angiotensin-converting enzyme; *ARB,* angiotensin II receptor blocker.
Sources: Canadian Hypertension Education Program (CHEP). (2015). *2015 Canadian Hypertension Education Program recommendations. Part 2, Recommendations for hypertension treatment* (Slide 32). Available at *http://guidelines.hypertension.ca/chep-resources/*; and Leung, A. A., Daskalopoulou, S. S., Dasgupta, K., et al. (2017). Hypertension Canada's 2017 guidelines for diagnosis, risk assessment, prevention, and treatment of hypertension in adults. *Canadian Journal of Cardiology, 33*(5), 557-576. doi: http://dx.doi.org/10.1016/j.cjca.2017.03.005.

TABLE 35-10 DRUG COMBINATIONS

To achieve optimal blood pressure targets:
- Multiple drugs are often required to reach target levels, especially in patients with type 2 diabetes.
- Replace multiple antihypertensive agents with single pill combination therapy.
- Low doses of multiple drugs may be more effective and better tolerated than higher doses of fewer drugs.
- Reassess patients with uncontrolled blood pressure at least every 2 months.
- A combination of two first-line agents may also be considered as initial treatment of hypertension.
- The combination of ACE inhibitors and ARBs should not be used.

ACEIs, angiotensin-converting enzyme inhibitors; *ARBs,* angiotensin II receptor blockers; *CCB,* calcium channel blocker.
Source: Hypertension Canada. (2017). *What's new? 2017 Hypertension Canada guidelines for the management of hypertension.* Retrieved from *https://www.hypertension.ca/images/CHEP_2017/HTN_Whats_New_2017_EN.pdf.*

After 1 year of optimum BP control, step-down therapy may be tried. The number of medications and their dosages are gradually decreased to the lowest amount that controls the BP. Regular follow-up is needed to detect any elevation of BP.

Adverse effects of antihypertensive drugs may be so severe or undesirable that the patient does not adhere to therapy. Table 35-8 describes the major adverse effects of antihypertensive drugs. Hyperuricemia, hyperglycemia, and hypokalemia are common adverse effects with both thiazide and loop diuretics. ACE inhibitors can lead to high levels of bradykinin, which can cause coughing. An individual who develops a cough with the use of ACE inhibitors may be switched to an A-II receptor blocker. Hyperkalemia can be a serious adverse effect of the potassium-sparing diuretics and ACE inhibitors.

Impotence may occur with some of the diuretics. Orthostatic hypotension and sexual dysfunction are two undesirable effects of adrenergic-inhibiting agents. Tachycardia and orthostatic hypotension are potential adverse effects of both vasodilators and angiotensin inhibitors.

Patient Teaching Related to Drug Therapy. Patient and caregiver teaching related to drug therapy is needed to identify and minimize adverse effects and to cope with therapeutic effects. Adverse effects of antihypertensive drug therapy are common. Adverse effects may be an initial response to a drug and may decrease with continued use of the drug. Informing the patient that adverse effects may lessen with time may enable the individual to continue taking the drug. The number or severity of adverse effects may be related to the dosage, and it may be necessary to change the drug or decrease the dosage. In this case, the patient should be advised to report the adverse effects to the health care provider who prescribed the medication.

A common adverse effect of several of these drugs is orthostatic hypotension. This condition is caused by an alteration of the autonomic nervous system's mechanisms for regulating BP, which are required for position changes. Consequently, the patient may feel dizzy, weak, and faint when assuming an upright position after sitting or lying down. (Specific measures to control or decrease orthostatic hypotension are presented later on in Table 35-15.)

Sexual dysfunction may occur with many of the antihypertensive drugs (see Table 35-8) and can be a major reason for nonadherence to the treatment plan. Often, the nurse must approach the patient on this sensitive subject and encourage discussion of any sexual dysfunction the patient may experience. It may be easier for the patient to discuss sexual problems once it has been explained that the drug may be the source of the problem and that the adverse effects can be decreased or eliminated by changing to another antihypertensive drug. The patient should be encouraged to discuss adverse effects with the health care provider who prescribed the medication. If the patient is reluctant to do so, the nurse may offer to alert the health care provider to the sexual adverse effect that the patient is experiencing. There are many options for treating hypertension; a plan that is acceptable to the patient should be achievable.

Some unpleasant effects of drugs result from their therapeutic effect, but the impact can be minimized. For example, dry mouth and frequent voiding are unpleasant effects of diuretics. Sugarless gum or candy may relieve the dry mouth. The nurse can assist the patient to develop a medication schedule to minimize unpleasant effects. When frequent urination interrupts sleep, taking the diuretic earlier in the day may be beneficial. Adverse effects of vasodilators and adrenergic inhibitors decrease if the drugs are taken in the evening. BP is lowest during the night and highest shortly after awakening; therefore, drugs with 24-hour duration of action should be taken as early in the morning as possible (e.g., 0400 or 0500 hours, if the patient awakens to void).

Resistant Hypertension. *Resistant hypertension* is the failure to reach goal BP in patients who are taking full doses of an appropriate three-drug therapy regimen that includes a diuretic. The nurse should carefully explore reasons why the patient is not at goal BP (Table 35-11). Studies have shown that the use of *renal denervation* (destruction of overactive renal nerves) reduces BP and muscle sympathetic nerve activity in patients with resistant hypertension. The exact mechanisms underlying sympathetic neural inhibition are not clear (Hering, Lambert, Marusic, et al., 2013).

TABLE 35-11 CAUSES OF RESISTANT HYPERTENSION

Improper BP measurement
- Volume overload
- Excess salt intake
- Volume retention from kidney disease
- Inadequate diuretic therapy

Drug-induced or other causes
- Nonadherence
- Illegal drugs (e.g., cocaine, amphetamines)
- Inadequate drug dosages
- Inappropriate combinations of drug therapy
- Nonsteroidal anti-inflammatory drugs
- Sympathomimetics (e.g., decongestants, diet pills)
- Oral contraceptives
- Corticosteroids
- Cyclosporin and tacrolimus (Prograf)
- Erythropoietin
- Licorice (including some chewing tobacco)
- Selected over-the-counter dietary or herbal supplements and medicines (e.g., ma huang, bitter orange)

Associated conditions
- Increasing obesity
- Excess alcohol consumption

Identifiable causes of secondary hypertension

Source: National Heart, Lung, and Blood Institute. (2004). *Seventh report of the Joint National Committee on Prevention, Detection, Evaluation, and Treatment of High Blood Pressure (JNC-7)*. NIH Publication No. 04-5230. Bethesda, MD: The Institute. Retrieved from *www.nhlbi.nih.gov/guidelines/hypertension/jnc7full.pdf*.

NURSING MANAGEMENT PRIMARY HYPERTENSION

NURSING ASSESSMENT
Subjective and objective data that should be obtained from a patient with hypertension are presented in Table 35-12.

NURSING DIAGNOSES
Nursing diagnoses and collaborative problems for the patient with hypertension include, but are not limited to, those presented in Table 35-13.

PLANNING
The overall goals for the patient with hypertension are that the patient will (1) achieve and maintain the individually determined target BP; (2) understand, accept, and implement the therapeutic plan; (3) experience minimal or no unpleasant adverse effects of therapy; and (4) be confident about the ability to manage and cope with this condition.

NURSING IMPLEMENTATION
HEALTH PROMOTION. Primary prevention of hypertension provides an attractive alternative to the costly cycle of managing hypertension and its complications. Current recommendations for primary prevention are based on lifestyle modifications that have been shown to prevent or delay the expected rise in BP in susceptible people. A diet rich in fruits, vegetables, and low-fat dairy foods, with reduced saturated and total fats, significantly lowers BP (see Table 35-7). This diet has been recommended for primary prevention in the general population. Dietary modifications that do not require active participation of the individual, such as a reduction in the amount of salt added to processed foods, may be even more effective.

TABLE 35-12 NURSING ASSESSMENT

Hypertension Data

Subjective Data
Important Health Information
Current health history: Family history of hypertension or cardiovascular disease; smoking or other tobacco use, alcohol use; sedentary lifestyle; usual salt and fat intake; weight gain or loss
Past health history: Known duration and past workup of high BP; cardiovascular, cerebro-vascular, renal, or thyroid disease; diabetes; pituitary disorders; obesity; dyslipidemia; menopause or hormone replacement status
Medications: Use of any prescription or over-the-counter, illicit, or natural health products; previous use of antihypertensive drug therapy

Symptoms
- Dyspnea on exertion, palpitations on exertion, anginal chest pain
- Fatigue
- Intermittent claudication, muscle cramps
- Nocturia
- Dizziness; blurred vision, paresthesias
- Erectile dysfunction, decreased libido

Objective Data
Cardiovascular
BP consistently >140 mm Hg systolic or 90 mm Hg diastolic, orthostatic change in BP and pulse; abnormal heart sounds; laterally displaced, sustained, forceful, apical pulse; diminished or absent peripheral pulses; carotid, kidney, ischial, or femoral bruits; presence of edema

Musculo-skeletal
Truncal obesity

Neurological
Mental status changes

Possible Findings
Abnormal serum electrolytes (especially potassium); increased creatinine, glucose, cholesterol, and triglyceride levels; proteinuria, microalbuminuria; evidence of ischemic heart disease and left ventricular hypertrophy on ECG

BP, blood pressure; *ECG,* electrocardiogram.

Individual Patient Evaluation. The majority of cases of hypertension are identified through routine screening procedures such as insurance and pre-employment or premilitary physical examinations. The nurse in these settings, as well as in most other practice settings, is in an ideal position to assess for the presence of hypertension, identify the risk factors for hypertension and coronary artery disease, and teach the patient about these conditions. In addition to BP determination, a complete health assessment should include such factors as age, sex, and race; diet history (including sodium and alcohol intake); weight patterns; and family history of heart disease, stroke, renal disease, and diabetes mellitus. Medications taken, both prescribed and over-the-counter, should be noted. The patient should be asked about a previous history of high BP and the results of treatment (if any) (see Table 35-12).

Initially, the BP is taken two or three times, at least 2 minutes apart, with the average pressure recorded as the value for that visit. Waiting for at least 2 minutes between readings allows the venous blood to drain from the arm and prevents inaccurate readings. Size and placement of the BP cuff are important

TABLE 35-13   NURSING ASSESSMENT

Hypertension

Nursing Diagnoses

- *Ineffective health maintenance* related to *insufficient resources* (lack of knowledge)
- *Anxiety* related to *stressors, threat to current status* (lifestyle changes associated with hypertension)
- *Sexual dysfunction* related to *vulnerability* (effects of antihypertensive medications)
- *Ineffective health management* related to:
  - *Insufficient knowledge of therapeutic regimen*
  - *Difficulty managing complex treatment regimen*
  - *Perceived barrier* (cost of medications)
  - *Insufficient social support*
  - *Difficulty navigating complex health care systems*
  - *Powerlessness*
- *Disturbed body image* related to *alteration in self-perception*
- *Ineffective peripheral tissue perfusion* related to *insufficient knowledge of disease process* (hypertension)

Collaborative Problems

- Potential complication: adverse effects from antihypertensive therapy
- Potential complication: hypertensive crisis
- Potential complication: stroke

TABLE 35-14   APPROPRIATE TECHNIQUE FOR MEASURING BLOOD PRESSURE

1. The use of electronic (oscillometric) measurement methods is preferred to manual measurement. The patient should be seated with the arm bared, supported, and positioned at heart level. The patient should have neither smoked nor ingested caffeine within 30 min before measurement. The patient should also not have used substances containing adrenergic stimulants, such as phenylephrine or pseudoephedrine, which may be found in decongestants or ophthalmic drops.
2. The patient's bowel and bladder should be comfortable. A quiet environment at a comfortable room temperature should be provided.
3. The patient should stay quiet before and during the procedure.
4. For initial readings, the nurse should take the blood pressure in both arms, and subsequently measure in the arm with the highest reading. Thereafter, two measurements should be taken on the side where the BP is highest. Out-of-office measurement should be performed to confirm the initial diagnosis of hypertension.
5. The appropriate cuff size must be used to ensure an accurate measurement. The rubber bladder should reach nearly around (at least 80% of the circumference) or completely encircle the arm. Cuff width should be at least 40% of the arm circumference. Several sizes of cuffs (e.g., child, adult, and large adult) should be available.
6. Measurements should be taken with a mercury sphygmomanometer, a recently calibrated anaeroid manometer, or a calibrated electronic device. Electronic measurement methods are preferred.
7. Both systolic and diastolic pressures should be recorded. The disappearance of sound should be used for the diastolic reading.
8. Two or more readings (taken at least 2 min apart) should be averaged. If the first two readings differ by >5 mm Hg, additional readings should be obtained.
9. The patient should be informed of the reading and advised of the need for periodic remeasurement.

BP, blood pressure.
Source: Adapted from Leung, A. A., Daskalopoulou, S. S., Dasgupta, K., et al. (2017). Hypertension Canada's 2017 Guidelines for diagnosis, risk assessment, prevention, and treatment of hypertension in adults. *Canadian Journal of Cardiology, 33*(5), 557-576. doi: http://dx.doi.org/10.1016/j.cjca.2017.03.005.

considerations for accurate measurement. The width of the inflatable bladder should be 40% of the upper arm circumference, and the length should be 80%. Use of a cuff that is too small or too large will result in readings that are falsely high or low, respectively. Ensure that the cuff is placed 2.5 cm above the antecubital fossa.

BP measurements of both arms should be performed initially to detect any differences between arms. Atherosclerotic narrowing of the subclavian artery can cause a falsely low reading on the side where the narrowing occurs. Therefore, the arm with the higher reading should be used for all subsequent BP measurements. The patient's arm is uncovered and placed at the level of the heart. The cuff should be inflated until no pulse is felt in the brachial artery located in the antecubital fossa of the arm being used. The cuff is then inflated an additional 10 to 20 mm Hg to ensure vascular occlusion. The pressure is released at 2 mm Hg per second. Releasing the pressure any more slowly or quickly may create inaccurate readings. Both SBP and DBP should be recorded, with the DBP recorded as the disappearance of sound (Table 35-14).

The BP and the pulse are initially measured with the patient in either the supine or the sitting position after at least 5 minutes of rest. BP and pulse should be measured again after 2 minutes, in the standing position. Usually, the SBP decreases on standing, whereas the DBP and the pulse increase. A decrease of more than 10 mm Hg in SBP, or any decrease in DBP when standing, is abnormal and should prompt further investigation. Common causes of abnormal postural BP values include intravascular volume loss (e.g., with diuretic therapy or dehydration) and inadequate vasoconstrictor mechanisms related to disease or medications. Postural changes in BP and pulse should be measured in older adults, people taking antihypertensive drugs, and when orthostatic hypotension is suspected. The common definition for

orthostatic hypotension is a decrease of 20 mm Hg (or more) in SBP or a decrease of 10 mm Hg (or more) in DBP that occurs when an individual assumes a standing position.

Screening Programs. Screening programs in the community are widely used to assess BP. At the time of the BP measurement, each person should be informed in writing of the numerical value of the reading and, if necessary, why further evaluation is important. Effort and resources should be focused on controlling BP in the person already identified as having hypertension; identifying and controlling BP in high-risk groups such as people who are Black or Southeast Asian, people who are obese, and blood relatives of people with hypertension; and screening those with limited access to the health care system.

Cardiovascular Risk Factor Modification. Education regarding cardiovascular risk factors is appropriate for individual and targeted screening programs. Modifiable cardiovascular risk factors include hypertension, obesity, diabetes mellitus, elevated serum lipids, tobacco use, and physical inactivity. Risk factors can easily be identified and modification discussed with the patient. (Health-promoting behaviours for cardiovascular risk factors are presented in Chapter 36, Table 36-4 and Figure 36-5.)

TABLE 35-15 PATIENT & CAREGIVER TEACHING GUIDE

Hypertension

When presenting information to the patient or caregiver, the nurse should do the following:

1. Provide the numerical value of the patient's BP and explain what it means.
2. Inform the patient that hypertension is usually asymptomatic and symptoms do not reliably indicate BP levels.
3. Explain that hypertension means elevated BP and does not relate to a "hyper" personality.
4. Explain that long-term follow-up and therapy are necessary to treat hypertension.
5. Explain that therapy will not cure, but should control, hypertension.
6. Tell the patient that controlled hypertension is usually compatible with an excellent prognosis and a normal lifestyle.
7. Explain the potential dangers of uncontrolled hypertension.
8. Be specific about the names, the actions, the dosages, and the adverse effects of prescribed medications.
9. Tell the patient to plan regular and convenient times for taking medications.
10. Tell the patient not to discontinue drugs abruptly because withdrawal may cause a severe hypertensive reaction.
11. Tell the patient not to double up on doses when a dose is missed.
12. Inform the patient that, if BP increases, the patient should not take an increased medication dosage before consulting with the health care provider.
13. Tell the patient not to take a medication belonging to someone else.
14. Inform the patient that adverse effects of medication often diminish with time.
15. Tell the patient to consult with the health care provider about changing drugs or dosages if impotence or other sexual problems develop.
16. Tell the patient to supplement the diet with foods high in potassium (e.g., citrus fruits and green leafy vegetables) if taking potassium-losing diuretics.
17. Tell the patient to avoid hot baths, excessive amounts of alcohol, and strenuous exercise within 3 hr of taking medications that promote vasodilation.
18. Explain that, to decrease orthostatic hypotension, the patient should arise slowly from bed, sit on the side of the bed for a few minutes, stand slowly, not stand still for prolonged periods, do leg exercises to increase venous return, sleep with the head of the bed raised or on pillows, and lie or sit down when dizziness occurs.
19. Caution about potentially high-risk over-the-counter medications, such as high-sodium antacids, appetite suppressants, and cold and sinus medications. Advise the patient to read warning labels and to consult with a pharmacist.

BP, blood pressure.

AMBULATORY AND HOME CARE. The primary nursing responsibilities for long-term management of hypertension are to assist the patient in reducing BP and adhering to the treatment plan. Nursing actions include patient and family teaching, detection and reporting of adverse treatment effects, adherence assessment and enhancement, and evaluation of therapeutic effectiveness (Table 35-15). Patient and caregiver teaching includes the following: (1) nutritional therapy, (2) drug therapy, (3) physical activity, (4) home monitoring of BP (if appropriate), (5) tobacco cessation (if applicable), and (6) stress management.

Physical Activity. *Physical activity* is bodily movement produced by skeletal muscles that requires energy expenditure.

♻ EVIDENCE-INFORMED PRACTICE

Translating Research Into Practice

The nurse is caring for Thao Nguyen, a 46-year-old man with a history of poorly controlled hypertension and chronic kidney disease. The nurse notes that he is taking three antihypertensive medications. He tells the nurse that he can no longer live with the adverse effects of these drugs (e.g., fatigue, dry mouth, erectile dysfunction). He states that he wants to stop taking the medications. He believes that if he changes his lifestyle by reducing salt from his diet, losing weight, and beginning exercise, he can control his hypertension.

Best Available Evidence	Clinician Expertise	Patient Preferences and Values
Uncontrolled BP places persons with concurrent risk for cardiovascular disease (e.g., diabetes, kidney disease) at highest risk for a cardiovascular event (e.g., stroke). Most patients with hypertension will need two or more medications to achieve their goal BP in addition to lifestyle changes.	The nurse knows that lifestyle changes can help reduce and control BP in many patients. However, patients with poorly controlled hypertension and target-organ disease require medications to control BP and prevent further complications.	Mr. Nguyen wishes to eliminate antihypertensive medications because of unpleasant and unacceptable adverse effects that are interfering with his quality of life.

Decision and Actions

The nurse discusses the role of lifestyle changes and medications in the treatment of hypertension and prevention of (further) target-organ disease with Mr. Nguyen. The nurse supports his intention to make lifestyle changes and validates his concerns regarding the adverse effects of the medications. They discuss these adverse effects, and the nurse explains that it may be possible to change some of his medications to eliminate or reduce the unpleasant adverse effects. However, given the severity of his hypertension and the chronic kidney disease, he will need to be on medications on a long-term basis. Any of his plans to discontinue medications need to be discussed with his health care provider.

Reference for Evidence

Daskalopoulou, S. S., Rabi, D. M., Zarnke, K. B., et al. (2015). The 2015 Canadian hypertension education program recommendations for blood pressure measurement, diagnosis, assessment of risk, prevention, and treatment of hypertension. *Journal of Cardiology, 31,* 549–568. doi:10.1016/j.cjca.2015.02.016.

INFORMATICS IN PRACTICE

Monitoring Blood Pressure

- Patients with hypertension who have a smartphone or computer access should be encouraged to use applications aimed at helping them manage their care, including BP self-monitoring and appointment tracking.
- Patients enter their SBP and DBP, heart rate, and other information, including the arm measured. They also indicate whether they were standing, sitting, or lying down as well as the time the BP was taken.
- At appointment time, the nurse can review the reports generated from the application to assist in determining how well the patient's BP has been controlled.

DBP, diastolic BP; *SBP,* systolic BP.

Health benefits from physical activity can be achieved with moderate-intensity activities. The goal for all adults is to accumulate 30 minutes of moderate-intensity activity daily. Generally, physical activity is more likely to be sustained if it is safe and enjoyable, fits easily into the daily schedule, and does not generate financial or social costs.

Shopping malls in many communities are open early in the morning (before shopping hours) and provide a warm, safe, flat area for walking. In some communities, health clubs offer special "off-peak" rates to encourage physical activity among older adults. Cardiac rehabilitation programs offer supervised exercise with education about reduction of cardiovascular risk factors. Nurses can assist people with hypertension to increase their physical activity by identifying and communicating the need for increased activity, explaining the difference between physical activity and exercise, assisting in initiating activity, and following up appropriately.

Home Blood Pressure Monitoring. Some patients benefit from regularly monitoring their BP at home. Home BP measurement may give a more valid indication of the BP because the patient is more relaxed. It is important to emphasize to the patient that a single reading is not as important as a series of readings over time. The patient should be instructed to take BP readings weekly (unless otherwise instructed), once the BP has stabilized. A log of the BP measurements should be maintained by the patient and brought to office visits.

Home BP readings may help achieve patient adherence by reinforcing the need to continue therapy. A patient may become excessively concerned with the BP readings when using home monitoring. Generally, however, this practice should reassure the patient that the treatment is effective.

Patient Adherence. A major challenge in the long-term management of the patient with hypertension is poor adherence with the prescribed treatment plan. The reasons are many and include inadequate patient teaching, unpleasant adverse effects of drugs, return of BP to normal range while on medication, lack of motivation, high cost of drugs, and lack of a trusting relationship between the patient and the health care provider. In addition to using BP determinations as an indicator of adherence, the nurse should also assess the patient's diet, activity level, and lifestyle.

Individual assessment to determine the reasons the patient does not adhere to the treatment plan as well as the development of an individualized plan with the patient's assistance are essential. The plan should be compatible with the patient's personality, habits, and lifestyle. Active patient participation increases the likelihood of adherence to the treatment plan. Measures such as involving the patient in scheduling medication convenient to a daily routine, helping the patient link pill-taking with another daily activity, and involving family members (if necessary) help increase patient adherence. Substituting combination tablets for multiple drugs once the BP is stabilized may also facilitate adherence because the patient has to take fewer pills each day and the cost may be less. It is important to help the patient and the family understand that hypertension is a chronic condition that cannot be cured but can be controlled with drug therapy, diet therapy, physical activity, periodic evaluation, and other relevant lifestyle changes (Table 35-16).

EVALUATION

The overall expected outcomes are that the patient with hypertension will (1) achieve and maintain desired BP as defined for

---

TABLE 35-16   RECOMMENDATIONS TO IMPROVE ADHERENCE TO ANTIHYPERTENSIVE PRESCRIPTIONS

Adherence can be improved by a multipronged approach. The nurse should:

- Assess adherence to pharmacological and nonpharmacological therapy at every physician visit.
- Simplify medication regimens to once-daily administration and utilize electronic medication adherence aids. Use fixed-dose combinations where available and appropriate.
- Tailor pill-taking to fit patient's daily habits.
- Encourage greater patient responsibility and autonomy in monitoring blood pressure and adjusting prescriptions.
- Coordinate with work-site health care providers to improve monitoring of adherence to pharmacological and lifestyle modification prescriptions.
- Educate patients and families about disease or treatment regimens.

---

the individual; (2) understand, accept, and implement the therapeutic plan; and (3) experience minimal or no unpleasant adverse effects of therapy.

AGE-RELATED CONSIDERATIONS

HYPERTENSION

Hypertension is common in people 60 years of age and older in industrialized countries. The SBP rises throughout the lifespan and DBP rises until age 55 or 60 years and then levels off. The following age-related physical changes play a role in the pathophysiology of hypertension in the older adult: (1) loss of tissue elasticity; (2) increased collagen content and stiffness of the myocardium; (3) increased peripheral vascular resistance; (4) decreased β-adrenergic receptor sensitivity; (5) blunting of baroreceptor reflexes; (6) decreased kidney function; and (7) decreased renin response to sodium and water depletion (Acelajado & Oparil, 2009).

In older adults taking antihypertensive medication, absorption of some drugs may be altered as a result of decreased splanchnic blood flow. Metabolism and excretion of drugs may also be prolonged.

Careful technique is important in assessing BP in older adults. In some older people, there is a wide gap between the first Korotkoff sound and subsequent beats. This is called the *auscultatory gap.* Failure to inflate the cuff enough may result in seriously underestimating the SBP. This problem can be avoided by palpating the brachial or radial artery while inflating the cuff to a level above the disappearance of the pulse.

Older adults are sensitive to BP changes; therefore, reducing SBP to less than 120 mm Hg in a person with longstanding hypertension could lead to inadequate cerebral blood flow. Medical therapy should be considered for adults when DBP is ≥100 mm Hg or SBP is ≥160 mm Hg regardless of age but excluding those with macrovascular tent organ damage or other cardiovascular risks (Leung, Daskalopoulou, Dasgupta, et al., 2017).

Because of varying degrees of impaired baroreceptor reflex mechanisms, orthostatic hypotension occurs often in older adults, especially in those with ISH. Orthostatic hypotension in this age group is often associated with volume depletion or chronic disease states, such as decreased renal and hepatic function or electrolyte imbalance. To reduce the likelihood of orthostatic hypotension, antihypertensive drugs should be started at low doses and increased cautiously. BP and pulse should be measured in the sitting and standing positions at every visit.

HYPERTENSIVE CRISIS

Hypertensive crisis is a severe and abrupt elevation in BP, arbitrarily defined as a DBP above 120 to 130 mm Hg. The rate of the rise of BP is more important than the absolute value in determining the need for emergency treatment. Prompt recognition and management of hypertensive crisis is essential to decrease the threat to organ function and life.

Hypertensive crisis occurs most commonly in patients with a history of hypertension who have failed to adhere to their prescribed medication regimen or who have been undermedicated. In this setting, rising BP is thought to trigger endothelial damage and the release of vasoconstrictor substances. A vicious cycle of BP elevation ensues, leading to life-threatening damage to target organs. Hypertensive crisis related to cocaine or crack use is becoming a more frequent problem. Other drugs, such as amphetamines, phencyclidine (PCP), and lysergic acid diethylamide (LSD), may also precipitate hypertensive crisis that may be complicated by drug-induced seizures, stroke, MI, or encephalopathy. Hypertensive crisis is classified by the degree of organ damage and the rapidity with which the BP must be lowered. *Hypertensive emergency,* which develops over hours to days, is a situation in which a patient's BP is severely elevated, with evidence of acute target-organ damage, especially damage to the central nervous system. Hypertensive emergencies include hypertensive encephalopathy, intracranial or subarachnoid hemorrhage, acute left ventricular failure with pulmonary edema, MI, renal failure, and dissecting aortic aneurysm. *Hypertensive urgency,* which develops over days to weeks, is a situation in which a patient's BP is severely elevated but there is no clinical evidence of target-organ damage.

Clinical Manifestations

A hypertensive emergency may be manifested as *hypertensive encephalopathy,* a syndrome in which a sudden rise in BP is associated with headache, nausea, vomiting, seizures, confusion, stupor, and coma. Other common manifestations are blurred vision and transient blindness. The manifestations of encephalopathy are probably the results of cerebral edema and spasms of cerebral vessels.

Renal insufficiency ranging from minor impairment to complete renal shutdown may occur. Rapid cardiac decompensation, ranging from unstable angina to infarction and pulmonary edema, is also possible with associated chest pain and dyspnea. Aortic dissection causes excruciating chest and back pain, often accompanied by diaphoresis and the loss of pulses in an extremity.

Patient assessment is extremely important, especially monitoring for signs of neurological dysfunction, retinal damage, heart failure, pulmonary edema, and renal failure. The neurological manifestations are often similar to the presentation of a stroke. However, a hypertensive crisis does not show the focal or lateralizing signs often seen with a stroke.

NURSING AND COLLABORATIVE MANAGEMENT HYPERTENSIVE CRISIS

BP level alone is a poor indicator of the seriousness of the patient's condition and is not the major factor in deciding the treatment for a hypertensive crisis. The association between elevated BP and signs of new or progressive end-organ damage (e.g., cerebrovascular, cardiac, retinal, or renal involvement) determines the seriousness of the situation.

Hypertensive emergencies necessitate hospitalization, parenteral administration of antihypertensive drugs, and intensive care monitoring. Generally, the initial treatment goal is to decrease mean arterial pressure (MAP) 10% to 20% in the first 1 to 2 hours, with further gradual reduction over the next 24 hours. Lowering the BP too far or too fast may decrease cerebral perfusion and could precipitate a stroke. A patient who has aortic dissection, unstable angina, or signs of MI must have the SBP lowered to 100 to 120 mm Hg as quickly as possible.

The intravenous (IV) drugs used for hypertensive emergencies include vasodilators (e.g., sodium nitroprusside, nitroglycerin, diazoxide [Proglycem], hydralazine hydrochloride [Apresoline]), adrenergic inhibitors (e.g., phentolamine mesylate [Rogitine], labetalol [Trandate], esmolol hydrochloride [Brevibloc]), and the ACE inhibitor enalapril (Vasotec). Sodium nitroprusside is the most effective parenteral drug for the treatment of hypertensive emergencies. Oral agents may be administered in addition to the parenteral drugs to help make an earlier transition to long-term therapy. The mechanisms of action and the adverse effects of these drugs are shown in Table 35-8.

Administered intravenously, the drugs have a rapid (within seconds to minutes) onset of action. The patient's BP and pulse should be taken every 2 to 3 minutes during the initial administration of these drugs. The use of an arterial line (see Chapter 68) or an automated BP monitoring machine (e.g., Dynamap) to monitor the BP is ideal. The rate of drug administration is titrated according to the level of BP. It is important to prevent hypotension and its effects in a person whose body has adjusted to hypertension. An excessive reduction in BP may cause stroke, MI, or visual changes. Frequently, continual ECG monitoring is done to observe for cardiac dysrhythmias. Extreme caution is needed in treating the patient with coronary artery disease or cerebro-vascular insufficiency. Hourly urinary output should be measured to assess renal perfusion. Careful monitoring of vital signs and urinary output provides information regarding the effectiveness of these drugs and the patient's response to therapy. Patients receiving IV antihypertensive drugs may be restricted to bed; getting up (e.g., to use the commode) may cause severe cerebral ischemia and fainting.

Regular, ongoing assessment is essential to evaluate the patient with severe hypertension. Frequent neurological checks, including level of consciousness, pupillary size and reaction, movement of extremities, and reactions to stimuli help detect any changes in the patient's condition. Cardiac, pulmonary, and renal systems should be monitored for decompensation caused by the severe elevation in BP (e.g., pulmonary edema, heart failure, angina, renal failure).

Hypertensive urgencies usually do not necessitate IV administration of medications but can be managed with oral agents. The patient with a hypertensive urgency may not need hospitalization, but requires frequent follow-up. The oral drugs most frequently used for hypertensive urgencies are captopril and clonidine (Catapres) (see Table 35-8). The disadvantage of oral medications is the inability to regulate the dosage from moment to moment, as can be done with IV medications. If a patient with hypertensive urgency is not hospitalized, outpatient follow-up should be arranged within 24 hours.

A patient with severe elevation of BP but without target-organ damage may not require emergent drug therapy or hospitalization. Allowing the patient to sit for 20 or 30 minutes in a quiet environment may significantly reduce BP. Oral drugs may then be instituted or adjusted. Additional nursing interventions include encouraging the patient to verbalize fears, answering questions concerning the hypertension, and eliminating excess noise in the patient's environment.

Once the hypertensive crisis is resolved, it is important to determine the cause. The patient will need appropriate management and extensive education to avoid future crises.

CASE STUDY

Primary Hypertension

Source: Mona Makela/ Shutterstock .com.

Patient Profile

Frank Windsong is a 45-year-old man who has no previous history of hypertension. At a screening clinic, his BP was found to be 180/120 mm Hg.

Subjective Data

- Father died of stroke at age 60
- Mother is alive but has type 2 diabetes
- States that he feels fine and is not a "hyper" person
- Smokes one pack of cigarettes daily
- Drinks a six-pack of beer on Friday and Saturday nights
- Does not enjoy physical activity
- Has had type 2 diabetes for 5 years and is nonadherent to his diabetic treatment plan
- Has been told that some medications interfere with sexual relationships

Objective Data

Physical Examination

- Moderately obese male
- Sustained apical impulse palpable in the fourth intercostal space, just lateral to the midclavicular line

Diagnostic Studies

- ECG: left ventricular hypertrophy
- Urinalysis: protein 0.3 g/L
- Serum creatinine level: 141 mmol/L

Collaborative Care

- Low-sodium diet
- Hydrochlorothiazide (HCTZ) 12.5 mg daily PO
- Enalapril sodium (Vasotec) 5 mg daily PO

Discussion Questions

1. What risk factors for hypertension does Mr. Windsong have?
2. What evidence of target-organ damage is present?
3. What misconceptions about hypertension should be corrected?
4. What are the nursing priorities for Mr. Windsong? What resources are available to assist in promoting health for Mr. Windsong?
5. ***Priority decision:*** Based on the assessment data presented, what are the priority nursing diagnoses? Are there any collaborative problems? How will they affect Mr. Windsong's treatment?
6. ***Evidence-informed practice:*** Mr. Windsong wants to know the most effective nonpharmacological strategies to lower his BP. What should the nurse tell him?

℮volve

Answers are available at *http://evolve.elsevier.com/Canada/Lewis/medsurg.*

■ REVIEW QUESTIONS

The number of the question corresponds to the same-numbered objective at the beginning of the chapter.

1. Which BP-regulating mechanism(s) can result in the development of hypertension if defective? *(Select all that apply)*
   a. Release of norepinephrine
   b. Secretion of prostaglandins PGE_2 and PGI_2
   c. Stimulation of the sympathetic nervous system
   d. Stimulation of the parasympathetic nervous system
   e. Activation of the renin–angiotensin–aldosterone system
2. While obtaining subjective assessment data from a client with hypertension, the nurse recognizes which of the following as a modifiable risk factor for the development of hypertension?
   a. Hyperlipidemia
   b. Excessive alcohol intake
   c. A family history of hypertension
   d. Consumption of a high-carbohydrate, high-calcium diet

3. The nurse includes which of the following ideas in teaching a client with hypertension about controlling the condition?
   a. All clients with elevated BP require medication.
   b. It is not necessary to limit salt in the diet if taking a diuretic.
   c. Obese people must achieve a normal weight in order to lower BP.
   d. Lifestyle modifications are indicated for all people with elevated BP.
4. What is a major consideration in the management of an older adult with hypertension?
   a. Prevent pseudohypertension from converting to true hypertension.
   b. Recognize that older adults are less likely to adhere to the drug therapy than younger adults.
   c. Ensure that the client receives larger initial doses of antihypertensive drugs because of impaired absorption.
   d. Use careful technique in assessing the BP of the client because of the possible presence of an auscultatory gap.

5. A client with newly diagnosed hypertension has a blood pressure of 158/98 mm Hg after 12 months of exercise and diet modifications. How does the nurse advise the client?
   a. Medication may be required because the BP is still not within the normal range.
   b. Continued monitoring of the BP every 3 to 6 months is all that will be necessary for treatment.
   c. Because lifestyle modifications were not effective, they do not need to be continued and drugs will be used.
   d. The client will have to make more vigorous changes in lifestyle if the client wants to stay off medication for hypertension.
6. A patient is admitted to the hospital in hypertensive emergency (BP 244/142 mm Hg). Sodium nitroprusside is started to treat the elevated BP. Which management strategy(ies) would be appropriate for this patient? *(Select all that apply)*
   a. Measuring hourly urine output.
   b. Decreasing the MAP by 50% within the first hour.
   c. Continuous BP monitoring with an intraarterial line.
   d. Maintaining bed rest and providing sedation to lower the BP.
   e. Assessing the patient for signs and symptoms of heart failure and changes in mental status.

1. a, c, e; 2. b; 3. d; 4. d; 5. a; 6. a, c, e.

⊖volve

For even more review questions, visit *http://evolve.elsevier.com/Canada/ Lewis/medsurg.*

REFERENCES

Acelajado, M. C., & Oparil, S. (2009). Hypertension in the elderly. *Clinics in Geriatric Medicine, 25*(3), 391–412. doi:10.1016/j.cger.2009.06.001. (Seminal).

Campbell, N. R. C., & Chen, G. (2010). Canadian efforts to prevent and control hypertension. *The Canadian Journal of Cardiology, 26,* 14C–17C. (Seminal).

Campbell, N. R. C., Lackland, D. T., & Niebylski, M. L. (2014). 2014 dietary salt fact sheet of the World Hypertension League, International Society of Hypertension, Pan American Health Organization technical advisory group on cardiovascular disease prevention through dietary salt reduction, the World Health Organization collaborating centre on population salt reduction, and World Action on Salt and Health. *The Journal of Clinical Hypertension, 17*(1), 7–10. doi:10.111/jch12402.

Campbell, N. R. C., & Niebylski, M. L. (2014). Prevention and control of hypertension: Developing a global agenda. *Current Opinion in Cardiology, 29*(4), 324–330. doi:10.1097/HCO.0000000000000067.

Dai, S., Robitaille, C., Bancej, C., et al. (2010). Executive summary—Report from the Canadian chronic disease surveillance system: Hypertension in Canada, 2010. *Chronic Diseases and Injuries in Canada, 31*(1).

Daskalopoulou, S. S., Rabi, D. M., Zarnke, K. B., et al. (2015). The 2015 Canadian hypertension education program recommendations for blood pressure measurement, diagnosis, assessment of risk, prevention, and treatment of hypertension. *Journal of Cardiology, 31,* 549–568. doi:10.1016/j.cjca.2015.02.016.

Geller, D. S. (2015). New developments in the genetics of hypertension: What should clinicians know? *Current Cardiology Reports, 17*(12), 2–8. doi:10.1007/s11886-015-0664-y.

Gilbert, R. E., Rabi, D., LaRochelle, P., et al. (2013). Treatment of hypertension. *Canadian Journal of Diabetes, 37,* S117–S118. doi:10.1016/j.jcjd.2013.01.033.

Heart and Stroke Foundation. (2015). *Statistics.* Retrieved from *http://www.heartandstroke.com/site/c.ikIQLcMWJtE/b.3483991/k.34A8/Statistics.htm.*

Hering, D., Lambert, E. A., Marusic, P., et al. (2013). Substantial reduction in single sympathetic nerve firing after renal denervation in patients with resistant hypertension. *Hypertension, 61,* 457–464. DOI: *http://dx.doi.org/10.1161/hypertensionaha.111.00194.*

Hypertension Canada. (2014). *Fact Sheet January.* Retrieved from *https://www.hypertension.ca/images/whatsnew/Final%20hypertension%20Fact%20Sheet%201.pdfhypertension.*

Hypertension Canada. (2017). *About CHEP.* Retrieved from *https://www.hypertension.ca/en/926-public/211-about-chep.*

Leung, A. A., Daskalopoulou, S. S., Dasgupta, K., et al. (2017). Hypertension Canada's 2017 guidelines for diagnosis, risk assessment, prevention, and treatment of hypertension in adults. *Canadian Journal of Cardiology, 33*(5), 557–576. doi: *http://dx.doi.org/10.1016/j.cjca.2017.03.005.*

McAlister, F. A., Wilkins, K., Joffres, M., et al. (2011). Changes in the rates of awareness, treatment and control of hypertension in Canada over the past two decades. *Canadian Medical Association Journal, 183*(9), 1007–1013. doi:10.1503/cmaj.101767.

Padwal, R. S., Bienek, A., McAlister, F. A., et al. (2015). Epidemiology of hypertension in Canada: An update. *Canadian Journal of Cardiology.* Retrieved from *http://dx.doi.org/10.1016/j.cjca.2015.07.734.*

Riaz, K., Dreisbach, A. W., Madhur, M. S., et al. (2012). *Hypertension.* Retrieved from *http://emedicine.medscape.com/article/241381-overview.*

Robitaille, C., Dai, S., Waters, C., et al. (2012). Diagnosed hypertension in Canada: Incidence, prevalence, and associated mortality. *Canadian Medical Association Journal, 184*(1), E49–E56. doi:10.1503/cmaj.101863.

Singh, M., Mensah, G. A., & Bakris, G. (2010). Pathogenesis and clinical physiology of hypertension. *Cardiology Clinics, 28*(4), 545–559. doi:10.1016/j.ccl.2010.07.001. (Seminal).

Sliwa, K., Stewart, S., & Gersh, B. (2011). Hypertension: A global perspective. *Circulation, 123,* 2892–2896. doi:10.1161/CIRCULATIONAHA.110.992362.

World Health Organization. (2013). *A global brief on hypertension. Silent killer, global public health crisis.* Retrieved from *http://www.who.int/cardiovascular_diseases/publications/global_brief_hypertension/en.*

World Health Organization. (2014). *Salt Reduction Fact Sheet.* Retrieved from *http://www.who.int/mediacentre/factsheets/fs393/en/.*

RESOURCES

Government of Canada Recommended intake of sodium
https://www.canada.ca/en/health-canada/services/food-nutrition/healthy-eating/sodium.html

Heart and Stroke Foundation Blood Pressure Action Plan
https://ehealth.heartandstroke.ca/heartstroke/bpap.net/ ?pgSrc=bpvanity

Heart and Stroke Foundation DASH diet
https://www.heartandstroke.ca/get-healthy/healthy-eating/dash-diet

Heart and Stroke Foundation of Canada
http://www.heartandstroke.ca

Hypertension Canada. Hypertension Canada's most recent guidelines for the diagnosis, assessment, prevention, and treatment of hypertension, along with summary documents, including downloadable slide kits, are available free of charge on the website.
www.hypertension.ca
www.hypertension.qc.ca
Video: "How to measure my blood pressure"
https://www.hypertension.ca/en/hypertension/what-do-i-need-to-know/how-to-measure-my-blood-pressure

Myhealthcheckup.com: Do you know your cardiovascular age? Programs that compare risk by using terms such as *cardiovascular age, vascular age,* and *heart age* have been shown to improve risk perception by patients and risk facto management by physicians.
http://www.myhealthcheckup.com

Registered Nurses' Association of Ontario: Nursing management of hypertension. (2005). *Best Practice Guideline.*
www.rnao.org/Storage/11/607_BPG_Hypertension.pdf

SCORE (Systematic Cerebrovascular and Coronary Risk Evaluation) Canada Risk Calculator: The SCORE risk calculator uses Canadian data.
http://www.score-Canada.ca

Sodium 101
http://www.sodium101.ca

Tobacco Free RNAO
http://tobaccofreernao.ca/en
http://tobaccofreernao.ca/en/treatment/intervention-strategies

---

World Health Organization
http://www.who.int/mediacentre/factsheets/fs393/en/

World Hypertension League
http://www.whleague.org/

For additional Internet resources, see the website for this book at *http://evolve.elsevier.com/Canada/Lewis/medsurg.*

Nursing Management

Coronary Artery Disease and Acute Coronary Syndrome

Written by: Rose Shaffer and Linda Bucher
Adapted by: Sandra Goldsworthy

eVolve WEBSITE

http://evolve.elsevier.com/Canada/Lewis/medsurg

- Review Questions
  (Online Only)
- Key Points
- Answer Guidelines for Case Study

- Conceptual Care Map Creator
  - Conceptual Care Map for Textbook Case Study
- Audio Glossary
- Content Updates

LEARNING OBJECTIVES

1. Describe the prevalence of heart disease in Canada.
2. Explain the etiology and the pathophysiology of coronary artery disease (CAD), angina, and acute coronary syndrome (ACS).
3. Identify risk factors for CAD and the nursing role in the promotion of therapeutic lifestyle changes for patients at risk.
4. Differentiate the precipitating factors, the clinical manifestations, and the collaborative care and nursing management of patients with CAD and ACS.
5. Explain the clinical manifestations, complications, diagnostic study results, and collaborative care of patients with ACS.

6. Describe the pathophysiology of myocardial infarction from the onset of injury through the healing process.
7. Evaluate drug therapy commonly used in treating patients with CAD and ACS.
8. Prioritize key components to include in the rehabilitation of patients recovering from ACS and coronary revascularization procedures.
9. Describe the precipitating factors, the clinical presentation, and the collaborative care of patients who are at risk for or have experienced sudden cardiac death.

KEY TERMS

acute coronary syndrome (ACS), p. 827	collateral circulation, p. 815	myocardial infarction (MI), p. 828	silent ischemia, p. 837
angina, p. 820	coronary artery disease (CAD), p. 813	percutaneous coronary	sudden cardiac death (SCD), p. 841
atherosclerosis, p. 814	coronary revascularization,	intervention (PCI), p. 829	unstable angina (UA), p. 827
chronic stable angina, p. 821	p. 833	Prinzmetal's angina, p. 824	

Heart disease is the second major cause of death in Canada, accounting for 19.8% (49 891) of all deaths in 2013 (Statistics Canada, 2017). In Canada, 70 000 people per year will have a myocardial infarction (MI), and, of those, 14 000 will not survive (Heart and Stroke Foundation of Canada, 2016a).

Patients with coronary artery disease (CAD) can be asymptomatic or can develop chronic stable angina. Unstable angina (UA) and MI, more serious manifestations of CAD, are termed *acute coronary syndrome* (ACS). Cardiovascular disease is the most common reason for hospitalization in Canada (Heart and Stroke Foundation of Canada, 2016a). Circulatory diseases are the leading cause of death among Indigenous peoples in

Canada (Heart and Stroke Foundation of Canada, 2016a). The "Determinants of Health" box discusses culture and social status as determinants of CAD in Canada.

CORONARY ARTERY DISEASE

Coronary artery disease (CAD) is a type of blood vessel disorder that is included in the general category of atherosclerosis; it may affect the heart's arteries and produce various pathological effects, especially the reduced flow of oxygen and nutrients to the myocardium. The term *atherosclerosis* is derived from two Greek words: *athere*, meaning "fatty mush," and *skleros*,

DETERMINANTS OF HEALTH

Coronary Artery Disease in Canada

Culture

- Immigrants to Canada tend to have better cardiovascular health than do native-born Canadians.
- Immigrants from South Asia have a higher risk for cardiovascular disease. Cardiovascular risk increases proportionally with length of stay in Canada.*

Income and Social Status

- Members of minority and low-income populations experience a disproportionate burden of death and disability from cardiovascular disease.†

References

*Tu, J. V., Chu, A., Rezai, M. R., et al. (2015). Incidence of major cardiovascular events in immigrants to Ontario, Canada: The CANHEART Immigrant Study. *Circulation, 132*(16), 1549–1559. doi:10.1161/CIRCULATIONAHA .115.015345.

†Franks, P., Winters, P. C., Tancredi, D. J., et al. (2011). Do changes in traditional coronary heart disease risk factors over time explain the association between socio-economic status and coronary heart disease? *BMC Cardiovascular Disorders, 11*(1), 1. doi:10.1186/1471-2261-11-28.

meaning "hard." This word combination indicates that atherosclerosis begins as soft deposits of fat that harden with age. Atherosclerosis is often referred to as "hardening of the arteries." Although this condition can occur in any artery in the body, the atheromas have a preference for the coronary arteries. *Arteriosclerotic heart disease (ASHD), cardiovascular heart disease (CVHD), ischemic heart disease,* and *coronary heart disease* are synonymous terms used to describe CAD.

ETIOLOGY AND PATHOPHYSIOLOGY

Atherosclerosis is the major cause of CAD. It is characterized by deposits of lipids within the intima of the artery. Endothelial injury and inflammation play a central role in the development of atherosclerosis.

The endothelium (the inner lining of the vessel wall) is normally nonreactive to platelets and leukocytes, as well as to coagulation, fibrinolytic, and complement factors. However, the endothelial lining can be injured as a result of tobacco use, hyperlipidemia, hypertension, toxins, diabetes, hyperhomocysteinemia, and infection causing a local inflammatory response (Huether & McCance, 2012) (Figure 36-1, *A*).

C-reactive protein (CRP), a protein produced by the liver, is a nonspecific marker of inflammation. It is increased in many patients with CAD (Strang & Schunkert, 2014) (see Chapter 34, Table 34-6). The level of CRP rises when there is systemic inflammation. Chronic elevations of CRP are associated with unstable plaques and the oxidation of low-density lipoprotein (LDL) cholesterol.

Developmental Stages

CAD is a progressive disease that develops over many years. By the time it becomes symptomatic, the disease process is usually well advanced. The stages of development in atherosclerosis are (a) fatty streak, (b) fibrous plaque, and (c) complicated lesion.

Fatty Streak. *Fatty streaks,* the earliest lesions of atherosclerosis, are characterized by lipid-filled smooth muscle cells. As streaks of fat develop within the smooth muscle cells, a yellow

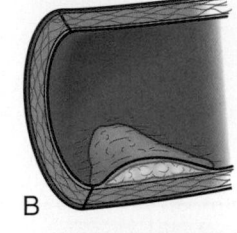

Chronic Endothelial Injury
- Hypertension
- Tobacco use
- Hyperlipidemia
- Hyperhomocysteinemia
- Diabetes
- Infections
- Toxins
- **Damaged endothelium**

Fatty Streak
- Lipids accumulate and migrate into smooth muscle cells

Fibrous Plaque
- Collagen covers the fatty streak
- Vessel lumen is narrowed
- Blood flow is reduced
- Fissures can develop

Complicated Lesion
- Plaque rupture
- Thrombus formation
- Further narrowing or total occlusion of vessel

FIGURE 36-1 Pathogenesis of atherosclerosis. **A,** Damaged endothelium. **B,** Fatty streak and lipid core formation. **C,** Fibrous plaque. Raised plaques are visible: some are yellow; others are white. **D,** Complicated lesion: thrombus is red; collagen is blue. Plaque is complicated by red thrombus deposition.

tinge appears (Huether & McCance, 2012). Fatty streaks can be seen in the coronary arteries by age 15 and involve an increasing amount of surface area as one ages. Treatment that lowers LDL cholesterol may reverse this process (Figure 36-1, *B*).

Fibrous Plaque. The *fibrous plaque* stage is the beginning of progressive changes in the endothelium of the arterial wall. These changes can appear in the coronary arteries by age 30 and increase with age.

Normally, the endothelium repairs itself immediately. However, this does not happen in people with CAD. LDLs and growth factors from platelets stimulate smooth muscle proliferation and thickening of the arterial wall. Once endothelial injury has taken place, lipoproteins (carrier proteins within the bloodstream) transport cholesterol and other lipids into the arterial intima. Collagen covers the fatty streak and forms a fibrous plaque that has a greyish or whitish appearance. These plaques can form on one portion of the artery or in a circular fashion involving the entire lumen. The borders can be smooth or irregular with rough, jagged edges. The result is a narrowing of the vessel lumen and a reduction in blood flow to the distal tissues (Figure 36-1, *C*).

FIGURE 36-2 Vessel occlusion with collateral circulation. **A,** Open, functioning coronary artery. **B,** Partial coronary artery closure with collateral circulation being established. **C,** Total coronary artery occlusion with collateral circulation bypassing the occlusion to supply the myocardium.

Complicated Lesion. The final stage in the development of the atherosclerotic lesion is the most dangerous. As the fibrous plaque grows, continued inflammation can result in plaque instability, ulceration, and rupture. Once the integrity of the artery's inner wall is compromised, platelets accumulate in large numbers, leading to a thrombus. The thrombus may adhere to the wall of the artery, leading to further narrowing or total occlusion of the artery. Activation of the exposed platelets causes expression of the glycoprotein IIb/IIIa receptors that bind fibrinogen. This, in turn, leads to further platelet aggregation and adhesion, further enlarging the thrombus. At this stage, the plaque is referred to as a *complicated lesion* (Figure 36-1, *D*).

Collateral Circulation

Normally, some arterial anastomoses or connections, termed collateral circulation, exist within the coronary circulation. Two factors contribute to the growth and extent of collateral circulation: (a) the inherited predisposition to develop new blood vessels *(angiogenesis)* and (b) the presence of chronic ischemia. When an atherosclerotic plaque occludes the normal flow of blood through a coronary artery and the resulting ischemia is chronic, increased collateral circulation develops (Figure 36-2). When occlusion of the coronary arteries occurs slowly over a long period, there is a greater chance that adequate collateral circulation will gradually develop, and the myocardium may continue receiving an adequate amount of blood and oxygen.

However, when CAD has a rapid onset (as in familial hypercholesterolemia) or coronary spasm occurs, there is not enough time for collateral circulation development, and the diminished arterial blood flow results in more severe ischemia or infarction.

CAD usually develops over many years, and clinical manifestations are not apparent in the early stages of the disease. Therefore, it is extremely important to identify people at risk and initiate therapeutic lifestyle changes and treatment strategies early.

RISK FACTORS FOR CORONARY ARTERY DISEASE

Many risk factors—characteristics or conditions that are statistically associated with a high incidence of a disease—have been associated with CAD. Cardiac risk factors are categorized as either *nonmodifiable* or *modifiable* (Table 36-1).

Nonmodifiable Risk Factors

Age, Sex, and Ethnicity. Genetic predisposition is an important factor in the occurrence of CAD, although the exact mechanism of inheritance is not fully understood. Some congenital defects

TABLE 36-1	RISK FACTORS FOR CORONARY ARTERY DISEASE
Nonmodifiable Risk Factors	**Modifiable Risk Factors**
Increasing age Sex (men > women until 65 yr of age) Ethnicity (White people > Black people) Genetic predisposition and family history of heart disease	**Major** Serum lipid alterations: elevated triglyceride and LDL cholesterol levels, decreased HDL levels Blood pressure ≥140/90 mm Hg Diabetes mellitus Tobacco use Physical inactivity Obesity: waist circumference ≥102 cm (40 inches) in men and ≥88 cm (35 inches) in women **Contributing** Fasting blood glucose level >10 mmol/L Psychosocial risk factors (e.g., depression, hostility and anger, stress) Elevated homocysteine levels

HDL, High-density lipoprotein; *LDL,* low-density lipoprotein.

🧬 **GENETICS IN CLINICAL PRACTICE**

Familial Hypercholesterolemia

Genetic Basis
- Autosomal dominant disorder
- Mutation in gene coding for the LDL receptor
- Multiple mutant alleles

Incidence
- Heterozygotes: 1 per 500
- Homozygotes: rare

Genetic Testing
- Disorder characterized by elevated serum LDL level
- Serum lipid profile can be used to measure total cholesterol, triglyceride, LDL, and HDL levels
- DNA testing available

Clinical Implications
- Common genetic disease
- Leading cause of coronary artery disease
- High cholesterol levels are a result of defective function of the LDL receptors
- Plasma levels of LDL remain elevated throughout life
- Those affected develop severe atherosclerosis in early to middle years

DNA, deoxyribonucleic acid; *HDL,* high-density lipoprotein; *LDL,* low-density lipoprotein.

in coronary artery walls predispose some people to the formation of plaques. Familial hypercholesterolemia, an autosomal dominant disorder, has been strongly associated with CAD at early ages (see the "Genetics in Clinical Practice" box). In most cases, patients with angina or MI can identify a parent or sibling who has died of CAD.

Major Modifiable Risk Factors

Elevated Serum Lipid Levels. An elevated serum lipid level is one of the four most firmly established risk factors for CAD (Anderson, Grégoire, Hegele, et al., 2013). The various types of

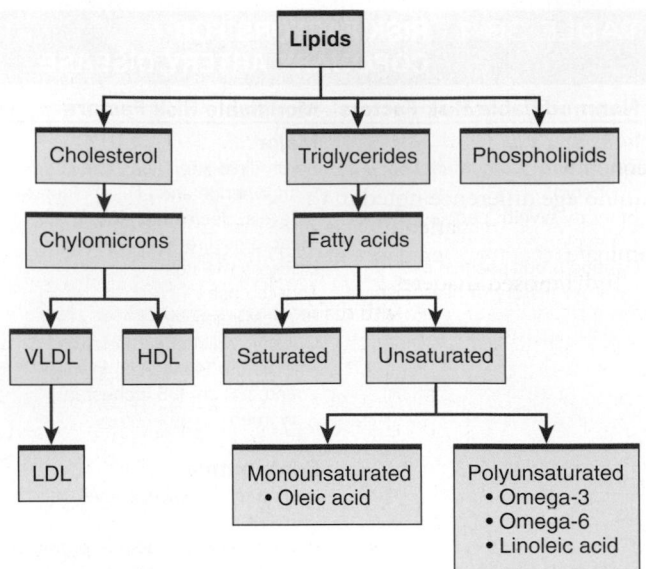

FIGURE 36-3 Types of serum lipids. *HDL,* high-density lipoprotein; *LDL,* low-density lipoprotein; *VLDL,* very-low-density lipoprotein.

Who to screen

Men ≥ 40 years of age; women ≥ 50 years of age or postmenopausal (consider screening earlier in ethnic groups at increased risk, such as South Asian or First Nations individuals); and all patients with any of the following conditions, regardless of age:

- Current cigarette smoking
- Diabetes
- Arterial hypertension
- Family history of premature CVD
- Family history of hyperlipidemia
- Erectile dysfunction
- Chronic kidney disease

- Inflammatory disease*
- HIV infection
- Chronic obstructive pulmonary disease
- Clinical evidence of atherosclerosis or abdominal aneurysm
- Clinical manifestation of hyperlipidemia
- Obesity (body mass index > 27)

How to screen

For all: history and examination, LDL, HDL, TG, non-HDL (will be calculated from profile), glucose, eGFR
Optional: apoB (instead of standard lipid panel), urine albumin : creatinine ratio (if eGFR < 60, hypertension, diabetes)

| Framingham risk score < 5%
Repeat every 3–5 years | Framingham risk score ≥ 5%
Repeat every year |

FIGURE 36-4 Patients whose plasma lipid profile should be screened. Source: Reprinted from *Journal of Cardiology,* 29(2), Anderson, T., Grégoire, J., Hegele, R., et al., Society Guidelines 2012 Update of the Canadian Cardiovascular Society Guidelines for the Diagnosis and Treatment of Dyslipidemia for the Prevention of Cardiovascular Disease in the Adult, pp. 151–167, Copyright 2013, with permission from Elsevier.
*Data on inflammatory bowel diseases are lacking.

serum lipids are presented in Figure 36-3. Approximately 40% of Canadians have high blood cholesterol (>5.2 mmol/L) (Heart and Stroke Foundation of Canada, 2016a). In Canada, clinical practice guidelines for the diagnosis, treatment, and prevention of dyslipidemia are available (Anderson, Grégoire, Hegele, et al., 2013). These guidelines incorporate (a) a description of patients whose lipid profile should be screened and (b) a classification of metabolic syndrome to evaluate central obesity (waist circumference plus two of the following: plasma triglyceride levels, high-density lipoprotein [HDL] cholesterol level, blood pressure [BP], and fasting plasma glucose level).

The current Canadian guidelines for treating dyslipidemia include a description of patients whose plasma lipid profile should be screened (Figure 36-4) and target lipid levels associated with risk level (Anderson, Grégoire, Hegele, et al., 2013). In the summary of these 2012 guidelines, recommended treatment includes smoking cessation, diet modification (reduced consumption of both saturated fats and refined sugars), weight reduction and maintenance, daily exercise, stress management, and (in patients at high risk) pharmacological therapy.

Hypertension. The second major risk factor in CAD is hypertension, which is defined as a BP of 140/90 mm Hg or higher. The Hypertension Canada recommendations for diagnosis of hypertension and follow-up are presented in Figure 35-2 in Chapter 35.

The stress of a constantly elevated BP increases the rate of atherosclerotic development. The pressure in the vessel is related to the shearing stress that causes endothelial injury. Atherosclerosis, in turn, causes narrowing and thickening of the arterial walls and decreases the distensibility and elasticity of vessels. More force is required to pump blood through diseased arterial vasculature, and this increased force is reflected in a higher BP. This increased workload is also manifested by left ventricular hypertrophy and decreased stroke volume with each contraction. Salt intake is positively correlated with elevated BP, adding volume and increasing systemic vascular resistance (SVR) to the cardiac workload. (See Chapter 35 for a complete discussion of hypertension.) Lifestyle modifications are a critical component of

hypertension management. Lifestyle factors that increase risk for hypertension include obesity, poor dietary habits, high sodium intake, low activity levels, high alcohol consumption, and high stress levels (Hypertension Canada, 2015).

Tobacco Use. A third major risk factor in CAD is tobacco use. The risk of developing CAD is two to six times higher in those who smoke tobacco or use smokeless tobacco than in those who do not. Further, tobacco smoking decreases estrogen levels, placing premenopausal women at greater risk for CAD. Risk is proportional to the number of cigarettes smoked. Changing to lower nicotine or filtered cigarettes does not affect risk.

Nicotine in tobacco smoke causes catecholamine (e.g., epinephrine, norepinephrine) release. These neurohormones cause an increased heart rate (HR), peripheral vasoconstriction, and increased BP. These changes increase the cardiac workload. Tobacco smoke is also related to an increase in LDL level, a decrease in HDL level, and a release of toxic oxygen radicals. All of these add to vessel inflammation and thrombosis (Huether & McCance, 2012).

Carbon monoxide, a byproduct of combustion found in tobacco smoke, affects the oxygen-carrying capacity of hemoglobin by reducing the sites available for oxygen transport. Thus the effects of an increased cardiac workload, combined with the oxygen-depleting effect of carbon monoxide, significantly decrease the oxygen available to the myocardium. There is also some indication that carbon monoxide is a chemical irritant and causes injury to the endothelium.

The benefits of smoking cessation are dramatic and almost immediate. CAD mortality rates drop to those of nonsmokers within 12 months. However, nicotine is highly addictive, and often intensive intervention is required to assist people to quit. Individual and group counselling sessions, nicotine replacement therapy, smoking cessation medications (e.g., bupropion [Zyban], varenicline [Champix]), and hypnosis are examples of smoking cessation strategies. (For information on smoking cessation, see Chapter 11, Tables 11-10 and 11-11, and the Resources at the end of the chapter.)

Chronic exposure to environmental tobacco (second-hand smoke) also increases the risk for CAD (Smith, Benjamin, Bonow, et al., 2011). People who live in the same household as the patient should be encouraged to stop smoking. By doing so, they reinforce the patient's effort and decrease the risk for ongoing exposure to environmental smoke. Pipe and cigar smokers, who often do not inhale, have an increased risk of CAD similar to those exposed to environmental tobacco smoke.

Physical Inactivity. Physical inactivity is the fourth major modifiable risk factor. Physical inactivity implies a lack of adequate physical exercise on a regular basis. An example of health-promoting regular physical activity is brisk walking (3 to 4 miles per hour) for at least 30 minutes five or more times a week (James, Oparil, Carter, et al., 2014).

The mechanism by which physical inactivity predisposes a person to CAD is mostly still unknown. Physically active people have increased HDL levels, and exercise improves thrombolytic activity, thus reducing the risk for clot formation. Exercise may also encourage the development of collateral circulation in the heart.

Exercise training for those who are physically inactive decreases the risk for CAD through more efficient lipid metabolism, increased HDL production, and more efficient oxygen extraction by the working muscles, thereby decreasing the cardiac workload. For those individuals with CAD, regular physical activity reduces symptoms, improves functional capacity, and improves other risk factors such as insulin resistance and glucose intolerance.

Obesity. The mortality rate from CAD is statistically higher among obese individuals, and the risk for CAD is proportional to a person's degree of obesity. *Obesity* is defined as a body mass index (BMI) of more than 30 kg/m² and a waist circumference of 102 cm or larger for men and 88 cm or larger for women (Heart and Stroke Foundation of Canada, 2016b). BMI is a calculation of body fat based on height and weight and can be calculated online (see the Resources section at the end of this chapter). In the past, BMI was the key indicator of health risk related to obesity, but waist circumference is now regarded as the factor that indicates the greatest health risk related to obesity (Smith, Benjamin, Bonow, et al., 2011). Obese persons may produce more LDLs and triglycerides, which are strongly related to atherosclerosis. Obesity is also often associated with hypertension. As well, evidence suggests that people who tend to store fat in the abdomen (i.e., have an "apple" figure) rather than in the hips and buttocks (i.e., have a "pear" figure) have a higher incidence of CAD; see Table 43-2. As obesity increases, the heart grows and uses more oxygen. In addition, there is an increase in insulin resistance in obese individuals (Huether & McCance, 2012).

Modifiable Contributing Risk Factors

Diabetes Mellitus. The incidence of CAD is two to four times greater among persons who have diabetes, even those with well-controlled blood glucose levels, than in the general population. Patients with diabetes manifest CAD not only more frequently but also at a younger age (Huether & McCance, 2012), with no age difference noted in the onset of symptoms between male and female patients. The presence of diabetes virtually eliminates the lower incidence of CAD in premenopausal women.

Undiagnosed diabetes is frequently discovered at the time a person has an MI. People with diabetes have an increased tendency toward endothelial dysfunction, which may account for the development of fatty streaks in these patients. Diabetic patients also have alterations in lipid metabolism and tend to have high cholesterol and triglyceride levels. Management of diabetes should include lifestyle changes and drug therapy to achieve a glycosylated hemoglobin (A1C or Hb A1C) level of less than 7% (Imran, Rabasa-Lhoret, & Ross, 2013).

Metabolic Syndrome. *Metabolic syndrome* refers to a cluster of risk factors for CAD whose underlying pathophysiology may be related to insulin resistance. These risk factors include obesity as defined by large waist circumference, hypertension, abnormal serum lipids, and an elevated fasting blood glucose (Huether & McCance, 2012) (see Table 43-5). These interrelated risk factors of metabolic origin appear to promote the development of CAD. (Chapter 43 discusses metabolic syndrome.)

Psychological States. The Framingham study provided early evidence that certain behaviours and lifestyles contribute to the development of CAD and correlate with CAD. However, the study of these behaviours remains controversial and complex. One type of behaviour, referred to as *type A*, includes perfectionism and a hardworking, driven personality. Type A people often suppress anger and hostility, feel a sense of time urgency, are impatient, and create stress and tension. These people may be more prone to MIs than those who are *type B*, characterized by being more easygoing, taking upsets in stride, knowing personal limitations, taking time to relax, and not being overachievers. However, findings from studies regarding these relationships are inconsistent.

Studies now are focusing on specific psychological risk factors thought to increase risk for CAD. These include depression; acute and chronic stress (e.g., poverty, serving as a caregiver); anxiety, hostility, and anger; and lack of social support (Burg, Edmondson, Shimbo, et al., 2013; Cohen, Edmondson, & Kronish, 2015). In particular, depression is a risk factor for both the development of and the worsening of CAD. Patients with depression have elevated levels of circulating catecholamines that may contribute to endothelial injury and inflammation and platelet activation. Depression is also a risk factor for adverse outcomes post-ACS (Lichtman, Froelicher, Blumenthal, et al., 2014). More research on the treatment of depression and other negative psychological states (e.g., anger) in patients with or at risk for CAD is needed to improve the emotional and physical health of these patients.

Stressful states correlate with the development of CAD (Jhamnani, Patel, Heimlich, et al., 2015). Sympathetic nervous system (SNS) stimulation—and its effect on the heart—is the physiological mechanism by which stress predisposes one to the development of CAD. SNS stimulation causes an increased release of catecholamines (e.g., epinephrine, norepinephrine). This stimulation increases HR and intensifies the force of myocardial contraction, resulting in increased myocardial oxygen demand.

Also, stress-induced mechanisms can cause elevated lipid and glucose levels and changes in blood coagulation, which can lead to increased atherogenesis.

Homocysteine. High homocysteine levels in the blood have been linked to an increased risk for CAD and other cardiovascular diseases (Burg, Edmonson, Shimbo, et al., 2013). Homocysteine is produced by the breakdown of the essential amino acid methionine, which is found in dietary protein. High homocysteine levels possibly contribute to atherosclerosis by (a) damaging the inner lining of blood vessels, (b) promoting plaque buildup, and (c) altering the clotting mechanism to make clots more likely to occur (see Chapter 34, Table 34-6).

Research is ongoing to determine whether a decline in homocysteine can reduce the risk for heart disease. B-complex vitamins (B_6, B_{12}, folic acid) have been shown to lower blood levels of homocysteine. Generally, a screening test for homocysteine is limited to those suspected of having elevated levels, such as older patients with pernicious anemia or people who develop CAD at an early age.

Substance Use. The use of illicit drugs, such as cocaine and methamphetamine, can produce coronary spasm resulting in myocardial ischemia and chest pain. Most people who are seen in the emergency department (ED) with drug-induced chest pain are initially indistinguishable from those with CAD. Although MI can occur, these patients more often have sinus tachycardia, high BP, angina, and anxiety (National Institute on Drug Abuse, 2016).

Health Promotion

The appropriate management of risk factors in CAD may prevent, modify, or retard the progression of the disease. Emphasis on prevention and early treatment of heart disease must be ongoing.

Identification of High-Risk People. Clinical manifestations of CAD are not apparent in the early stages of the disease. Therefore, regardless of the health care setting, it is extremely important to identify people at risk for CAD. Risk screening involves obtaining a thorough health history that includes questioning the patient about (a) family history of heart disease in parents and siblings; (b) the presence of any cardiovascular symptoms; (c) environmental factors, such as eating habits, type of diet, and level of exercise; (d) psychosocial factors, such as tobacco use, alcohol ingestion, recent stressful events (e.g., loss of a spouse), and any negative psychological states (e.g., anxiety, depression, anger); and (e) the place and type of employment to determine the kind of activities performed, exposure to pollutants or noxious chemicals, and the degree of stress associated with work.

Identifying the patient's attitudes and beliefs about health and illness can give some indication of how disease and lifestyle changes may affect the patient and can also reveal possible misconceptions about heart disease. Knowledge of the patient's educational background can help to determine teaching needs. If the patient is taking medications, it is important to know the names and dosages and whether the patient is compliant with the medication regimen.

Management of High-Risk People. Preventive measures should be recommended for all persons at risk for CAD. Risk factors such as age, sex, ethnicity, and genetics cannot be modified. However, people with these risk factors can still reduce their risk for CAD by controlling the additive effects of modifiable risk factors. For example, a young man with a family history of heart disease can decrease his risk by maintaining an ideal body

TABLE 36-2   PATIENT & CAREGIVER TEACHING GUIDE

Decreasing Risk Factors for Coronary Artery Disease

Risk Factor	Health-Promoting Behaviours
Hypertension	• Have regular BP checkups. • Take prescribed medications for BP control. • Reduce salt intake. • Never smoke or stop smoking. • Control or reduce weight. • Exercise regularly.
Elevated serum lipids	• Reduce total fat intake. • Reduce animal (saturated) fat intake. • Adjust total caloric intake to achieve and maintain ideal body weight. • Engage in a regular exercise program. • Increase amount of complex carbohydrates and vegetable proteins in diet.
Smoking*	• Enroll in program to stop smoking. • Change daily routines associated with smoking to reduce desire to smoke. • Substitute other activities for smoking. • Ask family members to support efforts to stop smoking.
Physical inactivity	• Develop and maintain routine for physical activity that is performed at least three or four times a week. • Increase activities to a level compatible with physical fitness.
Stressful lifestyle	• Increase awareness of behaviours that are detrimental to health. • Alter patterns that are conducive to stress and rushing (e.g., get up 30 min earlier so that breakfast is not eaten on way to work). • Set realistic goals for self. • Reassess priorities in view of health needs. • Learn effective coping strategies. • Avoid excessive and prolonged stress. • Take 20 min/day to meditate. • Plan time for adequate rest and sleep.
Obesity	• Change eating patterns and habits. • Reduce caloric intake. • Exercise regularly to increase caloric expenditure. • Avoid fad and crash diets, which are not effective over the long term. • Avoid large, heavy meals.
Diabetes mellitus†	• Follow the recommended diet. • Reduce weight and control diet. • Monitor blood glucose levels regularly.

BP, blood pressure.
*See Registered Nurses' Association of Ontario. (2007). *Integrating smoking cessation into daily nursing practice: Nursing Best Practices Guideline.* Toronto: Author. Available at *http://rnao.ca/bpg/guidelines/integrating-smoking-cessation-daily-nursing-practice.*
†See Chapter 52 for additional health-promoting behaviours.

weight, getting adequate physical exercise, reducing intake of saturated fats, and avoiding tobacco use.

Nurses can play a major role in teaching health-promoting behaviours and in encouraging patients who have modifiable risk factors to make lifestyle changes to reduce their risk for CAD (Table 36-2). Highly motivated people may just need to know how to reduce their risk in order to get started. For people who are less motivated to take charge of their health, the idea of reducing risk factors may be so remote that they are unable to perceive a threat of CAD. Few people want to make lifestyle changes, especially in the absence of symptoms. First, the nurse should assist these patients in clarifying their personal values. Then, by explaining the risk factors, the nurse may help them recognize their susceptibility to CAD. This information may help patients set realistic goals and allow them to choose which risk factor(s) to change first. Some people are reluctant to change until they begin to manifest overt symptoms or actually suffer an MI. Others, having suffered an MI, may find the idea of changing lifelong habits still unacceptable. Help them identify such choices and respect their final decision.

Physical Activity. A physical activity program should be designed to improve physical fitness by following the FITT formula: **f**requency (how often), **i**ntensity (how hard), **t**ime (how long), and **t**ype (isotonic). Everyone should aim for at least 30 minutes of moderate physical activity on most days of the week (James, Oparil, Carter, et al., 2014). In addition, adding weight training to an exercise program two days a week can help treat metabolic syndrome and improve muscle strength. Examples of moderate physical activity include brisk walking, hiking, biking, and swimming. Regular physical activity contributes to weight reduction, a reduction in systolic BP, and, in men more than in women, an increase in HDL cholesterol. The American Heart Association (AHA) has developed a program to encourage people, especially women, to increase their daily physical activity. (See the Resources at the end of this chapter.)

In Canada, the interest in attaining and maintaining health has made physical activity a field of major importance. Communities are developing or promoting exercise programs, such as aerobic exercise classes and cardiac walking and jogging groups, for people of all ages and with varying health needs. Local YMCAs often sponsor jogging, bicycling, swimming, and related courses. Many shopping malls open their doors in the early morning to allow people to walk indoors. The Heart and Stroke Foundation of Canada organizes many events that emphasize the need for physical activity in the promotion of health. Many large corporations provide gymnasiums in which their employees can exercise. For many people, running may be inadvisable; however, these people should be encouraged to pursue walking, swimming, or whatever exercise will accommodate their individual physical abilities.

Health Education in Schools. Awareness of the body and the maintenance of physical health is also emphasized in Canada's school systems. Schoolteachers play an important role in educating children and youths about good health practices. Besides teaching physical fitness topics, teachers often instruct students in how the body functions and responds to daily living. Lifestyle habits can be positively influenced at an early age to decrease the need for drastic changes later in life, such as those that may confront the students' parents. Teachers are largely taking advantage of the social climate that promotes health and health practices by finding innovative ways to present these values to a receptive, youthful audience before habits become ingrained. The Heart and Stroke Foundation of Canada has established school programs such as "Heart Smart," which provides teaching materials for teachers to incorporate into their curriculum. Printed and electronic materials are also available to help teachers educate students about healthy habits for better cardiac health.

Nutritional Therapy. The National Heart, Lung, and Blood Institute recommends *therapeutic lifestyle changes* for all people to reduce the risk of CAD by lowering LDL cholesterol. These recommendations, as well as recommendations from the Heart and Stroke Foundation of Canada, emphasize decreasing intake

TABLE 36-3 NUTRITIONAL THERAPY

Therapeutic Lifestyle Changes Diet

Nutrient	Recommended Daily Intake
Total fat (includes saturated-fat calories)	25%–35% of total daily calories
Saturated fat	<7% of total daily calories
Cholesterol	<200 mg
Plant stanols or sterols (e.g., margarines, nuts, seeds, legumes, vegetable oils)*	2 g
Dietary fibre*	10–25 g of soluble fibre
Total calories	Only enough calories to reach or maintain a healthy weight
Physical activity	At least 30 min of a moderate-intensity physical activity (e.g., brisk walking) on most, or preferably all, days of the week

*Diet options for additional lowering of low-density lipoprotein (LDL).
Source: National Heart, Blood, and Lung Institute. (2005). *Your guide to lowering your cholesterol with TLC.* Retrieved from *https://www.nhlbi.nih.gov/files/docs/public/heart/chol_tlc.pdf.*

of saturated fats and cholesterol and increasing intake of complex carbohydrates (e.g., whole grains, fruit, vegetables) and fibre (Eckel, Jakicic, Ard, et al., 2014; Heart and Stroke Foundation of Canada, 2016c) (Tables 36-3 and 36-4). Fat intake should account for about 30% of calories, with most coming from mono- and polyunsaturated fats (Figure 36-5). Red meat, egg yolks, and whole milk products are major sources of saturated fat and cholesterol and should be reduced or eliminated from diets. If a person's serum triglyceride level is elevated, the guidelines recommend reducing or eliminating alcohol intake and simple sugars.

Omega-3 fatty acids, when eaten regularly, reduce the risks associated with CAD. For individuals without CAD, the AHA recommends eating fatty fish twice a week because fatty fish such as salmon and tuna contains two types of omega-3 fatty acids: eicosapentaenoic acid (EPA) and docosahexaenoic acid (DHA). Patients with CAD are encouraged to take EPA and DHA supplements with their diet. The AHA also recommends eating tofu and other forms of soybean, canola, walnut, and flaxseed because these products contain alpha-linolenic acid, which becomes omega-3 fatty acid in the body. (For more information on the AHA's nutritional recommendations, see its website, listed in the Resources at the end of this chapter.)

Lifestyle changes, including eating a low-saturated-fat, high-fibre diet, avoiding tobacco, and increasing physical activity, can promote the reversal of CAD and reduce coronary events.

Cholesterol-Lowering Drug Therapy

An estimated 10 million Canadians have high cholesterol levels (≥5.2 mmol/L) (Heart and Stroke Foundation of Canada, 2016a). A complete lipid profile should be obtained every 5 years beginning at age 20. A person with a serum cholesterol level exceeding 5.2 mmol/L is at risk for CAD and should be treated. The Canadian guidelines for treatment focus on LDL levels (Figure 36-6). Treatment usually begins with smoking cessation, dietary caloric restriction (if overweight), decreased dietary fat and cholesterol intake, increased physical activity, and stress management (Smith, Benjamin, Bonow, et al., 2011). Serum cholesterol levels are reassessed after 6 months of diet therapy. If they remain

TABLE 36-4   NUTRITIONAL THERAPY

Tips to Implement Diet and Lifestyle Recommendations

General Tips

- Know your caloric needs to achieve and maintain a healthy weight.
- Know the calorie content of the foods and beverages you consume.
- Track your weight, physical activity, and caloric intake.
- Prepare and eat smaller, more frequent meals.
- Track your activities and, whenever possible, decrease sedentary activities (e.g., television watching, computer time).
- Incorporate physical movement into daily activities (e.g., take extra steps when possible).
- Do not smoke or use tobacco products.
- If you consume alcohol, do so in moderation (i.e., no more than one drink for women or two drinks for men a day).

Tips Related to Food Choices and Preparation

- Use the Nutrition Facts panel on food labels and ingredients list when choosing foods to buy.
- Select frozen and canned vegetables and fruits without high-calorie sauces or added salt and sugars.
- Replace high-calorie foods with fresh fruits and vegetables.
- Increase fibre intake by eating beans (legumes), whole-grain products, fruits, and vegetables.
- Use liquid vegetable oils in place of solid fats.
- Limit beverages and foods high in added sugars (e.g., sucrose, glucose, fructose, maltose, dextrose, corn syrups, concentrated fruit juice, honey).
- Choose foods made with whole grains (e.g., whole wheat, oats/oatmeal, rye, barley, corn, popcorn, brown rice, wild rice, buckwheat, cracked wheat, sorghum).
- Eliminate pastries and high-calorie bakery products (e.g., muffins, doughnuts).
- Select milk and dairy products that are either fat free or low fat.
- Reduce salt intake by:
  - Comparing the sodium content of similar products (e.g., different brands of tomato sauce) and choosing products with less sodium
  - Choosing versions of processed foods that are reduced in salt, including cereals and baked goods
  - Limiting condiments (e.g., soy sauce, ketchup)
- Use lean cuts of meat and remove skin from poultry before cooking or eating.
- Avoid processed meats that are high in saturated fat and sodium (e.g., deli meats).
- Grill, bake, or broil fish, meat, and poultry.
- Incorporate vegetable-based meat substitutes into favourite recipes (e.g., soy).
- Consume whole vegetables and fruits in place of juices.

Source: Adapted from Gidding, S. S., Lichtenstein, A. H., Faith, M. S., et al. (2009). Implementing American Heart Association pediatric and adult nutrition guidelines. *Circulation, 119*(8), 1161–1175. doi:10.1161/CIRCULATIONAHA.109.191856.

elevated, additional dietary options or drug therapy may be started (Table 36-5).

Drugs That Restrict Lipoprotein Production. The "statin" drugs (e.g., lovastatin, pravastatin [Pravachol], simvastatin [Zocor], atorvastatin [Lipitor], and rosuvastatin [Crestor]) are the most widely used and studied lipid-lowering drugs. These drugs inhibit the synthesis of cholesterol in the liver by blocking 3-hydroxy-3-methylglutaryl coenzyme A (HMG-CoA) reductase. An unexplained result of the inhibition of cholesterol synthesis is an increase in hepatic LDL receptors. Consequently, the liver is able to remove more LDLs from the blood. In addition, levels of HDLs increase slightly with the use of statins (Pagana, Pagana,

& Pike-MacDonald, 2013). Serious adverse effects of these drugs can include liver damage and myopathy that can progress to rhabdomyolysis (breakdown of skeletal muscle), but these are rare. Liver enzymes (e.g., aspartate aminotransferase, alanine aminotransferase) must be monitored regularly and checked any time dosage is increased. Creatine kinase (CK) enzymes are assessed if symptoms of myopathy (e.g., muscle aches, weakness) occur (Pagana, Pagana, & Pike-MacDonald, 2013).

Drugs That Increase Lipoprotein Removal. The major process of cholesterol elimination begins with its conversion to bile acids in the liver. Bile acid sequestrants such as cholestyramine and colestipol (Colestid) increase conversion of cholesterol to bile acids and decrease hepatic content of total cholesterol and LDLs.

Complaints associated with these drugs are related to palatability and a variety of upper and lower GI symptoms, including belching, heartburn, nausea, abdominal pain, and constipation. Bile acid sequestrants may interfere with absorption of other drugs (e.g., warfarin [Coumadin], thiazides, thyroid hormones, β-adrenergic blockers). Administering these drugs at a different time than other drugs may decrease this adverse effect (Pagana, Pagana, & Pike-MacDonald, 2013).

Drugs That Decrease Cholesterol Absorption. Drug therapy for hyperlipidemia is likely to be prolonged, perhaps continuing for a lifetime. It is essential that diet be modified in order to minimize the need for drug therapy. The patient must fully understand the rationale and goals of treatment, as well as the safety and adverse effects of lipid-lowering drug therapy (Pagana, Pagana, & Pike-MacDonald, 2013).

Antiplatelet Therapy

Acetylsalicylic acid (ASA; Aspirin) is recommended for most people at risk for cardiovascular disease. Low-dose ASA (81 mg) is recommended for adults 50 to 59 years old who have a calculated 10-year cardiovascular disease risk of 10% or more, are not at increased risk for bleeding (e.g., history of gastro-intestinal bleeding), have a life expectancy of at least 10 years, and are willing to take low-dose ASA for at least 10 years. For adults 60 to 69 years old who have a calculated 10-year cardiovascular disease risk of 10% or more, the decision to take low-dose ASA is an individual one. Adults who have no contraindications (e.g., history of stroke), have a life expectancy of at least 10 years, and are willing to take low-dose ASA daily for at least 10 years are more likely to benefit. Currently, there is insufficient evidence to recommend low-dose ASA for those younger than 50 or older than 70 (Bibbins-Domingo, Grossman, Curry, et al., 2016).

CHRONIC STABLE ANGINA

CAD is a progressive disease, and patients may be asymptomatic for many years, or they may develop chronic but stable chest pain syndromes. When the demand for myocardial oxygen exceeds the ability of the coronary arteries to supply the heart with oxygen, myocardial ischemia occurs. Angina, or chest pain, is the clinical manifestation of reversible myocardial ischemia. Either an increased demand for oxygen or a decreased supply of oxygen can lead to myocardial ischemia (Table 36-6). The primary reason for insufficient blood flow is narrowing of coronary arteries by atherosclerosis (Huether and McCance, 2012).

On the cellular level, the myocardium becomes hypoxic within the first 10 seconds of coronary occlusion. With total occlusion of the coronary arteries, contractility ceases after several minutes, depriving the myocardial cells of oxygen and glucose for aerobic

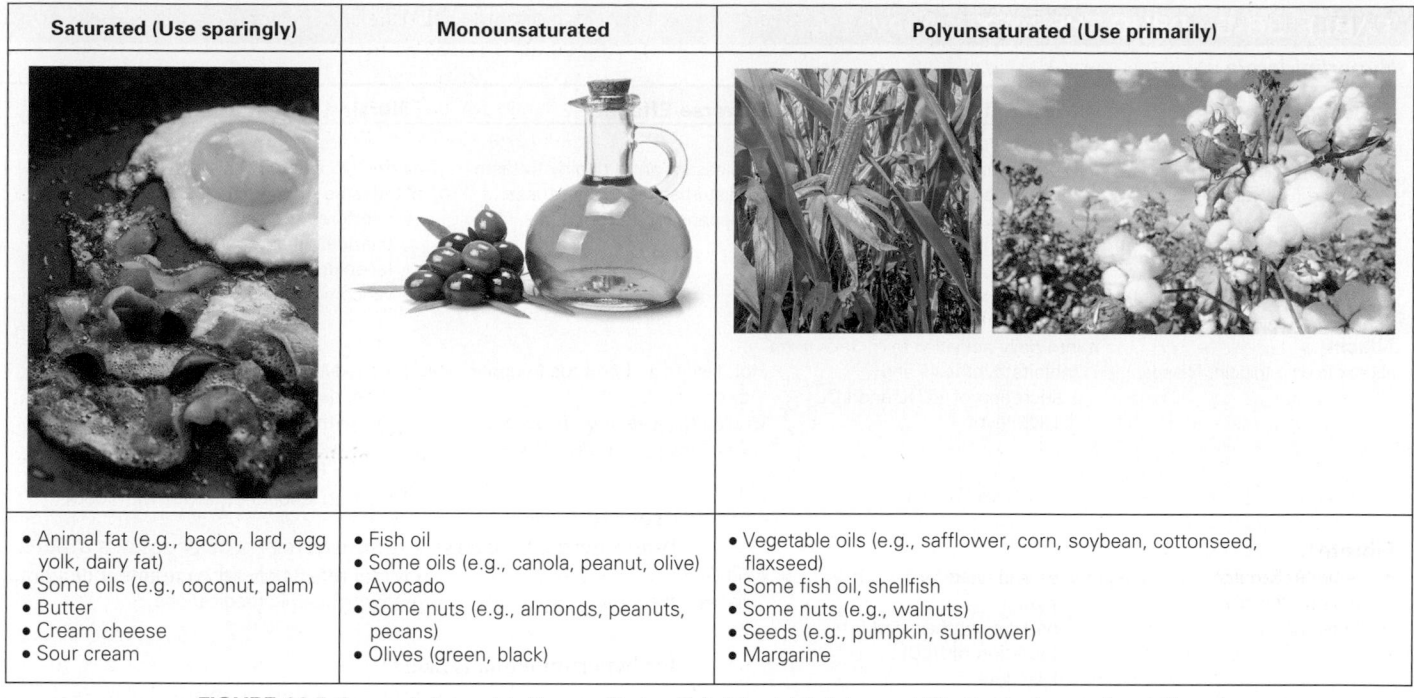

Saturated (Use sparingly)	Monounsaturated	Polyunsaturated (Use primarily)
• Animal fat (e.g., bacon, lard, egg yolk, dairy fat) • Some oils (e.g., coconut, palm) • Butter • Cream cheese • Sour cream	• Fish oil • Some oils (e.g., canola, peanut, olive) • Avocado • Some nuts (e.g., almonds, peanuts, pecans) • Olives (green, black)	• Vegetable oils (e.g., safflower, corn, soybean, cottonseed, flaxseed) • Some fish oil, shellfish • Some nuts (e.g., walnuts) • Seeds (e.g., pumpkin, sunflower) • Margarine

FIGURE 36-5 Types of dietary fat. Source: Photos © *(left to right):* Fotosearch/Shutterstock.com; Angel Simon/Shutterstock.com; petcharaPJ/Shutterstock.com; Jerry Horbert/Shutterstock.com.

FIGURE 36-6 Treatment decisions for high blood cholesterol, based on low-density lipoprotein levels. *FRS,* Framingham Risk Score; *LDL,* low-density lipoprotein. Source: Reprinted from *Journal of Cardiology,* 29(2), Anderson, T., Grégoire, J., Hegele, R., et al., Society Guidelines 2012 Update of the Canadian Cardiovascular Society Guidelines for the Diagnosis and Treatment of Dyslipidemia for the Prevention of Cardiovascular Disease in the Adult, pp. 151–167, Copyright 2013, with permission from Elsevier.
*Not all subjects with diabetes are at high 1-year risk; included for treatment based on randomized studies and high long-term risk.

metabolism. Anaerobic metabolism begins, and lactic acid accumulates. Myocardial nerve fibres are irritated by the increased lactic acid and transmit a pain message to the cardiac nerves and the upper thoracic posterior nerve roots. This is the reason for referred cardiac pain to the left shoulder and arm. In ischemic conditions, cardiac cells are viable for approximately 20 minutes. With restoration of blood flow, aerobic metabolism resumes, contractility is restored, and cellular repair begins.

Chronic stable angina refers to chest pain that occurs intermittently over a long period with the same pattern of onset, duration, and intensity of symptoms. When questioned (Table 36-7), some patients may deny feeling pain but describe a pressure or ache in the chest. It is an unpleasant feeling, often described as a "constrictive," "squeezing," "heavy," "choking," or "suffocating" sensation. Angina is rarely sharp or stabbing, and it usually does not change with position or breathing. Many people with angina

TABLE 36-5   DRUG THERAPY

Hyperlipidemia

Type and Name	Mechanism of Action	Adverse Effects	Nursing Considerations
Bile Acid Sequestrants and Cholesterol Absorption Inhibitors			
Colestipol (Colestid) Ezetimibe (Ezetrol)	Binds with bile acids in intestine, forming insoluble complex, and is excreted in feces	Unpleasant gritty quality to taste GI disturbances (e.g., nausea, dyspepsia, constipation)	Effective and safe for long-term use; adverse effects diminish with time; interferes with absorption of digoxin, thiazides, β-adrenergic blockers, fat-soluble vitamins, folic acid, vancomycin (Vancocin)
Niacin			
Nicotinic acid (niacin, Niaspan)	Inhibits synthesis and secretion of VLDL and LDL ↑ HDL level	Hot flashes and pruritus in upper torso and face GI disturbances (e.g., nausea and vomiting, dyspepsia, diarrhea)	Most adverse effects subside with time; decreased liver function and dysrhythmias may occur with high doses Acetylsalicylic acid (ASA; Aspirin) 30 min to 1 hr before niacin may prevent flushing; should be taken with food
Fibrates			
Bezafibrate (Bezalip) Fenofibrate (Lipidil) Gemfibrozil	↓ triglycerides by ↓ VLDL level ↓ hepatic synthesis and secretion of VLDL ↑ HDL level	Mild GI disturbances (e.g., nausea, diarrhea)	May ↑ effects of anticoagulants and hypoglycemic medications
Statins			
Atorvastatin (Lipitor) Fluvastatin (Lescol) Lovastatin Pravastatin (Pravachol) Rosuvastatin (Crestor) Simvastatin (Zocor)	Block synthesis of cholesterol ↓ LDL and triglyceride levels ↑ HDL level	Rash, mild GI disturbances, insomnia, elevated liver enzyme levels, lens opacities, rhabdomyolysis (specifically with lovastatin)	Well tolerated with few adverse effects Monitoring includes liver function tests and eye examinations

GI, gastro-intestinal; *HDL,* high-density lipoprotein; *LDL,* low-density lipoprotein; *VLDL,* very-low-density lipoprotein.

🔍 EVIDENCE-INFORMED PRACTICE

Research Highlight

Does Dietary Fat Modification Improve Cardiovascular Disease Outcomes?
Clinical Question
For adults (P), what is the effect of dietary fat modification or reduction (I) versus placebo, usual, or control diet (C) on overall mortality and cardiovascular morbidity and mortality (O)?

Best Available Evidence
Systematic review of randomized controlled trials (RCTs)

Critical Appraisal and Synthesis of Evidence
- 48 RCTs with 60 comparisons (*n* = 81 327) of adults with or without existing cardiovascular disease. Intervention was reduced or modified dietary fat intake compared with placebo, usual, or control diet.
- Low-fat diet reduced energy intake to <30% from fat and partially replaced fats with carbohydrates (simple or complex), protein, or fruit and vegetables.
- Modified-fat diet had 30% or more energy intake from total fats, with more monounsaturated or polyunsaturated fats than usual diet.

Conclusions
- Reducing saturated fat by reducing or modifying dietary fat reduced the risk of cardiovascular events.
- Risk for cardiovascular disease decreased in men (not women) by dietary fat modification.

Implications for Nursing Practice
- Counsel patients on modifying dietary fat intake by substituting mono-unsaturated or polyunsaturated fats for saturated fats.
- Assist the patient in collaboration with the dietitian to maintain long-term dietary fat changes.

Reference for Evidence
Hooper, L., Summerbell, C. D., Thompson, R., et al. (2011). Reduced or modified dietary fat for preventing cardiovascular disease. *The Cochrane Database of Systematic Reviews,* No. 7, Article CD002137. doi:10.1002/14651858 .CD002137.pub2.

P, patient population of interest; *I,* intervention or area of interest; *C,* comparison of interest or comparison group; *O,* outcomes of interest (see Chapter 1).

complain of indigestion or a burning sensation in the epigastric region. Although most of the pain experienced by people with angina is substernal, the sensation may occur in the neck or radiate to various locations, including the jaw, the shoulders, and down the arms (Figure 36-7). Sometimes the person may complain of pain between the shoulder blades and dismiss it as not being related to their heart.

The pain is usually brief (lasting 3 to 5 minutes) and commonly subsides when the precipitating factor is relieved (Table 36-8). Pain at rest is unusual. Electrocardiography (ECG) usually reveals

TABLE 36-6 FACTORS DETERMINING MYOCARDIAL OXYGEN NEEDS

Decreased Oxygen Supply	Increased Oxygen Demand or Consumption
Noncardiac Factors	
Anemia	Anxiety
Hypoxemia	Cocaine use
Pneumonia	Hypertension
Asthma	Hyperthermia
Chronic obstructive pulmonary disease	Hyperthyroidism
Low blood volume	Physical exertion
Cardiac Factors	
Coronary artery spasm	Aortic stenosis
Coronary artery thrombosis	Cardiomyopathy
Dysrhythmias	Dysrhythmias
Heart failure	Tachycardia
Valve disorders	

TABLE 36-7 "PQRST" ASSESSMENT OF ANGINA

"PQRST" can be used as a mnemonic to assist in obtaining information from the patient who has chest pain, as follows:

	Factor	Questions to Ask Patient
P	Precipitating events	What events or activities precipitated the pain/discomfort (e.g., argument, exercise, resting)?
Q	Quality of pain	What does the pain/discomfort feel like (e.g., pressure, dull, aching, tight, squeezing)?
R	Radiation of pain	Where is the pain/discomfort located? Does the pain radiate to other areas (e.g., back, arms, jaw, teeth, shoulder, elbow)?
S	Severity of pain	On a scale of 0 to 10, with 10 being the most severe pain you could imagine, how would you rate the pain/discomfort?
T	Timing	When did the pain/discomfort begin? Has the pain/discomfort changed since this time? Have you had pain like this before?

TABLE 36-8 FACTORS PRECIPITATING ANGINA

Physical Exertion
- Increased HR reduces the time the heart spends in diastole (the time of greatest coronary blood flow) and results in an increase in myocardial oxygen demand.
- Isometric exercise of the arms (e.g., raking, lifting heavy objects, or shovelling snow) can cause exertional angina.

Temperature Extremes
- Workload of the heart is increased.
- Blood vessels constrict in response to a cold stimulus.
- Blood vessels dilate and blood pools in the skin in response to a hot stimulus.

Strong Emotions
- The sympathetic nervous system is stimulated.
- The workload of the heart is increased.

Consumption of Heavy Meal
- The workload of the heart may be increased.
- During the digestive process, blood is diverted to the GI system, which reduces blood flow in the coronary arteries.

Tobacco Use
- Nicotine stimulates catecholamine release, causing vasoconstriction and an increase in HR.
- Tobacco diminishes available oxygen by increasing the level of carbon monoxide.

Sexual Activity
- The cardiac workload and sympathetic stimulation are increased.
- In a person with CAD, the extra cardiac workload may precipitate angina.

Stimulants*
- HR and subsequent myocardial oxygen demand are increased.

Circadian Rhythm Patterns
- These patterns are related to the occurrence of chronic stable angina, Prinzmetal's angina, myocardial infarction, and sudden cardiac death.
- Manifestations of CAD tend to occur in the early morning after the patient awakens.

CAD, coronary artery disease; *GI*, gastro-intestinal; *HR*, heart rate.
*For example, cocaine and amphetamines.

- Midsternal
- Left shoulder and down both arms
- Neck and arms

- Substernal radiating to neck and jaw
- Substernal radiating down left arm

- Epigastric
- Epigastric radiating to neck, jaw, and arms

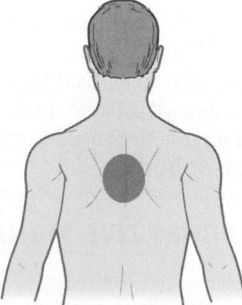
- Intrascapular

FIGURE 36-7 Common locations of pain during angina or myocardial infarction.

TABLE 36-9 COMPARISON OF MAJOR TYPES OF ANGINA

Type	Etiology	Characteristics
Chronic stable angina	Myocardial ischemia, usually secondary to CAD	• Episodic pain lasting 5–15 min • Provoked by exertion • Relieved by rest or nitroglycerin
Prinzmetal's angina	Coronary vasospasm	• Occurs primarily at rest • Triggered by smoking and increased levels of some substances (e.g., histamine, epinephrine) • May occur in presence or absence of CAD
Microvascular angina	Myocardial ischemia secondary to microvascular disease affecting the small, distal branches of the coronary arteries	• More common in women • Triggered by activities of daily living (e.g., shopping, work) vs. physical exercise (exertion) • Treatment may include nitroglycerin
Unstable angina	Rupture of thickened plaque, exposing thrombogenic surface	• New-onset angina • Chronic stable angina that increases in frequency, duration, or severity • Occurs at rest or with minimal exertion • Pain refractory to nitroglycerin

transient ST-segment depression, indicative of ischemia (see Chapter 38).

Chronic stable angina can be controlled with medications on an outpatient basis. Because episodes of chronic stable angina are often predictable, medications can be timed to provide peak effects during the time of day when angina is likely to occur. For example, if angina occurs on arising, the patient can take medication upon awakening and wait 30 minutes to 1 hour before engaging in activity. (The different types of angina are compared in Table 36-9.)

PRINZMETAL'S ANGINA

Prinzmetal's angina (also called *variant angina*) often occurs at rest, usually in response to spasm of a major coronary artery. It is a rare form of angina and occurs in many patients with a history of migraine headaches and Raynaud's phenomenon. The spasm may occur in the absence of CAD, as well as with documented disease. Prinzmetal's angina is not usually precipitated by increased physical demand. Coronary spasm can be described as a strong contraction of smooth muscle in the coronary artery caused by an increase in intracellular calcium.

Factors that may precipitate coronary artery spasm include increased myocardial oxygen demand and increased levels of certain substances (e.g., histamine, angiotensin, epinephrine, norepinephrine, prostaglandins). When spasm occurs, the patient experiences angina, and the ECG demonstrates transient ST-segment elevation (see Chapter 38). The pain may occur during rapid eye movement (REM) sleep, when myocardial oxygen consumption increases. The pain may be relieved by moderate exercise, or it may disappear spontaneously. Cyclic, short bursts of pain at a consistent time each day may also occur with this type of angina. It is usually treated with calcium channel blockers, nitrates, or both.

COLLABORATIVE MANAGEMENT

The treatment of chronic stable angina is aimed at decreasing oxygen demand, increasing oxygen supply, or both. Continued emphasis on the reduction of risk factors is a priority and should include those strategies discussed for patients with CAD (see pp. 818–820). In addition to antiplatelet and cholesterol-lowering drug therapy, the most common therapeutic intervention

TABLE 36-10 MAJOR TREATMENT ELEMENTS OF CHRONIC STABLE ANGINA

Strategies for the patient with chronic stable angina should address all of the treatment elements in the "ABCDEF" mnemonic:

A	Antiplatelet agent Antianginal therapy ACE inhibitor*
B	β-Adrenergic blocker Blood pressure
C	Cigarette smoking Cholesterol
D	Diet Diabetes
E	Education Exercise
F	Flu vaccination*

ACE, angiotensin-converting enzyme.
*Source: Smith, S., Benjamin, E., Bonow, R., et al. (2011). AHA/ACCF secondary prevention and risk reduction therapy for patients with coronary and other atherosclerotic vascular disease: 2011 update. Retrieved from *http://circ.ahajournals.org/content/124/22/2458*.

for the management of chronic stable angina is the use of nitrate therapy to enhance coronary blood flow (Table 36-10, Figure 36-8).

Drug Therapy

Drug therapy for chronic stable angina is aimed at preventing MI and death and reducing symptoms. Acetylsalicylic acid (ASA; Aspirin) (previously discussed) is recommended in the absence of contraindications (Table 36-11).

Short-Acting Nitrates. Short-acting nitrates are first-line therapy for the treatment of angina. Nitrates produce their principal effects by the following mechanisms:

1. Dilating peripheral blood vessels. This results in decreased SVR, venous pooling, and decreased venous blood return to the heart. Because of the reduced cardiac workload, myocardial oxygen demand is decreased.
2. Dilating coronary arteries and collateral vessels. This may increase blood flow to the ischemic areas of the heart. However, when the coronary arteries are severely atherosclerotic, coronary dilation is difficult to achieve.

Diagnostic

History and physical examination
ECG (12-lead)
Chest radiograph
Exercise stress tests
Echocardiogram
Nuclear imaging studies
Electron beam CT scan
Positron emission tomography
Coronary angiography
Laboratory studies:
- Cardiac troponin
- CK-MB
- Myoglobin
- Lipid panel
- CBC
- C-reactive protein
- Homocysteine

Collaborative Therapy

Chronic Stable Angina
Drug therapy*
- Antiplatelet therapy (e.g., ASA [Aspirin], clopidogrel [Plavix])
- Nitroglycerin
- ACE inhibitors, ARBs
- β-adrenergic blockers
- Calcium channel blockers
- Lipid-lowering drugs†
Management of risk factors for coronary artery disease‡
Coronary revascularization
- PCI
- CABG surgery

Acute Coronary Syndrome
12-lead and continuous ECG monitoring
IV access
O_2 therapy
Drug therapy*
- Nitroglycerin
- Morphine sulfate
- ASA
- β-adrenergic blockers
- ACE inhibitors, ARBs

Unstable Angina/ Non–ST-Segment-Elevation MI (NSTEMI)
Acute intensive drug therapy*
- Nitroglycerin
- Antiplatelet therapy (e.g., ASA, clopidogrel, glycoprotein IIb/IIIa inhibitors)
- Anticoagulation therapy (e.g., heparin, direct thrombin inhibitors)
Coronary angiography
- PCI

ST-Segment-Elevation MI (STEMI)
Emergent reperfusion therapy
- PCI
- Thrombolytic therapy*
- CABG surgery
Concurrent drug therapy
- Antiplatelet therapy
- Anticoagulation therapy

FIGURE 36-8 Collaborative care: chronic stable angina and acute coronary syndrome. *ACE,* angiotensin-converting enzyme; *ARBs,* angiotensin II receptor blockers; *ASA,* acetylsalicylic acid; *CABG,* coronary artery bypass graft; *CBC,* complete blood cell count; *CK-MB,* creatine kinase, muscle and brain; *CT,* computed tomography; *ECG,* electrocardiogram; *IV,* intravenous; O_2, oxygen; *PCI,* percutaneous coronary intervention. *See Table 36-11. †See Table 36-5. ‡See Tables 36-2, 36-3, and 36-4.

Sublingual Nitroglycerin. Nitroglycerin administered sublingually (Nitrostat) or by translingual spray (Nitrolingual) usually relieves pain in approximately 3 minutes, and its action has a duration of approximately 30 to 60 minutes. The recommended dosage for symptoms of angina is one tablet taken sublingually (SL) or one metered spray. If symptoms are unchanged or worse after 5 minutes, the patient should be instructed to contact the emergency medical services (EMS) system.

Nitroglycerin should be easily accessible to the patient at all times, and the patient must be instructed in its proper use: place a tablet under the tongue and allow it to dissolve, or, if using the spray, direct the spray under the tongue (do not inhale it). Nitroglycerin should cause a tingling sensation. If tingling is not felt and chest pain persists, the patient should know to contact EMS. The patient should be warned that HR may increase and a pounding headache, dizziness, or flushing may occur. The patient should be cautioned against quickly rising to a standing position because orthostatic hypotension may occur after nitroglycerin use.

Nitroglycerin tablets are marketed in light-resistant bottles with metal caps and, for protection from degradation, should be kept in the tightly closed bottle. Because they tend to lose potency once a bottle has been opened, the patient should be advised to purchase a new supply every 6 months.

Long-Acting Nitrates. Nitrates, such as isosorbide dinitrate and isosorbide mononitrate (Imdur), are longer-acting than SL or translingual nitroglycerin and can be used to reduce the

incidence of anginal attacks (Pagana, Pagana, & Pike-MacDonald, 2013). The predominant adverse effect of all nitrates is headache, caused by the dilation of cerebral blood vessels. Patients can be advised to take acetaminophen (Tylenol) with their nitrate to relieve the headache. Over time, the headaches may decrease, but the principal antianginal effect remains the same.

Orthostatic hypotension is a complication of all nitrates. Nurses should monitor BP after the initial dose because the venous dilation that occurs may cause a drop in BP, especially in volume-depleted patients. In addition, tolerance to nitroglycerin-induced vasodilation can develop. It is recommended that patients schedule an 8-hour nitrate-free period every day, usually during the night, except for patients who experience nocturnal angina (Pagana, Pagana, & Pike-MacDonald, 2013).

Transdermal Controlled-Release Nitrates. Currently, two systems are available for transdermal nitroglycerin drug administration: reservoir and matrix. The reservoir system delivers the medication using a rate-controlled permeable membrane. The matrix system provides for a slow delivery of the medication through a polymer matrix. Both reservoir and matrix delivery systems offer the advantages of steady plasma levels within the therapeutic range during 24 hours; thus only one application a day is necessary. The reservoir system has the disadvantage of dose dumping if the reservoir seal is punctured or broken; the matrix system, in contrast, avoids this problem. Both systems achieve steady-state plasma drug levels within 2 hours.

TABLE 36-11   DRUG THERAPY

Chronic Stable Angina and Acute Coronary Syndrome

Drug Classification	Mechanism of Action and Comments	Nursing Considerations	Drug Classification	Mechanism of Action and Comments	Nursing Considerations
Antiplatelet Agents			**Angiotensin-Converting Enzyme (ACE) Inhibitors***		
Acetylsalicylic acid (ASA; Aspirin)	• Inhibit cyclo-oxygenase (which produces thromboxane A_2, a potent platelet activator) • Should be administered as soon as acute coronary syndrome is suspected		Captopril Enalapril (Vasotec)	• Prevent conversion of angiotensin I to angiotensin II • Decrease endothelial dysfunction • Useful in treatment of heart failure, tachycardia, MI, hypertension, diabetes, and chronic kidney disease	
Adenosine Diphosphate Receptor Antagonists					
Clopidogrel (Plavix)	• Inhibit platelet aggregation • Alternative for patient who cannot use ASA • Oral clopidogrel, 75 mg/day, should be added to ASA therapy in patients with STEMI, regardless of whether they undergo reperfusion therapy)	Assess for signs of bleeding, stroke, thrombo-cytopenia, renal dysfunction, fever. Monitor CBC with differential and platelet count, serum bilirubin.	**Unfractionated Heparins†**		
			Heparin	• Prevent conversion of fibrinogen to fibrin and of prothrombin to thrombin	Monitor for signs of bleeding (bleeding gums, epistaxis, black tarry stools).
Nitrates			**Low-Molecular-Weight Heparins†**		
Sublingual nitroglycerin (Nitrostat) Translingual spray nitroglycerin (Nitrolingual) Transdermal nitroglycerin (Transderm-Nitro, Minitran) Extended-release buccal tablets Isosorbide mononitrate (Imdur) IV nitroglycerin (Nitroject)	• Promote peripheral vasodilation, decreasing preload and afterload • Promote coronary artery vasodilation	Assess for headache, dizziness, and hypotension.	Dalteparin (Fragmin) Enoxaparin (Lovenox)	• Bind to antithrombin III, enhancing its effect • Heparin–antithrombin III complex inactivates activated factor X and thrombin • Prevent conversion of fibrinogen to fibrin	Monitor for signs of bleeding.
			Glycoprotein IIB and IIIA Inhibitors		
			Abciximab (ReoPro) Eptifibatide (Integrilin) Tirofiban (Aggrastat)	• Prevent the binding of fibrinogen to platelets, thereby blocking platelet aggregation • Standard antiplatelet therapy in combination with ASA for patients at high risk for unstable angina	Monitor for signs of bleeding.
β-Adrenergic Blockers*			**Opioid Analgesics**		
Atenolol (Tenormin) Carvedilol Esmolol (Brevibloc) Metoprolol (Lopresor) Nadolol Propranolol (Inderal)	• Inhibit sympathetic nervous stimulation of the heart • Reduce both heart rate and contractility • Decrease afterload	Monitor apical heart rate and BP prior to administration. Assess for hypotension, dizziness, and signs of heart failure (dyspnea, crackles, weight gain, peripheral edema).	Morphine, morphine sulphate	• Function as analgesic and sedative • Act as vasodilator to reduce preload and myocardial O_2 consumption	Monitor respiratory rate; assess for respiratory depression, CNS depression, and hypotension.
			Fibrinolytic Therapy		
Calcium Channel Blockers*			Tissue plasminogen activator (t-PA; alteplase [Activase]) Tenecteplase (TNK, TNKase)	• Break up fibrin meshwork in clots • Used only in STEMI	Monitor for signs of bleeding.
Amlodipine (Norvasc) Diltiazem (Cardizem) Felodipine (Plendil) Nifedipine Verapamil (Isoptin)	• Prevent calcium entry into vascular smooth muscle cells and myocytes (cardiac cells) • Promote coronary and peripheral vasodilation • Reduce both heart rate and contractility	Monitor BP and pulse prior to administration. Monitor ECG. Assess for signs of heart failure (dyspnea, peripheral edema, crackles).			

BP, blood pressure; *CBC*, complete blood cell count; *ECG*, electrocardiogram; *IV*, intravenous; *MI*, myocardial infarction; *STEMI*, ST-segment elevation myocardial infarction.
*See Chapter 35, Table 35-8.
†See Chapter 40, Table 40-10.

β-Adrenergic Blockers. β-Adrenergic blockers (e.g., propranolol [Inderal], metoprolol [Lopresor], nadolol, atenolol [Tenormin], and carvedilol) are the preferred drugs for the management of chronic stable angina (Pagana, Pagana, & Pike-MacDonald, 2013). These drugs cause decreases in myocardial contractility, HR, SVR, and BP, all of which reduce the myocardial oxygen demand. β-Adrenergic blockers also have been shown to decrease morbidity and mortality in patients with CAD, especially following MI (Pagana, Pagana, & Pike-MacDonald, 2013).

β-Adrenergic blockers have many adverse effects and are sometimes poorly tolerated. Adverse effects may include bradycardia, hypotension, wheezing, and GI complaints. Many patients also complain of weight gain, depression, and sexual dysfunction. β-Adrenergic blockers should be avoided by patients with asthma and used cautiously by patients with diabetes because their effects mask signs of hypoglycemia. Abrupt discontinuation of β-adrenergic blockers may precipitate an increase in the frequency and intensity of angina attacks, so medical supervision during discontinuation is necessary (Pagana, Pagana, & Pike-MacDonald, 2013).

Calcium Channel Blockers. If use of β-adrenergic blockers is contraindicated or if they are poorly tolerated or do not control anginal symptoms, calcium channel blockers (e.g., nifedipine, verapamil, diltiazem [Cardizem]) are used (Pagana, Pagana, & Pike-MacDonald, 2013). These medications are also used to manage Prinzmetal's angina. Most of these drugs are available in sustained-release formulations for longer action, which has the advantages of helping increase patient adherence to therapy and of stabilizing blood levels of the drug. The three primary effects of calcium channel blockers are (a) systemic vasodilation with decreased SVR, (b) decreased myocardial contractility, and (c) coronary vasodilation.

Cardiac muscle and vascular smooth muscle cells are more dependent on extracellular calcium than are skeletal muscles and are therefore more sensitive to calcium channel blockers. Calcium channel blockers cause smooth muscle relaxation and relative vasodilation of coronary and systemic arteries, thus increasing blood flow.

Calcium channel blockers potentiate the action of digoxin by increasing serum digoxin levels during the first week of therapy. Therefore, serum digoxin levels should be closely monitored after starting this therapy. Normal digoxin levels are 0.6–1.3 nmol/L (0.8–2 ng/mL). The patient should be taught the signs and symptoms of digoxin toxicity.

Angiotensin-Converting Enzyme Inhibitors. Certain high-risk patients with chronic stable angina may benefit from the addition of an angiotensin-converting enzyme (ACE) inhibitor (e.g., captopril) to the drug regimen (Pagana, Pagana, & Pike-MacDonald, 2013). Such patients include those with diabetes, significant CAD as determined by coronary angiography (e.g., multivessel disease), or previous history of MI with left ventricular dysfunction. (ACE inhibitors are discussed further later in this chapter and in Chapter 35 and Table 35-8.)

Diagnostic Studies

When a patient has a history of CAD or if CAD is suspected, the physician orders a variety of studies (see Figure 36-8). After a detailed health history is documented and a physical examination is performed, a chest radiograph is usually taken to look for cardiac enlargement, aortic calcifications, and pulmonary congestion. A 12-lead ECG is obtained and, when possible, compared with an earlier tracing. Certain laboratory tests (e.g.,

lipid profile) and diagnostic studies (e.g., Holter monitoring, echocardiography) are ordered to confirm CAD and identify specific risk factors for CAD.

For patients with known CAD and chronic stable angina, common diagnostic studies include 12-lead ECG, echocardiography, exercise stress testing, pharmacological nuclear imaging, and coronary angiography (Pagana, Pagana, & Pike-MacDonald, 2013). (See Chapter 34 and Table 34-6 for a discussion of these studies, including nursing considerations.) Electrocardiography and coronary angiography are discussed in further detail in the section "Diagnostic Studies of the Cardiovascular System" in Chapter 34.

ACUTE CORONARY SYNDROME

When myocardial ischemia is prolonged and not immediately reversible, acute coronary syndrome (ACS) develops; this syndrome encompasses the spectrum of unstable angina, non–ST-segment elevation myocardial infarction (NSTEMI), and ST-segment elevation myocardial infarction (STEMI). Although each remains a distinct diagnosis, this nomenclature (ACS) reflects the relationships among pathophysiology, diagnosis, prognosis, and interventions for these disorders.

ETIOLOGY AND PATHOPHYSIOLOGY

ACS is associated with deterioration of an atherosclerotic plaque that was once stable. The plaque ruptures, exposing the intima to blood and stimulating platelet aggregation and local vasoconstriction with thrombus formation. This unstable lesion may be partially occluded by a thrombus (manifesting as UA or NSTEMI) or totally occluded by a thrombus (manifesting as STEMI). What causes a coronary plaque to suddenly become unstable is not well understood, but systemic inflammation (described earlier) is thought to play a role. Patients with suspected ACS require immediate hospitalization.

MANIFESTATIONS OF ACUTE CORONARY SYNDROME

Unstable Angina

Chest pain that is new in onset, occurs at rest, or has a worsening pattern is called unstable angina (UA). Patients with chronic stable angina may develop UA, or UA may be the first clinical manifestation of CAD. Unlike chronic stable angina, UA is unpredictable and represents an emergency. Patients with previously diagnosed chronic stable angina describe a significant change in the pattern of angina. It occurs with increasing frequency and is easily provoked by minimal or no exertion, during sleep, or even at rest. Patients without previously diagnosed angina describe anginal pain that has progressed rapidly in the past few hours, days, or weeks, often culminating in pain at rest.

Women with symptoms of UA seek medical attention more often than do men. Studies have shown that women have prodrome symptoms that are early manifestations of CAD, but because they are not recognized as such, what brings these women to first seek care is UA, before CAD is diagnosed. These symptoms include fatigue, shortness of breath, indigestion, and anxiety. Fatigue is the most prominent symptom. Because fatigue can be a symptom of many different diseases and syndromes, a thorough history of CAD risk factors should be obtained to identify these women.

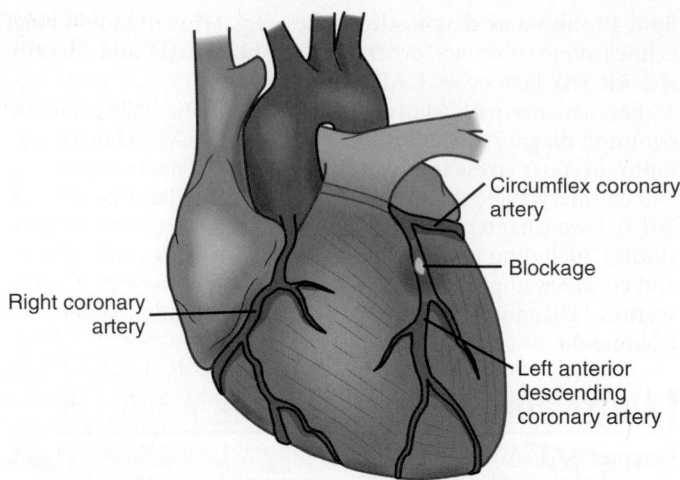

FIGURE 36-9 Diagram of occlusion of the left anterior descending coronary artery, resulting in a myocardial infarction.

FIGURE 36-10 Acute myocardial infarction in the posterolateral wall of the left ventricle, demonstrated by the absence of staining in the areas of necrosis *(white arrow)*. Note the scarring from a previous anterior wall myocardial infarction *(black arrow)*. Source: Kumar, V., Abbas, A. K., Fausto, N., et al. (2010). *Robbins and Cochran pathologic basis of disease* (8th ed., p. 6). Philadelphia: W. B. Saunders.

MYOCARDIAL INFARCTION

A myocardial infarction (MI) occurs as a result of sustained ischemia, causing irreversible myocardial cell death (necrosis; Figures 36-9 and 36-10). Between 80% and 90% of all acute MIs occur secondary to thrombus formation. When a thrombus develops, perfusion to the myocardium distal to the occlusion is halted, resulting in necrosis. Contractile function of the heart stops in the necrotic areas. The degree of altered function depends on the area of the heart involved and the size of the infarction. Most MIs involve some portion of the left ventricle.

The acute MI process takes time. Cardiac cells can withstand ischemic conditions for approximately 20 minutes before cellular death begins. The tissue to become ischemic earliest is the subendocardium (the innermost layer of tissue in the cardiac muscle). If ischemia persists, the entire thickness of the heart muscle becomes necrosed in approximately 5 to 6 hours.

Descriptions of infarctions are usually based on the location of damage (e.g., anterior, inferior, lateral, or posterior wall infarction). Damage can occur in more than one location (e.g., anterolateral MI, anteroseptal MI). The location of the infarction correlates with the involved coronary circulation. For example, inferior wall infarctions result from occlusions in the right coronary artery. Anterior wall infarctions result from occlusions in the left anterior descending artery. Occlusions in the left circumflex artery usually cause MIs in the lateral or posterior wall or both.

The degree of pre-established collateral circulation also influences the severity of infarction (see Figure 36-2). In an individual with a history of CAD, collateral circulation may be established, and so the area surrounding the infarction site develops a blood supply. This is one explanation for why a younger person who has an MI often experiences a more serious impairment than an older person with the same degree of occlusion.

Clinical Manifestations of Myocardial Infarction

Pain. Severe, immobilizing chest pain not relieved by rest, position change, or nitrate administration is the hallmark of an MI. Persistent and unlike any other pain, it is usually described as a feeling of heaviness, pressure, tightness, burning, or constriction or as a crushing sensation. Common locations are substernal, retrosternal, and epigastric areas. The pain may radiate to the neck, the jaw, and the arms or to the back (see Figure 36-7). It may occur while the patient is active or at rest or when the patient is asleep or awake. However, it commonly occurs in the early morning hours. It usually lasts for 20 minutes or more and is described as more severe than usual anginal pain. When epigastric pain is present, the patient may relate it to indigestion and take antacids without relief.

Not everyone has classic symptoms. Some patients may not experience pain but may have "discomfort," weakness, or shortness of breath. Although symptoms of an acute MI in women and men have more similarities than differences, some women may experience atypical discomfort, shortness of breath, or fatigue. Patients with diabetes are more likely to experience silent (asymptomatic) MIs as a result of cardiac neuropathy and seek care with atypical symptoms (e.g., dyspnea). Older patients may experience a change in mental status (e.g., confusion), shortness of breath, pulmonary edema, dizziness, or a dysrhythmia.

Sympathetic Nervous System Stimulation. During the initial phase of MI, catecholamines (norepinephrine and epinephrine) are released from the ischemic myocardial cells that normally contain varying quantities of these substances. The increased SNS stimulation results in release of glycogen, diaphoresis, and vasoconstriction of peripheral blood vessels. On physical examination, the patient's skin may be ashen, clammy, and cool to the touch.

Cardiovascular Manifestations. In response to the release of catecholamines, the BP and HR may initially be elevated. Later, the BP may drop because of decreased cardiac output (CO). If the drop is severe enough, renal perfusion and urine output may decrease. Crackles may be noted in the lungs, persisting for several hours to several days and suggesting left ventricular dysfunction. Jugular venous distension, hepatic engorgement, and peripheral edema may indicate right ventricular dysfunction.

Cardiac examination may reveal abnormal heart sounds that may seem distant. Careful auscultation may reveal splitting of heart sounds. Other abnormal sounds suggestive of ventricular dysfunction are the third heart sound (S_3) and the fourth heart sound (S_4). In addition, a loud holosystolic murmur may develop and may indicate a septal defect or mitral valve dysfunction.

Nausea and Vomiting. Nausea and vomiting can result in some patients due to reflex stimulation of the vomiting centre by the severe pain. These symptoms can also result from vasovagal reflexes initiated in the area of the infarcted myocardium.

Fever. The patient's temperature may increase within the first 24 hours up to 38°C and occasionally as high as 39°C. The temperature elevation may last for as long as 1 week. This increase in temperature is a systemic manifestation of the inflammatory process caused by myocardial cell death.

Healing Process

The body's response to cell death is the inflammatory process (see Chapter 14). Within 24 hours, leukocytes infiltrate the area. Enzymes are released from the dead cardiac cells and are important diagnostic indicators of MI. (See the section "Serum Cardiac Markers" later in this chapter.) The proteolytic enzymes of the neutrophils and macrophages remove all necrotic tissue by the second or third day. During this time, the necrotic muscle wall is thin. The development of collateral circulation improves areas of poor perfusion and may limit the zones of injury and infarction. Once infarction takes place, catecholamine-mediated lipolysis and glycogenolysis occur. These processes allow the increased amounts of plasma glucose and free fatty acids to be used by the oxygen-depleted myocardium for anaerobic metabolism. For this reason, serum glucose levels are frequently elevated after MI.

The necrotic zone is identifiable by ECG changes (e.g., ST-segment elevation, pathological Q wave) and on nuclear scanning after the onset of symptoms. At this point, the neutrophils and monocytes have cleared the necrotic debris from the injured area, and the collagen matrix that will eventually form scar tissue is laid down.

Ten to 14 days after MI, the scar tissue beginning to form is still weak. The myocardium is considered to be especially vulnerable to increased stress because of the unstable state of the healing heart wall. It is also at this time that the patient's activity level may be increasing, and so special caution and assessment are necessary. By 6 weeks after MI, scar tissue has replaced necrotic tissue. At this time, the injured area is said to be healed. The scarred area is often less malleable than the surrounding fibres. This condition may be manifested by uncoordinated wall motion, ventricular dysfunction, or pump failure.

These changes in the infarcted muscle also cause changes in the unaffected myocardium. In an attempt to compensate for the infarcted muscle, the normal myocardium hypertrophies and dilates. This process is called *ventricular remodelling*. Remodelling of normal myocardium can lead to the development of late heart failure (HF), especially in individuals with atherosclerosis of other coronary arteries, an anterior MI, or both.

Complications of Myocardial Infarction

Dysrhythmias. The most common complication after an MI is a dysrhythmia, which is present in 80% of patients who have had an MI. Dysrhythmias are the most common cause of death in patients in the pre-hospitalization period. Dysrhythmias are caused by any condition that affects the myocardial cell's sensitivity to nerve impulses, such as ischemia, electrolyte imbalances, and SNS stimulation. The intrinsic rhythm of the heartbeat is disrupted, causing a fast HR (tachycardia), a slow HR (bradycardia), or an irregular beat, any of which adversely affects the ischemic myocardium.

Life-threatening dysrhythmias occur most often with anterior wall infarction, HF, or shock. Complete heart block can occur in massive infarction. Ventricular fibrillation, a common cause of

sudden cardiac death (SCD), is a lethal dysrhythmia that most often occurs within the first 4 hours after the onset of pain. Premature ventricular contractions (PVCs) may precede ventricular tachycardia and fibrillation. Life-threatening ventricular dysrhythmias must be treated immediately. (See Chapter 38 for a detailed description of dysrhythmias and their management.)

Heart Failure. Heart failure is a complication of MI in which the pumping power of the heart has diminished. Depending on the severity and extent of the injury, HF occurs initially with subtle signs such as mild dyspnea, restlessness, agitation, or slight tachycardia. Other signs indicating the onset of HF include pulmonary congestion, seen on chest radiograph; S_3 or S_4 heart sounds, heard on auscultation; crackles, heard on auscultation of breath sounds; and jugular vein distension, caused by right-sided HF. (The treatment of acute decompensated HF is discussed in Chapter 37.)

Cardiogenic Shock. Cardiogenic shock is a condition in which inadequate oxygen and nutrients are supplied to the tissues because of severe left ventricular failure. Cardiogenic shock has occurred less often since the advent of early and rapid treatment of MI with fibrinolytic therapy and percutaneous coronary intervention (PCI), an intervention in which a catheter equipped with an inflatable balloon tip is inserted into a narrowed coronary artery and the balloon is inflated. The rate of mortality from cardiogenic shock is high. Cardiogenic shock necessitates aggressive management, including control of dysrhythmias, intra-aortic balloon pump (IABP) therapy, and support of contractility with the use of vasoactive drugs. The goal of therapy is to maximize oxygen delivery, reduce oxygen demand, and prevent complications such as acute kidney injury. (Cardiogenic shock is discussed in Chapter 69.)

Papillary Muscle Dysfunction. Papillary muscle dysfunction may occur if the infarcted area includes or is adjacent to the papillary muscle that attaches to the mitral valve (see Figure 34-2). Papillary muscle dysfunction causes mitral valve regurgitation, which increases the volume of blood in the left atrium. This condition aggravates an already compromised left ventricle by reducing CO even further. Papillary muscle dysfunction is detected by a systolic murmur at the cardiac apex radiating toward the axilla.

Papillary muscle rupture is a rare but life-threatening complication that causes massive mitral valve regurgitation, which results in dyspnea, pulmonary edema, and decreased CO. The patient's condition deteriorates rapidly. Treatment consists of rapid afterload reduction with nitroprusside, IABP therapy and immediate open-heart surgery with mitral valve replacement, or both. (See Chapter 39 for discussion of valvular disorders.)

Ventricular Aneurysm. Ventricular aneurysm results when the infarcted myocardial wall becomes thinned and bulges out during contraction. The patient with a ventricular aneurysm may experience refractory HF, dysrhythmias, and angina. Besides ventricular rupture, which is fatal, ventricular aneurysms harbour thrombi, which can cause an embolic stroke.

Pericarditis. Acute pericarditis—an inflammation of the visceral or parietal pericardium or both—may result in cardiac compression, decreased ventricular filling and emptying, and HF. It may occur 2 to 3 days after an acute MI as a common complication. Pericarditis is characterized by chest pain, which may vary from mild to severe, and is aggravated by inspiration, coughing, and movement of the upper body. The pain may be relieved by sitting in a forward position. The pain is usually different from the pain associated with an MI.

Assessment of a patient with pericarditis may reveal a friction rub over the pericardium. The sound may be best heard with the diaphragm of the stethoscope at the midsternal to lower sternal border. It may be persistent or intermittent. Fever may also be present.

Diagnosis of pericarditis can be made with serial 12-lead ECGs. Characteristic ECG changes are diffuse and reflect the inflammation of the pericardium. Treatment may include pain relief by ASA, corticosteroids, or nonsteroidal anti-inflammatory drugs (NSAIDs). (Pericarditis is discussed further in Chapter 39.)

Dressler's Syndrome. Dressler's syndrome is characterized by pericarditis with effusion and fever that develops 4 to 6 weeks after MI. It may also occur after open-heart surgery. It is thought to be caused by an antigen–antibody reaction to the necrotic myocardium. The patient experiences pericardial pain, fever, a friction rub, pleural effusion, and arthralgia. Laboratory findings include an elevated white blood cell count and an elevated sedimentation rate. Short-term courses of corticosteroids are used to treat this condition. (Dressler's syndrome is discussed further in Chapter 39.)

DIAGNOSTIC STUDIES

Unstable Angina and Myocardial Infarction

In addition to the patient's history of pain, risk factors, and health history, the primary diagnostic studies used to determine whether a person has UA or an MI include an ECG and measurement of serum cardiac markers (see Figure 36-8).

Electrocardiographic Findings. ECG is the primary tool to rule out or confirm UA or an MI. Changes in the QRS complex, the ST segment, and the T wave caused by ischemia and infarction can develop quickly with UA and MI. For diagnostic and treatment purposes, it is important to distinguish among STEMI, UA, and NSTEMI. Patients with STEMI tend to have a more extensive MI associated with prolonged and complete coronary occlusion and the development of a pathological Q wave on the ECG. Patients with UA or NSTEMI usually have transient thrombosis or incomplete coronary occlusion and usually do not develop pathological Q waves. Areas of ischemia or infarction may be noted on the ECG. Because MI is a dynamic process that evolves with time, the ECG often reveals the time sequence of ischemia, injury, infarction, and resolution of the infarction.

The ECG may also be normal or nondiagnostic when the patient comes to the ED with a complaint of chest pain. Within a few hours, the ECG may change to reflect the infarction process. These changes take place when cellular damage has occurred, interrupting the normal electrical depolarization of the ventricles. When the initial ECG is nondiagnostic, serial ECGs are obtained every 2 to 4 hours (Aehlert, 2013). (See Chapter 38 for discussion of ECG changes associated with ischemia and MI.)

Serum Cardiac Markers. After an MI, certain proteins called *serum cardiac markers* are released into the blood in large quantities from necrotic heart muscle. These markers, specifically serum cardiac enzymes and troponin, are important in the diagnosis of MI. When cardiac cells die, their intracellular enzymes are released into circulation. The increase in serum cardiac markers that occurs after cellular death can indicate whether cardiac damage is present and the approximate extent of the damage. CK and troponin are typically measured to diagnose an MI. Figure 36-11 indicates the peak levels and durations of these markers in the presence of MI.

FIGURE 36-11 Levels of serum cardiac markers in the blood after myocardial infarction. *CK-MB,* MB isoenzyme of creatine kinase.

CK levels begin to rise approximately 3 to 12 hours after an MI, peak in 24 hours, and return to normal within 2 to 3 days. The CK enzymes may be fractionated into bands, including the MB band. The MB isoenzyme of creatine kinase (CK-MB) band is specific to myocardial cells and can help quantify myocardial damage.

Cardiac-specific troponin is a myocardial muscle protein released into circulation after myocardial injury. In the heart, there are two subtypes: cardiac-specific troponin T (cTnT) and cardiac-specific troponin I (cTnI). These markers are highly specific indicators of MI, and their tests have greater sensitivity and specificity for myocardial injury than that for CK-MB (Pagana, Pagana, & Pike-MacDonald, 2013). The troponin level rises as quickly as the CK level. Troponins are usually measured for diagnostic purposes in conjunction with total CK and the MB fraction. Serum levels of cTnI and cTnT increase 3 to 12 hours after the onset of MI, peak at 24 to 48 hours, and return to baseline over 5 to 14 days.

Myoglobin is released into circulation within a few hours after an MI. Although it is one of the first serum cardiac markers whose levels increase after an MI, it lacks cardiac specificity. In addition, it is rapidly excreted in urine so that blood levels return to normal range within 24 hours after an MI (see Chapter 34, Table 34-6).

Coronary Angiography. The patient with UA or NSTEMI may undergo coronary angiography to evaluate the extent of the disease and to determine the most appropriate therapeutic modality. If appropriate, PCI may be performed at this time. Other patients may be treated with conservative medical management. Coronary angiography is the only way to confirm the diagnosis of Prinzmetal's angina.

Other Measures

When the ECG and serum cardiac marker levels do not confirm MI, other measures for diagnosing UA may be considered (see Chapter 34, Table 34-6). Exercise stress testing and echocardiography may be conducted when a patient has an abnormal but nondiagnostic baseline ECG. Dobutamine stress echocardiography can be performed in patients unable

✚ TABLE 36-12 EMERGENCY MANAGEMENT

Chest Pain

Etiology	Assessment Findings	Interventions
Cardiovascular • Angina • Myocardial infarction • Dysrhythmia • Pericarditis • Aortic aneurysm • Aortic valve disease **Respiratory** • Costochondritis • Pleurisy • Pneumonia • Pneumothorax • Pulmonary edema • Pulmonary embolus **Chest Trauma** • Rib or sternal fracture • Flail chest • Cardiac tamponade • Pneumothorax • Pulmonary contusion • Great vessel injury **Gastro-Intestinal** • Esophagitis • GERD • Hiatal hernia • Peptic ulcer • Cholecystitis **Others** • Stress • Strenuous exercise • Drugs • Acute anxiety	• Pain in chest, neck, arm, or shoulder • Cold, clammy skin • Diaphoresis • Nausea and vomiting • Epigastric pain • Indigestion or heartburn • Dyspnea • Weakness • Anxiety • Feeling of impending doom • Tachycardia • Irregular HR, murmurs • Palpitations • Dysrhythmias • Decreased BP • Narrowed pulse pressure • Unequal BP readings in upper extremities • Syncope, loss of consciousness • Decreased O$_2$ saturation • Decreased or absent breath sounds • Crackles, wheezes • Pericardial friction rub	**Initial** • Ensure patent airway. • Administer O$_2$ by nasal cannula or nonrebreather mask. • Obtain 12-lead ECG. • Insert two IV catheters. • Assess pain, using "PQRST" mnemonic (see Table 36-7). • Medicate for pain as ordered (e.g., morphine, nitroglycerin). • Initiate continuous ECG monitoring and identify underlying rhythm. • Obtain baseline blood test results (e.g., cardiac markers). • Obtain portable chest radiograph. • Assess for antiplatelet, anticoagulation, or fibrinolytic therapy or for PCI as appropriate. • Administer ASA (Aspirin) and β-adrenergic blockers for cardiac-related chest pain unless contraindicated. • Administer antidysrhythmic medications as indicated. **Ongoing Monitoring** • Monitor vital signs, level of consciousness, cardiac rhythm, and O$_2$ saturation. • Monitor response to medications (e.g., decrease in chest pain) and readminister or titrate medications (e.g., nitroglycerin) as needed. • Provide reassurance and emotional support to patient and family. • Explain all interventions and procedures to patient in simple terms. • Anticipate need for intubation if respiratory distress is evident. • Prepare for CPR, defibrillation, transcutaneous pacing, or cardioversion.

ASA, acetylsalicylic acid; *BP,* blood pressure; *CPR,* cardiopulmonary resuscitation; *GERD,* gastro-esophageal reflux disease; *HR,* heart rate; *IV,* intravenous; *O$_2$,* oxygen; *PCI,* percutaneous coronary intervention.

to exercise. (See Chapter 34 for additional information on cardiac assessment.)

COLLABORATIVE CARE

It is extremely important that ACS be rapidly diagnosed and treated to preserve cardiac muscle. Initial management of chest pain most often occurs in the ED. Emergency care of patients with chest pain is described in Table 36-12. An intravenous (IV) route is established to provide an accessible means for emergency drug therapy. Sublingual nitroglycerin and chewable ASA (Aspirin) are administered if not done by emergency medical personnel before arrival at the ED. Morphine sulphate is given by IV route for pain unrelieved by nitroglycerin. Oxygen is administered by nasal cannula at a rate of 2 to 4 L/min. Patients usually receive ongoing care in an intensive care unit or telemetry unit, in which continuous ECG monitoring is available. Dysrhythmias may be detected, and appropriate treatment can be instituted. The collaborative care of ACS is described in Figure 36-8.

Vital signs, including pulse oximetry, are monitored frequently during the first few hours after admission and are monitored closely thereafter. Bed rest and limitation of activity for 12 to 24 hours are initially ordered, with a gradual increase in activity unless it is contraindicated.

For patients with UA or NSTEMI who have increased levels of cardiac markers and ongoing angina, a combination of ASA (Aspirin), heparin (unfractionated [UH] or low-molecular-weight [LMWH]), and a glycoprotein IIb/IIIa inhibitor (e.g., abciximab [ReoPro], eptifibatide [Integrilin], tirofiban [Aggrastat]) is recommended. PCI is a common elective procedure considered once the patient is stabilized and angina is controlled or if angina returns or increases in severity.

For patients with STEMI or NSTEMI with elevated levels of cardiac markers, reperfusion therapy is initiated (see Figure 36-8). Reperfusion therapy—therapy to open the coronary artery that was occluded and restore blood flow to the myocardium—can include emergent PCI or fibrinolytic (thrombolytic) therapy. The goal in the treatment of MI is to salvage as much myocardial muscle as possible.

Emergent Percutaneous Coronary Intervention

In centres that perform at least 200 PCI procedures a year and have trained interventional cardiologists and cardiac surgical capability, emergent PCI is recommended as the first line of treatment for patients with confirmed MI (i.e., definitive ECG changes, presence of cardiac markers, or both). The goal is to open the affected artery within 90 minutes of the patient's arrival at the ED. In this situation, the patient undergoes cardiac catheterization to locate the blockage or blockages, to assess the severity of the blockages, to determine the presence of collateral circulation, and to evaluate left ventricular function. With actual visualization of the coronary artery system and left ventricular function, treatment modalities most beneficial to the patient can be selected. Usually PCI with the placement of one or more drug-eluting stents will be performed. Patients with severe left ventricular dysfunction may require the addition of IABP therapy, and a small percentage of patients may require emergency coronary artery bypass graft (CABG) surgery.

The advantages of PCI are that (a) it is an alternative to surgical intervention; (b) it is performed with the use of local anaesthetic; (c) the patient is ambulatory 24 hours after the procedure; (d) the length of hospital stay is approximately 1 to 3 days compared with the 4- to 6-day stay necessary with CABG surgery, thus reducing hospital costs; and (e) the patient can make a rapid return to work (approximately 5 to 7 days after PCI) instead of the 2- to 8-week convalescence period after CABG.

PCI is performed more frequently than CABG surgery. Techniques have been developed to provide blood flow to the distal myocardium during balloon inflation, which increases the safety of the procedure. Dilation may also be performed for stenotic grafts from previous CABG surgery.

The most serious complication of PCI is dissection of the newly dilated coronary artery. If the damage is extensive, the coronary artery could rupture, which would cause cardiac tamponade, ischemia and infarction, decreased CO, and possibly death. There is also danger of infarction if the lesion is calcified and a portion of the plaque becomes dislodged and occludes the vessel distal to the catheter. Coronary spasm can occur from the mechanical irritation of the catheter or the balloon or from chemical irritation from the contrast medium used to visualize the artery. Abrupt closure is a complication that can occur in the first 24 hours after PCI. Re-stenosis after PCI can also occur, and risk is greatest in the first 30 days after the procedure. Nursing care of the patient after PCI is similar to that after cardiac catheterization (see Chapter 34, Table 34-6).

Fibrinolytic Therapy

Fibrinolytic therapy offers the advantages of availability and rapid administration for patients who attend facilities without an interventional cardiac catheterization laboratory or for patients who are too far from such a facility for safe transfer. Treatment of MI with fibrinolytic therapy is aimed at stopping the infarction process by dissolving the thrombus in the coronary artery and reperfusing the myocardium. To be of most benefit, fibrinolytic therapy must be given as soon as possible, ideally within the first hour, and preferably within the first 6 hours, after the onset of symptoms. When reperfusion occurs within 6 hours, the mortality rate is reduced by 25%.

Indications and Contraindications. All fibrinolytics are given by IV (see Table 36-11). The choice of a thrombolytic agent is guided by considerations of cost, efficacy, and ease of administration. Although these drugs have different mechanisms of action and different pharmacokinetics, they all open the artery by lysis of the thrombus in the coronary artery. Administration of a fibrinolytic is targeted to occur within 30 minutes of the patient's arrival at the ED. Optimal outcomes can be achieved if the

TABLE 36-13	CONTRAINDICATIONS FOR THE USE OF FIBRINOLYTIC THERAPY
Absolute Contraindications	**Relative Contraindications**
• Active internal bleeding or bleeding diathesis (except for menstruation) • Known history of cerebral aneurysm or arteriovenous malformation • Known intracranial neoplasm (primary or metastatic) • Previous cerebral hemorrhage • Ischemic stroke within past 3 mo • Significant closed head or facial trauma within past 3 mo • Suspected aortic dissection	• Active peptic ulcer disease • Current use of anticoagulants • Pregnancy • Prior ischemic stroke not within past 3 mo; dementia; or known intracranial disease not covered under absolute contraindications • Surgery (including laser eye surgery) or puncture of noncompressible vessel within past 3 wk • Internal bleeding within past 2–4 wk • Serious systemic disease (e.g., advanced or terminal cancer, severe liver or kidney disease) • Severe uncontrolled hypertension (BP >180/110 mm Hg) on patient's arrival for care or chronic, severe, poorly controlled hypertension • Traumatic or prolonged (>10 min) cardiopulmonary resuscitation

BP, blood pressure.

fibrinolytic is administered within 60 minutes after onset of symptoms (Pagana, Pagana, & Pike-MacDonald, 2013).

Because all the fibrinolytics produce lysis of the pathological clot, they may also lyse other clots (e.g., a postoperative site). Therefore, patient selection is important because minor or major bleeding can be a complication of therapy (Pagana, Pagana, & Pike-MacDonald, 2013). Inclusion criteria for fibrinolytic therapy include (a) chest pain typical of acute MI and less than 6 hours in duration, (b) 12-lead ECG findings consistent with acute MI, and (c) no absolute contraindications (Table 36-13).

Procedure. Each hospital has its own protocol to follow for administration of fibrinolytic therapy. However, all protocols have several common factors. Blood for baseline laboratory studies is collected, two to three lines for IV therapy are started, and all other invasive procedures are performed before the fibrinolytic agent is given. This sequence reduces the possibility of bleeding in the patient.

Depending on the drug selected, therapy may be administered in one IV bolus or over time (30 to 90 minutes). The time at which therapy begins is noted, and the patient is monitored during and after administration. ECG, vital signs measurement, pulse oximetry, and heart and lung assessments are completed frequently to evaluate the patient's response to therapy. When reperfusion occurs, several clinical markers may change. The most reliable marker is the return of the ST segment to baseline values on the ECG. Other markers include a resolution of chest pain and a rapid rise of the CK-MB enzyme levels that occurs within 3 hours of therapy and peaks within 12 hours. The CK-MB levels increase as the necrotic myocardial cells release CK-MB enzymes into the circulation after perfusion has been restored to the area. The presence of reperfusion dysrhythmias (e.g., accelerated idioventricular rhythm) is a less reliable marker of reperfusion. These dysrhythmias are generally self-limiting and do not necessitate aggressive treatment. (See Chapter 38 for management of dysrhythmias.)

A major concern with fibrinolytic therapy is reocclusion of the artery. The site of the thrombus is unstable, and another clot may form, or spasm of the artery may occur. Because of these possibilities, most physicians begin IV heparin therapy. If another clot develops, the patient reports similar complaints of chest pain, and ECG changes return. The patient is re-evaluated and may receive a second dose of the fibrinolytic or be transferred to a cardiac catheterization laboratory for rescue PCI.

The major complication with fibrinolytic therapy is bleeding. Ongoing nursing assessment is essential. Minor bleeding (e.g., surface bleeding from IV sites or gingival bleeding) is expected and can be controlled by applying a pressure dressing or ice packs. If signs and symptoms of major bleeding occur (e.g., a drop in BP, an increase in HR, a sudden decrease in the patient's level of consciousness, blood in the urine or stool), the physician should be notified, and the therapy should be stopped.

Drug Therapy

IV nitroglycerin, ASA, β-adrenergic blockers, and systemic anticoagulation with either subcutaneous LMWH or IV UH are the initial drug treatments of choice for ACS (Pagana, Pagana, & Pike-MacDonald, 2013). IV antiplatelet drugs (e.g., glycoprotein IIb/IIIa inhibitor) may also be used if PCI is anticipated. ACE inhibitors are added for select patients after MI (discussed in the section "Angiotensin-Converting Enzyme Inhibitors"). Calcium channel blockers or long-acting nitrates can be added if the patient is already receiving adequate doses of β-adrenergic blockers, cannot tolerate β-adrenergic blockers, or has Prinzmetal's angina (Pagana, Pagana, & Pike-MacDonald, 2013).

Drug therapy for patients with ACS is described in Table 36-11. These drugs are discussed on pp. 824–827. ACS-specific drugs are discussed in the following sections.

Intravenous Nitroglycerin. IV nitroglycerin is used in the initial treatment of patients with ACS. The goal of therapy is to reduce anginal pain and improve coronary blood flow. Nitroglycerin has an immediate onset of action and can be titrated to prevent, treat, and stop UA (Pagana, Pagana, & Pike-MacDonald, 2013).

IV nitroglycerin is used to decrease preload and afterload while increasing the myocardial oxygen supply. The dose is usually titrated to relieve pain. Because hypotension is a common adverse effect, BP is closely monitored during this time. Tolerance is another adverse effect of IV nitroglycerin therapy. An effective strategy to manage this phenomenon is to administer a lower dosage at night and during sleep and a higher dosage during the day.

Morphine Sulphate. Morphine is given for chest pain that is unrelieved by nitroglycerin. As a vasodilator, it decreases cardiac workload by lowering myocardial oxygen consumption, reducing contractility, and decreasing BP and HR. In addition, morphine can help reduce anxiety and fear. In rare situations, morphine can depress respiration. Patients should be monitored for signs of bradypnea or hypoxia, a condition to be prevented when at all possible in myocardial ischemia and infarction.

β-Adrenergic Blockers. IV β-adrenergic blockers should not be given to patients with STEMI. They may be considered for treatment of hypertension in patients with no contraindications such as HF or low CO. Oral β-adrenergic blocker therapy should be initiated within 24 hours of STEMI in patients with no

contraindications. β-Adrenergic blockers are used to decrease myocardial oxygen demand by reducing HR, BP, and contractility. (See Table 36-11 and Chapter 35, Table 35-8 for a discussion of β-adrenergic blockers.)

Angiotensin-Converting Enzyme Inhibitors. ACE inhibitors (e.g., captopril) are recommended after anterior wall MIs or MIs that result in decreased left ventricular function (ejection fraction <40%) or pulmonary congestion. The use of ACE inhibitors can help prevent ventricular remodelling and prevent or slow the progression of HF. ACE inhibitor therapy should be continued indefinitely. For patients who cannot tolerate ACE inhibitors, angiotensin receptor blockers (e.g., losartan [Cozaar]) should be considered. (See Table 36-11 and Chapter 35, Table 35-8.)

Antidysrhythmia Medications. Dysrhythmias are the most common complications after an MI. In general, they are not treated aggressively unless they are life-threatening. (The medications used in the treatment of dysrhythmias are discussed in Chapter 38.)

Cholesterol-Lowering Drugs. A fasting lipid panel should be obtained for all patients admitted with ACS. Cholesterol-lowering drugs are recommended for all patients with elevated LDL cholesterol levels (see Figure 36-6 and Table 36-5).

Stool Softeners. After an MI, patients may be predisposed to constipation as a result of bed rest and opioid administration. Stool softeners such as docusate sodium (Colace) are given to facilitate and promote the comfort of bowel evacuation. These medications prevent straining and the resultant vagal stimulation from the Valsalva manoeuvre. Vagal stimulation produces bradycardia and can provoke dysrhythmias.

Nutritional Therapy

Initially, patients may be kept NPO (nothing by mouth) except for sips of water until stable (e.g., pain alleviated, nausea resolved). Diet is advanced as tolerated to one of low salt, low saturated fats, and low cholesterol.

Coronary Surgical Revascularization

Coronary revascularization (an intervention to restore blood flow to the affected myocardium) with CABG surgery is recommended for patients who (a) fail medical management, (b) have left main coronary artery or three-vessel disease, (c) are not candidates for PCI (e.g., lesions are long or difficult to access), (d) have failed PCI and continue to have chest pain, (e) have diabetes mellitus, or (f) are expected to have longer-term benefits with CABG than with PCI.

Coronary Artery Bypass Graft Surgery. CABG surgery consists of the placement of conduits to transport blood between the aorta or other major arteries and the myocardium distal to the blocked coronary artery (or arteries). The procedure may involve one or more grafts using the internal mammary artery (IMA), saphenous vein, radial artery, gastro-epiploic artery, inferior epigastric artery, or a combination of these (Figure 36-12).

CABG surgery requires a sternotomy (opening of the chest cavity) and *cardiopulmonary bypass* (CPB). During CPB, blood is diverted from the patient's heart to a machine, where it is oxygenated and returned (via a pump) to the patient. This allows the surgeon to operate on a quiet, nonbeating, bloodless heart while perfusion to vital organs is maintained.

The IMA is the most common artery used for bypass graft. It is left attached to its origin (the subclavian artery) but then dissected from the chest wall. Next, it is *anastomosed* (connected with sutures) to the coronary artery distal to the blockage.

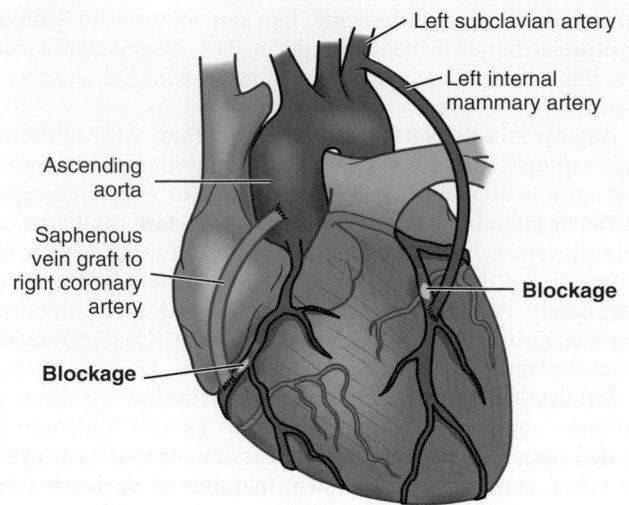

Left subclavian artery

Left internal mammary artery

Ascending aorta

Saphenous vein graft to right coronary artery

Blockage

Blockage

FIGURE 36-12 The distal end of the left internal mammary artery is grafted below the area of blockage in the left anterior descending artery. The proximal end of the saphenous vein is grafted to the aorta, and the distal end is grafted below the area of blockage in the right coronary artery.

When using the saphenous vein for a bypass graft, the surgeon removes the vein from one or both legs endoscopically. Sections are attached to the ascending aorta and then to a coronary artery distal to the blockage. Saphenous vein grafts do develop diffuse intimal hyperplasia, which contributes to future stenosis and graft occlusions. The use of antiplatelet therapy and statins after surgery improves vein graft patency. Patency rates of these grafts are 50% to 60% at 10 years (Hillis, Smith, Anderson, et al., 2011).

The radial artery is a thick, muscular artery that is prone to spasm. Perioperative calcium channel blockers and long-acting nitrates can control the spasms. Patency rates at 5 years are as high as 84%. There have been no reports of extremity complications (e.g., hand ischemia, wound infection) after removal of this artery (Hillis, Smith, Anderson, et al., 2011).

The gastro-epiploic and inferior epigastric artery are rarely used because the dissection of these arteries is extensive, increasing the length of surgery and the risk for wound complications at the harvest site, especially in an obese or diabetic patient (Hillis, Smith, Anderson, et al., 2011). Like the radial artery, these are prone to spasms. One-year patency rate for the epigastric artery is 90%, and 10-year patency rate for the gastro-epiploic artery is 62% (Hillis, Smith, Anderson, et al., 2011).

CABG surgery remains a palliative treatment for CAD and not a cure. Studies have shown improved patient outcomes, quality of life, and survival after CABG surgery. However, postoperative complications and mortality increase with age.

Women have higher operative mortality rates than men. This has been attributed to the late treatment of CAD in women because women first present with the disease at an older age and are more ill (e.g., decreased left ventricular function) at the time of surgery. Other possible factors include smaller-diameter coronary vessels and the less frequent use of the IMA.

Minimally Invasive Direct Coronary Artery Bypass. *Minimally invasive direct coronary artery bypass* (MIDCAB) offers patients with limited disease an approach to surgical treatment that does not involve a sternotomy and CPB. In many cases, these patients are too high risk for traditional bypass surgery (Bojar, 2011). The technique requires several small incisions between the ribs. A thoracoscope is used to dissect the IMA. The heart is slowed

using a β-adrenergic blocker (e.g., esmolol [Brevibloc]) or stopped temporarily with adenosine. A mechanical stabilizer immobilizes the operative site. The IMA is then sutured to the left anterior descending or right coronary artery. A radial artery or saphenous vein graft can be used if the IMA is not available.

Off-Pump Coronary Artery Bypass. The *off-pump coronary artery bypass* (OPCAB) procedure uses full or partial sternotomy to access all coronary vessels. OPCAB is performed on a beating heart using mechanical stabilizers and without CPB. It is usually reserved for patients who have limited disease but are at high risk for traditional surgery secondary to multiple comorbidities. Patients who are typically candidates for OPCAB have a very low ejection fraction, severe lung disease, acute or chronic kidney disease, a high risk for stroke, or a calcified aorta (Bojar, 2011).

Robot-Assisted Cardiothoracic Surgery. This technique incorporates the use of a robot in performing CABG or mitral valve replacement. The benefits of robotic surgery include increased precision, smaller incisions, decreased blood loss, less pain, and shorter recovery time.

Transmyocardial Laser Revascularization. *Transmyocardial laser revascularization* (TMR) is an indirect revascularization procedure. It is used for patients with advanced CAD who are not candidates for traditional CABG surgery and who have persistent angina after maximum medical therapy. The procedure involves the use of a high-energy laser to create channels in the heart to allow blood flow to ischemic areas. The procedure is performed during cardiac catheterization as a percutaneous TMR or during surgery using a left anterior thoracotomy incision as an adjunct to CABG.

NURSING MANAGEMENT
CHRONIC STABLE ANGINA AND ACUTE CORONARY SYNDROME

NURSING ASSESSMENT

Subjective and objective data that should be obtained from a patient with ACS are listed in Table 36-14.

NURSING DIAGNOSES

Nursing diagnoses for the patient with ACS may include but are not limited to those presented in Nursing Care Plan (NCP) 36-1.

PLANNING

The overall goals for a patient with ACS include (a) relief of pain, (b) preservation of the myocardium, (c) immediate and appropriate treatment of ischemia, (d) effective coping with illness-associated anxiety, (e) participation in a rehabilitation plan, and (f) reduction of risk factors.

NURSING IMPLEMENTATION: CHRONIC STABLE ANGINA

HEALTH PROMOTION. Behaviours to reduce the risk for CAD are presented in Table 36-2 and discussed on pp. 818–820.

ACUTE INTERVENTION. If a nurse is present during an anginal attack, the following measures should be instituted: (a) administration of supplemental oxygen; (b) measurement of vital signs; (c) 12-lead ECG; (d) prompt pain relief, first with a nitrate and then, if necessary, an opioid analgesic; (e) auscultation of heart sounds; and (f) comfortable positioning of the patient. The patient is likely to appear distressed and to have pale, cool, clammy skin. The BP and HR are probably elevated, and an atrial gallop sound (S_4) may be heard. A ventricular gallop sound (S_3) may indicate left ventricular dysfunction. A murmur heard during an anginal

TABLE 36-14 NURSING ASSESSMENT

Acute Coronary Syndrome

Subjective Data
Important Health Information
Current health history: Family history of heart disease; sedentary lifestyle; tobacco use
Past health history: Previous history of CAD, angina, MI, aortic stenosis, HF, or cardiomyopathy; hypertension; diabetes; anemia; lung disease; hyperlipidemia
Medications: Use of ASA (Aspirin), nitrates, β-adrenergic blockers, calcium channel blockers, ACE inhibitors, antihypertensive drugs, cholesterol-lowering drugs, vitamin or herbal supplements

Symptoms
- Substernal chest pain or pressure (squeezing, constricting, aching, sharp, tingling), possible radiation to jaw, neck, shoulders, back, or arms
- Indigestion, heartburn, nausea, belching, vomiting
- Palpitations, dyspnea, dizziness, weakness
- Fatigue, anxiety, feeling of impending doom

Objective Data
General
Anxiety, fear, restlessness

Integumentary
Cool, clammy, pale skin

Cardiovascular
Tachycardia or bradycardia, pulsus alternans (alternating weak and strong heartbeats), dysrhythmias (especially ventricular), S₃, S₄, higher or lower BP, murmur

Possible Findings
Elevated or nonelevated levels of serum cardiac markers, increased levels of serum lipids; increased WBC count; positive results of exercise stress test and thallium scans; ST-segment and T-wave abnormalities on ECG; cardiac enlargement, calcifications, or pulmonary congestion on chest radiograph; evidence of abnormal wall motion on stress echocardiogram; positive findings on coronary angiogram

ACE, angiotensin-converting enzyme; *ASA,* acetylsalicylic acid; *BP,* blood pressure; *CAD,* coronary artery disease; *ECG,* electrocardiogram; *HF,* heart failure; *MI,* myocardial infarction; *S₃,* third heart sound; *S₄,* fourth heart sound; *WBC,* white blood cell.

attack may be secondary to ischemia of a papillary muscle of the mitral valve. The murmur is likely to be transient and to disappear with the cessation of symptoms.

The nurse should ask the patient to rate the pain on a scale of 0 to 10 before and after treatment, to evaluate the effectiveness of the interventions. It is important to use the same words that patients use to describe their pain. Some patients may not always verbalize pain. The nurse must be attuned to other manifestations of pain, such as restlessness; elevated HR, respiratory rate, or BP; clutching of the bedclothes; or other nonverbal cues. Supportive and realistic reassurance and a calm, soothing manner help reduce the patient's anxiety during an anginal attack.

AMBULATORY AND HOME CARE. Patients with a history of angina should be reassured that a long, productive life is possible. Prevention of angina is preferable to its treatment, and this is why teaching is important. Patients should be provided information regarding CAD, angina, precipitating factors for angina, risk-factor reduction, and medications.

Patient teaching can be handled in a variety of ways. One-to-one contact between the nurse and the patient is often the most effective strategy. The time spent providing daily care is often an ideal teaching period. Teaching tools such as pamphlets, video recordings, heart models, and especially written information are necessary components of patient and family teaching (see Chapter 4).

Patients should be assisted in identifying factors that precipitate angina (see Table 36-8) and given instruction on how to avoid or control precipitating factors. For example, patients should be taught to avoid exposure to extremes of weather and to avoid consumption of large, heavy meals. If a heavy meal is ingested, adequate rest should be planned for 1 to 2 hours after the meal because blood is shunted to the GI tract to aid in digestion and absorption.

Patients should be assisted in identifying personal risk factors for CAD. Once these are known, methods of decreasing any modifiable risk factors should be discussed (see Table 36-2).

Teaching the patient and the family or caregivers about diets with low sodium and saturated-fat content may be appropriate (see Tables 36-3 and 36-4). Maintaining ideal body weight is important in controlling angina because weight above this level increases the myocardial workload.

Adhering to a regular, individualized program of physical activity that conditions the heart rather than overstressing the myocardium is important. As well, the patient and the caregivers must be instructed in the proper use of nitroglycerin (see pp. 824–825). Nitroglycerin tablets or ointments may be used prophylactically before an emotionally stressful situation, sexual intercourse, or physical exertion (e.g., climbing a long flight of stairs).

Counselling should be provided to assess the psychological adjustment of the patient and the family to the diagnosis of CAD and the resulting angina. Many patients feel a threat to their identity and self-esteem and may be unable to fill their usual roles in society. These emotions are normal and real.

NURSING IMPLEMENTATION: ACUTE CORONARY SYNDROME

ACUTE INTERVENTION. Priorities for nursing interventions in the initial phase of ACS include pain assessment and relief, physiological monitoring, promotion of rest and comfort, alleviation of stress and anxiety, and understanding of the patient's emotional and behavioural reactions. Proper management of these priorities decreases the oxygen needs of a compromised myocardium and reduces the risk for complications. In addition, the nurse should institute measures to avoid the hazards of immobility and yet encourage rest.

Pain. Nitroglycerin, morphine sulphate, and supplemental oxygen should be provided as needed to eliminate or reduce chest pain. Ongoing evaluation and documentation of the effectiveness of the interventions is important. Once pain is relieved, the nurse may have to deal with denial in a patient who interprets the absence of pain as an absence of cardiac disease.

Monitoring. Patients undergo continuous ECG monitoring while in the ED and the intensive care unit and usually after transfer to a step-down or general unit. The nurse should be educated in interpretation of the ECG so that dysrhythmias causing further deterioration of the cardiovascular status can be identified and treated. During the initial period after MI, ventricular fibrillation is the most common lethal dysrhythmia. In many patients, this dysrhythmia is often preceded by PVCs or

◎ NURSING CARE PLAN 36-1

Acute Coronary Syndrome

| NURSING DIAGNOSIS | **Decreased cardiac output** (related to altered contractility and altered heart rate and rhythm as evidenced by decrease in BP, elevation in HR, dyspnea, dysrhythmias, diminished pulses, peripheral edema, pulmonary edema, or a combination of these). |

Expected Patient Outcomes

- Maintains stable signs of effective cardiac perfusion

Nursing Interventions and *Rationales*

Cardiac Care
- Monitor vital signs frequently *to determine baseline and ongoing changes.*
- Monitor for cardiac dysrhythmias, including disturbances of both rhythm and conduction, *to identify and treat significant dysrhythmias.*
- Monitor respiratory status for symptoms of heart failure *to maintain appropriate levels of oxygenation and to detect signs of pulmonary edema.*
- Monitor fluid balance (e.g., intake and output, daily weight) *to monitor renal perfusion and observe for fluid retention.*
- Arrange exercise and rest periods *to prevent fatigue and decrease the oxygen demand on the myocardium.*

| NURSING DIAGNOSIS | **Acute pain** related to *biological injury agent* (imbalance between myocardial O_2 supply and demand) as evidenced by *self-report of pain characteristics using standard pain instrument* |

Expected Patient Outcomes

- Reports relief of pain

Nursing Interventions and *Rationales*

Cardiac Care
- Evaluate chest pain (e.g., PQRST [see Table 36-7]) *to accurately evaluate, treat, and prevent further ischemia.*
- Monitor vital signs frequently *to determine baseline and detect ongoing changes.*
- Obtain 12-lead ECG during pain episode *to help differentiate angina from extension of MI or pericarditis.*

Pain Management
- Provide optimal pain relief with prescribed analgesics *because pain exacerbates tachycardia and increases BP.*
- Consider the type and source of pain when selecting pain relief strategy *because angina responds to opioids and measures that increase myocardial perfusion.*

| NURSING DIAGNOSIS | **Anxiety** related to *threat of death, threat to current status* (pain, lifestyle changes) as evidenced by *restlessness, distress, helplessness* |

Expected Patient Outcomes

- Reports decreased anxiety and increased sense of self-control

Nursing Interventions and *Rationales*

Anxiety Reduction
- Observe for verbal and nonverbal signs of anxiety.
- Identify changes in level of anxiety *because anxiety increases the need for oxygen.*
- Use a calm, reassuring approach *so as not to increase patient's anxiety.*
- Instruct patient in use of relaxation techniques (e.g., relaxation breathing, imagery) *to enhance the patient's self-control.*
- Encourage family members to stay with patient *to provide comfort.*
- Encourage verbalization of feelings, perceptions, and fears *to decrease anxiety and stress.*
- Provide factual information concerning diagnosis, treatment, and prognosis *to decrease fear of the unknown.*

Coping Enhancement
- Provide the patient with realistic choices about certain aspects of care *to support decision making.*
- Assist the patient in identifying positive strategies *to deal with limitations and manage needed lifestyle or role changes.*
- Help the patient to grieve and work through the losses of chronic illness *to provide support.*

| NURSING DIAGNOSIS | **Activity intolerance** related to *physical deconditioning* (decreased cardiac output, poor lung perfusion) as evidenced by *fatigue, generalized weakness, abnormal heart rate response to activity* |

Expected Patient Outcomes

- Achieves a realistic program of activity that balances physical activity with energy-conserving activities

Nursing Interventions and *Rationales*

Cardiac Care
- Monitor patient's response to antidysrhythmic medications before activity *because these medications affect blood pressure and pulse.*
- Arrange exercise and rest periods *to prevent fatigue and to increase activity tolerance without rapidly increasing cardiac workload.*

Energy Management
- Assist patient to understand energy conservation principles (e.g., the requirement for restricted activity) *to promote healing by conserving energy.*
- Teach patient and significant others techniques of self-care that will minimize oxygen consumption (e.g., self-monitoring and pacing techniques for performance of activities of daily living) *to promote independence as well as minimize O_2 consumption.*

⊚ NURSING CARE PLAN 36-1

Acute Coronary Syndrome—cont'd

NURSING DIAGNOSIS	**Ineffective health management** related to *insufficient knowledge of therapeutic regimen* (rehabilitation process, home activities, medications) as evidenced by *difficulty with prescribed regimen*
Expected Patient Outcomes	**Nursing Interventions and *Rationales***

• Describes risk factors, the disease process, and rehabilitation activities necessary to manage the therapeutic regimen	*Cardiac Care: Rehabilitative* • Encourage realistic expectations for the patient, caregiver(s), and family member(s) *to promote realistic decision making.* • Instruct patient, caregiver(s), and family member(s) on appropriate prescribed and over-the-counter drugs *to promote adherence to drug regimens.* • Instruct the patient and caregiver on cardiac risk-factor modification (e.g., smoking cessation, diet, exercise) *to increase patient's control of the illness.* • Instruct the patient on self-care of chest pain (e.g., take sublingual nitroglycerin every 5 minutes three times; if chest pain unrelieved, seek emergency medical care). • Instruct the patient and caregiver on the exercise regimen, including warm-up, endurance, and cool-down, *to reduce cardiac risk factors.* • Instruct the patient and caregiver on wound care and precautions (e.g., sternal incision or catheterization site), if appropriate, *to prevent infection and promote healing after invasive therapies.* • Instruct the patient and caregiver on access to emergency services available in their community *to enable them to obtain immediate care if needed.*

ventricular tachycardia. The nurse should also monitor the patient for the presence of silent ischemia by monitoring the ST segment for shifts above or below the baseline of the ECG. **Silent ischemia** occurs without clinical symptoms such as chest pain. It is noted by ST-segment changes only and may place a patient at higher risk for adverse outcomes and even death (Conti, Bavry, & Petersen, 2012). If episodes of silent ischemia are observed, the physician should be notified. (See Chapter 38 for a complete discussion of ECG monitoring.)

In addition to frequent assessment of vital signs, intake and output should be evaluated at least once per shift, and physical assessment should be carried out to detect deviations from a patient's baseline parameters. Included is an assessment of lung sounds and heart sounds and inspection for evidence of early HF (e.g., dyspnea, tachycardia, pulmonary congestion, distended neck veins).

Assessment of the patient's oxygenation status is important, especially if the patient is receiving oxygen. Also, the nares should be checked for irritation or dryness, which can cause considerable discomfort if the nasal route is used for oxygen administration.

Rest and Comfort. With a severe insult to the myocardium, as in the case of ACS, it is important for the nurse to promote rest and comfort. Bed rest may be ordered for the first few days after an MI involving a large portion of the ventricle. A patient with an uncomplicated MI (e.g., angina resolved, no signs of complications) may rest in a chair within 8 to 12 hours after the event. The use of a commode or bedpan is based on patient preference.

When sleeping or resting, the body requires less work from the heart than it does when active. It is important to plan nursing and therapeutic actions to ensure adequate rest periods free from interruption. Comfort measures that can promote rest include frequent oral care, adequate warmth, a quiet atmosphere, use of relaxation therapy (e.g., guided imagery), and assurance that personnel are nearby and responsive to the patient's needs.

It is important that patients understand the reasons for limited activity. However, in spite of this limitation, patients are not completely restricted. Gradually, the cardiac workload is increased through more demanding physical tasks so that patients can

TABLE 36-15	PHASES OF REHABILITATION AFTER ACUTE CORONARY SYNDROME

Phase I: Hospital
• Occurs while the patient is still hospitalized.
• Activity level depends on severity of angina or MI.
• Patient may initially sit up in bed or chair, perform range-of-motion exercises and self-care (e.g., washing, shaving), and progress to ambulation in hallway and limited stair climbing.
• Attention focuses on management of pain, anxiety, dysrhythmias, and complications.

Phase II: Early Recovery
• Phase begins after the patient is discharged.
• Phase usually lasts 2–12 wk and is conducted in an outpatient facility.
• Activity level is gradually increased under the supervision of the cardiac rehabilitation team and with electrocardiographic monitoring.
• Team may suggest that physical activity (e.g., walking) be initiated at home.
• Information regarding risk-factor reduction is provided at this time.

Phase III: Late Recovery
• Long-term maintenance program is followed.
• Individual physical activity programs are designed and implemented at home, a local gym, or the rehabilitation centre.
• Patient and family may restructure lifestyles and roles as possible.
• Lifestyle changes should become lifelong habits.
• Medical supervision is still recommended.

MI, myocardial infarction.

achieve a discharge activity level adequate for home care. Phases of cardiac rehabilitation are outlined in Table 36-15.

Anxiety. Anxiety is present to various degrees in all patients with ACS. The nurse's role is to identify the source of anxiety and assist the patient in reducing anxiety. If the patient is afraid of being alone, a family member should be allowed to sit quietly by the bedside or to check in with the patient frequently. If a source of anxiety is fear of the unknown, the nurse should explore these concerns with the patient and help with appropriate reality testing.

If anxiety is caused by lack of information, the nurse should provide teaching appropriate to the patient's stated need and level of understanding. The nurse should answer the patient's questions with clear, simple explanations sufficient to reduce the patient's anxiety.

It is important to start teaching at the patient's level rather than to present a prepackaged protocol. Many patients are not yet ready to hear about the pathogenesis of CAD. The earliest questions usually relate to how the disease affects perceived control and independence. These questions include the following:

- When will I leave the intensive care unit?
- When can I be out of bed?
- When will I be discharged?
- When can I return to work?
- How much change will I have to make in my life?
- Will this happen again?

The nurse should advise patients to begin a more complete teaching program once they are feeling stronger. Many patients may not be able to consciously examine the most pervasive and typical concern: "Am I going to die?" Even if a patient denies this concern, it is helpful for the nurse to initiate conversation by remarking that fear of dying is a common concern reported by most patients who have experienced ACS. This information gives the patient "permission" to talk about an uncomfortable and frightening topic (Table 36-16).

Emotional and Behavioural Reactions. The emotional and behavioural reactions of a patient are varied and frequently follow a predictable response pattern (see Table 36-16). The role of the nurse is to understand what the patient is currently experiencing, to assist the patient in testing reality, and to support the use of constructive coping styles, recognizing that denial may be a positive coping style in the early phase of recovery from ACS.

The nurse has a duty to maximize and enhance the patient's social support systems. This entails assessing the support structure of the patient and family and allowing it to function. Often the patient is separated from the most significant support system at the time of hospitalization. The nurse's role can include talking with the family members, allowing the patient and the family to interact as necessary, and supporting the family members who will be able to provide the necessary support to the patient. Open visitation is helpful in decreasing anxiety and increasing support for the patient with ACS. It is important for the nurse to help the patient identify additional support systems (e.g., spiritual care) that can help the patient after discharge.

CORONARY REVASCULARIZATION. Patients with ACS may undergo coronary revascularization with PCI or CABG surgery. The major nursing responsibilities for the care of the patient after PCI involve monitoring for signs of recurrent angina; frequently assessing vital signs, including HR and rhythm; evaluating the groin site for signs of bleeding; and maintaining bed rest per institution policy.

Patients undergoing CABG surgery receive care in the intensive care unit for the first 24 to 36 hours. Ongoing and intensive monitoring of patients' hemodynamic status is critical. For such patients, much invasive equipment for monitoring cardiac status and other vital organs is present (see Chapter 68). This equipment includes a pulmonary artery catheter for measuring CO and other hemodynamic parameters, an intra-arterial line for continuous BP monitoring, pleural and mediastinal chest tubes for chest drainage, ECG leads for continuous monitoring to detect

TABLE 36-16	EMOTIONAL AND BEHAVIOURAL RESPONSES TO ACUTE CORONARY SYNDROME

Denial
- May have history of ignoring symptoms related to heart disease
- Minimizes severity of medical condition
- Ignores activity restrictions
- Avoids discussing illness or its significance

Anger
- Is commonly expressed as "Why did this happen to me?"
- Possibly directed at family, staff, or medical regimen

Anxiety and Fear
- Fears long-term disability and death
- Overtly manifests apprehension, restlessness, insomnia, tachycardia
- Less overtly manifests increased verbalization, projection of feelings to others, hypochondriasis
- Fears activity
- Fears recurrent angina, heart attacks, and sudden death

Dependency
- Is totally reliant on staff
- Is unwilling to perform tasks or activities unless approved by health care provider
- Wants to be monitored by ECG at all times
- Is hesitant to leave the intensive care unit or hospital

Depression
- Mourns loss of health, altered body function, and changes in lifestyle
- Realizes seriousness of situation
- Begins to worry about future implications of health problem
- Shows manifestations of withdrawal, apathy
- May be more evident after hospital discharge

Realistic Acceptance
- Focuses on optimum rehabilitation
- Plans changes compatible with altered cardiac function

ECG, electrocardiogram.

dysrhythmias, an endotracheal tube connected to mechanical ventilation, epicardial pacing wires for emergency pacing of the heart, a urinary catheter to monitor urine output, and a nasogastric tube for gastric decompression. Most patients are extubated within 12 hours after surgery and transferred to a step-down unit within 24 hours for continued monitoring of cardiac status.

Many of the postoperative complications that develop after CABG surgery are related to the use of CPB. Major consequences of CPB include bleeding and anemia from damage to red blood cells and platelets, fluid and electrolyte imbalances, and hypothermia because blood is cooled as it passes through the CPB machine. Nursing care focuses on assessing the patient for bleeding (e.g., chest tube drainage, incision sites), monitoring fluid status, replacing electrolytes as needed, and restoring temperature (e.g., with use of warming blankets).

Postoperative dysrhythmias, specifically atrial dysrhythmias, are common in the first 3 days after CABG surgery. Between 20% and 40% of patients develop postoperative atrial fibrillation. Discharge is often delayed in these patients as a result of the need for anticoagulation. (See Chapter 38 for information on treatment of atrial fibrillation.)

Nursing care for patients with a CABG also involves caring for the surgical sites: the chest, the arm, the leg, the abdomen, or some combination of these. Care of the radial artery harvest site includes careful observation of the incision site, as well as monitoring of sensory and motor function of the distal thumb and fingers. The patient with radial artery harvest should receive therapy with a calcium channel blocker for approximately 3 months to decrease the incidence of arterial spasm at the arm or the anastomosis site.

The care of the leg wound is similar to the postoperative care after the stripping of varicose veins (see Chapter 40). The management of the chest wound, which involves a sternotomy, is similar to that for other chest surgical procedures (see Chapter 30).

Elective CABG is generally well tolerated by older patients. However, the nurse caring for older adults must be aware that although the benefits of treatment may outweigh risks in this population, the incidence of complications—including dysrhythmias, stroke, and infection—is higher than that in younger individuals.

Postoperative nursing care of patients who have undergone a MIDCAB or OPCAB procedure is similar to that of patients who have undergone CABG surgery. Pain management is essential because patients with thoracotomy incisions report higher levels of pain than those with sternotomy incisions. The recovery time is somewhat shorter with these procedures, and patients often resume routine activities sooner than do patients who have CABG surgery.

AMBULATORY AND HOME CARE. *Rehabilitation* may be defined as the process of helping the patient adjust to a disability by teaching integration of all resources and concentrating more on existing abilities than on permanent disabilities. *Cardiac rehabilitation* is the restoration of a person to an optimal state of function in six areas: physiological, psychological, mental, spiritual, economic, and vocational. Many people recover from ACS physically, but they may never attain psychological well-being because of misconceptions about the illness or a need to practise illness behaviours. Returning to work and resuming all activities have long been outcome measures of cardiac rehabilitation and are important in terms of the cost-effectiveness of cardiac care and rehabilitation. (See the "Evidence-Informed Practice" box.)

In considering rehabilitation, the nurse and the patient must recognize that CAD is a chronic disease. It will not be cured, nor will it disappear by itself. Therefore, basic changes in lifestyle must be made to promote recovery and health. In many cases, these changes must be made at a time when the patient is middle-aged or older. The patient must also realize that recovery takes time. Resumption of physical activity after ACS or CABG surgery is slow and gradual. However, with appropriate and adequate supportive care, recovery is likely.

PATIENT TEACHING. Patient teaching begins with the nurse in the ED, progresses through the care provided by the staff nurse, and continues with the community health nurse. The purpose of teaching is to give the patient and the family the tools they need to make informed decisions about attainment of health. For teaching to be meaningful, the patient must be aware of the need to learn. Careful assessment of the patient's learning needs helps the nurse set goals and objectives that are realistic.

The timing of the teaching is important. When patients or families are in crisis (either physiological or psychological), they may not be able to learn new information. It is important to remember that early questions should be answered initially in simple, brief terms, without detailed elaboration, and that the

EVIDENCE-INFORMED PRACTICE
Research Highlight

What Is the Most Effective Cardiac Rehabilitation Program?
Clinical Question
In patients with coronary CAD (P), are comprehensive cardiac rehabilitation programs (I) more effective than exercise-only cardiac rehabilitation programs (C) in reducing mortality (O)?

Best Available Evidence
Systematic review of randomized controlled trials

Critical Appraisal and Synthesis of Evidence
- 47 randomized controlled trials ($n = 10\,794$).
- Reduction in overall and cardiovascular mortality.
- Reduction in hospital readmissions.
- Comprehensive cardiac rehabilitation (e.g., exercise in addition to psychosocial and educational interventions): 13%.
- Of 10 trials, 7 revealed significantly higher quality of life with exercise-based cardiac rehabilitation than with usual care.

Conclusions
- Exercise-based cardiac rehabilitation is effective in reducing cardiac deaths and other causes of mortality in patients with CAD.
- A broader sample that includes more women and is more ethnically diverse is needed for subsequent studies.

Implications for Nursing Practice
- Counsel patients at risk for CAD on the benefits of exercise.
- Include an exercise component in health and wellness programs for patients with CAD and those who have suffered a cardiac event.

Reference for Evidence
Heran, B., Ebrahim, S., Moxham, T., et al. (2011). Exercise-based rehabilitation for coronary heart disease. *The Cochrane Database of Systematic Reviews*, No. 7, Article CD001800. doi:10.1002/14651858.CD001800.pub2.

CAD, coronary artery disease; *PICO: P*, patient population of interest; *I*, intervention or area of interest; *C*, comparison of interest or comparison group; *O*, outcome(s) of interest (see Chapter 1).

answers to these questions often require repetition with elaboration later. When the shock and disbelief accompanying a crisis subside, the patient and the family are better able to focus on new information.

In addition to teaching the patient and the family what they wish to know, the nurse should recognize that several types of information are necessary for achieving optimal health. A teaching guide for the patient with ACS is presented in Table 36-17.

When medical terminology is used, its meaning should be explained in lay terms. For example, it can be explained that the heart, a four-chambered pump, is a muscle that, like all other muscles, needs oxygen to work properly. When blood vessels supplying the heart muscle with oxygen become narrowed by atherosclerosis, less oxygen reaches the heart muscle. It is a good idea for the nurse to have a model of the heart or to use a pad and pencil to sketch what is being explained. Literature written for a nonmedical audience is available through the Heart and Stroke Foundation of Canada. Video recordings are also helpful tools that can be used to teach patients.

Anticipatory guidance involves preparing the patient and the family for what to expect in the course of recovery and rehabilitation. By learning what to expect during treatment and recovery, the patient gains a sense of control over life. This sense of perceived control allows the patient to consciously consider stressors and thus possibly to promote recovery.

TABLE 36-17 PATIENT & CAREGIVER TEACHING GUIDE

Acute Coronary Syndrome

The following guidelines should be included when teaching the patient and caregiver about acute coronary syndrome.
- Signs and symptoms of angina and MI and reasons why they occur*
- Anatomy and physiology of the heart and vessels
- Cause and effect of atherosclerosis
- Definitions of terms (e.g., CAD, angina, MI, sudden cardiac death, HF)
- Healing after MI
- Identification of risk factors and ways to decrease risk* (see Table 36-2)
- Rationale for tests and treatments, including ECG, blood tests, and angiography, and for monitoring, rest, diet, and medications*
- Appropriate expectations about recovery and rehabilitation (anticipatory guidance)
- Resumption of work, physical activity, sexual activity
- Measures to take to promote recovery and health
- Importance of the gradual, progressive resumption of activity*
- When and how to seek help (e.g., contact EMS)

CAD, coronary artery disease; *ECG,* electrocardiogram; *EMS,* emergency medical services; *HF,* heart failure; *MI,* myocardial infarction.
*Identified by patients as most important to learn before discharge.

TABLE 36-18 PATIENT & CAREGIVER TEACHING GUIDE

FITT Physical Activity Guidelines After Acute Coronary Syndrome

Warm-Up and Cool-Down
Mild stretching for 3–5 min before the physical activity and 5 min after the activity is important. Activity should not be started or stopped abruptly.

Frequency
The patient should perform physical activity five or more times per week.

Intensity
Activity intensity should be determined by the patient's HR. If a treadmill test has not been performed, the person recovering from MI should not exceed 20 beats/min over the resting HR.

Type of Physical Activity
Physical activity should be regular, rhythmic, and repetitive; large muscles should be used to build up endurance (as in walking, cycling, swimming, and rowing).

Time
Duration of physical activity can be 30–60 min. It is important to begin slowly according to personal tolerance (perhaps only 5–10 min) and build up to 30 min.

FITT, frequency, intensity, time, and type; *HR,* heart rate; *MI,* myocardial infarction.

Physical Activity. Physical activity is an integral part of the rehabilitation program. It is necessary for optimal physiological functioning and psychological well-being. It has a direct, positive effect on maximal oxygen uptake, increasing CO, decreasing blood lipids, decreasing BP, increasing blood flow through the coronary arteries, increasing muscle mass and flexibility, improving the psychological state, and assisting in weight loss and control. A regular schedule of physical activity, even when begun after many years of sedentary living, is beneficial. The Canadian Guidelines for Physical Activity outline recommended activities and duration for all ages (Canadian Society for Exercise Physiology, 2011).

In the hospital, the patient's activity level is gradually increased so that by the time of discharge, the patient can tolerate moderate-energy activities of 3 to 6 metabolic equivalents (METs). Many patients with UA that has resolved or with an uncomplicated MI are in the hospital for approximately 3 to 4 days. By day 2, patients can ambulate in the hallway and begin limited stair climbing (e.g., three to four steps). Because of the short hospital stay, it is critical to give patients specific guidelines for physical activity so as to avoid overexertion. The nurse should stress to patients that they must "listen to what the body is saying"—the most important facet of recovery.

Teaching patients to check their pulse rate is a nursing responsibility. Patients should be taught the parameters within which to exercise. They should be told the maximum rate that the heart should beat at any point. If the HR exceeds this level or does not return to the rate of the resting pulse within a few minutes, patients should stop and rest. Patients should also be instructed to stop exercising if angina or dyspnea occurs. Basic physical activity guidelines for patients after ACS are based on the formula for frequency, intensity, time, and type (FITT) and are presented in Table 36-18.

The basic categories of physical activity are static *(isometric)* and dynamic *(isotonic).* Most daily activities are a mixture of the two. Static activities involve the development of tension during muscular contraction but produce little or no change in muscle length or joint movement. Lifting, carrying, and pushing heavy objects are primarily isometric activities. Because the HR and BP increase rapidly during isometric work, exercise programs involving isometric exercises should be limited.

Isotonic activities involve changes in muscle length and joint movement with rhythmic contractions at relatively low muscular tension. Walking, jogging, swimming, bicycling, and jumping rope are examples of activities that are predominantly isotonic. Isotonic exercise can put a safe, steady load on the heart and lungs and improve the circulation in many organs.

Many patients are referred to an outpatient cardiac rehabilitation program (see Table 36-15). These programs have been found to be beneficial to patients, but not all patients choose or are able to participate in them. Home-based cardiac rehabilitation programs have been developed as an alternative. Maintaining contact with patients appears to be the key to the success of these programs.

Older women (65 years or older) who experience MI frequently have poor adherence to a regular physical activity program. These women often describe a continued post-MI fatigue that is poorly understood. Another factor that has been linked to poor adherence to a physical activity program after MI is depression. Depression is common among patients with CAD, especially women (European Society of Cardiology, 2014). All patients with CAD should routinely be screened for depression and treatment recommended as appropriate.

The "Evidence-Informed Practice" box "What Is the Most Effective Cardiac Rehabilitation Program?" outlines recent research on cardiac rehabilitation.

Resumption of Sexual Activity. It is important to include sexual counselling for cardiac patients and their partners. This often-neglected area of discussion may be difficult for both the patient and the health care provider to approach. However, the patient's concern about resumption of sexual activity after hospitalization for ACS often produces more stress than the physiological act itself. Most of these patients change their sexual behaviour not because of physical problems but because they are concerned about sexual inadequacy, death during intercourse, and impotence. A concerned and knowledgeable health care provider could clarify any misconceptions with specific counselling.

Before providing guidelines on resumption of sexual activity, the nurse must know the patient's physiological status, the physiological effects of sexual activity, and the psychological effects of having a heart attack. Sexual activity for most middle-aged men and women with their usual partners is considered a moderate-energy activity equivalent to climbing two flights of stairs (Levine, Steinke, Bakaeen, et al., 2012).

Nurses may feel uncertain about how and when to begin counselling about resumption of sex. It is helpful to consider sex a physical activity and to discuss or explore feelings about it when discussing other physical activities with the patient. The dialogue may be opened with, for example, "Many people who have had a heart attack wonder when they will be able to resume sexual activity. Has this been of concern to you?" The nurse might also state, "Sexual activity is like other forms of activity and should be gradually resumed after MI. If your ability to perform sexually is concerning you, the energy you use is no more than that when walking briskly." Providing the patient with reading material on resumption of sexual activity can also facilitate discussion, introduced as so: "If resuming sexual activity has been of concern to you, this information should be helpful." This type of nonthreatening statement brings up the topic, allows the patient to explore personal feelings, and gives the patient an opportunity to raise questions with you or another health care provider (European Society of Cardiology, 2014). Common guidelines are presented in Table 36-19.

EVALUATION

The expected outcomes for the patient with an ACS are presented in NCP 36-1.

SUDDEN CARDIAC DEATH

Sudden cardiac death (SCD) is unexpected death resulting from various causes, including cardiac arrest. In many cases, SCD is not actually sudden. Teaching people about the symptoms of impending cardiac arrest and the actions to take can save lives. Rapid cardiopulmonary resuscitation (CPR) and defibrillation with an automated external defibrillator (AED), in combination with early advanced cardiac life support, can enhance the chances for long-term survival after a witnessed arrest.

Etiology and Pathophysiology

In SCD, cardiac function is disrupted abruptly, causing immediate loss of CO and cerebral blood flow. The affected person may or may not have a known history of CAD. SCD is the first sign of illness for 25% of people who die from heart disease (Mitrani & Myerburg, 2016). Death usually occurs within 1 hour of the onset of acute symptoms (e.g., angina, palpitations).

Acute ventricular dysrhythmias (e.g., ventricular tachycardia, ventricular fibrillation) cause the majority of cases of SCD. Less commonly, SCD occurs because of a primary left ventricular outflow obstruction (e.g., aortic stenosis, hypertrophic cardiomyopathy) or extreme slowing of the heart (bradycardia).

People who experience SCD because of CAD are categorized as (a) those who did not have an acute MI and (b) those who

---

TABLE 36-19 SEXUAL ACTIVITY AFTER ACUTE CORONARY SYNDROME

- When planning for resumption of sexual activity, the patient's goal should correspond to sexual activity before hospitalization for acute coronary syndrome.
- Physical training seems to improve the physiological response to coitus; therefore, daily physical activity during recovery should be encouraged.
- Consumption of food and alcohol should be reduced before intercourse is anticipated (e.g., waiting 3 to 4 hr after ingesting a large meal before engaging in sexual activity).
- Familiar surroundings and a familiar partner reduce anxiety.
- Masturbation may be a useful sexual outlet and may reassure the patient that sexual activity is still possible.
- Hot or cold showers should be avoided just before and just after intercourse.
- Foreplay is desirable because it allows a gradual increase in heart rate before orgasm.
- Positions during intercourse are a matter of individual choice.
- Orogenital sex places no undue strain on the heart.
- A relaxed atmosphere free of fatigue and stress is optimal.
- Prophylactic use of nitrates is effective in decreasing angina during sexual activity.
- Use of erectile agents (e.g., sildenafil [Viagra]) is contraindicated if the patient is taking nitrates in any form.
- Anal intercourse may cause undue cardiac stress because of the possibility of inducing a vasovagal response.

---

did have an acute MI. The first group accounts for the majority of cases of SCD. In this instance, victims usually have no warning signs or symptoms. Patients who survive are at risk for another episode of SCD because of the continued electrical instability of the myocardium that led to the initial event.

The second, smaller group of patients includes those who have had an MI and have suffered SCD. In these cases, patients usually do have prodrome symptoms, such as chest pain, palpitations, and dyspnea.

It is difficult to predict who is at risk for SCD. Risk factors for SCD include (a) male sex (especially Black men), (b) family history of premature atherosclerosis, (c) tobacco use, (d) diabetes mellitus, (e) hypercholesterolemia, (f) hypertension, and (g) cardiomyopathy.

NURSING AND COLLABORATIVE MANAGEMENT SUDDEN CARDIAC DEATH

People who survive an episode of SCD generally require a diagnostic workup to determine whether they have had an MI. Thus serial analyses of cardiac markers and ECGs are done, and treatment is planned accordingly. (See section on collaborative care of ACS.) In addition, because most people with SCD have CAD, cardiac catheterization is indicated to determine the possible location and extent of coronary artery occlusion. PCI or CABG surgery may also be indicated.

Most patients with SCD have a lethal ventricular dysrhythmia that has a high incidence of recurrence. Thus it is useful to know when those people are most likely to have a recurrence and what drug therapy is the most effective treatment. Assessment of dysrhythmias in these patients includes 24-hour Holter monitoring or other type of event recorder, exercise stress testing, signal-averaged ECG, and electrophysiological study (EPS) performed with fluoroscopy. Pacing electrodes are placed in select intracardiac areas, and stimuli are selectively used to attempt to produce dysrhythmias. The patient's response to various antidysrhythmic medications is determined and monitored in a controlled environment. (EPS is discussed in Chapters 34 and 38.)

The most common approach to preventing a recurrence is the use of an implantable cardioverter–defibrillator (ICD). Drug therapy with amiodarone may be used in conjunction with an ICD to decrease episodes of ventricular dysrhythmias.

When caring for these patients, the nurse should be alert to the patient's psychosocial adaptation to this sudden "brush with death." Many of these patients develop a "time bomb" mentality. They fear the recurrence of cardiopulmonary arrest and may become anxious, angry, and depressed. Their caregivers are likely to experience the same feelings.

Patients and caregivers may need to deal with additional issues, such as possible driving restrictions and change in occupation. The grief response varies among patients and caregivers. The nurse should be attuned to the specific needs of the patient and caregiver and teach them accordingly while providing appropriate emotional support.

CASE STUDY

Myocardial Infarction

Patient Profile

Owen Matthews, a 51-year-old successful executive, is rushed to the hospital by ambulance after experiencing crushing substernal chest pain that radiates down his left arm. He also complains of dizziness and nausea.

Source: Sergey Furtaev/ Shutterstock .com.

Subjective Data

- Has a history of chronic stable angina and hypertension
- States that he is "borderline diabetic"
- Overweight but recently lost 10 pounds
- Rarely exercises
- Has three teenage children who are causing "problems"
- Recently experienced loss of best friend and business partner, who died from cancer

Objective Data
Physical Examination

- Diaphoresis, shortness of breath, nausea
- BP, 165/100 mm Hg; pulse rate, 120; respiratory rate, 26/min

Diagnostic Studies

- ECG shows occasional premature ventricular contractions and ST elevation in leads II, III, aV_F, V_5, and V_6.
- Cardiac-specific troponin I level is elevated.
- Cholesterol level is 9.1 mmol/L.
- Hb A1C level is 9.0%.
- Inferolateral wall MI is diagnosed.

Collaborative Care
Emergency Department

- Oxygen, 2 L/min via nasal cannula, titrated to keep O_2 saturation >93%
- Continuous ECG monitoring
- ASA, 324 mg (chewable)
- Eptifibatide (Integrilin), IV
- Weight-based heparin, IV
- Nitroglycerin intravenously, titrated to relieve chest pain; withheld for systolic BP <100 mm Hg
- Morphine, 2 to 4 mg, IV q5min PRN for chest pain unrelieved by nitroglycerin
- Metoprolol (Lopresor), 5 mg IV q5min × 3 doses
- Vital sign measurements and pulse oximetry q10min
- Preparation of patient for transfer to cardiac catheterization laboratory for possible PCI

Discussion Questions

1. Which coronary arteries are probably occluded in Mr. Matthews's coronary circulation?
2. What risk factors contribute to its development? What risk factors were present in Mr. Matthews's life?
3. What is angina? How does angina differ from myocardial infarction?
4. What is the pathophysiological basis for the clinical manifestations that Mr. Matthews exhibited?
5. What is the significance of the results of the laboratory tests and ECG findings?
6. What is the rationale for each treatment measure ordered for Mr. Matthews?
7. ***Priority decision:*** What are the priority nursing interventions for Mr. Matthews immediately after his MI?
8. ***Priority decision:*** Based on the assessment data presented, what are the priority nursing diagnoses? Identify any collaborative problems.
9. ***Evidence-informed practice:*** Two days after an uncomplicated PCI and the placement of two stents, Mr. Matthews wants to know what the most effective strategies are to prevent another MI. Based on his clinical situation, what should the nurse recommend?

*e*volve

Answers are available at *http://evolve.elsevier.com/Canada/Lewis/medsurg*

REVIEW QUESTIONS

The number of the question corresponds to the same-numbered objective at the beginning of the chapter.

1. How many people in Canada will experience a myocardial infarction in a given year?
   a. 20 000
   b. 50 000
   c. 70 000
   d. 100 000
2. A nurse is teaching a client about coronary artery disease. Which changes occur in this disorder and should be included in the explanation? *(Select all that apply)*
   a. Diffuse involvement of plaque formation in coronary veins
   b. Abnormal levels of cholesterol, especially low-density lipoproteins

   c. Accumulation of lipid plaques or calcification within the coronary arteries
   d. Development of angina due to a decreased blood supply to the heart muscle
   e. Chronic vasoconstriction of coronary arteries leading to permanent vasospasm
3. Which statement indicates that the client requires additional instruction in reducing cardiac risk factors?
   a. "I would like to add weightlifting to my exercise program."
   b. "I can't keep my blood pressure normal without medication."
   c. "I can change my diet to decrease my intake of saturated fats."
   d. "I will change my lifestyle to reduce activities that increase my stress."

4. A hospitalized client with angina tells the nurse that she is having chest pain. What best describes the nature of anginal pain?
   a. It will be relieved by rest, nitroglycerin, or both.
   b. It is less severe than the pain of a myocardial infarction.
   c. It indicates that irreversible cellular damage is occurring.
   d. It is frequently associated with vomiting and extreme fatigue.

5. What does the clinical spectrum of ACS include?
   a. Unstable angina and STEMI
   b. Unstable angina and NSTEMI
   c. Stable angina and sudden cardiac death
   d. Unstable angina, STEMI, and NSTEMI

6. In a client recovering from an MI, in which period is the heart most vulnerable to stress?
   a. 3 weeks after the infarction
   b. 4 to 6 days after the infarction
   c. 10 to 14 days after the infarction
   d. When healing is complete, at 6 to 8 weeks

7. A client is admitted to the ED with chest pain of 2 hours' duration, ECG findings consistent with an acute MI, and occasional ventricular dysrhythmias. With what pharmacological therapy would the nurse expect the client to be managed initially?
   a. Diuretics
   b. Nitroglycerin spray

c. β-Adrenergic blockers
   d. Thrombolytic therapy with tissue plasminogen activator

8. Five days after an MI, a client is restless and apprehensive. How can the nurse assist the client?
   a. By providing all care and doing everything for the client
   b. By structuring the environment and the routine so that the client can rest
   c. By allowing the client to participate in planning and carrying out activities
   d. By encouraging the family to provide for the client's physical care and give emotional support

9. What is the most common pathological finding in individuals experiencing SCD?
   a. Cardiomyopathies
   b. Mitral valve disease
   c. Atherosclerotic heart disease
   d. Left ventricular hypertrophy

1. c; 2. b, c, d; 3. a; 4. a; 5. d; 6. c; 7. b; 8. c; 9. c.

ⒺVolve

For even more review questions, visit *http://evolve.elsevier.com/Canada/ Lewis/medsurg.*

REFERENCES

Aehlert, B. (2013). *ECGs made easy* (5th ed.). St. Louis: Elsevier.

Anderson, T., Grégoire, J., Hegele, R., et al. (2013). 2012 update of the Canadian Cardiovascular Society guidelines for the diagnosis and treatment of dyslipidemia for the prevention of cardiovascular disease in the adult. *Journal of Cardiology, 29*(2), 151–167. doi:10.1016/j.cjca.2012.11.032.

Bibbins-Domingo, K., Grossman, D. C., Curry, S. J., et al. (2016). Aspirin use for the primary prevention of cardiovascular disease and colorectal cancer: U.S. Preventive Services Task Force recommendation statement. *Annals of Internal Medicine, 164*(12), 836–845. doi:10.7326/M16-0577.

Bojar, R. (2011). *Manual of perioperative care in adult cardiac surgery* (5th ed.). Hoboken, NJ: Wiley-Blackwell.

Burg, M. M., Edmondson, D., Shimbo, D., et al. (2013). The "perfect storm" and acute coronary syndrome onset: Do psychosocial factors play a role? *Progressive Cardiovascular Disorders, 55*(6), 601–610. doi:10.1016/j.pcad.2013.03.003.

Canadian Society for Exercise Physiology. (2011). *Canadian physical activity guidelines*. Retrieved from *http://www.csep.ca/CMFiles/ Guidelines/PAGuidelinesBackgrounder_E.pdf.*

Cohen, B. E., Edmondson, D., & Kronish, I. M. (2015). State of the art review: Depression, stress, anxiety, and cardiovascular disease. *American Journal of Hypertension, 28*(11), 1295–1302. doi:10.1093/ajh/hpv047.

Conti, C. R., Bavry, A. A., & Petersen, J. W. (2012). Silent ischemia. *Journal of the American College of Cardiology, 59*(5), 435–441. doi:10.1016/j.jacc.2011.07.050.

Eckel, R. H., Jakicic, J. M., & Ard, J. D. (2014). 2013 AHA/ACC guideline on lifestyle management to reduce cardiovascular risk: A report of the American College of Cardiology/American Heart Association Task Force on Practice Guidelines. *Circulation, 129*(25), S76–S99.

European Society of Cardiology. (2014). *Women more likely to develop anxiety and depression after heart attack*. Retrieved from

https://www.escardio.org/The-ESC/Press-Office/Press-releases/Women -more-likely-to-develop-anxiety-and-depression-after-heart-attack.

Heart and Stroke Foundation of Canada. (2016a). *2016 report on the health of Canadians*. Retrieved from *http://www.heartandstroke .ca/-/media/pdf-files/canada/2017-heart-month/heartandstroke -reportonhealth-2016.ashx?la=en.*

Heart and Stroke Foundation. (2016b). *Healthy weight and waist*. Retrieved from *https://www.heartandstroke.ca/get-healthy/ healthy-weight/healthy-weight-and-waist.*

Heart and Stroke Foundation. (2016c). *Healthy eating*. Retrieved from *https://www.heartandstroke.ca/get-healthy/healthy-eating.*

Hillis, L. D., Smith, P. K., Anderson, J. L., et al. (2011). 2011 ACCF/ AHA guideline for coronary artery bypass graft surgery: Executive summary. *Circulation, 124*(23), 2610–2642. doi:10.1161/ CIR.0b013e31823b5fee.

Huether, S. E., & McCance, K. L. (2012). *Understanding pathophysiology* (5th ed.). St. Louis: Elsevier.

Hypertension Canada. (2015). *Hypertension Canada guidelines*. Retrieved from *http://guidelines.hypertension.ca/.*

Imran, A., Rabasa-Lhoret, R., & Ross, S. (2013). *Targets for glycemic control. Diabetes Canada Clinical Practice Guidelines*. Retrieved from *http://guidelines.diabetes.ca/executivesummary/ch8.*

James, P., Oparil, S., Carter, B., et al. (2014). 2014 evidence-based guideline for the management of high blood pressure in adults: Report from the panel members appointed to the eighth Joint National Committee (JNC 8). *Journal of the American Medical Association, 311*(5), 507–520. doi:10.1001/jama.2013.284427.

Jhamnani, S., Patel, D., Heimlich, L., et al. (2015). Meta-analysis of the effects of lifestyle modifications on coronary and carotid atherosclerotic burden. *American Journal of Cardiology, 115*(2), 268–275. doi:10.1016/j.amjcard.2014.10.035.

Levine, G. N., Steinke, E. E., Bakaeen, F. G., et al. (2012). Sexual activity and cardiovascular disease: A scientific statement from the American Heart Association. *Circulation, 125*(8), 1058–1072. doi:10.1161/CIR.0b013e3182447787.

Lichtman, J. H., Froelicher, E. S., Blumenthal, J. A., et al. (2014). Depression as a risk factor for poor prognosis among patients with acute coronary syndrome: Systematic review and recommendations. *Circulation, 129*(12), 1350–1369. doi:10.1161/CIR.0000000000000019.

Mitrani, R. D., & Myerburg, R. J. (2016). Ten advances defining sudden cardiac death. *Trends in Cardiovascular Medicine, 26*(1), 23–33. doi:10.1016/j.tcm.2015.03.017.

National Institute on Drug Abuse. (2016). *Drug facts: Cocaine.* Retrieved from *http://www.drugabuse.gov/publications/drugfacts/cocaine.*

Pagana, K., Pagana, T., & Pike-MacDonald, S. (2013). *Mosby's Canadian manual of diagnostic and laboratory tests.* Toronto: Elsevier.

Smith, S., Benjamin, E., Bonow, R., et al. (2011). *AHA/ACCF secondary prevention and risk reduction therapy for patients with coronary and other atherosclerotic vascular disease: 2011 update.* Retrieved from *http://circ.ahajournals.org/content/124/22/2458.*

Statistics Canada. (2017). *Leading causes of death, by sex.* Retrieved from *http://www.statcan.gc.ca/tables-tableaux/sum-som/l01/cst01/hlth36a-eng.htm.*

Strang, F., & Schunkert, H. (2014). C-reactive protein and coronary heart disease: All said—is not it? *Mediators of Inflammation,* doi:10.1155/2014/757123. article ID757123.

RESOURCES

Canadian Association of Critical Care Nurses
http://www.caccn.ca

Canadian Council of Cardiovascular Nurses
http://www.cccn.ca

Heart and Stroke Foundation of Canada
http://www.heartandstroke.ca

Hypertension Canada
guidelines.hypertension.ca

Public Health Agency of Canada: Substance Use/Addictions
http://www.phac-aspc.gc.ca/chn-rcs/saa-toxicomanie-eng.php

Registered Nurses' Association of Ontario Best Practice Guideline: Integrating Smoking Cessation Into Daily Nursing Practice
http://rnao.ca/sites/rnao-ca/files/Integrating_Smoking_Cessation_into_Daily_Nursing_Practice.pdf

---

American College of Cardiovascular Nurses (ACCN)
http://www.accn.net

American Heart Association
http://www.heart.org

American Heart Association Walking Program
http://startwalkingnow.org

Framingham Heart Study
http://www.framingham.com/heart/index.htm

Health Central: Heart Disease
https://www.healthcentral.com/heart-disease

National Heart, Lung, and Blood Institute: BMI Calculator
https://www.nhlbi.nih.gov/health/educational/lose_wt/BMI/bmicalc.htm

Sudden Cardiac Arrest Network
http://www.sca-aware.org/sca-survivor-network

For additional Internet resources, see the website for this book at *http://evolve.elsevier.com/Canada/Lewis/medsurg.*

Nursing Management
Heart Failure

Written by: Carolyn Moffa
Adapted by: Annemarie F. Kaan

ⓔvolve WEBSITE

http://evolve.elsevier.com/Canada/Lewis/medsurg

- Review Questions (Online Only)
- Key Points
- Answer Guidelines for Case Study
- Customizable Nursing Care Plan
  - Heart Failure
- Conceptual Care Map Creator
  - Conceptual Care Map for Textbook Case Study
- Audio Glossary
- Content Updates

LEARNING OBJECTIVES

1. Compare the pathophysiology of heart failure with preserved and reduced ejection fraction.
2. Relate the compensatory mechanisms involved in heart failure to the development of acute decompensated heart failure and chronic heart failure.
3. Select the appropriate nursing and collaborative interventions to manage a patient with acute decompensated heart failure.
4. Select the appropriate nursing and collaborative interventions to manage a patient with chronic heart failure.
5. Describe the indications for cardiac transplantation and the nursing management of cardiac transplant recipients.

KEY TERMS

cardiac transplantation, p. 854
heart failure (HF), p. 845

heart failure with preserved ejection fraction (HF-PEF), p. 846

heart failure with reduced ejection fraction (HF-REF), p. 846

paroxysmal nocturnal dyspnea, p. 849
pulmonary edema, p. 848

HEART FAILURE

Heart failure (HF) is an abnormal clinical syndrome involving impaired cardiac pumping or filling, or both. *Heart failure,* formerly called *congestive heart failure,* is the term preferred today because not all patients with HF have pulmonary congestion or volume overload. HF is associated with numerous types of cardiovascular diseases, particularly longstanding hypertension, coronary artery disease (CAD), and myocardial infarction (MI) (Table 37-1). HF is characterized by ventricular dysfunction, reduced exercise tolerance, diminished quality of life, and shortened life expectancy.

Globally, HF has become a major health problem. In contrast to other cardiovascular diseases, HF is projected to increase in incidence. The prevalence of HF increases with age, which is of particular concern to Canada's aging population (Braunwald, 2015).

In Canada, it is estimated that one in five people older than 40 will suffer from HF during their lifetime.

The burden of HF will continue to rise with the growing population. It was projected that between 1994 and 2050, readmissions to hospital for HF would triple. Multiple hospitalizations translate to a significant economic burden on communities (O'Meara, Thibodeau-Jarry, Ducharme, et al., 2014).

Despite improvements in therapy since the late 1980s, the mortality rate 1 year after diagnosis remains high, at 23.4% (O'Meara, Thibodeau-Jarry, Ducharme, et al., 2014).

Etiology and Pathophysiology

Coronary artery disease (CAD) and hypertension are the primary risk factors for HF. In Canada, CAD and hypertension are responsible for up to 47.7% and 26% of patients, respectively (Yeung, Van Dyke, Maclagan, et al., 2013).

Diabetes mellitus predisposes an individual to HF regardless of the presence of concomitant CAD or hypertension. The etiology is thought to be complex and related in part to insulin resistance and its effect on ventricular remodelling (Blair,

TABLE 37-1	COMMON CAUSES OF HEART FAILURE

Chronic	Acute
Coronary artery disease	Acute myocardial infarction
Hypertension	Dysrhythmias
Rheumatic heart disease	Pulmonary embolus
Congenital heart disease	Thyrotoxicosis
Ventricular septal defect	Hypertensive crisis
Pulmonary disease	Rupture of papillary muscle
Cardiomyopathy	Myocarditis
Anemia	Bacterial endocarditis
Bacterial endocarditis	
Valvular disorders	

TABLE 37-2	PRECIPITATING CAUSES OF HEART FAILURE

Cause	Mechanism
Anemia	↓ Oxygen-carrying capacity of the blood, stimulating ↑ in CO to meet tissue demands
Infection	↑ Oxygen demand of tissues, stimulating ↑ CO
Thyrotoxicosis	Changes in the tissue metabolic rate; ↑ HR and workload of the heart
Hypothyroidism	Indirectly predisposes to ↑ atherosclerosis; severe hypothyroidism decreases myocardial contractility
Dysrhythmias	May ↓ CO and ↑ workload and oxygen requirements of myocardial tissue
Bacterial endocarditis	Infection: ↑ metabolic demands and oxygen requirements
	Valvular dysfunction: causes stenosis and regurgitation
Myocarditis	↑ HR, ↓ CO, acute right and left ventricular failure
Pulmonary embolism	↑ Pulmonary pressure and exerts pressure on the RV, leading to right ventricular hypertrophy and failure
Pulmonary disease	↑ Pulmonary pressure and exerts a pressure load on the RV, leading to right ventricular hypertrophy and failure
Paget's disease	↑ Workload of the heart by ↑ vascular bed in the skeletal muscle
Nutritional deficiencies	May ↓ cardiac function by ↓ myocardial muscle mass and myocardial contractility
Hypervolemia	↑ Preload, causing volume load on the RV

CO, cardiac output; HR, heart rate; LV, left ventricle; RV, right ventricle.

Huffman, & Shah, 2013). Other risk factors for the development of HF include cigarette smoking, obesity, and high serum levels of cholesterol (Liu, Arnold, Howlett, et al., 2015).

HF may be caused by any interference with the normal mechanisms regulating cardiac output (CO). CO depends on (a) preload, (b) afterload, (c) myocardial contractility, and (d) heart rate (HR). (Preload, afterload, and other hemodynamic parameters are discussed in Chapter 34.) Any alteration in these factors can lead to decreased ventricular function and the resultant manifestations of HF.

In general, major causes of HF may be divided into two subgroups: primary causes (see Table 37-1) and precipitating causes (Table 37-2). Precipitating causes often increase the workload of the ventricles, which results in a decompensated condition that leads to decreased myocardial function.

Pathology of Ventricular Failure. HF is described as being accompanied by either reduced ejection fraction (systolic) or preserved ejection fraction (diastolic) (McKelvie, Moe, Ezekowitz, et al., 2013).

Heart Failure With Reduced Ejection Fraction. Heart failure with reduced ejection fraction (HF-REF), the most common form of HF, results from an inability of the heart to pump blood effectively. It is caused by impaired contractile function (e.g., myocardial ischemia), increased afterload (e.g., hypertension), cardiomyopathy, and mechanical abnormalities (e.g., valvular heart disease). The left ventricle (LV) loses its ability to generate enough pressure to eject blood forward through the aorta. The hallmark of HF-REF is a reduction in the left ventricular ejection fraction (EF; the percentage of total amount of end-diastolic blood volume that is ejected during each systole). Normal EF is higher than 55% of the ventricular volume. Patients with HF-REF requiring specialist intervention generally have an EF of 40% or lower (Arnold, Liu, Demers, et al., 2006).

Heart Failure With Preserved Ejection Fraction. Heart failure with preserved ejection fraction (HF-PEF)—often referred to as diastolic HF—is the inability of the ventricles to relax and fill during diastole. Decreased filling of the ventricles results in decreased stroke volume and cardiac output (CO). HF-PEF is characterized by high filling pressures, which are increased because of poorly compliant ventricles. This results in venous engorgement in both the pulmonary and systemic vascular systems. HF-PEF is often the result of left ventricular hypertrophy from hypertension (most common), myocardial ischemia, valve disease (e.g., aortic, mitral), or cardiomyopathy. However, many affected patients do not have an identifiable heart disease. The diagnosis

of HF-PEF is based on the presence of HF symptoms with a normal EF (Huether & McCance, 2012).

Mixed Heart Failure. HF of mixed origin occurs in disease states such as dilated cardiomyopathy. Dilated cardiomyopathy is a condition in which poor systolic function (weakened muscle function) is further compromised by dilated left ventricular walls that are unable to relax and hence fill effectively. Affected patients often have an extremely poor EF (<35%), high pulmonary pressures, and biventricular failure (both ventricles may be dilated and have poor filling and emptying capacity).

Patients with HF of any type have low systemic arterial blood pressure (BP), low CO, and poor renal perfusion. Poor exercise tolerance and ventricular dysrhythmias are also common. Whether a patient arrives at this point acutely as a result of myocardial infarction (MI) or chronically from worsening cardiomyopathy or hypertension, the body's response to this low CO is to mobilize its compensatory mechanisms to maintain CO and BP.

Compensatory Mechanisms. HF can have an abrupt onset, as with acute MI, or it can be a subtle process resulting from slow, progressive changes. The overloaded heart uses compensatory mechanisms to try to maintain adequate CO. The main compensatory mechanisms include (a) sympathetic nervous system (SNS) activation, (b) neuro-hormonal responses, (c) ventricular dilation, and (d) ventricular hypertrophy.

Sympathetic Nervous System Activation. SNS activation is often the first mechanism triggered in low-CO states. However, it is the least effective compensatory mechanism. In response to an inadequate stroke volume and CO, SNS activation increases,

DETERMINANTS OF HEALTH

Heart Disease Rehabilitation

- Barriers to cardiac rehabilitation utilization include lack of time, work, family responsibilities, and distance to facility.*

Gender
- Women are 36% less likely to enroll in cardiac rehabilitation programs.†
- Use of cardiac rehabilitation is associated with a more significant reduction in mortality among women than among men.‡

Culture
- Use of cardiac rehabilitation is lower among members of minority groups because of variations in cultural beliefs, diet, and exercise.*

Education and Literacy
- The educated and higher income individuals are more likely to use cardiac rehabilitation because of availability of resources and motivation.*

Personal Health Practice and Coping Skills
- After diagnosis of a cardiovascular related illness, fewer than 5% of Canadians who smoked quit.†

Health Services
- Use of cardiac rehabilitation is associated with a 50% reduction in mortality.†
- Only 40% of participants eligible to receive cardiac rehabilitation enroll in such programs.†

*Data from Mead, H., Ramos, C., & Grantham, S. C. (2016). Drivers of racial and ethnic disparities in cardiac rehabilitation use: Patient and provider perspectives. *Medical Care Research and Review, 73*(3), 251–282. doi:10.1177/1077558715606261.
†Heart and Stroke Foundation of Canada. (2015). Heart failure. Retrieved from *http://www.heartandstroke.ca/heart/conditions/heart-failure.*
‡Colbert, J. D., Martin, B. J., Haykowsky, M. J., et al. (2015). Cardiac rehabilitation referral, attendance and mortality in women. *European Journal of Preventive Cardiology, 22*(8), 979–986.

resulting in the increased release of catecholamines (epinephrine and norepinephrine). This results in increased HR, increased myocardial contractility, and peripheral vasoconstriction. Initially, this increase in HR and contractility improves CO. Over time, however, these factors are harmful, inasmuch as they increase the already failing heart's workload and need for oxygen. The vasoconstriction causes an immediate increase in preload, which may initially increase CO; but an increase in venous return to the heart, which is already volume overloaded, actually worsens ventricular performance.

Neuro-hormonal Responses. As the CO falls, blood flow to the kidneys decreases. This is sensed by the juxtaglomerular apparatus in the kidneys as decreased volume. In response, the kidneys release renin, which converts angiotensinogen to angiotensin I (see Chapter 47 and Figure 47-6). Angiotensin I is subsequently converted to angiotensin II by angiotensin-converting enzyme (ACE) made in the lungs. Angiotensin II causes (a) the adrenal cortex to release aldosterone, which results in sodium and water retention, and (b) increased peripheral vasoconstriction, which increases BP. This response is known as the *renin-angiotensin-aldosterone system* (RAAS).

Low CO causes a decrease in cerebral perfusion pressure. In response, the posterior pituitary gland secretes antidiuretic hormone (ADH; also called *vasopressin*). ADH increases water reabsorption in the kidneys, which causes water retention. As a result, blood volume is increased when a volume overload state already exists.

Other factors also contribute to the development of HF. The production of endothelin, a potent vasoconstrictor produced by the vascular endothelial cells, is stimulated by ADH, catecholamines, and angiotensin II. Endothelin results in further arterial vasoconstriction and an increase in cardiac contractility and hypertrophy.

Locally, proinflammatory cytokines are released by heart cells in response to various forms of cardiac injury (e.g., MI). Two cytokines, tumour necrosis factor (TNF) and interleukin-1 (IL-1), further depress heart function by causing hypertrophy, contractile dysfunction, and cell death. Over time, a systemic inflammatory response also occurs. This accounts for the cardiac and skeletal muscle myopathy and fatigue that accompany advanced HF.

Activation of the SNS and the neuro-hormonal response lead to elevated levels of norepinephrine, angiotensin II, aldosterone, ADH, endothelin, and proinflammatory cytokines. Together, these factors result in an increase in cardiac workload, myocardial dysfunction, and ventricular remodelling. Remodelling involves hypertrophy of the ventricular myocytes, which causes contractile cells to become enlarged and abnormally shaped. This altered geometric shape of the ventricles eventually leads to increased ventricular mass, increased wall tension, increased oxygen consumption, and impaired contractility. Although the ventricles become larger, they become less effective pumps. Ventricular remodelling is a risk factor for life-threatening dysrhythmias and sudden cardiac death.

Ventricular Dilation. Dilation is an enlargement of the chambers of the heart. It occurs when pressure in the heart chambers (usually the left ventricle) becomes chronically elevated. The muscle fibres of the heart stretch in response to the volume of blood in the heart at the end of diastole. The degree of stretch is directly related to the force of the contraction (systole), according to Starling's law. Initially, dilation is an adaptive mechanism to cope with increasing blood volume, and this increased contraction leads to increased CO and maintenance of arterial BP and perfusion. Eventually, this mechanism becomes inadequate because the elastic elements of the muscle fibres are overstretched and can no longer contract effectively, and CO diminishes (Figure 37-1, *A*).

Ventricular Hypertrophy. Hypertrophy is an increase in the muscle mass and cardiac wall thickness in response to overwork and strain (see Figure 37-1, *B*). It develops slowly because it takes time for muscle tissue to thicken. Initially, the increased contractile power of the muscle fibres leads to an increase in CO and maintenance of tissue perfusion. Over time, hypertrophic heart muscle has poor contractility and requires more oxygen to perform work, coronary artery circulation becomes poor (tissue becomes ischemic more easily), and the heart is prone to dysrhythmias.

Counter-Regulatory Mechanisms. The body's attempts to maintain balance are demonstrated by several counter-regulatory processes. Natriuretic peptides (atrial natriuretic peptide and brain, or B-type, natriuretic peptide [BNP]) are hormones produced by the heart muscle. Atrial natriuretic peptide is released from the atria and BNP is released from the ventricles in response to increased blood volume in the heart (Nawarskas, Bowman, & Anderson, 2015).

The natriuretic peptides have renal, cardiovascular, and hormonal effects. Renal effects include (a) increased glomerular filtration rate and diuresis and (b) excretion of sodium (natriuresis). Cardiovascular effects include vasodilation and decreased BP. Hormonal effects include (a) inhibition of aldosterone and

Enlarged atria

Enlarged ventricles

Thickened heart muscle

FIGURE 37-1 A, Dilated heart chambers. **B,** Hypertrophied heart chambers.

renin secretion and (b) interference with ADH release. The combined effects of atrial natriuretic peptide and BNP help counter the adverse effects of the SNS and RAAS in patients with HF (Huether & McCance, 2012).

Cardiac compensation occurs when compensatory mechanisms succeed in maintaining a CO that is adequate for essential tissue perfusion. Cardiac decompensation occurs when these mechanisms can no longer maintain adequate CO and tissue perfusion becomes insufficient.

Types of Heart Failure

HF is usually evidenced by biventricular failure, although one ventricle may become dysfunctional before the other. Normally, the pumping actions of the left and right sides of the heart complement each other, producing a continuous flow of blood. However, as a result of pathological conditions, one side may fail, and the other side continues to function normally for a time. Because of the prolonged strain, both sides of the heart eventually fail, resulting in biventricular failure.

Left-Sided Heart Failure. The most common form of initial heart failure is left-sided failure (Figure 37-2). Left-sided failure results from left ventricular dysfunction, which causes blood to back up through the left atrium and into the pulmonary veins. The increased pulmonary pressure causes fluid extravasation from the pulmonary capillary bed into the interstitium and then the alveoli, which is manifested as pulmonary congestion and edema.

Right-Sided Heart Failure. Right-sided heart failure causes backward blood flow to the right atrium and venous circulation. Venous congestion in the systemic circulation results in peripheral edema, hepatomegaly, splenomegaly, vascular congestion of the gastro-intestinal tract, and jugular venous distension. The primary cause of right-sided failure is left-sided failure. In this situation, left-sided failure results in pulmonary congestion and increased pressure in the blood vessels of the lungs (pulmonary hypertension). Eventually, chronic pulmonary hypertension results in right-sided hypertrophy and failure. Cor pulmonale (right ventricular dilation and hypertrophy caused by pulmonary disease) can also cause right-sided failure. (Cor pulmonale is discussed in Chapter 30.) Right ventricular infarction may also cause right ventricular failure.

Clinical Manifestations of Heart Failure

Regardless of etiology, acute decompensated heart failure (ADHF) typically manifests as pulmonary edema, an abnormal, life-threatening accumulation of fluid in the alveoli and interstitial spaces of the lungs (Figure 37-3). The most common cause of pulmonary edema is acute left ventricular failure secondary to acute myocardial ischemia. (Other etiological factors for pulmonary edema are listed in Chapter 30, Table 30-24.)

In most cases of ADHF, the pulmonary venous pressure increases as a result of decreased efficiency of the left ventricle. This results in engorgement of the pulmonary vascular system. As a result, the lungs become less compliant, and there is increased resistance in the small airways. In addition, the lymphatic system increases its flow to help maintain a constant volume of the pulmonary extravascular fluid. This early stage is clinically associated with a mild increase in the respiratory rate and a decrease in partial pressure of arterial oxygen (PaO₂).

If pulmonary venous pressure continues to increase, the increase in intravascular pressure causes more fluid to move into the interstitial space than the lymphatic vessels can drain. Interstitial edema occurs at this point. Tachypnea develops, and the patient becomes symptomatic (short of breath out of proportion to activity level). If the pulmonary venous pressure increases further, the tight alveoli lining cells are disrupted, and a fluid containing red blood cells moves into the alveoli (alveolar edema). As the disruption becomes worse from further increases in the pulmonary venous pressure, the alveoli and the airways are flooded with fluid (see Figure 37-3). This is accompanied by a worsening of the blood gas values (i.e., lower PaO₂ and possible increase in partial pressure of arterial carbon dioxide [PaCO₂] and progressive respiratory acidemia).

Clinical manifestations of pulmonary edema are distinct. Most affected patients are anxious, pale, and possibly cyanotic. The skin is clammy and cold from vasoconstriction caused by stimulation of the SNS. The patient has severe dyspnea, as evidenced by the use of accessory muscles of respiration, a respiratory rate greater than 30 breaths per minute, and orthopnea. There may be wheezing and coughing with the production of frothy, blood-tinged sputum. Auscultation of the lungs may reveal crackles, wheezes, and rhonchi throughout the lungs. The patient's

PATHOPHYSIOLOGY MAP

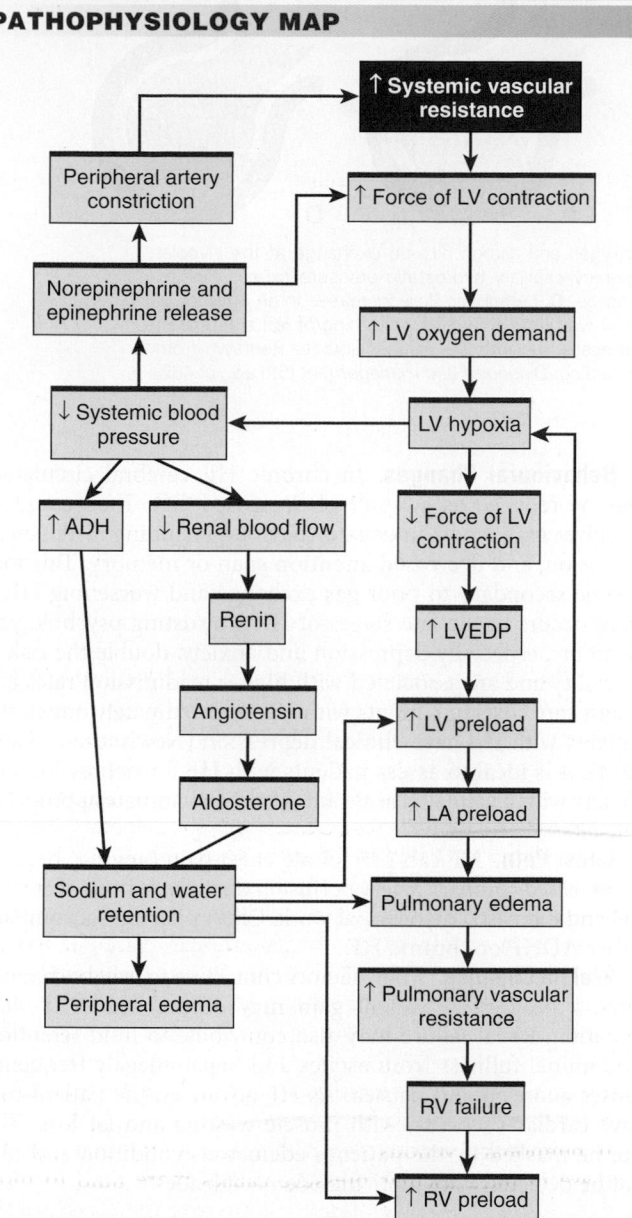

FIGURE 37-2 Illustration of how left-sided heart failure results from elevated systemic vascular resistance. Left-sided heart failure leads to right-sided heart failure. Systemic vascular resistance and preload are exacerbated by renal and adrenal mechanisms. *ADH,* antidiuretic hormone; *LA,* left atrial; *LV,* left ventricular; *LVEDP,* left ventricular end-diastolic pressure; *RV,* right ventricular. Source: Adapted from Huether, S. E., & McCance, K. L. (2004). *Understanding pathophysiology* (3rd ed.). St. Louis: Mosby.

HR is rapid, and BP may be elevated or decreased, depending on the severity of the HF.

ADHF can be categorized into one of four groups on the basis of hemodynamic and clinical status: dry-warm, dry-cold, wet-warm, and wet-cold (Figure 37-4). The most common presentation is the wet-warm status. Affected patients have adequate perfusion (warm) but volume overload (e.g., congestion, dyspnea, edema; McKelvie, Moe, Ezekowitz, et al., 2013).

Clinical Manifestations of Chronic Heart Failure

Chronic HF is characterized as a progressive worsening of ventricular function and chronic neuro-hormonal activation that

TABLE 37-3   CLINICAL MANIFESTATIONS OF HEART FAILURE

Right-Sided Heart Failure	Left-Sided Heart Failure
Signs	
RV heaves	LV heaves
Murmurs	Cheyne-Stokes respirations
Peripheral edema	Pulsus alternans (alternating
Weight gain	pulses: strong, weak)
↑ HR	↑ HR
Edema of dependent body parts	PMI displaced inferiorly and
(sacrum, anterior tibias, pedal	posteriorly (LV hypertrophy)
edema)	↓ PaO_2, slight ↑ $PaCO_2$ (poor O_2
Ascites	exchange)
Anasarca (massive generalized body	Crackles (pulmonary edema)
edema)	S_3 and S_4 (see Easy Auscultation
Jugular venous distension	website listed in the
Hepatomegaly (liver enlargement)	Resources at the end of this
Right-sided pleural effusion	chapter)
Symptoms	
Fatigue	Fatigue
Dependent edema	Dyspnea (shallow respirations
Right upper quadrant pain	≤32–40/min)
Anorexia and GI bloating	Orthopnea (shortness of breath
Nausea	in recumbent position)
	Dry, hacking cough
	Pulmonary edema
	Nocturia
	Paroxysmal nocturnal dyspnea

GI, gastro-intestinal; *HR,* heart rate; *LV,* left ventricular; *PaO₂,* arterial partial pressure of oxygen; *PaCO₂,* arterial partial pressure of carbon dioxide; *PMI,* point of maximal impulse; *RV,* right ventricle/ventricular; *S₃ and S₄,* third and fourth heart sounds.

results in ventricular remodelling. This process involves changes in the size, shape, and mechanical performance of the ventricle. The clinical manifestations of chronic HF depend on the patient's age, the underlying type and extent of heart disease, and which ventricle is failing to pump effectively. Table 37-3 lists the manifestations of right-sided HF and left-sided HF. Patients with chronic HF usually have manifestations of biventricular failure.

Fatigue. Fatigue is one of the earliest symptoms of chronic HF. The patient notices fatigue after activities that normally are not tiring. The fatigue is caused by decreased CO, impaired perfusion to vital organs, decreased oxygenation of the tissues, and anemia. Anemia can result from poor nutrition, renal disease, or drug therapy (e.g., ACE inhibitors).

Dyspnea. Dyspnea (shortness of breath) is a common manifestation of chronic HF. It is caused by increased pulmonary pressures secondary to interstitial and alveolar edema. Dyspnea can occur with mild exertion or at rest. Orthopnea is shortness of breath that occurs when the patient is in a recumbent position.

Paroxysmal Nocturnal Dyspnea. Paroxysmal nocturnal dyspnea occurs when the patient is asleep. It is caused by the reabsorption of fluid from dependent body areas when the patient is flat. The patient awakens in a panic, has feelings of suffocation, and has a strong desire to sit or stand up.

A cough is often associated with HF and may be the first clinical symptom. It begins as a dry, nonproductive cough and may be misdiagnosed as asthma or other lung disease. The cough is not relieved by position change or over-the-counter cough medicine.

FIGURE 37-3 As pulmonary edema progresses, it inhibits oxygen and carbon dioxide exchange at the alveolar capillary interface. **A,** Normal relationship. **B,** Increased pulmonary–capillary hydrostatic pressure causes fluid to move from the vascular space into the pulmonary interstitial space. **C,** Lymphatic flow increases in an attempt to pull fluid back into the vascular or lymphatic space. **D,** Failure of lymphatic flow and worsening of left-sided heart failure result in further movement of fluid into the interstitial space and into the alveoli. Source: Redrawn from Urden, L. D., Stacy, K. M., & Lough, M. E. (2010). *Critical care nursing: Diagnosis and management* (6th ed., p. 462, Figure 19-17). St. Louis: Mosby.

FIGURE 37-4 Categories of acute decompensated heart failure (ADHF). Source: Reprinted from *Canadian Journal of Cardiology*, 29(2), McKelvie, R. S., Moe, G. W., Ezekowitz, J. A., et al., The 2012 Canadian Cardiovascular Society heart failure management guidelines update: Focus on acute and chronic heart failure, pp. 168–181, Copyright 2013, with permission from Elsevier.

Tachycardia. Tachycardia is an early clinical sign of HF. One of the body's first mechanisms to compensate for a failing ventricle is to increase the HR. Because of diminished CO, SNS stimulation increases, which in turn increases HR. However, many patients with chronic HF take β blocker medications and may not show an increase in response to SNS stimulation.

Edema. Edema is a common sign of HF. It may occur in dependent body areas (peripheral edema), the liver (hepatomegaly), the abdominal cavity (ascites), and the lungs (pulmonary edema and pleural effusion). If the patient is in bed, sacral and scrotal edema may develop. Pressing on the edematous skin may leave a transient indentation (pitting edema). The development of dependent edema or a sudden weight gain of more than 2 kg (4 lb) in 2 days is often indicative of exacerbated HF.

Nocturia. A patient with chronic HF who has decreased CO also has impaired renal perfusion and decreased urine output during the day. However, when the patient lies down at night, fluid moves from the interstitial spaces back into the circulatory system. In addition, cardiac workload is decreased at night during rest. These combined effects result in increased renal blood flow and diuresis. The patient may complain of having to void frequently throughout the night.

Skin Changes. Because tissue capillary oxygen extraction is increased in a patient with chronic HF, the skin may appear dusky. Often the lower extremities are shiny and swollen, and hair growth on them is diminished or absent. Chronic swelling may result in pigment changes. This causes the skin to appear brown or brawny in areas covering the ankles and lower legs (hemosiderin staining).

Behavioural Changes. In chronic HF, cerebral circulation may be reduced as a result of decreased CO. The patient or caregiver may report unusual behaviour, including restlessness, confusion, and decreased attention span or memory. This may also be secondary to poor gas exchange and worsening HF. It often occurs in the late stages of HF. Coexisting psychological disorders, especially depression and anxiety, double the risk of mortality and are associated with higher readmission rates and health care costs in patients with HF. Approximately one in five patients with HF have clinical depression (Newhouse & Jiang, 2014). It is ideal to assess patients with HF for depression and anxiety with a validated scale and, if needed, initiate appropriate consults.

Chest Pain. HF can precipitate chest pain (angina) because of decreased coronary artery perfusion that results from decreased CO and increased myocardial work. Chest pain may accompany either ADHF or chronic HF.

Weight Changes. Many factors contribute to weight changes. First, a progressive weight gain may occur because of fluid retention. Renal failure may also contribute to fluid retention. Abdominal fullness from ascites and hepatomegaly frequently causes anorexia and nausea. As HF advances, the patient may have cardiac cachexia, with muscle wasting and fat loss. This can be masked by the patient's edematous condition and may not be detected until after the edema subsides.

Complications of Heart Failure

Pleural Effusion. Pleural effusion results from increasing pressure in the pleural capillaries. Transudative pleural effusion, commonly associated with HF, occurs as a result of the increased pressure in blood vessels or low albumin levels in the blood, which cause fluid to leak into the pleural space. (Pleural effusion is discussed in Chapter 30.)

Dysrhythmias. Chronic HF causes enlargement of the chambers of the heart. This enlargement (stretching of the atrial and ventricular walls) can cause changes in the normal electrical pathways. When numerous sites in the atria fire spontaneously and rapidly (atrial fibrillation), the organized atrial depolarization (contraction, or "atrial kick") no longer occurs. Atrial fibrillation also promotes thrombus formation within the atria. Thrombi may break loose and form emboli. This increases the risk for stroke in patients with atrial fibrillation. They require treatment with cardioversion, antidysrhythmics, anticoagulants, or a combination of these (see Chapter 38).

Patients with HF are also at risk for ventricular dysrhythmias (e.g., ventricular tachycardia, ventricular fibrillation). Ventricular tachycardia and fibrillation can lead to sudden cardiac death. (Sudden cardiac death is discussed in Chapter 36, and dysrhythmias are discussed in Chapter 38.)

Left Ventricular Thrombus. With ADHF or chronic HF, the enlargement of the LV and the decrease in CO combine to increase the chance of thrombus formation in the LV. Once a thrombus has formed, its volume may decrease the area of the LV, reducing left ventricular contractility, and cause a decrease in CO and worsening of the patient's perfusion. The development of emboli from the thrombus also increases the patient's risk for stroke.

Hepatomegaly. HF can lead to severe hepatomegaly, especially with right ventricular failure. Because the venous system is backed up, the liver lobules become congested with venous blood. The hepatic congestion leads to impaired liver function. Eventually, liver cells die, fibrosis occurs, and cirrhosis can develop (see Chapter 46).

Renal Failure. The decreased CO that accompanies acute and chronic HF results in decreased perfusion to the kidneys and can lead to renal insufficiency or failure (see Chapter 49).

Classification of Heart Failure

The New York Heart Association (NYHA) has developed a system for classifying symptoms experienced by patients with HF. The classification is widely used across Canada and the United States (Table 37-4).

TABLE 37-4 NEW YORK HEART ASSOCIATION FUNCTIONAL CLASSIFICATION OF PEOPLE WITH CARDIAC DISEASE

Class I	No limitation of physical activity. Ordinary physical activity does not cause fatigue, dyspnea, palpitations, or anginal pain.
Class II	Slight limitation of physical activity. No symptoms at rest. Ordinary physical activity results in fatigue, dyspnea, palpitations, or anginal pain.
Class III	Marked limitation of physical activity. Usually comfortable at rest. Ordinary physical activity causes fatigue, dyspnea, palpitations, or anginal pain.
Class IV	Inability to carry on any physical activity without discomfort. Symptoms of cardiac insufficiency or of angina may be present even at rest. If any physical activity is undertaken, discomfort is increased.

Source: From Criteria Committee of the New York Heart Association. (1994). Functional capacity and objective assessment. In M. Dolgin (Ed.), *Nomenclature and criteria for diagnosis of diseases of the heart and great vessels* (9th ed., pp. 253–255). Boston: Little, Brown.

Diagnostic Studies

Diagnosing HF is often difficult because neither the signs nor symptoms are highly specific, and both may mimic many other medical conditions, such as anemia or lung disease. The primary goal in diagnosis is to determine the underlying etiology of HF. Measures to assess the cause and degree of HF are included in Figure 37-5 (McKelvie, Moe, Ezekowitz, et al., 2013). Echocardiography and measurement of EF can be used to differentiate between HF-REF and HF-PEF, an important distinction to make in the early treatment of HF.

Measurement of either BNP or N-terminal–pro-BNP (NT–pro-BNP) levels is recommended to assist in the diagnosis of HF; in general, levels are positively correlated with the degree of left ventricular dysfunction and can help to differentiate dyspnea caused by HF from other causes of dyspnea (Moe, Ezekowitz, O'Meara, et al., 2015; Table 37-5).

NURSING AND COLLABORATIVE MANAGEMENT ACUTE DECOMPENSATED HEART FAILURE

The goal of therapy is to improve left ventricular function by decreasing intravascular volume, decreasing venous return (preload), decreasing afterload, improving gas exchange and oxygenation, and increasing CO (McKelvie, Moe, Ezekowitz, et al., 2013).

DECREASING INTRAVASCULAR VOLUME

Decreasing intravascular volume with the use of diuretics reduces venous return. A loop diuretic (e.g., furosemide [Lasix]) may be used to decrease volume because it may be administered by intravenous push, and its action within the kidney occurs rapidly. By decreasing venous return to the LV and thereby reducing preload, the overfilled LV may contract more efficiently and thus contribute to improving CO. This improves left ventricular function, decreases pulmonary vascular pressures, and improves gas exchange.

Ultrafiltration may be an option for a patient with volume overload. Ultrafiltration has generally been achieved through hemodialysis or with ultrafiltration by way of central venous access. (Ultrafiltration is discussed in Chapter 49.)

DECREASING VENOUS RETURN

Decreasing venous return (preload) reduces the amount of volume returned to the LV during diastole. This can be accomplished by placing the patient in high Fowler's position with the feet horizontal in the bed or dangling at the bedside. This position helps decrease venous return because of the pooling of blood in the extremities. This position also increases the thoracic capacity by decreasing intra-abdominal pressure on the lungs, allowing

TABLE 37-5 NATRIURETIC PEPTIDES CUT POINTS FOR THE DIAGNOSIS OF HEART FAILURE*

Peptide	Age in Years	HF Unlikely	HF Possible	HF Probable
BNP	All	<100 pg/mL	100–500 pg/mL	>500 pg/mL
NT–pro-BNP	<50	<300 pg/mL	300–450 pg/mL	>450 pg/mL
	50–75	<300 pg/mL	450–900 pg/mL	>900 pg/mL
	>75	<300 pg/mL	900–1800 pg/mL	>1800 pg/mL

Source: Reprinted from *Canadian Journal of Cardiology*, 31(1), Moe, G.W., Ezekowitz, J.A., O'Meara, E., et al., The 2014 Canadian Cardiovascular Society heart failure management guidelines focus update: Anemia, biomarkers, and recent therapeutic trial implications, pp. 3–16, Copyright 2015, with permission from Elsevier.
*Levels can be increased in the presence of renal dysfunction or sepsis and be decreased in obese patients.
BNP, B-type natriuretic peptide; *HF*, heart failure; *NT–pro-BNP*, N-terminal pro-BNP.

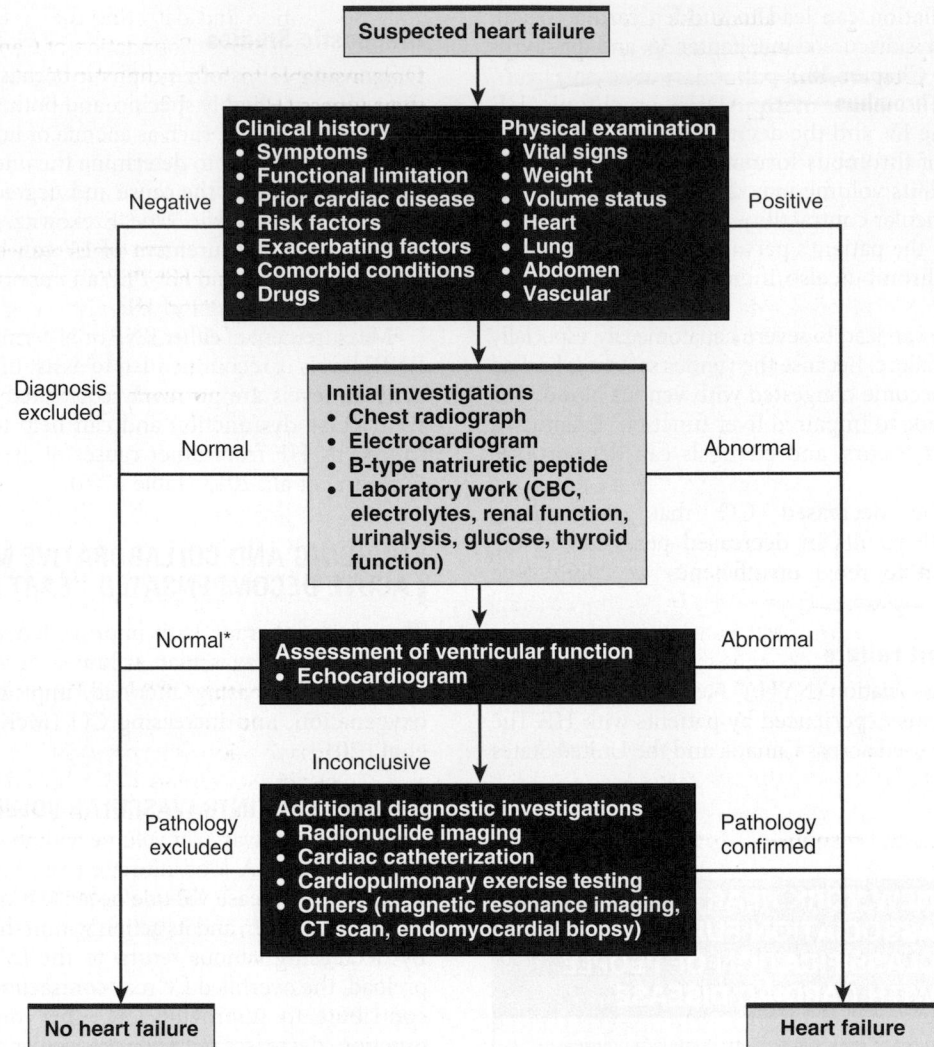

FIGURE 37-5 Algorithm for diagnosis of heart failure. *Normal ejection fraction does not rule out heart failure with preserved ejection fraction. *CBC,* complete blood count; *CT,* computed tomography. Source: Reprinted from *Canadian Journal of Cardiology,* 29(2), McKelvie, R. S., Moe, G. W., Ezekowitz, J. A., et al., The 2012 Canadian Cardiovascular Society heart failure management guidelines update: Focus on acute and chronic heart failure, pp. 168–181, Copyright 2013, with permission from Elsevier.

for improved ventilation. Intravenous nitroglycerine is a vasodilator used in the treatment of ADHF. It reduces circulating volume by decreasing preload and also increases coronary artery circulation by dilating the coronary arteries. In addition to reducing preload, it slightly reduces afterload (in high doses) and increases myocardial oxygen supply.

DECREASING AFTERLOAD

Afterload is the resistance against which the LV must pump; that is, it is the amount of work it takes for the LV to eject blood into the systemic circulation. Systemic vascular resistance (SVR) is a determinant of afterload, as is left ventricular filling. If afterload is reduced, the CO improves, and pulmonary congestion thereby decreases. Great care should be taken to ensure the patient's BP is adequate to provide cerebral and renal perfusion. Careful monitoring of vital signs is crucial.

IMPROVING GAS EXCHANGE AND OXYGENATION

Gas exchange may be improved by several measures. Intravenous morphine reduces preload and afterload and may decrease

myocardial oxygen demands, which can be raised as a result of anxiety and subsequent increased musculo-skeletal and respiratory activity. Administration of oxygen could be considered if the O_2 saturation falls below 90% (McKelvie, Moe, Ezekowitz, et al., 2013). Care must be taken to avoid oxygen if it is not required because it can reduce CO and increase SVR. (Oxygen therapy is discussed in Chapter 31.) In severe pulmonary edema, the patient may need noninvasive ventilatory support (e.g., bilevel positive airway pressure) or intubation and mechanical ventilation. (Ventilatory support is discussed in Chapter 68.)

IMPROVING CARDIAC FUNCTION

In a patient who is or becomes hemodynamically unstable—that is, becomes progressively hypotensive, has an HR that is abnormally fast or slow, develops dysrhythmias, or becomes hypoxic with cool and clammy skin—nursing care is more urgent, and treatment protocols may call for aggressive, complex therapies. The use of diuretics, morphine sulphate, and vasodilators may not be sufficient to control symptoms. The addition of positive inotropic therapy may be warranted, as well as the initiation of hemodynamic monitoring to evaluate the effectiveness of interventions. Once a pulmonary artery catheter is in position, CO, pulmonary artery pressure, and pulmonary artery occlusive pressure should be measured, and therapy should be instituted and titrated to maximize CO. A pulmonary artery occlusive pressure of 14 to 18 mm Hg generally achieves the goal of increasing CO. (Hemodynamic monitoring is discussed in Chapter 68.)

Inotropic drugs (e.g., dobutamine, milrinone) that increase myocardial contractility without increasing oxygen consumption may be effective. Dobutamine and milrinone also increase peripheral vasodilation. There is no evidence that inotropic drugs improve mortality rates. Milrinone has been linked to more frequent atrial arrhythmias, increased hypotension, and worsening HF. Therefore, use of inotropic drugs should be reserved for hemodynamically unstable patients only (McKelvie, Moe, Ezekowitz, et al., 2013).

REDUCING ANXIETY

Anxiety is reduced by the sedative action of morphine administered intravenously. When morphine is used, the patient must be watched closely for respiratory depression. In addition, a calm approach in providing care helps reduce anxiety.

Once the patient is more stable, the cause of pulmonary edema should be determined. Diagnosis of HF-REF or HF-PEF then guides further management protocols. Aggressive drug therapy may continue with intravenous forms of diuretics, inotropic drugs, vasodilators, and oral ACE inhibitors. Nursing care focuses on continual physical assessment, hemodynamic monitoring, and monitoring the patient's response to treatment.

COLLABORATIVE CARE: CHRONIC HEART FAILURE

The main goal in the management of HF is to treat the underlying cause and contributing factors, maximize CO, and alleviate symptoms. The management of dysrhythmias is discussed in Chapter 38, hypertension in Chapter 35, valvular disorders in Chapter 39, and coronary artery disease in Chapter 36.

Referral to Multidisciplinary Clinics or Specialist Care for Heart Failure

It is recommended that patients with newly diagnosed HF and patients at higher risk for the development of heart failure should be referred to a multidisciplinary heart failure clinic. These clinics, in Canada often referred to as *heart function clinics,* consist of a multidisciplinary team providing self-management coaching and a mechanism for assessment for more advanced therapies (Arnold, Liu, Demers, et al., 2006). It is recognized that these services are not accessible to some patients, and so many centres provide remote monitoring, whereby telehealth technologies are used to provide care.

Nonpharmacological Therapies

Oxygen. In a patient with HF, oxygen saturation of the blood may be reduced because the blood is not adequately oxygenated in the lungs. If oxygen saturation is less than 90%, administration of oxygen can improve tissue oxygenation. Thus appropriate use of oxygen therapy helps relieve dyspnea and fatigue. Pulse oximetry should be used to monitor the effectiveness of oxygen therapy.

Self-Management Teaching. An important part of HF care is helping the patient and family understand that HF is a chronic condition and become proficient in avoiding risks for

decompensation and detecting the early signs and symptoms. The Heart and Stroke Foundation of Canada makes many useful tools available to help support patients in learning to manage their illness (Heart and Stroke Foundation of Canada, 2015; see the Resources at the end of this chapter).

Exercise and Activity. Regular activity and exercise periods should be prescribed for all patients with stable chronic HF. Even patients with NYHA class III symptoms (see Table 37-4) should exercise three to five times per week for 30 to 45 minutes at a time. A cardiac rehabilitation program provides the patient with an individualized exercise regimen (Moe, Ezekowitz, O'Meara, et al., 2014). To ensure the patient's adherence to regular exercise, the medical team must be realistic about what the patient can achieve and must work around possible barriers to enable the patient to succeed.

Devices

Cardiac Resynchronization Therapy. For patients with HF who are receiving maximum medical therapy, continue to have NYHA functional class III or intravenous symptoms (see Table 37-4), and have a widened QRS interval, one therapy is biventricular pacing and cardiac resynchronization therapy (CRT). Traditional pacemakers pace one or two chambers (e.g., atrium or ventricle, or both). CRT coordinates contractility of the right ventricle (RV) and LV through biventricular pacing. Normal electrical conduction within the RV and LV improves left ventricular performance and CO. This additional therapy allows patients to increase their exercise capacity and decrease their overall symptoms. CRT has been shown to prolong life and improve quality of life in patients with NYHA functional class III and class IV HF (Howlett, McKelvie, Arnold, et al., 2009). CRT can be combined with traditional pacing capability, as well as with defibrillator technology.

Implantable Cardioverter–Defibrillator. If a patient has NYHA functional class II or III HF, is on optimal medical therapy, and has an EF of less than 35%, the implementation and use of an implantable cardioverter–defibrillator (ICD) with CRT may be warranted. Life-threatening ventricular dysrhythmias (e.g., ventricular tachycardia) are a complication of the ischemic myocardium and can cause sudden cardiac death. The addition of the ICD in these patients has reduced the overall rate of mortality from sudden cardiac death (Howlett, McKelvie, Arnold, et al., 2009). (Pacemakers and defibrillators are discussed in Chapter 38.)

Mechanical Circulatory Support. Several devices are available to sustain patients with HF in deteriorating conditions, especially those awaiting cardiac transplantation. The intra-aortic balloon pump is used for short-term support for HF patients with acute decompensation. However, the limitations of bed rest, infection, and vascular complications preclude its long-term use (see Chapter 68 for nursing management of circulatory assist devices).

Extracorporeal membrane oxygenation is a support device similar to a bypass machine used in cardiac surgery procedures. This system can be used to support critically ill patients with HF who are being assessed for more advanced therapy such as a ventricular assist device (VAD) (Figure 37-6). In Canada, VADs are used in carefully selected patients primarily as a bridge to cardiac transplantation. They provide highly effective long-term support for more than 2 years, allowing patients to live at home and even return to work while waiting for a transplant, and their use has become standard care for candidates for cardiac transplantation with acute decompensation. (Intra-aortic balloon

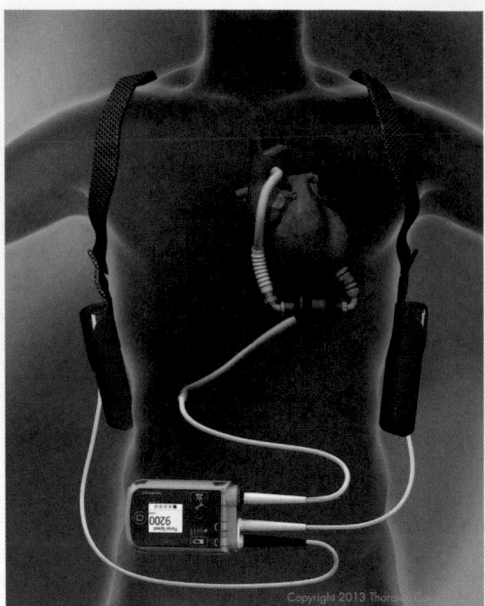

FIGURE 37-6 The HeartMate II ventricular assist device (Thoratec Corp., Pleasanton, CA), one of the devices used in transplantation centres across Canada as a bridge to heart transplantation. Source: HeartMate II and St. Jude are trademarks of St. Jude Medical, LLC or its related companies. Reproduced with permission of St. Jude Medical, © 2018. All rights reserved.

pumps, extracorporeal membrane oxygenation, and VADs are discussed further in Chapter 68.)

Cardiac Transplantation

Cardiac transplantation—the transfer of a heart from one person to another—is the treatment of choice in carefully selected patients with end-stage HF. Because of the lack of donor hearts, however, it is an option for only a small number of patients with HF. (Cardiac transplantation is discussed later in this chapter.)

Advance Care Planning and Goals of Care

HF is a chronic condition suffered primarily by older adults, and the prognosis is worse than that of most cancers. For many patients, therapies such as mechanical support and cardiac transplantation are not indicated.

HF is typically characterized by periods of stability interspersed with exacerbations and readmissions to hospital. In the end stages, the patient's quality of life can be limited by the symptoms, and many patients and families are not prepared for death.

The goal of care should be directed toward optimizing guideline-driven therapies outlined in this chapter and, in addition, early discussions with the patient and their loved ones about advance care planning (Figure 37-7). This includes goal setting in terms of patient's preferences, as well as planning for end of life. The role of the ICD and other life-prolonging interventions should be discussed regularly between the HF team and the patient.

Early intervention with palliative care support has shown to be effective at improving quality of life, helping patients and their families through these final stages (LeMond, Camacho, & Goodlin, 2015).

DRUG THERAPY: CHRONIC HEART FAILURE

General therapeutic objectives for drug management of chronic HF include the following: (a) identification of the type of HF

and the underlying causes, (b) correction of sodium and water retention and volume overload, (c) reduction of cardiac workload, (d) improvement of myocardial contractility, and (e) control of precipitating and complicating factors. The aims of treating HF are to improve symptoms, minimize adverse effects of treatment, prevent morbidity, and prolong survival. Current therapeutic approaches stress the importance of diuretics, ACE inhibitors, β-adrenergic blockers and mineralocorticoid receptor antagonists (previously known as *aldosterone antagonists;* Howlett, Chan, Ezekowitz, et al., 2016) (see Figure 37-7).

Diuretics

Diuretics are used in patients with HF to mobilize edematous fluid, reduce pulmonary venous pressure, and reduce preload (see Chapter 35, Table 35-8). If excess extracellular fluid is excreted, blood volume returning to the heart can be reduced and cardiac function improved.

Diuretics act on the kidneys by promoting excretion of sodium and water. Many varieties of diuretics are available, and some have specific indications for use. Thiazide diuretics may be the first choice for chronic HF because of their convenience, safety, low cost, and effectiveness. They are particularly useful in treating edema secondary to HF and in controlling hypertension. The thiazides inhibit sodium reabsorption in the distal tubule, thus promoting excretion of sodium and water.

Loop diuretics (e.g., furosemide [Lasix]) are potent diuretics. These drugs act on the ascending loop of Henle to promote sodium, chloride, and water excretion. Furosemide is more commonly used in cases of acute HF and pulmonary edema because its effects are slightly more predictable. Problems in using loop diuretics include reduction in serum potassium levels, ototoxicity, and possible allergic reaction in patients who are sensitive to sulpha-containing drugs (sulphonamides).

In patients who are not responsive to high-dose loop diuretics, metolazone (Zaroxolyn) or a thiazide diuretic can be added to the treatment regimen (Arnold, Liu, Demers, et al., 2006).

Angiotensin-Converting Enzyme Inhibitors

ACE inhibitors are useful in both systolic and diastolic HF, and they are the first-line therapy in the treatment of HF. Examples of ACE inhibitors include ramipril (Altace) and enalapril (Vasotec). Other examples of ACE inhibitors are discussed in Chapter 35 and listed in Table 35-8.

The conversion of angiotensin I to the potent vasoconstrictor angiotensin II requires the presence of ACE (see Chapter 47, Figure 47-6). ACE inhibitors exert their effects by blocking production of this enzyme, which results in decreased levels of angiotensin II. As a result, plasma aldosterone levels are also reduced.

Because CO is dependent on afterload in chronic HF, the reduction in SVR seen with the use of ACE inhibitors produces a significant increase in CO. Furthermore, the improvement of CO and the redistribution of regional blood flow that result from the use of ACE inhibitors help maintain tissue perfusion, even though BP may be decreased. Other hemodynamic changes include reductions in pulmonary artery pressure, right arterial pressure, and left ventricular filling pressure. Adverse effects of ACE inhibitors include symptomatic hypotension, chronic cough, and, when it is used in high doses, renal insufficiency. Aging and baseline renal insufficiency slow the metabolism of ACE inhibitors, and their toxicity may therefore be increased (Arnold, Liu, Demers, et al., 2006). It is recommended that these drugs

FIGURE 37-7 Therapeutic approach to patients with heart failure (HF) and reduced ejection fraction. *ACEi*, angiotensin-converting enzyme inhibitor; *AF*, atrial fibrillation; *ARB*, angiotensin receptor blocker; *BB*, β blocker; *BNP*, brain natriuretic peptide; *bpm*, beats per minute; *CRT*, cardiac resynchronization therapy; *HR*, heart rate; *ICD*, implantable cardioverter–defibrillator; *LVEF*, left ventricular ejection fraction; *MRA*, mineralocorticoid receptor antagonist; *NP*, natriuretic peptides; *NT-pro-BNP*, N-terminal pro–b-type natriuretic peptide; *NYHA*, New York Heart Association class; *SR*, sinus rhythm. Source: Reprinted from *Canadian Journal of Cardiology*, 32(3), Howlett, J. G., Chan, M., Ezekowitz, J. A., et al., The Canadian Cardiovascular Society Heart Failure Companion: Bridging Guidelines to Your Practice, pp. 296–310, Copyright 2016, with permission from Elsevier.

be started at the lowest dose and slowly increased over a 2- to 3-month period and that BP and renal function be monitored at regular intervals. Overall, ACE inhibitors are well tolerated by patients.

In patients who are unable to tolerate the ACE inhibitors because of angioedema or cough, angiotensin II receptor blockers (ARBs) such as losartan (Cozaar) or valsartan (Diovan) may be prescribed (see Chapter 35, Table 35-8). If a patient is already

taking an ACE inhibitor and a β-adrenergic blocker, an ARB can be added to the combination (Arnold, Liu, Demers, et al., 2006).

Neprilysin Inhibitors

A relatively new combination drug is available in Canada containing an ARB (valsartan) and a new class of HF medication called a neprilysin inhibitor (sacubitril). This drug combination has shown that it can significantly reduce rates of death from and rehospitalizations for heart failure in selected patients with HF. This drug replaces the use of ACE inhibitors (McMurray, Packer, Desai, et al., 2014).

β-Adrenergic Blockers

The use of β-adrenergic blockers (or β blockers) in combination with ACE inhibitors in the management of HF has become standard therapy for most patients. Examples include carvedilol and metoprolol (Lopressor). Marked improvement in rates of patient survival has been shown with the use of β-adrenergic blockers. β-Adrenergic blockers directly block the negative effects of the SNS on the failing heart, such as increased HR. Because β-adrenergic blockade can reduce myocardial contractility, care must be taken to start gradually, the dosage being increased slowly (typically every 2 weeks) as tolerated by the patient, until it reaches the maximum. Major adverse effects include edema, hypotension, fatigue, asthma exacerbations, and bradycardia.

DRUG ALERT—β-Adrenergic Blockers
- Overdosage can produce profound bradycardia, hypotension, broncho-spasm, and cardiogenic shock.
- Abrupt withdrawal may result in sweating, palpitations, and headaches.

Mineralocorticoid Receptor Antagonists

Spironolactone (Aldactone) is a potassium-sparing diuretic that promotes sodium and water excretion but blocks potassium excretion by blocking the action of aldosterone. Spironolactone appears to be additive to the benefits of ACE inhibitors, and renal function and potassium levels must be monitored carefully.

DRUG ALERT—Spironolactone (Aldactone)
- Potassium levels must be monitored during treatment.
- It must be used with caution in patients taking digoxin, inasmuch as hyperkalemia may reduce the effects of digoxin.
- Patients must avoid foods with high potassium content (e.g., bananas, oranges, dried apricots).
- Male patients must be assessed for gynecomastia, a common side effect of long-term use of spironolactone.

Eplerinone (Inspra) is a newer mineralocorticoid receptor antagonist that has effects similar to those of spironolactone; however, hyperkalemia seems to be less associated with this drug, as may sexual effects (e.g., gynacomastia; Barnes & Howard, 2005).

Inotropic Drugs

The use of inotropic drugs in patients with HF is directed at improving cardiac contractility to increase CO, decrease left ventricular diastolic pressure, and decrease SVR. Dobutamine and milrinone are the two agents most commonly used. Patients should be monitored carefully because these drugs may increase the risk of sudden death due to arrhythmia. Inotropic drugs are reserved primarily for hemodynamically unstable patients with ADHF (McKelvie, Moe, Ezekowitz, et al., 2013).

Sympathomimetic Agents. Sympathomimetic agents (or β-adrenergic agonists) include dopamine, dobutamine, epineph-rine (Adrenalin), and norepinephrine (Levophed). Stimulation of β-adrenergic receptors results in an increase in cyclic adenosine monophosphate within the myocardial cells and an increase in contractility (inotropic effect). The β-adrenergic agents are typically used as a short-term treatment of acute exacerbations of HF in the critical care environment. However, their role in

long-term therapy for HF is controversial (McKelvie, Moe, Ezekowitz, et al., 2013). Potential problems related to long-term treatment with these agents include tolerance (tachyphylaxis), increased ventricular irritability, limb ischemia, and increased myocardial oxygen demand.

Phosphodiesterase Inhibitors. Inhibition of phosphodiesterase enhances calcium entry into the cell and improves myocardial contractility. Phosphodiesterase inhibitors are also potent vasodilators. They increase CO and reduce arterial pressure (decrease afterload).

Milrinone increases myocardial contraction, increases CO, promotes peripheral vasodilation, and decreases SVR, thus augmenting performance of the LV. Adverse reactions include dysrhythmias, thrombo-cytopenia, and gastro-intestinal effects.

There is little evidence that inotropic drugs have a beneficial effect on mortality rates. Therefore, their use should be confined to short-term therapy only in patients in cardiogenic shock with volume overload and who have diuretic resistance (McKelvie, Moe, Ezekowitz, et al., 2013).

Vasodilator Drugs. Vasodilator drugs are a class of drugs that have shown to improve survival in ADHF. The goals of vasodilator therapy in the treatment of HF include (a) increasing venous capacity, (b) improving EF through improved ventricular contraction, (c) slowing the process of ventricular dysfunction, (d) decreasing heart size, and (e) avoiding stimulation of the neuro-hormonal responses initiated by the compensatory mechanisms of HF.

Nitrates cause vasodilation by acting directly on the smooth muscle of the vessel wall. Their effects primarily involve increasing venous capacitance, dilating the pulmonary vasculature, and improving arterial compliance. Therefore, the major hemodynamic effect of nitrates is to decrease preload. Nitrates are of particular benefit in the management of myocardial ischemia related to HF because they promote vasodilation of the coronary arteries. Men with HF who take nitrates should not also take an erectile agent (e.g., sildenafil [Viagra]) to manage erectile dysfunction because together these drugs could precipitate profound hypotension.

NUTRITIONAL THERAPY: CHRONIC HEART FAILURE

Diet education and weight management are critical in the patient's control of chronic HF. The nurse or the dietitian should obtain a detailed diet history, determining not only what foods the patient eats and when but also the sociocultural value of food for the patient. The nurse can use this information to assist the patient in solving problems and working with a dietitian to develop an individualized diet plan. The patient should be taught what foods have low and which have high sodium content and ways to enhance food flavours without the use of salt (e.g., substituting lemon juice and various spices).

The edema of chronic HF is often treated by dietary restriction of sodium. The degree of sodium restriction depends on the severity of the HF and the effectiveness of diuretic therapy. Diets that are severely restricted in sodium are rarely prescribed because they are unpalatable and patient adherence is poor. The Dietary Approach to Stop Hypertension (DASH) diet is effective as a first-line therapy for many patients with isolated systolic hyper-tension (see Chapter 35, Table 35-7). A commonly prescribed diet for a patient with mild HF is a 2-g/day sodium diet. All foods with high sodium content should be eliminated. For more severe HF or with concurrent diagnosis of hypertension, sodium intake is restricted to 1.5 g/day (Heart and Stroke Foundation of Canada, 2017; see also the Heart and Stroke Foundation website listed in the Resources at the end of this chapter). The patient and caregivers should be instructed on how to read labels to look for sodium as an ingredient (Table 37-6).

Typically, a low-sodium diet is unpalatable. In order to increase compliance with a low-sodium diet, the Heart and Stroke Foundation of Canada (2014) recommends that patients be advised to do the following:

- Stop using the salt shaker (remove it from the dinner table).
- Do not add salt to food during preparation.
- Read food labels carefully and look for foods that claim lower sodium content.
- Eat fresh fruit and vegetables whenever possible, and try to avoid pre-prepared and processed food.
- When eating out, ask about sodium content, and choose foods with less sodium.

The Canadian Cardiovascular Society recommends that all patients with fluid retention or congestion not responsive to diuretic therapy and patients with renal dysfunction or hyponatremia should restrict fluid intake to 1.5 to 2 L/day (Arnold, Liu, Demers, et al., 2006). That equates to six to eight glasses of fluid per day. Patients should be reminded that fluid is hidden in foods such as fruits and ice cream. In practice, most Canadian HF clinics advise fluid restriction for all HF patients.

It is vital that patients weigh themselves daily to monitor fluid retention. Patients should be instructed to weigh themselves at the same time each day, preferably before breakfast, while wearing the same type of clothing. This helps ensure valid comparisons from day to day and helps reveal early signs of fluid retention. If a patient experiences a weight gain of 2 kg (4 lb) over a 2-day period or 2.5 kg (5 lb) over a 5-day period, the patient should contact the primary care provider.

General Principles

According to *Eating Well with Canada's Food Guide* (Health Canada, 2011), which contains dietary recommendations endorsed by Health Canada in 2011, all Canadians should follow a diet with low sodium content. The guide recommends that the patient read the "Nutrition Facts" label, which is mandatory on all packaged foods, before purchasing foods (see Chapter 42, Figure 42-4).

Only a small amount of sodium occurs naturally in foods. Most sodium is added during processing. Table 37-7 gives examples of varying amounts of sodium in Western foods before and after processing.

The Chinese diet is usually very high in sodium. Patients with HF who adhere to a Chinese diet should be taught to consider the advice in Table 37-8. When teaching the patient with HF who adheres to an East Indian diet, the nurse should take into account the considerations presented in Table 37-9.

TABLE 37-6 NUTRITIONAL THERAPY

Sodium Label Language*

Claim	What It Means
Free of sodium or salt	The food contains <5 mg of sodium per serving.
Low in sodium or salt	The food contains ≤140 mg of sodium per serving (or per 100 g, if the food is a prepackaged meal).
Reduced or lower in sodium or salt	The food is processed, formulated, reformulated, or otherwise modified so that it contains at least 25% less sodium than regular foods of its type.
No added sodium or salt	The food contains no added salt, other sodium salts, or ingredients that contain sodium that functionally substitute for added salt.
Lightly salted	The food contains at least 50% less sodium added than the sodium added to the similar reference food.
Words to the effect that the food is "for use in a sodium-restricted diet"	The food meets the criteria for the first three claims in this table.
Words to the effect that the food is "for special dietary use" with respect to the sodium (salt) content	The food meets the criteria for either of the first two items in this table.

Source: Adapted from Canadian Food Inspection Agency. (2015). *Sodium (salt) claims* [summary table]. Retrieved from *http://www.inspection.gc.ca/food/labelling/food-labelling-for-industry/nutrient-content/specific-claim-requirements/eng/1389907770176/1389907817577?chap=9.*
*Products advertised as salt replacements should be used with caution: they may contain high quantities of potassium.

TABLE 37-7 NUTRITIONAL THERAPY:

Sodium Content in Different Food Groups

Food Groups	Sodium (mg)
Grains and Grain Products	
Cooked cereal, rice, pasta, unsalted, ½ cup	0–5
Ready-to-eat cereal, 1 cup	100–360
Bread, 1 slice	110–175
Vegetables	
Fresh or frozen, cooked without salt, ½ cup	1–70
Canned or frozen with sauce, ½ cup	140–460
Tomato juice, canned, ¾ cup	820
Fruit	
Fresh, frozen, or canned, ½ cup	0–5
Low-Fat or Fat-Free Dairy Foods	
Milk, 1 cup	120
Yogourt, 250 mL	160
Natural cheeses, 45 g	110–450
Processed cheeses, 45 g	600
Nuts, Seeds, and Dry Beans	
Peanuts, salted, ⅓ cup	120
Peanuts, unsalted, ⅓ cup	0–5
Beans, cooked from dried or frozen, without salt, ½ cup	400
Meats, Fish, and Poultry	
Fresh meat, fish, and poultry, 85-g serving	30–90
Tuna, canned, water pack, no salt added, 85-g serving	34–45
Tuna, canned, water pack, 85-g serving	250–350
Ham (lean) roasted, 85-g serving	1020

TABLE 37-8 CONSIDERATIONS FOR SODIUM INTAKE IN THE CHINESE DIET

Consideration	High Sodium Content	Recommended Alternatives
Protein	Barbecued meats, Chinese sausages, salted fish, dried shrimp, salted eggs, century eggs, canned fish with black beans	Fresh or frozen unsalted meats, fish, poultry, seafood, eggs, tofu
Condiments and sauces	Monosodium glutamate (MSG), soy sauce, oyster sauce, fish sauce, shrimp paste, Hoisin sauce, Teriyaki sauce, Chinese cooking wine, bean paste, miso, fermented tofu, ketchup	Fresh herbs, spices, and other flavoured substances, such as ginger, onion, garlic, garlic powder, green onion, curry powder, pepper, lemon, vinegar, honey, sesame oil, low-sodium soy sauce
Other foods	Instant noodles, instant rice with seasonings, salty soups, bouillon (cubes or powder)	Unprocessed grain products (e.g., fresh rice, rice noodles, udon noodles, congee, pasta, bread), low-sodium soups
Dining-out tips	Most food served in Chinese restaurants has high sodium content; eat in restaurants only occasionally	Plain rice rather than rice or noodles mixed with sauces (especially soy sauce or teriyaki sauce)

TABLE 37-9 CONSIDERATION FOR SODIUM INTAKE IN THE EAST INDIAN DIET

Consideration	High Sodium Content	Recommended Alternatives
Protein	Canned beans and lentils	Fresh beans and lentils to make daal
Condiments and sauces	Achaars (pickles); chutneys (made with salt); relish; tomato, curry, or mustard paste; black salt	Fresh herbs and spices: curry powder, turmeric, chili powder, mustard seeds, ginger, garlic, pepper, cumin, fenugreek (methi), garam masala
Dining out tips	Most food served in East Indian restaurants is high in sodium; eat in restaurants only occasionally	Ask for foods prepared without salt. Avoid salty chutneys or relishes

NURSING MANAGEMENT CHRONIC HEART FAILURE

NURSING ASSESSMENT

Subjective and objective data that should be obtained from a patient with HF include those listed in Table 37-10.

TABLE 37-10 NURSING ASSESSMENT

Heart Failure

Subjective Data
Important Health Information
Family, cultural and psychosocial history: availability of caregivers, living situation, pets at home, smoking, alcohol, illicit drug use, advance directives if available
Past health history: CAD (including recent MI), hypertension, cardiomyopathy, valvular or congenital heart disease, diabetes mellitus, thyroid or lung disease, rapid or irregular heart rate
Medications: use of and adherence to any cardiac medications; use of diuretics, estrogens, corticosteroids, nonsteroidal anti-inflammatory drugs, over-the-counter drugs, herbal supplements

Symptoms
Fatigue, depression, anxiety
Nausea, vomiting, anorexia, stomach bloating
Weight gain, ankle swelling, nocturia, decreased daytime urinary output
Dyspnea, orthopnea, cough
Chest pain or heaviness; palpitations, dizziness, fainting
RUQ pain, abdominal discomfort, constipation
Behavioural changes, visual changes

Objective Data
Integumentary
Cool, diaphoretic skin; cyanosis or pallor, peripheral edema (right-sided heart failure)

Respiratory
Tachypnea, crackles particularly at the bases, rhonchi, wheezes; frothy, blood-tinged sputum (see Chapter 28 for detailed respiratory assessment)

Cardiovascular
Tachycardia, S_3, S_4, murmurs, PMI displaced inferiorly and posteriorly, jugular vein distension (see Chapter 34 for detailed cardiac assessment)

Gastro-intestinal
Abdominal distension, hepatosplenomegaly, ascites

Neurological
Restlessness, confusion, decreased attention or memory

Possible Findings
Altered levels of serum electrolytes (especially Na^+ and K^+), ↑ BUN, ↑ BNP or NT–pro-BNP, creatinine, or liver function test results; chest radiograph demonstrating cardiomegaly, pulmonary congestion, and interstitial pulmonary edema; echocardiogram showing increased chamber size and decreased wall motion; ECG showing atrial and ventricular enlargement; ↓ O_2 saturation

BNP, brain or B-type natriuretic peptide; *BUN,* blood urea nitrogen; *CAD,* coronary artery disease; *ECG,* electrocardiogram; *MI,* myocardial infarction; *NT–pro-BNP,* N-terminal pro-BNP; *PMI,* point of maximal impulse; *RUQ,* right upper quadrant; *S3,* and *S4,* third and fourth heart sounds.

NURSING DIAGNOSES

Nursing diagnoses for patients with HF include, but are not limited to, those presented in Nursing Care Plan (NCP) 37-1.

PLANNING

The overall goals are that the patient with HF will (a) have decreased peripheral edema, (b) have decreased shortness of breath, (c) have increased exercise tolerance, (d) adhere to drug regimen, and (5) have no complications related to HF.

EVIDENCE-INFORMED PRACTICE

Translating Research Into Practice

Tara Fahed is a 62-year-old female patient recovering from an episode of acute decompensated heart failure (ADHF). Her HF is class III according to the New York Heart Association Functional Classification of Heart Disease (see Table 37-4). Her physician has recommended biventricular pacing (cardiac resynchronization therapy) for treatment of her HF symptoms. She tells the nurse that she does not want any artificial implants and that she has researched the use of hawthorn for treatment of her heart disease.

Best Available Evidence	Clinician Expertise	Patient Preferences and Values
Strong evidence supports the use of biventricular pacing (cardiac resynchronization therapy) to improve symptoms, exercise capacity, quality of life, ejection fraction, and survival and to decrease hospitalizations in patients like Ms. Fahed.	The nurse knows the benefits of and possible complications related to biventricular pacing in patients with Ms. Fahed's situation. The nurse also knows that there is strong evidence supporting the use of hawthorn in patients with mild to moderate HF.	Patient does not want any artificial implants. She wants to consider alternative (herbal) therapy.

Decision and Action

The nurse reviews the risks and benefits of biventricular pacing and herbal (hawthorn) therapy for the treatment of HF with Ms. Fahed. Ms. Fahed remains committed to the use of hawthorn—at least for a trial period. The nurse supports her decision and informs the physician of her wishes.

Reference for Evidence

Yancy, C. W., Jessup, M., Bozkurt, B., et al. (2013). 2013 ACCF/AHA guideline for the management of heart failure: Executive summary: A report of the American College of Cardiology Foundation/American Heart Association Task Force on Practice Guidelines. *Circulation, 128*(16), 1810–1852. http://dx.doi.org/10.1161/CIR.0b013e31829e8807.

NURSING IMPLEMENTATION

HEALTH PROMOTION. An important measure used to prevent HF is the treatment or control of the underlying heart disease. For example, in valvular disease, valve replacement should be planned before lung congestion develops. Coronary revascularization procedures should be performed in patients with CAD. Another important preventive measure concerns early and continued treatment of hypertension. Hyperlipidemic states in people with CAD should be managed with diet, exercise, and medication. The use of antidysrhythmic agents or an ICD–pacemaker is indicated for people with continuing low EF even if they are receiving optimal medical therapy or are at risk for sudden cardiac death. In addition, patients with HF should be counselled to quit smoking and obtain yearly vaccinations against the flu.

When HF is diagnosed, preventive care should focus on slowing the progression of the disease. The patient must understand the importance of following the medication, diet, and exercise regimens. Exercise training (e.g., cardiac rehabilitation) improves symptoms of chronic HF but is often underprescribed.

ACUTE INTERVENTION. Successful HF management depends on several important principles: (a) HF is a progressive disease, and treatment plans are established with quality-of-life goals; (b) symptoms are managed by the patient with self-management tools (daily weights, drug regimens, exercise plans); (c) salt and water must be restricted; (d) a regular, prescribed level of exercise should be maintained; and (e) use of support systems is essential to the success of the entire treatment plan (Arnold, Liu, Demers, et al., 2006).

Many patients with HF experience one or more episodes of acute decompensation. When they do, they may be initially managed in a critical care area and later transferred to a general medical or cardiology unit when their condition has stabilized. Nursing Care Plan 37-1 for patients with HF applies to patients with stabilized acute or chronic HF.

AMBULATORY AND HOME CARE. HF is a chronic illness. Important nursing responsibilities are (a) teaching the patient about the physiological changes that have occurred, (b) assisting the patient to adapt to both the physiological and the psychological changes, and (c) integrating the patient and the patient's family or support system in the overall care plan (Arnold, Liu, Demers, et al., 2006). It is known that patients with HF are at risk for depression and that those who are depressed are more likely to be rehospitalized and die prematurely (Newhouse & Jiang, 2014). Depression should be treated appropriately in order for patients to adhere to medical therapy. It must be emphasized to the patient and the patient's caregivers that it is possible to live productively with this chronic illness. Managing patients with HF out of the hospital setting is a priority of care. A patient and caregiver teaching guide for the patient with HF is presented in Table 37-11.

Patients with chronic HF are required to take medication for the rest of their lives. This often becomes difficult because a patient may be asymptomatic when HF is under control. It must be stressed that the disease is chronic and that medication administration must be continued even through stable periods to prevent acute decompensation.

The patient and caregivers should learn to evaluate how the patient is feeling, to recognize symptoms of possible decompensation, and to report them early. They need to understand that the medications the patient is taking may cause adverse effects that—especially in the initiation phase—can make the patient feel worse for some weeks after initiation and upward titration. The patient, caregivers, and primary health providers need to know that simply stopping some HF medications may not be appropriate. For example, a reported pulse rate of 50 bpm (especially in a patient who is also taking β-adrenergic blockers) may be acceptable and does not necessarily mean that the patient should stop taking the prescribed medication.

The home health nurse, the physiotherapist, or the occupational therapist can instruct the patient in energy-saving and energy-efficient behaviours after daily activities have been evaluated. The nurse can help link the patient with a cardiac rehabilitation or chronic disease program in the community to facilitate the recommended weekly exercise (30–40 minutes, three to five times per week, including aerobic activity and resistance training).

Using home health care services is essential in the care of HF patients and their caregivers. Many patients have multiple comorbidities conditions, and a degree of cognitive impairment is common. Frequent physical assessments, including vital signs and weight, are extremely important. The home care nurse can coach the patient and the patient's caregivers to implement systems to remember medications and times; identify problems, such as an increase in weight as evidence of worsening failure; and

⊚ NURSING CARE PLAN 37-1

Heart Failure

NURSING DIAGNOSIS	**Impaired gas exchange** (related to increased preload and alveolar–capillary membrane changes as evidenced by abnormal O_2 saturation, hypoxemia, dyspnea, tachypnea, tachycardia, restlessness, and patient's statement about being short of breath).

Expected Patient Outcomes	**Nursing Interventions and *Rationales***
• Maintains adequate O_2/CO_2 exchange at the alveolar–capillary membrane to meet O_2 needs of the body	*Respiratory Monitoring* • Monitor pulse oximetry, respiratory rate, rhythm, depth, and effort of respirations *to detect changes in respiratory status.* • Auscultate breath sounds, noting areas of decreased or absent ventilation and presence of adventitious sounds *to detect presence of pulmonary edema.* • Monitor for increased restlessness, anxiety, and work of breathing *to detect increasing hypoxemia.* *Oxygen Therapy* • Administer supplemental O_2 or other noninvasive ventilator support (e.g., bilevel positive airway pressure) as needed *to maintain adequate O_2 levels.* • Monitor the O_2 litre flow rate and placement of O_2 delivery device *to ensure O_2 is adequately delivered.* • Change O_2 delivery device from mask to nasal prongs during meals as tolerated *to sustain O_2 levels while patient is eating.* • Monitor the effectiveness of O_2 therapy *to identify hypoxemia and establish range of O_2 saturation.* *Positioning* • Position patient to alleviate dyspnea (e.g., semi-Fowler's position), as appropriate, *to improve ventilation by decreasing venous return to the heart and increasing thoracic capacity.*

NURSING DIAGNOSIS	**Decreased cardiac output** (related to altered contractility, altered preload, altered stroke volume, or a combination of these as evidenced by decreased ejection fraction, increased CVP, decreased peripheral pulses, jugular venous distension, orthopnea, chest pain, S_3 and S_4, and oliguria).

Expected Patient Outcomes	**Nursing Interventions and *Rationales***
• Maintains adequate blood pumped by the heart to meet metabolic demands of the body	*Cardiac Care* • Perform a comprehensive assessment of peripheral circulation (e.g., check peripheral pulses, edema, capillary refill, colour, and temperature of extremity) *to determine circulatory status.* • Note signs and symptoms of decreased cardiac output (e.g., chest pain, S_3, S_4, jugular venous distension) *to detect changes in status.* • Monitor fluid balance (e.g., input/output and daily weight) *to evaluate patient's fluid status.* • Monitor cardiac rhythm *to detect dysrhythmias.* • Monitor respiratory status for symptoms of heart failure (e.g., dyspnea, fatigue, tachypnea, orthopnea) *to identify involvement of respiratory system.* • Instruct patient and caregivers about activity restriction and progression *to allay fears and anxiety.* • Establish a supportive relationship with patient and caregivers *to promote adherence to the treatment plan.* • Inform patient of the purpose and benefits of the prescribed activity and exercise *to enhance adherence.*

NURSING DIAGNOSIS	**Excess fluid volume** related to *excessive fluid intake, excessive sodium intake* (decreased renal perfusion secondary to heart failure) as evidenced by *weight gain over short period of time, edema, adventitious breath sounds, oliguria*

Expected Patient Outcomes	**Nursing Interventions and *Rationales***
• Experiences reduction or absence of edema and stable baseline weight	*Hypervolemia Management* • Administer prescribed medications to reduce preload (e.g., furosemide, spironolactone, morphine, and nitroglycerine) *to treat hypervolemia.* • Monitor for therapeutic effects of medications (e.g., increased urine output, decreased CVP, decreased adventitious breath sounds) *to assess response to treatment.* • Monitor potassium levels after diuretic medications *to detect hypokalemia.* • Weigh patient daily and monitor trends *to evaluate effect of treatment.* • Monitor intake and output *to assess fluid status.* • Monitor respiratory pattern for symptoms anxiety, air hunger, orthopnea, dyspnea, tachypnea, cough, frothy sputum production, and shortness of breath *to detect signs and symptoms of pulmonary edema.* • Monitor hemodynamic status, including HR, BP, MAP, PAP, PAWP, CO, and CI, if available, *to evaluate effectiveness of therapy.* • Monitor adventitious breath sounds, adventitious heart sounds, JVD, and peripheral edema *to assess response to treatment.*

◎ NURSING CARE PLAN 37-1

Heart Failure—cont'd

NURSING DIAGNOSIS	*Activity intolerance* related to *imbalance between oxygen supply/demand* as evidenced by *abnormal heart rate response to activity, exertional dyspnea, and fatigue.*

Expected Patient Outcomes	Nursing Interventions and *Rationales*
• Achieves a realistic program of activity that balances physical activity with energy-conserving activities • Vital signs, O₂ saturation, and colour are within normal limits in response to activity	**Energy Management** • Encourage alternating rest and activity periods *to reduce cardiac workload and conserve energy.* • Provide calming diversionary activities to promote relaxation *to reduce O₂ consumption and to relieve dyspnea and fatigue.* • Monitor patient's O₂ response (e.g., pulse rate, cardiac rhythm, and respiratory rate) to self-care or nursing activities *to determine level of activity that can be tolerated.* • Teach patient and caregiver techniques of self-care (e.g., self-monitoring and pacing techniques for performance of ADLs) *to minimize O₂ consumption.* • Teach patient to change positions slowly from lying/sitting to standing because patient may experience a postural BP drop that causes dizziness and increases risk of falling. **Activity Therapy** • Collaborate with occupational and physical therapists *to plan and monitor activity or exercise program.* • Determine patient's commitment to increasing frequency and range of activities or exercise *to provide patient with obtainable goals.*

ADLs, activities of daily living; *BP,* blood pressure; *CI,* cardiac index; *CO,* cardiac output; *CVP,* central venous pressure; *HR,* heart rate; *JVD,* jugular venous distension; *MAP,* mean arterial pressure; *PAP,* pulmonary artery pressure; *PAWP,* pulmonary artery wedge pressure.

🔍 EVIDENCE-INFORMED PRACTICE

Research Highlight

Can Exercise Help Alleviate Depression in Patients With Heart Failure?

Clinical Question

For patients with heart failure (P), what is the effect of aerobic exercise (I) versus usual care (C) on depressive symptoms (O) at 3 and 12 months (T)?

Best Available Evidence

Randomized controlled trial (RCT)

Critical Appraisal and Synthesis of Evidence

RCT of 82 medical centres (*N* = 2 322) of patients with stable chronic heart failure.

• Intervention was aerobic exercise with a goal of 90 min/wk for months 1–3, followed by home exercise for ≥120 min/wk for months 4–12. Usual care was education and guideline-based heart failure care.
• Outcome measure was depressive symptoms.
• Patients engaged in aerobic exercise had fewer depressive symptoms at 3 and 12 months than did patients receiving usual care.

Conclusion

• Exercise resulted in a significant decrease in depressive symptoms.

Implications for Nursing Practice

• The nurse should encourage patients with heart failure to discuss with their health care provider reasonable exercise goals.
• The nurse should emphasize the mental and physical benefits to patients of engaging in supervised regular aerobic exercise.

Reference for Evidence

Blumenthal, J., Babyak, M., O'Connor, C., et al. (2012). Effects of exercise training on depressive symptoms in patients with chronic heart failure: The HF-ACTION randomized trial. *Journal of the American Medical Association, 308,* 465.

P, Patient population of interest; *I,* intervention or area of interest; *C,* comparison of interest or comparison group; *O,* outcomes of interest; *T,* timing (see Chapter 1).

institute interventions to prevent hospitalization. This may include altering medications and fluid restrictions. The home care nurse can also help identify the need for respite services to reduce caregiver burden.

▌EVALUATION

The expected outcomes for the patient with HF are presented in Nursing Care Plan 37-1.

CARDIAC TRANSPLANTATION

Heart transplantation was first performed in 1967. Since that time, cardiac transplantation has become the treatment of choice for carefully selected patients with end-stage HF. The main indications for transplantation are ischemic heart disease and dilated cardiomyopathy. Indications for and contraindications to heart transplantation are listed in Table 37-12.

Among the patients who meet the criteria for cardiac transplantation, the goal of the evaluation process is to identify patients who would most benefit from a new heart. After a complete physical examination and diagnostic workup, the patient and family undergo a comprehensive psychological profile that includes assessment of coping skills, family support systems, and motivation to follow the rigorous regimen that is essential to a successful transplantation. The complexity of the transplantation process may be overwhelming to a patient with inadequate support systems and a poor understanding of the lifestyle changes required after transplantation.

Once an individual is accepted as a transplantation candidate (this may happen rapidly during an acute illness or over a longer period, depending on the patient's condition), he or she is placed on a transplant list. Patients may wait at home and receive ongoing medical care if their medical condition is stable. If their condition is not stable, they may require hospitalization for more intensive therapy, including long-term mechanical cardiac support with a VAD. Unfortunately, the overall waiting period for a cardiac

TABLE 37-11   PATIENT & CAREGIVER TEACHING GUIDE

Heart Failure

What Is Heart Failure?

1. Provide individually tailored information about what heart failure is and how it is treated.
2. Discuss how people make the most of life with a chronic illness.

Health Promotion

1. Instruct patient to obtain annual flu vaccination.
2. Instruct patient to obtain pneumococcal vaccine (e.g., Pneumovax) and revaccination after 5 yr (for people at high risk of infection or serious disease).
3. Provide counselling regarding smoking cessation and weight reduction, if relevant.

Exercise and Rest

1. Once patient is cleared by physician, discuss the benefits of regular exercise and dispel myths.
2. Instruct patient to plan a regular activity program and scheduled rest periods throughout the day.
3. Encourage communication of concerns and fears and provide encouragement.

Drug Therapy

1. Teach patient to take each drug as prescribed by the physician or nurse practitioner.
2. Help patient develop a system (e.g., daily chart) to ensure medications have been taken.
3. Instruct patient to take pulse and BP each day before taking medications. Know what is normal for the patient.
4. Ensure that patient knows signs and symptoms of orthostatic hypotension and how to prevent them.
5. Ensure that patient knows own INR if taking warfarin (Coumadin) and how often to have blood monitored.
6. If relevant, teach patient signs and symptoms of overadministration of anticoagulation agents.

Dietary Therapy

1. Instruct patient to consult the written diet plan and list of permitted and restricted foods.

2. Teach patient to examine labels to determine sodium content and examine the labels of over-the-counter drugs such as laxatives, cough medicines, and antacids.
3. Encourage patient not to use salt in cooking or at the dining table.
4. Instruct patient to measure weight in the early morning every day after emptying bladder. Ensure that the patient knows to use the same scale and wear similar clothes.
5. Help patient keep track of daily weight and report weight gain of more than 2–2.5 kg (4–5 lb) in the course of 2 to 5 days.
6. Instruct patient to restrict fluid intake to no more than 6 to 8 cups per day and to remember that fluid can be hidden in many foods. These hidden fluids should be counted in the daily restriction.

Other Topics

1. If adverse effects are bothersome, discuss ways in which timing of medications may help to manage them.
2. Instruct patient to avoid extremes of heat and cold.
3. Encourage patient to keep regular appointments with health care provider.
4. Discuss end-of-life planning and the importance of advance directives.

Ongoing Monitoring

1. Educate patient about the signs and symptoms of recurring or progressing heart failure.
2. Instruct patient to report immediately to health care provider he development or worsening of any of the following:
   - Difficulty breathing, especially with exertion or when lying flat
   - Waking up breathless at night
   - Frequent dry, hacking cough, especially when lying down
   - Fatigue, weakness
   - Swelling of ankles, feet, or abdomen
   - Nausea with abdominal swelling, pain, and tenderness
   - Dizziness or fainting
3. Encourage patient to join local support networks such as cardiac rehabilitation or "Chronic Disease Management" programs.
4. Recognize depression as a major issue, and help patient seek treatment if signs and symptoms of depression occur.
5. Teach caregivers to recognize signs of cognitive impairment.

BP, blood pressure; *INR*, international normalized ratio.

transplant is difficult to define but is usually between 6 and 9 months, depending on donor availability.

Donor and recipient matching is based on body and heart size and ABO blood type. Negative lymphocyte crossmatch (explained in Chapter 16) is also important.

Most donor hearts are obtained at sites away from the institution where the transplantation is performed. The maximum acceptable ischemic time for cardiac transplantation is 4 to 6 hours.

The recipient is prepared for surgery, and cardiopulmonary bypass is used. The usual surgical procedure involves removing the recipient's heart, except for the posterior right and left atrial walls and their venous connections. The recipient's heart is then replaced with the donor heart, which has been trimmed to match. Care is taken to preserve the integrity of the donor sinoatrial node so that a sinus rhythm may be achieved postoperatively.

Immuno-suppressive therapy begins in the operating room. Some transplantation centres administer drugs to rapidly induce immuno-suppression in the operating room and critical care area because the regimens most commonly used are nephrotoxic and, hence, cannot be started for a few days after the surgery.

This induction therapy (usually with a monoclonal antibody) buys time to allow the kidneys to recover from the insult of surgery. (The mechanisms of action and adverse effects of these and other immuno-suppressants are discussed in Chapter 16 and Table 16-16.) Regimens vary, but tacrolimus [Prograf]) with mycophenolate mofetil (Cellcept) and prednisolone are most frequently used for maintenance immuno-suppression. In many Canadian programs, cardiac transplant recipients are weaned off prednisolone over a number of months, and after a year, it is uncommon for such patients to be taking prednisolone. The use of today's immuno-suppressants has resulted not only in reduced rates of rejection but also in slowing the rejection process so that early treatment can be instituted. Because of the use of immuno-suppressants, however, infection is a major complication after transplantation.

Endomyocardial biopsies via the right internal jugular vein are performed at repeated intervals to detect rejection in the first year. After 3 months, the incidence of acute rejection decreases dramatically; however, a type of CAD known as cardiac allograft vasculopathy (also known as *chronic rejection*) develops in a significant proportion of heart transplant recipients over the

TABLE 37-12 INDICATIONS FOR AND CONTRAINDICATIONS TO CARDIAC TRANSPLANTATION

Indications: Transplantation Centre–Specific
- End-stage heart disease refractory to medical therapy
- Refractory, life-threatening cardiac dysrhythmias
- Functional NYHA class III or IV status with demonstrated poor exercise capacity

Contraindications
- Pulmonary hypertension unrelieved with medication
- Primary systemic disease that would limit survival (e.g., malignancies)
- Renal dysfunction (creatinine level >200 mmol/L): patient could be considered for combined transplantation
- Active infection
- Technical issues
- Current tobacco use (6-month abstinence required)
- Illicit drug or excessive alcohol use (3-month abstinence required)
- Unstable psychiatric conditions
- Documented life-threatening nonadherence to medical regimen
- Malignancy (generally must be cancer free for 5 yr)
- Severe osteoporosis
- Significant peripheral vascular disease
- Diabetes mellitus with end-organ damage

Source: From Haddad, H., Isaac, D., Legare, J., et al. (2009). Canadian Cardiovascular Society consensus conference update on cardiac transplantation 2008: Executive summary. *Canadian Journal of Cardiology, 25*(4), 197–205.
NYHA, New York Heart Association.

long term. As a result, regular surveillance of the transplanted heart by means of diagnostic tests such as coronary angiography and echocardiography is performed for the rest of the recipient's life.

Advances in surgical technique and postoperative care have improved survival rates after cardiac transplantation. It is estimated that 50% of transplant recipients will be living after 10 years. This number is an overall average and varies greatly, depending on such factors as age at transplantation, severity of illness, adherence to medication regimens and risk factor modification, and social support systems. In the first year after transplantation, the major causes of death are acute rejection and infection. Later on, malignancy (especially lymphoma) and allograft vasculopathy are major causes of death.

One factor that may affect morbidity and mortality in heart transplantation is the patient's ability to adhere to medication regimens. To determine the scope of this problem, as well as attempting to identify some of the factors related to nonadherence, the BRIGHT study (Building research initiative group: chronic illness management and adherence in transplantation) is expected to provide important information for nurses when planning the care of these patients. The research team administered questionnaires to patients, nurses, and medical directors to explore demographics, practice patterns, self-reported adherence, and clinician-reported adherence. The study included approximately 40 heart transplantation centres in 11 countries and was completed in 2015 (Berben, Denhaerynck, Dobbels, et al., 2015).

Nursing management throughout the post-transplantation period focuses on promoting patient adaptation to the transplantation process, monitoring health, managing lifestyle changes, and ongoing teaching of the patient and caregivers.

Mechanical Cardiac Support Devices

Temporary support of one or both failed ventricles has been available for many years in the form of intra-aortic balloon pumps or extracorporeal membrane oxygenation. These circulatory support devices are designed for short-term use (days to weeks).

More recently, longer-term devices (for use over months to years) are being used in Canada as a bridge to heart transplantation or recovery of the native heart. These pumps are called *ventricular assist devices* (VADs). A number of VADs are available in Canada. Some examples include the HeartMate II (made by Thoratec Corp., Pleasanton, California; see Figure 37-6) and HeartWare HVAD (made by HeartWare Inc., Framingham, Massachusetts) electronic devices. These pumps are designed to support the LV. In many carefully selected patients, support of the LV alone will alleviate symptoms of right-sided HF by unloading the left side.

Patients carry around a battery pack with a small computer attached to their belt. With adequate social support, patients are able to live at home with these devices and, in some cases, return to work while waiting for a heart transplant. This improved mobility—the ability to live out of the hospital—and the improvement that results in the patient's nutritional state allow the patient to undergo transplantation in much improved physical condition. In the United States and Europe, instead of a transplant, some patients who are ineligible for transplantation use these devices. This practice is commonly referred to as *destination therapy*.

A totally artificial heart is available; however, it is not currently in use in Canada. For more information on mechanical cardiac support, see Chapter 68.

ETHICAL DILEMMAS
Transplant Recipient Requests

Situation
A 60-year-old woman has been awaiting heart transplantation for 6 months. At her recent clinic appointment, she asks if there is any possibility of receiving only a woman's heart. She tells the nurse that she does not want to receive a man's heart as she feels her personality would change.

Important Points for Consideration
- Hearts are not allocated on the basis of gender except as determined by size matching. Specifically, a large man is unlikely to receive a woman's heart because women in general are smaller; however a woman could receive a man's heart if they are the same size.
- There is no evidence that people assume the personalities of their donor.
- Heart transplantation programs do not respond to requests for specific attributes of organ donors such as race, gender, or cultural or religious practices.
- Heart transplantation programs do not give heart transplant recipients information about the characteristics of their donors.
- When heart transplantation candidates make these requests, it is often due to misinformation that has been published in the media. The nurse should explore with the patient her concerns and work with the psychosocial team to help her address them.

Clinical Decision-Making Questions
1. How might the nurse respond to the patient about such a request?
2. What supports should the nurse offer to the patient to assist her in working through her concerns?

CASE STUDY

Heart Failure

Source: Geo Martinez/ Shutterstock .com.

Patient Profile

Ms. Estrela, a 70-year-old woman, was admitted to the medical unit with complaints of increasing dyspnea on exertion.

Subjective Data

- Had a myocardial infarction (MI) at 58 years of age
- Has a 25-year history of hypertension
- Has experienced increasing dyspnea on exertion during the last 2 years
- Recently had a respiratory tract infection
- Has moist, productive cough
- Has edema in both legs up to the knees
- Cannot walk two blocks without getting short of breath
- Has to sleep with head elevated on three pillows
- Does not always remember to take medication
- 5-kg weight gain in 3 days

Objective Data

Physical Examination

- In respiratory distress; use of accessory muscles; respiratory rate, 36 breaths/min
- Moist crackles at both lung bases
- Skin cool and diaphoretic
- 2+ Pitting edema in both legs
- HR, 95 bpm and regular
- BP, 160/90 mm Hg
- Oxygen saturation, 88%

Diagnostic Studies

- Chest radiographic examination results: cardiomegaly; fluid in lower lung fields
- Echocardiogram results: ejection fraction (EF), 20%

Collaborative Care

- Enalapril, 5 mg PO (orally) daily
- Furosemide (Lasix), 40 mg PO bid
- Potassium, 40 mEq PO bid
- 2-g sodium diet
- Oxygen, 6 L/min to maintain O_2 saturation >90%
- Daily weight measurements
- Daily 12-lead electrocardiography (ECG); cardiac enzyme measurements, q8h three times
- Continuous cardiac monitoring
- Measurements of serum electrolytes, urea, creatinine, and BNP; complete blood cell count (CBC)

Discussion Questions

1. Explain the probable pathophysiological process of Ms. Estrela's heart disease.
2. What clinical manifestations of heart failure did Ms. Estrela exhibit?
3. What is the significance of the findings of the diagnostic studies?
4. Explain the rationale for each of the medical orders prescribed for Ms. Estrela.
5. *Priority decision:* What are the nurse's priority nursing interventions for Ms. Estrela?
6. *Priority decision:* What priority patient teaching measures should be instituted to prevent recurrence of an acute episode of heart failure?
7. *Priority decision:* On the basis of the assessment data presented, write one or more appropriate nursing diagnoses. Are there any collaborative problems?
8. *Evidence-informed practice:* Mrs. Estrela asks the nurse why it is so important to "watch her salt." She tells the nurse that food tastes better with salt. How might the nurse respond to her?

evolve

Answers are available at *http://evolve.elsevier.com/Canada/Lewis/medsurg*

REVIEW QUESTIONS

The number of the question corresponds to the same-numbered objective at the beginning of the chapter.

1. What are the manifestations of HF-REF that the nurse should recognize?
   a. ↓ Afterload and ↓ left ventricular end-diastolic pressure (LVEDP)
   b. ↓ Ejection fraction (EF) and ↑ pulmonary artery occlusive pressure (PAOP)
   c. ↓ PAOP and ↑ left ventricular EF
   d. ↑ Pulmonary hypertension associated with normal EF

2. Which compensatory mechanism leads to inappropriate sodium and fluid retention?
   a. Ventricular dilation
   b. Ventricular hypertrophy
   c. Neuro-hormonal response
   d. Sympathetic nervous system activation

3. Which drug used in the management of a client with acute pulmonary edema will decrease both preload and afterload and provide relief of anxiety?
   a. Morphine
   b. Amiodarone
   c. Dobutamine
   d. Aminophylline

4. How can a client with chronic HF best decrease the chances of having an acute decompensation?
   a. Resting and not making any exertions except under medical supervision
   b. Documenting fluid intake and urinary output each day
   c. Monitoring weight daily and reporting changes outside of recommended parameters
   d. Taking extra furosemide when shortness of breath occurs

5. Clients with a heart transplant are at risk for which complications in the first year after transplantation? *(Select all that apply)*
   a. Cancer
   b. Infection
   c. Rejection
   d. Vasculopathy
   e. Sudden cardiac death

1. b; 2. c; 3. a; 4. c; 5. b, c, e.

evolve

For even more review questions, visit *http://evolve.elsevier.com/Canada/ Lewis/medsurg.*

REFERENCES

Arnold, J. M., Liu, P., Demers, C., et al. (2006). Canadian Cardiovascular Society consensus conference recommendations on heart failure 2006: Diagnosis and management. *The Canadian Journal of Cardiology, 22*(1), 23–45. *http://dx.doi.org/10.1016/ S0828-282X(06)70237-9.* (Seminal).

Barnes, B. J., & Howard, P. A. (2005). Eplerenone: A selective aldosterone receptor antagonist for patients with heart failure. *The Annals of Pharmacotherapy, 39*(1), 68–76. *http:// dx.doi.org/10.1345/aph.1e306a.* (Seminal).

Berben, L., Denhaerynck, K., Dobbels, F., et al. (2015). Building research initiative group: Chronic Illness management and adherence in Transplantation (BRIGHT) study: Study protocol. *Journal of Advanced Nursing, 71*(3), 642–654. *http:// dx.doi.org/10.1111/jan.12519.*

Blair, J. E., Huffman, M., & Shah, S. J. (2013). Heart failure in North America. *Current Cardiology Reviews, 9*(2), 128–146. *http:// dx.doi.org/10.2174/1573403x11309020006.*

Braunwald, E. (2015). The war against heart failure: The Lancet lecture. *Lancet, 385*(9970), 812–824. *http://dx.doi.org.ezproxy .library.ubc.ca/10.1016/S0140-6736(14)61889-4.Canadian.*

Health Canada. (2011). *Eating well with Canada's food guide—A resource for educators and communicators.* Retrieved from *https:// www.canada.ca/en/health-canada/services/food-nutrition/ reports-publications/eating-well-canada-food-guide-resource- educators-communicators-2007.html.*

Heart and Stroke Foundation of Canada. (2014). *Dietary sodium, heart disease and stroke.* Retrieved from *http://www .heartandstroke.ca/-/media/pdf-files/canada/2017-position -statements/dietary-sodium-ps-eng.ashx.*

Heart and Stroke Foundation of Canada. (2015). *Managing your heart failure.* Retrieved from *http://www.heartandstroke.com/ site/c.ikIQLcMWJtE/b.3484065/k.9224/Heart_ failure.htm#managing-tab.*

Heart and Stroke Foundation of Canada. (2017). *Heart failure.* Retrieved from *https://www.heartandstroke.ca/heart/conditions/ heart-failure.*

Howlett, J. G., Chan, M., Ezekowitz, J. A., et al. (2016). The Canadian Cardiovascular Society heart failure companion: Bridging guidelines to your practice. *The Canadian Journal of Cardiology, 32*(3), 296–310. doi:10.1016/j.cjca.2015.06.019.

Howlett, J. G., McKelvie, R. S., Arnold, J. M., et al. (2009). Canadian Cardiovascular Society consensus conference guidelines on heart failure, update 2009: Diagnosis and management of right-sided heart failure, myocarditis, device therapy and recent important clinical trials. *The Canadian Journal of Cardiology, 25*(2), 85–105. *http://dx.doi.org/10.1016/S0828 282X(09)70477-5.* (Seminal).

Huether, S. E., & McCance, K. L. (Eds.). (2012). *Understanding pathophysiology* (5th ed.). St. Louis: Elsevier/Mosby.

LeMond, L., Camacho, S. A., & Goodlin, S. J. (2015). Palliative care and decision making in advanced heart failure. *Current Treatment Options in Cardiovascular Medicine, 17*(2), 359. *http:// dx.doi.org/10.1007/s11936-014-0359-5.*

Liu, P., Arnold, J. M., Howlett, J. G., et al. (2015). *CCS heart failure recommendations compendium.* Retrieved from *http://ccs.ca/ images/Guidelines/PocketGuides_EN/Pocket_Guides/HF_ Compendium_2013/index.html.*

McKelvie, R. S., Moe, G. W., Ezekowitz, J. A., et al. (2013). The 2012 Canadian Cardiovascular Society heart failure management guidelines update: Focus on acute and chronic heart failure. *The Canadian Journal of Cardiology, 29*(2), 168–181. *http:// dx.doi.org/10.1016/j.cjca.2012.10.007.*

McMurray, J. J. V., Packer, M., Desai, A. S., et al. (2014). Angiotensin-neprilysin inhibition versus enalapril in heart failure. *The New England Journal of Medicine, 371*(11), 993–1004. *http:// dx.doi.org/10.1056/NEJMoa1409077.*

Moe, G. W., Ezekowitz, J. A., O'Meara, E., et al. (2014). The 2013 Canadian Cardiovascular Society heart failure management guidelines update: Focus on rehabilitation and exercise and surgical coronary revascularization. *Canadian Journal of Cardiology, 30*(3), 249–263. *http://dx.doi.org/10.1016/j.cjca .2013.10.010.*

Moe, G. W., Ezekowitz, J. A., O'Meara, E., et al. (2015). The 2014 Canadian Cardiovascular Society heart failure management guidelines focus update: Anemia, biomarkers, and recent therapeutic trial implications. *Canadian Journal of Cardiology, 31*(1), 3–16. *http://dx.doi.org/10.1016/j.cjca .2014.10.022.*

Nawarskas, J. J., Bowman, B. N., & Anderson, J. R. (2015). Ivabradine. *Cardiology in Review, 23*(4), 201–211. *http:// dx.doi.org/10.1097/crd.0000000000000070.*

Newhouse, A., & Jiang, W. (2014). Heart failure and depression. *Heart Failure Clinics, 10*(2), 295–304. *http:// dx.doi.org/10.1016/j.hfc.2013.10.004.*

O'Meara, E., Thibodeau-Jarry, N., Ducharme, A., et al. (2014). The epidemic of heart failure: A lucid approach to stemming the rising tide. *The Canadian Journal of Cardiology, 30*(12 Suppl.), S442–S454. *http://dx.doi.org.ezproxy.library.ubc .ca/10.1016/j.cjca.2014.09.032.*

Yeung, D. F., Van Dyke, N. K., Maclagan, L. C., et al. (2013). A comparison of Chinese and non-Chinese Canadian patients hospitalized with heart failure. *BMC Cardiovascular Disorders, 13*, 114. *http://dx.doi.org/10.1186/1471-2261-13-114.*

RESOURCES

Canadian Association of Cardiovascular Prevention and Rehabilitation (CACPR)
http://www.cacpr.ca

Canadian Cardiovascular Society (CCS)
http://www.ccs.ca

Canadian Council of Cardiovascular Nurses
http://www.cccn.ca

Easy Auscultation: Extra Heart Sounds (S3 and S4)
http://www.easyauscultation.com/course-contents?courseid=25

The Heart and Stroke Foundation of Canada tools for patients learning to manage their illness
http://www.heartandstroke.ca/get-healthy/health-etools

For additional Internet resources, see the website for this book at *http://evolve.elsevier.com/Canada/Lewis/medsurg*

38

Nursing Management

Dysrhythmias

Written by: Linda Bucher
Adapted by: Sandra Goldsworthy

⊖volve WEBSITE

http://evolve.elsevier.com/Canada/Lewis/medsurg

- Review Questions (Online Only)
- Key Points
- Answer Guidelines for Case Study
- Student Case Study
  - Atrial Fibrillation
- Conceptual Care Map Creator
- Audio Glossary
- Content Updates

LEARNING OBJECTIVES

1. Describe the nursing management of patients requiring continuous electrocardiographic (ECG) monitoring.
2. Identify the clinical characteristics and ECG patterns of normal sinus rhythm, common dysrhythmias, and acute coronary syndrome (ACS).
3. Describe the nursing and collaborative management of patients with common dysrhythmias and ECG changes associated with ACS.
4. Differentiate between defibrillation and cardioversion, identifying indications for their use and nursing implications.
5. Describe the management of patients with temporary and permanent pacemakers.
6. Describe the management of patients with implantable cardioverter–defibrillators.
7. Explain the management of patients undergoing electrophysiological testing and radiofrequency ablation therapy.

KEY TERMS

asystole, p. 879
atrial fibrillation, p. 875
atrial flutter, p. 875
automatic external
    defibrillators (AEDs), p. 880

automaticity, p. 870
cardiac pacemaker, p. 882
complete heart block,
    p. 878
dysrhythmias, p. 866

electrocardiogram (ECG),
    p. 867
premature atrial
    contraction (PAC),
    p. 874

premature ventricular
    contraction (PVC), p. 878
ventricular fibrillation, p. 879
ventricular tachycardia (VT),
    p. 878

RHYTHM IDENTIFICATION AND TREATMENT

The ability to recognize normal and abnormal cardiac rhythms is an essential nursing skill. Cardiac monitoring is now used in a wide range of hospital, clinic, and home settings. Prompt assessment of abnormal cardiac rhythms, called dysrhythmias, and of the patient's response to them is critical. This chapter describes basic principles of electrocardiographic (ECG) monitoring and recognition of common dysrhythmias, as well as ECG changes that are associated with acute coronary syndrome (ACS). For more detailed information on ECG interpretation, the reader should refer to dedicated texts on this topic.

Conduction System

Four properties of cardiac cells enable the conduction system to initiate an electrical impulse, which is transmitted through the cardiac tissue and stimulates muscle contraction (Table 38-1). The conduction system of the heart is made up of specialized neuro-muscular tissue located throughout the heart (see Chapter 34, Figure 34-4). A normal cardiac impulse begins in the sinoatrial (SA) node in the upper right atrium. It is transmitted over the atrial myocardium via the bundle of Bachmann and internodal pathways, which causes atrial contraction. The impulse then travels to the atrioventricular (AV) node through the bundle of His and down the left and

TABLE 38-1	PROPERTIES OF CARDIAC CELLS
Automaticity	Ability to initiate an impulse spontaneously and continuously
Contractility	Ability to respond mechanically to an impulse
Conductivity	Ability to transmit an impulse along a membrane in an orderly manner
Excitability	Ability to be electrically stimulated

right bundle branches, ending in the Purkinje fibres, which transmit the impulse to the ventricles.

Conduction to the point just before the impulse leaves the Purkinje fibres takes place within the time of the PR interval of the ECG. When the impulse emerges from the Purkinje fibres, ventricular depolarization occurs, producing mechanical contraction of the ventricles and the QRS complex on the ECG. The electrical activity of the heart is illustrated in Chapter 34, Figure 34-4.

Nervous Control of the Heart

The autonomic nervous system plays an important role in the rate of impulse formation, the speed of conduction, and the strength of cardiac contraction. The components of the autonomic nervous system that affect the heart are the right and left vagus nerve fibres of the parasympathetic nervous system and the fibres of the sympathetic nervous system.

Stimulation of the vagus nerve causes a decrease in the rate of firing of the sinoatrial node, a slowing of impulse conduction of the atrioventricular node, and a decrease in the force of cardiac muscle contraction. Stimulation of the sympathetic nerves that supply the heart has essentially the opposite effect on the heart.

Electrocardiographic Monitoring

The electrocardiogram (ECG) is a graphic tracing of the electrical impulses produced in the heart. The waveforms on the ECG are produced by the movement of charged ions across the membranes of myocardial cells, representing depolarization and repolarization.

The membrane of a cardiac cell is semipermeable, allowing the intracellular concentration of potassium to remain high and the intracellular concentration of sodium to remain low. A high concentration of sodium and a low concentration of potassium are maintained outside the cell. The inside of the cell, when the cell is at rest or in the polarized state, is negative compared with the outside. When a cell or groups of cells are stimulated, each cell membrane changes its permeability and allows sodium to move rapidly into the cell, making the inside of the cell positive compared with the outside (*depolarization*). A slower movement of ions across the membrane restores the cell to the polarized state; this restoration is called *repolarization*. As shown in Figure 38-1, the phases of the cardiac action potential are as follows: phase 0 is the upstroke of rapid depolarization; phases 1, 2, and 3 represent repolarization; and phase 4 is a polarized state. Antidysrhythmia drugs have a direct effect on the various phases of the action potential. When antidysrhythmia drugs are used in a clinical setting, it is important to understand the ionic shifts in the cardiac cell and the action potential mechanism.

Conventionally, there are 12 recording leads in the ECG. Six of the 12 ECG leads (leads I, II, III, aV_R, aV_L, and aV_F) measure

FIGURE 38-1 Phases of the cardiac action potential on an electrocardiogram (ECG). The electrical potential, measured in millivolts, is indicated along the vertical axis of the graph. Time, measured in milliseconds, is indicated along the horizontal axis. The action potential *(black line)* has five phases, labelled *0* through *4*. Each phase represents a particular electrical event or combination of electrical events. Phase 0 is the upstroke of rapid depolarization and corresponds with ventricular contraction. Phases 1, 2, and 3 represent repolarization. Phase 4 is known as *complete repolarization* (or *the polarized state*) and corresponds to diastole. *RP*, resting membrane potential; *TP*, threshold membrane potential.

electrical forces in the frontal plane (Figure 38-2). The remaining six leads (V_1 through V_6) measure the electrical forces in the horizontal plane (precordial leads). The 12-lead ECG may show changes that are indicative of structural changes or damage such as ischemia, infarction, enlarged cardiac chambers, electrolyte imbalance, or drug toxicity (Goldsworthy, 2016). Obtaining 12 ECG views of the heart is also helpful in the assessment of dysrhythmias. An example of a normal 12-lead ECG appears in Figure 38-3.

When a patient's ECG is being continuously monitored, between 1 and 12 ECG leads may be used. The leads most commonly selected are leads II, V_1, and a modified chest lead—MCL_1—(Figure 38-4), which is similar to V_1 and is used when only three leads are available for monitoring.

The ECG can be visualized continuously on a monitor oscilloscope. A recording of the ECG (i.e., rhythm strip) is obtained on ECG paper attached to the monitor. The recording provides documentation of the patient's rhythm. It also allows for measurement of complexes and intervals and for assessment of dysrhythmias.

To correctly interpret an ECG, the nurse must know how to measure time and voltage on the ECG paper. ECG paper consists of large squares (heavy lines) and small squares (light lines; see Figure 38-5). Each large square incorporates 25 smaller squares (five horizontal and five vertical). Each small square represents 0.04 seconds horizontally and 0.1 millivolt (mV) vertically. This means that the large square represents 0.20 seconds and that 300 large squares represent 1 minute. Vertically, one large square is equal to 0.5 mV. These squares are used to calculate the heart rate (HR) and intervals between different ECG complexes.

A variety of methods can be used to calculate the HR from an ECG. Probably the most accurate way is to count the number of QRS complexes in 1 minute. However, this method is time

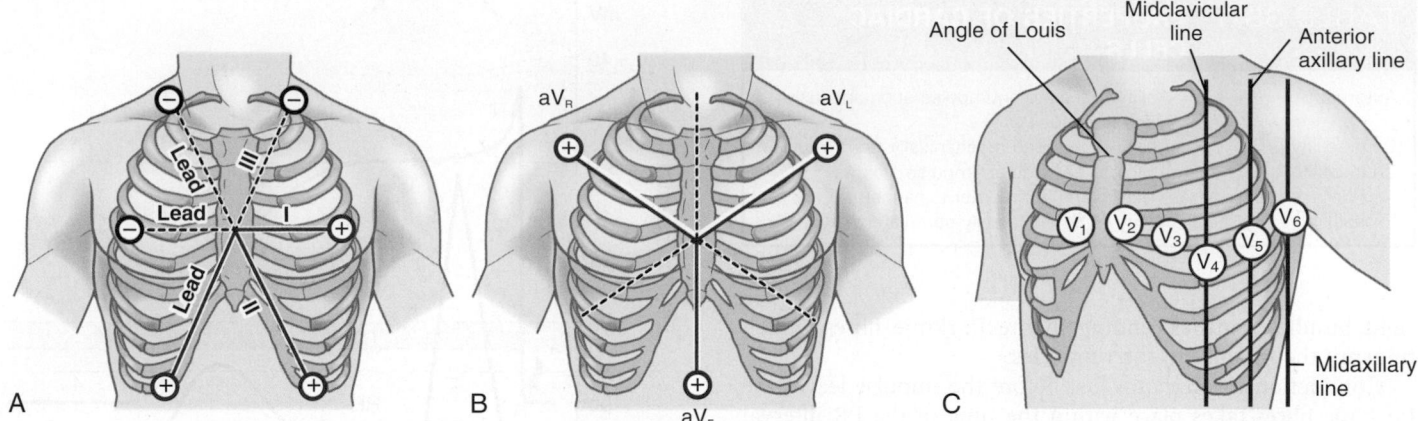

FIGURE 38-2 A, Limb leads I, II, and III. These bipolar leads are located on the extremities. Illustrated are the angles from which these leads view the heart. **B,** Limb leads aV_R, aV_L, and aV_F. These unipolar leads use the centre of the heart as their negative electrode. **C,** Placement for the unipolar chest leads: V_1, fourth intercostal space at the right sternal border; V_2, fourth intercostal space at the left sternal border; V_3, halfway between V_2 and V_4; V_4, fifth intercostal space at the left midclavicular line; V_5, fifth intercostal space at the left anterior axillary line; V_6, fifth intercostal space at the left midaxillary line.

FIGURE 38-3 Twelve-lead electrocardiogram showing a normal sinus rhythm.

consuming. If the rhythm is regular, a simpler process can be used: Every 3 seconds, a marker appears on the ECG paper. An R wave is the first upward (or positive) deflection of the QRS complex. The nurse can count the number of R–R intervals in 6 seconds and multiply that number by 10. This calculation yields the approximate number of beats per minute (Figure 38-6).

Another rapid method for calculating the HR when the rhythm is regular is to count the number of small squares within one R–R interval. Dividing this number by 1 500 yields the HR. The number of large squares within one R–R interval can also be counted and divided by 300 (see Figure 38-6). These methods are accurate only if the rhythm is regular.

An additional way to measure distances on the ECG strip is to use calipers. Calipers are used for fine measurements, especially for points of a specific wave or interval. Many times, a P or R wave does not fall directly on a light or heavy line. The fine points of the calipers can be placed exactly on the components to be measured and then moved to another part of the strip for time measurement.

ECG leads are attached to the patient's chest wall by means of an electrode pad fixed with electrical conductive gel. Before placing these on a patient, the nurse must properly prepare the patient's skin. Excessive hair on the chest wall should be clipped with scissors. The nurse should prepare the skin by rubbing

FIGURE 38-4 A, Lead placement for MCL₁ when a three-lead system is used. **B,** Lead placement for V₁ or V₆ when a five-lead system is used. **C,** Typical electrocardiographic tracing for lead MCL₁. *C,* chest; *LA,* left arm; *LL,* left leg; *RA,* right arm; *RL,* right leg. Source: Adapted from Urden, L. D., Stacy, K. M., & Lough, M. E. (2010). *Critical care nursing: Diagnosis and management* (6th ed., p. 370). St. Louis: Mosby.

FIGURE 38-5 Time and voltage on the electrocardiogram. Source: Adapted from Wesley, K. (2011). *Huszar's basic dysrhythmias and acute coronary syndromes: Interpretation and management* (4th ed., p. 19). St. Louis: Mosby.

gently with dry gauze until the skin is slightly pink. If the skin is oily, alcohol may be used first. In the case of a diaphoretic patient, a skin protectant should be applied before the electrode is placed. If leads and electrodes are not firmly placed, or if there is muscle activity or electrical interference from an outside source, an artifact may be seen on the monitor. An *artifact* is a distortion of the baseline and waveforms seen on the ECG (Figure 38-7). Accurate interpretation of cardiac rhythm is difficult when an artifact is present. If artifacts occur, the nurse should check for loose connections in the equipment. The electrodes on the patient

may need to be removed and replaced more securely or moved to areas that are less affected by movement (Goldsworthy, 2016).

Telemetry Monitoring. Telemetry monitoring is the observation of a patient's HR and rhythm to rapidly diagnose dysrhythmias, ischemia, or infarction. Two types of systems are used for telemetry monitoring. The first type, a centralized monitoring system, requires a nurse or telemetry technician to continuously observe all patients' rhythms at a central location. The second system of telemetry monitoring does not require constant surveillance by the nurse or technician. These systems have the capability of detecting and storing data. Sophisticated alarm systems provide different levels of detection of dysrhythmias, ischemia, or infarction, depending on the severity of each. However, computerized monitoring systems are not fail-proof. Frequent nursing assessment is important in caring for monitored patients.

INFORMATICS IN PRACTICE

Wireless ECG Monitoring

- Wireless electrocardiogram (ECG) monitoring systems continuously monitor and interpret the findings, sending an alert when patient rhythm or measurements (or both) fall outside of set parameters.
- Early detection of abnormal heart rhythms allows time to assess the patient for signs of hemodynamic instability (e.g., chest pain, hypotension, palpitations, dyspnea) and determine the need to intervene (e.g., call the rapid response team).
- These systems can automatically save the pre-event portion of the ECG while continuing to record the post-event portion and send all of the information to the health care provider.
- Computerized monitoring systems are not fail-proof. The nurse must frequently assess all monitored patients for any signs of hemodynamic instability.

FIGURE 38-6 The heart rate is calculated according to the interval between first upward (or positive) deflection (R wave) of one QRS complex to the R wave of the next. When the rhythm is regular, heart rate can be determined at a glance. The estimated heart rate is 80. The actual heart rate is 86. Source: Adapted from Wesley, K. (2011). *Huszar's basic dysrhythmias and acute coronary syndromes: Interpretation and management* (4th ed., p. 56). St. Louis: Mosby.

FIGURE 38-7 A, Electrocardiogram (ECG) demonstrating muscle tremor. **B,** ECG reflecting loose electrodes.

FIGURE 38-8 Electrocardiogram depicting normal sinus rhythm in lead II.

FIGURE 38-9 The ECG tracing as seen in normal sinus rhythm. 1, P wave; 2, PR interval; 3, QRS complex: Q wave, R wave, S wave; 4, ST segment; 5, T wave; 6, QT interval. Isoelectric (flat) line or baseline represents the absence of electrical activity in the heart cells.

Assessment of Cardiac Rhythm

When assessing the cardiac rhythm, the nurse must make an accurate interpretation and immediately evaluate the consequences of the findings for an individual patient. Assessment of the patient's hemodynamic response to any change in rhythm is essential because this information guides the selection of therapeutic interventions. Determination of the cause of dysrhythmias should be a priority. For example, tachycardias may be the result of fever and may cause a decrease in cardiac output (CO) and hypotension. Certain dysrhythmias may be a result of electrolyte disturbances and may lead to a life-threatening dysrhythmia. At all times, the patient must be assessed and abnormalities treated.

Normal sinus rhythm is a rhythm that originates in the SA node and follows the normal conduction pattern of the cardiac cycle (Figure 38-8). Figure 38-9 shows the normal electrical pattern of the cardiac cycle. Table 38-2 provides a description of ECG waveforms and intervals and possible sources of disturbances in these features. The P wave represents the depolarization of the atria (passage of an electrical impulse through the atria), causing atrial contraction. The PR interval represents the

period when the impulse spreads through the atria, the AV node, the bundle of His, and the Purkinje fibres. The QRS complex represents depolarization of the ventricles (ventricular contraction), and the QRS interval represents the time it takes for depolarization. The ST segment represents the time between ventricular depolarization and repolarization. This segment should be flat, or isoelectric, representing the absence of any electrical activity between these two events. The T wave represents repolarization of the ventricles. The QT interval represents the total time for depolarization and repolarization of the ventricles.

Electrophysiological Mechanisms of Dysrhythmias

Disorders of impulse formation can cause dysrhythmias. The heart has specialized cells found in the SA node, parts of the atria, the AV node, and the bundle of His and Purkinje fibres (His–Purkinje system) that are able to discharge spontaneously. This situation is termed automaticity. Normally, the main pacemaker of the heart is the SA node, which spontaneously discharges 60 to 100 times per minute (Table 38-3). A pacemaker from another site may be discharged in two ways. If the SA node discharges more slowly than a secondary pacemaker, the electrical discharges from the secondary pacemaker may passively "escape." The secondary pacemaker then discharges automatically at its intrinsic rate. These secondary pacemakers may originate from the AV node or the His–Purkinje system at rates of 40 to 60 times per minute and 20 to 40 times per minute, respectively.

TABLE 38-2   DEFINITION AND SOURCES OF VARIATION IN ECG WAVEFORMS AND INTERVALS*

Description	Normal Duration (sec)	Source of Possible Variation
P wave: Represents time for the electrical impulse that causes atrial depolarization (contraction) to pass through the atrium; should be upright	0.06–0.12	Disturbance in conduction within atria
PR interval: Measured from beginning of P wave to beginning of QRS complex; represents time taken for impulse to spread through the atria, the AV node and bundle of His, the bundle branches, and Purkinje fibres to a point immediately before ventricular contraction	0.12–0.20	Disturbance in conduction usually in AV node, bundle of His, or bundle branches but can be in atria as well
QRS interval: Measured from beginning to end of QRS complex; represents time taken for depolarization (contraction) of both ventricles (systole)	0.06–0.10	Disturbance in conduction in bundle branches or in ventricles
ST segment: Measured from the S wave of the QRS complex to the beginning of the T wave; represents the time between ventricular depolarization and repolarization (diastole); should be isoelectric (flat)	N/A	Disturbances usually caused by ischemia, injury, or infarction
T wave: Represents time for ventricular repolarization; should be upright	N/A	Disturbances usually caused by electrolyte imbalances, ischemia, or infarction
QT interval: Measured from beginning of QRS complex to end of T wave; represents time taken for entire electrical depolarization and repolarization of the ventricles	0.34–0.43	Disturbances usually affecting repolarization more than depolarization and caused by drugs, electrolyte imbalances, and changes in heart rate

AV, atrioventricular; *ECG,* electrocardiogram; *N/A,* not applicable.
*Heart rate influences the duration of these intervals, especially those of the PR and QT intervals (e.g., QT interval decreases in duration as heart rate increases).

TABLE 38-3   RATES OF THE CONDUCTION SYSTEM

SA node	60–100 times/min
AV junction	40–60 times/min
Purkinje fibres	20–40 times/min

AV, atrioventricular; *SA,* sinoatrial.

Another way that secondary pacemakers can originate is when they discharge more rapidly than the normal pacemaker of the SA node. Early or late beats may be triggered at an ectopic focus (area outside the normal conduction pathway) in the atria, the AV node, or the ventricles. This may result in a dysrhythmia, which replaces the normal sinus rhythm.

The impulse started by the SA node or an ectopic focus must be conducted to the entire heart chamber. The property of myocardial tissue that allows it to be depolarized by a stimulus is called *excitability*. This is an important part of the transmission of the impulse from one fibre to another. The level of excitability is determined by the length of time after depolarization that the tissues can be reactivated. The recovery period after stimulation is called the *refractory phase* or *refractory period*. The absolute refractory phase or period occurs when excitability is zero and heart tissue cannot be stimulated. The relative refractory period occurs slightly later in the cycle, and excitability is more likely to occur. In states of full excitability, the heart is completely recovered. Figure 38-10 shows the relationship between the refractory period and the ECG.

If conduction is depressed, and if some areas of the heart are blocked (e.g., by necrosis), the unblocked areas are activated earlier than the blocked areas. When the block is unidirectional, this uneven conduction may allow the initial impulse to re-enter areas that were previously not excitable but have recovered. The re-entering impulse may be able to depolarize the atria and ventricles, causing a premature beat. If the re-entrant excitation continues, tachycardia occurs (Aehlert, 2013).

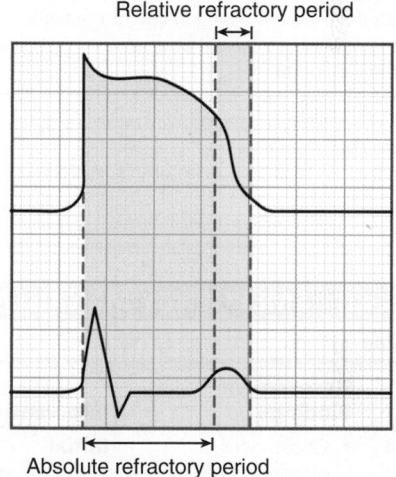

Relative refractory period

Absolute refractory period

FIGURE 38-10 Diagram of absolute and relative refractory periods correlated with the cardiac muscle's action potential and with an ECG tracing. Source: Adapted from Urden, L. D., Stacy, K. M., & Lough, M. E. (2010). *Critical care nursing: Diagnosis and management* (6th ed., p. 368). St. Louis: Mosby.

Evaluation of Dysrhythmias

Dysrhythmias occur as the result of various abnormalities and disease states (Aehlert, 2013). The cause of a dysrhythmia influences the treatment of the patient. Common causes of dysrhythmias are listed in Table 38-4. In Table 38-5, a systematic approach to assessing a cardiac rhythm is presented.

Dysrhythmias occurring in out-of-hospital settings present problems of management. Determination of the rhythm by cardiac monitoring is a high priority. If indicated, the emergency medical services (EMS) system is contacted after the patient has been assessed. Emergency care of the patient with a dysrhythmia is outlined in Table 38-6.

In addition to continuous ECG monitoring during hospitalization, several other methods are used to evaluate cardiac

TABLE 38-4   COMMON CAUSES OF DYSRHYTHMIAS

Cardiac Conditions	Other Conditions
• Accessory pathways	• Acid–base imbalances
• Conduction defects	• Alcohol
• Heart failure	• Coffee, tea, tobacco
• Hypertrophy of cardiac muscle	• Connective tissue disorders
• Myocardial cell degeneration	• Drug effects or toxicity
• Myocardial infarction	• Electric shock
	• Electrolyte imbalances
	• Emotional crisis
	• Hypoxia, shock
	• Metabolic conditions (e.g., thyroid dysfunction)
	• Near-drowning
	• Poisoning

TABLE 38-5   SYSTEMATIC APPROACH TO ASSESSING CARDIAC RHYTHMS

When assessing a cardiac rhythm, always assess the patient first, and then proceed with a systematic approach to interpreting the rhythm. A recommended approach is as follows:
1. Evaluate the rhythm (ventricular and atrial).
2. Determine the rate (ventricular and atrial).
3. Assess the presence and configuration of P waves.
4. Calculate the duration of the PR interval.
5. Calculate the QRS duration.
6. Calculate the QT interval.
7. Assess for changes in ST segment, T wave, or both.
8. Interpret the rhythm (e.g., atrial fibrillation).
9. Determine the clinical significance of this rhythm. Is the patient stable or unstable?
10. Determine the treatment for the rhythm.

TABLE 38-6   EMERGENCY MANAGEMENT

Dysrhythmias

Etiology	Assessment Findings	Interventions
See Table 38-4	• Chest, neck, shoulder, or arm pain • Cold, clammy skin • Decreased blood pressure • Decreased level of consciousness • Decreased O₂ saturation • Diaphoresis • Dizziness, syncope • Dyspnea • Extreme restlessness • Feeling of impending doom • Irregular rate and rhythm, palpitations • Nausea and vomiting • Numbness, tingling of arms • Pallor • Weakness and fatigue	**Initial** • Ensure patent airway • Administer O₂ via nasal cannula • Establish IV access • Apply cardiac monitoring electrodes • Identify underlying rhythm • Identify ectopic beats **Ongoing Monitoring** • Monitor vital signs, level of consciousness, O₂ saturation, and cardiac rhythm • Anticipate need for intubation if respiratory distress is evident • Prepare to initiate CPR or defibrillation, or both

CPR, cardiopulmonary resuscitation; *IV,* intravenous.

dysrhythmias and the effectiveness of antidysrhythmia drug therapy. An electrophysiological test (an invasive method) and Holter monitoring, event recorder monitoring, exercise treadmill testing, and signal-averaged ECG (all noninvasive methods) can be performed on both an inpatient and an outpatient basis.

An electrophysiological study (EPS) is performed to identify different mechanisms of tachydysrhythmias (dysrhythmias with rates >100), as well as heart blocks, bradydysrhythmias (dysrhythmias with rates <100), and causes of syncope. It can also be used to identify locations of accessory pathways and to determine the effectiveness of antidysrhythmia drugs. It involves introducing several electrode catheters transvenously through the femoral vein to the right side of the heart with fluoroscopic guidance. Electrical stimulation to various areas of the atrium and the ventricle is performed to induce the dysrhythmia. Immediate cardioversion or defibrillation may be required because serious dysrhythmias can be provoked during the procedure.

Preprocedure anxiety is common for patients undergoing EPS. Emotional support from the nurse is important. Patients should be told that they will be sedated but conscious during the procedure. Nursing care before and after the procedure is similar to that for cardiac catheterization (see Chapter 34). (EPS is also discussed in Chapter 34.)

The Holter monitor is a device that records the ECG while the patient is ambulatory. The device can record heart rhythm for 24 to 48 hours while the patient performs daily activities. The patient maintains a diary in which activities and any symptoms are recorded. Events in the diary can later be correlated with any dysrhythmias observed on the recording. The monitor is generally a useful device for detecting significant dysrhythmias and evaluating the effects of drugs during a patient's normal activities. It can also be used for detecting ischemia by analyzing ST segments. A limitation of the device is that patients who have frequent ventricular dysrhythmias, some of which may be lethal, may not have these dysrhythmias during the monitored time. (Holter monitoring is also discussed in Chapter 34.)

Use of event monitors has greatly improved the evaluation of outpatient dysrhythmias. Event monitors are recorders that are activated by the patient and can be used only at the time the patient experiences symptoms. The recorder is placed over the patient's chest during symptoms. The patient then transmits the rhythm to a central monitoring company via telephone. This is an easier method of documenting a dysrhythmia than the 24-hour monitor, especially if symptoms are not occurring daily. (Ambulatory ECG monitoring is discussed in Chapter 34.)

Exercise treadmill testing is used for evaluation of cardiac rhythm response to exercise. Exercise-induced dysrhythmias can be reproduced and analyzed, and drug therapy can be evaluated. These tests are performed with routine treadmill testing protocols. Diagnostic procedures for assessment of the cardiovascular system are presented in Chapter 34, Table 34-6.

Types of Dysrhythmias

Examples of the ECG tracings of common dysrhythmias are presented in Figures 38-11 through 38-19. Descriptive characteristics of common dysrhythmias are presented in Table 38-7.

Sinus Bradycardia. In sinus bradycardia, the conduction pathway is the same as that in sinus rhythm, but the SA node fires at a rate less than 60 beats/minute. This is referred to as *absolute bradycardia* (Figure 38-11, *A*). Relative bradycardia is an HR that is less than expected for the patient's condition, causing symptoms (Aehlert, 2013).

TABLE 38-7   CHARACTERISTICS OF COMMON DYSRHYTHMIAS

Pattern	Rate and Rhythm	P Wave	PR Interval	QRS Complex
Normal sinus rhythm	60–100 beats/min and regular	Normal	Normal	Normal
Sinus bradycardia	<60 beats/min and regular	Normal	Normal	Normal
Sinus tachycardia	>100 beats/min and regular	Normal	Normal	Normal
Premature atrial contraction	Usually 60–100 beats/min and irregular	Abnormal shape	Normal or variable	Normal (usually)
Paroxysmal supraventricular tachycardia	150–250 beats/min and regular	Abnormal shape, may be hidden	Variable	Normal (usually)
Atrial flutter	*Atrial:* 250–350 beats/min and regular *Ventricular:* >100 beats/min and irregular	Sawtooth shape	Variable	Normal (usually)
Atrial fibrillation	*Atrial:* 350–600 beats/min and irregular *Ventricular:* >100 beats/min and irregular or possibly any rate	Chaotic, fibrillatory	Not present	Normal (usually)
Junctional rhythms	40–140 beats/min and regular	Inverted (may be hidden)	Variable	Normal (usually)
First-degree AV heart block	Normal and regular	Normal	>0.20 sec, constant	Normal
Second-degree AV heart block				
Type I (Mobitz I, Wenckebach's)	*Atrial:* Normal and regular *Ventricular:* Slower and irregular	Normal	Progressively lengthened	Normal width, with pattern of one nonconducted QRS complex
Type II (Mobitz II)	*Atrial:* Usually normal and regular or irregular *Ventricular:* Slower and regular or irregular	More P waves than QRS complexes	Normal or prolonged	Widened, preceded by two or more P waves
Third-degree AV heart block	Ventricular rate 20–40 beats/min and regular	Normal, but no connection with QRS complex	None; PR interval not related to QRS complex; more P waves than QRS complexes	Normal or widened; no connection with P waves
Premature ventricular contraction	60–100 beats/min and irregular	None	Not present	Wide and distorted
Ventricular tachycardia	100–250 beats/min and regular or irregular	None	None	Wide and distorted
Ventricular fibrillation	Not measurable and irregular	Absent	Not present	Not measurable

AV, atrioventricular.

FIGURE 38-11 A, ECG demonstrating sinus bradycardia. **B,** ECG demonstrating sinus tachycardia.

Clinical Associations. Sinus bradycardia may be a normal sinus rhythm in aerobically trained athletes and in other individuals during sleep. It also occurs in response to carotid sinus massage, the Valsalva manoeuvre, hypothermia, increased intraocular pressure, increased vagal tone, and administration of parasympathomimetic drugs (e.g., bethanechol [Duvoid]).

Disease states associated with sinus bradycardia are hypothyroidism, increased intracranial pressure, obstructive jaundice, and inferior wall myocardial infarction (MI).

Electrocardiographic Characteristics. In sinus bradycardia, the HR is less than 60 beats/minute, and the rhythm is regular. The P wave precedes each QRS complex and has a normal shape and duration. The PR interval is normal, and the QRS complex has a normal shape and duration.

Clinical Significance. The clinical significance of sinus bradycardia depends on how the patient tolerates it hemodynamically. Signs of symptomatic bradycardia can include pale, cool skin; hypotension; weakness; angina; dizziness or syncope; confusion or disorientation; and shortness of breath.

Treatment. Treatment of sinus bradycardia consists of administration of atropine (an anticholinergic drug) for the patient with symptoms. Pacemaker therapy may be required.

Sinus Tachycardia. The conduction pathway is the same in sinus tachycardia as that in normal sinus rhythm. The discharge rate from the sinus node is increased as a result of vagal inhibition or sympathetic stimulation. The sinus rate is greater than 100 beats/minute (see Figure 38-11, *B*).

Clinical Associations. Sinus tachycardia is associated with physiological and psychological stressors such as exercise, fever, pain, hypotension, hypovolemia, anemia, hypoxia, hypoglycemia,

FIGURE 38-12 ECG demonstrating premature atrial contractions *(arrows)*.

FIGURE 38-13 Electrocardiogram demonstrating paroxysmal supraventricular tachycardia (PSVT). Arrows indicate beginning and ending of PSVT.

myocardial ischemia, heart failure (HF), hyperthyroidism, anxiety, and fear. It can also be an effect of drugs such as epinephrine (EpiPen), norepinephrine (Levophed), atropine, caffeine, theophylline, nifedipine, or hydralazine (Apresoline). In addition, many over-the-counter cold remedies have active ingredients (e.g., pseudoephedrine [Sudafed]) that can cause tachycardia.

Electrocardiographic Characteristics. In sinus tachycardia, the HR is greater than 100 beats/minute and the rhythm is regular. The P wave is normal, precedes each QRS complex, and has a normal shape and duration. The PR interval is normal, and the QRS complex has a normal shape and duration.

Clinical Significance. The clinical significance of sinus tachycardia depends on the patient's tolerance of the increased HR. The patient may have symptoms of dizziness, dyspnea, and hypotension. Increased myocardial oxygen consumption is associated with an increased HR. Angina or an increase in infarction size may accompany persistent sinus tachycardia in patients with an acute MI.

Treatment. Treatment is based on the underlying cause. For instance, if the patient is experiencing tachycardia from pain, tachycardia should resolve with effective pain management.

Premature Atrial Contraction. A **premature atrial contraction (PAC)** is a contraction originating from an ectopic focus in one atrium in a location other than the sinus node. The ectopic signal originates in the left or the right atrium and travels across both atria by an abnormal pathway, causing the P wave to be distorted (Figure 38-12). At the AV node, it may be stopped (nonconducted PAC), delayed (lengthened PR interval), or conducted normally. If the signal moves through the AV node, in most cases it is conducted normally through the ventricles.

Clinical Associations. In a normal heart, a PAC can result from emotional stress, physical fatigue, or the use of caffeine, tobacco, or alcohol. A PAC can also result from hypoxia, electrolyte imbalances, and disease states such as hyperthyroidism, chronic obstructive pulmonary disease (COPD), and heart disease, including coronary artery disease (CAD) and valvular disease.

Electrocardiographic Characteristics. Heart rate varies with the underlying rate and frequency of the PAC, and the rhythm is irregular. The P wave has a different shape from that of the P wave originating from the SA node. It may be notched or have downward (or negative) deflection, or it may be hidden in the preceding T wave. The PR interval may be shorter or longer than the PR interval originating from the SA node, but its length is within normal limits. The QRS complex is usually normal. If the QRS interval is 0.12 seconds or longer, conduction through the ventricles is abnormal.

Clinical Significance. In people with healthy hearts, isolated PACs are not significant. In people with heart disease, frequent PACs may indicate enhanced automaticity of the atria or a re-entry mechanism. Such PACs may warn of or initiate more serious dysrhythmias (e.g., supraventricular tachycardia).

Treatment. Treatment of PAC depends on the patient's symptoms. Withdrawal of sources of stimulation such as caffeine or sympathomimetic drugs may be warranted.

Paroxysmal Supraventricular Tachycardia. Paroxysmal supraventricular tachycardia (PSVT) is a dysrhythmia originating in an ectopic focus anywhere above the bifurcation of the bundle of His (Figure 38-13). Identification of the ectopic focus is often difficult even with 12-lead ECG because the dysrhythmia must be recorded as it is initiated.

PSVT occurs because of a re-entrant phenomenon (re-excitation of the atria when there is a one-way block). Usually, a PAC triggers a run of repeated premature beats. *Paroxysmal* refers to an abrupt onset and termination. The termination is sometimes followed by a brief period of asystole. Some degree of AV block may be present. PSVT can occur in the presence of Wolff–Parkinson–White (WPW) syndrome, or "pre-excitation." In this syndrome, extra conduction pathways or accessory pathways are present.

Clinical Associations. In the normal heart, PSVT is associated with overexertion, emotional stress, deep inspiration, and stimulants such as caffeine and tobacco. PSVT is also associated with rheumatic heart disease, digitalis toxicity, CAD, and cor pulmonale.

Electrocardiographic Characteristics. In PSVT, the HR is 100 to 300 beats/minute, and rhythm is regular or slightly irregular. The P wave is often hidden in the preceding T wave, but if seen, it may have an abnormal shape. The PR interval may be shortened or normal, and the QRS complex is usually normal.

Clinical Significance. The clinical significance of PSVT depends on symptoms and HR. A prolonged episode and heart rate greater than 180 beats/minute may precipitate a decrease in CO, resulting in hypotension, dyspnea, and angina.

Treatment. Treatment for PSVT includes vagal stimulation and drug therapy. Common vagal manoeuvres include Valsalva manoeuvres and coughing. Intravenous (IV) adenosine is the drug of first choice to convert PSVT to a normal sinus rhythm. This drug has a short half-life (1.5–10 seconds) and is well tolerated by most patients (Lehne, 2016). IV β-adrenergic blockers, calcium channel blockers (e.g., diltiazem [Cardizem]), and amiodarone can also be used. For a patient with WPW syndrome, amiodarone should be used. If vagal stimulation and drug therapy are ineffective and the patient becomes hemodynamically unstable, direct-current (DC) cardioversion may be used. (Cardioversion is discussed on p. 881.) If PSVT recurs in patients with WPW syndrome, they may ultimately be treated with radiofrequency ablation of the accessory pathway. (Radiofrequency ablation therapy is discussed on p. 884.)

DRUG ALERT—Adenosine (Adenocard)
- Injection site should be as close to the heart as possible (e.g., antecubital area).
- IV dose should be given rapidly (over 1–2 seconds) and followed with a rapid 20-mL normal saline flush.

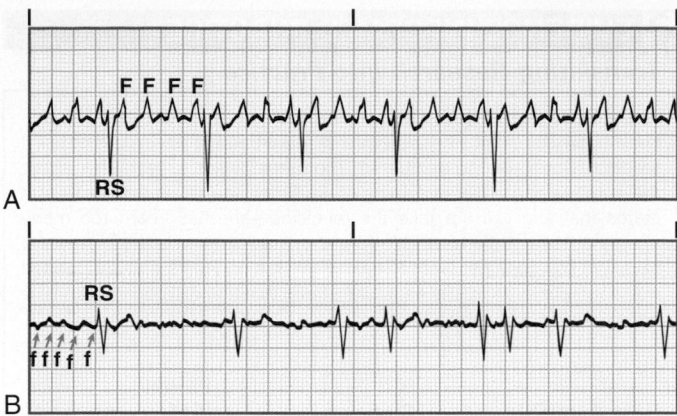

FIGURE 38-14 A, Atrial flutter with a 4:1 conduction (four flutter [F] waves to each QRS complex). **B,** Atrial fibrillation with a controlled ventricular response. Note the chaotic fibrillatory (f) waves (arrows) between the RS complexes. NOTE: Recorded from lead V₁.

- Patient's ECG must be monitored continuously. Brief period of asystole can occur.
- Patient should be observed for flushing, dizziness, chest pain, or palpitations.

Atrial Flutter. Atrial flutter is an atrial tachydysrhythmia identified by recurring, regular, sawtooth-shaped flutter (F) waves that originate from a single ectopic focus in the right atrium (Figure 38-14, A).

Clinical Associations. Atrial flutter rarely occurs in a normal heart. It is associated with disease states such as CAD, hypertension, mitral valve disorders, pulmonary embolus, chronic lung disease, cor pulmonale, cardiomyopathy, and hyperthyroidism and with the use of drugs such as digoxin, quinidine, and epinephrine.

Electrocardiographic Characteristics. In atrial flutter, atrial rate is 250 to 350 beats/minute. The ventricular rate varies according to the conduction ratio. In 2:1 conduction, the ventricular rate is typically found to be approximately 150 beats/minute. Atrial rhythm is regular, and ventricular rhythm is usually regular. The atrial flutter waves represent atrial depolarization followed by repolarization. The PR interval is variable and cannot be measured. The QRS complex is usually normal. Because of the ability of the AV node to delay signals from the atria, there is usually some AV block in a fixed ratio of flutter waves to QRS complexes (e.g., 2:1, 3:1).

Clinical Significance. The high ventricular rates (>100 beats/minute) and loss of the atrial "kick" (atrial contraction reflected by a sinus P wave) that are associated with atrial flutter can decrease CO and cause serious consequences such as HF, especially in the patient with underlying heart disease. Patients with atrial flutter are at increased risk for stroke because of the risk for thrombus formation in the atria from the stasis of blood. Warfarin (Coumadin) is used to prevent stroke in patients with atrial flutter of longer than 48 hours' duration (American Heart Association [AHA], 2015).

Treatment. The primary goal in treatment of atrial flutter is to slow the ventricular response by increasing AV block. Drugs used to control ventricular rate include calcium channel blockers and β-adrenergic blockers. Electrical cardioversion may be used to convert the atrial flutter to sinus rhythm in an emergency situation (i.e., the patient is hemodynamically unstable) and electively. Antidysrhythmia drugs used to convert atrial flutter

to sinus rhythm or to maintain sinus rhythm include amiodarone, propafenone (Rythmol), and ibutilide (Corvert) (Lehne, 2016).

Radiofrequency ablation is increasingly being used as curative therapy for atrial flutter. The procedure is performed in the electrophysiology laboratory and involves positioning a catheter in the right atrium between the inferior vena cava and the tricuspid valve. With the use of a low-voltage, high-frequency form of electrical energy, the tissue is ablated (or destroyed), the dysrhythmia is terminated, and normal sinus rhythm is restored in most cases (Greenberg & Chandrakantan, 2015). (Radiofrequency ablation in discussed on p. 884.)

Atrial Fibrillation. Atrial fibrillation is characterized by a total disorganization of atrial electrical activity caused by multiple ectopic foci, resulting in loss of effective atrial contraction (see Figure 38-14, B). Atrial fibrillation is the most common dysrhythmia encountered in the emergency department, and the focus of treatment is the rapid assessment of potential hemodynamic instability and identification and treatment of the underlying cause (Stiell & Macle, 2011). The dysrhythmia may be chronic or intermittent. Atrial fibrillation is the most common dysrhythmia in Canada, affecting approximately 350 000 people (Heart and Stroke Foundation, 2017). Its prevalence increases with age.

Clinical Associations. Atrial fibrillation usually occurs in patients with underlying heart disease, such as CAD, rheumatic heart disease, cardiomyopathy, hypertensive heart disease, HF, and pericarditis. It is often acutely caused by factors such as thyrotoxicosis, alcohol intoxication, caffeine use, electrolyte disturbances, stress, and cardiac surgery.

Electrocardiographic Characteristics. During atrial fibrillation, the atrial rate may be as high as 600 beats/minute. Ventricular rate can vary from as low as 50 beats/minute to as high as 180 beats/minute. Atrial fibrillation with ventricular rates greater than 100 are described as atrial fibrillation with a rapid ventricular response. When ventricular rates are less than 100, the condition is described as atrial fibrillation with a slow or controlled ventricular response. P waves are replaced by chaotic, fibrillatory waves in atrial fibrillation. The ventricular rhythm is usually irregular. The PR interval is not measurable, but the QRS complex usually has a normal shape and duration. At times, atrial flutter and atrial fibrillation may coexist.

Clinical Significance. Atrial fibrillation can often result in a decrease in CO because of ineffective atrial contractions or loss of atrial kick, a rapid ventricular response, or both. Thrombi may form in the atria as a result of blood stasis. An embolized clot may develop and travel to the brain, causing a stroke. Overall risk for stroke is increased three to five times with atrial fibrillation (Heart and Stroke Foundation, 2017).

Treatment. The goals of treatment for atrial fibrillation include a decrease in ventricular response (to <100/minute) and prevention of cerebral embolic events (Stiell & Macle, 2011). Ventricular rate control is a priority for patients with atrial fibrillation. Drugs used for rate control include calcium channel blockers (e.g., diltiazem) and β-adrenergic blockers (e.g., metoprolol).

For some patients, conversion of atrial fibrillation to a normal sinus rhythm may be a consideration (e.g., reduced exercise tolerance with rate control drugs, contraindications to warfarin). Antidysrhythmia drugs used for conversion to and maintenance of sinus rhythm include medications such as amiodarone in the stable patient (AHA, 2015). In unstable patients with severe left ventricular dysfunction or HF, amiodarone or DC cardioversion should be used (AHA, 2015).

FIGURE 38-15 Electrocardiogram demonstrating junctional escape rhythm. The P wave is hidden in the QRS complex. NOTE: Recorded from lead V_1.

Cardioversion may be used to convert atrial fibrillation to a normal sinus rhythm. Before proceeding to cardioversion, in the absence of systemic anticoagulation, the nurse must determine that the patient has had atrial fibrillation or atrial flutter for less than 48 hours (Stiell & Macle, 2011). The cardioversion procedure can cause clots to dislodge, which increases the patient's risk for stroke. If clots are present, the procedure is contraindicated.

If drugs or cardioversion do not convert atrial fibrillation to normal sinus rhythm, long-term anticoagulation therapy is required. Long-term follow-up with patients experiencing atrial fibrillation or flutter is recommended to assess the need for long-term antithrombotic therapy or antiarrhythmic therapy. (See Chapter 40 for discussion of anticoagulation therapy.)

Other treatment strategies exist for drug-refractory atrial fibrillation and for patients who cannot or choose not to have long-term anticoagulation. These include the use of radiofrequency ablation, which is similar to the procedure for atrial flutter (Canadian Cardiovascular Society, 2011).

Junctional Dysrhythmias. Junctional dysrhythmias are dysrhythmias that originate in the area of the AV node, primarily because the SA node has failed to fire or the signal has been blocked. In this situation, the AV node becomes the pacemaker of the heart. The impulse from the AV node usually moves in a retrograde (backward) manner that produces an abnormal P wave occurring just before or after the QRS complex or that is hidden in the QRS complex. The impulse usually moves normally through the ventricles. Junctional premature beats may occur, and they are treated in a manner similar to that for PACs. Other junctional dysrhythmias include junctional escape rhythm (Figure 38-15), accelerated junctional rhythm, and junctional tachycardia. These dysrhythmias are treated according to the patient's tolerance of the rhythm and the patient's clinical condition.

Clinical Associations. Junctional dysrhythmias are often associated with CAD, HF, cardiomyopathy, electrolyte imbalances, inferior MI, and rheumatic heart disease. Certain drugs (e.g., digoxin, amphetamines, caffeine, nicotine) can also cause junctional dysrhythmias (Aehlert, 2013).

Electrocardiographic Characteristics. In junctional escape rhythm, the HR is 40 to 60 beats/minute; in accelerated junctional rhythm, it is 61 to 100 beats/minute; and in junctional tachycardia, it is 101 to 150 beats/minute. Rhythm is regular. The P wave is abnormal in shape and inverted, or it may be hidden in the QRS complex (see Figure 38-15). The PR interval is less than 0.12 seconds when the P wave precedes the QRS complex. The QRS complex is usually normal.

Clinical Significance. Junctional escape rhythms serve as a safety mechanism for when the SA node has not been effective in firing. Escape rhythms such as this should not be suppressed.

⟲ EVIDENCE-INFORMED PRACTICE

Translating Research Into Practice

Geena Dodd is an 82-year-old woman with a new onset of atrial fibrillation and a history of mitral stenosis (high-risk factor). Her physician has ordered warfarin (Coumadin) to be started. The nurse begins to teach her about the purpose and adverse effects of warfarin. She stops the nurse and states that she will not take the medicine—she has heard too many stories about people bleeding from this medication. Furthermore, she says that she does not want to deal with the blood tests that are needed nor worry about what she eats. She states that she will continue to take her aspirin once a day as usual.

Best Available Evidence	Clinician Expertise	Patient Preferences and Values
Warfarin (Coumadin) is the drug of choice to treat patients with atrial fibrillation who have one or more high-risk factors, in order to prevent stroke. For patients for whom oral anticoagulation with warfarin is considered unsuitable (e.g., patient preference), the addition of clopidogrel (Plavix) to ASA (Aspirin) reduces the risk for major vascular events (especially stroke) but increases the risk for major hemorrhage.	Bleeding is a potential and serious adverse effect of warfarin and of dual antiplatelet therapy (ASA; Aspirin and clopidogrel). When taking warfarin, INR blood levels need to be checked on a regular basis. Patients should avoid drastic changes in diet, especially foods high in vitamin K (interfere with the action of warfarin).	Mrs. Dodd does not want to take warfarin or clopidogrel because she is afraid of bleeding. In addition, she does not want to change her lifestyle to accommodate the changes that would be needed to use warfarin.

Decision and Action

The nurse explains the risks of not taking the prescribed medicine (warfarin) or adequate medication (adding clopidogrel to her ASA [Aspirin] therapy). She tells the nurse that she understands completely. The nurse supports her choice and informs the physician of Mrs. Dodd's decision.

Reference for Evidence

Wann, L. S., Curtis, A. B., January, C. T., et al. (2011). 2011 ACCF/AHA/HRS focused update on the management of patients with atrial fibrillation (updating the 2006 guideline): A report of the American College of Cardiology Foundation/American Heart Association Task Force on Practice Guidelines. *Journal of the American College of Cardiology, 57,* 223. DOI: *http://dx.doi.org/10.1161/cir.0b013e3181fa3cf4.*

ASA, Acetylsalicylic acid; *INR,* international normalized ratio.

Accelerated junctional rhythm and junctional tachycardia, however, indicate a more serious problem with the sinoatrial node. These rhythms may result in a reduction of CO, causing the patient to become hemodynamically unstable (e.g., hypotensive).

Treatment. Treatment varies according to the type of junctional dysrhythmia. If a patient has symptoms with an escape junctional rhythm, atropine can be administered. In accelerated junctional rhythm and junctional tachycardia caused by digoxin toxicity, the digoxin is withheld. In the absence of digoxin toxicity,

A

PR interval

Blocked QRS

P   P   P

B

PR interval PR interval
0.24 sec   0.32 sec

Blocked QRS   Blocked QRS

P   P   P   P   P   P

C

P P   P P   P P   P P   P P

D

FIGURE 38-16 Heart block. **A,** First-degree atrioventricular (AV) block with a PR interval of 0.40 seconds. **B,** Second-degree AV block, type I, with progressive lengthening of the PR interval until a QRS complex is blocked. **C,** Second-degree AV block, type II, with constant PR intervals and variable blocked QRS complexes. **D,** Third-degree AV block. Note that there is no relationship between P waves and QRS complexes.

β-adrenergic blockers, calcium channel blockers, and amiodarone are used for rate control.

First-Degree Atrioventricular Block. *First-degree atrioventricular (AV) block* is a type of AV block in which every impulse is conducted to the ventricles but the duration of AV conduction is prolonged (Figure 38-16, *A*). After the impulse moves through the AV node, it is usually conducted normally through the ventricles.

Clinical Associations. First-degree AV block is associated with MI, CAD, rheumatic fever, hyperthyroidism, vagal stimulation, and drugs such as digoxin, β-adrenergic blockers, calcium channel blockers, and flecainide.

Electrocardiographic Characteristics. In first-degree AV block, the HR is normal, and the rhythm is regular. The P wave is normal, the PR interval is prolonged to more than 0.20 seconds, and the QRS complex usually has a normal shape and duration.

Clinical Significance. First-degree AV block is usually not serious but can be a precursor of higher degrees of AV block. Patients with first-degree AV block have no symptoms.

Treatment. There is no treatment for first-degree AV block. Modifications to causative medications may be considered. Patients should continue to be monitored for any new changes in heart rhythm.

Second-Degree Atrioventricular Block, Type I. *Type I second-degree AV block (Mobitz I or Wenckebach's heart block)* includes a gradual lengthening of the PR interval. It occurs because of a prolonged AV conduction time until an atrial impulse is not conducted and a QRS complex is blocked (missing) (see Figure 38-16, *B*). Type I AV block most commonly occurs in the AV node, but it can also occur in the His–Purkinje system.

Clinical Associations. Type I AV block may result from the use of drugs such as digoxin or β-adrenergic blockers. It may also be associated with CAD and other diseases that can slow AV conduction.

Electrocardiographic Characteristics. The atrial rate is normal, but the ventricular rate may be slower as a result of nonconducted atrial impulses or blocked QRS complexes. Once a ventricular beat is blocked, the cycle repeats itself with progressive lengthening of the PR intervals, until another QRS complex is blocked. The rhythm appears on the ECG in a pattern of grouped beats. Ventricular rhythm is irregular. The P wave has a normal shape. The QRS complex has a normal shape and duration.

Clinical Significance. Type I AV block is usually a result of myocardial ischemia or infarction. It is almost always transient and is usually well tolerated. However, in some patients (e.g., after an MI), it may be a warning signal of a more serious AV conduction disturbance.

Treatment. If the patient has symptoms, atropine is used to increase the HR, or a temporary pacemaker may be needed, especially if the patient has experienced an MI. If the patient has no symptoms, the rhythm should be closely observed with a transcutaneous pacemaker on standby. Bradycardia is more likely to become symptomatic when one or more of the following are present: (a) hypotension, (b) HF, or (c) shock.

Second-Degree Atrioventricular Block, Type II. In *type II second-degree AV block (Mobitz II heart block),* a P wave is not conducted without progressive antecedent PR lengthening. This almost always occurs when a block in one of the bundle branches is present (see Figure 38-16, *C*). On conducted beats, the PR interval is constant. Type II second-degree AV block is a more serious type of block, in which a certain number of impulses from the SA node are not conducted to the ventricles. This occurs in ratios of 2 : 1, 3 : 1, and so on (i.e., two P waves to one QRS complex, three P waves to one QRS complex). It may occur with varying ratios. Type II AV block almost always originates in the His–Purkinje system.

Clinical Associations. Type II AV block is associated with rheumatic heart disease, CAD, anterior MI, and digitalis toxicity.

Electrocardiographic Characteristics. The atrial rate is usually normal. The ventricular rate depends on the intrinsic rate and the degree of AV block. The atrial rhythm is regular, but the ventricular rhythm may be irregular. The P wave has a normal shape. The PR interval may be normal or prolonged in duration and remains constant on conducted beats. The QRS complex is usually more than 0.12 seconds because of bundle-branch block.

Clinical Significance. Type II AV block often progresses to third-degree AV block and is associated with a poor prognosis. The reduced HR often results in decreased CO with subsequent hypotension and myocardial ischemia. Type II AV block is an indication for therapy with a permanent pacemaker.

Treatment. Temporary treatment before the insertion of a permanent pacemaker may be necessary if the condition becomes symptomatic (e.g., hypotension, angina). Such treatment involves the use of a temporary transvenous or transcutaneous pacemaker (Aehlert, 2013).

Third-Degree Atrioventricular Block. Third-degree AV block, or complete heart block, constitutes one form of AV dissociation, in which no impulses from the atria are conducted to the ventricles (see Figure 38-16, *D*). The atria are stimulated and contract independently of the ventricles. The ventricular rhythm is an escape rhythm, and the ectopic pacemaker may be above or below the bifurcation of the bundle of His.

Clinical Associations. Third-degree AV block is associated with severe heart disease, including CAD, MI, myocarditis, cardiomyopathy, and some systemic diseases such as amyloidosis and progressive systemic sclerosis (scleroderma). Some medications can also cause third-degree AV block, such as digoxin, β-adrenergic blockers, and calcium channel blockers.

Electrocardiographic Characteristics. The atrial rate with third-degree AV block is usually a sinus rate of 60 to 100 beats/minute. The ventricular rate depends on the site of the block. If it is in the AV node, the rate is 40 to 60 beats/minute, and if it is in the His–Purkinje system, it is 20 to 40 beats/minute. Atrial and ventricular rhythms are regular but unrelated to each other. The P wave has a normal shape. The PR interval is variable, and there is no time relationship between the P wave and the QRS complex. The QRS complex is normal if an escape rhythm is initiated at the bundle of His or above. It is widened if an escape rhythm is initiated below the bundle of His.

Clinical Significance. Third-degree AV block almost always results in reduced CO with subsequent ischemia, HF, and shock. Syncope from third-degree AV block may result from severe bradycardia or even periods of asystole.

Treatment. When patients are unstable in the presence of a bradycardia, a transcutaneous pacemaker is typically used as first-line treatment (AHA, 2015). The use of drugs such as atropine, epinephrine, isoproterenol, and dopamine is a temporary measure to increase the HR and support blood pressure (BP) until temporary pacing is initiated. Patients need a permanent pacemaker implanted as soon as possible.

Premature Ventricular Contractions. A premature ventricular contraction (PVC) is a contraction originating in an ectopic focus in the ventricles. It is the premature occurrence of a QRS complex, which is wide and whose shape is distorted in comparison with a QRS complex initiated from the normal conduction pathway (Figure 38-17). PVCs that are initiated from different foci appear different in shape from each other and are called *multifocal* PVCs. PVCs that appear to have the same shape are called *unifocal* PVCs. When every other beat is a PVC, it is called *ventricular bigeminy.* When every third beat is a PVC, it is called *ventricular trigeminy.* Two consecutive PVCs are called a *couplet.* When three or more consecutive PVCs occur, it is called *ventricular tachycardia.* A PVC that falls on the T wave of a preceding beat is called the *R-on-T phenomenon.* This phenomenon is considered especially dangerous because the PVC is occurring during the relative refractory phase of ventricular repolarization. Excitability of the cardiac cells is increased during this time, and the risk for the PVC to initiate ventricular tachycardia or ventricular fibrillation is high.

Clinical Associations. PVCs are associated with stimulants such as caffeine, alcohol, nicotine, aminophylline, epinephrine, isoproterenol, and digoxin. They are also associated with electrolyte imbalances, hypoxia, fever, exercise, and emotional stress. Disease states associated with PVCs include MI, mitral valve prolapse, HF, and CAD.

Electrocardiographic Characteristics. HR varies according to intrinsic rate and number of PVCs. The rhythm is irregular

FIGURE 38-17 Various forms of premature ventricular contractions (PVCs).

because of premature beats. The P wave is absent in a PVC. The QRS complex is wide and distorted in shape, lasting more than 0.12 seconds. The T wave is generally large and opposite in direction to the major direction of the QRS complex.

Clinical Significance. PVCs are usually a benign finding in the patient with a normal heart. In heart disease, depending on frequency, PVCs may reduce the CO and precipitate angina and HF if they are frequently occurring (>10/minute). Because PVCs in CAD or acute MI represent ventricular irritability, the patient's physiological response to PVCs must be monitored.

Treatment. Treatment is often based on the cause of the PVCs (e.g., oxygen therapy for hypoxia, electrolyte replacement); however, infrequent PVCs are not typically treated. Assessment of the patient's hemodynamic status is important to guide treatment. Most importantly, the patient must be assessed for signs of decreased CO and whether the PVCs are causing the patient to be symptomatic (e.g., chest pain, dizziness) to determine whether treatment is indicated.

Ventricular Tachycardia. The diagnosis of ventricular tachycardia (VT) is made when a run of three or more PVCs occurs. It occurs when an ectopic focus or foci fire repetitively and the ventricle takes control as the pacemaker. VT appears in different forms, depending on the QRS configuration. Monomorphic VT (Figure 38-18, *A*) has QRS complexes that are the same in shape, size, and direction. In polymorphic VT, the QRS complexes gradually change back and forth from one shape, size, and direction to another over a series of beats. *Torsades de pointes* (French, "twisting of the points") is polymorphic VT associated

FIGURE 38-18 ECGs demonstrating ventricular tachycardia. **A,** Monomorphic. **B,** Torsades de pointes (polymorphic).

FIGURE 38-19 ECG demonstrating ventricular fibrillation.

with a prolonged QT interval of the underlying rhythm (see Figure 38-18, *B*).

Ventricular tachycardia may be sustained or nonsustained. Sustained VT lasts for more than 30 seconds. Nonsustained VT lasts for 30 seconds or less. The development of VT is an ominous sign. It is considered to be a life-threatening dysrhythmia because of decreased CO and the possibility of deterioration to ventricular fibrillation, which is a lethal dysrhythmia.

Clinical Associations. Ventricular tachycardia is associated with MI, CAD, significant electrolyte imbalances, cardiomyopathy, mitral valve prolapse, long QT syndrome, digitalis toxicity, and central nervous system disorders. This dysrhythmia has also been observed in patients who have no evidence of cardiac disease.

Electrocardiographic Characteristics. The ventricular rate in VT is 150 to 250 beats/minute. The rhythm is regular.

The QRS complex is distorted in appearance, with a duration exceeding 0.12 seconds and with the ST–T wave in the opposite direction to that of the QRS complex (see Figure 38-18). The R–R interval may be irregular or regular.

Clinical Significance. Ventricular tachycardia can be stable (patient has a pulse) or unstable (patient is pulseless). Sustained VT causes a severe decrease in CO as a result of decreased ventricular diastolic filling times and loss of atrial contraction. Results include hypotension, pulmonary edema, decreased cerebral blood flow, and cardiopulmonary arrest. The dysrhythmia must be treated quickly, even if it occurs only briefly and stops abruptly, because episodes may recur if prophylactic treatment is not begun. Ventricular fibrillation may also develop.

Treatment. Precipitating causes of VT must be identified and treated (e.g., electrolyte imbalances, ischemia). If the VT is monomorphic and the patient is hemodynamically stable (e.g., pulse is present) and has preserved left ventricular function, IV amiodarone is typically used. If the patient becomes hemodynamically unstable or has poor left ventricular function, IV amiodarone is given, followed by cardioversion if the original drug therapy alone is ineffective.

If the VT is polymorphic with a normal baseline QT interval, any one of the following medications is used: β-adrenergic blockers, amiodarone, or sotalol. Cardioversion is performed if drug therapy is ineffective.

If the VT is polymorphic with a prolonged baseline QT interval, therapies include IV magnesium and antitachycardia pacing (discussed later in this chapter). Drugs that prolong the QT interval should be discontinued. If the rhythm is not converted, cardioversion may be needed.

VT without a pulse is a life-threatening situation and is treated in the same manner as ventricular fibrillation—cardiopulmonary resuscitation (CPR) and rapid defibrillation are the first lines of treatment, followed by the administration of epinephrine if defibrillation is unsuccessful (AHA, 2015).

An *accelerated idioventricular rhythm* (AIVR) can develop when the intrinsic pacemaker rate (SA node or AV node) becomes lower than that of a ventricular ectopic pacemaker; the rate is between 40 and 100 beats/minute. It is most commonly associated with acute MI and reperfusion of the myocardium after fibrinolytic therapy or angioplasty of coronary arteries. It can also occur with digitalis toxicity. In the setting of acute MI, AIVR is usually self-limiting and well tolerated and necessitates no treatment. If it becomes symptomatic (e.g., hypotension, angina), atropine can be considered. Temporary pacing may be required. Drugs that suppress ventricular rhythms (e.g., lidocaine) should not be used because they can terminate the ventricular rhythm and further reduce the HR.

Ventricular Fibrillation. Ventricular fibrillation is a severe derangement of the heart rhythm, characterized by irregular undulations of varying shapes and amplitude on the ECG (Figure 38-19). This presentation represents the firing of multiple ectopic foci in the ventricle. Mechanically, the ventricle is simply "quivering," and no effective contraction—and consequently no cardiac output—occurs.

Clinical Associations. Ventricular fibrillation occurs in acute MI and myocardial ischemia and in chronic diseases such as CAD and cardiomyopathy. It may occur during cardiac pacing or cardiac catheterization procedures as a result of catheter stimulation of the ventricle. It may also occur with coronary reperfusion after fibrinolytic therapy. Other clinical associations are accidental electric shock, hyperkalemia, hypoxemia, acidosis, and drug toxicity.

Electrocardiographic Characteristics. In ventricular fibrillation, the HR is not measurable. The rhythm is irregular and chaotic. The P wave is not detectable, and the PR and the QRS intervals are not measurable.

Clinical Significance. Ventricular fibrillation results in an unresponsive, pulseless, and apneic state. If it is not rapidly treated, the patient will die.

Treatment. Treatment consists of assessment of circulation, airway, and breathing (CAB), and if no pulse is found, high quality CPR and advanced cardiac life support (ACLS) measures are initiated immediately with the use of defibrillation and definitive drug therapy. If a defibrillator is immediately available, it must be used without delay (AHA, 2015).

Asystole. Asystole represents the total absence of ventricular electrical activity. On occasion, P waves are detected. No ventricular contraction occurs because depolarization does not occur.

Patients are unresponsive, pulseless, and apneic. This is a lethal dysrhythmia that necessitates immediate treatment. Ventricular fibrillation may masquerade as asystole; thus the rhythm should be assessed in more than one lead. The prognosis of a patient with asystole is extremely poor.

Clinical Associations. Asystole is usually a result of advanced cardiac disease, a severe cardiac conduction system disturbance, or end-stage HF.

Clinical Significance. In general, patients with asystole have end-stage cardiac disease or have a prolonged cardiac arrest and cannot be resuscitated.

Treatment. Treatment consists of high quality CPR with initiation of ACLS measures, which include: IV/IO access, epinephrine 1 mg every 3 to 5 minutes, consider advanced airway, and capnography (AHA, 2015).

Pulseless Electrical Activity. Pulseless electrical activity (PEA) is a situation in which electrical activity can be observed on the ECG, but there is no mechanical activity of the ventricles and the patient has no pulse. The prognosis is poor unless the underlying cause can be identified and quickly corrected. The most frequent causes of PEA include hypovolemia, hypoxia, metabolic acidosis, hyperkalemia or hypokalemia, hypothermia, drug overdose, cardiac tamponade, MI, tension pneumothorax, and pulmonary embolus. Treatment begins with assessment of CAB and if no pulse is detected, high quality CPR is initiated and followed by IV/IO access, epinephrine 1 mg every 3 to 5 minutes, consider advanced airway, and capnography. Treatment is aimed at potential treatable causes (e.g., hypovolemia) (AHA, 2015).

Sudden Cardiac Death. The term *sudden cardiac death (SCD)* refers to death from a cardiac cause. The majority of SCDs result from ventricular dysrhythmias, specifically VT or ventricular fibrillation. (SCD is discussed further in Chapter 36.)

Antidysrhythmia Drugs

An increasing number of antidysrhythmia drugs have become available. Table 38-8 categorizes major drug classes by primary effects on the cardiac cells.

Defibrillation

Defibrillation is the most effective method of terminating ventricular fibrillation and pulseless VT. It is most effective when the myocardial cells are not anoxic or acidotic, making rapid defibrillation crucial for a successful patient outcome. Defibrillation is accomplished by the passage of a DC electric shock through the heart that is sufficient to depolarize the cells of the myocardium. The intent is that subsequent repolarization of myocardial cells allows the SA node to resume the role of pacemaker (AHA, 2015).

Research has shown that biphasic defibrillators are preferred over monophasic defibrillators and deliver successful shocks at lower energies and with fewer post-shock ECG abnormalities than monophasic defibrillators (Figure 38-20) (AHA, 2015).

The output of a defibrillator is measured in joules (J), or watts per second. The recommended energy for initial shocks in defibrillation depends on the type of defibrillator. Biphasic defibrillators deliver all shocks of 150 to 200 J. After the initial shock, CPR should be started immediately, beginning with chest compressions.

Rapid defibrillation can be performed with a manual or automatic device (Figure 38-21). Manual defibrillators require health care providers to interpret cardiac rhythms, determine

TABLE 38-8   DRUG THERAPY

Antidysrhythmia Drugs: Classifications, Actions, and Effects on ECG

Classification	Actions	Effects on ECG
Class I: Sodium channel blockers	Decrease conduction velocity in the atria, ventricles, and His–Purkinje system	—
Class IA • Procainamide (Procan) • Quinidine	Delay repolarization	Widened QRS and prolonged QT interval
Class IB • Lidocaine (Xylocaine) • Mexiletine • Phenytoin (Dilantin)	Accelerate repolarization	Little or none
Class IC • Flecainide (Tambocor) • Propafenone (Rythmol)	Decrease impulse conduction	Pronounced prodysrhythmic actions, widened QRS, prolonged QT interval
Class II: β-Adrenergic blockers • Atenolol (Tenormin) • Carvedilol • Esmolol (Brevibloc) • Metoprolol (Lopressor) • Sotalol*	Decrease automaticity of the SA node; decrease conduction velocity in AV node; reduce atrial and ventricular contractility	Bradycardia, prolonged PR interval, AV block
Class III: Potassium channel blockers • Amiodarone • Ibutilide (Corvert) • Sotalol*	Delay repolarization, which results in prolonged duration of action potential and prolonged refractory period	Prolonged PR and QT intervals, widened QRS, bradycardia
Class IV: Calcium channel blockers • Diltiazem (Cardizem) • Verapamil	Decrease automaticity of SA node; delay AV node conduction; reduce myocardial contractility	Bradycardia, prolonged PR interval, AV block
Other antidysrhythmia drugs • Adenosine (Adenocard) • Digoxin • Magnesium	Decrease conduction through AV node; reduce automaticity of SA node	Prolonged PR interval, AV block

AV, atrioventricular; *ECG,* electrocardiogram; *SA,* sinoatrial.
*Sotalol has both class II and class III properties.

the need for a shock, and deliver a shock. **Automatic external defibrillators (AEDs)** are defibrillators that have rhythm detection capability and the ability to advise the operator to deliver a shock with hands-free defibrillator pads. Proficiency in use of the AED is incorporated in the basic life support course for health care providers (AHA, 2015). The nurse should be familiar with the operation of the type of defibrillator that is used in the clinical setting and must be certified to use this equipment. The Heart and Stroke Foundation of Ontario has implemented a public access defibrillation (PAD) program in communities in order to enhance the provision of early advanced cardiac care to save lives (Heart and Stroke Foundation, 2012). Through this program,

FIGURE 38-20 Paddle placement and current flow in monophasic defibrillation **(A)** and biphasic defibrillation **(B)**.

FIGURE 38-21 The LifePak device contains a monitor, a defibrillator, and a transcutaneous pacemaker. Source: Science History Images/Alamy Stock Photo.

AEDs are placed in public places such as arenas, pools, and community centres.

Upon defibrillation, the operator calls, "All clear" and looks to see that personnel are not touching the patient or the bed at the time of defibrillator discharge. It is essential that the operator ensures that all personnel are clear before the defibrillator is discharged.

Synchronized Cardioversion. *Synchronized cardioversion is the therapy of choice for patients with hemodynamically unstable*

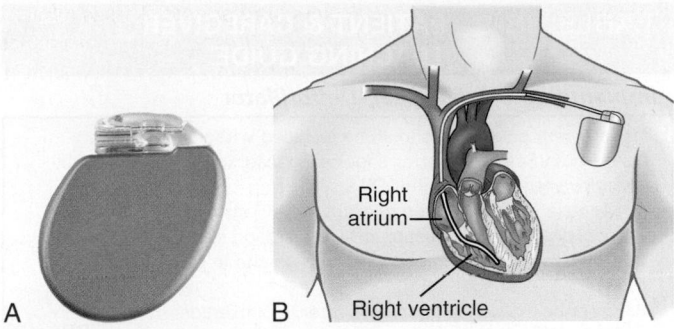

FIGURE 38-22 A, The implantable cardioverter–defibrillator (ICD) pulse generator. **B,** The ICD is placed in a subcutaneous pocket over the pectoral muscle. A single-lead system is placed transvenously from the pulse generator to the endocardium. The single lead detects dysrhythmias and delivers an electric shock to the heart muscle. Source: A, © Can Stock Photo/ CarolinaSmith.

ventricular or supraventricular tachydysrhythmias. A synchronized circuit in the defibrillator is used to deliver a countershock that is programmed to occur on the R wave of the QRS complex. The synchronizer switch must be turned on when cardioversion is planned.

The procedure for synchronized cardioversion is the same as for defibrillation, with the following exceptions. If synchronized cardioversion is performed on a nonemergency basis (i.e., the patient is awake and hemodynamically stable), the patient is sedated (e.g., IV midazolam) before the procedure. Strict attention to maintenance of a patent airway is important in this situation. When a patient with supraventricular tachycardia or VT with a pulse is hemodynamically unstable, synchronized cardioversion is performed as quickly as possible. In addition, the energy needed for synchronized cardioversion is generally less than the energy needed for defibrillation. Energy levels are started at 50 J on a defibrillator and increased (e.g., 100 J, 200 J) if needed.

Implantable Cardioverter–Defibrillator. The implantable cardioverter–defibrillator (ICD) is important technology for patients who (a) have survived SCD, (b) have spontaneous sustained VT, (c) demonstrate syncope with inducible VT or fibrillation during EPS, and (d) are at high risk for future life-threatening dysrhythmias (e.g., have cardiomyopathy). Use of the ICD has significantly decreased cardiac mortality rates among such patients and has added a new dimension to the management of life-threatening dysrhythmias and the prevention of SCD (AHA, 2015).

The ICD consists of a lead system placed via a subclavian vein to the endocardium. A battery-powered pulse generator is implanted subcutaneously, usually over the pectoral muscle on the patient's nondominant side. The pulse generator is similar in size to a cardiac pacemaker. The newest systems are single-lead systems instead of earlier multi-lead or patch systems (Figure 38-22). The ICD sensing system monitors the HR and the rhythm and identifies VT or ventricular fibrillation. Approximately 25 seconds after the sensing system detects a lethal dysrhythmia, the defibrillating mechanism delivers a 25-J or milder shock to the patient's heart. If the first shock is unsuccessful, the generator recycles and can continue to deliver shocks.

In addition to defibrillation capabilities, ICDs are equipped with antitachycardia and antibradycardia pacemakers. These sophisticated devices use dysrhythmia algorithms that detect dysrhythmias and determine the appropriate programmed response.

TABLE 38-9   PATIENT & CAREGIVER TEACHING GUIDE

Implantable Cardioverter–Defibrillator

The following guidelines should be included when teaching the patient and caregiver after undergoing insertion of an implantable cardioverter–defibrillator (ICD):

1. Maintain close follow-up with the physician for testing of ICD function and for inspection of ICD insertion site.
2. Watch for signs of infection at incision site (e.g., redness, swelling, drainage).
3. Keep the incision dry for 1 wk after ICD insertion.
4. Avoid lifting the operative-side arm above the shoulder for 1 wk.
5. Avoid direct blows to ICD site.
6. When travelling by airplane, inform airport security of the presence of the ICD because it may set off the metal detector. If a handheld screening wand is used, it should not be placed directly over the ICD.
7. When the ICD fires:
   - Lie down.
   - If you lose consciousness or if there is repetitive firing, someone should call 911.
   - If you are feeling well and there is repetitive firing, contact your physician's office for ICD interrogation, including battery checks and safety and diagnostic checks.
8. Ensure routine ICD check with interrogator–programmer device, which is needed every 2 to 3 months.
9. Wear a medical alert bracelet at all times.
10. Make sure an information card about the ICD is easily accessible in your wallet.
11. Ensure that your family members learn CPR.
12. Speak with your nurse, who should assist you with the development of positive coping strategies to reduce stress.
13. Avoid large electromagnetic and vibratory forces because they may turn off the device.
14. In general, do not drive until cleared by your physician. The approval to drive is based on the presence of dysrhythmias, the frequency of ICD firings, your overall health, and provincial or territorial laws regarding drivers with ICDs.

CPR, cardiopulmonary resuscitation; *ICD,* implantable cardioverter–defibrillator.

Pacemaker spike

FIGURE 38-23 ECG demonstrating ventricular capture (depolarization) secondary to signal (pacemaker spike) from pacemaker lead in the right ventricle.

A

B   Right ventricle

Right atrium

FIGURE 38-24 A, A dual-chamber rate-responsive pacemaker from Medtronic, Inc., is designed to treat patients with chronic heart problems in which the heart beats too slowly to adequately support the body's circulation needs. **B,** Pacing leads in both the atrium and the ventricle enable a dual-chamber pacemaker to sense and pace in both heart chambers. Source: *A,* © 2017 Medtronic.

These devices can initiate overdrive pacing of supraventricular and ventricular tachycardias, sparing the patient painful defibrillator shocks. They also provide backup pacing for bradydysrhythmias that may occur after defibrillation discharges. Preprocedure and post-procedure nursing care of patients undergoing ICD placement is similar to the care of patients undergoing permanent pacemaker implantation (see pp. 883 to 884).

Education of patients who receive an ICD is of extreme importance. Patients experience a variety of emotions, including fear of body image change, fear of recurrent dysrhythmias, expectation of pain with ICD discharge (described as a feeling of a blow to the chest), and anxiety about going home. Table 38-9 describes the teaching guidelines for the patient with an ICD and the patient's caregivers. Participation in an ICD support group should be encouraged. Online resources for patients with an ICD include support groups and the Sudden Cardiac Arrest Network (see the Resources at the end of Chapter 36.)

Pacemakers

The artificial **cardiac pacemaker** is an electronic device used to pace the heart when the normal conduction pathway is damaged or diseased. The basic pacing circuit consists of a power source (battery-powered pulse generator), one or more conducting leads (pacing leads), and the myocardium. The electrical signal (stimulus) travels from the pacemaker, through the leads, to the wall of the myocardium. The myocardium is "captured" and stimulated to contract (Figure 38-23).

Advances in technology have been applied extensively to pacemakers. This advancement has resulted in sophisticated, noninvasive, programmable single- and dual-chambered pacemakers with specialized circuits. The newer pacemakers are more physiologically accurate, pacing the atrium and one or both of the ventricles (Aehlert, 2013). Pacemakers were initially indicated for symptomatic bradydysrhythmias. However, advances now include pacing for antitachycardia and overdrive pacing. Antitachycardia pacing involves the delivery of a stimulus to the ventricle to terminate tachydysrhythmias (e.g., VT). Overdrive pacing involves pacing the atrium at rates of 200 to 500 impulses per minute in an attempt to terminate atrial tachycardias (e.g., atrial flutter, atrial fibrillation). Multiple other indications for pacemakers have evolved. A permanent pacemaker is one that is implanted totally within the body (Figure 38-24). The permanent pacemaker power source is implanted subcutaneously, usually over the pectoral muscle on the patient's nondominant side. It is attached to pacing leads, which are threaded transvenously to the right atrium and one or both ventricles. Indications for insertion of permanent pacemakers are listed in Table 38-10.

A specialized type of cardiac pacing has been developed for the management of HF. More than 50% of patients with HF have intraventricular conduction delays that cause abnormal ventricular activation and contraction and subsequent asynchrony between the right and left ventricles. This asynchrony can result in reduced systolic function, pump inefficiency, and worsened HF. Cardiac

FIGURE 38-25 Temporary external, dual-chamber demand pacemaker. Source: © 2017 Medtronic.

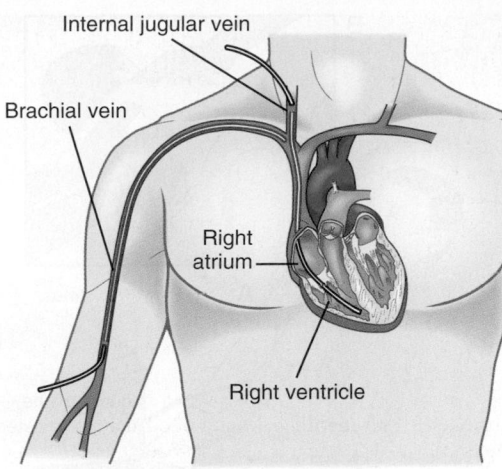

FIGURE 38-26 Temporary transvenous pacemaker catheter insertion. A single lead is positioned in the right ventricle through the brachial, subclavian, jugular, or femoral vein.

TABLE 38-10	INDICATIONS FOR PERMANENT PACEMAKER THERAPY

- Chronic atrial fibrillation with slow ventricular response
- Fibrosis or sclerotic changes of cardiac conduction system
- Hypersensitive carotid sinus syndrome
- Sick sinus syndrome
- Sinus node dysfunction
- Tachydysrhythmias
- Third-degree AV block

TABLE 38-11	INDICATIONS FOR TEMPORARY PACING

- Maintenance of adequate HR and rhythm during special circumstances such as surgery and postoperative recovery, cardiac catheterization, or coronary angioplasty; during drug therapy that may cause bradycardia; and before implantation of a permanent pacemaker
- As prophylaxis after open-heart surgery
- Acute anterior MI with second- or third-degree AV block or bundle-branch block
- Acute inferior MI with symptomatic bradycardia and AV block
- Termination of AV nodal re-entry or reciprocating tachycardia associated with WPW syndrome, atrial flutter, or ventricular tachycardia
- Suppression of ectopic atrial or ventricular rhythm
- EPS to evaluate patient with bradydysrhythmias and tachydysrhythmias

AV, atrioventricular; *EPS*, electrophysiology study; *MI*, myocardial infarction; *WPW*, Wolff–Parkinson–White.

resynchronization therapy (CRT) is a pacing technique that resynchronizes the cardiac cycle by pacing both ventricles, thus promoting improvement in ventricular function. Several devices are available in which CRT is combined with an ICD for maximum therapy. (HF is discussed in Chapter 37.)

Temporary Pacemaker. A temporary pacemaker is one whose power source is outside the body (Figure 38-25). There are three types of temporary pacemakers: transvenous, epicardial, and transcutaneous. Indications for temporary pacing are listed in Table 38-11.

A transvenous pacemaker consists of a lead or leads that are threaded transvenously to the right atrium, the right ventricle, or both and attached to the external power source (Figure 38-26). Most temporary transvenous pacemakers are inserted in critical care units in emergency situations. They are used until a permanent pacemaker can be inserted or the underlying cause of the dysrhythmia has been resolved.

To achieve epicardial pacing, an atrial pacing lead and a ventricular pacing lead are attached to the epicardium during heart surgery. The leads are passed through the chest wall and attached to the external power source. Epicardial pacing leads are placed prophylactically in case any bradydysrhythmias or tachydysrhythmias occur postoperatively.

A transcutaneous pacemaker (TCP) is used to maintain adequate HR and rhythm in an emergency situation. Placement of the transcutaneous pacemaker is a noninvasive procedure, and this pacemaker is used temporarily until a transvenous pacemaker can be inserted or until more definitive therapy is available.

The TCP consists of a power source and a rate- and voltage-control device that is attached to two large, multifunction electrode pads. One pad is positioned on the anterior part of the chest, usually at the V_2 or V_5 lead position, and the other pad is placed on the back between the spine and the left scapula at the level of the heart (Figure 38-27).

Before TCP therapy is initiated, the patient must be told what to expect. The uncomfortable muscle contractions that the pacemaker creates when the current passes through the chest wall should be explained. The patient should be reassured that the therapy is temporary and that the TCP will be replaced with a transvenous pacemaker as soon as possible. Whenever possible, an analgesic, sedative, or both should be provided.

Patient Monitoring. Patients with temporary or permanent pacemakers are monitored by ECG to evaluate the status of the pacemaker. Pacemaker malfunction is manifested primarily by a failure to sense or a failure to capture. *Failure to sense* is the situation in which the pacemaker fails to recognize spontaneous atrial or ventricular activity, and it fires inappropriately. Failure to sense may be caused by pacer lead damage, battery failure, or dislodgement of the electrode. *Failure to capture* is the situation in which the electrical charge to the myocardium is insufficient

FIGURE 38-27 Transcutaneous pacemaker. Pacing electrodes are placed on the patient's anterior **(A)** and posterior **(B)** chest walls and attached to an external pacing unit **(C)**.

TABLE 38-12   PATIENT & CAREGIVER TEACHING GUIDE

Pacemaker

The following guidelines should be included when teaching the patient and caregiver after undergoing insertion of a pacemaker:

1. Maintain follow-up care plan with a physician to check the pacemaker site and begin regular pacemaker function checks with interrogator or programmer device.
2. Watch for signs of infection at incision site, for example, redness, swelling, or drainage.
3. Keep the incision dry for 1 wk after pacemaker implantation.
4. Avoid lifting operative-side arm above shoulder level for 1 wk.
5. Avoid direct blows to generator site.
6. Avoid close proximity to high-output electrical generators or large magnets such as an MRI scanner. These devices can reprogram a pacemaker.
7. Don't be concerned about microwave ovens, which are safe to use and do not threaten pacemaker function.
8. Be aware that you may travel without restrictions. The small metal case of an implanted pacemaker rarely sets off an airport security alarm.
9. Ensure that you are taught how to take your pulse.
10. Carry a pacemaker information card at all times.
11. Watch for return of preimplantation symptoms (i.e., chest pain, excessive sweating, dizziness).

MRI, magnetic resonance imaging.

to produce atrial or ventricular contraction. Failure to capture may also be caused by pacer lead damage, battery failure, or dislodgement of the electrode, as well as by fibrosis at the electrode tip.

Complications of invasive temporary (i.e., transvenous) or permanent pacemaker insertion include infection and hematoma formation at the site of insertion of the pacemaker power source or leads; pneumothorax; failure to sense or capture with possible symptomatic bradycardia; perforation of the atrial or the ventricular septum by the pacing lead; and appearance of "end-of-life" battery parameters when the pacemaker is tested.

Several measures are taken to prevent or assess for complications, including prophylactic IV antibiotic therapy before and after insertion, post-insertion chest radiographic study to check lead placement and to rule out the presence of a pneumothorax; careful observation of insertion site; and continuous ECG monitoring of the patient's rhythm. After pacemaker insertion, the patient is permitted out of bed once the HR and rhythm are stable. Arm and shoulder activity is limited to prevent dislodgement of the newly implanted pacing leads. The nurse observes the insertion site for signs of bleeding and to check that the incision is intact. Any temperature elevation should be noted, and pain at the insertion site should be treated. Most patients are discharged the next day if the HR and rhythm are stable.

The nurse must provide patient teaching in addition to observing for complications after pacemaker insertion. The patient with a newly implanted pacemaker may have questions about activity restrictions and concerns about body image after the procedure. The goal of pacemaker therapy should be to enhance physiological functioning and the quality of life. This should be emphasized to the patient, and the nurse should give specific advice about activity restrictions. Patient and caregiver teaching for the patient with a pacemaker is outlined in Table 38-12.

After discharge, pacemaker function should be checked regularly during outpatient visits to a pacemaker interrogator or programmer or by home monitoring using telephone transmitter devices. Another method to evaluate pacemaker performance is noninvasive program stimulation, which is done on an outpatient basis in the electrophysiology laboratory.

Radiofrequency Ablation Therapy

Radiofrequency ablation (RFA) therapy is a relatively new development in the area of antidysrhythmia therapy. Radiofrequency energy (produced by a low-voltage, high-frequency form of electrical energy) is used to "burn" or ablate areas of the conduction system as definitive treatment of tachydysrhythmias.

Ablation therapy is performed after EPS has identified the source of the dysrhythmia. An electrode-tipped ablation catheter is used to ablate accessory pathways or ectopic sites in the atria, the AV node, and the ventricles. Catheter ablation is considered the nonpharmacological treatment of choice for AV nodal re-entrant tachycardia or for re-entrant tachycardia related to accessory bypass tracts, and to control the ventricular response of certain tachydysrhythmias. In some cases of uncontrolled ventricular response in atrial fibrillation or of atrial flutter that is unresponsive to medical therapy, the AV node or bundle of His may be ablated completely. If this is done, the patient must have a permanent pacemaker inserted at the same time. The ablation procedure is a successful therapy with a low complication rate. Care of the patient undergoing ablation therapy is similar to that of a patient undergoing cardiac catheterization (see Chapter 34).

ELECTROCARDIOGRAPHIC CHANGES ASSOCIATED WITH ACUTE CORONARY SYNDROME

The 12-lead ECG is the primary diagnostic tool used to evaluate patients receiving care for acute coronary syndrome (ACS). Many treatment decisions are directed by the ECG changes that occur with ACS. These definitive changes are in response to ischemia, injury, or infarction of myocardial cells and are detected in the leads that face the area of involvement (Figure 38-28). Reciprocal (opposite) ECG changes are often detected in the leads facing opposite the area involved in ACS. In addition, the pattern of

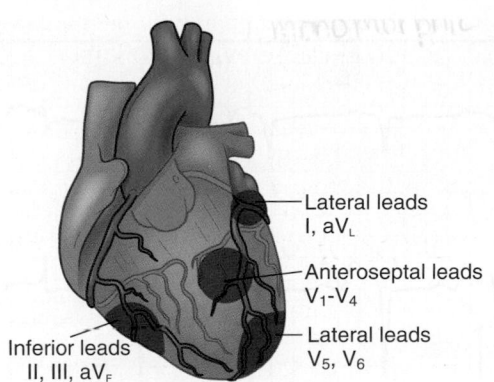

FIGURE 38-28 Diagram showing where leads detect ECG changes. Definitive ECG changes occur in leads that face the area of ischemia, injury, or infarction. Reciprocal changes may occur in leads facing opposite the area of ischemia, injury, or infarction.

FIGURE 38-29 Diagrams of changes in ST segment, T wave, and Q wave in association with myocardial ischemia **(A)**, injury **(B)**, and infarction **(C)**.

ECG changes provides information on the coronary artery involved in ACS (Table 38-13).

Ischemia

Typical ECG changes that are seen in myocardial ischemia include ST-segment depression, T-wave inversion, or both (Figure 38-29, A). ST-segment depression is significant if it is at least 1 mm (one small box) below the isoelectric line (see Figure 38-5). The isoelectric line is flat and represents the normal times in the cardiac cycle when the ECG is not recording any electrical activity in the heart. These times are as follows: (a) from the end of the P wave to the start of the QRS complex, (b) the entire ST segment, and (c) from the end of the T wave to the start of the next P wave (see Figure 38-9). ST-segment depression, T-wave inversion, or both occur in response to the electrical disturbance in the myocardial cells that is caused by an inadequate supply of blood and oxygen. Once the cause of the disturbance is treated (adequate blood flow is restored), the ECG changes resolve, and the ECG returns to the patient's baseline. (See Chapter 36 for a complete discussion of ACS.)

Injury and Infarction

Myocardial injury represents a stage of worsening ischemia that is potentially reversible but may evolve to infarction (necrosis) of myocardial cells. The typical ECG change seen during injury

TABLE 38-13	ECG EVIDENCE AND ASSOCIATED CORONARY ARTERY IN ACUTE CORONARY SYNDROME		
Area of Involvement of Left Ventricle	**ECG Evidence**		
	Leads Facing Area	**Leads Opposite Area**	**Associated Coronary Artery**
Septal wall	V_1, V_2	II, III, aV_F	Left anterior descending
Anterior wall	V_2, V_3, V_4	II, III, aV_F	Left anterior descending
Lateral wall, low	V_5, V_6	II, III, aV_F	Left anterior descending or circumflex
Lateral wall, high	I, aV_L	II, III, aV_F	Circumflex
Inferior wall	II, III, aV_F	I, aV_L, V_5, V_6	Right coronary artery

is ST-segment elevation. ST-segment elevation is significant if it is at least 1 mm above the isoelectric line (see Figure 38-29, B). If treatment is prompt and effective, it is possible to restore oxygen to the myocardium and avoid infarction. Avoidance of infarction is confirmed by the absence of serum cardiac markers. If serum cardiac markers are present, infarction has occurred and is referred to as an *ST-segment–elevation myocardial infarction* (STEMI).

In addition to ST-segment elevation, a pathological Q wave may be seen on the ECG with infarction (see Figure 38-29, C). A physiological Q wave is the first negative deflection (wave) after the P wave (see Figure 38-9). It is normally very small and narrow (<0.04 seconds in duration). A pathological Q wave that develops during infarction is deep and more than 0.03 seconds in duration. If it does appear, it indicates that at least half the thickness of the heart wall is involved, which is referred to as a *Q-wave MI* (Aehlert, 2013). The pathological Q wave may be present on the ECG indefinitely.

T-wave inversion related to infarction occurs within hours after an infarction and may persist for months. The ECG changes seen in injury and infarction reflect electrical disturbances in the myocardial cells that are caused by a prolonged lack of blood and oxygen leading to necrosis (Figure 38-30).

Patient Monitoring

Monitoring guidelines for patients with suspected ACS include continuous, multi-lead ECG and ST-segment monitoring (Pelter et al., 2014). The leads selected for monitoring should minimally include the leads that reflect the area of ischemia, injury, or infarction.

SYNCOPE

Syncope—a brief lapse in consciousness accompanied by a loss in postural tone (fainting)—is a common diagnosis in the emergency department and the hospital. The causes of syncope can be categorized as cardiovascular or noncardiovascular. The most common cardiovascular causes of syncope include (a) neuro-cardiogenic syncope or "vasovagal" syncope (e.g., carotid sinus sensitivity) and (b) primary cardiac dysrhythmias (e.g., tachycardias, bradycardias). Other causes can be related to

FIGURE 38-30 ECG findings with anteroseptal lateral wall myocardial infarction. Normally, leads I, aV$_L$, and V$_1$ to V$_3$ have a positive R wave. Note the pathological Q waves in these leads and the ST-segment elevation in leads V$_2$ to V$_5$ *(arrows)*.

prosthetic valve malfunction, pulmonary emboli, aortic dissection, and hypertrophic cardiomyopathy. Noncardiovascular causes are varied and can include hypoglycemia, hysteria, unwitnessed seizure, and vertebrobasilar transient ischemic attack (Jarvis et al., 2013).

A diagnostic workup for a patient with syncope from a suspected cardiac cause begins with ruling out structural or ischemic heart disease or both. This is done with echocardiography and stress testing. In older-adult patients, who are more likely to have ischemic and structural heart disease, EPS is used to diagnose atrial and ventricular tachydysrhythmias, as well as conduction system disease causing bradydysrhythmias, all of which can cause syncope. These problems can be treated with antidysrhythmia drug therapy, pacemakers, ICDs, catheter ablation therapy, or a combination.

In patients without structural heart disease or in whom the results of EPS testing are not diagnostic, head-upright tilt-table testing may be performed. Normally, an upright position results in gravity displacing 300 to 800 mL of blood to the lower extremities. Specialized nerve fibres called *mechanoreceptors* are located throughout the vascular system. These receptors respond to the increased blood volume by initiating a reflex increase in sympathetic stimulation and decrease in parasympathetic output. The end results are slight increases in HR and diastolic BP and a slight decrease in systolic BP.

In neuro-cardiogenic syncope, the increase in venous pooling that occurs in the upright position reduces venous return to the heart. This results in a sudden, compensatory increase in ventricular contraction. This reaction is misinterpreted by the

brain as a hypertensive state, and sympathetic stimulation is consequently withdrawn. This produces a paradoxical vasodilation and bradycardia (vasovagal response). The end results are bradycardia, hypotension, cerebral hypoperfusion, and syncope.

In the head-upright tilt-table test, the patient is placed supine on a table and supported by belts across the torso and the feet. Baseline ECG, BP, and HR are obtained in the horizontal position. Next, the table is tilted 60 to 80 degrees, and the patient is maintained in this upright position for 20 to 60 minutes. The ECG and HR are recorded continuously, and BP is measured every 3 minutes throughout the test. In healthy individuals, venous pooling activates the mechanoreceptors, resulting in the normal response just described.

If the patient's BP and HR responses are abnormal and clinical symptoms are reproduced (e.g., faintness), the test result is considered positive. If after 30 minutes there is no response, the table is returned to the horizontal position and an intravenous infusion of low-dose isoproterenol may be started in an attempt to provoke a response. Neuro-cardiogenic syncope that recurs frequently and interferes with normal activities can be treated with a variety of drugs (e.g., metoprolol).

Other diagnostic tests for syncope include various recording devices. Holter monitors and event monitors are used and are discussed in this chapter and Chapter 34. A subcutaneously implanted loop-recording device can also be used to record the ECG during presyncopal and syncopal events. The device can be interrogated after a syncopal event in order to determine the ECG rhythm at the time of the event.

CASE STUDY

Dysrhythmia

Source: © elbud/ Shutterstock .com.

Patient Profile

Jacob Singer, a 68-year-old retired postal worker, is admitted to the cardiac care unit after cardiac arrest. Defibrillation was performed by paramedics at his home. Mr. Singer is awake and lethargic but responding appropriately.

Subjective Data
- Has had two MIs and a history of HF
- Has shortness of breath, even in a sitting position

Objective Data

Physical Examination
- Appears anxious
- BP 92/60 mm Hg, pulse 98/min, respirations 28/min
- Lungs: bilateral coarse crackles
- Heart: S₃ gallop at apex

Diagnostic Studies
- ECG: frequent PVCs
- Echocardiogram: severe left ventricular dysfunction with ejection fraction (EF) of 20%
- Serum potassium level: 2.9 mmol/L

Collaborative Care
- Amiodarone infusion
- Scheduled for electrophysiology study (EPS)

Discussion Questions
1. Why is Mr. Singer at risk for ventricular fibrillation?
2. Why is amiodarone used after ventricular fibrillation?
3. What methods may be used to assess the effectiveness of an antidysrhythmia drug?
4. Would Mr. Singer be a candidate for an ICD?
5. If ventricular fibrillation recurred while Mr. Singer was receiving amiodarone infusion, what other IV medications would be tried?
6. What is the significance of the serum potassium value?
7. **Priority decision:** On the basis of these nursing diagnoses, what are the priority nursing interventions for Mr. Singer?
8. **Evidence-informed practice:** Once Mr. Singer is stable, he is scheduled for the insertion of a CRT/ICD. On the nurse's rounds, he asks why he needs two devices.

🅔volve

Answers are available at *http://evolve.elsevier.com/Canada/Lewis/medsurg.*

REVIEW QUESTIONS

The number of the question corresponds to the same-numbered objective at the beginning of the chapter.

1. A client with a stable blood pressure and no symptoms has the following ECG characteristics: atrial rate, 74 beats/minute and regular; ventricular rate, 62 beats/minute and irregular; P wave, normal contour; PR interval, lengthens progressively until a P wave is not conducted; QRS complex, normal contour. What would be the appropriate treatment for this rhythm?
   a. Epinephrine, 1 mg IV push
   b. Isoproterenol, IV continuous drip
   c. Immediate insertion of a temporary pacemaker
   d. Careful observation for signs of further heart block

2. The nurse is monitoring the ECG of a client admitted with ACS. Which of the following ECG characteristics would be most suggestive of ischemia?
   a. Sinus rhythm with a pathological Q wave
   b. Sinus rhythm with an elevated ST segment
   c. Sinus rhythm with a depressed ST segment
   d. Sinus rhythm with premature atrial contractions

3. The cardiac monitor of a client in the cardiac care unit after an acute myocardial infarction indicates ventricular bigeminy. What would be the most appropriate intervention from the following list?
   a. Performing defibrillation
   b. Treatment with intravenous amiodarone
   c. Insertion of a temporary pacemaker
   d. Continuing to monitor and attempt to determine the underlying cause

4. How does defibrillation differ from cardioversion?
   a. Defibrillation requires a greater dose of electrical current.
   b. Defibrillation is synchronized to countershock during the QRS complex.
   c. Cardioversion is indicated only for treatment of atrial tachydysrhythmias.
   d. Cardioversion may be done on a nonemergency basis with sedation of the client.

5. Which client teaching points should the nurse include when providing discharge instructions to a client with a new permanent pacemaker and the caregiver? *(Select all that apply)*
   a. Avoid or limit air travel.
   b. Take and record a daily pulse rate.
   c. Obtain and wear a medical alert bracelet at all times.
   d. Avoid lifting the arm on the side of the pacemaker above shoulder height.
   e. Avoid microwave ovens because they interfere with pacemaker function.

6. Which of the following is true when the client has an implantable cardiac defibrillator?
   a. Antidysrhythmia drugs can be discontinued.
   b. All members of the client's family should learn CPR.
   c. The client should not drive until the physician approves it after the ICD has been implanted.
   d. The client is usually relieved to have the device implanted to prevent dysrhythmias.

7. Which of the following would be essential to teach a client about before electrophysiological monitoring?
   a. A catheter will be placed in each of the femoral arteries to allow double-catheter use.
   b. The client will be given a general anaesthetic to prevent the awareness of "near-death" experiences.
   c. Ventricular tachycardia and ventricular fibrillation may be induced and treated during the procedure.
   d. The procedure is used to "burn" or ablate areas of the conduction system that are causing tachydysrhythmias.

1. d; 2. c; 3. d; 4. d; 5. b, c, d; 6. c; 7. d.

🅔volve

For even more review questions, visit *http://evolve.elsevier.com/Canada/ Lewis/medsurg.*

REFERENCES

Aehlert, B. (2013). *ECGs made easy* (5th ed.). St. Louis: Mosby.

American Heart Association. (2015). 2015 American Heart Association Guidelines for cardiopulmonary resuscitation and emergency cardiovascular care science. *Circulation, 122*(18), S639. doi:10.1161/CIR.0b013e3181fdf7aa.

Canadian Cardiovascular Society. (2011). Canadian Cardiovascular Society atrial fibrillation guidelines 2010. *Canadian Journal of Cardiology, 27*(2011), 27–97. doi:10.1016/j.cjca.2010.11.003.

Goldsworthy, S. (2016). *Compact clinical guide to arrhythmia and 12-lead EKG interpretation.* New York, NY: Springer.

Greenberg, M. L., & Chandrakantan, A. (2015). *Catheter ablation.* New York: eMedicine. Retrieved from *http://www.emedicine.com/med/topic2957.htm.*

Heart and Stroke Foundation. (2012). *Public access defibrillation (PAD) programs.* Retrieved from *http://restart.heartandstroke.ca/public-access-defibrillation-pad-programs.*

Heart and Stroke Foundation. (2017). *Atrial Fibrillation* Retrieved from *https://www.heartandstroke.ca/heart/conditions/atrial-fibrillation.*

Jarvis, C., Browne, A. J., MacDonald-Jenkins, J., et al. (2013). *Physical Examination and Health Assessment* (2nd ed.). St. Louis: Elsevier.

Lehne, R. (2016). *Pharmacology for nursing care* (9th ed.). St. Louis: Elsevier.

Pelter, M. M., Kozik, T. M., Al-Zaiti, S. S., and Carey, M. G. (2014). Acute coronary syndrome ST-segment monitoring. *American Journal of Critical Care, 23*(6), 503–504. doi:10.4037/ajcc2014847.

Stiell, I. G., Macle, L., & CCS Atrial Fibrillation Guidelines Committee. (2011). Canadian Cardiovascular Society Atrial Fibrillation Guidelines 2010: Management of Recent-Onset Atrial Fibrillation and Flutter in the Emergency Department. *Canadian Journal of Cardiology, 27*(1), 38–46.

RESOURCES

Resources for this chapter are listed in Chapter 36.

Nursing Management

Inflammatory and Structural Heart Disorders

Written by: Nancy Kupper and De Ann F. Mitchell
Adapted by: Sheila Rizza

⊜volve WEBSITE

http://evolve.elsevier.com/Canada/Lewis/medsurg

- Review Questions (Online Only)
- Key Points
- Answer Guidelines for Case Study
- Student Case Study
  - Rheumatic Fever and Heart Disease
- Conceptual Care Map Creator
- Supporting Media—Audio
  - Pericardial Friction Rub
- Customizable Nursing Care Plans
  - Infective Endocarditis
  - Valvular Heart Disease
- Audio Glossary
- Content Updates

LEARNING OBJECTIVES

1. Describe the etiology, pathophysiology, and clinical manifestations of infective endocarditis and pericarditis.
2. Discuss the collaborative care and nursing management of infective endocarditis and pericarditis.
3. Explain the importance of prophylactic antibiotic therapy in infective endocarditis.
4. Explain the etiology and clinical manifestations of myocarditis, along with the collaborative care and nursing management of patients with myocarditis.
5. Describe the etiology, pathophysiology, and clinical manifestations of rheumatic fever and rheumatic heart disease.
6. Discuss the collaborative care and nursing management of patients with rheumatic fever and rheumatic heart disease.
7. Identify the etiologies of congenital and acquired valvular heart diseases.
8. Discuss the pathophysiology and clinical manifestations of the various types of valvular heart problems and the diagnostic studies used in connection with them.
9. Describe the collaborative care and nursing management of patients with valvular heart disease.
10. Describe surgical interventions used in management of patients with valvular heart problems.
11. Describe the pathophysiology and clinical manifestations of the different types of cardiomyopathies.
12. Discuss the nursing care and collaborative management of patients with different types of cardiomyopathies.

KEY TERMS

acute rheumatic fever (ARF) p. 898
aortic stenosis, p. 904
aortic valve regurgitation (AR), p. 904
Aschoff bodies, p. 899
cardiac tamponade, p. 895

cardiomyopathy, p. 908
dilated cardiomyopathy (DCM), p. 909
endomyocardial biopsy (EMB), p. 898
hypertrophic cardiomyopathy (HCM), p. 910

infective endocarditis (IE), p. 889
Janeway's lesions, p. 892
mitral valve prolapse (MVP), p. 903
myocarditis, p. 897
Osler's nodes, p. 892

pericardial effusion, p. 895
pericardial friction rub, p. 895
pericardiocentesis, p. 897
pericarditis, p. 894
regurgitation, p. 901
rheumatic fever, p. 898
rheumatic heart disease, p. 898

INFLAMMATORY DISORDERS OF THE HEART

INFECTIVE ENDOCARDITIS

Infective endocarditis (IE), previously known as *bacterial endocarditis*, is an infection of the heart valves or the endocardial surface of the heart. The name of this disorder has changed because it is now recognized that organisms other than bacteria may cause the disease (Heart and Stroke Foundation of Canada, 2017a). The endocardium, the inner layer of the heart (Figure 39-1), is contiguous with the valves of the heart. Therefore, inflammation from IE affects the cardiac valves.

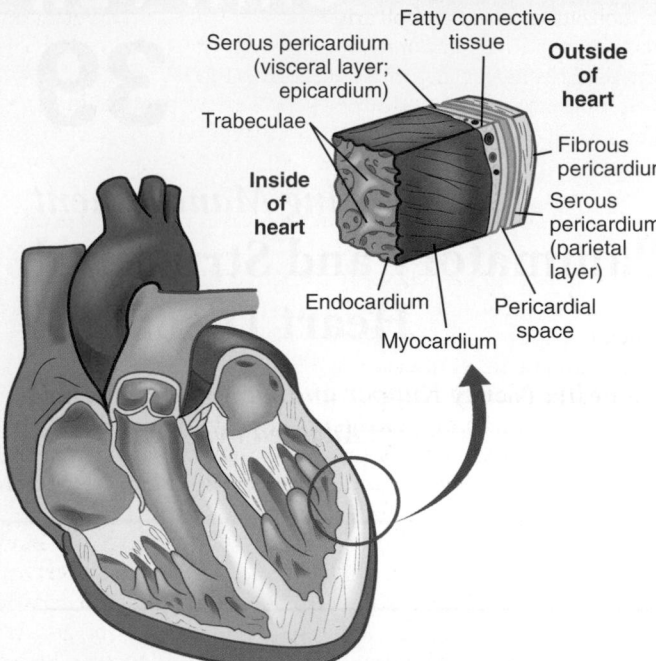

FIGURE 39-1 Layers of the heart muscle and pericardium. Source: Adapted from Patton, K. T., & Thibodeau, G. A. (2014). *The human body in health and disease* (6th ed., p. 371). St Louis: Mosby.

Before the era of antibiotics, IE was almost always fatal. The advent of penicillin therapy changed the prognosis dramatically, and mortality rates decreased appreciably.

Classification

Four different categories of IE describe the site of infection, the presence of cardiovascular devices, and how the individual acquired the infection: left-sided native valve IE, left-sided prosthetic valve IE, right-sided IE (includes intravenous [IV] drug use), and intracardiac and intravascular devices (e.g., pacemaker/defibrillator wires, hemodialysis). IE is identified as being community-acquired IE or health care–associated IE (Habib, Lancellotti, Antunes, et al., 2015; Que & Moreillon, 2011).

Etiology and Pathophysiology

The most common causative organisms of IE, *Staphylococcus aureus,* oral *Streptococcus,* and *Enterococci* are Gram-positive bacterial organisms responsible for more than 80% of IE cases (Table 39-1). Other possible pathogens include fungi and viruses. Newly identified pathogens, which are difficult to cultivate (e.g., *Bartonella, Tropheryma whippelii*), have been found to cause IE. Resistant organisms (e.g., methicillin-resistant *S. aureus*) also cause IE and are challenging conventional antibiotic therapy (Que & Moreillon, 2011; Baddour, Wilson, Bayer, et al., 2015).

IE occurs when blood flow turbulence within the heart allows the causative organism to infect previously damaged valves or other endothelial surfaces. It can occur in individuals with a variety of underlying cardiac conditions. The principal risk factors for IE are prior endocarditis, prosthetic valves, acquired valvular disease, and cardiac lesions. Several noncardiac conditions and procedures also can allow large numbers of organisms to enter the bloodstream and initiate the infectious process (Tables 39-2 and 39-3).

TABLE 39-1   CAUSATIVE ORGANISMS ASSOCIATED WITH INFECTIVE ENDOCARDITIS

Bacteria
- *Bartonella quintana*
- *Chlamydiae*
- Coagulase-negative staphylococci
- *Enterococci*
- HACEK group (*Haemophilus, Actinobacillus, Cardiobacterium, Eikenella, Kingella* species)
- Methicillin-resistant *Staphylococcus aureus*
- Vancomycin-resistant *S. aureus*
- *Rickettsiae*
- *S. aureus*
- *Staphylococcus epidermidis*
- *Streptococcus bovis*
- Groups A, B, and C streptococci
- *Streptococcus pneumoniae*
- Viridans streptococci
- *Tropheryma whippelii*

Fungi
- *Candida albicans*
- *Candida parapsilosis*
- *Aspergillus*

Viruses
- Coxsackievirus B

TABLE 39-2   PREDISPOSING CONDITIONS FOR THE DEVELOPMENT OF INFECTIVE ENDOCARDITIS

Cardiac Conditions
- Prior endocarditis
- Prosthetic valves
- Cardiac valvulopathy in cardiac transplant recipients
- Rheumatic heart disease (e.g., mitral valve regurgitation)
- Unrepaired cyanotic congenital heart disease, including palliative shunts and conduits
- Repaired congenital heart defect with prosthetic material or device, surgically or through catheterization, during the first 6 months when endothelialization occurs

Noncardiac Conditions
- Intravenous drug abuse
- Hospital-acquired bacteremia

Procedure-Associated Risks
- Intravascular devices (e.g., hemodialysis catheters)
- Procedures listed in Table 39-3

TABLE 39-3   PROCEDURES NECESSITATING ANTIBIOTIC PROPHYLAXIS TO PREVENT INFECTIVE ENDOCARDITIS*

Oropharyngeal
- All dental procedures likely to produce gingival or mucosal bleeding (not simple adjustment of orthodontic appliances or shedding of deciduous teeth), including professional cleaning
- Tonsillectomy or adenoidectomy

Respiratory
- Surgical procedures or biopsy involving respiratory mucosa

Integument
- Procedures on infected skin, skin structures, or musculo-skeletal tissues with incision of the tissue
- Prophylactic administration of antimicrobial agents to prevent infective endocarditis in patients undergoing genito-urinary or gastro-intestinal procedures no longer recommended (Baddour, Wilson, Bayer, et al., 2015)

*This table lists select procedures but is not all-inclusive.

Vegetations, the primary lesions of IE, consist of fibrin, leukocytes, platelets, and microbes that adhere to the valve surface or the endocardium (Figure 39-2). The loss of portions of these friable vegetations into the circulation results in *emboli.* As many as 22% to 50% of patients with IE will experience systemic

FIGURE 39-2 Bacterial endocarditis of the mitral valve. The valve is covered with large, irregular vegetations (*arrow*). Source: Damjanov, I., & Linder, J. (2000). *Pathology: A color atlas.* St. Louis: Mosby.

embolization. These emboli arise from left-sided heart vegetations and progress to various organs (particularly the brain, the kidneys, and the spleen), causing infarction, and to the extremities, causing limb infarction. Right-sided heart lesions embolize to the lungs. The risk of embolization is greatest within the first few days of commencing antimicrobial therapy (Habib, Lancellotti, Antunes, et al., 2015).

The infection may spread locally to cause damage to the valves or to their supporting structures. This damage results in dysrhythmias, valvular incompetence, and eventual invasion of the myocardium, leading to heart failure (HF), sepsis, and heart block (Figure 39-3).

Rheumatic heart disease was, at one time, the most common cause of IE; it now accounts for fewer than 20% of cases. Currently, the main contributing factors include (1) degenerative valve sclerosis; (2) recreational IV drug use; (3) use of prosthetic valves; (4) proliferation of intravascular device placement, resulting in health care–associated infections; and (5) renal dialysis (Habib, Lancellotti, Antunes, et al., 2015). Left-sided endocarditis is more common in patients with bacterial infections and underlying heart disease. The primary cause of right-sided endocarditis is IV use of illicit drugs. However, the incidence of affected left-sided valves has increased, especially with cocaine abuse. *S. aureus* is the most common causative organism in IV drug use IE.

PATHOPHYSIOLOGY MAP

Damage to endothelial surface from anatomic or traumatic changes

Primary focus of infection from causative organisms adhering to valve surface

Bacteria   Fungi   Viruses

Left-sided heart embolizations

Formation of vegetations consisting of fibrin, leukocytes, platelets, and microbes on valve surface and endocardium

Right-sided heart embolizations

Brain   Limb   Kidney   Liver   Spleen

Management with antibiotics

Local valve damage

Lungs

Healing

Infiltration to supporting structures

Sepsis   Heart failure   Heart block

FIGURE 39-3 Pathogenesis of infective endocarditis.

Clinical Manifestations

The findings in IE are nonspecific and can involve multiple organ systems. Low-grade fever occurs in more than 90% of patients but may be absent in older adults and in immuno-compromised patients. Other nonspecific manifestations include chills, weakness, malaise, fatigue, and anorexia. Arthralgias, myalgias, back pain, abdominal discomfort, weight loss, headache, and clubbing of fingers may occur in subacute forms of endocarditis.

Vascular manifestations of IE include *splinter hemorrhages* (longitudinal black streaks) that occur in the nail beds. Petechiae may occur as a result of fragmentation and microembolization of vegetative lesions and are common in the conjunctivae, the lips, the buccal mucosa, and the palate, and over the ankles, the feet, and the antecubital and popliteal areas. Osler's nodes (painful, tender, red or purple, pea-size lesions that last 1 to 2 days) may be found on the fingertips or the toes. Janeway's lesions (flat, painless, small, red spots) may be found on the palms and the soles. Funduscopic examination may reveal hemorrhagic retinal lesions called *Roth's spots.*

The onset of a new or changing murmur is noted in most patients with IE, with the aortic and mitral valves most commonly affected. The mitral murmur of endocarditis is generally a mid-to-late systolic regurgitant type. The aortic murmur may be early diastolic. Murmurs are often absent in tricuspid endocarditis because right-sided heart pressures are too low to be heard. HF is observed in 42% to 60% of patients with IE, more often in those with aortic valve endocarditis (29%) than in patients with mitral valve endocarditis (20%) (Habib, Lancellotti, Antunes, et al., 2015).

Clinical manifestations secondary to embolization in various body organs may also be present. Embolization to the spleen may result in sharp, left upper quadrant pain and splenomegaly. Local tenderness and abdominal rigidity may be present. Embolization to the kidneys may cause pain in the flank, hematuria, and azotemia. Emboli may lodge in small peripheral blood vessels of the arms and legs and may cause gangrene. Embolization to the brain may cause neurological problems such as hemiplegia, ataxia, aphasia, visual changes, and change in the level of consciousness. Pulmonary emboli may occur in right-sided endocarditis.

Diagnostic Studies

Obtaining the patient's recent health history is important in assessing IE. Inquiry should be made regarding any recent (within the past 3–6 months) dental, urological, surgical, or gynecological procedures, including normal or abnormal obstetrical delivery. Previous history of use of illicit IV drugs, previous valvular or congenital heart disease, intracardiac prosthetic device, recent cardiac catheterization, and skin, respiratory, or urinary tract infections should be documented.

Laboratory data, especially blood cultures, should also be assessed. Two blood cultures drawn 60 minutes apart will be positive in more than 90% of patients. Culture-negative endocarditis is often associated with antibiotic usage within the previous 2 weeks or caused by a pathogen not easily detected by standard culture procedures (e.g., *Bartonella* species). Negative cultures should be kept for 3 weeks if the clinical diagnosis remains endocarditis because of the possibility that a slow-growing causative organism may be detected.

A mild leukocytosis occurs in acute endocarditis (but is uncommon in the subacute form), with average white blood cell (WBC) counts ranging from 10 to 11×10^9/L. The erythrocyte

TABLE 39-4	COLLABORATIVE CARE

Cardiac Conditions Necessitating Antibiotic Prophylaxis to Prevent Infective Endocarditis*

- Prosthetic cardiac valves
- History of endocarditis
- Surgically constructed systemic–pulmonary shunts
- Complex cyanotic congenital heart disease
- Vascular grafts (first 6 mo after implantation)
- Cardiac transplantation requiring valvulopathy

*This table lists common cardiac conditions associated with high risk for infective endocarditis but is not all-inclusive.
Source: Habib, G., Lancellotti, P, Antunes, M., et al. (2015). Guidelines for the management of infective endocarditis. *European Heart Journal, 36*(44), 3075–3128. doi:10.1093/eurheartj/ehv319

sedimentation rate (ESR) and C-reactive protein (CRP) levels may be elevated.

Echocardiography is valuable in the diagnostic workup for a patient with IE when the blood cultures are negative or for the patient who is a surgical candidate and has an active infection. Transesophageal echocardiograms and digital imaging using two-dimensional transthoracic echocardiograms can detect vegetation, destructive lesions, and abscesses on valves (Habib, Lancellotti, Antunes, et al., 2015). A chest radiograph is done to detect the presence of *cardiomegaly* (an enlarged heart). An electrocardiogram (ECG) may show first- or second-degree atrioventricular (AV) block because the cardiac valves lie in proximity to cardiac conductive tissue, especially the AV node. Cardiac catheterization may be used to evaluate coronary artery patency and valvular function when surgical intervention is being considered for patients with IE.

Collaborative Care

Prophylactic Treatment. Antibiotic prophylaxis is recommended for patients with specific cardiac conditions before they undergo certain dental or surgical procedures (Baddour, Wilson, Bayer et al., 2015; Habib, Lancellotti, Antunes, et al., 2015). Procedures for which endocarditis prophylaxis is recommended are summarized in Table 39-4. Specific antibiotic regimens are recommended for dental procedures that require manipulation of the gingival or periapical region of the teeth or perforation of the oral mucosa and respiratory tract. Current guidelines suggest that routine activities of oral hygiene contribute to bacteremia that may result in IE (Habib, Lancellotti, Antunes, et al., 2015).

Drug Therapy. Accurate identification of the infecting organism is the key to successful treatment of IE. Long-term treatment is necessary to kill dormant bacteria clustered within the valvular vegetations. Complete eradication of the organism generally takes weeks to achieve, and relapses are common. Initially, patients are hospitalized and IV antibiotic therapy is started. Table 39-5 outlines suggested antibiotic regimens for patients with IE from various causative organisms and with different clinical circumstances.

Subsequent blood cultures may be performed to evaluate the effectiveness of antibiotic therapy. Blood cultures that remain positive indicate inadequate or inappropriate antibiotic administration, aortic root or myocardial abscess, or the wrong diagnosis (e.g., an infection elsewhere). Serum antibiotic drug levels are often monitored to establish therapeutic dosages. Finally, renal function is monitored when antibiotics are used that are

TABLE 39-5   **DRUG THERAPY**

Treatment of Infective Endocarditis With Outpatient Antibiotic Therapy*

Causative Agent	Antibiotic Regimen Options
Streptococcal endocarditis involving native valve	IV penicillin G or IV or IM ceftriaxone; IV penicillin G or IV or IM ceftriaxone plus IV or IM gentamicin; or IV vancomycin (Vancocin)
Enterococcal endocarditis involving native or prosthetic valve	IV ampicillin plus IV or IM gentamicin; or IV penicillin G plus IV or IM gentamicin; or IV vancomycin plus IV or IM gentamicin
Staphylococcal endocarditis in absence of prosthetic materials	IV cloxacillin or IV cefazolin for penicillin allergy
Fungal endocarditis in native or prosthetic valves	IV amphotericin B (Fungizone)

IM, intramuscular; *IV,* intravenous.
*This table lists common drug regimens but is not all-inclusive.

nephrotoxic (e.g., vancomycin [Vancocin]) and for patients with poor kidney function.

Fungal infection and prosthetic valve endocarditis (PVE) are most frequently observed in IV drug users and immuno-compromised patients and respond poorly to antibiotic therapy alone. Early prolonged (≥6 weeks) drug therapy is recommended in these situations (Habib, Lancellotti, Antunes, et al., 2015). Valve replacement has become an important adjunct procedure in the management of IE. It is used in more than 25% of cases. (Valve replacement is discussed later in this chapter.)

Fever may persist for 5 to 10 days after treatment has been started and can be treated with acetylsalicylic acid (ASA; Aspirin), acetaminophen (Tylenol), ibuprofen (Motrin), fluids, and rest. Complete bed rest is usually not indicated unless the temperature remains elevated or there are signs of HF. Endocarditis coupled with HF responds poorly to both drug therapy and valve replacement and is often life-threatening.

NURSING MANAGEMENT INFECTIVE ENDOCARDITIS

NURSING ASSESSMENT
Subjective and objective data that should be obtained from a patient with IE are presented in Table 39-6. Heart sounds should be assessed together with vital signs to detect a murmur or a change in the character of a pre-existing murmur and the presence of extradiastolic sounds.

Arthralgia is common, may involve multiple joints, and may be accompanied by myalgias. The patient should be assessed for joint tenderness, decreased range of motion, and muscle tenderness. The oral mucosa, conjunctivae, upper chest, and lower extremities should be examined for petechiae. A general systems assessment should be completed to facilitate recognition of hemodynamic and embolic complications.

NURSING DIAGNOSES
Nursing diagnoses for the patient with IE may include but are not limited to the following:

TABLE 39-6   **NURSING ASSESSMENT**

Infective Endocarditis

Subjective Data
Important Health Information
Past health history: Valvular, congenital, or syphilitic cardiac disease (including valve repair or replacement); previous endocarditis, childbirth, staphylococcal or streptococcal infections, health care–associated bacteremia
Medications: Immuno-suppressive therapy, recreational IV drug use
Surgery or other treatments: Recent obstetrical or gynecological procedures; invasive techniques including catheterization, cystoscopy, intravascular procedures; recent dental or surgical procedure; GI procedures (endoscopy)

Symptoms
- Exercise intolerance, generalized weakness, fatigue, malaise
- Cough, dyspnea on exertion, orthopnea
- Palpitations, night sweats
- Chest, back, or abdominal pain
- Headache, joint tenderness, muscle tenderness
- Weight gain or loss; anorexia
- Chills, diaphoresis
- Bloody urine

Objective Data
General
Fever

Integumentary
Osler's nodes on extremities; splinter hemorrhages under nail beds; Janeway's lesions on palms and soles; petechiae of skin, mucous membranes, or conjunctivae; purpura; peripheral edema, finger clubbing

Respiratory
Tachypnea, crackles

Cardiovascular
Dysrhythmias, tachycardia, new or enhanced murmurs, S_3, S_4, retinal hemorrhages

Possible Findings
Leukocytosis, anemia, ↑ ESR, ↑ CRP and cardiac enzymes; positive blood cultures; microscopic hematuria; echocardiogram showing chamber enlargement, valvular dysfunction, and vegetations; chest radiograph showing cardiomegaly and pulmonary infiltrates; ECG demonstrating ischemia and conduction defects, signs of systemic embolization or pulmonary embolism

CRP, C-reactive protein; *ECG,* electrocardiogram; *ESR,* erythrocyte sedimentation rate; *GI,* gastro-intestinal; *IV,* intravenous; *S_3,* third heart sound; *S_4,* fourth heart sound.

- *Decreased cardiac output* (related to altered heart rhythm, valvular insufficiency, and fluid overload)
- *Activity intolerance* related to *physical deconditioning* (generalized weakness, arthralgia, valvular dysfunction)

Additional information on nursing diagnoses for the patient with IE is presented in Nursing Care Plan 39-1, available on the Evolve website for this chapter.

PLANNING
The overall goals for the patient with IE include (a) normal or baseline cardiac function, (b) performance of activities of daily living without fatigue, and (c) knowledge of the therapeutic regimen to prevent recurrence of endocarditis.

NURSING IMPLEMENTATION

HEALTH PROMOTION. The incidence and the recurrence of IE can be decreased by identifying individuals who are at risk for the development of endocarditis (see Tables 39-2 and 39-4) and those who have had IE in the past and providing teaching to them. Assessment of a patient's history and an understanding of the disease process are crucial for planning and implementing appropriate health-promotion strategies. Teaching is crucial for patients with IE so that they understand and adhere to the planned treatment regimen. Patients should understand the need to avoid people with infection, especially upper respiratory infection, and to report cold, flu, and cough symptoms. The importance of avoiding excessive fatigue and the need to plan rest periods before and after activity should be carefully explained to patients. Good oral hygiene, including daily care and regular dental visits, is also important. Patients must inform all health care providers performing dental, medical, or surgical procedures of their history of IE. Patients should understand the significance of the prescribed prophylactic antibiotic therapy before any invasive procedure. Patients with a history of IV drug use should be referred for drug treatment.

AMBULATORY AND HOME CARE. Patients with IE will require nursing management (see NCP 39-1 for nursing diagnoses and interventions, available on the Evolve website for this chapter). IE generally requires treatment with antibiotics for 4 to 6 weeks, depending on the results of blood cultures (see Table 39-5). After initial treatment in the hospital, a patient who is hemodynamically stable and compliant may continue treatment in the home setting. The adequacy of the home environment in terms of in-home support and hospital access must be determined for successful management. Patients who receive outpatient IV antibiotics will require vigilant home nursing care.

Assessment findings are often nonspecific (see Table 39-6) but can help assist with the treatment plan. Fever, chronic or intermittent, is a common early sign. The patient or the caregiver needs instructions about the importance of monitoring body temperature because persistent, prolonged temperature elevations may mean that the drug therapy is ineffective. Patients with IE are at risk for life-threatening complications, such as cerebral emboli, pulmonary edema, and HF. Patients and caregivers must be taught to recognize signs and symptoms of these complications (e.g., change in mental status, dyspnea, chest pain).

Patients with IE need adequate periods of physical and emotional rest. Bed rest may be necessary when fever is present or when there are complications (e.g., heart damage). Otherwise, the patient may ambulate and perform moderate activity. To prevent problems because of immobility, the patient should wear elastic compression stockings, perform range-of-motion exercises, and cough and deep-breathe every 2 hours. Patients may experience anxiety and fear associated with the illness. The nurse must recognize such feelings and implement strategies to help the patient cope with the illness.

Laboratory data should be monitored to determine the effectiveness of the antibiotic therapy. Ongoing monitoring of blood cultures is necessary to ensure eradication of the infecting organism. IV lines should be monitored for patency, and antibiotics should be given according to schedule. Patients should be monitored continuously for adverse drug reactions.

During the course of therapy in either the home or the hospital setting, management will also focus on teaching the patient about the nature of the disease and on reducing the risk for reinfection. The nurse must explain to the patient the relationship of follow-up care, good nutrition, and early treatment of common infections (e.g., colds) to maintain good health. The patient should be instructed about symptoms that may indicate recurrent infection, such as fever, fatigue, malaise, and chills. If any of these symptoms occur, the patient should be aware of the importance of notifying a health care provider. Finally, the patient must be instructed about the need for and importance of prophylactic antibiotic therapy before invasive procedures (see Table 39-3).

EVALUATION

Expected outcomes for the patient with IE are presented in NCP 39-1.

ACUTE PERICARDITIS

Pericarditis, which may occur on an acute basis, is a condition caused by inflammation of the pericardial sac (the pericardium). The pericardium is composed of the inner serous membrane (visceral pericardium), which closely adheres to the epicardial surface of the heart and the outer fibrous (parietal) layer (see Figure 39-1). The pericardial space is the cavity between these two layers, and in the normal state, it contains 10 to 30 mL of serous fluid. Although the pericardium may be congenitally absent or surgically removed, it serves a useful anchoring function, provides lubrication to decrease friction during systolic and diastolic heart movements, and assists in preventing excessive dilation of the heart during diastole.

Etiology and Pathophysiology

The common causes of acute pericarditis are listed in Table 39-7. Acute pericarditis most often (80%–85% of the time) is idiopathic, with a variety of suspected viral causes. The coxsackievirus B group is the most commonly identified virus. In addition to idiopathic or viral pericarditis, causes of this syndrome include bacterial infection, fungal infection, acute myocardial infarction (MI), tuberculosis, neoplasm, autoimmune conditions, drug reactions, metabolic disorders, and trauma (Adler, Charron, Imazio, et al., 2015; Imazio, Gaita, & LeWinter, 2015).

Pericarditis in the acute MI patient may be described as two distinct syndromes: (a) *acute pericarditis*, which may occur within the initial 48 to 72 hours after an MI, and (b) *Dressler's syndrome* (late pericarditis), which appears 4 to 6 weeks after an MI (see Chapter 36).

An inflammatory response—including an influx of neutrophils, increased pericardial vascularity, and eventually fibrin deposition on the visceral pericardium—is the characteristic pathological finding in acute pericarditis (Figure 39-4).

Clinical Manifestations

Characteristic clinical manifestations found in acute pericarditis include progressive, frequently severe chest pain that is sharp and pleuritic in nature. The pain is generally worse with deep inspiration and when lying supine. It is relieved by sitting upright. The pain may radiate to the neck, arms, or left shoulder, making it difficult to differentiate from angina. One distinction is that the pain from pericarditis can be referred to the trapezius muscle (shoulder, upper back) because the phrenic nerve innervates these two regions. Pericarditis is diagnosed in 5% of people presenting to the emergency department with chest pain (Imazio, Gaita, & LeWinter, 2015; Adler, Charron, Imazio, et al., 2015). The dyspnea that accompanies acute pericarditis is related to the patient's need to breathe in rapid, shallow

TABLE 39-7 ETIOLOGIES OF PERICARDITIS

Infectious
- Viral: coxsackievirus A and B, echovirus, adenovirus, mumps, rubella, Epstein-Barr, varicella-zoster, hepatitis B, hepatitis C, human immunodeficiency virus
- Bacterial: *Mycobacterium tuberculosis* (most common; rarely other bacteria); pneumococci, staphylococci, streptococci, *Neisseria gonorrhoeae, Legionella pneumophila*, septicemia from Gram-negative organisms
- Fungal: *Histoplasma, Candida* species
- Infections: toxoplasmosis, Lyme disease

Noninfectious
- Uremia
- Myxedema
- Acute myocardial infarction
- Neoplasms: lung cancer, breast cancer, leukemia, Hodgkin's lymphoma, non-Hodgkin's lymphoma
- Trauma: thoracic surgery, pacemaker insertion, cardiac diagnostic procedures
- Radiation
- Dissecting aortic aneurysm

Hypersensitive or Autoimmune
- Delayed post–myocardial-pericardial injury
- Post–myocardial infarction (Dressler's) syndrome
- Postpericardiotomy syndrome
- Rheumatic fever
- Drug reactions: procainamide, hydralazine (Apresoline), isoniazid, doxorubicin, and daunorubicin (often associated with cardiomyopathy)
- Rheumatological diseases: rheumatoid arthritis, systemic lupus erythematosus, systemic sclerosis (scleroderma), ankylosing spondylitis

TABLE 39-8 MEASUREMENT OF PULSUS PARADOXUS

1. Make determination during quiet breathing with stable rhythm.
2. Determine systolic blood pressure.
3. Inflate blood pressure cuff until no sounds are heard with stethoscope.
4. Deflate cuff slowly until systolic sounds are heard on expiration, and note the pressure.
5. Deflate cuff until systolic sounds are heard throughout the respiratory cycle, and note the pressure.
6. Determine the difference between the measurements taken in Steps 4 and 5. This will equal the amount of paradox:

Sounds heard in expiration at	110 mm Hg
Sounds heard throughout cycle at	82 mm Hg
Amount of paradox	28 mm Hg

The difference is usually <10 mm Hg. If the difference is >10 mm Hg, cardiac tamponade may be present.

FIGURE 39-4 Acute pericarditis. Note the shaggy coat of fibrin covering the surface of the heart. Source: Damjanov, I., & Linder, J. (2000). *Pathology: A color atlas.* St. Louis: Mosby.

breaths to avoid chest pain and may be aggravated by fever and anxiety.

The hallmark finding in acute pericarditis is the **pericardial friction rub**. The rub is a scratching, grating, high-pitched sound believed to arise from friction between the roughened pericardial and epicardial surfaces. It is best heard with the stethoscope placed at the lower left sternal border of the chest with the patient leaning forward. Since it is difficult to tell a pericardial friction rub from a pleural friction rub, patients can be asked to hold their breath. If the rub is still heard, then it is cardiac. Pericardial friction rubs may require frequent attempts to identify because they are often intermittent and short-lived.

Complications

Two major complications that may result from acute pericarditis are pericardial effusion and cardiac tamponade. **Pericardial effusion** is an accumulation of excess fluid in the pericardium. It can occur rapidly (e.g., chest trauma) or slowly (e.g., tuberculous pericarditis). Large effusions may compress adjoining structures. Pulmonary tissue compression can cause cough, dyspnea, and tachypnea. Phrenic nerve compression can induce hiccups, and compression of the recurrent laryngeal nerve may result in hoarseness. Heart sounds are generally distant and muffled, although blood pressure (BP) is usually maintained by compensatory mechanisms.

Cardiac tamponade, also referred to as *pericardial tamponade*, develops as fluid accumulates in the pericardial sac (pericardial effusion), causing an increase in intrapericardial pressure and producing compression of the heart. The speed of fluid accumulation affects the severity of clinical manifestations. Cardiac tamponade can occur acutely (e.g., rupture of heart, trauma) or subacutely (e.g., secondary to uremia, malignancy). The patient with cardiac tamponade may report chest pain and is often confused, anxious, and restless. As the compression of the heart increases, heart sounds become muffled and the pulse pressure is narrowed. The patient will develop tachypnea, tachycardia, and a decreased cardiac output (CO). The neck veins are usually markedly distended because of increased jugular venous pressure, and a significant pulsus paradoxus is present. *Pulsus paradoxus* is a decrease in systolic BP with inspiration that is exaggerated in cardiac tamponade. (See Table 39-8 for the measurement technique.) In a patient with a slow onset of a cardiac tamponade, dyspnea may be the only clinical manifestation.

Diagnostic Studies

The ECG is useful in the diagnosis of acute pericarditis, with changes noted in approximately 90% of cases. The most sensitive ECG changes include diffuse (widespread) ST-segment elevations.

FIGURE 39-6 Pericardiocentesis performed under sterile conditions in conjunction with electrocardiogram (ECG) and hemodynamic measurements.

FIGURE 39-5 A, Radiograph of a normal chest. **B,** Pericardial effusion is present and the cardiac silhouette is enlarged with a globular shape (*arrows*). Source: Guzetta, C. E., & Dossey, B. M. (1992). *Cardiovascular nursing: Holistic practice.* St. Louis: Mosby.

TABLE 39-9 **COLLABORATIVE CARE**

Acute Pericarditis

Diagnostic	**Collaborative Therapy**
• History and physical examination	• Treatment of underlying disease
• Auscultation of chest	• Bed rest
• ECG	• ASA (Aspirin)
• Laboratory: CRP, ESR, white blood cell count, BUN,* serum creatinine	• NSAIDs
	• Colchicine
• TB test	• Corticosteroids
• Chest radiographic examination	• Pericardiocentesis (for large pericardial effusion or tamponade)
• Echocardiogram	• Pericardial window (for tamponade or ongoing pericardial effusion)
• Pericardiocentesis	
• Pericardial biopsy	
• CT scan	
• Cardiac nuclear scan	

ASA, acetylsalicylic acid; *BUN*, blood urea nitrogen; *CRP*, C-reactive protein; *CT*, computed tomography; *ECG*, electrocardiogram; *ESR*, erythrocyte sedimentation rate; *NSAIDs*, nonsteroidal anti-inflammatory drugs; *TB*, tuberculosis.
*Serum urea (nitrogen).

This reflects the abnormal repolarization that develops secondary to the pericardial inflammation. It is important to differentiate these changes from the ST changes seen in MI. (See Chapter 38 for more information on ECG monitoring.) The chest radiographic findings are generally normal, but cardiomegaly may be seen in a patient who has a large pericardial effusion (Figure 39-5). Echocardiographic findings are more useful in determining the presence of a pericardial effusion or cardiac tamponade. Newer methods such as tissue Doppler imaging and colour M-mode Doppler imaging of early left ventricular flow help to assess diastolic function and diagnose constrictive pericarditis (discussed later in the chapter). Computed tomography (CT) and cardiac magnetic resonance imaging (CMRI) provide for visualization of the pericardium and pericardial space (Imazio, Gaita, & LeWinter, 2015).

Common laboratory findings include leukocytosis and elevation of CRP and ESR. Troponin levels may be elevated in patients with ST-segment elevation and acute pericarditis, a reading that would indicate concurrent myocardial damage. The fluid obtained during pericardiocentesis (Figure 39-6) or the tissue from a pericardial biopsy may also be analyzed to determine the cause of the pericarditis.

Collaborative Care

Management of acute pericarditis is directed toward identification and treatment of the underlying problem (Table 39-9). Antibiotics should be used to treat bacterial pericarditis. Corticosteroids are generally reserved for patients with pericarditis secondary to systemic lupus erythematosus, patients already taking corticosteroids for a rheumatological or other immune system condition, or patients who do not respond to nonsteroidal anti-inflammatory drugs (NSAIDs). When necessary, prednisone is usually given according to a tapering dosage schedule. Corticosteroids are administered cautiously because of their numerous adverse effects, such as upper gastro-intestinal bleeding, sodium retention, hyperglycemia, hypokalemia, and Cushing's syndrome (see Chapter 51).

The pain and inflammation of acute pericarditis are usually treated with NSAIDs (e.g., ibuprofen) or high-dose salicylates (e.g., ASA [Aspirin]). Colchicine, an anti-inflammatory medication used for gout and previously used for recurrent pericarditis, is now recommended in the treatment of acute pericarditis (Adler, Charron, Imazio, et al., 2015). The COPE trial (**col**chicine for acute **pe**ricarditis) demonstrated that the use of colchicine with ASA reduced recurrence rates by 10.7% (from 32.3% to 21.6%) and reduced symptoms at 72 hours to 11.7% from 36.7% compared with conventional therapy (Imazio, Gaita, & LeWinter, 2015).

If surgical drainage is necessary, a **pericardiocentesis** may be performed. During this procedure, a 16- to 18-gauge needle is inserted into the pericardial space to remove fluid for analysis and to relieve cardiac pressure. The procedure is rapid and safe and done using a percutaneous approach that is guided by ECG and echocardiography. It is usually performed for pericardial effusion with acute cardiac tamponade, purulent pericarditis, and a high index of suspicion of neoplasm (see Figure 39-6). Hemodynamic support for the patient being prepared for the pericardiocentesis may include administration of volume expanders and inotropic drugs (e.g., dopamine) and the discontinuation of any anticoagulants. Complications from pericardiocentesis include dysrhythmias, further cardiac tamponade, pneumomediastinum, pneumothorax, myocardial laceration, and coronary artery laceration.

NURSING MANAGEMENT
ACUTE PERICARDITIS

The management of the patient's pain and anxiety during acute pericarditis is a primary nursing consideration. Assessment of the amount, the quality, and the location of the pain is important, particularly in distinguishing the pain of myocardial ischemia (angina) from the pain of pericarditis. Pericarditic pain is usually located in the precordium or left trapezius ridge and has a sharp, pleuritic quality that increases with inspiration. Pain is often relieved by sitting or leaning forward, and the pain is worsened when lying supine. ECG monitoring can aid in distinguishing these types of pain because ischemia usually involves localized ST-segment changes, as compared with the diffuse ST-segment changes present in acute pericarditis.

Pain relief measures include maintaining the patient on bed rest with the head of the bed elevated to 45 degrees and providing an overbed table for support. Anti-inflammatory medications help alleviate the patient's pain; however, in high doses, they can cause upper gastro-intestinal bleeding. Nursing interventions, therefore, should be directed toward identification and management of this potential problem. Specific interventions include administering these drugs with food or milk and instructing the patient to avoid any alcoholic beverages while taking the medications.

Other drugs, such as misoprostol, or a proton pump inhibitor may be ordered to protect the gastric mucosa. Anxiety-reducing measures for patients with acute pericarditis include providing simple, complete explanations of all procedures performed and the possible cause of the pain. These explanations are particularly important for patients whose diagnosis of acute pericarditis is being established and for patients who have already experienced angina or an acute MI.

The potential for decreased CO exists for patients with acute pericarditis because of the possibility of cardiac tamponade. Monitoring for the signs and symptoms of tamponade and preparing for possible pericardiocentesis are important nursing responsibilities.

CHRONIC CONSTRICTIVE PERICARDITIS
Etiology and Pathophysiology

Chronic constrictive pericarditis results from scarring with consequent loss of elasticity of the pericardial sac. It usually begins with an initial episode of acute pericarditis (often secondary to idiopathic causes, cardiac surgery, or radiation) and is characterized by fibrin deposition with a clinically undetected pericardial effusion. Resorption of the effusion slowly follows, with progression toward the chronic stage of fibrous scarring, thickening of the pericardium from calcium deposition, and eventual obliteration of the pericardial space. The fibrotic, thickened, and adherent pericardium encases the heart, thereby impairing the ability of the atria and ventricles to stretch adequately during diastole.

Clinical Manifestations

Manifestations of chronic constrictive pericarditis occur over an extended period and mimic those of HF and cor pulmonale. Many of the clinical manifestations are related to decreased CO. They include dyspnea on exertion, peripheral edema, ascites, fatigue, anorexia, and weight loss. The most prominent finding upon physical examination is elevated jugular venous pressure. Unlike with cardiac tamponade, the presence of significant pulsus paradoxus is uncommon. Auscultatory findings include a *pericardial knock,* which is a loud early diastolic sound often heard along the left sternal border.

Diagnostic Studies

ECG results are often nonspecific in chronic constrictive pericarditis. The cardiac silhouette on the chest radiograph may be normal or enlarged depending on the degree of pericardial thickening and the presence of a coexisting pericardial effusion. Two-dimensional echocardiography is insensitive for determining pericardial thickness but may inform the health care provider about the physiology. Colour M-mode and tissue Doppler imaging are used to confirm constrictive pericarditis. CT and MRI provide measurement of pericardial thickness and assessment of diastolic filling patterns. Cardiac catheterization is indicated when noninvasive investigation such as Doppler echocardiography, CT, or MRI do not provide definitive diagnosis (Adler, Charron, Imazio, et al., 2015).

NURSING AND COLLABORATIVE MANAGEMENT
CHRONIC CONSTRICTIVE PERICARDITIS

Unless the patient is free of symptoms or the condition is inoperable, the treatment of choice for chronic constrictive pericarditis is a *pericardiectomy.* This procedure involves complete resection of the pericardium through a median sternotomy with the use of cardiopulmonary bypass. Some patients show immediate improvement after surgery, but others may take weeks. The postoperative prognosis is improved when the surgery is performed before severe clinical disability has developed.

MYOCARDITIS
Etiology and Pathophysiology

Myocarditis is a focal or diffuse inflammation of the myocardium. Possible causes include viruses, bacteria, fungi, parasites, radiation therapy, and pharmacological and chemical factors. Viruses, particularly coxsackievirus types A and B, are the most common causative agents of myocarditis in Canada and the United States. Autoimmune disorders (e.g., polymyositis) also have been associated with the development of myocarditis. In some cases, no causative agent or factor can be identified (i.e., idiopathic myocarditis). Myocarditis is frequently associated with acute pericarditis, particularly when it is caused by coxsackievirus B strains or echoviruses (Caforio, Pankuweit, Arbustini et al., 2013). When the myocardium becomes infected, the causative agent invades the myocytes and causes cellular damage and necrosis. The immune response is activated, and cytokines and oxygen free radicals are released. As the infection progresses, an auto-immune response is activated, leading to further destruction of myocytes. Myocarditis results in cardiac dysfunction and has been linked to the development of dilated cardiomyopathy (DCM) (discussed later in this chapter).

Clinical Manifestations

The clinical features of myocarditis are variable, ranging from a benign course without any overt manifestations to severe heart involvement or sudden cardiac death (SCD). Fever, fatigue, malaise, myalgias, pharyngitis, dyspnea, lymphadenopathy, and nausea and vomiting are early systemic manifestations of the viral illness.

Early cardiac manifestations appear 7 to 10 days after viral infection. These include pleuritic chest pain with a pericardial friction rub and effusion, because pericarditis often accompanies myocarditis. Late cardiac signs relate to the development of HF and may include a third heart sound (S_3), crackles, jugular venous distension, syncope, peripheral edema, and angina.

Diagnostic Studies

The ECG changes for a patient with myocarditis are often nonspecific and reflect associated pericardial involvement (e.g., diffuse ST-segment abnormalities). Dysrhythmias and conduction disturbances may be present. Laboratory findings are also often inconclusive. They may include mild to moderate leukocytosis and atypical lymphocytes, increased ESR and CRP levels, elevated levels of myocardial markers such as troponin, and elevated viral titres (virus is generally present in tissue and fluid samples only during the initial 8–10 days of illness). Histological confirmation of myocarditis is done through endomyocardial biopsy (EMB). This technique involves removing several small pieces of myocardial tissue percutaneously from the right ventricle with a special instrument called a *bioptome* and microscopically examining the samples (Caforio, Pankuweit, Arbustini, et al., 2013). A biopsy done during the initial 6 weeks of acute illness is most diagnostic because, in this period, lymphocytic infiltration and myocyte damage indicative of myocarditis are present. Other studies to evaluate cardiac function include echocardiography, nuclear scans, and MRI.

Collaborative Care

The treatment for myocarditis in patients with fulminant HF includes cardiovascular support with inotropic or vasopressor therapy or both and mechanical circulatory support (e.g., left ventricular assist device [LVAD]). Care of patients with both myocarditis and HF is the same usual care for HF patients: beta blockers, angiotensin-converting enzyme (ACE) inhibitors, and diuretic therapy, the last of which may help to reduce fluid volume and decrease preload (Howlett, Chan, Exekoitz, et al., 2016).

Immuno-suppressive therapy with drugs such as prednisone, azathioprine (Imuran), and cyclosporine is not routinely recommended in the management of the patient with myocarditis but may be trialled in patients with an autoimmune disorder and those who are severely hemodynamically compromised and not responding to treatment. Intravenous immunoglobulin (IVIG) has not demonstrated improved outcomes but may be of use for the pediatric population (Kindermann, Barth, Mahfoud, et al., 2012). Antiviral and immuno-suppressive agents remain controversial, but these drugs have been shown to improve New York Heart Association (NYHA) functional classification (Kindermann, Barth, Mahfoud, et al., 2012; Caforio, Pankuweit, Arbustini, et al., 2013). Oxygen therapy, bed rest, restricted activity, and maintenance of standby emergency equipment are general supportive measures in the management of myocarditis.

NURSING MANAGEMENT
MYOCARDITIS

Decreased CO is an ongoing nursing diagnosis in the care of the patient with myocarditis. Interventions focus on assessment for the signs and symptoms of HF. Important nursing measures to decrease cardiac workload include using semi-Fowler's position, spacing out activity and rest periods, and providing a quiet environment. Prescribed medications that increase the heart's contractility and decrease the preload, the afterload, or both require careful monitoring. Ongoing evaluation of the effectiveness of these interventions is necessary.

Patients may be anxious about the diagnosis of myocarditis, recovery from myocarditis, and the therapeutic plan. Nursing measures include assessing the level of anxiety, instituting measures to decrease anxiety, and keeping the patient and caregivers informed about therapeutic measures.

Patients who receive immuno-suppressive therapy have additional problems of alterations in the immune response with the potential for infection and complications related to the therapy. Guidelines for care include monitoring for complications and providing the patient with a clean, safe environment by following proper infection-control procedures. Most patients with myocarditis recover spontaneously, although some may develop DCM. If severe HF occurs, the patient may require heart transplantation.

RHEUMATIC FEVER AND HEART DISEASE

Rheumatic fever is defined by the Heart and Stroke Foundation of Canada (2017b) as "an inflammatory disease that may affect several connective tissues of the body, especially those of the heart, brain, joints, or skin." Rheumatic fever potentially involves all layers of the heart (endocardium, myocardium, and pericardium). Rheumatic heart disease is a chronic condition resulting from rheumatic fever that is characterized by scarring and deformity of the heart valves.

Etiology and Pathophysiology

Acute rheumatic fever (ARF) is a complication that occurs as a delayed result (usually after 2–3 weeks) of group A streptococcal pharyngitis (Burke, 2015). Manifestations of ARF appear to be related to an abnormal immunological response to group A streptococcal cell membrane antigens. ARF has declined in developed countries as a result of the effective use of antibiotics to treat streptococcal infections. However, it remains an important public health problem in developing countries. The sequela of ARF, rheumatic heart disease, is found primarily in young adults.

Cardiac Lesions and Valvular Deformities. About 40% of ARF episodes are marked by carditis, and all layers of the heart (endocardium, myocardium, and pericardium) may be involved (see Figure 39-1). This generalized involvement gives rise to the term *rheumatic pancarditis*.

Rheumatic endocarditis is found primarily in the valves, with swelling and erosion of the valve leaflets. Vegetations form from deposits of fibrin and blood cells in areas of erosion. The lesions initially create fibrous thickening of the valve leaflets, fusion of commissures and chordae tendineae, and fibrosis of the papillary muscle. Valve leaflets may fuse and become thickened or even calcified, resulting in stenosis. Reduction in the mobility of valve leaflets may occur with failure of the leaflets, resulting in regurgitation. The mitral and aortic valves are most commonly affected.

Myocardial involvement is characterized by **Aschoff bodies**, which are tiny, rounded or spindle-shaped nodules formed by a reaction to inflammation with accompanying swelling and fragmentation of collagen fibres. As the Aschoff bodies age, they become more fibrous, and scar tissue forms in the myocardium. In addition to Aschoff bodies, a diffuse cellular infiltrate is present in interstitial tissues. Rheumatic pericarditis affects both layers of the pericardium, which become thickened and covered with a fibrinous exudate, and a serosanguineous pericardial effusion may develop. When healing occurs, fibrosis and adhesions develop that partially or completely obliterate the pericardial sac, but constrictive pericarditis does not occur.

These pathophysiological changes in the heart may occur as a result of an initial attack of rheumatic fever. However, recurrent infections may cause further structural damage.

Extracardiac Lesions. The lesions of rheumatic fever are systemic, involving the connective tissues especially. The joints (polyarthritis), skin (subcutaneous nodules), and central nervous system may be involved in rheumatic fever.

Clinical Manifestations

Symptoms of ARF can include chest pain, excessive fatigue, heart palpitations (the heart fluttering or missing beats), a thumping sensation in the chest, shortness of breath, and swollen ankles, wrists, or stomach (Heart and Stroke Foundation of Canada, 2017a). The diagnosis of ARF is suggested by a clustering of signs and symptoms as well as by laboratory findings. When not observed in its most severe form, the disease may be difficult to differentiate from many illnesses with similar clinical manifestations. Criteria established by T. D. Jones in 1944 have been revised by the American Heart Association and provide a basis for diagnosis (Gewitz, Baltimore, Tani, et al., 2015) (Table 39-10). The presence of two major criteria or one major and two minor criteria plus evidence of a preceding group A streptococcal infection indicates a high probability of ARF.

Major Criteria. *Carditis* is the most important manifestation of ARF and results in three signs: (a) an organic heart murmur or murmurs of mitral or aortic regurgitation or mitral stenosis; (b) cardiac enlargement and HF occurring secondary to myocarditis; and (c) pericarditis resulting in muffled heart sounds, chest pain, a pericardial friction rub, or signs of effusion.

Mono- or *polyarthritis* is the most common finding in rheumatic fever. The inflammatory process affects the synovial membranes of the joints, causing swelling, heat, redness, tenderness, and limitation of motion. The larger joints are most frequently affected, particularly knees, ankles, elbows, and wrists.

TABLE 39-10	**MODIFIED JONES CRITERIA FOR ACUTE RHEUMATIC FEVER**	
Major Criteria	**Minor Criteria**	**Evidence of Group A Streptococcal Infection**
• Carditis • Mono- or polyarthritis • Sydenham chorea • Erythema marginatum • Subcutaneous nodules	• Clinical findings: fever, polyarthralgia • Laboratory findings: ↑ ESR, ↑ WBC count, ↑ CRP • ECG findings: prolonged PR interval	• Laboratory findings: ↑ antistreptolysin O titre, positive throat culture, positive rapid antigen test for group A streptococci

CRP, C-reactive protein; *ECG*, electrocardiogram; *ESR*, erythrocyte sedimentation rate; *WBC*, white blood cell.

Chorea (Sydenham chorea) is the major central nervous system manifestation of ARF, often a delayed sign occurring several months after the initial infection. It is characterized by involuntary movements, especially of the face and the limbs, muscle weakness, and disturbances of speech and gait.

Erythema marginatum lesions are a less common feature of ARF. The bright pink maplike macular lesions occur mainly on the trunk and the proximal extremities and may be exacerbated by heat (e.g., warm bath). Subcutaneous nodules, usually associated with severe carditis, are firm, small, hard, painless swellings located over extensor surfaces of the joints, particularly knees, wrists, and elbows.

Minor Criteria. Minor clinical manifestations (see Table 39-10) are frequently present and are helpful in diagnosing the disease. The minor criteria are used as supplemental data to confirm the presence of rheumatic fever when only one major criterion is present.

Complications

A complication that can result from ARF is *chronic rheumatic carditis*. It results from changes in valvular structure that may occur months to years after an episode of ARF. Rheumatic endocarditis can result in fibrous tissue growth in valve leaflets and chordae tendineae with scarring and contractures. The mitral valve is most frequently involved; the aortic or tricuspid valve or both may also be affected.

Diagnostic Studies

No single diagnostic test exists for rheumatic fever (see Table 39-10). An echocardiogram may show valvular insufficiency and pericardial fluid or thickening. A chest radiographic study may show an enlarged heart if HF is present. The most consistent ECG change is delayed AV conduction as evidenced by prolongation of the PR interval.

Collaborative Care

Treatment consists of drug therapy and supportive measures (Table 39-11). Antibiotic therapy does not modify the course of the acute disease or the development of carditis. It does eliminate residual group A streptococci remaining in the tonsils and the pharynx and prevent the spread of organisms to close contacts.

TABLE 39-11   COLLABORATIVE CARE
Rheumatic Fever

Diagnostic	Collaborative Therapy
• History and physical examination	• Bed rest (modified)
• Laboratory findings (see Table 39-10)	• Benzathine penicillin (1.2 million units IM) daily for 10 days
• Throat culture	• Acetylsalicylic acid
• Chest radiograph	• Corticosteroids
• Echocardiogram	• Codeine
• ECG	• Carbamazepine, valproic acid, phenobarbital

ECG, electrocardiogram; IM, intramuscularly.

Salicylates, NSAIDs, and corticosteroids are the anti-inflammatory drugs most widely used in the management of ARF. All are effective in controlling the fever and joint manifestations. Salicylates or NSAIDs are used when arthritis is the main manifestation, and corticosteroids are used if severe carditis is present.

NURSING MANAGEMENT
RHEUMATIC FEVER AND HEART DISEASE

NURSING ASSESSMENT

Subjective and objective data that should be obtained from a patient with rheumatic fever and heart disease are presented in Table 39-12. It is important to note that rheumatic fever is more likely to reoccur in a person with a previous history of rheumatic fever than to occur in the general population. The skin of the patient should be assessed for subcutaneous nodules and erythema marginatum. The procedure involves palpation for subcutaneous nodules over all bony surfaces and along extensor tendons of the hands and feet. The nodules range in size from 1 to 4 cm and are hard, painless, and freely movable. Erythema marginatum can occur on the trunk and the inner aspects of the upper arm and the thigh. The erythematous maplike macules do not itch and are not raised. The possible presence of these bright pink macules should be assessed in good light because the rash is difficult to observe, especially if the patient is dark skinned.

NURSING DIAGNOSES

Nursing diagnoses for the patient with rheumatic fever and heart disease may include but are not limited to the following:
- *Decreased cardiac output* (related to valve dysfunction or HF)
- *Activity intolerance* related to *physical deconditioning* (arthralgia, arthritis, pain from pericarditis)
- *Ineffective health management* related to *insufficient knowledge of therapeutic regimen* (need for long-term prophylactic antibiotic therapy)

PLANNING

The overall goals for a patient with rheumatic fever include (a) normal or baseline heart function, (b) resumption of daily activities without joint pain, and (c) verbalization of the ability to manage the disease.

NURSING IMPLEMENTATION

HEALTH PROMOTION. Rheumatic fever is a preventable cardiovascular disease. Prevention involves early detection and immediate treatment of group A β-hemolytic streptococcal

TABLE 39-12   NURSING ASSESSMENT
Rheumatic Fever and Rheumatic Heart Disease

Subjective Data
Important Health Information
Past health history: Recent β-hemolytic streptococcal infection, previous rheumatic fever or rheumatic heart disease, family history of rheumatic fever

Symptoms
- Malaise, generalized weakness, fatigue
- Anorexia; weight loss
- Palpitations
- Ataxia; migratory joint pain and tenderness (especially large joints)
- Chest pain

Objective Data
General
Low-grade fever

Integumentary
Subcutaneous nodules and erythema marginatum

Cardiovascular
Tachycardia, pericardial friction rub, distant heart sounds; gallop rhythm, diastolic and systolic murmurs, peripheral edema

Neurological
Chorea (involuntary, purposeless, rapid motions; facial grimaces)

Musculo-Skeletal
Signs of polyarthritis including swelling, heat, redness, limitation of motion (especially of knees, ankles, elbows, shoulders, and wrists)

Possible Findings
Cardiomegaly on chest radiographic study; delayed AV conduction on ECG; valve abnormalities, chamber dilation, and pericardial effusion on echocardiogram; ↑ ASO titre, ↑ ESR, ↑ CRP, leukocytosis

ASO, antistreptolysin O; AV, atrioventricular; CRP, C-reactive protein; ECG, electrocardiogram; ESR, erythrocyte sedimentation rate.

pharyngitis. Adequate treatment of streptococcal pharyngitis prevents initial attacks of rheumatic fever. Treatment consists of intramuscular injection of penicillin G benzathine (Bicillin L-A) or oral penicillin V potassium. If the patient is allergic to penicillin, erythromycin or azithromycin (Zithromax) may be substituted. Oral therapy requires faithful adherence to the full course of treatment. The nurse's role is to educate people in the community to seek medical attention for symptoms of streptococcal pharyngitis and to emphasize the need for adequate treatment of this infection.

ACUTE INTERVENTION. The primary goals of managing a patient with ARF are to control and eradicate the infecting organism; prevent cardiac complications; relieve joint pain, fever, and other symptoms; and support the patient psychologically and emotionally. The nurse should administer antibiotics as ordered to treat the streptococcal infection and should teach the patient that oral antibiotic therapy requires faithful adherence to the full course of therapy. Antipyretics, NSAIDs, and corticosteroids should be administered as prescribed, and fluid intake monitored. Promotion of optimal rest is essential to reduce the cardiac workload and to diminish the metabolic needs of the body. Relief of joint pain is an important nursing goal. Painful joints should be positioned for comfort and proper alignment. Heat may be applied, and salicylates or NSAIDs administered to relieve joint pain. After the acute symptoms have subsided, the patient without carditis should ambulate. If the patient has carditis with HF, bed rest restrictions should be applied. (See Chapter 37 for care of a patient with HF.) Nonstrenuous activities should be encouraged once recovery has begun.

AMBULATORY AND HOME CARE. Secondary prevention aims to prevent the recurrence of rheumatic fever. The patient with a previous history of rheumatic fever should be taught about the disease process, possible sequelae, and the ongoing or permanent need for prophylactic antibiotics. Prior history of rheumatic fever makes the patient more susceptible to a second attack after a streptococcal infection. The best prevention is monthly injections of long-acting penicillin. Alternative treatment is administration of oral penicillin or erythromycin one or two times a day. Rheumatic fever without carditis after age 18 may require only 5 years of prophylactic antibiotic therapy, or therapy may continue indefinitely in patients with frequent exposure to group A streptococcus. Prophylactic treatment should continue for 10 years or until the age of 40 in individuals who develop residual rheumatic heart disease (Nishimura, Otto, Bonow, et al., 2014).

The dosage of antibiotics used in maintenance prophylaxis of rheumatic fever is not adequate to prevent IE when invasive procedures are performed. Additional prophylaxis is necessary if a patient with known rheumatic heart disease has a dental procedure or an invasive respiratory tract procedure (e.g., tonsillectomy) that involves perforation of the mucosa (see Table 39-3). The nurse must explain the difference between these two prophylactic programs.

Patient teaching should encourage good nutrition, hygienic practices, and adequate rest. The patient should also be cautioned about the possibility of developing valvular heart disease. The nurse should teach the patient to seek medical attention if symptoms such as excessive fatigue, dizziness, palpitations, or exertional dyspnea develop.

❙ EVALUATION

The following are expected outcomes for patients with rheumatic fever and heart disease:
- Ability to perform activities of daily living with minimal fatigue and pain
- Adherence to treatment regimen
- Expression of confidence in managing disease
- Prevention of complications

❙ VALVULAR HEART DISEASE

The heart contains two AV valves, the mitral and the tricuspid, and two semilunar valves, the aortic and the pulmonic, that are located in four strategic locations to control unidirectional blood flow (see Figure 34-2). Valvular heart disease is defined according to the valve or valves affected and the types of functional alteration: stenosis or regurgitation.

The pressure on either side of an open valve is normally equal. However, in a stenotic valve, the valve orifice is restricted, impeding the forward flow of blood and creating a pressure gradient across an open valve. The degree of stenosis (constriction or narrowing) is reflected in the degree of the pressure gradient (i.e., the higher the gradient, the greater the stenosis). In **regurgitation** (also called *valvular incompetence* or *insufficiency*), incomplete closure of the valve leaflets results in the backward flow of blood.

Valve disorders occur in children and adolescents primarily when congenital conditions such as tricuspid atresia, pulmonary stenosis, and aortic stenosis are present. Valvular heart disease has remained prevalent because of an increase in the number of older adults, many of whom have some form of cardiovascular disease. Aortic stenosis and mitral regurgitation (MR) are common valve disorders in older adults. Other causes of valve disease in adults include disorders related to acquired immune deficiency syndrome and the use of some antiparkinsonian drugs (Surapaneni, Vinales, Najib, et al., 2011).

MITRAL VALVE STENOSIS

Etiology and Pathophysiology

Most cases of adult mitral valve stenosis result from rheumatic heart disease; rheumatic mitral stenosis is most prevalent in developing countries (Lung & Vahanian, 2011). Less common causes include congenital mitral stenosis, rheumatoid arthritis, and systemic lupus erythematosus. Rheumatic endocarditis causes scarring of the valve leaflets and the chordae tendineae. Contractures and adhesions develop between the commissures (the junctional areas) of the two leaflets (Figure 39-7). These structural deformities cause obstruction of blood flow and create a pressure difference between the left atrium and the left ventricle during diastole. Left atrial pressure and volume elevations cause increased pulmonary vasculature pressure and subsequent hypertrophy of the pulmonary vessels. In chronic mitral stenosis, pressure overload occurs in the left atrium, the pulmonary bed, and the right ventricle.

FIGURE 39-7 Valvular stenosis and regurgitation. **A,** Normal position of the valve leaflets, or cusps, when the valve is open and closed. **B,** Open position of a stenosed valve (left) and closed position of regurgitant valve (right). **C,** Hemodynamic effect of mitral stenosis. The stenosed valve is unable to open sufficiently during left atrial systole, inhibiting left ventricular filling. **D,** Hemodynamic effect of mitral regurgitation. The mitral valve does not close completely during left ventricular systole, permitting blood to re-enter the left atrium. At the same time, blood is moving forward through the aortic valve. Source: Huether, S. E., McCance, K. L., Brashers, V. L., et al. (2014). *Pathophysiology: The biologic basis for disease in adults and children* (7th ed., p. 1167). St. Louis: Mosby.

TABLE 39-13   CLINICAL MANIFESTATIONS AND DIAGNOSTIC FINDINGS OF VALVULAR HEART DISEASES

	Clinical Manifestations	Electrocardiogram	Echocardiogram	Cardiac Catheterization
Mitral valve stenosis	Exertional dyspnea, hemoptysis; fatigue; palpitations; loud, accentuated S_1; opening snap; low-pitched, rumbling diastolic murmur	Right axis deviation, left atrial enlargement, right ventricular hypertrophy, P mitrale (wide, M-shaped P wave), atrial flutter or fibrillation	Restricted movement of mitral valve leaflets; decreased size of orifice; diastolic turbulence	Left atrial pressure increased at end of diastole, reduction in CO
Mitral valve regurgitation	*Acute:* generally poorly tolerated with fulminating pulmonary edema and shock developing rapidly; systolic murmur	Left atrial enlargement, atrial fibrillation	Hyperdynamic left ventricular contraction in association with shock; regurgitant jets and flail* chordae or leaflets	Contrast medium injection in left ventricle showing regurgitation of blood into left atrium
	Chronic: weakness, fatigue, exertional dyspnea, palpitations; an S_3 gallop, holosystolic or pansystolic murmur	P mitrale, left ventricular hypertrophy, atrial flutter or fibrillation	Left atrial enlargement; left ventricular hypertrophy; flail leaflets	Contrast medium injection in left ventricle showing regurgitation of blood into left atrium
Mitral valve prolapse	Palpitations, dyspnea, chest pain, activity intolerance, syncope; mobile midsystolic nonejection click and a late or holosystolic murmur	Usually normal; occasionally T-wave inversion or biplasticity in leads II, III, and aVf are noted; PVCs and tachydysrhythmias possible	On the M-mode echo, late-systolic posterior motion or holosystolic billowing of the mitral leaflets; on two-dimensional echo, systolic billowing of the mitral leaflets	Left ventricular angiogram reveals mitral leaflets with prominent scalloping as the leaflets billow into the left atrium during systole
Aortic valve stenosis	Angina pectoris, syncope, heart failure, normal or soft S_1, prominent S_4, crescendo–decrescendo murmur	Left ventricular hypertrophy, left bundle branch block, complete atrioventricular heart block	Restricted movement of aortic valve; diminished orifice; systolic turbulence	Left ventricular systolic pressure increased, reduction in CO
Aortic valve regurgitation	*Acute:* abrupt onset of profound dyspnea, transient chest pain, progression to shock	Left ventricular strain	Normal-sized left ventricle with hyperdynamic systolic contraction; aortic dissection can be seen, if cause of acute process	Significant elevation of left ventricular diastolic pressure
	Chronic: fatigue, exertional dyspnea; water-hammer pulse; heaving precordial impulse; diastolic high-pitched soft decrescendo diastolic murmur, characteristic Austin Flint murmur at diastolic rumble, systolic ejection click	Left ventricular hypertrophy	Enlarged left ventricle and dilated aortic root	Increase in left ventricular diastolic pressure, aortic root contrast medium injection demonstrating regurgitation of blood into left ventricle
Tricuspid stenosis and regurgitation	Peripheral edema, ascites, hepatomegaly; diastolic low-pitched decrescendo murmur with increased intensity during inspiration (stenosis); pansystolic murmur with increased intensity at inspiration (regurgitation)	Tall, peaked P waves; atrial fibrillation	Right ventricular dilation and paradoxical septal motion; usually poor visualization of tricuspid valve itself	Pressure gradient across tricuspid valve and increased right atrial pressure (stenosis); reflux of contrast medium into right atrium (regurgitation)

aVF, augmented vector foot; *CO*, cardiac output; *PVCs*, premature ventricular contractions; S_1, first heart sound; S_3, third heart sound; S_4, fourth heart sound.
*Flail mitral leaflet is a complication of mitral valve prolapse, which can lead to severe mitral regurgitation and left ventricular dysfunction.

Clinical Manifestations

The primary symptom of mitral stenosis is exertional dyspnea owing to reduced lung compliance (Table 39-13). Fatigue and palpitations from atrial fibrillation may occur. Heart sounds include a loud first heart sound and a low-pitched, rumbling diastolic murmur (best heard at the apex with the stethoscope bell). Less frequently, patients may have hoarseness (from atrial enlargement pressing on the laryngeal nerve), hemoptysis (from pulmonary hypertension), chest pain (from decreased CO), and

seizures or a stroke (from emboli). Emboli can arise from blood stasis in the left atrium.

MITRAL VALVE REGURGITATION

Etiology and Pathophysiology

Mitral valve function depends on intact mitral leaflets, mitral annulus, chordae tendineae, papillary muscles, left atrium, and left ventricle. A defect in any of these structures can result in regurgitation. Most cases of MR are caused by MI, chronic rheumatic heart disease, mitral valve prolapse (MVP), ischemic papillary muscle dysfunction, or IE. MI with left ventricular failure increases the risk for rupture of the chordae tendineae and for acute MR.

MR allows blood to flow backward from the left ventricle to the left atrium because of incomplete valve closure during systole. The left ventricle and the left atrium both work harder to preserve an adequate CO. In chronic MR, the additional volume load results in atrial enlargement, ventricular dilation, and eventual ventricular hypertrophy. In acute MR, the left atrium and ventricle do not abruptly dilate. The sudden increase in pressure and volume is transmitted to the pulmonary bed, resulting in pulmonary edema and shock.

Clinical Manifestations

The clinical course of MR is determined by the nature of its onset (see Table 39-13). Patients with acute MR will have thready peripheral pulses and cool, clammy extremities. A low CO may obscure a new systolic murmur. Rapid assessment (e.g., cardiac catheterization) and intervention (e.g., valve repair or replacement) are critical for a positive outcome.

Patients with chronic MR may remain asymptomatic for many years until the development of some degree of left ventricular failure. Initial symptoms of left ventricular failure may include weakness, fatigue, palpitations, and dyspnea that gradually progress to orthopnea, paroxysmal nocturnal dyspnea, and peripheral edema. Accentuated left ventricular filling leads to an audible S_3, even with normal left ventricular function. The murmur is a loud holosystolic or pansystolic murmur at the apex radiating to the left axilla. Patients with asymptomatic MR should be monitored carefully because the natural history for MR can be variable, and surgery (valve repair or replacement) should be considered before significant left ventricular failure or pulmonary hypertension develops (Nishimura, Otto, Bonow, et al., 2014).

MITRAL VALVE PROLAPSE

Etiology and Pathophysiology

Mitral valve prolapse (MVP) is a structural abnormality of the mitral valve leaflets and the papillary muscles or chordae that allows the leaflets to prolapse, or buckle, back into the left atrium during ventricular systole (Figure 39-8). The etiology of MVP is unknown but is related to diverse pathogenic mechanisms of the mitral valve apparatus. The term *prolapse* is misleading because, in some cases, the valvular anomaly permits normal function. MVP is one of the most common forms of valvular heart disease.

MVP is usually benign, but serious complications can occur, including MR, IE, SCD, and cerebral ischemia. There is an increased familial incidence (autosomal dominant) among some patients.

Clinical Manifestations

MVP covers a broad spectrum of severity. Most patients are asymptomatic and remain so for their entire lives. A characteristic of MVP is a murmur from regurgitation that gets more intense through systole. This could be a late or holosystolic murmur. Another major sign is one or more clicks usually heard in midsystole to late systole. MVP does not alter the first (S_1) or second (S_2) heart sounds. Severe MR is an uncommon complication of MVP.

FIGURE 39-8 Mitral valve prolapse. In this valvular abnormality, the mitral leaflets have prolapsed back into the left atrium. They also demonstrate hooding (*arrow*). The left ventricle is on the right. Source: Kumar, V., Abbas, A. K., & Aster, J. (2013). *Robbins basic pathology* (9th ed., p. 391). Philadelphia: Elsevier Saunders.

M-mode echocardiography confirms MVP by demonstrating late-systolic prolapse, and two-dimensional echocardiography reveals leaflet billowing into the left atrium. Dysrhythmias, most commonly ventricular premature contractions, paroxysmal supraventricular tachycardia, and ventricular tachycardia, may cause palpitations, light-headedness, and dizziness. IE may occur in patients with MR associated with MVP.

Patients may or may not have chest pain. The cause of the chest pain is not known, but it may be caused by abnormal tension on the papillary muscles. If chest pain occurs, it tends to occur in clusters, especially during periods of emotional stress. Dyspnea, palpitations, and syncope may occasionally accompany the chest pain and do not respond to antianginal treatment (e.g., nitrates). β-Adrenergic blockers may be prescribed to control palpitations and chest pain. Patients with MVP generally have a benign, manageable course unless problems associated with MR are present. A teaching plan for patients with MVP appears in Table 39-14.

AORTIC VALVE STENOSIS

Etiology and Pathophysiology

Congenitally abnormal stenotic aortic valves are generally discovered in childhood, adolescence, or young adulthood. In older patients, aortic stenosis is a result of rheumatic fever or degeneration that may have an etiology similar to that of coronary artery disease. In rheumatic valvular disease, fusion of the commissures and secondary calcification cause the valve leaflets to stiffen and retract, resulting in stenosis. If aortic stenosis does occur owing to rheumatic heart disease, mitral valve disease accompanies it. Isolated aortic valve stenosis is almost always nonrheumatic in origin. The incidence of rheumatic aortic valvular disease has been decreasing, but senile or degenerative stenosis is expected to increase as the population ages.

TABLE 39-14   PATIENT & CAREGIVER TEACHING GUIDE

Mitral Valve Prolapse

The following information should be included in the teaching plan for a patient with mitral valve prolapse (MVP) and the patient's caregiver.

• Take medications as prescribed (e.g., β-adrenergic blockers to control palpitations, chest pain).
• Adopt healthy eating patterns and avoid caffeine, which is a stimulant and may exacerbate symptoms.
• If using diet pills or other over-the-counter drugs, check for common ingredients that are stimulants (e.g., caffeine, ephedrine) because these will exacerbate symptoms.
• Implement an exercise program, in consultation with a health care provider, to maintain optimal health.
• Contact Emergency Medical Services or health care provider if symptoms develop or worsen (e.g., palpitations, fatigue, shortness of breath, anxiety).

An **aortic stenosis** causes obstruction of blood flow from the left ventricle to the aorta during systole. The effect is left ventricular hypertrophy and increased myocardial oxygen consumption because of the increased myocardial mass. As the disease course progresses and compensatory mechanisms fail, reduced CO leads to decreased tissue perfusion, pulmonary hypertension, and HF.

Clinical Manifestations

Symptoms of aortic stenosis (see Table 39-13) develop when the valve orifice becomes approximately one-third its normal size. Symptoms include the classic triad of angina, syncope, and exertional dyspnea, reflecting left ventricular failure. The prognosis is poor for a patient with symptoms and whose valve obstruction is not relieved. Use of nitroglycerin is contraindicated for patients with significant aortic stenosis because it would reduce preload, and preload is necessary to help open the stiffened aortic valve. Auscultation of aortic stenosis typically reveals a normal or soft S_1; a diminished or absent S_2; a systolic, crescendo–decrescendo murmur that ends before S_2; and a prominent S_4.

> **DRUG ALERT—Nitroglycerin**
> • This drug must be used cautiously in patients with aortic stenosis because it may cause significant hypotension.
> • Chest pain can worsen due to decrease in preload and drop in BP.

AORTIC VALVE REGURGITATION

Etiology and Pathophysiology

Aortic valve regurgitation (AR) may be the result of a primary disease of the aortic valve leaflets, of the aortic root, or of both. Acute AR is caused by IE, trauma, or aortic dissection and constitutes a life-threatening emergency. Chronic AR is generally the result of rheumatic heart disease, a congenital bicuspid aortic valve, syphilis, or chronic rheumatic conditions such as ankylosing spondylitis or Reiter's syndrome.

AR entails retrograde blood flow from the ascending aorta into the left ventricle when the valve should be closed, resulting in volume overload. The left ventricle initially compensates for chronic AR through dilation and hypertrophy. Myocardial contractility eventually declines, and blood volumes increase in the left atrium and the pulmonary bed. This increase results in pulmonary hypertension and right ventricular failure.

Clinical Manifestations

Patients with acute AR have sudden clinical manifestations of cardiovascular collapse (see Table 39-13). The left ventricle is exposed to aortic pressure during diastole. The patient develops severe dyspnea, chest pain, hypotension (indicating left ventricular failure), and shock, all of which constitute a medical emergency.

Patients with chronic, severe AR develop a *water-hammer pulse* (a strong, quick beat that collapses immediately). Heart sounds may include a soft or absent S_1, presence of S_3 or S_4, and a soft, decrescendo, high-pitched diastolic murmur. A systolic ejection click may also be heard as well as a low-frequency diastolic murmur known as an *Austin Flint murmur*.

The patient with chronic AR generally remains asymptomatic for years and is seen with exertional dyspnea, orthopnea, and paroxysmal nocturnal dyspnea only after considerable myocardial dysfunction has occurred (see Table 39-13). Angina occurs less frequently with AR than with aortic stenosis.

TRICUSPID AND PULMONIC VALVE DISEASE

Etiology and Pathophysiology

Diseases of the tricuspid and pulmonic valves are uncommon, with stenosis occurring more frequently than regurgitation. *Tricuspid valve stenosis* occurs almost exclusively in patients who have had rheumatic fever, have used IV drugs, have had multiple myocardial biopsies, have had radiation treatment, have used anorectic drugs, or have been treated with a dopamine receptor agonist (e.g., pergolide) (Nishimura, Otto, Bonow, et al., 2014). *Pulmonic valve stenosis* is almost always congenital.

Tricuspid and pulmonic stenosis both result in an increase in blood volume in the right atrium and the right ventricle, respectively. Tricuspid stenosis results in right atrial enlargement and elevated systemic venous pressures. Pulmonic stenosis results in right ventricular hypertension and hypertrophy (see Table 39-13).

DIAGNOSTIC STUDIES FOR VALVULAR HEART DISEASE

Diagnosis of valvular heart disease is generally based on the results of history, physical examination, echocardiogram, and cardiac catheterization (especially if surgery is considered) (Table 39-15). Chest radiograph results, ECG findings, and the clinical manifestations exhibited by the patient also aid in establishing the correct diagnosis.

An echocardiogram reveals valve structure, function, and chamber size. Transesophageal echocardiography and Doppler colour-flow imaging are valuable in diagnosing and monitoring the progression of valvular heart disease. Real-time three-dimensional echocardiography may be helpful in qualitative assessments of mitral valve and congenital heart disease. Cardiac catheterization detects pressure changes in the cardiac chambers, measures pressure gradients across the valves, and quantifies the size of valve openings. An ECG shows heart rate and rhythm and provides information about any ischemia or chamber enlargement. Chest radiograph reveals the heart size, alterations in pulmonary circulation, and calcification of valves.

Collaborative Care of Valvular Heart Disease

Conservative Therapy. An important aspect of conservative management of valvular heart disease is prevention of recurrent

TABLE 39-15 COLLABORATIVE CARE

Valvular Heart Disease

Diagnostic
- History and physical examination
- Chest radiograph
- CBC
- ECG
- Echocardiogram
- Cardiac catheterization

Collaborative Therapy
Nonsurgical
- Prophylactic antibiotic therapy
  - Rheumatic fever
  - Infective endocarditis (see Table 39-5)
- Medications to treat or control HF
  - Vasodilators* (e.g., nitrates, ACE inhibitors)
  - Positive inotropes (e.g., digoxin)
  - Diuretics (see Chapter 35, Table 35-8)
  - β-Adrenergic blockers (see Chapter 35, Table 35-8)
- Sodium restriction

- Anticoagulation therapy (see Table 40-13)
- Antidysrhythmia drugs
- Percutaneous transluminal balloon valvuloplasty
- Percutaneous valve replacement

Surgical
- Valve repair
  - Commissurotomy (valvulotomy)
  - Valvuloplasty
  - Annuloplasty
- Valve replacement

*Use cautiously in patients with aortic stenosis.
ACE, angiotensin-converting enzyme; *CBC*, complete blood cell count; *ECG*, electrocardiogram; *HF*, heart failure.

rheumatic fever and IE (see Table 39-15). Treatment depends on the valve involved and the severity of the disease. It focuses on preventing exacerbations of HF, acute pulmonary edema, thrombo-embolism, and recurrent endocarditis. If manifestations of HF develop, vasodilators, positive inotropes, β-adrenergic blockers, diuretics, and a low-sodium diet are recommended (see Chapter 37). Anticoagulant therapy is used to prevent and treat systemic or pulmonary embolization, and it is also used prophylactically for stroke prevention in patients with atrial fibrillation. Atrial dysrhythmias are common and are treated with digoxin, antidysrhythmia drugs, or electrical cardioversion. β-Adrenergic blockers may be used to slow the ventricular response in patients with atrial fibrillation. (Dysrhythmias are discussed in Chapter 38.)

Percutaneous Aortic Valve Replacement. Percutaneous aortic valve replacement is an alternative for select patients with severe symptomatic aortic stenosis who are at high risk and cannot be treated with traditional surgical intervention. Canada has been a world leader in this technique (Webb, Rodes-Cabau, Fremes, et al., 2012). The procedure, performed in the cardiac catheterization laboratory, involves inserting a bioprosthetic valve, which is advanced over a stiff guide wire using a femoral arterial approach.

Percutaneous Transluminal Balloon Valvuloplasty. An alternative treatment for some patients with valvular heart disease is the *percutaneous transluminal balloon valvuloplasty* (PTBV) procedure, which splits open the fused commissures. PTBV is used for mitral, tricuspid, and pulmonic stenosis, and less often for aortic stenosis. The procedure, performed in the cardiac catheterization laboratory, involves threading a balloon-tipped catheter from the femoral artery or vein to the stenotic valve so that the balloon may be inflated in an attempt to separate the valve leaflets. A single- or double-balloon technique may be used for the PTBV procedure. Currently, the use of a single Inoue balloon with hourglass configuration allows sequential inflation. This technique is the most popular because it is easy, has good results, and has fewer complications (e.g., left ventricular perforation) (Nishimura, Otto, Bonow, et al., 2014). The PTBV procedure is generally indicated for older-adult patients and for patients who are poor surgery candidates. PTBV has fewer complications than valve replacement. The long-term results of PTBV are similar to those of surgical commissurotomy (Nishimura, Otto, Bonow, et al., 2014).

Surgical Therapy. The decision for surgical intervention is based on the clinical state of the patient. The type of surgery used for a particular patient depends on the valves involved, the valvular pathology, the severity of the disease, and the patient's clinical condition. All types of valve surgery are palliative, not curative, and patients will require lifelong health care. Valve repair is typically the surgical procedure of choice. It is often used in mitral or tricuspid valvular heart disease and has a lower operative mortality rate than replacement. Mitral *commissurotomy (valvulotomy)* is the procedure of choice for patients with pure mitral stenosis. The less precise closed method of commissurotomy has generally been replaced by the open method in Canada, the United States, and Western Europe. The direct vision, or open, procedure requires the use of cardiopulmonary bypass, removal of thrombi from the atrium, excision of the left atrial appendage, commissure incision, and, as indicated, separation of fused chordae, splitting of underlying papillary muscle, and debriding of calcification of the valve. In contrast, the closed procedure is usually performed with the aid of a transventricular dilator inserted through the apex of the left ventricle into the ostium of the mitral valve.

Open surgical *valvuloplasty* involves repairing the valve by suturing the torn leaflets, chordae tendineae, or papillary muscles. It is primarily used to treat mitral or tricuspid regurgitation. Valve repair avoids the risks of replacement but may not establish total valvular competence. *Minimally invasive valvuloplasty* surgery, using mini-sternotomy or parasternal approaches, has shown results comparable with those of the open procedure; it also decreases length of hospitalization, use of blood transfusions, and postoperative atrial fibrillation (Schmitto, Mokashi, & Cohn, 2010).

Further repair or reconstruction of the valve may be necessary and can be achieved by annuloplasty, a procedure also used in cases of mitral or tricuspid regurgitation. *Annuloplasty* entails reconstruction of the annulus, with or without the aid of prosthetic rings.

INFORMATICS IN PRACTICE

Heart Surgery DVD or CD

- To learn about a procedure, many patients prefer to watch a DVD or listen to a CD instead of reading a pamphlet. A video can be an effective tool for the nurse to use in teaching the patient facing heart surgery and the patient's caregiver what to expect before and after the procedure.
- The nurse should remember that the DVD or CD is not the teacher.
- Before providing the patient with the DVD or CD, the nurse should discuss with the patient what the DVD or CD will cover and encourage the patient and caregiver to write down questions or to note what they do not understand.
- After the patient and caregiver view or listen to the material, the nurse should be available to answer any questions they have. The nurse should also reinforce important information from the DVD or CD.

Prosthetic Valves. Valvular replacement may be required for treating mitral, aortic, tricuspid, and occasionally pulmonic valvular disease. This procedure is the surgical treatment of choice for combined aortic stenosis and AR.

A wide variety of prosthetic valves are available. Desirable valves are nonthrombogenic and durable and create minimal stenosis. Prosthetic valves are categorized as mechanical or biological (tissue) valves (Table 39-16 and Figure 39-9).

Mechanical valves are manufactured from artificial materials and consist of combinations of metal alloys, Pyrolite carbon, and Dacron. *Biological valves* are constructed from bovine, porcine, and human cardiac tissue and usually contain some artificial materials. Innovations in freezing and thawing techniques have enabled human grafts to be preserved for extensive periods while retaining viability. Mechanical prosthetic valves are more durable and last longer than biological valves; however, they create an increased risk for thrombo-embolism, necessitating long-term anticoagulation therapy. The main complication of mechanical valves is hemorrhage from the use of anticoagulants (Nishimura, Otto, Bonow, et al., 2014). Biological valves do not necessitate anticoagulation therapy because of their low thrombogenicity. However, they are less durable because of the tendency

TABLE 39-16   TYPES OF CARDIAC PROSTHETIC AND TISSUE VALVES

Type	Description	Advantages	Disadvantages
Mechanical			
Caged-ball valve (Starr–Edwards, Magovern–Cromie)	Metal cage with several struts mounted on a circular ring; hollow metal or plastic ball (poppet) inside of cage	High durability (≤20 yr)	Possibility of blood clots forming on or around valve (thrombogenic) with risk for embolism Need for long-term anticoagulation therapy Very large
Tilting-disc valve (Lillehei–Kaster therapy, Medtronic Hall)	Mobile, lens-shaped disc attached to a circular sewing ring by two offset transverse struts; Pyrolite carbon composition	Hemodynamic efficiency High durability Low thrombogenicity	Need for long-term anticoagulation
Bileaflet valve (St. Jude Medical, Edwards Duromedics, Carbomedics)	Two pivoting semicircular discs that open centrally, mounted directly onto a sewing ring	Compact Successful use in children and patients with small aortic roots	Possibility of thrombogenicity and embolism Need for long-term anticoagulation therapy
Biological			
Porcine heterograft (Carpentier–Edwards, Medtronic Hancock)	Harvested aortic valve of pig that is preserved in glutaraldehyde and mounted on specially designed sewing ring	Low thrombogenicity Need for anticoagulation therapy for only 3 mo after placement	Limited durability (failure rate increases sharply after 5–7 yr) Cumbersome structural design
Pericardial heterograft (Carpentier–Edwards, Ionescu–Shiley)	Three leaflets composed of pericardium from 16- to 18-mo-old calves that are preserved in glutaraldehyde and mounted on a Dacron-covered frame	Low thrombogenicity Need for only short-term anticoagulation therapy Less resistance to blood flow; useful in patients with small aortic roots Outstanding durability	Early valve failure secondary to calcification and degeneration
Homograft (cadaver valve)	Harvested aortic valve from human cadaver that is initially frozen until needed for valve replacement, and then thawed, trimmed, and sewn into place with special mounting material	Excellent hemodynamics No hemolysis and low risk for embolism Only rare need for anticoagulation therapy	Limited durability Not useful for mitral or tricuspid valve replacement

A   B   C   D

FIGURE 39-9 Different types of prosthetic heart valves. **A,** Starr-Edwards caged ball valve. **B,** St. Jude bi-leaflet valve. **C,** Carpentier-Edwards porcine valve. **D,** CoreValve transcatheter aortic valve (CoreValve Evolut R). Sources: *A to C,* Bonow, R. O., Mann, D. L., Zipes, D. P., et al (2012). *Braunwald's heart disease: a textbook of cardiovascular medicine,* ed. 9, Philadelphia: Saunders; *D,* © Medtronic 2017.

for early calcification, tissue degeneration, and stiffening of the leaflets. Risks with both types of prosthetic valves include paravalvular leaks and endocarditis.

Long-term anticoagulation therapy is recommended for all patients with mechanical valves and for those with biological valves and atrial fibrillation. Some patients with biological valves or annuloplasty with prosthetic rings may need anticoagulation therapy for the first few months after surgery, until the suture lines are covered by endothelial cells (endothelialized).

The choice of valves depends on many factors. For example, if a patient cannot take an anticoagulant (e.g., women of child-bearing age), a biological valve may be considered. A mechanical valve may be best for a younger patient because it is more durable. For patients older than age 65, durability is less important than the risk for hemorrhage from anticoagulants.

NURSING MANAGEMENT VALVULAR DISORDERS

NURSING ASSESSMENT

Subjective and objective data should be obtained from patients with valvular disease and are presented in Table 39-17.

NURSING DIAGNOSES

Nursing diagnoses for the patient with valvular heart disease may include but are not limited to the following:

- *Decreased cardiac output* (related to valvular incompetence)
- *Excess fluid volume* related to *excessive fluid intake, excessive sodium intake* (fluid retention secondary to valvular-induced heart failure)
- *Activity intolerance* related to *imbalance between oxygen supply/demand*

Additional information on nursing diagnoses is presented in NCP 39-2, available on the website for this chapter.

PLANNING

The overall goals for the patient with valvular heart disease include (a) normal cardiac function, (b) improved activity tolerance, and (c) an understanding of the disease process and health maintenance measures.

NURSING IMPLEMENTATION

HEALTH PROMOTION. Diagnosing and treating streptococcal infections and providing prophylactic antibiotics for patients with a history of rheumatic fever are critical to preventing acquired rheumatic valvular disease. Patients at high risk for endocarditis and those with valvular prostheses must also be treated with prophylactic antibiotics (see Table 39-4).

Patients must adhere to recommended therapies. Individuals with a history of rheumatic fever, endocarditis, or congenital heart disease should know the symptoms suggestive of valvular heart disease so that early medical treatment may be obtained. The nurse's role is to educate individuals about their condition and the importance of adherence to prescribed therapies. Patient- and family-centred care is important. It is important for patients and caregivers to be well informed about their condition and options for treatment and actively involved in decision making.

ACUTE INTERVENTION AND AMBULATORY AND HOME CARE. Patients with progressive valvular heart disease may require hospitalization or outpatient care for management of HF, endocarditis, embolic disease, or dysrhythmias. HF is the most common reason for an ongoing need for medical care.

TABLE 39-17 NURSING ASSESSMENT

Valvular Heart Disease

Subjective Data
Important Health Information
Past health history: Rheumatic fever, endocarditis, congenital defects, myocardial infarction, chest trauma, cardiomyopathy, syphilis, Marfan syndrome, staphylococcal or streptococcal infections, HIV infection, or compromised immune system.

Medications
IV drug abuse

Symptoms
- Fatigue, generalized weakness, activity intolerance
- Palpitations, dizziness, fainting
- Dyspnea on exertion, cough, hemoptysis, orthopnea, paroxysmal nocturnal dyspnea
- Anginal or atypical chest pain

Objective Data
General
Fever

Integumentary
Diaphoresis, flushing, cyanosis, clubbing; peripheral edema

Respiratory
Crackles, wheezes, hoarseness

Cardiovascular
Abnormal heart sounds, including opening snaps, clicks, thrills, systolic and diastolic murmurs, S_3, and S_4; dysrhythmias, including premature atrial contraction, atrial fibrillation; tachycardia; ↑ or ↓ in pulse pressure; hypotension, water-hammer or thready peripheral pulses, brisk carotid pulses

Gastro-Intestinal
Ascites, hepatomegaly

Possible Diagnostic Findings
Cardiomegaly on chest radiograph; ECG abnormalities specific to involved valve; echocardiogram (valve abnormalities and chamber dilation); cardiac catheterization (abnormalities in valves, chamber pressures, gradients, cardiac output, and blood flow depending on involved valve)

ECG, electrocardiogram; *HIV,* human immunodeficiency virus; *IV,* intravenous; S_3, third heart sound; S_4, fourth heart sound.

The role of the nurse is to implement and evaluate the effectiveness of therapeutic management. Activity should be designed after considering the patient's limitations. An appropriate exercise plan can increase cardiac tolerance. However, activities that regularly produce fatigue and dyspnea should be restricted, and an explanation should be provided to the patient. Smoking cessation should be discussed and encouraged. Strenuous physical exercise should be avoided because damaged valves may not be able to handle the required increase in CO. Patients should be assisted in planning activities of daily living, with an emphasis on conserving energy, setting priorities, and taking planned rest periods. Referral to a vocational counsellor may be necessary for patients with a physically or emotionally demanding job.

Auscultation of the heart should be performed to monitor the effectiveness of digoxin, β-adrenergic blockers, and antidysrhythmic drugs. Teaching regarding the actions and adverse effects of drugs is important to achieve compliance. Patients must understand the importance of prophylactic antibiotic therapy to prevent IE (see Table 39-4). If the valve disease was caused by rheumatic fever, ongoing prophylaxis to prevent recurrence is necessary.

When valvular heart disease can no longer be managed medically, surgical intervention becomes necessary. Patients who are on anticoagulation therapy after surgery for valve replacement must have their international normalized ratio (INR) checked regularly (usually monthly) to assess the adequacy of therapy. The INR is a standardized system of reporting prothrombin time. Values of 2.5 to 3.5 are therapeutic for patients with mechanical valves.

Patients must realize that valve surgery is not a cure and that regular follow-up examinations by the health care provider will be required. The nurse also must teach the patient about when to seek medical care. Any manifestations of infection or HF, any signs of bleeding, and any planned invasive or dental procedures require the patient to notify the health care provider. Finally, patients should be encouraged to wear medical alert identification (e.g., bracelet).

EVALUATION

The expected outcomes for a patient with valvular heart disease are addressed in NCP 39-2, available on the website for this chapter.

ETHICAL DILEMMAS

Do Not Resuscitate

Situation
A 68-year-old man has been admitted for a second mitral valve surgery and coronary artery bypass graft surgery. He did not adhere to the treatment plan following his original surgery 7 years ago. The nurse is worried about his future adherence to medication, diet, and exercise regimens. His kidneys are failing, and he is on dialysis, making him a high-risk surgical patient. The patient and caregivers want all possible treatment and refuse to discuss do-not-resuscitate (DNR) orders.

Important Points for Consideration
- Nonadherence to the treatment plan in the past does not always indicate the patient will not follow the plan of care in the future. Many circumstances related to nonadherence are outside the patient's control such as finances, transportation, availability of assistance, and declining physical and mental capabilities.
- A competent patient can decide whether he wants continued treatment so as to be able to fight to live. This is even more important when family members support the patient's decision.
- Health care providers have an obligation to respect the patient's request for treatment unless there is no clear benefit to continued treatment. Patients' choices to continue or end treatment are based on their values and beliefs, which may not always coincide with those of the health care provider or team.
- DNR orders should reflect the patient's expressed wishes. These wishes can be expressed either through conversation, advance directives, or a surrogate decision maker.
- DNR orders should be re-evaluated periodically with the patient and family, especially before major diagnostic procedures or treatments.
- A nurse who does not agree with a patient's treatment choice should nevertheless respect the patient's choice and ask the patient to explain more about their situation and decision. The nurse should communicate the patient's choice to the health care team and a referral should be made to an ethics committee or similar group as appropriate.

Discussion Questions
1. What type of information should be provided to a patient and family in discussions about DNR orders? Who should provide this information?
2. What measures or strategies would be beneficial to assist the patient to better adhere to the treatment plan?
3. Who can initiate a referral to an ethics committee?

CARDIOMYOPATHY

Cardiomyopathy comprises a group of diseases that directly affect the structural or functional ability of the myocardium. A diagnosis of cardiomyopathy is made based on the patient's clinical manifestations and noninvasive and invasive diagnostic procedures.

Cardiomyopathy can be classified as primary or secondary. *Primary cardiomyopathy* refers to those conditions in which the etiology of the heart disease is unknown (idiopathic). The heart muscle in this case is the only portion of the heart involved; other cardiac structures are unaffected. In *secondary cardiomyopathy*, the cause of the myocardial disease is known and is secondary to another disease process. Common causes of secondary cardiomyopathy are listed in Table 39-18. Each type has its own pathogenesis, clinical presentation, and treatment protocols (Tables 39-19 and 39-20). Cardiomyopathies can lead

TABLE 39-18	CAUSES OF SECONDARY CARDIOMYOPATHY
Dilated	**Hypertrophic**
• Cardiotoxic agents—alcohol, cocaine, doxorubicin	• Aortic stenosis
• Genetic (autosomal dominant) or familial	• Genetic (autosomal dominant)
• Hypertension	• Hypertension
• Ischemia (coronary artery disease)	**Restrictive**
• Metabolic disorders	• Amyloidosis
• Muscular dystrophy	• Endomyocardial fibrosis
• Myocarditis	• Neoplastic tumour
• Pregnancy	• Post–radiation therapy
• Valve disease	• Sarcoidosis
	• Ventricular thrombus

TABLE 39-19	COMPARISON OF CARDIOMYOPATHIES	
Dilated	**Hypertrophic**	**Restrictive**
Major Manifestations		
Fatigue, weakness, palpitations, dyspnea	Exertional dyspnea, fatigue, angina, syncope, palpitations	Dyspnea, fatigue
Cardiomegaly: moderate to marked	Mild to moderate	Mild
Contractility		
↓	↑ or ↓	Normal or ↓
Valvular Incompetence		
Atrioventricular valves, particularly mitral	Mitral valve	Atrioventricular valves
Dysrhythmias		
Sinoatrial tachycardia, atrial and ventricular dysrhythmias	Atrial and ventricular dysrhythmias	Atrial and ventricular dysrhythmias
Cardiac Output		
↓	Normal or ↓	Normal or ↓
Outflow Tract Obstruction		
None	↑	None

TABLE 39-20 COLLABORATIVE CARE

Cardiomyopathy

Diagnostic	Collaborative Therapy
• History and physical examination	• Treatment of underlying cause
• Electrocardiogram	• Drug therapy
• B-type natriuretic peptide (BNP)	• Nitrates (except in HCM)
• Chest radiograph	• β-Adrenergic blockers
• Echocardiogram	• Antidysrhythmics
• Nuclear imaging studies	• ACE inhibitors
• Cardiac catheterization	• Diuretics
• Endocardial biopsy	• Mineralocorticoid receptor antagonist
	• Digitalis (except in HCM) unless used to treat atrial fibrillation)
	• Anticoagulants (if indicated)
	• Sacubitril valsartan (Entresto)
	• Ventricular assist device
	• Cardiac resynchronization therapy
	• Implantable cardioverter–defibrillator
	• Surgical correction
	• Cardiac transplant

ACE, angiotensin-converting enzyme; HCM, hypertrophic cardiomyopathy.

FIGURE 39-10 Dilated cardiomyopathy. The dilated left ventricular wall has thinned, and the chamber size and volume are increased. Source: Kumar, V., Abbas, A. K., & Aster, J. (2013). *Robbins basic pathology* (9th ed., p. 399). Philadelphia: Elsevier Saunders.

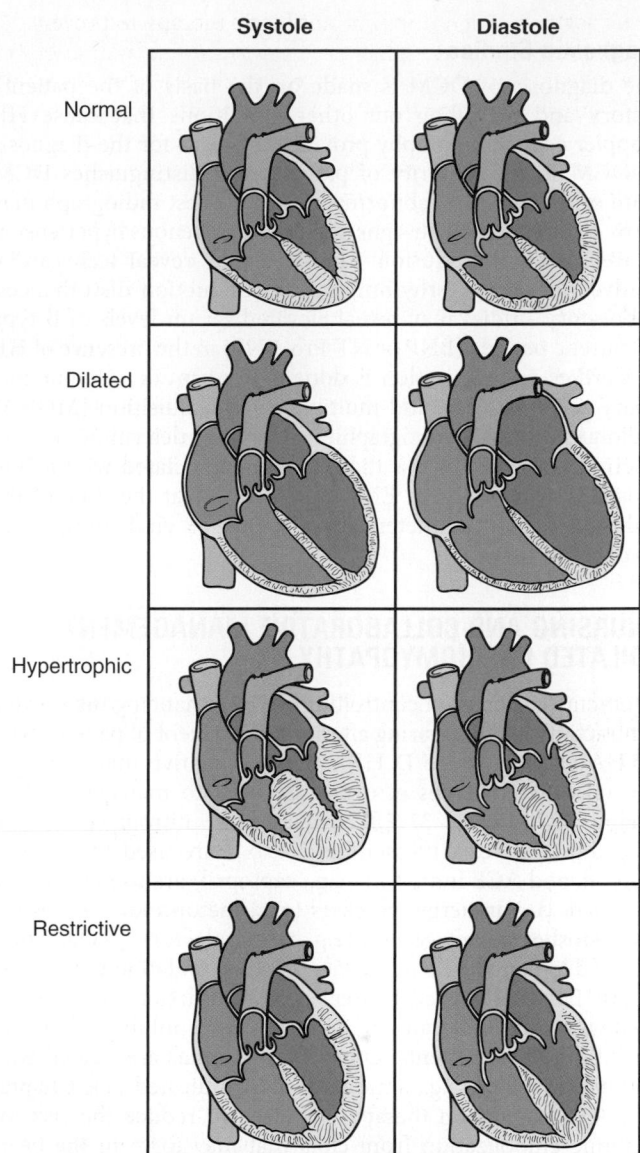

FIGURE 39-11 Types of cardiomyopathies and the differences in ventricular diameter during systole and diastole, compared with a normal heart. Source: Adapted from Urden, L. D., Stacy, K. M., & Lough, M. E. (2014). *Critical care nursing: Diagnosis and management* (7th ed., p. 376). St. Louis: Mosby.

to cardiomegaly and HF and are the leading reason for heart transplantation.

DILATED CARDIOMYOPATHY

Etiology and Pathophysiology

Dilated cardiomyopathy (DCM) is the most common type of cardiomyopathy. It causes HF in 25% to 40% of cases and has a genetic link in 40% of cases (Hershberger, Hedges, & Morales, 2013). DCM is characterized by a diffuse inflammation and rapid degeneration of myocardial fibres. These changes result in ventricular dilation, impairment of systolic function, atrial enlargement, and stasis of blood in the left ventricle. Cardiomegaly results from ventricular dilation (Figure 39-10) and causes contractile dysfunction in spite of an enlarged chamber size. In contrast to HF, the walls of the ventricles do not hypertrophy (Figure 39-11).

DCM often follows an infectious myocarditis. Other common causes of DCM are listed in Table 39-18.

Clinical Manifestations

The signs and symptoms of DCM may develop acutely after an infectious process or insidiously over time. Most people eventually develop HF. Symptoms can include decreased exercise capacity, fatigue, dyspnea at rest, paroxysmal nocturnal dyspnea, and orthopnea. As the disease progresses, the patient may experience dry cough, palpitations, abdominal bloating, nausea, vomiting, and anorexia. Signs can include an irregular heart rate with an abnormal S_3 or S_4 or both, tachycardia or bradycardia, pulmonary crackles, edema, weak peripheral pulses, pallor, hepatomegaly, and jugular venous distension. Heart murmurs and dysrhythmias are common. Decreased blood flow through an enlarged heart promotes stasis and blood clot formation and may lead to systemic embolization.

Diagnostic Studies

The diagnosis of DCM is made on the basis of the patient's history and by ruling out other conditions that cause HF. Doppler echocardiography provides the basis for the diagnosis of DCM in the majority of patients and distinguishes DCM from other structural abnormalities. The chest radiograph may show cardiomegaly with signs of pulmonary venous hypertension as well as pleural effusion. The ECG may reveal tachycardia, bradycardia, and dysrhythmias with conduction disturbances. Laboratory studies may reveal elevated serum levels of B-type natriuretic peptide (BNP or NT-Pro-BNP) in the presence of HF.

Cardiac catheterization is done to confirm or rule out coronary artery disease, and multiple gated acquisition (MUGA) radionuclide angiocardiographies are done to determine ejection fraction (EF). EFs of less than 20% are associated with a 50% mortality within 1 year. EMB may be done at the time of the right-sided heart catheterization to detect viral antigens in myocardial tissue.

NURSING AND COLLABORATIVE MANAGEMENT DILATED CARDIOMYOPATHY

Interventions focus on controlling HF by enhancing myocardial contractility and decreasing afterload. Treatment of patients with NYHA class IV, stage D HF is more palliative than curative. Several different types of drugs are used to manage HF (see Chapter 37, Figure 37-7). Nitrates (e.g., nitroglycerin) and loop diuretics (e.g., furosemide [Lasix]) are used to decrease preload, and ACE inhibitors (e.g., captopril) are used to reduce afterload. β-Adrenergic blockers (e.g., metoprolol [Lopresor]) and aldosterone antagonists (e.g., spironolactone [Aldactone]) are used to control the neuro-hormonal stimulation that occurs in HF. Digoxin is used to treat atrial fibrillation but must be used with caution because of increased susceptibility to digoxin toxicity in these patients. Other dysrhythmias are treated with antidysrhythmics (e.g., amiodarone) as indicated (see Chapter 38). Anticoagulation therapy is started to reduce the risk for systemic embolization from clots that may form in the heart chambers.

Drug and nutritional therapy and cardiac rehabilitation may help alleviate symptoms of HF as well as improve CO and quality of life. Patients with secondary DCM must be treated for the underlying disease process. For example, a patient with alcohol-related DCM must abstain from all alcohol intake. (See Chapter 37 for a complete discussion of HF.)

Unfortunately, DCM does not respond well to therapy, and patients may experience multiple episodes of HF. Intermittent dobutamine or milrinone infusions can be used, with patients' often being admitted to the hospital for a continuous infusion followed by aggressive diuresis. Alternatively, these infusions are done as an outpatient treatment or in the home under supervision of a home care nurse. After infusion, many patients experience an improvement in symptoms that lasts for several weeks.

Patients also may benefit from nonpharmacological therapies such as cardiac resynchronization therapy (Howlett, Chan, Ezekoitz, et al., 2016) or a ventricular assist device (VAD) that may allow the heart to rest and recover from acute HF or be a bridge to heart transplantation. Patients with terminal end-stage cardiomyopathy may be considered for heart transplantation or destination therapy with a permanent or implantable VAD (see Chapter 37). Currently, approximately 50% of heart transplantations are performed for treatment of cardiomyopathy. Heart transplant recipients have a good prognosis for survival. However, donor hearts are difficult to obtain, and many patients with DCM die while awaiting heart transplantation.

Patients with DCM are very ill people with a grave prognosis who need expert nursing care. Patients' families must learn cardiopulmonary resuscitation (CPR) and know how to access emergency care. The nurse should include family members and other support systems when planning a patient's care.

Home health and hospice nursing can provide the patient and the family with the continuous assessments and therapeutic interventions that are required to maximize and maintain functional status or prepare for a peaceful death. Observing for signs and symptoms of worsening HF, dysrhythmias, and embolic formation is paramount in this patient, as is monitoring drug responsiveness. The goal of therapy is to keep the patient at an optimal level of function and out of the hospital.

HYPERTROPHIC CARDIOMYOPATHY

Etiology and Pathophysiology

Hypertrophic cardiomyopathy (HCM)—formerly called *hypertrophic subaortic stenosis, asymmetrical septal hypertrophy (ASH),* or *hypertrophic obstructive cardiomyopathy (HOCM)*—is asymmetrical left ventricular hypertrophy without ventricular dilation. (HOCM was a misleading term because one-third of all patients with HCM have a nonobstructive left ventricular outflow tract (LVOT) at rest or with exertion.) In one form of the disease, the septum between the two ventricles becomes enlarged and obstructs the blood flow from the left ventricle. HCM can be idiopathic, although about one-half of all cases have a genetic basis characterized by inappropriate myocardial hypertrophy (see Table 39-18). HCM occurs less commonly than DCM and is more common in men aged 30 to 40 than in women. In one study, HCM occurred more frequently in young Black male athletes than in young White male athletes. The four main characteristics of HCM are (a) massive ventricular hypertrophy; (b) rapid, forceful contraction of the left ventricle; (c) impaired relaxation (diastolic dysfunction); and (d) obstruction of LVOT (not present in all patients). Ventricular hypertrophy is associated with a thickened intraventricular septum and ventricular wall (Figure 39-12). The end result is impaired ventricular filling as the ventricle becomes noncompliant and unable to relax. The primary defect of HCM is diastolic dysfunction from left ventricular stiffness. Decreased ventricular filling and obstruction to outflow can result in decreased CO, especially during exertion. HCM is the most common cause of SCD in otherwise healthy young people. It accounts for 3% of deaths in young competitive athletes (usually diagnosed in young adulthood) and is often seen in active, athletic individuals (Gersh, Maron, Bonow, et al., 2011; Wilson, Chandra, Papadakis, et al., 2011).

Clinical Manifestations

Patients with HCM may be asymptomatic or may have exertional dyspnea, fatigue, angina, and syncope. The most common symptom is dyspnea, which is caused by an elevated left ventricular diastolic pressure. Fatigue occurs because of the resultant decrease in CO and in exercise-induced flow obstruction. Angina can occur and is most often caused by the increased left ventricular muscle mass or compression of the small coronary arteries by the hypercontractile ventricular myocardium. The patient may also

Left ventricular hypertrophy

FIGURE 39-12 Hypertrophic cardiomyopathy. There is marked left ventricular hypertrophy, and the chamber size and volume are decreased. Source: Kumar, V., Abbas, A. K., & Aster, J. (2013). *Robbins basic pathology* (9th ed., p. 400). Philadelphia: Elsevier Saunders.

have syncope, especially during exertion. Syncope is most often caused by an increase in obstruction to aortic outflow during increased activity, resulting in decreased CO and cerebro-vascular circulation. Syncope can also be caused by dysrhythmias. Common dysrhythmias include supraventricular tachycardia, atrial fibrillation, ventricular tachycardia, and ventricular fibrillation. Any of these dysrhythmias may lead to loss of consciousness or SCD (SCD is discussed in Chapter 36).

Diagnostic Studies

Clinical findings on examination may be unremarkable. However, on palpation of the chest, there may be a forced apical impulse that may be displaced laterally. Auscultation may reveal an S_4 and a systolic ejection murmur between the apex and the sternal border at the fourth intercostal space. ECG findings usually indicate ventricular hypertrophy, ST–T-wave abnormalities, prominent Q waves in the inferior or precordial leads, left-axis deviation, and ventricular and atrial dysrhythmias (see Chapter 38).

The echocardiogram is the primary diagnostic tool to confirm the classic feature of HCM, which is left ventricular hypertrophy. The echocardiogram may also demonstrate wall motion abnormalities and diastolic dysfunction. Cardiac catheterization may also be helpful in the diagnosis of HCM.

NURSING AND COLLABORATIVE MANAGEMENT HYPERTROPHIC CARDIOMYOPATHY

Goals of intervention are to improve ventricular filling by reducing ventricular contractility and relieving LVOT obstruction. These can be accomplished with the use of β-adrenergic blockers, such as metoprolol (Lopresor), or calcium channel blockers, such as verapamil. Use of digitalis preparations is contraindicated unless they are used to treat atrial fibrillation. Antidysrhythmics, such as amiodarone or sotalol, are effective medications for dysrhythmias. However, their use has not been shown to prevent SCD. For patients at risk for SCD, the implantation of a cardioverter–defibrillator is recommended (see Chapter 38).

It has been found that AV pacing can be beneficial for patients with HCM and LVOT obstruction. By pacing the ventricles from the apex of the right ventricle, septal depolarization occurs first, allowing the septum to move away from the left ventricular wall and reducing the degree of obstruction of the LVOT.

Some patients may be candidates for surgical treatment of their hypertrophied septum. The indications for surgery include severe symptoms refractory to therapy with marked obstruction to aortic outflow (>50 mm Hg) while at rest. The surgery is termed a *ventriculomyotomy and myectomy*. It involves incision of the hypertrophied septal muscle and resection of some of the hypertrophied ventricular muscle. Most patients have good symptomatic improvement and improved exercise tolerance after surgery.

An alternative, nonsurgical procedure to reduce symptoms and the LVOT obstruction is alcohol-induced percutaneous transluminal septal myocardial ablation (PTSMA). Through this procedure, alcohol is administered into the first septal artery branching off the left anterior descending artery, causing ischemia and septal wall MI. Ablation of the septal wall decreases the flow obstruction, and the patient's symptoms decrease. The procedure improves HF symptoms and exercise capacity about 3 months after ablation. Mortality rates for the procedure are approximately 1% depending on the age and condition of the patient. Information on long-term effects of PTSMA in treated patients is lacking because the procedure is still new. Potential complications of PTSMA include conduction disturbances (e.g., heart block) and MI beyond the intended septum.

Nursing interventions for HCM focus on relieving symptoms, observing for and preventing complications, and providing emotional and psychological support. Teaching should focus on helping patients adjust their lifestyle to avoid strenuous activity and dehydration. Any activity, such as competitive sports, that causes an increase in systemic vascular resistance (thus increasing the obstruction to forward flow) is dangerous and should be avoided. HCM patients who experience chest pain need to rest and elevate their feet to improve venous return to the heart. Vasodilators such as nitroglycerin may worsen the chest pain by decreasing venous return to the heart, which can further obstruct blood flow from the heart.

RESTRICTIVE CARDIOMYOPATHY

Etiology and Pathophysiology

Restrictive cardiomyopathy (RCM) is the least common of the cardiomyopathic conditions. It is a disease of the heart muscle that impairs diastolic filling and stretch (see Figure 39-11). Systolic function remains unaffected. Although the specific etiology of RCM is unknown, a number of pathological processes may be involved in its development. Myocardial fibrosis, hypertrophy, and infiltration produce stiffness of the ventricular wall with loss of ventricular compliance. Secondary causes of RCM include amyloidosis, endocardial fibrosis, sarcoidosis, fibrosis of different etiology, and radiation to the thorax. With RCM, the ventricles are resistant to filling and, therefore, demand high diastolic filling pressures to maintain CO.

Clinical Manifestations

Classic symptoms of RCM are fatigue, exercise intolerance, and dyspnea because the heart cannot increase CO by increasing the heart rate without further compromising ventricular filling. Additional symptoms may include angina, orthopnea, syncope, and palpitations. The patient may have signs of HF, including dyspnea, peripheral edema, ascites, hepatomegaly, and jugular venous distension.

Diagnostic Studies

The chest radiograph may be normal, or it may show cardiomegaly from right and left atrial enlargement. Pleural effusions and pulmonary congestion may be evident in patients with progression to HF. The ECG may reveal a mild tachycardia at rest. The most common dysrhythmias are supraventricular (atrial fibrillation) and AV block. Echocardiography may reveal a left ventricle that is of normal size with a thickened wall, slightly dilated right ventricle, and dilated atria. EMB, CT, and nuclear imaging may be helpful in the diagnosis.

NURSING AND COLLABORATIVE MANAGEMENT RESTRICTIVE CARDIOMYOPATHY

Currently, no specific treatment for RCM exists. Interventions are aimed at improving diastolic filling and the underlying disease process. Treatment includes conventional therapy for HF and dysrhythmias. Heart transplantation may also be considered. Nursing care is similar to the care of a patient with HF. As in the treatment of patients with HCM, the patient should be taught to avoid situations that impair ventricular filling (e.g., strenuous activity, dehydration, and increases in systemic vascular resistance).

Nursing care of a patient with cardiomyopathy includes individualized teaching based on the patient's clinical manifestations.

All patients with cardiomyopathy are at risk for IE from any procedure that may cause bacteremia and should be instructed on the need for prophylactic antibiotics (see Table 39-3). A general patient and caregiver teaching guide is presented in Table 39-21.

TABLE 39-21   PATIENT & CAREGIVER TEACHING GUIDE
Cardiomyopathy

The following information should be included in the teaching plan for a patient with cardiomyopathy and the patient's caregiver.
- Take all medications as prescribed and follow up with health care provider.
- Use a low-sodium diet (if ordered) and read all product labels (food and over-the-counter drugs) for sodium content.
- Unless fluids are restricted, drink six to eight glasses of water a day.
- Achieve and maintain a reasonable weight, and avoid large meals.
- Avoid alcohol, caffeine, diet pills, and over-the-counter cold medicines that may contain stimulants.
- Balance activity and rest periods.
- Avoid heavy lifting or vigorous isometric exercises, and check with health care provider for exercise guidelines.
- Use stress-reduction activities: relaxation to relieve tension, guided imagery, diversional activities (see Chapter 8).
- Report to health care provider any signs of heart failure, including weight gain, edema, shortness of breath, and increased fatigue.
- Consider having family members learn CPR because of the potential for sudden cardiac arrest.
- Notify health care provider or dentist before any invasive medical or dental procedures since patients with cardiomyopathy are at risk for endocarditis (see Table 39-3).

CPR, cardiopulmonary resuscitation.

CASE STUDY

Valvular Heart Disease

Patient Profile

Ronald Balderson, a 50-year-old man, is admitted to the hospital for valvular heart disease.

Subjective Data
- Reports history of IV drug use
- Prior current regular alcohol intake of approximately 475 mL of whisky per day
- Complains of chest pain with minimal exertion
- Recently unemployed
- States he is short of breath and cannot sleep lying flat
- States he is tired and irritable all the time
- States he cannot afford medications
- Smokes a pack of cigarettes a day

Source: travleview/ Shutterstock .com.

Objective Data
Physical Examination
- Third heart sound (S_3)
- Loud holosystolic murmur of MR
- Wears dentures (teeth removed due to periodontal disease)
- Vital signs: temperature 37.2°C; pulse 110, irregular; respirations 24; BP 104/58

Diagnostic Studies
- ECG shows atrial fibrillation and a rapid ventricular response.
- Chest radiograph reveals pulmonary congestion and cardiomegaly.
- Transesophageal echocardiography shows left atrial and ventricular hypertrophy and mitral and aortic regurgitation.

Discussion Questions
1. Identify the cause and course of Mr. Balderson's disease based on his history and current examination.
2. Differentiate between mitral and aortic regurgitation.
3. What medical treatments or surgical procedures will Mr. Balderson probably require as his condition worsens?
4. ***Priority decision:*** On the basis of the assessment data provided, what are the priority nursing diagnoses?
5. ***Priority decision:*** Identify the priority nursing interventions for Mr. Balderson.
6. ***Evidence-informed practice:*** Mr. Balderson asks why he needs to be on "blood thinners" after his valves are replaced.

⊘volve
Answers are available at *http://evolve.elsevier.com/Canada/Lewis/medsurg*

REVIEW QUESTIONS

The number of the question corresponds to the same-numbered objective at the beginning of the chapter.

1. Assessment of an IV cocaine user with infective endocarditis should focus on which of the following signs and symptoms? *(Select all that apply)*
   a. Retinal hemorrhages
   b. Splinter hemorrhages
   c. Presence of Osler's nodes
   d. Painless nodules over bony prominences
   e. Painless erythematous macules on the palms and soles

2. Which of the following are nursing assessment findings for acute pericarditis?
   a. Wheezing and dull precordial pain
   b. Bradycardia, tachypnea, and murmur
   c. Chest pain, dyspnea, and pericardial friction rub
   d. Respiratory stridor, dull chest pain, and abdominal discomfort

3. Which of the following at-risk individuals need prophylactic antibiotics to prevent IE?
   a. Those with a history of IE.
   b. Those having a viral respiratory infection.
   c. Those entering the third trimester of pregnancy.
   d. Those exposed to human immunodeficiency virus.

4. A client is admitted with myocarditis. Which of the following clinical signs and symptoms might the nurse find while performing the initial assessment? *(Select all that apply)*
   a. Angina
   b. Pleuritic chest pain
   c. Splinter hemorrhages
   d. Pericardial friction rub
   e. Presence of Osler's nodes

5. When teaching a client about the long-term consequences of rheumatic fever, what possibilities should the nurse discuss?
   a. Valvular heart disease
   b. Pulmonary hypertension
   c. Superior vena cava syndrome
   d. Hypertrophy of the right ventricle

6. A client with rheumatic fever should be taught about the need for which of the following?
   a. Regular exercise
   b. Antibiotic therapy
   c. A high-protein diet
   d. Anticoagulant therapy

7. What is a common cause of aortic valve stenosis in older adults?
   a. Rheumatic fever
   b. Cardiomyopathy
   c. Congenital heart disease
   d. Acute infective endocarditis

8. Which of the following findings is indicative of left ventricular overload in a client with chronic aortic regurgitation?
   a. Dehydration and a pericardial friction rub
   b. An audible third heart sound and a midsystolic murmur
   c. Exertional dyspnea and a diastolic high-pitched murmur
   d. An audible third heart sound and a pansystolic or holosystolic murmur

9. A client hospitalized with aortic stenosis has a nursing diagnosis of *activity intolerance* related to *imbalance between oxygen supply/demand*. Which of the following is an appropriate nursing intervention for this client?
   a. Monitoring electrocardiogram to assess cardiac output
   b. Maintaining client on bed rest to reduce tissue oxygen demands
   c. Progressively increasing activity to increase cardiac tolerance
   d. Using semi-Fowler's position to decrease venous return and increase respiratory excursion.

10. What should the nurse caring for a client scheduled for a mitral valve replacement with a mechanical valve understand about this procedure?
    a. It is similar to a commissurotomy.
    b. It requires long-term anticoagulation therapy.
    c. It is the treatment of choice for an older-adult client with a history of falling.
    d. It involves the insertion of a transventricular dilator into the opening of the valve.

11. Which of the following assessment findings would the nurse expect in a client with dilated cardiomyopathy?
    a. Dyspnea and fatigue
    b. Wheezing and epigastric pain
    c. Palpitations and left lower quadrant tenderness
    d. Excessive sputum and lower abdominal cramping

12. The nurse plans care for a client with dilated cardiomyopathy based on what knowledge?
    a. Family members may be at risk because of the infectious nature of the disease.
    b. Medical management of the disorder focuses on treatment of the underlying cause.
    c. The prognosis of the client is poor, and emotional support is a high priority of care.
    d. The condition may be successfully treated with surgical ventriculomyotomy and septal ablation.

1. a, b, c, e; 2. c; 3. a; 4. a, b, d; 5. a; 6. b; 7. a; 8. c; 9. c; 10. b; 11. a; 12. c.

⊖volve

For even more review questions, visit *http://evolve.elsevier.com/Canada/Lewis/medsurg*.

REFERENCES

Adler, Y., Charron, P., Imazio, M., et al. (2015). 2015 ESC guidelines for the diagnosis and management of pericardial diseases. *European Heart Journal, 7*(36), 2921–2964. doi:10.1093/eurheart/ehv318.

Baddour, L. M., Wilson, W. R., Bayer, A. S., et al. (2015). Infective endocarditis in adults: Diagnosis, antimicrobial therapy, and management of complications. A scientific statement for healthcare professionals from the American Heart Association. *Circulation, 132*(15), 1435–1486. doi:10.1161/CIR.0000000000000296.

Burke, A. P. (2015). *Pathology of rheumatic heart disease.* Retrieved from *http://emedicine.medscape.com/article/1962779-overview*.

Caforio, A., Pankuweit, S., Arbustini, E., et al. (2013). Current state of knowledge on aetiology, diagnosis, management and therapy of myocarditis. *European Heart Journal, 34*(33), 2636s–2648d. doi:10.1093/eurheart/eht210.

Gersh, B. J., Maron, B. J., Bonow, R. O., et al. (2011). 2011 ACCF/AHA guidelines for the diagnosis and treatment of hypertrophic cardiomyopathy. *Circulation, 124*, e783–e831. doi:10.1161/CIR.0b013e318223e2bd.

Gewitz, M., Baltimore, R., Tani, L., et al. (2015). Revision of the Jones criteria for the diagnosis of acute rheumatic fever in the era of Doppler echocardiography: A scientific statement from the American Heart Association. *Circulation, 131*(20), 1806–1818. doi:10.1161/CIR.0000000000000205.

Habib, G., Lancellotti, P., Antunes, M., et al. (2015). 2015 ESC guidelines for the management of infective endocarditis. *European Heart Journal, 36*(44), 3075–3128. doi:10.1093/eurheartj/ehv319.

Heart and Stroke Foundation of Canada. (2017a). *Infective (bacterial) endocarditis.* Retrieved from *https://www.heartandstroke.ca/heart/conditions/infective-endocarditis.*

Heart and Stroke Foundation of Canada. (2017b). *What is rheumatic heart disease?* Retrieved from *https://www.heartandstroke.ca/heart/conditions/rheumatic-heart-disease.*

Hershberger, R. E., Hedges, D. J., & Morales, A. (2013). Dilated cardiomyopathy: The complexity of a diverse genetic architecture. *Nature Reviews Cardiology, 10*(9), 531–547. doi:10.1038/nrcardio.2013.105.

Howlett, J., Chan, M., Ezekoitz, J., et al. (2016). The Canadian Cardiovascular Society heart failure companion: Bridging guidelines to your practice. *Canadian Journal of Cardiology, 32*(3), 296–310. doi:10.1016/j.cjca.2015.06.019.

Imazio, M., Gaita, F., & LeWinter, M. (2015). Evaluation and treatment of pericarditis: A systematic review. *Journal of American Medical Association, 314*(14), 1498–1506. doi:10.1001/jama.2015.12763.

Kindermann, I., Barth, C., Mahfoud, F., et al. (2012). Update on myocarditis. *Journal of American College of Cardiology, 59*(9), 779–792. doi:10.1016/j.jacc.2011.09.074.

Lung, B., & Vahanian, A. (2011). Epidemiology of valvular heart disease in the adult. *Nature Reviews in Cardiology, 8*(3), 162–172. doi:10.1038/nrcardio.2010.202.

Nishimura, R., Otto, C., Bonow, R., et al. (2014). 2014 AHA/ACC guideline for the management of vascular health disease. *Journal of the American College of Cardiology, 63*(22), e57–e185. doi:10.1016/j.jacc.2014.02.536.

Que, Y., & Moreillon, P. (2011). Infective endocarditis. *Nature Reviews: Cardiology, 8*(6), 322–336. doi:10.1038/nrcardio.2011.43.

Schmitto, J. D., Mokashi, S. A., & Cohn, L. H. (2010). Minimally-invasive valve surgery. *Journal of the American College of Cardiology, 56*(6), 455–462. doi:10.1016/j.jacc.2010.03.053.

Surapaneni, P., Vinales, K. L., Najib, M. Q., et al. (2011). Valvular heart disease with the use of fenfluramine-phentermine. *Texas Heart Institute Journal, 38*(5), 581–583.

Webb, J., Rodes-Cabau, J., Fremes, S., et al. (2012). Transcatheter aortic valve implantation: A Canadian Cardiovascular Society position statement. *Canadian Journal of Cardiology, 28*(5), 520–528. doi:10.1016/j.cjca.2012.04.015.

Wilson, M., Chandra, N., Papadakis, M., et al. (2011). Hypertrophic cardiomyopathy and ultra-endurance running—two incompatible entities? *Journal of Cardiovascular Magnetic Resonance, 13*(77), doi:10.1186/1532-429X-13-77.

RESOURCES

Resources for this chapter are listed in Chapter 36 and Chapter 37.

Nursing Management
Vascular Disorders

Written by: Deidre D. Wipke-Tevis and Kathleen A. Rich
Adapted by: Phil Bourget

⊖volve WEBSITE

http://evolve.elsevier.com/Canada/Lewis/medsurg

- Review Questions (Online Only)
- Key Points
- Answer Guidelines for Case Study
- Student Case Studies
  - Abdominal Aortic Aneurysm
  - Chronic Peripheral Artery Disease

- Customizable Nursing Care Plans
  - Peripheral Artery Disease of the Lower Extremities
  - Patient after Surgical Repair of the Aorta

- Conceptual Care Map Creator
- Audio Glossary
- Content Updates

LEARNING OBJECTIVES

1. Relate the major risk factors to the etiology and pathophysiology of peripheral artery disease (PAD).
2. Describe the clinical manifestations, collaborative care and surgical and nursing management of PAD of the lower extremities.
3. Plan appropriate nursing interventions for the patient with acute arterial ischemic disorders of the lower extremities.
4. Differentiate the pathophysiology, clinical manifestations, and nursing management of thromboangiitis obliterans (Buerger's disease) and Raynaud's phenomenon.
5. Differentiate the pathophysiology, clinical manifestations, and collaborative care of different types of aortic aneurysms.
6. Select appropriate nursing interventions for a patient undergoing an aortic aneurysm repair.

7. Differentiate the pathophysiology, clinical manifestations, collaborative care, and nursing management of aortic dissection.
8. Evaluate the risk factors predisposing patients to the development of superficial vein thrombosis and venous thrombo-embolism (VTE).
9. Discriminate between the clinical characteristics of superficial vein thrombosis and VTE.
10. Compare and contrast the collaborative care and nursing management of patients with superficial vein thrombosis and VTE.
11. Prioritize the key aspects of nursing management of the patient receiving anticoagulant therapy.
12. Relate the pathophysiology and clinical manifestations to the collaborative care of patients with varicose veins, chronic venous insufficiency, and venous leg ulcers.

KEY TERMS

acute arterial ischemia, p. 921	deep vein thrombosis (DVT), p. 930	post-thrombotic syndrome, p. 933	thromboangiitis obliterans (Buerger's disease), p. 922
aneurysm, p. 924			
aortic dissection, p. 928	intermittent claudication, p. 916	Raynaud's phenomenon, p. 923	varicose veins, p. 939
chronic venous insufficiency (CVI), p. 940	peripheral artery disease (PAD), p. 915	superficial vein thrombosis (SVT), p. 930	venous thrombo-embolism (VTE), p. 930
critical limb ischemia, p. 919			Virchow's triad, p. 930

Problems of the vascular system include disorders of the arteries, veins, and lymphatic vessels. Arterial disorders are classified as aneurysmal, atherosclerotic, and nonatherosclerotic vascular diseases. Atherosclerotic vascular disease is divided into coronary, cerebral, peripheral, mesenteric, and renal artery disease (Creager, Belkin, Bluth, et al., 2012). This chapter is a discussion of peripheral artery disease (PAD), aortic aneurysm and dissection, and venous diseases.

PERIPHERAL ARTERY DISEASE

Peripheral artery disease (PAD) is a condition that involves thickening of artery walls, which results in a progressive narrowing of the arteries of the upper and lower extremities. The risk of developing PAD increases with age, increasing substantially after age 70. In people with diabetes mellitus, PAD occurs much earlier.

PAD is strongly related to other types of cardiovascular disease (CVD) and their risk factors. Patients with PAD are at significantly higher risk of premature mortality in general, death from CVD, major coronary events, and stroke (Mozaffarian, Benjamin, Go, et al., 2016). Thus PAD is a marker of advanced systemic atherosclerosis. Patients with PAD are more likely to have coronary artery disease, cerebral artery disease, or both. Many individuals are not familiar with or aware of PAD risk factors and complications (Hirsch, Allison, Gomes, et al., 2012).

ETIOLOGY AND PATHOPHYSIOLOGY OF PERIPHERAL ARTERY DISEASE

The leading cause of PAD is *atherosclerosis,* a gradual thickening of the *intima* (the innermost layer of the arterial wall) and the *media* (middle layer of the arterial wall) that leads to progressive narrowing of the artery lumen (see Figure 36-1 for diagrams of progression of atherosclerosis). Although the exact cause or causes of atherosclerosis are unknown, inflammation and endothelial injury play a major role (see Chapter 36).

Significant risk factors for PAD include tobacco use, diabetes, hyperlipidemia, elevated C-reactive protein levels, and uncontrolled hypertension. The use of tobacco is one of the main risk factors for PAD. Nicotine is a vasoconstrictor, and tobacco smoke impairs transport and cellular use of oxygen and increases blood viscosity and homocysteine levels. Other risk factors include family history, hypertriglyceridemia, increasing age, hyperhomocysteinemia, hyperuricemia, obesity, sedentary lifestyle, and stress (Ix, Biggs, Kizer, et al., 2011). Women with low lifetime recreational activity are at greater risk for PAD than are similarly sedentary men (Wilson, Sadrzadeh-Rafie, Myers, et al., 2011).

Atherosclerosis more commonly affects certain segments of the arterial tree. These include the coronary (see Chapter 36), carotid (see Chapter 60), common iliac, superficial femoral, popliteal, and tibial arteries (Figure 40-1). Clinical symptoms occur when vessels are 60% to 75% blocked.

PERIPHERAL ARTERY DISEASE OF THE LOWER EXTREMITIES

Lower extremity PAD may affect the aortoiliac, femoral, popliteal, tibial, or peroneal arteries or any combination of these (see Figure 40-1). The femoral popliteal area is the site most commonly affected in nondiabetic patients. Patients with diabetes mellitus tend to develop PAD in the arteries below the knee. In advanced PAD, occlusions are found at multiple levels.

Clinical Manifestations

In general, the severity of the clinical manifestations depends on the site and extent of the obstruction and the amount of collateral circulation. The classic symptom of lower extremity PAD is **intermittent claudication**, an ischemic muscle ache or pain that is precipitated by a consistent level of exercise, resolves within 10 minutes or less with rest, and is reproducible (McDermott, Kibbe, Guralnik, et al., 2013). The ischemic pain is a result of the accumulation of end products of anaerobic cellular metabolism, such as lactic acid. Once the patient stops exercising, the metabolites are cleared and the pain subsides. PAD of the aortoiliac arteries produces claudication in the buttocks and thighs, whereas calf claudication indicates femoral or popliteal artery involvement. Only about 10% of patients with PAD display the well-known symptom of intermittent claudication (McDermott,

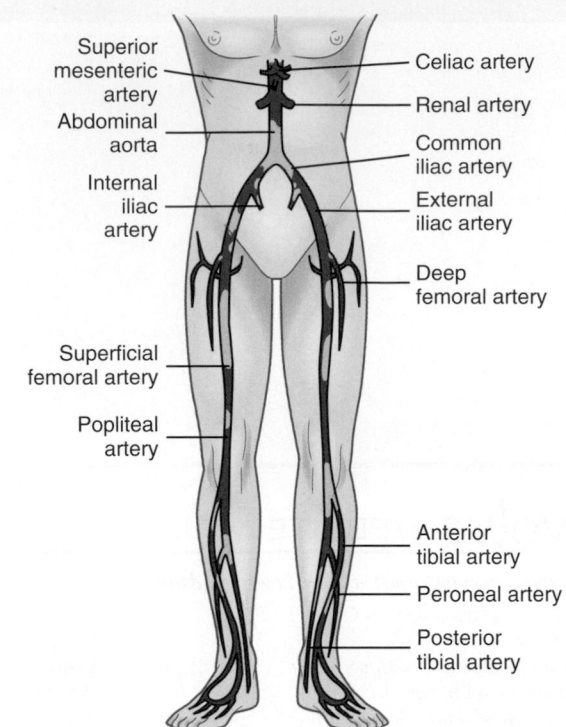

FIGURE 40-1 Common anatomical locations (shown in *yellow*) of atherosclerotic lesions of the abdominal aorta and lower extremities.

Kibbe, Guralnik, et al., 2013). If PAD involves the internal iliac (hypogastric) arteries, erectile dysfunction may result.

Paresthesia, manifested as numbness or tingling in the toes or feet, may result from nerve tissue ischemia. True peripheral neuropathy occurs more commonly in patients with diabetes (see Chapter 52) and in those with longstanding ischemia. Neuropathy produces excruciating shooting or burning pain in the extremity, does not follow particular nerve roots, and may be present near ulcerated areas. Gradually diminishing perfusion to neurons obviates sensations of both pressure and deep pain. Thus affected patients may not notice lower extremity injuries.

The physical appearance of the limb provides important information about blood flow. The skin becomes thin, shiny, and taut, and hair loss occurs on the lower legs. Pedal, popliteal, or femoral pulses are diminished or absent. Pallor (blanching of the foot) develops in response to leg elevation (*elevation pallor*). In dark-skinned patients with pallor, normal brown skin appears to be yellow-brown, and normal black skin often appears to be ashen grey. Assessment of limb pallor in the dark-skinned patient requires observation of less pigmented areas such as the nailbeds or sole of the foot. Conversely, *reactive hyperemia* (redness of the foot) develops when the limb is in a dependent position (*dependent rubour;* Table 40-1). It is difficult to observe erythema in the dark-skinned patient but the limb colour would be darker than other skin areas, often purple, blue or eggplant in colour.

As PAD progresses and involves increasing numbers of arterial segments, continuous pain at rest develops. *Rest pain* most often occurs in the forefoot or toes and is aggravated by limb elevation. Rest pain occurs when blood flow is insufficient to meet basic metabolic requirements of the distal tissues. Rest pain occurs more often at night because cardiac output tends to drop during sleep and the limbs are at the level of the heart. Affected patients often try to partially relieve pain by dangling the leg over the

TABLE 40-1   COMPARISON OF PERIPHERAL ARTERY AND VENOUS DISEASE

Characteristic	Peripheral Artery Disease	Venous Disease
Peripheral pulses	Decreased or absent	Present; may be difficult to palpate with edema
Capillary refill	>3 sec	<3 sec
Ankle–brachial index	≤0.90	>0.90
Edema	Absent unless leg is constantly in dependent position	Lower leg edema
Hair	Loss of hair on legs, feet, toes	Hair may be present or absent
Ulcer location	Tips of toes, foot, or lateral malleolus	Near medial malleolus
Ulcer margin	Rounded, smooth, looks "punched out"	Irregularly shaped
Ulcer drainage	Minimal	Moderate to large amount
Ulcer tissue	Black eschar or pale pink granulation	Yellow slough or dark red, "ruddy" granulation
Pain	Intermittent claudication or rest pain in foot; ulcer may or may not be painful	Dull ache or sensation of heaviness in calf or thigh; ulcer often painful
Nails	Thickened; brittle	Normal or thickened
Skin colour	Dependent rubour; elevation pallor	Bronze-brown pigmentation; varicose veins may be visible
Skin texture	Thin, shiny, taut	Skin thick, hardened, and indurated
Skin temperature	Cool, temperature gradient down the leg	Warm, no temperature gradient
Dermatitis	Rare	Frequent
Pruritus	Rare	Frequent

TABLE 40-2   COLLABORATIVE CARE

Peripheral Artery Disease

Diagnostic
- Health history and physical examination, including palpation of peripheral pulses
- Angiography
- Ankle–brachial index (ABI)
- Doppler ultrasound studies
- Duplex imaging
- Magnetic resonance angiography (MRA)
- Segmental blood pressures

Collaborative Therapy
- Achieve/maintain ideal body weight
- Angiotensin-converting enzyme inhibitors (see Table 35-8)
- Antiplatelet agent (ASA [Aspirin] or clopidogrel [Plavix])
- Cardiovascular disease risk factor modification
- Endarterectomy (for localized stenosis but rarely done)
- Follow Dietary Approaches to Stop Hypertension (DASH) diet (see Table 35-7)
- Nutritional therapy
- Patch graft angioplasty, often in conjunction with bypass surgery
- Pentoxifylline (Trental)
- Percutaneous transluminal atherectomy
- Percutaneous transluminal balloon angioplasty with or without stent
- Percutaneous transluminal cryoplasty
- Peripheral artery bypass surgery
- Proper foot care (see Chapter 52, Table 52-20)
- Regular physical exercise
- Structured walking/exercise program
- Sympathectomy (for pain management only)
- Thrombolytic therapy (for acute ischemia only)
- Tight blood pressure control
- Tight glucose control in diabetic patients
- Tobacco cessation
- Treatment of claudication symptoms
- Treatment of hyperlipidemia (see Table 36-5) and hypertriglyceridemia
- Amputation

side of the bed or sleeping in a chair to allow gravity to maximize blood flow.

Chronic rest pain, ulceration, or gangrene is characteristic of *critical limb ischemia*. Critical limb ischemia often necessitates amputation within 6 months if untreated (McDermott, Kibbe, Guralnik, et al., 2013). Every attempt is made to save the limb, and surgical or endovascular revascularization is indicated. If a patient is not a candidate for revascularization, or if revascularization is not technically possible, medical treatment is indicated (Jones, Dolor, Hasselblad, et al., 2014).

Complications

Lower extremity PAD progresses slowly. Prolonged ischemia leads to atrophy of the skin and underlying muscles. Because of the decreased arterial blood flow, even minor trauma to the feet (e.g., stubbing one's toe, blister from ill-fitting shoes) may result in delayed healing, wound infection, and tissue necrosis, especially in diabetic patients. Arterial (ischemic) ulcers most commonly occur over bony prominences on the toes, feet, and lower leg (see Table 40-1). Nonhealing arterial ulcers and gangrene are the most serious complications. Amputation may be needed if blood flow is not restored adequately or if severe infection occurs.

If PAD has been present for an extended period, collateral circulation may prevent gangrene of the extremity. Uncontrolled pain and severe, spreading infection are indicators that an amputation is required in individuals who are not candidates for revascularization.

Diagnostic Studies

Various tests are used to assess blood flow and outline the vascular system (Table 40-2). In Doppler ultrasonography, a probe is used to direct high-frequency sound waves toward the vessel being examined. Duplex imaging involves a colour Doppler system to systematically map blood flow throughout the entire region of an artery. When palpation of a peripheral pulse is difficult because of severe PAD, the Doppler imaging can determine the degree of blood flow. A palpable pulse and a pulse acquired through the use of Doppler ultrasonography (Doppler pulse) are not equivalent, and the terms are not interchangeable. *Segmental blood pressures* are measured (with Doppler ultrasonography and a sphygmomanometer) at the thigh, below the knee, and at ankle level while the patient is supine. A drop in segmental BP of greater than 30 mm Hg suggests PAD. Angiography and magnetic resonance angiography delineate the location and extent of PAD. They also provide information on inflow and outflow vessels to plan for surgery (see Table 34-6).

The *ankle–brachial index* (ABI) is a PAD screening tool. It is measured with a handheld Doppler probe. To calculate the ABI, the ankle systolic blood pressures (BPs) are divided by the higher of the left and right brachial systolic BP (Lin, Olson, Johnson, et al., 2013). A normal ABI is 1.00 to 1.40 and indicates adequate

TABLE 40-3	INTERPRETATION OF ANKLE–BRACHIAL INDEX RESULTS
Ankle–Brachial Index (ABI)	**Clinical Significance**
≥1.40	Noncompressible arteries
1.00–1.40	Normal ABI
0.91–0.99	Borderline ABI
≤0.90	Abnormal ABI
Classification of PAD Severity	
0.90–0.71	Mild PAD
0.71–0.41	Moderate PAD
≤40	Severe PAD

PAD, peripheral artery disease.

BP in the extremities. An ABI between 0.91 and 0.99 is considered borderline, a value of 0.90 or less is abnormal, and values greater than 1.40 indicate noncompressible arteries (Rooke, Hirsch, Misra, et al., 2011; Table 40-3). An ABI has limited usefulness when arteries are calcified and noncompressible, as occurs in patients with diabetes mellitus and PAD. In such patients, the ABI frequently is falsely elevated. ABI measurement is not recommended immediately after revascularization surgery or on distal bypass grafts because of the risk of graft thrombosis (Aboyans, Criqui, Abraham, et al., 2012).

Collaborative Care

Table 40-2 summarizes the collaborative care for a patient with PAD.

Risk Factor Modification. Patients who have diabetes and atherosclerotic vascular disease such as coronary artery disease or PAD are at the highest risk for cardiovascular events such as myocardial infarction (MI), ischemic stroke, and CVD-related death. The Clinical Practice Guidelines of the Canadian Diabetes Association Clinical Practice Guidelines Expert Committee (2013) stress the importance of lifestyle modifications such as achieving and maintaining a healthy body weight, regular physical activity, smoking cessation, optimal BP control, and optimal glycemic control to reduce CVD risk factors. Risk factors may be modified with drug therapy and lifestyle changes on the part of the patient and caregiver (see Tables 36-1 through 36-5). Tobacco cessation is essential in the management of patients with PAD to reduce the risk of CVD events, PAD progression, and death. Tobacco cessation is a complex and difficult process with a high incidence of relapse. All patients with PAD should have access to comprehensive smoking cessation interventions (see the Resources at the end of Chapter 11).

Canadian lipid guidelines recommend aggressive management with a low-density lipoprotein cholesterol level of 2.0 mmol/L or less, and a total cholesterol and high-density lipoprotein cholesterol ratio less than 4.0 mmol/L (Pike-MacDonald, 2013). Although dietary change is also recommended, this alone is unlikely to achieve these goals. Research indicates that in patients with PAD, treatment with a statin (e.g., simvastatin [Zocor]) not only lowers cholesterol levels but also reduces risks of CVD-related morbidity and mortality. Table 36-5 lists medications to lower cholesterol.

Hypertension is a major risk factor for PAD progression, as well as for other CVD events (e.g., stroke, MI, heart failure). The Canadian Hypertension Education Program (2015) recommendations for the management of hypertension in patients with PAD and CVD include BP lower than 140/90 mm Hg. In such patients

who also have diabetes mellitus, BP lower than 130/80 mm Hg is recommended. Initial antihypertensive drug therapy includes thiazides, angiotensin-converting enzyme inhibitors, and angiotensin II receptor blockers. Lifestyle changes are encouraged and include reducing dietary sodium and following the Dietary Approaches to Stop Hypertension (DASH) diet. (Hypertension is discussed in Chapter 35.)

Diabetes is a well-known risk factor for PAD and increases the risk of needing amputation in these patients. It is recommended that patients with diabetes maintain a glycosylated hemoglobin (hemoglobin A_{1c}) below 7.0% and, optimally, as close as possible to 6.0%. (Diabetes mellitus is discussed in Chapter 52.)

Drug Therapy. Antiplatelet agents are considered crucial for reducing the risks of CVD events and death in patients with PAD. Guidelines for oral antiplatelet therapy recommend acetylsalicylic acid (ASA; Aspirin) (75–325 mg/day). For patients who are ASA (Aspirin) intolerant, clopidogrel (Plavix; 75 mg/day) is indicated. Combination antiplatelet therapy with ASA (Aspirin) and clopidogrel is not recommended. Likewise, anticoagulants (e.g., warfarin [Coumadin]) are not recommended for the prevention of CVD events in patients with PAD. The use of angiotensin-converting enzyme inhibitors (e.g., ramipril [Altace]) decreases risks of morbidity and mortality (Rooke, Hirsch, Misra, et al., 2011).

Pentoxifylline (Trental) is used to treat intermittent claudication. It improves peripheral blood flow by increasing red blood cell flexibility and reducing blood viscosity. Anticoagulants, oral vasodilator prostaglandins, and chelation are not recommended for the treatment of claudication symptoms (McDermott, Kibbe, Guralnik, et al., et al., 2013). One promising approach to claudication treatment under investigation is levocarnitine (Carnitor), a naturally occurring derivative of the amino acid lysine. Carnitine improves initial and maximal treadmill walking distance and quality of life (Delaney, Spark, Thomas, et al., 2013).

> **DRUG ALERT—Clopidogrel (Plavix) and Omeprazole (Losec)**
> - Antiplatelet effect of clopidogrel is reduced by about half when given with omeprazole.
> - This increases the risk of myocardial infarction and stroke.

Exercise Therapy. The primary nondrug treatment for intermittent claudication is tobacco cessation in combination with a formal, supervised exercise-training program. Lack of exercise in patients with PAD is related to low quality of life, particularly in men (Parmenter, Dieberg, Phipps, et al., 2015). Walking is the most effective exercise for patients with PAD. A supervised, hospital-based PAD rehabilitation program is an effective means of improving exercise performance. Such programs typically include exercise for 30 to 60 minutes a day, three to five times a week, for 3 to 6 months. Supervised, treadmill exercise training improves walking performance and quality of life in patients with PAD regardless of whether they have claudication (McDermott, Kibbe, Guralnik, et al., 2013). A home exercise program is an alternative to a formal program. The nurse should encourage slow, progressive physical activity after a warm-up period. The patient is instructed to walk until the point of discomfort, stop and rest, and then resume walking until the discomfort recurs. Walking should be done for 30 to 40 minutes a day, three to five times a week, for at least 6 months. An exercise therapy program should also be implemented in patients with PAD after surgical interventions (discussed later in this chapter).

Nutritional Therapy. Patients with PAD should be taught to adjust their dietary intake so that their body mass index is less than 25 kg/m² and their waist circumference is less than 101.6 cm (40 inches) for men and less than 89 cm (35 inches) for women (Heart and Stroke Foundation of Canada, 2017). A diet high in fruits, vegetables, and whole grains and low in cholesterol, saturated fat, and salt is recommended. Dietary cholesterol intake should be less than 200 mg/day, saturated fat intake should be substantially reduced, and dietary sodium should be 2 g/day or less (see Chapter 37, Table 37-11).

Complementary and Alternative Therapies. A number of vitamin, mineral, dietary, and herbal supplements have been investigated in the treatment of intermittent claudication. Currently data are insufficient to support the efficacy of supplemental fish oil, ginkgo biloba, L-arginine, or homocysteine-lowering vitamins (e.g., folate, vitamin B₆, cobalamin) in the treatment of claudication (Brass, 2013). Vitamin E is not recommended to treat claudication (McDermott, Kibbe, Guralnik, et al., 2013). Patients taking antiplatelet agents (e.g., ASA [Aspirin]), nonsteroidal anti-inflammatory agents (NSAIDs; e.g., ibuprofen [Motrin]), and anticoagulants (e.g., warfarin) should consult with their health care provider before taking any dietary or herbal supplements because of potential interactions and bleeding risks (see the "Complementary & Alternative Therapies: Natural Health Products That May Affect Clotting" box later in the chapter; Grant, Bin, Kiat, et al., 2012).

Care of the Leg With Critical Limb Ischemia. Critical limb ischemia is a condition characterized by chronic ischemic rest pain lasting more than 2 weeks, arterial leg ulcers, or gangrene of the leg as a result of PAD (Rooke, Hirsch, Misra, et al., 2011). Optimal therapy is revascularization through surgery or endovascular procedure. Although aggressive CVD risk factor modification and antiplatelet therapy are palliative in nature, all patients with critical limb ischemia should undergo these to decrease the risk of a CVD event (Jones, Dolor, Hasselblad, et al., 2014).

Conservative management goals include protecting the extremity from trauma, decreasing ischemic pain, preventing and controlling infection, and maximizing perfusion. The patient should carefully inspect, cleanse, and lubricate both feet to prevent cracking of the skin and infection. The patient must avoid soaking feet to prevent skin *maceration* (or breakdown). If ulceration is present, the affected foot must be kept clean and dry. Any ulcers should be covered with a dry, sterile dressing to maintain cleanliness and protect the limb. Ulcers with significant depth may be treated with a variety of wound care products, but healing is unlikely without increased blood flow. The nurse should encourage the patient to select soft, roomy, and protective footwear and avoid extremes of heat and cold. The patient's heels should be kept free of pressure. This may be accomplished by placing a pillow under the calves so that the heels are off the bed. Commercially available devices can also provide heel protection. Opioid analgesia and placing the bed in the reverse Trendelenburg position may control pain and facilitate perfusion to the lower extremities (Jones, Dolor, Hasselblad, et al., 2014).

Some evidence indicates that spinal cord stimulation or hyperbaric oxygen therapy may be helpful in preventing the need for amputation in patients with critical limb ischemia (Benoit, O'Donnell, Kitsios, et al., 2012). Another promising strategy under investigation is gene therapy to stimulate blood vessel growth (angiogenesis; Grochot-Przeczek, Dulak, & Jozkowicz, 2013).

Interventional Radiological Catheter-Based Procedures. Interventional radiology catheter-based procedures are alternatives to open surgical approaches for treatment of PAD in the lower extremity. These procedures take place in a catheterization

laboratory rather than an operating room. Determining which intervention to use depends on stenosis location, along with type and severity of the lesion. After the procedure, most patients can ambulate the same day and return to normal activity within 24 to 48 hours. All of these procedures are similar to angiography in that they involve the insertion of a specialized catheter into the femoral artery. The *percutaneous transluminal angioplasty* procedure involves the use of a catheter that contains a cylindrical balloon at the tip. The end of the catheter is advanced to the narrowed (stenotic) area of the artery. When in position, the balloon is inflated, compressing the confining atherosclerotic intimal lining while also stretching the underlying media.

Stents, expandable metallic devices, are positioned within the artery immediately after the balloon angioplasty is performed. The stent acts as a scaffold to keep the artery open and is used as a treatment for peripheral artery dissection (Deiter & Nanjundappa, 2012). Dissection is a tear in the inner arterial wall that causes blood to flow between the layers of the artery, separating or dissecting the layers and often causing a false lumen. Stents may be covered with Dacron or a drug-eluting agent (e.g., paclitaxel) to minimize re-stenosis by reducing the amount of new tissue growth in the stent.

Atherectomy is the removal of the obstructing plaque. In directional atherectomy, a high-speed cutting disc built into the catheter end cuts long strips of the atheroma. In laser atherectomy, ultraviolet energy is used to break the molecular bonds of the atheroma to reduce the stenosis (Ahmed, 2015). Orbital or rotational atherectomy catheters have a diamond-coated tip that rotates at high speed (similar to a dentist drill) to pulverize the calcium within the atheroma into particles smaller than a blood cell.

Cryoplasty is a combination of two procedures: balloon angioplasty and cold therapy. The specialized balloon is inflated with liquid nitrous oxide that changes from liquid to gas as it enters the balloon. Expansion of the gas results in cooling to −10°C. The cold minimizes re-stenosis through reduction of smooth muscle cell activity (Dominguez, Bahadorani, Reeves, et al., 2015). Preprocedure and post-procedure nursing care are the same as those for diagnostic angiography. Antiplatelet agents are necessary after the procedure to reduce the risk of re-stenosis. Long-term, low-dose ASA (Aspirin) therapy is recommended after the procedure (Brass, 2013). Re-stenosis rates depend on the procedure performed, lesion type and length, and characteristics of the target vessel. Immediate post-procedure success rates are high (>95%) for iliac and femoral interventions (Ahmed, 2015).

Surgical Therapy. Various surgical approaches can be used to improve blood flow beyond a stenotic or occluded artery. The most common is a peripheral artery bypass operation with autogenous (native) vein or synthetic graft material to bypass or carry blood around the lesion (Figure 40-2). Synthetic grafts (expanded polytetrafluoroethylene or Dacron) typically are used for long bypasses such as axillary–femoral or axillary–popliteal bypasses. When a patient's own vein is not available, human umbilical vein, cryopreserved vein, or a composite sequential bypass graft is an alternative. Percutaneous transluminal angioplasty with stenting also may be used in combination with bypass surgery. Other surgical options include *endarterectomy* (opening the artery and removing the obstructing plaque) and *patch graft angioplasty* (opening the artery, removing plaque, and sewing a patch to the opening to widen the lumen).

Amputation may be required if tissue necrosis is extensive, if infectious gangrene or osteomyelitis (infection in the bone)

FIGURE 40-2 A, Femoral–popliteal bypass graft around an occluded superficial femoral artery. **B,** Femoral–posterior tibial bypass graft around occluded superficial femoral, popliteal, and proximal tibial arteries.

develops, or if all major arteries in the limb are occluded, all of which preclude the possibility of successful reparative surgery (Benoit, O'Donnell, Kitsios, et al., 2012). Every effort is made to preserve as much of the limb as possible so that the potential for rehabilitation is optimized. Implementation of an amputee mobility protocol after surgery can increase functional mobility of patients with a lower limb amputation and maximize their rehabilitation potential (Benoit, O'Donnell, Kitsios, et al., 2012). (Amputation is discussed in Chapter 65.)

COMPLEMENTARY & ALTERNATIVE THERAPIES
Natural Health Products That May Affect Clotting

Anticoagulant Effects
Increased
Angelica, anise, bilberry, bromelain, celery, chamomile, devil's claw, dong quai, fenugreek, feverfew, garlic, ginger, *Ginkgo biloba,* goldenseal, horse chestnut, licorice root, lovage root, meadowsweet, motherwort, parsley, passionflower, red clover, rue, turmeric, willow bark

Decreased
Coenzyme Q_{10}, ginseng, green tea, St. John's wort

Nursing Implications
- In general, these natural products should be used with caution or not at all by patients with bleeding or clotting disorders or those taking anticoagulant and antiplatelet drugs (e.g., warfarin [Coumadin], heparin, low-molecular-weight heparin, ASA [Aspirin], ticlopidine, or clopidogrel [Plavix]). These patients should consult with a health care provider before using any of these natural products.
- These natural health products should be discontinued at least 2 to 3 wk before surgery to avoid potential complications. If this is not possible, the herbal product in its original container should be brought to the health care provider or the surgery site so the anaesthesia care provider knows exactly what the patient is taking.
- One common mechanism of these products is to inhibit platelet aggregation.

TABLE 40-4 NURSING ASSESSMENT
Peripheral Artery Disease

Subjective Data
Important Health Information
Past health history: Diabetes mellitus, tobacco use, hypertension, hyperlipidemia, hypertriglyceridemia, hyperuricemia, impaired renal function, obesity; ↑ high-sensitivity C-reactive protein, homocysteine or lipoprotein (a) levels; positive family history; exposure to environmental smoke; sedentary lifestyle; stress
High intake of sodium, saturated fat, and cholesterol; elevated hemoglobin A_{1c} level
Exercise intolerance

Symptoms
- Buttock, thigh, or calf pain that is precipitated by exercise and that subsides with rest (intermittent claudication) or progresses to pain at rest; burning pain in feet and toes at rest; numbness, tingling, sensation of cold in legs or feet; progressive loss of sensation and deep pain in extremities
- Erectile dysfunction

Objective Data
Integumentary
Loss of hair on legs and feet; thick toenails; pallor with elevation; dependent rubour; thin, cool, shiny skin with muscle atrophy; skin breakdown and arterial ulcers, especially over bony areas; gangrene

Cardiovascular
Decreased or absent peripheral pulses; feet cool to touch; capillary refill >3 sec; possible presence of bruits at pulse sites

Neurological
Mobility or sensation impairment

Possible Diagnostic Findings
Arterial stenosis evident with duplex imaging, ↓ segmental limb pressures (Doppler ultrasound pressures combined with blood pressure measurements), ↓ ankle–brachial index (ABI), angiogram indicative of peripheral atherosclerosis

---

NURSING MANAGEMENT
LOWER EXTREMITY PERIPHERAL ARTERY DISEASE

NURSING ASSESSMENT
Table 40-4 lists subjective and objective data that the nurse should obtain from a patient with PAD.

NURSING DIAGNOSES
Nursing diagnoses for a patient with PAD of the lower extremities (who has not undergone surgery) may include, but are not limited to, the following:
- *Ineffective peripheral tissue perfusion* related to *insufficient knowledge of disease process*
- *Activity intolerance* related to *imbalance between oxygen supply/demand*
- *Chronic pain* related to *injury agent* (ischemia, inflammation, and swelling)
- *Ineffective health management* related to *insufficient knowledge of therapeutic regimen, difficulty managing complex treatment regimen*

Additional information on nursing diagnoses for the patient with PAD of the lower extremities is presented in Nursing Care Plan (NCP) 40-1, available on the Evolve website for this chapter.

PLANNING

The overall goals for a patient who has lower extremity PAD include (a) adequate tissue perfusion; (b) relief of pain; (c) increased exercise tolerance; and (d) intact, healthy skin on extremities.

NURSING IMPLEMENTATION

HEALTH PROMOTION. The nurse assesses the patient for CVD risk factors and provides instructions on how to control them (see Chapter 36, Tables 36-1 and 36-2). The nurse also teaches diet modification to reduce the intake of cholesterol, saturated fat, and refined sugars; proper care of the feet; and the avoidance of injury to the extremities. Patients with positive family histories of cardiac, diabetic, or vascular disease are encouraged to obtain regular follow-up care.

ACUTE INTERVENTION. After surgical or radiological intervention, the patient is moved to a recovery area for observation. The nurse checks the operative extremity every 15 minutes initially and then hourly for colour, temperature, capillary refill, presence of peripheral pulses, and sensation and movement. If the nurse observes loss of palpable pulses or a change in the Doppler sound over a pulse, or both, the physician or radiologist must be notified immediately and prompt intervention undertaken. ABI measurements may be ordered, and the indexes should be higher than the patient's baseline and should remain stable if the bypass (or stent) remains patent. The nurse compares all assessment findings with the patient's baseline and with findings in the opposite limb (Jarvis, Browne, Macdonald-Jenkins, et al., 2014). Many patients with PAD have a history of chronic ischemic rest pain and may have developed a tolerance to opioids. Therefore, aggressive pain management may be needed postoperatively.

After the patient leaves the recovery area, the nurse continues to monitor perfusion to the extremities and to assess for potential complications such as bleeding, hematoma, thrombosis, embolization, and compartment syndrome. A dramatic increase in pain, loss of previously palpable pulses, extremity pallor or cyanosis, decreasing ABIs, numbness or tingling, or a cold extremity suggests occlusion of the graft or stent. The nurse must report these findings to the physician immediately.

The patient should not be placed in a knee-flexed position except for exercise. The patient should be turned and repositioned frequently with pillows to avoid strain on the incision. On postoperative day 1, the nurse assists the patient out of bed several times daily. Short periods of different leg and body positions will not impair postoperative skin oxygen levels. Prolonged sitting with leg dependency should be discouraged because it may cause pain and edema, increase the risk of venous thrombosis, and place stress on the suture lines. If edema develops, the nurse positions the patient supine and elevates the edematous leg above heart level. On occasion, graduated compression stockings are used to help control leg edema. Walking even short distances is desirable. The use of a walker may be helpful, especially in frail older adult patients. Although graft patency and mortality rates are equivalent for men and women after lower extremity revascularization, women are more likely to develop wound complications than are men (Lo, Bensley, Hamdan, et al., 2013).

Surgical site infection after lower extremity revascularization occurs in about 11% of cases. Women develop such infections more often than do men. Careful postoperative assessment and wound care are important. Surgical site infections are associated with early graft loss, reoperation, and sepsis (Greenblatt, Rajamanickam, & Mell, 2011). If no complications are present, discharge from the hospital can be anticipated 3 to 5 days postoperatively.

AMBULATORY AND HOME CARE. The nurse should assess for CVD risk factors and be alert for opportunities to teach health promotion strategies to patients and their caregivers (see Chapters 4 and 36). Tobacco use in any form (including environmental smoke) is contraindicated. Nicotine exerts vasoconstrictive effects, and tobacco smoke impairs transport and cellular utilization of oxygen and increases blood viscosity and homocysteine levels. Continued tobacco use dramatically decreases the long-term patency rates of grafts and stents and increases the risk of an MI or stroke. The nurse should encourage physical activity and explain that it improves a number of CVD risk factors, including hypertension, hyperlipidemia, obesity, and glucose levels. Physical activity also improves peripheral circulation and increases walking distance (Parmenter, Dieberg, Phipps, et al., 2015).

The nurse should teach foot care to all patients with PAD. Meticulous foot care is especially important in diabetic patients with PAD (see Table 52-20). Diabetic neuropathy increases the patient's susceptibility to traumatic injury and results in delay in seeking treatment. Patients are instructed to inspect their legs and feet daily for mottling, changes in skin colour, skin texture, amount of subcutaneous fat, and reduction in hair growth. The nurse can also teach patients to check skin temperature and capillary refill and to palpate pulses. The nurse should emphasize that patients must report any changes in these findings or the development of any ulceration or inflammation to their health care provider. Thick or overgrown toenails and calluses are potentially serious and require regular attention by a skilled health care provider (e.g., podiatrist). Patients who have poor eyesight, back problems, obesity, or arthritis may need assistance with foot care. Patients are encouraged to wear clean, all-cotton or all-wool socks and comfortable shoes with rounded (not pointed) toes and soft insoles. Shoes should be laced loosely, and patients should break in new shoes gradually (Table 40-5).

EVALUATION

NCP 40-1, available on the Evolve website, addresses the expected outcomes for the patient with PAD of the lower extremities.

ACUTE ARTERIAL ISCHEMIC DISORDERS

Etiology and Pathophysiology

Acute arterial ischemia is a sudden interruption in the arterial blood supply to a tissue, organ, or extremity that, if left untreated, can result in tissue death. It is caused by embolism, thrombosis of a pre-existing atherosclerotic artery, or trauma. Embolization of a thrombus (clot) from the heart is the most frequent cause of acute arterial occlusion. Heart conditions in which thrombi can develop include infective endocarditis, MI, mitral valve disease, chronic atrial fibrillation, and cardiomyopathies; thrombi can also develop in prosthetic heart valves. Noncardiac sources of emboli include aneurysms, ulcerated atherosclerotic plaque, and venous thrombi. Emboli can also develop as a result of recent endovascular procedures, and, in rare cases, arteritis.

Thrombi become dislodged and may travel anywhere in the systemic circulation if they originate in the left side of the heart. The majority of emboli obstruct an artery of the lower extremity (e.g., iliofemoral, popliteal, tibial) (Anderson, Halperin, Albert, et al., 2013).

Arterial emboli tend to lodge at sites of arterial branching or in areas of atherosclerotic narrowing. An acute arterial occlusion

TABLE 40-5   PATIENT & CAREGIVER TEACHING GUIDE

Peripheral Artery Bypass Surgery

The following information should be included in the teaching plan for a patient undergoing peripheral artery bypass surgery and the patient's caregiver:

1. Patients can reduce risk factors by stopping the use of tobacco products, by controlling blood pressure and blood glucose levels (if diabetic), by lowering cholesterol and triglyceride levels, by achieving/maintaining ideal body weight, and by exercising regularly.
2. Patients should be provided rationales, basic mechanism of action, and anticipated duration of medications such as antiplatelets, antihypertensives, anticholesterol therapy, and pain medication.
3. Diet must be healthy—it is essential to recovery. Patients should drink plenty of fluids, follow a well-balanced diet (e.g., foods high in protein, vitamins C and A, and zinc; high-fibre foods; fresh fruits and vegetables), eat fewer high-fat foods, and reduce salt intake.
4. Patients should participate in a supervised exercise program, take a daily walk, or both. In the beginning, patients may take several short walks a day and rest between activities. Walking is gradually increased to 30–40 min/day, 3–5 days/wk.
5. Patients should care for their feet and legs; inspect feet and wash them daily; wear clean cotton or wool socks and well-fitting shoes; file toenails straight across; and avoid sitting with legs crossed, extreme hot and cold temperatures, and prolonged standing.
6. Routine postoperative wound care includes keeping incision clean and dry; Steri-Strips (if present) should not be disturbed.
7. Patients should monitor for signs and symptoms of impaired healing and infection of the leg incision, and they should notify the health care provider if any of the following occur:
   • Prolonged drainage or pus from the incision
   • Increased redness, warmth, pain, or hardness along incision
   • Separation of wound edges
   • Body temperature greater than 37.8°C
8. Patients must keep all follow-up appointments with their health care provider.
9. The health care provider should be notified if the patient experiences increased leg or foot pain or a change in the colour or temperature of the foot and leg.

causes the oxygen and blood supply distal to the embolus to decrease suddenly, producing ischemia. The amount of tissue and muscle at risk, degree of the ischemia, and extent of the symptoms depend on several factors, including (a) the location and size of the occlusion, (b) the occurrence of clot fragmentation with embolism to smaller vessels, (c) the degree of PAD already present, and (d) the presence of collateral vessels around the acute obstruction.

Sudden local thrombosis may occur at the site of an atherosclerotic plaque. States of hypovolemia (e.g., resulting from shock), hyperviscosity (e.g., resulting from polycythemia), and hypercoagulability (e.g., resulting from chemotherapy) predispose an individual to thrombotic arterial occlusion (Ouriel & Kasyap, 2011).

Traumatic injury to the extremity itself may cause partial or total occlusion. Acute arterial occlusion may also develop as a result of arterial dissection in the carotid artery or aorta or as a result of iatrogenic arterial injury (e.g., after angiography).

Clinical Manifestations

Clinical manifestations of acute arterial ischemia include the "six *Ps*": **p**ain, **p**allor, **p**aralysis, **p**ulselessness, **p**aresthesia, and **p**oikilothermia (adaptation of the limb to the environmental

temperature, most often cool). Without immediate intervention, ischemia may progress quickly to tissue necrosis and gangrene within a few hours. If the nurse detects these signs, the nurse should immediately notify the physician. Paralysis is a very late sign of acute arterial ischemia and signals the death of nerves supplying the extremity. Footdrop occurs as a result of nerve damage. Because nerve tissue is extremely sensitive to hypoxia, limb paralysis or ischemic neuropathy may be permanent even after revascularization.

Collaborative Care

Early treatment is essential to keep the affected limb viable during acute arterial ischemia. Anticoagulant therapy with continuous intravenous (IV) unfractionated heparin is started to prevent thrombus enlargement and inhibit further embolization (Schulman, 2014). In patients undergoing embolectomy, unfractionated heparin should be followed by long-term anticoagulation with warfarin (see discussion of other anticoagulant options later in this chapter). To restore blood flow, the embolus/thrombus is removed as soon as possible. Options for embolus/thrombus removal include percutaneous catheter-directed thrombolytic therapy, percutaneous mechanical thrombectomy with or without thrombolytic therapy, surgical thrombectomy, or surgical bypass (Jones, Dolor, Hasselblad, et al., 2014). Catheter-directed intra-arterial thrombolytic therapy (e.g., tissue plasminogen activator [tPA], or alteplase) is recommended for patients with short-term (<14 days) thrombo-embolic disease (Schulman, 2014). A percutaneous catheter is inserted into the femoral artery and threaded to the site of the clot, and the thrombolytic drug is infused. Thrombolytic agents work by directly dissolving the clot over a period of 24 to 48 hours. (Thrombolytic therapy is discussed in Chapter 36.) The catheter may act as a mechanical thrombectomy device; that is, it is also designed to remove or fragment the thrombus (Jones, Dolor, Hasselblad, et al., 2014).

Surgical intervention is recommended for some patients (e.g., those with ischemia for more than 14 days when catheter-based interventions are not possible, as with inability of the guide wire to transverse the thrombus) (Jones, Dolor, Hasselblad, et al., 2014). Direct arteriotomy may be necessary to remove the clot. Surgical revascularization may be used in a patient with trauma (e.g., laceration of the artery) or with significant arterial occlusion. Amputation is reserved for patients with ischemic rest pain and tissue loss, for whom limb salvage is not possible. If the patient remains at risk for further embolization from a persistent source (e.g., chronic atrial fibrillation), long-term oral anticoagulation is recommended to prevent further acute arterial ischemic episodes (see Table 40-10 later in this chapter) (Jones, Dolor, Hasselblad, et al., 2014).

THROMBOANGIITIS OBLITERANS

Thromboangiitis obliterans (Buerger's disease) is a nonatherosclerotic, segmental, recurrent inflammatory disorder of the small and medium-sized arteries and veins of the upper and lower extremities. In rare cases, systemic manifestations of the disease may involve cerebral, mesenteric, or coronary arteries. The disorder occurs predominantly in young men (<45 yr) with a long history of tobacco or marihuana use (or both), but without other CVD risk factors (e.g., hypertension, hyperlipidemia, diabetes mellitus) (Vijayakumar, Tiwari, & Prabhuswamy, 2013).

In Buerger's disease, an inflammatory process damages the blood vessel wall. Lymphocytes and giant cells infiltrate the vessel wall, and fibroblasts proliferate (Vijayakumar, Tiwari, & Prabhuswamy, 2013). Ultimately, thrombosis and fibrosis occur in the vessel, causing tissue ischemia. Patients with Buerger's disease have a high rate of periodontitis and the presence of *Porphyromonas gingivalis* (a periodontal pathogen) in the occluded blood vessels (Vijayakumar, Tiwari, & Prabhuswamy, 2013). This suggests that bacterial infection plays a role in the pathogenesis of Buerger's disease. Researchers are examining genetic factors in susceptible individuals (Vijayakumar, Tiwari, & Prabhuswamy, 2013). The symptom complex of Buerger's disease often is confused with PAD and other inflammatory or autoimmune diseases (e.g., scleroderma). Patients may have intermittent claudication of the feet, hands, or arms. As the disease progresses, rest pain and ischemic ulcerations develop. Other signs and symptoms may include colour and temperature changes of the limbs, paresthesia, superficial vein thrombosis, and cold sensitivity. There are no laboratory or diagnostic tests specific to Buerger's disease. Diagnosis is based on age at onset; history of tobacco use; clinical symptoms; involvement of distal vessels; presence of ischemic ulcerations; and exclusion of diabetes mellitus, autoimmune disease, thrombophilia (inherited tendency to clot), and proximal source of emboli (Vijayakumar, Tiwari, & Prabhuswamy, 2013).

Patients with Buerger's disease have red blood cell rigidity, elevated hematocrit, and increased blood viscosity (Vijayakumar, Tiwari, & Prabhuswamy, 2013). The mainstay of treatment for Buerger's disease is the complete cessation of tobacco and marihuana use in any form. Use of nicotine replacement products is contraindicated. Conservative management includes the use of antibiotics to treat any infected ulcers and analgesics to manage the ischemic pain. Patients must avoid trauma to the extremities. A variety of novel drug therapies to treat Buerger's disease have been studied, but the results have been marginal; one therapy with modest effectiveness in Europe has been IV iloprost (a prostaglandin analogue). Another promising area of research is the intramuscular gene transfer of vascular growth factors.

Surgical options include *sympathectomy* (transection of a nerve, ganglion, or plexus of the sympathetic nervous system, or a combination of these), implantation of a spinal cord stimulator, and bypass surgery. Sympathectomy and implantation of a spinal cord stimulator are useful in improving distal blood flow and reducing pain, but neither alters the inflammatory process. Bypass surgery typically is not an option, owing to the involvement of smaller, distal vessels, but may be used in selected patients with severe ischemia (Vijayakumar, Tiwari, & Prabhuswamy, 2013).

Painful ulcerations may necessitate finger or toe amputations. Amputation below the knee may be necessary in severe cases. The rate of amputation in patients who continue tobacco or marihuana use after diagnosis is much higher than in those who stop (Vijayakumar, Tiwari, & Prabhuswamy, 2013).

RAYNAUD'S PHENOMENON

Raynaud's phenomenon is an episodic vasospastic disorder of small cutaneous arteries, most frequently involving the fingers and toes. It occurs primarily in young women (typically between 15 and 40 years of age) and it is more common in women than in men (Prete, Fatone, Favoino, et al., 2014). The exact etiology of Raynaud's phenomenon remains unknown. One theory is that the vasospasm results from an exaggerated response to sympathetic nervous system stimulation. Other contributing factors include occupation-related trauma and pressure to the

FIGURE 40-3 Raynaud's phenomenon. Source: Kamal, A., & Brockelhurst, J. C. (1991). *Color atlas of geriatric medicine* (2nd ed.). St. Louis: Mosby–Year Book.

fingertips, as noted in typists, pianists, and people who use handheld vibrating equipment. Exposure to heavy metals (e.g., lead) may also be a contributing factor.

Primary Raynaud's phenomenon, the more common form of the disease, is associated with significantly poorer physical and mental health–related quality of life (Prete, Fatone, Favoino, et al., 2014). When symptoms occur in association with autoimmune diseases (e.g., rheumatoid arthritis, systemic lupus erythematosus), the disorder is called *secondary Raynaud's phenomenon*.

Raynaud's phenomenon is characterized by vasospasm-induced colour changes of the fingers, toes, ears, and nose (white, blue, and red). Decreased perfusion results in pallor (white). The digits then appear cyanotic (bluish-purple) (Figure 40-3). These changes are followed by rubour (redness), caused by the hyperemic response that occurs when perfusion is restored. The patient usually describes coldness and numbness in the vasoconstrictive phase, followed by throbbing, aching pain; tingling; and swelling in the hyperemic phase. An episode usually lasts only minutes but, in severe cases, may persist for several hours. Exposure to cold, emotional upset, tobacco use, and caffeine usually precipitate symptoms. After frequent, prolonged attacks, the skin may become thickened and the nails brittle. On occasion, complications include punctate (small hole) lesions of the fingertips and superficial gangrenous ulcers in advanced stages. Diagnosis is based on persistence of symptoms for at least 2 years. The primary focus of nursing management of Raynaud's phenomenon is patient education.

Instructions should focus on preventing recurrent episodes. Patients should wear loose, warm clothing as protection from the cold, including gloves when using the refrigerator or freezer or when handling cold objects. At all times, patients should avoid temperature extremes. Immersing hands in warm water often decreases the vasospasm. Patients should stop using all tobacco products and avoid caffeine and other drugs that have vasoconstrictive effects (e.g., amphetamines, cocaine, ergotamine, pseudoephedrine).

Patients with Raynaud's phenomenon often describe themselves as anxious or depressed, or both (Prete, Fatone, Favoino, et al., 2014). Biofeedback, relaxation training, and stress management may be useful. If these options are appropriate, the nurse should encourage patients to explore them. When a patient's episodes are severe and other therapies are ineffective, drug therapy is considered. Calcium channel blockers (e.g., diltiazem [Cardizem]) are the first-line drug therapy (Herrick, 2012). Calcium channel blockers relax smooth muscles of the arterioles by blocking the influx of calcium into the cells, thus reducing the frequency and severity of vasospastic attacks.

Sympathectomy is considered only in advanced cases. Patients with Raynaud's phenomenon should receive routine follow-up to monitor for development of connective tissue or autoimmune diseases because Raynaud's phenomenon may be an early sign of scleroderma (Merritt, 2015).

AORTIC ANEURYSMS

The aorta is the largest artery and supplies oxygen and blood to all vital organs. One of the most common problems affecting the aorta is an aneurysm, a permanent, localized outpouching or dilation of the vessel wall (either congenital or acquired). Aneurysms occur in men more often than in women, and their incidence increases with age. Peripheral artery aneurysms also develop but are less common.

Etiology and Pathophysiology

Aortic aneurysms may involve the aortic arch, thoracic aorta, abdominal aorta, or a combination. Most aneurysms, however, are found in the abdominal aorta below the level of the renal arteries. The growth rate of aneurysms is unpredictable, but the larger the aneurysm, the greater the risk of rupture. The dilated aortic wall becomes lined with thrombi that can embolize, leading to acute ischemic symptoms to distal (downstream) branches. Of true aortic aneurysms, 75% occur in the abdomen (Figure 40-4) and 25% in the thoracic aorta. Popliteal artery aneurysms rank third in frequency. Patients may have more than one aneurysm, in different locations.

Although various disorders are associated with aortic aneurysms, the primary cause may be classified as degenerative, congenital, mechanical, inflammatory, or infectious. The most common etiology of aneurysms of the aorta is atherosclerosis (Copstead & Banasik, 2013). It is known that atherosclerotic plaques are deposited beneath the *intima* (the innermost layer of the arterial wall). This plaque formation is thought to cause degenerative changes in the *media* (middle layer of the arterial wall), leading to loss of elasticity, weakening, and eventual dilation of the aorta.

Male sex, age of 65 years or older, and tobacco use are the major risk factors for abdominal aortic aneurysms (AAAs) of atherosclerotic origin. Other risk factors include the presence of coronary artery disease or PAD, hypertension, and high cholesterol levels (Copstead & Banasik, 2013). Studies have shown a strong genetic component in AAA development. The familial tendency is related to a number of congenital anomalies, including specific collagen defects (e.g., Ehlers-Danlos syndrome) and premature breakdown of vascular elastic tissue (Marfan syndrome; Copstead & Banasik, 2013). Less common causes of AAAs include penetrating or blunt trauma from motor vehicle collisions, inflammatory aortitis (e.g., Takayasu's or giant cell arteritis), and infectious aortitis (e.g., from syphilis or *Salmonella* or human immunodeficiency virus infection).

Classification

Aneurysms are classified as true or false (Figure 40-5, *A* to *D*). A *true aneurysm* is one in which the wall of the artery forms the aneurysm, with at least one vessel layer still intact. True aneurysms can be further subdivided into fusiform and saccular dilations. A *fusiform aneurysm* is circumferential and relatively uniform in shape. A *saccular aneurysm* is pouchlike with a narrow neck connecting the bulge to one side of the arterial wall.

A *false aneurysm,* or *pseudoaneurysm,* is not an aneurysm but a disruption of all layers of the arterial wall, resulting in bleeding that is contained by surrounding structures. False aneurysms may result from trauma or infection or occur after peripheral artery bypass graft surgery at the site of the graft-to-artery

FIGURE 40-4 Angiogram demonstrates a fusiform abdominal aortic aneurysm. Note calcification of the aortic wall *(arrows)* and extension of the aneurysm into the common iliac arteries. Source: Courtesy James O. Menzoian, Boston.

FIGURE 40-5 A, True fusiform abdominal aortic aneurysm. **B,** True saccular aortic aneurysm. **C,** False aneurysm, or pseudoaneurysm. **D,** Aortic dissection.

anastomosis. They may also result from arterial leakage after removal of cannulas such as lower extremity arterial catheters and intra-aortic balloon pump devices.

Clinical Manifestations

Thoracic aortic aneurysms are often asymptomatic. When they are symptomatic, the most common symptom is deep, diffuse chest pain extending to the interscapular area. Aneurysms located in the ascending aorta and the aortic arch can produce hoarseness in the patient as a result of pressure on the recurrent laryngeal nerve. Pressure on the esophagus can cause dysphagia. If the aneurysm presses on the superior vena cava, it can cause a decrease in venous drainage, resulting in jugular venous distension (distended neck veins) and edema of the head and the arms.

AAAs are often asymptomatic and frequently detected on routine physical examination or when the patient is examined for an unrelated problem (e.g., on abdominal radiographic examination, ultrasound study, computed tomography [CT] scan, or IV pyelography, or during abdominal surgery). On physical examination, a pulsatile mass in the periumbilical area slightly to the left of the midline may be detected. Bruits may be audible through a stethoscope placed over the aneurysm. These physical findings may be more difficult to detect in obese individuals.

Symptoms of an AAA may mimic pain associated with any abdominal or back disorder. Symptoms may result from compression of nearby anatomical structures. These include back pain caused by lumbar nerve compression and epigastric discomfort with or without alteration in bowel elimination, as a result of compression on the bowel. On occasion, embolization is caused by plaque released by an aneurysm, even a small one. This can cause the "blue toe syndrome," in which patchy mottling of the feet and toes occurs in the presence of palpable pedal pulses.

Complications

The most serious complication is rupture of the aneurysm. If blood from a rupture leaks into the retroperitoneal space, bleeding may be controlled by surrounding anatomical structures, preventing exsanguination and death. In such cases, many patients have severe back pain and may or may not have back or flank ecchymosis (Grey Turner's sign). In cases in which blood from a rupture leaks into the thoracic or abdominal cavity, more than 90% of patients die from massive hemorrhage (Go, Mozaffarian, Roger, et al., 2013). Such a patient who reaches the hospital is in hypovolemic shock with tachycardia, hypotension, pale clammy skin, decreased urine output, altered level of consciousness, and abdominal tenderness. (Shock is discussed in Chapter 69.) In this situation, simultaneous resuscitation and immediate surgical repair are necessary.

Diagnostic Studies

Chest radiographs reveal abnormal widening of the thoracic aorta. An abdominal radiograph may show calcification within the aortic wall. Because symptoms of thoracic aneurysm can mimic angina, electrocardiography is performed to rule out evidence of MI. Echocardiography is performed to assess the function of the aortic valve. Ultrasonography is useful for aneurysm screening and monitoring aneurysm size. A CT scan is the most accurate test for determining the length and cross-sectional diameter and the presence of thrombus in the aneurysm. Three-dimensional CT scans can assist in determining what type of surgical repair should be done. Magnetic resonance imaging (MRI) also may be used to diagnose and assess the location and severity of aneurysms.

Angiography, anatomical mapping of the aortic system by contrast imaging, provides information about the involvement of intestinal, renal, or distal vessels. Angiography is also useful if a suprarenal or thoraco-abdominal aneurysm is suspected. (Angiography is discussed in Chapter 34 and Table 34-6.)

Collaborative Care

The goal of management is to prevent aneurysm rupture and extension of dissection. Early detection and prompt treatment are essential. A careful review of body systems is necessary to identify any comorbid conditions, especially of the lungs, heart, or kidneys, because they may influence the patient's risk for surgical complications. Existing carotid and coronary artery obstructions may need to be corrected before the aneurysm is repaired. Conservative therapy of small, asymptomatic AAAs (4.0–5.5 cm) is the best practice (Filardo, Powell, Martinez, et al., 2012). This consists of risk factor modification (ceasing tobacco use, decreasing BP, optimizing lipid profile) and annual monitoring of aneurysm size with ultrasonography, CT, or MRI (Copstead & Banasik, 2013). Surgical intervention may be undertaken sooner if (a) the patient is a younger patient at low risk for surgical complications, (b) the aneurysm expands rapidly (i.e., >1-cm diameter increase per year), (c) the patient develops symptoms, or (d) the risk of rupture is high (Anderson, Halperin, Albert, et al., 2013).

Surgical Therapy. Before elective surgery, the patient is hydrated, and any electrolyte, coagulation, and hematocrit abnormalities are corrected. If the aneurysm has ruptured, emergency surgical intervention is required. With ruptured AAAs, the mortality rate is as high as 90%; the rate of survival is lowest in women and older adult patients (Lo, Bensley, Hamdan, et al., 2013).

The open aneurysm repair involves a large abdominal incision through which the surgeon (a) incises the diseased aortic segment, (b) removes any thrombus or plaque, (c) sutures a synthetic graft to the aorta proximal and distal to the aneurysm, and (d) sutures the native aortic wall around the graft to act as a protective cover (Figure 40-6). If the iliac arteries are also aneurysmal, a bifurcated graft replaces the entire diseased segment. With saccular aneurysms, it may be possible to excise only the bulbous lesion, the artery being repaired by primary closure (suturing the artery together) or by application of an autogenous or synthetic patch graft. Autotransfusion, which recycles the patient's own blood, reduces the need for blood transfusions during AAA surgery. (Autotransfusion is discussed in Chapter 33.)

All AAA resections necessitate aortic cross-clamping proximal and distal to the aneurysm. Most resections are performed in 30 to 45 minutes, after which time the clamps are removed and blood flow is restored. If the cross-clamp must be applied above the renal arteries, adequate renal perfusion after clamp removal should be ensured before the abdominal incision is closed. The risk of postoperative renal complications such as acute renal failure increases significantly when surgical repair of AAAs is above the level of the renal arteries.

Endovascular Graft Procedure. Minimally invasive endovascular aneurysm repair (EVAR) is an alternative to open aneurysm repair. EVAR involves the placement of a sutureless aortic graft into the abdominal aorta inside the aneurysm via femoral artery cutdowns. The graft, a Dacron cylinder consisting of several sections, is supported with multiple rings of flexible wire (Figure 40-7).

FIGURE 40-6 Surgical repair of an abdominal aortic aneurysm. **A,** Incising the aneurysmal sac. **B,** Insertion of synthetic graft. **C,** Suturing native aortic wall over synthetic graft.

FIGURE 40-7 Bifurcated (two-branched) endovascular stent grafting of an aneurysm. **A,** Insertion of a woven polyester tube (graft) covered by a tubular metal web (stent). **B,** The stent graft is inserted through a large blood vessel (e.g., femoral artery) by a delivery catheter. The catheter is positioned below the renal arteries in the area of the aneurysm. **C,** The stent graft is slowly released (deployed) into the blood vessel. When the stent comes in contact with the blood vessel, it expands to a preset size. **D,** A second stent graft can be inserted in the contralateral (opposite) vessel if necessary. **E,** Fully deployed bifurcated stent graft.

The main section of the graft is bifurcated and delivered through a femoral artery catheter. The second part of the graft is inserted through the opposite femoral artery. When all graft components are in place, they are released (deployed) against the vessel wall by balloon inflation (which creates a circumferential seal). The blood then flows through the endovascular graft, thus preventing further expansion of the aneurysm (Nienaber, Kische, Rousseau, et al., 2013). The aneurysmal wall shrinks over time because the blood is now being diverted through the endograft.

Patients must meet certain eligibility criteria to be candidates for EVAR. These include iliofemoral vessels that will allow for safe graft insertion and vessels of sufficient length and width to support the graft (Park, Azefor, Huang, et al., 2013). The benefits of EVAR include decreased anaesthesia and operative time, limited blood loss, decreased morbidity and mortality risks, small bilateral groin incisions, more rapid resumption of physical activity, shortened length of hospital stays, quicker recovery, higher patient satisfaction, and reduction in overall costs (Di Minno, Sparadella, Petitto, et al., 2014).

Complications. EVAR is less invasive than open aneurysm repair. EVAR also has fewer complications, and reports from non-randomized studies suggest that it may reduce early negative outcomes such as long hospital stays, paraplegia, and death (Abraha, Romagnoli, Montedori, et al., 2016). Women have a higher rate of complications after EVAR than do men; however, there are no sex differences in mortality rates (Gloviczki, Huang, Oderich, et al., 2015).

The most common complication is *endoleak,* the seepage of blood back into the old aneurysm. This may result from inadequacy of the seal at either graft end, a tear through the graft fabric, or leakage between overlapping graft segments, and coil embolization (insertion of beads) may be necessary for hemostasis (Park, Azefor, Huang, et al., 2013). Other potential complications include aneurysm growth above or below the graft aneurysm rupture, aortic dissection, bleeding, stent migration, renal artery occlusion caused by stent migration, graft thrombosis, incisional site hematoma, and incisional infection.

Graft dysfunction may necessitate conversion to an open surgical repair. Patients must have regular follow-up visits with their health care provider and routine CT scans for the rest of their lives to monitor for complications (e.g., stent migration, aneurysm recurrence).

A potentially lethal complication in an emergency repair of a ruptured AAA is the development of *intra-abdominal hypertension* with associated *abdominal compartment syndrome.* Persistent intra-abdominal hypertension reduces blood flow to the viscera. Abdominal compartment syndrome is the condition of impaired organ perfusion caused by intra-abdominal hypertension and resulting multisystem organ failure (Rubenstein, Bietz, Davenport, et al., 2015). Intra-abdominal hypertension is confirmed by measurement of the patient's intra-abdominal pressure indirectly through a catheter and transducer system, typically with an indwelling urinary catheter.

Treatment goals include control of situations that lead to intra-abdominal hypertension. Interventions include open (surgical) decompression, percutaneous drainage, and percutaneous drainage combined with infusion of tissue plasminogen activator. Conservative measures such as intubation, ventilation, patient positioning, gastric decompression, cautious fluid resuscitation, pain management, and temporary hemofiltration are also used.

NURSING MANAGEMENT
AORTIC ANEURYSMS AND AORTOILIAC DISEASE

NURSING ASSESSMENT

The nurse should obtain a thorough history and perform a thorough physical assessment. Because atherosclerosis is a systemic disease, the nurse should look for signs of coexisting cardiac, pulmonary, cerebral, and lower extremity vascular problems.

The patient is monitored for signs of aneurysm rupture, such as diaphoresis; pallor; weakness; tachycardia; hypotension; abdominal, back, groin, or periumbilical pain; changes in level of consciousness; or a pulsating abdominal mass.

Establishing baseline data is critical for comparison with later postoperative assessments. The nurse must pay special attention to the character and quality of the patient's peripheral pulses and renal and neurological status. Before surgery, the nurse should mark and document pedal pulse sites (dorsalis pedis and posterior tibial) and any skin lesions on the lower extremities.

PLANNING

The overall goals for a patient undergoing aortic surgery include (a) normal tissue perfusion, (b) intact motor and sensory function, and (c) no complications related to surgical repair, such as thrombosis, infection, or rupture.

NURSING IMPLEMENTATION

HEALTH PROMOTION. To promote overall health, the nurse encourages the patient to reduce CVD risk factors (see Table 36-2), including BP control, tobacco cessation (see Chapter 11), increasing physical activity, and maintaining normal body weight and serum lipid levels. These measures also help ensure continued graft patency after surgical repair.

ACUTE INTERVENTION. During the preoperative period, the nurse should provide emotional support and education to the patient and caregiver and thoroughly assess all body systems. Preoperative teaching includes a brief explanation of the disease process, the planned surgical procedures, preoperative routines, what to expect immediately after surgery (e.g., recovery room, the presence of tubes and drains), and usual postoperative timelines. Specific preoperative routines vary by institution and surgeon. In general, patients undergoing aortic surgery have a bowel preparation (e.g., laxatives, enemas) and skin cleansing with an antimicrobial agent the day before surgery, receive nothing by mouth (NPO status) after midnight the day of surgery, and receive IV antibiotics immediately before the incision is made. If appropriate, a preoperative visit to the intensive care unit may be helpful to the patient and caregiver. Patients with a history of CVD should receive a beta blocker (e.g., metoprolol [Lopressor]) preoperatively to reduce the risk of morbidity and mortality.

After aortic surgery, patients typically go to an intensive care unit for 24 to 48 hours for close monitoring. When the patient arrives in the intensive care unit, various devices are in place, including an endotracheal tube for mechanical ventilation; an arterial line; a central venous pressure (CVP) or pulmonary artery catheter; peripheral IV lines; an indwelling urinary catheter; and, depending on the approach and the surgeon's preference, a nasogastric tube. If the thorax is opened during surgery, chest tubes are in place. The patient needs continuous electrocardiographic and pulse oximetry monitoring. Pain medication is administered via epidural catheter or patient-controlled analgesia. In addition to the usual goals of care for a postoperative patient (e.g., maintaining adequate respiratory function, fluid and electrolyte balance, and pain control; see Chapter 22), the nurse should monitor graft patency and renal perfusion. The nurse should also monitor for and intervene to limit or treat dysrhythmias, infections, and neurological complications. See NCP 40-2, available on the Evolve website for this chapter, for care of the patient with an aneurysm repair or other aortic surgery.

Graft Patency. An adequate BP is important for maintaining graft patency. Prolonged hypotension may result in graft thrombosis.

Administration of IV fluids and blood components (as indicated) is essential for adequate blood flow. CVP readings or pulmonary artery pressures and urinary output are monitored hourly in the immediate postoperative period to help assess the patient's hydration and perfusion status.

Severe hypertension must be prevented because it may cause undue stress on the arterial anastomoses, resulting in leakage of blood or rupture at the suture lines. Drug therapy with IV diuretics (e.g., furosemide [Lasix]) or IV antihypertensive agents (e.g., nitroprusside [Nipride], esmolol [Brevibloc], and labetalol [Trandate]) may be indicated (Dasgupta, Quinn, Zarnke, et al., 2014).

Cardiovascular Status. Myocardial ischemia or infarction may occur in the perioperative period because of decreased myocardial oxygen supply or increased myocardial oxygen demands. Cardiac dysrhythmias may occur because of electrolyte imbalances, hypoxemia, hypothermia, or myocardial ischemia. Nursing interventions include continuous electrocardiographic monitoring; frequent electrolyte and arterial blood gas determinations; administration of oxygen, IV antidysrhythmic and antihypertensive medications, and electrolytes as needed; adequate pain control; and resumption of cardiac medications.

Infection. A prosthetic vascular graft infection is a relatively rare but potentially life-threatening complication. Nursing interventions to prevent infection should include ensuring that the patient receives a broad-spectrum antibiotic as prescribed. The nurse should assess body temperature regularly and report elevations promptly. Laboratory data should be monitored for an elevated white blood cell (WBC) count, which may be the first indication of an infection. The nurse should ensure adequate nutrition and assess the surgical incision for signs of infection (e.g., redness, swelling, drainage). All IV, arterial, and CVP or pulmonary artery catheter insertion sites should be cared for with strict aseptic technique because they are ports of entry for bacteria. Meticulous perineal care for the patient with an in-dwelling urinary catheter is essential to minimize the risk of urinary tract infection. Surgical incisions must be kept clean and dry.

Gastrointestinal Status. After open abdominal aortic surgery, paralytic ileus may develop as a result of anaesthesia and the handling of the bowel during surgery. The intestines may become swollen and bruised, and peristalsis ceases for variable intervals. A retroperitoneal surgical approach can be used to decrease the risk of bowel complications.

An nasogastric tube may be placed during surgery and arranged with low, intermittent suction to decompress the stomach, prevent aspiration of stomach contents, and decrease pressure on suture lines. The nurse records the amount and character of the nasogastric output. While the patient is NPO, oral care should be provided frequently. Ice chips or lozenges may be used to soothe a dry or irritated throat. The nurse assesses for bowel sounds; the passing of flatus signals returning bowel function and should be noted. Early ambulation should be encouraged because this promotes the return of bowel functioning. A paralytic ileus rarely lasts beyond the fourth postoperative day.

If the blood supply to the bowel is disrupted during surgery, temporary ischemia or infarction (leading to death) of intestinal tissue may result. Clinical manifestations of this rare but serious complication include absence of bowel sounds, fever, abdominal distension, diarrhea, and bloody stools. If bowel infarction occurs, immediate reoperation is necessary to restore blood flow, with probable resection of the infarcted bowel.

Neurological Status. Neurological complications can occur after aortic surgery. When the ascending aorta and the aortic arch are involved, the nurse assesses the patient's level of consciousness, pupil size and response to light, facial symmetry, tongue deviation, speech, ability to move upper extremities, and quality of hand grasps (see Chapter 58). When the descending aorta is involved, neuro-vascular assessment of the lower extremities is important. The nurse must record all assessments and report changes from baseline to the physician immediately.

Peripheral Perfusion Status. The aneurysm's anatomical location indicates the areas of interest related to peripheral perfusion. The nurse should check and record all peripheral pulses hourly for several hours and then routinely, according to institutional policy. When the ascending aorta and aortic arch are involved, the nurse assesses the carotid, radial, and temporal artery pulses. For surgery of the descending aorta, the nurse assesses the femoral, popliteal, posterior tibial, and dorsalis pedis pulses (see Chapter 34, Figure 34-6).

When checking pulses, the nurse should mark the locations with a felt-tip pen so that other medical staff can locate them easily. In some cases, a Doppler ultrasound study may be needed to assess peripheral pulses. The nurse checks skin temperature and colour, capillary refill time, and sensation and movement of the extremities (see Chapter 34).

On occasion, lower extremity pulses may be absent for a short time after surgery because of vasospasm and hypothermia. Decrease in or absence of the pulse accompanied by coolness, pallor, or mottling of the extremity or pain in the extremity may indicate embolization or graft occlusion. The nurse must report these findings to the physician immediately. Graft occlusion necessitates reoperation if identified early. Thrombolytic therapy may also be considered. In some patients, pulses may have been absent before surgery owing to coexistent PAD. It is essential to compare findings with those of the preoperative status to determine the cause of a decrease in or absence of pulse and the proper treatment.

Renal Perfusion Status. Postoperatively, the patient has an indwelling urinary catheter. In the immediate postoperative period, the nurse records urine output hourly, and urinary output is maintained at 0.5 to 1 mL/kg/hr. The nurse maintains accurate fluid intake and output and records daily weights until the patient resumes a regular diet. CVP and pulmonary artery pressures also provide important information about hydration status. The nurse evaluates renal function by monitoring daily blood urea nitrogen and serum creatinine levels. (For signs and symptoms of acute kidney injury, see Chapter 49.) Irreversible renal failure may occur after aortic surgery, particularly in individuals at high risk for complications (e.g., patients with diabetes). Renal perfusion can decrease as a result of embolization of the aortic thrombus/plaque to one or both renal arteries. This causes ischemia of one or both kidneys. Hypotension, dehydration, prolonged aortic clamping during surgery, or blood loss also can lead to a decrease in renal perfusion.

AMBULATORY AND HOME CARE. The nurse instructs the patient and caregiver to increase activities gradually after the patient returns home. Fatigue, poor appetite, and irregular bowel habits are common. The patient should avoid heavy lifting for 6 weeks after surgery. Any redness, swelling, increased pain, drainage from incisions, or fever greater than 37.8°C should be reported to a health care provider.

The nurse teaches the patient and caregiver to look for changes in colour or warmth of the extremities. Patients and caregivers can learn to palpate peripheral pulses to assess changes in their quality.

Sexual dysfunction in male patients is common after aortic surgery. Preoperatively, the nurse should document baseline sexual function and recommend counselling as appropriate. A referral to an urologist may be useful if erectile dysfunction occurs.

EVALUATION

Expected outcomes for the patient who undergoes aortic surgery include the following:

- Patent arterial graft with adequate distal perfusion
- Adequate urine output
- No signs of infection

AORTIC DISSECTION

Aortic dissection, often misnamed "dissecting aneurysm," is not a type of aneurysm. Rather, dissection (tearing of the inner layer of the vessel) results from the creation of a false lumen (between the intima and the media) through which blood flows (see Figure 40-5). Classification is based on anatomical location (ascending versus descending aorta) and duration of onset (acute versus chronic). Approximately 60% to 70% of aortic dissections involve the ascending aorta and are acute in onset (Copstead & Banasik, 2013). Acute aortic dissections (i.e., diagnosed within 14 days of symptom onset) carry a mortality rate as high as 1% per hour (Estrera, Azam, Shalhub, et al., 2015). Chronic dissections almost exclusively involve the descending aorta.

Etiology and Pathophysiology

Most experts attribute nontraumatic aortic dissection to the degeneration of the elastic fibres in the medial layer. Chronic hypertension accelerates the degradation process. Aortic dissection is believed to arise from an intimal tear. Intimal tears typically occur in areas with the greatest rate of rise of BP: for example, immediately above the aortic valve and just distal to the left subclavian artery. As the heart contracts, each systolic pulsation causes increased pressure on the damaged area, which further increases the dissection. Extension of the dissection may cut off blood supply to critical areas such as the brain, kidneys, spinal cord, and extremities. The false lumen may remain patent, become thrombosed (clotted), rejoin the true lumen by way of a distal tear, or rupture.

Aortic dissection affects two to five times more men than women and occurs mostly in the sixth and seventh decades of life (Conrad & Cambria, 2014). Approximately half of all dissections in women younger than 40 years occur during pregnancy (Lo, Bensley, Hamdan, et al., 2013). Predisposing factors include age, aortic diseases (e.g., aortitis, coarctation, arch hypoplasia), atherosclerosis, blunt or iatrogenic trauma, tobacco use, cocaine or methamphetamine use, congenital heart disease (e.g., bicuspid aortic valve), connective tissue disorders (e.g., Marfan or Ehlers-Danlos syndrome), family history, history of heart surgery, male sex, pregnancy, and poorly controlled hypertension (Erbel, Aboyans, Boileau, et al., 2014). Younger patients are more likely to have a bicuspid aortic valve or Marfan syndrome, to have undergone prior aortic valve surgery, or to have suffered recent trauma (Wojnarski, Svensson, Roselli, et al., 2015).

Clinical Manifestations

The majority of patients with an acute ascending aortic dissection report sudden, severe onset of excruciating chest pain, back pain, or both, radiating to the neck or shoulders. The pain is frequently described as "sharp" and "worst ever" followed less frequently by "tearing" or "ripping." Patients with acute descending aortic dissection are more likely to report pain in their back, abdomen, or legs. Dissection pain can be differentiated from MI pain, whose onset is more gradual and of increasing intensity. As the dissection progresses, pain may migrate. Older patients are less likely to have abrupt onset of chest or back pain (in their back, abdomen, or legs) and more likely to have hypotension and vague symptoms. Some patients have a painless aortic dissection, which emphasizes the importance of the physical examination (Wojnarski, Svensson, Roselli, et al., 2015).

If the aortic arch is involved, the patient may exhibit neurological deficits, such as altered level of consciousness, weakened or absence of carotid and temporal pulses, and dizziness or syncope. An ascending aortic dissection usually produces some degree of disruption in blood flow in the coronary arteries and aortic valve insufficiency. The patient may develop angina, MI, and a new high-pitched, diastolic heart murmur. If severe enough, these complications can result in left ventricular failure with the development of dyspnea, orthopnea, and pulmonary edema. When either subclavian artery is involved, radial, ulnar, and brachial pulse quality and BP readings may be different between the left and the right arms. As the dissection progresses down the aorta, the abdominal organs and lower extremities demonstrate evidence of decreased tissue perfusion.

Complications

A severe and life-threatening complication of an acute ascending aortic dissection is cardiac tamponade, which occurs when blood from the dissection leaks into the pericardial sac. Clinical manifestations of tamponade include hypotension, narrowed pulse pressure, jugular venous distension, muffled heart sounds, and pulsus paradoxus (see Chapter 39). The aorta may rupture because it is weakened by the dissection. Hemorrhage may occur into the mediastinal, pleural, or abdominal cavities. Aortic rupture typically results in exsanguination and death. Dissection can lead to occlusion of the blood supply to vital organs. Symptoms of spinal cord ischemia range from weakness and decreased sensation to complete lower extremity paralysis. Renal ischemia can lead to renal failure. Manifestations of abdominal (mesenteric) ischemia include abdominal pain, decreased bowel sounds, altered bowel function, and bowel necrosis.

Diagnostic Studies

Diagnostic studies to detect aortic dissection are similar to those performed for suspected aneurysms (Table 40-6). A chest radiograph may show a widening of the mediastinum and pleural effusion. Three-dimensional CT scanning, MRI, and transesophageal echocardiography are equally reliable for the diagnosis of acute aortic dissection (Copstead & Banasik, 2013). A CT scan or MRI can provide more detailed information on the presence and severity of the dissection. Transesophageal echocardiography is preferred in very unstable patients or those with contraindications to CT or MRI (e.g., those with metal implants, allergies to contrast material) (Erbel, Aboyans, Boileau, et al., 2014).

Collaborative Care

Patients with acute aortic dissection are managed in the intensive care unit. The initial goals of therapy for acute aortic dissection without complications are heart rate and BP control and pain management. Heart rate and BP control reduces stress on the aortic

TABLE 40-6 **COLLABORATIVE CARE**

Aortic Dissection

Diagnostic	**Collaborative Therapy**
• Health history and physical examination	• Bed rest
• Chest radiography	• Blood transfusion (if necessary)
• CT scan with three-dimensional reconstruction	• Pain relief with opioids
• Electrocardiography	***Drug Therapy*** (see Table 35-8)
• Magnetic resonance imaging	• ACE inhibitors
• Transesophageal echocardiography	• IV β-blockers (e.g., esmolol [Brevibloc])
	• IV calcium channel blockers
	• Sodium nitroprusside (Nipride)
	Surgical Therapy
	• Surgical aortic resection and repair
	• Endovascular aortic dissection repair

ACE, angiotensin-converting enzyme; *CT,* computed tomography; *IV,* intravenous.

wall by reducing systolic BP and myocardial contractility (see Table 40-6). An IV beta-adrenergic blocker (e.g., esmolol [Brevibloc]) is titrated to effect a target heart rate of 60 beats/minute or less. A calcium channel blocker (e.g., diltiazem [Cardizem], verapamil [Calan]) can be used to lower heart rate if a beta-adrenergic blocker is contraindicated. An IV angiotensin-converting enzyme inhibitor (e.g., enalapril [Vasotec]) may also be used. Reducing the heart rate, BP, and myocardial contractility limits extension of the dissection. Morphine is the preferred analgesic because it decreases sympathetic nervous system stimulation and relieves pain. Supportive treatment for an acute aortic dissection serves as a bridge to surgery.

Conservative Therapy. A patient with an acute descending aortic dissection without complications can be treated conservatively. Supportive treatment includes pain relief and BP control. Conservative treatment includes pain relief, heart rate and BP control, and CVD risk factor modification.

Endovascular Dissection Repair. Endovascular repair of chronic descending aortic dissection is an effective treatment option (Antoniou, Georgiadis, Antoniou et al., 2013; Park, Azefor, Huang, et al., 2013). Endovascular repair is the standard modality to treat acute descending aortic dissections with complications (e.g., hemodynamic instability, peripheral ischemia) (Park, Azefor, Huang, et al., 2013). Endovascular dissection repair is similar to EVAR. However, a temporary lumbar drain may be inserted for cerebro-spinal fluid removal to reduce spinal cord edema and help prevent paralysis (Nienaber, Kische, Rousseau, et al., 2013).

Surgical Therapy. An acute ascending aortic dissection is considered a surgical emergency. Otherwise, surgery is indicated when drug therapy is ineffective or when complications (e.g., heart failure) occur. Because the aorta is fragile after dissection, surgery is delayed for as long as possible to allow time for edema to decrease and to enable clotting of the blood in the false lumen. Surgery involves resection of the aortic segment containing the intimal tear and replacement with a synthetic graft. Even with prompt surgical intervention, the in-hospital rate of mortality from acute aortic dissection remains high. Women experience poorer surgical outcomes and higher mortality rates than do men (Lo, Bensley, Hamdan, et al., 2013). Causes of in-hospital mortality include aortic rupture, mesenteric ischemia, sepsis, and multiorgan failure.

NURSING MANAGEMENT AORTIC DISSECTION

Preoperatively, nursing management includes keeping the patient in bed in a semi-Fowler's position and maintaining a quiet environment. These measures help to keep the systolic BP at the lowest possible level that maintains vital organ perfusion (typically between 110 and 120 mm Hg); the desired outcome is to maintain a mean arterial pressure of greater than 65 mm Hg. In order to maintain the mean arterial pressure, the minimal diastolic pressure ought to be approximately 44 mm Hg (Dasgupta, Quinn, Zarnke, et al., 2014). Opioids and sedatives are administered as ordered. The nurse must manage pain and anxiety for patient comfort and because these symptoms can cause elevations in the systolic BP.

Administration of IV antihypertensive agents requires careful supervision. This entails continuous electrocardiographic and intra-arterial BP monitoring (see Chapters 35 and 68). The nurse should monitor vital signs frequently, sometimes as often as every 2 to 3 minutes, until target BP is reached. The nurse should observe for changes in peripheral pulses and signs of increasing pain, restlessness, and anxiety. If the arteries branching off the aortic arch are involved, decreased cerebral blood flow may alter the patient's level of consciousness. Postoperative care is similar to that after aortic aneurysm repair (see the "Nursing Management: Aortic Aneurysms and Aortoiliac Disease" section earlier in this chapter, and NCP 40-1 on the Evolve website).

In preparation for discharge, the nurse should focus on patient and caregiver teaching. All patients with a history of aortic dissection, regardless of anatomic location or treatment modality, require long-term medical therapy to control BP. Patients need to understand that antihypertensive drugs must be taken daily for the rest of their lives. Beta-adrenergic blockers (e.g., metoprolol [Lopressor]) are used to control BP and decrease myocardial contractility. It is important that patients understand the drug regimen and potential adverse effects (e.g., dizziness, depression, fatigue, erectile dysfunction). The nurse must tell the patient to discuss any adverse effects with the health care provider before discontinuing the drug. Follow-up with regularly scheduled MRI or CT is essential. The most common cause of death in long-term survivors is aortic rupture from redissection or aneurysm formation. The nurse must instruct patients that, if the pain or other symptoms return, they should contact emergency medical services for immediate care.

VENOUS DISORDERS

PHLEBITIS

Phlebitis is the inflammation (e.g., redness, tenderness, warmth, mild edema) of a superficial vein without the presence of a thrombus (Mackman, 2012). It occurs in about 65% of all patients receiving IV therapy. It is rarely infectious and usually resolves quickly with removal of the IV catheter.

VENOUS THROMBO-EMBOLISM

Venous thrombo-embolism (VTE), also known as *venous thrombosis,* is a condition in which a thrombus forms in association with inflammation of the vein. It is the most common disorder of the veins and is classified as either superficial vein thrombosis or deep vein thrombosis. Superficial vein thrombosis (SVT) is the formation of a thrombus in a superficial vein, usually the greater or lesser saphenous vein. Deep vein thrombosis (DVT) is a disorder involving a thrombus in a deep vein, most commonly the iliac and femoral veins (Copstead & Banasik, 2013). VTE represents the spectrum of pathology from DVT to pulmonary embolism (Cosmi, 2015; Table 40-7). (Pulmonary embolism is discussed in Chapter 30.)

SVT is generally a benign disorder. However, nearly 25% of patients with SVT also have VTE at the time of diagnosis. There is a risk for extension of the clot to deeper veins if the thrombus involves the superficial femoral vein or is near the saphenofemoral junction (Mackman, 2012).

Etiology

Three important factors (called Virchow's triad) in the etiology of venous thrombosis are (a) venous stasis, (b) damage of the endothelium (inner lining of the vein), and (c) hypercoagulability

TABLE 40-7	COMPARISON OF SUPERFICIAL VEIN THROMBOSIS AND VENOUS THROMBO-EMBOLISM	
Characteristic	**Superficial Vein Thrombosis**	**Venous Thrombo-embolism**
Usual location	Typically, superficial leg veins (e.g., varicosities); occasionally, superficial arm veins.	Deep veins of arms (e.g., axillary, subclavian), legs (e.g., femoral), and pelvis (e.g., iliac or inferior or superior vena cava) and pulmonary system.
Clinical findings	Tenderness, rubour, warmth, pain, inflammation and induration along the course of the superficial vein. Vein appears as palpable cord. Edema rarely occurs.	Tenderness to pressure over involved vein, induration of overlying muscle, venous distension. Edema. Mild to moderate pain possible. Deep rubour in area caused by venous congestion. Systemic temperature possibly greater than 38°C. Note: Some patients may have no obvious physical changes in the affected extremity.
Sequelae	If left untreated, clot may extend to deeper veins and VTE may occur.	Embolization to lungs (pulmonary embolism) may occur and may result in death.* Pulmonary hypertension and post-thrombotic syndrome with or without venous leg ulceration may develop.

*See Chapter 30 for clinical findings related to pulmonary embolism.
IV, intravenous; *VTE,* venous thrombo-embolism.

PATHOPHYSIOLOGY MAP

FIGURE 40-8 Pathophysiology of venous thrombo-embolism. *RBCs,* red blood cells; *WBCs,* white blood cells.

of the blood (Figure 40-8). The patient at risk for the development of venous thrombosis usually has conditions predisposing to these three disorders (Table 40-8).

Venous Stasis. Normal blood flow in the venous system depends on the action of muscles in the extremities and the functional adequacy of venous valves, which allow unidirectional flow. *Venous stasis* occurs when the valves are dysfunctional or the muscles of the extremities are inactive. Venous stasis occurs more frequently in people who are obese or pregnant, have heart failure or atrial fibrillation, have been on long trips without regular exercise, have a prolonged surgical procedure, or are immobile for long periods (e.g., with spinal cord injury, fractured hip, limb paralysis) (Reitsma, Versteeg, & Middeldorp, 2012).

Endothelial Damage. Damage to the endothelium of the vein may be caused by direct (e.g., surgery, intravascular catheterization, trauma, fracture, burns) or indirect (chemotherapy, vasculitis, sepsis, hyperhomocysteinemia, diabetes) injury to the vessel (Anderson, Halperin, Albert, et al., 2013). Damaged endothelium stimulates platelet activation and initiates the coagulation cascade. This results in decreased fibrinolytic capabilities and predisposes the patient to thrombus development.

Hypercoagulability of Blood. Hypercoagulability of blood occurs in many hematological disorders, particularly polycythemia, severe anemias, malignancies (e.g., cancers of the breast, brain, pancreas, and gastro-intestinal tract), nephrotic syndrome, antithrombin III deficiency, elevated lipoprotein (a) levels, elevated (clotting) factor VIII levels, hyperhomocysteinemia, protein C deficiency, and protein S deficiency (Rattan, Jones, & Namias, 2015). A patient with sepsis is predisposed to hypercoagulability because of endotoxins that are released. Some medications (e.g., corticosteroids, estrogens) predispose a patient to thrombus formation.

TABLE 40-8 RISK FACTORS FOR VENOUS THROMBO-EMBOLISM

Venous Stasis
- Advanced age
- Atrial fibrillation
- Bed rest
- Chronic heart failure
- Fractured leg or hip
- Long trips without adequate exercise
- Obesity
- Orthopedic surgery (especially lower extremity)
- Pregnancy and postpartum period
- Prolonged immobility
- Spinal cord injury or limb paralysis
- Stroke
- Varicose veins

Hypercoagulability of Blood
- Antiphospholipid antibody syndrome
- Antithrombin III deficiency
- Dehydration or malnutrition
- Elevated (clotting) factor VIII or lipoprotein (a) level
- Erythropoiesis-stimulating drugs (e.g., epoetin alfa [Eprex])
- Factor V Leiden or prothrombin gene mutation
- High altitudes
- Hormone replacement therapy

- Hyperhomocysteinemia
- Malignancies (especially breast, brain, hepatic, pancreatic, and gastro-intestinal)
- Nephrotic syndrome
- Oral contraceptives, especially in women >35 yr of age who use tobacco
- Polycythemia vera
- Pregnancy and postpartum period
- Protein C deficiency
- Protein S deficiency
- Sepsis
- Severe anemia
- Tobacco use

Endothelial Damage
- Abdominal and pelvic surgery (e.g., gynecological or urological surgery)
- Caustic or hypertonic intravenous medications
- Fractures of pelvis, hip, or leg
- History of previous venous thrombo-embolism (VTE)
- In-dwelling, peripherally inserted central vein catheter
- Intravenous drug abuse
- Trauma

Women of child-bearing age who take estrogen-based oral contraceptives, as well as postmenopausal women receiving oral hormone replacement therapy are at increased risk for VTE (Reitsma, Versteeg, & Middeldorp, 2012). Women who use oral contraceptives and tobacco double their risk because of the vasoconstricting effects of nicotine. Smoking causes hypercoagulability by increasing plasma fibrinogen and homocysteine levels and activating the intrinsic coagulation pathway. Women who use tobacco and oral contraceptives, are older than 35 years, and have a family history of VTE are at extremely high risk for VTE. In women with known thrombophilia, the benefits of hormone replacement therapy, tamoxifen (Nolvadex-D), or raloxifene (Evista) must be weighed against the risk for VTE (Rattan, Jones, & Namias, 2015). Transdermal or intranasal hormone replacement therapy may be safer than oral hormone replacement therapy with respect to risk for VTE (Rockman, Maldinado, Jacobowitz, et al., 2012).

Pathophysiology

Localized platelet aggregation and fibrin entrap RBCs, WBCs, and more platelets to form a thrombus. A frequent site of thrombus formation is the valve cusps of veins, where venous stasis occurs. As the thrombus enlarges, increased numbers of blood cells and fibrin collect behind it, producing a larger clot with a "tail" that eventually occludes the lumen of the vein.

If a thrombus only partially occludes the vein, endothelial cells cover the thrombus and stop the thrombotic process. If the thrombus does not become detached, it undergoes lysis or becomes firmly organized and adherent within 5 to 7 days. Organized thrombi may detach and result in emboli. Turbulence of blood flow is a major factor contributing to embolization. A thrombus can become an embolus that flows through the venous circulation to the heart and lodges in the pulmonary circulation, becoming a pulmonary embolism (see Chapter 30, Figure 30-11).

Superficial Vein Thrombosis

Clinical Manifestations. The patient with SVT may have a palpable, firm, subcutaneous cordlike vein (see Table 40-7). The area surrounding the vein may be tender to the touch, reddened, and warm (Figure 40-9). A mild systemic temperature elevation and leukocytosis may be present. Extremity edema may or may not occur. The most common cause of upper extremity SVT is vein trauma caused by cannulation of a vein or IV therapy. It is more likely to occur if the catheter is located in a small vein or is left in place for more than 48 hours or if the IV solutions administered are caustic or hyperosmolar (Scott, Mahdi, & Alikhan, 2015).

In rare cases, infectious or suppurative SVT occurs at an IV site. Unfortunately, there may not be any local signs or symptoms. A high-grade fever or pulmonary embolism may be the first indication of infectious SVT (Cosmi, 2015). An elevated WBC count, positive blood cultures, or both, may also be present. The most common causative organism is *Staphylococcus aureus*.

Risk factors for SVT include increased age; pregnancy; obesity; malignancy; thrombophilia; estrogen therapy; recent sclerotherapy (e.g., treatment for varicose veins); long-distance travel; and a history of CVI, SVT, or VTE (van Langevelde, Lijfering, Rosendaal, et al., 2011). SVT also can occur in persons with endothelial alterations (e.g., Buerger's disease). It also may be unprovoked.

Collaborative Care. The initial treatment of infusion-related SVT involves the immediate removal of the IV catheter. If edema is present, the extremity should be elevated to promote reabsorption of fluid from the interstitial space into the vasculature. The application of warm, moist heat may help relieve pain and inflammation. Oral NSAIDs (e.g., diclofenac [Voltaren]), topical NSAIDs (e.g., diclofenac gel), or topical heparin gels are used to treat symptoms for a maximum of 2 weeks (Di Nisio & Middeldorp, 2014). Suppurative infusion-related SVT typically necessitates drainage of the abscess, excision of the affected tissue, and administration of systemic antibiotics (Di Nisio & Middeldorp, 2014). Systemic anticoagulants are not recommended for infusion-related SVT (Scott, Mahdi, & Alikhan, 2015).

Duplex ultrasonography is used to confirm the diagnosis (clot with a 5-cm diameter or larger) and to rule out clot extension to a deep vein (Kearon, Akl, Comerota, et al., 2012). For patients with a lower extremity SVT involving the greater saphenous vein or the sapheno-femoral junction, initial treatment consists of low-molecular-weight heparin (LMWH) or unfractionated heparin, followed by warfarin (Scott, Mahdi, & Alikhan, et al., 2015). Use of oral NSAIDs in combination with anticoagulants is not recommended. If the SVT affects a very short vein segment and is not near the sapheno-femoral junction, anticoagulants are not necessary, and oral or topical NSAIDs are appropriate. Additional interventions for SVT include educating the patient to wear graduated compression stockings and perform mild exercise such as walking.

Compression helps reduce edema, and walking increases endogenous fibrinolysis (Pavon, Adam, Razouki, et al. 2016; Rattan, Jones, & Namias. 2015).

Venous Thrombo-embolism

Clinical Manifestations. Patients with lower extremity VTE may or may not have unilateral leg edema, pain, tenderness with palpation, dilated superficial veins, a sense of fullness in the thigh or the calf, paresthesias, warm skin, erythema, or a systemic temperature greater than 38°C (see Table 40-7). A positive Homans sign (pain on forced dorsiflexion of the foot when the leg is raised) is a classic sign but very unreliable because false positive findings are common (Whitehead, Stephen, & Stansby, 2015). If the inferior vena cava is involved, the legs may be edematous and cyanotic. About 5% to 10% of VTEs involve the upper extremity veins and may extend into the internal jugular vein or superior vena cava (Kearon, Akl, Comerota, et al., 2012). If the superior vena cava is involved, symptoms may occur in the arms, neck, back, and face. Diagnosis of an initial VTE is based on clinical assessment combined with D-dimer

FIGURE 40-9 Superficial vein thrombosis of the hand following intravenous therapy. Source: Grieg, J. D., & Garden, O. J. (1996). *Color atlas of surgical diagnosis.* London: Times Mirror International.

testing and duplex ultrasonography (Bates, Jaeschke, Stevens, et al., 2012).

Complications. The most serious complications of VTE are pulmonary embolism, post-thrombotic syndrome, and phlegmasia cerulea dolens (described later in this chapter). Pulmonary embolism is a potentially life-threatening complication of VTE (see Chapter 30).

Post-thrombotic syndrome occurs in 20% to 50% of patients with VTE despite adequate anticoagulant therapy. It results from chronic venous hypertension caused by valvular destruction (from inflammation and scarring), stiffness and noncompliance of vein walls, and persistent venous obstruction. Symptoms include pain, aching, sensation of heaviness, swelling, cramps, itching, and tingling (Crumley, 2011; Henke & Comerota, 2011). Clinical signs include persistent edema, increased pigmentation, eczema, secondary varicosities, and *lipodermatosclerosis* (Figure 40-10). Venous ulceration can occur with severe post-thrombotic syndrome. Manifestations of post-thrombotic syndrome typically begin within 2 years of a VTE (Crumley, 2011; Henke & Comerota, 2011). Risk factors include persistent leg symptoms 1 month after VTE, location of VTE near the iliofemoral junction, extensive VTE, recurrent VTE, obesity, older age, and female sex. Sequential compression devices may be used for patients with severe post-thrombotic syndrome (Cohen, Akl, & Kahn, 2012).

Phlegmasia cerulea dolens (swollen, blue, painful leg), a very rare complication, may develop in the advanced stages of cancer. It results from one or more severe lower extremity VTEs that involve the major leg veins, causing near-total occlusion of venous outflow. Patients typically experience sudden, massive swelling, deep pain, and intense cyanosis of the extremity. If untreated, the venous obstruction causes arterial occlusion and gangrene and necessitates amputation.

Diagnostic Studies. Table 40-9 lists the various diagnostic studies used to determine the site or location and extent of a VTE.

Collaborative Care

Prevention and Prophylaxis. VTE prophylaxis is a core measure of quality health care in hospitalized patients undergoing surgery. In addition, it is recommended that hospitals have a formal, hospital-wide thromboprophylaxis policy that addresses VTE prevention on admission of all adult patients.

FIGURE 40-10 Lipodermatosclerosis. Skin on lower leg becomes scarred, and the leg becomes tapered like an "inverted bottle." Hallmark signs of lipodermatosclerosis are leathery skin, brown discoloration, hyperpigmentation and hypopigmentation, and circumferential or near-circumferential scarring and shrinking of the extremity. Source: From Etufugh, C. N., & Phillips, T. J. (2007). Venous ulcers. *Clinics in Dermatology, 25*(1), 125. doi:10.1016/j.clindermatol.2006.09.004.

In patients at risk for VTE, various interventions are used. Their use is based on such factors as bleeding and thrombosis risk, past medical history, current medications, medical diagnoses, scheduled procedures, and patient preferences (Kahn, Lim, Dunn, et al., 2012). Early and aggressive mobilization based on the patient's condition is the easiest and most cost-effective method to decrease VTE risk (Christakou & Zakyntinos, 2014). Patients on bed rest need to change position every 2 hours. Unless it is contraindicated, the nurse should teach patients to flex and extend their feet, knees, and hips every 2 to 4 hours while awake. Patients who are able to get out of bed need to be in a chair for meals and ambulate at least four to six times per day as tolerated. The nurse must reinforce the importance of these measures to the patient and caregiver. Research has shown that patients want additional information on VTE and prevention of VTE (Christakou & Zakyntinos, 2014). Early and frequent ambulation is sufficient prophylaxis for low-risk patients who are undergoing minor surgical procedures and have no additional VTE risk factors (Parmenter, Dieberg, Phipps, et al., 2015).

Graduated compression (antiembolism) stockings (e.g., thromboembolic deterrent hose) are a part of VTE prevention in hospitalized patients. When fitted and worn properly, these stockings increase venous blood flow velocity, prevent venous wall dilation, improve venous valve function, and stimulate endothelial fibrinolytic activity (Pavon, Adam, Razouki, et al., 2016). The patient's legs must be measured accurately, the stocking size and length (thigh-high or knee-high) must be the correct size, the stockings should be applied properly, and the patient and caregiver need to be educated regarding proper use (Pavon, Adam, Razouki, et al., 2016). "Correct use" means the toe hole is under the toes, the heel patch is over the heel, the thigh gusset is on the inner thigh (thigh length only), and there are no wrinkles. The stockings are not to be rolled down, cut, or otherwise altered. Venous return is impeded by the stockings if the top elastic band is too tight or the stockings are rolled down. This actually increases the risk of VTE and skin damage (Li, Yuan, & Qi, 2012). The nurse should monitor patients regularly to ensure that the stockings are being worn properly, the size is still appropriate, and peripheral perfusion is adequate (Pavon, Adam, Razouki, et al., 2016). If the patient's legs are swollen after surgery, remeasurement is necessary, and a larger stocking size may be needed. The nurse must thoroughly assess the skin with the stockings off at least once a day or more frequently, depending on the patient's condition.

Sequential compression devices (SCDs) are inflatable garments wrapped around the legs that apply intermittent external pressure to the lower extremities. They are often used in combination with graduated compression stockings (Li, Yuan, & Qi, 2012). Benefits are similar to those provided by stockings. As with graduated compression stockings, the nurse must accurately measure the extremities to ensure correct fit. SCDs do not provide effective VTE prophylaxis if they are not applied correctly, if the fit is incorrect, or if the patient does not wear the device continuously except during bathing, skin assessment, and ambulation (Li, Yuan, & Qi, 2012). SCDs are not to be worn when a patient has an active VTE because of the risk of pulmonary embolism. Preventive anticoagulation is recommended for many patients; the recommendation depends on the patient's risk for VTE (Schulman, 2014). VTE prevention is enhanced if SCDs are used along with anticoagulation.

Drug Therapy. Anticoagulants are used routinely for VTE prevention and treatment. The regimen depends on the patient's

TABLE 40-9   DIAGNOSTIC STUDIES

Venous Thrombo-embolism*

Study	Description and Abnormal Findings
Blood Laboratory Studies	
ACT, aPTT, INR, bleeding time, Hb, Hct, platelet count	Alterations if patient has underlying blood dyscrasia (e.g., increased Hb and Hct in patient with polycythemia).
D-dimer	Fragment of fibrin formed as result of fibrin degradation and clot lysis. Elevated results suggest venous thrombo-embolism (VTE). *Normal results:* 3.0 mmol/L (<50 ng/mL)
Fibrin monomer complex	Forms when concentration of thrombin exceeds that of antithrombin. Presence is evidence of thrombus formation and suggests VTE. *Normal results:* <10 mg/dL (<10 mcg/mL)
Noninvasive Venous Studies	
Venous compression ultrasonography	Evaluation of deep femoral, popliteal, and posterior tibial veins. *Normal finding:* Veins collapse with application of external pressure *Abnormal finding:* Veins fail to collapse with application of external pressure; failure to collapse suggests a thrombus
Duplex ultrasonography	Combination of compression ultrasonography with spectral and colour flow Doppler study. Veins are examined for respiratory variation, compressibility, and intraluminal filling defects to help determine location and extent of thrombus (most widely used test to diagnose VTE).
Invasive Venous Studies	
Computed tomography venography (CTV)	Spiral CT used to evaluate veins in the pelvis, thighs, and calves after injection of venous phase contrast material; involves less contrast material than does traditional venography; may be performed simultaneously with CT angiography of pulmonary vessels for patients being evaluated for VTE.
Magnetic resonance venography	MRI with specialized software to evaluate blood flow through veins; can be performed with or without contrast material; highly accurate for pelvic and proximal veins; less accurate for calf veins; can distinguish acute and chronic thrombus.
Contrast venography (phlebography)	Radiographic determination of location and extent of clot with contrast media to outline filling defects; identifies the presence of collateral circulation; once the "gold standard" of invasive venous studies but currently rarely performed

*See Table 30-25 for diagnostic studies for pulmonary embolism.
ACT, activated clotting time; *aPTT*, activated partial thromboplastin time; *CT*, computed tomography; *Hb*, hemoglobin; *Hct*, hematocrit; *INR*, international normalized ratio; *MRI*, magnetic resonance imaging.

VTE risk. The goal of anticoagulant therapy for VTE prophylaxis is to prevent clot formation. The goals for treatment of a confirmed VTE are to prevent new clot development, prevent spread of the clot, and prevent embolization.

Three major classes of anticoagulants are available: (a) vitamin K antagonists, (b) thrombin inhibitors (both indirect and direct), and (c) factor Xa inhibitors (Ageno, Gallus, Wittkowsky, et al., 2012; Table 40-10). The use of ASA (Aspirin) alone for VTE thromboprophylaxis is not recommended for any patient group (Brotons, Benamouzig, Filipiak et al., 2015). Anticoagulant therapy does not dissolve the clot. Lysis of the clot begins spontaneously through the body's intrinsic fibrinolytic system (see Chapter 32).

Vitamin K Antagonists. The oral anticoagulant for long-term or extended anticoagulation is warfarin, a vitamin K antagonist. Warfarin inhibits activation of the vitamin K–dependent coagulation factors II, VII, IX, and X, as well as the anticoagulant proteins C and S (Schulman, 2014). (Figure 32-4 displays the clotting pathways, and clotting factors are listed in Table 32-3.) Warfarin begins to take effect in 48 to 72 hours. It then takes several more days to achieve a maximum effect. Thus an overlap of a parenteral anticoagulant (e.g., unfractionated heparin or LMWH) and warfarin typically is required for 5 days. The level of anticoagulation is monitored daily with the international normalized ratio (INR). The INR is a standardized system of reporting prothrombin time (Table 40-11).

The nurse should carefully document the patient's history before warfarin therapy is started. Antiplatelet agents (e.g., ASA [Aspirin]) generally are not given with warfarin because they increase bleeding risk (Schulman, 2014). Other drugs that

interact with warfarin include NSAIDs; phenytoin (Dilantin); barbiturates; and many vitamin, mineral, dietary, and herbal supplements (see the "Complementary & Alternative Therapies: Natural Health Products That May Affect Clotting" box). A diet that frequently varies in vitamin K intake (e.g., green leafy vegetables) can make it difficult to achieve and maintain a therapeutic INR level.

Genetic variants in the genes *VKORC1* and *CYP2C9* (cytochrome P450 2C9) may influence how some people respond to warfarin. Although genetic testing is available, pharmacogenetic-based dosing is currently not recommended in clinical practice (Guyatt, Akl, Crowther, et al., 2012).

Thrombin Inhibitors: Indirect. Indirect thrombin inhibitors are divided into two major classes: unfractionated heparin and LMWHs. Unfractionated heparin (e.g., heparin) affects both the intrinsic and the common pathways of blood coagulation by way of antithrombin found in blood plasma. Antithrombin is a natural anticoagulant that inhibits the activated coagulation factors II (prothrombin), IX, X, XI, and XII (see Figure 32-4). Heparin increases the inhibition rate significantly.

Heparin can be given subcutaneously for VTE prophylaxis or by continuous IV infusion for VTE treatment. When heparin is given intravenously, clotting status, as measured by activated partial thromboplastin time (aPTT), must be monitored frequently (see Table 40-11). One serious adverse effect of heparin is *heparin-induced thrombo-cytopenia* (HIT). HIT is an immune reaction to heparin in which the platelet count diminishes severely and suddenly, along with a paradoxical increase in venous or arterial thrombosis (Sartori, Favaretto, Migliaccio, et al., 2016).

TABLE 40-10 DRUG THERAPY

Anticoagulant Therapy

Anticoagulant	Drug	Route of Administration	Comments
Vitamin K antagonists	Warfarin (Coumadin)	PO	INR is used for monitoring therapeutic levels. Drugs are administered at the same time each day. Variations of certain genes (e.g., *CYP2CP, VKORC1*) may influence response to the drug. Antidote: Vitamin K
Thrombin Inhibitors: Indirect			
Unfractionated heparin	Heparin sodium	Continuous IV Intermittent IV Subcut	Therapeutic effects measured at regular intervals by the aPTT or ACT. CBC is monitored at regular intervals. If administered subcutaneously, drug should be injected deep into subcutaneous tissue (preferably into the abdominal fatty tissue or above the iliac crest), inserting the entire length of the needle. Skinfold is held during injection but released before needle is removed. The nurse should not aspirate, not inject intramuscularly, and not rub site after injection. Sites should be rotated. Antidote: Protamine
Low-molecular-weight heparin (LMWH)	Enoxaparin (Lovenox) Tinzaparin (Innohep) Dalteparin (Fragmin) Nadroparin (Fraxiparine)	Subcut	Routine coagulation tests typically not required. CBC is monitored at regular intervals. Air bubble should not be expelled before drug is administered subcutaneously. The nurse should follow remaining administration guidelines as described for unfractionated heparin. Dosage should be reduced in patients with renal impairment. Extreme caution should be used in patients with a history of HIT. *Antidote*: Protamine
Thrombin Inhibitors: Direct			
Hirudin derivatives	Lepirudin (Refludan)	IV or subcut IV	Therapeutic effect measured by ACT or aPTT. Used in patients with HIT when anticoagulation is still required.
	Bivalirudin (Angiomax)	IV or subcut	*Antidote*: None
Synthetic thrombin inhibitors	Argatroban	IV	Therapeutic effect measured by aPTT. Used in patients at risk for or with HIT.
	Dabigatran (Pradaxa)	Subcut	*Antidote:* None
Factor Xa Inhibitors			
	Fondaparinux (Arixtra) Rivaroxaban (Xarelto)	Subcut and IV PO	Routine coagulation tests not required. CBC and creatinine are monitored at regular intervals. Air bubble should not be expelled before drug is administered. The nurse should follow remaining administration guidelines as described for unfractionated heparin. Approved for VTE prophylaxis and treatment. For patients undergoing surgery, initial dose should be given no earlier than 6 hr postoperatively. Should be administered with caution in elderly patients and patients with impaired renal function. May cause thrombo-cytopenia. If uncontrollable bleeding occurs, treatment with recombinant factor VIIa may be effective. *Antidote*: None

ACT, activated clotting time; *aPTT*, activated partial thromboplastin time; *CBC*, complete blood count; *HIT*, heparin-induced thrombo-cytopenia; *INR*, international normalized ratio; *IV*, intravenous; *PO*, oral; *Subcut*, subcutaneous; *VTE*, venous thrombo-embolism.

HIT is diagnosed by measurements for the presence of heparin antibodies in the blood. Treatment requires immediately stopping heparin therapy and, if further anticoagulation is required, using a nonheparin anticoagulant (Schulman, 2014). Another adverse effect of long-term heparin therapy is osteoporosis (Tufano, Coppola, Contaldi, et al., 2015).

LMWHs (e.g., enoxaparin [Lovenox] and dalteparin [Fragmin]) are derived from heparin, but the molecule size is about one-third that of unfractionated heparin (Schulman, 2014). They have more bioavailability, more predictable dose effects, longer half-life, and fewer bleeding complications than does unfractionated heparin. LMWHs also are less likely than heparin to cause HIT and osteoporosis. LMWHs typically do not necessitate anticoagulant monitoring and dose adjustment. Protamine neutralizes the effect of LMWH.

Thrombin Inhibitors: Direct. *Direct thrombin inhibitors* are classified as hirudin derivatives or synthetic thrombin inhibitors.

Hirudin is manufactured through recombinant DNA technology. It binds specifically with thrombin and directly inhibits its function without causing plasma protein and platelet interactions. Hirudin derivatives (e.g., lepirudin [Refludan] and bivalirudin [Angiomax]) are administered by continuous IV infusion. Lepirudin is approved for prophylaxis or treatment of HIT, whereas bivalirudin is approved for patients with HIT who undergo percutaneous coronary angioplasty. Anticoagulant activity is monitored according to aPTT or activated clotting time (see Table 40-11). There is no antidote for hirudin derivatives if bleeding occurs.

Argatroban, a synthetic direct thrombin inhibitor, inhibits thrombin. It is used as an alternative to heparin for the prevention and treatment of HIT and for patients known to have HIT who require percutaneous coronary interventions. Dabigatran (Pradaxa), an oral direct thrombin inhibitor, is used for VTE prevention after elective joint replacement, for stroke prevention in nonvalvular atrial fibrillation, and as a treatment option for

TABLE 40-11	TESTS OF BLOOD COAGULATION		
Drugs Monitored		**Normal Value**	**Therapeutic Value**
International normalized ratio (INR)		0.75–1.25	2–3
• Vitamin K antagonists (e.g., warfarin [Coumadin])			
Activated partial thromboplastin time (aPTT)		25–35 sec	46–70 sec
• Unfractionated heparin (e.g., heparin)			
• Hirudin derivatives (e.g., bivalirudin [Angiomax])			
• Synthetic thrombin inhibitors (e.g., argatroban; dabigatran (Pradaxa)			
Activated clotting time (ACT)		70–120 sec*	>300 sec
• Unfractionated heparin			
• Hirudin derivatives			
• Synthetic thrombin inhibitors			
Anti–factor Xa			
• Low-molecular-weight heparin (e.g., enoxaparin [Lovenox])		0 U/mL	U/mL
• Factor Xa inhibitors (e.g., fondaparinux [Arixtra])		0 U/mL	0.2–1.5 U/mL

*Varies based on type of system and test reagent or activator used.

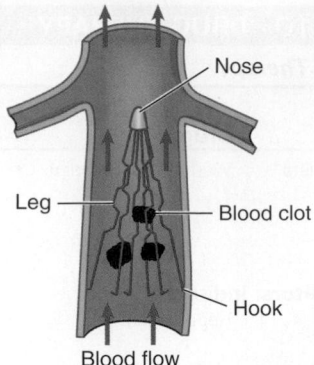

FIGURE 40-11 Inferior vena caval interruption technique with a Greenfield stainless steel filter to prevent pulmonary embolism. As blood travels up the vena cava, clots are trapped in the filter.

VTE. The effects of argatroban and dabigatran are not reversible. Anticoagulant effect is monitored for both medications according to aPTT or activated clotting time.

Factor Xa Inhibitors. *Factor Xa inhibitors* (e.g., fondaparinux [Arixtra]) inhibit factor Xa directly or indirectly, producing rapid anticoagulation. Fondaparinux is recommended for both treatment and prophylaxis of VTE. It is given subcutaneously. Coagulation monitoring or dose adjustment is not needed, although its anticoagulant activity can be measured with anti–factor Xa assays (see Table 40-11). If uncontrollable bleeding occurs, recombinant factor VIIa may be useful. Fondaparinux is contraindicated in patients with renal insufficiency. Rivaroxaban (Xarelto) is an oral factor Xa inhibitor used for VTE prevention.

Anticoagulation Therapy for VTE Prophylaxis. For VTE prophylaxis in hospitalized patients at risk for thrombosis who are not bleeding, low-dose unfractionated heparin, LMWH, or fondaparinux is prescribed. Patients with moderate VTE risk (e.g., those undergoing general, gynecological, or urological surgery; those with acute medical problems) should receive unfractionated heparin, LMWH, or fondaparinux (Khan, 2015). Patients with high VTE risk (e.g., those who have sustained trauma) should receive VTE prophylaxis with LMWH, fondaparinux, or warfarin until discharge (Khan, 2015). It is recommended that patients undergoing high-risk gynecological surgery (e.g., for cancer) and major orthopedic surgery (e.g., total knee or hip replacement) be prescribed VTE prophylaxis up to 35 days after discharge. Similarly, all critically ill patients (e.g., those who have sustained trauma) should receive VTE prophylaxis while hospitalized (Rattan, Jones, & Namias, 2015).

Anticoagulation Therapy for Venous Thrombo-embolism Treatment. Patients with confirmed VTE should receive initial treatment with LMWH, unfractionated heparin, or fondaparinux, as well as warfarin, for at least 5 days or until the INR is 2.0 or higher for 24 hours. Patients with one or more of multiple comorbid conditions, complex medical issues, or a very large VTE usually are hospitalized for treatment and typically receive

IV unfractionated heparin LMWH is recommended over unfractionated heparin for most patients with acute VTE. Depending on clinical presentation, many of these patients can be managed safely and effectively as outpatients (Whayne, 2012). Fondaparinux may be particularly useful for VTE treatment in patients with a history of HIT.

Thrombolytic Therapy for Venous Thrombo-embolism. Another treatment option for patients with a thrombus is catheter-directed administration of a thrombolytic drug (e.g., urokinase, recombinant tissue plasminogen activator [recombinant alteplase]) (Kearon, Akl, Comerota, et al., 2012). Catheter-directed thrombolytic drugs directly dissolve clots, reduce the acute symptoms, and decrease the incidence of postphlebitic vein problems. Additional catheter-based interventions such as angioplasty, stents, or mechanical thrombectomy with a high-speed impeller to fragment the thrombus can be used in conjunction with the thrombolytic drug (Kearon, Akl, Comerota, et al., 2012). (Thrombolytic therapy is discussed in Chapter 36.)

Surgical Therapy. Although most cases of VTE are managed medically, a small number of patients undergo surgery. Surgical options include open venous thrombectomy and inferior vena cava interruption. Venous thrombectomy involves the removal of a thrombus through an incision in the vein (Panico, Jafferani, Shah, et al., 2015). Vena cava interruption devices (e.g., Greenfield, VenaTech, or TrapEase filters) can be inserted percutaneously through the right femoral or right internal jugular veins. The filter device is opened, and the spokes penetrate the vessel walls (Figure 40-11). This results in "sieve-type" obstruction, allowing filtration of clots without interruption of blood flow. Complications after the insertion of the device are rare but include air embolism, improper placement, migration of the filter, and perforation of the vena cava with retroperitoneal bleeding (Dominguez, Bahadorani, Reeves, et al., 2015). Over time, venous congestion can occur from accumulation of trapped clots. These can clog the filter and completely occlude the vena cava, necessitating filter removal and replacement. A filter device is recommended if anticoagulant therapy is contraindicated because of an increased risk of bleeding.

NURSING MANAGEMENT
VENOUS THROMBO-EMBOLISM

NURSING ASSESSMENT

Table 40-12 lists the subjective and objective data to obtain from a patient with VTE.

EVIDENCE-INFORMED PRACTICE

Translating Research Into Practice

The nurse is caring for Hana Bercier, a 78-year-old woman who is being discharged with a prescription for enoxaparin (Lovenox) after a knee replacement. Her granddaughter will be her primary caregiver. Because arthritis limits dexterity in Ms. Bercier's hands, the nurse is preparing to teach her granddaughter how to inject the medication. Her granddaughter tells the nurse that Ms. Bercier is a modest woman and will not permit her abdomen to be exposed. She asks if the injection can be given in her arm.

Best Available Evidence	Clinician Expertise	Patient Preferences and Values
Enoxaparin (per the package literature) should be administered by deep subcutaneous injection in the abdomen. Injection sites should be rotated.	Some patients have told the nurse that they used alternate sites for injection of enoxaparin, specifically the thighs and upper arms. The nurse has no evidence about the efficacy of the drug when alternate sites are used.	Ms. Bercier states she does not want to expose herself to her granddaughter. The granddaughter expresses a desire to support her grandmother's need for modesty.

Decision and Action

The nurse discusses the importance of following the drug manufacturer's recommendations regarding site selection with Ms. Bercier and her granddaughter. The nurse further explains that there is no evidence on whether alternate sites are equally effective. Ms. Bercier's granddaughter states that she is the only one available to do this and she needs to respect her grandmother's wishes. The nurse teaches the granddaughter how to inject enoxaparin in Ms. Bercier's upper arms and to alternate the sites and arms. The nurse informs the physician of Ms. Bercier's decision and documents the teaching and related conversation.

Reference for Evidence

Sanofi-Aventis. (2013). *Lovenox: Prescribing information.* Retrieved from *http:// products.sanofi.us/lovenox/lovenox.html#section-5.1.*

NURSING DIAGNOSES

Nursing diagnoses and collaborative problems for a patient with VTE include, but are not limited to, the following:

- *Acute pain* related to *physical injury agent* (venous congestion, impaired venous return, and inflammation)
- *Ineffective health maintenance* related to *insufficient resources* (lack of knowledge about disorder and its treatment)
- *Risk for impaired skin integrity* related to *alteration in fluid volume* (altered peripheral tissue perfusion)
- Potential complication: bleeding related to anticoagulant therapy
- Potential complication: pulmonary embolism related to embolization of thrombus, dehydration, and immobility

PLANNING

The overall goals for the patient with VTE include (a) pain relief, (b) decreased edema, (c) no skin ulceration, (d) no bleeding complications, and (e) no evidence of pulmonary embolism.

NURSING IMPLEMENTATION

ACUTE INTERVENTION. Nursing care for the patient with VTE is directed toward the prevention of emboli formation and the

TABLE 40-12 NURSING ASSESSMENT

Venous Thrombo-embolism

Subjective Data
Important Health Information
Past health history: Trauma to vein, intravascular catheter (e.g., peripherally inserted central catheter), varicose veins, pregnancy or recent childbirth, bacteremia, obesity, prolonged bed rest, irregular heartbeat (e.g., atrial fibrillation), COPD, HF, cancer, coagulation disorders and hypercoagulable states, systemic lupus erythematosus, MI, spinal cord injury, stroke, prolonged air travel, recent bone fracture, dehydration
Medications: Use of estrogens (including oral contraceptives, hormone replacement therapy), tamoxifen (Nolvadex-D), raloxifene (Evista), corticosteroids, excessive amounts of vitamin E, IV use of recreational drugs
Surgery or other treatments: Any recent surgery, especially orthopedic, gynecological, gastric, or urological; previous surgery involving veins; central venous catheter

Symptoms
- Pain in area on palpation or ambulation

Objective Data
General
Fever, anxiety, pain

Integumentary
Increased size of affected extremity in comparison with opposite extremity; taut, shiny, warm skin; erythematous skin; tenderness to palpation. Some patients may have no physical changes in the affected extremity.

Cardiovascular
Distension and warmth of superficial veins in affected area; edema and cyanosis of extremities, neck, back, and face (if superior vena cava involvement)

Possible Findings
Leukocytosis, abnormal coagulation, anemia or ↑ hematocrit and RBC count, ↑ D-dimer level, positive venous compression on duplex ultrasound study; positive findings on CTV, magnetic resonance venography, or contrast venography.

COPD, chronic obstructive pulmonary disease; *CTV,* computed tomography venography; *HF,* heart failure; *IV,* intravenous; *MI,* myocardial infarction; *RBC,* red blood cell.

reduction of inflammation. Because effective anticoagulation is essential, the nurse should review with the patient any medications, vitamins, minerals, and dietary and natural health products being taken that may interfere with anticoagulation therapy (Grant, Bin, Kiat, et al., 2012) (see the "Complementary and Alternative Therapies: Natural Health Products That May Affect Clotting" box). Depending on the anticoagulant ordered, the nurse should monitor INR, aPTT, activated clotting time, anti–factor Xa levels, complete blood cell count, creatinine, factor X levels, hemoglobin, hematocrit, platelet levels, and liver enzyme levels (Holbrook, Schulman, Witt, et al., 2012). Platelet counts in patients receiving unfractionated heparin or LMWH should be monitored to assess for HIT. Doses of unfractionated heparin, warfarin, and direct thrombin inhibitors should be titrated on the basis of results of clotting studies and physician-established parameters. Dosages of direct thrombin inhibitors may need adjustment for patients with impaired renal or liver function. The nurse should always check the results of appropriate tests before initiating, administering, or adjusting anticoagulant therapy.

DRUG ALERT—Anticoagulant Therapy

- Patients taking coagulants should avoid taking ASA (Aspirin), nonsteroidal anti-inflammatory drugs (NSAIDs), fish oil supplements, garlic supplements, ginkgo biloba, and certain antibiotics (e.g., sulfamethoxazole and trimethoprim [Bactrim]).
- Patients should be instructed to report any signs of bleeding (e.g., black or bloody stools, bloody urine, coffee-ground or bloody vomit, nosebleeds).
- The nurse should assess for signs of bleeding (e.g., hypotension, tachycardia, hematuria, melena, hematemesis, petechiae, ecchymosis).

The nurse should monitor for bleeding and reduce the risk of bleeding that may rise with anticoagulant therapy (Table 40-13). The nurse must be aware that the risk of bleeding is greater in persons receiving LMWH or unfractionated heparin who have an

---

TABLE 40-13 NURSING INTERVENTIONS FOR PATIENTS RECEIVING ANTICOAGULANTS

Assessment
- Evaluating appropriate laboratory coagulation tests for target therapeutic levels
- Evaluating lower extremity for ecchymosis/hematoma development if intermittent compression device is used
- Evaluating platelet count for signs of heparin-induced thrombocytopenia (HIT)
- Examining urine and stool for overt signs of blood
- Inspecting skin frequently, especially under any splinting devices
- Monitoring vital signs as indicated
- Notifying the health care provider of any abnormalities in assessments, vital signs, or laboratory values
- Performing assessment of risk for falling per institutional policy, and implementing safety measures as needed
- Performing assessments frequently to observe for signs and symptoms of bleeding (e.g., hypotension, tachycardia), clotting, or both

Injections
- Applying manual pressure for at least 10 min (or longer if needed) on venipuncture sites
- Avoiding intramuscular injections
- Minimizing venipunctures
- Using small-gauge needles for venipunctures unless ordered therapy necessitates the use of a larger gauge

Routine Care and Patient Education
- Administering stool softeners to avoid hard stools and straining
- Applying graduated compression stockings or sequential compression devices as ordered and with attention to proper size, application, and use
- Applying moisturizing lotion to skin
- Avoiding removal or disruption of established clots
- Avoiding restraints if possible; using only soft, padded restraints if needed
- Instructing patient not to forcefully blow nose
- Instructing patient to avoid restrictive clothing
- Instructing patient to use electric razors, not straight razors
- Instructing patient to use soft toothbrushes or foam swabs for oral care
- Limiting tape application; using paper tape as appropriate
- Lubricating tubes (e.g., suction catheter) adequately before insertion
- Performing physical care in a gentle manner
- Repositioning the patient carefully at regular intervals
- Using humidified O_2 source
- Using support pads, mattresses, bed cradles, and therapeutic beds as indicated

---

active gastro-duodenal ulcer, prior bleeding history, low platelet count, hepatic or renal failure, rheumatic disease, and cancer and those older than 85 years (Decousus, Tapson, Bergmann, et al., 2011). Patients receiving warfarin with an INR of 5.0 or more are also at increased risk for bleeding. In the event of anticoagulation above target goals, the nurse should give reversal agents (e.g., protamine, vitamin K) or make dosage adjustments as ordered. In the event of major vitamin K antagonist–related bleeding, rapid treatment with four-factor prothrombin complex concentrate and IV vitamin K is recommended over fresh-frozen plasma.

SAFETY ALERT
- The nurse should observe the patient closely for the following events:
  - Any overt or occult bleeding
  - Epistaxis and bleeding gingivae
  - Blood (visible or occult) in emesis, urine, stool, and sputum
  - Oozing or visible bleeding from trauma site or surgical incision
  - Excessive menstrual bleeding
- The nurse should monitor vital signs for changes: decreased blood pressure, increased heart rate
- Intramuscular injections should be avoided
- The patient should be assessed for mental status changes, especially in the older patient, because they may indicate cerebral bleeding.

Early exercise, in comparison with bed rest, does not increase the short-term risk of a pulmonary embolism in patients with VTE (Hillegass, Puthoff, Frese, et al., 2015). In addition, early exercise after VTE results in a more rapid decrease in edema and limb pain (McDermott, Kibbe, Guralnik, et al., 2013). The nurse should emphasize to the patient and caregiver the importance of exercise and assist the patient to ambulate several times a day. For patients who have acute VTE with severe edema and limb pain, bed rest with limb elevation may initially be prescribed.

AMBULATORY AND HOME CARE. The nurse should focus discharge teaching on modification of VTE risk factors, use of graduated compression stockings, importance of monitoring laboratory values, medication instructions, and guidelines for follow-up. Once the edema is resolved, the patient should be measured for custom-fit, graduated compression stockings. Stocking use (or sleeves in the case of an upper extremity VTE) is recommended for at least 2 years after a VTE to support the vein walls and valves and decrease swelling and pain (Bernstein, Kristianson, Akl, et al., 2016; Pavon, Adam, Razouki, et al., 2016). Regular use of graduated compression stockings reduces the occurrence of post-thrombotic syndrome (which leads to chronic venous insufficiency) (Pavon, Adam, Razouki, et al., 2016).

If appropriate, patients should be instructed to stop smoking, to avoid all nicotine products, and to avoid constrictive clothing. If appropriate, women with a history of VTE should be instructed to stop using birth control pills or oral hormone replacement therapy (Rockman, Maldinado, Jacobowitz, et al., 2012). Patients need to avoid standing or sitting in a motionless, leg-dependent position. Frequent knee flexion, ankle rotation, and active walking during long periods of sitting or standing, as on car or airplane trips, should be encouraged. For patients at high risk for VTE who are planning a long trip, knee-high graduated compression stockings or one dose of LMWH before departure should be recommended (Schulman, 2014).

The patient and caregiver should be taught the signs and symptoms of pulmonary embolism such as sudden onset of dyspnea, tachypnea, and pleuritic chest pain. (Pulmonary embolism is discussed in Chapter 30.) They should contact emergency medical services if these symptoms occur. However, adults older than 70 years are less likely to have calf or thigh swelling or pleuritic pain, two of the classic symptoms of VTE (Copstead & Banasik, 2013).

The patient and caregiver need thorough education regarding medication dosage, actions, and adverse effects, the need for routine blood tests, and what symptoms to report to the health care provider (Table 40-14). Devices are available for home monitoring of INR. Patients taking LMWH or fondaparinux or their caregivers should be taught how to administer the medication subcutaneously. Active or young patients need to avoid contact sports and activities with high risk for trauma (e.g., skiing). Older patients need to know to take safety precautions to prevent falls (e.g., avoid use of throw rugs). The nurse must instruct the patient and caregiver to apply pressure for 10 to 15 minutes if bleeding occurs (e.g. nosebleeds). If the bleeding persists, they should contact emergency medical services.

A well-balanced diet, including calcium and vitamin E, is important because these affect coagulation. Patients taking warfarin should be taught to follow a consistent diet of foods containing vitamin K, to avoid taking any supplements containing vitamin K, and to avoid excessive amounts of vitamin E and alcohol. Proper hydration to prevent additional hypercoagulability of the blood, which may occur with dehydration, should be encouraged.

Patients who are overweight not only need to limit caloric intake but also must increase physical activity to achieve and maintain desired weight. A balanced program of rest and exercise also improves venous return. The nurse should assist the patient to develop an exercise program with an emphasis on walking and swimming. Water exercise is particularly beneficial because of the gentle, even pressure of the water. A 6-month exercise program of daily walking improves calf muscle flexibility, strength, and pump function and reduces post-thrombotic syndrome (Christakou & Zakyntinos, 2014).

EVALUATION

The expected outcomes for the patient with VTE include the following:

- Minimal to no pain
- Intact skin
- No signs of hemorrhage or occult bleeding
- No signs of respiratory distress

VARICOSE VEINS

Varicose veins, or *varicosities*, are dilated, tortuous subcutaneous veins most commonly found in the saphenous vein system. Varicosities may be small and innocuous or large and bulging. *Primary varicose veins* (idiopathic) are caused by a congenital weakness of the veins and are more common in women. *Secondary varicose veins* typically result from a previous VTE. Secondary varicose veins also may occur in the esophagus (esophageal varices), vulva, spermatic cords (varicoceles), and anorectal area (hemorrhoids), and as abnormal arteriovenous connections. Reticular veins are smaller varicose veins that appear flat, less tortuous, and bluish green. Telangiectasias (often referred to as *spider veins*) are very small visible vessels (generally <1 mm in diameter) that appear bluish-black, purple, or red.

Etiology and Pathophysiology

The etiology of varicose veins is multifactorial in nature. Superficial veins in the lower extremities become dilated and tortuous in response to increased venous pressure. Risk factors include family history of chronic venous disease, weakness of the vein structure, female sex, Latin American ethnicity, tobacco use, increasing age, obesity, multiparity, history of VTE, venous obstruction resulting from extrinsic pressure by tumours, thrombophilia, phlebitis, previous leg injury, and occupations that require prolonged standing or sitting (Wittens, Davies, Baekgaard, et al., 2015). Although the exact etiology remains unknown, it is thought that the vein valve leaflets are stretched and become incompetent (do not fit together properly). Incompetent vein valves allow retrograde blood flow, particularly when the patient is standing, which results in increased venous pressure and further venous distension.

Clinical Manifestations and Complications

Discomfort from varicose veins varies among people and tends to be worse after episodes of SVT. Many patients are concerned about cosmetic disfigurement. The most common varicose vein symptom is a heavy, achy feeling or pain after prolonged standing, which is relieved by walking or limb elevation. Some patients feel pressure or complain of an itchy, burning, or cramplike sensation

---

TABLE 40-14   PATIENT & CAREGIVER TEACHING GUIDE

Anticoagulant Therapy

The following information should be included in the teaching plan for a patient receiving anticoagulant therapy and for the patient's caregiver.

1. Reasons for and basic mechanism of action of anticoagulant therapy and how long the anticipated therapy will last
2. The need to take medication at same time each day (preferably in afternoon or evening)
3. Depending on medication prescribed, the need for frequent follow-up with blood tests to assess therapeutic effect of the drug and whether change in drug dosages is required
4. Adverse effects of drug therapy that necessitate medical attention:
   - Any bleeding that does not stop after a reasonable amount of time (usually 10–15 min)
   - Blood in urine or stool, or black, tarry stools
   - Chest pain, shortness of breath, palpitations (heart racing)
   - Cold, blue, or painful feet
   - Severe headaches or stomach pains
   - Unusual bleeding from gums, throat, skin, or nose, or heavy menstrual bleeding
   - Vomiting blood or coffee-ground emesis
   - Weakness, dizziness, mental status changes
5. Avoidance of any trauma or injury that might cause bleeding (e.g., vigorous brushing of teeth, contact sports, in-line roller skating, use of straight razor)
6. Avoidance of all ASA (Aspirin)-containing drugs or nonsteroidal anti-inflammatory drugs
7. Limiting alcohol intake to small to moderate amount (341 mL [12 oz] of beer, 118 mL [4 oz] of wine, or 30 mL [1 oz of hard liquor per day)
8. Wearing a MedicAlert bracelet or necklace indicating what anticoagulant is being taken
9. Avoiding frequent changes in eating habits, such as dramatically increasing foods high in vitamin K (e.g., broccoli, spinach, kale, greens); avoiding supplemental vitamin K
10. Consulting with health care provider before beginning or discontinuing any medication, vitamin, mineral, or dietary or herbal supplement (see the "Complementary and Alternative Therapies: Natural Health Products That May Affect Clotting" box)
11. Informing all health care providers, including dentist, of anticoagulant therapy
12. The necessity of correct dosing; supervision may be required (e.g., patients experiencing confusion or cognitive impairment; Whayne, 2012)

in the affected leg. Swelling or nocturnal leg cramps also may occur. SVT is the most frequent complication of varicose veins and may occur spontaneously or after trauma, surgical procedures, or pregnancy. Rare complications include rupture of the varicose veins, resulting in external bleeding and skin ulcerations.

Diagnostic Studies and Collaborative Care

Superficial varicose veins can be diagnosed by appearance. Duplex ultrasonography can reveal obstruction and reflux in the venous system with considerable accuracy. It is the test most widely used to diagnose deep varicose veins.

Treatment usually is not indicated if varicose veins are only a cosmetic problem. If venous insufficiency develops, collaborative care involves rest with limb elevation, graduated compression stockings and exercise, such as walking. Two herbal therapies used for varicose vein treatment are horse chestnut seed extract (*Aesculus hippocastanum*) and butcher's broom (*Ruscus aculeatus*; Grant, Bin, Kiat, et al., 2012). (See the "Chronic Venous Insufficiency and Venous Leg Ulcers" section later in this chapter.)

Sclerotherapy involves the injection of a substance that obliterates venous telangiectasias, reticular veins, and small, superficial varicose veins 5 mm or larger in diameter (Marsden, Perry, Kelley, et al., 2013) (Figure 40-12). Commonly used sclerosing agents include hypertonic saline, polidocanol, and glycerine. Direct IV injection of a sclerosing agent induces inflammation and results in eventual thrombosis of the vein. This procedure is performed in an office setting and causes minimal discomfort. Potential complications include itching, pain, blistering, edema, hyperpigmentation, necrosis, recurrence of varicosities, SVT, visual disturbances, and VTE (Marsden, Perry, Kelley, et al., 2013). After injection, a thigh-high graduated compression stocking is worn or an elastic bandage is applied to the leg for several days to maintain pressure over the vein. Long-term compression therapy is advised to help prevent the development of further varicosities.

Newer, more costly, but noninvasive options for the treatment of venous telangiectasias include laser therapy and high-intensity pulsed-light therapy (Marsden, Perry, Kelley, et al., 2013). Laser or light therapy is indicated for isolated small telangiectasias or for patients in whom sclerotherapy is contraindicated or has been previously ineffective. Laser treatment typically requires more

than one session, scheduled at 6- to 12-week intervals. Vascular lasers work by heating the hemoglobin in the vessels, which leads to thermocoagulation and results in vessel sclerosis (Marsden, Perry, Kelley, et al., 2013). Pulsed-light therapy is similar to laser therapy, but a spectrum of light, rather than a single wavelength, is used. Potential complications of these therapies include pain, blistering, hyperpigmentation, and superficial erosions.

Surgical intervention is indicated for recurrent superficial venous thrombosis or when chronic venous insufficiency cannot be controlled with conservative therapy. The traditional surgical intervention involves ligation of the entire vein (usually the greater saphenous vein) and dissection and removal of its incompetent tributaries. An alternative but time-consuming technique is ambulatory phlebectomy. This procedure involves pulling the varicosity through a stab incision followed by excision of the vein. Potential complications include bleeding, bruising, and infection. In up to 30% of patients, a new vein forms to replace the one removed (Marsden, Perry, Kelley, et al., 2013).

A newer, less invasive procedure is endovenous ablation of the saphenous vein. Ablation involves the insertion of a catheter that emits energy. This causes collapse and sclerosis of the vein (Rasmussen, Lawaetz, Bjoern, et al., 2013). Potential complications include bruising, tightness along the vein, recanalization (reopening of the vein), and paresthesia (Rasmussen, Lawaetz, Bjoern, et al., 2013). Endovenous ablation also may be done in combination with saphenofemoral ligation or phlebectomy.

NURSING MANAGEMENT
VARICOSE VEINS

Prevention is a key factor related to varicose veins. The patient should be instructed to avoid sitting or standing for long periods, maintain ideal body weight, take precautions against injury to the extremities, avoid wearing constrictive clothing, and walk daily.

After vein ligation surgery, the patient should be encouraged to practise deep breathing, which promotes venous return. It is important to check the extremities regularly for colour, movement, sensation, temperature, edema, and quality of pedal pulses. Bruising and discoloration are considered normal. Postoperatively, the legs should be elevated 15 degrees to limit edema. Graduated compression stockings should be applied, removed every 8 hours for short periods, and then reapplied.

Long-term management of varicose veins is directed toward improving circulation and cosmetic appearance, relieving discomfort, and avoiding complications and ulceration. Varicose veins can recur in other locations after vein ligation. The patient needs to learn the proper use and care of custom-fitted graduated compression stockings. The patient should apply stockings in bed, before rising in the morning. In some instances, patients also use SCDs at home to control edema (Pavon, Adam, Razouki, et al., 2016). The importance of periodic positioning of the legs above the heart should be stressed. An overweight patient may need assistance with weight loss. A patient with a job that requires long periods of standing or sitting needs to frequently flex and extend her or his hips, legs, and ankles and change positions.

FIGURE 40-12 A, Lateral aspect of varicose veins before treatment. **B,** Lateral aspect of varicose veins 2 years after initial treatment with sclerotherapy. Source: Goldman, M. P., Guex, J. J., & Weiss, R.A. (2011). *Sclerotherapy: Treatment of varicose and telangiectatic leg veins* (5th ed.). Philadelphia: Mosby.

CHRONIC VENOUS INSUFFICIENCY AND VENOUS LEG ULCERS

Chronic venous insufficiency (CVI), a common problem in women and older adults, is a condition in which leg veins and valves fail to keep blood moving forward. This results in *ambulatory venous hypertension*. CVI can lead to *venous leg ulcers* (formerly called *venous stasis ulcers* or *varicose ulcers*). Although CVI and venous leg ulcers are not life-threatening diseases, they are painful, debilitating, and costly chronic conditions that adversely affect the quality of patients' lives (O'Donnell, Passman, Marsten, et al., 2014).

Etiology and Pathophysiology

Both long-standing primary varicose veins and post-thrombotic syndrome can progress to CVI. The causes of CVI include vein valve incompetence, deep vein obstruction, congenital venous malformation, and arteriovenous fistula (Copstead & Banasik, 2013). The basic problem is incompetent valves of the deep veins. As a result, hydrostatic pressure in the veins increases and serous fluid and RBCs leak from the capillaries and venules into the tissue, which results in edema. Enzymes in the tissue eventually break down RBCs, causing the release of *hemosiderin,* which causes a brownish skin discoloration. Over time, the skin and subcutaneous tissue around the ankle are replaced by fibrous tissue, which results in thick, hardened, contracted skin. Although the causes of CVI are known, the exact pathophysiology of venous leg ulcers is not known

Clinical Manifestations and Complications

In individuals with CVI, the skin of the lower leg is leathery, with a characteristic brownish or "brawny" appearance from the hemosiderin deposition. Edema usually has been persistent for a prolonged period. Eczema, or "stasis dermatitis," is often present, and itching is a common complaint (see Table 40-1).

Venous ulcers classically are located above the medial malleolus (Figure 40-13; see Table 40-1). Many such ulcers are quite painful, particularly when edema or infection is present (Maddox, 2012). Pain may be worse when the leg is in a dependent position. If the venous ulcer is untreated, the wound becomes more extensive, eroding wider and deeper and increasing the likelihood of wound infection and cellulitis. Recurrent episodes of cellulitis may lead

FIGURE 40-13 Venous leg ulcer. Source: Kamal, A., & Brocklehurst, J. C. (1991). *Color atlas of geriatric medicine* (2nd ed.). St. Louis: Mosby–Year Book.

to destruction of the superficial lymphatic vessels, causing a secondary lymphedema to develop (Maddox, 2012). On very rare occasions, severe CVI with longstanding nonhealing venous ulcers may result in the need for amputation.

Collaborative Care

Compression is essential for CVI treatment, venous ulcer healing, and prevention of ulcer recurrence. A variety of options are available for compression therapy, including elastic wraps, custom-fitted graduated compression stockings, elastic tubular support bandages, a Velcro wrap (CircAid), SCDs, a paste bandage (Unna boot) with an elastic wrap, and multilayer (three or four) bandage systems (e.g., Profore) (Woo, Alavi, Evans, et al., 2013). There are benefits to each type of compression therapy. Each patient should be evaluated individually when an extrinsic compression method is chosen. Before instituting compression therapy, the nurse should assess the arterial status to make sure that coexistent PAD is not present. An ABI of less than 0.9 suggests PAD, and levels of compression should not be high.

Moist environment dressings are the basis of wound care. A variety of these dressings are available and include transparent film dressings, hydrocolloids, hydrogels, foams, calcium alginates, impregnated gauze, gauze moistened with saline, and combination dressings. When used in conjunction with compression, moist environment dressings are more effective than dry dressings in hastening the healing of venous leg ulcers. (Hydrocolloid and other dressings are discussed in Chapter 14 and Table 14-11.)

The nurse should evaluate the nutritional status of a patient with a venous ulcer. A balanced diet with adequate protein, calories, and micronutrients is essential for healing. Nutrients most important for healing include protein, vitamins A and C, and zinc. Foods high in protein (e.g., meat, beans, cheese, tofu), vitamin A (green leafy vegetables), vitamin C (citrus fruits, tomatoes, cantaloupe), and zinc (meat, seafood) must be provided.

For patients with diabetes mellitus, maintaining normal blood glucose levels assists the healing process. For overweight individuals with CVI and no active venous ulcer, a weight loss diet should be considered (O'Donnell, Passman, Marsten, et al., 2014). Routine antibiotic therapy is not indicated. Clinical signs of infection in a venous ulcer include change in quantity, colour, or odour of the drainage; presence of pus; erythema of the wound edges; change in sensation around the wound; warmth around the wound; increased local pain or edema, or both; dark-coloured granulation tissue; induration around the wound; delayed healing; and cellulitis. If signs of infection are present, the nurse should obtain a wound culture before instituting antibiotic therapy. The usual treatment for infection is debridement, wound excision, and systemic antibiotics. A number of antimicrobial dressings (e.g., cadexomer iodine, silver) are available for use on contaminated or infected venous ulcers.

If the ulcer does not heal with conservative therapy, drug therapy should be considered. Pentoxifylline or micronized purified flavonoid fraction (Daflon) is recommended with compression therapy to improve healing (Kahn, Comerota, Cushman, et al., 2014). Pentoxifylline minimizes WBC activation and adhesion to capillary endothelium and decreases oxidative stress. Micronized purified flavonoid fraction acts on WBCs to decrease inflammation and edema (Raffetto & Eberhardt, 2014).

Alternative treatments include coverage with a split-thickness skin graft, cultured epithelial autograft, allograft, or bioengineered skin such as Dermagraft (O'Donnell, Passman, Marsten, et al., 2014). Before the graft is applied, the ulcer is debrided, varicosities in the area are removed, and veins are ligated. (Skin grafting is discussed in Chapter 27.) Although grafts may assist with healing, they do not replace the need for lifelong compression therapy.

A natural health product used for CVI treatment is horse chestnut seed extract (HCSE). Escin (the active ingredient) reduces leg pain, itching, and swelling (Pittler & Ernst, 2012). Minor adverse effects associated with HCSE include dizziness, gastro-intestinal complaints, headache, and pruritus. The efficacy of HCSE in venous ulcer healing and recurrence has not been determined.

NURSING MANAGEMENT
CHRONIC VENOUS INSUFFICIENCY AND VENOUS LEG ULCERS

Long-term management of venous leg ulcers should focus on teaching the patient about self-care measures because the ulcers often recur (Weller & Evans, 2012). The nurse should instruct the patient and caregiver to avoid trauma to the limbs and should teach them proper skin care. The nurse should also demonstrate the correct application of graduated compression stockings and stress the importance of regular replacement.

It is important to discuss activity guidelines and proper limb positioning. Proper foot and leg care is essential to avoid additional skin trauma. In patients with CVI, the skin is dry, flaky, and itchy as a result of stasis dermatitis. Daily moisturizing decreases itching and prevents cracking of the skin. Venous dermatitis may result from contact with sensitizing products such as antibacterial agents (e.g., gentamicin, neomycin); additives in bandages or dressings (e.g., adhesives); ointments containing lanolin, alcohols, benzocaine, or balsam of Peru; and over-the-counter creams or lotions with fragrance or preservatives (Weller & Evans, 2012). With each dressing change, the nurse must assess the wound for signs of infection.

Patients with CVI with or without a venous ulcer should be instructed to avoid standing or sitting for long periods. Standing or sitting with the legs in a dependent position decreases periulcer skin blood perfusion and oxygen levels. Patients with venous ulcers should elevate their legs above the level of the heart to reduce edema. Patients should begin a daily walking program once an ulcer heals. Prescription graduated compression stockings should be worn daily and replaced every 4 to 6 months to reduce the occurrence of CVI (Nelson & Bell-Syer, 2014).

CASE STUDY

Peripheral Artery Disease

Source: Air Images/ Shutterstock .com.

Patient Profile

Leo Ducharme, a 76-year-old man, was admitted to the hospital with rest pain in both legs and a nonhealing ulcer of the big toe on the right foot.

Subjective Data
- History of a myocardial infarction, stroke, hypertension, arthritis, and type 1 diabetes mellitus
- Underwent a left femoral–popliteal bypass 5 years ago
- Has a 45-pack-yr history of tobacco use
- Has been using insulin for 30 years
- Complains of sudden, intense increase in right foot pain for past 2 hr
- Has slept in recliner with right leg in dependent position for several months

Current Medications
- Furosemide (Lasix), 40 mg/day PO
- Enalapril (Vasotec), 5 mg/day PO
- Aspart (NovoRapid) insulin with meals
- Glargine insulin (Lantus), 50 units daily subcutaneously
- Diltiazem sustained-release (Tiazac), 240 mg/day PO
- ASA (Aspirin), 325 mg/day PO
- Fish oil daily (self-prescribed)

Objective Data
Physical Examination
- BP, 148/92 mm Hg; irregular apical heart rate, 90/min; respiratory rate, 22/min; temperature, 36.6°C
- Alert and oriented but anxious, no apparent physical or mental deficits from previous stroke
- Diminished right femoral pulse, popliteal pulse detected only with use of a Doppler probe, posterior tibial pulse detected with use of Doppler probe, and dorsalis pedis pulse absent (not palpable or visible on Doppler study); left leg pulses are weakly palpable

- Right leg ABI: 0.20; left leg ABI: 0.68
- Has a 2-cm necrotic ulcer on tip of right big toe
- Has thickened toenails; shiny, thin skin on legs; and hair absent on both lower legs
- Right foot is very cool, pale, and mottled in colour with decreased sensation
- No peripheral edema present
- Bedside glucose measurement 16 mmol/L (last meal 4 hr before admission)

Discussion Questions
1. What are Mr. Ducharme's risk factors for peripheral artery disease (PAD)?
2. Differentiate Mr. Ducharme's signs and symptoms of chronic PAD from those of acute arterial ischemia.
3. Identify the possible cause or causes for the sudden, intense increase in right foot pain.
4. How would the nurse interpret Mr. Ducharme's ABI findings?
5. What additional diagnostic tests can be performed to assess the extent of Mr. Ducharme's PAD?
6. Given the physical examination data, what initial medications might the physician prescribe?
7. What treatment modalities are possible for Mr. Ducharme?
8. **Priority decision:** What are the priority nursing responsibilities in caring for Mr. Ducharme?
9. **Priority decision:** On the basis of the assessment data presented, what are the priority nursing diagnoses? Are there any collaborative problems?
10. **Evidence-informed practice:** In patient education for Mr. Ducharme, what evidence-informed advice should the nurse give him regarding the use of dietary supplements such as fish oil?

𝒆volve

Answers are available at http://evolve.elsevier.com/Canada/Lewis/medsurg

REVIEW QUESTIONS

The number of the question corresponds to the same-numbered objective at the beginning of the chapter.

1. A 50-year-old woman weighs 95 kg and has a history of tobacco use, high blood pressure, high sodium intake, and sedentary lifestyle. When an individualized care plan is developed for this client, which of the following risk factors related to PAD would the nurse determine need to be modified?
   a. Weight and diet
   b. Activity level and diet
   c. Tobacco use and high blood pressure
   d. Sedentary lifestyle and high blood pressure

2. Rest pain is a manifestation of PAD that results from which chronic condition?
   a. Vasospasm of small cutaneous arteries in the feet
   b. Increase in retrograde venous blood flow in the legs
   c. Decrease in arterial blood flow to the nerves of the feet
   d. Decrease in arterial blood flow to the leg muscles during exercise

3. A client with infective endocarditis develops sudden left leg pain with pallor, paresthesia, and a loss of peripheral pulses. What should the nurse's initial action be?
   a. To elevate the leg to promote venous return
   b. To start anticoagulant therapy with IV heparin
   c. To notify the physician of the change in peripheral perfusion
   d. To place the bed in reverse Trendelenburg position to promote perfusion

4. Which clinical manifestations are seen in clients with either Buerger's disease or Raynaud's phenomenon? *(Select all that apply)*
   a. Intermittent fevers
   b. Sensitivity to cold temperatures
   c. Gangrenous ulcers on fingertips
   d. Colour changes of fingers and toes
   e. Episodes of superficial vein thrombosis

5. A client is admitted to the hospital with a diagnosis of abdominal aortic aneurysm. Which signs and symptoms would suggest that his aneurysm has ruptured?
   a. Sudden shortness of breath and hemoptysis
   b. Sudden, severe low back pain and bruising along his flank
   c. Gradually increasing substernal chest pain and diaphoresis
   d. Sudden, patchy blue mottling on feet and toes and rest pain

6. Which of the following are priority nursing measures after an abdominal aortic aneurysm repair?
   a. Assessment of cranial nerves and mental status
   b. Administration of IV heparin and monitoring of aPTT
   c. Administration of IV fluids and monitoring of kidney function
   d. Elevation of the legs and application of graduated compression stockings

7. What is the first priority of collaborative care of a client with a suspected acute aortic dissection?
   a. To reduce anxiety
   b. To control blood pressure
   c. To monitor for chest pain
   d. To increase myocardial contractility

8. Which of the following clients has the highest risk for venous thrombo-embolism (VTE)?
   a. A 62-year-old man with spider veins who is having arthroscopic knee surgery.
   b. A 32-year-old woman who smokes, takes oral contraceptives, and is planning a trip to Europe.
   c. A 26-year-old woman who is 3 days postpartum and received maintenance IV fluids for 12 hours during her labour.
   d. An active 72-year-old man at home recovering from transurethral resection of the prostate for benign prostatic hyperplasia.

9. Which of the following are probable clinical findings in a person with an acute lower extremity VTE? *(Select all that apply)*
   a. Pallor and coolness of foot and calf
   b. Mild to moderate calf pain and tenderness
   c. Grossly diminished or absent pedal pulses
   d. Unilateral edema and induration of the thigh
   e. Palpable cord along a superficial varicose vein

10. The recommended treatment for an initial VTE in an otherwise healthy person with no significant comorbid conditions would include which of the following?
    a. IV argatroban while the person is an inpatient
    b. IV unfractionated heparin while the person is an inpatient
    c. Subcutaneous unfractionated heparin while the person is an outpatient
    d. Subcutaneous low-molecular-weight heparin while the person is an outpatient

11. Which of the following is a key teaching instruction for the client who is receiving anticoagulant therapy?
    a. Monitor for and report any signs of bleeding.
    b. Do not take acetaminophen (Tylenol) for a headache.
    c. Decrease your dietary intake of foods containing vitamin K.
    d. Arrange to have blood drawn routinely to check drug levels.

12. Which of the following is the most important intervention in healing and control of venous leg ulcers?
    a. Sclerotherapy
    b. Using moist environment dressings
    c. Taking horse chestnut seed extract daily
    d. Applying elastic compression stockings

1. c; 2. d; 3. c; 4. b, c, d; 5. b; 6. c; 7. b; 8. b; 9. b, c; 10. d; 11. a; 12. d.

ⓔvolve

For even more review questions, visit *http://evolve.elsevier.com/Canada/Lewis/medsurg.*

REFERENCES

Aboyans, V., Criqui, M. H., Abraham, P., et al. (2012). Measurement and interpretation of the ankle–brachial index: A scientific statement from the American Heart Association. *Circulation, 126*(24), 2890–2909. doi:10.1161/CIR.0b013e318276fbcb.

Abraha, I., Romagnoli, C., Montedori, A., et al. (2016). Thoracic stent graft versus surgery for thoracic aneurysm. *Cochrane Database of Systematic Reviews*, (6), Article CD006796, doi:10.1002/14651858.CD006796.pub4.

Ageno, W., Gallus, A. S., Wittkowsky, A., et al. (2012). Oral anticoagulant therapy: Antithrombotic Therapy and Prevention of Thrombosis, 9th ed: American College of Chest Physicians evidence-based clinical practice guidelines. *Chest, 141*(Suppl. 2), e44S–e88S. doi:10.1378/chest.11-2292.

Ahmed, S. M. (2015). Role of atherectomy devices in the treatment of lower extremity peripheral arterial disease. *EC Cardiology, 1*(1), 1–9.

Anderson, J. L., Halperin, J. L., Albert, N. B., et al. (2013). Management of patients with peripheral artery disease (compilation of 2005 and 2001 ACCF/AHA guideline recommendations): A report of the American College of Cardiology Foundation/American Heart Association Task Force on Practice Guidelines. *Circulation, 127*(13), 1425–1443. doi:10.1161/CIR.0b013e31828b82aa.

Antoniou, G., Georgiadis, G., Antoniou, S., et al. (2013). Endovascular repair for ruptured abdominal aortic aneurysm confers an early survival benefit over repair. *Journal of Vascular Surgery, 58*(4), 1091–1105. doi:10.1016/j.jvs.2013.07.109.

Bates, S. M., Jaeschke, R., Stevens, S., et al. (2012). Diagnosis of DVT: Antithrombotic Therapy and Prevention of Thrombosis, 9th ed: American College of Chest Physicians evidence-based clinical practice guidelines. *Chest, 141*(Suppl. 2), e351S–e418S. doi:10.1378/chest.11-2299.

Benoit, E., O'Donnell, T. F., Jr., Kitsios, G., et al. (2012). Improved amputation free survival in unreconstructable critical limb ischemia and its implications for clinical trial design and quality measurement. *Journal of Vascular Surgery, 55*(3), 781–789. doi:10.1016/j.jvs.2011.10.089.

Bernstein, C. F., Kristianson, A., Akl, E. A., et al. (2016). Compression stockings for preventing the post-thrombotic syndrome in patients with deep vein thrombosis. *American Journal of Medicine, 129*(4), 447.e1–447.e20. doi:10.1016/j.amjmed.2015.11.031.

Brass, E. P. (2013). Intermittent claudication: New targets for drug development. *Drugs, 73*(10), 999–1014. doi:10.1007/s-40265-013-0078-3.

Brotons, C., Benamouzig, R., Filipiak, K., et al. (2015). A systematic review of aspirin in primary prevention: Is it time for a new approach? *American Journal of Cardiovscular Drugs, 15*(2), 113–133. doi:10.1007/s40256.014-0100-5.

Canadian Diabetes Association Clinical Practice Guidelines Expert Committee. (2013). Canadian Diabetes Association 2013 clinical practice guidelines for the prevention and management of diabetes in Canada. *Canadian Journal of Diabetes, 37*(Suppl. 1), S1–S212.

Canadian Hypertension Education Program. (2015). *Criteria for diagnosis of hypertension and recommendations for follow-up.* Retrieved from *http://guidelines.hypertension.ca/diagnosis-assessment/diagnosis/.*

Christakou, A., & Zakyntinos, S. (2014). The effectiveness of early mobilization in hospitalized patients with deep venous thrombosis. *Hospital Chronicles, 9*(1), 11–16. doi:*http://dx.doi.org/10.2015/hc.v9i1.553.*

Cohen, J., Akl, E., & Kahn, S. (2012). Pharmacologic and compression therapies for postthrombotic syndrome: A systematic review of randomized controlled trials. *Chest, 141*(2), 308–320. doi:10.1378/chest.11-1175.

Conrad, M. F., & Cambria, R. P. (2014). Aortic dissection. In J. L. Cronenwett & K. W. Johnston (Eds.), *Rutherford's vascular surgery* (8th ed.). Philadelphia: Saunders.

Copstead, L. E., & Banasik, J. (2013). *Pathophysiology* (5th ed.). St. Louis: Elsevier Saunders.

Cosmi, B. (2015). Management of superficial vein thrombosis. *Journal of Thrombosis and Haemostasis, 13*(7), 1175–1183. doi:10.111/jth.12986.

Creager, M. A., Belkin, B., Bluth, E. I., et al. (2012). ACCF/AHA/ACR/SCAI/SIR/STS/SVM/SVN/SVS key data elements and definitions for peripheral atherosclerotic vascular disease: A report of the American College of Cardiology Foundation/American Heart Association Task Force on Clinical Data Standards. *Journal of American College of Cardiology, 49*(3), 294–357. doi:10.1016/j.jacc.2011.10.860. (Seminal).

Crumley, C. (2011). Post-thrombotic syndrome patient education based on the health belief model: Self-reported intention to comply with recommendations. *Journal of Wound, Ostomy, and Continence Nursing, 38*(6), 648–654. doi:10.1097/WON.0b013e31822efc86.

Dasgupta, K., Quinn, R. R., Zarnke, K. B., et al. (2014). The 2014 Canadian Hypertension Education Program recommendations for blood pressure management, diagnosis, assessment of risk, prevention and treatment of hypertension. *Canadian Journal of Cardiology, 30*(5), 485–501. doi:10.1016/j.cjca.2014.02.002.

Decousus, H., Tapson, V. F., Bergmann, J. F., et al. (2011). Factors at admission associated with bleeding risk in medical patients: Findings from the IMPROVE investigators. *Chest, 139*(1), 69–79. doi:10.1378/chest.09-3081.

Deiter, P., & Nanjundappa, A. (2012). Ask the experts: A focus on stenting for lower peripheral artery disease. *Clinical Practice, 9*(5), 499–501. doi:10.221/cpr.12.45.

Delaney, C. L., Spark, J. I., Thomas, J., et al. (2013). A systematic review to evaluate the effectiveness of carnitine supplementation in improving walking performance among individuals with intermittent claudication. *Atherosclerosis, 229*(1), 1–9. doi:10.1016/j.atherosclerosis.2013.03.004.

Di Minno, G., Sparadella, G., Petitto, M., et al. (2014). Systematic reviews and meta-analysis for more profitable strategies in peripheral artery disease. *Annals of Medicine, 46*(7), 475–489. doi:10.3109/07853890.2014.932618.

Di Nisio, M. E., & Middeldorp, S. (2014). Treatment of lower extremity superficial thrombophlebitis. *Journal of the American Medical Association, 311*(7), 729–730. doi:10.1001/j.jama.2014.520.

Dominguez, A., Bahadorani, J., Reeves, R., et al. (2015). Endovascular therapy for critical limb ischemia. *Expert Review of Cardiovascular Therapy, 13*(4), 429–444. doi:10.1586/14779072.2015.1019472.

Erbel, R., Aboyans, V., Boileau, C., et al. (2014). 2014 ESC guidelines on the diagnosis and treatment of aortic diseases. *European Heart Journal, 35*(41), 2873–2926. doi:10.1093/eurheartj/ehu281.

Estrera, A. L., Azam, J., Shalhub, H., et al. (2015). Outcomes of open repair for chronic descending thoracic aortic dissection. *Annals of Thoracic Surgery, 99*(3), 786–793. doi:10.1016/j.atoracsur.2014.08.077.

Filardo, G., Powell, J. T., Martinez, M. A., et al. (2012). Surgery for small asymptomatic abdominal aortic aneurysms. *The Cochrane Database of Systematic Reviews,* (3), Article CD001835. doi:10.1002/14651858.CD001835.pub3.

Gloviczki, P., Huang, Y., Oderich, G. S., et al. (2015). Clinical presentation, comorbidities, and age, but not female gender predict survival after endovascular repair of abdominal aortic aneurysm. *Journal of Vascular Surgery, 61*(4), 853–861.e2. doi:10.1016/j.jvs.2014.12.004.

Go, A. S., Mozaffarian, D., Roger, V. L., et al. (2013). Heart disease and stroke statistics—2013 update: A report from the American Heart Association. *Circulation, 127,* e6–e245. doi:10.1161/cir.0b013e31828124ad.

Grant, S. J., Bin, Y. S., Kiat, H., et al. (2012). The use of complementary and alternative medicine by people with cardiovascular disease: A systematic review. *BMC Public Health, 12,* 299. doi:10.1186/1471-2458-12-299.

Greenblatt, D. Y., Rajamanickam, V., & Mell, M. W. (2011). Predictors of surgical site infection after open lower extremity revascularization. *Journal of Vascular Surgery, 54*(2), 433–439. doi:10.1016/j.jvs.2011.01.034.

Grochot-Przeczek, A., Dulak, J., & Jozkowicz, A. (2013). Therapeutic angiogenesis for revascularization in peripheral artery disease. *Gene, 525*(2), 220–228. doi:10.1016/j.gene.2013.03.097.

Guyatt, G. H., Akl, E. A., Crowther, M., et al. (2012). Executive summary: Antithrombotic Therapy and Prevention of Thrombosis, 9th ed: American College of Chest Physicians evidence-based clinical practice guidelines. *Chest, 141*(Suppl. 2), 7S–47S. doi:10.1378/chest.1412S3.

Heart and Stroke Foundation of Canada. (2017). *Healthy weight and waist.* Retrieved from *https://www.heartandstroke.ca/get-healthy/healthy-weight/healthy-weight-and-waist.*

Henke, P. K., & Comerota, A. J. (2011). An update on etiology, prevention, and therapy of postthrombotic syndrome. *Journal of Vascular Surgery, 53*(2), 500–509. doi:10.1016/j.jvs.2010.08.050.

Herrick, A. L. (2012). The pathogenesis, diagnosis and treatment of Raynaud's phenomenon. *Nature Reviews. Rheumatology, 8*(8), 469–479. doi:10.1038/nrrheum.2012.96.

Hillegass, E., Puthoff, M., Frese, E., et al. (2015). Role of physical therapists in the management of individuals at risk for or diagnosed with thromboembolism: Evidence-based clinical practice guideline. *Physical Therapy, 96*(2), 143–166. doi:10.2522/ptj.20150264.

Hirsch, A. T., Allison, M. A., Gomes, A. S., et al. (2012). A call to action: Women and peripheral artery disease: A scientific statement from the American Heart Association. *Circulation, 125*(11), 1449–1472. doi:10.1161/CIR.0b013e31824c39ba.

Holbrook, A., Schulman, S., Witt, D. M., et al. (2012). Evidence-based management of anticoagulant therapy: Antithrombotic Therapy and Prevention of Thrombosis, 9th ed: American College of Chest Physicians evidence-based clinical practice guidelines. *Chest, 141*(Suppl. 2), e152S–e184S. doi:10.1378/chest.11-2295.

Ix, J. H., Biggs, M. L., Kizer, J. R., et al. (2011). Association of body mass index with peripheral arterial disease in older adults: The Cardiovascular Health Study. *American Journal of Epidemiology, 174*(9), 1036–1043. doi:10.1093/aje/kwr228.

Jarvis, C., Browne, A., Macdonald-Jenkins, J., et al. (2014). *Physical examination and health assessment* (2nd ed.). St. Louis: Elsevier.

Jones, W. S., Dolor, R. J., Hasselblad, V., et al. (2014). Comparative effectiveness of endovascular and surgical revascularization for patients with peripheral artery disease and critical limb ischemia: Systematic review of revascularization in critical limb ischemia. *American Heart Journal, 167*(4), 489–498.e7. doi:10.1016/j.ahj.2013.12.012.

Kahn, S. R., Comerota, A. J., Cushman, M., et al. (2014). The postthrombotic syndrome: Evidence-based prevention, diagnosis, and treatment strategies: A scientific statement from the American Heart Association. *Circulation, 130*(18), 1636–1661. doi:10.1161/CIR.0000000000000130.

Kahn, S. R., Lim, W., Dunn, A. S., et al. (2012). Prevention of VTE in nonsurgical patients: Antithrombotic Therapy and Prevention of Thrombosis, 9th ed: American College of Chest Physicians evidence-based clinical practice guidelines. *Chest, 141*(Suppl. 2), e195S–226S. doi:10.1378/chest.11-2296.

Kearon, C., Akl, E. A., Comerota, A. J., et al. (2012). Antithrombotic therapy for VTE disease: Antithrombotic Therapy and Prevention of Thrombosis, 9th ed: American College of Chest Physicians evidence-based clinical practice guidelines. *Chest, 141*(Suppl. 2), e419S–e496S. doi:10.1378/chest.11-2301.

Khan, N. (2015). Developments and risk analysis in anticoagulation. *British Journal of Cardiac Nursing, 10*(2), 66–73. doi:10.12968/bjca.2015.10.2.66.

Li, G. M., Yuan, T. M., & Qi, G. W. (2012). Implementation of best practice evidence in the nursing management of graduated compression stockings (GCS) in the prevention of venous thromboembolism in an adult surgical setting. *PACEsetterS, 9*(3), 35–42. doi:10.1097/01.jbi.0000419757.e8.

Lin, J., Olson, C. M., Johnson, E. S., et al. (2013). The ankle–brachial index for peripheral artery disease screening prediction among asymptomatic adults: A systematic evidence review for the U.S. Preventive Services Task Force. *Annals of Internal Medicine, 159*(5), 333–341. doi:10.7326/0003-4819-159-5-201309030-00007.

Lo, R. C., Bensley, R. P., Hamdan, A. D., et al. (2013). Gender differences in abdominal aortic aneurysm presentation, repair and mortality in the Vascular Study Group of New England. *Journal of Vascular Surgery, 57*(5), 1261–1268. doi:10.1016/j.jvs.2012.11.039.

Mackman, N. (2012). New insights into the mechanisms of venous thrombosis. *Journal of Clinical Investigation, 122*(7), 2331–2336. doi:10.1172/jci60229.

Maddox, D. (2012). Effects of venous leg ulcer on patient's quality of life. *Nursing Standard, 26*(38), 42–49. doi:10.7748/ns.2012.05.06.26.38.42c9111.

Marsden, G., Perry, M., Kelley, K., et al. (2013). Diagnosis and management of varicose veins: Summary of NICE guidelines. *British Medical Journal, 347*, f4279. doi:10.1136/bmj.f4279.

McDermott, M., Kibbe, M., Guralnik, J. M., et al. (2013). Comparative effectiveness study of self-directed walking exercise, lower extremity revascularization, and functional decline in peripheral artery disease. *Journal of Vascular Surgery, 57*(4), 990–996. doi:10.1016/j.jvs.2012.09.068.

Merritt, W. (2015). Role and rationale for extended periarterial sympathectomy in the management of severe Raynaud's syndrome: Techniques and results. *Hand Clinics, 31*(1), 101–120. doi:10.1016/j.hcl.2014.09.011.

Mozaffarian, D., Benjamin, E. J., Go, A. S., et al. (2016). Heart disease and stroke statistics—2016 Update: A report from the American Heart Association. *Circulation, 133*(4), e38–e360. doi:10.1161/CIR.0000000000000350.

Nelson, E., & Bell-Syer, S. E. M. (2014). Compression for preventing recurrence of venous ulcers. *The Cochrane Database of Systematic Reviews*, (9), Article CD002303. doi:10.1002/14651858.CD002303.pub3.

Nienaber, C. A., Kische, S., Rousseau, H., et al. (2013). Endovascular repair of type B aortic dissection: Long-term results of the randomized investigation of stent grafts in aortic dissection trial. *Circulation: Cardiovascular Interventions, 6*, 407–416. doi:10.1161/CIRCINTERVENTIONS.113.000463.

O'Donnell, T. F., Passman, M. A., Marsten, W. A., et al. (2014). Management of venous leg ulcers: Clinical practice guidelines of the Society for Vascular Surgery and the American Venous Forum. *Journal of Vascular Surgery, 60*(Suppl. 2), 3S–59S. doi:10.1016/j.jvs.2014.04.049.

Ouriel, K., & Kasyap, V. (2011). Acute limb ischemia. In M. Jaff & C. White (Eds.), *Vascular disease: Diagnostic and therapeutic approaches* (pp. 245–254). Minneapolis: Cardiotext.

Panico, A., Jafferani, A., Shah, F., et al. (2015). Advances in peripheral arterial disease endovascular revascularization. *Cardiology Clinics, 33*(1), 89–98. doi:10.1016/j.ccl.2014.09.002.

Park, B. D., Azefor, N., Huang, C., et al. (2013). Trends in treatment of ruptured abdominal aortic aneurysm: Impact of endovascular repair and implications for future care. *Journal of the American College of Surgeons, 216*(4), 745–754. doi:10.1016/j.jamcollsurg.2012.12.028.

Parmenter, B. J., Dieberg, G., Phipps, G., et al. (2015). Exercise training for health-related quality of life in peripheral artery disease: A systematic review and meta-analysis. *Vascular Medicine, 20*(1), 30–40. doi:10.1177/1358863X14559092.

Pavon, J. M., Adam, S. S., Razouki, Z. A., et al. (2016). Effectiveness of intermittent pneumatic compression devices for venous thromboembolism prophylaxis in high-risk surgical patients: A systematic review. *Journal of Arthroplasty, 31*(2), 524–532. doi:10.1016/j.arth.2015.09.043.

Pike-MacDonald, S. A. (Ed.), (2013). *Mosby's Canadian manual of diagnostic and laboratory tests* (1st Canadian ed.). Toronto: Elsevier.

Pittler, M. H., & Ernst, E. (2012). Horse chestnut seed extract for chronic venous insufficiency. *The Cochrane Database of Systematic Reviews,* (11), Article CD003230. doi:10.1002/14651858. CD003230.pub4.

Prete, M., Fatone, M. C., Favoino, E., et al. (2014). Raynaud's phenomenon: From molecular pathogenesis to therapy. *Autoimmunity Reviews, 13*(6), 655–667. doi:10.1016/j.autrev .2013.12.001.

Raffetto, J. D., & Eberhardt, R. T. (2014). Chronic venous disorders. In J. L. Cronenwett & K. W. Johnston (Eds.), *Rutherford's vascular surgery* (8th ed.). Philadelphia: Saunders.

Rasmussen, L., Lawaetz, M., Bjoern, L., et al. (2013). Randomized clinical trial comparing endovenous laser ablation and stripping of the great saphenous vein with clinical and duplex outcome after 5 years. *Journal of Vascular Surgery, 58*(2), 421–426. doi:10.1016/j.jvs.2012.12.048.

Rattan, R., Jones, K. M., & Namias, N. (2015). Management of lower extremity vascular injuries: State of the art. *Current Surgery Reports, 3*(11), 1–9. doi:10.1007/s40137-015-0118-x.

Reitsma, P. H., Versteeg, H. H., & Middeldorp, S. (2012). Mechanistic view of risk factors for venous thromboembolism. *Arteriosclerosis, Thrombosis, and Vascular Biology, 32*(3), 563–568. doi:10.1161/ ATVBAHA.111.242818.

Rockman, C., Maldonado, T. C., Jacobowitz, G. R., et al. (2012). Hormone replacement therapy is associated with a decreased prevalence of peripheral artery disease in postmenopausal women. *Annals of Vascular Surgery, 26*(3), 411–418. doi:10.1016/ j.avsg.2011.10.012.

Rooke, T. W., Hirsch, A. T., Misra, S., et al. (2011). 2011 ACCF/AHA focused update of the guidelines for the management of patients with peripheral artery disease (updating the 2005 guideline): A report of the American College of Cardiology Foundation/American Heart Association task force on practice guidelines. *Circulation, 124*(18), 2020–2045. doi:10.1161/CIR.0b013e31822e80c3.

Rubenstein, C., Bietz, G., Davenport, D., et al. (2015). Abdominal compartment syndrome associated with endovascular and open repair of ruptured abdominal aortic aneurysms. *Journal of Vascular Surgery, 61*(3), 648–654. doi:10.1016/j.jvs.2014.10.011.

Sartori, M., Favaretto, E., Migliaccio, L., et al. (2016). The incidence of heparin-induced thrombocytopenia in patients treated with low molecular weight heparin for superficial vein thrombosis. *Thrombosis Research, 139*, 154–157. doi:10.1016/j.thromres.2016.02.004.

Schulman, S. (2014). Advantages and limitations of the new anticoagulants. *Journal of Internal Medicine, 275*(1), 1–11. doi:10.1111/joim.12138.

Scott, G., Mahdi, A. J., & Alikhan, R. (2015). Superficial vein thrombosis: A current approach to management. *British Journal of Hematology, 168*(5), 639–645. doi:10.1111/bjh.13255.

Tufano, A., Coppola, A., Contaldi, P., et al. (2015). Oral anticoagulants and the risk of osteoporosis: New anticoagulants better than old? *Seminars in Thrombosis and Hemostasis, 41*(4), 382–388. doi:10.1055/s-00341543999.

van Langevelde, K., Lijfering, W. M., Rosendaal, F. R., et al. (2011). Increased risk of venous thrombosis in persons with clinically diagnosed superficial vein thrombosis: Results from the MEGA study. *Blood, 118*(15), 4239–4241. doi:10.1182/blood-2011-05 -356071.

Vijayakumar, A., Tiwari, R., & Prabhuswamy, V. K. (2013). Thromboangiitis obliterans (Buerger's disease)—Current practices. *International Journal of Inflammation, 2013*, 156905. doi:10.1155/2013/156905.

Weller, C., & Evans, S. (2012). Venous leg ulcer management in general practice: Practice nurses and evidence-based guidelines. *Australian Family Physician, 41*(5), 331–337.

Whayne, T. F. (2012). A review of the role of anticoagulation in the treatment of peripheral artery disease. *International Journal of Angiology, 21*(4), 187–194. doi:10.1055/s-0032-1330232.

Whitehead, I., Stephen, E., & Stansby, G. (2015). Diagnosing deep vein thrombosis. In V. Bhattacharya, G. Stansby, & P. Kesteyen (Eds.), *Prevention and management of venous thromboembolism* (pp. 51–63). London: Imperial College Press.

Wilson, A. M., Sadrzadeh-Rafie, A. H., Myers, J., et al. (2011). Low lifetime recreational activity is a risk factor for peripheral arterial disease. *Journal of Vascular Surgery, 54*(2), 427–432, 432.e1-4. doi:10.1016/j.jvs.2011.02.052.

Wittens, C., Davies, A. H., Baekgaard, R., et al. (2015). Management of chronic venous disease: Clinical practice guidelines of the European Society for Vascular Surgery (ESVS). *European Journal of Vascular and Endovascular Surgery, 49*(6), 678–737. doi:10.1016/j.ejvs.2015.02.007.

Wojnarski, C. M., Svensson, L. G., Roselli, E. E., et al. (2015). Aortic dissection in patients with bicuspid aortic valve–associated aneurysms. *Annals of Thoracic Surgery, 100*(5), 1666–1674. doi:10.1016/j.athoracsur.2015.04.126.

Woo, K. Y., Alavi, A., Evans, R., et al. (2013). New advances in compression therapy for venous leg ulcers. *Surgical Technology International, 23*, 61–68.

RESOURCES

Canadian Cardiovascular Society
https://www.cccn.ca/

Canadian Council of Cardiovascular Nurses
http://www.cccn.ca/index2.cfm

Canadian Patient Safety Institute: Venous Thromboembolism (VTE)
http://www.patientsafetyinstitute.ca/en/Topic/Pages/Venous -Thromboembolism-(VTE).aspx?k=Venous%20 Thromboembolism%20(VTE)

Canadian Society for Vascular Surgery
https://canadianvascular.ca

Canadian Society of Vascular Nursing
https://csvn.ca/

Heart and Stroke Foundation of Canada
http://www.heartandstroke.ca

Hypertension Canada
https://www.hypertension.ca/en/

For additional Internet resources, see the website for this book at *http://evolve.elsevier.com/Canada/Lewis/medsurg.*

Problems of Ingestion, Digestion, Absorption, and Elimination

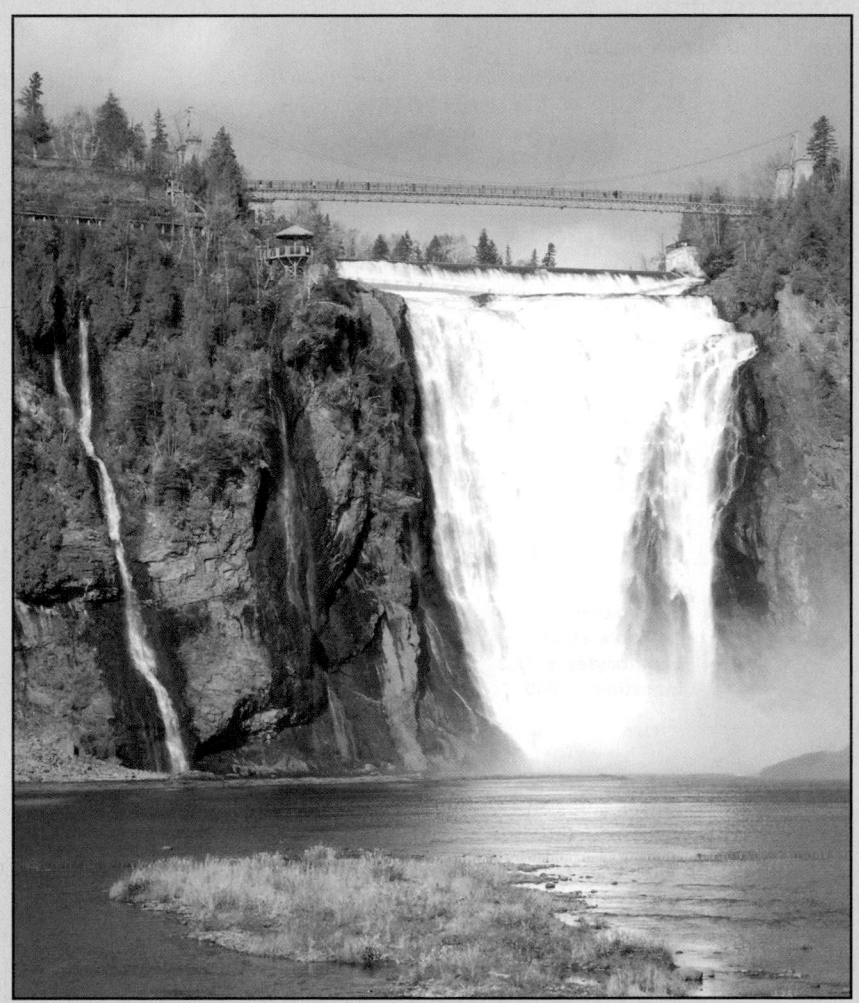

Source: FLX2/Shutterstock.com.

Nursing Assessment
Gastro-Intestinal System

Written by: Paula Cox-North
Adapted by: Shohreh Abrouie

evolve WEBSITE

http://evolve.elsevier.com/Canada/Lewis/medsurg

- Review Questions (Online Only)
- Key Points

- Answer Guidelines for Case Study
- Conceptual Care Map Creator
- Audio Glossary

- Supporting Media—Animations
  - Rectal Examination
- Content Updates

LEARNING OBJECTIVES

1. Describe the structures and functions of the organs of the gastro-intestinal tract.
2. Describe the structures and functions of the liver, the gallbladder, the biliary tract, and the pancreas.
3. Differentiate between the processes of ingestion, digestion, absorption, and elimination.
4. Relate the age-related changes in the gastro-intestinal system to differences in assessment findings.
5. Select the significant subjective and objective data related to the gastro-intestinal system that should be obtained from a patient.

6. Describe the appropriate techniques used in the physical assessment of the gastro-intestinal system.
7. Differentiate normal from abnormal findings of a physical assessment of the gastro-intestinal system.
8. Describe the purpose, significance of results, and nursing responsibilities related to diagnostic studies of the gastro-intestinal system.

KEY TERMS

absorption, p. 951
bilirubin, p. 954
defecation, p. 952
deglutition, p. 949
digestion, p. 950

endoscopy, p. 966
hematemesis, p. 961,
   Table 41-11
hepatocytes, p. 953
ingestion, p. 949

Kupffer cells, p. 953
melena, p. 962, Table 41-11
pyrosis, p. 961, Table 41-11
steatorrhea, p. 962,
   Table 41-11

tenesmus, p. 962,
   Table 41-11
Valsalva manoeuvre, p. 952
villi, p. 950

The main function of the gastro-intestinal (GI) system is to supply nutrients to body cells. This function is accomplished through the processes of *ingestion* (taking in food), *digestion* (breakdown of food), and *absorption* (transfer of food products into circulation). *Elimination* is the process of excreting the waste products of digestion.

The GI system (also called the *digestive system*) consists of the GI tract and its associated organs and glands. Included in the GI tract are the mouth, the esophagus, the stomach, the small intestine, the large intestine, the rectum, and the anus. The associated organs are the liver, the pancreas, and the gallbladder (Figure 41-1).

Factors outside the GI tract can influence its functioning. Both psychological and emotional factors, such as stress and anxiety, influence GI functioning in many people. Stress may

be manifested as anorexia, nausea, epigastric and abdominal pain, or diarrhea. However, GI problems should never be attributed solely to psychological factors. Organic and psychologically based problems can exist independently or concurrently. Physical factors such as dietary intake, ingestion of alcohol and caffeine-containing products, cigarette smoking, and fatigue may also affect GI function. Some organic diseases of the GI system, such as peptic ulcer disease and ulcerative colitis, may be aggravated by stress.

STRUCTURES AND FUNCTIONS OF THE GASTRO-INTESTINAL SYSTEM

The GI tract is a tube approximately 9 m long, extending from the mouth to the anus. The entire tract is composed of four

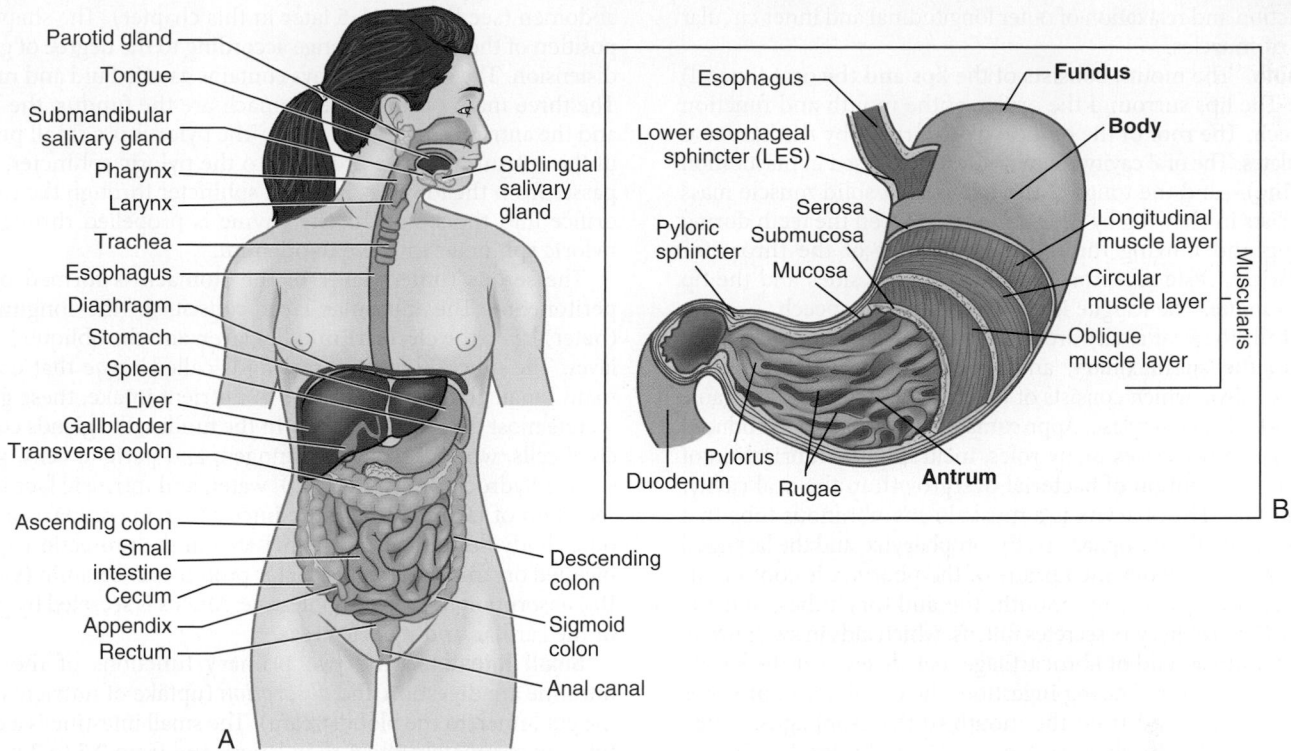

FIGURE 41-1 Location of organs of the gastro-intestinal system.

common layers. From the inside to the outside, these layers are (a) mucosa, (b) submucosa, (c) muscle, and (d) serosa (see Figure 41-1). In the esophagus, the outer coat is fibrous tissue rather than serosa. The muscular coat consists of two layers: the circular (inner) and the longitudinal (outer).

The GI tract is innervated by the parasympathetic and the sympathetic branches of the autonomic nervous system. The parasympathetic system is mainly excitatory, and the sympathetic system is mainly inhibitory. For example, peristalsis is increased by parasympathetic stimulation and decreased by sympathetic stimulation. Sensory information is relayed via both sympathetic and parasympathetic afferent fibres.

The GI tract and accessory organs receive approximately 25% to 30% of the cardiac output. Circulation in the GI system is unique in that venous blood that drains from the GI tract organs empties into the portal vein, which then perfuses the liver. The upper portion of the GI tract receives its blood supply from the splanchnic artery. The small intestine receives its blood supply from branches of the hepatic and superior mesenteric arteries. The large intestine receives its blood supply mainly from the superior and inferior mesenteric arteries. Because such a large percentage of the cardiac output is used to perfuse these organs, the GI tract is a major source from which blood flow can be diverted during exercise or stress.

The two types of movement of the GI tract are *mixing* (segmentation) and *propulsion* (peristalsis). The secretions of the GI system consist of enzymes and hormones for digestion, mucus to provide protection and lubrication, and water and electrolytes.

The abdominal organs are almost completely covered by the peritoneum. The two layers of the peritoneum are the parietal, which lines the abdominal cavity wall, and the visceral, which covers the abdominal organs. The peritoneal cavity is the potential space between the parietal and visceral layers. The two folds

of the peritoneum are the mesentery and the omentum. The mesentery is the attachment of the small intestine and part of the large intestine to the posterior abdominal wall and contains blood and lymph vessels. The lesser omentum extends from the lesser curvature of the stomach and the upper duodenum to the liver, and the greater omentum hangs from the stomach over the intestines like an apron. The omentum contains fat and lymph nodes.

The primary functions of the GI system are (a) ingestion and propulsion (movement) of food; (b) secretion of mucus, water, and enzymes; (c) digestion; (d) absorption; and (e) elimination. Each part of the GI system performs different activities to accomplish these functions.

Ingestion and Propulsion of Food

Ingestion is the intake of food. A person's appetite or desire to ingest food is a significant factor in how much food is eaten. Multiple factors are involved in the control of appetite. An appetite centre is located in the hypothalamus. It is directly or indirectly stimulated by hypoglycemia, an empty stomach, decrease in body temperature, and input from higher brain centres. The hormone *ghrelin*, released from the stomach mucosa, plays a role in appetite stimulation. Another hormone, *leptin*, is involved in appetite suppression (see Chapter 43, Table 43-3). The sight, smell, and taste of food frequently stimulate appetite. Appetite may be inhibited by stomach distension, illness (especially accompanied by fever), hyperglycemia, nausea and vomiting, certain drugs (e.g., amphetamines), and psychological factors, such as depression.

Swallowing (**deglutition**) is the mechanical component of ingestion. The organs involved in the swallowing of food are the mouth, the pharynx, and the esophagus. Swallowed food is moved to the stomach by means of peristalsis, the coordinated, sequential contraction and relaxation of outer longitudinal and inner circular layers of muscles.

Mouth. The mouth consists of the lips and the oral (buccal) cavity. The lips surround the orifice of the mouth and function in speech. The roof of the oral cavity is formed by the hard and soft palates. The oral cavity contains the teeth—used in mastication (chewing)—and the tongue. The tongue is a solid muscle mass and assists in chewing by keeping food between the teeth during chewing and moving the food to the back of the throat for swallowing. Taste receptors are found on the sides and the tip of the tongue. The tongue is also important in speech.

Within the oral cavity are three pairs of salivary glands: the parotid, the submaxillary, and the sublingual. These glands produce saliva, which consists of water, protein, mucin, inorganic salts, and salivary amylase. Approximately 1 L of saliva is produced each day. Saliva serves many roles, including the lubrication of food and prevention of bacterial overgrowth in the oral cavity.

Pharynx. The pharynx is a musculo-membranous tube that is divided into the nasopharynx, the oropharynx, and the laryngeal pharynx. The mucous membrane of the pharynx is continuous with the nasal cavity, the mouth, the auditory tubes, and the larynx. The oropharynx secretes mucus, which aids in swallowing. The epiglottis is a lid of fibrocartilage that closes over the larynx during swallowing. During ingestion, the oropharynx provides a route for the food from the mouth to the esophagus. When receptors in the oropharynx are stimulated by food or liquid, the swallowing reflex is initiated.

Esophagus. The esophagus is a hollow, muscular tube that receives food from the pharynx and moves it to the stomach by peristaltic contractions. It is 23 to 25 cm long and 2 cm in diameter. The esophagus is located in the thoracic cavity; it starts behind the trachea at the lower end of the pharynx and extends to the stomach. The upper one-third of the esophagus is composed of striated skeletal muscle, and the distal two-thirds are composed of smooth muscle.

With swallowing, the upper esophageal sphincter (cricopharyngeal muscle) relaxes, and a peristaltic wave moves the bolus into the esophagus. Between swallows, the esophagus is collapsed. It is structurally composed of four layers: the inner mucosa, submucosa, muscularis propria, and outermost adventitia. The muscular layers contract (peristalsis) and propel the food to the stomach. The lower esophageal sphincter (LES) at the distal end of the esophagus remains contracted except during swallowing, belching, or vomiting. The LES is an important barrier that prevents reflux of acidic gastric contents into the esophagus.

Digestion and Absorption

Mouth. Digestion begins in the mouth. *Digestion* involves both a mechanical process (mastication) and a chemical process. Saliva is the first secretion involved, and its main function is to lubricate and soften the food mass, thus facilitating swallowing. Saliva contains amylase (ptyalin), which hydrolyzes starches to maltose. However, salivary amylase is not necessary for the digestion of carbohydrates.

Stomach. The functions of the stomach are to store food, secrete digestive juices, mix the food with gastric secretions, and empty the resulting content (called *chyme*) into the small intestine at a rate at which digestion can occur. The stomach absorbs only small amounts of water, alcohol, electrolytes, and certain drugs.

The stomach is usually J-shaped and lies obliquely in the epigastric, umbilical, and left hypochondriac regions of the abdomen (see Figure 41-5 later in this chapter). The shape and position of the stomach change according to the degree of gastric distension. The stomach always contains gastric fluid and mucus. The three main parts of the stomach are the fundus, the body, and the antrum (see Figure 41-1). The pylorus is a small portion of the antrum that lies proximal to the pyloric sphincter. Food passes from the lower esophageal sphincter through the cardiac orifice into the stomach. The chyme is propelled through the pyloric sphincter into the duodenum.

The serous (outer) layer of the stomach is formed by the peritoneum. The muscular layer consists of the longitudinal (outer) layer, the circular (middle) layer, and the oblique (inner) layer. The mucosal layer forms folds called *rugae* that contain many small glands. In response to nutrient intake, these glands secrete most of the gastric juice. In the fundus, the glands contain chief cells, which secrete pepsinogen, and parietal cells, which secrete hydrochloric acid (HCl), water, and intrinsic factor. The secretion of HCl makes gastric juice acidic in comparison with other body fluids. This acidic pH aids in the protection against ingested organisms. Intrinsic factor promotes cobalamin (vitamin B_{12}) absorption in the small intestine. Mucus is secreted by glands in the cardiac and pyloric areas.

Small Intestine. The two primary functions of the small intestine are digestion and *absorption* (uptake of nutrients from the gut lumen to the bloodstream). The small intestine is a coiled tube approximately 5 to 6 m in length and from 2.5 to 2.8 cm in diameter, diminishing in diameter at the lower end. It extends from the pylorus to the ileocecal valve. The small intestine is composed of the duodenum, the jejunum, and the ileum. The ileocecal valve, which separates the small intestine from the large intestine, prevents reflux of large intestine contents into the small intestine.

The serous coat of the small intestine is formed by the peritoneum. The mucosa is thick, vascular, and glandular. Folds in the mucosa slow the passage of food and provide a greater surface area for digestion and absorption.

Absorption occurs through the villi, which are functional units present throughout the entire small intestine. **Villi** are minute, finger like projections in the mucous membrane. They contain goblet cells that secrete mucus and epithelial cells that produce the intestinal digestive enzymes. The epithelial cells on the villi also have *microvilli*, which compose the brush border. Thus the presence of villi and microvilli also greatly increases the surface area for absorption.

The digestive enzymes on the brush border of the microvilli chemically break down nutrients so that they can be absorbed. The villi are surrounded by the crypts of Lieberkühn, which contain the multipotent stem cells for the other epithelial cell types. (Stem cells are discussed in Chapter 16.) Brunner's glands in the submucosa of the duodenum secrete mucus.

Physiology of Digestion. Digestion is the physical and chemical breakdown of food into absorbable substances. Digestion in the GI tract is facilitated by the timely movement of food through the various organs and the secretion of specific enzymes. These enzymes break down foodstuffs to particles of appropriate size for absorption (Table 41-1).

The process of digestion begins in the mouth, where the food is chewed, mechanically broken down, and mixed with saliva. The saliva lubricates the food. In addition, salivary amylase begins the breakdown of starch. Salivary gland secretion is stimulated by chewing movements and the sight, the smell, the thought, and the taste of food. The food is swallowed and passes into the

TABLE 41-1	GASTRO-INTESTINAL SECRETIONS RELATED TO DIGESTION	
Daily Amount (mL)	**Secretions or Enzymes**	**Action**
Salivary Glands		
1 000–1 500	Salivary amylase (ptyalin)	Initiation of starch digestion
Stomach		
2 500	Pepsinogen	Protein digestion
	HCl acid	Activation of pepsinogen to pepsin
	Lipase	Fat digestion
	Intrinsic factor	Essential for absorption of cobalamin in the ileum
Small Intestine		
3 000	Enterokinase	Activation of trypsinogen to trypsin
	Amylase	Carbohydrate digestion
	Peptidases	Protein digestion
	Aminopeptidase	Protein digestion
	Maltase	Maltose to two glucose molecules
	Sucrase	Sucrose to glucose and fructose
	Lactase	Lactose to glucose and galactose
	Lipase	Fat digestion
Pancreas		
700	Trypsinogen	Protein digestion
	Chymotrypsin	Protein digestion
	Amylase	Starch to disaccharides and trisaccharides
	Lipase	Fat digestion
Liver and Gallbladder		
700–1 200	Bile	Emulsification of fats and aid in absorption of fatty acids and fat-soluble vitamins (A, D, E, and K)

TABLE 41-2	PHASES OF GASTRIC SECRETION	
Phase	**Stimulus to Secretion**	**Secretion**
Cephalic (nervous)	Sight, smell, taste of food (before food enters stomach); initiated in the CNS and mediated by the vagus nerve	HCl, pepsinogen, mucus
Gastric (hormonal and nervous)	Food in antrum of stomach, vagal stimulation	Release of gastrin from antrum into circulation to stimulate gastric secretions and motility
Intestinal (hormonal)	Presence of acidic chyme (pH <2) in small intestine stimulates release of secretin, gastric inhibitory polypeptide, and cholecystokinin into circulation to decrease acid secretion	Chyme (pH >3) stimulates release of duodenal gastrin to increase acid secretion

CNS, central nervous system; *HCl,* hydrochloric acid.

esophagus, where peristaltic waves propel it to the stomach. No digestion or absorption occurs in the esophagus.

In the stomach, the digestion of proteins begins with the release of pepsinogen from chief cells. The acidic environment of the stomach results in the conversion of pepsinogen to its active form, pepsin. Pepsin begins the initial breakdown of proteins. In the stomach, digestion of starches and fats is minimal. The food is mixed with gastric secretions, which are under neural and hormonal control (Tables 41-2 and 41-3). The stomach also serves as a reservoir for food, which is slowly expelled into the small intestine. The length of time that food remains in the stomach depends on the composition of the food, but average meals remain from 3 to 4 hours.

Digestion is completed in the small intestine, where carbohydrates are hydrolyzed to monosaccharides, fats to glycerol and fatty acids, and proteins to amino acids. The physical presence of *chyme* (food mixed with gastric secretions), along with its chemical nature in the small intestine, stimulates motility and secretion. Secretions involved in digestion include enzymes from the pancreas, bile from the liver (see Table 41-1), and intestinal

secretions from glands in the small intestine. Both secretion and motility are under neural and hormonal control.

When food enters the stomach and small intestine, hormones are released into the bloodstream (see Table 41-3). The hormone *secretin* stimulates the pancreas to secrete fluid with a high concentration of bicarbonate. This alkaline secretion enters the duodenum and neutralizes acid in the chyme. The duodenal mucosa also secretes mucus to protect against the HCl acid. In response to the presence of chyme, the hormone *cholecystokinin* (CCK), produced by the duodenal mucosa, enters the bloodstream and stimulates contraction of the gallbladder and relaxation of the sphincter of Oddi. These actions enable bile to flow from the common bile duct into the duodenum. Bile is necessary for the digestion of fats. CCK also stimulates the pancreas to synthesize and secrete enzymes for enzymatic digestion of carbohydrates, fats, and proteins.

Enzymes on the brush border of the microvilli complete the digestion process. These enzymes hydrolyze disaccharides to monosaccharides and peptides to amino acids for absorption.

Absorption is the transfer of the end products of digestion across the intestinal wall to the circulation. Most absorption occurs in the small intestine. The surface area of the small intestine is greatly increased by its circular folds, villi, and microvilli. The movement of the villi enables the end products of digestion to come in contact with the absorbing membrane. Monosaccharides (from carbohydrates), fatty acids (from fats), amino acids (from proteins), water, electrolytes, and vitamins are absorbed.

Elimination

Large Intestine. The large intestine is a hollow, muscular tube approximately 1.5 to 2 m long and 5 cm in diameter. The four parts of the large intestine are (a) the cecum and the appendix, a narrow tube at the end of the cecum; (b) the colon (ascending colon on the right side, transverse colon across the abdomen,

TABLE 41-3 MAJOR HORMONES CONTROLLING GASTRO-INTESTINAL SECRETION AND MOTILITY

Hormone	Source	Activating Stimuli	Function
Gastrin	Gastric and duodenal mucosa	Stomach distension, partially digested proteins in pylorus	Stimulates gastric acid secretion and motility; maintains lower esophageal sphincter tone
Secretin	Duodenal mucosa	Acid entering small intestine	Inhibits gastric motility and acid secretion; stimulates pancreatic bicarbonate secretion
Cholecystokinin	Duodenal mucosa	Fatty acids and amino acids in small intestine	Causes contraction of gallbladder and relaxation of sphincter of Oddi, allowing increased flow of bile into duodenum; stimulates release of pancreatic digestive enzymes
Gastric inhibitory peptide	Duodenal mucosa	Fatty acids and lipids in small intestine	Inhibits gastric acid secretion and gastric motility

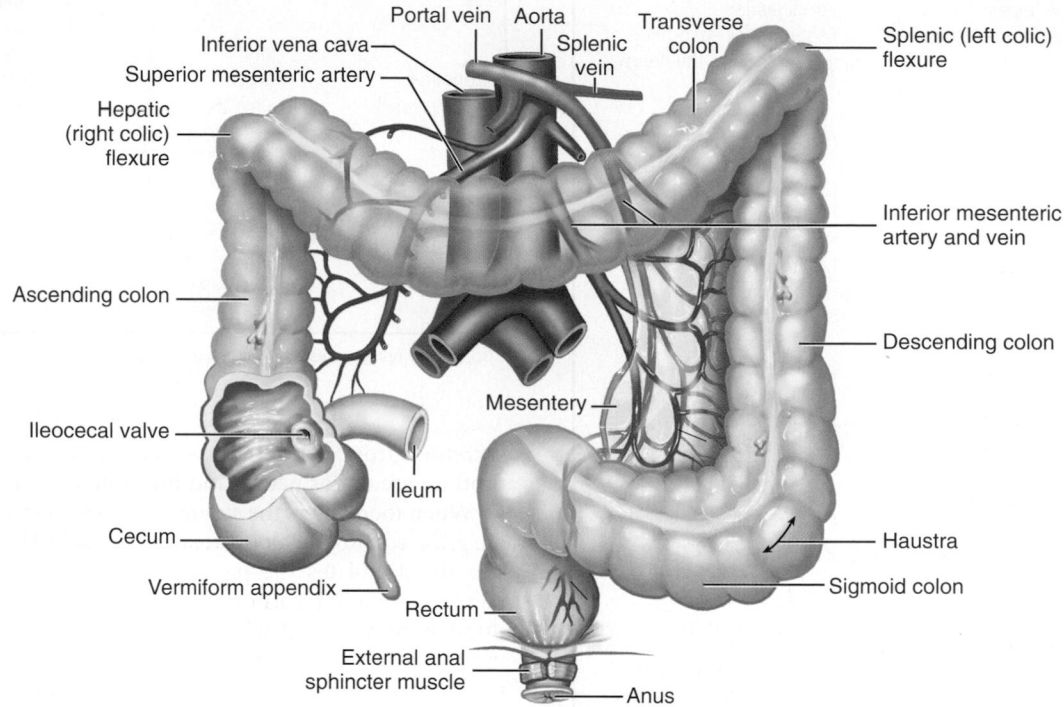

FIGURE 41-2 Anatomical locations of the large intestine. Source: Patton, K. T., & Thibodeau, G. A. (2013). *Anatomy and physiology* (8th ed., p. 885). St. Louis: Mosby.

descending colon on the left side, and the sigmoid colon); (c) the rectum; and (d) the anus, the terminal portion of the large intestine (Figure 41-2).

The most important function of the large intestine is the absorption of water and electrolytes. It also forms feces and serves as a reservoir for the fecal mass until defecation occurs. Feces are composed of water, bacteria, food residue, unabsorbed GI secretions, and desquamated epithelial cells. The large intestine secretes mucus, which acts as a lubricant and protects the mucosa.

Microorganisms in the colon play an important role in metabolism of bile salts, estrogens, androgens, lipids, carbohydrates, various nitrogenous substances, and drugs, as well as in protecting against infection. Intestinal bacteria are responsible for the breakdown of proteins not digested or absorbed in the small intestine. These amino acids are deaminated by the bacteria, leaving ammonia, which is carried to the liver and converted to urea. Bacteria in the colon also synthesize vitamin K and some of the B vitamins. In addition, bacteria play a part in the production of flatus.

The movements of the large intestine are usually slow. When the circular muscles contract, they produce a kneading action

termed *haustral churning*. Propulsive mass movement (peristalsis) also occurs. When food enters the stomach and the duodenum, the gastro-colic and duodeno-colic reflexes are initiated, resulting in peristalsis in the colon. These reflexes are more active after the first daily meal and frequently result in bowel evacuation.

Defecation, the discharge of feces from the rectum, is a reflex action involving voluntary and involuntary control. Feces in the rectum stimulate sensory nerve endings that produce the urge to defecate. The reflex centre for defecation is in the sacral portion of the spinal cord (parasympathetic nerve fibres). These fibres produce contraction of the rectum and relaxation of the internal anal sphincter. Defecation is controlled voluntarily by relaxing the external anal sphincter when the urge to defecate is felt. An acceptable environment for defecation is usually necessary; otherwise the urge to defecate is suppressed. If defecation is suppressed over long periods, problems can occur, such as constipation or stool impaction.

Defecation can be facilitated by appropriate positioning (sitting or squatting) or by the **Valsalva manoeuvre.** This manoeuvre involves contraction of the chest muscles on a closed glottis with simultaneous contraction of the abdominal muscles. These actions

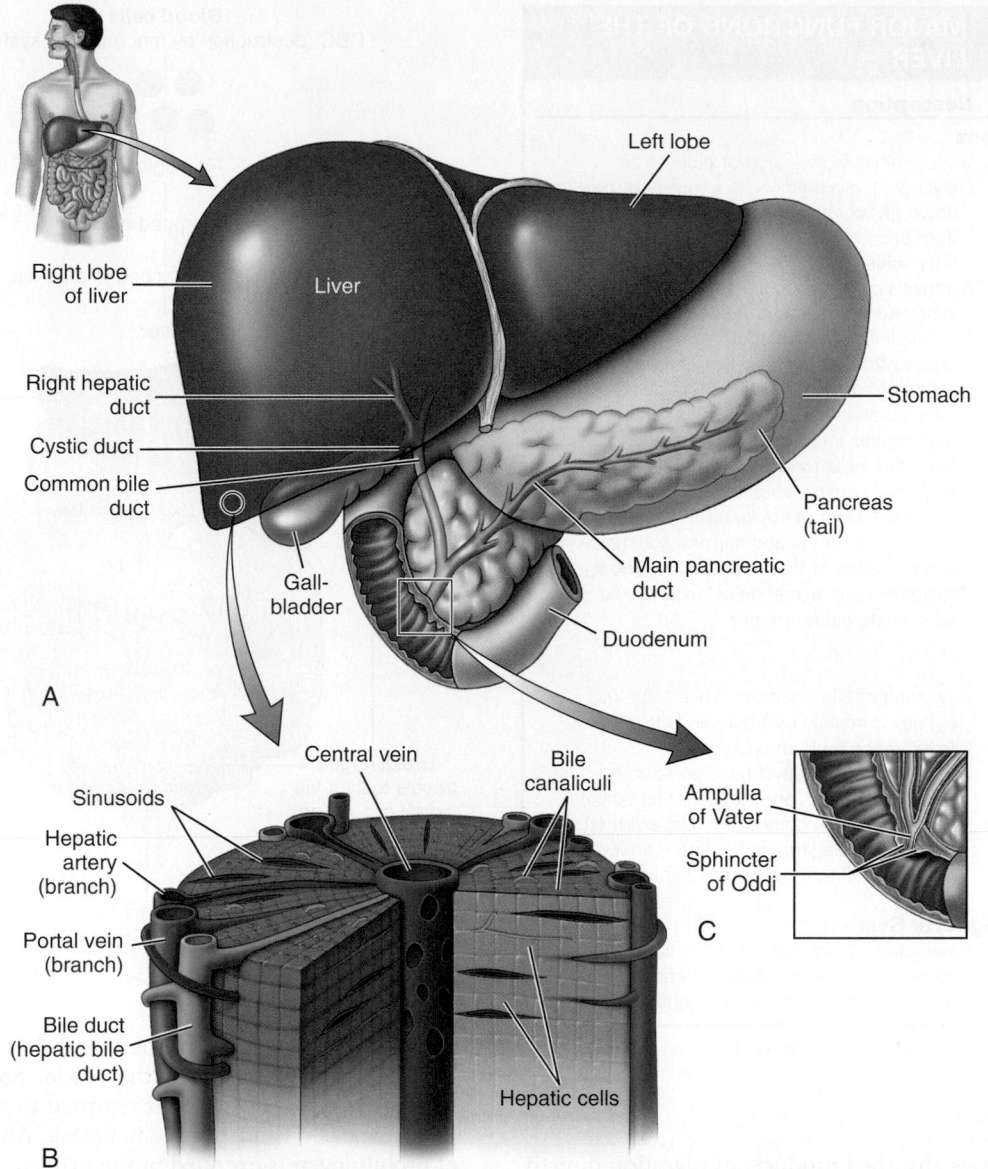

FIGURE 41-3 A, Gross structure of the liver, gallbladder, pancreas, and duct system. **B,** Liver lobule. **C,** Entrance of the common bile duct into the duodenum.

result in increased intra-abdominal pressure. The Valsalva manoeuvre may be contraindicated in patients with head injury, cardiac problems, hemorrhoids, or liver cirrhosis with portal hypertension and in those who have undergone recent eye or abdominal surgery.

Liver, Biliary Tract, and Pancreas

Liver. The liver is the largest internal organ in the body, weighing approximately 1 200 to 1 600 g in adults. It lies in the right hypochondriac and epigastric regions (see Figure 41-5 later in chapter) and is divided into right and left lobes (Figure 41-3). Glisson's capsule, which contains blood vessels, lymphatic vessels, and nerves, covers the liver. Liver disease or swelling may cause this capsule to become distended, leading to pain and oozing of lymphatic fluid into the peritoneal space.

The functional units of the liver are lobules. The lobule consists of plates of specialized hepatic cells (**hepatocytes**) arranged around

a central vein. The capillaries (sinusoids) are located between the plates of hepatocytes and are lined with **Kupffer cells,** which carry out phagocytic activity (removal of bacteria and toxins from the blood). Kupffer cells also ingest aged red blood cells, breaking down hemoglobin into heme and globin. The heme is further broken down into iron and bilirubin, which is secreted into the bile. Interlobular bile ducts form from bile capillaries (*canaliculi*). The hepatic cells secrete bile into the canaliculi.

The nerve supply to the liver is from the left vagus and the sympathetic celiac plexus. The liver receives both arterial and venous blood. About one-third of the blood supply comes from the hepatic artery (branch of the celiac artery), and two-thirds comes from the portal vein.

A large amount of blood is required for the liver to fulfill its metabolic functions. The portal (enterohepatic) circulatory system brings blood to the liver from the stomach, intestines, spleen, and pancreas. This blood enters the liver through the portal vein.

TABLE 41-4 MAJOR FUNCTIONS OF THE LIVER

Function	Description
Metabolic Functions	
Carbohydrate metabolism	Glycogenesis (conversion of glucose to glycogen), glycogenolysis (process of breaking down glycogen to glucose), gluconeogenesis (formation of glucose from amino acids and fatty acids)
Protein metabolism	Synthesis of nonessential amino acids, synthesis of plasma proteins (except γ-globulin), urea formation from NH_3 (NH_3 formed from deamination of amino acids by action of bacteria on proteins in colon)
Fat metabolism	Synthesis of lipoproteins, breakdown of triglycerides into fatty acids and glycerol, formation of ketone bodies, synthesis of fatty acids from amino acids and glucose, synthesis and breakdown of cholesterol
Detoxification	Inactivation of drugs and harmful substances and excretion of their breakdown products
Steroid metabolism	Conjugation and excretion of gonadal and adrenal steroid hormones
Bile Synthesis	
Bile production	Formation of bile, containing bile salts, bile pigments (mainly bilirubin), and cholesterol
Bile excretion	Bile excretion by liver ($\cong$1 L/day)
Storage	Glucose in form of glycogen; fat-soluble vitamins (A, D, E, and K) and water-soluble vitamins (B_1, B_2, cobalamin, folic acid); fatty acids; minerals (iron and copper); amino acids in form of albumin and β-globulins
Mononuclear Phagocyte System	
Kupffer cells	Breakdown of old RBCs, WBCs, bacteria, and other particles; breakdown of hemoglobin from old RBCs to bilirubin and biliverdin

NH₃, ammonia; *RBC*, red blood cell; *WBC*, white blood cell.

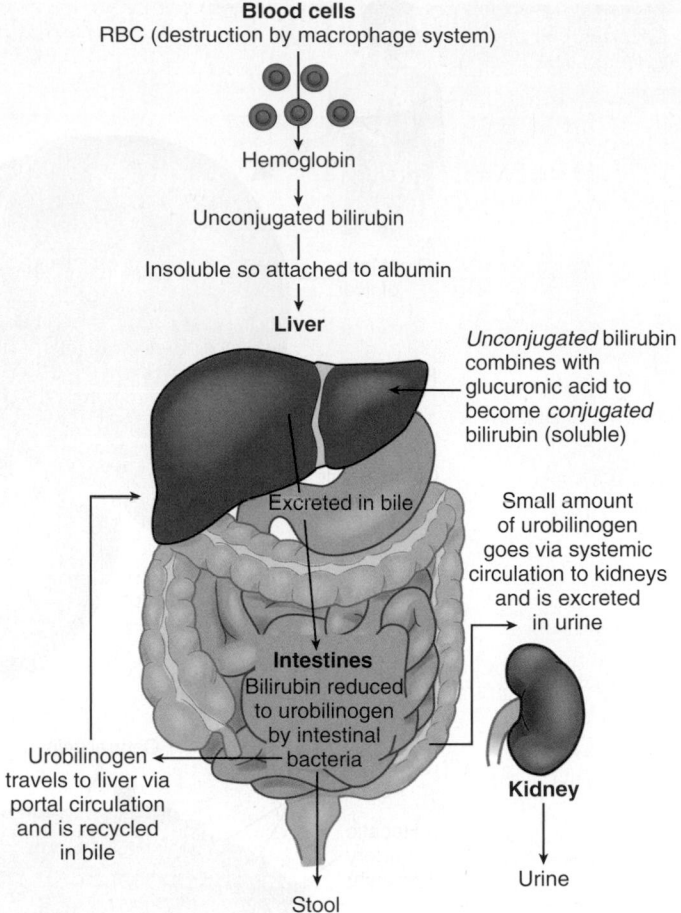

FIGURE 41-4 Bilirubin metabolism and conjugation. *RBC*, red blood cell.

The portal vein carries absorbed products of digestion directly to the liver. In the liver, the portal vein branches and comes into contact with each lobule. The blood in the sinusoids is a mixture of arterial and venous blood.

The liver is essential for life. It functions in the manufacture, the storage, the transformation, and the excretion of a number of substances involved in metabolism. The functions of the liver are numerous but can be classified into three main areas, as identified in Table 41-4.

Biliary Tract. The biliary tract consists of the gallbladder and the duct system. The gallbladder is a pear-shaped sac located below the liver. The function of the gallbladder is to concentrate and store bile. It can hold approximately 45 mL of bile.

Bile is produced by the hepatic cells and secreted into the biliary canaliculi of the lobules. Bile then drains into the interlobular bile ducts, which unite into the two main left and right hepatic ducts. The hepatic ducts merge with the cystic duct from the gallbladder to form the common bile duct (see Figure 41-3). Most bile is stored and concentrated in the gallbladder. It is then released into the cystic duct and moves down the common bile duct to enter the duodenum at the ampulla of Vater. In the intestines, most of the bilirubin is reduced to stercobilinogen and urobilinogen by bacterial action. Stercobilinogen accounts

for the brown colour of stool. A small amount of conjugated bilirubin is reabsorbed by the blood. Some urobilinogen is reabsorbed by the blood and returned to the liver through the portal circulation and excreted in the bile. An insignificant amount of urobilinogen is excreted in the urine.

Bilirubin Metabolism. Bilirubin, a pigment derived from the breakdown of aged red blood cells, is produced constantly (Figure 41-4). Because it is insoluble in water, it is bound to albumin for its transport to the liver. This form of bilirubin is referred to as *unconjugated*. In the liver, bilirubin is conjugated with glucuronic acid. Conjugated bilirubin is water soluble and is excreted in bile. Bile also consists of water, cholesterol, bile salts, electrolytes, and phospholipids. Bile salts are needed for fat emulsification and digestion.

Pancreas. The pancreas is a 20-cm long, slender gland lying behind the stomach and in front of the first and second lumbar vertebrae. It consists of a head, a body, and a tail. The anterior surface is covered by peritoneum. The pancreas contains lobes and lobules. The pancreatic duct extends along the gland and enters the duodenum through the common bile duct (see Figure 41-3). The pancreas has both exocrine and endocrine functions. The exocrine function of the pancreas contributes to the process of digestion. Exocrine cells in the pancreas secrete pancreatic enzymes (see Table 41-1). The endocrine function occurs in the islets of Langerhans, whose beta cells secrete insulin; alpha cells secrete glucagon; delta cells secrete somatostatin; and F cells secrete pancreatic polypeptide.

TABLE 41-5   AGE-RELATED DIFFERENCES IN ASSESSMENT

Gastro-Intestinal System

Potential Changes	Differences in Assessment Findings
Mouth	
Periodontal disease	Red, swollen, bleeding gums; painful chewing; loose or sensitive teeth
Loss of teeth	Presence of dentures, difficulty chewing
Decreased sensitivity of taste buds, decreased sense of smell	Diminished sense of taste (especially saltiness and sweetness)
Decreased volume of saliva	Dry oral mucosa
Atrophy of gingival tissue	Poorly fitting dentures
Esophagus	
Decreased tone and motility	Complaints of pyrosis (heartburn), dysphagia, eructation (belching); potential for hiatal hernia and aspiration
Stomach	
Atrophy of gastric mucosa, decreased blood flow	Food intolerances; signs of anemia as result of cobalamin malabsorption; slower gastric emptying
Small Intestine	
Slightly decreased secretion of most digestive enzymes, decreased motility	Complaints of indigestion; slowed intestinal transit; delayed absorption of fat-soluble vitamins
Liver, Gallbladder, Pancreas	
Decreased size and lowered position	Easier palpation because lower border extends past costal margin
Decreased protein synthesis, decreased ability to regenerate cells	Decreased drug and hormone metabolism
Distension of pancreatic ducts, decreased lipase production, impairment of pancreatic reserve	Impaired fat absorption, decreased glucose tolerance
Large Intestine, Anus, Rectum	
Decreased anal sphincter tone and nerve supply to rectal area	Increased possibility of fecal incontinence
Decreased muscular tone, decreased motility	Flatulence, abdominal distension, relaxed perineal musculature
Increased transit time, decreased sensation to defecation	Constipation, fecal impaction

AGE-RELATED CONSIDERATIONS

EFFECTS OF AGING ON THE GASTRO-INTESTINAL SYSTEM

The process of aging causes changes in the functional ability of the GI system, although to a lesser extent than in other organ systems (Table 41-5). Diet, alcohol intake, and obesity affect organs of the GI system, making it challenging to distinguish the effects of aging from lifestyle. Tooth enamel and dentin wear down, making the teeth susceptible to caries. Periodontal disease can lead to the loss of teeth. Xerostomia (decreased saliva production), or "dry mouth," affects many older adults and may be associated with difficulty swallowing (dysphagia). Dysphagia is characterized by abnormal passage of food from the mouth to the stomach. It may involve oral, pharyngeal, or esophageal processes of swallowing. Dysphagia is more common in older adults because of inadequate chewing or insufficient lubrication. The number of taste buds decreases, the sense of smell diminishes, and salivary secretions lessen, all of which can lead to a decrease in appetite and make eating less pleasurable.

Age-related changes in the esophagus include delayed emptying caused by smooth muscle weakness and an incompetent lower esophageal sphincter (Miller, 2012). Motility of the GI system decreases with age, but secretion and absorption are affected to a lesser extent. Many older adults experience a decrease in HCl secretion (hypochlorhydria), delayed gastric emptying, and constipation. With chronic atrophic gastritis, the number of parietal cells decreases, and the amount of acid and intrinsic factor secreted is subsequently reduced. Intestinal villi are shortened and become more convoluted. Intestinal absorption, motility, and blood flow decrease, thus hampering nutrient absorption.

Liver mass decreases after the age of 40 years, but results of liver function tests remain within normal ranges. Age-related enzyme changes in the liver decrease the liver's ability to metabolize drugs and hormones. Blood flow to the liver decreases, which affects the efficiency of drug metabolism. The size of the pancreas is unaffected by aging, but it does undergo structural changes such as fibrosis, fatty acid deposits, and atrophy. Secretion of digestive enzymes decreases. Aging does not cause changes in the structure and function of the gallbladder and bile ducts, although the incidence of gallstones increases (Heuman, 2017).

Rectal muscle mass is reduced, and the anal sphincter weakens. Changes in the enteric nervous system and a reduction in dietary fibre, along with reduced fluid intake and decreased physical activity, all contribute to constipation in older adults.

Older adults, especially those older than 85, are at risk for decreased food intake, as a result of financial, environmental, and social circumstances (Miller, 2012). Financial constraints can affect both the quality and quantity of food available. Age-related changes in the GI system and differences in assessment findings are presented in Table 41-5.

ASSESSMENT OF THE GASTRO-INTESTINAL SYSTEM

Subjective Data

Important Health Information

Past Health History. Patients should be asked about changes in weight. Any unexplained or unplanned weight loss or weight gain within the past 12 months should be explored in detail. A history of chronic dieting and repeated weight loss and gain should also be documented. Usual patterns of elimination should be noted.

Information should be gathered about the history or existence of the following problems related to GI functioning: abdominal pain, nausea and vomiting, diarrhea, constipation, abdominal distension, jaundice, anemia, heartburn, dyspepsia, changes in appetite, hematemesis, food intolerance (including lactose) or allergies, dysphagia, indigestion, excessive gas, bloating, melena, hemorrhoids, and rectal bleeding. In addition, patients should be asked about the frequency of bowel movements, use of laxatives and antacids, and history or existence of diseases such as gastritis, hepatitis, colitis, gallbladder disease, peptic ulcer, cancer, hernias (especially hiatal hernias), or infection with *Clostridium difficile*. (*C. difficile* is discussed in Chapter 45.)

TABLE 41-6 POTENTIALLY HEPATOTOXIC DRUGS

Dosage-Related	Idiosyncratic/Rare
• Acetaminophen (Tylenol)	• Amiodarone (Cordarone)
• ddl/d4T for HIV	• Alcohol
• Isoniazid (INH)	• Amoxicillin-clavulanic acid (Clavulin)
• Methotrexate	• Carbamazepine
	• Ketoconazole
	• NSAIDs
	• Ramipril (Altace)
	• Statins
	• Sulphonamides
	• Thiazolidinediones

d4T, stavudine; *ddl,* didanosine; *HIV,* human immunodeficiency virus; *NSAIDs,* nonsteroidal anti-inflammatory drugs.

TABLE 41-7 SURGICAL PROCEDURES INVOLVING THE GASTRO-INTESTINAL SYSTEM

Surgical Procedure	Description
Antrectomy	Removal of antrum portion of stomach
Appendectomy	Removal of appendix
Cecostomy	Opening into cecum
Cholecystectomy	Removal of gallbladder
Cholecystostomy	Opening into gallbladder
Choledochojejunostomy	Opening between common bile duct and jejunum
Choledocholithotomy	Opening into common bile duct for removal of stones
Colectomy	Removal of colon
Colostomy	Opening into colon
Gastrectomy	Removal of stomach
Gastrostomy	Opening into stomach
Glossectomy	Removal of tongue
Hemiglossectomy	Removal of half of tongue
Ileostomy	Opening into ileum
Pyloroplasty	Enlargement and repair of pyloric sphincter area
Vagotomy	Resection of branch of vagus nerve

CASE STUDY

Patient Introduction

Source: Anton_Ivanov/ Shutterstock .com.

Lyle Collins is a 58-year-old man from Drury, Ontario. Mr. Collins's wife and family drove 50 kilometres to take him to the hospital because of his deteriorating health. He comes into the emergency department (ED) doubled over in pain. He is grimacing and holding his abdomen with both arms and presents to the triage nurse.

Critical Thinking

Throughout this assessment chapter, think about Mr. Collins with the following questions in mind:

1. What are the possible causes for Mr. Collins's acute abdominal pain?
2. What would be the nurse's priority assessment?
3. What questions should the nurse ask Mr. Collins?
4. What should be included in the physical assessment? What would the nurse be looking for?
5. What diagnostic studies might be ordered?

evolve

Answers are available at *http://evolve.elsevier.com/Canada/Lewis/medsurg.*

Medications. The health history should include an assessment of the patient's past and current use of medications. The names of all drugs, their frequency of use, and their duration of use are important. This is a critical aspect of history taking because many medications not only may have an effect on the GI system but also may be affected by abnormalities of the GI system and surrounding organs. The medication assessment should include information about the use of over-the-counter (OTC) drugs, prescription drugs, and herbal products and nutritional supplements (see Chapter 12). Many chemicals and drugs are potentially hepatotoxic (Table 41-6) and can result in significant harm to the patient unless their use is monitored closely. For example, chronic high doses of acetaminophen may be hepatotoxic. Nonsteroidal anti-inflammatory drugs (NSAIDs) (including acetylsalicylic acid [Aspirin]) may predispose patients to upper GI bleeding if not taken cautiously with food or if a patient has severe liver disease. Antibiotics can cause changes in the normal bacterial composition in the GI tract that result in diarrhea. The nurse should ask patients about laxative or antacid use, including the type and the frequency.

Surgery or Other Treatments. Information should be obtained about hospitalizations for any problems related to the GI system, particularly any abdominal or rectal surgery, including the year, the reason for surgery, the postoperative course, and any blood transfusions. Terms related to surgery of the GI system are listed in Table 41-7.

CASE STUDY—cont'd

Subjective Data

Source: Anton_Ivanov/ Shutterstock .com.

A focused subjective assessment of Mr. Collins reveals the following information:

History of current illness: Mr. Collins states he has not been feeling well for the past several weeks. He feels weak and is easily fatigued. Denies exposure to chemicals. No recent travel outside of Canada. Rates pain as a 9 on a scale of 0–10. States pain comes and goes in waves. Prefers to lie still with knees flexed and drawn into his abdomen. States has had alternating episodes of constipation and diarrhea. He noticed some bright red blood in stools. Has not had a bowel movement for 4 days.

Past medical history: Negative history for medical or surgical problems.

Medications: None.

Functional assessment: Mr. Collins is 175 cm tall and weighs 64 kg (BMI: 20.9 kg/m²). States has been losing weight over the past several months and does not have an appetite. No food allergies. Smokes approximately 1 pack of cigarettes/day for 20 yr. Drinks beer on a daily basis, typically three or four bottles per day.

See pp. 960 and 967 for more information on Mr. Collins.

Objective Data

In addition to collecting subjective data related to the patient's diet history and overall health (Table 41-8), objective data related to a nutritional assessment should be obtained. Examples of objective data include anthropometric measurements (height, weight, skinfold thickness), results of blood studies such as serum protein, albumin, and hemoglobin levels, as well as a physical examination.

TABLE 41-8 HEALTH HISTORY

Gastro-Intestinal System: Questions for Obtaining Subjective Data

Appetite
- Any change in appetite?* Are you more or less hungry?
- Any change in weight?* Do your clothes still fit the same as they used to? How much weight have you gained or lost? Over what time frame? Is the change in weight intentional?

Dysphagia
- Any problems swallowing?* How long have you had this problem?

Food Intolerance or Allergies
- Are there any foods you cannot eat?* What happens when you do eat them (e.g., heartburn, gas, bloating, indigestion, allergic reaction)?

Abdominal Pain
- Do you have any abdominal pain?*
- Is the pain in one spot, or does it move around?
- How long have you had this pain?
- Does it come and go, or is it constant? Does it get worse before or after meals? When is the pain worst (e.g., position, stress, activity)?
- Can you describe how it feels (e.g., cramping, burning, stabbing, aching)?
- What brings on the pain (e.g., menstruation, stress, overeating, fatigue)?
- Do any other symptoms occur when you have the pain (e.g., nausea and vomiting, gas, rectal bleeding, frequent urination, vaginal or penile discharge)?*
- What works to relieve the pain (e.g., rest, heat, walking, change of position, medication)?*

Nausea and Vomiting
- Any nausea or vomiting?* How much comes up?
- What colour is it? Is it bloody? Is there a particular odour?
- Do you have pain, diarrhea, fever, or chills at the same time as the nausea and vomiting?
- Does anyone else you have been in contact with over the past 24 hours have the same symptoms? Have you eaten any foods in the past 24 hours that you suspect may be the cause?

Bowel Habits
- How often do you have a bowel movement?
- Any recent changes in colour, consistency, or frequency?
- Any problems with diarrhea or constipation?
- Do you use laxatives or stool softeners? Which ones? How often?

Past History
- Any past problems with your digestive system (e.g., ulcer, gallbladder problems, hepatitis, appendicitis, colitis, hernia)?*
- Any surgical procedures on your abdomen?*
- Do you know the results of any tests that were done relating to your abdomen?*

Medications
- What medications are you currently taking?
- How much alcohol do you drink each day? When was your last alcoholic drink?
- Do you smoke? How many packs a day?

Nutrition Assessment
- Describe your usual daily food and fluid intake.

*If yes, describe.
Source: Based on Jarvis, C., Browne, A. J., MacDonald-Jenkins, J., et al. (Eds.). (2014). *Physical examination and health assessment* (2nd Canadian ed., 553–554). Toronto: W. B. Saunders.

Physical Examination
Mouth

Inspection. The lips should be inspected for symmetry, colour, and size and for abnormalities such as pallor or cyanosis, cracking, ulcers, or fissures. The dorsum (top) of the tongue should have a thin white coating; the undersurface should be smooth. The nurse should observe for any lesions. Using a tongue blade, the nurse should inspect the buccal mucosa and note the colour, any areas of pigmentation, and any lesions. Dark-skinned individuals normally have patchy areas of pigmentation. When assessing the teeth and gums, the nurse should look for caries; loose teeth; abnormal shape and position of teeth; and swelling, bleeding, discoloration, or inflammation of the gingivae. Any distinctive breath odour should be noted.

The pharynx is inspected by tilting the patient's head back and depressing the tongue with a tongue blade. The tonsils, the uvula, the soft palate, and the anterior and posterior pillars should be observed. The nurse should have the patient say, "Ah." The uvula and the soft palate should rise and remain in the midline.

Palpation. The nurse should palpate any suspect areas in the mouth such as ulcers, nodules, indurations, and areas of tenderness.

In older adults, the mouth must be assessed carefully. Particular attention should be given to the condition of the gums and the tongue, the fit and the condition of dentures (if present), the ability to swallow, and the presence of lesions. A patient who has dentures must remove the dentures during an oral examination to allow for adequate visualization and palpation of the area.

FIGURE 41-5 A, Abdominal quadrants. **B,** Abdominal regions. *LLQ,* left lower quadrant; *LUQ,* left upper quadrant; *RLQ,* right lower quadrant; *RUQ,* right upper quadrant.

Abdomen. Two anatomical systems are used to describe the surface of the abdomen. In one system, the abdomen is divided into four quadrants by a vertical line from the sternum to the pubic bone and by a perpendicular line across the abdomen at the umbilicus (Figure 41-5, *A;* Table 41-9). In the other system, the abdomen is divided into nine regions (see Figure 41-5, *B*), but only the epigastric, umbilical, and suprapubic or hypogastric regions are commonly addressed.

Good lighting is required for the abdominal examination. The patient should be in the supine position and as relaxed as

TABLE 41-9	ABDOMINAL STRUCTURES IN REGIONS OF ABDOMEN		
Right Upper Quadrant	**Left Upper Quadrant**	**Right Lower Quadrant**	**Left Lower Quadrant**
• Liver and gallbladder • Pylorus • Duodenum • Head of pancreas • Right adrenal gland • Portion of right kidney • Hepatic flexure of colon • Portion of ascending and transverse colon	• Left lobe of liver • Spleen • Stomach • Body of pancreas • Left adrenal gland • Portion of left kidney • Splenic flexure of colon • Portion of transverse and descending colon	• Lower pole of right kidney • Cecum and appendix • Portion of ascending colon • Bladder (can be palpated only if distended) • Right ovary and salpinx • Uterus (can be palpated only if enlarged) • Right spermatic cord • Right ureter	• Lower pole of left kidney • Sigmoid flexure • Portion of descending colon • Bladder (can be palpated only if distended) • Left ovary and salpinx • Uterus (can be palpated only if enlarged) • Left spermatic cord • Left ureter

possible. To help relax the abdominal muscles, the patient should slightly flex the knees, and the head of the bed should be raised slightly. The patient should have an empty bladder. The nurse's hands should be warm when the abdominal examination is performed, to avoid eliciting muscle guarding. The patient should be instructed to breathe slowly through the mouth.

Inspection. The nurse should assess the abdomen for skin changes (colour, texture, scars, striae, dilated veins, rashes, and lesions), umbilicus (location and contour), symmetry, contour (flat, rounded [convex], concave, protuberant, distended), observable masses (hernias or other masses), and movement (pulsations and peristalsis). A normal aortic pulsation may be visible in the epigastric area. The nurse should look across the abdomen tangentially (across the abdomen in a line) for peristalsis. Peristalsis is not normally visible in an adult but may be visible in a thin person.

Auscultation. During examination of the abdomen, the nurse should auscultate before percussion and palpation because these latter procedures may alter the bowel sounds. Auscultation of the abdomen includes listening for increased or decreased bowel sounds and vascular sounds. The diaphragm of the stethoscope is used to auscultate bowel sounds because they are relatively high pitched. The bell of the stethoscope is used to detect lower-pitched sounds. Normal bowel sounds occur 5 to 35 times per minute and sound like high-pitched clicks or gurgles. Warming the stethoscope in the hands before auscultation helps prevent abdominal muscle contraction. The nurse should listen in the epigastrium and in all four quadrants (starting in the lower right quadrant) for bowel sounds for 2 to 5 minutes. A perfectly "silent abdomen" is uncommon (Jarvis, Browne, MacDonald-Jenkins, et al., 2014). After listening for several minutes, the nurse frequently finds that the sounds are not absent but hypoactive. If the nurse does not hear bowel sounds, the amount of time listened in each quadrant without hearing bowel sounds should be noted.

The frequency and intensity of bowel sounds vary, depending on the phase of digestion. Normally, they sound relatively high pitched and gurgling. Loud gurgles indicate hyperperistalsis and are termed *borborygmi* (stomach growling). The bowel sounds are more high pitched (rushes and tinkling) when the intestines are under tension, such as in intestinal obstruction. The nurse should listen for decreased or absent bowel sounds. Terms used to describe bowel sounds include *present, absent, increased, decreased, high pitched, tinkling, gurgling,* and *rushing.* Normally, no aortic bruits should be heard. A bruit, best heard with the bell of the stethoscope, is a swishing or buzzing sound and indicates turbulent blood flow.

Percussion. The purpose of percussion of the abdomen is to determine the presence of fluid, distension, and masses. Sound

waves vary according to the density of underlying tissues. The presence of air produces a higher-pitched, hollow sound, termed *tympany,* and the presence of fluid or masses produces a short, high-pitched sound with little resonance, termed *dullness.* The nurse should lightly percuss all four quadrants of the abdomen and assess the distribution of tympany and dullness. Tympany is the predominant percussion sound of the abdomen.

Dullness in the dependent parts of the abdomen may reflect ascites (see Table 41-11). Percussion for *shifting dullness* is a test used to assess for ascites. With the person in supine position, the nurse percusses from the top of the abdomen down the sides of the abdomen and marks the border between tympany and dullness. Then the person is turned onto the side and the nurse percusses from the upper side of the abdomen downward. The sound changes from tympany to dullness as the fluid level is reached (Jarvis et al., 2014).

To percuss the liver, the nurse should start below the umbilicus in the right midclavicular line and percuss lightly upward until dullness is heard, thus determining the lower border of liver dullness. After determining the lower border of the liver, the nurse should start at the nipple line in the right midclavicular line and percuss downward between ribs to the area of dullness, which indicates the upper border of the liver. The height or vertical space between the two areas should be measured to determine the size of the liver. The height of the person correlates directly with the span of the liver. The normal range of liver span is 6 to 12 cm. A liver span greater than 12 cm may indicate liver enlargement.

Palpation. *Light palpation* is used to detect tenderness or cutaneous hypersensitivity, muscular resistance, masses, and swelling. It also helps patients to relax for deeper palpation. The nurse should keep fingers together and press gently with the pads of the fingertips, depressing the abdominal wall about 1 cm. Smooth movements should be used and all quadrants palpated (Figure 41-6, *A*). *Voluntary guarding* occurs when the person is ticklish, cold, or tense, and it occurs bilaterally. The nurse should help the person to relax because guarding interferes with deep palpation.

Deep palpation is used to delineate abdominal organs and masses (see Figure 41-6, *B*). The palmar surfaces of the fingers should be used to press more deeply. Again, all quadrants should be palpated. When palpating masses, note the location, the size, the shape, and the presence of tenderness. The patient's facial expression should be observed during these manoeuvres because it will provide nonverbal cues of discomfort or pain.

An alternative method for deep abdominal palpation is the two-hand method. One hand is placed on top of the other. The fingers of the top hand apply pressure to the bottom hand.

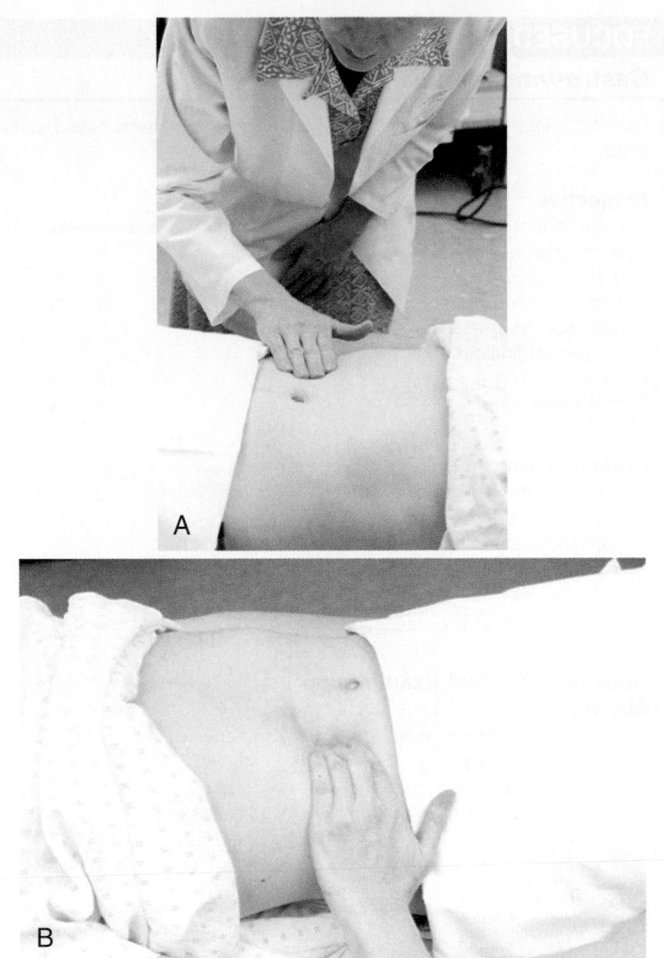

FIGURE 41-6 Palpation of the abdomen. **A,** Technique for light palpation. **B,** Technique for deep palpation. Source: Doughty, D. B., & Jackson, D. B. (1993). *Mosby's clinical nursing series: Gastrointestinal disorders.* St. Louis: Mosby.

FIGURE 41-7 Liver palpation. **A,** Technique with one hand under the patient. **B,** Alternative technique to palpate liver with fingers hooked over the costal region. Source: Jarvis, C., Browne, A. J., MacDonald-Jenkins, J., et al. (Eds.). (2014). *Physical examination and health assessment* (2nd Canadian ed.). (5th ed., p. 578). Toronto: Elsevier.

The fingers of the bottom hand feel for organs and masses. This method may be more effective with an obese abdomen.

Check any areas of concern for rebound tenderness by pressing in slowly and firmly over the painful site. The palpating fingers are withdrawn quickly. Pain on withdrawal of the fingers indicates peritoneal inflammation. Because assessing for rebound tenderness may produce pain and severe muscle spasm, it should be performed at the end of the examination and only by an experienced practitioner. The iliopsoas muscle test is performed when an acute or perforated appendix is suspected. With the patient in the supine position and the hip flexed, the right leg is lifted up. As the patient tries to keep the leg up, push the leg down over the lower part of the right thigh. Pain is felt in the right lower quadrant when the iliopsoas muscle is inflamed, which occurs with appendix inflammation or perforation.

To palpate the liver, the nurse's left hand is placed beneath the supine patient to support the right eleventh and twelfth ribs (Figure 41-7). The patient may relax on the nurse's hand. The nurse should press the left hand forward and place the right hand on the patient's right abdomen, lateral to the rectus muscle. The fingertips should be below the lower border of liver dullness and pointed toward the right costal margin. The nurse should gently press in and up. The patient should take a deep breath with the abdomen so that the liver drops and is in a better position

to be palpated. The nurse should try to feel the liver edge as it comes down to the fingertips. During inspiration, the liver edge should feel firm, sharp, and smooth. The nurse should document the description of the surface, contour, and any tenderness.

To palpate the spleen, the nurse moves to the left side of the patient. The nurse places the right hand under the patient and supports and presses the patient's left lower rib cage forward. The left hand is placed below the left costal margin and presses it in toward the spleen. The nurse should ask the patient to breathe deeply. The nurse's fingertips can feel the tip or edge of an enlarged spleen. The spleen is not normally palpable. If it is palpable, the nurse should not continue because manual compression of an enlarged spleen may cause it to rupture.

Rectum and Anus. The nurse should inspect the perianal and anal areas for colour, texture, lumps, rashes, scars, erythema, fissures, and external hemorrhoids. Any lumps or unusual areas should be palpated with a gloved hand.

For the digital examination of the rectum, the gloved, lubricated index finger is placed against the anus while the patient strains (Valsalva manoeuvre). Then, as the sphincter relaxes, the nurse inserts the gloved, lubricated finger. The finger is pointed toward the umbilicus. The nurse should try to get the patient to relax. The finger is inserted into the rectum as far as possible, and all surfaces are palpated. Nodules, tenderness, or any irregularities should be assessed. A sample of stool can be removed with the gloved finger and checked for occult blood. However, a single guaiac-based fecal occult blood test has limited sensitivity in detecting colorectal cancer.

TABLE 41-10   NORMAL FINDINGS IN PHYSICAL ASSESSMENT OF THE GASTRO-INTESTINAL SYSTEM

Mouth
- Moist, pink lips
- Moist, pink buccal mucosa and gingivae without plaques or lesions
- Teeth in good repair
- Protrusion of tongue in midline without deviation or fasciculations
- Pink uvula in midline, soft palate, tonsils, and posterior pharynx
- Smooth swallowing without coughing or gagging

Abdomen
- Flat without masses or scars
- No abdominal tenderness
- No bruises
- Bowel sounds in all quadrants
- Nonpalpable liver and spleen
- Liver 10 cm in right midclavicular line
- Generalized tympany

Anus
- Absence of lesions, fissures, and hemorrhoids
- Good sphincter tone
- Rectal walls smooth and soft
- No masses
- Stool soft, brown, and heme negative

Documentation of a normal physical assessment of the GI system is described in Table 41-10. Age-related differences in the GI system and differences in assessment findings are described in Table 41-5. Assessment abnormalities are listed in Table 41-11. A focused assessment is used to evaluate the status of previously identified GI problems and to monitor for signs of new problems (see Table 3-6). A focused assessment of the GI system is presented in the "Focused Assessment" box.

DIAGNOSTIC STUDIES OF THE GASTRO-INTESTINAL SYSTEM

Diagnostic studies provide objective data for monitoring the patient's condition and planning appropriate interventions. Table 41-12 lists common diagnostic studies of the GI system. For most diagnostic studies, the nurse should make sure that a signed consent form for the procedure has been completed and is in the patient's health care record. It is the responsibility of the health care provider performing the procedure to explain the procedure and obtain the written consent. However, nurses play an important role in educating patients regarding the procedures. When preparing patients, the nurse must ask about any known allergies to drugs or contrast media.

Many of the diagnostic procedures of the GI system necessitate measures to cleanse the GI tract, as well as the ingestion or injection of a contrast medium or a radiopaque tracer. Often, the patient undergoes a series of GI diagnostic tests. The patient is monitored closely to ensure adequate hydration and nutrition during the testing period. Some diagnostic studies of the GI system are especially difficult and uncomfortable for older adults. It may be necessary to individualize care and make adjustments. Many radiological studies use either barium sulphate or diatrizoate meglumine and diatrizoate sodium (Gastrografin) as a contrast medium. Barium sulphate is more effective for visualizing mucosal

FOCUSED ASSESSMENT

Gastro-Intestinal (GI) System

Use this checklist to make sure the key assessment steps have been done.

Subjective
Ask the patient about any of the following and note the responses:

Loss of appetite	Y	N
Abdominal pain	Y	N
Changes in stools; if so, check colour, consistency, frequency, for presence of blood and any other unexpected findings	Y	N
Nausea, vomiting	Y	N
Painful swallowing	Y	N

Objective: Diagnostic
Check the following laboratory results for critical values:

Endoscopy: colonoscopy, sigmoidoscopy, esophago-gastro-duodenoscopy	✓
Radiology: upper GI series, lower GI series	✓
Stool for occult blood or ova and parasites	✓
Liver function tests	✓

Objective: Physical Examination
Inspect

Skin for colour, lesions, scars, petechiae, and any other unexpected findings	✓
Abdominal contour for symmetry and distension	✓
Anus and rectum for intact skin, presence or absence of hemorrhoids	✓

Auscultate*

Bowel sounds	✓

Palpate

Abdominal quadrants with light touch	✓
Abdominal quadrants with deep technique	✓

*Note: Perform auscultation before palpation.

CASE STUDY

Objective Data: Physical Examination

A focused assessment of Mr. Collins reveals the following: BP 120/74, heart rate 110, respiratory rate 24, temp 38°C. Abdomen firm and slightly distended. High-pitched bowel sounds in upper quadrants. No bowel sounds auscultated in left lower quadrant. Mild abdominal palpation elicits pain.

As you continue to read this chapter, consider diagnostic studies that may be ordered for Mr. Collins.

Source: Anton_Ivanov/ Shutterstock .com.

See pp. 956 and 967 for more information on Mr. Collins.

detail. Gastrografin is water soluble and rapidly absorbed, so it is preferred when a perforation is suspected. If barium escapes into the peritoneal cavity, it can cause peritonitis. However, if the patient is at high risk for aspiration, use of water-soluble media is contraindicated and barium is preferred.

Radiological Studies

Upper Gastro-Intestinal Series. An upper GI series with small bowel follow-through enables visualization of the esophagus,

Text continued on p. 966

TABLE 41-11 ASSESSMENT ABNORMALITIES

Gastro-Intestinal System

Finding	Description	Possible Etiology and Significance
Mouth		
Ulcer, plaque on lips or in mouth	Sore or lesion	Carcinoma, viral infections
Cheilosis	Softening, fissuring, and cracking of lips at angles of mouth	Riboflavin deficiency
Cheilitis	Inflammation of lips (usually lower) with fissuring, scaling, crusting	Often unknown
Geographic tongue	Scattered red, smooth (loss of papillae) areas on dorsum of tongue	Unknown
Smooth tongue	Red, slick appearance	Cobalamin deficiency
Leukoplakia	Thickened white patches	Premalignant lesion
Pyorrhea	Recessed gingivae, purulent pockets	Periodontitis
Herpes simplex	Benign vesicular lesion	Herpesvirus
Candidiasis	White, curdlike lesions surrounded by erythematous mucosa	*Candida albicans*
Glossitis	Reddened, ulcerated, swollen tongue	Exposure to streptococci, irritation, injury, vitamin B deficiencies, anemia
Acute marginal gingivitis	Friable, edematous, painful, bleeding gingivae	Irritation from ill-fitting dentures, calcium deposits on teeth, food impaction
Esophagus and Stomach		
Dysphagia	Difficulty swallowing, sensation of food sticking in esophagus	Esophageal problems, cancer of esophagus
Hematemesis	Vomiting of blood	Esophageal varices, bleeding peptic ulcer (bleeding in upper GI tract)
Pyrosis	Heartburn, burning in epigastric or substernal area	Hiatal hernia, esophagitis, incompetent lower esophageal sphincter
Dyspepsia	Burning or indigestion	Peptic ulcer, gallbladder disease
Odynophagia	Painful swallowing	Cancer of esophagus, esophagitis
Eructation	Belching	Gallbladder disease
Nausea and vomiting	Feeling of impending vomiting, expulsion of gastric contents through mouth	GI infections, common manifestation of many GI diseases; stress, fear, and pathological conditions
Abdomen		
Distension	Excessive gas accumulation, enlarged abdomen; generalized tympany	Obstruction, paralytic ileus
Ascites	Accumulated fluid within abdominal cavity; eversion of umbilicus (usually)	Peritoneal inflammation, heart failure, metastatic carcinoma, cirrhosis
Bruit	Humming or swishing sound heard through stethoscope over vessel	Partial arterial obstruction (narrowing of vessel), turbulent flow (aneurysm)
Hyper-resonance	Loud, tinkling rushes	Intestinal obstruction
Borborygmi	Audible waves of loud, gurgling abdominal sounds produced by hyperactive bowel	Hyperactive intestinal peristalsis; result of eating, inflammatory bowel disease, infectious enteritis, mesenteric ischemia
Reduced or absent bowel sounds	No auscultation of bowel sounds	Peritonitis, paralytic ileus, obstruction; hypoactive bowel sounds are normal immediately post-op
Absence of liver dullness	Tympany on percussion	Air from viscus (e.g., perforated ulcer)
Masses	Lump on palpation	Tumours, cysts
Rebound tenderness	Sudden pain when examiner's fingers are withdrawn quickly (Blumberg sign)	Peritoneal inflammation, appendicitis
Inspiratory arrest	Sharp pain stops inspiration when the liver is palpated during a deep breath (Murphy sign)	Cholecystitis
Nodular liver	Enlarged, hard liver with irregular edge or surface	Cirrhosis, carcinoma
Hepatomegaly	Enlargement of liver, liver edge >1–2 cm below costal margin	Metastatic carcinoma, hepatitis, venous congestion
Splenomegaly	Enlargement of spleen	Chronic leukemia, hemolytic states, portal hypertension, some infections
Hernia	Bulge or nodule in abdomen, usually appearing on straining	Inguinal (in inguinal canal), femoral (in femoral canal), umbilical (herniation of umbilicus), or incisional (defect in muscles after surgery)

Continued

TABLE 41-11 ASSESSMENT ABNORMALITIES

Gastro-Intestinal System—cont'd

Finding	Description	Possible Etiology and Significance
Rectum and Anus		
Hemorrhoids	Thrombosed veins in rectum and anus (internal or external)	Portal hypertension, chronic constipation, prolonged sitting or standing, pregnancy
Mass	Firm, nodular edge	Tumour, carcinoma
Pilonidal cyst	Opening of sinus tract, cyst in midline just above coccyx	Probably congenital
Fissure	Ulceration in anal canal	Straining, irritation
Melena	Abnormal, black, tarry stool containing digested blood	Cancer, bleeding in upper GI tract from ulcers, varices
Tenesmus	Spasmodic contraction of the anal sphincter with pain and persistent desire to empty the bowel; painful and ineffective straining at stool	Ulcerative colitis, diarrhea secondary to GI infection such as food poisoning
Steatorrhea	Passage of large amounts of fat as a fatty, frothy, foul-smelling stool	Chronic pancreatitis, biliary obstruction, malabsorption problems (result of failure to digest and absorb fat)

GI, gastro-intestinal.

TABLE 41-12 DIAGNOSTIC STUDIES

Gastro-Intestinal (GI) System

Study	Description and Purpose	Nursing Responsibility
Radiology		
Upper GI series or barium swallow study	Fluoroscopic radiographic study using contrast medium Used to diagnose structural abnormalities of the esophagus, the stomach, and the duodenal bulb	Explain procedure to patient, including the need to drink contrast medium and to assume various positions on radiographic study examination table. Keep patient NPO for 8–12 hr before procedure. Instruct patient to avoid smoking after midnight the night before the study. After radiograph, take measures to prevent contrast medium impaction (fluids, laxatives). Warn patient that stool may be white for up to 72 hr after test.
Small bowel series	Fluoroscopic radiographic study using contrast medium Images are obtained q30 min until medium reaches terminal ileum	Same as for upper GI series.
Lower GI series or barium enema study	Fluoroscopic radiographic examination of colon using contrast medium, which is administered rectally (enema) Double-contrast or air-contrast barium enema is test of choice Air is infused after thick barium flows through transverse colon Endoscopic procedures have made necessity for this test less common than in the past	The evening before the procedure, administer purgatives, laxatives, enemas, or a combination of these until colon is clear of stool. The patient is put on a clear liquid diet the evening before procedure. Keep patient NPO for 8 hr before test. Instruct patient about being given barium by enema. Explain that cramping and urge to defecate may occur during procedure and that patient may be placed in various positions on tilt table. After the procedure, administer fluids, laxatives, or suppositories to assist in expelling barium. Observe stool for passage of contrast medium.
Cholangiography		
• Percutaneous transhepatic cholangiography (PTC)	Fluoroscopic radiographic study used to determine filling of hepatic and biliary ducts After local anaesthesia is induced and with monitored anaesthesia care (formerly called *conscious sedation*), liver is entered with long needle (under fluoroscopy), bile duct is entered, bile withdrawn, and radiopaque contrast medium injected IV antibiotics are administered prophylactically	Observe patient for signs of hemorrhage, bile leakage, and infection. Assess patient's medications for possible contraindications, precautions, or complications with the use of contrast medium.
• Surgical cholangiography	Study performed during surgery on biliary structures, such as gallbladder Contrast medium is injected into common bile duct	Explain to patient that anaesthetic and contrast medium will be used. Assess patient's medications for possible contraindications, precautions, or complications with the use of contrast medium.
• Magnetic resonance cholangiopancreatography (MRCP)	MRI technology used to obtain images of biliary and pancreatic ducts	Explain procedure to patient. Contraindicated in patient with metal implants (e.g., pacemaker) or who is pregnant.

TABLE 41-12 DIAGNOSTIC STUDIES

Gastro-Intestinal (GI) System—cont'd

Study	Description and Purpose	Nursing Responsibility
Ultrasonography	Nonradiographic study used to show the size and configuration of organs Noninvasive procedure in which high-frequency sound (ultrasound) waves are passed into body structures and recorded as they are reflected (bounded)	
• Abdominal ultrasonography	Ultrasound study used to detect abdominal masses (tumours and cysts), biliary and liver disease, gallstones A conductive gel (lubricant jelly) is applied to the skin and a transducer is placed on the area	Keep patient NPO for 8–12 hr before procedure. Air or gas can reduce quality of images. Food intake can cause gallbladder contraction, resulting in suboptimal study results.
• Endoscopic ultrasonography (EUS)	Ultrasound study using a small transducer installed on tip of endoscope Because EUS transducer gets close to the organs being examined, images obtained are often more accurate and detailed than images provided by traditional ultrasonography Detects and helps stage esophageal, gastric, rectal, biliary, and pancreatic tumours and abnormalities Also used to guide fine-needle aspiration to diagnose cancer or dysplasia	Same as for esophago-gastro-duodenoscopy.
Nuclear imaging scans (scintigraphy)	Radionuclide studies used to show size, shape, and position of organ Functional disorders and structural defects may be identified Radionuclide (radioactive isotope) is injected IV, and a counter (scanning) device picks up radioactive emission, which is recorded on paper Only tracer doses of radioactive isotopes are used	Tell patient that substance to be ingested contains only traces of radioactivity and poses little to no danger. Schedule no more than one radionuclide test per day. Explain to patient the need to lie flat during the scan.
• Gastric emptying studies	Radionuclide studies used to assess ability of stomach to empty solids or liquids in patients with emptying disorders resulting from peptic ulcer, ulcer surgery, diabetes, gastric malignancies, or functional disorders • Solid-emptying study: cooked egg white containing ^{99m}Tc is eaten • Liquid-emptying study: orange juice with ^{99m}Tc is swallowed Sequential images from gamma camera are recorded q2min for up to 60 min	Same as for nuclear imaging scans.
• Hepatobiliary (HIDA) scintigraphy	Radionuclide study used to identify obstructions of bile ducts (e.g., gallstones, tumours), diseases of gallbladder, and bile leaks Patient is given ^{99m}Tc IV and positioned under camera to record distribution of tracer in the liver, biliary tree, gallbladder, and proximal small bowel	Same as for nuclear imaging scans.
• Scintigraphy of GI bleeding	Radionuclide study used to reveal exact site of active GI blood loss Patient is given ^{99m}Tc-labelled sulphur colloid or patient's own red blood cells (RBCs) labelled with ^{99m}Tc, and images of the abdomen are obtained at intermittent intervals	Same as for nuclear imaging scans.
Computed tomographic (CT) scan	Noninvasive radiological examination allows exposures at different depths Used to detect biliary tract, liver, and pancreatic disorders Use of oral and IV contrast media accentuates density differences	Explain procedures to patient. Determine sensitivity to iodine if contrast material is used.
Magnetic resonance imaging (MRI)	Noninvasive procedure using radiofrequency waves and a magnetic field Used to detect hepatobiliary disease, hepatic lesions, and sources of GI bleeding and to stage colorectal cancer IV contrast medium (gadolinium) may be used	Explain procedure to patient. Contraindicated in patients with metal implants (e.g., pacemaker) or who are pregnant.

Continued

TABLE 41-12   **DIAGNOSTIC STUDIES**

Gastro-Intestinal (GI) System—cont'd

Study	Description and Purpose	Nursing Responsibility
Virtual colonoscopy	Combines CT scanning or MRI with computer virtual reality software to detect colon and bowel diseases and conditions, including polyps, colorectal cancer, diverticulosis, and lower GI bleeding Air is introduced via a tube placed in rectum to enlarge colon to enhance visualization Images obtained while patient is on back and stomach Computer combines images to form two- and three-dimensional images, which are viewed on monitor	Bowel preparation similar to that for colonoscopy (see below under "Endoscopy"). Unlike conventional colonoscopy, virtual colonoscopy necessitates no sedatives and no endoscope. Procedure takes about 15–20 min.

Endoscopy

Study	Description and Purpose	Nursing Responsibility
Esophago-gastro-duodenoscopy (EGD)	Enables direct visualization of mucosal lining of esophagus, stomach, and duodenum with flexible endoscope Video imaging may be used to visualize stomach motility Inflammations, ulcerations, tumours, varices, or Mallory–Weiss tear may be detected Biopsy samples may be obtained, and varices can be treated with band ligation or sclerotherapy	Before the procedure: Keep patient on NPO status for 8 hr. Make sure signed consent is obtained. Give preoperative medication if ordered. Explain to patient that local anaesthetic may be sprayed on throat before insertion of endoscope and that patient will be sedated during the procedure. After the procedure: Keep patient NPO until gag reflex returns (usually 2–4 hr); gently tickle back of patient's throat to determine return of reflex. Instruct patient to use warm saline gargles for relief of sore throat. Check temperature q15–30 min for 1–2 hr (sudden temperature spike is sign of perforation).
Colonoscopy	Enables direct visualization of entire colon up to ileocecal valve with flexible fibre-optic endoscope Patient's position is changed frequently during procedure to assist with advancement of endoscope to cecum Used to detect and diagnose inflammatory bowel disease, polyps, tumours, and diverticulosis and to dilate strictures Procedure allows for removal of colonic polyps without laparotomy	Before the procedure: Bowel preparation is completed. Procedure varies with physician preference. For example, patient may be kept on clear fluids 1–2 days before procedure, and cathartic or enema (or both) administered the night before. An alternative is to give 4.5 L (1 gal) of polyethylene glycol (Colyte) the evening before (8-oz glass q10min). Purgatives such as PICO-SALAX may be administered. Explain to patient that a flexible endoscope will be inserted while patient is in side-lying position and that sedative will be given. After procedure: Be aware that patient may experience abdominal cramps caused by stimulation of peristalsis because bowel is constantly inflated with air during procedure. Observe for rectal bleeding and signs of perforation (e.g., malaise, abdominal distension, tenesmus). Check vital signs.
Capsule endoscopy	Study most commonly used to visualize small intestine and diagnose diseases such as Crohn's disease, small bowel tumours, celiac disease, and malabsorption syndrome and to identify sources of possible GI bleeding in areas not accessible by upper endoscopy or colonoscopy Patient swallows a capsule (approximately the size of a large vitamin) with a camera that provides endoscopic observation of GI tract (see Figure 41-10); camera takes >50 000 images during 8-hr examination Capsule relays images to monitoring device that patient wears on belt After examination, images are downloaded to a workstation Not used in patients with suspected intestinal strictures	Dietary preparation: similar to that for colonoscopy. The video capsule is swallowed, and patient is usually kept NPO until 4–6 hr later. Procedure is comfortable for most patients. Eight hours after swallowing the capsule, the patient returns to have the monitoring device removed. Peristalsis causes passage of the disposable capsule with a bowel movement.

TABLE 41-12 DIAGNOSTIC STUDIES

Gastro-Intestinal (GI) System—cont'd

Study	Description and Purpose	Nursing Responsibility
Sigmoidoscopy	Enables direct visualization of rectum and sigmoid colon with lighted flexible endoscope Sometimes special table is used to tilt patient into knee–chest position Used to detect tumours, polyps, inflammatory and infectious diseases, fissures, hemorrhoids	Administer enemas evening before and morning of procedure. Make sure signed consent is obtained. Patient may have clear liquids day before, or no dietary restrictions may be necessary. Explain to patient knee–chest position (unless patient is older adult or very ill), need to take deep breaths during insertion of scope, and possible urge to defecate as scope is passed. Encourage patient to relax and let abdomen go limp. Observe for rectal bleeding after polypectomy or biopsy.
Endoscopic retrograde cholangiopancreatography (ERCP)	Endoscopic technique enables direct visualization of structures Fibre-optic endoscope (using fluoroscopy) is inserted through the oral cavity into descending duodenum, and then common bile and pancreatic ducts are cannulated Contrast medium is then injected into ducts Technique can also be used to retrieve a gallstone from distal common bile duct, dilate strictures, obtain biopsy of tumours, or diagnose pseudocysts	Before the procedure, explain procedure to patient, including patient's role. Keep patient NPO for 8 hr before procedure. Make sure signed consent is obtained. Administer sedative immediately before and during procedure. Administer antibiotics if ordered. After the procedure, check vital signs. Check for signs of perforation or infection. Be aware that ERCP-induced pancreatitis is most common complication; this complication manifests as abdominal pain, nausea, and vomiting. Check for return of gag reflex.
Endoscopic ultrasonography	Combined use of endoscopy and ultrasonography with the use of an ultrasound transducer attached to an endoscope Enables visualization of esophagus, stomach, intestine, liver, pancreas, and gallbladder	Similar to that for esophago-gastro-duodenoscopy.
Laparoscopy (peritoneoscopy)	Enables visualization of peritoneal cavity and contents with laparoscope Biopsy specimen may be obtained Performed with patient under general anaesthesia in operating room Double-puncture peritoneoscopy enables better visualization of abdominal cavity, especially liver Can eliminate need for exploratory laparotomy in many patients	Keep patient on NPO status for 8 hr before study. Make sure signed consent is obtained. Administer preoperative sedative. Ensure that bladder and bowel are emptied. Inform patient that local anaesthetic is used before laparoscope insertion. Observe for possible complications of bleeding and bowel perforation after the procedure.
Blood Studies		
Amylase	Measures secretion of amylase by pancreas Is important in diagnosing acute pancreatitis Level peaks in 24 hr and then drops to normal in 48–72 hr Depending on method, reference range is 100–300 U/L (60–120 SU/dL)	Obtain blood sample in acute attack of pancreatitis. Explain procedure to patient.
Lipase	Measures secretion of lipase by pancreas. Level stays elevated longer than that of serum amylase Reference range is <160 U/L	Explain procedure to patient.
Gastrin	Measures secretion of gastrin by the cells of the antrum of the stomach and by the pancreatic islets of Langerhans Reference interval: 0–180 ng/L (0–180 pg/mL) during fasting	Explain procedure to patient.

Continued

TABLE 41-12   DIAGNOSTIC STUDIES

Gastro-Intestinal (GI) System—cont'd

Study	Description and Purpose	Nursing Responsibility
Liver Biopsy	Percutaneous procedure uses needle inserted between sixth and seventh or between eighth and ninth intercostal spaces on the right side to obtain specimen of hepatic tissue Often performed under ultrasound or CT guidance	Before procedure, check patient's coagulation status (prothrombin time, clotting or bleeding time). Ensure that patient's blood is typed and crossmatched. Measure vital signs as baseline data. Explain holding of breath after expiration when needle is inserted. Make sure signed consent is obtained. After procedure, check vital signs to detect internal bleeding q15min × 2, q30min × 4, q1hr × 4. Keep patient lying on right side for a minimum of 2 hr to splint puncture site. Keep patient in bed in flat position for 12–14 hr. Assess patient for complications such as bile peritonitis, shock, and pneumothorax.
Fecal Tests		
Fecal immunochemical test	Tests for the presence of blood in stool Possible indicator of colorectal cancer	Explain procedure and indication to patient. No medical or dietary restrictions
Fecal analysis	Form, consistency, and colour of fecal sample are noted Specimen examined for mucus, blood, pus, parasites, and fat content Fecal occult blood test (FOBT): guaiac test, Hemoccult, Hemoccult II, Hemoccult-SENSA, Hematest are performed Single DNA test (PreGen-Plus) is a panel of DNA markers used to detect and monitor colorectal cancer	Observe patient's stools. Collect stool specimens. Check stools for blood. Keep diet free of red meat for 24–48 hr before occult blood test.
Stool culture	Tests for presence of bacteria, including *Clostridium difficile*	Collect stool specimen.

GI, gastro-intestinal; *IV*, intravenously; *ng/L*, nanograms per litre; *NPO*, nothing by mouth; *pg/mL*, pictograms per millilitre; *RBCs*, red blood cells; *SU*, Somogyi units; *^{99m}Tc*, technetium-99m; *U/L*, units per litre; *WBCs*, white blood cells.

the stomach, and the small intestine by means of fluoroscopy and radiographic examination. A barium swallow study is used to identify esophageal, stomach, and small intestine disorders such as esophageal strictures, varices, polyps, tumours, hiatal hernia, and foreign bodies, as well as peptic ulcers in the stomach or duodenum. The barium swallow study begins with the patient swallowing a thick barium solution (contrast medium). The patient then assumes different positions on the radiographic study examination table. The movement of the contrast medium through the upper GI tract is observed with fluoroscopy, and several radiographic images are obtained (see Table 41-12).

Lower Gastro-Intestinal Series. The purpose of a lower GI series (barium enema radiograph) is to observe by means of fluoroscopy the filling of the colon with contrast medium and to observe by radiograph the filled colon. This procedure helps identify polyps, tumours, and other lesions in the colon. The patient is administered an enema of contrast medium. The air-contrast barium enema provides better visualization of inflammatory bowel disease, polyps, tumours, and gallstones (Figure 41-8). Because the patient must retain the barium, this study is not tolerated well by patients who are older or immobile.

Abdominal Ultrasonography. Ultrasonography is a noninvasive, nonradiographic approach used to show the size and the configuration of organs. It is the diagnostic procedure of choice for detecting cholelithiasis (gallstones). Ultrasonography is also used for detecting appendicitis, acute cholecystitis, and other changes in abdominal organs (see Table 41-12).

Endoscopy

Endoscopy is the direct visualization of a body structure through a lighted fibre-optic instrument (endoscope). The GI structures

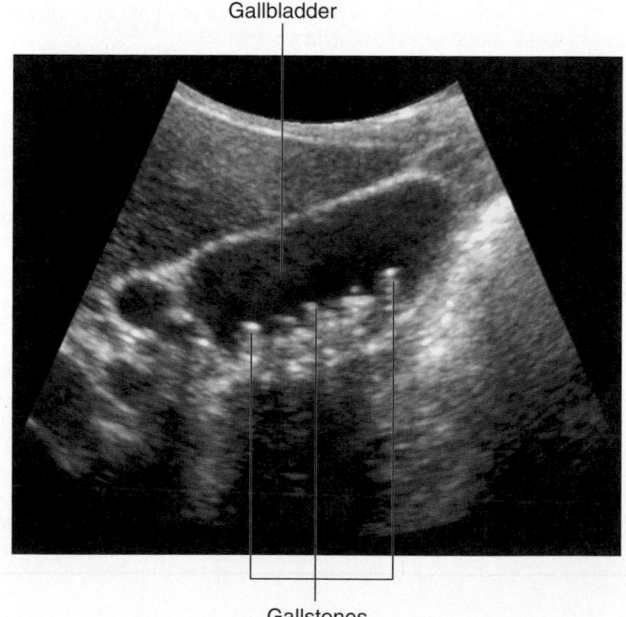

Gallblader

Gallstones

FIGURE 41-8 Ultrasound image of gallbladder, showing multiple gallstones. Source: Drake, R. L., Vogl, W., & Mitchell, A. W. M. (2010). *Gray's anatomy for students* (2nd ed., p. 326). Edinburgh: Churchill Livingstone.

that can be examined through endoscopy include the esophagus, the stomach, the duodenum, the colon, and, with the aid of fluoroscopy and radiographs, the pancreas and the biliary tree. The pancreatic, hepatic, and common bile ducts can be visualized with side-viewing flexible endoscopes. This procedure is called

The endoscope is passed though the mouth to the opening of pancreatic duct in the duodenum

Gallbladder

Pancreatic duct

Common hepatic duct

Common bile duct

Endoscope

Contrast media is injected into the common bile duct and pancreatic duct

Duodenum

FIGURE 41-9 Endoscopic retrograde cholangiopancreatography. Source: Nucleus Medical Media Inc./Alamy Stock Photo.

endoscopic retrograde cholangiopancreatography (ERCP) and is illustrated in Figure 41-9.

The endoscope is an instrument channel through which biopsy forceps and cytology brushes may be passed. Cameras may be attached to take video recordings and still pictures. Endoscopy of the GI tract is often performed in combination with biopsy and cytological studies. The major complication of GI endoscopy is perforation through the structure being viewed. The incidence of this complication is decreased with the use of the flexible fibre-optic endoscopes.

For all endoscopic procedures, informed written consent is required. Specific endoscopy procedures are discussed in Table 41-12. In addition to diagnostic procedures, many invasive and therapeutic procedures may be performed with endoscopes. These include procedures such as polypectomy, sclerosis of varices, laser treatment, cauterization of bleeding sites, papillotomy, removal of stones in the common bile duct, and balloon dilations. For many endoscopic procedures, patients require intravenous short-acting sedatives.

Endoscopic Ultrasonography. Endoscopic ultrasound (EUS) is a relatively new endoscopic technique that provides highly accurate images of the esophagus, GI tract, pancreas, and liver. EUS provides high-resolution imaging of the GI tract because of its unique ability to differentiate the histological layers of the GI tract wall. It is most often used for preoperative staging of esophageal, gastric, pancreatic, and colorectal cancers. It can also be used to detect gallstones.

Capsule Endoscopy. In capsule endoscopy, the patient swallows a capsule containing a disposable video camera (Figure 41-10). As the video camera passes through the intestine, images are

CASE STUDY

Objective Data: Diagnostic Studies

Source: Anton_Ivanov/ Shutterstock .com.

The ED physician performs a rectal examination and finds a palpable mass. The following diagnostic tests are ordered:
- CBC
- Electrolytes
- Liver function tests
- Urinalysis
- CT scan of the abdomen
- Colonoscopy

The CBC reveals an Hb of 68 mmol/L and an Hct of 20%. The white blood cell count is normal. The electrolytes, liver function tests, and urinalysis are within normal limits. The CT scan reveals pockets of gas and fluid in the ascending colon and two medium-sized tumours in the transverse colon.

See pp. 956 and 960 for more information on Mr. Collins.

transmitted by radiofrequency. This procedure is particularly useful in visualization of the portion of the small bowel that is not within reach of standard upper and lower endoscopy. It allows more access to the small bowel for patients with an obscure source of GI bleeding. This technology may be particularly helpful in discovering the cause of GI bleeding when results of standard upper endoscopy and colonoscopy are normal.

Liver Biopsy

A liver biopsy is performed when hepatic tissue is needed to establish a diagnosis such as fibrosis, cirrhosis, hepatitis, and

FIGURE 41-10 Capsule endoscopy. **A,** The pill-sized video capsule has its own camera and light source. **B,** As it travels through the GI tract, it sends messages through sensing electrodes placed on the chest and abdomen to a data recorder worn on a waist belt. **C,** After the test, the images are viewed on a computer. Source: Dye, C. E., Gaffney, R. R., Dykes, T. M., et al. (2012). Endoscopic and radiographic evaluation of the small bowel in 2012. *The American Journal of Medicine, 125*(12), 1228.e1–1288.e12.

neoplasms. It may also be used for monitoring the progress of liver disease.

Liver biopsy may be performed as an open or closed procedure. The *open method* involves making an incision and removing a wedge of tissue. It is performed in the operating room, often concurrently with another surgical procedure, with the patient under general anaesthesia. The *closed*, or *needle*, *biopsy* is a percutaneous procedure in which the site is infiltrated with a local anaesthetic and a needle is inserted between the sixth and seventh or between the eighth and ninth intercostal spaces on the right side. The patient lies supine with the right arm over the head. The patient should be instructed to exhale fully and not breathe while the needle is inserted (see Table 41-12). It is important to perform a nursing assessment before and after a liver biopsy.

Liver Function Studies

Liver function tests are usually described separately from other GI diagnostic studies. Liver function tests are laboratory (blood) studies that reflect hepatic disease. Table 41-13 lists some common liver function tests.

TABLE 41-13   DIAGNOSTIC STUDIES

Liver Function Tests

Test	Description and Purpose	Test	Description and Purpose
Bile Formation and Excretion		**Hemostatic Functions**	
Serum bilirubin	Measurement of ability of liver to conjugate and excrete bilirubin; enables differentiation between unconjugated (indirect) and conjugated (direct) bilirubin in plasma	Prothrombin	Determination of prothrombin activity Reference range: 11–12.5 sec
• Total	Measurement of direct and indirect total bilirubin Reference range: 5.1–17 mcmol/L	Vitamin K	Essential cofactor for many clotting factors Reference range: 0.22–4.88 nmol/L
• Direct	Measurement of conjugated bilirubin; level is elevated in obstructive jaundice Reference range: 1.7–5.1 mcmol/L	**Serum Enzyme Tests**	
		Alkaline phosphatase (ALP)	Origination in bone and liver; serum level elevated when excretion is impaired as a result of obstruction in the biliary tract Reference range: 35–120 U/L
• Indirect	Measurement of unconjugated bilirubin; level is elevated in hepatocellular (hepatitis, cirrhosis, neoplasm or hepatic congestion) and hemolytic conditions Reference range: 3.4–12 mcmol/L	Aspartate aminotransferase (AST)	Serum level elevated in liver damage and inflammation Reference range: 0–35 U/L Women's values are slightly lower than men's
Urinary bilirubin	Measurement of urinary excretion of conjugated bilirubin Normal finding: 0–0.034 mcmol/L (negative)	Alanine aminotransferase (ALT)	Serum level elevated in liver damage and inflammation Reference range: 4–36 U/L
Protein Metabolism		γ-Glutamyl transpeptidase (GGT)	Present in biliary tract (not in skeletal muscle or cardiac tissue); serum level elevated in hepatitis and alcoholic liver disease; more sensitive for detecting biliary obstruction, cholangitis, or cholecystitis than ALP Reference ranges: 8–38 IU/L
Serum protein levels	Measurement of serum proteins manufactured by the liver Albumin reference range: 35–50 g/L; globulin reference range: 23–34 g/L; total protein reference range: 64–83 g/L Normal A/G ratio: 1.5:1–2.5:1		
α-Fetoprotein	Tumour marker, especially for hepatic cancer Reference range: <40 mcg/L	**Lipid Metabolism**	
Ammonia	Conversion of ammonia to urea normally occurs in the liver; elevated ammonia level can result in hepatic encephalopathy secondary to liver cirrhosis Reference range: 6–47 mcmol/L	Serum cholesterol	Synthesis and excretion by liver; serum level elevated in biliary obstruction, lowered in extensive liver disease and malnutrition Reference range: <5.0 mmol/L, age dependent HDL reference range: >1.55 mmol/L LDL reference range: <2.59 mmol/L

HDL, high-density lipoprotein; *IU/L,* international units per litre; *LDL,* low-density lipoprotein; *U/L,* units per litre.

REVIEW QUESTIONS

The number of the question corresponds to the same-numbered objective at the beginning of the chapter.

1. A client is admitted to the hospital with a diagnosis of diarrhea with dehydration. The nurse recognizes that increased peristalsis resulting in diarrhea can be related to which of the following mechanisms?
   a. Sympathetic inhibition
   b. Mixing and propulsion
   c. Sympathetic stimulation
   d. Parasympathetic stimulation

2. A client has an elevated blood level of indirect (unconjugated) bilirubin. Which of the following might cause this finding?
   a. The gallbladder is unable to contract to release stored bile.
   b. Bilirubin is not being conjugated and excreted into the bile by the liver.
   c. The Kupffer cells in the liver are unable to remove bilirubin from the blood.
   d. There is an obstruction in the biliary tract preventing flow of bile into the small intestine.

3. Which of the following normally protects the bowel from the acidity of gastric contents as they move into the small intestine?
   a. Inhibition of secretin release
   b. Release of bicarbonate by the pancreas
   c. Release of pancreatic digestive enzymes
   d. Release of gastrin by the duodenal mucosa

4. An 80-year-old man states that although he adds a lot of salt to his food, it still does not have much flavour. Which of the following factors related to aging would account for this finding?
   a. Some disorder; he should not experience changes in the ability to taste
   b. Loss of taste buds, especially for sweetness and saltiness
   c. Some loss of taste sensation but no difficulty chewing food
   d. Loss of the sense of taste because the ability to smell is decreased

5. Which of the following questions is appropriate to initiate a GI assessment?
   a. "What is your usual bowel elimination pattern?"
   b. "What percentage of your income is spent on food?"
   c. "Have you travelled to a foreign country in the past year?"
   d. "Does stress give you diarrhea?"

6. Which of the following is appropriate for the nurse to undertake during an examination of the abdomen?
   a. Position the client in the supine position with the bed flat and knees straight.
   b. Listen in the epigastrium and all four quadrants for 2 to 5 minutes for bowel sounds.
   c. Use the following order of techniques: inspection, palpation, percussion, auscultation.
   d. Describe bowel sounds as absent if no sound is heard in the lower right quadrant after 2 minutes.

7. Which of the following findings would be considered a normal physical assessment finding of the GI system? *(Select all that apply)*
   a. Nonpalpable liver and spleen
   b. Borborygmi in upper right quadrant
   c. Tympany on percussion of the abdomen
   d. Liver edge 2 to 4 cm below the costal margin
   e. Finding of a firm, nodular edge on the rectal examination

8. Which of the following is correct in preparing a client for a colonoscopy?
   a. A signed consent form is not necessary.
   b. Sedation may be used during the procedure.
   c. Only one cleansing enema is necessary for preparation.
   d. A light meal should be eaten the day before the procedure.

1. d; 2. b; 3. b; 4. b; 5. a; 6. a; 7. a, b, and c; 8. b.

⊖volve

For even more review questions, visit *http://evolve.elsevier.com/Canada/Lewis/medsurg*.

REFERENCES

Heuman, D. M. (2017). *Gallstones (Cholelithiasis)*. Retrieved from *https://emedicine.medscape.com/article/175667-overview#a5*,

Jarvis, C., Browne, A. J., MacDonald-Jenkins, J., et al. (Eds.). (2014). *Physical examination and health assessment* (2nd Canadian ed.). Toronto: Elsevier.

Miller, C. A. (2012). *Nursing for wellness in older adults* (5th ed.). Philadelphia: Wolters Kluwer Health Lippincott, Williams & Wilkins.

RESOURCES

Resources for this chapter are listed in Chapters 42, 44, 45, and 46.

Nursing Management
Nutritional Problems

Written by: Rose DiMaria-Ghalili
Adapted by: Ellen Vogel, Christina Vaillancourt,
Andrea Miller, and Maysam Youssef

evolve WEBSITE

http://evolve.elsevier.com/Canada/Lewis/medsurg

- Review Questions (Online Only)
- Key Points
- Answer Guidelines for Case Study
- Customizable Nursing Care Plans
- Enteral Nutrition
- Parenteral Nutrition
- Conceptual Care Map Creator
- Audio Glossary
- Content Updates

LEARNING OBJECTIVES

1. Relate the essential components of a well-balanced diet to their impact on health outcomes.
2. Describe the common etiological factors, clinical manifestations, and management of malnutrition.
3. Describe the components of a nutritional assessment.
4. Explain the indications, complications, and nursing management principles related to the use of enteral nutrition.

5. Explain the indications, complications, and nursing management related to the use of parenteral nutrition.
6. Compare the etiological factors, clinical manifestations, and nursing management of eating disorders.

KEY TERMS

anorexia nervosa, p. 976
bulimia nervosa, p. 976
enteral nutrition (EN), p. 983
food security, p. 975

malabsorption syndrome, p. 975
malnutrition, p. 974
nutrition, p. 970
optimal nutritional status, p. 971

overnutrition, p. 971
parenteral nutrition (PN), p. 987
protein–calorie malnutrition (PCM), p. 974
undernutrition, p. 971

This chapter focuses on problems related to nutrition. A review of normal nutrition provides a basis for evaluating nutritional status. Malnutrition, eating disorders, and types of supplemental nutrition, including enteral and parenteral nutrition, are discussed.

NUTRITIONAL PROBLEMS

As one of the fundamental requirements for sustaining life, eating is a highly symbolic and culturally meaningful act. It is unusual to hear a newscast that does not have several stories relating to the food we eat. Newspapers and bestseller lists frequently highlight nutrition- and food-related books, illustrating the importance of food and eating to Canadians. Nutrition is also inextricably linked to the development of and the recovery from illness.

Nurses, as the first point of contact for patients, frequently initiate patient referrals to dietitians. Thus, knowledge and skills

in nutrition and nutritional screening are essential to effective patient care. Dietitians and nurses often collaborate in the development and implementation of nutritional care plans.

Dietitians, as part of the multidisciplinary team, provide expertise in the assessment of the nutritional status of individuals throughout the life cycle and in development of nutritional care plans for wide-ranging health concerns. Dietitians have extensive knowledge in the biochemical and nutritional components of foods and how these influence metabolic and physiological processes. Importantly, dietitians understand the feeding environment and underlying psychosocial, economic, and health determinants that influence food intake at individual, family, and societal levels (Dietitians of Canada, 2016).

Nutrition is the process by which the body uses food for energy, growth, maintenance, and repair of body tissues. Nutritional status can be viewed as a continuum from undernutrition to optimal nutrition to overnutrition. Any alteration in the process of nutrient intake or use can potentially cause nutritional problems. Nutritional problems can occur in all age groups, cultures, ethnic groups, and socioeconomic classes and across all educational levels. Attitudes toward the importance of food and eating habits are established early. Cultural or religious preferences and requirements are frequently reflected in dietary intakes. The financial status of a family or an individual may influence the type and amount of nutritionally sound food that can be purchased (Tarasuk, Mitchell, & Dachner, 2016).

Today there is much interest in understanding the link between nutrition and the onset of chronic diseases. Numerous reports have shown that a significant portion of morbidity and mortality among Canadians is related to chronic diseases. In 2013, the Public Health Agency of Canada stated in its strategic plan for preventing chronic disease that three of every five Canadians over 20 live with a chronic disease and four of five are at risk of developing a chronic disease (Public Health Agency of Canada [PHAC], 2013). Internationally, Canada's health care spending is among the highest in the world, representing approximately 11% of the gross domestic product in 2016 (Canadian Institute for Health Information, 2017). Poor nutrition is a key preventable risk factor for many of the chronic diseases that influence morbidity, disability, and premature death in Canada.

NORMAL NUTRITION

Undernutrition occurs when nutritional reserves become depleted or when nutrient intake is inadequate to meet daily requirements or metabolic demands. Undernutrition affects vulnerable groups, including infants, children, pregnant women, new immigrants, individuals living in rural or remote communities, individuals with low incomes, hospitalized people, and older adults. Undernutrition

increases the risk for impaired growth and development, lowers resistance to infection and disease, delays wound healing, results in longer hospital stays, and increases health-related expenses.

Optimal nutritional status is achieved when nutrients consumed meet daily requirements and metabolic demands, including any increased demands related to growth, pregnancy, or illness. Individuals with optimal nutritional status have a lower risk of developing chronic diseases and generally live longer than those with a chronic illness.

Overnutrition results from the consumption of nutrients—most frequently, calories, sodium, and fat—in excess of requirements. A major nutritional problem today, overnutrition results in the development of chronic diseases including obesity, some cancers, and type 2 diabetes.

The nutrients required to optimize health over a lifetime are the same for all healthy individuals; however, the amount required of each nutrient differs based on stages of the life cycle. Nutritional needs can be viewed as a continuum across the lifespan: they change as individuals grow, age, and respond to variations in their environment, physical activity, and health. Optimal nutrition is essential for its contribution to overall health and well-being and to the prevention of chronic conditions.

Optimal nutrition in the absence of any underlying disease process results from the ingestion of a balanced diet. *Eating Well With Canada's Food Guide,* commonly referred to as "Canada's Food Guide," provides Canadians with recommendations for healthy eating (Health Canada, 2011) (Figure 42-1). The guide is based on current nutritional science and defines four major foods groups. This standardization ensures that a diet based on the food guide will provide an adequate intake to support optimal nutritional status. The information contained in Canada's Food

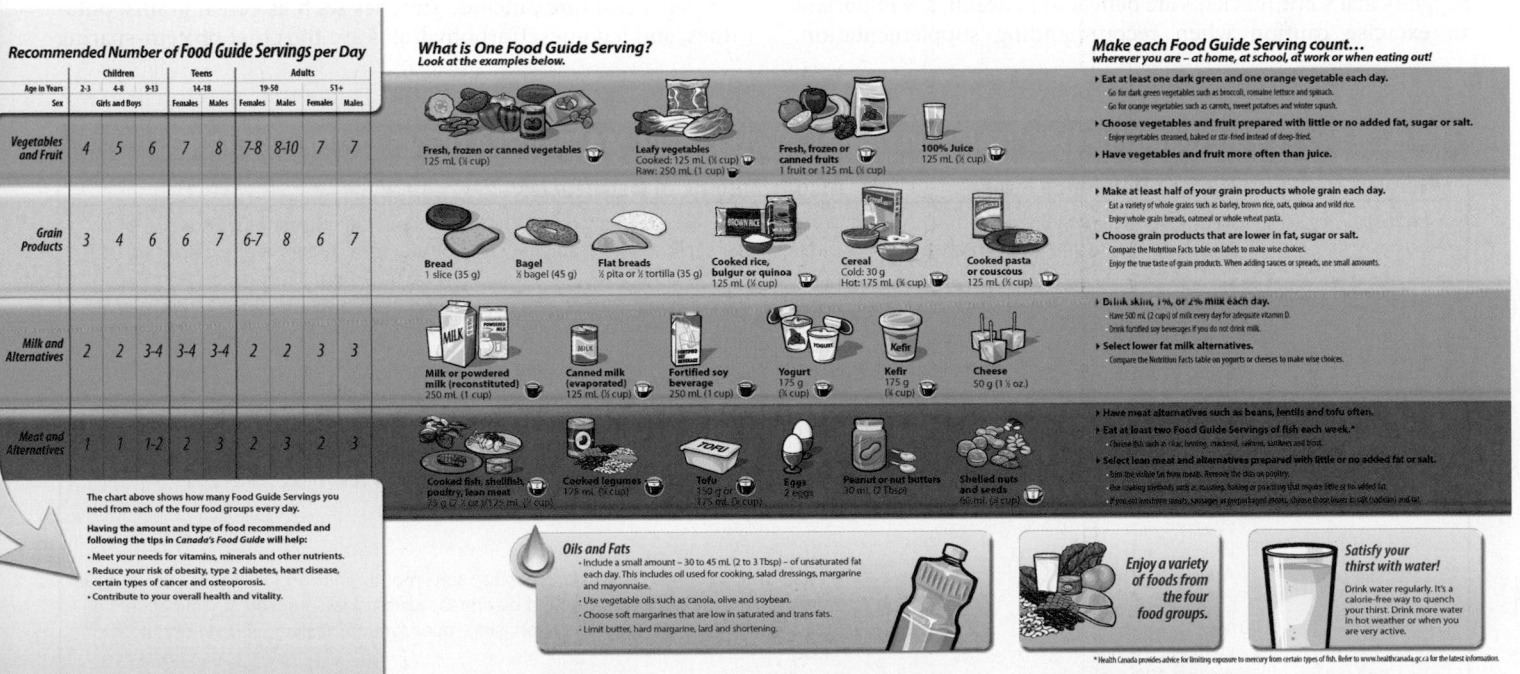

FIGURE 42-1 *Eating Well With Canada's Food Guide.* The Resources at the end of this chapter provide a link to the guide and interactive tools ("My Food Guide") that allow nurses and their patients to personalize the information in Canada's Food Guide. Source: © All rights reserved. *Eating Well with Canada's Food Guide.* Health Canada, 2011. Adapted and reproduced with permission from the Minister of Health, 2017.

Guide is based on the most up-to-date evidence at the time of publication. The Food Guide is reviewed and updated periodically based on current evidence and public health priorities. At the time of writing, a new Food Guide is due to be released in 2018 and is expected to contain significant changes.

Canada's Food Guide can be used by anyone to plan a healthy diet; it is flexible and can be adapted to include combination foods and ethnically diverse foods that reflect the country's multicultural profile. (In addition to English and French, the guide is available in 10 other languages: Arabic, Chinese, Farsi [Persian], Korean, Punjabi, Russian, Spanish, Tagalog, Tamil, and Urdu [Health Canada, 2013].) The food guide also provides alternative choices for meat, milk, and other animal-based foods.

Eating Well With Canada's Food Guide—First Nations, Inuit and Métis is a food guide tailored to reflect traditions and food choices of a specific population group (Health Canada, 2010). This guide includes traditional and store-bought foods that are generally available, affordable, and accessible to Indigenous people across Canada.

Canada's Food Guide was developed in accordance with the daily dietary reference intake (DRI) requirements, a comprehensive set of nutrient reference values for healthy populations (Table 42-1). There is a DRI set for each nutrient. These nutrient reference values are intended to help individuals optimize their health, prevent disease, and avoid overconsumption of any single nutrient. The reference values include the estimated average requirement (EAR), the recommended dietary allowance (RDA), the adequate intake (AI) and the tolerable upper limit (UL) (Institute of Medicine, 2005). The DRI values are designed to maintain health and prevent disease, not to restore health. Nutrient needs may exceed DRIs during times of acute stress or chronic illness.

In recent years, there has been considerable interest in vitamin and mineral supplementation as a means of prevention and treatment of acute and chronic diseases. Although evidence suggests that some nutrients are beneficial to health, it is important to exercise caution when recommending supplementation.

Exceeding the UL can increase a person's risk for nutrient toxicity. As well, consumption of high levels of one vitamin or mineral may interfere with the absorption of another. For example, ingestion of high levels of zinc can interfere with the absorption of calcium; ingestion of high levels of vitamin C enhances the absorption of iron, which can lead to iron toxicity. To avoid harmful adverse effects, patients should be encouraged to discuss vitamin and mineral supplementation with their primary care provider before using.

Major Nutrients

The major nutritional constituents of foods are carbohydrates (and fibre), fats, proteins, vitamins, minerals, and water. Carbohydrates, fats, and proteins provide energy. Vitamins, minerals, and water do not provide energy; some serve as structure (e.g., calcium in bones), and all assist in body processes such as food digestion, muscle movement, waste disposal, growth of new tissues (e.g., wound healing), and energy production (from carbohydrates, proteins, and fats). An individual's daily calorie requirements are influenced by body composition, age, gender, and physical activity. Adjustments in caloric intake are necessary when there are changes in a person's health status and daily activity level. An average adult requires an estimated 20 to 35 kcal/kg of body weight per day, leaning toward the higher end if the person is critically ill or very active and the lower end if the person is sedentary (American Society of Parenteral and Enteral Nutrition [ASPEN], 2016). (*Kilocalorie* is the correct unit to designate caloric intake and expenditure; however, *calorie* is the term more commonly used.)

Carbohydrates, the body's primary source of energy, yield approximately 4 kcal/g. Carbohydrates are classified as simple or complex. Simple carbohydrates include *monosaccharides* (e.g., glucose and fructose), found in fruits and honey, and *disaccharides* (e.g., sucrose, maltose, and lactose), found in foods such as table sugar and milk. Complex carbohydrates, or *polysaccharides*, include starches such as cereal grains, potatoes, and legumes. Carbohydrates are the chief protein-sparing

TABLE 42-1	RECOMMENDED DAILY VITAMIN INTAKE AND MANIFESTATIONS OF DEFICIENCIES	
Vitamin	**Dietary Reference Intake**	**Manifestations of Deficiencies**
A (retinol)	*Men:* 900 mcg/retinol equivalents* *Women:* 700 mcg/retinol equivalents	Dry, scaly skin; increased susceptibility to infection; night blindness; anorexia; eye irritation; keratinization of respiratory and GI mucosa; bladder stones; anemia; retarded growth
D	*Adults age 19–70:* 600 IU *Adults age >70:* 800 IU	Muscular weakness, excessive sweating, diarrhea and other GI disturbances, bone pain, active or healed rickets, osteomalacia
E	*Adults:* 15 mg	Neurological deficits
K	*Men:* 120 mcg *Women:* 90 mcg	Defective blood coagulation
B₁ (thiamine)	*Men:* 1.2 mg *Women:* 1.1 mg	Anorexia, fatigue, nervous irritability, constipation, paresthesias, insomnia
B₆ (pyridoxine)	*Men age 19–50:* 1.3–1.7 mg *Men age >51:* 1.7 mg *Women age 19–50:* 1.3–1.5 mg *Women age >51:* 1.5 mg	Seizures, dermatitis, anemia, neuropathy with motor weakness, anorexia
B₁₂ (cobalamin)	*Adults:* 2–4 mcg	Megaloblastic anemia, anorexia, glossitis, sore mouth and tongue, pallor, neurological problems such as depression and dizziness, weight loss, nausea, constipation
C	*Men:* 90 mg *Women:* 75 mg	Bleeding gums, loose teeth, easy bruising, poor wound healing, scurvy, dry, itchy skin
Folate (folic acid)	*Adults:* 400 mcg	Impaired cell division and protein synthesis, megaloblastic anemia, anorexia, fatigue, sore tongue, diarrhea, forgetfulness

GI, gastro-intestinal.

*1 retinol equivalent = 10 international units vitamin A activity from β-carotene or 3.33 international units vitamin A activity from retinol.

TABLE 42-2	DIETARY REFERENCE INTAKE (DRI) FOR FIBRE
	Grams of Fibre per Day
Men 19–50 years of age	38
Men ≥51 years of age	30
Women 19–50 years of age	25
Women ≥51 years of age	21

TABLE 42-3 GOOD SOURCES OF PROTEIN

Complete Proteins	Incomplete Proteins
• Milk and milk products (e.g., cheese)	• Grains (e.g., corn)
• Eggs	• Legumes (e.g., navy beans, soybeans, peas)
• Fish	• Nuts (e.g., peanuts)
• Meats	• Seeds (e.g., sesame seeds, sunflower seeds)
• Poultry	

ingredients in a nutritionally sound diet. Canada's Food Guide recommends that 55% of daily energy needs be supplied by carbohydrates, especially foods rich in complex carbohydrates and fibre. The rainbow design of the Food Guide places grain products, vegetables, and fruit in the outermost arcs to ensure that Canadians eat the recommended amount of carbohydrates (Health Canada, 2011).

Fibre is the indigestible parts of plant foods. Diets rich in fibre are associated with improved blood cholesterol and blood glucose levels, healthy bowel function, and healthy body weight (Table 42-2).

Fats are stored in adipose tissue and in the abdominal cavity. Besides being a major source of energy, fats act as insulation, which reduces loss of body heat in cold environments and provides padding and protection for vital organs. Fats also act as carriers of essential fatty acids (linoleic and alpha-linolenic) and fat-soluble vitamins (A, D, E, and K). Fats provide a feeling of satiety after eating. Canada's Food Guide recommends that approximately 30% of total energy come from fat, including 10% from saturated fat (Health Canada, 2012). One gram of fat yields 9 calories. A total fat intake of 30% or less equates to an intake of 60 g to 105 g of fat per day (Health Canada, 2015a).

Dietary fat is composed of four types of fatty acids: polyunsaturated, monounsaturated, saturated, and trans fats. Monounsaturated and polyunsaturated fats lower the risk for heart disease. Polyunsaturated fats, including omega-3 and omega-6 fats, are essential to good health. These fatty acids are not synthesized by the body and must be obtained from the diet. Omega-6 essential fatty acids are found in vegetable oils such as corn, sunflower, and soybean oils; primary sources of omega-3 fatty acids are fatty fish, flaxseed, and some nuts. Monounsaturated fats are found in vegetable oils, including olive and canola oils.

Saturated fats are found naturally in both vegetable- and animal-based foods, including coconut and palm oil and butter and full-fat dairy products. Trans fats are found naturally in some animal-based foods. Trans fats are formed when liquid oils are made into semisolid fats like shortening and hard margarine. Saturated and trans fats increase the risk for heart disease because they raise serum low-density lipoprotein (LDL) cholesterol levels (the so-called bad cholesterol) (Health Canada, 2012). Trans fats are particularly dangerous because they also reduce levels of high-density lipoprotein (HDL) cholesterol (the so-called good cholesterol) (Health Canada, 2012).

Proteins, another essential component of a well-balanced diet, can be obtained from both animal and plant sources. Proteins are essential for tissue growth, repair, and maintenance; body regulatory functions; and energy production. Ideally, proteins provide 15% to 20% of daily caloric needs. The recommended daily intake (RDI) for protein is 0.8 to 1 g/kg of body weight. One gram of protein yields 4 calories. Proteins are complex nitrogenous organic compounds, of which amino acids are the fundamental units of structure. The 22 amino acids can be classified as essential

and nonessential. The body is capable of synthesizing nonessential amino acids if an adequate supply of protein is available. The nine essential amino acids must be provided through dietary sources. Protein sources containing all the essential amino acids are considered to be high-quality proteins that are easier to digest. Generally, animal-based proteins are easier to digest and are often referred to as *complete proteins* because they contain all essential amino acids (Institute of Medicine, 2005).

Grain products also contribute to protein intake. Plant-based proteins such as legumes and grains lack one or more of the essential amino acids and are more difficult to digest. These types of proteins are called *incomplete proteins*. The digestion difficulty can be overcome by combining high-protein plant-based foods. This concept is called *mutual supplementation*. Mutual supplementation is the strategy of combining two incomplete protein sources so that the amino acids in one food compensate for the missing ones in the other food. See Table 42-3 for a list of good sources of protein.

Vitamins are organic compounds required in small amounts for normal metabolism. Vitamins function primarily in enzyme reactions that facilitate the metabolism of amino acids, fats, and carbohydrates. Vitamins are divided into two categories: water-soluble vitamins (vitamin C and the B-complex vitamins) and fat-soluble vitamins (vitamins A, D, E, and K). Vitamin D, in particular, has recently received widespread attention because of a growing body of evidence that suggests it may have a beneficial effect on some types of cancer, in particular colorectal cancer, and other immune-related diseases (Dietitians of Canada, 2013). Since the body stores fat-soluble vitamins, consuming too much can result in toxicity. Upper limits have been established for vitamins A, D, and E.

Mineral salts (e.g., magnesium, iron, calcium) make up approximately 4% of total body weight. Minerals present in minute amounts are referred to as *trace elements*. Minerals required in amounts greater than 100 mg/day are called *major minerals*. Minerals are necessary to build tissues, regulate body fluids, and assist in various body functions. Some minerals are stored and can be toxic if taken in excess amounts. The daily requirement for minerals varies greatly, from a few micrograms of trace minerals to 1 g or more of the major minerals, such as calcium, phosphorus, and sodium. Table 42-4 lists the major minerals and trace elements. A well-balanced diet based on Canada's Food Guide will typically meet the daily requirements for minerals.

Vegetarian Diet

The common element among all vegetarians is the exclusion of meat, poultry, game, fish, shellfish or crustaceans, and meat by-products from the diet. Vegetarians base their diet on convictions founded in religious or cultural beliefs, a respect for all living beings, ethical–ecological ideals, economics, or

TABLE 42-4	MAJOR MINERALS AND TRACE ELEMENTS

Major Minerals	Trace Elements
• Calcium	• Chromium
• Chloride	• Copper
• Magnesium	• Fluoride
• Phosphorus	• Iodine
• Potassium	• Iron
• Sodium	• Manganese
• Sulphur	• Molybdenum
	• Selenium
	• Zinc

TABLE 42-5 NUTRITIONAL THERAPY

Foods High in Iron

These foods provide 25%–39% of the dietary reference intake (DRI) of iron.

Food	Serving Size
Breads, Cereals, and Grain Products	
Farina, regular or quick-cooked (enriched)	157 mL (⅔ cup)
Oatmeal, instant, fortified, prepared (enriched)	157 mL (⅔ cup)
Ready-to-eat cereals, fortified (enriched)	30 g
Meat, Poultry, Fish, and Alternatives	
Beef liver, braised	90 g
Pork liver, braised	90 g
Chicken or turkey liver, braised	118 mL (½ cup), diced
Clams: steamed, boiled, or canned (drained)	90 g
Oysters: baked, broiled, steamed, or canned (undrained)	90 g
Soybeans, cooked	118 mL (½ cup)

food preferences. *Vegans* eat only plant-based food, whereas *lacto-ovo-vegetarians* eat plant-based foods as well as dairy products and eggs.

Vegetarians can be at risk for vitamin, mineral, or protein deficiencies unless their diets are well planned. Plant protein, although of a lesser quality than that of animal origin, fulfills most of the protein requirements in a vegetarian diet. Combinations of vegetable-protein foods (e.g., rice and kidney beans) can increase digestibility and nutritional quality. Lacto-ovo-vegetarians obtain additional protein from dairy products and eggs. Soy milk fortified with calcium and vitamin D is a good source of protein and can be an alternative to cow's milk. Many palatable meat analogue products are now available for individuals following a vegetarian diet.

The primary risk for nutrient deficiency in a strict vegan is lack of cobalamin (vitamin B_{12}). Vegans not taking cobalamin supplements or consuming foods fortified with cobalamin are susceptible to the development of megaloblastic anemia and the neurological signs of cobalamin deficiency. Strict vegetarians and lacto-ovo-vegetarians are also at risk for iron deficiency. The iron in plant-based foods such as legumes, dark-green leafy vegetables, iron-fortified cereals, and whole grains and cereals is poorly absorbed. Table 42-5 lists examples of foods high in iron. Consuming foods rich in vitamin C (e.g., citrus fruits, tomatoes, potatoes, peppers, and strawberries) will enhance the absorption of iron from plant-based iron-rich foods.

CULTURALLY COMPETENT CARE

People's unique cultural heritages may affect their eating customs and nutritional status. Each culture has its own beliefs and behaviours related to food and the role that food plays in the etiology and treatment of disease. In addition, culture and religion can influence what food is considered edible as well as how it is prepared and when it is eaten. It is important to consider cultural, religious, and ethnic influences when assessing a patient's nutritional status and suggesting interventions requiring dietary changes. Additionally, the nurse should avoid *cultural stereotyping* by making assumptions or generalizations about diet based on an individual's cultural background. Dietary habits differ considerably within and among ethnic groups (Colby, 2013). Acculturation, the extent to which immigrants adopt attributes of a new culture, can also affect dietary practices (Deng, Zhang, & Chan, 2013).

MALNUTRITION

Malnutrition is a deficit, excess, or imbalance of the essential components of a balanced diet. Malnutrition can refer to alterations in macronutrients (carbohydrates, proteins, and fat) or micronutrients (electrolytes, minerals, and vitamins). The terms *undernutrition* and *overnutrition* are also used to describe malnutrition.

Undernutrition affects body tissues, functional ability, and overall health (Allard, Keller, Jeejeebhoy, et al., 2015). Undernutrition does exist in Canada, where income-related food insecurity is increasingly acknowledged as a key social determinant of health. Between 2013 and 2014, about 12% of all Canadian households experienced food insecurity (Tarasuk, Mitchell, & Dachner, 2016). The food insecurity rate was lower among households with children than those with only adults. In many food-insecure households in Canada, adults were protecting children by compromising their own nutrition. Lone-parent families with children under 18 years and households in Nunavut reported the highest rates of food insecurity in Canada (15.7% and 46.8% respectively) (Tarasuk, Mitchell, & Dachner, 2016).

Malnutrition is a problem in both developing and developed countries and across the continuum of care (community, hospital, long-term care). Prevalence of malnutrition in Canadian hospitals has been reported to be 15% to 75% (Allard, Keller, Jeejeebhoy, et al., 2015).

Etiology of Malnutrition

Several terms describe the types and causes of adult malnutrition. Protein–calorie malnutrition (PCM) is the most common form of undernutrition. The following etiology-based terms are preferred for use in clinical practice settings, as they indicate the interaction and importance of inflammation on nutritional status (White, Guenter, Jensen, et al., 2012).

• *Starvation-related malnutrition*, or primary PCM, occurs when nutritional needs are not met (Figure 42-2). In primary PCM, there is chronic starvation without inflammation (e.g., anorexia nervosa).

• *Chronic disease–related malnutrition*, or secondary PCM, is associated with conditions that have sustained mild to moderate inflammation. It occurs when dietary intake does not meet tissue needs because of disease, although it would under normal conditions. Examples of conditions associated

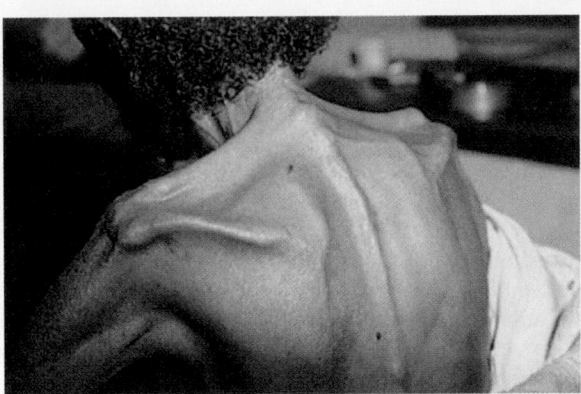

FIGURE 42-2 Patient with malnutrition. Source: Morgan, S. L., & Weiniser, R. (1998). *Fundamentals of clinical nutrition* (2nd ed.). St. Louis: Mosby.

TABLE 42-6	CONDITIONS THAT INCREASE THE RISK FOR MALNUTRITION

- Dementia
- Depression
- Alcohol use disorder
- Excessive dieting to lose weight
- Swallowing disorders (e.g., neurological conditions, head and neck cancer, stroke)
- Decreased mobility that limits access to food or its preparation
- Nutrient losses from malabsorption, dialysis, fistulas, or wounds
- Drugs with antinutrient or catabolic properties, such as corticosteroids and oral antibiotics
- Extreme need for nutrients because of hypermetabolism or stresses such as infection, burns, trauma, or fever
- No oral intake, receiving standard intravenous solutions (e.g., 5% dextrose), or both for 5 days

with this type of malnutrition include organ failure, cancer, rheumatoid arthritis, obesity, and metabolic syndrome.

- *Acute disease– or injury-related malnutrition* is associated with acute disease or injury states with marked inflammatory response (e.g., major infection, burns, trauma, surgery).

Many factors contribute to the development of malnutrition, including socioeconomic factors, physical illnesses, incomplete diets, food–drug interactions, and psychological illness such as eating disorders. Table 42-6 lists conditions that increase the risk for malnutrition.

Socioeconomic Factors. At every stage of the life cycle, health is directly or indirectly influenced by key determinants of health such as education and literacy, income and social status, employment and working conditions, and social environments (PHAC, 2014). Although the health of Canadians is considered to be very good by international standards, a number of factors influence overall quality of life, including the aging of the population; increasing survival rates for potentially fatal conditions; and changes in behaviours related to eating, physical activity, and the use of substances such as drugs, tobacco, and alcohol.

The Food and Agriculture Organization (FAO) of the United Nations (1996) defines **food security** as "when all people, at all times, have physical and economic access to sufficient, safe and nutritious food to meet their dietary needs and food preferences for an active and healthy life." Individuals or families with limited financial resources may have *food insecurity* (inadequate access). Food insecurity is problematic, as it affects the overall quality

(i.e., nutritional value) and quantity of food that is available. Families with food insecurity often choose less expensive "filling" foods, which are more energy dense (high fat) and less nutritious. This type of diet increases the risk for nutrient deficiencies.

Individuals and families may use "safety net programs," including food-assistance programs, housing and energy subsidies, and in-kind contributions from relatives, friends, food pantries, or charitable organizations to help them obtain food. Many families with limited economic resources struggle through the "heat or eat" phenomenon: trying both to pay household utility bills and to put food on the table but sometimes having to choose one or the other. Older adults on a fixed income may have an added burden of deciding whether to pay for medications or buy food. The nurse and the dietitian can assist patients in making food choices that meet nutritional requirements while staying within their limited resources.

Individuals and families with lower social economic status are less likely to consume the nutrients needed for proper health and well-being than those earning higher incomes (Health Canada, 2015b). Studies have also linked food insecurity to the prevalence of unhealthy weights. Lower-income families consume more energy-dense, nutrient-poor diets, whereas families with higher income consume more whole grains, lean meats, low-fat dairy products, and fresh vegetables and fruit.

Physical Illnesses. Regardless of the illness, an individual who is ill has increased nutritional needs. Pathological conditions are frequently aggravated by undernutrition, and an existing nutrient deficiency is likely to become more severe during illness. Malnutrition is a common consequence of illness, surgery, injury, or hospitalization. Hospitalized patients, especially older adults, are at risk of becoming malnourished. Prolonged illness, major surgery, sepsis, draining wounds, burns, hemorrhage, fractures, and immobilization can all contribute to malnutrition.

Anorexia, nausea, vomiting, diarrhea, abdominal distension, and cramping may accompany diseases of the gastro-intestinal (GI) system. Any combination of these symptoms interferes with usual food consumption and metabolism. Whereas *anorexia* is a loss of normal appetite and may occur as a result of physical or mental illness, *cachexia* refers to a wasting syndrome that causes weakness and loss of weight, fat, and muscle. Cachexia is a major cause of morbidity and mortality in patients with cancer, human immunodeficiency virus (HIV), or other serious long-term illnesses such as chronic obstructive pulmonary disease.

Fever accompanies many illnesses, injuries, and infections, with a concomitant increase in the body's basal metabolic rate (BMR) and nitrogen loss. Each degree of temperature increase on the Celsius scale raises the BMR by about 13%. Without an increase in caloric intake, the body uses protein stores to supply calories, and protein depletion develops. After the body temperature returns to normal, the rate of protein breakdown and resynthesis may be increased for several weeks.

Consider the nutritional requirements of a patient who is not overtly ill but is undergoing diagnostic studies. This patient may be nutritionally fit on entering the hospital but can become malnourished because of the dietary restrictions imposed by multiple diagnostic studies.

Malabsorption syndrome is the impaired absorption of nutrients from the GI tract. Decreases in digestive enzymes or in bowel surface area can quickly lead to a deficiency state. Many medications have undesirable GI adverse effects and alter normal digestive and absorptive processes. Antibiotic use appears to modify the intestinal microbiome in the normal state. New research suggests that the microbiome likely plays a critical role in the healthy human immune system and metabolism (Tuddenham & Sears, 2015).

Use of Probiotics. The FAO of the United Nations and the World Health Organization define probiotics as "living microorganisms, which when administered in adequate amounts confer health benefits on the host" (Morelli & Capurso, 2012). Recent research suggests that changes in the gut microbiota may increase a person's predisposition to certain diseases (Zhang, Li, Gan, et al., 2015). Dietary nutrients may be converted into metabolites by intestinal microbes that serve as biologically active molecules, which affect regulatory functions in the host. Probiotics may restore the composition of the gut microbiome and introduce beneficial functions to gut microbial communities, resulting in amelioration or prevention of gut inflammation (Hemarajata & Versalovic, 2013).

Incomplete Diets. Vitamin deficiencies are rare in most developed countries. When present, vitamin deficiencies usually involve several vitamins. When vitamin imbalances occur because of incomplete diets, they are often found among people with a pattern of alcohol or drug use, people who are chronically ill, such as patients on hemodialysis or those receiving cancer treatment, and individuals who maintain poor dietary practices. People who have had GI surgery may be at risk for vitamin deficiencies. For example, resection of the terminal ileum poses a risk for deficiencies of fat-soluble vitamins. After a gastrectomy, patients require cobalamin (vitamin B_{12}) supplementation. Individuals following fad diets or those with poorly planned vegetarian diets are also at risk.

Clinical manifestations of vitamin imbalances are most commonly exhibited as neurological manifestations. In the growing child, the central nervous system (CNS) is primarily involved, whereas the peripheral nervous system is most often affected in adults. The recommended DRIs and manifestations of deficiencies are presented in Table 42-1.

Drug–Nutrient Interactions. A *drug–nutrient interaction* occurs when a medication affects the use of nutrients in the body. Many medications may interact with food or beverages. Potential adverse interactions include incompatibilities, altered drug effectiveness, and impaired nutritional status. For example, many medications produce adverse effects such as changes in taste, changes in appetite, and nausea. Grapefruit juice can increase the absorption of some drugs, enhancing their effect. Recently, individuals taking thyroid replacement hormone (e.g., levothyroxine [Synthroid]) have been instructed to avoid taking dairy products, antacids, or iron preparations within one hour of taking their medication.

Drug–nutrient interactions can also occur with over-the-counter medications and herbs and dietary supplements. The role of the interdisciplinary team is to monitor and prevent these potential interactions for patients while in the hospital and before discharge.

Eating Disorders. Eating disorders are complex psychiatric disorders strongly associated with other mental illnesses, such as mood, personality, and anxiety disorders. Society's promotion of an ideal body image has also been implicated. Eating disorders have the highest mortality rate of any mental illness. Data provided to the Standing Committee on the Status of Women suggest that as many as 600 000 to 900 000 Canadians meet the diagnostic criteria for an eating disorder, with an even larger number of individuals reporting symptoms that are seriously debilitating but insufficient for diagnosis (LeBlanc, 2014). Eating disorders involve a serious disturbance in eating behaviour in addition to disturbances in perception of body size and shape. There is increasing evidence to suggest that up to 20% of all patients with an eating disorder are male (LeBlanc, 2014). Male and female patients have similar psychological comorbidities, including depression and anxiety. The manifestation of eating disorders in boys and men may be different than those in girls and women. Some men may pursue weight loss, while others may seek to increase their weight through weightlifting (LeBlanc, 2014).

The *female athlete triad* is a syndrome in which eating disorders, amenorrhea, and osteoporosis are present (De Souza, Nattiv, Joy, et al., 2014). The triad is seen in females participating in sports that emphasize leanness and low body weight.

Anorexia Nervosa. Anorexia nervosa is a serious, often chronic, and life-threatening eating disorder characterized by self-imposed weight loss, endocrine dysfunction, and a distorted psychopathological attitude toward weight and eating (National Eating Disorder Information Centre [NEDIC], 2014). It manifests clinically as abnormal weight loss, deliberate self-starvation, intense fear of gaining weight or becoming fat, lanugo (soft, downy hair covering the body except the palms and soles), refusal to eat, continuous dieting, hair loss, sensitivity to cold, compulsive exercising, absent or irregular menstruation, dry skin, and constipation. Diagnostic studies often show iron-deficiency anemia and an elevated serum urea (nitrogen) level that reflects marked intravascular volume depletion and prerenal azotemia. A lack of potassium in the diet and loss of potassium in the urine lead to potassium deficiency resulting in muscle weakness, cardiac dysrhythmias, and renal failure. If the eating pattern continues for a prolonged time, body wasting with signs of severe malnutrition become evident, and death may be imminent.

Multidisciplinary treatment must involve a combination of nutritional support and psychiatric care. Although most of the treatment for an eating disorder is provided in the community, hospitalization may be necessary for patients with severe physical complications that cannot be managed in an outpatient setting. Nutritional replenishment must be closely supervised to ensure consistent and ongoing weight gain. Refeeding syndrome (discussed later in the chapter) is a rare but serious complication of refeeding programs. The use of enteral or parenteral feedings may be necessary. Improved nutrition is not a cure for anorexia nervosa; the underlying psychiatric problem must be identified and addressed.

Bulimia Nervosa. Bulimia nervosa is an eating disorder characterized by frequent binge eating, self-induced vomiting associated with loss of control over eating, and a persistent concern with body image (NEDIC, 2014). Individuals with bulimia nervosa may have a normal body mass index (BMI) but weight that fluctuates with bingeing and purging. They may abuse diet drugs, laxatives, or diuretics, or they may exercise excessively. Signs of frequent vomiting—such as macerated knuckles, swollen salivary glands, broken blood vessels in the eyes, and dental problems—are common. Abnormal laboratory parameters, including hypokalemia, metabolic alkalosis, and elevated serum amylase, may occur with frequent vomiting (Westmoreland, Krantz, & Mehler, 2016).

The cause of bulimia remains unclear. It is thought to be similar to that of anorexia nervosa. Substance abuse, anxiety, affective disorders, and personality disturbances have been reported among persons with bulimia. Patients with bulimia often go to great lengths to conceal abnormal eating habits. As the behaviour persists, many problems associated with the

EVIDENCE-INFORMED PRACTICE

Research Highlight

What Is the Effect of Internet-Based Interventions on Eating Disorders?
Clinical Question
In persons with eating disorders (P), are Internet-based interventions (I) effective in the treatment of eating-disorder behaviours (O)?

Synthesis of Best Available Evidence
- Systematic review of randomized controlled trials (RCTs) and nonrandomized controlled studies.
- Eight studies of persons (n=609) diagnosed with bulimia nervosa, binge eating, or more than one eating disorder. Participants were mainly females (97%) with average age of 24 to 45 years old. In most studies, cognitive behavioural therapy (CBT) with a guided self-help component was the basis of the intervention. Planned contact between coach and participant averaged once per week. Outcomes were symptoms of eating-disorder behaviours (e.g., binge eating and purging), anxiety, depression, and quality of life.
- Significant reductions were noted in binge eating and purging. Improvements in depressive symptoms, anxiety, and quality of life were also reported.

Conclusions
- Internet-based interventions using CBT have positive effects on reducing bulimia nervosa and binge eating.

Implications for Nursing Practice
- Why is it important for health care providers to facilitate alternative methods of treatment delivery other than face-to-face?
- How can a nurse help a patient with an eating disorder who resides in a rural area and regularly misses clinic appointments because of transportation problems?

Reference for Evidence
Dölemeyer, R., Tietjen, A., Kersting, A., et al. (2013). Internet-based interventions for eating disorders in adults: A systematic review. *BMC Psychiatry, 13*, 207. doi:10.1186/1471-244X-13-207.

P, patient population of interest; *I*, intervention or area of interest; *O*, outcome(s) of interest (see Chapter 1).

condition become increasingly hard for patients to deal with effectively.

As with anorexia, a treatment combination of psychological counselling and diet therapy is essential, as are education and emotional support for the patient and the family. Fluoxetine (Prozac) is the only Health Canada–approved antidepressant for treating bulimia nervosa. However, it may not be appropriate in all patients with bulimia. Support groups such as the National Eating Disorder Information Centre (see the Resources at the end of this chapter) are helpful to those affected by these disorders.

Pathophysiology of Starvation

Knowledge of the pathophysiology of the starvation process is useful in understanding the physiological changes that occur in PCM. Initially, the body selectively uses carbohydrates (glycogen) rather than fat and protein to meet metabolic needs. These carbohydrate stores, found in the liver and muscles, are minimal and may be depleted within 18 hours. During this early phase of starvation, the only use of protein is in its obligatory participation in cellular metabolism. However, once carbohydrate stores are depleted, protein begins to be converted to glucose for energy. The resulting available plasma glucose allows the metabolic processes to continue. As the body uses amino acids for energy, a negative nitrogen balance (greater nitrogen excretion) occurs. However, within 5 to 9 days, body fat is fully mobilized to supply much of the needed energy.

In prolonged starvation, up to 97% of calories are provided by fat, and protein is conserved. Depletion of fat stores depends on the amount available; fat stores are generally exhausted within 4 to 6 weeks. Once fat stores are depleted, protein, including that from internal organs and plasma, can no longer be spared and rapidly decreases, as it is the only remaining source of energy.

If malnourished patients have surgery, experience bodily trauma, or have an infection, the stress response, with concomitant increase in energy expenditure, is superimposed on the starvation response, resulting in an increase in the metabolic rate and a subsequent increase in energy requirements. Protein stores are no longer spared and are used with increasing frequency to meet the demands of the increased metabolic needs.

As protein depletion continues, liver function becomes impaired, and synthesis of protein decreases. As a result of this decrease, the plasma oncotic pressure lowers. A major function of plasma proteins, primarily of albumin, is to maintain the osmotic pressure of the blood. Because of this decreased plasma oncotic pressure, body fluids shift from the vascular space into the interstitial compartment. As protein ingestion decreases and body stores are depleted, albumin eventually leaks into the interstitial space along with the fluid. Edema becomes clinically observable, and when present in the face and the legs of a patient, it often masks underlying wasting of muscle.

As total blood volume is reduced, the skin appears dry and wrinkled. With the shift of fluids to the interstitial space, ions also move. Sodium (a predominant extracellular ion) is found in increased amounts within the cell, and potassium (a predominant intracellular ion) and magnesium shift to the extracellular space. The sodium–potassium exchange pump has high energy needs, using 20% to 50% of all calories ingested. When the diet is extremely deficient in calories and essential proteins, the pump will fail, leaving sodium inside the cell (along with water), and the cell will expand, resulting in edema.

The liver is the organ that loses the most mass during protein deprivation. It gradually becomes infiltrated with fat, secondary to decreased synthesis of lipoproteins. Immediate intervention is required, or death will rapidly ensue.

Impact of Inflammation. Inflammation affects nutrient metabolism and is an important component of nutritional status. During the starvation process, there is a decreased BMR, sparing of skeletal muscle, and decreased protein breakdown. However, in inflammatory states, there are alterations in the expression of proinflammatory (e.g., interleukin-6) and anti-inflammatory cytokines (e.g., interleukin-10). These cytokine changes result in increased protein and skeletal muscle breakdown, increased BMR, increased glucose turnover, decreased negative acute-phase protein (albumin, prealbumin) production, and increased positive acute-phase protein (e.g., C-reactive protein [CRP]) production (Jensen, 2015; Jensen, Hsiao, & Wheeler, 2012).

Clinical Manifestations

The clinical manifestations of malnutrition range from mild to emaciation and death. The most obvious signs on physical examination are apparent in the skin (dry and scaly skin, brittle nails, rashes, hair loss), mouth (crusting and ulceration, changes in tongue), muscles (decreased mass and weakness), and CNS (mental changes such as confusion, irritability). The speed at which malnutrition develops depends on the quantity and quality of the protein intake, caloric value, illness, and the person's age.

The manifestations of malnutrition result from numerous interactions at the cellular level. As protein intake declines, the muscles (which are the largest store of protein in the body) become wasted and flabby. This wasting away leads to weakness and fatigability. Decreased protein is available for tissue repair, causing delayed wound healing. The person becomes more susceptible to infections. Both humoral and cell-mediated immunity are deficient. Leukocytes in the peripheral blood decrease. Impaired phagocytosis occurs because of the lack of energy needed to drive the process. Many malnourished people are anemic, generally because of nutritional deficiencies in iron and folic acid (necessary building blocks for red blood cells [RBCs]).

NURSING MANAGEMENT
HIGH-RISK NUTRITIONAL STATUS

NURSING ASSESSMENT

Regardless of setting, the nurse must be aware of the nutritional status of the patient. The nurse is often the first-line health care provider dealing with a patient. The patient's height, weight, and diet history are important components of any nursing assessment.

Nutritional status may well be a major factor in the outcome of, and perhaps the underlying reason for, many illnesses.

In many institutions, nurses are responsible for initial nutrition screening to identify individuals who are malnourished or at risk for malnutrition. Results of nutrition screening determine whether a more detailed nutrition assessment is necessary (Table 42-7).

Nutrition screening, the first step in assessing nutritional status, can be completed in any setting (e.g., clinic, home, hospital, long-term care facilities). Based on readily obtained data, nutrition screening is an efficient way to identify individuals at nutrition risk, including those who have experienced unintentional weight loss, inadequate food intake, or recent illness. A variety of valid tools, such as the Canadian Nutrition Screening Tool (CNST), is available for screening different populations (Figure 42-3).

ASSESSMENT OF NUTRITIONAL INTAKE. Individuals identified as being at nutritional risk during screening should be referred, when possible, to a dietitian to undergo a *comprehensive nutritional assessment*, which includes evaluation of dietary history and clinical information, physical examination, and anthropometric measures.

Various methods for collecting current dietary intake information are available, including the 24-hour recall, food frequency questionnaire, and food diary. Documentation of nutritional

TABLE 42-7 NURSING ASSESSMENT

Malnutrition

Subjective Data **Important Health Information** *Current health:* ↑ or ↓ weight, weight problems; ↑ or ↓ appetite, typical dietary intake; food preferences and aversions; food allergies or intolerances; ill-fitting or absent dentures; dry mouth, difficulty in chewing or swallowing; bloating or gas; ↑ sensitivity to cold; delayed wound healing; constipation, diarrhea, nocturia, decreased urinary output *Past health history:* Severe burns, major trauma, hemorrhage, draining wounds, bone fractures with prolonged immobility, chronic renal or liver disease, cancer, malabsorption syndrome, GI obstruction, infectious diseases (e.g., TB, AIDS), acute (e.g., trauma, sepsis) or chronic (e.g., rheumatoid arthritis) inflammatory condition *Medications:* Corticosteroids, chemotherapeutic agents, diet pills *Surgery or other treatments:* Recent surgery, radiation *Functional assessment:* ↑ or ↓ activity patterns; weakness, fatigue, ↓ endurance; alcohol or drug abuse; change in family (e.g., loss of a spouse); financial resources **Objective Data** **General** Listless, cachectic; underweight for height **Integumentary** Dry, brittle, sparse hair with colour changes and lack of lustre, alopecia; dry, scaly lips, fever blisters, angular crusts and lesions at corners of mouth (cheilosis); brittle, ridged nails; ↓ tone and elasticity of skin; cool, rough, dry, scaly skin with brown-grey pigment changes; reddened, scaly dermatitis, scrotal dermatitis; slight cyanosis; peripheral edema **Eyes** Pale or red conjunctivae, grey keratinized epithelium on conjunctiva (Bitot's spots); dryness and dull appearance of conjunctiva and cornea, soft cornea; blood vessel growth in cornea; redness and fissuring of eyelid corners	**Respiratory** ↓ respiratory rate, ↓ vital capacity, crackles, weak cough **Cardiovascular** ↑ or ↓ heart rate, ↓ BP, dysrhythmias **Gastro-Intestinal** Swollen, smooth, raw, beefy red tongue (glossitis), hypertrophic or atrophic papillae; dental caries, absent or loose teeth, discoloured tooth enamel; spongy, pale, receded gums with a tendency to bleed easily, periodontal disease; ulcerations, white patches or plaques, redness, swelling of oral mucosa; distended, tympanic abdomen; ascites, hepatomegaly, ↓ bowel sounds; steatorrhea **Neurological** Decreased or loss of reflexes, tremor; inattention, irritability, confusion, syncope **Musculo-Skeletal** ↓ muscle mass with poor tone, "wasted" appearance; bow legs, knock knees, beaded ribs, chest deformity, prominent bony structures **Possible Diagnostic Findings** ↓ hemoglobin and hematocrit; ↓ MCV, MCH, or MCHC (iron deficiency); ↑ MCV or MCH (folic acid or cobalamin deficiency); altered serum electrolyte levels, especially hyperkalemia; ↓ BUN (serum urea [nitrogen]) and creatinine; ↓ serum albumin, transferrin, and prealbumin; ↓ lymphocytes; ↑ liver enzymes; ↓ serum vitamin levels

AIDS, acquired immune deficiency syndrome; *BP,* blood pressure; *BUN,* blood urea nitrogen; *GI,* gastro-intestinal; *MCH,* mean corpuscular hemoglobin; *MCHC,* mean corpuscular hemoglobin concentration; *MCV,* mean corpuscular volume; *TB,* tuberculosis.

Ask the patient the following questions*	Date:		Date:	
	Admission		Rescreening	
	Yes	No	Yes	No
Have you lost weight in the past 6 months **WITHOUT TRYING** to lose this weight? If the patient reports a weight loss but gained it back, consider it as NO weight loss.				
Have you been eating less than usual **FOR MORE THAN A WEEK**?				
Two "YES" answers indicate nutrition risk				

* If the patient is unable to answer the questions, a knowledgeable informant can be used to obtain the information. If the patient is uncertain regarding weight loss, ask if clothing is now fitting more loosely.

FIGURE 42-3 Canadian Nutrition Screening Tool (CNST). Source: Canadian Malnutrition Task Force. (March 2014). *Canadian nutrition screening tool.* Retrieved from *http://nutritioncareincanada.ca/sites/default/uploads/files/CNST.pdf.*

intake for hospitalized patients can best be achieved through calorie counts of nutrients consumed or infused.

The 24-Hour Recall. The most common method of obtaining information about dietary intake is the *24-hour recall*. The individual or family member is asked to recall everything eaten within the past 24 hours. It is important to be aware of potential information gaps when this method is used: (a) the individual or family member may not be able to recall type or amount of food eaten; (b) intake within the past 24 hours may be atypical of usual intake; (c) the individual or family member may alter the truth for a variety of reasons; and (d) snack items and use of gravies, sauces, and condiments may be under-reported.

The Food Frequency Questionnaire. To counter some of the challenges inherent in the 24-hour recall method, a *food frequency questionnaire* may also be completed. Information is collected related to how many times per day, week, or month an individual eats particular foods. The food frequency questionnaire does not quantify amount of food eaten, and, similar to the 24-hour recall, it relies on the individual's or family member's memory.

The Food Diary. Food diaries require the individual or family member to write down everything consumed for a certain period of time. Three days—2 working and 1 nonworking day—are customarily used. A food diary is most accurate if the individual is instructed to record information immediately after eating. Potential challenges with the food diary include (a) nonadherence, (b) inaccurate recording, (c) atypical intake on the recording days, and (d) conscious alteration of diet during the recording period.

Direct Observation. *Direct observation* of the feeding and eating process can lead to detection of problems not readily identified through standard nutrition interviews. For example, observing the typical feeding techniques used by a parent or caregiver and the interaction between the individual and the caregiver can be of value when assessing failure to thrive in children or unintentional weight loss in older adults.

ANTHROPOMETRIC MEASUREMENTS. *Anthropometric measurements* are gross measures of fat and muscle contents. These measurements are most beneficial when done serially and by well-trained anthropometrists to evaluate long-term effects of malnutrition or responses to nutritional interventions. They consist of measures of skinfold thickness at various sites, which are indicators of subcutaneous fat stores, and midarm muscle circumference, an indicator of protein stores. These measurements are then compared with standards for healthy people of the same age and gender.

The sites most reflective of body fat are those over the biceps and the triceps, below the scapula, above the iliac crest, and over the upper thigh. Both skinfold thickness and midarm circumference are decreased in malnutrition. These measurements may also be influenced by shifts in hydration status. The exact relationship of the midarm circumference measure to body composition of functional protein, both muscle and nonmuscle, remains to be established.

LABORATORY STUDIES. The diagnosis of PCM is best determined by laboratory studies of body composition, including a thorough history of weight loss, dietary history, and measures of functional status and inflammation. Serum albumin has a half-life of approximately 20 to 22 days. In the absence of marked fluid loss, such as from hemorrhage or burns, the serum albumin value lags behind actual protein changes by more than 2 weeks and therefore is not a good indicator of acute changes in nutritional status. Prealbumin, a protein synthesized by the liver, has a half-life of 2 days and is a better indicator of recent or current nutritional status.

However, the extent to which visceral proteins, including albumin, prealbumin, and transferrin, are true markers of malnutrition is questionable. Albumin, prealbumin, and transferrin are *negative acute-phase proteins,* which means that during an inflammatory response, the synthesis of these proteins in the liver is decreased. Therefore, low or below-normal levels of these negative acute-phase proteins correspond to an inflammatory state rather than accurately indicating nutritional status.

CRP, which is a *positive acute-phase protein,* is typically elevated during inflammation and predicts morbidity and mortality. Serum electrolyte levels reflect changes between the intracellular and extracellular spaces. Serum potassium level is often elevated. The RBC count and the hemoglobin level indicate the presence and degree of anemia. The total lymphocyte count decreases with malnutrition. Liver enzyme levels, a reflection of liver function, may be elevated during malnutrition. Serum levels of fat- and water-soluble vitamins are usually decreased. The lowered serum levels of the fat-soluble vitamins correlate with the clinical signs of steatorrhea (fatty stools).

NURSING DIAGNOSES

Nursing diagnoses for the patient with malnutrition include but are not limited to the following:

- *Imbalanced nutrition: less than body requirements* related to *insufficient dietary intake* (decreased access, ingestion, digestion, or absorption of food)

- *Feeding self-care deficit* related to *fatigue, weakness, discomfort*
- *Deficient fluid volume* related to *insufficient fluid intake* (access to or absorption of fluids)
- *Risk for impaired skin integrity* as evidenced by *inadequate nutrition*
- *Ineffective health maintenance* related to *ineffective coping strategies, insufficient resources*

PLANNING

The overall goals are that the patient with malnutrition will (a) achieve weight gain, (b) consume a specified number of calories per day (with a diet individualized for the patient), and (c) have no adverse consequences related to malnutrition or nutrition therapies.

NURSING IMPLEMENTATION

HEALTH PROMOTION. Nurses are in an ideal position to teach and reinforce healthy eating habits with individuals and groups of persons throughout the lifespan. Nurses often collaborate with other health care providers (e.g., dietitians, social workers, physicians) in the nutritional assessment and health education of patients. They may use or refer patients to free nutrition resources from Eat Smart Meet Smart (Saskatchewan) or another provincial or territorial source (see the Resources at the end of this chapter).

As part of the health care team, the nurse can support a patient in improving her or his health status by reinforcing healthy eating habits throughout the lifespan. Encouraging healthy eating by teaching Canada's Food Guide and encouraging patients to read food labels will support the patient in making positive changes. Nutrition labelling is mandatory on all prepared foods. The nutrition facts table (Figure 42-4) provides the information needed to make informed food choices; the table includes the amounts of 13 core nutrients and the calories in each serving.

This information allows for the comparison of food products to facilitate healthier food purchases.

ACUTE CARE. Nurses collaborate with the health care provider and dietitian to identify malnutrition and implement appropriate interventions to meet the patient's nutritional needs. The patient's nutritional state, including risk factors for malnutrition, should be assessed during the nurse's physical evaluation.

With increased stress, such as surgery, severe trauma, and sepsis, the patient needs more calories and protein. Wound healing requires increased protein synthesis. The patient who is malnourished or is at risk for malnutrition and is undergoing major surgery needs several weeks of increased protein and calorie intake preoperatively to promote healing and replenish body stores postoperatively. When fever is present, the metabolic rate increases and nitrogen loss accelerates. Despite the return of body temperature to normal, the rate of protein breakdown and resynthesis may be accelerated for several weeks.

A patient's weight and height should be recorded on admission, and the weight routinely assessed and documented throughout a hospital stay. To ensure accuracy, the nurse should weigh the patient at the same time each day, on the same scale, with the same type or amount of clothing, and with an empty bladder. Before discharge, the patient and caregiver need to be taught the importance of good nutrition and the rationale for recording the daily weight, intake, and output. Daily weights give an ongoing record of body weight gain or loss. Rapid gains and losses are usually the result of shifts in fluid balance. In conjunction with accurate recording of food and fluid intake, the body weight provides a clearer picture of the patient's fluid and nutritional state.

If the patient is able to take food by mouth, obtaining a daily calorie count and diet diary can help ensure an accurate record of food intake. The nurse and the dietitian can assist the patient and family in selecting high-calorie and high-protein foods (unless medically contraindicated). Offering foods preferred by the patient enhances intake, so the family should be encouraged to bring the patient's favourite foods from home.

The environment should be conducive to eating: quiet, with the bedside table cleared of clutter and set at the appropriate height, and urinals, bedpans, and emesis basins placed out of sight. The patient should be offered oral hygiene and hand hygiene and assisted into a comfortable position. If the patient needs help, the nurse should open cartons and packages. Nonurgent care should be performed before or after mealtime to avoid unnecessary interruptions.

Undernourished patients usually need between-meal supplements. These may consist of items prepared in the dietary department or commercially prepared products. These items provide extra calories, proteins, fluids, and nutrients. In addition, offering small, frequent meals may improve a patient's tolerance for food intake by distributing the amount of food more evenly throughout the day. If a patient is unable to consume enough nutrition with a high-calorie, high-protein diet, oral liquid nutritional supplements may be added. The protein and calorie intake required by a malnourished patient depends on the cause of the malnutrition, treatments, and stressors affecting the patient.

Some patients may benefit from appetite stimulants such as megestrol acetate (Megace OS) to improve nutritional intake. If the patient is still unable to take in enough calories, enteral feedings may be considered. Contraindications for enteral nutrition (EN) include GI obstruction, prolonged ileus, severe diarrhea or vomiting, and enterocutaneous fistula. If enteral feedings are not feasible, parenteral nutrition (PN) may be initiated.

Nutrition Facts
Per 3/4 cup (175g)

Amount		% Daily Value	
Calories 160			
Fat 2.5 g		**4** %	
Saturated 1.5 g		**8** %	
+ Trans 0 g			
Cholesterol 10 mg			
Sodium 75 mg		**3** %	
Carbohydrate 25 g		**8** %	
Fibre 0 g		**0** %	
Sugars 24 g			
Protein 8 g			
Vitamin A	2 %	Vitamin C	0 %
Calcium	20 %	Iron	0 %

FIGURE 42-4 Nutrition facts table. An interactive version of this table with explanations of the components and other information are available at the Health Canada Food and Nutrition website (see Resources at the end of this chapter). Source: © All rights reserved. *Nutrition Facts Table*. Health Canada, 2012. Adapted and reproduced with permission from the Minister of Health, 2017.

AMBULATORY AND HOME CARE. Patients may be discharged with instructions for a therapeutic diet regimen. Discharge preparation for a patient and family is important. They must be aware of the cause of the undernourished state and strategies to avoid the problem in the future. The patient must be made aware that undernourishment, whatever the cause, can recur and that a diet high in protein and calories for a few weeks cannot fully restore a normal nutritional state; many months are needed to reach this goal. Diet instruction is usually carried out by the dietitian, but it is important for the nurse to assess the patient's understanding and reinforce the information whenever possible. The ability of the patient to follow dietary instructions must be examined in light of past eating habits, religious and ethnic preferences, age, income, community or other resources, and state of health.

The need for continual follow-up care to accomplish and maintain rehabilitation must be emphasized. Discharge planning should include visits by the home health nurse and outpatient dietitian referrals.

EVALUATION

The following are expected outcomes for a patient who is malnourished:

- The patient will achieve and maintain optimal body weight.
- The patient will consume a well-balanced diet.
- The patient will experience no adverse outcomes related to malnutrition.
- The patient will maintain optimal physical functioning.

AGE-RELATED CONSIDERATIONS

MALNUTRITION

Older adults are particularly vulnerable to malnutrition, which increases their rate of hospitalization and care cost. Older hospitalized patients with malnutrition are more likely to have poor wound healing, pressure injuries, infections, decreased muscle strength, postoperative complications, and increased morbidity and mortality risks (DiMaria-Ghalili, 2014). (Pressure injuries are discussed in Chapter 14.) Older adults commonly report a decreased appetite, problems with chewing or swallowing, inadequate nutrient intake, and consumption of only one meal per day. Being on a limited income may play a role in the number of meals eaten per day or the dietary quality of meals. Social isolation is another problem for many older adults. Those who live alone may lose their desire to cook and often report a decrease in appetite. Some older adults may have functional limitations that can affect their ability to purchase food as well as cook and prepare meals. Furthermore, older adults may lack access to transportation to buy food. For a complete list of factors affecting nutritional intake of older adults, see Table 42-8.

Chronic illnesses associated with aging can also affect nutritional status. For example, depression and dysphagia can affect intake. Poor oral health from cavities, gum disease, and missing teeth as well as xerostomia (dry mouth) can impair the older adult's ability to lubricate, masticate, and swallow food. Medications (e.g., antidepressants, antihypertensives, bronchodilators) can cause dry mouth, alter the taste of food, or decrease appetite.

Physiological changes associated with aging include a decrease in lean body mass and redistribution of fat around internal organs, which can decrease caloric requirements. Sarcopenia (loss of lean body mass with aging) affects muscle strength and function (Litchford, 2014). Older adults on bed rest or prolonged inactivity

TABLE 42-8	AGE-RELATED DIFFERENCES IN ASSESSMENT

Factors Affecting Nutritional Intake in Older Adults

Physical Factors	
- Age	- Mental awareness
- Anorexia	- Social isolation
- Decreased number of taste buds	**Socioeconomic Factors**
- Dental problems	- Availability of desired foods
- Food intolerances	- Availability of transportation to food stores
- Health status	- Available time for food preparation and eating
- Physical disability	- Education level and nutritional knowledge
- Prescribed diets	- Financial status
- Prescribed or over-the-counter drugs	- Food restrictions (intentional or unintentional)
Psychosocial Factors	- Lack of food preparation equipment
- Importance of food in the past	
- Loneliness or loss	

lose more lean body mass than younger adults on bed rest do. Changes in odour and taste perception (due to medications, nutrient deficiencies, or taste-bud atrophy) can also alter nutritional status.

Lifestyle changes such as retirement or relocation to residence living can have a significant impact on the eating habits of older adults. Other factors to assess include ethnic background, previous dietary practices, food preferences, knowledge of proper diet, food availability, accessibility of safe food storage, transportation, and health status. Problems related to any or all of these areas can alert the nurse to the possibility of a nutritional problem. For older adult patients living in long-term care establishments, eating with others, having the freedom to choose the menu and one's table companions, having appropriate feeding assistance available, and enjoying a calm atmosphere contribute to residents' experiencing more pleasure and gaining more nutrition from their meals.

Some of the physiological changes associated with aging affect the nutritional status of older adults. The following changes are of particular interest:

1. Changes in the oral cavity (e.g., change in bite surfaces of the teeth, periodontal disease, drying of the mucous membranes of the mouth and tongue, poorly fitting dentures, decreased muscle strength for chewing, decreased number of taste buds, decreased saliva production)
2. Changes in digestion and motility (e.g., decreased absorption of cobalamin, vitamin A, and folic acid and decreased GI motility)
3. Changes in the endocrine system (e.g., decreased tolerance to glucose)
4. Changes in the musculo-skeletal system (e.g., decreased bone density, degenerative joint changes)
5. Decrease in vision and hearing (e.g., procurement and preparation of food are more difficult)

Certain illnesses that are more prevalent in the older population are considered to be diet related. These include atherosclerosis, osteoporosis, diabetes mellitus, dementia, cancer, and diverticulosis. Multiple drugs are often required to treat these and other common chronic illnesses of older patients, and many of these drugs have an adverse effect on the appetite, increasing the possibility of inadequate nutrition.

Daily requirements for healthy older adults to maintain their weight include 30 kcal/kg of body weight and 0.8 to 1 g/kg of protein per day, with no more than 30% of calories coming from fat. Requirements may differ among individuals, depending on the degree of malnutrition and physiological stress. To prevent loss of muscle mass and maintain function, older adults should consume a moderate amount of high-quality protein at each meal (Litchford, 2014). Daily vitamin D requirements are also higher for older adults.

Malnutrition can occur in an older person independent of changes in weight and energy requirements. Special strategies, such as adaptive devices (e.g., large-handled eating utensils), often are helpful in increasing dietary intake. Some older people may require nutritional support therapies until their strength and general health improve. Before starting any nutritional support therapy (e.g., EN or PN), the nurse should review the older adult's advance directives regarding the use of artificial nutrition and hydration.

Some communities offer community nutrition programs for older people as well as home-delivered meal programs such as Meals on Wheels. However, these programs alone may not be able to fully support older adults in accessing adequate nutritious food. It is not uncommon for older adults to access food banks.

Dysphagia

Dysphagia, or difficulty in swallowing, is a symptom of disease or dysfunction and can result from a number of medical conditions. Among adults, the prevalence of dysphagia ranges from 12% to 13% in acute-care facilities and up to 60% in long-term care facilities (Touhy, Jett, Boscart, et al., 2012). Dysphagia increases the risk for malnutrition, dehydration, choking episodes, aspiration, chest infections or pneumonia, and death; in addition, it can cause psychosocial problems, such as social isolation and embarrassment, which may reduce quality of life (Dietitians of Canada, 2015).

Nurses must carefully assess all patients for signs of dysphagia (Table 42-9). A swallowing assessment, performed by a speech–language pathologist can help identify patients at risk for aspiration, including the location of the swallowing problem and which food consistencies are safest. The speech–language pathologist may also determine swallowing exercises, appropriate head positioning, and swallowing techniques.

The goal of nutrition intervention in dysphagia management should be to minimize weight loss (through adequate energy and protein intakes) and maintain hydration. Diet texture and fluid consistency modifications may be required for patient safety. Food texture may be modified with the addition of sauces or gravies and through mechanical alteration such as mincing or puréeing. The consistency of beverages may also be modified through the use of thickening agents. Thickened fluids range in consistency from nectar-like to honey-like to pudding-like consistency.

SPECIALIZED NUTRITION SUPPORT

Oral Nutrition

If patients are unable to maintain or achieve adequate nutritional status, nutrition support may be necessary. High-calorie oral supplements can help improve the nutritional status of older adults. It is important to note that these supplements should not be used as meal substitutes but between meals as snacks. In some hospitals and long-term care facilities, these beverages are used

---

TABLE 42-9   INDICATORS OF DYSPHAGIA

Obvious Indicators of Dysphagia
- Difficult, painful chewing or swallowing
- Regurgitation of undigested food
- Difficulty controlling food or liquid in the mouth
- Drooling
- Hoarse voice
- Coughing or choking before, during, or after swallowing
- Globus sensation (lump in the throat)
- Nasal regurgitation
- Feeling of obstruction
- Unintentional weight loss—for example, in people with dementia

Less Obvious Indicators of Dysphagia
- Change in respiration pattern
- Unexplained temperature spikes
- Wet voice quality
- Tongue fasciculation (may indicate motor neuron disease)
- Xerostomia
- Heartburn
- Change in eating—for example, eating slowly or avoiding social occasions
- Frequent throat clearing
- Recurrent chest infections
- Atypical chest pain

Source: University of Maryland Medical Centre. (2016). *Dysphagia*. Retrieved from *http://www.umm.edu/health/medical/altmed/condition/dysphagia*.

🔍 EVIDENCE-INFORMED PRACTICE
Research Highlight

Does Nutritional Education Improve Functional Outcomes in Older Adults?
Clinical Question
In older adults (P), what is the effect of nutritional education (I) on diet, physical and emotional functioning, and quality of life (O)?

Best Available Evidence
- Systematic review of RCTs

Critical Appraisal and Synthesis of Evidence
- Twenty-three RCTs (n = 12 610) of community-dwelling older adults (65 yr and older) with various diseases. Five trials with nutritional education only; remaining trials with nutritional and lifestyle advice, exercise advice, or screening. Education varied in format and intensity.
- Outcomes included diet, functional outcomes (e.g., strength, balance), hospital readmissions, depression, anxiety, and quality of life.
- Results showed improved body mass index, weight loss, and physical health with decreased depression.
- Brief interventions were as effective as more lengthy ones.

Conclusion
- Nutritional education alone or in combination with other interventions positively influences physical and emotional health.

Implications for Nursing Practice
- Locate nutritional educational resources for older patients residing at home.
- Help patients identify community programs to make positive changes in lifestyle and exercise.

Reference for Evidence
Young, K., Bunn, F., Trivedi, D., et al. (2011). Nutritional education for community dwelling older people: A systematic review of randomised controlled trials. *International Journal of Nursing Studies, 48*(6), 751–780. doi:10.1016/j.ijnurstu.2011.03.007.

P, patient population of interest; *I*, intervention or area of interest; *O*, outcomes of interest (see Chapter 1).

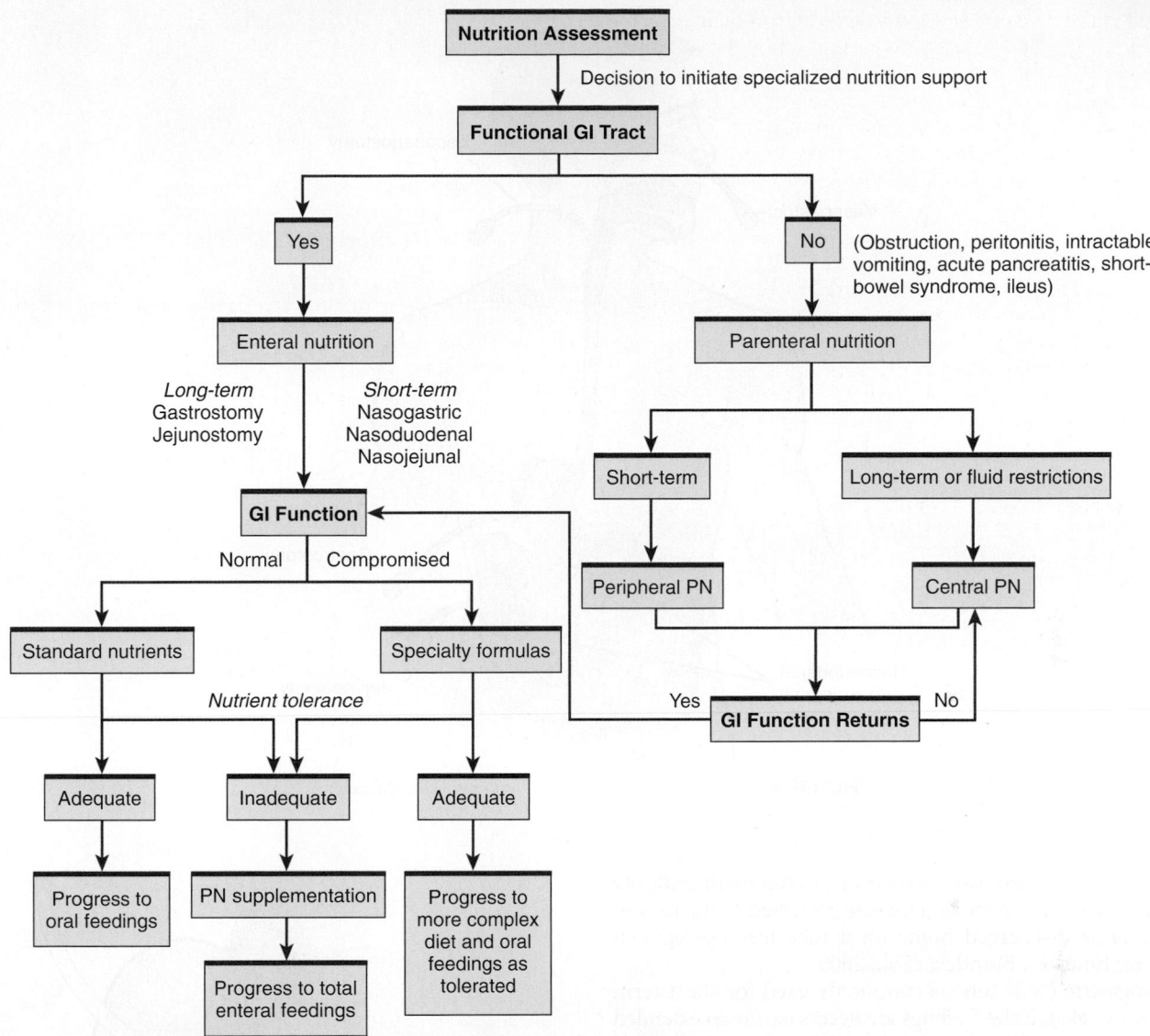

FIGURE 42-5 Nutrition support algorithm. *GI*, gastro-intestinal, *PN*, parenteral nutrition. Source: Adapted with permission of the American Society for Parenteral and Enteral Nutrition (ASPEN). ASPEN Board of Directors. (2002). Guidelines for the use of parenteral and enteral nutrition in adult and pediatric patients. *Journal of Parenteral and Enteral Nutrition, 26*(Suppl. 1), 8SA.

instead of water with oral medication administration to increase caloric or protein intake (often referred to as *Med Pass*).

For patients who are unable to consume enough nutrition orally with a high-calorie, high-protein diet (food and supplements), nutrition support such as EN (also called *tube feeding*) may be considered. If EN is not feasible, PN may be considered. For a decision-making plan related to nutrition support, see the algorithm in Figure 42-5.

Enteral Nutrition

Enteral nutrition (EN), also known as *tube feeding,* is nutrition (e.g., a nutritionally balanced liquefied food or formula) delivered through the GI tract distal to the oral cavity via a tube, catheter, or stoma (Boullata, Carney, & Guenter, 2010). EN may be ordered for the patient who has a functioning GI tract but is unable to take any or enough oral nourishment.

Indications for EN may include anorexia, orofacial fractures, head and neck cancer, neurological or psychiatric conditions that prevent oral intake, extensive burns, critical illness, mechanical ventilation, and chemotherapy or radiation therapy. EN is considered to be more easily administered, safer, more physiologically efficient, and less expensive than PN. EN is used to provide nutrients by way of the GI tract either alone or as a supplement to oral nutrition or PN.

There are a wide variety of enteral formulas. Formula concentration, flavour, osmolality, and amounts of protein, sodium, and fat vary. There are special formulas for patients with diabetes and liver, kidney, or lung disease. Most enteral formulas are lactose free. Most standard formulas provide between 1 and 1.5 kcal/mL; high-energy formulas provide 2 kcal/mL. The more calorically dense the formula, the less water it contains. The number and size of particles in the formula determines its osmolality. The more hydrolyzed or broken down the nutrients, the greater the osmolality.

Common delivery options are continuous or cyclical infusion by pump, intermittent infusion by gravity, or by bolus with a

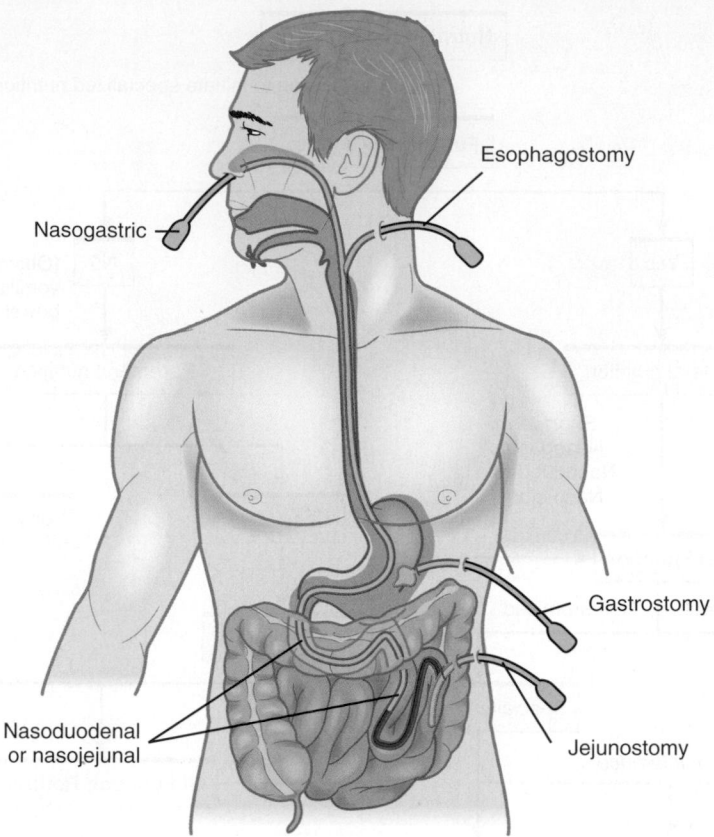

FIGURE 42-6 Common enteral feeding tube placement locations.

syringe. Continuous infusion is used most often with critically ill patients. Intermittent feeding may be preferred as the patient improves or is discharged home on a tube-feeding regimen (Bankhead, Boulatta, Brantley, et al., 2009).

Λ nasogastric (NG) tube is commonly used for short-term feeding (<4 weeks). If the feedings are necessary for an extended time, other means of feeding may be used, such as an esophagostomy tube, a gastrostomy tube, or a jejunostomy tube that delivers nutrients directly into the jejunum. Transpyloric (nasointestinal) tube placement or placement into the jejunum is used when physiological conditions warrant feeding the patient below the pyloric sphincter. Figure 42-6 shows the locations of commonly used enteral feeding tubes.

Orogastric, Nasogastric, and Nasointestinal Tubes. Polyurethane or silicone feeding tubes are long, small in diameter, soft, and flexible, thereby decreasing the risk for mucosal damage from prolonged placement. Polyurethane and silicone tubes are radiopaque, making their position readily identified by radiograph. Placement into the small intestine decreases the likelihood of regurgitation of contents into the esophagus and subsequent aspiration. With the use of a stylet, these tubes can be placed in a comatose patient because the ability to swallow is not essential during insertion.

Although the smaller feeding tubes (12-8 French) have advantages over wider-lumen tubes (≥14 French), such as the standard decompression NG tube, there are some disadvantages. Because of the small diameter, these tubes are more easily occluded, and it can be more problematic to check for gastric residual volumes. They are particularly prone to obstruction when oral drugs have not been thoroughly crushed and dissolved

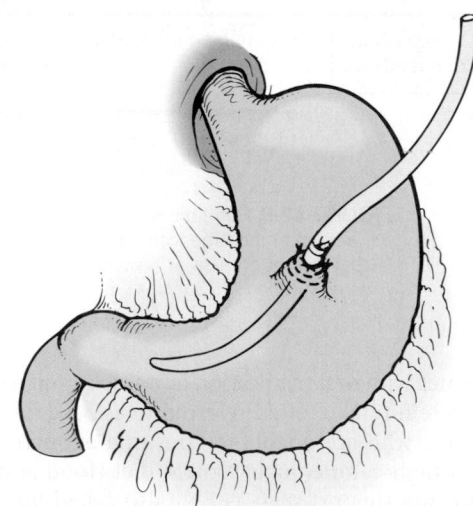

FIGURE 42-7 Placement of a gastrostomy tube. Source: Redrawn from Mahan, L. K., & Arlin, M. (1992). *Krause's food, nutrition, and diet therapy* (8th ed.). Philadelphia: Saunders.

in water before administration. Failure to flush the tubing after both drug administration and residual volume determinations can result in tube clogging. Clogging of the tube may necessitate removal and insertion of a new tube, adding to cost and patient discomfort.

Gastrostomy and Jejunostomy Tubes. A gastrostomy tube may be used for a patient who requires EN over an extended time (>4–6 weeks) (Figure 42-7).

FIGURE 42-8 Percutaneous endoscopic gastrostomy. **A,** Gastrostomy tube placement via percutaneous endoscopy. Using endoscopy, a gastrostomy tube is inserted through the esophagus into the stomach and then pulled through a stab wound made in the abdominal wall. **B,** A retention disc and bumper secure the tube.

Gastrostomy tubes can be placed surgically, radiologically, or endoscopically. The placement of a percutaneous endoscopic gastrostomy (PEG) tube is shown in Figure 42-8. The patient must have an intact, unobstructed GI tract, and the esophageal lumen must be wide enough to pass the endoscope for PEG tube placement. A PEG tube and a radiologically placed gastrostomy tube have several advantages. These procedures have fewer risks than surgical placement. They require IV sedation and local anaesthesia, a technique that can be done at a lower cost. IV antibiotics are given before the procedure.

For the patient with chronic reflux, a jejunostomy tube with continuous feedings may be appropriate to reduce the risk for aspiration (Bankhead, Boullata, Brantley, et al., 2009). Jejunostomy tubes are placed either endoscopically or with open or laparoscopic surgery. Combination gastro-jejunostomy (GJ) tubes allow for simultaneous gastric decompression and small bowel feeding. When a patient has a GJ tube, it is important to know which port is the gastric and which is the jejunal.

Enteral feedings can be started within 24 to 48 hours after surgical placement of a gastrostomy or jejunostomy tube, without waiting for flatus or a bowel movement. Most PEG tube feeding can start within 2 hours of insertion, although institutional policies may vary (Boullata, Carney, & Guenter, 2010). The feeding tube is either premarked or marked at the skin insertion site. At regular intervals, the tube insertion length should be rechecked. The tube is most often connected to a pump for continuous feeding.

Tube Feedings and Safety. Nurses play a critical role in ensuring that tube feedings are administered safely. Aspiration and dislodged tubes are two important safety concerns. Nursing management of tube feedings is addressed in Table 42-10.

Accidental tube removal can result in delayed feedings and potential discomfort because of tube replacement. The management of common problems in patients receiving tube feedings is presented in Table 42-11. A nursing care plan (NCP) 42-1 for the patient receiving enteral nutrition is available on the Evolve website.

Specific care and teaching related to feeding tubes and enteral nutrition are summarized in the following section. Remember

TABLE 42-10 **NURSING MANAGEMENT: FEEDING TUBES**
1. The nurse should check tube placement before feeding and before each drug administration.
2. GI contractility factors should be evaluated when initiating EN; however, overt signs of contractility should not be required prior to initiation of EN.
3. Liquid medications should be used rather than pills, as appropriate.   • Viscous liquid medications should be diluted.   • The nurse should confirm whether medications are intended to be taken with meals.   • Medications should not be added to enteral feeding formula.
4. If it is necessary to use tablets, they should be crushed to a fine powder to prevent clogging feeding tubes.
5. General principles of tube feeding (e.g., bed elevation, checking gastric residual volume, and flushing tube with water) must be followed.
6. The nurse should assess regularly for complications (e.g., aspiration, diarrhea, abdominal distension, hyperglycemia, constipation, and fecal impaction).

EN, enteral nutrition; *GI,* gastro-intestinal.

that it is important to teach the patient and caregiver how to care for the feeding tube and how to properly administer enteral nutrition.

Patient Position. Proper patient positioning decreases the risk for aspiration. To prevent aspiration, the nurse should elevate the head of the bed to a minimum of 30 degrees, but preferably 45 degrees. If the patient does not tolerate a backrest elevation, the reverse Trendelenburg position should be used to elevate the head of the bed unless contraindicated. If the head of the bed needs to be lowered for a procedure, the patient should be returned to an elevated position as soon as possible. Institution policy should be followed for suspending feeding while the patient is supine. If intermittent delivery is used, the head should remain elevated for 30 to 60 minutes after feeding.

Aspiration Risk. All enterally fed patients should be evaluated for risk of aspiration. Before starting tube feedings, the nurse

TABLE 42-11 COMMON PROBLEMS OF PATIENTS RECEIVING TUBE FEEDINGS

Problems and Possible Causes	Corrective Measures	Problems and Possible Causes	Corrective Measures
Vomiting and Aspiration		Contamination of formula or tubing	Change tubing q24h
Improper tube placement	Replace tube in proper position and check tube position before beginning feeding and q8h if feedings are continuous		Follow manufacturer's guidelines for maximum length of time formula can be at room temperature
Delayed gastric emptying, increased residual volume	Hold feeding for 1 hr; then, if residual volume is less than before, resume feeding	Low-fibre formula	Change to formula with more fibre
Aspiration risk	Keep head of bed elevated to 30- to 45-degree angle	Tube moving distally	Properly secure tube before beginning feeding
	Have patient sit up on side of bed or in chair		Check tube position before each feeding or at least q24h if feedings are continuous
	Encourage ambulation unless contraindicated	**Constipation**	
Contamination of formula	Refrigerate unused formula and recording date opened; discard outdated formula every 24 hr	Low fibre	Consult health care provider for change in formula to one with higher fibre content
	Discard formula left standing for longer than manufacturer's guidelines: 8–12 hr for ready-to-feed formulas (cans) or 4 hr for reconstituted formula or closed system as per manufacturer's guidelines		Obtain bowel routine order
		Poor fluid intake	Increase fluid intake if not contraindicated
			Give free water, as well as formula, to a total fluid intake of 30 mL/kg body weight
		Medications	Check for medications that may be constipating
Diarrhea		Impaction	Perform rectal examinations to check for and manually remove feces if present
Feeding too fast, hypertonic formula, or medications	Evaluate number and volume of stools (if greater than three to five per day or >500 mL), consider patient's medical history, and assess abdomen for distension or pain	**Dehydration**	
		Excessive diarrhea, vomiting	Decrease rate or changing formula
	Contact physician, consider medications, and rule out infection (*Clostridium difficile*)		Check drugs that patient is receiving, especially antibiotics
			Take care to prevent bacterial contamination of formula and equipment
	Decrease rate of feeding	Poor fluid intake	Increase intake, if appropriate, and check amount and number of feedings
	Change to continuous drip feedings	High-protein formula	Change formula
	Check for drugs that may cause diarrhea (e.g., antibiotics)	Hyperosmotic diuresis	Check blood glucose levels frequently
			Change formula

should ensure the tube is in the proper position and maintain head-of-bed elevation as described above. Checking gastric residual volumes is important when giving feedings into the stomach. An increased residual volume increases the risk for aspiration of the formula into the lungs (Boullata, Carney, & Guenter, 2010).

Gastric residual volumes should be checked every 4 hours during the first 48 hours for gastrically fed patients. After attaining the enteral feeding rate goal, gastric residual monitoring can be decreased to every 6 to 8 hours in non–critically ill patients or continued every 4 hours in critically ill patients. Promotility drugs such as erythromycin or metoclopramide improve gastric emptying and may reduce aspiration risk. Feeding tubes may need to be advanced below the ligament of Treitz (jejunostomy) if gastric residual volumes consistently measure more than 500 mL. The nurse should not obtain residual volumes for EN delivered through a jejunostomy tube.

Tube Position. Radiographic confirmation of proper positioning in the GI tract needs to be obtained for newly inserted nasal or orogastric tubes (small-bore or large-bore) before administering feedings or medications. Smaller feeding tubes can pass directly

into the bronchus on insertion without any obvious respiratory manifestations. The nurse should not rely on the auscultation method to differentiate between gastric and respiratory or gastric and small bowel placement.

Proper placement of the tube needs to be maintained after starting feedings. A small bowel tube may dislocate upward into the stomach, or the tube's tip can dislocate upward into the esophagus. To determine if a feeding tube is still in the proper position, the nurse should mark the exit site of the feeding tube at the time of the initial radiograph and check the tube's external length regularly.

The nurse should observe for negative pressure when attempting to withdraw fluid from the feeding tube (Boullata, Carney, & Guenter, 2010). Negative pressure is more likely to be felt during attempts to aspirate fluid from a small bowel tube than from a gastric tube. The nurse also needs to observe for unexpected changes in residual volume. An increase in gastric residual volume may indicate displacement of a small intestine tube into the stomach (Boullata, Carney, & Guenter, 2010). If a significant increase is observed in the external length, other bedside tests should be used to help determine whether the tube has become dislocated. These measures include assessing aspirate colour and pH. Because each of these measures has limitations, placement should be confirmed with more than one test. The nurse should consider applying a nasal bridle in patients who attempt to pull out a tube or for whom taping the nose is difficult.

Site Care. Skin care around gastrostomy and jejunostomy tube sites is important because the action of digestive juices irritates the skin. The skin around the feeding tube should be assessed daily for signs of redness and maceration. The nurse needs to monitor bumper tension and routinely check for pressure injury.

To keep the skin clean and dry, the nurse should initially rinse it with sterile water, dry it, and apply a dressing until the site is healed. After that, the site can be washed with mild soap and water. A protective ointment (zinc oxide, petroleum gauze) or a skin barrier may be used on the skin around the tube. If the skin is irritated, the nurse should consider using other types of drain or tube pouches. A wound, ostomy, and continence nurse can provide assistance if issues arise.

Tube Patency. All enteral feeding tubes require routine flushing. They should be flushed with 30 mL of warm tap water every 4 hours during continuous feedings or before and after each intermittent feeding. Sterile water should be used in immuno-compromised and critically ill patients. Tubes must be flushed between each medication and after all medications are given. The nurse should try to only use liquid medications and not mix medications (Boullata, Carney, & Guenter, 2010). Clogged tubes should be flushed with warm water, using a back-and-forth motion.

Misconnection. An *enteral feeding misconnection* is an inadvertent connection between an enteral feeding system and a nonenteral system such as an IV line, a peritoneal dialysis catheter, or a tracheostomy tube cuff. With an enteral feeding misconnection, nutritional formula intended for administration into the GI tract is administered via the wrong route, resulting in serious and potentially life-threatening consequences. Nursing interventions aimed at decreasing the risk for enteral feeding misconnections are found in Table 42-12. (See also NCP 42-1, available on the Evolve website, for patients receiving EN.)

AGE-RELATED CONSIDERATIONS

ENTERAL FEEDS

EN feeding strategies are used in older patients to improve nutritional status. Because of physiological changes associated with aging, older adults are more vulnerable to complications associated with nutritional interventions, especially fluid and electrolyte imbalances. Complications such as diarrhea can leave the patient dehydrated. Decreased thirst perception or impaired cognitive function decreases the patient's ability to seek additional fluids.

With aging comes an increased risk for glucose intolerance. As a result, older patients may be more susceptible to hyperglycemia in response to the high carbohydrate load of some EN formulas. Older adults with compromised cardiovascular function (e.g., heart failure) will have a decreased ability to handle large volumes of formula. If this happens, the patient may need a more concentrated formula (2.0 kcal/mL). Older adults have an increased risk for aspiration caused by gastro-esophageal reflux disease (GERD), delayed gastric emptying, hiatal hernia, or diminished gag reflex. Physical mobility, fine motor movement, and visual system changes associated with aging may contribute to difficulties in managing EN in the home setting.

TABLE 42-12 NURSING MANAGEMENT: DECREASE RISK FOR ENTERAL FEEDING MISCONNECTIONS

To decrease the risk for enteral feeding misconnections, the nurse should do the following:
1. Teach visitors and nonclinical staff to notify a nurse if an enteral feeding line becomes disconnected.
2. Teach visitors and nonclinical staff not to reconnect enteral feeding lines.
3. Never modify or adapt IV or feeding devices, because doing so may compromise the safety features incorporated into their design.
4. When making a reconnection, routinely trace lines back to their origins and then ensure that they are secure.
5. Never force connections if the device parts do not seem to fit properly. Ill-fitting pieces indicate a problem.
6. When a patient arrives on a new unit or in a new setting, or during shift-to-shift hand-off, recheck connections and trace all tubes.
7. Route tubes and catheters that have different purposes in distinct and standardized directions (e.g., IV lines should be routed toward the patient's head, enteral lines should be routed toward the feet).
8. Package together all parts needed for enteral feeding and reduce the availability of additional adapters and connectors so as to minimize the presence of dissimilar tubes or catheters that could be improperly connected.
9. Label or colour-code feeding tubes and connectors and educate staff about the labelling or colour-coding process in the institution's enteral feeding system.
10. Always identify and confirm the solution's label, because a three-in-one parenteral nutrition solution can appear similar to an enteral nutrition formulation bag. The bags should be labelled with large, bold statements such as "WARNING! For Enteral Use Only—NOT for IV Use."
11. Make all connections under proper lighting conditions.
12. Follow the facility's protocol for reporting adverse events and near misses.

IV, intravenous.

Source: Reprinted from *The Joint Commission Journal on Quality and Patient Safety*, 34(5), Peggi Guenter, Rodney W. Hicks, Debora Simmons, Jay Crowley, Stephanie Joseph, Richard Croteau, Cathie Gosnell, Nancy G. Pratt, Timothy W. Vanderveen, Enteral feeding misconnections: A consortium position statement, pp. 289–290, Copyright 2008, with permission from Elsevier.

Parenteral Nutrition

Parenteral nutrition (PN) refers to the administration of nutrients by a route other than the GI tract (e.g., the bloodstream). (Parenteral nutrition was formerly called total parenteral nutrition [TPN].) PN is used when the GI tract cannot be used for the ingestion, digestion, and absorption of essential nutrients. PN is a relatively safe method of providing complete nutritional support.

PN is customized to meet the needs of each patient. The composition is reformulated as the patient's condition changes. The nurse, therefore, must collaborate with the interprofessional team in delivering PN to the patient.

Composition. Commercially prepared PN base solutions are available. These solutions contain dextrose and protein in the form of amino acids. The pharmacy adds prescribed electrolytes (e.g., sodium, potassium, chloride, calcium, magnesium, and phosphate), vitamins, and trace elements (e.g., zinc, copper, chromium, and manganese) to meet the patient's needs. A three-in-one or total nutrient admixture containing an IV fat emulsion (lipids), dextrose, and amino acids is widely used. Premixed PN solutions are relatively new and require manipulation of the dextrose and amino acids prior to use. Standard electrolytes are available

TABLE 42-13	COMMON INDICATIONS FOR PARENTERAL NUTRITION*

- Chronic severe diarrhea and vomiting
- Complicated surgery or trauma
- Gastro-intestinal obstruction
- Gastro-intestinal tract anomalies and fistulas
- Intractable diarrhea
- Severe anorexia nervosa
- Severe malabsorption
- Short bowel syndrome

*This list is not all-inclusive.

in premixed solutions, and multivitamins are added prior to use (Ayers, Holcombe, Plogsted, et al., 2014). Table 42-13 lists common indications for the use of PN. NCP 42-2, available on the Evolve website, presents nursing diagnoses and care for patients undergoing parenteral nutrition.

Calories. Calories in PN are supplied primarily by carbohydrates in the form of dextrose and by fat in the form of fat emulsion. The administration of between 100 and 150 g of dextrose (1 g provides ≈3.4 kcal, as opposed to oral carbohydrates, which provide 4 kcal) has a protein-sparing effect. Providing adequate nonprotein calories in the form of glucose and fat allows the use of amino acids for wound healing and not for energy. However, overfeeding can lead to metabolic complications. To minimize these problems, an energy intake of 25 to 35 kcal/kg/day in a nonobese patient is often recommended.

Fat-emulsion solutions of 10%, 20%, and 30% are available. Fat emulsions provide approximately 1 kcal/mL (10% solution) or 2 kcal/mL (20% solution). Fat emulsions primarily contain soybean or safflower triglycerides with egg phospholipids added as an emulsifier. They provide a large number of calories in a relatively small amount of fluid. This is beneficial when the patient is at risk for fluid overload.

IV fat emulsions should provide up to 30% of total calories. Most stable patients receive 1 g/kg/day, and the maximum daily lipid dose is 2.5 g/kg. Critically ill patients may not tolerate this dose and may receive less than 1 g/kg/day. Serum triglyceride levels are determined at the beginning of PN and then monitored closely after that. IV fat emulsions administered separately should be administered over a course of 8 to 10 hours, and infusion rates should not exceed 0.11 g/kg/hour (Ayers, Holcombe, Plogsted, et al., 2014).

Nausea, vomiting, and elevated temperature may occur, especially when lipids are infused quickly. Fat emulsions are contraindicated in the patient with a disturbance in fat metabolism, such as hyperlipidemia. They are used cautiously in the patient at risk for fat embolism (e.g., fractured femur) and the patient with an allergy to eggs or soybeans. Lipid emulsions are also used cautiously in patients with pancreatitis, bleeding disorders, liver failure, or respiratory disease.

Protein. The normal healthy person of average body size needs approximately 45 to 65 g (0.8–1 g/kg/day) of protein daily. Protein should be provided at the rate of 1 to 1.5 g/kg/day depending on the patient's needs. In a nutritionally depleted patient who is also under the stress of illness or surgery, protein requirements can exceed 150 g/day (1.5 to 2 g/kg/day) to ensure positive nitrogen balance. Burn patients, who are often on PN, EN, and oral food, may need upward of 2 g/kg/day. Protein needs may be lower than 1 g/kg/day and restricted in individuals with end-stage renal disease who are not on dialysis.

Electrolytes. The exact amount of electrolytes needed depends on the patient's health problem and on serum electrolyte levels. The assessment of individual requirements should take place daily at the beginning of therapy and then several times a week as the treatment progresses. The following are ranges for average daily electrolyte requirements for adult patients without renal or hepatic impairment (Ayers, Holcombe, Plogsted, et al., 2014).
Sodium: 1 to 2 mmol/kg/day
Potassium: 1 to 2 mmol/kg/day
Chloride: as needed to maintain acid–base balance
Magnesium: 8 to 20 mmol/day
Calcium: 10 to 15 mmol/day
Phosphate: 20 to 40 mmol/day

The exact amount of electrolytes needed depends on the patient's health problem and on electrolyte levels as determined by blood testing.

Trace Elements and Vitamins. Zinc, copper, chromium, manganese, selenium, molybdenum, and iodine supplements may be added according to the patient's condition and needs. Levels of these elements are monitored in the patient receiving PN. The health care provider may order additional amounts of these elements to be added to the solutions according to the patient's requirements.

The daily addition of a multivitamin preparation to the PN generally meets the vitamin requirements.

Methods of Administration. PN may be administered as central parenteral nutrition (CPN) or peripheral parenteral nutrition (PPN). Both CPN and PPN are used in a patient who is not a candidate for EN.

Central Parenteral Nutrition. *Central peripheral nutrition* is indicated when long-term support is necessary or when the patient has high protein and caloric requirements. CPN is administered through a central venous catheter or a peripherally inserted central catheter (PICC) whose tip lies in the superior vena cava (see Chapter 19). CPN solutions are hypertonic, measuring at least 1600 mmol/L. The high glucose content ranges from 20% to 50%. CPN must be infused in a large central vein so that rapid dilution can occur. The use of a peripheral vein for hypertonic CPN solutions would cause irritation and thrombo-phlebitis.

CPN may be given through a central venous catheter that originates at the subclavian or jugular vein and whose tip lies in the superior vena cava (see Figure 42-9). It can also be given using a PICC that is placed into the basilic or cephalic vein and then advanced into the distal end of the superior vena cava (see Figure 19-19).

Peripheral Parenteral Nutrition. *Peripheral parenteral nutrition* is administered through a peripherally inserted catheter or vascular access device, which uses a large vein. PPN is used when (a) nutritional support is needed for only a short time, (b) protein and caloric requirements are not high, (c) the risk of a central catheter is too great, or (d) PN is used to supplement inadequate oral intake.

Comparison of Central and Peripheral Parenteral Nutrition. Compared with CPN, PPN contains fewer nutrients. Although having fewer nutrients makes PPN less hypertonic, it still has an osmolality of up to 800 mmol/L. This level of osmolality increases the risk for phlebitis. Another potential complication of PPN is fluid overload. PPN requires large volumes of fluid, which many patients cannot tolerate.

Complications. Complications associated with PN are related either to the catheter or to the PN infusion itself (Table 42-14).

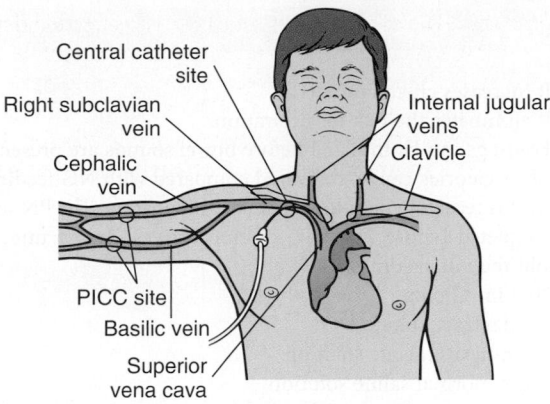

FIGURE 42-9 Placement of a catheter for central parenteral nutrition using the subclavian vein. Peripherally inserted central catheters (PICCs) are inserted using the basilic or the cephalic vein. Source: Redrawn from Mahan, L. K., & Arlin, M. (1992). *Krause's food, nutrition, and diet therapy* (8th ed.). Philadelphia: Saunders.

Refeeding syndrome is characterized by fluid retention and electrolyte imbalances (hypophosphatemia, hypokalemia, hypomagnesemia). Hypophosphatemia is the hallmark of refeeding syndrome and is associated with serious outcomes, including cardiac dysrhythmias, respiratory arrest, and neurological disturbances (e.g., paresthesias). Conditions that predispose patients to refeeding syndrome include longstanding malnutrition states, such as alcohol use disorder, vomiting and diarrhea, chemotherapy, and major surgery. Refeeding syndrome can occur any time a malnourished patient starts aggressive nutritional support.

NURSING MANAGEMENT
PARENTERAL NUTRITION

HOME NUTRITION SUPPORT

Home PN or EN is an accepted mode of nutritional therapy for the person who does not require hospitalization but requires

TABLE 42-14	COMPLICATIONS OF PARENTERAL NUTRITION

Infection
- Fungal
- Gram-positive bacteria
- Gram-negative bacteria

Metabolic
- Hyperglycemia; hypoglycemia; and hyperosmolar, hyperglycemic state
- Altered renal function (prerenal azotemia)
- Essential fatty acid deficiency
- Electrolyte and vitamin excesses and deficiencies
- Trace mineral deficiencies
- Dyslipidemia

Catheter-Related Problems
- Air embolus
- Pneumothorax, hemothorax, and hydrothorax
- Hemorrhage
- Dislodgement
- Thrombosis of great vein
- Phlebitis

continued nutrition support. Some patients have been successfully treated at home for many months and even years. It is important for the nurse to educate the patient or caregiver about catheter or tube care, proper technique in mixing and handling of the solutions and tubing, and adverse effects and complications.

Home nutritional therapies are expensive, and specific criteria must be met for these expenses to be reimbursed by provincial, territorial, or private health insurance programs. The discharge planning team needs to be involved early in the admission to help plan for discharge. Home nutrition support may also be a burden on the patient and caregivers and may affect quality of life.

CASE STUDY

Undernutrition

Source: Tolikoff Photography/ Shutterstock .com.

Patient Profile
Mrs. Mary Smith is a 70-year-old woman who is 162.5 cm tall and weighs 45.4 kg. She was recently admitted to the medical unit at a community hospital in Yellowknife, Northwest Territories.

Subjective Data
- Reports 13.5-kg weight loss during past 2 months
- Has recently had a thrombotic stroke with hemiparesis and dysphagia
- Has a history of rheumatoid arthritis
- Has had nothing by mouth for the past 24 hours and just started enteral nutrition via a PEG tube
- Lives with her daughter, who is at her bedside

Objective Data
Physical Examination
- Has left-sided weakness
- Blood pressure is 150/90 mm Hg
- A PEG tube was recently placed

Laboratory Results
- Serum albumin 29 g/L
- Prealbumin 1.1 g/L

Discussion Questions
1. What are Mrs. Smith's risk factors for malnutrition?
2. What is her BMI?
3. What factors increase her risk for developing dysphagia and malnutrition?
4. What should the nurse include in a successful weight-gain program for Mrs. Smith?
5. What possible complications of enteral nutrition could Mrs. Smith be at risk for developing?
6. **Priority decision:** What is the priority of the nursing care for Mrs. Smith?
7. **Priority decision:** Based on the assessment data presented, what are the priority nutrition-related problems and the issues that the multidisciplinary team could collaborate on to improve Mrs. Smith's nutritional status?
8. **Evidence-informed practice:** Mrs. Smith's daughter tells the nurse that her mother's abdomen appears bloated, and she wonders if she should massage it.

evolve
Answers are available at *http://evolve.elsevier.com/Canada/Lewis/medsurg*.

REVIEW QUESTIONS

The number of the question corresponds to the same-numbered objective at the beginning of the chapter.

1. The percentage of daily calories (acceptable macronutrient ranges) for healthy adults (≥19 yr) as described in Canada's Food Guide consists of which of the following?
   a. 10%–20% carbohydrate, 30%–45% protein, 10%–25% fat
   b. 30%–45% carbohydrate, 15%–30% protein, 25%–40% fat
   c. 5%–15% carbohydrate, 35%–55% protein, 5%–20% fat
   d. 55% carbohydrate, 15%–20% protein, 30% fat

2. During starvation, in what order does the body obtain substrate for energy?
   a. Glycogen, skeletal protein, fat, visceral protein
   b. Visceral protein, fat stores, glycogen
   c. Fat stores, skeletal protein, visceral protein
   d. Liver protein, muscle protein, visceral protein

3. For which type of client is a complete nutritional assessment including anthropometric measurements important? *(Select all that apply)*
   a. A client with a BMI of 17.5 kg/m^2
   b. A client complaining of frequent nocturia
   c. A client who reports a 5-year history of constipation
   d. A client who reports an unintentional weight loss of 5 kg in 2 months

4. What is one advantage of a percutaneous endoscopic gastrostomy (PEG) tube placement relative to nasogastric (NG) feedings for the client receiving long-term enteral nutrition?

   a. It increases client comfort.
   b. It eliminates the risk for aspiration.
   c. Feedings can be initiated before bowel sounds are present.
   d. More calories can be delivered compared with NG feeding.

5. A client is receiving peripheral parenteral nutrition. The PN solution is completed before the new solution arrives on the unit. What should the nurse administer?
   a. 20% intralipids
   b. 5% dextrose solution
   c. 5% Ringer's lactate solution
   d. 0.45% normal saline solution

6. A client with anorexia nervosa shows signs of malnutrition. During initial refeeding, what does the nurse carefully assess the client for?
   a. Hyperkalemia
   b. Hypoglycemia
   c. Hypercalcemia
   d. Hypophosphatemia

1. d; 2. a; 3. a, d; 4. a; 5. b; 6. a.

⊜volve

For even more review questions, visit *http://evolve.elsevier.com/Canada/Lewis/medsurg*.

REFERENCES

Allard, J. P., Keller, H., Jeejeebhoy, K. N., et al. (2015). Malnutrition at hospital admission—Contributors and effect on length of stay: A prospective cohort study from the Canadian Malnutrition Task Force. *Journal of Parenteral and Enteral Nutrition*, doi:10.1177/0148607114567902. 0148607114567902.

American Society for Parenteral and Enteral Nutrition (ASPEN). (2016). Guidelines for the provision and assessment of nutrition support therapy in the adult critically ill patient. *Journal of Parenteral and Enteral Nutrition*, 40(2), 159–211. doi:10.1177/0148607115621863.

Ayers, P., Holcombe, B., Plogsted, S., et al. (2014). *A.S.P.E.N. Parental nutrition handbook* (2nd ed.). Silver Spring, MD: A.S.P.E.N.

Bankhead, R., Boullata, J., Brantley, S., et al. (2009). A.S.P.E.N. enteral nutrition practice recommendations. *Journal of Enteral and Parenteral Nutrition*, 33(2), 122–167. doi:10.1177/0148607108330314. (Seminal).

Boullata, J., Carney, L. N., & Guenter, P. (Eds.), (2010). *A.S.P.E.N. enteral nutrition handbook*. Silver Spring, MD: A.S.P.E.N. (Seminal).

Canadian Institute for Health Information. (2017). *Health spending data*. Retrieved from *https://www.cihi.ca/en/spending-and-health-workforce/spending*.

Colby, S. E. (2013). Multicultural food perspectives: Strategies for health care providers. *American Journal of Lifestyle Medicine*, 7(1), 13–19. doi:10.1177/1559827612461898.

Deng, F., Zhang, A., & Chan, C. B. (2013). Acculturation, dietary acceptability, and diabetes management among Chinese in North America. *Frontiers in Endocrinology*, 4, 108. doi:10.3389/fendo.2013.00108.

De Souza, M. J., Nattiv, A., Joy, E., et al. (2014). 2014 Female Athlete Triad Coalition Consensus Statement on treatment and return to play of the female athlete triad: 1st International Conference held in San Francisco, California, May 2012 and 2nd International Conference held in Indianapolis, Indiana, May 2013. *British Journal of Sports Medicine*, 48, 289. doi:10.1136/bjsports-2013-093218.

Dietitians of Canada. (2013). *Vitamin D: What you need to know*. Retrieved from *https://www.dietitians.ca/Downloads/Factsheets/Vitamin-D-What-you-need-to-know.aspx*.

Dietitians of Canada. (2015). *Defining the role of the dietitian in dysphagia assessment and management*. Retrieved from *http://www.dietitians.ca/Downloads/Public/Dysphagia-Role-Paper-2015.aspx*.

Dietitians of Canada. (2016). *What does a dietitian do?* Retrieved from *http://www.dietitians.ca/Become-a-Dietitian/What-Does-a-Dietitian-Do.aspx*.

DiMaria-Ghalili, R. A. (2014). Integrating nutrition in the comprehensive geriatric assessment. *Nutrition in Clinical Practice*, 29(4), 420–427. doi:10.1177/0884533614537076.

Food and Agriculture Organization of the United Nations (FAO). (1996). *The Rome declaration on world food security*. Retrieved from *http://www.fao.org/wfs*. (Seminal).

Health Canada (2010). *Eating well with Canada's food guide—First Nations, Inuit and Métis*. Ottawa: Author. Retrieved from *https://www.canada.ca/en/health-canada/services/food-nutrition/reports-publications/eating-well-canada-food-guide-first-nations-inuit-metis.html*. (Seminal).

Health Canada (2011). *Eating well with Canada's food guide*. Ottawa: Author. Retrieved from *https://www.canada.ca/content/dam/hc-sc/migration/hc-sc/fn-an/alt_formats/hpfb-dgpsa/pdf/food-guide-aliment/view_eatwell_vue_bienmang-eng.pdf*.

Health Canada. (2012). *Fats*. Retrieved from *https://www.canada.ca/en/health-canada/services/nutrients/fats.html?_ga=1.132236814.1469460016.1447943329*.

Health Canada (2013). *Canada's food guide: Translated versions of the guide.* Ottawa: Author. Retrieved from *http://www.hc-sc.gc.ca/fn-an/food-guide-aliment/order-commander/guide_trans-trad-eng.php.*

Health Canada. (2015a). *What type and amount of fat do I need?* Retrieved from *https://www.canada.ca/en/health-canada/services/food-nutrition/canada-food-guide/choosing-foods/oils-fats/what-type-amount-need.html.*

Health Canada. (2015b). *Health at a glance: Food insecurity in Canada.* Retrieved from *http://www5.statcan.gc.ca/olc-cel/olc.action?lang=en&ObjId=82-624-X201500114138&ObjType=47.*

Hemarajata, P., & Versalovic, J. (2013). Effects of probiotics on gut microbiota: Mechanisms of intestinal immunomodulation and neuromodulation. *Therapeutic Advances in Gastroenterology, 6*(1), 39–51. doi:10.1177/1756283X12459294.

Institute of Medicine (2005). *Dietary reference intakes for energy, carbohydrate, fat, fatty acids, cholesterol, protein and amino acids.* Washington, DC: National Academies Press. (Seminal).

Jensen, G. L. (2015). Malnutrition and inflammation—"Burning down the house": Inflammation as an adaptive physiologic response versus self-destruction? *Journal of Parenteral and Enteral Nutrition, 39*(1), 56–62. doi:10.1177/0148607114529597.

Jensen, G. L., Hsiao, P. Y., & Wheeler, D. (2012). Adult nutrition assessment tutorial. *Journal of Parenteral and Enteral Nutrition, 36*(3), 267–274. doi:10.1177/0148607112440284.

LeBlanc, H. (2014) *Eating disorders among girls and women in Canada. Report of the Standing Committee on the Status of Women.* Retrieved from *http://www.parl.gc.ca/content/hoc/Committee/412/FEWO/Reports/RP6772133/feworp04/feworp04-e.pdf.*

Litchford, M. D. (2014). Counteracting the trajectory of frailty and sarcopenia in older adults. *Nutrition in Clinical Practice, 29*(4), 428–434. doi:10.1177/0884533614536231.

Morelli, L., & Capurso, L. (2012). FAO/WHO guidelines on probiotics 10 years later. *Journal of Clinical Gastroenterology, 46*(Suppl. 1), s1–s2. doi:10.1097/MCG.0b013e318269fdd5.

National Eating Disorder Information Centre (NEDIC). (2014). *Know the facts.* Retrieved from *http://nedic.ca/clinical-definitions.*

Public Health Agency of Canada (PHAC). (2013). *Preventing chronic disease strategic plan 2013–2016.* Retrieved from *http://publications.gc.ca/collections/collection_2014/aspc-phac/HP35-39-2013-eng.pdf.*

Public Health Agency of Canada (PHAC). (2014). *The chief public health officer's report on the state of public health in Canada, 2014: Public health in the future.* Retrieved from *http://www.phac-aspc.gc.ca/cphorsphc-respcacsp/2014/app-ann-a-eng.php.*

Tarasuk, V., Mitchell, A., & Dachner, N. (2016). *Household food insecurity in Canada, 2014.* Toronto: Research to identify policy options to reduce food insecurity (PROOF). Retrieved from *http://proof.utoronto.ca/wp-content/uploads/2016/04/Household-Food-Insecurity-in-Canada-2014.pdf.*

Touhy, T., Jett, K., Boscart, V., et al. (2012). *Ebersole and Hess' gerontological nursing and healthy aging* (1st Canadian ed.). Toronto: Elsevier.

Tuddenham, S., & Sears, C. L. (2015). The intestinal microbiome and health. *Current Opinion in Infectious Diseases, 28*(5), 464–470. doi:10.1097/QCO.0000000000000196.

Westmoreland, P., Krantz, M., & Mehler, P. (2016). Medical complications of anorexia nervosa and bulimia. *The American Journal of Medicine, 129*(1), 30–37. doi:10.1016/j.amjmed.2015.06.031.

White, J. V., Guenter, P., Jensen, G., et al. (2012). Consensus statement of the Academy of Nutrition and Dietetics/American Society for Parenteral and Enteral Nutrition: Characteristics recommended for the identification and documentation of adult malnutrition (undernutrition). *Journal of the Academy of Nutrition and Dietetics, 112*(11), 730–738. doi:10.1016/j.jand.2012.03.012.

Zhang, Y. J., Li, S., Gan, R. Y., et al. (2015). Impacts of gut bacteria on human health and diseases. *International Journal of Molecular Sciences, 16*(4), 7493–7519.

RESOURCES

Canadian Malnutrition Task Force
http://nutritioncareincanada.ca

Canadian Mental Health Association
http://www.cmha.ca

Canadian Nutrition Society
http://www.cns-scn.ca

Canadian Vascular Access Association
http://cvaa.info

Diabetes Canada
http://www.guidelines.diabetes.ca

Dietitians of Canada
http://www.dietitians.ca

EatRight Ontario
http://www.eatrightontario.ca

Eat Smart Meet Smart (Saskatchewan)
https://www.saskatchewan.ca/residents/health/wellness-and-prevention/nutrition-and-exercise/eat-smart-meet-smart

Government of Canada: Dietary Reference Intakes Tables
https://www.canada.ca/en/health-canada/services/food-nutrition/healthy-eating/dietary-reference-intakes/tables.html

Government of Canada: Health
https://www.canada.ca/en/services/health.html

Health Canada: Eating Well With Canada's Food Guide
https://www.canada.ca/en/health-canada/services/canada-food-guides.html

Health Canada: Interactive Nutrition Facts Table
https://www.canada.ca/en/health-canada/services/understanding-food-labels/nutrition-facts-tables.html#a4

Health Canada: Therapeutic Products Directorate
https://www.canada.ca/en/health-canada/corporate/about-health-canada/branches-agencies/health-products-food-branch/therapeutic-products-directorate.html

Healthy Eating (British Columbia)
https://www.healthyfamiliesbc.ca/work/healthy-eating

Healthy Eating (New Brunswick)
http://www2.gnb.ca/content/gnb/en/departments/social_development/wellness/content/healthy_living/healthy_eating.html

Heart and Stroke Foundation of Canada
http://www.heartandstroke.ca

National Eating Disorder Information Centre
http://www.nedic.ca

Oley Foundation
http://www.oley.org

Public Health Agency of Canada
http://www.phac-aspc.gc.ca

Academy for Eating Disorders
http://www.aedweb.org

American Society for Parenteral and Enteral Nutrition (ASPEN)
http://www.nutritioncare.org

Critical Care Nutrition
http://www.criticalcarenutrition.com

European Society for Parenteral and Enteral Nutrition and Metabolism (ESPEN)
http://www.espen.org

National Association of Anorexia Nervosa and Associated Disorders (ANAD)
http://www.anad.org

For additional Internet resources, see the website for this book at *http://evolve.elsevier.com/Canada/Lewis/medsurg.*

Nursing Management
Obesity

Written by: Sharon L. Lewis
Adapted by: Kathy G. Danzinger and Jenifer R. Bennett

℮volve WEBSITE

http://evolve.elsevier.com/Canada/Lewis/medsurg

- Review Questions (Online Only)
- Key Points
- Answer Guidelines for Case Study
- Student Case Study
  - Obesity and Osteoarthritis
- Conceptual Care Map Creator
- Audio Glossary
- Content Updates

LEARNING OBJECTIVES

1. Discuss the epidemiology and etiology of obesity.
2. Describe the classification systems for determining a person's body size and associated health risks.
3. Explain the health risks associated with obesity.
4. Discuss nutritional, physical activity, and behaviour-modification therapies for patients who are obese.
5. Describe the different bariatric surgical procedures used to treat obesity.
6. Describe the nursing management related to conservative and surgical therapies for obesity.
7. Describe the etiology, the clinical manifestations, and the nursing and collaborative management of metabolic syndrome.

KEY TERMS

bariatric surgery, p. 1004
body mass index (BMI), p. 994
lipectomy, p. 1007

metabolic syndrome, p. 998
morbidly obese, p. 995
obese, p. 995

obesity, p. 993
overweight, p. 994
waist-to-hip ratio (WHR), p. 995

OBESITY

Obesity is a complex, chronic, multifactorial disease that develops from the interaction between genetics and the environment. It manifests as an abnormal increase in the proportion of fat cells in the body. Weight gain in which the body is moving toward an overweight or obese state is characterized predominantly by adipocyte hypertrophy and hyperplasia. Through this process, adipocytes can increase their volume several thousand times to accommodate large increases in lipid storage. In addition, preadipocytes are triggered to become adipocytes. This process occurs primarily in the visceral (intra-abdominal) and subcutaneous tissues of the body (Cornier, Després, Davis, et al., 2011).

Overweight and obesity result from a complex interaction of genetic, nutritional, physiological, psychological, behavioural, environmental, and social factors that create an imbalance between energy intake and energy expenditure. There is increasing evidence that obesity is not a problem resulting from a lack of willpower and self-control but, instead, is a pervasive, progressive, and serious chronic condition that is strongly associated with a variety of comorbid conditions and that has a major effect on the physical, mental, social, cultural, and economic health of those affected (Williams, Mesidor, Winters, et al., 2015). The Canadian Medical Association's having recognized obesity as a chronic disease will lead to enhanced funding for research, prevention, and treatment (Rich, 2015). Interventions to address obesity must account for the complexity and progressive nature of the chronic condition and support appropriate lifelong management, which often necessitates sustained contact and support from trained health care providers (Kirk, Penney, McHugh, et al., 2011).

Classifications of Body Weight and Obesity

The majority of people with obesity have *primary obesity,* which is calorie intake that exceeds the body's metabolic demands. Others have *secondary obesity,* which can result from various congenital anomalies, chromosomal anomalies, metabolic problems, or lesions and disorders of the central nervous system. The first step in the treatment of obesity is to determine whether the patient has any physical conditions that may be causing or contributing to the obesity. A thorough history and physical examination are necessary and will reveal the extent and duration of the obesity.

The degree to which a patient is classified as underweight, healthy (normal) weight, overweight, or obese is assessed with the use of a **body mass index (BMI)** chart (Figure 43-1). BMI is calculated by dividing weight (in kilograms) by height (in metres squared). Research studies in large groups of people have shown that the BMI can be classified into ranges associated with health risk (Table 43-1). Individuals with a BMI of 25 to 29.9 kg/m^2 are classified as being **overweight**, those with a BMI

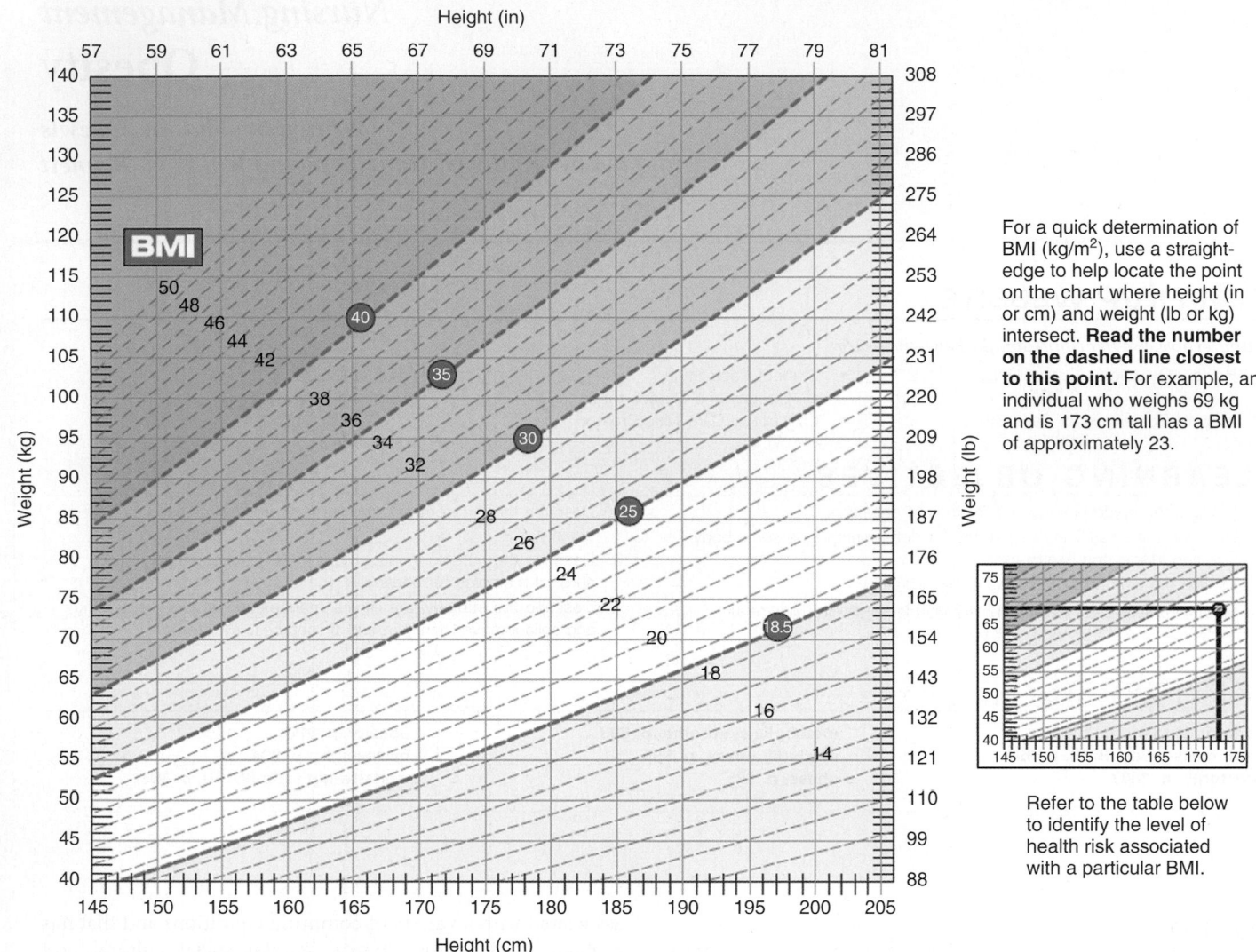

For a quick determination of BMI (kg/m^2), use a straight-edge to help locate the point on the chart where height (in or cm) and weight (lb or kg) intersect. **Read the number on the dashed line closest to this point.** For example, an individual who weighs 69 kg and is 173 cm tall has a BMI of approximately 23.

Refer to the table below to identify the level of health risk associated with a particular BMI.

FIGURE 43-1 Body mass index chart. Source: Health Canada. (2003). *Canadian guidelines for body weight classification in adults* (Cat. no. H49-179/2003E). Ottawa: Author. Retrieved from *http://www.hc-sc.gc.ca/fn-an/alt_formats/hpfb-dgpsa/ pdf/nutrition/cg_quick_ref-ldc_rapide_ref-eng.pdf.*

TABLE 43-1 CLASSIFICATION OF OVERWEIGHT AND OBESITY

| | BMI (kg/m^2) | Obesity Class | Disease Risk Based on Waist Circumference* | |
			Men ≤102 cm Women ≤89 cm	Men >102 cm Women >89 cm
Underweight	<18.5	—	—	—
Normal†	18.5–24.9	—	—	—
Overweight	25.0–29.9	—	Increased	High
Obese	30.0–34.9	Class I	High	Very high
	35.0–39.9	Class II	Very high	Very high
Morbidly obese	≥40.0	Class III	Extremely high	Extremely high

BMI, body mass index.
*Disease risk for type 2 diabetes, hypertension, and cardiovascular disease.
†Increased waist circumference can also be a marker for increased risk in persons of normal weight.
Source: Adapted from National Heart, Lung, and Blood Institute: Classification of overweight and obesity by BMI, waist circumference, and associated disease risks. (n.d.) Retrieved from *http://www.nhlbi.nih.gov/health/public/heart/obesity/lose_wt/bmi_dis.htm.*

of 30 to 40 kg/m² are classified as obese, and those with a BMI of more than 40 kg/m² are classified as morbidly obese.

Waist circumference is another way to assess and classify a person's weight (see Table 43-1). Health risks increase with a waist circumference greater than 101.6 cm in men and greater than 88.9 cm in women (Ford, Maynard, & Li, 2014). People who have visceral fat with truncal obesity are at an increased risk for cardiovascular disease and metabolic syndrome (discussed later in this chapter).

The waist-to-hip ratio (WHR) is another method used to assess obesity. This ratio is a method of describing the distribution of both subcutaneous and visceral adipose tissue. The ratio is calculated by dividing the waist measurement by the hip measurement. A WHR less than 0.8 is optimal. A WHR greater than 0.8 indicates more truncal fat, which puts the individual at a greater risk for health complications.

Body shape is another method of identifying those who are at a higher risk for health problems (Table 43-2). Individuals with fat located primarily in the abdominal area, an *apple-shaped body*, have *android obesity*. Those with fat distribution in the upper legs, a *pear-shaped body*, have *gynoid obesity*. Genetics has an important role in determining a person's body shape and weight (Wei, Hemani, Gyenesei, et al., 2012). Gynoid obesity carries a better prognosis but is more difficult to treat. It is believed that abdominal fat is more readily available and can be mobilized to maintain elevated triglyceride and lipid levels. Individuals with an apple shape carry more visceral fat than people with a pear shape and have increased amounts of fat around the organs. Pear-shaped individuals carry more subcutaneous fat, which causes more cellulite to appear. Abdominal and visceral fat have been linked to metabolic syndrome, a major complication of obesity (Tchernof & Després, 2013). Visceral fat actively harms the body by decreasing insulin sensitivity and levels of high-density lipoprotein (HDL) cholesterol and increasing blood pressure. Visceral fat also releases more free fatty acids into the bloodstream.

TABLE 43-2 RELATIONSHIP BETWEEN BODY SHAPE AND HEALTH RISKS

Body Shape	Health Risks
Gynoid (pear)	• Osteoporosis • Varicose veins • Cellulite • Subcutaneous fat traps and stores of dietary fat • Trapped fatty acids stored as triglycerides

Android (apple)	• Heart disease
	• Diabetes mellitus
	• Breast cancer
	• Endometrial cancer
	• Visceral fat more active, causing:
	  • ↓ insulin sensitivity
	  • ↑ triglycerides
	  • ↓ HDL cholesterol
	  • ↑ BP
	  • ↑ free fatty acid release into blood

BP, blood pressure; *HDL*, high-density lipoprotein.

Epidemiology of Obesity

In developed and developing countries, obesity has reached epidemic proportions. The prevalence of overweight and obesity among Canadians has approximately doubled since the early 1980s. In 2014, approximately 40% of Canadians self-reported as overweight or obese (Statistics Canada, 2014). About one in four adult Canadians were obese in 2011–2012. The proportion of Canadians who are obese has increased 17.5% since 2003. In general, more men than women are obese, and obesity rates have increased more for men than for women since 2003. The highest proportions of people with obesity are found in Atlantic Canada, the Prairie provinces, the Northwest Territories, Nunavut, Yukon, and smaller cities in northern and southwestern Ontario. The lowest proportions of people with obesity are found in Toronto, Montreal, Vancouver, and areas of southern British Columbia (Navaneelan & Janz, 2014).

Obesity in adulthood is often a problem that begins in childhood or adolescence. Between 2009 and 2011, 31.5% (1.6 million) of Canadian children aged 5 to 17 were classified as overweight or obese (Roberts, Shields, de Groh, et al., 2012). Reversing the childhood obesity crisis is key to addressing the overall obesity epidemic.

In Indigenous populations, 26% of off-reserve adults and 36% of on-reserve First Nations people are estimated to be obese (Canadian Institute for Health Information [CIHI] & Public Health Agency of Canada [PHAC], 2011). Although data examining changes in obesity prevalence among Indigenous peoples are limited, obesity remains more prominent among adults and children in this population than among non-Indigenous populations.

Obesity is a societal problem as much as a complex medical concern, because of the adverse health conditions related to weight gain and the associated expenses for health care. Obesity costs the Canadian economy somewhere between $4.6 billion and $7.1 billion a year. Those costs are split evenly between direct health care costs and indirect costs such as lost productivity of people unable to work either because of disability or because they are unable to find employment due to discrimination (CIHI & PHAC, 2011).

Etiology and Pathophysiology

In one sense, the etiology of obesity can be considered simplistically. It occurs because energy intake exceeds energy output. However, the processes leading to obesity are much more complex and still undergoing investigation. The causes of obesity involve significant genetic–biological susceptibility factors that are highly influenced by environmental and psychosocial factors.

Genetic–Biological Basis. Studies of twins suggest the existence of genetic factors in obesity (Naukkarinen, Rissanen, Kaprio, et al., 2012). Estimates suggest obesity is inherited in more than 50% of cases (Malis, Rasmussen, Poulsen, et al., 2005). However, genetic factors do not totally account for the etiology of obesity.

A number of genes have been linked to obesity. Genes actually may influence how calories are stored and energy released. "Energy-thrifty" genes, once protective against long periods when food was not available, are now maladaptive in societies in which food availability is no longer a primary issue. Genes may be responsible for why two individuals living in the same environment can vary considerably in body size.

A strong link exists between a gene known as *FTO* (fat mass and obesity-associated gene) and a person's BMI. Variants of this gene may explain why some people become overweight, whereas others do not. People with two copies of a certain allele at the *FTO* gene weigh 3 kg more and have a greater risk for obesity than those who do not have the risk allele (Tung, Yeo, O'Rahilly, et al., 2014). More research is needed to better understand the role of genes in obesity.

Regulation of eating behaviour, energy metabolism, and body fat metabolism are controlled by signals from the periphery that act on the hypothalamus (Figure 43-2). Appetite is influenced by many factors that are integrated by the brain, most importantly within the hypothalamus. Input to the hypothalamus is received from the periphery from many different hormones and peptides (Table 43-3). Interaction of these hormones and peptides at the level of the hypothalamus may be an important determinant in factors contributing to obesity.

Adipocytes are not just a storage unit for triglycerides; they are also endocrine cells known to produce at least 100 different proteins. These proteins are secreted as enzymes, adipokines, growth factors, and hormones that contribute to the development of insulin resistance and atherosclerosis.

Environmental Factors. Environmental factors play an important role in obesity. In today's culture, there is greater access to food, particularly prepackaged and fast foods, as well as soft drinks, all of which have poor nutritional quality. Portion size of meals has also increased (Table 43-4). Individuals with obesity tend to underestimate food and caloric intake. Eating outside of the home impedes the ability to control the composition and the quality of food.

Lack of physical activity is another factor that contributes to weight gain and obesity. The amount of physical activity people engage in has decreased, both in the workplace and at home. With increases in technology and labour-saving devices, Canadians are expending less energy in their everyday lives. Numerous initiatives have been enacted in Canada to address inactivity and resultant obesity throughout the lifespan, such as Partici-pACTION (see the Resources at the end of the chapter), but further measures are needed.

Socioeconomic status can affect obesity in a variety of indirect ways. People with low incomes may buy food that is less expensive but often has poorer nutritional quality and greater caloric content,

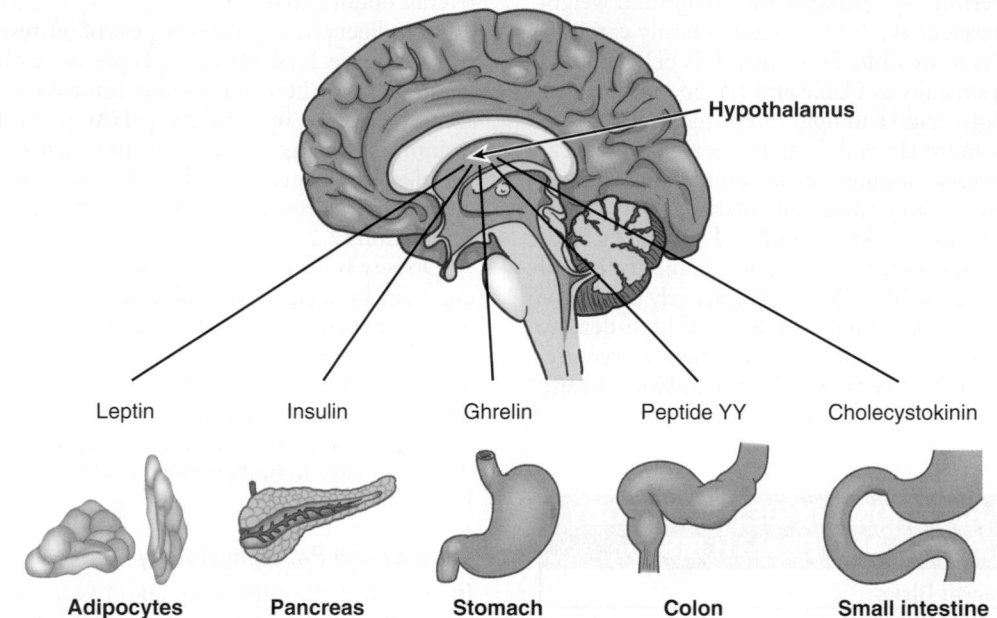

FIGURE 43-2 Some of the common hormones and peptides that interact with the hypothalamus to control and influence eating patterns, metabolic activities, and digestion. Obesity causes a disruption in this balance (see Table 43-3).

TABLE 43-3   HORMONES AND PEPTIDES IN OBESITY

Hormone or Peptide	Where Produced	Normal Function	Alteration in Obesity
Leptin	Adipocytes	Suppresses appetite and hunger Regulates eating behaviour	Obesity is associated with high leptin levels, and when leptin levels are high, leptin resistance develops; thus people who are obese may lose the effect of appetite suppression.
Insulin	Pancreas	Decreases appetite	Circulating levels are frequently high.
Ghrelin	Stomach (primarily)	Stimulates appetite ↑ after food deprivation ↓ in response to the presence of food in the stomach	Normal postprandial decline does not occur; increased appetite and overeating may result.
Peptide YY	Descending colon and rectum	Inhibits appetite by slowing GI motility and gastric emptying	Circulating levels are decreased; release is decreased after eating.
Cholecystokinin	Duodenum Jejunum	Inhibits gastric emptying and sends satiety signals to hypothalamus	Role is unknown.

GI, gastro-intestinal.

TABLE 43-4 PORTION SIZES: PAST VERSUS PRESENT

Food	20 Years Ago	Today
Turkey sandwich	320 cal	820 cal
Bagel	7.6 cm diameter: 140 cal	15.2 cm diameter: 350 cal
Cheeseburger	333 cal	590 cal
Soft drink	237 mL: 105 cal	591 mL: 250 cal

for example, prepackaged foods rather than fresh meats and produce. This population may also live in environments that do not accommodate outdoor activities (e.g., safe playgrounds, walking tracks, tennis courts, swimming pools). Gyms tend to be attended by more affluent individuals.

Psychosocial Factors. People use food for many reasons beyond nutritional maintenance. Many food associations begin in childhood, such as using food for comfort and reward. Furthermore, when overeating begins in childhood and continues into adulthood, a person's ability to sense fullness, or *satiety,* is compromised. Whether the desire to eat is triggered by specific foods or by the availability of a wide variety, some people consume food beyond their body's needs. The social component of eating occurs due to the association of food with pleasure. Food has become the central focus of most social events and celebrations. All these factors must be included when considering the etiology and treatment of obesity.

Health Risks Associated With Obesity

Many health conditions are more prevalent among people with obesity (Figure 43-3). The mortality rate rises as the rate of obesity increases, especially when obesity is associated with visceral fat. Among people with a BMI of 30 kg/m² or higher, the mortality

Psychosocial
• Depression
• Low self-esteem
• Risk for suicide
• Discrimination
• Social isolation

Endocrine/Metabolic
• Type 2 diabetes mellitus
• Metabolic syndrome
• Polycystic ovary syndrome

Respiratory
• Obesity hypoventilation syndrome
• Sleep apnea
• Asthma
• Pulmonary hypertension
• Exercise intolerance

Reproductive (Women)
• Menstrual irregularities
• Infertility
• Gestational diabetes

Reproductive (Men)
• Hypogonadism
• Gynecomastia
• Sexual dysfunction

Musculo-skeletal
• Osteoarthritis
• Impaired mobility and flexibility
• Gout
• Lumbar disk disease
• Chronic low back pain

Cardiovascular
• Hyperlipidemia
• Sudden cardiac death
• Right-sided heart failure
• Left ventricular hypertrophy
• Coronary artery disease
• Deep venous thrombosis
• Atrial fibrillation
• Hypertension
• Cardiomyopathy
• Venous stasis
• Varicose veins

Gastro-Intestinal
• Nonalcoholic steatohepatitis (NASH)
• Gallstones
• Gastro-esophageal reflux disease (GERD)

Genito-Urinary
• Kidney cancer
• Chronic kidney disease
• Stress incontinence

Cancer
• Esophagus, pancreas, thyroid, colorectal, and gallbladder cancer (both genders)
• Endometrial, breast, and ovarian cancer (women)

FIGURE 43-3 Health risks associated with obesity.

TABLE 43-5	DIAGNOSTIC CRITERIA FOR METABOLIC SYNDROME*
Measurement	**Categorical Cutoff Point**
Waist circumference	Men: ≥102 cm
	Women: ≥88 cm
Triglyceride levels	≥1.7 mmol/L
	or
	Drug treatment for elevated triglyceride levels
HDL cholesterol level	Men: <1.0 mmol/L
	Women: <1.3 mmol/L
	or
	Drug treatment for reduced HDL cholesterol level
BP	≥130 mm Hg systolic
	or
	≥85 mm Hg diastolic
	or
	Drug treatment for hypertension
Fasting glucose level	≥5.6 mmol/L
	or
	Drug treatment for elevated glucose level

BP, blood pressure; *HDL,* high-density lipoprotein.
*At least three of the five measures must exceed the cutoff level for a diagnosis of metabolic syndrome.
Source: Alberti, K. G., Eckel, R. H., Grundy, S. M., et al. (2009). Joint scientific statement: Harmonizing the metabolic syndrome: A joint interim statement of the International Diabetes Federation Task Force on Epidemiology and Prevention; National Heart, Lung, and Blood Institute; American Heart Association; World Heart Federation; International Atherosclerosis Society; and International Association for the Study of Obesity. *Circulation, 120,* 1640–1645.

rates from all causes—especially from cardiovascular disease—are generally 50% to 100% higher than the rates for people with BMIs in the normal range. The number of years lived with obesity also has a direct link to the risk for mortality (Abdullah, Wolfe, Stoelwinder, et al., 2011). In addition to these problems, patients with obesity have a reduced quality of life. Fortunately, most of these conditions can improve with weight loss. Loss of 5% to 10% of excess body weight can significantly improve obesity-related comorbid conditions (Lau, 2007).

METABOLIC SYNDROME

Metabolic syndrome—also known as *syndrome X, insulin resistance syndrome,* and *dysmetabolic syndrome*—is a collection of risk factors that increase an individual's chance of developing cardiovascular disease and diabetes mellitus. The Canadian Heart Health Surveys, completed between 1986 and 1992, remain the most recent representative Canadian source of measured anthropometry and cardiovascular risk factors. Metabolic syndrome is diagnosed if an individual has three or more of the conditions listed in Table 43-5.

Etiology and Pathophysiology

The main underlying risk factor for metabolic syndrome is insulin resistance related to excessive visceral fat (Figure 43-4). In a person with insulin resistance, the body's cells have a diminished ability to respond to the actions of insulin. To compensate, the pancreas secretes more insulin, which results in hyperinsulinemia.

Other characteristics associated with metabolic syndrome include hypertension, increased risk of clotting, and abnormalities in cholesterol levels. Most people with metabolic syndrome are overweight or obese; however, genetics and environment

PATHOPHYSIOLOGY MAP

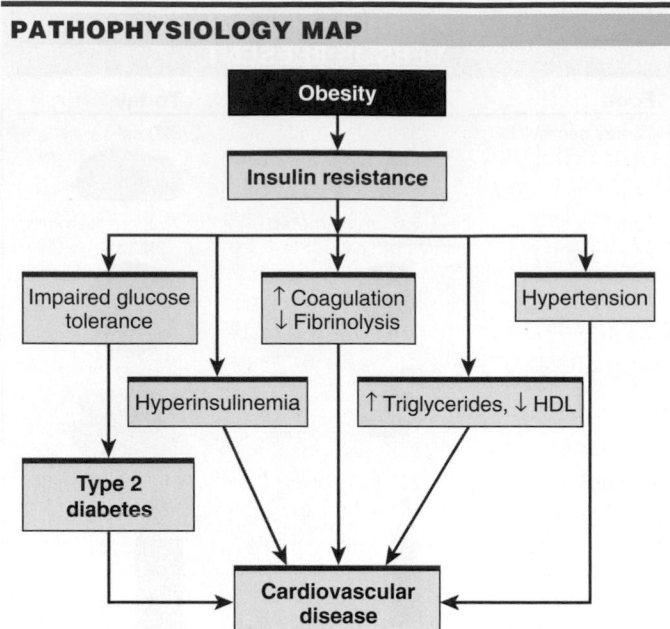

FIGURE 43-4 Relationships among insulin resistance, obesity, diabetes mellitus, and cardiovascular disease. *HDL,* high-density lipoprotein.

also have important roles in the development of metabolic syndrome.

Patients diagnosed with metabolic syndrome typically have diabetes and cannot maintain a proper level of glucose, have hypertension and secrete a large amount of insulin, or they have survived a heart attack and have hyperinsulinemia.

NURSING AND COLLABORATIVE MANAGEMENT METABOLIC SYNDROME

Lifestyle therapies are the first-line interventions to reduce the risk factors for metabolic syndrome. Management or reversal of metabolic syndrome can be achieved by reducing the major risk factors of cardiovascular disease: lowering low-density lipoprotein (LDL) cholesterol level, quitting smoking, lowering blood pressure (BP), and reducing glucose levels. For long-term reduction of risk, weight should be decreased, physical activity increased, and healthy dietary habits established.

No specific treatment for metabolic syndrome is available. Nurses can assist patients by providing information on healthy diets, physical activity, and positive lifestyle changes. The diet should be low in saturated fats and promote weight loss. Although low-carbohydrate diets may offer short-term weight loss, there is no strong evidence to support long-term weight loss with such diets. Weight reduction and maintenance of a lower weight should be the first priority in patients with abdominal obesity and metabolic syndrome.

Because sedentary lifestyles contribute to metabolic syndrome, increasing regular physical activity reduces a patient's risk factors. In addition to assisting in weight reduction, regular physical activity has been found to decrease the triglyceride level and increase the HDL cholesterol level in patients with metabolic syndrome.

Patients who are unable to reduce their risk factors with lifestyle therapies alone and those at high risk for a coronary event or diabetes may be considered for drug therapy. Although there is no medication for metabolic syndrome, cholesterol-lowering medication and antihypertensives can be used. Metformin (Glucophage) has also been used to prevent diabetes by lowering glucose levels and enhancing the cells' sensitivity to insulin.

Cardiovascular Problems. Obesity is a significant risk factor for predicting cardiovascular disease in both men and women. The WHR is the best predictor of these risks. Obesity, especially android obesity, is connected with increased levels of LDLs and triglycerides and decreased levels of HDLs. Obesity is also associated with hypertension. Hypertension can occur because of increased circulating blood volume, abnormal vasoconstriction, decreased vascular relaxation, and increased cardiac output. Measurement of BP in a patient with obesity requires the use of a larger cuff size to avoid artifactual increases.

Respiratory Problems. Severe obesity may be connected with sleep apnea and obesity hypoventilation syndrome. Affected patients also have reduced chest wall compliance, increased work in breathing, and decreased total lung capacity and functional residual capacity. Weight loss can bring substantial improvement in lung function.

Diabetes Mellitus. Hyperinsulinemia and insulin resistance are common features of obesity. Insulin resistance is more strongly related to visceral fat than to fat in other locations. Obesity is a major risk factor for type 2 diabetes (see Figure 43-4). As many as 90% of cases of type 2 diabetes are associated with excess weight (Wilding, 2014). Weight loss and exercise are linked with improved glucose control in diabetes.

Musculo-Skeletal Problems. Obesity is correlated with an increased incidence of osteoarthritis as a result of stress put on weight-bearing joints. Hyperuricemia and gout are often found in people who are obese and in those who have metabolic syndrome.

Gastro-Intestinal and Liver Problems. Gastro-esophageal reflux disease (GERD; also called *acid reflux*) and gallstones are prevalent among people with obesity. Gallstones occur when bile becomes supersaturated with cholesterol. Nonalcoholic steatohepatitis (NASH) is more common in people with obesity. In people with NASH, lipids are deposited in the liver, resulting in a fatty liver. NASH is associated with increased production of hepatic glucose and can eventually progress to cirrhosis and be fatal. Weight loss can improve NASH.

Cancer. Overweight and obesity not only increase the risk for cardiovascular disease and type 2 diabetes mellitus but also are now known risk factors for a variety of cancer types (Schmandt, Iglesias, Co, et al., 2011). The risk for breast, endometrial, ovarian, and cervical cancer is increased in women with obesity, possibly because of the increased estrogen levels (estrogen is stored in fat cells) associated with obesity in postmenopausal women. Colorectal cancer has been linked to hyperinsulinemia. Increased waist circumference and WHR, indicators of abdominal obesity, are associated with increased risk for colon cancer in both men and women. Men with obesity have higher mortality rates with cancer of the prostate. Obesity often leads to GERD, which increases the risk for esophageal cancer because of the irritation and inflammation caused by frequent or constant exposure of the esophageal lining to stomach acid and bile.

Psychosocial Issues. The consequences of obesity extend beyond physical changes and often affect the individual's emotional well-being. Clear and consistent stigmatization of people with obesity and, in some cases, discrimination occur in three important areas of living: employment, education, and health care (Budd & Peterson, 2014). In addition to dealing with the negative social impact, many people with obesity have low self-esteem, withdraw from social interaction, and experience major depression.

NURSING AND CONSERVATIVE COLLABORATIVE MANAGEMENT
PATIENTS WITH OBESITY

NURSING ASSESSMENT

The nurse, working closely with the health care team, plays a major role in the planning and management of care for patients with obesity. Information that can assist nurses in understanding patients with obesity and provide a basis for intervention is presented in Table 43-6. Because many individuals with obesity have experienced weight bias in the past, nurses should ensure that their approach and actions are free of any possible interpretation of continued insensitivity. By being sensitive when asking specific and leading questions, nurses can often obtain information that patients may otherwise withhold out of embarrassment or shyness (Table 43-7). Nurses must provide acceptable reasons for asking personally intrusive questions, respond to patients' concerns about diagnostic tests, and interpret test outcomes. A patient's answers to questions must be treated with respect, understanding, and a nonjudgemental attitude. Knowledge regarding assessment and stepwise management for the treatment of obesity (Figure 43-5) can help nurses, in conjunction with the interdisciplinary team, to guide patients and their families through weight-loss interventions.

The health care provider should explore genetic and endocrine factors such as hypothyroidism, hypothalamic tumours, Cushing's syndrome, hypogonadism in men, and polycystic ovary disease in women. Laboratory tests of liver function, fasting glucose level, lipid panel (triglyceride level and LDL and HDL cholesterol levels) assist in evaluating the cause and effects of obesity.

As part of the initial nursing history and physical examination, each body system should be examined, with particular attention to the organ system in which the patient has expressed a problem or concern. Measurements used with people with obesity may include skin fold thickness, height, weight, and BMI. Specific documentation of these measurements assists the health care provider with a more in-depth history and physical examination.

NURSING DIAGNOSES

Nursing diagnoses for the patient with obesity include but are not limited to the following:

- *Ineffective breathing pattern* related to *obesity* (decreased lung expansion)
- *Obesity* related to *energy expenditure below energy intake based on standard assessment*
- *Impaired skin integrity* related to *moisture, pressure over bony prominence*
- *Chronic low self-esteem* related to *cultural incongruence, inadequate respect from others, inadequate belonging*
- *Impaired physical mobility* related to *body mass index (BMI) >75th percentile appropriate for age and gender*
- *Disturbed body image* related to *alteration in self-perception*

PLANNING

The overall goals are that the patient with obesity will (a) modify eating patterns, (b) participate in a program of regular physical activity, (c) achieve weight maintenance (stop historic pattern of continued weight gain over time) or achieve weight loss to a

TABLE 43-6 NURSING ASSESSMENT
Patient With Obesity

Subjective Data
Important Health Information
Past health history: Time of obesity onset; diseases related to metabolism and obesity (e.g., hypertension, cardiovascular problems, stroke, cancer, chronic joint pain, respiratory problems, diabetes mellitus, cholelithiasis, metabolic syndrome); family history of obesity; history of weight gain and loss
Medications: Prescription and over-the-counter (including supplements and herbal products)
Surgery or other treatments: Prior bariatric surgery, other weight-reduction procedures, or other major surgical procedures related to risk factors precipitated by obesity

Medical History
- Comorbid conditions (time since diagnosis, current treatment, and current symptoms)
- Drowsiness, somnolence; dyspnea on exertion, orthopnea, paroxysmal nocturnal dyspnea
- History or symptoms of mental illness (feelings of depression, guilt, rejection, isolation)
- Psychosocial history (income, housing, supports)
- Menstrual irregularity, heavy menstrual flow in women, infertility
- Altered sexual activity or function
- Barriers to performing activities of daily living
- Nutritional status

Objective Data
General
BMI ≥30 kg/m^2; waist circumference: woman, >88 cm; man, >102 cm

Respiratory
Increased work in breathing; wheezing; rapid, shallow breathing, sleep apnea, neck circumference (<42 cm=low risk)

Cardiovascular
Hypertension, tachycardia, dysrhythmias, hyperlipidemia

Musculo-Skeletal
Decreased joint mobility and flexibility; knee, hip, and low back pain

Reproductive
Menstrual irregularities and infertility in women; gynecomastia and hypogonadism in men

Possible Findings
Elevated levels of serum glucose, cholesterol, triglycerides, and A$_{1c}$; chest radiograph demonstrating an enlarged heart; ECG tracing showing dysrhythmia; abnormal results of liver function tests, radiograph evidence of osteoarthritis

BMI, body mass index; *ECG,* electrocardiogram.

TABLE 43-7 ASSESSING A PATIENT WITH OBESITY

When assessing a patient with obesity, the nurse should consider asking several different types of questions, such as the following:
- What is the patient's history with weight gain and weight loss?
- Is the patient interested in losing weight or managing weight differently?
- What does the patient think contributes to his or her weight?
- What barriers does the patient feel impede weight-loss efforts?
- What does food mean to the patient? How does the patient use food (e.g., to relieve stress, provide comfort)?
- Is the patient's food intake influenced by hunger?
- Are other family members overweight?
- Are there environmental or genetic factors influencing the weight gain?

obesity, often citing a lack of time during appointments, lack of professional reward for weight management, lack of reimbursement for weight-management services, and a lack of knowledge of or faith in the effectiveness of weight-management interventions. If a health care provider associates obesity with lack of willpower and with overindulgence, patients can experience shame in a setting that claims to be a caring one. Nurses are in a pivotal position to help people with overweight and obesity deal with negative experiences and to educate other health care providers to eliminate their bias.

Before selecting a weight-loss strategy with the patient, the following questions should be asked:
- What is the patient's motivation for losing weight?
- Is the patient experiencing any major stresses that will make it difficult to focus on weight control?
- Does the patient have any psychiatric illnesses—such as severe depression, substance abuse, or a binge-eating disorder—that will derail weight-loss efforts?
- Can the patient devote the minimal amount of time for physical activity (e.g., at least 15 to 30 minutes per day for the next 6 months) that is needed for a serious weight-loss effort?

A patient's motivation should be assessed because it is essential for a favourable outcome. Lack of motivation is a huge barrier to change. However, patients should be encouraged to focus on the reasons for wanting to lose weight as they face the challenges in dealing with obesity.

When no organic cause for obesity (e.g., hypothyroidism) can be found, it should be considered a complex, chronic illness. A multipronged approach with attention to multiple factors—including nutrition therapy, physical activity, cognitive–behavioural therapy, and perhaps pharmacotherapy and bariatric surgery—should be used (see Figure 43-5). Focusing on more than one aspect probably provides better balance to weight-loss and weight-control efforts. All opportunities for patient education should stress healthy eating habits and adequate physical activity as lifestyle patterns. A comprehensive, patient-centred, and collaborative approach should be the goal of the health care team (Lau, Douketis, Morrison, et al., 2007).

Even with a comprehensive action plan, there is a high rate of weight regain among people in all age groups, which is discouraging considering the amount of time and effort expended in the process of attempting to lose weight. For successful management of obesity, it helps to view obesity as a chronic condition that necessitates day-to-day attention to losing weight and maintaining weight loss. It is essential that the nurse take a

specified level, (d) maintain weight loss at a specified level, and (e) minimize or prevent health problems related to obesity.

NURSING IMPLEMENTATION
The nurse, working closely with the other members of the health care team, plays a major role in the planning and management of the care of a patient with obesity. To be effective, nurses must be aware of their own perceptions of and beliefs about obesity and obesity interventions. Although health care for patients with obesity has inherently greater demands, health care providers often fail to address these needs, and people with obesity under-utilize health care opportunities available to them. In addition, health care providers are reluctant to counsel patients about

FIGURE 43-5 Algorithm for the assessment and stepwise management of adults who are overweight or obese. *BMI,* body mass index; *HDL,* high-density lipoprotein; *LDL,* low-density lipoprotein. Source: Adapted from Lau, D. C. W. (2007). Synopsis of the 2006 Canadian clinical practice guidelines on the management and prevention of obesity in adults and children. *Canadian Medical Association Journal, 176*(8), 1103–1106. Copied under licence from Access Copyright. Further reproduction, distribution or transmission is prohibited except as otherwise permitted by law.

nonjudgemental approach in helping patients manage their problems related to obesity.

NUTRITIONAL THERAPY. Restricted food intake is a cornerstone for any weight loss or maintenance program. A good weight-loss plan should promote healthy eating using Canada's Food Guide (Health Canada, 2011; see Chapter 42, Figure 42-1). Nutrition interventions should be developed with a qualified and experienced health care provider, preferably a registered dietitian (Lau, 2007). To support a negative energy balance, it is recommended that energy intake be reduced by 500 to 1 000 kcal per day below estimated energy needs to achieve a 0.5 to 1 kg weight loss per week (Lau, Douketis, Morrison, et al., 2007). Diets may be classified as low-calorie (800–1 200 kcal/day) or very-low-calorie (less than 800 kcal/day). Although an example of a low-calorie diet is presented in Table 43-8, it is important for the nurse to be aware that dietitians work with patients to develop diets that are based on the patients' current caloric consumption, with subsequent incremental reductions, because the diet must be sustainable over time for the resultant weight loss to be maintained. Once the patient has achieved one goal, subsequent progressive goals are set.

People on low-calorie and very-low-calorie diets need frequent professional monitoring because the severe energy restriction places them at risk for deficiency of multiple nutrients. A diet that includes adequate amounts of fruits and vegetables provides enough bulk to prevent constipation and meets daily vitamin A and vitamin C requirements. Lean meat, fish, and eggs provide sufficient protein, as well as B-complex vitamins. Restricting dietary intake so that it is below energy requirements is an effective way to reduce body weight.

TABLE 43-8 NUTRITIONAL THERAPY

Sample 1 200-Calorie Weight Reduction Diet*

General Principles

1. Eat regularly. Do not skip meals.
2. Measure foods to determine the correct portion size.
3. Avoid concentrated sweets, such as sugar, candy, honey, pies, cakes, cookies, and regular soft drinks.
4. Reduce fat intake by baking, broiling, or steaming foods.
5. Maintain a regular physical activity program for successful weight loss.

Meal	Menu Plan
Breakfast	30 g (¾ cup) dry cereal (unsweetened)
	1 small banana
	250 mL (1 cup) non-fat milk
	Coffee, black, unsweetened
Lunch	Beef and cheese enchiladas (made with 35 g cheese and 57 g lean ground beef)
	2 corn tortillas with shredded lettuce
	10 mL (2 tsp) chili sauce
	175 g (1 cup) sliced tomatoes and cucumbers
	30 mL (1 tbsp) low-fat salad dressing
	90 g (approx 12) grapes
	500 mL (2 cups) water
Dinner	75 g baked chicken breast (no skin)
	5 mL (1 tsp) margarine
	350 g (2 cups) tossed salad and 30 mL (1 tbsp) low-fat salad dressing
	90 g (½ cup) strawberries
	90 g (½ cup) whole grain rice
	250 mL (1 cup) non-fat milk

*For 1 500 calories, add one meat and alternatives serving and two vegetable and fruit servings, and include one serving of the daily recommended oil and fats. For 1 800 calories, add one grain product serving, one milk and alternative, two meat and alternative servings, two vegetable and fruit servings, and an additional serving of oil and fats.

Most overweight people have at some time attempted to lose weight. Some have had limited and temporary success, and others have met only with failure. Many individuals attempt weight loss by trying out a least one of the many fad diets that offer the enticement of quick weight loss with little effort. Often these fad diets advocate for the elimination of one or more categories of foods (e.g., carbohydrates) and should not be followed. Low-carbohydrate diets, for example, do produce a rapid weight loss, but they also may not allow for adequate amounts of fibre, vitamins, and minerals. These diets are difficult to maintain in the long term because of their restrictive nature. It is best to recommend a dietary approach in which caloric restriction includes all food groups. Patients find it easier to incorporate such changes into their lifestyles and do not become bored with their food options. The nurse must work to support patients' understanding that following a well-balanced, low-calorie diet is an essential part of weight loss and is superior to fad diets in achieving and supporting weight loss and sustained weight maintenance. The degree of success of any reducing diet depends in part on the amount of weight to be lost. People with moderate obesity attain the goal more easily than people with morbid obesity. Perhaps because men have a higher percentage of lean body mass, men are able to lose weight more quickly than women. Women have a higher percentage of body fat, which is metabolically less active than muscle tissue. Postmenopausal women are particularly prone to weight gain, including increased abdominal fat.

Assessing and supporting readiness for change and patient motivation are essential steps in successful weight-loss interventions. The patient must understand the need for weight loss and weight control and the advantages that will occur. The nurse can assist by helping the patient track eating patterns with a diet diary. A frank discussion of eating habits helps the patient realize that eating is often the result of bad habits picked up with time and not the result of hunger. The bad habits must be changed, or weight loss will be only temporary.

Setting a realistic and healthy goal, such as losing 0.5 to 1 kg per week, must be mutually agreed on at the outset. Trying to lose too much too fast usually results in a sense of frustration and failure for the patient. The nurse can help the patient understand that losing large amounts of weight in a short period causes skin and underlying tissue to lose elasticity and tone, resulting in loose folds of skin and tissue. Inevitably, the patient reaches plateau periods during which no weight is lost. These plateaus may last from several days to several weeks. It is especially important for the patient to realize that these are normal occurrences during weight reduction so as to prevent discouragement, frustration, and giving up of the prescribed dietary plan. A weekly check of body weight is a good method of monitoring progress. Daily weighing is not recommended because of the frequent fluctuations resulting from retained water (including urine) and elimination of feces. Instruct the patient to record his or her weight at the same time of the day, wearing the same type of clothing.

There is no firm agreement on the number of meals to be eaten when a person is on a diet; however, breakfast should not be missed. Some nutritionists advocate several small meals per day because the body's metabolic rate is temporarily increased immediately after eating. However, when several small meals are ingested per day, more calories may be consumed. The patient should be instructed to carefully adhere to portion sizes and stay within the total daily calorie allotment. There seems to be general agreement that consumption of most of the daily caloric intake at a large evening meal results in less weight loss than when the calories are evenly distributed throughout the day.

When a person first begins a weight reduction program, food portion sizes must be carefully determined to stay within the dietary guidelines. Portion sizes have increased considerably since the 1990s (Wright & Aronne, 2012; see Table 43-4). Food portions can be weighed on a scale, or everyday objects can be used as a visual cue to determine portion sizes; for example, the size of a woman's fist or a baseball is equivalent to one serving of vegetables or fruit. A serving of meat is about the size of an adult's palm or a deck of cards. A serving of cheese is about the size of a thumb or six dice (see the Alberta Health Services website listed in the Resources section at the end of this chapter for a sample patient teaching tool). A test on portion sizes is also available online (see the Resources at the end of this chapter). A food journal is an important tool for understanding eating habits and bringing awareness to the patient regarding actual food consumed. Journalling also aids the dietitian in setting goals when working with patients learning proper eating habits.

As identified in Chapter 42, Canada's Food Guide provides a solid example of a balanced diet and instruction to assist individuals with making healthy choices, with appropriate portions from each of the food groups. Patients can be further assisted in understanding and exercising good portion control and choosing appropriate proportions from each of the food groups by describing a healthy meal by how portions fit on a plate (Figure 43-6). Half of a "healthy plate" consists of vegetables and fruit, one-fourth consists of meat and meat alternatives, and one-fourth consists of grain products.

A list of healthy, low-calorie foods serves as a good reference and enables patients to eat an occasional meal at a restaurant. Patients who carefully follow the prescribed diet may not need to take vitamin supplements. Appropriate fluid intake should be encouraged. Alcoholic beverages are usually not permitted on a reducing diet because they increase the caloric intake and have low nutritional value.

PHYSICAL ACTIVITY. Physical activity is an essential part of a weight-control program. Current recommendations state that, to achieve health benefits, people need 150 minutes of moderate to vigorous aerobic activity per week (Canadian Society for Exercise Physiology, 2012). There is no evidence that increased activity promotes an increase in appetite or leads to dietary excess. In fact, physical activity frequently has the opposite effect. The addition of physical activity produces more weight loss than does dieting alone. Increasing physical activity has a favourable effect on body fat distribution with a reduction in WHR. Physical activity is especially important in maintaining weight loss in people with overweight and obesity.

The nurse and the patient should explore possible ways to increase physical activity in daily routines. It may be as simple as parking farther from a patient's place of employment or taking the stairs rather than the elevator. The patient should be encouraged to wear a pedometer to track daily activity, with a goal of 10 000 steps a day. However, initial success may be walking a third of the recommended steps, with incremental increases over time.

Joining a health club can be one mechanism of getting physical activity. Walking, swimming, and cycling are sensible forms of physical activity and have long-term benefits. Engaging in weekend exercise only or in spurts of strenuous activity is not advantageous and can actually be dangerous. When large muscles are involved in the physical activity program, a primary benefit is cardio-vascular conditioning. Overweight men and women who are active and fit have lower rates of morbidity and mortality than overweight people who are sedentary and unfit. Therefore, physical activity is of benefit to overweight people even if it does not make them lean.

An increased physical activity program offers many psychological benefits. Patients can achieve reduction in tension and stress, better-quality sleep and rest, increased stamina and energy, improved self-concept and self-confidence, better attitudes toward work and play, and increased optimism about the future.

BEHAVIOUR MODIFICATION. The assumption behind cognitive–behavioural modification is two-fold: (a) that obesity is a learned disorder caused by overeating and (b) that the critical difference between a person with obesity and a person of normal weight is in the cues that regulate eating behaviour. Therefore, most behaviour-modification programs de-emphasize the diet and focus on how and when the person eats. Participants often are taught to restrict their eating to designated meals and to increase the amount of physical activity in their lives. People who have undergone behaviour therapy are more successful in maintaining their losses over an extended time than are those who do not participate in such training.

Common behavioural techniques included in weight-management interventions are (a) self-monitoring, (b) stimulus control, and (c) rewards. *Self-monitoring* may involve the person keeping a record of what and when foods are eaten, as well as how the person was feeling when the foods were consumed. *Stimulus control* is aimed at separating events that trigger eating from the act of eating. *Rewards* may be used as incentive for weight loss. Short- and long-term goals are useful benchmarks for earning rewards. It is important that the reward for a specified weight loss not be associated with food, such as dinner out or a favourite treat. Reward items do not have to have a monetary component. For example, time for a hot bath or an hour of pleasure reading would be an enjoyable reward for many people. People may participate in group or individual sessions or both as they work toward their goals.

SUPPORT GROUPS. Patients may benefit from joining a support group that includes professional counselling. Many self-help groups are available to people who want to learn more about successful dieting and who like the support of others who have the

HEALTHY PLATE

1/2 VEGETABLES & FRUIT
Choose variety of colors. Green, yellow orange and red are the best choices

1/4 GRAIN FOOD
Try to avoid refined (white) grains and prefer whole (brown) grains

1/4 PROTEIN
Fish, poultry, nuts, dairy are ideal sources of protein

WATER
Avoid sugary drinks

FIGURE 43-6 The sizes of healthy portions on a plate. Source: medejaja/Shutterstock.com.

same problems and similar experiences. Take Off Pounds Sensibly (TOPS) is the oldest nonprofit organization of this type in the world. Behaviour modification is an integral part of the program, along with nutrition education. Weight Watchers International, Inc. is probably the most successful commercial weight-reduction enterprise. Weight Watchers offers a food plan that is nutritionally balanced and practical to follow and its programs have included behaviour-modification techniques since 1974.

Commercial weight-reduction centres have proliferated across the nation. Many of these programs are staffed by nurses or dietitians or both, and candidates must undergo an initial physical examination by a health care provider before being accepted for weight reduction. Although behaviour-modification training is often incorporated within these programs, they are often costly, and the cost may be prohibitive for people with limited financial resources. In addition, many of these programs offer special prepackaged foods and supplements that must be purchased as part of the weight-reduction plan. Only these prescribed foods and drinks are to be consumed until an agreed-on amount of weight is lost. The patient is encouraged to buy the same type of foods for the maintenance phase of the program, which lasts from 6 months to 1 year. This is problematic for reasons beyond just the associated costs. Obesity, as with all chronic diseases, resumes its course when the intervention stops. Patients are often frustrated to find that the weight they lost is regained once they stop participating in the commercial program. Individuals who discontinue such programs must be supported to learn to adjust their diet appropriately to maintain their intervention and the resultant weight loss.

Many places of employment have started programs on health teaching and maintenance. The rationale for such programs is that better health repays the cost of the programs through improved work performance, decreased absenteeism, and eventually less hospitalization. Weight-reduction and hypertension-reduction programs have been instituted and are popular with employees.

DRUG THERAPY

Drugs have been used to treat obesity but only as adjuncts to nutrition, physical activity, and behaviour-modification therapies. Pharmacotherapy should be reserved for patients with a BMI ≥ 27 kg/m^2 who have existing comorbid conditions (e.g., hypertension, dyslipidemia, coronary artery disease, type 2 diabetes mellitus, and sleep apnea) and for those with a BMI ≥ 30 kg/m^2. Currently, drugs approved for weight loss in Canada are the kind that decrease nutrient absorption. Drugs that decrease food intake by reducing appetite or increasing satiety (e.g., sibutramine [Meridia]) and drugs that increase energy expenditure (e.g., ephedrine) are not approved for weight loss in Canada at this time.

Nutrient Absorption–Blocking Drugs

Orlistat (Xenical), a drug that was developed for weight loss and maintenance, works by blocking fat breakdown and absorption in the intestine. It inhibits the action of intestinal lipases. The undigested fat is excreted in the feces. Although this medication has a high safety profile, levels of some fat-soluble vitamins may decrease, and those vitamins may have to be supplemented. Orlistat is associated with leakage of stool, flatulence, diarrhea, and abdominal bloating, which is accentuated if a high-fat diet is consumed. These adverse effects limit its acceptance as a weight-loss tool (Kang & Park, 2012). Liraglutide (Saxenda) is an injectable drug newly used for weight management. It works by blocking GLP1 (glucagon-like peptide). Normally, liraglutide is used for the treatment of type 2 diabetes, but higher doses have been found to help with weight loss in those following a calorie-reduced diet and a physical activity regimen (Pi-Sunyer, Astrup, Fujioka, et al., 2015). In February 2015, Health Canada approved the use of liraglutide (Saxenda) for weight management in patients with BMI >27 kg/m^2 and one or more health-related comorbidities or with a BMI >30 kg/m^2. Adverse effects of liraglutide include nausea and diarrhea as well as increased risk for pancreatitis and gallbladder disease (Novo Nordisk, 2016).

Drugs do not cure obesity, and the patient must understand that without substantial changes in food intake and increased physical activity, weight will be regained when short-term drug therapy is stopped. Supervised long-term drug therapy with safe compounds can contribute to weight management as well as weight loss. As with any pharmacological treatment, there are adverse effects. Careful evaluation for the presence of other medical conditions can help determine which drugs, if any, would be advisable for a given patient.

The role of the nurse in relation to drug therapy should centre on teaching the patient about proper administration and adverse events and how the drug fits into the larger weight-loss plan. Modifying the dosage without consulting a health care provider can have detrimental effects. The nurse should re-emphasize that the diet and physical activity regimens are the cornerstones of permanent weight loss. Drugs may be helpful, but they do not change the patient's eating behaviour. The purchase of over-the-counter diet aids should be discouraged.

COLLABORATIVE SURGICAL THERAPY

Bariatric surgery is an invasive procedure used to treat morbid obesity. Bariatric surgery is currently the only treatment that has been found to help sustain weight loss in individuals who are severely obese. The majority of patients who undergo bariatric surgery have successfully improved their overall quality of life. A great deal of excess weight is lost, comorbid conditions resolve, and patients' appearance, social opportunities, and economic opportunities are improved (Dunham, 2013).

Criteria guidelines for bariatric surgery include having a BMI of 40 kg/m^2 or higher or a BMI of 35 kg/m^2 or higher plus one or more severe obesity-related comorbid conditions (e.g., hypertension, type 2 diabetes mellitus, heart failure, or sleep apnea). Many adults meet these criteria, and additional recommendations must be taken into account, including a documented history of conventional weight loss attempts that have been unsuccessful over time; a demonstrated history of accountability and responsibility marked by attending appointments regularly, practising self-monitoring, completing laboratory tests, regularly taking medications, and making time for healthy eating and activity. The patient must have full understanding of the benefits and limitations of a surgical procedure to assist with the management of obesity, and the risk of the surgical procedure must be lower than the risks of not providing the treatment (Karmali, Johnson Stoklossa, Sharma, et al., 2010). Table 43-9 describes exclusion criteria for bariatric surgery.

Patients are not good candidates for bariatric surgery if they (a) are obese as a result of a treatable disorder (e.g., hypothyroidism); (b) have untreated depression or psychosis, binge-eating disorder, or bulimia; (c) currently abuse drugs or alcohol; (d) have severe cardiac disease with prohibitive anaesthetic-related risks; (e) have severe coagulopathy; or (f) are unable to comply

TABLE 43-9 EXCLUSION CRITERIA FOR BARIATRIC SURGERY

Patients *who are* or *who have* any of the following characteristics should not be offered bariatric surgery:

- BMI <35 kg/m^2
- Age <18 yr or >65 yr
- A medical condition that makes surgery too risky
- Clinically significant or unstable mental-health concerns
- An unrealistic postsurgical target weight
- Unrealistic expectations of a surgical procedure
- Not tried or optimized lifestyle or medical treatments
- A history of poor compliance with lifestyle, medical, or mental health interventions
- Pregnant, lactating, or plan for pregnancy within 2 yr of potential surgical treatment
- Lack of safe access to abdominal cavity or gastro-intestinal tract
- Smokers (All smokers, regardless of their weight status, should quit smoking for at least 8 weeks before surgery as a goal of risk-factor management. All patients should be encouraged to remain nonsmokers or participate in smoking cessation programs.)

BMI, body mass index.
Source: Karmali, S., Johnson Stoklossa, C., Sharma, A., et al. (2010). Bariatric surgery: A primer. *Canadian Family Physician, 56,* 874.

with nutritional requirements. Bariatric surgeries fall into one of three broad categories: restrictive, malabsorptive, or a combination of malabsorptive and restrictive (Table 43-10 and Figure 43-7). In restrictive procedures, the stomach is reduced in size (less food eaten), and in malabsorptive procedures, the length of the small intestine is decreased (less food absorbed).

Restrictive Surgeries

Restrictive bariatric surgery reduces either the size of the stomach, which causes the patient to feel full more quickly, or the amount allowed to enter the stomach. The stomach and the intestine digest and absorb food normally when restrictive gastro-intestinal surgery is performed. Because digestion is not altered, the risk for anemia or cobalamin deficiency is low. These procedures can be performed using a laparoscopic approach, which decreases the rate of wound infection and hernia formation. Weight loss is typically more gradual with these procedures. Several restrictive procedures are available. The most common are discussed below.

Vertical Banded Gastroplasty. *Vertical banded gastroplasty* involves partitioning the stomach into a small pouch in the upper portion along the lesser curvature of the stomach. This small pouch drastically limits capacity. In addition, the stoma opening

FIGURE 43-7 Bariatric surgical procedures. **A,** Vertical banded gastroplasty involves creating a small gastric pouch. **B,** Adjustable gastric banding involves the use of a band to create a gastric pouch. **C,** Vertical sleeve gastrectomy involves creating a sleeve-shaped stomach by removing approximately 85% of the stomach. **D,** Biliopancreatic diversion with duodenal switch procedure involves creating an anastomosis between the stomach and intestine. **E,** Roux-en-Y gastric bypass procedure involves constructing a gastric pouch whose outlet is a Y-shaped limb of small intestine.

TABLE 43-10 SURGICAL INTERVENTIONS FOR MORBID OBESITY*

Procedure	Anatomical Changes	Advantages	Complications
Restrictive Surgery			
Adjustable gastric banding (AGB) (Lap-Band, Realize band)	Band encircles the stomach, creating a stoma and a gastric pouch with 10- to 15-mL capacity	Food digestion occurs through normal process Band can be adjusted to ↑ or ↓ restriction Surgery can be reversed Absence of dumping syndrome Lack of malabsorption	Low complication rate Some nausea and vomiting initially Problems with adjustment device Band may slip or erode into stomach wall Gastric perforation
Vertical sleeve gastrectomy	About 85% of stomach removed, leaving a sleeve-shaped stomach with 60- to 150-mL capacity	Function of stomach preserved No bypass of intestine Avoids complications of obstruction, anemia, vitamin deficiencies	Possible limitation to weight loss Leakage related to stapling
Vertical banded gastroplasty (VBG)	Band placed around stomach, and staples used above band to create a small gastric pouch	No surgical anastomosis More normal anatomy and physiology maintained Lower risk for infection	High complication rate Slow weight loss Rupture of staple line Dilated pouch Dumping syndrome (nausea, vomiting, diarrhea, or a combination of these related to ingestion of sweets, high-calorie liquids, or dairy products)
Malabsorptive Surgery			
Biliopancreatic diversion (BPD) with or without duodenal switch	70% of the stomach removed horizontally Anastomosis between the stomach and the intestine Decreases the amount of small intestine available for nutrient absorption Duodenal switch cuts the stomach vertically so stomach is shaped like a tube	Increased amount of food intake Less food intolerance Greater long-term weight loss Rapid weight loss	Abdominal bloating, diarrhea, and foul-smelling gas (steatorrhea) Three or four loose bowel movements a day Malabsorption of fat-soluble vitamins Iron deficiency Protein-calorie malnutrition† Dumping syndrome†
Combination of Restrictive and Malabsorptive Surgery			
Roux-en-Y gastric bypass (RYGB)	Restrictive surgery on stomach, creating small gastric pouch connected to jejunum Remaining stomach and first segment of small intestine are bypassed	Better weight loss results than with gastric restrictive procedures Lower incidence of malnutrition and diarrhea Rapid improvement of weight-related comorbidities	Leak at site of anastomosis Anemia: iron deficiency, cobalamin deficiency, folic acid deficiency Calcium deficiency Dumping syndrome

*See Figure 43-7.
†Less common with duodenal switch.

to the rest of the stomach is banded to delay emptying of solid food from the proximal pouch. This procedure has been replaced by other procedures because of lack of sustained or desired weight loss and the high incidence of complications.

Adjustable Gastric Banding. With *adjustable gastric banding*, the stomach size is limited by an inflatable band placed around the fundus of the stomach. This restrictive procedure can be done using the Lap-Band system or the Realize band system. The band is connected to a subcutaneous port and can be inflated or deflated (by fluid injection in the health care provider's office) to change the stoma size to meet the patient's needs as weight is lost. The procedure can be done laparoscopically and can be modified or reversed after the initial procedure. Adjustable gastric banding is the procedure most commonly performed, and it is the preferred option for patients who are at surgical risk because it is a less invasive approach.

Malabsorptive Surgery

In malabsorptive surgery to reduce weight, the surgeon bypasses various lengths of the small intestine so that less food is absorbed.

Biliopancreatic Diversion. Biliopancreatic diversion (BPD) involves removing approximately 75% of the stomach to produce both restriction of food intake and reduction of acid output. The remaining portion of the stomach is connected to the lower portion of the small intestine. Nutrients pass without being digested. The patient loses weight because most of the calories and nutrients are routed into the colon, where they are not absorbed.

This procedure can increase the risk for gallstone formation and may necessitate removal of the gallbladder. Patients should be aware of the possibilities of intestinal irritation and ulcers. Other risks from BPD include abdominal bloating and foul-smelling stool or gas. During the period when the intestines adjust, bowel movements can be very liquid and frequent. This condition may lessen over time, but it may be a lifelong condition. Patients should also monitor their protein, iron, and cobalamin intake to ensure that they do not develop malnutrition or anemia. Supplements and vitamins should be taken to offset these risks.

Biliopancreatic Diversion With Duodenal Switch. A variation of the BPD procedure involves a duodenal switch in which the surgeon leaves intact a larger portion of the stomach, as well as a small part of the duodenum. This procedure also enables sparing of the pyloric valve, which helps prevent dumping syndrome. (Dumping syndrome is discussed in the next section and in Chapter 44.)

Combination of Restrictive and Malabsorptive Surgery

Roux-en-Y Surgical Procedure. The Roux-en-Y gastric bypass procedure is a combination of restrictive and malabsorptive surgery. Complication rates with this procedure are low, patient tolerance is excellent, and the procedure has proved to sustain long-term weight loss. Because of this, the Roux-en-Y gastric bypass procedure is the bariatric surgery most commonly performed. In this procedure, the stomach size is decreased with a gastric pouch anastomosis that empties directly into the jejunum. This surgery can be performed through an open abdominal incision or through laparoscopy. Variations of this procedure include (a) stapling the stomach without transection to create a small gastric pouch (capacity of 20–30 mL); (b) creating an upper and a lower gastric pouch that are totally disconnected from each other; and (c) creating an upper gastric pouch and completely removing the lower pouch. After the procedure, food bypasses 90% of the stomach, the duodenum, and a small segment of jejunum.

Weight loss is usually greatest during the first year after surgery. Weight tends to stabilize after 18 months. Outcomes include increased glucose tolerance, decreased BP, decreased levels of cholesterol and triglycerides, decreased incidence of GERD, and decreased sleep apnea. A complication of this procedure is *dumping syndrome,* in which gastric contents empty too rapidly into the small intestine, overwhelming its ability to digest nutrients (see Chapter 44). Symptoms can include vomiting, nausea, weakness, sweating, faintness, and, on occasion, diarrhea. To avoid dumping syndrome, patients are discouraged from eating sugary foods after surgery. Because sections of the small intestine are bypassed, poor absorption of iron can cause iron-deficiency anemia. The patient needs to take a multivitamin with iron and calcium supplements. Chronic anemia caused by cobalamin deficiency may also occur. This problem usually can be managed with cobalamin injections or intranasal cobalamin preparations.

Cosmetic Surgeries to Reduce Fatty Tissue and Skin Folds

Lipectomy. Lipectomy (adipectomy) is performed to remove unsightly loose folds of adipose tissue for cosmetic reasons. In some patients, up to 15% of the total fat cells can be removed from the breasts, the abdomen, and the lumbar and femoral areas. There is no evidence that adipose tissue regenerates at the surgical sites. However, it must be emphasized to the patient that surgical removal does not prevent obesity from recurring, especially if lifetime eating habits remain the same. Although body image and self-esteem may be enhanced by such procedures, these operations are not without complications. In patients with obesity, the effects of anaesthetics can be dangerous, and wound healing has the potential to be poor. It is more useful for the majority of patients contemplating a lipectomy to be instructed in preventive health measures, such as slow weight reduction to maintain and preserve tissue integrity, the value of physical activity, and behaviour-modification techniques.

Liposuction. Another surgical procedure is *liposuction,* or suction-assisted lipectomy. The current use is for cosmetic purposes and not for weight reduction. This surgical intervention helps improve facial appearance and body contours. A good candidate for this type of surgery is a person who has achieved weight reduction but has excess fat under the chin, along the jawline, in the nasolabial folds, over the abdomen, or around the waist and upper thighs. A long, hollow, stainless steel cannula is inserted through a small incision over the fatty tissue to be suctioned. The purpose of this type of surgery is to improve body appearance, thereby enhancing body image and self-concept. It is not usually recommended for older patients because the skin is less elastic and does not accommodate the new underlying shape.

NURSING MANAGEMENT
PATIENT WITH OBESITY UNDERGOING SURGERY

NURSING IMPLEMENTATION

PERIOPERATIVE CARE. Many patients with a BMI greater than 35 kg/m^2 have several other medical conditions related to obesity that increase their surgical risk factors and affect their care before, during, and after surgery. This section discusses general nursing considerations for the care of patients with obesity who are having surgery. (General care of patients before, during, and after surgery is discussed in Chapters 20 to 22.)

PREOPERATIVE CARE. There are special care considerations for patients with obesity admitted to the hospital for surgical treatment, especially the ones who have morbid obesity. Before surgery, it is important to conduct a preoperative interview with the patient to obtain past and current health information and to ensure that the patient understands the surgical procedure that he or she is scheduled to undergo. If the patient has a disease other than obesity, care may need to be coordinated with the patient's cardiologist, pulmonologist, gynecologist, gastro-enterologist, or other specialist.

Every effort should be made to ensure the patient's dignity and privacy before admission. Most nursing units are not prepared to meet the needs of a patient who may be too large for a typical hospital bed or who does not fit into standard patient care gowns. To eliminate embarrassment for the patient and frustration for the staff, plans should be made to meet particular needs. Oversized BP cuffs should be ready for use when the patient arrives. A single-bed room may be necessary for the privacy of the patient and to accommodate the bed and sitting arrangements. A strongly reinforced trapeze bar should be placed over the bed to facilitate movement and positioning. In some cases, a bariatric chair may have to be built and beds joined together to allow the patient to sit and sleep in comfort.

The nurse must consider how the patient will be weighed and transported within the hospital and in what ways simple physical assessment strategies may have to be adjusted. Bariatric equipment such as an oversized wheelchair, bariatric bed, walker, and various lifting devices should be made available in the hospital and used.

Bathing, turning, and ambulating the patient may require extra staff, and a plan to meet this need should be in place before the patient's admission. Routine physical assessment strategies do not work well with patients with morbid obesity, who have numerous layers of skin folds covering areas that must be assessed. If alternative or unique methods of dealing with this problem are not identified, assessment of respiratory status and bowel sounds or even wound inspection could be awkward for the nurse and embarrassing for the patient. Wound infection is one of the most common complications after surgery. Because of the many layers of skin folds, especially in the abdominal area, preoperative skin preparation is important. Many patients are instructed to take several showers a day for a few days before admission to the hospital. Careful cleansing with soap and warm water of the abdominal area from the breasts to below the waist is emphasized.

Obesity can cause a patient's breathing to become shallow and rapid. The extra adipose tissue in the chest and the abdomen compresses the diaphragmatic, thoracic, and abdominal structures. This compression restricts the chest's ability to expand, causing the lungs to not work as efficiently as they would otherwise. Thus, the patient retains more carbon dioxide. In addition, less oxygen is delivered to the lungs, resulting in hypoxemia, pulmonary hypertension, and polycythemia. Instruct the patient in the proper coughing technique, deep breathing, and methods of turning and positioning to prevent pulmonary complications after surgery. Introduce the use of spirometry before surgery. Use of the spirometer helps prevent and alleviate postoperative lung congestion. Practising these strategies preoperatively can aid the patient in performing them correctly after surgery. Furthermore, if the patient uses a continuous positive airway pressure (CPAP) device at home for sleep apnea, make arrangements for use of a CPAP machine while the patient is in the hospital. (See Chapter 68 for further discussion on CPAP; see Chapter 9 for more information on sleep apnea and the use of CPAP.)

Obtaining venous access may also be complicated by excess adipose tissue. An assistant may be needed to help. If a patient has pitting edema or excess fat, the nurse should firmly, with pressure, hold a finger over the spot. The nurse may also want to mark the spot of injection with a sterile skin marker once a vein is found. Edema can become worse if the nurse chooses to anchor the catheter by taping the arm. This action can further impede venous return, causing venous stasis, pooling of intravenous fluids, extravasation, or infiltration. The nurse may also want to use multiple tourniquets to distend veins and hold back excess tissue. To avoid aggravating the edema, the tourniquet should be removed as soon as it is no longer needed. The nurse may also need a longer catheter (longer than 2.5 cm) to traverse overlying tissue. The cannula must reach far enough into the vein to ensure that it does not become dislodged or cause infiltration.

The use of anaesthetic agents during the surgery increases the patient's risk for failure to wean from mechanical ventilation. The patient must be informed of this risk so that he or she can know what to expect upon waking up from the anaesthesia.

Special Considerations for Bariatric Surgery. The hospital experience will depend on the type of procedure and the surgical approach. The nurse should prepare the patient before surgery for the possibility of returning to the room with one or more of the following: urinary catheter, intravenous (IV) catheter, compression stockings, and a nasogastric (NG) tube. The nurse should emphasize that vital signs will be checked and general assessment conducted frequently to monitor for immediate complications. Furthermore, the patient must understand that he or she will be assisted with ambulation soon after surgery and encouraged to deep-breathe to prevent pulmonary complications. Liquids will be started soon after surgery but only after the patient is fully awake and no anastomotic leaks are found.

POSTOPERATIVE CARE. The initial postoperative care focuses on careful assessment and immediate intervention for cardiopulmonary complications, thrombus formation, anastomotic leaks, and electrolyte imbalances. The transfer of the patient from surgery may require many trained staff members. During the transfer, the patient's airway should remain stabilized, and

pain should be managed at a tolerable level. Maintain the head of the patient at a 35- to 40-degree angle to reduce abdominal pressure and increase tidal flow. If the patient has severe obesity, the nursing team should closely monitor for rapid oxygen desaturation. The body stores anaesthetic agents in adipose tissue; thus the patient with excess adipose tissue is at risk for resedation. As adipose cells release anaesthetic back into the bloodstream, the patient may become sedated after surgery. If this happens, the nursing care team should be prepared to perform a head-tilt or jaw-thrust manoeuvre and keep the patient's oral and nasal airways opened. Early ambulation is essential for the postoperative bariatric patient. Preoperative teaching facilitates the patient's cooperation with what will be an uncomfortable activity. The patient should be informed that typically the evening after surgery, he or she will be assisted to walk and then be ambulated at least three or four times each day. The dangers of thrombo-phlebitis and the measures to counteract its development are a routine part of preoperative teaching. The patient should know that sequential compression devices or elastic compression stockings will be applied to the legs and that active and passive range-of-motion exercises will be a frequent part of daily care. Low-dose heparin may be ordered. Depending on the size of the patient and the amount of pain he or she is experiencing, the patient may not be able to assist the nurse in turning. Extra nurses may be needed to help turn the patient safely.

The patient should also be informed that the nursing care team will assess the patient's skin for delayed wound healing and the development of seromas, hematomas, wound dehiscence, wound evisceration, and wound infection. Skin folds should be kept clean and dry to prevent dermatitis and secondary bacterial or fungal infections.

Special Considerations for Bariatric Surgery. The patient experiences considerable abdominal pain after bariatric surgery. Pain medications should be given as frequently as necessary during the immediate postoperative period (first 24 hours). The nurse must be diligent in assessing pain and be aware that pain could be caused by an anastomotic leak rather than typical surgical pain.

Abdominal wounds must be observed frequently for the amount and type of drainage, condition of the sutures, and signs of infection. The nurse must protect the incision against undue straining that accompanies turning and coughing. Wound dehiscence and impaired wound healing are potential problems for patients with obesity. Monitoring the vital signs assists in identifying problems such as infection.

If an NG tube is inserted, the nurse must monitor it for correct positioning. However, the NG tube must never be inserted or repositioned by the nurse. Vomiting with an NG tube in place requires repositioning the tube, so the surgeon should be notified immediately. The upper gastric pouch is small, and irrigating the tube with too much solution or manipulating tube position can lead to disruption of the anastomosis or the staple line.

Skin care should be performed several times each shift. Perspiration may be excessive at times. The many layers of skin should be kept clean and dry so that this source of irritation is eliminated. For the patient who has an in-dwelling catheter, perineal care is important to prevent urinary tract infection.

During the immediate postoperative period (first 24 hours), water and sugar-free clear liquids are administered (30 mL every 2 hours while the patient is awake). Before discharge, the patient should be instructed about a measured amount of a high-protein liquid diet. The patient is taught to eat slowly and to stop when feeling full and not to consume liquids with solid food. Vomiting is a common complication during this time. A dietitian is typically a part of the bariatric team and assists with the patient's transition to the new diet.

AMBULATORY AND HOME CARE

Special Considerations for Bariatric Surgery. The patient who has undergone major surgical treatment for obesity has not, in the past, been successful in following or maintaining a prescribed diet. Now the patient is forced to reduce the oral intake as a result of the anatomical changes brought about by the operation. The patient finds that adherence to a regimen of reduced intake is necessary because of the concern for abdominal distension, cramping abdominal pain, and perhaps diarrhea.

Weight loss is considerable during the first 6 to 12 months. During this time, the patient must learn to adjust intake sufficiently to maintain a stable weight. Although behaviour modification was not an intended outcome when these surgical procedures were devised, it has become an unexpected and beneficial secondary benefit. The diet generally prescribed should be high in protein and low in carbohydrates, fat, and roughage, and consist of six small feedings daily. Fluids should not be ingested with the meal, and, in some cases, fluids should be restricted to less than 1 000 mL per day. Fluids and foods high in carbohydrates tend to promote diarrhea and symptoms of dumping syndrome. In general, calorically dense foods (foods high in fat) should be avoided to enable more nutritionally sound food to be consumed.

Proper diet must be clearly understood by the patient. Late complications can be anticipated after gastric bypass or gastroplasty, including anemia, vitamin deficiencies, diarrhea, and psychiatric problems. Failure to lose weight or loss of too much weight may be caused by the surgical formation of a stomach pouch that is too large or of an outlet that is much too small, respectively. Peptic ulcer formation, dumping syndrome, and small bowel obstruction may occur late in the recovery and rehabilitative stages.

Long-term follow-up care must be stressed, in part because of complications late in the recovery period. Encourage the patient to adhere strictly to the prescribed diet and to keep the health care provider informed of any changes in physical or emotional condition. Some patients have been known to overeat when they return home and gain rather than lose weight.

The nurse must anticipate and recognize several potential psychological problems after surgery. Some patients express guilt because the only way they could lose weight was by surgical means rather than by the "sheer willpower" of reduced dietary intake. The nurse should be ready to provide support so that such patients do not dwell on negative feelings.

Many patients with morbid obesity who blamed their feelings of social inferiority or inadequacies on their appearance before bypass surgery may suffer from episodes of depression (see the "Evidence-Informed Practice" box). By 6 to 8 months after surgery, considerable weight loss will have occurred, and patients are able to see clearly how much their appearance has changed. Massive weight loss often leaves the patient with large quantities of loose skin that can cause problems related to altered body image. Reconstructive surgery at least 1 full year after the initial surgery may alleviate this situation. Reduction of breasts, upper arms, thighs, and excess abdominal skin folds are possible solutions. Discussion of this possible outcome with the patient before surgery and again during the rehabilitation phase of recovery helps facilitate the patient's adjustment to a new body image and social reintegration.

⟳ EVIDENCE-INFORMED PRACTICE

Translating Research Into Practice

William Giles is a 35-yr-old male patient weighing 166.4 kg with a BMI of 54.3 kg/m². He underwent gastric bypass surgery and is now ready for discharge. The bariatric program at the hospital he is in recommends attendance at support groups after surgery. Mr. Giles informs the nurse that he does not feel comfortable in group settings and will not be attending these meetings.

Best Available Evidence	Clinician Expertise	Patient Preferences and Values
Patients attending psychotherapeutic interventions or support groups in combination with bariatric surgery experience greater weight-loss results than patients treated with only bariatric surgery.	The nurse has heard from several former bariatric patients who have maintained their weight loss after surgery and attributed this success, in part, to their participation in the support group offered at the facility.	Patient does not feel comfortable in group settings.

Decision and Action

The nurse explores Mr. Giles's feelings about groups and shares the reports from former patients with him. He continues to be firm about his unwillingness to attend any support groups. The nurse discusses with him that it is his decision and assures him that his progress will be monitored. The nurse also gently reminds him that he can change his decision at any time. The physician is informed of the patient's choice.

Reference for Evidence

Beck, N. N., Johannsen, M., Støving, R. K., et al. (2012). Do postoperative psychotherapeutic interventions and support groups influence weight loss following bariatric surgery? A systematic review and meta-analysis of randomized and nonrandomized trials. *Obesity Surgery, 22*(11), 1790–1797.

▌EVALUATION

The following outcomes are expected for patients with obesity after surgery:

- The patient will experience long-term weight loss.
- The patient will experience improvement in obesity-related comorbid conditions.
- The patient will integrate healthy practices into daily routines.
- The patient will monitor for adverse effects of surgical therapy.
- The patient will have an improved self-image.

▌AGE-RELATED CONSIDERATIONS

OBESITY IN OLDER ADULTS

The prevalence of obesity is increasing in all age groups, including older people (CIHI & PHAC, 2011). The number of older adults with obesity has risen markedly because of both an increase in the total number of older people and an increase in the percentage of people who are obese. Obesity is more common in older women than in older men. A decrease in energy expenditure is an important contributor to a gradual increase in body fat with increasing age.

Obesity in older adults can exacerbate age-related declines in physical function and lead to frailty and disability. Excess body weight places more demands on arthritic joints; mechanical strain on weight-bearing joints can lead to premature immobility.

Older adults may find that excess intra-abdominal weight causes urinary incontinence. Excess weight may also contribute to hypoventilation and sleep apnea. Obesity is associated with shortened lifespan: individuals who are obese live 6 to 7 years less than do people of normal weight.

Obesity affects quality of life for older adults. Weight loss can improve quality of life and physical function and lessen obesity-related health complications. The same therapeutic approaches to obesity discussed earlier also apply to older adults.

CASE STUDY

Obesity

Source: Antonio Gravante/ Shutterstock .com.

Patient Profile
Mrs. Stella Roman is a 60-year-old woman.

Subjective Data
- Reports gradual weight gain of 30 kg during past 40 years
- Spends most of her free time watching television
- Reports health problems related to type 2 diabetes mellitus, shortness of breath, hypertension, chest pressure, and osteoarthritis
- Underwent knee replacement surgery at age 56 for osteoarthritis

Objective Data
Physical Examination
- Height: 162.5 cm; weight: 105 kg
- Has obese, nontender, soft abdomen
- Blood pressure: 160/100 mm Hg

Laboratory Results
- Fasting blood glucose level: 13.9 mmol/L
- Total cholesterol level: 5.3 mmol/L
- Triglyceride level: 3.36 mmol/L
- HDL cholesterol level: 0.8 mmol/L

Discussion Questions
1. What are Mrs. Roman's risk factors for obesity?
2. What is her estimated BMI?
3. Of the possible complications of obesity, which ones does Mrs. Roman have? Why did she develop them?
4. *Priority decision:* How would the nurse assist Mrs. Roman in designing a successful program for weight loss and weight management?
5. What are Mrs. Roman's risk factors for metabolic syndrome?
6. Is Mrs. Roman a candidate for surgical intervention for obesity? If so, why? If not, why not?
7. *Priority decision:* On the basis of the assessment data presented, what are the priority nursing diagnoses? Are there any collaborative problems?

evolve

Answers are available at *http://evolve.elsevier.com/Canada/Lewis/medsurg.*

REVIEW QUESTIONS

The number of the question corresponds to the same-numbered objective at the beginning of the chapter.

1. Which of the following statements best describes the etiology of obesity?
   a. Obesity results primarily from a genetic predisposition.
   b. Psychosocial factors can override the effects of genetics in the etiology of obesity.
   c. Obesity is the result of complex interactions between genetic and environmental factors.
   d. Genetic factors are more important than environmental factors in the etiology of obesity.

2. Which obesity classification is *most* often associated with cardio-vascular health problems?
   a. Primary obesity
   b. Secondary obesity
   c. Gynoid fat distribution
   d. Android fat distribution

3. Health risks associated with obesity include which of the following? *(Select all that apply)*
   a. Colorectal cancer
   b. Rheumatoid arthritis
   c. Polycystic ovary disease
   d. Nonalcoholic steatohepatitis
   e. Systemic lupus erythematosus

4. What is the best nutritional therapy for a person with obesity?
   a. Low-carbohydrate diet
   b. High-protein diet
   c. Low-sugar diet
   d. Foods from the basic food groups

5. Which bariatric surgical procedure involves creating a stoma and gastric pouch that is reversible and does not involve malabsorption?
   a. Vertical gastric banding
   b. Biliopancreatic diversion
   c. Roux-en-Y gastric bypass
   d. Adjustable gastric banding

6. A client with obesity has undergone Roux-en-Y gastric bypass surgery. In planning postoperative care, what should the nurse anticipate?
   a. The client may have severe diarrhea early in the postoperative period.
   b. The client will not be allowed to ambulate for 1 to 2 days postoperatively.
   c. The client will require nasogastric suction until healing of the incision occurs.
   d. The client may have only liquids orally, and in very limited amounts, during the early postoperative period.

7. Which of the following criteria must be met for a diagnosis of metabolic syndrome? *(Select all that apply)*
   a. Hypertension
   b. Elevated triglyceride levels
   c. Elevated plasma glucose level
   d. Increased waist circumference
   e. Decreased LDL levels

1. c, 2. d, 3. a, c, d, 4. d, 5. d, 6. d, 7. a, b, c, d.

evolve

For even more review questions, visit *http://evolve.elsevier.com/Canada/ Lewis/medsurg.*

REFERENCES

Abdullah, A., Wolfe, R., Stoelwinder, J. U., et al. (2011). The number of years lived with obesity and the risk of all-cause and cause-specific mortality. *International Journal of Epidemiology*, *40*(4), 985–986. doi:10.1093/ije/dyr018.

Budd, G. M., & Peterson, J. A. (2014). CE: The obesity epidemic, part 1: Understanding the origins. *The American Journal of Nursing*, *114*(12), 40–46. doi:10.1097/01.NAJ.0000457410.83963.4b.

Canadian Institute for Health Information (CIHI) & Public Health Agency of Canada (PHAC). (2011). *Obesity in Canada: A joint report from the Public Health Agency of Canada and the Canadian Institute for Health Information*. Retrieved from *https:// secure.cihi.ca/free_products/Obesity_in_canada_2011_en.pdf*.

Canadian Society for Exercise Physiology. (2012). *Canadian physical activity guidelines and Canadian sedentary behaviour guidelines*. Retrieved from *http://www.csep.ca/cmfiles/guidelines/csep _guidelines_handbook.pdf*.

Cornier, M. A., Després, J. P., Davis, N., et al. (2011). Assessing adiposity: A scientific statement from the American Heart Association. *Circulation*, *124*(18), 1996–2019. doi:10.1161/ CIR.0b013e318233bc6a.

Dunham, M. (2013). Caring for patients undergoing bariatric surgery. *Nursing*, *43*(10), 44–50. doi:10.1097/01.NURSE .0000432118.12880.ff.

Ford, E. S., Maynard, L. M., & Li, C. (2014). Trends in mean waist circumference and abdominal obesity among US adults, 1999–2012. *Journal of the American Medical Association*, *312*(11), 1151–1153. doi:10.1001/jama.2014.8362.

Health Canada (2011). *Eating well with Canada's food guide*. Ottawa: Author. Retrieved from *https://www.canada.ca/en/health-canada/ services/canada-food-guides.html*.

Kang, J. G., & Park, C. Y. (2012). Anti-obesity drugs: A review about their effects and safety. *Diabetes & Metabolism Journal*, *36*(1), 13–25. doi:10.4093/dmj.2012.36.1.13.

Karmali, S., Johnson Stoklossa, C., Sharma, A., et al. (2010). Bariatric surgery: A primer. *Canadian Family Physician*, *56*, 873–879. (Seminal).

Kirk, S. F., Penney, T. L., McHugh, T. L., et al. (2011). Effective weight management practice: A review of the lifestyle intervention evidence. *International Journal of Obesity*, *36*, 178–185. doi:10.1038/ijo.2011.80.

Lau, D. C. W. (2007). Synopsis of the 2006 Canadian clinical practice guidelines on the management and prevention of obesity in adults and children. *Canadian Medical Association Journal*, *176*(8), 1103–1106. doi:10.1503/cmaj.070306. (Seminal).

Lau, D. C. W., Douketis, J. D., Morrison, K. M., et al. (2007). 2006 Canadian clinical practice guidelines on the management and prevention of obesity in adults and children [summary]. *Canadian Medical Association Journal*, *176*(8), S1–S13. doi:10.1503/cmaj.061409. (Seminal).

Malis, C., Rasmussen, E. L., Poulsen, P., et al. (2005). Total and regional fat distribution is strongly influenced by genetic factors in young and elderly twins. *Obesity Research*, *13*(12), 2139–2145. doi:10.1038/oby.2005.265. (Seminal).

Naukkarinen, J., Rissanen, A., Kaprio, J., et al. (2012). Causes and consequences of obesity: The contribution of recent twin studies. *International Journal of Obesity*, *36*(8), 1017–1024. doi:10.1038/ ijo.2011.192.

Navaneelan, T., & Janz, T. (2014). *Adjusting the scales: Obesity in the Canadian population after correcting for respondent bias*. Statistics Canada. Retrieved from *http://www.statcan.gc.ca/pub/82-624-x/ 2014001/article/11922-eng.htm*.

Novo Nordisk. (2016). *Saxenda*. Retrieved from *https://www .saxenda.com*.

Pi-Sunyer, X., Astrup, A., Fujioka, K., et al. (2015). A randomized, controlled trial of 3.0 mg of liraglutide in weight management. *N Engl J Med*, *373*(1), 11–22. doi:10.1056/NEJMoa1411892.

Rich, P. (2015). *CMA recognizes obesity as a disease*. Retrieved from *https://www.cma.ca/En/Pages/cma-recognizes-obesity-as-a -disease.aspx*.

Roberts, K. C., Shields, M., de Groh, M., et al. (2012). Overweight and obesity in children and adolescents: Results from the 2009 to 2011 Canadian Health Measures Survey. *Health Reports*, *23*(3), 37–41.

Schmandt, R. E., Iglesias, D. A., Co, N. N., et al. (2011). Understanding obesity and endometrial cancer risk: Opportunities for prevention. *American Journal of Obstetrics and Gynecology*, *205*(6), 518–525. doi:10.1016/j.ajog.2011.05.042.

Statistics Canada. (2014). *Body mass index, overweight or obese, self-reported, adult, by age group and sex (Number of persons)*. Retrieved from *http://www.statcan.gc.ca/tables-tableaux/sum-som/ l01/cst01/health81a-eng.htm*.

Tchernof, A., & Després, J. P. (2013). Pathophysiology of human visceral obesity: An update. *Physiological Reviews*, *93*(1), 359–404. doi:10.1152/physrev.00033.2011.

Tung, Y. L., Yeo, G. S., O'Rahilly, S., et al. (2014). Obesity and FTO: Changing focus at a complex locus. *Cell Metabolism*, *20*(5), 710–718. doi:10.1016/j.cmet.2014.09.010.

Wei, W. H., Hemani, G., Gyenesei, A., et al. (2012). Genome-wide analysis of epistasis in body mass index using multiple human populations. *European Journal of Human Genetics*, *20*(8), 857–862. doi:10.1038/ejhg.2012.17.

Wilding, J. P. H. (2014). The importance of weight management in type 2 diabetes mellitus. *International Journal of Clinical Practice*, *68*(6), 682–691. doi:10.1111/ijcp.12384.

Williams, E. P., Mesidor, M., Winters, K., et al. (2015). Overweight and obesity: Prevalence, consequences, and causes of a growing public health problem. *Curr Obes Rep*, *4*(3), 363–370. doi:10.1007/s13679-015-0169-4.

Wright, S. M., & Aronne, L. J. (2012). Causes of obesity. *Abdominal Imaging*, *37*(5), 730–732. doi:10.1007/s00261-012-9862-x.

RESOURCES

Alberta Health Services: Healthy Eating Starts Here
http://www.albertahealthservices.ca/nutrition/page5623.aspx

Canadian Association of Bariatric Physicians and Surgeons
http://www.cabps.ca

Canadian Cancer Society Research Institute
http://www.cancer.ca/Research.aspx

Canadian Guidelines for Body Weight Classification in Adults
http://www.hc-sc.gc.ca/fn-an/alt_formats/hpfb-dgpsa/pdf/nutrition/ cg_quick_ref-ldc_rapide_ref-eng.pdf

Canadian Institutes of Health Research: Institute of Nutrition, Metabolism & Diabetes (INMD)
http://www.cihr-irsc.gc.ca/e/13521.html

Canadian Obesity Network
http://www.obesitynetwork.ca

Canadian Physical Activity Guidelines
http://www.csep.ca/cmfiles/guidelines/csep_guidelines_handbook.pdf

Canadian Society for Exercise Physiology
http://www.csep.ca/home

Dietitians of Canada
http://www.dietitians.ca

Health Canada
http://www.hc-sc.gc.ca

National Eating Disorder Information Centre
http://www.nedic.ca

Public Health Agency of Canada: Physical Activity
http://www.phac-aspc.gc.ca/pau-uap/paguide/index.html

Academy for Eating Disorders
http://www.aedweb.org

National Eating Disorders Association
http://www.nationaleatingdisorders.org

National Heart, Lung, and Blood Institute: Portion Distortion
https://www.nhlbi.nih.gov/health/educational/wecan/eat-right/portion-distortion.htm

Overeaters Anonymous Headquarters
http://www.overeatersanonymous.org

Take Off Pounds Sensibly (TOPS)
http://www.tops.org

Weight Watchers International, Inc.
http://www.weightwatchers.com

For additional Internet resources, see the website for this book at *http://evolve.elsevier.com/Canada/Lewis/medsurg*.

Nursing Management

Upper Gastro-Intestinal Problems

Written by: Paula P. Cox-North
Adapted by: Françoise Verville

eVolve WEBSITE

http://evolve.elsevier.com/Canada/Lewis/medsurg

- Review Questions (Online Only)
- Key Points
- Answer Guidelines for Case Study
- Student Case Studies
  - Oral Cancer
  - Peptic Ulcer Disease

- Customizable Nursing Care Plans
  - Nausea and Vomiting
  - Peptic Ulcer Disease
- Conceptual Care Map Creator
- Audio Glossary
- Content Updates

LEARNING OBJECTIVES

1. Describe the etiology, complications, collaborative care, and nursing management of nausea and vomiting.
2. Describe the etiology, clinical manifestations, and treatment of common oral inflammations and infections.
3. Describe the etiology, clinical manifestations, complications, collaborative care, and nursing management of oral cancer.
4. Explain the types, pathophysiology, clinical manifestations, complications, and collaborative care, including surgical therapy, and nursing management of gastro-esophageal reflux disease and hiatal hernia.
5. Describe the pathophysiology, clinical manifestations, complications, and collaborative care of esophageal cancer, diverticula, achalasia, and esophageal strictures.

6. Differentiate between acute and chronic gastritis, including the etiology, pathophysiology, collaborative care, and nursing management.
7. Explain the common etiology, clinical manifestations, collaborative care, and nursing management of upper gastro-intestinal bleeding.
8. Compare and contrast gastric and duodenal ulcers, including the etiology and pathophysiology, clinical manifestations, complications, collaborative care, and nursing management.
9. Describe the clinical manifestations, collaborative care, and nursing management of gastric cancer.
10. Identify the common types of food poisoning and the nursing responsibilities related to food poisoning.

KEY TERMS

achalasia, p. 1029
Barrett's esophagus, p. 1023
dysphagia, p. 1019
esophageal cancer, p. 1026
esophageal diverticula,
   p. 1029

esophagitis, p. 1022
gastric cancer, p. 1032
gastritis, p. 1030
gastro-esophageal reflux
   disease (GERD),
   p. 1022

hiatal hernia, p. 1025
leukoplakia, p. 1019
Mallory-Weiss tear, p. 1036
nausea, p. 1013
peptic ulcer disease (PUD),
   p. 1040

physiological stress ulcer,
   p. 1043
vomiting, p. 1013

NAUSEA AND VOMITING

Nausea and vomiting are the most common manifestations of gastro-intestinal (GI) diseases. **Nausea** is a feeling of discomfort in the epigastrium with a conscious desire to vomit. **Vomiting** is the forceful ejection of partially digested food and secretions *(emesis)* from the upper GI tract. Vomiting is a complex act that requires the coordinated activities of several structures: closure of the glottis, deep inspiration with contraction of the diaphragm in the inspiratory position, closure of the pylorus, relaxation of the stomach and lower esophageal sphincter (LES),

and contraction of the abdominal muscles with increasing intra-abdominal pressure. These simultaneous activities force the stomach contents up through the esophagus, into the pharynx, and out the mouth. Although nausea and vomiting can occur independently, they are usually closely related and usually treated as one problem.

Etiology and Pathophysiology

Nausea and vomiting occur in a wide variety of GI disorders, as well as in conditions that are unrelated to GI disease. Such conditions include pregnancy, infectious diseases, central

1013

nervous system (CNS) disorders (e.g., meningitis, CNS tumour), cardiovascular problems (e.g., myocardial infarction, heart failure), metabolic disorders (e.g., Addison's disease, uremia), adverse effects of drugs (e.g., opioids digitalis), allergies, and psychological factors (e.g., stress, fear).

In general, nausea occurs before vomiting and is characterized by contraction of the duodenum and by slowing of gastric motility and emptying. A single episode of nausea accompanied by vomiting may not be significant. However, if vomiting occurs several times, it is important that the cause be identified.

A vomiting centre in the brainstem coordinates the multiple components involved in emesis. This centre receives input from various stimuli. Neural impulses reach the vomiting centre via afferent pathways through branches of the autonomic nervous system. Visceral receptors for these afferent fibres are located in the GI tract, the kidneys, the heart, and the uterus. When stimulated, these receptors relay information to the vomiting centre, which then initiates the vomiting reflex (Figure 44-1).

In addition, the chemoreceptor trigger zone (CTZ), located on the floor of the fourth ventricle in the brain, responds to chemical stimuli of drugs and toxins. The CTZ also plays a role in emesis when it is caused by labyrinthine stimulation (e.g., motion sickness). Once stimulated, the CTZ transmits impulses directly to the vomiting centre.

Vomiting also can occur when the GI tract becomes overly irritated, excited, or distended. It can be a protective mechanism to rid the body of spoiled or irritating foods and liquids. Immediately before the act of vomiting, the person becomes aware of the need to vomit. The autonomic nervous system is activated, resulting in both parasympathetic and sympathetic nervous system stimulation. Sympathetic activation produces tachycardia, tachypnea, and diaphoresis. Parasympathetic stimulation causes relaxation of the lower esophageal (cardiac) sphincter, an increase in gastric motility, and a pronounced increase in salivation. These manifestations are experienced immediately before emesis.

Clinical Manifestations

Nausea is a subjective complaint. *Anorexia* (lack of appetite) usually accompanies nausea and is brought on by unpleasant stimulation involving any of the five senses. When nausea and vomiting are prolonged, dehydration can develop rapidly. In addition to water, essential electrolytes (e.g., potassium, sodium, chloride, hydrogen) are also lost. As vomiting persists, the patient may suffer severe electrolyte imbalances, loss of extracellular fluid volume, decreased plasma volume, and eventually circulatory failure. Metabolic alkalosis can result from loss of gastric hydrochloric acid (HCl). (The word *acid* contained in the shorthand of the chemical formula is a concept important for an understanding of GI chemistry and function.) Metabolic acidosis can occur because of the loss of bicarbonate when contents from the small intestine are vomited. However, metabolic acidosis is a less common result of severe vomiting than is metabolic alkalosis. Weight loss resulting from fluid loss is evident in a short time when vomiting is severe.

The threat of pulmonary aspiration is a concern when vomiting occurs in a patient who is an older adult, is unconscious, or has other conditions that impair the gag reflex. A patient who cannot adequately manage self-care should be put in a semi-Fowler's or side-lying position to prevent aspiration.

Collaborative Care

The goals of collaborative care are to determine and treat the underlying cause of the nausea and vomiting and to provide symptomatic relief. Determining the cause is often difficult because nausea and vomiting are manifestations of many conditions of the GI tract and of disorders of other body systems. An interprofessional approach to management of patients involving pharmacists, dietitians, and social workers should be considered.

The history must include important information regarding times when the vomiting occurs, precipitating factors, and a description of the contents of the vomitus or emesis. There are sex-related differences in risk for nausea and vomiting associated with both surgical procedures and motion sickness. Women are more likely than men to experience nausea and vomiting (Kovac, 2013). In all patients, vomiting, regurgitation, and projectile vomiting must be differentiated. *Regurgitation* is a process in which partially digested food is slowly brought up from the stomach. Retching or vomiting seldom precedes it. *Projectile vomiting* is a very forceful expulsion of stomach contents without nausea and is a characteristic of CNS tumours.

The presence of fecal odour and bile after prolonged vomiting indicates intestinal obstruction below the level of the pylorus. The presence of bile in the emesis may suggest obstruction below the ampulla of Vater or bile reflux gastritis. The presence of partially digested food several hours after a meal is indicative of gastric outlet obstruction or delay in gastric emptying.

The colour of the emesis aids in determining the presence and the source of bleeding. Vomitus with a "coffee grounds" appearance is associated with bleeding in the stomach, where blood changes to dark brown as a result of its interaction with gastric acid. Bright red blood indicates active bleeding, which is suggestive of a tear in the mucosal lining of the lower esophagus or the fundus of stomach, bleeding gastric or duodenal ulcer or neoplasm, or bleeding esophageal varices.

Drug Therapy. The choice of drugs in the treatment of nausea and vomiting depends on the cause of the problem. Many different drugs can be used (Table 44-1). Because the cause cannot always

FIGURE 44-1 Stimuli involved in the act of vomiting. *CTZ,* chemoreceptor trigger zone; *GI,* gastro-intestinal. Source: Modified from McKenry, L., Tessier, E., & Hogan, M. (2006). *Mosby's pharmacology in nursing* (22nd ed.). St. Louis: Mosby.

TABLE 44-1 DRUG THERAPY

Nausea and Vomiting

Classification	Drug
Dopamine antagonists	• Domperidone (Motilium) • Haloperidol (Haldol) • Metoclopramide
Antihistamine	• Cyclizine • Dimenhydrinate (Gravol) • Diphenhydramine (Benadryl)
Serotonin antagonist	• Dolasetron (Anzemet) • Granisetron (Kytril) • Ondansetron (Zofran)
Antimuscarinic (anticholinergic)	• Scopolamine (hyoscine)
Phenothiazine	• Chlorpromazine (Largactil) • Prochlorperazine (Stemetil) • Promethazine (Phenergan)
Benzodiazepine	• Clonazepam (Clonapam) • Diazepam (Valium) • Lorazepam (Ativan)
Others	• Aprepitant (Emend) • Corticosteroids • Dexamethasone (Decadron)

be readily determined, drugs must be administered with caution. Antiemetics used before the cause of the vomiting is established can mask the underlying disease process and delay diagnosis and treatment. Many of the antiemetic drugs act on the CNS at the level of the CTZ. In general, they block the neurochemicals that appear to trigger nausea and vomiting.

Many drugs that control nausea and vomiting—antimuscarinics, antihistamines, and phenothiazines—have anticholinergic actions, and their use is contraindicated in patients with glaucoma, prostatic hyperplasia, pyloric or bladder neck obstruction, or biliary obstruction. They share many common adverse effects, which include dry mouth, hypotension, sedative effects, rashes, and GI disturbances such as constipation. Consultation with a pharmacist may be indicated before these drugs are administered to a patient with multiple medical problems.

Metoclopramide and domperidone (Motilium) act both centrally and peripherally on dopamine receptors. Peripherally, they enhance the release of acetylcholine, which results in increased gastric emptying. Because of this effect, these drugs are considered prokinetics. However, about 10% to 20% of patients taking metoclopramide experience adverse CNS effects ranging from anxiety to hallucinations. Extrapyramidal adverse effects, including tremor and dyskinesias similar to those of Parkinson's disease, may also occur. Domperidone does not cross the blood–brain barrier and thus produces fewer adverse effects than does metoclopramide.

DRUG ALERT—Metoclopramide
- Chronic use or high doses of metoclopramide carry the risk of tardive dyskinesia.
- Tardive dyskinesia is a neurological condition characterized by involuntary and repetitive movements of the body (e.g., extremity movements, lip smacking).
- With discontinuation of the drug, the tardive dyskinesia persists.

Antagonists to specific serotonin (5-HT) receptors have been found to act both centrally and peripherally to reduce nausea and vomiting. In particular, antagonists to the 5-HT3 receptor are effective in reducing cancer chemotherapy–induced vomiting, vomiting caused by total body irradiation, GI motility disturbances, carcinoid syndrome, and nausea and vomiting related to migraine headache and anxiety. Serotonin antagonists, including ondansetron (Zofran), granisetron (Kytril), and dolasetron (Anzemet), act both centrally in the vomiting centre and peripherally to enhance gastric emptying.

Dexamethasone is used in the management of cancer chemotherapy–induced emesis, usually in combination with other antiemetics. Dexamethasone alone or in combination with ondansetron reduces both acute and delayed chemotherapy-induced nausea and vomiting. Aprepitant (Emend), a substance P/neurokinin-1 receptor antagonist, is used for the prevention of chemotherapy-induced nausea and vomiting, as well as prevention of postoperative nausea and vomiting. Coadministration with warfarin results in decreased prothrombin time, and so the international normalized ratio (INR) must be closely monitored. The efficacy of hormonal contraceptives may also be reduced, which necessitates an alternative method during treatment and for 1 month after the last dose. Benzodiazepines have no direct antiemetic effect but may be useful as adjunct therapy in the treatment of chemotherapy-induced nausea and vomiting.

Nutritional Therapy. Patients with severe vomiting require intravenous (IV) fluid therapy with electrolyte and glucose replacement until they are able to tolerate oral intake. In some cases, a nasogastric (NG) tube and suction are used to decompress the stomach. Keeping the stomach empty reduces the stimulus to vomit. The NG tube should be stabilized to eliminate its movement in the nose and back of the throat because this can stimulate nausea and vomiting.

Once the symptoms have subsided, oral nourishment is started with clear liquids. Extremely hot or cold liquids are not usually well tolerated. Carbonated beverages, at room temperature and with the carbonation gone, and warm tea are more easily tolerated. The addition of dry toast or crackers may alleviate the feeling of nausea and help prevent vomiting. Water is the initial fluid of choice for rehydration by mouth.

As the patient's condition improves, a diet high in carbohydrates and low in fatty foods should be provided. Items such as a baked potato, plain gelatin, cereal with milk and sugar, and hard candy may be added. Foods that are known to be poorly tolerated include coffee, spicy foods, and highly acidic foods. Food should be eaten slowly and in small amounts to prevent overdistension of the stomach. When solid foods have been reintroduced, fluids should be taken between meals rather than with meals. It is advised that the patient avoid physical activity and sit upright for approximately 1 hour after meals. A dietitian may be consulted about appropriate foods that will maintain nutritional health and are well tolerated by the patient during the recovery process.

NURSING MANAGEMENT
NAUSEA AND VOMITING

NURSING ASSESSMENT

Each patient with a history of prolonged and persistent nausea or vomiting requires a thorough nursing assessment before a specific plan of care is developed. Although the conditions associated with nausea and vomiting are numerous, the nurse should have a basic understanding of the more common conditions and should be able to identify a patient who is at high risk of complications from nausea and vomiting. Knowledge of the physiological mechanisms involved in nausea and vomiting

TABLE 44-2 NURSING ASSESSMENT

Nausea and Vomiting

Subjective Data
Important Health Information
Past health history: GI disorders, chronic indigestion, food allergies, pregnancy, infection, CNS disorders, recent travel, bulimia, metabolic disorders, cancer, cardiovascular disease, renal disease
Medications: Use of antiemetics, digitalis, opioids, ferrous sulphate, ASA (Aspirin), aminophylline, alcohol, antibiotics; general anaesthetic; chemotherapy
Surgery or other treatments: Recent surgery

Symptoms
- Emesis, dry heaves, dry mouth, anorexia, weight loss
- Weakness, fatigue
- Abdominal tenderness or pain

Objective Data
General
Lethargy, sunken eyeballs

Integumentary
Pallor, dry mucous membranes, poor skin turgor

Gastro-intestinal
Amount, frequency, character (e.g., projectile), content (undigested food, blood, bile, feces), and colour of vomitus (red, "coffee grounds," green-yellow)

Urinary
Decreased output, concentrated urine

Possible Findings
Altered serum electrolyte levels (especially hypokalemia), metabolic alkalosis, abnormal upper GI findings on endoscopy or abdominal radiographs

ASA, acetylsalicylic acid; *CNS,* central nervous system; *GI,* gastro-intestinal.

and the demonstration of a genuine regard for the patient are essential. Table 44-2 lists subjective and objective data that should be obtained from a patient with nausea and vomiting, regardless of the underlying cause.

NURSING DIAGNOSES

Nursing diagnoses for the patient with nausea and vomiting may include, but are not limited to, the following:

- *Nausea* related to *noxious environmental stimuli, noxious taste, unpleasant visual stimuli*
- *Deficient fluid volume* related to *insufficient fluid intake* (prolonged vomiting)
- *Imbalanced nutrition: less than body requirements* related to *insufficient dietary intake* (nausea and vomiting)

Additional information on nursing diagnoses is presented in Nursing Care Plan (NCP) 44-1, available on the Evolve website.

PLANNING

The overall goals are that the patient with nausea and vomiting will (a) experience minimal or no nausea and vomiting, (b) have normal electrolyte levels and hydration status, and (c) return to a normal pattern of fluid balance and nutrient intake.

NURSING IMPLEMENTATION

ACUTE INTERVENTION. The majority of individuals with nausea and vomiting can be managed at home. However, when nausea

COMPLEMENTARY & ALTERNATIVE THERAPIES

Nausea and Vomiting

A number of studies have demonstrated that acupressure or acupuncture at specific points is effective in reducing postoperative nausea and vomiting (Holmér Pettersson & Wengström, 2012).

Some patients use herbs such as ginger and peppermint oil for nausea and vomiting. Breathing exercises, massage, changing body position, self-hypnosis, guided imagery, biofeedback, music therapy, or exercise may be helpful for some patients (Canadian Cancer Association, 2015a).

Nursing Implications
- Patients taking anticoagulant therapy, digoxin, or hypoglycemic agents should not use ginger. Ginger also should not be used if a patient has gallstones or heart failure.

and vomiting persist regardless of home treatment strategies, hospitalization may be necessary for diagnosis of the underlying problem. Until a diagnosis is confirmed, the patient is kept on nothing-by-mouth (NPO) status and given IV fluids. An NG tube connected to suction may be necessary for a patient with persistent vomiting and for a patient in whom the possible diagnosis may be bowel obstruction or paralytic ileus.

With prolonged vomiting, there is a probability of dehydration and of acid–base and electrolyte imbalances. The nurse plans care that includes accurate recording of intake and output, monitoring vital signs, assessing for signs of dehydration, proper positioning to prevent possible aspiration by a susceptible patient, and observing for changes in the patient's general physical comfort and mentation. The nurse takes responsibility for providing physical and emotional support; maintaining a quiet, odour-free environment; and giving explanations regarding any diagnostic tests or procedures performed.

Patients who are hospitalized for other health problems may be prone to episodes of nausea and vomiting. These individuals include patients who are recovering immediately after surgery from the effects of the procedure, anaesthesia, and pain. Nausea and vomiting are common adverse effects in patients with cancer receiving chemotherapeutic drugs. (Nursing care of patients with cancer is discussed in Chapter 18 and in NCP 18-2, available on the Evolve website.)

AMBULATORY AND HOME CARE. The patient and caregiver may need instructions on (a) how to deal successfully with the unpleasant sensations of nausea, (b) methods of preventing nausea and vomiting, and (c) strategies to maintain fluid and nutritional intake. The occurrence of nausea or vomiting may be minimized if measures are taken to keep the immediate environment quiet, free of noxious odours, and well ventilated. Sudden changes of position and unnecessary activity should be avoided. Use of relaxation techniques, acupressure, frequent rest periods, and diversional tactics help prevent nausea and vomiting and facilitate a more rapid recovery from their effects. Cleansing the face and the hands with a cool washcloth and mouth care between episodes increase the person's comfort level. When the symptoms occur, all foods and drugs should be stopped until the acute phase is past.

If a medication is suspected as the cause, the health care provider should be notified immediately so that either the dosage can be altered or a different drug can be prescribed. The patient should be reminded that stopping a prescribed drug without consulting the health care provider may eliminate the immediate cause of the nausea and vomiting but may also have detrimental effects on health or the disease state.

When food is identified as the precipitating cause of nausea and vomiting, the nurse should help the patient solve the problem. What food was it? When was it eaten? Has this food caused problems in the past? Is anyone else in the family sick?

When the patient believes some foods and fluids can be tolerated, the nurse might suggest that it would be helpful to begin with clear liquids or warm beverages, Gatorade, tea or broth, dry crackers or toast, and then plain gelatin. Bland foods, such as pasta, rice, and cooked chicken, are generally well tolerated in small amounts. An antiemetic drug should be taken only if prescribed by the health care provider. Taking over-the-counter (OTC) drugs for relief of symptoms may make the condition worse. Patients should be asked to describe any use of nontraditional preparations.

EVALUATION

The following are expected outcomes for the patient with nausea and vomiting:

- The patient will be comfortable with minimal or no nausea and vomiting.
- The patient will maintain body weight.
- The patient's electrolyte levels will be within normal range.
- The patient will be able to maintain adequate intake of fluids and nutrients.
- The patient will maintain normal urine volume.

AGE-RELATED CONSIDERATIONS

NAUSEA AND VOMITING

Older adult patients experiencing nausea and vomiting require careful assessment and monitoring, particularly during periods of fluid loss and subsequent rehydration therapy. Older adults are more likely to have cardiac or renal insufficiency, which increases their risk for life-threatening fluid and electrolyte imbalances. In addition, excessive replacement of fluid and electrolytes may result in adverse consequences for an older adult who has heart failure or renal disease. Moreover, older adults with a decreased level of consciousness may be at high risk for aspiration of vomitus. Close monitoring of the patient's physical status and level of consciousness during episodes of vomiting must be a primary concern for the nurse.

In addition, older adults are particularly susceptible to the CNS adverse effects of antiemetic drugs; these drugs may produce confusion. Dosages should be reduced and efficacy closely evaluated. Safety precautions also should be instituted for these patients.

FOODBORNE ILLNESS

Foodborne illness and *food poisoning* are nonspecific terms that describe acute GI symptoms such as nausea, vomiting, diarrhea, and colicky abdominal pain caused by the intake of contaminated food. Food most commonly causes illness if it is contaminated with microorganisms or their products. The GI tract is frequently the portal of entry for the microorganisms. The epidemiology of foodborne illness is changing. There are new organisms, and many have spread worldwide. The two main types of food poisoning are (a) acute gastro-enteritis from bacteria and (b) neurological symptoms from botulism. Bacteria account for most foodborne illnesses. Raw foods that have become contaminated during growing, harvesting, processing, storing, shipping, or final preparation are the most common source. When food is uncooked

and left out for more than 2 hours at room temperature, bacteria can multiply quickly. The most common bacterial causes of food poisoning are listed in Table 44-3.

Poisonous chemicals, such as mercury, arsenic, zinc, and potassium chlorate, may contaminate foods. Poisoning can also occur from ingestion of poisonous plants (e.g., certain mushroom species).

Prevention of occurrence is the focus of interventions. Teaching should include correct food preparation and cleanliness, adequate cooking, and refrigeration. If the patient is hospitalized, care focuses on correction of fluid and electrolyte imbalance from diarrhea and vomiting. With botulism, additional assessment and care relative to neurological symptoms are indicated (see Chapter 63).

Escherichia coli O157:H7 Poisoning

Escherichia coli O157:H7 causes hemorrhagic colitis and kidney failure, and in young children and older adults, *E. coli* O157:H7 infection can be life-threatening (Centers for Disease Control and Prevention, 2015). *E. coli* O157:H7 is found primarily in undercooked meats, particularly poultry and hamburger. *E. coli* outbreaks have also been observed with contaminated leafy vegetables, fruits, and nuts. Person-to-person contact in families, nursing homes, and child care centres is also an important mode of transmission. Infection can also occur after drinking raw milk, unpasteurized juice, or contaminated fruit juices and after swimming in or drinking sewage-contaminated water.

Most strains of *E. coli* are harmless and live in the intestines of healthy humans and animals. *E. coli* O157:H7 produces a powerful toxin and can cause severe illness. The clinical manifestations of *E. coli* O157:H7 infection include diarrhea and abdominal cramping pain for 2 to 8 days (on average, 3–4 days) after the organism is swallowed. The diarrhea is variable, ranging from mild to bloody. The diarrhea may start out as watery but may progress to bloody. Systemic complications, including hemolytic uremia and thrombo-cytopenic purpura, and even death can occur.

Infection with *E. coli* O157:H7 is diagnosed when the bacteria are detected in the stool. All people who suddenly have diarrhea with blood should get their stool tested (stool culture) for *E. coli* O157:H7.

Treatment involves supportive care to maintain blood volume. The use of antibiotics remains controversial. Most affected people recover without antibiotics or other specific treatment. Patients should avoid antidiarrheal agents, such as loperamide (Imodium). Other therapies may include dialysis and plasmapheresis.

In approximately 2% to 7% of infections, particularly in young children and older adults, hemolytic uremic syndrome (HUS) occurs, in which the red blood cells (RBCs) are destroyed and kidney function fails. HUS is a life-threatening condition and approximately 3% to 5% of patients with HUS die. About one third of people with HUS have abnormal kidney function many years after the onset, and a few require long-term dialysis. Additional long-term complications of HUS include hypertension, seizures, blindness, and paralysis.

ORAL INFLAMMATIONS AND INFECTIONS

Oral infections and inflammations may be manifestations of specific mouth diseases, or they may occur in the presence of some systemic diseases such as leukemia or vitamin deficiency. Oral inflammations and infections can severely impair the

TABLE 44-3 BACTERIAL FOOD POISONING

Causative Agent	Sources	Onset of Symptoms	Clinical Manifestations	Treatment	Prevention
Staphylococcal					
Toxin from *Staphylococcus aureus*	Meat, bakery products, cream fillings, salad dressings, milk; skin and respiratory tract of food handlers	30 min–7 hr	Vomiting, nausea, abdominal cramping, diarrhea	Symptomatic, fluid and electrolyte replacement, antiemetics	Immediate refrigeration of foods, monitoring of food handlers
Clostridial					
Clostridium perfringens	Meat or poultry dishes cooked at lower temperature (stew or pot pie), rewarmed meat dishes, gravies, improperly canned vegetables	8–24 hr	Diarrhea, nausea, abdominal cramps, vomiting (rare); midepigastrium pain	Symptomatic, fluid replacement	Correct preparation of meat dishes, serving of food immediately after cooking, or rapid cooling of food
***Salmonella* Organisms**					
Salmonella typhimurium (grows in gut)	Improperly cooked poultry, pork, beef, lamb, and eggs	8 hr to several days	Nausea and vomiting, diarrhea, abdominal cramps, fever and chills	Symptomatic, fluid and electrolyte replacement	Correct preparation of food
Botulism					
Toxin from *Clostridium botulinum;* ingested toxin is absorbed from gut and blocks acetylcholine at neuro-muscular junction	Improperly canned or preserved food, home-preserved vegetables, preserved fruits and fish, canned commercial products	12–36 hr	GI symptoms: nausea, vomiting, abdominal pain, constipation, distension Central nervous system symptoms: headache, dizziness, muscular incoordination, weakness, inability to talk or swallow, diplopia, breathing difficulties, paralysis, delirium, coma	Maintenance of ventilation, polyvalent antitoxin, guanidine HCl (enhances acetylcholine release)	Correct processing of canned foods, discarding suspect canned goods
Escherichia coli					
E. coli serotype O157:H7	Contaminated beef, pork, milk, cheese, fish, prepackaged cookie dough	Varies by strain: 8 hr–1 wk	Bloody stools, hemolytic uremic syndrome, abdominal cramping, profuse diarrhea	Symptomatic, fluid and electrolyte replacement	Correct preparation of food
***Listeria* Organisms**					
Gram-positive rod-shaped bacterium	Most cases associated with ingesting contaminated dairy products, poultry, and meat	1–90 days	In immuno-competent host: fever, diarrhea Immuno-compromised host (pregnant women, older adults, immuno-compromised persons at greatest risk): meningitis ± septicemia	Ampicillin and trimethoprim-sulphamethoxazole or erythromycin	Pasteurization, proper washing, refrigeration, and cooking of foods potentially contaminated with animal manure or sewage

GI, gastro-intestinal.

ingestion of food and fluids. Common inflammations and infections of the oral cavity are listed in Table 44-4. Patients who are immuno-suppressed (e.g., those with acquired immune deficiency syndrome [AIDS] and those receiving chemotherapy) are most susceptible to oral infections. Patients receiving corticosteroid inhalant treatment for asthma are at risk for oral infections, especially candidiasis.

Oral infections may predispose to infections in other body organs. For example, the oral cavity can be considered a potential reservoir for respiratory pathogens. Oral pathogens have also been associated with heart disease.

An important element in reducing the incidence of oral infections and inflammation is good oral hygiene. Management of oral infections and inflammation is focused on identification of the cause, elimination of infection, provision of comfort measures, and maintenance of nutritional intake.

ORAL CANCER

Oral (or oropharyngeal) cancer may occur on the lips or anywhere within the mouth (e.g., tongue, floor of the mouth, buccal mucosa, hard palate, soft palate, pharyngeal walls, tonsils). It was estimated

TABLE 44-4	INFECTIONS AND INFLAMMATION OF THE MOUTH		
Condition	**Etiology**	**Clinical Manifestations**	**Treatment**
Gingivitis	Neglected oral hygiene, malocclusion, missing or irregular teeth, faulty dentistry, eating of soft rather than fibrous foods	Inflamed gingivae and interdental papillae; bleeding during toothbrushing; development of pus; formation of abscess with loosening of teeth (periodontitis)	Prevention through health teaching, dental care, gingival massage, professional cleaning of teeth, fibrous foods, conscientious brushing habits with flossing
Vincent's infection (acute necrotizing ulcerative gingivitis, trench mouth)	Fusiform bacteria; Vincent's spirochetes; predisposing factors of stress, excessive fatigue, poor oral hygiene, nutritional deficiencies (vitamins B and C)	Painful, bleeding gingivae; eroding necrotic lesions of interdental papillae; ulcerations that bleed; increased saliva with metallic taste; fetid mouth odour; anorexia, fever, and general malaise	Rest (physical and mental); avoidance of smoking and alcoholic beverages; soft, nutritious diet; correct oral hygiene habits; topical applications of antibiotics; mouth rinses with hydrogen peroxide and saline solutions
Oral candidiasis (moniliasis or thrush)	*Candida albicans* (a yeastlike fungus), debilitation, prolonged high-dose antibiotic or corticosteroid therapy	Pearly, bluish-white "milk-curd" membranous lesions on mucosa of mouth and larynx; sore mouth; yeasty halitosis	Nystatin suspension or fluconazole as oral therapy, good oral hygiene
Herpes simplex (cold sore, fever blister)	Herpes simplex virus type 1 or 2; factors predisposing to upper respiratory infections, excessive exposure to sunlight, food allergies, emotional tension, onset of menstruation	Lip lesions, mouth lesions, vesicle formation (single or clustered); shallow, painful ulcers	Spirits of camphor, corticosteroid cream, mild antiseptic mouthwash, viscous lidocaine; removal or control of predisposing factors, antiviral agents (e.g., acyclovir [Zovirax])
Aphthous stomatitis (canker sore)	Recurrent and chronic form of infection secondary to systemic disease, trauma, stress, or unknown causes	Ulcers of mouth and lips, causing extreme pain; ulcers surrounded by erythematous base	Corticosteroids (topical or systemic), tetracycline oral suspension
Parotitis (inflammation of parotid gland, surgical mumps)	Usually *Staphylococcus* species, occasionally *Streptococcus* species, debilitation and dehydration with poor oral hygiene, NPO status for an extended time	Pain and swelling in area of gland and ear, absence of salivation, purulent exudate from gland, erythema, ulcers	Antibiotics, mouthwashes, warm compresses; preventive measures such as chewing gum, sucking on hard candy, adequate fluid intake
Stomatitis (inflammation of mouth)	Trauma; pathogens; irritants (tobacco, alcohol); renal, liver, and hematological diseases; adverse effect of many cancer chemotherapy drugs and irradiation	Excessive salivation, halitosis, sore mouth	Removal or treatment of cause, oral hygiene with soothing solutions, topical medications; soft, bland diet

NPO, nothing by mouth.

that 4 700 new cases of oral cancer would be diagnosed in Canada in 2017, and that 1 250 persons would die from the disease (Canadian Cancer Society, 2017). It is more common after 45 years of age. It is more common in men (male-to-female ratio, 2:1). Squamous cell carcinoma is the most common oral malignant tumour (95% of cases of oral cancer). Mortality rates have been decreasing since the early 1980s. The rate of 5-year survival for all stages of cancer of the oral cavity and pharynx combined is 63%.

Most of the oral malignant lesions occur on the lower lip. Other common sites are the lateral border and undersurface of the tongue, the labial commissure, and the buccal mucosa. Carcinoma of the lip has the most favourable prognosis of any of the oral tumours. This is probably because lip lesions are more apparent to the patient than other oral lesions and are usually diagnosed earlier.

Etiology and Pathophysiology

Although the definitive cause of oral cancer is unknown, there are a number of predisposing factors (Table 44-5). Factors that influence the development of oral cancer include tobacco use (e.g., cigar, cigarette, pipe, snuff), excessive alcohol intake, human papillomavirus infection, chewing betel quid or areca nut, precancerous conditions of the oral cavity (e.g., leukoplakia), and a family history of squamous cell carcinoma. A positive history of tobacco and alcohol use, in the past or currently, is the most significant etiological factor in oral cancer. Constant overexposure to ultraviolet radiation from the sun is also a factor in the development of cancer of the lip. Irritation from the pipe stem resting on the lip is a factor in pipe smokers.

Clinical Manifestations

The common manifestations of oral cancer are leukoplakia, erythroplakia, ulcerations, a sore that bleeds easily and does not heal, and a rough area (felt with the tongue). **Leukoplakia,** called "white patch" or "smoker's patch," is often considered a precancerous lesion; approximately 3% to 17.5% of these lesions actually transform into malignant cells within 15 years. It is a whitish patch on the mucosa of the mouth or the tongue that results from chronic irritation, especially from smoking. The patch becomes *keratinized* (hard and leathery) and is sometimes described as *hyperkeratosis. Erythroplasia* (erythroplakia), which is seen as a red velvety patch on the mouth or tongue, is also considered a precancerous lesion. Areas of erythroplakia have a 51% chance of becoming malignant. Later symptoms of oral cancer are pain, **dysphagia** (difficulty swallowing), and difficulty in moving the jaw (e.g., chewing and speaking).

Cancer of the lip usually appears as an indurated, painless ulcer on the lip. The first sign of carcinoma of the tongue is an ulcer or area of thickening. Soreness or pain of the tongue may occur, especially when hot or highly seasoned foods are eaten. Cancerous lesions are most likely to develop in the proximal

TABLE 44-5 TYPES AND CHARACTERISTICS OF ORAL CANCER

Location	Predisposing Factors	Clinical Manifestations	Treatment
Lip	Constant overexposure to sun, ruddy and fair complexions, recurrent herpetic lesions, irritation from pipe stem, syphilis, immuno-suppression	Indurated, painless ulcer	Surgical excision, radiation therapy
Tongue	Tobacco, alcohol, chronic irritation, syphilis	Ulcer or area of thickening; soreness or pain; increased salivation, slurred speech, dysphagia, toothache, earache (later signs)	Surgery (hemiglossectomy or glossectomy), radiation therapy
Oral cavity	Poor oral hygiene, tobacco usage (pipe and cigar smoking, snuff, chewing tobacco), chewing betel nut, chronic alcohol intake, chronic irritation (jagged tooth, ill-fitting prosthesis, chemical or mechanical irritants), exposure to HPV	Leukoplakia; erythroplakia; ulcerations; sore spot; rough area; pain, dysphagia, difficulty in chewing and speaking (later signs)	Surgery (mandibulectomy, radical neck dissection, resections of buccal mucosa), internal and external radiation therapy

HPV, human papillomavirus.

TABLE 44-6 COLLABORATIVE CARE

Oral Cancer

Diagnostic	Collaborative Therapy*
• History and physical examination	• Surgery
• Biopsy	• Surgical excision of the tumour
• Oral exfoliative cytological study	• Radical neck dissection
• Radiographs, CT, and MRI	• Radiation therapy (internal or external)
	• Combined surgical resection with radiation therapy
	• Chemotherapy

*Any of these approaches may be used, depending on the primary lesion and the extent of metastasis.
CT, computed tomography; *MRI,* magnetic resonance imaging.

half of the tongue. Some patients experience limitation of movement of the tongue. Later symptoms of cancer of the tongue include increased salivation, slurred speech, dysphagia, toothache, and earache. Approximately 30% of patients with oral cancer have an asymptomatic neck mass.

Diagnostic Studies

Endoscopic examination in combination with biopsy of the suspected lesion with cytological examination is the best definitive diagnostic study for oral cancer. Oral exfoliative cytological study involves scraping the suspect lesion and spreading this scraping on a slide. In contrast to biopsy, a negative result of a cytological smear does not reliably rule out the possibility of a malignant condition, but it may be used as an initial screening test. The definitive diagnosis of cancer is based on biopsy and histological findings. Once cancer is diagnosed, radiographs, computed tomography, and magnetic resonance imaging (MRI) are useful in the staging of oral cancer (Canadian Cancer Society, 2015b).

Collaborative Care

Collaborative care of patients with oral carcinoma usually consists of surgery, radiation therapy, chemotherapy, or a combination of these (Table 44-6).

Surgical Therapy. Surgery remains the most effective treatment, especially for removing the central core of the tumour. Various surgical procedures may be performed, depending on the location and the extent of the tumour. Many of the operations are radical procedures involving extensive resections. Some examples are partial *mandibulectomy* (removal of the mandible), *hemiglossectomy* (removal of half of the tongue), *glossectomy* (removal of the tongue), resections of the buccal mucosa and the floor of the mouth, and radical neck dissection. Composite resections, which are combinations of the various surgical procedures, may be performed.

Because cancers of the oral cavity metastasize early to the cervical lymph nodes, a radical neck dissection is commonly performed. It includes wide excision of the involved primary lesion with removal of the regional lymph nodes, the deep cervical lymph nodes, and their lymphatic channels. In addition, the following structures may also be removed or transected (depending on the extent of the primary lesion): sternocleidomastoid muscle and other closely associated muscles, internal jugular vein, mandible, submaxillary gland, part of the thyroid and parathyroid glands, and spinal accessory nerve. A tracheostomy is commonly performed along with the radical neck dissection. Drainage tubes are inserted into the surgical area and connected to the suction device to remove fluid and blood.

Nonsurgical Therapy. Chemotherapy and radiation therapy are used together when the lesions are more advanced or involve several structures of the oral cavity. Chemotherapy may also be used when surgery and radiation therapy fail or as the initial therapy for smaller tumours (see Chapter 18).

Palliative treatment may be the best management when the prognosis is poor, the cancer is inoperable, or the patient decides against surgery. The aim of palliation is to treat the symptoms and make the patient more comfortable. If it becomes difficult for the patient to swallow, a gastrostomy may be performed to allow for adequate nutritional intake. (Gastrostomy is discussed in Chapter 42.) Analgesic medication should be given freely to such a patient. Frequent suctioning of the oral cavity becomes necessary when swallowing becomes difficult. (Other nursing measures for terminally ill patients are discussed in Chapter 13.)

Nutritional Therapy. Because of depression, alcoholism, or presurgery radiation treatment, patients may be malnourished even before surgery. After radical neck surgery, the patient may be unable to take in nutrients through the normal route of ingestion because of swelling, location of sutures, or difficulty with swallowing. Parenteral fluids are given for the first 24 to 48 hours. After this time, tube feedings are usually given via an NG tube or a nasointestinal tube that was placed during surgery.

Sometimes a temporary feeding gastrostomy may be used. (NG and gastrostomy feedings are described in Chapter 42.) Cervical esophagostomy and pharyngostomy have also been used. The nurse must observe for tolerance of the feedings and (in consultation with a dietitian) adjust the amount, the time, and the formula if nausea, vomiting, diarrhea, or distension occurs. The patient is instructed about the tube feedings. When the patient can swallow, small amounts of water are given. Close observation for choking is essential. Suctioning may be necessary to prevent aspiration.

NURSING MANAGEMENT
ORAL CANCER

NURSING ASSESSMENT

Subjective and objective data that should be obtained from a patient with oral cancer are listed in Table 44-7.

NURSING DIAGNOSES

Nursing diagnoses for patients with oral cancer may include, but are not limited to, the following:

- *Imbalanced nutrition: less than body requirements* related to *insufficient dietary intake* (oral pain, difficulty chewing and swallowing, surgical resection, and radiation treatment)
- *Chronic pain* related to *injury agent* (tumour, surgery, or radiation treatment)
- *Anxiety* related to *stressors, threat of death, threat to current status* (diagnosis of cancer, potential for disfiguring surgery)

TABLE 44-7   NURSING ASSESSMENT

Oral Cancer

Subjective Data
Important Health Information
Current health history: Use of alcohol or tobacco, pipe smoking, poor oral hygiene
Past health history: Recurrent oral herpetic lesions, syphilis, exposure to sunlight, HPV infection or vaccination
Medications: Immuno-suppressants
Surgery or other treatments: Removal of prior tumours or lesions

Symptoms
- Reduced oral intake, weight loss, difficulty in chewing or swallowing food; increased salivation; intolerance to certain foods or temperatures of food
- Mouth or tongue soreness or pain, toothache, earache, neck stiffness, difficulty speaking

Objective Data
Integumentary
Indurated, painless ulcer on lip; painless neck mass

Gastro-intestinal
Areas of thickening or roughness, ulcers, leukoplakia, or erythroplakia on the tongue or the oral mucosa; limited movement of the tongue; increased salivation, drooling; slurred speech; poor oral hygiene, foul breath odour

Possible Findings
Positive result of exfoliative cytological smear (microscopic examination of cells removed by scraping); positive biopsy findings

HPV, human papillomavirus.

PLANNING

The overall goals are that the patient with carcinoma of the oral cavity will (a) have a patent airway, (b) be able to communicate, (c) have adequate nutritional intake to promote wound healing, and (d) have relief of pain and discomfort.

NURSING IMPLEMENTATION

HEALTH PROMOTION. The nurse has a significant role in early detection and treatment of oral cancer. The nurse must provide the patient with information regarding predisposing factors, such as constant overexposure to the sun, tobacco, and other irritants, such as chewing betel nuts. Smoking and the long-term use of smokeless tobacco are the major risk factors for oral cancer. A patient identified as a smoker should be informed about smoking cessation programs available in the community. (Smoking cessation is discussed in Chapter 11. See also the link to the CAN-ADAPTT *Canadian Smoking Cessation Clinical Practice Guideline* in the Resources at the end of this chapter.)

It is important that adolescents and teenagers be informed about the danger of using snuff and chewing tobacco. In addition, oral cancers have an increased chance of recurrence if risk factors are not reduced. The nurse should also teach correct oral hygiene and dental care and encourage the patient to seek preventive dental care. Risk factors should be identified. Because early detection of oral cancer is important, the patient should be taught to examine the mouth and to recognize danger signals of oral cancer. If any of these signals are present, the patient should be instructed to visit a health care provider. Danger signals include unexplained pain or soreness in the mouth, unusual bleeding from the oral cavity, dysphagia, and swelling or lump in the neck.

Any individual with an ulcerative lesion that does not heal within 2 to 3 weeks should be referred to a health care provider, and a biopsy of the lesion should probably be performed. The nurse should inspect the patient's oral cavity to detect suspect lesions.

ACUTE INTERVENTION. Preoperative care for a patient who is to undergo a radical neck dissection involves consideration of the patient's physical and psychosocial needs. Physical preparation is the same as for any major surgery, with special emphasis on oral hygiene. Alcohol intake should be assessed thoroughly, and measures should be implemented early to assess and treat withdrawal if it is a problem. Explanations and emotional support are of special significance and should include postoperative measures relating to communication and feeding. The surgical procedure should be explained to the patient, and the nurse should make sure that the patient understands the information. (Radical neck dissection and related nursing management are discussed in Chapter 29 and in NCP 29-2, available on the Evolve website.)

EVALUATION

The following are expected outcomes for the patient with oral cancer:
- The patient will have no respiratory complications.
- The patient will be able to communicate.
- The patient will participate in regular follow-up examinations.
- The patient will maintain adequate nutritional intake to promote wound healing and overall health.
- The patient will experience minimal pain and discomfort with eating, drinking, and talking.

ESOPHAGEAL DISORDERS

GASTRO-ESOPHAGEAL REFLUX DISEASE

Etiology and Pathophysiology

Gastro-esophageal reflux disease (GERD) is not a disease but a syndrome. GERD is defined as any clinically significant symptomatic condition or histopathological alteration presumed to be secondary to reflux of gastric contents into the lower esophagus. In Canada, GERD is the most prevalent acid-related disorder; for approximately 13% of Canadians, GERD symptoms occur at least once a week (Canadian Society of Intestinal Research, 2015).

There is no single cause of GERD. Several factors or a combination of factors can be involved (Figure 44-2). It results when the defences of the lower esophagus are overwhelmed by the reflux of stomach acidic contents into the esophagus. Predisposing conditions include hiatal hernia, incompetent LES, decreased esophageal clearance (ability to clear liquids or food from the esophagus into the stomach) as a result of impaired esophageal motility, and decreased gastric emptying. The acidic gastric secretions that are regurgitated up into the lower esophagus result in esophageal irritation and inflammation (esophagitis). In addition, the presence of the gastric enzyme pepsin, intestinal enzymes (e.g., trypsin), and bile salts is corrosive to the esophageal mucosa. The degree of inflammation depends on the amount and the composition of gastric reflux and on the ability of the esophagus to clear the acidic contents.

One of the primary factors in GERD is incompetence of the LES. An incompetent LES results in a decrease in pressure in the distal portion of the esophagus. As a result, gastric contents are able to move from an area of higher pressure (stomach) to an area of lower pressure (esophagus) when the patient is in a supine position or has an increase in intra-abdominal pressure. Decreases in LES pressure can be caused by certain foods (e.g., caffeine, chocolate) and drugs (e.g., anticholinergics). A common cause of GERD is a hiatal hernia, which is discussed in the next section.

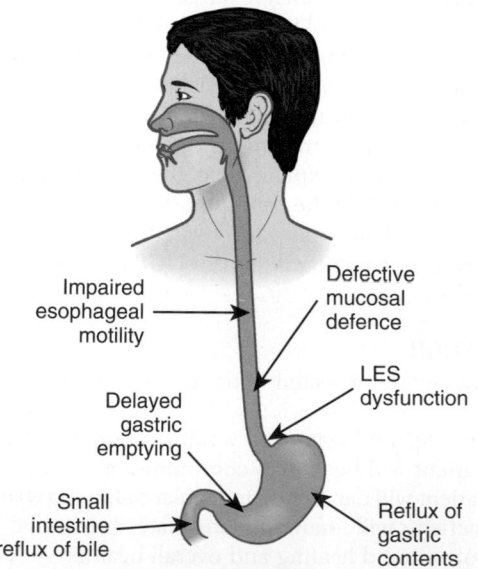

FIGURE 44-2 Factors involved in the pathogenesis of gastro-esophageal reflux disease (GERD). *LES,* lower esophageal sphincter.

Clinical Manifestations

The symptoms of GERD vary from individual to individual, but the diagnosis can usually be made on the basis of history and physical examination. Heartburn *(pyrosis)* from gastro-esophageal reflux is the most common clinical manifestation. It is caused by irritation of the esophagus by the gastric secretions. Heartburn is described as a burning, tight sensation that is felt intermittently beneath the lower sternum and spreads upward to the throat or the jaw. Approximately once a week, the majority of patients with GERD have mild symptoms, including heartburn, after a meal, with no evidence of mucosal damage.

Heartburn may occur after ingestion of food or drugs that decrease the LES pressure or are directly irritating to the esophageal mucosa (Table 44-8). An individual with GERD may also report respiratory symptoms, including wheezing, coughing, and dyspnea. Otolaryngological symptoms include hoarseness, sore throat, a globus sensation (sensation of a lump in the throat), and choking. *Regurgitation* (effortless return of food or gastric contents from the stomach into the esophagus or mouth) is a fairly common manifestation of GERD. It is often described as hot, bitter, or sour liquid coming into the throat or mouth. Gastric symptoms—including early satiety, bloating after a meal, nausea, and vomiting—are related to delayed gastric emptying. Symptoms that would prompt endoscopic evaluation include dysphagia (solid food, progressive), odynophagia (painful swallowing), bleeding and subsequent anemia, weight loss, and persistent vomiting. Further investigation is indicated if suspected GERD symptoms are actually cardiac in origin, if the patient has respiratory symptoms secondary to reflux, or for individuals who do not respond to medical therapy after 8 weeks (Richter, 2014).

Complications

Complications of GERD are related to the direct local effects of gastric acid on the esophageal mucosa. Esophagitis (inflammation of the esophagus) is a frequent complication of GERD. Other risk factors for esophagitis include hiatal hernia, chemical irritation from lye, and physical irritants such as smoking, cold or hot liquids, and excessive alcoholic intake. Trauma to the esophagus may also produce inflammation. The appearance of esophagitis with esophageal ulcerations is shown in Figure 44-3.

Repeated exposure may cause scar tissue formation and decreased distensibility of the esophagus *(esophageal stricture).* This may result in dysphagia.

TABLE 44-8	COMMON FOODS/DRUGS AFFECTING LOWER ESOPHAGEAL SPHINCTER PRESSURE

Increase Pressure
• Bethanechol (Duvoid)
• Metoclopramide
 	
Decrease Pressure
• Alcohol
• Chocolate (theobromine)
• Fatty foods
• Nicotine
• Peppermint, spearmint
	• Tea, coffee (caffeine)
	• Drugs
	  • Anticholinergics
	  • β-Adrenergic blockers
	  • Calcium channel blockers
	  • Diazepam (Valium)
	  • Morphine sulphate
	  • Nitrates
	  • Progesterone
	  • Theophylline

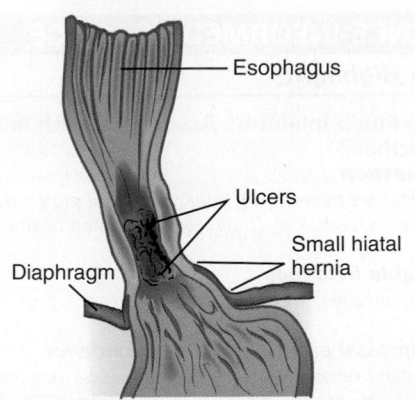

FIGURE 44-3 Esophagitis with esophageal ulcerations.

TABLE 44-9 COLLABORATIVE CARE

Gastro-Esophageal Reflux Disease and Hiatal Hernia

Diagnostic	Drug Therapy
• History and physical examination	• Antacids
• Barium swallow	• Antisecretory agents
• Motility (manometry) studies	• Cholinergic drugs
• pH monitoring (laboratory or 24-hr ambulatory)	• H₂-receptor blockers*
• Upper GI endoscopy with biopsy and cytological analysis	• Proton pump inhibitors*
	• Prokinetic drug therapy*
Collaborative Therapy	**Surgical Therapy**
Conservative	• Belsey fundoplication
• Elevation of head of bed on 10- to 15-cm blocks	• Hill gastropexy
• High-protein, low-fat diet with avoidance of foods and fluids that decrease LES pressure or irritate acid-sensitive esophagus	• Nissen fundoplication
	• Toupet fundoplication
	Endoscopic Therapy
	• Intraluminal valvuloplasty
	• Radiofrequency therapy
	• Stretta device

*See Table 44-10.
GI, gastro-intestinal; *LES,* lower esophageal sphincter.

Another complication of GERD is Barrett's esophagus (esophageal metaplasia). Barrett's esophagus is considered a precancerous lesion and increases the risk for esophageal cancer. In Barrett's esophagus, the normal squamous epithelium of the esophagus is replaced with columnar epithelium. These cell changes are thought to be related to chronic reflux esophagitis. Signs and symptoms of Barrett's esophagus can range from none to mild to bleeding and perforation. Because patients with Barrett's esophagus are at higher risk for adenocarcinoma, they may need to be monitored on a regular basis (every 2.5 years) with endoscopy and biopsy (Almond & Barr, 2014).

Respiratory complications of GERD include bronchospasm, laryngospasm, and cricopharyngeal spasm. These complications are caused by irritation of the upper airway by gastric secretions. With GERD, there is also the potential for pneumonia as a result of aspiration of gastric contents into the respiratory system. Dental erosion, especially in the posterior teeth, may result from acid reflux into the mouth.

Diagnostic Studies

Diagnostic studies are performed to determine the cause of the GERD, such as hiatal hernia (Table 44-9). Barium swallow studies may be done to determine whether there is protrusion of the upper part of the stomach (called the *gastric fundus*). Endoscopy is useful in assessing the competence of the LES and the extent of inflammation (if present), potential scarring, and strictures (Canadian Society of Intestinal Research, 2014). Biopsy and cytological specimens can be obtained to differentiate carcinoma of the stomach or esophagus from Barrett's esophagus. Esophageal manometric studies can be performed to measure pressure in the esophagus, as well as in the LES. The pH may be determined with the use of specially designed probes in the laboratory or ambulatory monitoring systems, which may demonstrate the presence of acid in the normally alkaline esophagus. Radionuclide tests may also be performed to detect reflux of gastric contents and the rate of esophageal clearance.

Collaborative Care

Most cases of GERD can be successfully managed by lifestyle modifications and drug therapy. These are long-term approaches requiring patient education and adherence to therapeutic regimens. When these therapies are ineffective, surgery is an option (see Table 44-9).

Lifestyle Modifications. Patients with GERD are taught to avoid factors that aggravate symptoms. Particular attention is given to diet and drugs that may affect the LES, acid secretion, or gastric emptying. Patients who are overweight or obese are encouraged to lose weight. Patients who smoke are encouraged to stop.

Nutritional Therapy. Diet does not cause GERD, but food can aggravate symptoms. No specific diet is necessary, but foods that cause reflux should be avoided. Fatty foods stimulate the release of cholecystokinin, a hormone from the duodenum that decreases LES pressure. High-fat foods also decrease the rate of gastric emptying. Foods that decrease LES pressure, such as chocolate, peppermint, and caffeinated beverages (coffee, cola, and tea; see Table 44-8), should be avoided because they are conducive to reflux. Milk products should be avoided, especially at bedtime, because milk increases gastric acid secretion. To prevent overdistension of the stomach, small, frequent meals are advised. The patient should avoid late-evening meals and nocturnal snacking. Fluids should be taken between rather than with meals to reduce gastric distension. Certain foods (e.g., tomato-based products, orange juice) may irritate the acid-sensitive esophagus and may have to be avoided. To reduce intra-abdominal pressure, weight reduction is recommended if the patient is overweight.

Drug Therapy. Drug therapy for GERD is focused on improving LES function, increasing esophageal clearance, decreasing volume and acidity of reflux, and protecting the esophageal mucosa (Table 44-10). There are two approaches to drug therapy. In the "step-up" approach, therapy starts with antacids and OTC histamine (H₂)-receptor (H₂R) blockers; then prescription H₂R blockers and, finally, proton pump inhibitors (PPIs) are included. The "step-down" approach involves starting with a PPI and, over time, titrating down to prescription H₂R blockers and, finally, to OTC H₂R blockers and antacids.

Antacids produce quick but short-lived relief of heartburn. They act by neutralizing HCl. They should be taken 1 to 3 hours after meals and at bedtime. OTC antacids with or without alginic acid (e.g., Gaviscon) may be useful in patients with mild, intermittent heartburn. The alginic acid reacts with sodium bicarbonate and forms a viscous solution that floats to the surface of the gastric contents and coats the esophagus, acting as a mechanical barrier to reflux. However, in patients with moderate to severe or frequent symptoms or patients with documented esophagitis,

TABLE 44-10 DRUG THERAPY

Gastro-Esophageal Reflux Disease (GERD)

Mechanism of Action	Examples
Increase Lower Esophageal Sphincter Pressure	
Cholinergic	Bethanechol (Duvoid)
Promotility	
Prokinetic	Metoclopramide
Acid-Neutralizing	
Antacids	Aluminum hydroxide and magnesium hydroxide (Maalox, Mylanta)
Antisecretory	
H₂-receptor blockers	Famotidine (Pepcid)
	Nizatidine (Axid)
	Ranitidine (Zantac)
Proton pump inhibitors	Esomeprazole (Nexium)
	Dexlansoprazole (Dexilant)
	Lansoprazole (Prevacid)
	Omeprazole (Losec)
	Pantoprazole (Pantoloc)
	Rabeprazole (Pariet)
Cytoprotective	
Alginic acid-antacid	Aluminum hydroxide + magnesium trisilicate (Gaviscon)
Acid-protective	Sucralfate

these regimens are not effective in relieving symptoms or healing erosive lesions.

Antisecretory agents decrease the secretion of HCl by the stomach. H₂R blockers (e.g., ranitidine [Zantac]) are available in OTC and prescription formulations. Some formulations include combinations of H₂R blockers and antacids; for example, Pepcid Complete includes famotidine, calcium carbonate, and magnesium hydroxide. In prescription-strength doses, H₂R blockers reduce symptoms and promote esophageal healing in approximately 50% of patients. Many patients experience relapse (i.e., GERD symptoms return) with discontinuation of the drug.

PPIs also decrease stomach HCl secretion. These drugs act by inhibiting the proton pump mechanism responsible for the secretion of hydrogen ions (H⁺). PPIs promote esophageal healing in approximately 80% to 90% of patients but are more expensive than H₂R blockers. PPIs may also be beneficial in decreasing the incidence of esophageal strictures, a complication of chronic GERD. Long-term use of PPIs has been associated with decreased bone density, chronic hypochlorhydria, increased risk of infection with *Clostridium difficile* in hospitalized patients, and pneumonia (Owen, Panesar, Marks, et al., 2014).

Another drug that may be used to treat GERD is sucralfate, an antiulcer drug used for its cytoprotective properties. Cholinergic drugs, such as bethanechol (Duvoid), may be used to increase LES pressure, improve esophageal emptying in the supine position, and increase gastric emptying. However, the value of current cholinergic agents is limited because they also stimulate HCl secretion. Prokinetic (motility-enhancing) drugs such as metoclopramide promote gastric emptying and reduce the risk of gastric acid reflux (see Table 44-10).

Surgical Therapy. Surgical therapy (antireflux surgery) may be necessary if long-term conservative therapy fails, in the presence of a hiatal hernia, or in the presence of complications, such as esophageal stricture and stenosis (narrowing), chronic

EVIDENCE-INFORMED PRACTICE

Research Highlight

Are Proton Pump Inhibitors Associated With Increased Risk of Diarrhea?
Clinical Question
Among hospitalized patients (P), does the use of proton pump inhibitor drugs (I) increase the risk of *C. difficile*–associated diarrhea (O)?

Best Available Evidence
Meta-analysis of case-control and cohort studies

Critical Appraisal and Synthesis of Evidence
- In 23 studies, researchers examined medical records of 300 000 hospitalized patients for proton pump inhibitor (PPI) exposure and confirmation of acute diarrhea due to *C. difficile*.
- Patients taking PPIs have a greater risk (65%) of *C. difficile*–associated diarrhea (CDAD).

Conclusion
- There is a significant positive association between PPIs and the incidence of CDAD.

Implications for Nursing Practice
- Advise patients taking PPIs of the risk for diarrhea and to contact their health care provider if it does not improve.
- Inform patients that CDAD symptoms include watery stool, abdominal pain, and fever.
- Institute infection control procedures in hospitalized patients suspected of having *C. difficile* infection.

Reference for Evidence
Janarthanan, S., Ditah, I., Adler, D. G., et al. (2012). *Clostridium difficile*–associated diarrhea and proton pump inhibitor therapy: A meta-analysis. *Am J Gastroenterol*, 107(7), 1001–1010. doi:10.1038/ajg.2012.179.

P, Patient population of interest; *I*, intervention or area of interest; *O*, outcomes of interest (see Chapter 1).

esophagitis, and bleeding. Many surgical procedures are performed laparoscopically. The objective of surgical interventions for GERD is to reduce reflux of gastric contents by enhancing the integrity of the LES. Surgical interventions for GERD are called *antireflux procedures*. In these procedures, the fundus of the stomach is wrapped around the lower portion of the esophagus in varying positions.

A diagram of the Nissen fundoplication is shown in Figure 44-4. Laparoscopically performed Nissen and Toupet fundoplications have become the standard antireflux surgical procedures. The use of laparoscopic antireflux surgery for GERD has reduced complications, overall morbidity, and the cost of hospitalization in comparison with a thoracic or open abdominal approach (Funk, Kanji, Scott Melvin, et al., 2014).

Endoscopic Therapy. Alternatives to surgical therapy include endoscopic mucosal resection, photodynamic therapy, cryotherapy, and radiofrequency ablation (image-guided technique that kills cells through heating). For patients with high-grade dysplasia, endoscopic mucosal resection can also be used as a diagnostic test to obtain biopsy samples.

NURSING MANAGEMENT
GASTRO-ESOPHAGEAL REFLUX DISEASE

Patients with GERD must avoid factors that cause reflux. A patient teaching guide is provided in Table 44-11. Patients who smoke should stop. Smoking causes an almost immediate drop in LES

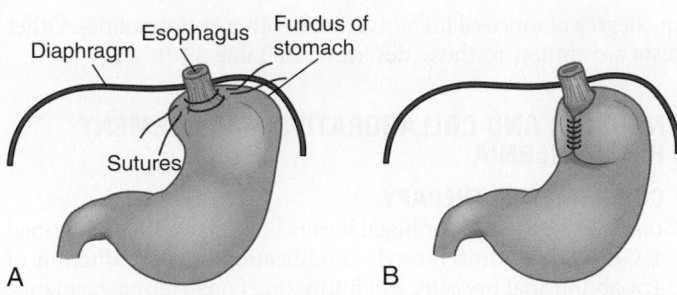

FIGURE 44-4 Nissen fundoplication for repair of hiatal hernia. **A,** The fundus of the stomach is wrapped around the distal esophagus. **B,** The fundus is then sutured to itself. Source: Modified from Doughty, D. B., & Jackson, D. B. (1993). *Mosby's clinical nursing series: Gastrointestinal disorders*. St. Louis: Mosby.

TABLE 44-11   PATIENT & CAREGIVER TEACHING GUIDE

Prevention of Gastro-Esophageal Reflux Disease

The following guidelines should be included when teaching the patient and caregiver about prevention of gastro-esophageal reflux disease. The nurse should:

1. Explain the rationale for a high-protein, low-fat diet. If the patient is overweight or obese, the need for weight loss should be discussed.
2. Encourage the patient to eat small, frequent meals to prevent gastric distension.
3. Explain the rationale for avoiding alcohol, smoking (which causes an almost immediate, marked decrease in LES pressure), and beverages that contain caffeine.
4. Teach the patient not to lie down for 2–3 hrs after eating, not to wear tight clothing around the waist, and not to bend over (especially after eating).
5. Encourage the patient to sleep with head of bed elevated 30 degrees (gravity fosters esophageal emptying).
6. Teach information regarding drugs, including rationale for their use and common adverse effects.
7. Discuss strategies for weight reduction, if appropriate.
8. Encourage patient and caregiver to share concerns about lifestyle changes and living with a chronic problem.

LES, lower esophageal sphincter.

pressure and decreases the ability to clear acid from the esophagus. Patients may need to be referred to other members of the health care team or to community resources for assistance in stopping smoking. (See Chapter 11 for additional information related to smoking cessation.) Substances that decrease LES pressure and tone should be avoided (see Table 44-8). If stress seems to cause symptoms, measures to cope with stress should be discussed. (See Chapter 8 for stress management techniques.) The patient should also be taught possible adverse effects of drugs.

Nursing care for the patient who is having acute symptoms consists mainly of encouraging the patient to follow the necessary regimen, as described in Table 44-11. The patient may be taking drugs to relieve heartburn, and so the nurse must both observe for adverse effects and evaluate the drugs' effectiveness. Even when symptoms are brought under control, the patient may need to continue taking the drugs because the underlying problem is still present. Because of the link between GERD and metaplastic changes in the lower esophagus (Barrett's esophagus), patients are instructed to see their health care provider if symptoms persist.

The nurse must observe for and instruct the patient about adverse effects of the drugs being taken. Adverse effects with H₂R

blockers and PPIs are rare. Antacids have minimal adverse effects: Those that contain aluminum tend to cause constipation, whereas those that contain magnesium tend to cause diarrhea. Several of the antacids are combinations of aluminum and magnesium designed to minimize these adverse effects. If the patient is taking bethanechol (Duvoid), adverse effects to observe for include urinary urgency, increased salivation, and abdominal cramping with diarrhea, nausea, vomiting, and hypotension. Such adverse effects often limit the effectiveness of cholinergic agents in the treatment of GERD. Adverse effects of metoclopramide include restlessness, anxiety, insomnia, and hallucinations. Adverse effects of sucralfate include drowsiness, dizziness, nausea, vomiting, constipation, urticaria, and other types of rash.

Postoperative care focuses on concerns related to prevention of respiratory complications, maintenance of fluid and electrolyte balance, and prevention of infection. If a thoracic approach is used, a chest tube is inserted. Assessment and management related to closed chest drainage are important (see Chapter 30).

If an open abdominal incision is used, respiratory complications can occur in a patient because it is a high abdominal incision. Respiratory assessment should include respiratory rate and rhythm, pulse rate and rhythm, and signs of pneumothorax (e.g., dyspnea, chest pain, cyanosis). Deep breathing is essential to fully expand the lungs.

The patient receives IV fluids and electrolytes until the return of peristalsis. Care should be taken to maintain patency of the NG tube (if present) to prevent the need to reinsert the tube. It is dangerous to attempt to replace the tube because the surgical repair can be perforated. Immediately after the surgical procedure, the patient cannot voluntarily vomit or belch, and this may cause bloating and abdominal discomfort. When peristalsis returns, only fluids are given initially. Solids are added gradually so that the stomach is not overdistended. The nurse must maintain an accurate recording of intake and output and observe for fluid and electrolyte imbalances (see Chapter 19). (Care of the patient after a laparotomy procedure is described in Chapter 45 and NCP 45-2, available on the Evolve website.)

After surgical therapy, there should be no symptoms of gastric reflux. However, the recurrence rate may range from 10% to 30% over a 20-year period after surgery. The patient should be instructed to report symptoms such as heartburn and regurgitation. Such problems may be temporary and resolve with time. The patient should report persistent dysphagia, sense of epigastric fullness, and bloating. A normal diet is gradually resumed. The patient should avoid foods that are gas forming and should try to prevent gastric distension. Food should be chewed thoroughly.

HIATAL HERNIA

Hiatal hernia is herniation of a portion of the stomach into the esophagus through an opening (hiatus) in the diaphragm. It is also referred to as *diaphragmatic hernia* and *esophageal hernia*. The incidence of hiatal hernia is difficult to determine. However, it is the most common abnormality found on radiographic examination of the upper GI tract. Hiatal hernias are common in older adults and are more common in women than in men.

Types

Hiatal hernias are classified into the following two types (Figure 44-5):

1. *Sliding:* The junction of the stomach and the esophagus is above the hiatus of the diaphragm, and a part of the stomach

FIGURE 44-5 A, Sliding hiatal hernia. **B,** Para-esophageal (rolling) hiatal hernia.

slides through the hiatal opening in the diaphragm. The stomach "slides" into the thoracic cavity when the patient is supine and usually goes back into the abdominal cavity when the patient is standing upright. This is the most common type of hiatal hernia.

2. *Para-esophageal* or *rolling:* The esophagogastric junction remains in the normal position, but the fundus and the greater curvature of the stomach roll up through the diaphragm, forming a pocket alongside the esophagus.

Etiology and Pathophysiology

Many factors contribute to the development of hiatal hernia. Structural changes, such as weakening of the muscles in the diaphragm around the esophagogastric opening, are usually contributing factors. Factors that increase intra-abdominal pressure, including obesity, pregnancy, ascites, tumours, tight corsets, intense physical exertion, and heavy lifting on a continual basis, may also predispose to development of a hiatal hernia. Other predisposing factors are increased age, trauma, poor nutrition, and a forced recumbent position, as when a prolonged illness confines the person to bed. In some cases, congenital weakness is a contributing factor.

Clinical Manifestations

Hiatal hernia may be asymptomatic. The signs and symptoms of hiatal hernia, when present, are similar to those described for GERD. Heartburn, especially after a meal or after lying supine, is a common symptom. Affected patients may report dysphagia. Frequently, the symptoms of hiatal hernia mimic those of gallbladder disease, peptic ulcer disease (PUD), and angina. Reflux and discomfort are also associated with position, occurring soon or several hours after the person lies down. Bending over may cause a severe burning pain, which is usually relieved by sitting or standing. Other common precipitating factors of pain include consumption of large meals and alcohol and smoking. Nocturnal symptoms of heartburn are common, especially if the person has eaten before going to sleep.

Complications

Complications that may occur with hiatal hernia include GERD, hemorrhage from erosion, stenosis (narrowing of the esophagus), ulcerations of the herniated portion of the stomach, strangulation of the hernia, and regurgitation with tracheal aspiration.

Diagnostic Studies

A barium swallow study is an important diagnostic measure that may reveal the protrusion of gastric mucosa through the esophageal hiatus in a patient with hiatal hernia. Endoscopic visualization of the lower esophagus provides information on the degree of mucosal inflammation or other abnormalities. Other tests are similar to those described in Table 44-9.

NURSING AND COLLABORATIVE MANAGEMENT HIATAL HERNIA

CONSERVATIVE THERAPY

Conservative therapy for hiatal hernia is similar to that described for GERD, including lifestyle modifications (e.g., reduction of intra-abdominal pressure by eliminating constricting garments, avoiding lifting and straining, eliminating alcohol and smoking, elevating the head of the bed) and the use of antacids and antisecretory agents (i.e., PPIs, H_2R blockers). Elevation of the head of the bed on 10- to 15-cm blocks assists gravity in maintaining the stomach in the abdominal cavity and also helps prevent reflux and tracheal aspiration. If the patient is overweight, the patient should be encouraged to lose weight.

SURGICAL THERAPY

The objective of surgical interventions for hiatal hernia is to reduce reflux by enhancing the integrity of the LES. There are four slightly varied procedures: the Nissen fundoplication, the Toupet fundoplication or technique, the Hill gastropexy, and the Belsey fundoplication. These surgical procedures are all variations of fundoplication, which involves wrapping the fundus of the stomach around the lower portion of the esophagus in varying positions. These procedures reduce the hernia, help maintain an acceptable LES pressure, and prevent movement of the gastro-esophageal junction. The Nissen fundoplication is illustrated in Figure 44-4. As with GERD, laparoscopically performed Nissen and Toupet techniques have become the standard antireflux surgeries for hiatal hernia (Funk, Kanji, Scott Melvin, et al., 2014). A thoracic or open abdominal approach may also be used in selected cases.

AGE-RELATED CONSIDERATIONS

GASTRO-ESOPHAGEAL REFLUX DISEASE AND HIATAL HERNIA

Both the incidence of GERD and that of hiatal hernia increase with age. They are associated with weakening of the diaphragm, obesity, kyphosis, and use of corsets or other factors that increase intra-abdominal pressure. In some older adults, hiatal hernia is asymptomatic. The first indications may include esophageal bleeding secondary to esophagitis or respiratory complications (e.g., aspiration pneumonia) related to aspiration of gastric contents. The LES may become less competent with aging in some individuals.

The clinical course and the management of GERD and hiatal hernia in older adults are similar to those for the younger adult. With the increased use of laparoscopic procedures, surgical risks have been reduced. However, an older adult with cardiovascular and pulmonary problems may not be a good candidate for surgical intervention. In addition, changes in lifestyle, including elimination of dietary factors such as caffeine-containing beverages and chocolate, and elevating the head of the bed on blocks, may be more difficult for the older adult.

ESOPHAGEAL CANCER

Esophageal cancer is a rare malignant neoplasm of the esophagus. There are two main types: squamous cell carcinoma and adenocarcinoma. The rate of 5-year survival is 14% despite multimodal treatment options. Cancer of the esophagus occurs in three times as many men than in women, and the rate has remained relatively stable since the mid-1980s. The incidence of one type of esophageal cancer (esophageal adenocarcinoma), although it is still relatively rare in Canada, doubled from 1986 to 2006 (Otterstatter, Brierley, De, et al., 2012). This may be because of the rising prevalence of obesity and GERD. It was estimated that 2 300 new cases of esophageal cancer would be diagnosed in Canada during 2017 (Canadian Cancer Society, 2017). Adenocarcinomas arise from the glands lining the esophagus and resemble cancers of the stomach and the small intestine, whereas squamous cell carcinoma starts in the squamous cells that line the esophagus. The incidence of esophageal cancer increases with age.

Etiology and Pathophysiology

The cause of esophageal cancer is unknown. Important risk factors are smoking and excessive alcohol intake, chewing betel quid, GERD, tylosis, achalasia, Plummer-Vinson syndrome, chemical injury to the esophagus, exposure to ionizing radiation, and a personal history of oral cancer or a family history of esophageal cancer (Canadian Cancer Society, 2015c). One risk factor for esophageal adenocarcinoma is Barrett's esophagus. (Barrett's esophagus is described in the earlier "Complications" section under "Gastro-esophageal Reflux Disease.")

The majority of esophageal tumours are located in the middle and lower portions of the esophagus. The malignant tumour usually appears as an ulcerated lesion and has often advanced by the time the patient experiences symptoms. The tumour may penetrate the muscular layer and even extend outside the wall of the esophagus. Obstruction of the esophagus occurs in the later stages.

Clinical Manifestations

The onset of symptoms is usually late in relation to the extent of the tumour. Progressive dysphagia is the most common symptom and may be expressed as a substernal feeling as if food is not passing (globus sensation). Initially, the dysphagia occurs only with meat, then with soft foods, and eventually with liquids.

Pain develops late in the course of the disease and is described as occurring in the substernal, epigastric, or back areas and usually increases with swallowing. The pain may radiate to the neck, the jaw, the ears, and the shoulders. If the tumour is in the upper third of the esophagus, symptoms such as sore throat, choking, and hoarseness may occur. Weight loss is fairly common. When esophageal stenosis is severe, regurgitation of blood-flecked esophageal contents is common.

Complications

Hemorrhage may occur if the cancer erodes through the esophagus and into the aorta. Esophageal perforation with fistula formation into the lung or the trachea sometimes develops. The tumour may enlarge enough to cause esophageal obstruction. Metastases spread via the lymph system, the liver and the lungs being common sites of metastasis.

Diagnostic Studies

A barium swallow study with fluoroscopy may demonstrate a narrowing of the esophagus at the site of the tumour (Table 44-12). Sometimes a crater is visible. Endoscopy with biopsy is necessary to make a definitive diagnosis of carcinoma by

TABLE 44-12 COLLABORATIVE CARE

Esophageal Cancer

Diagnostic Studies	Collaborative Therapy

• History and physical examination
 • Barium swallow study
 • Bronchoscopy
 • CT, MRI
 • Endoscopic ultrasonography
 • Endoscopy of esophagus with biopsy
	• Surgical resection
	   • Esophagectomy
	   • Esophagogastrostomy
	   • Esophagoenterostomy
	   • Gastrostomy
	 • Chemotherapy
	 • Dilation
	 • Laser therapy
	 • Palliative therapy
	 • Radiation
	 • Stent or prosthesis

CT, computed tomography; *MRI,* magnetic resonance imaging.

identification of malignant cells. Endoscopic ultrasonography is an important tool used to stage esophageal cancer. A bronchoscopic examination may be performed to detect malignant involvement of the lung. Computed tomography and MRI are also used to assess the extent of the disease.

Collaborative Care

The treatment of esophageal cancer depends on the location of the tumour and whether invasion or metastasis has occurred (see Table 44-12). Esophageal cancer has a poor prognosis, mainly because it is not usually diagnosed until the disease is advanced. The best results may be obtained with a combination of surgery, chemotherapy, and radiation.

The types of surgical procedures that can be performed are (a) removal of part or all of the esophagus (*esophagectomy*) with use of a Dacron graft to replace the resected part, (b) resection of a portion of the esophagus and anastomosis of the remaining portion to the stomach (*esophagogastrostomy*), and (c) resection of a portion of the esophagus and anastomosis of a segment of colon to the remaining portion (*esophagoenterostomy*). The surgical approaches may be thoracic or both abdominal and thoracic. In comparison with the other procedures, minimally invasive esophagectomy (laparoscopic vagal nerve–sparing surgery) has the advantages of smaller incisions, shorter hospital stays, and fewer pulmonary complications. Overall outcomes appear to be similar to open resections of the esophagus. Chemotherapy in combination with radiation treatment before or after surgery is currently used (Canadian Cancer Society, 2015d). Current treatment regimens can be found through the Canadian Cancer Society. If the tumour is in the cervical section (upper third) of the esophagus, radiation treatment is usually indicated. A tumour in the lower third of the esophagus is usually resected surgically.

Palliative therapy consists of restoration of the swallowing function and maintenance of nutrition and hydration. Dilation, stent placement, or both can relieve obstruction. Dilation is accomplished with various types of dilators (e.g., Celestin's tube). Dilation often relieves dysphagia and allows for improved nutrition. Placement of a stent or prosthesis may help when dilation is no longer effective. The prostheses are composed of silicone rubber or nylon-reinforced latex tubes with distal and proximal collars. The prosthesis is placed in the esophagus so that food and fluids can pass through the stenotic segment of the esophagus. The prosthesis can be placed endoscopically.

Endoscopic laser therapy or vaporization of the tumour may be used in combination with dilation. Obstruction recurs as the tumour grows, but laser therapy can be repeated. Sometimes these procedures are combined with radiation therapy. Other measures for palliation include gastrostomy or esophagostomy tube placements for nutritional support and pain management.

Nutritional Therapy. After esophageal surgery, parenteral fluids are given. When fluids are allowed, 30 to 60 mL of water is given hourly, with gradual progression to small, frequent bland meals. The patient should be in an upright position to prevent regurgitation of the fluid. The patient is observed for signs of intolerance to the feeding or leakage of the feeding into the mediastinum. Symptoms that indicate leakage are pain, increased temperature, and dyspnea. Symptoms of food intolerance include vomiting and abdominal distension. A gastrostomy may be performed for the purpose of feeding the patient. (Gastrostomy and tube feedings are discussed in Chapter 42.)

NURSING MANAGEMENT
ESOPHAGEAL CANCER

NURSING ASSESSMENT

The patient should be asked about any history of GERD, hiatal hernia, achalasia, or Barrett's esophagus. The patient is also questioned regarding tobacco and alcohol use. The patient should be assessed for progressive dysphagia and *odynophagia* (burning, squeezing pain during swallowing). The nurse should question the patient regarding the type of substances ingested that cause dysphagia, such as meat, soft foods, and liquids. The patient is also assessed for pain (substernal, epigastric, or back areas), choking, heartburn, hoarseness, cough, anorexia, weight loss, and regurgitation (sometimes bloody).

NURSING DIAGNOSES

Nursing diagnoses for the patient with esophageal cancer include, but are not limited to, the following:

- *Chronic pain* related to *injury agent* (compression of tumour on surrounding tissues)
- *Imbalanced nutrition: less than body requirements* related to *insufficient dietary intake* (dysphagia, odynophagia, weakness)
- *Risk for aspiration* related to *decrease in gastro-intestinal motility* (difficulty swallowing and regurgitation)
- *Anxiety* related to *threat to current status, threat of death*

PLANNING

The overall goals are that the patient with esophageal cancer will (a) have relief of symptoms, including pain and dysphagia; (b) achieve optimal nutritional intake; (c) understand the prognosis of the disease; and (d) experience the best possible quality of life during disease progression.

NURSING IMPLEMENTATION

HEALTH PROMOTION. Patients with diagnosed GERD and hiatal hernia need to be counselled regarding regular follow-up evaluation. Health counselling should focus on elimination of smoking and excessive alcohol intake, as well as other risk factors for GERD. Maintenance of good oral hygiene and dietary habits (intake of fresh fruits and vegetables) may also be helpful.

Patients with Barrett's esophagus need to be monitored because this is considered a premalignant condition. Early diagnosis of esophageal tumours is important but difficult because the onset of symptoms is usually late in the course of the disease. Patients are encouraged to seek medical attention for any esophageal problems, especially dysphagia. Patients who are at risk for esophageal adenocarcinoma, such as those with evidence of Barrett's esophagus and a diagnosis of achalasia (discussed later in the "Other Esophageal Disorders" section), may need regular endoscopic screening with biopsy and cytological study.

ACUTE INTERVENTION

Preoperative Care. In addition to general preoperative teaching and preparation, particular attention to the patient's nutritional needs and oral care is important. Many patients are poorly nourished because of the inability to ingest adequate amounts of food and fluids before surgery. A high-calorie, high-protein diet is recommended. It may have to be in liquid form. Some patients may need IV fluid replacement or parenteral nutrition. The patient and the family member are instructed on how to keep an intake and output record and how to assess for signs of fluid and electrolyte imbalance. Some treatment protocols necessitate preoperative radiation treatment and chemotherapy.

Meticulous oral care is essential. The mouth, including tongue, gingivae, and teeth or dentures, must be cleaned thoroughly. Milk of magnesia with mineral oil may be used to remove any crusting that has formed. A mixture of mouthwash (nonalcohol), ice, and water makes a refreshing rinse for the patient.

Teaching should include information about chest tubes (if a thoracic approach is used), IV lines, NG tubes, gastrostomy feeding, turning, coughing, and deep breathing. (General preoperative care is presented in Chapter 20.)

Postoperative Care. After surgery for esophageal cancer, most patients have an NG tube in place, and there may be bloody drainage for 8 to 12 hours. The drainage gradually changes to greenish yellow. Assessment of the drainage, maintenance of the tube, and oral and nasal care are nursing responsibilities. The nurse should not reposition or reinsert the NG tube without consulting with the surgeon.

Because of the location of the incision and the general condition of the patient, special emphasis must be placed on prevention of respiratory complications. Turning and deep breathing should be done every 2 hours. Use of an incentive spirometer helps to prevent respiratory complications.

The patient should be positioned in semi-Fowler's or Fowler's position to prevent reflux and aspiration of gastric secretions. When the patient can drink fluids or eat, the upright position should be maintained for at least 2 hours after eating in order to assist the movement of food through the GI tract.

AMBULATORY AND HOME CARE. Many patients require long-term follow-up care after surgery for esophageal cancer. Patients may undergo chemotherapy and radiation treatment after surgery. Such patients need encouragement and assistance in maintaining adequate nutrition. A permanent feeding gastrostomy may be necessary. Most of these patients have fears and anxieties about a diagnosis of cancer. The nurse should know what the health care provider has told the patient regarding the prognosis and then provide appropriate counselling.

Referral to a home health nurse may be necessary for continued care of the patient (e.g., gastrostomy teaching, follow-up wound care). (See Chapter 13 for management of terminally ill patients, and Chapter 18 for that of patients with cancer.)

EVALUATION

The following are expected outcomes for the patient with esophageal cancer:

- The patient will maintain a patent airway.
- The patient will have relief of pain.
- The patient will be able to swallow comfortably.
- The patient will consume adequate nutritional intake.
- The patient will understand the prognosis of the disease.
- The patient will experience the best possible quality of life during disease progression.

OTHER ESOPHAGEAL DISORDERS

Eosinophilic Esophagitis

Eosinophilic esophagitis is characterized by swelling of the esophagus caused by an infiltration of *eosinophils*. Many people with this condition have a personal or family history of other allergic diseases. The most common food triggers are milk, egg, wheat, rye, and beef. Environmental allergens—such as pollens; moulds; cat, dog, and dust mite allergens—may be involved in the development of eosinophilic esophagitis.

Clinical manifestations include severe heartburn, difficulty swallowing, food impaction in the esophagus, nausea, vomiting, and weight loss. The diagnosis is based on the symptoms and biopsy findings of eosinophils infiltrating the esophageal tissue obtained from endoscopy.

Allergy skin testing helps determine the person's allergens. A trial of avoidance of the foods to which the person's allergy test results are positive is the initial form of treatment for eosinophilic esophagitis. A variety of treatment approaches, including acid suppression, corticosteroids, and endoscopic dilation, can be used alone or in combination.

Corticosteroids are frequently used to treat eosinophilic esophagitis when avoidance of allergic triggers does not relieve symptoms. Corticosteroids may be used orally (prednisone) or as a topical therapy, as with inhaled corticosteroids (e.g., fluticasone [Flovent]). In asthma, for which fluticasone is typically used, corticosteroids are inhaled. In eosinophilic esophagitis, they are swallowed, and this results in the delivery of the drug directly to the esophagus.

Esophageal Diverticula

Esophageal diverticula are saclike outpouchings of one or more layers of the esophagus. They occur in three main areas: (a) above the upper esophageal sphincter *(Zenker's diverticulum)*, which is the most common location; (b) near the esophageal midpoint *(traction diverticulum)*; and (c) above the LES *(epiphrenic diverticulum)* (Figure 44-6). Pharyngeal pouches (Zenker's diverticula) occur most commonly in older adults (age >70 yr), and typical symptoms include dysphagia, regurgitation, chronic cough, aspiration, and weight loss. Traction diverticulum may not cause signs and symptoms. However, many affected patients report a sour taste in the mouth and halitosis (bad breath) caused by the decomposition of stagnant food in the diverticulum. Complications include malnutrition, aspiration, and perforation. A diagnosis is easily established by barium studies.

There is no specific treatment for diverticula. Some patients find they can empty the pocket of food that collects by applying pressure at a point on the neck. The diet may have to be limited to foods that pass more readily (e.g., blenderized foods). Treatment of the diverticulum may be necessary if nutrition becomes

FIGURE 44-6 Possible sites for the occurrence of esophageal diverticula. These hollow outpouchings may occur just above the upper esophageal sphincter (Zenker's, the most common type of diverticulum), near the midpoint of the esophagus (traction), and just above the lower esophageal sphincter (epiphrenic). Source: Modified from Price, S. A., & Wilson, L. M. (2003). *Pathophysiology: Clinical concepts of disease processes* (6th ed.). St. Louis: Mosby.

disrupted. Treatment is surgical via an endoscopic or external cervical approach and should include a cricopharyngeal myotomy. Open approaches have been associated with significant morbidity because the majority of affected patients are older adults, many of whom have general medical problems.

Esophageal Strictures

The most common cause of esophageal strictures (narrowing) is chronic GERD. The ingestion of strong acids or alkalis, external beam radiation, and surgical anastomosis can also lead to the development of strictures. In addition, trauma such as throat lacerations and gunshot wounds may lead to strictures as a result of scar formation (collagen deposition) from healing. The strictures usually develop over a long time. Strictures can be dilated endoscopically with *bougies* (dilating instruments). Another technique is balloon dilation, which is done under endoscopic guidance and does not necessitate fluoroscopy. Surgical excision with anastomosis is sometimes necessary. The patient may have a temporary or permanent gastrostomy.

Achalasia

Achalasia is the absence of peristalsis of the lower two thirds (smooth muscle) of the esophagus. Pressure in the LES is increased, and relaxation of the LES is incomplete. Obstruction of the esophagus at or near the diaphragm occurs. Food and fluid accumulate in the lower esophagus. The result of this condition is dilation of the lower esophagus (Figure 44-7). The altered peristalsis is a result of impairment of the neurons that innervate the lower esophagus. There is a selective loss of inhibitory neurons, which results in unopposed excitation of the LES. Achalasia affects people of all ages and both sexes. The course of the disease is chronic.

Dysphagia (difficulty swallowing) is the most common symptom and occurs with both liquids and solids. Patients may report a globus sensation. Substernal chest pain (similar to the pain of angina) occurs during or immediately after a meal. *Halitosis* (foul-smelling breath) and the inability to eructate (belch)

FIGURE 44-7 Esophageal achalasia. **A,** Early stage, showing tapering of lower esophagus. **B,** Advanced stage, showing dilated, tortuous esophagus.

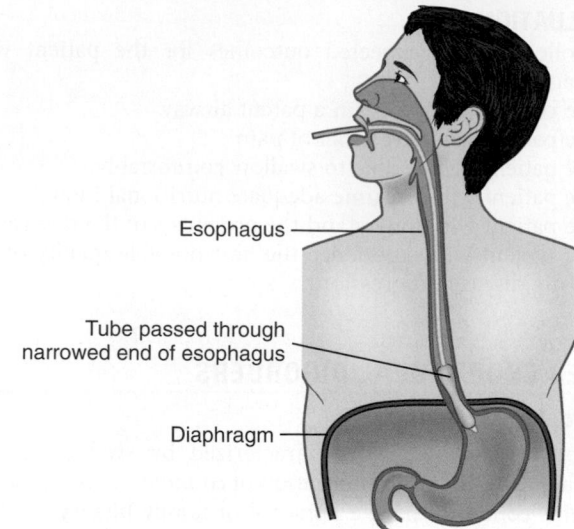

FIGURE 44-8 Pneumatic dilation attempts to treat achalasia by maintaining an adequate lumen and decreasing lower esophageal sphincter tone. Source: Modified from Price, S. A., & Wilson, L. M. (2003). *Pathophysiology: Clinical concepts of disease processes* (6th ed.). St. Louis: Mosby.

are other symptoms. Another common symptom is regurgitation of sour-tasting food and liquids, especially when the patient is in a horizontal position. Patients with achalasia also report symptoms (e.g., heartburn) of GERD. Weight loss is typical.

Diagnosis usually involves manometric studies of the lower esophagus and/or endoscopy. The exact cause of achalasia is not known, and so treatment is focused on symptom management. Treatment consists of dilation, surgery, and use of drugs. All these therapies are directed at relieving the stasis caused by the increased LES pressure, the nonrelaxing LES, and the aperistaltic esophagus. Treatment of symptoms consists of a semisoft bland diet, eating slowly and drinking fluid with meals, and sleeping with the head elevated.

Drug therapy is used to manage early achalasia when there is no significant esophageal dilation. Drug therapy is used as a short-term measure and is considered as an alternative only in patients unable to undergo pneumatic dilation or surgery. Endoscopic injection of botulinum toxin (Botox) into the LES can be offered for initial relief of symptoms, but the effects are short term, and symptoms are likely to recur within 1 year. It works by inhibiting the release of acetylcholine from nerve endings, thereby promoting relaxation of the smooth muscle. This treatment does not carry the risk of perforation that can occur with pneumatic dilation. Repeated injections are required, or the patient must be switched to other therapy. However, there may be subsets of patients, such as older adult patients or those with multiple medical problems, who are poor candidates for more invasive procedures, for whom botulinum toxin injection is the preferred approach. Other classes of drugs used in the management of achalasia include anticholinergics, calcium channel blockers, and long-acting nitrates, which act by relaxing the smooth muscle.

Esophageal dilation *(bougienage)* is an effective treatment measure for many patients. The LES is usually pneumatically dilated with a balloon-tipped dilator passed orally. A variety of different dilators are available for this procedure. All depend on forcible expansion of a balloon in the LES (Figure 44-8). The forceful dilation does not restore normal esophageal motility, but it does provide for emptying of the esophagus into the stomach.

Surgical intervention may become necessary. An esophagomyotomy may be performed. In this procedure, the muscle fibres that enclose the narrowed area of the esophagus are divided. This allows the mucosa to pouch out through the division in the muscle layer so that food can be swallowed without obstruction.

A similar procedure is the Heller myotomy (cardiomyotomy), which disrupts the LES and reduces LES pressure. An antireflux procedure is often performed with the myotomy. The Heller myotomy can be performed laparoscopically, which reduces the potential for postoperative complications.

Esophageal Varices

Esophageal varices are veins in the lower portion of the esophagus that become dilated and tortuous as a result of portal hypertension. Esophageal varices are a common complication of liver cirrhosis and are discussed further in Chapter 46.

DISORDERS OF THE STOMACH AND UPPER SMALL INTESTINE

GASTRITIS

Types

Gastritis, an inflammation of the gastric mucosa, is one of the most common problems affecting the stomach. Gastritis may be acute or chronic and may be diffuse or localized. Chronic gastritis has been further divided into three subtypes: (a) autoimmune, which involves the body and the fundus of the stomach; (b) diffuse antral, which affects primarily the antrum; and (c) multifocal, which is diffuse throughout the stomach. The causes of gastritis and its relationship to other gastric disorders, such as *Helicobacter pylori* infection and gastric cancer, are the focus of ongoing research.

Etiology and Pathophysiology

Gastritis occurs as the result of a breakdown in the normal gastric mucosal barrier. This mucosal barrier normally protects the stomach tissue from autodigestion by HCl and the proteolytic enzyme pepsin. When the barrier is broken, HCl can diffuse back into the mucosa. The backward diffusion of acid results in tissue edema, disruption of capillary walls with loss of plasma into the gastric lumen, and possibly hemorrhage.

TABLE 44-13   CAUSES OF GASTRITIS

Drugs	Pathophysiological Conditions
• acetylsalicylic acid (ASA; Aspirin)	• Burns
• Corticosteroid drugs	• Crohn's disease
• Nonsteroidal anti-inflammatory drugs	• Large hiatal hernia
	• Physiological stress
	• Reflux of bile and pancreatic secretions
Diet	• Renal failure (uremia)
• Alcohol	• Sepsis
• Spicy, irritating food	• Shock
Microorganisms	**Other Factors**
• *Helicobacter pylori*	• Endoscopic procedures
• Salmonella organisms	• Nasogastric suction
• Staphylococcus organisms	• Psychological stress
Environmental Factors	
• Radiation	
• Smoking	

Causes of gastritis are listed in Table 44-13. Drugs such as acetylsalicylic acid (ASA: Aspirin), nonsteroidal anti-inflammatory drugs (NSAIDs), and digitalis have direct irritating effects on the gastric mucosa. In addition, corticosteroids and NSAIDs are known to inhibit the synthesis of prostaglandins that are protective of the gastric mucosa. This leaves the gastric mucosa more susceptible to mucosal damage. NSAID-related gastritis is associated with many of the older drugs, including piroxicam (Pirox), naproxen (Naprosyn), sulindac (Sulin), indomethacin, diclofenac (Voltaren), and ibuprofen (Motrin, Advil). The use of cyclo-oxygenase–2 (COX-2) inhibitors has been associated with fewer GI adverse effects than the nonselective use of NSAIDs. However, even these agents are associated with an increased risk of upper GI inflammation and bleeding.

Dietary indiscretions can also result in acute gastritis. After an alcoholic drinking binge, acute damage to the gastric mucosa can range from local destruction of superficial epithelial cells to desquamation and destruction of the mucosa, with mucosal congestion, edema, and hemorrhage. Prolonged damage induced by repeated alcohol abuse can result in chronic gastritis. Eating large quantities of spicy, irritating foods and metabolic conditions such as uremia can also cause acute gastritis.

An important causative factor in chronic gastritis, in particular in the diffuse antral and multifocal types, is *H. pylori* infection. *H. pylori*–associated gastritis is a common problem in adults, many of whom do not have symptoms of gastritis. It is currently thought that *H. pylori* infection is acquired in childhood. For reasons not clearly understood, *H. pylori* is capable of promoting the breakdown of the gastric mucosal barrier, given certain "triggers" or conditions. Thus, given time, *H. pylori* will eventually have a destructive effect on its host environment. *H. pylori* has been linked to gastric cancer and mucosa-associated lymphoid tissue (MALT) lymphoma of the stomach. (The role of *H. pylori* in ulcer development is discussed in greater detail later in the "Duodenal Ulcers" section.)

Autoimmune atrophic gastritis is a form of chronic gastritis that affects both the fundus and the body of the stomach and is associated with an increased risk of gastric cancer. Approximately 30% of patients with *H. pylori* infection are found to have antigastric antibodies as well. Thus there may be a link between the host's response to the presence of *H. pylori* and the development of autoimmune chronic gastritis.

Other causes of chronic gastritis, although not as common, have been identified. Infections with bacteria, viruses, and fungi, including *Mycobacterium*, *Cytomegalovirus*, and *Treponema pallidum*, are associated with chronic gastritis. Gastritis can result from reflux of bile salts from the duodenum into the stomach as a result of anatomical changes after surgical procedures such as gastro-duodenostomy and gastro-jejunostomy. Prolonged vomiting may also cause reflux of bile salts. In addition, intense emotional responses and CNS lesions may produce inflammation of the mucosal lining as a result of hypersecretion of HCl or corticosteroids (Cushing's syndrome).

Progressive gastric mucosal atrophy from chronic alterations in the protective mucosal barrier causes the gastric chief and parietal cells to die eventually. With the decrease in the number of acid-secreting parietal cells and atrophy of the gastric mucosa, *hypochlorhydria* (decreased acid secretion) or *achlorhydria* (lack of acid secretion) occurs.

Clinical Manifestations

The symptoms of acute gastritis include anorexia, nausea and vomiting, epigastric tenderness, and a feeling of fullness. Hemorrhage is commonly associated with alcohol abuse and at times may be the only symptom. Acute gastritis is self-limiting, lasting from a few hours to a few days, and the mucosa is expected to heal completely.

The manifestations of chronic gastritis are similar to those described for acute gastritis. Some affected patients have no symptoms directly associated with the gastric lesion. However, when the acid-secreting cells are lost or do not function as a result of atrophy, the source of *intrinsic factor* is also lost. The loss of intrinsic factor, a substance secreted by the gastric mucosa that is essential for the absorption of cobalamin (vitamin B_{12}, which is essential for the growth and maturation of RBCs) in the terminal ileum, ultimately results in cobalamin deficiency. Over time, the body's storage of cobalamin in the liver is depleted, and a deficiency state exists. Lack of this important vitamin results in the development of anemia and neurological complications. (Cobalamin deficiency anemia is discussed in Chapter 33.)

Diagnostic Studies

Diagnosis of acute gastritis is most often based on a history of drug and alcohol use. The diagnosis of chronic gastritis may be delayed or completely missed because the symptoms are nonspecific. Endoscopic examination with biopsy is necessary to obtain a definitive diagnosis. Breath, urine, serum, and gastric tissue biopsy tests are available for the determination of *H. pylori*. These tests are described later in this chapter in the "Diagnostic Studies" section under "Peptic Ulcer Disease." Radiological studies are not helpful because the superficial mucosa is generally involved, and changes are not clearly visible on radiographs. A complete blood cell count (CBC) may demonstrate the presence of anemia that results from blood loss or lack of intrinsic factor. Stools are tested for the presence of occult blood. A gastric analysis, although currently not used as much, demonstrates the amount of HCl present; achlorhydria is a common sign of severe atrophic gastritis. Serum tests for antibodies to parietal cells and intrinsic factor may be performed. Tissue biopsy with cytological examination is necessary to rule out gastric carcinoma.

NURSING AND COLLABORATIVE MANAGEMENT GASTRITIS

ACUTE GASTRITIS

Eliminating the cause and preventing or avoiding it in the future are generally all that is needed to treat acute gastritis. The plan of care is supportive and similar to that described for nausea and vomiting. If vomiting accompanies acute gastritis, bed rest, NPO status, and IV fluids may be prescribed. Dehydration can occur rapidly in patients with acute gastritis with vomiting. Fluids and electrolytes lost through vomiting and occasionally diarrhea are replaced. Antiemetics are given for nausea and vomiting (see Table 44-1). In severe cases of acute gastritis, an NG tube may be used, either for lavage of the precipitating agent from the stomach or in conjunction with suction to keep the stomach empty and free of noxious stimuli. Clear liquids are resumed when acute symptoms have subsided, with gradual reintroduction of solid, bland foods.

If hemorrhage is considered likely, vital signs must be checked frequently and the vomitus tested for blood. All of the management strategies discussed later in the "Upper Gastro-intestinal Bleeding" section also apply to severe gastritis.

Drug therapy is focused on reducing irritation of the gastric mucosa and providing relief of symptoms. Antacids are beneficial in the relief of abdominal discomfort by raising intragastric pH to above 6. H_2R blockers or PPIs may be used to reduce gastric HCl secretion. The nurse must have knowledge of the action and the therapeutic effects of PPIs and H_2R blockers to teach the patient and to monitor the effects of the drugs.

CHRONIC GASTRITIS

The treatment of chronic gastritis focuses on evaluating and eliminating the specific cause (e.g., cessation of alcohol intake, abstinence from drugs, *H. pylori* eradication). Currently, antibiotic and antisecretory agent combinations are used to eradicate infection with *H. pylori* (Table 44-14). For patients with pernicious anemia, oral or parenteral administration of cobalamin is needed (see Chapter 33). Discussion of the continued need for this essential vitamin must be included in the plan of care.

The patient undergoing treatment for chronic gastritis may have to adapt to many lifestyle changes and adhere strictly to a drug regimen. A nonirritating diet consisting of six small meals a day and the use of an antacid after meals may help provide relief from symptoms. Smoking is contraindicated. An interdisciplinary team approach in which the physician, the nurse, the dietitian, and the pharmacist provide consistent information and support may increase the patient's success in making these alterations. Because the incidence of gastric cancer is higher among patients who have a history of chronic gastritis, especially atrophic gastritis, close medical follow-up should be emphasized.

GASTRIC CANCER

Gastric cancer (also called *stomach cancer*) is an adenocarcinoma of the stomach wall (Figure 44-9). It is the second most frequent cause of cancer death worldwide (Thomson & Young, 2011). Although less common in Canada, it was estimated that 3 500 new gastric cancer cases would be diagnosed in 2017 (Canadian Cancer Society, 2017). Gastric cancer is more prevalent in men of the lower socioeconomic class, primarily those living in urban areas. Gastric cancer is typically at an advanced stage when diagnosed and is not usually amenable to surgical resection. The

TABLE 44-14   DRUG THERAPY

Helicobacter pylori *Infection*

Treatment	Duration	Eradication Rate
Triple-Drug Therapy (Recommended as First-Line Therapy)		
Proton pump inhibitor* Amoxicillin Clarithromycin (Biaxin)	7–14 days	>70%–85%
Quadruple Therapy		
Proton pump inhibitor* Bismuth subsalicylate Tetracycline Metronidazole (Flagyl)	10–14 days	85%

*See Table 44-10.

FIGURE 44-9 Gastric cancer. Gross photograph shows an ill-defined, excavated central ulcer surrounded by irregular, heaped-up borders. Source: Kumar, V., Abbas, A. K., Fausto, N., et al. (2010). *Robbins and Cotran pathologic basis of disease* (8th ed.). Philadelphia: Saunders.

disease is confined to the stomach in only 10% to 20% of affected patients. The rate of 5-year survival is 25%.

Etiology and Pathophysiology

Many factors have been implicated in the development of gastric cancer: *H. pylori* infection; smoking; family history of gastric cancer; inherited conditions (e.g., hereditary diffuse gastric cancer); certain stomach conditions, including gastritis; previous stomach surgery; infection with the Epstein-Barr virus; exposure to ionizing radiation; and type A blood (Canadian Cancer Society, 2015e).

Gastric carcinogenesis probably begins with a nonspecific mucosal injury as a result of aging, autoimmunity, or repeated exposure to irritants such as bile, anti-inflammatory agents, or alcohol. Nutritional or other undetermined genetic deficiencies may impede mucosal repair, which results in chronic gastritis and subsequent proliferation of *H. pylori*. Infection with *H. pylori*, especially at an early age, is considered a definite risk factor for gastric cancer. It is possible that *H. pylori* and resulting metabolic changes can induce a sequence of transitions from dysplasia to carcinoma in situ. Individuals with MALT lymphoma are at higher risk for gastric cancer.

Other predisposing factors associated with a high incidence of gastric cancer are atrophic gastritis, pernicious anemia, adenomatous polyps, hyperplastic polyps, and achlorhydria. The relationship between chronic gastric ulcers and the development of gastric cancer is still controversial. Malignant transformation of a benign chronic ulcer does occur but accounts for fewer than 5% of all gastric cancers. It is known that people with achlorhydria or pernicious anemia are more likely to develop gastric cancer than are people with normal gastric acid production.

Gastric cancers often spread to adjacent organs before any distressing symptoms occur. The tumour may grow to large dimensions without obstructing the lumen of the stomach simply because the lumen itself is so large. The interval from onset of symptoms to consultation with a health care provider may be as long as 6 months. This long delay is largely attributed to the vague, intermittent abdominal distress experienced by the patient. Unfortunately, these symptoms are nonspecific; most healthy persons at one time or another experience them as a result of dietary indiscretions, nervous tension, and anxiety.

Gastric cancer can occur in any portion of the stomach. Tumours located at the cardia and the fundus are associated with a poor prognosis. These tumours typically infiltrate rapidly to the surrounding tissue, regional lymph nodes, and liver. Patients with tumour growth along the lesser curvature have a better survival rate. Adenocarcinomas account for more than 95% of the cancers, and sarcomas (comprising lymphomas and leiomyomas) make up the rest.

The tumour growth is insidious and follows a pattern of continuous infiltration. Gastric cancer may spread by direct extension along the mucosal surface and infiltrate through the stomach wall. The rich lymphatic plexuses in the stomach facilitate distant metastasis. Seeding of tumour cells into the peritoneal cavity may occur late in the course of the disease.

Clinical Manifestations

The clinical manifestations exhibited by persons with gastric cancer can be categorized by signs and symptoms of anemia, PUD, or indigestion. Anemia is a common occurrence with gastric cancer. It is caused by chronic blood loss that occurs as the lesion erodes through the mucosa or as a direct result of pernicious anemia, which develops when intrinsic factor is lost. The affected person appears pale and weak and reports fatigue, weakness, dizziness, and in extreme cases, shortness of breath. The stool specimen may be positive for occult blood.

The symptoms of gastric cancer are sometimes identical to those of PUD. The pain and discomfort may be alleviated by belching and by the use of antacids, antisecretory agents, and diet modifications. Manifestations related to indigestion include vague feeling of epigastric fullness with feelings of early satiety after meals. Weight loss, dysphagia, and constipation frequently accompany epigastric distress. When nausea, vomiting, and hematemesis occur, they may indicate gastric outlet obstruction or may be a warning of impending hemorrhage.

With more advanced disease, the physical examination may reveal that the patient is pale and lethargic if anemia is present. When the appetite has been poor and weight loss has been considerable, the patient may appear cachectic. A mass may be detected beneath the abdominal wall and is seen to move with each inspiration. On palpation, the mass may be felt in the epigastrium. Masses that are predominantly in the antrum of the stomach are generally found to the left of the midline. Masses located to the right of midline usually tend to be metastases to the liver or indicate involvement of the perigastric lymph nodes. Supraclavicular lymph nodes that are hard and enlarged and located on the left side are suggestive of metastasis via the thoracic duct from the stomach lesion. The presence of ascites is a poor prognostic sign.

TABLE 44-15 COLLABORATIVE CARE

Gastric Cancer

Diagnostic Studies	Collaborative Therapy
• History and physical examination	**Surgical Therapy**
• Alpha-fetoprotein measurement	• Subtotal gastrectomy: Billroth I or II procedure
• Carbohydrate antigen (CA-) 19-9, CA-125, CA 72-4 assessments	• Total gastrectomy with esophago-jejunostomy
• Carcinoembryonic antigen (CEA) assessment	
• Complete blood cell count	**Adjuvant Therapy**
• Endoscopic ultrasonography	• Radiation therapy
• Endoscopy and biopsy	• Chemotherapy
• Exfoliative cytological study	• Combination radiation therapy and chemotherapy
• Liver enzyme measurements	
• Serum amylase measurement	
• Stool examination	
• Tumour marker assessment	
• Upper GI barium study	
• Urinalysis	

GI, gastro-intestinal.

Diagnostic Studies

The diagnostic studies for gastric cancer are presented in Table 44-15.

Endoscopic examination of the stomach remains the best diagnostic tool. Lesions that go undetected on the radiograph can be viewed more easily and a biopsy performed when endoscopy is used. The stomach can be distended with air during the procedure so that the mucosal folds can be stretched. Fixation of the mucosa is indicative of malignancy.

Upper GI barium studies may demonstrate alterations in gastric contractility and emptying but do not always reveal small lesions of the cardia and fundus.

Blood chemistry studies assist in the determination of anemia and its severity. Elevations in liver enzymes and serum amylase levels may indicate liver and pancreatic involvement. Stool examination provides evidence of occult or gross bleeding.

Several tumour markers are often present in patients with gastric cancer (see Table 44-15). Serum tests for these markers are commonly performed before surgery for this disease. Serum markers are not used as the only diagnostic tools for gastric cancer because elevations may be related to other factors such as smoking and the presence of benign lesions. (Carcinoembryonic antigen and other tumour markers are discussed in Chapter 18.)

Collaborative Care

When the diagnosis of gastric cancer has been confirmed, the treatment of choice is surgical removal of the tumour. The preoperative management of the patient with gastric cancer focuses on the correction of nutritional deficits, treatment of anemia, and replacement of blood volume.

Transfusions of packed RBCs correct the anemia. If a gastric lesion has been located at or near the pylorus and is causing gastric outlet obstruction, gastric decompression may be necessary before surgery. When the tumour has extended into the transverse colon, and if partial colon resection is also required, special preparation of the bowel is necessary. This preparation may include a low-residue diet, enemas to cleanse the bowel, and the use of antibiotics to reduce the intestinal bacteria. Correction of malnutrition is important if surgery is planned. Malnutrition is associated with increased rates of postoperative complications and mortality.

Surgical Therapy. The surgical intervention used in the treatment of gastric cancer may be the same surgical procedures used for PUD. The location and the extent of the lesion, the patient's physical condition, and the preference of the surgeon determine the specific surgery employed. When metastasis is widespread at the time of diagnosis, surgical intervention may be only palliative.

The surgical aim is to remove the tumour by resecting as much of the stomach as necessary and a margin of normal tissue. When the lesion is located in the cardia or high in the fundus, a total gastrectomy with esophago-jejunostomy is performed. This combination of procedures involves anastomosis of the lower end of the esophagus to the jejunum (Figure 44-10). Lesions located in the antrum or the pyloric region are generally treated in either a Billroth I or a Billroth II procedure. When the tumour has metastasized to adjacent organs, such as the spleen, ovaries, or bowel, the surgical procedures must be modified and extended as necessary.

The chance of a complete cure by surgical means is decreased considerably when the lymph nodes are involved. Survival is shortened when organs adjacent to the stomach show evidence of invasion at the time of surgery.

Adjuvant Therapy. Surgery is the only definitive means of achieving a cure. However, when the patient cannot physically withstand a surgical procedure or when surgical cure is not feasible, radiation therapy or chemotherapy alone or in combination may be used. Neither radiation therapy nor chemotherapeutic agents have been very successful when used as the primary mode of treatment. Because the radiosensitivity of gastric cancers is low, radiation therapy has proved to be of little value.

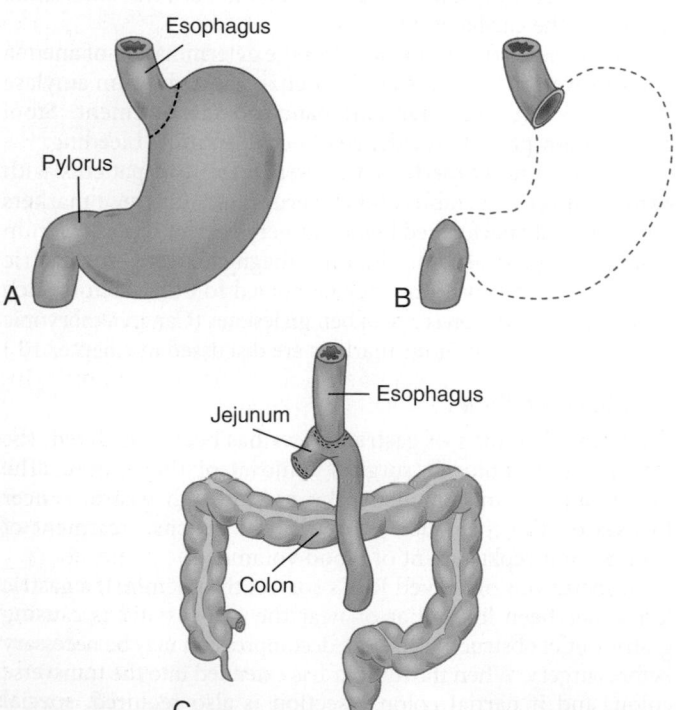

FIGURE 44-10 Total gastrectomy for gastric cancer. **A,** Normal anatomical structure of the stomach. **B,** Removal of the stomach (total gastrectomy). **C,** Anastomosis of the esophagus with the jejunum (esophago-jejunostomy).

When it is used as a palliative measure, the tumour mass can be decreased, with temporary relief of the cardia or pyloric obstruction.

The combination of chemotherapy and radiation therapy is now being used for patients who are at high risk for disease recurrence after surgery. Single-agent chemotherapy for gastric cancer has traditionally been of little value. Agents that have been identified as having some effect on gastric cancer are a combination of 5-fluorouracil and cisplatin (BC Cancer Agency, 2012). The combination of radiation therapy with chemotherapy involving 5-fluorouracil and leucovorin after surgical resection increases survival. Additional therapies, including intraperitoneal administration of chemotherapeutic agents, are undergoing evaluation. The role of biological therapy is still under investigation for use in gastric cancer. (These therapies are discussed in Chapter 18.)

NURSING MANAGEMENT
GASTRIC CANCER

NURSING ASSESSMENT

The assessment of a person with possible gastric cancer is similar to that done for PUD (see Table 44-25). Important information that should be obtained from the patient and the family include data from a nutritional assessment, a psychosocial history, the patient's perceptions of the health problem and the need for hospitalization, and the physical examination of the patient.

The nutritional assessment must elicit information regarding appetite and changes in eating patterns over the previous 6 months. It is necessary to determine the patient's normal weight and any changes that may have occurred in the preceding few months. Unexplained weight loss is common in many types of cancer before diagnosis. A history of vague symptoms of dyspepsia, early satiety, feeling full after consuming even a small amount of food, or symptoms of gas pain should help the nurse differentiate these typical gastric cancer symptoms from those of peptic ulcer. The nurse should determine whether pain is present, where and when it occurs, and how it is relieved. When the pain has been controlled with ingestion of foods, fluids, or antacids for a time but now continues or worsens regardless of interventions, gastric cancer may be the underlying cause.

Psychosocial and demographic data include the patient's age, present or previous occupation, and financial status. Gastric cancer can occur at any age, but the risk increases with age. The majority of new cases occur in people older than 65. A family history of cancer, especially gastric cancer, confers a greater than normal risk.

It is important to determine the patient's personal perception of the health problem and method of coping with hospitalization, diagnostic tests, and procedures. The possibility of a diagnosis of cancer and a treatment regimen that may include surgery, chemotherapy, or radiation treatment is predictive of a prolonged stressful period and a possibly fatal outcome. Therefore, it is important for the nurse to support the patient and the family if tests result in an unfavourable diagnosis and complex treatment interventions are planned. If surgery is probable, the nurse should assess what the patient expects from surgery (cure or palliation) and how that patient has responded to any previous surgical procedures.

A complete physical examination reveals the patient's current functional abilities, the presence of other health problems, and an estimate of how well the patient may respond to therapy. Cachexia may be evident if the nutritional state has been compromised for an extended time. A malnourished patient does not respond well to chemotherapy or radiation therapy and is a poor candidate for surgery.

NURSING DIAGNOSES

Nursing diagnoses for the patient with gastric cancer include, but are not limited to, the following:

- *Imbalanced nutrition: less than body requirements* related to *insufficient dietary intake* (inability to ingest, digest, or absorb nutrients)
- *Acute pain* related to *biological injury agent* (underlying disease process)
- *Anxiety* related to *threat to current status, threat of death*

PLANNING

The overall goals are that the patient with gastric cancer will (a) experience minimal discomfort, (b) achieve optimal nutritional status, and (c) maintain a degree of spiritual and psychological well-being appropriate to the disease stage.

NURSING IMPLEMENTATION

HEALTH PROMOTION. The nursing role in the early detection of cancer of the stomach is focused primarily on identification of the patient at risk because of specific disorders such as pernicious anemia and achlorhydria. The nurse should be aware of symptoms associated with gastric cancer, its pattern of spread, and the significant findings on physical examination. The nurse should understand that the cure rate is often quite dismal because symptoms do not arise until late in the course of the disease process, are vague, and often mimic other conditions, such as PUD.

The nurse must be alert to problems suggesting gastric cancer, such as poor appetite, weight loss, fatigue, and persistent gastric distress. If any of these manifestations are present, medical attention should be obtained and the necessary diagnostic tests performed.

In addition, any patient with a positive family history of gastric cancer should be encouraged to undergo diagnostic evaluation if manifestations of anemia, peptic ulcer, or vague epigastric distress are present. It is important that the nurse recognize the possibility of gastric cancer in a patient in whom 3 weeks of prescribed therapy for peptic ulcer fails to provide relief.

ACUTE INTERVENTION

Preoperative Care. When the diagnostic tests confirm the presence of a malignancy, patients and their families generally react with shock, disbelief, and depression, regardless of how thoroughly they may have been prepared for this possible outcome. Throughout this period, the nurse must give emotional and physical support, provide information, clarify test results, and maintain a positive attitude with respect to the patient's immediate recovery and long-term survival.

On admission to hospital, the patient may be in poor physical condition. Surgery may have to be delayed while the patient becomes more physically able to withstand the strain of a major operation. A positive nutritional state enhances wound healing, as well as the ability to withstand infection and other possible postoperative complications. Often, the patient is better able to tolerate several small meals a day than three regular meals. The diet may be supplemented by a variety of commercial liquid supplements (see Chapter 42) and vitamins. The nurse is challenged to find innovative ways of persuading the patient to eat when lack of appetite and state of mind make eating difficult and unrewarding. Enlisting the family's assistance with meals

and encouraging intake may be beneficial. If the patient is unable to ingest oral feedings, it may be necessary to provide for nutritional needs with tube feedings or parenteral nutrition.

If needed, blood replacement and fluid volume restoration may be carried out in the preoperative period. Because anemia is usually present, packed RBCs may be administered. Close observation for reactions to the transfusions is important. The hemoglobin and hematocrit levels provide information on the progress of therapy.

The preoperative teaching plan before gastric surgery for cancer is much the same as that for peptic ulcer surgery (see the previous "Collaborative Therapy: Surgical Therapy for Peptic Ulcer Disease" section under "Peptic Ulcer Disease").

Postoperative Care. Postoperative care of the patient with gastric cancer is similar to that after a Billroth I or II procedure (see the previous "Collaborative Therapy: Surgical Therapy for Peptic Ulcer Disease" section under "Peptic Ulcer Disease"). When the surgical intervention has involved a total gastrectomy, the plan of care is somewhat different. The operation performed usually requires resection of some of the lower esophagus along with the removal of the entire stomach and anastomosis of the esophagus to the jejunum. The chest cavity must be entered, and drainage is accomplished by the insertion of chest tubes. (Chest surgery and drainage tubes are discussed in Chapter 30.) After total gastrectomy, the NG tube does not drain a large quantity of secretions because removal of the stomach has eliminated the reservoir capacity. The NG tube is removed after several days, when intestinal peristalsis has resumed. Small amounts of clear fluid may then be started. The patient requires close observation for signs of leakage of the fluids at the anastomosis, as evidenced by an elevation in body temperature and increasing dyspnea. When fluids are well tolerated without distress, the amount may be increased and some solid foods added.

As a consequence of a total gastrectomy, patients experience the symptoms of dumping syndrome. Unfortunately, weight loss is very common among such patients, and poor nutritional intake often contributes. Postoperative wound healing may be impaired because of inadequate dietary intake. This necessitates parenteral or oral replacement of vitamins C, D, and K; the B-complex vitamins; and cobalamin. Because these vitamins (with the exception of cobalamin) are absorbed primarily in the upper part of the small intestine, they must be replaced because the duodenum has been bypassed in the surgical procedure.

Postoperative care after a Billroth I or II operative procedure should be the same as that after peptic ulcer surgery. Patients who have undergone these procedures are also subject to the same type of postgastrectomy complications such as dumping syndrome and postprandial hypoglycemia.

Patients with advanced malignant disease can be offered only palliative treatment. When chemotherapy is prescribed, the nurse must have current information regarding the action and adverse effects of the drugs. Patients should be made aware of the potential benefits and hazards that can result from the chemotherapy. Radiation therapy can be used as an adjuvant to surgery or for palliation. In general, patients are quite fearful of radiation therapy and may have many misconceptions regarding its value and dangers. To reassure the patient and ensure completion of the designated number of treatments, the nurse must provide detailed instruction. Because most therapy is completed on an outpatient basis, the nurse should assess each patient's knowledge of radiation therapy, care of the skin, the need for good nutrition and fluid intake during therapy, and the appropriate use of antiemetic drugs. (Specific care of patients receiving chemotherapy and radiation therapy is discussed in Chapter 18 and in NCP 18-1 and NCP 18-2, available on the Evolve website.)

AMBULATORY AND HOME CARE. Before the patient is discharged, the need for teaching should be reviewed. Most dietary measures useful after peptic ulcer surgery are applicable after surgery for gastric cancer. Plans should be made for the relief of pain, including comfort measures and the judicious use of analgesics. Wound care, if needed, must be taught to the primary caregiver in the home situation. Dressings, special equipment, or special services may be required for the patient's continued care at home. A list of community agencies that are available for assistance can be provided before the patient goes home. The services of the Canadian Cancer Society are especially helpful.

When chemotherapy or radiation therapy is to be continued after discharge, a referral for a home health nurse may be beneficial. The home health nurse can assist with recovery, determine the degree of patient adherence, and be a sympathetic health care provider with whom the patient can consult.

Long-term follow-up must be stressed. The patient must be encouraged to comply with the prescribed dietary and drug regimens, to keep appointments for chemotherapy administration or radiation treatments, and to keep the physician informed of changes in physical condition. (Long-term management of patients with cancer is discussed in Chapter 18.)

EVALUATION

Expected outcomes are the following for the patient with gastric cancer:

- The patient will experience no or minimal discomfort, pain, or nausea.
- The patient will achieve optimal nutritional status.
- The patient will maintain a degree of psychological well-being appropriate to the disease stage.

UPPER GASTRO-INTESTINAL BLEEDING

Upper GI bleeding represents a significant clinical and societal burden because of the associated morbidity, mortality, and financial implications. Despite advances in critical care, hemodynamic monitoring, and endoscopy, there has been little change in the mortality rate for upper GI bleeding, which has remained approximately 6% to 10% since the 1960s. This is partly because the incidence of upper GI bleeding is higher among older adults, men, and individuals in lower socioeconomic groups (Kurian & Lobo, 2015).

Etiology and Pathophysiology

Although the most serious loss of blood from the upper GI tract is characterized by a sudden onset, insidious occult bleeding can also be a major problem. The severity of bleeding depends on whether the origin is venous, capillary, or arterial. (Types of upper GI bleeding are listed in Table 44-16.) Bleeding from an arterial source is profuse, and the blood is bright red. The bright red colour indicates that the blood has not been in contact with the stomach's acid secretions. In contrast, "coffee grounds" vomitus reveals that the blood and other contents have been in the stomach for some time and have been changed by contact with gastric secretions. A massive upper GI hemorrhage is generally defined as a loss of more than 1 500 mL of blood or of 25% of intravascular blood volume. *Melena* (black, tarry stools) indicates slow bleeding from an upper GI source. The longer the passage of blood through

TABLE 44-16	TYPES OF UPPER GASTRO-INTESTINAL BLEEDING	
Type	**Clinical Manifestations**
Obvious bleeding	
• Hematemesis	Bloody vomitus appearing as fresh, bright red blood or "coffee grounds" appearance (dark, grainy digested blood)
• Melena	Black, tarry stools (often foul smelling) caused by digestion of blood in the gastro-intestinal tract; the discoloration is caused by the presence of iron
Occult bleeding	Small amounts of blood in gastric secretions, vomitus, or stools not apparent by appearance; detectable by guaiac test

TABLE 44-17	COMMON CAUSES OF UPPER GASTRO-INTESTINAL BLEEDING	
Drug-Induced	**Stomach and Duodenum**
• Corticosteroids	• Gastric cancer
• Nonsteroidal anti-inflammatory drugs	• Hemorrhagic gastritis
• Salicylates	• Peptic ulcer disease
	• Polyps
Esophagus	• Stress-related mucosal disease
• Esophageal varices	
• Esophagitis	**Systemic Diseases**
• Mallory–Weiss tear	• Blood dyscrasias (e.g., leukemia, aplastic anemia)
	• Liver failure (cirrhosis)
	• Renal failure (uremia)

the intestines, the darker the colour of the stool as a result of the degradation of hemoglobin and the release of iron.

Discovering the cause of the bleeding is not always an easy task. A variety of areas in the GI tract may be involved, and there may be many different reasons for the blood loss. Table 44-17 lists the common causes of bleeding. Although systemic diseases (e.g., leukemia, blood dyscrasias) that interfere with normal blood clotting must be considered whenever upper GI bleeding occurs, the most common sites are the esophagus, stomach, and duodenum.

Esophageal Origin. Bleeding from an esophageal source is probably the result of chronic esophagitis, a Mallory–Weiss tear, or esophageal varices. Chronic esophagitis can be caused by the ingestion of chemicals, including drugs irritating to the mucosa. Alcohol and smoking are known irritants of the esophageal mucosa. GERD with or without a hiatal hernia can lead to chronic irritation and erosion. A **Mallory–Weiss tear** is usually caused by severe retching and vomiting. This tear occurs in the esophageal mucosa at the junction of the esophagus and the stomach and results in severe bleeding.

Esophageal varices are usually secondary to cirrhosis of the liver. Anything that may increase the pressure (e.g., coughing, sneezing, trauma) or cause mechanical irritation (e.g., vomiting, irritation, erosion) may result in sudden, massive bleeding. (Esophageal varices are discussed in Chapter 46.)

Stomach and Duodenal Origin. Bleeding ulcers account for 36% of cases of upper GI bleeding (Mitra, Marrow, & Nayar, 2012). Erosion of a blood vessel by an ulcer located in the stomach

FIGURE 44-11 Multiple stress ulcers of the stomach, highlighted by dark digested blood on their surfaces. Source: Kumar, V., Abbas, A. K., & Fausto, N. (2005). *Robbins and Cotran pathologic basis of disease* (7th ed.). Philadelphia: Saunders.

or duodenum must always be considered as a possible cause of upper GI bleeding. A gastric ulcer may penetrate the left gastric artery, and a duodenal ulcer may penetrate the superior pancreatico-duodenal artery.

Acute gastritis produced by ingestion of drugs or alcohol or the reflux of bile from the small intestine can result in bleeding. Drugs, either prescribed by the health care provider or OTC, are a major cause of upper GI bleeding. For example, a patient who regularly takes ASA (Aspirin) or ASA-containing compounds may be at risk for bleeding episodes. ASA (Aspirin), NSAIDs (e.g., ibuprofen), and corticosteroids can cause irritation and disruption of the gastric mucosal barrier. ASA-containing products are sold without prescriptions as OTC drugs. A thorough history of all commonly used drugs is therefore necessary whenever upper GI bleeding is suspected.

Stress-related mucosal disease (SRMD), also called *physiological stress ulcers,* occurs in patients who have sustained severe burns or trauma or had major surgery. In SRMD, there is either diffuse superficial mucosal injury or discrete deeper ulcers in the fundus and body portions of the stomach (Figure 44-11). Patients with coagulopathy and those who experience respiratory failure that necessitates mechanical ventilation for more than 48 hours are at highest risk (Pilkington, Wagstaff, & Greenwood, 2012).

Emergency Assessment and Management

In approximately 80% to 85% of patients who have massive upper GI hemorrhage, the bleeding stops spontaneously; however, the cause must be identified and treatment initiated immediately. Although a complete history of events leading to the bleeding episode is important in discovering the cause of the blood loss, its documentation should be deferred until emergency care has been initiated. The immediate physical examination must include a systematic evaluation of the patient's condition with emphasis on blood pressure, rate and character of pulse, peripheral perfusion with capillary refill, and observation for the presence or absence of neck vein distension. Vital signs should be monitored every 15 to 30 minutes. Signs and symptoms of shock must be evaluated, and treatment should be started as soon as possible if it occurs (see Chapter 69). The patient's respiratory status is carefully assessed, along with a thorough abdominal examination. The presence or absence of bowel sounds should be assessed and noted. A tense, rigid, boardlike abdomen may indicate the presence of a perforation and peritonitis.

Once the immediate interventions have begun, the patient or the family should answer the following questions: Does the patient have a history of previous bleeding episodes? Has weight loss been a recent problem? Has the patient received blood transfusions in the past, and were there any transfusion reactions? Does the patient have a religious preference that prohibits the use of blood or blood products? Does the patient have any other illnesses that may contribute to bleeding or interfere with treatment (e.g., heart failure, diabetes mellitus)?

Laboratory studies are ordered, including a CBC; prothrombin time measurement; measurements of blood urea nitrogen (BUN), serum electrolytes, blood glucose, liver enzymes, and arterial blood gases; and a type and crossmatch for possible blood transfusions. Vomitus and stools can be tested for the presence of gross and occult blood. A urinalysis provides information on the presence of blood in the urine, and the specific gravity gives an immediate indication of the patient's hydration status.

Intravenous lines, preferably two, with a 16- or 18-gauge needle, should be established for fluid and blood replacement. The type and amount of fluids infused is dictated by physical and laboratory findings. It is generally best to begin with an isotonic crystalloid solution (e.g., lactated Ringer's solution). Whole blood, packed RBCs, and fresh-frozen plasma may be used to replace lost volume in massive hemorrhage. Because of the potential for fluid overload and immunological reactions, packed RBCs are often preferred over whole blood. (The use of blood transfusions is discussed in Chapter 33.) The hemoglobin and hematocrit values are not of immediate assistance in estimating the degree of blood loss, but they provide a baseline for guiding further treatment. The initial hematocrit may be normal and may not reflect the loss until 4 to 6 hours after fluid replacement has taken place because initially the loss of plasma and RBCs is equal. When upper GI bleeding is less profuse, infusion of isotonic saline solution followed by packed RBCs helps restore the hematocrit more quickly and does not create complications related to fluid volume overload. The use of supplemental oxygen may help increase blood oxygen saturation.

For most patients with profuse bleeding, an indwelling urinary catheter is inserted so that urine volume can be accurately assessed every hour. A central venous pressure line may be inserted so that the patient's fluid volume status can be monitored easily. Empirical PPI therapy with high-dose bolus and subsequent infusion is often started before endoscopy.

Diagnostic Studies

Endoscopic procedures allow physicians to identify sources of GI bleeding through direct visualization. For example, the site of bleeding from severe gastritis, an esophageal varix, a gastric or duodenal ulcer, or angiodysplasia can be determined easily and treated effectively. The endoscope is designed to facilitate the passing of various instruments, sclerosing drugs, and probes to control and stop GI bleeding. In addition to using endoscopic procedures to stop bleeding, these procedures also allow direct visualization of the bleeding site. Angiography is used in diagnosing upper GI bleeding only when endoscopy cannot be done. It is an invasive procedure for which preparation and setup time are required, and it may not be appropriate for a patient at high risk for complications whose condition is unstable. In this procedure, a catheter is placed into the left gastric or superior mesenteric artery and advanced until the site of bleeding is discovered.

TABLE 44-18   DRUG THERAPY

Gastro-Intestinal Bleeding

Drug	Source of Gastro-Intestinal Bleeding	Mechanism of Action
Antacids*	Duodenal ulcer, gastric ulcer, acute gastritis (corrosive, erosive, and hemorrhagic)	Neutralize acid and maintain gastric pH >5.5; elevated pH inhibits activation of pepsinogen
H_2-receptor blockers: cimetidine, famotidine (Pepcid), nizatidine (Axid), ranitidine (Zantac)	Duodenal ulcer, gastric ulcer, esophagitis, acute gastritis (especially hemorrhagic)	Inhibit action of histamine at H_2 receptors on parietal cells and decrease HCl secretion
Proton pump inhibitors: omeprazole (Losec), esomeprazole (Nexium), lansoprazole (Prevacid), pantoprazole (Pantoloc)	—	Inhibit the cellular pump, which is necessary for secretion of HCl
Vasopressin	Acute gastritis (corrosive, erosive, and hemorrhagic), esophageal varices	Causes vasoconstriction and increases smooth muscle activity of the GI tract; reduces pressure in the portal circulation and arrests bleeding
Octreotide (Sandostatin)	Upper gastro-intestinal bleeding, esophageal varices	Somatostatin analogue that decreases splanchnic blood flow; decreases HCl secretion via decrease in release of gastrin

*See Table 44-23.
GI, gastro-intestinal; *HCl,* hydrochloric acid.

Collaborative Care

Endoscopic Therapy. Endoscopic hemostasis is used to identify and stop bleeding. Endoscopy performed within the first 24 hours of bleeding is important for diagnosis and determining the need for surgical or radiologic intervention.

The goal of endoscopic hemostasis is coagulation or thrombosis in the bleeding vessel. Several techniques are used, including (a) thermal (heat) probe, (b) multipolar and bipolar electrocoagulation probe, (c) argon plasma coagulation (APC), and (d) neodymium:yttrium–aluminum–garnet (Nd:YAG) laser. Multipolar electrocoagulation and thermal probe are the two most commonly used procedures. The heat probe causes tissue coagulation by directly applying a heating element to the bleeding site. Argon plasma coagulation is a noncontact method in which monopolar current is delivered to tissue. For variceal bleeding, other strategies include variceal ligation, injection sclerotherapy, and balloon tamponade.

Surgical Therapy. Surgical intervention is indicated when bleeding continues despite the therapy provided and when the site of the bleeding has been identified. The site of the hemorrhage determines the choice of operation. In addition, the surgeon must consider the age of the patient because mortality rates are considerably higher among patients older than 60 years.

Drug Therapy. During the acute phase, drugs are used to decrease bleeding, decrease HCl secretion, and neutralize the HCl that is present. Drug therapy to decrease bleeding is administered during endoscopy. Injection therapy with epinephrine (1 : 10 000 dilution) is effective for acute hemostasis. These agents produce tissue edema and, ultimately, pressure on the source of bleeding. To prevent rebleeding, injection therapy is often combined with other therapies (e.g., thermocoagulation or laser treatment). A sclerosant (an agent that produces inflammation and results in fibrosis of the tissues) such as ethanolamine may be used, especially if the cause of bleeding is esophageal varices.

Antidiuretic hormone, a chemical released from the posterior pituitary, can be used for the management of variceal bleeding because it promotes vasoconstriction. It is used to treat upper GI bleeding in patients who do not respond to other therapies and are poor candidates for surgery. It is administered systemically through a vein or intra-arterially at the local site of actual bleeding.

Adverse effects of intravenously administered vasopressin include decreased myocardial contractility and decreased coronary blood flow. The patient undergoing vasopressin therapy must be closely monitored for its myocardial, visceral, and peripheral ischemic adverse effects. Vasopressin should be used with caution in patients with a known history of vascular disease.

Efforts are made to reduce acid secretion because the acidic environment can alter platelet function and interfere with clot stabilization. H_2R blockers (e.g., ranitidine [Zantac]) or PPIs (e.g., pantoprazole [Pantoloc]) are administered intravenously to decrease acid secretion. Table 44-18 reviews the mechanism of action of H_2R blockers and PPIs. Although these drugs have no proven ability to control active bleeding, they have become part of standard treatment protocols.

In patients with upper GI bleeding, early administration of the somatostatin analogue octreotide (Sandostatin) may be used. The drug reduces splanchnic blood flow, as well as acid secretion. This drug is given in IV boluses up to 5 to 6 days after the onset of bleeding.

Antacids have long been known to neutralize HCl and continue to be used as an adjunct therapy for PUD. Because antacids neutralize HCl and increase the pH of gastric contents to above 5, the conversion of pepsinogen to its active form, pepsin, is inhibited. The most frequently used antacid preparations are magnesium hydroxide, magnesium trisilicate, aluminum hydroxide, calcium carbonate, and sodium bicarbonate (see Table 44-23 later in this chapter). Aluminum hydroxide and magnesium trisilicate are the most useful because they are nonabsorbable. Calcium carbonate and sodium bicarbonate are absorbable, and prolonged use can lead to systemic alkalosis.

Sedatives to control agitation and restlessness should be administered cautiously. They make accurate assessment of the patient's condition more difficult. Anticholinergic drugs are contraindicated for use in acute upper GI bleeding episodes.

NURSING MANAGEMENT
UPPER GASTRO-INTESTINAL BLEEDING

NURSING ASSESSMENT

As the nurse begins care of a patient admitted with upper GI bleeding, a thorough and accurate nursing assessment is an

TABLE 44-19 NURSING ASSESSMENT

Upper Gastro-Intestinal Bleeding

Subjective Data
Important Health Information
Past health history: Precipitating events before bleeding episode, previous bleeding episodes and treatment, peptic ulcer disease, esophageal varices, esophagitis, acute and chronic gastritis, stress-related mucosal disease; family history of bleeding; history of smoking or heavy alcohol use
Medications: Use of ASA (Aspirin), nonsteroidal anti-inflammatory drugs, corticosteroids, anticoagulants

Symptoms
- Nausea, vomiting, weight loss; thirst
- Diarrhea; black, tarry stools; decreased urinary output; sweating
- Weakness, dizziness, fainting
- Epigastric pain, abdominal cramps

Objective Data
General
Fever

Integumentary
Clammy, cool, pale skin; pale mucous membranes, nail beds, and conjunctivae; spider angiomas; jaundice; peripheral edema

Respiratory
Rapid, shallow respirations

Cardiovascular
Tachycardia, weak pulse, orthostatic hypotension, slow capillary refill

Gastro-intestinal
Red or "coffee grounds" vomitus; tense, rigid abdomen, ascites; hypoactive or hyperactive bowel sounds; black, tarry stools

Urinary
Decreased urinary output, concentrated urine

Neurological
Agitation, restlessness; decreasing level of consciousness

Possible Findings
↓ Hematocrit and hemoglobin; hematuria; guaiac-positive stools, emesis, or gastric aspirate; ↓ levels of clotting factors; ↑ liver enzymes; abnormal results of upper GI studies or endoscopy

ASA, acetylsalicylic acid; *GI,* gastro-intestinal.

essential first step. Subjective and objective data that should be obtained from the patient or significant others are listed in Table 44-19.

The patient experiencing upper GI bleeding may not be able to provide specific information about the cause of the bleeding until the immediate physical needs are met. An immediate nursing assessment is performed while the patient is being prepared for initial treatment. The assessment includes the patient's level of consciousness, vital signs, appearance of neck veins and skin colour, and capillary refill. The abdomen is checked for distension, guarding, and peristalsis. Immediate determination of vital signs indicates whether the patient is in shock from blood loss and also provides a baseline blood pressure and pulse by which to monitor the progress of treatment. Signs and symptoms of hypovolemic shock include low blood pressure; rapid, weak pulse; increased thirst; cold, clammy skin; and restlessness. Vital signs

are monitored every 15 to 30 minutes, and the health care provider should be informed of any significant changes.

NURSING DIAGNOSES

Nursing diagnoses for the patient with upper GI bleeding include, but are not limited to, the following:

- *Risk for decreased cardiac output* (related to loss of blood)
- *Deficient fluid volume* related to *insufficient fluid intake, excessive fluid loss through abnormal route* (acute loss of blood and gastric secretions)
- *Ineffective peripheral tissue perfusion* related to *insufficient knowledge of modifiable factors* (loss of circulatory volume)
- *Anxiety* related to *threat to current status, threat of death*

PLANNING

The overall goals are that the patient with upper GI bleeding will (a) have no further GI bleeding, (b) have the cause of the bleeding identified and treated, (c) experience a return to a normal hemodynamic state, (d) experience minimal or no symptoms of pain or anxiety, and (e) be able to verbalize causative and preventive measures.

NURSING IMPLEMENTATION

HEALTH PROMOTION. Although not all cases of upper GI bleeding can be anticipated and prevented, the nurse shares responsibility with the health care provider in trying to identify the patient who is at high risk. Patients with a history of chronic gastritis or PUD should always be considered in the high-risk category because of the increased incidence of bleeding associated with chronic irritation or chronic ulcers. Patients who have had one major bleeding episode are more likely than others to have another. Patients are instructed to avoid gastric irritants such as alcohol and smoking, to prevent or decrease stress-inducing situations at home or at work, and to take only prescribed medications. OTC drugs can be harmful because they may contain ingredients (e.g., ASA [Aspirin]) that have potentially irritating effects on the mucosa.

Patients who require regular administration of ulcerogenic drugs, such as ASA (Aspirin), corticosteroids, or NSAIDs, need instruction regarding the potential adverse effects that these drugs may have on the GI mucosa. These drugs are avoided if at all possible. However, if ASA (Aspirin) must be prescribed, enteric-coated tablets can be substituted for regular tablets. Taking the drugs with meals or snacks lessens the potential irritating effects. For patients who must take NSAIDs, a change to a preparation with less GI toxicity may be considered. COX-2 inhibitors (e.g., celecoxib [Celebrex]) have less of an effect on the production of tissue prostaglandins and are associated with fewer GI adverse effects, although cardiac risks are associated with COX-2 inhibitors. The coadministration of an NSAID with a PPI can reduce bleeding risk. For the patient at risk for gastric ulcers because of NSAID use, misoprostol may also be prescribed. This prostaglandin analogue inhibits acid secretion and reduces the incidence of upper GI bleeding episodes associated with NSAID use. However, the drug has several important adverse effects, including uterine cramping in women and diarrhea. Because of its effects on the uterus, its use is contraindicated in women of child-bearing age.

When the nurse is working with a patient who has a history of liver cirrhosis with esophageal varices, the instructions must be specific about the importance of avoiding known irritants, such as alcohol and smoking. The prompt treatment of an upper respiratory tract infection should be stressed. Severe coughing or sneezing can create increased pressure on the already fragile varices and may result in massive hemorrhage.

Patients who are known to have blood dyscrasias (e.g., aplastic anemia) or liver dysfunction or who are taking cancer chemotherapeutic drugs have a potential for a bleeding problem because of altered hemostasis caused by a decrease in clotting factors and platelets. When such patients also have a history of ulcer disease, gastritis, varices, or drug and alcohol abuse, they should be carefully instructed regarding their disease process and drugs, and they should be closely observed for bleeding.

ACUTE INTERVENTION. Patients should be approached in a calm and assured manner to help decrease their level of anxiety. Caution should be used before sedatives are administered for restlessness because it is one of the warning signs of shock and may be masked by the drugs.

Once an infusion has been started, the IV line must be maintained for fluid or blood replacement. An accurate intake and output record is essential so that the patient's hydration status can be assessed. Urine output should be measured hourly. A rate of at least 0.5 mL/kg/hr indicates adequate renal perfusion. Lesser amounts may indicate renal insufficiency secondary to loss of blood volume. Specific gravity readings consistently greater than 1.030 (normal is 1.005–1.030) indicate that the urine is extremely concentrated and that the blood volume is probably low. The health care provider must be kept informed of these important parameters so that the IV solutions can be increased or decreased accordingly. If a patient has a central venous pressure line in place, readings should be recorded every 1 to 2 hours. Hemodynamic monitoring provides an accurate and quick assessment of blood flow and pressure within the cardiovascular system (see Chapter 68).

Older adult patients and patients with a history of cardiovascular problems should be observed closely for signs of fluid overload. However, the threat of volume overload and pulmonary edema must be a constant concern in all patients who are receiving large amounts of IV fluids within a short time. Therefore, auscultation of breath sounds and close observation of respiratory effort are important. Electrocardiographic monitoring can also be used to evaluate cardiac function.

Foods such as beets or even swallowed mouthwash can give vomitus a bloody appearance. Unless the contents of the vomitus are checked for occult blood, recorded observations gleaned from appearance alone may be false. Swallowed blood from a nosebleed must also be accurately noted to avoid misdiagnosis of an upper GI bleeding episode. When an NG tube is inserted, the nurse must pay special attention to keeping it in proper position and observing the aspirate for blood.

The nurse caring for a patient with upper GI bleeding should be well informed as to what constitutes blood in the stools. Black, tarry stools are not usually associated with a brisk hemorrhage but are indicative of the presence of bleeding of prolonged duration. Bright red blood in the stool is usually from a source in the lower bowel. (Lower GI bleeding is discussed in Chapter 45.) Menses and bleeding hemorrhoids should be ruled out as possible sources of blood in the stools. When vomitus contains blood but the stool contains no gross or occult blood, the hemorrhage is considered to have been of short duration.

By monitoring results of the patient's laboratory studies, the nurse can estimate the effectiveness of therapy. The hemoglobin and hematocrit are usually evaluated about every 4 to 6 hours if the patient is actively bleeding. At first, the hematocrit level may not accurately reflect the amount of blood lost or the amount of blood replaced and will appear falsely high or low. The patient's BUN level is assessed. It is generally elevated with a significant hemorrhage because blood proteins are broken down by bacteria in the GI tract. However, renal disease may also result in an elevated BUN level. Many patients receive oxygen by mask or nasally to ensure that the circulating blood has an adequate oxygen content.

When oral nourishment is begun, the patient is observed for symptoms of nausea and vomiting and a recurrence of bleeding. Feedings initially consisting of clear fluids are given hourly until tolerance is determined. These feedings help neutralize the gastric secretions and assist in the mucosal repair. Foods are then introduced gradually if the patient exhibits no signs of discomfort. Consultation with a dietitian ensures the introduction of appropriate foods and support for the patient's nutrition.

The patient in whom hemorrhage was the result of chronic alcohol abuse requires close observation for the beginning of delirium tremens as withdrawal from alcohol takes place. Symptoms indicating the beginning of delirium tremens are agitation, uncontrolled shaking, sweating, and vivid hallucinations. (Alcohol withdrawal is discussed in Chapter 11.)

AMBULATORY AND HOME CARE. Patients and caregivers must be taught how to avoid future bleeding episodes. Ulcer disease, drug or alcohol abuse, and liver and respiratory diseases can all result in upper GI bleeding. Patients and caregivers must be made aware of the consequences of nonadherence to diet and drug therapy. It must be emphasized that no drugs (especially ASA [Aspirin] and NSAIDs) other than those prescribed by the health care provider should be taken. With the assistance of programs for smoking or alcohol cessation or rehabilitation, smoking and alcohol should be eliminated because they are sources of irritation and interfere with tissue repair. The need for long-term follow-up care may be necessary because of the possibility of another bleeding episode. The patient and the family should be instructed on what to do if an acute hemorrhage occurs in the future.

❚ EVALUATION

The following are expected outcomes for the patient with upper GI bleeding:

- The patient will have no upper GI bleeding.
- The patient will maintain normal fluid volume.
- The patient will experience a return to a normal hemodynamic state.
- The patient will experience absence of or tolerable levels of pain and will be comfortable.
- The patient will understand potential etiological factors and make appropriate lifestyle modifications.

PEPTIC ULCER DISEASE

Peptic ulcer disease (PUD) is a condition characterized by erosion of the GI mucosa that results from the digestive action of HCl and pepsin. Any portion of the GI tract that comes into contact with gastric secretions is susceptible to ulcer development, including the lower esophagus, stomach, duodenum, and margin of gastro-jejunal anastomosis after surgical procedures.

Types

Peptic ulcers can be classified as acute or chronic, depending on the degree and duration of mucosal involvement

(Figure 44-12), and as gastric or duodenal, according to the location. Acute ulcers (see Figure 44-12) are characterized by superficial erosion and minimal inflammation. They are of short duration and resolve quickly when the cause is identified and removed. Chronic ulcers (Figure 44-13) are of long duration, eroding through the muscular wall with the formation of fibrous tissue. They are present continuously for many months or intermittently throughout the lifetime. Chronic ulcers are at least four times as common as acute ulcers.

Gastric and duodenal ulcers, although defined as peptic ulcers, have different causes and incidences (Table 44-20). In general, treatment is similar for all types of ulcers.

Etiology and Pathophysiology

Peptic ulcers develop only in the presence of an acidic environment. In typical cases, a person with a gastric ulcer has normal to less-than-normal gastric acidity in comparison with the person with a duodenal ulcer. However, some intraluminal acid does seem to be essential for a gastric ulcer to occur.

Pepsinogen, the precursor of pepsin, is activated to pepsin in the presence of HCl and a pH of 2 to 3. The HCl secreted by the parietal cells has a pH of 0.8. After HCl mixes with the stomach contents, the pH reaches 2 to 3, a range of acidity highly favourable for pepsin activity. When the stomach acid level is neutralized by the presence of food or antacids, or acid secretion is blocked by drugs, the pH is increased to 3.5 or more. At a pH of 3.5 or more, pepsin has little or no proteolytic activity.

The stomach is normally protected from autodigestion by the gastric mucosal barrier. The GI tract has a high rate of cell turnover, and the surface mucosa of the stomach is renewed

FIGURE 44-12 Peptic ulcers, including an erosion, an acute ulcer, and a chronic ulcer. Both the acute and the chronic ulcers may penetrate the entire wall of the stomach. Source: Modified from Price, S. A., & Wilson, L. M. (2003). *Pathophysiology: Clinical concepts of disease processes* (6th ed., p. 331). St. Louis: Mosby.

FIGURE 44-13 Peptic ulcer of the duodenum. Source: Kumar, V., Abbas, A. K., Fausto, N., et al. (2010). *Robbins and Cotran pathologic basis of disease* (8th ed.). Philadelphia: Saunders.

TABLE 44-20	COMPARISON OF GASTRIC AND DUODENAL ULCERS	
Characteristic	**Gastric Ulcers**	**Duodenal Ulcers**
Lesion	Superficial; smooth margins; round, oval, or cone shaped	Penetrating (associated with deformity of duodenal bulb from healing of recurrent ulcers)
Location of lesion	Predominantly in the antrum; also in body and fundus of stomach	First 1–2 cm of duodenum
Gastric secretion	Normal to decreased	Increased
Incidence	• Greater in women	• Greater in men, but increasing in women, especially postmenopausal
	• Peak age, 50–60 yr	• Peak age, 35–45 yr
	• Increased with smoking, drug, and alcohol use	• Increased with smoking, drug, and alcohol use
	• More common among persons of lower socioeconomic status and in unskilled labourers	• Associated with psychological stress
	• Increased with incompetent pyloric sphincter and bile reflux	• Associated with other diseases (e.g., chronic obstructive pulmonary disease, pancreatic disease, hyperparathyroidism, Zollinger–Ellison syndrome, chronic renal failure)
	• Increased with stress ulcers after severe burns, head trauma, and major surgery	
Clinical manifestations	• Burning or gaseous pressure in high left epigastrium and back and upper abdomen	• Pain 2–4 hr after meals and midmorning, midafternoon, middle of night; pain is periodic and episodic
	• Burning, cramping, pressure-like pain across midepigastrium and upper abdomen; back pain with posterior ulcers	• Pain relief with antacids and food; occasional nausea and vomiting
	• Pain 1–2 hr after meals; if penetrating ulcer, aggravation of discomfort with food	
	• Occasional nausea and vomiting, weight loss	
Recurrence rate	High	High
Complications	Hemorrhage, perforation, outlet obstruction, intractability	Hemorrhage, perforation, obstruction

PATHOPHYSIOLOGY MAP

FIGURE 44-14 Disruption of gastric mucosa and pathophysiological consequences of backwards diffusion of acids. *ASA,* acetylsalicylic acid; *NSAIDs,* nonsteroidal anti-inflammatory drugs.

PATHOPHYSIOLOGY MAP

FIGURE 44-15 Relationship between mucosal blood flow and disruption of the gastric mucosal barrier.

about every 3 days. As a result of this high turnover rate, the mucosa can continually repair itself except in extreme instances, when the cell breakdown rate surpasses the cell renewal rate. Normally, water, electrolytes, and water-soluble substances (e.g., glucose) can easily pass through the barrier. However, the mucosal barrier prevents the backwards diffusion of acid from the gastric lumen through the mucosal layers to the underlying tissue.

Under specific circumstances, the mucosal barrier can be impaired, and backwards diffusion of acid can occur (Figure 44-14). When the barrier is broken, HCl freely enters the mucosa and injury to the tissues occurs. This results in cellular destruction and inflammation. Histamine is released from the damaged mucosa, resulting in vasodilation and increased capillary permeability. The released histamine is then capable of stimulating further secretion of acid and pepsin.

As described in the "Gastritis" section, a variety of agents are known to destroy the mucosal barrier. By generating ammonia in the mucous layer, *H. pylori* may create a condition of chronic inflammation, rendering the mucosa especially vulnerable to other noxious substances. Ulcerogenic drugs, such as ASA (Aspirin) and NSAIDs, inhibit synthesis of prostaglandins and cause abnormal permeability of the mucosal barrier. Corticosteroids have the ability to decrease the rate of mucosal cell renewal and thereby decrease its protective effects. Lipid-soluble cytotoxic drugs can pass through the barrier and destroy it.

When the mucosal barrier is disrupted, there is a compensatory increase in blood flow (Figure 44-15). This phenomenon can occur in several ways. Prostaglandin-like substances and histamine act as vasodilators, thus increasing capillary blood flow. As blood flow increases within the affected mucosa, H$^+$ are rapidly removed

from the area, buffers are delivered to help neutralize the H$^+$ present, nutrients necessary for cell function arrive, and the rate of mucosal cell replication increases. When the increase is sufficient to dilute, buffer, and remove the excess H$^+$, tissue damage may be minimal or not occur at all. When blood flow is not sufficient to carry out these events, tissue injury results. Figure 44-15 shows a representation of the interrelationship between the mucosal blood flow and disruption of the gastric mucosal barrier.

Two mechanisms protect against damage. First, mucus is secreted by superficial mucous cells and forms a layer that can entrap or slow the diffusion of H$^+$ across the mucosal barrier in the stomach. Second, bicarbonate is secreted by the gastric and duodenal mucosa, and this helps neutralize HCl in the lumen of the GI tract.

Increased vagal nerve stimulation from a variety of causes (e.g., emotions) results in hypersecretion of HCl. Increased concentrations of HCl can alter the mucosal barrier. Duodenal ulcers are associated with high acid content. It has been suggested that the continual response of the parietal cells to maximal stimulation results in hyperplasia of the cells.

Gastric Ulcers. Although gastric ulcers can occur in any portion of the stomach, they are most commonly found on the lesser curvature close to the antral junction. Gastric ulcers are less common than duodenal ulcers. Gastric ulcers are more prevalent among women and in older adults. The rate of mortality from gastric ulcers is greater than that from duodenal ulcers because the incidence of gastric ulcers peaks in persons older than 50 years. Persons from the lower socioeconomic class and manual or unskilled workers are more prone to gastric ulcers.

Although gastric ulcers are characterized by normal to low secretion of gastric acid, the backwards diffusion of acid is greater with chronic gastric ulcers than with duodenal ulcers or in the healthy person. Therefore, the critical pathological process in gastric ulcer formation may not be the amount of acid that is secreted but the amount that is able to penetrate the mucosal barrier.

Gastric ulcers have also been attributed to various factors that can lead to acute episodes or to chronic involvement. The role of *H. pylori* in ulcer development is discussed in the following "Duodenal Ulcers" section. It is thought that destruction of the gastric mucosa by noxious agents such as drugs or smoking may be enhanced by the presence of *H. pylori,* which further promotes gastric mucosal destruction.

Drugs can cause acute gastric ulcers and, in some cases, can lead to the development of chronic ulcers. The drugs most often implicated include ASA (Aspirin), corticosteroids, NSAIDs (e.g., ibuprofen), and reserpine (Serpasil) (not commercially available in Canada). It is estimated that 1% to 3% of patients taking NSAIDs for 1 year experience serious GI complications, including gastritis, gastric ulcer, upper GI hemorrhage, or ulcer perforation. Other known causes of gastric ulcer formation are chronic alcohol abuse, chronic gastritis, and bile reflux gastritis that results from an incompetent pyloric sphincter. Cigarette smoking is positively linked with gastric ulcers. Nicotine seems to enhance reflux of duodenal contents into the antrum of the stomach. The ingestion of hot, rough, or spicy foods has been suggested as a cause, but there is no evidence to substantiate this claim.

Duodenal Ulcers. Duodenal ulcers account for about 80% of all peptic ulcers. Although duodenal ulcers still affect more men than women, the incidence of duodenal ulcers has followed a downward trend among men and steadily increased among women. The explanation for this change has not been clearly identified. Duodenal ulcers may occur at any age, but the incidence is especially high between the ages of 35 and 45 years. Duodenal ulcers can develop in anyone, regardless of occupation or socioeconomic group.

The development of duodenal ulcers is associated with high HCl secretion. Several diseases have been identified with a high risk of duodenal ulcer development, including chronic obstructive pulmonary disease, cirrhosis of the liver, chronic pancreatitis, hyperparathyroidism, chronic renal failure, and Zollinger–Ellison syndrome. (*Zollinger–Ellison syndrome* is a rare condition characterized by severe peptic ulceration, gastric acid hypersecretion, elevated serum gastrin levels, and gastrinoma of the pancreas or the duodenum.) The treatments used for these conditions may also promote ulcer development. Alcohol ingestion and heavy smoking habits are also associated with duodenal ulcer formation, inasmuch as both are known stimulants of acid secretion.

Although many factors are thought to contribute to the formation of duodenal ulcers, *H. pylori* has been identified as playing a key role. *H. pylori* is found in approximately 90% to 95% of patients with duodenal ulcers. However, a clear-cut direct causal relationship between *H. pylori* and duodenal ulcer formation has not yet been proved. Not all individuals with evidence of *H. pylori* go on to develop ulcers, which suggests that additional factors are needed to produce these conditions. *H. pylori* survives in the human upper GI tract for a long time because of its ability to move in mucus and attach to mucosal cells. In addition, it secretes a substance called *urease,* which buffers the area around the bacterium and protects it from destruction in an acidic environment.

Infection with *H. pylori* is most common in underdeveloped countries and among persons of low socioeconomic status. Although the routes of transmission are largely unknown, it is thought that infection occurs during childhood via transmission from family members to the child, possibly through a fecal–oral route, an oral–oral route, or both. In Canada and the United States, persons born before 1940 have a significantly higher risk of carrying *H. pylori* than do younger persons. This enhanced prevalence in older persons has been attributed to the presence of crowded living conditions and poor sanitation practices, which were more common in the first half of the twentieth century.

Research into a genetic cause for ulcers has shown that some members of the same family are more prone than others to develop gastric or duodenal ulcers. Supporting a genetic etiology is the fact that persons with blood group O have an increased incidence of duodenal ulcers. Evidence is not complete, however, and the ulcer development could just as well be the result of sharing the same environment.

Stress-Related Mucosal Disease. *Stress-related mucosal disease* (SRMD) is a condition of acute ulcers that develop after a major physiological insult such as trauma or surgery. A physiological stress ulcer is a form of erosive gastritis. It is believed that the gastric mucosa of the body of the stomach undergoes a period of transient ischemia in association with hypotension, severe injury, extensive burns, and complicated surgery. The ischemia is caused by decreased capillary blood flow or shunting of blood away from the GI tract so that blood flow bypasses the gastric mucosa. This occurs as a compensatory mechanism in hypotension or shock. The decrease in blood flow produces an imbalance between the destructive properties of HCl and pepsin and the protective factors of the stomach's mucosal barrier, especially in the fundic portion, and this imbalance results in ulceration. Multiple superficial erosions result, and these may bleed. Risk factors for development of stress ulcer bleeding are respiratory failure and coagulopathy. Patients with those conditions should receive prophylaxis with antisecretory agents. Stress gastritis is diagnosed with endoscopy, and treatment is with aggressive reduction of gastric acid secretions by means of H_2R blockers or PPIs.

Clinical Manifestations

It is common for patients with gastric or duodenal ulcers to have no pain or other symptoms. The gastric and duodenal mucosae are not rich in sensory pain fibres, which may account for this phenomenon. When pain does occur with duodenal ulcer, it is described as "burning" or "cramplike," and it is most often located in the midepigastric region beneath the xiphoid process. In contrast, the pain associated with gastric ulcers is located high in the epigastrium; it occurs spontaneously about 1 to 2 hours after meals and is described as "burning" or "gaseous." The pain can occur when the stomach is empty or when food has been ingested. If the ulcer has eroded through the gastric mucosa, food tends to aggravate rather than alleviate the pain. Some persons do not experience any pain until the presence of the ulcer is demonstrated through a serious complication such as hemorrhage or perforation.

Ulcers located on the posterior aspect of the duodenum can be manifested by back pain. The pain usually occurs 2 to 4 hours after meals. It is relieved by antacids alone or in combination with an H_2R blocker or PPI and sometimes by foods that neutralize and dilute the HCl. A characteristic of duodenal ulcer is its tendency to occur continuously for a few weeks or months and then disappear for a time, only to recur some months later.

Complications

The three major complications of chronic PUD are hemorrhage, perforation, and gastric outlet obstruction. All are considered emergency situations and are initially treated conservatively.

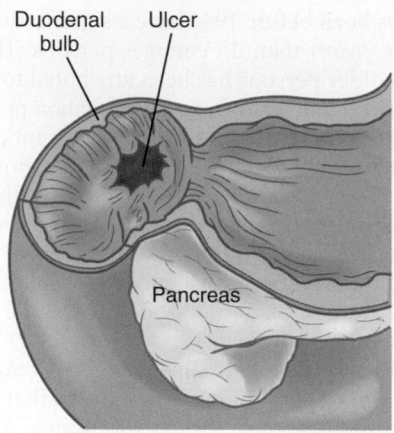

Duodenal bulb   Ulcer   Pancreas

FIGURE 44-16 Duodenal ulcer of the posterior wall penetrating into the head of the pancreas, resulting in walled-off perforation.

However, surgery may become necessary at any time during the course of the therapy.

Hemorrhage. Hemorrhage is the most common complication of PUD. It develops as a result of erosion of the granulation tissue at the base of the ulcer during healing or erosion of the ulcer through a major blood vessel. Duodenal ulcers account for a greater percentage of upper GI bleeding episodes than do gastric ulcers.

Perforation. Perforation of an ulcer is considered the most lethal complication of peptic ulcer. Perforation is common in large penetrating duodenal ulcers that have not healed and are located on the posterior mucosal wall (Figure 44-16). Perforated gastric ulcers are most often located on the lesser curvature of the stomach. Even though duodenal ulcers are more prevalent and perforate more frequently, mortality rates associated with perforation of gastric ulcers are higher.

Perforation of a peptic ulcer occurs when the ulcer penetrates the serosal surface, with spillage of either gastric or duodenal contents into the peritoneal cavity. The size of the perforation is directly proportional to the length of time the patient has had the ulcer: the larger the perforation, the longer the history of the ulcer. Small perforations seal themselves and result in a cessation of symptoms; larger perforations necessitate immediate surgical closure. Spontaneous sealing occurs as a result of large amounts of fibrin being produced in response to the perforation. This leads to fibrinous fusion of the duodenum or the gastric curvature to adjacent tissue, mainly the liver.

The clinical manifestations of perforation are characterized by their sudden and dramatic onset. The patient experiences sudden, severe upper abdominal pain that quickly spreads throughout the abdomen. The visceral and parietal layers of the peritoneum have an abundance of pain receptors, and this contributes to the abruptness and intensity of the pain experienced. There may be shoulder pain if the spillage causes irritation to the phrenic nerve. The abdominal muscles contract, appearing rigid and boardlike as they attempt to protect the abdomen from further injury. The patient's respirations become shallow and rapid. Bowel sounds are usually absent. Nausea and vomiting may occur but are generally absent. Many affected patients report a history of ulcer disease or recent symptoms of indigestion.

The contents entering the peritoneal cavity from the stomach or the duodenum contain a variety of ingredients that include air, saliva, food particles, HCl, pepsin, bacteria, bile, and pancreatic fluid and enzymes. Bacterial peritonitis may occur within 6 to 12 hours. The intensity of the peritonitis is proportional to the amount and the duration of the spillage through the perforation. It is difficult to determine from the sudden onset of symptoms whether gastric or duodenal ulcer is the cause because the clinical characteristics of intestinal perforation are the same (see Chapter 45).

Gastric Outlet Obstruction. Ulcers located in the antrum and the prepyloric and pyloric areas of the stomach and the duodenum can predispose to gastric outlet obstruction. In the early phase of obstruction (often referred to as the *compensated phase*), gastric emptying is normal to near normal. Over time, the increase in contractile force needed to empty the stomach results in hypertrophy of the stomach wall. After longstanding obstruction, the stomach enters the decompensated phase, which results in dilation and atony. The obstruction is not totally the result of fibrous scar tissue because active ulcer formation is associated with edema, inflammation, and pylorospasm, all of which contribute to the narrowing of the pylorus.

Patients with gastric outlet obstruction generally have a long history of ulcer pain. Ulcer-like pain of short duration or complete absence of pain is more indicative of a malignant obstruction. The pain progresses to a more generalized upper abdominal discomfort that becomes worse toward the end of the day as the stomach fills and dilates. Relief may be obtained by belching or by self-induced vomiting. Involuntary vomiting is common and often projectile. The vomitus contains food particles that were ingested many hours or even a day or two before the vomiting episode. There is often an offensive odour if the contents have been dormant in the stomach for a time. Affected patients who vomit frequently are anorexic, with evident weight loss, and report thirst and an unpleasant taste in the mouth.

Patients with gastric outlet obstruction may have a swelling in the upper abdomen that indicates dilation of the stomach. Peristalsis is loud, and visible peristaltic waves are often observed passing across the abdomen from left to right. If the stomach is grossly dilated, it is possible to palpate it as well.

Diagnostic Studies

The diagnostic measures used to determine the presence and location of a peptic ulcer are similar to those used for acute upper GI bleeding. Endoscopy is the procedure most often used because of the manoeuvrability of fibre-optic endoscopes for viewing the entire gastric and duodenal mucosa (Figure 44-17). This procedure can also be used to determine the degree of ulcer healing after treatment. During endoscopy, tissue specimens can be obtained for identification of *H. pylori* and to rule out gastric cancer.

Currently, several diagnostic tests are available to confirm *H. pylori* infection. These are classified as noninvasive and invasive. *Noninvasive tests* include serum or whole blood antibody tests, particularly immunoglobulin G (IgG). However, because of the length of time that IgG levels remain elevated in the blood after the infection, the serological tests do not help distinguish active from recently treated disease. The urea breath test can determine the presence of active infection. Urea is a by-product of the metabolism of *H. pylori* bacteria. *Invasive tests* involve biopsy of the stomach and include the rapid urease test and tests of other histological markers of infection. These tests have greater sensitivity and specificity but involve an endoscopic procedure.

Barium studies are of benefit in the diagnosis of gastric outlet obstruction. Barium normally should pass from the stomach

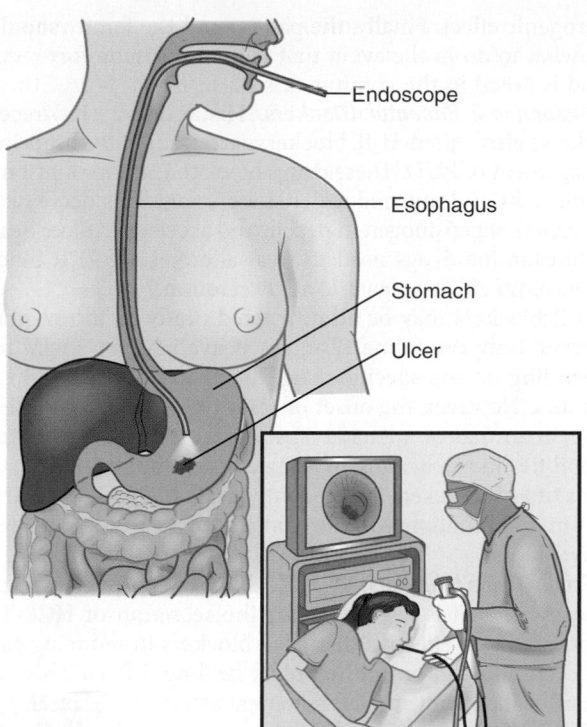

Endoscope

Esophagus

Stomach

Ulcer

FIGURE 44-17 Esophago-gastro-duodenoscopy (EGD) enables the examiner to directly visualize the mucosal lining of the stomach with a flexible endoscope. Ulcers or tumours can be directly visualized and biopsy samples taken.

TABLE 44-21 COLLABORATIVE CARE

Peptic Ulcer Disease

Diagnostic
- History and physical examination
- Complete blood cell count
- *Helicobacter pylori* testing of breath, urine, blood, tissue
- Liver enzyme measurements
- Serum electrolyte measurements
- Upper GI endoscopy with biopsy
- Urinalysis

Collaborative Therapy
Conservative Therapy
- Adequate rest
- Bland diet (six small meals a day)
- Cessation of smoking
- Drug therapy
  - Antacids (see Table 44-23)
  - Antibiotics for *H. pylori* infection (see Table 44-14)
  - Anticholinergics
  - Cytoprotective drugs
  - H₂-receptor blockers (see Table 44-22)
  - Proton pump inhibitors (see Table 44-22)
- Stress reduction

Acute Exacerbation
Without Complications
- Adequate rest
- Cessation of smoking
- IV fluid replacement
- NPO
- Drug therapy
  - Antacids
  - Anticholinergics
  - H₂-receptor blockers
  - Proton pump inhibitors
  - Sedatives

Acute Exacerbation With Complications (Hemorrhage, Perforation, Obstruction)
- Bed rest
- Blood transfusions
- IV fluid replacement (lactated Ringer's solution)
- NG suction
- NPO
- Stomach lavage (possible)

Surgical Therapy
- Billroth I and II procedures
- Gastric outlet obstruction: pyloroplasty and vagotomy
- Perforation: simple closure with omentum graft
- Ulcers: removal or reduction
- Vagotomy and pyloroplasty

GI, gastro-intestinal; *IV*, intravenous; *NG*, nasogastric; *NPO*, nothing by mouth.

within 2 hours, but with gastric outlet obstruction, 50% of the barium remains on follow-up films up to 6 hours later.

Gastric analysis has questionable value in the diagnosis of PUD because, in many patients, gastric secretions are normal in amount and composition. However, it can provide important data for (a) identifying a possible gastrinoma (Zollinger–Ellison syndrome), (b) determining the degree of gastric hyperacidity, and (c) evaluating the results of therapy such as vagotomy and antisecretory drug therapy. Gastric analysis procedure is described in Chapter 41.

Laboratory analyses, including a CBC, urinalysis, liver enzyme studies, serum amylase determination, and stool examination, should be performed. A CBC may indicate the presence of anemia secondary to bleeding from the ulcer. Liver enzyme studies help determine any liver problems, such as cirrhosis, that may complicate the treatment of the ulcer. Urine and stool are routinely tested for the presence of blood. A serum amylase determination frequently provides information on pancreatic function in patients in whom posterior penetration of the pancreas is suspected.

Collaborative Care: Conservative Therapy

When the patient's clinical manifestations and health history suggest the diagnosis of PUD and diagnostic studies confirm it, a medical regimen is instituted (Table 44-21). The regimen consists of adequate rest, dietary modifications, drug therapy, elimination of smoking, and long-term follow-up care. The aim of the treatment program is to decrease the degree of gastric acidity, enhance mucosal defence mechanisms, and minimize the harmful effects on the mucosa.

Patients are generally treated in ambulatory care clinics. Pain disappears after 3 to 6 days, but ulcer healing is much slower. Complete healing may take 3 to 9 weeks, depending on ulcer

size and the treatment regimen employed. Healing of the ulcer should be assessed by means of radiographic or endoscopic examination. Endoscopic examination is the only accurate method by which to monitor ulcer healing; follow-up examinations are performed 3 to 6 months after diagnosis and treatment.

Adequate rest, both physical and emotional, is important in the treatment process. A quiet, calm environment at home or on the job is not easy to achieve, and some modifications in the patient's daily routine may be needed. The elimination or reduction of stressors helps decrease the stimulus for overproduction of HCl. Moderation in daily activity is essential.

When ASA (Aspirin) or nonselective NSAIDs must be continued, enteric-coated preparations or coadministration with a PPI or misoprostol should be considered. Patients with *H. pylori* infection are treated as per established protocols.

As mentioned previously, smoking has an irritating effect on the mucosa, increases gastric motility, and delays mucosal healing. It should be eliminated completely or drastically reduced. The combination of adequate rest and abstinence from smoking accelerates ulcer healing.

Drug Therapy. Drugs are a vital part of therapy. The patient must be well informed about each drug prescribed, why it is ordered, and the expected benefits. Strict adherence to the prescribed regimen of drugs is important. Drug therapy includes the use of antacids, H₂R blockers, PPIs, antibiotics, anticholinergics, and cytoprotective therapy (Tables 44-22 through 44-24).

TABLE 44-22   DRUG THERAPY

Peptic Ulcer Disease

Antisecretory
- H₂-receptor blockers
  - Famotidine (Pepcid)
  - Nizatidine (Axid)
  - Ranitidine (Zantac)
- Proton pump inhibitors
  - Dexlansoprazole (Dexilant)
  - Esomeprazole (Nexium)
  - Lansoprazole (Prevacid)
  - Omeprazole (Losec)
  - Pantoprazole (Pantoloc)
- Anticholinergics

Antisecretory and Cytoprotective
- Misoprostol

Cytoprotective
- Sucralfate bismuth subsalicylate (Pepto-Bismol)

Neutralizing
- Antacids*

Antibiotics for *Helicobacter pylori* Infection
- Amoxicillin
- Clarithromycin (Biaxin)
- Metronidazole (Flagyl)
- Tetracycline

Others
- Tricyclic antidepressants
  - Doxepin (Sinequan)
  - Imipramine

*See Table 44-23.

TABLE 44-23   DRUG THERAPY

Antacid Preparations

Ingredient	Trade Name
Single substance	
• Aluminum carbonate	Basaljel
• Aluminum hydroxide gel tablets	Amphojel
• Aluminum phosphate	Phosphalugel
• Calcium carbonate	Alka-2, Tums
• Dihydroxyaluminum sodium carbonate	Rolaids
• Magaldrate	Riopan
• Magnesium hydroxide	Milk of magnesia
• Sodium bicarbonate	Alka-Seltzer
Mixtures of aluminum hydroxide and magnesium salts	Gaviscon, Maalox/Diovol

TABLE 44-24   DRUG THERAPY

Adverse Effects of Antacid Therapy

Antacid	Reactions
Aluminum hydroxide gels	Constipation, phosphorus depletion with chronic use
Calcium carbonate	Constipation or diarrhea, hypercalcemia, milk-alkali syndrome, renal calculi
Magnesium preparations	Diarrhea, hypermagnesemia
Sodium preparations	Milk–alkali syndrome if used with large amounts of calcium; used with caution in patients with sodium restrictions

Because recurrence of peptic ulcer is frequent, interruption or discontinuation of therapy can have detrimental results. The patient must be encouraged to comply with therapy and continue with follow-up care for at least 1 year. If changes in lifestyle are part of the prescribed therapy, they should be maintained. Antacids, H₂R blockers, and PPIs may be stopped after the ulcer has healed or may be prescribed in the form of low-dose maintenance therapy. No other drugs, unless prescribed by the health care provider, should be taken because they may have an ulcerogenic effect. Finally, the patient and the family should be told what to do in the event that pain and discomfort recur or blood is noted in the vomitus or stools.

Histamine-2 Receptor Blockers. Histamine-2 (H₂)-receptor blockers, also called H₂R blockers, are frequently used in the management of PUD. These drugs block the action of histamine on the H₂Rs and thus reduce HCl secretion. This decreases the conversion of pepsinogen to pepsin and accelerates ulcer healing. (Antihistamine drugs used to treat allergies are H₁R blockers and have no effect on gastric acid secretion.)

H₂R blockers may be administered orally or intravenously; however, only ranitidine (Zantac) is available in an IV form. Depending on the specific drug, therapeutic effects last up to 12 hours. However, the onset of action (i.e., symptom relief) is longer than that of antacids. H₂R blockers have demonstrated capabilities in the healing of gastric and duodenal ulcers. OTC forms of H₂R blockers are currently available. H₂R blockers are used in combination with antibiotics to treat ulcers related to *H. pylori.*

Proton Pump Inhibitors. PPIs block the adenosine triphosphatase enzyme that is important for the secretion of HCl. These agents are more effective than H₂R blockers in reducing gastric acid secretion and promoting ulcer healing. PPIs are also used in combination with antibiotics to treat ulcers caused by *H. pylori.*

Antibiotic Therapy. Antibiotics are prescribed to eradicate *H. pylori* infection. The treatment of *H. pylori* is the most important element of treating ulcer disease in patients with *H. pylori* infection. When *H. pylori* is present, ulcer recurrence rates can be as high as 75% to 90% when H₂R blockers are taken alone, whereas with antibiotic treatment, the recurrence rate may be less than 10%. Antibiotic therapy for *H. pylori* is detailed in Table 44-14.

Once the presence of *H. pylori* has been determined, antibiotic treatment is instituted. The regimen of choice is based on the antibiotic susceptibility of the *H. pylori* organism, allergies, patient adherence, adverse effects, and costs. Most drug regimens involve treatment for 7 to 14 days (Rx Files Academic Detailing Program, 2014).

Antacids. Antacids are used as adjunct therapy for PUD. They increase gastric pH by neutralizing the acid. As a result, the acid content of chyme reaching the duodenum is reduced. In addition, some antacids, such as aluminum hydroxide, can bind to bile salts, thus decreasing the detrimental effects of bile on the gastric mucosa. Patients who are vulnerable to SRMD may be treated prophylactically with antacids along with an antisecretory agent.

Antacids consist of systemic and nonsystemic types. *Systemic antacids,* such as sodium bicarbonate, are extremely soluble and are absorbed into the circulation. Their long-term use can lead to systemic alkalosis; therefore, they are rarely used in ulcer treatment. The *nonsystemic antacids* are insoluble and poorly absorbed. The common commercial nonsystemic antacids consist of magnesium hydroxide or aluminum hydroxide as single preparations or in various combinations (see Table 44-23). The antacid preparation may be in liquid or tablet form. The neutralizing effects of antacids taken on an empty stomach last only 20 to 30 minutes because they are quickly evacuated. When antacids are taken after meals, the effects may last as long as 3 to 4 hours. With therapy regimens that call for frequent administration (e.g., hourly), adherence is often poor.

The type and dosage of the antacid prescribed depends on adverse effects (see Table 44-24), as well as potential drug interactions. Preparations with high sodium content should be administered with caution in older adults and in patients with liver cirrhosis, hypertension, heart failure, or renal disease. Magnesium preparations should not be prescribed for patients with renal failure because of the risk of magnesium toxicity. The most frequent adverse effect experienced with magnesium antacids is diarrhea. Aluminum hydroxide causes constipation. An antacid combination of aluminum and magnesium salts seems to lessen the adverse effects of both.

Antacids have the capacity to interact unfavourably with some drugs. They can enhance the absorption of drugs such as dicumarol and amphetamines. The action of digitalis preparations can be potentiated when taken in combination with calcium or magnesium antacids. In some instances, antacids may decrease the absorption rates of prescribed drugs, such as tetracycline. Therefore, it is important to inform the health care provider of any drugs that the patient is taking before antacid therapy is begun.

Anticholinergic Drugs. Anticholinergic drugs (e.g., scopolamine [hyoscine]) are only occasionally ordered in the treatment of PUD. These drugs decrease cholinergic (vagal) stimulation of HCl secretion. Opinion is divided with regard to their efficacy in preventing recurrences and their therapeutic effectiveness in alleviating symptoms and preventing complications. Because of their tendency to decrease gastric motility, they should not be used for gastric ulcers in which stasis of secretions increases the patient's pain and discomfort. Anticholinergics are associated with a number of adverse effects, such as dry mouth and skin, flushing, thirst, tachycardia, dilated pupils, blurred vision, and urine retention. Anticholinergics must be prescribed with caution in patients with narrow-angle glaucoma, benign prostatic hyperplasia, and gastric outlet obstruction.

Cytoprotective Drug Therapy. Sucralfate is used for the short-term treatment of ulcers. It has proved to be cytoprotective of the esophagus, the stomach, and the duodenum. Its ability to accelerate ulcer healing is thought to be a result of the formation of an ulcer-adherent complex covering the ulcer and thereby protecting it from erosion caused by pepsin, acid, and bile salts. Sucralfate does not have acid-neutralizing capabilities. Its action is most effective at a low pH, and it should be given at least 30 minutes before or after an antacid. Adverse effects are minimal. However, it does bind with digoxin, warfarin (Coumadin), phenytoin (Dilantin), and tetracycline, which reduces the bioavailability of these drugs.

Misoprostol is a synthetic prostaglandin analogue. It has protective and some antisecretory effects on gastric mucosa. It is used for the prevention of gastric ulcers induced by NSAIDs and ASA (Aspirin). A major advantage of misoprostol is that it does not interfere with the therapeutic effects of ASA (Aspirin) and NSAIDs. Persons who require ongoing NSAID therapy, such as those with osteoarthritis, may benefit from the use of misoprostol. All NSAIDs, even COX-2 inhibitors, impair ulcer healing.

Other Drugs. Tricyclic antidepressants (e.g., imipramine, doxepin [Sinequan]) and serotonin reuptake inhibitors may be prescribed for patients with ulcer disease. Antidepressants may contribute to overall pain relief through their effects on pain transmission by afferent fibres. In addition, tricyclic antidepressants have, to varying degrees, some anticholinergic properties, which result in reduced acid secretion. Selective serotonin reuptake inhibitors are associated with a slight increase in risk of upper GI bleeding.

Nutritional Therapy. Dietary modifications may be necessary so that foods and beverages irritating to the patient can be avoided or eliminated. Alcohol and caffeine-containing products should be eliminated because of their irritating effects.

Dietary instructions should include a sample diet with a list of foods that usually cause distress and should, therefore, be eliminated from the diet. Foods known to irritate the gastric mucosa include hot, spicy foods and pepper, alcohol, carbonated beverages, tea, coffee, and broth (meat extract). These foods also have limited buffering ability in addition to stimulating gastric acid secretion. Foods high in roughage, such as raw fruit, salads, and vegetables, may irritate an inflamed mucosa. If these foods are well chewed, this seems to be less of a problem.

Protein is considered the best neutralizing food, but it also stimulates gastric secretions. Carbohydrates and fats are the least stimulating to HCl secretion, but they do not neutralize acid well. The patient must determine a suitable combination of these essential nutrients that does not cause undue distress.

Milk can neutralize gastric acidity and contains prostaglandins and growth factors, both of which may protect the GI mucosa from injury.

Therapy Related to Complications of Peptic Ulcer Disease

Acute Exacerbation. An acute exacerbation of peptic ulcer can usually be treated with the same regimen used for conservative therapy. However, the situation is considered more serious because of the possible complications of perforation, hemorrhage, and gastric outlet obstruction.

Bleeding, increased pain and discomfort, and nausea and vomiting frequently accompany an acute exacerbation. If the patient experiences recurrent vomiting or gastric outlet obstruction, an NG tube may be placed into the stomach with intermittent suction for about 24 to 48 hours.

If the patient has a history of an incompetent pyloric sphincter that allows reflux of duodenal contents into the stomach, an NG tube is used to remove intestinal contents from the stomach. This period of stomach rest eliminates any causative factors that may have precipitated the acute exacerbation and enables the resolution of edema and inflammation of the mucosa. Fluids and electrolytes are replaced by IV infusion until the patient is able to tolerate oral feedings without distress.

Management is similar to that described for upper GI bleeding. Blood or blood products may be administered. Careful monitoring of the vital signs, intake and output, laboratory study results, and signs of impending shock is important during this acute episode.

Endoscopic evaluation is performed to reveal the degree of inflammation or bleeding, as well as the ulcer location. It is important to ascertain the presence of a prepyloric or pyloric ulcer that can cause gastric outlet obstruction. When endoscopic examination reveals no major problems and the patient's physical condition stabilizes, the plan of care for the patient should follow the same regimen of diet, activity, and drugs used in conservative therapy. A 5-year follow-up program is recommended after acute exacerbation. An increase in the healing rate is achieved after conservative treatment, but the treatment plan cannot prevent the scar formation that can result in gastric outlet obstruction.

Perforation. The immediate focus of management of a patient with a perforation is to stop the spillage of gastric or duodenal contents into the peritoneal cavity and restore blood volume. An NG tube is inserted into the stomach to provide continuous aspiration and gastric decompression to halt spillage through the perforation. Although duodenal aspiration is not achieved as promptly, placement of the tube as near to the perforation site as possible facilitates decompression.

Circulating blood volume must be replaced with lactated Ringer's and albumin solutions. These solutions substitute for the fluids lost from the vascular and interstitial space as the peritonitis develops. Blood replacement in the form of packed RBCs may be necessary. A central venous pressure line and an indwelling urinary catheter, unless contraindicated, should be inserted and monitored hourly. Broad-spectrum antibiotic therapy should be started immediately to treat bacterial peritonitis. Administration of pain medications provides comfort.

The operative procedure involving the least risk to the patient is simple oversewing of the perforation and reinforcement of the area with a graft of omentum. The excess gastric contents are suctioned from the peritoneal cavity during the surgical procedure. There is controversy over whether more definitive surgical treatment of a perforated ulcer achieves better results than does simple closure. Other types of surgical procedures depend on the location of the peptic ulcer and the surgeon's preference. If cure of the ulcer is the ultimate goal, the surgical procedures may include gastric resection or vagotomy and pyloroplasty.

Gastric Outlet Obstruction. The aim of therapy for obstruction is to decompress the stomach, correct any existing fluid and electrolyte imbalances, and improve the patient's general state of health. An NG tube is inserted into the stomach and attached to continuous suction to remove excess fluids and undigested food particles. With continuous decompression for several days, the stomach has the opportunity to regain its normal muscle tone, the ulcer can begin healing, and the inflammation and edema will subside.

The tube is clamped after several days of suction, and gastric residue is measured periodically. The frequency and amount of time the tube remains clamped are proportional to the amount of aspirate obtained and the comfort level of the patient. A method commonly followed is to clamp the tube overnight for approximately 8 to 12 hours and to measure the gastric residue in the morning. When the aspirate falls below 200 mL, it is considered to be within a normal range, and the patient can begin oral intake of clear liquids. Initially, oral fluids are begun at 30 mL/hr and then gradually increased in amount. The patient must be watched carefully for signs of distress or vomiting. As the amount of gastric residue decreases, solid foods are added and the tube is removed.

IV fluids and electrolytes are administered according to the degree of dehydration, vomiting, and electrolyte imbalance indicated by laboratory studies. Pain relief results from the decompression measures, and analgesics are usually not necessary. Antacids and antisecretory drug therapy (i.e., H₂R blockers, PPIs) are an integral part of treatment if the obstruction has been determined on endoscopic examination to be the result of an active ulcer. Pyloric obstruction may be treated nonsurgically by balloon dilations performed through the endoscope. Surgical intervention may be necessary to remove scar tissue.

NURSING MANAGEMENT
PEPTIC ULCER DISEASE

NURSING ASSESSMENT
Subjective and objective data that should be obtained from a patient with PUD are presented in Table 44-25.

NURSING DIAGNOSES
Nursing diagnoses related to PUD may include, but are not limited to, the following.

TABLE 44-25   NURSING ASSESSMENT
Peptic Ulcer Disease

Subjective Data
Important Health Information
Current health history: Chronic alcohol abuse, smoking, caffeine use
Past health history: Chronic kidney disease, pancreatic disease, chronic obstructive pulmonary disease, serious illness or trauma, hyperparathyroidism, cirrhosis of the liver, Zollinger–Ellison syndrome; family history of peptic ulcer disease
Medications: Use of acetylsalicylic acid (ASA: Aspirin), corticosteroids, nonsteroidal anti-inflammatory drugs
Surgery or other treatments: Complicated or prolonged surgery

Symptoms
- Black, tarry stools
- Common: burning midepigastric or back pain occurring 2–4 hrs after meals and relieved by food (duodenal ulcers), nocturnal pain; high epigastric pain occurring 1–2 hrs after meals (gastric ulcers); pain may be precipitated or aggravated by food
- Weight loss, anorexia; nausea and vomiting, hematemesis; dyspepsia, heartburn, belching

Objective Data
General
Anxiety, irritability

Gastro-intestinal
Epigastric tenderness

Possible Findings
Anemia; guaiac-positive stools; positive blood, urine, breath, or stool tests for *Helicobacter pylori*; abnormalities revealed by upper gastro-intestinal endoscopic and barium studies

---

- *Acute pain* related to *biological injury agent* (increased gastric secretions)
- *Ineffective health management* related to *insufficient knowledge of therapeutic regimen*
- *Nausea* related to *anxiety, fear, gastro-intestinal irritation*

Additional information on nursing diagnoses for the patient with PUD is presented in NCP 44-2, available on the Evolve website.

PLANNING
Overall goals are that the patient with PUD will (a) comply with the prescribed therapeutic regimen, (b) experience a reduction in or absence of discomfort related to PUD, (c) exhibit no signs of GI complications related to the ulcerative process, (d) have complete healing of the peptic ulcer, and (e) make appropriate lifestyle changes to prevent recurrence.

NURSING IMPLEMENTATION
HEALTH PROMOTION. Nurses must be involved in identifying patients at risk for ulcer development. Early detection and treatment of ulcers are important aspects of reducing morbidity associated with ulcers. Patients with PUD who are taking ulcerogenic drugs such as ASA (Aspirin) and NSAIDs are at risk for ulcer development. Patients need to be encouraged to take these drugs with food. Patients should be taught to report symptoms related to gastric irritation, including epigastric pain, to their health care provider.

ACUTE INTERVENTION. During the acute exacerbation of an ulcer, patients generally report increased pain and nausea and vomiting, and some may have evidence of bleeding. Initially, many patients attempt to cope with the symptoms at home before seeking medical assistance.

During this acute phase, the patient may be maintained on NPO status for a few days, an NG tube is inserted and connected to intermittent suction, and fluids are replaced intravenously. The rationale for this therapy must be conveyed to the anxious patient and caregiver. They must understand that the advantages far outweigh any temporary discomfort imposed by the presence of the tube. Regular mouth care alleviates the dry mouth. Cleansing and lubrication of the nares facilitates breathing and decreases soreness. When the stomach is kept empty of gastric secretions, the ulcer pain diminishes and ulcer healing begins. Usually, this form of intervention is effective.

Because the patient is on NPO status, IV fluids are ordered. The type and amount administered are directly related to the fluid lost, the manifestations exhibited by the patient, and the results of the hemoglobin, hematocrit, and electrolyte determinations. The nurse should be aware of any other current health problem that could be adversely affected by the type of fluid used or the rate of the infusion. Repeated monitoring of these parameters provides information on the hydration status and the effectiveness of treatment. Vital signs are initially measured at least hourly so that shock can be detected and treated.

Physical and emotional rest are conducive to ulcer healing. The patient's immediate environment should be quiet and restful. The use of a mild sedative or tranquilizer has beneficial effects when the patient is anxious and apprehensive. The nurse must use good judgement before sedating a person who is becoming increasingly restless. There is danger that the drug will mask the signs of shock secondary to upper GI bleeding.

If the patient's condition improves without progression of symptoms (e.g., increased pain, vomiting, and hemorrhage), the regimen outlined for conservative therapy is followed. However, complications such as hemorrhage, perforation, and obstruction can occur.

Hemorrhage. Changes in the vital signs and an increase in the amount and redness of the aspirate often signal massive upper GI bleeding. When there is an increased amount of blood in the gastric contents, the patient's pain is often decreased because the blood helps to neutralize the acidic gastric contents. It is important to maintain the patency of the NG tube so that blood clots do not obstruct the tube. If the tube becomes blocked, the patient can develop abdominal distension. Similar interventions are used to those described for upper GI bleeding in the section "Nursing Management: Upper Gastro-intestinal Bleeding." The nurse must monitor the results of the hemoglobin and hematocrit determinations.

Perforation. When there is sudden, severe abdominal pain unrelated in intensity and location to the pain that brought the patient to the hospital, the nurse must recognize the possibility of ulcer perforation. When any patient with an ulcer, particularly a chronic duodenal ulcer, demonstrates these manifestations, perforation should be suspected and the health care provider notified immediately.

Patients with perforation demonstrate a rigid, boardlike abdomen; have severe generalized abdominal and shoulder pain; draw up the knees; and have shallow, grunting respirations. The bowel sounds that may have been previously normal or hyperactive may diminish and disappear.

Vital signs are important parameters and should be promptly recorded every 15 to 30 minutes. The nurse should temporarily stop all oral or NG drugs and feedings until the health care provider can be notified and a definitive diagnosis made. If perforation has taken place, anything taken internally can add to the spillage into the peritoneal cavity and increase discomfort. If IV fluids are being administered at the time of the perforation, the rate should be maintained or increased to replace the depleted plasma volume.

When perforation is confirmed, antibiotic therapy is usually started, and careful observation for allergic reactions must be made. When the perforation fails to seal spontaneously, surgical closure is necessary and is performed as soon as possible. There is often little time to prepare the patient and caregiver thoroughly for the surgical intervention, but some instructions can be conveyed while the immediate therapy is begun. If major reconstructive surgery is anticipated, the patient and caregiver may question the need when the problem is only a small hole.

Gastric Outlet Obstruction. Gastric outlet obstruction can occur at any time and is most likely to occur in patients in whom the ulcer is located close to the pylorus. Because the onset of symptoms is usually gradual, the condition is not generally as serious an emergency as hemorrhage or perforation. Relief of symptoms may be achieved by constant NG aspiration of stomach contents. This allows edema and inflammation to subside and then enables normal flow of gastric contents through the pylorus.

Obstruction can also occur during the treatment of an acute episode of peptic ulcer exacerbation. If these symptoms are experienced while the patient is still on NPO status, the patency of the NG tube should be investigated. Regular irrigation of the tube with a saline solution facilitates proper functioning. It may be helpful to reposition the patient from side to side so that the tube tip is not constantly lying against the mucosal surface.

When oral feedings have been resumed and symptoms of obstruction are observed, the health care provider should be promptly informed. In general, all that is necessary to treat the problem is to resume gastric aspiration so that the edema and inflammation resulting from the acute episode have time to resolve. IV fluids with electrolyte replacement keep the patient hydrated during this period. The NG tube can be clamped, and gastric fluids can be aspirated to check for retention. It is important to maintain accurate intake and output records, especially of the gastric aspirate. The patient should be kept aware of why these symptoms are being experienced. In some instances in which treatment is not successful, surgery may be performed after the acute phase has passed.

Ambulatory and Home Care. Patients in whom PUD has been diagnosed have specific needs that must be met to prevent and avoid recurrence or complications. General instructions should cover aspects of the disease process itself, drugs, possible changes in lifestyle (including diet), and regular follow-up care. Table 44-26 provides a patient and caregiver teaching guide for patients with PUD.

Knowing the cause of the ulcer and understanding the disease process may motivate a patient to become more involved in care and to adhere to the therapy regimen. The patient must understand the dietary modifications and why they are important for recovery and health maintenance. The nurse and the dietitian should elicit a dietary history from the patient and plan for ways that dietary modifications can be easily incorporated into the patient's home and work setting. The patient who is following a diet prescribed for another illness needs to know how to balance the two so that neither condition is harmed by dietary interventions.

Patients do not always give the health care provider accurate information regarding habitual use of alcohol or cigarettes. The

TABLE 44-26   PATIENT & CAREGIVER TEACHING GUIDE

Peptic Ulcer Disease

The following guidelines should be included when teaching the patient and caregiver about peptic ulcer disease. The nurse should:

1. Describe dietary modifications, including avoidance of foods that cause epigastric distress. These foods may include black pepper, spicy foods, and acidic foods. Carbonated beverages and caffeine should also be avoided.
2. Explain the rationale for avoiding cigarettes. In addition to promoting ulcer development, smoking delays ulcer healing.
3. Emphasize the need to reduce or eliminate alcohol ingestion.
4. Explain the rationale for avoiding OTC drugs unless approved by the patient's health care provider. Many preparations contain ingredients, such as ASA (Aspirin), that should not be taken unless approved by the health care provider. The patient should check with the health care provider regarding the use of nonsteroidal anti-inflammatory drugs.
5. Explain the rationale for not interchanging brands of antacids and H_2-receptor blockers that can be purchased OTC without checking with the health care provider. Doing so can lead to harmful adverse effects.
6. Emphasize the need to take all medications as prescribed, including both antisecretory and antibiotic drugs. Failure to take medications as prescribed can result in relapse.
7. Explain the importance of reporting any of the following:
   • Bloody emesis or tarry stools
   • Increase in epigastric pain
   • Increased nausea or vomiting
8. Describe the relationship between symptoms and stress. Stress-reducing activities and relaxation strategies are encouraged.
9. Encourage patient and caregiver to share concerns about lifestyle changes and living with a chronic illness.

ASA, acetylsalicylic acid; *OTC,* over-the-counter.

nurse should provide useful information about the detrimental effects of alcohol and cigarettes on ulcer disease and ulcer healing and provide resources on cessation and rehabilitation programs.

The nurse should teach the patient about prescribed drugs, including their actions, adverse effects, and inherent dangers if omitted for any reason. The patient should know why OTC drugs (e.g., ASA [Aspirin]) should not be taken unless approved by the health care provider. Because antacids and some H_2R blockers may be bought without a prescription, the patient must be informed that interchanging brands without checking with the health care provider or nurse can lead to harmful adverse effects.

Efforts should be made to obtain more information about the patient's psychosocial status. Knowledge of lifestyle, occupation, and coping behaviours can be helpful to the plan of care. The patient may be reluctant to talk about personal subjects, the stress experienced at home or on the job, the usual methods of coping, or dependence on drugs or alcohol. Unfortunately, the patient often does not recognize the relationship between lifestyle or occupation and ulcer disease. It is important to listen for subtle clues from the patient's statements and to observe for behaviours that broaden the database of what is known about the patient.

The need for long-term follow-up care must be stressed. Because successful treatment is frequently followed by a recurrence of the ulcer disease, patients should be encouraged to seek immediate intervention if symptoms of the disease come back.

Patients who have recurrence of ulcer disease after initial healing must learn to live with a disease that is chronic. They may be angry and frustrated, especially if the prescribed mode of therapy has been faithfully followed and yet has failed to prevent the recurrence or extension of the disease process.

Unfortunately, many patients do not comply with the plan of care originally designed, and they experience repeated exacerbations. Patients quickly learn that they often experience no discomfort when they omit prescribed drugs or indulge in occasional dietary indiscretions. Consequently, they make no or little alteration in lifestyle. After an acute exacerbation, the patient is often more amenable to following the plan of care and open to suggestions for changes in lifestyle. Changes, such as smoking cessation and alcohol abstinence, are difficult for many people, and the idea of making them may be met with resistance. The patient may fare better from a reduction in his or her use of these substances rather than from total elimination. Although alcohol and smoking are known to interfere with ulcer healing, they frequently serve as coping mechanisms. From the patient's point of view, the distress caused by their total elimination may outweigh the benefits to be gained from abstention. The goal, however, should always be total cessation. A patient with chronic ulcers must be aware of the complications that may result from the disease, the clinical manifestations indicating their presence, and what to do about them until the health care provider can be seen.

EVALUATION

Expected outcomes for the patient with PUD are addressed in NCP 44-2 on the Evolve website.

Collaborative Therapy: Surgical Therapy for Peptic Ulcer Disease

Because of the use of antisecretory and antibiotic agents, surgery for PUD is uncommon. Surgery is performed on patients with complications that are unresponsive to medical management or who have concerns about gastric cancer.

A variety of surgical procedures are used to treat ulcer disease. They usually involve a partial gastrectomy, vagotomy, or pyloroplasty. Partial gastrectomy with removal of the distal two-thirds of the stomach and anastomosis of the gastric stump to the duodenum is called a *gastro-duodenostomy,* or *Billroth I* operation (Figure 44-18). Partial gastrectomy with removal of the distal two-thirds of the stomach and anastomosis of the gastric stump to the jejunum is called a *gastro-jejunostomy,* or *Billroth II* operation. In both procedures, the antrum and the pylorus are removed. Because the duodenum is bypassed, the Billroth II operation is the preferred surgical procedure to prevent recurrence of duodenal ulcers.

Vagotomy is the severing of the vagus nerve, either totally (truncal) or selectively at some point in its innervation to the stomach. In a truncal vagotomy, both the anterior and the posterior trunks are severed. *Selective vagotomy* consists of cutting the nerve at a particular branch of the vagus nerve, resulting in denervation of only a portion of the stomach, such as the antrum or the parietal cell mass.

Pyloroplasty consists of surgical enlargement of the pyloric sphincter to facilitate the easy passage of contents from the stomach. It is most commonly done after vagotomy or to enlarge an opening that has been constricted from scar tissue. A vagotomy decreases gastric motility and, subsequently, gastric emptying. A pyloroplasty accompanying vagotomy increases gastric emptying.

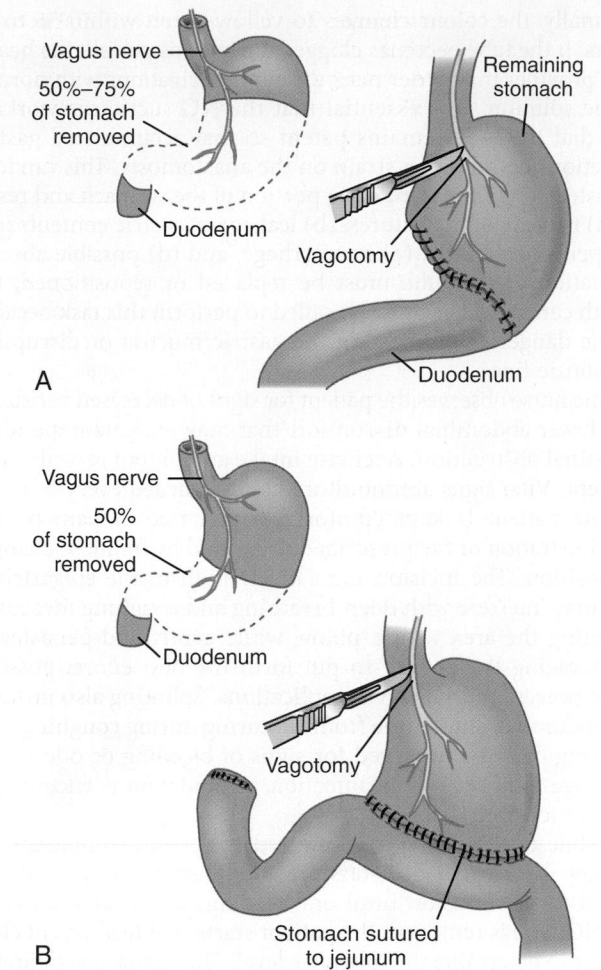

Vagus nerve

50%–75% of stomach removed

Duodenum

Remaining stomach

Vagotomy

Duodenum

A

Vagus nerve

50% of stomach removed

Duodenum

Vagotomy

Stomach sutured to jejunum

B

FIGURE 44-18 A, Billroth I procedure (subtotal gastric resection with gastro-duodenostomy anastomosis). **B,** Billroth II procedure (subtotal gastric resection with gastro-jejunostomy anastomosis).

Postoperative Complications. The most common postoperative complications from peptic ulcer surgery are dumping syndrome, postprandial hypoglycemia, and bile reflux gastritis.

Dumping Syndrome. *Dumping syndrome,* in which patients experience vagal symptoms after a meal, such as generalized weakness or dizziness, is the direct result of surgical removal of a large portion of the stomach and the pyloric sphincter. These changes drastically reduce the reservoir capacity of the stomach. Although dumping syndrome is more commonly experienced after a Billroth II procedure, it can occur after any gastric reconstruction and vagotomy.

Dumping syndrome is associated with meals having a hyperosmolar composition. Normally, gastric chyme enters the small intestine in small amounts, and shifts in fluid from the extracellular space are minimal. After surgery, however, the stomach no longer has control over the amount of gastric chyme entering the small intestine. Consequently, a large bolus of hypertonic fluid enters the intestine and results in fluid being drawn into the bowel lumen. This creates a decrease in plasma volume. A secondary consequence of this fluid shift is distension of the bowel lumen, which stimulates intestinal motility and the urge to defecate.

Approximately one-third to one-half of patients experience dumping syndrome after peptic ulcer surgery. The onset of symptoms occurs at the end of a meal or within 15 to 30 minutes after eating. The patient usually describes feelings of generalized weakness, sweating, palpitations, and dizziness. These symptoms are attributed to the sudden decrease in plasma volume. The patient reports abdominal cramps, borborygmi (audible abdominal sounds produced by hyperactive intestinal peristalsis), and the urge to defecate. These manifestations usually last for no longer than an hour after meals.

Postprandial Hypoglycemia. *Postprandial hypoglycemia* is considered a variant of the dumping syndrome because it is the result of uncontrolled gastric emptying of a bolus of fluid high in carbohydrate into the small intestine. The bolus of concentrated carbohydrate results in hyperglycemia and the release of excessive amounts of insulin into the circulation. A secondary hypoglycemia then occurs, with symptoms appearing about 2 hours after meals. The symptoms experienced are the ones observed in any hypoglycemic reaction and include sweating, weakness, mental confusion, palpitations, tachycardia, and anxiety.

Bile Reflux Gastritis. Gastric surgery that involves the pylorus, either reconstruction or removal, can result in reflux alkaline gastritis. Prolonged contact with bile, especially bile salts, causes damage to the gastric mucosa. Chronic gastritis of this form may result in the backwards diffusion of H^+ through the gastric mucosa. Paradoxically, peptic ulcer may recur after surgical treatment that was intended as a cure.

The symptoms associated with reflux alkaline gastritis are continuous epigastric distress that increases after meals. Vomiting relieves the distress but only temporarily. The administration of cholestyramine, either before or with meals, has met with success. Cholestyramine binds with the bile salts that are the source of irritation in this condition. Aluminum hydroxide antacids have also been used in the treatment of this condition.

Nutritional Therapy. Discharge planning and instruction should be started as soon as the immediate postoperative period is successfully passed. Dietary instructions may be given by the dietitian and reinforced by the nursing staff. Because the stomach's reservoir has been greatly diminished after gastric resection, the meal size must be reduced accordingly. The patient should be advised to stop drinking fluids with meals. Dry foods with a low-carbohydrate content and moderate protein and fat content are better tolerated initially. These dietary changes, with the incorporation of a short rest period after each meal, reduce the likelihood of dumping syndrome. Reassurance that following these dietary measures will result in cessation of these symptoms within a few months is essential for long-term adherence to instructions.

Postprandial hypoglycemic reaction can be avoided if these dietary instructions are followed. The immediate ingestion of sugared fluids or candy relieves the hypoglycemic symptoms. The treatment of this type of hypoglycemia is similar to that of dumping syndrome. To avoid similar occurrences, the patient should be instructed to limit the amount of sugar consumed with each meal and to eat small, frequent meals with moderate amounts of protein and fat. Although only a small percentage of patients experience bile reflux gastritis, all patients must be cautioned to notify the health care provider of any continuous epigastric distress after meals that is similar to that felt before surgery.

With regard to dumping syndrome, the symptoms are self-limiting and often disappear within several months to a year after surgery. Interventions prescribed are diet instruction, rest, and reassurance. As mentioned previously, the diet should consist of small dry feedings daily that are low in carbohydrate, are

TABLE 44-27 NUTRITIONAL THERAPY

Postgastrectomy Dumping Syndrome

Purpose

To slow the rapid passage of food into the intestine; to control symptoms of the dumping syndrome (dizziness, sense of fullness, diarrhea, tachycardia), which sometimes occur after a partial or total gastrectomy

Diet Principles

1. Meals are divided into six small feedings to avoid overloading intestines at mealtimes.
2. Fluids should not be taken with meals but at least 30–45 min before or after meals; this helps prevent distension or a feeling of fullness.
3. Concentrated sweets (e.g., honey, sugar, jelly, jam, candies, sweet pastries, sweetened fruit) are avoided because they sometimes cause dizziness, diarrhea, and a sense of fullness.
4. Protein and fats are increased to promote rebuilding of body tissues and to meet energy needs. Meat, cheese, eggs, and milk products are specific foods to increase in the diet.
5. The amount of time these restrictions should be followed varies. The health care provider decides the proper amount of time to remain on this prescribed diet according to the patient's clinical condition and progress.

restricted in refined sugars, and contain moderate amounts of protein and fat (Table 44-27). Fluids should be taken between meals but not with the meal, and the patient should plan rest periods of at least 30 minutes after each meal. The recumbent position is the most beneficial if the patient can arrange it. Reassuring the patient that the unpleasant symptoms are usually of short duration is helpful in gaining cooperation. A small percentage of patients experience long-term problems and may require further reconstructive surgery.

NURSING MANAGEMENT
SURGICAL THERAPY FOR PEPTIC ULCER DISEASE

PREOPERATIVE CARE

When surgery is planned with the goal of curing the ulcer disease, the surgeon should provide necessary information about the procedure and the expected outcome so that the patient can make an informed decision. The nurse can help the patient and the family by clarifying and interpreting their questions. A discussion of the surgical procedure accompanied by a diagram or picture showing the anatomical changes that will result should be incorporated into the preoperative teaching plan. Instructions should be clear on what to expect after surgery, including comfort measures, pain relief, coughing and breathing exercises, use of an NG tube, and IV fluid administration (see Chapter 20).

POSTOPERATIVE CARE

Care of the patient after major abdominal surgery is similar to the postoperative care after abdominal laparotomy (see Chapter 45 and NCP 45-2). An NG tube is used to decompress the remaining portion of the stomach to decrease pressure on the suture line and to allow for resolution of edema and inflammation resulting from surgical trauma.

The gastric aspirate must be carefully observed for colour, amount, and odour during the immediate postoperative period. The colour of the aspirate is expected to be bright red at first, with a gradual darkening within the first 24 hours after surgery.

Normally, the colour changes to yellow-green within 36 to 48 hours. If the tube becomes clogged during this period, the health care provider may order periodic gentle irrigations with normal saline solution. It is essential that the NG suction is working and that the tube remains patent so that accumulated gastric secretions do not put a strain on the anastomosis. This can lead to distension of the remaining portion of the stomach and result in (a) rupture of the sutures, (b) leakage of gastric contents into the peritoneal cavity, (c) hemorrhage, and (d) possible abscess formation. If the tube must be replaced or repositioned, the health care provider must be called to perform this task because of the danger of perforating the gastric mucosa or disrupting the suture line.

The nurse observes the patient for signs of decreased peristalsis and lower abdominal discomfort that may indicate impending intestinal obstruction. Accurate intake and output records must be kept. Vital signs are monitored and recorded every 4 hours.

The patient is kept comfortable and free of pain by the administration of the prescribed drugs and by frequent changes in position. The incision is relatively high in the epigastrium and may interfere with deep-breathing and coughing measures. Splinting the area with a pillow while gently and persistently encouraging the patient to put forth the best efforts possible helps prevent pulmonary complications. Splinting also protects the abdominal suture line from rupturing during coughing. The dressing must be observed for signs of bleeding or odour and drainage indicative of an infection. Ambulation is encouraged and is increased daily.

While the NG tube is connected to suction equipment, IV therapy is maintained. Potassium and vitamin supplements are added to the infusion until oral feedings are resumed. Before the NG tube is removed, the patient starts oral feedings of clear liquids to determine the tolerance level. The stomach is aspirated within 1 or 2 hours to assess the amount remaining and its colour and consistency. When fluids are well tolerated, the tube is removed, and fluids are increased in frequency with a slow progression to regular foods. The regimen of six small meals a day is begun.

Pernicious anemia is a long-term complication of total gastrectomy and may occur after partial gastrectomy. Pernicious anemia is caused by the loss of intrinsic factor, which is produced by the parietal cells. Depending on the amount of parietal cell mass removed in surgery, the patient may eventually require regular administration of cobalamin (vitamin B_{12}). (Cobalamin deficiency and pernicious anemia are discussed in Chapter 33.)

PUD is a chronic problem, and ulcers can recur, especially at the site of the anastomosis. Adequate rest, nutrition, and avoidance of known irritants and stressors are keys to complete recovery. Avoiding the use of drugs not prescribed by the health care provider is re-emphasized, along with restrictions on smoking and alcohol use. If the patient is willing to make these kinds of adjustments in lifestyle, rehabilitation is more likely to be successful.

AGE-RELATED CONSIDERATIONS

PEPTIC ULCER DISEASE

The incidence of peptic ulcers and, in particular, gastric ulcers in patients older than 60 years is increasing. This is related to the increased use of NSAIDs. In older adults, pain may not be the first symptom associated with an ulcer. For some patients, the first manifestation may be frank gastric bleeding (e.g., hematemesis, melena) or a decrease in hematocrit. The rates of morbidity and mortality associated with gastric ulcers are higher in older adults than in younger adults because of concomitant health problems (e.g., cardiovascular, pulmonary) and a decreased ability to withstand hypovolemia.

The treatment and management of ulcers in older adults are similar to that in younger adults. An emphasis is placed on

prevention of both gastritis and peptic ulcers. This includes teaching patients to take NSAIDs and other gastric-irritating drugs with food, milk, or antacids. Patients may be treated with antisecretory agents (i.e., PPIs or H_2R blockers). They should be instructed to avoid irritating substances, such as alcohol and smoking, and to report abdominal pain or discomfort to the health care provider.

CASE STUDY

Hiatal Hernia

Source: Blend Images/ Shutterstock .com.

Patient Profile

Ishleen Chaudry, a 45-year-old elementary school teacher, has had a sliding hiatal hernia for 10 years. Mrs. Chaudry is admitted to the hospital for a hiatal hernia repair.

Subjective Data
- Reports increasing heartburn, especially at night
- Is currently on a bland diet and taking antacids
- Reports of substernal pain and heartburn
- Reports some problems with regurgitation

Objective Data
Physical Examination
- 157 cm tall and weighs 88 kg

Diagnostic Study
- Barium swallow study and an endoscopy revealed a large sliding hiatal hernia.

Collaborative Care
- Mrs. Chaudry underwent a Nissen fundoplication through a laparoscopic approach.

Discussion Questions
1. Explain the pathophysiology of a hiatal hernia. What is the difference between a sliding and a paraesophageal hiatal hernia?
2. What are the characteristic symptoms of a hiatal hernia? Which of these did Mrs. Chaudry have?
3. Describe a Nissen fundoplication procedure. What is the objective of this surgical procedure? Why was a laparoscopic approach used?
4. What are potential postoperative complications, and what nursing measures prevent them?
5. What should be included in a teaching plan for Mrs. Chaudry?
6. **Priority decision:** On the basis of the assessment data presented, what are the priority nursing diagnoses? Are there any collaborative problems?

e)volve

Answers are available at *http://evolve.elsevier.com/Canada/Lewis/medsurg*

REVIEW QUESTIONS

The number of the question corresponds to the same-numbered objective at the beginning of the chapter.

1. The daughter of a client calls to tell the nurse that her 85-year-old mother has been nauseated all day and has vomited twice. Before the nurse hangs up and telephones the health care provider to communicate the assessment data, what does the nurse instruct the client's daughter to do?
   a. Administer antispasmodic drugs and observe skin turgor.
   b. Give her mother sips of water and elevate the head of her bed to prevent aspiration.
   c. Offer her mother a high-protein liquid supplement to drink to maintain her nutritional needs.
   d. Offer her mother large quantities of Gatorade to drink because older adults are at risk for sodium depletion.
2. The nurse explains to a patient with Vincent's infection that treatment will include which of the following?
   a. Smallpox vaccinations
   b. Viscous lidocaine rinses
   c. Amphotericin B suspension
   d. Topical application of antibiotics
3. The nurse is involved in health promotion related to oral cancer. Which behaviours are included in the teaching of adolescents with regard to behaviours that put them at risk for oral cancer? *(Select all that apply)*

   a. Avoiding use of perfumed lip gloss
   b. Discouraging use of chewing gum
   c. Avoiding use of smokeless tobacco
   d. Discouraging drinking of carbonated beverages
   e. Avoiding excessive alcohol consumption
4. What information is included when the nurse is explaining gastro-esophageal reflux disease (GERD) to a client with GERD?
   a. Results in acid erosion and ulceration of the esophagus caused by frequent vomiting
   b. Will require surgical wrapping or repair of the pyloric sphincter to control the symptoms
   c. Is the protrusion of a portion of the stomach into the esophagus through an opening in the diaphragm
   d. Often involves relaxation of the lower esophageal sphincter, allowing stomach contents to back up into the esophagus
5. A client who has undergone an esophagectomy for esophageal cancer develops increasing pain, fever, and dyspnea when a full liquid diet is started postoperatively. What are these symptoms most indicative of?
   a. An intolerance to the feedings
   b. Extension of the tumour into the aorta
   c. Leakage of fluid or foods into the mediastinum
   d. Esophageal perforation with fistula formation into the lung

6. The pernicious anemia that may accompany gastritis is caused by which of the following?
   a. Chronic autoimmune destruction of cobalamin stores in the body
   b. Progressive gastric atrophy from chronic breakage in the mucosal barrier and blood loss
   c. A lack of intrinsic factor normally produced by acid-secreting cells of the gastric mucosa
   d. Hyperchlorhydria resulting from an increase in acid-secreting parietal cells and degradation of red blood cells

7. For the client being discharged after an acute episode of gastro-intestinal (GI) bleeding, what information would the nurse's teaching plan include?
   a. Taking only drugs prescribed by the health care provider
   b. Avoiding taking ASA (Aspirin) with acidic beverages such as orange juice
   c. Taking all drugs 1 hour before mealtime to prevent further bleeding
   d. Reading all over-the-counter (OTC) drug labels to avoid those containing stearic acid and calcium

8. The nurse is teaching the client and her family about possible causes of peptic ulcers. How does the nurse explain ulcer formation?
   a. Caused by a stressful lifestyle and other acid-producing factors such as *Helicobacter pylori*
   b. Inherited within families and reinforced by bacterial spread of *Staphylococcus aureus* in childhood
   c. Promoted by factors that tend to cause oversecretion of acid, such as excess dietary fats, smoking, and *H. pylori*

   d. Promoted by a combination of possible factors that may result in erosion of the gastric mucosa, including certain drugs and alcohol

9. What information should be included in an optimal teaching plan for an outpatient with gastric cancer who is receiving radiation therapy?
   a. Cancer support groups, alopecia, and stomatitis
   b. Avitaminosis, ostomy care, and community resources
   c. Prosthetic devices, skin conductance, and grief counselling
   d. Wound and skin care, nutrition, drugs, and community resources

10. Several clients are seen at an urgent care centre with symptoms of nausea, vomiting, and diarrhea that began 2 hours ago while they were attending a large family reunion potluck dinner. What kinds of foods that were ingested should the nurse question the patients specifically about? *(Select all that apply)*
    a. Beef
    b. Meat and milk
    c. Poultry and eggs
    d. Home-preserved vegetables
    e. Potato salad

1. b; 2. d; 3. c, e; 4. d; 5. c; 6. c; 7. a; 8. d; 9. d; 10. b, e.

⊖volve

For even more review questions, visit *http://evolve.elsevier.com/Canada/Lewis/medsurg*.

REFERENCES

Almond, L. M., & Barr, H. (2014). Management controversies in Barrett's oesophagus. *Journal of Gastroenterology, 49*(2), 195–205. doi:10.1007/s00535-013-0816-z.

BC Cancer Agency (2012). *Chemotherapy protocols: Gastrointestinal.* Retrieved from *http://www.bccancer.bc.ca/HPI/Chemotherapy Protocols/Gastrointestinal/default.htm#Esophagus,Stomach*.

Canadian Cancer Society (2015a). *Nausea and vomiting.* Retrieved from *http://www.cancer.ca/en/cancer-information/diagnosis-and-treatment/managing-side-effects/nausea-and-vomiting/?region=sk*.

Canadian Cancer Society (2015b). *Oral cancer: Diagnosing oral cavity cancer.* Retrieved from *http://www.cancer.ca/en/cancer-information/cancer-type/oral/diagnosis/?region=on*.

Canadian Cancer Society (2015c). *Esophageal cancer: Risk factors for esophageal cancer.* Retrieved from *http://www.cancer.ca/en/cancer-information/cancer-type/esophageal/risks/?region=bc*.

Canadian Cancer Society (2015d). *Esophageal cancer: Treatments for esophageal cancer.* Retrieved from *http://www.cancer.ca/en/cancer-information/cancer-type/esophageal/treatment/?region=bc*.

Canadian Cancer Society (2015e). *Stomach cancer: Stomach cancer statistics.* Retrieved from *http://www.cancer.ca/en/cancer-information/cancer-type/stomach/statistics/?region=on*.

Canadian Cancer Society's Advisory Committee on Cancer Statistics (2017). *Canadian cancer statistics 2017.* Toronto: Canadian Cancer Society. Retrieved from *http://www.cancer.ca/~/media/cancer.ca/CW/cancer%20information/cancer%20101/Canadian%20cancer%20statistics/Canadian-Cancer-Statistics-2017-EN.pdf?la=en*.

Canadian Society of Intestinal Research (2014). *Gastroesophageal reflux disease (GERD).* Retrieved from *http://www.badgut.org/wp-content/uploads/GIS-PIH-GE.pdf*.

Canadian Society of Intestinal Research (2015). *Report card: Acid reflux and GERD.* Retrieved from *http://www.badgut.org/about-us/newsroom/report-cards/gerd-report-card/*.

Centers for Disease Control and Prevention (2015). *E. coli (Escherichia coli).* Retrieved from *http://www.cdc.gov/ecoli/general/index.html*.

Funk, L. M., Kanji, A., Scott Melvin, W., et al. (2014). Elective antireflux surgery in the US: an analysis of national trends in utilization and inpatient outcomes from 2005 to 2010. *Surgical Endoscopy, 28*(5), 1712–1719. doi:10.1007/s00464-013-3380-y.

Holmér Pettersson, P., & Wengström, Y. (2012). Acupuncture prior to surgery to minimise postoperative nausea and vomiting: A systematic review. *Journal of Clinical Nursing, 21*(13/14), 1799–1805. doi:10.1111/j.1365-2702.2012.04114.x.

Kovac, A. (2013). Update on the management of postoperative nausea and vomiting. *Drugs, 73*(14), 1525–1547. doi:10.1007/s40265-013-0110-7.

Kurian, M., & Lobo, A. (2015). Acute upper gastrointestinal bleeding. *Clinical Medicine, 15*(5), 481–485. doi:10.7861/clinmedicine.15-5-481.

Mitra, V., Marrow, B., & Nayar, M. (2012). Management of acute upper gastrointestinal bleeding. *Gastrointestinal Nursing, 10*(7), 34–41.

Otterstatter, M. C., Brierley, J. D., De, P., et al. (2012). Esophageal cancer in Canada: Trends according to morphology and anatomical location. *Canadian Journal of Gastroenterology, 26*(10), 723–727. doi:10.1155/2012/649108.

Owen, C., Panesar, P., Marks, D. J. B., et al. (2014). The dangers of proton pump inhibitor therapy. *British Journal of Hospital Medicine, 75*(7), C108–C112.

Pilkington, K., Wagstaff, M., & Greenwood, J. (2012). Prevention of gastrointestinal bleeding due to stress ulceration: A review of current literature. *Anaesth Intensive Care, 40*(2), 253–259.

Richter, J. E. (2014). Current diagnosis and management of suspected reflux symptoms refractory to proton pump inhibitor therapy. *Gastroenterology Hepatology, 10*(9), 547–555.

Rx Files Academic Detailing Program (2014). *Rx files: Drug comparison charts.* Saskatoon, SK: Saskatoon Health Region.

Thomson, G., & Young, K. G. (2011). *Cancer in Canada: Framing the crisis and previewing the opportunity for donors.* Retrieved from *http://www.charityintelligence.ca/cancer-in-canada.*

RESOURCES

CAN-ADAPTT Canadian Smoking Cessation Clinical Practice Guideline
https://www.nicotinedependenceclinic.com/English/CANADAPTT/ Documents/CAN-ADAPTT%20Canadian%20Smoking%20 Cessation%20Guideline_website.pdf

Canadian Association of Gastroenterology
https://www.cag-acg.org

Canadian Cancer Society
http://www.cancer.ca

Canadian Society of Gastroenterology Nurses and Associates
https://csgna.com

Canadian Society of Intestinal Research
http://www.badgut.org/

For additional Internet resources, see the website for this book at *http://evolve.elsevier.com/Canada/Lewis/medsurg*

Nursing Management

Lower Gastro-Intestinal Problems

Written by: Diana L. Gallagher and Mariann M. Harding
Adapted by: Françoise Verville

evolve WEBSITE

http://evolve.elsevier.com/Canada/Lewis/medsurg

- Review Questions (Online Only)
- Key Points
- Answer Guidelines for Case Study
- Student Case Study
  - Ulcerative Colitis

- Customizable Nursing Care Plans
  - Acute Infectious Diarrhea
  - Colostomy/Ileostomy
  - Inflammatory Bowel Disease
  - Laparotomy

- Conceptual Care Map Creator
- Audio Glossary
- Content Updates

LEARNING OBJECTIVES

1. Explain the common etiologies, collaborative care, and nursing management of diarrhea, fecal incontinence, and constipation.
2. Describe the common causes of acute abdominal pain and nursing management of the patient following an exploratory laparotomy.
3. Describe the collaborative care and nursing management of acute appendicitis, peritonitis, and gastro-enteritis.
4. Compare and contrast ulcerative colitis and Crohn's disease, including pathophysiology, clinical manifestations, complications, collaborative care, and nursing management.
5. Differentiate among mechanical, neurogenic, and vascular bowel obstructions, including causes, collaborative care, and nursing management.
6. Describe the clinical manifestations and collaborative management of colorectal cancer.

7. Explain the anatomical and physiological changes and nursing management of the patient with an ileostomy and the patient with a colostomy.
8. Differentiate between diverticulosis and diverticulitis, including clinical manifestations, collaborative care, and nursing management.
9. Compare and contrast the types of hernias, including etiology and surgical and nursing management.
10. Describe the types of malabsorption syndrome and collaborative care.
11. Describe the types, clinical manifestations, collaborative care, and nursing management of anorectal conditions.

KEY TERMS

anal fissure, p. 1096
anal fistula, p. 1097
appendicitis, p. 1068
celiac disease, p. 1079
colorectal cancer, p. 1084
constipation, p. 1061
Crohn's disease, p. 1076

diarrhea, p. 1056
diverticulum, p. 1093
fecal impaction, p. 1060
fecal incontinence, p. 1060
gastro-enteritis, p. 1070
hemorrhoids, p. 1095
hernia, p. 1094

inflammatory bowel disease (IBD), p. 1071
intestinal obstruction, p. 1081
irritable bowel syndrome (IBS), p. 1068
lactase deficiency, p. 1080
ostomy, p. 1089

peritonitis, p. 1069
pilonidal sinus, p. 1097
pseudo-obstruction, p. 1081
short bowel syndrome (SBS), p. 1081
ulcerative colitis (UC), p. 1071

DIARRHEA

Diarrhea—the frequent passage of loose, watery stools—is not a disease but a symptom. The term *diarrhea* may mean different things to different patients. It is commonly used to denote an increase in stool frequency or volume and an increase in the looseness of stool.

Etiology and Pathophysiology

Causes of diarrhea can be divided into general classifications of decreased fluid absorption, increased fluid secretion, motility disturbances, or a combination of these (Table 45-1). Causes of acute infectious diarrhea are listed in Table 45-2.

Ingestion of infectious organisms is the primary cause of acute diarrhea. Viruses cause most cases of infectious diarrhea.

Although viral infections can be deadly, they are usually short lived (48 hours) and mild. Therefore most patients rarely seek treatment.

Infectious organisms attack the intestines in different ways. Some organisms (e.g., *Rotavirus A, Norovirus, G. lamblia*) alter secretion or absorption (or both) of the enterocytes of the small intestine without causing inflammation. Other organisms (e.g.,

Clostridium difficile) impair absorption by destroying cells, cause inflammation in the colon, and produce toxins that also cause damage.

Organisms enter the body in contaminated food (e.g., *Salmonella* organisms in undercooked eggs and chicken) or contaminated drinking water (e.g., *G. lamblia* in contaminated lakes or pools). Travellers often get diarrhea, especially if they travel to countries with poorer sanitation than their own. An infection can also be transmitted from one individual to another via the fecal–oral route. For example, adult day care workers can transmit infection from one resident to another if they do not wash their hands thoroughly after changing soiled linen.

An individual's susceptibility to pathogenic organisms is influenced by age, gastric acidity, intestinal microflora, and immuno-competence. Older adults are most likely to suffer life-threatening diarrhea. Since stomach acid kills ingested pathogens, medications designed to decrease stomach acid (e.g., proton pump inhibitors and histamine [H_2]-receptor blockers) increase the likelihood that pathogens will survive (Blush & Matzo, 2012).

The healthy human colon contains short-chain fatty acids and bacteria such as *E. coli*. These organisms aid in fermentation and provide a microbial barrier against pathogenic bacteria. Antibiotics kill off the normal flora, making the individual more susceptible to pathogenic organisms. For example, patients receiving broad-spectrum antibiotics (e.g., clindamycin, cephalosporins, fluoroquinolones) are susceptible to pathogenic strains of *C. difficile*. *C. difficile* is the most serious antibiotic-associated diarrhea and is becoming more prevalent. Probiotics, in particular *Saccharomyces boulardii* and *Lactobacillus*, may be helpful in preventing antibiotic-induced diarrhea in some patients (Johnston, Ma, Goldenberg, et al., 2012).

People who are immuno-compromised because of disease (e.g., human immunodeficiency virus [HIV]) or immuno-suppressive medications are susceptible to gastro-intestinal (GI) tract infection.

TABLE 45-1   CAUSES OF DIARRHEA

Decreased Fluid Absorption
- Oral intake of poorly absorbable solutes (e.g., laxatives)
- Maldigestion and malabsorption
- Mucosal damage: celiac disease, inflammatory bowel disease, radiation injury, ischemic bowel
- Pancreatic insufficiency (e.g., cystic fibrosis)
- Intestinal enzyme deficiencies (e.g., lactase)
- Bile salt deficiency
- Decreased surface area (e.g., intestinal resection, short gut syndrome)

Increased Fluid Secretion
- Infectious: bacterial endotoxins (e.g., cholera, *Escherichia coli, Shigella, Salmonella, Staphylococcus, Clostridium difficile,* viral agents [rotavirus], and parasitic agents [*Giardia lamblia*])
- Drugs: laxatives, antibiotics, suspensions, or elixirs containing sorbitol
- Foods: candy, gum, and mints containing sorbitol
- Hormonal: vasoactive intestinal polypeptide secretion from adenoma of the pancreas; gastrin secretion caused by Zollinger–Ellison syndrome; calcitonin secretion from carcinoma of the thyroid
- Tumour: villous adenoma

Motility Disturbances
- Irritable bowel syndrome: ↑ visceral sensitivity and transit
- Diabetic enteropathy: ↑ transit secondary to autonomic neuropathy
- Gastrectomy: ↑ transit as a result of dumping syndrome

TABLE 45-2   CAUSES OF ACUTE INFECTIOUS DIARRHEA

	Onset	Duration	Symptoms and Signs
Viral			
Rotavirus	18–24 hr	3–8 days	Fever, vomiting, and profuse watery diarrhea
Norwalk virus	18–24 hr	24–48 hr	Nausea, vomiting, diarrhea, stomach cramping
Bacterial			
Escherichia coli	4–24 hr	3–4 days	Four or five loose stools per day, nausea, malaise, low-grade fever
Enterohemorrhagic E. coli (O157:H7)	4–24 hr	4–9 days	Bloody diarrhea, severe cramping, fever
Shigella	24 hr	7 days	Watery stools containing blood and mucus; tenesmus, urgency, severe cramping, fever
Salmonella	6–48 hr	2–5 days	Watery diarrhea, nausea, vomiting, abdominal cramps, fever
Campylobacter species	24 hr	<7 days	Profuse, watery diarrhea; malaise, nausea, abdominal cramps, low-grade fever
Clostridium perfringens	8–12 hr	24 hr	Watery diarrhea, abdominal cramps, vomiting
Clostridium difficile	4–9 days after start of antibiotics	24 hr	Associated with antibiotic treatment; symptoms range from mild, watery diarrhea to severe abdominal pain, fever, leukocytosis, leukocytes in stool
Parasitic			
Giardia lamblia	1–3 wk	Few days to 3 months	Sudden onset; malodorous, explosive, watery diarrhea; flatulence, epigastric pain and cramping, nausea
Entamoeba histolytica	4 days	Weeks to months	Frequent soft stools with blood and mucus (in severe cases, watery stools), flatulence, distension, abdominal cramps, fever, leukocytes in stool
Cryptosporidium	2–10 days	1–6 months	Watery diarrhea, nausea, vomiting, abdominal cramps, weight loss in AIDS

AIDS, acquired immune deficiency syndrome.

Not all diarrhea is due to infection. For example, drugs and specific food intolerances can cause diarrhea. Also, large amounts of undigested carbohydrate in the bowel produce an osmotic diarrhea that promotes rapid transit and prevents absorption of fluid and electrolytes. Lactose intolerance and certain laxatives (e.g., lactulose, sodium phosphate, magnesium citrate) produce an osmotic diarrhea. Bile salts and undigested fats also lead to excessive fluid secretion in the GI tract. The diarrhea from celiac disease and short bowel syndrome results from malabsorption in the small intestine.

Clinical Manifestations

Diarrhea may be acute or chronic. Acute diarrhea most commonly results from infection. Bacterial or viral infection of the intestine may result in explosive watery diarrhea, tenesmus (spasmodic contraction of the anal sphincter, with pain and persistent desire to defecate), and cramping abdominal pain. Perianal skin irritation may also develop. Systemic manifestations include fever, nausea, vomiting, and malaise. Leukocytes, blood, and mucus may be present in the stool, depending on the causative agent (see Table 45-2). Acute diarrhea is often self-limiting in the adult. Symptoms continue until the irritant or the causative agent is excreted. The mucous membrane lining of the GI tract is composed of epithelial cells, which regenerate following the inflammatory response.

Diarrhea is considered chronic when it persists for at least 2 weeks or when it subsides and returns more than 2 to 4 weeks after the initial episode. Severe diarrhea may be debilitating and life-threatening. A patient may have severe dehydration (water and sodium loss) and electrolyte disturbances (e.g., hypokalemia). Malabsorption and malnutrition are also sequelae of chronic diarrhea. Throughout the world, diarrhea is one of the major causes of death.

Diagnostic Studies

Accurate diagnosis and management of diarrhea require a thorough history, physical examination, and when indicated, laboratory tests. A thorough history, including history of travel, medication use, diet and food allergies, previous surgery and adjunctive therapies, interpersonal contacts, and family history should be obtained. Blood tests may identify anemia, elevated white blood cell (WBC) count, iron and folate deficiencies, elevated liver enzyme levels, and electrolyte disturbances. Stools may be examined for the presence of blood, mucus, WBCs, and ova and parasites. Stool cultures help to identify infectious organisms.

In a patient with chronic diarrhea, measurement of stool electrolytes, pH, and osmolality may help determine whether the diarrhea is related to decreased fluid absorption or increased fluid secretion (secretory diarrhea). Measurement of stool fat and undigested muscle fibre may indicate fat and protein malabsorption conditions, including pancreatic insufficiency. Elevated serum levels of GI hormones such as vasoactive intestinal polypeptide and gastrin may be present in some patients with secretory diarrhea. Endoscopy may be used to examine the mucosa and to obtain specimens via biopsy for examination. Upper and lower radiographic studies with barium contrast may be helpful in detecting mucosal disease as well as structural abnormalities.

Collaborative Care

The treatment of diarrhea is based on the cause and aimed at replacing fluid and electrolytes and decreasing the number, volume, and frequency of stools. Oral solutions containing glucose and electrolytes (e.g., Pedialyte) may be sufficient to replace losses

TABLE 45-3 DRUG THERAPY

Antidiarrheal Drugs

Type	Mechanism of Action	Examples
Demulcent	Soothes, coats, and protects mucous membranes	bismuth subsalicylate* (Pepto-Bismol); calcium polycarbophil
Anticholinergic (combination products)	Inhibits GI motility	diphenoxylate with atropine sulphate (Lomotil), loperamide (Imodium)†‡
Antisecretory	Decreases intestinal secretion	octreotide (Sandostatin), a synthetic analogue of somatostatin
Opioid	Decreases CNS stimulation of GI tract motility and secretion; directly inhibits GI motility	codeine
Probiotics	Alters balance of intestinal flora	*Saccharomyces*, *Lactobacillus*

CNS, central nervous system; *GI*, gastro-intestinal.
*Also inhibits bacterial activity.
†Also absorbent, which contributes to the adhesiveness of the stool.
‡Has cholinergic and noncholinergic actions.

from mild diarrhea. In situations of severe diarrhea, parenteral administration of fluids, electrolytes, vitamins, and nutrition is warranted.

Once the cause of the diarrhea has been determined, pharmaceutical agents may be given to coat and protect mucous membranes, absorb irritating substances, inhibit GI motility, decrease intestinal secretions, and decrease central nervous system stimulation of the GI tract (Table 45-3). Patients with infectious diarrhea are not given antidiarrheal agents because of the potential of prolonging exposure to the infectious agent. Regardless of the cause of diarrhea, antidiarrheal drugs should not be given for a prolonged time.

Antibiotics are reserved for treating specific bacterial organisms. Antibiotics can cause diarrhea by altering the normal bowel flora. Patients receiving antibiotics (e.g., clindamycin) are susceptible to *Clostridium difficile (C. difficile)* infection.

C. difficile is a Gram-positive, spore-forming bacterium that causes diarrhea and serious intestinal problems such as pseudomembranous colitis (Goldberg, Bhalodia, Jacob, et al., 2015). *C. difficile* is the most common cause of infectious diarrhea in the developed world and one of the most common infections in both hospitals and long-term care facilities in Canada. Health care workers should follow infection control precautions to prevent transmission of *C. difficile* from patient to patient (Table 45-4). Symptoms of *C. difficile* include watery diarrhea with or without blood (at least three bowel movements per day for 2 or more days), fever, loss of appetite, nausea, and abdominal pain or tenderness.

This bacterium has been found to be present in normal bowel flora as well as in the genito-urinary tract, in abdominal wounds, and on the skin of hospital workers. Patients entering hospitals may already be colonized with *C. difficile,* although healthy people are not usually vulnerable to the organism. Prolonged antibiotic therapy, cytotoxic chemotherapy, and advanced age are risk factors that may affect the bowel's resistance to colonization or its ability to suppress competing organisms, thus enhancing the growth of *C. difficile.* Laboratory confirmation may be made on the basis

TABLE 45-4	HANDWASHING TO PREVENT HEALTH CARE–ASSOCIATED INFECTIONS

The Four Moments for Hand Hygiene in Health Care
1. BEFORE initial patient–patient environment contact
2. BEFORE aseptic procedure
3. AFTER body fluid exposure risk
4. AFTER patient–patient environment contact

Source: Adapted from Public Health Ontario. (2016). Just clean your hands—your 4 moments for hand hygiene. Retrieved from *http://www.publichealthontario.ca/en/ BrowseByTopic/InfectiousDiseases/JustCleanYourHands/Pages/Just-Clean-Your-Hands.aspx?_ga=1.252110089.1468344323.1452279958.*

of a single, unpreserved stool sample. Metronidazole (Flagyl) is the first-line therapy for this infection, followed by vancomycin. Fidaxomicin (Dificid) is also approved to treat *C. difficile*, but the cost precludes its use as a first line agent (Leong & Zelenitsky, 2013).

NURSING MANAGEMENT
ACUTE INFECTIOUS DIARRHEA

NURSING ASSESSMENT

Nursing assessment should begin with a thorough history and physical examination (Table 45-5). The patient should be asked to describe the stool pattern and associated symptoms. Questions should focus on duration of diarrhea and frequency, character, and consistency of stool. A medication history should include use of antibiotics, laxatives, and other drugs known to cause diarrhea. Recent travel, stress, and health and family illnesses should be discussed. Dietary history should include questions about eating habits, appetite, and food intolerances, especially milk and dairy products, as well as food preparation practices.

Physical examination begins with obtaining vital signs, height, and weight. The patient's skin should be inspected for decreased turgor, dryness, and areas of breakdown. The abdomen should be inspected for distension, auscultated for bowel sounds, and palpated for tenderness.

NURSING DIAGNOSES

Nursing diagnoses for the patient with acute infectious diarrhea may include, but are not limited to, the following:
- *Diarrhea* related to *infection*
- *Deficient fluid volume* related to *insufficient fluid intake, excessive fluid loss through abnormal route*

For additional information on nursing diagnoses for diarrhea, see those presented in Nursing Care Plan (NCP) 45-1, available on the Evolve website.

PLANNING

The overall goals are that the patient with diarrhea will (1) not transmit the microorganism causing the infectious diarrhea, (2) cease having diarrhea and resume normal bowel patterns, (3) have normal fluid and electrolyte and acid–base balance, (4) have normal nutritional intake, and (5) have no perianal skin breakdown.

NURSING IMPLEMENTATION

Adherence to appropriate infection control practices and precautions (see Chapter 17, Table 17-8) is important, and all cases

TABLE 45-5	NURSING ASSESSMENT

Diarrhea

Subjective Data
Important Health Information
Past health history: Recent travel, infections, stress; diverticulitis or malabsorption; metabolic disorders; inflammatory bowel disease; irritable bowel syndrome; chronic laxative abuse
Medications: Use of laxatives, magnesium-containing antacids, sorbitol-containing suspensions or elixirs, antibiotics, methyldopa, digitalis, colchicine; OTC antidiarrheal medications
Surgery or other treatments: Stomach or bowel surgery, radiation

Symptoms
- Malaise
- Food intolerances; anorexia, nausea, vomiting; weight loss; thirst
- Increased stool frequency, volume and looseness; change in colour and character of stools; steatorrhea, abdominal bloating; decreased urinary output
- Abdominal tenderness, abdominal pain and cramping; tenesmus

Objective Data
General
Lethargy, sunken eyeballs, fever, malnutrition

Integumentary
Pallor, dry mucous membranes, poor skin turgor, perianal irritation

Gastro-Intestinal
Frequent soft to liquid stools that may alternate with constipation; altered stool colour; abdominal distension, hyperactive bowel sounds; presence of pus, blood, mucus, or fat in stools; fecal impaction

Urinary Tract
Decreased output, concentrated urine

Possible Findings
Abnormal serum electrolyte levels; anemia; leukocytosis; eosinophilia; hypoalbuminemia; positive stool cultures; presence of ova, parasites, leukocytes, blood, or fat in stool; abnormal sigmoidoscopic or colonoscopic findings; abnormal lower GI series (barium enema study)

GI, gastro-intestinal; OTC, over-the-counter.

of acute diarrhea should be considered infectious until the cause is determined. The use of precautions is effective in reducing the spread of infectious diarrhea.

Handwashing is the most important measure in preventing the transfer of microorganisms. Hands should be washed before and after contact with each patient and when body fluids of any kind are handled. The patient should be taught the principles of hygiene, infection control practices and precautions, and the potential dangers of an illness that is infectious to themselves and others. Family and visitors should also be advised of precautions. Proper handling, cooking, and storage of food should be discussed with the patient suspected of having infectious diarrhea.

Best practice guidelines for the management of *C. difficile* (see the Resources at the end of this chapter) state that all patients suspected of having *C. difficile* should be placed in a single room with dedicated toileting facilities such as a private bathroom or individual commode chair. When the number of patients with *C. difficile* exceeds the institution's single-room capacity, those patients with confirmed *C. difficile* may share a room. For patients in multi-bed rooms, the following precautions should be observed:

1. Signage indicating the precautions to be used should be visibly displayed.
2. A barrier supply cart should be easily accessible.
3. A laundry hamper should be placed as close to the patient's bed space as possible.
4. A commode chair should be dedicated for the patient's use.

Signage indicating that contact precautions are to be used should be posted on the door of any room of a patient with suspected or confirmed *C. difficile*. The nurse should ensure that appropriate environmental cleaning is taking place, including twice-daily cleaning with a hospital-grade disinfectant of all horizontal surfaces in the room and all items within reach of patients with suspected or confirmed *C. difficile*. Visitors should receive instruction from the nurse regarding the nature of *C. difficile* and the importance of hand hygiene and how to properly carry it out. Soap and warm water is recommended because alcohol-based hand sanitizers do not effectively destroy *C. difficile* spores. If a visitor is providing care for a patient or having significant contact with the patient's immediate environment, the visitor should wear gloves and gown. The visitor should also receive instruction from the nurse on the correct use of personal protective equipment and be instructed not to use the patient's toilet or go into other patients' rooms. Chapter 17 discusses contact precautions.

FECAL INCONTINENCE

Etiology and Pathophysiology

Fecal incontinence, or the involuntary passage of stool, may result from multiple causes (Table 45-6). It is important to have an understanding of normal fecal continence to understand fecal incontinence. Normally, fecal contents pass from the sigmoid colon into the rectum, causing rectal distension. Sensory (stretch) receptors in the muscles surrounding the rectum provide the sensation of rectal filling. This causes a reflex relaxation of the internal anal sphincter and contraction of the external anal sphincter. Sensory receptors in the epithelium of the anal canal can usually distinguish among solid, liquid, and gas. The combination of contraction of the abdominal muscles, relaxation of the pelvic muscles, squatting (which straightens the anorectal angle), and voluntary relaxation of the external anal sphincter allows for elimination of feces. Therefore, motor (contraction of muscles) or sensory (ability to perceive presence of stool or to experience the urge to defecate) problems or their combination can result in fecal incontinence. In addition, fecal incontinence can be secondary to **fecal impaction**, which is an accumulation of hardened feces in the rectum or the sigmoid colon that the individual is unable to move. Fecal incontinence caused by fecal impaction is a common problem in older adults.

Diagnostic Studies and Collaborative Care

The diagnosis and effective management of fecal incontinence require a thorough health history and physical examination, with appropriate diagnostic studies. In all cases, a rectal examination should be performed, followed by examination with a flexible sigmoidoscope. Fecal impaction, internal prolapse, increased perineal descent, and rectocele may be identified by rectal examination. If the impaction is higher in the colon, an abdominal radiograph may be helpful. Flexible sigmoidoscopy may identify inflammation, tumours, fissures, and other sigmoid–rectal pathological conditions. Other studies may include barium enema, colonoscopy, endorectal ultrasound, and anorectal manometry.

Treatment of incontinence depends on the cause. If fecal incontinence is related to noninfectious diarrhea, dietary changes may be advised, and antidiarrheal agents may be prescribed. In contrast, the management of rectoceles (a defect of the recto-vaginal septum) may include teaching the patient exercises to strengthen the muscles of the pelvic floor (Kegel exercises), insertion of a vaginal pessary, and in some cases, surgery.

Fecal impaction usually resolves after manual disimpaction and use of lubricants and cleansing enemas. To prevent recurrence, a high-fibre diet (see Table 45-9, later in this chapter), along with increased fluid intake, should be given unless contraindicated. Dietary fibre supplements or bulk-forming laxatives (e.g., psyllium) can improve continence by increasing stool bulk, firming consistency, and promoting sensation of rectal filling. Protection of perianal skin and the use of appropriate fecal containment devices (e.g., perianal pouches or adult briefs) will help to protect skin and promote patient comfort and dignity.

Biofeedback therapy may be an option for the patient. This therapy is intended to (1) improve awareness of rectal sensation and coordination of the internal and external anal sphincters and (2) increase the strength of contraction of the external sphincter (Fargo & Latimer, 2012). Biofeedback training requires adequate mental status and motivation to learn. It is a safe, painless, and inexpensive treatment for fecal incontinence. (Biofeedback is discussed further in Chapter 12.)

Surgery (e.g., sphincter repair procedures, diverting ostomy) should be considered only when conservative treatment fails.

NURSING MANAGEMENT
FECAL INCONTINENCE

NURSING ASSESSMENT

Fecal incontinence is not only an embarrassment to the patient but also a potential hazard to the patient's normal skin integrity.

TABLE 45-6 CAUSES OF FECAL INCONTINENCE

Traumatic
- Anorectal surgery
- Fistulectomy
- Hemorrhoidectomy
- Abdominal surgery (e.g., nerve injury)
- Traumatic injuries (e.g., gunshot wounds, impalements, foreign body insertion)
- Traumatic childbirth
- Sexual abuse
- Anal intercourse

Neurological
- Degenerative diseases
- Dementia
- Diabetes mellitus (secondary to neuropathic changes)
- Multiple sclerosis
- Spinal cord injuries
- Spinal cord tumour
- Stroke

Inflammatory
- Infection
- Radiation
- Inflammatory bowel disease

Other
- Diarrhea
- Fecal impaction
- Loss of rectal elasticity

Pelvic Floor Dysfunction
- Medications
- Rectal prolapse

Functional
- Physical or mobility impairments affecting toileting ability

An assessment of the patient's general condition is necessary to identify the best alternative for managing the patient with fecal incontinence. The health care provider should identify normal bowel habits and current symptoms, including stool frequency and consistency. Information about the passage of blood or mucus, pain during defecation, and a feeling of incomplete evacuation is sought. The health care provider determines whether the patient has defecation urgency and is aware of leaking stool. It should be determined whether there is coexisting urinary incontinence.

Assessment should also include history of multiple or traumatic childbirths, previous anorectal surgery, and injury. A neurological assessment that includes evaluation of mental status can be helpful in identifying the most effective treatment for the patient.

NURSING DIAGNOSES

Nursing diagnoses for the patient with fecal incontinence include, but are not limited to, the following:

- *Bowel incontinence* related to *generalized decline in muscle tone* (dysfunctional rectal sphincter)
- *Risk for falls* related to *diarrhea, incontinence*
- *Toileting self-care deficit* related to *impaired ability to transfer, impaired mobility*
- *Risk for situational low self-esteem* related to *decrease in control over environment* (inability to control bowel movements, hospital isolation protocols)
- *Risk for impaired skin integrity* as evidenced by *excretions* (incontinence of stool)
- *Social isolation* related to *social behaviour incongruent with norms* (bowel incontinence)

PLANNING

The overall goals are that the patient with fecal incontinence will (1) have normal bowel control, (2) maintain perianal skin integrity, and (3) not suffer any self-esteem problems related to problems with bowel control.

NURSING IMPLEMENTATION

If appropriate, prevention and treatment of fecal incontinence may be managed by implementing a bowel training program. Bowel training is effective in many patients because, once the bowel is empty, the rectum does not fill until the next day. The lack of stool in the rectum reduces the likelihood of incontinence. The patient should be assisted to a commode or bathroom at a regular time daily to assist with re-establishment of bowel regularity. A good time to establish this pattern is within 30 minutes after breakfast. Most individuals experience an urge to defecate following the first meal of the day because of the gastrocolic reflex. If the usual bowel habits differ from this pattern, efforts should be made to adhere to the patient's individual timing. Patients are at risk for injury owing to falls related to their inability to control bowel evacuation and attempting to reach a bathroom in time. Safety measures should be implemented to prevent this. Best practice guidelines on the prevention of falls are available from the Registered Nurses' Association of Ontario (RNAO) (2011a).

If these techniques are ineffective in re-establishing bowel regularity, a bisacodyl (Dulcolax) or glycerin suppository or a small phosphate enema may be administered 15 to 30 minutes before the usual evacuation time. These preparations stimulate the anorectal reflex and often can be discontinued when a regular pattern is re-established.

Maintenance of skin integrity is important, especially in patients who are bedridden or older-adult patients. Nursing management may necessitate the use of fecal containment devices, incontinence briefs, and meticulous skin care. Rectal tubes and catheters are usually not recommended because their use for an extended period may decrease responsiveness of the rectal sphincter and cause ulceration or perforation of the rectal mucosa. Use of incontinence briefs may be helpful in maintaining skin integrity if changed frequently. Meticulous cleaning after each stool is required. Gentle washing, rinsing, thorough drying, and application of a protective barrier cream with each bowel movement are essential to the maintenance of skin integrity. Monitor the skin for the development of yeast or fungal infections.

Perianal pouching is an alternative in the management of fecal incontinence. These are pouches similar in appearance to one-piece ostomy pouches that are designed to be applied over the anus, allowing for the collection of stool. Pouching provides skin protection, odour control, fecal containment, comfort, and dignity. Because odour is often a problem, deodorant sprays and room deodorizers may be used. For the patient who is ambulatory, a regular chair or special tilt commode wheelchair may be used. Regardless of the patient's mobility, the nurse must make sure the skin is clean and intact and the odour is controlled.

CONSTIPATION

Constipation is a decrease in frequency of bowel movements from what is "normal" for the individual; hard, difficult-to-pass stools; a decrease in stool volume; retention of feces in the rectum; or some combination of these problems. Because individuals vary, it is important to compare current symptoms with the patient's normal pattern of elimination. It is also important to remember that changes in bowel habits may indicate bowel obstruction produced by an underlying disease process, such as a tumour.

Etiology and Pathophysiology

Constipation may be caused by insufficient dietary fibre, inadequate fluid intake, medications, and lack of exercise. If proper preventive measures are subsequently taken, constipation should not recur. Constipation may also occur as a result of behaviours related to sociocultural beliefs, environmental constraints, ignoring the urge to defecate, chronic laxative abuse, and multiple organic causes. Changes in diet, mealtime, or daily routines are a few environmental factors that may cause constipation. Depression and stress can also result in constipation.

Some patients believe that they are constipated if they do not have a daily bowel movement. This can result in chronic laxative use and subsequent cathartic colon syndrome. In this condition, the colon becomes dilated and *atonic* (lacking muscle tone).

Ignoring the urge to defecate for a time causes the muscles and mucosa in the rectal area to become insensitive to the presence of feces. In addition, the prolonged retention of feces in the rectum results in drying of the stool because of the absorption of water. The harder and drier the feces, the more difficult they are to expel.

Clinical Manifestations

The clinical presentation of constipation may vary from a chronic discomfort to an acute event mimicking an "acute abdomen." Other clinical manifestations are presented in Table 45-7. Hemorrhoids, or dilated hemorrhoidal veins or varicosities, are the most common complication of chronic constipation. They result from venous engorgement caused by repeated executions

TABLE 45-7	CLINICAL MANIFESTATIONS OF CONSTIPATION
• Abdominal distension or bloating • Abdominal pain • Anorexia • Decreased frequency of bowel movements • Hard, dry stool • Headache • Increased flatulence	• Increased rectal pressure • Nausea • Palpable mass • Stone- or rock-shaped stool (fecalith) • Stool with blood • Straining • Tenesmus

of the Valsalva manoeuvre (straining) and venous compression from hard, impacted stool. (Hemorrhoids are further discussed later in this chapter, in the section on anorectal problems.)

The Valsalva manoeuvre is a manoeuvre that involves contraction of the chest muscles on a closed glottis with simultaneous contraction of the abdominal muscles; it is used during straining to pass a hardened stool and may cause serious problems in patients with heart failure, cerebral edema, hypertension, and coronary artery disease. During straining, the patient takes a deep inspiration, the breath is held, and the glottis closes and traps the air. Simultaneously with the contraction of the chest muscles against the closed airway, the abdominal muscles contract and try to push against the colon. Increases in intra-abdominal pressure and intrathoracic pressure occur, reducing venous return to the heart. The heart slows (bradycardia) temporarily, cardiac output is decreased, and there is a transient drop in arterial pressure. When the patient relaxes, there is decreased thoracic pressure and a sudden flow of blood into the heart, causing distension and an increase in heart rate. Immediately, arterial pressure rises momentarily. These changes may be fatal for the patient who cannot compensate for sudden overload of blood flow returning to the heart.

Constipation may contribute to diverticulosis. Diverticula are thought to be caused by increased intraluminal pressure and decreased intestinal compliance. Diverticulosis and diverticulitis are described later in this chapter.

In the presence of *obstipation,* or fecal impaction secondary to constipation, colonic perforation may occur. Perforation, which is life-threatening, causes abdominal pain, nausea, vomiting, fever, and an elevated WBC count. An abdominal radiograph shows the presence of free air, which is diagnostic of perforation. Anal fissures and rectal mucosal ulcers may also occur as a result of stool stasis or straining.

Diagnostic Studies and Collaborative Care

A thorough history and physical examination should be performed to determine the underlying cause of constipation and initiate treatment. Abdominal radiographs, barium enema, colonoscopy, sigmoidoscopy, and anorectal manometry may be helpful in the diagnosis. Many cases of constipation can be managed with diet therapy, including increased intake of fibre and fluids and an exercise program. Consult a dietitian to review dietary influences. Laxatives (Table 45-8) should be used cautiously because with chronic overuse, they may contribute to ongoing constipation. A stepwise approach for laxative use that progresses from bulk-forming fibre preparations to stimulants is recommended, depending on the acuteness of the constipation episode. Enemas are fast-acting and are beneficial in the immediate treatment of constipation, but their use for long-term treatment of constipation

should be limited. Soapsuds enemas should be avoided because they may lead to inflammation of colonic mucosa. Excessive hypotonic enemas with tap water can cause water excess, and sodium phosphate enemas have been associated with electrolyte imbalances. Oil-retention enemas may be used to soften fecal impactions. Biofeedback therapy may benefit patients who are constipated as a result of *anismus* (uncoordinated contraction of the anal sphincter during straining). Methylnaltrexone (Relistor) is a peripheral μ-opiate receptor antagonist that decreases constipation caused by opioid use. The drug is administered subcutaneously. This agent does not block the analgesic effects (Rx Files Academic Detailing Program, 2014).

Nurses must educate patients in whom the perception of constipation is related to beliefs and misinformation about bowel function. Appropriate information on normal bowel function must be given and discussed along with information on the adverse consequences of excessive use of laxatives and enemas.

A patient with severe constipation related to bowel motility or mechanical disorders may require more intensive treatment. Diagnostic studies such as anorectal manometry, GI tract transit studies, and sigmoidoscopic rectal biopsies should be performed before treatment.

Nutritional Therapy. Diet is an important factor in the prevention of constipation. Many patients experience an improvement in their symptoms when they simply increase their intake of dietary fibre and fluids. Dietary fibre is found in two forms: insoluble and soluble in water. Both are contained in most foods, but some foods are higher in soluble fibre (Table 45-9).

Insoluble fibre, which is found in higher concentrations in whole wheat and bran, remains essentially unchanged by the time it reaches the colon. Soluble fibres form gel-like substances that add viscosity to the digested contents, causing decreased gastric emptying and increased transit in the small intestine. When these fibres ferment and form gas, the gas increases stool bulk, promoting defecation and sequestering fluid, which softens stools. Soluble fibre is found in oat bran, fruits, vegetables, and psyllium. Patients should be told that fibre will increase gas production initially but that this effect decreases with time.

The diet should also include a fluid intake of at least 3 000 mL/day, unless contraindicated by cardiac or renal disease. Increasing fibre intake without increasing fluids may predispose the patient to worsening constipation, impaction, or obstruction. The nurse should consult a dietitian to help with patient food preferences and access. The patient's understanding of the diet and the importance of dietary fibre is important for ensuring compliance.

NURSING MANAGEMENT CONSTIPATION

NURSING ASSESSMENT

Subjective and objective data that should be obtained from a patient with constipation are presented in Table 45-10.

NURSING DIAGNOSES

Nursing diagnoses for the patient with constipation can include, but are not limited to, the following:

• *Constipation* related to *decrease in gastrointestinal motility, dehydration*

PLANNING

The overall goals are that the patient with constipation will (1) increase dietary intake of fibre and fluids; (2) have the passage

TABLE 45-8 DRUG THERAPY

Cathartic Agents

Category	Mechanisms of Action	Example	Onset of Action	Comments
Bulk-forming	Absorb water; increase bulk-stimulating peristalsis	Psyllium: Metamucil	Usually within 24 hr	Must be taken with adequate fluids; can increase gas; contraindicated in patients with possible obstruction or known strictures
Stool softeners and lubricants	Lubricate intestinal tract and soften feces, making hard stools easier to pass; do not affect peristalsis	Mineral oil, docusate calcium, docusate sodium (Colace)	Softeners up to 72 hr; lubricants up to 8 hr	Can block absorption of fat-soluble vitamins A, D, E, and K
Saline and osmotic solutions	Cause retention of fluid in intestinal lumen due to osmotic effect	Magnesium salts: magnesium citrate, magnesium hydroxide (milk of magnesia) Sodium phosphates: Fleet enema, Fleet Phospho-Soda oral solution Lactulose Polyethylene glycol saline solutions: PegLyte, GoLYTELY, Colyte	15 min–3 hr	Magnesium-containing products may cause hypermagnesemia in patients with renal insufficiency; sodium phosphate products may cause electrolyte imbalances in patients with renal insufficiency (increased sodium, increased phosphate, decreased calcium)
Stimulants	Increase peristalsis by irritating colon wall and stimulating enteric nerves	Anthraquinone drugs: cascara sagrada, senna (Senokot) bisacodyl (Dulcolax)	Usually within 12 hr	Can cause melanosis coli (brown or black pigmentation of colon); are most widely abused laxatives; should not be used in patients with impaction or obstipation
Selective chloride channel activator	Increases intestinal fluid secretion and motility	lubiprostone (Amitiza)	Usually within 24 hr	Used in the treatment of idiopathic constipation and irritable bowel syndrome with constipation (women only) Contraindicated in patients with history of mechanical GI obstruction
Intestinal secretagogue	Increases fluid secretion and accelerates intestinal transit	linaclotide (Constella)	Usually within 24 hr	Used in the treatment of idiopathic constipation and irritable bowel syndrome with constipation (men and women)

of soft, formed stools; and (3) not have any complications, such as bleeding hemorrhoids.

NURSING IMPLEMENTATION

Nursing management should be based on the patient's symptoms (see Table 45-7) and the assessment of the patient (see Table 45-10). An important role of the nurse is teaching the patient the importance of dietary measures to prevent constipation. A patient and caregiver teaching guide for constipation is presented in Table 45-11. Additional constipation guidelines are readily available, including those developed by the Registered Nurses' Association of Ontario (2011b). Emphasis should be placed on maintenance of a high-fibre diet, increased fluid intake, and a regular exercise program. The patient should be taught to (1) establish a regular meal pattern, (2) maintain a regular time to defecate, and (3) avoid suppressing the urge to defecate. In many people, the urge to defecate occurs after breakfast because of the stimulation of the gastrocolic reflex. The patient should be discouraged from using laxatives and enemas to achieve and maintain fecal elimination.

Proper position is important when defecating. For a patient in bed, the bedpan should be placed and the head of the bed should be elevated as high as the patient can tolerate. For the person who can sit on a toilet, a footstool may be placed in front of the toilet. Placing the feet on the footstool promotes flexion of the hips, which assists in defecation. For those requiring commodes, tilt commodes may provide proper positioning.

The patient with poor muscle tone should be assessed by a physiotherapist for abdominal muscle strength and taught to contract the abdominal muscles several times a day. Sit-ups and straight leg raises can also be used to improve abdominal muscle tone.

ACUTE ABDOMINAL PAIN

Etiology and Pathophysiology

The causes of an acute onset of abdominal pain ("acute abdomen") are varied and can include conditions related to inflammation, peritonitis, obstruction, and internal bleeding (Table 45-12).

TABLE 45-9 NUTRITIONAL THERAPY

High-Fibre Foods*

	Fibre per Serving (g)	Size of Serving	Calories of Serving
Vegetables			
Asparagus	3.5	½ cup	18
Beans			
• Navy	8.4	½ cup	80
• Kidney	9.7	½ cup	94
• Lima	8.3	½ cup	63
• Pinto	8.9	½ cup	78
• String	2.1	½ cup	18
Broccoli	3.5	½ cup	18
Carrots, raw	1.8	½ cup	15
Corn	2.6	½ medium ear	72
Peas, canned	6.7	½ cup	63
Potatoes			
• Baked	1.9	½ medium	72
• Sweet	2.1	½ medium	79
Squash, acorn	7.0	1 cup	82
Tomato, raw	1.5	1 small	18
Fruits			
Apple	2.0	½ large	42
Banana	1.5	½ medium	48
Blackberries	6.7	¾ cup	40
Orange	1.6	1 small	35
Peach	2.3	1 medium	38
Pear	2.0	½ medium	44
Raspberries	9.2	1 cup	42
Strawberries	3.1	1 cup	45
Grain Products			
Bread			
• Rye	0.8	1 slice	62
• White	0.7	1 slice	64
• Whole wheat	1.3	1 slice	59
Cereal			
• All-Bran (100%)	8.4	⅓ cup	70
• Corn Flakes	2.6	¾ cup	70
• Shredded Wheat	2.8	1 biscuit	70
Crackers, Graham	1.4	2 squares	53
Popcorn	3.0	3 cups	62
Rice			
• Brown	1.6	⅓ cup	72
• White	0.5	⅓ cup	76

*Recommended for patients with diverticulosis, irritable bowel syndrome, constipation, hemorrhoids, atherosclerosis, dyslipidemia, and diabetes mellitus.

Clinical Manifestations

Pain is the presenting symptom of greatest relevance for acute abdominal pain. The patient may also complain of abdominal tenderness, nausea, vomiting, diarrhea, constipation, flatulence, fatigue, fever, and abdominal distension.

Diagnostic Studies and Collaborative Management

Many disorders must be ruled out before a diagnosis is confirmed. Diagnosis begins with a complete history and physical examination. Physical examination should include a rectal and pelvic examination. A complete blood cell count (CBC), urinalysis, an abdominal radiographic examination, and an electrocardiogram (ECG) are done initially. In women of child-bearing age who have acute abdominal pain, pregnancy tests should be performed

TABLE 45-10 NURSING ASSESSMENT

Constipation

Subjective Data
Important Health Information
Current health history: Chronic laxative or enema abuse; rigid beliefs regarding bowel routine; changes in diet or mealtime; inadequate fibre and fluid intake; immobility; change in daily activity routines; sedentary lifestyle
Past health history: Colorectal disease, neurological dysfunction, bowel obstruction, environmental changes, cancer, irritable bowel syndrome; history of chronic laxative or enema abuse
Medications: Use of aluminum and calcium antacids, anticholinergics, antidepressants, antihistamines, antipsychotics, diuretics, opioids, iron, laxatives, enemas

Symptoms
• Malaise
• Anorexia, nausea
• Hard, difficult-to-pass stool, decrease in frequency and amount of stools; flatus, abdominal distension; tenesmus, rectal pressure; fecal incontinence (if impacted)
• Dizziness, headache, anorectal pain; abdominal pain on defecation

Objective Data
General
Lethargy

Integumentary
Anorectal fissures, hemorrhoids

Gastro-Intestinal
Abdominal distension; hypoactive or absent bowel sounds; palpable abdominal mass, usually in LLQ; fecal impaction; small, hard, dry stool; stool streaked with blood

Possible Findings
Positive FOB; abdominal radiograph demonstrating stool in lower colon

FOB, fecal occult blood test; *LLQ,* left lower quadrant.

to rule out ectopic pregnancy. The findings of these studies may provide some information about the cause of the acute abdomen.

Emergency management of the patient with acute abdominal pain is presented in Table 45-13. The goal of management is to stabilize the patient's condition and to identify and treat the cause. When the patient is seen with an acute condition in the abdomen, the health care provider attempts to make a differential diagnosis because some causes of abdominal pain do not necessitate surgery (see Table 45-12). It was previously thought that pain medication should be withheld because analgesics might obscure progression of clinical manifestations and impede diagnosis. In fact, appropriate pain management that does not result in altered consciousness can decrease diffuse pain and abdominal rigidity and help localize the pain, leading to earlier diagnosis and treatment.

In addition to being a therapeutic measure, surgery can also be diagnostic. Operative exploration is done, usually after a careful examination, a review of the patient status, and a review of diagnostic test results. Surgical exploration may be done laparoscopically or through an open midline abdominal wound (laparotomy). Direct examination may permit the cause to be identified and allow for completion of the definitive procedure.

TABLE 45-11 PATIENT & CAREGIVER TEACHING GUIDE

Constipation

The following guidelines should be included when teaching the patient and caregiver(s) about constipation.

1. **Eat dietary fibre.**
   Eat 20 to 30 g of fibre per day. Gradually, over 1 to 2 weeks, increase the amount of fibre eaten. Fibre softens hard stools and adds bulk to stool, promoting evacuation.
   - Foods high in fibre: raw vegetables and fruits, beans, breakfast cereals (All-Bran, oatmeal)
   - Fibre supplements: Metamucil, Citrucel, FiberCon

2. **Drink fluids.**
   Drink 3 L/day. Drink water or fruit juices; avoid large volumes of caffeinated coffee, tea, and cola. Fluids soften hard stools; caffeine promotes fluid loss through urination.

3. **Exercise regularly.**
   Walk, swim, or bike at least three times per week. Contract and relax abdominal muscles when standing or by doing sit-ups to strengthen muscles and prevent straining. Exercise stimulates bowel motility and moves stool through the intestine.

4. **Establish a regular time to defecate.**
   First thing in the morning or after the first meal of the day is a good time because people often have the urge to defecate at this time.

5. **Do not delay defecation.**
   Respond to the urge to have a bowel movement as soon as possible. Persistently delaying defecation results in hard stools and a decreased "urge" to defecate. More water is absorbed from stool by the intestine over time. The intestine becomes less sensitive to the presence of stool in the rectum.

6. **Record your bowel elimination pattern.**
   Record bowel movements on a calendar. Regular monitoring of bowel movement will assist in early identification of a problem.

7. **Avoid laxatives and enemas.**
   Do not overuse laxatives and enemas. They may actually promote constipation because the normal motility of the bowel is interrupted and bowel habituation cannot occur.

TABLE 45-12 CAUSES OF ACUTE ABDOMINAL PAIN

• Abdominal penetrating trauma	• Mesenteric adenitis
• Acute ischemic bowel injury	• Pancreatitis
• Appendicitis	• Pelvic inflammatory disease
• Blunt abdominal trauma	• Peptic ulcer
• Bowel obstruction with perforation or necrosis	• Perforated gastro-intestinal malignancy
• Cholecystitis	• Peritonitis
• Crohn's disease	• Postcolonoscopy bowel perforation
• Diverticulitis ± peritonitis	• Ruptured abdominal aneurysm
• Foreign body perforation	• Ruptured ectopic pregnancy
• Gastritis	• Ruptured ovarian cyst
• Gastro-enteritis	• Ulcerative colitis ± toxic megacolon
• Incarcerated or strangulated hernias	• Uterine rupture
	• Volvulus

NURSING MANAGEMENT ACUTE ABDOMINAL PAIN

NURSING ASSESSMENT

Vital signs, including blood pressure and pulse rate, should be taken immediately to determine hypovolemic changes. An elevated temperature may indicate an inflammatory or infectious process. The abdomen should be inspected for distension, masses, abnormal pulsation, rashes, scars, and pigmentation changes. Bowel sounds should be auscultated. Bowel sounds that are diminished, absent, or hyperactive in a quadrant may indicate a complete bowel obstruction, acute peritonitis, or paralytic ileus. Palpation should be gentle.

A thorough assessment of the patient's symptoms should be made to determine onset, location, intensity, duration, frequency, and character of pain. The nurse should determine whether the pain has spread or moved to new locations (quadrants) as well as what makes the pain worse or better. It should also be determined whether the pain is associated with other symptoms, such as nausea, vomiting, changes in bowel and bladder habits, or vaginal discharge in women. Assessment of vomiting should include amount, colour, consistency, and odour of the vomitus. Bowel patterns and habits should also be assessed carefully.

NURSING DIAGNOSES

Nursing diagnoses for the patient with acute abdominal pain include, but are not limited to, the following:

- *Acute pain* related to *biological injury agent* (inflammation of the peritoneum, abdominal distention)
- *Risk for deficient fluid volume* as evidenced by *insufficient fluid intake* (inflammation or infection)
- *Anxiety* related to *threat to current status, threat of death*

PLANNING

The overall goals are that the patient with acute abdominal pain will have (1) resolution of the underlying process, (2) relief of abdominal pain, (3) freedom from complications (especially hypovolemic shock), and (4) normal nutritional status.

NURSING IMPLEMENTATION

Nursing interventions are based on the diagnosis and medical or surgical management of the patient. General care for the patient involves management of fluid and electrolyte imbalances, pain, and anxiety.

ACUTE INTERVENTION

Preoperative Care. Emergency preparation of the patient with acute abdominal pain is usually limited to a CBC, typing and crossmatching of blood, and clotting studies. Catheterization, administration of medications (e.g., antibiotics), and the passage of a nasogastric (NG) tube may be done in the emergency department or operating room. (General care of the preoperative patient is discussed in Chapter 20.)

Postoperative Care. Postoperative care depends on the type of surgical procedure performed. The increased use of laparoscopic procedures has reduced the risk for potential postoperative complications related to wound care and altered GI motility. These newer procedures generally result in shorter hospital stays. A general NCP for the postoperative patient is available on the Evolve website for Chapter 22. Nursing care for the patient following a laparotomy is presented in NCP 45-2, also on the Evolve website.

An NG tube may or may not be present in the patient returning from surgery. If present, the NG tube is connected to suction as ordered. The purpose of the NG tube is to empty the stomach of secretions and gas to prevent gastric distension. GI peristaltic activity is often impaired because of the manipulative procedures of the surgery and anaesthesia.

TABLE 45-13 EMERGENCY MANAGEMENT

Acute Abdominal Pain

Etiology	Assessment Findings	Interventions
Inflammation	**Abdominal and Gastro-Intestinal Findings**	**Initial**
• Appendicitis	• Diffuse, localized, dull, burning, or sharp abdominal pain or tenderness	• Ensure patent airway.
• Cholecystitis	• Rebound tenderness and guarding	• Administer oxygen via nasal cannula or nonrebreather mask if O$_2$ saturation <94%.
• Crohn's disease	• Abdominal distension	• Establish IV access with large-bore catheter and infuse warm normal saline or lactated Ringer's solution. Insert additional large-bore catheter if shock is present, as ordered.
• Diverticulitis	• Abdominal rigidity	
• Gastritis	• Nausea and vomiting	
• Pancreatitis	• Diarrhea	
• Ulcerative colitis	• Hematemesis	• Obtain blood for CBC and serum electrolytes assessment.
	• Melena	• Consider ECG.
Vascular Problems		• Anticipate order for amylase level, pregnancy tests, clotting studies, and type and crossmatch as appropriate.
• Ruptured aortic aneurysm	**Hypovolemic Shock**	
• Mesenteric vascular occlusion or ischemia	• ↓ Blood pressure	
	• ↓ Pulse pressure	• Insert indwelling urinary catheter.
Gynecological Problems	• Tachycardia	• Obtain urine R&M, C&S.
• Pelvic inflammatory disease	• Cool, clammy skin	• Insert NG tube as needed.
• Ruptured ectopic pregnancy	• ↓ Level of consciousness	• Keep patient on NPO status.
• Ruptured ovarian cyst		• Assess bowel sound characteristics.
Infectious Diseases		**Ongoing Monitoring**
• Giardiasis		• Monitor vital signs, level of consciousness, O$_2$ saturation, and intake–output.
• Salmonellosis		• Assess pain characteristics.
		• Assess amount and character of emesis.
Other		Anticipate diagnostic tests.
• Obstruction or perforation of abdominal organ		Anticipate surgical intervention.
• Gastro-intestinal bleeding		• Maintain NPO status.
• Trauma		

CBC, complete blood cell count; *C&S*, culture and sensitivity; *ECG*, electrocardiogram; *IV*, intravenous; *NG*, nasogastric; *NPO*, nothing by mouth; *R&M*, routine and microscopic.

If the upper GI tract has been entered, drainage from the NG tube may be dark brown to dark red for the first 12 hours. Later, it should be light yellowish-brown, or it may have a greenish tinge because of the presence of bile. If a dark red colour continues or if bright red blood is observed, the health care provider should be notified at once of the possibility of hemorrhage. The "coffee grounds" appearance of the drainage is owing to the presence of small amounts of blood that have been chemically altered by gastric secretions.

The NG tube is checked regularly for patency. The tube may become obstructed with mucus, sediment, or blood clots. An order is usually written to irrigate the tube with 20 to 30 mL of tap or sterile water or normal saline solution if needed. An accurate record of intake and output, including emesis and gastric drainage, is essential. The nurse assesses serum electrolyte values and acid–base balance because prolonged gastric suctioning can result in loss of sodium, chloride, potassium, water, and hydrochloric acid.

The NG tube is removed when intestinal peristalsis returns, usually 24 to 72 hours after surgery. Motility of the stomach normally returns within 24 to 48 hours. Motility of the small intestine usually resumes within 12 to 24 hours, whereas return of large intestine motility may take as long as 3 to 5 days. Peristaltic activity can be assessed by auscultation for bowel sounds.

Mouth care and nasal care are essential. The patient tends to breathe through the mouth while the NG tube is in place. In addition, increased nasal secretions and crusting result from mechanical stimulation of the NG tube.

Parenteral fluids are administered to provide the patient with fluids and electrolytes until bowel sounds return. Ice chips may be ordered because they aid in the flow of saliva and prevent a dry mouth and sore throat. When bowel sounds return, fluids and food are increased gradually. Nausea and vomiting are not uncommon after abdominal surgery and are often self-limiting. Observation is important in determining the cause. Antiemetics such as dimenhydrinate (Gravol), ondansetron (Zofran), or metoclopramide may be ordered.

Abdominal distension and gas pains are also common after surgery; these are owing to swallowed air and impaired peristalsis resulting from immobility, manipulation of abdominal contents during surgery, and adverse effects of anaesthesia. The health care provider should be informed of abdominal distension and rigidity and worsening abdominal pain. Gradually, as intestinal activity increases, distension and gas pains decrease.

CARE OF NASOGASTRIC AND NASOINTESTINAL TUBES. Nurses may be instructed to insert NG tubes. Insertion is easier if the patient relaxes, takes deep breaths, and swallows when instructed. Once the tube is in place, it is extremely important to (1) confirm placement of the tube (e.g., by aspiration of gastric contents), (2) ensure the tube is properly secured to prevent dislodgement, and (3) provide appropriate nasal and mouth care. When an NG tube is in place, the patient breathes through the mouth, drying the mouth and lips. The nurse should encourage and assist the patient to brush the teeth frequently. Mouthwash and water for the patient to use in rinsing the mouth and petroleum jelly (if the patient is not on oxygen) or water-soluble lubricant for the lips should be provided at the bedside.

The patient's nose should be checked for signs of irritation from the NG tube. This area should be cleaned and dried daily with application of a water-soluble lubricant and retaping of the tube. NG tubes should be checked every 4 hours for patency. Characteristics of the NG losses may differ depending upon the underlying reason for the tube placement. Pale yellow to dark green bile drainage is more likely after abdominal surgery, whereas odoriferous thick drainage with food particles may be seen with bowel obstructions. Hemolyzed sanguineous drainage (often called "coffee grounds" owing to its dark brown, granular appearance) or fresh sanguineous drainage should be reported immediately to the physician or surgeon. The volume of NG losses should also be monitored. Excessive losses (>500–1 000 mL/24 hr) may have to be replaced with intravenous (IV) fluids and electrolytes to maintain adequate hydration. Generally, NG tubes can be removed once normal bowel function returns (passing of gas and stool) and the patient is no longer vomiting.

AMBULATORY AND HOME CARE. Preparation for discharge begins when the patient returns from the operating room. Instructions to the patient and family should include any modifications in activity, care of the incision, diet, and drug therapy. Small, frequent meals high in calories should be taken initially, with a gradually increased intake of food as tolerated.

Normal activities should be resumed gradually. Some activity restrictions may be required for 6 to 8 weeks. The patient should be aware of possible complications after surgery and should notify the health care provider immediately if vomiting, fever, pain, weight loss, incisional drainage, or changes in bowel function occur.

EVALUATION

The expected outcomes are that the patient with acute abdominal pain will have (1) resolution of the cause of the acute abdominal pain; (2) relief of abdominal pain and discomfort; (3) freedom from complications (especially hypovolemic shock and septicemia); and (4) normal fluid, electrolyte, and nutritional status.

ABDOMINAL TRAUMA

Etiology and Pathophysiology

Injuries to the abdominal area occur most often as a result of blunt trauma (e.g., motor vehicle accident) or penetration injuries, primarily gunshot wounds or stab wounds to the abdomen. Blunt trauma is most common. Regardless of whether it is a blunt or penetration injury, the result is often the same: damage to or alteration of the internal organs.

Common injuries of the abdomen include lacerated liver, ruptured spleen, pancreatic trauma, mesenteric artery tears, diaphragmatic rupture, urinary bladder rupture, great vessel tears, renal injury, and stomach or intestinal rupture. These injuries may result in massive blood loss and hypovolemic shock. Surgery must be performed as early as possible to repair the damaged organs and to stop the bleeding. Common sequelae of intra-abdominal trauma are peritonitis and sepsis, particularly when the bowel is perforated.

Clinical Manifestations

Clinical manifestations of abdominal trauma are (1) guarding and splinting of the abdominal wall; (2) a hard, distended abdomen (may indicate intra-abdominal bleeding); (3) decreased or absent bowel sounds; (4) contusions, abrasions, or bruising over the flanks or the abdomen; (5) severe abdominal pain; (6) pain over the scapula caused by irritation of the phrenic nerve by free blood in the abdomen; (7) hematemesis or hematuria; and (8) signs of hypovolemic shock (Table 45-14). An ecchymotic discoloration around the umbilicus (Cullen's sign) can indicate intra-abdominal or retroperitoneal hemorrhage.

TABLE 45-14 EMERGENCY MANAGEMENT

Abdominal Trauma

Etiology	Assessment Findings	Interventions
Blunt	**Hypovolemic Shock**	**Initial**
• Falls	• ↓ Level of consciousness	• Ensure patent airway.
• Motor vehicle collisions	• Tachypnea	• Administer O₂ via face mask.
• Pedestrian accidents	• Tachycardia	• Control external bleeding with direct pressure or sterile
• Assault with blunt object	• ↓ Blood pressure	pressure dressing.
• Crush injuries	• ↓ Pulse pressure	• Establish IV access with two large-bore catheters, and infuse
• Explosions		warm normal saline or lactated Ringer's solution.
	Surface Findings	• Obtain blood for type and crossmatch and CBC.
Penetrating	• Abrasions or ecchymoses on abdominal wall,	• Remove clothing.
• Knife	flank, or perineum	• Stabilize impaled objects with bulky dressing—do not remove.
• Gunshot wounds	• Open wounds: lacerations, eviscerations,	• Cover protruding organs or tissue with sterile, saline dressing.
• Other missiles	puncture wounds, gunshot wounds	• Insert indwelling urinary catheter if there is no blood at the
	• Impaled object	meatus, pelvic fracture, or boggy prostate.
	• Healed incisions or old scars	• Obtain urine for urinalysis.
		• Insert NG tube if no evidence of facial or neck trauma.
	Abdominal and Gastro-Intestinal	• Anticipate diagnostic peritoneal lavage.
	Findings	
	• Nausea and vomiting	**Ongoing Monitoring**
	• Bloody urine	• Monitor vital signs, level of consciousness, O₂ saturation, and
	• Abdominal pain	urine output.
	• Abdominal distension	• Maintain patient warmth using blankets, warm IV fluids
	• Abdominal rigidity	(40–45°C), or warm humidified oxygen.
	• Guarding	
	• Rebound tenderness	
	• Pain with radiation to shoulder and back	

CBC, complete blood cell count; *IV,* intravenous; *NG,* nasogastric.

Intra-abdominal injuries can also be associated with low rib fractures, fractured femur, fractured pelvis, and thoracic injury. If any of these injuries are present, the patient should be observed for abdominal trauma.

Diagnostic Studies

Specific diagnostic procedures include CBC, urinalysis, radiographs of the abdomen and the chest, high-resolution computed tomographic (CT) scan, and abdominal ultrasound. With the availability of emergency department ultrasound and CT, peritoneal lavage is rarely performed as a diagnostic tool and is contraindicated in pregnant women or patients with pelvic fractures. If performed, the fluid is observed for gross abnormalities—such as the presence of blood, bile, feces, or food fibres—and is sent to the laboratory for microscopic evaluation.

NURSING AND COLLABORATIVE MANAGEMENT ABDOMINAL TRAUMA

Emergency management of abdominal trauma focuses on establishing a patent airway and adequate breathing, fluid replacement, and prevention of hypovolemic shock (see Table 45-14). IV lines are inserted, and volume expanders or blood is given if the patient is hypotensive. An NG tube is inserted to decompress the stomach and prevent the aspiration of vomitus.

Regardless of the mechanism of injury, physical evidence of abdominal trauma in a patient who is hemodynamically unstable mandates immediate laparotomy. In other cases, the indications for laparotomy must be correlated with the mechanism of injury. For example, if an individual has a gunshot wound or impaled object, surgery is usually indicated. An impaled object should never be removed until skilled surgical care is available. Removal may cause further injury and bleeding. If surgery is performed, the postoperative nursing care is similar to the care of the patient after laparotomy (see NCP 45-2, available on the Evolve website).

CHRONIC ABDOMINAL PAIN

Chronic abdominal pain may originate from abdominal structures or may be referred from a site with the same or a similar nerve supply. Some common causes are irritable bowel syndrome (IBS), peptic ulcer disease, diverticulitis, chronic pancreatitis, hepatitis, cholecystitis, pelvic inflammatory disease, and vascular insufficiency.

Diagnosis of chronic abdominal pain presents a challenge. Assessment should begin with a thorough history and identification of the specific pain pattern. Character and severity of pain, location, duration, and onset should be determined. The assessment should also include the relationship of pain to meals, defecation, and activity and factors that increase or decrease the pain. Chronic abdominal pain can be described as dull, aching, or diffuse.

Endoscopy, CT scans, magnetic resonance imaging (MRI), laparoscopy, and radiological barium studies have decreased the need for exploratory laparotomy. Treatment for chronic abdominal pain is comprehensive and directed toward palliation of symptoms using appropriate medications, such as analgesics and antiemetics, as well as psychological or behavioural therapies (e.g., relaxation therapies).

IRRITABLE BOWEL SYNDROME

Irritable bowel syndrome (IBS) is a chronic functional disorder characterized by intermittent and recurrent abdominal pain associated with an alteration in bowel function (diarrhea or constipation or both). Other symptoms commonly found include abdominal distension, excessive flatulence, bloating, urge to defecate, urgency, and sensation of incomplete evacuation. IBS is a common problem affecting approximately 5 million Canadians (Canadian Digestive Health Foundation, 2016). Neurological hypersensitivity within the GI (enteric) nerves, physical or emotional stress (or both), dietary issues such as food allergies or sensitivities, antibiotic use, GI infection, bile acid malabsorption, chronic alcohol abuse, abnormalities in GI secretions or digestive muscle contractions (peristalsis) (or both), acute infection or inflammation of the intestine (enteritis) have been identified as factors that precipitate IBS symptoms (Thompson & Read, 2015). IBS is not a psychological disorder, even though stress, depression, panic, or anxiety may aggravate bowel symptoms.

The key to accurate diagnosis is a thorough history and physical examination. Emphasis should be on symptoms, past health history (including psychosocial aspects such as physical or sexual abuse), family history, and drug and dietary history. Diagnostic tests should be used to rule out more serious life-threatening disorders with symptoms similar to those of IBS, such as colorectal cancer (CRC), peptic ulcer disease, inflammatory bowel disease (IBD), and malabsorption disorders. Symptom-based criteria for IBS have been standardized and are referred to as the Rome III criteria. The Rome III criteria include abdominal discomfort or pain for at least 3 months, with onset at least 6 months before, that has at least two of the following characteristics: (1) relieved with defecation, (2) onset associated with a change in stool frequency, and (3) onset associated with a change in stool appearance (Ishihara, Yashima, & Kushiyama, et al., 2012).

The health care provider should encourage the patient to verbalize concerns and anxiety. A diet containing at least 20 g/day of dietary fibre should be initiated (see Table 45-9). This may also include the addition of psyllium-containing products (e.g., Metamucil).

The patient whose primary symptoms are abdominal distension and increased flatulence should be advised to eliminate common gas-producing foods such as broccoli and cabbage from the diet and to use lactose-free products if there is lactose intolerance. Various medications are available and choice will depend on whether the patient has diarrhea or constipation. Other therapies include relaxation and stress management techniques, antidepressants, acupuncture, and herbal therapy, although no single therapy has been found to be effective for all patients. Patients should be referred to a dietitian to review dietary practices. Maintaining a healthy diet according to Canada's Food Guide (see Chapter 42) should be encouraged.

INFLAMMATORY DISORDERS

APPENDICITIS

Appendicitis is an inflammation of the appendix, a narrow blind tube that extends from the inferior part of the cecum. Appendicitis occurs in approximately 7% of the world's population. It can

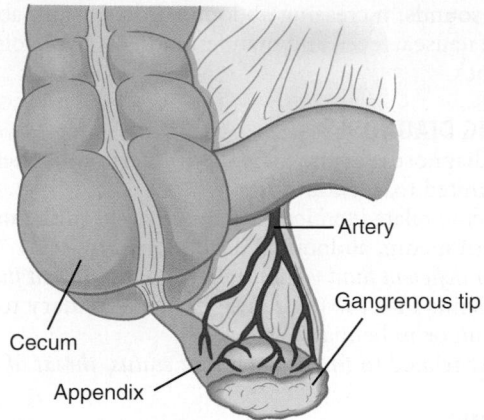

FIGURE 45-1 In appendicitis, the blood supply of the appendix is impaired by inflammation and bacterial infection in the wall of the appendix, which may result in gangrene.

occur at any age but is most common in young adults (Pickhardt, Lawrence, Pooler, et al., 2011).

Etiology and Pathophysiology

The most common causes of appendicitis are occlusion of the appendiceal lumen by a *fecalith* (accumulated feces) (Figure 45-1) and intramural thickening caused by hypergrowth of lymphoid tissue. Obstruction results in edema, venous engorgement, and the invasion by bacteria, which can lead to gangrene and perforation.

Clinical Manifestations

Appendicitis typically begins with periumbilical pain, followed by anorexia, nausea, and vomiting. The pain is persistent and continuous, eventually shifting to the right lower quadrant and localizing at the McBurney point (located halfway between the umbilicus and the right iliac crest). The iliopsoas and obturator tests may further support a diagnosis of appendicitis. Further assessment of the patient reveals localized tenderness, rebound tenderness (Blumberg sign), and muscle guarding. The patient usually prefers to lie still, often with the right leg flexed. Low-grade fever may or may not be present, and coughing aggravates pain. Older adults may report less severe pain, slight fever, and discomfort in the right iliac fossa. The Rovsing sign may be elicited by palpation of the left lower quadrant, causing pain to be felt in the right lower quadrant. Complications of acute appendicitis are perforation, peritonitis, and abscesses.

Diagnostic Studies and Collaborative Care

Examination of the patient includes a complete history and physical examination (particularly palpation of the abdomen) and a differential WBC count. A urinalysis may be done to rule out genito-urinary conditions that mimic the manifestations of appendicitis. CT scan is the preferred diagnostic procedure, but ultrasound is also used.

The treatment of appendicitis may include surgical removal (appendectomy) if the inflammation is localized. If the appendix has ruptured and there is evidence of peritonitis or an abscess, conservative treatment, consisting of antibiotic therapy and parenteral fluids, may be used to prevent sepsis and dehydration for 6 to 8 hours before an appendectomy is performed.

TABLE 45-15	CAUSES OF PERITONITIS
Primary • Bloodborne organisms • Genital tract organisms • Cirrhosis with ascites • GI tract organisms **Secondary** • Appendicitis with rupture • Blunt or penetrating trauma to abdominal organs	• Diverticulitis with rupture • Ischemic bowel disorders • Obstruction in the gastro-intestinal tract • Pancreatitis • Perforated peptic ulcer • Peritoneal dialysis • Postoperative anastomotic leak

GI, gastro-intestinal.

NURSING MANAGEMENT APPENDICITIS

The patient with abdominal pain is encouraged to see a health care provider and to avoid self-treatment, particularly the use of laxatives and enemas. The increased peristalsis from these may cause perforation of the appendix. Until the patient is seen by a health care provider, nothing should be taken by mouth (NPO) to ensure that the stomach is empty in the event that surgery is needed. Local application of heat is never used because it may cause the appendix to rupture. In addition, the patient should be observed for evidence of peritonitis. Usually, surgery is performed as soon as a diagnosis is made.

Postoperative nursing management is similar to postoperative care of the patient after laparotomy (see NCP 45-2 on the Evolve website). Ambulation begins the day of surgery or the first postoperative day. The diet is advanced as tolerated. The patient is usually discharged on the first or second postoperative day, and normal activities are resumed 2 to 3 weeks after surgery.

PERITONITIS

Etiology and Pathophysiology

Peritonitis results from a localized or generalized inflammatory process of the peritoneum. Causes of peritonitis are listed in Table 45-15. Peritonitis may appear in acute and chronic forms; trauma or rupture of an organ containing chemical irritants or bacteria (which are released into the peritoneal cavity) may cause it. Examples of a chemical peritonitis include peptic ulcer perforation and ruptured ectopic pregnancy. A chemical peritonitis is commonly followed by bacterial invasion. Bacterial peritonitis can be caused by a traumatic injury (e.g., gunshot wound, ruptured appendix), or it can be secondary to other diseases or conditions (e.g., pancreatitis, peritoneal dialysis).

The response of the peritoneum to the leakage of GI contents is to attempt to localize the offending agent by "walling it off" by exuding fibrin-containing fluids and swelling. Adhesions may form. These adhesions may reduce or disappear when the infection is eliminated. Normally, peritoneal injuries heal without formation of adhesions unless other factors—such as infection, ischemia, or foreign substances—are present.

Clinical Manifestations

Abdominal pain is the most common symptom of peritonitis. A universal sign of peritonitis is tenderness over the involved area. Rebound tenderness, muscular rigidity, and spasm are other major signs of irritation of the peritoneum. Abdominal distension

TABLE 45-16 COLLABORATIVE CARE

Peritonitis

Diagnostic
- History and physical examination
- CBC
- Serum electrolytes
- Abdominal radiographic examination
- Abdominal paracentesis and culture of fluid
- CT scan or ultrasound
- Peritoneoscopy

Collaborative Therapy
Preoperative or Nonoperative
- NPO status
- Oxygen support
- Fluid replacement
- Antibiotic therapy

- NG suction
- Analgesics
- Preparation for surgery to include the above and nutritional support

Postoperative
- NPO status
- NG tube to suction
- Semi-Fowler's position
- IV fluids with electrolyte replacement
- Nutritional support as needed
- Antibiotic therapy
- Blood transfusions as needed
- Sedatives and opioids

CBC, complete blood cell count; *CT,* computed tomographic (scan); *IV,* intravenous; *NG,* nasogastric; *NPO,* nothing by mouth.

or ascites, fever, tachycardia, tachypnea, nausea, vomiting, and altered bowel habits may also be present. These manifestations vary depending on severity and acuteness of the underlying cause. Complications of peritonitis include hypovolemic shock, septicemia, intra-abdominal abscess formation, paralytic ileus, and organ failure.

Diagnostic Studies

A CBC is done to determine elevations in WBC count and hemoconcentration (Table 45-16). Peritoneal aspiration may be performed and the fluid analyzed for blood, bile, pus, bacteria, fungus, and amylase content. A radiograph of the abdomen may show dilated loops of bowel consistent with paralytic ileus, free air if perforation has occurred, or air–fluid levels if an obstruction is present. Ultrasound and CT scans may identify the presence of ascites and abscesses. *Peritoneoscopy* (an endoscope is placed through a stab wound in the abdomen to inspect the peritoneum) may be helpful in the patient without ascites. Direct examination of the peritoneum can be obtained along with biopsy specimens for diagnosis.

Collaborative Care

The goals of the management of peritonitis are to identify and eliminate the cause, combat infection, and prevent complications. Patients with milder cases of peritonitis or those who are poor surgical risks may be managed nonsurgically. Treatment consists of antibiotics, NG suction, analgesics, and IV fluid administration. Patients who require surgery need preoperative preparation as previously described. Those patients may be placed on parenteral nutrition (PN) because of increased nutritional requirements. (PN, formerly called *total parenteral nutrition* [TPN], is discussed in Chapter 42.)

NURSING MANAGEMENT
PERITONITIS

NURSING ASSESSMENT

Assessment of the patient's pain, including the location, is important and may help in determining the cause of peritonitis. The patient should be assessed for the presence and the quality

of bowel sounds, increasing abdominal distension, abdominal guarding, nausea, fever, and manifestations of hypovolemic and septic shock.

NURSING DIAGNOSES

Nursing diagnoses for the patient with peritonitis include, but are not limited to, the following:
- *Acute pain* related to *biological injury agent* (inflammation of the peritoneum, abdominal distention)
- *Risk for deficient fluid volume* related to *insufficient fluid intake* (fluid shifts into the peritoneal cavity secondary to trauma, infection or ischemia)
- *Anxiety* related to *threat to current status, threat of death*

PLANNING

The overall goals for the patient with peritonitis are for (1) resolution of inflammation, (2) relief of abdominal pain, (3) freedom from complications, and (4) normal nutritional status.

NURSING IMPLEMENTATION

The patient with peritonitis is extremely ill and needs skilled supportive care. The patient is monitored for signs of sepsis, pain, and response to analgesic therapy. The patient may be positioned with knees flexed to increase comfort. The nurse should provide rest and a quiet environment. Sedatives may be given to allay anxiety.

Accurate monitoring of fluid intake and output and electrolyte status is necessary to determine replacement therapy. Vital signs are monitored frequently. Antiemetics may be administered to decrease nausea and vomiting and further fluid losses. The patient is on NPO status and may have an NG tube in place to decrease gastric distension.

If the patient has an open surgical procedure, drains are inserted to remove purulent drainage and excessive fluid. Postoperative care of the patient is similar to the care of the patient with an exploratory laparotomy (see NCP 45-2, on the Evolve website).

GASTRO-ENTERITIS

Gastro-enteritis is an inflammation of the mucosa of the stomach and the small intestine. Clinical manifestations include nausea, vomiting, diarrhea, abdominal cramping, and distension. Fever, increased WBC counts, and blood or mucus in the stool may be present. Causative agents are varied (see Table 45-2). Most cases are self-limiting and do not necessitate hospitalization. However, older-adult patients and patients who are chronically ill may be unable to consume sufficient fluids orally to compensate for fluid loss. Until vomiting has ceased, the patient should be on NPO status. If dehydration has occurred, IV replacement of fluids may be necessary. As soon as tolerated, oral fluids containing glucose and electrolytes should be given. If the causative agent is identified, appropriate pharmacologic therapy is initiated.

NURSING MANAGEMENT
GASTRO-ENTERITIS

Accurate monitoring of intake and output is important for successful replacement of lost fluid. Strict medical asepsis and infection control precautions should be instituted when indicated. The patient should be instructed in the importance of proper food handling and preparation of food to prevent infections such as salmonellosis and botulism (see Chapter 44, Table 44-3).

Symptomatic nursing care is given for nausea, vomiting, and diarrhea. The importance of rest and increased fluid intake should be stressed. The nurse should assess complaints of pain, vomiting, and diarrhea because, often, gastro-enteritis is confused with appendicitis. To allay the patient's apprehension, the nurse should explain that gastro-enteritis usually runs an acute course with no sequelae.

INFLAMMATORY BOWEL DISEASE

Inflammatory bowel disease (IBD) is an autoimmune disease that currently refers to two disorders of the GI tract (Crohn's disease and ulcerative colitis [UC]) characterized by idiopathic inflammation and ulceration. Multiple factors are likely involved in the etiology of IBD, including environmental factors, genetic predisposition, and alterations in the function of the immune system (Leone, Chang, & Devkota, 2013). Both UC and Crohn's disease commonly occur during the teenage years and early adulthood, but both have a second peak from ages 50 to 70. Both are more prevalent in industrialized regions of the world. Epidemiological studies show a higher incidence of IBD in White people (particularly those of Jewish descent) (see the "Determinants of Health" box) and in family members (especially monozygotic compared with dizygotic twins). For both conditions, the clinical manifestations are varied, with unpredictable periods of remission interspersed with episodes of acute inflammation (Figure 45-2). Both diseases can be debilitating. In Canada, about 10 000 new cases of IBD are diagnosed annually (Canadian Society of Intestinal Research, 2014).

ULCERATIVE COLITIS

Ulcerative colitis (UC) is a chronic IBD characterized by inflammation and ulceration of the rectum and the colon. It may occur at any age but peaks between the ages of 15 and 25 years. There is a second, smaller peak onset between 50 and 70 years of age. UC equally affects both sexes (Rocchi, Benchimol, Bernstein, et al., 2012).

Etiology and Pathophysiology

The inflammation of UC is diffuse and involves the mucosa and the submucosa, with alternate periods of exacerbations and remissions (see Table 45-24 later in the chapter). The disease begins in the rectum and spreads proximally along the colon in a continuous fashion.

The mucosa of the rectum and the colon is hyperemic and edematous in the affected area. Multiple abscesses develop in the crypts of Lieberkühn (intestinal glands). As the disease advances, the abscesses break through the crypts into the submucosa, leaving ulcerations. These ulcerations also destroy the mucosal epithelium, causing bleeding and diarrhea. Losses of fluid and electrolytes occur because of the decreased mucosal surface area for absorption. Breakdown of cells results in protein loss through the stool. Areas of inflamed mucosa can form pseudopolyps—tonguelike projections into the bowel lumen. Granulation tissue develops, and the mucosa musculature becomes thickened, shortening the colon.

Although the precipitating factors involved in UC are poorly understood, it is clear that the disease onset involves an inflammatory response. Specific proinflammatory cytokines such as

Inflammatory bowel disease (IBD)

Crohn's disease   Ulcerative colitis

FIGURE 45-2 Comparison of distribution patterns of Crohn's disease and ulcerative colitis.

DETERMINANTS OF HEALTH

Colon Disorders

Physical Environment
- Inflammatory bowel disease (IBD) is more common in temperate regions of North America, South Africa, and Australia.*
- The prevalence of colorectal cancer is highest in Canada and the United States, northwestern Europe and Australia.†

Biology and Genetic Endowment: Culture
- Familial adenomatous polyposis (FAP) is a genetic condition that causes adenomatous polyps to develop on the inner lining, or mucosa, of the colon and rectum. If untreated, most people with FAP will develop colorectal cancer by age 30.
- IBD is more common among Ashkenazi Jewish people and those of Scandinavian descent.*

Gender
- Men are at greater risk of developing colorectal cancer. The risk for colorectal cancers also increases with age. Most people who are diagnosed are older than 50.

References

*Crohn's and Colitis Canada. (2014). Risk factors. Retrieved from *http://www. crohnsandcolitis.ca/site/c.dtJRL9NUJmL4I I/b.0221447/k.9BC5/Risk_Factors. htm.*
†Canadian Cancer Society. (2016). Risk factors for colorectal cancer. Retrieved from *http://www.cancer.ca/en/cancer-information/cancer-type/colorectal/ risks/?region=on.*

tumour necrosis factor–alpha (TNF-α) have been implicated in promoting this inflammatory response.

Clinical Manifestations

UC may appear as an acute fulminating crisis or, more commonly, as a chronic disorder with mild to severe acute exacerbations that occur at unpredictable intervals over many years. The major symptoms of UC are bloody diarrhea and abdominal pain. Pain may vary from the mild lower abdominal cramping associated with diarrhea to the severe, constant abdominal pain that may be associated with toxic megacolon and acute perforations. With mild disease, diarrhea may consist of one or two semiformed stools, containing small amounts of blood, per day. The patient may have no other systemic manifestations. In moderate UC, there is increased stool output (four to five stools per day), increased bleeding, and systemic symptoms (e.g., fever, malaise, anorexia). In severe cases, diarrhea is bloody, contains mucus, and occurs 10 to 20 times a day. In addition, fever, weight loss greater than 10% of total body weight, anemia, tachycardia, and dehydration are present.

Complications

Complications of UC may be classified into those that are intestinal and those that are extraintestinal. Intestinal complications of UC include hemorrhage, perforation, toxic megacolon, and colonic dilation. Hemorrhage is a result of inflamed, ulcerated mucosa and is usually controlled with conservative medical therapy. Massive hemorrhage is unusual and requires emergency surgery. *Toxic megacolon* (extensive dilation and paralysis of the colon), bleeding, and fulminant colitis are the most common complications associated with UC. Colonic dilation, most often in the transverse colon, occurs as a result of severe acute inflammation of the entire colon wall. Perforation is most often associated with toxic megacolon but may occur alone. Most cases of perforation occur in the left side of the colon.

A patient who has had UC for more than 10 years is at greater risk for colorectal cancer. The risk for cancer depends on age at onset, duration, and extent of disease. The patient should be regularly screened with colonoscopy. Extraintestinal manifestations of the disease may be directly related to the colitis, or they may be nonspecific complications mediated by a disturbance in the immune system (Table 45-17). Colitis-related complications are associated with active inflammation and may respond to treatment of the underlying bowel disease. These manifestations can involve the joints, the skin, the mouth, and the eyes as well as disturbances of the hematological system, including anemia, leukocytosis, and thrombocytosis. Skin lesions such as erythema nodosum and pyoderma gangrenosum are among the most

frequently seen extraintestinal manifestations. Uveitis is the most common eye problem (Crohn's and Colitis Canada, 2016).

Diagnostic Studies

Several studies are appropriate for diagnosis of UC (Table 45-18). Blood studies should include a CBC, serum electrolyte levels, and serum protein levels. A CBC typically shows iron-deficiency anemia from blood loss. An elevated WBC count may indicate toxic megacolon or perforation. Elevated erythrocyte sedimentation rate and C-reactive protein reflect inflammation. Decreases in serum electrolytes, such as sodium, potassium, chloride, bicarbonate, and magnesium, are caused by fluid and electrolyte losses from diarrhea. Hypoalbuminemia is present with severe disease and results from protein loss from the bowel. The stool should be examined for blood, pus, and mucus. Stool cultures should be obtained to rule out infectious causes of inflammation.

Imaging studies include double-contrast barium enema, small bowel series (small bowel follow-through), transabdominal ultrasound, CT, and MRI. Examinations with a sigmoidoscope and a colonoscope allow direct examination of the mucosa of the lower GI tract. Using a sigmoidoscope, the health care provider can view the rectum, the sigmoid colon, and the distal descending colon. The colonoscope allows for examination of the entire large intestine. The extent of inflammation, ulcerations, pseudopolyps, strictures, and lesions may be identified. Biopsy specimens should be taken for definitive diagnosis. Scopes should not be used when the rectum and the colon are severely inflamed because of the risk for perforation.

Collaborative Care

The goals of treatment are to (1) rest the bowel, (2) control the inflammation, (3) manage fluids and nutrition, (4) manage patient stress, (5) provide education about the disease and treatment, and (6) provide symptomatic relief. The mainstays of drug therapy

---

TABLE 45-17 EXTRAINTESTINAL MANIFESTATIONS OF INFLAMMATORY BOWEL DISEASE

Musculo-skeletal	**Metastatic Crohn's Disease**
• Peripheral arthritis (colitic)	**Mouth**
• Ankylosing spondylitis	• Aphthous ulcers (stomatitis)
• Sacroiliitis	
• Osteoporosis	**Ophthalmological**
• Finger clubbing	• Conjunctivitis
	• Uveitis
Dermatological	• Episcleritis
• Erythema nodosum	
• Pyoderma gangrenosum	**Hepatobiliary**
	• Gallstones
Other	• Primary sclerosing cholangitis
• Thrombo-embolism	• Portal vein thrombosis
• *Clostridium difficile*	
	Genito-Urinary
	• Kidney stones

TABLE 45-18 COLLABORATIVE CARE

Ulcerative Colitis

Diagnostic	**Severe (Fulminant) Disease**
• History and physical examination	• IV fluids with electrolytes
• Colonoscopy	• Blood transfusions
• Sigmoidoscopy	• NPO status
• Barium enema	• Nutritional support (parenteral therapy)
• CBC, ESR, electrolytes, BUN,* creatinine, albumin	• Antimicrobial therapy†
• Culture and sensitivity testing of stool (including *Clostridium difficile*)	• Immuno-suppressants†
	• Immuno-modulators†
• Stool for occult blood	• Corticosteroids†
	• Surgery if no improvement
Collaborative Therapy	
Mild and Moderate Disease	
• Nutritional support (low-residue diet and no dairy products)	
• Antimicrobial therapy†	
• 5-Aminosalicylates†	
• Corticosteroids†	
• Antidiarrheal agents†	

BUN, blood urea nitrogen; *CBC,* complete blood cell count; *IV,* intravenous; *NPO,* nothing by mouth; *ESR,* erythrocyte sedimentation rate.
*Serum urea (nitrogen).
†See Table 45-19.

TABLE 45-19 DRUG THERAPY

Inflammatory Bowel Disease

Category	Action	Examples
Antimicrobial	Prevent or treat secondary infection	metronidazole (Flagyl), ciprofloxacin (Cipro)
5-Aminosalicylates (5-ASA)	Decrease GI inflammation*	*Systemic:* sulphasalazine (Salazopyrin), mesalazine (Asacol, Pentasa), olsalazine (Dipentum) *Rectal suppository:* mesalazine (Salofalk)
Corticosteroids	Decrease inflammation	*Systemic:* corticosteroids (cortisone, prednisone, budesonide) *Enemas:* hydrocortisone (Cortenema), budesonide (Entocort) *Rectal foam:* hydrocortisone (Cortifoam)
Antidiarrheal	Decrease GI motility†	diphenoxylate (Lomotil), loperamide (Imodium)
Immuno-suppressants	Suppress immune response	azathioprine (Imuran), cyclosporine (Neoral)
Immuno-modulators	Inhibit the cytokine tumour necrosis factor–alpha (TNF-α)	infliximab (Remicade), adalimumab (Humira)
Hematinics and vitamins	Correct iron deficiency anemia and promote healing	*Oral iron:* ferrous sulphate, ferrous gluconate *Iron injection:* iron dextran (DexIron), iron sucrose (Venofer)

GI, gastro-intestinal.
*Mechanism of action unknown, possibly antimicrobial as well as anti-inflammatory.
†Used with caution during severe disease because of potential to produce toxic megacolon.

are sulphasalazine (Salazopyrin) and corticosteroids. Hospitalization is indicated if the patient fails to respond to corticosteroid therapy or if complications are suspected.

Drug Therapy. Drug therapy is an extremely important aspect of treatment (Table 45-19) (Rx Files Academic Detailing Program, 2014). The principal drug used is sulphasalazine (Salazopyrin), a combination of sulphapyridine and 5-aminosalicylic acid (5-ASA). It is effective in the maintenance of clinical remission and in the treatment of mild to moderately severe disease episodes. After remission is obtained, therapy is continued with a gradual reduction over several months. The maintenance dose is usually continued for at least 1 year.

DRUG ALERT—Sulphasalazine (Salazopyrin)
- May cause yellowish-orange discoloration of skin and urine.
- Avoid exposure to sunlight and ultraviolet light until photosensitivity is determined.

During active disease, 5-ASA (the active form of sulphasalazine) and corticosteroid enemas are effective in the treatment of left-sided UC and proctitis. Topical salicylate therapy is the treatment of choice in patients with localized disease. 5-ASA

(mesalazine) can also be administered orally. The acrylic-coated tablets provide delivery of the drug more distally in the intestine.

Corticosteroids are of proven benefit in the management of active UC. Oral prednisone or prednisolone is effective in treatment of mild to moderate disease without systemic manifestations. If remission is not achieved, the patient requires hospitalization and IV corticosteroid therapy. The patient is placed on a regimen of bowel rest. Fluids and electrolytes are administered intravenously. For *proctitis* (inflammation of the rectum and the anus), hydrocortisone enemas, rectal foams, or suppositories can be effective in the treatment of inflammation. Rectal foams are usually administered in 5-mL volumes, and patients can generally administer this themselves. Enemas are the preferred choice if the disease spreads beyond the rectum. Retention enemas have been shown to deliver drugs into the descending colon and beyond in patients with active disease. Patients taking corticosteroids need to be monitored for common adverse effects such as Cushing's syndrome, hypertension, hirsutism, and mood swings.

Immuno-suppressive drugs (e.g., cyclosporin) have been used in severe cases of UC, when a patient has failed to respond to any of the usual drugs and before surgery is considered. Adverse effects of cyclosporin include renal dysfunction, hypertension, headache, and muscle cramps. Regular cyclosporin trough levels should be determined to ensure proper dosing of this medication. Therapeutic response to IV cyclosporin usually allows for conversion to an oral preparation for long-term therapy. Anti–TNF-α blocking agents (e.g., infliximab [Remicade]) were previously considered for use more with Crohn's disease; they are now also considered valuable in the management of moderate to severe refractory UC (Rx Files Academic Detailing Program, 2014).

Surgical Therapy. Approximately 80% to 85% of patients with UC go into remission with conservative therapy and nursing management, but 15% to 20% require surgery. Surgery is indicated if (1) the patient fails to respond to treatment; (2) exacerbations are frequent and debilitating; (3) massive bleeding, perforation, strictures, or obstruction occurs; (4) there are tissue changes that suggest that dysplasia is occurring; or (5) carcinoma develops.

Surgical procedures used to treat chronic UC include (1) total proctocolectomy with permanent ileostomy and (2) total proctocolectomy with ileoanal reservoir.

Total Proctocolectomy With Permanent Ileostomy. Total proctocolectomy with a permanent ileostomy is a one-stage operation involving the removal of the colon, the rectum, and the anus, with closure of the anus. The end of the terminal ileum is brought out through the abdominal wall and forms a stoma, or ostomy. The stoma is usually placed in the right lower quadrant within the rectus muscle.

Total Proctocolectomy With Ileoanal Reservoir. A more widely performed procedure involves total proctocolectomy with the formation of an ileal reservoir and anal anastomosis (Figure 45-3). The ileoanal reservoir surgical procedure is usually a staged approach, encompassing a combination of one to three procedures, performed approximately 12 weeks apart. The initial procedure generally includes a colectomy with temporary end ileostomy and a possible mucous fistula. The second surgery involves a takedown of the ileostomy and mucous fistula, resection of the rectal stump to just above the anal sphincters, and formation of the ileal reservoir and subsequent anastomosis to the anus, with a diverting temporary loop ileostomy (to protect the reservoir during healing). The final, third, surgery involves a takedown

FIGURE 45-3 Ileoanal reservoir. **A,** Formation of a reservoir. **B,** Posterior suture lines completed. **C,** J-shaped configuration for an ileoanal reservoir. **D,** S-shaped configuration for an ileoanal reservoir.

of the loop ileostomy, which functionalizes the reservoir. Depending upon the preoperative health of the patient, these staged surgeries may be combined into a two-stage procedure or a single operation. Adaptation to the reservoir occurs over the next 3 to 6 months, which usually results in a bowel movement frequency of four to eight pasty stools per day and good daytime continence.

Patient selection includes absence of colorectal cancer, small intestine free of disease (e.g., Crohn's disease), competent anorectal sphincter, and physical status adequate to permit lengthy surgery. In addition, the patient needs to be motivated and capable of understanding self-care instructions.

Postoperative Care. *Postoperative* care following surgical procedures to treat UC includes routine observations for patients who have had abdominal surgery. Stoma viability, mucocutaneous border (the area where the mucous membrane of the bowel is sutured to the skin), and peristomal skin integrity must be monitored. Because a more proximal portion of the bowel is used to create the diverting loop ileostomy in the second stage, stomal output may be as high as 1 500 to 2 000 mL/24 hr. Intra-venous fluid support is important, including replacements for excessive ileostomy losses (>1 200 mL/24 hr). The patient must be observed for signs of hemorrhage, abdominal abscesses, small bowel obstruction, dehydration, and other related complications. If an NG tube is used, it will be removed when bowel function returns. Drainage of serosanguineous fluid from the abdominal drain site may vary from 100 to 150 mL/24 hr. The drain is usually removed within 3 to 4 days of surgery. The urinary catheter is removed 2 to 4 days after surgery. Systemic antibiotics are discontinued within 24 hours of the operation, and corticosteroids, if used, are tapered.

Transient incontinence of mucus from the reservoir is a result of intraoperative manipulation of the anal canal and the effects of some medications (opioids, sedatives). The patient should be reassured before and after the operation regarding this potential but transient problem. Kegel exercises may be recommended several weeks postoperatively to strengthen the pelvic floor and the sphincter muscles. They are not recommended in the immediate postoperative period. Perianal skin care must be implemented with the first bowel movement to protect the epidermis from frequent pericare and stool irritation. The patient should be instructed to gently rinse the skin with water or a spray cleanser with a surfactant and dry thoroughly. A barrier cream should be used, and a perineal pad may be required.

The most frequent type of ileostomy that is constructed is a loop. This can present as a pouching challenge because the os (opening) may tilt down and drain inferiorly such that stool causes irritation to the surrounding skin. An enterostomal therapy (ET) nurse will help with these challenging problems. Self-care instructions should be taught and reviewed, and written information with discharge supplies should be provided before discharge. Stoma care is presented later in this chapter (see Nursing Management: Ostomy Surgery).

Nutritional Therapy. An important component in the treatment of UC is diet. The dietitian is an important member of the team and should be consulted regarding dietary recommendations. The goals of diet management are to provide adequate nutrition without exacerbating symptoms, to correct and prevent malnutrition, to replace fluid and electrolyte losses, and to prevent weight loss. The diet for each patient must be individualized.

Traditionally, during the acute phase, the patient may be on NPO status. When food is permitted, a high-calorie, high-protein, low-residue diet with vitamin and iron supplements is frequently prescribed. (A low-residue diet is presented in Table 45-20.) Special dietary restrictions are not usually necessary. Some health care providers allow the patient to eat anything that does not cause symptoms. Cold foods, high-residue foods (e.g., whole wheat bread, cereal with bran, nuts, raw fruit), and smoking increase GI motility and should be avoided. Fish oil preparations have been evaluated for their ability to reduce inflammation in active UC. However, their palatability is low.

Often, enteral supplements and parenteral nutrition are necessary. Patients with systemic manifestations, significant fluid and electrolyte losses, or malabsorption may need parenteral nutrition or enteral feedings, such as elemental diets. Elemental diets are high in calories and nutrients, lactose free, and absorbed in the proximal small intestine.

Parenteral nutrition allows for a positive nitrogen balance. Vitamins, minerals, electrolytes, and other important nutrients (e.g., glucose, amino acids) can be administered to promote healing and correct nutritional deficiencies. (PN is discussed in Chapter 42.)

Supplemental iron (ferrous sulphate or ferrous gluconate) may be necessary to prevent or treat iron-deficiency anemia resulting from chronic blood loss. Parenteral iron may be needed for patients who cannot tolerate oral iron. Iron dextran (DexIron) administered intramuscularly by Z-track or intravenously may be necessary if anemia is severe. In patients receiving long-term sulphasalazine therapy, folic acid deficiency may develop, and supplementation may be necessary. Potassium supplements may be necessary if corticosteroid therapy is used because retention of sodium and loss of potassium can result in hypokalemia and subsequent toxic megacolon. Zinc deficiency can result

TABLE 45-20 NUTRITIONAL THERAPY

Low-Residue Diet

Purpose

Low-residue diet provides foods low in fibre, which will result in a reduced amount of fecal material in the lower intestinal tract.

General Principles

1. This diet eliminates foods that are indigestible or stimulating to the intestinal tract to reduce the amount of residue in the colon. Foods should be included or excluded according to the following list.
2. Hot and cold foods should be eaten slowly.
3. Milk products are limited to 2 cups daily. For a more restricted-residue diet, milk should be eliminated.

Food	Foods Included	Foods Excluded
Beverages	Carbonated drinks, coffee, tea, cocoa, strained fruit juices	Alcohol, fruit juices with pulp
Bread	White bread, rolls, rusks, melba toast, crackers	Bread and crackers containing whole grain flour or bran; any hot breads such as biscuits, muffins, waffles, or pancakes
Cereals	Cooked, refined, or strained cereals: cream of wheat, cream of rice, farina, grits, dry cereals without bran; noodles; spaghetti; macaroni	Whole grain cereals; cereals containing bran, nuts, and raisins; Shredded Wheat
Meat	Lean, tender ground beef, lamb, pork, veal or fish, broiled, stewed, or baked; canned tuna or salmon; shellfish; crisp bacon, chicken or turkey without skin, liver; creamy peanut butter	Fried, smoked, pickled, or cured meats; highly seasoned ham; fried fish; luncheon meats
Egg	All but fried	Fried or uncooked eggs
Cheese	Milk, cheese (aged cheddar), cottage cheese	All other cheeses
Milk	Limit to 1–2 cups (if tolerated), including that used in cooking; plain yogourt	Fruit yogourt
Fats	Butter, margarine, cream, oil, crisp bacon, mayonnaise, plain gravy	Any other; rich or spiced gravies
Soup	Cream and vegetable soups made from foods allowed and with quantity of milk allowed, bouillon, broth; strained vegetable juices	Cream and vegetable soups from foods not allowed (peas and dried beans)
Vegetables	Cooked or canned vegetables; strained vegetables; potatoes without skins; vegetable juices	Raw vegetables, all vegetables not strained, dried beans, peas, and legumes
Fruits	Strained fruit juices, cooked or canned fruits; ripe bananas, applesauce, pears, peaches, peeled apricots, Napoleon cherries, baked apple (no skin)	Raw fruits, fruits with skins, seeds
Desserts	Plain desserts (custards and puddings, plain ice cream for milk allowance), sherbet, plain gelatin desserts, angel food cake, sponge cake, plain butter cake, plain cookies	Nuts, coconut, raisins, rich desserts (pies, rich cakes, cobblers)
Condiments	Allspice, cinnamon, mace, paprika, salt, ground thyme, sugar, vinegar, lemon juice	All others

from severe or chronic diarrhea, and supplementation may be necessary.

NURSING MANAGEMENT
ULCERATIVE COLITIS

NURSING ASSESSMENT

Subjective and objective data that should be obtained from a patient with UC are presented in Table 45-21.

NURSING DIAGNOSES

Nursing diagnoses for the patient with UC include, but are not limited to, the following:

- *Diarrhea* related to *increase in stress level* (bowel inflammation and intestinal hyperactivity)
- *Imbalanced nutrition: less than body requirements* related to *insufficient dietary intake* (decreased absorption, increased nutrient loss through diarrhea)
- *Ineffective coping* related to *insufficient sense of control, inadequate confidence in ability to deal with situation*

For additional information on nursing diagnoses on IBD, see NCP 45-3, available on the Evolve website.

PLANNING

The overall goals are that the patient with UC will (1) respond to medical management, (2) maintain normal fluid and electrolyte balance, (3) be free from pain or discomfort, (4) participate in medical and surgical management, and (5) maintain nutritional balance.

NURSING IMPLEMENTATION

During the acute phase, attention is focused on hemodynamic stability, pain control, fluid and electrolyte balance, and nutritional support. Accurate intake and output records must be maintained. The number and characteristics of stools are monitored. Nursing care of the patient with UC is directed toward an intensive therapeutic and supportive program (see NCP 45-3). It is important for the nurse to establish a good working relationship and encourage the patient to talk about himself or herself and daily activities. An explanation of all procedures and treatment is necessary and may allay some apprehension.

Psychosocial support may be indicated if the patient is experiencing emotional problems, but the nurse must recognize that the patient's behaviour may result from factors other than emotional ones. Any person who has 10 to 20 bowel movements a day and has rectal discomfort may be anxious, frustrated, discouraged, and depressed. Along with other team members, the nurse can assist the patient to accept the chronic condition and to have an optimistic view with the possibility of cure after surgery. The nurse may find that inadequate coping mechanisms in the patient with UC are owing to early onset of the disease (often at 10–15 years of age), which

TABLE 45-21   NURSING ASSESSMENT

Ulcerative Colitis

Subjective Data

Important Health Information

Past health history: Infection; autoimmune disorders; family history of inflammatory bowel disease

Medications: Use of antidiarrheal medications, steroids, other immuno-suppressives; herbal, homeopathic, or naturopathic remedies

Symptoms

- Fatigue, malaise
- Nausea, vomiting, anorexia; weight loss; dietary intolerances
- Frequent bloody stools containing mucus and pus
- Lower abdominal pain (worse before defecating), cramping, tenesmus

Objective Data

General

Intermittent fever; emaciated appearance

Integumentary

Pale skin with poor turgor, dry mucous membranes; rash, nodules (on lower legs), or blisters; anorectal irritation

Gastro-Intestinal

Abdominal distension, hyperactive bowel sounds, abdominal cramps

Cardiovascular

Tachycardia, hypotension (including postural)

Possible Findings

Anemia; leukocytosis; electrolyte imbalance; hypoalbuminemia; vitamin and trace metal deficiencies; abnormal sigmoidoscopic, colonoscopic, and barium enema findings

---

may have interfered with usual growth, development, and maturation.

Restricted physical activity and possibly bedrest may be ordered if the patient has a severe exacerbation. Nursing interventions to prevent complications of immobility should be instituted. Teaching related to treatment, drugs, diet, diagnostic tests, and the disease and its management is important.

Rest is important in the management of UC. Patients may lose much sleep because of frequent episodes of diarrhea and abdominal pain. Nutritional deficiencies and anemia leave the patient feeling weak and listless. Activities should be scheduled around rest periods. Nurses can provide physical and emotional support to the patient during acute exacerbations.

Until diarrhea is controlled, the patient must be kept clean, dry, and free of odour. Facilitating management of bowel movements, including close proximity to a bathroom or a bedside commode, is helpful. A deodorizer should be placed in the room. Antidiarrheal agents should be administered as ordered. If the patient has continuous diarrhea, the ET nurse may give helpful suggestions. Meticulous perianal skin care using plain water or a skin cleanser (no harsh soap) is necessary to treat and prevent skin breakdown. Use of skin barrier creams may help to protect perianal skin.

EVALUATION

The expected outcomes for the patient with UC are presented in NCP 45-3, available on the Evolve website.

CROHN'S DISEASE

Crohn's disease is a chronic IBD of unknown origin that can affect any part of the GI tract from the mouth to the anus. Crohn's disease occurs most often between the ages of 15 and 30 years. When it occurs in older adults, the morbidity and mortality rates are higher because of other chronic problems that may be present. Both sexes are affected, with a slightly higher incidence in women. Similar to UC, it occurs more often in Jewish and upper–middle-class urban populations. Canada may have one of the highest incidence rates of both Crohn's disease and UC in the world.

Etiology and Pathophysiology

Crohn's is a systemic autoimmune disorder with significant abnormal inflammation of the GI tract (Mazal, 2014). Recently, the first gene associated with Crohn's disease, the *NOD2* gene, was identified. Research is ongoing to understand how defects in the *NOD2* gene lead to Crohn's disease and into finding the other genes that cause IBD. It can affect any part of the GI tract but is most often seen in the terminal ileum and the colon. Approximately 5% of patients with Crohn's disease have ileojejunitis. Involvement of the esophagus, the stomach, or the duodenum is uncommon. The inflammation involves all layers of the bowel wall (i.e., it is transmural). Areas of involvement are usually discontinuous *skip lesions,* with segments of normal bowel occurring between diseased portions (see Table 45-24). Typically, ulcerations are deep and longitudinal and penetrate between islands of inflamed edematous mucosa, causing the classic cobblestone appearance. Thickening of the bowel wall occurs as well as narrowing of the lumen with stricture development. Abscesses or fistula tracts that communicate with other loops of bowel, the skin, the bladder, the rectum, or the vagina may develop. Histologically, granulomas (chronic inflammatory lesions) are present in 50% of patients and may be located in any layer of the bowel wall.

Clinical Manifestations

The manifestations of Crohn's disease depend largely on the anatomical site of involvement, the extent of the disease process, and the presence or absence of complications. The onset of Crohn's disease is usually insidious, with nonspecific complaints such as diarrhea, fatigue, abdominal pain, weight loss, and fever. Early diagnosis may be more difficult than for UC. The principal manifestations of Crohn's disease are diarrhea and abdominal pain. Diarrhea is usually nonbloody and is a result of the inflammatory process or malabsorption. Pain may be severe and intermittent or constant, depending on the cause. Other manifestations include abdominal cramping and tenderness, abdominal distension, fever, and fatigue. Similar to UC, extraintestinal complications may be directly related to the GI inflammation and small intestinal pathological conditions (malabsorption), or they may be nonspecific complications mediated by a disturbance in the immune system. Extraintestinal manifestations, such as arthritis and finger clubbing, may precede the onset of bowel disease. As the disease progresses, there is weight loss, malnutrition, dehydration, electrolyte imbalances, anemia, increased peristalsis, pain around the umbilicus and right lower quadrant, and possible perianal disease.

Crohn's disease is a chronic disorder with unpredictable periods of recurrence and remission. Attacks are intermittent, usually recurring over a period of several weeks to months.

Complications

Complications, both GI and extraintestinal, are common in Crohn's disease. Scar tissue from the inflammation and ulceration narrows the lumen of the intestine and may cause strictures and obstruction, a frequent complication. Fistulas are a cardinal feature and may develop between segments of bowel. Cutaneous fistulas, common in the perianal area, and recto-vaginal fistulas also occur. Fistulas communicating with the urinary tract may cause urinary tract infections. Inflammation of the intestines may involve all layers, predisposing the patient to perforation and the formation of intra-abdominal abscesses and peritonitis (Mazal, 2014).

Impaired absorption causing various nutritional abnormalities may occur as a result of damage to areas of the intestinal mucosa. Fat malabsorption causes a deficiency in the fat-soluble vitamins (A, D, E, and K). The patient may have an intolerance to gluten (a protein found in barley, rye, and wheat).

Systemic complications are similar to those of UC and include arthritis, liver disease, cholelithiasis (especially with ileal involvement), ankylosing spondylitis, pyoderma gangrenosum, erythema nodosum, and uveitis. Renal disorders are common, especially nephrolithiasis (kidney stones) secondary to increased oxalate absorption.

Diagnostic Studies

Diagnosis of Crohn's disease can be made by means of a thorough history and physical examination, to establish clinical signs and symptoms; barium studies; and endoscopy with biopsy (Table 45-22). Laboratory studies may determine electrolyte disturbances and the presence of anemia. Barium studies are useful in determining location and extent of the disease and may reveal classic findings, such as stricture formations in the ileum (string sign), cobblestoning of the mucosa, fistulas, and areas of abnormal and normal mucosa. Endoscopic studies, such as colonoscopy and sigmoidoscopy, are useful in detecting such early mucosal changes as patchy inflammation, small ulcerations, and skip areas that may not be seen radiologically. Biopsies may be performed to determine the presence of granulomas. Barium studies are performed to determine the degree of ileal involvement. Upper GI barium studies are done to diagnose upper gastro-duodenal disease. Because an endoscope can enter only the distal ileum, capsule endoscopy may be used in the diagnosis of small intestine disease. Capsule endoscopy is a useful diagnostic test, but the high cost of the procedure limits its use (Mazal, 2014).

Collaborative Care

The goal of collaborative care is to control the inflammatory process, relieve symptoms, correct metabolic and nutritional problems, and promote healing. Drug therapy and nutritional support are the mainstays of treatment.

Drug Therapy. Drug therapy for Crohn's disease is presented in Table 45-19. Sulphasalazine (Salazopyrin) is effective when the disease involves the large intestine but is much less effective when only the small intestine is involved. Corticosteroid therapy is effective in reducing inflammation and suppressing disease. The dosage and the route of administration depend on severity of the illness and the area involved. Once clinical symptoms subside, the dosage should be tapered. Immuno-suppressive agents (azathioprine) may be tried if repeated trials with corticosteroids fail. Patients require close monitoring because of the serious adverse effects of these drugs. Metronidazole (Flagyl) is useful in treating Crohn's disease of the perianal area. Marked exacerbations have been reported when the drug is stopped. In patients with Crohn's disease in remission, fish oil preparations have been evaluated for their ability to prevent recurrence of inflammation; however, their palatability is low.

Biological drug therapies of Crohn's disease include monoclonal antibodies to TNF-α (infliximab [Remicade]), adalimumab [Humira]), and to a leukocyte adhesion molecule (natalizumab [Tysabri]). Infliximab has been shown to reduce the degree of inflammation in patients who are refractory to other drug therapies. However, not all patients with Crohn's disease respond to infliximab.

Nutritional Therapy. Elemental diets and parenteral nutrition may be used in patients with Crohn's disease (see Chapter 42). Parenteral nutrition may be given to patients with severe disease, small bowel fistulas, or short bowel syndrome (described later in this chapter). It is given before and after surgery to promote wound healing, reduce complications, and hasten recovery. The elemental diet provides a high-calorie, high-nitrogen, fat-free, no-residue substrate that is absorbed in the proximal small bowel. This diet can be given to most patients with Crohn's disease, even during acute exacerbations.

The diet should otherwise be low in residue, roughage, and fat but high in calories and protein. It may be difficult to maintain adequate absorption during periods of disease exacerbation and even during periods of remission. Milk and milk products may have to be excluded from the diet. Lactose, the primary disaccharide found in milk, may not be adequately digested because of the inability of the damaged intestinal mucosa to produce sufficient amounts of lactase. High-fat diets are poorly tolerated because of the loss of absorbing mucosa and altered bile salt metabolism and absorption.

Vitamin deficiencies may develop as a result of malabsorption. Cobalamin (vitamin B_{12}) injections every month may be needed because of the inability of the terminal ileum (if affected) to absorb this vitamin.

Surgical Therapy. Surgery is used in patients with severe symptoms that are unresponsive to therapy and in those with life-threatening complications. The majority of patients with Crohn's disease eventually require surgery at least once in the course of their disease. Indications for surgery are outlined in

TABLE 45-22 COLLABORATIVE CARE

Crohn's Disease

Diagnostic	Collaborative Therapy
• History and physical examination	• High-calorie, high-vitamin, high-protein, low-residue, dairy-free diet
• CBC, ESR	• Antimicrobial agents*
• Serum chemistries	• Corticosteroid drugs*
• Testing of stool for occult blood	• Immuno-suppressants*
• Radiological studies with barium contrast	• Immuno-modulators*
• Sigmoidoscopy and colonoscopy with biopsy	• Supplementary PN
	• Elemental diet
	• Physical and emotional rest
	• Surgery†

CBC, complete blood cell count; *ESR*, erythrocyte sedimentation rate; *PN*, parenteral nutrition.
*See Table 45-19.
†See Table 45-23.

TABLE 45-23 INDICATIONS FOR SURGICAL THERAPY FOR CROHN'S DISEASE

- Drainage of abdominal abscess
- Failure to respond to conservative therapy
- Fistulas
- Inability to decrease corticosteroids
- Intestinal obstruction
- Massive hemorrhage
- Perforation
- Secondary hydronephrosis
- Severe anorectal disease
- Suspicion of carcinoma

Table 45-23. Unlike UC, Crohn's disease is not cured by surgery. The recurrence rate after surgery is high. The surgical procedure depends on the affected area and the condition of the patient. Conservative intestinal resection with anastomosis of healthy bowel is the procedure of choice.

NURSING MANAGEMENT CROHN'S DISEASE

Care of patients with Crohn's disease is similar to that of patients with UC (see NCP 45-3, available on the Evolve website). As the patient's condition improves, the nurse should allow for more self-care, provide frequent rest periods, and advise the patient of the importance of rest and avoidance or control of emotional stress. This may be difficult for the patient when told the nature of the disease and the limitations of the treatment. Patients who have perianal fistulas or abscesses may need special skin care. Postoperative care should be the same as for laparotomy.

In the majority of patients with Crohn's disease, the course is chronic and intermittent. The patient and significant others may need help in setting realistic short- and long-term goals. Teaching is important and should include (1) the importance of rest and diet management, (2) perianal care, (3) action and adverse effects of drugs, (4) symptoms of recurrence of disease, (5) when to seek medical care, and (6) use of stress management techniques.

AGE-RELATED CONSIDERATIONS

INFLAMMATORY BOWEL DISEASE

Although IBDs (i.e., UC and Crohn's disease) are considered diseases of young adults, a second peak in the distribution of these inflammatory conditions occurs around the ages of 50 to 70 years. The pathogenesis, natural history, and clinical course of UC and Crohn's disease in older adults are similar to those observed in younger patients. However, the distribution of the inflammation appears to be somewhat different. In older-adult patients with UC, the distal colon is usually involved (proctitis). In older adults with Crohn's disease, the colon rather than the small intestine tends to be involved. There is less recurrence of Crohn's disease in older adults treated with surgical resection. The degree of inflammation associated with both conditions tends to be less in older-adult patients than in younger patients.

Collaborative care of older-adult patients with one of these conditions is similar to care of younger patients. However, because of increased risk for cardiovascular and pulmonary complications, older adults tend to have increased morbidity associated with surgical procedures.

TABLE 45-24 COMPARISON OF ULCERATIVE COLITIS AND CROHN'S DISEASE

Characteristic	Ulcerative Colitis	Crohn's Disease
Clinical		
Usual age at onset	Teens to mid-30s	Teens to mid-30s
Diarrhea	Common	Common
Abdominal cramping pain	Common	Common
Fever (intermittent)	During acute episodes	Common
Weight loss	Rare	Severe
Rectal bleeding	Common	Fairly common
Tenesmus	Severe	Infrequent
Malabsorption and nutritional deficiencies	Minimal incidence	Common
Pathological		
Location	Starts distally in the rectum and spreads proximally in a continuous fashion up the colon	Can occur anywhere along GI tract from mouth to anus, with characteristic skip lesions; most frequent site is terminal ileum
Distribution	Continuous	Segmental (skip lesions)
Depth of involvement	Mucosa and submucosa	Entire thickness of bowel wall (transmural)
Granulomas	Occasional	Common
Cobblestoning of mucosa	Rare	Common
Pseudopolyps	Common	Rare
Small bowel involvement	Minimal (backwash ileitis)	Common
Complications		
Fistulas	Rare	Common
Strictures	Occasional	Common
Anal abscesses	Rare	Common
Perforation	Common	Common
Toxic megacolon	Common	Rare
Carcinoma	Increased incidence after 10 yrs of disease	Slightly greater than general population
Recurrence after surgery	Cure with proctocolectomy	40–60% or more recurrence after segmental resections of small or large intestine

GI, gastro-intestinal.

In addition to Crohn's disease and UC, older adults are also vulnerable to inflammation of the colon (colitis) from medication use and systemic vascular disease. Drugs such as nonsteroidal anti-inflammatory drugs (NSAIDs), digitalis, vasopressin, estrogen, and allopurinol (Zyloprim) have been associated with colitis development in older-adult patients. Colitis may also be secondary to ischemic bowel disease related to atherosclerosis and heart failure.

Inflammation of the colon as a result of Crohn's disease or UC results in diarrhea, which may be bloody. The loss of fluid and electrolytes and possibly blood may leave older adults more vulnerable to problems related to volume depletion and dehydration. This may be particularly problematic in patients with diminished renal and cardiovascular function. Thus, nursing management is focused on careful assessment of fluid and electrolyte status and evaluation of the replacement therapies.

MALABSORPTION SYNDROME

Malabsorption results from impaired absorption of fats, carbohydrates, proteins, minerals, and vitamins. The stomach, small intestine, liver, and pancreas regulate normal digestion and absorption. Digestive enzymes ordinarily break down nutrients so that absorption can take place through the intestinal mucosa and nutrients can get into the bloodstream. If there is an interruption in this process at any point, malabsorption may occur. Several problems can cause malabsorption (Table 45-25). They can be classified into malabsorption caused by (1) biochemical or enzyme deficiencies, (2) bacterial proliferation, (3) disruption of small intestine mucosa, (4) disturbed lymphatic and vascular circulation, or (5) surface area loss. Lactose intolerance is the most common malabsorption disorder, followed by IBD, celiac disease, tropical sprue, and cystic fibrosis.

The most common clinical manifestation of malabsorption is steatorrhea, which is the passage of large amounts of fat as bulky, fatty, frothy, foul-smelling, yellow-grey, greasy stools with putty-like consistency that float in water and are difficult to flush (Table 45-26).

Tests used to determine the cause of malabsorption include qualitative examination of stool for fat (e.g., Sudan III stain), a 72-hour stool collection for quantitative measurement of fecal fat, serological testing for celiac disease, and fecal elastase testing to determine if there is pancreatic insufficiency. Other diagnostic studies include a CT scan and endoscopy to obtain a small bowel biopsy specimen for diagnosis. A small bowel barium enema is performed to identify abnormal mucosal patterns. Capsule endoscopy can be used to assess the small intestine for alterations in mucosal integrity and inflammation.

Tests for carbohydrate malabsorption include the D-xylose test and the lactose tolerance test. Laboratory studies that are frequently ordered include a CBC, measurement of prothrombin time (to see if vitamin K absorption is adequate), serum vitamin A and carotene levels, serum electrolytes, cholesterol, and calcium.

TABLE 45-25 COMMON CAUSES OF MALABSORPTION

Biochemical or Enzyme Deficiencies
- Lactase deficiency
- Biliary tract obstruction
- Pancreatic insufficiency
- Cystic fibrosis
- Chronic pancreatitis
- Zollinger–Ellison syndrome

Bacterial Proliferation
- Tropical sprue
- Parasitic infection

Small Intestinal Mucosal Disruption
- Celiac disease
- Whipple's disease
- Crohn's disease

Disturbed Lymphatic and Vascular Circulation
- Lymphoma
- Ischemia
- Lymphangiectasia
- Heart failure

Surface Area Loss
- Billroth II gastrectomy
- Gastro-jejunal bypass surgery for obesity
- Short bowel syndrome
- Distal ileal resection, disease, or bypass

CELIAC DISEASE

Celiac disease is an autoimmune disease characterized by damage to the small intestinal mucosa from the ingestion of wheat, barley, and rye in genetically susceptible individuals (Lowth, 2014). It was previously considered a rare intestinal disease that began in childhood, accompanied by symptoms of diarrhea, malabsorption, and malnutrition. We now know that it is relatively common, occurs at all ages, and has a wide variety of symptoms. *Celiac sprue* and *gluten-sensitive enteropathy* are other names for celiac disease. Celiac disease is not the same disease as *tropical sprue,* a chronic disorder acquired in tropical areas that is characterized by progressive disruption of jejunal and ileal tissue

TABLE 45-26 CLINICAL MANIFESTATIONS OF MALABSORPTION

Clinical Manifestations	Pathophysiology
Gastro-Intestinal	
Weight loss	Malabsorption of fat, carbohydrates, and protein leading to loss of calories; marked reduction in caloric intake or increased use of calories
Diarrhea	Impaired absorption of water, sodium, fatty acids, bile, or carbohydrates
Flatulence	Bacterial fermentation of unabsorbed carbohydrates
Steatorrhea	Undigested and unabsorbed fat
Glossitis, cheilosis, stomatitis	Deficiency of iron, riboflavin, cobalamin, folic acid, and other vitamins
Hematological	
Anemia	Impaired absorption of iron, cobalamin, and folic acid
Hemorrhagic tendency	Vitamin C deficiency
	Vitamin K deficiency inhibiting production of clotting Factors II, VII, IX, and X
Musculo-Skeletal	
Bone pain	Osteoporosis from impaired calcium absorption
	Osteomalacia secondary to hypocalcemia, hypophosphatemia, inadequate vitamin D
Tetany	Hypocalcemia, hypomagnesemia
Weakness, muscle cramps	Anemia, electrolyte depletion (especially potassium)
Muscle wasting	Protein malabsorption
Neurological	
Altered mental status	Dehydration
Paresthesias	Cobalamin deficiency
Peripheral neuropathy	Cobalamin deficiency
Night blindness	Thiamine deficiency, vitamin A deficiency
Integumentary	
Bruising	Vitamin K deficiency
Dermatitis	Fatty acid deficiency, zinc deficiency, niacin and other vitamin deficiencies
Brittle nails	Iron deficiency
Hair thinning and loss	Protein deficiency
Cardiovascular	
Hypotension	Dehydration
Tachycardia	Hypovolemia, anemia
Peripheral edema	Protein malabsorption, protein loss in diarrhea

resulting in nutritional difficulties. Tropical sprue is treated with folic acid and tetracycline. Celiac disease is most common in people of European ancestry, and it is estimated that approximately 1 in every 133 people in Canada is affected by celiac disease (Canadian Celiac Association, 2014).

Etiology and Pathophysiology

Three factors necessary for developing celiac disease are genetic predisposition, gluten ingestion, and an immune-mediated response. As with other autoimmune diseases, the tissue destruction that occurs with celiac disease is the result of chronic inflammation. Inflammation is activated by the ingestion of gluten found in wheat, rye, and barley. Gluten contains specific peptides called *prolamines*. In genetically susceptible individuals, partial digestion of gluten releases prolamine peptides, which are absorbed into the lamina propria in the intestinal submucosa.

Once in the lamina propria, peptides bind to human leukocyte antigen (HLA)-DQ2 and HLA-DQ8 (or both) antigens and activate an inflammatory response. Inflammation damages the microvilli and brush border of the small intestine, decreasing the amount of surface area available for nutrient absorption (Mavrinac, Ohannessian, Dowling, et al., 2014). Damage is most severe in the duodenum, probably related to the greater exposure to gluten. The intestinal damage decreases distal to the duodenum. The inflammation continues until gluten ingestion ceases.

Clinical Manifestations

Classic signs of celiac disease include foul-smelling diarrhea, steatorrhea, flatulence, abdominal distension, and symptoms of malnutrition. Some people have no obvious GI symptoms, and may have atypical symptoms such as decreased bone density and osteoporosis, dental enamel hypoplasia, iron and folate deficiencies, peripheral neuropathy, and reproductive problems (Mavrinac et al., 2014). A pruritic, vesicular skin lesion, called *dermatitis herpetiformis*, is sometimes present and occurs as a rash on the buttocks, scalp, face, elbows, and knees. Celiac disease is also associated with autoimmune diseases, particularly rheumatoid arthritis, type 1 diabetes mellitus, and thyroid disease. Protein, fat, and carbohydrate absorption is affected, leading to poor growth, weight loss, muscle wasting, and other signs of malnutrition. Abnormal folate, iron, and cobalamin levels can occur. Iron-deficiency anemia is one of the most common manifestations of celiac disease. Patients may exhibit lactose intolerance and should eliminate lactose-containing products until the disease is under control. Inadequate calcium intake and vitamin D absorption can lead to decreased bone density and osteoporosis. Poor nutrition leads to reproductive problems.

Diagnostic Studies and Collaborative Care

Celiac disease is confirmed when (1) there is histological evidence of the disease following biopsy from the small intestine and (2) the symptoms and histological evidence disappear when the person eats a gluten-free diet (Mavrinac et al., 2014). Diagnostic testing must be done before the person is placed on a gluten-free diet because the diet will alter the results. Biopsies show flattened mucosa and noticeable losses of villi. Celiac disease should be ruled out during a diagnostic workup of IBS because the symptoms are similar. Many people spend years seeking treatment for nonspecific complaints before celiac disease is diagnosed (thus the large number of people who are diagnosed in adulthood). Treatment with a gluten-free diet halts the process. Most patients recover completely within 3 to 6 months of treatment, but they need to maintain a gluten-free diet for life. Wheat, barley, oats, and rye products must be avoided. Although pure oats do not contain gluten, oat products can become contaminated with wheat, rye, and barley during the milling process. Gluten is also found in some medications and in many food additives, preservatives, and stabilizers. A combination of corticosteroids and a gluten-free diet is used to treat individuals who do not respond to the gluten-free diet alone. If the disease is untreated, chronic inflammation and hyperplasia continue. Individuals with celiac disease have an increased risk for non-Hodgkin's lymphoma and GI cancers.

LACTASE DEFICIENCY

Lactase deficiency is a condition in which the lactase enzyme is deficient or absent. *Lactase* is the enzyme that breaks down lactose into two simple sugars—glucose and galactose. Although primary lactase deficiency seems to be hereditary, milk intolerance may not become clinically evident until late adolescence or early adulthood. About 5% of the adult population has primary lactase deficiency. The highest incidence in Canada is found in people who are Black, Indigenous, Latin American, Asian, and of Jewish descent. Often, acquired lactase deficiency is seen in conjunction with other GI diseases in which the mucosa has been damaged, including UC, Crohn's disease, gastro-enteritis, and celiac disease.

Clinical Manifestations

The symptoms of lactose intolerance include bloating, flatulence, crampy abdominal pain, and diarrhea. They may occur within a half hour to several hours after drinking a glass of milk or ingesting a milk product. The diarrhea of lactose intolerance results from fluid secretion into the small intestine, a response to the osmotic action of undigested lactose.

NURSING AND COLLABORATIVE MANAGEMENT LACTASE DEFICIENCY

Many people who are lactose-intolerant are aware of their milk intolerance and avoid milk. A lactose intolerance test can be performed to rule out milk allergies. The patient is given 50 g of lactose orally. Blood samples are drawn before the consumption of lactose and at 15-, 30-, 60-, and 90-minute intervals. Failure of the blood glucose level to increase more than 20 mg/dL is suggestive of lactase deficiency. Results of the hydrogen breath test after ingestion of lactose are abnormal.

Treatment consists of eliminating lactose from the diet by avoiding milk and milk products. A lactose-free diet is given initially and is gradually advanced to a low-lactose diet, as tolerated by the patient. Many people who are lactose-intolerant may not exhibit symptoms if lactose is taken in small amounts. In some people, lactose may be tolerated better if taken with meals.

The patient needs to be aware that milk, ice cream, cottage cheese, and cheese have a high lactose content. If the milk has been fermented (e.g., cultured buttermilk, yogourt, sour cream), the patient with low lactase levels may tolerate it better.

Lactase enzyme (Lactaid) is available commercially as an over-the-counter (OTC) product. It is mixed with milk and breaks down the lactose before the milk is ingested. Lactase tablets can also be taken with the ingestion of other dairy products. Since avoidance of milk and milk products can lead to calcium deficiency, supplements may be necessary to prevent osteoporosis.

SHORT-BOWEL SYNDROME

Short bowel syndrome (SBS) results from extensive resection of the small intestine. Rapid intestinal transit, impaired digestive and absorption processes, and fluid and electrolyte losses characterize the syndrome. In adults, extensive resection of the small intestine may be necessary for bowel infarction because of vascular thrombosis or insufficiency, abdominal trauma, cancer, radiation enteritis, or Crohn's disease.

The length and the portions of small bowel resected are associated with the number and severity of symptoms. Resections of up to 50% of the small intestine cause little disturbance of bowel function, especially if the terminal ileum and the ileocecal valve remain intact. After large resections, the remaining intestine undergoes adaptive changes that are more pronounced in the ileum. The villi and the crypts increase in size, and absorptive capacity of the remaining intestine increases. Intestinal adaptation is enhanced by the presence of food, fibre, bile, and pancreatic secretions in the lumen and continues for up to 2 years. Resection of the ileum, the ileocecal valve, or the colon results in a rapid intestinal transit, decreasing absorption time. Ileal resection causes malabsorption of cobalamin, bile salts, and fat, resulting in steatorrhea.

Clinical Manifestations

The predominant manifestations of SBS are diarrhea, steatorrhea, and weight loss. There may be signs of malnutrition and multiple vitamin and mineral deficiencies (e.g., cobalamin and zinc deficiency, hypocalcemia). The patient may develop lactase deficiency and bacterial overgrowth. Oxalate kidney stones may form from increased colonic absorption of oxalate.

Collaborative Care

The overall goals are that the patient with SBS will have fluid and electrolyte balance, normal nutritional status, and control of diarrhea. In the period immediately following massive bowel resection, patients receive PN to replace fluid, electrolyte, and nutrient losses. Hypersecretion of gastric acid, for which the cause is unknown, is reduced by proton pump inhibitors (e.g., omeprazole [Losec]).

A high-carbohydrate, low-fat diet supplemented with soluble fibre and pectin may slow transit time and improve nutrient absorption, decrease stool output, and enable patients to wean off parenteral nutrition. The patient with SBS is encouraged to eat at least six to eight meals per day to increase the overall time food is present in and in contact with the intestine. Oral intake can be supplemented with elemental nutrient formulas and tube feeding during the night. For patients with severe malabsorption, PN may be reinstituted. Oral supplements of calcium, zinc, and multivitamins are typically recommended.

Opioid antidiarrheal drugs are the most effective in decreasing intestinal motility (see Table 45-3). For patients with limited ileal resections (<100 cm), cholestyramine reduces diarrhea resulting from unabsorbed bile acids and increases their excretion in feces. Bile acids stimulate intestinal fluid secretion and reduce colonic fluid absorption.

Intestinal transplantation is a procedure performed at a few specialized transplant centres. Candidates for this procedure are patients with SBS, dependence on parenteral nutrition, and chronic liver disease. It is often considered a last-resort treatment option for patients with intestinal failure who develop life-threatening complications from parenteral nutrition. Transplantation may include the intestine alone, liver and intestine, or multivisceral combinations (stomach, duodenum, jejunum, ileum, colon, and pancreas).

INTESTINAL OBSTRUCTION

Intestinal obstruction occurs when a partial or complete obstruction of the intestine prevents intestinal contents from passing through the GI tract; it requires prompt treatment. The causes of intestinal obstruction can be classified as mechanical or nonmechanical.

Types of Intestinal Obstruction

Mechanical. *Mechanical obstruction* may be caused by an occlusion of the lumen of the intestinal tract (Figure 45-4). Most intestinal obstructions occur in the small intestine and are usually due to adhesions. Adhesions can develop after abdominal surgery. Obstruction can occur within days of surgery or years later. Carcinoma is the most common cause of large bowel obstruction, followed by volvulus and diverticular disease.

Nonmechanical. A *nonmechanical obstruction* may result from a neuro-muscular or vascular disorder. Paralytic (adynamic) ileus is an impairment of intestinal motility (ileus that persists for more than 2 to 3 days), and is the most common form of nonmechanical obstruction. It can occur after any abdominal surgery. Other causes of paralytic ileus include peritonitis, inflammatory responses (e.g., acute pancreatitis, acute appendicitis), electrolyte abnormalities, and thoracic or lumbar spinal fractures.

Pseudo-obstruction is an apparent mechanical obstruction of the intestine without demonstration of obstruction by radiological methods. Collagen vascular diseases and neurological and endocrine disorders may cause pseudo-obstruction, but mostly, it is found to be idiopathic.

Vascular obstructions are rare and are due to an interference with the blood supply to a portion of the intestines. The most common causes are emboli and atherosclerosis of the mesenteric arteries. The celiac, inferior, and superior mesenteric arteries supply blood to the bowel. Emboli may originate from thrombi in patients with chronic atrial fibrillation, diseased heart valves, and prosthetic valves. Venous thrombosis may be seen in low–blood flow states, such as heart failure and shock.

Etiology and Pathophysiology

Normally, 6 to 8 L of fluid enters the small bowel daily. Most of the fluid is absorbed before it reaches the colon. Approximately 75% of intestinal gas is swallowed air. Bacterial metabolism produces methane and hydrogen gases. Fluid, gas, and intestinal contents accumulate proximal to the intestinal obstruction. This causes distension, and the distal bowel may collapse. The distension reduces the absorption of fluids and stimulates intestinal secretions. As the fluid increases, so does the pressure in the lumen of the bowel. The increased pressure leads to an increase in capillary permeability and extravasation of fluids and electrolytes into the peritoneal cavity. Edema, congestion, and necrosis from impaired blood supply as well as possible rupture of the bowel may occur. The retention of fluid in the intestine and the peritoneal cavity can lead to a severe reduction in circulating blood volume and result in hypotension and hypovolemic shock.

The electrolyte-rich fluids, which are normally absorbed in the bowel, are retained in the bowel and subsequently lost into

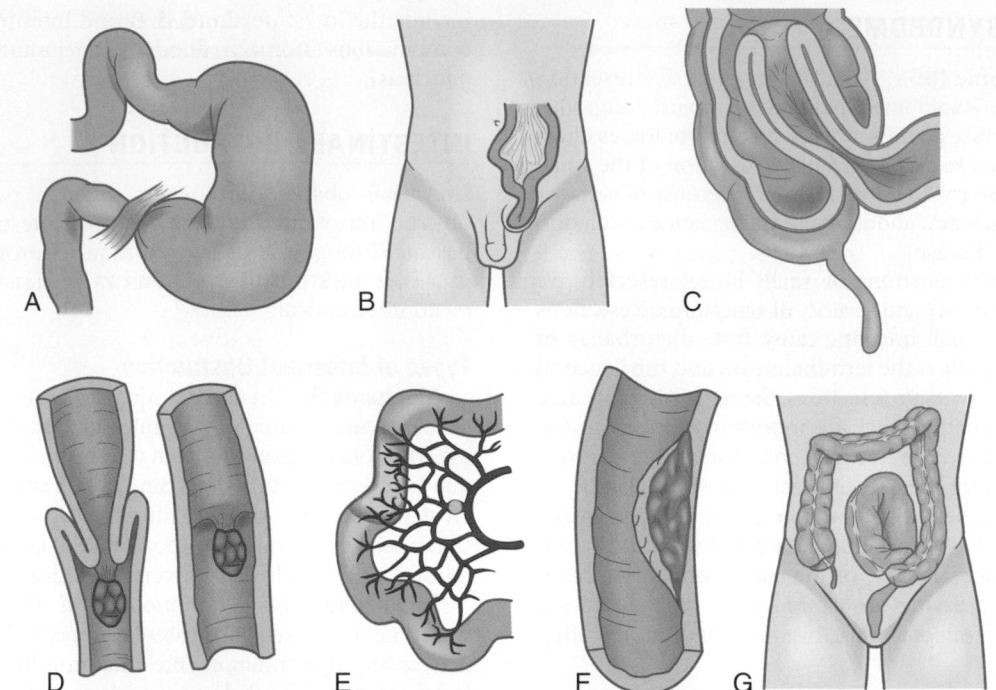

FIGURE 45-4 Bowel obstructions. **A,** Adhesions. **B,** Strangulated inguinal hernia. **C,** Ileocecal intussusception. **D,** Intussusception from polyps. **E,** Mesenteric occlusion. **F,** Neoplasm. **G,** Volvulus of the sigmoid colon.

the peritoneal cavity. The location of the obstruction determines the extent of fluid, electrolyte, and acid–base imbalances. If the obstruction is high, as in an obstruction in the pylorus, metabolic alkalosis may result from the loss of hydrochloric acid from the stomach through vomiting or NG intubation.

When the obstruction is located in the small bowel, dehydration occurs rapidly. Dehydration and electrolyte imbalances do not occur early in large bowel obstruction. If the obstruction is below the proximal colon, most GI fluids have been absorbed before reaching the point of the obstruction. Solid fecal material accumulates until symptoms of discomfort appear. Reverse peristalsis may cause vomiting of fecal material very late in the bowel obstruction.

Simple obstructions of the intestine involve blockage of the lumen in one spot. A closed-loop obstruction occurs when the lumen is blocked in two different spots (e.g., volvulus). This results in an isolated segment of bowel and obstruction proximal to that segment. Strangulation and gangrene are likely to develop if treatment is not immediate. A strangulated obstruction occurs when the circulation to the obstructed intestine is impaired. This is the most dangerous form of obstruction because it may lead to necrosis of the intestine (incarcerated). Volvulus, hernias, or adhesions are the most common causes.

Clinical Manifestations

The clinical manifestations of intestinal obstruction vary, depending on the location of the obstruction, and include nausea, vomiting, abdominal pain, distension, inability to pass flatus, and obstipation (Table 45-27). Obstruction located high in the small intestine produces rapid-onset, sometimes projectile vomiting with bile-containing vomitus. Vomiting from more distal obstructions of the small intestine is more gradual in onset. The vomitus may be orange-brown and foul smelling because of bacterial overgrowth. Vomiting may be entirely absent in large

TABLE 45-27	CLINICAL MANIFESTATIONS OF SMALL AND LARGE INTESTINAL OBSTRUCTIONS	
Clinical Manifestations	Small Intestine	Large Intestine
Onset	Rapid	Gradual
Vomiting	Frequent and copious	Late manifestation
Pain	Colicky, cramplike, intermittent	Low-grade, cramping abdominal pain
Bowel movement	Feces for a short time	Absolute constipation
Abdominal distension	Dependent upon location of obstruction, minimal to greatly increased	Greatly increased

bowel obstruction if the ileocecal valve is competent; otherwise, the patient may eventually vomit fecal material.

Vomiting usually relieves abdominal pain in high intestinal obstructions. Persistent, colicky abdominal pain is seen with lower intestinal obstruction. A characteristic sign of mechanical obstruction is pain that comes and goes in waves. This is caused by intestinal peristalsis working to move bowel contents past the obstructed area. In contrast, paralytic ileus produces a more constant generalized discomfort. Strangulation causes severe, constant pain that is rapid in onset. Abdominal distension is a common manifestation of intestinal obstructions. It is usually absent or minimally noticeable in proximal obstructions of the small intestine and greatly increased in lower intestinal obstructions. Abdominal tenderness and rigidity are usually absent unless strangulation or peritonitis has occurred.

Auscultation of bowel sounds reveals high-pitched sounds above the area of obstruction. The patient often notes borborygmi (audible abdominal sounds produced by hyperactive intestinal motility). The patient's temperature rarely rises above 37.8°C unless strangulation or peritonitis has occurred.

Diagnostic Studies

A thorough history and physical examination should be performed for patients with intestinal obstruction. CT scan and abdominal radiographic studies are the most useful diagnostic aids. Upright and lateral abdominal radiographs show the presence of gas and fluid in the intestines (air–fluid levels). The presence of intraperitoneal air indicates perforation. Sigmoidoscopy or colonoscopy may provide direct visualization of an obstruction in the colon.

Laboratory tests are important and provide essential information. A CBC and serum electrolyte, amylase, and blood urea nitrogen (BUN) determinations should be performed. An elevated WBC count may indicate strangulation or perforation; elevated hematocrit values may reflect hemoconcentration. Decreased hemoglobin and hematocrit values may indicate bleeding from a neoplasm or strangulation with necrosis. Serum electrolytes should be monitored to assess the patient's fluid and electrolyte balance. Serum sodium, potassium, and chloride concentrations are decreased in small-bowel obstruction. The BUN value may be increased because of dehydration. The stool should be checked for occult blood.

Collaborative Care

Treatment for intestinal obstruction is directed toward decompression of the intestine by removal of gas and fluid, correction and maintenance of fluid and electrolyte balance, and relief or removal of the obstruction. NG tubes may be used to decompress the bowel. NG tubes may be inserted before surgery to empty the stomach and relieve distension. NG or venting percutaneous tubes are effective in the treatment of patients with neurogenic obstruction who do not require surgery.

Sigmoidoscopy may successfully reduce a sigmoid volvulus. Colon-decompression catheters may be passed through partially obstructed areas via a colonoscope to decompress the bowel before surgery.

Intravenous infusions that contain normal saline solution and potassium should be given to maintain fluid and electrolyte balance. PN may be necessary in some cases to correct nutritional deficiencies, improve the patient's nutritional status before surgery, and promote postoperative healing.

Most mechanical obstructions are treated surgically. Surgery may involve resecting the obstructed segment of bowel and anastomosing the remaining healthy bowel. Partial or total colectomy, colostomy, or ileostomy may be required when extensive obstruction or necrosis is present. Occasionally, obstructions can be removed nonsurgically. A colonoscope can be used to remove polyps, dilate strictures, and remove and destroy tumours with a laser.

NURSING MANAGEMENT
INTESTINAL OBSTRUCTION

NURSING ASSESSMENT

Intestinal obstruction is a potentially life-threatening condition. Nursing assessment must begin with a detailed patient history and physical examination. The type and the location of obstruction usually cause characteristic symptoms. The nurse should determine location, duration, intensity, and frequency of abdominal pain and whether abdominal tenderness or rigidity is present. For vomiting, the onset, frequency, colour, odour, and amount

of vomitus should be recorded. Bowel function, including passage of flatus, should be determined. The nurse auscultates for bowel sounds and documents the character and the location; inspects the abdomen for scars, palpable masses, and distension; and observes for muscle guarding and tenderness.

NURSING DIAGNOSES

Nursing diagnoses for patients with intestinal obstructions include, but are not limited to, the following:

- *Acute pain* related to *biological injury agent* (abdominal distention and increased peristalsis)
- *Deficient fluid volume* related to *insufficient fluid intake* (decrease in intestinal fluid absorption, third space fluid shifts, NG suction)

PLANNING

The overall goals are that the patient with an intestinal obstruction will have (1) relief of the obstruction and return to normal bowel function, (2) minimal to no discomfort, (3) normal fluid and electrolyte status, and (4) maintenance of adequate nutrition.

NURSING IMPLEMENTATION

The patient should be monitored closely for signs of dehydration and electrolyte imbalance. A strict intake and output record should be maintained. Intravenous fluids should be administered as ordered. Serum electrolyte levels should be monitored. A patient with a high obstruction is more likely to have metabolic alkalosis; a patient with a low obstruction is at greater risk for metabolic acidosis. The patient is often restless and constantly changes position to relieve the pain. The nurse should provide comfort measures, promote a restful environment, and keep distractions and visitors to a minimum. Nursing care of the patient after surgery for an intestinal obstruction is similar to care of the patient after a laparotomy (see NCP 45-2, available on the Evolve website).

POLYPS OF THE LARGE INTESTINE

Colonic polyps arise from the mucosal surface of the colon and project into the lumen. They may be *sessile* (flat, broad based, and attached directly to the intestinal wall) or *pedunculated* (attached to the intestinal wall by a stalk). Polyps tend to be sessile when small and become pedunculated as they enlarge, especially if they are in the left or descending colon (Figure 45-5). They may be found anywhere in the large intestine but are most commonly found in the rectosigmoid area. Although most polyps are asymptomatic, rectal bleeding or occult blood in the stool are the most common manifestations.

Types of Polyps

The most common types of polyp are hyperplastic and adenomatous. *Hyperplastic polyps* originate from the epithelium and are non-neoplastic growths. They rarely grow larger than 5 mm and never cause clinical symptoms. Other benign (non-neoplastic) polyps include inflammatory polyps, lipomas, and juvenile polyps (Table 45-28).

Adenomatous polyps are characterized by neoplastic changes in the epithelium. They are closely linked to colorectal adenocarcinoma. Structurally, there are three types, with tubular adenomas being the most prevalent. The risk for cancer in the polyp increases with polyp size and villous structure. Villous adenomas have a higher risk of turning cancerous than tubular

FIGURE 45-5 Endoscopic image of a pedunculated polyp in the descending colon. Source: David Musher/Science Source.

TABLE 45-28	TYPES OF POLYPS OF THE LARGE INTESTINE
Neoplastic	**Non-Neoplastic**
• Epithelial polyps (adenomatous)	• Epithelial polyps (hyperplastic)
• Tubular adenoma	• Hereditary polyposis syndromes
• Tubular villous adenoma	• Familial juvenile polyposis
• Villous adenoma	• Inflammatory polyps
• Hereditary polyposis syndromes (adenomatous polyposis syndrome)	• Pseudopolyps
• Familial adenomatous polyposis (FAP)	• Benign lymphoid polyps
	• Submucosal
	• Lipomas
	• Leiomyomas
	• Fibromas

GENETICS IN CLINICAL PRACTICE
Familial Adenomatous Polyposis (FAP)

Genetic Basis
- Autosomal dominant disorder
- Mutation in *APC* gene located on chromosome 5

Incidence
- 1 in 5 000–7 500 people
- Men and women affected equally

Genetic Testing
- DNA testing available to detect *APC* gene mutation

Clinical Implications
- FAP is characterized by the presence of colorectal polyps (usually >1 000).
- Polyps are not present at birth but appear during adolescence and early adulthood.
- FAP accounts for at least 1% of all colorectal cancers.
- If untreated, FAP almost always results in the development of colon cancer before the age of 40.
- With FAP, there is also increased incidence of gastric and small intestinal polyps.
- Many deaths related to FAP could be prevented with early and aggressive monitoring and treatment, including frequent colonoscopies and total colectomy.
- Individuals with a family history of FAP could benefit from genetic counselling and teaching.

APC, adenomatous polyposis coli; *FAP*, familial adenomatous polyposis.

adenomas. Removing adenomatous polyps decreases the occurrence of colorectal cancer.

Although there are several polyposis syndromes, they are relatively rare. Of these, *familial adenomatous polyposis* (FAP) is the most common (see the "Genetics in Clinical Practice" box). This disorder is characterized by multiple polyps that at times number in the thousands and that are located in the large intestine and sometimes in other areas of the GI tract. Patients with a history of FAP have a lifetime risk of developing colorectal cancer that approaches 100%. They also develop cancer at an earlier age (i.e., <40 years of age) than patients with non-FAP colorectal cancer. For children of patients with FAP, screening must be initiated at puberty and then conducted annually. These children have a 50% risk of developing FAP. When there is indication of disease, total colectomy with ileostomy is the treatment of choice. Patients with FAP are also at risk for cancers of the thyroid, small bowel, liver, and brain, so lifetime cancer surveillance is essential (Suhaimi, Nazri, Latar, et al., 2015).

Diagnostic Studies and Collaborative Care

Barium enema, sigmoidoscopy, colonoscopy and CT/MRI colonography (virtual colonoscopy) are used to diagnose polyps. All polyps are considered abnormal and should be removed. In patients whose polyps are identified through barium enema, removal (polypectomy) should be done through a colonoscope or a sigmoidoscope. If the polyp is not removable, a biopsy specimen should be taken for tissue examination. Surgery is not indicated unless carcinoma is present or certain cases of polyposis syndromes warrant it. The patient should be observed for rectal bleeding, fever, severe abdominal pain, and abdominal distension, which may indicate hemorrhage or perforation.

COLORECTAL CANCER

Colorectal cancer (a malignant disease of the colon, the rectum, or both) is the second-most common cause of cancer death in Canada. In 2015, it was estimated that there would be 25 100 new cases of colorectal cancer diagnosed in Canada, and that 9 300 people would die from it (Colorectal Cancer Association of Canada, 2016a).

The incidence of colorectal cancer at specific sites varies (Figure 45-6). In both sexes, the incidence of right colon cancers has increased, and cancers in the rectum have decreased. The highest percentages of colorectal cancers in Canada are currently located in the rectum, the ascending colon, and the sigmoid colon. Approximately 20% of colorectal cancers are within reach of the examining finger, and 50% are within reach of the sigmoidoscope.

Etiology and Pathophysiology

Risk factors for CRC include a diet high in red or processed meat, obesity, physical inactivity, alcohol, long-term smoking, and low intake of fruits and vegetables. Groups at high risk for colorectal cancer have been identified (Table 45-29), and genetic conditions such as FAP and a personal history of IBD place an individual at risk for CRC. About one-third of cases of CRC occur in patients with a family history of CRC. (See the two "Genetics in Clinical Practice" boxes in this chapter.) Age is a risk factor in both men and women. The risk for development

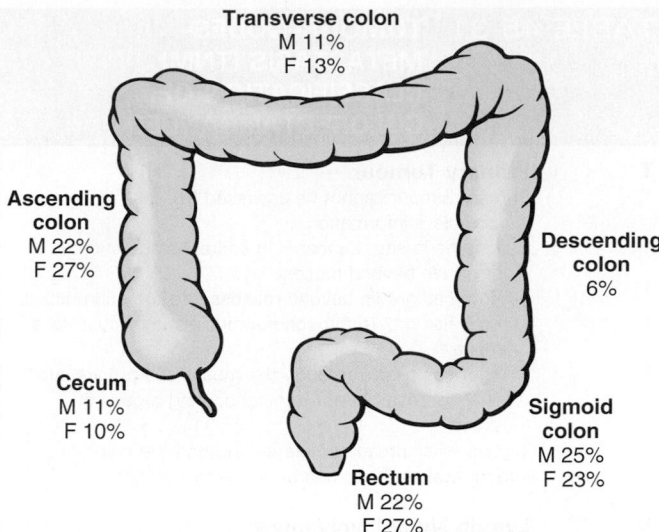

FIGURE 45-6 Incidence of colorectal cancer. Approximately one-half of all colon cancers occur in the rectosigmoid area. Percentages are listed for males *(M)* and females *(F)*.

TABLE 45-29	RISK FACTORS FOR COLORECTAL CANCER

- Age >50 years
- Alcohol (over 4 drinks per week)
- Chronic inflammatory bowel disease
- Cigarette smoking
- Colorectal polyps
- Familial adenomatous polyposis (FAP)
- Family history of colorectal cancer or adenomas
- History of ovarian, endometrial, or breast cancer (women)
- Increased consumption of red meat
- Obesity
- Previous history of colorectal cancer

in the general population increases slightly after the age of 50 years and then rises rapidly in the following decades.

Adenocarcinoma is the most common type of colorectal cancer. Most colorectal cancers begin as adenomatous polyps that arise from the mucosa lining the lumen of the colon and the rectum. As it grows, the cancer progresses down from the tip of the polyp through the body and stalk. It becomes invasive and penetrates the muscularis mucosae. Once through the muscularis mucosae, tumour cells gain access to the regional lymph nodes and the vascular system and can spread to distant sites. The most common sites of metastasis are the regional lymph nodes, liver, lungs, and peritoneum. Because venous blood leaving the colon and rectum flows through the portal vein and inferior rectal vein, the liver and lung are common sites of metastasis. The cancer spreads from the liver to other sites, including the lungs, bones, and brain. The cancer can also spread directly into adjacent structures. The growing tumour can obstruct the bowel. Other complications include bleeding, perforation, peritonitis, and fistula formation.

Clinical Manifestations

Clinical manifestations of colorectal cancer are usually nonspecific or do not appear until the disease is advanced. Rectal bleeding is the most common symptom of colorectal cancer but it may

GENETICS IN CLINICAL PRACTICE

Hereditary Nonpolyposis Colorectal Cancer

Genetic Basis
- Autosomal dominant disorder
- Mutations in *MSH2, MLH1, MSH6, PMS2* genes
- Mutations in genes that error-check DNA (repair genes)

Incidence
- 1 in 500–2000 people

Genetic Testing
- DNA testing available

Clinical Implications
- HNPCC accounts for 5% of all colorectal cancers.
- Individuals with gene mutation have 80%–90% lifetime risk of developing colorectal cancer.
- Average age of diagnosis is in the mid-40s.
- Cancer arises from single colorectal lesion in absence of polyposis.
- Cancers tend to occur on right side of colon.
- HNPCC is less aggressive and is associated with longer survival rates than colon cancers that develop without known risk factors.
- People with gene mutation are at high risk of developing other cancers, including uterine, ovarian, ureter, pancreas, stomach, and small intestinal cancer.
- Individuals with known gene mutations should be monitored with colonoscopy every year.
- Examination by pelvic ultrasound and endometrial biopsy should also be considered for women.

HNPCC, hereditary nonpolyposis colorectal cancer.

not be visible to the naked eye Other commonly seen manifestations include alternating constipation and diarrhea, abdominal cramps, gas or bloating, change in stool calibre (narrow, ribbon-like), loss of appetite, early satiety, weight loss, lethargy and sensation of incomplete evacuation (Figure 45-7) (Colorectal Cancer Association of Canada, 2016b).

Iron-deficiency anemia and occult bleeding dictate further investigation. Due to increased emphasis on screening practices, colon cancer is now often detected during screening procedures.

Diagnostic Studies

A thorough history, with close attention to family history, should be obtained, and a physical examination should be performed (Table 45-30). The digital rectal examination is the most important aspect of the physical examination because many rectal cancers are within reach of the finger. In the asymptomatic person who is 50 years or older with no risk factors (other than age), a *fecal occult blood test* (FOBT) or *fecal immunochemical test* (FIT) once a year and flexible sigmoidoscopy every 5 years beginning at age 50 are important aspects of the examination. Fecal occult blood tests have been used for more than 30 years to screen for colorectal cancer and continue to be widely used in North America. Patients need to be taught to abstain from red meat, acetylsalicylic acid (ASA; Aspirin) and NSAIDs (if medically safe) before testing, to avoid false positives. The FIT uses antibodies to detect human hemoglobin protein in stool. It is performed in much the same way as the FOBT, but there are no drug or dietary restrictions. The Septin9 blood test is another screening tool for CRC. It detects the presence of methylated Septin9 DNA, which is correlated with an increased risk for CRC (Colorectal Cancer Association of Canada, 2016c).

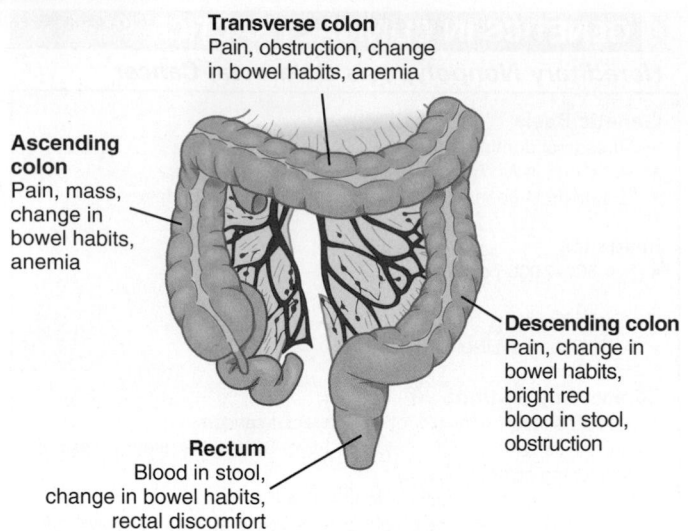

Transverse colon
Pain, obstruction, change
in bowel habits, anemia

Ascending colon
Pain, mass,
change in
bowel habits,
anemia

Descending colon
Pain, change in
bowel habits,
bright red
blood in stool,
obstruction

Rectum
Blood in stool,
change in bowel habits,
rectal discomfort

FIGURE 45-7 Signs and symptoms of colorectal cancer by location of primary lesion. Source: Modified from McCance, K. L., & Huether, S. E. (2010). *Pathophysiology: The biologic basis for disease in adults and children* (6th ed., p. 1502). St. Louis: Mosby.

TABLE 45-30 COLLABORATIVE CARE

Colorectal Cancer

Diagnostic	Collaborative Therapy
• History and physical examination	• Surgery
• Digital rectal examination	• Right hemicolectomy
• Sigmoidoscopy	• Left hemicolectomy
• Colonoscopy	• Abdominal–perineal resection
• Barium enema	• Laparoscopic colectomy
• CBC	• Radiation
• Liver function tests	• Chemotherapy
• Testing of stool for occult blood	
• Carcinoembryonic antigen (CEA) test	
• CT scan of abdomen	
• Ultrasound (including endorectal)	
• MRI	

CBC, complete blood cell count; *CT*, computed tomographic (scan); *MRI*, magnetic resonance imaging.

TABLE 45-31 TUMOUR–NODES–METASTASIS (TNM) CLASSIFICATION OF COLORECTAL CANCER

T	**Primary Tumour**
T_x	Primary tumour cannot be assessed because of incomplete information.
T_{is}	Carcinoma in situ. Cancer is in earliest stage and has not grown beyond mucosa layer.
T_1	Tumour has grown beyond mucosa into the submucosa.
T_2	Tumour has grown through submucosa into muscularis propria.
T_3	Tumour has grown through the muscularis propria into the subserosa but not to neighbouring organs or tissues.
T_4	Tumour has spread completely through the colon or rectal wall and into nearby tissues or organs.
N	**Lymph Node Involvement**
N_x	Lymph nodes cannot be assessed.
N_0	No regional lymph node involvement is found.
N_1	Cancer is found in one to three nearby lymph nodes.
N_2	Cancer is found in four or more nearby lymph nodes.
M	**Metastasis**
M_x	Presence of distant metastasis cannot be assessed.
M_0	No distant metastasis is seen.
M_1	Distant metastasis is present.

Stage	TNM		
0	T_{is}	N_0	M_0
IA	T_1	N_0	M_0
IB	T_2	N_0	M_0
II	T_1	N_2	M_0
	T_2	N_1	M_0
	T_3	N_0	M_0
IIIA	T_2	N_2	M_0
	T_3	N_{1-2}	M_0
IIIB	T_4	N_{0-1}	M_0
IV	T_4	N_2	M_0
	T_{1-4}	N_{0-2}	M_1

Colonoscopy is the procedure of choice. Synchronous lesions may be present at other sites in the colon, and tissue diagnosis may be made by biopsy during the procedure. Other procedures include endorectal ultrasonography and *CT colonography (virtual colonoscopy)* to localize the lesion and determine its size or the presence of metastases.

Laboratory studies should include a CBC to check for anemia, clotting studies, and liver function tests. A CT scan of the abdomen may be helpful in detecting liver metastases, retroperitoneal and pelvic disease, and depth of penetration of the tumour into the bowel wall. A CT scan should be done before surgery. Liver function tests are performed to determine the presence of liver metastases.

A carcinoembryonic antigen (CEA) test is often performed, although it is not specific for colorectal cancer. A normal level of CEA does not exclude the possibility of a malignant condition. This test is used most effectively in following the progress of a patient after surgery. Return to normal of a previously elevated CEA indicates successful removal of the tumour. In contrast, postoperative CEA levels that are persistently elevated or that increase suggest the presence of residual tumour or tumour spread.

Collaborative Care

Prognosis and treatment correlate with pathological staging of the disease. Several methods of staging are available, with the TNM (tumour–nodes–metastasis) system (Table 45-31) being the most widely used. It describes a patient's cancer based on the degree of invasion of the primary tumour, lymph node involvement, and presence of metastasis. The stage at diagnosis is key in determining prognosis and appropriate treatment.

Several noninvasive procedures may be performed through a colonoscope to effectively treat certain types of colorectal cancer. Endoscopic polypectomy is a highly effective and safe procedure. Adequate treatment can be obtained if the resected margin of the polyp is free of cancer, the cancer is well differentiated, and there is no apparent lymphatic or blood vessel involvement. Laser therapy may be used to ablate nonresectable tumours. This is usually used only as palliative therapy in patients with obstructive symptoms.

Surgical Therapy. The location and the extent of the cancer determine the type of surgery performed. Success of surgery depends on resection of the tumour with an adequate margin of healthy bowel and resection of the regional lymph nodes.

Right hemicolectomy is performed when the cancer is located in the cecum, the ascending colon, the hepatic flexure, or the transverse colon to the right of the middle colic artery. A portion of the terminal ileum, the ileocecal valve, and the appendix are removed, and an ileotransverse anastomosis is performed. A left hemicolectomy involves resection of the left transverse colon, the splenic flexure, the descending colon, the sigmoid colon, and the upper portion of the rectum.

Clear margins are most difficult to obtain with rectal carcinoma. Location of the rectal lesion determines the surgical procedure to be performed. There must be enough rectum left to ensure a secure anastomosis and preservation of anal sphincter function, or an abdominal–perineal resection is indicated. Abdominal–perineal resection is most often performed when the cancer is located within 5 cm of the anus, although ultra-low anterior resections can be performed (within 1 to 2 cm of the anus) by skilled surgeons.

In the abdominal–perineal resection, an abdominal incision is made, and the proximal sigmoid is brought through the abdominal wall as a permanent colostomy. The distal sigmoid, rectum, and anus are removed through a perineal incision. The perineal wound may be primarily closed with a drain or left open with appropriate dressings to allow healing by secondary intention. Complications that can occur are delayed wound healing, hemorrhage, persistent perineal sinus tracts, infections, and urinary tract and sexual dysfunctions.

Low anterior resection may be indicated for tumours of the rectosigmoid and the mid-to-upper rectum. The use of EEA (end-to-end anastomosis) staplers has allowed lower and more secure anastomoses. The stapler is passed through the anus, where the colon is stapled to the rectum. This technique has made it possible to resect lesions to a point as low as 1 to 2 cm from the anus.

Sphincter-sparing procedures are being performed on patients who are a poor operative risk and on patients with early disease. The number of these procedures may increase with continued early detection and surveillance. In these procedures, a local resection is performed, and the anal sphincters are left intact.

Laparoscopic colectomy may be an option in earlier stage cancers. Potential benefits are faster return of bowel function, fewer incisional infections, shortened hospital stay, and improved cosmetic appearance (Colorectal Cancer Association of Canada, 2016d).

Chemotherapy and Radiation Therapy. Chemotherapy is recommended when a patient has positive lymph nodes at the time of surgery or has metastatic disease. Chemotherapy is used both as an adjuvant therapy following colon resection and as primary treatment for nonresectable colorectal cancer. Various chemotherapy agents including Capecitabine (Xeloda), Fluorouracil (Efudex), folinic acid (leucovorin), and other drugs are used, with choice being based on the stage of the disease (Colorectal Cancer Association of Canada, 2016d).

> **DRUG ALERT—Capecitabine (Xeloda)**
> - Nurse instructs patient not to get immunizations without physician's approval.
> - Nurse reports temperature of >38°C immediately.

Radiation may be used preoperatively as an adjuvant to colon resection and chemotherapy or as a palliative measure for patients with advanced lesions. As a palliative measure, its primary objective is to reduce tumour size and provide symptomatic relief. (For a discussion of radiation therapy, see Chapter 18.)

NURSING MANAGEMENT COLORECTAL CANCER

NURSING ASSESSMENT

Subjective and objective data that should be obtained from a patient with colorectal cancer are presented in Table 45-32.

NURSING DIAGNOSES

Nursing diagnoses for the patient with cancer of the colon or the rectum include, but are not limited to, the following:
- *Constipation* related to *decrease in gastro-intestinal motility*
- *Anxiety* related to *threat to current status, threat of death*
- *Ineffective coping* related to *inadequate opportunity to prepare for stressor, insufficient sense of control* (diagnosis of cancer, adverse effects of treatment)

PLANNING

The overall goals are that the patient with colorectal cancer will have (1) appropriate treatment (removal of tumour, adjunctive therapy), (2) normal bowel elimination patterns, (3) quality of life appropriate to disease prognosis, (4) relief of pain, and (5) feelings of comfort and well-being.

TABLE 45-32 NURSING ASSESSMENT
Colorectal Cancer

Subjective Data
Important Health Information
Past health history: Previous breast or ovarian cancer, familial adenomatous polyposis (FAP), callous adenoma, adenomatous polyps, inflammatory bowel disease; family history of colorectal, breast, or ovarian cancer
Medications: Use of any medication affecting bowel function (e.g., cathartics, antidiarrheal agents)

Symptoms
- Weakness, fatigue
- Anorexia, weight loss; nausea and vomiting
- Change in bowel habits; alternating diarrhea and constipation, defecation urgency; rectal bleeding; mucoid stools; black, tarry stools; increased flatus, decrease in stool calibre; feelings of incomplete evacuation
- Abdominal and low back pain, tenesmus

Objective Data
General
Pallor, cachexia, lymphadenopathy (later signs)

Gastro-Intestinal
Palpable abdominal mass (late sign), distension, ascites, and hepatomegaly (liver metastasis)

Possible Findings
Anemia; positive fecal occult blood; palpable mass on digital rectal examination; positive sigmoidoscopy, colonoscopy, barium enema, or CT scan; positive biopsy

CT, computed tomographic (scan).

NURSING IMPLEMENTATION

HEALTH PROMOTION. The current recommendations from the Canadian Cancer Society (2016) for colorectal cancer screening in patients who are not at high risk include FOBT or FIT performed every 2 years starting at the age of 50. Positive findings should be followed with flexible sigmoidoscopy, colonoscopy, or double-contrast barium enema.

Screening for high-risk patients should begin before age 50, usually beginning with colonoscopy and continuing at more frequent intervals that vary according to risk factors (Canadian Cancer Society, 2016).

A number of epidemiology studies reported that use of NSAIDs (e.g., ibuprofen [Advil]) or long-term use of ASA (Aspirin) may reduce the development of adenomatous colorectal polyps and reduce the risk for colorectal cancer (Friis, Riis, Erichsen, et al., 2015).

ACUTE INTERVENTION

Preoperative Care. Acute nursing care for the patient with a colon resection is similar to the care of the patient having a laparotomy (see NCP 45-2, available on the Evolve website). In addition to general preoperative teaching and ostomy care instructions, the patient undergoing abdominal–perineal resection should be informed of the extent of the surgical procedure and the potential for sexual dysfunction after surgery. Comfortable positioning may be difficult with either an open or a closed perineal wound. Side-to-side positioning in bed and the use of pressure-reducing support surfaces for the bed and chair may be helpful. Doughnut cushions should not be used because these delay wound healing. The patient may experience phantom rectal sensation because the sympathetic nerves responsible for rectal control are not severed during the surgery. The nurse must be astute in distinguishing phantom sensations from perineal abscess pain.

Postoperative Care. After an abdominal–perineal resection, there are two wounds, and a stoma is surgically constructed in the left lower quadrant. There is an abdominal incision through which the colon is resected, and an incision is made in the perineum. The management of a perineal incision differs according to the type of wound. Different approaches may be taken with the perineal wound: (1) packing of the entire open wound or (2) primary closure of the perineal wound with closed-suction drainage of the pelvic cavity. The type of management of the perineal wound is individualized. The open and packed method is used in patients with extensive bleeding in the perineal wound or when there are concerns about local wound infection. A Jackson-Pratt or a Hemovac suction device placed through the buttocks into the pelvic cavity is commonly used to provide drainage of the operative site during the early postoperative period.

A patient who has open and packed wounds requires meticulous postoperative care. During the immediate postoperative period, the perineal dressing may quickly become saturated with serosanguineous drainage. Proper containment of the drainage with appropriate topical dressings such as calcium alginates or hydrofibres will assist in the management of the wound. All drainage is carefully assessed for amount, colour, and consistency.

The nurse should examine the wound regularly and record bleeding, excessive drainage, and unusual odour. The perineal wound is usually irrigated with a normal saline solution when the dressings are changed. Topical dressing selection should be made applying wound care principles: reduce bacterial burden, facilitate moist wound healing, contain drainage, and protect periwound skin. Negative-pressure therapy may be an option to enhance wound healing. Aseptic technique is always used.

When the perineal wound is closed, the drains are left in place for approximately 3 to 5 days. During this time, the drainage is examined and observations recorded. The area around the drains is observed for signs of inflammation and is kept clean and dry. The nurse should observe for signs of induration, erythema, purulent drainage around the suture line, fever, and elevated WBC count. Perineal wound closure may be done with removable or dissolvable sutures. If removable sutures are used, these are generally left in place for 2 to 3 weeks.

If the patient complains of pain and itching in and around the wound, carefully inspect the wound for signs of local infection, maceration from wound drainage, or yeast. Use of a pressure-reducing chair cushion provides comfort when sitting, and side-to-side positioning in bed will help with comfort.

Sexual dysfunction is a possible complication of an abdominal–perineal resection and should be included in the plan of care. Although the effect of the procedure depends on the extent of pelvic dissection, the surgeon must inform the patient of the risk preoperatively. The nurse should understand that erection, ejaculation, and orgasm involve different nerve pathways and that a dysfunction of one does not mean total sexual dysfunction. The ET nurse is an important member of the team and can often provide factual information concerning sexual dysfunction and management options.

AMBULATORY AND HOME CARE. Psychological support for the patient and family is important. The relative 5-year survival rate for patients with colorectal cancer is 64%. This presents a problem for the patient and health care providers because of the often painful, debilitating, and demoralizing manifestations produced by the recurrent disease and the lack of any effective palliative therapy. Chemotherapy may be used as an adjuvant measure for the patient with evidence of local or distant metastasis. (The special needs of the patient with cancer are discussed in Chapter 18.)

The open perineal wound may not be completely healed before discharge. After discharge, the health care provider, home health nurse, and ET nurse usually see the patient. Regular reassessment of the wound to determine progress and ideal topical dressing management should be done. Clipping the buttock hair close to the perineal wound will aid dressing adherence and prevent wound bed irritation from long hairs. The nurse should report persistent drainage or prolonged wound healing because it may also indicate the presence of a foreign body, fistula, or rectal tissue not removed during surgery. The patient and significant others may be taught assessment and management of the wound. The patient and the family should be aware of all community services available for assistance.

Patients with colostomies need to know how to care for them. Even when patients do not have stomas, they may experience diarrhea, constipation, incontinence, or difficulty passing stool, depending on the section of the colon removed and the surgical procedure performed. Patients need to know about diet; incontinence products; and strategies for managing bloating, diarrhea, and bowel evacuation. Often, a combination of dietary changes and drugs is used to control diarrhea and constipation.

Patients with sphincter-sparing surgery frequently experience diarrhea and incontinence of feces and gas. They often need antidiarrheal drugs or bulking agents to control the diarrhea, but may overuse them and become constipated. Consultation with a dietitian would help patients and caregivers understand

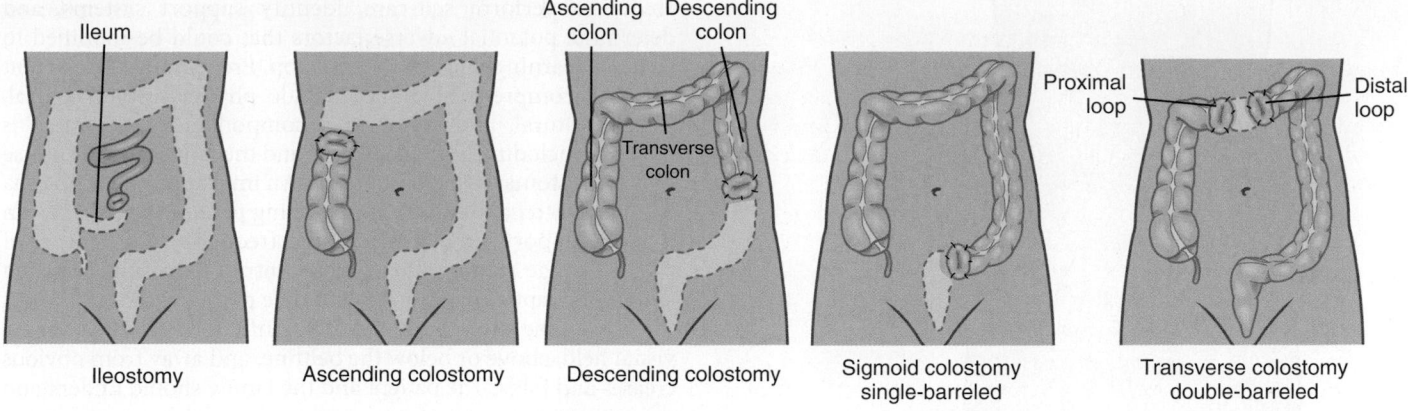

FIGURE 45-8 Types of ostomies.

how to choose foods that are less likely to cause diarrhea and odour and could help them discover which foods are problematic for them.

EVALUATION

The following are expected outcomes for the patient with colorectal cancer:

- The patient will have regular bowel elimination patterns.
- The patient will have relief of pain.
- The patient will have balanced nutritional intake.
- The patient will have quality of life appropriate to disease prognosis.
- The patient will have feelings of comfort and well-being.

OSTOMY SURGERY

Types

The creation of an **ostomy** is a surgical procedure in which an opening is made to allow passage of urine from the bladder, or intestinal contents from the bowel, to an incision or stoma surgically created in the wall of the abdomen. In the context of intestinal reconstruction, the bowel is brought through an opening in the abdominal wall. The edges of the bowel are sutured to the surrounding skin, exposing the inner lining of the bowel (mucosa); this opening is the stoma. Bowel excretion will now occur through the stoma. The stoma may be permanent or temporary, depending upon the underlying reason for the surgery.

When the ileum is brought through the abdominal wall, it is called an *ileostomy* (Figure 45-8). It is commonly used in surgical treatment of UC, Crohn's disease, and FAP and may be used to temporarily protect distal anastomoses, such as in a low anterior resection.

A *colostomy* describes the colon being brought through the abdominal wall. *Colostomy* is a generic term and may be used to describe any part of the colon (large intestine) that is brought to the surface. Locations for colostomies are shown in Figure 45-8. A temporary colostomy may be created as an emergency measure following bowel obstruction (e.g., malignant tumour), abdominal trauma (e.g., gunshot wound), or a perforated diverticulum. A loop colostomy (see Figure 45-9) and double-barrelled colostomy (see Figure 45-8) may be created as temporary colostomies, but they may be permanent if the reason for surgery is palliation for obstructing cancer. A comparison of colostomies and ileostomy is shown in Table 45-33.

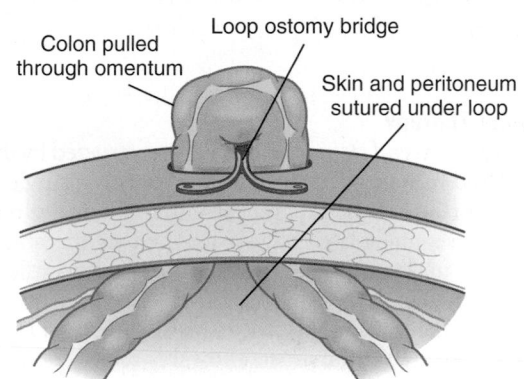

FIGURE 45-9 Loop colostomy.

TABLE 45-33	COMPARISON OF COLOSTOMIES AND ILEOSTOMY		
	Colostomy		
	Transverse	**Sigmoid**	**Ileostomy**
Stool consistency	Semiliquid to semiformed	Formed	Liquid to pasty
Fluid requirement	Possibly increased	No change	Increased
Bowel regulation	No	Yes (if there is a history of a regular bowel pattern)	No
Pouch and skin barriers	Yes	Dependent on regulation	Yes
Irrigation	No	Possible every 24–48 hr (if patient meets criteria)	No
Indications for surgery	Palliation for distal, nonoperable obstructing cancers; trauma	Cancer of the rectum or rectosigmoid area; perforated diverticulitis; trauma; invading gynecological cancers	Ulcerative colitis, Crohn's disease, diseased or injured colon, birth defect, familial adenomatous polyposis; trauma; cancer; ischemic colitis

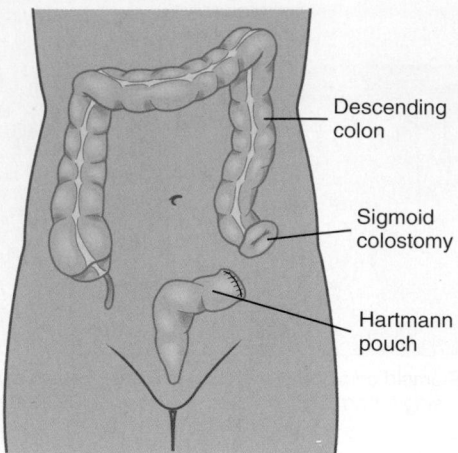

FIGURE 45-10 Sigmoid colostomy. Distal bowel is oversewn and left in place to create a Hartmann pouch.

Surgical Therapy

End Stoma. An *end stoma* is surgically constructed by dividing the bowel and bringing out the proximal end as a single stoma. The distal portion of the GI tract is either surgically removed or the distal segment is oversewn and left in the abdominal cavity with its mesentery intact. An end colostomy or ileostomy is then constructed. When the distal bowel is oversewn rather than removed, the result of the procedure is known as a *Hartmann pouch* (Figure 45-10). If the distal bowel is removed, the stoma is permanent; if the distal bowel remains intact and oversewn, the potential exists for the bowel to be reanastomosed and the stoma to be closed (referred to as a *takedown*).

Loop Stoma. A *loop stoma* is constructed by bringing a loop of bowel to the abdominal surface and then opening the anterior wall of the bowel to provide fecal diversion. This results in one stoma with a proximal and distal opening as well as an intact posterior wall that separates the two openings. The loop of bowel may be supported by a plastic rod for 3 to 7 days after surgery to prevent it from slipping back into the abdominal cavity (see Figure 45-9). A loop stoma is usually temporary.

Double-Barrelled Stoma. When the bowel is divided, both the proximal and the distal ends are brought through the abdominal wall as two separate stomas (see Figure 45-8). The proximal one is the functioning stoma; the distal stoma is referred to as the mucous fistula. The double-barrelled stoma is usually temporary.

Ileoanal Reservoir. As described in the section on UC earlier in this chapter, this procedure involves total colectomy and ileoanal anastomosis, with the formation of an ileal reservoir (see Figure 45-3).

NURSING MANAGEMENT OSTOMY SURGERY

PREOPERATIVE CARE

It is important to review the information the patient has received from the health care provider. Psychological preparation and support are very important. The family and the patient usually have many questions concerning the procedures. If available, an ET nurse should visit with the patient and the family. An ET nurse is a nurse with additional education and training who specializes in the care and management of individuals with ostomies. The nurse or the ET nurse must determine the patient's

ability to perform self-care, identify support systems, and determine potential adverse factors that could be modified to facilitate learning during rehabilitation. Preoperative assessment must be comprehensive and include physical, psychological, social, cultural, and educational components. Assessment is ongoing, including both the patient and the family. The ET nurse marks the stoma site before surgery. An improperly placed stoma complicates rehabilitation by increasing patient dependency on nursing support and increasing time, frequency, and expense of pouch change routine. It can also contribute to skin irritation and poor adaptation. Stomas should be placed within the rectus muscle, on the superior aspect of a skinfold, within the patient's visual field, above or below the beltline, and away from obvious creases and folds. The patient and the family should understand the extent of surgery, the type of stoma, and its care. Trained visitors from ostomy support groups may also provide reassurance and guidance for the patient and family. The patient and family have the opportunity to see a person who has adjusted well and who has experienced some of the same feelings and concerns. Bowel preparation before surgery may be required. Orally administered osmotic lavages (e.g., GoLYTELY) have shortened the classic 72-hour preparation with clear liquids, cathartics, and enemas. Preoperative IV antibiotics are given.

COLOSTOMY CARE

Postoperative nursing care should focus on assessing the stoma, protecting the skin and the stoma, selecting the pouch, providing patient education on ostomy self-care, and assisting the patient to adapt psychologically to a changed body. Nursing care for the patient with a colostomy is presented in NCP 45-4, available on the Evolve website.

The stoma should be pink or red. A dusky purple stoma indicates ischemia, and a brown-black stoma indicates necrosis. The nurse should assess and document stoma colour every 4 to 8 hours for the first 72 hours after surgery, when necrosis is more likely to occur. There is initial mild to moderate swelling of the stoma, which will settle 4 to 6 weeks after surgery (Table 45-34). Application of an appropriate skin barrier is important to protect the peristomal skin. Several pouching options are available from ostomy supply companies. The peristomal skin should be cleansed with warm water and dried thoroughly before the new barrier is applied.

Principles of ostomy care and pouching selection include (1) protection of peristomal skin from effluent, trauma, or both; (2) protection of the stoma from trauma; (3) secured containment of odour and effluent; (4) preservation of patient dignity; and (5) cost containment of pouching system. An ET nurse can assist with the education of the patient and selection of the most appropriate appliance. Openings to the traditional skin barrier should be cut 3 to 4 mm larger than the base of the stoma to allow for normal stomal peristalsis. Newer, mouldable barriers eliminate the need for precise measuring and simplify the care for patients.

The volume, colour, and consistency of the drainage are recorded. Each time the pouch is changed, the condition of the skin and stoma are observed. If any abnormalities are noted (rash, blisters, ulcers), an ET nurse should be consulted for assessment and management.

A colostomy in the transverse colon has semiliquid to pasty stools and moderate to large volumes of flatus. A colostomy in the sigmoid or the descending colon has semiformed or formed stools and can sometimes be regulated by the irrigation method.

TABLE 45-34 POSTOPERATIVE CHARACTERISTICS OF STOMA

Characteristic	Description or Cause
Colour*	
Pink, rose to brick red	Viable stoma mucosa
Pale pink	May indicate anemia
Blanching, dark red to purple	May indicate inadequate blood supply to the stoma, low flow state, excessive tension on the bowel mesentery at the time of construction, or venous congestion; usually occurs in the first 72 hr after surgery
Edema†	
Mild to moderate edema	Normal in the initial postoperative period
	Trauma to the stoma
	Any medical condition that results in edema
Moderate to severe edema	Obstruction proximal to the stoma
Bleeding	
Small amount	Oozing from the stomal mucosa when touched or cleansed is normal because of its vascularity
Moderate to large amount‡	Moderate to large amount of bleeding from stomal mucosa could indicate coagulation factor deficiency; trauma to the stoma
	Moderate to large amount of bleeding from intestinal stoma could indicate lower gastro-intestinal bleeding

*Sustained colour changes must be reported to surgeon.
†Closely observe, monitor, and report to the surgeon.
‡Report moderate to large amounts of bleeding to surgeon.

TABLE 45-35 NUTRITIONAL THERAPY

Effects of Food and Liquids on Stoma Output

Odour Producing*
- Eggs
- Garlic
- Onions
- Fish
- Asparagus
- Cabbage
- Broccoli
- Cauliflower
- Alcohol
- Spicy foods

Gas Forming*
- Beans and legumes
- Cabbage family
- Onions
- Beer
- Carbonated beverages
- Cheeses (strong)
- Asian vegetables

Diarrhea Causing*
- Alcohol
- Beer
- Cabbage family
- Spinach
- Green beans
- Coffee
- Spicy foods
- Fruits and vegetables (raw)

Potential Obstruction in Ileostomy†
- Nuts
- Raisins
- Popcorn
- Seeds
- Fruits and vegetables (raw)

*The effect of food on stoma output is individual. Patients are not discouraged from eating the above-listed foods and beverages.
†Patients are encouraged to chew high-roughage food well, or cook the foods and limit the amounts in the initial postoperative period (4–6 wk after surgery), and to drink increased amounts of fluids.

Patients may choose to use drainable, closed-end pouches or pouch liners to manage the stool.

For most patients with colostomies, there are few, if any, dietary restrictions. A well-balanced diet and adequate fluid intake are important. The patient's medical and surgical history must be considered when individualizing dietary instructions. Table 45-35 lists foods and their effects on stoma output.

COLOSTOMY IRRIGATIONS. Colostomy irrigations can be used to regulate bowel function, treat constipation, or prepare the bowel for surgery. When done to achieve a regular bowel pattern, the irrigations habituate the bowel to function at a specific time every day or every other day. If control is achieved, there should be little or no spillage between irrigations. The patient who establishes regularity may need to wear only a pad or small pouch over the stoma. Not all patients can be managed with irrigations. An ET nurse can help to assess whether this is an appropriate management technique. The patient who is not eligible for irrigations or chooses not to establish regularity by irrigations must wear a pouch at all times.

All equipment should be assembled before irrigation. Usually, a commercially obtained irrigation set has all the equipment needed. The nurse should encourage the patient to watch the procedure and should explain each step to the patient. The cone tip on the tubing controls the depth of insertion and prevents the water from prematurely coming out from the stoma. If resistance is met, force should not be used because perforation

of the intestine can result. However, this occurrence is unlikely when using a stoma cone. A hard plastic catheter is not recommended because of the risk for intestinal perforation. The procedure should not be rushed; the patient should feel relaxed. The patient or a family member must be instructed in the procedure and must be able to demonstrate the ability to irrigate before doing so independently. This can be done in the outpatient setting. Habituation of the bowel takes 3 to 6 weeks.

The patient should be able to perform a pouch change, care for skin and stoma, control odour, and identify signs and symptoms of complications. The patient should know the importance of fluids and food in the diet, have access to community resources, and know when to seek medical care. Home care and outpatient follow-up by an ET nurse are highly recommended. Patients should be discharged with written instructions for pouch change, teaching literature relevant to the type of stoma they have, a list and samples of products they use, a list of product retailers (including names and phone numbers), outpatient follow-up appointments with the surgeon and the ET nurse, and the phone numbers of the surgeon and the nurse. The patient and caregiver teaching guidelines are included in Table 45-36.

ILEOSTOMY CARE

Care of the ileostomy is presented in NCP 45-4, available on the Evolve website. Ileostomy stomal protrusion of at least 2 cm makes care easier. When the stoma is flat, stool can undermine the seal and cause altered skin integrity. Stomal function is frequent, and the stool is extremely irritating to the skin. Regularity cannot be established, so a pouch must be worn at all times. An open-ended, drainable pouch is worn by the patient so that effluent can be emptied when the pouch is one-third full. Usually, the drainable pouch is worn for 4 to 7 days before being changed, as long as leakage does not occur

TABLE 45-36	PATIENT & CAREGIVER TEACHING GUIDE

Ostomy Self-Care

The following guidelines should be included when teaching the patient and caregiver about ostomy care. The nurse should:

1. Explain the following principles of ostomy care:
   - Routinely change appliances, cleanse skin, and inspect stoma and skin.
   - Empty pouch before it is one-third full.
   - Use deodorants as needed.
   - The nurse should explain how to contact the enterostomal therapy nurse.
   - The nurse should explain how to obtain additional supplies or accessories.
   - Ensure access to home health services.
2. Identify a well-balanced diet and dietary supplements if necessary to prevent nutritional deficiencies, and teach the following dietary and fluid intake guidelines:
   - Identify foods to reduce diarrhea, gas, or obstruction (with ileostomy).
   - Identify foods to reduce constipation and gas (with colostomy).
   - Drink at least 1 500–3 000 mL/day of fluid to prevent dehydration (unless contraindicated).
   - Increase fluid intake during hot weather, excessive perspiration, or diarrhea to replace losses and prevent dehydration.
   - Get to know the signs and symptoms of dehydration and when to seek help from a health care provider.
   - Contact your registered dietitian with any questions.
3. Describe potential resources to assist with emotional and psychological adjustment, and teach the patient to:
   - Identify people available to provide emotional support.
   - Identify community resources for psychosocial support.
   - Contact local ostomy support groups for information or peer support.
4. Explain the importance of follow-up care and reporting any signs and symptoms of the following:
   - Fluid and electrolyte deficits (dehydration)
   - Fever
   - Diarrhea
   - Constipation
   - Other stoma problems, including a change in appearance of the stoma or its function, a change in the peristomal skin, tenderness, erythema, or pain

under the pouching system. If pouch leakage occurs, the pouch should be promptly removed, the skin should be cleansed, and a new pouching system applied. Frequent leaks of the appliance warrant assessment of appropriateness of the pouching by an ET nurse. A transparent pouch may be used in the initial postoperative period to facilitate assessment of stoma viability and stoma function, but opaque pouches for discharge and home enhance aesthetics.

Immediately after surgery, intake and output must be accurately monitored. The patient should be observed for signs and symptoms of fluid and electrolyte imbalance, particularly potassium, sodium, and fluid deficits. In the first 24 to 48 hours after surgery, the amount of drainage from the stoma may be negligible. A person with an ileostomy has lost the absorptive functions provided by the colon as well as the delay feature provided by the ileocecal valve. Once peristalsis returns, the patient may experience a period of high-volume bilious output of 1 200 to 1 800 mL/day. Later, the amount can average 800 mL daily because the proximal small bowel adapts and absorbs more fluid. If the small bowel has been shortened as a result of surgical resections, the drainage from the ileostomy may be greater. The patient

must understand the importance of fluid and electrolyte balance. A dietitian is helpful in assessing and determining patient food and fluid requirements.

The patient should be instructed to drink at least 1.5 to 2 L of fluid daily; more may be necessary when diarrhea occurs and when perspiration is increased. Diarrhea from an ileostomy can produce dehydration and acidosis from the loss of bicarbonate. The patient may require brief hospitalization for IV fluid rehydration if large volumes of diarrhea occur.

Usually a low-residue diet is ordered initially. Insoluble fibre–containing foods are reintroduced gradually. Later, there are few dietary restrictions. It is important to limit the amount of high-roughage foods (e.g., popcorn), chew them well, and accompany them with fluids. The goal for the patient is a return to a normal, presurgical diet.

The stoma may bleed easily when it is touched or cleansed because it has a high vascular supply. The patient should be told that minimal oozing of blood is normal. If the terminal ileum has been removed, the patient may need cobalamin (vitamin B_{12}) supplementation.

ADAPTATION TO AN OSTOMY

Adaptation to the ostomy is a gradual process. The patient experiences a grief reaction to the loss of a body part and an alteration in body image. Each person uses different coping mechanisms. The adjustment period for the person depends on the individual. Psychological support during the grieving process is needed. There are many concerns, including body image, sexual activity, family responsibilities, and changes in lifestyle. The patient may become resentful and have fears of odour or leakage. Supportive measures by nurses include helping the patient acquire knowledge, providing or recommending support services, and identifying coping mechanisms that are effective. The nurse provides support by responding to the physiological needs of stoma care and psychosocial needs related to self-esteem.

Gradual involvement of the patient in self-care of the ostomy should be encouraged. Although initial visualization of the stoma and participation in care is distressing, supportive teaching from the nurse will enhance confidence and independence in care. Teaching at the appropriate time is an important part of the care and can contribute to a smooth adjustment process.

Gradual resumption of activities of daily living can occur within 2 to 3 weeks. Heavy lifting, physical exertion, and participation in sports should be avoided for 6 to 8 weeks. The patient's physical condition determines when sexual activity may be resumed. Bathing and swimming are not prohibited. Refer patients to the Ostomy Canada Society for information and support (www.ostomycanada.ca).

SEXUAL DYSFUNCTION AFTER OSTOMY SURGERY

Discussion of sexuality and sexual function must be incorporated in the plan of care. The nurse can help the patient understand that sexual function or sexual activity may be affected but that sexuality does not have to be altered.

Pelvic surgery can disrupt nerve and vascular supply to the genitals. Radiation, chemotherapy, and medications can also alter sexual function. Hormones and overall physical health of the patient influence desire. Certain pain medications and antiemetics can lower libido. Generalized fatigue caused by illness can also influence desire. By communicating this information to patients, they can plan sexual activity around a drug schedule and energy levels. Any pelvic surgery that removes the rectum has the potential of damaging the parasympathetic nerve plexus. Erection in men depends on the parasympathetic nerves that control blood flow and vascular supply to the pelvis and the pudendal nerves that transmit sensory responses from the genital area. Nerve-sparing surgical techniques are used when possible to preserve sexual function. Radiation therapy to the pelvis can reduce blood vascularity to the pelvis by causing scarring in the small blood vessels. Pelvic surgery usually does not affect a woman's arousal unless part of or the entire vagina is removed. Radiation therapy can affect vaginal expansion and lubrication.

Muscular contraction and the genital pleasure that occur during orgasm are not disrupted by pelvic surgery. If the sympathetic nerves in the presacral area are damaged, the male mechanism of emission can be disrupted. This can occur with an abdominal–perineal resection. Orgasms can occur in both men and women who have had stoma surgery, although other aspects of the sexual response may be affected.

The psychological impact of the stoma and how it affects the patient's body image and self-esteem must be discussed. Emotional factors can contribute to sexual problems. A life-threatening illness can override concerns about sexual function. The nurse can assist a patient to identify ways of coping with depression and anxiety resulting from illness, surgery, or postoperative problems.

The social impact of the stoma is interrelated with its psychological, physical, and sexual aspects. Concerns of people with stomas include the ability to resume sexual activity, altering clothing styles, the effect on daily activities, sleeping while wearing a pouch, passing gas, the presence of odour, cleanliness, and deciding when or whether to tell others about the stoma. The fear of rejection from a partner or the fear that others will not find them desirable as a sexual partner can be a concern. The nurse should encourage open communication about feelings and should realize that the patient needs time to adjust to the pouch and to body changes before feeling secure in her or his sexual functioning.

Pregnancy is possible with an ostomy. As the abdomen expands in the second and third trimesters, the stoma may retract and alternate pouching may be required. A woman with an ostomy who becomes pregnant should have regular medical care and assessment by an ET nurse.

DIVERTICULOSIS AND DIVERTICULITIS

A **diverticulum** is an outpouching of the mucosa through the circular smooth muscle of the intestinal wall. Diverticula may occur at any point within the GI tract but are most commonly found in the sigmoid colon. Clinically, diverticular disease occurs in two forms: diverticulosis and diverticulitis. With *diverticulosis*, multiple noninflamed diverticula are present; the patient is most often free of symptoms or may have alternating periods of constipation and diarrhea. In *diverticulitis*, inflammation of the diverticula occurs (Figure 45-11).

Etiology and Pathophysiology

Diverticular disease is a common GI disorder that affects over 50% of Canadians over the age of 80 (Canadian Digestive Health Foundation, 2017). A diverticulum is a saccular dilation or outpouching of the mucosa through the circular smooth muscle of the intestinal wall. It affects men and women equally, but men seem to have a higher rate of complications. Most people with diverticular disease are asymptomatic and are unaware that they have the disease.

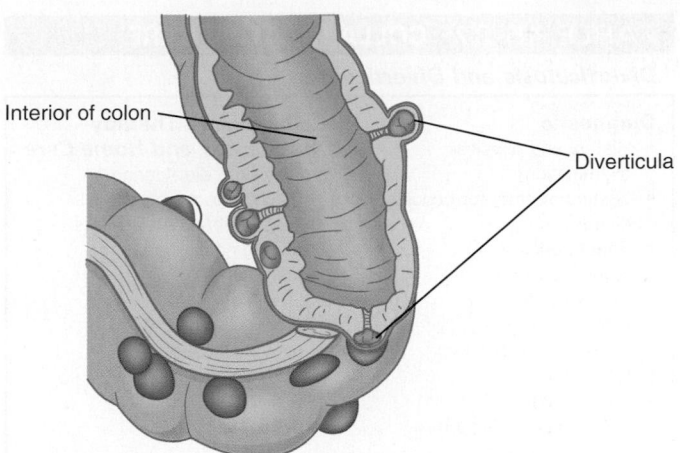

FIGURE 45-11 Diverticula are outpouchings of the colon. When they become inflamed, the condition is diverticulitis. The inflammatory process can spread to the surrounding area in the intestine.

PATHOPHYSIOLOGY MAP

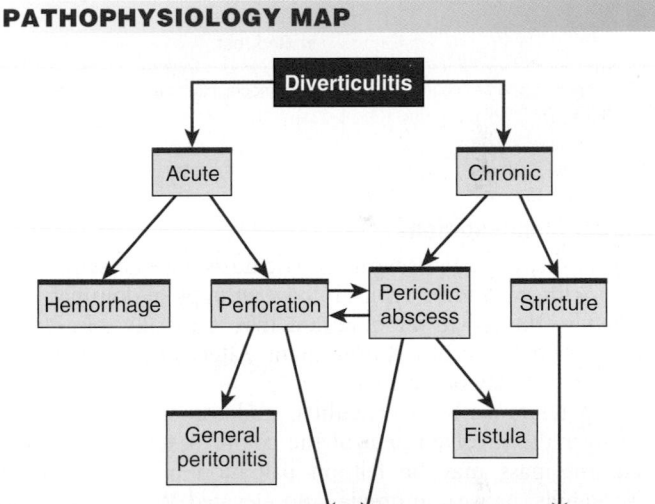

FIGURE 45-12 Complications of diverticulitis.

There is no known cause of diverticular disease, but deficiency in dietary fibre has been associated with it. The disease is more prevalent in Western populations that consume diets low in fibre and high in refined carbohydrates.

When diverticula form, the smooth muscle of the colon wall becomes thickened. Lack of dietary fibre slows transit time, and more water is absorbed from the stool, making its passage through the lumen more difficult. Decreased bulk of the stool, combined with a more acutely narrowed lumen in the sigmoid colon, causes high intraluminal pressures. These factors are believed to contribute to the formation of diverticula.

The cause of diverticulitis is related to the retention of stool and bacteria in the diverticulum, forming a hardened mass called a *fecalith*. This occurrence causes inflammation and usually small perforations. Inflammation of the diverticulum spreads to the surrounding tissues (Figure 45-12), causing it to become edematous. Abscesses may form, or complete perforation with peritonitis may occur.

TABLE 45-37   COLLABORATIVE CARE

Diverticulosis and Diverticulitis

Diagnostic	Collaborative Therapy
• History and physical examination	**Ambulatory and Home Care**
• Testing of stool for occult blood	• High-fibre diet (during nonsymptomatic periods)
• Barium enema	• Dietary fibre supplements (during nonsymptomatic periods)
• Sigmoidoscopy	• Stool softeners
• Colonoscopy	• Clear liquid diet
• CBC	• Oral antibiotics
• CT scan with contrast	• Bulk laxatives
• Urinalysis	• Weight reduction (if overweight)
• Blood culture	
• Abdominal radiograph	**Acute Care: Diverticulitis**
• Chest radiograph	• IV antibiotics
	• NPO status
	• IV fluids
	• Possible colon resection for perforation, obstruction, or hemorrhage
	• Bed rest

CBC, complete blood cell count; *CT,* computed tomographic (scan); *IV,* intravenous; *NPO,* nothing by mouth.

Clinical Manifestations

The majority of patients with diverticulosis have no symptoms. Those with symptoms typically have crampy abdominal pain located in the left lower quadrant that is usually relieved by passage of flatus or bowel movement. Alternating constipation and diarrhea may be present.

In patients with diverticulitis, abdominal pain is localized over the involved area of the colon. A tender left lower quadrant mass may be felt on palpation of the abdomen. Fever, chills, nausea, anorexia, and elevated WBC count may be present. Older adults with diverticulitis are frequently afebrile, with a normal WBC count and little, if any, abdominal tenderness.

Complications of diverticulitis include perforation with peritonitis, abscess and fistula formation, bowel obstruction, ureteral obstruction, and bleeding. Diverticular bleeding is the most common cause of lower GI bleeding. Bleeding usually stops spontaneously.

Diagnostic Studies

A CT scan with oral contrast is the test of choice for diverticulitis. A CBC, urinalysis, and FOBT should be performed (Table 45-37). A barium enema is used to determine narrowing or obstruction of the colonic lumen. A colonoscopy may be performed to rule out possible hidden polyps or lesions. A patient with acute diverticulitis should not have a barium enema or colonoscopy because of the possibility of perforation and peritonitis.

NURSING AND COLLABORATIVE MANAGEMENT DIVERTICULOSIS AND DIVERTICULITIS

Uncomplicated diverticular disease is treated with a high-fibre diet (see Table 45-9) and bulk laxatives, such as psyllium hydrophilic mucilloid (Metamucil). In acute diverticulitis, the goal of treatment is to allow the colon to rest and the inflammation to subside. The patient is kept on NPO status with parenteral fluids for hydration. The patient should be observed for signs of possible peritonitis. In acute diverticulitis, broad-spectrum antibiotic therapy is required. The temperature and the WBC count are monitored.

When the acute attack subsides, oral fluids are allowed, progressing to a semisolid diet. At this stage, the patient should be observed for a recurrent attack. If the patient has a bowel resection or colostomy, the nursing care is the same as for these procedures.

Surgical intervention is necessary to drain abscesses and to resect an obstructing inflammatory mass or perforated segment. The usual surgical procedures involve resection of the involved colon with a temporary diverting colostomy. The bowel is reanastomosed after the colon has healed.

The patient should be provided with a full explanation of the condition. Consultation with a dietitian regarding high-fibre diets is recommended.

HERNIAS

A **hernia** is a protrusion of a viscus through an abnormal opening or a weakened area in the wall of the cavity in which it is normally contained. If the hernia can be placed back into the abdominal cavity, it is known as *reducible*. The hernia can be reduced by manipulation, or reduction can occur spontaneously when the person lies down. If the hernia cannot be placed back into the abdominal cavity, it is known as *irreducible or* incarcerated, and the intestinal flow may be obstructed. When the hernia is irreducible and the intestinal flow and blood supply are obstructed, the hernia is *strangulated*. The result is an acute intestinal obstruction and ischemia, necessitating surgery.

Types

The *inguinal hernia* is the most common type of hernia and occurs at the point of weakness in the abdominal wall where the spermatic cord emerges in men and the round ligament in women (Figure 45-13). When the protrusion escapes through the inguinal ring and follows the spermatic cord or the round ligament, it is termed an *indirect* hernia. When it escapes through the posterior inguinal wall, it is a *direct* hernia. An inguinal hernia is more common in men.

A *femoral hernia* occurs when there is a protrusion through the femoral ring into the femoral canal. It occurs below the inguinal (Poupart) ligament as a bulge. It becomes strangulated easily and occurs more often in women. The umbilical hernia occurs when the rectus muscle is weak or the umbilical opening fails to close after birth.

Ventral, or incisional, hernia is caused by weakness of the abdominal wall at the site of a previous incision. It is found most commonly in patients who are obese, who have had multiple surgical procedures in the same area, and who have had inadequate wound healing because of poor nutrition or infection.

Clinical Manifestations

Commonly, a hernia occurs over the involved area when the patient stands or strains. Severe pain is caused if the hernia becomes strangulated. In this situation, the clinical manifestations of a bowel obstruction, such as vomiting, crampy abdominal pain, and distension, are found.

FIGURE 45-13 Types of hernias. **A,** Umbilical hernia. **B,** Femoral hernias (note swelling below the inguinal ligaments). **C,** Indirect inguinal hernia. Source: **A** and **B,** from Zitelli, B. J., McIntire, S. C., & Nowalk, A. J. (2012). *Zitelli and Davis' atlas of pediatric physical diagnosis* (6th ed.), Philadelphia: Saunders; **C,** from Swartz, M. H. (2010). *Textbook of physical diagnosis: History and examination* (6th ed., p. 545). Philadelphia: Saunders.

NURSING AND COLLABORATIVE MANAGEMENT HERNIAS

Diagnosis is based on history and physical examination findings. Surgery is the treatment of choice for hernias to prevent the possible complication of strangulation. The surgical repair of a hernia is known as a *herniorrhaphy.* The reinforcement of the weakened area with fascia or mesh is known as a *hernioplasty.* When there is strangulation, necrosis and gangrene may develop if immediate care is not given. A bowel resection of the involved area or a temporary ostomy may be needed to treat a strangulated hernia.

Some patients with inguinal hernias wear a truss, a firm pad placed over the hernia and held in place with a belt. The truss is worn to keep the hernia from protruding. The truss should be applied when the hernia is reduced. If the hernia cannot be reduced, the truss should not be used. If a patient wears a truss, the nurse should check for skin irritation caused by the continual rubbing and pressure of the truss.

After an inguinal hernia repair, the patient may have difficulty voiding; thus, the nurse should observe for a distended bladder. An accurate intake and output record is important. Scrotal edema is a painful complication after an inguinal hernia repair. A scrotal support may help relieve discomfort. Coughing is not encouraged, but deep breathing and turning should be done. If the patient needs to cough or sneeze, the incision should be splinted during these functions. After discharge, the patient may be restricted from heavy lifting or activities for 6 to 8 weeks. Some surgeons do not put any limitations on physical activities.

ANORECTAL PROBLEMS

HEMORRHOIDS

Hemorrhoids are varicosities in the lower rectum or the anus caused by congestion in the veins of the hemorrhoidal plexus. They may be *internal* (occurring above the internal sphincter) or *external* (occurring outside the external sphincter) (Figures 45-14 and 45-15). Symptoms of hemorrhoids, including bleeding, pruritus, prolapse, and pain, are common in all age groups. In affected people, hemorrhoids appear periodically, depending on the amount of anorectal pressure.

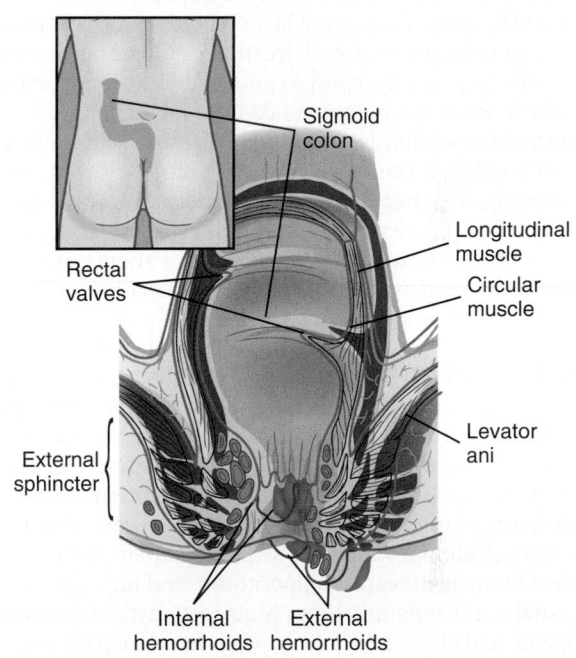

FIGURE 45-14 Anatomical structures of the rectum and the anus with external and internal hemorrhoids.

FIGURE 45-15 Thrombosed external hemorrhoids. Source: Townsend, C. M., Beauchamp, R. D., Evers, B. M., et al. (Eds.). (2012). *Sabiston textbook of surgery: The biological basis of modern surgical practice* (19th ed.). Saunders: Philadelphia.

Etiology and Pathophysiology

Hemorrhoids are thought to develop as a result of shearing forces during defecation. This force damages supporting muscles. When supporting tissues in the anal canal weaken, usually as a result of straining at defecation, venules become dilated. In addition, blood flow through the veins of the hemorrhoidal plexus is impaired. An intravascular clot in the venule results in a thrombosed external hemorrhoid. They are the most common cause of bleeding with defecation. The amount of blood lost at one time may be small but may lead to iron-deficiency anemia over time.

Hemorrhoids may be precipitated by many factors, including pregnancy, prolonged constipation, straining in an effort to defecate, heavy lifting, prolonged standing and sitting, and portal hypertension (as found in cirrhosis).

Clinical Manifestations

The patient with internal hemorrhoids may be asymptomatic. However, when internal hemorrhoids become constricted, the patient will report pain. Internal hemorrhoids can bleed, resulting in blood on toilet paper after defecation or blood on the outside of stool. The patient may report a chronic, dull, aching discomfort, particularly when the hemorrhoids have prolapsed.

External hemorrhoids are reddish blue and seldom bleed or cause pain unless a vein ruptures. If the blood clots in external hemorrhoids, they become inflamed and painful and are said to be thrombosed. External hemorrhoids cause intermittent pain, pain on palpation, itching, and burning. Patients also report bleeding associated with defecation. Constipation or diarrhea can aggravate these symptoms.

Diagnostic Studies and Collaborative Care

Internal hemorrhoids are diagnosed by digital examination, anoscopy, or sigmoidoscopy. External hemorrhoids can be diagnosed by visual inspection and digital examination. Therapy should be directed toward the causes and the patient's symptoms. A high-fibre diet and increased fluid intake prevent constipation and reduce straining, which allows engorgement of the veins to subside. Ointments, creams, suppositories, and impregnated pads that contain anti-inflammatory agents (e.g., hydrocortisone), or astringents and anaesthetics (e.g., witch hazel, benzocaine) may be used to shrink the mucous membranes and relieve discomfort. Stool softeners may be ordered to keep the stools soft; sitz baths may be ordered to relieve pain.

Surgical excision and clot removal are generally recommended for thrombosed external hemorrhoids. For internal hemorrhoids, one of four nonsurgical approaches can be used. The first is *band ligation*. Through an anoscope, the hemorrhoid is identified and then ligated with a rubber band. The constrictive effect impairs circulation, and the tissue becomes necrotic, separates, and sloughs off. There is some local discomfort with this procedure, but no anaesthetic is required. *Infrared coagulation* can be used to treat bleeding internal hemorrhoids. In this procedure, either infrared or electrical current reduces local inflammation. *Cryotherapy* involves rapid freezing of the hemorrhoid. Because this method can result in acute pain, it is used less often. Finally, *laser treatment* can be used to treat internal hemorrhoids. This procedure involves expensive equipment and tends to be more costly than band ligation and coagulation therapies.

A *hemorrhoidectomy* is the surgical excision of hemorrhoids. Surgery is indicated when there is prolapse, excessive pain or bleeding, or large hemorrhoids. In general, hemorrhoidectomy is reserved for patients with severe symptoms related to multiple thrombosed hemorrhoids or marked protrusion. Surgical removal may be done by cautery, clamp, or excision. One surgical approach is to leave the area open so that healing takes place by secondary intention. In another approach, the hemorrhoids are removed, the tissue is sutured, and healing takes place by primary intention wound healing.

NURSING MANAGEMENT HEMORRHOIDS

Conservative nursing management for the patient with hemorrhoids includes teaching measures regarding prevention of constipation, avoidance of prolonged standing or sitting, proper use of OTC drugs available for hemorrhoidal symptoms, and the need to seek medical care for severe symptoms of hemorrhoids (e.g., excessive pain and bleeding, prolapsed hemorrhoids) when necessary. Sitz baths (15–20 minutes), two to three times each day for 7 to 10 days, may be helpful to reduce the discomfort and swelling associated with hemorrhoids.

Pain caused by sphincter spasm is a common problem after a hemorrhoidectomy. The nurse must be aware that, although the procedure is minor, the pain is severe. Opioids are usually given initially. Sitz baths are started 1 to 2 days after surgery. A warm sitz bath provides comfort and keeps the anal area clean. Initially, the patient should not be left alone because of the possibility of weakness or fainting.

Packing may be inserted into the rectum to absorb drainage. A T-binder may hold the dressing in place. If packing is inserted, it usually is removed on the first or second postoperative day. The nurse should assess for rectal bleeding. The patient may be embarrassed when the dressing is changed, and privacy should be provided. The patient usually dreads the first bowel movement and often resists the urge to defecate. Pain medication may be given before the bowel movement to reduce discomfort.

A stool softener such as docusate (Colace) is usually ordered for the first few postoperative days. If the patient does not have a bowel movement within 2 to 3 days, other oral laxatives may be given.

Patients are taught the importance of diet, care of the anal area, symptoms of complications (especially bleeding), and avoidance of constipation and straining. Sitz baths are recommended for 1 to 2 weeks. The health care provider may order a stool softener to be taken for a time. Hemorrhoids may recur. Occasionally, anal strictures develop and dilation is necessary. Regular checkups are important in the prevention of any further problems.

ANAL FISSURE

An **anal fissure** is a skin ulcer or a crack in the lining of the anal wall that is caused by trauma, local infection, or inflammation. Fissures are considered either primary or secondary, based on their etiology. *Primary fissures* usually occur as a result of local trauma associated with defecation or anal intercourse. When there is high pressure in the internal anal sphincter, it can result in ischemia, which can lead to fissuring. Thus, sexual practices and conditions that promote constipation are likely to be associated with fissure development. *Secondary fissures* are caused by a variety of conditions, including IBD, prior anal surgery, infection (syphilis, tuberculosis, chlamydia, gonorrhea, herpes simplex virus), and human immunodeficiency virus (HIV) infection.

The most common clinical manifestations are painful spasms of the anal sphincter and severe, burning pain during defecation. Some bleeding may occur, and constipation results because of fear of pain associated with bowel movements.

Anal fissures are diagnosed through physical examination. Treatment of anal fissures is directed at correcting the underlying conditions, such as hard stools. Most acute fissures require 2 to 4 weeks to heal. Conservative treatment consists of bowel regulation with mineral oil and stool softeners. Warm sitz baths (15–20 minutes, three times a day) and anal anaesthetic suppositories (Anusol) are also ordered. Topical preparations, including nitrates and calcium channel blockers, are used to decrease rectal and anal pressure to allow the fissure to heal without sphincter damage. Local injections of botulinum toxin are also used to decrease rectal and anal pressure and are most effective when combined with nitrates.

For chronic fissures, other invasive procedures may be needed. These include coagulation therapy or surgical treatment (sphincterotomy). Surgical treatment involves excision of the fissure. Postoperative nursing care is the same as the care for the patient who has had a hemorrhoidectomy.

ANORECTAL ABSCESS

Anorectal abscesses are undrained collections of perianal pus (Figure 45-16). They are the result of obstruction of the anal glands, leading to infection and subsequent abscess formation. Abscess formation can occur secondary to anal fissures, trauma, or IBD.

The most common causative organisms are *Escherichia coli*, staphylococci, and streptococci. Clinical manifestations include local pain and swelling, foul-smelling drainage, tenderness, and elevated temperature. Sepsis can occur as a complication. Anorectal abscesses are diagnosed by rectal examination.

Surgical therapy consists of drainage of abscesses. The wound will be left open and allowed to heal by secondary intention. Topical dressing selection is determined based on wound care principles (maintain moist wound environment, manage bacterial burden, protect from further trauma). Care must be taken to avoid soiling the dressing during urination or defecation. A low-residue diet is given. Discharge teaching should include access to home health care, wound care, and the importance of sitz baths; thorough cleaning after bowel movements; and follow-up visits to a health care provider.

ANAL FISTULA

An **anal fistula** is an abnormal tunnel leading out from the anus or the rectum. It may extend to the outside of the skin, the vagina, or the buttocks. Anal fistulas are a complication of Crohn's disease (occurring in the perianal area). This condition often precedes an anorectal abscess.

Feces enter the fistula and may cause a localized infection. There may be persistent, blood-stained, purulent discharge or stool leakage from the fistula. The patient may need to use dressings to contain the drainage and protect perifistular skin.

Surgical therapy may involve a fistulotomy or a fistulectomy. In a *fistulotomy*, the fistula is opened and healthy tissue is allowed to granulate. A *fistulectomy* is an excision of the entire fistulous tract. Appropriate topical therapy is used, and the wound is allowed to heal by secondary intention. In severe cases of perianal disease caused by Crohn's disease, a diverting loop ileostomy may be required to manage the fistulas. Care is the same as that given after a hemorrhoidectomy.

ANAL CANCER

Anal cancer is uncommon in the general population, but the incidence is increasing. Human papillomavirus (HPV) is associated with about 80% of the cases of anal cancer. Risk factors include having many sexual partners, genital warts (which are caused by HPV), smoking, receptive anal sex, and HIV infection.

Most frequently, the initial symptom is rectal bleeding. Other symptoms include rectal pain and sensation of a rectal mass. Some patients have no symptoms, which leads to delayed diagnosis and treatment.

It is especially important to screen high-risk individuals. A swab of the anal mucosa can be obtained during a digital rectal examination. Identification of cell changes (e.g., dysplasia, neoplasia) can be determined. High-resolution anoscopy allows for visualization of the mucosa and biopsy. An endo-anal *(endorectal) ultrasound* may also be done.

The use of condoms to reduce the transmission of HPV is recommended. The HPV vaccine Gardasil is used for the prevention of anal cancer and associated precancerous lesions caused by HPV types 6, 11, 16, and 18. Another HPV vaccine, Cervarix, may also be useful in the prevention of HPV-associated anal cancer. After vaccination with HPV vaccine, patients at risk need to continue their recommended screening program.

Treatment of anal cancer depends on the size and depth of the lesions. Topical therapy with bichloroacetic or trichloroacetic acid may be used to kill the HPV virus. Imiquimod (Aldara), an immuno-modulator, is also used as a topical agent. Therapy also includes surgery, radiation, and chemotherapy.

PILONIDAL SINUS

A **pilonidal sinus** is a small tract under the skin between the buttocks in the sacrococcygeal area. It is thought to be of congenital origin. It may have several openings and is lined with epithelium and hair, thus given the name *pilonidal* ("a nest of hair").

The skin in the sacrococcygeal region is moist, and the movement of the buttocks causes the short, wiry hair to penetrate

Pelvirectal abscess
Submucosal abscess
Ischiorectal abscess
Perianal abscess
Anal crypt
Openings of anorectal fistulas

FIGURE 45-16 Common sites of anorectal abscesses and fistula formation.

the skin. The irritated skin becomes infected and forms a pilonidal cyst or abscess. There are no symptoms unless there is an infection. If it becomes infected, the patient complains of pain and swelling at the base of the spine, and there may be spontaneous drainage of pus.

The formed abscess requires incision and drainage. The wound may be primarily closed or left open to heal by secondary intention. The wound is packed with appropriate topical therapeutic material. The wounds are often very painful, and the patient

may require premedication before dressing changes. The patient is usually more comfortable lying on the abdomen or side. Sitting for prolonged periods of time may be difficult. Activities that contribute to shear in the area (running, sports, long walks) should be avoided until the wound heals. Because the area is poorly vascularized, healing of open pilonidal wounds may be prolonged. Ensuring that surrounding hair is clipped and kept out of the wound bed is imperative. Unfortunately, despite excision of the tract, pilonidal cysts or abscesses may reoccur.

CASE STUDY

Colorectal Cancer

Source: Anton_Ivanov/ Shutterstock .com.

Patient Profile

Lyle Collins, a 58-year-old man, is from Drury, Ontario. Mr. Collins's wife and family drove 50 kilometres to take him to the hospital because of his deteriorating health (see the case study in Chapter 41).

Subjective Data

See the case study in Chapter 41.

Objective Data
Physical Examination

See the case study in Chapter 41.

Laboratory Tests
- CT scan and colonoscopy show two medium-sized tumours in the transverse colon.

Collaborative Care
Surgical Procedure
- Transverse hemicolectomy performed and lymph node biopsies taken.
- Pathology results indicate that the adenocarcinoma tumour has invaded the muscle wall of the colon, and two out of five lymph nodes are positive for cancer.

Postoperative
- Feels like his life has ended and does not want to leave hospital.
- States that there is no one to take care of him at his home and he is far away from the hospital.

Follow-Up Treatment
- Scheduled for outpatient chemotherapy.

Discussion Questions
1. What are the signs and symptoms of colorectal cancer that Mr. Collins has manifested (see the case study in Chapter 41)?
2. What types of diagnostic information are available from a colonoscopy versus a sigmoidoscopy?
3. What stage of CRC does Mr. Collins probably have? What treatment is recommended for this stage of CRC?
4. How could the nurse provide emotional support to Mr. Collins and his family?
5. What is a culturally sensitive way for the nurse to support Mr. Collins and his family in making decisions about his continued health care?
6. **Priority decision:** Based on the assessment data, what are the priority nursing diagnoses? Are there any collaborative problems?
7. **Priority decision:** What are the priority nursing interventions for Mr. Collins at this stage of his illness?
8. **Evidence-informed practice:** Mr. Collins had not had a previous colonoscopy. He is worried that other members of his family may have colon cancer. What can the nurse tell him about the recommendations for colorectal cancer screening?

⊝volve

Answers available at *http://evolve.elsevier.com/Canada/Lewis/medsurg*.

REVIEW QUESTIONS

The number of the question corresponds to the same-numbered outcome at the beginning of the chapter.

1. The appropriate collaborative therapy for the client with acute diarrhea caused by a viral infection is to do which of the following?
   a. Increase fluid intake
   b. Administer an antibiotic
   c. Administer antimotility drugs
   d. Quarantine the client to prevent spread of the virus
2. When a 35-year-old female client is admitted to the emergency department with acute abdominal pain, which possible diagnosis should the nurse consider that may be the cause of her pain? (*Select all that apply*)
   a. Gastro-enteritis
   b. Ectopic pregnancy
   c. Gastro-intestinal bleeding
   d. Irritable bowel syndrome
   e. Inflammatory bowel disease

3. Assessment findings suggestive of peritonitis include which of the following?
   a. Rebound abdominal pain
   b. A soft, distended abdomen
   c. Dull, continuous abdominal pain
   d. Restlessness
4. In planning care for the client with Crohn's disease, the nurse recognizes which major factor about Crohn's disease that differentiates it from ulcerative colitis?
   a. It frequently results in toxic megacolon.
   b. It causes fewer nutritional deficiencies than ulcerative colitis.
   c. It often recurs after surgery, whereas ulcerative colitis is curable with a colectomy.
   d. It is manifested by rectal bleeding and anemia more frequently than ulcerative colitis is.

5. The nurse performs a detailed assessment of the abdomen of a client with a possible bowel obstruction, knowing that which of the following are manifestations of an obstruction in the large intestine? *(Select all that apply)*
   a. Persistent abdominal pain
   b. Marked abdominal distention
   c. Diarrhea that is loose or liquid
   d. Colicky, severe, intermittent pain
   e. Profuse vomiting that relieves abdominal pain

6. A client with stage I colorectal cancer is scheduled for surgery. Teaching for this client would include an explanation of which of the following?
   a. That chemotherapy will begin after recovery from the surgery
   b. That both chemotherapy and radiation can be used as palliative treatments
   c. That follow-up colonoscopies will be needed to ensure that the cancer does not recur
   d. That a wound nurse, ostomy nurse, and continence nurse will visit to identify an abdominal site for the ostomy

7. The nurse explains to the client undergoing ostomy surgery that the procedure that maintains the most normal functioning of the bowel is which of the following?
   a. A sigmoid colostomy
   b. A transverse colostomy
   c. A descending colostomy
   d. An ascending colostomy

8. In contrast to the client with diverticulitis, which of the following is true for the client with diverticulosis?
   a. Has rectal bleeding
   b. Often has no symptoms
   c. Has localized cramping pain
   d. Frequently develops peritonitis

9. Which of the following is a nursing intervention that is most appropriate to decrease postoperative edema and pain after an inguinal herniorrhaphy?
   a. Applying a truss to the hernia site
   b. Allowing the client to stand to void
   c. Supporting the incision during coughing
   d. Applying a scrotal support with ice bag

10. The nurse determines that the goals of dietary teaching have been met when the client with celiac disease selects which of the following from the menu?
    a. Scrambled eggs and sausage
    b. Buckwheat pancakes with syrup
    c. Oatmeal, skim milk, and orange juice
    d. Yogourt, strawberries, and rye toast with butter

11. What should a client be taught after a hemorrhoidectomy?
    a. Take mineral oil before bedtime.
    b. Eat a low-fibre diet to rest the colon.
    c. Administer oil-retention enema to empty the colon.
    d. Use prescribed pain medication before a bowel movement.

1. a, 2. a, b, c, d, e, 3. a, 4. c, 5. a, b, c, 6. c, 7. a, 8. b, 9. d, 10. a, 11. d.

⊖volve

For even more review questions, visit *http://evolve.elsevier.com/Canada/ Lewis/medsurg*.

REFERENCES

Blush, R. R., & Matzo, M. (2012). Acute infectious diarrhea. *AJN, American Journal of Nursing, 112*(8), 65–68. doi:10.1097/01 .NAJ.0000418105.99929.4f.

Canadian Cancer Society. (2016). *Screening for colorectal cancer*. Retrieved from *http://www.cancer.ca/en/prevention-and-screening/ early-detection-and-screening/screening/screening-for-colorectal -cancer/?region=sk*.

Canadian Celiac Association. (2014). *About celiac disease*. Retrieved from *http://www.celiac.ca/?page_id=882*.

Canadian Digestive Health Foundation. (2016). *Irritable bowel syndrome*. Retrieved from *http://cdhf.ca/en/disorders/details/id/12*.

Canadian Digestive Health Foundation. (2017). *Statistics: diverticular disease*. Retrieved from *http://www.cdhf.ca/en/statistics*.

Canadian Society of Intestinal Research. (2014). *Inside facts*. Retrieved from *http://www.badgut.org/information-centre/ fast-facts/*.

Colorectal Cancer Association of Canada. (2016a). *Just the facts: Canadian cancer statistics 2015*. Retrieved from *http:// www.colorectal-cancer.ca/en/just-the-facts/colorectal/*.

Colorectal Cancer Association of Canada. (2016b). *Just the facts: Symptoms*. Retrieved from *http://www.colorectal-cancer.ca/en/ just-the-facts/symptoms/*.

Colorectal Cancer Association of Canada. (2016c). *Screening and diagnostics: Septin9 blood tests*. Retrieved from *http:// www.colorectal-cancer.ca/en/screening/septin9-test/*.

Colorectal Cancer Association of Canada. (2016d). *Treatments and side-effects: Treatment options*. Retrieved from *http://*

www.colorectal-cancer.ca/en/treating-cancer/treatment-cancer/ #LAPCCY.

Crohn's and Colitis Canada. (2016). *Health issues outside the gut*. Retrieved from *http://www.crohnsandcolitis.ca/site/ c.dtJRL9NUJmL4H/b.9012451/k.4898/Health_Issues_Outside_the_ Gut.htm*.

Fargo, M. V., & Latimer, K. M. (2012). Evaluation and management of common anorectal conditions. *American Family Physician, 85*(6), 624–630.

Friis, S., Riis, A. H., Erichsen, R., et al. (2015). Low-dose Aspirin or nonsteroidal anti-inflammatory drug use and colorectal cancer risk: A population-based, case-control study. *Annals of Internal Medicine, 163*(5), 347–355. doi:10.7326/M15-0039.

Goldberg, E. J., Bhalodia, S., Jacob, S., et al. (2015). Clostridium difficile infection: A brief update on emerging therapies. *American Journal of Health-System Pharmacy, 72*(12), 1007–1012. doi:10.2146/ajhp140645.

Ishihara, S., Yashima, K., Kushiyama, Y., et al. (2012). Prevalence of organic colonic lesions in patients meeting Rome III criteria for diagnosis of IBS: A prospective multi-center study utilizing colonoscopy. *Journal of Gastroenterology, 47*(10), 1084–1090. doi:10.1007/s00535-012-0573-4.

Johnston, B. C., Ma, S. S., Goldenberg, J. Z., et al. (2012). Probiotics for the prevention of Clostridium difficile–associated diarrhea: A systematic review and meta-analysis. *Annals of Internal Medicine, 157*(12), 878–888. doi:10.7326/0003-4819-157-12-201212180 -00563.

Leone, V., Chang, E. B., & Devkota, S. (2013). Diet, microbes, and host genetics: The perfect storm in inflammatory bowel diseases.

Journal of Gastroenterology, 48(3), 315–321. doi:10.1007/s00535-013-0777-2.

Leong, C., & Zelenitsky, S. (2013). Treatment strategies for recurrent *Clostridium difficile* infection. *The Canadian Journal of Hospital Pharmacy, 66*(6), 361–368.

Lowth, M. (2014). Coeliac disease: Clinical features, diagnosis and management. *Practice Nurse, 44*(8), 36–40.

Mavrinac, M. A., Ohannessian, A., Dowling, E. P., et al. (2014). Why celiac disease is so easy to miss. *Journal of Family Practice, 63*(9), 508–513.

Mazal, J. (2014). Crohn disease: Pathophysiology, diagnosis, and treatment. *Radiologic Technology, 85*(3), 297–322.

Pickhardt, P., Lawrence, E., Pooler, B., et al. (2011). Diagnostic performance of multidetector computed tomography for suspected acute appendicitis. *Annals of Internal Medicine, 154*(12), 789–796. doi:10.7326/0003-4819-154-12-201106210-00006.

Registered Nurses' Association of Ontario (RNAO). (2011a). *Prevention of falls and fall injuries in the older adult.* Retrieved from *http://rnao.ca/sites/rnao-ca/files/Prevention_of_Falls_and_Fall_Injuries_in_the_Older_Adult.pdf.*

Registered Nurses' Association of Ontario (RNAO). (2011b). *Prevention of constipation in the older adult population.* Retrieved from *http://rnao.ca/sites/rnao-ca/files/Constipation_supplement_2011.pdf.*

Rocchi, A., Benchimol, E. I., Bernstein, C. N., et al. (2012). Inflammatory bowel disease: A Canadian burden of illness review. *Canadian Journal of Gastroenterology, 26*(11), 811. doi:10.1155/2012/984575.

Rx Files Academic Detailing Program. (2014). *Rx Files: Drug comparison charts.* Saskatoon, SK: Saskatoon Health Region.

Suhaimi, S. N. A., Nazri, N., Latar, N. H. M., et al. (2015). Familial adenomatous polyposis–associated papillary thyroid cancer. *Malaysian Journal of Medical Sciences, 22*(4), 69–72.

Thompson, J., & Read, N. (2015). Managing the symptoms of irritable bowel syndrome. *Nurse Prescribing, 13*(5), 230–234. doi:10.12968/npre.2015.13.5.230.

RESOURCES

Canadian Association of Gastroenterology
http://www.cag-acg.org

Canadian Cancer Society
http://www.cancer.ca

Canadian Celiac Association
http://www.celiac.ca/

Canadian Society for Enterostomal Therapy
http://www.caet.ca/

Canadian Society of Gastroenterology and Associates
http://www.csgna.com

The Canadian Society of Intestinal Research
http://www.badgut.com

Colorectal Cancer Association of Canada
http://www.colorectal-cancer.ca

Crohn's & Colitis Foundation of Canada (CCFC)
http://www.ccfc.ca

For additional Internet resources, see the website for this book at *http://evolve.elsevier.com/Canada/Lewis/medsurg*

Nursing Management

Liver, Pancreas, and Biliary Tract Problems

Written by: Kathy H. Wu
Adapted by: Colina Yim

℮volve WEBSITE

http://evolve.elsevier.com/Canada/Lewis/medsurg

- Review Questions (Online Only)
- Key Points
- Answer Guidelines for Case Study
- Student Case Studies
  - Acute Pancreatitis and Septic Shock
  - Cholelithiasis and Cholecystitis
  - Hepatitis

- Customizable Nursing Care Plans
  - Acute Viral Hepatitis
  - Advanced Cirrhosis
  - Acute Pancreatitis

- Conceptual Care Map Creator
  - Conceptual Care Map for Textbook Case Study
- Audio Glossary
- Content Updates

LEARNING OBJECTIVES

1. Define *jaundice*, and describe the manifestations associated with the different causes of jaundice.
2. Differentiate among the types of viral hepatitis, including etiology, pathophysiology, clinical manifestations, complications, and collaborative care.
3. Describe the nursing management of patients with viral hepatitis.
4. Explain the etiology, pathophysiology, clinical manifestations, complications, collaborative care, and nursing management of patients with cirrhosis.
5. Describe the pathophysiology, clinical manifestations, complications, and collaborative care of patients with nonalcoholic fatty liver disease.

6. Describe the clinical manifestations and management of hepato-cellular carcinoma.
7. Differentiate between acute and chronic pancreatitis related to the pathophysiology, clinical manifestations, complications, collaborative care, and nursing management.
8. Explain the clinical manifestations, collaborative care, and nursing management of patients with pancreatic cancer.
9. Explain the pathophysiology, clinical manifestations, complications, and collaborative care, including surgical therapy, of patients with gallbladder disorders.
10. Describe the nursing management of patients undergoing surgical treatment of cholecystitis and cholelithiasis.

KEY TERMS

acute liver failure, p. 1123
acute pancreatitis, p. 1126
ascites, p. 1115
asterixis, p. 1117
cholecystitis, p. 1132
cholelithiasis, p. 1132
chronic pancreatitis, p. 1129

cirrhosis, p. 1113
esophageal varices, p. 1115
fetor hepaticus, p. 1117
fulminant hepatitis, p. 1104
hepatic encephalopathy, p. 1117
hepatitis, p. 1102

hepato-renal syndrome (HRS), p. 1117
jaundice, p. 1101
nonalcoholic fatty liver disease (NAFLD), p. 1111
nonalcoholic steatohepatitis (NASH), p. 1111

paracentesis, p. 1118
portal hypertension, p. 1115
pseudocyst, p. 1127
spider angiomas, p. 1114

The liver, the pancreas, and the biliary tract are critical organs that are responsible for many functions vital to life. Nursing management of patients with liver, pancreatic, and gallbladder problems is the focus of this chapter. Viral hepatitis, cirrhosis, acute pancreatitis, cholecystitis, and cholelithiasis are described in detail.

JAUNDICE

Jaundice, a yellowish discoloration of body tissues, results when the concentration of bilirubin in the blood becomes abnormally increased. It is a symptom rather than a disease. The term *jaundice* is often used interchangeably with *hyperbilirubinemia.* However, a careful clinical examination cannot detect jaundice

FIGURE 46-1 Patient with jaundice. Source: Butcher, G. P. (2004). *Gastroenterology: An illustrated colour text*. London, UK: Churchill Livingstone.

until the serum bilirubin level is higher than 34 mcmol/L, twice the normal upper limit. Jaundice is usually first observed in the sclera and later in the skin (Figure 46-1).

Most of the body's bilirubin is formed from the breakdown of hemoglobin (from red blood cells) by macrophages (see Chapter 41, Figure 41-4). This unconjugated (indirect) bilirubin is released into the blood circulation tightly bound to albumin and is not water soluble. Because the unconjugated bilirubin is not water soluble, it cannot be filtered in the kidneys and is not excreted in the urine. In the liver, the unconjugated bilirubin is conjugated with glucuronic acid to form conjugated (direct) bilirubin, which is water soluble. Conjugated bilirubin is secreted into bile, which flows through the hepatic and the biliary duct systems into the small intestine. In the large intestine, bilirubin is converted to stercobilinogen and urobilinogen by bacterial action. Stercobilinogen is responsible for the characteristic brown colour of feces. Some urobilinogen is reabsorbed into the portal circulation and returned to the liver. Normally, a very small amount of urobilinogen is excreted in urine.

Jaundice can be classified as prehepatic, hepatic, and posthepatic (or cholestatic). There is, however, much overlap, particularly between the hepatic and posthepatic varieties.

Prehepatic Jaundice

Prehepatic jaundice results from an increase in the load of bilirubin before the bile arrives at the liver. The most common cause of this increased load is overproduction of unconjugated bilirubin, as in hemolysis (excessive breakdown of red blood cells). Hemolysis can be related to blood transfusion reactions, sickle cell crisis, and hemolytic anemia. In benign hereditary conditions, such as Gilbert syndrome, the amount of unconjugated bilirubin in the blood is increased. The liver is unable to handle this increased bilirubin load. Bilirubin cannot be detected in the urine.

Hepatic Jaundice

Hepatic jaundice results from an alteration in the liver's ability to take up bilirubin from the blood or to conjugate or excrete it into bile. In hepato-cellular disease, the hepatocytes are damaged and leak bilirubin; thus levels of conjugated bilirubin are increased. In severe liver injuries, levels of both unconjugated and conjugated bilirubin are elevated as a result of both the inability of hepatocytes to conjugate bilirubin and the continued leaking of conjugated bilirubin from cells. Through reflux, conjugated bilirubin returns to the circulation and is excreted in urine because it is water soluble. The most common causes of hepatic jaundice are hepatitis, cirrhosis, and hepato-cellular carcinoma (HCC).

Posthepatic (Cholestatic) Jaundice

Posthepatic jaundice is caused by failure of bile to reach the duodenum, mostly because of obstruction of bile flow through the liver or through the biliary duct system. The obstruction may be intrahepatic or extrahepatic. Intrahepatic obstructions result from swelling or fibrosis of the liver's canaliculi and bile ducts. The swelling can be caused by damage from liver tumours, hepatitis, or cirrhosis. Causes of extrahepatic obstruction include obstruction of the common bile duct by a stone, sclerosing cholangitis, and pancreatic cancer. Laboratory findings show an elevation of levels of both unconjugated and conjugated bilirubin and urine bilirubin.0 Because bilirubin does not enter the intestines, the level of fecal or urinary urobilinogen is decreased or nonexistent. When obstruction is complete, the stools are clay coloured.

DISORDERS OF THE LIVER

VIRAL HEPATITIS

Hepatitis is a broad term meaning inflammation of the liver. The most common cause of hepatitis is a viral infection. The common types of viral hepatitis are A, B, C, D, and E. Other viruses—such as cytomegalovirus, Epstein-Barr virus, herpesvirus, coxsackievirus, and rubella virus—may cause hepatitis, but the liver is usually not the primary infected organ. Hepatitis may also be caused by chemicals and drugs (including alcohol; see Chapter 41, Table 41-6), autoimmune diseases, metabolic disorders, and genetic abnormalities.

Viral hepatitis is a major public health concern. Surveillance of these viruses is carried out by the National Notifiable Disease Reporting System of Health Canada, and confirmed cases must therefore be reported. The only definitive way to distinguish among the various forms of viral hepatitis is by the presence of the antigens and the subsequent development of antibodies to them. However, the person who is immune to one virus can still develop another type of viral hepatitis. The major characteristics of the hepatitis viruses are presented in Table 46-1. Each type of viral hepatitis is discussed in detail later in this chapter.

Pathophysiological Features

Liver. The pathophysiological changes in the various types of viral hepatitis are similar. Hepatitis involves widespread inflammation of liver tissue. During an acute viral hepatitis infection, liver damage is mediated by cytotoxic cytokines and natural killer cells that cause lysis of infected hepatocytes (liver cells). Liver cell damage results in liver cell necrosis (death). Inflammation may interrupt bile flow, causing cholestasis (impaired flow of bile). Liver cells can normally regenerate through cellular replication, and if no complications occur, they should resume their normal function. If liver cell loss is massive, cellular replication may not be possible.

A chronic viral hepatitis infection causes chronic inflammation and can cause fibrosis that, over decades, can progress to cirrhosis. (Cirrhosis is discussed later in this chapter.)

Systemic Effects. The antigen–antibody complexes between the virus and its corresponding antibody form a circulating immune complex in the early phases of hepatitis. The circulating immune complexes activate the complement system (see Chapter 16). The clinical manifestations of this activation are rash, angioedema, arthritis, fever, and malaise. *Cryoglobulinemia* (presence of abnormal proteins in the blood), glomerulo-nephritis,

TABLE 46-1 CHARACTERISTICS OF HEPATITIS VIRUSES

Incubation Period and Mode of Transmission	Sources of Infection	Infectivity
Hepatitis A Virus (HAV)		
15–50 days (average 28) Fecal–oral route (primarily fecal contamination and oral ingestion)	Crowded conditions (e.g., day care, nursing home). Poor personal hygiene. Poor sanitation. Contaminated food, water, shellfish. Persons with subclinical infections, infected food handlers. Sexual contact with infected partner. IV drug users.	Most infectious during 2 wk before onset of symptoms. Infectious until 1–2 wk after the start of symptoms.
Hepatitis B Virus (HBV)		
45–180 days (average 56–96) Percutaneous (parenteral) or permucosal exposure to blood or blood products Sexual contact Perinatal transmission	Contaminated needles, syringes, and blood products. Sexual activity with infected partner. Contact with asymptomatic carrier. Tattoos or body piercing with contaminated needles.	Before and after symptoms appear. Infectious for 4–6 mo. Carriers continue to be infectious for life.
Hepatitis C Virus (HCV)		
14–180 days (average 56) Percutaneous (parenteral) or mucosal exposure to blood or blood products High-risk sexual contact Perinatal contact	Blood and blood products. Needles and syringes. Sexual activity with infected partners.	1–2 wk before symptoms appear. Continues during clinical course. 75%–85% go on to develop chronic hepatitis C and remain infectious.
Hepatitis D Virus (HDV)		
2–26 wk HBV must precede HDV Chronic carriers of HBV always at risk	Same as HBV. Can cause infection only when HBV is present. Routes of transmission same as for HBV.	Blood infectious at all stages of HDV infection.
Hepatitis E Virus (HEV)		
15–64 days (average 26–42 days) Fecal–oral route Outbreaks associated with contaminated water supply in developing countries	Contaminated water, poor sanitation. Found in Asia, Africa, and Mexico. Not common in United States.	Not known. May be similar to HAV.

IV, intravenous.

DETERMINANTS OF HEALTH

Hepatitis C Virus (HCV) Infection

Culture and Ethnicity

- The incidence of acute hepatitis C infection among Indigenous males is 1.5 times higher than in the non-Indigenous Canadian-born population; the incidence rate for Indigenous females is 3.9 times higher.*

Personal Health Practices and Coping Skills

- Due to their tendency to engage in high-risk behaviours, prison inmates are at greater risk for HCV exposure than the general Canadian population is.†
- Injection drug users who shared drug preparation equipment are more likely than people who do not use injection drugs to contract HCV infection.‡

Gender

- The rates of HCV infection are higher in younger women. In Canadian street youth, the incidence of HCV was doubled in females due to concurrent high-risk behaviours (e.g., unprotected sex, drug use).¶

References

*Uhanova, J., Tate, R. B., Tataryn, D. J., et al. (2013). The epidemiology of hepatitis C in a Canadian Indigenous population. *Canadian Journal of Gastroenterology and Hepatology, 27*(6), 336–340.

†Kouyoumdjian, F. G., & McIsaac, K. E. (2015). Persons in correctional facilities in Canada: A key population for hepatitis C prevention and control. *Canadian Journal of Public Health, 106*(6), E454. doi:10.17269/cjph.106.5132.

‡Myers, R. P., Krajden, M., Bilodeau, M., et al. (2014). Burden of disease and cost of chronic hepatitis C virus infection in Canada. *Canadian Journal of Gastroenterology and Hepatology, 28*(5), 243–250.

¶Puri, N., DeBeck, K., Feng, C., et al. (2014). Gender influences on hepatitis C incidence among street youth in a Canadian setting. *Journal of Adolescent Health, 55*(6), 830–834.

and vasculitis have also been found secondary to immune complex activation.

Clinical Manifestations

The clinical manifestations of viral hepatitis can be classified into acute and chronic hepatitis (Table 46-2). Many individuals with acute hepatitis have no symptoms. Individuals who are immuno-suppressed may also have no symptoms. As a result, many acute infections are often not diagnosed.

The clinical symptoms, if present, in acute infections are similar across all types of hepatitis viruses. However, the course of infections varies among the types of hepatitis (discussed in detail in individual sections on viral hepatitis).

Acute Phase. The acute phase of a viral hepatitis infection usually lasts 1 to 4 months. During the incubation period, symptoms may include anorexia, nausea, occasional vomiting, and right upper quadrant discomfort. The infected person may find food or alcohol repugnant and, if a smoker, may develop a

TABLE 46-2	**CLINICAL MANIFESTATIONS OF HEPATITIS**

Acute
- Altered taste and smell
- Anorexia
- Arthralgias
- Constipation or diarrhea
- Dark urine
- Fatigue
- Fever
- Headache
- Hepatomegaly
- Jaundice
- Light stools
- Malaise
- Nausea, vomiting
- Pruritus
- Right upper quadrant discomfort
- Splenomegaly
- Urticaria
- Weight loss

Chronic
- Easy fatigability
- Hepatomegaly
- Malaise
- Myalgia and arthralgia

distaste for cigarettes. Other symptoms may include malaise, fatigue, headache, low-grade fever, arthralgias, and skin rashes. Physical examination may reveal hepatomegaly, lymphadenopathy, and sometimes splenomegaly. The acute phase is the period of maximal infectivity.

The acute phase may be icteric (jaundice) or anicteric (no jaundice). Jaundice results when bilirubin diffuses into the tissues. The urine may darken because of excretion of excess bilirubin by the kidneys. If conjugated bilirubin cannot flow out of the liver because of obstruction or inflammation of the bile ducts, the stools become light or clay coloured. Pruritus sometimes accompanies the jaundice and occurs as a result of the accumulation of bile salts beneath the skin.

The convalescent phase begins as jaundice is disappearing and lasts from weeks to months; the average is 2 to 4 months. During this period, the patient's major complaint is malaise and easy fatigability. Hepatomegaly remains for several weeks, but splenomegaly usually subsides.

Chronic Phase. The disappearance of jaundice does not mean resolution of the virus infection. Many hepatitis B and C infections result in chronic, lifelong disease. Almost all cases of acute hepatitis A resolve with no progression to a chronic state. Most patients with chronic viral hepatitis B or C have no symptoms. Others may have nonspecific symptoms, including malaise, fatigue, myalgias, arthralgias, and hepatomegaly (see Table 46-2). Chronic hepatitis B and C can progress to severe scarring of the liver (cirrhosis) and liver failure if left untreated.

Complications

The overall mortality rate for acute viral hepatitis is less than 1%. The risk for death is higher in older adults and those with underlying debilitating illnesses, including existing liver disease. Complications that can occur include acute liver failure, chronic hepatitis, cirrhosis of the liver, hepato-cellular carcinoma, and fulminant hepatitis.

Fulminant hepatitis is an acute clinical syndrome that results in severe impairment or necrosis of liver cells and potential liver failure. It occurs only in a small percentage of patients. It may develop in co-infection with HBV and HDV. It is less frequent with acute HCV infection and rarely occurs with acute HAV. Liver failure usually causes death unless liver transplantation is performed. (Fulminant hepatitis is further discussed later in this chapter.)

Diagnostic Studies

Viral Serological Tests. The viral antigens and antibodies are serological markers used to diagnose the different types of viral hepatitis. The specific markers and their interpretations for each type of viral hepatitis are explained under the headings of the particular viruses.

Serum Liver Enzymes. These tests cannot differentiate one type of hepatitis from another, but they are helpful in determining the type of liver injury, whether it is related to liver cell injury or bile duct abnormalities.

Aspartate aminotransferase (AST) and alanine aminotransferase (ALT) are liver enzymes whose levels can indicate liver cell injury. In severe acute viral hepatitis, the levels can be markedly increased to more than 1 000 U/L. Elevated levels of alkaline phosphatase (ALP) and γ-glutamyl transpeptidase (GGT) are usually associated with bile duct injuries, but these levels can rise to a lesser extent in viral hepatitis infections.

Liver Function Tests. The term *liver function tests* (LFTs) has often been used broadly to include liver enzyme measurements, but that use is misleading. The LFTs that more accurately reflect liver function are serum albumin, serum bilirubin, and prothrombin time, which is standardized to the international normalized ratio (INR). In mild acute viral hepatitis, serum albumin, serum bilirubin, and INR remain normal. When jaundice is detectable on physical examination, the serum bilirubin level is usually at least twice the normal upper limit (>34 mcmol/L). Deteriorating liver function is demonstrated by increased INR and serum bilirubin and decreased serum albumin.

Hepatitis A

Canada has a relatively low incidence of hepatitis A (World Health Organization [WHO], 2010), and it has been slowly decreasing since the introduction of hepatitis A vaccine in 1996. The World Health Organization estimates an annual total of 1.5 million cases of hepatitis A worldwide (WHO, 2013), but seroprevalence data imply there are tens of millions of HAV infections annually (Public Health Agency of Canada [PHAC], 2011). In developing countries, hepatitis A infection is nearly universal during childhood.

Hepatitis A Virus (HAV). HAV is an RNA virus. The virus is found in feces 2 weeks or more before the onset of symptoms and up to 1 week after the onset of jaundice (Figure 46-2). Anti-HAV immunoglobulin M (IgM) appears in the serum as the stool becomes negative for the virus. The presence of anti-HAV IgM indicates acute hepatitis. A positive anti-HAV IgG indicates a past infection or an immune response as a result of vaccination. Its presence provides lifelong immunity (Table 46-3).

The mode of transmission of HAV is usually fecal–oral (mainly by ingesting food or liquid infected with the virus) and rarely parenteral. Poor hygiene, improper handling of food, crowded situations, and poor sanitary conditions are related factors. Foodborne hepatitis A outbreaks usually result from contamination of food during preparation by an infected food handler. The risk for transmission is highest before clinical symptoms are apparent. The virus can also be transmitted by patients with anicteric (asymptomatic) hepatitis A.

Clinical Manifestations. Hepatitis A usually causes acute symptoms in adults but not in younger children. Typical symptoms include anorexia, nausea, fatigue, fever, and jaundice (see Table 46-2). The symptom severity increases with age. Fewer than 10% of affected children younger than 6 years develop jaundice. Recovery usually takes 4 to 6 weeks, but it may take months. Hepatitis A does not lead to chronicity and rarely causes fulminant hepatic failure. There is no specific treatment for hepatitis A. Hospitalization is normally unnecessary unless the patient is

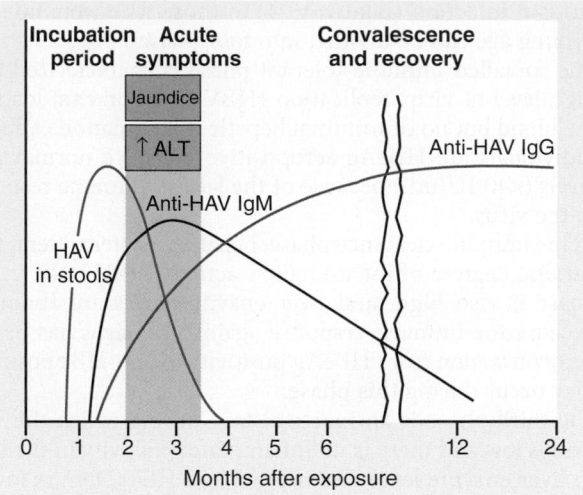

FIGURE 46-2 Course of infection with hepatitis A virus (HAV). *ALT,* alanine aminotransferase; *anti-HAV IgG,* immunoglobulin G class antibody to hepatitis A virus; *anti-HAV IgM,* immunoglobulin M class antibody to hepatitis A virus. Source: McCance, K. L., & Huether, S. E. (2010). *Pathophysiology: The biologic basis for disease in adults and children* (6th ed., p. 1488). St. Louis: Mosby.

TABLE 46-4	SEROLOGY TESTS FOR HBV INFECTION
Test	**Significance of a Positive Finding**
HBsAg (hepatitis B surface antigen)	Infection; persistence of positive result >6 months indicates chronic infection
HBeAg (hepatitis B e antigen)	High virus activity and high degree of infectiousness
Anti-HBe (antibody to hepatitis B e antigen)	Associated with lower rate of virus replication and less infectious state; in cases of mutated viruses, positive result can be associated with active virus replication and high infectivity
Anti-HBc total (total antibody to hepatitis B core antigen)	Past or ongoing infection; seropositivity persists for life; does not appear after vaccination
Anti-HBc IgM (IgM class antibody to hepatitis B core antigen)	Acute infection
Anti-HBs (antibody to hepatitis B surface antigen)	Protective antibody produced with recovery from infection or in response to vaccination

HBV, hepatitis B virus; *IgM,* immunoglobulin M.

TABLE 46-3	SEROLOGY TESTS FOR HAV INFECTION
Tests	**Significance of a Positive Finding**
Anti-HAV IgM (antibody to HAV, immunoglobulin M)	Acute infection
Anti-HAV IgG (antibody to HAV, immunoglobulin G)	Long-term immunity, due to either a past infection or vaccination

HAV, Hepatitis A virus.

severely dehydrated. Management is focused on relief of symptoms. Recovery from HAV infection confers lifelong immunity against the virus.

Hepatitis B

Hepatitis B is an important vaccine-preventable infectious disease in Canada. Worldwide, nearly 2 billion people are infected with HBV and, of these, 350 million have been unable to clear the infection and have become chronically infected. In Canada, the overall reported incidence of HBV was 0.6 cases per 100 000 people (PHAC, 2014a). Because of the heterogeneity of the Canadian population, immigrants—particularly those from regions highly endemic for hepatitis B—constitute the largest group of carriers of chronic hepatitis B.

Hepatitis B Virus (HBV). HBV is a deoxyribonucleic acid (DNA) virus that is far more infectious than the human immunodeficiency virus (HIV). It can live outside a human body for up to 7 days.

HBV has a complex structure. It expresses a few viral proteins or antigens that can be measured in blood. Each antigen has a corresponding antibody that may develop in response to the HBV infection. Hepatitis B surface antigen (HBsAg) represents the outer protein coat of the virus. The persistence of HBsAg in the blood for 6 to 12 months or longer indicates a chronic hepatitis B state. Development of antibody toward HBsAg (anti-HBs) signifies immunity. The HBV core antigen (HBcAg) can be observed only in the liver and not in blood, but its antibody

(anti-HBc) can be measured, and its presence in blood indicates infection. Hepatitis B e antigen (HBeAg) is a third viral protein excreted by the virus. Its presence is associated with an active viral replication state and high infectivity. The absence of HBeAg, however, does not always rule out active disease, because some people can have mutant viruses that cannot express e antigen, and hence they have active e antigen negative chronic hepatitis B. The different serological markers of hepatitis B are explained in Table 46-4.

HBV is transmitted perinatally by mothers who have the viral infection; percutaneously (e.g., intravenous [IV] drug use, accidental needle-stick punctures, tattoos); sexually; or horizontally by permucosal exposure to infectious blood, blood products, or other body fluids (e.g., semen, vaginal secretions). Transmission occurs when infected blood or other body fluids enter the body of a person who is not immune to the virus.

In people with HBV, HBsAg has been detected in almost every bodily fluid. Infected semen and saliva contain much lower concentrations of HBV than blood, and the risk of virus transmission via these secretions is very low. There is no evidence that urine, feces, tears, and sweat are infective.

Breastfeeding is safe and is not a risk factor for mother-to-child transmission (Chen, Chen, Wen, et al., 2013). All infants born to HBsAg-infected mothers must receive both vaccination and immune globulins at birth. All breastfeeding mothers should take good care of their nipples to avoid cracking and bleeding. Kissing, hugging, sharing food, and casual contacts with infected individuals does not transmit HBV infection.

According to the *Primary Care Management of Hepatitis B Guide* (PHAC, 2014b), the at-risk groups that should be screened and tested for hepatitis B include injection or inhalation drug users, people who have unprotected sex with multiple sexual partners, those who have spent time in prison, homosexual men, and individuals from areas of the world where the virus is common.

Acute Hepatitis B. Most acutely infected individuals, especially neonates and young children born to mothers with hepatitis B, have no symptoms. Fulminant hepatitis is uncommon.

FIGURE 46-3 Course of a resolved hepatitis B (HBV) infection. *ALT,* alanine aminotransferase; *anti-HBc,* antibody to hepatitis B core antigen; *anti-HBe,* antibody to HBeAg; *anti-HBs,* antibody to HBsAg; *HBeAg,* hepatitis B e antigen; *HBsAg,* hepatitis B surface antigen; *HBV,* hepatitis B virus; *IgG,* immunoglobulin G; *IgM,* immunoglobulin M. Source: McCance, K. L., & Huether, S. E. (2014). *Pathophysiology: The biologic basis for disease in adults and children* (7th ed., p. 1458). St. Louis: Mosby.

FIGURE 46-4 Phases of chronic hepatitis B infection. *ALT,* alanine aminotransferase; *Anti-HBe,* antibody to hepatitis B e antigen (HBeAg); *HBV,* hepatitis B virus. Source: From Dooley, J. S., Lok, A. S. F., Burroughs, A., & Heathcote, E. J. (2011). *Sherlock's diseases of the liver and biliary system* (12th ed., p. 378). Copyright © 2011, John Wiley and Sons.

The course of an acute HBV infection that spontaneously resolves is shown in Figure 46-3. After an acute infection, the percentage of infected people in whom the infection does not resolve and becomes chronic varies with age. Up to 90% of neonates who contract HBV at birth become chronically infected. In contrast, more than 95% of adults can clear the HBV infection except for those who are immuno-compromised, such as those with HIV co-infection. Children under age 6 with HBV have a 30% to 50% risk of it developing into a chronic infection (WHO, 2017).

Acute hepatitis B normally does not necessitate antiviral treatment. Management focuses on relief of symptoms and counselling to prevent virus transmission, including contacts tracing.

Chronic Hepatitis B. The course of chronic hepatitis B is highly variable and rather complex. Some infected individuals may have exacerbations and remissions of inflammatory activity in the liver, some have continuous active inflammation, and others have no inflammation whatsoever for life. The course of a chronic

hepatitis B infection (Figure 46-4) in those who were infected at a young age can be divided into four phases:

1. The so-called immune-tolerant phase is characterized by a high level of virus replication (HBV DNA or viral load) in the blood but no or minimal hepatic inflammation. Affected individuals are HBeAg seropositive but have normal ALT levels (<40 IU/mL) because of the lack of immune response to the virus.
2. In the immune clearance phase, hepatitis is intermittent, with varying degrees of inflammatory activity. HBV DNA in this phase is also high, and liver enzyme levels are abnormal because the immune response against the virus has begun. Seroconversion from HBeAg positivity to anti-HBe positivity may occur during this phase.
3. The third phase is an inactive stage during which the viral load is low and there is no inflammatory activity in the liver, so liver enzyme levels are normal and HBV DNA is low or undetectable. Some individuals remain in this phase and have inactive hepatitis B throughout life.
4. Others progress to the final phase. They develop a high viral load and abnormal liver enzyme levels, signalling the reactivation of HBV infection.

Every year, about 1% of patients become cleared of HBsAg. Patients with chronic hepatitis B are at risk for the development of hepato-cellular carcinoma.

Drug Therapy. Drug therapy for chronic HBV includes interferon (IFN) and oral antiviral agents. Therapy focuses on decreasing the viral load and liver enzymes and slowing the rate of disease progression. The long-term goals are to prevent cirrhosis, liver failure, and hepato-cellular carcinoma. Current drug therapies for chronic HBV suppress but do not eradicate the virus (Terrault, Bzowej, Chang, et al., 2016).

Interferon. IFN has both antiviral and immuno-modulatory activity. IFN is available in two forms: conventional (Intron A) and pegylated. Conventional IFN has a short half-life, which necessitates frequent subcutaneous administrations, and is rarely used these days. Pegylated IFN, a long-acting weekly subcutaneous injection, is preferred over the conventional IFN for simplicity (Terrault, Bzowej, Chang, et al., 2016). The long-acting preparations are made by conjugating a conventional IFN with polyethylene glycol (PEG) in a process known as *pegylation.*

In patients with HBV who are receiving IFN, one-third exhibit a significant reduction of viral load, normalization of ALT levels, and loss of HBeAg. The response to treatment may vary on the basis of viral genotype. IFN treatment is associated with a number of adverse drug events (Table 46-5). These adverse events are dosage related and tend to decrease in severity with continued treatment. For patients receiving IFN, blood cell counts and liver enzyme levels should be measured at least every 4 weeks, but more often if needed. Treatment duration of 48 weeks is recommended (Terrault, Bzowej, Chang, et al., 2016).

Nucleoside and Nucleotide Analogues. The oral nucleoside analogue classes of antiviral agents used to treat HBV infection include lamivudine (Heptovir), telbivudine (Sebivo), and entecavir (Baraclude); the nucleotide analogues are adefovir (Hepsera) and tenofovir (Viread). These drugs are given when there is evidence of active viral replication. They inhibit viral DNA synthesis and thereby reduce the amount of virus in the blood, decreasing liver damage and normalizing liver enzymes. Most patients with HBV infection require long-term treatment with these medications.

TABLE 46-5 HCV DRUG THERAPY: MOST COMMON ADVERSE EFFECTS

Interferon	Ribavirin
Influenza-Like Symptoms	• Anemia
• Arthralgia	• Anorexia
• Asthenia	• Cough
• Chills	• Dyspnea
• Fatigue	• Insomnia
• Headache	• Pruritus
• Low-grade fever	• Rash
• Nausea	• Teratogenicity (interferes with normal fetal
Other Effects	development)
• Depression	
• Thinning hair	
• Insomnia	
• Irritability	
• Itching or dry skin	
• Mood swings	
• Thyroid dysfunction	
• Weight loss	

HCV, hepatitis C virus.

TABLE 46-6 SEROLOGY TESTS FOR HCV INFECTION

Test	Significance
Anti-HCV (antibody to hepatitis C virus)	Positive result indicates either past exposure or current infection
	An initial screening test for HCV
HCV RNA	Quantitative result indicates active ongoing viral multiplication, also referred to as *viral load*

HCV, hepatitis C virus; *RNA,* ribonucleic acid.

Development of drug resistance is an issue with oral antiviral drugs. Of patients who take lamivudine for more than 3 years, up to 70% develop resistance. Patients with lamivudine-resistant HBV infection can be treated with another class of drugs (i.e., adefovir or tenofovir). Because adefovir is considerably less potent and associated with an increasing rate of resistance, it is no longer commonly prescribed. Adefovir and entecavir should not be taken by women who are pregnant. Tenofovir demonstrated no drug resistance development in a 7-year follow-up study (Buti, Tsai, Petersen, et al., 2015). Acute, severe exacerbations of hepatitis B have been reported after discontinuation of these drugs. If these drugs are discontinued, liver function should be monitored closely for several months.

> **DRUG ALERT—Adefovir (Hepsera) and Tenofovir (Viread)**
> • These drugs can cause nephrotoxicity.
> • Serum creatinine levels should be monitored, especially in patients at risk, including those with pre-existing renal disease and those taking nephrotoxic drugs (e.g., cyclosporine, aminoglycoside, vancomycin).

> **DRUG ALERT—Adefovir (Hepsera) and Entecavir (Baraclude)**
> • These drugs should not be taken by pregnant women.

Hepatitis C

Approximately 138 600 Canadians (0.5% of the population) are affected by hepatitis C (Myers, Shah, Burak, et al., 2015). These figures are likely an underestimate because the Canadian Health Survey excluded several high-risk groups, including incarcerated persons, Indigenous peoples, and persons who inject drugs (PWIDs).

Of all the forms of hepatitis, hepatitis C is the most likely to cause long-term liver damage; up to 80% of people with HCV infection develop a chronic infection. Although the overall prevalence of chronic hepatitis C is declining, its complications are increasing due to aging of the infected population and the progression of the disease. Modelling data suggest that cases of decompensated cirrhosis, hepato-cellular carcinoma, and liver-related mortality is expected to rise through 2025 (Myers, Shah, Burak, et al., 2015).

Hepatitis C Virus (HCV). HCV is an ribonucleic acid (RNA) virus that is primarily transmitted percutaneously. In Canada, the most common mode of HCV transmission is the sharing of contaminated needles and equipment among PWIDs. Transmission during blood transfusion has been eliminated. The proportion of cases related to high-risk sexual behaviour (unprotected sex, multiple partners) has increased in recent years. However, sexual transmission among monogamous heterosexual partners remains rare. The risk for perinatal transmission is approximately 5% but is higher in women with HIV–HCV co-infection. People who were born in regions where HCV is common are also at risk because of the lack of universal precautions and medical practices in which contaminated equipment is used (e.g., during childhood immunization). Other transmission risks are related to needle-stick injuries and hemodialysis.

Diagnostic Tests. The initial test for HCV infection is antibody testing. Unlike antibodies to HAV and HBV, antibodies to HCV are not protective and their presence in the blood does not indicate immunity. A positive result of an anti-HCV test can be related to either a past or current exposure (Table 46-6). To confirm if disease is active or not, HCV RNA (the presence of replicating HCV) should be tested. In those whose HCV infection has resolved, anti-HCV results remain positive but HCV RNA are negative.

After initial exposure to the virus, HCV RNA appears in blood earlier than anti-HCV, and patients can test positive at approximately 2 weeks after exposure. Therefore, HCV RNA helps identify the presence of the virus in exposed individuals (e.g., health care workers) before antibodies develop. HCV RNA detection is particularly useful in immuno-compromised patients (e.g., patients with HIV) who have active disease but whose anti-HCV is negative because antibody production is very low (below the detection level of the antibody tests).

HCV has six genotypes and more than 50 subtypes. In Canada, 75% of HCV infections are caused by HCV genotype 1. Genotyping currently plays an important role in the management of patients receiving treatment, but it may not have any impact once a pan-genotypic treatment becomes available.

Drug Therapy

Acute Hepatitis C. The rate of spontaneous clearance of acute hepatitis C (AHC) has been reported as more than 50% in some studies. The younger the patient is when infected, the higher the likelihood of spontaneous clearance. Patients with symptoms also have a higher chance of eliminating the infection.

Chronic Hepatitis C. Unlike hepatitis B, chronic hepatitis C can be cured with drug therapy (Table 46-6) that can completely eradicate the virus, termed a sustained virological response (SVR), and thus prevent HCV-related complications. The treatment landscape of hepatitis C has changed rapidly since the introduction of direct-acting antiviral agents (DAAs) in 2011. Before then, the standard therapy was a combination of pegylated IFN-α-2a (Pegasys) plus ribavirin (combination was Pegasys

RBV) or IFN-α-2b (PEG-Intron) plus ribavirin (combination is Pegetron), which can cause many intolerable adverse effects. These combination therapies are now rarely used. The second wave of newer DAAs introduced in 2014 have much improved efficacy and tolerability and shorter treatment durations and provide the option of IFN- and ribavirin-free therapy. In contrast to the many adverse effects from IFN, the newer DAAs have only a few common adverse effects, including headaches and fatigue. The all-oral DAAs therapy is a major advance in the field of viral hepatitis. Currently, the most commonly used DAAs in Canada include sofosbuvir (Sovaldi), sofosbuvir/ledipasvir (Harvoni), ombitasvir/paritaprevir/ritonavir/dasabuvir (Holkira pak), daclatasvir (Daklinza), and elbasvir/grazoprevir (Zepatier). The treatment choice depends very much on patients' access to third-party insurance coverage, the severity of their liver disease, and the HCV genotypes. Detailed treatment regimens, dosing schedule, duration, and monitoring can be found in the 2015 Canadian guidelines on the management of chronic hepatitis C (Myers, Shah, Burak, et al., 2015).

The currently approved medications for HCV and their most common adverse effects are listed in Table 46-6.

> **DRUG ALERT—Ribavirin**
> • During treatment, pregnancy must be avoided, both by women taking the drug and by women whose male partners are taking the drug.

Many patients with HIV infection also have HCV infection. Patients who have stable HIV infection and relatively intact immune systems (CD4$^+$ counts >200/mcL) are treated for hepatitis C with the goal of eradicating HCV infection and reducing the risk for progression to cirrhosis. Their treatment cure rates in the era of DAAs are comparable to those with non–HIV-infected individuals (Karageorgopoulos, Allen, Bhagani, et al., 2015).

Hepatitis D

Hepatitis D virus (HDV), also called *delta virus*, is a defective single-stranded RNA virus that cannot survive on its own. Of the 350 million people infected with HBV worldwide, 15 million are co-infected with HDV. Although the prevalence of HDV in Canada is extremely low, people who are at risk for HBV infection (e.g., people who use injection drugs) should also be screened for HDV.

HDV requires HBV to replicate. It can be acquired at the same time as HBV (co-infection) or at a later time in an existing HBV infection (super-infection). HBV–HDV co-infection can cause fulminant hepatitis and more severe disease than HBV infection alone. A positive anti-HDV (hepatitis D antibody) test indicates exposure to HDV whereas HDV RNA confirms active disease. Currently in Canada, HDV RNA testing can be performed only in government-approved laboratories.

HDV, similar to HBV, is transmitted percutaneously. HDV is rarely acquired through sexual transmission. The symptoms of acute infection are the same as those of other viral hepatitis infection. People at risk for HDV infection are only those at risk for HBV. No vaccine for HDV is available; however, vaccination against HBV reduces risk for HDV co-infection. Treatment of HDV infection is with IFN-α. However, response rates are poor (<30%), and relapse is common.

Hepatitis E

Hepatitis E virus (HEV) is an RNA virus transmitted via the fecal–oral route, most commonly through drinking contaminated water. Infection with HEV, initially thought to occur primarily in developing countries, has been reported in increasing numbers

---

TABLE 46-7 COLLABORATIVE CARE

Viral Hepatitis

Diagnostic
- History and physical examination
- Liver enzyme measurements
  - Alanine aminotransferase (ALT)
  - Aspartate aminotransferase (AST)
- Liver function tests
  - Albumin, bilirubin, INR
- Hepatitis tests
  - Anti-HAV: IgM or IgG
  - HBsAg
  - Anti-HBs
  - Anti-HBc: IgM or total (IgM + IgG)
  - HBV DNA
  - Anti-HCV
  - HCV RNA
- Genotyping for HBV, HCV
  - Anti-HDV

Collaborative Therapy
Acute and Chronic
- Well-balanced diet
- Vitamin supplements if needed
- Rest (degree of strictness varies)
- Avoidance of alcohol and hepatotoxic drugs

Chronic HBV
- Interferon therapy
  - Conventional IFN (Intron A), pegylated IFN-α-2a (Pegasys), pegylated IFN-α-2b
- Oral antiviral agents
  - Lamivudine (Heptovir), adefovir (Hepsera), telbivudine (Sebivo), entecavir (Baraclude), tenofovir (Viread)

Chronic HCV
- Pegylated IFN-α-2a (Pegasys) + ribavirin (combination is Pegasys RBV), pegylated IFN α-2b (PegIntron) + ribavirin (combination is Pegetron)
- Sofosbuvir (Sovaldi), sofosbuvir/ledipasvir (Harvoni), ombitasvir/paritaprevir/ritonavir/dasabuvir (Holkira pak), daclatasvir (Daklinza), elbasvir/grazoprevir (Zepatior)

Anti-HBc, antibody to hepatitis B core antigen; *anti-HBs,* antibody to surface antigen; *DNA,* deoxyribonucleic acid; *HAV,* hepatitis A virus; *HBsAg,* hepatitis B surface antigen; *HBV,* hepatitis B virus; *HCV,* hepatitis C virus; *HDV,* hepatitis D virus; *IgG,* immunoglobulin G; *IgM,* immunoglobulin M; *IFN,* interferon; *INR,* international normalized ratio; *RNA,* ribonucleic acid.

---

in many developed countries, including the United States (Kamar, Dalton, Abravanel, et al., 2014). Current prevalence of hepatitis E in Canada remains unknown, and the virus has not been reported as a public health threat. HEV infection causes acute self-limiting hepatitis. Pregnant women, however, are at risk for more severe disease. In immuno-suppressed people, hepatitis E may progress to a chronic infection and even cirrhosis. The diagnosis is confirmed through detection of IgM anti-HEV antibodies.

Table 46-7 shows the collaborative care for viral hepatitis.

NURSING MANAGEMENT
VIRAL HEPATITIS

NURSING ASSESSMENT

Subjective and objective data that should be obtained from a person with hepatitis are presented in Table 46-8.

TABLE 46-8 NURSING ASSESSMENT

Hepatitis

Subjective Data
Important Health Information
Past health history: Family history of or exposure to person infected with viral hepatitis; exposure to benzene, carbon tetrachloride or other hepatotoxic agents; recent travel; ingestion of contaminated food or water; exposure to contaminated needles including medical or dental equipment; hemodialysis; blood or blood product transfusions; organ transplantation; misuse of alcohol; previous injection drug use; previous cocaine use; smoking history; high-risk sexual behaviour; exposure as health care worker; chronic care institution resident; incarceration
Medications: Exposure to new drug therapies; misuse of acetaminophen, new prescriptions, over-the-counter or herbal medications or supplements

Symptoms
• Weight loss, anorexia, vomiting, feeling of fullness in right upper quadrant
• Malaise; taste change
• Skin rashes or hives, pruritus
• Right upper quadrant pain and tenderness
• Jaundice, dark urine; light-coloured stools
• Fatigue, arthralgias, myalgias

Objective Data
General
Low-grade fever, lethargy, lymphadenopathy

Integumentary
Rash, other skin changes, jaundice, icteric sclera, interferon injection sites

Gastro-Intestinal
Hepatomegaly, splenomegaly

Possible Diagnostic Findings
Abnormal results of liver enzyme studies: ↑ serum total bilirubin level, hypoalbuminemia, anemia, bilirubin in urine, and ↑ urobilinogen; prolonged prothrombin time (INR); positive test results for hepatitis, including anti-HAV IgM, anti-HAV IgG, HBsAg, HBeAg, anti-HBc IgM, HBV DNA, anti-HCV, HCV RNA, and anti-HDV; abnormal findings on radiological imaging

DNA, deoxyribonucleic acid; *HAV,* Hepatitis A virus; *HBc,* hepatitis B core antigen; *HBeAg,* hepatitis B e antigen; *HBsAg,* hepatitis B surface antigen; *HBV,* hepatitis B virus; *HCV,* hepatitis C virus; *HDV,* hepatitis D virus; *IgG,* immunoglobulin G; *IgM,* immunoglobulin M; *INR,* international normalized ratio; *RNA,* ribonucleic acid.

NURSING DIAGNOSES

Nursing diagnoses for the patient with hepatitis may include but are not limited to the following:
• *Imbalanced nutrition: less than body requirements* related to *insufficient dietary intake* (anorexia and nausea)
• *Activity intolerance* related to *physical deconditioning* (fatigue and weakness)
• *Risk for impaired liver function* (as evidenced by viral infection)
Additional information on nursing diagnoses for the patient with hepatitis is presented in Nursing Care Plan (NCP) 46-1, available on the Evolve website.

PLANNING

The overall goals are that the patient with viral hepatitis will (a) have relief of discomfort, (b) be able to resume normal activities, and (c) experience a return to normal liver function without complications.

NURSING IMPLEMENTATION

HEALTH PROMOTION. Viral hepatitis is a public health problem. The nurse has a significant role in the control and prevention of this infectious disease. The nurse must first understand the epidemiology of the different types of viral hepatitis, including risk factors for acquisition, before considering appropriate control measures.

Hepatitis A. HAV is usually the cause of outbreaks of viral hepatitis. Preventive measures include personal and environmental hygiene and health education to promote good sanitation. Careful handwashing, especially after bowel movements and before eating, is probably the most important precaution. Both hepatitis A vaccine and immune globulin are administered for prevention. (See Table 46-9 for more information on hepatitis A health promotion and prevention.)

From a public health perspective, vaccination, or active immunization, is an effective means of controlling hepatitis A and the best protection against HAV infection. Canada currently does not have a universal HAV immunization program. Adults at risk are advised to receive the vaccine as pre-exposure prophylaxis. These include people who travel to HAV-endemic regions, illicit drug users, men who have sex with men, persons with chronic liver disease, persons with clotting factor disorders (e.g., hemophilia), and residents of communities where hepatitis A is highly endemic (PHAC, 2016).

The HAV vaccine is inactivated hepatitis A virus and is currently available in several forms, including Havrix, Vaqta, and Avaxim. Primary immunization consists of a single dose administered intramuscularly in the deltoid muscle. A booster is recommended between 6 and 12 months after the primary dose to ensure adequate antibody titres and long-term protection. The primary immunization provides immunity within 30 days after a single dose in more than 95% of those vaccinated. Twinrix, a combined HAV and HBV vaccine, is available for children and adults. The primary immunization consists of three doses, given on a 0-, 1-, and 6-month schedule, the same schedule used for the single HBV vaccine. Booster doses are not needed in people who completed the primary three doses. Twinrix may be given to individuals at high risk for hepatitis infection, as previously mentioned. The adverse effects of the vaccine are mild and are usually limited to soreness and redness at the injection site.

Hepatitis A immune globulin can be administered either before or after exposure. Immune globulin provides temporary (6 to 8 weeks) passive immunity and is effective for preventing hepatitis A if given within 1 to 2 weeks after exposure. Immune globulin is recommended for those without anti-HAV antibodies who are exposed to hepatitis A by close contact (e.g., household, day care centre) with people who have HAV or through foodborne exposure. Although immune globulin may not prevent infection in all persons, it may modify the illness to a subclinical infection. It may also be administered as a prophylactic measure for travellers to countries that have a high incidence of hepatitis A.

The patient with acute hepatitis A is hospitalized only when symptoms are severe. Isolation is generally not required for hepatitis A; however, infection-control precautions must be used (see Chapter 17, Table 17-8). A private room is indicated if the patient is incontinent of stool or has poor personal hygiene.

Hepatitis B. The best way to reduce HBV infection is to identify those at risk, screen them for HBV, and vaccinate those who are not infected (see Table 46-9). The nurse must be aware of which individuals are at risk for contracting hepatitis B and teach ways to reduce risks of transmission.

Hepatitis B vaccine is the most effective means of prevention. Since the late 1990s, universal immunization against HBV has been part of the vaccine programs offered by all provinces and territories in Canada. Although different jurisdictions offer the vaccines for people of different ages, the HBV vaccine programs ensure that every child is vaccinated by the end of high school. It is also important to vaccinate adults in at-risk groups, including people who use injection or inhalation drugs, those who live with or have sexual contact with hepatitis B carriers, persons with chronic liver disease, people with hemophilia, persons with chronic renal disease or undergoing dialysis, individuals infected with HIV, and health care providers (Government of Canada, 2016).

Hepatitis B vaccine is produced through recombinant DNA technology. The vaccines are Recombivax HB, Engerix-B, and Twinrix. These are given in a series of three injections in the deltoid muscle. The second dose is administered within 1 month of the first one, and the third one within 6 months of the first. A newer hepatitis B–containing vaccine, Infanrix Hexa, also contains diphtheria, tetanus toxoids, pertussis, poliomyelitis, and *Haemophilus influenzae* type b (DTap-HB-IPV-Hib vaccine) and is given at 2, 4, 6, and 12 to 23 months of age. Hepatitis B vaccine is more than 95% effective. Successful vaccination should result in anti-HBs titres of 10 IU/mL or greater. Boosters (additional doses) to increase the antibody levels are generally not recommended. Only minor adverse reactions have been reported with vaccination, including transient fever and soreness at the injection site. The vaccine is not contraindicated during pregnancy.

For postexposure prophylaxis, the vaccine and hepatitis B immune globulin (HBIG) are administered. HBIG contains antibodies to HBV and confers temporary passive immunity. It is prepared from plasma of donors with a high titre of anti-HBs and is expensive. HBIG is recommended for postexposure prophylaxis in cases of needle-stick, mucous membrane contact, or sexual exposure and for infants born to mothers who are positive for HBsAg. It should be given after exposure, preferably within 24 hours. The vaccine series should also be started.

Preventive measures should also include teaching individuals at high risk of contracting HBV to reduce risks. Good hygienic practices, including handwashing and using gloves when expecting contact with blood, are important. HBV-infected individuals should not share razors, toothbrushes, and other personal items. Practising safer sex should be strongly recommended, particularly if the sexual partner's hepatitis B status is unknown.

Hepatitis C. No vaccine is currently available for hepatitis C. The primary measures to prevent HCV transmission include screening of blood, organ, and tissue donors; use of infection-control precautions; and modification of high-risk behaviour. As with HBV prevention, the nurse should identify individuals at high risk for contracting HCV and teach methods to reduce risks. Individuals at risk include those who use injection drugs (or have used them in the past, even once or many years ago), people who received blood or blood products before 1992, patients who are or have been undergoing hemodialysis, workers in hemodialysis units and laboratories in which blood is handled, people with multiple sexual partners, prisoners, and sexual partners of individuals with HCV infection. Because of the number of people with hepatitis C who have not been diagnosed, birth-cohort screening (1945–1975) regardless of risk-factor status is cost-effective (Shah, Heathcote, & Feld, 2013).

Currently, the Public Health Agency of Canada does not recommend immune globulin for postexposure prophylaxis (e.g., needle-stick exposure from an infected person) for HCV infection. After an acute exposure (e.g., through needle-stick), baseline anti-HCV and ALT levels should be measured in both the person already infected (i.e., the source) and the person exposed to HCV. Follow-up testing for anti-HCV and ALT activity should be performed 4 to 6 months later. If the source is someone with known HCV infection, HCV RNA should be measured 2 weeks later to confirm viral transmission.

As with hepatitis B prevention, the use of universal precautions is important. The use of a condom is advised for sexual intercourse with an individual with HCV, and razors, toothbrushes, and other personal items should not be shared. Health promotion and preventive measures for hepatitis A, B, and C are summarized in Table 46-9.

TABLE 46-9 VIRAL HEPATITIS: HEALTH PROMOTION AND PREVENTATIVE MEASURES

Hepatitis A
General Measures
- Good handwashing
- Proper personal hygiene
- Environmental sanitation
- Control and screening (signs, symptoms) of food handlers
- Serological screening
- Active immunization for people in at-risk groups

Use of Immune Globulin
- Early administration (1–2 wk after exposure) to those exposed
- Prophylaxis for travellers to areas where hepatitis A is common if they have not previously received HAV vaccine

Special Considerations for Health Care Providers
- Wash hands after contact with an affected patient or after removal of gloves
- Use infection-control precautions

Hepatitis B and C Percutaneous Transmission
- Screening of donated blood
  - Hepatitis B: HBsAg
  - Hepatitis C: anti-HCV
- Use of disposable needles and syringes

Sexual Transmission
- Acute exposure: HBIG administration to sexual partner of HBsAg-positive person
- Administration of HBV vaccine series to uninfected sexual partners
- Use of condoms for sexual intercourse

General Measures
- Good handwashing
- Avoidance of sharing toothbrushes and razors
- HBIG administration for one-time exposure (needle-stick, contact of mucous membranes with infectious material)
- Active immunization: HBV vaccine

Special Considerations for Health Care Providers
- Using infection-control precautions
- Considering the blood of all patients potentially infectious
- Disposing of needles properly
- Using needleless IV access devices when possible

HAV, hepatitis A virus; *HBIG,* Hepatitis B immunoglobulin; *HBsAg,* hepatitis B surface antigen; *HBV,* hepatitis B virus; *HCV,* hepatitis C virus; *IV,* intravenous.

ACUTE INTERVENTION

Jaundice. In patients with acute hepatitis, assess for jaundice. In light-skinned people, jaundice is usually observed first in the sclera of the eyes and later in the skin. In dark-skinned people, jaundice is observed in the hard palate of the mouth and the inner canthus of the eyes. The urine may be dark brown or brownish red because of the presence of bilirubin. Comfort measures should be used to relieve fatigue, weakness, headache, and arthralgias (see NCP 46-1, available on the Evolve website).

Ensuring that the patient receives adequate nutrition can be a challenge. Anorexia and a distaste for food can cause nutritional problems. Dietary assessment should be performed. Small, frequent meals may be preferable to three large ones and may help prevent nausea. Measures to stimulate the appetite—such as mouth care, antiemetics, and attractively served meals in pleasant surroundings—should be included in the nursing care plan. Carbonated beverages, ginger, and avoidance of very hot or very cold foods may help counteract the symptom of nausea. Adequate hydration is important.

Rest. Patients with symptomatic acute viral hepatitis have fatigue and decreased energy. Rest is important to help conserve energy. The nurse should help the patient space activities both to conserve energy and to avoid overexertion; assess the patient's response to the rest and activity plan; and modify it accordingly. Assessment of symptoms and liver function tests can be used as a guide to activity.

AMBULATORY AND HOME CARE. Most individuals with acute viral hepatitis are cared for at home, and so the nurse needs to assess patients' knowledge of nutrition and provide the necessary dietary teaching. Rest and adequate nutrition are important for those with impaired liver synthetic functions. Patients should be cautioned about overexertion and the need to follow the health care provider's advice about when to return to work. Patients and their families should be taught how to prevent transmission among household members and what symptoms should be reported to the health care provider. Symptoms of worsening liver function include bleeding tendencies (caused by increased INR), abdominal swelling (from ascites), and confusion (caused by encephalopathy). Patients should be instructed to have regular follow-up for at least 1 year after the diagnosis of acute viral hepatitis. Those who are unable to resolve the acute infection and become chronic HBV or HCV carriers should be assessed for the need of a referral to a hepatologist, if it is not already done. All patients with chronic HBV or HCV infection should avoid excessive use of alcohol to prevent acceleration of disease progression.

Patients who remain seropositive for HBsAg should not donate blood, semen, or organs. Patients who receive IFN for the treatment of hepatitis B or C require education regarding this drug and its adverse effects. Patients and caregivers need to be taught how to administer a subcutaneous injection. They must also be informed about the numerous adverse effects with the therapy, including influenza-like symptoms (e.g., fever, malaise, fatigue, chills; see Table 46-6). (Additional information on interferon is presented in Chapters 16 and 18.)

| EVALUATION

Expected outcomes for the patient with viral hepatitis are addressed in NCP 46-1, available on the Evolve website.

Control of Viral Hepatitis in Health Care Providers

Hepatitis A. Hepatitis A is rarely transmitted from patients to health care providers. When transmission does occur, it is

TABLE 46-10	**MEASURES TO PREVENT TRANSMISSION OF HEPATITIS VIRUSES FROM PATIENTS TO HEALTH CARE PERSONNEL***
HAV	**HBV and HCV**
• Maintenance of good personal hygiene • Handwashing after contact with a patient or after removal of gloves • Use of infection-control precautions†	• Use of infection-control precautions† • Frequent handwashing and after each patient contact • Avoidance of direct contact with blood or blood-containing secretions • Handling the blood of all patients as potentially infective • Proper disposal of needles • Vaccination against HBV • Using needleless IV access devices when they are available

HAV, hepatitis A virus; *HBV,* hepatitis B virus; *HCV,* hepatitis C virus; *IV,* intravenous.
*To prevent the contraction of viral hepatitis from patients with diagnosed and undiagnosed hepatitis, health care providers should wear disposable gloves, goggles, and gown (sometimes) when fecal or blood contamination is likely in handling (a) soiled bedpans, urinals, and catheters and (b) patient's bed linens soiled by body excreta or secretions.
†See Chapter 17, Table 17-8.

associated with undiagnosed hepatitis A in patients who are being treated for other problems. If the patient is incontinent of stool, infection-control precautions must be strictly enforced to prevent transmission.

Hepatitis B. Health care workers may be exposed to HBV from needle sticks, blood contamination, or transmission through mucous membranes or nonintact skin. After a needle-stick injury, the chance that the health care worker will become infected with HBV is 6% to 30% (Centers for Disease Control and Prevention, 2013). Vaccination is the most effective method of preventing HBV. All health care workers in Canada are strongly advised to be immunized against HBV. Many health care organizations provide free hepatitis B vaccinations through the occupational health department to their at-risk employees.

Hepatitis C. Transmission usually results from percutaneous needle exposure or other blood exposure and undetected parenteral transmission. Measures to prevent transmission of the viruses from patients to health care providers are presented in Table 46-10. Of particular concern to the public has been the issue of health care workers infected with bloodborne agents such as hepatitis virus and HIV. Many Canadian hospitals have committees that advise on the practice modifications needed for infected workers.

NONALCOHOLIC FATTY LIVER DISEASE AND NONALCOHOLIC STEATOHEPATITIS

Nonalcoholic fatty liver disease (NAFLD) refers to a spectrum of disease that ranges from simple fatty liver that causes no hepatic inflammation (steatosis) to nonalcoholic steatohepatitis (NASH) to severe liver scarring (cirrhosis). This spectrum of liver disease occurs in people who drink little or no alcohol and is characterized by the accumulation of fat in liver cells. In the case of NASH, this fat buildup causes inflammation and liver cell injury.

NASH is diagnosed histologically by evidence of liver cell ballooning and presence of Mallory bodies. NASH can progress and cause cirrhosis, which can lead to liver cancer and liver failure. When the liver fails, liver transplantation is the only treatment alternative.

Causes

NAFLD is a growing concern around the globe (Mahady & George, 2016). The most common cause of fatty liver disease is obesity. According to the *Obesity in Canada* report (Public Health Agency of Canada & Canadian Institute for Health Information, 2011), one in four Canadians is obese. Obesity rates almost doubled among both sexes in most age groups in the adult and youth categories. Obesity is linked to many chronic diseases, and fatty liver disease is one of them. About 75% of obese people are at risk of developing simple fatty liver, and, of those, up to 25% are at risk of developing fatty liver with inflammation (i.e., NASH).

NAFLD also occurs in patients with metabolic syndrome.

Clinical Manifestations and Diagnostic Studies

Most patients with NAFLD have no symptoms. NAFLD is usually diagnosed during routine medical checkup or during evaluation of other health problems such as hypertension, diabetes, or obesity. Elevations in liver enzyme levels (ALT, AST) are often the first signs of NAFLD. However, such elevations may be associated with other liver disorders. Symptoms, if present, are nonspecific and may include fatigue, malaise, and vague pain in the right upper abdominal quadrant. Enlarged liver (hepatomegaly) and enlarged spleen (splenomegaly) may be detected on first examination of the patient. Only a small number of patients exhibit signs of serious liver disease (e.g., ascites, anasarca, variceal hemorrhage). Jaundice occurs late in NASH and indicates advanced liver disease. As the disease progresses, serum albumin level decreases and serum bilirubin level and prothrombin time increase.

Definitive diagnosis is by liver biopsy. Ultrasonography and computed tomography (CT) are also used to diagnose NAFLD.

Collaborative Care

Patients with NAFLD who are older, are obese, or have diabetes are at risk for advanced liver disease. Currently, there is no definitive treatment available. Therapy is directed at reduction of risk factors, including treatment of diabetes, reduction in body weight, and elimination of harmful medications. No specific dietary therapy is recommended; however, a heart-healthy diet is appropriate. Lifestyle counselling interventions that focused on physical activities and eating behaviours have enabled significant improvement in liver function test results.

Health promotion and patient education are important in preventing the development of NAFLD. Ways to prevent fatty liver include maintaining a healthy body mass index (≤25), avoiding increased abdominal fat (for men, keeping waist circumference <102 cm; for women, <88 cm), eating a heart-healthy diet, exercising at least three times weekly, limiting alcohol to no more than two drinks at a time, taking only medications that are needed, and following physicians' recommendations.

ALCOHOL AND DRUG-INDUCED HEPATITIS

Alcohol Hepatitis

Alcohol consumption, frequently the cause of acute or chronic liver disease, can produce a spectrum of symptoms, ranging from mild elevation in liver enzymes (AST and ALT) to acute alcoholic hepatitis to advanced fibrosis and cirrhosis, which usually occur after decades of excessive alcohol intake. Patients may have serious liver disease caused by another chronic disease (e.g., chronic HCV infection) in combination with alcoholic liver disease.

Acute alcoholic hepatitis is a syndrome of hepatomegaly, jaundice, elevation in liver enzyme tests (AST, ALT, alkaline phosphate), low-grade fever, and possibly ascites and prolonged prothrombin time. These symptoms may improve with cessation of alcohol intake.

Patients may have undetected liver disease and be seen with complications of cirrhosis. Even at this stage, abstinence can result in significant reversal in some patients. If liver function does not recover after abstaining from alcohol for several months or longer, liver transplantation may be considered.

Drug-Induced Liver Injury (DILI)

Drug-induced liver injury (DILI) is one of the more common causes of jaundice. Many medications (prescription, over-the-counter [OTC], and herbal supplements) can cause an increase in liver enzymes and, in severe cases, jaundice and acute liver failure (Chalasani, Hayashi, Bonkovsky, et al., 2014). The pattern of injury depends on the drug causing the reaction. The most common cause of DILI is acetaminophen.

> **DRUG ALERT—Acetaminophen (Tylenol)**
> - Drug is safe if taken at recommended levels and not combined with alcohol. It is also present in a variety of pain relievers, fever reducers, and cough medicines as a somewhat "hidden" ingredient; thus patients taking several drugs may not realize that they are taking a higher amount of acetaminophen.
> - Its toxic effects are dose related. Ingestion of more than 10 g/day leads to acute liver failure.
> - Combining the drug with alcohol increases risk for liver injury.

The pathophysiological changes in the liver and the clinical manifestations of toxic and drug-induced hepatitis are similar to those of viral hepatitis. The usual presenting clinical findings are anorexia, nausea, vomiting, hepatomegaly, splenomegaly, and abnormal results of liver function studies. Treatment is largely supportive, as in acute viral hepatitis. Recovery may be rapid if the hepatotoxin is identified and removed. Liver transplantation may be necessary in cases with severe liver injuries.

AUTOIMMUNE AND GENETIC LIVER DISEASES

Autoimmune Hepatitis

Autoimmune hepatitis (AIH) is a chronic inflammatory disorder of the liver that occurs when the body's immune system attacks its own liver cells. The cause is unknown, but its occurrence may be related to genetic and environmental factors or to drug, virus, or toxin exposure that triggers the activation of the immune system. However, the immune system remains activated after the trigger is removed. The majority (70% to 80%) of patients with AIH are women, and many affected patients have other autoimmune diseases such as celiac disease or hypothyroidism.

The course of AIH is variable. Some patients have no symptoms, whereas others have an acute presentation with symptoms similar to those of acute viral hepatitis. Symptoms include fatigue, arthralgia, abdominal pain, and occasionally jaundice. Diagnosis is usually based on the presence of autoantibodies (i.e., antinuclear antibodies [ANA] and anti–smooth muscle antibodies

[ASMA]), high levels of serum immunoglobulins, and elevated liver enzymes. Liver cancer develops in approximately 6% of patients with AIH.

Treatment with prednisone alone or in combination with azathioprine (Imuran) induces remission in approximately 80% of patients. If these drugs are not effective, other immuno-suppressive therapies (e.g., cyclosporine, tacrolimus [Prograf], or mycophenolate mofetil [CellCept]) are administered. Many patients who stop treatment experience relapse; therefore, treatment is usually lifelong to maintain remission. The most common cause of relapse is failure to adhere to the treatment regimen. Patients who do adhere and respond do not have a shortened life expectancy. However, liver transplantation is indicated for those with liver failure.

Wilson's Disease

Wilson's disease is an autosomal recessive gene disorder of copper metabolism that affects mainly the liver but also the brain, eyes, and kidneys. It is associated with increased storage of copper. Mutations in the affected gene, *ATP7*, lead to decreased biliary excretion of copper and result in its accumulation in the liver, which causes liver cell injury. Wilson's disease has an average worldwide prevalence of 1 per 30 000.

The hallmark of the disease is corneal Kayser–Fleischer rings, which are brownish-red rings seen in the cornea near the limbus. In addition to liver disease, many affected patients also have neurological dysfunction, including movement disorders (tremor, involuntary movements), drooling, dysarthria, rigid dystonia, seizures, migraine headaches, and insomnia.

Diagnosis is based on clinical findings, including the corneal rings and neurological symptoms. Serum ALT and AST levels are elevated, serum ceruloplasmin levels are low, serum uric acid levels are decreased, and urinary copper excretion levels are increased. Measurable copper concentrations from liver biopsy samples can also be present.

The mainstay initial treatment of symptomatic patients or those with active disease is with chelating agents such as D-penicillamine or high-dose zinc that promote the excretion. Treatment is lifelong. Liver transplantation is reserved for acute liver failures or for treatment failures.

Hereditary Hemochromatosis

Hereditary hemochromatosis (HH) is a genetic disorder that affects the liver, heart, pancreas, and endocrine system. It is an inherited condition that is related to the mutation in the *HFE* gene, causing an increase and inappropriate absorption of dietary iron. Prolonged increased iron absorption can lead to complications such as cirrhosis, hepato-cellular carcinoma, diabetes, and heart disease. (Hemochromatosis is discussed further in Chapter 33.)

Primary Biliary Cholangitis

Until 2015, *primary biliary cholangitis (PBC)* was termed *primary biliary cirrhosis* (Beuers, Gershwin, Gish, et al., 2015). It is a chronic and slowly progressive disease caused by inflammation and destruction of small bile ducts in the liver. A T-cell–mediated attack on the small bile duct epithelial cells results in the loss of bile ducts and ultimately in *cholestasis* (blockage of bile flow). Over time, cholangitis, along with the associated inflammation and destruction of the bile ducts, leads to liver fibrosis and cirrhosis. Although the etiology of PBC is not completely understood, it appears that both genetic and environmental factors such as chemical exposure and infection may play a role.

Most patients (95%) diagnosed with PBC are women between ages 30 and 60. The disease is associated with other autoimmune disorders such as rheumatoid arthritis, Sjögren syndrome, and scleroderma.

In the early stages, patients may have no symptoms and may present with generalized pruritus, hepatomegaly, hyperpigmentation of the skin, and fatigue. Jaundice is a sign of late-stage disease. Osteoporosis is also found in a significant number of patients with PBC, and they may also have signs of fat malabsorption, including low levels of fat-soluble vitamins, which occur because of decreased bile secretion. Levels of serum alkaline phosphatase, antimitochondrial antibodies, antinuclear antibodies, and serum lipid levels are also elevated in patients with PBC. Histological evidence of disease is found on liver biopsy.

The goals of treatment are suppression of ongoing liver damage, prevention of complications, and symptom management. The only drug approved for treatment of PBC in Canada is ursodiol (Urso). This drug increases the rate of bile acid secretion and appears to have a cytoprotective effect. Management focuses on malabsorption, skin disorders such as pruritus and xanthomas (cholesterol deposits in the skin), hyperlipidemia, vitamin deficiencies, anemia, and fatigue. Cholestyramine is administered to treat pruritus. Patients are monitored for progression to cirrhosis. Liver transplantation is a treatment option for end-stage liver disease in patients with PBC.

Primary Sclerosing Cholangitis

Primary sclerosing cholangitis (PSC) is a disease of unknown etiology characterized by chronic inflammation, fibrosis, and strictures (narrowing) of the medium and large bile ducts. The majority of patients with PSC also have ulcerative colitis. Complications of PSC can include cholangitis, cholestasis with jaundice, cholangiocarcinoma (bile duct cancer), and cirrhosis.

Drug therapy has not been beneficial. Treatment is directed at reducing the incidence of biliary complications and at screening for bile duct and colorectal cancer, which is related to the high incidence of ulcerative colitis. Patients with advanced liver disease may require liver transplantation.

CIRRHOSIS OF THE LIVER

Cirrhosis is a diffuse pathological process, characterized by fibrosis (scar tissue) and conversion of normal liver architecture to abnormal nodules (Figure 46-5). Fibrosis occurs when the liver cells attempt to regenerate after liver injuries but the regenerative process is disorganized. The overgrowth of new and fibrous connective tissue distorts the normal lobular structure, resulting in lobules of irregular size and shape with impeded blood flow. Eventually, irregular and disorganized regeneration, poor cellular nutrition, and hypoxia caused by inadequate blood flow and scar tissue result in decreased functioning of the liver. Cirrhosis is the final stage of chronic liver disease.

Cirrhosis is a significant cause of morbidity and mortality. It is ranked as the tenth leading cause of death in Canadians (Statistics Canada, 2017); the incidence is highest between ages 40 and 60. It is twice as common in men as in women.

Etiology

Any chronic liver disease—including chronic viral hepatitis, NAFLD, and autoimmune hepatitis—as well as excessive alcohol intake can cause cirrhosis. However, excessive alcohol ingestion remains one of the most common causes of cirrhosis. Alcohol

FIGURE 46-5 Cirrhosis that developed secondary to alcoholism. The characteristic diffuse nodularity of the surface is caused by the combination of regeneration and scarring of the liver. Source: Kumar, V., Abbas, A. K., Fausto, J. N., et al. (2010). *Robbins and Cotran pathologic basis of disease* (8th ed., p. 858). Philadelphia: W. B. Saunders.

has a direct hepatotoxic effect, and it causes cell necrosis and fatty infiltration in the liver. Some controversy continues as to whether the cause of cirrhosis is alcohol or the malnutrition that frequently coexists with chronic ingestion of alcohol. A common problem in people with alcohol use disorder is protein malnutrition. Cases of nutrition-related cirrhosis have resulted from extreme dieting, malabsorption, and obesity.

Approximately 20% of patients with chronic hepatitis C and 25% of those with chronic hepatitis B develop cirrhosis. Chronic inflammation and cell necrosis result in fibrosis and, ultimately, cirrhosis. The combination of chronic hepatitis and excessive alcohol use exacerbates the degree of liver damage.

Biliary causes of cirrhosis include PBC and PSC (both described above).

Cardiac cirrhosis includes a spectrum of hepatic derangements that result from longstanding, severe right-sided heart failure. The treatment is aimed at managing the underlying heart failure.

Clinical Manifestations

Cirrhosis can be classified as *compensated* or *decompensated*. In well-compensated cirrhosis, the liver is able to continue to function normally despite severe hepatic cell injury. Results of liver function tests—including albumin level, bilirubin level, and prothrombin time—are normal. In decompensated cirrhosis, one or more of the complications from cirrhosis (discussed in the following section) occurs.

The onset of cirrhosis is usually insidious. Most patients with early compensated cirrhosis have no specific physical symptoms. Some patients may complain of abdominal pain, described as a dull, heavy feeling in the right upper quadrant or epigastrium. The pain may be caused by swelling and stretching of the liver capsule, spasm of the biliary ducts, intermittent vascular spasm, or a combination of these. Other early manifestations are non-specific, including lassitude, fatigue, slight weight loss, and enlargement of the liver and the spleen.

Early symptoms of decompensated cirrhosis that leads to liver failure can be abrupt. Symptoms may include anorexia, dyspepsia, nausea and vomiting, weakness, muscle loss, and diarrhea or constipation. These symptoms occur as a result of the liver's altered metabolism of carbohydrates, fats, and proteins.

Manifestations of Advanced Cirrhosis. Late symptoms result from the complications of portal hypertension and liver failure.

Jaundice, peripheral edema, and ascites develop gradually as the liver's synthesis function deteriorates. Other late symptoms include skin lesions, hematological disorders, endocrine disturbances, and peripheral neuropathies (Figure 46-6). In the advanced stages, the liver becomes small and nodular and feels firm on palpation.

Jaundice. Jaundice occurs as a result of the liver's decreased ability to excrete conjugated bilirubin (hepatic jaundice). The jaundice may be minimal or severe, depending on the degree of liver damage. If obstruction of the biliary tract occurs, obstructive jaundice may also occur and is usually accompanied by pruritus. The pruritus is caused by an accumulation of bile salts underneath the skin.

Skin Lesions. Various skin manifestations are commonly seen in cirrhosis. Spider angiomas *(telangiectasia* or *spider nevi)* are small, dilated blood vessels with a bright-red centre and spider-like branches. They occur on nose, cheeks, upper trunk, neck, and shoulders. *Palmar erythema* (a red area that blanches with pressure) appears on the palms of the hands. Both of these abnormalities are attributed to an increase in circulating estrogen as a result of the damaged liver's inability to metabolize steroid hormones.

Hematological Problems. Hematological problems include thrombo-cytopenia, leukopenia, anemia, and coagulation disorders. Thrombo-cytopenia is the strongest indicator of cirrhosis. Thrombo-cytopenia, leukopenia, and anemia are probably caused by splenomegaly, which results from backup of blood from the portal vein into the spleen. Overactivity of the enlarged spleen results in increased removal of blood cells, particularly the platelets, from circulation. The anemia also results from inadequate red blood cell production and survival. Other factors involved in the anemia are related to poor diet, poor absorption of folic acid, and bleeding from varices (enlarged veins).

The coagulation problems result from the liver's inability to produce prothrombin and other factors essential for blood clotting. Coagulation problems are manifested by hemorrhagic phenomena or bleeding tendencies, such as epistaxis, purpura, petechiae, easy bruising, gingival bleeding, and heavy menstrual bleeding.

Endocrine Disturbances. Normally, the liver metabolizes hormones including adrenocortical hormones, estrogen, and testosterone. When the damaged liver is unable to do so, various manifestations occur. In men, gynecomastia, loss of axillary and pubic hair, testicular atrophy, and impotence with loss of libido may occur as a result of estrogen accumulation. Younger women with cirrhosis may develop amenorrhea, and older women may have vaginal bleeding. The liver fails to metabolize aldosterone adequately, which results in hyperaldosteronism with subsequent sodium retention, water retention, and potassium loss.

Peripheral Neuropathy. Peripheral neuropathy is a common finding in alcoholic cirrhosis and is probably caused by a dietary deficiency of thiamine, folic acid, and cobalamin (vitamin B_{12}). The neuropathy usually results in mixed neurological symptoms, but sensory symptoms may predominate (see Figure 46-6).

Complications

Major complications of cirrhosis are portal hypertension with resultant esophageal or gastric varices or both, peripheral edema and ascites, hepatic encephalopathy (mental status changes including coma), and hepato-renal syndrome. One or more of these complications are suggestive of disease decompensation.

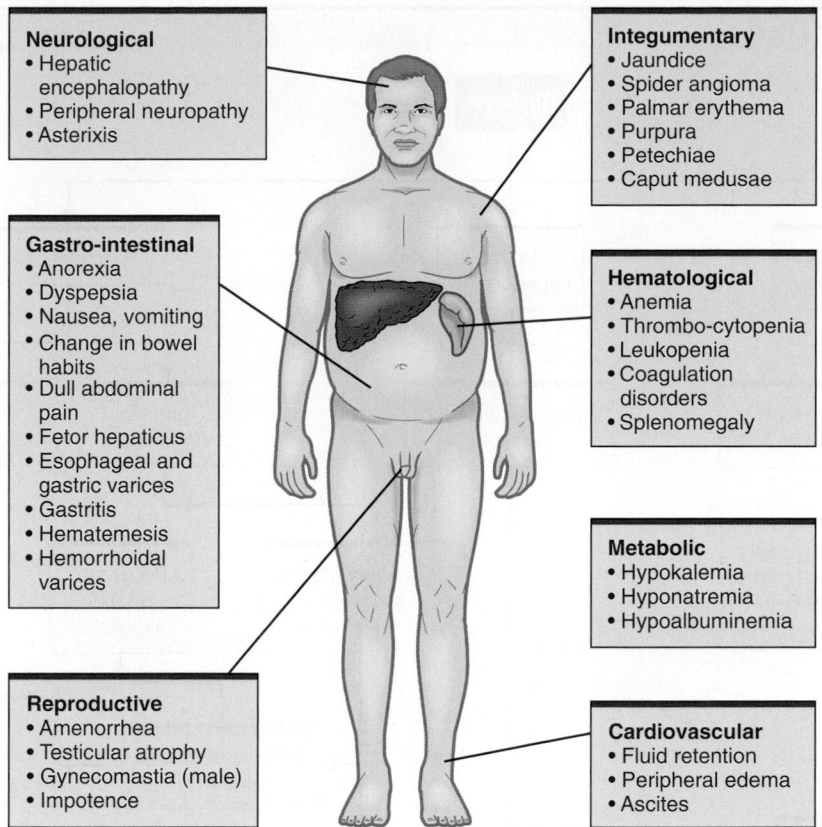

Neurological
- Hepatic encephalopathy
- Peripheral neuropathy
- Asterixis

Integumentary
- Jaundice
- Spider angioma
- Palmar erythema
- Purpura
- Petechiae
- Caput medusae

Gastro-intestinal
- Anorexia
- Dyspepsia
- Nausea, vomiting
- Change in bowel habits
- Dull abdominal pain
- Fetor hepaticus
- Esophageal and gastric varices
- Gastritis
- Hematemesis
- Hemorrhoidal varices

Hematological
- Anemia
- Thrombo-cytopenia
- Leukopenia
- Coagulation disorders
- Splenomegaly

Metabolic
- Hypokalemia
- Hyponatremia
- Hypoalbuminemia

Reproductive
- Amenorrhea
- Testicular atrophy
- Gynecomastia (male)
- Impotence

Cardiovascular
- Fluid retention
- Peripheral edema
- Ascites

FIGURE 46-6 Systemic clinical manifestations of advanced liver cirrhosis.

Portal Hypertension and Esophageal and Gastric Varices. Because of the structural changes in the liver as a result of the cirrhotic process, the portal and hepatic veins and sinusoids are compressed and damaged. These changes result in obstruction to the normal flow of blood through the portal system, which causes portal hypertension.

Portal hypertension is characterized by increased venous pressure in the portal circulation, as well as by splenomegaly, large collateral veins, ascites, systemic hypertension, and esophageal varices. Collateral circulation develops in an attempt both to reduce this high portal pressure and to reduce the increased plasma volume and lymphatic flow. The collateral channels are commonly formed in the lower esophagus (the anastomosis of the left gastric vein and the azygos veins), anterior abdominal wall, parietal peritoneum, and rectum. Varicosities may develop in areas where the collateral and systemic circulations communicate, resulting in esophageal and gastric varices, *caput medusae* (ring of varices around the umbilicus), and hemorrhoids.

Esophageal varices are complexes of tortuous veins located at the lower end of the esophagus. They are enlarged and swollen as a result of portal hypertension. Gastric varices are located in the upper portion (fundus) of the stomach. These collateral vessels contain little elastic tissue and are quite fragile. They tolerate the high pressure poorly, and therefore bleed easily. Large varices are more likely to bleed.

Bleeding esophageal varices are the most life-threatening complication of cirrhosis. The patient may have melena or hematemesis. Hemorrhage may be slow and oozing or massive. Massive hemorrhage is a medical emergency.

Peripheral Edema and Ascites. Peripheral edema sometimes precedes ascites, but in some patients, its development coincides with or occurs after ascites. Edema is caused by decreased colloidal oncotic pressure as a result of impaired liver synthesis of albumin and by increased portacaval pressure from portal hypertension. Peripheral edema manifests as ankle and presacral edema.

Ascites is the accumulation of serous fluid in the peritoneal or the abdominal cavity. When the portal pressure is elevated in the liver, as occurs in cirrhosis, proteins shift from the blood vessels via the larger pores of the sinusoids (capillaries) into the lymph space (Figure 46-7). When the lymphatic system is unable to carry off the excess proteins and water, they leak through the liver capsule into the peritoneal cavity. The osmotic pressure of the proteins pulls additional fluid into the peritoneal cavity (Table 46-11).

A second mechanism of ascites formation is hypoalbuminemia, which results from the inability of the liver to synthesize albumin. The hypoalbuminemia results in decreased colloidal oncotic pressure. A third mechanism of ascites, hyperaldosteronism, results when aldosterone is not metabolized by damaged hepatocytes. The increased level of aldosterone causes an increase in sodium reabsorption by the renal tubules. This retention of sodium, as well as an increase in antidiuretic hormone, causes additional water retention in affected patients. Because of edema formation, intravascular volume and, subsequently, renal blood flow and glomerular filtration are decreased.

Ascites is manifested by abdominal distension with weight gain (Figure 46-8). If the ascites is severe, the umbilicus may be everted. Abdominal striae with distended abdominal wall veins may be present. Urinary output is decreased, and signs of dehydration (e.g., dry tongue and skin, sunken eyeballs, muscle weakness) are manifested. Hypokalemia is common and results from an excessive loss of potassium caused by the increased

PATHOPHYSIOLOGY MAP

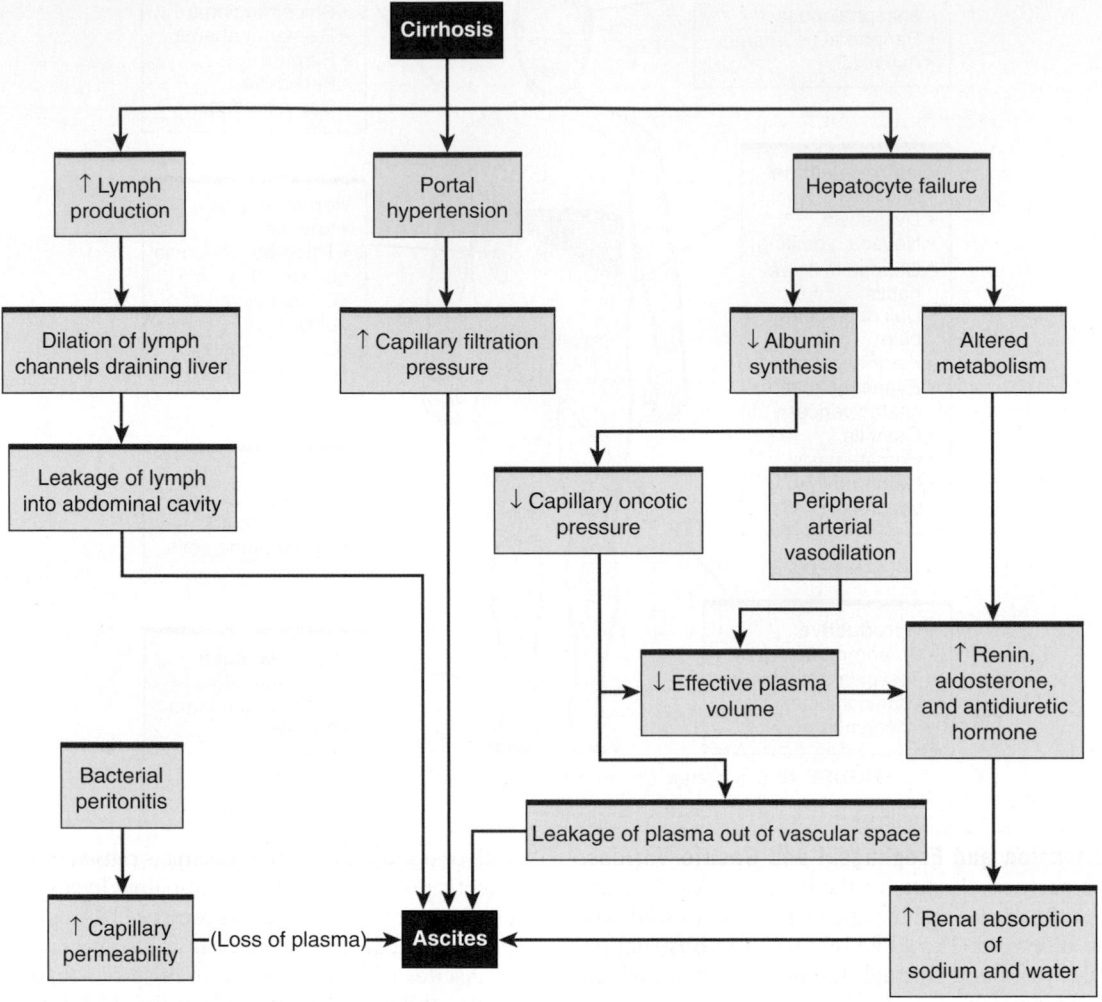

FIGURE 46-7 Mechanisms for development of ascites. Source: Adapted from McCance, K. L., & Huether, S. E. (2014). *Pathophysiology: The biologic basis for disease in adults and children* (7th ed., p. 1454). St. Louis: Mosby.

TABLE 46-11   FACTORS INVOLVED IN THE DEVELOPMENT OF ASCITES

Factor	Mechanism
Portal hypertension	Increase in resistance of blood flow through liver
Increased flow of hepatic lymph	Leaking of protein-rich lymph from surface of cirrhotic liver; intrahepatic blockage of lymph channels
Decreased serum colloidal oncotic pressure	Impairment of liver synthesis of albumin; loss of albumin into peritoneal cavity
Hyperaldosteronism	Increase in aldosterone secretion, stimulated by decreased renal blood flow; decreased liver metabolism of aldosterone
Impaired water excretion	Reduction in renal vascular flow and excessive serum levels of antidiuretic hormone

FIGURE 46-8 Gross ascites. Source: Butcher, G. P. (2004). *Gastroenterology: An illustrated colour text.* London: Churchill Livingstone.

aldosterone. Lowering of potassium levels can also result from diuretic therapy administered to treat the ascites.

Hepatic Encephalopathy. Hepatic encephalopathy is a neuropsychiatric manifestation of advanced liver disease. The pathogenesis of hepatic encephalopathy is multifactorial and includes the neurotoxic effects of ammonia, abnormal neurotransmission, astrocyte swelling, and inflammatory cytokines. A major source of ammonia is the bacterial and enzymatic deamination of amino acids in the intestines. The ammonia that results from this deamination process normally goes to the liver via the portal circulation and is converted to urea, which is then excreted by the kidneys. When the blood is shunted past the liver via the collateral anastomoses, or when the liver is unable to convert ammonia to urea, ammonia levels in the systemic circulation rise. The ammonia crosses the blood–brain barrier and produces neurotoxic manifestations. Factors that increase ammonia in circulation may precipitate hepatic encephalopathy (Table 46-12). Hepatic encephalopathy can also occur after placement of transjugular intrahepatic portosystemic shunt (TIPS), which is used to treat portal hypertension (Riggio, Nardelli, Moscucci, et al., 2012).

Clinical manifestations of encephalopathy are changes in neurological and mental responsiveness, ranging from sleep disturbances to lethargy to deep coma. Changes may occur suddenly because of an increase in ammonia in response to bleeding varices, or they may occur gradually as blood ammonia levels slowly increase. A grading system is used to classify the stages of hepatic encephalopathy (Table 46-13). A characteristic symptom of hepatic encephalopathy is asterixis (flapping tremors) involving the arms and hands. When asked to stretch out the arms and hands, the patient is unable to hold this position, and the hands exhibit a series of rapid flexion and extension movements. Impairments in writing involve difficulty in moving the pen or pencil from left to right and *constructional apraxia* (the inability to construct simple figures). Other signs include hyperventilation, hypothermia, and grimacing and grasping reflexes.

Fetor hepaticus—a musty, sweet odour of the patient's breath—occurs in some patients with encephalopathy. This odour results from the accumulation of digestive by-products that the liver is unable to degrade.

Hepato-Renal Syndrome. Hepato-renal syndrome (HRS) is a serious complication of decompensated cirrhosis. It is a type of kidney failure with advancing azotemia, oliguria, and intractable ascites. In this syndrome, the kidneys have no structural abnormality. The etiology is complex, but the final common pathway is likely to be portal hypertension along with liver decompensation that results in splanchnic and systemic vasodilation and decreased arterial blood volume. As a result, renal vasoconstriction occurs, leading to kidney failure. This kidney failure can be reversed by liver transplantation. In patients with cirrhosis, HRS frequently follows diuretic therapy, GI hemorrhage, or paracentesis.

Diagnostic Studies

In patients with decompensated cirrhosis, most of the liver function studies (see Table 46-7 for tests) will be abnormal.

Enzymes levels including AST, ALT, alkaline phosphatase, and γ-glutamyl transpeptidase are elevated because of their release from damaged liver cells and bile ducts. However, in end-stage liver disease, AST and ALT levels may be normal. Patients with cirrhosis have decreased total protein, decreased albumin, increased serum bilirubin, and increased globulin levels. Fat

TABLE 46-12	FACTORS PRECIPITATING HEPATIC ENCEPHALOPATHY
Factor	**Mechanism**
Cerebral depressants (e.g., opioids)	Decrease in drug metabolism by liver, which causes higher drug levels and cerebral depression
Constipation	Increase in ammonia from bacterial action on feces
Dehydration	Potentiation of ammonia toxicity
GI hemorrhage	Increase in ammonia in GI tract
Hypokalemia	Potassium ions are needed by brain to metabolize ammonia
Hypovolemia	Increase in blood ammonia, caused by hepatic hypoxia; impairment of cerebral, hepatic, and renal function because of decreased blood flow
Increased metabolism	Increase in workload of liver
Infection	Increase in catabolism; increase in cerebral sensitivity to toxins
Metabolic alkalosis	Facilitation of transport of ammonia across blood–brain barrier; increase in renal production of ammonia
Paracentesis	Loss of sodium and potassium ions; decrease in blood volume
Uremia (kidney failure)	Retention of nitrogenous metabolites

GI, gastro-intestinal.

TABLE 46-13	GRADING SCALE FOR HEPATIC ENCEPHALOPATHY		
Grade	**Level of Consciousness**	**Intellectual Function**	**Neurological Findings**
0	Insomnia, sleep disturbances	Subtle change in computational skills	Impaired handwriting, tremor
1	Lack of awareness, personality change	Short attention span, mild confusion, depression	Incoordination, asterixis
2	Lethargy, drowsiness, inappropriate behaviour	Disorientation	Asterixis, abnormal reflexes
3	Asleep, rousable	Loss of meaningful conversation, marked confusion, incomprehensible speech	Asterixis, abnormal reflexes
4	Not rousable	Absent	Decerebrate May be responsive to painful stimuli

metabolism abnormalities are reflected by decreased cholesterol levels. The prothrombin time or INR is prolonged, and bilirubin metabolism is altered.

Liver Biopsy. Liver biopsy may be done to confirm the underlying causes of the liver disease. Liver biopsy is unnecessary to confirm cirrhosis if cirrhosis is clinically evident (e.g., nodular appearance of the liver on ultrasonography, presence of thrombo-cytopenia).

Liver biopsy is normally performed percutaneously. In patients with abnormal coagulation, biopsy must be performed via the transjugular vein. The most common risk of liver biopsy is bleeding.

Noninvasive Fibrosis Markers. Transient elastography (FibroScan) is a noninvasive imaging technique by which the degree of hepatic fibrosis is measured. Its use in Canada was approved in 2010. It is an ultrasonography-based imaging technique for detecting liver stiffness. It has excellent diagnostic accuracy for the diagnosis of cirrhosis, regardless of the underlying causes of the liver disease (Wilder, & Patel, 2014).

Models of serum markers (e.g., FibroTest) are also noninvasive tests that can be performed with blood samples. FibroTest is most commonly used in Canada. In this model, five parameters are used (bilirubin, γ-glutamyl transpeptidase, haptoglobin, apolipoprotein, and α₂-macroglobulin), in addition to patient's age and sex, to calculate a fibrosis score for predicting the degree of liver fibrosis.

Collaborative Care in Advanced Cirrhosis of the Liver

The goal of therapy for patients with cirrhosis is to slow the disease progression and to treat symptoms associated with decompensation. Collaborative care measures are listed in Table 46-14. Management of specific complications related to decompensated cirrhosis is described next.

Ascites. The presence of ascites indicates disease decompensation. Management is focused on sodium restriction, diuretics, and fluid removal. Affected patients are encouraged to limit sodium intake to 2 g (88 mmol) per day. More stringent sodium restriction is no longer recommended because it can result in reduced nutritional intake and subsequent malnutrition problems. Fluid restriction is usually not necessary unless severe ascites develops. Fluid and electrolyte balance should be accurately assessed and controlled. Albumin infusions are used to help maintain intravascular volume and adequate urinary output by increasing plasma colloid osmotic pressure.

Diuretic therapy is an important part of ascites management. A combination of drugs that work at multiple sites in the nephron is often more effective. Spironolactone (Aldactone) is an effective diuretic. It is an antagonist of aldosterone and is potassium sparing. Other potassium-sparing diuretics include amiloride (Apo-Amilzide) and triamterene (Teva-Triamterene). A high-potency loop diuretic, such as furosemide (Lasix), is frequently administered in combination with a potassium-sparing drug. Hydrochlorothiazide is rarely administered because it is not as potent as the loop diuretics.

Paracentesis (needle puncture of the abdominal cavity) may be performed to remove ascitic fluid or to test the fluid for infection (spontaneous bacterial peritonitis). However, it is indicated only when the diuretic therapy fails and to relieve symptoms such as abdominal pain or difficulty breathing. The relief provided by paracentesis is only temporary because the fluid reaccumulates.

TIPS (discussed later in this section) is used to alleviate ascites that does not respond to diuretics.

Esophageal and Gastric Varices. The main therapeutic goal for esophageal and gastric varices is prevention of bleeding. All patients with cirrhosis should have an upper endoscopy (esophago-gastro-duodenoscopy [EGD]) to screen for varices (Garcia-Tsao, Sanyal, Grace, et al., 2007). Risk factors for esophageal bleeding include variceal size (the largest varices are at highest risk of bleeding), decreased wall thickness, and degree of liver dysfunction (associated with increased portal hypertension). Patients who have esophageal varices should avoid ingesting

---

TABLE 46-14 COLLABORATIVE CARE
Advanced Cirrhosis of the Liver

Diagnostic
- History and physical examination
- CBC
- Computed tomography
- Endoscopy (esophago-gastro-duodenoscopy)
- Liver biopsy (if indicated)
- Liver enzyme measurements (AST, ALT, ALP, GGT)
- Liver function studies (albumin, bilirubin, INR)
- Liver stiffness measurement (FibroScan)
- Liver ultrasonography
- Magnetic resonance imaging
- Serum electrolyte measurements
- Serum fibrosis markers (FibroTest)

Collaborative Therapy
Conservative Therapy
- Avoidance of alcohol, acetylsalicylic acid (Aspirin), sedatives, and nonsteroidal anti-inflammatory drugs
- Rest (in decompensated cirrhosis)

Ascites
- Diuretics
- Low-sodium diet
- Paracentesis (if indicated)
- TIPS

Esophageal and Gastric Varices
- Balloon tamponade
- Drugs
  - Nonselective β-blockers (e.g., nadolol)
  - Octreotide (Sandostatin)
  - Vasopressin
- Endoscopic sclerotherapy or band ligation
- TIPS

Hepatic Encephalopathy
- Antibiotics (rifaximin [Zaxine])
- Lactulose

ALP, alkaline phosphatase; *ALT*, alanine aminotransferase; *AST*, aspartate aminotransferase; *CBC*, complete blood cell count; *GGT*, γ-glutamyl transpeptidase; *INR*, international normalized ratio; *TIPS*, transjugular intrahepatic portosystemic shunt.

---

alcohol, acetylsalicylic acid (ASA; Aspirin), and nonsteroidal anti-inflammatory drugs (NSAIDs). For patients who have esophageal varices that have not bled, prophylactic treatment with nonselective beta blockers (e.g., propranolol or nadolol) has been shown to reduce the risk of bleeding, as well as the number of bleeding-related deaths. Nonselective beta blockers reduce portal venous pressure by decreasing cardiac output and possibly by constricting splanchnic vessels.

When variceal bleeding occurs, the first step is to stabilize the patient and manage the airway. IV therapy is initiated and may include administration of blood products. Variceal bleeding is diagnosed on endoscopic examination. Management that involves a combination of drug therapy and endoscopic therapy is more successful than either approach alone.

Drug therapy may include octreotide (Sandostatin), vasopressin, and β-adrenergic blockers. The main goal of drug therapy is to stop the bleeding. IV administration of vasopressin produces vasoconstriction of the splanchnic arterial bed, decreases portal blood flow, and decreases portal hypertension. Because vasopressin has adverse effects (including decreased coronary blood flow and heart rate and increased blood pressure), nitroglycerin is often administered in combination with vasopressin for reducing the detrimental effects of the vasopressin while enhancing its beneficial effect. Vasopressin should be avoided or administered cautiously in older adults because of the risk of cardiac ischemia.

Endoscopic therapies include sclerotherapy and ligation of varices. Endoscopic sclerotherapy involves injecting a sclerosing agent into the varices to thrombose and obliterate the distended veins. Endoscopic ligation or banding of the varices is performed by placing a small rubber band (elastic O-ring) around the base of the varix. Endoscopic ligation is as effective as endoscopic sclerotherapy with fewer complications.

Balloon tamponade may be used in patients with brisk esophageal or gastric variceal hemorrhage that cannot be controlled on initial endoscopy. Balloon tamponade controls the hemorrhage by mechanical compression of the varices. Either the Minnesota or Sengstaken–Blakemore tube (Figure 46-9) is used for this purpose. These tubes have two balloons, one gastric and one esophageal. The Sengstaken–Blakemore tube has three lumens: one for the gastric balloon, one for the esophageal balloon, and one for gastric aspiration. The Minnesota tube has an esophageal aspiration port. When inflated, the gastric and esophageal balloons put mechanical compression on the varices. The gastric balloon anchors the tube in position and also applies pressure to any bleeding gastric varices.

Supportive measures during an acute variceal bleed include administration of fresh-frozen plasma and packed red blood cells, vitamin K, and proton pump inhibitors. Lactulose may be administered to prevent hepatic encephalopathy from breakdown of blood and the release of ammonia in the intestine. Antibiotics such as norfloxacin are given prophylactically to prevent bacterial infections.

Long-Term Management. Because of the high incidence of recurrent bleeding and the mortality risk with each bleeding episode, continued therapy is necessary. Long-term management of patients who have had an episode of bleeding includes the use of nonselective beta blockers, repeated endoscopic ligation, and portosystemic shunts.

Shunting Procedures. Surgical and nonsurgical methods of shunting blood away from the esophageal varices are available. Shunting procedures tend to be used more after a second major bleeding episode than after an initial bleeding episode. In TIPS, a tract (shunt) between the systemic and portal venous systems is nonsurgically created to redirect portal blood flow (Figure 46-10).

Under radiological guidance, the catheter is placed in the jugular vein and then threaded through the superior and inferior venae cavae to the hepatic vein. The wall of the hepatic vein is punctured, and the catheter is directed to the portal vein. Stents are positioned along the passageway, overlapping in the liver tissue and extending into both veins.

This procedure reduces portal venous pressure and decompresses the varices, thus controlling bleeding. This procedure does not interfere with future liver transplantation. Limitations of the TIPS procedure include the increased risk for hepatic encephalopathy and stenosis of the stent. TIPS is contraindicated in patients with severe hepatic encephalopathy, hepato-cellular carcinoma, severe hepato-renal syndrome, and portal vein thrombosis. Various surgical shunting procedures are no longer in common use but may be used to decrease portal hypertension by diverting some of the portal blood flow and simultaneously allowing adequate liver perfusion. The surgical shunts still in use are the portacaval shunt and the distal splenorenal shunt (Figure 46-11). Surgical shunts are more likely to be used in emergency situations. Although a prophylactic portacaval shunt decreases bleeding episodes, it does not prolong life. Patients

1 Esophageal balloon tube
2 Gastric aspirating tube
3 Gastric balloon tube
4 Esophageal balloon
5 Gastric balloon

FIGURE 46-9 A, Diagram of Sengstaken–Blakemore tube. **B,** Diagram of tube inserted into esophagus and stomach.

FIGURE 46-10 Total portal diversion after insertion of a transjugular intrahepatic portosystemic shunt (TIPS). **A,** Portal venogram before TIPS insertion shows filling of large esophageal varices *(arrows).* **B,** After TIPS insertion, flow to varices is eliminated. The direction of intrahepatic portal vein flow is now reversed, toward the TIPS. Source: Reprinted from *Journal of Vascular Surgery,* Volume 16(2), Jeanne M. LaBerge, Ernest J. Ring, John R. Lake, Linda D. Ferrell, Margaret M. Doherty, Roy L. Gordon, John P. Roberts, Marc Y. Peltzer, Nancy L. Ascher, "Transjugular intrahepatic portosystemic shunts: Preliminary results in 25 patients," pp. 258–267, Copyright 1992, with permission from Elsevier.

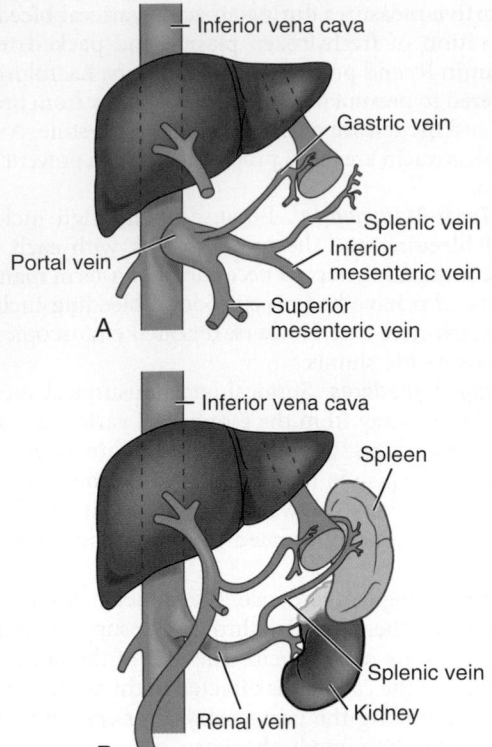

FIGURE 46-11 Portosystemic shunts. **A,** Portacaval shunt. The portal vein is anastomosed to the inferior vena cava, diverting blood from the portal vein to the systemic circulation. **B,** Distal splenorenal shunt. The splenic vein is anastomosed to the renal vein. The portal venous flow remains intact, and esophageal varices are selectively decompressed (by decompression of the short gastric veins). The spleen conducts blood from the high pressure of the esophageal and gastric varices to the low-pressure renal vein.

can develop hepatic encephalopathy as a result of the diversion of the ammonia past the liver and into the systemic circulation.

Hepatic Encephalopathy. The goal of the management of hepatic encephalopathy is the reduction of ammonia formation. Ammonia formation in the intestines is reduced with lactulose, a drug that traps the ammonia in the gut. The laxative effect of lactulose expels the ammonia from the colon. It is usually administered orally to prevent encephalopathy but can be given as an enema or via a nasogastric (NG) tube.

Antibiotics such as rifaximin (Zaxine) may also be given concomitantly in patients who do not respond to lactulose alone. Constipation should be prevented.

Control of hepatic encephalopathy also involves treatment of precipitating causes (see Table 46-12). One strategy involves controlling GI hemorrhage and removing the blood from the GI tract to decrease the protein in the intestine. Electrolyte disorders, acid–base imbalances, and infections should also be treated.

Liver transplantation may be considered in patients with recurring hepatic encephalopathy and end-stage liver disease. The decision to perform liver transplantation depends on a number of factors, including the cause of the cirrhosis and other systemic medical problems.

Drug Therapy. There is no specific drug therapy for cirrhosis. However, a number of drugs are used to treat symptoms and complications of advanced liver disease (Table 46-15).

TABLE 46-15   DRUG THERAPY

Advanced Cirrhosis

Drug	Mechanism of Action
Diuretics	
• Spironolactone (Aldactone)	Blocking action of aldosterone; potassium sparing
• Amiloride (Apo-Amilzide)	Inhibition of reabsorption of sodium and secretion of potassium
• Furosemide (Lasix)	Rapid action on distal tubule and loop of Henle to prevent reabsorption of sodium and water
• Triamterene (Teva-Triamterene)	Inhibition of reabsorption of sodium and secretion of potassium
Lactulose	Acidification of feces in bowel and trapping of ammonia, causing its elimination in feces
Propranolol (Inderal) or nadolol	Reduction of portal venous pressure
Proton pump inhibitors (e.g., pantoprazole [Pantoloc])	Decrease in gastric acidity
Rifaximin (Zaxine)	Decrease in bacterial flora,
Neomycin sulphate	decrease in formation of ammonia
Vasopressin	Hemostasis and control of bleeding
Octreotide (Sandostatin)	in esophageal varices; constriction of splanchnic arterial bed
Vitamin K	Correction of clotting abnormalities

Nutritional Therapy. The diet for a patient with cirrhosis without complications is high in calories (3 000 kcal/day) with high carbohydrate content and moderate to low fat levels. Protein restriction may be appropriate in some patients immediately after a severe flare of symptoms (i.e., episodic hepatic encephalopathy). However, protein restriction is rarely justified in patients with cirrhosis and persistent hepatic encephalopathy. Indeed, malnutrition is a more serious clinical problem than hepatic encephalopathy for many of these patients.

Many patients with alcoholic cirrhosis have protein–calorie malnutrition and may benefit from receiving enteral formulas containing protein from branched-chain amino acids that are metabolized by the muscles. They provide protein that is more easily metabolized by the liver. Total parenteral nutrition or tube feedings may be required.

In patients with ascites and edema, diet must be low in sodium. The degree of sodium restriction depends on the patient's condition. Table salt is a common, well-known source of sodium, but sodium is also present in baking soda and baking powder. Other foods that are high in sodium content include canned soups and vegetables, salted snacks such as potato chips, nuts, smoked meats and fish, crackers, breads, olives, pickles, ketchup, and beer. Sodium is also present in many OTC drugs (e.g., antacids); however, most antacids now have a lower sodium content than they did in the past. Carbonated beverages tend to be high in sodium, but low-sodium and sodium-free carbonated drinks are also available. Patients should be advised to read food labels; foods high in protein usually have large amounts of sodium. Alternative protein supplements that are low in sodium may have to be administered. Food can be made more palatable by the use of seasonings such as garlic, parsley, onion, lemon juice, and spices.

NURSING MANAGEMENT CIRRHOSIS

NURSING ASSESSMENT

Subjective and objective data that should be obtained from an individual with cirrhosis are presented in Table 46-16.

NURSING DIAGNOSES

Nursing diagnoses for the patient with advanced cirrhosis include but are not limited to the following:

- *Imbalanced nutrition: less than body requirements* related to *insufficient dietary intake* (anorexia, nausea, impaired utilization and storage of nutrients)
- *Impaired skin integrity* related to *moisture, pressure over bony prominence* (peripheral edema, ascites, pruritus)

TABLE 46-16   NURSING ASSESSMENT

Cirrhosis

Subjective Data

Important Health Information

Past health history: Previous viral, toxic, or idiopathic hepatitis; chronic biliary obstruction and infection; severe right-sided heart failure; chronic alcohol use disorder

Medications: Adverse reaction to any medication; use of anticoagulants, acetylsalicylic acid (Aspirin), nonsteroidal anti-inflammatory drugs, acetaminophen (Tylenol)

Symptoms

- Weakness, fatigue, difficulty with concentration
- Change in sleep–wake pattern
- Anorexia, muscle loss
- Gum bleeding
- Yellow sclera or skin; pruritus; easy bruising
- Dull pain in right upper quadrant or epigastric region
- Erectile dysfunction; amenorrhea

Objective Data

General

Fever, cachexia, muscle wasting

Integumentary

Icteric sclera, jaundice, petechiae, ecchymoses, spider angiomas, palmar erythema, alopecia, clubbing, peripheral edema

Respiratory

Shallow, rapid respirations, epistaxis

Gastro-Intestinal

Abdominal distension, ascites, distended abdominal wall veins, palpable liver and spleen, foul breath; hematemesis; black, tarry stools; hemorrhoids; fetor hepaticus

Neurological

Confusion, asterixis

Reproductive

Gynecomastia and testicular atrophy (men), erectile dysfunction (men), loss of libido (men and women), amenorrhea or heavy menstrual bleeding (women)

Possible Findings

Anemia, thrombo-cytopenia; leukopenia; ↓ serum albumin level; abnormal liver function studies; ↑ INR and bilirubin levels; abnormal abdominal ultrasound or MRI results

INR, international normalized ratio; *MRI,* magnetic resonance imaging.

- *Excess fluid volume* related to *compromised regulatory mechanism* (portal hypertension and hyperaldosteronism)
- *Ineffective health maintenance* related to *ineffective coping strategies* (alcohol use)

Additional information on nursing diagnoses for the patient with cirrhosis is presented in NCP 46-2, available on the Evolve website.

PLANNING

The overall goals are that the patient with cirrhosis will (a) have relief of discomfort, (b) have minimal to no complications (ascites, esophageal varices, hepatic encephalopathy), and (c) maintain as normal a lifestyle as possible.

NURSING IMPLEMENTATION

HEALTH PROMOTION. The common causes of cirrhosis are alcohol, viral hepatitis, biliary obstruction, obesity, and right-sided heart failure. Prevention and early treatment of cirrhosis must focus on eliminating the primary cause. Alcohol use disorder must be treated. Patients should be urged to avoid alcohol ingestion, and their efforts should be supported. Adequate nutrition, especially for those at risk for cirrhosis, is essential to prevent muscle loss. Acute and chronic viral hepatitis must be identified and treated early so that it does not progress to cirrhosis or liver failure. Biliary disease should be treated to avoid biliary obstruction and infection. The underlying cause (e.g., chronic lung disease) of right-sided heart failure must be treated so that the heart failure does not lead to cirrhosis.

Acute Intervention. The focus of nursing care for a patient with advanced cirrhosis is on conserving the patient's energy and strength (see NCP 46-2). Patients should be provided rest periods for recovery but be allowed to engage in activities as tolerated. The nurse should modify the patient's activity and rest schedule according to signs of clinical improvement (e.g., decreasing jaundice, improvement in results of liver function studies).

Anorexia, nausea and vomiting, pressure from ascites, and poor eating habits create problems in maintaining adequate nutrition. Oral hygiene before meals may improve the patient's taste sensation. Between-meal nourishments should be available at times when the patient can best tolerate them. Foods the patient prefers should also be available whenever possible. The nurse should explain to the patient and caregivers the reason for any dietary restrictions.

Nursing assessment and care should include the patient's physiological response to cirrhosis. If jaundice is present, the nurse should document where it is observed—sclera, skin, hard palate. If the jaundice is accompanied by pruritus, cholestyramine may be ordered to help relieve the pruritus. Other measures to help alleviate pruritus include baking soda baths, lotions containing antihistamines and calamine, the use of soft linens, and control of extreme hot and cold temperatures. The patient's nails should be kept short and clean.

The colour of the urine and stools should be noted. When jaundice is present, the urine is often dark brown and foamy when shaken. The stool is grey or tan.

Edema and ascites are frequent manifestations of decompensated cirrhosis and necessitate nursing assessment and interventions. Accurate calculation and recordings of intake and output, as well as daily body weights, help in the ongoing assessment of the location and the extent of the edema.

When paracentesis is required, the patient should void immediately before the procedure to prevent puncture of the bladder. After the procedure, the nurse should monitor vital signs for hypovolemia and check the dressing for bleeding and leakage from the puncture site.

Dyspnea is a frequent problem for patients with ascites, which can often lead to pleural effusion. A semi-Fowler's or Fowler's position allows for maximal respiratory efficiency. Pillows can be used to support the arms and the chest and may increase the patient's comfort and ability to breathe.

Meticulous skin care is essential because the edematous tissues are prone to breakdown. An alternating–air pressure mattress or other special mattress should be used, if possible. A turning schedule (minimum of every 2 hours) must be adhered to rigidly. The patient's abdomen should be supported with pillows. If the abdomen is taut, cleansing must be done very gently. Patients with ascites tend to move very little because of the abdominal discomfort and dyspnea, so range-of-motion, deep-breathing, and coughing exercises are helpful in preventing respiratory problems. The lower extremities may be elevated. If scrotal edema is present, a scrotal support provides some comfort.

When the patient is taking diuretics, monitor serum levels of sodium, potassium, chloride, bicarbonate, and creatinine, especially with any changes in the diuretic dosage. The nurse should observe for signs of fluid and electrolyte imbalance. Hypokalemia may be manifested by cardiac dysrhythmias, hypotension, tachycardia, and generalized muscle weakness. Water excess is manifested by muscle cramping, weakness, lethargy, and confusion.

Observations and nursing care in relation to hematological disorders (bleeding tendencies, anemia, increased susceptibility to infection) are the same as for patients with advanced liver disease (see NCP 46-2 on the Evolve website).

The nurse must assess the patient's response to altered body image resulting from jaundice, spider angiomas, palmar erythema, ascites, and gynecomastia. The patient may experience anxiety and embarrassment regarding these changes. The nurse should explain these phenomena and be a supportive listener. Nursing care with concern and warmth helps the patient maintain self-esteem.

Bleeding Esophageal Varices. If the patient has esophageal or gastric varices, the nurse should observe for signs of bleeding from the varices, such as hematemesis and melena. If hematemesis occurs, the nurse must call the physician and be ready to assist with treatment used to control the bleeding. The patient may be admitted to the critical care unit. The patient's airway must be maintained.

To stop the bleeding, the physician may perform sclerotherapy or ligation procedures. Balloon tamponade may be used in cases of refractory bleeding that is unresponsive to sclerotherapy or ligation. When balloon tamponade is used, the initial nursing task is to explain to the patient the use of the tube and how it will be inserted. The balloons should be checked for patency. It is usually the physician's responsibility to insert the tube via the nose or the mouth (see Figure 46-9). Then the gastric balloon is inflated with approximately 250 mL of air, and the tube is retracted until resistance (gastro-esophageal junction) is felt. The tube is secured by placing a piece of sponge or foam rubber at the nostrils (nasal cuff). For continued bleeding, the esophageal balloon is then inflated. A sphygmomanometer is used to measure and maintain the desired pressure at 20 to 40 mm Hg. The positions of the balloons are verified radiologically.

Nursing care includes monitoring for complications of rupture or erosion of the esophagus, regurgitation and aspiration of gastric contents, and occlusion of the airway by the balloon. If the gastric balloon breaks or is deflated, the esophageal balloon will slip upward, obstructing the airway and causing asphyxiation. If this happens, the nurse must cut the tube or deflate the esophageal balloon; thus scissors should be kept at the patient's bedside. Regurgitation is minimized by oral and pharyngeal suctioning and by keeping the patient in a semi-Fowler's position.

The patient is unable to swallow saliva because the esophagus is occluded by the inflated esophageal balloon. The patient should be encouraged to expectorate, and an emesis basin and tissues should be provided. Frequent oral and nasal care provides relief from the taste of blood and irritation from mouth breathing.

Hepatic Encephalopathy. The focus of nursing care of the patient with hepatic encephalopathy is on maintaining a safe environment, sustaining life, and assisting with measures to reduce episodes of drowsiness. The nurse should assess (a) the patient's level of responsiveness (e.g., reflexes, pupillary reactions, orientation), (b) sensory and motor abnormalities (e.g., hyper-reflexia, asterixis, motor coordination), (c) fluid and electrolyte imbalances, (d) acid–base imbalances, and (e) the effect of treatment measures.

Assessment of the neurological status should be performed at least every 2 hours and should include an exact description of the patient's behaviour. The care of the patient with neurological problems is based on the severity of the encephalopathy.

Constipation, which is a common precipitating factor for encephalopathy, should be prevented. Drugs, laxatives, and enemas should be given as ordered. Any GI bleeding may worsen encephalopathy. Patients who are taking lactulose for diarrhea and excessive fluid and electrolyte losses must be evaluated. It is desirable for the patient to have two to three loose bowel movements per day to promote elimination of toxins.

AMBULATORY AND HOME CARE. The patient with advanced cirrhosis may face a prolonged course and the possibility of serious, life-threatening problems and complications. The patient and the caregivers need to understand the importance of continuous health care and medical supervision and ways to reduce mortality risk (Table 46-17).

Patients with cirrhosis should receive vaccination for hepatitis A and B if they are not already immune. Infection with these viruses in patients with cirrhosis can lead to fulminant hepatitis. Patients should avoid ASA, NSAIDs, and aminoglycosides, which can cause bleeding, edema, and renal complications. Patients should also avoid sleeping pills or sedatives that contain codeine because they can lead to encephalopathy. Total abstinence from alcohol is mandatory. A low-sodium diet should be followed at home. Patients with cirrhosis have higher risks for infection and surgical complications, and so any infections must be promptly treated, and surgical procedures that necessitate general anaesthesia must first be discussed with the liver specialist. Patients with cirrhosis are at high risk for hepato-cellular carcinoma. The current recommendation is hepatoma surveillance with abdominal ultrasonography every 6 months. Hepato-cellular carcinoma, when small, is curable.

Cirrhosis is a chronic disorder. The patient is affected not only physically but also psychologically, socially, and economically. Major lifestyle changes may be required, especially if alcohol use is the primary cause. The nurse should provide information regarding community support programs, such as Alcoholics Anonymous, for help with alcohol use disorder. Other health teaching should include information about early signs of disease decompensation such as black stools and abdominal swelling.

TABLE 46-17 PATIENT & CAREGIVER TEACHING GUIDE

Cirrhosis in Ambulatory and Home Care Setting

The following guidelines should be included when teaching the patient and caregiver. The nurse should:

1. Explain the importance of continuous medical care with the goal of prolonging survival and avoiding disease complications.
2. Teach patients and caregivers the symptoms of complications (e.g., black stools, confusion) and when to seek medical attention to enable prompt treatment of complications.
3. Teach about the importance of a low-sodium diet and how to make food more palatable by using herbs and spices.
4. Teach patients to avoid certain drugs:
   - ASA (Aspirin): increases risk of bleeding
   - NSAIDs: increase risk of bleeding, edema
   - ASA, NSAIDs, aminoglycoside: increase risk of renal impairment
   - ACE inhibitors: cause fluid retention
   - Sleeping pills, sedatives, and cough syrups that contain opioids may cause confusion
5. Encourage complete abstinence from alcohol because alcohol can further injure the liver.
6. Teach patients to seek medical attention promptly for any type of infections to avoid complications.
7. Teach patients to avoid heavy lifting (e.g., Valsalva manoeuvre), which increases portal pressure and heightens risk of hemorrhage.
8. Encourage patients to receive hepatitis A and B vaccine, if the patient is not immune, to prevent risk for fulminant hepatitis when exposed to these viruses.
9. Ensure that patients undergo ultrasound surveillance every 6 months for early detection of liver cancer.

ACE, angiotensin-converting enzyme; *ASA,* acetylsalicylic acid; *NSAID,* nonsteroidal anti-inflammatory drug.

Counselling information regarding sexual problems may be needed. The emphasis of home care for patients with cirrhosis should focus on helping patients maintain the highest level of wellness possible and initiate and maintain necessary lifestyle changes.

EVALUATION

Expected outcomes for patients with advanced cirrhosis are addressed in NCP 46-2, available on the Evolve website.

ACUTE LIVER FAILURE

Acute liver failure is a clinical condition characterized by rapid deterioration of liver function resulting in encephalopathy and coagulopathy in persons with no known history of liver disease. It is a broad term that encompasses *fulminant hepatic failure,* which describes development of encephalopathy within 8 weeks of the onset of the illness. In general, the disease runs its course over 8 weeks, but it can last as long as 26 weeks. Depending on the cause, survival rates range from 10% to 40% with intensive support.

The most common cause of acute liver failure is drugs, usually acetaminophen, in combination with alcohol (Lee, Larson, Stravitz, et al., 2011). People with alcohol use disorder are particularly susceptible to the detrimental effects of acetaminophen on the liver. Other drugs that can cause acute liver failure include isoniazid, halothane, sulpha-containing drugs, and NSAIDs. Drugs can cause liver cell failure by disrupting essential intracellular processes or causing an accumulation of toxic metabolic products.

Hepatic failure may also occur rarely with HAV infection. Mushroom poisoning is also associated with fulminant liver failure. The majority of mushroom poisonings occur with *Amanita phalloides* (also known as "death cap").

Clinical Manifestations and Diagnostic Studies

Manifestations of acute liver failure include jaundice, coagulation abnormalities, and encephalopathy; changes in mentation are the first clinical sign. Patients with acute liver failure are susceptible to a wide variety of complications, including cerebral edema, renal failure, hypoglycemia, metabolic acidosis, sepsis, and multiorgan failure.

Acute liver failure is identified in most patients by abnormalities in laboratory values and clinical manifestations resulting from hepatic necrosis and fibrosis. Most often, serum bilirubin levels are elevated and the prothrombin time is prolonged. Liver enzyme levels (AST, ALT) are often markedly elevated. Additional laboratory tests include blood chemistry evaluation (especially glucose because hypoglycemia may be present and require correction); complete blood cell counts (CBCs); screening for acetaminophen and other drugs and toxins; viral hepatitis serological testing (especially for HAV and HBV); and measurements of serum ceruloplasmin (enzyme synthesized in liver) levels, α_1-antitrypsin levels, iron levels, and autoantibodies (ANA and ASMA). Plasma ammonia levels may also be measured.

Liver biopsy may be performed via the transjugular route because of coagulopathy, when a condition such as autoimmune hepatitis, metastatic liver disease, or lymphoma is suspected. In addition, ultrasonography, CT, or magnetic resonance imaging (MRI) is helpful in providing information about the liver size and contour, presence of ascites, presence of tumours, and patency of the blood vessels.

NURSING AND COLLABORATIVE MANAGEMENT ACUTE LIVER FAILURE

Because acute liver failure may progress rapidly, with hour-by-hour changes in consciousness, early transfer to the critical care unit is preferred once the diagnosis is made. Planning for transfer to a transplantation centre should begin in patients with grade 1 or 2 encephalopathy because the condition may worsen rapidly. Early transfer is important because the risks involved with patient transport may increase or even preclude transfer once stage 3 or 4 encephalopathy develops (see Table 46-13).

Renal failure is a frequent complication in patients with liver failure and may be caused by dehydration, hepato-renal syndrome, or acute tubular necrosis. The probability of renal failure may be even greater with acetaminophen overdose or other toxins, in which direct renal toxicity occurs. Although few patients die of renal failure alone, it often contributes to mortality risk and may worsen the prognosis.

The nurse should protect a patient's renal function by maintaining adequate fluid balance, withholding nephrotoxic agents (e.g., aminoglycosides, NSAIDs), and promptly identifying and treating infection. Liver transplantation is the treatment of choice for acute liver failure. Cerebral edema, cerebellar herniation, and brain stem compression are the most common causes of death. (Treatment of cerebral edema is described in Chapter 59.)

The nurse checks a patient's mental status frequently if the level of consciousness declines. To minimize agitation, the patient's environment should be kept quiet. Additional measures include padding bedrails to avoid injury from possible seizures, observing the patient closely to avoid injuries, monitoring intake and output for renal function, and providing good skin and oral care to avoid breakdown and infection.

Monitoring and management of hemodynamic and renal parameters, glucose levels, electrolyte levels, and acid–base status are critical. The nurse should conduct frequent neurological evaluations for signs of elevated intracranial pressure. The patient should be positioned with the head elevated at 30 degrees. Stimulation of the patient should be avoided. Manoeuvres that cause straining, or Valsalva-like movements, may increase intracranial pressure. The use of any sedatives should be avoided because of their effects on mental status, and the use of benzodiazepines because of the increased risk of encephalopathy.

Alterations in level of consciousness may compromise nutritional intake. Factors such as coagulation problems may influence whether enteral nutrition is initiated. An NG tube may irritate the nasal and esophageal mucosa and thus cause bleeding.

LIVER CANCER

Hepato-cellular carcinoma (HCC), the primary liver cancer, is the third most common cancer in the world. It is also the fifth most common cause of cancer-related death in men and the seventh in women (Sherman, Burak, Maroun, et al., 2011). The Multidisciplinary Canadian Consensus for the Management and Treatment of Hepatocellular Carcinoma reported that the incidence rate among men 40 to 84 years old was 15.4 per 100 000 in the years 2006 to 2010. The incidence rate for women is four to eight times lower but has also shown an increasing trend (Sherman, Burak, Maroun, et al., 2011).

About 80% to 90% of people with HCC have cirrhosis of the liver. Cirrhosis is therefore a major risk factor regardless of the cause of cirrhosis. In North America, chronic HCV infection is the major underlying cause of HCC. Among those with chronic HBV infection, the risk for HCC is further increased if they are male, are older, have a family history of HCC, or are infected with HBV genotype C. NAFLD is also a well-established risk factor for HCC although to a lesser extent than HBV and HCV infections.

In liver cancer, hemorrhage and necrosis in the liver are common. Single or multiple tumours can occur; they can be well defined or diffusely spread over the entire liver. Some tumours infiltrate other organs, such as the gallbladder, or move to the peritoneum or the diaphragm. The liver is a common site of metastatic growth because of its high rate of blood flow and extensive capillary network. Cancer cells in other parts of the body are commonly carried to the liver via the portal circulation (Figure 46-12). Primary liver tumours commonly metastasize to the lungs.

Clinical Manifestations and Diagnostic Studies

Liver cancers usually produce no symptoms until they become very large. Diagnosing small liver cancers in the presence of cirrhosis is sometimes a challenge when the liver is nodular and severely scarred. Clinical manifestations in later stages of cancer include weight loss, epigastric or right upper quadrant pain, anorexia, nausea and vomiting, weakness, and jaundice. More severe clinical symptoms such as ascites, peripheral edema, encephalopathy, and variceal bleeding occur in the setting of decompensated liver disease. A hemorrhagic tumour can cause blood clots to form, leading to pulmonary emboli as a complication.

FIGURE 46-12 Multiple hepatic metastases from a primary colon cancer. Source: Kumar, V., Abbas, A. K., & Fausto, N. (2005). *Robbins and Cotran pathologic basis of disease* (7th ed.). Philadelphia: W. B. Saunders.

Liver cancer can be diagnosed with ultrasound, CT, and MRI. A percutaneous biopsy is performed when the results of diagnostic imaging studies are inconclusive or tissue is needed to guide treatment. Risks of biopsy include bleeding and potential tumour cell spread. Serum alpha-fetoprotein (AFP) levels are elevated in approximately 60% of patients with HCC. The level of elevation may not correlate with the clinical features of HCC (e.g., stage or prognosis). (Alpha-fetoprotein is discussed in Chapter 18.)

NURSING AND COLLABORATIVE MANAGEMENT
LIVER CANCER

Treatment of liver cancer depends on the size and number of tumours, presence of spread beyond of the liver, and the age and overall health of the patient. Surgical resection (partial hepatectomy) is performed when there is no evidence of invasion of hepatic blood vessels. Hepatectomy offers the best chance for cure of liver cancer. Liver transplantation can be an option when the tumour is localized. Other treatment options are radiofrequency ablation (RFA), chemoembolization, and chemotherapies.

RFA has become the most frequently used modality for treating tumours that are less than 2 to 3 cm in diameter. The overall survival rates are 100% and 98% at 1 and 2 years, but the 5-year recurrence rates are as high as 70% (El-Serag, 2011). In RFA, a thin needle is inserted into the core of the tumour. Electrical energy is then used to create heat in a specific location for a limited time. The end result is destruction of tumour cells. Complications are uncommon but can include infection, bleeding, dysrhythmias, and skin burn.

Chemoembolization (sometimes called *transarterial chemoembolization [TACE]*) is a minimally invasive procedure performed in the interventional radiology department. A catheter is placed in the arteries to the tumour, and an embolic agent is administered, mixed with one or more chemotherapeutic agents. The embolic agent reduces the blood supply to the tumour, thus allowing greater exposure of liver cells to the chemotherapy drugs. A postembolization syndrome of fever and abdominal pain related to liver ischemia occurs in up to 50% of patients receiving chemoembolization.

Systemic chemotherapy is not used for patients with HCC because of the poor response rates. Sorafenib (Nexavar), a targeted therapy, is now used to treat HCC. It is taken orally and works by inhibiting new blood vessels' growth to tumours. It has many adverse effects, including rash on the hands and feet, diarrhea, and fatigue.

Nurses play a very important role in health promotion and health teaching for prevention of HCC. HBV vaccination for people at high risk for HBV infection can drastically reduce the occurrence of liver cancer. Early treatment for chronic hepatitis B and C viral infections before the establishment of cirrhosis also helps decrease risk for liver cancer. For patients at risk of developing HCC (e.g., those with cirrhosis), cancer surveillance with ultrasound every 6 months is a recommended clinical practice as small cancers are potentially curable (Sherman, Burak, Maroun, et al., 2011).

The prognosis for patients with liver cancer depends on how early the tumour is detected. Nursing interventions for patients with liver cancer focus on keeping patients as comfortable as possible. (See Chapter 18 for care of patients with cancer.)

LIVER TRANSPLANTATION

Canada's first liver transplantation was performed in Montreal in 1970. In 2015, 533 liver transplantations were performed in Canada (Canadian Institute for Health Information, 2017), up to 35% of which were for hepatitis C–related liver disease.

Liver transplantation has become an acceptable therapeutic option for many people with end-stage liver disease or localized and recurrent HCC. It improves overall health and quality of life. Liver transplantation is contraindicated in patients with widespread malignant disease. Among recipients, 1-year survival rates are 85% to 95%, and 5-year survival rates are 75% (Haque, Scudamore, Steinbrecher, et al., 2010).

Liver transplant candidates undergo a rigorous pretransplantation assessment to confirm the diagnosis of end-stage liver disease and to assess for other comorbid conditions (e.g., cardiovascular disease, chronic kidney disease) that may affect the patient's surgical outcome. The evaluation includes physical examination, laboratory tests (CBC, liver function tests), cardiac and pulmonary evaluations, endoscopy, CT scan, and psychological testing. Contraindications for liver transplantation include severe extrahepatic disease, advanced hepato-cellular carcinoma or other cancer, ongoing drug or alcohol use, and inability to comprehend or comply with the rigorous post-transplantation course.

Liver transplantation is performed using either a deceased-(cadaver) or living-donor liver (see Chapter 49 for a general discussion of organ transplants). For a living-donor liver transplantation, a living person donates a portion of his or her liver to another. However, live liver donation poses potential risks to the donor, including biliary problems, hepatic artery thrombosis, wound infection, postoperative ileus, and pneumothorax.

Postoperative complications of liver transplantation include bleeding, infection, and rejection. Rejection is the most feared but the most easily treated complication. It often necessitates only adjustment of immuno-suppressive drug dosages. Cyclosporine, the original immuno-suppressant drug, improved the rates of success of liver transplantation. Tacrolimus (Prograf) is currently the first-line immuno-suppressive drug in most programs. Both these drugs are calcineurin inhibitors. The mechanism of action and adverse effects of cyclosporine are discussed in Chapter 16 and Table 16-16. Other immuno-suppressants used include mycophenolate mofetil (CellCept), azathioprine (Imuran),

corticosteroids, and sirolimus (Rapamune) (see Chapter 16, Table 16-16). The interleukin-2 receptor antagonist basiliximab (Simulect) and polyclonal antilymphocyte antibodies, such as thymoglobulin, may be administered to patients at high risk for complications.

Almost all liver diseases may recur after transplantation. Because of the effective antiviral agents for HBV infection and the concurrent use of hepatitis B immune globulin, HBV reinfection is rare. Patients with HCV have lower survival rates than do other patient groups. Factors that may contribute to recurrent HCV include the donor's advanced age, HCV genotype 1, high HCV RNA levels before the transplantation, and co-infection with other viruses (e.g., cytomegalovirus). Although the recurrence of HCV is nearly universal after liver transplantation, avoidance of changes in immuno-suppressive regimen helps to prevent clinically aggressive disease. Antiviral therapy for HCV after transplantation is initiated on an individual basis. Overall, liver transplantation provides good long-term survival.

The patient who has undergone liver transplantation requires highly skilled nursing care, either in the intensive care unit or in a dedicated transplantation unit. Common respiratory problems are pneumonia, atelectasis, and pleural effusions, so measures such as coughing, deep breathing, incentive spirometry, and repositioning are needed to prevent complications. Drainage from the Jackson-Pratt drain, the NG tube, and the T-tube should be measured, and the colour and the consistency of drainage noted. Postoperative nursing care also includes assessing neurological status; monitoring for signs of hemorrhage; preventing pulmonary complications; assessing drainage, electrolyte levels, and urine output; and monitoring for signs and symptoms of infection and rejection.

Monitoring for infection is a critical aspect of nursing care after liver transplantation because infection is the most common cause of mortality and morbidity. Infections can be viral, fungal, or bacterial. Fever may be the only sign of infection. Nutrition, physiotherapy, and patient education focused on medication regimens, signs and symptoms of infection, and lifestyle practices are all key to lifelong success in transplant recipients. Emotional support for the patient and family is also essential for successful transplantation outcomes.

AGE-RELATED CONSIDERATIONS

LIVER DISEASE IN OLDER ADULTS

The incidence of liver disease increases with age. With aging, the liver size decreases, drug metabolism slows, and hepato-biliary function is altered. The liver's ability to respond to injury, particularly to regenerate after injury, decreases (Carrion & Martin, 2012). As well, transplanted livers take longer to regenerate in older adults than in younger adults.

Older patients are particularly vulnerable to drug-induced hepatitis. This vulnerability is due to several factors, including decline in body weight and increased use of prescription and OTC drugs, which can lead to drug interactions and potential drug toxicity. Age-related decreases in liver function caused by decreased liver blood flow and enzyme activity result in decreased drug metabolism. In addition, with aging, the liver's ability to recover from drug-induced injury is reduced.

A growing number of older adults have chronic hepatitis C and subsequent cirrhosis. The presence of HCV and elevated liver enzyme levels are often found during a routine health assessment. Because older adults have more comorbid conditions,

PATHOPHYSIOLOGY MAP

FIGURE 46-13 Pathogenic process of acute pancreatitis. *GI,* gastro-intestinal.

liver transplantation may not be an option in the case of liver failure.

Lifetime health behaviours may also influence the development of chronic liver disease in the older adult. Chronic alcohol use and obesity can contribute to alcoholic cirrhosis, NASH, and subsequent liver failure. Older adults with comorbid cardiovascular and pulmonary diseases are less able to tolerate variceal bleeding. In older adults with liver disease, hepatic encephalopathy may be misdiagnosed as dementia.

DISORDERS OF THE PANCREAS

ACUTE PANCREATITIS

Acute pancreatitis is an acute inflammation of the pancreas. The degree of inflammation varies from mild edema to severe hemorrhagic necrosis. Acute pancreatitis is most common in middle-aged men and women.

Etiology and Pathophysiology

Many factors can cause injury to the pancreas. In Canada, the most common cause is gallbladder disease (gallstones), followed by alcohol use disorder. Acute pancreatitis attacks are also associated with hypertriglyceridemia (serum triglyceride level >11 mmol/L). Less common causes include trauma (postsurgical, abdominal), viral infections (mumps, coxsackievirus), penetrating duodenal ulcer, cysts, abscesses, cystic fibrosis, certain drugs (azathioprine, corticosteroids, thiazides, estrogens, sulphonamides, HIV medications, anti-inflammatory drugs), metabolic disorders (hyperparathyroidism, renal failure), and vascular disease. Pancreatitis may occur after surgical procedures on the pancreas, stomach, duodenum, or biliary tract. Pancreatitis can also develop following endoscopic retrograde cholangiopancreatography (ERCP). In some cases, the cause is unknown (idiopathic).

The most common pathogenic mechanism is believed to be autodigestion of the pancreas (Figure 46-13). Injury to pancreatic cells or activation of the pancreatic enzymes is caused in the pancreas rather than in the intestine. The activation of pancreatic enzymes may be due to reflux of bile acids into the pancreatic ducts through an open or distended sphincter of Oddi. This reflux may result from blockage created by gallstones. Obstruction of a pancreatic duct results in pancreatic ischemia.

Trypsinogen is an inactive proteolytic enzyme produced by the pancreas. It is released into the small intestine via the

FIGURE 46-14 In acute pancreatitis, the pancreas appears edematous and is commonly hemorrhagic (*H*). Source: Stevens, A., & Lowe, J. (2000). *Pathology: Illustrated review in colour* (2nd ed.). London: Mosby.

pancreatic duct. In the intestine, it is activated to trypsin by enterokinase. Normally, trypsin inhibitors in the pancreas and the plasma bind and inactivate any trypsin that is inadvertently produced. In pancreatitis, activated trypsin is present in the pancreas and can digest the pancreas and produce bleeding.

It is not entirely clear how chronic alcohol use causes acute pancreatitis. It is thought that alcohol increases the production of digestive enzymes in the pancreas. However, because only 5% to 10% of people with alcohol use disorder develop pancreatitis, it is believed that other factors such as environment (high-fat diet, smoking) and genetics also contribute to the cause.

The pathophysiological involvement of acute pancreatitis ranges from mild (*edematous* or *interstitial pancreatitis*) to severe (*necrotizing pancreatitis;* Figure 46-14). In mild pancreatitis, the functions of the gland return to normal upon recovery. In severe pancreatitis, approximately half of patients have a permanent decrease in endocrine and exocrine function. Such patients are also at risk of developing pancreatic necrosis, organ failure, septic complications, or a combination of these, all of which are associated with higher mortality rates (Tenner, Baillie, DeWitt, et al., 2013).

Clinical Manifestations

Abdominal pain is the predominant symptom of acute pancreatitis. The pain is caused by distension of the pancreas, peritoneal irritation, and obstruction of the biliary tract.

The pain is usually located in the left upper quadrant, but it may be in the midepigastrium. It commonly radiates to the back because of the retroperitoneal location of the pancreas. The pain has a sudden onset and is described as severe, deep, piercing, and continuous or steady. It is aggravated by eating and frequently occurs when the patient is recumbent. It is not relieved by vomiting. The pain may be accompanied by flushing, cyanosis, and dyspnea. The patient may assume various positions involving flexion of the spine in an attempt to relieve the severe pain.

Other manifestations of acute pancreatitis include nausea and vomiting, low-grade fever, leukocytosis, hypotension, tachycardia, and jaundice. Abdominal tenderness with muscle guarding is common. Bowel sounds may be decreased or absent. Paralytic ileus may occur and causes marked abdominal distension. The lungs are frequently involved, with crackles present. Intravascular damage from circulating trypsin may cause areas of cyanosis or greenish to yellow-brown discoloration of the abdominal wall. Other areas of ecchymoses are the flanks (*Grey Turner's spots* or *sign,* a bluish flank discoloration) and the periumbilical area (*Cullen's sign,* a bluish periumbilical discoloration). These ecchymoses may occur in severe cases as a result of seepage of blood-stained exudate from the pancreas.

Shock is possible as a result of hemorrhage into the pancreas, toxemia from the activated pancreatic enzymes, or hypovolemia as a result of massive shift of exudates of blood and plasma proteins into the retroperitoneal space.

Complications

The severity of the disease varies according to the extent of pancreatic destruction. Some patients recover completely, some have recurring attacks, and some develop chronic pancreatitis. Acute pancreatitis can be life-threatening.

Two significant local complications of acute pancreatitis are pseudocyst and abscess. A pancreatic pseudocyst is a cavity continuous with or surrounding the outside of the pancreas. It is filled with necrotic products, plasma, pancreatic enzymes, and inflammatory exudates. Manifestations of pseudocyst are abdominal pain, palpable epigastric mass, nausea, vomiting, and anorexia. The serum amylase level frequently remains elevated. These cysts usually resolve spontaneously within a few weeks, but they may perforate, causing peritonitis, or they may rupture into the stomach or duodenum. Treatment consists of an internal drainage procedure with an anastomosis between the pancreatic duct and the jejunum.

A pancreatic abscess is a large collection of pus within the pancreas. It results from extensive necrosis in the pancreas. It may become infected or perforate into adjacent organs. Manifestations of an abscess include upper abdominal pain, abdominal mass, high fever, and leukocytosis. Pancreatic abscesses require prompt surgical drainage to prevent sepsis.

The main systemic complications of acute pancreatitis are pulmonary (pleural effusion, atelectasis, and pneumonia), cardiovascular (hypotension), and tetany caused by hypocalcemia. The pulmonary complications are likely caused by the passage of exudate containing pancreatic enzymes from the peritoneal cavity through transdiaphragmatic lymph channels. Enzyme-induced inflammation of the diaphragm reduces diaphragm movement, which leads to atelectasis. Trypsin can activate prothrombin and plasminogen, increasing the patient's risk for intravascular thrombi, pulmonary emboli, and disseminated intravascular coagulation. Hypocalcemia is a sign of severe disease, caused in part by the combining of calcium and fatty acids during fat

necrosis. The exact mechanisms of how or why hypocalcemia occurs are not well understood.

Diagnostic Studies

The primary diagnostic tests for acute pancreatitis are measurements of serum amylase and lipase. The serum amylase level is usually elevated early and remains so for 24 to 72 hours. The serum lipase level is also elevated and is an important test for differentiating acute pancreatitis from other disorders such as mumps and cerebral trauma. Other abnormal findings include an increase in liver enzymes, triglycerides, glucose, and bilirubin and a decrease in calcium.

Abdominal ultrasound, radiograph, or CT scan can be used to identify pancreatic problems. Contrast-enhanced CT and magnetic resonance cholangiopancreatography (MRCP) are used for detecting pancreatitis-related complications such as pseudocysts and abscesses. MRCP often replaces the use of ERCP, which itself can cause acute pancreatitis.

Collaborative Care

Objectives of collaborative care for acute pancreatitis include (a) relief of pain; (b) prevention or alleviation of shock; (c) reduction of pancreatic secretions; (d) control of fluid and electrolyte imbalance; (e) prevention or treatment of infections; and (f) removal of the precipitating cause, if possible (Table 46-18).

Conservative Therapy. Treatment is primarily focused on supportive care, including aggressive hydration, pain management, management of metabolic complications, and minimization of pancreatic stimulation. Relief and control of pain are very important. IV morphine may be administered. Pain medications may be combined with an antispasmodic agent. However, atropine-like drugs should be avoided when paralytic ileus is present because they may decrease GI motility and further contribute to the problem. Other medications that relax smooth muscles (spasmolytics), such as nitroglycerin or papaverine, may be used.

If shock is present, plasma or plasma volume expanders such as dextran or albumin may be given. Fluid and electrolyte imbalances are corrected with lactated Ringer's solution. Central

---

TABLE 46-18 COLLABORATIVE CARE

Acute Pancreatitis

Diagnostic	Collaborative Therapy
• History and physical examination	• Albumin (if shock is present)
• Abdominal ultrasound	• Antibiotics (if necrotizing
• Blood glucose	pancreatitis is present)
• Chest radiograph	• IV calcium gluconate, 10%
• Contrast-enhanced CT	(if tetany is present)
• Endoscopic ultrasound	• Lactated Ringer's solution
• ERCP	• NPO with NG tube to
• Flat-plate radiograph of the	suction
abdomen	• Pain medication (e.g.,
• MRCP	morphine)
• Serum amylase	• Proton pump inhibitors (e.g.,
• Serum calcium	omeprazole [Losec])
• Serum lipase	
• Triglycerides	

CT, computed tomography; *ERCP,* endoscopic retrograde cholangiopancreatography; *IV,* intravenous; *MRCP,* magnetic resonance cholangiopancreatography; *NG,* nasogastric; *NPO,* nothing by mouth.

venous pressure readings may be used to assist in determining requirements to increase systemic vascular resistance in patients with ongoing hypotension.

Pancreatic enzyme secretion must be reduced or suppressed in order to decrease stimulation of the pancreas and allow it to rest. Suppression of pancreatic secretion is accomplished by keeping the patient on nothing-by-mouth (NPO) and by using NG suction to reduce vomiting and gastric distension and to prevent gastric acidic contents from entering the duodenum. Certain drugs may also be administered for this purpose (Table 46-19). With resolution of the pancreatitis, the patient resumes oral intake. For the patient with severe acute pancreatitis who does not resume oral intake, enteral nutrition support may be initiated.

The inflamed and necrotic pancreatic tissue is a good medium for bacterial growth. In patients with acute necrotizing pancreatitis, infection is the leading cause of morbidity and mortality. Therefore, it is important to prevent infections. The prophylactic use of antibiotics is somewhat controversial. The patient should be monitored closely so that antibiotic therapy can be instituted early if infection occurs.

Surgical Therapy. When the acute pancreatitis is related to gallstones, urgent ERCP and endoscopic sphincterotomy may be performed and followed by laparoscopic cholecystectomy to reduce the potential for recurrence. Surgical intervention may also be indicated when the diagnosis is uncertain and for patients who do not respond to conservative therapy. Patients with severe acute pancreatitis may require drainage of necrotic fluid collections. Drainage can be accomplished either surgically under CT guidance or endoscopically. A pseudocyst can be drained percutaneously, and a drainage tube is left in place.

Drug Therapy. Several different drugs are used to treat problems associated with pancreatitis (see Table 46-19). Currently there are no drugs that cure pancreatitis.

Nutritional Therapy. Initially, patients with acute pancreatitis are kept on NPO status to reduce pancreatic secretion. In cases of moderate to severe pancreatitis, the patient may require enteral feeding via a jejunal feeding tube. When food is allowed, small, frequent feedings are given. The diet is usually high in carbohydrate content because that is the least stimulating to the exocrine portion of the pancreas. Intolerance to oral foods should be suspected if a patient reports pain, has increasing abdominal girth, or has elevated amylase and lipase levels. The patient needs to abstain from alcohol. Supplemental fat-soluble vitamins may be administered (see Chapter 42).

NURSING MANAGEMENT ACUTE PANCREATITIS

NURSING ASSESSMENT

Subjective and objective data that should be obtained from a person with acute pancreatitis are presented in Table 46-20.

TABLE 46-19 DRUG THERAPY

Acute and Chronic Pancreatitis

Drug	Mechanism of Action or Rationale
Acute Pancreatitis	
Antacids	Neutralization of gastric HCl secretion and subsequent decrease in secretin, which stimulates production and secretion of pancreatic secretions
Antispasmodics (e.g., dicyclomine [Bentylol]*)	Decrease of vagal stimulation, motility, and pancreatic outflow (through inhibition of volume and concentration of bicarbonate and enzymatic secretion)
Carbonic anhydrase inhibitor (acetazolamide)	Reduction in volume and bicarbonate concentration of pancreatic secretion
Morphine, meperidine (Demerol)	Relief of pain
Nitroglycerin or papaverine	Relaxation of smooth muscles and relief of pain
Proton pump inhibitors (omeprazole [Losec])	Decrease in HCl secretion (HCl stimulates pancreatic activity)
Chronic Pancreatitis	
Insulin	Treatment for diabetes mellitus, if it occurs, or for hyperglycemia
Pancreatin, pancrelipase	Replacement therapy for pancreatic enzymes

HCl, Hydrochloric acid.
*Contraindicated in patients with paralytic ileus.

TABLE 46-20 NURSING ASSESSMENT

Acute Pancreatitis

Subjective Data
Important Health Information
Past health history: Biliary tract disease, alcohol use, abdominal trauma, duodenal ulcers, infection, metabolic disorders
Medications: Thiazides, anti-inflammatory drugs
Surgery or other treatments: Surgical procedures on the pancreas, stomach, duodenum, or biliary tract; ERCP

Symptoms
- Dyspnea
- Nausea, vomiting, or both; anorexia
- Severe abdominal pain that may radiate to the back and is aggravated by food, alcohol, or both
- Weakness or lassitude

Objective Data
General
Restlessness, anxiety, low-grade fever

Integumentary
Flushing, diaphoresis, discoloration of abdomen and flanks, cyanosis, jaundice; decreased skin turgor; dry mucous membranes

Respiratory
Tachypnea, basilar crackles

Cardiovascular
Tachycardia, hypotension

Gastro-Intestinal
Abdominal distension, tenderness, and muscle guarding; diminished bowel sounds

Possible Findings
↑ Serum amylase and lipase levels, leukocytosis, hyperglycemia, dyslipidemia, hypocalcemia, abnormal findings on ultrasound and CT scan of pancreas, abnormal findings on ERCP or MRCP

CT, computed tomographic; *ERCP,* endoscopic retrograde cholangiopancreatography; *MRCP,* magnetic resonance cholangiopancreatography.

NURSING DIAGNOSES

Nursing diagnoses for patients with acute pancreatitis may include but are not limited to the following:

- *Acute pain* related to *biological injury agent* (distention of pancreas, peritoneal irritation, obstruction of biliary tract)
- *Deficient fluid volume* related to *insufficient fluid intake* (vomiting, restricted oral intake, fluid shift into the retroperitoneal space)
- *Imbalanced nutrition: less than body requirements* related to *insufficient dietary intake* (anorexia, dietary restrictions, nausea)
- *Ineffective health management* related to *insufficient knowledge of therapeutic regimen* (diet restrictions), *ineffective coping strategies* (alcohol intake)

Additional information on nursing diagnoses for the patient with pancreatitis is presented in NCP 46-3, available on the Evolve website for this chapter.

PLANNING

The overall goals are that patients with acute pancreatitis will have (a) relief of pain, (b) normal fluid and electrolyte balance, (c) minimal to no complications, and (d) no recurrent attacks.

NURSING IMPLEMENTATION

HEALTH PROMOTION. Health promotion is focused on the assessment of the predisposing and etiological factors of pancreatitis and on encouragement of early intervention to prevent occurrence of acute pancreatitis. The patient should be advised to eliminate alcohol intake, especially if there have been any previous episodes of pancreatitis. Attacks of pancreatitis become milder or disappear when alcohol use is discontinued.

ACUTE INTERVENTION. During the acute phase, it is important to monitor vital signs. Hemodynamic stability may be compromised by hypotension, fever, and tachypnea. A vital part of the nursing care plan for patients with acute pancreatitis is monitoring for electrolyte imbalances and response to IV fluids. Frequent vomiting, along with gastric suction, may cause electrolyte levels to decrease. Respiratory failure may develop in patients with severe acute pancreatitis. It is important to assess respiratory function (e.g., breath sounds, oxygen saturation levels). If acute respiratory distress syndrome develops, the patient may require intubation and mechanical ventilatory support. Because hypocalcemia can also occur, the nurse must observe for symptoms of tetany, such as jerking, irritability, and muscular twitching. Numbness or tingling around the lips and in the fingers is an early indicator of hypocalcemia. The patient should be assessed for a positive Chvostek's or Trousseau's sign (see Chapter 19). Calcium gluconate (as ordered) should be given to treat symptomatic hypocalcemia. In addition, hypomagnesemia may develop, necessitating the observation of serum magnesium levels.

Because abdominal pain is a prominent symptom of pancreatitis, a major focus of nursing care is the relief of pain (see NCP 46-3). Pain and restlessness can increase body metabolism and subsequent stimulation of pancreatic secretions. Morphine or meperidine (Demerol) may be used for pain relief. The nurse should assess and document the duration of pain relief. Measures such as comfortable positioning, frequent changes in position, and relief of nausea and vomiting assist in reducing the restlessness that usually accompanies the pain. Assuming positions that flex the trunk and draw the knees up to the abdomen may decrease pain. A side-lying position with the head elevated 45 degrees decreases tension on the abdomen and may also help ease the pain.

Nursing measures for the patient who is kept NPO or has an NG tube should include frequent oral and nasal care to relieve the dryness of the mouth and nose. Oral care is essential to prevent parotitis. If the patient is taking anticholinergics to decrease GI secretions, dryness of the mouth is exacerbated. If antacids are taken to neutralize gastric acid secretions, they should be sipped slowly or administered through the NG tube. The patient with acute pancreatitis is susceptible to infections. The nurse should monitor for fever and other manifestations of infection. Respiratory infections are common because the retroperitoneal fluid raises the diaphragm, which causes the patient to take shallow, guarded abdominal breaths. Measures to prevent respiratory tract infections include frequent turning, coughing, deep breathing, and assuming a semi-Fowler's position. Other important assessments are for signs of paralytic ileus, renal failure, and mental changes. The blood glucose level should be monitored to assess damage to the beta cells of the islets of Langerhans in the pancreas.

After pancreatic surgery, the patient may require special wound care for an anastomotic leak or a fistula. To prevent skin irritation, measures such as skin barriers (Stomahesive or Karaya paste), pouching, and drains should be used. In addition to protecting the skin, pouching also provides a more accurate determination of fluid and electrolyte losses and increases patient comfort.

AMBULATORY AND HOME CARE. After acute pancreatitis, most patients may need home care follow-up to prevent infection, monitor pain, and detect complications. Physiotherapy may be needed if the patient has lost physical reserve and muscle strength. Patient counselling should include that directed toward alcohol abstinence and cigarette smoking cessation. Abstinence from alcohol prevents future pancreatitis attacks. Because tobacco can stimulate the pancreatic enzyme secretions, smoking should be avoided. Counselling recommendations and strategies for smoking cessation, including resources, can be referenced from the *Integrating Smoking Cessation Into Daily Nursing Practice* best practice guideline by the Registered Nurses' Association of Ontario, listed in the Resources at the end of this chapter.

Dietary teaching should include restriction of fats because they stimulate the secretion of cholecystokinin, which then stimulates the pancreas. Carbohydrates are less stimulating to the pancreas. The patient should be advised to avoid crash dieting and bingeing because they can precipitate attacks. The patient and the caregivers should be taught the symptoms of infection, diabetes mellitus, and steatorrhea (foul-smelling, frothy stools). These changes indicate possible ongoing destruction of pancreatic tissue. The patient and the caregivers should also be educated about the prescribed regimen, including the importance of taking the required medications and following the recommended diet.

EVALUATION

Expected outcomes for patients with acute pancreatitis are presented in NCP 46-3, available on the Evolve website.

CHRONIC PANCREATITIS

Chronic pancreatitis is a continuous, prolonged inflammatory and fibrosing process of the pancreas. The pancreas becomes progressively destroyed as it is replaced with fibrotic tissues. Strictures and calcifications may also occur in the pancreas.

Etiology and Pathophysiology

In Western countries, 70% of cases of chronic pancreatitis are associated with alcohol use disorder. However, not all people who overuse alcohol develop chronic pancreatitis, which suggests that affected people have cofactors that predispose them to the direct toxic effect of the alcohol on the pancreas. In some patients, an identifiable cause may not be found (*idiopathic pancreatitis*). Chronic pancreatitis may follow acute pancreatitis, but it may also occur in the absence of any history of acute episodes.

Chronic pancreatitis can be classified into *obstructive* and *nonobstructive*. In nonobstructive pancreatitis, there is inflammation and sclerosis, mainly in the head of the pancreas and around the pancreatic duct. The ducts are obstructed with protein precipitates. These precipitates block the pancreatic duct and eventually calcify. This process is followed by fibrosis and glandular atrophy. Pseudocysts and abscesses commonly develop. Alcohol use disorder is the most common cause of nonobstructive calcifying pancreatitis.

Obstructive pancreatitis is associated with biliary disease. The most common cause is inflammation of the sphincter of Oddi associated with cholelithiasis. Cancer of the ampulla of Vater, the duodenum, or the pancreas can also cause this type of chronic pancreatitis.

Clinical Manifestations

As with acute pancreatitis, a major manifestation of chronic pancreatitis is abdominal pain. The patient may have episodes of acute pain, but it usually is chronic (recurrent attacks at intervals of months or years). The attacks may become more and more frequent until they are almost constant, or they may diminish as pancreatic fibrosis develops. The pain is located in the same areas as in acute pancreatitis but is usually described as a heavy, gnawing feeling or sometimes as burning and cramplike. The pain is not relieved with food or antacids.

Other clinical manifestations are symptoms of pancreatic insufficiency, including malabsorption with weight loss, constipation, mild jaundice with dark urine, steatorrhea, and diabetes mellitus. The steatorrhea may become severe, with voluminous, foul-smelling, fatty stools. Urine and stool may be frothy. Some abdominal tenderness may be present. Chronic pancreatitis is also associated with a variety of complications, including pseudocyst formation, bile duct or duodenal obstruction, diabetes mellitus, pancreatic ascites or pleural effusion, splenic vein thrombosis, pseudoaneurysms, and pancreatic cancer.

Diagnostic Studies

The diagnosis is based on the patient's signs and symptoms, laboratory studies, and imaging. In chronic pancreatitis, the levels of serum amylase and lipase may be elevated slightly or not at all, depending on the degree of pancreatic fibrosis. Serum bilirubin and alkaline phosphatase levels may be increased. Mild leukocytosis is usually present, and the sedimentation rate is usually elevated.

Stool samples are examined for fecal fat content. Deficiencies of fat-soluble vitamins and cobalamin, glucose intolerance, and possibly diabetes may also be found in patients with chronic pancreatitis. ERCP is used to visualize the pancreatic and common bile ducts, as well as changes in the pancreatic ductal system, such as gross dilation and microcysts. Other imaging studies such as CT, MRI, MRCP, transabdominal ultrasound, and endoscopic ultrasound are useful in patients with chronic pancreatitis. These tests show a variety of changes, including calcifications, ductal dilation, pseudocysts, and pancreatic enlargement. The secretin stimulation test, although not widely used, may help to assess pancreatic function.

Collaborative Care

When a patient with chronic pancreatitis experiences an acute attack, the therapy is identical to that for acute pancreatitis. At other times, the focus is on prevention of further attacks, relief of pain, and control of pancreatic exocrine and endocrine insufficiency. Sometimes, doses of analgesics must be large and frequent to relieve the pain.

Diet, pancreatic enzyme replacement, and control of diabetes are measures used to control the pancreatic insufficiency. The diet should be bland and low in fat. Small, frequent meals should be encouraged. Fatty, rich, and stimulating foods should be avoided in order to decrease pancreatic secretions. Alcohol must be totally eliminated from the diet. Smoking should be stopped as it is associated with accelerated progression of chronic pancreatitis.

Pancreatic enzyme products (e.g., pancreatin and pancrelipase) containing amylase, lipase, and trypsin are administered to replace the deficient pancreatic enzymes. They are usually enteric coated to prevent their breakdown or inactivation by gastric hydrochloric acid. Bile salts are sometimes administered to facilitate the absorption of the fat-soluble vitamins (A, D, E, and K) and to prevent further fat loss. If diabetes develops, it is controlled with insulin or oral hypoglycemic agents. Acid-neutralizing (e.g., antacids) and acid-inhibiting drugs (e.g., proton pump inhibitors) may be administered to decrease hydrochloric acid levels, but they have little overall effect on the outcome of the disease.

When biliary disease is present or if obstruction or pseudocyst develops, surgery may be indicated. Surgical procedures can divert bile flow or relieve ductal obstruction. A choledochojejunostomy diverts bile around the ampulla of Vater, where spasm or hypertrophy of the sphincter may be present. In this procedure, the common bile duct is anastomosed into the jejunum. One type is the Roux-en-Y pancreatojejunostomy, in which the pancreatic duct is opened and an anastomosis is made with the jejunum. Pancreatic drainage procedures relieve ductal obstruction. Some patients may undergo ERCP with either sphincterotomy or stent placement at the site of obstruction, or both. These patients require follow-up ERCP to either exchange or remove the stent.

NURSING MANAGEMENT
CHRONIC PANCREATITIS

Except during an acute episode, the focus of nursing management is on chronic care and health promotion. Patients must be instructed to take measures to prevent further attacks. Dietary control, along with adherence to pancreatic enzyme treatment regimens, is essential. The pancreatic enzymes are taken with meals or snacks. Patients' stools should be examined for steatorrhea to help determine the effectiveness of the enzyme treatment. Patients and caregivers must be given clear instructions on stool assessment.

If diabetes has developed, patients need instruction about testing of blood glucose levels and medications (see Chapter 52). Patients who are taking antisecretory agents must take them as ordered to control gastric acidity. Antacids should be taken after meals and at bedtime.

Alcohol must be avoided. Patients who have developed a dependence on alcohol may need referral to other agencies or resources to help with this problem (see Chapter 11).

PANCREATIC CANCER

Pancreatic cancer is a disease with a dismal outcome. In Canada, it was estimated that 1 in 79 Canadians will have pancreatic cancer, making it the twelfth most common fatal disease (Kanji & Gallinger, 2013). Pancreatic cancer affects older people; the incidence peaks among those 65 to 75 years of age. The prognosis of pancreatic cancer is poor. The majority of patients die within 5 to 12 months of the initial diagnosis, and the overall 5-year survival rate is about 6%.

Etiology and Pathophysiology

The cause of pancreatic cancer remains unknown. Cigarette smoking is the most established environmental risk factor for pancreatic cancer (Kanji & Gallinger, 2013). Active smokers are twice as likely as nonsmokers to develop pancreatic cancer. The risk is related to both duration and number of cigarettes smoked. Other risk factors are obesity (BMI >35), heavy alcohol use, and genetic dispositions.

Most pancreatic tumours are adenocarcinomas originating from the epithelium of the ductal system. More than half the tumours occur in the head of the pancreas. As the tumour grows, the common bile duct becomes obstructed, and obstructive jaundice develops. Tumours starting in the body or the tail often do not produce symptoms until their growth is advanced. The majority of cancers have metastasized at the time of diagnosis. Metastases to the lymph nodes are common.

Clinical Manifestations

Common manifestations of pancreatic cancer include abdominal pain (dull, aching), anorexia, nausea, and rapid and progressive weight loss. Jaundice occurs when the cancer is in the head of the pancreas because of the ductal obstruction. Pruritus may accompany obstructive jaundice.

Pain is common and is related to the location of malignancy. Extreme, unrelenting pain is related to extension of the cancer into the retroperitoneal tissues and nerve plexuses. The pain is frequently located in the upper abdomen or the left hypochondrium and often radiates to the back. Its onset is commonly related to eating, and it also occurs at night. Weight loss results from poor digestion and absorption caused by lack of digestive enzymes from the pancreas.

Diagnostic Studies

Endoscopic ultrasonography, CT scan, ERCP, MRI, and MRCP are the most commonly used imaging techniques for diagnosing pancreatic diseases, including cancer. Endoscopic ultrasonography involves imaging the pancreas with the use of an endoscope positioned in the stomach and duodenum. It also allows for fine-needle aspiration of the tumour. CT scan is often the initial study and provides information on metastasis and vascular involvement. ERCP allows visualization of the pancreatic duct and the biliary system. When ERCP is used, pancreatic secretions and tissue can be collected for analysis of different tumour markers. MRI and MRCP can also be used for diagnosing and staging the cancer.

Tumour markers are used both for establishing the diagnosis of pancreatic adenocarcinoma and for monitoring the response

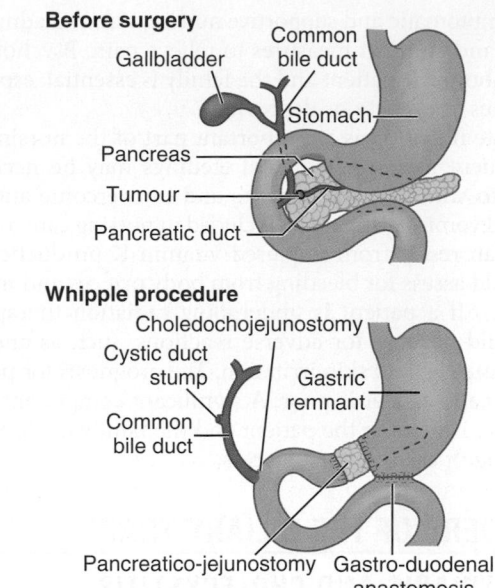

FIGURE 46-15 Whipple procedure, or radical pancreatico-duodenectomy. This surgical procedure involves resection of the proximal pancreas, adjoining duodenum, distal portion of the stomach, and distal segment of the common bile duct, and the removal of the gallbladder. An anastomosis of the pancreatic duct, common bile duct, and stomach to the jejunum is created.

to treatment. Cancer-associated antigen (CA-19-9) is elevated in pancreatic cancer and is the most commonly used tumour marker.

Collaborative Care

Surgery is the most effective treatment for cancer of the pancreas. Only 15% to 20% of affected patients have resectable tumours. The classic surgical procedure is a *radical pancreatico-duodenectomy*, or *Whipple procedure* (Figure 46-15). This procedure involves resection of the proximal pancreas (proximal pancreatectomy), the adjoining duodenum (duodenectomy), the distal portion of the stomach (partial gastrectomy), and the distal segment of the common bile duct, and removal of the gallbladder. An anastomosis of the pancreatic duct, the common bile duct, and the stomach to the jejunum is created. A total pancreatectomy is performed in some institutions. Sometimes, a simple bypass procedure, such as a cholecystojejunostomy to relieve biliary obstruction, may be used as a palliative measure. Some surgeons suggest a more radical resection, such as a total pancreatico-duodenectomy with splenectomy. Biliary stents can be used as a palliative measure when tumours compress the bile duct. Common postsurgical complications include delayed gastric emptying and pancreatic anastomotic leaks.

Adjuvant treatment with chemotherapy or radiotherapy is often used postsurgery. Chemotherapy usually consists of 5-fluorouracil (5-FU) and gemcitabine, either alone or in combination with agents such as capecitabine (Xeloda) or erlotinib (Tarceva). Erlotinib is a targeted therapy.

NURSING MANAGEMENT
PANCREATIC CANCER

Because patients with pancreatic cancer have many of the same problems as patients with pancreatitis, nursing care includes the same measures (see NCP 46-3, Patient With Acute Pancreatitis, available on the Evolve website for this chapter). The nurse should provide symptomatic and supportive nursing care and administer analgesics and comfort measures to relieve pain. Psychological support to both the patient and the family is essential, especially during times of anxiety or depression.

Adequate nutrition is an important part of the nursing care plan. Frequent and supplemental feedings may be necessary. Measures to stimulate the appetite and to overcome anorexia, nausea, and vomiting should be included in nursing care. Because bleeding can result from impaired vitamin K production, the nurse should assess for bleeding from body orifices and mucous membranes. If a patient is undergoing radiation therapy, the nurse should observe for adverse reactions, such as anorexia, nausea, vomiting, and skin irritation. The prognosis for patients with pancreatic cancer is poor. A significant component of the nursing care is helping the patient and the family or significant others through the grieving process.

DISORDERS OF THE BILIARY TRACT

CHOLELITHIASIS AND CHOLECYSTITIS

The most common disorder of the biliary system is cholelithiasis (stones in the gallbladder) (Figures 46-16 and 46-17). The stones may be lodged in the neck of the gallbladder or in the cystic duct. Cholecystitis (inflammation of the gallbladder) is usually associated with cholelithiasis. Cholecystitis may be acute or chronic.

Cholelithiasis occurs in 10% to 15% of adults in developed countries. The prevalence is highest in Indigenous populations,

FIGURE 46-16 Cholesterol gallstones in a gallbladder that was removed. Source: Kumar, V., Abbas, A. K., Aster, J. C., et al. (2010). *Robbins and Cotran pathologic basis of disease* (8th ed.). Philadelphia: W. B. Saunders.

FIGURE 46-17 Radiograph of a gallbladder with gallstones.

affecting about 64% of women and 30% of men in certain communities (Stinton & Shaffer, 2012). *Cholecystectomy* (removal of the gallbladder) ranks among the most common surgical procedures. Although gallstones are common, more than 80% of affected patients have no symptoms. The incidence of cholelithiasis is higher in women, particularly multiparous women, and in people older than 40 years. Postmenopausal women on estrogen therapy are at somewhat greater risk than are women who are taking birth control pills. Oral contraceptives alter the character of bile, resulting in increased cholesterol saturation. Other factors that increase the occurrence of gallbladder disease are a sedentary lifestyle, a familial tendency, and obesity. Obesity causes increased secretion of cholesterol in bile. The incidence of gallstones in industrialized and developing societies will probably escalate because of the increase in dietary fat and carbohydrate intake coupled with reductions in dietary fibre intake.

Etiology and Pathophysiology

Cholelithiasis. The cause of gallstones is unknown. Gallstones develop when the balance that keeps cholesterol, bile salts, and calcium in solution is altered so that these substances precipitate. Conditions that upset this balance include infection and disturbances in the metabolism of cholesterol. When the bile secreted by the liver is supersaturated with cholesterol (lithogenic bile), the bile in the gallbladder also becomes supersaturated with cholesterol. When that happens, precipitation of cholesterol occurs. The cholesterol type of gallstone accounts for 90% of all gallstones. Risk factors for developing cholesterol gallstones can be genetic, dietary, and medication related.

Black pigment gallstones account for 2% of gallstones, and they consist of polymerized calcium bilirubinate. Patients with hemolytic anemia, cirrhosis, and ileal diseases are at highest risk for developing black pigment stones.

Brown pigment gallstones are infrequent and usually form in the bile ducts as a result of stasis of bile and infection. These stones consist of unconjugated bilirubin and calcium salts. People at risk include those with duodenal diverticula, bile duct strictures, or parasitic diseases.

The stones may remain in the gallbladder or migrate to the cystic duct or to the common bile duct. They cause pain as they pass through the ducts, and they may lodge in the ducts and produce an obstruction. Small stones are more likely to move into a duct and cause obstruction. Table 46-21 lists the changes and the manifestations that occur when the stones obstruct the common bile duct. If the blockage occurs in the cystic duct, the bile can continue to flow into the duodenum directly from the liver. However, when the bile in the gallbladder cannot escape, this stasis of bile may lead to cholecystitis.

Cholecystitis. Cholecystitis is most commonly associated with obstruction caused by gallstones or biliary sludge. Cholecystitis in the absence of obstruction (acalculous cholecystitis) occurs most commonly in older adults and in patients who have trauma or extensive burns or have recently undergone surgery. Acalculous cholecystitis can also occur as a result of prolonged immobility and fasting, prolonged total parenteral nutrition, and diabetes mellitus. Bacteria (reaching the gallbladder via the vascular or the lymphatic route) or chemical irritants in the bile can also produce cholecystitis. *Escherichia coli, Streptococci,* and *Salmonellae* are common causative bacteria.

Inflammation is the major pathophysiological process in cholecystitis; it may be confined to the mucous lining, or it may

TABLE 46-21	CLINICAL MANIFESTATIONS CAUSED BY OBSTRUCTED BILE FLOW
Clinical Manifestation	**Etiology**
Bleeding tendencies	Lack of or decreased absorption of vitamin K, resulting in decreased production of prothrombin
Clay-coloured stools	Blockage of flow of bile salts out of the liver
Dark amber urine, which foams when shaken	Soluble bilirubin in urine
Intolerance of fatty foods (nausea, sensation of fullness, anorexia)	No bile in small intestine for fat digestion
No urobilinogen in urine	No bilirubin reaching small intestine to be converted to urobilinogen
Obstructive jaundice	No bile flow into duodenum
Pruritus	Deposition of bile salts in skin tissues
Steatorrhea	No bile salts in duodenum, preventing fat emulsion and digestion

involve the entire wall of the gallbladder. During an acute attack of cholecystitis, the gallbladder is edematous and hyperemic. It may be distended with bile or pus. The cystic duct is also involved and may become occluded. The wall of the gallbladder becomes scarred after an acute attack. Functioning decreases if large amounts of tissue undergo fibrosis.

Clinical Manifestations

Cholelithiasis may produce severe symptoms or none at all *(silent cholelithiasis)*. The severity of symptoms depends on whether the stones are stationary or mobile and whether obstruction is present. When a stone is lodged in the ducts or when stones are moving through the ducts, spasms may result. The gallbladder spasms occur in response to the stone. The spasms sometimes produce severe pain, which is termed *biliary colic* even though the pain is rarely colicky; it is more often steady. The pain can be excruciating and accompanied by tachycardia, diaphoresis, and prostration. The severe pain may last up to an hour, and when it subsides, there is residual tenderness in the right upper quadrant. The attacks of pain frequently occur 3 to 6 hours after a high-fat meal or when the patient lies down. When total obstruction occurs, symptoms related to bile duct blockage manifest (see Table 46-21).

Manifestations of cholecystitis vary from indigestion to moderate to severe pain, fever, and jaundice. Initial symptoms of acute cholecystitis include pain and tenderness in the right upper quadrant (which may be referred to the right shoulder and scapula) and indigestion. The pain may be acute and be accompanied by nausea and vomiting, restlessness, and diaphoresis. Manifestations of inflammation include leukocytosis and fever. Physical findings include a positive Murphy sign, a manoeuvre that elicits a painful response when the right subcostal region is palpated. The manoeuvre may cause a sudden stop of inspiration as the inflamed gallbladder reaches the examiner's fingers (inspiratory arrest). Symptoms of chronic cholecystitis include fat intolerance, dyspepsia, heartburn, and flatulence.

Complications

Complications of cholelithiasis and cholecystitis include gangrenous cholecystitis, subphrenic abscess, acute pancreatitis, *cholangitis* (inflammation of bile ducts), biliary cirrhosis, fistulas, and rupture of the gallbladder, which can cause bile peritonitis. In older patients and those with diabetes, gangrenous cholecystitis and bile peritonitis are the most common complications of cholecystitis. *Choledocholithiasis* (stone in the common bile duct) may occur, producing symptoms of obstruction.

Diagnostic Studies

Ultrasound is 90% to 95% accurate in detecting stones. It is especially useful for patients who are allergic to contrast medium. ERCP allows for visualization of the gallbladder, the cystic duct, the common hepatic duct, and the common bile duct. Bile samples taken during ERCP are sent for culture to identify possibly infecting organisms. Laboratory tests may reveal elevations in some liver enzymes, such as alkaline phosphatase, ALT, and AST. The white blood cell (WBC) count is increased as a result of inflammation. Both the direct and indirect bilirubin levels are elevated, as is the urinary bilirubin level if an obstructive process is present. If the common bile duct is obstructed, no bilirubin reaches the small intestine to be converted to urobilinogen. The serum amylase is increased if the pancreas is involved.

Collaborative Care

Once gallstones become symptomatic, definitive surgical intervention with cholecystectomy is usually indicated. However, in some cases, conservative therapy may be considered.

Conservative Therapy

Cholelithiasis. The treatment of gallstones depends on the stage of the disease. Bile acids (cholesterol solvents) such as ursodeoxycholic acid are administered to dissolve stones. However, the gallstones may recur. Gallstones are not usually treated with drugs because of the high use and success of laparoscopic cholecystectomy.

Standard ERCP clears stones from the common bile duct in approximately 90% of patients (Figure 46-18). This procedure allows for visualization of the biliary system, placement of stents, and sphincterotomy (papillotomy) if warranted. In this procedure, the endoscope is passed through the duodenum. With an electrodiathermy knife attached to the endoscope, the sphincter of Oddi is widened (sphincterotomy). A basket is used to retrieve the stone. The stone may be removed in the basket, but more commonly it is left in the duodenum and will be passed naturally in the stool.

Extracorporeal shock-wave lithotripsy (ESWL) is another nonsurgical treatment for gallstones. In ESWL, a lithotripter uses high-energy shock waves to disintegrate gallstones once they have been located by ultrasound. It usually takes 1 to 2 hours to disintegrate the stones. After they are broken up, the fragments pass through the common bile duct and into the small intestine. Usually ESWL and oral dissolution therapy are used together.

Cholecystitis. During an acute episode of cholecystitis, the focus of treatment is on control of pain, control of possible infection with antibiotics, and maintenance of fluid and electrolyte balance (Table 46-22). If nausea and vomiting are severe, an NG tube may be inserted, and gastric decompression may be used to prevent further gallbladder stimulation. Anticholinergics are administered to decrease secretion and counteract smooth muscle spasms. Analgesics are given for pain relief.

Surgical Therapy.
Laparoscopic cholecystectomy is the treatment of choice for symptomatic cholelithiasis. Approximately 92% of all cholecystectomies are performed laparoscopically. In

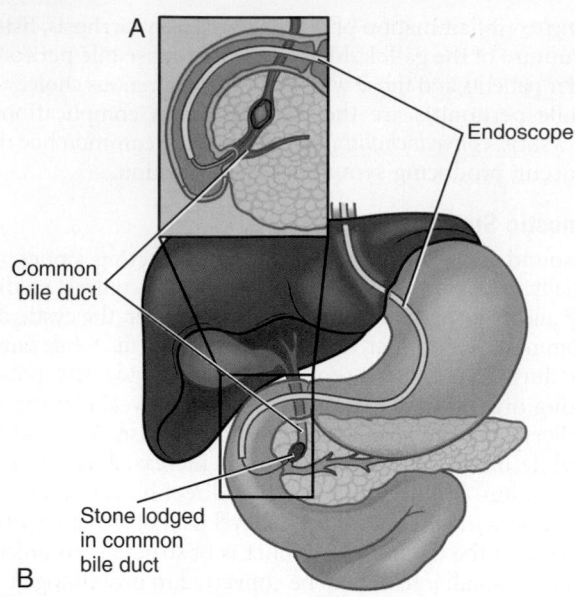

FIGURE 46-18 Standard endoscopic retrograde cholangiopancreatography (ERCP). **A,** During endoscopic sphincterotomy, an endoscope is advanced through the mouth and stomach until its tip sits in the duodenum opposite the common bile duct. **B,** After widening the duct mouth by incising the sphincter muscle, the physician advances a basket attachment into the duct and snags the stone.

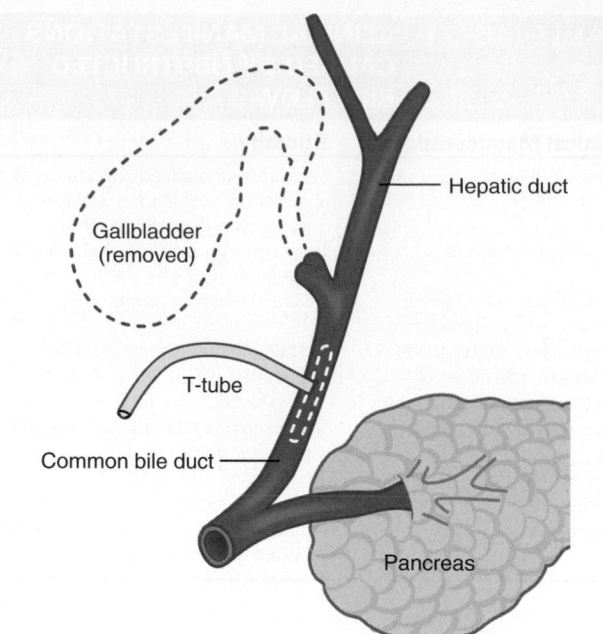

FIGURE 46-19 Placement of T-tube during cholecystectomy. *Dotted lines* indicate parts removed.

TABLE 46-22   **COLLABORATIVE CARE**

Cholelithiasis and Acute Cholecystitis

Diagnostic	• ERCP with sphincterotomy (papillotomy)
• History and physical examination	• Extracorporeal shock-wave lithotripsy
• ERCP	• Fat-soluble vitamins (A, D, E, and K)
• Liver enzyme measurements	• IV fluids
• Serum bilirubin	• NPO with NG tube, later progressing to low-fat diet
• Ultrasound	
• WBC count	**Dissolution Therapy**
Collaborative Therapy	• Ursodeoxycholic acid
Conservative Therapy	**Surgical Therapy***
• Analgesics	• Incisional cholecystectomy
• Antiemetics	• Laparoscopic cholecystectomy
• Antibiotics (for secondary infection)	
• Anticholinergics (antispasmodics)	

ERCP, endoscopic retrograde cholangiopancreatography; *IV,* intravenous; *NG,* nasogastric; *NPO,* nothing by mouth; *WBC,* white blood cell.
*See Table 46-23.

this procedure, the gallbladder is removed through one to four small punctures in the abdomen. A 1-cm puncture is made slightly above the umbilicus, and the surgeon inflates the abdominal cavity with 3 to 4 L of CO_2 to improve visibility. A laparoscope that has a camera attached is inserted into the abdomen. Two additional punctures made just below the ribs are used for insertion of grasping forceps. A dissection laser is inserted into the fourth puncture. (The incision sites may vary.) Using closed-circuit monitors to view the abdominal cavity, the surgeon retracts and dissects the gallbladder and removes it with grasping forceps.

This procedure is relatively minor and entails few complications. Most patients have minimal postoperative pain and are

discharged the day of or the day after surgery. In most cases, patients are able to resume normal activities and return to work within 1 week. The main complication is injury to the common bile duct. The few contraindications to laparoscopic cholecystectomy include peritonitis, cholangitis, gangrene or perforation of the gallbladder, portal hypertension, and serious bleeding disorders.

On select patients, an incisional (open) cholecystectomy may be performed. This procedure involves removal of the gallbladder through a right subcostal incision. A T-tube is inserted into the common bile duct during surgery when a common bile duct exploration is part of the surgical procedure (Figure 46-19). This ensures patency of the duct until the edema produced by the trauma of exploring and probing the duct has subsided. It also allows the excess bile to drain while the small intestine is adjusting to receiving a continuous flow of bile.

Transhepatic Biliary Catheter. The transhepatic biliary catheter can be used preoperatively in biliary obstruction and in hepatic dysfunction secondary to obstructive jaundice. It can also be inserted for palliative care when inoperable carcinoma of the liver, pancreatic duct, or bile duct obstructs bile flow. Under fluoroscopic guidance, the catheter is percutaneously inserted across the liver parenchyma into the common bile duct and duodenum. It decompresses obstructed extrahepatic bile ducts so that bile can flow freely. After insertion, the catheter is connected to a drainage bag. The skin around the catheter insertion site has to be cleansed daily with an antiseptic. It is important to observe for bile leakage at the insertion site. Depending on the reason for the catheter, the patient may be discharged with it in place.

Drug Therapy. The most common drugs used in the treatment of gallbladder disease are analgesics, anticholinergics (antispasmodics), fat-soluble vitamins, and bile salts. Morphine or meperidine (Demerol) may be administered for pain management. Anticholinergics such as atropine and other antispasmodics may be administered to relax the smooth muscle and decrease ductal tone. If a patient has chronic gallbladder disease or any biliary tract obstruction, fat-soluble vitamins (A, D, E, and K) will probably be given. Bile salts may be administered to facilitate digestion and vitamin absorption. For treatment of pruritus, cholestyramine may provide relief. Cholestyramine is a resin that binds bile salts in the intestine, increasing their excretion in the feces. It is administered in powder form and should be mixed with milk or juice. Adverse effects include nausea, vomiting, diarrhea or constipation, and skin reactions.

Nutritional Therapy. Many patients have fewer problems if they eat smaller, more frequent meals, with some fat at each meal to promote gallbladder emptying. If obesity is a problem, a reduced-calorie diet is indicated. The diet should be low in saturated fats (e.g., butter, shortening) and high in fibre and calcium. Rapid weight loss should be avoided because it can promote gallstone formation. After a laparoscopic cholecystectomy, the patient should have liquids for the rest of the day and eat light meals for a few days. If an incisional cholecystectomy is performed, the patient may progress from liquids to a bland diet once bowel sounds have returned. The amount of fat in the postoperative diet depends on the patient's tolerance of fat. A low-fat diet may be helpful if the flow of bile is reduced (usually only in the early postoperative period) or if the patient is overweight. Some patients need to restrict fats for 4 to 6 weeks. Otherwise, no special dietary instructions are needed other than to eat nutritious meals and avoid excessive fat intake.

NURSING MANAGEMENT GALLBLADDER DISEASE

NURSING ASSESSMENT
Subjective and objective data that should be obtained from a person with gallbladder disease are presented in Table 46-23.

NURSING DIAGNOSES
Nursing diagnoses for patients with gallbladder disease treated surgically include but are not limited to the following:
- *Acute pain* related to physical injury agent (surgical procedure)
- *Ineffective health management* related to *insufficient resources* (lack of knowledge of diet and postoperative management)

PLANNING
The overall goals are that the patient with gallbladder disease will have (a) relief of pain and discomfort, (b) no complications postoperatively, and (c) no recurrent attacks of cholecystitis or cholelithiasis.

NURSING IMPLEMENTATION
HEALTH PROMOTION. The nurse should recognize the predisposing factors for gallbladder disease in general health screening. Patients at risk should be taught initial clinical manifestations and be instructed to seek medical care if these manifestations occur. Patients with chronic cholecystitis do not have acute symptoms and may not seek help until jaundice and biliary obstruction occur. Earlier detection in these patients is beneficial so that the condition can be managed with lifestyle modifications (e.g., a low-fat diet).

ACUTE INTERVENTION. Nursing objectives for the patient undergoing conservative therapy include managing pain, relieving

---

TABLE 46-23 NURSING ASSESSMENT

Cholecystitis or Cholelithiasis

Subjective Data
Important Health Information
Past health history: Obesity, multiparity, infection, cancer, extensive fasting, pregnancy; positive family history; sedentary lifestyle
Medications: estrogen or oral contraceptives
Surgery or other treatments: Previous abdominal surgery

Symptoms
- Clay-coloured stools, steatorrhea, flatulence; dark urine
- Moderate to severe pain in right upper quadrant that may radiate to the back or scapula
- Positive Murphy sign
- Pruritus
- Weight loss, anorexia; indigestion, fat intolerance, nausea and vomiting, dyspepsia; chills

Objective Data
General
Fever, restlessness

Integumentary
Jaundice, icteric sclera; diaphoresis

Respiratory
Tachypnea, splinting during respirations

Cardiovascular
Tachycardia

Gastro-Intestinal
Palpable gallbladder, abdominal guarding and distension

Possible Findings
↑ Serum liver enzymes and bilirubin; absence of urobilinogen in urine; ↑ urinary bilirubin; leukocytosis; abnormal ultrasound findings

---

nausea and vomiting, providing comfort and emotional support, maintaining fluid and electrolyte balance, maintaining nutrition, making accurate assessments of effectiveness of treatment, and observing for complications.

Many patients with acute cholecystitis or cholelithiasis have severe pain. The medications ordered to relieve the pain should be administered as required by patients and before the pain becomes more severe. The nurse should determine what medications relieve the pain and how much medication is required. The nurse must also observe for adverse effects of the medications. Nursing comfort measures, such as a clean bed, comfortable positioning, and oral care, are appropriate.

For patients who have severe nausea and vomiting, insertion of an NG tube and gastric decompression may be necessary. Eliminating food and fluid intake also prevents further stimulation of the gallbladder. Oral hygiene, care of nares, accurate intake and output measurements, and maintenance of suction should be a part of the nursing care plan for such patients. For patients with less severe nausea and vomiting, antiemetics are usually adequate. When a patient is vomiting, comfort measures such as frequent mouth rinses should be provided. Any vomitus must be removed immediately from the patient's view.

If pruritus occurs with jaundice, measures to relieve itching include baking soda or oatmeal baths; lotions, such as those containing calamine; antihistamines; soft, old linen; and control of the temperature (not too hot and not too cold). The patient's nails should be kept short and clean. Patients should be taught to rub with their knuckles rather than scratch with their nails when they cannot resist scratching.

The nursing care plan for such patients also includes assessment of progression of the symptoms and development of complications. The nurse should observe for signs of bile duct obstructions: jaundice; clay-coloured stools; dark, foamy urine; steatorrhea; fever; and increased WBC count.

When symptoms of obstruction are present (see Table 46-21), the nurse must be aware of possible bleeding as a result of decreased prothrombin production. Common sites to observe for bleeding are the mucous membranes of the mouth, the nose, the gingivae, and injection sites. If injections are given, a small-gauge needle should be used and gentle pressure applied after the injection. The nurse should know the patient's prothrombin time and use this as a guide in the assessment process.

Assessment for infections includes monitoring of vital signs. Fever with chills and jaundice may indicate choledocholithiasis. Nursing care of the patient after ERCP with papillotomy includes assessment to detect complications such as pancreatitis, perforation, infection, and bleeding. Abdominal pain and fever may indicate pancreatitis. The patient should be rested for several hours and ingest nothing by mouth until the gag reflex returns.

Postoperative Care. Postoperative nursing care after a laparoscopic cholecystectomy includes monitoring for complications such as bleeding, making the patient comfortable, and preparing the patient for discharge. A common postoperative problem is referred pain to the shoulder because of the carbon dioxide (CO_2) that is used to inflate the abdominal cavity during surgery. CO_2 may not be released or absorbed by the body. The CO_2 can irritate the phrenic nerve and the diaphragm, causing some difficulty breathing. Placing the patient in a Sims position (left side with right knee flexed) helps move the gas pocket away from the diaphragm. Deep breathing and early ambulation should be encouraged. Severe pain can be relieved by opioid analgesics such as oxycodone or codeine. The patient is allowed clear liquids and can walk to the bathroom to void. Many patients go home the same day as the procedure.

Postoperative nursing care for incisional cholecystectomy is the same as general postoperative nursing care (see Chapter 22). The goal is to prevent postoperative complications. If the patient has a T-tube (see Figure 46-19), the nursing care plan should focus on maintaining bile drainage and observing for the T-tube functioning and drainage. The T-tube is connected to a closed gravity drainage system. If the Penrose or Jackson-Pratt drain or the T-tube is draining large amounts, a sterile pouching system should be used to protect the skin.

AMBULATORY AND HOME CARE. For patients who have conservative therapy, long-term nursing management depends on symptoms and on whether surgical intervention is planned. Dietary teaching is usually necessary. The food should be low in fat. A weight-reduction program should be recommended for patients with obesity. Patients may need to take fat-soluble vitamin supplements. The nurse should instruct patients about symptoms that indicate obstruction (stool and urine changes, jaundice, and pruritus). The nurse should explain the importance of continued follow-up care. Patients who undergo a laparoscopic cholecystectomy are discharged soon after the surgery; therefore, home care is important. Teaching is essential; a teaching guide is presented in Table 46-24.

TABLE 46-24 PATIENT & CAREGIVER TEACHING GUIDE

Laparoscopic Cholecystectomy: Postoperative Care

The following guidelines should be included when teaching the patient and caregiver about postoperative care following laparoscopic cholecystectomy.

1. Remove the bandages on the puncture site the day after surgery, and bathe or shower.
2. Notify the surgeon of any of the following signs and symptoms:
   • Redness; swelling; bile-coloured drainage or pus from any incision
   • Severe abdominal pain, nausea, vomiting, fever, chills
3. Resume normal activities gradually.
4. Return to work within 1 week of surgery if no complications ensue.
5. Resume normal diet; a low-fat diet, however, is usually better tolerated for several weeks after surgery.

After an incisional cholecystectomy, the patient is usually discharged in 2 to 3 days. The patient must avoid heavy lifting for 4 to 6 weeks. Usual sexual activities, including intercourse, can be resumed as soon as the patient feels ready, unless the physician instructs otherwise. If the patient is required to remain on a low-fat diet for 4 to 6 weeks, a dietary teaching plan is necessary. A weight-reduction program may be helpful if the patient is overweight. Most patients tolerate a regular diet with no difficulties but should avoid excessive fats.

EVALUATION

The overall expected outcomes are that the patient with gallbladder disease will (a) be comfortable and free of pain and (b) will verbalize understanding of activity level and dietary restrictions.

GALLBLADDER CANCER

Primary cancer of the gallbladder is uncommon. The majority of gallbladder carcinomas are adenocarcinomas. A relationship exists between cancer of the gallbladder and chronic cholecystitis and cholelithiasis. The early symptoms of carcinoma of the gallbladder are insidious and are similar to those of chronic cholecystitis and cholelithiasis, which makes diagnosis difficult. Later symptoms are usually those of biliary obstruction.

Diagnosis and staging of gallbladder cancer are done using endoscopic ultrasound, transabdominal ultrasound, CT, MRI, MRCP, or a combination of these methodologies. Unfortunately, gallbladder cancer often is not detected until the advanced stage. When it is found early, surgery can be curative. Several factors influence successful surgical outcomes, including the depth of cancer invasion, extent of liver involvement, presence of venous or lymphatic invasion, and lymph node metastasis. Extended cholecystectomy with lymph node dissection has improved the outcomes for patients with gallbladder cancer.

When surgery is not an option, endoscopic implantation of stents in the biliary tree to reduce obstructive jaundice can be done. Adjuvant therapies, including radiation therapy and chemotherapy, may be used, depending on the disease state. Overall, cancer of the gallbladder has a poor prognosis.

Nursing management involves supportive care with special attention to nutrition, hydration, skin care, and pain relief. Many of the nursing care measures used for patients with cholecystitis and cholelithiasis are frequently applied, as are nursing care measures for patients with cancer (see Chapter 18).

CASE STUDY

Cirrhosis of the Liver

Source: triocean/ Shutterstock .com.

Patient Profile

Mr. Arnold Bisson is a 55-year-old man admitted with a diagnosis of an upper GI bleed secondary to cirrhosis of the liver.

Subjective Data

- Has been vomiting for 2 days, noticed blood in the toilet when he vomits
- Was informed 10 years ago that he had cirrhosis
- Had a blood transfusion 25 years ago after a car accident
- Acknowledges that he has been drinking heavily for more than 30 years
- Complains of anorexia, nausea, and abdominal discomfort

Objective Data
Physical Examination

- Is thin and malnourished
- Has moderate ascites
- Has jaundice of sclera and skin
- Has 4+ pitting edema of the lower extremities
- Has palpable liver and spleen

Laboratory Values

- Total bilirubin: 150 mcmol/L
- Albumin: 26 g/L
- AST: 210 U/L
- ALT: 190 U/L
- Hb 60 g/L and Hct of 20%
- Platelet count: 75 × 10⁹/L
- INR: 2.1
- Anti-HCV (antibody to hepatitis C) positive and HCV RNA negative
- HBsAg (hepatitis B surface antigen) negative and anti-HBs (antibody to hepatitis B surface antigen) positive

Discussion Questions

1. What are the possible causes of cirrhosis? What is the most likely etiology responsible for Mr. Bisson's cirrhosis?
2. Describe the pathophysiological changes that occur in the liver as cirrhosis develops.
3. List Mr. Bisson's clinical manifestations of liver failure. For each manifestation, explain the pathophysiological basis.
4. Explain the significance of the results of his laboratory values.
5. If Mr. Bisson begins to manifest signs and symptoms of hepatic encephalopathy, what would the nurse monitor? What measures should be instituted to control or decrease encephalopathy?
6. Mr. Bisson was being closely observed for the possibility of gastro-intestinal bleeding. Why is this considered a possible complication?
7. **Priority decision:** On the basis of the assessment data presented, what are the nursing diagnoses? Are there any collaborative problems?
8. **Priority decision:** What are the priority nursing interventions for the patient at this stage of his illness?

evolve

Answers are available on *http://evolve.elsevier.com/Canada/Lewis/medsurg*

REVIEW QUESTIONS

The number of the question corresponds to the same-numbered objective at the beginning of the chapter.

1. During assessment of a client with posthepatic (cholestatic) jaundice, which of the following would the nurse expect to find?
   a. Clay-coloured stools
   b. Dark urine and stools
   c. Pyrexia and severe pruritus
   d. Elevated urinary urobilinogen level
2. A client with hepatitis A is in the acute phase. Which of the following should the nurse's plan of care consider?
   a. Pruritus is a common problem with jaundice in this phase.
   b. The client is most likely to transmit the disease during this phase.
   c. Gastro-intestinal symptoms are not as severe in hepatitis A as they are in hepatitis B.
   d. Extrahepatic manifestations of glomerulonephritis and polyarteritis are common in this phase.
3. A client with acute hepatitis B is being discharged in 2 days. Which of the following instructions should the nurse include in the discharge teaching plan?
   a. Resume alcohol as soon as he is symptom free.
   b. Use a condom during sexual intercourse.
   c. Have family members get an injection of immune globulin.
   d. Follow a low-protein, moderate-carbohydrate, moderate-fat diet.
4. A client with advanced cirrhosis asks the nurse why his abdomen is so swollen. The nurse's response is based on the knowledge of which of the following?
   a. A lack of clotting factors promotes the collection of blood in the abdominal cavity.

   b. Portal hypertension and hypoalbuminemia cause a fluid shift into the peritoneal space.
   c. Decreased peristalsis in the gastro-intestinal tract contributes to gas formation and distension of the bowel.
   d. Bile salts in the blood irritate the peritoneal membranes, causing edema and pocketing of fluid.
5. A client has been told that she has elevated liver enzyme caused by NAFLD. Which of the following instructions should the nurse's teaching plan include?
   a. Have genetic testing performed.
   b. Follow a heart-healthy diet and regular exercise program.
   c. Lose weight quickly within the next 4 weeks.
   d. Avoid alcohol until the liver enzyme levels return to normal.
6. In caring for a client with metastatic liver cancer, which of the following should the nurse perform?
   a. Focus primarily on symptomatic and comfort measures
   b. Reassure the client that chemotherapy offers a good prognosis for recovery
   c. Promote the client's confidence that surgical excision of the tumour will be successful
   d. Provide information necessary for the client to make decisions regarding liver transplantation
7. Nursing management of a client with acute pancreatitis includes which of the following? *(Select all that apply)*
   a. Checking for signs of hypocalcemia
   b. Observing stools for signs of steatorrhea
   c. Providing a diet low in carbohydrates with moderate fat
   d. Giving insulin based on a sliding scale
   e. Monitoring for infection, particularly respiratory tract infection

8. A client with pancreatic cancer is admitted to the hospital for evaluation for treatment. The client asks the nurse to describe Whipple procedure, which the surgeon has planned. Which of the following would the nurse include in her explanation?
   a. Creation of a bypass around the obstruction caused by the tumour by joining the gallbladder to the jejunum
   b. Resection of the entire pancreas and the distal portion of the stomach, with anastomosis of the common bile duct and the stomach into the duodenum
   c. Removal of part of the pancreas, part of the stomach, the duodenum, and the gallbladder, with joining of the pancreatic duct, the common bile duct, and the stomach to the jejunum
   d. Radical removal of pancreas, duodenum, and spleen, and attachment of the stomach to the jejunum, which requires oral supplementation of pancreatic digestive enzymes and insulin replacement therapy

9. The nursing management of a client with cholecystitis in association with cholelithiasis should include which of the following?

a. Recommendation of a diet low in saturated fat
b. Information that gallstones once removed tend not to recur
c. Avoidance of morphine in the management of pain
d. Treatment with oral bile salts that dissolve gallstones

10. What information should be included in teaching about home management after a laparoscopic cholecystectomy?
   a. Keeping the bandages on the puncture sites for 48 hours
   b. Reporting any bile-coloured drainage or pus from any incision
   c. Using over-the-counter antiemetics if nausea and vomiting occur
   d. Emptying and measuring the contents of the bile bag from the T-tube every day

1. a; 2. b; 3. b; 4. b; 5. b; 6. a; 7. a; 8. c; 9. a; 10. b.

ⓔvolve

For even more review questions, visit *http://evolve.elsevier.com/Canada/ Lewis/medsurg.*

REFERENCES

Beuers, U., Gershwin, M. E., Gish, R. G., et al. (2015). Changing nomenclature for PBC: From "cirrhosis" to "cholangitis.". *Gastroenterology, 149*(6), 1627–1629. doi:10.1053/j. gastro.2015.08.031.

Buti, M., Tsai, N., Petersen, J., et al. (2015). Seven-year efficacy and safety of treatment with tenofovir disoproxil fumarate for chronic hepatitis B virus infection. *Digestive Diseases and Sciences, 60*(5), 1457–1464. doi:10.1007/s10620-014-3486-7.

Canadian Institute for Health Information. (2017). *CORR annual statistics 2017*. Retrieved from *https://www.cihi.ca/en/corr-annual -statistics-2017.*

Carrion, A. F., & Martin, P. (2012). Viral hepatitis in the elderly. *American Journal of Gastroenterology, 107*(5), 691–697. doi:10.1038/ajg.2012.7.

Centers for Disease Control and Prevention. (2013). *Bloodborne pathogens—Occupational exposure*. Retrieved from *https:// www.cdc.gov/oralhealth/infectioncontrol/bloodborne_exposures .htm.*

Chalasani, N. P., Hayashi, P. H., Bonkovsky, H. L., et al. (2014). ACG clinical guideline: The diagnosis and management of idiosyncratic drug-induced injury. *American Journal of Gastroenterology, 109*(7), 950–966. doi:10.1038/ajg.2014.131.

Chen, X., Chen, J., Wen, J., et al. (2013). Breastfeeding is not a risk factor for mother-to-child transmission of hepatitis B virus. *PLoS ONE, 8*(1), e55303. doi:10.1371/journal.pone.0055303.

El-Serag, H. B. (2011). Hepatocellular carcinoma. *New England Journal of Medicine, 365*, 1118–1127. doi:10.1056/ NEJMra1001683.

Garcia-Tsao, G., Sanyal, A. J., Grace, N. D., et al. (2007). Prevention and management of gastroesophageal varices and variceal hemorrhage in cirrhosis. *Hepatology (Baltimore, Md.), 46*, 922–938. doi:10.1002/hep.21907. (Seminal).

Government of Canada. (2016). *Part IV: Active vaccines. Canadian immunization guide*. Retrieved from *http://www.phac-aspc.gc.ca/ publicat/cig-gci/p04-hepb-eng.php.*

Haque, M., Scudamore, C. H., Steinbrecher, U. P., et al. (2010). Liver transplantation: Current status in British Columbia. *British Columbia Medical Journal, 52*(4), 203–210. Retrieved from *http://www.bcmj.org/article/liver-transplantation-current -status-british-columbia.* (Seminal).

Kamar, N., Dalton, H. R., Abravanel, F., et al. (2014). Hepatitis E virus infection. *Clinical Microbiology Reviews, 27*(1), 116–138. doi:10.1128/CMR.00057-13.

Kanji, Z. S., & Gallinger, S. (2013). Diagnosis and management of pancreatic cancer. *Canadian Medical Association Journal, 185*(14), 1219–1226. doi:10.1503/cmaj.121368.

Karageorgopoulos, D. E., Allen, J., & Bhagani, S. (2015). Hepatitis C in human immunodeficiency virus co-infected individuals: Is this still a "special population"? *World Journal of Hepatology, 7*(15), 1936–1952. doi:10.4254/wjh.v7.i15.1936.

Lee, W. M., Larson, A. M., & Stravitz, T. R. (2011). *AASLD position paper: The management of acute liver failure: An update 2011*. Retrieved from *https://www.aasld.org/sites/default/files/guideline _documents/141022_Position_ALF_4UFb.pdf.*

Mahady, S. E., & George, J. (2016). Exercise and diet in the management of nonalcoholic fatty liver disease. *Metabolism: Clinical and Experimental, 65*(8), 1172–1182. doi:10.1016/j. metabol.2015.10.032.

Myers, R. P., Shah, H., Burak, K. W., et al. (2015). An update on the management of chronic hepatitis C: 2015 Consensus guidelines from the Canadian Association for the Study of the Liver. *Canadian Journal of Gastroenterology Hepatology, 29*(1), 19–34. doi:10.1155/2015/692408.

Public Health Agency of Canada (PHAC). (2014a). *Hepatitis B—Get the facts*. Retrieved from *http://www.phac-aspc.gc.ca/hcai-iamss/ bbp-pts/hepatitis/hep_b-eng.php.*

Public Health Agency of Canada (PHAC). (2014b). *Primary care management of hepatitis B—Quick reference*. Retrieved from *http://www.phac-aspc.gc.ca/publicat/hep/hbv-vhb/ index-eng.php#sec1-1.*

Public Health Agency of Canada (PHAC). (2016). *Canadian immunization guide: Part 4—Active vaccines*. Retrieved from *https://www.canada.ca/en/public-health/services/publications/ healthy-living/canadian-immunization-guide-part-4-active -vaccines/page-6-hepatitis-a-vaccine.html?=undefined&wbdisable =true.*

Public Health Agency of Canada (PHAC) & Canadian Institute for Health Information (CIHI). (2011). *Obesity in Canada report*. Retrieved from *http://www.phac-aspc.gc.ca/hp-ps/hl-mvs/oic-oac/ index-eng.php.*

Riggio, O., Nardelli, S., Moscucci, F., et al. (2012). Hepatic encephalopathy after transjugular intrahepatic portosystemic

shunt. *Clinics in Liver Disease, 16*(1), 133–146. doi:10.1016/
j.cld.2011.12.008.

Shah, A. H., Heathcote, J., & Feld, J. J. (2013). A Canadian screening
program for hepatitis C: Is now the time? *Canadian Medical
Association Journal, 185*(15), 1325–1328. doi:10.1503/
cmaj.121872.

Sherman, M., Burak, K., Maroun, J., et al. (2011). Multidisciplinary
Canadian consensus recommendations for the management and
treatment of hepatocellular carcinoma. *Current Oncology, 18,*
228–240. doi:10.3747/co.v18i5.952.

Statistics Canada. (2017). *Leading causes of death, total population, by
age group and sex, Canada.* CANSIM Table 102-0561. Retrieved
from *http://www5.statcan.gc.ca/cansim/a05?lang=eng
&id=1020561.*

Stinton, L. M., & Shaffer, E. A. (2012). Epidemiology of gallbladder
disease: Cholelithiases and cancer. *Gut and Liver, 6*(2), 172–187.
doi:10.5009/gnl.2012.6.2.172.

Tenner, S., Baillie, J., DeWitt, J., et al. (2013). American College of
Gastroenterology guideline: Management of acute pancreatitis.
American Journal of Gastroenterology, 108(9), 1400–1415.
doi:10.1038/ajg.2013.218.

Terrault, N. A., Bzowej, N. H., Chang, K. M., et al. (2016). AASLD
guidelines for treatment of chronic hepatitis B. *Hepatology
(Baltimore, Md.), 63*(1), 261–283. doi:10.1002/hep.28156.

Wilder, J., & Patel, K. (2014). The clinical utility of FibroScan® as a
noninvasive diagnostic test for liver disease. *Medical Devices
(Auckland, NZ), 7,* 107. doi:10.2147/MDER.S46943.

World Health Organization (WHO). (2010). *The global prevalence of
hepatitis A virus infection and susceptibility: A systematic review.*
Retrieved from *http://whqlibdoc.who.int/hq/2010/WHO_IVB
_10.01_eng.pdf.* (Seminal).

World Health Organization (WHO). (2013). *Hepatitis A.* Retrieved
from *http://www.who.int/biologicals/vaccines/hepatitis_A/en/
index.html.*

World Health Organization (WHO). (2017). *Hepatitis B.* Retrieved
from *http://www.who.int/mediacentre/factsheets/fs204/en.*

RESOURCES

BC Centre for Disease Control
http://www.bccdc.ca

Canadian Association for the Study of the Liver
http://www.hepatology.ca

Canadian Association of Gastroenterology
https://www.cag-acg.org

Canadian Hemophilia Society
http://www.hemophilia.ca

Canadian Liver Foundation
http://www.liver.ca

**CATIE: Canada's Source for HIV and Hepatitis C
Information**
http://www.hepcinfo.ca

Hepatitis Central: Hepatitis C Support Groups
http://www.hepatitis-central.com/hcv/support/canada/toc.html

Public Health Agency of Canada
http://www.phac-aspc.gc.ca/index-eng.php

**Registered Nurses' Association of Ontario: Integrating
Smoking Cessation Into Daily Nursing Practice**
*http://rnao.ca/sites/rnao-ca/files/Integrating_Smoking_Cessation
_into_Daily_Nursing_Practice.pdf*

For additional Internet resources, see the website for this book
at *http://evolve.elsevier.com/Canada/Lewis/medsurg.*

Problems of Urinary Function

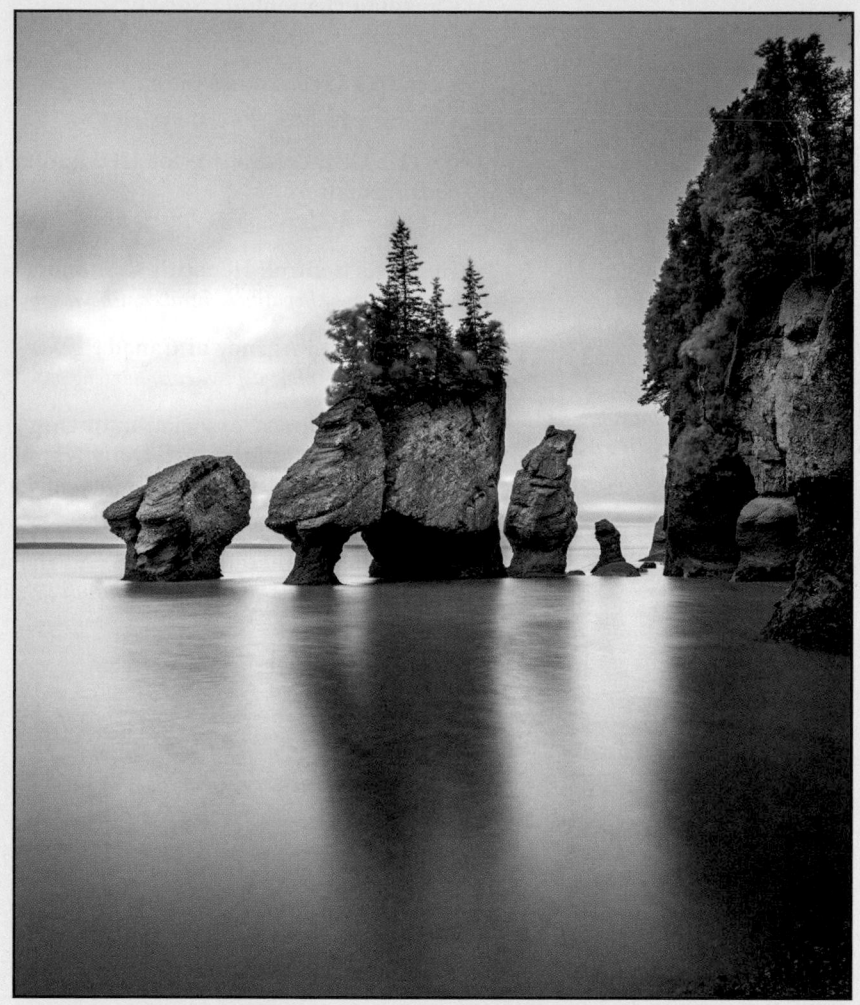

Source: Vincent St. Thomas/Shutterstock.com.

Nursing Assessment
Urinary System

Written by: Suzanne Teresa Parsell
Adapted by: Kathleen Rodger and Lynn Jansen

evolve WEBSITE

http://evolve.elsevier.com/Canada/Lewis/medsurg

- Review Questions (Online Only)
- Key Points
- Answer Guidelines for Case Study
- Conceptual Care Map Creator
- Audio Glossary
- Content Updates

LEARNING OBJECTIVES

1. Describe the anatomical location and functions of the kidneys, the ureters, the bladder, and the urethra.
2. Explain the physiological events involved in the formation and passage of urine, from glomerular filtration to voiding.
3. Identify relevant subjective patient information and objective data that should be collected to determine health history, health status, and clinical manifestations of patients with urinary disorders.
4. Describe age-related changes in the urinary system.
5. Describe the appropriate techniques used in the physical assessment of the urinary system.
6. Differentiate normal from common abnormal findings of a physical assessment of the urinary system.
7. Describe the range of tests performed in the analysis of urine.
8. Describe the normal physical and chemical characteristics of urine.

KEY TERMS

costovertebral angle, p. 1152
creatinine, p. 1157
cystometrography, p. 1161
cystoscopy, p. 1160
glomerular filtration rate (GFR), p. 1143

glomerulus, p. 1143
intravenous pyelography (IVP), p. 1158
nephron, p. 1142
renal arteriography, p. 1159
renal biopsy, p. 1160

retrograde pyelography, p. 1159
urinalysis, p. 1154
urodynamics testing, p. 1161

"Bones can break, muscles can atrophy, glands can loaf, even the brain can go to sleep without immediate danger to survival. But should the kidneys fail ... neither bone, muscle, gland, nor brain could carry on" (Smith, 1953). This statement underlines the importance of kidneys to our lives. Adequate functioning of the kidneys is essential to the maintenance of a healthy body. If the kidneys fail completely and treatment is not given, death is inevitable.

The primary functions of the kidneys are (a) to filter waste products from the bloodstream, (b) to maintain fluid and electrolyte and acid–base balance in the body, and (c) to excrete metabolic waste products. The two kidneys perform the primary physiological functions. Secondary functions of the kidneys are to regulate (a) blood pressure, (b) bone density, and (c) erythropoiesis. The kidneys are connected to two narrow tubules, the ureters, which reabsorb 99% of filtered products and transport urine from the kidney to the bladder. Urine flows from the bladder and from the body through the urethra (Figure 47-1).

STRUCTURES AND FUNCTIONS OF THE URINARY SYSTEM

Kidneys

Macrostructure. The paired kidneys are bean-shaped organs that are retroperitoneal (behind the peritoneum), on either side of the vertebral column at about the level of the twelfth thoracic (T12) vertebra to the third lumbar (L3) vertebra. Each kidney weighs 115 to 175 g and is about 12 cm long. With the liver above it, the right kidney is at the level of the twelfth rib, lower than the left kidney. An adrenal gland lies on top of each kidney.

Each kidney is surrounded by a considerable amount of fat and connective tissue that serve to support and maintain its

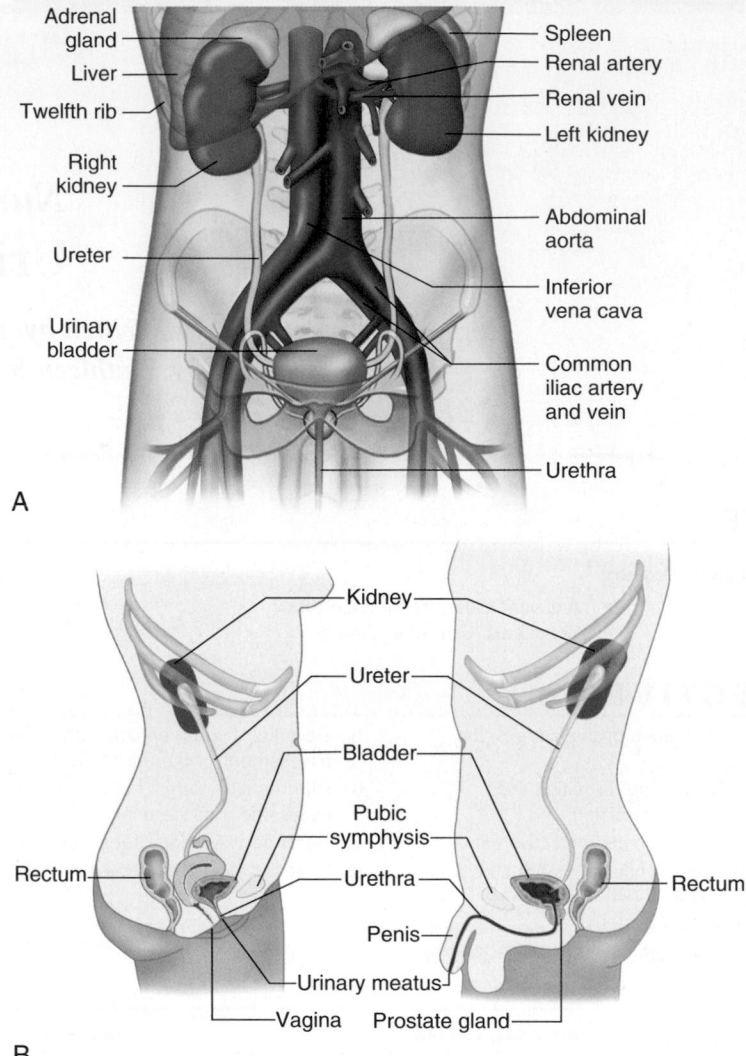

A

B

FIGURE 47-1 Illustrations of organs of the urinary system. **A,** Upper urinary tract in relation to other anatomical structures. **B,** Male urethra in relation to other pelvic structures and female urethra in relation to other pelvic structures. Source: From Patton, K. T., & Thibodeau, G. A., (2015). *Anatomy and physiology* (9th ed., p. 969, Figure 42-4). St. Louis: Mosby. Copyright Elsevier 2015.

position. The surface of the kidney is covered by a thin, smooth layer of fibrous membrane called the *capsule.* These structures protect the kidney and serve as a shock absorber should the kidney be subjected to a sudden force from a blunt object striking the abdomen or back. The *hilus* on the medial side of the kidney serves as the entry site for the renal artery and nerves, as well as the exit site for the renal vein and the ureter.

On a longitudinal section of the kidney (Figure 47-2), the parenchyma (actual tissue) of the kidney can be visualized. The outer layer is termed the *cortex,* and the inner layer is called the *medulla.* The medulla consists of a number of pyramids. The apices of these pyramids are called *papillae,* and urine passes through the papillae to enter the calyces. The minor calyces widen and merge to form major calyces, which form a funnel-shaped sac called the *renal pelvis.* The minor and major calyces transport urine to the renal pelvis in preparation for transportation to the bladder via the ureter. The renal pelvis can store a small volume of urine (3 to 5 mL).

Microstructure. The functional unit of the kidney is the **nephron.** Each kidney has about 1 million nephrons. A nephron is composed of a glomerulus, Bowman capsule, and the tubular system. The tubular system consists of the proximal convoluted tubule, the loop of Henle, and the distal convoluted tubule (Figure 47-3). The glomeruli, Bowman capsule, the proximal tubule, and the distal tubule are located in the cortex of the kidney. The loop of Henle and the collecting ducts are located in the medulla (Figure 47-4; see also Figure 47-2). Several nephrons converge into a collecting duct, which eventually merges into a pyramid and empties via the papilla into a minor calyx (see Figures 47-2 and 47-4).

Blood Supply. A blood supply of about 1200 mL/min, which is 20% to 25% of total cardiac output, flows to the two kidneys. Blood reaches the kidneys via the renal artery, which arises from the aorta and enters the kidney through the hilus. The renal artery divides into secondary branches and then into still smaller branches, each of which eventually forms an afferent arteriole. The afferent arteriole divides into a capillary network termed the *glomerulus,* which is a tuft of up to 50 capillaries. The capillaries of the glomerulus eventually unite in the efferent arteriole (Figure 47-5). This arteriole splits to form a capillary

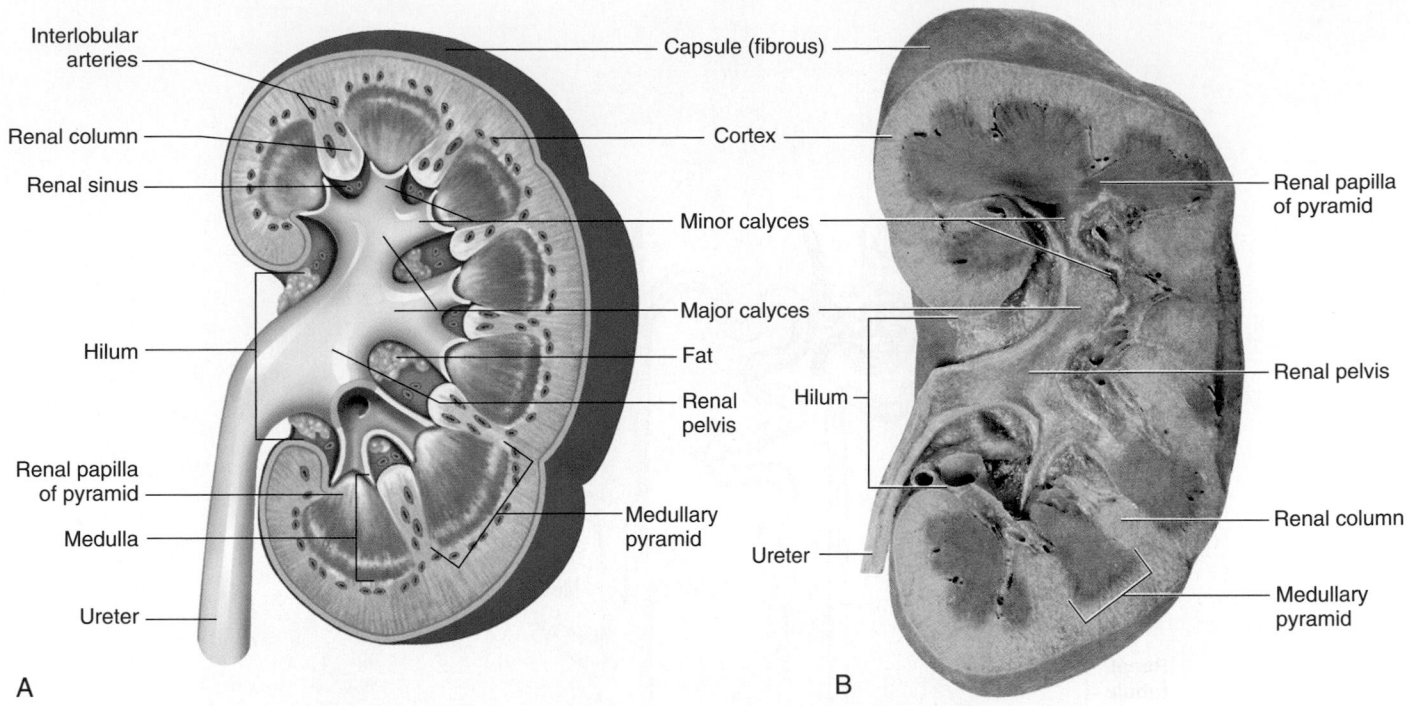

FIGURE 47-2 Illustration of a longitudinal section of the kidney. Source: From Patton, K. T., & Thibodeau, G. A., (2015). *Anatomy and physiology* (9th ed., p. 968, Figure 42-2). St. Louis: Mosby. Copyright Elsevier 2015. *A,* Adapted from Brundage DJ: *Renal disorders, Mosby's clinical nursing series,* St. Louis, 1992, Mosby.

network called the *peritubular capillaries,* which, as the name suggests, surround the tubular system. All peritubular capillaries eventually drain into the venous system. The renal vein empties into the inferior vena cava.

Physiology of Urine Formation. The process of urine formation is extremely complex. It represents the outcome of a multistep process of filtration, reabsorption, secretion, and excretion of water, electrolytes, and metabolic waste products. Although urine formation is the result of this process, the primary function of the kidneys is to filter the blood and maintain the body's internal homeostasis.

Glomerular Function. Urine formation starts at the glomerulus, where blood is filtered. The glomerulus, a capillary network within the kidneys that comprises up to 50 capillaries, is a semipermeable membrane and so allows for filtration (see Figure 47-3). The hydrostatic pressure of the blood within the glomerular capillaries causes a portion of blood to be filtered across the semipermeable membrane into Bowman capsule, where the filtered portion of the blood, called the *glomerular filtrate,* begins to pass down to the tubule. Filtration is more rapid in the glomerulus than in ordinary tissue capillaries because of the porosity of the glomerular membrane. The ultrafiltrate is similar in composition to blood except that it lacks blood cells, platelets, and large plasma proteins. Under normal conditions, the capillary pores are too small to allow the loss of these large blood components. Capillary permeability is increased in many renal diseases, enabling plasma proteins to pass into the urine.

The amount of blood filtered by the glomeruli in a given time is termed the **glomerular filtration rate (GFR).** The normal GFR is about 125 mL/min (Grossman & Porth, 2014). However, on average, only 1 mL is excreted as urine per minute because

TABLE 47-1	FUNCTIONS OF THE SEGMENTS OF THE NEPHRON
Component	**Function**
Glomerulus	Selective filtration of water and solutes from the blood
Proximal tubule	Reabsorption of 80% of electrolytes and water; reabsorption of all glucose and amino acids; reabsorption of HCO_3^-; secretion of H^+ and creatinine
Loop of Henle	Reabsorption of Na^+ and Cl^- in ascending limb; reabsorption of water in descending loop; concentration of filtrate
Distal tubule	Secretion of K^+, H^+, and ammonia; reabsorption of water (regulated by ADH); reabsorption of HCO_3^-; regulation of Ca^{2+} and PO_4^{2-} by parathyroid hormone, regulation of Na^+ and K^+ by aldosterone
Collecting duct	Reabsorption of water (ADH required)

ADH, antidiuretic hormone; *Ca^{2+},* calcium; *Cl^-,* chloride; *H^+,* hydrogen; *HCO_3^-,* bicarbonate; *K^+,* potassium; *Na^+,* sodium; *PO_4^{2-},* phosphate.

the peritubular capillary network reabsorbs most glomerular filtrate before it reaches the end of the collecting duct.

Tubular Function. Because the glomerular membrane is a selective filtration membrane that filters primarily by size, provision is made for the reabsorption of essential materials and the excretion of nonessential ones (Table 47-1).

In the proximal convoluted tubule, about 80% of the electrolytes are reabsorbed. Normally, all the glucose, amino acids, and small proteins are reabsorbed. For the most part, reabsorption occurs by active transport. Hydrogen ions (H^+) and creatinine are secreted into the filtrate (Grossman & Porth, 2014).

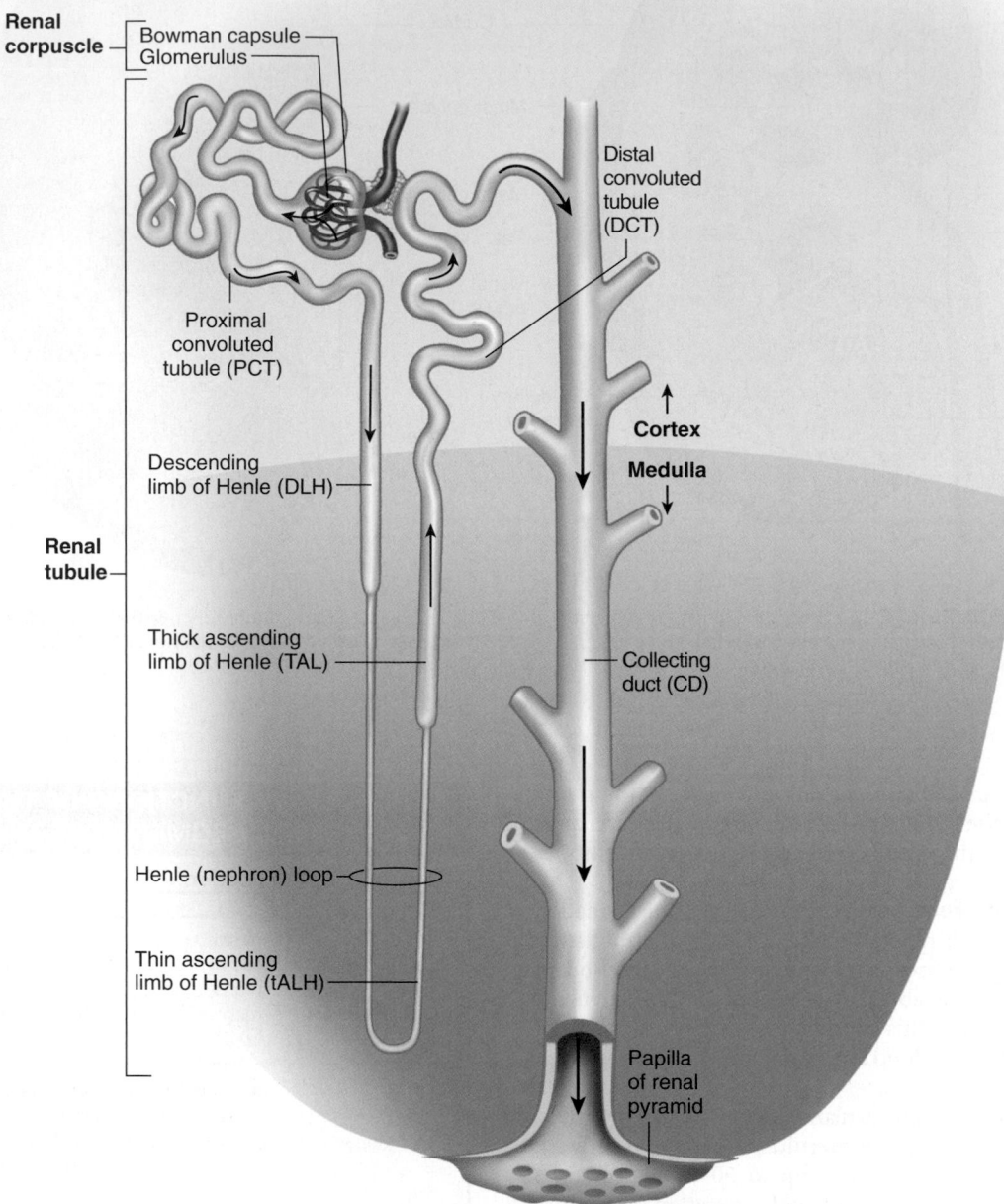

FIGURE 47-3 The nephron is the basic functional unit of the kidney. This illustration of a single nephron unit also shows the surrounding blood vessels. Source: From Patton, K. T., & Thibodeau, G. A., (2015). *Anatomy and physiology* (9th ed., p. 971, Figure 42-10). St. Louis: Mosby. Copyright Elsevier 2015. Adapted from Brundage DJ: *Renal disorders, Mosby's clinical nursing series,* St. Louis, 1992, Mosby.

The loop of Henle is important in conserving water and thus concentrating the filtrate. Reabsorption continues in the loop of Henle. The descending loop is permeable to water and moderately permeable to sodium, urea, and other solutes. In the ascending limb, chloride ions (Cl⁻) are actively reabsorbed, followed passively by sodium ions (Na⁺). About 25% of the filtered sodium is reabsorbed in the ascending limb.

Two important functions of the distal convoluted tubules are final regulation of water balance and acid–base balance (Grossman & Porth, 2014). Antidiuretic hormone (ADH), released by the

posterior portion of the pituitary gland, is required for water reabsorption. The stimuli for ADH release are increased serum osmolality and decreased blood volume. ADH makes the distal convoluted tubules and the collecting ducts permeable to water, allowing it to be reabsorbed into the peritubular capillaries and to be eventually returned to circulation. In the absence of ADH, the tubules are practically impermeable to water, and any water in the tubules leaves the body as urine.

In the presence of aldosterone (released from the adrenal cortex) acting on the distal tubule, reabsorption of Na⁺ and water

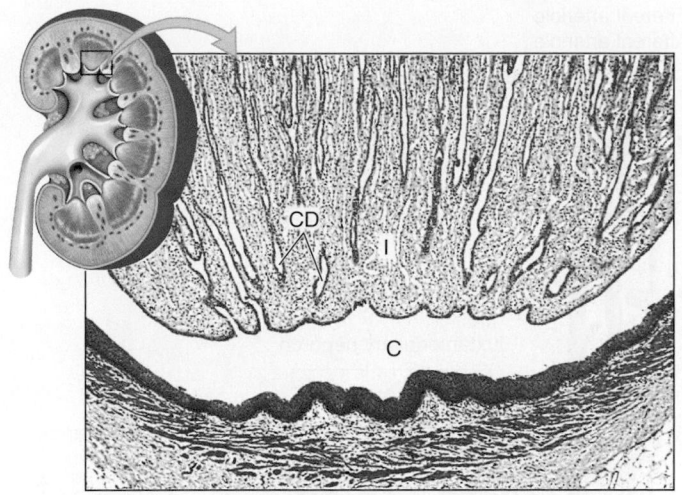

FIGURE 47-4 Illustration of collecting ducts *(CD)* seen opening into a calyx *(C)* at the papillary tip. The interstitial tissue *(I)* includes some loops of Henle. Source: From Patton, K. T., & Thibodeau, G. A. (2013). *Anatomy and physiology* (8th ed., p. 980, Figure 31-16). St. Louis: Mosby.

occurs. In exchange, potassium ions (K^+) are excreted. The secretion of aldosterone is influenced by both circulating blood volume and plasma concentrations of Na^+ and K^+.

Acid–base regulation involves reabsorbing and conserving most of the bicarbonate (HCO_3^-) and secreting excess H^+. The distal tubule functions in different ways to maintain the pH of extracellular fluid (ECF) volume within a range of 7.35 to 7.45 (see Chapter 19).

Atrial natriuretic factor (ANF) is a hormone secreted from cells in the right atrium when right atrial blood pressure increases. ANF inhibits the secretion and effect of ADH and results in a large volume of dilute urine.

Parathyroid hormone is released from the parathyroid gland in response to low serum calcium levels. It causes increased tubular reabsorption of calcium ions (Ca^{2+}) and decreased tubular reabsorption of phosphate ions (PO_4^{2-}). Therefore, serum Ca^{2+} levels are increased.

The basic function of nephrons is to cleanse or clear blood plasma of unnecessary substances. After the glomerulus has filtered the blood, the tubules separate the portions of tubular fluid that are useful to the body from those that are not. The necessary portions are returned to the blood, and the unnecessary portions pass into urine as waste.

Other Functions of the Kidney. In addition to their function of regulating the volume and the composition of ECF, the kidneys have other vital functions, including the production of erythropoietin, activation of vitamin D, and production and secretion of renin.

Production of Erythropoietin. Erythropoietin is a hormone produced by the kidney and released in response to hypoxia and decreased renal blood flow. Erythropoietin stimulates the production of red blood cells (RBCs) in the bone marrow. A deficiency of erythropoietin in renal failure leads to anemia.

Activation of Vitamin D. Vitamin D is a hormone that can be obtained in the diet or synthesized by the action of ultraviolet radiation on cholesterol in the skin. These forms of vitamin D are inactive and require two more steps to become metabolically active. The first step in activation occurs in the liver; the second step occurs in the kidneys. Active vitamin D is essential for the absorption of calcium from the gastro-intestinal (GI) tract. The

patient with kidney failure (also called *renal failure*) has a deficiency of the active metabolite of vitamin D and manifests as problems of altered calcium and phosphate balance.

Production and Secretion of Renin. Renin, an enzyme, is important in the regulation of blood pressure and is the first step in the RAA (renin–angiotensin–aldosterone) pathway. Renin is released from the *juxtaglomerular apparatus* of the nephron (Figure 47-6) in response to decreased arterial blood pressure, renal ischemia, ECF depletion, increased norepinephrine, and increased urinary Na^+ concentration. Renin catalyzes the splitting of the plasma protein angiotensinogen (from the liver) into angiotensin I, which is subsequently converted to angiotensin II by a converting enzyme made in the lungs. Angiotensin II stimulates the release of aldosterone from the adrenal cortex, which causes retention of Na^+ and water, leading to an increase in ECF. Angiotensin II also causes increases in peripheral vasoconstriction. The increases in ECF and vasoconstriction cause an elevation in blood pressure, which inhibits renin release. Excessive renin production caused by impaired renal perfusion may be a contributing factor in hypertension (see Chapters 35 and 49).

ANF acts directly on the medullary collecting ducts and indirectly on other tubular segments (by inhibiting several steps in the RAA pathway) to inhibit sodium reabsorption. It inhibits secretion of renin and aldosterone and causes an increase in GFR (through its effects on the renal arterioles), all of which increase excretion of sodium and water. Angiotensin converting enzyme (ACE) inhibitors and angiotensin receptor blockers (ARBs) are commonly used drugs to help control blood pressure in patients with hypertension. Since the mechanism of action works directly on RAA pathway, these drugs are also understood to cause adverse effects that can directly impact kidney function, such as proteinuria, increased serum creatinine, nephrotic syndrome, and renal failure (McCance & Huether, 2014).

Prostaglandins (PGs) are important regulators of cellular function. In the kidney, PG synthesis (primarily PGE_2 and PGI_2) occurs primarily in the medulla. These PGs have a vasodilating action in addition to increasing renal blood flow and promoting Na^+ excretion. They also counteract the vasoconstrictor effect of substances such as angiotensin and norepinephrine. Renal PGs may have a systemic effect in lowering blood pressure by decreasing systemic vascular resistance (McCance & Huether, 2014). In addition, they are associated with hypertension that develops in renal failure. When there is a loss of functioning tissue, these renal vasodilators are also lost (see Chapter 49).

Ureters

The ureters are tubes approximately 25 to 35 cm long and 2 to 8 mm in diameter that carry urine from the renal pelvis to the bladder (see Figure 47-1). The narrow area where the ureter joins the renal pelvis is termed the *uretero-pelvic junction*. After coursing down along the psoas muscle, the ureter crosses over the pelvic brim and the iliac artery and inserts into the base of the bladder at the *uretero-vesical junction* (UVJ). The ureteral lumen is narrowest at these junctions; consequently, they are often the sites of urinary stone (calculus) obstruction. Because the lumen of the ureter is narrow, it can be easily occluded internally (e.g., by calculi) or externally (e.g., by tumours, adhesions, or inflammation).

Sympathetic and parasympathetic nerves, along with the vascular supply, surround the mucosal lining of the ureter. Circular and longitudinal smooth muscle fibres are arranged in a meshlike outer layer and contract to promote the peristaltic one-way flow

FIGURE 47-5 Blood supply of nephrons. In this illustration, two types of nephrons (cortical and juxtaglomerular) are shown surrounded by the peritubular blood supply. Source: From Patton, K. T., & Thibodeau, G. A. (2013). *Anatomy and physiology* (8th ed., p. 981, Figure 31-17). St. Louis: Mosby.

of urine. These muscle contractions can be affected by distension as well as by neurological, endocrine, and pharmacological factors. Stimulation of these nerves during passage of a stone or clot may cause acute, severe pain, termed *renal colic*.

Because the renal pelvis holds only 3 to 5 mL of urine, kidney damage can result from a backflow of more than that amount

of urine. The UVJ relies on the ureter's angle of bladder penetration and muscle fibre attachments with the bladder to prevent the backflow of urine (reflux) and ascending infection. The distal ureter entering the bladder has more longitudinal muscle fibres than the upper ureter. This segment enters the bladder laterally at its base, courses along obliquely through the bladder wall for

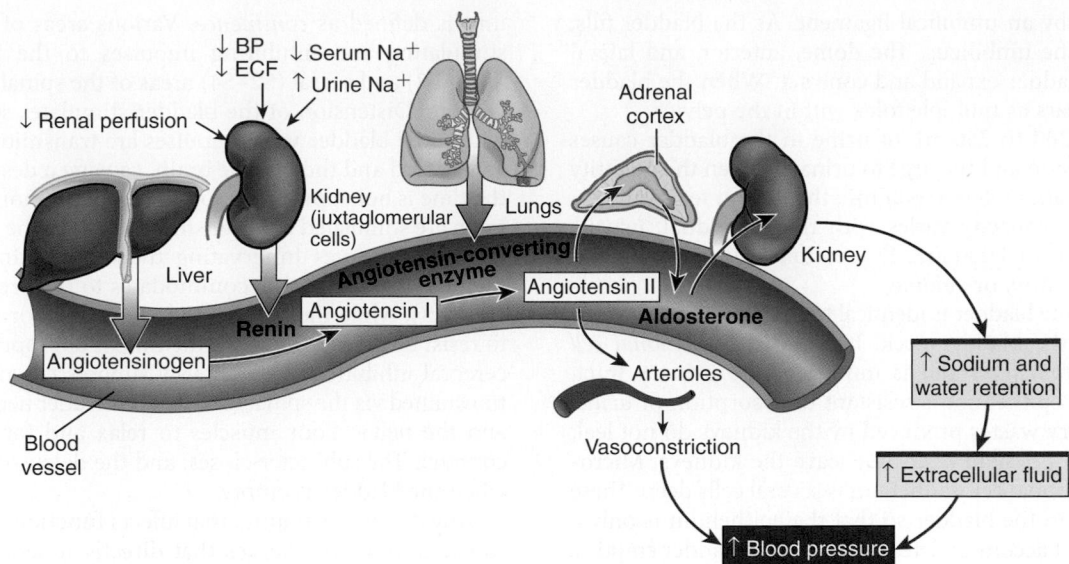

FIGURE 47-6 Renin–angiotensin–aldosterone system. Source: Adapted from Herlihy, B. (2014). *The human body in health and illness* (5th ed., p. 466, Figure 24-3). Philadelphia: W. B. Saunders.

FIGURE 47-7 Illustration of the male urinary bladder. Source: Patton, K. T., & Thibodeau, G. A. (2013). *Anatomy and physiology* (8th ed., p. 974, Figure 31-5). St. Louis: Mosby.

about 1.5 cm, and intermingles with muscle fibres of the bladder base. Circular and longitudinal bladder muscle fibres adjacent to the embedded ureter help secure it. When bladder pressure rises (e.g., during voiding or coughing), muscle fibres that the ureter shares with the bladder base contract first to help promote urethral lumen closure. The bladder then contracts against its base to further close the UVJ and prevent urine from moving back through the junction.

Bladder

The urinary bladder is a distensible organ positioned behind the symphysis pubis and is anterior to the vagina and the rectum. (Figure 47-7 shows the male urinary bladder.) Its primary functions are to serve as a reservoir for urine and to help the body eliminate waste products. Normal adult urine output is approximately 1 500 mL/day, which varies with food and fluid intake. The volume of urine produced at night is less than half of that formed during the day because of hormonal influences (e.g., ADH). This diurnal pattern of urination is normal. Most people urinate five to six times during the day and only occasionally at night.

The triangular area formed by the two ureteral openings and the bladder neck at the base of the bladder is the *trigone*. It is affixed to the pelvis by many ligaments, and it does not change its shape during bladder filling or emptying. The bladder muscle, the *detrusor*, is composed of layers of intertwined smooth muscle fibres and is capable of considerable distension during bladder filling and contraction during emptying. It is affixed to the abdominal wall by an umbilical ligament. As the bladder fills, it rises toward the umbilicus. The dome, anterior, and lateral aspects of the bladder expand and contract. When the bladder is empty, it appears as multiple folds within the pelvis.

On average, 200 to 250 mL of urine in the bladder causes moderate distension and the urge to urinate. When the quantity of urine reaches about 400 to 600 mL, the person feels uncomfortable. Bladder capacity varies with the individual, usually ranging from 600 to 1 000 mL. Evacuation of urine is termed *urination, micturition,* or *voiding.*

The lining of the bladder is identical to that of the renal pelvis, the ureter, and the bladder neck. It is called *transitional cell epithelium* or *urothelium* and is unique to the urinary tract. Transitional cell epithelium is resistant to absorption of urine. Therefore, urinary wastes produced by the kidneys do not leak out of the urinary system after they leave the kidneys. Microscopically, transitional cell epithelium is several cells deep. These cells stretch out in the bladder so that the epithelium is only a few cells deep as it accommodates filling. As the bladder empties, the epithelium resumes its multicellular layer formation.

Because the linings of these organs are similar, transitional cell tumours that occur in one section of the urinary tract can easily metastasize to other urinary tract areas. Malignant cells may move down from upper urinary tract tumours and become established in the bladder, or large bladder tumours can invade the ureter. Tumour recurrence within the bladder is common.

Urethra

The urethra is a small muscular tube that leads from the bladder neck to the external meatus. Its primary function is to serve as a conduit for urine to the bladder and then to the outside of the body.

The urothelium and submucosal layers are the same as those of the bladder. Smooth muscle fibres extend from the bladder neck down into the urethra and are further supported by circular smooth muscle fibres around the urethra. Special C-shaped striated muscle fibres (the rhabdo-sphincter or external sphincter) surround a portion of the urethra and, when bladder pressure increases, voluntarily contract and prevent leaking.

The female urethra is 3 to 5 cm long and lies behind the symphysis pubis but anterior to the vagina (see Figure 47-1, *B*). The rhabdo-sphincter encircles the middle third of the urethra. The shortness of the urethra is a contributing factor to the increased incidence of urinary tract infections in women.

The male urethra, which is about 20 to 25 cm long, originates at the bladder neck and extends the length of the penis (see Figure 47-1, *B*). It is often viewed as consisting of three parts. The prostatic urethra extends from the bladder neck through the prostate to the urogenital diaphragm. The membranous urethra passes through the urogenital diaphragm. The rhabdo-sphincter encircles this portion. Because of the concentrated muscular support, this short portion is not very expandable. As a consequence, stricture formation in this area after instrumentation is common. The penile urethra continues through the corpus spongiosum, a cavernous penile body, through the urogenital diaphragm to a distal dilated area, the fossa navicularis, before terminating at the meatus.

Urethro-Vesical Unit Function

Together, the bladder, the urethra, and the pelvic floor muscles form the *urethro-vesical unit.* Normal voluntary control of this unit is defined as *continence.* Various areas of the brain send stimulating and inhibiting impulses to the thoraco-lumbar (T11–L2) and sacral (S2–S4) areas of the spinal cord to control voiding. Distension of the bladder stimulates stretch receptors within the bladder wall. Impulses are transmitted to the sacral spinal cord and then to the brain, causing a desire to urinate. If the time is not appropriate for voiding, inhibitor impulses in the brain are stimulated and transmitted back to the thoraco-lumbar and sacral nerves innervating the bladder. In a coordinated manner, the detrusor accommodates to the pressure (does not contract), while the sphincter and pelvic floor muscles tighten to resist bladder pressure. If the time is appropriate for voiding, cerebral inhibition is voluntarily suppressed, and impulses are transmitted via the spinal cord for the bladder neck, the sphincter, and the pelvic floor muscles to relax and for the bladder to contract. The sphincter closes, and the detrusor muscle relaxes when the bladder is empty.

Any disease or trauma that affects function of the brain, the spinal cord, or the nerves that directly innervate the bladder, the bladder neck, the external sphincter, or the pelvic floor can affect bladder function. These conditions include diabetes mellitus, paraplegia, and tetraplegia (quadriplegia). Drugs affecting nerve transmission also can affect bladder function.

AGE-RELATED CONSIDERATIONS

EFFECTS OF AGING ON THE URINARY SYSTEM

Anatomical changes in the aging kidney include a 20% to 30% decrease in size and weight between the ages of 30 and 90 years. This loss in renal mass is predominantly in the cortex. The aging nephron fails as a unit because glomerular and tubular function appears to decrease at the same rate. By the seventh decade of life, 30% to 50% of glomeruli have lost their function. Despite losing this original kidney volume, older individuals maintain body fluid homeostasis unless they encounter diseases or other physiological stressors (Nguyen & Goldfarb, 2012).

Blood flow to and within the kidneys also decreases with age. There is no evidence, however, that atherosclerotic vascular disease is primarily responsible for the age-related changes in the kidneys.

Physiological changes in the aging kidney include a decrease in renal blood flow; a decrease in GFR; and decreases in the abilities to conserve Na^+, dilute or concentrate urine, and excrete an acid load. Under normal conditions, the aging kidney is able to maintain homeostasis, but after abrupt changes in blood volume, acid load, or other insults, the kidney may not be able to function effectively because much of its renal reserve has been lost (McCance & Huether, 2014).

Physiological changes also occur in the aging bladder and urethra. Estrogen receptors exist in the female urethra, bladder, vagina, and pelvic floor. As estrogen levels decrease with age, tissues become less elastic, thin, and less vascular. Estrogen replacement may be prescribed to minimize these changes. Periurethral striated muscle fibres and muscles supporting the bladder relax. Consequently, older women are more prone to urethral irritation, urinary incontinence, and urethral and bladder infections (Eriksson, Olofsson, Gustafson, et al., 2014). Although urinary incontinence in older women has long been associated with diminished estrogen levels, the incidence of incontinence has been found to be higher in menopausal women who use hormone therapy. These findings may promote changes in therapy for postmenopausal urinary incontinence.

TABLE 47-2 AGE-RELATED DIFFERENCES

Urinary System

Changes	Differences in Assessment Findings
Kidney	
↓ Amount of renal tissue	Less palpable
↓ Number of nephrons and renal blood vessels; thickened basement membrane of Bowman capsule and glomeruli	↓ Creatinine clearance, ↑ BUN level
↓ Function of loop of Henle and tubules	Alterations in drug excretion; nocturia; loss of normal diurnal excretory pattern because of ↓ ability to concentrate urine; less concentrated urine
Ureter, Bladder, and Urethra	
↓ Elasticity and muscle tone	Palpable bladder after urination because of retention
Weakening of urinary sphincter	Stress incontinence (especially during Valsalva manoeuvre), dribbling of urine after urination
↓ Bladder capacity and sensory receptors	Frequency, urgency, nocturia, overflow incontinence
Estrogen deficiency, leading to thinning and dryness of vaginal tissue	Stress or overactive bladder, dysuria
↑ Prevalence of unstable bladder contractions	Overactive bladder
Prostatic enlargement	Hesitancy, frequency, urgency, nocturia, straining to urinate, retention, dribbling

BUN, blood urea nitrogen.

TABLE 47-3 POTENTIALLY NEPHROTOXIC AGENTS

Antibiotics
- Amikacin
- Amphotericin B
- Bacitracin
- Cephalosporins
- Gentamicin
- Neomycin
- Polymyxin B
- Streptomycin
- Sulphonamides
- Tobramycin
- Vancomycin

Other Agents
- Anaesthetics
- Acetylsalicylic acid (ASA; Aspirin)
- Captopril
- Cimetidine
- Cisplatin
- Cocaine
- Contrast medium
- Cyclosporin (Neoral, Sandimmune)
- Ethylene glycol
- Gold
- Heavy metals
- Heroin
- Lithium
- Methotrexate
- Nonsteroidal anti-inflammatory drugs (e.g., ibuprofen, indomethacin, naproxen)
- Quinine
- Rifampin
- Salicylate (large quantities)

Eriksson, Olofsson, Gustafson, and colleagues (2015) report that approximately one-third of older women suffer from urinary tract infections each year. In a qualitative descriptive study, they found that these women struggled with activities of daily life and felt miserable and restricted when the urinary tract infection was acute. Many of these women were identified as having other health conditions and were frail and thus vulnerable to disease. It is important to adapt supportive nursing strategies to both assess and intervene with this population.

Men's prostates enlarge as they age, and because the prostate surrounds the proximal urethra, increasing prostate size may affect urinary patterns in men, causing hesitancy, retention, slow stream, and bladder infections. Constipation, a complaint often expressed by older adults, can also affect urination. Partial urethral obstruction may occur because of the rectum's close proximity to the urethra (Registered Nurses' Association of Ontario, 2011).

A summary of age-related changes in the urinary system and differences in assessment findings is presented in Table 47-2.

ASSESSMENT OF THE URINARY SYSTEM

Subjective Data

Important Health Information

Past Health History. The patient should be questioned about the presence or history of diseases that are known to be related to renal or other urological problems. Some of these diseases are hypertension, diabetes mellitus, gout and other metabolic problems, connective tissue disorders (e.g., systemic lupus erythematosus, systemic sclerosis [scleroderma]), skin or upper respiratory infections of streptococcal origin, tuberculosis, viral hepatitis, congenital disorders, neurological conditions (e.g., stroke, back injury), and trauma. Specific urinary problems such as cancer, infections, benign prostatic hyperplasia, and calculi should be noted.

Medications. An assessment of the patient's current and past use of medications is important. This list should include over-the-counter drugs, prescription medications, and herbs. Drugs affect the urinary tract in several ways. Many drugs are known to be nephrotoxic (Table 47-3). Certain drugs may alter the quantity and the character of urine output (e.g., diuretics). Numerous drugs, such as nitrofurantoin, change urine colour. Anticoagulants may cause hematuria. Many antidepressants, calcium channel blockers, antihistamines, and drugs used to treat neurological and musculo-skeletal disorders affect the ability of the bladder or the sphincter to contract or relax normally.

Surgery and Other Treatments. The patient should also be questioned about any previous hospitalizations related to renal or urological diseases, and women should be asked about all urinary problems during past pregnancies. The duration, the severity, and the patient's perception of any problem and its treatment should be sought. Past surgical procedures, particularly pelvic surgery, and urinary tract instrumentation should be documented. Information should be obtained from the patient about any radiation or chemotherapy treatment for cancer.

Key Questions. Nurses must convey sensitivity and understanding while asking urinary health assessment questions to maintain the patient's physical and emotional comfort. Key questions to ask a patient with problems related to the urinary system are listed in Table 47-4.

Health History. The nurse should ask about the patient's general health, particularly when disease affecting the kidneys is suspected. Sometimes responses such as "feeling tired all the time"; changes in weight or appetite; excess thirst; fluid retention; and complaints of headache, pruritus, or blurred vision may be related to abnormal kidney function. Similarly, in older patients, malaise and non-localized abdominal discomfort may be the only symptoms of a urinary tract infection (Wagner & Hardin-Pearce, 2014).

TABLE 47-4 HEALTH HISTORY

Urinary System: Questions for Obtaining Subjective Data

Health History

- How is your energy level compared to how it was a year ago?
- Have you ever smoked? If yes, how many packs per day?
- What occupations or work positions have you held?
- Do you have any history of kidney disease, kidney stones, urinary tract infections?*
- Have you had any tests or surgical procedures on your kidney, bladder, or [in men] prostate?*
- Do certain activities aggravate any urinary problems you might have?*
- Have urinary problems caused you to alter or stop any activity or exercise?*
- How do you move or get to the bathroom?*
- What medications are you currently taking?*
- Do you take vitamin or mineral supplements?*

Nutritional Assessment

- How much and what kinds of fluids do you drink daily? Describe when fluid intake occurs over a day.
- Do you drink coffee? Colas? Alcohol? How often? How much?
- Do you eat chocolate? How often? How much?
- Do you spice your food heavily?*

Elimination Assessment

- Do you ever have difficulty holding your urine (water) long enough to get to the toilet? (or) How long can you hold your urine after you first feel the need to go to the bathroom?
- Do you ever leak urine? If so, what causes urine leakage? Do you leak when you cough or sneeze, laugh, walk, run, or lift a heavy object? Do you leak when you touch a doorknob or attempt to open the bathroom door or if you are unable to reach a toilet right away? When did the leaking begin?
- What have you done to manage the problem of leaking? (Have you cut down on the amount of fluids that you drink? Do you empty your bladder as a precautionary measure?)
- Are there certain things that make the problem worse or better?
- Does it happen all of the time, or just at certain times?
- Are you able to sit through a 2-hour meeting or ride in a car for 2 hours without urinating?
- Do you ever leak urine at night? If so, how often and how much do you leak? (If the response is affirmative, the nurse should try to differentiate between this symptom and the habit of going to the bathroom after waking up for some other reason.)
- Do you ever find that you have leaked without awareness of doing so?
- Do you use special devices or supplies for urine elimination or control? If so, (a) What types of devices or supplies do you use?

(b) How often do you use these devices or supplies? (c) How many of these devices or supplies do you use on a daily basis?
- Immediately after urinating (passing your water), does it feel as if you have not emptied your bladder completely? Do you experience any hesitancy and straining? A weakened force of stream? Any dribbling?
- Do you have to exert pressure during urination to feel as if your bladder is being completely emptied?
- [Men] When you urinate (pass water), do you have any difficulty starting the stream or keeping the stream going?
- Do you ever notice blood in your urine?* If so, at what point in the urination does it occur?
- How often do you move your bowels? Do you ever experience constipation (hardened stools that are difficult to pass or a sensation that you are unable to completely evacuate your bowels)?

Activity Assessment

- Have you changed any of your activities because you need to stay near a toilet?
- Do you avoid going to certain places because of difficulty holding your urine (water)?

Pain Assessment

- Do you ever have pain when you urinate?* If so, where is the pain?
- [Women] Do you feel any pressure in your pelvic area?

Self-Concept Assessment

- How does the urinary problem make you feel about yourself?
- Have you been perceiving your body differently since the urinary problem developed?
- Does the urinary problem interfere with your relationships with family or friends?*
- Has the urinary problem caused a change in your job status or affected your ability to carry out job-related responsibilities?*

Sexuality Assessment

- Has the urinary problem caused any change in your sexual pleasure or performance?*
- Do you ever notice any blood or red-tinged urine when you urinate after intercourse?

Coping Assessment

- Have you ever sought help or talked to a primary care provider or other health care professional about this problem?
- Do you feel able to manage the problems associated with your urinary problem? If not, explain.
- What strategies are you using to cope with your urinary problem?

*Describe.

Source: Adapted from Jarvis, C., Browne, A. J., MacDonald-Jenkins, J., et al. (Eds.). (2014). *Physical examination and health assessment* (1st Canadian ed., pp. 749–751). Toronto: Elsevier Canada; and Miller, C. A. (2009). Urinary function. In C. A. Miller (Ed.), *Nursing for wellness in older adults* (5th ed., pp. 390–416). Philadelphia: Lippincott Williams & Wilkins.

An occupational history should be taken. Exposure to certain chemicals can affect the kidneys and the urinary tract system. Phenol and ethylene glycol are examples of nephrotoxic chemicals. Aromatic amines and certain organic chemicals may increase the risk for bladder cancers. Textile workers, painters, hairdressers, and industrial workers have a higher incidence of bladder tumours.

A smoking history should be obtained. Cigarette smoking is a major factor in the risk for bladder cancer. Bladder tumours occur four times more frequently in cigarette smokers than in nonsmokers.

Places where a patient has lived may affect the incidence and prevalence of renal disease. Higher mineral content of the soil and water may be a contributing factor. People living in Middle Eastern countries or Africa can acquire certain parasites that can cause cystitis or bladder cancer.

A family history of certain renal or urological problems increases the likelihood that similar problems will occur in the patient. The nurse should ask about family members who have had any of the diseases referred to in the past health history, as well as polycystic renal disease and congenital urinary tract abnormalities such as Alport syndrome (congenital nephritis).

Nutritional Assessment. The usual quantity and types of fluid that a patient drinks are important information in relation to urinary tract disease. Dehydration may contribute to urinary infections, calculi formation, and renal failure. Large intake of particular foods, such as dairy products or foods high in proteins, may also lead to calculi formation. Asparagus may cause the urine to smell musty, and redness of urine caused by beet ingestion may be mistaken for blood. Coffee, alcohol, carbonated beverages, or spicy foods often aggravate urinary inflammatory diseases. An unexplained weight gain may be the result of fluid retention secondary to a renal problem. Anorexia, nausea, and vomiting can dramatically affect fluid status and require careful assessment. Information on vitamin and mineral supplements and herbal therapies should be obtained. The patient may not think of these supplements and therapies when listing over-the-counter drugs; supplements are often considered part of nutritional intake.

Elimination Assessment. Questions about urine elimination patterns are the cornerstone of the health history in patients with a lower urinary tract disorder. This line of inquiry begins with a question about how patients manage urine elimination. The majority of patients eliminate urine by spontaneous voiding, and they should be asked about daytime (diurnal) voiding frequency and the frequency of nocturia. Patients should also be queried about additional bothersome lower urinary tract symptoms, including urgency, incontinence, or urinary retention. Table 47-5 lists some of the common clinical manifestations of urinary tract disorders. Changes in the colour and the appearance of urine are often significant and should be evaluated. If blood is visible in the urine, it should be determined whether it occurs at the beginning, throughout, or at the end of urination.

Bowel function should also be investigated. Problems with fecal incontinence may signal neurological causes of bladder problems because of shared nerve pathways. Constipation and fecal impaction can partially obstruct the urethra, causing inadequate bladder emptying, overflow incontinence, and infection.

The nurse should find out patients' methods of handling a urinary problem. A patient may already be using a catheter or collection device. Sometimes a patient has to assume a particular position to urinate or must perform such manoeuvres as pressing on the lower abdomen (Credé method), straining (Valsalva manoeuvre), or stretching the rectum to empty the bladder.

Activity Assessment. The patient's level of activity should be assessed. A sedentary person is more likely than an active individual to have stasis of urine, which can predispose to infection and calculi. Demineralization of bones in a person with limited physical activity causes increased urine calcium precipitation.

An active person may find that increasing activity aggravates a urinary problem. A patient who has had prostate surgery or who has weakened pelvic floor muscles may leak urine when attempting particular activities such as running. Some men may develop chronic inflammatory prostatitis or epididymitis after heavy lifting or long-distance driving.

Nocturia is a common and a particularly bothersome lower urinary tract symptom that often leads to sleep deprivation, daytime sleepiness, and fatigue. It occurs in multiple disorders affecting the lower urinary tract, including urinary incontinence, urinary retention, and interstitial cystitis. Nocturia also may be attributable to polyuria from renal disease, poorly controlled diabetes mellitus, alcoholism, excessive fluid intake, or obstructive sleep apnea. When the nurse asks the patient about nocturia, it is helpful to determine whether the desire to urinate is what causes the patient to arise from sleep or whether pain or some

TABLE 47-5	CLINICAL MANIFESTATIONS OF DISORDERS OF THE URINARY SYSTEM

General Manifestations
- Anorexia
- Blurred vision
- Chills
- Change in body weight
- Change in mentation
- Excess thirst
- Fatigue
- Headaches
- Hypertension
- Itching
- Nausea and vomiting

- Incontinence
- Nocturia
- Overactive bladder
- Retention
- Stress incontinence
- Urgency

Urinary System Symptoms
Pain
- Dysuria
- Flank or costovertebral angle
- Groin
- Suprapubic

Changes in Patterns of Urination
- Change in stream
- Dribbling
- Dysuria
- Frequency
- Hesitancy of stream

Changes in Urine Output
- Anuria
- Oliguria
- Polyuria

Changes in Urine Composition
- Colour (red, brown, yellowish-green)
- Increased concentration
- Dilution
- Hematuria
- Pyuria

Edema
- Anasarca
- Ankle
- Ascites
- Facial (periorbital)
- Sacral

CASE STUDY

Patient Introduction

Source: Jean-Philippe Menard/ Shutterstock .com.

Amal Malcolm is a 28-yr-old man who comes to the emergency department (ED) in acute distress, with complaints of severe abdominal pain. The pain began about 6 hr ago after he finished a 10-mile (16K) run as part of his training for a marathon. He says that the pain has steadily increased, he is nauseated, and his urine is a dark, smoky colour.

Critical Thinking

Throughout this assessment chapter, think about Mr. Malcolm's symptoms with the following questions in mind:

1. What are the possible causes of Mr. Malcolm's abdominal pain, nausea, and urine colour?
2. What would be the priority assessment of Mr. Malcolm?
3. What questions should be asked of Mr. Malcolm?
4. What should be included in the physical assessment? What should be looked for?
5. What diagnostic studies should be ordered?

Mr. Malcolm and his condition will be followed throughout this assessment chapter. See pp. 1152 and 1154 for more information on Mr. Malcolm.

ⓔvolve

Answers available at *http://evolve.elsevier.com/Lewis/medsurg*.

other symptom interrupts sleep and the person urinates as a matter of habit before returning to bed. Up to one episode of nocturia is considered normal in younger adults, and up to two episodes are considered acceptable among adults age 65 years or older. Sleep problems associated with a urinary disorder should be documented. Older adults may awaken several times during the night to urinate and may need to be assured that this may be normal. However, a complete assessment should be made to rule out any problem.

Pain Assessment. Pain is a frequent symptom of urinary tract disease. Types of pain associated with renal and urological problems include dysuria, groin pain, costovertebral pain, and suprapubic pain. If pain is present, the location, the character, and the duration should be assessed. The absence of pain when other urinary symptoms exist is also significant. Many urinary tract tumours are painless in the early stages.

Self-Concept Assessment. Problems associated with the urinary system—such as incontinence, urinary diversion procedures, and chronic fatigue—can result in loss of self-esteem and a negative body image. Sensitive questioning may elicit cues to problems in this area.

Relationship and Sexuality Assessment. Urinary problems can affect many aspects of a person's life, including the ability to work and relationships with others. These factors have important implications for future treatment and management. The nurse must be alert to cues from the patient.

Urinary system problems may be serious enough to cause problems in job-related and social situations. Chronic dialysis therapy often makes regular employment or full-time homemaking difficult. Also, concurrent poor health and negative body image can seriously alter existing roles. The nurse should assess this area to plan appropriate interventions.

The nurse should ask about the effect of a renal or urological problem on the patient's sexual patterns and satisfaction. Problems related to personal hygiene and fatigue can seriously affect a sexual relationship. Although urinary incontinence is not directly associated with sexual dysfunction, it often has a devastating effect on self-esteem and on social and intimate relationships. Counselling of both the patient and the partner may be indicated.

Objective Data
Physical Examination

Inspection. The nurse should assess for changes in the following:

Skin: Pallor, yellow-grey cast, excoriations, changes in turgor, bruises, texture (e.g., rough, dry skin)

Mouth: Stomatitis, ammonia breath odour

Face and extremities: Generalized edema, peripheral edema, bladder distension, masses, enlarged kidneys

Abdomen: Skin changes described earlier, as well as striae, abdominal contour for midline mass in lower abdomen (may indicate urinary retention) or unilateral mass (occasionally observed in adults, indicating enlargement of one or both kidneys from large tumour or polycystic kidney)

Weight: Weight gain secondary to edema; weight loss and muscle wasting in renal failure.

General state of health: Fatigue, lethargy, and diminished alertness

Palpation. The kidneys are posterior organs protected by the abdominal organs, the ribs, and the heavy back muscles. A landmark useful in locating the kidneys is the **costovertebral angle** (CVA) formed by the rib cage and the vertebral column. The normal-sized left kidney is rarely palpable because the spleen lies directly on top of it. On occasion, the lower pole of the right kidney is palpable.

To palpate the right kidney, the examiner's left hand is placed behind and supports the patient's right side between the rib cage

CASE STUDY

Subjective Data

Source: Jean-Philippe Menard/ Shutterstock .com.

A focused subjective assessment of Amal Malcolm revealed the following information.

Past Medical History: History of one isolated incidence of possible gout 6 yr ago. He stopped drinking alcohol with no further occurrence. Appendectomy 12 yr ago.

Medications: None.

Overall Health Management: Mr. Malcolm states that he is usually healthy. He does not smoke or drink alcohol. He believes he is able to monitor self and maintain healthy lifestyle. He has never experienced this type of pain before. Describes the pain as being sharp and colicky (coming in waves). Rates the pain as 9 on a scale of 0 to 10.

Functional Assessment

Nutrition and Metabolic History: Mr. Malcolm is currently on a high-protein diet as he trains for the marathon. He eats a lot of chicken, beef, and seafood. He drinks milk-based protein shakes and water after exercising but admits that he thinks he does not drink enough to replace fluid loss in perspiration. He drinks coffee for energy but denies eating chocolate or other sweets. He also avoids sodas.

Elimination: He denies any history of difficulty or pain upon urination. No identified constipation or diarrhea. This is the first time he has ever noticed a change of colour in his urine.

Self-Care History: Prides himself in his ability to exercise and run without difficulty.

Coping and Stress Management: Worried that this pain may interfere with his marathon training.

See pp. 1151 and 1154 for more information on Mr. Malcolm.

and the iliac crest (Figure 47-8). The patient's right flank is elevated with the examiner's left hand, and the examiner's right hand is used to palpate deeply for the patient's right kidney. The lower pole of the right kidney may feel like a smooth, rounded mass that descends on inspiration. If the kidney is palpable, its size, contour, and tenderness should be noted. Kidney enlargement is suggestive of neoplasm or other serious renal pathological conditions.

The urinary bladder is normally not palpable unless it is distended with urine. If the bladder is full, it may feel like a smooth, round, firm organ and is sensitive to palpation.

Percussion. Tenderness in the flank area may be detected by fist percussion. This technique is performed by striking the fist (kidney punch) of one hand against the dorsal surface of the other hand, which is placed flat on the patient along the posterior CVA margin. Normally, a firm blow in the flank area should not elicit pain. Tenderness and pain at the CVA may indicate a kidney infection or polycystic kidney disease.

Normally, a bladder is not percussible until it contains at least 150 mL of urine. If the bladder is full, dullness is heard above the symphysis pubis. A distended bladder may be percussed as high as the umbilicus.

Auscultation. The diaphragm of the stethoscope may be used to auscultate over both CVAs and in the upper abdominal quadrants. With this technique, the abdominal aorta and the renal arteries are auscultated for a bruit (an abnormal murmur), which indicates impaired blood flow to the kidneys.

Table 47-6 lists the normal physical assessment findings in the urinary system. Table 47-7 lists common assessment abnormalities of the urinary system. Variations in assessment findings

FIGURE 47-8 Palpating the right kidney. Source: From Brundage, D. J. (1992). *Renal disorders.* St. Louis: Mosby.

TABLE 47-6	EVIDENCE OF NORMAL PHYSICAL FINDINGS

- No costovertebral angle tenderness
- Nonpalpable kidney and bladder
- No palpable masses

may be normal in older adults. Table 47-2 shows the age-related changes in the urinary system and differences in assessment findings. The nurse should use a focused assessment to evaluate the status of previously identified urinary system problems and to monitor for signs of new problems. A focused assessment of the urinary system is presented in the "Focused Assessment: Urinary System" box.

DIAGNOSTIC STUDIES

Table 47-8 lists and describes diagnostic tests common to the urinary system. It is important to conduct appropriate diagnostic tests to locate, understand, and manage urinary problems. The accuracy of the results is influenced by (a) adherence to the proper procedures related to the study and (b) cooperation of the patient in restricting fluids, collecting urine specimens, lying quietly on the examination table, and following other instructions.

For many radiological investigations, a bowel preparation must be used the evening before the study to clear the lower GI tract of feces and flatus. Because the kidneys lie in a retroperitoneal location, the contents of the colon may obstruct visualization of the urinary tract. If a bowel preparation is not properly performed, a test may be unsuccessful and must be rescheduled. Commonly used bowel preparations include enemas, castor oil, magnesium citrate, and bisacodyl (Dulcolax) tablets or suppositories. Some

TABLE 47-7	ASSESSMENT ABNORMALITIES

Urinary System

Finding	Description	Possible Etiology and Significance
Anuria	Technically no urination (24-hr urine output of <100 mL)	Acute renal failure, end-stage renal disease, bilateral ureteral obstruction
Burning on urination	Stinging pain in urethral area	Urethral irritation, urinary tract infection
Dysuria	Painful or difficult urination	Sign of urinary tract infection, interstitial cystitis, and a wide variety of pathological conditions
Enuresis	Involuntary nocturnal urinating	Symptom of lower urinary tract disorder
Frequency	Increased incidence of urinating	Acutely inflamed bladder, retention with overflow, excess fluid intake
Hematuria	Blood in the urine	Cancer of genito-urinary tract, blood dyscrasias, renal disease, urinary tract infection, stones in kidney or ureter, medications (anticoagulants)
Hesitancy	Delay or difficulty in initiating urination	Partial urethral obstruction
Incontinence	Inability to voluntarily control discharge of urine	Neurogenic bladder, bladder infection, injury to external sphincter
Nocturia	Frequency of urination at night	Renal disease with impaired concentrating ability, bladder obstruction, heart failure, diabetes mellitus
		May occur after renal transplantation
Oliguria	Diminished amount of urine in a given time (24-hr urine output of 100–400 mL)	Severe dehydration, shock, transfusion reaction, kidney disease, end-stage renal disease
Pain	Presence of pain over suprapubic area (related to bladder), urethral pain (irritation of bladder neck), flank (CVA) pain	Infection, urinary retention, foreign body in urinary tract, urethritis, pyelonephritis, renal colic or stones
Pneumaturia	Passage of urine containing gas	Fistula connections between bowel and bladder, gas-forming urinary tract infections
Polyuria	Large volume of urine in a given time	Diabetes mellitus, diabetes insipidus, chronic renal failure, diuretics, excess fluid intake
Retention	Inability to urinate, even though bladder contains excessive amount of urine	Urethral stricture or obstruction; neurogenic bladder; postanaesthesia status
		May occur after pelvic surgery, childbirth, catheter removal
Stress incontinence	Involuntary urination with increased pressure (sneezing or coughing)	Weakness of sphincter control
Urgency	Strong desire to urinate	Inflammatory lesions in bladder or urethra, acute bacterial infections

CVA, costovertebral angle.

FOCUSED ASSESSMENT
Urinary System

Use this checklist to ensure that the key assessment steps have been performed.

Subjective
Ask the patient about experiencing any of the following, and note responses.

Painful urination	Y	N
Changes in colour of urine (blood, cloudy)	Y	N
Change in characteristics of urination (diminished, excessive)	Y	N
Problems with frequent nighttime urination (nocturia)	Y	N

Objective: Diagnostic
Check the following laboratory results for critical values

Blood urea nitrogen	✓
Serum creatinine	✓
Urinalysis	✓
Urine culture and sensitivity	✓

Objective: Physical Examination
Inspect

Abdomen	
Urinary meatus for inflammation or discharge	✓
Palpate	
Abdomen for bladder distention, masses, or tenderness	✓
Percuss	
Costovertebral angle for tenderness	✓
Auscultate	
Renal arteries for bruits	✓

CASE STUDY
Objective Data: Physical Examination

Source: Jean-Philippe Menard/ Shutterstock .com.

A focused assessment of Amal Malcolm revealed the following information.

Mr. Malcolm is lying on the ED stretcher with his knees bent and drawn to his abdominal area. He appears restless and keeps moving from back to side in an effort to reduce his discomfort. Vital signs as follows: BP 156/70, apical pulse 108, respiratory rate 24, temperature 37.4°C, O₂ saturation 96% on room air. Awake, alert, and oriented ×3. Lungs clear to auscultation. Apical pulse regular. Abdomen nondistended with + bowel sounds in all four quadrants. No rebound tenderness. Positive costovertebral tenderness. Voiding small amounts of dark, smoky urine.

As you continue to read this chapter, consider which diagnostic studies would likely be performed for Mr. Malcolm.

See pp. 1151 and 1152 for more information on Mr. Malcolm.

bowel preparations, such as magnesium citrate and Fleet enema, are contraindicated for use in patients with renal failure—magnesium cannot be excreted by patients with renal failure (see Chapter 49).

When a patient has repeated diagnostic studies on consecutive days, it is important to prevent dehydration. It is not uncommon for a patient to take nothing by mouth (NPO) after midnight, spend all morning in the radiology department, be too tired to eat, sleep all afternoon, and be on NPO status after midnight again because of studies scheduled for the next day. Severe dehydration, especially in a patient who is diabetic or debilitated, or in an older-adult patient, may lead to acute renal failure. The nurse is responsible for ensuring that a patient undergoing diagnostic studies is properly hydrated and given adequate nourishment between studies. The nurse should also check with the health care provider regarding the insulin dose for patients with diabetes who are NPO.

CASE STUDY
Objective Data: Diagnostic Studies

Source: Jean-Philippe Menard/ Shutterstock .com.

The health care provider orders the following initial diagnostic studies for Amal Malcolm:
- CBC, basic metabolic panel (electrolytes, BUN, creatinine)
- Urinalysis, culture if indicated
- Renal ultrasound

Although Mr. Malcolm's laboratory results are all within normal limits, his renal ultrasound identifies calculi in the left ureter. There is currently no hydronephrosis. The health care provider prescribes parenteral opioids for pain management and admits Mr. Malcolm to a medical unit for further observation.

See pp. 1151 and 1152 for more information on Mr. Malcolm.

Analysis of Urine

Urinalysis. In evaluating disorders of the urinary tract, one of the first studies performed is a **urinalysis** (Table 47-9; see Table 47-8). This test is a general examination of urine for routine and microscopic findings and may establish baseline information, provide information about possible abnormalities, indicate what further studies need to be done, and supply information on the progression of a diagnosed disorder.

For a routine urinalysis, a specimen may be collected at any time of the day. However, it is best to obtain the first specimen urinated in the morning. This concentrated specimen is more likely to contain abnormal constituents if they are present in the urine. The specimen should be examined within 1 hour of urination. If it is not, bacteria multiply rapidly, RBCs hemolyze, casts (moulds of renal tubules) disintegrate, and the urine becomes alkaline as a result of urea-splitting bacteria. If it is not possible to send the specimen to the laboratory immediately, it should be refrigerated. However, to obtain the best results, the nurse should coordinate specimen collection with routine laboratory hours.

Multiple reagent strips (also called *urine dipsticks*) are commonly used by laboratories and in outpatient settings to provide chemical analysis of urine, along with a microscopic interpretation. The results of a urinalysis usually include a description of the appearance, specific gravity (mass and density), pH, glucose, ketones, and protein in the urine and a microscopic examination of urine sediment for white blood cells (WBCs), RBCs, crystals, and casts (see Table 47-9).

Composite Urine Collections. Composite urine specimens are collected over a period that may range from 2 to 24 hours. The purpose of a composite specimen is to examine or measure specific components, such as electrolytes, glucose, protein, 17-ketosteroids, catecholamines, creatinine, and minerals. These specimens may have to be refrigerated, or preservatives may have to be added to the container used for collecting urine.

TABLE 47-8 DIAGNOSTIC STUDIES

Urinary System

Study	Description and Purpose	Nursing Responsibility
Urine Tests		
Urinalysis	This is a general examination of urine for routine and microscopic evaluation, to establish baseline information or provide data to establish a tentative diagnosis and determine whether further tests are to be ordered (see Table 47-9).	Usually the first urinated morning specimen is required, but it may not be appropriate for all diagnostic purposes. Ensure that the specimen is examined within 1 hr of urinating. Wash patient's perineal area if soiled with menses or fecal material.
Creatinine clearance	Creatinine is a waste product of protein breakdown (primarily body muscle mass). Clearance of creatinine by the kidney approximates the GFR. Normal creatinine clearance varies with age and is approximately 20% higher in men than in women. Normal finding is 1.42–2.25 mL/sec (85–135 mL/min).	Collect 24-hr urine specimen. Discard sample from first urination when test is started. Save urine from all subsequent urinations for 24 hr. Instruct patient to urinate at end of 24 hr and add that specimen to collection. Ensure that serum creatinine clearance is determined during 24-hr period.
Urine for culture and sensitivity (C&S) ("clean catch," "midstream")	Test is performed to confirm suspected urinary tract infection and identify causative organisms. Normally, the bladder is sterile, but the urethra contains bacteria and a few WBCs. If specimen is properly collected, stored, and handled, the following can be expected: <10 000 organisms/mL usually indicates no infection; 10 000–100 000/mL is usually not diagnostic, and test may have to be repeated; and >100 000/mL indicates infection.	Use sterile container for collection of urine. Touch only outside of container. For women, separate labia with one hand and clean meatus with other hand, using at least three sponges (saturated with cleansing solution) in a front-to-back motion. For men, retract foreskin (if present) and cleanse glans with at least three cleansing sponges (saturated with cleansing solution). After cleaning, instruct patient to start urinating and then continue voiding in sterile container. (The initial voided urine flushes out most contaminants in the urethra and the perineal area.) Catheterization may be needed if patient is unable to cooperate with this procedure.
Concentration test	Study is an evaluation of renal concentration ability. Concentration is measured from specific gravity readings. Normal finding is 1.020–1.035.	Instruct patient to fast after a given time in evening (in usual procedure). Collect three urine specimens at hourly intervals in morning.
Residual urine	Test is a determination of amount of urine left in bladder after urination. Finding may be abnormal in patients who have problems with bladder enervation, sphincter impairment, BPH, equine syndrome (nerve compression), or urethral strictures. Normal finding is ≤50 mL urine (increases with age).	If residual urine test is ordered, catheterize patient immediately after patient urinates, or use bladder ultrasonography equipment, including portable scanner. If a large amount of residual urine is obtained, health care provider may order catheter to be left in bladder.
Protein dipstick determination (Albustix, Combistix)	Test detects protein (primarily albumin) in urine. Normal finding is grade 0 to trace amounts.	Dip end of stick in urine, and read result by comparison with colour chart on label as directed. Grading is from 0 to 4+. Interpret with caution. A positive result may not indicate significant proteinuria; some medications may produce false-positive readings.
Quantitative test for protein	A 12- or 24-hr collection yields a more accurate indication of the amount of protein in urine. Persistent proteinuria usually indicates glomerular renal disease. Normal finding is <0.15 g/24 hr (<150 mg/24 hr), and protein consists mainly of albumin.	Perform 12- or 24-hr urine collection.
Urine cytology	Test is used to identify changes in cellular structure indicative of malignancy, especially bladder cancer.	Obtain urine and send immediately to laboratory. The first morning specimen should not be used.
Blood Tests		
Bicarbonate (HCO$_3^-$)	Most patients in renal failure have metabolic acidosis and low serum HCO$_3^-$ levels. Normal finding is 21–28 mmol/L.	Explain the test and watch for postpuncture bleeding.
BUN	Test is most commonly used to identify presence of renal problems. Concentration of urea in blood is regulated by rate at which kidney excretes urea. Normal finding is 3.6–7.1 mmol/L.	When interpreting BUN, the nurse should be aware that nonrenal factors (e.g., rapid cell destruction from infections, fever, GI bleeding, trauma, athletic activity and excessive muscle breakdown, corticosteroid therapy) may cause increase in BUN level. A low BUN level could result from overhydration or advanced liver disease.
Creatinine	Study is more reliable than BUN as a determinant of renal function. Creatinine is end product of muscle and protein metabolism and is liberated at a constant rate. Normal values: 53–106 mcmol/L for men, 44–97 mcmol/L for women. Normal finding is 44–133 mcmol/L.	Explain the test and watch for postpuncture bleeding.
Urea-to-creatinine ratio	Normal finding is 10:1.	—
Calcium (Ca^{2+})	Calcium is main mineral in bone and aids in muscle contraction, neurotransmission, and clotting. In renal disease, decreased reabsorption of Ca^{2+} leads to renal osteodystrophy. Normal calcium levels in adults range from 2.25–2.75 mmol/L.	Explain the test and watch for postpuncture bleeding.

Continued

TABLE 47-8   DIAGNOSTIC STUDIES

Urinary System—cont'd

Study	Description and Purpose	Nursing Responsibility
Potassium (K⁺)	Kidneys are responsible for excreting majority of body's potassium. In renal disease, K⁺ determinations are critical because K⁺ is one of the first electrolytes whose levels become abnormal. Highly elevated K⁺ levels (>6 mmol/L) can lead to muscle weakness and cardiac dysrhythmias. Normal values are 3.5–5 mmol/L.	Explain the test and watch for postpuncture bleeding.
Phosphorus	Phosphorus balance is inversely related to Ca²⁺ balance. In renal disease, phosphorus levels are elevated because the kidney is the primary excretory organ. Normal values are 0.97–1.45 mmol/L.	Explain the test and watch for postpuncture bleeding.
Sodium (Na⁺)	Sodium is the main extracellular electrolyte determining blood volume. Values usually stay within normal range until late stages of renal failure. Normal finding is 135–145 mmol/L.	Explain the test and watch for postpuncture bleeding.
Uric acid	Study is used as a screening test primarily for disorders of purine metabolism but can indicate kidney disease as well. Values depend on renal function and rate of purine metabolism and dietary intake of food rich in purines. Normal findings are 160–430 mcmol/L for women and 340–501 mcmol/L for men.	Explain the test and watch for postpuncture bleeding.

Radiological Procedures

Kidneys, ureters, bladder (KUB)	Study involves radiographic examination of abdomen and pelvis and delineates size, shape, and position of kidneys.	Perform bowel preparation (if ordered).
Intravenous pyelography (IVP)	Radiographic examination visualizes urinary tract after IV injection of contrast material.	Assess renal function. If BUN and creatinine levels are elevated, use of contrast dye in diagnostic procedure may not be safe. Evening before procedure, administer cathartic or enema to empty colon of feces and gas. Keep patient on NPO status 8 hr before procedure. Before procedure, assess patient for iodine sensitivity to avoid anaphylactic reaction. Inform patient that procedure involves lying on table and having serial radiographs taken. After procedure, encourage fluids (if permitted) to flush out contrast material.
Nephro-tomography	Radiograph is performed with rotating tubes. Test delineates segments of the kidney at different levels. Multiple exposures are obtained to visualize specific sections of the kidney after IV injection of contrast material.	Explain the procedure and prepare the patient as for IVP.
Retrograde pyelography	Radiograph of urinary tract is performed after injection of contrast material into kidneys. Cystoscope is inserted, and ureteral catheters are inserted through it into renal pelvis. Contrast material is injected through catheters.	Prepare patient as for IVP. Inform patient that pain may be experienced from distension of pelvis and discomfort from cystoscope. Inform patient that anaesthetic may be administered for procedure.
Renal arteriography (angiography)	Study helps visualize renal blood vessels. Contrast material is injected into renal artery via catheter inserted into femoral artery.	Prepare patient evening before procedure by administering cathartic or enema. Before injection of contrast material, test for iodine sensitivity. After procedure, check insertion site for bleeding, and measure peripheral pulses in involved leg every 30–60 min to detect occluded blood flow, if any.
Renal ultrasonography	Small external ultrasound probe is placed on patient's skin. Conductive gel is applied to the skin. Noninvasive procedure involves passing sound waves into body structures and recording images as the waves are reflected back. Computer interprets tissue density on the basis of sound waves and displays it in picture form. Study is most valuable in detection of renal or perirenal masses and in differential diagnosis of renal cysts, solid masses, and identification of obstructions. It can be used safely in patients with renal failure.	Explain procedure to patient.
CT	Study provides excellent visualization of kidneys. Kidney size can be evaluated; tumours, abscesses, suprarenal masses (e.g., adrenal tumours, pheochromocytomas), and obstructions can be detected. Advantage of CT over ultrasonography is its ability to distinguish subtle differences in density. Use of IV-administered contrast media during CT accentuates density of renal tissue and helps differentiate masses.	Explain procedure to patient and ask patient about iodine sensitivity before injection of contrast material.

TABLE 47-8 DIAGNOSTIC STUDIES

Urinary System—cont'd

Study	Description and Purpose	Nursing Responsibility
MRI	Computer-generated images rely on radiofrequency waves and alteration in magnetic field. Useful for visualization of kidneys. Not proven useful for detecting urinary calculi or calcified tumours.	Explain procedure to patient. Have patient remove all metal objects. Patients with a history of claustrophobia may need to be sedated.
Cystography	Purpose of study is to visualize bladder and evaluate vesico-ureteral reflux. Contrast material is instilled into bladder via cystoscope or catheter.	Explain procedure to patient. If procedure is performed via cystoscope, follow nursing care related to cystoscopy.
Renal Radionuclide Imaging		
Renal scan	Purpose of scan is to show blood flow, glomerular filtration, tubular function, and excretion. Radioactive isotopes are injected by IV route. Radiation detector probes are placed over kidney, and scintillation counter monitors radioactive material in kidney. Radioisotope distribution in kidney is scanned and mapped. Test is useful in showing location, size, and shape of kidney and, in general, assessing blood perfusion and kidney's ability to secrete urine. Abscesses, cysts, and tumours may appear as cold spots because of presence of nonfunctioning tissue.	Requires no dietary or activity restriction. Inform patient that no pain or discomfort should be felt during test.
Surgical Study		
Renal biopsy	Purpose is to obtain renal tissue for examination to determine type of renal disease or to monitor progress of renal disease. This technique is usually performed percutaneously (skin biopsy) through needle insertion into lower lobe of kidney. Can be guided by CT or ultrasonography.	Before procedure, ascertain coagulation status through patient's history, medication history, CBC, hematocrit, prothrombin time, and bleeding and clotting times. Type and crossmatch for blood. Ensure consent form is signed. After procedure, apply pressure dressing to biopsy site and check frequently for bleeding. Measure vital signs frequently. Observe urine for gross bleeding. Determine microscopic bleeding by use of dipstick. Assess patient for flank pain. Monitor hematocrit levels.
Endoscopy		
Cystoscopy	Study involves use of tubular lighted cystoscope to inspect bladder. Lithotomy position is used. Study may be performed while patient receives local or general anaesthesia, depending on needs and condition of patient.	Before procedure, force fluids or administer IV fluids if general anaesthesia is to be used. Ensure that consent form is signed. Explain procedure to patient. Administer preoperative medication. After procedure, explain that burning on urination, pink-tinged urine, and urinary frequency are expected effects after cystoscopy. Do not let patient walk alone immediately after procedure because orthostatic hypotension may occur. Offer warm sitz baths, heat, and mild analgesics to relieve discomfort.
Urodynamics Testing		
Cystometrography	Purpose of study is to evaluate bladder tone, sensations of filling, and bladder (detrusor) stability. Study involves insertion of catheter and instillation of water or saline solution into bladder. Measurements of pressure exerted against bladder wall are recorded.	Explain procedure to patient and observe patient for manifestations of urinary infection after procedure.

BPH, benign prostatic hyperplasia; *BUN*, blood urea nitrogen; *CBC*, complete blood cell count; *CT*, computed tomographic (scan); *GFR*, glomerular filtration rate; *eGFR*, estimated glomerular filtration rate; *GI*, gastro-intestinal; *IV*, intravenous; *MRI*, magnetic resonance imaging; *NPO*, nothing by mouth; *WBC*, white blood cell.

For collection of a composite urine specimen, the patient is instructed to urinate and discard this first urine specimen. This time is noted as the start of the test. All urine from subsequent urinations is saved in a container for the designated period. Finally, at the end of the period, the patient is asked to urinate, and this urine sample is added to the container. Incomplete collections do not provide valid results. Reminding the patient to save all urine during the study period is critical.

Creatinine Clearance. One of the most common composite indicators used to analyze urinary system disorders is creatinine clearance. Creatinine is a waste product produced by protein breakdown (primarily body muscle mass). Urinary excretion of creatinine is a measure of the amount of active muscle tissue in the body, not of body weight; therefore, people with larger muscle mass have higher values. Because almost all creatinine in the blood is normally excreted by the kidneys, creatinine clearance is the most accurate indicator of renal function. The result of a creatinine clearance test closely approximates that of the GFR (National Kidney Foundation, 2016). A blood specimen for serum creatinine determination should be obtained during the period of urine collection.

Creatinine levels remain remarkably constant for each person because they are not significantly affected by protein ingestion, muscular exercise, water intake, or rate of urine production.

TABLE 47-9   URINALYSIS FINDINGS

Evaluation	Normal Finding	Abnormal Findings and Significance
Colour	Amber yellow	Dark, smoky colour suggests hematuria. Yellow-brown to olive green indicates excessive bilirubin. Cloudiness of freshly voided urine indicates infection. Colourless urine indicates excessive fluid intake, renal disease, or diabetes insipidus.
Smell	Aromatic	After urine has been standing, smell becomes more ammonia-like. In urinary tract infections, urine smells unpleasant.
Protein	<0.15 g/day	Persistent proteinuria is characteristic of acute and chronic renal disease, especially involving glomeruli. In absence of disease, positive reading may be caused by high-protein diet, strenuous exercise, dehydration, fever, or emotional stress. Vaginal secretions may contaminate urine specimen and produce positive reading.
Glucose	None	Glycosuria indicates diabetes mellitus or low renal threshold for glucose reabsorption (if blood glucose level is normal). Small amounts may be found after glucose loading (e.g., glucose tolerance test).
Ketones	None	Altered carbohydrate and fat metabolism indicates diabetes mellitus and starvation. Findings can also occur in dehydration, vomiting, and severe diarrhea.
Bilirubin	None	Bilirubinuria is as significant as jaundice in detection of liver disorders. Bilirubin may appear in urine before jaundice becomes visible or may be present in persons with hepatic disorders who do not have recognizable jaundice.*
Specific gravity	1.005–1.030 Maximum concentrating ability of kidney (1.025–1.030)	*Low:* dilute urine and possibly excessive diuresis. *High:* dehydration. *Fixed at about 1.010:* kidneys are unable to concentrate urine, which suggests that kidneys are progressing to end-stage renal disease.
Osmolality (random specimen)	50–1200 mmol/kg	Measurement of osmolality is more accurate than measurement of specific gravity for determining diluting and concentrating ability of kidneys. Deviations from normal indicate tubular dysfunction. Findings indicate whether kidney has lost ability to concentrate or dilute urine. (Not part of routine urinalysis.)
pH	4.6–8.0 (average, 6.0)	A pH of >8.0 may be the result of standing of urine or urinary tract infection because bacteria decompose urea to form ammonia. A pH of <4.0 may indicate respiratory or metabolic acidosis.
RBC	0–4/hpf	Bleeding in urinary tract is caused by calculi, cystitis, neoplasm, glomerulo-nephritis, tuberculosis, kidney biopsy, or trauma.
WBC	0–5/hpf	Increased number of WBCs in urine (pyuria) indicates urinary tract infection or inflammation.
Casts	None; occasional hyaline casts	Casts are moulds of the renal tubules and may contain protein, WBCs, RBCs, or bacteria. Noncellular casts are hyaline in appearance, and a few may be found in normal urine. Casts indicate renal dysfunction or upper urinary tract infection.
Culture for organisms	No organisms in bladder; count of <10^5 CFU/L organisms/mL is result of normal urethral flora	Bacteria counts >10^8 CFU/L indicate urinary tract infection. Organisms most commonly found in urinary tract infections are *Escherichia coli, enterococci, Klebsiella* species, *Proteus* species, and *streptococci*.

CFU, colony-forming unit; *hpf*, high-powered field (or what can be seen in one view of the slide through the microscope); *RBC*, red blood cells; *WBC*, white blood cells.
*See Chapter 46 for further discussion.

Normal creatinine clearance values range from 1.42 to 2.25 mL/sec (85–135 mL/min). After age 40, the creatinine clearance rate decreases at a rate of about 1 mL/min/yr.

Urine Cytology. Urine can be checked for abnormal cellular structures that occur with bladder cancer. Specimens may be obtained from voiding, catheterization, or bladder irrigation (bladder washing). The first morning's voided specimen should not be used because epithelial cells may change in appearance in urine held in the bladder overnight. As with urinalysis, the specimen should be fresh or brought to the laboratory within the hour. An alcohol-based fixative is then added to preserve the cellular structure. Urine cytological study is used for detection and monitoring the prognosis of bladder cancer.

Radiological Studies

Diagnostic urine studies are summarized in Table 47-8.

Kidney, Ureter, and Bladder Radiography. The kidney, ureter, and bladder (KUB) radiograph is an abdominal view obtained without use of a contrast medium to show the renal outline, the psoas shadow, and the full bladder. Radiopaque stones and foreign bodies can be seen on this radiograph. The form, the size, and the position of the kidneys can also be seen. Abscesses, tumours, and cysts may distort anatomical relationships on the KUB image. Sometimes nephrotomography (sectional views that focus on a single plane of the kidney) is ordered at the same time as the KUB study to maximize visualization of the kidneys.

Intravenous Pyelography. Intravenous pyelography (IVP), or excretory urography, enables visualization of the urinary tract. The presence, the position, the size, and the shape of the kidneys, the ureters, and the bladder can be evaluated. Cysts, tumours, lesions, and obstructions cause a distortion in the normal appearance of these structures.

The procedure consists of injecting an IV dose of contrast material, which circulates in the blood and is excreted by the kidneys into the urine. As with all contrast studies, possible iodine and shellfish allergies should be determined before the study. During injection, the patient may experience sensations of warmth, facial flushing, and a salty taste. After injection, radiographs are taken sequentially. The sequencing of images is planned so that contrast excretion can be followed from the cortex of the kidney to the bladder. The presence of bladder atony or outlet obstruction also can be detected by an image obtained after urination, which shows the residual volume of urine in the bladder.

Patients with significantly decreased renal function should not undergo IVP because the contrast material is not properly excreted by the kidneys. Contrast medium can also be nephrotoxic and can worsen renal function.

Retrograde Pyelography. Retrograde pyelography is the radiographic visualization of the kidneys, the ureter, and the bladder after direct injection of contrast material into the kidney via a ureteral catheter introduced through a cystoscope. It may be performed if the urinary tract cannot be visualized using IVP or if the patient is allergic to IV contrast material or has decreased renal function. The risks associated with retrograde pyelography are similar to those related to cystoscopy, including the risk for infection and the use of anaesthetics.

Antegrade Pyelography. Antegrade pyelography is performed to evaluate the upper urinary tract when the patient has an allergy to contrast media, when renal function is decreased, or when abnormalities prevent passage of a ureteral catheter. Contrast media may be injected percutaneously into the renal pelvis or via a nephrostomy tube that is already in place (this method is also called *nephrostography*) when tube function or ureteral integrity must be determined after trauma or surgery. Complications of antegrade pyelography include hematuria, infection, and hematoma.

Renal Ultrasonography. Renal ultrasonography uses high-frequency sound waves to image the kidneys, the ureter, and the bladder. Because radiation exposure is avoided, a number of images can be obtained, and studies can be repeated over a brief period. Images can be obtained with the patient in both the prone and the supine positions. A bowel preparation is not required for renal ultrasonography.

Computed Tomography. Computed tomographic (CT) scan of the abdomen and the pelvis may be performed to detect tumours and possible metastases. CT can differentiate these from cysts or abscesses. Contrast material may be used to help visualize urinary structures more clearly in the computer-generated images. The patient is instructed to lie very still during the procedure while the machine takes precise transaxial images. Sedation may be required if the patient is unable to cooperate.

Renal Arteriography. The purpose of renal arteriography (angiography) is to visualize the renal blood vessels. In this radiological study, contrast material is injected into the renal artery via a catheter inserted into the femoral artery. The findings in arteriography can assist in diagnosing renal artery stenosis (Figure 47-9), additional or missing renal blood vessels, and renovascular hypertension and can assist in differentiating between a renal cyst and a renal tumour. Renal arteriography is also included in the workup of a potential renal transplant donor.

The patient is given a local anaesthetic at the site of catheter insertion. Usually, a catheter is inserted into the femoral artery and passed up the aorta to the level of the renal arteries (Figure 47-10). Contrast media is then injected to outline the renal blood supply, and radiographic images are taken.

The patient may experience a transient warm feeling along the course of the blood vessel when the contrast material is injected. After the catheter is removed, a pressure dressing is placed over the femoral injection site. It is important to observe the site for bleeding. Usually, bed rest with the affected leg kept straight is prescribed. Peripheral pulses in the involved leg should be measured at least every 30 to 60 minutes to detect occlusion of blood flow caused by a thrombus, if any. Complications that may result from renal arteriography include thrombus, embolus, local inflammation, and hematoma. Patients with baseline renal

FIGURE 47-9 Renal arteriogram showing stenosis *(arrow)* of the right renal artery. Source: From Brundage, D. J. (1992). *Renal disorders.* St. Louis: Mosby.

FIGURE 47-10 Diagram of catheter insertion for renal arteriography.

insufficiency may experience a decrease in renal function secondary to the nephrotoxic contrast material.

Cystography. The purpose of cystography is to outline and visualize the bladder and evaluate the UVJ for reflux. In addition to suspected vesico-ureteral reflux, indications for cystography include a neurogenic bladder and recurrent urinary tract infections. Cystography can also delineate abnormalities of the bladder, such as diverticula, calculi, and tumours. In this procedure, a contrast material is instilled via a cystoscope or catheter into the bladder.

Voiding cysto-urethrography (VCUG) is a voiding study of the bladder opening (bladder neck) and urethra. The bladder is filled with contrast material. During urination, images are obtained to visualize the bladder and the urethra. After urination, another image is obtained to assess for residual urine. VCUG can detect abnormalities of the lower urinary tract, urethral stenosis, bladder neck obstruction, and prostatic enlargement (Rosier, Kuo, de Gennaro, et al., 2013).

Urethrography. Urethrography is similar to cystography. Contrast material is injected in a retrograde manner into the urethra to identify strictures, diverticula, or other urethral pathological conditions. When urethral trauma is suspected, urethrography is performed before catheterization.

Loopography. Loopography is used to detect obstructions, anastomotic leaks, stones, reflux, and other uropathological features when a patient has a urinary pouch or ileal conduit. Because urinary diversions are created with sections of bowel, contrast absorption is a risk. The patient should be closely monitored for reactions to the contrast media.

Renal Radionuclide Imaging. Renal scans involving the use of radionuclides are useful in evaluating the anatomical structures, perfusion, and function of the kidneys. The results reveal the difference between the two kidneys in regard to blood flow, tubular function, and excretion. A normal scan shows symmetrical functioning of both kidneys. Normally, the distribution of activity is recorded throughout the kidneys. A lesion (e.g., a tumour) is indicated by the absence of radioactivity in the involved area and the appearance of the resultant defect on the scan. This study is particularly useful in detecting renal vascular disease, acute renal failure, and upper urinary tract obstruction. It is also useful in monitoring the function of a transplanted kidney.

Renal Biopsy. The purpose of renal biopsy is to obtain renal tissue for examination to establish a diagnosis or to monitor progress of renal disease. Biopsy material can be obtained through open biopsy or closed percutaneous needle biopsy. Open biopsy is rarely performed because it is a surgical procedure that necessitates general anaesthesia. Percutaneous needle biopsy, conducted through needle insertion into the lower lobe of the kidney, is more common.

Absolute contraindications to a percutaneous renal biopsy are bleeding disorders, the presence of a single kidney, and uncontrolled hypertension. Relative contraindications include suspected renal infection, hydronephrosis, and possible vascular lesions. Patients about to undergo biopsy should stop taking acetylsalicylic acid (ASA; Aspirin) or warfarin (Coumadin) before the procedure as advised by their physicians.

In this procedure, the patient lies prone with a pillow or sandbag to elevate the abdomen and the kidneys. The position of the kidney is marked on the body, under guidance with CT, IVP, or ultrasonography. Local anaesthetic is used, and a biopsy needle is inserted into the kidney just below the twelfth rib. The patient is instructed to hold his or her breath while the biopsy specimen is being taken.

After the procedure, a pressure dressing is applied, and the patient is kept prone for 30 to 60 minutes. Usually bed rest is prescribed for 24 hours. Vital signs should be measured every 5 to 10 minutes during the first hour and then, if no problems are noted, with decreasing frequency. The biopsy site should be inspected frequently for bleeding. Serial urine specimens should be assessed for gross and microscopic hematuria. A dipstick can be used to test for bleeding, even when hematuria is not obvious. The physician may order all urine sent for laboratory analysis to detect possible hematuria. The patient should be assessed for flank pain, hypotension, decreasing hematocrit, and temperature elevation and should also be observed for chills, urinary frequency, and dysuria.

Complications of a renal biopsy include renal hemorrhage, hematoma, and infection. Even if no complications occur, the patient should be instructed to avoid lifting heavy objects for 5 to 7 days. The patient should be instructed not to take any anticoagulant drugs until permission is given by the physician who performed the biopsy.

Endoscopy

Cystoscopy. Cystoscopy is a radiological bladder procedure in which contrast material is instilled into the bladder. The main purpose is to inspect the interior of the bladder and evaluate the vesico-ureteral reflux with a tubular lighted endoscope called a *cystoscope* (Figure 47-11).

Cystoscopes can be used to insert ureteral catheters, remove calculi, obtain biopsy specimens of bladder lesions, and treat bleeding lesions. In most cases, bladder disorders can be determined by cystoscopic examination.

Cystoscopy is usually performed in a cystoscopy room in the radiology department, in a urology clinic, or in the operating room. Most of the pain associated with cystoscopy results from spasms and contractions of bladder and sphincter. Some of the bladder and sphincter spasms may be alleviated if the patient uses relaxation and deep breathing. A local anaesthetic is instilled into the urethra before cystoscope insertion. During the examination, saline solution is instilled slowly to distend the bladder. This improves visualization but causes an urge to urinate.

After the procedure, the patient can expect to have some burning on urination, blood-tinged urine, and urinary frequency from the irritation of cystoscope insertion and manipulation. The nurse should observe for bright red bleeding, which is not normal. After the procedure, the nurse is responsible for keeping the patient well hydrated, administering mild analgesics, providing sitz baths, and applying heat to decrease the patient's discomfort. Complications that may result from cystoscopy include urinary retention, urinary tract hemorrhage, bladder infection, and perforation of the bladder.

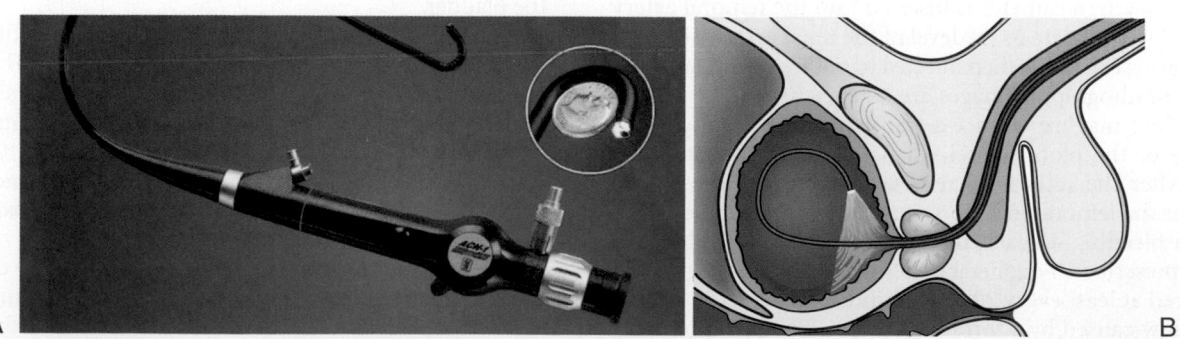

FIGURE 47-11 Cystoscopic examination of the bladder. **A,** Flexible cystonephroscope. **B,** Illustration of nephroscope inserted into male bladder. Source: Courtesy Circon Corp, Santa Barbara, California.

Urodynamics Testing

Urodynamics testing is a set of studies designed to measure urinary tract function. Urodynamic tests entail study of the storage of urine within the bladder and the flow of urine through the urinary tract to the outside of the body. A combination of techniques may be used to provide a detailed assessment of urinary incontinence.

Urinary Flow Study. The urinary flow study (uroflow) entails measurement of urine volume in a single voiding, expelled in a specified time and expressed in millilitres per second. As the patient voids, the stream pattern is depicted graphically on a printout.

The patient is asked to start the test with a reasonably full bladder, urinate into a special container, and try to empty the bladder completely. The container generates a graph in which flow rate is compared to time. This test is used to (a) assess the degree of outflow obstruction caused by such conditions as benign prostatic hyperplasia or stricture; (b) assess bladder or sphincter dysfunction effects on voiding such as occurs with neuropathological conditions; and (c) evaluate the effects of treatment for lower urinary tract problems. Residual urine volume should be measured immediately after a urinary flow study to help identify the degree of chronic urinary retention that is often associated with abnormal flow patterns.

A normal maximum flow rate is about 20 to 25 mL/sec for men and about 25 to 30 mL/sec for women. However, the volume voided and the patient's age can affect the flow rate; thus variations are normal and common. Graphic displays can illustrate straining and intermittent flow patterns or other abnormal voiding disorders.

Cystometrography. **Cystometrography** is an evaluation of the compliance (elastic property) and stability of the detrusor muscle of the bladder, as well as bladder tone, sensations of filling, and bladder (detrusor) instability. It is a measurement of intravesical pressure during the course of bladder filling. Usually, it is ordered if a patient has incontinence or neurogenic bladder. The procedure consists of insertion of a specially designed catheter while the patient is in a supine position. If abdominal pressure is also to be measured, a second tube is inserted into the rectum or the vagina. This tube is typically attached to a small, fluid-filled balloon to allow pressure recording. Saline or sterile water for irrigation, or contrast used for cystography, is infused into the bladder, and pressures are measured. During the infusion, the patient is asked about sensations of bladder filling, usually including the first urge to urinate, a strong urge to urinate, and perception of bladder fullness.

Sphincter Electromyography. In electromyography (EMG), the electrical activity created when the nervous system stimulates motor units within a muscle is recorded. Through the placement of needles, percutaneous wires, or patches near the urethra, the pelvic floor muscle activity can be assessed. During filling cystometrography, sphincter EMG is used to identify voluntary pelvic floor muscle contractions and the response of these muscles to bladder filling, coughing, and other provocative manoeuvres.

Voiding Pressure Flow Study. The voiding pressure flow study combines a urinary flow rate, cystometric pressures (intravesical, abdominal, and detrusor pressures), and a sphincter EMG for detailed evaluation of micturition. It is completed by assisting the patient to a specialized toilet and allowing him or her to urinate while the various pressure tubes and EMG apparatus remain in place.

Video-Urodynamics Testing. Video-urodynamics testing is a combination of the filling cystometrography, sphincter EMG, or urinary flow study (or both of the latter tests) with anatomical imaging of the lower urinary tract, typically via fluoroscopy. This combination is used in selected cases to identify an obstructive lesion and characterize anatomical changes in the bladder and lower urinary tract.

Radionuclide Cystography. Radionuclide cystography is used to detect and grade vesico-ureteral reflux. Similar to VCUG, a small dose of radioisotope tracer is instilled into the bladder via urethral catheter. The procedure is more sensitive than VCUG, and the radiation dose is one-thousandth that used in VCUG.

Whitaker Test. Whitaker test is used to measure the pressure differential between the renal pelvis and the bladder. The presence of a ureteral obstruction can be assessed. Percutaneous access to the renal pelvis is achieved by placement of a catheter in the renal pelvis. A catheter is also placed in the bladder. Fluid is perfused through the percutaneous tube or needle at a rate of 10 mL/min. Pressure data are then collected. These pressure measurements are studied in combination with fluoroscopic imaging to identify the level of obstruction.

■ REVIEW QUESTIONS

The number of the question corresponds to the same-numbered objective at the beginning of the chapter.

1. Which of the following is affected by a renal stone in the pelvis of the kidney?
   a. The structural support of the kidney
   b. Regulation of the concentration of urine
   c. The entry and exit of blood vessels at the kidney
   d. Collection and drainage of urine from the kidney
2. A client with renal disease has oliguria and a creatinine clearance rate of 40 mL/min. Which of the following functions of the kidney is most directly implicated in these abnormal findings?
   a. Tubular secretion
   b. Glomerular filtration
   c. Capillary permeability
   d. Concentration of filtrate
3. Which of the following conditions might place a client at risk for urinary calculi?
   a. Adrenal insufficiency
   b. Serotonin deficiency
   c. Hyperaldosteronism
   d. Hyperparathyroidism
4. Which of the following are normal changes associated with aging of the urinary system that the nurse would assess in an older adult?
   a. Decreased levels of blood urea nitrogen
   b. Postvoiding residual urine
   c. Increased bladder capacity
   d. More easily palpable kidneys

5. Which of the following does the nurse undertake during physical assessment of the urinary system?
   a. Percussion of the flank area with a firm blow
   b. Palpation of an empty bladder as a small nodule
   c. Prone positioning of the client to palpate the kidneys
   d. Auscultation to determine the level of urine in the bladder
6. Which of the following are normal findings, expected by the nurse on physical assessment of the urinary system? *(Select all that apply)*
   a. Nonpalpable left kidney
   b. Auscultation of renal artery bruit
   c. CVA tenderness elicited by a kidney punch
   d. No CVA tenderness elicited by a kidney punch
   e. Palpable bladder to the level of the symphysis pubis
7. Which of the following is an important nursing responsibility after IVP?
   a. Assessment of the client for flank pain
   b. Encouragement of extra oral fluid intake

c. Observation of urine for remaining contrast material
d. Encouragement of ambulation 2 to 3 hours after the study

8. Which of the following would the nurse expect to find on reading the urinalysis results of a dehydrated client?
   a. A pH of 8.4
   b. RBC measurement of 4 per high-powered field
   c. Colour and appearance: yellow, cloudy
   d. Specific gravity of 1.035

1. d; 2. b; 3. d; 4. b; 5. a; 6. a, d; 7. b; 8. d.

⊖volve

For even more review questions, visit *http://evolve.elsevier.com/Canada/Lewis/medsurg*.

REFERENCES

Eriksson, I., Olofsson, B., Gustafson, Y., et al. (2014). Older women's experiences of suffering from urinary tract infections. *Journal of Clinical Nursing, 23*(9-10), 1385–1394. doi:10.1111/jocn.12422.

Grossman, S., & Porth, C. M. (2014). *Essentials of Pathophysiology: Concepts of Altered Health States* (9th ed.). Philadelphia: Lippincott.

McCance, K. L., & Huether, S. E. (2014). *Pathophysiology: The biologic basis for disease in adults and children* (7th ed.). St. Louis: Mosby.

National Kidney Foundation. (2016). *Frequently asked questions about GFR estimates*. Retrieved from *https://www.kidney.org/content/ckd-epi-creatinine-equation-2009*.

Nguyen, T. V., & Goldfarb, D. S. (2012). The older adult patient and kidney function. *The Consultant Pharmacist: The Journal of the American Society of Consultant Pharmacists, 27*(6), 431–444. doi:10.4140/TCP.n.2012.431.

Registered Nurses' Association of Ontario. (2011). *Nursing best practice guidelines: Promoting continence using prompted voiding.* Retrieved from *http://rnao.ca/sites/rnao-ca/files/Promoting_Continence_Using_Prompted_Voiding.pdf*.

Rosier, P. F. W. M., Kuo, H.-C., de Gennaro, M., et al. (2013). Urodynamic Testing. In P. Abrams, L. Cardozo, S. Khoury, et al. (Eds.), *5th International Consultation on Incontinence* (5th ed., pp. 420–506). Paris: International Consultation on Urological Diseases—European Association of Urology.

Smith, H. W. (1953). *Fish to philosopher*. Boston: Little, Brown. (Seminal).

Wagner, K., Johnson, K., & Hardin-Pierce, M. (2014). *High Acuity Nursing* (6th ed.). Englewood Cliffs, NJ: Prentice-Hall.

RESOURCES

Resources for this chapter are listed in Chapters 48 and 49.

Nursing Management
Renal and Urological Problems

Written by: Suzanne Teresa Parsell
Adapted by: Kathleen Rodger and Lynn Jansen

evolve WEBSITE

http://evolve.elsevier.com/Canada/Lewis/medsurg

- Review Questions (Online Only)
- Key Points
- Answer Guidelines for Case Study
- Student Case Studies
  - Bladder Cancer With Urinary Diversion
  - Glomerulo-Nephritis and Acute Kidney Injury

- Customizable Nursing Care Plans
  - Acute Renal Lithiasis
  - Ileal Conduit
  - Urinary Tract Infection
- Conceptual Care Map Creator
- Audio Glossary
- Content Updates

LEARNING OBJECTIVES

1. Describe the pathophysiology, clinical manifestations, collaborative care, and drug therapy of cystitis, urethritis, and pyelonephritis.
2. Explain the nursing management of urinary tract infections.
3. Describe the immunological mechanisms involved in glomerulo-nephritis.
4. Explain the clinical manifestations and the nursing and collaborative management of acute poststreptococcal glomerulo-nephritis, Goodpasture's syndrome, and chronic glomerulo-nephritis.
5. Describe the common causes, clinical manifestations, collaborative care, and nursing management of nephrotic syndrome.
6. Compare and contrast the etiology, clinical manifestations, collaborative care, and nursing management of various types of urinary calculi.

7. Explain the common causes and management of renal trauma, renal vascular problems, and hereditary renal problems.
8. Describe the mechanisms of renal involvement in metabolic and connective tissue disorders.
9. Describe the clinical manifestations and collaborative care of kidney and bladder cancers.
10. Describe the common causes and management of bladder dysfunctions.
11. Differentiate among ureteral, suprapubic, nephrostomy, and urethral catheters with regard to indications for use and nursing responsibilities.
12. Explain the nursing and collaborative management of the patient undergoing nephrectomy or urinary diversion surgery.

KEY TERMS

calculus, p. 1176
cystitis, p. 1164
glomerulo-nephritis, p. 1172
Goodpasture's syndrome, p. 1173
hydronephrosis, p. 1175

hydroureter, p. 1175
ileal conduit, p. 1194
interstitial cystitis (IC), p. 1170
lithotripsy, p. 1178
nephrolithiasis, p. 1176
nephrosclerosis, p. 1181

nephrotic syndrome, p. 1174
polycystic kidney disease (PKD), p. 1182
pyelonephritis, p. 1164
renal artery stenosis, p. 1181
renal vein thrombosis, p. 1181

stricture, p. 1180
urethritis, p. 1164
urinary incontinence (UI), p. 1186
urinary retention, p. 1186

Renal and urological disorders encompass a wide spectrum of clinical problems. The diverse causes of these disorders may involve infectious, immunological, obstructive, metabolic, collagen-related and vascular, traumatic, congenital, neoplastic, and neurological mechanisms. This chapter discusses specific disorders of the kidneys, ureters, bladder, and urethra. Acute kidney injury and chronic kidney disease are discussed in Chapter 49. Female reproductive problems are discussed in Chapter 56. Male reproductive problems are discussed in Chapter 57.

INFECTIOUS AND INFLAMMATORY DISORDERS OF THE URINARY SYSTEM

URINARY TRACT INFECTION

Urinary tract infections (UTIs) are the most common bacterial infection in women. During their lifetime, more than half of women will have a UTI (Al-Badr & Al-Shaikh, 2013), and up to 50% of these will have another infection within a year

TABLE 48-1	COMMON MICRO-ORGANISMS CAUSING URINARY TRACT INFECTIONS
• *Escherichia coli** • *Candida* • *Enterobacter* • *Enterococcus* • *Klebsiella*	• *Proteus* • *Pseudomonas* • *Serratia* • *Staphylococcus*

*Causes about 80% of infections in persons who do not have urinary tract structural abnormalities or calculi.

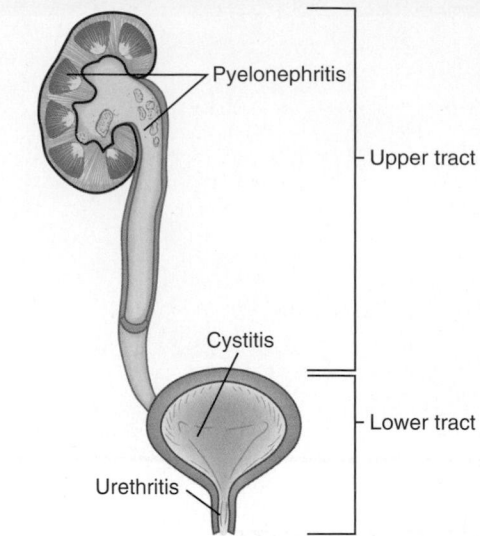

FIGURE 48-1 Sites of infectious processes in the urinary tract.

(Zak, 2014). In the older-adult population, the prevalence of UTI varies from 30% to 50% in women and 25% to 40% in men. In some cases, patients who develop Gram-negative bacteremia die, and one-third of these cases are caused by bacterial infections originating in the urinary tract (National Institute of Diabetes and Digestive and Kidney Diseases [NIDDK], 2017).

Inflammation of the urinary tract may be attributable to a variety of disorders, but bacterial infection is by far the most common (Nicolle, 2013). In the majority of healthy persons, the bladder and its contents are free from bacteria. Nevertheless, a number of otherwise healthy individuals, including many young-adult women and older women and men, have some bacteria colonizing the bladder. This condition is called *asymptomatic bacteriuria* and does not warrant treatment. In contrast, an infection of the urinary system is diagnosed when bacterial invasion of the urinary tract occurs. Bacterial counts of 10^5 colony-forming units per millilitre (CFU/mL) or higher typically indicate a clinically significant UTI. However, counts as low as 10^2 to 10^3 CFU/mL in a person with signs and symptoms are indicative of UTI.

Escherichia coli (*E. coli*) (Table 48-1) is the most common pathogen leading to a UTI. Although fungal and parasitic infections may also cause UTIs, they are uncommon. UTIs from these causes are sometimes observed in immuno-suppressed patients, patients with diabetes mellitus, or patients who have undergone multiple courses of antibiotic therapy. They also may be seen in persons living in or having travelled to certain developing countries. Recurrent UTIs are one of the most common bacterial infections in women. Increased antibiotic resistance may be making treatment and prevention of UTIs difficult (Chisholm, 2015).

Classification

Several classification systems can be used for UTIs (Nicolle, 2013). For example, a UTI can be broadly classified as an upper or a lower UTI according to its location within the urinary system (Figure 48-1). Infection of the upper urinary tract (involving the renal parenchyma, renal pelvis, and ureters) typically causes fever, chills, and flank pain, whereas a UTI confined to the lower urinary tract does not usually have systemic manifestations. Specific terms are used to further delineate the location of a UTI or inflammation. For example, **pyelonephritis** implies inflammation (usually caused by infection) of the renal parenchyma and the collecting system. **Cystitis** indicates an inflammatory condition of the urinary bladder, characterized by pain, urgency and frequency of urination, and hematuria. **Urethritis** means inflammation of the urethra.

Classifying a UTI as complicated or uncomplicated is also useful. *Uncomplicated infections* are those that occur in an otherwise normal urinary tract (Nicolle, 2013). *Complicated infections* include those that occur concurrently with obstruction, stones, or catheters; those that occur in patients with existing diabetes or neurological diseases; and recurrent infections. Patients with a complicated infection are at risk for renal damage.

UTIs can also be classified according to their natural history. An *initial infection* (sometimes called a first or an isolated infection) refers to an uncomplicated UTI in a person who has never had an infection or who experiences one that is remote from any previous UTI (usually separated by a period of years). In contrast, a *recurrent UTI* is a reinfection in a person who experienced a previous infection that was successfully eradicated. A recurrent UTI that occurs because the original infection was not adequately eradicated is classified as unresolved bacteriuria or bacterial persistence. *Unresolved bacteriuria* occurs when bacteria are initially resistant to the antibiotic used to treat an infection, when the antibiotic agent fails to achieve adequate concentrations in the urine or the bloodstream to kill bacteria, or when the antibiotic is discontinued before the underlying bacteriuria is completely eradicated. *Bacterial persistence* also may occur when bacteria develop resistance to the antibiotic agent selected for treatment or when a foreign body in the urinary system serves as a harbour or anchor allowing bacteria to survive despite appropriate therapy.

Etiology and Pathophysiology

The urinary tract above the urethra is normally sterile. Several physiological and mechanical defence mechanisms assist in maintaining sterility and preventing UTIs. These defences include normal voiding with complete emptying of the bladder, normal antibacterial capability of the bladder mucosa and urine, uretero-vesical junction (UVJ) competence, and peristaltic activity that propels urine toward the bladder. An alteration in any of these defence mechanisms increases the risk of contracting a UTI. Table 48-2 lists predisposing factors to UTIs.

The organisms that usually cause UTIs are introduced via the ascending route from the urethra. Other, less common routes are via the bloodstream or the lymphatic system. Most infections are caused by Gram-negative bacilli normally found in the gastro-intestinal (GI) tract, although Gram-positive organisms

TABLE 48-2 PREDISPOSING FACTORS TO URINARY TRACT INFECTIONS

Factors Increasing Urinary Stasis
- Extrinsic obstruction (tumour, fibrosis compressing urinary tract)
- Intrinsic obstruction (stone, tumour of urinary tract)
- Urinary retention (including neurogenic bladder and low bladder-wall compliance)

Foreign Bodies
- In-dwelling catheter
- Ureteral stent (proximity of urethral and anal orifices)
- Urinary calculi

Anatomical Factors
- Congenital defects leading to obstruction or urinary stasis
- Fistula (abnormal opening) exposing urinary stream to skin, vagina, or fecal stream
- Shorter female urethra (proximity of urethral and anal orifices)

Factors Compromising Immune Response
- Diabetes mellitus
- Human immunodeficiency virus infection

Functional Disorders
- Constipation
- Voiding dysfunction with detrusor sphincter dyssynergia

TABLE 48-3 LOWER URINARY TRACT SYMPTOMS

Emptying Symptoms
- Dysuria—difficulty voiding
- Hesitancy—difficulty starting the urine stream, resulting in a delay between initiation of urination by relaxation of the urethral sphincter and the actual start of the urine stream
- Intermittency—interruption of the urinary stream while voiding
- Pain on urination
- Postvoid dribbling—urine loss after completion of voiding
- Urinary retention or incomplete emptying—inability to empty urine from the bladder, which can be caused by atonic bladder or obstruction of the urethra; can be acute or chronic
- Weak urinary stream

Storage Symptoms
- Incontinence—involuntary or unwanted loss or leakage of urine
- Nocturia—waking up two or more times at night because of the need or the urge to void
- Nocturnal enuresis—complaint of loss of urine during sleep; called *bedwetting* in children
- Urgency—a sudden, strong or intense desire to void immediately, usually accompanied by frequency
- Urinary frequency—an abnormally frequent (usually eight times in a 24-hr period) desire to void, often of only small quantities (e.g., <200 mL)

such as streptococci, enterococci, and *Staphylococcus saprophyticus* can also cause urinary infections. A common factor contributing to ascending infection is urological instrumentation (e.g., catheterization, cystoscopic examinations). Instrumentation allows bacteria that are normally present at the opening of the urethra to enter the urethra or the bladder. Sexual intercourse promotes "milking" of bacteria from the vagina and the perineum and may cause minor urethral trauma that predisposes women to UTIs.

Rarely do UTIs result from a hematogenous route, where bloodborne bacteria secondarily invade the kidneys, the ureters, or the bladder from elsewhere in the body. For a kidney infection to occur from hematogenous transmission, there must be prior injury to the urinary tract, such as obstruction of a ureter, damage caused by stones, or renal scars.

An important source of UTIs is health care–acquired, or health care–associated, infection. The cause of health care–associated infection is often *E. coli* and, less frequently, *Pseudomonas* organisms. Urological instrumentation, particularly with an in-dwelling urinary catheter, is the most common predisposing factor.

Clinical Manifestations

Bothersome lower urinary tract symptoms (LUTS) are seen in UTIs of the upper urinary tracts as well as those confined to the lower tract. These symptoms are related to either bladder storage or bladder emptying. These symptoms are defined in Table 48-3.

These symptoms include dysuria, frequency of urination (>q2h), urgency, and suprapubic discomfort or pressure. The urine may contain grossly visible blood (hematuria) or sediment, giving it a cloudy appearance. Flank pain, chills, and the presence of a fever indicate an infection involving the upper urinary tract (pyelonephritis). It is important to remember that these symptoms, considered characteristic of a UTI, are often absent in older adults. Older adults tend to experience nonlocalized abdominal

discomfort rather than dysuria and suprapubic pain (Arinzon, Shabat, Peisakh, et al., 2012). In addition, they may have cognitive impairment, delirium, and falls. Older adults are also less likely to experience a fever with infection of the upper urinary tract. Patients older than age 80 may experience a slight decline in temperature. People with significant bacteriuria may have no symptoms or may have nonspecific symptoms such as fatigue or anorexia.

Multiple factors may produce bothersome LUTS like those that can accompany a UTI. For example, patients with bladder tumours or those receiving intravesical chemotherapy or pelvic radiation usually experience urinary frequency, urgency, and dysuria. Interstitial cystitis, discussed later in this chapter, is a chronic inflammatory condition of unknown etiology also producing bothersome urinary symptoms that sometimes cause it to be confused with a UTI.

Diagnostic Studies

Dipstick urinalysis should be obtained initially to identify the presence of nitrites (indicating bacteriuria), white blood cells (WBCs), and leukocyte esterase (an enzyme present in WBCs). These findings can be confirmed by microscopic urinalysis. Following confirmation of bacteriuria and pyuria, a urine culture may be obtained. A urine culture is indicated in complicated or health care–associated UTIs, persistent bacteria, or frequently recurring UTIs (more than two to three episodes per year). Urine also may be cultured when the infection is unresponsive to empirical therapy or the diagnosis is questionable. A voided midstream technique yielding a clean-catch urine sample is preferred for obtaining a urine culture in most circumstances. (See Chapter 47, Table 47-8, for a description of this technique.) However, a specimen obtained by catheterization or suprapubic needle aspiration provides more accurate results and may be necessary when an adequate clean-catch specimen cannot be readily obtained.

A urine culture is accompanied by *sensitivity testing* to determine the bacteria's susceptibility to a variety of antibiotic drugs. The results of this test allow the health care provider to select an antibiotic known to be capable of destroying the bacterial strain producing a UTI in a specific patient.

Imaging studies of the urinary tract are indicated in select cases. For example, an intravenous pyelogram (IVP) or abdominal computed tomographic (CT) scan may be obtained when obstruction of the urinary system is suspected of causing a UTI.

Collaborative Care and Drug Therapy

Once a UTI has been diagnosed, appropriate antimicrobial therapy is initiated. An antibiotic may be selected based on the health care provider's best judgement (empirical therapy) or the results of sensitivity testing. The collaborative care and drug therapy of cystitis are summarized in Table 48-4. Uncomplicated cystitis can be treated by a short-term course of antibiotics, typically for 1 to 3 days. In contrast, complicated UTIs require longer-term treatment, lasting 7 to 14 days or even longer (Hooton, 2012).

Trimethoprim–sulphamethoxazole (TMP-SMX) or nitrofurantoin is often used empirically to treat uncomplicated or initial UTIs. TMP-SMX has the advantages of being relatively inexpensive and being taken only twice daily. Nitrofurantoin is normally given three to four times daily, but a long-acting preparation (MacroBid) is available that is taken twice daily. Ampicillin or amoxicillin is not frequently selected when empirically treating an uncomplicated UTI because these antibiotics must be administered three to four times daily. In addition to these drugs, the fluoroquinolones (including ciprofloxacin [Cipro], levofloxacin, and norfloxacin) may be used to treat complicated UTIs (Nicolle, 2013). *Prophylactic*, or *suppressive*, *antibiotics* are sometimes administered to patients who experience repeated UTIs.

DRUG ALERT—Nitrofurantoin (MacroBid)
- Avoid sunlight. Use sunscreen, and wear protective clothing.
- Notify health care provider immediately if fever, chills, cough, chest pain, dyspnea, rash, or numbness or tingling of fingers or toes develops.

A low dose of TMP-SMX, nitrofurantoin, or another antibiotic, such as ciprofloxacin, may be administered on a daily basis in an attempt to prevent recurring UTIs, or a single dose may be taken before an event likely to provoke a UTI, such as intercourse. However, although suppressive therapy is often effective on a short-term basis, this strategy is limited because of the risk for antibiotic resistance, ultimately leading to breakthrough infections with increasingly virulent pathogens.

NURSING MANAGEMENT
URINARY TRACT INFECTION

NURSING ASSESSMENT

Subjective and objective data that should be obtained from a patient with a UTI are presented in Table 48-5.

NURSING DIAGNOSES

Nursing diagnoses for the patient with a UTI may include but are not limited to the following:
- *Impaired urinary elimination* related to *multiple causality* (effects of UTI)
- *Readiness for enhanced health management* as evidenced by *expressed desire to enhance management of risk factors*

Additional information on nursing diagnoses for the patient with a UTI is presented in Nursing Care Plan (NCP) 48-1, available on the Evolve website.

TABLE 48-4 COLLABORATIVE CARE

Urinary Tract Infection

Diagnostic
- History and physical examination
- Imaging studies of urinary tract (e.g., IVP, cystoscopy) (if indicated)
- Urinalysis
- Urine for culture and sensitivity (if indicated)

Collaborative Therapy
Uncomplicated UTI
- Adequate fluid intake
- Antibiotic: 1- to 3-day treatment regimen
  - Nitrofurantoin (MacroBid)
  - Trimethoprim–sulphamethoxazole (Septra)
- Counselling about risk for recurrence and reduction of risk factors

Recurrent, Uncomplicated UTI
- Repeated urinalysis and consideration of need for urine culture and sensitivity testing
- Antibiotic: 3- to 5-day treatment regimen
  - Nitrofurantoin (MacroBid)
  - Sensitivity-guided antibiotic (ampicillin, amoxicillin, first-generation cephalosporin, fluoroquinolone)
  - Trimethoprim–sulphamethoxazole (Septra)
- Consideration of 3- to 6-mo trial of suppressive antibiotics
- Adequate fluid intake
- Counselling about risk for recurrence and reduction of risk factors
- Imaging study of urinary tract in select cases

IVP, intravenous pyelogram; *UTI,* urinary tract infection.

TABLE 48-5 NURSING ASSESSMENT

Urinary Tract Infection

Subjective Data
Important Health Information
Past health history: Previous UTIs; urinary calculi, stasis, reflux, strictures, or retention; neurogenic bladder; pregnancy; prostatic hyperplasia; sexually transmitted infection; bladder cancer
Medications: Use of antibiotics, anticholinergics, antispasmodics
Surgery or other treatments: Recent urological instrumentation (catheterization, cystoscopy, surgery)

Symptoms
- Lassitude, malaise
- Nausea, vomiting, and anorexia; chills
- Suprapubic or low back pain, pressure in bladder area, costovertebral tenderness; bladder spasms, dysuria, burning on urination, sense of incomplete emptying
- Urinary frequency, urgency, hesitancy; nocturia

Objective Data
General
Fever

Urinary
Hematuria; cloudy, foul-smelling urine; tender, enlarged kidney

Possible Findings
Leukocytosis; urinalysis positive for bacteria, pyuria, RBCs, and WBCs; positive urine culture; IVP, CT scan, ultrasound, voiding cysto-urethrogram and cystoscopy demonstrating abnormalities of urinary tract

CT, computed tomography; *IVP,* intravenous pyelogram; *RBCs,* red blood cells; *UTI,* urinary tract infection; *WBCs,* white blood cells.

PLANNING

The overall goals are (a) that the patient with a UTI will have relief from bothersome LUTS, (b) prevention of upper urinary tract involvement, and (c) prevention of recurrence.

NURSING IMPLEMENTATION

HEALTH PROMOTION. Health-promotion measures include recognizing individuals who are at risk for a UTI. Debilitated persons, older adults, patients with underlying diseases (e.g., cancer, human immunodeficiency virus [HIV], or diabetes mellitus) that compromise host immune responses, and patients treated with immuno-suppressive drugs or corticosteroids are at high risk for UTIs. Especially for these individuals, health-promotion activities can help decrease the frequency of infections and promote early detection of infection. Health-promotion activities include educating the patient about preventive measures, such as (a) emptying the bladder regularly and completely, (b) evacuating the bowel regularly, (c) wiping the perineal area from front to back after urination and defecation, and (d) drinking an adequate amount of liquid each day. The recommended daily liquid intake for the ambulatory adult is approximately 33 mL/kg of body weight per day. Thus, a 70-kg person would require 2 310 mL each day. The person will obtain approximately 20% of this fluid from food, leaving 1 848 mL, or nearly eight 236-mL glasses of fluid, to be obtained by drinking. Although suppressive antibiotics are not generally recommended, daily intake of cranberry juice (consumed as pure juice, 236 mL twice daily) or cranberry essence tablets may reduce the risk for certain UTIs (Wang, Fang, Chen, et al., 2012) (see the "Evidence-Informed Practice" box). In addition, it is important to advise the patient to seek early treatment once symptoms are identified.

The nurse can play a major role in the prevention of health care–associated infections. Avoidance of unnecessary catheterization and early removal of in-dwelling catheters are the most effective means for reducing health care–associated UTIs. All patients undergoing instrumentation of the urinary tract are at risk of developing a health care–associated UTI. Aseptic technique must always be followed during these procedures. Washing hands before and after contact with each patient and wearing gloves for care involving the urinary system are especially important. When a catheter has been inserted, special measures must be employed, as explained in the section on urethral catheterization later in this chapter.

Routine and thorough perineal hygiene is important for all hospitalized patients, especially when a bedpan is used. Answering the call light quickly or offering the bedpan or urinal at frequent intervals to a bedridden patient should reduce the number of incontinent episodes.

ACUTE INTERVENTION. Acute intervention for a patient with a UTI includes ensuring adequate fluid intake if it is not contraindicated. It is sometimes difficult to get the patient to maintain an adequate fluid intake because the person may think it will worsen the discomfort and frequency associated with a UTI. The patient needs to be told that fluids will increase frequency of urination at first but will also dilute the urine, making the bladder less irritable. Fluids will help flush out bacteria before they have a chance to colonize in the bladder. Caffeine, alcohol, citrus juices, chocolate, and highly spiced foods or beverages should be avoided because they are potential bladder irritants.

Local application of heat to the suprapubic area or lower back may relieve the discomfort associated with a UTI. The

patient can be advised to apply a heating pad (turned to its lowest setting) to these areas. A warm shower can also be effective in providing temporary relief. The patient should be instructed about the prescribed drug therapy, including adverse effects. The nurse should emphasize the importance of taking the full course of antibiotics. Often patients stop antibiotic therapy once symptoms disappear. This practice can lead to inadequate treatment and recurrence of infection or to bacterial resistance to antibiotics. Sometimes a second drug or a reduced dose of drug is ordered after the initial course to suppress bacterial growth in certain patients susceptible to recurrent UTIs. The patient should be advised to watch for any changes in the colour or the consistency of the urine and for a decrease in or cessation of symptoms as a sign of the effectiveness of therapy. The patient should be counselled that persistence of bothersome LUTS beyond the antibiotic treatment course or the onset of flank pain or fever should be reported promptly to a health care provider.

AMBULATORY AND HOME CARE. The nurse's responsibility in ambulatory and home care settings is to work with the patient

---

🔍 EVIDENCE-INFORMED PRACTICE

Research Highlight

Do Cranberry Products Prevent Urinary Tract Infections?

Clinical Question
Among adults and children (P), what is the effect of cranberry-containing products (I) vs. placebo vs. nonplacebo control (C) in preventing urinary tract infections (O)?

Best Available Evidence
Systematic review of randomized controlled trials (RCTs)

Critical Appraisal and Synthesis of Evidence
- Thirteen RCTs ($n = 1616$) of patients at high risk for recurrent urinary tract infections (UTIs), including women, older adults, patients with neuropathic bladder, and pregnant women. Children were also studied.
- Cranberry products were juice, capsules, or tablets given for 6 mo in most cases.
- Cranberry-containing products had a positive effect in preventing symptomatic UTIs.
- These products showed greater effect in women (especially those with recurrent UTIs), children, cranberry juice drinkers, and those taking the products more than twice daily.

Conclusions
- Cranberry-containing products can prevent UTIs.
- Cranberry juice was more effective than cranberry capsules. This difference may be due to increased hydration from the juice.

Implications for Nursing Practice
- Inform patients who are at an increased risk for recurrent UTIs that cranberry products have a protective effect in reducing UTIs.
- Cranberry juice works by preventing the attachment of bacteria to the epithelial cells in the bladder wall.
- Emphasize the importance of adequate fluid intake, including drinking cranberry juice.

Reference for Evidence
Wang, C., Fang, C., Chen, N., et al. (2012). Cranberry-containing products for prevention of urinary tract infections in susceptible populations: A systematic review and meta-analysis of randomized controlled trials. *Archives of Internal Medicine, 172*(13), 988–996.

P, Patient population of interest; *I*, intervention or area of interest; *C*, comparison of interest or comparison group; *O*, outcomes of interest (see Chapter 1).

TABLE 48-6   PATIENT & CAREGIVER TEACHING GUIDE

Urinary Tract Infection

The following information should be included when teaching the patient and caregiver about UTI to prevent recurrence:

1. The patient must take all antibiotics as prescribed. Symptoms may improve after 1 to 2 days of therapy, but organisms may still be present.
2. The patient must be instructed about appropriate hygiene, including the following:
   a. Careful cleansing of perineal region
   b. Wiping from front to back after urinating
   c. Cleansing with soap and water after each bowel movement
3. The patient should be taught about the importance of emptying the bladder before and after intercourse, which may help flush out bacteria introduced during intercourse. The patient should wash the genital area with warm water before having sex.
4. The patient should be advised to urinate regularly, approximately q2–4 hr during the day.
5. The patient should be advised about how to maintain adequate fluid intake (33 mL [1 oz] per kilogram of body weight per day).
6. The patient should understand why harsh soaps, bubble baths, powders, and sprays should not be applied in the perineal area.
7. The patient should be advised to report symptoms or signs of recurrent UTI (e.g., cloudy urine, pain on urination, urgency, frequency).

UTI, urinary tract infection.

FIGURE 48-2 Acute pyelonephritis. Cortical surface shows greyish-white areas of inflammation and abscess formation. Source: Kumar, V., Abbas, A. K., & Aster, J. (2015). *Robbins and Cotran pathologic basis of disease* (9th ed., p. 931, Figure 20-27). Philadelphia: Saunders.

to promote understanding about the need for ongoing care (Table 48-6).

The patient must understand the need for follow-up care with urine culture to determine if the infection has been adequately treated. Recurrent symptoms caused by bacterial persistence or inadequate treatment typically occur within 1 to 2 weeks after completion of therapy. If the patient has been adherent, a relapse indicates the need for further evaluation.

▎EVALUATION

The expected outcomes for the patient with a UTI are presented in NCP 48-1, available on the Evolve website.

ACUTE PYELONEPHRITIS

Etiology and Pathophysiology

Pyelonephritis is an inflammation of the renal parenchyma (Figure 48-2) and collecting system (including the renal pelvis). The most common cause is bacterial infection, but fungi, protozoa, or viruses sometimes infect the kidney (Kumar, Ankur, Wolf, et al., 2015).

Urosepsis is a systemic infection arising from a urological source. Its prompt diagnosis and effective treatment are critical because, unless promptly eradicated, it leads to septic shock and death in 15% of cases. Septic shock is the outcome of unresolved bacteremia involving a Gram-negative organism. (Septic shock is discussed in Chapter 69.)

Pyelonephritis usually begins with colonization and infection of the lower urinary tract via the ascending urethral route. Bacteria normally found in the intestinal tract, such as *E. coli, Proteus, Klebsiella,* or *Enterobacter* species, frequently cause pyelonephritis. A pre-existing factor is often present, such as *vesico-ureteral reflux* (retrograde or backward movement of urine from lower to upper urinary tract) or dysfunction of lower urinary tract function such as obstruction from benign prostatic hyperplasia (BPH), a stricture, or a urinary stone.

Acute pyelonephritis commonly starts in the renal medulla and spreads to the adjacent cortex. Recurring episodes of pyelonephritis, especially in the presence of obstructive abnormalities, can lead to a scarred, poorly functioning kidney and a condition called *chronic pyelonephritis.*

Clinical Manifestations and Diagnostic Studies

The clinical manifestations of acute pyelonephritis vary from mild fatigue to the sudden onset of chills, fever, vomiting, malaise, flank pain, and the bothersome LUTS characteristic of cystitis. *Costovertebral tenderness* is typically present on the affected side. The clinical manifestations usually subside within a few days, even without specific therapy, but bacteriuria and pyuria usually persist.

Urinalysis shows pyuria, bacteriuria, and varying degrees of hematuria. WBC casts may be found in the urine, indicating involvement of the renal parenchyma. A complete blood cell count (CBC) will show leukocytosis and a shift to the left with an increase in immature neutrophils (bands). Urine cultures must be obtained when pyelonephritis is suspected. In patients with more severe illness who are hospitalized, blood cultures are also obtained.

Imaging studies, such as an IVP or CT scan, requiring intravenous injection of contrast materials are usually not obtained in the early stages of pyelonephritis so as to prevent the possible spread of infection. Alternatively, ultrasonography of the urinary system may be obtained to identify anatomical abnormalities or the presence of an obstructing stone and reduce the need for catheterization. Imaging studies are also used to assess for complications of pyelonephritis such as impaired renal function, scarring, chronic pyelonephritis, or abscesses.

Urosepsis is characterized by bacteriuria and bacteremia (presence of bacteria in blood). If bacteremia is a possibility, close observation and monitoring of vital signs are essential. Prompt recognition and treatment of septic shock may prevent irreversible damage or death.

TABLE 48-7 COLLABORATIVE CARE

Acute Pyelonephritis

Diagnostic
- History and physical examination
- Blood culture (if bacteremia is suspected)
- CBC count with WBC differential
- Palpation for flank pain
- Ultrasound (initially), IVP, VCUG, radionuclide imaging, CT scan
- Urinalysis
- Urine for culture and sensitivity

Collaborative Therapy
Mild Symptoms
- Adequate fluid intake
- Follow-up urine culture and imaging studies
- Nonsteroidal anti-inflammatory drugs or antipyretic drugs
- Outpatient management or short hospitalization for IV antibiotics:
  - Empirically selected broad-spectrum antibiotics (ampicillin, vancomycin) combined with an aminoglycoside (e.g., tobramycin, gentamicin)
  - Switch to sensitivity-guided therapy (when results available) for 14–21 days
  - Trimethoprim–sulphamethoxazole (Septra)
  - Fluoroquinolones (e.g., ciprofloxacin [Cipro], norfloxacin)

Severe Symptoms
- Adequate fluid intake (initially parenteral; switched to oral fluids as nausea, vomiting, and dehydration subside)
- Hospitalization
- Nonsteroidal anti-inflammatory or antipyretic drugs to reverse fever and relieve discomfort
- Parenteral antibiotics:
  - Empirically selected broad-spectrum antibiotics (e.g., ampicillin, vancomycin) combined with an aminoglycoside (e.g., tobramycin, gentamicin)
  - Switch to sensitivity-guided antibiotic therapy when results of urine and blood cultures are available
  - Oral antibiotics when patient tolerates oral intake; administer for 7–21 days
- Urinary analgesics (e.g., to relieve bothersome lower urinary tract symptoms)
- Follow-up urine culture and imaging studies

CBC, complete blood count; *CT,* computed tomography; *IV,* intravenous; *IVP,* intravenous pyelogram; *VCUG,* voiding cysto-urethrogram; *WBC,* white blood cell.

Collaborative Care and Drug Therapy

The diagnostic tests and the collaborative therapy of acute pyelonephritis are summarized in Table 48-7. Patients with severe infections or complicating factors, such as nausea and vomiting with dehydration, require hospital admission.

Patients with mild symptoms may be treated on an outpatient basis with antibiotics for 14 to 21 days (see Table 48-7). Parenteral antibiotics are often given initially in the hospital to rapidly establish high serum and urinary drug levels. When initial treatment resolves acute symptoms and the patient is able to tolerate oral fluids and drugs, the person may be discharged on a regimen of oral antibiotics for an additional 14 to 21 days. Symptoms and signs typically improve or resolve within 48 to 72 hours after starting therapy (Grabe, Bartoletti, Bjerklund-Johansen, et al., 2014).

Relapses may be treated with a 6-week course of antibiotics. Reinfections may be treated as individual episodes of disease or managed with long-term antibiotic therapy. Antibiotic prophylaxis may also be used for recurrent infections. The effectiveness of therapy is evaluated in accordance with the presence or absence of bacterial growth on a urine culture.

NURSING MANAGEMENT ACUTE PYELONEPHRITIS

NURSING ASSESSMENT
Subjective and objective data that should be obtained from a patient with pyelonephritis are presented in Table 48-5.

NURSING DIAGNOSES
Nursing diagnoses for a patient with pyelonephritis include but are not limited to those for a patient with a UTI (see NCP 48-1).

PLANNING
The overall goals are that the patient with pyelonephritis will have (a) relief of pain, (b) normal body temperature, (c) no complications, (d) normal renal function, and (e) no recurrence of symptoms.

NURSING IMPLEMENTATION
HEALTH PROMOTION. Health promotion and maintenance measures are similar to those for cystitis (see "Nursing Management: Urinary Tract Infection," earlier in this chapter). In addition, it is important that patients receive early treatment for cystitis to prevent ascending infections. The need for regular medical care should be stressed to patients with structural abnormalities of the urinary tract because these patients are at high risk for infection.

ACUTE INTERVENTION AND HOME CARE. Nursing interventions vary depending on the severity of symptoms. Interventions include teaching and working with the patient to promote understanding about the disease process with emphasis on (a) the need to continue drugs as prescribed, (b) the need for a follow-up urine culture to ensure proper management, and (c) identification of risk for recurrence or relapse (see Table 48-5 and NCP 48-1). In addition to antibiotic therapy, patients should be encouraged to drink at least eight glasses of fluid every day, even after the infection has been treated. Rest is often indicated to increase patient comfort. Patients with frequent relapses or reinfections may be treated with long-term, low-dose antibiotics. Understanding the rationale for therapy is important to enhance patient application of knowledge for disease management.

EVALUATION
The expected outcomes for patients with pyelonephritis are presented in NCP 48-1, available on the Evolve website.

CHRONIC PYELONEPHRITIS

Chronic pyelonephritis is a term used to describe a kidney that has become shrunken and has lost function owing to scarring or fibrosis (Davis, Brady, & Creagh, 2014). It usually occurs as the outcome of recurring infections involving the upper urinary tract. However, it also may occur in the absence of an existing infection and a recent or remote history of UTIs. Alternative terms used to describe this condition include *interstitial nephritis, chronic atrophic pyelonephritis,* or *reflux nephropathy* (when scarring occurs in the presence of vesico-ureteral reflux).

Chronic pyelonephritis is diagnosed by radiological imaging and histological testing rather than assessment of clinical features. Imaging studies reveal a small, contracted kidney with a thinned parenchyma. The collecting system may be small or hydronephrotic. Pathological analysis reveals loss of functioning nephrons, infiltration of the parenchyma with inflammatory cells, and fibrosis.

The level of renal function in chronic pyelonephritis varies, depending on whether one or both kidneys are affected, the magnitude of scarring, and the presence of coexisting infection. Chronic pyelonephritis often progresses to end-stage renal disease when both kidneys are involved, even if the underlying infection is successfully eradicated. (Nursing and collaborative management of patients with chronic kidney disease are discussed in Chapter 49.)

URETHRITIS

Urethritis is an inflammation of the urethra. Causes of urethritis include a bacterial or viral infection, *Trichomonas* and monilial infection (especially in women), chlamydia, and gonorrhea (especially in men). In men, urethritis usually arises from sexual transmission; purulent discharge usually indicates a gonococcal urethritis, whereas a clear discharge typically signifies a nongonococcal urethritis. (Sexually transmitted infections are discussed in Chapter 55.) Urethritis also produces bothersome LUTS, including dysuria and frequent urination, similar to those seen with cystitis.

Urethritis is difficult to diagnose in women, as urethral discharge may not be present. Cultures on split urine collections (taken at beginning of urine flow and then midstream) or any urethral discharge may confirm a diagnosis of urethral infection.

Treatment is based on identifying and treating the cause and providing symptomatic relief. Sulphamethoxazole with trimethoprim or nitrofurantoin are examples of drugs used for bacterial infections. Metronidazole (Flagyl) and clotrimazole may be used for treating *Trichomonas*. Drugs such as fluconazole (Diflucan) may be prescribed for monilial infections. In chlamydial infections, doxycycline may be used. Women with negative urine cultures and no pyuria do not usually respond to antibiotics. Hot sitz baths may temporarily relieve symptoms. Patients should be instructed to avoid the use of vaginal deodorant sprays, to properly cleanse the perineal area after bowel movements and urination, and to avoid intercourse until symptoms subside. Patients with sexually transmitted urethritis should be instructed to refer their sex partners for evaluation and testing if they had sexual contact in the 60 days preceding onset of symptoms or diagnosis.

URETHRAL DIVERTICULA

Urethral diverticula are the result of obstruction and subsequent rupture of the periurethral glands into the urethral lumen with epithelialization (regrowth of tissue) over the opening of the resulting periurethral cavity (Urology Care Foundation, n.d.). Urethral diverticula are much more common in females than in males, with an incidence in women of 1% to 5%. Urethral diverticula occur mostly in the area of the periurethral glands. These glands are found along the entire length of the urethra, with the majority draining into the distal third of the urethra; Skene glands are the largest and most distal. A person may have more than one diverticulum, caused by urethral trauma from child-bearing, urethral instrumentation, dilation or infection with gonococcal organisms, or normal vaginal flora. Urethral diverticula present some of the more challenging diagnostic and reconstructive cases in urology.

Symptoms include dysuria, postvoid dribbling, frequent urination (>q2h), urgency, suprapubic discomfort or pressure, dyspareunia, a feeling of incomplete bladder emptying, and urinary incontinence. As well, the urine may contain gross hematuria or sediment, giving it a cloudy appearance. However, one in four women have no symptoms. An anterior vaginal wall mass may be noted on physical examination, which, upon palpation, may be quite tender and express purulent discharge through the urethra. Radiographic studies such as voiding cysto-urethrography (VCUG) should be used to confirm the diagnosis. Additional studies include ultrasound and magnetic resonance imaging (MRI) to determine the size of the diverticulum in relation to the urethral lumen.

Surgical options include transurethral incision of the diverticular neck, marsupialization (creation of a permanent opening) of the diverticular sac into the vagina (often referred to as a *Spence procedure*), and surgical excision. Surgical excision of a urethral diverticulum should be performed with caution because the diverticular sac may be adherent to the adjacent urethral lumen, and careless excision of the sac may result in a large urethral defect requiring construction of a neourethra (new urethra). Other important considerations during surgery include identification and closure of the diverticular neck, complete removal of the mucosal lining of the diverticular sac to prevent recurrence, and a multiple-layered closure to prevent postoperative urethro-vaginal fistula formation. A complication of the surgery may be stress urinary incontinence.

INTERSTITIAL CYSTITIS

Interstitial cystitis (IC) is a chronic, painful inflammatory disease of the bladder believed to be associated with an autoimmune or allergic response. It is thought to affect as many 101 228 Canadians (3%). IC is most frequently diagnosed in midlife (Davis, Brady, & Creagh, 2014). The ratio of women to men with IC is 10 to 12:1 (NIDDK, 2011). Although the etiology of IC remains unknown, probable contributing factors include chronic inflammation with mast cell invasion of the bladder wall (possibly provoked by an infection or an autoimmune disorder), defects of the glycosaminoglycan layer that protects the bladder mucosa from the irritating effects of urine exposure, abnormal constituents in the urine, and neurological dysfunction (Gish, 2011).

The two primary clinical manifestations that characterize IC are pain and bothersome LUTS (e.g., frequency, urgency). The pain associated with IC is usually located in the suprapubic area but may involve the vagina, labia, or entire perineal region. It varies from moderate to severe in intensity and is exacerbated by bladder filling, postponing urination, physical exertion, pressure against the suprapubic area, dietary intake of certain foods, and emotional distress. The pain is transiently relieved by urination. Bothersome LUTS are very similar to those of a UTI, and the condition is often misdiagnosed as a recurring or chronic UTI. The pain and voiding symptoms produced by IC remit and exacerbate over time. Some patients experience an onset of symptoms that disappear altogether after a period of weeks to months, whereas others have persistent symptoms over a period of months to years.

IC is a diagnosis of exclusion. The condition is suspected whenever a patient experiences symptoms of a UTI despite the absence of bacteriuria, pyuria, or a positive urine culture. A careful history and physical examination are necessary to exclude a variety of disorders that may produce somewhat similar symptoms, such as UTI or endometriosis. This evaluation must include at least one negative urine culture during a period of active symptoms. Cystoscopic examination may reveal a small bladder capacity and superficial ulcerations with bladder filling called *glomerulations,* but these findings are frequently absent and are not unique to IC. Criteria for diagnosing IC are presented in Table 48-8.

Collaborative Care and Drug Therapy

Because the etiology of IC is unknown, no single treatment has been identified that consistently reverses or relieves symptoms. Various therapies have been effective in alleviating or relieving uncomfortable symptoms in most patients (Gish, 2011; Quillin & Erickson, 2012). Dietary and lifestyle alterations are used to relieve pain and diminish voiding frequency and nocturia. Dietary alterations include elimination of foods and beverages likely to exacerbate the symptoms. Eating a diet low in acidic foods and avoiding consumption of beverages such as coffee, tea, and carbonated and alcoholic drinks can be helpful in reducing IC symptoms. Patients may be advised that an over-the-counter dietary supplement called calcium glycerophosphate alkalinizes the urine and can provide relief from the irritating effects of certain foods. This agent may be particularly helpful when dining away from home where the patient has less control over the preparation of foods.

A number of tricyclic antidepressants, including amitriptyline (Elavil) and doxepin, are used to reduce the burning pain and urinary frequency. Pentosan (Elmiron) is a drug used to enhance the protective effects of the glycosaminoglycan layer of the bladder. It is thought to relieve pain associated with IC by reducing the irritating effects of urine on the bladder wall. Medications that may provide modest relief from IC symptoms include nifedipine, which is a calcium channel blocker. Although these drugs are effective over time (weeks to months), they do not provide the immediate relief that may be needed when a patient experiences an acute exacerbation of symptoms. For this relief, a short course of opioid analgesics may be given.

Several drugs may be instilled directly into the bladder through a small catheter. Dimethyl sulphoxide probably acts by desensitizing pain receptors in the bladder wall. Heparin and hyaluronic acid also may be instilled into the bladder to relieve IC symptoms. Like pentosan, they are thought to enhance the protective properties of the glycosaminoglycan layer of the bladder. These medications are often administered with lidocaine, which rapidly desensitizes the bladder wall, rendering the patient better able to tolerate instillation of additional heparin or hyaluronic acid and providing transient relief from pain. The bacille Calmette–Guérin (BCG) vaccine, an attenuated form of *Mycobacterium bovis* administered intravesically, is now in clinical trials. The mechanism of action of BCG is unclear, but it may alleviate a possible autoimmune disorder provoking the chronic inflammation characteristic of the disorder.

Distension of the bladder during endoscopic examination relieves IC-related pain and voiding frequency, probably by temporarily disrupting sensory nerve endings in the bladder wall. Several surgical procedures have been used in an attempt to relieve severe, debilitating pain. Urinary diversion, the surgical removal of the bladder and rerouting flow of urine to an ostomy on the abdomen, is an approach that can be used when other measures fail. Unfortunately, some patients have reported pain within the urinary diversion, possibly indicating that components of the urine may contribute to IC in certain cases.

NURSING MANAGEMENT
INTERSTITIAL CYSTITIS

Assessment focuses on characterization of the pain associated with IC. The patient is asked about specific dietary or lifestyle factors known to exacerbate or alleviate pain and about the intensity of the pain. Objective data collection includes a bladder log or voiding diary kept over a period of at least 3 days to determine diurnal voiding frequency and patterns of nocturia. A simultaneous pain record may be useful.

Reassurance that IC is a real condition experienced by others and that it can be effectively treated may relieve the anxiety, anger, guilt, and frustration related to experiences of chronic pain and voiding dysfunction in the absence of a clear-cut diagnosis and treatment strategy.

A UTI may occur during the course of IC management. A UTI is likely to produce an acute exacerbation of bothersome LUTS and urinary frequency as well as dysuria (not typically associated with IC) and odorous urine, possibly with hematuria.

Broad dietary restrictions are often necessary to control IC-related pain. Patients must be given instruction about the need to maintain good nutrition. Specifically, they may be advised to take a multivitamin containing no more than the recommended dietary allowance for essential vitamins and to avoid high-potency vitamins, because these formulations may irritate the bladder. Patients are also advised to obtain information, including recipes and menus for a well-balanced diet specifically designed to avoid bladder-irritating foods and beverages, from support organizations such as the Women's College Hospital in Toronto and the Interstitial Cystitis Association in the United States (see the Resources at the end of this chapter). Elimination of a variety of foods and beverages from the diet that are likely to irritate the bladder typically provides modest to profound relief from symptoms. Typical bladder irritants include caffeine, alcohol, citrus products, aged cheeses, nuts, foods containing vinegar, curries or hot peppers, and foods or beverages likely to lower urinary pH. In addition, the patient should be taught to self-manage the use of calcium glycerophosphate or pantoprazole (Pantoloc). The patient is advised to avoid clothing that creates

TABLE 48-8	CLINICAL CRITERIA FOR THE DIAGNOSIS OF INTERSTITIAL CYSTITIS

Inclusion Criteria
- Bothersome urinary urgency
- Cystoscopic evidence of ulcerations or glomerulations (not specific to interstitial cystitis)
- Pain with bladder filling or postponing urination
- Small bladder capacity on urodynamic testing

Exclusion Criteria
- Active genital herpes
- Bladder capacity >350 mL on urodynamic testing
- Bladder tumour
- Daytime voiding frequency (eight or more times per day)
- History of chemotherapy, particularly if treated with cyclophosphamide (Procytox)
- History of pelvic irradiation
- Overactive bladder contractions on urodynamic testing
- Tubercular cystitis

suprapubic pressure, including pants with tight belts or restrictive waistlines.

Written educational materials concerning diet, coping with the need for frequent urination, and strategies for coping with the emotional burden of IC are available from the Interstitial Cystitis Association. Providing such materials affords an excellent opportunity for the nurse to introduce the patient to the existence of this patient advocacy group.

RENAL TUBERCULOSIS

Renal tuberculosis (TB) is rarely a primary lesion. It is usually secondary to TB of the lung. In a small percentage of patients with pulmonary TB, the tubercle bacilli reach the kidneys via the bloodstream. Onset occurs 5 to 8 years after the primary infection. The patient is often asymptomatic when the kidney is initially infiltrated with bacilli. Sometimes, the patient complains of fatigue and develops a low-grade fever. As the lesions ulcerate, infection descends to the bladder, and the patient experiences frequent urination, burning on voiding, and epididymitis (in men). Symptoms of a UTI are the first sign in the majority of patients with renal TB. Renal lesions may calcify as they heal. Infrequently, renal colic, lumbar and iliac pain, and hematuria may be present. A diagnosis is based on localization of tubercle bacilli in the urine and on IVP findings.

Long-term complications of renal TB depend on the duration of the disease before treatment. The renal parenchyma become scarred, and ureteral strictures develop. The earlier treatment is initiated, the less likely renal failure is to develop. Reduced bladder volume may be irreversible in advanced disease. The patient may require long-term urological follow-up. (Nursing and collaborative management for the patient with TB are discussed in Chapter 30.)

IMMUNOLOGICAL DISORDERS OF THE KIDNEY

GLOMERULO-NEPHRITIS

Immunological processes involving the urinary tract predominantly affect the renal glomerulus. The disease process results in glomerulo-nephritis, an immune-related inflammation of the glomeruli characterized by proteinuria, hematuria, decreased urine production, and edema. The condition affects both kidneys equally. Although the glomerulus is the primary site of inflammation, tubular, interstitial, and vascular changes also occur. Glomerulo-nephritis is divided into a number of classifications, which may describe (a) the extent of damage (diffuse or focal), (b) the initial cause of the disorder (e.g., systemic lupus erythematosus, systemic sclerosis [scleroderma], streptococcal infection), or (c) the extent of changes (minimal or widespread).

Clinical Manifestations

Clinical manifestations of glomerulo-nephritis include varying degrees of hematuria (ranging from microscopic to gross) and urinary excretion of various formed elements, including red blood cells (RBCs), WBCs, and casts. Proteinuria and elevated serum urea (blood urea nitrogen [BUN]) and serum creatinine levels are other manifestations. In most cases, recovery from the acute illness is complete. However, if progressive involvement occurs, the result is destruction of renal tissue and marked renal insufficiency.

A patient's history provides important information related to glomerulo-nephritis. It is necessary to assess exposure to drugs, immunizations, microbial infections, and viral infections such as hepatitis. It is also important to evaluate the patient for more generalized conditions involving immune disorders, such as systemic lupus erythematosus and systemic sclerosis.

ACUTE POSTSTREPTOCOCCAL GLOMERULO-NEPHRITIS

Acute poststreptococcal glomerulo-nephritis (APSGN) is most common in children and young adults, but all age groups can be affected. APSGN develops 5 to 21 days after an infection of the pharynx or the skin (e.g., streptococcal sore throat, impetigo) by certain nephrotoxic strains of group A β-hemolytic streptococci. The patient produces antibodies to the streptococcal antigen. Although the specific mechanism is not known, the antigen–antibody complexes are deposited in the glomeruli and activate complement (Doig & Huether, 2014). Complement activation (discussed in Chapter 14) causes an inflammatory reaction to the injury. The response to the injury is also a decrease in the filtration of metabolic waste products from the blood and an increase in the permeability of the glomerulus to larger protein molecules.

Clinical Manifestations and Complications

The clinical manifestations of APSGN appear as a variety of signs and symptoms, which may include generalized body edema, hypertension, oliguria, hematuria with a smoky or rusty appearance, and proteinuria. Fluid retention occurs as a result of decreased glomerular filtration. The edema appears initially in low-pressure tissues, such as around the eyes (periorbital edema), but later progresses to involve the total body as ascites or peripheral edema in the legs. Smoky urine indicates bleeding in the upper urinary tract. The degree of proteinuria varies with the severity of the glomerulo-nephropathy. Hypertension primarily results from increased extracellular fluid volume. Patients with APSGN may have abdominal or flank pain. Some, however, will have no symptoms, and the problem is found on routine urinalysis.

More than 95% of patients with APSGN recover completely or improve rapidly with conservative management. Chronic glomerulo-nephritis develops in 5% to 15% of affected persons, and irreversible renal failure occurs in less than 1% of patients (Ralph & Carapetis, 2013).

Diagnostic Studies

The diagnosis of APSGN is based on a complete history and physical examination and laboratory studies (Table 48-9) to determine the presence or history of a group A β-hemolytic streptococcus in a throat or skin lesion. An immune response to the streptococcus is often demonstrated by assessment of antistreptolysin O titres. The finding of decreased complement components (especially C3 and CH50) indicates an immune-mediated response. A renal biopsy may be performed to confirm the presence of the disease.

Dipstick and urine sediment microscopy will reveal the presence of erythrocytes in significant numbers. Erythrocyte casts are highly suggestive of acute glomerulo-nephritis. Proteinuria may range from mild to severe. Screening blood tests

TABLE 48-9   COLLABORATIVE CARE

Acute Glomerulo-Nephritis

Diagnostic	Collaborative Therapy
• History and physical examination	• Adjustment of dietary protein intake to level of proteinuria and uremia
• BUN, serum creatinine, and albumin	• Antihypertensive therapy
• CBC	• Diuretics
• Complement levels and ASO titre	• Rest
• Renal biopsy (if indicated)	• Sodium and fluid restriction
• Urinalysis	

ASO, antistreptolysin O; *BUN,* blood urea nitrogen; *CBC,* complete blood cell count.

include BUN and serum creatinine to assess the extent of renal impairment.

NURSING AND COLLABORATIVE MANAGEMENT ACUTE POSTSTREPTOCOCCAL GLOMERULO-NEPHRITIS

The management of APSGN focuses on symptomatic relief (see Table 48-9). Rest is recommended until the signs of glomerular inflammation (proteinuria, hematuria) and hypertension subside. Edema is treated by restricting sodium and fluid intake and by administering diuretics. Severe hypertension is treated with antihypertensive drugs. Dietary protein intake may be restricted if there is evidence of an increase in nitrogenous wastes (e.g., elevated BUN). The restriction varies with the degree of proteinuria. (Low-protein, low-sodium, fluid-restricted diets are discussed in Chapter 49.) Antibiotics should be given only if the streptococcal infection is still present. Corticosteroids and cytotoxic drugs have not been shown to be of value.

One of the most important ways to prevent the development of APSGN is to encourage early diagnosis and treatment of sore throats and skin lesions. If streptococci are found in the culture, treatment with appropriate antibiotic therapy (usually penicillin) is essential. The patient must be encouraged to take the full course of antibiotics to ensure that the bacteria have been eradicated. Good personal hygiene is an important factor in preventing the spread of cutaneous streptococcal infections. (The Kidney Foundation of Canada website [see the Resources at the end of this chapter] provides information on the management of kidney disease and support groups.)

GOODPASTURE'S SYNDROME

Goodpasture's syndrome is an autoimmune disease characterized by the presence of antibodies circulating against the glomerular and alveolar basement membranes. Damage to the kidneys and lungs results when binding of the antibody causes an inflammatory reaction mediated by complement activation (see Chapter 14).

Goodpasture's syndrome is a rare disease that is seen mostly in young male smokers. The clinical manifestations include hemoptysis, pulmonary insufficiency, crackles, wheezes, renal involvement with hematuria and renal failure, weakness, pallor, and anemia. Pulmonary hemorrhage usually occurs and may precede glomerular abnormalities by weeks or months. Abnormal diagnostic findings include low hematocrit and hemoglobin levels, elevated BUN and serum creatinine levels, hematuria, and proteinuria. Circulating serum anti–glomerular basement membrane (anti-GBM) antibodies parallel the activity of the renal disease and are diagnostic of this syndrome.

NURSING AND COLLABORATIVE MANAGEMENT GOODPASTURE'S SYNDROME

Until recently, the prognosis for patients with Goodpasture's syndrome was poor. However, with the development of immuno-suppressive therapy and advances in transplantation techniques, the outlook has improved. Management consists of corticosteroids, immuno-suppressive drugs (e.g., cyclophosphamide [Procytox], azathioprine [Imuran]), plasmapheresis (see Chapter 16), and dialysis.

Nursing management appropriate for a critically ill patient who is experiencing symptoms of acute kidney injury and respiratory distress is instituted. Death is often secondary to hemorrhage in the lungs and respiratory failure. (Nursing interventions for a patient in acute kidney injury are discussed in Chapter 49, and nursing interventions for a patient with respiratory failure are discussed in Chapter 70.)

RAPIDLY PROGRESSIVE GLOMERULO-NEPHRITIS

Rapidly progressive glomerulo-nephritis (RPGN) is glomerular disease associated with rapid, progressive loss of renal function over days to weeks. Renal failure may occur within weeks to months, in contrast to chronic glomerulo-nephritis, in which it develops insidiously and progresses over many years. The manifestations of RPGN are hypertension, edema, proteinuria, hematuria, and RBC casts.

RPGN can occur in a variety of situations: (a) as a complication of inflammatory or infectious disease (e.g., APSGN), (b) as a complication of a multisystemic disease (e.g., systemic lupus erythematosus, Goodpasture's syndrome), (c) as an idiopathic disease, or (d) in association with the use of certain drugs (e.g., penicillamine).

Treatment is directed toward correction of fluid overload, hypertension, uremia, and inflammatory injury to the kidney. Treatment includes corticosteroids, cytotoxic agents, and plasmapheresis. Dialysis therapy and transplantation are used as maintenance therapy for the patient with RPGN. Following renal transplantation, RPGN may recur.

CHRONIC GLOMERULO-NEPHRITIS

Chronic glomerulo-nephritis is a syndrome that reflects the end stage of glomerular inflammatory disease. Most types of glomerulo-nephritis and nephrotic syndrome can eventually lead to chronic glomerulo-nephritis.

The syndrome is characterized by proteinuria, hematuria, and the slow development of uremic syndrome as a result of decreasing renal function. Chronic glomerulo-nephritis does not usually follow an acute course; it progresses insidiously toward renal failure over a few to as many as 30 years.

Chronic glomerulo-nephritis is often found coincidentally as an abnormality on a urinalysis or when elevated blood pressure is detected. It is common to find that the patient has no recollection or history of acute nephritis or any renal problems. A renal biopsy may be performed to determine the exact cause and nature of the glomerulo-nephritis. However, ultrasound and CT scanning are generally preferred as diagnostic measures.

TABLE 48-10	CAUSES OF NEPHROTIC SYNDROME

Primary Glomerular Disease
- Primary nephrotic syndrome
- Focal glomerulo-nephritis
- Inherited nephrotic disease

Extrarenal Causes
Multisystem Disease
- Amyloidosis
- Diabetes mellitus
- Systemic lupus erythematosus

Infections
- Bacterial (streptococcal, syphilis)
- Protozoal (malaria)
- Viral (hepatitis, human immunodeficiency virus infection)

Neoplasms
- Hodgkin's disease
- Leukemias
- Solid tumours of lungs, colon, stomach, breast

Drugs
- Captopril
- Heroin
- Nonsteroidal anti-inflammatory drugs
- Penicillamine

Allergens (e.g., bee sting, pollen)

Treatment is supportive and symptomatic. Hypertension and UTIs should be treated vigorously. Protein and phosphate restrictions may slow the rate of progression of kidney disease. (Management of chronic kidney disease is discussed in Chapter 49.)

NEPHROTIC SYNDROME

Etiology and Clinical Manifestations

Nephrotic syndrome describes a clinical course that can be associated with a number of disease conditions. Some of the more common causes of nephrotic syndrome are listed in Table 48-10. In adults, about one-third of patients with nephrotic syndrome will have a systemic disease such as diabetes or systemic lupus erythematosus. The remainder will be categorized as having idiopathic nephrotic syndrome.

The characteristic manifestations include peripheral edema, massive proteinuria, dyslipidemia, and hypoalbuminemia. Characteristic blood chemistries include decreased serum albumin, decreased total serum protein, and elevated serum cholesterol. The increased glomerular membrane permeability found in nephrotic syndrome is responsible for the massive excretion of protein in the urine. This excretion results in decreased serum protein and subsequent edema formation. Ascites and anasarca develop if there is severe hypoalbuminemia.

The diminished plasma oncotic pressure from the decreased serum proteins stimulates hepatic lipoprotein synthesis, which results in dyslipidemia. Initially, cholesterol and low-density lipoproteins are elevated. Later, the triglyceride level also increases. Fat bodies (fatty casts) commonly appear in the urine.

Immune responses, both humoral and cellular, are altered in nephrotic syndrome. As a result, infection is an important cause of morbidity and mortality. Calcium and skeletal abnormalities may occur, including hypocalcemia, blunted calcemic response to parathyroid hormone, hyperparathyroidism, and osteomalacia.

With nephrotic proteinuria, loss of clotting factors can result in a relative hypercoagulable state. Hypercoagulability with thrombo-embolism is potentially the most serious complication of nephrotic syndrome. The renal vein is the most common site for thrombus formation. Pulmonary emboli occur in about 40% of nephrotic patients with thrombosis.

Collaborative Care

Treatment of nephrotic syndrome is symptomatic (Mayo Clinic Staff, 2012). The goals are to relieve edema and cure or control the primary disease. Management of the edema includes the cautious use of angiotensin-converting enzyme inhibitors, nonsteroidal anti-inflammatory drugs, and a low-sodium (2–3 g/day), low- to moderate-protein (0.5–0.6 g/kg of body weight per day) diet. Dietary salt restrictions are a key to managing edema. In some individuals, thiazide or loop diuretics may be needed. If urine protein loss exceeds 10 g/24 hr, additional dietary protein may be needed.

The treatment of dyslipidemia is often unsuccessful. However, treatment with lipid-lowering agents, such as colestipol (Colestid) and lovastatin, may result in moderate decreases in serum cholesterol levels. If thrombosis is detected, anticoagulant therapy may be necessary for up to 6 months.

Corticosteroids and cyclophosphamide (Procytox) may be used to treat severe cases of nephrotic syndrome. Management of diabetes and treatment of edema are the only measures used for nephrotic syndrome related to diabetes.

NURSING MANAGEMENT NEPHROTIC SYNDROME

A major nursing intervention for patients with nephrotic syndrome is related to edema. It is important to assess the edema by weighing the patient daily, accurately recording intake and output, and measuring abdominal girth or extremity size. Comparing this information daily provides the nurse with a tool for assessing the effectiveness of treatment. The edematous skin must be cleaned carefully. Trauma should be avoided, and the effectiveness of diuretic therapy must be monitored.

Patients with nephrotic syndrome have the potential to become malnourished or anorexic from the excessive loss of protein in the urine. Maintaining a low- to moderate-protein diet that is also low in sodium is not always easy. Serving small, frequent meals in a pleasant setting may encourage better dietary intake.

Because these patients are susceptible to infection, measures should be taken to avoid exposure to persons with known infections. People with nephrotic syndrome are often ashamed of an edematous appearance and need support in dealing with an altered body image.

OBSTRUCTIVE UROPATHIES

Urinary obstruction refers to any anatomical or functional condition that blocks or impedes the flow of urine (Figure 48-3). It may be congenital or acquired. Obstruction may be the result of (a) intrinsic causes such as anomalies, diverticula, tumours, or benign growth within the urinary tract; (b) extrinsic causes such as tumours, adhesions, retroperitoneal fibrosis, or prolapsed

FIGURE 48-3 Common causes of urinary tract obstruction.

FIGURE 48-4 Hydronephrosis of the kidney with marked dilation of the pelvis and the calyces and thinning of the renal parenchyma. Source: Kumar, V., Abbas, A. K.., & Aster, J. (2015). *Robbins and Cotran pathologic basis of disease* (9th ed., p. 950, Figure 20-48). Philadelphia: Saunders.

adjacent organs; or (c) functional causes as a result of neurological or psychogenic factors. Some common intrinsic obstructions are narrowing of the uretero-pelvic junction (UPJ), bladder neck contracture, BPH, urethral stricture, and urethral meatal stenosis. Common extrinsic causes include pelvic and abdominal tumours or a prolapsed uterus. Examples of functional causes are neurogenic bladder and vesico-sphincter dyssynergia (disturbance in muscle coordination) after spinal cord injury.

Damage from urinary tract obstruction affects the system above the level of the obstruction. The severity of these effects depends on location, duration of obstruction, amount of pressure or dilation, presence of urinary stasis, and the presence of infection. Infection increases the risk of irreversible damage.

Although obstruction distal to the prostate in men or the bladder neck in women causes mucosal scarring and a slower stream, it rarely results in major obstructive uropathy because the urethral wall pressure is less than that of the bladder neck and bladder. Urethral obstruction may contribute to outlet resistance and cause lower or upper urinary tract damage when other obstructive or dysfunctional factors are also present. For example, there is an increased risk for compromised renal function in a patient with a spinal cord injury with vesico-sphincter dyssynergia.

When obstruction occurs at the level of the bladder neck or the prostate, significant bladder changes can occur. Detrusor muscle fibres hypertrophy (increase in size) to contract harder-to-push urine out a narrower pathway. Over a long period, the detrusor loses its ability to compensate for this resistance. Muscle bundles separate and become less compliant. This separation is called *trabeculation*. Trabeculation is caused by the deposition of collagen in the bladder wall that separates the smooth muscle fascicles. Trabeculation may hasten the decompensation of the detrusor. The areas between these muscle bundles are called *cellules*. Because these areas have no muscle support, the bladder mucosa can herniate between detrusor muscle bundles, forming sacs that drain poorly, called *diverticula*. The amount of residual urine in a noncompensating bladder can be very high.

Pressure increases during bladder filling or storage and can be transmitted to the ureter when *bladder outlet obstruction* is present. This pressure overcomes the normal peristaltic pressure and leads to *reflux* (a backflow of urine), which in turn causes ureteral dilation, kinking, and tortuosity; **hydroureter** (dilation of the renal pelvis); vesico-ureteral reflux (backflow or backward movement of urine from the lower to upper urinary tracts); and **hydronephrosis** (dilation or enlargement of the renal pelvis and the calyces; Figure 48-4) and consequent chronic pyelonephritis and renal atrophy. If only one kidney is obstructed, the other kidney may try to compensate by hypertrophy, but the ureter will not be dilated on this contralateral side.

Partial obstruction may occur in the ureter or at the UPJ. If the pressure remains low or moderate, the kidney may continue to dilate with no noticeable loss of function. There is an increased risk of pyelonephritis because of urinary stasis and reflux. If only one kidney is involved and the other kidney is functioning, the patient may be free of symptoms. If both kidneys or only one functioning kidney is involved (e.g., if the patient has only one kidney), alterations in renal function (e.g., increased BUN or serum creatinine levels) are found. If the obstruction progresses, oliguria or anuria develops. Often, episodes of oliguria are followed by polyuria if the obstruction is a stone that becomes dislodged. Treatment calls for location and relief of the blockage. This can include insertion of a tube (e.g., urethral or ureteral), surgical correction of the disease process, or diversion of the urinary stream above the level of blockage.

URINARY TRACT CALCULI

One in 10 Canadians will have a kidney stone at some point in life (Canadian Urological Association, 2014). Many of these people require hospitalization. In Canada, the incidence of kidney stones is highest in the East and decreases to the West. Except for struvite (magnesium–ammonium phosphate) stones associated with UTI, stone disorders are more common in men than in women (Canadian Urological Association, 2014).

The majority of patients with stones are between 20 and 55 years of age. The incidence is also higher in persons with a family history of stone formation. Recurrence of stones can affect up to 50% of patients (Canadian Urological Association, 2014). There is seasonal variation, with stone formation occurring more often in the summer months in Canada, thus supporting the role of dehydration in this process. Stone formation in the kidney seems to increase in incidence as countries become more industrialized whereas the incidence of bladder stones decreases.

Etiology and Pathophysiology

Many factors affect the incidence and the type of stone formation, including metabolic, dietary, genetic, climatic, lifestyle, and occupational influences (Table 48-11). Various theories have been proposed to explain the formation of stones in the urinary tract; however, no single theory can account for stone formation in all cases. Crystals, when in a supersaturated concentration, can precipitate and unite to form a stone. Keeping urine dilute and free flowing reduces the risk for recurrent stone formation in many individuals. It is known that a *mucoprotein* (the matrix for the stone) is formed in the kidney that forms stones. Urinary pH, solute load, and inhibitors in the urine affect the formation of stones. The lower the pH is, the less soluble uric acid and cystine are. The higher the pH, the less soluble calcium and phosphate.

Other important factors in the development of stones include obstruction with urinary stasis and urinary infection with urea-splitting bacteria (e.g., *Proteus, Klebsiella, Pseudomonas,* and some species of staphylococci). These bacteria cause the urine to become alkaline and contribute to the formation of struvite (magnesium–ammonium phosphate) stones (Flannigan, Choy, Chew, et al., 2014).

Infected stones, when they are entrapped in the kidney, may assume a staghorn configuration as they enlarge (Figure 48-5). Infected stones are frequent in patients with an external urinary diversion, long-term in-dwelling catheter, neurogenic bladder, or urinary retention. Genetic factors may also contribute to urine stone formation. Cystinuria is an autosomal recessive disorder. In this disorder, there is a marked increased excretion of cystine.

Types

A **calculus** is an abnormal stone formed in body tissues by an accumulation of mineral salts. The term *calculus* refers to the stone, and *lithiasis* refers to stone formation (**nephrolithiasis** thus indicates the formation of stones in the urinary tract). The five major categories of stones are (a) calcium phosphate, (b) calcium oxalate, (c) uric acid, (d) cystine, and (e) struvite (magnesium–ammonium phosphate) (Table 48-12). Stone composition may be mixed, although calcium stones are the

TABLE 48-11	RISK FACTORS FOR THE DEVELOPMENT OF URINARY TRACT CALCULI

Metabolic
- Abnormalities that result in increased urine levels of calcium, oxaluric acid, uric acid, or citric acid

Climate
- Warm climates that cause increased fluid loss, low urine volume, and increased solute concentration in urine

Diet
- Excessive amounts of tea or fruit juices that elevate urinary oxalate level
- Large intake of calcium* and oxalate
- Large intake of dietary proteins that increase uric acid excretion
- Low fluid intake that increases urinary concentration

Genetic
- Family history of stone formation, cystinuria, gout, or renal acidosis

Lifestyle
- Sedentary occupation, immobility

*Recent research suggests that a high dietary calcium intake, which was previously thought to contribute to kidney stones, may actually lower the risk by reducing the urinary excretion of oxalate, a common factor in many stones (National Kidney Foundation, 2015a).
Source: National Institute of Diabetes and Digestive and Kidney Diseases. (2013). *Eating, diet & nutrition for kidney stones.* Retrieved from http://kidney.niddk.nih.gov/KUDiseases/pubs/kidneystonediet/index.aspx#calcium.

FIGURE 48-5 A, Renal staghorn calculus. A large calculus fills the renal pelvis, shaped to its contours and resembling the horn of a stag *(S).* **B,** Embedded staghorn calculus *(yellow arrow)* in a hydronephrotic, infected, nonfunctioning kidney. Sources: *A,* Stevens, A., Lowe, J., & Scott, I. (2009). *Core pathology: Illustrated review in color* (3rd ed.). London: Mosby; *B,* Bullock, N., Doble, A., Turner, W., et al. (2008). *Urology: An illustrated colour text.* London: Churchill Livingstone.

TABLE 48-12   TYPES OF URINARY TRACT CALCULI

Urinary Stone	Incidence (%)	Characteristics	Predisposing Factors	Therapeutic Measures
Calcium oxalate*	35–40	Small, often possible to get trapped in ureter; more frequent in men than in women	Idiopathic hypercalciuria; hyperoxaluria; family history; independent of urinary pH	Increase hydration. Reduce dietary oxalate.† Give thiazide diuretics. Give cellulose phosphate to chelate calcium and prevent GI absorption. Give potassium citrate to maintain alkaline urine. Give cholestyramine to bind oxalate. Give calcium lactate to precipitate oxalate in GI tract.
Calcium phosphate	8–10	Mixed stones (typically); occur with struvite or oxalate stones	Alkaline urine, primary hyperparathyroidism	Treat underlying causes and other stones.
Struvite ($MgNH_4PO_4$)	10–15	Three to four times more common in women than men; always in association with urinary tract infections; large staghorn type (usually)‡	Urinary tract infections (usually *Proteus* organisms)	Administer antimicrobial agents, acetohydroxamic acid (Lithostat). Use surgical intervention to remove stone. Take measures to acidify urine.
Uric acid	5–8	Predominant in men, high incidence in Jewish men	Gout; acidic urine; inherited condition	Reduce urinary concentration of uric acid. Alkalinize urine with potassium citrate. Administer allopurinol. Reduce dietary purines.†
Cystine	1–2	Genetic autosomal recessive defect, defective absorption of cystine in GI tract and kidney, excess concentrations causing stone formation	Acidic urine	Increase hydration. Give penicillamine and tiopronin to prevent cystine crystallization. Give potassium citrate to maintain alkaline urine.

GI, gastro-intestinal.
*Calcium stones can exist as calcium oxalate, calcium phosphate, or a mixture of both. Calcium stones account for the majority of all stones.
†See Table 48-13.
‡See Figures 48-5 and 48-6.

most common. Calculi can be found in various locations in the urinary tract.

Clinical Manifestations

Urinary stones cause clinical manifestations when they obstruct urinary flow. Common sites of complete obstruction are at the UPJ (the point where the ureter crosses the iliac vessels) and the UVJ. Symptoms include abdominal or flank pain (usually severe), hematuria, and renal colic. The pain may be associated with nausea and vomiting. The type of pain is determined by the location of the stone. If the stone is nonobstructing, pain may be absent. If the obstruction is in a calyx or at the UPJ, the patient may experience dull costovertebral flank pain or even colic. Pain resulting from the passage of a calculus down the ureter is intense and colicky. The patient may be in mild shock with cool, moist skin. As a stone nears the UVJ, pain will be felt in the lateral flank and sometimes down into the testicles, the labia, or the groin. Other clinical manifestations include the presence of urinary infection accompanied by fever, vomiting, nausea, and chills.

Diagnostic Studies

Diagnostic studies useful in the evaluation and management of renal lithiasis include urinalysis, urine culture, IVP, retrograde pyelogram, ultrasound, and cystoscopy. A plain film of the abdomen and renal ultrasound will identify larger, radiopaque stones. An IVP or retrograde pyelogram is used to localize the degree and the site of obstruction or to confirm the presence of a radiolucent stone, such as a uric acid or cystine calculus (see Figure 48-5, *B*). Ultrasonography can be used to identify a radiopaque or radiolucent calculus in the renal pelvis, the calyx, or the proximal ureter. It is less useful when attempting to locate

stones trapped in the midureter. A CT scan may be used to differentiate a nonopaque stone from a tumour.

Retrieval and analysis of the stones are important in the diagnosis of the underlying problem contributing to stone formation. The patient's BUN and serum creatinine levels are also measured to assess renal function. A careful history, including previous stone formation, prescribed and over-the-counter medications and dietary supplements, and family history of urinary calculi, is useful. Measurement of urine pH can aid in the diagnosis of struvite stones and renal tubular acidosis (tendency to alkaline pH) and uric acid stones (tendency to acidic pH).

Collaborative Care

Evaluation and management of patients with renal lithiasis consist of two concurrent approaches. The first approach is directed toward management of the acute attack. This involves treating the symptoms of pain, infection, or obstruction as indicated for the individual patient. Opioids are typically required at frequent intervals for relief of renal colic pain. Many stones pass spontaneously. However, stones larger than 4 mm are unlikely to pass through the ureter.

The second approach is directed toward evaluation of the cause of the stone formation and the prevention of further development of stones. Information to be obtained from the patient includes family history of stone formation, geographic residence, nutritional assessment including the intake of vitamins A and D, activity pattern (active or sedentary), history of periods of prolonged illness with immobilization or dehydration, and any history of disease or surgery involving the GI or genito-urinary tract.

Therapy for people who are active stone formers requires a concerted management approach, with primary emphasis on teaching and on developing a therapeutic regimen that the patient can manage. Adequate hydration, dietary sodium restrictions, dietary changes (Table 48-13), and the use of medications keep urinary stone formation to a minimum. The medications prescribed depend on the specific problem underlying stone formation. These drugs prevent stone formation in various ways, including altering urine pH, preventing excessive urinary excretion of a substance, or correcting a primary disease (e.g., hyperparathyroidism).

Treatment of struvite stones calls for control of infection, which may be difficult if the stone remains in place. In addition to antibiotics, acetohydroxamic acid (Lithostat) may be used in the treatment of kidney infections that result in the continual formation of struvite stones. Acetohydroxamic acid (Lithostat), an inhibitor of the chemical action caused by the persistent bacteria, can be used effectively to retard struvite stone formation (Flannigan, Choy, Chew, et al., 2014). This medication is available in Canada through the Special Access Drug Program at Health Canada. If the infection cannot be controlled, the stone may have to be removed surgically.

Indications for endo-urological, lithotripsy, or open surgical stone removal include the following:

- Stones too large for spontaneous passage
- Stones associated with bacteriuria or symptomatic infection
- Stones causing impaired renal function
- Stones causing persistent pain, nausea, or ileus
- Inability of patient to be treated medically
- Patient with one kidney

Endo-Urological Procedures. To remove a small stone located in the bladder, a cystoscopy is done. For large stones (Figure 48-6), a *cystolitholapaxy* is done. In this procedure, large stones are broken up with an instrument called a *lithotrite* (stone crusher). The bladder is then irrigated and the crushed stones washed out. A *cystoscopic lithotripsy* uses an ultrasonic lithotrite to pulverize stones. Complications associated with these cystoscopic procedures include hemorrhage, retained stone fragments, and infection.

Flexible *ureteroscopes*, inserted via a cystoscope, can be used to remove stones from the renal pelvis and the upper urinary tract. Ultrasonic, laser, or electrohydraulic lithotripsy can be used in conjunction with the ureteroscope to pulverize and break the stone into fragments.

In *percutaneous nephrolithotomy*, a nephroscope is inserted through a sinus tract from the skin into the kidney pelvis. Stones can be fragmented using ultrasound, electrohydraulic, or laser lithotripsy. The stone fragments are removed and the pelvis irrigated. A percutaneous nephrostomy tube is usually left in place to ensure that the ureter is not obstructed. Complications include bleeding, injury to adjacent structures, and infection.

Lithotripsy. Lithotripsy involves the use of sound waves to break renal stones into small particles that can be eliminated from the urinary tract. Lithotripsy techniques include percutaneous ultrasonic lithotripsy, electrohydraulic lithotripsy, laser lithotripsy, and extracorporeal shock-wave lithotripsy (Ordon, Andonian, Blew, et al., 2015).

Extracorporeal shock-wave lithotripsy and laser lithotripsy are the most common. In *percutaneous ultrasonic lithotripsy*, an ultrasonic probe is placed in the renal pelvis via a percutaneous nephroscope (inserted through a small incision in the flank)

TABLE 48-13 NUTRITIONAL THERAPY

Urinary Tract Calculi

Depending on the type of calculi, the diet should be modified to decrease foods that are high in the substance that is the cause of the calculi. Listed below are foods that are moderate or high in purine, calcium, or oxalate content.

Purine
- *High:* Sardines, herring, mussels, liver, kidney, goose, venison, meat soups, sweetbreads
- *Moderate:* Chicken, salmon, crab, veal, mutton, bacon, pork, beef, ham

Calcium
- Milk, cheese, ice cream, yogourt, sauces containing milk; all beans (except green beans), lentils; fish with fine bones (e.g., sardines, kippers, herring, salmon); dried fruits, nuts; chocolate, cocoa, Ovaltine

Oxalate
- Spinach, rhubarb, asparagus, cabbage, tomatoes, beets, nuts, celery, parsley, runner beans; chocolate, cocoa, instant coffee, Ovaltine, tea; Worcestershire sauce

---

FIGURE 48-6 A, Calcium oxalate stones. **B,** Plain abdominal radiograph shows a large bladder calculus. Source: Bullock, N., Doble, A., Turner, W., et al. (2008). *Urology: An illustrated colour text.* London: Churchill Livingstone.

and is positioned against the stone. The patient is given general or spinal anaesthesia for this procedure. The probe produces ultrasonic waves, which break the stone into sandlike particles. Percutaneous lithotripsy is not often used as a primary approach to a renal or upper ureteral stone unless the stone is large and other lithotripsy procedures have failed.

The *electrohydraulic lithotripsy* probe is also placed directly on a stone, but it breaks the stone into small fragments that are removed by forceps or suction. A continuous saline irrigation flushes out the stone particles, and all outflow drainage is strained so that the particles can be analyzed. Forceps or basket extraction can also be used to remove the calculi. Complications are rare but include hemorrhage, sepsis, and abscess formation. Postoperatively, the patient usually complains of moderate to severe colicky pain. The first few voids are bright red; as the bleeding subsides, the urine becomes dark red or turns a smoky colour. Antibiotics are usually given for 2 weeks to reduce the risk for infection.

Laser lithotripsy probes are used to fragment lower ureteral and large bladder stones. A holmium laser medium is preferred; it fragments stones but does not injure the surrounding tissue.

In *extracorporeal shock-wave lithotripsy,* a noninvasive procedure, the patient is anaesthetized (spinal or general) and placed in a water bath. Anaesthesia is necessary to keep the patient very still during the procedure. Some of the newer-generation lithotripters do not require submersion and use other means of initiating shock waves.

Fluoroscopy or ultrasound is used to focus the lithotripter on the affected kidney, and a high-voltage spark generator produces high-energy acoustic shock waves that shatter the stone without damaging the surrounding tissues. The stone is broken into fine sand, which is excreted into the patient's urine within a few days after the procedure.

Hematuria is common after lithotripsy procedures. A self-retaining ureteral stent is often placed after the procedure to promote passage of sand from the fragmented stone and to prevent obstruction caused by its buildup in the ureter. The stent is removed 1 to 2 weeks after lithotripsy. A primary advantage of these techniques compared with open surgery is the decrease in the length of hospitalization and the patient's earlier return to normal activities. Additional treatment may be necessary, especially if a stone is large and in the midureter or the distal ureter.

Surgical Therapy. A small group of select patients need open surgical procedures, such as patients with morbid obesity or those with complex abnormalities in the calyces or at the UPJ. The type of open surgery performed depends on the location of the stone. A *nephrolithotomy* is an incision into the kidney to remove a stone. A *pyelolithotomy* is an incision into the renal pelvis to remove a stone. If the stone is located in the ureter, a *uretero-lithotomy* is performed. A *cystotomy* may be indicated for bladder calculi. For open surgery on the kidney or ureter, a flank incision directly below the diaphragm and across the side is usually the preferred surgical approach. The most common complication following these surgical procedures is hemorrhage.

Nutritional Therapy. Patients with an obstructing stone should be advised to drink adequate fluids to avoid dehydration. Forcing fluids is avoided because this strategy has not proved effective in assisting patients to spontaneously "pass" (excrete) the stone via the urine. In addition, forcing fluids may exacerbate the colic associated with this episode.

After an episode of urolithiasis, however, a high fluid intake (≈3 000 mL/day) is recommended to produce a urine output of at least 2 L/day. High urine output prevents supersaturation of minerals (i.e., dilutes the concentration) and promotes excretion of minerals within the urine, thus preventing stone formation. Increasing the fluid intake is especially important for patients who are active in sports, live in a dry climate, perform physical exercise, have a family history of stone formation, or work in an occupation that requires outdoor labour or a great deal of physical activity that can lead to dehydration. Water is the preferred fluid, and consumption of colas, coffee, and tea should be limited because high intake of these beverages tends to increase rather than diminish the risk for recurring urinary calculi (Ferraro, Taylor, Gambaro, et al., 2013).

Dietary intervention may be important in the management of urolithiasis. In the past, calcium intake was routinely restricted for patients with kidney stones. However, more recent research suggests that a high dietary calcium intake, which was previously thought to contribute to kidney stones, may actually lower the risk by reducing the urinary excretion of oxalate, a common factor in many stones (Canadian Urological Association, 2014). Initial nutritional management should include limiting oxalate-rich foods and thereby reducing oxalate excretion. Foods high in calcium, oxalate, and purines are presented in Table 48-13.

NURSING MANAGEMENT RENAL CALCULI

NURSING ASSESSMENT
Subjective and objective data that should be obtained from a patient with urinary tract lithiasis are presented in Table 48-14.

NURSING DIAGNOSES
Nursing diagnoses for the patient with urinary tract lithiasis include but are not limited to the following:

- *Impaired urinary elimination* related to *multiple causality* (trauma or obstruction)
- *Acute pain* related to *physical injury agent, biological injury agent* (effects of stones)
- *Deficient knowledge* related to *insufficient information* (unfamiliarity with information resources, lack of experience with urinary stones)

Additional information on nursing diagnoses for the patient with urinary tract lithiasis is presented in NCP 48-2, available on the Evolve website.

PLANNING
The overall goals are that the patient with urinary tract calculi will have (a) relief of pain, (b) no urinary tract obstruction, and (c) an understanding of measures to prevent further recurrence of stones.

NURSING IMPLEMENTATION
A program to prevent stone recurrence always includes adequate fluid intake to produce a urine output of approximately 2 L/day. The nurse should consult with the health care provider concerning recommendations for fluid intake in a given patient. A modestly active, ambulatory patient would be required to drink about 2 000 to 2 200 mL/day with the residual 20% to 30% of fluids gained through consumption of foods. The volume of necessary fluids will be higher in the highly active patient who works outdoors or who regularly engages in demanding athletic activities. In contrast, fluid intake will be less for the very sedentary or immobile person. Preventive measures for the person who is on

TABLE 48-14 NURSING ASSESSMENT

Urinary Tract Calculi

Subjective Data
Important Health Information
Current health history: Dietary intake of purines, calcium, oxalates, phosphates; fluid intake
Past health history: Recent or chronic UTI; bed rest or sedentary lifestyle; immobilization; previous urinary tract stones, obstruction, or kidney disease with urinary stasis; gout; prostatic hyperplasia; hyperparathyroidism; family history of renal calculi
Medications: Prior use of medication for prevention of stones or treatment of UTI; allopurinol, analgesics
Surgery or other treatments: External urinary diversion, long-term in-dwelling urinary catheter

Symptoms
- Acute, severe, colicky pain in flank, back, abdomen, groin, or genitalia; burning on urination, dysuria, anxiety
- Decreased urinary output, urinary urgency, urinary frequency, feeling of bladder fullness
- Nausea, vomiting; chills

Objective Data
General
Guarding, fever

Integumentary
Warm, flushed skin or pallor with cool, moist skin (mild shock)

Gastro-Intestinal
Abdominal distension, absence of bowel sounds

Urinary
Oliguria, hematuria, tenderness on palpation of renal areas, passage of stone or stones

Possible Findings
↑ Serum urea (BUN) and serum creatinine levels; RBCs, WBCs, pyuria, crystals, casts, minerals, bacteria on urinalysis; ↑ uric acid, calcium, phosphorus, oxalate, or cystine values on 24-hr urine sample; calculi or anatomical changes on IVP or KUB radiographic study; direct visualization of obstruction on cysto-ureteroscopy

BUN, blood urea nitrogen; *IVP,* intravenous pyelogram; *KUB,* kidneys, ureters, bladder; *RBCs,* red blood cells; *UTI,* urinary tract infection; *WBCs,* white blood cells.

bed rest or is relatively immobile for a prolonged time include maintaining an adequate fluid intake, turning the patient every 2 hours, and helping the patient to sit or stand, if possible, to maximize urinary flow.

Additional preventive measures focus on reducing metabolic or secondary risk factors. For example, dietary restriction of purines may be helpful to patients at risk for developing uric acid stones. Reduced intake of oxalates may be indicated in patients with recurring calcium oxalate calculi. Patients are taught about dosage, scheduling, and potential adverse effects of medications used to reduce the risk for stone formation. Select patients may be taught to self-monitor urinary pH or be asked to measure urinary output.

Pain management and patient comfort are primary nursing responsibilities when managing an obstructing stone and renal colic (see NCP 48-2). It is important to ensure that the patient retrieves any spontaneously passed stones. All urine voided by the patient should be strained through gauze or a special urine strainer in an effort to detect the stone. The high fluid intake

necessary for stone prevention is suspended, but consumption should be adequate to meet daily needs and prevent dehydration. Ambulation is generally encouraged to promote the movement of the stone from the upper to the lower urinary tract, but the patient should not walk unattended when experiencing acute colic, particularly if opioid analgesics are being used.

EVALUATION

The expected outcomes for the patient with urinary calculi are presented in NCP 48-2, available on the Evolve website.

STRICTURES

A **stricture** is an abnormal temporary or permanent narrowing of the lumen of a hollow organ, in this context, of the ureter or the urethra.

Ureteral Strictures

Ureteral strictures can affect the entire length of the ureter, from the UPJ to the UVJ. These strictures are usually an unintended result of surgical intervention, usually secondary to adhesions or scar formation. Depending on its severity, ureteral obstruction can threaten the function of the kidney. Clinical manifestations of a ureteral stricture include mild to moderate colic; this pain may be of moderate to severe intensity if the patient consumes a large volume of fluids (alcohol, in particular) over a brief period. Infection is unusual unless a calculus or foreign object such as a stent or nephrostomy tube is present.

The discomfort and obstruction of a ureteral stricture may be temporarily bypassed by placing a stent under endoscopic control or by diverting urinary flow via a nephrostomy tube inserted into the renal pelvis of the affected kidney. Definitive correction requires dilation with a balloon or catheter. If the stricture is severe or recurs after initial balloon or catheter dilation, it may be incised under endoscopic control (*endo-ureterotomy*). In select cases, an open surgical approach may be required to excise the stenotic area and reanastomose the ureter to the contralateral ureter (*uretero-ureterostomy*) or to the renal pelvis. Alternatively, distal ureteral strictures may be managed by a *uretero-neocystostomy* (reimplantation of the ureter into the bladder wall).

Urethral Stricture

A *urethral stricture* is the result of fibrosis or inflammation of the urethral lumen (Urology Care Foundation, n.d.). Causes of urethral strictures include trauma, urethritis (particularly following gonococcal infection), and a congenital defect in the canalization of the urethra; causes can also be iatrogenic (following surgical intervention). Once the process of inflammation and fibrosis begins, the lumen of the urethra narrows, and its compliance (ability to close or open in response to bladder filling or micturition) is compromised. Meatal stenosis, a narrowing of the urethral opening, is also common.

Clinical manifestations associated with a urethral stricture include a diminished force of the urinary stream, spraying, or a split urine stream. The patient may report feelings of incomplete bladder emptying with urinary frequency and nocturia. Moderate to severe obstruction of the bladder outlet may lead to acute urinary retention. The patient may report a history of urethritis, difficulty with placement of a urinary catheter, or trauma involving the penis or the perineum. However, many patients are unable to recall any such events, thus leading to a diagnosis of an idiopathic stricture. A history of a UTI is not uncommon, particularly if the stricture involves the distal urethra.

Initial management of a stricture may be based on dilation. A metal instrument (urethral sound) or a series of progressively enlarging stents can be placed into the urethra (filiforms and followers) to expand its lumen in a stepwise fashion. Although this procedure may be initially successful, recurring stenosis is frequent. Recurrences may be managed by teaching the patient to repeatedly dilate the urethra by self-catheterization every few days. Alternatively, an endoscopic or open surgical procedure may provide a more durable solution to an obstructive urethral stricture. Shorter strictures may be managed by resection of the fibrotic area with primary reanastomosis. Longer strictures may require autotransplantation of a substitute segment such as a skin flap.

RENAL TRAUMA

A rise in the incidence of traumatic renal injuries is related to an increase in the mechanization and speed of transportation and to the increase in violent crimes and injuries (da Costa, Amend, Stenzl, et al., 2016). Blunt trauma is the most common cause. Injury to the kidney should be considered in cases of multiple injuries, sports injuries, traffic accidents, and falls. It is especially likely when the patient injures the abdomen, the flank, or the back. Penetrating injuries may result from violent encounters (e.g., gunshot or stabbing incidents) or may be of iatrogenic origin.

Clinical findings include a history of trauma to the area of the kidneys. Gross or microscopic hematuria may be present. Diagnostic studies include urinalysis, IVP with cystography, ultrasound, CT scan, or MRI evaluation. Renal arteriography may also be used. Both the injured kidney and the uninvolved kidney should be evaluated to provide information for further management.

The severity of renal trauma depends on the extent of the injury. Treatments range from bed rest, fluids, and analgesia to surgical exploration and repair or nephrectomy.

Nursing interventions vary with the type and the extent of associated injuries. Specific interventions related to renal trauma include ensuring increased fluid intake, providing comfort measures, monitoring for shock (e.g., penetrating injury), monitoring intake and output, observing for hematuria, determining the presence of myoglobinuria, assessing the cardiovascular status, and monitoring the use of potentially nephrotoxic antibiotics.

RENAL VASCULAR PROBLEMS

Vascular problems involving the kidney include (a) nephrosclerosis, (b) renal artery stenosis, and (c) renal vein thrombosis.

NEPHROSCLEROSIS

Nephrosclerosis is sclerosis of the small arteries and arterioles of the kidney, resulting in renal tissue destruction. The decreased blood flow results in patchy necrosis of the renal parenchyma. Ischemic necrosis and destruction of glomeruli with subsequent fibrosis also occur.

Benign nephrosclerosis usually occurs in adults 30 to 50 years of age. It is caused by vascular changes resulting from hypertension and from the process of atherosclerosis. Atherosclerotic vascular changes account for most of the loss of renal function associated with aging. There is a direct relation between the degree of nephrosclerosis and the severity of hypertension. The patient with benign nephrosclerosis may have normal renal function in the early stages. The only detectable abnormality may be hypertension.

Accelerated nephrosclerosis, or *malignant nephrosclerosis,* is associated with malignant hypertension, a complication of hypertension characterized by a sharp increase in blood pressure with a diastolic pressure greater than 130 mm Hg (Linas, 2011). The patient is usually a young adult, with a male-to-female predominance of 2 : 1. Renal insufficiency progresses rapidly.

Treatment for benign nephrosclerosis is the same as that for essential hypertension (see Chapter 35). Malignant nephrosclerosis is treated with aggressive antihypertensive therapy (see Chapter 35). The availability and use of antihypertensives have improved the prognosis for patients with benign and malignant nephrosclerosis. Renal dysfunction and renal failure (in some persons) constitute two of the major complications of hypertension. The prognosis for patients with malignant hypertension is poor, with the major cause of death related to renal failure.

Diabetic patients who have renal complications such as diabetic nephropathy often suffer progressive impairment of renal function (see Chapter 52).

RENAL ARTERY STENOSIS

Renal artery stenosis, a partial occlusion of one or both renal arteries and their major branches, is a major cause of abrupt-onset hypertension. It can be caused by atherosclerotic narrowing or fibromuscular hyperplasia. Renal artery stenosis accounts for 1% to 2% of all cases of hypertension.

When hypertension develops rather abruptly, renal artery stenosis should be considered as a possible cause, especially in patients younger than 30 or older than 50 years and in patients with no familial history of hypertension. This contrasts with the age distribution for essential hypertension, which peaks between 30 and 50 years of age. A renal arteriogram is the best diagnostic tool for identifying renal artery stenosis.

The goals of therapy are control of blood pressure and restoration of perfusion to the kidney. Percutaneous transluminal renal angioplasty is the procedure of choice, especially in older patients who are poor surgical risks. Surgical revascularization of the kidney is indicated when blood flow is decreased enough to cause renal ischemia or when evidence indicates that renovascular hypertension is present and might be resolved by surgical intervention. The surgical procedure usually involves anastomoses between the kidney and another major artery, usually the splenic artery or the aorta. In select cases of unilateral renal involvement with high renin production, unilateral nephrectomy may be indicated.

RENAL VEIN THROMBOSIS

Renal vein thrombosis, an embolus occurring in the renal vein, may occur unilaterally or bilaterally. Trauma, extrinsic compression (e.g., tumour, aortic aneurysm), renal cell carcinoma, pregnancy, contraceptive use, and nephrotic syndrome are associated with renal vein thrombosis.

Symptoms include flank pain, hematuria, or fever or nephrotic syndrome. Anticoagulation is important in treatment because there is a high incidence of pulmonary emboli. Corticosteroids may be used for patients with nephrosis. Surgical thrombectomy may be performed instead of or along with anticoagulation (Barbour, Greenwald, Djurdjev, et al., 2012).

HEREDITARY RENAL DISEASES

Hereditary renal diseases involve developmental abnormalities of the renal parenchyma. These abnormalities are either isolated or part of more complex malformation syndromes. The majority of inherited structural abnormalities are cystic. However, cysts may also develop as a result of obstructive uropathies, metabolic derangements, or neurological diseases. Cysts may be evaluated to rule out any tumour content.

POLYCYSTIC KIDNEY DISEASE

Polycystic kidney disease (PKD) is one of the most common genetic diseases in Canada. It may first become apparent in either childhood or adulthood. It involves both kidneys and occurs in both men and women. The cortex and the medulla are filled with thin-walled cysts that are several millimetres to several centimetres in diameter (Figure 48-7). The cysts enlarge and destroy surrounding tissue by compression. They are filled with fluid and may contain blood or pus.

There are two forms of hereditary polycystic renal disease. The adult form of PKD is an autosomal dominant disorder. It is latent for many years and is usually evidenced between the ages 30 and 40. However, PKD has also been found in newborns. The childhood form of PKD is a rare autosomal recessive disorder that is often rapidly progressive (see the "Genetics in Clinical Practice" box).

Clinical Manifestations

In the patient with PKD (Figure 48-8), symptoms appear when the cysts begin to enlarge. A common early symptom of adult PKD is abdominal or flank pain, which is steady and dull or abrupt in onset as well as episodic and colicky. This pain is often caused by bleeding into the cysts. On physical examination, palpable bilateral enlarged kidneys are often found. Other clinical manifestations include hematuria (from rupture of cysts), UTI, and hypertension.

Diagnosis is based on clinical manifestations, family history, IVP, ultrasound, or CT scan. Usually, the disease progresses to end-stage renal failure, although some individuals have relatively mild disease and die from unrelated problems. Loss of kidney function to the point of end-stage renal disease occurs by age 60 in 50% of patients (Mayo Clinic Staff, 2014).

Collaborative Care

There is no specific treatment for PKD. A major aim of treatment is to prevent infections of the urinary tract or to treat them with appropriate antibiotics if they occur. Nephrectomy may be necessary if pain, bleeding, or infection becomes a chronic, serious problem.

When the patient begins to experience progressive renal failure, the interventions are determined by the remaining renal function. Nursing measures are those used for management of end-stage renal disease (see Chapter 49). They include diet modification; fluid restriction; medications (e.g., antihypertensives); assisting the patient to accept the chronic disease process; and assisting the patient and family to deal with physical, socioeconomic, and emotional reactions to the disease.

GENETICS IN CLINICAL PRACTICE

Polycystic Kidney Disease

	Adult	Child
Genetic basis	• Autosomal dominant	• Autosomal recessive
Incidence	• 1 in 500 to 1 000	• 1 in 6 000 to 40 000
Gene location	• Chromosomes 4 and 16	• Chromosome 6
Genetic testing	• DNA testing available	• DNA testing available
Age of onset	• Usually between the ages of 30 and 40 yr, but can begin earlier	• Infancy or childhood
Clinical implications	• Multisystem involvement • Systemic hypertension occurs in 60%–80% of patients • Families at risk should be screened	• 30%–50% of affected newborns die shortly after birth

FIGURE 48-7 Comparison of polycystic kidney with normal kidney. Source: Brundage, D. J. (1992). *Renal disorders*. St. Louis: Mosby.

FIGURE 48-8 Man with an 11-kg polycystic kidney. Source: Lemmi, F. O., & Lemmi, C. A. E. (2000). *Physical assessment findings* (CD-ROM). Philadelphia: Saunders.

Patients with adult PKD often have children by the time the disease is diagnosed. Each child of a parent with PKD has a 50% chance of having the disease. Patients will need appropriate counselling regarding plans for having more children. In addition, genetic counselling resources should be provided for the children.

MEDULLARY CYSTIC DISEASE

Medullary cystic disease is a hereditary disorder that occurs in two forms. The *autosomal recessive form* is associated with renal failure before age 20; the *autosomal dominant form* is associated with renal failure after age 20. Most cysts are located in the medulla. The kidneys are asymmetrical, are significantly scarred, and have defects in their concentration ability. Polyuria, progressive renal failure, severe anemia, metabolic acidosis, and poor sodium conservation are common. Hypertension in patients with this disease can be a terminal event. Genetic counselling may be helpful in family planning. Treatment measures are those related to end-stage renal disease (see Chapter 49).

ALPORT SYNDROME

Alport syndrome is also known as *chronic hereditary nephritis*. Two forms of the disease exist: (a) classic Alport syndrome, which is inherited as a sex-linked disorder with hematuria, sensorineural deafness, and deformities of the anterior surface of the lens, and (b) nonclassic Alport syndrome, which is inherited as an autosomal trait that causes hematuria but not deafness or lens deformities (National Kidney Foundation, 2015b). The disease affects males earlier and more severely than females and is often diagnosed in the first decade of life. The basic defect is altered synthesis of the GBM, and patients most commonly have hematuria and progressive uremia. Treatment is supportive, although the disease will not recur after kidney transplantation. Corticosteroids and cytotoxic drugs are not effective.

RENAL INVOLVEMENT IN METABOLIC AND CONNECTIVE TISSUE DISEASES

Various metabolic and connective tissue disease processes may have an effect on renal function. The pathophysiological effects on the renal parenchyma are not always specific to each process. The clinical course of renal involvement is that of chronic progressive nephropathy, which can result in uremia and death. Management includes treatment of the primary disorder along with symptomatic relief of renal involvement. If renal involvement progresses to end-stage renal disease, management includes dialysis or transplantation (see Chapter 49). Nursing interventions include teaching the patient about the primary disease process, the renal involvement, and the resulting need to comply with dietary and fluid restrictions and drug regimens.

Diabetic nephropathy is the primary cause of end-stage renal failure in Canada (Canadian Diabetes Association Clinical Practice Guidelines Expert Committee, 2013). Diabetes mellitus may affect the kidneys in several ways. Microangiopathic changes in diabetes consist of diffuse glomerulo-sclerosis, involving thickening of the GBM, and nodular glomerulo-sclerosis (Kimmelstiel–Wilson syndrome), which is characterized by nodular lesions. Nodular glomerulo-sclerosis is reasonably specific for type 1 diabetes mellitus. Patients with diabetes who are prone to glomerulo-nephropathy (i.e., the presence of trace proteinuria or retinopathy) require careful monitoring of glucose levels and insulin requirements. (Diabetes mellitus is discussed in Chapter 52.)

Gout is a syndrome of acute attacks of arthritis caused by hyperuricemia (see Chapter 67). Monosodium urate crystals deposited in joints are responsible for the syndrome. Renal disease may develop as a result of damage caused by deposition of uric acid crystals in the renal interstitium and the tubules.

Amyloidosis is a group of disorders evidenced by impaired organ function from the infiltration of tissues with a hyaline substance (amyloid). The hyaline consists largely of protein. Kidney involvement is common in amyloidosis. Proteinuria is often the first clinical manifestation.

Systemic lupus erythematosus is a connective tissue disorder characterized by the involvement of several tissues and organs, particularly the joints, the skin, and the kidneys. (Systemic lupus erythematosus is discussed in Chapter 67.) Clinical manifestations of lupus nephritis are similar to those of other forms of glomerulo-nephritis. Renal failure frequently occurs in systemic lupus erythematosus and has a poor prognosis.

Systemic sclerosis (scleroderma) is a disease of unknown etiology characterized by widespread alterations of connective tissue and vascular lesions in many organs (see Chapter 67). In the kidney, vascular lesions are associated with fibrosis. An immune complex mechanism has been postulated as a possible etiological factor. The severity of renal involvement varies. Patients who develop severe renal lesions have a poor prognosis.

URINARY TRACT TUMOURS

KIDNEY CANCER

The incidence of kidney cancer in Canada is rising. In 2012, it was estimated that 5 600 new cases would be diagnosed across the country that year and that 1 700 people would die from it. Kidney cancers arise from the cortex or the pelvis (and the calyces). Tumours arising from both areas may be benign or malignant. However, malignant tumours are more frequent. Adenocarcinoma (renal cell carcinoma) is the most common type. Adenocarcinoma occurs twice as often in men as in women and is typically discovered when the person is 50 to 70 years old. Cigarette smoking is the most significant risk factor for the development of adeno-carcinoma (Canadian Cancer Society, 2016). Other risk factors are obesity, the use of phenacetin-containing analgesics, and exposure to asbestos, cadmium, and gasoline (Nogueras, Thomas, & Porter, 2015).

There are no characteristic early symptoms. Generalized symptoms of weight loss, weakness, and anemia are the earliest manifestations. The classic manifestations of gross hematuria, flank pain, and a palpable mass are those of advanced disease. The most common sites of metastases include the lungs, liver, and long bones. Local extension of kidney cancer into the renal vein and the vena cava is common (Figure 48-9). Renal cystic disease and renal-associated carcinomas may develop in patients with end-stage renal disease who are receiving maintenance renal dialysis (see Chapter 49).

Several studies are used to diagnose kidney cancer. IVP with nephrotomography is the primary examination by which most masses are detected and evaluated. Ultrasounds have improved the ability to differentiate between a tumour and a cyst.

FIGURE 48-9 Adenocarcinoma. Cross-section shows yellowish cancer in one pole of the kidney. The tumour also involves the dilated thrombosed renal vein. Source: Kumar, V., Abbas, A. K., & Aster, J. (2015). *Robbins and Cotran pathologic basis of disease* (9th ed., p. 954, Figure 20-51). Philadelphia: Saunders.

TABLE 48-15	ROBSON'S SYSTEM OF STAGING RENAL CARCINOMA
Stage	**Description**
I	Limitation to renal capsule
II	Spreading to perirenal fat but confined within fascia; includes metastasis to adrenal gland
III	Regional lymph node involvement, tumour thrombus in renal vein or vena cava, involvement of renal vein or vena cava
IV	Presence of distant metastases

Angiography, percutaneous needle aspiration, CT, and MRI are also used in the diagnosis of renal tumours. Small renal tumours are found earlier because of the increased use of CT scans and MRI. Radionuclide isotope scanning is used to detect metastases.

Robson's system of staging renal carcinoma is presented in Table 48-15. The treatment of choice is a radical nephrectomy, which is the removal of the kidney, the adrenal gland, the surrounding fascia, part of the ureter, and the draining lymph nodes. Radiation therapy is used palliatively in inoperable cases and when there are metastases to bone or lungs.

Chemotherapy using 5-fluorouracil (5-FU) and gemcitabine is used to treat metastatic disease. However, renal cell carcinoma is refractory to most chemotherapy drugs. Biological therapy, including interferon-alfa (IFN-α) and interleukin-2 (IL-2), is most promising in the treatment of metastatic disease (North, Basappa, Bjarnason, et al., 2013). Adverse effects of IL-2 include capillary leakage syndrome, fever, chills, fatigue, and hypotension.

The 5-year survival rate of patients with early-stage kidney cancer is 60% to 70% after undergoing radical nephrectomy. The

FIGURE 48-10 A, A papillary transitional cell carcinoma is seen arising from the dome of the bladder as a cauliflower-like lesion. **B,** Opened bladder shows a bladder cancer at an advanced stage. The yellow areas represent ulcerations and necrosis. Source: *A,* Stevens, A., & Lowe, J. (2000). *Pathology: Illustrated review in color* (2nd ed.). London: Mosby; *B,* Kumar, V., Abbas, A. K., & Aster, J. (2015). *Robbins and Cotran pathologic basis of disease* (9th ed., p. 967, Figure 21-12). Philadelphia: Saunders.

5-year survival rate for patients with metastatic disease is only 3% to 10%. However, patients with metastatic disease often remain stable for a prolonged period (North, Basappa, Bjarnason, et al., 2013).

BLADDER CANCER

It was estimated that 8 900 Canadians would be diagnosed with bladder cancer in 2017 and that 2 400 Canadians would die from this disease (Canadian Cancer Society's Advisory Committee on Cancer Statistics, 2017). Bladder cancer is the sixth most common type of cancer diagnosed in Canadians. The most frequent malignant tumour of the urinary tract is transitional cell carcinoma of the bladder. Most bladder tumours are papillomatous growths within the bladder (Figure 48-10). Cancer of the bladder is most common between the ages of 60 and 70 years and is at least three times more common in men than in women. Risk factors for bladder cancer include cigarette smoking, exposure to dyes used in the rubber and cable industries, and chronic use of phenacetin-containing analgesics (Canadian Cancer Society, 2016). Women treated with radiation for cervical cancer and patients receiving cyclophosphamide (Procytox) also have increased risk, but the reason is unknown.

Individuals with chronic, recurrent stones (often bladder) and chronic lower urinary infections have an increased risk for squamous cell cancer of the bladder. Patients who have in-dwelling catheters for long periods can develop these chronic conditions.

Clinical Manifestations and Diagnostic Studies

Gross, painless hematuria (chronic or intermittent) is the most common clinical finding. Bladder irritability with dysuria, urinary frequency, and urinary urgency may also occur. When cancer is suspected, urine specimens for cytology can be obtained to determine the presence of neoplastic or atypical cells. Exfoliated cells from the epithelial surface of the bladder can readily be detected in voided specimens. Other recent urine tests assess for specific factors associated with bladder cancer, such as bladder tumour antigens. Bladder cancers can be detected using IVP, ultrasound, CT, or MRI. However, the presence of cancer is confirmed by cystoscopy and biopsy.

The depth of invasion of the bladder wall and surrounding tissue determines the clinical staging of carcinoma of the bladder. The Jewett–Strong–Marshall classification system broadly classifies bladder cancer as superficial (carcinoma in situ, O, A), invasive (B_1, B_2, C), or metastatic (D_1–D_4) disease. Pathological grading systems are also used to classify the malignant potential of tumour cells, indicating a scale from well-differentiated to anaplastic categories. Low-stage, low-grade bladder cancers are the most responsive to treatment and are more easily cured.

NURSING AND COLLABORATIVE MANAGEMENT BLADDER CANCER

Collaborative care of the patient with bladder cancer is outlined in Table 48-16.

SURGICAL THERAPY

Surgical therapies include a variety of procedures. *Transurethral resection with fulguration* (electrocautery) is used for the diagnosis and treatment of superficial lesions with a low recurrence rate. This procedure is also used to control bleeding in the patient who is a poor operative risk or who has advanced tumours. With this technique, the tumour mass is excised by means of a blade inserted through the cystoscope. The remaining portions of the tumour are cauterized.

A second technique, *laser photocoagulation*, is also used to treat superficial bladder cancers. This procedure can be repeated a number of times to manage recurrences. The advantages of laser include bloodless destruction of the lesion, minimal risk for perforation, and lack of need for a urinary catheter. The primary disadvantage is that, owing to destruction of the tumour, pathological evaluation for grading and staging cannot be completed.

A third technique used is *open loop resection* (snaring of polyp types of lesion) *with fulguration*. It is used for the control of bleeding, for large superficial tumours, and for multiple lesions.

TABLE 48-16 COLLABORATIVE CARE

Bladder Cancer

Diagnostic
- History and physical examination
- CT scan
- Cystoscopy with biopsy
- Cytology studies
- Intravenous pyelogram
- Ultrasound
- Urinalysis

Collaborative Therapy
- Surgical treatment
  - Laser photocoagulation
  - Open loop resection or fulguration
  - Radical cystectomy
  - Segmental cystectomy
  - Transurethral resection with fulguration
- Radiation
- Intravesical immunotherapy
  - Bacille Calmette–Guérin
  - Interferon alfa
- Intravesical chemotherapy
  - Doxorubicin
  - Mitomycin
  - Thiotepa
- Systemic chemotherapy

CT, computed tomography.

Treatment of large lesions entails a segmental resection of the bladder *(segmental cystectomy).*

Postoperative instructions for any of these procedures includes drinking a large volume of fluid each day for the first week following the procedure and avoiding intake of alcoholic beverages. Patients are taught to self-monitor their urine. It is anticipated to be pink during the first several days after the procedure, but it should not be bright red or contain blood clots. Approximately 7 to 10 days following tumour resection or ablation, the patient may observe dark-red or rust-coloured flecks in the urine. These are anticipated and represent scabs from the healing tumour resection sites. Opioid analgesics may be required for a brief period after the procedure, along with stool softeners. Patients can be encouraged to take a 15- to 20-minute sitz bath two or three times a day to promote muscle relaxation and to reduce the risk for urinary retention. The nurse should also help the patient and family cope with fears about cancer, surgery, and sexuality and should emphasize the importance of regular follow-up care. Frequent routine cystoscopies are required.

When the tumour is invasive or when it involves the trigone (the area where the ureters insert into the bladder) and the patient is free from metastasis beyond the pelvic area, a partial or radical cystectomy with urinary diversion is the treatment of choice (see the section on urinary diversion later in the chapter). A *partial cystectomy* includes resection of that portion of the bladder wall containing the tumour, along with a margin of normal tissue. A *radical cystectomy* involves removal of the bladder, the prostate, and the seminal vesicles in men and the bladder, the uterus, the cervix, the urethra, and the ovaries in women (Kassouf, Traboulsi, Kulkarni, et al., 2015).

RADIATION THERAPY AND CHEMOTHERAPY

Radiation therapy is used with cystectomy or as the primary therapy when the cancer is inoperable or when surgery is refused. Increasingly, radiation therapy is being combined with systemic chemotherapy. Sometimes, combination systemic chemotherapy is used for bladder cancer, usually preoperatively or before radiation therapy, or is used to treat distant metastases. Chemotherapy drugs used in treating invasive bladder cancer include cisplatin, vinblastine, and methotrexate.

INTRAVESICAL THERAPY

Chemotherapy with local instillation of chemotherapeutic or immune-stimulating agents can be delivered directly into the bladder by a urethral catheter. Protocols vary, but intravesical therapy is usually initiated at weekly intervals for 6 to 12 weeks. The chemotherapeutic drugs are instilled directly into the patient's bladder and retained for about 2 hours. The patient's position may be changed every 15 minutes for maximum contact in all areas of the bladder, especially if the tumour occurred on the bladder dome. The use of maintenance therapy after the initial induction regimen may be beneficial.

BCG, a weakened strain of *Mycobacterium bovis,* is the treatment of choice for carcinoma in situ. BCG stimulates the immune system rather than acting directly on cancer cells in the bladder. When BCG alone fails, IFN-α may be used in addition to BCG. Other treatments that can be used when BCG fails include thiotepa, an alkylating agent.

Most patients have irritation upon voiding and hemorrhagic cystitis following intravesical therapy. Thiotepa, when absorbed into circulation from the bladder wall, can significantly reduce

WBC and platelet counts in some individuals. BCG may cause flulike symptoms, hematuria, or systemic infection. Other adverse effects usually associated with chemotherapy, such as nausea, vomiting, and hair loss, are not experienced with intravesical chemotherapy.

Nursing responsibilities include encouraging the patient to increase the daily fluid intake and to quit smoking, assessing the patient for secondary UTI, and stressing the need for routine urological follow-up. The patient may have fears or concerns about sexual activity or bladder function that will have to be addressed.

URINARY INCONTINENCE AND RETENTION

Urinary incontinence (UI) is an uncontrolled loss of urine that is of sufficient magnitude to be a problem. Approximately 3.3 million Canadians experience incontinence, including 10% of children 6 years of age and up, 25% of women middle-aged and older, and 15% of men aged 60 years and older (Canadian Continence Foundation, 2016). Among younger adults, more women than men are affected by UI. Although UI has traditionally been viewed as a social or hygienic problem, it is now known to affect quality of life as well as contribute to morbidity in older adults. (UI is not a natural consequence of aging.)

Causes of UI may be transient (e.g., caused by confusion or depression, infection, medications, restricted mobility, or stool impaction). Acquired disorders are described in Table 48-17. Patients may have more than one type of incontinence and may not disclose UI symptoms because of associated stigma.

Urinary retention is the inability to empty the bladder despite micturition or the accumulation of urine in the bladder because of the inability to urinate. It may be associated with dribbling urinary leakage called *overflow UI. Acute urinary retention* is the total inability to pass urine via micturition; it is a medical emergency. *Chronic urinary retention* is defined as incomplete bladder emptying despite urination. Postvoid residual volumes in patients with chronic urinary retention vary widely; values of 150 to 200 mL or higher generally necessitate further evaluation. Smaller volumes may justify evaluation when they produce LUTS or occur in a context of recurring UTIs. Urinary retention is caused by two different dysfunctions of the urinary system: bladder outlet obstruction and deficient detrusor contraction strength. Obstruction leads to urinary retention when the blockage prevents bladder evacuation of its contents despite a detrusor contraction. A common cause of obstruction in men is an enlarged prostate. Urinary retention also results when the detrusor muscle no longer has the strength to contract with enough force or for long enough to completely empty the bladder.

Common causes of deficient detrusor muscle contraction strength are neurological diseases affecting sacral segments 2, 3, and 4; longstanding diabetes mellitus; overdistension; chronic alcoholism; and drugs (e.g., anticholinergic drugs).

NURSING MANAGEMENT
URINARY INCONTINENCE

Nurses' relational care approaches through listening to patients' questions and valuing patients' knowledge about UI are required to address socioemotional well-being and promote application of UI management techniques. The majority of UI symptoms can be managed conservatively with the following interventions:

hydration; reduction in consumption of caffeine and alcohol (bladder irritants); smoking cessation (smoking increases the risk of stress incontinence); and constipation management, which includes adequate fluid intake, increase in dietary fibre, light exercise, and judicious use of stool softeners. (The management of constipation is discussed in Chapter 45.) As well, continence strategies can assist in preventing falls and fall-related injuries in older adults (Registered Nurses' Association of Ontario [RNAO], 2011).

Habit training or prompted toileting is useful for patients with urge, mixed, and functional UI. Habit training uses the results of a voiding diary or bladder log to determine patterns of daytime voiding frequency. A goal is then established for voiding frequency, usually ranging from 2 to 3 hours. Voiding is scheduled rigidly during waking hours according to the baseline urinary frequency identified on the bladder log. At night, the person is advised to urinate as normal if awakened from sleep with the desire to void. Habit training may be combined with pelvic muscle training, focusing on techniques such as urge suppression. Prompted toileting is indicated for patients with altered cognitive function and functional UI (usually coexisting with urge UI). Specifically, caregivers are taught to remind the patient to toilet on a regular basis (usually q2–3h), and the patient is assisted to the toilet and given praise for successful toileting. A trial of prompted toileting, in conjunction with a urological evaluation, is used to predict the ultimate success of such a program.

In the hospital, nursing management includes maximizing toilet access and promoting privacy when offering the urinal or bedpan or assisting the patient to the bathroom every 2 to 3 hours or at scheduled times.

When attempting to manage UI, many women use feminine hygiene pads, and many men and women use household products such as rags, paper towels, or folded toilet tissue. None of these products is adequately designed to wick urine away from the skin, prevent soiling of clothing, and reduce or eliminate odour. The nurse should share information on products specifically designed to contain urine. For example, patients with mild to moderate UI often benefit from incontinence pads containing a material specifically designed to absorb many times its weight in water. Patients with higher volume urine loss or those with double urinary and fecal incontinence may benefit from disposable or reusable incontinence briefs or pad–pant systems.

Diagnostic Studies

The basic evaluation for UI and urinary retention includes a focused history, physical assessment, and a bladder log or voiding record whenever possible. Information should be obtained regarding the onset of UI, factors that provoke urinary leakage, and associated conditions. The nurse should pay special attention to factors known to produce transient UI, particularly when a relatively sudden onset of urine loss is reported. The physical examination begins with an assessment of general health and functional issues associated with urinary function, including mobility, dexterity, and cognitive function. A pelvic examination includes careful inspection of the perineal skin for signs of erosion or rashes related to UI. Local innervation and pelvic muscle strength should also be evaluated. Whenever possible, the patient is asked to keep a bladder log or voiding diary documenting the timing of urinations, episodes of urinary leakage, and frequency of nocturia for a period of 1 to 7 days. This record can be kept by nursing staff if the person is in an inpatient facility.

TABLE 48-17	ACQUIRED DISORDERS CAUSING URINARY INCONTINENCE	
Type and Description	**Causes**	**Treatment**
Stress Incontinence* Sudden increase in intra-abdominal pressure causes involuntary passage of urine. It can occur during coughing, heavy lifting, straining, or laughing.	*Females:* Condition is found most commonly in women with relaxed pelvic musculature (frequently from obstetrical complications or multiple pregnancies). Structures of the female urethra atrophy when estrogen decreases. *Males:* Prostate surgery for benign prostatic hyperplasia or prostatic carcinoma.	Perineal muscle exercises (e.g., Kegel exercises), weight loss if patient is obese, insertion of vaginal pessary, estrogen (vaginal creams, tablets, or vaginal ring) Condom catheters or penile clamp, surgery Urethral inserts, patches, or bladder neck support devices to correct underlying problem
Urge Incontinence* Condition occurs randomly when involuntary urination is preceded by warning a few seconds to a few minutes in advance. Leakage is periodic but frequent. Nocturnal frequency and incontinence are common. Condition may appear with varying severity during psychological stress.	Condition is caused by uncontrolled contraction or overactivity of detrusor muscle. Bladder escapes central inhibition and contracts reflexively. Conditions include central nervous system disorders (e.g., cerebro-vascular disease, Alzheimer's disease, brain tumour, Parkinson's disease), bladder disorders (e.g., carcinoma in situ, radiation effects, interstitial cystitis), interference with spinal inhibitory pathways (e.g., malignant growth in spinal cord, spondylosis), and bladder outlet obstruction, as well as conditions of unknown etiology.	Treatment of underlying cause, instruction to have patient urinate more frequently or on time schedule, anticholinergic drugs (e.g., imipramine) at bedtime, calcium channel blockers, condom catheters, vaginal estrogen
Overflow Incontinence Pressure of urine in overfull bladder overcomes sphincter control. Urination may also occur frequently in small amounts during the night. Bladder remains distended and is usually palpable.	Disorder is caused by outlet obstruction (prostatic hyperplasia, bladder neck obstruction, urethral stricture) or by underactive detrusor muscle caused by myogenic or neurogenic factors (e.g., herniated disk, diabetic neuropathy). It may also occur after anaesthesia and surgery (especially procedures such as hemorrhoidectomy, herniorrhaphy, cystoscopy). Neurogenic bladder (flaccid type) is another cause.	Urinary catheterization to decompress bladder, implementation of Credé or Valsalva manoeuvre, α-adrenergic blocker (e.g., prazosin) to decrease outlet resistance, bethanechol (Duvoid) to enhance bladder contractions, intermittent catheterization, surgery to correct underlying problem
Reflex Incontinence No warning or stress precedes periodic involuntary urination. Urination is frequent, is moderate in volume, and occurs equally during the day and night.	Spinal cord lesion above S2 interferes with central nervous system inhibition. Disorder results in detrusor hyper-reflexia and interferes with pathways coordinating detrusor contraction and sphincter relaxation.	Treatment of underlying cause, bladder decompression to prevent ureteral reflux and hydronephrosis, intermittent self-catheterization, α-adrenergic blocker (e.g., prazosin) to relax internal sphincter, diazepam or baclofen to relax external sphincter, prophylactic antibiotics, surgical sphincterotomy
Incontinence After Trauma or Surgery Vesico-vaginal or urethro-vaginal fistula may occur in women. Alteration in continence control in men involves proximal urethral sphincter (bladder neck and prostatic urethra) and distal urethral sphincter (external striated muscle).	Fistulas may occur during pregnancy, after delivery of baby, as a result of hysterectomy or invasive cancer of cervix, or after radiation therapy. Incontinence is found as postoperative complication after transurethral, perineal, or retropubic prostatectomy.	Surgery to correct fistula, urinary diversion surgery to bypass urethra and bladder, external condom catheter, penile clamp, placement of artificial implantable sphincter
Functional Incontinence Loss of urine resulting from problems of patient mobility or environmental factors.	Older adults often have problems that affect balance and mobility.	Modifications of environment or care plan that facilitate regular, easy access to toilet and promote patient safety (e.g., better lighting, ambulatory assistance equipment, clothing alterations, timed voiding, different toileting equipment)

*Patients can have a combination of stress and urge incontinence that is referred to as *mixed incontinence*.

TABLE 48-18 INTERVENTIONS FOR URINARY INCONTINENCE

Intervention	Description
Lifestyle Modifications	Self-management strategies to reduce or eliminate risk factors, including the following: • Smoking cessation • Weight reduction • Good bowel regimen • Reduction of bladder irritants such as caffeine • Fluid modifications for those with urge incontinence
Scheduling Voiding Regimens	
• Timed voiding	Toileting on a fixed schedule (typically q2–3h during waking hours)
• Habit retraining	Scheduled toileting with adjustments of voiding intervals (longer or shorter) based on the individual's voiding pattern
• Prompted voiding	Scheduled toileting that requires prompts to void from a caregiver (typically q3h); used in conjunction with operant conditioning techniques for rewarding individuals for maintaining continence and appropriate toileting
• Bladder retraining and urge-suppression strategies	Scheduled toileting with progressive voiding intervals; includes teaching of urge-control strategies using relaxation and distraction techniques, self-monitoring, use of reinforcement techniques, and other strategies such as conscious contraction of pelvic floor muscles
Pelvic Floor Muscle Rehabilitation	
• Pelvic floor muscle (Kegel) exercises or training	See Table 48-19
• Vaginal weight training	Active retention of increasing vaginal weights at least twice a day; typically used in combination with pelvic floor muscle exercises
• Biofeedback	See "Complementary & Alternative Therapies" box
• Electrical stimulation	Application of low-voltage electric current to sacral and pudendal afferent fibres through vaginal, anal, or surface electrodes; used to inhibit bladder overactivity and improve awareness, contractility, and efficiency of pelvic muscle contraction
Anti-Incontinence Devices	
• Intravaginal support devices (pessaries and bladder neck support prostheses)	Devices to support bladder neck, relieve minor pelvic organ prolapse, and change pressure transmission to the urethra
• Transvaginal sling device	Prevents involuntary release of urine through urethral support
• Intraurethral occlusive device (urethral plug)	Single-use device that is worn in the urethra to provide mechanical obstruction to prevent urine leakage; removed for voiding
• Penile compression device	Mechanical fixed compression applied to the penis to prevent any flow or leakage via the urethra; must be released hourly to void
Containment Devices	
• External collection devices	External catheter (condom) systems (i.e., penile sheaths) direct urine into a drainage bag; most commonly used by men
• Absorbent products	Variety of reusable and disposable pads and pant systems

The urinalysis is used to identify possible factors contributing to transient UI or urinary retention (e.g., urinary infection, diabetes mellitus). A postvoid residual urine must be measured in the patient undergoing evaluation for urinary retention and UI. The postvoid residual volume is obtained by asking the patient to urinate, followed by catheterization within a relatively brief period (preferably 5–10 min). Alternatively, a bladder scan device can be used to estimate the residual volume. Although less accurate than the catheterized residual measurement, this technique avoids catheterization with its associated discomfort and risk for UTI. Urodynamic testing is indicated in select cases of UI and urinary retention (Bettez, Tu, Carlson, et al., 2012). Imaging studies of the upper urinary tract (e.g., ultrasound, IVP) are obtained when retention or UI is associated with UTIs or when there is evidence of upper urinary tract involvement.

Collaborative Care: Urinary Incontinence

An estimated 80% of incontinence can be cured or significantly improved. Transient, reversible factors are corrected initially, followed by management of established UI (see Table 48-17). In general, less invasive treatments are attempted before more invasive methods (e.g., surgery) are used. Nevertheless, the choice of initial treatment is highly individualized and based on patient preference, the type and severity of UI, and associated anatomical defects.

Several therapies may be employed to improve urinary continence. These interventions are outlined in Table 48-18. Pelvic muscle training (Kegel exercises) is used to manage stress, urge, or mixed UI (Table 48-19). Biofeedback is used to assist the patient to identify, isolate, contract, and relax the pelvic muscles (see the "Complementary & Alternative Therapies" box). Strength training is used to improve the efficiency of the sphincter. Neuro-muscular education is used to teach patients how and when to contract the pelvic floor muscles to maximize continence. Bladder training or habit training involves rigidly scheduled toileting intervals designed to enhance bladder capacity and reduce the frequency and volume of urine loss. *Prompted toileting* is a behavioural technique used in patients with functional UI. In this case, patients with impaired cognitive function are regularly reminded to urinate, assisted to the toilet, and offered praise for successful toileting.

TABLE 48-19 PATIENT & CAREGIVER TEACHING GUIDE

Pelvic Floor Muscle (or Kegel) Exercises

What Is the Pelvic Floor Muscle?
Your pelvic floor muscle provides support for your bladder and rectum and, in women, the vagina and the uterus. If it weakens or is damaged, it cannot support these organs and their position can change. This causes problems with the normal bladder and rectal function. If you have a weak pelvic floor muscle, you might want to do special exercises to make the muscle stronger, prevent unwanted urine leakage, and lessen urinary urgency.

MALE

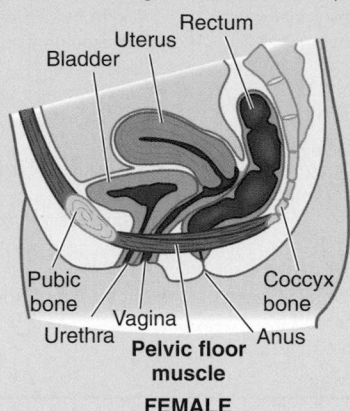

FEMALE

Finding the Pelvic Floor Muscle
Without tensing the muscles of your leg, buttocks, or abdomen, imagine that you are trying to control the passing of gas or pinching off a stool. Or imagine you are in an elevator full of people and you feel the urge to pass gas. What do you do? You tighten or pull in the ring of muscle around your rectum—your pelvic floor muscle. You should feel a lifting sensation in the area around the vagina or a pulling in of your rectum.

How to Do the Exercises
There are two different kinds of exercises—short squeezes and long squeezes.
1. To do the *short squeezes*, tighten your pelvic floor muscle quickly, squeeze hard for 2 sec, and then relax the muscle. Also, when you have strong urinary urges, try to tighten your pelvic floor muscle quickly and hard several times in a row until the urge passes.
2. To do the *long squeezes*, tighten the muscle for 5–10 sec before you relax. Do both of these exercises 40–50 times each day.

When to Do These Exercises
You can do these exercises anytime and anywhere. You can do these exercises in any position, but sitting or lying down may be the easiest.

How Long Does It Take Before You Notice a Change?
After 4–6 wk of doing these exercises, you should start to see less urine leakage and urinary urgency.

Source: Courtesy of Diane Newman.

 COMPLEMENTARY & ALTERNATIVE THERAPIES

Biofeedback for Urinary Incontinence in Women

Clinical Uses
Kegel exercises help to strengthen the pelvic floor muscles. Biofeedback helps to isolate muscle groups in the pelvis.

Effects
Sensors for biofeedback are placed in the vagina or on the skin outside of the vagina. These sensors measure electrical signals produced when muscles contract. Biofeedback training develops an awareness of and control of the pelvic floor muscles.

Nursing Implications
- If done correctly, pelvic floor muscle exercise is effective treatment for mild to moderate UI and other conditions related to pelvic floor muscle weakness. Unfortunately, many women do not do these exercises correctly. Biofeedback is a tool to make sure that these exercises are done correctly. Most supplementary insurance plans cover the cost of biofeedback.

Electrical stimulation of the pelvic floor muscles relies on very-low-voltage and low-frequency pulses to stimulate muscle contraction and diminish overactive bladder contractions. It can be used as monotherapy for the treatment of urge or mixed UI or in conjunction with pelvic muscle training in the management of stress UI. Minimally invasive electrical stimulation uses a transvaginal or transrectal probe, or a device can be surgically implanted near the pelvic nerve roots.

Drug Therapy. Drug therapy varies according to the UI type (Table 48-20). Drugs have a very limited role in the management of stress UI. α-Adrenergic agonists can be used to increase urethral resistance at the level of the sphincter mechanism. Unfortunately, they exert a limited beneficial effect, and they are associated with adverse effects including exacerbation of hypertension and tachycardia. Drugs play a more central role in the management of urge or reflex UI. Antimuscarinic (also called anticholinergic or antispasmodic) drugs relax the bladder muscle and inhibit overactive detrusor contractions. Two preparations, long-acting tolterodine (Detrol LA) and oxybutynin in a releasing capsule (Ditropan XL), are preferred because of their efficacy and the modest incidence of their adverse effects compared with older antimuscarinic agents.

TABLE 48-20   DRUG THERAPY

Voiding Dysfunction*

Drug Class and Mechanism of Action	Drug	Drug Class and Mechanism of Action	Drug
Muscarinic Receptor Antagonists and Anticholinergics Reduce overactive bladder contractions in urge urinary incontinence and overactive bladder	• Oxybutynin (Ditropan XL, Oxytrol transdermal system) • Tolterodine (Detrol, Detrol LA) • Dicyclomine (Bentylol)	**Tricyclic Antidepressants** Reduce sensory urgency and burning pain of interstitial cystitis Reduce overactive bladder contractions	• Imipramine • Amitriptyline (Elavil)
α-Adrenergic Antagonists Reduce urethral sphincter resistance to urinary outflow	• Doxazosin (Cardura) • Terazosin • Tamsulosin (Flomax CR)	**Calcium Channel Blockers** Reduce smooth muscle contraction strength May reduce burning pain of interstitial cystitis	• Nifedipine (Adalat) • Diltiazem • Verapamil (Isoptin)
5α-Reductase Inhibitors Androgen suppression that results in epithelial atrophy and a decrease in total prostate size	• Finasteride (Proscar)	**Hormone Therapy** Local application reduces urethral irritation and increases host defences against UTI	• Estrogen cream (Premarin, Estrace) • Estrogen vaginal ring (Estring) • Estrogen vaginal tablets (Vagifem)

UTI, urinary tract infection.
*The type of drug therapy depends on the type of incontinence.

DRUG ALERT—Tolterodine (Detrol)
• Overdosage can result in severe anticholinergic effects.
• These effects include GI cramping, diaphoresis, blurred vision, and urinary urgency.

Surgical Therapy. Surgical techniques also vary according to the type of UI (Bettez, Tu, Carlson, et al., 2012). The Marshall–Marchetti–Krantz procedure involves suspending the urethra and the bladder neck by suturing the anterior vaginal wall on each side to the periosteum of the pubic bones and the lower rectum through an abdominal incision. The Pereyra procedure and subsequent modifications involve suspending the tissues adjacent to the bladder neck to the abdominal fascia, mainly through a transvaginal approach. Placement of a suburethral sling, using autologous fascia, cadaveric fascia, or a synthetic material, can also correct stress UI in women. An artificial urethral sphincter can be used in women or men with intrinsic sphincter deficiency and severe stress UI. Bolsters can also be implanted in men with stress UI to increase urethral resistance. This procedure is technically similar to the suburethral sling surgery often performed in women. A tension-free synthetic vaginal tape also can be used to treat stress UI. This transvaginal slinglike material is placed under the midurethra through incisions in the abdominal and vaginal wall (Kociszewski, Rautenberg, Kuszka, et al., 2012). Alternatively, one of several bulking agents can be injected underneath the mucosa of the urethra to correct stress UI in women or men (Bettez, Tu, Carlson et al., 2012).

Bulking agents include glutaraldehyde cross-linked bovine collagen (GAX collagen), small silicone beads (Durasphere), or polytetrafluoroethylene (Teflon). Because of the risk of migration of Teflon particles, GAX collagen or Durasphere injections are most commonly used today.

Collaborative Care: Urinary Retention

Scheduled toileting and double voiding may be effective in chronic urinary retention with moderate postvoid residual volumes. However, for acute or chronic urinary retention, intermittent catheterization may be required. It allows the patient to remain free of an in-dwelling catheter with its associated risk of UTI and urethral irritation. However, an in-dwelling catheter is used when urethral obstruction renders intermittent catheterization uncomfortable or unfeasible, or when a patient is unwilling or unable to perform intermittent catheterization.

Drug Therapy. Several drugs may be administered to promote bladder evacuation. For patients with obstruction at the level of the bladder neck, an α-adrenergic blocker may be prescribed. These drugs relax the smooth muscle of the bladder neck, the prostatic urethra, and possibly the dually innervated rhabdo-sphincter, diminishing urethral resistance. Examples of α-adrenergic blocking agents are listed in Table 48-20. They are indicated for use in patients with BPH, bladder neck dyssynergia, or detrusor sphincter dyssynergia. Finasteride (Proscar) is a 5α-reductase enzyme inhibitor that reduces prostate size by inhibiting the conversion of testosterone to dihydrotestosterone. Finasteride is also useful for the hematuria that occasionally complicates symptomatic BPH in older men. Bethanechol chloride (Duvoid) is sometimes prescribed to promote contractility in the weakened detrusor muscle (Bettez, Tu, Carlson, et al., 2012).

Surgical Therapy. Surgical interventions are often useful when managing urinary retention caused by obstruction. Transurethral or open surgical techniques are used in select patients to treat benign or malignant prostatic enlargement, bladder neck contracture, urethral strictures, or dyssynergia of the bladder neck. Pelvic reconstruction using an abdominal or transvaginal approach can be used to correct bladder outlet obstruction in women with severe pelvic organ prolapse.

Unfortunately, surgery plays little role in the management of urinary retention caused by deficient detrusor contraction strength. Attempts to create a bladder stimulator (implanted device capable of stimulating micturition) have proved largely unsuccessful because of the difficulty in achieving a coordinated detrusor contraction associated with pelvic muscle and striated sphincter relaxation.

NURSING MANAGEMENT
URINARY RETENTION

Acute urinary retention is a medical emergency that requires prompt recognition and bladder drainage. The nurse should insert a catheter (as prescribed) unless otherwise directed. A catheter with a retention balloon is used in anticipation of the need for an in-dwelling catheter.

Patients with acute urinary retention (as well as patients predisposed to these episodes) should be taught strategies to minimize risk, including avoiding intake of large volumes of fluid over a brief period. Instead, patients should be advised to drink small volumes throughout the day. Patients are advised to warm up before attempting urination when chilled and to avoid large volumes of alcohol intake because it leads to polyuria and a diminished awareness of the need to urinate until the bladder is distended. Patients who are unable to urinate are advised to drink a cup of coffee or brewed tea containing caffeine to create or maximize urinary urgency and to take a warm shower and attempt to urinate while in the bathtub or shower, with reassurance that they can easily bathe immediately following bladder evacuation. If these strategies do not lead to successful urination, patients are advised to seek immediate care.

Patients with chronic urinary retention may be managed by behavioural methods, in-dwelling or intermittent catheterization (Table 48-21), surgery, or drugs (Bettez, Tu, Carlson, et al., 2012). Scheduled toileting and double voiding are the primary behavioural interventions used for chronic retention. Scheduled toileting is used to reduce rather than expand bladder capacity. In this case, patients are asked to void every 3 to 4 hours regardless of the desire to urinate. This intervention is particularly useful in patients with chronic overdistension, diabetes mellitus, or chronic alcohol use characterized by a large bladder capacity and diminished or delayed sensations of bladder filling and urgency. Double voiding is an attempt to maximize bladder evacuation. The patient is asked to urinate, sit on the toilet for 3 to 4 minutes, and urinate again before exiting the bathroom.

INSTRUMENTATION

Reasons for short-term urinary catheterization are listed in Table 48-21. Two reasons that are not valid indications for catheterization are (1) routine acquisition of a urine specimen for laboratory analysis and (2) convenience of the nursing staff or the patient's family. The risks for health care–associated infection are too high to allow catheterization of a patient for the convenience of health care providers or family members. Catheterization to obtain sterile urine specimens may occasionally be indicated when patients have a history of complicated urinary infection. These specimens have to be as free of contaminants as possible. A catheter should be the final means of providing the patient with a dry environment for prevention of skin breakdown and protection of dressings or skin lesions.

Urinary catheterization is used when indicated in the management of hospitalized patients. However, it is not without serious risks. The urinary tract is the most common site of health care–associated infections. Urinary catheterization is a major cause of UTIs. Strict aseptic technique is mandatory when a urinary catheter is inserted. After insertion, maintenance and protection of the closed drainage system are major nursing responsibilities. Irrigation of the catheter should not be routinely performed.

While a patient has a catheter in place, nursing actions should include maintaining patency of the catheter, managing fluid intake, providing for the comfort and safety of the patient, and preventing infection. Attention should be given to the psychological implications of urinary drainage. Patient concerns can include embarrassment related to exposure of the body, an altered body image, and fear concerning the care of the catheter, which results in increased dependency.

Catheters vary in construction materials, tip shape (Figure 48-11), and size of the lumen. Catheters are sized according to the French scale. Each French unit equals 0.33 mm of diameter. The diameter measured is the internal diameter of the catheter. The size used varies with the size of the individual and the purpose for catheterization. In women, urethral catheter sizes 12 to 14F are the most common; in men, sizes 14 to 16F are used. The primary problem resulting from too large a catheter is tissue erosion secondary to excessive pressure on the meatus or the urethra. Four routes are used for urinary tract catheterization: urethral, ureteral, suprapubic, and via a nephrostomy tube.

Urethral Catheterization

The most common route of catheterization is through the external meatus into the urethra, past the internal sphincter, and into the bladder. Principles that should be considered in the management of patients with a urethral catheter include the following:

- Catheterized patients, particularly those who are ambulatory, should receive appropriate instruction regarding catheter care.
- A sterile, closed drainage system should always be used in short-term catheterization. The distal urinary catheter and the proximal drainage tube should not be disconnected except for necessary catheter irrigation. The catheter should be taped to the leg. Unobstructed downhill flow must be maintained. The collecting bag should be emptied regularly and kept below the level of the bladder. A poorly functioning catheter should

---

TABLE 48-21   INDICATIONS FOR URINARY CATHETERIZATION

In-Dwelling Catheter
- Accurate measurement of urinary output in critically ill patient
- Bladder decompression preoperatively and operatively for lower abdominal or pelvic surgery
- Facilitation of surgical repair of urethra and surrounding structures
- Measurement of residual urine after urination (referred to as postvoid residual [PVR]) if portable ultrasound not available
- Relief of urinary retention caused by lower urinary tract obstruction, paralysis, or inability to void
- Splinting of ureters or urethra to facilitate healing after surgery or other trauma in area
- Terminal illness or severe impairment that makes positioning or clothing changes uncomfortable or that is associated with intractable pain
- Urine contamination of stage 3 or 4 pressure injuries that has impeded healing, despite appropriate personal care for the incontinence

Straight (In-and-Out) Catheter
- Collection of sterile urine sample in select situations
- Instillation of medications into bladder
- Study of anatomical structures of urinary system
- Urodynamic testing

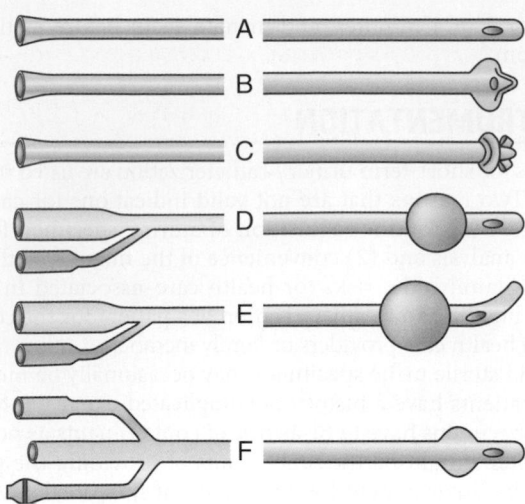

FIGURE 48-11 Different types of commonly used catheters. **A,** Simple urethral catheter. **B,** Mushroom or Pezzar (can be used for suprapubic catheterization). **C,** Winged-tip or Malecot catheter. **D,** In-dwelling with inflated balloon. **E,** In-dwelling with coudé tip or Tiemann tip. **F,** Three-way in-dwelling (the third lumen is used for irrigation of the bladder).

be replaced. A leg bag should not be used for patients in a hospital setting on a short-term basis because the risk for bacterial infection is great when the catheter is disconnected and the drainage bags are exchanged.

- Perineal care (one to two times per day and when necessary) should include cleaning of the meatus–catheter junction with soap and water. Following this, an antimicrobial ointment may be applied. Lotion or powder should not be used near the catheter. The catheter should be properly secured to the leg to prevent movement and urethral traction.

- Sterile technique must be used whenever the collecting system is opened. Catheter irrigation is performed only when obstruction or blood clots are suspected or, in the case of long-term catheterization, to reduce sediment buildup. If frequent irrigations are necessary in short-term catheterization for catheter patency, a triple-lumen catheter may be preferable, permitting continuous irrigations within a closed system. Small volumes of urine for culture can be aspirated from the distal catheter by means of a sterile syringe and a 21-gauge needle after the drainage tubing is clamped. The puncture site must first be prepared with a tincture of iodine or alcohol solution. Many drainage systems are now equipped with a sampling port. Silicone or plastic catheters do not self-seal. Urine for chemical analysis (e.g., electrolytes) can be obtained from the drainage bag.

- When a patient is catheterized for less than 2 weeks, routine catheter change is not necessary. For long-term use of an in-dwelling catheter, regular replacement is necessary. With long-term use of a catheter, a leg bag may be used. If the collection bag is reused, it should be washed with soap and water and rinsed thoroughly. When not reused immediately, it should be filled with 0.5 cup of vinegar and drained. The vinegar is effective against *Pseudomonas* and other organisms and eliminates odours.

Ureteral Catheters

The ureteral catheter is placed through the ureters into the renal pelvis. The catheter is inserted either (a) by being threaded up the urethra and bladder to the ureters under cystoscopic observation or (b) by surgical insertion through the abdominal wall into the ureters. The ureteral catheter is used after surgery to splint the ureters and to prevent them from being obstructed by edema. The urine volume from the ureteral catheter should be recorded separately from other urinary catheters. The patient is usually kept on bed rest while a ureteral catheter is in place until specific orders indicate that ambulation is permissible. The self-retaining ureteral catheter is often inserted after a lithotripsy procedure or when ureteral obstruction from adjacent tumours or fibrosis threatens renal function. The double-J ureteral catheter is often used and allows the patient to ambulate. One end coils up in the kidney pelvis, and the other coils in the bladder.

The placement of the ureteral catheter should be checked frequently, and tension on the catheter should be prevented. The catheter drains urine from the renal pelvis, which has a capacity of 3 to 5 mL. If the volume of urine in the renal pelvis increases, the additional pressure will cause tissue damage to the pelvis. Therefore, the ureteral catheter should not be clamped. If the physician orders irrigation of the ureteral catheter, strict aseptic technique is required. If output is decreased, the physician should be notified immediately. Drainage should be checked often (at least q1–2h). It is normal for some urine to drain around the ureteral catheter into the bladder. Accurate recording of urine output from both the ureters and the urethral catheter is essential. Sometimes, a ureteral catheter may be used as a stent and is not expected to drain. It is important to check with the physician as to the type of catheter and what to expect.

Suprapubic Catheters

Suprapubic catheterization is the simplest and oldest method of urinary diversion. The two methods of insertion of a suprapubic catheter into the bladder are (a) through a small incision in the abdominal wall and (b) by the use of a trocar. A suprapubic catheter is placed while the patient is under general anaesthesia for another surgical procedure or at the bedside with a local anaesthetic. The catheter may be sutured into place. The nursing responsibility includes taping the catheter to prevent dislodgement. The care of the tube and catheter is similar to that of the urethral catheter. A pectin-based skin barrier (e.g., Stomahesive) is effective around the insertion site in protecting the skin from breakdown.

The suprapubic catheter is used in temporary situations such as bladder, prostate, and urethral surgery. The suprapubic catheter is also used long-term in select patients (e.g., male patient with tetraplegia [quadriplegia] who tends to form penoscrotal fistulas).

A suprapubic catheter is prone to poor drainage because of mechanical obstruction of the catheter tip by the bladder wall, sediment, and clots. Nursing interventions to ensure patency of the tube include (a) preventing tube kinking by coiling the excess tubing and maintaining gravity drainage, (b) having the patient turn from side to side, and (c) milking the tube. If these measures are not effective, the catheter is irrigated with sterile technique after a physician's order has been obtained.

If the patient experiences bladder spasms that are difficult to control, urinary leakage may result. Oxybutynin (Ditropan XL) or other oral antispasmodics or belladonna and opium (B&O) suppositories may be prescribed to decrease bladder spasms.

Nephrostomy Tubes

The nephrostomy tube (catheter) is inserted on a temporary basis to preserve renal function when a complete obstruction of the ureter is present. It is inserted directly into the pelvis of the kidney and attached to connecting tubing for closed drainage. The principle is the same as with the ureteral catheter; that is, the catheter should never be kinked, lain or leaned on, or clamped. If the patient complains of excessive pain in the area or if there is excessive drainage around the tube, the catheter should be checked for patency. If irrigation is ordered, strict aseptic technique is required. No more than 5 mL of sterile saline solution is gently instilled at one time to prevent overdistension of the kidney pelvis and renal damage. Infection and secondary stone formation are complications associated with the insertion of a nephrostomy tube.

Intermittent Catheterization

An alternative approach to a long-term in-dwelling catheter is *intermittent catheterization* (Newman & Willson, 2011). It is being used with increasing frequency in conditions characterized by neurogenic bladder (e.g., spinal cord injuries, chronic neurological diseases) or bladder outlet obstruction in men and can be self-managed. This type of catheterization may also be used in the oliguric and anuric phases of acute kidney injury to reduce the possibility of infection from an in-dwelling catheter. Intermittent catheterization is also used postoperatively, often after a surgical procedure for female incontinence or radioactive seed implantation into the prostate for cancer. The main goal of intermittent catheterization is to prevent urinary retention, stasis, and compromised blood supply to the bladder caused by prolonged pressure.

The technique consists of inserting a urethral catheter into the bladder every 3 to 5 hours. Some patients do intermittent catheterization only once or twice a day to measure residual urine and to ensure an empty bladder. Patients should be instructed to wash and rinse the catheter and their hands with soap and water before and after catheterization. Lubricant is necessary for men and may make catheterization more comfortable for women. The catheter may be inserted by the patient or the care provider. Once the bladder is emptied, the catheter is removed. The catheter can be dried and placed in a carrying pouch or purse or folded in a paper towel until it is next needed. The same catheter can be used for weeks at a time. In general, patients should change the catheter every 2 to 4 weeks.

In the hospital, sterile technique is used. For home care, a clean technique that includes good handwashing with soap and water is used. There has been no significant increase in infection with the use of an appropriate clean technique as compared with sterile technique. Several patients living in the community have permanent in-dwelling catheters, which can pose risks for infection, as well as limit the patient's ability to lead an active life. Community patients who are candidates for clean intermittent self-catheterization need personal instruction and support to become comfortable with the procedure. Patients need to demonstrate the desire, motivation, and manual dexterity required to manage the procedure, and commit to assimilating it into regular activities of daily living. They may feel anxious about performing such an intimate and possibly uncomfortable procedure. The nurse may need to balance the risks versus benefits of implementing the self-catheterization procedure for the patient.

Instructing the patient to learn the proper clean procedure, in a logical step-by-step fashion, is recommended to support patients so that they can achieve independence (Woodward, Steggal, and Tinhunu, 2013). The patient is taught to observe for signs of UTI so that treatment can be instituted early. If indicated, some patients are placed on a regimen of prophylactic antibiotics.

SURGERY OF THE URINARY TRACT

RENAL AND URETERAL SURGERY

The most common indications for nephrectomy are a renal tumour, polycystic kidneys that are bleeding or severely infected, massive traumatic injury to the kidney, and the elective removal of a kidney from a donor. Surgery involving the ureters and the kidneys is most commonly performed to remove calculi that become obstructive, correct congenital anomalies, and divert urine when necessary.

Preoperative Management

The basic needs of the patient undergoing renal and ureteral surgery are similar to those of any patient who experiences surgery (see Chapters 20 through 22). In addition, it is especially important preoperatively to ensure adequate fluid intake and a normal electrolyte balance. The patient should be told that there will probably be a flank incision on the affected side and that surgery will require a hyperextended, side-lying position. This position frequently causes the patient to experience muscle aches after surgery. If a nephrectomy is planned, the patient must be assured that one working kidney is sufficient to maintain normal renal function.

Postoperative Management

Specific postoperative needs of a patient are related to urine output, respiratory status, and abdominal distension.

Urine Output. In the immediate postoperative period, urine output should be determined at least every 1 to 2 hours. Drainage from various catheters should be recorded separately. The catheter or tube should not be clamped or irrigated without a specific order. The total urine output should be at least 0.5 mL/kg/hr. Peak flow rates can be measured with a urometer. It is also important to assess for urine drainage on the dressing and to estimate the amount. Daily weighing of the patient is important. The same scale should be used and properly balanced, and the patient should wear similar clothing and dressings each time.

It is important to observe and monitor the colour and the consistency of urine. Urine with increased amounts of mucus, blood, or sediment may occlude the drainage tubing or catheter.

Respiratory Status. Renal surgery is often performed through a flank incision just below the diaphragm and often involves removal of the twelfth rib. Postoperatively, it is important to ensure adequate ventilation. The patient is often reluctant to turn, cough, and deep breathe because of the incisional pain. Adequate pain medication should be given to ensure the patient's comfort and ability to perform coughing and deep-breathing exercises. Frequently, additional respiratory devices such as an incentive spirometer are used every 2 hours while the patient is awake. In addition, early and frequent ambulation assists in maintaining adequate respiratory function.

Abdominal Distension. Abdominal distension is present to some degree in most patients who have had surgery on their kidneys or ureters. It is most commonly the result of paralytic ileus caused by manipulation and compression of the bowel during surgery. Oral intake is restricted until bowel sounds are present (usually 24–48 hr after surgery). Intravenous fluids are given until the patient can take oral fluids. Progression to a regular diet follows.

Laparoscopic Nephrectomy

Laparoscopic nephrectomy can be performed in select situations to remove a diseased kidney. It can also be used to obtain a kidney from a living donor to be transplanted into a person with end-stage renal disease. In contrast to the open incision of about 18 cm required in a conventional nephrectomy, a laparoscopic nephrectomy is performed using five puncture sites. One incision is to view the kidney and another is to dissect it. The laparoscope contains a miniature camera so that the surgeons can watch what they are doing on a video monitor. Once dissected, the kidney is manoeuvred into a nylon impermeable sack, and its contents can then be safely removed from the patient. Compared with conventional nephrectomy, the laparoscopic approach is less painful and requires no sutures or staples, involves a shorter hospital stay, and has a much faster recovery. NCP 48-3, regarding care of patients with an ileal conduit, identifies key nursing diagnoses that apply to caring for patients with a nephrectomy pertaining to (a) management of anxiety related to lack of knowledge regarding a major surgical procedure, (b) knowledge deficits about preoperative, operative, and postoperative procedures, (c) risks for infection related to the surgical procedure, and (d) deficient fluid volume.

URINARY DIVERSION

Urinary diversion may be performed with and without cystectomy. Urinary diversion procedures are performed to treat cancer of the bladder, neurogenic bladder, congenital anomalies, strictures, trauma to the bladder, and chronic infections with deterioration of renal function. Numerous urinary diversion techniques and bladder substitutes are possible, including an incontinent urinary diversion, continent urinary diversion catheterized by patient, or an orthotopic bladder so that the patient voids urethrally. Types of these surgical procedures are presented in Table 48-22 and Figure 48-12.

Incontinent Urinary Diversion

Incontinent urinary diversion is diversion to the skin, requiring an appliance. The simplest form is the cutaneous ureterostomy, but scarring and strictures of the ureter have led to the use of ileal or colonic conduits. The most commonly performed incontinent urinary diversion procedure is the **ileal conduit** (ileal loop). In this procedure, a 15- to 20-cm segment of the ileum is converted into a conduit for urinary drainage. The colon (colon conduit) can be used instead of the ileum. The ureters are anastomosed into one end of the conduit, and the other end of the bowel is brought out through the abdominal wall to form a stoma (Figure 48-13). Although the segment of bowel remains supported by the mesentery, it is completely isolated from the intestinal tract. The bowel is anastomosed and continues to function normally. Because there is no valve and no voluntary control over the stoma, drops of urine flow from the stoma every few seconds, requiring the use of a permanent external collecting device. The visible stoma and the need for external collection devices are obvious disadvantages of this procedure. The lifelong care and dealing with the stoma and collection devices may be psychologically difficult. These problems have stimulated the increasing use of continent diversions and orthotopic bladder substitutes.

Continent Urinary Diversions

A *continent urinary diversion* is an intra-abdominal urinary reservoir that is catheterizable or has an outlet controlled by the

---

TABLE 48-22   TYPES OF URINARY DIVERSION SURGERY REQUIRING COLLECTION DEVICES

Description	Advantages	Disadvantages	Special Considerations
Ileal			
Conduit ureters are implanted into part of ileum or colon that has been resected from intestinal tract. Abdominal stoma is created.	Relatively good urine flow with few physiological alterations	External appliance necessary to continually collect urine	Surgical procedure is more complex. Postoperative complications may be increased. Reabsorption of urea by ileum occurs. Meticulous attention is necessary to care for stoma and collecting device.
Cutaneous Ureterostomy			
Ureters are excised from bladder and brought through abdominal wall, and stoma is created. Ureteral stomas may be created from both ureters, or ureters may be brought together and one stoma created.	No need for major surgery as required with ileal conduit	External appliance necessary because of continuous urine drainage; possibility of stricture or stenosis of small stoma	Periodic catheterizations may be required to dilate stomas to maintain patency.
Nephrostomy			
Catheter is inserted into pelvis of kidney. Procedure may be done to one or both kidneys and may be temporary or permanent. It is most frequently done in advanced disease as palliative procedure.	No need for major surgery	High risk for renal infection; predisposition to calculus formation from catheter	Nephrostomy tube may have to be changed every month. Catheter must never be clamped.

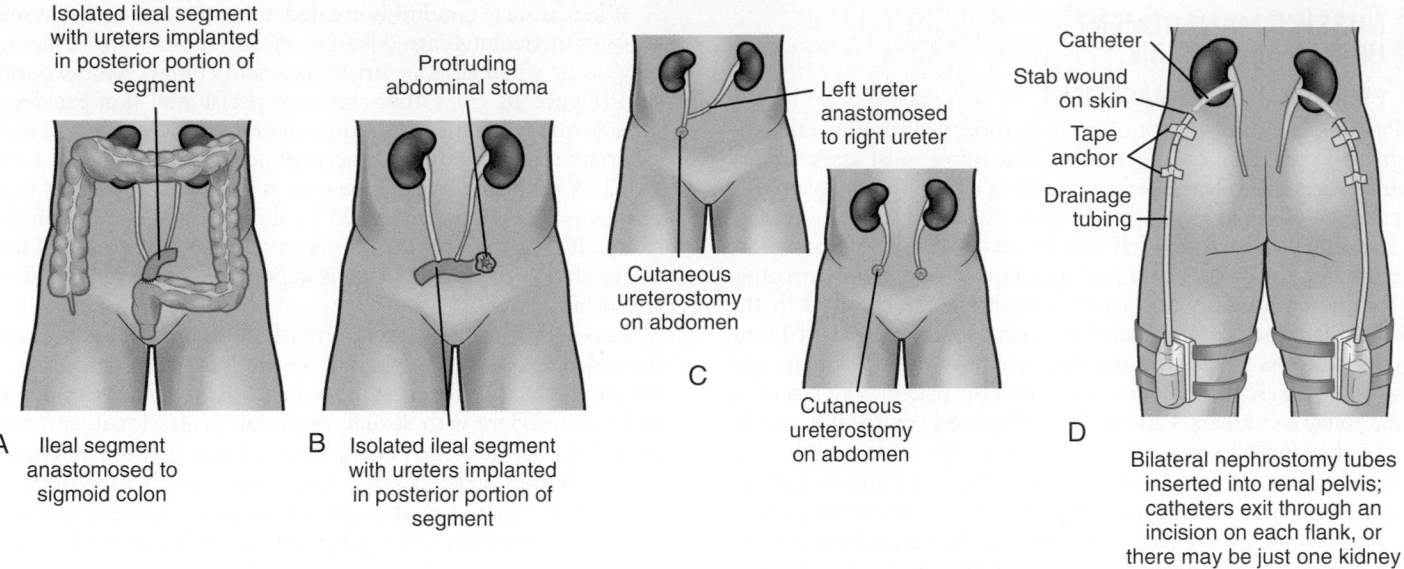

FIGURE 48-12 Methods of urinary diversion. **A,** Uretero-ileo-sigmoidostomy. **B,** Ileal loop (or ileal conduit).
C, Ureterostomy (transcutaneous ureterostomy and bilateral cutaneous ureterostomies). **D,** Nephrostomy.

FIGURE 48-13 Ideal urinary stoma. It is symmetrical, has no skin breakdown, and protrudes about 1.5 cm. The mucosa is a healthy red, and the configuration is flat when the patient is upright and supine. Source: Courtesy Lynda Brubacher, Virginia Mason Hospital, Seattle, WA.

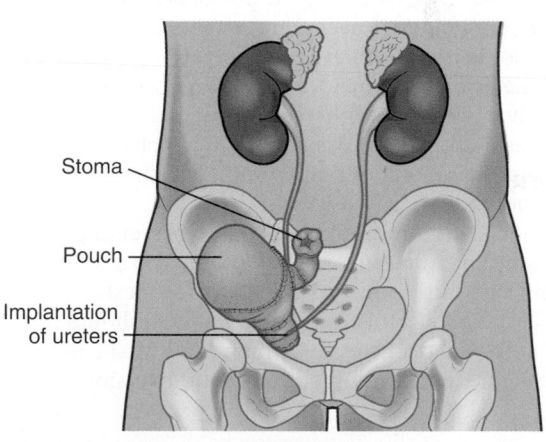

FIGURE 48-14 Creation of a Kock pouch with implantation of ureters into one intussuscepted portion of the pouch and creation of a stoma with the other intussuscepted portion.

anal sphincter. Continent diversions are internal pouches created similarly to the ileal conduit. Reservoirs have been constructed from the ileum, ileocecal segment, or colon. Large segments of bowel are altered to prevent peristaltic action. A continence mechanism is formed between this large, low-pressure reservoir and the stoma by intussuscepting a portion of bowel. In this way, a patient does not leak involuntarily. The patient with a continent reservoir needs to self-catheterize every 4 to 6 hours but does not need to wear external attachments. Examples of continent diversions are the Kock (Figure 48-14), Mainz, Indiana, and Florida pouches. A main difference among these diversions is the segment of bowel used. For example, the Indiana pouch uses the right colon as a reservoir and has become a popular form of continent urinary diversion.

Orthotopic Bladder Substitution

Orthotopic bladder substitutes can be derived from various segments of the intestines. An isolated segment of the distal ileum is often preferred. Various procedures include the hemi-Kock pouch, Studer pouch, and the ileal W-neobladder. In these procedures, the bowel is surgically reshaped to become a neobladder. The ureters and urethra are sutured into the neobladder. Orthotopic bladder reconstruction has become a more viable option for both men and women if cancer does not involve the bladder neck or urethra (Park & Ahn, 2011). The advantage of orthotopic bladder substitution is that it allows for natural micturition. Incontinence is a possible problem with this technique, and intermittent catheterization may be required.

NURSING MANAGEMENT
URINARY DIVERSION

PREOPERATIVE MANAGEMENT

Patients awaiting cystectomy and urinary diversion must be given a great deal of information. The nurse must assess ability and readiness to learn before initiating a teaching program. If a patient is not ready to learn, the teaching plan should be adjusted. The patient's anxiety and fear may be decreased by the information. However, the anxiety and fear may also interfere with learning. The patient's family and caregivers should be involved in the teaching process. A discussion of the social aspects of living with a stoma (including clothing, changes in body image and sexuality, exercise, and odour) provides the patient with facts that may allay some fears. Patients who will have a continent diversion must be taught to catheterize and irrigate the pouch and be able to adhere to a strict catheterization schedule. Patients with an orthotopic neobladder may have problems with incontinence. Concerns about the effect on sexual activities should be discussed. The enterostomal therapy nurse should be involved in the preoperative phase of the patient's care. A visit from an ostomate or enterostomal therapy nurse can be helpful. Additional interventions are presented in NCP 48-3, available on the Evolve website.

POSTOPERATIVE MANAGEMENT

Nursing interventions during the postoperative period (see NCP 48-3 for care after an ileal conduit) should be planned to prevent surgical complications such as postoperative atelectasis and shock (see Chapter 22). The incidence of thrombo-phlebitis increases after pelvic surgery. With removal of part of the bowel, the incidence of paralytic ileus and small bowel obstruction increases, the patient is kept on nothing-by-mouth status, and a nasogastric tube is necessary for 3 to 5 days.

Specific attention should be given to preventing injury to the stoma and maintaining urine output. Mucus is present in the urine because it is secreted by the intestines as a result of the irritating effect of the urine. Patients should be told that this is a normal occurrence. A high fluid intake is encouraged to "flush" the ileal conduit or continent diversion.

When an ileal conduit is created, the skin around the stoma requires meticulous care. Alkaline encrustations with dermatitis may occur when alkaline urine comes in contact with exposed skin (Figure 48-15). Other common peristomal skin problems include yeast infections, product allergies, and shearing-effect excoriations. Changing appliances (pouches) is described in Table 48-23. A properly fitting appliance is essential to prevent skin problems. The appliance should be about 0.2 cm larger than the stoma. It is normal for the stoma to shrink within the first few weeks after surgery. The urine is kept acidic to prevent alkaline encrustations.

Acceptance of the surgery and of alterations in body image is needed to ensure the patient's best adjustment. Concerns of the patient include fear that the stoma will be offensive to others and will interfere with sexual, personal, professional, and recreational activities. The patient should know that few activities, if any, will be restricted as a result of the urinary diversion.

Discharge planning after an ileal conduit includes teaching the patient symptoms of obstruction or infection and care of

FIGURE 48-15 Ammonia salt encrustation secondary to alkaline urine. Source: Courtesy Lynda Brubacher, Virginia Mason Hospital, Seattle, WA.

TABLE 48-23   PATIENT & CAREGIVER TEACHING GUIDE

Changing Ileal Conduit Appliances

Temporary Appliance	Permanent Appliance*
1. Cut hole in pouch to fit over stoma (pouch 3.2 mm [⅛ inch] larger than stoma).	1. Keep appliance in place for 2–14 days.
2. Remove old pouch.	2. Change appliance when fluid intake has been restricted for several hours.
3. Clean area gently, and remove old adhesive.	3. Sit or stand in front of mirror.
4. Wash area with warm water.	4. Moisten edge of faceplate with adhesive solvent and gently remove.
5. Place wick (rolled-up 4 × 4–inch) over stoma to keep area dry during rest of procedure.	5. Clean skin with adhesive solvent.
6. Dry skin around stoma.	6. Wash skin with warm water. (Patient may shower.)
7. Apply a prescribed skin protectant around stoma to area where pouch will be placed.	7. Dry skin and inspect.
8. Apply pouch by first smoothing its edges toward side and lower portion of body.	8. Place wick (rolled-up 4 × 4–inch) over stoma to keep skin free of urine.
9. Remove wick and complete application of bag.	9. Apply skin cement to faceplate and skin.
10. For a patient who is usually in bed: Apply bag so that it lies toward side of body.	10. Place appliance over stoma.
11. For a patient who is ambulatory: Apply bag so that it lies vertically.	11. Wash removed appliance with soap and lukewarm water; soak in distilled vinegar; rinse with lukewarm water and air dry.
12. Connect drainage tubing to pouch.	
13. Keep drainage pouch on same side of bed as stoma.	

*Many disposable appliances with self-adhesive backing are used as permanent appliances.

the ostomy. The patient with an ileal conduit is fitted for a permanent appliance 7 to 10 days after surgery and may need to be refitted at a later time, depending on the degree of stoma shrinkage. Appliances are made of a variety of products, including natural and synthetic rubbers, plastics, and metals. Most appliances have a faceplate that adheres to the skin, a collecting pouch, and an opening to drain the pouch. The faceplate may be secured to the skin with glues, adhesives, or adhering synthetic wafers. Some appliances do not require adhesives, but their design relies on pressure to keep the pouch in place. If improperly fitted or applied, the faceplate may cause skin problems (Figure 48-16). A bag may be used for night drainage. The patient needs information on where to purchase supplies, emergency telephone numbers, location of ostomy support groups, and follow-up visits with an enterostomal therapist. Physician follow-up is imperative to monitor and correct homeostatic abnormalities and to prevent complications and renal function deterioration.

FIGURE 48-16 Retracted urinary stoma with pressure sore from faceplate above stoma. Source: Courtesy Lynda Brubacher, Virginia Mason Hospital, Seattle, WA.

CASE STUDY

Urinary Tract Infection

Source: Syda Productions/ Shutterstock .com.

Patient Profile
Maria Guinto, a 28-year-old woman with diabetes, was seen in the nurse practitioner's office for a history of painful, frequent urination.

Subjective Data
• Has had history of painful, frequent urination with passage of small volumes of urine for 3 days
• Has had intermittent fever, chills, and back pain during these 3 days
• Was frightened when she saw blood in her urine
• Is anxious because her father died of kidney cancer
• Has a history of recurrent UTIs

Objective Data
Physical Examination
• Complains of bilateral flank pain and abdominal tenderness to palpation
• Temperature is 38°C

Diagnostic Study
• Urinalysis: pyuria and hematuria

Discussion Questions
1. What are the most common organisms that cause UTIs?
2. What factors predispose a patient to a UTI?
3. What is the difference between upper and lower UTIs?
4. ***Priority decision:*** What are the priority nursing interventions that will help Ms. Guinto cope with her symptoms?
5. What can the nurse do to help Ms. Guinto prevent another UTI?
6. Why might she be having recurrent bouts of UTIs? What other diagnostic tests may be indicated?
7. ***Priority decision:*** Based on the data presented, write one or more appropriate nursing diagnoses. Are there any collaborative problems?

evolve
Answers are available on *http://evolve.elsevier.com/Canada/Lewis/medsurg*.

REVIEW QUESTIONS

The number of the question corresponds to the same-numbered objective at the beginning of the chapter.

1. Organisms that cause pyelonephritis most commonly reach the kidneys through which means?
   a. The bloodstream
   b. The lymphatic system
   c. A descending infection
   d. An ascending infection

2. What should the nurse teach the female client who has frequent urinary tract infections (UTIs)?
   a. Urinate after sexual intercourse.
   b. Take tub baths with bubble bath.
   c. Take prophylactic sulphonamides for the rest of her life.
   d. Restrict fluid intake to prevent the need for frequent voiding.

3. Which of the following immunological mechanisms are involved in glomerulo-nephritis?
   a. Tubular blocking by precipitates of bacteria and antibody reactions

   b. Deposition of immune complexes and complement along the glomerular basement membrane (GBM)
   c. Thickening of the GBM from autoimmune microangiopathic changes
   d. Destruction of glomeruli by proteolytic enzymes contained in the GBM

4. What is one of the most important roles of the nurse in relation to acute poststreptococcal glomerulo-nephritis (APSGN)?
   a. To promote early diagnosis and treatment of sore throats and skin lesions
   b. To encourage clients to request antibiotic therapy for all upper respiratory infections
   c. To teach clients with APSGN that long-term prophylactic antibiotic therapy is necessary to prevent recurrence
   d. To monitor clients for respiratory symptoms that indicate that the disease is affecting the alveolar basement membrane

5. Why does edema occur in nephrotic syndrome?
   a. Decreased aldosterone secretion from adrenal insufficiency
   b. Increased hydrostatic pressure caused by sodium retention
   c. Increased fluid retention caused by decreased glomerular filtration
   d. Decreased colloidal osmotic pressure caused by loss of serum albumin

6. A client is admitted to the hospital with severe renal colic caused by renal lithiasis. What is the nurse's first priority in management of the client?
   a. To administer opioids as prescribed
   b. To obtain supplies for straining all urine
   c. To encourage fluid intake of 3 to 4 L/day
   d. To keep the client on nothing-by-mouth status in preparation for surgery

7. In which of the following conditions should the nurse recommend genetic counselling for the client's children?
   a. Nephrotic syndrome
   b. Chronic pyelonephritis
   c. Malignant nephrosclerosis
   d. Adult-onset polycystic renal disease

8. The nurse instructs a client with diabetes to maintain careful control of his blood glucose levels related to which disease-related complication?
   a. Uric acid calculi and nephrolithiasis
   b. Renal sugar-crystal calculi and cysts
   c. Lipid deposits in the glomeruli and the nephrons
   d. Thickening of the GBM and glomerulo-sclerosis

9. Which of the following conditions would the nurse identify as a risk factor for kidney and bladder cancers? *(Select all that apply)*
   a. acetylsalicylic acid (ASA: Aspirin) use
   b. Tobacco use
   c. Chronic alcohol abuse
   d. Use of artificial sweeteners
   e. Chronic use of phenacetin-containing analgesics

10. Which nursing interventions are most important in order to increase bladder control in a client with urinary incontinence? *(Select all that apply)*
    a. Restricting fluids to diminish the risk for urinary leakage
    b. Counselling the client to maintain a regular voiding schedule
    c. Clamping and releasing a catheter to increase bladder tone
    d. Teaching the client biofeedback mechanisms to suppress the urge to void

11. A client with a uretero-lithotomy returns from surgery with a nephrostomy tube in place. What is the priority nursing action related to caring for this client?
    a. Encouraging the client to drink fruit juices and milk
    b. Forcing fluids of at least 2 to 3 L/day after nausea has subsided
    c. Notifying the physician if nephrostomy tube drainage is more than 30 mL/hr
    d. Irrigating the nephrostomy tube with 10 mL of normal saline solution as needed

12. A client has had a cystectomy and ileal conduit diversion performed. Four days postoperatively, mucous shreds are seen in the drainage bag. Which action should the nurse undertake?
    a. Notify the physician.
    b. Notify the charge nurse.
    c. Irrigate the drainage tube.
    d. Chart it as a normal observation.

1. d; 2. a; 3. b; 4. a; 5. d; 6. a; 7. d; 8. d; 9. b, e; 10. a, b; 11. b; 12. d.

Ⓔvolve

For even more review questions, visit *http://evolve.elsevier.com/Canada/Lewis/medsurg.*

REFERENCES

Al-Badr, A., & Al-Shaikh, G. (2013). Recurrent urinary tract infections management in women: A review. *Sultan Qaboos University Medical Journal, 13*(3), 359–367.

Arinzon, Z., Shabat, S., Peisakh, A., et al. (2012). Clinical presentation of urinary tract infection (UTI) differs with aging in women. *Archives of Gerontology and Geriatrics, 55*(1), 145–147. doi:10.1016/j.archger.2011.07.012.

Barbour, S. J., Greenwald, A., Djurdjev, O., et al. (2012). Disease-specific risk of venous thromboembolic events is increased in idiopathic glomerulonephritis. *Kidney International, 81*(2), 190–195. doi:10.1038/ki.2011.312.

Bettez, M., Tu, L. M., Carlson, K., et al. (2012). 2012 update: Guidelines for adult urinary incontinence collaborative consensus document for the Canadian Urological Association. *Canadian Urological Association Journal, 6*(5), 354–363. doi:10.5489/cuaj.12248.

Canadian Cancer Society. (2016). *Kidney cancer statistics.* Retrieved from *http://www.cancer.ca/en/cancer-information/cancer-type/kidney/statistics/?region=on.*

Canadian Cancer Society's Advisory Committee on Cancer Statistics (2017). *Canadian cancer statistics 2017.* Toronto: Canadian Cancer Society. Retrieved from *http://www.cancer.ca/~/media/cancer.ca/CW/cancer%20information/cancer%20101/Canadian%20cancer%20statistics/Canadian-Cancer-Statistics-2017-EN.pdf?la=en.*

Canadian Continence Foundation. (2016). *Facts on incontinence.* Retrieved from *http://www.canadiancontinence.ca/EN/what-is-urinary-incontinence.php.*

Canadian Diabetes Association Clinical Practice Guidelines Expert Committee. (2013). Canadian Diabetes Association clinical practice guidelines for the prevention and management of diabetes in Canada. *Canadian Journal of Diabetes, 37*(Suppl. 1), S1–S212.

Canadian Urological Association. (2014). *Kidney stones.* Retrieved from *https://www.cua.org/themes/web/assets/files/patient_info/secured/en/35e-kidney_stones_s.pdf.*

Chisholm, A. H. (2015). Probiotics in preventing recurrent urinary tract infections in women: A literature review. *Urologic Nursing, 35*(1), 18–21, 29. doi:10.7257/1053-816X.2015.35.1.18.

da Costa, I. A., Amend, B., Stenzl, A., et al. (2016). Contemporary management of acute kidney trauma. *Journal of Acute Disease, 5*(1), 29–36. doi:10.1016/j.joad.2015.08.003.

Davis, N. F., Brady, C. M., & Creagh, T. (2014). Interstitial cystitis/painful bladder syndrome: Epidemiology, pathophysiology and evidence-based treatment options. *European Journal of Obstetrics, Gynecology, and Reproductive Biology, 175*, 30–37. doi:10.1016/j.ejogrb.2013.12.041.

Doig, A. K., & Huether, S. E. (2014). Alterations of renal and urinary tract function. In K. L. McCance & S. E. Huether (Eds.),

Pathophysiology: The biologic basis for disease in adults and children (7th ed., pp. 1340–1375). St. Louis, MO: Elsevier Mosby.

Ferraro, P. M., Taylor, E. N., Gambaro, G., et al. (2013). Soda and other beverages and the risk of kidney stones. *Clinical journal of the American Society of Nephrology, 8*(8), 1389–1395. doi:10.2215/CJN.11661112.

Flannigan, R., Choy, W. H., Chew, B., et al. (2014). Renal struvite stones—Pathogenesis, microbiology, and management strategies. *Nature Reviews. Urology, 11*(6), 333–341. doi:10.1038/nrurol.2014.99.

Gish, B. A. (2011). Interstitial cystitis/bladder pain syndrome: Symptoms, screening and treatment. *Nursing for Womens Health, 15*(6), 496–507.

Grabe, M., Bartoletti, R., Bjerklund-Johansen, T. E., et al. (2014). Guidelines on urological infections. *European Association of Urology.* Retrieved from *http://uroweb.org/wp-content/uploads/19-Urological-infections_LR.pdf.*

Hooton, T. M. (2012). Clinical practice: Uncomplicated urinary tract infection. *New England Journal of Medicine, 366*(11), 1028–1037. doi:10.1056/NEJMcp1104429.

Kassouf, W., Traboulsi, S. L., Kulkarni, G. S., et al. (2015). CUA guidelines on the management of non-muscle invasive bladder cancer. *Canadian Urological Association Journal, 9*(9-10), E690–E704. doi:10.5489/cuaj.3320.

Kociszewski, J., Rautenberg, O., Kuszka, A., et al. (2012). Can we place tension-free vaginal tape where it should be? The one-third rule. *Ultrasound in Obstetrics and Gynecology, 39,* 210–214. doi:10.1002/uog.10050.

Kumar, S., Ankur, D., Wolf, B., et al. (2015). Urinary tract infections. *Disease-A-Month, 61*(2), 45–59. doi:10.1016/j.disamonth.2014.12.002.

Linas, S. L. (2011). Hypertensive crisis: Emergency and urgency. In J.-L. Vincent, E. Abraham, F. A. Moore, et al. (Eds.), *Textbook of Critical Care* (6th ed., pp. 662–670). Philadelphia: Elsevier Saunders.

Mayo Clinic Staff. (2012). *Nephrotic syndrome.* Retrieved from *http://www.mayoclinic.com/health/nephrotic-syndrome/DS01047.*

Mayo Clinic Staff. (2014). *Polycystic kidney disease: Symptoms and causes.* Retrieved from *http://www.mayoclinic.org/diseases-conditions/polycystic-kidney-disease/basics/complications/con-20028831.*

National Institute of Diabetes and Digestive and Kidney Diseases (NIDDK). (2011). *Interstitial cystitis/Painful bladder syndrome* (NIH Publication No. 11–3220). Retrieved from *http://www.niddk.nih.gov/health-information/health-topics/urologic-disease/interstitial-cystitis-painful-bladder-syndrome/Documents/IC_PBS_T_508.pdf.*

National Institute of Diabetes and Digestive and Kidney Diseases (NIDDK). (2017). *Bladder infection (urinary tract infection—UTI) in adults.* Retrieved from *https://www.niddk.nih.gov/health-information/urologic-diseases/bladder-infection-uti-in-adults.*

National Kidney Foundation (2015a). *6 easy ways to prevent kidney stones.* Retrieved from *https://www.kidney.org/atoz/content/kidneystones_prevent.*

National Kidney Foundation. (2015b). *Alport syndrome.* Retrieved from *https://www.kidney.org/atoz/content/alport.*

Newman, D. K., & Willson, M. M. (2011). Review of intermittent catheterization and current best practices. *Urologic Nursing, 31*(1), 12–28.

Nicolle, L. E. (2013). Urinary tract infection. *Critical Care Clinics, 29*(3), 699–715. doi:10.1016/j.ccc.2013.03.014.

Nogueras, D. J., Thomas, D. J., & Porter, B. O. (2015). Renal problems. In L. M. Dunphy, J. E. Winland-Brown, B. O. Porter, et al. (Eds.), *Primary care: The art and science of advanced practice nursing* (4th ed., pp. 596–641). Philadelphia: F. A. Davis Company.

North, S., Basappa, N., Bjarnason, G., et al. (2013). Management of advanced kidney cancer: Canadian Kidney Cancer Forum 2013 consensus update. *Canadian Urological Association Journal, 7*(7-8), 238–243. doi:10.5489/cuaj.536.

Ordon, M., Andonian, S., Blew, B., et al. (2015). *Canadian urological association guideline: Management of ureteral calculi.* Retrieved from *https://www.cua.org/themes/web/assets/files/cua_guideline_management_of_ureteral_calculi_-_approved.pdf.*

Park, J., & Ahn, H. (2011). Radical cystectomy and orthotopic bladder substitution using ileum. *Korean Journal of Urology, 52*(4), 233–240. doi:10.4111/kju.2011.52.4.233.

Quillin, R. B., & Erickson, D. R. (2012). Management of interstitial cystitis/bladder pain syndrome: A urology perspective. *Urologic Clinics of North America, 39*(3), 389–396. doi:10.1016/j.ucl.2012.05.007.

Ralph, A. P., & Carapetis, J. R. (2013). Group A streptococcal diseases and their global burden. *Current Topics in Microbiology and Immunology, 368,* 1–27.

Registered Nurses' Association of Ontario. (2011). *Prevention of falls and fall injuries in the older adult. Registered Nurses' Association of Ontario Best Practice Guideline Supplement.* Retrieved from *http://rnao.ca/sites/rnao-ca/files/Prevention_of_Falls_and_Fall_Injuries_in_the_Older_Adult.pdf.*

Urology Care Foundation. (n.d.). *What is urethral diverticulum?* Retrieved from *http://www.urologyhealth.org/urologic-conditions/urethral-diverticulum.*

Wang, C. H., Fang, C. C., Chen, N. C., et al. (2012). Cranberry-containing products for prevention of urinary tract infections in susceptible populations: A systematic review and meta-analysis of randomized controlled trials. *Archives of Internal Medicine, 172*(13), 988–996. doi:10.1001/archinternmed.2012.3004.

Woodward, S., Steggal, M., & Tinhunu, J. (2013). Clean intermittent self catheterization: Improving quality of life. *British Journal of Nursing, 22*(9), 1212–1218.

Zak, D. (2014). Managing uncomplicated urinary tract infections in reproductive-aged women: A primary care approach. *Journal of the American Association of Nurse Practitioners, 26*(12), 658–663. doi:10.1002/2327-6924.12110.

RESOURCES

Canada IC, Bladder & Pelvic Pain Support Groups
https://www.ic-network.com/ic-support-center/canada-ic-bladder-pelvic-pain-support-groups/?

Canadian Association of Nephrology Nurses and Technologists
http://cannt.ca

Canadian Kidney Foundation Educational Resources
https://www.kidney.ca/resources

Canadian Urological Association
http://www.cua.org

Cancer Care Ontario Toolbox: Evidence-Based Guidelines
https://www.cancercare.on.ca/toolbox/qualityguidelines

Kidney Foundation of Canada
http://www.kidney.ca/

Ostomy Canada Society
http://www.ostomycanada.ca

Registered Nurses' Association of Ontario Best Practice Guidelines
http://www.rnao.org/Page.asp?PageID=924&ContentID=1274

Women's College Hospital: Coping
http://www.womenshealthmatters.ca/health-centres/pelvic-health/interstitial-cystitis/coping

Women's College Hospital: Interstitial Cystitis
http://www.womenshealthmatters.ca/health-centres/pelvic-health/interstitial-cystitis

American Cancer Society
http://www.cancer.org

American Urological Association: Bladder Health
http://www.auanet.org/advocacy/advocacy-by-topic/bladder-health

International Continence Society (ICS)
http://www.icsoffice.org

Interstitial Cystitis Association
http://www.ichelp.com

Wound, Ostomy and Continence Nurses Society
http://www.wocn.org

For additional Internet resources, see the website for this book at *http://evolve.elsevier.com/Canada/Lewis/medsurg*.

Nursing Management

Acute Kidney Injury and Chronic Kidney Disease

Written by: Hazel A. Dennison
Adapted by: Debbie Rickeard

⊝volve WEBSITE

http://evolve.elsevier.com/Canada/Lewis/medsurg.

- Review Questions (Online only)
- Key Points
- Answer Guidelines for Case Study
- Student Case Studies
  - Kidney Transplant
  - Glomerulo-nephritis and Acute Kidney Injury

- Customizable Nursing Care Plan
  - Chronic Kidney Disease
- Conceptual Care Map Creator
- Audio Glossary
- Content Updates

LEARNING OBJECTIVES

1. Differentiate between acute kidney injury and chronic kidney disease.
2. Identify criteria used in the classification of acute kidney injury using the acronym RIFLE (risk, injury, failure, loss, end-stage kidney disease).
3. Describe the clinical course of acute kidney injury.
4. Explain the collaborative care and nursing management of a patient with acute kidney injury.
5. Define chronic kidney disease and delineate the five stages of chronic kidney disease based on the glomerular filtration rate.
6. Select risk factors that contribute to the development of chronic kidney disease.
7. Summarize the significance of cardiovascular disease in individuals with chronic kidney disease.
8. Explain the collaborative care and related nursing management of the patient with chronic kidney disease.
9. Differentiate among renal replacement therapies for individuals with chronic kidney disease.
10. Discuss the role of the nurse in the management of individuals who receive a renal transplant.

KEY TERMS

acute kidney injury (AKI), p. 1202
acute renal failure (ARF), p. 1202
acute tubular necrosis (ATN), p. 1203
arteriovenous fistula (AVF), p. 1221
arteriovenous graft (AVG), p. 1221
azotemia, p. 1202
automated peritoneal dialysis (APD), p. 1219

chronic kidney disease (CKD), p. 1208
chronic kidney disease–mineral and bone disorder (CKD–MBD), p. 1211
continuous ambulatory peritoneal dialysis (CAPD), p. 1219
continuous renal replacement therapy (CRRT), p. 1224
dialysis, p. 1217

end-stage renal disease (ESRD), p. 1208
hemodialysis (HD), p. 1217
oliguria, p. 1203
paired organ donation, p. 1227
peritoneal dialysis (PD), p. 1217
renal osteodystrophy, p. 1211
renal replacement therapy (RRT), p. 1201
uremia, p. 1208

Kidney disease may cause the partial or complete impairment of kidney function. It results in an inability to excrete metabolic waste products and water, as well as functional disturbances of all body systems. This impairment may be acute or chronic in nature (Table 49-1). Acute kidney injury (AKI) has a rapid onset. Chronic kidney disease (CKD) usually develops slowly over months to years. If CKD progresses to stage 5 (worst functioning), **renal replacement therapy (RRT)** (dialysis or transplantation) is necessary for long-term survival. Early CKD care focuses on prevention and delaying progression of

disease and educating patients about the treatment options for RRTs so an informed decision can be made when the time comes. As with other chronic illnesses in Canada, CKD is much more common in the older-adult population. Between 2003 and 2013, the number of Canadians aged 45 to 64 with CKD increased by 46%, while Canadians 65 and older saw a 66% increase. During the same time period, the number of Canadians aged 45 and older with diabetes also increased by more than 60% (Canadian Institute for Health Information [CIHI], 2014).

TABLE 49-1	COMPARISON OF ACUTE KIDNEY INJURY AND CHRONIC KIDNEY DISEASE	
	Acute Kidney Injury	**Chronic Kidney Disease**
Onset	Sudden	Gradual, often over many years
Most common cause	Acute tubular necrosis	Diabetic nephropathy
Diagnostic criteria	Acute reduction in urine output, elevation in serum creatinine, or both	GFR <60 mL/min/1.73 m^2 for >3 mo, kidney damage >3 mo, or both
Reversibility	Potentially	Progressive and irreversible
Mortality	High (~60%)	19%–24% (patients on dialysis)
Primary cause of death	Infection	Cardiovascular disease

GFR, glomerular filtration rate.
Source: Kellum, J., Bellomo, R., & Ronco, C. (2008). Definition and classification of acute kidney injury. *Nephron Clinical Practice, 109*(4), 182–187. doi:10.1159/000142926; and U.S. Renal Data System. (2008). USRDS 2008 annual data report: Atlas of end-stage renal disease. Bethesda, MD: National Institute of Diabetes and Digestive and Kidney Diseases.

FIGURE 49-1 RIFLE (risk, injury, failure, loss, end-stage kidney disease) Criteria. *AKI*, acute kidney injury; *ESRD*, end-stage renal disease; *GFR*, glomerular filtration rate; *UO*, urine output. Williams, L. (2014). Take aim at acute kidney injury with RIFLE criteria. *Nursing, 44*(7), 50–55 6p. doi:10.1097/01.NURSE.0000445730.84886.88

In 2012, 41 252 Canadians were being treated for kidney failure, with 23 814 on dialysis and 17 438 with a functioning kidney transplant (CIHI, 2014).

ACUTE KIDNEY INJURY

Acute kidney injury (AKI), previously known as **acute renal failure (ARF)**, is a more inclusive term encompassing a broader subset of patients with varying degrees of kidney injury (Moreland & Phiri, 2015). AKI is characterized by an abrupt decline in kidney function, leading to a rise in serum creatinine or a reduction in urine output, or both (Moreland & Phiri, 2015). The severity of dysfunction can range from a small increase in serum creatinine or reduction in urine output to the development of **azotemia** (an accumulation of nitrogen waste products [urea nitrogen, creatinine] in the blood).

Although AKI is potentially reversible, despite advances in its treatment, the mortality rate is high (Libório, Leite, Neves, et al., 2015). Usually, AKI affects people with other life-threatening conditions. Most commonly, AKI follows severe, prolonged hypotension or hypovolemia or exposure to a nephrotoxic agent.

The ARF associated with AKI usually develops over hours or days, with progressive elevations of blood urea nitrogen (BUN), creatinine, and potassium, with or without oliguria. Severe AKI develops in over 60% of intensive care unit (ICU) patients, with mortality rates of 70% to 80%.

One of the most commonly used classification systems for AKI uses serum creatinine, glomerular filtration rate (GFR), and urine output to identify **r**isk, **i**njury, **f**ailure, **l**oss, and **e**nd-stage kidney disease (the RIFLE Criteria) (Figure 49-1) (Williams, 2014). The criteria for evaluating AKI have been found to correlate with outcome and are a good predictor of mortality in hospitalized patients (Liborio et al., 2015).

Etiology and Pathophysiology

AKI is a complex disorder, with many etiological factors and varied clinical manifestations that range from minimal elevation in serum creatinine to anuric renal failure (Ellis, 2013; Williams, 2014). The causes leading to AKI with renal failure are divided into prerenal, intrarenal (or intrinsic), and postrenal categories (Table 49-2).

Prerenal causes of AKI are factors external to the kidneys. These factors reduce systemic circulation, causing a reduction in renal blood flow and lead to decreased glomerular perfusion and filtration. Although renal tubular and glomerular function is preserved, glomerular filtration is reduced as a result of decreased perfusion. Hypovolemia, decreased cardiac output, decreased peripheral vascular resistance, and vascular obstruction can all decrease the effective circulating volume of the blood. With a decrease in circulating blood volume, autoregulatory mechanisms that increase angiotensin II, aldosterone, norepinephrine, and antidiuretic hormone attempt to preserve blood flow to essential organs. Prerenal azotemia results in a reduction in the excretion of sodium (<20 mmol/L), increased salt and water retention, and decreased urine output.

Prerenal AKI can also be caused by vasoactive medications such as angiotensin-converting enzyme (ACE) inhibitors, angiotensin receptor blockers (ARBs), epinephrine, and large doses of dopamine that cause intrarenal vasoconstriction leading to hypoperfusion of the glomeruli (Ellis, 2013). AKI associated with prerenal causes is usually reversible. If the course of prerenal failure is prolonged, intrarenal damage may ensue, usually resulting in acute tubular necrosis.

Intrarenal causes include conditions that cause direct damage to the renal tissue (parenchyma), resulting in impaired nephron function. Intrarenal causes of AKI are usually owing to prolonged ischemia or the presence of nephrotoxins, hemoglobin released from hemolyzed red blood cells (RBCs), or myoglobin released from necrotic muscle cells. Nephrotoxins can cause obstruction of intrarenal structures by crystallization or by actually damaging the epithelial cells of the tubules. Hemoglobin and myoglobin block the tubules and cause renal vasoconstriction. Primary renal diseases such as acute glomerulo-nephritis and systemic lupus erythematosus may also cause AKI.

TABLE 49-2	COMMON CAUSES OF ACUTE KIDNEY INJURY

Prerenal
- Anaphylaxis
- Antihypertensive drugs
- Bilateral renal vein thrombosis
- Burns
- Cardiac dysrhythmias
- Cardiogenic shock
- Decreased cardiac output
- Decreased peripheral vascular resistance
- Decreased renovascular blood flow
- Dehydration
- Embolism
- Excessive diuresis
- GI losses (diarrhea, vomiting)
- Heart failure
- Hemorrhage
- Hepatorenal syndrome
- Hypoalbuminemia
- Hypovolemia
- Myocardial infarction
- Neurological injury
- Pericardial tamponade
- Pulmonary edema
- Renal artery thrombosis
- Septic shock
- Valvular heart disease

Intrarenal
- Acute glomerulo-nephritis
- Allergies (antibiotics [sulphonamides, rifampin], nonsteroidal anti-inflammatory drugs, ACE inhibitors)
- Chemical exposure (ethylene glycol, lead, arsenic, carbon tetrachloride)
- Drugs (aminoglycosides [gentamicin, amikacin], amphotericin B)
- Hemolytic blood transfusion reaction
- Infections (bacterial [acute pyelonephritis], viral [CMV], fungal [candidiasis])
- Interstitial nephritis
- Malignant hypertension
- Nephrotoxic injury
- Prolonged prerenal ischemia
- Radiocontrast agents
- Severe crush injury
- Systemic lupus erythematosus
- Thrombotic disorders
- Toxemia of pregnancy

Postrenal
- Benign prostatic hyperplasia
- Calculi formation
- Cancer (bladder, prostate, cervical, colorectal)
- Neuro-muscular disorders
- Spinal cord disease
- Strictures
- Trauma (back, pelvis, perineum)

ACE, angiotensin-converting enzyme; *CMV,* cytomegalovirus; *GI,* gastro-intestinal.

FIGURE 49-2 Acute tubular necrosis. In acute tubular necrosis, the kidneys are swollen and pale. Source: Stevens, A., & Lowe, J. (2000). *Pathology: Illustrated review in color* (2nd ed.). London: Mosby.

Acute tubular necrosis (ATN) is the most common intrarenal cause of AKI and is primarily the result of ischemia, nephrotoxins, or sepsis (Figure 49-2). Severe renal ischemia causes a disruption in the basement membrane and patchy destruction of the tubular epithelium. Nephrotoxic agents cause necrosis of tubular epithelial cells, which slough off and plug the tubules. ATN is potentially reversible if the basement membrane is not destroyed and the tubular epithelium regenerates.

Possible pathological processes involved in ATN include the following:

1. Hypovolemia and decreased renal blood flow stimulate renin release, which activates the renin–angiotensin–aldosterone system (see Chapter 47, Figure 47-6) and results in constriction of the peripheral arteries and the renal afferent arterioles. With decreased renal blood flow, there is decreased glomerular capillary pressure and GFR as well as tubular dysfunction and, ultimately, oliguria.
2. Ischemia alters glomerular epithelial cells and decreases glomerular capillary permeability. This reduces the GFR, which significantly reduces blood flow and leads to tubular dysfunction.
3. When tubules are damaged, interstitial edema occurs, and necrotic epithelial cells accumulate in the tubules. The debris lowers the GFR by obstructing the tubules and increasing intratubular pressure.
4. Glomerular filtrate leaks back into plasma through holes in the damaged tubular membranes, which decreases intratubular fluid flow.

Postrenal causes of AKI involve mechanical obstruction of urinary outflow. As the flow of urine is obstructed, urine refluxes into the renal pelvis, impairing kidney function. The most common causes are benign prostatic hyperplasia, prostate cancer, calculi, trauma, and extrarenal tumours. Postrenal AKI is almost always treatable if identified before permanent kidney damage occurs.

Clinical Manifestations

Prerenal or postrenal AKI that has not caused intrarenal damage usually resolves quickly with correction of the cause. However, if parenchymal damage has occurred from either cause, or from intrarenal causes, ATN results or the course of AKI is prolonged. Clinically, ATN progresses through three phases: initiation, maintenance, and recovery (Lang, 2014). In some situations, the patient does not recover from AKI, and CKD results.

Initiation Phase. The initiation phase of ATN is characterized by an increase in serum creatinine and BUN and a decrease in urine output (Murphy & Byrne, 2010).

Maintenance Phase. The maintenance phase of ATN may last from days to weeks. During this phase, patients may be anuric, oliguric, or nonoliguric. In the case of patients who are nonoliguric, a dilute urine (low specific gravity) is made, but uremic toxins are not removed. The oliguric phase usually lasts 10 to 14 days, but it can last for months in some cases. The longer the oliguric phase lasts, the poorer the prognosis for recovery of complete renal function.

The manifestations of the oliguric phase are changes in urinary output, fluid and electrolyte abnormalities, and uremia. (For a definition of *uremia,* see the discussion of the clinical manifestations of CKD, later in this chapter.) The nurse must be alert for the signs and symptoms of these changes.

Urinary Changes. The most common initial manifestation of ATN is **oliguria,** in which urine output generally decreases to less than 400 mL/24 hr. If ATN is caused by ischemia, oliguria will occur within 24 hours. If ATN is caused by nephrotoxic drugs, the onset may be delayed for as long as a week. The duration of the oliguric phase is generally 10 to 14 days, but it can last months in some cases.

Oliguria associated with ATN is characterized by urine with a normal specific gravity (1.010) and a high sodium concentration (>40 mmol/L), and urine osmolality at about 300 mmol/kg, indicating that the injured tubules cannot respond to autoregulatory mechanisms. The urine sediment may show RBCs and white blood cells (WBCs), casts, and proteinuria. The casts are formed from mucoprotein impressions of the necrotic renal tubular epithelial cells, which detach or slough into the tubules.

Fluid Volume Excess. When urinary output decreases, fluid retention occurs. The severity of the symptoms depends on the extent of the fluid overload. The neck veins may become distended with a bounding pulse. Edema and hypertension may develop. Fluid overload can eventually lead to heart failure, pulmonary edema, and pericardial and pleural effusions.

Metabolic Acidosis. In renal failure, the kidneys cannot synthesize ammonia, which is needed for hydrogen ion excretion or to excrete acid products of metabolism. The serum bicarbonate level decreases because bicarbonate is used up in buffering hydrogen ions. In addition, defective reabsorption and regeneration of bicarbonate occurs. The patient may develop Kussmaul's respirations (rapid, deep respirations) to increase the excretion of carbon dioxide. Lethargy and stupor will occur if treatment is not started.

Sodium Balance. Damaged tubules cannot conserve sodium. Consequently, the urinary excretion of sodium may increase, resulting in normal or below-normal levels of serum sodium. Excessive intake of sodium should be avoided because it can lead to volume expansion, hypertension, and heart failure. Uncontrolled hyponatremia or water excess can lead to cerebral edema.

Potassium Excess. Hyperkalemia is a common, life-threatening complication seen in patients with oliguria. Serum potassium levels increase because the normal ability of the kidneys to regulate and excrete potassium is impaired. Hyperkalemia associated with AKI may be precipitated by a number of causes. Massive tissue trauma may result in the release of additional potassium into the extracellular fluid by the damaged cells. Bleeding and blood transfusions may cause cellular destruction, releasing more potassium into the extracellular fluid. Acidosis worsens hyperkalemia as hydrogen ions enter the cells and potassium is driven out of the cells into the extracellular fluid.

Most often, patients with hyperkalemia are asymptomatic. Some patients may complain of weakness with severe hyperkalemia. Severe hyperkalemia requires immediate treatment. Before clinical signs of hyperkalemia are apparent, the electrocardiogram (ECG) will show tall, peaked T waves; widening of the QRS complex; and ST depression. Progressive changes in the ECG that are related to increasing potassium levels are depicted in Chapter 19, Figure 19-14. Because cardiac muscle is very intolerant of acute increases in potassium, treatment is essential when hyperkalemia develops.

Hematological Disorders. Several hematological disorders are seen in connection with AKI. Anemia occurs because renal failure results in impaired erythropoietin production. Uremia decreases platelet adhesiveness and can lead to bleeding from multiple sources (e.g., intestines, brain). WBCs are also altered, causing immunodeficiency. This leaves the patient susceptible to numerous systemic and local infections. Infection (sepsis) in combination with AKI is associated with double the mortality rate, and half of the survivors suffer permanent kidney damage or chronic kidney disease (Emlet, Shaw, & Kellum, 2015).

Calcium Deficit and Phosphate Excess. Activated vitamin D must be present for calcium absorption from the gastro-intestinal

(GI) tract to occur. Only functioning kidneys can activate vitamin D. Thus, in the presence of kidney failure, GI absorption of calcium decreases, and a low serum calcium level results. When hypocalcemia occurs, the parathyroid gland secretes parathyroid hormone (PTH), which stimulates bone demineralization and causes calcium to be released from the bones. Phosphate is released as well, leading to hyperphosphatemia, which is worsened by the decreased excretion of phosphate by the kidneys. Normally, plasma calcium is found ionized or free (physiologically active form) or bound to protein. In the acidotic state associated with renal failure, more calcium is in the ionized form. Although it is unusual for hypocalcemia to be symptomatic in renal failure, an ionized calcium level that does decrease significantly can lead to tetany.

Waste Product Accumulation. The kidneys are the primary excretory organs for urea, an end product of protein metabolism, and creatinine, an end product of endogenous muscle metabolism. The BUN and creatinine levels are elevated in kidney failure. An elevated BUN level must be interpreted with caution because dehydration, corticosteroids, catabolism resulting from infections, fever, severe injury, and GI bleeding can also elevate BUN. The best serum indicator of renal failure is creatinine because it is not significantly altered by other factors. Measuring creatinine clearance by using radioactive tracer (inulin) is the most accurate method for assessing renal function, but it is expensive and impractical. Clinically, the recommended method to evaluate kidney function is with an estimated glomerular filtration rate (eGFR) (Baron, Cheng, Bazari, et al., 2015).

Neurological Disorders. Neurological changes can occur as nitrogenous waste products accumulate in the brain and other nervous tissue. The symptoms can be as mild as fatigue and difficulty concentrating or can escalate to seizures, stupor, and coma.

Eventually, all body systems become involved in the acute uremic syndrome. The extrarenal manifestations are generally similar to those found in the patient with chronic uremia (see the discussion of CKD later in this chapter).

Recovery Phase. The recovery phase of AKI is marked by a return of BUN, creatinine, and GFR toward normal ranges (Baron et al., 2015). During this phase, patients may experience a diuretic phase that can result in fluid and electrolyte abnormalities. The diuretic phase begins with a gradual increase in daily urine output to 1 to 3 L/day, but it may reach 3 to 5 L or more per day. Although urine output increases, the nephrons are still not fully functional. The high urine volume is caused by osmotic diuresis from the high urea concentration in the glomerular filtrate and the inability of the tubules to concentrate the urine. In this phase, the kidneys have recovered their ability to excrete wastes but not to concentrate the urine. Hypovolemia and hypotension can occur from massive fluid losses. Because of the large losses of fluid and electrolytes, the patient must be monitored for hyponatremia, hypokalemia, and dehydration. The diuretic phase may last 1 to 3 weeks. Near the end of this phase, the patient's acid–base, electrolyte, and waste product (BUN, creatinine) values begin to normalize. Although the major improvements occur in the first 1 to 2 weeks of this phase, renal function may take up to 12 months to stabilize.

The outcome of AKI is influenced by the patient's overall health, the severity of renal failure, and the number and type of complications. Some individuals do not recover and progress to CKD. The older-adult patient is less likely to recover full kidney function than the younger patient. Among the individuals who recover, the majority achieve clinically normal kidney function with no complications (e.g., hypertension).

Diagnostic Studies. Urinalysis is an important diagnostic test. Urine sediment containing abundant cells, casts, or proteins suggests intrarenal disorders. The urine osmolality, sodium content, and specific gravity help to differentiate the types of AKI. Urine sediment may be normal in both prerenal and postrenal AKI. Hematuria, pyuria, and crystals may be seen with postrenal AKI.

To establish a diagnosis of AKI, other testing may be required. A renal ultrasound is often the first test done and provides information about anatomy and function. Ultrasound does not require the use of nephrotoxic contrast agents. A renal scan can assess renal blood flow and the integrity of the collecting system. A computed tomographic (CT) scan can identify lesions and masses as well as obstruction, but exposure to radiation is higher and it may involve contrast that can be nephrotoxic. Magnetic resonance imaging (MRI) and magnetic resonance angiography (MRA) are not recommended—gadolinium, a contrast medium used with MRI and MRA, has been associated with the development of *nephrogenic systemic fibrosis* in patients with compromised renal function.

Collaborative Care

Because AKI is potentially reversible, the primary goals of treatment are to eliminate the cause, manage the signs and symptoms, and prevent complications while the kidneys recover (Table 49-3). The first step is to determine whether there is sufficient intravascular volume and cardiac output to ensure adequate perfusion of the kidneys. Diuretic therapy is often administered along with volume expanders to prevent fluid overload. Diuretic therapy usually includes loop diuretics (e.g., furosemide [Lasix]) or an osmotic diuretic (e.g., mannitol). If AKI is already established, forcing fluids and diuretics will not be effective and may, in fact, be harmful. Medical management without RRT may be all that is necessary until renal function improves. The general trend is to initiate early and frequent RRT to minimize symptoms and prevent complications.

Fluid intake must be closely monitored during the oliguric phase. The general rule for calculating the permitted fluid intake is to add all losses for the previous 24 hours (e.g., urine, diarrhea, emesis, blood) plus 600 mL for insensible losses (e.g., respiration, diaphoresis). For example, if a patient excreted 300 mL of urine on Tuesday with no other losses, the fluid intake on Wednesday would be restricted to 900 mL.

Hyperkalemia is one of the most serious complications of AKI because it can cause life-threatening cardiac dysrhythmias. The various therapies used to treat elevated potassium levels are listed in Table 49-4. Both insulin and salbutamol temporarily shift potassium into the cells, but it eventually shifts back out. Calcium gluconate raises the threshold at which dysrhythmias will occur, serving to temporarily stabilize the myocardium. Only cation exchange resins, such as sodium polystyrene sulphonate (Kayexalate) or calcium resonium, and dialysis actually remove potassium from the body. Sodium polystyrene sulphonate should not be given, or mixed with sorbitol, to patients who do not have normal bowel function because of associated bowel necrosis (Batterink, Lin, Au-Yeung, et al., 2015).

The most common indications for RRT in AKI include (1) volume overload resulting in compromised cardiac or pulmonary status, or both; (2) elevated potassium levels; (3) metabolic acidosis (serum bicarbonate level <15 mmol/L); (4) BUN level greater than 43 mmol/L; (5) significant change in mental status; and (6) pericarditis, pericardial effusion, or cardiac tamponade. Although laboratory values provide rough parameters, the best guide to treatment is good clinical assessment.

TABLE 49-3 COLLABORATIVE CARE

Acute Kidney Injury

Diagnostic	Collaborative Therapy
• History and physical examination	• Treatment of precipitating cause
• Identification of precipitating cause	• Fluid restriction (allowance = 600 mL + previous 24-hr fluid loss)
• Serum creatinine and BUN levels	• Nutritional therapy
• Serum electrolytes	• Adequate protein intake (0.6–2 g/kg/day), depending on degree of catabolism
• Urinalysis	• Potassium restriction
• Renal ultrasound	• Phosphate restriction
• Renal scan (as indicated)	• Sodium restriction
• CT scan (as indicated and without contrast if possible)	• Measures to lower potassium (if elevated)*
• Retrograde pyelogram (as indicated)	• Calcium supplements or phosphate-binding agents
	• Parenteral nutrition (if indicated)†
	• Enteral nutrition (if indicated)†
	• Initiation of renal replacement therapy (if necessary)

BUN, blood urea nitrogen; *CT,* computed tomographic.
*See Table 49-4.
†Renal formulations of these two forms of nutrition are available.

TABLE 49-4 TREATMENT OF HYPERKALEMIA

Stabilize Myocardium
• If the ECG shows hyperkalemia-related abnormalities, *calcium gluconate IV* is given. Calcium raises the threshold potential, thus counteracting the toxic effect of potassium on the myocardium, which can induce life-threatening dysrhythmias.

Shift Potassium Into Cells
• *Regular IV insulin administration* causes potassium to move into cells. Glucose is given concurrently to prevent hypoglycemia. When effects of insulin diminish, potassium shifts back out of cells.
• *Salbutamol* will also temporarily shift potassium back into cells.
• *Sodium bicarbonate* can correct acidosis and causes shift of potassium into cells.

Enhance Potassium Removal
• *Cation exchange resins* such as *sodium polystyrene sulphonate (Kayexalate)* are administered by mouth or retention enema. When resin is in the bowel, potassium is exchanged for sodium. Therapy removes 1 mmol of potassium/g of drug. *Calcium resonium* is another such resin.
• Loop diuretics such as *furosemide* can increase potassium excretion in the urine if the patient has any urine output.
• *Dialysis,* particularly *hemodialysis,* can bring potassium levels to normal within 30 min to 2 hr.

Long-Term Treatment
• *Restrict intake of dietary potassium* to 40 mmol/day and avoid potassium-containing salt substitutes.
• Limit or discontinue medications that can precipitate or exacerbate hyperkalemia such as ACE inhibitors, ARBs, and potassium-sparing diuretics.

ACE, angiotensin-converting enzyme; *ARBs,* angiotensin receptor blockers; *ECG,* electrocardiogram; *IV,* intravenous.

If RRT is required, many options are available, but there is no consensus regarding the best approach. Even though peritoneal dialysis (PD) is considered a viable option for RRT, it is rarely used. Intermittent hemodialysis (HD) (e.g., at intervals of 4 hr, either daily or every other day, or three to four times per week) and continuous renal replacement therapy (CRRT) have both been used effectively. CRRT is provided continuously over approximately 24 hours and has much slower blood flow rates than intermittent HD.

HD is the method of choice when rapid changes are required in a short time. It is technically more complicated because specialized staff and equipment are required. It also requires anticoagulation to prevent the patient's blood from clotting when it contacts the foreign material in the dialysis circuit. Rapid fluid shifts during HD may cause hypotension.

RRT, PD, HD, and CRRT are discussed later in this chapter.

Nutritional Therapy. The challenge of nutritional management in AKI is to provide adequate calories to prevent catabolism despite the restrictions required to prevent electrolyte and fluid disorders and azotemia. Adequate energy should be provided from carbohydrate and fat sources to prevent ketosis from endogenous fat breakdown and gluconeogenesis from muscle-protein breakdown. The daily caloric intake for patients with AKI should be about 25 to 35 kcal/kg, based on estimated metabolic stress and protein energy requirements (Fiaccadori, Maggiore, Cabassi, et al., 2013). Protein dosage varies from 1.5 to 2.5 g/kg/day, depending on the stage of AKI and whether or not RRT is required (Fiaccadori et al., 2013).

Potassium and sodium are regulated in accordance with plasma levels. Sodium is restricted as needed to prevent edema, hypertension, and heart failure. Hyperphosphatemia, hypocalcemia, and hypermagnesemia are common and must be monitored and regulated (Fiaccadori et al., 2013). Dietary fat intake is increased so that the patient receives at least 30% to 40% of total calories from fat. Fat-emulsion intravenous (IV) infusions can also be given as a nutritional supplement and provide a good source of nonprotein calories (see Chapter 42). If a patient cannot maintain adequate oral intake, enteral nutrition is the preferred route for nutritional support (see Chapter 42). When the GI tract is not functional, parenteral nutrition (PN) is necessary for the provision of adequate nutrition. The patient treated with PN may need daily HD or CRRT to remove the excess fluid. Concentrated PN formulas are available to minimize fluid volume (Baron et al., 2015).

NURSING MANAGEMENT
ACUTE KIDNEY INJURY

NURSING ASSESSMENT

An assessment of the patient with AKI includes the specific areas presented in Table 49-5. It is important to monitor the vital signs and intake and output. The urine should be examined for colour, specific gravity, glucose, protein, blood, and sediment. The patient's general appearance should be assessed, including skin colour, peripheral edema, neck vein distension, and bruises.

If the patient is receiving RRT, the access site should be observed for signs of inflammation. Evaluate the patient's mental status and level of consciousness. Examine the oral mucosa for dryness and inflammation. Auscultate the lung fields for crackles and wheezes or diminished breath sounds. Monitor the heart for the presence of a third heart sound (S₃ or gallop), murmurs, or a pericardial friction rub. Assess ECG readings for the presence

TABLE 49-5	MANIFESTATIONS OF ACUTE KIDNEY INJURY
Body System	**Clinical Manifestations**
Urinary	Casts
	↓ Osmolality
	Proteinuria
	↓ Specific gravity
	Urinary output
	↑ Urinary sodium
Cardiovascular	Dysrhythmias
	Heart failure
	Hypertension (after development of fluid overload)
	Hypotension (early)
	Pericardial effusion
	Pericarditis
	Volume overload
Respiratory	Kussmaul's respirations
	Pleural effusions
	Pulmonary edema
Gastro-intestinal	Anorexia
	Bleeding
	Constipation
	Diarrhea
	Nausea and vomiting
	Stomatitis
Hematological	Anemia (development within 48 hr)
	Defect in platelet functioning
	Leukocytosis
	↑ Susceptibility to infection
Neurological	Asterixis
	Lethargy
	Memory impairment
	Seizures
Metabolic	↑ BUN
	↑ Creatinine
	↑ Phosphate
	↑ Potassium
	↓ Bicarbonate
	↓ Calcium
	↓ pH
	↓ Sodium

BUN, blood urea nitrogen.

of dysrhythmias. Review laboratory values and diagnostic test results. All of the previous data are essential for developing a collaborative plan of care.

NURSING DIAGNOSES

Nursing diagnoses and potential complications for the patient with AKI include, but are not limited to, the following:

- *Risk for infection* as evidenced by *alteration in skin integrity* (invasive lines)
- *Excess fluid volume* related to *excessive fluid intake* (kidney injury and fluid retention)
- *Fatigue* related to *malnutrition, physical deconditioning* (anemia, metabolic acidosis, uremic toxins)
- *Anxiety* related to *threat to current status, threat of death* (disease processes, therapeutic interventions, uncertainty of prognosis)
- Potential complication: dysrhythmias related to electrolyte imbalances

PLANNING

The overall goals for the patient with AKI are to (1) completely recover without any loss of kidney function, (2) maintain normal fluid and electrolyte balance, (3) have decreased anxiety, and (4) understand and adhere to the treatment plan and follow-up care.

NURSING IMPLEMENTATION

HEALTH PROMOTION. Prevention of AKI is essential because of the high mortality rate associated with it and is primarily directed toward identifying and monitoring high-risk populations, controlling nephrotoxic drugs and industrial chemicals, and preventing prolonged episodes of hypotension and hypovolemia. In the hospital, the factors that increase the risk of developing AKI are advanced age, massive trauma, major surgical procedures, extensive burns, cardiac failure, sepsis, obstetrical complications, and baseline renal insufficiency caused by hypertension or diabetes mellitus. Careful monitoring of intake and output and of fluid and electrolyte balance is essential. Extrarenal losses of fluid should be assessed and recorded from vomiting, diarrhea, hemorrhage, and increased insensible losses. Prompt replacement of significant fluid losses will help prevent ischemic tubular damage associated with trauma, burns, and extensive surgery. Intake and output records and the patient's weight provide valuable indicators of fluid volume status. Aggressive diuretic therapy for the patient with fluid overload resulting from any cause can lead to decreased renal blood flow.

For patients with any level of renal insufficiency—and particularly patients with diabetes or older-adult patients with renal insufficiency—who are undergoing diagnostic studies requiring IV contrast media, special attention must be given to prevent a nephrotoxic injury secondary to the dye. Adequate hydration before and after the test is critical. The use of acetylcysteine may be helpful in providing added protection to the kidneys (Quintavalle, Donnarumma, Fiore, et al., 2013). Patients with urinary tract infections need prompt treatment and careful follow-up care. Chemotherapeutic drugs that cause hyperuricemia also can put a patient at risk for renal injury.

Individuals taking drugs that are potentially nephrotoxic (see Chapter 47, Table 47-3) must have renal function monitored. Nephrotoxic drugs should be used sparingly in high-risk patients. When these drugs must be used, they should be given in the smallest effective doses for the shortest possible periods. The patient should be cautioned about the abuse of over-the-counter analgesics (especially nonsteroidal anti-inflammatory drugs [NSAIDs]) because some of these may worsen renal function in the patient with borderline renal insufficiency by decreasing glomerular pressure or causing interstitial nephritis. ACE inhibitors can also decrease perfusion pressure and cause hyperkalemia, and their use may be contraindicated in renal insufficiency. Industrial and agricultural chemicals and products (e.g., organic solvents, insecticides, cleaning agents) must be monitored regularly to assess their safety for employees and the general population.

ACUTE INTERVENTION. The patient with AKI is most often critically ill and often has a high burden of comorbid illness (e.g., diabetes, cardiovascular disease) that also affects renal function. The nurse needs to focus on the patient holistically because there are many physical and emotional needs. Usually, the changes caused by AKI arise suddenly. Both the patient and the family need assistance in understanding that the functioning of the whole body can be disrupted by renal failure.

The nurse has an important role in managing fluid and electrolyte balance during the oliguric and diuretic phases. Observing and recording accurate intake and output are essential.

It is important to measure weights daily, with the same scale and at the same time each day, to allow for the evaluation and detection of excessive gains or losses of body fluid (1 kg is equivalent to 1 000 mL of fluid). The nurse needs to be knowledgeable about the common signs and symptoms of hypervolemia (in the oliguric phase) or hypovolemia (in the diuretic phase), potassium and sodium disturbances, and other electrolyte imbalances that may occur in AKI (see Chapter 19).

Because infection is the leading cause of death in AKI, meticulous aseptic technique is critical. The patient must be protected from other individuals with infectious diseases. The nurse should be alert for local manifestations of infection (e.g., swelling, redness, pain) as well as systemic manifestations (e.g., malaise, leukocytosis) but should realize that an elevated temperature may not be present. Patients with renal failure have a blunted febrile response to an infection (e.g., pneumonia). If antibiotics are used to treat an infection, the type, frequency, and dosage must be carefully considered because the kidneys are the primary route of excretion for many antibiotics. Dosages and dosing intervals need to be considered in relation to the patient's level of kidney function if the drug is primarily eliminated by the kidneys. Nephrotoxic drugs (see Chapter 47, Table 47-3) should be avoided.

Skin care and measures to prevent pressure injuries should be performed because the patient usually develops edema as well as decreased muscle tone. Mouth care is important to prevent stomatitis, which develops when ammonia (produced by bacterial breakdown of urea) in saliva irritates the mucous membranes.

INFORMATICS IN PRACTICE

Computer Monitoring of Antibiotic Safety

- Many patients receiving antibiotic therapy are at risk for kidney failure.
- The computer should be set to send an alert about elevated creatinine levels and, if possible, send a text message.
- With earlier notification of the health care provider, medications can be stopped or doses adjusted and the patient's kidney function preserved.

AMBULATORY AND HOME CARE. Recovery from AKI is highly variable and depends on the underlying illness, the general condition and the age of the patient, the length of the oliguric phase, and the severity of nephron damage. Good nutrition, rest, and activity are necessary. Dietary restrictions should be regulated in accordance with kidney function. Follow-up care and regular evaluation of renal function are necessary. Teach the patient the signs and symptoms of recurrent kidney disease. Emphasize measures to prevent the recurrence of AKI.

The long-term convalescence of 3 to 12 months may cause psychosocial and financial hardships for the family. Make referrals for counselling as appropriate. If the kidneys do not recover, the patient will need to transition to life on chronic dialysis or possible future transplantation.

EVALUATION

The following are expected outcomes for the patient with AKI:
- Regain and maintain normal fluid and electrolyte balance.
- Comply with treatment regimen.
- Experience no infectious complications.
- Have complete recovery.

AGE-RELATED CONSIDERATIONS

ACUTE KIDNEY INJURY

Older adults are more susceptible than younger adults to AKI because the number of functioning nephrons decreases with age. Impaired function of other organ systems (e.g., cardiovascular disease, impaired pancreas function) can increase the risk of developing AKI. The aging kidney is less able to compensate for changes in fluid volume, solute load, and cardiac output. Common causes of AKI in the older adult include dehydration, hypotension, diuretic therapy, aminoglycoside therapy, obstructive disorders (e.g., prostatic hyperplasia), surgery, infection, and radiocontrast agents.

CHRONIC KIDNEY DISEASE

Chronic kidney disease (CKD) involves the progressive, irreversible loss of kidney function. The Kidney Disease Outcomes Quality Initiative (KDOQI) defines CKD as either kidney damage or GFR <60 mL/min/1.73 m² for 3 months or longer. CKD is classified as one of five stages, depending on the level of severity based on GFR (Table 49-6). CKD involves progressive, irreversible destruction of the nephrons in both kidneys. Not all people with CKD will progress to stage 5, in which RRT would be necessary; however, all those affected will require ongoing monitoring.

Identifying the stage of CKD allows for early intervention to reduce cardiovascular risk, delay progression, and prevent the need for RRT (Grams, Chow, Segev, et al., 2013). RRTs include PD, HD, and renal transplantation. Stage 5 CKD, often referred to as end-stage renal disease (ESRD), is advanced kidney disease with GFR less than 15 mL/min/1.73 m², when most patients with CKD require some form of RRT. At this point, RRT (dialysis or transplantation) is usually required. In 2012, there were 5 431

new patients on dialysis in Canada. Of these, over half (53%) were older than 65 years (CIHI, 2014). Although there are many causes of CKD, the leading causes of CKD in Canada are diabetes mellitus (38%) and renal vascular disease (15%) (CIHI, 2014).

The kidneys have remarkable functional reserve. Up to 80% of the GFR (reflected in creatinine clearance measurements) may be lost with few overt changes in the functioning of the body. A person is born with about 2 million nephrons and can survive without RRT until almost 90% of the nephrons are lost. In the majority of cases, the individual passes through the early stages of CKD without recognizing the disease state because the remaining nephrons hypertrophy to compensate. The prognosis and the course of CKD are highly variable, depending on the etiology, the individual's condition and age, and the adequacy of medical follow-up. Some individuals live normal, active lives with compensated renal failure, whereas others may rapidly progress to ESRD.

Since 1973, many deaths have been prevented through the use of RRTs. Dialysis modalities remain the most common RRT for people with stage 5 CKD because of (1) a lack of donated organs, (2) medical conditions that preclude transplantation, or (3) personal reasons, in which an individual may decline transplantation as a treatment option. With the advances made in medical science, an increasing number of individuals are receiving RRTs, including older adults and those with complex medical problems. All people with advanced CKD, regardless of age, should be offered RRT unless it is medically contraindicated.

TABLE 49-6 STAGES* AND DESCRIPTIONS OF CHRONIC KIDNEY DISEASE†

	Description	GFR (mL/min/1.73 m²)	Action‡
Stage 1	Kidney damage with normal or ↑ GFR	≥90	Diagnosis and treatment of comorbid conditions CVD risk reduction
Stage 2	Kidney damage with mild ↓ GFR	60–89	Estimation of progression
Stage 3	Moderate ↓ GFR	30–59	Evaluation and treatment of complications
Stage 4	Severe ↓ GFR	15–29	Preparation for renal replacement therapy
Stage 5	Kidney failure	<15 (or dialysis)	Renal replacement therapy (if uremia present and patient desires treatment)

CVD, cardiovascular disease; GFR, glomerular filtration rate.
*Stages 1 to 5 identify patients who have chronic kidney disease.
†Chronic kidney disease is defined as either kidney damage or GFR <60 mL/min/1.73 m² for 3 mo. Kidney damage is defined as pathological abnormalities or markers of damage, including abnormalities in blood or urine tests or imaging studies.
‡Includes actions from preceding stages.
Source: Reprinted from National Kidney Foundation. KDOQI Clinical Practice Guidelines for Chronic Kidney Disease: Evaluation, Classification and Stratification. Am J Kidney Dis 39:S1-S000, 2002 (suppl 1), with permission from Elsevier.

DETERMINANTS OF HEALTH

Chronic Kidney Disease

Culture; Biology and Genetic Endowment
- Chronic kidney disease (CKD) has a disproportionate impact on certain ethnic groups in Canada, related to the higher incidence of diabetes and hypertension within these populations. These groups include Canadians who are of Indigenous, Asian, South Asian, Pacific Island, African/Caribbean, and Latin American origin.*
- The rate of CKD is six times higher among Indigenous people with diabetes than among other ethnic groups with diabetes.
- The specific causes of cultural and ethnic differences in occurrence of CKD are not clear. However, it appears that genetic factors contribute to differences in diabetic nephropathy among ethnic groups.

Reference
*The Kidney Foundation of Canada. (2006). *Living with kidney disease* (4th ed., pp. 2–4). Montreal: Author. Retrieved from http://www.kidney.ca/document.doc?id=237.

Clinical Manifestations

As renal function progressively deteriorates, excretory, regulatory, and endocrine function are lost, and these effects are manifested in every body system, no matter what the underlying cause of CKD. These excretory, regulatory, and endocrine functional impairments are manifested in retained substances, including urea, creatinine, phenols, hormones, electrolytes, water, and many other substances. Uremia is a constellation of signs and symptoms resulting from the buildup of waste products and excess fluid associated with kidney failure. These signs and symptoms may include, but are not limited to, elevated serum creatinine and BUN, abnormal electrolytes, acidosis, anemia, fluid volume excess, nausea, loss of appetite, fatigue, decreased cognition, pruritus,

Psychological
• Anxiety
• Depression

Cardiovascular
• Hypertension
• Heart failure
• Coronary artery disease
• Pericarditis
• Peripheral artery disease

Gastro-intestinal
• Anorexia
• Nausea
• Vomiting
• Gastro-intestinal bleeding
• Gastritis

Endocrine/Reproductive
• Hyperparathyroidism
• Thyroid abnormalities
• Amenorrhea
• Erectile dysfunction

Metabolic
• Carbohydrate intolerance
• Hyperlipidemia

Hematological
• Anemia
• Bleeding
• Infection

Neurological
• Fatigue
• Headache
• Sleep disturbances
• Encephalopathy

Ocular
• Hypertensive retinopathy

Pulmonary
• Pulmonary edema
• Uremic pleuritis
• Pneumonia

Integumentary
• Pruritus
• Ecchymosis
• Dry, scaly skin

Musculo-skeletal
• Vascular and soft tissue
  calcifications
• Osteomalacia
• Osteitis fibrosa

Peripheral neuropathy
• Paresthesias
• Restless legs syndrome

FIGURE 49-3 Clinical manifestations of chronic uremia.

and neuropathy (Figure 49-3). It is important to recognize that the manifestations of uremia vary among patients, according to the cause of the kidney disease, comorbid conditions, age, and degree of adherence to the prescribed medical regimen. Many patients are very tolerant of the changes that occur because the changes develop gradually. Uremia often occurs when the GFR is 10 mL/min/1.73 m² or lower.

Urinary System. In the early stage of CKD, polyuria results from the inability of the kidneys to concentrate urine. This happens most often at night, and the patient must arise several times to urinate (nocturia). Because of the decrease in renal concentrating ability, the specific gravity of urine gradually becomes fixed at around 1.010 (the osmolar concentration of plasma). As CKD worsens, oliguria develops, and eventually anuria (urine output 40 mL/24 hr) develops. If the patient is still producing urine, proteinuria, casts, pyuria, and hematuria could be present, depending on the cause of the kidney disease.

Metabolic Disturbances

Waste Product Accumulation. As GFR declines, the serum creatinine and BUN levels increase. Accumulation of nitrogenous waste products in advanced stages of CKD is often manifested by symptoms of nausea, vomiting, lethargy, fatigue, impaired thought processes, and headaches as a result of the multisystemic involvement of CKD.

Serum creatinine continues to be the most common biochemical parameter to estimate the GFR, but it alone is not an accurate measure of GFR (Baron et al., 2015) (Serum creatinine tends to be an ineffective marker of early as well as advanced

kidney disease. The eGFR is a better measure of overall kidney function than creatinine or BUN. The eGFR may be calculated by the laboratory using mathematical formulas. If this method is not available, GFR calculators and tables can be used (see link to the MDRD [modification of diet in renal disease] calculator in Table 49-8). The serum creatinine level in an older-adult patient with ESRD will be lower than it is in a younger person with the same degree of renal dysfunction. Decreased muscle mass and decreased muscle activity from aging account for this finding because creatinine is an end product of muscle metabolism.

Altered Carbohydrate Metabolism. Defective carbohydrate metabolism is caused by impaired glucose use resulting from cellular insensitivity to the normal action of insulin. The exact nature of this insulin resistance is unclear, but it may be related to circulating insulin antagonists, alterations in hormone receptors, or abnormalities of transport mechanisms. Moderate hyperglycemia, hyperinsulinemia, and abnormal glucose tolerance tests may be seen. Insulin and glucose metabolism may improve (but not to normal values) after the initiation of dialysis.

Patients with diabetes who become uremic may require less insulin than before the onset of CKD. This is because insulin, which is dependent on the kidneys for excretion, remains in circulation longer. The insulin regimen must be individualized and glucose levels monitored carefully.

Elevated Triglycerides. Hyperinsulinemia stimulates hepatic production of triglycerides. Almost all patients with uremia develop dyslipidemia, with elevated very-low-density lipoproteins, normal or decreased low-density lipoproteins, and lowered high-density lipoproteins. The altered lipid metabolism is related to decreased levels of the enzyme lipoprotein lipase, which is important in the breakdown of lipoproteins.

Electrolyte and Acid–Base Imbalances

Potassium. Hyperkalemia is a serious electrolyte disorder associated with kidney disease. Fatal dysrhythmias can occur when the serum potassium level reaches 7 to 8 mmol/L. Hyperkalemia results from the decreased excretion by the kidneys, the breakdown of cellular protein, bleeding, and metabolic acidosis. The most common causes of hyperkalemia in CKD are associated with diet, dietary supplements, drugs, and IV infusions.

Sodium. Sodium may be normal or low in renal failure. Because of impaired sodium excretion, sodium is retained along with water. If large quantities of body water are retained, dilutional hyponatremia occurs. Sodium retention can contribute to edema, hypertension, and heart failure. Sodium intake must be individually determined but is generally restricted to 2 g/24 hr.

Calcium and Phosphate. Calcium and phosphate alterations are in the Musculo-Skeletal System section, later in this chapter.

Magnesium. Magnesium is excreted primarily by the kidneys. It is sometimes used as a phosphate-binding agent in patients with CKD. Hypermagnesemia is generally not a problem unless the patient is ingesting magnesium (e.g., milk of magnesia, magnesium citrate, antacids containing magnesium). Clinical manifestations of hypermagnesemia can include absence of reflexes, decreased mental status, cardiac dysrhythmias, hypotension, and respiratory failure.

Metabolic Acidosis. Metabolic acidosis results from the impaired ability of the kidneys to excrete the acid load (primarily ammonia) and from defective reabsorption and regeneration of bicarbonate. The average adult produces 80 to 90 mmol/day of acid. In renal failure, plasma bicarbonate, which is an indirect measure of acidosis, usually falls to a new steady state at around 16 to 20 mmol/L. It generally does not progress below this level because hydrogen ion production is usually balanced by buffering from demineralization of the bone (the phosphate buffering system). Although Kussmaul's respiration is uncommon in CKD, this breathing pattern reduces the severity of acidosis by increasing carbon dioxide excretion.

Hematological System

Anemia. Anemia is very common in CKD. A normocytic, normochromic anemia is associated with CKD and is a result of decreased production of the hormone erythropoietin by the kidneys, resulting in decreased erythropoiesis by the bone marrow (Wittwer, 2013). Erythropoietin stimulates precursor cells in the bone marrow to produce RBCs. Other factors contributing to anemia are nutritional deficiencies, decreased RBC lifespan, increased hemolysis of RBCs, frequent blood samplings, and bleeding from the GI tract. For patients receiving maintenance HD, blood loss in the dialyzer may also contribute to the anemic state. Elevated levels of PTH (produced to compensate for low serum calcium levels) can inhibit erythropoiesis, shorten survival of RBCs, and cause bone marrow fibrosis, which can result in decreased numbers of hematopoietic cells.

Sufficient iron stores are needed for erythropoiesis. Many patients with renal failure are iron deficient and require iron replacement. Folic acid, which is water soluble and essential for RBC maturation, is removed with dialysis and needs to be replaced in the diet with supplementation (1 mg/day).

Bleeding Tendencies. The most common cause of bleeding in uremia is a qualitative defect in platelet function. This dysfunction is caused by impaired platelet aggregation and impaired release of platelet factor III. In addition, alterations in the coagulation system with increased concentrations of both factor VIII and fibrinogen are found in the serum of these patients. The altered platelet function, hemorrhagic tendencies, and GI bleeding can usually be corrected with regular HD or PD.

Infection. Patients with advanced CKD have an increased susceptibility to infection. Infectious complications are caused by changes in leukocyte function and altered immune response and function. Both cellular and humoral immune responses are suppressed. Other factors contributing to the increased risk for infection include malnutrition, hyperglycemia, and external trauma (e.g., catheters, needle insertions into vascular access sites).

Cardiovascular System. Morbidity and mortality from cardiovascular disease are high in patients with CKD, and the presence of CKD worsens the outcomes of cardiovascular disease (Sarafidis & Bakris, 2015). Many patients will die from cardiovascular disease before CKD stage 5 requiring dialysis develops (Sarafidis & Bakris, 2015). Management of cardiovascular risk factors in patients with CKD should be a focus of care (Sarafidis & Bakris, 2015).

The most common cardiovascular abnormality is hypertension, which usually exists before ESRD sets in and is worsened by sodium retention and increased extracellular fluid volume. In some individuals, increased renin production contributes to the problem (see Chapter 47, Figure 47-6). Hypertension accelerates atherosclerotic vascular disease, produces intrarenal arterial spasm, and eventually leads to left ventricular hypertrophy and heart failure (Sarafidis & Bakris, 2015). Hypertension also causes retinopathy, encephalopathy, and nephropathy.

The vascular changes from longstanding hypertension and the accelerated atherosclerosis from elevated triglyceride levels are responsible for many cardiovascular complications (e.g., myocardial infarction, stroke). Diabetes mellitus is a major risk factor for the development of vascular problems.

Heart failure from left ventricular hypertrophy can lead to pulmonary edema. Peripheral edema is often present. Cardiac dysrhythmias may result from hyperkalemia, hypocalcemia, and decreased coronary artery perfusion.

Uremic pericarditis can develop and occasionally progresses to pericardial effusion and cardiac tamponade. Pericarditis is manifested by a friction rub, chest pain, and low-grade fever.

Respiratory System. Respiratory changes include dyspnea from fluid overload, pulmonary edema, uremic pleuritis (pleurisy), pleural effusion, a predisposition to respiratory infections, and in very advanced CKD, Kussmaul's respiration. "Uremic lung," or uremic pneumonitis, is typically found in CKD and shows up as interstitial edema on chest radiograph. This condition usually responds to vigorous fluid removal during dialysis treatments.

Gastro-Intestinal System. Every part of the GI system is affected with CKD, as a result of inflammation of the mucosa caused by excessive urea. Stomatitis with exudates and ulcerations, a metallic taste in the mouth, and *uremic fetor* (a urinous odour of the breath) are commonly found. As CKD progresses, anorexia, nausea, and vomiting caused by irritation of the GI tract by waste products may be present. Patients are also at risk for weight loss and malnutrition. Diabetic gastroparesis (delayed gastric emptying) can compound these problems for patients with diabetes. GI bleeding is also a risk because of irritation of the mucosa by waste products, coupled with the platelet defect. Constipation may be caused by the ingestion of iron salts or calcium-containing phosphate binders, or both. Constipation can be made worse by the limited fluid intake and inactivity.

Neurological System. Neurological changes are expected as renal failure progresses. They are attributed to increased nitrogenous waste products, electrolyte imbalances, metabolic acidosis, and axonal atrophy and demyelination of nerve fibres (Walton, 2015). High levels of uremic toxins have been implicated in axonal damage.

The central nervous system (CNS) becomes depressed, resulting in lethargy, apathy, decreased ability to concentrate, fatigue, irritability, and altered mental ability. Although uncommon, seizures and coma may result from a rapidly increasing BUN and hypertensive encephalopathy.

Peripheral neuropathy is initially manifested by a slowing of nerve conduction to the extremities. The patient complains of restless legs syndrome and may describe it as "bugs crawling inside the leg." Paresthesias occur most often in the feet and legs and may be described by the patient as a burning sensation. Eventually, motor involvement may lead to bilateral foot drop, muscular weakness and atrophy, and loss of deep tendon reflexes. Muscle twitching, jerking, asterixis (hand-flapping tremor), and nocturnal leg cramps also occur. In patients with diabetes, uremic neuropathy is compounded by the neuropathy associated with diabetes mellitus.

The treatment for neurological problems is dialysis or transplantation. Dialysis should improve the general CNS symptoms and may slow or halt the progression of neuropathies. However, motor neuropathy may not be reversible.

Musculo-Skeletal System. Chronic kidney disease–mineral and bone disorder (CKD–MBD) is a term used to describe the systemic components of this clinical syndrome that include characteristic bone abnormalities, changes in mineral balance (calcium, phosphorus, PTH, and vitamin D), and vascular and other soft tissue calcification (Felsenfeld, Levine, & Rodriguez, 2015). These manifestations develop owing to progressive deterioration in kidney function (Figure 49-4). As kidney function declines, phosphorus elimination decreases and less vitamin D is converted to its active form, resulting in decreased serum levels (Felsenfeld et al., 2015). To absorb calcium from the GI tract, activated vitamin D is necessary. Thus, decreased active vitamin D levels result in less calcium absorption from the intestine and, therefore, decreased serum calcium levels (Alshayeb, Josephson, & Sprague, 2013). When hypocalcemia occurs, the parathyroid gland secretes PTH, which stimulates bone demineralization with the release of calcium from the bones. Phosphate is released as well, leading to elevated serum phosphate levels. Hyperphosphatemia has been shown to directly decrease serum calcium levels and further reduce the ability of the kidneys to activate vitamin D (Felsenfeld et al., 2015).

Hyperphosphatemia, decreased vitamin D level, and hypocalcemia lead to overstimulation of the parathyroid glands, resulting in excess secretion of PTH (Felsenfeld et al., 2015). PTH that remains elevated for long periods of time leads to hypertrophy of the parathyroid gland and bone disease (Felsenfeld et al., 2015).

CKD–MBD is a common complication of CKD and results in both skeletal (renal osteodystrophy) and extraskeletal complications (vascular and soft tissue complications). Renal osteodystrophy includes a number of skeletal disorders: (1) *osteitis fibrosa,* in which there is an increased number of osteoclasts and osteoblasts, high bone turnover, and fibrosis of the marrow; (2) *osteomalacia,* with low bone turnover and abnormal mineralized bone; (3) *adynamic bone disorder,* in which there is low bone turnover with normal mineralization; and (4) *mixed*

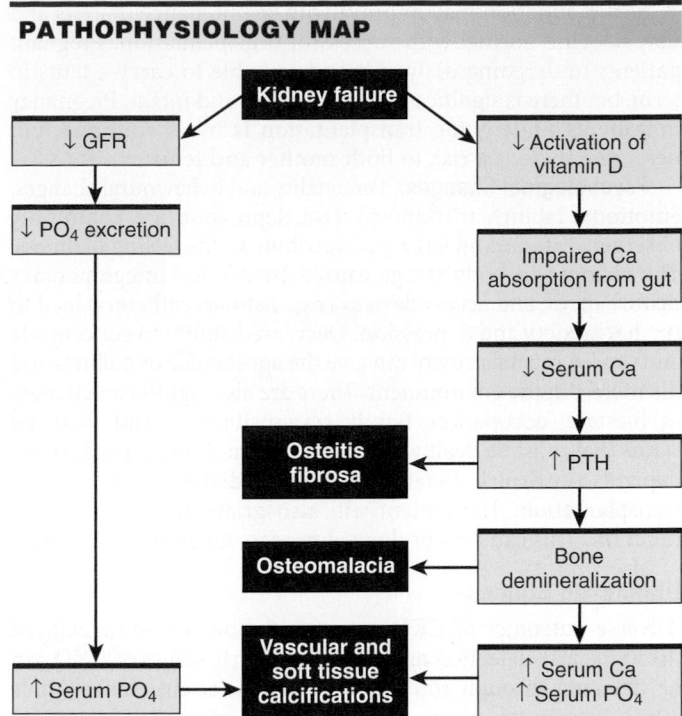

PATHOPHYSIOLOGY MAP

FIGURE 49-4 Mechanisms of chronic kidney disease–mineral and bone disorder (CKD–MBD). *Ca,* calcium; *GFR,* glomerular filtration rate; *PO₄,* phosphate; *PTH,* parathyroid hormone.

osteodystrophy, with high bone turnover and abnormal mineralization (Miller, 2014).

Extraskeletal complications include vascular and soft tissue calcification (Felsenfeld et al., 2015). The excess phosphate binds with calcium, leading to the formation of insoluble calcifications that are deposited in the vascular walls and soft tissue. Common sites are blood vessels, GI tract, lungs, muscles, skin, subcutaneous tissues, myocardium, and eyes (Zyga & Kolovos, 2013). Cardiovascular calcification is an important contributor to cardiovascular disease in people with CKD and CKD–MBD (Hain & Haras, 2015), and vascular calcification is the likely cause of high cardiovascular morbidity and mortality in patients with CKD (Zyga & Kolovos, 2013).

Integumentary System. Pruritus is highly prevalent in patients with CKD. It most commonly results from a combination of the dry skin, calcium–phosphate deposition in the skin, and sensory neuropathy. The itching may be so intense that it can lead to bleeding or infection secondary to scratching. Uremic frost is a rare condition in which urea crystallizes on the skin and is usually seen only when BUN levels are extremely high.

Reproductive System. Both men and women can experience infertility and a decreased libido in CKD. Women usually have decreased levels of estrogen, progesterone, and luteinizing hormone, causing anovulation and menstrual changes (usually amenorrhea). Menses and ovulation may return after dialysis is started. Men experience loss of testicular consistency, decreased testosterone levels, and low sperm counts. Sexual dysfunction in both sexes may also be caused by anemia, which causes fatigue and decreased libido. In addition, peripheral neuropathy can cause impotence in men and anorgasmy in women. Additional factors that may cause changes in sexual function are psychological problems (e.g., anxiety, depression), physical stress, and adverse effects of drugs.

Sexual function may improve with maintenance dialysis and may become normal with successful transplantation. Pregnant patients undergoing dialysis have been able to carry a fetus to term, but there is significant risk to mother and infant. Pregnancy in patients undergoing transplantation is more common, but here, too, there is a risk to both mother and fetus.

Psychological Changes. Personality and behavioural changes, emotional lability, withdrawal, and depression are commonly observed. Fatigue and lethargy contribute to the feeling of illness. The changes in body image caused by edema, integumentary disturbances, and access devices (e.g., fistulas, catheters) lead to further anxiety and depression. Decreased ability to concentrate and slowed mental activity can give the appearance of dullness and disinterest in the environment. There are also significant changes in lifestyle, occupation, family responsibilities, and financial status that must be dealt with by the patient. Long-term survival depends on drugs, dietary restrictions, dialysis, and possibly transplantation. The patient will also grieve the loss of renal function. This can be a prolonged process for some individuals.

Diagnostic Studies

Adverse outcomes of CKD can often be prevented or delayed through early detection and treatment. Early stages of CKD can be detected through routine laboratory measurements (Table 49-7). Proteinuria is one of the most important risk factors for the progression of CKD leading to dialysis and is the earliest marker of kidney damage (Sarafidis & Bakris, 2015). Patients at high risk for kidney disease, such as those with diabetes, hypertension, vascular disease, autoimmune disease, GFR less than 60 mL/min/1.73 m², and edema should be screened for proteinuria (Sarafidis & Bakris, 2015). The preferred method for screening for proteinuria is the measurement of the urine

protein-to-creatinine ratio or the albumin-to-creatinine ratio (Sarafidis & Bakris, 2015). A dipstick evaluation for protein in the urine may be done but is not as accurate. Patients with diabetes need to have examination of their urine for microalbuminuria if none is detected on routine urinalysis. The presence of proteinuria in two or three consecutive urine samples is needed to determine persistent proteinuria (Sarafidis & Bakris, 2015). A person with persistent proteinuria (1+ protein on standard dipstick testing, two or more times, over a 3-month period) should have further assessment of risk factors and a diagnostic workup with blood and urine tests. A urine test for albumin-to-creatinine ratio provides an accurate estimate of the protein and albumin excretion rate. A ratio greater than 300 mg albumin/1 g creatinine signals CKD (Bakker, 2013).

A urinalysis can detect RBCs, WBCs, protein, casts, and glucose. Imaging of the kidneys to exclude obstruction and note the size of the kidneys is usually done by ultrasound. Other diagnostic studies (see Table 49-7) help establish the diagnosis and cause of CKD.

Serum creatinine alone poorly reflects kidney function, and a rise in blood creatinine is observed only after significant loss of functioning nephrons (National Institute of Diabetes and Digestive and Kidney Diseases, 2013). GFR is the preferred measure used to determine kidney function. Several GFR calculators are available. The two equations used most frequently to estimate GFR are the Cockcroft–Gault formula and the Modification of Diet in Renal Disease (MDRD) Study equation (Table 49-8). The National Kidney Foundation KDOQI guidelines recommend the MDRD Study equation to estimate GFR (McAlister, Exekowitz, Grisolia, et al., 2015).

Collaborative Management: Chronic Kidney Disease

The focus in CKD is on prevention and early identification to deter the progression of kidney disease. When a patient is diagnosed as having CKD, every effort is made to detect and treat potentially reversible causes (e.g., cardiac failure, dehydration, infections, nephrotoxins, urinary tract obstruction, renal artery stenosis). A renal biopsy may be necessary to provide a definitive diagnosis. The goals of CKD care are to preserve existing renal function, delay progression of renal disease, treat clinical manifestations,

---

TABLE 49-7 COLLABORATIVE CARE

Management of Chronic Kidney Disease

Diagnostic
- BUN, serum creatinine, and eGFR
- CT scan
- History and physical examination
- Identification of reversible renal disease
- Protein-to-creatinine ratio in first, morning-voided specimen
- Renal biopsy
- Renal scan
- Renal ultrasound
- Serum calcium, phosphorous, albumin, and parathyroid hormone levels
- Serum electrolytes
- Serum hemoglobin level and iron indices
- Urinalysis and urine culture

Collaborative Therapy
- Adjustment of drug dosages according to degree of renal function
- Antihypertensive therapy
- Calcium supplementation, phosphate binders, or both
- Correction of extracellular fluid volume overload or deficit
- Erythropoietin therapy
- Measures to lower potassium*
- Nutritional therapy†
- Renal replacement therapy (dialysis, kidney transplantation)

BUN, blood urea nitrogen; *CT,* computed tomographic (scan); *eGFR,* estimated glomerular filtration rate.
*See Table 49-4.
†See Tables 49-9 and 49-10.

TABLE 49-8 SERUM CREATININE IS A POOR INDICATOR OF KIDNEY FUNCTION

Calculation of GFR is considered the best index to estimate kidney function, as indicated by the following example.

	Type of Patient	
Estimation of GFR	**76-Year-Old White Woman (Weight 56 kg)**	**28-Year-Old White Man (Weight 74 kg)**
SCr	155 mmol/L	155 mmol/L
GFR—estimated by the Cockcroft-Gault formula*	28.4 mL/min	65.7 mL/min
GFR—estimated by MDRD equation†	30 mL/min/1.73 m²	49 mL/min/1.73 m²

GFR, glomerular filtration rate; *MDRD,* modification of diet in renal disease; *SCr,* serum creatinine.
*Cockcroft-Gault GFR = [(140 − age) × (weight in kg) × 1.2]/(SCr (mmol/L). For women, multiply the result by 0.85 (Flamant et al., 2012).
†GFR as estimated by MDRD and Cockcroft-Gault equation calculator can be accessed at *http://www.mdcalc.com/mdrd-gfr-equation/.*

prevent complications, educate patients and families regarding kidney disease and options for care, and prepare patients for RRT (Chenoweth, Hines, Hall, et al., 2015). The care of the patient with CKD must be tailored to the stage of CKD. Early CKD care can lead to effective planning and appropriate timing of dialysis start and creation of the dialysis access. In the early stages of CKD, pharmacological and nutritional therapy and supportive care are essential components of the CKD care plan.

Drug Therapy

Hyperkalemia. There are multiple strategies for managing hyperkalemia (see Table 49-4). Every effort is made to control it with the restriction of high-potassium foods and drugs. Acute hyperkalemia may require urgent intervention. The level of potassium that should be treated has not been firmly established; however, based on a systematic review (Kovesdy, 2015), it is suggested that nonpharmacological steps be instituted for management of potassium levels above 5.5 mmol/L and pharmacological intervention at potassium levels of 6.0 mmol/L or greater. An ECG should be considered to assess for cardiac dysrhythmias that may require treatment. Common ECG changes associated with hyperkalemia include peaked T waves and widened QRS complexes. Patients with ECG changes consistent with severe hyperkalemia should be treated with IV calcium-based salts such as calcium gluconate or calcium chloride (Chih-Hung, Chien-Hua, We-Tien, et al., 2016). Acute hyperkalemia may require treatment with IV glucose and insulin and/or β$_2$-adrenergic agonists such as salbutamol to shift potassium into the cells. Rebound after potassium-shifting therapy occurs within 2 hours if steps have not been taken to reduce potassium either through urine excretion or HD (Chih-Hung et al., 2016). A cation exchange resin, such as sodium polystyrene sulphonate (Kayexalate), is commonly used to lower potassium levels and can be administered on an outpatient basis. Cation exchange resins take hours to days to reduce potassium.

Because sodium polystyrene sulphonate exchanges sodium ions for potassium ions, the patient should be observed for sodium and water retention. If life-threatening dysrhythmias are present, dialysis may be required.

Hypertension. The progression of CKD can be delayed by controlling hypertension (Ritchie, Rainone, Green, et al., 2013). Treatment of hypertension consists of lifestyle modifications (e.g., exercise, weight reduction, avoidance of alcohol, stress management), dietary sodium and fluid restriction, and the administration of antihypertensive drugs (Judd & Calhoun, 2015). The Canadian Hypertension Education Program (CHEP, 2015) recommends a target blood pressure for patients with nondiabetic CKD of less than 140/90 mm Hg; for those with diabetes mellitus, it should be less than 130/80 mm Hg.

For patients with nondiabetic CKD and proteinuria, ACE inhibitors (e.g., ramipril [Altace], enalapril [Vasotec]) or ARBs (e.g., irbesartan [Avapro], losartan [Cozaar]) are recommended as initial therapy (CHEP, 2015). ACE inhibitors and ARBs decrease proteinuria and delay the progression of renal failure. For additional therapy, the use of thiazide diuretics (e.g., hydrochlorothiazide) or loop diuretics (e.g., furosemide [Lasix]) for volume overload is suggested (CHEP, 2015).

For patients with renovascular disease, CHEP suggests cautious use of ACE inhibitors and ARBs as patients with bilateral disease or a solitary kidney are at increased risk for AKI (CHEP, 2015).

For patients with diabetes, CHEP (2015) suggests use of ACE inhibitors or ARBs as initial therapy. Other antihypertensive drugs commonly used include dihydropyridine calcium channel blockers (nifedipine [Adalat], amlodipine [Norvasc] and thiazide or thiazide-like diuretics).

ACE inhibitors and ARBs must be used cautiously in CKD because they can further decrease the GFR and increase serum potassium levels. Most people require a number of antihypertensives to achieve target blood pressure, and regimens must be individualized based on other existing comorbidities.

Blood pressure (BP) should periodically be measured in supine, sitting, and standing positions to effectively monitor the effect of antihypertensive drugs. The patient should be taught how to monitor the BP at home and taught what BP readings require immediate intervention. BP control is essential to slow atherosclerotic changes that could further impair renal function.

Chronic Kidney Disease–Mineral and Bone Disorder. Interventions for CKD–MBD include limiting dietary phosphorus, administering phosphate binders, and supplementing vitamin D. Phosphate intake is generally restricted to less than 1 000 mg/day, but usually dietary control is not adequate. Calcium-based phosphate binders such as calcium carbonate and calcium acetate are used to bind the phosphate, which is then excreted in the stool. Giving a calcium-based binder when the phosphate levels are still high (1.98 mmol/L) may cause the formation of calcium–phosphate deposits. Sevelamer (Renagel) is a phosphate binder that contains neither calcium nor aluminum.

Because dementia (aluminum toxicity) and bone disease (osteomalacia) are associated with excessive absorption of aluminum, aluminum preparations should be avoided if possible and used with caution in patients with renal failure. Magnesium-containing antacids (Maalox, Mylanta) are used in moderation because magnesium is dependent on the kidneys for excretion. Phosphate binders should be administered with each meal to be effective because most phosphate is absorbed within 1 hour after eating. Hypercalcemia may occur with calcium supplementation and is associated with increased cardiac calcifications and mortality in patients with ESRD. Calcium binders are generally limited to a maximum of 1 500 mg/day with the total daily calcium intake including diet not exceeding 2 g. Constipation is a frequent adverse effect of phosphate binders and may necessitate the use of stool softeners.

Hypocalcemia is often a problem because of the inability of the GI tract to absorb calcium in the absence of vitamin D. If hypocalcemia persists even when serum phosphate levels are controlled and supplemental calcium is given, the active form of vitamin D should be given. It is commercially available in oral preparations such as calcitriol (Rocaltrol). It is important to lower the phosphate level before administering calcium or vitamin D because these drugs may contribute to soft tissue calcification if both calcium and phosphate levels are elevated. Calcimimetics such as cinacalcet (Sensipar) may be prescribed to lower PTH and may also cause hypocalcemia (Felsenfeld et al., 2015).

If renal osteodystrophy remains severe despite medical management, a subtotal parathyroidectomy may be performed to decrease the synthesis and secretion of PTH. In some situations, a total parathyroidectomy is performed, and some parathyroid tissue is transplanted into the forearm. The transplanted cells produce PTH as needed. If production of PTH becomes excessive, some of the cells can be removed from the forearm under local anaesthesia.

The most common methods for evaluating the status of the bone disease are skeletal radiographs, bone scans, bone biopsy, and bone densitometry. PTH and alkaline phosphatase levels should also be measured. Alkaline phosphatase is elevated when there is demineralization of the bone but can also be increased by liver disease.

Anemia. The most important cause of anemia in CKD is a decreased production of erythropoietin. With the use of recombinant DNA technology, erythropoiesis-stimulating agents (ESAs) are available for the treatment of anemia. ESAs can be administered intravenously or subcutaneously. They have been very effective in treating anemia. A significant increase in hemoglobin is usually not seen for 2 to 3 weeks. The patient who is receiving erythropoietin has improved exercise tolerance and an enhanced quality of life.

Significant morbidity and mortality have been associated with trying to normalize hemoglobin levels (Sarafidis & Bakris, 2015). The Canadian Society of Nephrology (CSN) *Guidelines for the Management of Chronic Kidney Disease* recommend a target hemoglobin of 110 g/L, with an acceptable range between 100 and 120 g/L (Sarafidis & Bakris, 2015; Hung & Tarng, 2014). A common adverse effect of ESAs is the development or acceleration of hypertension. The underlying mechanism is related to the hemodynamic changes (e.g., increased whole blood viscosity) that occur as the anemia is corrected. Patients with significantly elevated BP should not receive ESAs.

Another adverse effect of ESA therapy is the development of functional iron deficiency resulting from the increased demand for iron to support erythropoiesis. The CSN *Guidelines for the Management of Chronic Kidney Disease* recommend a target ferritin level greater than 100 ng/mL and a transferring saturation level greater than 20% (Sarafidis & Bakris, 2015; Hung & Tarng, 2014). Most patients receive iron supplements. The GI adverse effects of oral iron, including gastric irritation and constipation, may lead to nonadherence to therapy. Orally administered iron should not be taken at the same time as phosphate binders because calcium binds the iron, preventing absorption. The patient should be advised that iron may make the stool a dark colour.

Most patients on HD receive IV iron. Supplemental folic acid is usually given because it is needed for RBC formation and is removed by dialysis.

Blood transfusions should be avoided in treating anemia unless the patient experiences an acute blood loss or has symptomatic anemia (e.g., dyspnea, excess fatigue, tachycardia, palpitations, chest pain). Undesirable effects of transfusions are the suppression of erythropoiesis as a result of a decrease in the hypoxic stimulus, the possible transmission of hepatitis B or C or human immunodeficiency virus (HIV), the possibility of developing antibodies that may affect transplantation, and the possibility of iron overload because each unit of blood contains about 250 mg of iron.

Dyslipidemia. There is a high prevalence of dyslipidemia for patients with CKD (Levin, Hemmelgarn, Culleton, et al., 2008). Currently, good evidence-informed research is lacking to guide the management of dyslipidemia in CKD. The National Kidney Foundation Kidney Disease Outcomes Quality Initiative (NKF KDOQI) recommends the use of statins in patients with stages 1 to 3 CKD, per guidelines for the general population (Kim, Langworthy, & Hennessey, 2014).

Complications of Drug Therapy. Because the kidneys play a large role in the absorption, distribution, metabolism, and elimination of drugs, people with CKD are at risk for medication-related problems that can lead to increased morbidity and mortality (Liles, 2014). Many drugs are partially or totally excreted by the kidneys. Delayed and decreased elimination lead to an accumulation of drugs in the body and potential for drug toxicity. Dialysis may remove or lower drug levels. Drug doses and frequency of administration must be adjusted based on the level of kidney function and whether or not the patient is receiving dialysis. Drugs of particular concern include digoxin, oral glycemic agents (e.g., metformin, glyburide), antibiotics, and opioid medication (e.g., hydromorphone [Dilaudid], morphine).

Patients should be advised to avoid NSAIDs. These drugs block the synthesis of the renal prostaglandins that promote vasodilation. This can worsen renal hypoperfusion and cause interstitial nephritis. Many NSAIDs are available over the counter, so it is essential that the patient be cautioned. Acetaminophen can be substituted.

Nutritional Therapy

Protein Restriction. The diet is designed to be as normal as possible to maintain good nutrition (Table 49-9). All patients with CKD should be seen by a dietitian. Protein energy wasting in CKD is a strong predictor of mortality (Ikizler, Cano, Franch, et al., 2013). Protein is moderately restricted because BUN is an end product of protein metabolism. For the patient who is not undergoing dialysis, one guide is to restrict protein intake to 0.6 to 0.75 g/kg of ideal body weight (IBW)/day when the creatinine clearance is less than 25 mL/min (Goldstein-Fuchs

---

TABLE 49-9   NUTRITIONAL THERAPY

Daily Requirements for the Patient With Chronic Kidney Disease

	CKD Stages 3–4 Management	Hemodialysis	Peritoneal Dialysis
Fluid allowance	Urine output + 600 mL	Urine output + 600 mL	Often no restriction
Protein*	0.6–0.75 g/kg body weight	1.2–1.3 g/kg IBW	≥1.2–1.3 g/kg IBW
Calories	30–35 kcal/kg EDW	30–35 kcal/kg EDW†	30–35 kcal/kg IBW†
Fat	Determined by caloric requirement	Determined by caloric requirement	Determined by caloric requirement
Carbohydrate	Unlimited intake of sugars, starches; bread and cereal products limited owing to protein restriction	Same as for conservative management	Dependent on individual patient needs
Iron	Variable	Variable	Variable
Potassium	2–3 g	2–3 g	3–4 g, no restrictions
Sodium	2–3 g	2–3 g	2–4 g
Phosphorus	800–1 000 mg	1 000 mg	1 000 mg
Calcium	Variable	1 000–1 500 mg	1 000–1 500 mg
Folic acid	1-mg supplement	1-mg supplement	1-mg supplement

CKD, chronic kidney disease; *EDW*, estimated dry weight; *IBW*, ideal body weight.
*At least 50% of protein intake should be of high biological value (e.g., coming from eggs, milk, meat).
†Includes dialysate calories.

& Kalantar-Zadeh, 2015). This moderate restriction may slow progression of CKD for these patients. For patients with more severe renal insufficiency, low-protein diets should be used with caution because these patients are at risk of developing malnutrition.

Once the patient starts dialysis, protein intake can be increased to 1.2 to 1.3 g/kg of IBW/day. Dietary protein guidelines for PD differ from those for HD because excessive amounts of protein are lost in the dialysate. The protein intake must be high enough to compensate for the losses so that the nitrogen balance is maintained. The recommended protein intake is at least 1.2 g/kg of IBW/day and can be increased depending on the individual needs of the patient. At least 50% of protein intake should have high biological value, containing all of the essential amino acids (e.g., eggs, milk, meat, poultry).

Sufficient calories from carbohydrates and fat are needed to minimize catabolism of body protein and to maintain body weight. Therefore, 100 g of carbohydrates and an appropriate amount of fat are prescribed to maintain an intake of 30 to 35 kcal/kg body weight/day. See Table 49-9 for specific guidelines.

For patients with malnutrition or inadequate caloric intake, commercially prepared products that are high in calories and low in protein, sodium, and potassium are available.

Because the diet for CKD is deficient in vitamins, and water-soluble vitamins are lost through dialysis, multivitamins are prescribed.

Sodium and Fluid Restriction. Fluid intake for patients with CKD depends on the daily urine output and overall fluid balance. For patients not yet on dialysis, fluids are generally not restricted and diuretics and a low-sodium diet help to manage fluid retention. For patients receiving HD, fluids are generally restricted as urine output begins to decline. Generally, 600 mL (from insensible loss) plus an amount equal to the previous day's urine output is allowed for a patient receiving dialysis. Foods that are liquid at room temperature (e.g., gelatin, ice cream) should be counted as fluid intake. The fluid allotment should be spaced throughout the day so that the patient does not become thirsty. For the patient receiving long-term HD, fluid intake is adjusted so that weight gains are no more than 1 to 3 kg between dialyses.

To achieve the optimal fluid balance, sodium must also be restricted. Sodium-restricted diet allowances may vary from 2 to 4 g, depending on the degree of edema and hypertension. Sodium and salt should not be equated because the sodium content in 1 g of sodium chloride is equivalent to 400 mg of sodium. The patient should be instructed to avoid high-sodium foods such as cured meats, pickled foods, canned soups and stews, frankfurters, cold cuts, soy sauce, and salad dressings. Most salt substitutes should not be used because they contain potassium chloride.

Potassium Restriction. The potassium restriction depends on the ability of the kidneys to excrete this electrolyte. Dietary allowances for potassium range from about 2 to 4 g. Some patients on PD do not need potassium restrictions. Some foods with high potassium content that should be avoided are oranges, bananas, melons, tomatoes, prunes, raisins, deep green and yellow vegetables, beans, and legumes (Table 49-10).

Phosphate Restriction. CKD alters the homeostasis of calcium, phosphorus, and vitamin D (Felsenfeld et al., 2015). As CKD progresses, phosphorus excretion diminishes, resulting in hyperphosphatemia. Phosphate should be limited to approximately 1 000 mg/day. Foods that are high in phosphate include dairy

TABLE 49-10 NUTRITIONAL THERAPY

High-Potassium Foods

Fruits and Fruit Juices	Vegetables	Cereal
• Apple juice	• Beans, white and pinto*	• All-Bran*
• Avocados*	• Broccoli	• Raisin Bran*
• Bananas*	• Carrots	
• Grapefruit juice	• Lima beans, cooked*	**Meat and Poultry**
• Honeydew melons*	• Mushrooms, fresh*	• Beef,* pork, cooked
• Orange juice*	• Potato, baked*	• Chicken
• Oranges	• Squash, baked*	• Turkey
• Prune juice*	• Spinach, cooked*	
• Prunes*		**Miscellaneous**
• Raisins*	**Dairy**	• Chocolate
• Tomato juice*	• Milk*	• Molasses
• Tomatoes	• Yogourt*	• Sunflower seeds*

*>10 mmol of potassium per serving.

products (e.g., milk, ice cream, cheese, yogourt) and foods containing dairy products (pudding). Most foods that are high in phosphate are also high in calcium. Restricting phosphate will restrict calcium intake.

NURSING MANAGEMENT CHRONIC KIDNEY DISEASE

NURSING ASSESSMENT

The nurse should obtain a complete history of any existing renal disease or family history of renal disease because some renal disorders have a hereditary basis (e.g., polycystic kidney disease, Alport's syndrome). Information on long-term health problems such as hypertension, diabetes, recurrent urinary tract infections, and systemic lupus erythematosus should be obtained because these conditions can lead to CKD. Because the kidneys play a large role in the absorption, distribution, metabolism, and elimination of drugs and because many drugs are potentially nephrotoxic, both current and past use of prescription and over-the-counter drugs must be reviewed.

The nurse should assess the patient's dietary habits and discuss any problems. The height and weight should be measured, and any recent weight changes must be evaluated.

Clinical manifestations of CKD are apparent in multiple body systems (see Figure 49-3). Fatigue, lethargy, and pruritus are often the early symptoms of CKD. Hypertension and changes in urine characteristics are often the first signs.

CKD is a lifelong and life-limiting illness. The chronicity of renal disease and the long-term nature of treatment modalities affect every area of a person's life, including family relationships, social and work activities, and self-image and emotional state. Support systems should be assessed. The choice of treatment modality may be related to support systems available to the patient.

It is important to respect a patient's choice not to receive treatment. Many times, patients will initiate the conversation about palliative care themselves. The discussion needs to focus on moving from the curative approach to promotion of comfort care and consideration for end-of-life care. The nurse should listen to the patient and caregiver, allowing them to do most of the talking, and pay special attention to their hopes and fears (Schell & Holley, 2013) (Table 49-11). (Palliative and end of-life care is discussed in Chapter 13.)

TABLE 49-11	SUMMARY OF RECOMMENDATIONS FOR DECISION SUPPORT FOR ADULTS LIVING WITH CHRONIC KIDNEY DISEASE

Practice Recommendations
Patient Decision-Making Needs
1.0   Nurses know the common decisions faced by an adult with CKD.
   Nursing Actions:
   • Nurses identify the decision the patient is facing at a particular point in time.
2.0   Nurses screen the patient for decisional conflict at initial contact and as the patient's situation and condition changes.
   Nursing Actions:
   • Nurses screen for decisional conflict.
3.0   Nurses determine the source of the patient's decisional conflict.
   Nursing Actions:
   • Nurses assess the patient's knowledge and expectations about the options.
   • Nurses assess and discuss the availability of resources.
   • Nurses objectively measure the patient's confidence and ability for making decisions and self-managing their CKD.
   • Nurses assist the patient to clarify his or her values.
   • Nurses clarify the patient's preferred role in decision making and who else the patient wants to involve in the decision-making process.

Decision Support Interventions
4.0   Nurses understand the difference between providing patient education and providing decision support.
   Nursing Actions:
   • Nurses describe patient education.
   • Nurses describe the additional elements involved with decision support.
5.0   Nurses use patient decision aids and other tools to provide decision support.
   Nursing Actions:
   • Nurses remain neutral when supporting the patient in the decision-making process.
   • Nurses use validated tools to provide decision support.
   • Nurses help the patient to build confidence in participation in decision making.
   • Nurses meet the patient's knowledge needs.
   • Nurses help the patient clarify his or her values.
   • Nurses help the patient mobilize resources.
   • Nurses help the patient to communicate with others during the decision-making process.
   • Nurses obtain commitment from the patient for the next decision-making step(s).

CKD, chronic kidney disease.
Source: Registered Nurses' Association of Ontario. (2009). *Decision Support for Adults Living with Chronic Kidney Disease.* Toronto, Canada. Registered Nurses' Association of Ontario.

NURSING DIAGNOSES

Nursing diagnoses for the patient with CKD in stage 4 may include, but are not limited to, the following:

• *Excess fluid volume* related to *excessive fluid intake* (impaired kidney function)
• *Risk for electrolyte imbalance* as evidenced by *excessive fluid volume* (impaired kidney function)
• *Imbalanced nutrition: less than body requirements* related to *insufficient dietary intake* (restricted intake of nutrients, nausea, vomiting, anorexia, stomatitis)

Additional information on nursing diagnoses for the patient with CKD is presented in Nursing Care Plan (NCP) 49-1, available on the Evolve website.

PLANNING

The majority of CKD care occurs in the ambulatory care setting. The overall goals are that a patient with CKD will (1) demonstrate knowledge and ability to comply with the therapeutic regimen, (2) participate in decision making for the plan of care and future treatment modality, (3) demonstrate effective coping strategies, and (4) continue with activities of daily living within physiological limitations.

NURSING IMPLEMENTATION

HEALTH PROMOTION.   Identify individuals at risk for CKD. These include people with a history (or a family history) of renal disease, hypertension, diabetes mellitus, and repeated urinary tract infection. These individuals should have regular checkups, including assessments of serum creatinine and BUN and urinalysis. People with diabetes should have their urine checked for microalbuminuria if routine urinalysis is negative for protein. They should be advised that any changes in urine appearance (colour, odour), frequency, or volume must be reported to the health care provider. If a patient must be prescribed a potentially nephrotoxic drug, it is important to monitor renal function with serum creatinine and BUN.

Individuals who have been identified as being at risk need to take measures to prevent or delay the progression of CKD and reduce the risk for cardiovascular disease. These measures include glycemic control for patients with diabetes (see Chapter 52), optimizing BP control, and lifestyle modifications, including smoking cessation.

CARE CONSIDERATIONS FOR CHRONIC KIDNEY DISEASE IN STAGES 4 TO 5.   The specific nursing management of the patient with CKD in stages 4 to 5 is detailed in NCP 49-1, available on the Evolve website. It is important to teach the patient and the family because diet, drugs, and follow-up medical care are the responsibilities of the patient (Table 49-12). The patient should check weight daily, learn to take daily BPs, and be able to identify signs and symptoms of fluid overload, hyperkalemia, and other electrolyte imbalances. The patient and the family must understand the importance of strict dietary adherence. A registered dietitian should meet with the patient and the family on a regular basis for diet planning. A diet history and consideration of cultural variations will facilitate diet planning and adherence.

The patient needs a complete understanding of prescribed drugs, the dosages, and the common adverse effects. It may be helpful to make a list of the drugs and the times of administration that can be posted in the home. The patient must be instructed to avoid certain over-the-counter drugs such as NSAIDs and natural and herbal preparations. ACE inhibitors may have to be discontinued if they are contributing to hyperkalemia or decreased GFR.

Motivation on the part of the patient to assume the primary role in the management of the disease is essential. The period of predialysis care provides an opportunity to evaluate each patient's ability to manage the disease. This knowledge will be helpful when determining the treatment modality.

AMBULATORY AND HOME CARE.   The length of time that a patient with CKD can be managed without RRT is highly variable and depends on the progression of renal failure and the presence of other comorbid conditions. When RRT is required, HD, PD, and transplantation are the available treatment options.

TABLE 49-12 PATIENT & CAREGIVER TEACHING GUIDE

Chronic Kidney Disease in Stages 4 and 5

When teaching the patient and caregiver about management of chronic kidney disease, the nurse should:

1. Explain dietary (protein, sodium, potassium, phosphate) and fluid restrictions incorporating the patient's own cultural dietary patterns.
2. Encourage discussion of difficulties in modifying diet and fluid intake.
3. Explain signs and symptoms of electrolyte imbalance, especially high potassium.
4. Teach alternative ways of reducing thirst, such as sucking on ice cubes, lemon, or hard candy.
5. Explain the rationale for prescribed drugs and common adverse effects.
   Examples
   • Phosphate binders should be taken with meals.
   • Iron supplements should be taken between meals.
6. Explain the importance of reporting any of the following:
   • Weight gain >2 kg
   • Increasing blood pressure
   • Shortness of breath
   • Edema
   • Increasing fatigue or weakness
   • Confusion or lethargy
7. Encourage patient and caregiver(s) to share concerns about lifestyle changes, living with a chronic illness, and decisions about type of dialysis or transplantation.

TABLE 49-13 COMPARISON OF PERITONEAL DIALYSIS AND HEMODIALYSIS

Peritoneal Dialysis
Advantages
• Fewer dietary restrictions
• Home dialysis possible
• Less cardiovascular stress
• Less complicated than hemodialysis
• Portable system with CAPD
• Preferable for the diabetic patient
• Relatively short training time
• Usable in the patient with vascular access problems

Disadvantages
• Catheter can migrate
• Contraindication in the patient with multiple abdominal surgeries, trauma, unrepaired hernia
• Protein loss into dialysate
• Risk for aggravated dyslipidemia
• Risk for bacterial or chemical peritonitis
• Risk for exit-site and tunnel infections
• Risk for hyperglycemia
• Risk for self-image problems with catheter placement
• Surgery for catheter placement

Hemodialysis
Advantages
• Effective potassium removal
• Home dialysis possible
• Less protein loss than with peritoneal dialysis
• Lowering of serum triglycerides
• Rapid fluid removal
• Rapid removal of urea and creatinine
• Temporary access can be placed at bedside

Disadvantages
• Added blood loss that contributes to anemia
• Dietary and fluid restrictions
• Extensive equipment necessary
• Heparinization may be necessary
• Hypotension during dialysis
• Longer training time for home hemodialysis vs. peritoneal
• Self-image problems with permanent access
• Specially trained personnel necessary (if in-centre option chosen)
• Surgery for permanent access placement
• Vascular access problems

CAPD, continuous ambulatory peritoneal dialysis.

Extensive and ongoing teaching and discussion about RRTs should occur early (CKD in stage 3) in order for the patient to make an informed decision about future therapies, including RRT and advanced directives.

The patient and the family need a clear explanation of what is involved in dialysis and transplantation. The patient should be informed that, if dialysis is chosen, the option of transplantation still remains, if the patient is medically suitable. It should be emphasized that, if a transplanted organ fails, the patient can return to dialysis. The patient should also be counselled that retransplantation may also be an option.

EVALUATION

The expected outcomes for the patient with CKD are presented in NCP 49-1, available on the Evolve website.

DIALYSIS

Dialysis is the movement of fluid and molecules across a semipermeable membrane from one compartment to another. Clinically, dialysis is a technique in which substances move from the blood through a semipermeable membrane (dialyzer) and into a dialysis solution (dialysate). It is used to correct fluid and electrolyte imbalances and to remove waste products in renal failure. It can also be used to treat drug overdoses. The two methods of dialysis available are PD and HD (Table 49-13). **Peritoneal dialysis (PD)** is a method of removing waste products and excess fluid from the blood using a natural semipermeable membrane, the peritoneum. Dialysis fluid is infused into the peritoneal cavity, and excess fluid and waste products pass across the membrane into the fluid, which is then drained and discarded. In **hemodialysis (HD)**, waste products and excess fluid are removed from the blood using a machine to pump the blood through an artificial semipermeable membrane (usually made of cellulose-based or synthetic materials).

When CKD progresses to the point that the patient's symptoms, fluid volume status, or both can no longer be managed without dialysis, dialysis therapy is initiated. Generally, dialysis is initiated when the GFR (or creatinine clearance) is less than 15 mL/min/1.73 m². This criterion can vary widely in different clinical situations. Certain uremic complications, including encephalopathy, neuropathies, uncontrolled hyperkalemia, pericarditis, and accelerated hypertension, indicate a need for immediate dialysis.

GENERAL PRINCIPLES OF DIALYSIS

Solutes and water move across the semipermeable membrane from the blood to the dialysate or from the dialysate to the blood, in accordance with concentration gradients. The principles of diffusion, osmosis, and ultrafiltration are involved in dialysis (Figure 49-5). *Diffusion* is the movement of solutes from an area of greater concentration to an area of lesser concentration. In renal failure, urea, creatinine, uric acid, and electrolytes (potassium, phosphate) move from the blood to the dialysate with the net effect of lowering their concentration in the blood. RBCs, WBCs, and plasma proteins are too large to diffuse through the pores of the membrane. Bacteria and viruses that may be present in the dialysate are too large to migrate through the pores into the blood.

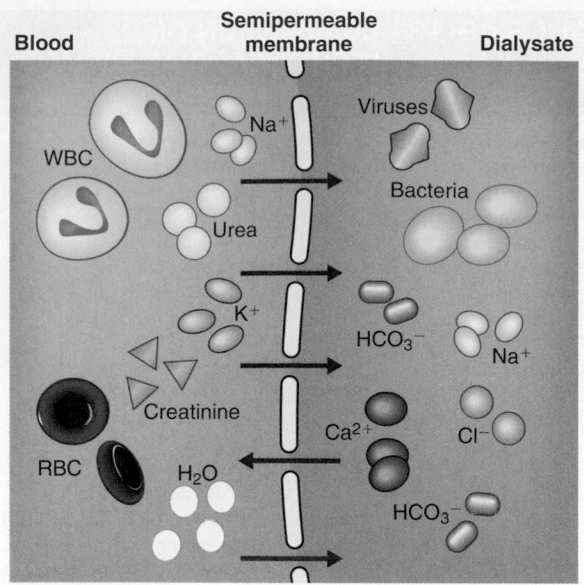

FIGURE 49-5 Osmosis and diffusion across a semipermeable membrane. *Ca*, calcium; *Cl*, chlorine; *HCO₃*, bicarbonate; *H₂O*, water; *K*, potassium; *Na*, sodium; *RBC*, red blood cell; *WBC*, white blood cell.

Osmosis is the movement of fluid from an area of lesser to an area of greater concentration of solutes. Glucose is added to the dialysate and creates an osmotic gradient across the membrane, pulling excess fluid from the blood.

Ultrafiltration (water and fluid removal) results when there is an osmotic gradient or pressure gradient across the membrane. In PD, excess fluid is removed by increasing the osmolality of the dialysate (osmotic gradient) with the addition of glucose. In HD, the gradient is created by increasing pressure in the blood compartment (positive pressure) or decreasing pressure in the dialysate compartment (negative pressure). Extracellular fluid moves into the dialysate because of the pressure gradient. The excess fluid is removed by creating a pressure differential between the blood and the dialysate solution, with a combination of positive pressure in the blood compartment and negative pressure in the dialysate compartment.

PERITONEAL DIALYSIS

Although PD was first used in 1923, it did not come into widespread use for chronic treatment until the 1970s with the development of soft, pliable peritoneal solution bags and the introduction of the concept of continuous PD. In Canada, 19% of patients were receiving peritoneal dialysis compared with 79% who were receiving HD in 2012 (CIHI, 2014).

Catheter Placement

Peritoneal access is obtained by inserting a catheter through the anterior abdominal wall (Figure 49-6). Most catheter exit sites are in the abdomen; however, some catheters are inserted using a presternal technique, where the catheter exits on the chest (Crabtree, 2015). The catheters vary in length and have one or two Dacron cuffs on the subcutaneous and peritoneal portions of the catheter that act as anchors and prevent the migration of microorganisms down the shaft from the skin. Within a few weeks of insertion, fibrous tissue grows into the Dacron cuff, holding the catheter in place and preventing bacterial penetration into the peritoneal cavity. The tip of the catheter rests in the

FIGURE 49-6 Peritoneal dialysis showing a peritoneal catheter inserted into the peritoneal cavity.

peritoneal cavity and has many perforations spaced along the distal end of the tubing to allow fluid to flow in and out of the catheter. There are numerous types of PD catheters.

The technique for catheter placement varies. Although it is possible to place a permanent catheter in the peritoneal cavity at the bedside with a trocar, it is usually done via surgery so that its placement can be directly visualized, minimizing potential complications. Preparation of the patient for catheter insertion includes emptying the bladder and the bowel, weighing the patient, and obtaining a signed consent form.

In the nonsurgical (bedside) approach, an area approximately 2 cm below the umbilicus is numbed with a local anaesthetic, and a small stab wound is made. A stylet is inserted, and the abdomen is distended with dialysis solution. The catheter is then placed into the peritoneal cavity. When the patient feels pressure in the rectal area and has the urge to defecate, the catheter is in place.

In the surgical approach, a midline umbilical incision is made, and a small puncture is made to one side and below this incision. The distal end of the catheter is placed in the peritoneum, and it is tunnelled under the skin to the puncture site. The tunnel helps prevent peritonitis. After the catheter is inserted, the skin is cleaned with an antiseptic solution, and a sterile dressing is applied. Complications of catheter insertion include perforation of the bladder, the bowel, or a blood vessel and the introduction of bacteria.

The catheter is connected to a sterile tubing system and secured to the abdomen with tape. The catheter is irrigated immediately with heparinized dialysate (usually 500 mL) to clear blood and fibrin from it. Prophylactic antibiotics may also be given. Catheter placement is usually done with same-day surgery, and the patient is discharged home with a sterile dressing covering the PD catheter. The patient needs instructions on keeping the dressing dry, avoiding accidentally pulling the catheter, and receiving follow-up care.

Before starting PD, it is preferable to allow a waiting period of 7 to 14 days for proper sealing of the catheter and for tissue to grow into the cuffs. Postoperative exit-site care should be restricted to trained staff (Young, Chan, Blagg, et al., 2012). About 2 to 4 weeks after catheter implantation, the exit site should be clean, dry, and free of redness and tenderness (Figure 49-7). Once the catheter incision site is healed, routine care should be done daily or every other day. This care includes the use of antibacterial soap or mild, medical-grade disinfectants as well as examination of the catheter site for signs of infection. Each centre will have a policy about exit-site care, and patients are taught how to examine and care for their PD catheter and exit site by the PD nursing staff.

Dialysis Solutions and Cycles

PD is accomplished by putting dialysis solution into the peritoneal space. The three phases of the PD cycle are *inflow* (fill), *dwell* (equilibration), and *drain*. The three phases are called an *exchange*. The dialysis prescription is tailored to the patient's needs. During inflow, a prescribed amount of solution, usually 2 L, is infused through an established catheter over about 10 minutes. After the solution has been infused, the inflow clamp is closed before air enters the tubing.

During the dwell phase, or equilibration phase, diffusion and osmosis occur between the patient's blood and the peritoneal cavity. The dwell time can last from 20 to 30 minutes to 8 or more hours, depending on the goals of PD.

Drain time takes 15 to 30 minutes. The cycle starts again with the infusion of another 2 L of solution. For manual PD, a period of about 30 to 50 minutes is required to complete an exchange.

Dialysis solutions vary, and the choice of exchange volume is primarily determined by the size of the peritoneal cavity. A larger person may tolerate a 3-L volume without any difficulty, whereas an average-size person usually tolerates a 2-L exchange.

Ultrafiltration (fluid removal) during PD depends on osmotic forces, with glucose being the most effective agent available. Dextrose remains the most commonly used osmotic agent available in PD solutions. It is relatively safe but has been associated with high rates of peritoneal glucose absorption leading to hypertriglyceridemia, hyperglycemia, and long-term peritoneal membrane dysfunction. The amount of dextrose in the solution varies among 0.5%, 1.5%, 2.5%, and 4.25%, depending on the fluid volume goal. Alternate osmotic agents include icodextrin and amino acid solutions.

Peritoneal Dialysis Systems

Two types of PD currently being used are automated peritoneal dialysis (APD) and continuous ambulatory peritoneal dialysis (CAPD).

Automated Peritoneal Dialysis. Automated peritoneal dialysis (APD), also called *continuous cycling peritoneal dialysis*, is a popular form of PD that is done while the patient sleeps. An automated device called a *cycler* is used to perform the dialysis exchanges (Figure 49-8). The automated cycler times and controls the fill, dwell, and drain phases. The machine cycles four or more exchanges per night, with 1 to 2 hours per exchange. Alarms and monitors are built into the system to make it safe for the patient to dialyze while sleeping. The patient disconnects from the machine in the morning and usually leaves fluid in the abdomen during the day. One to two daytime manual exchanges may also be prescribed to ensure adequate dialysis.

Continuous Ambulatory Peritoneal Dialysis. Continuous ambulatory peritoneal dialysis (CAPD) is a type of PD that is done during the day and consists of a minimum of four exchanges of dialysis fluid per day. CAPD exchanges are carried out manually by exchanging 1.5 to 3 L of peritoneal dialysate at least four times daily, with dwell times averaging 4 hours. For example, one schedule starts the exchanges at 0700 hours, 1200 hours, 1700 hours, and 2200 hours.

Dialysis fluid is instilled into the peritoneal cavity and remains (dwells) there for a specified period, allowing for the removal

FIGURE 49-7 Peritoneal catheter exit site. Source: Mediscan/Alamy Stock Photo.

FIGURE 49-8 Automated peritoneal dialysis cycler, which can be used while the patient is sleeping at night or for hospitalized patients who require frequent exchanges. Source: © Can Stock Photo/rob3000.

of waste products and excess fluid; it is then drained and fresh fluid is instilled. It is continuous in that dialysis fluid is always in the peritoneal cavity so dialysis is continuously going on. After the equilibration period, the dialysate (effluent) is drained from the peritoneal cavity, and a new 2-L bag of dialysate solution is infused. It is critical in PD to maintain aseptic technique to avoid peritonitis. Several tubing connections and devices are commercially available to help maintain an aseptic system.

Potential contraindications for PD include the following:
1. History of multiple abdominal surgical procedures or severe abdominal pathological condition (e.g., severe pancreatitis, diverticulitis).
2. Recurrent abdominal wall or inguinal hernias.
3. Excessive obesity with large abdominal wall and fat deposits.
4. Pre-existing vertebral disease (e.g., chronic back problems).
5. Severe obstructive pulmonary disease.

Complications of Peritoneal Dialysis

Exit-Site Infection. Infection of the peritoneal catheter exit site is most commonly caused by *Staphylococcus aureus* or *Staphylococcus epidermidis* (from skin flora). Superficial exit-site infections caused by these organisms are generally resolved with antibiotic therapy. Clinical manifestations of an exit-site infection include redness at the site, tenderness, and drainage. If not treated immediately, subcutaneous tunnel infections usually result in abscess formation and may cause peritonitis, necessitating catheter removal.

Peritonitis. Peritonitis results from contamination or from progression of an exit-site or tunnel infection. Most frequently, peritonitis occurs because of improper technique in making or breaking connections for exchanges. Less commonly, peritonitis results from bacteria in the intestine crossing over into the peritoneal cavity. Peritonitis is usually caused by *S. aureus* or *S. epidermidis*.

The primary clinical manifestation of peritonitis is a cloudy peritoneal effluent that has a WBC count of over 0.1×10^9/L (particularly neutrophils) or demonstration of bacteria in the peritoneal effluent by Gram stain or culture. GI manifestations may also be present, including diffuse abdominal pain, diarrhea, vomiting, abdominal distension, and hyperactive bowel sounds. Fever may or may not be present. Cultures, Gram stain, and a cell count with WBC differential of the peritoneal effluent are used to confirm the diagnosis of peritonitis. Antibiotics can be given by mouth or by IV or intraperitoneal route. The patient is usually treated on an outpatient basis. Repeated infections may necessitate the removal of the peritoneal catheter and termination of PD. The formation of adhesions in the peritoneum can result from repeated infections and interferes with the peritoneal membrane's ability to act as a dialyzing surface.

Abdominal Pain. Although not severe, pain is a common complication, caused by the low pH of the dialysate solution, peritonitis, intraperitoneal irritation (which usually subsides in 1 to 2 weeks), and placement of the catheter. Pain can also occur when the tip of the catheter touches the bladder, the bowel, or the peritoneum. A change in the position of the catheter should correct this problem. Accidental infusion of air or infusing the dialysate too rapidly may cause referred pain in the shoulder. If the infusion rate is decreased, the pain usually subsides.

Outflow Problems. It is expected that at least 80% of the volume instilled in the peritoneal cavity is returned when draining the cavity after an exchange. Causes of poor outflow include constipation, a kink in the catheter or transfer set, omentum wrapped around the catheter, and migration of the catheter out of the pelvic region. Laxatives and stool softeners can be used to relieve constipation and promote regular bowel movements. Outflow problems related to omental entrapment or migration may necessitate radiological intervention, surgical manipulation of the catheter, or both.

Hernias. Because of increased intra-abdominal pressure secondary to the dialysate infusion, umbilical or inguinal hernias or diastasis recti can develop in predisposed individuals such as multiparous women and older men. However, in most situations after hernia repair, PD can be resumed after several days, using small dialysate volumes and keeping the patient supine.

Lower Back Problems. Increased intra-abdominal pressure can cause or aggravate lower back pain. The lumbosacral curvature is increased by intraperitoneal infusion of dialysate. Orthopedic binders and a regular exercise program for strengthening the back muscles have been beneficial for some patients.

Bleeding. Effluent drained after the first few exchanges may be pink or slightly bloody because of the trauma of catheter insertion. Bloody effluent over several days or the new appearance of blood in the effluent can indicate active intraperitoneal bleeding. If this occurs, BP and hemoglobin should be checked. Blood may also be present in the effluent of women who are menstruating or ovulating; this occurrence necessitates no intervention.

Pulmonary Complications. Atelectasis, pneumonia, and bronchitis may occur from repeated upward displacement of the diaphragm, resulting in decreased lung expansion. The longer the dwell time, the greater the likelihood of pulmonary problems. Frequent repositioning and deep-breathing exercises can help. When the patient is lying in bed, elevation of the head of the bed may prevent these problems.

Protein Loss. The peritoneal membrane is permeable to plasma proteins, amino acids, and polypeptides. These substances are lost in the dialysate fluid. The amount of loss may be as much as 5 to 15 g/day. This loss may increase to up to 40 g/day during episodes of peritonitis as the membrane becomes more permeable. Positive nitrogen balance can be maintained with adequate protein intake.

Carbohydrate and Lipid Abnormalities. Dialysate glucose is absorbed via the peritoneum in quantities that may be as high as 100 to 150 g/day. Continuous absorption of glucose results in increased insulin secretion and increased plasma insulin levels. The hyperinsulinemia stimulates hepatic production of triglycerides.

Effectiveness of and Adaptation to Chronic Peritoneal Dialysis

Learning the self-management skills required to do PD involves a relatively short training program. PD provides independence and flexibility with treatment, and travelling is easier. A major advantage of PD is its simplicity and that it is a home-based treatment that allows the patient to be in control.

Clinically, the patient receiving PD does as well as the patient receiving HD and sometimes better. There are fewer dietary restrictions, and greater mobility is possible than with conventional HD. The major disadvantage is the possibility of developing peritonitis.

PD is especially indicated for the individual who has vascular access problems or responds poorly to the hemodynamic stresses of HD (e.g., the older-adult patient with diabetes and cardiovascular disease). The diabetic patient with ESRD does better with PD than with HD. The advantages of PD for the diabetic

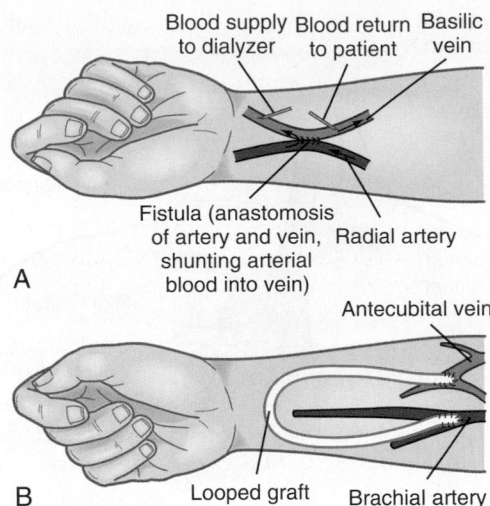

FIGURE 49-9 Vascular access for hemodialysis. **A,** Arteriovenous fistula. **B,** Arteriovenous graft.

FIGURE 49-10 Arteriovenous fistula created by anastomosing an artery and a vein. Source: Courtesy Dr. Stephen Van Voorst, MD.

patient include better BP control, less hemodynamic instability because fluid shifts are gradual, and prevention of retinal hemorrhage because heparin is not required as it is in HD.

HEMODIALYSIS

HD is a method of removing waste products and excess fluid from the blood using a machine to pump the blood through an artificial semipermeable membrane (dialyzer).

Vascular Access Sites for Hemodialysis

Obtaining vascular access is one of the greatest challenges associated with HD. To carry out HD, a very rapid blood flow is required, and access to a large blood vessel is essential. The types of vascular access in current use include arteriovenous fistulas (AVFs) and grafts (AVGs), and tunnelled and nontunnelled central venous catheters (CVCs). AVFs are superior to synthetic AVGs and CVCs and are associated with better long-term survival, lower infection and complication rates, and lower health care expenditure (Gowda, Pavan, & Babu, 2014; Kuhan, Antoniou, Nikam, et al., 2013).

Arteriovenous Fistulas and Grafts. A native **arteriovenous fistula (AVF)** is the preferred HD access, created by surgically connecting a vein and an artery, usually in the forearm (Gowda et al., 2014; Kuhan et al., 2013) (Figures 49-9, *A* and 49-10). The preferred sites for creating an AVF are the wrist (radiocephalic) and the elbow (brachiocephalic) (Gowda et al., 2014). The fistula provides for arterial blood flow through the vein. The increased pressure of the arterial blood flow through the vein causes the vein to dilate and become tough, making it amenable to repeated venipuncture. The vein is accessed using two large-gauge needles.

AVFs have the best overall patency rates and the least number of complications (e.g., thrombosis, infection) of all vascular accesses. The CSN *Clinical Practice Guidelines for Vascular Access* suggest that the AVF should be created at least 3 to 4 months before starting dialysis (Canadian Society of Nephrology, 2012) The AVF requires 4 to 6 weeks, and preferably 3 months, to mature (dilate and toughen) sufficiently for use. AVFs are more difficult to create in people with severe peripheral vascular disease, diabetes, prolonged IV drug use, or previous multiple IV

procedures in the forearm. For these individuals, a synthetic graft may be required.

An **arteriovenous graft (AVG)** is an HD access created with a synthetic graft that is attached to an artery and a vein. It is used for people who do not have suitable vessels for an AVF. The preferred site for a synthetic graft is a forearm, using a curved loop radiocephalic graft. The graft is a surgically created anastomosis between an artery (usually radial) and a vein (usually cephalic) (see Figure 49-9, *B*). An interval of 3 to 6 weeks is usually necessary to allow the graft to heal, but some centres may use it earlier (Canadian Society of Nephrology, 2012). The graft, like the fistula, is under the skin and is accessed using two large-gauge needles. The graft material is self-healing, meaning it should close over any puncture site after the needle is removed. Infections in other parts of the body can result in infection and damage to the graft and have a tendency to be thrombogenic (Gowda et al., 2014).

Normally, a *thrill* can be felt by palpating the area of anastomosis, and a bruit can be heard with a stethoscope. The bruit and the thrill are created by the turbulence of arterial blood rushing into the vein. BPs, IV insertion, and venipuncture should not be performed on an extremity with an AVF or AVG. This is to prevent thrombosis and infection in the vascular access. Protection of the vascular access site is of paramount importance.

An AVF is much less likely to clot and become infected than a graft. Thrombosis in AVGs is common but can often be corrected using interventional radiology techniques or a surgical procedure. AVFs and AVGs can cause the development of distal ischemia (steal syndrome) because too much of the arterial blood is being shunted or "stolen" from the distal extremity. This is usually seen soon after surgery and may require surgical correction. Aneurysms can also develop at the fistula site and can rupture if left untreated. AVG infections are not uncommon, and immediate treatment is essential to salvage the graft and prevent bacteremia. Severe AVG infections may necessitate graft removal.

Central Venous Catheters. In some situations when immediate vascular access is required, a temporary CVC is placed by percutaneous cannulation of the internal jugular or the femoral vein. Internal jugular vein cannulation is associated with a low incidence of thrombosis, which is the primary reason this method is preferred over subclavian cannulation. In addition to vessel thrombosis and stenosis, subclavian vein cannulation has been associated with pneumothorax and brachial plexus; therefore, this site should be used as a last resort. A flexible

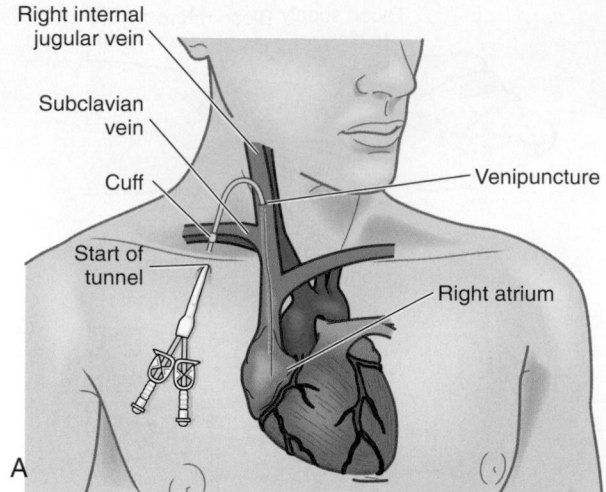

FIGURE 49-11 Temporary double-lumen vascular access catheter for acute hemodialysis. **A,** Soft, flexible dual-lumen tube is attached to a Y hub. **B,** Blood is withdrawn continuously through the red lumen (upstream) and returned through the blue lumen (downstream), thus reducing recirculation. Source: *A,* © Can Stock Photo/Terrapanthera.

Teflon, silicone rubber, or polyurethane catheter can be inserted at the bedside into the internal jugular vein and provides access to circulation without surgery (Figure 49-11, *A*). The catheters usually have a double external lumen with an internal septum separating the two internal segments (see Figure 49-11, *B*). One lumen is used for blood removal and the other for blood return. Femoral catheters should be sutured into place and can be left in place as long as there are no complications (Jin, Wang, Wu, et al., 2015).

Disadvantages of femoral vessel cannulation include the following: (1) the location encourages catheter kinking and (2) the groin is not a clean site. Potential complications of femoral catheterization are femoral vein thrombosis with pulmonary emboli (especially if the treatment is prolonged), infections, immobility, and inadvertent blood vessel punctures with hematoma formation. Temporary catheters are generally stiff and inflexible. They can cause trauma to the vessel, so bedrest is recommended. Temporary catheters in the internal jugular vein should be sutured in place and should be replaced as soon as possible by a tunnelled catheter that can be left in place for several weeks. Proper catheter position should be confirmed using radiography before use (Jin et al., 2015). Temporary catheters are generally left in place only for short periods or until a tunnelled catheter can be inserted.

Tunnelled catheters, which are soft and flexible, may be an option for patients who have exhausted all other vascular access sites. These catheters can be used as temporary access while awaiting fistula placement and development or as long-term access when other forms of access have failed. This type of catheter exits on the upper chest wall and is tunnelled subcutaneously to the internal jugular vein (Figure 49-12). The catheter tip rests in the right atrium. It has one or two subcutaneous Dacron cuffs that prevent infection from tracking along the catheter and anchor the catheter, eliminating the need for sutures.

For CVCs, no drugs should be administered or blood withdrawn via the catheter by nondialysis staff. This is to minimize the risk for infection, catheter loss, and accidental injection of heparin. Trained dialysis staff will instill heparin into the lumens

FIGURE 49-12 A, Right internal jugular placement for a tunnelled, cuffed semipermanent catheter. **B,** Temporary hemodialysis catheter in place. **C,** Long-term cuffed hemodialysis catheter. Source: *B* and *C,* Courtesy Dr. Stephen Van Voorst, MD.

of the catheter at the end of each treatment to ensure patency and withdraw it before the next treatment.

Dialyzers

The dialyzer is a long plastic cartridge that contains thousands of parallel hollow tubes or fibres (Figure 49-13). The fibres are the semipermeable membrane, made of cellulose-based or other synthetic materials. The blood is pumped into the top of the cartridge and is dispersed into all of the fibres. Dialysis fluid (dialysate) is pumped into the bottom of the cartridge and bathes the outside of the fibres. Ultrafiltration, diffusion, and osmosis

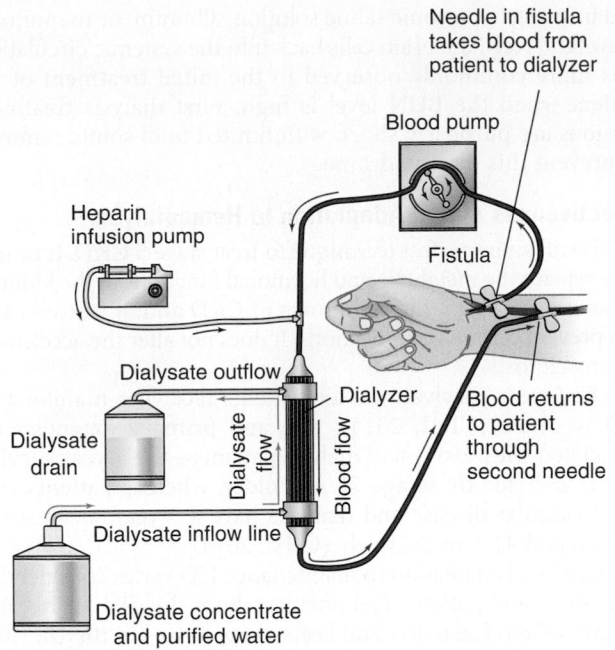

FIGURE 49-13 Components of a hemodialysis system. Blood is removed via a needle inserted in a fistula or via catheter lumen. It is propelled to the dialyzer by a blood pump. Heparin is infused to prevent clotting. Dialysate is pumped in and flows in the opposite direction to that of the blood. The dialyzed blood is returned to the patient through a second needle or catheter lumen. Old dialysate and ultrafiltrate are drained and discarded.

FIGURE 49-14 Patient receiving in-centre hemodialysis. Source: © Can Stock Photo/PicsFive.

occur across the pores of this semipermeable membrane. When the dialyzed blood reaches the end of the semipermeable fibres, it converges into a single tube that returns it to the patient. Available dialyzers differ in regard to surface area, membrane composition and thickness, clearance of waste products, and removal of fluid.

Procedure

To initiate chronic dialysis in a patient with an AVG or AVF, two needles are placed in the fistula or graft. One needle is used to draw blood from the patient and circulate it through the extracorporeal circuit and dialyzer, and the other needle is used to return the blood. If the patient has a catheter, the two blood lines are attached to the two catheter lumens, and blood is circulated through the dialysis blood circuit similar to that of the AVF and is sent to the dialyzer with the assistance of a blood pump. Heparin is added to the blood as it flows into the dialyzer because any time blood contacts a foreign substance it has a tendency to clot. When the blood enters the extracorporeal circuit, it is propelled through the top of the dialyzer by a blood pump at a flow rate of 200 to 500 mL/min, while the dialysate circulates in the opposite direction at a rate of 300 to 900 mL/min. Blood is returned from the dialyzer to the patient through the second needle or the blue (venous) catheter lumen.

In addition to the dialyzer, there is a dialysate delivery and monitoring system (Figure 49-14). This system pumps the dialysate through the dialyzer in the direction opposite to that of the blood flow.

Before beginning treatment, the nurse must complete an assessment of the patient that includes fluid status (weight, BP, peripheral edema, lung and heart sounds), condition of vascular access, temperature, and general skin condition. The difference between the last postdialysis weight and the present predialysis weight represents the amount of fluid weight gained since the last treatment. This information is used to determine the ultrafiltration or the amount of fluid to be removed. Each kilogram represents approximately 1 L of fluid. Ideally, no more than 1 to 1.5 kg should be gained between treatments to prevent the hypotension associated with the removal of larger volumes of fluid. Many patients gain 2 to 3 kg between treatments, and this volume usually can be removed if their BP is not labile. While the patient is on dialysis, vital signs should be taken at least every 30 to 60 minutes because rapid changes may occur in the BP.

Most maintenance dialysis units use reclining chairs that allow for elevation of the feet if hypotension develops. Most people sleep, read, talk, or watch television during dialysis. Treatments usually last 3 to 5 hours and are done a minimum of three times per week to achieve adequate clearance and maintain fluid balance.

Settings for Hemodialysis. HD units and treatments are performed in a variety of settings. Acutely ill patients may require dialysis in the ICU setting. Most large teaching hospitals in Canada have dialysis units that accommodate patients who are in hospital as well as a chronic outpatient population. Many satellite and outpatient clinics provide chronic HD treatments. The patient may choose to do self-care with backup support from trained personnel if needed. Self-care patients generally put in their dialysis needles, set up the machine, and monitor the course of their treatment. Patients receiving HD are able to travel if dialysis treatments can be arranged at another dialysis unit.

Dialysis done at home is an optimal option for patients requiring RRT. Treatments are more cost effective and have many benefits for the patient (Czajkowski, Pienkos, Schiller, et al., 2013). HD can also be done at home. Today, in Canada, almost 20% of patients receiving HD use it at home (Johnson, 2014; Young et al., 2012). One of the main advantages of home HD is that it allows greater freedom in choosing dialysis times. Some modifications for a special electrical outlet, plumbing, and water treatment are necessary to accommodate the HD machine in the home setting.

Complications of Hemodialysis

Hypotension. Hypotension that occurs during HD primarily results from rapid removal of vascular volume (hypovolemia), decreased cardiac output, and decreased systemic intravascular resistance. The drop in BP during dialysis may precipitate lightheadedness, nausea, vomiting, seizures, vision changes, and chest pain from cardiac ischemia. The usual treatment for hypotension includes decreasing the volume of fluid being removed and infusion of 0.9% saline solution (100–300 mL). If a patient experiences recurrent hypotensive episodes, a reassessment may have to be done of dry weight and BP drugs. BP drugs should be held before dialysis if there are frequent episodes of hypotension during dialysis.

Muscle Cramps. Painful muscle cramps are a common problem with HD. They result from rapid removal of sodium and water or from neuro-muscular hypersensitivity. Treatment includes reducing the ultrafiltration rate and infusing hypertonic saline or a normal saline bolus. The nurse should also educate the patient about restricting salt and fluid in the diet to reduce weight gains between dialysis treatments.

Loss of Blood. Blood loss may result from blood not being completely rinsed from the dialyzer, accidental separation of blood tubing, dialysis membrane rupture, or bleeding after the removal of needles at the end of dialysis. If a patient has received too much heparin or has clotting problems, there can be significant postdialysis bleeding. It is essential to rinse back all blood, to closely monitor heparinization to prevent excess anticoagulation, and to hold firm but nonocclusive pressure on access sites until the risk of bleeding has passed.

Hepatitis. A common cause of hepatitis B and C in dialysis patients includes transmission of health care–associated infection within hemodialysis units. As blood is screened for hepatitis B and C, blood transfusions are an unlikely source for the hepatitis infection. Dialysis patients may contract the bloodborne pathogen of hepatitis B and C as the general population does, through IV drug use or unprotected sex. (See Chapter 17 for infection control precautions and Chapter 46 for more detailed discussion on hepatitis.)

Sepsis. Sepsis is most often related to infections of vascular access sites. Bacteria can also be introduced during the dialysis treatment as a result of poor technique or interruption of blood tubing or dialyzer membranes. Bacterial endocarditis can occur because of the frequent and prolonged access to the vascular system. Aseptic technique is essential to prevent this problem. Nurses must monitor patients for signs and symptoms of sepsis, such as fever, hypotension, and an elevated WBC count. (See Chapter 69 for nursing management of septic shock.)

Disequilibrium Syndrome. *Disequilibrium syndrome* is a rare complication of modern HD and develops as a result of very rapid changes in the composition of the extracellular fluid. Urea, sodium, and other solutes are removed more rapidly from the blood than from the cerebro-spinal fluid and the brain. This rapid removal creates a high osmotic gradient in the brain, resulting in the shift of fluid into the brain, causing cerebral edema. Manifestations include nausea, vomiting, confusion, restlessness, headaches, twitching and jerking, and seizures. The rapid changes in osmolality may cause muscle cramps and worsen hypotension. Treatment consists of slowing or stopping dialysis and infusing hypertonic saline solution, albumin, or mannitol to draw fluid from the brain cells back into the systemic circulation. It is more commonly observed in the initial treatment of the patient when the BUN level is high. First dialysis treatment sessions are purposely short, with limited total solute removal, to prevent this rare syndrome.

Effectiveness of and Adaptation to Hemodialysis

HD is still an imperfect technique to treat stage 5 CKD. It cannot fully replace the metabolic and hormonal functions of the kidneys. It can ease many of the symptoms of CKD and, if started early, can prevent certain complications. It does not alter the accelerated atherosclerosis.

The 5-year survival rate for patients receiving maintenance HD is 41.4% (CIHI, 2014). Age and primary diagnosis are associated with survival of dialysis patients—the 5-year survival rate is 26% for those age 75 and older, whereas patients with renal vascular disease and diabetes have a 5-year survival rate of 37% and 41% respectively (CIHI, 2014).

Individual adaptation to maintenance HD varies considerably. Initially, many patients feel positive about the dialysis because it makes them feel better and keeps them alive, but there is often great ambivalence about whether it is worthwhile. Dependence on a machine is a reality, and some have dreams about being tied to the machine. In response to their illness, patients undergoing dialysis may demonstrate nonadherence to medical therapy, depression, and suicidal tendencies. The primary nursing goals are to help patients regain or maintain positive self-esteem and control of their lives and continue to be productive in society.

Continuous Renal Replacement Therapy

Continuous renal replacement therapy (CRRT) is an alternative or adjunctive method for treating AKI. It provides a means by which uremic toxins and fluids are removed from a patient who is hemodynamically unstable, while acid–base status and electrolytes are adjusted slowly and continuously. Patients selected for this treatment are usually those who do not respond to dietary interventions or pharmacological agents.

Various types of CRRT are available, such as continuous venovenous hemofiltration (CVVH), continuous venovenous hemodialysis (CVVHD), and continuous venovenous hemodiafiltration (CVVHDF) (Claure-Del Grando, Macedo, & Mehta, 2012) (Table 49-14). Various hybrid modalities that combine aspects of conventional HD and CRRT can be used and are

TABLE 49-14	TYPES OF CONTINUOUS RENAL REPLACEMENT THERAPIES	
Therapies	**Abbreviation**	**Purpose**
Continuous venovenous hemofiltration*	CVVH	Solute loss via convection; hemodilution using replacement fluid
Continuous venovenous hemodialysis*	CVVHD	Solute loss via convection and diffusion
Continuous venovenous hemodiafiltration	CVVHDF	—
Slow continuous ultrafiltration	SCUF	Fluid removal via ultrafiltration
Slow low-efficiency dialysis	SLED	—

*Most commonly used therapies.

FIGURE 49-15 Basic schematic of continuous venovenous therapies. Blood pump is required to pump blood through the circuit. Replacement ports are used for continuous venovenous hemofiltration (CVVH) and continuous venovenous hemodialysis (CVVHD) only; replacements can be given prefilter or postfilter. Dialysate port is used for CVVHD only. Regardless of modality, ultrafiltrate is drained via the ultrafiltration drain port.

determined based on the needs of the patient. Some common hybrid modalities include slow low-efficiency dialysis (SLED) and slow continuous ultrafiltration (SCUF) (Claure-Del Grando et al., 2012).

Vascular access for CRRT is achieved through the use of a double-lumen catheter (as used in HD, noted in Figure 49-13, A) placed in the femoral or the jugular vein. The subclavian vein should be used only if no other access site is available, owing to the increased complication rates of pneumothorax, hemorrhage, and stenosis (Claure-Del Grando et al., 2012). Under the influence of hydrostatic pressure and osmotic pressure, water and nonprotein solutes pass out of the filter into the extracapillary space and drain through the ultrafiltrate port into a collection device (Foley bag) (Figure 49-15). The remaining fluid continues through the filter and returns to the patient via the return port of the double-lumen catheter. While the ultrafiltrate drains out of the hemofilter, fluid and electrolyte replacements can be infused into the infusion port located after the filter, as the blood returns to the patient. This fluid is designed to replace volume and solutes such as sodium, chloride, bicarbonate, and glucose. It will also further dilute intravascular fluid, decreasing the concentration of unwanted solutes such as BUN, creatinine, and potassium. The infusion rate of replacement fluid is determined by the degree of the fluid and electrolyte imbalance. Replacement fluid may also be infused into the infusion port before the hemofilter. This method allows for greater clearance of urea and can decrease filter clotting.

Anticoagulation (e.g., heparin) is needed to prevent blood clotting during CRRT. Heparin dosage is based on the patient's activated clotting time (ACT), partial prothrombin time (PPT), or prothrombin time (PT).

Several features of CRRT differ from those of HD:

1. It is continuous rather than intermittent. Large volumes of fluid can be removed over days (24 hr to >2 wk) versus hours (3 to 4 hr).

2. Solute removal can occur by convection (no dialysate required) in addition to osmosis and diffusion.
3. It causes less hemodynamic instability (e.g., hypotension).
4. It does not require constant monitoring by a specialized HD nurse but does require a trained ICU nurse.
5. It does not require complicated HD equipment, but a blood pump is needed for venovenous therapies.

The type of CRRT is customized to the needs of the patient. Some types involve the use of replacement fluids. Large volumes of fluid may be removed hourly (200–800 mL), and then a portion of this fluid is replaced. The type of fluid replacement is dependent on the stability of the patient's condition and the patient's individualized needs. Ultrafiltration and convective losses occur, and solute concentrations in the blood are diluted with the replacement fluid.

CRRT can be continued as long as 30 to 40 days, but the hemofilter should be changed every 24 to 48 hours because of loss of filtration efficiency and the potential for clotting.

The nurse responsible for the care of the patient with AKI who is receiving CRRT may be a critical care nurse or a nephrology nurse specialist, working in collaboration with other health care providers. Specific nursing interventions include obtaining weights and monitoring and documenting laboratory values daily to ensure adequate fluid and electrolyte balance. Hourly intake–output measurements and monitoring of vital signs and hemodynamic status are essential. Although reductions in central venous pressure and pulmonary artery pressure are expected, there should be little change in mean arterial pressure or cardiac output. Patency of the CRRT system is assessed and maintained, and the patient's vascular access site is cared for to prevent infection. Treatment is discontinued and the vascular access is removed once the patient's AKI is resolved or there is a decision to withdraw treatment owing to patient deterioration.

KIDNEY TRANSPLANTATION

Major progress has been made in organ transplantation since the first kidney transplantation was performed in 1954 in Boston between identical twins. The advances made in organ procurement and preservation, surgical techniques, tissue typing and matching, understanding the immune system, immuno-suppressant therapy, and preventing and treating rejection have dramatically increased the success of organ transplantation.

The disparity between the supply and the demand for organs is significant. In Canada, over 23 000 patients received dialysis in 2012, a level that has remained virtually unchanged since 2003. Over 17 438 patients were living with a kidney transplant in 2012, almost triple the number in 1993 (CIHI, 2014). According to CIHI data, 10 641 adult patients received renal transplants between 2000 and 2009. Transplantation from a deceased donor usually requires a prolonged waiting period, with median waiting times between 2010 and 2012 of 3.9 years (CIHI, 2014). By province, the longest median wait time was in British Columbia (5.0 years), while the shortest median wait time was in Saskatchewan, at just 2.2 years (CIHI, 2014).

Kidney transplantation is extremely successful, with 1-year graft survival rates of about 93% for deceased donor transplants and greater than 97.5% for living donor transplants (CIHI, 2014). An advantage of kidney transplantation when compared with dialysis is that when normal kidney function is restored, many of the pathophysiological changes associated with renal failure are reversed. It also eliminates the dependence on dialysis and the

ETHICAL DILEMMAS
Allocation of Resources

Situation

A transplantation nurse coordinator is considering her feelings about two patients who are being evaluated for placement on the waiting list for a deceased donor kidney transplantation. One patient is a 40-year-old school teacher. She is married and has two children. The other patient is a 22-year-old unemployed man who is actively using cocaine. He misses three to four dialysis treatments per month and does not take his phosphate binders or antihypertensive drugs consistently.

Important Points for Consideration

- Psychological, physiological, and adherence factors are included in the assessment process for eligibility for organ transplantation.
- In kidney transplantation, the organ is transplanted into the patient who has received the most points based on a scoring system, regardless of the health care provider's opinion of the patient's worth. If a patient is denied transplantation candidacy on this basis, he or she must be given a chance to change or improve the problem or condition in a specified period.
- The national organ procurement system is designed to be unbiased about the patient in all respects. Once a patient is placed on the list for transplantation, that patient is deemed of no greater or lesser worth than any other patient.
- Because organ donation is voluntary in Canada, any concerns that the system of procurement and transplantation is not fair may negatively affect the pool of available organs.

Clinical Decision-Making Questions

1. What guidance is provided by the Canadian Nurses Association (CNA) *Code of Ethics for Registered Nurses* (2017) to help nurses address kidney transplantation issues?
2. What might be the nurse's feelings about which of the patients should receive the next available organ?

accompanying dietary and lifestyle restrictions. Transplantation is also less expensive than dialysis after the first year.

Ethical Issues

Transplantation health care in Canada is governed by laws and statutes. It is complex and involves many people, professionals, services, functions, and levels of government. Voluntary consent must be given by the donor (Gill, Klarenbach, Barnieh, et al., 2014); in some provinces, one can provide advance written consent on a driver's licence or in a will (although permission from the donor's legal next of kin is still required after brain death is determined). In the absence of formal written consent at death, family or significant others can donate organs of the deceased if they had prior knowledge of the donor's intent. Kidneys may be obtained from deceased or living donors. It is illegal to buy or sell organs in Canada. (See the "Ethical Dilemmas" box in this chapter and in Chapter 16.)

Recipient Selection

Appropriate recipient selection is important for a successful outcome. Candidacy is determined by a variety of medical and psychosocial factors that vary among transplantation centres. A careful evaluation is completed in an attempt to identify and minimize potential complications after transplantation. Certain patients, particularly those with cardiovascular disease and diabetes mellitus, are considered high risk. With careful evaluation and monitoring, high-risk patients can achieve the same success rates as other patients. Some patients who are approaching ESRD can receive a transplant before dialysis is required if they have

a living donor. This approach is most advantageous for patients with diabetes, who have a much higher mortality rate on dialysis than people who do not have diabetes.

Contraindications to transplantation include disseminated malignancies, refractory or untreated cardiac disease, chronic respiratory failure, extensive vascular disease, chronic infection, and unresolved psychosocial disorders (e.g., alcoholism, drug addiction) and nonadherence to medical regimens. The presence of hepatitis B or C is not a contraindication to transplantation.

Surgical procedures may be required before transplantation based on the results of the recipient evaluation. Coronary artery bypass graft surgery may be indicated for advanced coronary artery disease. Cholecystectomy may be necessary for patients with a history of gallstones, biliary obstruction, or cholecystitis. On rare occasions, bilateral nephrectomies may be done for patients with refractory hypertension, recurrent urinary tract infections, or grossly enlarged kidneys resulting from polycystic kidney disease.

Histocompatibility Studies

Histocompatibility testing is discussed in Chapter 16.

Donor Sources

Kidneys for transplantation may be obtained from compatible blood–type deceased donors, blood relatives, emotionally related living donors (e.g., spouses, friends), and altruistic living donors who are unknown to the recipient. Expanding the living donor pool is one of the best possibilities for decreasing the size of the deceased donor waiting list and reducing waiting times.

Living Donors. Living donors must undergo an extensive multidisciplinary evaluation to be certain they are in good health and have no history of disease that would place them at risk of developing kidney failure or operative complications. Psychosocial and financial evaluations are done as well. Crossmatches are done at the time of the evaluation and about a week before the transplantation to ensure that no antibodies to the donor are present or that the antibody titre is below the allowed level. Advantages of a living donor transplantation include better patient and graft survival rates regardless of histocompatibility match, immediate organ availability, immediate function because of minimal "cold time" (kidney out of the body and not getting blood supply), and the opportunity to have the recipient in the best possible medical condition because the surgery is elective.

The potential donor will see a nephrologist for a complete history and physical and laboratory and diagnostic studies. Laboratory studies include a 24-hour urine study for creatinine clearance and total protein, complete blood count, and chemistry and electrolyte profiles. Hepatitis B and C, HIV, and cytomegalovirus (CMV) testing are done to assess for the presence of any transmissible diseases. An ECG and chest radiography are also obtained. A renal ultrasound and a renal arteriogram or three-dimensional CT are performed to ensure that the blood vessels supplying each kidney are adequate and that there are no anomalies and to determine which kidney will be removed.

A transplantation psychologist or social worker will determine whether the individual is emotionally stable and able to deal with the issues related to organ donation. All donors must be informed about the risks and benefits of donation, the potential short- and long-term complications, and what can be expected during the hospitalization and recovery phases. Although the cost of the evaluation and surgery are covered by the recipient's insurance, there is no compensation available for lost wages during the posthospitalization recovery period. This period can last 6 weeks or longer.

Incompatibility between a potential transplant recipient and a prospective donor is a major barrier to living donor transplantations. **Paired organ donation** is another option that allows a living donor to donate a kidney to a different compatible recipient, with the intent that another donor will donate to the first donor's designated recipient (Paramesh, 2013). In 2009, the Canadian Blood Services launched a pilot project for a living donor paired exchange (LDPE) registry that is now available to every province (The Organ Registry Team [ORT] [Ottawa] & The Organ and Tissue Donation and Transplantation [OTDT] Team [Ottawa and Edmonton], 2015). The registry is designed to facilitate transplants between recipients and living donors who have an incompatible match with other recipient donor pairs in the same situation (ORT & OTDT, 2015). The recipient–donor pairs in the LDPE registry are entered in a complex computer algorithm that identifies opportunities for transplants between them (ORT & OTDT, 2015).

Deceased Donors. Deceased (cadaver) kidney donors are relatively healthy individuals who have suffered an irreversible brain injury with a declaration of brain death. The most common causes of injury are cerebral trauma from motor vehicle accidents or gunshot wounds, intracerebral or subarachnoid hemorrhage, and anoxic brain damage caused by cardiac arrest. The donor must have effective cardiovascular function and be supported on a ventilator to preserve the organs. The age range of most suitable kidney donors is from 2 to 70 years. The age of the donor is less important than the quality of kidney function. The donor must be free of active IV drug use; severe hypertension; longstanding diabetes mellitus; malignancies; sepsis; and communicable diseases, including HIV, hepatitis B and C, syphilis, and tuberculosis. Permission from the donor's legal next of kin is required after brain death is determined, even if the donor carried a signed donor card.

The kidneys are removed and preserved. They can be preserved for up to 72 hours, but most transplantation surgeons prefer to transplant kidneys before the cold time reaches 24 hours. Experience has shown that prolonged cold time increases the likelihood that the kidney will not function immediately and the transplant recipient will require dialysis until the ATN from the extended cold time resolves.

In Canada, patients who receive a kidney from deceased donors are selected from provincial waiting lists that use an objective computerized point system. ABO group, human lymphocyte antigen (HLA) typing, age, antibody level, and length of time waiting are entered into the computer matching program as each candidate is listed. When a donor becomes available, the donor's HLA data, ABO type, and other key information is compared with the data of all patients awaiting transplantation locally. Donors and recipients must have the same blood type. The kidney is offered to the recipient with the most points. If there are no patients in the local area who are suitable, the organ is then offered in the region, and then to the nation. When a kidney arrives at the recipient's transplantation centre, a final crossmatch is done. The final crossmatch must be negative for the deceased donor transplantation to proceed. (Crossmatching is discussed in Chapter 16.)

Surgical Procedure

Living Donor. The donor nephrectomy is performed by a urologist or transplantation surgeon. The donor's surgery begins 1 to 2 hours before the recipient's surgery is started. The recipient is surgically prepared for the kidney transplantation in a nearby operating room.

Laparoscopic donor nephrectomy is the most common approach to removing a kidney from a living donor. (Laparoscopic nephrectomy is discussed in Chapter 48.) The laparoscopic approach significantly decreases the hospital stay, pain, operative blood loss, debilitation, and length of time off work.

For a conventional nephrectomy, the donor is placed in the lateral decubitus position on the operating table so that the flank is presented laterally. An incision is made at the level of the eleventh rib. The rib may have to be removed to provide adequate visualization of the kidney.

Kidney Transplant Recipient. The transplanted kidney is usually placed extraperitoneally in the iliac fossa. The right iliac fossa is preferred to facilitate anastomoses and minimize the occurrence of ileus.

Before any incisions are made, a urinary catheter is placed into the bladder. An antibiotic solution is instilled to distend the bladder and decrease the risk for infection. A crescent-shaped incision is made, extending from the iliac crest to the symphysis pubis (Figure 49-16). The peritoneum is left intact. The iliac and the hypogastric vessels are dissected free.

Rapid revascularization is critical to prevent ischemic injury to the kidney. The donor artery is anastomosed to the recipient's internal iliac (hypogastric) or external iliac artery. The donor vein is anastomosed to the recipient's external iliac vein. Kidney transplants with living donors can be technically more difficult

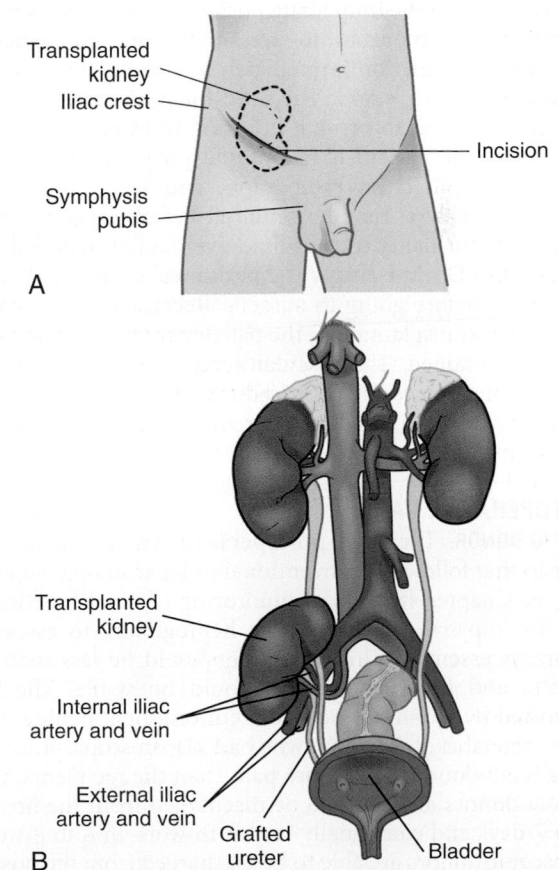

FIGURE 49-16 A, Surgical incision for a renal transplantation. **B,** Surgical placement of a transplanted kidney.

because the blood vessel lengths can be shorter than in cadaveric transplants.

When the anastomoses are complete, the clamps are released, and blood flow to the kidney is re-established. The kidney should become firm and pink. Urine may begin to flow from the ureter immediately. Mannitol or furosemide (Lasix) may be administered to promote diuresis.

The donor ureter in most cases is then tunnelled through the bladder submucosa before entering the bladder cavity and being sutured in place. This approach is called a *ureteroneocystostomy*. This approach allows the bladder wall to compress the ureter as it contracts for micturition, thereby preventing reflux of urine up the ureter into the transplanted kidney. The transplantation surgery takes approximately 3 to 4 hours.

NURSING MANAGEMENT
KIDNEY TRANSPLANT RECIPIENT

The successful recovery and rehabilitation of the recipient are made possible with careful nursing assessment, diagnosis, intervention, and evaluation of all body systems. With a length of hospital stay averaging 4 to 5 days, discharge planning and teaching needs must be identified and addressed early in the hospital course.

PREOPERATIVE CARE

Nursing care of the patient in the preoperative phase includes emotional and physical preparation for surgery. Because the patient and the family may have been waiting years for the kidney transplantation, a review of the operative procedure and what can be expected in the immediate postoperative recovery period is necessary. It is important to stress that there is a chance the kidney may not function immediately and that dialysis may be required for days to weeks. The need for immuno-suppressive drugs and measures to prevent infection must be reviewed.

To ensure the patient is in optimal physical condition for surgery, an ECG, chest radiograph, and laboratory studies are ordered. Dialysis may be required before surgery for any significant abnormality such as fluid overload or hyperkalemia. A patient on PD must empty the peritoneal cavity of all dialysate solution before going to surgery. Because dialysis may be required after transplantation, the patency of the vascular access must be maintained. The vascular access extremity should be labelled "dialysis access, no procedures" to prevent use of the affected extremity for BP measurement, blood drawing, or IV infusions.

POSTOPERATIVE CARE

LIVING DONOR. The usual postoperative care for the donor is similar to that following conventional or laparoscopic nephrectomy (see Chapter 48). Close monitoring of renal function, to assess for impairment, and of the hemoglobin, to assess for bleeding, is essential. The creatinine should be less than 124 mcmol/L, and the hemoglobin should be stable. The pain experienced by a donor who had a conventional nephrectomy is greater than that of the donor who had a laparoscopic procedure. Generally, all donors have more pain than the recipients. Conventional donors are ready to be discharged from the hospital in 4 to 7 days and can usually return to work in 6 to 8 weeks. Laparoscopic donors are able to be discharged from the hospital in 2 to 4 days and can return to work in 4 to 6 weeks. The donor is seen by the surgeon 1 to 2 weeks after discharge.

Nurses caring for the living donor need to acknowledge the precious gift that this person has given. The donor has taken physical, emotional, and financial risks to assist the recipient. It is vital that this individual not be forgotten after surgery. The donor will need even greater support if the donated organ either does not work immediately or, for some reason, fails.

KIDNEY TRANSPLANT RECIPIENT. The first priority during this period is maintenance of fluid and electrolyte balance. In some centres, kidney transplant recipients spend the first 12 to 24 hours in the ICU because of the close monitoring required. Very large volumes of urine may be produced soon after the blood supply to the transplanted kidney is re-established. This diuresis is owing to (1) the new kidney's ability to filter BUN, which acts as an osmotic diuretic; (2) the abundance of fluids administered during the operation; and (3) initial renal tubular dysfunction, which inhibits the kidney from concentrating urine normally. Urine output during this phase may be as high as 1 L/hr and gradually decreases as the BUN and creatinine levels become more normal. Urine output is replaced, millilitre for millilitre, hourly for the first 12 to 24 hours. Central venous pressure readings are essential for monitoring postoperative fluid status. Dehydration must be prevented to prevent subsequent renal hypoperfusion and renal tubular damage. Electrolyte monitoring is critical to assess for the hyponatremia and hypokalemia often associated with rapid diuresis. Treatment with potassium supplements or 0.9% normal saline solution infusion may be indicated. IV sodium bicarbonate may also be required if the patient becomes acidotic.

ATN is becoming more common because of prolonged cold times and the use of marginal deceased donors (those who are medically suboptimal)—the ischemic damage from extended cold times causes ATN. While ATN is present, dialysis may be required to maintain fluid and electrolyte balance. If high-output ATN is present, the ability to excrete fluid is intact but not the ability to regulate metabolic wastes or electrolytes. If oliguric or anuric ATN is present, there is risk for fluid overload in the immediate postoperative period, and the patient must be assessed closely for the need for dialysis. The period of ATN can last anywhere from days to weeks, with gradually improving kidney function. Most patients experiencing ATN will be discharged from the hospital on dialysis. This is extremely discouraging for the patient, who will need reassurance that renal function usually improves. Dialysis will be discontinued when urine output increases and kidney function begins to normalize.

A sudden decrease in urine output in the early postoperative period is a cause for concern. It may be owing to dehydration, rejection, a urine leak, or obstruction. A common cause of early obstruction is a blood clot in the urinary catheter. Catheter patency must be maintained because the catheter remains in the bladder for 3 to 5 days to allow the bladder anastomosis to heal. If blood clots are suspected, gentle catheter irrigation with an order from the health care provider can re-establish patency.

Postoperative teaching should include the prevention and treatment of rejection, infection, and complications of surgery and the purpose and adverse effects of immuno-suppression (Trevitt, Dunsmore, Murphy, et al., 2012). Frequent blood tests and clinic visits help detect rejection early. Patient education to ensure a smooth transition from hospital to home is an integral part of the nursing care.

Immuno-suppressive Therapy

The goal of immuno-suppression is to adequately suppress the immune response to prevent rejection of the transplanted kidney while maintaining sufficient immunity to prevent overwhelming infection. Immuno-suppressive therapy is discussed in Chapter 16 and in Table 16-16.

Complications of Transplantation

Rejection. Rejection is one of the major problems following kidney transplantation. Rejection can be hyperacute or acute or chronic. (These types of rejection are discussed in Chapter 16.) Prevention and early diagnosis of rejection is essential for long-term graft function.

Infection. Infection remains a significant cause of morbidity and mortality after transplantation (Hoffart, 2014; Trevitt et al., 2012). The transplant recipient is at risk for infection because of suppression of the body's normal defence mechanisms by surgery, immuno-suppressive drugs, and the effects of ESRD. Underlying systemic illness such as diabetes mellitus or systemic lupus erythematosus, malnutrition, and advanced age can further compound the negative effects on the immune response. At times, the signs and symptoms of infection can be subtle. Nurses caring for transplant recipients must be astute in their observation and assessment because prompt diagnosis and treatment of infections will improve patient outcomes.

The most common infections observed in the first month after transplantation are similar to those acquired by any postoperative patient, such as pneumonia, wound infections, IV line and drain infections, and urinary tract infections. Fungal and viral infections are not uncommon because of the patient's immuno-suppressed state. Fungal infections can include *Candida, Cryptococcus, Aspergillus,* and *Pneumocystis jiroveci.* Fungal infections are difficult to treat, require prolonged treatment periods, and often involve the administration of nephrotoxic drugs. Transplant recipients usually receive prophylactic antifungal drugs to prevent these infections, such as nystatin, fluconazole (Diflucan), and sulphamethoxazole-trimethoprim.

Viral infections, including CMV, Epstein-Barr virus, herpes simplex virus (HSV), varicella-zoster virus, and polyomavirus (e.g., BK virus) can be primary or reactivation of existing disease (Hoffart, 2014; Trevitt et al., 2012). Primary infections occur as new infections after transplantation from an exogenous source such as the donated organ or blood transfusion. Reactivation occurs when a virus exists in a patient and becomes reactivated after transplantation because of immuno-suppression.

CMV is one of the most common viral infections. If a recipient has never had CMV and receives an organ from a donor with a history of CMV, antiviral prophylaxis will be administered (IV ganciclovir, valganciclovir). If a primary active CMV infection is diagnosed or there is symptomatic reactivation of CMV, IV ganciclovir will be given along with an immune globulin that contains CMV antibodies. To prevent HSV infections, oral acyclovir is given for several months after the transplantation.

Cardiovascular Disease. Transplant recipients have an increased incidence of atherosclerotic vascular disease. Cardiovascular disease is the leading cause of death after renal transplantation (Parnham, Gleadle, Leong, et al., 2015). Hypertension, dyslipidemia, diabetes mellitus, smoking, rejection, infections, and increased homocysteine levels can all contribute to cardiovascular disease. Immuno-suppressants can worsen hypertension and dyslipidemia. It is important that the patient be taught to control risk factors such as elevated cholesterol, triglycerides, and blood glucose and weight gain. Adherence to the prescribed antihypertensive and dyslipidemia regimen is essential not only to prevent cardiovascular events but also to prevent damage to the new kidney. (Hypertension is discussed in Chapter 35.)

Malignancies. The overall incidence of malignancies in kidney transplant recipients is about 6%, which is 100 times greater than in the general population. The primary cause of this increased incidence is the immuno-suppressive therapy. Not only do immuno-suppressants suppress the immune system, but they also suppress the ability to fight infection and the production of abnormal cells such as cancer cells. The malignancies include cancers of the skin, lips, kidney, hepato-biliary system, vulva, and perineum; lymphomas; and Kaposi's sarcoma and other sarcomas. Regular screening for cancer is an important part of the transplant recipient's preventive care. The patient must also be advised to avoid sun exposure by using protective clothing and sunscreens to minimize the incidence of skin cancers and to check the skin regularly and report any suspicious lesions.

Recurrence of Original Renal Disease. Recurrence of the original disease that destroyed the native kidneys occurs in some kidney transplant recipients. It is most common with certain types of glomerulo-nephritis, immunoglobulin A nephropathy, diabetes mellitus, and focal segmental sclerosis. Disease recurrence can result in the loss of a functioning kidney transplant. Patients must be advised before transplantation if they have a disease known to recur.

Corticosteroid-Related Complications. Aseptic necrosis of the hips, the knees, and other joints can result from chronic corticosteroid therapy and renal osteodystrophy. Most transplant recipients receive calcium supplements, vitamin D, and bisphosphonates in an effort to prevent or minimize the bone disorders associated with corticosteroid use. Patient teaching should include the importance of regular bone mineral density testing, weight-bearing exercise, smoking cessation, and limiting alcohol consumption. Other significant problems related to corticosteroids include peptic ulcer disease, glucose intolerance and diabetes, cataracts, dyslipidemia, and an increased incidence of infections and malignancies. In the first year after transplantation, corticosteroid doses are usually decreased to 5 to 10 mg a day. The use of tacrolimus and cyclosporin has allowed for the corticosteroid doses to be much lower than they were in the past. Some patients have been successfully withdrawn from corticosteroids 1.5 to 2 years after transplantation, thus eliminating these problems. Vigilant monitoring for adverse effects of corticosteroids and early treatment are essential.

AGE-RELATED CONSIDERATIONS

CHRONIC KIDNEY DISEASE

The incidence of stage 5 CKD in Canada is increasing most rapidly in older-adult patients. At the end of 2012, 41 252 Canadians were living with stage 5 CKD. Since 2003, this number has grown 40% from 29 540. More than half (53%) of newly diagnosed patients with CKD were 65 years of age or older as compared to 33% in 1990 (CIHI, 2014). The most common diseases leading to renal failure in older adults are diabetes and hypertension. HD is the predominant RRT for older-adult patients starting dialysis. In 2012, 84% of those age 65 years or older were started with HD compared to other RRTs (CIHI, 2014). Expenditures can be expected to increase as the CKD-affected population ages and has a correspondingly greater number of comorbid conditions.

The care of the older adult with CKD is particularly challenging, not only because of the normal physiological changes of aging that occur but also because of the number of comorbid conditions that develop (Stevens, Lamb, & Levin, 2015). Physiological changes of clinical importance in the older-adult patient with CKD include diminished cardiopulmonary function, bone loss, immunodeficiency, altered protein synthesis, impaired cognition, and altered drug metabolism. Malnutrition is common in the older-adult patient with CKD for a variety of reasons, including lack of mobility, lack of understanding of basic nutritional requirements, social isolation, physical disability, impaired cognitive function, and malabsorption problems (Stevens, Lamb, & Levin, 2015).

The older-adult patient needs to consider the best option for treatment modality based on his or her health, personal preferences, and the support available. Home PD allows the patient to be more mobile and to enjoy an increased sense of control over the illness. PD causes less hemodynamic instability than HD but does require self-care or assistance from another person. The older adult may not have adequate help in the home to provide assistance. Establishing vascular access for HD may be difficult in an older-adult patient because of atherosclerotic changes. Travel to and from the HD unit may also be problematic if the patient does not drive or have access to reliable public transportation. Although transplantation is an option, older-adult patients must be carefully screened to ensure that the benefits outweigh the risks. A living donor is preferable so that there is not a prolonged waiting time.

The most common cause of death in the older-adult patient with CKD is cardiovascular disease (myocardial infarction, stroke), followed by withdrawal from dialysis. If a competent patient decides to withdraw from dialysis, it is essential to support the patient and the family. Ethical issues (see the "Ethical Dilemmas" box) to be considered in this situation include patient competency, benefit versus burden of treatment, and futility of treatment. Withdrawal from treatment is not a failure if the patient is well informed and comfortable with the decision.

The increasing number of debilitated older-adult patients with CKD receiving dialysis has raised a number of ethical concerns about the use of scarce resources in a population with a limited life expectancy. Substantial evidence exists showing success of dialysis (especially PD) in older adults. Quality of life has also been reported to be good to excellent in many older-adult patients with CKD. There appears to be no justification for excluding older adults from dialysis programs. Rationing dialysis on the basis of age alone is not supported based on current outcome and quality-of-life data.

ETHICAL DILEMMAS

Withdrawing Treatment

Situation

A 70-year-old patient with diabetes mellitus and chronic renal failure who has been receiving dialysis for 10 years tells the nurse that he wants to discontinue his dialysis. His quality of life has diminished during the past 2 years since his wife died. He is not a prospective transplantation patient.

Important Points for Consideration

- Quality of life is an important consideration for patients when evaluating whether to begin or discontinue treatment.
- Quality-of-life decisions often weigh the benefit of treatment against the burden of treatment. When a treatment becomes too burdensome, the patient (if competent) may request to withdraw the treatment.
- A determination must be made whether there is some other treatable problem such as depression that may be clouding the patient's judgement.
- Patient autonomy, or the patient's right to self-determination regarding treatment decisions, applies to both initiating and discontinuing treatment.
- If a decision is made to withdraw treatment, the health care team, the patient, and the family should develop an appropriate follow-up plan that includes palliative care and hospice support.

Clinical Decision-Making Questions

1. How should the nurse respond to the patient's request?
2. What is the position of the Canadian Nurses Association (CNA) on withdrawing or withholding treatment that no longer benefits the patient or causes suffering?

CASE STUDY

Chronic Kidney Disease

Patient Profile

Natalia Battong, a 42-year-old schoolteacher, has been treated for type 2 diabetes mellitus since the age of 25. Her nephrologist has observed her for the past several years for manifestations of progressive chronic kidney disease. Eight weeks ago, she had an arteriovenous fistula created in preparation for starting hemodialysis. Over the past week, she has experienced anorexia, nausea, vomiting, problems with concentration, and pruritus.

Source: iofoto/
Shutterstock
.com.

Subjective Data

- Complains of swelling in her feet and hands
- Has gained 4.5 kg in the past 2 weeks
- Complains of dyspnea and weakness when walking

Objective Data
Laboratory Data

- Estimated glomerular filtration rate (eGFR): 8.0 mL/min/1.73 m²
- Serum creatinine: 560 mmol/L
- Blood urea nitrogen (BUN): 32 mmol/L
- Potassium: 6 mmol/L
- Hemoglobin: 95 g/L

Chest Radiograph

- Pulmonary edema

Discussion Questions

1. Explain the basic pathophysiological changes that resulted in the development of Mrs. Battong's diabetic nephropathy.
2. What are the indications for dialysis in this patient?
3. Identify the abnormal diagnostic study results, and explain why each would occur.
4. Explain why Mrs. Battong developed each of the clinical manifestations she shows.
5. **Priority decision:** What are the priority nursing interventions for Mrs. Battong and her family?
6. **Priority decision:** Based on the assessment data provided, what are the priority nursing diagnoses? Are there any collaborative problems?

evolve
Answers are available at *http://evolve.elsevier.com/Canada/Lewis/medsurg.*

REVIEW QUESTIONS

The number of the question corresponds to the same-numbered objective at the beginning of the chapter.

1. Which of the following characterizes acute kidney injury? *(Select all that apply)*
   a. Primary cause of death is infection.
   b. An abrupt decline in kidney function with a rise in serum creatinine
   c. Disease course is potentially reversible.
   d. Cardiovascular disease is the most common cause of death

2. The RIFLE Criteria define three stages of AKI based on changes in which of the following?
   a. Blood pressure (BP) and urine osmolality
   b. Urine output and urinary creatinine
   c. Fractional excretion of urinary sodium and glomerular filtration rate (GFR)
   d. Baseline serum creatinine and urine output

3. In the oliguric phase of acute kidney injury (AKI), for which symptoms does the nurse monitor the client?
   a. Hypotension
   b. Pulmonary edema
   c. Hypernatremia
   d. Hypokalemia

4. The nurse monitors the client in the diuretic phase of AKI for which serum electrolyte imbalances?
   a. Hyperkalemia and hyponatremia
   b. Hyperkalemia and hypernatremia
   c. Hypokalemia and hyponatremia
   d. Hypokalemia and hypernatremia

5. Which systemic effect best characterizes chronic kidney disease (CKD)?
   a. Progressive irreversible damage of the kidneys
   b. Rapid decrease in urinary output with an elevated blood urea nitrogen (BUN)
   c. Progressive increase in creatinine clearance
   d. Rapid rise in serum creatinine from baseline

6. Nurses need to educate clients at risk for developing CKD. Which of the following individuals are considered to be at increased risk? *(Select all that apply)*
   a. Older-adult Canadians who are Black
   b. People who are older than 60 years
   c. Clients with a history of pancreatitis
   d. Individuals who are obese

7. Clients with CKD experience an increased incidence of cardiovascular disease related to which of the following? *(Select all that apply)*
   a. Vascular calcification
   b. Genetic predisposition
   c. Hypertension
   d. Increased high-density lipoproteins

8. Clients with CKD stages 3–4 require a collaborative approach to care that focuses on delaying the progression of CKD by which of the following?
   a. Educating clients and caregivers about BP control
   b. Instructing clients to significantly restrict protein in their diet
   c. Instructing clients that radiocontrast agents are not harmful at this stage of CKD
   d. Educating clients to restrict their sodium intake to 3.5 g/day

9. Which of the following interventions should the nurse undertake to assess the patency of a newly placed arteriovenous graft for dialysis?
   a. Irrigate the graft daily with low-dose heparin.
   b. Monitor for any increase in blood pressure in the affected arm.
   c. Listen with a stethoscope over the graft for the presence of a bruit.
   d. Frequently monitor the pulses and the neuro-vascular status distal to the graft.

10. Following a kidney transplantation, which signs of rejection would the nurse include in her or his client education?
    a. Fever, weight loss, increased urinary output, increased BP
    b. Fever, weight gain, increased urinary output, increased BP
    c. Fever, weight loss, decreased urinary output, decreased BP
    d. Fever, weight gain, decreased urinary output, increased BP

1. a, b, c; 2. d; 3. b; 4. c; 5. a; 6. a, b, & d; 7. a & c; 8. a; 9. c; 10. d.

evolve

For even more review questions, visit *http://evolve.elsevier.com/Canada/Lewis/medsurg.*

REFERENCES

Alshayeb, H., Josephson, M., & Sprague, S. (2013). CKD-mineral and bone disorder management in kidney transplant recipients. *American Journal of Kidney Diseases, 61*(2), 310–325. doi:10.1053/j.ajkd.2012.07.022.

Bakker, S. L. (2013). Chronic kidney disease: Defining clinical cut-offs for albumin:creatinine ratio. *Nature Reviews. Nephrology, 9*(12), 710–712. doi:10.1038/nrneph.2013.233.

Baron, J. M., Cheng, X. S., Bazari, H., et al. (2015). Enhanced creatinine and estimated glomerular filtration rate reporting to facilitate detection of acute kidney injury. *American Journal of Clinical Pathology, 143*(1), 42–49. doi:10.1309/AJCP05XBCQPHTLGQ.

Batterink, J., Lin, J., Au-Yeung, S. H. M., et al. (2015). Effectiveness of sodium polystyrene sulfonate for short-term treatment of hyperkalemia. *The Canadian Journal of Hospital Pharmacy, 68*(4), 296–303.

Canadian Hypertension Education Program (CHEP). (2015). *The 2015 Canadian hypertension education program recommendations for blood pressure measurement, diagnosis, assessment of risk, prevention, and treatment of hypertension.* Retrieved from *http://www.onlinecjc.ca/article/S0828-282X%2815%2900130-0/pdf.*

Canadian Institute for Health Information (CIHI). (2014). *2003 to 2012 Annual report—Treatment of end-stage organ failure in Canada, 2003–2012.* Retrieved from *https://secure.cihi.ca/free_products/2014_CORR_Annual_Report_EN.pdf.*

Canadian Nurses Association. (2017). *Code of ethics for registered nurses.* Retrieved from *https://www.cna-aiic.ca/html/en/Code-of-Ethics-2017-Edition/files/assets/basic-html/page-1.html#.*

Canadian Society of Nephrology. (2012). Report of the Canadian Society of Nephrology vascular access working group. *Seminars in Dialysis, 25*(1), 22–25. doi:10.1111/j.1525-139X.2011.01009.x.

Chenoweth, C. E., Hines, S. C., Hall, K. K., et al. (2015). Variation in infection prevention practices in dialysis facilities: Results from the national opportunity to improve infection control in ESRD (end-stage renal disease) project. *Infection Control and Hospital Epidemiology, 36*(7), 802–806. doi:10.1017/ice.2015.55.

Chih-Hung, W., Chien-Hua, H., We-Tien, C., et al. (2016). The effects of calcium and sodium bicarbonate on severe hyperkalaemia during cardiopulmonary resuscitation: A retrospective cohort study of adult in-hospital cardiac arrest. *Resuscitation, 98,* 105–111. doi:10.1016/j.resuscitation.2015.09.384.

Claure-Del Grando, R., Macedo, E., & Mehta, R. (2012). Management options: Continuous renal replacement therapy. In E. Lerma & A. Nissenson (Eds.), *Nephrology secrets* (3rd ed.). Philadelphia: Mosby.

Crabtree, J. H. (2015). Peritoneal dialysis catheter implantation: Avoiding problems and optimizing outcomes. *Seminars in Dialysis, 28*(1), 12–15. doi:10.1111/sdi.12299.

Czajkowski, T., Pienkos, S., Schiller, B., et al. (2013). First exposure to home therapy options—Where, when, and how. *Nephrology Nursing Journal, 40*(1), 29–34.

Ellis, P. (2013). Back to basics: Acute kidney injury. *Journal of Renal Nursing, 5*(1), 38–39.

Emlet, D. R., Shaw, A. D., & Kellum, J. A. (2015). Sepsis-associated AKI: Epithelial cell dysfunction. *Seminars in Nephrology, 35*(1), 85–95. doi:10.1016/j.semnephrol.2015.01.009.

Felsenfeld, A. J., Levine, B. S., & Rodriguez, M. (2015). Pathophysiology of calcium, phosphorus, and magnesium dysregulation in chronic kidney disease. *Seminars in Dialysis, 28*(6), 564–577. doi:10.1111/sdi.12411.

Fiaccadori, E., Maggiore, U., Cabassi, A., et al. (2013). Nutritional evaluation and management of AKI patients. *Journal of Renal Nutrition, 23*(3), 255–258. doi:10.1053/j.jrn.2013.01.025.

Gill, J. S., Klarenbach, S., Barnieh, L., et al. (2014). Financial incentives to increase Canadian organ donation: Quick fix or fallacy? *American Journal of Kidney Diseases, 63*(1), 133–140. doi:10.1053/j.ajkd.2013.08.029.

Goldstein-Fuchs, J., & Kalantar-Zadeh, K. (2015). Nutrition intervention for advanced stages of diabetic kidney disease. *Diabetes Spectrum, 28*(3), 181–186. doi:10.2337/diaspect.28.3.181.

Gowda, A., Pavan, M., & Babu, K. (2014). Vascular access profile in maintenance hemodialysis patients. *Iranian Journal of Kidney Diseases, 8*(3), 218–224.

Grams, M. E., Chow, E. H., Segev, D. L., et al. (2013). Lifetime incidence of CKD stages 3–5 in the United States. *American Journal of Kidney Diseases, 62*(2), 245–252. doi:10.1053/j.ajkd.2013.03.009.

Hain, D. J., & Haras, M. S. (2015). Chronic kidney disease. In C. S. Counts (Ed.), *Core curriculum for nephrology nursing* (5th ed.). Pitman, NJ: Anthony J. Jannetti.

Hoffart, N. (2014). The development of kidney transplant nursing. *Nephrology Nursing Journal, 41*(6), 127–138.

Hung, S., & Tarng, D. (2014). ESA and iron therapy in chronic kidney disease: A balance between patient safety and hemoglobin target. *Kidney International, 86*(4), 676–678. doi:10.1038/ki.2014.179.

Ikizler, T. A., Cano, N. J., Franch, H., et al. (2013). Prevention and treatment of protein energy wasting in chronic kidney disease patients: A consensus statement by the International Society of Renal Nutrition and Metabolism. *Kidney International, 84*(6), 1096–1107. doi:10.1038/ki.2013.147.

Jin, L., Wang, J., Wu, C., et al. (2015). Femoral arteriovenous fistula associated with leg swelling 6 months after removal of a hemodialysis catheter: A case report. *Medicine, 94*(40), 1–3. doi:10.1097/MD.0000000000001738.

Johnson, S. R. (2014). Home dialysis grows despite cost and logistical hurdles. *Modern Healthcare, 44*(41), 23–24.

Judd, E., & Calhoun, D. A. (2015). Management of hypertension in CKD: Beyond the guidelines. *Advances in Chronic Kidney Disease, 22*(2), 116–122. doi:10.1053/j.ackd.2014.12.001.

Kim, J. J., Langworthy, D. R., & Hennessey, E. K. (2014). Clinical implications of statin therapy in patients undergoing hemodialysis. *American Journal of Health-System Pharmacy, 71*(9), 703–710. doi:10.2146/ajhp130305.

Kovesdy, C. (2015). Management of hyperkalemia: An update for the internist. *American Journal of Medicine, 128*(12), 1281–1287. doi:10.1016/j.amjmed.2015.05.040.

Kuhan, G., Antoniou, G. A., Nikam, M., et al. (2013). A meta-analysis of randomized trials comparing surgery versus endovascular therapy for thrombosed arteriovenous fistulas and grafts in hemodialysis. *Cardiovascular & Interventional Radiology, 36*(3), 699–705. doi:10.1007/s00270-013-0564-8.

Lang, J. (2014). Taking action against acute kidney injury in primary care. *Clinical Advisor, 17*(11), 41–48.

Levin, A., Hemmelgarn, B., Culleton, B., et al. (2008). Guidelines for the management of chronic kidney disease. *Canadian Medical Association Journal, 179*(11), 1154–1162.

Libório, A. B., Leite, T. T., Neves, F. O., et al. (2015). AKI complications in critically ill patients: Association with mortality rates and RRT. *Clinical Journal of the American Society of Nephrology, 10*(1), 21–28. doi:10.2215/CJN.04750514.

Liles, A. M. (2014). Medication pitfalls in the CKD clinic: Case presentations. *Advances in Chronic Kidney Disease, 21*(4), 349–354. doi:10.1053/j.ackd.2014.03.014.

McAlister, F. A., Ezekowitz, J. A., Grisolia, E. F., et al. (2015). Clinical implications of the CKD epidemiology collaboration (CKD-EPI) equation compared with the modification of diet in renal disease (MDRD) study equation for the estimation of renal dysfunction in patients with cardiovascular disease. *Internal & Emergency Medicine, 10*(8), 955–963. doi:10.1007/s11739-015-1260-2.

Miller, P. D. (2014). Bone disease in CKD: A focus on osteoporosis diagnosis and management. *American Journal of Kidney Diseases, 64*(2), 290–304. doi:10.1053/j.ajkd.2013.12.018.

Moreland, J., & Phiri, E. (2015). Developing an interactive booklet for patients with acute kidney injury. *Journal of Renal Nursing, 7*(3), 138–141.

Murphy, F., & Byrne, G. (2010). The role of the nurse in the management of acute kidney injury. *British Journal of Nursing, 19*(3), 146–152.

National Institute of Diabetes and Digestive and Kidney Diseases. (2013). *Frequently asked questions about GFR.* Retrieved from *http://www.niddk.nih.gov/health-information/health-communication-programs/nkdep/lab-evaluation/faqs/Pages/faqs.aspx.*

Organ Registry Team (ORT) (Ottawa) & the Organ and Tissue Donation and Transplantation (OTDT) Team (Ottawa and Edmonton). (2015). Living donor paired exchange registry helps kidney patients get the transplants they need. *CANNT, 21*(1), 12.

Paramesh, A. S. (2013). What's new in the transplant OR? *AORN Journal, 97*(4), 435–447. doi:10.1016/j.aorn.2013.01.016.

Parnham, S., Gleadle, J. M., Leong, D., et al. (2015). Myocardial perfusion is impaired in asymptomatic renal and liver transplant recipients: A cardiovascular magnetic resonance study. *Journal of

Cardiovascular Magnetic Resonance (Biomed Central), 17(1), 1–9. doi:10.1186/s12968-015-0166-5.

Quintavalle, C., Donnarumma, E., Fiore, D., et al. (2013). Therapeutic strategies to prevent contrast-induced acute kidney injury. *Current Opinion in Cardiology, 28*(6), 676–682. doi:10.1097/HCO.0b013e3283653f41.

Ritchie, J., Rainone, F., Green, D., et al. (2013). Extreme elevations in blood pressure and all-cause mortality in a referred CKD population: Results from the CRISIS Study. *International Journal of Hypertension,* 1–8. doi:10.1155/2013/597906.

Sarafidis, P. A., & Bakris, G. L. (2015). Cardiovascular disease in CKD in 2014: New insights into cardiovascular risk factors and outcomes. *Nature Reviews. Nephrology, 11*(2), 70–72. doi:10.1038/nrneph.2014.242.

Schell, J. O., & Holley, J. L. (2013). Opportunities to improve end-of-life care in ESRD. *Clinical Journal of the American Society of Nephrology, 8*(12), 2028–2030. doi:10.2215/CJN.10321013.

Stevens, P. E., Lamb, E. J., & Levin, A. (2015). Integrating guidelines, CKD, multimorbidity, and older adults. *American Journal of Kidney Diseases, 65*(3), 494–501. doi:10.1053/j.ajkd.2014.09.024.

Trevitt, R., Dunsmore, V., Murphy, F., et al. (2012). Pre- and post-transplant care: Nursing management of the renal transplant recipient: Part 2. *Journal of Renal Care, 38*(2), 107–114. doi:10.1111/j.1755-6686.2012.00302.x.

Walton, B. (2015). Chronic kidney diseases: Stages and nursing care. *Ohio Nurses Review, 8*(3), 5–11.

Williams, L. (2014). Take aim at acute kidney injury with RIFLE criteria. *Nursing, 44*(7), 50–55. doi:10.1097/01.NURSE.0000445730.84886.88.

Wittwer, I. (2013). Iron deficiency anaemia in chronic kidney disease. *Journal of Renal Care, 39*(3), 182–188. doi:10.1111/j.1755-6686.2013.12026.x.

Young, B., Chan, C., Blagg, C., et al. (2012). How to overcome barriers and establish a successful home HD program. *Clinical Journal of the American Society of Nephrology, 7*(12), 2023–2032. doi:10.2215/CJN.07080712.

Zyga, S., & Kolovos, P. (2013). Cardiovascular disease and chronic inflammation in end stage kidney disease. *International Journal of Caring Sciences, 6*(1), 29–36.

RESOURCES

Canadian Association of Nephrology Nurses and Technologists (CANNT)
http://www.cannt.ca/

Canadian Institute for Health Information
http://www.cihi.ca

Canadian Organ Replacement Register (CORR)
*http://www.cihi.ca/CIHI-ext-portal/internet/en/document/
types+of+care/specialized+services/organ+replacements/
services_corr*

Canadian Society of Nephrology (CSN)
https://www.csnscn.ca/

Hypertension Canada
http://www.hypertension.ca/

The Kidney Foundation of Canada
http://www.kidney.ca/

International Society of Nephrology (ISN)
http://www.isn-online.org

International Transplant Nurses Society
http://www.itns.org

National Kidney Foundation
http://www.kidney.org

National Kidney Foundation: Calculators for Health Care Professionals
http://www.kidney.org/professionals/kdoqi/gfr_calculator.cfm

RenalWEB Patient Education
http://www.renalweb.com/topics/patiented/patiented.htm

United Network for Organ Sharing (UNOS)
http://www.unos.org

For additional Internet resources, see the website for this book at *http://evolve.elsevier.com/Canada/Lewis/medsurg.*

SECTION 10

Problems Related to Regulatory and Reproductive Mechanisms

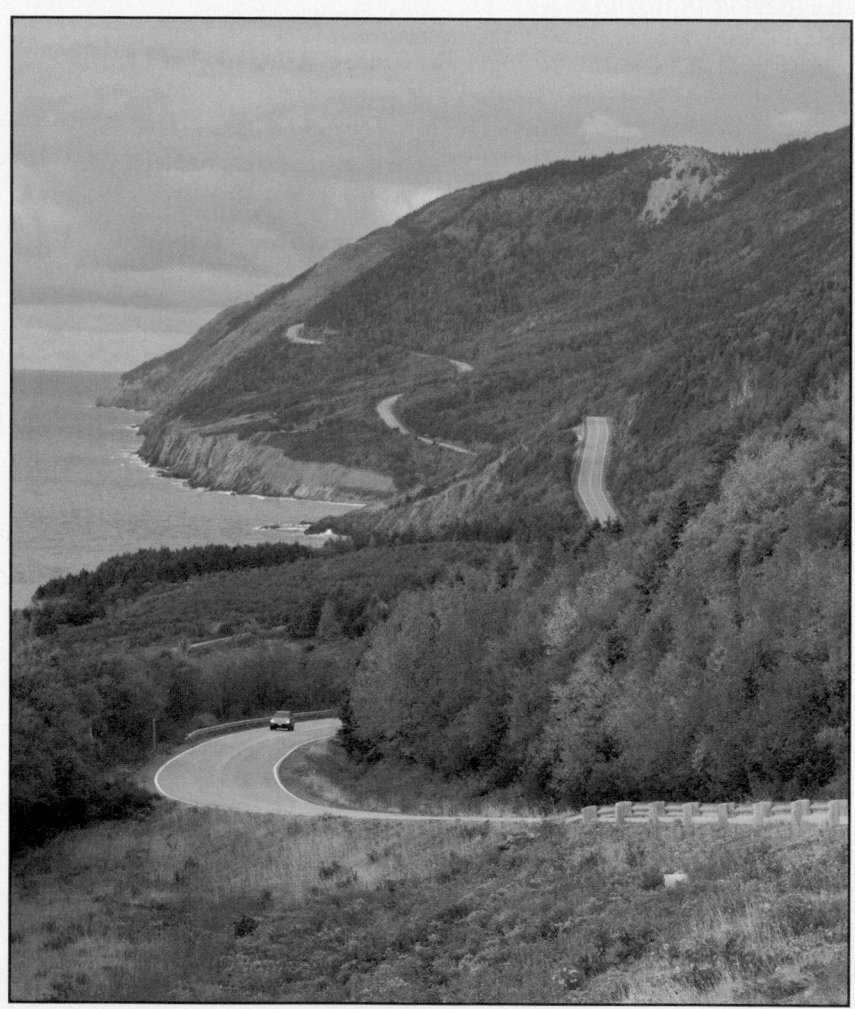

Source: Steve Smith/Shutterstock.com.

Nursing Assessment
Endocrine System

Written by: Katherine A. Kelly
Adapted by: Daphne Connolly

evolve WEBSITE

http://evolve.elsevier.com/Canada/Lewis/medsurg
- Review Questions (Online Only)
- Key Points
- Answer Guidelines for Case Study
- Conceptual Care Map Creator
- Audio Glossary
- Content Updates

LEARNING OBJECTIVES

1. Describe the common characteristics and the functions of hormones.
2. Identify the locations of the endocrine glands.
3. Describe the functions of hormones secreted by the pituitary, thyroid, parathyroid, and adrenal glands and the pancreas.
4. Describe the locations and the roles of hormone receptors.
5. Identify the significant subjective and objective assessment data related to the endocrine system that should be obtained from a patient through an interview, examination, and review of the relevant documentation.
6. Identify the appropriate technique to use in the physical assessment of the thyroid gland.
7. Relate age-related changes in the endocrine system to differences in assessment findings.
8. Differentiate normal from common abnormal findings in the physical assessment of the endocrine system.
9. Describe the purpose, significance of results, and nursing responsibilities related to diagnostic studies of the endocrine system.

KEY TERMS

aldosterone, p. 1242
antidiuretic hormone (ADH), p. 1240
catecholamines, p. 1241

corticosteroid, p. 1242
cortisol, p. 1242
glucagon, p. 1242
growth hormone (GH), p. 1239

hormone, p. 1236
insulin, p. 1242
islets of Langerhans, p. 1242
negative feedback, p. 1236

positive feedback, p. 1238
thyroxine (T$_4$), p. 1241
triiodothyronine (T$_3$), p. 1241
tropic hormones, p. 1239

The endocrine system and the nervous system are two of the primary communicating and coordinating systems in the body. The nervous system communicates through nerve impulses; the endocrine system communicates through chemical substances known as *hormones*, and it plays a role in reproduction, growth and development, and regulation of energy. The endocrine glands include the hypothalamus, pituitary gland, thyroid, parathyroids, adrenal glands, pancreas, ovaries, testes, and pineal gland (Figure 50-1). The pineal gland secretes melatonin and is involved in regulation of gonadal function and development, as well as chronobiological rhythms (Ben-Moshe, Foulkes, & Gothilf, 2014). In addition to the endocrine glands, other body organs secrete hormones. For example, the kidneys secrete erythropoietin, the heart secretes atrial natriuretic peptide, and the gastro-intestinal tract secretes numerous peptide hormones (e.g., gastrin). These hormones are discussed in their respective assessment chapters.

STRUCTURES AND FUNCTIONS OF THE ENDOCRINE SYSTEM

Glands

The organs of the endocrine system are referred to as *glands*. Endocrine glands produce chemical substances called *hormones* and secrete them into the blood, by which they eventually affect specific target tissues. A *target tissue* is the body tissue or organ on which the hormone has its effect. For example, the thyroid (the gland) synthesizes thyroxine (the hormone), which influences all body tissues (target tissue). It is important to note that not all glands in the body belong to the endocrine system. There are two types of glands: *Exocrine glands* secrete their substances into ducts that then empty into a body cavity or onto a surface (e.g., skin). For example, salivary glands produce saliva, which is secreted through salivary ducts into the mouth. *Endocrine glands,* in contrast, secrete their substances directly into the blood, not into ducts.

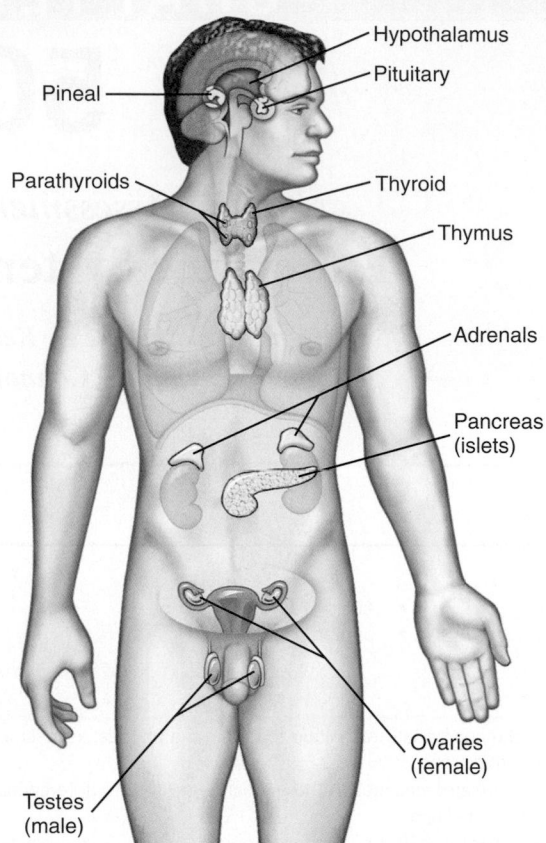

FIGURE 50-1 Location of the major endocrine glands. The parathyroid glands lie on the posterior surface of the thyroid. Source: Modified from Patton, K. T., & Thibodeau, G. A. (2013). *Anatomy and physiology.* (8th ed., p. 564, Figure 25-2). St Louis: Mosby.

Hormones

Classifications and Functions. A hormone is a chemical substance synthesized and secreted by a specific organ or tissue. Most hormones have common characteristics, including (a) secretion in small amounts at variable but predictable rates, (b) circulation through the blood, and (c) binding to specific cellular receptors either in the cell membrane or within the cell.

Hormones are classified by their chemical structure: *lipid-soluble hormones* and *water-soluble* (protein-based) *hormones.* Lipid-soluble hormones include steroid hormones (all hormones produced by the adrenal cortex and the sex glands) and thyroid hormones. All other hormones are water soluble (Ojeda & Kovacs, 2012). The differences in solubility are important for understanding how the hormone interacts with the target cell.

Hormones control a number of physiological activities. Important hormonal functions are related to reproduction, response to stress and injury, electrolyte balance, energy metabolism, growth, maturation, and aging. Hormones also play a role in the function of the nervous system. Some hormones have a regulatory effect on nervous tissue. For example, catecholamines are hormones when they are secreted by the adrenal medulla, but they act as neurotransmitters when secreted by nerve cells in the brain and the peripheral nervous system. When epinephrine travels through the blood, it is a hormone and affects target tissues. When it travels across synaptic junctions, it acts as a neurotransmitter (Barnes, Carson, & Nair, 2015). Hormones can also influence behaviour. For example, excess growth hormone,

cortisol, and parathyroid hormone can cause mood swings. Depression has been associated with adrenal insufficiency and hypothyroidism. Table 50-1 summarizes the major hormones, glands, or tissues from which they are synthesized, target organs or tissues, and functions.

Hormone Transport. Hormones are carried by the blood to other sites in the body where their actions are exerted. Some hormones (e.g., steroids and thyroid hormones) are not water soluble. Therefore, these types of hormones are bound to plasma proteins for transport in the blood. Although hormones are inactive when bound to plasma proteins, they can be released when appropriate and immediately exert their action at the target tissue. Water-soluble hormones (e.g., protein hormones, catecholamines) circulate freely in the blood and are not dependent on proteins for transport.

Targets and Receptors. As mentioned, hormones exert their effects on target tissue. The hormone recognizes the target tissue by attaching to receptors (the site that interacts with the hormone) in the cell membrane (e.g., protein-type hormone receptors) or within cells of the target tissue (e.g., thyroid and steroid hormone receptors). The specificity of hormone–target cell interaction is determined by receptors in a "lock-and-key" type of mechanism. Thus, a hormone acts only on cells that have a receptor specific for that hormone (Figure 50-2). The location of the receptor sites affects the mechanism of action for the hormone.

Protein Hormone Receptors. Protein hormone action is a two-step process. The receptor is located in the target cell membrane; thus the hormone itself acts as a "first messenger." The hormone–receptor interaction stimulates the production of a "second messenger" such as cyclic adenosine monophosphate (cAMP). cAMP works by activating enzymes to regulate intracellular activity (Figure 50-3).

Steroid Hormone Receptors. Steroid and thyroid hormone receptors are located inside the cell. Because these hormones are lipid soluble, they pass through the target cell membrane by passive diffusion and bind to receptor sites located in the cytoplasm or nucleus of the target cell (Molina, 2013). Intracellular hormone–receptor complexes, such as those observed in steroid hormone action, bind to specific sites on DNA to stimulate or inhibit the synthesis of messenger RNA. When new messenger RNA is synthesized, it migrates to the cytoplasm, where it stimulates the synthesis of new protein. These new proteins produce specific effects in the target cell (see Figure 50-3).

Regulation of Hormonal Secretion. Endocrine activity is regulated by specific mechanisms of varying levels of complexity. These mechanisms stimulate or inhibit hormone synthesis and secretion and include simple feedback, complex feedback, nervous system control, and physiological rhythms.

Simple Feedback. The regulation of hormone levels in the blood depends on a highly specialized mechanism called *feedback.* Feedback is based on the blood level of a particular substance. The substance may be a hormone or another chemical compound regulated by, or responsive to, a hormone. In negative feedback, the most common type of feedback system, the gland responds by increasing or decreasing the secretion of a hormone on the basis of feedback from various factors (Molina, 2013). Negative feedback is similar to the functioning of a thermostat in which cold air in a room activates the thermostat to release heat and hot air turns off the thermostat to prevent more hot air from entering the room.

The pattern of insulin secretion is a physiological example of negative feedback between glucose and insulin. Elevated blood

TABLE 50-1   MAJOR ENDOCRINE GLANDS AND HORMONES

Hormones	Target Tissue	Functions
Anterior Pituitary (Adenohypophysis)		
Growth hormone (GH) or somatotropin	All body cells	Promotes protein anabolism (growth, tissue repair) and lipid mobilization and catabolism
Thyroid-stimulating hormone (TSH) or thyrotropin	Thyroid gland	Stimulates synthesis and release of thyroid hormones, growth and function of thyroid gland
Adrenocorticotrophic hormone (ACTH)	Adrenal cortex	Fosters growth of adrenal cortex; stimulates secretion of corticosteroids
Gonadotropic hormones • Follicle-stimulating hormone (FSH) • Luteinizing hormone (LH)*	Reproductive organs	Stimulates sex hormone secretion, reproductive organ growth, reproductive processes
Melanocyte-stimulating hormone (MSH)	Melanocytes in skin	Increases melanin production in melanocytes to make skin darker in colour
Prolactin	Ovary and mammary glands in girls and women	Stimulates milk production in lactating women; increases response of follicles to LH and FSH.
	Testes in men	Stimulates testicular function in men.
Posterior Pituitary (Neurohypophysis)		
Oxytocin	Uterus; mammary glands	Stimulates milk secretion, uterine contractility
Antidiuretic hormone (ADH; vasopressin)	Renal tubules, vascular smooth muscle	Promotes reabsorption of water, vasoconstriction
Thyroid		
Thyroxine (T_4)	All body tissues	Precursor to T_3
Triiodothyronine (T_3)	All body tissues	Regulates metabolic rate of all cells and processes of cell growth and tissue differentiation
Calcitonin	Bone tissue	Regulates calcium and phosphorus blood levels; decreases serum Ca^{2+} levels
Parathyroids		
Parathyroid hormone (PTH), or parathormone	Bone, intestine, kidney tissues	Regulates calcium and phosphorus blood levels; promotes bone demineralization and increases intestinal absorption of Ca^{2+}; increases serum Ca^{2+} levels
Adrenal Medulla		
Epinephrine (adrenaline)	Sympathetic effectors	Increases in response to stress; enhances and prolongs effects of sympathetic nervous system
Norepinephrine (noradrenaline)	Sympathetic effectors	Increases in response to stress; enhances and prolongs effects of sympathetic nervous system
Adrenal Cortex		
Corticosteroids (e.g., cortisol, hydrocortisone)	All body tissues	Promotes metabolism, response to stress; anti-inflammatory
Androgens (e.g., DHEA androsterone) and estradiol	Reproductive organs	Promotes masculinization in men, growth and sexual activity in women
Mineralocorticoids (e.g., aldosterone)	Kidney	Regulates sodium and potassium balance and thus water balance
Pancreas (Islets of Langerhans)		
Insulin (from beta cells)	General	Promotes movement of glucose out of blood and into cells
Amylin (from beta cells)	Liver, stomach	Decreases gastric motility, glucagon secretion, and endogenous glucose release from liver; increases satiety
Glucagon (from alpha cells)	General	Stimulates glycogenolysis and gluconeogenesis
Somatostatin	Pancreas	Inhibits insulin and glucagon secretion
Pancreatic polypeptide	General	Influences regulation of pancreatic exocrine function and metabolism of absorbed nutrients
Gonads		
Women: Ovaries		
Estrogen	Reproductive system, breasts	Stimulates development of secondary sex characteristics, preparation of uterus for fertilization, and fetal development; stimulates bone growth
Progesterone	Reproductive system	Maintains lining of uterus necessary for successful pregnancy
Men: Testes		
Testosterone	Reproductive system	Stimulates development of secondary sex characteristics, spermatogenesis

*In men, sometimes referred to as interstitial cell-stimulating hormone (ICSH).
DHEA, dehydroepiandrosterone.

glucose levels stimulate the secretion of insulin from the pancreas. As blood glucose levels decrease, the stimulus for insulin secretion also decreases. The homeostatic mechanism is considered negative feedback because it reverses the change in blood glucose level. Another example of negative feedback is the relationship between calcium and parathyroid hormone (PTH). Low blood levels of calcium stimulate the parathyroid gland to release PTH, which acts on bone, the intestine, and the kidneys to increase blood calcium levels. The increased blood calcium levels then inhibit further PTH release (Figure 50-4).

Positive feedback is a second method of regulation of hormone secretion. The positive feedback mechanism increases the target organ action beyond normal. The action of oxytocin during childbirth is an example. The hormone oxytocin from the posterior pituitary gland stimulates and increases uterine contractions. The release of oxytocin is stimulated by pressure receptors in the vagina. As the fetus enters the vagina during childbirth, the pressure receptors sense increased pressure and signal the brain to release more oxytocin. Oxytocin release leads to stronger uterine contractions. When birth is finished, the stimulus to the pressure receptors in the vagina ends, and thus oxytocin secretion decreases.

Nervous System Control. In addition to chemical regulation, some endocrine glands are directly affected by the activity of the nervous system. Pain, emotion, sexual excitement, and stress can stimulate the nervous system to modulate hormone secretion. Neural involvement is initiated by the central nervous system and implemented by the sympathetic nervous system. For example, stress is sensed by the central nervous system, and the sympathetic nervous system secretes catecholamines that increase heart rate and blood pressure to deal with stress more effectively. (Effects of stress are discussed further in Chapter 8.)

Rhythms. Another regulatory mechanism affecting many hormonal secretions involves the rhythms of secretions. These

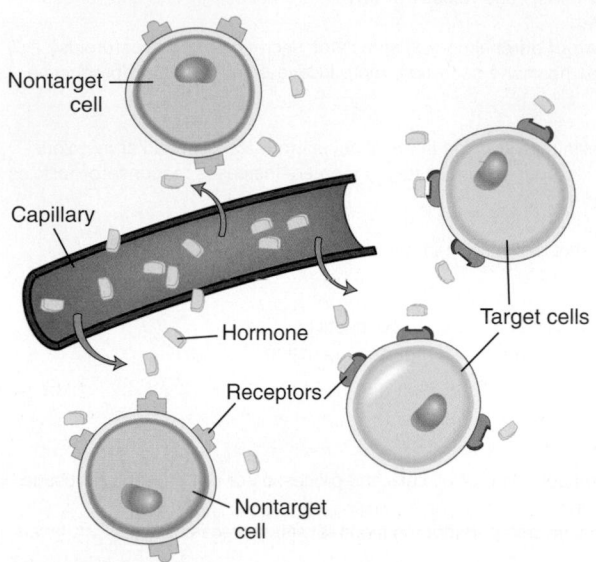

FIGURE 50-2 The target cell concept. Hormones act only on cells that have receptors specific to that hormone because the shape of the receptor determines which hormone can react with it. This is an example of the lock-and-key model of biochemical reactions.

FIGURE 50-3 Actions of protein and steroid hormones. **A,** Protein hormones bind to receptors located on the surface of the cell membrane. The hormone–receptor interaction stimulates the formation of cyclic adenosine monophosphate (cAMP), thereby activating various cell processes. Source: Herlihy, B. (2014). *The human body in health and illness.* (5th ed., p. 261, Figure 14-2 B & C). St. Louis: Elsevier Saunders.

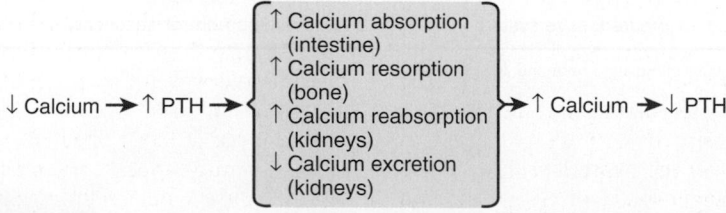

FIGURE 50-4 Feedback mechanism between parathyroid hormone (PTH) and calcium.

FIGURE 50-5 Circadian rhythm of cortisol secretion.

TABLE 50-2	HORMONES OF THE HYPOTHALAMUS

The following hormones from the hypothalamus target the anterior pituitary.

Releasing Hormones
- Corticotropin-releasing hormone (CRH)
- Gonadotropin-releasing hormone (GnRH)
- Growth hormone–releasing factor (GHRH), or somatotropin-releasing hormone
- Prolactin-releasing hormone (PRF)
- Thyrotropin-releasing hormone (TRH)

Inhibiting Hormones
- Prolactin-inhibiting hormone (PIH)
- Somatostatin (inhibits growth hormone release)

rhythms originate in brain structures. A common physiological rhythm is the *circadian rhythm,* in which a hormone level fluctuates predictably during a 24-hour period (Markova-Car, Jurišić, Ilić, et al., 2014). These rhythms may be related to sleep–wake or dark–light cycles. For example, in a person who sleeps at night, the cortisol level rises early in the day, declines toward evening, and rises again toward the end of sleep to peak by morning (Figure 50-5). Secretion of growth hormone and prolactin peaks during sleep. Thyroid-stimulating hormone (TSH) secretion is also maximal during sleep and ebbs 3 hours after a person awakens in the morning. The menstrual cycle is an example of a body rhythm that is longer than 24 hours *(infradian).* These rhythms must be considered when hormone levels on laboratory results are interpreted. (See the Diagnostic Studies of the Endocrine System section in this chapter and additional diagnostic studies sections in Chapter 51.)

Hypothalamus

The relationship between the hypothalamus and the pituitary gland is one of the most important aspects of the endocrine system. Although the pituitary gland has been referred to as the "master gland," most of its functions rely on an interrelationship with the hypothalamus. The hypothalamus and the pituitary gland integrate communication between the nervous and endocrine systems. Thus, neuroendocrinology is the study of the interactions between these two systems (McEwen, Gray, & Nasca, 2015). The hypothalamus is located in the most central part of the diencephalon area of the brain (see Figure 50-1). Although it is part of the brain, the hypothalamus secretes many hormones. Two important groups of hormones from the hypothalamus are releasing hormones and inhibiting hormones (Molina, 2013). The function of these hormones is to either stimulate (release) or inhibit the secretion of hormones from the anterior pituitary (Table 50-2).

The hypothalamus also contains neurons, which receive input from the brain stem and limbic system. These neurons influence the limbic system, brain stem, and spinal cord. This creates a circuit to facilitate the coordination of the endocrine system, the autonomic nervous system, and the expression of complex behavioural responses, such as anger and feelings of fear and pleasure.

Pituitary Gland

The pituitary gland *(hypophysis)* is very small: about the size of a pea. It is located in the sella turcica, under the hypothalamus, at the base of the brain above the sphenoid bone (see Figure 50-1). The pituitary gland is connected to the hypothalamus by the infundibular *(hypophyseal)* stalk. This stalk serves as a communication mechanism between the hypothalamus and the pituitary gland. The pituitary gland consists of two parts, the *anterior* lobe *(adenohypophysis)* and the *posterior* lobe *(neurohypophysis).* Hormones secreted from each of these pituitary lobes serve very different functions.

Anterior Pituitary Gland. The anterior lobe accounts for 80% of the gland by weight. As mentioned previously, the anterior pituitary is regulated by the hypothalamus through releasing and inhibiting hormones. These hypothalamic hormones reach the anterior pituitary through a network of capillaries known as the *hypothalamus–hypophyseal portal system.* The releasing and inhibiting hormones in turn affect the secretion of six hormones from the anterior pituitary gland (Figure 50-6; see Table 50-2).

Tropic Hormones. Several hormones secreted by the anterior pituitary gland are referred to as **tropic hormones.** These hormones control the secretion of hormones by other glands. TSH stimulates the thyroid gland to secrete thyroid hormones. Adrenocorticotrophic hormone (ACTH) stimulates the adrenal cortex to secrete corticosteroids. Follicle-stimulating hormone stimulates secretion of estrogen and the development of ova in the female and sperm in the male. Luteinizing hormone stimulates ovulation in girls and women and secretion of sex hormones in both sexes.

Growth Hormone. **Growth hormone (GH)** has effects on all body tissue. GH, as its name suggests, affects the growth and development of skeletal muscles and long bones, thereby affecting a person's size and height. It also has numerous biological actions, including a role in the metabolism of protein, fat, and carbohydrate (Molina, 2013).

Prolactin. Prolactin is a hormone that stimulates the breast development necessary for lactation after childbirth. Prolactin is also referred to as *lactogenic hormone.*

Posterior Pituitary Gland. The posterior pituitary is composed of nerve tissue and is essentially an extension of the hypothalamus. The communication between the hypothalamus and the posterior pituitary gland occurs through nerve tracts known as the *median eminence.* The hormones secreted by the posterior pituitary

FIGURE 50-6 Relationship among the hypothalamus, the pituitary, and the target organs. The hypothalamus communicates with the anterior pituitary via a capillary system and with the posterior pituitary via nerve tracts. The anterior and posterior pituitary hormones are shown with their target tissues. *FSH,* follicle-stimulating hormone; *LH,* luteinizing hormone. Source: Adapted from Patton, K. T., Thibodeau, G. A., & Douglas, M. M. (2012). *Essentials of anatomy & physiology* (p. 332, Figure 15-8). St. Louis: Elsevier Mosby.

gland—antidiuretic hormone and oxytocin—are actually produced in the hypothalamus. These hormones travel down the nerve tracts from the hypothalamus to the posterior pituitary gland and are stored until their release is triggered by the appropriate stimuli (see Figure 50-6).

Antidiuretic Hormone. The major physiological role of **antidiuretic hormone (ADH)**—also called *vasopressin*—is regulation of fluid volume by stimulating reabsorption of water in the renal tubules. ADH is also a potent vasoconstrictor.

The most important stimulus of ADH secretion is *plasma osmolality,* a measure of solute concentration of circulating blood (Figure 50-7). Plasma osmolality increases when there is a decrease in extracellular fluid or an increase in solute concentration. The increased plasma osmolality activates osmoreceptors, which are extremely sensitive, specialized neurons in the hypothalamus. These activated osmoreceptors stimulate ADH release (Molina, 2013). Table 50-3 lists factors that affect ADH release. When ADH is released, the renal tubules reabsorb water, causing urine to be more concentrated. When ADH release is inhibited, renal tubules do not reabsorb water, causing urine to be more dilute.

Oxytocin. Oxytocin stimulates both ejection of milk into mammary ducts and contraction of uterine smooth muscle. Oxytocin secretion is increased by stimulation of touch receptors in the nipples of lactating women and of vaginal pressure receptors.

Pineal Gland. The pineal gland is located in the brain and is composed of photoreceptive cells. The secretion of the hormone melatonin is its primary function. Melatonin secretion is increased in response to exposure to the dark and decreased in response

FIGURE 50-7 Relationship of plasma osmolality to antidiuretic hormone (ADH) release and action.

to light. The gland helps to regulate circadian rhythms and the reproductive system at the onset of puberty.

Thyroid Gland

The thyroid gland is located in the anterior portion of the neck, in front of the trachea. It consists of two encapsulated lateral lobes

TABLE 50-3	FACTORS AFFECTING RELEASE OF ANTIDIURETIC HORMONE
Stimulate Release	**Inhibit Release**
• Decreased fluid volume	• β-Adrenergic agonists
• Hypotension	• Alcohol
• Increased plasma osmolality	• Decreased plasma osmolality
• Nausea and vomiting	• Increased fluid volume
• Pain	

FIGURE 50-9 The adrenal gland is composed of the adrenal cortex and the adrenal medulla.

FIGURE 50-8 Thyroid and parathyroid glands. Note the surrounding structures. Source: Thibodeau, G. A., & Patton, K. T. (2010). *The human body in health and disease* (5th ed., p. 321, Figure 11-7). St. Louis: Mosby.

connected by a narrow isthmus (Figure 50-8). The thyroid is a highly vascular organ and is regulated by TSH from the anterior pituitary. The three hormones produced and secreted by the thyroid gland are thyroxine, triiodothyronine, and calcitonin.

Thyroxine and Triiodothyronine. The major function of the thyroid gland is the production, storage, and release of the thyroid hormones: **thyroxine (T_4)** and **triiodothyronine (T_3)**. T_4 is by far the most abundant thyroid hormone, accounting for 90% of thyroid hormone produced by the thyroid gland. T_3, however, is much more potent and has greater metabolic effects. About 20% of circulating T_3 is secreted directly by the thyroid gland, and the remainder is obtained by peripheral conversion of T_4 (Molina, 2013). Iodine is necessary for the synthesis of thyroid hormones. T_4 and T_3 affect metabolic rate, caloric requirements, oxygen consumption, carbohydrate and lipid metabolism, growth and development, brain function, and nervous system activity. More than 99% of thyroid hormones are bound to plasma proteins, especially T_4-binding globulin synthesized by the liver. Only the unbound "free" hormones are biologically active.

Thyroid hormone production and release is stimulated by TSH from the anterior pituitary gland. When circulating levels of thyroid hormone are low, the hypothalamus releases thyrotropin-releasing hormone (TRH), which in turn causes the anterior pituitary gland to release TSH. High levels of circulating thyroid hormone have an inhibitory effect on the secretion of both TRH from the hypothalamus and TSH from the anterior pituitary gland (Molina, 2013).

Calcitonin. Calcitonin is a hormone produced by C cells (parafollicular cells) of the thyroid gland in response to high circulating calcium levels. Calcitonin inhibits calcium resorption (loss of substance) from bone, increases calcium storage in bone,

and increases renal excretion of calcium and phosphorus, thereby lowering serum calcium levels. Although it provides a counter-mechanism to PTH, calcitonin does not play a critical role in calcium balance (Molina, 2013).

Parathyroid Glands

The parathyroid glands are small, oval structures usually arranged in pairs behind each thyroid lobe (see Figure 50-8). Most people have four such glands. The major cell type of the glands is epithelial, and the glands are richly supplied with blood from the inferior and superior thyroid arteries.

Parathyroid Hormone. The parathyroids secrete parathyroid hormone (PTH) (also called *parathormone*). Its major role is to regulate the blood level of calcium. PTH acts on bone, the kidneys, and indirectly, the gastro-intestinal tract. In bone, PTH stimulates bone resorption and inhibits bone formation, which results in the release of calcium and phosphate into the blood. In the kidneys, PTH increases calcium reabsorption and phosphate excretion. In addition, PTH stimulates the renal conversion of vitamin D to its most active form (1,25-dihydroxyvitamin D_3). This active form then enhances the intestinal absorption of calcium.

The secretion of PTH is directly regulated by a feedback system (see Figure 50-4) and is not under pituitary and hypothalamic control. When the serum calcium level is low, PTH secretion increases; when the serum calcium level rises, PTH secretion falls. In addition, high levels of active vitamin D inhibit PTH secretion, and low levels of magnesium stimulate PTH secretion.

Adrenal Glands

The adrenal glands are small, paired, highly vascularized glands located on the upper portion of each kidney. Each gland consists of two parts: the medulla and the cortex (Figure 50-9). Each part has distinct functions, and the glands act independently of one another.

Adrenal Medulla. The adrenal medulla is the inner part of the gland and consists of sympathetic postganglionic neurons. The medulla secretes the catecholamines *epinephrine* (adrenalin), *norepinephrine* (noradrenaline), and *dopamine*. **Catecholamines**, usually considered neurotransmitters, are hormones when secreted by the adrenal medulla because they are released into the circulation and transported to their target organs. Catecholamines exert their effects after binding to adrenergic receptors on cells, and they have widespread effects on all body systems. Catecholamines are an essential part of the body's response to stress (see Chapter 8).

Adrenal Cortex. The adrenal cortex is the outer part of the adrenal gland. It secretes more than 50 steroid hormones, which are classified as *glucocorticoids, mineralocorticoids,* and *androgens.* Cholesterol is the precursor for steroid hormone synthesis. Glucocorticoids (e.g., cortisol) are named for their effects on glucose metabolism. Mineralocorticoids (e.g., aldosterone) are essential for the maintenance of fluid and electrolyte balance. Adrenal androgens are produced and secreted in small but significant amounts. The term corticosteroid refers to any of the hormones synthesized by the adrenal cortex (excluding androgens).

Cortisol. Cortisol, the most abundant and potent glucocorticoid, is necessary to maintain life. One major function of cortisol is the regulation of blood glucose concentration. Cortisol increases blood glucose through stimulation of hepatic gluconeogenesis (conversion of amino acids to glucose) and inhibiting protein synthesis (Molina, 2013). Cortisol also decreases peripheral glucose use in the fasting state.

Another major effect of glucocorticoids is their anti-inflammatory action and supportive actions in response to stress. A marked increase in the rate of cortisol secretion by the adrenal cortex aids the body in coping more effectively with stressful situations (see Chapter 8). Cortisol decreases the inflammatory response by stabilizing the membranes of cellular lysosomes and preventing increased capillary permeability. The lysosomal stabilization reduces the release of proteolytic enzymes and thereby limits their destructive effect on surrounding tissue. Cortisol can also inhibit production of prostaglandins, thromboxanes, and leukotrienes and alter the cell-mediated immune response.

Cortisol helps maintain vascular integrity and fluid volume. It has a mineralocorticoid effect because it can bind to mineralocorticoid receptors.

Cortisol is secreted in a diurnal pattern (see Figure 50-5). The major control of cortisol is by means of a negative feedback mechanism that involves the secretion of corticotropin-releasing hormone from the hypothalamus. This hormone stimulates the secretion of ACTH by the anterior pituitary. Cortisol levels are also increased by surgical stress, burns, infection, fever, psychoses, acute anxiety, and hypoglycemia.

Aldosterone. Aldosterone is a potent mineralocorticoid that maintains extracellular fluid volume. It acts at the renal tubule to promote renal reabsorption of sodium and excretion of potassium and hydrogen ions. Aldosterone synthesis and secretion are stimulated by angiotensin II, hyponatremia, and hyperkalemia and inhibited by atrial natriuretic peptide and hypokalemia.

Adrenal Androgens. The third class of steroids synthesized and secreted by the adrenal cortex are the androgens. Normally, the adrenal cortex secretes small amounts of androgens. Adrenal androgens stimulate pubic and axillary hair growth and sex drive in women. In girls and women, androgens are converted to estrogen in the peripheral tissues. In postmenopausal women, the major source of estrogen is from the peripheral conversion of adrenal androgen to estrogen. The effects of adrenal androgen in men are negligible in comparison with testosterone secreted by the testes.

Pancreas

The pancreas is a long, tapered, lobular, soft gland located behind the stomach and anterior to the first and second lumbar

vertebrae. The pancreas has both exocrine and endocrine functions. The hormone-secreting portion of the pancreas is referred to as the islets of Langerhans. The islets account for less than 2% of the gland and consist of four types of hormone-secreting cells: α, β, delta, and F cells. α Cells produce and secrete the hormone glucagon. Insulin and amylin are produced and secreted by β cells. Somatostatin is produced and secreted by the delta cells. Pancreatic polypeptide is secreted by the F (or PP) cells.

Glucagon. Glucagon is synthesized and released from pancreatic α cells in response to low levels of blood glucose, to protein ingestion, and to exercise. Glucagon increases blood glucose levels by stimulating glycogenolysis, gluconeogenesis, and ketogenesis. Usually, glucagon and insulin function in a reciprocal manner to maintain normal blood glucose levels. The exception is after ingestion of a high-protein, carbohydrate-free diet, in which case both hormones are secreted. In this instance, glucagon counteracts the inhibitory effect of insulin on gluconeogenesis, and normal blood glucose levels are maintained.

Insulin. Insulin is the principal regulator of the metabolism and storage of ingested carbohydrates, fats, and proteins. Insulin facilitates glucose transport across cell membranes in most tissues. However, the brain, nerves, lens of the eye, hepatocytes, erythrocytes, and cells in the intestinal mucosa and kidney tubules are not dependent on insulin for glucose uptake. An increased blood glucose level is the major stimulus for insulin synthesis and secretion. Other stimuli to insulin secretion are increased amino acid levels and vagal stimulation. Insulin secretion is usually inhibited by low blood glucose levels and by glucagon, somatostatin, hypokalemia, and catecholamines (Table 50-4).

A major effect of insulin on glucose metabolism occurs in the liver, where the hormone enhances glucose incorporation into glycogen and triglycerides by altering enzymatic activity and inhibiting gluconeogenesis. Another major effect occurs in peripheral tissues, where insulin facilitates glucose transport into cells, transport of amino acids across muscle membranes and their synthesis into protein, and transport of triglycerides into adipose tissue. Thus, insulin is a storage, or *anabolic,* hormone.

The endocrine system functions to regulate body processes and maintain internal homeostasis despite vastly changing substrates, as is observed in glucose homeostasis after food ingestion. After a meal, insulin is responsible for the storage of nutrients *(anabolism).* In the fasting state (during which ingested glucose is not readily available), hormones such as catecholamines, cortisol, and glucagon break down stored complex fuels *(catabolism)* to provide simple glucose as fuel for energy.

TABLE 50-4	FACTORS INFLUENCING SECRETION OF INSULIN
Stimulate Secretion	**Inhibit Secretion**
↑ Glucose levels	↓ Glucose levels
↑ Amino acid levels	↓ Amino acid levels
↑ Gastro-intestinal hormone levels	↓ Potassium levels
↑ Vagal stimulation	↑ Corticosteroid hormone levels
↑ Fats	↑ Catecholamine levels
	↑ Somatostatin levels
	↑ Glucagon levels (usually)
	↑ Insulin levels

AGE-RELATED CONSIDERATIONS

THE ENDOCRINE SYSTEM

Normal aging has many effects on the endocrine system (Table 50-5). These include (a) decreased hormone production and secretion, (b) altered hormone metabolism and biological activity, (c) decreased responsiveness of target tissues to hormones, and (d) alterations in circadian rhythms.

Assessment of the effects of aging on the endocrine system is difficult because the subtle changes of aging often mimic manifestations of endocrine disorders. Some endocrine changes associated with aging are obvious; others are subtle. The nurse must be aware that endocrine problems may manifest differently in an older adult than in a younger person. Older adults may have multiple comorbid conditions and take multiple medications that alter the body's usual response to endocrine dysfunction. Symptoms of endocrine dysfunction such as fatigue, constipation, or mental impairment in older adults are often missed because they are attributed solely to aging. It is important that the nurse consider age-related endocrine changes when assessing an older adult (Saxon, Etten, & Perkins, 2014).

ASSESSMENT OF THE ENDOCRINE SYSTEM

Hormones affect every body tissue and system, causing great diversity in the signs and symptoms of endocrine dysfunction. Therefore, assessment of the endocrine system is often difficult, and keen clinical skills are required to detect manifestations of disorders. Endocrine dysfunction may result from deficient or excessive hormone secretion, transport abnormalities, an inability of the target tissue to respond to a hormone, or inappropriate stimulation of the target-tissue receptor.

Endocrine disorders may have specific or nonspecific (vague) clinical manifestations. When signs and symptoms are specific, such as the classic "polys" (polyuria, polydipsia, and polyphagia) in diabetes mellitus, the assessment is easier; nonspecific signs and symptoms, such as tachycardia, palpitations, fatigue, or altered mood, are more problematic. Nonspecific changes should alert the health care provider to the possibility of an endocrine disorder. The most common nonspecific symptoms, fatigue and depression, often are accompanied by other manifestations such as changes in energy level, alertness, sleep patterns, mood, affect, weight, skin, hair, personal appearance, and sexual function.

Subjective Data

The lack of clear-cut manifestations of endocrine problems necessitates a conscientious and detailed health history. A thorough health history yields data to help sort out possible causes and the effect of the problem on the person's life (Table 50-6).

Important Health Information

Past Health History. During an assessment, the patient should be questioned about the general state of health and whether any changes in it have occurred. In addition, the patient or significant other should be specifically questioned about previous or current endocrine abnormalities and abnormal patterns of growth and development.

Family History. Heredity can play a major role in the occurrence of endocrine problems. The patient should be questioned about conditions in family members such as diabetes mellitus or insipidus; hyperthyroidism or hypothyroidism; or goiter (see Table 50-6 for more examples). Such questioning frequently elicits information about a familial tendency.

Medications. The patient should be questioned about the use of all medications (both prescription and over-the-counter drugs) and the use of herbs and dietary supplements. The patient should be asked the reason for taking the drug, the dosage, and the length of time taken. The patient should specifically be asked about the use of hormone replacements. Information that the patient is currently taking hormone replacements such as insulin, thyroid hormone, or corticosteroids (e.g., prednisone) helps direct the nurse in regard to possible problems associated with the use of these agents. For example, corticosteroids may cause glucose intolerance in susceptible patients by increasing

TABLE 50-5 AGE-RELATED DIFFERENCES IN ASSESSMENT

Endocrine System

Changes	Clinical Significance
Thyroid	
Atrophy of thyroid gland; decrease in TSH and T_3 secretion; increased nodules	Increased incidence of hypothyroidism with aging; however, most older adults maintain adequate thyroid function. Thyroid hormone replacement dose lower in older adults.
Parathyroid	
Increased secretion of PTH and increased basal level of PTH	Increased calcium resorption from bone (demineralization); hypercalcemia, hypercalciuria (may reflect defective renal mechanism)
Adrenal Cortex	
Adrenal cortex: more fibrotic and slightly smaller	Decreased metabolic clearance rate for glucocorticoids
Decreased metabolism of cortisol	
Decreased plasma levels of adrenal androgens and aldosterone	
Adrenal Medulla	
Increased secretion and basal level of norepinephrine. No change in plasma epinephrine levels.	Decreased responsiveness to β-adrenergic agonists and receptor blockers
Decreased β-adrenergic receptor response to norepinephrine	May partly explain increased incidence of hypertension with aging
Pancreas	
Increase in fibrosis and fatty deposits in pancreas. Increased glucose intolerance and decreased sensitivity to insulin.	May partly contribute to increased incidence of diabetes mellitus with advanced aging
Gonads	
Women: decline in estrogen secretion	Women experience symptoms associated with menopause and have increased risk for atherosclerosis and osteoporosis
Men: decline in testosterone secretion	Men may or may not experience symptoms

PTH, parathyroid hormone; T_3, triiodothyronine; T_4, thyroxine; *TSH,* thyroid-stimulating hormone.

TABLE 50-6   HEALTH HISTORY

Endocrine System: Questions for Obtaining Subjective Data

Past History
- Do you have any previous or current problems with your endocrine system (e.g., problems with thyroid, diabetes, changes in facial or body hair)?
- Have you had any previous hospitalizations, surgical procedures, or treatments for endocrine problems?
- Are you currently taking or have you ever taken medications for an endocrine problem such as a thyroid disorder or diabetes?

Family History
- Is there any family history of diabetes mellitus or insipidus; hyperthyroidism or hypothyroidism; goitre; hypertension or hypotension; obesity; infertility; growth problems; pheochromocytoma (neoplastic tumour of the adrenal medulla or sympathetic ganglia); autoimmune diseases (e.g., Addison's disease); or adrenal hyperplasia?
- Have any other members of your family ever had a problem similar to your problem today?

Review of Systems
Overall Health Status
- How do you feel generally? Have you had any changes recently to your health?
- Have there been any changes in your appetite or weight?*
- Have you noticed any changes in your ability to perform your usual activities in comparison with last year? Five years ago?*
- Do you experience fatigue with or without activity?*

Eyes, Ears, Nose, Mouth, and Throat
- Have you experienced any blurring or double vision?* When was your last eye examination?
- Have you noticed any difficulty swallowing?*
- Are your shirts harder to button at the neck?

Cardiovascular System
- Do you experience heart palpitations?*

Musculo-Skeletal System
- Do you have difficulty holding things because of shakiness of your hands?*

Gastro-Intestinal System
- Describe your usual bowel pattern. Have you noted any bowel changes?*
- Do you use anything, such as laxatives, to help you move your bowels?*

Genito-Urinary System
- Do you have to get up at night to urinate? If so, how many times? Do you keep water by your bed at night?
- Have you ever had a kidney stone?*

Neurological System
- Do you feel more nervous than you used to? Do you notice your heart pounding or that you sweat at times when you do not think you should be sweating?
- How is your memory? Have you noticed any changes?
- How long can you concentrate on any one thing? Has this changed lately?

Endocrine System
- Do you feel that most rooms are too hot or too cold? Do you frequently have to put on a sweater, or do you feel as though you need to open windows when others in the room seem comfortable?*

Integumentary System
- Have you noticed any changes in the distribution of the hair anywhere on your body?*
- Have you noticed any changes in the colour of your skin, particularly on your face, neck, hands, or body creases?*
- Has the texture of your skin changed? For example, does it seem thicker and drier than it used to?*

Sexual and Reproductive History
Women
- When did you start to menstruate? Was this earlier or later than other women in your family? If you still menstruate, do you have scant, heavy, or irregular menstrual flows?
- How many children have you had? How much did they weigh at birth? Were you told you had diabetes during any pregnancy?*
- Were you able to nurse your children if you wanted to?
- Are you menopausal? If so, for how long?
- Are you attempting to get pregnant but cannot?* Are you in treatment to become pregnant? * Are you using birth control? *
- Are you postmenopausal? If so, do you have any vaginal bleeding?

Men
- Have you noticed any changes in your ability to have an erection?*
- Are you trying to have children but cannot?*

Functional Assessment (Including Activities of Daily Living)
Activity and Mobility
- Do you have a planned exercise program? If yes, what is it, and have you had to make any changes in this routine lately? If so, why and what kinds of changes?

Sleep and Rest
- How many hours do you sleep at night? Do you feel rested on awakening?
- Are you ever awakened by sweating during the night?*
- Do you have nightmares?*
- Does anyone in your family complain about your snoring?*

Nutrition and Elimination
- What is your weight and height?
- How much do you want to weigh?
- Have there been any changes in your appetite or weight?*

Interpersonal Relationships
- Are you in a relationship? Are you able to take care of any significant others that need your assistance? Are you able to take care of your home? If not, why not?

Coping and Stress Management
- What kind of stressors do you have?
- How do you deal with stress or problems?
- What is your support system? To whom do you turn when you have a problem?
- Do you feel sad or uninterested in life?*

Occupational Health
- Where do you work? What kind of work do you do? Are you able to do what is expected of you and what you expect of yourself?
- If you are retired, what do you do with your time? What did you do before you retired?
- If you are unemployed, are you looking for work?

Self-Care and Health Promotion Activities
- Women: Have you had a mammogram or Pap smear recently?
- Men: Have you had a prostate examination recently?
- Both: If so, what were the results and dates of these tests? How often do you have these tests?

*If yes, describe.

Source: Adapted from Jarvis, C., Browne, A. J., MacDonald-Jenkins, J., et al. (Eds.). (2014). *Physical examination and health assessment.* (2nd Canadian ed.). (pp. 66–73). Toronto: Elsevier Canada.

glycogenolysis and insulin resistance. The adverse effects of many nonhormone medications can contribute to problems affecting endocrine function. For example, many drugs can affect blood glucose levels.

Surgery and Other Treatments. The nurse should inquire about previous hospitalizations, surgery, chemotherapy, and radiation therapy (especially irradiation of the neck). Surgery of the brain or a severe blow to the head could have resulted in pituitary or hypothalamic alterations.

Objective Data

Most endocrine glands are inaccessible for direct examination. With the exception of the thyroid and the male gonads, the glands are deeply encased in the body, protected against injury and trauma. However, assessment can be accomplished with a variety of objective data. The nurse must understand the actions of hormones so that by monitoring the target tissue, he or she can assess the function of a gland.

Physical Examination. The nurse must remember that the endocrine system affects every body system. Clinical manifestations of endocrine function vary significantly, depending on the gland involved. Specific clinical findings for the various endocrine problems are discussed in Chapters 51 and 52. Regardless of the type of endocrine dysfunction, the following general examination procedure should be followed.

Vital Signs. All vital signs are measured at the beginning of the examination. Variations in temperature may be associated with thyroid dysfunction. Cardiovascular changes such as tachycardia, bradycardia, hypotension, or hypertension may occur with a variety of endocrine-related problems.

Height and Weight. Assessment of the endocrine system includes a history of growth and development patterns, weight distribution and changes, and comparisons of these factors with normal findings. Growth pattern abnormalities are suggestive of problems associated with growth hormone. Changes in weight also may be associated with endocrine dysfunction. Thyroid disorders and diabetes mellitus are examples of endocrine disorders that can affect body weight. Body mass index is a height-to-weight ratio used to assess nutritional status (see Chapter 43, Figure 43-1).

CASE STUDY

Patient Introduction

Source: aastock/ Shutterstock .com.

Lydia Mollon is a 35-yr-old woman who comes to the clinic complaining of "just not feeling well." She is accompanied by her partner, Holly. She states that she has gained a lot of weight despite trying to watch her diet and just seems to be getting more and more tired. Holly voices concerns about changes in her partner's energy level.

Critical Thinking

Throughout this assessment chapter, think about Ms. Mollon's concerns with the following questions in mind:

1. What are the possible causes of Ms. Mollon's weight gain, fatigue, and irritability?
2. What would be the priority assessment of Ms. Mollon?
3. What questions should be asked of Ms. Mollon?
4. What should be included in the physical assessment? What should be looked for?
5. What diagnostic studies should be ordered?

Ms. Mollon and her condition will be followed throughout this assessment chapter. See below and pp. 1247 and 1254 for more information on Ms. Mollon.

evolve

Answers available at *http://evolve.elsevier.com/Canada/Lewis/medsurg.*

CASE STUDY

Subjective Data

Source: aastock/ Shutterstock .com.

A focused subjective assessment of Lydia Mollon revealed the following information.

Past Medical History: Denies any medical or surgical history. Has not seen a health care provider (HCP) for 8 years.

Medications: None.

Overall Health Management: Ms. Mollon works as a receptionist for a local law firm and states it is all she can do some days to make it through the workday.

Functional Assessment

Sleep and Rest: Ms. Mollon states that she frequently wakes up with a headache and goes to bed with the same headache, describing it as a dull, throbbing ache between her eyes. She sleeps 10+ hr at night but does not feel rested on awakening.

She definitely does not have the energy she had 5 yr ago or even 6 mo ago. She used to enjoy gardening and going out with their friends but now can barely manage work and coming home.

Ms. Mollon states that she has no ambition to exercise. She is just too tired at the end of the workday and has no energy on the weekends either. She also complains of leg cramps with walking.

Nutrition, Elimination and Metabolic History: Ms. Mollon reports a steady weight gain over the past 6 mo, mainly in her abdominal area. She feels as if she looks pregnant but knows that is not possible. Her appetite has actually decreased but she has not been able to lose any weight. She

says she feels "bloated." She also complains of facial hair growth and has noticed that she bruises easily. Whenever she gets a bug bite, it seems to take forever to heal. Ms. Mollon denies difficulty with swallowing, hoarseness, palpitations, or tremors. She also denies any changes or difficulty with urination or bowel movements.

Coping and Stress Management: Ms. Mollon is worried she is going crazy. She finds herself easily angered and irritable, frequently snapping at co-workers and her partner. She states this is not her usual self and she at first thought it was because she was dealing with a constant, dull headache.

Lately, she has noticed that her vision is blurry and that is making work and life even more difficult and stressful. When asked about her headache, she states it hurts between her eyes. She rates the pain as a 4 on a scale of 0 to 10 and states that acetaminophen or ibuprofen does not alleviate the pain. The pain is typically worse on arising in the morning and slowly decreases during the day.

Ms. Mollon hates the way she looks. She says when she looks in the mirror, she can't believe what she sees. She feels as if she has aged 10 yr over the past 6 mo and has gained weight in her face, neck, and trunk. She is concerned that her scalp hair is thinning and she is growing a beard. She states that she is beginning to wonder if she is "turning into a man!"

Ms. Mollon states that she is finding it more and more difficult to cope with the stresses of her job, her relationship with her partner, and life in general. She believes her emotions are very "raw and labile," totally different from the easy-going, smiling person she had once prided herself in being.

See pp. 1247 and 1254 for more information on Ms. Mollon.

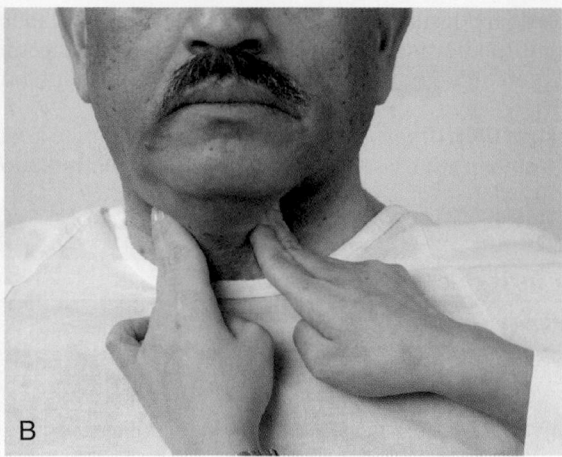

FIGURE 50-10 Palpation of the thyroid gland. **A,** Posterior approach. **B,** Anterior approach. Source: Wilson, S., & Giddens, J. F. (2013). *Health assessment for nursing practice* (5th ed., p. 177, Figure 19-53). St. Louis: Mosby Elsevier.

It may also be helpful to compare the patient's current body weight to the usual body weight in order to assess changes. Weight change (percentage) is calculated by subtracting the current body weight from the usual weight, dividing by the usual body weight, and multiplying by 100.

Mental–Emotional Status. Throughout the examination, the patient's orientation, alertness, memory, affect, personality, anxiety, appropriateness of dress, and speech pattern should be assessed objectively. Endocrine disorders can commonly cause changes in mental and emotional status.

Integument. The nurse should note the colour and the texture of skin, hair, and nails. The overall skin colour should be noted, as should pigmentation, and any ecchymosis should be documented. Hyperpigmentation, or "bronzing," of the skin (particularly on knuckles, elbows, knees, genitalia, and palmar creases) is a classic finding in Addison's disease but also is present with ACTH-producing tumours and acromegaly (Jarvis, Browne, MacDonald-Jenkins, et al., 2014). The nurse should palpate the skin for texture and presence of moisture. The nurse should also examine the hair distribution, not only on the head but also on the face, the trunk, and the extremities. The appearance and texture of the hair should be examined. Dull, brittle hair; excessive hair growth; or hair loss may indicate endocrine dysfunction.

Head. The size and contour of the head are inspected. Facial features should be symmetrical. Inspect the eyes for position, symmetry, shape, movement, opacity over the lens, eyelid lag, and edema. Visual acuity should also be checked because changes may be associated with a pituitary tumour or diabetic retinopathy. In the mouth, the buccal mucosa, the condition of the teeth (malocclusion and mottling), and tongue size should be inspected, and fasciculations (localized, unco-ordinated, uncontrollable twitching of a single muscle group) documented.

Neck. When inspecting the thyroid gland, the nurse should make observations first in the normal position (preferably with side lighting), then with the patient's neck in slight extension, and then as the patient swallows some water. The trachea should be midline, and the neck should appear symmetrical. Any unusual bulging over the thyroid area should be noted. If enlargement of the thyroid gland is not noticeable, palpation can be performed.

(Because palpation can trigger the release of thyroid hormones, palpation should be deferred in patients with a visibly enlarged thyroid gland.) When the thyroid is enlarged, the lateral lobes should be auscultated with the stethoscope bell to determine the presence of a bruit.

The thyroid gland is difficult to palpate. Thyroid palpation requires considerable practice, as well as validation by a more experienced examiner. Water should always be available for the patient to swallow as part of this examination. There are two acceptable approaches to thyroid palpation: anterior and posterior. For *anterior palpation,* the nurse stands in front of the patient, with the patient's neck flexed (Figure 50-10, *B*). The nurse places a thumb horizontally with the upper edge along the lower border of the patient's cricoid cartilage. The thumb is then moved over the isthmus as the patient swallows water. The fingers are then placed laterally to the anterior border of the sternocleidomastoid muscle, and each lateral lobe is palpated before and while the patient swallows water.

For *posterior palpation,* the nurse stands behind the patient (Figure 50-10, *A*). With the thumbs of both hands resting on the nape of the patient's neck, the nurse uses the index and middle fingers of both hands to feel for the thyroid isthmus and for the anterior surfaces of the lateral lobes. To facilitate the examination of each lobe and to relax the neck muscles, the nurse asks the patient to flex the neck slightly forward and to the right. The thyroid cartilage is displaced to the right by the nurse's left hand and fingers. The nurse palpates with the right hand after placing the thumb deep and behind the sternocleidomastoid muscle with the index and middle fingers in front of it; the area is palpated with the right hand (Figure 50-10). While this is done, the patient is asked to swallow water. This procedure is repeated on the left side. The thyroid is palpated for its size, shape, symmetry, and tenderness and for any nodules.

The thyroid is often not palpable. If palpable, it usually feels smooth, with a firm consistency, and is not tender with gentle pressure. Nodules, enlargement, asymmetry, or hardness is abnormal, and the patient should be referred for further evaluation.

Thorax. The thorax should be inspected for shape and characteristics of the skin. The presence of gynecomastia in men should be noted. The nurse auscultates lung sounds and heart

CASE STUDY

Objective Data: Physical Examination

Source: aastock/ Shutterstock .com.

A focused assessment of Lydia Mollon reveals the following:

Ms. Mollon is sitting on the edge of the examination table. She appears somewhat anxious. Her BP is 190/80, heart rate 84, respiratory rate 20, temp 37°C. Her weight is 82.6 kg, and she is 160 cm tall.

Ms. Mollon's face is reddened and puffy, and she appears to have a lump on the back of her neck and shoulders. She has some acne on her face, along with some hair growth on her upper lip and chin area. Her abdomen is protruding but her arms and legs are thin. She has +1 edema in her ankles bilaterally. There are several ecchymotic areas on her upper and lower extremities, as well as purple stretch marks on her abdomen.

Throughout this chapter, consider which diagnostic studies would likely be performed for Ms. Mollon. See pp. 1245 and 1254 for more information on Ms. Mollon.

---

sounds, noting the presence of adventitious lung sounds or extra heart sounds.

Abdomen. No abdominal examination findings are specific for endocrine dysfunction other than skin characteristics and hyperactive or hypoactive bowel sounds.

Extremities. The nurse assesses the size, shape, symmetry, and general proportion of hands and feet. The skin is inspected for changes in pigmentation and presence of lesions and edema. Muscle strength is evaluated, as are deep tendon reflexes. In the upper extremities, the nurse assesses for the presence of tremors by placing a piece of paper in the patient's outstretched fingers, palm down.

Genitalia. The nurse inspects the hair distribution pattern. A diamond pubic hair distribution pattern in women or a triangular pattern in men are abnormal findings and might indicate endocrine dysfunction. For men, the testes should be palpated; for women, any clitoral enlargement should be noted.

Common assessment abnormalities related to the endocrine system are presented in Table 50-7. A focused assessment is used to evaluate the status of previously identified endocrine problems and to monitor for signs of new problems (see Chapter 3, Table 3-6). A focused assessment of the endocrine system is described in the "Focused Assessment" box at right.

DIAGNOSTIC STUDIES OF THE ENDOCRINE SYSTEM

Accurately performed laboratory tests and radiological examinations contribute to the diagnosis of an endocrine problem. Laboratory tests usually involve blood and urine testing. Ultrasonography may be used as a screening tool to localize endocrine growths such as thyroid nodules. Radiological tests include regular radiography, computed tomography, and magnetic resonance imaging. For all diagnostic testing, the nurse is responsible for explaining the procedure to the patient and family. Diagnostic studies common to the endocrine system are described in Table 50-8.

Laboratory Studies

Laboratory studies used to diagnose endocrine problems may include direct measurement of the hormone level or an indirect

---

FOCUSED ASSESSMENT

Endocrine System

Use this checklist to ensure the key assessment steps have been performed.

Subjective

Ask the patient about experiencing any of the following, and note responses.

Excessive or increased thirst	Y	N
Excessive or decreased urination	Y	N
Excessive hunger	Y	N
Intolerance of heat or cold	Y	N
Excessive sweating	Y	N
Recent weight gain or loss	Y	N

Objective: Diagnostic

Check the following laboratory results for critical values

Potassium level	✓
Glucose level	✓
Sodium level	✓
Glycosylated hemoglobin (A$_{1C}$) level	✓
Thyroid studies: TSH, (T$_3$, and T$_4$ levels [if ordered])	✓

Objective: Physical Examination
Inspect/Measure

Body temperature	✓
Height and weight	✓
Alertness and emotional state	✓
Skin, for changes in colour and texture	✓
Hair, for changes in colour, texture, and distribution	✓

Auscultate

Heart rate, blood pressure	✓

Palpate

Extremities, for edema	✓
Skin, for texture and temperature	✓
Neck, for thyroid size, shape	✓

TSH, thyroid-stimulating hormone; *T$_3$*, triiodothyronine; *T$_4$*, thyroxine.

---

indication of gland function by evaluation of blood or urine components affected by the hormone (e.g., electrolytes).

Hormones with fairly constant basal levels (e.g., T$_4$) need be measured only once. Notation of sample time on the laboratory slip and sample is important for hormones with circadian or sleep-related secretion (e.g., cortisol). Evaluation of other hormones may require multiple blood sampling, as in suppression tests (e.g., dexamethasone) and stimulation tests (e.g., glucose tolerance). In these situations, it is often necessary to obtain intravenous access to administer medications and fluids and to collect multiple blood samples.

Pituitary Studies. Disorders associated with the pituitary gland can manifest in a wide variety of ways because of the number of hormones produced. Many diagnostic studies are available to evaluate these hormones either directly or indirectly (see Table 50-8).

Thyroid Studies. There are a number of tests available to evaluate thyroid function. The most sensitive and accurate laboratory test is measurement of TSH; thus it is often recommended as a first diagnostic test for evaluation of thyroid function (Thyroid

Text continued on p. 1253

TABLE 50-7 ASSESSMENT ABNORMALITIES

Endocrine System

Finding	Description	Possible Etiology and Significance
Integument		
Hyperpigmentation	Darkening of the skin, particularly in creases and skinfolds	Addison's disease, caused by increased secretion of melanocyte-stimulating hormone
Depigmentation (vitiligo)	Patchy areas of light skin	May be a marker of autoimmune endocrine disorders
Striae	Purplish-red marks below the skin surface, usually observed on abdomen, breasts, and buttocks (see Chapter 51, Figure 51-11)	Cushing's syndrome
Changes in skin texture	Thick, cold, dry skin	Hypothyroidism
	Thick, leathery, oily skin	Growth hormone excess (acromegaly)
	Warm, smooth, moist skin	Hyperthyroidism
Changes in hair distribution	Hair loss	Hypothyroidism, hyperthyroidism, decreased pituitary secretion
	Diminished axillary and pubic hair	Cortisol deficiency
	Hirsutism (excessive facial hair on women)	Cushing's syndrome, prolactinoma (a pituitary tumour)
Skin ulceration	Areas of ulcerated skin, most commonly observed on legs and feet	Peripheral neuropathy and peripheral vascular disease, which are contributory factors in the development of diabetic foot ulcers
Edema	Generalized edema	Mucopolysaccharide accumulation in tissue in hypothyroidism
Head and Neck		
Visual changes	Decreased visual acuity or decreased peripheral vision	Pituitary gland enlargement or tumour, which leads to pressure on optic nerve
Exophthalmos	Protrusion of eyeballs from orbits	Hyperthyroidism; results from fluid accumulation in eye and retro-orbital tissue
Moon facies	Periorbital edema and facial fullness	Increased cortisol secretion as a result of Cushing's syndrome
Myxedema	Puffiness, periorbital edema, masklike affect	Infiltration of dermis by hydrophilic mucopolysaccharides in hypothyroidism
Goitre	Generalized enlargement of thyroid gland	Hyperthyroidism, hypothyroidism, iodine deficiency
Thyroid nodule (one or more)	Localized enlargement of thyroid gland	May be benign or malignant
Cardiovascular		
Chest pain	Angina caused by increased metabolic demands	Hyperthyroidism, hypothyroidism
Dysrhythmias	Tachycardia, atrial fibrillation	Hypothyroidism or hyperthyroidism, hypoparathyroidism or hyperparathyroidism, pheochromocytoma
Hypertension	Elevation in blood pressure caused by increased metabolic demands and catecholamines	Hyperthyroidism, pheochromocytoma, Cushing's syndrome
Musculo-Skeletal		
Changes in muscular strength or muscle mass	Generalized weakness, fatigue, or both	Common symptoms associated with many endocrine problems, including pituitary, thyroid, parathyroid, and adrenal dysfunction; diabetes mellitus; diabetes insipidus
	Decreased muscle mass	Specifically observed in growth hormone deficiency and in Cushing's syndrome secondary to protein wasting
Enlargement of bones and cartilage	Coarsening of facial features; increases in size of hands and feet over a period of several years	Growth hormone excess in adults, as in acromegaly
Nutrition		
Changes in weight	Weight loss	Hyperthyroidism; caused by increases in metabolism, diabetic ketoacidosis
Altered glucose levels	Weight gain	Hypothyroidism, Cushing's syndrome, type 2 diabetes mellitus
	Increased serum glucose level	Diabetes mellitus, Cushing's syndrome, growth hormone excess
Neurological		
Lethargy	State of mental sluggishness or somnolence	Hypothyroidism
Tetany	Intermittent involuntary muscle spasms, usually involving the extremities	Severe calcium deficiency that can occur with hypoparathyroidism
Seizure	Sudden involuntary contraction of muscles	Consequence of a pituitary tumour; fluid and electrolyte imbalance associated with excessive ADH secretion; complications of diabetes mellitus; severe hypothyroidism
Increased deep tendon reflexes	Hyper-reflexia	Hyperthyroidism, hypoparathyroidism
Gastro-Intestinal		
Constipation	Passage of infrequent, hard stools	Hyperthyroidism or calcium imbalances caused by hyperparathyroidism

TABLE 50-7 ASSESSMENT ABNORMALITIES

Endocrine System—cont'd

Finding	Description	Possible Etiology and Significance
Reproductive		
Changes in reproductive function	Menstrual irregularities, decreased libido, decreased fertility, erectile dysfunction	Various endocrine abnormalities, including pituitary hypofunction, growth hormone excess, thyroid dysfunction, and adrenocortical dysfunction
Other		
Polyuria	Excessive urinary output	Diabetes mellitus (secondary to hyperglycemia) or diabetes insipidus (associated with decreased ADH secretion)
Polydipsia	Excessive thirst	Extreme water losses in diabetes mellitus (with severe hyperglycemia) or diabetes insipidus (associated with decreased ADH)
Decreased urine output	ADH leading to reabsorption of water from kidney tubules	Syndrome of inappropriate antidiuretic hormone (SIADH)
Thermoregulation	Cold sensitivity	Hypothyroidism caused by a slowing of metabolic processes
	Heat intolerance	Hyperthyroidism caused by excessive metabolism

ADH, antidiuretic hormone.

TABLE 50-8 DIAGNOSTIC STUDIES

Endocrine System

Study	Description and Purpose	Normal Values	Nursing Responsibility
Pituitary Studies **Blood Studies**			
Growth hormone (GH) (somatotropin)	Evaluation of GH secretion Used to identify GH deficiency or excess; GH levels are affected by time of day, food intake, and stress	Male: <5 mcg/L Female: <10 mcg/L	Make sure that patient has been fasting and has not recently been emotionally or physically stressed. Indicate patient fasting status and recent activity level on the laboratory slip. Send blood sample to laboratory immediately.
Somatomedin C (insulin-like growth factor [IGF-1])	Evaluation of GH secretion Provides an accurate reflection of mean plasma concentration of GH because it is not subject to circadian rhythm and fluctuations	5.5–14.4 nmol/L Low levels indicate GH deficiency; high levels indicate GH excess	Note if patient has fasted overnight, as overnight fasting is preferred.
Growth hormone (GH) stimulation	Needed to adequately diagnose GH deficiency Measurement of GH secretion in response to stimulation (insulin, arginine) For insulin, baseline blood levels for GH, glucose, and cortisol are obtained; insulin is then administered IV; blood samples for GH are obtained at 0, 60, and 90 min after insulin is administered; blood glucose levels are monitored at 15- to 30-min intervals; blood glucose should drop to less than 2.2 mmol/L for effective test results, and GH level should rise two-fold to three-fold over baseline levels Response is subnormal or absent in GH deficiency	Growth hormone levels >10 mcg/L	Ensure that patient or family understands this procedure. Patient must be on NPO status after midnight. Water is permitted on morning of the test. IV access is established for administration of medications and frequent blood sampling. Continually assess for hypoglycemia and hypotension. After test, provide a sweet snack or IV glucose infusion as physician orders.
Gonadotropins • Follicle-stimulating hormone (FSH) • Luteinizing hormone (LH)	Useful in distinguishing primary gonadal problems from pituitary insufficiency Normal levels vary according to age and sex Levels are low in pituitary insufficiency and high in primary gonadal failure	*FSH* Male: <22 IU/L Female: • Follicular phase: <20 IU/L • Ovulatory peak: <40 IU/L • Luteal phase: <20 IU/L • Postmenopause levels: 40–160 IU/L *LH* Male: 1–9 IU/L Female: • Follicular phase: 1–18 IU/L • Ovulatory peak: 20–80 IU/L • Luteal phase: 0.5–18 IU/L • Postmenopause levels: 12–55 IU/L	There is no special preparation of the patient. Note on the laboratory slip time of menstrual cycle or whether female patient is postmenopausal.

Continued

TABLE 50-8 DIAGNOSTIC STUDIES

Endocrine System—cont'd

Study	Description and Purpose	Normal Values	Nursing Responsibility
Water deprivation (restriction) (ADH stimulation)	Used to differentiate causes of polyuria, including neurogenic DI, nephrogenic DI, and psychogenic polydipsia ADH or vasopressin is administered subcutaneously	Neurogenic DI: >9% increase in urine osmolality Nephrogenic DI: <9% increase in urine osmolality Psychogenic polydipsia: <9% increase in osmolality	Caution: Severe dehydration may occur with neurogenic or nephrogenic DI during this test. Test lasts 6 hr, usually from 0600 to 1200 hours. Obtain baseline weight and urine and plasma osmolality. Send hourly samples for measuring urine osmolality. Discontinue test and rehydrate if patient's weight drops more than 2 kg at any time. Rehydrate with oral fluids. Check orthostatic BP and pulse after rehydration to ensure adequate fluid volume.
Prolactin level	Diagnose and monitor prolactin-secreting pituitary adenomas	Male: <20 mcg/L Female: • Nonlactating: <25 mcg/L • Pregnant: 20–400 mcg/L Levels above normal reflect potential pituitary tumour; levels below may be pituitary apoplexy	Draw blood within 3–4 hr after patient awakens. Specimen must be sent to the laboratory immediately. If there is a delay, the specimen is placed in water and crushed ice.

Radiology

Study	Description and Purpose	Normal Values	Nursing Responsibility
Magnetic resonance imaging (MRI)	Most common uses are visualization of the CNS, bony spine, joints, extremities, and breasts	—	Inform patient of the need to lie as still as possible during the test; explain that tests are painless and noninvasive.
Computed tomographic (CT) scan with contrast media	Used to detect presence and size of tumour Oral or IV contrast medium (or both) may be used	—	Inform patient of the need to lie still during the procedure. If IV contrast medium is to be used, check for iodine allergy before test.

Thyroid Studies
Blood Studies

Study	Description and Purpose	Normal Values	Nursing Responsibility
Thyroid-stimulating hormone (TSH)	Measurement of TSH levels Considered the most sensitive method for evaluating thyroid disease Generally recommended as first diagnostic test for thyroid dysfunction	2–10 mIU/L	Explain blood collection procedure to patient. No specific preparations are necessary.
Thyroxine (T_4), total	Measurement of total serum level of T_4 Useful in evaluating thyroid function and monitoring thyroid therapy	Male: 51–154 nmol/L Female: 64–154 nmol/L	Same as for TSH measurement.
Triiodothyronine (T_3)	Measurement of serum levels of T_3 Helpful in diagnosing hyperthyroidism if T_4 levels are normal	Adult: 1.7–5.2 pmol/L	Same as for TSH measurement.
Free T_4	Measurement of active component of total T_4 Because level remains constant, this is considered better indication of thyroid function than total T_4	10–36 pmol/L	Same as for TSH measurement.
T_3 uptake (T_3RU)	Indirect measurement of binding capacity of thyroid-binding globulin	24%–34% uptake	Same as for TSH measurement.
Thyroid antibodies (Ab) • Thyroid peroxidase (TPO) Ab • Thyroglobulin Ab • Thyroid-stimulating Ab	Measurements of levels of thyroid antibodies Assists in the diagnosis of an autoimmune thyroid disease and distinguishes it from thyroiditis One or more antibody tests may be ordered, depending on symptoms	—	Same as for TSH measurement.
Thyroglobulin	Test to identify the presence of functioning thyroid tissue or thyroid cancer cells; result used primarily as a tumour marker for patients being treated for thyroid cancer	Male: 0.5–53 mcg/L Female: 0.5–43 mcg/L	Same as for TSH measurement.

Radiology

Study	Description and Purpose	Normal Values	Nursing Responsibility
Ultrasonography	Evaluation of thyroid nodule or nodules to determine whether they are fluid filled (cystic) or solid tumour	—	Explain that gel and a transducer will be used over the neck. Neither fasting nor sedation is required.

TABLE 50-8   DIAGNOSTIC STUDIES

Endocrine System—cont'd

Study	Description and Purpose	Normal Values	Nursing Responsibility
Thyroid scan and uptake	Scan: Used to evaluate nodules of the thyroid. Radioactive isotopes are given PO or IV. Scanner passes over thyroid and makes graphic record of radiation emitted. Normal thyroid scan reveals homogeneous pattern with symmetrical lobes. Benign nodules appear as warm spots because they take up the radionuclide; malignant tumours appear as cold spots because they tend not to take up the radionuclide. Radioactive iodine uptake (RAIU): Provides direct measurement of thyroid activity. Useful for evaluation of functional activity of solitary thyroid nodules. Patient is given radioactive iodine either PO or IV. The uptake by the thyroid gland is measured with a scanner at several time intervals such as 2- to 4-hr intervals and at 24 hr. The values of RAIU are expressed in percentage of uptake.	—	Explain procedure to the patient. Check for iodine and shellfish allergy before test. Be sure patient understands that radioactive iodine taken orally is harmless. No special preparation is required. Patient should not have supplemental iodine for several weeks before the test. Thyroid medications interfere with test results.
Parathyroid Studies ***Blood Studies*** Parathyroid hormone (PTH)	Measurement of PTH level in serum to evaluate hypercalcemia or hypocalcemia Results must be interpreted in terms of concomitantly measured serum calcium level	Intact (whole): 10–65 ng/L	Fasting specimen preferred. Inform patient that blood sample will be collected. Sample may need to be kept on ice. Apply pressure to venipuncture site.
Total serum calcium	Measurement of total serum calcium to help detect bone and parathyroid disorders Hypercalcemia can indicate primary hyperparathyroidism, and hypocalcemia can indicate hypoparathyroidism	2.25–2.75 mmol/L	Inform patient that blood sample will be collected. Avoid prolonged tourniquet application. Apply pressure to venipuncture site.
Ionized calcium	Measurement of free form of calcium unaffected by variable serum albumin levels	1.05–1.3 mmol/L	Same as for total serum calcium.
Serum phosphate	Measurement of inorganic phosphorus Hyperphosphatemia indicates primary hypoparathyroidism or secondary causes (e.g., renal failure); hypophosphatemia indicates hyperparathyroidism Phosphorus and calcium levels are inversely related	0.97–1.45 mmol/L	Fasting preferred. Inform patient that blood sample will be collected. Take specimen to laboratory immediately. Apply pressure to venipuncture site.
Adrenal Studies ***Blood Studies*** Cortisol	Measures amount of total cortisol in serum and evaluation of status of adrenal cortex function	138–635 nmol/L at 0800 hr 83–359 nmol/L at 1600 hr	Cortisol has diurnal variation: levels are higher in the morning than in evening. Sample should be collected in morning; evening samples may also be ordered. Mark time of blood collection on laboratory slip. Patient's anxiety should be minimized.
Aldosterone	Measurement of aldosterone levels to evaluate for hyperaldosteronism	Upright posture (at least 2 hr): <0.03–1.05 nmol/L Supine position: Peak 0.35 nmol/L Nadir 0.14 nmol/L	Usually, morning blood sample is preferred. On laboratory slip, indicate patient position (supine, sitting, standing) during venipuncture.
Adrenocorticotrophic hormone (ACTH) (corticotropin)	Measurement of the plasma level of ACTH Although ACTH is a pituitary hormone, it controls adrenal cortex secretion; this value helps determine whether underproduction or overproduction of cortisol is caused by dysfunction of the adrenal gland or pituitary gland	Morning: <18 pmol/L Evening: <11 pmol/L	Patient should be on NPO status after midnight before morning blood collection. Minimize patient's stress. Diurnal levels correspond with variation of cortisol levels; that is, levels are higher in morning, lower in evening. ACTH is very unstable; blood tube must be placed on ice and sent to laboratory immediately.

Continued

TABLE 50-8 DIAGNOSTIC STUDIES

Endocrine System—cont'd

Study	Description and Purpose	Normal Values	Nursing Responsibility
ACTH stimulation with cosyntropin	Used to evaluate adrenal function Baseline plasma cortisol levels are measured; IV cosyntropin (synthetic ACTH) is administered; samples are collected 30 and 60 min after bolus	For the rapid stimulation test, cortisol levels increase more than 267 nmol/L above baseline	Inject cosyntropin with a plastic syringe, and collect blood samples in plastic heparinized tubes. Ensure sample collection at appropriate times.
ACTH suppression (dexamethasone suppression)	Assessment of adrenal function; especially helpful if hyperactivity is suspected Useful in evaluation of Cushing's syndrome Dexamethasone is administered at 2300 hr to suppress secretion of corticotropin-releasing hormone; plasma cortisol sample is collected at 0800 hr	Cortisol level <138 nmol/L indicates normal adrenal response (50% decrease in cortisol production)	Ensure that patient has fasted. Inform patient that blood sample will be collected. Observe venipuncture site for bleeding and hematoma formation. Do not test acutely ill patients; those under stress are not tested. ACTH may override suppression. Screen patient for drugs such as estrogen and glucocorticoids, which may produce false-positive results. Ensure accurate timing of medication and sample collection.
Metanephrine	Screening for pheochromocytoma; more accurate than urinary vanillylmandelic acid (VMA) and catecholamine measurements	12–60 pg/mL Normetanephrine: 18–111 pg/mL Results may vary by laboratory	Ask about recent history of vigorous exercise, high levels of stress, or starvation (may artificially ↑ levels). Ingestion of caffeine, alcohol, levodopa, lithium, nitroglycerin, acetaminophen, and medications containing epinephrine or norepinephrine can alter test results.

Urine Studies

17-Ketosteroids	Measurement of androgen metabolites in urine and evaluation of adrenocortical and gonadal function	Male: 20–70 mcmol/day Female: 20–60 mcmol/day	Instruct patient regarding 24-hr urine collection. Tell patient that specimen must be kept refrigerated or on ice during collection. Determine whether preservative is required for method used.
Aldosterone	Measurement of urinary aldosterone level to diagnose hyperaldosteronism	0.11–0.86 nmol	Ensure that patient is on unrestricted diet with normal salt intake and no medication for 3 wk before collection. Instruct patient regarding 24-hr urine collection.
Cortisol, urine (free cortisol)	Measurement of free (unbound) cortisol for patients with suspected hyper- or hypofunction of the adrenal gland Preferred test for evaluating hypercortisolism	0800 hr: 138–635 nmol/L 1600 hr: 83–359 nmol/L	Instruct patient about 24-hr urine collection and avoidance of stressful situations and excessive physical exercise. Some drugs may alter levels. Ensure that patient is on low-sodium diet.
Vanillylmandelic acid (VMA)	Measurement of urinary excretion of catecholamine metabolite; helpful in diagnosing pheochromocytoma	<35 mcmol/24 hr Elevated values indicate pheochromocytoma	Collect specimen with a preservative. Keep on ice. Consult with laboratory or physician about whether patient should discontinue any drugs 3 days before urine collection and a VMA-restricted diet.

Radiology

Abdominal computed tomographic (CT) scan	The radiological examination of choice for the adrenal gland Used to detect tumour and size of tumour mass or metastatic spread Oral or IV contrast medium, or both, may be used	—	Inform patient of the need to lie still during the procedure. If IV contrast medium is to be used, check for iodine and shellfish allergy before test.

Pancreatic Studies
Blood Studies

Fasting blood glucose (FBG) level	Measurement of circulating glucose level	4–6 mmol/L	Ensure that patient fasts for at least 4–8 hr; water intake is permitted.

TABLE 50-8 DIAGNOSTIC STUDIES

Endocrine System—cont'd

Study	Description and Purpose	Normal Values	Nursing Responsibility
Oral glucose tolerance test (OGTT)	2-hr test: Used to diagnose diabetes mellitus if FBG result is equivocal; patient drinks 75 g of glucose. Samples for glucose are collected immediately and at 30, 60, and 120 min 5-hr test: Used to evaluate hypoglycemia. Patient drinks 100 g of glucose; samples of glucose are collected immediately and at 30, 60, 90, 120, 180, 240, and 300 min	<11.1 mmol/L at 30 and 60 min <7.8 mmol/L at 120 min <6.4 mmol/L at 3 and 4 hr	Instruct patient to fast (unless otherwise ordered), refrain from smoking and ingesting caffeine, and fast for 12 hr before test. Ensure that patient's diet 3 days before test included 150–300 g of carbohydrate. Simultaneously monitor glucose levels with capillary glucose monitoring if the patient is symptomatic. Encourage water during the test. Collect urine samples hourly. Allow patient to eat after test. Administer medications as ordered, after the test.
Capillary glucose monitoring	Provides immediate glucose values with glucose oxidase or electrochemical methods	Capillary values (whole blood): 10%–15% less than serum values Most capillary blood glucose meters automatically accommodate for this discrepancy	Obtain large drop of blood from clean finger, touch strip to drop of blood (not finger), time accurately, and compare colours in good lighting if visual method is used. Use digital readout if it is available. Use automatic finger-puncture device if it is available. Be sure to change section of device that touches patient's fingers between uses.
Glycosylated or hemoglobin (A$_{1c}$)	Measurement of degree of glucose control during previous 3 mo (lifespan of hemoglobin molecule)	<6% for patients without diabetes <7% for patients with good diabetic control (values vary; check with laboratory)	Inform patient that fasting is not necessary and that blood sample will be collected. Observe venipuncture site for bleeding or hematoma formation.
Urine Studies			
Glucose	Estimation of amount of glucose in urine through use of an enzymatic method Dipstick is dipped into the urine and read for colour changes after 1 min	Random: negative 24-hr: <2.78 mmol/24 hr (<0.5 g/24 hr)	Use freshly voided urine specimen collected at appropriate time. Know that many different drugs alter glucose readings and that errors are great if directions for timing are not followed exactly. Follow package directions.
Ketones	Measurement of amount of acetone excreted in urine as result of incomplete fat metabolism Tested with a dipstick as described for glucose study	Negative or trace amount of ketone is normal Positive result can indicate lack of insulin and diabetic ketoacidosis	Use freshly voided urine specimen. Test is often performed with glucose test. Directions must be followed exactly. Certain drugs can produce false-positive and false-negative results.
Radiology			
Abdominal computed tomographic (CT) scan	The radiological examination of choice for pancreas Used to identify tumours or cysts Oral or IV contrast medium (or both) may be ordered	—	Inform patient of the need to lie still during the procedure. If IV contrast is to be used, check for iodine allergy before test.

ADH, antidiuretic hormone; *AU,* arbitrary units (T$_3$RU). *BP,* blood pressure; *DI,* diabetes insipidus; *IV,* intravenous; *NPO,* nothing by mouth; *PO,* by mouth.

Foundation of Canada, 2015). Common additional tests ordered in the presence of abnormal TSH levels include measurements of total serum T$_4$, free T$_4$, and total serum T$_3$. The Canadian Society of Endocrinology and Metabolism (CSEM, 2015) in conjunction with Choosing Wisely Canada (2014) has recommended that free T$_4$ or T$_3$ not be used to screen for hypothyroidism or to monitor and adjust levothyroxine (L-T$_4$, Synthroid) dose in patients with known primary hypothyroidism.

Free T$_4$ is the unbound T$_4$, and its level is a more accurate reflection of thyroid function than that of total T$_4$. Less common

tests that help in the differentiation of various types of thyroid disease include measurement of T$_3$, assessment of free T$_3$ resin uptake, measurement of thyroid autoantibodies, thyroid scanning, ultrasonography, and biopsy. CSEM (2015) does not recommend ultrasound as a routine evaluation of abnormal thyroid function tests. These tests are performed to help differentiate various types of thyroid disorders.

Parathyroid Studies. The only hormone secreted by the parathyroid glands is PTH. Because the function of PTH is to regulate serum calcium and phosphate levels, abnormalities in

CASE STUDY

Objective Data: Diagnostic Studies

Source: aastock/ Shutterstock .com.

The health care provider orders the following initial diagnostic studies to be drawn in the morning after an 8-hr fast:
- CBC, basic metabolic panel (electrolytes, BUN, creatinine)
- Fasting blood glucose (FBG)
- TSH, free T₄
- Plasma cortisol levels
- Plasma ACTH levels

CBC results reveal a WBC of 12.2×10⁹/L and a decreased lymphocyte count at 8×10⁹/L. The rest of the CBC is within normal limits (WNL).

The FBG is 7.2 mmol/L. The plasma cortisol and ACTH levels are elevated. Thyroid studies are within normal limits. Based on findings, the health care provider diagnoses Ms. Mollon with Cushing's syndrome.

See pp. 1245 and 1247 for more information on Ms. Mollon.

PTH secretion are reflected in the calcium and phosphate levels. For this reason, diagnostic tests for the parathyroid gland typically include measurements of PTH, serum calcium, and serum phosphate.

Adrenal Studies. Diagnostic tests associated with the adrenal glands focus on the three types of hormones secreted: glucocorticoids, mineralocorticoids, and androgens. These hormone levels can be measured both in blood plasma and in urine. Urine studies are usually performed as 24-hour urine collections. The major advantage of a 24-hour urine sample is that the short-term fluctuations in hormone levels seen in plasma samples are eliminated (Pagana & Pagana, 2013).

Pancreatic Studies. The tests found in Table 50-8 are geared toward evaluating the metabolism of glucose. They are important in the diagnosis and management of diabetes. (Diagnostic studies for diabetes are discussed in Chapter 52.)

REVIEW QUESTIONS

The number of the question corresponds to the same-numbered objective at the beginning of the chapter.

1. Which of the following is a characteristic common to all hormones?
   a. They circulate in the blood bound to plasma proteins.
   b. They influence cellular activity of specific target tissues.
   c. They accelerate the metabolic processes of all body cells.
   d. They enter cells to alter the cell's metabolism or gene expression.

2. A client is receiving radiation therapy for cancer of the kidney. The nurse monitors the client for signs and symptoms of damage to which of the following organ(s)?
   a. Pancreas
   b. Thyroid
   c. Adrenal glands
   d. Posterior pituitary gland

3. A client has a serum sodium level of 152 mmol/L. What is the normal hormonal response to this situation?
   a. Release of ADH
   b. Release of renin
   c. Secretion of aldosterone
   d. Secretion of corticotropin-releasing hormone

4. All cells in the body are believed to have intracellular receptors for which of the following?
   a. Insulin
   b. Glucagon
   c. Growth hormone
   d. Thyroid hormone

5. When obtaining subjective data from a client during assessment of the endocrine system, the nurse asks specifically about which of the following?
   a. Energy level
   b. Intake of vitamin C
   c. Employment history
   d. Frequency of sexual intercourse

6. What is an appropriate technique to use during physical assessment of the thyroid gland?
   a. Ask the client to hyperextend the neck during palpation.
   b. Percuss the neck for dullness to define the size of the thyroid.
   c. Have the client swallow water during inspection and palpation of the gland.
   d. Use deep palpation to determine the extent of a visibly enlarged thyroid gland.

7. Why do endocrine disorders often go unrecognized in older adults?
   a. Symptoms are often attributed to aging.
   b. Older adults rarely have identifiable symptoms.
   c. Endocrine disorders are relatively rare in the older adult.
   d. Older adults usually have subclinical endocrine disorders that minimize symptoms.

8. Which of the following would the nurse consider an abnormal finding during an endocrine assessment? *(Select all that apply)*
   a. Blood pressure of 100/70
   b. Soft, formed stool every other day
   c. Excessive facial hair on a woman
   d. 1.5-kg weight gain over the last 6 months
   e. Hyperpigmented coloration in lower legs

9. A client has a total serum calcium level of 0.75 mmol/L. If this finding reflects hypoparathyroidism, what would the nurse expect further diagnostic testing to reveal?
   a. Decreased serum PTH
   b. Increased serum ACTH
   c. Increased serum glucose
   d. Decreased serum cortisol levels

1. b; 2. c; 3. a; 4. d; 5. a; 6. c; 7. a; 8. c, e; 9. a.

ⓔvolve

For even more review questions, visit *http://evolve.elsevier.com/Canada/ Lewis/medsurg*.

REFERENCES

Barnes, M. A., Carson, M. J., & Nair, M. G. (2015). Non-traditional cytokines: How catecholamines and adipokines influence macrophages in immunity, metabolism and the central nervous system. *Cytokine, 72*(2), 210–219. doi:10.1016/j.cyto.2015.01.008.

Ben-Moshe, Z., Foulkes, N. S., & Gothilf, Y. (2014). Functional development of the circadian clock in the zebrafish pineal gland. *BioMed Research International*, 235781. doi:10.1155/2014/235781.

The Canadian Society of Endocrinology and Metabolism (CSEM). (2015). *Clinical practice guidelines and quality improvement.* Retrieved from *http://www.endo-metab.ca/cpgs-qi.*

Choosing Wisely Canada. (2014). *Endocrinology and metabolism: Five things physicians and patients should question.* Retrieved from *http://www.choosingwiselycanada.org/recommendations/endocrinology-and-metabolism/.*

Jarvis, C., Browne, A. J., MacDonald-Jenkins, J., et al. (Eds.), (2014). *Physical examination and health assessment* (2nd Canadian ed.). Toronto: Elsevier Canada.

Markova-Car, E. P., Jurišić, D., Ilić, N., et al. (2014). Running for time: Circadian rhythms and melanoma. *Tumour Biology, 35*(9), 8359–8368. doi:10.1007/s13277-014-1904-2.

McEwen, B., Gray, J. D., & Nasca, C. (2015). Redefining neuroendocrinology: Stress, sex and cognitive and emotional regulation. *The Journal of Endocrinology*, JOE-15. doi:10.1530/JOE-15-0121.

Molina, P. (2013). *Endocrine physiology* (4th ed.). New York: McGraw-Hill Medical.

Ojeda, S. R., & Kovacs, W. J. (2012). Organization of the endocrine system. In W. J. Kovacs & S. R. Ojeda (Eds.), *Textbook of endocrine physiology* (pp. 3–20). New York: Oxford University Press.

Pagana, K. D., & Pagana, T. J. (2013). *Mosby's Canadian manual of diagnostic and laboratory tests* (1st ed.). S.A. Pike-MacDonald (Canadian ed.). New York: Springer Publishing Company.

Saxon, S. V., Etten, M. J., & Perkins, E. A. (2014). *Physical change and aging: A guide for the helping professions* (6th ed.). New York: Springer Publishing Company.

Thyroid Foundation of Canada. (2015). *Thyroid Foundation of Canada*. Retrieved from *http://www.thyroid.ca/clinical_diagnosis.php.*

RESOURCES

Resources for this chapter are listed in Chapter 51 and Chapter 52.

Nursing Management
Endocrine Problems

Written by: Katherine A. Kelly
Adapted by: Daphne Connolly

evolve WEBSITE

http://evolve.elsevier.com/Canada/Lewis/medsurg

- Review Questions (Online Only)
- Key Points
- Answer Guidelines for Case Study
- Student Case Studies
  - Addison's Disease
  - Cushing's Syndrome
  - Hyperthyroidism

- Customizable Nursing Care Plans
  - Hyperthyroidism
  - Hypothyroidism
  - Cushing's Syndrome
- Conceptual Care Map Creator
- Audio Glossary
- Content Updates

LEARNING OBJECTIVES

1. Describe the pathophysiology, clinical manifestations, collaborative care, and nursing management of the patient with an imbalance of hormones produced by the anterior pituitary gland.

2. Describe the pathophysiology, clinical manifestations, collaborative care, and nursing management of the patient with an imbalance of hormones produced by the posterior pituitary gland.

3. Describe the pathophysiology, clinical manifestations, collaborative care, and nursing management of the patient with thyroid dysfunction.

4. Describe the pathophysiology, clinical manifestations, collaborative care, and nursing management of the patient with an imbalance of the hormone produced by the parathyroid glands.

5. Describe the pathophysiology, clinical manifestations, collaborative care, and nursing management of the patient with an imbalance of hormones produced by the adrenal cortex.

6. Describe the pathophysiology, clinical manifestations, collaborative care, and nursing management of the patient with an excess of hormones produced by the adrenal medulla.

7. Explain the adverse effects of corticosteroid therapy.

8. Describe common nursing assessments, interventions, rationales, and expected outcomes related to patient teaching for management of chronic endocrine problems.

KEY TERMS

acromegaly, p. 1256
Addison's disease, p. 1279
cretinism, p. 1270
Cushing's syndrome, p. 1275
diabetes insipidus (DI), p. 1261
exophthalmos, p. 1265

goitre, p. 1263
Graves' disease, p. 1265
hyperaldosteronism, p. 1282
hyperparathyroidism, p. 1272
hyperthyroidism, p. 1265
hypoparathyroidism, p. 1274

hypopituitarism, p. 1259
hypothyroidism, p. 1270
myxedema, p. 1270
myxedema coma, p. 1271
pheochromocytoma, p. 1283

syndrome of inappropriate
    antidiuretic hormone
    (SIADH), p. 1260
thyroiditis, p. 1264
thyrotoxicosis, p. 1265

DISORDERS OF THE ANTERIOR PITUITARY GLAND

ACROMEGALY

Etiology and Pathophysiology

Acromegaly is a condition caused by excessive secretion of growth hormone (GH) and characterized by an overgrowth of the bones and soft tissues in the hands, feet, and face. It occurs most often as a result of a benign pituitary tumour (adenoma). Because the problem develops after epiphyseal closure, the bones of the arms and legs do not grow longer. Acromegaly is relatively rare. The estimated annual incidence is about 3 to 4 cases per 1 million population (Puig, 2015). Both sexes are affected in equal numbers.

Clinical Manifestations

Manifestations of acromegaly begin gradually, usually in the third and fourth decades of life. Typically, the time between the initial onset of symptoms and the final diagnosis is an average of 7 to

FIGURE 51-1 Example of progressive changes in facial features in acromegaly. Source: Courtesy Linda Haas, Seattle, Washington.

Pituitary gland
Sella turcica
Sphenoid sinus

FIGURE 51-2 Surgery on the pituitary gland is most commonly performed with the trans-sphenoidal approach. An incision is made in the inner aspect of the upper lip and gingiva. The sella turcica is entered through the floor of the nose and the sphenoid sinuses.

10 years (Miller, Learned-Miller, Trainer, et al., 2011). Individuals experience enlargement of the hands and feet. The enlargement of the bones and cartilage may cause symptoms that range from mild joint pain to deforming, crippling arthritis. Changes in physical appearance occur, with thickening and enlargement of bony and soft tissue on the face and head (Figure 51-1). Enlargement of the mandible causes the jaw to jut forward. The paranasal and the frontal sinuses enlarge, as does the bony tissue of the forehead. Enlargement of soft tissue around the eyes, nose, and mouth results in a coarsening of facial features. Enlargement of the tongue results in speech difficulties, and the voice deepens as a result of hypertrophy of the vocal cords.

Sleep apnea may also occur and is thought to be related to upper airway narrowing that results from changes in pharyngeal soft tissues (Melmed & Kleinberg, 2016). The skin becomes thick, leathery, and oily. People with acromegaly may also experience peripheral neuropathy and proximal muscle weakness. Women may develop menstrual disturbances. Individuals with acromegaly are more likely to develop polyps in the colon and colon cancer.

The enlarged pituitary gland can exert pressure on surrounding structures within the brain, leading to visual disturbances and headaches. Because GH mobilizes stored fat for energy, it increases free fatty acid levels in the blood, which predisposes patients to atherosclerosis. The hormone also antagonizes the action of insulin and causes hyperglycemia. Manifestations of diabetes mellitus may occur, including *polydipsia* (increased thirst) and *polyuria* (increased urination). Prolonged secretion of GH leads to glucose intolerance.

Untreated acromegaly leads to a number of changes in the body. Effects on the cardiovascular system include cardiomegaly, left ventricular hypertrophy, angina pectoris, and hypertension. For this reason, disease of the cardiovascular system is associated with increased mortality rates among these individuals. Other systems that undergo changes include the gastro-intestinal (GI), genito-urinary, musculo-skeletal, and nervous systems.

Diagnostic Studies

In addition to the history and physical examination, diagnosis of GH excess requires evaluation of plasma insulin-like growth factor (IGF-1) levels and GH response to an oral glucose tolerance test (OGTT). A single measurement of serum GH is of limited value in the diagnosis of acromegaly because GH levels normally fluctuate. IGF-1 levels are more constant and thus provide a more reliable measure. A preferred test for acromegaly is the OGTT. Normally, GH concentration falls during an OGTT. In acromegaly, these levels do not fall (Turbow & Patterson, 2014).

Magnetic resonance imaging (MRI) is indicated for the identification and the localization of the pituitary tumour and the determination of its extension into surrounding tissue. High-resolution computed tomographic (CT) scan with contrast media may also be used to localize the tumour. A complete ophthalmological examination, including evaluation of visual fields, is performed if the tumour lies adjacent to the optic chiasm or the optic nerves (Katznelson, Laws, Jr., Melmed, et al., 2014).

Collaborative Care

The therapeutic goal in acromegaly is to return GH levels to normal. This is accomplished by surgery, radiation therapy, drug therapy, or a combination of these therapies. The prognosis depends on age at onset, age when treatment is initiated, and tumour size. Usually, bone growth can be arrested and soft tissue hypertrophy can be reversed. However, sleep apnea and diabetic and cardiac complications may persist in spite of treatment.

Surgical Therapy. Surgery is the treatment of choice and offers the best hope for a cure, especially for smaller tumours. The *trans-sphenoidal approach* is recommended (Katznelson et al., 2014; Figure 51-2). Surgery produces an immediate reduction in GH levels, followed by a drop in IGF-1 levels within a few weeks. Patients with larger tumours or those with GH levels higher than 50 mcg/L may require adjuvant radiation or drug therapy.

When the entire pituitary gland is removed during surgery *(hypophysectomy),* the loss of pituitary hormones is permanent. Rather than replacing the pituitary (tropic) hormones, which requires parenteral administration, the essential hormones produced by target organs (glucocorticoids, thyroid hormone, and sex hormones) can be replaced orally. Hormone replacement must be continued throughout life.

Radiation Therapy. Radiation therapy is considered when surgery has failed to produce complete remission and for patients considered to be at high risk for surgical complications. The long delay before GH levels normalize limits its usefulness in treating symptoms (Turbow & Patterson, 2014). Radiation therapy is usually offered in combination with drugs that reduce GH levels. Radiation therapy has also been used to reduce the size of a tumour before surgery. (Radiation therapy is discussed in Chapter 18.) Hypopituitarism commonly results from radiation therapy and necessitates hormone therapy.

Stereotactic radiosurgery (gamma-knife surgery, proton beam, linear accelerator) may be used for small, surgically inaccessible pituitary tumours (see Chapter 59). This procedure consists of a single dose of radiation delivered to one site from multiple angles.

Drug Therapy. Three groups of drugs are used in the treatment of acromegaly: somatostatin analogues, dopamine agonists, and GH-receptor antagonists. These drugs reduce GH levels and can be used as initial treatment or as adjunct therapy with surgery or radiation. The most common drug used for acromegaly is octreotide (Sandostatin), a somatostatin analogue that reduces GH levels to within the normal range in many patients. Octreotide is given by subcutaneous injection three times a day. Two long-acting analogues, octreotide (Sandostatin LAR), and lanreotide (Somatuline Autogel), are available as intramuscular (IM) injections every 2 to 4 weeks. Dopamine agonists, such as cabergoline (Dostinex) and bromocriptine mesylate (Apo-bromocriptine), may also be used in the treatment of acromegaly to suppress GH secretion. They are not commonly used as sole therapy; rather, they are combined with somatostatin analogues. A GH receptor antagonist, pegvisomant (Somavert), has been developed for use in the treatment of acromegaly and directly blocks GH action, resulting in decreased levels of IGF-1. It is recommended for patients in whom surgery, somatostatin analogues, and dopamine agonists have failed (Puig, 2015).

NURSING MANAGEMENT
ACROMEGALY

NURSING ASSESSMENT

The nurse must assess for signs and symptoms of abnormal tissue growth and evaluate changes in the physical size of each patient. Patients should be questioned about increases in hat, ring, glove, and shoe sizes and about changes in appearance. Photographs are helpful for evaluating any changes (Figure 51-1). Because physical changes occur slowly and over a long time, it is possible that the individual is not even aware of them.

NURSING IMPLEMENTATION

After surgery in which a trans-sphenoidal approach has been used, the head of the patient's bed should be elevated at a 30-degree angle at all times. This elevation prevents pressure on the sella turcica and decreases the incidence of headaches, a frequent postoperative problem. Neurological status, including pupillary response, should be monitored in order to detect neurological complications. Patients should be instructed to avoid vigorous coughing, sneezing, and straining at stool (Valsalva manoeuvre) to prevent leakage of cerebro-spinal fluid from the point at which the sella turcica was entered.

Any clear nasal drainage should be sent to the laboratory to be tested for glucose. A glucose level higher than 1.67 mmol/L indicates leakage of cerebro-spinal fluid from an open connection to the brain. If this happens, the patient is at an increased risk for meningitis. Complaints of persistent and severe generalized or supraorbital headache may indicate leakage of cerebro-spinal fluid into the sinuses. A cerebro-spinal fluid leak usually resolves within 72 hours when treated with head elevation and bedrest. If the leak persists, daily spinal taps may be performed to reduce pressure to below-normal levels and allow the fossa to heal. When a patient has a cerebro-spinal fluid leak, intravenous (IV) antibiotics should be administered as ordered to prevent meningitis. If the leak does not respond to treatment within 72 hours, surgical intervention may be required.

Mild analgesics are given for headaches. The nurse should perform mouth care every 4 hours to keep the surgical area clean and free of debris and to promote patient comfort. Tooth brushing should be avoided for at least 10 days to prevent disrupting the suture line and to avoid discomfort.

If stereotactic radiosurgery is performed, the patient is usually moved from the specialized radiation centre to the neurosurgical nursing unit for overnight observation. The patient is in a stereotactic head frame. Vital signs, neurological status, and fluid volume status must be carefully monitored. Possible complications include increased headaches, seizures, nausea, and vomiting. A patient with a history of seizures is at increased risk for seizures for at least 24 hours after the procedure. All staff should know how to remove a stereotactic frame in case of an emergency. The patient may experience discomfort at the pin sites. Pin site care should be performed according to institutional policy. Family members can be instructed in pin site care if the patient is discharged with pins in place.

A possible postoperative complication is transient diabetes insipidus (DI). This complication may occur because of the loss of antidiuretic hormone (ADH), which is stored in the posterior lobe of the pituitary gland, or because of cerebral edema related to manipulation of the pituitary gland during surgery. To assess for DI, urine output and serum and urine osmolarity must be closely monitored. Clinical manifestations and treatment of DI are discussed in more detail later in this chapter.

If a hypophysectomy is performed or the pituitary gland is damaged, replacement of ADH, cortisol, and thyroid hormone is necessary. These medications must be taken for life; therefore, careful patient teaching is essential.

Surgery may result in permanent loss or deficiencies in follicle-stimulating hormone (FSH) and luteinizing hormone (LH). This can lead to decreased fertility for both sexes. The nurse should assist patients in working through the grieving process associated with these losses.

The need for continued drug therapy reduces the patient's perception of independence and requires considerable emotional adjustment. The teaching plan should include self-administration of subcutaneous injections if prescribed. Cost issues related to the expense of ongoing medication, as well as other therapies, may be another area for nursing intervention.

The nurse must consider the emotional impact of a hypophysectomy when counselling patients and planning the educational program related to hormone replacement. Serial photographs to show improvement may be helpful. Psychological support from the nurse and from the patient's family and friends is needed to promote positive mental health outcomes for a patient with acromegaly. Patients with acromegaly may be at higher risk for colon polyps and colorectal cancer, and screening for colon neoplasia with colonoscopy at diagnosis is suggested (Katznelson et al., 2014).

EXCESSES OF OTHER TROPIC HORMONES

Excesses of tropic hormones and overproduction of a single anterior pituitary hormone usually cause syndromes related to hormone excess from the target organ. If the adrenocorticotrophic hormone (ACTH) level is increased, Cushing's disease results; if the thyroid-stimulating hormone (TSH) level is excessive, hyperthyroidism develops.

Prolactinomas (prolactin-secreting adenomas) are the most frequently occurring pituitary tumours (Turbow & Patterson, 2014). Common manifestations experienced by women with prolactinomas include galactorrhea, ovulatory dysfunction (anovulation, infertility), menstrual dysfunction (oligomenorrhea or amenorrhea), decreased libido, and hirsutism. In men, erectile dysfunction and decreased libido and sperm density may result. Headaches and visual problems may also occur. The visual problems are secondary to pressure on the optic chiasm. Because prolactinomas do not typically enlarge, drug therapy is usually the first-line treatment (Yang, Hong, Lee, et al., 2011). Dopamine agonists such as cabergoline (Dostinex) and bromocriptine have been used successfully to treat this disorder. Surgery with the trans-sphenoidal approach discussed previously may be considered, depending on the size and extent of the tumour. Radiation therapy for treatment of prolactinomas has been used to a somewhat limited degree, mainly in patients in whom the tumour has failed to respond to medical or surgical therapy.

HYPOFUNCTION OF THE PITUITARY GLAND

Hypopituitarism is a rare disorder that involves a decrease in one or more of the pituitary hormones; signs and symptoms relate to the underlying disorder and to the specific pituitary hormones that are deficient or absent. The anterior pituitary gland secretes ACTH, TSH, FSH, LH, GH, and prolactin; the posterior pituitary gland secretes ADH and oxytocin. A deficiency of only one pituitary hormone is referred to as *selective hypopituitarism*. Total failure of the pituitary gland results in deficiency of all pituitary hormones; this condition is referred to as *panhypopituitarism*. The hormone deficiencies most commonly associated with hypopituitarism involve GH and the gonadotropins (e.g., LH, FSH).

Etiology and Pathophysiology

The most common cause of pituitary hypofunction is a pituitary tumour. Autoimmune disorders, infections, pituitary infarction (Sheehan's syndrome), or destruction of the pituitary gland (as a result of trauma, irradiation, or surgical procedures) can also cause hypopituitarism. *Sheehan's syndrome* is a postpartum condition of pituitary necrosis and hypopituitarism after circulatory collapse resulting from uterine hemorrhaging.

Hormone deficiencies involving anterior pituitary hormones lead to end-organ failure; thus the effects of hypopituitarism depend on the specific pituitary hormone or hormones that are lacking. For example, infertility may be the first indication of pituitary hypofunction associated with a pituitary tumour. Deficiencies of TSH and ACTH are life-threatening. ACTH deficiency causes a tendency toward shock and may result in an episode of acute adrenal insufficiency (refractory and life-threatening shock from sodium and water depletion). (Adrenal shock is discussed later in this chapter.)

Clinical Manifestations and Diagnostic Studies

The manifestations associated with pituitary hypofunction vary with the type and degree of dysfunction. Early manifestations associated with a space-occupying lesion include headaches, visual changes (decreased visual acuity or decreased peripheral vision), loss of smell, nausea and vomiting, and seizures. Manifestations associated with hyposecretion of the target glands vary widely (Table 51-1).

In addition to a history and physical examination, diagnostic studies such as MRI and CT are used to identify a pituitary tumour. Laboratory tests for diagnosing hypopituitarism vary widely but generally involve the direct measurement of pituitary hormones (e.g., TSH) or an indirect determination of the target organ hormones (e.g., triiodothyronine [T_3], thyroxine [T_4]). (See Chapter 50 for more information regarding diagnostic studies.)

TABLE 51-1	CLINICAL MANIFESTATIONS OF HYPOPITUITARISM
Hormone Deficiency	**Clinical Manifestations**
Growth hormone (GH)	Subtle, nonspecific findings. Truncal obesity, decreased muscle mass and strength, weakness, fatigue, depression or flat affect
Follicle-stimulating hormone (FSH) and luteinizing hormone (LH)	*Women:* Menstrual irregularities, loss of libido, changes in secondary sex characteristics such as decreased breast size *Men:* Testicular atrophy, diminished spermatogenesis, loss of libido, impotence, decreased facial hair and muscle mass
Thyroid-stimulating hormone (TSH)	Mild form of primary hypothyroidism: fatigue, cold intolerance, constipation, lethargy, weight gain
Adrenocorticotrophic hormone (ACTH)	Involves a deficiency of cortisol: weakness, fatigue, headache, dry and pale skin, diminished axillary and pubic hair, lowered resistance to infection, fasting hypoglycemia

NURSING AND COLLABORATIVE MANAGEMENT HYPOPITUITARISM

Treatment of hypopituitarism consists of surgery or radiation therapy for tumour removal, followed by permanent hormone replacement. Surgery and radiation therapy for pituitary tumours are discussed earlier in this chapter. Hormone therapy is carried out with the appropriate pituitary hormone (e.g., GH, corticosteroids, thyroid hormone, and sex hormones). Hormone therapies for thyroid hormone and corticosteroids are discussed later in this chapter.

A primary nursing role in anterior pituitary insufficiency is the assessment and recognition of signs and symptoms associated with hypopituitarism. Nursing management is directed at problems that result from hormone deficiency. The nurse also plays a pivotal role in teaching patients about diagnostic procedures, the disease process, and collaborative care options. Because the need for hormone therapy is lifelong, patient teaching must cover hormonal administration, adverse drug effects, and follow-up therapy.

Somatropin (Humatrope) is used for GH replacement therapy. Adults with GH deficiency respond well to GH replacement and experience increased energy, increased lean body mass, a feeling of well-being, and improved body image. The adverse drug effects most commonly reported by adults include swelling in the feet and the hands, pain in the joints, and headache. Somatropin is given as a subcutaneous injection. The dosage and administration is variable because it is adjusted according to the degree of relief from symptoms, IGF-1 levels, and the development of adverse effects.

Although gonadal deficiency is not life-threatening, replacement therapy is offered to improve sexual function and general well-being. This therapy, however, is contraindicated in individuals with certain medical conditions, such as breast cancer, phlebitis, pulmonary embolism in women, and prostate cancer in men. Estrogen and progesterone replacement therapy may be indicated for hypogonadal women to treat hot flashes, vaginal dryness, and decreased libido. Hormone therapy for women is discussed in greater detail in Chapter 56. Testosterone is used to treat men with gonadotropin deficiency. The benefits achieved with testosterone therapy include a return of male secondary sex characteristics; improvement in libido; and increased muscle mass, bone mass, and bone density.

DISORDERS OF THE POSTERIOR PITUITARY GLAND

The hormones secreted by the posterior pituitary—ADH and oxytocin—are actually produced in the hypothalamus and then transported to and stored in the posterior pituitary gland. ADH, also referred to as *arginine vasopressin* (AVP) or *vasopressin,* plays a major role in the regulation of water balance and osmolarity (see Chapter 50).

The two primary conditions associated with ADH secretion are a result of either overproduction or underproduction of ADH. Overproduction or oversecretion of ADH results in the syndrome of inappropriate antidiuretic hormone (SIADH). Underproduction or undersecretion of ADH results in a condition referred to as *diabetes insipidus.*

SYNDROME OF INAPPROPRIATE ANTIDIURETIC HORMONE

Etiology and Pathophysiology

SIADH occurs when ADH is released despite normal or low plasma osmolarity (Figure 51-3). SIADH results from an abnormal production or sustained secretion of ADH and is characterized by fluid retention, serum hypo-osmolality, dilutional hyponatremia, hypochloremia, concentrated urine in the presence of normal or increased intravascular volume, and normal renal function. This syndrome occurs more commonly in older adults (Runkle, Gomez-Hoyos, Cuesta-Hernández, et al., 2015).

The abnormal production or sustained secretion of ADH that leads to SIADH has various causes (Table 51-2). The most common cause is malignancy, especially small cell lung cancer. SIADH tends to be self-limiting when caused by head trauma or drugs but is chronic in nature when associated with tumours or metabolic diseases.

PATHOPHYSIOLOGY MAP

FIGURE 51-3 Pathophysiology of syndrome of inappropriate antidiuretic hormone (SIADH). Source: Redrawn from Urden, L. D., Stacy, K. M., & Lough, M. E. (2014). *Critical care nursing: Diagnosis and management* (7th ed., p. 838, Figure 33-6). St. Louis: Mosby.

Clinical Manifestations and Diagnostic Studies

Excess ADH increases both permeability of the distal tubules and collecting ducts and reabsorption of water into the circulation. Consequently, extracellular fluid volume expands, plasma osmolality declines, the glomerular filtration rate (GFR) increases, and sodium levels decline (dilutional hyponatremia) (Hong, 2012). Hyponatremia causes muscle cramps and weakness. Patients with SIADH experience low urinary output and increased body weight (Robinson & Verbalis, 2016). As the serum sodium level falls (usually to less than 120 mmol/L), manifestations become more severe and include vomiting, abdominal cramps, muscle twitching, and seizures. As plasma osmolality and serum sodium levels continue to decline, cerebral edema may occur, leading to lethargy, anorexia, confusion, headache, seizures, and coma.

SIADH is diagnosed from simultaneous measurements of urine and serum osmolality. The dilutional hyponatremia is indicated by a serum sodium level of less than 134 mmol/L, serum osmolality of less than 280 mmol/kg, and a urine specific gravity greater than 1.005. A serum osmolality much lower than the urine osmolality indicates the inappropriate excretion of concentrated urine in the presence of dilute serum.

Collaborative Care

Once SIADH is identified, treatment is directed at the underlying cause of the disorder. Medications that stimulate the release of ADH should be avoided or discontinued (see Table 51-2). The immediate treatment goal is to restore normal fluid volume and osmolality. If symptoms are mild and the serum sodium level exceeds 125 mmol/L, the only treatment may be restriction of fluids to between 800 and 1 000 mL/day. This restriction should result in gradual, daily reductions in weight, a progressive rise in serum sodium concentration and osmolality, and improvement in symptoms.

TABLE 51-2	CAUSES OF SYNDROME OF INAPPROPRIATE ANTIDIURETIC HORMONE

Malignant Tumours	**Drug Therapy**
• Colorectal cancer	• Antineoplastic agents (vincristine, vinblastine, cyclophosphamide [Procytox])
• Lymphoid cancers (Hodgkin's disease, non-Hodgkin's lymphoma, lymphocytic leukemia)	• Carbamazepine (Tegretol)
• Pancreatic cancer	• Chlorpropamide
• Prostate cancer	• General anaesthetic agents
• Small cell carcinoma of the lung	• Opioids
• Thymus cancer	• Oxytocin
	• SSRI antidepressants
Central Nervous System Disorders	• Thiazide diuretics
• Brain tumours	• Tricyclic antidepressants
• Cerebral atrophy	
• Cerebro-vascular injury	**Miscellaneous Conditions**
• Guillain-Barré syndrome	• Adrenal insufficiency
• Head injury (skull fracture, subdural hematoma, subarachnoid hemorrhage)	• Chronic obstructive pulmonary disease
• Infection (encephalitis, meningitis)	• HIV infection
• Systemic lupus erythematosus	• Hypothyroidism
	• Lung infection (pneumonia, tuberculosis, lung abscess)
	• Positive pressure mechanical ventilation

HIV, human immunodeficiency virus; *SSRI,* selective serotonin reuptake inhibitor.

In cases of severe hyponatremia (serum sodium level <120 mmol/L), especially in the presence of neurological symptoms such as seizures, IV hypertonic saline solution (3% to 5%) may be administered. Hypertonic saline must be administered very slowly on an infusion pump to avoid too rapid a rise in sodium. A diuretic such as furosemide (Lasix) may be used to promote diuresis, but only if the serum sodium level is at least 125 mmol/L because it may promote further loss of sodium. Because furosemide increases potassium, calcium, and magnesium losses, supplements may be needed. A fluid restriction of 500 mL/day is also indicated for patients with severe hyponatremia.

In chronic SIADH, water restriction of between 800 and 1 000 mL/day is recommended. Because this degree of restriction may not be tolerated, agents that block the effect of ADH on the renal tubules may be prescribed, thereby allowing more dilution of urine. Tolvaptan (Samsca), a vasopressin receptor antagonist, is used to treat euvolemic hyponatremia in hospitalized patients. This medication should be initiated in a closely monitored setting to prevent rapid correction of the serum sodium level.

NURSING MANAGEMENT
SYNDROME OF INAPPROPRIATE
ANTIDIURETIC HORMONE

The nurse can be instrumental in the early detection and treatment of SIADH. An appropriate nursing assessment (Table 51-3) should be conducted for patients at risk for SIADH and those who have confirmed SIADH. Specifically, the nurse should be alert for low urinary output with a high specific gravity, a sudden weight gain, or a decline in serum sodium level. Nursing management of acute onset of SIADH is presented in Table 51-3.

When SIADH is chronic, patients must learn to self-manage treatment regimens. Fluids are restricted to between 800 and

1 000 mL/day. Ice chips or sugarless chewing gum can help decrease thirst. If drinking liquids is an aspect of socialization, patients should be assisted in planning fluid intake so that liquid allowances are saved for social occasions. Patients may be treated with a diuretic to remove excess fluid volume. The diet should be supplemented with sodium and potassium, especially if diuretics are prescribed. Solutions of these electrolytes must be well diluted to prevent gastro-intestinal irritation or damage. They are best taken at mealtime to allow mixing with and dilution by food. Patients should be taught the symptoms of fluid and electrolyte imbalances, especially those involving sodium and potassium, so that responses to treatment can be monitored (see Chapter 19).

DIABETES INSIPIDUS

Etiology and Pathophysiology

Diabetes insipidus (DI) is a group of conditions associated with a deficiency of production or secretion of ADH or with a decreased renal response to ADH caused by injury to the neurohypophyseal system. The decrease in ADH results in fluid and electrolyte imbalances caused by increased urinary output and increased plasma osmolality (Figure 51-4). Depending on the cause, DI may be transient or a chronic lifelong condition.

Diabetes insipidus has several classifications (Table 51-4). *Central DI* is the most common form.

Clinical Manifestations

DI is characterized by increased thirst (polydipsia) and increased urination (polyuria; see Figure 51-4) (John & Day, 2012). The primary characteristic of DI is the excretion of large quantities of urine (5–20 L per day) with a very low specific gravity (<1.005) and urine osmolality of less than 100 mmol/kg. Serum osmolality is elevated (usually >300 mmol/kg) as a result of hypernatremia caused by pure water loss in the kidneys. Most affected patients compensate for fluid loss by drinking great amounts of water so that serum osmolality is normal or only moderately elevated. Patients may be fatigued from nocturia and may experience generalized weakness.

Central DI usually occurs suddenly with excessive fluid loss. After intracranial surgery, DI usually has a triphasic pattern: the

---

TABLE 51-3 NURSING ASSESSMENT

Syndrome of Inappropriate Antidiuretic Hormone

Assessment
- Daily weight measurement
- Frequent measurement of intake (oral and parenteral) and output
- Frequent measurement of urine specific gravity
- Frequent measurement of vital signs
- Monitoring of heart and lung sounds
- Monitoring of level of consciousness
- Observation for signs of hyponatremia (e.g., decreased neurological function, seizures, nausea and vomiting, muscle cramping)

Management
- Frequent oral hygiene
- Frequent turning, positioning, and range of motion exercise (if patient is bedridden)
- Positioning of head of bed flat or with no more than 10 degrees of elevation to enhance venous return to heart and increase left atrial filling pressure, thereby reducing ADH release
- Protection from injury (e.g., assist with ambulation, bed alarm) because of potential alterations in mental status
- Provision of distractions to decrease the discomfort of thirst related to fluid restrictions
- Provision of support for patient and significant others regarding diagnosis and any mental status changes
- Restricting total fluid intake to no more than 1 000 mL/day (including that taken with medications)
- Seizure precautions

ADH, antidiuretic hormone.

PATHOPHYSIOLOGY MAP

FIGURE 51-4 Pathophysiology of diabetes insipidus. Source: Redrawn from Urden, L. D., Stacy, K. M., & Lough, M. E. (2014). *Critical care nursing: Diagnosis and management* (7th ed., p. 833, Figure 33-5). St. Louis: Mosby.

TABLE 51-4	TYPES AND CAUSES OF DIABETES INSIPIDUS
Types	**Causes**
Central (neurogenic) DI	Results from an interference with ADH synthesis or release. Multiple causes include brain tumour, head injury, brain surgery, CNS infections.
Nephrogenic DI	Results from inadequate renal response to ADH despite presence in adequate levels. Causes include drug therapy (especially lithium), renal damage, or hereditary renal disease.
Primary DI	Results from excessive water intake. Causes are structural lesion in thirst centre and psychological disorder.

ADH, antidiuretic hormone; *CNS*, central nervous system; *DI*, diabetes insipidus.

acute phase, with abrupt onset of polyuria; an interphase, in which urine volume apparently normalizes; and a third phase, in which central DI is permanent. The third phase is usually apparent within 10 to 14 days postoperatively. Central DI that results from head trauma is usually self-limiting and improves with treatment of the underlying problem. DI following cranial surgery is more likely to be permanent. Although the clinical manifestations of nephrogenic DI are similar, the onset and the amount of fluid losses are less dramatic.

If oral fluid intake cannot keep up with urinary losses, a severe fluid volume deficit results. This deficit is manifested by weight loss, constipation, poor tissue turgor, hypotension, tachycardia, and shock. In addition, affected patients show central nervous system (CNS) manifestations, ranging from irritability and mental dullness to coma. These manifestations are related to increasing serum osmolality and hypernatremia. Because of the polyuria, severe dehydration and hypovolemic shock may occur.

Diagnostic Studies

Because DI may be central, nephrogenic, or psychogenic in origin, identification of the cause is the initial step. A complete history is documented, and a thorough physical examination is performed. Primary or psychogenic DI is associated with overhydration and hypervolemia rather than with the dehydration and hypovolemia seen in other forms of DI. A water deprivation test is usually performed to confirm the diagnosis of central DI. Before the water deprivation test, the patient's baseline weight, pulse, urine and plasma osmolalities, specific gravity of urine, and blood pressure (BP) are measured. All fluids are withheld for 8 to 16 hours. Patients may be anxious and should be reassured that the test will be stopped if fluid volume deficit becomes severe. Patients should be observed throughout the test because of the craving to drink. During the test, the patient's BP, weight, and urine osmolality are assessed hourly. The test continues until urine osmolality stabilizes (hourly increase of <30 mmol/kg in 3 consecutive hours), body weight declines by 3%, or orthostatic hypotension develops. ADH is then given, and urine osmolality is measured 1 hour later. In central DI, the rise in urinary osmolality after vasopressin administration exceeds 9%. Individuals with nephrogenic DI will have no response (Pagana & Pagana, 2013).

Collaborative Care

Determining and treating the primary cause is central in the collaborative management of DI. The therapeutic goal is maintenance of fluid and electrolyte balance.

For central DI, fluid and hormonal replacement is the cornerstone of treatment. In acute DI, hypotonic saline is administered IV and titrated to replace urinary output (Gardner, 2011). Hormone replacement is necessary because of the lack of ADH production or secretion. Desmopressin acetate (DDAVP), an analogue of ADH, is the hormone replacement of choice for central DI. DDAVP can be administered orally, IV, or as a nasal spray. Another drug available for ADH replacement is vasopressin. Several drugs can be used for the treatment of partial central DI, including carbamazepine (Tegretol).

Hormone replacement has little effect in the treatment of nephrogenic DI because the kidney is unable to respond to ADH. Instead, the treatment for nephrogenic DI revolves around dietary measures (low-sodium diet) and thiazide diuretics. Limiting sodium intake to no more than 3 g per day is thought to help decrease urine output. Thiazide diuretics (e.g., hydrochlorothiazide) are able to slow the GFR and allow the kidneys to reabsorb more water in the loop of Henle and the distal tubules. When low-sodium diet and thiazides are not effective, indomethacin (Indocin) may be prescribed. Indomethacin, a nonsteroidal anti-inflammatory drug (NSAID), helps increase renal responsiveness to ADH.

NURSING MANAGEMENT
DIABETES INSIPIDUS

Nursing management of patients with DI revolves around early detection, maintenance of adequate hydration, and patient teaching for long-term management.

Acute DI is treated with fluids and hormone replacement. Fluids are replaced orally or IV, depending on the patient's condition and ability to drink copious amounts of fluids. Adequate amounts of fluids should be kept at the patient's bedside. If IV glucose solutions are used, the serum glucose level should be monitored because hyperglycemia and glucosuria can lead to osmotic diuresis, which increases the fluid volume deficit. Monitoring of blood pressure (BP), heart rate, and urine output and specific gravity is essential and may be required hourly in the patient who is acutely ill. Level of consciousness must also be monitored, as well as signs of acute dehydration, by assessing alertness, response to stimuli, mucous membranes, tachycardia, and skin turgor. Accurate records of intake and output, urine specific gravity, and daily weights are mandatory in the assessment of fluid volume status.

Nursing interventions also include the administration of DDAVP. Patients should be assessed for weight gain, headache, restlessness, and signs of hyponatremia and water intoxication. By monitoring fluid intake and output and the urine specific gravity, the nurse can assess the adequacy of treatment. The health care provider should be notified immediately if the patient with DI develops increased urine volume with a low specific gravity because this may indicate the need to change the dosage of DDAVP.

The patient with chronic DI requiring long-term ADH replacement needs instruction in self-management. DDAVP can be taken orally or intranasally. Nasal irritation may result from nasal administration. Headache, nausea, and other signs of hyponatremia may indicate overdosage, whereas failure to improve may indicate underdosage. The patient should be instructed to report any of these symptoms. Patients taking DDAVP should be instructed to monitor their weight daily; increases in weight may indicate fluid retention. The need for close follow-up, including laboratory studies, is an essential part of the teaching plan.

Table 51-5 compares diabetes insipidus and SIADH.

TABLE 51-5 COMPARISON OF DIABETES INSIPIDUS AND SIADH

Feature	Diabetes Insipidus	SIADH
Definition	Deficiency of ADH results in inability to conserve water.	Excessive amounts of ADH are secreted from posterior pituitary and other ectopic sources.
Pathophysiological features	With ADH deficiency, permeability of water is diminished, which results in excretion of large volumes of hypotonic fluid. Three patterns may develop: (a) transient diabetes insipidus—abrupt onset within first few days after neurosurgery, resolves; (b) permanent diabetes insipidus—abrupt and early onset, persists for several weeks or for life; (c) triphasic diabetes insipidus—an acute phase with abrupt onset of polyuria; an interphase, in which urine volume apparently normalizes; and a third phase, in which central diabetes insipidus is permanent.	Key features of ADH excess are (a) water retention, (b) hyponatremia, and (c) hypo-osmolality. Continual release of ADH causes water retention from renal tubules and collecting ducts; extracellular fluid volume increases with dilutional hyponatremia; and hyponatremia suppresses renin and aldosterone secretions, which causes decrease in proximal tubule reabsorption of Na^+.
Clinical manifestations	Genito-urinary: polyuria: 5 to 18 L/day; clear urine; urinary frequency; nocturia Gastro-intestinal: weight loss; polydipsia (if thirst mechanism intact) Integumentary: dry skin and mucous membranes Neurological: mentation changes as electrolyte imbalance and hypotension worsen	Related to degree of hyponatremia: confusion, lethargy, irritability, seizures, coma Gastro-intestinal: decreased motility with anorexia, nausea, vomiting; abrupt weight gain *without edema* in 5%-10% of affected patients

ADH, antidiuretic hormone; *SIADH,* syndrome of inappropriate antidiuretic hormone.
Source: Adapted from Black, J. M., & Hawks, J. H. (2009). *Medical-surgical nursing: Clinical management for positive outcomes* (8th ed., pp. 1058–1059). St. Louis: Saunders Elsevier.

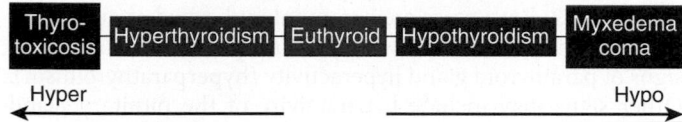

FIGURE 51-5 Continuum of thyroid dysfunction.

DISORDERS OF THE THYROID GLAND

The thyroid hormones—thyroxine (T_4) and triiodothyronine (T_3)—regulate energy metabolism, growth, and development. Disorders of the thyroid gland include enlargement, benign and malignant nodules, inflammation, and hyperfunctioning and hypofunctioning states (Figure 51-5).

GOITRE

A goitre is an enlarged thyroid gland. In a person with a goitre, the thyroid cells are stimulated to grow, which may result in an overactive thyroid (hyperthyroidism) or an underactive one (hypothyroidism). Goitres are common in patients with Graves' disease (Figure 51-6). A goitre that produces excess thyroid hormone is called a *toxic goitre.* A nontoxic goitre produces normal levels of thyroid hormone. Goitre as a clinical manifestation of thyroid disorders is further discussed in the following sections.

The most common cause of goitre worldwide is a lack of iodine in the diet. In Canada, where most people use iodized salt, goitre is more often caused by the overproduction or underproduction of thyroid hormones or by nodules that develop in the gland itself. Foods or drugs that contain thyroid-inhibiting substances (goitrogens) can cause goitre (Table 51-6).

In a person with a goitre, TSH and T_4 levels are measured to determine whether a goitre is associated with hyperthyroidism, hypothyroidism, or normal thyroid function. Thyroid antibodies are measured to assess for thyroiditis (inflammation of the thyroid). Treatment with thyroid hormone may prevent further thyroid enlargement. Large goitres are removed surgically.

FIGURE 51-6 Exophthalmos and goitre of Graves' disease. Source: Forbes, C. D., & Jackson, W. F. (2003). *Color atlas and text of clinical medicine* (3rd ed., p. 309, Figure 7.55). London: Mosby.

THYROID NODULES AND CANCER

A *thyroid nodule,* a palpable deformity of the thyroid gland, may be benign or malignant. More than 95% of all thyroid nodules are benign. The incidence of thyroid nodules increases with age. Benign nodules are usually not dangerous, but they can cause tracheal compression if they become too large. Nodules should be assessed and evaluated (discussed in the section Diagnostic Studies).

Thyroid cancer is the most common endocrine-related carcinoma. It was estimated that 5 600 new cases of thyroid cancer would be diagnosed in Canada in 2012 (Canadian Cancer Society's Steering Committee on Cancer Statistics, 2012), the majority of these in women. The primary sign of thyroid cancer is the

TABLE 51-6	**GOITROGENS**	
Thyroid Inhibitors	**Other Drugs**	**Foods***
• Iodine in large doses	• Amiodarone	• Broccoli
• Methimazole	• Lithium	• Brussels sprouts
(Tapazole)	• Para-aminosalicylic	• Cabbage
• Propylthiouracil	acid	• Cauliflower
	• Salicylates	• Kale
	• Sulphonamides	• Mustard
		• Peanuts
		• Turnips

*List is not all-inclusive.

presence of a painless, palpable nodule or nodules in an enlarged thyroid gland. Patients or health care providers discover most of these nodules during routine palpation of the neck.

Types of Thyroid Cancer

The four main types of thyroid cancer include papillary, follicular, medullary, and anaplastic. *Papillary* thyroid cancer is the most common type, accounting for about 70% to 80% of all thyroid cancers. Papillary cancer tends to grow slowly and spreads initially to lymph nodes in the neck.

Follicular thyroid cancer, which accounts for approximately 10% to 15% of all thyroid cancers, tends to occur in older adults. Follicular cancer first grows into the cervical lymph nodes. Follicular cancer is more likely than papillary cancer to grow into blood vessels and, from there, to spread to the lungs and bones.

Medullary thyroid cancer, which accounts for 5% to 10% of all thyroid cancers, is more likely to occur in families and to be associated with other endocrine problems. It can be diagnosed through genetic testing for a proto-oncogene called *RET*. In family members of a person with medullary thyroid cancer, a positive finding of the *RET* proto-oncogene can enable early diagnosis and treatment of medullary thyroid cancer.

Anaplastic thyroid cancer, which accounts for less than 5% of all thyroid cancers, is the most advanced and aggressive thyroid cancer. It is the least likely to respond to treatment.

Diagnostic Studies

Nodular enlargement of the thyroid gland or palpation of a mass usually necessitates radiological evaluation. Ultrasonography is often the first radiological test used in the diagnostic workup of a thyroid nodule. CT, MRI, and ultrasonography-guided fine-needle aspiration (FNA) are other diagnostic options. FNA is indicated when a tissue sample is necessary for pathological examination. A thyroid scan may also be performed to evaluate for possible malignancy. The scan shows whether nodules on the thyroid are "hot" or "cold." Thyroid tumours may or may not take up radioactive iodine (RAI). Tumours that take up the RAI are called "hot" nodules and are nearly always benign. If the nodule does not take up the radioactive iodine, it appears as "cold" and has a higher risk of being malignant. Measurement of serum calcitonin is also helpful in diagnosis because increased levels are associated with medullary thyroid carcinoma.

NURSING AND COLLABORATIVE CARE THYROID CANCER

Surgical removal of the tumour is usually indicated in the treatment of thyroid cancer. Surgical procedures may range from unilateral total lobectomy to total thyroidectomy with bilateral lobectomy. RAI may be given to some patients to destroy any remaining cancer cells after surgery but is not commonly used (Lamartina, Durante, Filetti, et al., 2015). In addition, many thyroid cancers are TSH dependent, and thyroid hormone in high doses is often prescribed to inhibit pituitary secretion of TSH. Radiation therapy is rarely used (Thyroid Foundation of Canada, 2016). Chemotherapy may be used in advanced disease. Nursing care for patients with thyroid tumours is similar to care for patients who have undergone thyroidectomy and should also include general nursing measures for patients with cancer (see Chapter 18 and NCPs 18-1 and 18-2 for the care of patients undergoing radiation and chemotherapy, available on the Evolve website).

MULTIPLE ENDOCRINE NEOPLASIA

Multiple endocrine neoplasia is an inherited condition characterized by hormone-secreting tumours (Clark, 2015). Multiple endocrine neoplasia is caused by the mutation of one of two genes, *MEN1* or *RET,* that normally control cell growth. Tumours may develop in childhood or later in life.

The two major types of multiple endocrine neoplasia are type 1 and type 2. Both types are commonly inherited as autosomal dominant disorders. People with type 1 neoplasia commonly show signs of parathyroid gland hyperactivity (hyperparathyroidism). Other signs may include hyperactivity of the pituitary gland (prolactinoma) and pancreas (gastrinomas). In most cases, the tumours are initially benign, and some tumours later become malignant. People with type 2 neoplasia often have clinical manifestations of medullary thyroid carcinoma. They may also develop pheochromocytoma (tumour of the adrenal glands). (Pheochromocytoma is discussed later in this chapter.)

Treatment of the tumour(s) may include conservative management (watchful waiting), medication to block the effects of excess hormone, and surgical removal of the gland or tumour (or both). It is important for patients with multiple endocrine neoplasia to have regular screening visits with their health care provider so that new tumours may be detected early and existing tumours carefully monitored.

THYROIDITIS

Thyroiditis is an inflammation of the thyroid gland that can have several causes. *Subacute granulomatous thyroiditis* is thought to be caused by a viral infection. *Acute thyroiditis* is caused by a bacterial or fungal infection. Subacute and acute forms of thyroiditis have abrupt onsets and usually a recent viral infection. The thyroid gland is tender and enlarged, and the patient often has neck pain and fatigue (Lian-Xi, Xing, Bing, et al., 2014). *Chronic autoimmune thyroiditis* (Hashimoto's thyroiditis) can lead to hypothyroidism. *Hashimoto's thyroiditis* is a chronic autoimmune disease in which thyroid tissue is replaced by lymphocytes and fibrous tissue (Figure 51-7). It is the most common cause of goitrous hypothyroidism and is most common in women. *Silent thyroiditis,* a form of lymphocytic thyroiditis, has a variable onset and no apparent symptoms. *Postpartum thyroiditis* occurs frequently in women with a history of thyroid disease who have recently given birth. In most respects, silent and postpartum thyroiditis resemble Hashimoto's thyroiditis, except that the gland tends to recover and thyroid hormone treatment needs to be administered for only a few weeks (Thyroid Foundation of Canada, 2016).

FIGURE 51-7 Appearance of the neck in Hashimoto's thyroiditis. Source: Belchetz, P. E., & Hammond, P. (2003). *Mosby's color atlas and text of diabetes and endocrinology.* London: Mosby.

T_4 and T_3 levels are initially elevated in subacute, acute, and silent thyroiditis but may become depressed over time. TSH levels are initially low and then elevated. Thyroid hormone levels are usually low in chronic Hashimoto's thyroiditis, but the TSH level is high. Radioactive iodine uptake (RAIU) is suppressed in subacute and silent thyroiditis. Antithyroid antibodies are present in patients with Hashimoto's thyroiditis.

Recovery from thyroiditis may be complete in weeks or months without treatment. If the condition is bacterial in origin, treatment may include specific antibiotics or surgical drainage. In subacute and acute forms, salicylates and NSAIDs are administered. If patients do not respond to these drugs in 48 hours, corticosteroids are administered. Propranolol (Inderal) or atenolol (Tenormin) may be used for the cardiovascular symptoms of a hyperthyroid condition. Thyroid hormone replacement is indicated if a patient is hypothyroid.

Nursing care of patients with thyroiditis involves teaching about treatment and encouraging adherence to the treatment regimen. Patients are instructed to remain under close health care supervision so that progress can be monitored and any change in symptoms can be reported immediately to the health care provider.

Patients with thyroiditis of autoimmune origin may be susceptible to other autoimmune disorders such as Addison's disease, pernicious anemia, premature gonadal failure, or Graves' disease (Hubbard, 2011). Patients should be taught the signs and symptoms of these disorders, particularly Addison's disease. A patient receiving thyroid hormone replacement must be taught the expected adverse effects of these drugs and how to manage them. Patients treated surgically need care similar to that given to patients undergoing thyroidectomy.

HYPERTHYROIDISM

Hyperthyroidism is hyperactivity of the thyroid gland with sustained increase in synthesis and release of thyroid hormones. Thyrotoxicosis is the clinical syndrome of hypermetabolism caused by excess circulating levels of T_4, T_3, or both. Hyperthyroidism and thyrotoxicosis usually occur together, as in Graves' disease. However, in some forms of thyroiditis, thyrotoxicosis may occur without hyperthyroidism (Vaidya & Pearce, 2014).

Hyperthyroidism is more prevalent among women than among men; the frequency is highest among people 20 to 40 years old. The most common form of hyperthyroidism is Graves' disease. Other causes include toxic nodular goitre, thyroiditis, exogenous iodine excess, pituitary tumours, and thyroid cancer.

Etiology and Pathophysiology

Graves' Disease. Graves' disease is an autoimmune disease of unknown etiology marked by diffuse thyroid enlargement and excessive thyroid hormone secretion. Precipitating factors such as insufficient iodine supply, infections, and stressful life events may interact with genetic factors to cause Graves' disease. In Canada, Graves' disease accounts for 90% of the cases of hyperthyroidism and is more common in females (Thyroid Foundation of Canada, 2016). Cigarette smoking increases the risk for the development of eye problems associated with the disease (Strianese, Piscopo, Elefante, et al., 2013). Patients with this disease develop antibodies to the TSH receptor. These antibodies attach to the receptors and stimulate the thyroid gland to release T_3, T_4, or both. The excessive release of thyroid hormones leads to the clinical manifestations associated with thyrotoxicosis. The disease is characterized by remissions and exacerbations, with or without treatment. It may progress to destruction of thyroid tissue, which causes hypothyroidism.

Toxic Nodular Goitres. Nodular goitres are characterized by thyroid hormone–secreting nodules that are independent of TSH stimulation. If associated with signs of hyperthyroidism, a nodule is termed *toxic.* A goitre may have multiple nodules (multinodular goitre) or a single nodule (solitary autonomous nodule). The nodules are usually benign follicular adenomas. Toxic nodular goitres occur equally in men and women. Although they can appear at any age, the frequency of toxic multinodular goitre is highest among people older than 40 years.

Clinical Manifestations

The clinical manifestations of hyperthyroidism are related to the effects of excess amounts of thyroid hormones. Excess amounts of circulating thyroid hormone directly increase metabolism. They also increase tissue sensitivity to stimulation by the sympathetic nervous system.

Palpation of the thyroid gland may reveal a goitre. When the thyroid gland is excessively large, a goitre may be visible. Auscultation of the thyroid gland may reveal bruits, a reflection of increased blood supply. Another common finding associated with hyperthyroidism is *ophthalmopathy,* a term used to describe abnormal eye appearance or function. A classic finding in Graves' disease is exophthalmos, a protrusion of the eyeballs from the orbits (see Figure 51-6). Exophthalmos is a type of infiltrative ophthalmopathy that results from impairment of venous drainage from the orbit, which causes increased fat deposits and fluid (edema) in the retro-orbital tissues. Because of increased pressure, the eyeballs are forced outward and protrude. This sign is seen in 20% to 50% of patients with Graves' disease. It is usually bilateral but can be unilateral or asymmetrical. In ophthalmopathy, the upper eyelids are usually retracted and elevated, with the sclera visible above the iris. When the eyelids do not close completely, the exposed corneal surfaces become dry and irritated. Serious consequences, such as corneal ulcers and eventual loss of vision, can occur. The changes in the ocular muscles result in muscle weakness, causing diplopia.

Other common manifestations of thyroid hyperfunction are summarized in Table 51-7. A patient with advanced disease may exhibit many of the manifestations, whereas a patient in the early stages of hyperthyroidism may exhibit only weight loss and increased nervousness. Manifestations of hyperthyroidism (e.g., palpitations, tremors, weight loss) in older adults do not differ significantly from those in younger adults. In some instances in

TABLE 51-7   CLINICAL MANIFESTATIONS OF THYROID DYSFUNCTION

Hypofunction	Hyperfunction	Hypofunction	Hyperfunction
Cardiovascular System		**Musculo-Skeletal System**	
• Anemia	• Angina	• Arthralgia	• Dependent edema
• Cardiac hypertrophy	• Atrial fibrillation (more common	• Fatigue	• Fatigue
• Decreased rate and force of	in older adults)	• Muscular aches and pains	• Muscle weakness
cardiac contractions	• Bounding, rapid pulse	• Slow movements	• Osteoporosis
• Distant heart sounds	• Cardiac hypertrophy	• Weakness	• Proximal muscle wasting
• Increased capillary fragility	• Dysrhythmias		
• Tendency to develop heart	• Increased cardiac output	**Nervous System**	
failure, angina, myocardial	• Increased rate and force of	• Anxiety, depression	• Depression, fatigue, apathy (in
infarction	cardiac contractions	• Apathy	older adults)
• Varied changes in blood	• Palpitations	• Delayed relaxation of deep	• Difficulty in focusing eyes
pressure	• Systolic hypertension	tendon reflexes	• Exhaustion
	• Systolic murmurs	• Fatigue	• Fine tremor (of fingers and
		• Forgetfulness	tongue)
Respiratory System		• Hoarseness	• Hyper-reflexia of tendon reflexes
• Decreased breathing capacity	• Dyspnea on mild exertion	• Lethargy	• Inability to concentrate
• Dyspnea	• Increased respiratory rate	• Paresthesias	• Insomnia
		• Polyneuropathy	• Lability of mood, delirium
Gastro-Intestinal System		• Slow, slurred speech	• Nervousness
• Celiac disease	• Diarrhea, frequent defecation	• Slowed mental processes	• Personality changes: irritability,
• Constipation	• Hepatomegaly	• Stupor, coma	agitation
• Decreased appetite	• Increased appetite, thirst		• Restlessness
• Distended abdomen	• Increased bowel sounds		• Stupor, coma
• Enlarged, scaly tongue	• Increased peristalsis		
• Nausea and vomiting	• Splenomegaly	**Reproductive System**	
• Weight gain	• Weight loss	• Decreased libido	• Amenorrhea
		• Infertility	• Decreased fertility
Integumentary System		• Prolonged menstrual periods or	• Decreased libido
• Decreased sweating	• Clubbing of fingers (thyroid	amenorrhea	• Erectile dysfunction in men
• Dry, sparse, coarse hair	acropachy)		• Gynecomastia in men
• Dry, thick, inelastic, cold skin	• Diaphoresis		• Menstrual irregularities
• Generalized interstitial edema	• Fine, silky hair		
• Pallor	• Hair loss (may be patchy)	**Other**	
• Poor turgor of mucosa	• Palmar erythema	• Decreased hearing	• Elevated basal temperature
• Puffy face	• Premature greying (in men)	• Goitre	• Exophthalmos
• Thick, brittle nails	• Pretibial myxedema (infiltrative	• Increased sensitivity to opioids,	• Eyelid lag, stare
	dermopathy)	barbiturates, anaesthetics	• Eyelid retraction
	• Thin, brittle nails detached from	• Increased susceptibility to	• Goitre
	nail bed (onycholysis)	infection	• Increased sensitivity to stimulant
	• Warm, smooth, moist skin	• Intolerance of cold	drugs
		• Sleepiness	• Intolerance of heat
			• Rapid speech

which confusion and agitation are reported, dementia may be suspected and may delay the diagnosis. In Table 51-8, features of hyperthyroidism in younger- and older-adult patients are compared.

Complications

Thyrotoxic crisis (also called *thyroid storm*) is a rare, acute condition in which all hyperthyroid manifestations are intensified. Although thyrotoxic crisis is considered a life-threatening emergency, death is rare when treatment is initiated early. The cause is thought to be stressors (e.g., infection, trauma, surgery) in a patient with pre-existing hyperthyroidism, either diagnosed or undiagnosed. Heart and nerve tissues become more sensitive to sympathetic nervous system activation because more binding sites for epinephrine and norepinephrine are present.

Manifestations include severe tachycardia, heart failure, shock, hyperthermia (temperature up to 40.7°C), restlessness, agitation, seizures, abdominal pain, nausea, vomiting, diarrhea, delirium, and coma. Treatment is aimed at reducing circulating thyroid hormone levels and the clinical manifestations of this disorder by appropriate drug therapy. Supportive therapy is directed at managing respiratory distress, fever reduction, fluid replacement, and elimination or management of the initiating stressor or stressors.

Diagnostic Studies

The two primary laboratory findings used to confirm the diagnosis of hyperthyroidism are decreased TSH levels and elevated free T_4 levels. Total T_3 and T_4 levels may also be assessed, but these are not as definitive. Measurements of total T_3 and T_4 include both free and bound (to protein) hormone levels. The free hormone is the only form of the hormone that is biologically active.

The radioactive iodine uptake test is indicated to differentiate Graves' disease from other forms of thyroiditis. The 24-hour test of radioiodine uptake in patients with Graves' disease reveals a diffuse, homogeneous uptake of 35% to 90%, whereas in patients with thyroiditis, the amount of uptake is less than 20%. Patients with nodular goitre demonstrate uptake in the high-normal range (see Table 51-8).

TABLE 51-8 COMPARISON OF HYPERTHYROIDISM IN YOUNGER AND OLDER ADULTS

Features	Younger Adults	Older Adults
Common causes	Graves' disease in >90% of cases	Graves' disease or toxic nodular goitre
Common symptoms	Nervousness; irritability; weight loss; heat intolerance; warm, moist skin	Anorexia, weight loss, apathy, lassitude, depression, confusion
Goitre	Present in >90% of cases	Present in ~50% of cases
Ophthalmopathy	Exophthalmos present in 20%–50% of cases	Occasional exophthalmos
Cardiac features	Tachycardia and palpitations common, but without heart failure	Angina, dysrhythmias (especially atrial fibrillation), or heart failure may occur

TABLE 51-9 COLLABORATIVE CARE

Hyperthyroidism

Diagnostic
- History and physical examination
- Electrocardiography
- Laboratory tests
  - Serum free T$_4$, TSH levels
  - TRH stimulation test
- Ophthalmological examination
- Radioactive iodine uptake (RAIU)

Collaborative Therapy
Drug Therapy
- Antithyroid drugs
  - Methimazole (Tapazole)
  - Propylthiouracil (Propyl-Thyracil)

- Iodine
- β-Adrenergic blockers (e.g., propranolol [Inderal])

Radiation Therapy
- Radioactive iodine

Surgical Therapy
- Subtotal thyroidectomy

Nutritional Therapy
- Frequent meals
- High-calorie diet
- High-protein diet

T$_4$, thyroxine; *TRH*, thyrotropin-releasing hormone; *TSH*, thyroid-stimulating hormone.

Collaborative Care

The overall goal in the treatment of hyperthyroidism is to block the adverse effects of thyroid hormones and stop their oversecretion. The three primary treatment options for patients with hyperthyroidism are antithyroid medications, radioactive iodine therapy, and subtotal thyroidectomy (Table 51-9). However, the choice of treatment is influenced by the patient's age, the severity of the disorder, complicating features (including pregnancy), and the patient's preferences.

Drug Therapy. Drugs used in the treatment of hyperthyroidism include antithyroid drugs, iodine, and β-adrenergic blockers. It is important to note that although these drugs are useful in the treatment of thyrotoxic states, they are not considered curative. Radiation therapy or surgery may ultimately be required.

Antithyroid Drugs. The first-line antithyroid drugs used in the treatment of hyperthyroidism are thioamides, such as propylthiouracil (Propyl-Thyracil) and methimazole (Tapazole). These drugs inhibit the synthesis of thyroid hormones. Propylthiouracil also blocks peripheral conversion of T$_4$ to T$_3$. Individual response is considerably varied; however, improvement usually begins 1 to 2 weeks after the initiation of therapy, and good results are seen within 4 to 8 weeks. Therapy is usually continued for 6

months to 2 years to allow for spontaneous remission. The major disadvantages of these drugs are possible nonadherence to the regimen and a high rate of recurrence of hyperthyroidism when the drugs are discontinued. Indications for use of antithyroid drugs include Graves' disease in young patients, hyperthyroidism during pregnancy, and the need to attain a euthyroid state before surgery or radiation therapy.

Iodine. Iodine is used with other antithyroid drugs in the preparation of a patient for thyroidectomy or for treatment of thyrotoxic crisis. The administration of iodine in large doses rapidly inhibits synthesis of T$_3$ and T$_4$ and blocks the release of these hormones into the circulation. It also decreases the vascularity of the thyroid gland, which makes surgery safer and easier. The effect of iodine is usually maximal within 1 to 2 weeks. Because the therapeutic effect lessens, long-term iodine therapy is not effective in controlling hyperthyroidism. Iodine is available in the form of Lugol's solution (Health Canada, 2016).

β-Adrenergic Blockers. β-Adrenergic blockers are used for symptomatic relief of thyrotoxicosis that results from increased β-adrenergic receptor stimulation caused by excess thyroid hormones. Propranolol (Inderal) is usually administered with other antithyroid agents and rapidly provides symptomatic relief. Atenolol (Tenormin) is the preferred β-adrenergic blocker for use in hyperthyroid patients with asthma or heart disease.

Radioactive Iodine Therapy. Radioactive iodine (RAI) therapy is the treatment of choice for most nonpregnant adults. (Before initiation of therapy, a pregnancy test is performed on all women who menstruate.) RAI damages or destroys thyroid tissue, thus limiting thyroid hormone secretion. Patients should be instructed that radiation-related thyroiditis and parotiditis are possible and may cause dryness and irritation of the mouth and throat. Relief may be obtained with frequent sips of water, ice chips, or the use of normal saline or a baking soda solution (e.g., 10 mL of baking soda in 250 mL of water) to gargle three or four times per day. The discomfort should subside in 3 to 4 days. If dryness and irritation persist, patients should contact the health care provider. The response to radioactive iodine is delayed, and the effect may not be maximal for 2 to 3 months. For this reason, patients are usually treated with antithyroid drugs and propranolol before and during the first 3 months after the initiation of RAI, until the effects of irradiation become apparent. Although this method of treatment is usually effective, there is a high incidence of post-treatment hypothyroidism, which results in the need for lifelong thyroid hormone replacement. Patients and the family or caregiver should be taught about the symptoms of hypothyroidism and instructed to seek medical help if these symptoms occur.

Surgical Therapy. Thyroidectomy is indicated when a large goitre causes tracheal compression, when patients do not respond to antithyroid therapy, and in patients with thyroid cancer. In addition, surgery may be performed when an individual is not a candidate for RAI. One advantage of thyroidectomy over RAI is a more rapid reduction in T$_3$ and T$_4$ levels. A *subtotal thyroidectomy* is the preferred surgical procedure and involves the removal of a significant portion (90%) of the thyroid gland. If too much tissue is taken, the gland does not regenerate after surgery, and hypothyroidism results.

Endoscopic thyroidectomy is a minimally invasive procedure. In this procedure, several small incisions are made through which an endoscope and other instruments can be passed to remove thyroid tissue or nodules. It is an appropriate procedure for patients with small nodules (<3 cm in diameter) in whom there is no evidence of malignancy. Advantages of endoscopic thyroidectomy over the traditional approach are less scarring, less pain, and a faster return to normal activity.

Before surgery, antithyroid drugs, iodine, and β-adrenergic blockers may be administered to achieve a euthyroid state and to control symptoms. Iodine reduces vascularization of the gland, thereby reducing the risk for hemorrhage. Postoperative complications include hypothyroidism, damage to or inadvertent removal of parathyroid glands (causing hypoparathyroidism and hypocalcemia), hemorrhage, injury to the recurrent or the superior laryngeal nerve, thyrotoxic crisis, and infection.

Nutritional Therapy. The potential for nutritional deficits is high when the metabolic rate is increased. A high-calorie diet (4000 to 5000 kcal/day) may be ordered to satisfy hunger and prevent tissue breakdown. This is accomplished with six full meals a day and snacks high in protein, carbohydrates, minerals, and vitamins, particularly vitamin A, thiamine, vitamin B$_6$, and vitamin C. The protein allowance should be 1 to 2 g/kg of ideal body weight. Increased carbohydrates should compensate for disturbed metabolism, provide energy, and spare body protein stores. Highly seasoned and high-fibre foods should be avoided because they can further stimulate the already hyperactive GI tract. Substitutes should be provided for caffeine-containing beverages such as coffee, tea, and cola because their stimulating effects increase restlessness and sleep disturbances. The nurse should consult a dietitian for guidance in meeting the nutritional needs of a patient with hyperthyroidism.

NURSING MANAGEMENT HYPERTHYROIDISM

NURSING ASSESSMENT

Subjective and objective data that should be obtained from an individual with hyperthyroidism are presented in Table 51-10.

NURSING DIAGNOSES

Nursing diagnoses for patients with hyperthyroidism include, but are not limited to, the following:
- *Activity intolerance* related to *physical deconditioning* (fatigue, exhaustion, heat intolerance secondary to hypermetabolism)
- *Imbalanced nutrition: less than body requirements* related to *insufficient dietary intake* (hypermetabolism)

Additional information on nursing diagnoses for the patient with hyperthyroidism are presented in Nursing Care Plan (NCP) 51-1, available on the Evolve website.

PLANNING

The overall goals are that patients with hyperthyroidism will (a) experience relief from symptoms, (b) have no serious complications related to the disease or treatment, (c) maintain nutritional balance, and (d) adhere to the therapeutic plan.

NURSING IMPLEMENTATION

ACUTE INTERVENTION. Individuals who have hyperthyroidism are usually treated in an out-patient setting. However, patients who develop acute thyrotoxicosis and those who undergo thyroidectomy require hospitalization and acute care.

Acute Thyrotoxicosis. Acute thyrotoxicosis is a systemic syndrome that necessitates aggressive treatment, often in a critical care unit. Medications that block thyroid hormone production and the sympathetic nervous system (see previous discussion) should

---

TABLE 51-10 NURSING ASSESSMENT

Hyperthyroidism

Subjective Data
Important Health Information
Past health history: Pre-existing goitre; recent infection or trauma; immigration from iodine-deficient area; autoimmune disease; positive family history of thyroid or autoimmune disorders
Medications: Use of thyroid hormones or herbal therapies that may contain thyroid hormone

Symptoms
- Chest pain; dyspnea on exertion; palpitations
- Decreased libido; erectile dysfunction, gynecomastia (in men); amenorrhea (in women)
- Diarrhea; polyuria
- Emotional lability, irritability, restlessness, personality changes, delirium, nervousness
- Heat intolerance; pruritus; sweating
- Insomnia
- Insufficient iodine intake; weight loss; increased appetite or thirst; nausea
- Muscle weakness, fatigue

Objective Data
General Observation
Agitation, rapid speech and body movements; hyperthermia, enlarged or nodular thyroid gland

Eyes
Exophthalmos, eyelid retraction; infrequent blinking

Integumentary
Warm, diaphoretic, velvety skin; thin, loose nails; fine, silky hair and hair loss; palmar erythema; digital clubbing; white pigmentation of skin (vitiligo); diffuse edema of legs and feet

Respiratory
Tachypnea

Cardiovascular
Tachycardia, bounding pulse, systolic murmurs, dysrhythmias, hypertension

Gastro-Intestinal
Increased bowel sounds; hepatosplenomegaly

Neurological
Hyper-reflexia; diplopia; fine tremors of hands, tongue, eyelids; stupor; coma

Musculo-Skeletal
Muscle wasting

Reproductive
Menstrual irregularities, infertility in women; erectile dysfunction, gynecomastia in men

Possible Findings
↑ T$_3$ level, ↑ T$_4$ level; ↑ T$_3$ resin uptake; ↓serum TSH level; chest radiograph showing enlarged heart, findings of tachycardia, atrial fibrillation on ECG

ECG, electrocardiogram; *T$_3$,* triiodothyronine; *T$_4$,* thyroxine; *TSH,* thyroid-stimulating hormone.

be administered. Supportive therapy includes monitoring for cardiac dysrhythmias and decompensation, ensuring adequate oxygenation, and administering IV fluids to replace fluid and electrolyte losses. This is especially important in patients who develop vomiting and diarrhea.

The patient's room should be kept calm and quiet because increased metabolism causes sleep disturbances. Provision of adequate rest may be a challenge because of the patient's irritability and restlessness. Specific interventions may include (a) placing the patient in a cool room, away from very ill patients and noisy, high-traffic areas; (b) using lightweight bed coverings and changing the linen frequently if the patient is diaphoretic; (c) encouraging and assisting with exercise involving large muscle groups (tremors can interfere with small-muscle coordination) to allow the release of nervous tension and restlessness; and (d) establishing a supportive, trusting relationship to help the patient cope with aggravating events and to lessen anxiety.

Exophthalmos, when present, incurs a potential for corneal injury related to irritation and dryness. Affected patients may also have orbital pain. Nursing interventions to relieve eye discomfort and prevent corneal ulceration include applying artificial tears to soothe and moisten conjunctival membranes. Salt restriction may help reduce periorbital edema. Elevation of the patient's head promotes fluid drainage from the periorbital area—the patient should sit upright as much as possible. Dark glasses reduce glare and prevent irritation from air currents, dust, and dirt. If the eyelids cannot be closed, they should be lightly taped shut for sleep. To maintain flexibility, the patient should be taught to exercise the intraocular muscles several times a day by turning the eyes in the complete range of motion. Good grooming can be helpful in reducing the loss of self-esteem that can result from an altered body image. If the exophthalmos is severe, corticosteroids, radiation of retro-orbital tissues, orbital decompression, or corrective eyelid or muscle surgery may be helpful.

Thyroid Surgery. When subtotal thyroidectomy is the treatment of choice, patients must be adequately prepared in order to avoid postoperative complications. To alleviate thyrotoxicosis, iodine treatment or propylthiouracil may be given before surgery. Iodine is mixed with water or juice and sipped through a straw after meals. The nurse assesses patients for signs of iodine toxicity, such as swelling of buccal mucosa and other mucous membranes, excessive salivation, nausea and vomiting, and skin reactions. If toxicity occurs, iodine administration should be discontinued and the physician notified.

Preoperative teaching should include comfort and safety measures in which patients can participate. Coughing, deep breathing, and leg exercises should be practised and their importance explained. Patients should be taught how to support the head manually while turning in bed because this manoeuvre minimizes stress on the suture line after surgery. Range-of-motion exercises of the neck should be practised. The nurse should explain routine postoperative care such as IV infusions. Patients should be told that talking is likely to be difficult for a short time after surgery.

SAFETY ALERT
- Airway obstruction, although not common, may occur postoperatively.
- Airway obstruction is an emergency situation.
- Oxygen, suction equipment, and a tracheostomy tray should be readily available in the patient's room.

Recurrent laryngeal nerve damage leads to vocal cord paralysis. If both cords are paralyzed, spastic airway obstruction may occur, necessitating an immediate tracheostomy.

Respiration may also become difficult because of excess swelling of the neck tissues, hemorrhage, hematoma formation, and laryngeal stridor. *Laryngeal stridor* (harsh, vibratory sound) may occur during inspiration and expiration as a result of edema of the laryngeal nerve. Laryngeal stridor may also be related to tetany, which occurs if the parathyroid glands are removed or damaged during surgery, which leads to hypocalcemia. To treat tetany, calcium salts such as calcium gluconate and calcium chloride should be readily available for IV administration. After a thyroidectomy, the patient should be cared for as follows:

1. Assessment every 2 hours for 24 hours for signs of hemorrhage or tracheal compression, such as irregular breathing, neck swelling, frequent swallowing, sensations of fullness at the incision site, choking, and blood on the dressings.
2. Placement in a semi-Fowler's position, and support of the patient's head with pillows, with care to avoid flexion of the neck and any tension on the suture lines.
3. Monitoring of vital signs. The nurse completes the initial assessment by checking for signs of hypocalcemia and tetany secondary to hypoparathyroidism (e.g., tingling sensation in toes, in fingers, or around the mouth; muscular twitching; apprehension) and by evaluating difficulty in speaking and hoarseness. The nurse should also check for the presence of Trousseau's and Chvostek's signs for 72 hours (see Chapter 19, Figure 19-15). Some hoarseness is to be expected for 3 to 4 days after surgery because of edema.
4. Control of postoperative pain with medication.

If postoperative recovery is uneventful, patients are ambulated within hours after surgery, are permitted to take fluid as soon as tolerated, and may eat soft foods the day after surgery.

The appearance of the incision may be distressing to patients. They can be reassured that the scar will fade and eventually look like a normal neck wrinkle. A scarf, jewellery, a high collar, or other covering can effectively camouflage a fresh scar.

AMBULATORY AND HOME CARE
Postoperative Care. Patients and family members need to be aware that thyroid hormone balance should be monitored periodically to ensure that normal function has returned. Most patients experience a period of relative hypothyroidism soon after surgery because of the substantial reduction in the size of the thyroid. The remaining tissue usually hypertrophies, recovering the capacity to produce the hormone needed by the body, but this takes time. Thyroid hormone is not administered because exogenous hormone inhibits pituitary production of TSH and delays or prevents the restoration of normal gland function and thyroid tissue regeneration.

To prevent weight gain, caloric intake must be reduced substantially below the amount that was required before surgery. Adequate iodine is necessary to promote thyroid function, but excesses inhibit the thyroid. Seafood once or twice a week or normal use of iodized salt should provide sufficient iodine intake. Regular exercise stimulates the thyroid gland and should be encouraged. High environmental temperature should be avoided because it inhibits thyroid regeneration.

Regular follow-up care is necessary. Patients should be seen biweekly for a month and then at least semiannually to assess for the development of hypothyroidism. If a complete thyroidectomy has been performed, patients need instruction in lifelong thyroid replacement. Patients should be taught the signs and symptoms of progressive thyroid failure and instructed to seek medical care if these develop. Hypothyroidism is relatively easy to manage with oral administration of thyroid replacement.

EVALUATION

The following are expected outcomes for patients with hyperthyroidism:

- Relief from symptoms
- No serious complications related to the disease or the treatment
- Adherence to the therapeutic plan

HYPOTHYROIDISM

Etiology and Pathophysiology

Hypothyroidism affects approximately 2 per 100 people (Thyroid Foundation of Canada, 2016). Hypothyroidism results from insufficient circulating thyroid hormone as a result of various abnormalities. Hypothyroidism can be primary (related to destruction of thyroid tissue or defective hormone synthesis) or secondary (related to pituitary disease with decreased secretion of TSH or hypothalamic dysfunction with decreased secretion of thyrotropin-releasing hormone [TRH]). It may also be transient, related to thyroiditis or discontinuation of thyroid hormone therapy.

Iodine deficiency is the most common cause of hypothyroidism worldwide. In Canada, the most common cause of primary hypothyroidism in the adult is atrophy of the thyroid gland. This atrophy is the end result of Hashimoto's thyroiditis and Graves' disease. These autoimmune diseases destroy the thyroid gland. Hypothyroidism also may develop as a result of treatment for hyperthyroidism, specifically the surgical removal of the thyroid gland or radioactive iodine therapy. Drugs such as amiodarone (which contains iodine) and lithium (which blocks hormone production) are known to produce hypothyroidism.

Cretinism, hypothyroidism that develops in infancy, is caused by thyroid hormone deficiencies during fetal or early neonatal life. All infants in Canada are screened for decreased thyroid function at birth.

Clinical Manifestations

Regardless of the cause, hypothyroidism has common features. It has systemic effects, characterized by an insidious and non-specific slowing of body processes. The clinical presentation can range from no symptoms to classic symptoms and physical changes easily detected on examination. Unless hypothyroidism occurs after thyroidectomy or thyroid ablation, or during treatment with antithyroid drugs, the onset of symptoms may occur unnoticed over months to years. The severity of symptoms experienced depends on the degree of thyroid hormone deficiency and the long-term physiological effects of thyroid hormone deficiency. Long-term effects may involve any body system but are more pronounced in neurological, cardiovascular, GI, reproductive, and hematological systems.

Many affected patients are fatigued and lethargic and experience personality and mental changes. The mental changes observed in hypothyroidism include impaired memory, slowed speech, decreased initiative, and somnolence. Many individuals with hypothyroidism appear depressed.

Hypothyroidism is associated with decreased cardiac output and decreased cardiac contractility. The patient may experience low exercise tolerance and shortness of breath on exertion. In patients with a pre-existing cardiovascular condition, hypothyroidism may cause significant hemodynamic compromise (Grais & Sowers, 2014).

Anemia is a common feature of hypothyroidism. Erythropoietin levels may be low or normal. Oxygen demand is decreased, and the bone marrow is hypocellular; the result is a low hematocrit. Other hematological problems are related to cobalamin, iron, and folate deficiencies. The patient may bruise easily. Increased serum cholesterol and triglyceride levels and the accumulation of mucopolysaccharides in the intima of small blood vessels can result in coronary atherosclerosis. This accumulation is seldom symptomatic (i.e., characterized by angina) because of the decreased myocardial oxygen consumption that has been observed in hypothyroidism.

GI motility is decreased in hypothyroidism, and achlorhydria (absence or decrease of hydrochloric acid) is common. Constipation, which is a common complaint, may progress to obstipation and, in rare cases, to intestinal obstruction. Other physical changes include cold intolerance, hair loss, dry and coarse skin, brittle nails, hoarseness, muscle weakness and swelling, and weight gain. Weight gain is probably a result of decreased metabolic rate.

Patients with severe, longstanding hypothyroidism may display **myxedema,** the accumulation of hydrophilic mucopolysaccharides in the dermis and other tissues (Figure 51-8). This mucinous edema causes the characteristic facies of hypothyroidism (i.e., puffiness, periorbital edema, and masklike affect). Individuals with hypothyroidism may describe impaired self-image in regard to their disabilities and altered appearance.

Women with hypothyroidism frequently complain of menorrhagia. In addition, cycles may be anovulatory, and subsequent infertility may occur (Dittrich, Beckmann, Oppelt, et al., 2011).

In older adults, the typical manifestations of hypothyroidism (including fatigue, cold and dry skin, hoarseness, hair loss, constipation, and cold intolerance) may be attributed to normal aging. For this reason, these symptoms may not raise suspicion

FIGURE 51-8 Patient with myxedema, displaying the characteristic facies of hypothyroidism (i.e., puffiness, periorbital edema, and masklike affect). Source: Seidel, H. M., Ball, J., Dains, J., et al. (2015). *Mosby's guide to physical examination* (8th ed., p. 190, Figure 10-10). St. Louis: Mosby. (Originally from Lemmi, F. O., Lemmi, C. A. E. [2000]. *Physical assessment findings.* [CD-ROM]. Philadelphia: Saunders.)

about an underlying condition. Older adults who have confusion, lethargy, and depression should be evaluated for thyroid disease.

Complications

The mental sluggishness, drowsiness, and lethargy of hypothyroidism may progress gradually or suddenly to a notable impairment of consciousness or coma. This situation, myxedema coma, constitutes a medical emergency. Myxedema coma can be precipitated by infection, drugs (especially opioids, tranquilizers, and barbiturates), exposure to cold, and trauma. It is characterized by subnormal temperature, hypotension, and hypoventilation. For patients experiencing myxedema to survive, vital functions must be supported and IV thyroid hormone replacement must be administered.

Diagnostic Studies

The most common and reliable laboratory tests used to evaluate thyroid function are measurements of TSH and free T_4. These values, when correlated with symptoms evident in the history and physical examination, confirm the diagnosis. Serum TSH levels help determine the cause of hypothyroidism—they are high when the defect is in the thyroid and low when it is in the pituitary gland or hypothalamus. An increase in TSH level after injection of TRH suggests hypothalamic dysfunction, whereas no change suggests anterior pituitary dysfunction (Table 51-11). The presence of thyroid peroxidase antibodies suggests an autoimmune origin of the problem. Other abnormal laboratory findings are elevated cholesterol and triglyceride levels, anemia, and increased creatine kinase level.

Collaborative Care

The overall goal for treatment in a patient with hypothyroidism is restoration of a euthyroid state as safely and rapidly as possible with hormone replacement therapy. A low-calorie diet is indicated to promote weight loss.

Levothyroxine (Synthroid, Eltroxin) is the drug of choice to treat hypothyroidism. In young and otherwise healthy patients, the maintenance replacement dose is adjusted according to the patients' response and laboratory findings. In older-adult patients and in patients with compromised cardiac status, a lower initial dosage is recommended because the usual dosage may increase myocardial oxygen demand. The increased oxygen demand may cause angina and cardiac dysrhythmias. Any chest pain experienced by a patient starting thyroid replacement should be reported immediately; electrocardiography (ECG) must be performed and serum cardiac enzymes measured. In patients without adverse

TABLE 51-11 COLLABORATIVE CARE

Hypothyroidism

Diagnostic Studies	Collaborative Therapy
• History and physical examination • Serum T_3 and serum T_4 levels (if ordered) • Serum TSH and free T_4 levels • Thyroid peroxidase antibodies • TRH stimulation test	• Monitoring thyroid hormone levels and adjusting dosage (if needed) • Nutritional therapy to promote weight loss • Patient and caregiver teaching (see Table 51-12) • Thyroid hormone replacement (e.g., levothyroxine)

T_3, triiodothyronine; T_4, thyroxine; *TRH*, thyrotropin-releasing hormone; *TSH*, thyroid-stimulating hormone.

effects, the dose is increased at 4- to 6-week intervals. It is important that patients take replacement medication regularly. Lifelong thyroid replacement therapy is usually required.

DRUG ALERT—Levothyroxine (Synthroid)
- Patients with cardiovascular disease who take this drug must be carefully monitored.
- Heart rate must be monitored and pulse greater than 100 beats/min or an irregular heartbeat must be reported.
- Chest pain, weight loss, nervousness, tremors, or insomnia must be promptly reported.
- Multiple levothyroxine preparations are currently available. Patients taking levothyroxine must have serum TSH levels checked 4 to 6 weeks after changing levothyroxine preparation.

NURSING MANAGEMENT HYPOTHYROIDISM

NURSING ASSESSMENT

Careful assessment of patients suspected of having hypothyroidism may reveal the early and subtle changes that indicate dysfunction. Assessment should include questions about weight gain, mental changes, fatigue, slowed and slurred speech, cold intolerance, skin changes such as increased dryness or thickening, constipation, and dyspnea. Patients should be questioned about recent introduction of iodine-containing medications. They should be assessed for bradycardia; distended abdomen; dry, thick, cold skin; thick, brittle nails; paresthesias; and muscular aches and pains.

NURSING DIAGNOSES

Nursing diagnoses for patients with hypothyroidism may include, but are not limited to, the following:
- *Activity intolerance* related to *physical deconditioning* (weakness and fatigue)
- *Constipation* related to *decrease in gastro-intestinal motility*

Additional information on nursing diagnoses for the patient with hypothyroidism is presented in Nursing Care Plan (NCP) 51-2, available on the Evolve website.

PLANNING

The overall goals are that patients with hypothyroidism will (a) experience relief from symptoms, (b) maintain a euthyroid state, (c) maintain a positive self-image, and (d) adhere to a lifelong regimen of thyroid replacement therapy.

NURSING IMPLEMENTATION

HEALTH PROMOTION. There is currently no consensus regarding thyroid function screening. Although hypothyroidism is relatively common, particularly among women older than 50, screening of the general population is not strongly justified (Premawardhana, 2015). Research suggests that populations at high risk for thyroid dysfunction should be screened for subclinical (asymptomatic) thyroid disease. Individuals at risk include those with a family history of thyroid disease, those with a history of neck irradiation, women older than 50, and women who have just given birth.

ACUTE INTERVENTION. Most individuals with hypothyroidism do not require acute nursing care. However, a patient who develops myxedema coma does require acute nursing care, often in a critical care setting. Mechanical respiratory support and cardiac monitoring are frequently necessary. Thyroid hormone replacement therapy and all other medications should be administered IV because paralytic ileus may be present with myxedema coma. If the patient is hyponatremic, hypertonic saline may be administered until the serum sodium level reaches at least 130 mmol/L. Core temperature should be monitored because many patients with myxedema coma are hypothermic.

The nurse monitors a patient's progress by assessing vital signs, body weight, fluid intake and output, and visible edema. Cardiac assessment is especially important because the cardiovascular response to the hormone determines the medication regimen. Energy level and mental alertness should be noted. These should increase within 2 to 14 days and continue to rise steadily to normal levels.

AMBULATORY AND HOME CARE. Patient and caregiver teaching is essential for patients with hypothyroidism (Table 51-12). Initially, patients with hypothyroidism need more time than usual to comprehend all the necessary information. It is important to provide written instructions, repeat the information often, and assess the patient's comprehension level regularly.

The need for lifelong drug therapy must be stressed. Patients should be taught expected and unexpected adverse drug effects. Specifically, the signs and symptoms of hypothyroidism or hyperthyroidism that indicate hormone imbalance should be included in the teaching plan. Toxic symptoms should be clearly defined. Table 51-7 lists signs of hyperthyroidism that are the same as toxic symptoms of thyroid hormone replacement.

Patients must be taught to contact a health care professional immediately if signs of overdose—such as orthopnea, dyspnea, rapid pulse, palpitations, nervousness, or insomnia—appear. A patient with diabetes mellitus should test his or her capillary blood glucose level at least daily because return to the euthyroid state frequently increases insulin requirements. In addition, thyroid preparations potentiate the effects of anticoagulants and decrease the effect of digitalis compounds. Thus, the patient should be taught the toxic signs and symptoms of these medications and should remain under close medical observation until his or her condition is stable.

It is sometimes difficult for patients to recognize signs of overdosage or underdosage of drug therapy; therefore, a family member or friend should also receive instructions. Handouts

for patients should be written in understandable language and should accompany verbal instruction. The handouts should be reviewed with patients and the family to assess understanding, and information should be clarified when necessary.

With treatment, striking transformations occur in both appearance and mental function. In most adults, both return to normal. Cardiovascular conditions and (occasionally) psychosis may persist despite corrections of the hormonal imbalance. Relapses occur if treatment is interrupted.

EVALUATION

The following are expected outcomes for patients with hypothyroidism:

- Relief from symptoms
- Maintenance of a euthyroid state as evidenced by normal thyroid hormone and TSH levels
- Avoidance of complications of therapy
- Adherence to lifelong therapy

ETHICAL DILEMMAS
Alternative Healers

Situation
The nurse is caring for an Indigenous woman with thyroid disease. Thyroid replacement therapy is the planned treatment. The patient's traditional healer tells her not to take the medication and suggests that she should begin a herbal regimen instead. Should the nurse intervene?

Important Points for Consideration
- Culturally competent nursing care should incorporate the patient's cultural and religious values and beliefs.
- Patient autonomy, the patient's right to choose a treatment plan, should be respected.
- Having adequate, understandable information about available treatment options and their possible consequences facilitates an informed choice.

Clinical Decision-Making Questions
1. What information should the nurse obtain from the patient? What information should the nurse provide for the patient?
2. How should the nurse proceed? Should the nurse try to incorporate the healer's herbal regimen into the plan of care while attempting to persuade the woman of the need for the thyroid replacement therapy?

DISORDERS OF THE PARATHYROID GLANDS

HYPERPARATHYROIDISM

Etiology and Pathophysiology

Hyperparathyroidism is a condition involving increased secretion of parathyroid hormone (PTH). PTH helps regulate calcium and phosphate levels by stimulating bone resorption of calcium, renal tubular reabsorption of calcium, and activation of vitamin D. Thus oversecretion of PTH is associated with increased serum calcium levels. Hyperparathyroidism affects approximately 0.1% to 0.4% of the general population, it occurs more frequently among women, and the incidence increases with age (Pallan, Rahman, & Khan, 2012).

Hyperparathyroidism is classified as primary, secondary, or tertiary. *Primary hyperparathyroidism* results from an increased secretion of PTH, which leads to disorders of calcium, phosphate, and bone metabolism. The most common cause is a benign neoplasm or a single adenoma in the parathyroid gland. Primary hyperparathyroidism usually occurs between the ages of 30 and

---

TABLE 51-12 PATIENT & CAREGIVER TEACHING GUIDE

Hypothyroidism

The following instructions should be included when teaching the patient and caregiver about management of hypothyroidism. The nurse should:

1. Explain the nature of thyroid hormone deficiency and self-care practices necessary to prevent complications. Patient and family caregivers must understand thyroid replacement therapy. It is especially important to emphasize the need for lifelong replacement, the need to take the medication continually, and the need for regular follow-up care.
2. Emphasize the need for a comfortable, warm environment because of intolerance of cold.
3. Teach measures to prevent skin breakdown. Soap should be used sparingly and lotion applied to skin.
4. Caution patients, especially older adults, to avoid sedatives. If sedatives must be used, suggest that the lowest dose be used. Caregivers should closely monitor patient's mental status, level of consciousness, and respiration.
5. Discuss with patients measures to minimize constipation. Suggestions should include a gradual increase in activity and exercise, increased fibre in diet, use of stool softeners, and maintenance of a regular bowel elimination time. Enemas should not be used because they produce vagal stimulation, which can be hazardous if cardiac disease is present.

70 years. The incidence peaks in the fifth and sixth decades of life. Patients who have previously undergone head and neck irradiation may have an increased risk of developing a parathyroid adenoma.

Secondary hyperparathyroidism appears to be a compensatory response to states that induce or cause hypocalcemia, the main stimulus of PTH secretion. Disease conditions associated with secondary hyperparathyroidism include vitamin D deficiencies, malabsorption, chronic renal failure, and hyperphosphatemia.

Tertiary hyperparathyroidism occurs when the parathyroid glands become hyperplastic and negative feedback is lost from circulating calcium levels; thus, PTH is secreted autonomously, even with normal calcium levels. This condition is observed in patients who have undergone kidney transplantation after a long period of dialysis treatment for chronic renal failure. (Chapter 49 discusses parathyroid hormone and kidney function.)

Excessive levels of circulating PTH usually lead to hypercalcemia and hypophosphatemia, creating a multisystem effect (Table 51-13). In the skeleton, decreased bone density, cyst formation, and general weakness can occur as a result of the effect of PTH on osteoclastic activity (bone resorption) and osteoblastic activity (bone formation). In the kidneys, the excess calcium cannot be reabsorbed; as a result, levels of calcium in the urine increase (hypercalciuria). This urinary calcium level, along with a large amount of urinary phosphate, can lead to calculi formation (Cipriani, Biamonte, Costa, et al., 2015). In addition, PTH stimulates the synthesis of a biologically active form of vitamin D, a potent stimulator of calcium transport in the intestine. In this way, PTH indirectly increases GI absorption of calcium, contributing further to the high serum calcium levels.

Clinical Manifestations and Complications

Clinical manifestations of hyperparathyroidism range from no symptoms (the condition is diagnosed through testing for unrelated problems) to overt symptoms. Clinical manifestations are associated with hypercalcemia and are summarized in Table 51-13. The major manifestations include muscle weakness, loss of appetite, constipation, fatigue, emotional disorders, and shortened attention span. Major signs include loss of calcium from bones (osteoporosis), fractures, and kidney stones (nephrolithiasis). Neuro-muscular abnormalities are characterized by muscle weakness, particularly in the proximal muscles of the lower extremities. Asymptomatic cases are often identified through routine calcium screening. Serious complications of hyperparathyroidism are renal failure; pancreatitis; cardiac changes; and fractures of long bones, ribs, and vertebrae.

TABLE 51-13   CLINICAL MANIFESTATIONS OF PARATHYROID DYSFUNCTION

Hypofunction	Hyperfunction	Hypofunction	Hyperfunction
Cardiovascular		**Neurological**	
• Decreased cardiac output	• Dysrhythmias	• Disorientation, confusion (in older adults)	• Abnormalities of gait
• Decreased contractility of heart muscle	• Hypertension	• Headache	• Delirium, confusion, coma
• Dysrhythmias	• Shortened Q–T interval on ECG	• Hyperactive deep tendon reflexes	• Emotional irritability
• Prolongation of Q–T and ST intervals on ECG		• Irritability	• Headache
		• Memory impairment	• Hyperactive deep tendon reflexes
Gastro-Intestinal		• Paresthesias of perioral area, hands, and feet	• Memory impairment
• Abdominal cramps	• Anorexia	• Personality changes	• Paresthesias
• Fecal incontinence (in older adults)	• Cholelithiasis	• Positive Chvostek's or Trousseau's sign	• Personality disturbances
• Malabsorption	• Constipation	• Psychiatric manifestations of depression, anxiety, psychosis	• Poor coordination
	• Nausea and vomiting	• Seizures	• Psychomotor retardation
	• Pancreatitis	• Tremor	• Psychosis, depression
	• Peptic ulcer disease		
	• Vague abdominal pain		
	• Weight loss		
		Renal	
Integumentary		• Urinary frequency	• Hypercalciuria
• Brittle nails, transverse ridging	• Moist skin	• Urinary incontinence	• Kidney stones (nephrolithiasis)
• Changes in developing teeth, lack of tooth enamel	• Skin necrosis		• Polyuria
• Dry, scaly skin			• Urinary tract infections
• Hair loss on scalp and body			
		Other	
Musculo-Skeletal		• Eye changes, including lenticular opacities, cataracts, papilledema	• Corneal calcification on slit-lamp examination
• Difficulty in walking	• Backache		
• Fatigue	• Compression fractures of spine		
• Painful muscle cramps	• Decreased muscle tone, muscle atrophy		
• Skeletal radiograph changes, osteosclerosis	• Osteoporosis		
• Soft tissue calcification	• Pain on weight bearing		
• Weakness	• Pathological fractures of long bones		
	• Skeletal pain		
	• Weakness, fatigue		

ECG, electrocardiogram.

Diagnostic Studies

PTH levels are elevated in hyperparathyroidism. Serum calcium levels usually exceed 2.75 mmol/L. Because of its inverse relation with the calcium level, the serum phosphorus level is usually below 0.1 mmol/L. Elevations occur in other laboratory values: urine calcium, serum chloride, uric acid, creatinine, amylase (if pancreatitis is present), and alkaline phosphatase (if bone disease is present). Bone density measurements may also be used to detect bone loss. Imaging studies, such as MRI, CT, and ultrasonography, may help localize the adenoma.

Collaborative Care

The treatment objectives for hyperparathyroidism are to relieve the manifestations and prevent complications caused by excess PTH. The choice of therapy depends on the urgency of the clinical situation, the degree of hypercalcemia, and the underlying cause of the disorder.

Surgical Therapy. The most effective treatment of primary and secondary hyperparathyroidism is surgical intervention. Parathyroidectomy leads to rapid reduction of chronically high calcium levels. Criteria for surgery include serum calcium levels higher than 0.25 mmol/L above normal level; creatinine clearance rate of less than 60 mL/min; T-score lower than –2.5 at any site on bone mineral density testing, previous fracture fragility, or both; and age younger than 50 (Callender & Udelsman, 2014). The surgical procedure involves partial or complete removal of the parathyroid glands. The most common procedure involves use of an endoscope and is performed on an outpatient basis. Successful removal of the parathyroid glands is facilitated by preoperative nuclear scanning with technetium-99m (99mTc) (Callender & Udelsman, 2014).

Autotransplantation of normal parathyroid tissue in the forearm or near the sternocleidomastoid muscle may be performed, which allows PTH secretion to continue with normalization of calcium levels. If autotransplantation is not possible, or if it fails, patients need to take calcium supplements for the rest of their lives.

Nonsurgical Therapy. A conservative approach is often used in patients who are asymptomatic or have mild symptoms of hyperparathyroidism. This approach includes an annual examination with tests for serum calcium and creatinine clearance and evaluation of bone density every 1 to 2 years (three sites). Continued ambulation and the avoidance of immobility are critical aspects of management. Dietary measures also include maintenance of a high fluid intake and a moderate calcium intake.

Phosphorus intake is usually supplemented unless this is contraindicated by an increased risk for urinary calculi formation. Several drugs currently used in the treatment of hyperparathyroidism are helpful in lowering calcium levels but do not treat the underlying problem. Bisphosphonates (e.g., alendronate [Fosamax]) inhibit osteoclastic bone resorption and rapidly normalize serum calcium levels. Estrogen or progestin therapy can reduce serum and urinary calcium levels in postmenopausal women and may slow the demineralization of the skeleton. Oral phosphate may be used to inhibit the calcium-absorbing effects of vitamin D in the intestine. Phosphates should be used only if a patient has normal renal function and low serum phosphate levels. Calcimimetic agents (e.g., cinacalcet [Sensipar]) are a class of drugs that increase the sensitivity of the calcium receptor on the parathyroid gland, resulting in decreased PTH secretion and calcium blood levels and thus sparing calcium stores in the bone. Drugs in this class are currently indicated for secondary hyperparathyroidism in individuals with chronic kidney disease who are undergoing dialysis, for patients with parathyroid cancer, and for patients with symptomatic hypercalcemia in primary hyperparathyroidism.

NURSING MANAGEMENT
HYPERPARATHYROIDISM

Nursing care for patients after a parathyroidectomy is similar to that for patients after a thyroidectomy. The major postoperative complications are associated with hemorrhage and fluid and electrolyte disturbances. *Tetany,* a condition of neuro-muscular hyperexcitability associated with a sudden decrease in calcium levels, is another concern. It is usually apparent early in the postoperative period but may develop over several days. Mild tetany, characterized by an unpleasant tingling sensation of the hands and around the mouth, may be present but should abate without problems. If tetany becomes more severe (e.g., muscular spasms or laryngospasms develop), IV calcium may be given. IV calcium gluconate should be readily available for patients after parathyroidectomy in case acute tetany occurs.

The nurse monitors intake and output to evaluate fluid status. Calcium, potassium, phosphate, and magnesium levels are assessed frequently, as are Chvostek's and Trousseau's signs (see Chapter 19, Figure 19-15). The nurse also encourages mobility to promote bone calcification.

If surgery is not performed, treatment to relieve symptoms and prevent complications is initiated. The nurse can assist patients with hyperparathyroidism to adapt the meal plan to their lifestyle. A referral to a dietitian may be useful. Because immobility can aggravate the bone loss, the nurse must stress to patients the importance of an exercise program. Patients should be encouraged to keep the regular appointments, and the tests being performed should be explained. Patients should also be instructed in the symptoms of hypocalcemia or hypercalcemia and to report them, should they occur. Hypocalcemia and hypercalcemia are discussed in Chapter 19.

HYPOPARATHYROIDISM

Etiology and Pathophysiology

Hypoparathyroidism is an uncommon condition associated with inadequate levels of circulating PTH. It is characterized by hypocalcemia that results from a lack of PTH to maintain serum calcium levels. PTH resistance at the cellular level may also occur (pseudohypoparathyroidism). This condition is caused by a genetic defect that results in hypocalcemia in spite of normal or high PTH levels and is often associated with hypothyroidism and hypogonadism.

The most common cause of hypoparathyroidism is iatrogenic. This may include accidental removal of the parathyroid glands or damage to the vascular supply of the glands during neck surgery (e.g., thyroidectomy, radical neck surgery) (Gupta, Chaudhary, Durga, et al., 2015). Idiopathic hypoparathyroidism resulting from the absence, fatty replacement, or atrophy of the glands is a rare disease that usually occurs early in life and may be associated with other endocrine disorders. Affected patients may have antiparathyroid antibodies. Severe hypomagnesemia also leads to a suppression of PTH secretion (Famularo, Minisola, Bravi, et al., 2012).

Clinical Manifestations

The clinical features of acute hypoparathyroidism result from a low serum calcium level (see Table 51-13). Sudden decreases in calcium concentration cause tetany. This state is characterized by tingling sensations in the lips, the fingertips, and occasionally the feet and by increased muscle tension, which escalates to paresthesias and stiffness. Painful tonic spasms of smooth and skeletal muscles can cause dysphagia, a constricted feeling in the throat, and laryngospasms that can compromise breathing. Patients are usually anxious and apprehensive. Abnormal laboratory findings include decreased serum calcium and PTH levels and increased serum phosphate levels. Other causes of chronic hypocalcemia include chronic renal failure, vitamin D deficiency, and hypomagnesemia.

NURSING AND COLLABORATIVE MANAGEMENT HYPOPARATHYROIDISM

The primary treatment goals for a patient with hypoparathyroidism are to treat acute complications such as tetany, maintain normal serum calcium levels, and prevent long-term complications. Emergency treatment of tetany requires the administration of IV calcium. IV calcium chloride or calcium gluconate should be infused slowly because high blood levels of calcium can cause hypotension, serious cardiac dysrhythmias, or cardiac arrest; thus ECG monitoring is indicated when calcium is administered. Patients who take digoxin are particularly vulnerable. IV calcium can cause venous irritation and inflammation. Extravasation may cause cellulitis, necrosis, and tissue sloughing. IV patency should be assessed before administration.

Rebreathing may partially alleviate acute neuro-muscular symptoms associated with hypocalcemia, such as generalized muscle cramps or mild tetany. Patients who can cooperate should be instructed to breathe in and out of a paper bag or breathing mask. This reduces carbon dioxide excretion from the lungs, increases carbonic acid levels in the blood, and lowers the pH.

A lower pH (acidic environment) enhances the degree of ionization of calcium, causing an increase in the proportion of total body calcium available in the active form. This then temporarily alleviates the manifestations of hypocalcemia.

Patients with hypoparathyroidism need instruction in the management of long-term drug therapy and nutrition. Oral calcium supplements of at least 1.5 to 3 g/day in divided doses are usually prescribed. PTH replacement is not a recommended drug therapy because of the expense and the need for parenteral administration. Vitamin D is administered to patients with chronic and resistant hypocalcemia to enhance intestinal calcium absorption and bone resorption. The primary preparation is calcitriol (Rocaltrol). This drug raises calcium levels rapidly and is quickly metabolized. Rapid metabolism is desired because vitamin D is a fat-soluble vitamin, and toxicity can cause irreversible renal impairment.

A high-calcium meal plan includes foods such as dark green vegetables, soybeans, and tofu. Patients should be told to avoid foods containing oxalic acid (e.g., spinach, rhubarb), phytic acid (e.g., bran, whole grains), and phosphorus (e.g., protein-rich foods such as meats, poultry, fish, nuts, beans, and dairy products) because they reduce calcium absorption.

Patients should be instructed about the need for lifelong treatment and follow-up care, including the monitoring of calcium levels three to four times a year.

DISORDERS OF THE ADRENAL CORTEX

There are three main classifications of adrenal steroid hormones. *Glucocorticoids* regulate metabolism, increase blood glucose levels, and are critical in the physiological stress response. In humans, the primary glucocorticoid is cortisol. *Mineralocorticoids* regulate sodium and potassium balance. The primary mineralocorticoid is aldosterone. *Androgens* contribute to growth and development in both genders and to sexual desire and satisfaction in women. The term *corticosteroid* refers to any one of these three types of hormones produced by the adrenal cortex.

CUSHING'S SYNDROME

Etiology and Pathophysiology

Cushing's syndrome is a spectrum of clinical abnormalities caused by excess levels of corticosteroids, particularly glucocorticoids (Lacroix, Feelders, Stratakis, et al., 2015). Several conditions can cause this metabolic disorder (Table 51-14). The most common causes are iatrogenic administration of exogenous corticosteroids (e.g., prednisone) in large doses for several weeks or longer and the chronic and excessive production of cortisol by the adrenal cortex. Approximately 85% of cases of endogenous Cushing's syndrome result from an ACTH-secreting pituitary tumour (Cushing's disease). Other causes of Cushing's syndrome include adrenal tumours and ectopic ACTH production by tumours outside the hypothalamic-pituitary-adrenal axis (usually of the lung or the pancreas). Cushing's disease and primary adrenal tumours are most common in women age 20 to 40 years; ectopic ACTH production is more common in men.

Clinical Manifestations

The clinical manifestations of Cushing's syndrome can occur in most body systems and are related to excess levels of corticosteroids (Table 51-15). Although manifestations of glucocorticoid excess usually predominate, symptoms of mineralocorticoid and androgen excess may also appear.

Corticosteroid excess causes pronounced changes in physical appearance (Figure 51-9). Weight gain, the most common feature, results from the accumulation of adipose tissue in the trunk, the face, and the cervical area (see Figure 51-9). Transient weight gain from sodium and water retention may be present because of the mineralocorticoid effects of cortisol. Hyperglycemia occurs because of glucose intolerance (associated with cortisol-induced insulin resistance) and increased gluconeogenesis by the liver.

The catabolic effects of cortisol on peripheral tissue cause protein wasting. Muscle wasting leads to muscle weakness, especially in the extremities. Loss of protein matrix in bone leads to osteoporosis with subsequent pathological fractures (e.g., vertebral compression fractures) and bone and back pain. Loss

---

TABLE 51-14 CAUSES OF CUSHING'S SYNDROME

- ACTH-secreting pituitary tumour (Cushing's disease)
- Cortisol-secreting neoplasm within the adrenal cortex that can be either carcinoma or adenoma
- Excess secretion of ACTH from carcinoma of the lung or other malignant growth outside the pituitary or the adrenal glands
- Prolonged administration of high doses of corticosteroids

ACTH, adrenocorticotrophic hormone.

TABLE 51-15	CLINICAL MANIFESTATIONS: ADRENOCORTICAL HORMONE DYSFUNCTION	
Category	**Hypofunction (Addison's Disease)**	**Hyperfunction (Cushing's Syndrome)**
Glucocorticoids		
Cardiovascular	Hypotension, tendency to develop refractory shock, vasodilation	Hypervolemia, hypertension, edema of lower extremities
Fluids and electrolytes	Hyponatremia, hypovolemia, dehydration, hyperkalemia	Sodium and water retention, edema, hypokalemia
Gastro-intestinal	Anorexia, nausea and vomiting, cramping abdominal pain, diarrhea	Increase in secretion of pepsin and hydrochloric acid; anorexia
General appearance	Weight loss	Centripetal (truncal) obesity, thin extremities, rounding of face (moon facies), fat deposits on back of neck and on shoulders (buffalo hump)
Hematological system	Anemia, lymphocytosis	Leukocytosis, lymphopenia, polycythemia, increased coagulability
Immune system	Tendency for coexisting autoimmune diseases	Inhibition of immune response, suppression of allergic response, inhibition of inflammation
Integumentary system	Bronzed or smoky hyperpigmentation of face, neck, hands (especially creases), buccal membranes, nipples, genitalia, and scars (if pituitary function is normal); vitiligo, alopecia	Thin, fragile skin; purplish red striae (see Figure 51-11); petechial hemorrhages; bruises; florid cheeks (facial plethora); acne; poor wound healing
Mental and emotional state	Neurasthenia, depression, exhaustion or irritability, confusion, delusions	Euphoria, irritability, hypomania to depression, emotional lability
Metabolism	Hypoglycemia, insulin sensitivity, fever	Hyperglycemia, negative nitrogen balance, dyslipidemia
Musculo-skeletal	Fatigability	Muscle wasting in extremities, proximal muscle weakness, fatigue, osteoporosis, awkward gait, back and joint pain, weakness
Renal/urinary	—	Glycosuria, hypercalciuria, kidney stones
Mineralocorticoids		
Cardiovascular	Hypovolemia, tendency toward shock, decreased cardiac output, decrease in heart size	Hypertension, hypervolemia
Fluids and electrolytes	Sodium loss, decreased volume of extracellular fluid, hyperkalemia, salt craving	Marked sodium and water retention, tendency toward edema, marked hypokalemia, alkalosis
Androgens		
Integumentary	Decreased axillary and pubic hair (in women)	Hirsutism, acne, hyperpigmentation
Musculo-skeletal	Decrease in muscle size and tone	Muscle wasting and weakness
Reproductive	No effect in men; decreased libido in women	Menstrual irregularities and enlargement of clitoris in women; gynecomastia and testicular atrophy in men

FIGURE 51-9 Cushing's syndrome. Facies include a rounded face (moon facies) with thin, reddened skin. Hirsutism may also be present. Source: Seidel, H. M., Ball, J., Dains, J., et al. (2006). *Mosby's guide to physical examination* (6th ed., p. 272, Figure 10-17). St. Louis: Mosby.

of collagen makes the skin weaker and thinner; therefore, the skin bruises more easily. Catabolic processes predominate, and wound healing is delayed. Mood disturbances (e.g., irritability, anxiety, euphoria), insomnia, irrationality, and occasionally psychosis may occur.

Mineralocorticoid excess may cause hypertension (secondary to fluid retention), whereas adrenal androgen excess may cause pronounced acne, masculinization in women, and feminization in men. Menstrual disorders and hirsutism in women and gynecomastia and erectile dysfunction in men occur more commonly with adrenal carcinomas.

The clinical presentation is the first indication of Cushing's syndrome (Figure 51-10). Of particular importance are (a) centripetal (truncal) obesity or generalized obesity; (b) so-called moon facies (fullness of the face) with facial plethora; (c) purplish red striae, which are usually depressed below the skin surface, on the abdomen, the breasts, or the buttocks (Figure 51-11); (d) hirsutism in women; (e) menstrual disorders in women; (f) hypertension; and (g) unexplained hypokalemia.

Diagnostic Studies

When Cushing's syndrome is suspected, a 24-hour urine sample is collected to measure free cortisol (see Chapter 50). If the free cortisol results are borderline, a low-dose dexamethasone suppression

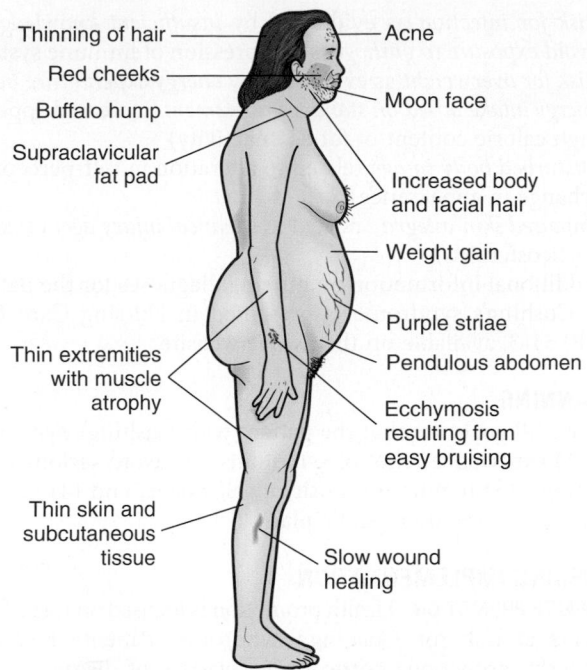

Thinning of hair

Red cheeks

Buffalo hump

Supraclavicular fat pad

Thin extremities with muscle atrophy

Thin skin and subcutaneous tissue

Acne

Moon face

Increased body and facial hair

Weight gain

Purple striae

Pendulous abdomen

Ecchymosis resulting from easy bruising

Slow wound healing

FIGURE 51-10 Common characteristics of Cushing's syndrome.

FIGURE 51-11 Cushing's syndrome. Truncal obesity; broad, purple striae; and easy bruising (left antecubital fossa). Source: Chew, S. L., & Leslie, D. (2006). *Clinical endocrinology and diabetes: An illustrated colour text.* (1st ed., p. 28, Figure 2). Edinburgh: Churchill Livingstone.

test is performed. Plasma cortisol (the primary glucocorticoid) levels may be elevated, with loss of diurnal variation. Elevation in the midnight serum cortisol level confirms the diagnosis of Cushing's syndrome with 100% sensitivity (Juszczak & Grossman, 2012). False-positive results can occur in patients with depression, those under acute stress, and those who are actively alcoholic. CT and MRI of the pituitary and adrenal glands may be used.

Plasma ACTH levels may be low, normal, or elevated, depending on the underlying problem. High or normal levels indicate ACTH-dependent Cushing's disease, whereas low or undetectable levels indicate an adrenal or exogenous etiology. Other findings on diagnostic tests associated with, but not diagnostic of, Cushing's syndrome include granulocytosis, lymphopenia, eosinopenia, hyperglycemia, glycosuria, hypercalciuria, and osteoporosis. Hypokalemia and alkalosis occur in ectopic ACTH syndrome and adrenal carcinoma.

TABLE 51-16 COLLABORATIVE CARE

Cushing's Syndrome

Diagnostic
- History and physical examination
- 24-hour urine collection for free cortisol measurement
- Blood chemistry evaluation for sodium, potassium, and glucose
- Complete blood cell count
- CT, MRI
- Dexamethasone suppression test
- Examination of visual field
- Measurement of plasma ACTH level
- Measurement of plasma cortisol levels for diurnal variations
- Mental status examination

Collaborative Therapy*

Adrenocortical Adenoma, Carcinoma, or Hyperplasia
- Adrenalectomy (open or laparoscopic)
- Drug therapy
  - Ketoconazole (Nizoral)
  - Mitotane (Lysodren)

Pituitary Adenoma
- Radiation therapy
- Trans-sphenoidal resection

Ectopic ACTH-Secreting Tumour
- Treatment of the tumour responsible (surgical removal or radiation therapy)

Exogenous Corticosteroid Therapy
- Discontinuance of or alteration in administration of exogenous corticosteroids

ACTH, adrenocorticotrophic hormone; *CT,* computed tomographic (scan); *MRI,* magnetic resonance imaging.
*Treatment is based on underlying cause.

Collaborative Care

The primary goal of treatment for Cushing's disease is to normalize hormone secretion. The specific treatment is dependent on the underlying cause (Table 51-16). If the underlying cause is a pituitary adenoma, the standard treatment is surgical removal of the tumour through the trans-sphenoidal approach (Dallapiazza & Jane, Jr., 2015). (The trans-sphenoidal approach is discussed earlier in this chapter.) Irradiation of the pituitary adenoma may be necessary if surgical outcomes are not optimal or if a patient is at high risk for surgical complications. Adrenalectomy is indicated for Cushing's syndrome caused by adrenal tumours or hyperplasia. On occasion, bilateral adrenalectomy is necessary.

Laparoscopic adrenalectomy is considered an appropriate surgical approach except for patients with known or suspected malignant adrenal tumours. An open surgical adrenalectomy is the treatment of choice for adrenal cancer. Patients with ectopic ACTH-secreting tumours are managed by treating the primary neoplasm.

Drug therapy is used when surgery is contraindicated or as an adjunct to surgery. The goal of drug therapy is the inhibition of adrenal function (medical adrenalectomy). Mitotane (Lysodren) suppresses cortisol production, alters peripheral metabolism of cortisol, and decreases plasma and urine corticosteroid levels. Ketoconazole can be used to inhibit cortisol synthesis. These drugs are used cautiously because they are often toxic at doses needed to reduce corticosteroid synthesis.

If Cushing's syndrome has developed during the course of prolonged administration of corticosteroids (e.g., prednisone), one or more of the following alternatives may be tried: (a) gradual discontinuance of corticosteroid therapy, (b) reduction of the corticosteroid dose, and (c) conversion to an alternate-day regimen. Gradual tapering of the corticosteroids is necessary to avoid potentially life-threatening adrenal insufficiency. An alternate-day regimen is one in which twice the daily dosage of a shorter-acting corticosteroid is given every other morning to minimize hypothalamic-pituitary-adrenal suppression, growth suppression, and altered appearance.

NURSING MANAGEMENT CUSHING'S SYNDROME

NURSING ASSESSMENT

Subjective and objective data that should be obtained from a patient with Cushing's syndrome are presented in Table 51-17.

NURSING DIAGNOSES

Nursing diagnoses for patients with Cushing's syndrome may include, but are not limited to, the following:

TABLE 51-17 NURSING ASSESSMENT

Cushing's Syndrome

Subjective Data

Important Health Information

Past health history: Pituitary tumour (Cushing's disease); adrenal, pancreatic, or pulmonary neoplasms; GI bleeding; frequent infections

Medications: Use of corticosteroids

Symptoms
- Amenorrhea, erectile dysfunction, decreased libido
- Anxiety, mood disturbances, emotional lability, psychosis
- Headache; back, joint, bone, and rib pain; poor concentration and memory
- Insomnia, poor sleep quality
- Malaise, weakness, fatigue
- Negative feelings regarding changes in personal appearance
- Polyuria
- Prolonged wound healing, easy bruising
- Weight gain, anorexia

Objective Data

General

Centripetal (truncal) obesity, supraclavicular fat pads, buffalo hump, moon facies

Integumentary

Facial plethora; hirsutism of body and face, thinning of head hair; thin, friable skin; acne; petechiae; purpura; hyperpigmentation; purplish red striae on breasts, buttocks, and abdomen; edema of lower extremities

Cardiovascular

Hypertension

Musculo-Skeletal

Muscle wasting, thin extremities, awkward gait

Reproductive

Gynecomastia, testicular atrophy (in men); enlarged clitoris (in women)

Possible Findings

Hypokalemia, hyperglycemia, dyslipidemia; polycythemia, granulocytosis, lymphocytopenia, eosinopenia; ↑ plasma cortisol level; high, low, or normal ACTH levels; abnormal result of dexamethasone suppression test; ↑ levels of urine free cortisol and 17-ketosteroids; glycosuria, hypercalciuria; osteoporosis on radiograph

ACTH, adrenocorticotrophic hormone; *GI,* gastro-intestinal.

- *Risk for infection* as evidenced by *insufficient knowledge to avoid exposure to pathogens* (suppression of immune system)
- *Risk for overweight* as evidenced by *energy expenditure below energy intake based on standard assessment* (increased appetite, high caloric content of foods, inactivity)
- *Disturbed body image* related to alteration in self-perception (change in appearance)
- *Impaired skin integrity* related to *chemical injury agent* (excess corticosteroids)

Additional information on nursing diagnoses for the patient with Cushing's syndrome is presented in Nursing Care Plan (NCP) 51-3, available on the Evolve website.

PLANNING

The overall goals are that the patient with Cushing's syndrome will (1) experience relief of symptoms, (2) avoid serious complications, (3) maintain a positive self-image, and (4) actively participate in the therapeutic plan.

NURSING IMPLEMENTATION

HEALTH PROMOTION. Health promotion is focused on identifying patients at risk for Cushing's syndrome. Patients receiving long-term, exogenous cortisol for a variety of diseases are at risk. Teaching patients about medication use and monitoring of adverse drug effects are important preventive measures.

ACUTE INTERVENTION. Patients with Cushing's syndrome are seriously ill. Because the therapeutic interventions produce many adverse drug effects, the focus of daily assessment is on signs and symptoms of hormone and drug toxicity and complicating conditions such as cardiovascular disease, diabetes mellitus, and infection. Nursing assessment should include monitoring of vital signs, daily weighing, and measuring glucose levels. Because signs and symptoms of inflammation such as fever and redness may be minimal or absent, the nurse must assess for pain, loss of function, and purulent drainage as signs of possible infection. The nurse also monitors for signs and symptoms of thrombo-embolic events (pulmonary emboli) such as sudden chest pain, dyspnea, or tachypnea.

Another important focus of nursing care is emotional support. Changes in appearance such as centripetal obesity, multiple bruises, hirsutism in women, and gynecomastia in men can be distressing. Patients may feel unattractive or unwanted. The nurse can help by remaining sensitive to patients' feelings and offering respect and unconditional acceptance. Patients can be reassured that the physical changes and much of the emotional lability will resolve when hormone levels return to normal.

If treatment involves surgical removal of a pituitary adenoma, an adrenal tumour, or one or both adrenal glands, nursing care has an additional focus on preoperative and postoperative care.

Preoperative Care. Before surgery, the patient should be brought to optimal physical condition. Hypertension and hyperglycemia must be controlled, and hypokalemia is corrected with diet and potassium supplements. A high-protein meal plan helps correct the protein depletion. Preoperative teaching depends on the type of surgical approach planned (hypophysectomy or adrenalectomy) but should include information regarding the postoperative care that patients should anticipate. Patients should be told that in the postoperative period (for both open and laparoscopic adrenalectomy), they will probably have a nasogastric tube, urinary catheter, IV therapy, central venous pressure monitoring, and leg sequential compression devices to prevent emboli. Preoperative management for patients undergoing a hypophysectomy is discussed earlier in this chapter.

Postoperative Care. Surgery on the adrenal glands poses risks beyond those of other types of operations. Because the glands are highly vascular, the risk for hemorrhage is increased. Manipulation of glandular tissue during surgery may cause the release of large amounts of hormone into the circulation that produce marked fluctuations in the metabolic processes affected by these hormones. After surgery, BP, fluid balance, and electrolyte levels tend to be unstable because of these hormone fluctuations.

High doses of corticosteroids (e.g., hydrocortisone [Solu-Cortef]) are administered IV during surgery and for several days afterward to ensure adequate responses to the stress of the procedure. If large amounts of endogenous hormone have been released into the systemic circulation during surgery, hypertension is likely to develop, increasing the risk for hemorrhage. High levels of corticosteroids also increase susceptibility to infection and delay wound healing.

Any significant changes in BP, respirations, or heart rate should be reported to the physician. Fluid intake and output should be monitored carefully and assessed for potential imbalances. The critical period for circulatory instability ranges from 24 to 48 hours after surgery. IV corticosteroids are given, and the dosage and the rate of flow are adjusted to the patient's clinical manifestations and fluid and electrolyte balances. Oral doses are given as tolerated. The IV line may be kept in place after IV corticosteroids are withdrawn to maintain access for quick administration of corticosteroids or vasopressors. Morning urine levels of cortisol (assessed at the same time each morning) are measured to evaluate the effectiveness of the surgery.

If the corticosteroid dosage is tapered too rapidly after surgery, acute adrenal insufficiency may develop. Vomiting, increased weakness, dehydration, and hypotension may indicate hypocortisolism. In addition, patients may complain of painful joints, pruritus, or peeling skin and may experience severe emotional disturbances. These signs and symptoms should be reported so that drug doses can be adjusted. The nurse must constantly be alert for signs of corticosteroid imbalance. After surgery, the patient is usually maintained on bedrest until the BP stabilizes. Because the usual inflammatory responses are suppressed, the nurse must be alert for subtle signs of postoperative infections. The nurse must use meticulous care when changing the dressing and during any other procedures that necessitate access to body cavities, circulation, or areas under the skin, so that infection is prevented. A nursing care plan for patients with Cushing's syndrome (NCP 51-3) is available on the Evolve website for this chapter.

AMBULATORY AND HOME CARE. Discharge instructions are based on the patient's lack of endogenous corticosteroids and resulting inability to react to stressors physiologically. The nurse should consider a referral for a visiting nurse, especially for older adults, because of the need for ongoing evaluation and education. Patients should wear medical alert bracelets at all times and carry medical identification and instructions in a wallet or purse. Exposure to extremes of temperature, infections, and emotional disturbances should be avoided as much as possible. Stress may produce or precipitate acute adrenal insufficiency because the remaining adrenal tissue cannot meet an increased hormonal demand. Many patients can be taught to adjust their corticosteroid replacement therapy in accordance with their stress levels. The nurse should consult with each patient's health care provider to determine the parameters for dosage changes if this plan is feasible. If a patient cannot adjust his or her own medication or if weakness, fainting, fever, or nausea and vomiting occur, the patient should contact the health care provider for a possible adjustment in corticosteroid dosage. Many patients require lifetime replacement therapy; however, it may take several months to adjust the hormone dose satisfactorily, and patients should be prepared for this.

EVALUATION

The expected outcomes for patients with Cushing's syndrome are as follows:

- No signs or symptoms of infection
- Appropriate weight for height
- Increased acceptance of appearance
- Healing and maintenance of intact skin

ADRENOCORTICAL INSUFFICIENCY

Etiology and Pathophysiology

Adrenocortical insufficiency (hypofunction of the adrenal cortex) may have a primary cause (known as *Addison's disease*) or a secondary cause (lack of pituitary ACTH secretion). In **Addison's disease,** the supply of all three classes of adrenal corticosteroids (glucocorticoids, mineralocorticoids, and androgens) is reduced. In secondary adrenocortical insufficiency, levels of corticosteroids and androgens are deficient, but those of mineralocorticoids rarely are. ACTH deficiency may be caused by pituitary disease or suppression of the hypothalamic-pituitary-adrenal axis as a result of the administration of exogenous corticosteroids.

The most common cause of Addison's disease in industrialized nations is an autoimmune response (Puttana, Cunningham, & Dainty, 2013). Adrenal tissue is destroyed by antibodies against the patient's own adrenal cortex. Susceptibility genes for Addison's disease are beginning to be identified (Napier, Mitchell, Gan, et al., 2015). Often, other endocrine conditions are present, and Addison's disease is considered a component of polyglandular autoimmune syndrome (Puttana, Cunningham, & Dainty, 2013). Tuberculosis causes Addison's disease worldwide, but it is now an uncommon cause in Canada. Other causes include infarction, fungal infections (e.g., histoplasmosis), acquired immune deficiency syndrome (AIDS), and metastatic cancer. Iatrogenic Addison's disease may be caused by adrenal hemorrhage, often related to anticoagulant therapy, antineoplastic chemotherapy, ketoconazole therapy for AIDS, or bilateral adrenalectomy. Adrenal insufficiency most often occurs in adults younger than 60 years and affects both sexes equally. Addison's disease, if caused by an autoimmune response, is most common in White women.

Clinical Manifestations

Because manifestations do not tend to become evident until 90% of the adrenal cortex is destroyed, the disease is often advanced before it is diagnosed. The manifestations have a very slow (insidious) onset and include progressive weakness, fatigue, weight loss, and anorexia as primary features. Skin hyperpigmentation, a striking feature, is observed primarily in sun-exposed areas of the body, at pressure points, over joints, and in creases (Figure 51-12); it is most likely caused by increased secretion of β-lipotropin (which contains melanocyte-stimulating hormone [MSH]). Secretion of this tropic hormone is increased because of decreased negative feedback and subsequent low corticosteroid levels. Other frequent manifestations of primary adrenal hypofunction are hypotension, hyponatremia, hyperkalemia, nausea and vomiting, and diarrhea. Irritability and depression may also occur.

FIGURE 51-12 Hyperpigmentation typically observed in Addison's disease. Source: Chew, S. L., & Leslie, D. (2006). *Clinical endocrinology and diabetes: An illustrated colour text*. Edinburgh: Churchill Livingstone.

TABLE 51-18 COLLABORATIVE CARE	
Addison's Disease	
Diagnostic	**Collaborative Therapy**
• History and physical examination • ACTH stimulation test • CT, MRI • Measurement of plasma cortisol levels • Measurement of serum electrolytes • Measurement of urine cortisol and aldosterone levels	• Daily glucocorticoid (e.g., hydrocortisone) replacement (two-thirds on awakening in morning, one-third in late afternoon)* • Daily mineralocorticoid (fludrocortisone acetate) replacement in morning* • Increased dose of cortisol for stress situations (e.g., surgery, hospitalization) • Salt additives for excess heat or humidity

ACTH, adrenocorticotrophic hormone; *CT,* computed tomographic (scan); *MRI,* magnetic resonance imaging.
*For conditions of normal daily stress, in individuals with usual daytime activity.

Secondary adrenocortical hypofunction shares many signs and symptoms in common with Addison's disease, but hyperpigmentation is not characteristic because ACTH and related peptide levels are low.

Complications

Patients with adrenocortical insufficiency are at risk for an acute adrenal insufficiency *(addisonian crisis),* a life-threatening emergency caused by insufficient adrenocortical hormones or a sudden sharp decrease in these hormones. Addisonian crisis is triggered by stress (e.g., from infection, surgery, trauma, hemorrhage, or psychological distress); by sudden withdrawal of corticosteroid hormone therapy (which often occurs when a patient who lacks knowledge of the importance of replacement therapy stops following the regimen); by adrenal surgery; or by sudden pituitary gland destruction.

During acute adrenal insufficiency, manifestations of glucocorticoid and mineralocorticoid deficiencies are severe and include hypotension (particularly postural), tachycardia, dehydration, hyponatremia, hyperkalemia, hypoglycemia, fever, weakness, and confusion. Hypotension may lead to shock. Circulatory collapse associated with adrenal insufficiency is often unresponsive to the usual treatment (vasopressors and fluid replacement). GI manifestations include nausea, vomiting, diarrhea, and pain in the abdomen. Pain may also occur in the lower back or the legs.

Diagnostic Studies

In addition to clinical features, cortisol levels that are subnormal or fail to rise over basal levels with an ACTH stimulation test can be diagnostic for Addison's disease. A failure of cortisol levels to rise in response to ACTH stimulation indicates primary adrenal disease. A positive response to ACTH stimulation indicates that the adrenal gland is functioning and that the probable cause is pituitary disease (see Chapter 50).

Other abnormal laboratory findings include hyperkalemia, hypochloremia, hyponatremia, hypoglycemia, anemia, and increased blood urea nitrogen levels. Urine levels of free cortisol are low, as is the urine level of aldosterone (Pagana & Pagana, 2013). An ECG may show low voltage and a vertical QRS axis. In addition, peaked T-waves caused by hyperkalemia may be evident. CT and MRI are used to localize tumours or identify adrenal calcifications or enlargement (Table 51-18).

Collaborative Care

Treatment of adrenocortical insufficiency is focused on management of the underlying cause when possible. The mainstay of treatment for adrenocortical insufficiency is replacement therapy (see Table 51-18). Hydrocortisone, the most commonly used form of replacement therapy, has both glucocorticoid and mineralocorticoid properties. During situations associated with physiological stress, glucocorticoid dosage must be increased to prevent addisonian crisis. Mineralocorticoid replacement with fludrocortisone acetate is administered daily, with increased salt in the diet.

Addisonian crisis is a life-threatening emergency requiring aggressive management. Treatment must be directed toward shock management and high-dose hydrocortisone replacement. Large volumes of 0.9% saline solution and 5% dextrose are administered to reverse hypotension and electrolyte imbalances until BP returns to normal.

NURSING MANAGEMENT
ADDISON'S DISEASE

NURSING IMPLEMENTATION

ACUTE INTERVENTION. When the patient with Addison's disease is hospitalized—whether for diagnosis, an acute crisis, or some other health problem—nursing management focuses on monitoring the patient while correcting fluid and electrolyte balance. Vital signs and signs of fluid volume deficit and electrolyte imbalance are assessed. Trends in serum glucose, sodium, and potassium are monitored. Baseline data are established regarding mental status, vital signs, and weight. A complete medication history is obtained to determine drugs that can potentially interact with corticosteroids. These drugs include oral hypoglycemics, cardiac glycosides, oral contraceptives, anticoagulants, and NSAIDs.

Changes are noted in BP, weight gain, weakness, or other manifestations of Cushing's syndrome. In addition, the patient must be protected against exposure to infection and assisted with daily hygiene. The patient must also be protected from noise, light, and environmental temperature extremes—the patient cannot cope with these stresses because of the inability to produce corticosteroids.

The patient who is hospitalized because of adrenal crisis usually responds by the second day and can start oral corticosteroid replacement. The patient must be instructed about the importance of keeping scheduled follow-up appointments.

TABLE 51-19 PATIENT & CAREGIVER TEACHING GUIDE

Addison's Disease

The following information should be included when teaching the patient and caregiver about management of Addison's disease:

1. Names, dosages, and actions of drugs
2. Symptoms of overdosage and underdosage
3. Conditions necessitating increased medication (e.g., trauma, infection, surgery, emotional crisis)
4. Course of action to take in regard to changes in medication
   - Increase in dose of corticosteroid
   - Administration of large dose of corticosteroid intramuscularly, including demonstration and return demonstration
   - Consultation with health care provider
5. Prevention of infection and need for prompt and vigorous treatment of existing infections
6. Need for lifelong replacement therapy
7. Need for lifelong medical supervision
8. Need for medical identification device
9. Prevention of falls
10. Adverse effects of corticosteroid therapy and prevention techniques
11. Special instruction for patients who are diabetic, and management of blood glucose when taking corticosteroids

TABLE 51-20 DRUG THERAPY

Diseases and Disorders Treated With Corticosteroids

Hormone Replacement
- Adrenal insufficiency
- Congenital adrenal hyperplasia

Therapeutic Effect
Allergic Reactions
- Anaphylaxis
- Bee stings
- Contact dermatitis
- Drug reactions
- Serum sickness
- Urticaria

Collagen Diseases
- Giant cell arteritis
- Mixed connective tissue disorders
- Polymyositis
- Polyarteritis nodosa
- Rheumatoid arthritis
- Systemic lupus erythematosus

Gastro-Intestinal Diseases
- Celiac disease
- Inflammatory bowel disease

Endocrine Diseases
- Hashimoto's thyroiditis
- Hypercalcemia
- Thyrotoxic crisis (thyroid storm)

Liver Diseases
- Alcohol-related hepatitis
- Autoimmune hepatitis

Neurological Diseases
- Head trauma
- Prevention of cerebral edema and increase in intracranial pressure

Pulmonary Diseases
- Aspiration pneumonia
- Asthma
- Chronic obstructive pulmonary disease

Other Diseases/Disorders
- Immuno-suppression
- Inflammation
- Malignancies, leukemia, lymphoma
- Nephrotic syndrome
- Skin diseases

AMBULATORY AND HOME CARE. The nurse has an important role in the long-term management of Addison's disease. The serious nature of the disease and the need for lifelong replacement therapy necessitate a well-organized and carefully presented teaching plan. Table 51-19 outlines the major areas that must be included in the teaching plan.

Glucocorticoids are usually given in divided doses, two-thirds in the morning and one-third in the afternoon. Mineralocorticoids are given once daily, preferably in the morning. This dosage schedule reflects normal circadian rhythm in endogenous hormone secretion and decreases the intensity of adverse effects associated with corticosteroid replacement therapy. Because the aim of replacement therapy is to return hormone levels to normal, nursing care is designed to help patients maintain hormone balance and manage the medication regimen.

Because the patient with Addison's disease is unable to tolerate physical or emotional stress without additional exogenous corticosteroids, long-term care revolves around recognizing the need for extra medication and techniques for stress management. The need for corticosteroid hormone is proportional to stress levels. A patient who cannot produce endogenous hormone must adjust the dose of exogenous hormone to the stress level. Examples of situations requiring corticosteroid adjustment are fever, influenza, extraction of teeth, and rigorous physical activity, such as playing tennis on a hot day or running a marathon. Doses are usually doubled in situations of minor stress (e.g., a respiratory infection, dental work) and tripled in situations of major stress (e.g., divorce, loss of parent). When the stress level is in doubt, it is better to err on the side of over-replacement. If vomiting or diarrhea occurs, as may happen with influenza, the health care provider must be notified immediately because electrolyte replacement may be necessary. In addition, these manifestations may be early indicators of crisis. Overall, patients who take their medications consistently can anticipate a normal life expectancy.

The patient must be taught the signs and symptoms of corticosteroid deficiency and excess and to report these signs to the health care provider so the dosage can be adjusted to each patient's needs. It is critical that patients wear a medical alert bracelet and carry a wallet card stating that they have Addison's disease so that appropriate therapy can be initiated in case of an unexpected stressful event. The patient should be instructed and given handouts related to other medications that cause a need to increase glucocorticoid dosage (e.g., phenytoin [Dilantin], barbiturates, rifampin [Rifadin], and antacids). Estrogen inhibits steroid metabolism. The nurse should instruct patients receiving mineralocorticoid therapy (fludrocortisone acetate) (a) on how to measure their BP, (b) to increase salt intake, and (c) to report significant changes to their health care provider. Changes may indicate a need for dosage adjustment.

Patients should carry an emergency kit at all times. The kit should consist of 100 mg of intramuscular (IM) hydrocortisone, syringes, and instructions for use. The patient and significant others should be instructed in how to administer an IM injection in case the replacement therapy cannot be taken orally. Patients should verbalize instructions, practise IM injections with saline, and receive written instructions about when to alter the dose (Quinkler, Beuschlein, Hahner, et al., 2013).

CORTICOSTEROID THERAPY

Corticosteroids are used to relieve the signs and symptoms associated with many diseases (Table 51-20). The long-term administration of corticosteroids in therapeutic dosages often leads to serious complications and adverse effects (Table 51-21). For this reason, corticosteroid therapy is not recommended for minor chronic conditions. Therapy should be reserved for diseases in which there is a risk for death or permanent loss of function and conditions in which short-term therapy is likely to produce

TABLE 51-21   DRUG THERAPY

Effects and Adverse Effects of Corticosteroids

- BP increases because of excess blood volume and potentiation of vasoconstrictor effects. Hypertension predisposes to heart failure.
- Fat from extremities is redistributed to trunk and face.
- Glucose intolerance predisposes to diabetes mellitus.
- Healing is delayed, and patient is at increased risk for wound dehiscence.
- Hypocalcemia related to anti–vitamin D effect may occur.
- Hypokalemia may develop.
- Manifestations of inflammation, including redness, tenderness, heat, swelling, and local edema, are suppressed.
- Mood and behaviour changes may be observed.
- Patient is predisposed to peptic ulcer disease.
- Protein depletion decreases bone formation, density, and strength; patient is thus predisposed to pathological fractures, especially compression fractures of the vertebrae (osteoporosis).
- Skeletal muscle atrophy and weakness occur.
- Suppression of pituitary ACTH synthesis occurs. Corticosteroid deficiency is likely if hormone treatment is withdrawn abruptly. Corticosteroid doses should be tapered.
- Susceptibility to infection is increased. Infection develops more rapidly and spreads more widely.

ACTH, adrenocorticotrophic hormone; *BP,* blood pressure.

remission or recovery. The potential benefits of treatment must always be weighed against the risks.

Effects of Corticosteroid Therapy

Corticosteroid therapy has multiple effects. Although these actions can prove to be beneficial and therapeutic in some situations, they can contribute to adverse effects as well. The expected effects of corticosteroid therapy include the following:

1. *Anti-inflammatory action.* Corticosteroids decrease the number of circulating lymphocytes, monocytes, and eosinophils. They enhance the release of polymorphonuclear leukocytes from bone marrow, inhibit the accumulation of leukocytes at the site of inflammation, and inhibit the release of substances involved in the inflammatory response (e.g., kinins, prostaglandins, histamine) from the leukocytes. As a result, manifestations of inflammation, including redness, tenderness, heat, swelling, and local edema, are suppressed.

2. *Immuno-suppression.* Corticosteroids cause atrophy of lymphoid tissue, suppress the cell-mediated immune responses, and decrease the production of antibodies.

3. *Maintenance of normal blood pressure.* Corticosteroids potentiate the vasoconstrictor effect of norepinephrine and act on the renal tubules to increase sodium reabsorption and enhance potassium and hydrogen excretion. Retention of sodium (and subsequently water) increases blood volume and helps maintain BP. Mineralocorticoids have a direct effect on sodium reabsorption in the distal tubules of the kidneys; as a result, sodium retention and water retention are increased.

4. *Carbohydrate and protein metabolism.* Corticosteroids antagonize the effects of insulin and can induce glucose intolerance by increasing hepatic glycogenolysis and insulin resistance. They also stimulate the breakdown of protein for gluconeogenesis, which can lead to skeletal muscle wasting. Although corticosteroids mobilize free fatty acids and cause redistribution of fat in Cushingoid patterns, the mechanism underlying this process is unknown.

Complications Associated With Corticosteroid Therapy

A beneficial effect in one situation may be a harmful one in another. For example, the vasopressive effect of a hormone is critical in enabling the organism to function in stressful situations, but it can produce hypertension when used for drug therapy. Suppression of inflammation and the immune response may help save the life of someone experiencing anaphylaxis or receiving a transplant, but it causes reactivation of latent tuberculosis and greatly reduces resistance to other infections and cancers. In addition, corticosteroids inhibit the antibody response to vaccines.

DRUG ALERT—Corticosteroids

The nurse should do the following:
- Instruct patients not to discontinue therapy abruptly.
- Monitor patients for signs of infection.
- Instruct patients with diabetes to closely monitor blood glucose levels.

NURSING AND COLLABORATIVE MANAGEMENT CORTICOSTEROID THERAPY

Many patients receive corticosteroid therapy, particularly glucocorticoid therapy, for nonendocrine reasons (see Table 51-20). Thorough instruction is necessary to ensure patient adherence to the regimen. When corticosteroids are used as nonreplacement therapy, they are taken once daily or once every other day. They should be taken early in the morning with food to decrease gastric irritation. Because exogenous corticosteroid administration may suppress endogenous ACTH and therefore endogenous cortisol (suppression is time and dose dependent), the danger of abrupt cessation of corticosteroid therapy must be emphasized to patients and significant others. When taken for longer than 1 week, corticosteroids suppress adrenal production, and oral steroids should be tapered. In acute care or home care situations, nurses must ensure that increased doses of steroid are prescribed with increased physical or emotional stress.

Because patients often receive corticosteroid treatment for prolonged periods (>3 months), corticosteroid-induced osteoporosis is an important concern (Clarke, 2012). Therapies to reduce the resorption of bone may include increased calcium intake, vitamin D supplementation, administration of bisphosphonates (e.g., alendronate [Fosamax]), and institution of a low-impact exercise program. Further instruction and interventions to minimize the adverse effects and complications of corticosteroid therapy are listed in Table 51-22.

HYPERALDOSTERONISM

Etiology and Pathophysiology

Hyperaldosteronism is characterized by excessive aldosterone secretion. The main effects of aldosterone are retention of sodium and excretion of potassium and hydrogen ion. Thus the hallmark of this disease is hypertension with hypokalemic alkalosis. *Primary hyperaldosteronism* (PA) is most commonly caused by a small, solitary adrenocortical adenoma. On occasion, multiple lesions are involved and are associated with bilateral adrenal hyperplasia. PA affects both sexes equally and occurs most frequently between the ages of 30 and 50 years. It is estimated that approximately 1% of cases of hypertension are caused by PA. *Secondary hyperaldosteronism* occurs in response to a nonadrenal cause of elevated aldosterone levels such as renal artery stenosis, renin-secreting tumours, or chronic renal disease.

TABLE 51-22   PATIENT & CAREGIVER TEACHING GUIDE

Corticosteroid Therapy

The following instructions should be included when teaching the patient and caregiver about management of corticosteroid therapy.

1. Plan a diet high in protein, calcium, and potassium but low in fat and concentrated simple carbohydrates such as sugar, honey, syrups, and candy.
2. Identify measures to ensure adequate rest and sleep, such as daily naps and avoidance of caffeine late in the day.
3. Develop and maintain an exercise program to help maintain bone integrity.
4. Recognize edema and ways to restrict sodium intake to less than 2 000 mg/day if edema occurs.
5. Monitor glucose levels and recognize symptoms and signs of hyperglycemia (e.g., polydipsia, polyuria, blurred vision) and glycosuria (glucose in the urine). Patients should be instructed to report hyperglycemic symptoms or capillary glucose levels higher than 10 mmol/L or urine findings that are positive for glucose.
6. Notify health care provider if patients are experiencing postprandial heartburn or epigastric pain that is not relieved by antacids.
7. See an eye specialist yearly to assess possible development of cataracts.
8. Use safety measures such as getting up slowly from a bed or a chair, and use good lighting to prevent accidental injury.
9. Maintain good hygiene practices and avoid contact with people with colds or other contagious illnesses to prevent infection.
10. Inform all health care providers about long-term corticosteroid use.
11. Realize that doses of corticosteroids may need to be increased in times of physical and emotional stress.
12. Never abruptly stop taking the corticosteroids because this could lead to addisonian crisis and possibly death.

Clinical Manifestations

Elevations in aldosterone levels are associated with retention of sodium and elimination of potassium. Sodium retention leads to hypernatremia, hypertension, and headache. Edema does not usually occur because the rate of sodium excretion increases, which prevents more severe sodium retention. The potassium wasting leads to hypokalemia, which causes generalized muscle weakness, fatigue, cardiac dysrhythmias, glucose intolerance, and metabolic alkalosis that may lead to tetany.

Diagnostic Studies

The diagnosis of hyperaldosteronism should be suspected in all hypertensive patients with hypokalemia that are not being treated with diuretics. PA is associated with elevations in plasma aldosterone levels and decreased plasma renin activity, elevated sodium levels, and decreased serum potassium levels. Adenomas are localized by means of CT or MRI. If a tumour is not found, plasma 18-hydroxycorticosterone is measured after overnight bedrest. A level higher than 1.38 nmol/L indicates the presence of an adenoma.

NURSING AND COLLABORATIVE MANAGEMENT PRIMARY HYPERALDOSTERONISM

The preferred treatment for PA is surgical removal of the adrenal gland that has the adenoma (adrenalectomy). A laparoscopic approach is most often used. Before surgery, patients should be treated with a low-sodium diet, potassium-sparing diuretics (spironolactone [Aldactone] or eplerenone [Inspra]), and

antihypertensive agents to normalize serum potassium levels and BP. Spironolactone and eplerenone block the binding of aldosterone to the mineralocorticoid receptor in the terminal distal tubules and collecting ducts of the kidneys, thus increasing the excretion of sodium and water and the retention of potassium. Oral potassium supplements and sodium restrictions may also be necessary. Potassium supplementation and a potassium-sparing diuretic should not be started simultaneously because of the danger of hyperkalemia. Patients taking eplerenone should be instructed to avoid grapefruit juice.

Patients with bilateral adrenal hyperplasia are treated with a potassium-sparing diuretic. Calcium channel blockers may also be used to control BP. Dexamethasone may be used to decrease the hyperplasia.

Nursing care includes careful assessment for signs of fluid and electrolyte imbalance (especially potassium imbalance) and cardiovascular status. BP should be monitored frequently before and after surgery because unilateral adrenalectomy is successful in controlling hypertension in only 80% of patients with adenoma. Patients receiving maintenance therapy with spironolactone need instruction about the possible adverse effects (gynecomastia, erectile dysfunction, and menstrual disorders), as well as knowledge about the signs and symptoms of hypokalemia and hyperkalemia. Patients should be taught how to monitor their own BP and the need for frequent monitoring. The need for continued health supervision should be stressed.

DISORDERS OF THE ADRENAL MEDULLA

PHEOCHROMOCYTOMA

Etiology and Pathophysiology

Pheochromocytoma is a rare condition characterized by a tumour of the adrenal medulla that arises from the chromaffin cells and produces excessive amounts of catecholamines (epinephrine, norepinephrine). The secretion of excessive catecholamines results in severe hypertension (Li, Spiler, Fahey, 3rd, et al., 2013). If left untreated, it may lead to hypertensive encephalopathy, diabetes mellitus, cardiomyopathy, and death. It is most commonly seen in young to middle-aged adults. Pheochromocytoma may be inherited in persons with multiple endocrine neoplasia.

Clinical Manifestations

The most striking clinical features of pheochromocytoma include severe, episodic hypertension accompanied by the classic manifestations of severe, pounding headache; tachycardia with palpitations; profuse sweating; and unexplained abdominal or chest pain. Such "attacks" may be provoked by many medications, including antihypertensives, opioids, radiological contrast media, and tricyclic antidepressants. The duration of the episodes varies from a few minutes to several hours.

Diagnostic Studies

Although pheochromocytoma is associated with a number of symptoms, the correct diagnosis is often missed. Pheochromocytoma is an uncommon cause of hypertension, accounting for only 0.1% of all cases. This condition should be considered in patients who do not respond to traditional hypertensive treatments.

The simplest and most reliable diagnostic test for pheochromocytoma is measurement of urinary fractionated metanephrines (catecholamine metabolites) and fractionated catecholamines and creatinine, usually done as a 24-hour urine collection. Serum catecholamines may be elevated during an "attack." CT scans and MRI are used for diagnosing tumours. Health care providers should avoid palpating the abdomen of a patient with suspected pheochromocytoma, since it may cause the sudden release of catecholamines and severe hypertension.

NURSING AND COLLABORATIVE MANAGEMENT PHEOCHROMOCYTOMA

The primary treatment for pheochromocytoma consists of surgical removal of the tumour. Treatment with α- and β-adrenergic receptor blockers is required preoperatively to control BP and prevent an intraoperative hypertensive crisis. The α-adrenergic receptor blocker prazosin (Minipress) is given up to 2 weeks preoperatively to reduce BP and alleviate other symptoms of catecholamine excess, but calcium channel blockers may also be effective (Shah & Ruan, 2014) After adequate α-adrenergic blockade, β-adrenergic receptor blockers (e.g., propranolol) are used to decrease tachycardia and other dysrhythmias. If beta blockers are started too early, unopposed α-adrenergic stimulation could precipitate a hypertensive crisis. Sympathetic blocking agents may result in orthostatic hypotension. Patients must be advised to make postural changes cautiously.

Surgery is more commonly performed via laparoscopic adrenalectomy than via open abdominal incision. Complete removal of the adrenal tumour cures the hypertension in the majority of affected individuals, but hypertension persists in approximately 10% to 30% of patients. For these individuals, BP management involves standard antihypertensive drug therapy. If surgery is not an option, medication is used to diminish catecholamine production by the tumour and simplify chronic management.

Case finding is an important nursing function. Any patient with hypertension accompanied by symptoms of sympathoadrenal discharge should be referred to a health care provider for definitive diagnosis. An important part of the nursing assessment is observation of patients for the classic triad of symptoms of pheochromocytoma—severe, pounding headache; tachycardia; and profuse sweating. BP should be monitored immediately if a patient is experiencing an attack. The nurse should be prepared to check BP when any of the drugs that might precipitate an attack are administered.

The nurse should attempt to make patients with pheochromocytoma as comfortable as possible. All diagnostic samples should be collected appropriately. Capillary blood glucose levels should be monitored to assess for diabetes mellitus. Patients need rest, nourishing food, and emotional support during this period.

Preoperative and postoperative care is similar to that for any patient undergoing adrenalectomy, except that BP fluctuations from catecholamine excesses tend to be severe and must be carefully monitored. Because hypertension may persist even when the tumour is removed, the nurse should stress the importance of follow-up care and routine BP monitoring. Patients taking catecholamine synthesis inhibitors should be instructed to rise slowly while holding on to a secure object because this medication can cause orthostatic hypotension.

CASE STUDY

Graves' Disease

Source: JPagetRF Photos/ Shutterstock .com.

Patient Profile

Ruth Delaware, a 47-year-old woman, was admitted to the hospital with a high fever. After an endocrine workup, she received a diagnosis of Graves' disease.

Subjective Data
- Reports recent job loss because of inability to cope with job stress
- Reports symptoms including fatigue, unintentional weight loss, insomnia, palpitations, and heat intolerance

Objective Data
Physical Examination
- Fever of 40°C
- BP of 150/78, pulse of 118, and respiratory rate of 24
- Hot, moist skin
- Fine tremors of the hands
- Grade 4+ deep tendon reflexes and muscle strength of grades 1 to 2

Collaborative Care
- Subtotal thyroidectomy planned for 2 months later
- Started on propylthiouracil and propranolol (Inderal)

Discussion Questions

1. What is the cause of Ms. Delaware's symptoms?
2. What diagnostic studies were probably ordered? What results have established the diagnosis of Graves' disease?
3. Why was surgery delayed?
4. What was the purpose of drug therapy for Ms. Delaware?
5. *Priority decision:* What are Ms. Delaware's priority learning needs? What teaching strategies would the nurse use if Ms. Delaware could not read?
6. What are the nursing interventions for successful long-term management of Ms. Delaware after the subtotal thyroidectomy?
7. *Priority decision:* On the basis of the assessment data presented, what are the priority nursing diagnoses pertinent to Ms. Delaware while she is hospitalized? Are there any collaborative problems?
8. *Evidence-informed practice:* Why is Ms. Delaware counselled to give up her longstanding cigarette smoking habit?

⊖volve

Answers are available at *http://evolve.elsevier.com/Canada/Lewis/medsurg.*

REVIEW QUESTIONS

The number of the question corresponds to the same-numbered objective at the beginning of the chapter.

1. After a hypophysectomy for acromegaly, which of the following should be the focus of postoperative nursing care?
   a. Frequent monitoring of serum and urine osmolarity
   b. Parenteral administration of a GH-receptor antagonist
   c. Keeping the client in a recumbent position at all times
   d. Client teaching regarding the need for lifelong hormone therapy

2. A client with a head injury develops SIADH. Which of the following manifestations of SIADH would the nurse expect to find?
   a. Hypernatremia and edema
   b. Muscle spasticity and hypertension
   c. Low urine output and hyponatremia
   d. Weight gain and decreased glomerular filtration rate (GFR)

3. The health care provider prescribes levothyroxine (Synthroid) for a client with myxedema. After teaching regarding this drug, the nurse determines that further instruction is needed when the client says which of the following?
   a. "I can expect the medication dose may need to be adjusted."
   b. "I only need to take this drug until my symptoms are improved."
   c. "I can expect to return to normal function with the use of this drug."
   d. "I will report any chest pain or difficulty breathing to the doctor right away."

4. Which of the following symptoms would lead the nurse to suspect damage or removal of the parathyroid glands after thyroid surgery?
   a. Muscle weakness and weight loss
   b. Hyperthermia and severe tachycardia
   c. Hypertension and difficulty swallowing
   d. Laryngospasms and tingling in the hands and feet

5. Which of the following are important nursing intervention(s) when caring for a client with Cushing's syndrome? *(Select all that apply)*
   a. Restricting protein intake
   b. Monitoring blood glucose levels
   c. Observing for signs of hypotension
   d. Administering medication in equal doses
   e. Protecting the client from exposure to infection

6. Which of the following is an important preoperative nursing intervention before an adrenalectomy for hyperaldosteronism?
   a. Monitor blood glucose levels
   b. Restrict fluid and sodium intake
   c. Administer potassium-sparing diuretics
   d. Advise the client to make postural changes slowly

7. How does the nurse instruct the client who is taking corticosteroids to control the adverse effects of drug therapy?
   a. Increase calcium intake to 1 500 mg/day
   b. Perform glucose monitoring for hypoglycemia
   c. Obtain immunizations due to high risk for infections
   d. Avoid abrupt position changes because of orthostatic hypotension

8. What does the nurse teach the client regarding the best time to take corticosteroids for replacement purposes?
   a. Once a day at bedtime
   b. Every other day on awakening
   c. On arising and in the late afternoon
   d. At consistent intervals every 6 to 8 hours

ⓔvolve

1. a, 2. c, 3. b, 4. d, 5. b, e, 6. c, 7. a, 8. c.

For even more review questions, visit *http://evolve.elsevier.com/Canada/Lewis/medsurg*.

REFERENCES

Callender, G. G., & Udelsman, R. (2014). Surgery for primary hyperparathyroidism. *Cancer, 120*(23), 3602–3616. doi:10.1002/cncr.28891.

Canadian Cancer Society's Steering Committee on Cancer Statistics. (2012). *Canadian Cancer Statistics 2012*. Toronto, ON: Canadian Cancer Society. Retrieved from *http://www.cancer.ca/~/media/cancer.ca/CW/cancer%20information/cancer%20101/Canadian%20cancer%20statistics/Canadian-Cancer-Statistics-2012-EN.pdf*.

Cipriani, C., Biamonte, F., Costa, A. G., et al. (2015). Prevalence of kidney stones and vertebral fractures in primary hyperparathyroidism using imaging technology. *Journal of Clinical Endocrinology & Metabolism, 100*(4), 1309–1315. doi:10.1210/jc.2014-3708.

Clark, P. (2015). Multiple endocrine neoplasia syndromes. *Journal of Infusion Nursing*, (Suppl. 6), S36–S42. doi:10.1097/NAN.0000000000000143.

Clarke, B. L. (2012). Corticosteroid-induced osteoporosis: An update for dermatologists. *American Journal of Clinical Dermatology, 13*(3), 167–190. doi:10.2165/11594250-000000000-00000.

Dallapiazza, R. F., & Jane, J. A., Jr. (2015). Outcomes of endoscopic transsphenoidal pituitary surgery. *Endocrinology & Metabolism Clinics of North America, 44*(1), 105–115. doi:10.1016/j.ecl.2014.10.010.

Dittrich, R., Beckmann, M. W., Oppelt, P. G., et al. (2011). Thyroid hormone receptors and reproduction. *Journal of Reproductive Immunology, 90*(1), 58–66. doi:10.1016/j.jri.2011.02.009.

Famularo, G., Minisola, G., Bravi, M., et al. (2012). Tetany, hypomagnesemia, and proton-pump inhibitors. *American Journal of Medicine, 125*(10), e7–e8. doi:10.1016/j.amjmed.2012.04.027.

Gardner, D. G. (2011). Endocrine emergencies. In D. Gardner & D. Shoback (Eds.), *Greenspan's basic and clinical endocrinology* (9th ed., pp. 763–787). New York: McGraw Hill.

Grais, I., & Sowers, J. (2014). Thyroid and the heart. *The American Journal of Medicine, 127*(8), 691–698. doi:10.1016/j.amjmed.2014.03.009.

Gupta, S., Chaudhary, P., Durga, C. K., et al. (2015). Validation of intra-operative parathyroid hormone and its decline as early predictors of hypoparathyroidism after total thyroidectomy: A prospective cohort study. *International Journal of Surgery, 18*, 150–153. doi:10.1016/j.ijsu.2015.04.074.

Health Canada. (2016). *Drug product database*. Retrieved from *http://webprod5.hc-sc.gc.ca/dpd-bdpp/index-eng.jsp*.

Hong, L. (2012). Management of hyponatremia associated with syndrome of inappropriate antidiuretic hormone secretion. *Topics in Clinical Nutrition, 29*(2), 187–196. doi:10.1097/01.TIN.000044590290393.82.

Hubbard, J. G. H. (2011). Thyrotoxicosis and thyroiditis. *Surgery (Oxford), 29*(9), 440–445. doi:10.1016/j.mpsur.2011.06.003.

John, C. A., & Day, M. W. (2012). Central neurogenic diabetes insipidus, syndrome of inappropriate secretion of antidiuretic hormone, and cerebral salt-wasting syndrome in traumatic brain injury. *Critical Care Nurse, 32*(2), e1–e8. doi:10.4037/ccn2012904.

Juszczak, A., & Grossman, A. (2012). The investigation of Cushing syndrome: Essentials in optimizing appropriate diagnosis and management. *Annals of Saudi Medicine, 32*(5), 455–461. doi:10.5144/0256-4947.2012.455.

Katznelson, L., Laws, E. R., Jr., Melmed, S., et al. (2014). Acromegaly: An endocrine society clinical practice guideline. *Journal of Clinical Endocrinology & Metabolism, 99*(11), 3933–3951. doi:10.1210/jc.2014-2700.

Lacroix, A., Feelders, R. A., Stratakis, C. A., et al. (2015). Cushing's syndrome. *Lancet, 386*(9996), 913–927. doi:10.1016/S0140-6736(14)61375-1.

Lamartina, L., Durante, C., Filetti, S., et al. (2015). Low-risk differentiated thyroid cancer and radioiodine remnant ablation: A systematic review of the literature. *Journal of Clinical Endocrinology & Metabolism, 100*(5), 1748–1761. doi:10.1210/jc.2014-3882.

Li, Y., Spiler, I. J., Fahey, T., 3rd, et al. (2013). A looming danger: Pheochromocytoma. *American Journal of Medicine, 126*(12), 1054–1056. doi:10.1016/j.amjmed.2013.08.023.

Lian-Xi, L., Xing, W., Bing, H., et al. (2014). Localized subacute thyroiditis presenting as a painful hot nodule. *BMC Endocrine Disorders, 14*(1), 106–115. doi:10.1186/1472-6823-14-4.

Melmed, S., & Kleinberg, D. (2016). Pituitary masses and tumors. In S. Melmed, K. S. Polonsky, P. R. Larsen, et al. (Eds.), *Williams textbook of endocrinology* (13th ed., pp. 232–299). Philadelphia: Elsevier.

Miller, R. E., Learned-Miller, E. G., Trainer, P., et al. (2011). Early diagnosis of acromegaly: Computers vs clinicians. *Clinical Endocrinology, 75*(2), 226–231. doi:10.1111/j.1365-2265.2011.04020.x.

Napier, C., Mitchell, A. L., Gan, E., et al. (2015). Role of the X-linked gene GPR174 in autoimmune Addison's disease. *Journal of Clinical Endocrinology & Metabolism, 100*(1), E187–E190. doi:10.1210/jc.2014-2694.

Pagana, K. D., & Pagana, T. J. (2013). Blood Studies: Overview and Tests. In S. A. Pike-MacDonald (Ed.), *Mosby's Canadian manual of diagnostic and laboratory tests* (1st Can. ed.). Toronto: Elsevier.

Pagana, K. D., & Pagana, T. J. (2013). Urine studies. In S. A. Pike-MacDonald (Ed.), *Mosby's Canadian manual of diagnostic and laboratory tests* (1st Can. ed.). Toronto: Elsevier.

Pallan, S., Rahman, M. O., & Khan, A. A. (2012). Diagnosis and management of primary hyperparathyroidism. *BMJ: British Medical Journal (Overseas & Retired Doctors Edition), 344*(7849), 55–60. doi:10.1136/bmj.e1013.

Premawardhana, L. (2015). Universal screening for hypothyroidism in pregnancy: Time for a paradigm shift? *Endocrine, 48*(1), 9–11. doi:10.1007/s12020-014-0512-7.

Puig, D. M. (2015). Treatment of acromegaly in the era of personalized and predictive medicine. *Clinical Endocrinology, 83*(1), 3–14. doi:10.1111/cen.12731.

Puttana, A., Cunningham, A. R., & Dainty, P. (2013). Addison's disease and its associations. *BMJ Case Reports, 1–3. doi:10.1136/bcr-2013-010473.

Quinkler, M., Beuschlein, F., Hahner, S., et al. (2013). Adrenal cortical insufficiency—A life threatening illness with multiple etiologies. *Deutsches Aerzteblatt International, 110*(51-52), 882–888. doi:10.3238/arztebl.2013.0882.

Robinson, A. G., & Verbalis, J. G. (2016). Posterior pituitary. In S. Melmed, K. S. Polonsky, P. R. Larsen, et al. (Eds.), *Williams textbook of endocrinology* (13th ed., pp. 300–332). Philadelphia: Elsevier.

Runkle, I., Gomez-Hoyos, E., Cuesta-Hernández, M., et al. (2015). Hyponatraemia in older patients: A clinical and practical approach. *Reviews in Clinical Gerontology, 25*(1), 31–52. doi:10.1017/S0959259814000197.

Shah, N. H., & Ruan, D. T. (2014). Pheochromocytoma: A devious opponent in a game of hide-and-seek. *Circulation, 130*(15), 1295–1298. doi:10.1161/CIRCULATIONAHA.114.008544.

Strianese, D., Piscopo, R., Elefante, A., et al. (2013). Unilateral proptosis in thyroid eye disease with subsequent contralateral involvement: Retrospective follow-up study. *BMC Ophthalmology, 13*(1), 21. doi:10.1186/1471-2415-13-21.

Thyroid Foundation of Canada. (2016). *Health guides on thyroid disease.* Retrieved from *http://www.thyroid.ca/educational_material.php.*

Turbow, S. D., & Patterson, B. C. (2014). Hypothalamic and pituitary disorders. In E. I. Felner & G. E. Umpierrez (Eds.), *Endocrine pathophysiology* (pp. 19–39). Philadelphia: Lippincott Williams & Wilkins.

Vaidya, B., & Pearce, S. S. (2014). Diagnosis and management of thyrotoxicosis. *BMJ: British Medical Journal (Clinical Research Edition), 349*, g5128. doi:10.1136/bmj.g5128.

Yang, M. S., Hong, J. W., Lee, S. K., et al. (2011). Clinical management and outcome of 36 invasive prolactinomas treated with dopamine agonist. *Journal of Neuro-Oncology, 104*(1), 195–204. doi:10.1007/s11060-010-0459-3.

RESOURCES

Canadian Addison Society
http://www.addisonsociety.ca

The Canadian Society of Endocrinology and Metabolism
http://www.endo-metab.ca/

Thyroid Foundation of Canada
http://www.thyroid.ca

American Association of Clinical Endocrinologists (AACE)
https://www.aace.com

American Society for Bone and Mineral Research
http://www.asbmr.org

Endocrine Nurses Society (ENS)
http://www.endo-nurses.org

Endocrine Society
http://www.endo-society.org

EndocrineWeb.com
http://www.endocrineweb.com/

National Endocrine and Metabolic Diseases Information Service
http://endocrine.niddk.nih.gov

Pituitary Network Association
https://www.pituitary.org

Society for Endocrinology
http://www.endocrinology.org/

For additional Internet resources, see the website for this book at *http://evolve.elsevier.com/Canada/Lewis/medsurg.*

Nursing Management
Diabetes Mellitus

Written by: Jane K. Dickinson
Adapted by: Tess Montada-Atin

evolve WEBSITE

http://evolve.elsevier.com/Canada/Lewis/medsurg

- Review Questions (Online Only)
- Key Points
- Answer Guidelines for Case Study
- Student Case Studies
  - Type 1 Diabetes Mellitus and Diabetic Ketoacidosis
- Customizable Nursing Care Plan
  - Diabetes Mellitus
- Conceptual Care Map Creator
  - Conceptual Care Map for Textbook Case Study
- Audio Glossary
- Content Updates

LEARNING OBJECTIVES

1. Describe the pathophysiology and clinical manifestations of diabetes mellitus.
2. Describe the differences between type 1 and type 2 diabetes mellitus.
3. Describe the collaborative care of the patient with diabetes mellitus.
4. Describe the role of nutrition and exercise in the management of diabetes mellitus.
5. Describe the nursing management of a patient with newly diagnosed diabetes mellitus.
6. Describe the nursing management of the patient with diabetes mellitus in the ambulatory and home care settings.
7. Identify the pathophysiology and clinical manifestations of acute and chronic complications of diabetes mellitus.
8. Explain the collaborative care and nursing management of the patient with acute and chronic complications of diabetes mellitus.

KEY TERMS

diabetes mellitus (DM), p. 1287
diabetic ketoacidosis (DKA), p. 1311
diabetic nephropathy, p. 1318
diabetic neuropathy, p. 1318
glycemic index (GI), p. 1302
hyperosmolar hyperglycemic state (HHS), p. 1313
insulin resistance, p. 1290
lipodystrophy, p. 1298
prediabetes, p. 1290
Somogyi effect, p. 1298

DIABETES MELLITUS

Diabetes mellitus (DM) is a multisystem disease related to abnormal insulin production, impaired insulin utilization, or both. DM is a serious health problem throughout the world. According to the World Health Organization (WHO), 347 million people have DM (WHO, 2015). By 2030, this figure is expected to top 366 million. Canadian data indicate that the estimated prevalence of diagnosed DM in adults is 9.3% (~3.4 million people) (Canadian Diabetes Association [CDA], 2015).

Approximately 65% to 80% of people with DM will die as a result of heart disease or stroke (Poirier, Dufour, Carpentier, et al., 2013). DM is a contributing factor in the deaths of approximately 41 500 Canadians each year. Canadian adults with DM are twice as likely as people without DM to die prematurely. For example, a 35-year-old Canadian with DM is four times more likely to die at that age than a 35-year-old without DM. Life expectancy for people with type 2 DM may be shortened by 5 to 10 years (Stone, Fitchett, Grover, et al., 2013). The financial burden of DM and its complications on people with the disease and on the Canadian health care system is enormous. A person with DM incurs medical costs that are two to three times higher than those of a person without DM. A person with DM can face direct costs for medication and supplies ranging from $1 000 to $15 000 per year. DM and its complications cost the Canadian health care system an estimated $11.7 billion in 2010 and this figure will rise to $16 billion by 2020 (CDA and Diabetes Quebec [DQ], 2011).

Approximately 10% of people with DM have type 1 DM. However, the number of people with type 2 DM is increasing dramatically owing to a number of factors—in the Western

DETERMINANTS OF HEALTH

Diabetes

Income and Social Status
- Low income and food insecurity appear to be associated with a higher prevalence of diabetes and diabetes-related complications.*

Biology and Genetics
- Indigenous people are among the highest risk populations for developing diabetes in Canada.†
- Almost 80% of new Canadians come from populations at high risk for developing type 2 DM (e.g., people of Latin American, Asian, South Asian, or African descent).‡

Personal Health Practices and Coping Skills
- Progression to type 2 DM can be prevented or delayed through lifestyle modifications such as weight loss and weight control, consuming a healthy diet, and exercising.¶
- Electronic mobile devices can be used to deliver educational and motivational text messages about lifestyle modification.¶

References

*Silverman, J., Krieger, J., Kiefer, M., et al. (2015). The relationship between food insecurity and depression, diabetes distress and medication adherence among low-income patients with poorly-controlled diabetes. *Journal of general internal medicine, 30*(10), 1476–1480.

†Harris, S. B., Bhattacharyya, O., Dyck, R., et al. (2013). Type 2 diabetes in Aboriginal peoples. *Canadian Journal of Diabetes, 37*(Suppl 1), S191–S196.

‡Canadian Diabetes Association (CDA). (2009). The prevalence and costs of diabetes facts. Retrieved from *http://www.diabetes.ca/documents/about-diabetes/PrevalanceandCost_09.pdf*.

¶Ramachandran, A., Snehalatha, C., Ram, J., et al. (2013). Effectiveness of mobile phone messaging in prevention of type 2 diabetes by lifestyle modification in men in India: A prospective, parallel-group, randomised controlled trial. *The Lancet Diabetes & Endocrinology, 1*(3), 191–198.

FIGURE 52-1 Normal endogenous insulin secretion. In the first hour or two after meals, insulin concentrations rise rapidly in blood and peak at about 1 hour. After meals, insulin concentrations promptly decline toward preprandial values as carbohydrate absorption from the gastro-intestinal tract declines. After carbohydrate absorption from the gastro-intestinal tract is complete and during the night, insulin concentrations are low and fairly constant, with a slight increase at dawn.

world, people are living longer, obesity rates are rising, and lifestyles are becoming increasingly sedentary. There is increased immigration from high-risk populations, with 77% of Canadians coming from populations that are at higher risk for type 2 DM. These populations include people of Latin American, Asian, South Asian, and African descent (CDA and DQ, 2011) (see Determinants of Health box). Risk levels for these groups are between two and six times higher than for White Canadians.

There are three recognized groups of Indigenous people in Canada: First Nations, Inuit, and Métis. These populations are three to five times more likely than the general population to develop type 2 DM (CDA, 2013a). An estimated 25% of individuals in First Nations communities on reserves who are over age 45 have DM. According to the CDA Clinical Practice Guidelines Expert Committee (CDA, 2013a), the prevalence of type 2 DM in Canadian Indigenous children 5 to 18 years of age is noted to be as high as 1%, with the highest in the Plains Cree people of Central Canada. Screening every 2 years should also be considered from age 10 or established puberty in Indigenous children with more than one additional risk factor (CDA, 2013a).

DM is a serious problem for the Métis, more frequently affecting women, older adults, people who are obese, and those with lower levels of education. The disease has a negative impact on quality of life and is associated with significant comorbidities in this population (Shah, Cauch-Dudek, & Pigeau, 2011; Martens et al., 2011). It has been documented that Indigenous communities in Canada experience prevalence rates of DM that are among the highest in the world (CDA and DQ, 2011). Comparing First

Nations with non–First Nations people in Manitoba, it was found that rates of DM and diabetes-related lower-limb amputations were higher (Martens, Barlett, Prior, et al., 2011).

Etiology and Pathophysiology

Current theories link the causes of DM, singly or in combination, to genetic, autoimmune, viral, and environmental factors (e.g., obesity, sedentary lifestyle, stress). Regardless of its cause, DM is primarily a disorder of glucose metabolism related to absent or insufficient insulin supply or poor utilization of the insulin that is available.

Although the *CDA 2013 Clinical Practice Guidelines* recognize 11 different classifications of the disease, most of these types are rarely encountered in routine nursing practice (CDA, 2013a). The two most common types of DM are classified as type 1 and type 2 DM (Table 52-1). Gestational diabetes mellitus (GDM), prediabetes, and secondary DM (discussed later in this chapter) are other classifications of DM commonly seen in clinical practice.

Normal Insulin Metabolism. Insulin is a hormone produced by the beta cells in the islets of Langerhans of the pancreas. Under normal conditions, insulin is continuously released into the bloodstream in small pulsatile increments (a basal rate), with increased release (bolus) when food is ingested (Figure 52-1). The activity of released insulin lowers blood glucose and facilitates a stable, normal glucose range of approximately 4 to 6 mmol/L. The average amount of insulin secreted daily by an adult is approximately 40 to 50 units, or 0.6 units/kg of body weight.

Other hormones (glucagon, epinephrine, growth hormone, and cortisol) work to oppose the effects of insulin and are often referred to as *counter-regulatory hormones*. These hormones work to increase blood glucose levels by stimulating glucose production and output by the liver and by decreasing the movement of glucose into the cells. Insulin and these counter-regulatory hormones provide a sustained but regulated release of glucose for energy during food intake and periods of fasting and usually maintain blood glucose levels within the normal range. An abnormal production of any or all of these hormones may be present in DM.

Insulin is released from the pancreatic beta cells as its precursor, proinsulin, and is then routed through the liver. Proinsulin is composed of two polypeptide chains, chain A and chain B, which are linked by the C-peptide chain. Insulin is formed when enzymes

TABLE 52-1 CHARACTERISTICS OF TYPE 1 AND TYPE 2 DIABETES MELLITUS

Factor	Type 1 Diabetes Mellitus	Type 2 Diabetes Mellitus	Factor	Type 1 Diabetes Mellitus	Type 2 Diabetes Mellitus
Age at onset	More common in young people but can occur at any age	Usually ≥35 yr but can occur at any age; Incidence is increasing in children	Endogenous insulin	Minimal or absent	Possibly excessive; adequate but delayed secretion or reduced utilization; secretions diminish over time
Type of onset	Signs and symptoms abrupt, but disease process may be present for several years	Insidious; may go undiagnosed for years	Nutritional status	Thin, normal, or obese	Obese or normal
			Symptoms	Thirst, polyuria, polyphagia, fatigue, weight loss	Frequently none, fatigue, recurrent infections
Prevalence	Accounts for 5%–10% of all types of diabetes	Accounts for 90% of all types of diabetes	Ketosis	Prone at onset or during insulin deficiency	Resistant except during infection or stress
Environmental factors	Viruses, toxins	Obesity, lack of exercise			
Primary defect	Absent or minimal insulin production due to an autoimmune process	Insulin resistance, decreased insulin production over time, and alterations in production of adipokines	Nutritional therapy	Essential	Essential
			Insulin	Required for all	Required for some
			Oral antihyperglycemic agents	Not indicated	Usually beneficial
			Vascular and neurological complications	Frequent	Frequent
Islet-cell antibodies	Often present at onset	Absent			

cleave C off, leaving the A and B chains. The presence of C peptide in serum is a useful indicator of beta-cell function.

Insulin facilitates glucose transport from the bloodstream across the cell membrane to the cytoplasm of the cell. The rise in plasma insulin after a meal stimulates storage of glucose as glycogen in liver and muscle, inhibits gluconeogenesis, enhances fat deposition in adipose tissue, and increases protein synthesis. The fall in insulin level during normal overnight fasting facilitates the release of stored glucose from the liver, protein from muscle, and fat from adipose tissue. For this reason, insulin is known as the *anabolic* or *storage hormone*.

Skeletal muscle and adipose tissue have specific receptors for insulin and are considered insulin-dependent tissues. Other tissues (e.g., brain, liver, blood cells) do not directly depend on insulin for glucose transport but require an adequate glucose supply for normal function. Although liver cells are not considered insulin-dependent tissue, insulin receptor sites on the liver facilitate the hepatic uptake of glucose and its conversion to glycogen.

Type 1 Diabetes Mellitus. Formerly known as "juvenile-onset" or "insulin-dependent" DM, *type 1 DM* most often occurs in people who are younger than 30 years, with a peak onset between ages 11 and 13. The rate of type 1 DM in children is highest in Europe (Finland and Sweden) (International Diabetes Federation [IDF], 2015). Most cases of type 1 DM are sporadic; only 10% to 15% of affected individuals have a first-degree relative with type 1 DM at the time of diagnosis. Typically, it is seen in people with a lean body type, although it can occur in people who are overweight. This form includes *latent autoimmune diabetes mellitus in adults* (LADA); the term is used to describe the small number of people with apparent type 2 DM who appear to have immune-mediated loss of pancreatic beta cells (CDA, 2013a).

Etiology and Pathophysiology. Type 1 DM results from progressive destruction of pancreatic beta cells owing to an autoimmune process in susceptible individuals. Autoantibodies to the islet cells cause a reduction of 80% to 90% of normal beta-cell function before hyperglycemia and other manifestations occur (Figure 52-2). A genetic predisposition and exposure to a virus are factors that may contribute to the pathogenesis of type 1

DM. Occasionally, type 1 DM may be caused by nonimmune factors of unknown (idiopathic) etiologies. This type of DM is known as *type 1B DM*. When type 1 DM is caused by an immune mechanism, the disease is known as *type 1A*.

Predisposition to type 1 DM is believed to be related to human leukocyte antigens (HLAs) (see Chapter 16 for a discussion of HLAs and disease associations). Theoretically, when an individual with certain HLA types is exposed to viral infections, the beta cells of the pancreas are destroyed, either directly or through an autoimmune process. The HLA types associated with an increased risk for type 1 DM include HLA-DR3 and HLA-DR4 (see the Genetics in Clinical Practice box, Types 1 and 2 Diabetes Mellitus).

Onset of Disease. Type 1 DM is associated with a long preclinical period. The islet-cell autoantibodies responsible for beta-cell destruction are present for months to years before the onset of symptoms. Manifestations of type 1 DM develop when the person's pancreas can no longer produce insulin. Once this occurs, the onset of symptoms is usually rapid, and the patient comes to the emergency department with impending or actual ketoacidosis. The patient usually has a history of recent and sudden weight loss as well as the classic symptoms of *polydipsia* (excessive thirst), *polyuria* (frequent urination), and *polyphagia* (excessive hunger).

The individual with type 1 DM requires a supply of insulin from an outside source (*exogenous insulin*), such as an injection, in order to sustain life. Without insulin, the patient will develop diabetic ketoacidosis (DKA), a life-threatening condition resulting in metabolic acidosis that, if untreated, could be fatal. Newly diagnosed patients with type 1 DM may experience a remission, or "honeymoon period," soon after treatment is initiated. During this time, the patient requires very little injected insulin because beta-cell mass remains sufficient for glucose control as the progressive destruction continues to occur. Eventually, as more beta cells are destroyed, blood glucose levels increase, more insulin is needed, and the honeymoon period ends. It is critical for the patient to monitor blood glucose very closely during this period. The honeymoon period usually lasts 3 to 12 months, after which the person will require insulin on a permanent basis.

Type 1 Diabetes Mellitus

Pancreas

- Autoimmune destruction of beta cells
- Autoantibodies present for months to years before clinical symptoms
- Insufficient production of insulin

Type 2 Diabetes Mellitus

Pancreas

- Defective beta cell secretion of insulin
- Insulin resistance stimulates ↑ insulin secretion
- Eventual exhaustion of beta cells in many people
- ↑ Glucagon secretion

Liver

- Excess glucose production
- Inappropriate regulation of glucose production

Adipose tissue

- ↓ Adiponectin and ↑ leptin
- Results in altered glucose and fat metabolism

Muscle

- Defective insulin receptors
- Insulin resistance
- Decreased uptake of glucose by cells resulting in hyperglycemia

FIGURE 52-2 Altered mechanisms in type 1 and type 2 diabetes mellitus.

Prediabetes. Prediabetes, also known as *impaired glucose tolerance* (IGT) or *impaired fasting glucose* (IFG), is noted when a fasting or a 2-hour plasma glucose level is higher than normal (6.1–6.9 mmol/L for IFG and 7.1–11 mmol/L for IGT) but lower than that considered diagnostic for DM. Up to 6 million Canadians have prediabetes, putting them at risk of developing DM and its complications, particularly cardiovascular disease. About 50% of Canadians with prediabetes develop type 2 DM in their lifetime (CDA and DQ, 2011).

Long-term damage to the body, especially the heart and blood vessels, may already be occurring in patients with prediabetes. People with prediabetes usually do not have symptoms. Individuals with prediabetes should have their blood glucose and A$_{1c}$ tested regularly and should watch for the symptoms of DM, such as polyuria, polyphagia, or polydipsia. If action is taken to manage blood glucose, patients with prediabetes can delay or prevent the development of type 2 DM. Maintaining a healthy weight, exercising regularly, eating a healthy diet, and using medication when required are measures found to reduce the risk of developing DM in people with prediabetes by almost 60% (CDA, 2013a).

Type 2 Diabetes Mellitus. Type 2 DM is, by far, the most prevalent type of DM, accounting for over 90% of patients with DM. Type 2 DM usually occurs in people older than 35 years, and 80% to 90% of patients are overweight at the time of diagnosis.

The most powerful risk factor is believed to be obesity, specifically abdominal and visceral adiposity. Visceral adipocytes release an excess amount of free fatty acids, which are associated with insulin resistance at the level of the liver, as well as several adipocytokines, which cause insulin resistance in the muscle (Neeland, Turer, Ayers, et al., 2012). Obesity has a tendency to run in families and probably has a genetic basis (see the Genetics in Clinical Practice box, Types 1 and 2 Diabetes Mellitus).

Other risk factors for type 2 DM are membership in a high-risk population (e.g., people of Indigenous, Latin American, South Asian, Asian, or African descent), history of IGT or IFG, presence of complications associated with DM, vascular disease, history of GDM, and history of delivery of an infant with macrosomia. Hypertension, dyslipidemia, being overweight, abdominal obesity, polycystic ovary syndrome (PCOS), and acanthosis nigricans are associated with insulin resistance and are also risk factors for type 2 DM. Insulin resistance with compensatory hyperinsulinemia is a common feature of PCOS, in both lean and obese women. The exact mechanisms for abnormalities of insulin action in PCOS are not fully understood (Rojas, Chavez, Olivar, et al., 2014). Acanthosis nigricans is a cutaneous sign of an underlying condition and is characterized by a velvety, light brown to black hyperpigmented thickening of the skin, usually on the back, the sides of the neck, the axillae, and flexural surfaces (Atwa, Emaraz, Balata, et al., 2014). The pathways that lead to acanthosis nigricans are not well known. However, the association of acanthosis nigricans with disorders such as DM characterized by insulin resistance suggests that hyperinsulinemia plays a key role in the development of acanthosis nigricans (Atwa et al., 2014). The incidence of type 2 DM is at least three times higher in people with schizophrenia than in the general population and is thought to be related to antipsychotic medications (CDA, 2013a; Moisan, Turgeon, Desjardins, et al., 2013) These medications have contributed to the prevalence of obesity in patients with schizophrenia, which is a known risk factor for insulin resistance and type 2 DM.

Prevalence of type 2 DM increases with age, with about half of the people diagnosed being older than 55. In the past, type 2 DM was known as "adult-onset" DM. This term is no longer considered appropriate because the disease is now being seen in a rapidly growing number of children and adolescents, particularly in the Indigenous population. In a large study, people at risk for type 2 DM were able to cut that risk by 58% by exercising moderately for 30 minutes a day and by losing 5% to 7% of their body weight (CDA, 2013a). Other large studies have shown similar results in reducing risk.

Etiology and Pathophysiology. In type 2 DM, the pancreas usually continues to produce some *endogenous* (self-made) insulin. However, the insulin that is produced is either insufficient for the needs of the body, poorly utilized by the tissues, or both. In contrast, there is a virtual absence of endogenous insulin in type 1 DM. The presence of endogenous insulin is the major pathophysiological distinction between type 1 and type 2 DM.

Genetic mutations that lead to insulin resistance and a higher risk for obesity have been found in many people with type 2 DM. It is likely that multiple genes are involved in this complex, multifactorial disorder (see the Genetics in Clinical Practice box).

Four major metabolic abnormalities have a role in the development of type 2 DM. The first factor is insulin resistance in glucose and lipid metabolism, which is a condition in which body tissues do not respond to the action of insulin. This lack of response is owing to insulin receptors that are unresponsive to the action of insulin, insufficient in number, or both. Most

GENETICS IN CLINICAL PRACTICE

Types 1 and 2 Diabetes Mellitus

	Type 1 Diabetes Mellitus	Type 2 Diabetes Mellitus	Maturity-Onset Diabetes of the Young (MODY)
Genetic basis	Associations between specific human leukocyte antigens (HLA-DR3, HLA-DR4)	Majority of cases are polygenic	Autosomal dominant, monogenic (single gene)
	As many as 40 genes (and maybe more) influence susceptibility	As many as 25 genes influence susceptibility	Caused by mutations in any of the MODY genes (types 1–11)
Incidence	Accounts for about 5%–10% of cases in Canada	Accounts for about 90% of cases in Canada	Accounts for 1%–5% of people with diabetes
Risk to offspring and twins	Risk to offspring of mothers with diabetes is only 1%–4% Risk to offspring of diabetic fathers is 5%–6%	Risk to offspring is 8%–14%	If one parent has MODY, the offspring has a 50% chance of developing the disease If one parent has MODY, the offspring has a 50% chance of being a carrier
	Identical twin concordance is 30%–40%	Identical twin concordance often exceeds 60%–75%	
Clinical implications	Disease is a result of complex interaction of genetic, autoimmune, and environmental factors	Disease is a result of complex genetic interactions, which are modified by environmental factors such as body weight and exercise	Characterized by young age of onset (often before 25), not associated with obesity or hypertension

insulin receptors are located on skeletal muscle, fat, and liver cells. Insulin mediates glucose uptake into fat tissue and skeletal muscle through GLUT4 glucose transporters. Insulin resistance in fat cells is associated with a decrease in the number of GLUT4 transporters and altered activity in individuals with type 2 DM (Ismail-Beigi, 2012). When insulin is not properly used, the entry of glucose into the cell is impeded, resulting in hyperglycemia. In the early stages of insulin resistance, the pancreas responds to high blood glucose by producing greater amounts of insulin (if beta-cell function is normal). This creates a temporary state of hyperinsulinemia that coexists with the hyperglycemia.

A second factor in the development of type 2 DM is a marked decrease in the ability of the pancreas to produce insulin, as the beta cells become fatigued from the compensatory overproduction of insulin or when beta-cell mass is lost. The resulting IFG and IGT place the individual at risk of developing DM and its complications. This does not necessarily mean that all people with prediabetes will progress to DM. A significant proportion will revert to normal blood glucose levels (CDA, 2013a). The underlying basis for the failure of beta cells to adapt is unknown. However, it may be linked to the adverse effects of chronic hyperglycemia or high circulating free fatty acids.

A third factor is inappropriate glucose production by the liver. Instead of properly regulating the release of glucose in response to blood levels, the liver does so in a haphazard way that does not correspond to the body's needs at the time. Furthermore, there is increased secretion of glucagon from the alpha cells of the pancreas that stimulates glucose production by the liver, adding to the increase in blood sugar. However, this is not considered a primary factor in the development of type 2 DM.

A fourth factor is alteration in the production of hormones and cytokines by adipose tissue (adipocytokines). Adipocytokines appear to play a role in glucose and fat metabolism and are likely to contribute to the pathophysiology of type 2 DM. The two main adipocytokines believed to affect insulin sensitivity are adiponectin and leptin. Others include tumour necrosis factor α (TNF-α), interleukin-6 (IL-6), and resistin. The role of resistin in the pathogenesis of obesity-mediated insulin resistance and type 2 DM, however, remains controversial (Beckers, De Freitas, Zegers, et al., 2011). Figure 52-2 depicts the altered mechanisms in type 1 and type 2 DM.

Metabolic syndrome (also known as *insulin resistance syndrome*) is a cluster of abnormalities that act synergistically to greatly increase the risk for cardiovascular disease. Metabolic syndrome is characterized by abdominal obesity, hypertension, dyslipidemia, insulin resistance, and dysglycemia. Patients with metabolic syndrome are at significant risk of developing DM and cardiovascular disease (CDA, 2013a). Lifestyle interventions have been shown to be highly effective in delaying or preventing the onset of DM in people with IGT. Risk factors for metabolic syndrome include, but are not limited to, abdominal obesity, sedentary lifestyle, urbanization and Westernization, and being Indigenous or of Latin American or African descent. Overweight individuals with metabolic syndrome can prevent or delay the onset of DM through a program of weight loss and regular physical activity. (Metabolic syndrome is discussed in further detail in Chapter 43.)

Onset of Disease. Disease onset in type 2 DM is usually gradual. The person may go for many years with undetected hyperglycemia that might produce few, if any, symptoms. Many people are diagnosed on routine laboratory testing. If the patient with type 2 DM has marked hyperglycemia (e.g., 28–55 mmol/L), a sufficient endogenous insulin supply may prevent DKA from occurring. However, osmotic fluid and electrolyte loss related to hyperglycemia may become severe and lead to hyperosmolar hyperglycemic state. (Complications of DM are discussed later in this chapter.)

Gestational Diabetes. Gestational diabetes mellitus (GDM) develops during pregnancy. In Canada, it occurs in about 3% of pregnancies in the non-Indigenous population (CDA, 2013a), and the rates are two to three times higher in Indigenous populations (CDA, 2013a). It is detected between 24 and 28 weeks of gestation, using a sequential screening method with a 50-g oral glucose challenge test, followed by a 75-g oral glucose tolerance test (OGGT). Women with multiple risk factors should be offered screening at any time during pregnancy (CDA, 2013a). Treatment of GDM reduces perinatal death and neonatal complications such as birth trauma, hypoglycemia, hyperbilirubinemia, and respiratory distress syndrome (CDA, 2013a). Nutritional counselling is considered to be the first-line therapy. Physical activity should be encouraged as tolerated. If nutritional counselling alone does not achieve target fasting, or postprandial blood glucose levels, or both, insulin therapy is usually indicated. Approximately 10% of patients progress to DM soon after pregnancy. Although most women with GDM will have normal glucose levels within 6 weeks postpartum, their risk of developing type 2 DM in 5 to 10 years is increased. Women should be screened postpartum to determine their glucose status. The 2013 CDA guidelines recommend a 75-g OGTT be done between 6 weeks and 6 months postpartum. Education on lifestyle modifications to prevent DM should continue postpartum. GDM and management of the pregnant patient with DM is a specialized area not covered in detail in this chapter. The reader is advised to consult a DM and obstetrics text for information about this subject.

Secondary Diabetes. In some people, DM occurs because of another medical condition or as a result of the treatment of a medical condition that causes abnormal blood glucose levels. Conditions that may cause secondary DM include schizophrenia, cystic fibrosis, Cushing's syndrome, hyperthyroidism, immunosuppressive therapy, and the use of parenteral nutrition. Commonly used medications that can induce DM in some people include corticosteroids (prednisone), phenytoin (Dilantin), and atypical antipsychotics (e.g., clozapine [Clozaril]). Secondary DM may resolve when the underlying condition is treated or the medication is discontinued.

Clinical Manifestations

Type 1 Diabetes Mellitus. Because the onset of type 1 DM is rapid, the initial manifestations are usually acute. The classic symptoms are *polyuria* (frequent urination), *polydipsia* (excessive thirst), and *polyphagia* (excessive hunger). The osmotic effect of glucose produces the manifestations of polydipsia and polyuria. Polyphagia is a consequence of cellular malnourishment when insulin deficiency prevents utilization of glucose for energy. Weight loss may occur because the body cannot get glucose and turns to other energy sources, such as fat and protein. Weakness and fatigue may also be experienced, because body cells lack needed energy from glucose. There may be pronounced changes in visual acuity owing to changes in the lens with hyperglycemia and fluid retention. Women may have vaginal yeast infections. Ketoacidosis, a complication associated with untreated type 1 DM, is associated with additional clinical manifestations that are discussed later in this chapter.

Type 2 Diabetes Mellitus. The clinical manifestations of type 2 DM are often nonspecific, although it is possible that an individual with type 2 DM will experience some of the classic symptoms associated with type 1. Some of the more common manifestations associated with type 2 DM include fatigue, recurrent infections, prolonged wound healing, visual acuity changes, and painful peripheral neuropathy in the feet. Unfortunately, the clinical manifestations appear so gradually that, before the person knows it, he or she may have complications.

Complications

Complications of DM are discussed in detail later in this chapter.

Diagnostic Studies. The 2013 CDA guidelines recommend any one of the following four methods and their criteria for the

diagnosis of DM and a repeat confirmatory test on another day in the absence of symptomatic hyperglycemia:

1. Glycated hemoglobin (A_{1c}) ≥6.5% (in adults), using a standardized, validated assay, in the absence of conditions that affect the accuracy of the A_{1c} and not for suspected type 1 DM or
2. Fasting blood glucose (FBG) level ≥7.0 mmol/L. (*Fasting* is defined as no caloric intake for at least 8 hours.) or
3. Random plasma glucose (RPG) measurement ≥11.1 mmol/L. (*Random* is defined as any time of day without regard to the interval since the last meal.) or
4. Two-hour plasma glucose (PG) level in a 75 g OGTT ≥11.1 mmol/L

It is preferable that the same test be repeated for confirmation, but an RPG level in an asymptomatic individual should be confirmed with any of the other tests (A_{1c}, FBG, or 2-hr PG in 75-g OGTT). When overt symptoms of hyperglycemia (polyuria, polydipsia, and polyphagia) are present, the diagnosis has been made and a confirmatory test is not required before treatment is initiated.

IFG, IGT, or A_{1c} of 6.0% to 6.4% each represent an intermediate stage between normal glucose homeostasis and DM. The stage is called *prediabetes* (see discussion on prediabetes earlier in this chapter). When the FBG level is 6.1 to 6.9 mmol/L, the individual is considered to have IFG. IGT is classified when a 2-hour PG in a 75-g OGTT level is 7.8 to 11.0 mmol/L (CDA, 2013a). The combination of IFG and an A_{1c} of 6.0% to 6.4% is predictive of 100% progression to type 2 DM over a 5-year period.

Measurement of glycated hemoglobin, also known as the *A_{1c} test,* is not only used for diagnosing diabetes but is also useful in determining glycemic control over time. The test works by showing the amount of glucose that has been attached to hemoglobin molecules, which are attached to the red blood cell (RBC) for the life of the cell (~120 days). Therefore, an A_{1c} test indicates the overall glucose control for the previous 90 to 120 days. All patients with DM should have regular assessments of A_{1c} every 3 to 6 months. Major studies have demonstrated that people with DM who can maintain near-normal A_{1c} levels over time have a greatly reduced risk for the development of retinopathy, nephropathy, and neuropathy. For most people with DM, the ideal A_{1c} goal is 7% or less. Normal range is 6% or less. A target A_{1c} of less than 6.5% can be considered in some patients with type 2 DM to further lower the risk for nephropathy but must be balanced against the risk for hypoglycemia and increased mortality in those at an elevated risk for cardiovascular disease (CDA, 2013a). Diseases affecting RBCs (e.g., sickle cell anemia, thalassemia trait) or recent blood transfusions can affect the A_{1c} results and should be taken into consideration in the interpretation of this test result. It is important to know where an individual is on the glucose continuum (Figure 52-3).

Collaborative Care

The goals of DM management are to promote well-being, reduce symptoms, prevent acute complications of hyperglycemia and hypoglycemia, and delay the onset and progression of long-term complications. These goals are most likely to be met when patients are able to maintain blood glucose levels as near to normal as possible. Patient teaching, which enables patients to become the most active participants in their own care, is essential for a successful treatment plan. Nutritional therapy, exercise, self-monitoring of blood glucose, and drug therapy are the tools used in the management of DM (Table 52-2). All individuals

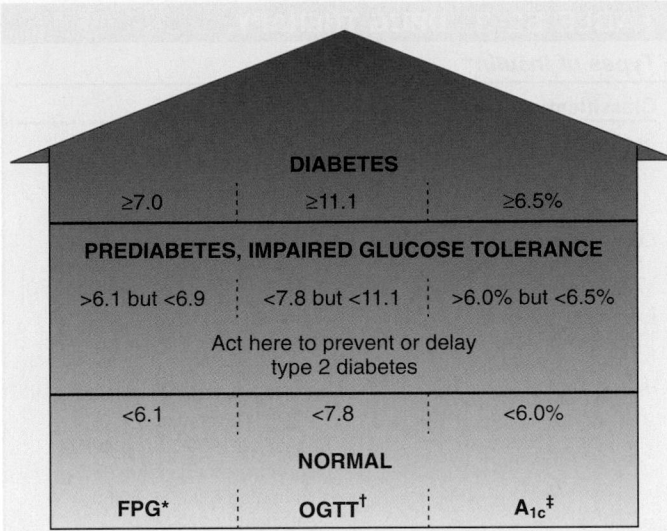

FIGURE 52-3 The glucose continuum. Numbers represent blood glucose levels in millimoles per litre (mmol/L).

*The fasting plasma glucose (FPG) test: After an overnight fast, blood glucose is measured in the morning.

†The 2-hour oral glucose tolerance test (OGTT): Includes a fasting blood glucose test and glucose measurements 2 hours after drinking a glucose-containing solution.

‡The glycated hemoglobin (A_{1c}) is a 2 to 3 month average blood glucose test that can be done at any time of the day.

Note: The Diabetes Canada believes that either test is appropriate to measure prediabetes (impaired glucose tolerance) and diabetes.

---

with type 1 DM require insulin from the time of diagnosis. For some people with type 2 DM, lifestyle modifications, including healthy eating, regular physical activity, and maintenance of desirable body weight will be sufficient to attain an optimal level of blood glucose control. For the majority, however, drug therapy with oral antihyperglycemic agents (OHAs), noninsulin injectable agents, or insulin, will be necessary.

Drug Therapy: Insulin

Exogenous (injected) insulin is needed when a patient has inadequate insulin to meet specific metabolic needs and a satisfactory blood glucose level cannot be maintained through the combination of nutritional therapy, exercise, and OHAs and noninsulin injectable agents. Exogenous insulin is always required for the management of type 1 DM. Individuals with type 2 DM may be treated with insulin alone or with insulin in combination with OHAs (CDA, 2013a). Insulin requirement may increase significantly during periods of severe stress, such as illness or surgery.

Types of Insulin. In Canada, beef insulin was withdrawn in 1999 but can still be bought from international sources. Human biosynthetic insulin is now the most widely used insulin. Human insulin is derived from common bacteria (e.g., *Escherichia coli*) or yeast cells using recombinant DNA technology. Insulin analogues are made by modifying the amino acid sequence of the insulin molecule (Cheng, 2011). Insulins differ in regard to onset, peak action, and duration (Figure 52-4). The specific properties and different combinations of these insulins can be used to tailor treatment to the patient's specific patterns of blood glucose levels, lifestyle, eating, and activity. Different types of insulin are listed in Table 52-3. Most insulin preparations start

TABLE 52-2 COLLABORATIVE CARE

Diabetes Mellitus

Diagnostic
- History and physical examination
- Blood pressure
- Blood tests: including FBG, postprandial blood glucose, glycated hemoglobin (A_{1c}), fasting lipid profile, serum creatinine, electrolytes, calculation of creatinine clearance, TSH
- Dental examination
- Doppler scan—ankle-brachial index (if indicated)
- ECG (if indicated)
- Foot (podiatric) examination
- Fundoscopic examination—dilated eye examination
- Monitoring of weight
- Neurological examination, including monofilament test for sensation to lower extremities
- Random urine for microalbuminuria (MAU), complete urinalysis, and acetone if indicated

Collaborative Therapy
- Oral antihyperglycemic agents and noninsulin injectable agents (see Table 52-7)
- Angiotensin-converting enzyme (ACE) inhibitors or angiotensin II receptor blockers (ARBs) (high risk for a cardiovascular event) (see Chapter 35, Table 35-8)
- Blood pressure control
  - Target <130/80 mm Hg
- Drug therapy
  - Enteric-coated acetylsalicylic acid (ASA; Aspirin) (80 mg or 325 mg)
  - Insulin (see Figure 52-4 and Tables 52-3 and 52-4)
  - Lipid-lowering therapy (high risk for a cardiovascular event) (see Chapter 36, Table 36-5)
- Exercise therapy (see Tables 52-9 and 52-10)
- Nutritional therapy (see Table 52-8)
- Patient and caregiver teaching and follow-up programs
- Self-monitoring of blood glucose (SMBG)
- Vascular protection

ECG, electrocardiogram; *FBG,* fasting blood glucose; *TSH,* thyroid-stimulating hormone.
Source: Canadian Diabetes Association (CDA) Clinical Practice Guidelines Expert Committee. (2013). Clinical practice guidelines for the prevention and management of diabetes in Canada. *Canadian Journal of Diabetes, 37*(Suppl 1), S197–S198.

---

with regular insulin as a base. By adding zinc, acetate buffers, and protamine to insulin in various ways, the onset of activity, peak, and duration times can be manipulated. Zinc and protamine are added to make NPH (neutral protamine Hagedorn). In rare instances, these additives may cause an allergic reaction at the injection site. Switching the brand or the type of insulin may alleviate this localized reaction.

Health care providers should refer to the most current edition of *Compendium of Pharmaceuticals and Specialties* (Canadian Pharmacists Association, Ottawa, Ontario, Canada) and product monographs for detailed information.

Insulin Regimens. Examples of insulin regimens ranging from one to four injections per day are presented in Table 52-4. The exogenous insulin regimen that most closely mimics endogenous insulin production is the basal–bolus regimen, which uses rapid- or short-acting (bolus) insulin before meals and intermediate- or long-acting (basal) background insulin once or twice a day. The basal–bolus regimen is *intensive insulin therapy,* which consists of multiple daily insulin (MDI). The goal is to achieve a near-normal glucose level of 4 to 7 mmol/L before meals, or 4 to 6 mmol/L if this can be reached safely without severe hypoglycemia. The Diabetes Control and Complications Trial (DCCT) Research

Rapid-acting: lispro, lispro U200, aspart

Onset: 10–15 minutes
Peak: 60–90 minutes
Duration: 3–5 hours

Short-acting: regular

Onset: ½–1 hour
Peak: 2–4 hours
Duration: 5–8 hours

Intermediate-acting: NPH

Onset: 1–3 hours
Peak: 6–8 hours
Duration: 12–16 hours

Extended long-acting: insulin glargine (Lantus), insulin detemir (Levemir)

Onset: 1–2 hours
Peak: no pronounced peak
Duration: 24+ hours

FIGURE 52-4 Commercially available insulin preparations showing onset, peak, and duration of action of relative plasma insulin level. *NPH*, neutral protamine Hagedorn.

TABLE 52-3 DRUG THERAPY

Types of Insulin*

Classification	Examples
Rapid-acting analogue (clear)	Lispro (Humalog)
	Lispro U200 (Humalog)
	Aspart (NovoRapid)
	Glulisine (Apidra)
Short-acting (clear)	Regular (Novolin ge Toronto, Humulin R)
Intermediate-acting (cloudy)	NPH (Humulin N, Novolin ge NPH)
Extended long-acting analogue (clear)	Glargine (Lantus)
	Glargine U300 (Toujeo)
	Detemir (Levemir)
Premixed (cloudy)	Regular/NPH 30/70† (Humulin 30/70, Novolin ge 30/70)
	Regular/NPH 50/50 and 40/60
	Lispro/lispro protamine 25/75 (Humalog Mix 25); 50/50 (Humalog Mix 50)
	Aspart/aspart protamine 30/70 (NovoMix 30)

NPH, neutral protamine Hagedorn.
*Insulin preparations are clear solutions except for NPH and protamine-containing insulin, which are cloudy.
†These numbers refer to percentages of each type of insulin.

have an onset of action of approximately 10 to 15 minutes (as compared with 30 to 60 minutes for regular insulin). Rapid-acting insulin is considered to be the type that best mimics natural insulin secretion in response to a meal. It should be administered 0 to 15 minutes before meals and can be given up to 15 minutes after meals. However, preprandial administration achieves better postprandial glycemic control. When rapid-acting insulin is used as mealtime coverage in people with type 1 DM, an additional and longer-acting insulin must also be used as basal background insulin because the duration of rapid-acting insulin is so short. Other benefits of rapid-acting insulin include decreased postmeal hyperglycemia, decreased hypoglycemic episodes, and increased flexibility compared with regular insulin (CDA, 2013a). Regular insulin is also a mealtime insulin and has an onset of action of 30 to 60 minutes; it should be injected 30 to 45 minutes before a meal to ensure that the onset of action coincides with meal absorption. Because timing an injection 30 to 45 minutes before a meal is difficult for people to incorporate into their lifestyles, the rapid-acting insulins are often preferred by people who take insulin with meals (CDA, 2013a).

Long- or Intermediate-Acting (Basal) Background Insulin. Insulin glargine (Lantus) and detemir (Levemir) are extended long-acting basal insulins that are released steadily and continuously over 24 hours. The duration of insulin glargine U300 (Toujeo) is up to 30 hours. These long-acting insulins do not have a peak of action (see Figure 52-4). They may be used for once-daily subcutaneous administration at bedtime in patients with type 1 and type 2 DM who require basal (long-acting) insulin for the control of hyperglycemia. Because they lack a peak action time, the risk for hypoglycemia is greatly reduced. They are clear, colourless insulins. The nurse should be aware of the potential danger of confusing glargine, glargine U300, and detemir with other clear insulins (rapid- or short-acting) (Registered Nurses' Association of Ontario [RNAO], 2009). Glargine, glargine U300, and detemir must not be diluted or mixed with any other insulin or solution as this action can change the time or action profile of these long-acting

Group demonstrated that people with type 1 DM who have tight glucose control through intensive management develop fewer and less severe complications (DCCT, 1993). Ideally, regimens should be collaboratively selected by the patient and the health care provider (CDA, 2013a). The criteria for selection are based on the type of DM and the required, desired, and feasible levels of glycemic control, in addition to economic factors and flexibility. Starting a multiple daily injection regimen with 3 to 4 injections per day may be overwhelming for patients. Depending on the patient's glycemic control, introducing a once or twice a day insulin regimen may be more manageable.

Mealtime Insulin (Bolus). Synthetic, rapid-acting insulins include lispro (Humalog), lispro U200 (Canadian Diabetes Association Clinical Practice Guidelines Expert Committee, 2016), aspart insulin (NovoRapid), and glulisine (Apidra). They

TABLE 52-4   DRUG THERAPY

Common Insulin Regimens

Regimen	Type of Insulin/Frequency	Action Profile*	Comments
Once a day Single dose	Intermediate (NPH) at bedtime *Or*	0700 1200 1800 2400 0700	One injection should cover nighttime coverage.
	Long-acting (glargine [Lantus], detemir [Levemir]) *In morning or at bedtime*	0700 1200 1800 2400 0700	One injection will last 24 hr with no peaks and less chance for hypoglycemia. Does not cover postprandial blood sugars.
Twice a day Split-mixed dose	NPH and regular *Or* NPH and rapid *Before breakfast and at dinner*	0700 1200 1800 2400 0700 (I + R) (I + R) (I + H) (I + H)	Two injections provide coverage for 24 hr. Patient must adhere to a set meal plan.
Three times a day Combination of mixed and single dose	NPH and regular *Or* NPH and rapid *Before breakfast* + Regular or rapid *Before dinner* + NPH *At bedtime*	0700 1200 1900 2100 2400 0700 (I + R) (R) (I) (I + H) (H)	Three injections provide coverage for 24 hr, particularly during early a.m. hours. Potential is reduced for hypoglycemia between 0200 and 0300 hours.
Basal-bolus Multiple dose	Regular or rapid *Before breakfast, lunch, and dinner* + NPH *Twice daily or at bedtime* Or	0700 1200 1900 2100 0700 (R) (R) (R) (I) (H) (H) (H)	More flexibility is allowed at mealtimes and for amount of food intake. Good postprandial control. Premeal blood glucose checks and establishing and following individualized algorithms are necessary. Patients with type 1 DM will require basal insulin to cover 24 hr.
Basal-bolus Multiple dose	Regular or rapid *Before breakfast, lunch, and dinner* + Long-acting (glargine or detemir) *Once a day, usually at bedtime*	0700 1200 1800 2400 0700	Four injections required per day. Most physiological approach, except for pump.

NPH, neutral protamine Hagedorn.

*Key:

———————Rapid-acting (lispro, aspart, glulisine) insulin

———————Short-acting (regular) insulin

- - - - - - - - -Intermediate-acting (NPH) or long-acting (glargine, detemir) insulin

---

analogues and cause precipitation (Sanofi-Aventis Canada, 2015; NovoNordisk, 2016b).

Intermediate-acting insulin NPH is also used as a basal insulin that has a duration of 10 to 16 hours. The disadvantage is that it has a peak at 4 to 10 hours, which can result in hypoglycemia. It is the only basal insulin that can be mixed with the short- and rapid-acting insulins. NPH is a cloudy insulin that must be gently agitated before administration (Forum for Injection Technique [FIT] Canada, 2011).

Combination Therapy. Two different insulin types are commonly used in combination to mimic normal endogenous insulin secretion (see Table 52-4). Short- or rapid-acting insulin is often mixed with an intermediate-acting insulin to provide both mealtime and basal coverage without having to administer two separate injections. Patients may mix the two types of insulin themselves or may use a commercially premixed formula (Figure 52-5; see also Table 52-3). It is important to teach patients to draw the clear (short- or rapid-acting) insulin first when mixing to avoid potential contamination with the cloudy (intermediate-acting) insulin. Introducing intermediate insulin into a rapid- or short-acting vial may increase its duration of action. The premixed formulas offer convenience to patients and are especially helpful to those who lack the visual, manual, or cognitive skills to mix insulin themselves. However, the convenience of these formulas

1 Wash hands.
2 Gently rotate NPH insulin bottle.
3 Wipe off tops of insulin vials with alcohol sponge.
4 Draw back amount of air into the syringe that equals total dose.

5 Inject air equal to NPH dose into NPH vial. Remove syringe from vial.

36 units

36 U Air NPH insulin (cloudy)

6 Inject air equal to regular dose into regular vial.

12 units

12 U Air Regular insulin (clear)

7 Invert regular insulin bottle and withdraw regular insulin dose.

Regular insulin (clear)

Regular insulin 12 units

8 Without adding more air to NPH vial, carefully withdraw NPH dose and add to regular insulin already in syringe.

NPH insulin (cloudy)

NPH insulin —
Regular — 36 units
insulin 48 units (total dose)

FIGURE 52-5 Mixing insulins. This stepwise process avoids the problem of contaminating regular insulin with intermediate-acting insulin. *NPH*, neutral protamine Hagedorn.

sacrifices the potential for optimal blood glucose control because there is less opportunity for flexible dosage and administration based on need.

Storage of Insulin. As a protein, insulin requires special storage considerations. Heat and freezing alter the insulin molecule. The insulin vial, cartridge, or disposable insulin pen that the patient is currently using may be left at room temperature for up to 4 weeks, unless the room temperature is higher than 30°C or below freezing (<2°C). Unopened vials, cartridges, and disposable insulin pens must be refrigerated. Prolonged exposure to direct sunlight should be avoided. Nondisposable insulin pens should not be stored in the refrigerator. The same principles apply for a patient who is travelling; insulin can be stored in a thermos or cooler to keep it cool (not frozen) if the patient is travelling in hot climates (RNAO, 2009).

Prefilled syringes containing two types of insulin are stable for up to 1 week when stored in the refrigerator, whereas syringes containing only one type of insulin are stable up to 30 days. Prefilled syringes may be beneficial to patients who are sight impaired or who lack the manual dexterity to fill their own syringes at home. In these cases, family members, friends, and caregivers may prefill syringes on a periodic basis. These should be stored in a vertical position with the needle pointed up to avoid clumping of suspended insulin binders in the needle (RNAO, 2009). Some insulin combinations, such as insulin lispro and NPH, are not appropriate for prefilling and storage because the

TABLE 52-5 **PATIENT & CAREGIVER TEACHING GUIDE**

Insulin Therapy

The following instructions should be included when teaching the patient and caregiver about insulin therapy.
1. Wash hands thoroughly.
2. Check insulin type and expiration date.
3. If a cloudy insulin is used, gently roll container to resuspend insulin. It should look uniformly milky.
4. Remove the cover from the needle.
5. Pull the plunger down until the tip of the plunger is at the line for the number of units required. Put the needle into the vial and push the air into the vial.
6. Turn the vial upside down and slowly push plunger up and down to get rid of air bubbles and then pull plunger down until it is at the line for the correct dose of insulin.
7. Check that the amount of insulin is correct and that there are no large air bubbles in the syringe. Remove the syringe.
8. Select proper injection site (see Figure 52-6) and inject into a skin lift (pinched skin) at 90 degrees. To prevent possible intramuscular injections, slim individuals may need to inject into the skin lift at 45 degrees. (The use of 8-mm needles is recommended.)
9. After injecting insulin, leave needle in place for 5 sec to ensure that all insulin has been injected and then remove needle and release skin lift.
10. Dispose of single-use syringe safely. *Note:* When instructing patient to self-inject insulin, use the following guidelines (if appropriate):
   • Inspect insulin for any changes before each use (i.e., clumping, precipitation, change in clarity or colour).
   • Aspiration does not need to be done before injection. The injection site does not need to be cleansed with alcohol.

onset, action, and peak times of the mixture of the two can differ from those of either of the types. Pharmacy references should be consulted as needed when mixing and prefilling different types of insulin. Prefilled syringes should be gently rolled between the palms to warm the refrigerated insulin and to resuspend the particles before injecting (RNAO, 2009). Lantus insulin cannot be stored in a prefilled syringe (RNAO, 2009).

Administration of Insulin. Because insulin is inactivated by gastric juices, it cannot be taken orally. The only route of administration currently approved for self-administration is subcutaneous injection by syringe or insulin pen or by continuous subcutaneous infusion (pump). Intravenous (IV) administration of regular insulin can be done with medical supervision when immediate onset of action is desired in the hospital setting.

Injection. The steps in administering a subcutaneous insulin injection are outlined in Table 52-5. The technique should be taught to new insulin users and reviewed periodically with long-term users. It should never be assumed that, because insulin is being used, the patient knows and practises the correct insulin injection technique. Inaccurate preparation is often caused by poor eyesight. Air bubbles in the syringe may not be seen, or the scale on the syringe may be read improperly.

The patient receiving mixed insulins (e.g., regular and an intermediate-acting insulin) needs to learn the proper technique for combining both in the same syringe if commercially prepared premixed insulins are not used (see Figure 52-5).

The speed with which peak serum concentrations are reached varies with the anatomical site used for injection. The fastest absorption is from the abdomen, followed by the arm, the thigh, and the buttock. Appropriate sites for insulin injection are noted in Figure 52-6, although the abdomen is the preferred site. The

FIGURE 52-6 Injection sites for insulin. The abdomen is the preferred site.

FIGURE 52-7 Parts of an insulin pen.

patient should be cautioned about injecting into a site that is to be exercised. For example, the patient should not inject insulin into the thigh and then go jogging. Exercise of the area containing the injection site together with the increased body heat generated by the exercise may increase the rate of absorption and speed the onset of insulin action.

Before purified human insulins were widely used, patients were advised to rotate anatomical injection sites to prevent *lipodystrophy,* a condition that produces lumps and dents in the skin from repeated injection in the same spot. The use of human insulin reduces the risk for lipodystrophy. Because of this, and because rotating sites causes variability in insulin absorption, rotation of injection sites to different anatomical sites is no longer the recommended practice. Instead, patients are advised to rotate the injection within one particular site, such as the abdomen. Sometimes, it is helpful to think of the entire abdomen as a checkerboard, with each square representing an injection site as the patient rotates sites systematically across the board.

Most commercial insulin is available as U100, indicating that 1 mL contains 100 units of insulin. U100 insulin must be used with a U100-marked syringe. Disposable, plastic insulin syringes are available in a variety of sizes, including 1, 0.5, and 0.3 mL. The 0.5-mL size may be used for doses of 50 units or less, and the 0.3-mL syringe can be used for doses of 30 units or less. Smaller syringes offer a number of advantages. The major benefit is increased accuracy and reliability when delivering smaller doses because wider line markings are easier to see. Patients should be cautioned to check dosage lines carefully when changing syringe types because some use a scale of 1-unit increments and others use 2-unit increments.

Recapping should be done only by the person using the syringe. The nurse must never recap a needle that has been used by a patient. The use of an alcohol swab on the site before self-injection is no longer recommended. Routine hygiene such as washing with soap and rinsing with water is adequate. This recommendation applies primarily to patient self-injection technique. When injection occurs in a health care facility, policy may dictate site preparation with alcohol to prevent hospital-acquired infection. Injection should be performed at a 45- to 90-degree angle, depending on the thickness of the patient's fat pad.

An insulin pen is a compact portable device that serves the same function as a needle and syringe but is handier to use (Figure 52-7). The insulin pen uses 300-unit cartridges, which are packaged in a box of five, for a total of 1 500 units. One of the advantages of insulin pens is that they are less "medical" looking. The insulin pen has a numerical dial-up device that clicks for each unit being dialled. The pen can dial up to a maximum of 60 to 70 units, depending on the device. This is a safer and more convenient option for most patients, especially those with visual impairment, dexterity problems, and peripheral neuropathy. Pen-needle tips are finer than syringe tips and must be changed with every injection. They are manufactured in a variety of sizes—4, 5, 6, 8, and 12 to 12.7 mm—for a variety of body-fat types (FIT Canada, 2011).

Alternate Delivery Methods. Continuous subcutaneous insulin infusion can be administered using an insulin pump, a small battery-operated device that holds and delivers insulin (Figure 52-8). Usually worn on the belt, under clothing, or directly affixed to the body, the pump is connected to a catheter inserted into the subcutaneous tissue in the abdominal wall. Every 2 to 3 days, the insertion site is changed and the pump is refilled with insulin and reprogrammed. The device is programmed to deliver a continuous infusion of rapid-acting insulin 24 hours a day, known as the *basal rate.* Basal insulin can be temporarily increased or decreased based on activity level changes or illness. At mealtime, the user programs the pump to deliver a bolus infusion of insulin appropriate to the amount of carbohydrate ingested and to bring down high premeal blood glucose, if necessary. A major advantage of the insulin pump is the reduction of hypoglycemia episodes. Pumps also offer the benefit of a more normal lifestyle, allowing users more flexibility with meal and activity patterns as insulin delivery becomes very similar to the normal physiological pattern. The insertion site should be checked daily for redness and swelling (Pickup, 2012; American Association of Diabetes Educators [AADE], 2011).

Problems With Insulin Therapy. Hypoglycemia, allergic reactions, lipodystrophy, and Somogyi effect are the problems associated with insulin therapy. Hypoglycemia is discussed in detail later in this chapter. (Guidelines for assessing patients treated with insulin are presented in Table 52-6.)

Allergic Reactions. Local inflammatory reactions to insulin, such as itching, erythema, and burning around the injection site, may occur. Local reactions may be self-limiting within 1 to 3 months or may improve with a low dose of antihistamine. A true insulin allergy is a systemic response with urticaria and possibly anaphylactic shock, generally resulting from the use of animal insulins. Fortunately, this type of allergy is rare, particularly since human insulin has become available. Zinc and protamine—used as preservatives in the insulin and the latex rubber stoppers on the vials—have been implicated in insulin reactions.

FIGURE 52-8 A, The Omnipod® Insulin Management System is a tubeless, wireless, and waterproof pump that is affixed directly to the body and holds and delivers insulin. **B,** The Personal Diabetes Manager (PDM) wirelessly programs insulin delivery via the Pod. The PDM has a built-in glucose meter. Source: Courtesy Insulet Canada Corporation.

TABLE 52-6 ASSESSING THE PATIENT TREATED WITH ANTIHYPERGLYCEMIC AGENTS	
For Patient With Newly Diagnosed Diabetes or Re-Evaluation of Medication Regimen	
Cognitive	Is patient or responsible other able to understand antihyperglycemic agents are being used as part of diabetes management?
	Is patient or responsible other able to understand concepts of asepsis, combining insulins, insulin–OHA actions, and adverse effects?
	Is patient able to remember to take >1 dose/day?
	Does patient take medications at right times in relation to meals?
Psychomotor	Is patient or responsible other physically able to prepare and administer accurate doses of the medication?
Affective	What emotions and attitudes are patient and responsible others displaying in regard to diagnosis of diabetes and antihyperglycemic treatment? Is the patient displaying acceptance of diagnosis of DM and readiness to learn?
For Follow-Up of Patient Treated With Antihyperglycemic Agents	
Effectiveness of therapy	Is patient having symptoms of hyperglycemia or hypoglycemia?
	Does blood glucose record show good or poor control?
	Is glycated hemoglobin (A_{1c}) consistent with glucose records?
Adverse effects of therapy	Has patient had hypoglycemic episodes? If so, how often? What time of day? What was the precipitating event? Inconsistent meal timing, meal carbohydrate content, alcohol, or exercise?
	Are there complaints of nightmares, night sweats, or early-morning headaches?
	Has patient had skin rash, gastro-intestinal upset, ankle edema, or weight gain since taking the antihyperglycemic agent?
	Is atrophy or hypertrophy present at injection sites?
Self-management behaviours	If patient is having hypoglycemic episodes, how are those episodes managed? Has the patient analyzed episodes to determine the cause?
	How much insulin, OHA, or noninsulin injectable is the patient taking and at what time of day? Is patient adjusting the medication dose? Under what circumstances and by how much?
	Has exercise pattern changed?
	Is patient adhering to healthy eating recommendations? Are meals taken at times corresponding to peak insulin action? Is patient performing SMBG?

GI, gastro-intestinal; *OHA,* oral antihyperglycemic agent; *SMBG,* self-monitoring of blood glucose.

Lipodystrophy. Lipodystrophy (hypertrophy or atrophy of subcutaneous tissue) may occur if the same injection sites are used frequently. Hypertrophy, a thickening of the subcutaneous tissue, eventually regresses if the patient does not use the site for at least 6 months. The use of hypertrophied sites may result in erratic insulin absorption. Lipodystrophies have been most commonly associated with beef, or beef and pork, insulin and rarely with human insulin.

Somogyi Effect and Dawn Phenomenon. Wide differences in early-morning (low) and fasting (high) glucose levels characterize the Somogyi effect. Usually occurring during the hours of sleep, the Somogyi effect produces a decline in blood glucose level in response to too much insulin. Counter-regulatory hormones are released, stimulating lipolysis, gluconeogenesis, and glycogenolysis, which in turn produce rebound hyperglycemia and ketosis. The danger of this effect is that, when blood glucose levels are measured in the morning, hyperglycemia is apparent, and the patient (or the health care provider) may, therefore, increase the insulin dose. The Somogyi effect is associated with the occurrence of undetected hypoglycemia during sleep, although it can happen at any time.

The patient may report headaches on awakening and may recall night sweats or nightmares. If the Somogyi effect is suspected as a cause for early-morning high blood glucose, the patient may be advised to check blood glucose levels between 0200 and 0400 hours to determine whether hypoglycemia is present at that time. If it is, the insulin dosage of administration affecting the early-morning blood glucose is reduced.

The *dawn phenomenon* is characterized by hyperglycemia that is present on awakening in the morning, owing to the release of counter-regulatory hormones in the predawn hours. It has been suggested that growth hormone and cortisol are possible factors in this occurrence. The dawn phenomenon affects the majority of people with DM and tends to be most severe when growth hormone is at its peak in adolescence and young adulthood.

Careful assessment is required to document each phenomenon because the treatment for each differs. The treatment for Somogyi effect is reduction of insulin dosage. The treatment for dawn phenomenon is an adjustment in the timing of insulin administration or an increase in insulin. The assessment must include insulin dose, injection sites, and variability in the time of meals or insulin administration. In addition, the patient is asked to measure and document bedtime, nighttime (between 0200 and 0400 hours), and morning FBG levels on several occasions. If the predawn levels are below 3.3 mmol/L and signs and symptoms of hypoglycemia are present, the insulin dosage should be reduced. If the 0200 to 0400–hour blood glucose level is high, the insulin dosage should be increased. In addition, the patient should be counselled on appropriate bedtime snacks.

Drug Therapy: Antihyperglycemic Agents

Oral antihyperglycemic agents and noninsulin injectables work to improve the mechanisms by which insulin and glucose are produced and used by the body. These medications work on three defects of type 2 diabetes: (1) insulin resistance, (2) decreased insulin production, and (3) increased hepatic glucose production. Oral antihyperglycemic agents and noninsulin injectables may be used in combination with agents from several classes or with insulin to achieve blood glucose targets. Guidelines for assessing patients receiving these medications are shown in Table 52-6.

Currently, many classes of antihyperglycemics are available to improve DM control for patients with type 2 DM (CDA, 2013a). These agents are listed in Table 52-7.

Insulin Secretagogues. *Sulphonylureas* have been widely used to treat type 2 DM since the 1950s. The primary action of the sulphonylureas is to increase beta-cell insulin production from the pancreas. Caution must be exercised in dosage determination in older adults and patients with renal impairment owing to the increased risk for hypoglycemia. Therapy with sulphonylureas is generally more effective early in the course of type 2 DM. According to one study, up to a third of patients on monotherapy with a sulphonylurea will require a second agent within 5 years (Kahn, Haffner, Heise, et al., 2006).

Meglitinides. Like the sulphonylureas, meglitinides (repaglinide [GlucoNorm]) increase insulin production from the pancreas. But because they are more rapidly absorbed and eliminated, they offer a reduced potential for hypoglycemia. When meglitinides are taken just before meals, pancreatic insulin production increases during and after the meal, mimicking the normal blood glucose response to eating. Patients should be instructed to take meglitinides anytime from 30 minutes before each meal right up to the time of the meal, and not to take a dose if they are not eating. They are safer to use in patients with irregular mealtimes.

Biguanides. Metformin (Glucophage) is the only biguanide glucose-lowering agent available worldwide. It can be used alone or with sulphonylureas, other OHAs, or insulin to treat type 2

DM. The primary action of metformin is to reduce glucose production by the liver. It also enhances insulin sensitivity at the tissue level and improves glucose transport into the cells. Metformin is recommended as the first-line medication for most people with type 2 DM (CDA, 2013a). Besides being an effective blood glucose–lowering agent, metformin has other advantages. Unlike insulin secretagogues and insulin, metformin does not promote weight gain. It also has beneficial effects on plasma lipids. Metformin is also used to treat prediabetes, especially in individuals who are obese and have impaired fasting glucose.

Patients who are undergoing surgery or any radiological procedures that involve the use of a contrast medium are instructed to temporarily discontinue metformin before surgery or the procedure. They should not resume the metformin until 48 hours afterward, once their serum creatinine has been checked and is found to be normal.

DRUG ALERT—Metformin
- Do not use in patient with kidney disease, liver disease, or heart failure. Lactic acidosis is a rare complication of metformin accumulation.
- IV contrast media that contain iodine pose a risk for acute kidney injury, which could exacerbate metformin-induced lactic acidosis.
- Avoid use in people who drink excessive amounts of alcohol.

α-Glucosidase Inhibitors. Also known as *starch blockers,* glucosidase inhibitors work by slowing down the absorption of carbohydrate in the small intestine. Acarbose (Glucobay) is the available drug in this class. Taken with the first bite of each main meal, they are most effective in lowering postprandial blood glucose. Effectiveness of these medications is measured by checking 2-hour postprandial glucose levels. Medications from this class are not effective against fasting hyperglycemia (CDA, 2013a).

Thiazolidinediones. Sometimes referred to as *insulin sensitizers,* thiazolidinediones include pioglitazone (Actos) and rosiglitazone (Avandia). They are most effective for people who have insulin resistance. They improve insulin sensitivity, transport, and utilization at target tissues.

Because they do not increase insulin production, thiazolidinediones will not cause hypoglycemia when used alone, but the risk is still present when a thiazolidinedione is used in combination with insulin or an insulin secretagogue. Patients taking these medications may experience a secondary benefit of improved triglyceride, high-density lipoprotein (HDL), and blood pressure levels (CDA, 2013a). Use with insulin is not approved in Canada because the combination potentiates the adverse effect of edema and subsequent weight gain.

Dipeptidyl Peptidase-4 Inhibitors. A newer class of glucose-lowering drugs available in Canada is the dipeptidyl peptidase-4 (DPP-4) inhibitors. This class of drugs includes sitagliptin (Januvia), saxagliptin (Onglyza), linagliptin (Trajenta) and alogliptin (Nesina). The incretin hormones, which are part of the physiological process that regulates glucose homeostasis, are normally inactivated by DPP-4. By inhibiting DDP-4, these medications slow the inactivation of incretin hormones. Incretin hormones are released by the intestines throughout the day, but levels increase in response to a meal. When glucose levels are normal or elevated, incretins increase insulin synthesis and release from the pancreas as well as decrease hepatic glucose production. DPP-4 inhibitors manage type 2 DM by increasing and prolonging increased incretin levels. These drugs are glucose-dependent (i.e., they respond to the presence of elevated glucose and result in insulin release only when needed), and therefore, they lower the potential for hypoglycemia. The main benefit of these drugs over

TABLE 52-7 DRUG THERAPY

Antihyperglycemic Agents for Diabetes Mellitus

Type	Mechanism of Action	Adverse Effects
Insulin Secretagogues: Sulphonylureas Gliclazide (Diamicron, Diamicron MR) Glimepiride (Amaryl) Glyburide (Diabeta) (chlorpropamide and tolbutamide are available in Canada but rarely used)	Stimulate release of insulin from beta cells; decrease glycogenolysis and gluconeogenesis; glimepiride may improve insensitivity in tissues	Weight gain, hypoglycemia
Meglitinide Repaglinide (GlucoNorm)	Stimulates a rapid and short-lived release of insulin from the pancreas	Less weight gain, decreased incidence of hypoglycemia compared with glyburide
Biguanide Metformin (Glucophage, Glumetza)	Inhibits hepatic glucose production; increases peripheral and liver sensitivity to insulin	Nausea, upset stomach, diarrhea; less weight gain than sulphonylureas and does not cause hypoglycemia; potential lactic acidosis in renal or hepatic impairment; has to be held at the time of or before procedures and held for 48 hr after administration of IV contrast media
α-Glucosidase Inhibitors Acarbose (Glucobay)	Delays absorption of glucose and digestion of CHO in small intestine, lowering after-meal blood glucose levels	Flatulence, abdominal pain, diarrhea
Thiazolidinediones Pioglitazone (Actos) Rosiglitazone (Avandia)	↑ Glucose uptake in muscle and fat; inhibit hepatic glucose production	Edema, weight gain, heart failure; causes ovulation in premenopausal women with PCOS; not recommended for patients with heart failure
Dipeptidyl Peptidase-4 Inhibitors Sitagliptin (Januvia) Saxagliptin (Onglyza) Linagliptin (Trajenta) Alogliptin (Nesina)	Enhance the incretin system, stimulate release of insulin from pancreatic beta cells, and inhibit hepatic glucose production	Upper respiratory tract infection, sore throat, headache, diarrhea
Noninsulin Injectable Agents: GLP-1 Receptor Agonists Liraglutide (Victoza) Exenatide (Byetta) Albiglutide (Eperzan) Dulaglutide (Trulicity)* Exenatide QW (Bydureon)*	Stimulate release of insulin; decrease glucagon secretion, increase satiety, decrease gastric emptying	Nausea, vomiting, hypoglycemia, diarrhea, headache
Sodium-Glucose Cotransporter Type 2 (SGLT2) Inhibitors Canagliflozin (Invokana) Dapagliflozin (Forxiga) Empagliflozin (Jardiance)	Enhance urinary glucose excretion	Genital infections, urinary tract infections, hypotension, increased lipids
Combination Therapy Avandamet (rosiglitazone [Avandia] and metformin [Glucophage]) Janumet/Janumet XR (sitagliptin [Januvia] and metformin/metformin XR [Glucophage/Glucophage XR]) Jentadueto (linagliptin [Trajenta] and metformin [Glucophage]) Kazano (alogliptin [Nesina] and metformin [Glucophage]) Komboglyze (metformin [Glucophage] and saxagliptin [Onglyza]) Oseni (alogliptin [Nesina] and pioglitazone [Actos])	See mechanism of action for individual drugs, above	See adverse effects for individual drugs, above

CHO, carbohydrates; *GI,* gastro-intestinal; *IV,* intravenous; *PCOS,* polycystic ovarian syndrome.
*Canadian Diabetes Association Clinical Practice Guidelines Expert Committee. (2016). Pharmacologic management of type 2 diabetes: 2016 interim update. *Canadian Journal of Diabetes, 40*(2016):193–195.

other medications for DM with similar effects is the absence of weight gain as an adverse effect. These drugs may be taken alone or in combination with other OHAs (CDA, 2013a; Bristol-Myers Squibb [BMS] Canada, 2011).

Sodium-Glucose Cotransporter Type 2 (SGLT2) Inhibitors. Canagliflozin (Invokana), dapagliflozin (Forxiga) and empagliflozin (Jardiance) are the medications in a new class of drugs known as sodium-glucose cotransporter Type 2 (SGLT2) inhibitors available in Canada. These drugs work by blocking the reabsorption of glucose by the kidney, increasing glucose excretion, and lowering blood glucose levels (Harper, Clement, Goldenberg, et al., 2015).

Combination Therapy. Many combination drugs are currently available. These drugs combine two different classes of medications to treat DM. These agents are listed in Table 52-7. One advantage of combined therapy is improved patient compliance.

Glucagon-Like Peptide (GLP)-1 Receptor Agonists (Incretin Mimetics). Liraglutide (Victoza), exenatide (Byetta), exenatide QW (Bydureon), albiglutide (Eperzan), and dulaglutide (Trulicity) are the GLP-1 receptor agonists available in Canada. These drugs stimulate GLP-1 (one of the incretin hormones), which is found to be decreased in people with type 2 DM. The mechanisms of action of these drugs are similar to those performed by the incretin hormone it mimics. They stimulate the release of insulin from the pancreatic beta cells. Other mechanisms of actions are (1) suppression of glucagon secretion from the pancreatic beta cells, which reduces glucose output from the liver; (2) reduction of food intake by increasing satiety, thereby reducing caloric intake; and (3) slowing gastric emptying. These drugs are not indicated for use with insulin. GLP-1 receptor agonists are administered using a subcutaneous injection in a prefilled pen (NovoNordisk, 2016a; Eli Lilly Canada, 2011).

DRUG ALERT—Exenatide (Byetta)
- Acute pancreatitis and kidney problems have been associated with its use.

DRUG ALERT—Liraglutide (Victoza)
- Avoid use in patients with a personal or family history of medullary thyroid cancer
- Acute pancreatitis has been associated with its use.

Other Drugs Affecting Blood Glucose Levels. Both the patient and the health care provider must be aware of drug interactions that can potentiate hypoglycemic and hyperglycemic effects. For example, β-adrenergic blockers can mask symptoms of hypoglycemia and prolong the hypoglycemic effects of insulin. Thiazide and loop diuretics can potentiate hyperglycemia by inducing potassium loss, although low-dose therapy with a thiazide is usually considered safe.

Nutritional Therapy

Although nutritional therapy is the cornerstone of care for the person with DM, it is also its most challenging aspect. Nutritional therapy can reduce A_{1c} by an absolute 1% to 2% with the greatest impact at the initial stages of DM (CDA, 2013a). Achieving nutritional goals requires a coordinated team effort that takes into account the behavioural, cognitive, socioeconomic, cultural, and spiritual aspects of the person. Because of these complexities, it is recommended that a DM nurse educator and a registered dietitian, with expertise in DM management, be members of the team.

Nutritional therapy for the management of DM is based on a plan of healthy eating that is appropriate and beneficial for all members of the general population, whether they have DM or

TABLE 52-8   NUTRITIONAL THERAPY
Diabetes Mellitus

Factor	Type 1 Diabetes Mellitus	Type 2 Diabetes Mellitus
Total calories	Increase in caloric intake possibly necessary to achieve desirable body weight and restore body tissues	Reduction in caloric intake desirable for overweight or obese patient
Effect of diet	Diet and insulin necessary for glucose control	Diet alone possibly sufficient for glucose control
Distribution of calories	Equal distribution of carbohydrates through meals or adjustment of carbohydrates for insulin activity	Equal distribution recommended; low-fat diet desirable; consistency of carbohydrate at meals desirable
Consistency in daily intake	Necessary for glucose control	Desirable for weight reduction and moderation of blood glucose levels
Uniform timing of meals	Crucial for NPH insulin programs; flexibility with multidose rapid-acting insulin	Desirable but not essential, unless using insulin or sulphonylureas
Intermeal and bedtime snacks	Frequently necessary	Is based on patient's eating habits and preferences; may be necessary if using insulin or sulphonylureas
Nutritional supplement for exercise programs	Carbohydrates 20 g/hr for moderate physical activities	May be necessary if patient's blood glucose levels are controlled on sulphonylureas or insulin

NPH, neutral protamine Hagedorn.

not. In an institutional setting, the prescribed diet is often labelled "diabetic diet" or "no added sugar," indicating that the meal plan follows the CDA's current nutritional recommendations.

Eating Well With Canada's Food Guide (see Chapter 42, Figure 42-1) summarizes and illustrates nutritional guidelines and nutrient needs. These are appropriate in guiding the food choices of people with DM. Nutritional therapy and meal planning should be individualized to accommodate the person's preferences, age, needs, culture, lifestyle, and readiness to change. Tools used to measure the effectiveness of nutritional therapy include blood glucose, A_{1c}, and lipid values; tests of renal status; and clinical measurements such as body weight, body mass index, waist circumference, and blood pressure (CDA, 2013a). Table 52-8 describes nutritional therapy for type 1 and type 2 DM.

The Canadian Diabetes Association was renamed Diabetes Canada in 2017; it continues to provide a variety of nutrition teaching tools to assist health care providers. These are accessible online at the Diabetes Canada website or through the Diabetes Canada office. The resource entitled *Just the Basics: Healthy Eating for Diabetes Management and Prevention* is an example of such a tool (CDA, 2013b). It provides tips for healthy eating, DM prevention, and management for support until the person can see a dietitian. This tool highlights the need for the following:

1. Eating three meals per day at regular times and eating at intervals no more than 6 hours apart
2. Limiting sugars and sweets such as sugar, regular pop, desserts, candies, jam, and honey
3. Limiting the amount of high-fat food such as fried foods, chips, and pastries
4. Eating more high-fibre foods (whole-grain breads and cereals, lentils, dried beans and peas, brown rice, fruits, and vegetables)
5. Drinking water if thirsty
6. Adding physical activity to the lifestyle (CDA, 2013a)

Type 1 Diabetes Mellitus. Meal planning should be based on the individual's usual food intake and balanced with insulin and exercise patterns. The insulin regimen should be developed with the patient's eating habits and activity pattern in mind. Patients using rapid-acting insulin can make adjustments in dosage before the meal, based on the current blood glucose level and the carbohydrate content of the meal or snack. Intensified insulin therapy, such as multiple daily injections or the use of an insulin pump, allows considerable flexibility in food selection and can be adjusted for deviations from usual eating and exercise habits. All people with type 1 DM should be seen by a registered dietitian to learn about carbohydrate-counting strategies.

Type 2 Diabetes Mellitus. The emphasis for nutritional therapy in type 2 DM should be placed on achieving glucose, lipid, and blood pressure goals. Because 80% to 90% of people with type 2 DM are overweight, calorie and fat reduction is a goal. Weight loss has been shown to improve glycemic control by increasing insulin sensitivity and glucose uptake and decreasing hepatic glucose output (CDA, 2013a).

There is no one proven strategy or method that can be uniformly recommended. A nutritionally adequate meal plan with a reduction of total fat (especially saturated fats), an increase of fibre, and a decrease in simple sugars can bring about decreased calorie and carbohydrate consumption. Eating many small meals is another strategy that can be adopted to spread nutrient intake throughout the day. A weight loss of 5% to 7% of body weight often improves glycemic control, even if desirable body weight is not achieved. Weight loss is best attempted by a moderate decrease in calories and an increase in caloric expenditure. Regular exercise and learning new behaviours and attitudes can help facilitate long-term lifestyle changes. Monitoring of blood glucose levels, A_{1c}, lipids, and blood pressure provides feedback on how well the goals of nutritional therapy are being met.

Food Composition. DM has been called a disease of carbohydrate metabolism, but it is actually a general metabolic disorder involving three categories of energy-providing nutrients: carbohydrates, fats, and proteins. Therefore, the nutrient balance of a diabetic diet is essential to maintenance of blood glucose levels. The nutritional energy intake should be constantly balanced with the energy output of the individual, taking into account exercise and metabolic work of the body. The following are general recommendations for nutrient balance; each patient's individual meal plan should be developed with a dietitian and with her or his lifestyle and health goals in mind and is based on Canada's food guide (Health Canada, 2011; CDA, 2013a; American Diabetes Association [ADA], 2013):

- *Protein:* 15% to 20% of energy. There is no evidence that usual protein intake (15%–20% of energy) should be modified. Those with diabetic nephropathy should limit protein intake to 15% of energy and be monitored closely by a registered dietitian.

- *Fat:* less than 35% of energy. Combined saturated fats and trans-fatty acids should be reduced to less than 7% of energy intake. Polyunsaturated fat should be limited to less than 10% of energy intake. Foods rich in polyunsaturated omega-3 fatty acids and plant oils should be included.
- *Fibre:* approximately 25 to 50 g/day from a variety of food sources, including soluble and cereal fibres.
- *Carbohydrate:* 45% to 60% of energy. Carbohydrates should include whole grains, fruits, vegetables, and low-fat milk. Patients should try to consume higher-fibre sources of carbohydrate. Less than 10% of daily energy should come from sucrose (sugar). Low-carbohydrate diets are not recommended for DM management.

Glycemic index (GI) is the term used to describe the rise in blood glucose levels after a person has consumed carbohydrate-containing food. The GI of foods was developed to compare the postprandial responses of the body with carbohydrate-containing foods. A GI of 100 refers to the response to 50 g of glucose or white bread in a normal person without DM. All other food with an equivalent carbohydrate value is measured against this standard. For example, the GI of an apple is 52, regular milk 27, baked potato 93, cornflake cereal 119, and baked beans 69 (ADA, 2008) (see the Resources at the end of this chapter for an online calculator for GI).

The GI of carbohydrates should be considered when choosing them in a meal plan. Foods with a high GI (e.g., potatoes, white bread) will cause a sharp rise in blood glucose, whereas those with a low GI (e.g., brown rice) steadily increase blood glucose over a longer period. Although the GI affects blood glucose, the total amount of carbohydrates is more important than the source (CDA, 2013a).

Nutritive and nonnutritive sweeteners may be included in a healthy meal plan, in moderation. Nonnutritive sweeteners approved by Health Canada include the sugar substitutes, saccharin, aspartame, sucralose, acesulphame-K, steviol glycosides, tagatose, thaumatin, and cyclamate (CDA, 2013a).

Alcohol. Alcohol is high in calories, has no nutritive value, and can be a partner in contributing to hypertriglyceridemia. In addition, it has detrimental effects on the liver (see Chapter 46). The inhibitory effect of alcohol on glucose production by the liver can cause severe hypoglycemia in patients taking insulin or OHAs that increase insulin secretion. Hypoglycemia may occur up to 24 hours after alcohol consumption in those with type 1 DM. Because alcohol consumption can make blood glucose more difficult to control, patients should be encouraged to discuss the use of alcohol honestly with their health care providers (CDA, 2013a).

Alcohol can also cause other serious adverse effects when used in conjunction with certain OHAs used to treat DM. For example, there is a risk for lactic acidosis in patients who have alcohol dependency and use metformin. Alcohol consumption should be limited to 1 to 2 standard drinks per day (e.g., 1 glass or 142 mL wine) or fewer than 14 standard drinks per week for men and fewer than 9 for women (CDA, 2013a). Alcohol can sometimes be incorporated into healthy eating if blood glucose is well controlled and if the patient is not on medications that will cause adverse effects. A patient can reduce the risk for alcohol-induced hyperglycemia or hypoglycemia by consuming alcohol with food, using sugar-free mixes, and drinking dry, light wines (CDA, 2013a).

Healthy Eating Education. Dietitians are the primary source of nutrition education. However, all members of the interdisciplinary team should be prepared to answer basic questions about healthy eating and DM. Access to a dietitian may not be possible for patients who live in remote areas, and nurses often assume responsibility for teaching basic dietary management. *Eating Well With Canada's Food Guide* (see Chapter 42, Figure 42-1) is a simple, accessible, and appropriate tool for health care team members to use to educate people with DM about nutrition.

An effective method of presenting the basics of meal planning is the *plate method*. This simple method helps the patient visualize the amount of vegetables, starch, and protein that should fill a dinner plate (CDA, 2013a). For lunch and dinner, one-half of the plate is filled with vegetables, one-fourth is filled with a starch, and one-fourth is filled with 60 to 90 g (2–3 oz) of lean meat or other protein source. A glass of low-fat milk and a small piece of fresh fruit complete the meal. The breakfast plate is filled halfway with starch, and one-fourth of the plate contains an optional protein. Low-fat milk and fresh fruit complete the breakfast. Assuming low-fat and nonfat foods are selected, following the plate method will provide a well-balanced diet.

Nutrition education should include the patient's family and significant others, and it is most effective to teach the person who will be cooking. However, it is important that the responsibility for making healthy food choices falls to the patient with DM. A support network of family and friends is the key to making successful and sustainable nutritional and lifestyle changes.

In an acute health care facility, the nutritional needs of the patient with DM vary slightly from the normal meal plans. Previously, standardized calorie-level meal patterns were used, but new alternatives are now being used, such as the consistent-carbohydrate DM meal plan. Under this system, meal plans are not created according to calorie levels, but instead are created with consistent carbohydrate content. For example, every day, each breakfast contains the same amount of carbohydrates as the previous day; the same method is used for lunch and dinner (CDA, 2013a).

Exercise

Regular, consistent exercise is considered an essential part of DM and prediabetes management. Exercise increases insulin sensitivity and can have a direct effect on lowering blood glucose levels. It also contributes to weight loss, which also decreases insulin resistance. The therapeutic benefits of regular physical activity may result in a decreased need for DM medicines in order to reach target blood glucose goals. Regular exercise may also help reduce triglyceride and low-density lipoprotein (LDL) cholesterol levels, reduce blood pressure, and improve circulation (CDA, 2013a; ADA, 2015). Any new exercise program in the person with DM should be started only after medical clearance and should be started slowly, with gradual progression toward the desired goal. People with type 2 DM should accumulate at least 150 minutes of moderate-intensity aerobic activity—such as brisk walking, cycling, or dancing—each week, spread over at least 3 separate days. Performance of resistance exercises three times per week should also be encouraged in addition to aerobic exercise (CDA, 2013a).

Before starting an exercise program, all patients with DM should undergo a pre-exercise assessment by a medical doctor and should be started slowly with gradual progression toward the desired goal (CDA, 2013a). Patients who use insulin and insulin secretagogues, such as sulphonylureas or meglitinides, are at increased risk for hypoglycemia when there is an increase

TABLE 52-9	ACTIVITIES THAT AFFECT CALORIC EXPENDITURE	
Light Activity (100–200 Kcal/Hr)	**Moderate Activity (200–350 Kcal/Hr)**	**Vigorous Activity (400–900 Kcal/Hr)**
• Driving a car • Fishing • Light housework • Secretarial work • Teaching • Walking casually	• Active housework • Bicycling (light) • Bowling • Dancing • Gardening • Golfing • Roller skating • Walking briskly	• Aerobic exercise • Bicycling (vigorous) • Hard labour • Ice skating • Outdoor sports • Running • Soccer • Tennis • Wood chopping

in physical activity, especially if the patient exercises at the time of peak drug action or if food intake has not been sufficient to maintain adequate blood glucose levels. Hypoglycemia can also occur if a normally sedentary patient with DM has an unusually active day. The glucose-lowering effects of exercise can last up to 48 hours after the activity, so it is possible for hypoglycemia to occur during that time. It is recommended that patients who use medications that can cause hypoglycemia schedule exercise about 1 hour after a meal or have a 10- to 15-g carbohydrate snack before exercising. Several small carbohydrate snacks can be taken every 30 minutes during exercise to prevent hypoglycemia. Patients using medications that place them at risk for hypoglycemia should always carry a fast-acting source of carbohydrate, such as juice, glucose tablets, or hard candies, when exercising. Table 52-9 gives guidelines on the number of calories burned per hour for different activities.

Although exercise is generally beneficial to blood glucose levels, strenuous activity can be perceived by the body as a stress, causing a release of counter-regulatory hormones, which results in a temporary elevation of blood glucose. As a result, hyperglycemia may occur in cases of poorly controlled type 2 DM or in patients with type 1 DM who exercise at a time of day when insulin action is waning. Some patients may have to inject a small bolus of rapid-acting or regular insulin if the blood glucose level is elevated before exercising to prevent progressive hyperglycemia. Furthermore, patients should exercise with caution if the blood glucose is elevated and there are no ketones. However, exercise should be postponed and the patient should take additional insulin when the blood sugar is elevated and urine ketones are present (CDA, 2013a).

Monitoring Blood Glucose

Self-monitoring of blood glucose (SMBG) is a cornerstone of DM management. By providing a "real-time" blood glucose reading, SMBG enables the patient to make self-management decisions regarding diet, exercise, and medication. SMBG is also important for detecting episodic hyperglycemia and hypoglycemia.

Portable blood glucose monitors are used at the hospital bedside and by patients who perform SMBG independently. A wide variety of blood glucose monitors are available (Figure 52-9). Usually, disposable lancets are used to obtain a small drop of capillary blood (usually from a finger stick) that is placed onto a glucose testing strip. After a specified time, the monitor displays a digital reading of the blood glucose. The technology of SMBG is a rapidly changing field, with more convenient systems

FIGURE 52-9 A blood glucose monitor (Accu-Chek Aviva) is used to measure blood glucose levels. Source: Courtesy Roche Diagnostics Canada, Laval, QC.

FIGURE 52-10 The MiniMed Paradigm® REAL-Time Revel™ Insulin Pump (A) delivers insulin through a thin plastic tubing to an infusion set, which has a cannula (B) that sits under the skin. Continuous glucose monitoring occurs through a tiny sensor (C) inserted under the skin. Sensor data are sent continuously to the insulin pump through wireless technology, giving a more complete picture of glucose levels, which can lead to better treatment decisions and better glucose control. Source: Phanie/Alamy Stock Photo.

being introduced every year. Newer systems allow the user to collect blood from alternative sites such as the forearm or the palm but will not register rapidly changing blood glucose readings. Therefore, finger sticks are still recommended if symptoms of low blood glucose are present. The most advanced systems require 4 seconds to provide results with only 0.3 µL of capillary blood.

Continuous glucose monitoring (CGM) systems provide another route for monitoring glucose. They measure glucose concentrations in the interstitial fluid. There are two devices available—the real-time CGM (personal) and the retrospective CGM (professional). The real-time CGM available in Canada is the Medtronic MiniMed Paradigm REAL-Time System (Figure 52-10). Using a sensor inserted under the skin, it displays glucose values continuously, with the values updating every 5 minutes. The sensor is inserted by the patient, using an automatic insertion device. Data are sent from the sensor to a transmitter, which displays the glucose value on an insulin pump. The patient is

TABLE 52-10   PATIENT & CAREGIVER TEACHING GUIDE

Obtaining a Capillary Sample for Blood Glucose Testing

The following instructions should be included when teaching the patient and caregiver about SMBG.
1. Wash hands with soap and warm water. It is not necessary to clean the site with alcohol, and it may interfere with test results by artificially lowering them.
2. If it is difficult to obtain an adequate drop of blood for testing, do any or all of the following: warm the hands in warm water, let the arm hang down for a few minutes before the finger puncture is made, use a new lancet with every puncture, or use a higher setting on the lancing device.
3. If the puncture is made on the finger, use the side of the finger pad rather than near the centre. There are fewer nerve endings along the side of the finger pad. If an alternative site is used (e.g., forearm), special equipment may be needed. Alternative-site testing is not recommended after a meal or for people with erratic blood glucose control experiencing hypoglycemia. Refer to manufacturer's instructions for alternative-site use.
4. The puncture should be only deep enough to obtain a sufficiently large drop of blood. Unnecessarily deep punctures may cause pain and bruising.
5. Lancets should be disposed of in designated "sharps" containers obtained from drug stores. Lancets and needles should not be placed in garbage cans, recycling bins, toilets, or glass jars.

alerted during episodes of hypoglycemia and hyperglycemia, allowing corrective action to be taken quickly. The retrospective CGM captures data but does not display. CGMs assist patients and health care providers to identify trends and track patterns. These data are particularly useful for the management of insulin therapy. These systems still require finger-stick measurements using a blood glucose monitor to calibrate the sensor and to make treatment decisions.

The blood glucose level reported by a laboratory is sometimes higher than that reported on the patient's home glucose monitor or the hospital's portable monitor. This is because some monitors give capillary blood glucose values from whole blood (via finger stick), whereas venous samples taken in the laboratory provide plasma readings. Plasma samples, or venous samples, are approximately 10% to 12% higher. Most monitors are automatically calibrated to give a "plasma" test result (even though whole blood was used for the sample) so that the home readings can be more readily compared with laboratory values. The literature accompanying a monitor will identify whether that particular monitor is calibrated to give plasma or whole blood readings.

Instructions for using a blood glucose monitor accompany each product. Because errors in monitoring technique can cause errors in management strategies, thorough patient education is crucial. Initial education should be followed up at regular intervals with reassessment. In addition, patients must be taught to use and interpret control solutions. Control solution should be used when first using a glucometer, when a new bottle of strips is used or when there is a reason to believe that the readings are not correct. Lab-to-meter correlation should be done between SMBG and simultaneous venous FBG, at least annually or when A_{1c} does not match SMBG readings, to ensure accuracy of SMBG. At blood glucose levels >4.2 mmol/L, a difference of <20% is considered acceptable (CDA, 2013a). Table 52-10 lists the steps that should be taught to the patient learning to perform SMBG.

The primary advantage of SMBG is that it supplies immediate information about blood glucose levels that can be used to make adjustments in food intake, activity patterns, and medication dosages. It also produces accurate records of daily glucose fluctuations and trends as well as alerting the patient to acute episodes of hyperglycemia and hypoglycemia. Furthermore, it provides patients with a tool for achieving and maintaining specific glycemic goals. SMBG is recommended as an essential part of daily DM management for all people using insulin or OHAs. The frequency of monitoring depends on several factors, including the patient's glycemic goals, the type of DM the patient has, the patient's ability and willingness to perform the test independently, and the treatment regimen. It is recommended that patients with type 1 DM test at least three times per day and include both preprandial and postprandial testing. Those using an insulin pump may test more frequently. People with type 2 DM treated with OHAs or lifestyle alone will have more variable and individualized testing regimens. For patients with type 2 DM treated with once-daily insulin and OHAs, monitoring at least once daily is recommended (CDA, 2013a).

Blood glucose testing should also be performed whenever hypoglycemia is suspected so that immediate action can be taken if necessary. When the person with DM is ill, the blood glucose should be tested at 4-hour intervals to determine the effects of this stressor on the blood glucose level.

SMBG is an empowering tool that allows the patient to be an active partner in the treatment of DM. Achieving the desired level of patient participation does require time and effort from the health care provider. The nurse involved in this aspect of management should anticipate a close working relationship with patients as they refine their techniques and learn appropriate decision making about managing their DM. A patient who is visually impaired, cognitively impaired, or limited in manual dexterity needs careful evaluation of the degree to which SMBG can be performed independently. Nurses working in home health and outpatient settings may need to identify caregivers who can assume this responsibility. Adaptive devices are available to help patients with certain limitations. These include "talking meters" and other equipment for people who are visually impaired as well as devices to stabilize insulin vials and syringes for those with limitations affecting dexterity.

Bariatric Surgery

Bariatric surgery may be considered for patients with type 2 diabetes who have a body mass index (BMI) >40.0 kg/m^2 (class III obesity) or BMI >35.0 to 39.9 kg/m^2 (class II obesity) and comorbidities, when lifestyle interventions are inadequate in achieving and maintaining healthy weight goals (CDA, 2013a) (see the "Evidence-Informed Practice" box). Patients with type 2 diabetes who have undergone bariatric surgery need lifelong monitoring and support. (Bariatric surgery is discussed in Chapter 43.)

CULTURALLY COMPETENT CARE

DIABETES MELLITUS

Because culture can have a strong influence on dietary preferences and meal preparation practices, culturally competent care has special relevance for the patient with diabetes. This is especially pertinent when considering the prevalence of diabetes in diverse Canadian cultural groups such as people of Indigenous, Latin American, South Asian, Asian, or African descent. The influence

EVIDENCE-INFORMED PRACTICE

Research Highlight

Bariatric Surgery for Adults With Type 2 Diabetes Who Are Obese

Clinical Question

In adults who are severely obese (P), how do gastric bypass and biliopancreatic diversion (I) compare with medical therapy (C) for remission from type 2 diabetes mellitus (O)?

Best Available Evidence

- Systematic review of randomized controlled trials (RCTs)

Critical Appraisal and Synthesis of Evidence

- Sixty adults with type 2 diabetes for ≥5 yr with a BMI ≥35 kg/m^2 and Hb A$_{1c}$ ≥7.0%
- Roux-en-Y gastric bypass (n=20), biliopancreatic diversion (n=20), or medical therapy (n=20)
- At 2 yr, more patients in the gastric bypass and biliopancreatic diversion groups achieved diabetes remission than in the medical therapy group
- Bypass and biliopancreatic diversion each reduced A$_{1c}$, glucose levels, and BMI more than medical therapy

Conclusion

- Bariatric surgery (gastric bypass and biliopancreatic diversion) decreases BMI, improves glycemic control, and increases remission from type 2 diabetes more than medical therapy does, in adults who are severely obese.

Implications for Nursing Practice

1. In addition to behavioural and medical approaches, bariatric surgery often normalizes blood glucose levels, reduces or avoids the need for drugs, and provides a potentially cost-effective approach to treating the disease.
2. Bariatric surgery is an appropriate treatment for people with type 2 diabetes and obesity who are not achieving recommended treatment targets with medical therapies, especially when there are other major comorbidities.

Reference for Evidence

Mingrone, G., Panunzi, S., De Gaetano, A., et al. (2012). Bariatric surgery versus conventional medical therapy for type 2 diabetes. *New England Journal of Medicine, 366*(17), 1577–1585. doi:10.1056/NEJMoa1200111.

P, Patient population of interest; *I*, intervention or area of interest; *C*, comparison of interest or comparison group; *O*, outcomes of interest.

of culture on food choices and meal planning should be explored with the patient as part of the health history. When giving diet instructions, efforts should be made to consider the food preferences of the cultural group. Nutritional resources specifically designed for members of different cultural groups are available from Diabetes Canada.

NURSING MANAGEMENT
DIABETES MELLITUS

NURSING ASSESSMENT

Table 52-11 provides initial subjective and objective data that might be obtained from a person with DM. After the initial assessment, periodic patient assessments should be done on a regular basis.

NURSING DIAGNOSES

Nursing diagnoses related to DM may include, but are not limited to, the following.

TABLE 52-11   NURSING ASSESSMENT

Diabetes Mellitus

Subjective Data
Important Health Information
Past health history: Mumps, rubella, coxsackievirus, or other viral infections; recent trauma, infection, or stress; pregnancy, gave birth to infant >4 kg; chronic pancreatitis; Cushing's syndrome, acromegaly; family history of type 1 or type 2 diabetes mellitus; obesity
Date of last eye and dental examination, compliance with diet in patients with previously diagnosed diabetes
Medications: Use of and compliance with insulin or OHAs; use of corticosteroids, diuretics, phenytoin (Dilantin)
Surgery or other treatments: Any recent surgery

Symptoms
- Constipation or diarrhea; frequent urination, nocturia, urinary incontinence
- Depression, irritability, apathy
- Erectile dysfunction; frequent vaginal infections; decreased libido
- Malaise
- Muscle weakness, fatigue
- Poor healing, especially involving the feet
- Thirst, hunger, nausea and vomiting
- Weight loss (type 1), weight gain (type 2)

Objective Data
Eyes
Vitreal hemorrhages; cataracts; soft, sunken eyeballs*

Integumentary
Dry, warm, inelastic skin; pigmented lesions (on legs); ulcers (especially on feet), loss of hair on toes; acanthosis nigricans

Respiratory
Rapid, deep respirations (Kussmaul's respiration)*

Cardiovascular
Hypotension*; weak, rapid pulse*, peripheral pulses diminished, feet pale and cool to touch

Gastro-Intestinal
Dry mouth, vomiting*, fruity breath*

Neurological
Altered reflexes, restlessness, confusion, stupor, coma, reduced sensation or vibration sense in feet

Musculo-Skeletal
Muscle wasting

Possible Findings
- Glucose level ≥7.0 mmol/L; glucose tolerance test ≥11.1 mmol/L; glycosylated hemoglobin ≥6%
- Urinalysis: glycosuria, ketonuria, microalbuminuria, or proteinuria
- Other: serum electrolyte abnormalities; acidosis; ↑ creatinine, ↑ total cholesterol, LDL, VLDL, and triglycerides; ↓ HDL; leukocytosis

HDL, high-density lipoprotein; *LDL,* low-density lipoprotein; *OHA,* oral antihyperglycemic agent; *VLDL,* very-low-density lipoprotein.
*Indicates manifestations of ketoacidosis.

- *Ineffective health management* related to *insufficient resources* (deficient knowledge of diabetes management)
- *Risk for unstable blood glucose levels* as evidenced by *insufficient diabetes management*
- *Risk for injury* as evidenced by *insufficient knowledge of modifiable factors* (resulting in episodes of hypoglycemia)

- *Risk for peripheral neurovascular dysfunction* (related to vascular effects of diabetes)

Additional information on nursing diagnoses for the patient with diabetes is also presented in Nursing Care Plan (NCP) 52-1, available on the Evolve website.

PLANNING

The overall goals for the patient with DM include the following: (1) to be an active participant in the management of the DM regimen; (2) to experience few or no episodes of hypoglycemia or acute hyperglycemic emergencies; (3) to maintain blood glucose levels at normal or near-normal levels; (4) to prevent, minimize, or delay the occurrence of chronic complications of DM; and (5) to adjust lifestyle to accommodate DM regimen with a minimum of stress.

NURSING IMPLEMENTATION

HEALTH PROMOTION. The role of the nurse in health promotion and maintenance relates to the identification, monitoring, and education of the patient at risk for the development of DM. Obesity is the number one predictor of type 2 DM. The Diabetes Prevention Program (DPP) found that a modest weight loss of 5% to 10% of body weight, from dietary modifications and regular exercise of 30 minutes five times a week, lowered the risk of developing type 2 DM up to 58% (DPP Research Group, 2002).

Diabetes Canada recommends screening every 3 years in individuals 40 years of age or older or in individuals at high risk using a risk calculator. It is important to screen earlier and more frequently in people with additional risk factors for diabetes or for those at very high risk using a risk calculator. The Canadian Diabetes Risk Assessment Questionnaire (CANRISK) is a statistically valid tool that may be suitable for diabetes risk assessment in the Canadian population and is available at *http://healthycanadians .gc.ca/diseases-conditions-maladies-affections/disease-maladie/ diabetes-diabete/canrisk/index-eng.php.*

The FBG, A_{1c}, or both are the preferred methods for screening in clinical settings; however, the 75-g OGTT is indicated in those with IFG or when A_{1c} is 6.0% to 6.4%. Screening should be considered at a younger age or be carried out more frequently in individuals who meet the criteria listed in Table 52-12 (CDA, 2013a).

ACUTE INTERVENTION. Acute situations involving the patient with DM include hypoglycemia, DKA, and hyperosmolar hyperglycemic state (HHS). Nursing management for these situations is discussed in more detail later in this chapter. Other areas of acute intervention relate to management during stress, such as during acute illness and surgery.

Stress of Acute Illness and Surgery. Both emotional and physical stress can increase the blood glucose level and result in hyperglycemia. Because it is impossible to totally avoid stress in life, certain situations may require more intense management, such as extra insulin, to maintain glycemic goals and prevent hyperglycemia.

Acute illness, injury, and surgery are situations that may evoke a counter-regulatory hormone response resulting in hyperglycemia. Even minor illnesses such as a viral upper respiratory infection or the flu can cause this. When patients with DM are ill, they should continue with the regular meal plan while increasing the intake of noncarbohydrate-containing fluids, such as broth, water, and other decaffeinated beverages. They should also continue taking OHAs and insulin as prescribed and check

TABLE 52-12   CRITERIA FOR SCREENING IN ASYMPTOMATIC, UNDIAGNOSED INDIVIDUALS

Type 1 Diabetes Mellitus

Screening presumably healthy individuals for the presence of any immune markers (e.g., HLA), outside of a clinical trial setting, is not recommended.

Type 2 Diabetes Mellitus

In asymptomatic, undiagnosed individuals, or those at high risk using a risk calculator, screening* for diabetes should be considered in all individuals at ≥40 yr and, if normal, should be repeated at 3-yr intervals.

Screening should be considered at a younger age, or be carried out more frequently, in individuals who are at very high risk using a risk calculator or who have the following additional risk factors:

- Are members of a high-risk ethnic population (Indigenous or of Latin American, South Asian, Asian, or African descent)
- Are overweight, particularly with abdominal obesity
- Have a first-degree relative with type 2 diabetes
- Have a history of gestational diabetes mellitus
- Have a history of impaired fasting glucose or impaired glucose tolerance
- Have acanthosis nigricans
- Have complications associated with diabetes
- Have delivered a macrosomic infant (>4.4 kg)
- Have dyslipidemia
- Have hypertension
- Have polycystic ovary syndrome
- Have schizophrenia
- Have vascular disease

HLA, human lymphocyte antigen.
*Screening may include fasting blood glucose (FBG), glycated hemoglobin (A$_{1c}$), or both. A 75-g oral glucose tolerance test (OGTT) is indicated when the FBG is 6.1 mmol/L to 6.9 mmol/L or A$_{1c}$ is 6.0% to 6.4%, or both.
Source: Adapted from Canadian Diabetes Association (CDA) Clinical Practice Guidelines Expert Committee. (2013). Clinical practice guidelines for the prevention and management of diabetes in Canada. *Canadian Journal of Diabetes Care, 37*(Suppl 1), S13.

blood glucose at least every 4 hours around the clock. With type 1 DM, if the glucose is greater than 14 mmol/L, urine should be tested for ketones every 3 to 4 hours. Patients should report moderate to large ketone levels to the health care provider.

When the illness causes the patient to eat less than normal, the patient should continue to take OHAs, noninsulin injectables, and insulin as prescribed, while supplementing food intake with carbohydrate-containing fluids. Examples include soups, juices, and regular decaffeinated soft drinks. The health care provider should be notified promptly if the patient is unable to keep anything down, and the patient should go to the emergency department if vomiting occurs more than twice in 12 hours. The patient should understand that medication for DM, including insulin, should not be withheld during times of illness because counter-regulatory mechanisms often increase the blood glucose level dramatically. Food intake is also important during this time because the body requires extra energy to deal with the stress of the illness. Extra insulin may be necessary to meet this demand and to prevent the onset of DKA in the patient with type 1 DM (CDA, 2013a).

During the perioperative period, adjustments in the DM regimen can be planned to ensure glycemic control. For patients undergoing major surgery who require insulin (type 1 or type 2 DM), IV fluids with dextrose and insulin are administered immediately before, during, and after surgery. For patients undergoing minor or moderate surgery who require insulin (type 1 or type 2 DM), recommendations are provided by the physician to reduce the insulin dosage the night before and the day of surgery. For patients taking OHAs who are undergoing major, moderate, or minor surgery, DM medications may be put on hold for as long as 24 hours before the day of surgery, and IV fluids with dextrose and insulin may be administered. The patient should understand that this is a temporary measure and is not to be interpreted as a worsening of DM. Patients who are undergoing surgery or any radiological procedures that involve the use of a contrast medium are instructed to hold their metformin (Glucophage) at the time of or before surgery or the procedure. They will also be instructed not to resume the metformin (Glucophage) until 48 hours after the surgery or the procedure and after their serum creatinine has been checked and is normal (Sanofi-Aventis, 2009).

The nurse caring for an unconscious surgical patient receiving insulin must be alert for signs of hypoglycemia, such as sweating, tachycardia, and tremors. Frequent monitoring of blood glucose will prevent episodes of severe hypoglycemia in such a patient (CDA, 2013a).

AMBULATORY AND HOME CARE. Successful management of DM requires ongoing interaction among the patient, the family, and the health care team. It is important that a DM nurse educator be involved in the care of the patient and the family. This person provides expertise in many areas of specialized care needs.

Because DM is a complex, chronic condition, a great deal of patient contact takes place in outpatient and home settings. The major goal of patient care in these settings is to enable the patient or caregiver to reach an optimal level of independence in self-care activities. Unfortunately, many patients with DM face challenges in reaching these goals. DM increases the risk for other chronic conditions that can affect self-care activities. These include visual impairment, lower extremity problems that affect mobility, and other functional limitations related to cardiovascular disease. Therefore, important nursing functions are to assess the ability of patients and caregivers in such activities as meal preparation, SMBG, safe administration of OHAs, and insulin injection techniques. Assistive devices for self-administration of insulin include syringe magnifiers, vial stabilizers, and dose-preparation aids for people who are visually impaired as well as pill organizers for those taking OHAs. In some cases, the nurse will make referrals to others who can help the patient achieve the self-care goals. These may include a community health nurse, pharmacist, dietitian, occupational therapist, or social worker.

A diagnosis of DM affects the patient in many profound ways. Patients with DM must continually contend with lifestyle choices that affect the food they eat, the activities they engage in, and the demands on their time and energy. In addition, they face the prospect of the devastating complications of this disease. Careful assessment of what it means to the patient to have DM should be the starting point of patient teaching. The nurse can help patients make adjustments by displaying an attitude that is supportive and nonjudgemental. The goals of teaching should be collaboratively determined by the patient and the nurse, based on individual needs as well as therapeutic requirements.

The patient's support system must be identified. The family or other members of the support system need to be involved in teaching so they can care for the patient when self-care is no longer possible. The family and significant others need to be encouraged to provide emotional support and encouragement as the patient deals with the reality of living with a chronic disease.

Insulin Therapy. Nursing responsibilities for the patient receiving insulin include proper administration, assessment of the patient's response to insulin therapy, and education of the patient regarding administration of, adjustment to, and adverse effects of insulin (RNAO, 2009) (Table 52-13). Table 52-6 lists guidelines for the nurse assessing a patient using OHAs and insulin.

Assessment of the patient who is new to insulin administration must include an evaluation of the patient's ability to manage this therapy safely. This includes the ability to understand the interaction of insulin, diet, and activity and to be able to recognize and treat the symptoms of hypoglycemia appropriately. If the patient does not have the cognitive skills to do these things, another responsible person must be identified and educated. The patient or caregiver must also have the cognitive and the manual skills needed to prepare and inject the insulin. If the patient or family lacks these, additional resources will be needed to assist the patient.

Many patients are fearful when they first begin using insulin. Some patients find it difficult to self-inject because they are afraid of needles or the pain associated with an injection. Some are afraid they will hurt themselves by giving too much or too little insulin. And in some cases, the patient believes that using insulin is a "last ditch" effort and that he or she is now in the final stages of the disease process. Therefore, it is important to explore the patient's underlying fears before beginning the teaching (Wang & Yeh, 2012; RNAO, 2009).

Follow-up assessment of the patient who has been using insulin therapy includes an inspection of injection sites for signs of lipodystrophy and other reactions; review of insulin preparation, storage, timing, and injection technique; a history of hypoglycemic episodes; and review of the patient's method for handling hypoglycemic episodes. A review of the patient's recorded blood glucose tests is also important in assessing overall glycemic control.

Oral and Noninsulin Injectable Agents. Nursing responsibilities for the patient taking OHAs and noninsulin injectables are similar to those for the patient taking insulin. Proper administration, assessment of the patient's use of and response to these medications, and education of the patient and the family about OHAs and noninsulin injectables are all part of the nurse's function.

The nurse's assessment can be extremely valuable in determining the most appropriate antihyperglycemic agent for a patient. Factors such as the patient's financial situation, cognitive status, eating habits, home environment, attitude toward DM, and medication history all play a significant role in determining the most appropriate OHA for the individual patient. For example, frail older adults who live alone are at high risk for severe hypoglycemia because low blood glucose is frequently undetected and untreated in this population. This is especially true if the patient has a short-term memory deficit. In these cases, an OHA that does not cause hypoglycemia, or a shorter-acting OHA, would be most appropriate.

Patient education is an essential nursing function when caring for the patient who uses OHAs for blood glucose control. Some patients may assume that their DM is not a serious condition if they are taking "only a pill" for glycemic control. Therefore, the patient should be instructed that these agents will help keep

---

TABLE 52-13 PATIENT & CAREGIVER TEACHING GUIDE

General Guidelines for the Management of Diabetes Mellitus

When teaching patients and caregivers about the management of diabetes mellitus, the nurse should:

Disease Process
- Determine the patient's readiness to learn.
- Include an introduction about the pancreas and the islets of Langerhans.
- Describe how insulin is made and what affects its production.
- Discuss the relationship between insulin and glucose.
- Explain the difference between type 1 and type 2 diabetes.

Physical Activity
- Determine patient's readiness to change.
- Help the patient identify realistic goals and barriers to physical activity.
- Discuss the importance of regular exercise on the management of blood glucose, improvement of cardiovascular function, and general health.

Menu Planning
- Individualize meal plans to accommodate the patient's age, type and duration of diabetes, concurrent medical therapies, treatment goals, values, preferences, needs, culture, lifestyle, economic status, activity level, readiness to change, and abilities.
- Educate the patient on the importance of a well-balanced diet as part of a diabetes management plan.
- Explain the impact of carbohydrates on the glycemic index and blood glucose levels.

Medication Adherence
- Ensure that the patient is well educated on the proper use of insulin (see Table 52-5) noninsulin injectables, and oral agents.
- Account for any limitations or inabilities for self-medication on the patient's part. If necessary, involve the family or caregiver in proper use of medication.
- Discuss all adverse effects and safety issues regarding medication.

Monitoring Blood Glucose
- Individualize the frequency of monitoring to the patient's unique circumstances.
- Teach how to correctly monitor blood glucose levels.
- Include when blood glucose levels should be checked, how to record them, and if appropriate, how to adjust insulin levels accordingly.
- Teach how behaviour and actions affect results.

Risk Reduction
- Ensure that the patient understands and appropriately responds to the signs and symptoms of hypoglycemia and hyperglycemia (see Table 52-15).
- Stress the importance of proper foot care (see Table 52-20), regular eye examinations, and consistent glucose monitoring.
- Inform the patient about the effect that stress can have on blood glucose.

Psychosocial
- Help the patient identify what is important to him or her.
- Advise the patient of resources that are available to facilitate the adjustment and answer questions about living with a chronic condition such as diabetes (see Resources at the end of this chapter).

blood glucose controlled and will help prevent serious long- and short-term complications of DM. Patients should be instructed that OHAs and noninsulin injectables are used in addition to healthy eating and activity as therapy for DM and that they should continue with their meal and activity plans. Patients should not take extra pills if overeating has occurred unless specifically instructed to do so by their health care provider. If the patient uses insulin secretagogues, instructions should be given in regard to prevention, symptom recognition, and management of hypoglycemia.

The patient should also be instructed to contact a health care provider if periods of illness or extreme stress occur. During such a period, insulin therapy may be required to prevent or treat hyperglycemic symptoms and avoid an acute hyperglycemic emergency.

Personal Hygiene. The potential for microvascular complications and infections necessitates diligent skin and dental hygiene practices on the part of the patient. Because of the susceptibility to periodontal disease, daily tooth brushing and flossing should be encouraged in addition to regular visits to the dentist. When dental work must be done, the dentist should be informed that the patient has DM.

Routine care should include an emphasis on foot care, including daily assessment of feet (RNAO, 2013; CDA, 2013a). Problems associated with the feet and the lower extremities are presented later in this chapter. If cuts, scrapes, or burns occur, they should be treated promptly and monitored carefully. The area should be washed, and a nonabrasive or nonirritating antiseptic ointment may be applied. The area should be covered with a dry, sterile pad. If the injury does not begin to heal within 24 hours, or if signs of infection develop, the health care provider should be notified immediately.

Medical Identification and Travel. Patients should be instructed to carry medical identification at all times indicating that they have DM (Figure 52-11). Police, paramedics, and many private citizens are aware of the need to look for this identification when working with someone who is sick or unconscious. Every person with DM should wear a medical alert bracelet or necklace. An identification card can supply valuable information, such as the name of the health care provider and the type and dose of insulin, noninsulin injectables, or OHA.

Travel for a patient with DM requires advance planning. The patient should have a full set of DM care supplies in the carry-on luggage when travelling by plane, train, or bus. This includes blood glucose monitoring equipment, insulin, and pen needles or syringes. When pen needles, syringes, and lancing devices are carried onto a commercial airliner, a letter from the prescribing

health care provider indicating medical necessity may prevent delays at security checkpoints. Screeners should be notified if an insulin pump is used so they can inspect it while it is on the body, rather than remove it.

For patients who use insulin or an OHA that can cause hypoglycemia, snack items and a fast-acting carbohydrate source for treating hypoglycemia should be included in the carry-on luggage and on the person at all times. Extra insulin should be available in case a vial or cartridge breaks or gets lost. In addition, the patient should carry a full day's supply of food to be prepared for possibly cancelled flights, delayed meals, and closed restaurants. If the patient is planning a trip out of the country, it is wise to have a letter from the health care provider explaining that the patient has DM and requires all the materials being transported, particularly pen needles and syringes, for ongoing health care.

Some travel involves significant time changes such as travelling coast to coast or across the International Date Line. The patient should contact the DM health care provider to plan an appropriate meal and insulin schedule. During travel, most patients find it helpful to keep watches set to the time of the city of origin until they reach their destination, and then switch to travel destination time as soon as possible. The key to travel when taking insulin is to know the type of insulin being taken, its onset of action, the anticipated peak time, and mealtimes.

Patient and Caregiver Teaching. The goals of DM self-management education are to enable the patient to become the most active participant in her or his care, while matching level of self-management to the ability of the individual patient. Patients who actively manage their DM care have better outcomes than those who do not. For this reason, an educational approach that facilitates informed decision making on the part of the patient is widely advocated. Sometimes, this is referred to as the *empowerment approach* to education.

Unfortunately, patients can encounter a variety of physical, psychological, emotional, and socioeconomic barriers when it comes to effectively managing their DM. These barriers may include feelings of inadequacy about one's own abilities, unwillingness to make the necessary behavioural changes, ineffective coping strategies, lack of resources, and cognitive deficits. If the patient is not able to manage the disease, a family member may be able to assume part of this role. If the patient or the family cannot make decisions related to DM management, the nurse may refer the patient to a social worker or other resources within the community. These resources can assist the patient and the family in outlining a feasible treatment program that meets their capabilities. Patient and health care provider resources are listed at the end of this chapter.

An assessment of the patient's knowledge of DM and lifestyle preferences is useful in planning a teaching program. Tables 52-13 and 52-14 present guidelines to use for patient and caregiver teaching (See the "Informatics in Practice" box on using gaming for patient teaching). The nurse should assess the patient's knowledge base frequently so that gaps in knowledge or incorrect or inaccurate ideas can be quickly corrected.

Diabetes Canada offers pamphlets, booklets, and a bimonthly magazine called *Diabetes Dialogue*. Chapters of Diabetes Canada are located in all major Canadian cities, and most can be reached by accessing Diabetes Canada online. Diabetes Canada also publishes research and education materials and sponsors conferences for health care providers concerned with DM education, research, and management of patients. The *2013 Clinical Practice*

I have DIABETES

If unconscious or behaving abnormally, I may be having a reaction associated with diabetes or its treatment.

If I can swallow, give me a sweet drink, orange juice, LifeSavers, or low-fat milk.

If I do not recover promptly, call a physician or send me to the hospital.

If I am unconscious or cannot swallow, do not attempt to give me anything by mouth, but call 911 or send me to the hospital immediately.

FIGURE 52-11 Medical Alerts. A patient with diabetes should carry a card and wear a bracelet or necklace that indicates diabetes. If the patient with diabetes is unconscious, these measures will ensure prompt and appropriate attention.

TABLE 52-14   **PATIENT & CAREGIVER TEACHING GUIDE**

Instructions for Patients With Diabetes Mellitus

Do	Do Not	Do	Do Not
Blood Glucose		**Nutrition**	
• Monitor your blood glucose at home and record results in a log. • Take your insulin, OHA, or noninsulin injectable (or any combination) as prescribed. • Rotate injection site areas weekly. • Obtain an A_{1c} blood test every 3–6 mo as an indicator of your long-term blood glucose control. • Know signs and symptoms of hypoglycemia and hyperglycemia. • Carry some form of rapid-acting glucose at all times so you can treat hypoglycemia quickly. • Instruct family members in the use of glucagon administration in the case of emergencies owing to severe hypoglycemia.	• Skip doses of your insulin, especially when you are sick. • Run out of insulin. • Ignore the symptoms of hypoglycemia and hyperglycemia.	• Follow a healthy eating plan, and eat regular meals at regular times. • Choose foods low in saturated and trans-fats and high in fibre. • Limit the amount of alcohol you drink. • Know your cholesterol level.	• Drink excessive amounts of alcohol because this may lead to unpredictable low blood glucose reactions and high triglycerides. • Follow a fad diet. • Drink regular pop or lots of fruit juices.
		Other Guidelines	
		• Obtain an annual eye examination by an ophthalmologist. • Obtain annual urine testing for protein. • Examine your feet at home, daily. • Change socks daily. • Trim nails straight across. • Wear well-fitting shoes to help prevent foot injury. Break in new shoes gradually. • Always carry identification that says you have diabetes. • Have other medical problems treated, especially high blood pressure and high cholesterol. • Quit smoking. • Have an annual influenza vaccination.	• Smoke cigarettes. • Go barefoot. • Put baby oil or lotion between your toes. • Ignore the signs of infection. • Apply hot or cold directly to your feet. • Wear tight socks, garters, or elastics or knee-highs.
Exercise			
• Learn how exercise and food affect your blood glucose levels. • Begin an exercise program after approval from a health care provider.	• Forget that exercise will lower your blood glucose level. • Exercise if your blood glucose levels are very elevated. This may lead to a temporary worsening of your blood glucose levels.		

OHA, oral antihyperglycemic agent.

Guidelines for the Prevention and Management of Diabetes in Canada were released in the spring of 2013 and updated guidelines are released every 5 years (see the Resources at the end of this chapter). Prepared under the leadership of the Clinical and Scientific Section of the Canadian Diabetes Association/Diabetes Canada, the guidelines represent the contributions of more than 99 experts from a broad range of health care disciplines. These experts have evaluated and graded the international literature on the best evidence to guide screening, prevention, diagnosis, care, management, and education for Canadians living with type 1 and type 2 DM and GDM. Diabetes Canada also gives recognition to education programs that meet the international standards of DM education and can provide a list of these programs. Pharmaceutical and diagnostic companies specializing in DM-related products also have promotions and free educational materials for patients and health care providers.

EVALUATION

The expected outcomes for the patient with DM are addressed in Nursing Care Plan (NCP) 51-1, available on the Evolve website.

COMPLEMENTARY & ALTERNATIVE THERAPIES

Herbs and Supplements That May Affect Glucose Levels

Possible Hypoglycemic Herbs and Supplements*
• Aloe, alpha-lipoic acid, fish oils, goldenseal, bilberry eleuthero, ginseng, milk thistle, Chinese cinnamon (Cinnamomum cassia) chromium, garlic, and sage

Possible Hyperglycemic Herbs and Supplements*
• St. John's wort, celery seed, rosemary, and melatonin

Nursing Implications
• It is very important that patients with diabetes consult with their health care providers before using natural health products such as herbs, probiotics, or nutritional supplements. Patients who use herbs should monitor their blood glucose levels carefully and regularly. The Canadian Diabetes Association (CDA) Clinical Practice Guidelines Expert Committee does not recommend the use of natural health products for the management of diabetes as there is insufficient evidence regarding its safety and efficacy (CDA, 2013a).

*www.naturalstandard.com

TABLE 52-15 COMPARISON OF HYPERGLYCEMIA AND HYPOGLYCEMIA

Hyperglycemia	Hypoglycemia	Hyperglycemia	Hypoglycemia
Manifestations*		**Treatment**	
• Abdominal cramps • Blurred vision • Elevated blood glucose† • Glycosuria • Headache • Increase in appetite followed by lack of appetite • Increase in urination • Nausea and vomiting • Progression to DKA or HHS • Weakness, fatigue	• Blood glucose <4.0 mmol/L • Changes in vision • Cold, clammy skin • Emotional changes • Faintness, dizziness • Headache • Hunger • Nervousness, tremors • Numbness of fingers, toes, mouth • Rapid heartbeat • Seizures, coma • Unsteady gait, slurred speech	• Check blood glucose frequently; check urine for ketones; record results • Continuance of OHA or insulin as ordered; may need increase in dose • Get medical care • Hourly drinking of fluids • IV fluids may be necessary	• Discussion with health care provider about insulin or OHA dosage • Follow-up with snack if regular meal more than 1 hr away, and contact health care provider if no effect • Immediate ingestion of 15–20 g of simple carbohydrates • Ingestion of another 15–20 g of simple carbohydrates in 15 min if no relief obtained
Causes		**Preventive Measures**	
• Corticosteroids • Emotional, physical stress • Illness, infection • Inactivity • Poor absorption or lack of insulin • Too little or no diabetes medication • Too much food	• Alcohol intake without food • Diabetes medication or food taken at wrong time • Loss of weight without change in medication • Too little food—delayed, omitted, inadequate intake • Too much diabetic medication • Too much exercise without compensation • Use of β-adrenergic blockers interfering with recognition of symptoms	• Accurate administration of insulin, noninsulin injectables, and OHA • Adherence to sick-day rules when ill • Checking of blood for glucose as ordered • Contacting of health care provider regarding ketonuria • Maintenance of diet • Maintenance of good personal hygiene • Taking prescribed dose of medication at proper time • Wearing medical alert bracelet (diabetes)	• Ability to recognize and know symptoms and treat them immediately • Accurate administration of insulin, noninsulin injectables, and OHA • Carrying a snack of simple carbohydrates • Checking blood glucose as ordered • Education of friends, family, fellow employees about symptoms and treatment • Ingestion of all recommended foods at proper time • Provision of compensation for exercise • Taking prescribed dose of medication at proper time • Wearing medical alert bracelet (diabetes)

DKA, diabetic ketoacidosis; *HHS*, hyperosmolar hyperglycemic state; *IV*, intravenous; *OHA*, oral antihyperglycemic agent.
*There is usually a gradual onset of symptoms in hyperglycemia and a rapid onset in hypoglycemia.
†Specific clinical manifestations related to elevated levels of blood glucose vary according to the patient.

INFORMATICS IN PRACTICE

Patient Teaching Using Gaming

- Teaching is a critical part of nursing care for patients with diabetes. It is possible to put some fun into patient teaching by using gaming applications.
- Patients can try an application with a quiz-show format. The patient answers questions about diabetes and then compares his or her answers in real time to those of other players. The questions (e.g., How does exercise affect insulin?) are written to help the patient learn to manage diabetes on a daily basis.
- Players in online simulations become either a caregiver to or a patient with type 1 DM. Players earn rewards by properly managing blood glucose levels.

ACUTE COMPLICATIONS OF DIABETES MELLITUS

Acute complications of DM arise from events associated with *hyperglycemia* or *hypoglycemia*. Hypoglycemia is also referred to as an *insulin reaction* or *low blood glucose*. It is important for the health care provider to be able to distinguish between hyperglycemia and hypoglycemia because hypoglycemia worsens rapidly and constitutes a serious threat if action is not immediately taken. Table 52-15 compares manifestations, causes, treatment, and prevention of hyperglycemia and hypoglycemia.

DIABETIC KETOACIDOSIS

Etiology and Pathophysiology

Diabetic ketoacidosis (DKA) is an acute metabolic complication of DM occurring when fats are metabolized in the absence of insulin. It is caused by a profound deficiency of insulin and is characterized by hyperglycemia, ketosis, metabolic acidosis, and dehydration (volume depletion). It is most likely to occur in people with type 1 DM but may be seen in type 2 DM in conditions of severe illness or stress, when the pancreas cannot meet the extra demand for insulin. Precipitating factors include illness, infection, inadequate insulin dosage, insulin omission, undiagnosed type 1 DM, and poor self-management.

When the circulating supply of insulin is insufficient, glucose cannot be properly used for energy, so the body breaks down fat stores as a secondary source of fuel (Figure 52-12). Ketones are acidic by-products of fat metabolism that can cause serious problems when they become excessive in the blood. Ketosis alters

PATHOPHYSIOLOGY MAP

FIGURE 52-12 Metabolic events leading to diabetic ketoacidosis. Source: Kumar, V., Abbas, A. K., Fausto, N., et al. (2010). *Robbins and Cotran pathologic basis of disease.* (8th ed., p. 1144, Figure 24-39). Philadelphia: Saunders.

the pH balance, causing metabolic acidosis to develop. Ketonuria is a process that begins when ketone bodies are excreted in the urine. During this process, electrolytes become depleted as cations (sodium, potassium, and ammonium salts) are eliminated along with the anionic ketones in an attempt to maintain electrical neutrality.

Insulin deficiency impairs protein synthesis and causes excessive protein degradation. This condition results in nitrogen losses from the tissues. Insulin deficiency also stimulates the production of glucose from amino acids (from proteins) in the liver and leads to further hyperglycemia. But because there is a deficiency of insulin, the additional glucose cannot be used and the blood glucose level rises further, adding to the osmotic diuresis. Untreated, this condition leads to severe depletion of sodium, potassium, chloride, magnesium, and phosphate. Potassium is most affected in DKA. Acidosis causes hydrogen ions to move from the extracellular fluid to the intracellular space. Hydrogen movement into the cell promotes potassium movement out of the cell into the extracellular compartment, resulting in severe potassium depletion in the intracellular space.

Most of the shifted extracellular potassium is lost in the urine because of osmotic diuresis. The serum potassium can be normal or even high, but this finding is misleading because there is an intracellular and total body loss of potassium (CDA, 2013a).

Vomiting caused by the acidosis results in more fluid and electrolyte losses. Eventually, hypovolemia, followed by shock, ensues.

Renal failure may eventually occur from hypovolemic shock. This result causes the retention of ketones and glucose, and the metabolic acidosis progresses. Untreated, the patient becomes comatose as a result of dehydration, electrolyte imbalance, and acidosis. If the condition is not treated, death is inevitable.

Clinical Manifestations

Signs and symptoms of DKA include polyuria and polydipsia, leading to dehydration. Dehydration is manifested by poor skin turgor, dry mucous membranes, tachycardia, and orthostatic hypotension. Early symptoms may include lethargy and weakness. As the patient becomes severely dehydrated, the skin becomes dry and loose, and the eye sockets become sunken. Nausea and vomiting are common symptoms. Abdominal pain is occasionally seen. This may be owing to dehydration of muscle tissue, delayed gastric emptying, and ileus induced by electrolyte disturbance and metabolic acidosis (Sanuth, Bidlencik, & Volk, 2014). Finally, Kussmaul's respiration (rapid, deep breathing associated with dyspnea) is the body's attempt to reverse metabolic acidosis through the exhalation of excess carbon dioxide. Acetone is noted on the breath as a sweet, fruity odour. (See Chapter 19 for a discussion of respiratory compensation of metabolic acidosis.) Laboratory findings include a blood glucose level above 14 mmol/L, arterial blood pH below 7.35, serum bicarbonate level less than 15 mmol/L, anion gap greater than 12 mmol/L, and ketones in the blood and urine (CDA, 2013a).

Collaborative Care

Before the advent of self-monitoring of blood glucose and β hydroxybutyrate (capillary blood ketones), all patients with DKA required hospitalization for treatment. Today, hospitalization may not be required. In instances in which fluid and electrolyte imbalances are not severe and blood glucose levels can be safely monitored at home, early stages of DKA may be managed on an outpatient basis (Table 52-16). However, the decision about where the patient is managed must also take other factors into consideration. These factors include the presence of fever, nausea, vomiting, and diarrhea; altered mental status; nature of the cause of the ketoacidosis; and availability of frequent communication (every few hours) with the health care provider.

Regardless of the setting in which it occurs, DKA is a serious condition that proceeds rapidly and must be treated promptly. (Table 52-17 describes the emergency management of a patient with DKA.) Because fluid imbalance is potentially life-threatening, the initial goal of therapy is to establish IV access and begin fluid and electrolyte replacement. Typically, the initial fluid therapy regimen comprises an infusion of 0.45% or 0.9% NaCl IV solution at a rate to restore urine output to 30 to 60 mL/hr and to raise blood pressure. When blood glucose levels approach 14 mmol/L, 5% dextrose is added to the fluid regimen to prevent hypoglycemia (Westerberg, 2013; CDA, 2013a).

The aim of fluid and electrolyte therapy is to replace extracellular and intracellular water and to correct deficits of sodium, chloride, bicarbonate, potassium, phosphate, magnesium, and nitrogen. Early potassium replacement is essential because hypokalemia is a significant cause of preventable death during treatment of DKA. Although initial serum potassium may be normal or high, levels can rapidly decrease once therapy starts because insulin drives potassium into the cells, leading to life-threatening hypokalemia.

IV insulin administration is therapy directed toward correcting hyperglycemia and hyperketonemia. Insulin therapy is withheld until fluid resuscitation is under way and serum potassium is greater than 3.3 mmol/L because insulin allows water and potassium to enter the cell along with glucose and can lead to a depletion of vascular volume and hypokalemia. Initially, a bolus of insulin is delivered, followed by a continuous infusion (CDA, 2013a).

TABLE 52-16 COLLABORATIVE CARE

Diabetic Ketoacidosis (DKA) and Hyperosmolar Hyperglycemic State (HHS)

Diagnostic
- History and physical examination
- Blood studies, including immediate blood glucose, complete blood count, ketones, pH, electrolytes, blood urea nitrogen, arterial blood gases
- Urinalysis, including specific gravity, pH, glucose, ketones

Collaborative Therapy
- Administration of IV fluids
- Assessment of blood and urine for ketones
- Assessment of blood glucose levels
- Assessment of cardiovascular and respiratory status
- Assessment of mental status
- Central venous pressure monitoring (if indicated)
- ECG monitoring
- Electrolyte replacement
- IV administration of short-acting insulin
- Recording of intake and output

ECG, electrocardiogram; IV, intravenous.

SAFETY ALERT
- Too-rapid administration of IV fluid and a rapid lowering of serum glucose can lead to cerebral edema.

HYPEROSMOLAR HYPERGLYCEMIC STATE

Hyperosmolar hyperglycemic state (HHS) is a life-threatening syndrome that can occur in the patient with DM who is able to produce enough insulin to prevent DKA but not enough to prevent severe hyperglycemia, osmotic diuresis, and extracellular fluid depletion (Figure 52-13). HHS is less common than DKA. The main difference between HHS and DKA is that the patient with HHS usually has enough circulating insulin so that ketoacidosis does not occur. Because HHS produces fewer symptoms in the earlier stages, blood glucose levels can climb quite high before the problem is recognized. The higher blood glucose levels increase serum osmolality and produce more-severe neurological manifestations, such as somnolence, coma, seizures, hemiparesis, and aphasia. HHS often occurs in the older-adult patient with type 2 DM and is often related to impaired thirst sensation, a functional inability to replace fluids, or both. There is usually a history of inadequate fluid intake, increasing mental depression, and polyuria. Laboratory values in HHS include blood glucose greater than 34 mmol/L and a marked increase in serum osmolality. Ketone bodies are absent or minimal in both blood and urine.

Collaborative Care

HHS constitutes a medical emergency and has a high mortality rate. Therapy is similar to that for the treatment of DKA and includes immediate IV administration of either 0.9% or 0.45% NaCl at a rate that is dependent on cardiac status and the degree of fluid volume deficit. Regular insulin is given by IV bolus, followed by an infusion after fluid replacement therapy is instituted to aid in reducing the hyperglycemia. When blood glucose levels fall to approximately 14 mmol/L, IV fluids containing glucose are administered to prevent hypoglycemia. Electrolytes are monitored and replaced as needed. Hypokalemia is not as

TABLE 52-17 EMERGENCY MANAGEMENT

Diabetic Ketoacidosis

Etiology	Assessment Findings	Interventions
- Change in diet, insulin, or exercise regimen - Dehydration owing to illness with vomiting or diarrhea - Inadequate treatment of existing diabetes mellitus - Infection - Insulin not taken as prescribed, or omitted - Undiagnosed diabetes mellitus	- Abdominal pain - Breath odour of acetone - Dry mouth - Eyes that appear sunken - Fever - Flushed, dry skin - Glucosuria and ketonuria - Gradually increasing restlessness, confusion, lethargy - Laboured breathing (Kussmaul's respiration) - Nausea and vomiting - Oral or vaginal *Candida albicans* (yeast infection) - Rapid, weak pulse; orthostatic hypotension - Serum glucose >14 mmol/L - Thirst - Urinary frequency	**Initial** - Administer IV sodium bicarbonate if severe acidosis (pH <7.0). - Administer oxygen as per physician's order. - Administer potassium IV to correct hypokalemia. - Begin continuous regular insulin drip 0.1 units/kg/hr, as needed. - Begin fluid resuscitation with 0.9% NaCl solution until BP stabilized and urine output 30–60 mL/hr. - Ensure patent airway. - Establish IV access with large-bore catheter. - Identify history of diabetes, time of last food, and time and amount of last insulin injection. **Ongoing Monitoring** - Assess breath sounds for fluid overload. - Monitor serum glucose, pH, and serum potassium. - Monitor vital signs, level of consciousness, cardiac rhythm, oxygen saturation, and urine output.

BP, blood pressure; IV, intravenous.

PATHOPHYSIOLOGY MAP

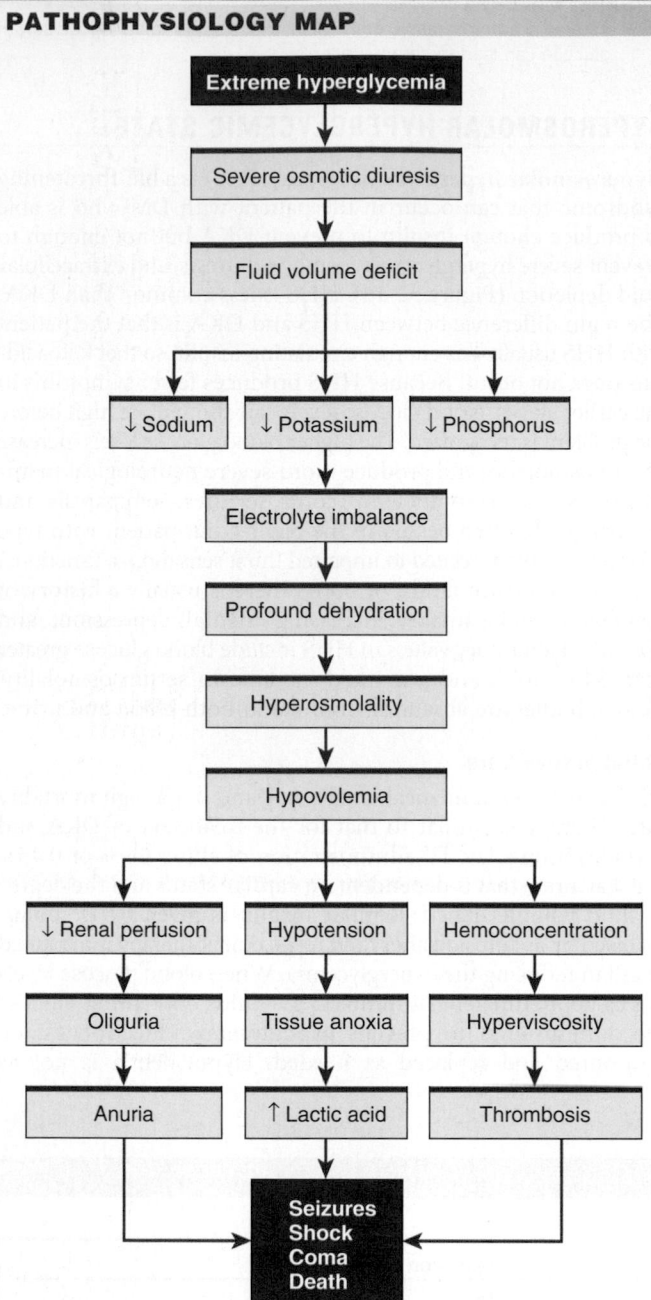

FIGURE 52-13 Pathophysiology of hyperosmolar hyperglycemic state (HHS). Source: Redrawn from Urden, L. D., Stacy, K. M., & Lough, M. E. (2014). *Critical care nursing: Diagnosis and management* (7th ed., p. 828, Figure 33-4). St. Louis: Mosby.

significant in HHS as it is in DKA, although fluid losses may result in milder potassium deficits that necessitate replacement. Vital signs, intake and output, tissue turgor, laboratory values, and cardiac monitoring are assessed to monitor the efficacy of fluid and electrolyte replacement. Patients with renal or cardiac compromise require special monitoring to avoid fluid overload during fluid replacement. This includes monitoring of serum osmolality and frequent assessment of cardiac, renal, and neurological status (CDA, 2013a).

The management for both DKA and HHS is similar, except that HHS necessitates greater fluid replacement (see Table 52-16).

Once the patient is stabilized, attempts to detect and correct the underlying precipitating cause should be initiated.

NURSING MANAGEMENT
DIABETIC KETOACIDOSIS AND HYPEROSMOLAR HYPERGLYCEMIC STATE

When hospitalized, the patient is closely monitored with appropriate blood and urine tests. The nurse is responsible for monitoring blood glucose and urine for output and ketones as well as for using laboratory data to support care.

Nursing responsibilities include monitoring the administration of IV fluids to correct dehydration, insulin therapy to reduce blood glucose and serum ketones, and electrolytes to correct electrolyte imbalance; assessment of renal status; assessment of the cardiopulmonary status related to hydration and electrolyte levels; and monitoring of the level of consciousness.

The nurse must also monitor the signs of potassium imbalance resulting from hypoinsulinemia and osmotic diuresis (see Chapter 19). When treatment for hyperglycemia is begun with insulin, serum potassium levels may decrease rapidly because potassium moves into the cells once insulin becomes available. This movement of potassium into and out of extracellular fluid influences cardiac functioning. Cardiac monitoring is a useful aid in detecting hyperkalemia and hypokalemia because characteristic changes indicating potassium excess or deficit are observable on electrocardiogram (ECG) tracings (see Chapter 19, Figure 19-14). Vital signs should be assessed often to determine the presence of fever, hypovolemic shock, tachycardia, and Kussmaul's respiration (Westerberg, 2013).

HYPOGLYCEMIA

Hypoglycemia, or low blood glucose, occurs when there is too much insulin in proportion to available glucose in the blood. This causes the blood glucose level to drop to less than 4 mmol/L. Once plasma glucose drops to this level, neuroendocrine hormones are released and the autonomic nervous system is activated. Suppression of insulin secretion and production of glucagon and epinephrine provide defence against hypoglycemia. Epinephrine release causes manifestations that include diaphoresis, tremors, hunger, nervousness, anxiety, pallor, and palpitations. As a primary energy source, the brain requires a constant supply of glucose in sufficient quantities to function properly; therefore, hypoglycemia can eventually affect cognitive functioning. These manifestations are referred to as *neuroglycopenic signs* and may include irritability, visual disturbances, difficulty speaking, stupor, confusion, and coma. Manifestations of hypoglycemia can mimic alcohol intoxication. Untreated hypoglycemia can progress to loss of consciousness, seizures, coma, and death.

Hypoglycemic unawareness (or *asymptomatic hypoglycemia*) is a condition in which patients do not experience the usual autonomic nervous system warning signs and symptoms of hypoglycemia, increasing their risk for dangerously low blood glucose levels. This condition is often related to autonomic neuropathy of DM that interferes with the secretion of counter-regulatory hormones that produce these symptoms. Older-adult patients and patients who use β-adrenergic blockers are also at risk for hypoglycemic unawareness. For patients with risk factors for hypoglycemic unawareness, it is usually not safe to aim for tight blood glucose control owing to the increased potential of hypoglycemia. They are usually managed with blood glucose goals that are somewhat higher than patients who are able to detect and manage the onset of hypoglycemia.

Hypoglycemic symptoms may occur when a very high blood glucose level falls too rapidly, for example, a blood glucose level of 16 mmol/L falling quickly to 8 mmol/L. Although the blood glucose level is above normal by definition and measurement, the sudden metabolic shift can evoke hypoglycemic symptoms. Too-vigorous management of hyperglycemia with insulin can induce this type of situation.

Causes of hypoglycemia are often related to a mismatch in the timing of food intake and the peak action of insulin or OHAs that increase endogenous insulin secretion. The balance between blood glucose and insulin can be disrupted by the administration of too much insulin or medication, the ingestion of insufficient carbohydrates, delaying the time of eating, and performing unusual amounts of exercise. Insulin reactions can occur at any time, but most occur when the OHA or insulin is at its peak of action. Although hypoglycemia is more common with insulin therapy, it can occur with OHAs and may be severe and persist for an extended time because of the longer duration of action.

NURSING AND COLLABORATIVE MANAGEMENT HYPOGLYCEMIA

Hypoglycemia can usually be quickly reversed with effective and rapid treatment. At the first sign of hypoglycemia, the blood glucose should be checked if possible (Table 52-18). If it is below

TABLE 52-18 COLLABORATIVE CARE

Hypoglycemia

Diagnostic
- Capillary blood glucose (evaluated and reported on an emergency basis)
- History (if possible) and physical examination

Collaborative Therapy
- Determination of cause of hypoglycemia (after correction of condition)

Conscious Patient With Mild to Moderate Hypoglycemia
- Administration of 15–20 g of fast-acting (simple) carbohydrate (e.g., commercial dextrose products [per label instructions]; 175 mL of fruit juice or regular soft drink; 6–8 Life Savers; for patient taking acarbose: 15 mL (1 tbsp) syrup or honey, or 125–150 mL low-fat milk, or dextrose tabs (because the absorption of glucose itself is not affected)*
- Recheck of blood glucose in 15 minutes; if no improvement, repetition of treatment of 15–20 g of carbohydrate
- Administration of additional food or longer-acting combination such as carbohydrate plus protein or fat (e.g., crackers with peanut butter or cheese) after symptoms subside, if meal is longer than 1 hr away
- Immediate notification of health care provider or emergency service (if patient is outside hospital) if symptoms do not subside after two or three administrations of fast-acting carbohydrate

Severe Hypoglycemia or Unconscious Patient
- Intravenous administration of 20–50 mL of dextrose 50% in water (D50W) given over 1–3 min
- Subcutaneous or intramuscular injection of 1 mg glucagon

*Canadian Diabetes Association (CDA) Clinical Practice Guidelines Expert Committee. (2013). 2013 Clinical practice guidelines for the prevention and management of diabetes in Canada. *Canadian Journal of Diabetes Care, 37*(Suppl), S70.

4 mmol/L, the patient should begin treatment immediately. If the blood glucose is above 4 mmol/L, other causes of the signs and symptoms should be investigated. If the patient has manifestations of hypoglycemia and monitoring equipment is not available, hypoglycemia should be assumed and treatment should be initiated.

Hypoglycemia is treated by ingesting 15 to 20 g of a simple (fast-acting) carbohydrate, such as three or four glucose tablets, 175 mL of fruit juice or regular soft drink, or six Life Savers candies. Commercial products such as gels or tablets containing specific amounts of glucose are convenient for carrying in a purse or pocket to be used in such situations.

Treatment with sweet foods containing fat, such as chocolate bars, cookies, and ice cream, should be avoided because fat will slow down the absorption of the sugar and delay the response to treatment. Overtreatment with large quantities of simple carbohydrates should be avoided to prevent a rapid fluctuation to hyperglycemia. A prompt but moderate approach is best. Blood glucose should be checked 15 minutes after the initial treatment and repeated if blood glucose remains lower than 4 mmol/L. Once the blood glucose is greater than 4 mmol/L, the patient should eat a snack if the next regularly scheduled meal is more than an hour away in order to prevent hypoglycemia from recurring. Good snacks include one protein and one starch choice such as a peanut butter sandwich, cheese and crackers, or cereal and milk. Blood glucose should also be checked again about 45 minutes after eating the snack to ensure that hypoglycemia is not recurring (CDA, 2013a).

If there is no significant improvement in the patient's condition after two to three doses of 15 to 20 g of simple carbohydrate or if the patient is not alert enough to swallow, 1 mg of glucagon may be administered by intramuscular or subcutaneous injection. Glucagon stimulates a strong hepatic response to convert glycogen to glucose, making glucose rapidly available. Rebound hypoglycemia is a potential adverse effect of glucagon. Having the patient ingest a starch snack after recovery may prevent this from happening. Patients with minimal glycogen stores will not respond to glucagon. These include patients with alcohol-related hepatic disease, starvation, and adrenal insufficiency. In an acute care setting, patients with hypoglycemia are treated with 20 to 50 mL of 50% dextrose by IV push.

Once the hypoglycemic episode has resolved, the nurse should explore with the patient the reasons why the situation developed. This assessment may indicate the need for additional education of the patient and the family to prevent future episodes of hypoglycemia. The danger of hypoglycemic episodes must be stressed; safety concerns include risks such as driving a motorized vehicle or bicycle, operating heavy machinery, and falls; these episodes also have a long-term impact upon memory.

CHRONIC COMPLICATIONS OF DIABETES MELLITUS

Chronic complications of DM are primarily those of end-organ disease that result from damage to the large and small blood vessels (angiopathy) secondary to chronic hyperglycemia (Figure 52-14). Angiopathy, or blood vessel disease, is estimated to account for the majority of deaths among patients with DM. These chronic blood vessel dysfunctions are divided into two categories: *macrovascular complications* and *microvascular complications*.

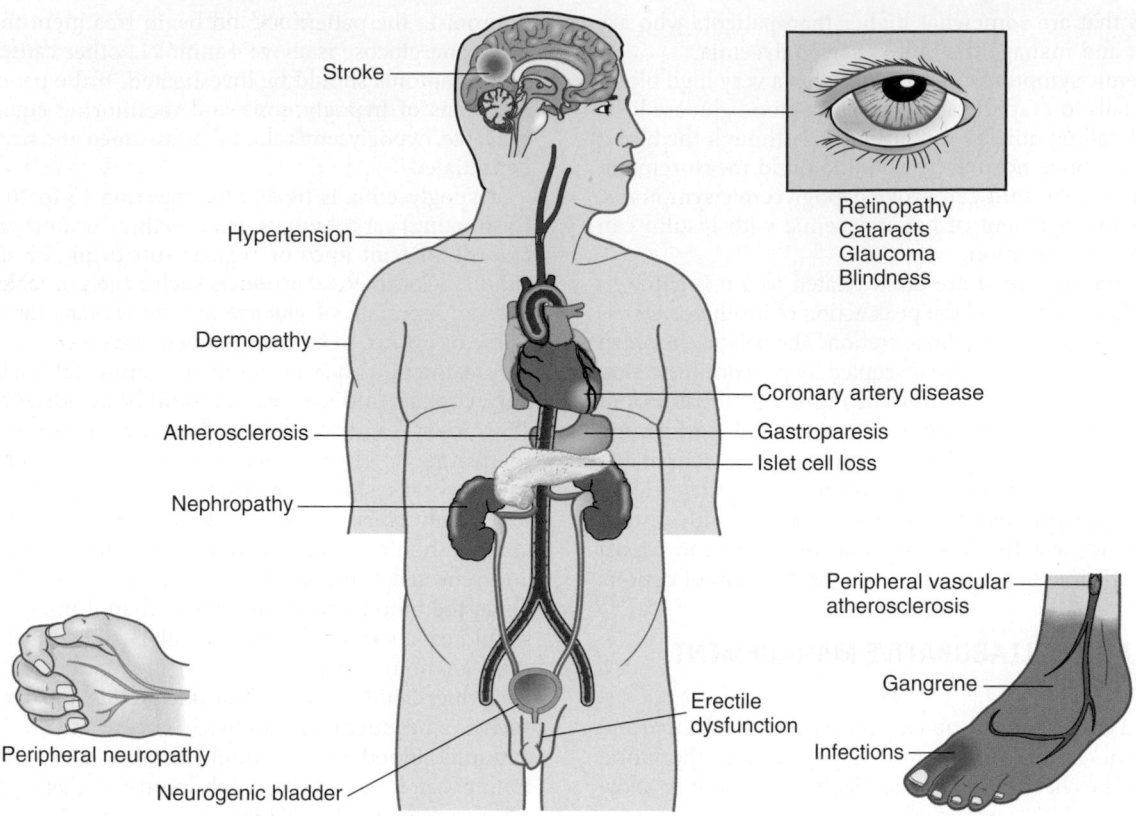

FIGURE 52-14 Long-term complications of diabetes mellitus. Source: Kumar, V., Abbas, A. K., & Aster, J. (2015). *Robbins and Cotran pathologic basis of disease* (9th ed., p. 1116, Figure 24-34). Philadelphia: Saunders.

Several theories exist as to how and why chronic hyperglycemia damages cells and tissues. Possible causes include (1) the accumulation of damaging by-products of glucose metabolism, such as sorbitol, which is associated with damage to nerve cells; (2) the formation of abnormal glucose molecules in the basement membrane of small blood vessels such as those that circulate to the eye and the kidney; and (3) a derangement called *oxidative stress* in RBC function that leads to a decrease in oxygenation to the tissues.

The Diabetes Control and Complication Trial (DCCT) was a landmark study that has greatly influenced DM management since its results were announced in 1993 (DCCT Research Group, 1993). This study demonstrated that, in patients with type 1 DM, the risk for microvascular complications could be significantly reduced by keeping blood glucose levels as near to normal as possible for as much of the time as possible (intensive insulin therapy). In this study, patients were randomly assigned to one of two groups: intensive or standard treatment. The intensive treatment group took three or more insulin injections a day or used an insulin pump and tested their blood glucose four to five times a day. The patients in the standard treatment group took one to two injections a day and tested their blood glucose once or twice a day. The average A_{1c} in the intensive treatment group was 7.2%; in the standard treatment group, it was 9%. (The normal range for A_{1c} in a person without DM is 4% to 6%.) The results showed that the subjects in the intensive therapy group reduced their risk for the development of retinopathy, nephropathy, and peripheral neuropathy. The adverse effects associated with intensive therapy were an increase in frequency of hypoglycemic episodes and weight gain.

Based on the findings of the DCCT Research Group (1993), the CDA *Clinical Practice Guidelines* (2013a) included recommendations for treatment goals to maintain blood glucose levels as near to normal as possible in most people with diabetes. Specific targets for individual patients must take into account the risk for severe or undetected hypoglycemia as an adverse effect of tight glucose control.

The United Kingdom Prospective Diabetes Study (UKPDS) demonstrated that intensive treatment of type 2 DM with OHAs alone, OHAs in combination with insulin, or insulin alone, can also significantly lower the risk of developing DM-related microvascular complications such as retinopathy, nephropathy, and neuropathy. The findings from this study showed a 25% reduction of microvascular disease in subjects who maintained long-term glycemic control, including a 1% reduction in A_{1c}, regardless of the initial value (UKPDS, 1998).

Because of the devastating effects of long-term complications, patients with DM require scheduled and ongoing monitoring for the detection and prevention of chronic complications. The recommendations for ongoing evaluation are listed in Table 52-19. It is imperative that patients understand the importance of regular follow-up examinations (CDA, 2013a).

Macrovascular Complications

Macrovascular complications are diseases of the large and medium-sized blood vessels; these complications occur with greater frequency and with an earlier onset in people with DM. Although atherosclerotic plaque formation is believed to have a genetic origin, its development seems to be promoted by the altered lipid metabolism common to DM. Tight glucose control

TABLE 52-19 MONITORING FOR LONG-TERM COMPLICATIONS OF DIABETES MELLITUS*

Complication	Type of Examination	Frequency
Retinopathy	Funduscopic–dilated-eye examination by experienced professional	*Type 1:* annually, starting 5 yr after onset of diabetes *Type 2:* at diagnosis; then every 1–2 yr if normal
Nephropathy	Random urinalysis for albumin-to-creatinine ratio (ACR), serum creatinine converted to eGFR	*Type 1:* annually; if no CKD, starting 5 yr after onset of diabetes *Type 2:* at diagnosis and then annually if normal; if CKD present, ACR and eGFR at least every 6 mo
Neuropathy (foot and lower extremities)	Visual examination of foot	Daily by patient Every visit by health care provider
	Comprehensive foot examination: assessment of structural abnormalities, neuropathy (monofilament, tuning fork), vascular disease (peripheral pulses), ulcerations, and evidence of infection	*Type 1:* annually, starting 5 yr after onset of diabetes *Type 2:* at diagnosis and annually
Cardiovascular disease	Blood pressure	Every visit
	Lipid panel	At the time of diagnosis, and then every 1–3 yr
	ECG	Baseline and every 2 yr if >40 yr; >30 yr and duration >15 yr; end organ damage; cardiac risk factors

CKD, chronic kidney disease; *ECG,* electrocardiogram; *eGFR,* estimated glomerular filtration rate.
*Based on the recommendations of the Canadian Diabetes Association (CDA) Clinical Practice Guidelines Expert Committee. (2013). 2013 Clinical practice guidelines for the prevention and management of diabetes in Canada. *Canadian Journal of Diabetes Care, 37*(Suppl 1), S199.

may help delay the atherosclerotic process (DCCT Research Group, 1993; UKPDS, 1998). Macrovascular diseases include cerebro-vascular, cardiovascular, and peripheral vascular disease. Adults with DM have two to three times the risk for heart and cerebro-vascular disease of those without DM (CDA, 2013a). Although genetic makeup cannot be altered, strategies for vascular protection are recommended and include health behaviour interventions such as healthy eating, weight modification, smoking cessation, and increased physical activity. Smoking is associated with significantly increased risks for total mortality, cardiovascular events, and lower extremity amputation in those with DM. The cessation of smoking reduces cardiovascular risk and the risk for renal disease and improves glycemic control (CDA, 2013a; Pan, Wang, Talaei, et al., 2015). (Smoking is discussed in Chapter 11.) The addition of an angiotensin-converting enzyme (ACE) inhibitor; antiplatelet therapy such as acetylsalicylic acid (ASA;

Aspirin); and lipid, blood pressure, and glycemic control are pharmacological interventions that protect the heart and will reduce mortality risk by 50% in patients with type 2 DM (Gaede, Lund-Anderson, Parving, et al., 2008). Optimizing blood pressure control in patients with DM is significant for the prevention of cardiovascular and renal disease. The target blood pressure for people with DM is 130/80 mm Hg.

Insulin resistance seems to play an important role in the development of cardiovascular disease and is implicated in the pathogenesis of essential hypertension and dyslipidemia. The term *metabolic syndrome* is applied to the clinical association of insulin resistance, hypertension, and increased very-low-density lipoprotein (VLDL) and decreased HDL cholesterol concentrations. The role of insulin resistance in the pathogenesis of cardiovascular disease is not well understood, but it seems to combine with dyslipidemia in contributing to greater risk for cardiovascular disease in patients with DM. All patients with DM should be screened for dyslipidemia at the time DM is diagnosed. Most people with DM are considered at high risk for a vascular event (CDA, 2013a).

Lifestyle changes such as healthy eating and exercise are first-line interventions to achieve an optimal lipid profile. If unsuccessful, lipid-lowering therapy such as statins, fibrates, or both may be added to optimize lipid levels, thereby reducing risk for a vascular event.

Microvascular Complications

Microvascular complications result from thickening of the vessel membranes in the capillaries and arterioles in response to conditions of chronic hyperglycemia. They differ from macrovascular complications in that they are specific to DM. Although microangiopathy can be found throughout the body, the areas most noticeably affected are the eyes (retinopathy), the kidneys (nephropathy), the nerves (neuropathy), and the skin (dermopathy). Thickening of the basement membrane has been found in some people with type 2 DM before or at the time of diagnosis or before the onset of symptoms of DM. However, clinical manifestations may not appear until 10 to 20 years after the onset of DM, depending on the glycemic control over that period of time as measured by A_{1c}.

DIABETIC RETINOPATHY

Etiology and Pathophysiology

Diabetic retinopathy refers to the process of microvascular damage to the blood vessels in the retina as a result of chronic hyperglycemia, presence of nephropathy, and hypertension in patients with DM. After 15 years with DM, nearly all patients with type 1 DM and 80% with type 2 DM will have some degree of retinal disease. Diabetic retinopathy is estimated to be the most common cause of new cases of blindness in people of working age (CDA, 2013a; ADA, 2011).

Retinopathy can be classified as nonproliferative or proliferative. In *nonproliferative retinopathy,* the most common form, partial occlusion of the small blood vessels in the retina causes the development of microaneurysms in the capillary walls. The walls of these microaneurysms are so weak that capillary fluid leaks out, causing retinal edema and eventually hard exudates or intraretinal hemorrhages. Vision may be affected if the macula is involved.

Proliferative retinopathy, the most severe form, involves the retina and the vitreous. When retinal capillaries become occluded, the body compensates by forming new blood vessels to supply the retina with blood, a pathological process known as *neovascularization*. These new vessels are extremely fragile and hemorrhage easily, producing vitreous contraction. Eventually, light is prevented from reaching the retina as the vessels become torn and bleed into the vitreous cavity. The patient sees black or red spots or lines. If these new blood vessels pull the retina while the vitreous contracts, causing a tear, partial or complete retinal detachment will occur. If the macula is involved, vision is lost. Without treatment, more than half of patients with proliferative diabetic retinopathy will be blind.

Collaborative Care

The earliest and most treatable stages of diabetic retinopathy often produce no changes in the vision. Because of this, the patient with DM must have regular dilated-eye examinations by an ophthalmologist or a specially trained optometrist for early detection and treatment. The best approach to the management of diabetic eye disease is to prevent it by maintaining good glycemic and blood pressure control.

The most common forms of treatment for diabetic retinopathy are early laser photocoagulation therapy of the retina, vitrectomy and intraocular injection of pharmacological agents. Photocoagulation by laser destroys the ischemic areas of the retina that produce growth factors that encourage neovascularization, thereby preventing further vision loss, and reduces legal blindness up to 90% in people with severe nonproliferative retinopathy and proliferative retinopathy (CDA, 2013a). (Photocoagulation is discussed in Chapter 24.)

Vitrectomy is the aspiration of blood, membrane, and fibres from the inside of the eye through a small incision just behind the cornea. Vitrectomy is indicated in patients with advanced proliferative retinopathy with vitreous hemorrhage or retinal detachment of the macula. (Vitrectomy is discussed in Chapter 24.)

Recent research has identified the importance of vascular endothelial growth factor (VEFG) in the development of diabetic retinopathy. Three anti-VEFG drugs are now widely used in Canada to treat diabetic retinopathy: aflibercept (Eylea), bevacizumab (Avastin), and ranibizumab (Lucentis) (Canadian Agency for Drugs and Technologies in Health [CADTH], 2016). Bevacizumab (Avastin) is used in an expanded or off-label manner but has not been approved by Health Canada for this purpose (CADTH, 2016).

People with DM are also prone to other visual problems. Glaucoma occurs as a result of the occlusion of the outflow channels, secondary to neovascularization. This type of glaucoma is difficult to treat and often results in blindness. Cataracts develop at an earlier age and progress more rapidly in people with DM.

NEPHROPATHY

Diabetic nephropathy is a microvascular complication associated with damage to the small blood vessels that supply the glomeruli of the kidney. It is the leading cause of end-stage renal disease (ESRD) in Canada. The risk for nephropathy is similar in patients with either type 1 or type 2 DM. Risk factors for the development of diabetic nephropathy include hypertension, genetic predisposition, smoking, and chronic hyperglycemia. Results of the DCCT and UKPDS studies have demonstrated that kidney disease can be significantly reduced when near-normal blood glucose

control is achieved and maintained (DCCT Research Group, 1993; UKPDS, 1998).

Hypertension significantly accelerates the progression of diabetic nephropathy and retinopathy and the risk for stroke. Therefore, aggressive blood pressure management is indicated for all patients with DM. ACE-inhibitor drugs (e.g., ramipril [Altace]) and angiotensin II receptor blockers (e.g., losartan [Cozaar]) are commonly prescribed to patients with DM because they are effective blood pressure–lowering agents with few adverse effects. In addition, both these drugs are often prescribed to patients with DM even when they are not hypertensive because drugs in either class have a protective effect on the kidney that prevents the progression of diabetic nephropathy independent of hypertension control (CDA, 2013a). (See Chapter 35 for a discussion of hypertension and Chapter 49 for a discussion of renal failure.)

Standards for the prevention and detection of nephropathy in patients with DM include yearly screening for the presence of microalbuminuria (MAU). This test detects kidney damage at an earlier stage than the standard dipstick test for macroprotein in the urine. Screening for MAU should be performed using a random urine for albumin-to-creatinine ratio (ACR) and serum creatinine for estimated glomerular filtration rate (eGFR). A 24-hour urine collection for determination of creatinine clearance and serum creatinine may be performed when there is doubt about the accuracy of an eGFR (CDA, 2013a).

NEUROPATHY

Diabetic neuropathy is nerve damage that occurs because of the metabolic derangements associated with DM. About 40% to 50% of patients with DM have some degree of neuropathy, with neurological complications occurring equally in type 1 and type 2 DM (CDA, 2013a). The most common type of neuropathy affecting people with DM is peripheral sensory neuropathy. This condition can lead to the loss of protective sensation in the lower extremities, and, coupled with other factors, peripheral sensory neuropathy significantly increases the risk for complications that can result in a lower limb amputation. Although, amputation rates for people with diabetes have decreased in the past decade, they remain very high compared with rates for those without diabetes. (CDA, 2013a).

Etiology and Pathophysiology

The pathophysiological processes of diabetic neuropathy are not well understood. Several theories exist, including metabolic, vascular, and autoimmune elements. The prevailing theory suggests that persistent hyperglycemia leads to an accumulation of sorbitol and fructose in the nerves that causes damage by an unknown mechanism. The result is reduced nerve conduction and demyelinization. Ischemia in blood vessels damaged by chronic hyperglycemia that supply the peripheral nerves is also implicated in the development of diabetic neuropathy. Neuropathy can precede, accompany, or follow the diagnosis of DM.

Classification

The two major categories of diabetic neuropathy affect the peripheral nervous system: sensory neuropathy (which affects the somatic division) and autonomic neuropathy (which affects the autonomic division). Each of these types can take on several forms.

Sensory Neuropathy. The most common form of sensory polyneuropathy is distal symmetrical neuropathy, which affects the hands, the feet, or both, bilaterally. This condition is sometimes referred to as *stocking-glove neuropathy*. Characteristics of distal symmetrical neuropathy include paresthesias, abnormal sensations, pain, and loss of sensation. The paresthesias may be associated with tingling, burning, and itching sensations. The patient may report a feeling of walking on pillows or numb feet. At times, the skin becomes so sensitive (hyperesthesia) that even light pressure from bed sheets cannot be tolerated. Complete or partial loss of sensitivity to touch and temperature is common. The pain, which is often described as burning, cramping, crushing, or tearing, is usually worse at night and may occur only at that time. Foot injury and ulcerations can occur without the patient ever having pain (Figure 52-15). Neuropathy can also cause atrophy of the small muscles of the hands and feet, causing deformity and limiting fine movement.

Control of blood glucose is the only treatment for diabetic neuropathy. It is effective in many, but not all, cases. Drug therapy may be used to treat neuropathic symptoms, particularly pain. Medications commonly used include topical creams (e.g., capsaicin), tricyclic antidepressants (e.g., amitriptyline [Elavil]), selective serotonin and norepinephrine reuptake inhibitors (e.g., duloxetine [Cymbalta]), and antiseizure medications (e.g., gabapentin [Neurontin]; pregabalin [Lyrica]). Capsaicin is a moderately effective topical cream made from chili peppers. It depletes the accumulation of pain-mediating chemicals in the peripheral sensory neurons. The cream is applied with gloves three to four times a day. There is usually an increase in symptoms at the start of therapy, which is followed by relief of pain in 2 to 3 weeks. Tricyclic antidepressants are also moderately effective in treating the symptoms of diabetic neuropathy. They work by inhibiting the reuptake of norepinephrine and serotonin, which are neurotransmitters that are believed to play a role in the transmission of pain through the spinal cord (Kaur, Hota, Bhansali, et al., 2011). Duloxetine is thought to relieve pain by increasing the levels of serotonin and norepinephrine, which improves the body's ability to regulate pain. Although gabapentin has been found to be effective in treating the pain of diabetic neuropathy, its mechanism of action is not well understood.

FIGURE 52-15 Neuropathy: neurotrophic ulceration. Source: Urden, L. D., Stacy, K. M., & Lough, M. E. (2009). *Thelan's critical care nursing: Diagnosis and management* (6th ed.). St. Louis: Mosby.

Autonomic Neuropathy. Autonomic neuropathy can affect nearly all body systems and lead to hypoglycemic unawareness, bowel incontinence and diarrhea, and urinary retention. Delayed gastric emptying (gastro-paresis) is a complication of autonomic neuropathy that can produce anorexia, nausea, vomiting, gastro-esophageal reflux, and persistent feelings of fullness. Gastro-paresis can trigger hypoglycemia by delaying food absorption. Cardiovascular abnormalities associated with autonomic neuropathy are postural hypotension, resting tachycardia, and "silent" or painless myocardial infarction. A patient with postural hypotension should be instructed to change slowly from a lying or sitting position to a standing position.

DM can affect sexual function in men and women. Erectile dysfunction in men with diabetes is well recognized and common, often being the first manifestation of autonomic failure. Erectile dysfunction associated with DM is believed to result from damage to the sacral parasympathetic nerves. Determining whether this problem is of organic or psychological origin is an important part of the assessment. Decreased libido is a problem for some women with DM. Monilial and nonspecific vaginitis are also common. Organic erectile dysfunction or sexual dysfunction in either the male or the female patient requires sensitive therapeutic counselling for both the patient and the patient's partner (Bella, Lee, Carrier, et al., 2015). (See Chapter 57 for a further discussion of erectile dysfunction.)

A neurogenic bladder may develop as sensation in the inner bladder wall decreases, causing urinary retention. A patient with retention has infrequent voiding, difficulty in voiding, and a weak stream of urine. Emptying the bladder every 3 hours in a sitting position helps prevent stasis and subsequent infection. Tightening the abdominal muscles during voiding and using Credé manoeuvre (mild massage downward over the lower abdomen and bladder) may also help with complete bladder emptying. Cholinergic agonist drugs such as bethanechol (Duvoid) may be used. The patient may also have to learn self-catheterization (see Chapter 48).

COMPLICATIONS OF THE FOOT AND THE LOWER EXTREMITY

In Canada, people with diabetes are approximately 20 times more likely to be hospitalized for nontraumatic lower limb amputations than those without diabetes (Kuhnke, Botros, Elliott, et al., 2013). The development of diabetic foot complications is a multifactorial process (RNAO, 2013). Complications result from a combination of microvascular and macrovascular diseases that place the patient at risk for injury and serious infection that may lead to amputation (Figure 52-16). Sensory neuropathy and peripheral vascular disease (PVD) are risk factors, and clotting abnormalities, impaired immune function, and autonomic neuropathy also play important roles. Smoking is deleterious to the health of lower extremity blood vessels and increases the risk for amputation.

Sensory neuropathy is a major risk factor for lower extremity amputation in the person with DM. Loss of protective sensation (LOPS) often prevents the patient from becoming aware that a foot injury has occurred. Improper footwear and injury from stepping on foreign objects while barefoot are common causes of undetected foot injury in the person with LOPS (Alexiadou & Doupis, 2012). Because the primary risk factor for lower extremity amputation is LOPS, annual screening using a *monofilament* is an extremely important preventive measure. This is done by applying a thin, flexible filament to several spots on the

FIGURE 52-16 The necrotic toe developed as a complication of diabetes. **A,** Before amputation. **B,** After amputation. Source: Chew, S. L., & Leslie, D. (2006). *Clinical endocrinology and diabetes: An illustrated colour text.* Edinburgh: Churchill Livingstone.

TABLE 52-20	PATIENT & CAREGIVER TEACHING GUIDE

Foot Care

The following instructions should be included when teaching the patient and caregiver about foot care

1. Wash feet daily with a mild soap and warm water. Test water temperature with a thermometer or hands first.
2. Pat feet dry gently, especially between toes.
3. Examine feet daily for cuts; blisters; swelling; and red, tender areas. Do not depend on feeling sores. If eyesight is poor, have others inspect feet.
4. Use lanolin on feet to prevent skin from drying and cracking. Do not apply between toes.
5. Do not use commercial remedies or sharp blades to remove calluses or corns.
6. Cleanse cuts with warm water and mild soap, covering with clean dressing. Do not use iodine, rubbing alcohol, or strong adhesives.
7. Report skin infections or nonhealing sores to health care provider immediately.
8. Cut and file toenails even, with the rounded contour of the toes. Do not cut down corners. The best time to trim nails is after a shower or bath. See a foot care specialist if advice or treatment is needed.
9. Separate overlapping toes with cotton or lamb's wool.
10. Avoid open-toe, open-heel, and high-heel shoes. Leather shoes are preferred to synthetic ones. Wear slippers at home and shoes on the beach. Do not go barefoot. Shake out shoes before putting on.
11. Wear clean, absorbent (cotton or wool) socks or stockings that have not been mended. Coloured socks must be colourfast.
12. Do not wear socks or stockings that leave impressions, hindering circulation.
13. Do not use hot water bottles or heating pads to warm feet. Wear socks for warmth.
14. Guard against frostbite.
15. Exercise feet daily either by walking or by flexing and extending feet in suspended position. Avoid prolonged sitting, standing, and crossing of legs.

Source: Canadian Diabetes Association (CDA) Clinical Practice Guidelines Expert Committee. (2013). 2013 Clinical practice guidelines for the prevention and management of diabetes in Canada. *Canadian Journal of Diabetes, 37*(Suppl.1), S1–S227.

plantar surface of the foot and toes and asking the patient to report if it is felt. Insensitivity to a 10-g Semmes-Weinstein monofilament has been shown to greatly increase the risk for diabetic foot ulcers that can lead to amputation. If the patient has LOPS, aggressive measures must be taken to teach the patient how to prevent foot ulceration. These measures include the selection of proper footwear, including prescription shoes. Other measures are to carefully avoid injury to the foot, practise diligent skin and nail care, inspect the foot thoroughly each day, and treat small problems promptly (CDA, 2013a; RNAO, 2013).

PVD increases the risk for amputation by causing a reduction in blood flow to the lower extremities. When blood flow is decreased, oxygen, white blood cells, and vital nutrients are not available to the tissues. Therefore, wounds take longer to heal and the risk for infection increases. Signs of PVD include intermittent claudication, pain at rest, cold feet, loss of hair, delayed capillary filling, and dependent rubor (redness of the skin that occurs when the extremity is in a dependent position). The disease is diagnosed by history, ankle–brachial index (ABI), and angiography. Management includes control or reduction of risk factors, particularly smoking, high saturated fat intake, and hypertension. Femoral bypass or graft surgery is indicated in some patients. Proper care of the feet is essential for patients with PVD. Guidelines for patient teaching are listed in Table 52-20.

The Doppler instrument is used to perform the ABI to diagnose the presence or degree of PVD. Similar to an electronic stethoscope, this device amplifies sound. The procedure is noninvasive and can measure blood pressure and blood flow velocity in the lower extremities. It can indicate areas of stenosis or occlusion and is useful as an indicator of the need for additional vascular tests. To determine location and extent of PVD, an angiography can be completed. Angiography is an invasive procedure and it provides information on the actual blood vessel condition.

Proper care of a diabetic foot ulcer is critical to prevention of infections. Management requires an interdisciplinary approach that addresses glycemic control, infection, lower extremity vascular status, and local wound care (CDA, 2013a). The fundamentals of good wound care involve an optimal wound environment, off-loading of the ulcer site, and in nonischemic wounds, regular debridement of nonviable tissue.

Neuropathic arthropathy, or *Charcot foot,* results in ligament softening and bony deformities that ultimately lead to joint dysfunction and foot drop. The pathogenesis of Charcot foot is not clear, but it is likely owing to a combination of mechanical and vascular factors resulting from peripheral neuropathy and is mediated through an uncontrolled inflammation in the foot (Hordon, 2011; Rogers, Frykberg, Armstrong, et al., 2011; CDA, 2013a). Changes that occur with Charcot foot happen gradually and create an abnormal distribution of weight over the foot, further increasing the chances of developing an ulcer on the plantar aspect of the foot as new pressure points emerge. Neuropathic ulcers resemble a "BB-shot" or "punched-out" wound and are usually painless. This high-risk foot complication requires immediate attention such as foot radiographic studies and referral to a high-risk foot team of chiropody, orthopedic surgery, and plastic surgery specialists. Infection and subsequent amputation is a danger and necessitates the long-term use of antibiotics and weeks of avoidance of weight bearing on the affected limb (CDA, 2013a). Foot deformity should be recognized early and proper footwear fitted before ulceration occurs.

INTEGUMENTARY COMPLICATIONS

The skin is often affected in patients with DM. *Acanthosis nigricans* is a dark, coarse, thickened skin predominantly seen in flexures and on the neck. Acanthosis nigricans is a risk factor for type 2 DM and is associated with hyperinsulinemia and insulin resistance (CDA, 2013a; Atwa et al., 2014). Skin disorders such as diabetic dermopathy and necrobiosis lipoidica diabeticorum are attributed to microangiopathy. Shin spots are brown spots located on the anterior surfaces of the lower extremities. They are harmless and painless and initially measure less than 1 cm in diameter. *Necrobiosis lipoidica diabeticorum* (Figure 52-17) is believed to be the result of the breakdown of collagen in the skin. It usually appears as red-yellow lesions, with atrophic skin that becomes shiny and transparent, revealing tiny blood vessels under the surface. Because the thin skin is prone to injury, special care must be taken to protect affected areas from injury and ulceration. This condition is not common, but it may appear before other clinical signs or symptoms of DM. It is more frequently seen in young women. *Granuloma annulare,* associated mainly with type 1 DM, is probably autoimmune in nature and forms partial rings of papules, often on the dorsal surface of hands and feet.

INFECTION

A patient with DM is more susceptible to infections than other patients are. The mechanisms for this phenomenon include a defect in the mobilization of inflammatory cells and an impairment of phagocytosis by neutrophils and monocytes. Organisms

FIGURE 52-17 Necrobiosis lipoidica diabeticorum. Source: Chew, S. L., & Leslie, D. (2006). *Clinical endocrinology and diabetes: An illustrated colour text.* Edinburgh: Churchill Livingstone.

such as yeast thrive in a high–blood glucose environment. Thus, recurring or persistent infections such as *Candida albicans,* as well as boils and furuncles, in the undiagnosed patient often lead the health care provider to suspect DM. Loss of sensation (peripheral neuropathy) may delay the detection of an infection in the feet.

Persistent glycosuria may predispose to bladder infections, especially in patients with a neurogenic bladder. Decreased circulation resulting from angiopathy can prevent or delay the immune response. Antibiotic therapy has prevented infection from being a major cause of death in patients with DM. The treatment of infections must be prompt and vigorous.

AGE-RELATED CONSIDERATIONS

DIABETES MELLITUS

The prevalence of DM increases with age. A major reason for this is that the process of aging is associated with a reduction in beta-cell function, decreased insulin sensitivity, altered carbohydrate metabolism, and a progressive increase in A_{1c} (CDA, 2013a). Aging is also associated with a number of conditions that are more likely to be treated with medications that impair insulin action (e.g., corticosteroids, antihypertensives, phenothiazines). Undiagnosed and untreated DM is more common in the older adult, partly because many of the normal physiological changes of aging, such as visual changes and decreased glomerular filtration, resemble those of DM.

Although good glycemic control is important to people of all ages with DM, several factors are taken into account when determining glycemic goals for an older adult. One is that hypoglycemic unawareness is more common in this age group, making these patients more likely to suffer adverse consequences from blood glucose–lowering therapy. They may also have delayed psychomotor function that could interfere with the ability to treat hypoglycemia. Other factors to consider in establishing glycemic goals for the older-adult patient include the patient's own desire for treatment and other coexisting medical problems such as cognitive impairment. Compounding the challenge is that DM has been found to contribute to a greater rate of decline of cognitive function. Although it is generally agreed that treatment aiming for the same glycemic targets is indicated for otherwise healthy older adults as well as younger persons with DM to prevent acute complications and avoid unpleasant symptoms, strict glycemic control should be based on the degree of frailty (CDA, 2013a). Patients with moderate or advanced frailty have a reduced life expectancy and thus should have a less stringent glycemic target A_{1c} of <8.5%, as recommended by CDA 2013 clinical practice guidelines.

As for any group, healthy eating and exercise are recommended as therapy for older-adult patients with DM. This plan should take into account functional limitations that may interfere with physical activity and the ability to prepare meals. Because of the physiological changes that occur with aging, the therapeutic outcome for the older adult with DM who receives OHAs may be altered. The short-acting insulin secretagogues (e.g., repaglinide [GlucoNorm]) are usually well tolerated and appear to have fewer adverse effects and fewer drug interaction problems than longer-acting insulin secretagogues (glyburide [Diabeta]). Other OHAs described earlier in this chapter may also be used in older-adult patients with DM. Insulin therapy may be instituted if OHAs are not effective. However, it is important to recognize that older-adult patients are more likely to have limitations in manual dexterity and visual acuity, both of which are necessary for accurate insulin administration (CDA, 2013a).

Patient teaching should be based on the individual's needs, using a slower pace with simple printed materials. It is important to include family or a support person in the teaching. The patient education issues for the older-adult patient include those related to vision, mobility, cognitive status, memory, functional ability, financial and social situation, the effect of multiple medications, eating habits, the potential for undetected hypoglycemia, and quality-of-life issues.

CASE STUDY

Diabetic Ketoacidosis

Patient Profile

Hector DeSouza, a 34-year-old male, was admitted to the emergency department after he was found unconscious in his apartment by his wife.

Source: KreativeKolors/ Shutterstock .com.

Subjective Data (Provided by Wife)
- Was diagnosed with type 1 DM 12 months ago
- Has had difficulty coping with the diagnosis and missed his last 2 follow-up appointments with his diabetes team.
- Was taking 50 units of insulin daily: 5 units of insulin lispro (Humalog) with breakfast, 5 units with lunch, and 10 units with dinner, plus 30 units of insulin glargine (Lantus) at bedtime
- Has history of gastro-enteritis for 1 week, with vomiting and anorexia
- Stopped taking insulin 2 days ago when he was unable to eat

Objective Data
Physical Examination
- Breathing is deep and rapid
- Acetone smell on breath
- Skin flushed and dry

Diagnostic Studies
- Blood glucose level of 40.5 mmol/L
- Blood pH of 7.26

Discussion Questions
1. Briefly explain the pathophysiology of the development of diabetic ketoacidosis (DKA) in this patient.
2. What clinical manifestations of DKA does Mr. DeSouza exhibit?
3. What factors precipitated Mr. DeSouza's DKA?
4. *Priority decision:* What is the priority nursing intervention for Mr. DeSouza?
5. What distinguishes this case history from one of hyperosmolar hyperglycemic state (HHS) or hypoglycemia?
6. *Priority decision:* What is the priority teaching that should be done with Mr. DeSouza and his family?
7. What role should Mr. DeSouza's wife have in the management of his diabetes?
8. *Priority decision:* Based on the assessment data presented, what are the priority nursing diagnoses? Are there any collaborative problems?
9. *Evidence-informed practice:* Mr. DeSouza's wife asks if she should have given her husband insulin when he got sick. How should the nurse respond?

evolve

Answers are available on *http://evolve.elsevier.com/Canada/Lewis/medsurg*

REVIEW QUESTIONS

The number of the question corresponds to the same-numbered objective at the beginning of the chapter.

1. Polydipsia and polyuria related to diabetes mellitus are primarily caused by which of the following?
   a. The release of ketones from cells during fat metabolism
   b. Fluid shifts resulting from the osmotic effect of hyperglycemia
   c. Damage to the kidneys from exposure to high levels of glucose
   d. Changes in red blood cells resulting from attachment of excessive glucose to hemoglobin

2. Which statement would be correct for a client with type 2 diabetes mellitus who is admitted to the hospital with pneumonia?
   a. The client must receive insulin therapy to prevent the development of ketoacidosis.
   b. The client has islet-cell antibodies that have destroyed the ability of the pancreas to produce insulin.
   c. The client has minimal or absent endogenous insulin secretion and requires daily insulin injections.
   d. The client may have sufficient endogenous insulin to prevent ketosis but is at risk for development of hyperosmolar hyperglycemic state.

3. Analyze the following diagnostic findings for a client with type 2 diabetes. Which of the following results will need further assessment?

   a. A$_{1c}$ 9.0%
   b. FBG 7.2 mmol/L
   c. BP 126/80
   d. LDL cholesterol of 2.1 mmol/L

4. Which statement by the client with type 2 diabetes is accurate?
   a. "I am supposed to have a meal or snack if I drink alcohol."
   b. "I am not allowed to eat any sweets because of my diabetes."
   c. "I do not need to watch what I eat because my diabetes is not the bad kind."
   d. "The amount of fat in my diet is not important. Only carbohydrates raise my blood sugar."

5. The nurse is caring for a client with newly diagnosed type 1 diabetes. What information is essential to include in the client teaching before discharge from the hospital? *(Select all that apply)*
   a. Insulin administration
   b. Elimination of sugar from diet
   c. Need to reduce physical activity
   d. Use of a portable blood glucose monitor
   e. Hypoglycemia prevention, symptoms, and treatment

6. What is the priority action for the nurse to take if the client with type 2 diabetes complains of blurred vision and irritability?
   a. Call the physician.
   b. Administer insulin as ordered.

c. Check the client's blood glucose level.

d. Assess for other neurological symptoms.

7. A client with diabetes has a serum glucose level of 36 mmol/L and is unresponsive. Following assessment of the client, the nurse suspects diabetic ketoacidosis (DKA) rather than hyperosmolar hyperglycemic state (HHS), based on which finding?

a. Polyuria

b. Severe dehydration

c. Rapid, deep respirations

d. Decreased serum potassium

8. Which of the following are appropriate therapies for clients with diabetes mellitus? *(Select all that apply)*

a. Use of diuretics to treat nephropathy

b. Use of angiotensin-converting enzyme inhibitors to treat nephropathy

c. Use of serotonin agonists to decrease appetite

d. Use of laser photocoagulation to treat retinopathy

e. Use of statins to treat dyslipidemia

1. b; 2. d; 3. a; 4. a; 5. a, d, e; 6. c; 7. c; 8. b, d, e.

ⓔvolve

For even more review questions, visit *http://evolve.elsevier.com/Canada/ Lewis/medsurg.*

REFERENCES

Alexiadou, K., & Doupis, J. (2012). Management of diabetic foot ulcers. *Diabetes Therapy, 3*(4), 1–15. doi:10.1007/ s13300-012-0004-9.

American Association of Diabetes Educators (AADE). (2011). *Insulin pump therapy: Best practices in choosing and using infusion devices.* 1–28. Retrieved from *http://www.infusion -set.com/media/12119192/12-30-11-aade_insulin_whitepaper _print.pdf.*

American Diabetes Association (ADA). (2008). Nutrition recommendations and interventions for diabetes. *Diabetes Care, 31*(Suppl. 1), S61–S78. doi:10.2337/dc08-S061. (Seminal).

American Diabetes Association (ADA). (2011). Position statement: Standards of medical care in diabetes. *Diabetes Care, 34*(Suppl. 1), S11–S61. doi:10.2337/dc11-S011.

American Diabetes Association (ADA). (2013). Position statement: Nutrition therapy recommendations for the management of adults with diabetes. *Diabetes Care, 36*(1), 3821–3842. doi:10.2337/dc13-2042.

American Diabetes Association (ADA). (2015). Standards of medical care in diabetes. *Diabetes Care, 38*(Suppl. 1), S1–S90. doi:10.2337/ dc15-S003.

Atwa, M., Emaraz, A., Balata, M., et al. (2014). Serum leptin, adiponectin, and resistin among adult patients with acanthosis nigricans: Correlations with insulin resistance and risk factors for cardiovascular disease. *International Journal of Dermatology, 53*(10), e410–e420. doi:10.1111/ijd.12340.

Beckers, S., De Freitas, F., Zegers, D., et al. (2011). Identification and functional characterization of a missense mutation in resistin in two patients with severe obesity and insulin resistance. *European Journal of Endocrinology, 164*(6), 927–936. doi:10.1530/ EJE-10-1080.

Bella, A., Lee, J., Carrier, S., et al. (2015). 2015 CUA Practice guidelines for erectile dysfunction. *Canadian Urological Association Journal, 9*(1-2), 23–29. doi:10.5489/cuaj.2699.

Bristol-Myers Squibb (BMS) Canada. (2011). *Product monograph: Onglyza.* Montreal: Author.

Canadian Agency for Drugs and Technologies in Health (CADTH). (2016). *Anti-vascular endothelial growth factor drugs for retinal conditions.* Retrieved from *https://www.cadth.ca/sites/default/files/ pdf/TR0009_anti-vegf-in-brief-e.pdf.*

Canadian Diabetes Association (CDA). (2013a). Clinical Practice Guidelines Expert Committee. 2013 Clinical practice guidelines for the prevention and management of diabetes in Canada. *Canadian Journal of Diabetes, 37*(Suppl. 1), S1–S227.

Canadian Diabetes Association (CDA). (2013b). *Just the basics: Tips for health eating. Diabetes prevention and management.* Toronto: Author. Retrieved from *http://guidelines.diabetes.ca/cdacpg/media/ documents/patient-resources/just-the-basics-healthy-eating.pdf.*

Canadian Diabetes Association (CDA). (2015). *Diabetes charter for Canada. Diabetes in Canada.* Retrieved from *https:// www.diabetes.ca/getmedia/513a0f6c-b1c9-4e56-a77c-6a492bf7350f/ diabetes-charter-backgrounder-national-english.pdf.aspx.*

Canadian Diabetes Association (CDA) and Diabetes Quebec (DQ). (2011). *Diabetes: Canada at the tipping point charting a new path.* Toronto: Author. Retrieved from *http://www.diabetes.ca/ documents/get-involved/WEB_Eng.CDA_Report_.pdf.*

Canadian Diabetes Association Clinical Practice Guidelines Expert Committee. (2016). Pharmacologic management of type 2 diabetes: 2016 interim update. *Canadian Journal of Diabetes, 40*(2016), 193–195.

Cheng, A. (2011). The rule of 3's: Insulin use in type 2 diabetes. *Canadian Diabetes, 24*(1), 3–9.

Diabetes Control and Complications Trial (DCCT) Research Group. (1993). The effect of intensive treatment of diabetes on the development and progression of long-term complications in insulin-dependent diabetes mellitus. *New England Journal of Medicine, 329*(14), 977–986. (Seminal).

Diabetes Prevention Program (DPP) Research Group. (2002). Reduction in the incidence of type 2 diabetes with lifestyle intervention or metformin. *New England Journal of Medicine, 346*(6), 393–403. doi:10.2337/diacare.25.12.2165. (Seminal).

Eli Lilly Canada. (2011). *Product monograph: Byetta.* Toronto: Author.

Forum for Injection Technique (FIT) Canada (2011). *Recommendations for best practice in injection technique.* Retrieved from *http://www.bd.com/resource.aspx?IDX =25063.*

Gaede, P., Lund-Anderson, H., Parving, H., et al. (2008). Effects of multifactorial intervention on mortality in type 2 diabetes. *New England Journal of Medicine, 358*(6), 580–591. doi:10.1056/ NEJMoa0706245. (Seminal).

Harper, W., Clement, M., Goldenberg, R., et al. (2015). Policies, guidelines and consensus statements: Pharmacologic management of type 2 diabetes—2015 interim update. *Canadian Journal of Diabetes, 39*(4), 250–252. doi:10.1016/j.jcjd.2015.05.009.

Health Canada. (2011). *Eating well with Canada's food guide.* Ottawa: Author. Retrieved from *http://www.hc-sc.gc.ca/fn-an/ food-guide-aliment/index-eng.php.*

Hordon, L. (2011). *Diabetic neuropathic arthropathy. 2012 UpToDate.* Philadelphia: Wolters-Kluwer Health. Retrieved from *http://*

www.uptodate.com/contents/diabetic-neuropathic-arthropathy *#H24803269.*

International Diabetes Federation (IDF). (2015). *Diabetes Atlas* (7th ed.). Retrieved from *http://www.diabetesatlas.org.*

Ismail-Beigi, F. (2012). Glycemic management of type 2 diabetes mellitus. *New England Journal of Medicine, 366*(14), 1319–1327. doi:10.1056/NEJMcp1013127.

Kahn, S., Haffner, S., Heise, M., et al. (2006). Glycemic durability of rosiglitazone, metformin or glyburide monotherapy. *New England Journal of Medicine, 355*(23), 2427–2443. doi:10.1056/ NEJMoa066224. (Classic).

Kaur, H., Hota, D., Bhansali, A., et al. (2011). A comparative evaluation of amitriptyline and duloxetine in painful diabetic neuropathy: A randomized, double-blind, cross-over clinical trial. *Diabetes Care, 34*(4), 818–822. doi:10.2337/dc10-1793.

Kuhnke, J., Botros, M., Elliott, J., et al. (2013). The case for diabetic foot screening. *Diabetic Foot Canada, 1*(2), 8–14.

Martens, P., Barlett, J., Prior, H., et al. (2011). What is the comparative health status and associated risk factors for the Métis? A population-based study in Manitoba, Canada. *BMC Public Health, 11*(1), 814. doi:10.1186/1471-2458-11-814.

Moisan, J., Turgeon, M., Desjardins, O., et al. (2013). Comparative safety of antipsychotics: Another look at the risk of diabetes. *Canadian Journal of Psychiatry, 58*(4), 218–224.

Neeland, I., Turer, A., Ayers, C., et al. (2012). Dysfunctional adiposity and the risk of prediabetes and type 2 diabetes in obese adults. *JAMA: The Journal of the American Medical Association, 308*(11), 1150–1159. doi:10.1001/2012.jama.11132.

NovoNordisk. (2016a). *Product monograph: Victoza.* Mississauga, ON: Novo-Nordisk Canada Inc. Retrieved from *http://www .novonordisk.ca/content/dam/Canada/AFFILIATE/www -novonordisk-ca/OurProducts/PDF/victoza-product-monograph .pdf.*

NovoNordisk. (2016b). *Product monograph: Levemir.* Mississauga, ON: NovoNordisk Canada Inc. Retrieved from *http:// www.novonordisk.ca/content/dam/Canada/AFFILIATE/ www-novonordisk-ca/OurProducts/PDF/levemir-product -monograph.pdf.*

Pan, A., Wang, Y., Talaei, M., et al. (2015). Relation of smoking with total mortality and cardiovascular events among patients with diabetes mellitus: A meta-analysis and systematic review. *Circulation, 132*(19), 1795–1804. doi:10.1161/ CIRCULATIONAHA.115.017926.

Pickup, J. C. (2012). Insulin pump therapy for type 1 diabetes. *New England Journal of Medicine, 366*(17), 1616–1624. doi:10.1056/ NEJMct1113948.

Poirier, P., Dufour, R., Carpentier, A., et al. (2013). Canadian Diabetes Association clinical practice guidelines for the prevention and management of diabetes in Canada: Screening for the presence of coronary artery disease. *Canadian Journal of Diabetes 2013, 37*(Suppl. 1), S105–S109.

Registered Nurses' Association of Ontario (RNAO). (2009). Subcutaneous administration of insulin in adults with type 2 diabetes—*Revision*. In RNAO (Ed.), *Nursing Best Practice Guidelines*. Toronto: Author. (Seminal).

Registered Nurses' Association of Ontario (RNAO). (2013). Assessment and management of foot ulcers for people with diabetes. In RNAO (Ed.), *Nursing Best Practice Guidelines* (2nd ed.). Toronto: Author.

Rogers, L., Frykberg, R., Armstrong, D., et al. (2011). The Charcot foot in diabetes. *Diabetes Care, 34*, 2123–2129. doi:10.2337/ dc11-0844.

Rojas, J., Chavez, M., Olivar, L., et al. (2014). Polycystic ovary syndrome, insulin resistance, and obesity: Navigating the pathophysiologic labyrinth. *International Journal of Reproductive Medicine,* 1–17. doi:10.1155/2014/719050.

Sanofi-Aventis Canada Inc. (2009). *Product monograph: Glucophage.* Laval, QC: Sanofi-Aventis Inc. Retrieved from *http:// products.sanofi.ca/en/glucophage.pdf.*

Sanofi-Aventis Canada Inc. (2015). *Product monograph: Lantus.* Laval, QC: Sanofi-Aventis Canada Inc. Retrieved from *http:// products.sanofi.ca/en/lantus.pdf.*

Sanuth, B., Bidlencik, A., & Volk, A. (2014). Management of acute hyperglycemic emergencies: Focus of diabetic ketoacidosis. *American Association of Critical Care Nurses, 25*(3), 197–202. doi:10.1097/NCI.0000000000000045.

Shah, B. R., Cauch-Dudek, K., & Pigeau, L. (2011). Diabetes prevalence and care in the Métis population of Ontario, Canada. *Diabetes Care, 34*(12), 2555–2556. doi:10.2337/dc11-0945.

Stone, J., Fitchett, D., Grover, S., et al. (2013). Canadian Diabetes Association clinical practice guidelines for the prevention and management of diabetes in Canada: Vascular protection in people with diabetes. *Canadian Journal of Diabetes 2013, 37*(Suppl. 1), S100–S104.

United Kingdom Prospective Diabetes Study (UKPDS). (1998). Intensive blood glucose control with sulphonylureas or insulin compared with conventional treatment and risk of complications in patients with type 2 diabetes. *Lancet, 352*(9131), 837–853. (Seminal).

Wang, H. F., & Yeh, M. C. (2012). Psychological resistance to insulin therapy in adults with type 2 diabetes: Mixed-method systematic review. *Journal of Advanced Nursing, 68*(4), 743–757. doi: 10.1111/j.1365-2648.2011.05853.

Westerberg, D. (2013). Diabetic ketoacidosis: Evaluation and treatment. *American Family Physician, 87*(5), 337–346.

World Health Organization (WHO). (2015). *Diabetes.* Geneva: Author. Retrieved from *http://www.who.int/mediacentre/factsheets/ fs312/en/.*

RESOURCES

Canadian Diabetes Association: *2013 Clinical Practice Guidelines for the Prevention and Management of Diabetes in Canada*
http://guidelines.diabetes.ca

Canadian Diabetes Association: Financial assistance programs
https://www.diabetes.ca/getmedia/4873c9cc-1105-4c11-9e90 -230ea52a9c60/ontario-financial-assistance-programs.pdf .aspx

Diabetes Canada (formerly Canadian Diabetes Association)
http://www.diabetes.ca

Dietitians of Canada
http://www.dietitians.ca

Heart and Stroke Foundation
http://www.heartandstroke.on.ca/

MedsCheck Diabetes Program
http://www.health.gov.on.ca/en/pro/programs/drugs/medscheck/ docs/diabetes.pdf

Public Health Agency of Canada

http://www.phac-aspc.gc.ca/cd-mc/diabetes-diabete/
pay-payer-eng.php
http://www.phac-aspc.gc.ca/cd-mc/publications/diabetes-diabete/
facts-figures-faits-chiffres-2011/highlights-saillants-eng.php
#chp5

Registered Nurses' Association of Ontario (RNAO) Nursing Best Practice Guidelines

http://rnao.ca/bpg

American Diabetes Association (ADA)

http://www.diabetes.org

Glycemic Index Calculator (University of Sydney)

http://www.glycemicindex.com

International Diabetes Federation (IDF)

http://www.idf.org

Joslin Diabetes Center

http://www.joslin.harvard.edu

National Diabetes Information Clearinghouse

http://www.niddk.nih.gov

For additional Internet resources, see the website for this book at *http://evolve.elsevier.com/Canada/Lewis/medsurg.*

Nursing Assessment

Reproductive System

Written by: Kim K. Choma
Adapted by: Maureen A. Barry

℮volve WEBSITE

http://evolve.elsevier.com/Canada/Lewis/medsurg

- Review Questions (Online Only)
- Key Points

- Answers Guidelines for Case Study
- Conceptual Care Map Creator
- Audio Glossary

- Supporting Media—Animations
  - Lymphatic Drainage of Breast
  - The Menstrual Cycle
- Content Updates

LEARNING OBJECTIVES

1. Describe the structures and functions of the male and female reproductive systems.
2. Summarize the functions of the major hormones essential for functioning of the male and female reproductive systems.
3. Explain the physiological changes during the stages of sexual response for both a man and a woman.
4. Link the age-related changes of the male and female reproductive systems to the differences in assessment findings.
5. Identify significant subjective and objective data related to the male and female reproductive systems and information about sexual function that should be obtained from a patient.

6. Select the appropriate techniques to use in the physical assessment of the male and female reproductive systems.
7. Differentiate normal from common abnormal findings of a physical assessment of the male and female reproductive systems.
8. Describe the purpose, significance of results, and nursing responsibilities related to diagnostic studies of the male and female reproductive systems.

KEY TERMS

amenorrhea, p. 1333
clitoris, p. 1330
ductus deferens (or vas deferens), p. 1327
dyspareunia, p. 1338

epididymis, p. 1327
gonads, p. 1326
menarche, p. 1332
menopause, p. 1333

menstrual cycle, p. 1332
mons pubis, p. 1330
nulliparous, p. 1329
spermatogenesis, p. 1326

STRUCTURES AND FUNCTIONS OF THE MALE AND FEMALE REPRODUCTIVE SYSTEMS

Both the male and female reproductive systems consist of primary (or essential) organs and secondary (or accessory) organs. The primary reproductive organs are referred to as gonads. The female gonads are the ovaries; the male gonads are the testes. The primary responsibility of the gonads is secretion of hormones and production of gametes (ova and sperm). Secondary or accessory organs are responsible for (a) transporting and nourishing the ova and sperm and (b) preserving and protecting the fertilized eggs.

Male Reproductive System

The three primary roles of the male reproductive system are (a) production and transportation of sperm, (b) deposit of sperm in the female reproductive tract, and (c) secretion of hormones. The primary reproductive organs in boys and men are the testes. Secondary reproductive organs include ducts (epididymis, ductus deferens, ejaculatory duct, and urethra), sex glands (prostate gland, Cowper's glands, and seminal vesicles), and the external genitalia (scrotum and penis) (Figure 53-1).

Testes. The paired testes are ovoid, smooth, firm organs measuring 3.5 to 5.5 cm long and 2 to 3 cm wide. They are within the scrotum, which is a loose protective sac composed of a thin, loose outer layer of skin over a tough connective tissue layer. Within the testes, coiled structures known as seminiferous tubules form *spermatozoa* (immature sperm). The process of sperm production is called spermatogenesis. Interstitial cells of the testes lie between the seminiferous tubules and produce the male sex hormone testosterone.

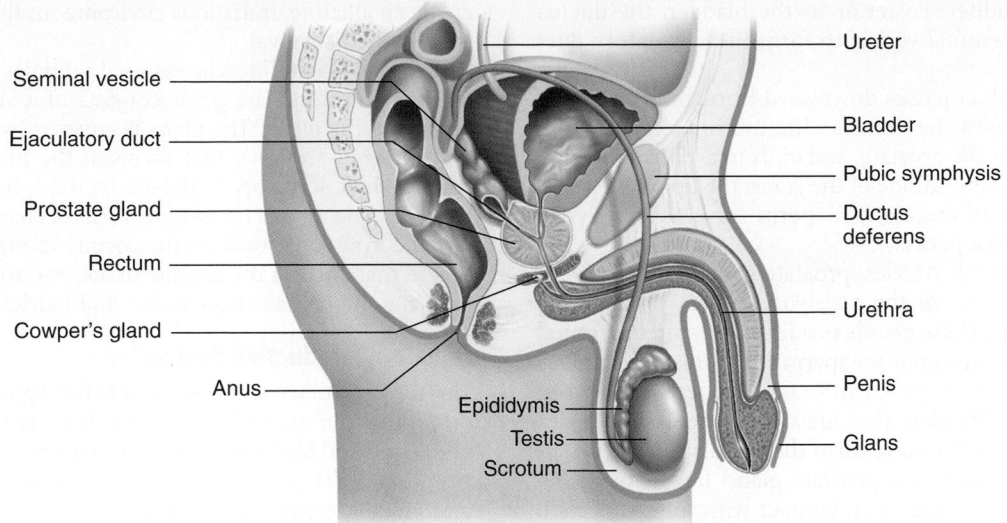

FIGURE 53-1 External and internal male sex organs. Source: Patton, K. T., & Thibodeau, G. A. (2013). *Anatomy and physiology* (8th ed., p. 1045, Figure 34-1). St. Louis: Mosby.

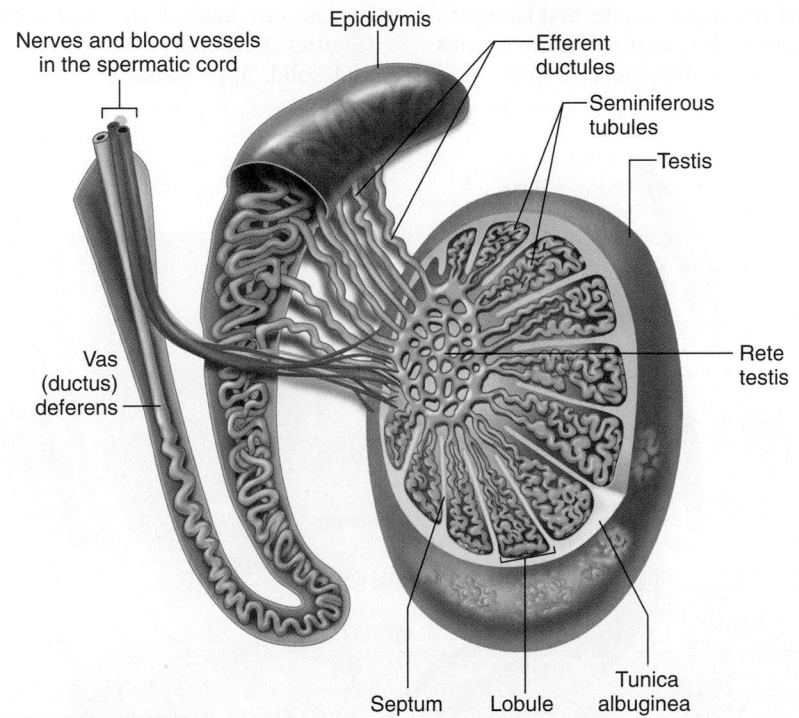

FIGURE 53-2 Seminiferous tubules, testis, epididymis, and ductus (vas) deferens in the male reproductive system. Source: Patton, K. T., & Thibodeau, G. A. (2013). *Anatomy and physiology* (8th ed., p. 1046, Figure 34-3B). St. Louis: Mosby.

Ducts. Sperm formed in the seminiferous tubules move through a series of ducts. These ducts transport the sperm from the testes to the outside of the body. As sperm exit the testes, they enter and pass through the epididymis, the ductus deferens, the ejaculatory duct, and the urethra.

The epididymis is a comma-shaped structure located on the posterior-superior aspect of each testis within the scrotum; it transports the sperm as they mature (Figure 53-2; see also Figure 53-1). It is a very long, tightly coiled tubular structure that measures about 6 m in length (Patton & Thibodeau, 2015). The epididymis transports the sperm as they mature. Sperm exit the epididymis through a long, thick tube known as the **ductus deferens (or vas deferens)**.

The ductus deferens is continuous with the epididymis within the scrotal sac. It travels upward through the scrotum and continues through the inguinal ring into the abdominal cavity. The spermatic cord is a connective tissue sheath that encloses the ductus deferens, arteries, veins, nerves, and lymph vessels as it ascends up through the inguinal canal (see Figure 53-2). In the abdominal cavity, the ductus deferens travels up, over, and behind the bladder. Posterior to the bladder, the ductus deferens joins the seminal vesicle to form the ejaculatory duct (see Figure 53-1).

The ejaculatory duct passes downward through the prostate gland, connecting with the urethra. The urethra extends from the bladder, through the prostate, and ends in a slitlike opening (the meatus) on the ventral side of the *glans,* the tip of the penis. During the process of ejaculation, sperm travels through the urethra and out of the penis.

Glands. The seminal vesicles, prostate gland, and Cowper's (bulbourethral) glands are the accessory glands of the male reproductive system. These glands produce and secrete seminal fluid (semen), which surrounds the sperm and forms the *ejaculate.*

The seminal vesicles lie posterior to the bladder and between the rectum and the bladder. The ducts of the seminal vesicles fuse with the ductus deferens to form the ejaculatory ducts that enter the prostate gland. The prostate gland lies beneath the bladder. Its posterior surface is in contact with the rectal wall. The prostate normally measures 2 cm wide and 3 cm long and is divided into right and left lateral lobes and an anteroposterior median lobe. Cowper's glands lie on each side of the urethra and slightly posterior to it, just below the prostate. The ducts of these glands enter directly into the urethra.

Secretions from the seminal vesicles, prostate, and Cowper's glands make up most of the fluid in the ejaculate. These various secretions serve as a medium for the transport of sperm and create an alkaline, nutritious environment that promotes sperm motility and survival.

External Genitalia. The external genitalia consist of the penis and the scrotum. The penis consists of a shaft, and the tip is known as the *glans.* The glans is covered by a fold of skin, the prepuce (or foreskin), that forms at the junction of the glans and the shaft of the penis. In circumcision, the prepuce has been removed. The shaft of the penis consists of erectile tissue composed of the corpus cavernosum, the corpus spongiosum, the fibrous sheath that encases the erectile tissue, and the urethra. The skin covering the penis is thin, loose, and hairless.

Female Reproductive System

The three primary roles of the female reproductive system are (a) production of ova (eggs), (b) secretion of hormones, and (c) protection and facilitation of the development of the fetus during gestation. Like males, females have primary and secondary reproductive organs. The primary reproductive organs in females are the paired ovaries. Secondary reproductive organs include ducts (Fallopian tubes), the uterus, the vagina, sex glands (Bartholin's glands and breasts), and the external genitalia (vulva).

Pelvic Organs

Ovaries. The ovaries are usually located on either side of the uterus, just behind and below the Fallopian (uterine) tubes (Figures 53-3 and 53-4). The almond-shaped ovaries are firm and solid, approximately 1.5 cm wide and 3 cm long. Their

Sacral promontory

Uterine tube

Ureter

Uterosacral ligament

Rectouterine pouch (of Douglas)

Cervix

Fornix of vagina

Coccyx

Anus

Vagina

Suspensory ligament (of uterine tube)

Ovarian ligament

Body of uterus

Fundus of uterus

Round ligament

Vesico-uterine pouch

Parietal peritoneum

Urinary bladder

Pubic symphysis

Urethra

Clitoris

Labium minus

Labium majus

FIGURE 53-3 Female reproductive tract and related organs. Source: Patton, K. T., & Thibodeau, G. A. (2013). *Anatomy and physiology* (8th ed., p. 1065, Figure 35-1A). St. Louis: Mosby.

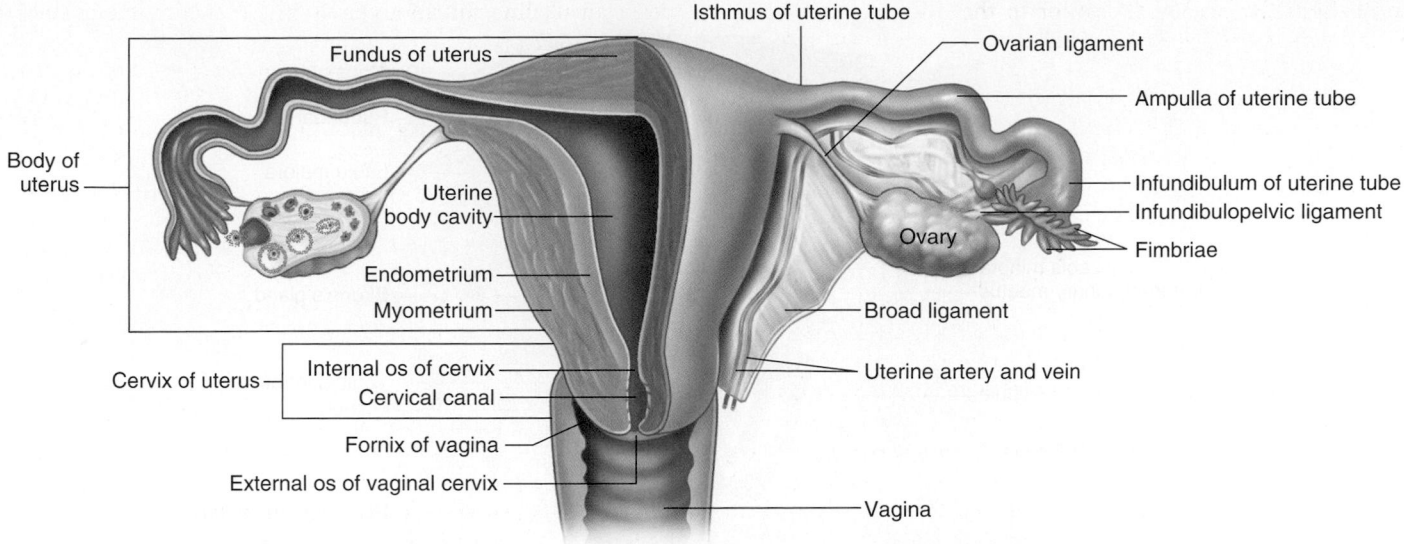

FIGURE 53-4 Female reproductive tract. Source: Modified from Patton, K. T., & Thibodeau, G. A. (2013). *Anatomy and physiology* (8th ed., p. 1066, Figure 35-3A). St. Louis: Mosby.

functions include *ovulation* and secretion of the two major reproductive hormones, estrogen and progesterone. The outer zone of the ovary contains follicles with germ cells, or *oocytes.* Each follicle contains a primordial (immature) oocyte surrounded by granulosa and theca cells. These two layers protect and nourish the oocyte until the follicle reaches maturity and ovulation occurs. However, not all follicles reach maturity. In a process termed *atresia,* most of the primordial follicles become smaller and are reabsorbed by the body. Thus the number of follicles declines from 2 to 4 million at birth to approximately 300,000 to 400,000 at menarche. This number continues to decrease throughout a woman's reproductive years. Fewer than 500 oocytes are actually released by ovulation during the reproductive years of a normal healthy woman.

Fallopian Tubes. Normally, each month during a woman's reproductive years, one ovarian follicle reaches maturity, and the ovum is ovulated, or expelled, from the ovary through the stimulus of the gonadotropic hormones: follicle-stimulating hormone (FSH) and luteinizing hormone (LH). The ovum then travels up a Fallopian tube, where fertilization by sperm may occur. An ovum can be fertilized up to 72 hours after its release from the ovary.

The distal ends of the Fallopian tubes consist of finger-like projections called *fimbriae* that "massage" the ovaries at ovulation to help extract the mature ovum. The tubes, which average 12 cm in length, extend from the fimbriae to the superior lateral borders of the uterus. Fertilization usually takes place within the outer third of the Fallopian tubes.

Uterus. The uterus is a pear-shaped, hollow, muscular organ (see Figures 53-3 and 53-4). It is located between the bladder and the rectum. In the mature **nulliparous** (never pregnant) woman, the uterus is approximately 6 to 8 cm long and 4 cm wide. The uterine walls consist of an outer serosal layer, the perimetrium; a middle muscular layer, the myometrium; and an inner mucosal layer, the endometrium.

The uterus consists of the fundus, the body (or corpus), and the cervix (see Figures 53-3 and 53-4). The body makes up about 80% of the uterus and connects with the cervix at the isthmus (or neck). The cervix is the lower portion of the uterus that

FIGURE 53-5 Cervical os and squamocolumnar junction (transformation zone). Courtesy Candy Tedschi, NP, Great Neck, NY.

projects into the anterior wall of the vaginal canal. It makes up about 15% to 20% of the uterus in the nulliparous female. The cervix consists of the *ectocervix,* the outer portion that protrudes into the vagina, and the *endocervix,* the canal in the opening of the cervix. The opening of the cervix is referred to as the *cervical os* (Figure 53-5).

The ectocervix is covered with squamous epithelial cells, which give it a smooth, pinkish appearance. The endocervix contains a lining of columnar epithelial cells, which give it a rough, reddened appearance. The junction at which the two types of epithelial cells meet is termed the *squamocolumnar junction* and contains the optimal types of cells needed for an accurate Papanicolaou (Pap) smear to screen for cervical cancer.

The cervical canal is 2 to 4 cm long and is relatively tightly closed. The cervix, however, allows sperm to enter the uterus and also allows menstruation to occur. The columnar epithelium, under hormonal influence, provides elasticity; thus the cervix can stretch to allow passage of a fetus during labour and the

FIGURE 53-6 External female genitalia. Source: Modified from Thibodeau, G. A., & Patton, K. T. (2013). *Anatomy and physiology* (8th ed., p. 1065, Figure 35-2). St. Louis: Mosby.

birth process. The entrance of sperm into the uterus is facilitated by mucus produced by the cervix under the influence of estrogen. Under normal conditions, the cervical mucus becomes watery, stretchy, and more abundant at ovulation. This mucus facilitates the passage of sperm into the uterus. The postovulatory cervical mucus, under the influence of progesterone, is thick and inhibits sperm passage.

Vagina. The vagina is a tubular structure 8 to 10 cm long that is lined with squamous epithelium. The secretions of the vagina consist of cervical mucus, desquamated epithelium, and during sexual stimulation, a watery secretion. These fluids protect against vaginal infection. The muscular and erectile tissue of the vaginal walls allows enough dilation and contraction to accommodate the passage of the fetus during labour, as well as penetration of the penis during intercourse. The anterior vaginal wall lies along the urethra and the bladder. The posterior vaginal wall is adjacent to the rectum.

Pelvis. The female pelvis consists of four bones (two pelvic bones, sacrum, and coccyx) held together by several strong ligaments. The sections of these bones that lie below the ilio-pectineal line play a very important role during birth: their ability to separate is often a factor in determining the ability of a woman to deliver a child vaginally.

External Genitalia. The external portion of the female reproductive system (Figure 53-6), commonly called the *vulva,* consists of the mons pubis, labia majora, labia minora, clitoris, urethral meatus, Skene's glands, vaginal introitus (opening), and Bartholin's glands.

The **mons pubis** is a fatty layer lying over the pubic bone. In female adults, it is covered by coarse hair that lies in a triangular pattern. (The pubic hair pattern in male adults is diamond-shaped.) The labia majora are folds of adipose tissue that form the outer borders of the vulva. The hairless labia minora form the borders of the vaginal orifice and extend anteriorly to enclose the clitoris (Hurt, Guile, Bienstock, et al., 2011).

The *vestibule* is a boat-shaped fossa between the labia minora, extending from the clitoris at the anterior end to the vaginal opening at the posterior end. The perineum is the area between the vagina and the anus. The vaginal introitus is surrounded by thin membranous tissue called the *hymen.* In female adults, the hymen usually appears as folds or hymenal tags and separates the external genitalia from the vagina. At the posterior aspect of the vagina, a tense band of mucous membrane connecting the posterior ends of the labia minora is referred to as the *posterior fourchette.*

The **clitoris** is erectile tissue that lies anterior to the urethral meatus and the vaginal orifice and becomes engorged during sexual excitation. It lies anterior to the urethral meatus and the vaginal orifice and is usually covered by the prepuce (McCance, Huether, Brashers, et al., 2014). Clitoral stimulation is an important part of sexual activity for many women.

Ducts of the Skene's glands lie alongside the urinary meatus and are thought to help lubricate the urinary meatus (McCance, Huether, Brashers, et al., 2014). Bartholin's glands, located at the posterior and lateral aspects of the vaginal orifice, secrete a thin, mucoid material believed to contribute slightly to lubrication during sexual intercourse. These glands are not usually palpable unless sebaceous-like cysts form or an infection is present, such as a sexually transmitted infection (STI).

Breasts. The breasts are a secondary sex characteristic; they develop during puberty in response to estrogen and progesterone. Cyclical hormonal changes lead to regular changes in breast tissue to prepare it for lactation when fertilization and pregnancy occur.

The breasts extend from the second to the sixth ribs, with an area called the *tail of Spence* reaching the axilla. The fully mature breast is dome-shaped and contains a pigmented centre termed the *areola.* The areolar region contains Montgomery's tubercles, which are similar to sebaceous glands and assist in lubricating the nipple. During lactation, the alveoli secrete milk (Figure 53-7). The milk then flows into a ductal system and is transported to the lactiferous sinuses. The nipple contains 15 to 20 tiny openings through which the milk flows during breastfeeding. The fibrous and fatty tissue that supports and separates the channels of the mammary duct system primarily accounts for the varying sizes and shapes of the breasts in different individuals.

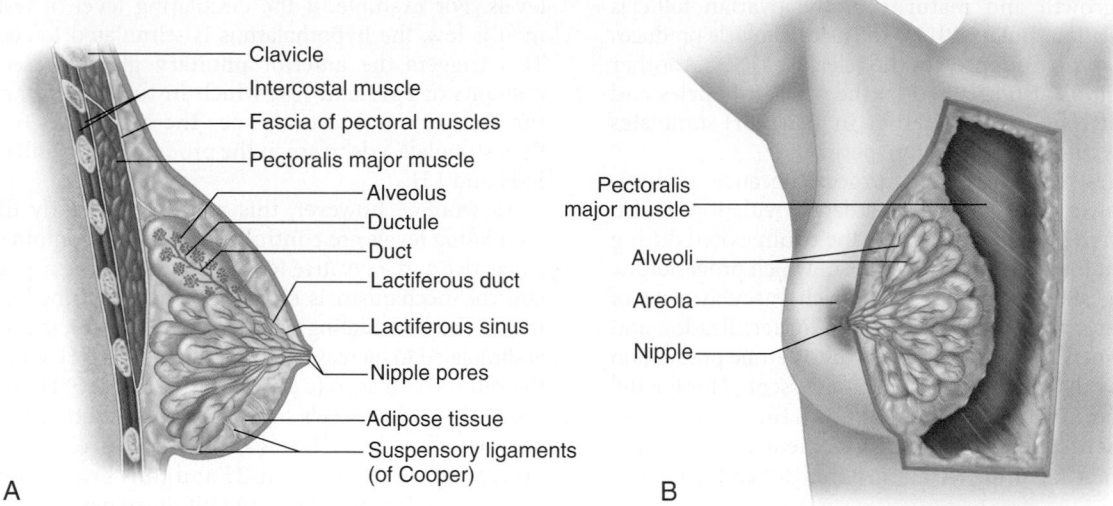

A

B

FIGURE 53-7 The lactating female breast. **A,** Illustration of a sagittal section of a lactating breast. Glandular structures are anchored to the overlying skin and to the pectoral muscle by suspensory ligaments of Cooper. Each lobule of glandular tissues is drained by a lactiferous duct that eventually opens through the nipple. **B,** Illustration of the anterior view of a lactating breast. In nonlactating breasts, the glandular tissue is much less evident; adipose tissue makes up most of each breast. Source: Thibodeau, G. A., & Patton, K. T. (2013). *Anatomy and physiology* (8th ed., p. 1083, Figure 36-16). St. Louis: Mosby.

CASE STUDY

Patient Introduction

Source: Dubova/ Shutterstock .com.

Anna Kaluza is a 68-year-old woman who comes to the breast centre because she found a large lump in her right breast while showering. She is somewhat anxious, stating, "My breasts are typically lumpy, but this feels different!"

Discussion Questions

Throughout this chapter, think about Mrs. Kaluza's concerns with the following questions in mind:
1. What are the possible causes for a lump in Mrs. Kaluza's breast?
2. What would be the priority assessment of Mrs. Kaluza?
3. What questions would the nurse ask Mrs. Kaluza?
4. What should be included in the physical assessment? What would the nurse be looking for?
5. What diagnostic studies would the nurse expect to be ordered?

Mrs. Kaluza and her condition will be followed throughout this assessment chapter. See pp. 1336, 1340, and 1347 for more information on Mrs. Kaluza.

evolve

Answers available at *http://evolve.elsevier.com/Lewis/medsurg*.

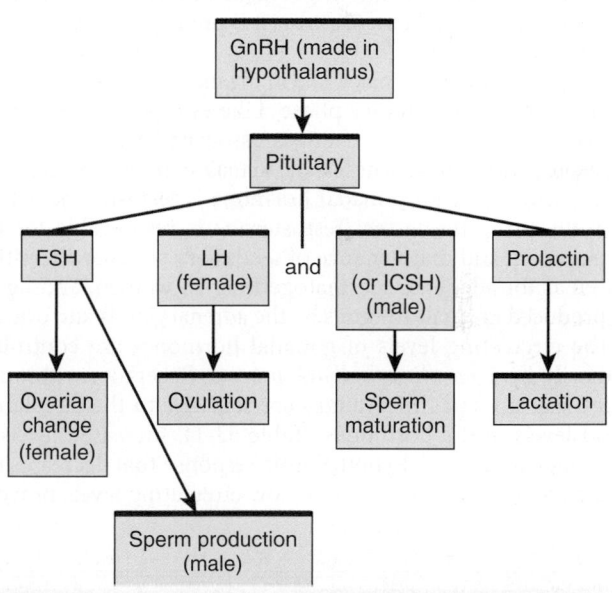

FIGURE 53-8 Hypothalamic–pituitary–gonadal axis. Only the major pituitary hormone actions are depicted. *FSH*, follicle-stimulating hormone; *GnRH*, gonadotropin-releasing hormone; *ICSH*, interstitial cell–stimulating hormone; *LH*, luteinizing hormone.

The breast has a rich lymphatic network that drains into the axillary and clavicular channels (see Chapter 54, Figure 54-7). Superficial lymph nodes are located in the axilla and are accessible to examination. This system is often responsible for the metastasis of a malignant tumour from the breast to other parts of the body.

Neuroendocrine Regulation of the Reproductive System

The hypothalamus, the pituitary gland, and the gonads secrete numerous hormones (Figure 53-8). (Endocrine hormones are discussed in Chapter 50.) These hormones regulate the processes of ovulation, spermatogenesis (process of sperm production), and fertilization and the formation and function of the secondary sex characteristics. In women, the hormones secreted by the anterior pituitary gland cause cyclical changes in the ovaries. The hypothalamus secretes gonadotropin-releasing hormone (GnRH), which stimulates the pituitary gland to secrete its hormones, including FSH and LH. LH in males is sometimes called *interstitial cell–stimulating hormone* (ICSH). The gonadal hormones are estrogen, progesterone, and testosterone.

In women, FSH production by the anterior pituitary gland stimulates the growth and maturity of the ovarian follicles necessary for ovulation (Bulun, 2011). The mature follicle produces estrogen, which in turn suppresses the release of FSH. Another hormone, inhibin, is also secreted by the ovarian follicles and inhibits both GnRH and FSH secretion. In men, FSH stimulates the seminiferous tubules to produce sperm.

LH contributes to the ovulatory process because it causes follicles to complete maturation and undergo ovulation. It also causes the ruptured follicle (area where the ovum exited during ovulation) to turn into a corpus luteum from which progesterone is secreted. Progesterone maintains the rich vascular state of the uterus (secretory phase) in preparation for fertilization and implantation. In men, LH (ICSH) triggers testosterone production by the interstitial cells of the testes and thus is essential for the full maturation of sperm. Prolactin has no known function in men. In women, prolactin stimulates the development and growth of the mammary glands. During lactation, it initiates and maintains milk production.

The gonadal hormones, estrogen and progesterone, are produced by the ovaries in women. Small amounts of an estrogen precursor are also produced in the adrenal cortices. Estrogen is essential to the development and maintenance of the secondary sex characteristics, the proliferative phase of the menstrual cycle immediately after menstruation, and the uterine changes essential to pregnancy. The role and importance of estrogen in men are not well understood. In men, estrogen is produced predominantly in the adrenal cortex.

Progesterone plays a major role in the menstrual cycle but most specifically in the secretory phase. Like estrogen, progesterone is involved in the bodily changes associated with pregnancy. Adequate progesterone is necessary to maintain an implanted egg.

In men, the major gonadal hormone is testosterone, which is produced by the testes. Testosterone is responsible for the development and maintenance of secondary sex characteristics, as well as for adequate spermatogenesis. In women, androgens are produced in small amounts by the adrenal glands and ovaries.

The circulating levels of gonadal hormones are controlled primarily by a *negative feedback process*. Receptors within the hypothalamus and the pituitary are sensitive to the circulating blood levels of the hormones (Table 53-1). Increased levels of hormones stimulate a hypothalamic response that decreases the high circulating levels. Likewise, low circulating levels provoke

a hypothalamic response that increases the low circulating levels. For example, if the circulating level of testosterone in men is low, the hypothalamus is stimulated to secrete GnRH. This triggers the anterior pituitary gland to secrete greater amounts of FSH and LH, which in turn set off an increase in the production of testosterone. The high levels of testosterone then stimulate a decrease in the production of GnRH and thus of FSH and LH.

In women, however, this process is slightly different. The circulating levels are controlled through a combination of both a negative and a positive feedback system. The negative feedback control mechanism is similar to that described previously in men. When circulating estrogen levels are low, the hypothalamus is stimulated to increase its production of GnRH. GnRH stimulates the pituitary to secrete greater amounts of FSH and LH, which results in higher levels of estrogen production by the ovaries. Reciprocally, higher levels of circulating estrogen result in a decreasing secretion of GnRH and thus bring about a decrease in the secretion of FSH by the pituitary gland.

A positive feedback control mechanism also exists in women: With the increased levels of circulating estrogen, GnRH is produced at a higher level, which results in an increased level of LH from the pituitary, which instigates ovulation. Likewise, lowered levels of estrogen result in a lowered level of LH.

Menarche

Menarche is the first episode of menstrual bleeding and indicates that a girl has reached puberty. Menarche usually occurs at approximately 12 to 13 years of age (Jameson, De Groot, de Kretser, et al., 2016). Menstrual cycles are often irregular for the first 1 to 2 years after menarche because of *anovulatory* cycles (cycles without ovulation).

Menstrual Cycle

The major functions of the ovaries are ovulation and the secretion of hormones. These functions are accomplished during the normal menstrual cycle, a monthly process mediated by the hormonal activity of the hypothalamus, the pituitary gland, and the ovaries. Menstruation occurs during each month in which an egg is not fertilized (Figure 53-9). The endometrial cycle is divided into three phases labelled in relation to uterine and ovarian changes: (a) the *proliferative* or *follicular phase,* (b) the *secretory* or *luteal phase,* and (c) the *menstrual* or *ischemic phase.* The length of the menstrual cycle ranges from 20 to 40 days, the average being 28 days.

The menstrual cycle begins on the first day of one menstrual period (menses), which usually lasts 4 to 6 days, and ends the day before the first day of the next. Table 53-2 includes characteristics of the menstrual cycle and related patient teaching. During this time, estrogen and progesterone levels are low, but FSH levels begin to increase. During the follicular phase, usually a single follicle matures fully under the stimulation of FSH. (The mechanism that ensures that usually only one follicle reaches maturity is not known.) The mature follicle stimulates estrogen production, causing the negative feedback that results in decreased FSH secretion.

Although the initial stage of follicular maturation is stimulated by FSH, complete maturation and ovulation occur only when LH is present. When estrogen levels peak on about the twelfth day of the cycle, there is a surge of LH, which triggers ovulation a day or two later. After ovulation (maturation and release of an ovum), LH promotes the development of the corpus luteum.

TABLE 53-1 GONADAL FEEDBACK MECHANISMS

Negative Feedback
Female
↓ Estrogen ⟶ ↑ GnRH ⟶ ↑ FSH (pituitary) ⟶ ↑ Estrogen
(hypothalamus) (ovaries)

Male
↓ Testosterone ⟶ ↑ GnRH ⟶ ↑ FSH and LH ⟶ ↑ Testosterone
(hypothalamus) (or ICSH) (testes)
(pituitary)

Positive Feedback
↑ Estrogen ⟶ ↑ GnRH ⟶ ↑ LH
(hypothalamus) (pituitary)

FSH, follicle-stimulating hormone; *GnRH,* gonadotropin-releasing hormone; *ICSH,* interstitial cell–stimulating hormone; *LH,* luteinizing hormone.

FIGURE 53-9 Events of the menstrual cycle. The various *lines* depict the changes in blood hormone levels, the development of the follicles, and the changes in the endometrium during the cycle. *FSH,* follicle-stimulating hormone; *LH,* luteinizing hormone. Source: Adapted from Thibodeau, G. A., & Patton, K. T. (2013). *Anatomy and physiology* (8th ed., p. 1079, Figure 35-14). St. Louis: Mosby.

The fully developed corpus luteum continues to secrete estrogen and initiates progesterone secretion. If fertilization occurs, high levels of estrogen and progesterone continue to be secreted owing to the continued activity of the corpus luteum from stimulation by human chorionic gonadotropin (hCG). If fertilization does not take place, estrogen production decreases, and progesterone secretion stops, and, accordingly, menses occurs.

During the *follicular phase,* the endometrial lining of the uterus also undergoes change. As larger amounts of estrogen are produced, the endometrial lining undergoes proliferative changes, and cellular growth, including the length of blood vessels and glandular tissue, increases.

With ovulation and the resulting increased levels of progesterone, the *luteal* (or *secretory*) phase begins. If the corpus luteum regresses (i.e., fertilization does not occur) and estrogen and progesterone levels fall, the endometrial lining can no longer be supported. As a result, the blood vessels contract, and tissue begins to slough (fall away). This sloughing results in the menses and the start of the menstrual cycle (Rebar & Erickson, 2011).

Menopause

Menopause is the physiological cessation of menses associated with declining ovarian function. It is usually considered complete after 1 year of amenorrhea (absence of menstruation; Hurt, Guile, Bienstock, et al., 2011). (Menopause is discussed in Chapter 56.)

Phases of the Sexual Response

The sexual response is a complex interplay of psychological and physiological phenomena and is influenced by a number of

TABLE 53-2 PATIENT & CAREGIVER TEACHING GUIDE

Characteristics of Menstruation

The following information should be included when teaching the patient and her family about menstruation.

Characteristic	Teaching
Menarche Occurs between ages 10 and 16 yr; average age at onset is 12 or 13 yr.	See health care provider regarding possible endocrine or developmental abnormality when menarche is delayed.
Interval Usually is 21–35 days, but regular cycles as short as 17 or as long as 45 days are considered normal if pattern is consistent for individual.	Keep written record to identify own pattern of menstrual cycle. Expect some irregularity in perimenopausal period. Be aware that drugs (phenothiazines, opioids, contraceptives) and stressful life events can result in missed periods.
Duration Menstrual flow generally lasts 2–8 days.	Realize that pattern is fairly constant but that wide variations do exist.
Amount Menstrual flow varies from 20 to 80 mL per menses; average is 30 mL. Amount varies among women and in the same woman at different times. It is usually heaviest first 2 days.	Count number of pads or tampons used per day. The average tampon or pad, when completely saturated, absorbs 20–30 mL. Very heavy flow is indicated by complete soaking of two pads in 1–2 hr. IUD or drugs such as anticoagulants and thiazides can produce heavy menses.
Composition Menstrual discharge is a mixture of endometrium, blood, mucus, and vaginal cells. It is dark red and less viscous than blood and usually does not clot.	Clots indicate heavy flow or vaginal pooling.

IUD, intrauterine device.

variables, including daily stress, illness, and crisis. The changes that occur during sexual excitement are similar for men and women. Masters and Johnson (1966) described the sexual response in terms of excitement, plateau, orgasmic, and resolution phases.

Male Sexual Response. The penis and the urethra are essential for the transport of sperm into the vagina and the cervix during intercourse. This transport is facilitated by penile erection in response to sexual stimulation during the *excitement phase.* Erection results from the filling of the large venous sinuses within the erectile tissue of the penis. In the flaccid state, these sinuses hold only a small amount of blood, but during the erection stage, they are congested with blood. Because the penis is richly endowed with sympathetic, parasympathetic, and pudendal nerve endings, it is readily stimulated to erection. The loose skin of the penis becomes taut as a result of the intense venous congestion. This erectile tautness allows for easy insertion during intercourse.

As the man reaches the *plateau phase*, the erection is maintained, and the penis increases in diameter as a result of a slight increase in vasocongestion. Testicle size also increases. Sometimes the glans penis becomes more reddish-purple.

The subsequent contraction of the penile and urethral musculature during the *orgasmic phase* propels the sperm outward through the meatus. In this process, termed *ejaculation,* sperm are released into the ductus deferens during contractions. Sperm advance through the urethra, where fluids from the prostate and the seminal vesicles are added to the sperm, forming the ejaculate. The sperm continue their path through the urethra, receiving a small amount of fluid from Cowper's glands, and are finally ejaculated through the urinary meatus. *Orgasm* is characterized by the rapid release of the vasocongestion and muscular tension (myotonia) that have developed. The rapid release of muscular tension (through rhythmic contractions) occurs primarily in the penis, prostate gland, and seminal vesicles. After ejaculation, a man enters the *resolution phase*. During this phase, the penis undergoes involution, gradually returning to its unstimulated, flaccid state.

Female Sexual Response.   The changes that occur in a woman during sexual excitation are similar to those in a man. In response to stimulation, the clitoris becomes congested and vaginal lubrication increases as a result of secretions from the cervix, Bartholin's glands, and vaginal walls. This initial response is the *excitation phase.*

As excitation is maintained in the *plateau phase*, the vagina expands and the uterus is elevated. In the *orgasmic phase*, contractions occur in the uterus from the fundus to the lower uterine segment. The cervical os relaxes slightly, which helps the sperm enter, and the vagina undergoes rhythmic contractions. Muscular tension is rapidly released through rhythmic contractions in the clitoris, the vagina, and the uterus. This phase is followed by a *resolution phase* in which these organs return to their pre-excitation state. However, women do not have to go through the resolution (refractory) recovery state before they can be orgasmic again. They can be multiorgasmic without resolution between orgasms.

AGE-RELATED CONSIDERATIONS

THE REPRODUCTIVE SYSTEM AND SEXUAL RESPONSE

With advancing age, changes occur in the male and female reproductive systems. In women, many of these changes are related to the altered estrogen production that is associated with menopause. A reduction in circulating estrogen along with an increase in androgens in postmenopausal women is associated with breast and genital atrophy, reduction in bone mass, and increased rate of atherosclerosis. Vaginal dryness may occur, which can lead to urogenital atrophy and changes in the quantity and composition of vaginal secretions (Kaunitz & Manson, 2015).

A gradual hormonal decline also occurs in elderly men. Manifestations of hormonal decline in men can be physical, psychological, or sexual. Some of the changes include an increase in prostate size and a decrease in testosterone level, sperm production, muscle tone of the scrotum, and size and firmness of the testicles (Laborde & Brannigan, 2011). Erectile dysfunction and sexual dysfunction occur in some men as a result of these changes. Age-related changes in the reproductive systems and differences in assessment findings are presented in Table 53-3.

TABLE 53-3   AGE-RELATED DIFFERENCES IN ASSESSMENT

Reproductive System

	Changes	Differences In Assessment Findings
Male		
Penis	Decreased subcutaneous fat, decreased skin turgor	Easily retractable foreskin (if uncircumcised); decrease in size; fewer sustained erections
Testes	Decreased testosterone production	Decrease in size; change in position (lower)
Prostate	Benign hyperplasia	Enlargement
Breasts	Enlargement	Gynecomastia (abnormal enlargement)
Female		
Breasts	Decreased subcutaneous fat, increased fibrous tissue, decreased skin turgor	Less resilient, looser, more pendulous tissue; decreased size; duct around nipple may feel like stringy strand
Vulva	Decreased skin turgor	Atrophy; decreased amount of pubic hair; decreased size of clitoris and labia
Vagina	Atrophy of tissue, decreased muscle tone, alkaline pH	Pale and dry mucosa; relaxation of outlet; mucosa thinning; narrowing and shortening of vagina; increased potential for infection
Urethra	Decreased muscle tone	Cystocele (protrusion of bladder through vaginal wall)
Uterus:	Decreased thickness of myometrium	Decrease in size, uterine prolapse
Ovaries	Decreased ovarian function	Nonpalpable ovaries; decreased size

TABLE 53-4   AGE-RELATED CHANGES IN SEXUAL FUNCTIONING

Men
- Increased stimulation necessary for erection
- Decreased force of ejaculation
- Decreased ability to attain or sustain erection
- Decreased size and rigidity of the penis at full erection
- Decreased libido and interest in sex

Women
- Decreased vaginal lubrication
- Decreased sensitivity with labia shrinking and more clitoris exposed
- Difficulty in maintaining arousal
- Difficulty in achieving orgasm after stimulation
- Decreased libido and interest in sex

Gradual changes resulting from advancing age occur in the sexual responses of men and women (Table 53-4). The cumulative effects of these changes, as well as the negative social attitude toward sexuality in older adults, can affect the sexual practices of older adults. Nurses have an important role in providing accurate and unbiased information about sexuality and age. Nurses should emphasize the normality of sexual activity in older adults.

ASSESSMENT OF THE MALE AND FEMALE REPRODUCTIVE SYSTEMS

Subjective Data

Important Health Information. In addition to general health information, the nurse must elicit information specifically relating to the reproductive system. Reproduction and sexual issues are often considered extremely personal and private. The nurse must develop trust to elicit such information. A professional demeanour is important when the nurse obtains a reproductive or sexual history. The nurse must be sensitive, ask gender-neutral questions when asking about partners, and maintain an awareness of a patient's culture and beliefs. It is helpful if the nurse begins with the least sensitive information (e.g., menstrual history) before asking questions about more sensitive issues, such as sexual practices or STIs.

Past Health History. The past health history should include information about major illnesses, hospitalizations, and surgeries. The nurse should inquire about any infections involving the reproductive system, including STIs. For women, a complete obstetrical and gynecological history should be documented.

Common pediatric illnesses that affect reproductive function are mumps and rubella. The occurrence of mumps in young men has been associated with an increase in sterility. Bilateral testicular atrophy can occur secondary to mumps-related orchitis. In the health history, the nurse should ask male patients whether they have had mumps, have been immunized with mumps vaccine, or have any indications of sterility.

Rubella is of primary concern to women of child-bearing age. If rubella occurs during the first 3 months of pregnancy, the fetus is at increased risk for congenital anomalies. For this reason, nurses should encourage immunization for all women of child-bearing age who have not yet been immunized for rubella or have not already had the disease. (Rubella immunity can be determined by antibody titres.) However, women should not be immunized if they are already pregnant (Centers for Disease Control and Prevention, 2014). Women are also advised not to conceive for at least 1 month after being immunized with the combination measles-mumps-rubella vaccine (Centers for Disease Control and Prevention, 2014).

The nurse should also ask about the patient's current health status and the presence of any acute or chronic health problems. Problems in other body systems are often related to problems with the reproductive system. The nurse must ask about possible endocrine disorders, particularly diabetes mellitus, hypothyroidism, and hyperthyroidism, because these disorders directly interfere with women's menstrual cycles and with sexual performance. Men who have diabetes mellitus may experience erectile dysfunction and retrograde ejaculation. In women with uncontrolled diabetes mellitus, pregnancy may incur significant health risks. Many other chronic illnesses such as cardiovascular disease, respiratory disorders, anemia, cancer, and kidney and urinary tract disorders may affect the reproductive system and sexual functioning.

A history of stroke should be determined. In men, strokes may cause physiological or psychological erectile dysfunction. Men who have suffered a myocardial infarction may experience erectile dysfunction because of the fear that sexual activity will precipitate another heart attack. Women share this concern, both as partners of someone who has had a myocardial infarction and as patients recovering from a myocardial infarction. Although most patients have concerns about sexual activity after a myocardial

infarction, many are not comfortable expressing these concerns to the nurse. The nurse must be sensitive to this concern. In women, a history of cardiovascular disease (e.g., hypertension, thrombo-phlebitis, angina) causes a higher incidence of morbidity and mortality with pregnancy or the use of oral contraceptives.

Family History. The nurse should inquire about a history of cancer, particularly cancer of the reproductive organs. Having a first-degree relative who has cancer of the breast, the ovaries, the uterus, or the prostate significantly increases the risk of cancer for the patient. It is also important to determine if the patient has a familial tendency for diabetes mellitus, hypothyroidism, hyperthyroidism, hypertension, stroke, angina, myocardial infarction, endocrine disorders, or anemia.

Medications. The nurse should document all prescription and over-the-counter medications that the patient is taking, as well as the reasons for using the medications, the dosages, and the lengths of time that the medications have been taken. All drugs taken by female patients of child-bearing age should be evaluated for possible teratogenic effects. The patient should also be asked about the use of herbal products and dietary supplements.

Particularly relevant in the assessment of the reproductive system is the use of diuretics (sometimes prescribed for premenstrual edema), psychotropic agents (which may interfere with sexual performance), and antihypertensives (some of which may cause erectile dysfunction). Patients who use certain cardiovascular and antihypertensive medications such as thiazide diuretics (e.g., hydrochlorthiazide), aldosterone receptor blockers (e.g., spironolactone [Aldactone]) or β-adrenergic receptor blockers (e.g., propranolol [Inderal]) must be closely assessed for problems that interfere with sexual performance (Chrysant, 2015). The nurse must also note the use of drugs such as alcohol, marijuana, barbiturates, amphetamines, and phencyclidine (PCP [also called "angel dust"]), which can have serious behavioural and physiological effects on the functioning of the reproductive system.

In women, the use of oral contraceptives or other hormone therapy should be noted. The long-term use of both estrogen and progesterone in hormone therapy appears to increase the risk of blood clots, cardiovascular disease, stroke, gallbladder disease, and breast and uterine cancer in postmenopausal women (American College of Obstetricians and Gynecologists, 2015). The short-term use of hormone therapy appears to be appropriate for certain women, depending on their risk factors. (Hormone therapy is discussed in Chapter 56.) Women who use tobacco have a much higher risk of clotting disorders than do women who do not use tobacco.

A history of cholecystitis and hepatitis is important information because these conditions may be contraindications to oral contraceptive use. Cholecystitis is often aggravated by oral contraceptives, and chronic active inflammation of the liver generally precludes the use of estrogen products because they are metabolized by the liver. Chronic obstructive pulmonary disease may be a contraindication to oral contraceptive use because progesterone thickens respiratory secretions.

Surgery or Other Treatments. Any surgical procedures should be noted in the health history. Surgical procedures involving the reproductive system are listed in Table 53-5. Therapeutic or spontaneous abortions should also be documented.

Documenting a Health History Related to a Reproductive Problem. When collecting information related to reproductive health, the nurse should start with questions of lesser sensitivity, proceeding to more sensitive issues after rapport has been

CASE STUDY

Subjective Data

Source: Dubova/ Shutterstock .com.

A focused assessment of Anna Kaluza revealed the following information.

Past Medical History: Type 2 diabetes for 5 yr, hypertension, stress incontinence, osteoarthritis. No surgical history. No personal history of breast cancer.

Family History: Her mother received a diagnosis of breast cancer at age 60, and her sister, at age 40.

Medications: Metformin (Glucophage), 500 mg PO bid for the past 4 yr; estradiol/norethisterone acetate (Activelle), 1 mg/0.5 mg/day PO for the past 14 yr; lisinopril (Prinivil), 10 mg/day PO for the past 3 yr.

Overall Health Management: Had onset of menarche at age 11, menopause at age 53. Has two daughters (aged 34 and 32) and a son (30). Mrs. Kaluza denies any breast pain. She is afraid that she may now have breast cancer because of her family history.

Functional Assessment

Activity and Mobility: Mrs. Kaluza does not exercise routinely. Occasionally takes a walk around the block with her husband. Otherwise, her life is fairly sedentary.

Nutrition and Metabolic History: Mrs. Kaluza is 158 cm tall and weighs 75 kg. She reports gaining most of her weight after menopause. She tries to eat a well-balanced meal and watch her carbohydrate intake because of her diabetes.

Elimination: Denies any changes or difficulty with urination or bowel movements except for stress incontinence when she coughs or laughs. States she always wears a panty liner "just in case."

Self-Care and Health Promotion Activities: Her last mammogram was obtained 2 years ago. She does not smoke but does enjoy one to two glasses of wine with her dinner every evening.

See pp. 1331, 1340, and 1347 for more information on Mrs. Kaluza.

TABLE 53-5 SURGICAL PROCEDURES INVOLVING THE REPRODUCTIVE SYSTEMS

Surgery	Description
Male	
Herniorrhaphy	Repair of hernia
Orchiectomy	Removal of one or both testes
Prostatectomy	Removal of prostate gland
Repair of testicular torsion	Correction of axial rotation of spermatic cord, which cuts off blood supply to the testicle, epididymis, and other structures
Transurethral resection of prostate (TURP)	Removal of prostate tissue via the urethra (e.g., obstructive benign prostatic hyperplasia)
Varicocelectomy	Repair of varicose vein of scrotum
Vasectomy	Removal of part of ductus (vas) deferens; can be an elective procedure for sterilization or contraception
Female	
Cryosurgery	Use of subfreezing temperature to destroy tissue, especially for treatment of abnormal cells in the cervix
Dilation and curettage (D&C)	Dilation of cervix and scraping of endometrium, performed to diagnose disease of uterus, to correct heavy or prolonged vaginal bleeding, or to empty uterus of products of conception; also used in the treatment of infertility to correlate state of endometrium and time of cycle
Hysterectomy	Removal of uterus
Mastectomy	Removal of one or both breasts
Oophorectomy	Removal of one or both ovaries
Repair of cystocele	Correction of protrusion of urinary bladder into vagina
Repair of rectocele	Correction of protrusion of rectum into vagina
Salpingectomy	Removal of one or both Fallopian tubes
Tubal ligation or sterilization	Ligation of Fallopian tubes

established. The nurse is also in a unique position to discuss general health issues related to women or men and to emphasize health promotion and self-care activities. The key questions to ask a patient with a reproductive problem are presented in Table 53-6 and discussed in more detail in the paragraphs below.

Menstrual History. The menstrual history includes the date of the beginning of the most recent menstrual period, description of menstrual flow, age at menarche, and, if applicable, age at menopause. Menstrual history data are used in the detection of pregnancy, infertility, and numerous other gynecological concerns. Changes in the usual menstrual pattern must be explicitly described to determine whether the change is transient and unimportant or connected with a more serious gynecological problem. *Metrorrhagia* (spotting or bleeding between menstruations), *menorrhagia* (excessive menstrual bleeding), *amenorrhea* (absence of menstruation), and *postcoital bleeding* are examples of such problems. Changes in menstrual patterns associated with the use of contraceptive pills, intrauterine devices (IUDs), birth control patches, or medroxyprogesterone (Depo-Provera) injections must be identified. Contraceptive pills usually decrease the amount and duration of flow, whereas some IUDs may cause an increase in the amount and duration. Some IUDs also increase the severity of dysmenorrhea. However, newer IUDs contain progestin and may be therapeutic.

Obstetrical History. The obstetrical history includes the number of pregnancies, full-term births, preterm births, and live births. Other obstetrical information should include information about any ectopic pregnancies or abortions, either spontaneous or therapeutic, and any problems that occurred with pregnancy.

Menopause. Obtaining a menopause history includes asking the date of the beginning of the most recent menstrual period and asking about any other symptoms of menopause such as hot flashes, heavy sweats, vaginal dryness, headaches, sleeping problems, mood changes, decreased libido, and urinary problems. Women should be asked whether they are using or have ever used hormone therapy. It is also important to explore how the woman feels about menopause because the drop in estrogen levels during perimenopause and menopause can lead to depression. Women are also more prone to osteoporosis and heart disease after menopause owing to the lower levels of estrogen, and the nurse must discuss ways to prevent and reduce the risk of these diseases.

Nutritional History. Anemia is a common problem in women in their reproductive years, particularly during pregnancy and the postpartum period. The adequacy of the diet should be evaluated with this condition in mind.

A thorough nutritional and psychological history should be taken to assess for the presence of an eating disorder. Anorexia

TABLE 53-6 HEALTH HISTORY

Reproductive System: Questions for Obtaining Subjective Data

Past History
- Are you having any problems in the area of your genitals?*
- Have you had treatment for such problems in the past, and how were those treated?
- Have you had any surgery on your uterus, ovaries, vagina, or prostate?*
- Any history of kidney disease, kidney stones, prostate problems?*
- Have you had bladder infections? If so, when? How often?

Family History
- Describe the health of your family members. Any history of breast, uterine, ovarian, or prostate cancer?

Review of Systems
Overall Health Status
- How do you feel in general? Have you had any changes recently in your health?
- What is your weight and height? Have there been any changes in your appetite or weight?*

Gastro-Intestinal System
- Describe your usual bowel pattern. Have you noted any bowel changes?*

Genito-Urinary System
- Do you experience problems with urination (e.g., pain; burning; dribbling; inability to control urine; frequency; small amounts; urinating at night; blood in the urine; urine that is dark, cloudy, or foul smelling)? Do you urinate when you sneeze or laugh or cough?
- Do you have any discharge from your vagina or penis?*
- Have you had bladder infections? If so, when? How often?

Sexual and Reproductive History†
Women
- *Menstrual history:* When did you start to menstruate? Was this earlier or later than other women in your family? Do you have scant, heavy, or irregular menstrual flows? On what date did your most recent menstrual period begin?
- *Obstetrical history:* How many children have you had? How many times were you pregnant? How many living children, miscarriages, or abortions? Could you be pregnant now? Are you trying to become pregnant?

- *Menopausal history:* Have your periods changed or stopped? Are you experiencing any of the symptoms of menopause—hot flashes, headaches, heavy sweats, vaginal dryness? Are you taking or have you taken HT? How are you feeling about menopause?
- Are you postmenopausal? If so, do you have any bleeding from your uterus?

Men
- Have you noticed any changes in your ability to have an erection?*
- Are you trying to have children but cannot?*

Functional Assessment (Including Activities of Daily Living)
Activity and Mobility
- Do you have a planned exercise program? If yes, what is it, and have you had to make any changes in this routine lately? If so, why and what kinds of changes?

Sleep and Rest
- How many hours do you sleep at night? Do you feel rested on awakening?
- Are you ever awakened by sweating during the night?*

Nutrition
- *Women:* Have you had any problems with anemia?* Have you had problems with eating disorders?*

Interpersonal Relationships
- Are you in a relationship? Are you able to take care of your significant others and your home? If not, why not?

Self-Care and Health Promotion Activities
- *Women:* Have you noticed anything different about your breasts? Have you had a Pap test or mammography recently? If so, what were the results and dates of these tests? How often do you have these checks?
- *Men:* Have you noticed anything different about your testes? Have you had a prostate examination recently? If so, what were the results and dates of these tests?

Adapted from Jarvis, C., Browne, A. J., MacDonald-Jenkins, J. & Luctkar-Flude, M. (Eds.). (2014). *Physical examination and health assessment.* (2nd Canadian ed.). (pp. 66–73). Toronto: Elsevier Canada.
*If yes, describe.
†See Table 53-7 for sexual history questions.
HT, hormone therapy; *Pap,* Papanicolaou.

can cause amenorrhea and the subsequent problems, such as osteoporosis, that are related to estrogen deficiency. From early adolescence, women can be counselled regarding adequate calcium intake and the role of calcium in the prevention of osteoporosis. The patient's daily calcium intake should be estimated to determine whether the patient needs supplementation. Folic acid intake for women in their reproductive years should be evaluated because a deficiency can result in spina bifida and other neural tube defects in the fetus (Cordero, Crider, Rogers, et al., 2015).

Self-Care History. It is important to establish the patient's perception of his or her own health and measures that the patient takes to maintain health. Specifically, it is important to ask about self-examination practices and screenings. Regular breast self-examination is no longer recommended but women are

encouraged to become familiar with their own breasts because they are often the ones who notice changes possibly indicative of breast cancer (Canadian Cancer Society, 2016a). Screening mammography according to age-specific guidelines (see Chapter 54), and Papanicolaou (Pap) tests are integral to a woman's health. Sexually active women older than 21 are also advised to have regular Pap tests every 1 to 3 years, depending on provincial/ territorial screening guidelines and previous test results (Canadian Cancer Society, 2016b). There is not enough evidence to support regular testicular self-examinations for men but it is important that they know what is normal for them because most testicular cancers are discovered first by men themselves (Canadian Cancer Society, 2016c). Men older than 50 years are advised to talk to their physician about their personal risk for prostate cancer and the advisability of them having screening tests for early detection of prostate cancer such as a digital rectal examination and a prostate-specific antigen test (Canadian Cancer Society, 2016d). Men at high risk for prostate cancer (i.e., Black men, men with first-degree relatives who have prostate cancer) should begin these discussions before age 50 with their health care provider (Canadian Cancer Society, 2016d).

Assessment of the reproductive system is incomplete without information about the patient's lifestyle choices. The nurse should know whether a woman uses cigarettes, alcohol, caffeine, or other drugs because these substances can be detrimental to both mother and fetus. Cigarette smoking may delay conception and can also increase the risk of morbidity in women using oral contraceptives. Early menopause is also associated with smoking in women. These substances may also adversely affect the sperm count in men and cause erectile dysfunction or decreased libido.

The nurse should also document whether the patient is allergic to sulfonamides, penicillin, rubber, or latex. Sulfonamides and penicillin are used frequently in the treatment of reproductive and genito-urinary problems such as vaginitis and gonorrhea. Rubber and latex are commonly used in diaphragms and condoms. An allergy to these substances precludes their use as contraceptive methods.

Elimination. Many gynecological problems can result in genito-urinary problems. Stress incontinence and urge incontinence are common in older women because the pelvic musculature relaxes as a result of multiple births or advancing age. Vaginal infections predispose patients to chronic or recurrent urinary tract infections. Metastasis of malignant tumours of the reproductive system to the genito-urinary system is possible because of their proximity. Benign prostatic hyperplasia is a common problem of older men. It can alter normal urination, causing retention and difficulty in initiating the urinary stream.

Sexual Health History. The extent and the depth of the interview about a patient's sexuality depend primarily on the expertise of the interviewer and on the needs and the willingness of the patient. Before obtaining a sexual history, interviewers should assess their comfort with their own sexuality because any discomfort in questioning becomes obvious to the patient. Interviews must be carried out in an environment that provides reassurance, confidentiality, and a nonjudgmental attitude. The nurse needs to explain that a sexual health history is a routine part of history taking for all patients and ask permission to ask questions related to sexual health.

There is evidence that older adults avoid seeking help for sexual concerns because of sexual stigma, including lack of knowledge about sexual problems, discomfort talking about sex, and beliefs that sexual activity in older persons is inappropriate (Syme & Cohn, 2016). Sexual history taking should be a routine part of periodic health examinations. According to Ports, Barnack-Tavlaris, Syme, and associates (2014), health care providers underestimate the prevalence of patients' sexual concerns and would benefit from more training in comprehensive sexual history taking, especially with older adults.

Table 53-7 outlines specific questions for a sexual history. A sexual history should include information regarding sexual activity, beliefs, and practices. Sexual preference (heterosexual, homosexual, bisexual), the frequency and type of sexual activity (e.g., penile–vaginal, penile–rectal, oral, etc), and the number of partners and protective measures against STIs and pregnancy should be explored. The patient's knowledge of safe sexual practices should be determined. A history of multiple sex partners and unprotected sex increases the risk of contracting an STI.

TABLE 53-7	SEXUAL HEALTH HISTORY FORMAT

- Are you currently in a sexual relationship? If yes, do you prefer relationships with men, women, or both? In which type of sex do you engage (e.g., penile–vaginal, penile–rectal, oral)?
- How frequently do you engage in sexual activities? Are you and your partner(s) satisfied with the sexual relationship? Do you communicate comfortably about sexual activity?
- Do you have a significant other? If yes, is this relationship satisfying? If no, explain.
- Do you or your partner(s) have multiple partners? How many sexual partners have you had in the past 3 months?
- Do you prefer relationships with men, women, or both? (If the patient is gay or lesbian, inquire whether he or she is in a significant relationship.)
- Has your sex life changed during the past year? If yes, how?
- What kind of sex do you engage in (e.g., oral, vaginal, rectal)?
- Are you experiencing any problems that are affecting your sexuality? If yes, describe.
- Have you ever had a sexually transmitted infection? If yes, what?
- How do you protect yourself from sexually transmitted infections? If protection is used, what type? Do you use protection every time you have intercourse?
- Are you currently using any birth control measures? If yes, what type(s)? How long have you been using this method? How effective do you feel this has been?
- How old were you when you first had intercourse? Was it by choice? Have you ever been forced into sexual acts as a child or an adult? If so, how has this affected you or your partner?
- How often have you experienced erectile dysfunction (male) or difficulty with vaginal lubrication (female) or pain with intercourse?
- Do you or your partner(s) frequently use drugs or alcohol before you engage in sexual activity?

Source: Adapted from Wilson, S. F., & Giddens, J. F. (2013). *Health assessment for nursing practice* (5th ed.). St. Louis: Mosby.

For a woman, this can increase the risk of pelvic inflammatory disease, which can compromise her ability to become pregnant.

Individuals should be asked about their general satisfaction with sexuality. The patient should be questioned about sexual beliefs and practices and whether orgasm is achieved. Any unexplained change in sexual practices or performance should be explored. Problems of the reproductive system can cause physiological or psychological problems that can lead to **dyspareunia** (painful intercourse), erectile dysfunction, sexual dysfunction, or infertility. Both the cause and the effect of such problems should be determined.

Inclusive and Appropriate Health Care for Sexual and Gender Minority Communities. People who identify themselves as lesbian, gay, bisexual, transgender, or queer (LGBTQ) account for approximately 5% to 10% of the population in the United States (Grant, Koskovich, Frazer, et al., 2010). In the Community Health Survey (Statistics Canada, 2014), 1.7% of Canadians aged 18 to 59 identified themselves as homosexual (gay or lesbian) and 1.3% as bisexual. Members of sexual and gender minority communities experience barriers to inclusive and appropriate health care (Rapid Response Service, 2014). Because prevailing attitudes in society discourage self-disclosure, members of the LGBTQ community often seek help later in the disease process. They underutilize the health care system because they often encounter insensitivity or homophobic attitudes, as well as discrimination, in some health care settings (Rainbow Health Ontario, 2014). A growing body of international research indicates that sexual- and gender-minority communities experience higher rates of cervical, breast, and anal cancer; eating disorders; depression and other mental health issues; and a higher incidence of smoking- and alcoholism-related health problems (Rainbow Health Ontario, 2014; Rapid Response Service, 2014).

Nurses must understand the unique needs of LGBTQ community members and provide inclusive and appropriate health care. Members of sexual- and gender-minority communities need to know that they are welcome, have rights, and are safe. The physical environment must acknowledge that LGBTQ people exist and are welcome (e.g., signage, posters, brochures, agency literature).

In language and agency forms and assessment tools, heterosexuality should not be assumed as the norm but should allow individuals to disclose their sexual identity, same-sex partnerships and sexual behaviour without fear of discrimination. Some examples of inclusive care are the use of the following language and concepts: *partner* or *spouse* instead of *husband* or *wife, significant relationships* instead of *next of kin,* and a broad definition of family that goes beyond traditional concepts to recognize as family whomever the patient considers that family to be.

Members of the LGBTQ community and their families also need affirmation that their identity is acknowledged and respected. In addition, the behaviour of the health care provider must demonstrate understanding of each person's unique needs.

Objective Data

Physical Examination: Male. The examination of the male external genitalia includes inspection and palpation. An examination may be performed with the patient lying or standing. The standing position is generally preferred. The examiner should be seated in front of the standing patient and should wear gloves during examination of the male genitalia.

Pubis. The nurse observes the distribution and general characteristics of the pubic hair and the skin. Normally, the hair is in a diamond-shaped pattern and is coarser than scalp hair. The absence of hair is not a normal finding unless the man is shaving or waxing the pubic hair.

Penis. The nurse notes the size and the skin texture of the penis and any lesions, scars, or swelling. In addition, the location of the urethral meatus, as well as the presence or absence of a foreskin, should be documented. The foreskin, if present, should be retracted to note any redness, discharge, irritation, or swelling and then replaced over the glans after observation. The glans is compressed to note any discharge and, if present, its amount, colour, and odour. The examiner palpates the penile shaft for tenderness or masses and observes the ventral and dorsal aspects.

Scrotum and Testes. This part of the examination is performed by a nurse with advanced skills. The nurse would start by performing a complete skin examination by lifting each testis to inspect all sides of the scrotal sac. The scrotum is palpated in order to note changes in consistency or the presence of masses. It is important to note whether the testes are descended. The left testis usually hangs lower than the right. An undescended testis is a major risk factor for testicular cancer, as well as a potential cause of male infertility (Zoltick, 2011).

Inguinal Region and Spermatic Cord. This part of the examination is performed by a nurse with advanced skills. The nurse first inspects the skin overlying the inguinal regions for rashes or lesions. The patient should be asked to bear down or cough. While he is straining, the inguinal area should be inspected for the presence of a bulge. No bulging should be seen.

Examination of the inguinal area continues with palpation. Using the index or the middle finger, the nurse palpates the right and left inguinal rings. The finger should be inserted into the lower aspect of the scrotum and should follow the spermatic cord upward through the triangular, slitlike opening of the inguinal ring. At this point, the patient should be asked to bear down and cough. The nurse determines whether the strain produces a bulging of the intestines through the ring, indicating the presence of a hernia, a condition that necessitates follow-up. The inguinal lymph nodes should also be palpated. Enlargement of the lymph nodes (termed *lymphadenopathy*) could suggest a pelvic organ infection or malignancy.

Anus and Prostate. The nurse inspects the anal sphincter and the perineal region for lesions, masses, and hemorrhoids. A digital rectal examination is required for all men who have symptoms of prostate trouble, such as difficulty in initiating the flow and the urge to void frequently. This examination should be performed annually for all men 50 years of age or older. This part of the examination is performed by a nurse with advanced skills.

Physical Examination: Female. Physical examination of female genitalia often begins with inspection and palpation of the breasts and then proceeds to the abdomen and the genitalia. Examination of the abdomen provides an opportunity to detect pain or any masses that may involve the genito-urinary system. (Abdominal examination is discussed in more detail in Chapter 41.) The nurse needs to assess the patient's comfort level and obtain consent before beginning an assessment of the reproductive system. It is also important to be sensitive to the patient's questions and needs during the procedure.

Breasts. A clinical breast examination is a thorough breast assessment performed by a trained health care provider. Clinical breast examination is not considered an effective screening procedure for breast cancer, and so it is not done routinely. It is performed if there is a lump or change in a woman's breasts or axillae area (Canadian Cancer Society, 2016a).

When performing a clinical breast examination, the nurse first examines the breasts by visual inspection. With the patient seated, the breasts are observed for symmetry, size, shape, skin colour and texture, vascular patterns, dimpling, and unusual lesions. The patient is asked to put her arms at her sides and then overhead, to lean forward, and to press hands on hips. The nurse observes for any abnormalities during these manoeuvres. The axillae and the clavicular areas are palpated for enlarged lymph nodes.

After the patient assumes a supine position, a pillow is placed under her back on the side to be examined. The nurse should asks the patient to put her arm above and behind her head. These manoeuvres flatten breast tissue and make palpation easier. Then the nurse palpates the breast in a systematic manner, using the distal finger pads for palpation. The area palpated includes the tail of Spence (the upper outer tail of breast tissue that extends into the axilla) because this region and the upper outer quadrant are the areas where most breast malignancies develop. Finally, the nurse palpates the area around the areolae for masses. The nipple is compressed to determine the presence of discharge or any masses. The colour, consistency, and odour of any discharge are documented.

External Genitalia. Gloves are used for examination of the female external genitalia. The nurse inspects the mons pubis, labia majora, labia minora, posterior fourchette, perineum, and anal region for characteristics of skin, hair distribution, and contour. Any lesions, inflammation, swelling, and discharge are

TABLE 53-8 PHYSICAL ASSESSMENT OF THE REPRODUCTIVE SYSTEM: NORMAL FINDINGS

Male	Female
Breasts	
Symmetrical. No masses or tenderness behind nipple. No drainage, retraction, or lesions noted. No lymphadenopathy.	Symmetrical without dimpling. No masses or tenderness behind nipple. Nipples soft; no drainage, retraction, or lesions noted. No lymphadenopathy.
External Genitalia	
Diamond-shaped hair distribution. No lesions or discharge noted. Scrotum symmetrical, testes descended; no masses. No inguinal hernia.	Triangular hair distribution. Genitalia dark pink; no lesions, redness, swelling, or inflammation in perineal region. No vaginal discharge noted. No tenderness with palpation of Skene's ducts and Bartholin's glands.
Anus	
No hemorrhoids, fissures, or lesions noted.	No hemorrhoids, fissures, or lesions noted.

CASE STUDY

Objective Data: Physical Examination

Source: Dubova/ Shutterstock .com.

Focused assessment of Anna Kaluza reveals the following:
A palpable, firm, fixed, 1.5-cm mass in upper, outer quadrant of right breast. No dimpling, redness, or swelling noted. No masses palpated in left breast. No lymphadenopathy noted.
Throughout this chapter, consider which diagnostic studies would be performed for Mrs. Kaluza. See pp. 1331, 1336, and 1347 for more information on Mrs. Kaluza.

FOCUSED ASSESSMENT

Reproductive System

Use this checklist to ensure the key assessment steps have been done.

Subjective
Ask the patient about any of the following and note responses

Vaginal discharge/itching, unusual bleeding	Y	N
Penile pain, lesions, discharge	Y	N
Medications: oral contraceptives, antihypertensives, psychotropics, hormones	Y	N
Clinical examinations of reproductive systems (breast, pelvis, testicles, prostate) and results	Y	N
Pain in the abdomen, pelvis, or genitalia	Y	N

Objective: Diagnostic
Check the following for results and critical values

Serum hCG	✓
Serum PSA	✓
Culture and sensitivity test results	✓
Hormone levels (testosterone, progesterone, estrogen) if done	✓
Screen for STIs (e.g., *Chlamydia*, gonorrhea)	✓
Laboratory reports: wet mounts, dark-field microscopy	✓
Radiograph of pelvis or breasts	✓
Ultrasound study of prostate	✓

Objective: Physical Examination
Inspect

External genitalia for redness, swelling, drainage	✓
Breasts for swelling, dimpling, retraction, drainage	✓

Palpate

Breast tissue for masses or inflammation	✓
Testicles for lumps	✓

hCG, human chorionic gonadotropin; *PSA*, prostate-specific antigen; *STIs*, sexually transmitted infections.

documented. The nurse separates the labia to fully inspect the clitoris, the urethral meatus, and the vaginal orifice.

Internal Pelvic Examination. This part of the examination is performed by a nurse with advanced skills. During the speculum examination, the nurse observes the walls of the vagina and the cervix for inflammation, discharge, polyps, and suspicious growths. During this examination, it is possible to obtain a Pap test and collect secretions for culture and microscopic examination. After the speculum examination, the nurse performs a bimanual examination to assess the size, the shape, and the consistency of the uterus, the ovaries, and the tubes. The tubes are not normally palpable.

Parts of the pelvic and bimanual examinations are not included in this text because they are considered advanced skills and are not usually within the scope of the nurse generalist.

Table 53-8 provides an example of a recording format for the physical assessment findings for the male and female reproductive systems. Tables 53-9 through 53-11 summarize common assessment abnormalities of the breasts, the female reproductive system, and the male reproductive system, respectively.

A *focused assessment* is used to evaluate the status of previously identified reproductive problems and to monitor for signs of new problems (see Table 3-6). This evaluation is described in the "Focused Assessment" box.

DIAGNOSTIC STUDIES OF REPRODUCTIVE SYSTEMS

The most commonly used diagnostic studies in the assessment of the reproductive systems are summarized in Table 53-12, and select studies (Figure 53-10) are described in more detail below.

Urine Studies

Pregnancy Testing. Pregnancy is generally validated by measuring human chorionic gonadotropin (hCG) in the urine (Office on Women's Health, 2014). A solution containing monoclonal antibodies specific for hCG is mixed with a small amount of urine. The presence of hCG causes a change in colour of the tested urine.

In home pregnancy test kits, the same assay principle is used. Positive results are based on the presence of hCG in urine. Some tests can detect pregnancy as early as the first day after a missed menstrual period. These tests are 99% accurate if the test is performed exactly per instructions (Office on Women's Health, 2014). A second test is recommended within a week if the first test result is negative (assuming menses have not yet occurred).

Hormone Studies. Although estrogen studies are performed on urine, the results are frequently inaccurate because estrogen

Text continued on p. 1346

TABLE 53-9 ASSESSMENT ABNORMALITIES

Breast

Finding	Description	Possible Etiology and Significance
Nipple inversion or retraction	Recent onset, erythematous, pain, unilateral.	Abscess, inflammation, cancer.
	Recent onset (usually within past year), unilateral, lack of tenderness.	Neoplasm.
Nipple secretions		
• Galactorrhea (female)	Milky, no relationship to lactation, unilateral or bilateral or intermittent or consistent presentation.	Drug therapy, particularly phenothiazines, tricyclic antidepressants, methyldopa. Hypofunction or hyperfunction of thyroid or adrenal glands. Tumours of hypothalamus or pituitary gland. Excessive estrogen. Prolonged suckling or breast foreplay.
• Galactorrhea (male)	Milky, bilateral presentation.	Chorioepithelioma of testes, manifestation of pituitary tumour.
• Purulent	Grey-green or yellow. Frequent unilateral presentation. Association with pain, erythema, induration, nipple inversion.	Puerperal (after birth) mastitis (inflammatory condition of breast) or abscess.
	Same description as mastitis or abscess but usually without nipple inversion.	Infected sebaceous cyst.
• Serous discharge	Clear appearance, unilateral or bilateral or intermittent or consistent presentation.	Intraductal papilloma.
• Dark green or multicoloured discharge	Thick, sticky, and frequently bilateral.	Ductal ectasia (dilation of mammary ducts).
• Serosanguineous or bloody drainage	Unilateral presentation.	Papillomatosis (widespread development of nipple-like growths), intraductal papilloma, carcinoma (male and female).
Scaling or irritation of nipple	Unilateral or bilateral presentation, crusting, possible ulceration.	Paget's disease, eczema, infection.
Nodules, lumps, or masses (male and female)	Multiple, bilateral, well-delineated, soft or firm, mobile cysts. Pain. Premenstrual occurrence.	Fibrocystic changes.
	Rubbery consistency, fluid-filled interior. Pain.	Ductal ectasia.
	Soft, mobile, well-delineated cyst. Absence of pain.	Lipoma, fibroadenoma.
	Erythema, tenderness, induration.	Infected sebaceous cysts, abscesses.
	Usually singular, hard, irregularly shaped, poorly delineated, nonmobile.	Neoplasm.
Dimpling of breast	Unilateral, recent onset, no pain.	Neoplasm.

TABLE 53-10 ASSESSMENT ABNORMALITIES

Female Reproductive System

Finding/Description	Possible Etiology and Significance	Finding/Description	Possible Etiology and Significance
Vulvar Discharge		Same as either of preceding descriptions, possible pain	Neoplasm
White, thick, curdy, frequent itching and inflammation, yeast-like smell or lack of odour	Candidiasis (candidal or yeast infection), vaginitis	Reddened base, vesicles, and small erosions; pain	Lymphogranuloma venereum, genital herpes, chancroid
Thin grey or white, copious flow; malodorous or "fishy" smell; vulvar irritation	Bacterial vaginosis infection	Indurated, firm ulcers; lack of pain	Chancre (syphilis), granuloma inguinale
Frothy green or yellow; malodorous	*Trichomonas vaginalis* infection	**Abdominal Pain or Tenderness**	
Bloody discharge	*Chlamydia trachomatis* or *Neisseria gonorrhoeae* infection, menstruation, trauma, cancer	Intermittent or consistent tenderness in right or left lower quadrant	Salpingitis (infection of Fallopian tube), ectopic pregnancy, ruptured ovarian cyst, PID, tubal or ovarian abscess
Vulvar Erythema		Periumbilical location, consistent occurrence	Cystitis, endometritis (inflammation of endometrium), ectopic pregnancy
Bright or beefy red colour, itching	*Candida albicans,* allergy, chemical vaginitis		
Reddened base, painful vesicles or ulcerations	Genital herpes	**Abnormal Vaginal Bleeding**	
Macules or papules, itching	Chancroid (STI), contact dermatitis, scabies, pediculosis	Unusual and inappropriate uterine bleeding	Dysfunctional uterine bleeding, usually anovulatory bleeding, menorrhagia (heavy menstrual bleeding), metrorrhagia (irregular, frequent bleeding), postmenopausal bleeding
Vulvar Growths			
Soft, fleshy growth; nontender	Condyloma acuminatum		
Flat and warty appearance, nontender	Condyloma latum		

PID, pelvic inflammatory disease; *STI,* sexually transmitted infection.

TABLE 53-11   ASSESSMENT ABNORMALITIES

Male Reproductive System

Finding	Description	Possible Etiology and Significance	Finding	Description	Possible Etiology and Significance
Penile growths or masses	Indurated, smooth, disclike appearance; absence of pain; singular presentation	Chancre	Scrotal masses	Localized swelling with tenderness, unilateral or bilateral presentation	Epididymitis (inflammation of epididymis), testicular torsion, orchitis (mumps)
	Papular to irregularly shaped ulceration with pus, lack of induration	Chancroid		Swelling, tenderness Unilateral or bilateral presentation; swelling without pain; translucent, cordlike or wormlike appearance	Incarcerated hernia Hydrocele (accumulation of fluid in outer covering of testes), spermatocele (firm, sperm-containing cyst of epididymis), varicocele (dilation of veins that drain testes), hematocele (accumulation of blood within scrotum)
	Ulceration with induration and nodularity	Cancer			
	Flat, wartlike nodule	Condyloma latum			
	Elevated, fleshy, moist, elongated projections with single or multiple projections	Condyloma acuminatum			
	Localized swelling with retracted, tight foreskin	Paraphimosis (inability to replace foreskin to its normal position after retraction), trauma		Firm, nodular testes or epididymis; frequent unilateral presentation	Tuberculosis, cancer
Vesicles, erosions, or ulcers	Painful, erythematous base; vesicular or small erosions	Genital herpes, balanitis (inflammation of glans penis), chancroid	Penile discharge	Clear to purulent colour, minimal to copious flow	Urethritis or gonorrhea, *Chlamydia trachomatis* infection, trauma
	Painless, singular, small erosion with eventual lymphadenopathy	Lymphogranuloma venereum, cancer	Penile or scrotal erythema	Macules and papules	Scabies, pediculosis
			Inguinal masses	Bulging, unilateral presentation during straining	Inguinal hernia
				1- to 3-cm nodules	Lymphadenopathy

TABLE 53-12   DIAGNOSTIC STUDIES

Male and Female Reproductive Systems

Study	Description and Purpose	Nursing Responsibility
Urine Studies		
Human chorionic gonadotropin (hCG)	Reveals pregnancy Also reveals hydatidiform mole and chorioepithelioma (in men and women) *Males and nonpregnant females:* negative	Obtain menstrual history from patient, including birth control methods. Determine presence or absence of presumptive signs of pregnancy (e.g., breast changes, increased whitish vaginal discharge).
Testosterone	Reveals tumours and developmental anomalies of the testes *Female:* 6.9–41.6 nmol/24 hr *Male:* 139–469 nmol/24 hr	Instruct patient to collect 24-hr urine specimen and to keep it refrigerated.
Follicle-stimulating hormone (FSH)	Indicates gonadal failure because of pituitary dysfunction *Female:* Follicular phase: 2–5 U/24 hr Midcycle: 8–60 U/24 hr Luteal phase: 2–10 U/24 hr Postmenopause: 35–100 U/24 hr *Male:* 3–11 U/24 hr	Instruct patient to collect 24-hr urine specimen; to indicate phase of menstrual cycle or if menopausal; and to indicate whether taking oral contraceptives or hormones.
Blood Studies		
Prolactin	Reveals pituitary dysfunction that can cause amenorrhea *Female:* <25 mcg/L *Male:* <20 mcg/L	Observe venipuncture site for bleeding or hematoma.
Prostate-specific antigen (PSA)	Reveals prostate cancer Also a sensitive test for monitoring response to therapy Reference interval: <2.5 mcg/L	Inform patient that there are no food or fluid restrictions. Collect 5 mL of blood. Observe venipuncture site for bleeding.

TABLE 53-12 DIAGNOSTIC STUDIES

Male and Female Reproductive Systems—cont'd

Study	Description and Purpose	Nursing Responsibility
hCG	Reveals pregnancy Can be used as a tumour marker for testicular malignancy Also used to detect hydatidiform mole *Males and nonpregnant females:* <5 IU/mL	Ask patient at point what she is in her menstrual cycle, whether she has missed menses, and, if so, how late menses are.
Testosterone	Indicates whether androgen levels are elevated because of testicular, adrenal, or ovarian dysfunction or pituitary tumours Serum levels also measured to assess male infertility and tumours of testicle or ovary *Male:* 9.75–38 nmol/L *Female:* <0.52–2.43 nmol/L	Collect health history to rule out potential sources of interference with accuracy of results (e.g., use of corticosteroids or barbiturates, presence of hypothyroidism or hyperthyroidism).
Progesterone	Indicates cause of infertility Used to monitor success of drugs for infertility or the effect of treatment with progesterone Indicates whether ovulation is occurring Helps diagnose problems with the adrenal glands and some types of cancer *Female:* Follicular phase: <1.6 nmol/L Luteal phase: 9.54–79.5 nmol/L After menopause: <1.27 nmol/L *Male:* 0.32–1.6 nmol/L	Include measurements during most recent menstrual period and trimester of pregnancy because progesterone levels vary with gestation.
Estradiol	Indicates ovarian function Useful in assessing estrogen-secreting tumours and states of precocious female puberty May be used to confirm perimenopausal status Increased serum estradiol levels in men may be indicative of testicular tumours *Female:* Follicular phase: 73.4–1284.9 pmol/L Luteal phase: 110–1652 pmol/L After menopause: ≤73.4 pmol/L *Male:* 37–183.5 pmol/L	Observe venipuncture site for bleeding or hematoma.
FSH	Indicates gonadal failure owing to pituitary dysfunction Used to validate menopausal status *Female:* Follicular phase: 1.37–9.9 IU/L Ovulatory peak: 6.7–17.2 IU/L Luteal phase: 1.09–9.2 IU/L Postmenopause: 19.3–100.6 IU/L *Male:* 1.42–15.4 IU/L	Inform patient that no food or fluid restrictions are required. Ask patient which phase of menstrual cycle she is in, whether she is menopausal, and whether she is taking oral contraceptive or hormone therapy.
Venereal Disease Research Laboratory (VDRL) test (flocculation)	Nonspecific antibody tests used to screen for syphilis Readings can be positive within 1–2 wk after appearance of primary lesion (chancre) or 4–15 wk after initial infection *Reference interval:* negative or nonreactive	
Rapid plasma reagin (RPR) assay (agglutination)	Nonspecific antibody tests used to screen for syphilis *Reference interval:* negative or nonreactive	Obtain data to identify conditions such as hepatitis, pregnancy, and autoimmune diseases that may interfere with accuracy of results.
Fluorescent treponemal antibody absorption (FTA-Abs) test	Reveals syphilis antibodies Also reveals early syphilis with great accuracy Usually performed if results of aforementioned nonspecific tests are equivocal *Reference interval:* negative or nonreactive	
Cultures and Smears		
Dark-field microscopy	Direct examination of specimen obtained from potential syphilitic lesion (chancre) to detect *Treponema pallidum*	Avoid direct skin contact with open lesion.
Wet mounts	Direct microscopic examination of specimen of vaginal discharge, performed immediately after collection Indicates presence or absence and number of *Trichomonas* organisms, bacteria, white and red blood cells, and candidal buds or hyphae May reveal other clues to or causes of inflammation or infection	Explain procedure and purpose to patient. Instruct patient not to use douche before examination. Prepare for collection of specimens (glass slide, 10%–20% potassium hydroxide [KOH] solution, sodium chloride [NaCl] solution, and cotton-tipped applicators).

Continued

TABLE 53-12   DIAGNOSTIC STUDIES

Male and Female Reproductive Systems—cont'd

Study	Description and Purpose	Nursing Responsibility
Cultures and Smears—cont'd		
Cultures	Specimens of vaginal, urethral, or cervical discharge that are cultured to assess presence of gonorrhea or *Chlamydia* Rectal and throat cultures may also be obtained, depending on data in sexual history	Obtain specific contact and sexual history inclusive of oral and rectal intercourse. Instruct patient against using douche before examination. Obtain urethral specimen from men before they void. Instruct women who are sexually active with multiple partners to have at least a yearly culture for gonorrhea and *Chlamydia*. Instruct sexually active men to have any discharge evaluated immediately to rule out gonorrhea strains that do not cause classic symptoms of dysuria.
Gram stain	Used for rapid detection of gonorrhea Presence of gram-negative intracellular diplococci generally warrants initiation of treatment Not highly accurate for women Also a valid alternative for *Chlamydia* testing	Same as for cultures
Cytological Studies		
Papanicolaou (Pap) smear	Microscopic study of exfoliated cells via special staining and fixation technique to detect abnormal cells Most commonly studies of cells obtained directly from the endocervix and ectocervix	Instruct women who are sexually active and who are between the ages of 21 and 69 to have Pap smears according to Canadian Cancer Society guidelines (every 1–3 yr, depending on provincial and territorial screening guidelines).* Instruct patients not to use douche for at least 24 hr before examination. Carefully document menstrual and gynecological history.
Nipple discharge test	Cytological study of nipple discharge	Ask whether patient is taking hormonal preparations or other drugs, is breastfeeding, or has a history of amenorrhea.
Radiological Studies		
Mammography • Screening • Diagnostic	X-ray image of breast tissue on radiographic film, used to assess breast tissue Reveals benign and malignant masses Performed when patient has suspect clinical symptoms or when an abnormality is found on screening mammogram Additional views of affected breast are taken	Instruct patient about advantages of the examination. Explain that the Canadian Cancer Society recommends screening with mammography every 2 yr for women who are 50–69 yr of age (see Chapter 54 for more information).†
Ultrasonography (abdominal and transvaginal)	Used to measure and record high-frequency sound waves as they pass through tissues of variable density In women, useful in detecting masses >3 cm, such as ectopic pregnancy, IUD, ovarian cyst, and hydatidiform mole In men, used to detect testicular torsion or masses	Instruct patient that a full bladder may be required, depending on the reason for the study.
Ultrasound-guided biopsy	Use of ultrasound guidance during a biopsy, usually done as an outpatient procedure Used to direct the biopsy needle into the region of interest and obtain a sample of tissue Small tissue sample is removed to diagnose infection, inflammation, or mass	Inform patient of purpose of this procedure. It is usually done as an outpatient procedure.
Computed tomography (CT) of pelvis	Reveals tumours within the pelvis	Explain procedure to patient. Instruct patient to lie still during the procedure. If IV contrast medium is used, check for iodine allergy.
Magnetic resonance imaging (MRI)	Use of radio waves and magnetic field to view soft tissue Useful if mammogram is abnormal or in presence of breast dysplasia Also used to diagnose abnormalities in the female and male reproductive systems	Screen patient for metal parts and pacemaker. Inform patient that the procedure is painless. Instruct patient to lie still during the procedure.
Invasive Procedures		
Breast biopsy	Histological examination of breast tissue excised either by needle aspiration or excisional biopsy	*Before biopsy:* Instruct patient about operative procedures and sedation. *After biopsy:* Perform wound care and instruct patient about breast self-examination.

TABLE 53-12   DIAGNOSTIC STUDIES

Male and Female Reproductive Systems—cont'd

Study	Description and Purpose	Nursing Responsibility
Hysteroscopy	Visualization of uterine lining through hysteroscope inserted through cervix Used mainly to diagnose and treat abnormal bleeding such as that caused by fibroids or polyps Biopsy sample may be taken during the procedure	Explain purpose and method of procedure and that it might be done in the physician's office. Inform patient that mild cramping and slight bloody discharge after procedure is normal.
Hysterosalpingography	Fluoroscopy with a contrast material injected into the uterine cavity via the cervix Used to check for blocked Fallopian tubes, adhesions near ovary, or abnormalities of the uterus	Inform patient about procedure and that it may be fairly uncomfortable. Check patient for iodine allergy.
Colposcopy	Direct visualization of cervix with binocular microscope that allows magnification and study of cellular dysplasia and cervix abnormalities Used as follow-up study for abnormal Pap test results and for examination of women exposed to DES in utero Biopsy sample from cervix may be taken during examination Valuable in decreasing number of false-negative results of cervical biopsies	Describe this outpatient procedure to patient. Inform patient that this examination is similar to speculum examination.
Conization	Removal of cone-shaped sample of squamocolumnar tissue of cervix for direct study	Explain purpose and method of procedure and that it requires use of surgical facilities and anaesthesia. Instruct patient to avoid sexual intercourse and tampons for about 3–4 wk. Also discuss necessity for 3-wk follow-up.
Loop electrosurgical excision procedure (LEEP)	Excision of cervical tissue via an electrosurgical instrument Helps diagnose and treat cervical dysplasia Minimizes amount of tissue removed and preserves child-bearing ability	Explain purpose and method of procedure and that it may be done in the physician's office. Inform patient that she may feel slight tingling or abdominal cramping during procedure. Inform patient that discharge, bleeding, and cramping may occur for 1–3 days after procedure.
Culdotomy, culdoscopy, and culdocentesis	*Culdotomy:* incision made through posterior fornix of cul-de-sac that allows visualization of peritoneal cavity (i.e., uterus, tubes, and ovaries) *Culdoscopy:* used after culdotomy to closely study these structures; valuable in fertility evaluations. *Culdocentesis:* withdrawal of fluid for examination	Explain purpose and method of procedure. Prepare patient for vaginal operation with preoperative instruction and sedation. Perform assessment of bleeding and discomfort after surgery.
Laparoscopy (peritoneoscopy)	Visualization of pelvic structures via fibre-optic endoscopes inserted through small abdominal incisions Instillation of CO_2 into cavity to improve visualization Used in diagnostic assessment of uterus, tubes, and ovaries (see Figure 53-10) Can be performed in conjunction with tubal sterilization	Before surgery, instruct patient about procedure, prepare patient's abdomen, and reassure patient about sedation. Inform patient of probability of shoulder pain owing to air in the abdomen.
Dilatation and curettage (D&C)	Operative procedure dilates cervix and allows curetting of endometrial lining Used in assessment of abnormal bleeding and cytological evaluation of lining.	Before surgery, instruct patient about procedure and sedation. Perform postoperative assessment of degree of bleeding (frequent perineal pad check during first 24 hr).

Fertility Studies

Study	Description and Purpose	Nursing Responsibility
Semen analysis	Assessment of semen for volume (2–5 mL), viscosity, sperm count (>20 million/mL), sperm motility (60% motile), and percentage of abnormal sperm (60% with normal structure).	Instruct patient to bring in fresh specimen within 2 hr of ejaculation.
Basal body temperature assessment	Indirectly indication of whether ovulation has occurred (temperature rises at ovulation and remains elevated during secretory phase of normal menstrual cycle)	Instruct woman to take her temperature with special basal temperature thermometer (calibrated in tenths of degrees) every morning before getting out of bed. Instruct woman to record temperature on graph.
Huhner, Sims-Huhner test	Examination of mucus sample of cervix within 2–8 hr after intercourse Assessment of total number of sperm in relation to number of live sperm Used to determine whether cervical mucus is "hostile" to passage of sperm from vagina into uterus	Instruct couples to have intercourse at estimated time of ovulation and be present for test within 2–8 hr after intercourse.

Continued

TABLE 53-12   DIAGNOSTIC STUDIES

Male and Female Reproductive Systems—cont'd

Study	Description and Purpose	Nursing Responsibility
Fertility Studies—cont'd		
Endometrial biopsy	Use of small curette to obtain piece of endometrial lining to assess endometrial changes common to progesterone secretion after ovulation Also used to assess abnormal menstrual or postmenopausal uterine bleeding	Tell patient that test must be performed after ovulation. Explain that procedure should cause only short period of uterine cramping and light, bloody vaginal discharge for about 24 hr.
Hysterosalpingography	See earlier section in table related to hysterosalpingography, under "Invasive Procedures."	See earlier section in table related to hysterosalpingography, under "Invasive Procedures."
Serum progesterone measurement	Same those of as blood studies.	Same as those of blood studies.
Genetic Studies		
DNA testing for *BRCA1* and *BRCA2* gene mutations (blood or saliva sample)	Testing for inherited mutations in breast cancer *(BRCA)* genes, which increase a female's susceptibility for the development of breast or ovarian cancer Recommended in cases of family history associated with an increased risk of a harmful mutation in either gene	Inform patient that results may take up to 1 month to be available. Advise genetic counselling before and after testing.

*Canadian Cancer Society. (2015). *Cervical cancer: Screening for cervical cancer.* Retrieved from *http://www.cancer.ca/en/cancer-information/cancer-type/cervical/screening/?region=on.*
†Canadian Cancer Society. (2015). *Breast cancer: Screening for breast cancer.* Retrieved from *http://www.cancer.ca/en/cancer-information/cancer-type/breast/screening/?region=on.*
DES, diethylstilbestrol; *FSH,* follicle-stimulating hormone; *hCG,* human chorionic gonadotropin; *IUDs,* intrauterine devices.

Round ligament
Uterus (fundus)
Uterine tube
Ovary
Sigmoid colon

Uterus (fundus)
Uterine tube (swollen)

FIGURE 53-10 Laparoscopic views of the female pelvis. **A,** Normal appearance. **B,** Pelvic inflammatory disease. Note the reddish inflammatory membrane covering and fixing the ovary and uterus to the surrounding structures. Source: Thibodeau, G. A., & Patton, K. T. (2013). *Anatomy and physiology* (8th ed., p. 1088, Figure 35-21). St. Louis: Mosby.

levels vary during the normal cycle and it is difficult to estimate the day of the cycle in women with irregular menses. Adrenal androgens are precursors of estrogens and can be measured in the urine of both men and women. For more information regarding hormone studies, see Chapter 50.

Blood Studies

Hormone Studies. Serum assays for hCG can detect pregnancy before a woman misses her menstrual period, as early as 10 days after conception (Pagana & Pagana, 2013). The prolactin assay is used primarily in the workup of a patient with amenorrhea. High levels of prolactin are normally associated with low levels of estrogen, such as those that occur during lactation. However, the same finding can occur with pituitary adenomas, especially with otherwise unexplained *galactorrhea* (excessive secretion of breast milk). Serum progesterone and estradiol are sometimes measured in ovarian function assessment, particularly for amenorrhea. In addition, hormonal blood studies are essential components of a thorough fertility workup.

Tumour Markers. Biological tumour markers are used to assess for malignant disease and to monitor therapy (marker levels rise as disease progresses and fall with disease regression). Alpha-fetoprotein, hCG, and cancer antigen 125 (CA-125) are sometimes used as tumour markers for reproductive system malignancies. A specific tumour antigen such as prostate-specific antigen is another type of tumour marker, frequently measured to determine the presence of prostate cancer.

Serological Tests for Syphilis. The Venereal Disease Research Laboratory (VDRL) test and the rapid plasma reagin (RPR) test are used to detect the presence of antibodies in the serum of patients thought to be infected with syphilis. These tests are inexpensive and reliable but yield high levels of false-positive results in patients with inflammatory disorders. The fluorescent treponemal antibody absorption test is a more specific treponemal assay and should be used after a positive finding on the VDRL or RPR test.

Cultures and Smears

Cultures and smears are most frequently employed in the diagnosis of STIs. Specimens for cultures and smears are most commonly taken from the vagina, endocervix, and rectum for females and the urethra and rectum for males. For a culture, the specimen is placed on a special culture medium. A smear involves rubbing the specimen on a slide for direct examination. Gram stain smears have been shown to be effective in the diagnosis of *Chlamydia* infection. A nucleic acid amplification test is used to screen for both gonorrhea and *Chlamydia* from a wide variety of samples, including vaginal, endocervical, urine, and urethral specimens.

Dark-field microscopy involves the direct examination of a specimen obtained from a syphilitic chancre for the diagnosis of syphilis.

Cytological Studies

Cytology is the study of cells under microscopic examination. The Pap smear is a screening test to detect abnormal cells obtained from the cervix or vagina. It involves obtaining cells from the cervical canal, preferably the endocervix, as well as from the vagina. The cells are placed in a fixative for examination by a cytologist for cellular abnormalities. Screening guidelines for the Pap test (also called a *smear*) are discussed in Chapter 56.

Cytological study is also indicated for nipple discharge. Cytological examination can detect the presence of malignant cells and distinguish the discharge with such cells from one associated with infection.

Radiological Studies

Mammography. Mammography, one of the most frequently used diagnostic tools to assess the reproductive system, is used to detect breast masses. Mammography and screening guidelines for mammography are discussed in Chapter 54.

Ultrasonography. Ultrasonography has many applications for diagnostic study. Pelvic ultrasonography is used to obtain images of the pelvic organs. Transvaginal ultrasonography can be used

to aid in diagnosing abnormalities of the ovaries or the uterus. These types of ultrasound studies are also used to detect pregnancy in the uterus, ectopic pregnancy, ovarian cysts, and other pelvic masses. Breast ultrasonography is useful in the detection of fluid-filled masses. In men, ultrasonography is used to detect testicular masses and testicular torsion. Transrectal ultrasonography is useful in locating prostate tumours.

CASE STUDY

Objective Data: Diagnostic Studies

Source: Dubova/ Shutterstock .com.

The breast specialist orders the following for Mrs. Kaluza:
- Digital mammography
- Ultrasonography of breasts
- Magnetic resonance imaging (MRI) of breasts

The mammography reveals an increased density in the right breast. The ultrasound study identifies the mass as solid and not fluid filled. The MRI confirms the presence of a suspicious mass in the right breast.

The health care provider schedules Mrs. Kaluza for a fine-needle aspiration (FNA) biopsy. The results of the ultrasonography-guided FNA biopsy reveal an adenocarcinoma. See pp. 1331, 1336, and 1340 for more information on Mrs. Kaluza.

▌REVIEW QUESTIONS

The number of the question corresponds to the same-numbered objective at the beginning of the chapter.

1. Which of the following is a normal reproductive function that may be altered in a client who undergoes a prostatectomy?
   a. Sperm production
   b. Production of testosterone
   c. Production of seminal fluid
   d. Release of sperm from the epididymis

2. What does estrogen production by the mature ovarian follicle cause?
   a. Decreased secretion of follicle-stimulating hormone (FSH) and luteinizing hormone (LH)
   b. Increased production of gonadotropin-releasing hormone (GnRH) and FSH
   c. Release of GnRH and increased secretion of LH
   d. Decreased release of FSH and decreased progesterone production

3. Female orgasm is the result of which of the following? *(Select all that apply)*
   a. Constriction of the cervical os
   b. Uterine and vaginal contractions
   c. Vaginal enlargement and uterine elevation
   d. Clitoral swelling and increased vaginal lubrication
   e. Rapid release of muscular tension in the reproductive structures

4. Which of the following is an age-related finding noted by the nurse during assessment of an older woman's reproductive system?
   a. Dyspareunia
   b. Vaginal dryness
   c. Nipple retraction
   d. Increased sensitivity of labia

5. Which of the following should be included as significant information about a client's past medical history in relation to the reproductive system?

   a. Extent of sexual activity
   b. General satisfaction with sexuality
   c. Previous sexually transmitted infections
   d. Self-image and relationships with others

6. Which of the following examination techniques is used to evaluate a client's breasts? *(Select all that apply)*
   a. Palpation
   b. Percussion
   c. Inspection
   d. Auscultation

7. Which of the following would be considered an abnormal finding during physical assessment of the male reproductive system?
   a. Slight clear urethral discharge
   b. The glans covered with prepuce
   c. Symmetrical scrotum
   d. Descended testes

8. The nurse is caring for a client scheduled for an endometrial biopsy who is having difficulty becoming pregnant. What will the nurse explain to the woman?
   a. That the outpatient procedure is usually performed before ovulation
   b. That bleeding and discharge are common 2 to 4 days after the procedure
   c. That a small sample of tissue is obtained to diagnose and treat cervical dysplasia
   d. That common changes in endometrial cells in relation to progesterone levels will be assessed

1. c; 2. c; 3. b, d, e; 4. b; 5. c; 6. a, c; 7. a; 8. d.

ⓔvolve

For even more review questions, visit *http://evolve.elsevier.com/Canada/ Lewis/medsurg.*

REFERENCES

American College of Obstetricians and Gynecologists. (2015, April). *Patient education fact sheet: Hormone therapy.* Retrieved from *http://www.acog.org/-/media/For-Patients/pfs003.pdf.*

Bulun, S. (2011). Physiology and pathology of the female reproductive axis. In S. Melmed, K. Polonsky, P. R. Larsen, et al. (Eds.), *Williams textbook of endocrinology* (12th ed.). St. Louis: Elsevier Saunders.

Canadian Cancer Society. (2016a). *Breast cancer: Screening for breast cancer.* Retrieved from *http://www.cancer.ca/en/cancer-information/cancer-type/breast/screening/?region=on.*

Canadian Cancer Society. (2016b). *Cervical cancer: Screening for cervical cancer.* Retrieved from *http://www.cancer.ca/en/cancer-information/cancer-type/cervical/screening/?region=on.*

Canadian Cancer Society. (2016c). *Testicular cancer: Finding testicular cancer early.* Retrieved from *http://www.cancer.ca/en/cancer-information/cancer-type/testicular/finding-cancer-early/?region=on.*

Canadian Cancer Society. (2016d). *Prostate cancer: Finding prostate cancer early.* Retrieved from *http://www.cancer.ca/en/cancer-information/cancer-type/prostate/finding-cancer-early/?region=on.*

Centers for Disease Control and Prevention. (2014). *Maternal vaccines: Part of a healthy pregnancy.* Retrieved from *http://www.cdc.gov/vaccines/adults/rec-vac/pregnant.html.*

Chrysant, S. G. (2015). Antihypertensive therapy causes erectile dysfunction. *Current Opinion in Cardiology, 30*(4), 383–390. doi:10.1097/HCO.0000000000000189.

Cordero, A. M., Crider, K. S., Rogers, L. M., et al. (2015). Optimal serum and red blood cell folate concentrations in women of reproductive age for prevention of neural tube defects: World Health Organization guidelines. *MMWR Morb Wkly Rep, 64*(15), 421–423. Retrieved from *http://www.cdc.gov/mmwr/preview/mmwrhtml/mm6415a5.htm?s_cid=mm6415a5_e.*

Grant, J. M., Koskovich, G., Frazer, M. S., et al. (2010). *Outing age 2010: Public policy issues affecting lesbian, gay, bisexual and transgender elders.* Washington, D.C: National Gay and Lesbian Task Force.

Hurt, K. J., Guile, M. W., Bienstock, J. L., et al. (2011). *The Johns Hopkins manual of gynecology and obstetrics* (4th ed.). Philadelphia: Lippincott Williams & Wilkins.

Jameson, J. L., De Groot, L. J., de Kretser, D. M., et al. (2016). *Endocrinology: Adult and pediatric* (7th ed., Vol. 2). Boston: Elsevier Saunders.

Kaunitz, A. M., & Manson, J. E. (2015). Management of menopausal symptoms. *Obstetrics & Gynecology, 126*(4), 859–876. doi:10.1097/AOG.0000000000001058.

Laborde, E., & Brannigan, R. E. (2011). Androgen deficiency in the aging male: The tip of the iceberg? *Urology Times, 38*(5), 44+.

Masters, W. H., & Johnson, E. (1966). *Human sexual response.* Boston: Little Brown. (Seminal).

McCance, K. L., Huether, S. E., Brashers, V. L., et al. (2014). *Pathophysiology: The biologic basis for disease in adults and children* (7th ed.). St. Louis: Mosby.

Office on Women's Health. (2014). *Pregnancy tests.* Retrieved from *http://www.womenshealth.gov/publications/our-publications/briefs/pregnancy-tests/OWH_FS_Pregnancy_Tests.pdf.*

Pagana, K. D., & Pagana, T. J. (2013). *Mosby's Canadian manual of diagnostic and laboratory tests* (1st ed.; S. A. Pike-MacDonald, Canadian ed.). St. Louis: Mosby.

Patton, K. T., & Thibodeau, G. A. (2015). *Structure and function of the body* (15th ed.). St. Louis: Mosby.

Ports, K. A., Barnack-Tavlaris, J. L., Syme, M. L., et al. (2014). Sexual health discussions with older adult patients during periodic health exams. *The Journal of Sexual Medicine, 11*(4), 901–908. doi:10.1111/jsm.12448.

Rainbow Health Ontario (2014). *About LGBTQ health.* Retrieved from *http://www.rainbowhealthontario.ca/about-lgbtq-health/.*

Rapid Response Service (2014). *Rapid response: Facilitators and barriers to health care for lesbian, gay and bisexual (LGB) people. Rapid Review # 79.* Toronto: Ontario HIV Treatment Network. Retrieved from *http://www.ohtn.on.ca/Pages/Knowledge-Exchange/Rapid-Responses/Documents/RR79.pdf.*

Rebar, R., & Erickson, G. (2011). Reproductive endocrinology and infertility. In C. Goldman & A. Schafer (Eds.), *Goldman's Cecil medicine* (24th ed.). St. Louis: Elsevier Saunders.

Statistics Canada. (2014). *Canadian Community Health Survey—Annual component (CCHS).* Retrieved from *http://www23.statcan.gc.ca/imdb/p2SV.pl?Function=getSurvey&SDDS=3226.*

Syme, M. L., & Cohn, T. J. (2016). Examining aging sexual stigma attitudes among adults by gender, age, and generational status. *Aging Ment Health, 20*(1), 36–45. doi:10.1080/13607863.2015.1012044.

Zoltick, B. (2011). Shedding light on testicular cancer. *Nurse Practitioner, 36*(7), 32–39. doi:10.1097/01.NPR.0000398870.16580.86.

RESOURCES

Resources for this chapter are listed in Chapters 56 and 57.

Nursing Management
Breast Disorders

Written by: Darcy Burbage
Adapted by: Jackie Hartigan-Rogers

⊖volve WEBSITE

http://evolve.elsevier.com/Canada/Lewis/medsurg

- Review Questions (Online Only)
- Key Points
- Answer Guidelines for Case Study

- Customizable Nursing Care Plan
  - Mastectomy or Lumpectomy
- Conceptual Care Map Creator
  - Conceptual Care Map for Textbook Case Study

- Audio Glossary
- Content Updates

LEARNING OBJECTIVES

1. Summarize screening guidelines for the early detection of breast cancer.
2. Describe the technique of breast self-awareness, including rationale and reasons for referral.
3. Explain the types, causes, clinical manifestations, collaborative care, and nursing management of common benign breast disorders.
4. Assess the risk factors for breast cancer.
5. Describe the pathophysiology and clinical manifestations of breast cancer.
6. Describe the collaborative care and the nursing management of breast cancer.
7. Specify the physical and psychological preoperative and postoperative aspects of nursing management for patients undergoing a mastectomy.
8. Explain the indications for reconstructive breast surgery; types, potential risks, and complications of reconstructive breast surgery; and nursing management after reconstructive breast surgery.

KEY TERMS

cyst, p. 1352, Table 54-1
fibroadenoma, p. 1353
fibrocystic changes, p. 1352

galactorrhea, p. 1353
gynecomastia, p. 1353
lumpectomy, p. 1359

lymphedema, p. 1359
mammoplasty, p. 1366
mastalgia, p. 1351

mastectomy, p. 1353
mastitis, p. 1351
Paget's disease, p. 1356

Breast disorders are a significant health concern for women. Most breast pain is of a benign nature, with the most frequently encountered breast disorders in women being nipple discharge, intraductal papilloma, duct ectasia, breast pain, and fibrocystic changes such as cysts and fibroadenomas (Onstad & Stuckey, 2013; "Managing Fibrocystic", 2015; Women's College Hospital, 2015). In men, gynecomastia is the most common breast disorder.

In Canada, there is a one in eight chance that a woman will receive a diagnosis of breast cancer in her lifetime (Canadian Cancer Society, 2017a). Whether the actual diagnosis is one of a benign condition or a malignancy, the initial discovery of a lump or change in the breast often triggers intense feelings of anxiety, fear, and denial. These feelings can be associated with both the fear of death and the possible loss of a breast. The potential loss of a breast, or part of a breast, may be devastating

because of the significant psychological, social, sexual, and body image implications associated with it.

ASSESSMENT OF BREAST DISORDERS

It is critical that breast disorders be detected early, diagnosed accurately, and treated promptly. The frequency of breast examinations is determined by a woman's age, the presence of significant risk factors, and her medical history. Guidelines established in Canada regarding breast surveillance practices include the following:

- Women of all ages should be familiar with their breasts and report any changes to their health care providers.
- Women ages 40 to 49 should discuss with a health care provider their individual risk for breast cancer, along with the risks and benefits of mammography.

- Women aged 50 to 69 should undergo mammography every 2 years.
- Women aged 70 or older should talk to a health care provider about an individualized screening program.
- A health care provider may also perform a physical examination of the breasts (clinical breast examination).
- Women who are at high risk for developing breast cancer should talk to their health care providers about a personal plan of testing (Canadian Cancer Society, 2017b).

It is recommended that all women discuss the risks and benefits of mammography with their health care providers (Canadian Cancer Society, 2017b). The benefits of early detection of breast cancer are well established. The use of screening mammography has significantly improved early and accurate detection of breast malignancies. Mammography can identify breast abnormalities that may be cancer before physical symptoms appear. Canada's national guidelines have been established on the basis of research that women aged 50 to 69 benefit most from regular breast screening (Canadian Cancer Society, 2017b).

There has been some confusion with regard to the value of breast self-examination (BSE) and screening mammography for younger women and its role in reducing rates of mortality from breast cancer (Canadian Task Force on Preventive Health Care, 2011; Silversides, 2012). The emphasis now is to assist women to become aware of how their breasts normally look and feel and to understand that there is no right or wrong way for them to check their breasts (Figure 54-1). Nurses should teach women that it is important to get to know the whole area of breast tissue including up to the collarbone and under armpits

and nipples (Canadian Cancer Society, 2017b). Women should be encouraged to report any new breast changes (e.g., nipple discharge, presence of a lump) to their health care providers (Canadian Cancer Society, 2017b).

If a woman decides she wants to practise BSE and undergo mammography screening, health care providers must ensure that the benefits and risks, as well as the woman's values and preferences, are discussed fully (Canadian Task Force on Preventive Health Care, 2011).

It is also important that nurses ensure patients' awareness of Canada's clinical practice guidelines for the care and treatment of breast cancer. All patients who have completed primary treatment for breast cancer should have regular follow-up surveillance that comprises a medical history, physical examination, and annual mammography. The frequency of visits must be adjusted according to the individual patient's needs. Special topics of concern that have to be addressed with patients who have breast cancer include cognitive functioning, fatigue, weight management, osteoporosis, sexual functioning, and pregnancy (Canadian Task Force on Preventive Health Care, 2011).

DIAGNOSTIC STUDIES

Radiological Studies

Several techniques can be used to screen for breast disorders or provide a diagnosis of a suspect physical finding. *Mammography* is a method used to visualize the internal structure of the breast with the use of radiography (Figure 54-2). This generally well-tolerated procedure can detect suspect findings that cannot be felt by palpation. Mammography has significantly improved the early and accurate detection of breast malignancies. Improved imaging technology has also reduced the amount of radiation used in mammography. Digital mammography, in which radiographic images are digitally coded into a computer, is an addition to screening programs (Canadian Partnership Against Cancer, 2013; Figure 54-2).

Three-dimensional (3-D) mammography is a new type of mammography; it provides a clearer 3-D view of overlapping breast tissue structures, which helps to accurately detect and diagnose breast cancer (Canadian Agency for Drugs and Technologies in Health [CADTH], 2015).

Calcifications are the abnormality most easily recognized on mammograms (see Figure 54-2). These deposits of calcium crystals

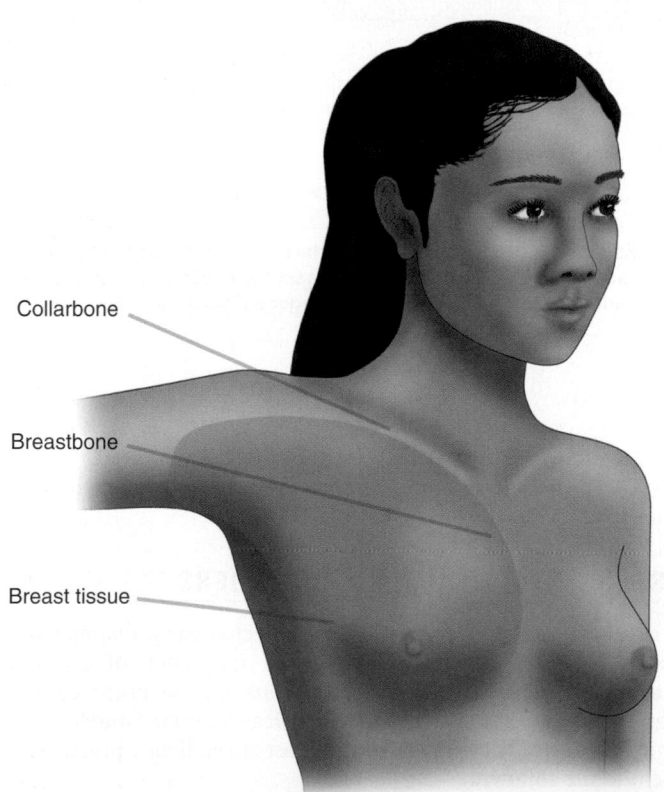

FIGURE 54-1 Every woman should know her breasts. She should be aware of what is normal by looking at and feeling her breasts any way that works best for her. She should get to know the whole area of her breast tissue: up to the collarbone, under the armpits, and including the nipples. Every woman should get to know her breasts well enough to notice changes. Source: Monica Schroeder/Science Source.

Collarbone

Breastbone

Breast tissue

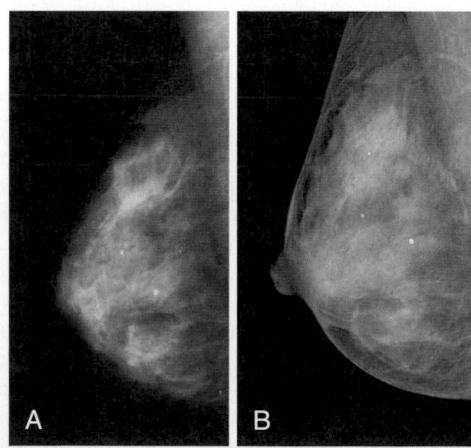

FIGURE 54-2 Screening mammograms showing dense breast tissue and benign, scattered microcalcifications of a 57-year-old. **A,** Image obtained with conventional radiography. **B,** Image obtained with digital radiography. Source: Adam, A. (2008). *Grainger and Allison's diagnostic radiology* (5th ed.). St. Louis: Churchill Livingstone.

form in the breast for many reasons, such as inflammation, trauma, and aging. Although most calcifications are benign, they also may be associated with preinvasive cancer.

A comparison of current and prior mammograms may reveal early cancerous tissue changes. Because some tumours metastasize late, early detection by mammography allows for earlier treatment and the prevention of metastasis of lesions that are smaller or less aggressive. In younger women, mammography is less sensitive because of the greater density of breast tissue and because developing breast tissue is radiosensitive, resulting in more false-negative results (CADTH, 2015). About 10% to 15% of all breast cancers cannot be seen on mammograms and are detected only by palpation. If the clinical findings are suspect, ultrasound or magnetic resonance imaging (MRI) may be used, and biopsy may be recommended based on the findings.

Ultrasonography is used in conjunction with mammography to differentiate a solid mass from a cystic mass, to evaluate a mass in a pregnant or lactating woman, or to locate and guide biopsy for a suspect lesion on breast MRI. Palpable masses should be investigated with both mammography and ultrasonography (CADTH, 2015).

MRI is recommended as a sensitive screening tool for women at high risk for breast cancer, for women whose findings on mammography or ultrasonography are suspect for malignancy, and for women in whom breast cancer was previously detected by mammography. Limitations of MRI include its high cost, which may result in less frequent use of this method of screening (CADTH, 2015).

Biopsies

A definitive diagnosis of a suspect area is made by means of histological examination of a biopsy sample of tissue. Biopsy techniques include fine-needle aspiration (FNA), core needle, stereotactic core needle, wire localization, and surgical biopsy (also called *open biopsy*).

In *FNA biopsy,* a thin, fine needle is inserted into the lesion and cellular fluid aspirated into a syringe. Three or four passes are usually made. FNA and cytological evaluation may be helpful in making a diagnosis and planning treatment. If the results are negative but the lesion is suspect, an additional biopsy may be necessary. Biopsy results are usually available within 24 to 48 hours.

A *core needle biopsy* is commonly used as a preferred method for obtaining and diagnosing a breast tissue specimen (Onstad & Stuckey, 2013). It involves removing samples of breast tissue using a hollow needle, which takes small cylinder shaped (core) samples.

Stereotactic core needle biopsy is a reliable diagnostic technique for obtaining a biopsy sample of an abnormality seen on a mammogram. The use of 3-D images assists in pinpointing the exact location of a lump or suspect lesion in order to guide the needle to obtain a sample of breast tissue. Patients should be informed that the procedure is uncomfortable. The patient is positioned lying face down on a table that has an opening for the breast. The skin is anaesthetized, and a small incision is made to allow the entrance of a biopsy needle that has a special cutting device. This process is repeated several times, and the core samples are sent for pathological analysis. Larger samples of tissue can be removed using a special *vacuum-assisted device* (VAD), which uses suction to collect the tissue sample. An advantage of VAD is that the needle is inserted only once into the breast and then can be rotated, which allows for multiple samples through a single needle insertion.

These outpatient techniques have advantages over a surgical biopsy, including minimal scarring, local anaesthesia, reduced cost, and shorter recovery time. A *surgical biopsy* involves removal of part or all of a suspect lesion through an incision into the breast. If the lesion is small, deep, and difficult to locate, a *wire localization biopsy* may be used during surgery. A special fine wire is placed into the lesion under radiographic guidance, and then the surgeon follows this wire to help locate the lesion.

BENIGN BREAST DISORDERS

Mastalgia

Mastalgia (breast pain) is the most common breast-related complaint in women. The most common form is *cyclic mastalgia*, which coincides with the menstrual cycle (Onstad & Stuckey, 2013). It is described as diffuse breast tenderness or heaviness. Breast pain may last 2 to 3 days or most of the month. The pain is related to hormonal sensitivity. The symptoms often decrease with menopause. *Noncyclic mastalgia* has no relationship to the menstrual cycle and can continue into menopause. It may be constant or intermittent throughout the month and last for several years. Symptoms include a burning sensation, aching, or soreness in the breast. The cause of the pain of noncyclic mastalgia is not known (Canadian Cancer Society, 2017c).

Mammography and targeted ultrasound are often performed to exclude cancer and provide etiology of mastalgia. Cyclic pain may be relieved somewhat by reductions in caffeine and dietary fat intake; by vitamins E, A, and B complex and gamma-linolenic acid (evening primrose oil); and by continual wearing of a support bra. Massage with ice or heat, analgesics, and anti-inflammatory medications may also help. Medications that might be recommended include oral contraceptives and danazol (Cyclomen). Because of the androgenic adverse effects of danazol (acne, edema, hirsutism), this therapy is unacceptable for many women.

Breast Infections

Mastitis. Mastitis is an inflammatory condition of the breast that occurs most frequently in lactating women (Table 54-1). *Lactational mastitis* manifests as a localized area that is erythematous, painful, and tender on palpation. Fever is often present. The infection develops when organisms, usually staphylococci, gain access to the breast through a cracked nipple. In its early stages, mastitis can be cured with antibiotics. Breastfeeding should continue unless an abscess is forming or a purulent drainage is noted. The mother may wish to use a nipple shield or to hand-express milk from the involved breast until the pain subsides. She should see her health care provider promptly to begin a course of antibiotic therapy. Any breast that remains red, tender, and not responsive to antibiotics necessitates follow-up care and evaluation for inflammatory breast cancer (Onstad & Stuckey, 2013).

Lactational Breast Abscess. If lactational mastitis persists after several days of antibiotic therapy, a lactational breast abscess may have developed. In this condition, the skin may become red and edematous over the involved breast, often with a corresponding palpable mass, and the patient may have a fever. Antibiotics alone constitute insufficient treatment for a breast abscess. Ultrasonography-guided drainage of the abscess or surgical incision and drainage are necessary (Onstad & Stuckey, 2013). The drainage is cultured, sensitivities are measured, and therapy with an appropriate antibiotic is begun. Breastfeeding can continue in most cases with ongoing treatment of the abscess (Irusen, Rohwer, Steyn, et al., 2015).

TABLE 54-1	SELECT BENIGN BREAST DISORDERS	
Disorder	**Incidence**	**Clinical Manifestations**
Lactational mastitis	Occurs in up to 10% of postpartum lactating mothers (both primipara and multipara), usually 2–4 wk after parturition	Warm to touch, indurated, painful, often unilateral; most commonly caused by *Staphylococcus aureus*
Fibrocystic changes	Most common between ages 35 and 50	Not usually discrete masses but nodularity instead (movable, soft); usually accompanied by cyclic pain and tenderness; mass(es) often cyclic in occurrence
Cyst	Most common after age 35, incidence decreases after menopause; develop in 1 per 14 women	Palpable fluid-filled mass (movable, soft); multiple cysts can occur and recur; rarely associated with breast cancer
Fibroadenoma	Occurs in 10% of all women aged 15–40	Palpable mass (movable, firm), usually 2–3 cm in size; rarely associated with breast cancer
Fat necrosis	Many women report previous history of trauma to breast	Usually a hard, very tender, mobile, indurated mass with irregular borders
Duct ectasia	Perimenopausal woman: most common in women in their 50s; previous lactation; inverted nipples	Fixation of nipple, usually accompanied by nipple discharge of thick, grey material; often associated with breast pain

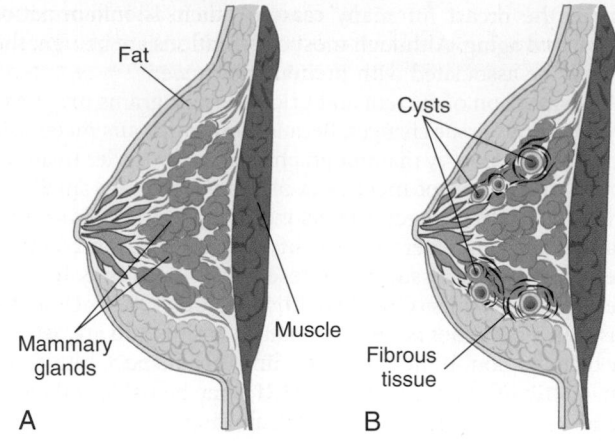

FIGURE 54-3 A, Normal breast tissue. **B,** Fibrocystic breast tissue.

Fibrocystic Changes

Fibrocystic changes in the breast constitute a benign condition characterized by changes in breast tissue (Figure 54-3). The changes include the development of excess fibrous tissue, hyperplasia of the epithelial lining of the mammary ducts, proliferation of mammary ducts, and cyst formation. Pain is caused by nerve irritation from edema in the connective tissue and by fibrosis from pinching of the nerve. Fibrocystic changes are not associated with increased risk for breast cancer. Masses or nodularities can appear in both breasts. They are often found in the upper, outer quadrants and usually occur bilaterally.

Fibrocystic changes are the most frequently occurring breast disorder. They occur most frequently in women between 35 and 50 years of age but often begin as early as 20 years of age. Pain and nodularity often increase over time but tend to subside after menopause unless high doses of estrogen replacement are used. Fibrocystic changes are thought to result from a heightened responsiveness of breast tissue to circulating estrogen and progesterone (Canadian Cancer Society, 2017d).

Fibrocystic changes most commonly occur in women with premenstrual abnormalities, nulliparous women, women with a history of spontaneous abortion, nonusers of oral contraceptives, and women with early menarche and late menopause. Symptoms related to fibrocystic changes often worsen in the premenstrual phase and subside after menstruation.

Manifestations of fibrocystic breast changes include one or more palpable lumps that are often round, well delineated, and freely movable within the breast (see Table 54-1). Discomfort ranging from tenderness to pain may also occur. The lump is usually observed to increase in size and perhaps in tenderness before menstruation. Cysts may enlarge or shrink rapidly, becoming larger before menstruation and shrinking afterward. Nipple discharge associated with fibrocystic breasts is often milky, watery-milky, yellow, or green.

Mammography may be helpful in distinguishing fibrocystic changes from breast cancer. However, in some women, the breast tissue is so dense that it is difficult to obtain a mammographic study. In these situations, ultrasonography may be more useful in differentiating a cystic mass from a solid mass.

NURSING AND COLLABORATIVE MANAGEMENT FIBROCYSTIC CHANGES

With the initial discovery of a discrete mass in the breast by a woman or her health care provider, aspiration or surgical biopsy may be indicated. If the nodularity is recurrent, a wait of 7 to 10 days may be planned in order to note any changes that may be related to the menstrual cycle. For large or frequent cysts, surgical removal may be favoured over repeated aspiration. An excisional biopsy would be recommended if (a) no fluid is found on aspiration, (b) the fluid that is found is hemorrhagic, or (c) a residual mass remains after fluid aspiration. Excisional biopsy is performed in an outpatient surgery unit.

Biopsy may be indicated for women with fibrocystic disorders who are at increased risk for breast cancer. Atypical hyperplasia, which is discovered on breast biopsy, increases a woman's risk for developing breast cancer later in life.

Women with cystic changes should be encouraged to return regularly for follow-up examinations throughout life. They may also be taught BSE to self-monitor changes. Severe fibrocystic changes may make palpation of the breast more difficult. Any changes in symptoms or changes found during the BSE should be reported and evaluated.

Treatment for a fibrocystic condition is similar to that described earlier for mastalgia. The nurse's role in the care of patients with fibrocystic breast changes is primarily one of teaching. Patients should be taught that the cysts may recur in one or both breasts until menopause and that the cysts may enlarge or become painful just before menstruation. In addition, patients should be reassured that the cysts do not "turn into" cancer. Patients should be advised that any new lump that does not respond in a cyclic manner over 1 to 2 weeks should be examined by a health care provider promptly.

Fibroadenoma

Fibroadenoma is a common cause of discrete benign breast lumps in young women, generally between 15 and 40 years of age. It is the most frequent cause of breast masses in women younger than 25 years. The possible cause of fibroadenoma may be increased estrogen sensitivity in a localized area of the breast. Fibroadenomas are usually small but can be large (2 to 3 cm) and are typically painless, round, well delineated, and very mobile. They may be soft but are usually solid, firm, and rubbery in consistency. There is no accompanying retraction or nipple discharge, and they are often painless. Fibroadenomas may appear as a single, unilateral mass, although multiple, bilateral fibroadenomas have been reported. Growth is slow and often ceases when the size reaches 2 to 3 cm. Size is not affected by menstruation. However, pregnancy can stimulate dramatic growth.

NURSING AND COLLABORATIVE MANAGEMENT FIBROADENOMA

Fibroadenomas are easily detected on physical examination and may be visible on mammography and ultrasonography. Definitive diagnosis, however, requires an image-guided core needle biopsy or excisional biopsy and tissue examination by a pathologist. Treatment of fibroadenomas can include observation with regular monitoring, after a malignancy has been ruled out, or surgical excision. In women older than 35 years, all new lesions should be evaluated with breast ultrasonography and, possibly, biopsy.

In some clinical settings, as an alternative to surgery, cryoablation can be used to remove tumours after an established diagnosis of a fibroadenoma. In *cryoablation,* a cryoprobe is inserted into the tumour under ultrasound guidance. Extremely cold gas is piped into the tumour. The frozen tumour dies and is either reduced in size or completely eliminated. Benefits include minimal scarring and quick recovery time.

The nurse needs to emphasize to patients with a fibroadenoma the benign nature of the lesion and encourage them to have follow-up examinations.

Nipple Discharge

Nipple discharge may occur spontaneously or as a result of nipple manipulation. A milky secretion constitutes inappropriate lactation (galactorrhea) and may be a result of drug therapy, endocrine problems, or a neurological disorder, or it may be idiopathic.

Secretions can also be serous, grossly bloody, or brown to green (Onstad & Stuckey, 2013). These secretions may be caused by either benign or malignant disease. Cytological study of the secretion may help determine the specific disease. Diseases associated with nipple discharge include intraductal papilloma, duct ectasia, cystic disease, and malignancies. Treatment depends on identification of the cause (Onstad & Stuckey, 2013). In most cases, nipple discharge is not related to malignancy.

Intraductal Papilloma. An *intraductal papilloma* is a benign, soft, wartlike growth found in the mammary ducts. It is usually unilateral. It is typically accompanied by a bloody discharge from the nipple that can be intermittent or spontaneous. Most intraductal papillomas are beneath the areola and cannot be palpated. They are usually found in women aged 40 to 60 years. A single duct or several ducts may be involved. Treatment includes excision of the papilloma and the involved duct or duct system. Papillomas may be associated with an increased risk for cancer.

Duct Ectasia. *Duct ectasia* (duct dilation) is a benign breast disorder of perimenopausal and postmenopausal women that involves the ducts in the subareolar area. Several bilateral ducts are usually involved. Multicoloured, sticky discharge is the primary symptom. Duct ectasia is initially painless but may progress to causing a burning sensation, itching, and pain around the nipple, as well as swelling in the areolar area. Inflammatory signs are often present, the nipple may retract, and the discharge may become bloody in more advanced disease. Duct ectasia is not associated with malignancy. If an abscess develops, warm compresses and antibiotics are usually effective treatments. Therapy consists of close follow-up examinations or surgical excision of the involved ducts.

Gynecomastia

Gynecomastia, a transient, noninflammatory enlargement of one or both breasts, is a common noncancerous breast problem in men (Canadian Cancer Society, 2017e). Gynecomastia by itself is not an established risk factor for breast cancer. Mammography may be completed to screen for malignancy. The most common cause of gynecomastia is a disturbance of the normal ratio of active androgen to estrogen in plasma or within the breast itself.

Gynecomastia may also be a manifestation of other problems. It may accompany developmental abnormalities of the male reproductive organs. Gynecomastia may occur as an adverse effect of drug therapy, particularly with administration of estrogens and androgens, digitalis, ranitidine (Zantac), and spironolactone (Aldactone). Use of heroin and marihuana can also cause gynecomastia.

Senescent Gynecomastia. *Senescent gynecomastia* occurs in up to 70% of older men (Deepinder & Braunstein, 2011). A probable cause is the elevation in plasma estrogen in older-adult men as the result of increased conversion of androgens to estrogens in peripheral circulation. Although initially unilateral, the tender, firm, centrally located enlargement may become bilateral. When gynecomastia is characterized by a discrete, circumscribed mass, it must be biopsied to differentiate it from the rarer breast cancer in men. Senescent gynecomastia necessitates no treatment and generally regresses within 6 to 12 months.

AGE-RELATED CONSIDERATIONS

BREAST CHANGES

The loss of subcutaneous fat and structural support and the atrophy of mammary glands often cause breasts to become pendulous in postmenopausal women. The nurse should encourage older women to wear a well-fitting bra. Adequate support can improve physical appearance and reduce pain in the back, shoulders, and neck. It can also prevent *intertrigo* (dermatitis caused by friction between opposing surfaces of skin). Surgical lifting of sagging breasts is possible and may be desirable when reconstruction is performed after a mastectomy (surgical removal of all or a portion of a breast).

The decrease in glandular tissue in older women makes a breast mass easier to palpate. This decreased density is probably age related and occurs to a lesser degree with women receiving hormone therapy. Rib margins may be palpable in older women and can be confused with a mass. As a woman becomes more familiar with her own breasts and is reassured about her findings, the anxiety about this finding should decrease. The nurse should encourage older women to continue examining their breasts and to talk to their health care providers about an individualized screening program, because the incidence of breast cancer increases with age.

BREAST CANCER

Breast cancer is the most common cancer in Canadian women, excluding nonmelanoma skin cancer. It is second only to lung cancer as the leading cause of death from cancer in women. It can occur in men, although less commonly (Canadian Cancer Society, 2017a). It was estimated that, in 2017, 26 300 new cases of breast cancer would be diagnosed in women in Canada, and approximately 230 new cases in men. Each year in Canada, approximately 5 060 deaths (5 000 women and 60 men) occur in relation to breast cancer (Canadian Cancer Society, 2017a). The number of deaths of women from breast cancer in every age group has declined, partly as a result of increased mammography screening and decreased use of hormone therapy (Canadian Cancer Society, 2017f). The five-year survival rate for women with breast cancer is 87% and 79% for men (Canadian Cancer Society, 2017a).

Etiology and Risk Factors

Although the etiology is not completely understood, a number of factors are thought to contribute to breast cancer (Table 54-2). Risk factors appear to be cumulative and interacting. Therefore, the presence of other risk factors may greatly increase the overall risk, especially for people with a positive family history. Identification of risk factors increases the need for careful clinical surveillance of a patient and for participation in cancer screening measures.

Risk Factors for Women. The identifiable risk factors most associated with breast cancer include female gender and advancing age. Women are at far greater risk than men because 99% of breast cancers occur in women. The incidence of breast cancer in women is very low before 25 years of age and increases gradually until age 60. After age 60, the incidence increases dramatically.

Hormonal regulation of the breast is related to the development of breast cancer, but the mechanisms are poorly understood. The hormones estrogen and progesterone may act as tumour promoters to stimulate breast cancer growth if malignant changes in the cells have already occurred. Data from the Women's Health Initiative study have shown that the use of combined hormone therapy (estrogen plus progesterone) increases breast cancer risk by 25% (Canadian Cancer Society, 2017g). The use of estrogen replacement therapy alone (for women who have had a prior hysterectomy) does not currently appear to increase breast cancer risk. Oral contraceptives that contain both estrogen and progesterone cause a slight increase in the risk of breast cancer, particularly for women who have used them for 10 years or longer (Canadian Cancer Society, 2017f). Modifiable risk factors include weight gain during adulthood, sedentary lifestyle, dietary fat intake, obesity, and alcohol intake (Canadian Cancer Society, 2017f). Environmental factors such as radiation exposure may also play a role.

Genetic Factors. Family history is an important risk factor, especially if the involved family member also had ovarian cancer, was premenopausal, had bilateral breast cancer, and is a first-degree

TABLE 54-2	RISK FACTORS FOR BREAST CANCER
Increased Risk	**Comments**
Female	Women account for 99% of breast cancer cases.
Age 50 or older	The majority of breast cancers are found in postmenopausal women. After age 60, the incidence is greatly elevated.
Family history	Breast cancer in a first-degree relative—particularly when the person is premenopausal or the tumour is bilateral—increases risk. Gene mutations (*BRCA1* or *BRCA2*) play a role in 5%–10% of breast cancer cases.
Hormone use	The use of estrogen, progesterone, or both as hormone therapy, especially in postmenopausal women, increases risk.
Personal history of breast cancer, colon cancer, endometrial cancer, ovarian cancer	Personal history significantly increases risk of breast cancer, risk of cancer in the other breast, and recurrence.
Early menarche (<age 12); late menopause (>age 55)	A long menstrual history increases the risk for breast cancer.
First full-term pregnancy after age 30; nulliparity	Prolonged exposure to unopposed estrogen increases risk for breast cancer.
Benign breast disorder with atypical epithelial hyperplasia, LCIS	Atypical changes in breast biopsy increase the risk for breast cancer.
Dense breast tissue	Mammograms are harder to read and interpret. Dense tissue may be associated with more aggressive tumours.
Weight gain and obesity after menopause	Fat cells store estrogen, which increases the likelihood of developing breast cancer.
Exposure to ionizing radiation	Radiation (e.g., prior treatment for Hodgkin's lymphoma) damages DNA.
Alcohol consumption	Women who drink ≥1 alcoholic beverage per day have an increased risk for breast cancer.
Physical inactivity	Breast cancer risk is decreased by 33% in physically active women in comparison with sedentary women.

DNA, deoxyribonucleic acid; *LCIS,* lobular carcinoma in situ.

relative (i.e., mother, sister, daughter). Having any first-degree relative with breast cancer increases a woman's risk for breast cancer 1.5 to 3 times, depending on age. (The Determinants of Health box discusses other factors contributing to breast cancer.)

As many as 5% to 10% of all patients with breast cancer may have inherited a specific genetic abnormality contributing to the development of their breast cancer (Canadian Cancer Society, 2017f). The *BRCA1* gene, located on chromosome 17, and the *BRCA2* gene, located on chromosome 11, are tumour suppressor genes that, when functioning normally, inhibit tumour development. Women with inherited *BRCA1* or *BRCA2* mutations have up to an 85% lifetime chance of developing breast cancer (Canadian Cancer Society, 2017f). These women are also at high risk for developing ovarian cancer (Canadian Cancer Society,

DETERMINANTS OF HEALTH

Breast Cancer

Personal Health Practices and Coping Skills
- Women with a higher body mass index (BMI) (>31.1) are at an increased risk for developing breast cancer.*
- Physical inactivity is a probable risk factor for breast cancer.*

Gender
- Breast cancer is more common in women; it can occur in men, although it is rare.†

Income
- Women with higher incomes have a slightly higher incidence of breast cancer, which may be related to having children later in life or having fewer children.*

Lifestyle
- Working at night may increase the risk of developing breast cancer.*

References

*Canadian Cancer Society. (2017). *Risk factors for breast cancer.* Retrieved from *http://www.cancer.ca/en/cancer-information/cancer-type/breast/risks/?region=on.*

†Canadian Cancer Society. (2017). *Know your risk: Gender and age.* Retrieved from *http://www.cbcf.org/central/AboutBreastHealth/KnowYourRisk/Pages/Gender-Age.aspx.*

TABLE 54-3	TYPES OF BREAST CANCER
Type	**Frequency of Occurrence**
Invasive/Infiltrating ductal carcinoma	70%–75%
• Colloid (mucinous)	
• Inflammatory	
• Paget's disease	
• Medullary	
• Tubular	
Invasive/Infiltrating lobular carcinoma	5%–10%
Noninvasive carcinoma	20%
• Ductal carcinoma in situ	

GENETICS IN CLINICAL PRACTICE

Breast Cancer

Genetic Basis
- Mutations in genes *BRCA1* and *BRCA2*
- Autosomal dominant transmission

Incidence
- Approximately 5% to 10% of breast cancers are related to *BRCA1* and *BRCA2* gene mutations.
- Women with *BRCA1* and *BRCA2* gene mutations have a 40% to 80% lifetime risk of developing breast cancer.
- *BRCA1* and *BRCA2* gene mutations are associated with early-onset breast cancer.
- Men with *BRCA1* and *BRCA2* gene mutations have an increased risk for breast and prostate cancer.
- Family history of both breast and ovarian cancer increases the risk of having a *BRCA1* mutation.

Genetic Testing
- DNA testing is available for *BRCA1* and *BRCA2* gene mutations.

Clinical Implications
- Most breast cancers (about 90%–95%) are not inherited. They are associated with genetic changes that occur after a person is born (somatic mutations).
- Bilateral oophorectomy, bilateral mastectomy, or both reduce the risk for breast cancer in women with *BRCA1* and *BRCA2* mutations.
- Mutations in the *BRCA1* and *BRCA2* genes increase the risk for ovarian cancer.
- Genetic counselling and testing for *BRCA* mutations should be considered for women whose personal or family history puts them at high risk for a genetic predisposition to breast cancer.

2017f). Routine screening for genetic abnormalities in women without evidence of a strong family history of breast cancer is not warranted (see the "Genetics in Clinical Practice: Breast Cancer" box). Research investigating the role of genes in the development of breast cancer continues.

Risk Factors for Men. Predisposing risk factors for breast cancer in men include hyperestrogenism, a family history of breast cancer, and radiation exposure. A thorough examination of the male breast should be a routine part of a physical examination for all men. Men in *BRCA*-positive families may consider genetic testing. Men with an abnormal *BRCA* gene also have an increased risk of developing prostate cancer.

Prophylactic Oophorectomy and Mastectomy. In women with *BRCA1* or *BRCA2* mutations, prophylactic bilateral oophorectomy can decrease the risk for breast cancer and ovarian cancer (Canadian Cancer Society, 2017h). In deciding whether and when to undergo this surgical procedure, women should receive counselling about the risks and benefits of prophylactic oophorectomy, including those related to fertility.

Women who have a high risk of developing breast cancer (i.e., related to factors such as family history and prior tissue biopsy findings) may, in consultation with their health care provider, choose to undergo prophylactic bilateral mastectomy. Research has shown that contralateral prophylactic mastectomy (mastectomy of the unaffected breast) can decrease the risk for contralateral breast cancer, but survival rates have not been determined (Chagpar, 2014).

Women with hereditary (non-*BRCA*) breast cancer have a higher risk of developing a secondary primary breast cancer in the unaffected (contralateral) breast. These women may also choose to have the unaffected breast removed prophylactically at the time of initial surgery for breast cancer or at a later time. The rate of contralateral prophylactic mastectomies in women has been steadily increasing (Chagpar, 2014).

Pathophysiology

Various types of breast cancer have been identified on the basis of their histological characteristics and growth patterns (Table 54-3). The main components of the breast are lobules (milk-producing glands) and ducts (milk passages that connect the lobules and the nipple). In general, breast cancer arises from the epithelial lining of the ducts *(ductal carcinoma)* or from the epithelium of the lobules *(lobular carcinoma)*. Breast cancers may be in situ (within the duct or lobule) or invasive (arising from the duct or lobule and invading through the wall of the duct or lobule).

Metastatic breast cancer is breast cancer that has spread to bone, the liver, the lungs, or the brain. Cancer growth rate can range from slow to rapid. Factors that affect cancer prognosis are tumour size, axillary node involvement (the more nodes involved, the worse the prognosis), tumour differentiation, estrogen and progesterone receptor status, and *human epidermal growth factor receptor 2* (HER2) status. HER2 is a transmembrane receptor that helps regulate cell growth. In many patients with breast cancer, it is overexpressed (Yeo, Turner, & Jones, 2014).

TYPES OF BREAST CANCER

Breast cancer can be classified as noninvasive or invasive, and as ductal or lobular (see Table 54-3).

Noninvasive Breast Cancer. An estimated 20% of all breast cancers are noninvasive. These intraductal cancers include *ductal carcinoma in situ* (DCIS) and *lobular carcinoma in situ* (LCIS). DCIS tends to be unilateral and may progress to invasive breast cancer if left untreated.

Although the management of DCIS can be controversial, patients should discuss all treatment options with their physician, including local excision, mastectomy with breast reconstruction, breast-conserving surgery (lumpectomy), radiation therapy, and tamoxifen (Nolvadex-D) therapy.

The term *lobular carcinoma in situ* is somewhat misleading. Although LCIS is a risk factor for developing breast cancer, it is not known to be a premalignant lesion. Although no treatment is necessary, patients with LCIS should increase their surveillance for breast cancer. Tamoxifen may be given to some patients as a chemopreventive drug.

Invasive (Infiltrating) Ductal Carcinoma. *Invasive (infiltrating) ductal carcinoma* is the most common type of breast cancer. It starts in the milk duct and then breaks through the wall of the duct, invading the surrounding tissue. From there it may metastasize to other parts of the body.

Types of invasive (infiltrating) ductal carcinoma include *medullary carcinoma,* which accounts for 15% of all breast cancers and most frequently occurs in women in their late 40s and 50s. *Tubular carcinoma* accounts for about 2% of all breast cancers, is usually found in women over 50 years of age, and has an excellent prognosis. *Colloid (mucinous) carcinoma* accounts for about 1% to 2% of all breast cancers and usually has a favourable prognosis.

Inflammatory Breast Cancer. *Inflammatory breast cancer,* the most malignant form of all breast cancers, is rare. It is an aggressive and fast-growing cancer with a high risk for metastasis. The skin of the breast looks red, feels warm, and has a thickened appearance that is often described as resembling an orange peel (*peau d'orange*). The inflammatory changes, often mistaken for an infection, are caused by blockage of lymph channels by cancer cells. Chemotherapy given before surgery is usually the first course of treatment, often followed by radiation. Hormonal therapy may also be indicated.

Paget's Disease. Paget's disease is a rare breast malignancy characterized by a persistent lesion of the nipple and areola with or without a palpable mass. (This is different from Paget's disease of the bone, which is discussed in Chapter 66.) Most women with Paget's disease have underlying ductal carcinoma. Only in rare cases is the cancer confined to the nipple itself. Itching, a burning sensation, bloody nipple discharge with superficial erosion, and ulceration may be present. Diagnosis of Paget's disease is confirmed by pathological examination of the erosion. Nipple changes are often diagnosed as an infection or dermatitis, which can lead to delays in proper treatment. The treatment of Paget's disease may include lumpectomy and radiation therapy or a simple or modified radical mastectomy. The prognosis is good when the cancer is confined to the nipple. The nursing

care for patients with Paget's disease is the same as the care for patients with breast cancer.

Invasive (Infiltrating) Lobular Carcinoma. *Invasive (infiltrating) lobular carcinoma* usually appears as a subtle thickening in the upper outer quadrant of the breast. Often positive for estrogen and progesterone receptors, these tumours respond well to hormone therapy.

Clinical Manifestations

Breast cancer is detected as a lump or mammographic abnormality in the breast. It occurs most often in the upper outer quadrant of the breast because this is the location of most of the glandular tissue (Figure 54-4). Breast cancers vary in growth rate. If palpable, breast cancer is characteristically hard and may be irregularly shaped, poorly delineated, nonmobile, and nontender.

A small percentage of breast cancers cause nipple discharge. The discharge is usually unilateral and may be clear or bloody. Nipple retraction may occur. *Peau d'orange* may result from the plugging of the dermal lymphatic vessels. With large cancers, infiltration, induration, and dimpling (pulling in) of the overlying skin may also be noted.

Complications

The main complication of breast cancer is recurrence (Table 54-4). Recurrence may be local or regional (skin or soft tissue near the mastectomy site, axillary or internal mammary lymph nodes) or distant (most commonly involving bone, the lung, the brain, or the liver). However, metastatic disease can be found in any distant site.

Metastatic disease involves the growth of colonies of cancerous breast cells in parts of the body distant from the breast. Metastases primarily occur through the lymphatic vessels, principally those of the axilla (see Figure 54-7, later in the chapter). However, the cancer can spread to other parts of the body without invading the axillary nodes even when the primary breast tumour is small. Even with node-negative breast cancer, there is a possibility of distant metastasis.

Diagnostic Studies

In addition to studies used to diagnose breast cancer (see discussion earlier in this chapter), other tests are useful in predicting the risk for local or systemic recurrence. These tests include axillary lymph node status, tumour size, estrogen and progesterone

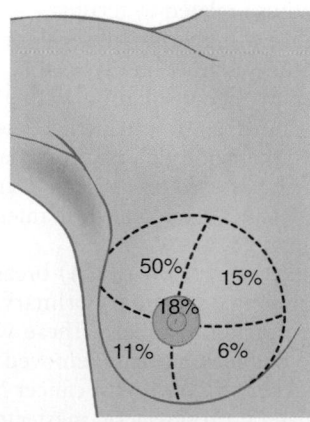

FIGURE 54-4 Distribution of where breast cancer occurs.

receptor status, and cell-proliferative indices. Results of many of these diagnostic studies are useful prognostic indicators of the disease.

Axillary lymph node involvement is one of the most important prognostic factors in breast cancer. An *axillary lymph node*

TABLE 54-4	COMMON SITES OF BREAST CANCER RECURRENCE AND METASTASIS
Site	**Clinical Manifestations**
Local Recurrence	
Skin, chest wall	Firm, discrete nodules; occasionally pruritic, usually painless; commonly in or near a scar
Regional Recurrence	
Lymph nodes	Enlarged nodes in axilla or supraclavicular area, usually nontender
Distant Metastases	
Skeletal	Localized pain of gradually increasing intensity; percussion tenderness at involved sites; pathological fracture caused by involvement of bone cortex
Spinal cord	Progressive back pain, localized and radiating; change in bladder or bowel function; loss of sensation in lower extremities
Brain	Headache described as "different"; unilateral sensory loss; focal muscular weakness, hemiparesis, incoordination (ataxia); nausea or vomiting unrelated to medication; cognitive changes
Pulmonary (including lung nodules and pleural effusions)	Shortness of breath, tachypnea, nonproductive cough (not present in all patients)
Liver	Abdominal distension; right lower quadrant abdominal pain, sometimes with radiation to scapular area; nausea and vomiting, anorexia, weight loss; weakness and fatigue; hepatomegaly, ascites, jaundice; peripheral edema; elevated liver enzyme levels
Bone marrow	Anemia; infection; increased bleeding, bruising, petechiae; weakness and fatigue; mild confusion, light-headedness; dyspnea

dissection (ALND) is often performed to determine whether cancer has spread to the axilla on the side of the breast cancer (Canadian Cancer Society, 2017i). The more nodes involved, the higher the risk for recurrence. Patients with four or more positive nodes have the highest risk for recurrence.

Lymphatic mapping and *sentinel lymph node biopsy (SLNB)* helps the surgeon identify the lymph node or nodes that drain first from the tumour site *(sentinel node)*. SLNB is less invasive than ALND (Canadian Cancer Society, 2017j). A radioisotope or blue dye is injected into the tumour site, and intraoperatively, it is determined in which sentinel lymph nodes the radioisotope or blue dye is located (Figure 54-5). A local incision is made in the axilla, and the surgeon dissects the blue-stained sentinel node or the radioactive lymph node. In general, in SLNB, one to four axillary lymph nodes are removed. The nodes are then sent for a frozen-section pathological analysis. If the results are negative, no further axillary surgery is required. If the results are positive, the surgeon may choose to remove additional lymph nodes during the same procedure or during a follow-up surgical procedure in consultation with the patient. SLNB has been associated with lower rates of lymphedema and other arm symptoms (Canadian Cancer Society, 2017j).

Tumour size is a valuable prognostic variable: the larger the tumour, the poorer the prognosis. The wide variety of histological types of breast cancer explains the heterogeneity of the disease. In general, the more well differentiated the tumour is, the less aggressive it is. Poorly differentiated tumours appear morphologically disorganized and are more aggressive.

Another diagnostic test useful for both treatment decisions and prediction of prognosis is measurement of estrogen and progesterone receptor status. Receptor-positive tumours (a) commonly show histological evidence of being well differentiated, (b) frequently have a diploid (more normal) deoxyribonucleic acid (DNA) content and low proliferative indices, (c) have a lower chance for recurrence, and (d) are frequently hormone dependent and responsive to hormone therapy. Receptor-negative tumours (a) are often poorly differentiated histologically, (b) have a high incidence of aneuploidy (abnormally high or low DNA content) and higher proliferative indices, (c) frequently recur, and (d) are usually unresponsive to hormonal therapy.

  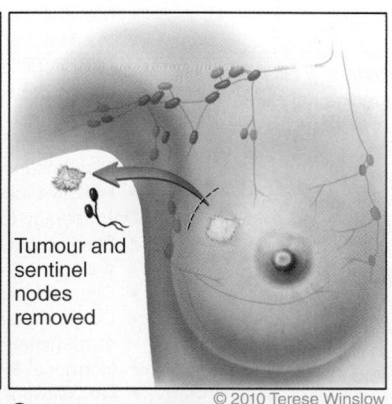

A   B   C

© 2010 Terese Winslow
U.S. Govt. has certain rights

FIGURE 54-5 Sentinel lymph node biopsy of the breast. **A,** A radioactive dye or blue dye is injected near the tumour. **B,** The injected material is detected visually or with a probe that detects radioactivity. **C,** The sentinel nodes (the first lymph nodes to take up the material) are removed and checked for cancer cells. Source: Ignatavicius, D., & Workman, M. L. (2016). *Medical-surgical nursing: Patient-centered collaborative care.* (8th ed., p. 1472, Figure 70-5). St. Louis: Saunders.

Ploidy status correlates with tumour aggressiveness. Diploid tumours have been shown to have a significantly lower risk for recurrence than aneuploid tumours.

Cell-proliferative indices indirectly measure the rate of tumour cell proliferation. The percentage of tumour cells in the synthesis (S) phase of the cell cycle (see Chapter 18, Figure 18-1) is another important prognostic indicator.

Another prognostic indicator is the marker HER2, which is a protein that can be measured in breast tissue. Overexpression of this receptor has been associated with a greater risk for recurrence and a poorer prognosis in breast cancer. Between 20% and 30% of metastatic breast cancers produce excessive HER2. High numbers of HER2 receptors are associated with unusually aggressive tumour growth. The presence of this marker assists in the selection and sequence of chemotherapy and the prediction of a patient's response to treatment (Canadian Cancer Society, 2017k).

Collaborative Care

Currently, a wide range of treatment options is available to patients and health care providers making critical decisions about how to treat breast cancer (Tables 54-5 and 54-6). Prognostic factors are considered when treatment decisions are made about a specific breast cancer. Some of these factors also enter into the staging of breast cancer. The most widely accepted staging method for breast cancer is the American Joint Committee on Cancer's TNM system (Canadian Cancer Society, 2017l). In this system, tumour size (T), nodal involvement (N), and presence of metastasis (M) are used to determine the stage of disease. The stage of a breast cancer describes its size and the extent to which it has spread (Table 54-7).

The stages range from I to IV, with stage I being very small tumours (<2 cm) with no lymph node involvement and no metastasis. Further classification within these stages depends on the size of the tumour and the number of lymph nodes involved. Stage IV indicates the presence of metastatic spread, regardless of tumour size or lymph node involvement.

The therapeutic regimen is often dictated by the clinical stage and biology of the cancer. (Adverse drug effects and appropriate nursing management of general treatment modalities for cancer are discussed in Chapter 18 and in Nursing Care Plan [NCP] 18-1, available on the Evolve website.)

In spite of the advent of new prognostic indicators such as determination of DNA content and analysis of cell-cycle phases, the presence or absence of malignant cells in lymph nodes remains

---

TABLE 54-5 COLLABORATIVE CARE

Breast Cancer

Diagnostic
Prediagnosis
- Health history, including risk factors
- Biopsy
- Breast MRI (if indicated)
- Mammography
- Physical examination, including breast and lymph nodes
- Ultrasonography

Postdiagnosis
- Cell-proliferative indices
- Estrogen and progesterone receptor status
- Genetic assays
- HER2 marker
- Lymphatic mapping and SNLD

Staging Workup
- Bone scan (if indicated)
- Calcium and phosphate levels
- Chest radiograph
- Complete blood cell count, platelet count
- CT scan of chest, abdomen, pelvis (if indicated)
- Liver function tests
- MRI (if indicated)
- PET (if indicated)

Collaborative Therapy
- Surgery
  - Breast-conserving (lumpectomy) with SNLD, ALND, or both
  - Modified radical mastectomy (may include reconstruction)
- Radiation therapy
  - Primary radiotherapy
  - Adjuvant radiotherapy
  - High-dose brachytherapy
  - Palliative radiotherapy
- Drug therapy (see Table 54-6)
  - Biological and targeted therapy
  - Chemotherapy
  - Chemotherapy for recurrent or metastatic disease
  - Hormonal therapy
  - Neoadjuvant or adjuvant chemotherapy

ALND, axillary lymph node dissection; *CT,* computed tomography; *HER2,* human epidermal growth factor receptor 2; *MRI,* magnetic resonance imaging; *PET,* positron emission tomography; *SNLD,* sentinel lymph node dissection.

TABLE 54-6 DRUG THERAPY

Breast Cancer

Drug Class	Mechanism of Action	Indications
Hormone Therapy		
Estrogen Receptor Blockers		
Tamoxifen (Nolvadex-D)	Blocks estrogen receptors (ERs)	ER-positive breast cancer in premenopausal and postmenopausal women Used as a preventive measure in high-risk premenopausal and postmenopausal women
Fulvestrant (Faslodex)	Blocks ERs	ER-positive breast cancer in postmenopausal women only
Aromatase Inhibitors		
Anastrozole (Arimidex) Letrozole (Femara) Exemestane (Aromasin)	Prevents production of estrogen by inhibiting aromatase	ER-positive breast cancer in postmenopausal women only
Estrogen Receptor Modulator		
Raloxifene (Evista)	In breast, blocks the effect of estrogen In bone, promotes the effect of estrogen and prevents bone loss	Postmenopausal women
Biological and Targeted Therapy		
Trastuzumab (Herceptin) Pertuzumab (Perjeta)	Blocks HER2 receptor	ER-positive breast cancer in postmenopausal women only
Lapatinib (Tykerb)	Inhibits HER2 tyrosine kinase and EGFR tyrosine kinase	ER-positive breast cancer in postmenopausal women only

EGFR, epidermal growth factor receptor; *HER2,* human epidermal growth factor receptor 2.

a powerful prognostic factor related to local recurrence or metastasis after primary therapy.

Surgical Therapy. Surgery is considered the primary treatment for breast cancer. Table 54-8 describes the most common surgical procedures used to treat breast cancer. Breast-conserving surgery with radiation therapy and modified radical mastectomy with or without reconstruction are currently the most common options for resectable breast cancer (Figure 54-6). Most women with a diagnosis of early-stage breast cancer (≤4 to 5 cm in size) are candidates for either treatment choice. The overall survival rate with lumpectomy and radiation is about the same as that with

TABLE 54-7	STAGING OF BREAST CANCER		
Stage	**Tumour Size**	**Lymph Node Involvement**	**Metastasis**
0	TIS*	No	No
I	<2 cm	No	No
II			
A	No evidence of tumour ranging to 5 cm	No, or 1–3 axillary nodes or internal mammary nodes or both	No
B	Ranging from 2 to >5 cm	No, or 1–3 axillary nodes or internal mammary nodes or both	No
III			
A	No evidence of tumour ranging to >5 cm	Yes, 4–9 axillary nodes or internal mammary nodes or both	No
B	Any size with extension to chest wall or skin	Yes, 4–9 axillary nodes or internal mammary nodes or both	No
C	Any size	Yes, ≥10 axillary nodes, internal mammary nodes, infraclavicular nodes, or a combination of these	No
IV	Any size	Any type of nodal involvement	Yes

TIS, tumour in situ.
Source: Adapted from Canadian Cancer Society. (2015). Stages of breast cancer. Retrieved from *http://www.cancer.ca/en/cancer-information/cancer-type/breast/staging/?region=on*; and American Joint Committee on Cancer. (2010). AJCC cancer staging manual (7th ed.). Retrieved from *https://cancerstaging.org/references-tools/deskreferences/Pages/AJCC-7th-Ed-Cancer-Staging-Manual.aspx.*

modified radical mastectomy (Hwang, Lichtensztajn, Gomez, et al., 2013).

Breast-Conserving Surgery. Breast-conserving surgery (also called **lumpectomy**) involves the removal of the entire tumour along with a margin of normal surrounding tissue (Figure 54-6, *A*). After surgery, radiation therapy is delivered to the entire breast, ending with a boost to the tumour bed. Depending on the staging of the disease, chemotherapy may be administered before radiation therapy. Contraindications to breast-conserving surgery include the following: breast size too small in relation to the tumour size to yield an acceptable cosmetic result, masses and calcifications that are multifocal (within the same breast quadrant), masses that are multicentric (in more than one quadrant), diffuse calcifications in more than one quadrant, or central location of tumour near the nipple. Contraindications to radiation therapy (e.g., active lupus or prior radiation therapy in the radiation field) may make mastectomy a better surgical option.

One of the main advantages of breast-conserving surgery and radiation therapy is that the breast, including the nipple, is preserved. The goal of the combined surgery and radiation is to both maximize the benefits of the cancer treatment and the cosmetic outcome and minimize the risks. Disadvantages of this approach include the increased cost of the surgery plus radiation therapy over surgery alone and the possible adverse effects of irradiation.

Axillary Node Dissection. ALND on the same side as the breast cancer is often performed and, until the early 2000s, was the standard of care for invasive breast cancer. In general, ALND typically involves the removal of 12 to 20 nodes. SLNB has replaced ALND for patients in whom malignant cells are not identified in the sentinel nodes (see Figure 54-5). Recent guidelines suggest that women with one or two positive sentinel lymph nodes who are having breast-conserving surgery followed by radiotherapy may not need ALND (Yeo, Turner, & Jones, 2014). Examination of the lymph nodes provides prognostic information and helps determine further treatment (chemotherapy, hormone therapy, or both).

Lymphedema (accumulation of lymph in soft tissue) can occur as a result of the excision or irradiation of lymph nodes (Nicholson, 2015) (Figure 54-7). When the axillary nodes cannot return lymph fluid to the central circulation, the fluid accumulates in the arm, causing obstructive pressure on the veins and impeding venous return (Figure 54-8). Patients may experience heaviness,

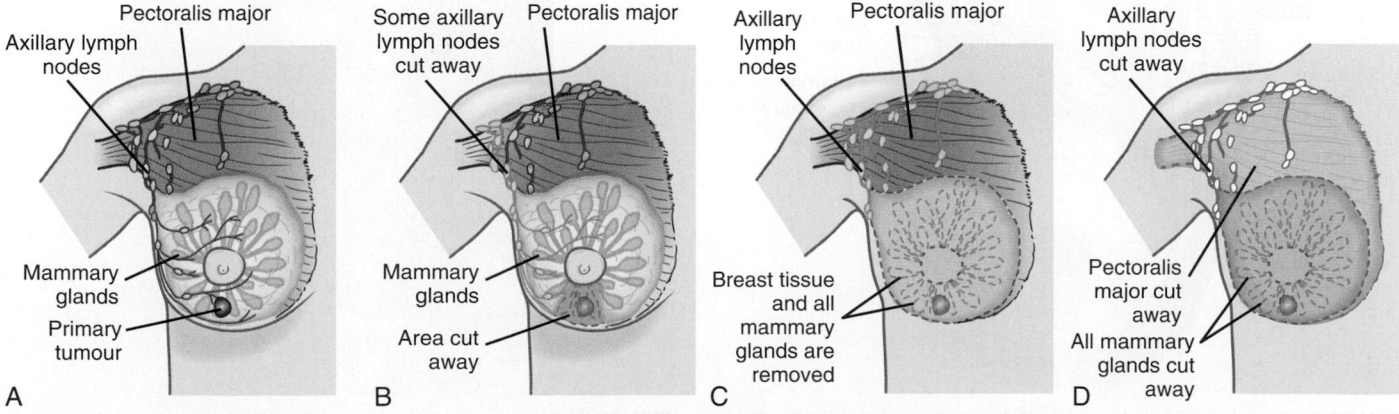

FIGURE 54-6 Breast cancer surgery. **A,** Preoperative. **B,** Lumpectomy. **C,** Simple mastectomy. **D,** Modified radical mastectomy.

TABLE 54-8 SURGICAL PROCEDURES FOR BREAST CANCER

Procedure	Description	Adverse Effects	Complications	Patient Issues
Breast-conserving surgery (lumpectomy) with radiation therapy	Wide excision of tumour, SLNB or ALND, radiation therapy	Breast soreness Breast edema Skin reactions Arm swelling Sensory changes in breast and arm	Short-term: moist desquamation,* hematoma, seroma, infection Long-term: fibrosis, lymphedema,† myositis, pneumonitis,* rib fractures*	Prolonged treatment* Impaired arm mobility† Change in texture and sensitivity of breast
Modified radical mastectomy	Removal of breast, preservation of pectoralis muscle, SLNB or ALND	Tightening of chest wall, scarring Phantom breast sensations Lymphedema Sensory changes Impaired range of motion	Short-term: skin flap necrosis, seroma, hematoma, infection Long-term: sensory loss, muscle weakness, lymphedema	Loss of breast Incision Body image Need for prosthesis Impaired arm mobility
Tissue expansion and breast implants	Expander used to slowly stretch tissue; saline gradually injected into reservoir over weeks to months Insertion of implant under musculo-fascial layer of chest wall	Discomfort Sensation of chest wall tightness	Short-term: skin flap necrosis, wound separation, seroma, hematoma, infection Long-term: capsular contractions, displacement of implant	Body image Prolonged physician visits to expand implants Potential additional surgical procedures for nipple construction, symmetry
Breast reconstruction tissue flap procedures	TRAM flap procedure‡: a musculo-cutaneous flap (muscle, skin, fat, blood supply) is transposed from abdomen to the mastectomy site	Pain related to two surgical sites and extensive surgery	Short-term: delayed wound healing, infection, skin flap necrosis, abdominal hernia, hematoma	Prolonged postoperative recovery
	DIEP flap procedure: a free flap that transfers skin and fat from the abdomen to the chest; differs from TRAM flap because no muscle is moved	Requires more time in surgery than TRAM flap Pain related to two surgical sites	If procedure fails, tissue flap may die and have to be completely removed If tissue dies, new reconstruction may not be done for 6–12 months	Patients may experience less pain and restriction of movement than with a TRAM flap

ALND, axillary lymph node dissection; *DIEP,* deep inferior epigastric artery perforator; *SLNB,* sentinel lymph node biopsy; *TRAM,* transverse rectus abdominis musculo-cutaneous.
*Specific to radiation therapy.
†If ALND is performed (less likely with SLNB).
‡May be performed concurrently with mastectomy.

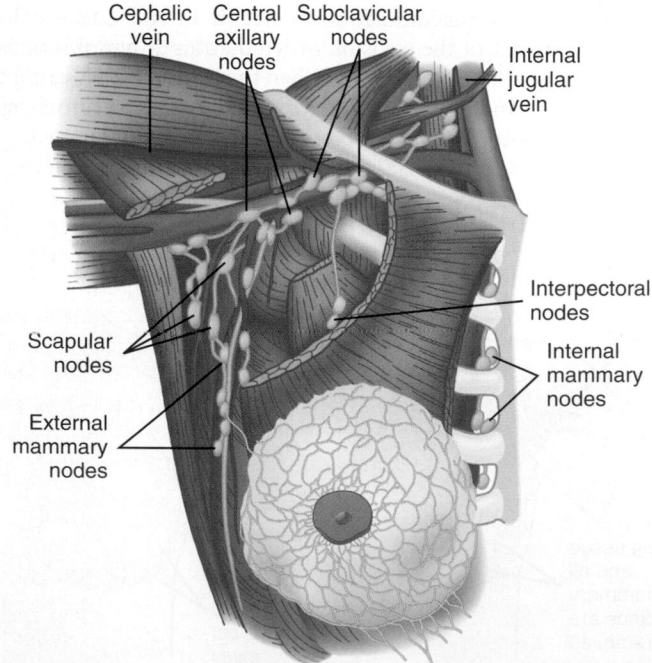

FIGURE 54-7 Illustration of lymph nodes and drainage in the axilla. The sentinel lymph node is usually found in the external mammary nodes. In a complete axillary dissection, all nodes would be removed. Source: Townsend, C. M., Beauchamp, R. D., Evers, B. M., et al. (2009). *Sabiston textbook of surgery* (18th ed.). St. Louis: Mosby.

FIGURE 54-8 Lymphedema. Accumulation of fluid in the tissue after excision of lymph nodes. Source: Swartz, M. H. (2010). *Textbook of physical diagnosis: History and examination* (6th ed., p. 443, Figure 15-3). Philadelphia: W. B. Saunders.

pain, impaired motor function in the arm, and numbness and paraesthesia in the fingers as a result of lymphedema. Cellulitis and progressive fibrosis can result from lymphedema. Although lymphedema is not always preventable, it can be controlled somewhat after surgery or radiation therapy (see discussion later in this chapter).

Modified Radical Mastectomy. A modified radical mastectomy includes removal of the breast and the axillary lymph nodes, but it spares the pectoralis major muscle. This surgery is preferred over breast-conserving surgery if the tumour is too large to excise with adequate margins, or if it is so large that excision would produce a poor cosmetic result. Some patients may select this surgical procedure over lumpectomy when presented with a choice.

When a modified radical mastectomy is performed, patients have the option of breast reconstruction. If a patient chooses to have reconstructive surgery, it can be performed immediately after the mastectomy, or it can be delayed until postoperative recovery is complete (Canadian Cancer Society, 2017m).

Postmastectomy Pain Syndrome. *Postmastectomy pain syndrome* can occur after a mastectomy or an axillary node dissection. Common symptoms include chest and upper arm pain, tingling sensations down the arm, numbness, shooting or pricking pain, and unbearable itching that persist beyond the normal 3-month healing time. The cause most commonly theorized about the onset of this syndrome is injury to intercosto-brachial nerves, which are sensory nerves that exit chest wall muscles and provide sensation to the shoulder and the upper arm.

Treatments include nonsteroidal anti-inflammatory drugs, antidepressants, topical lidocaine patches, eutectic mixture of local anaesthetics (lidocaine and prilocaine), and anticonvulsant drugs (e.g., gabapentin [Neurontin]). Other possible treatment modalities include imagery, biofeedback, physical therapy to prevent "frozen shoulder" syndrome as a result of inadequate movement, and psychological counselling with a person trained in the management of chronic pain syndromes.

Adjuvant Therapy. The decision to recommend adjuvant (additional) therapy after surgery depends on the stage of the disease (number of involved nodes and tumour size); the menstrual status, health, and age of the patient; cancer cell characteristics; and presence or absence of estrogen, progesterone, and HER2. Adjuvant therapies include local radiation therapy and systemic therapies such as chemotherapy and hormone therapy (Canadian Cancer Society, 2017n).

Radiation Therapy. Radiation therapy may be used as (a) primary treatment to prevent local breast recurrences after breast-conserving surgery (see the Evidence-Informed Practice: Translating Research Into Practice box), (b) adjuvant treatment after mastectomy to prevent local and nodal recurrences, and (c) palliative treatment for pain caused by local, regional, or distant recurrence.

Primary Radiation Therapy. When radiation therapy is the primary treatment, it is usually performed after local excision of the breast mass. The breast (and, in some cases, the regional lymph nodes) is irradiated 5 days per week over the course of approximately 4 to 6 weeks. An external beam of radiation is used to deliver an approximate total dose of 4 500 to 5 000 cGy (4 500 to 5 000 rd). During the final week or so, the patient receives a supplemental dose of radiation targeted directly to the area where the tumour was located. This dose is called a "boost" and is usually delivered in a method similar to the patient's regular radiation but to a smaller area. Fatigue, skin changes, and breast edema may be temporary adverse effects of external beam

---

EVIDENCE-INFORMED PRACTICE

Translating Research Into Practice

Maia Samsa is a 53-year-old woman who was diagnosed with breast cancer 2 weeks ago. She is recovering from a lumpectomy with negative lymph nodes. Her physician has recommended adjuvant therapy with radiation.

Best Available Evidence	Clinician Expertise	Patient Preferences and Values
The addition of radiation therapy to lumpectomy reduces the risk for local cancer recurrence.	Radiation is recommended even with negative lymph nodes after a lumpectomy. Many patients have minimal or no adverse effects from radiation therapy. The most common ones are fatigue, malaise, skin reactions, and ulcers or irritation of the skin.	She tells the nurse that she is not sure if she wants to have radiation treatment because she is afraid of the adverse effects.

Decision and Action

The nurse should review the possible adverse effects and how they can be managed and then explain to Ms. Samsa the risks of not taking the radiation treatment, which can include recurrence. Ms. Samsa tells the nurse that she will discuss it with her husband and possibly reconsider. The nurse understands the patient's concerns and informs the physician of her indecisiveness.

Reference for Evidence

Berrang, T. S., Olivotto, I., Kim, D. H., et al. (2011). Three-year outcomes of a Canadian multicenter study of accelerated partial breast irradiation using conformal radiation therapy. *International Journal of Radiation Oncology, Biology, Physical, 81*(5), 1220–1227. doi:10.1016/j.ijrobp.2010.07.2003.

---

radiation therapy. To decrease the risk for axillary recurrence, irradiation of the axilla or supraclavicular nodes or both may be indicated when lymph nodes are involved. Chemotherapy may be used systemically before radiation therapy to enhance the local effects of radiation. (Nursing management of patients receiving radiation therapy is discussed in Chapter 18, and in NCP 18-1.)

The decision to use radiation therapy after mastectomy is based on the probability that local residual cancer cells are present (related to tumour size and biology and number of involved lymph nodes). Irradiating the area does not prevent the appearance of distant metastasis at a later date. The site of the radiation therapy field (lymph nodes, chest wall, or both) depends on the risk for recurrence.

High-Dose Brachytherapy. *Brachytherapy* (internal radiation) is an alternative to traditional radiation treatment for early-stage breast cancer. For many years, internal radiation therapy has been delivered primarily through a multicatheter implant method that requires many catheters to be placed in the breast. After placement, a radioactive seed is delivered into each catheter to treat the target area.

Currently, the most widely practised method is balloon brachytherapy. Traditional radiation treatments can take 5 to 6 weeks; in contrast, high-dose brachytherapy with the balloon catheter may require only 5 days.

The MammoSite Radiation Therapy System (MammoSite RTS) is a minimally invasive method of delivering internal

FIGURE 54-9 High-dose brachytherapy for breast cancer. The MammoSite Radiation Therapy System involves the insertion of a single small balloon catheter *(B)* at the time of the lumpectomy or shortly thereafter into the tumour resection cavity (the space that is left after the surgeon removes the tumour). A tiny radioactive seed *(A)* is inserted into the balloon, connected to a machine called an *afterloader (C)*, and delivers the radiation therapy.

radiation therapy. In this technique, a balloon catheter is used to insert radioactive seeds into the breast after the tumour is removed (Figure 54-9). Radiation is emitted by a tiny radioactive seed attached by a wire on the way to an afterloader, a computer-controlled machine. The seed travels through the MammoSite RTS applicator into the inflated balloon. The radiation dose is focused on the area of the breast at highest risk for tumour recurrence.

Radiation therapy with the MammoSite RTS is performed over a 1- to 5-day period on an outpatient basis. Patients typically receive treatments twice a day for 5 days.

The MammoSite RTS may also be used as boost therapy in conjunction with external irradiation.

The source of radiation does not remain in the body between treatments or after the final treatment is over. The tiny radioactive seed is inserted only during treatment and then removed. Once the final session is completed, the balloon is deflated, and the system is removed.

Palliative Radiation Therapy. In addition to reducing the primary tumour mass with a resultant decrease in pain, radiation therapy is used to stabilize symptomatic metastatic lesions in such sites as bone, soft tissue organs, the brain, and the chest and is successful in controlling recurrent or metastatic disease.

Systemic Therapy. The goal of systemic therapy is to destroy tumour cells that may have spread to distant sites. Systemic therapy as an adjuvant to primary local treatment (in the absence of demonstrable metastases) can decrease the rate of recurrence and increase the length of survival. Because of the high risk for recurrent disease, nearly all women with evidence of node involvement, particularly those whose hormone receptor status is negative, have some type of systemic therapy. Some women, particularly those with a larger tumour or a more aggressive type of tumour, are at higher risk for recurrent or metastatic disease. Systemic therapy is often recommended for such women even when no evidence of node involvement is found. Weighing the risks and benefits of adjuvant therapy is a complex process.

Chemotherapy. *Chemotherapy* is the use of cytotoxic drugs to destroy cancer cells. Many breast cancers are responsive to chemotherapy. In some patients, chemotherapy is administered preoperatively. Preoperative (neoadjuvant) chemotherapy can decrease the size of the primary tumour, possibly enabling surgery to be less extensive. Breast cancer survival rates with preoperative

chemotherapy are no different from those with postoperative chemotherapy (Kong, Moran, Zhang, et al., 2011).

Combinations of drugs yield results superior to those of a single drug. The benefits of combination treatment result from the use of drugs that have different mechanisms of action and work at different parts of the cell cycle. The more common combination-therapy protocols are as follows:

- Cyclophosphamide (Procytox), methotrexate, and 5-fluorouracil (5-FU), referred to as *CMF*
- Doxorubicin and cyclophosphamide, with or without the addition of a taxane such as paclitaxel (Abraxane) or docetaxel (Taxotere)
- Cyclophosphamide, doxorubicin or epirubicin (Pharmorubicin PFS), and 5-FU, referred to as *CAF* or *CEF*

DRUG ALERT—Doxorubicin

- Patient should be monitored for signs of cardiotoxicity and heart failure (e.g., new onset of shortness of breath, pedal edema, decreased activity tolerance, dysrhythmias, ECG changes).
- Patient should not have immunizations without physician's approval.
- Patient must avoid contact with those who recently received live virus vaccine.

Certain drugs may be used alone to treat metastatic breast cancer. A medication used alone results in fewer adverse effects than do combinations. Docetaxel (Taxotere), capecitabine (Xeloda), and an albumin-bound form of paclitaxel (Abraxane) are used when metastatic breast cancer has not responded to standard chemotherapy (Canadian Cancer Society, 2017o). Vinorelbine (Navelbine), used to treat metastatic breast cancer, is better tolerated because it produces fewer and milder adverse effects than do other chemotherapeutic drugs.

Because healthy cells are also affected by chemotherapy, various adverse effects accompany this treatment modality. The incidence and severity of predictable and commonly observed adverse effects are influenced by the specific drug combination, drug schedule, and drug doses. Usually, body organs with rapidly dividing cells are the most strongly affected. The most common adverse effects involve the gastro-intestinal tract, bone marrow, and hair follicles, resulting in nausea, anorexia, weight gain, bone marrow suppression and subsequent fatigue, and alopecia (hair loss) (Canadian Cancer Society, 2017p).

Cognitive changes during and after treatment, especially with chemotherapy ("chemo brain"), have been reported in 30% to 60% of women with breast cancer. These changes include difficulties in concentration, memory, and maintaining focus and attention. Ongoing research is focusing on why the cognitive impairment occurs (Player, Mackenzie, Willis, et al., 2014).

Hormonal Therapy. Estrogen can promote the growth of breast cancer cells if the cells are estrogen receptor–positive. Hormonal therapy blocks the source of estrogen, thus promoting tumour regression (Canadian Cancer Society, 2017q). Hormonal therapy may be used as an adjuvant to primary treatment or in patients with recurrent or metastatic cancer. Two advances have increased the use of hormone therapy in breast cancer. First, hormone receptor assays, which are reliable diagnostic tests, identify women who are likely to respond to hormone therapy. Both the estrogen and progesterone receptor status of the tumour can be determined. The importance of these assays is their ability to predict whether hormonal therapy is a treatment option for women with breast cancer, either at the time of initial therapy or if the cancer recurs. Second, drugs have been developed that can inactivate the hormone-secreting glands as effectively as surgery or radiation. Chances of tumour regression are significantly greater in women whose tumours contain estrogen and progesterone receptors (Canadian Cancer Society, 2017q).

Estrogen deprivation can occur when ovarian function is damaged by surgery, radiation therapy, or drug therapy (see Table 54-6). Hormonal therapy can (a) block or destroy the estrogen receptors or (b) suppress estrogen synthesis through inhibiting aromatase, an enzyme needed for endogenous estrogen synthesis.

Estrogen Receptor Blockers. Tamoxifen (Nolvadex) has for many years been the hormonal agent of choice in estrogen receptor–positive women with breast cancer of all stages (Canadian Cancer Society, 2017q). Tamoxifen, an antiestrogen drug, blocks the estrogen receptor sites of malignant cells and thus inhibits the growth-stimulating effects of estrogen. It is commonly used in early-stage and advanced breast cancer and to treat recurrent disease. Tamoxifen may also be used to prevent breast cancer in individuals at high risk for its development. Adverse effects of tamoxifen may include hot flashes, mood swings, vaginal discharge and dryness, and other effects commonly associated with decreased estrogen levels. It also increases the risk for blood clots, cataracts, stroke, and endometrial cancer in postmenopausal women. Treatment with tamoxifen generally lasts 5 years (Canadian Cancer Society, 2017q).

DRUG ALERT—Tamoxifen (Nolvadex)
- Irregular vaginal bleeding or spotting may occur.
- Decreased visual acuity, corneal opacity, and retinopathy can occur in women receiving high doses (240–320 mg/day for >17 months). These problems may be irreversible.
- Patient should be instructed to report decreased visual acuity immediately.
- Patient should be monitored for signs of deep-vein thrombosis, pulmonary embolism, and stroke, including shortness of breath, leg cramps, and weakness.

Fulvestrant (Faslodex) may be administered when advanced breast cancer no longer responds to tamoxifen. This drug slows cancer progression by destroying estrogen receptors in the breast cancer cells. Fulvestrant is given intramuscularly on a monthly basis. Common adverse effects include fatigue, hot flashes, and nausea.

Aromatase Inhibitors. Aromatase inhibitor drugs interfere with the enzyme that synthesizes endogenous estrogen and are used in the treatment of breast cancer in postmenopausal women. These drugs include anastrozole (Arimidex), letrozole (Femara), and exemestane (Aromasin). Aromatase inhibitors do not block the production of estrogen by the ovaries; thus they are of little benefit and may be harmful in premenopausal women.

Clinical trials have demonstrated improved disease-free survival when these drugs are given after tamoxifen treatment has ended (Canadian Cancer Society, 2017q). They also appear to be more effective than tamoxifen in preventing breast cancer recurrence and possibly more effective in preventing contralateral disease. The adverse effects of aromatase inhibitors are different from those of tamoxifen. Aromatase inhibitors only rarely cause blood clots, and they do not cause endometrial cancer. Because they block the production of estrogen in postmenopausal women, osteoporosis and bone fractures may occur. These drugs have also been associated with night sweats, nausea, arthralgias, and myalgias.

Raloxifene (Evista), a drug used to prevent bone loss, is now being used to reduce the risk for breast cancer in postmenopausal women without stimulating endometrial growth. Raloxifene may act by blocking estrogen receptors in the breast, similar to its action in the bone. (Raloxifene is discussed in the section on osteoporosis in Chapter 66.)

Less common hormone-deprivation strategies include bilateral oophorectomy, adrenalectomy, and hypophysectomy.

Biological and Targeted Therapy. Some breast cancers make excessive amounts of the HER2 protein. For patients who are HER2 positive, trastuzumab (Herceptin) is a monoclonal antibody to HER2. After the antibody attaches to the antigen, it is taken into the cancer cells and eventually kills them. It can be used alone or in combination with other chemotherapy such as docetaxel (Taxotere) or paclitaxel (Abraxane) to treat patients whose tumours overexpress the *HER2* gene. Additional genetic testing may offer information on which patients are good candidates for treatment with trastuzumab.

DRUG ALERT—Trastuzumab (Herceptin)
- Drug should be used with caution in women with pre-existing heart disease.
- Patient should be monitored for signs of ventricular dysfunction and heart failure.

A new kind of targeted anticancer drug, trastuzumab emtansine (Kadcyla), is made up of the drugs trastuzumab and emtansine, which is an antibody-drug combination. Pertuzumab (Perjeta) is another new anti-HER2 therapy that is used for patients who have not received prior treatment for metastatic breast cancer with an anti-HER2 agent or chemotherapy.

Lapatinib (Tykerb) may be used in combination with capecitabine (Xeloda) for patients with advanced, metastatic disease whose tumours produce excessive HER2. The combination treatment is indicated for women in whom disease has become resistant to other cancer drugs (Canadian Cancer Society, 2017r). Lapatinib works inside the cell by blocking the function of the HER2 protein. Adverse effects can include diarrhea, nausea, vomiting, rash, and a syndrome of numbness, tingling, swelling, and pain in the hands and feet. Cardiotoxicity has also been reported.

Advanced breast cancer in postmenopausal women who are estrogen and progesterone receptor–positive and HER2 positive may be treated with lapatinib in combination with capecitabine (Xeloda) and letrozole (Femara). Denosumab (Prolia, Xgeva), a monoclonal antibody, may be used to increase bone mass in patients with metastasis to the bone and at high risk for fracture from aromatase inhibitor therapy. (The use of biological and targeted therapies is discussed further in Chapter 18.)

Follow-Up and Survivorship Care. After surgery, patients must be monitored for the rest of their life at regular intervals. Most have professional examinations every 6 months for 2 years and then annually thereafter. In addition, it is recommended that these patients perform monthly examinations on both breasts or on the remaining breast and the surgical site. The most common site of local recurrence of breast cancer is at the surgical site. These patients should also undergo appropriate breast imaging at regular intervals (usually 6 months to 1 year), as determined by their risk for recurrence and breast cancer history.

CULTURALLY COMPETENT CARE

BREAST CANCER

Among diverse ethnic groups, differences exist in the incidence, mortality rates, and relevant care issues related to breast cancer. In addition, cultural differences may involve gender roles, health beliefs, religion, and family structure. Other differences may relate to dietary factors and disparities in the access to and use

🔍 EVIDENCE-INFORMED PRACTICE

Research Highlight

What Is the Effect of Physical Activity in Cancer Survivors?

Clinical Question

For cancer survivors (P) does physical activity (I) improve physical and psychological outcomes (O) after primary treatment completion (T)?

Best Available Evidence

Systematic review of randomized controlled trials (RCTs)

Critical Appraisal and Synthesis of Evidence

- Thirty-four RCTs of cancer survivors: 22 studies were of breast cancer survivors. Intervention was mostly aerobic exercise. Duration of physical activity ranged from 3 to 60 wk (median of 13 wk). Control groups mainly were sedentary or assigned no exercise.
- Breast cancer survivors who did physical activity had an increased ability to bench and leg press, improved quality of life, and decreased fatigue and depression.
- Overall, cancer survivors who exercised showed improved BMI, body weight, peak oxygen consumption, distance walked in 6 min, handgrip strength, and quality of life.

Conclusion

- Physical activity has positive effects on physical and psychological outcomes and quality of life.

Implications for Nursing

- To help patients get interested in physical activity, nurses should discuss with them their favourite forms of exercise, hobbies, and activities.
- Nurses should help patients identify physical activity resources (e.g., walking paths, swimming pool, gym).
  - The patient's barriers to active participation in exercise should be assessed.
  - When possible, patients should be assisted in adhering to recommended activities.

Reference for Evidence

Fong, D., Ho, J., Hui, B., et al. (2012). Physical activity for cancer survivors: Meta-analysis of randomized controlled trials. *British Medical Journal, 344,* e70.

BMI, body mass index; *P,* patient population of interest; *I,* intervention or area of interest; *O,* outcome(s) of interest; *T,* timing (see Chapter 1).

of clinical breast examinations and screening mammography. Inequities in cancer care and outcomes exist among Canada's various ethnic and social groups despite universal health care (Ahmed & Shahid, 2012). Cultural values strongly influence how women respond to and cope with breast cancer and treatment. Nurses need to consider how health behaviours are influenced by cultural norms and, in particular, the cultural value of breasts and the cultural factors related to the disease of breast cancer. Immigrants to Canada often underutilize screening and prevention services. Women may delay screening or treatment for varying reasons, including an acceptance of disease as inevitable fate or "God's will," a mistrust of Western medicine, language barriers, lack of health care access, or the stigma of a cancer diagnosis. Among Indigenous populations, survival rates for preventable cancers are poorer than in the general population. Action strategies that eliminate cultural barriers to quality cancer care are essential, including integration of person-centred care and cultural competency as core values, to meet the needs of racially and ethnically diverse patients with breast cancer (Ahmed & Shahid, 2012).

NURSING MANAGEMENT BREAST CANCER

NURSING ASSESSMENT

Many factors need to be considered when a nurse is assessing a patient with a breast problem. The history of the breast disorder assists in establishing the diagnosis. The presence of nipple discharge, pain, rate of growth of the lump, breast asymmetry, and correlation with the menstrual cycle should all be investigated.

The size and location of the lump or lumps should be carefully documented. The physical characteristics of the lesion, such as consistency, mobility, and shape, should be assessed. If nipple discharge is present, the colour and consistency should be noted, as well as whether it occurs from one or both breasts.

Subjective and objective data that should be obtained from an individual with suspected or diagnosed breast cancer are presented in Table 54-9.

NURSING DIAGNOSES

Nursing diagnoses related to the care of a patient with diagnosed breast cancer vary. After diagnosis and before a treatment plan has been selected, the following diagnoses apply:

- *Decisional conflict* related to *insufficient information* (treatment options and their effects)
- *Anxiety* related to *threat to current status, threat of death* (diagnosis of cancer)
- *Disturbed body image* related to *alteration in self-perception*

If a mastectomy or lumpectomy is planned, the nursing diagnoses may include but are not limited to those presented in NCP 54-1, available on the Evolve website.

PLANNING

The overall goals are that patients with breast cancer will (a) actively participate in the decision-making process related to treatment options, (b) adhere to the therapeutic plan, (c) manage the adverse effects of adjuvant therapy, and (d) access and benefit from the support provided by significant others and health care providers.

NURSING IMPLEMENTATION

ACUTE INTERVENTION. The time between the diagnosis of breast cancer and the selection of a treatment plan can be a difficult period for a woman and her family. Although the primary care provider has discussed treatment options, patients often rely on a nurse to clarify and expand on these options. During this often stressful time, patients may not be coping effectively. Appropriate nursing interventions are to explore the patient's usual decision-making patterns, to help her accurately evaluate the advantages and disadvantages of the options, to provide information relevant to the decision, and to support the patient and family once the decision is made.

During this period, patients may exhibit signs of distress or tension—such as tachycardia, increased muscle tension, sleep disturbances, and restlessness—whenever they focus on the decision to be made. Nurses should assess the body language, motor activity, and affect of their patients during periods of high stress and indecision so that appropriate interventions can be used.

Regardless of the surgery planned, patients must be provided with sufficient information to ensure informed consent. Some patients seek extensive, detailed information, whereas others avoid information. Sensitivity to the individual's need for and type of information is essential. The information includes (a)

TABLE 54-9 NURSING ASSESSMENT

Breast Cancer

Subjective Data

Important Health Information

Past health history:
- Family history of breast cancer (especially mother or sister, young age at diagnosis)
- History of abnormal mammogram findings or atypical findings in prior biopsy
- Benign breast disorders with atypical changes
- Previous unilateral breast cancer
- Menstrual history (early menarche with late menopause)
- Pregnancy history (nulliparity or first full-term pregnancy after age 30)
- Previous endometrial, ovarian, or colon cancer
- Hyperestrogenism and testicular atrophy (in men)
- Dietary habits and history of alcohol use
- Level of usual physical activity, weight, and BMI

Medications: Use of hormones, especially as postmenopausal hormone therapy and in oral contraceptives; infertility treatments

Surgeries or other treatments: Exposure to therapeutic radiation (e.g., for Hodgkin's lymphoma or thyroid cancer)

Symptoms
- Palpable change found on self-examination
- Obesity; unexplained severe weight loss (possible indicator of metastasis)
- Changes in cognition; headache; bone pain (possible indicators of metastasis)
- Unilateral nipple discharge (clear, milky, or bloody)
- Change in breast contour, size, or symmetry
- Psychological stress
- Anxiety regarding threat to self-esteem

Objective Data

General

Axillary and supraclavicular lymphadenopathy

Integumentary

Firm, discrete nodules at mastectomy site (possible indicator of local recurrence); peripheral edema (possible indicator of metastasis)

Respiratory

Pleural effusions (possible indicator of metastasis)

Gastro-Intestinal

Hepatomegaly, jaundice; ascites (possible indicators of liver metastasis)

Reproductive

Hard, irregular, nonmobile breast lump, most often in upper outer sector, possibly fixated to fascia or chest wall; nipple inversion or retraction, erosion; edema (*peau d'orange* appearance), erythema, induration, infiltration, or dimpling (in later stages)

Possible Diagnostic Findings

Finding of mass or change in tissue on breast examination; abnormal findings on mammography, ultrasonography, or breast MRI; positive results of FNA or surgical biopsy or similar results with needle biopsy

BMI, body mass index; *FNA*, fine-needle aspiration; *MRI*, magnetic resonance imaging.

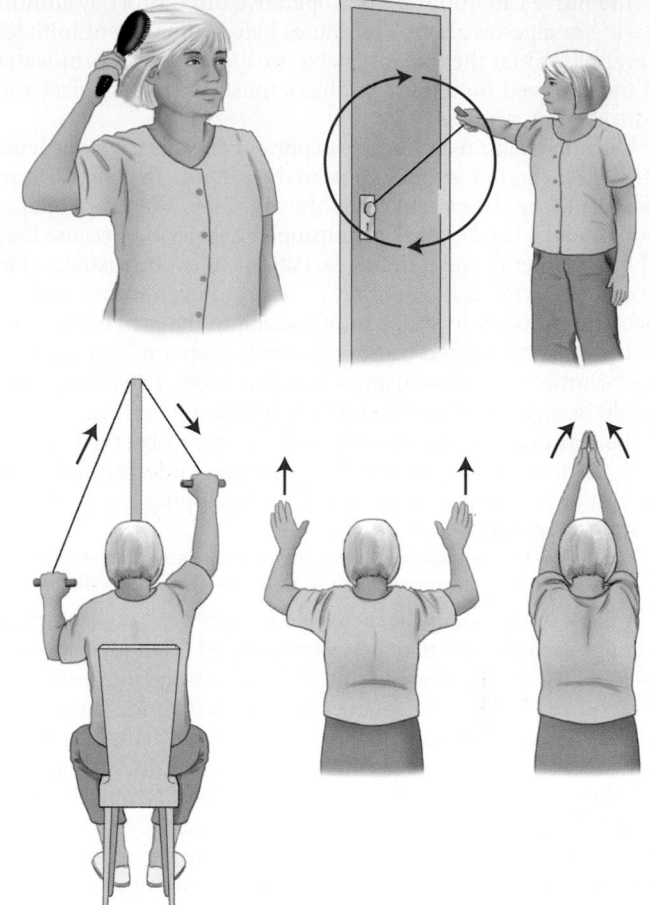

FIGURE 54-10 Postoperative exercises for patient with a mastectomy or lumpectomy with axillary lymph node dissection.

preoperative instructions on pain control, turning, coughing, and deep breathing; (b) a review of postoperative exercises; and (c) explanation of the recovery period from the time of surgery until discharge.

Many women who undergo breast-conserving surgery have an uncomplicated postoperative course with variable pain intensity. Pain is most affected by the extent of the lymph node dissection performed. If an ALND or a mastectomy has been performed, drains are generally left in place, and patients are discharged home with them. Patients and their families need to be taught, with a return demonstration, how to manage the drains at home.

Restoring arm function on the affected side after mastectomy and ALND is a key nursing goal. The patient should be placed in a semi-Fowler's position with the arm on the affected side elevated on a pillow. Flexing and extending the fingers should begin in the recovery room, with progressive increases in activity encouraged.

Postoperative arm and shoulder exercises are instituted gradually with a surgeon's direction (Figure 54-10). These exercises are designed to prevent contractures and muscle shortening, maintain muscle tone, and improve lymph and blood circulation. The difficulty and pain encountered by the patient in performing the previously simple tasks included in the exercise program may cause frustration and depression. The goal of all exercise is a gradual return to full range of motion within 4 to 6 weeks.

The nurse can minimize postoperative discomfort by administering analgesics about 30 minutes before the patient initiates exercises. When the patient is able to shower, the warm water on the involved shoulder often has a muscle-relaxing effect and reduces joint stiffness.

The nurse must use measures to prevent or reduce lymphedema after ALND and must teach these to the patient. The affected arm should not be dependent, even during sleep. Elastic bandages should not be used in the early postoperative period because they inhibit collateral lymph drainage. Patients must be instructed to protect the arm on the operative side from even minor trauma such as a pinprick or sunburn. If trauma to the arm occurs, the area should be washed thoroughly with soap and water, and a topical antibiotic ointment and a bandage or other sterile dressing should be applied. Patients must be taught to advise their surgeon of the trauma, and the site of injury must be observed closely for evidence of inflammation. Patients must understand that for the rest of their life, they are at risk of developing lymphedema.

SAFETY ALERT
- Blood pressure readings, venipunctures, and injections should not be performed on the affected arm so as to prevent lymphedema.

When lymphedema is acute (see Figure 54-8), complete decongestive therapy may be recommended (Canadian Cancer Society, 2017s). This therapy consists of a massage-like technique to mobilize the subcutaneous accumulation of fluid. This is then followed by compression bandaging and the wearing of a pneumatic compression sleeve. This sleeve intermittently applies mechanical massage to the arm and facilitates lymph drainage up toward the heart. Diuretics, isometric exercises, and elevation of the arm so that it is level with the heart may be recommended to reduce the fluid volume in the arm. The patient may need to wear a fitted elastic pressure-gradient sleeve (a) during waking hours to maintain maximum volume reduction and (b) preventively during air travel.

PSYCHOLOGICAL CARE. Effective care includes sensitivity to the woman's efforts to cope with a life-threatening disease. A relationship in which the woman can express her authentic feelings is therapeutic. The nurse can help to meet the woman's psychological needs in the following ways:

- Providing a safe environment for the expression of the full range of feelings
- Helping her identify sources of support and strength, such as her partner, family, and spiritual or religious practices
- Encouraging her to identify and learn individual coping strengths
- Promoting communication between the patient and her family, friends, or both
- Providing accurate and complete answers to her questions about the disease, treatment options, and reproductive, fertility, or lactation issues (if appropriate)
- Offering information about community resources, such as CancerConnection through the Canadian Cancer Society, CanSurmount, Look Good Feel Better, and local support organizations and groups
- Offering information about available resources for mental health counselling if needed

Nurses can promote a woman's recovery by referring her to peer support resources. The Reach to Recovery program of the Canadian Cancer Society is a rehabilitation program for women who have undergone breast surgery. It is designed to help them meet their psychological, physical, and cosmetic needs. The volunteers, who have had breast cancer, can answer questions about expectations, surgery, and recovery. The Canadian Cancer Society and the Canadian Cancer Society Research Institute can provide excellent materials to assist nurses in meeting the special needs of women with breast cancer.

It is important for health care providers to remain sensitive to the complex psychological effect that a diagnosis of cancer and subsequent breast surgery can have on a woman and her family (Astin, Shapiro, & Shapiro, 2013). Diverse emotional responses are common. The nurse's accepting attitude and the offering of resources can greatly alleviate the common feelings of fear, anger, anxiety, and depression experienced by many patients.

AMBULATORY AND HOME CARE. The nurse should explain the specific follow-up routine to patients and emphasize the importance of ongoing monitoring and breast self-awareness. To address needs for individual and family support in addition to coping needs, referral to a mental health care provider may be indicated. Immediately after surgery, symptoms that should be reported to the clinician include fever, inflammation at the surgical site, erythema, postoperative constipation, and unusual swelling. Changes to report beyond the immediate postsurgical period are new back pain, weakness, shortness of breath, and confusion.

For women who have undergone mastectomy without breast reconstruction, a variety of products are available to meet specific individual needs. These include garments ranging from camisoles with soft breast prosthetic inserts to a fitted prosthesis with bra. For women who choose a breast prosthesis, a certified fitter can help them select a comfortable, more permanent weighted prosthesis and bra, generally at 4 to 8 weeks postoperatively. The role of the nurse is to present the choices and resources without judgement.

The loss of a breast can have varying implications for women's sexual identity and relationships. The nurse can initiate a discussion of sexuality by inviting questions about relationships or intimacy concerns within the recovery framework (Dow & Kennedy Sheldon, 2015). To be effective sources of support for the patient, the spouse, sexual partner, or family members often need help in dealing with their emotional reactions to the diagnosis and surgery. There are no physical reasons for a mastectomy to prevent sexual satisfaction. Women taking hormonal therapy, however, may have a decreased sexual drive or vaginal dryness. They may need to use lubrication to prevent discomfort during intercourse. Concerns about sexuality are not well addressed by many health care providers (Dow & Kennedy Sheldon, 2015). If difficulty in adjustment or other problems develop, counselling may be necessary to deal with the emotional component of a mastectomy and the diagnosis of cancer.

Depression and anxiety may occur with the continued stress and uncertainty of a cancer diagnosis. Patients' self-esteem and identity may also be threatened. The support of family and friends and participation in a cancer support group are important aspects of care that are often helpful in improving quality of life.

EVALUATION

The expected outcomes for patients after a mastectomy or lumpectomy are presented in NCP 54-1, available on the Evolve website.

MAMMOPLASTY

Mammoplasty is the surgical change in the size or shape of the breast. It may be performed electively for cosmetic purposes to

FIGURE 54-11 Appearances after breast surgery. **A,** Appearance of chest after bilateral mastectomy. **B,** Postoperative breast reconstruction before nipple–areolar reconstruction. **C,** Postoperative breast reconstruction after nipple–areolar reconstruction. Source: Fortunato, N., & McCullough, S. M. (1998). *Plastic and reconstructive surgery.* St. Louis: Mosby. Courtesy Brian Davies, MD.

either enlarge or reduce the size of the breasts. It may also be performed to reconstruct the breast after a mastectomy.

A professional, nonjudgemental attitude and clear information about surgical breast options are most useful for women engaged in decision making about mammoplasty. It is important that patients set realistic expectations about what mammoplasty can accomplish and about possible complications, such as hematoma formation, hemorrhage, and infection. If an implant is involved, the woman must understand that capsular contracture (complication of internal scar tissue forming a constricting capsule around a breast implant) and the resultant loss of the implant are possible (Health Canada, 2012).

Breast Reconstruction

Breast reconstructive surgery may be performed simultaneously with a mastectomy or some time afterward to achieve symmetry and to restore or preserve body image. The timing of reconstruction surgery should be based on the psychological needs of individual patients. Immediate breast reconstruction after mastectomy is commonly performed. The advantages of immediate reconstruction are the need for only one surgical procedure, only one anaesthesia induction, and only one recovery period; also, reconstructive surgery takes place before the development of scar tissue or adhesions. Early reconstruction does not delay or influence further treatment or adversely affect predicted survival.

Indications. The main indication for breast reconstruction is to improve a woman's self-image and help her regain a sense of normality and assist her in coping with the loss of the breast. Current techniques cannot restore lactation, nipple sensation, or nipple erectility. Therefore, the erotic functions of the breast are not present. Although the breast will not fully resemble its premastectomy appearance, the reconstructed appearance usually represents an improvement over the mastectomy scar (Figure 54-11). The contour of the breast is restored without the use of an external prosthesis.

Types of Reconstruction

Breast Implants and Tissue Expansion. Breast implants are placed in a pocket under the pectoralis muscle, which protects the implant and provides soft tissue coverage over it. Implants can be placed either at the time of mastectomy or later. A small magnet is embedded in most expanders to help locate the port where the fluid is injected. Therefore, a woman with a magnet in place should not undergo MRI. Because many patients who have undergone mastectomy have insufficient tissue, simple placement of an implant may lead to small breast reconstruction

FIGURE 54-12 Tissue expansion. **A,** Diagram of tissue expander with gradual expansion. **B,** Tissue expander in place after mastectomy. Sources: **A,** Cameron, J. (1995). *Current surgical therapy* (5th ed.). St. Louis: Mosby. **B,** Fortunato, N., & McCullough, S. M. (1998). *Plastic and reconstructive surgery.* St. Louis: Mosby. Courtesy Brian Davies, MD.

that is tight or firm. Autologous (one's own) tissue reconstruction may then be recommended.

A tissue expander can be used to stretch the skin and muscle at the mastectomy site before implants are inserted (Figure 54-12). The use of tissue expanders and breast implants is the most common breast reconstruction technique currently used. Placement of the expander can be performed at the time of mastectomy or at a later date. The tissue expander, which is minimally inflated at the time of surgery, is gradually filled by weekly injections of sterile water or saline solution, which stretch the skin and muscle. Once the tissue is adequately stretched and the anticipated breast size is reached, the expander is surgically removed and a permanent implant is inserted. Some expanders are designed to remain in place and become the implant, eliminating the need for a second surgical procedure. Tissue expansion does not work well in individuals with extensive scar tissue from surgery or radiation therapy.

The body's natural response to the presence of a foreign substance is the formation of a fibrous capsule around the implant (Health Canada, 2012). If excessive capsular formation occurs as a result of infection, hematoma, trauma, or reaction to a foreign body, a contracture can develop, resulting in deformation of the breast. Surgeons differ in their approaches to the prevention of contracture formation, although gentle manual massage around the implant is routine. Prevention of the problems that cause excessive capsule formation is critical. Other postoperative

FIGURE 54-13 Diagrams of the transverse rectus abdominis musculo-cutaneous (TRAM) flap procedure. **A,** TRAM flap is planned. **B,** The abdominal tissue, while attached to the rectus muscle, nerve, and blood supply, is tunnelled through the abdomen to the chest. **C,** The flap is trimmed to shape the breast. The lower abdominal incision is closed. **D,** Nipple and areola are reconstructed after the breast is healed.

complications include skin ulceration, hypertrophic scar formation, intercostal neuralgia, and wound infection.

Tissue Flap Procedures. An additional choice for breast reconstruction is the use of autologous tissue to re-create a breast mound. If insufficient muscle is left after mastectomy or if the chest wall has been irradiated, the person's own tissue may be used to repair the soft tissue defects. Musculo-cutaneous flaps are most often taken from the back (latissimus dorsi muscle) or the abdomen (transverse rectus abdominis muscle). In the latissimus dorsi musculo-cutaneous flap, a block of skin and muscle from the patient's back is used to replace tissue removed during mastectomy. A small implant may be needed beneath the flap to obtain reasonable breast shape and size. A disadvantage of this technique is an additional scar on the back.

The *transverse rectus abdominis musculo-cutaneous (TRAM) flap* is the most frequently used flap operation (Canadian Cancer Society, 2017t). The rectus abdominis muscles are paired flat muscles running from the rib cage down to the pubic bone. Arteries running inside the muscles provide branches at many levels, and these branches supply the fat and skin across a large expanse of the abdomen. In this technique, the surgeon elevates a large block of tissue from the lower abdominal area but leaves it attached to the rectus muscle (Figure 54-13). This tissue is then tunnelled or placed as "free flaps" under the skin up to the area where the breast will be reconstructed. Then it is moulded and fashioned to form a breast. The abdominal incision is closed, which results in an appearance similar to that of an abdominoplasty. This surgical procedure can last 2 to 8 hours, and recovery can take at least 6 to 8 weeks. Some patients have reported persistent fatigue and reduced quality of life following surgery (Stagl, Antoni, Lechner, et al., 2014; Amaya, Hosokawa, Okamoto, et al., 2015). Complications include bleeding, seroma, hernia, infection, and low back pain. An implant may be used in addition to the flap if the flap does not provide the desired cosmetic result alone. Patients who smoke, who are too thin, or who are overweight are not good candidates for this type of procedure.

A *deep inferior epigastric artery perforator (DIEP) flap* is a version of the free flap that does not use muscle tissue. With the DIEP flap, only the skin and fat are taken from the same lower abdominal area as the TRAM flap. Patients may experience less pain and restriction of movement with this procedure.

Total skin-sparing mastectomy is the preservation of the skin of the nipple and areola with the removal of underlying breast tissue. It can be done at the same time as immediate breast reconstructive surgery.

Nipple–Areolar Reconstruction. The majority of patients who undergo breast reconstruction also receive nipple–areolar reconstruction. Nipple reconstruction gives the reconstructed breast a much more natural appearance. Nipple–areolar reconstruction is usually done a few months after breast reconstruction. Tissue to construct a nipple may be taken from the opposite breast or from a small flap of tissue on the reconstructed breast mound. The areola may be grafted from the labia, skin in the area of the groin, or lower abdominal skin, or it may be tattooed with a permanent pigmented dye. In some patients, a small implant may be placed under the completed nipple–areolar reconstruction to add additional projection.

Breast Augmentation

In augmentation mammoplasty (the procedure to enlarge the breasts), an implant is placed in a surgically created pocket between the capsule of the breast and the pectoral fascia or, ideally, under the pectoral muscle. Most implants are silicone envelopes filled with a fluid such as dextran, saline, or silicone. Because of their resemblance to the human breast, implants filled with silicone were the most widely used until 1992, when Health Canada asked manufacturers to stop the sale of silicone implants in Canada in response to potential health hazards related to silicone leakage. Currently in Canada, two types of breast implants (saline-filled and silicone gel–filled) have the required licensing from Health Canada. All implants contain an insert that identifies all potential risks related to breast implant surgery (Health Canada, 2012).

Breast Reduction

For some women, large breasts can be a source of physical and psychological discomfort. They can interfere with normal daily activities such as walking, typing, and driving a car. The weight of large breasts can lead to back, shoulder, and neck problems, including degenerative nerve changes. Overly large breasts can interfere with self-esteem and self-image, and the comfort in wearing some clothing may be affected. Reduction in the size of the breasts can have positive effects on both the psychological and physical health of the patient. Reduction mammoplasty is performed by resecting wedges of tissue from the upper and lower quadrants of the breast. The excess skin is removed, and the areola and nipple are relocated on the breast. Lactation can usually be accomplished if massive amounts of tissue are not removed and the nipples are left connected during surgery.

NURSING MANAGEMENT
BREAST AUGMENTATION AND REDUCTION

Breast augmentation and breast reduction may be performed in the outpatient surgical area, or they may involve overnight hospitalization. General anaesthesia is used. Drains are generally placed in the surgical site to prevent hematoma formation and then removed 2 to 3 days after surgery or when drainage is less than 20 to 30 mL per day. The drainage must be examined for colour and odour to detect postoperative infection or hemorrhage. The woman's temperature should also be monitored. Dressings should be changed as necessary, with sterile technique. After surgery, the woman should be assured that the appearance of the breast will improve once healing is complete. Depending on physician instructions, patients may be instructed to wear a bra that provides good support continuously for 2 to 3 days after breast reduction or augmentation. Depending on the extent of the operation, most women can resume normal activities within 2 to 3 weeks. Strenuous exercise may not be appropriate until several weeks later.

CASE STUDY

Breast Cancer

Source: Dubova/ Shutterstock .com

Patient Profile

Anna Kaluza, a 68-year-old married woman, has been diagnosed with breast cancer (see the case study in Chapter 53). She is scheduled for surgery in the morning for a lumpectomy and sentinel lymph node biopsy (SLNB) with possible axillary dissection.

Collaborative Care
Preoperative

- When she is seen in the preoperative clinic 1 week before surgery, Mrs. Kaluza is crying uncontrollably and says, "My husband does not want to look at me anymore. He is afraid of what I am going to look like with a flat chest."
- She says, "I cannot sleep, so I just pace the floor at night."
- She expresses concern that her two daughters (34 and 32) and their daughters are going to get "this horrible disease."

Operative Procedure

- A lumpectomy and SLNB are performed.
- Mrs. Kaluza has cancer cells in her sentinel lymph node.
- Axillary node dissection is then done involving the removal of 12 to 20 nodes.

Postoperative

- She does not want to leave hospital; she wants to stay in bed.
- She has fever with swelling and restricted range of motion in right arm.
- Pain is not controlled well with pain medication.

Follow-Up Findings and Treatment
- Two positive lymph nodes are found.
- She is scheduled for outpatient chemotherapy followed by external beam radiation.

Discussion Questions
1. What in Mrs. Kaluza's breast cancer experience with her family members (see the assessment case study in Chapter 53) might influence her coping response?
2. What information would the nurse provide to Mrs. Kaluza about her surgery?
3. What complication did she develop after her surgery?
4. Which common postoperative exercises will Mrs. Kaluza need to practise after her surgery?
5. What community resources are available to help Mrs. Kaluza and her family adjust to the change in her body and to cope with the diagnosis of cancer? How can the nurse access these resources?
6. What information about breast cancer risks is important to provide to Mrs. Kaluza about her radiation treatment and chemotherapy?
7. **Priority decision:** On the basis of the assessment data, what are the priority nursing diagnoses? Are there any collaborative problems?
8. What information is it important for the nurse to provide to Mrs. Kaluza and her daughters? What early-detection measures are important for them to know?
9. **Evidence-informed practice:** Mrs. Kaluza wants to know what the psychological benefit may be for her daughters if they decide on a breast cancer genetic risk assessment.

Answers are available at *http://evolve.elsevier.com/Canada/Lewis/medsurg*.

REVIEW QUESTIONS

The number of the question corresponds to the same-numbered objective at the beginning of the chapter.

1. An occupational health nurse is planning a program on breast screening practices for women in the company. Which method should the nurse use to promote learning and adherence among participants? (*Select all that apply*)
   a. An audiotape that describes the procedure of breast self-awareness
   b. Distribution of a packet of articles from the medical literature
   c. A discussion of the value of early detection of breast cancer
   d. Written guidelines for mammography and breast self-awareness
   e. Community resources where they can obtain an ultrasound and MRI

2. Which of the following techniques is the most appropriate way to teach a client how to know her breasts?
   a. Teach her palpation of cervical lymph nodes.
   b. Teach her to practise hard squeezing of the breast tissue.
   c. Teach her the importance of a mammogram to evaluate breast tissue.
   d. Teach her inspection of the whole area of breast tissue for any changes.

3. What explanation should the nurse provide when teaching a client with painful fibrocystic breast changes about the condition?
   a. All discrete breast lumps must be subjected to biopsy to rule out malignant changes.
   b. The symptoms will probably subside after menopause unless hormone replacement is used.
   c. The lumps will become progressively larger and more painful, eventually necessitating surgical removal.
   d. Restriction of coffee and chocolate and supplements of vitamin E can relieve the discomfort for many patients.

4. When discussing risk factors for breast cancer with a group of women, which of the following should the nurse stress as the greatest known risk factor for breast cancer?
   a. Being a woman older than 60 years
   b. Experiencing menstruation for 40 years or more
   c. Using estrogen replacement therapy during menopause
   d. Having a paternal grandmother with postmenopausal breast cancer

5. A client has a lumpectomy with sentinel lymph node biopsy that yields results positive for cancer. Which of the following results supports the most favourable prognosis? *(Select all that apply)*
   a. Well-differentiated tumour
   b. Estrogen receptor–positive tumour
   c. Involvement of two to four axillary nodes
   d. Overexpression of *HER2* cell marker
   e. Aneuploidy status from cell proliferation studies

6. A client with breast cancer has been scheduled for a modified radical mastectomy with an axillary node dissection. Which of the following should the nurse perform postoperatively to restore arm function on the affected side?
   a. Apply heating pads or blankets to increase circulation.
   b. Place daily ice packs to minimize the risk for lymphedema.
   c. Teach passive exercises with the affected arm in a dependent position.
   d. Emphasize regular exercises for the affected shoulder to increase range of motion.

7. Which of the following should the nurse implement preoperatively to meet the psychological needs of a woman scheduled for a modified radical mastectomy?
   a. Discuss the limitations of breast reconstruction.
   b. Include her significant other in all conversations.
   c. Promote an environment for expression of feelings.
   d. Explain the importance of regular follow-up screening.

8. Which of the following statements is suitable to make when teaching clients how to prevent capsular formation after breast reconstruction with implants?
   a. Gently massage the area around the implant.
   b. Bind the breasts tightly with elastic bandages.
   c. Exercise the arm on the affected side to promote drainage.
   d. Avoid strenuous exercise until implant healing has occurred.

1. c, d; 2. d; 3. d; 4. a; 5. a, b; 6. d; 7. c; 8. a.

⊝volve

For even more review questions, visit *http://evolve.elsevier.com/Canada/ Lewis/medsurg.*

REFERENCES

Ahmed, S., & Shahid, R. K. (2012). Disparity in cancer care: A Canadian perspective. *Current Oncology, 19*(6), e376–e382. doi:10.3747/co.19.1177.

Amaya, F., Hosokawa, T., Okamoto, A., et al. (2015). Can acute pain treatment reduce postsurgical comorbidity after breast cancer surgery? A literature review. *BioMed Research International, 2015,* 1–8. doi:10.1155/2015/641508.

Astin, J. A., Shapiro, J., & Shapiro, D. (2013). Psychological control and morbidity/mortality in breast cancer patients: A 20-year follow-up study. *Behavioral Medicine, 39*(1), 7–10. doi:10.108 0/08964289.2012.708683.

Canadian Agency for Drugs and Technologies in Health (CADTH). (2015). Tomosynthesis (3D mammography) for breast cancer screening. *Issues in Emerging Health Technologies, 135,* 1–10. Retrieved from *https://www.cadth.ca/tomosynthesis-3d -mammography-breast-cancer-screening.*

Canadian Cancer Society. (2017a). *Breast cancer statistics.* Retrieved from *http://www.cancer.ca/en/cancer-information/cancer-type/ breast/statistics/?region=bc.*

Canadian Cancer Society. (2017b). *Screening for breast cancer.* Retrieved from *http://www.cancer.ca/en/cancer-information/ cancer-type/breast/screening/?region=bc.*

Canadian Cancer Society. (2017c). *Breast pain.* Retrieved from *http://www.cancer.ca/en/cancer-information/cancer-type/breast/ breast-cancer/non-cancerous-conditions/breast-pain-mastalgia/ ?region=bc.*

Canadian Cancer Society. (2017d). *Fibrocystic breast changes.* Retrieved from *http://www.cancer.ca/en/cancer-information/ cancer-type/breast/breast-cancer/non-cancerous-conditions/ fibrocystic-changes/?region=bc.*

Canadian Cancer Society. (2017e). *Other non-cancerous breast conditions.* Retrieved from *http://www.cancer.ca/en/cancer -information/cancer-type/breast/breast-cancer/non-cancerous -conditions/other-non-cancerous-conditions/?region=on.*

Canadian Cancer Society. (2017f). *Risk factors for breast cancer.* Retrieved from *http://www.cancer.ca/en/cancer-information/ cancer-type/breast/risks/?region=on.*

Canadian Cancer Society. (2017g). *Hormone replacement therapy: HRT and cancer.* Retrieved from *http://www.cancer.ca/en/ prevention-and-screening/be-aware/artificial-hormones/hormone -replacement-therapy/?region=on#ixzz4sIjBXmnW.*

Canadian Cancer Society. (2017h). *Reducing your risk for breast cancer.* Retrieved from *http://www.cancer.ca/en/cancer-information/ cancer-type/breast/risks/reducing-your-risk/?region=on&p=1.*

Canadian Cancer Society. (2017i). *Axillary lymph node dissection (ALND).* Retrieved from *http://www.cancer.ca/en/ cancer-information/diagnosis-and-treatment/tests-and-procedures/ axillary-lymph-node-dissection/?region=on&p=1.*

Canadian Cancer Society. (2017j). *Sentinel lymph node dissection (ALND).* Retrieved from *http://www.cancer.ca/en/cancer -information/diagnosis-and-treatment/tests-and-procedures/sentinel -lymph-node-biopsy-slnb/?region=on.*

Canadian Cancer Society. (2017k). *HER2 status test.* Retrieved from *http://www.cancer.ca/en/cancer-information/diagnosis-and-treatment/ tests-and-procedures/her2-status-testing/?region=on&p=1.*

Canadian Cancer Society. (2017l). *Staging breast cancer.* Retrieved from *http://www.cancer.ca/en/cancer-information/cancer-type/ breast/staging/?region=on&p=1.*

Canadian Cancer Society. (2017m). *Surgery for breast cancer.* Retrieved from *http://www.cancer.ca/en/cancer-information/ cancer-type/breast/treatment/surgery/?region=on.*

Canadian Cancer Society. (2017n). *Risk of breast cancer recurrence and adjuvant therapy*. Retrieved from *http://www.cancer.ca/en/cancer-information/cancer-type/breast/treatment/risk-of-breast-cancer-recurrence-and-adjuvant-therapy/?region=on*.

Canadian Cancer Society. (2017o). *Chemotherapy for breast cancer*. Retrieved from *http://www.cancer.ca/en/cancer-information/cancer-type/breast/treatment/chemotherapy/?region=on*.

Canadian Cancer Society. (2017p). *Side effects of chemotherapy*. Retrieved from *http://www.cancer.ca/en/cancer-information/diagnosis-and-treatment/chemotherapy-and-other-drug-therapies/chemotherapy/side-effects-of-chemotherapy/?region=on*.

Canadian Cancer Society. (2017q). *Hormonal therapy for breast cancer*. Retrieved from *http://www.cancer.ca/en/cancer-information/cancer-type/breast/treatment/hormonal-therapy/?region=on*.

Canadian Cancer Society. (2017r). *Targeted therapy for breast cancer*. Retrieved from *http://www.cancer.ca/en/cancer-information/cancer-type/breast/treatment/targeted-therapy/?region=on*.

Canadian Cancer Society. (2017s). *Lymphedema*. Retrieved from *http://www.cancer.ca/en/cancer-information/diagnosis-and-treatment/managing-side-effects/lymphedema/?region=on*.

Canadian Cancer Society. (2017t). *Types of breast reconstruction*. Retrieved from *http://www.cancer.ca/en/cancer-information/cancer-type/breast/treatment/surgery/types-of-breast-reconstruction/?region=on*.

Canadian Partnership Against Cancer (2013). *Quality determinants of breast cancer screening with mammography in Canada*. Toronto: Author.

Canadian Task Force on Preventive Health Care. (2011). Recommendations on screening for breast cancer in average-risk women aged 40–74 years. *Canadian Medical Association Journal, 183*(17), 1991–2001. doi:10.1503/cmaj.110334.

Chagpar, A. B. (2014). Prophylactic bilateral mastectomy and contralateral prophylactic mastectomy. *Surgical Oncology Clinics of North America, 23*(3), 423–430, doi. *http://dx.doi.org/10.1016/j.soc.2014.03.008*.

Deepinder, F., & Braunstein, G. D. (2011). Gynecomastia: Incidence, causes and treatment. *Expert Review of Endocrinology and Metabolism, 6*(5), 723–730. doi:10.1586/eem.11.57.

Dow, J., & Kennedy Sheldon, L. (2015). Breast cancer survivors and sexuality: A review of the literature concerning sexual functioning, assessment tools, and evidence-based interventions. *Clinical Journal of Oncology Nursing, 19*(4), 456–461. doi:10.1188/15.CJON.456-461.

Health Canada. (2012). *It's your health: Breast implants*. Retrieved from *http://www.hc-sc.gc.ca/hl-vs/iyh-vsv/med/implants-eng.php*.

Hwang, E. S., Lichtensztajn, D. Y., Gomez, S. L., et al. (2013). Survival after lumpectomy and mastectomy for early stage invasive breast cancer. *Cancer, 119*(7), 1402–1411. doi:10.1002/cncr.27795.

Irusen, H., Rohwer, A., Steyn, D., et al. (2015). Treatments for breast abscesses in breastfeeding women. *The Cochrane Database of Systematic Reviews*, No. 8, Article CD010490. doi:10.1002/14651858.CD010490.pub2.

Kong, X., Moran, M. S., Zhang, N., et al. (2011). Meta-analysis confirms achieving pathological complete response after neoadjuvant chemotherapy predicts favourable prognosis for breast cancer patients. *European Journal of Cancer, 47*(14), 2084–2091. doi:10.1016/j.ejca.2011.06.014.

Managing fibrocystic breast changes and pain: Perspectives for the clinician. (2015). *Contemporary OB/GYN, 60*(5). Retrieved from *http://www.violetdaily.com/wp-content/uploads/2015/05/Managing-FBCPain_ClinicianPerspective.pdf*.

Nicholson, P. (2015). Lymphedema risk after breast cancer treatment. *Women's Health Matters. Women's College Hospital*. Retrieved from *http://www.womenshealthmatters.ca/feature-articles/feature-articles/Lymphedema-risk-after-breast-cancer-treatment/*.

Onstad, M., & Stuckey, A. (2013). Benign breast disorders. *Obstetrics & Gynecology Clinics of North America, 40*(3), 459–473. doi:10.1016/j.ogc.2013.05.004.

Player, L., Mackenzie, L., Willis, K., et al. (2014). Women's experiences of cognitive changes or "chemobrain" following treatment for breast cancer: A role for occupational therapy? *Australian Occupational Therapy Journal, 61*(4), 230–240. doi:10.1111/1440-1630.12113.

Silversides, A. (2012). Breast self-examination: What it means and why the thinking about it has changed. *Canadian Women's Health Network*. Retrieved from *http://www.cwhn.ca/en/network_magazine/breast_self-examination*.

Stagl, J. M., Antoni, M. H., Lechner, S. C., et al. (2014). Postsurgical physical activity and fatigue-related daily interference in women with breast cancer. *Psychology & Health, 29*(2), 177–198. doi:10.1080/08870446.2013.843682.

Women's College Hospital. (2015). *Benign breast tumours*. Retrieved from *http://www.womenshealthmatters.ca/health-centres/breast-cancer-info-reviewed-by-doctors-research-treatment-symptoms-and-amp-diagnosis/benign-breast-tumours*.

Yeo, B., Turner, N. C., & Jones, A. (2014). An update on the medical management of breast cancer. *British Medical Journal, 348*, 1–7. doi:10.1136/bmj.g3608.

RESOURCES

Breast Cancer Society of Canada
http://www.bcsc.ca

Canadian Association of Nurses in Oncology
http://www.cano-acio.ca/

Canadian Association of Provincial Cancer Agencies (CAPCA)
http://www.capca.ca

Canadian Breast Cancer Foundation (CBCF)
http://www.cbcf.org

Canadian Breast Cancer Network (CBCN)
http://www.cbcn.ca

Canadian Cancer Society
http://www.cancer.ca

Canadian Cancer Society Research Institute
http://www.cancer.ca/research

Canadian Oncology Societies (COS)
http://www.cos.ca

Canadian Partnership Against Cancer
http://www.partnershipagainstcancer.ca

American Cancer Society: Breast Cancer
http://www.cancer.org/cancer/breastcancer/index

Living Beyond Breast Cancer
http://www.lbbc.org

National Breast Cancer Coalition
http://www.natlbcc.org

National Cancer Institute & Breast Cancer Risk Assessment Tool
http://www.cancer.gov & http://www.cancer.gov/bcrisktool/

National Coalition for Cancer Survivorship (NCS)
http://www.canceradvocacy.org

National Lymphedema Network (NLN)
http://www.lymphnet.org

OncoLink (cancer information site of the Abramson Cancer Center, University of Pennsylvania)
http://www.oncolink.org

Oncology Nursing Society (ONS)
http://www.ons.org

Susan G. Komen
http://ww5.komen.org

For additional Internet resources, see the website for this book at *http://evolve.elsevier.com/Canada/Lewis/medsurg*.

Nursing Management
Sexually Transmitted Infections

Written by: Adena Bargad
Adapted by: Shelley L. Cobbett

⊘volve WEBSITE

http://evolve.elsevier.com/Canada/Lewis/medsurg
- Review Questions (Online Only)
- Key Points
- Answer Guidelines for Case Study
- Conceptual Care Map Creator
- Audio Glossary
- Content Updates

LEARNING OBJECTIVES

1. Assess the factors contributing to the high incidence of sexually transmitted infections (STIs).
2. Explain the etiology, clinical manifestations, complications, and diagnostic abnormalities of gonorrhea, syphilis, chlamydial infections, genital herpes, and genital warts.
3. Compare and contrast primary genital herpes with recurrent genital herpes.
4. Explain the collaborative care and the drug therapy for gonorrhea, syphilis, chlamydial infections, genital herpes, and genital warts.
5. Identify the nursing assessment and the nursing diagnoses for patients who have a sexually transmitted infection.
6. Describe the nursing role in the prevention and control of sexually transmitted infections.
7. Describe the nursing management of patients with sexually transmitted infections.

KEY TERMS

chancre, p. 1378, Table 55-3
chlamydial infections, p. 1379
genital herpes, p. 1380

gonorrhea, p. 1374
gummas, p. 1378,
    Table 55-3

sexually transmitted infections (STIs),
    p. 1373
syphilis, p. 1376

SEXUALLY TRANSMITTED INFECTIONS

Sexually transmitted infections (STIs) are infectious diseases that are commonly acquired through sexual contact (Table 55-1) but may also be contracted by other routes, such as through blood, blood products, perinatal transmission, and autoinoculation. STIs can be bacterial (gonorrhea, chlamydial infection, syphilis), viral (genital herpes, genital warts), or both. Most infections start as lesions on the genitalia and other sexually exposed mucous membranes.

Wide dissemination to other areas of the body can then occur. A latent or subclinical phase is present with all STIs. This can lead to a long-term persistent infection and the transmission of disease from an asymptomatic (but infected) person to another person. Having one STI increases the risk of acquiring another. A person can have different STIs at the same time.

In Canada, three nationally reportable STIs—gonorrhea, syphilis, and chlamydial infection—must be reported to the Communicable Disease Division in each province and territory (Public Health Agency of Canada [PHAC], 2013a). Since 1997, there has been a steady increase in the rates of all three of these infections (PHAC, 2013a) but it is not clear if this is an actual increase or just a result of changes in the diagnosing and reporting of STIs (PHAC, 2013b). Young Canadians have the highest reported rates of sexually transmitted infections, although the numbers of cases being reported among middle-aged and older adults is increasing (PHAC, 2013b). There are also some noteworthy trends related to populations at high risk for STIs, such as injection-drug users, sex workers, individuals who are homeless, and anonymous sexual partners (e.g., a person met online or at a bathhouse or rave party) (PHAC, 2013a).

The more commonly diagnosed STIs are discussed in this chapter. Human immunodeficiency virus (HIV) infection and related problems are discussed in Chapter 17. Hepatitis B & C infection and related problems are discussed in Chapter 46.

TABLE 55-1   CAUSES OF SEXUALLY TRANSMITTED INFECTIONS

Cause	Infection or Condition
Bacterial	
Chlamydia trachomatis	Nongonococcal urethritis; cervicitis; lymphogranuloma venereum
Neisseria gonorrhoeae	Gonorrhea
Treponema pallidum	Syphilis
Viral	
Cytomegalovirus	Encephalitis, esophagitis, retinitis, pneumonitis in immuno-compromised patients
Hepatitis B & C viruses	Hepatitis B and C (see Chapter 46)
Herpes simplex virus (HSV)	Genital herpes
Human immunodeficiency virus (HIV) (See Chapter 17)	HIV infection, acquired immune deficiency syndrome (AIDS)
Human papilloma virus (HPV)	Genital warts; cervical, vulvar, vaginal, penile, anal, and oropharyngeal cancers
Poxvirus*	Molluscum contagiosum
Other	
Trichomonas vaginalis	Trichomoniasis
Phthirus pubis (crab louse)*	Ectoparasitic infestation (pubic lice) See Chapter 26
Sarcoptes scabiei*	Ectoparasitic infestation (scabies) See Chapter 26

*Transmission through both intimate sexual and nonsexual contact

FACTORS AFFECTING INCIDENCE OF SEXUALLY TRANSMITTED INFECTION

Many factors contribute to the current STI rates. Earlier reproductive maturity and increased longevity have resulted in a longer sexual lifespan. The increase in the total population has resulted in an increase in the number of susceptible hosts. Other factors include greater sexual freedom, failure to use barrier methods (e.g., condom, dental dam) during sexual activity, and the media's increased emphasis on sexuality. Substance use contributes to unsafe sexual practices. In addition, increased leisure time, more national and international travel, and urbanization have brought together people with varying social behaviours and value systems.

Changes in the methods of contraception that are typically used are also reflected in the incidence of STIs. The condom is considered to be the best form of protection (other than abstinence) against STIs. However, among the 1.8 million sexually active Canadians aged 15 to 49 years who had two or more sexual partners, only 57.5% used a condom the last time they had sex (Statistics Canada, 2015). Males are more likely than females to use a condom, and condom use decreases with age (Statistics Canada, 2015). Commonly used oral contraceptives cause the secretions of the cervix and the vagina to become more alkaline. This change produces a more favourable environment for the growth of organisms that cause STIs at these sites. Women who take oral contraceptives have a lower risk for pelvic inflammatory disease (PID) as a result of the ability of the cervical mucus to act as a barrier against bacteria. However, the proliferation of *Chlamydia* organisms, the leading cause of nongonococcal PID, may be enhanced by oral contraceptive use. Whether users of intrauterine devices (IUDs) are at increased risk for PID is controversial, but IUDs do not confer protection from STIs.

Long-acting contraceptives such as levonorgestrel (Jaydess) and medroxyprogesterone (Depo-Provera) also confer no protection against STIs. Although these methods do not prevent transmission from partner to partner, they do prevent pregnancy and, therefore, transmission of the infection to a fetus.

Nurses need to strive to attend to the physiological and psychological needs of the large number of people living with incurable STIs in Canada. Chronic viral STIs can have longstanding negative effects on a patient's psychosocial well-being, highlighting the need for strengthened prevention efforts.

BACTERIAL INFECTIONS

GONORRHEA

Gonorrhea is the second-most frequently occurring STI. Between 2003 and 2012, the rate of reported cases of gonorrhea increased by 38.9%, from 26.0 to 36.2 per 100 000 (PHAC, 2012). Although rates of gonorrhea increased in both sexes and across all age groups (12 561 cases reported in 2012), a greater relative rate increase was observed in females (PHAC, 2012). Continued monitoring for antimicrobial resistance is important to prevent the spread of drug-resistant gonorrhea and to ensure successful cure rates for this treatable infection. Most provinces and territories have enacted laws that permit examination and treatment of minors without parental consent.

Etiology and Pathophysiology

Gonorrhea is caused by *Neisseria gonorrhoeae*, a gram-negative diplococcus bacterium. The infection is spread by direct physical contact with an infected host, usually during sexual activity (vaginal, oral, or anal). Mucosal tissues in the genitalia (urethra in men, cervix in women), rectum, and oropharynx are especially sensitive to gonococcal infection. Neonates can develop gonorrhea during delivery from an infected mother. The delicate gonococcus is easily killed by drying, heating, or washing with an antiseptic solution. As a consequence, indirect transmission by instruments or linens is rare.

The incubation period is 3 to 8 days. The disease confers no immunity to subsequent reinfection. Gonorrhea elicits an inflammatory response that, if left untreated, leads to the formation of fibrous tissue and adhesions, which increase a woman's risk of experiencing an ectopic pregnancy (PHAC, 2013a).

Clinical Manifestations

Men. The initial site of infection in men is usually the urethra. Symptoms of urethritis consist of dysuria and profuse, purulent urethral discharge that develops 2 to 5 days after infection (Figure 55-1). The testicles may also become painful or swollen. Men generally seek medical evaluation early in the infection because their symptoms are usually obvious and distressing. It is unusual for men with gonorrhea to be asymptomatic (PHAC, 2013a).

Women. Most women who contract gonorrhea are asymptomatic or have minor symptoms that are often overlooked, which makes it possible for them to remain a source of infection. A few affected women may complain of vaginal discharge, dysuria, or frequency of urination. Changes in menstruation may be a symptom, but many affected women disregard these changes. After the incubation period, redness and swelling occur at the site of contact, which is usually the cervix or the urethra (Figure 55-2). A greenish-yellow purulent exudate often develops, with a potential for abscess formation. The infection may remain local or

FIGURE 55-1 Profuse, purulent drainage in a patient with gonorrhea. Source: Marx, K., Walls, R., & Hockberger, R. (2010). *Rosen's emergency medicine: Concepts and clinical practice* (7th ed.). St Louis: Mosby.

FIGURE 55-2 Endocervical gonorrhea. Cervical redness and edema with discharge. Source: Morse, S., Moreland, A., & Holmes, K. (Eds.). (1996). *Atlas of sexually transmitted diseases and AIDS.* London: Mosby-Wolfe.

FIGURE 55-3 Skin lesions from disseminated gonococcal infection. **A,** On hand. **B,** On the fifth toe. Sources: **A,** Cohen, J., & Powderly, W. G. (2004). *Infectious diseases* (2nd ed.). St. Louis: Mosby. **B,** Mandell, G. L., Bennett, J. E., & Dolin, R. (2010). *Mandell, Douglas, and Bennett's principles and practice of infectious diseases* (7th ed.). Philadelphia: Churchill Livingstone.

can spread by direct tissue extension to the uterus, fallopian tubes, and ovaries. Although the vulva and the vagina are uncommon sites for a gonorrheal infection, they may become involved when little or no estrogen is present, as is the case in prepubertal girls and postmenopausal women. Because the vagina acts as a natural reservoir for infectious secretions, transmission is often more efficient from men to women than it is from women to men.

General. Anorectal gonorrhea may be present and is usually caused by anal intercourse. Symptoms may include soreness, itching, and mucopurulent anal discharge. In a small percentage of individuals, gonococcal pharyngitis results from orogenital sexual contact. Most patients with rectal infections and infections in the throat have few symptoms. When the gonococcus can be demonstrated by a laboratory culture, individuals of either sex can transmit the infection to their sexual partners.

Complications

Because men often seek treatment early in the course of the disease, they are less likely to develop complications. The complications that do occur in men are prostatitis, urethral strictures, and sterility from orchitis or epididymitis. Because women without symptoms seldom seek treatment, complications are more common and usually constitute the reason for seeking medical attention. PID, Bartholin abscess, ectopic pregnancy, chronic pelvic pain, and infertility are the main complications of gonorrhea in women. A small percentage of infected people may develop disseminated gonococcal infection (DGI). In DGI, the appearance of skin lesions, fever, arthralgia, arthritis, or endocarditis usually causes the patient to seek medical help (Figure 55-3).

Eye Infections in Newborns. Infants with untreated gonorrheal infection develop permanent blindness. Most provinces and territories require the instillation of a prophylactic drug such as erythromycin or tetracycline into the eyes of all newborns as a precaution (Perry, Hockenberry, Lowdermilk, et al., 2017). Gonococcal eye infections in newborns (ophthalmia neonatorum) are therefore relatively rare today.

Diagnostic Studies

For men, a presumptive diagnosis of gonorrhea is made if the man has a history of sexual contact with a new or infected partner followed within a few days by a urethral discharge. Typical clinical manifestations, combined with a positive finding in a Gram-stained smear of the purulent discharge from the penis, give an almost certain diagnosis. A culture of the discharge is indicated for men whose smears are negative in the presence of strong clinical evidence. The nucleic acid amplification test (NAAT) (using ligase or polymerase chain reaction) is a nonculture test with sensitivity similar to culture tests for *N. gonorrhoeae* and can be done on a wide variety of samples, including vaginal, endocervical, urethral, and urine specimens (Borhart & Birnbaumer, 2011).

Diagnosing gonorrhea in women on the basis of symptoms is difficult because most infected women are symptom-free or have complaints that may be confused with other conditions. Smears and purulent discharge do not establish a diagnosis of gonorrhea because the female genito-urinary tract normally harbours a large number of organisms that resemble *N. gonorrhoeae*. A culture must be performed to confirm the diagnosis. Although the cervix is the most common site of sampling, specimens for culture may also be taken from the urethra, anus, or oropharynx. A urine specimen can reveal gonorrhea if it is present in the cervix or urethra.

Collaborative Care

Collaborative care for the patient with a gonorrheal infection is presented in Table 55-2.

TABLE 55-2 COLLABORATIVE CARE

Gonorrhea

Diagnostic
- History and physical examination
- Gram-stained smears of urethral or endocervical exudate
- Cultures for *Neisseria gonorrhoeae*
- NAAT to detect *N. gonorrhoeae*
- Testing for other STIs (syphilis, HIV, chlamydial infection)

Collaborative Therapy
Drug Therapy
- Uncomplicated gonorrheal infections:
  - Cefixime (Suprax) 800 mg PO in a single dose (preferred) plus azithromycin (Zithromax) 1 g PO in a single dose OR
  - Ceftriaxone 250 mg IM in a single dose plus azithromycin (Zithromax) 1 g PO in a single dose
  - Alternate treatment with azithromycin (Zithromax) 2 g PO in a single dose
- Also treated for chlamydial infection, unless a *Chlamydia* test result is available and negative
- Gonococcal infections reportable to the public health department in all provinces and territories
- Treatment of sexual contacts
- Instruction on abstinence from sexual intercourse and alcohol during treatment
- Re-examination if symptoms persist or recur after completion of treatment

HIV, human immunodeficiency virus; *IM,* intramuscularly; *PO,* by mouth (per os); *NAAT,* nucleic acid amplification test; *STI,* sexually transmitted infection.
Source: Modified from Centers for Disease Control and Prevention. (2015). *Sexually transmitted diseases treatment guidelines, 2015. Morbidity and Mortality Weekly Report, 64*(3), 1–138. Retrieved from *http://www.cdc.gov/std/tg2015/tg-2015-print.pdf* and from Public Health Agency of Canada. (2013, updated 2016). *Canadian guidelines on sexually transmitted infections.* Ottawa: Author. Retrieved from *http://www.phac-aspc.gc.ca/std-mts/sti-its/cgsti-ldcits/section-5-6-eng.php.*

Drug Therapy. Because of a short incubation period and high infectivity, treatment is generally instituted before culture results are available, even in the absence of any signs or symptoms (PHAC, 2013a). Quinolones such as ciprofloxacin and ofloxacin are no longer preferred drugs for the treatment of gonorrhea in Canada because of the rapid increase in quinolone-resistant strains of *N. gonorrhoeae* (PHAC, 2013a). Patients with coexisting syphilis are likely to be treated with the same drugs used for gonorrhea.

All sexual contacts of patients with gonorrhea must be examined and treated to prevent reinfection after resumption of sexual relations. The "ping-pong" effect of re-exposure, treatment, and reinfection can cease only when infected partners are treated simultaneously. In addition, the patient should be counselled to abstain from sexual intercourse and alcohol during treatment. Sexual intercourse allows the infection to spread and can delay complete healing, and alcohol has an irritant effect on the healing urethral walls. Caution men against squeezing the penis to look for further discharge. Reinfection, rather than treatment failure, is the main cause for infections identified after treatment has ended.

SYPHILIS

The incidence of syphilis has steadily increased in Canada by 101.0% between 2003 and 2012, from 2.9 to 5.8 per 100 000 (PHAC, 2012). During this same time frame, rates increased among males by 128.3% and decreased among females by 40.9%,

and the rate of reported cases of infectious syphilis in males was markedly higher than that in females (11 as compared to 0.5 per 100 000) (PHAC, 2012). In males, rates of infectious syphilis were highest among those aged 25 to 29; in females, rates were highest among those aged 20 to 24. In 2012, infectious syphilis rates varied geographically, and the highest rates occurred in Quebec (PHAC, 2012). Syphilis remains an important health problem.

Etiology and Pathophysiology

Syphilis is caused by *Treponema pallidum,* a spirochete. This bacterium is thought to enter the body through very small breaks in the skin or mucous membranes. Its entry is facilitated by the minor abrasions that often occur during sexual intercourse. Syphilis is a complex disease in which many organs and tissues of the body can become infected with *T. pallidum.* The infection causes the production of antibodies that also react with normal tissues. Not all people who are exposed to syphilis acquire the disease. In about one-third of cases, infection is acquired after intercourse with an infected person; in addition to sexual contact, syphilis may be spread through contact with infectious lesions and sharing of needles among people who use intravenous (IV) drugs.

T. pallidum is extremely fragile and easily destroyed by drying, heating, or washing. The incubation period for syphilis ranges from 3 to 90 days (average, 21 days) (PHAC, 2013a). In congenital syphilis, the infection is transmitted from an infected mother to the fetus in utero after the tenth week of gestation. An infected pregnant woman has a high risk for a stillbirth or a baby dying shortly after birth (Hawkes, Matin, Broutet, et al., 2011). Universal screening of pregnant women has remained the standard of care in Canada (PHAC, 2013a).

People at high risk for acquiring syphilis are also at an increased risk for acquiring HIV infection. The presence of syphilitic lesions on the genitalia enhances HIV transmission. HIV-infected patients with syphilis appear to be at greatest risk for clinically significant central nervous system (CNS) involvement and may require more intensive treatment with penicillin than other patients with syphilis do. The treatment failure rate is higher in HIV-positive patients with syphilis than in HIV-negative patients who acquire syphilis (Lin, Zheng, Tong, et al., 2011). Therefore, the assessment of all patients with syphilis should also include testing for HIV (with the patient's consent). Conversely, patients with HIV should be tested at least annually for syphilis.

Clinical Manifestations

Syphilis has a variety of signs and symptoms that can mimic those of a number of other diseases (Da Silva Carneiro, Pirmez, de Hollanda, et al., 2013) (Figures 55-4, 55-5, and 55-6); thus in comparison with other STIs, it is more difficult to recognize syphilis. If it is not treated, specific clinical stages are characteristic of the progression of the disease (Table 55-3).

Complications

Complications of the disease occur mostly in the late stage of syphilis. The gummas of benign late syphilis may produce irreparable damage to bone, liver, or skin but seldom result in death. In cardiovascular syphilis, the resulting aneurysm may press on structures such as the intercostal nerves, causing pain. The possibility of a rupture rises as the aneurysm increases in size. Scarring of the aortic valve results in aortic valve insufficiency and, eventually, heart failure.

Neuro-syphilis causes degeneration of the brain with mental deterioration (Mehrabian, Raycheva, Traykova, et al., 2012).

FIGURE 55-4 Primary syphilis chancre. Source: Forbes, C. D., & Jackson, W. F. (2003). *Color atlas and text of clinical medicine.* (3rd ed.). London: Mosby.

FIGURE 55-5 Secondary syphilis. Bilateral, symmetrical cutaneous lesions. Source: Habif, T. (2004). *Clinical dermatology: A color guide to diagnosis and therapy* (4th ed., p. 319, Figure 10-9). St. Louis: Mosby.

FIGURE 55-6 Destructive skin gummas associated with tertiary syphilis. Source: Cohen, J., & Powderly, W. G. (2004). *Infectious diseases* (2nd ed.). St. Louis: Mosby.

Problems related to sensory nerve involvement are a result of tabes dorsalis (progressive locomotor ataxia). There may be sudden attacks of pain anywhere in the body, which can confuse the diagnosis with other conditions. Loss of vision and sense of position in the feet and legs can also occur. Walking may become even more difficult as joint stability is lost. (Neuro-syphilis is also discussed in Chapter 63.)

Diagnostic Studies

The first step in the diagnosis of syphilis is to obtain a detailed and accurate sexual history. Chapter 53 provides some guidelines for taking a sexual health history as well as examples of sexual health history questions in Chapter 53, Table 53-7.

When taking a sexual history, it is important to know the sexual orientation and gender identity of the patient, but is also important not to assume that the patient is heterosexual or clearly gendered. What is more helpful is to consider sexuality and gender as existing along a continuum rather than the limitations of terms such as *heterosexual* or *homosexual* and *male* or *female*. Questions such as, "Do you have sex with men or women or both?" are more inclusive and provide more useful information when questioning patients about their sexual practices. In addition, inquire about vaginal, oral, or anal sex. A physical examination should be done to identify any suspicious lesions or other significant signs and symptoms. Since syphilis is "the great imitator" of other conditions, it is easily missed. Oral sex is an important transmission route that is sometimes overlooked.

The presence of spirochetes on dark-field microscopic examination and direct fluorescent antibody (DFA) tests of lesion exudate or tissue can confirm a clinical diagnosis of syphilis. However, syphilis is more commonly diagnosed through a serological test. Tests for syphilis may be classified as those performed for screening and those performed for confirmation of a positive screening result. Nonspecific antitreponemal antibodies can be detected by tests such as the Venereal Disease Research Laboratory (VDRL) test and the rapid plasma reagin (RPR) test. These nontreponemal tests are suitable for screening purposes and usually yield positive results 10 to 14 days after the appearance of a chancre. The fluorescent treponemal antibody absorption (FTA-ABS) test and the *T. pallidum* particle agglutination (TP-PA) test detect specific antitreponemal antibodies and are suitable for confirming the diagnosis.

False-negative and false-positive results do occur with the nontreponemal tests (VDRL, RPR). A false-negative result may be obtained during primary syphilis if the test is performed before the individual has had time to produce antibodies. A false-positive finding may occur after smallpox vaccination or with other diseases or conditions such as hepatitis, infectious mononucleosis, collagen diseases (e.g., systemic lupus erythematosus), pregnancy, or aging. Positive nontreponemal test results should be confirmed by more specific treponemal tests to rule out other causes. In the cerebro-spinal fluid (CSF), changes such as increased white blood cell count, increased total protein levels, and a positive result of the treponemal antibody test are diagnostic of asymptomatic neuro-syphilis.

If a patient is treated with antibiotics early in the course of the disease on the basis of the history and the symptoms, the serological test may not indicate the presence of syphilis. Once a patient has positive serological findings for syphilis, indicating the presence of antibodies, these findings may remain positive for an indefinite period in spite of successful treatment.

TABLE 55-3 STAGES OF SYPHILIS

Manifestations	Communicability	Manifestations	Communicability
Primary Chancre (painless indurated lesion of penis, vulva, lips, mouth, vagina, and rectum) (Figure 55-4) occurs 3 to 90 days after inoculation Regional lymphadenopathy (draining of the microorganisms into the lymph nodes) Genital ulcers *Duration of stage:* 3–8 wk	Exudate from chancre highly infectious; blood is infectious Most infectious stage, but transmission can occur at any stage if there are moist lesions	**Latent** Absence of signs or symptoms Diagnosis based on positive specific treponemal antibody test together with normal CSF and absence of clinical manifestations *Duration of stage:* Throughout life or progression to late stage	Noninfectious after 4 yr; possible placental transmission Almost 25% of persons with latent syphilis develop late syphilis, in some cases many years later
Secondary Occurs a few weeks after chancre appears Systemic manifestations: flulike symptoms (e.g., malaise, fever, sore throat, headaches, fatigue, arthralgia, headache, generalized adenopathy) Cutaneous lesions bilateral; symmetric rash that begins on the trunk and involves the palms and soles (Figure 55-5); mucous patches in the mouth, tongue, or cervix; *Condylomata lata* (moist, weeping papules) in the anal and genital area Weight loss, alopecia *Duration of stage:* 1–2 yr	Exudate from skin and mucous membrane lesions highly infectious	**Late (Tertiary)*** Appearance 3–20 yr after initial infection Gummas (chronic, destructive lesions affecting any organ of body, especially skin, bone, liver, mucous membranes) (Figure 55-6) *Cardiovascular:* Aneurysms, aortic valve insufficiency, aortitis *Neuro-syphilis:* General paresis (personality changes from minor to extreme [psychosis], tremors, physical and mental deterioration), tabes dorsalis (ataxia, areflexia, paresthesias, lightning pains, damaged joints [Charcot's joints]), speech disturbances. *Duration of stage:* Chronic (without treatment), possibly fatal	Noninfectious Spinal fluid possibly containing organism

CSF, cerebro-spinal fluid.
*Several forms such as cardiovascular syphilis and neuro-syphilis occur together in approximately 25% of untreated cases.

TABLE 55-4 COLLABORATIVE CARE

Syphilis

Diagnostic	Collaborative Therapy

• History and physical examination
• Dark-field microscopy
• Nontreponemal or treponemal (or both) serological testing
• Testing for other STIs (HIV infection, gonorrhea, chlamydial infection)
	• Appropriate drug therapy (see Table 55-5)
	• Confidential counselling and testing for HIV infection
	• Case finding
	• Surveillance
	  • Repeat of quantitative nontreponemal tests at 6 and 12 months
	  • Examination of cerebro-spinal fluid at 1 year if treatment involves alternative antibiotics or treatment failure has occurred

HIV, human immunodeficiency virus; *STI*, sexually transmitted infections.

Collaborative Care

Drug Therapy. Management of syphilis is aimed at eradication of all syphilitic organisms (Table 55-4). However, treatment cannot reverse damage that is already present in the late stage of the disease. Benzathine penicillin G remains the treatment of choice for all stages of syphilis (PHAC, 2013a). Therapy for the various stages of syphilis that is in accordance with national STI guidelines provided by the PHAC (2013a) is described in Table 55-5. All stages of syphilis should be treated. When symptoms are chronic or recur after drug therapy has ended, the patient should undergo repeated treatment. All patients with neuro-syphilis must be carefully monitored, with periodic serological testing, clinical evaluation at 6-month intervals, and repeat CSF examinations for at least 3 years. Specific management is based on the symptoms. It is also very important that all sexual contacts in the previous 90 days be treated.

> **DRUG ALERT—Benzathine penicillin G (Bicillin L-A)**
> • Reports from some jurisdictions have indicated inappropriate use of short-acting benzylpenicillin (penicillin G) intramuscularly for the treatment of infectious syphilis rather than long-acting benzathine penicillin G (Bicillin L-A) (PHAC, 2013a).
> • Nurses need to be aware of the similar names of these two products to prevent and avoid inappropriate and inadequate treatment.

There are approximately 1.36 million pregnant women globally that have probable active syphilis (Newman, Kamb, Hawkes, et al., 2013). In pregnant women with syphilis, benzathine penicillin G, 2.4 million units IM weekly for one to three doses, is administered, depending on the stage of syphilis. Treatment administered in the second half of pregnancy may pose a risk for premature labour and fetal distress. Pregnant women receiving treatment should be advised to seek medical care if fetal movements decrease.

CHLAMYDIAL INFECTIONS

Chlamydial infections are the most prevalent bacterial STI in Canada today, with 103 716 cases reported in 2012 and with approximately 1 of every 2 cases reported in women (PHAC,

TABLE 55-5 DRUG THERAPY

Syphilis

Stage	Preferred Treatment	Alternative Treatment*
All nonpregnant adults: • Primary syphilis • Secondary syphilis • Early latent syphilis (<1 year duration)	Benzathine penicillin G (Bicillin L-A) 2.4 million units IM in a single dose	• Doxycycline (Vibramycin) 100 mg PO BID for 14 days • Alternate agent (to be used in exceptional circumstances)—ceftriaxone 1 g IV or IM daily for 10 days
All nonpregnant adults • Late latent syphilis • Latent syphilis of unknown duration • Cardiovascular syphilis and other tertiary syphilis not involving central nervous system	Benzathine penicillin G (Bicillin L-A) three doses of 2.4 million units each, IM, at 1-wk intervals (total dose, 7.2 million units)	• Consider penicillin desensitization • Doxycycline (Vibramycin) 100 mg PO BID for 28 days • Alternate agent (to be used in exceptional circumstances)—ceftriaxone 1 g IV or IM daily for 10 days
All adults • Neuro-syphilis	Penicillin G 3-4 million units every 4 hr IV for 10–14 days (total dose, 16–24 million units)	• Strongly consider penicillin desensitization followed by treatment with penicillin • Ceftriaxone 2 g IV or IM daily for 10–14 days

IM, intramuscularly; *IV,* intravenously; *PO,* by mouth (per os).
*Given when penicillin is contraindicated.
Source: © All rights reserved. Canadian *Guidelines on Sexually Transmitted Infections.* Public Health Agency of Canada, 2013. Adapted and reproduced with permission from the Minister of Health, 2017.

TABLE 55-6 RISK FACTORS FOR CHLAMYDIAL INFECTION

• Early age at first sexual intercourse
• History of STIs, coexisting and cervical ectopy
• Inconsistent or incorrect use of barrier contraception (condoms, dental dams)
• New or multiple sex partners
• Use of alcohol and drugs (indirect risk factors)
• Vulnerable populations (people who use injection drugs, incarcerated individuals, sex trade workers, street youth)
• Women and adolescents

STIs, sexually transmitted infections.
Source: Faber, M., Nielsen, A., Nygard, M., et al. (2011). Genital chlamydia, genital herpes, trichomonas vaginalis and gonorrhea prevalence, and risk factors among nearly 70,000 randomly selected women in 4 Nordic countries. *Sexually Transmitted Diseases, 38*(8), 727–734. doi:10.1097/OLQ.0b013e318214bb9b.

2012). In both sexes, rates of chlamydial infections were highest in those aged 20 to 24 years (PHAC, 2012). Under-reporting is substantial because most infected people have no symptoms and therefore do not seek testing. Chlamydial infections are a major contributor to PID, ectopic pregnancy, and infertility among women and to nongonococcal urethritis in men (Bender, Hermann, Anderson, et al., 2011).

Etiology and Pathophysiology

Chlamydial infections are caused by *Chlamydia trachomatis,* a Gram-negative bacterium, and can be transmitted during vaginal, anal, or oral sex. Numerous different serotypes, or strains, of *C. trachomatis* cause urogenital infections (e.g., nongonococcal urethritis [NGU] in men and cervicitis in women), ocular trachoma, and lymphogranuloma venereum. Table 55-6 lists the risk factors for chlamydial infection. Because of the high prevalence of asymptomatic infections, screening of populations at high risk is needed to identify those infected (see the "Evidence-Informed Practice" box).

Clinical Manifestations and Complications

Chlamydial infection is known as a silent disease because symptoms may be absent or minor in most infected women and

EVIDENCE-INFORMED PRACTICE

Research Highlight

What Strategies Improve Screening Rates for Repeat Chlamydial Infections?

Clinical Question

In patients with repeat chlamydial infections (P), what is the effect of reminders and mailed screening kits (I) versus no intervention (C) on rescreening rates (O)?

Best Available Evidence

Systematic review of randomized controlled trials (RCTs) and observational studies

Critical Appraisal and Synthesis of Evidence

• Eight trials (N=25 to 5 863/trial) compared patient rescreening rates for repeat chlamydial infections.
• Interventions were mailed screening kits, motivational interviewing, financial incentives, and reminders.
• Rescreening occurred 3 weeks to 12 months after the initial chlamydial infection.
• Mailed screening kits for sample self-collection and phone call, postcard, and email reminders significantly increased rescreening rates.

Conclusion

• Mailed screening kits, reminders, and a combination of both methods increased rescreening rates.

Implications for Nursing Practice

• Repeat chlamydial infections are common and increase the risk for complications.
• Remind patient of importance of rescreening.
• To increase rescreening rates, tailor interventions to meet patient needs and preferences.
• Text message and automated phone call reminders may also be effective.

Reference for Evidence

Guy, R., Hocking, J., Low, N., et al. (2012). Interventions to increase rescreening for repeat chlamydial infection. *Sexually Transmitted Diseases, 39*(2), 136–146. doi:10.1097/OLQ.0b013e31823ed4ec.

P, Patient population of interest; *I,* intervention or area of interest; *C,* comparison of interest or comparison group; *O,* outcomes of interest (see Chapter 1).

in many men (Champion & Collins, 2012). Signs and symptoms in men include urethritis (dysuria, urethral discharge), epididymitis (unilateral scrotal pain, swelling, tenderness, fever), and proctitis (rectal discharge and pain during defecation). In women, signs and symptoms include cervicitis (mucopurulent discharge, hypertrophic ectopy [area that is edematous and bleeds easily]), urethritis (dysuria, frequent urination, pyuria), bartholinitis (purulent exudate), dyspareunia (pain with intercourse), and menstrual abnormalities.

Complications often develop when chlamydial infections are poorly managed, inaccurately diagnosed, or undiagnosed. Because chlamydial infections are closely associated with gonococcal infections, clinical differentiation may be difficult. In men, urethritis, epididymitis, and proctitis may occur with both infections. In women, bartholinitis, cervicitis, and salpingitis (inflammation of the fallopian tube) can occur in both chlamydial and gonococcal infections. Therefore both infections are usually treated concurrently, even without diagnostic proof. The incubation period of 1 to 3 weeks for chlamydial infection is longer than that for gonorrhea, and the symptoms are often milder. If a pregnant woman has chlamydia, her baby may be born prematurely, have eye infections, or develop pneumonia (Government of Canada, 2013).

In men, epididymitis can lead to rare complications, including abscess, sepsis, and infertility. In women, chlamydial infections can cause fallopian tube damage, a leading cause of ectopic pregnancy and infertility. Complications from chlamydial infections in women may result in PID and scarring of the fallopian tubes, which can result in infertility and a higher risk for ectopic or tubal pregnancies (Government of Canada, 2013). Although it is rare, both sexes are at risk for a type of arthritis known as Reiter's syndrome, which causes inflammation and swelling of the joints (Government of Canada, 2013).

Diagnostic Studies and Collaborative Care

Chlamydial infections in men can be diagnosed by ruling out gonorrhea. The discharge in chlamydial infections (cervical in women; urethral in men and women) appears to be less purulent, less watery, and less painful than in gonorrhea. Culture is the preferred method of diagnosis for medicolegal purposes, and culture is recommended for throat specimens (PHAC, 2013a). NAATs are more sensitive and more specific than culture, enzyme immunoassay, and direct fluorescent antibody assay.

For nonmedicolegal purposes, NAATs should be used whenever possible for urine and for urethral or cervical specimens.

Drug Therapy. When diagnosed, chlamydial infection can be easily treated and cured. Chlamydial infections respond to treatment with doxycycline or azithromycin, with erythromycin or ofloxacin used as an alternative treatment regimen (PHAC, 2013a). Follow-up care should include advising the patient to return if the symptoms persist or recur, treatment of sex partners, and encouraging the use of condoms during all sexual contacts. The high incidence of recurrence may be due to failure to treat the sexual partners of infected people. Because of the high prevalence of asymptomatic infections, screening of high-risk populations is needed to identify those who are infected.

> **DRUG ALERT—Doxycycline**
> * Patients on this drug should avoid unnecessary exposure to sunlight.
> * Patients should not take this drug with antacids, iron products, or dairy products.

VIRAL INFECTIONS

GENITAL HERPES

Genital herpes is not a reportable infection in most provinces and territories, except the Atlantic provinces. The annual incidence of genital herpes in Canada is, therefore, not known. In the United States, approximately 15.5% of people aged 14 to 49 have genital herpes (Centers for Disease Control and Prevention, 2015).

Etiology and Pathophysiology

Genital herpes is a sexually transmitted infection caused by the herpes simplex virus (HSV), usually type 2. The virus enters through the mucous membranes or breaks in the skin during contact with an infected person (Figure 55-7). HSV then reproduces inside the cell and spreads to the surrounding cells. The virus next enters the peripheral or autonomic nerve endings and ascends to the sensory or autonomic nerve ganglion, where it often becomes dormant. Viral reactivation (recurrence) may occur when the virus descends to the initial site of infection, either the mucous membranes or the skin. When a person is infected with HSV, the infection is usually chronic within the individual for life. Transmission occurs through direct contact

| Inoculation of herpes viral particles into broken skin | Replication of virus in epidermal cells leads to swelling and tenderness | Vesicle formation as serum collects within damaged epidermis | Erosion and viral shedding (blister has lost roof); epidermis begins to heal |

FIGURE 55-7 Stages of infection with herpes simplex virus (HSV). Source: Morse, S., Moreland, A., & Holmes, K. (Eds.). (1996). *Atlas of sexually transmitted diseases and AIDS.* London: Mosby-Wolfe.

with skin or mucous membrane or through asymptomatic viral shedding (PHAC, 2013a).

Two different strains of HSV cause infection. In general, HSV type 1 (HSV-1) causes infection above the waist, involving the gingivae, the dermis, the upper respiratory tract, and the CNS. HSV-2 most frequently infects the genital tract and the perineum (i.e., locations below the waist). However, either strain can cause disease on the mouth or the genitals. The incidence and prevalence of HSV-1 genital infection are increasing globally, particularly among college students. The majority of genital herpes cases, however, are caused by HSV-2 infection (PHAC, 2013a).

Clinical Manifestations

In the primary (initial) episode of genital herpes, the patient may complain of burning, itching, or tingling at the site of inoculation. Multiple small, vesicular, and sometimes painless lesions may appear on the inner thigh, penis, scrotum, vulva, perineum, perianal region, vagina, or cervix (Roett, Mayor, & Uduhiri, 2012) and contain large quantities of infectious viral particles (Figure 55-8). The lesions rupture and form shallow, moist ulcerations. Finally, crusting and epithelialization of the erosions occur. Primary infections tend to be associated with local inflammation and pain, accompanied by systemic manifestations such as fever, headache, malaise, myalgia, and regional lymphadenopathy.

Urination may be painful from the urine touching active lesions. Urinary retention may occur as a result of HSV urethritis or cystitis. A purulent vaginal discharge may develop with HSV cervicitis. The duration of symptoms is longer and the frequency of complications is greater in women. Primary lesions are generally present for 17 to 20 days, but new lesions sometimes continue to develop for 6 weeks. The lesions heal spontaneously unless secondary infection occurs.

Recurrent genital herpes occurs in about 50% to 80% of individuals during the year after the primary episode. Stress, fatigue, sunburn, general illness, immuno-suppression, and menses are commonly noted triggers. Many patients can predict a recurrence by noticing the early prodrome symptoms of tingling, burning, and itching at the site where the lesions will eventually appear (Roett et al., 2012). The symptoms of recurrent episodes are less severe, and the lesions usually heal within 8 to 12 days. With time, the lesions generally recur less frequently.

Complications

Although most infections are of a relatively benign nature, complications of genital herpes may involve the CNS, causing aseptic meningitis and lower motor neuron damage. Neuron damage may result in atonic bladder, erectile dysfunction, and constipation. Another complication is *autoinoculation* of the virus to extragenital sites such as the lips (Figure 55-9), the breasts, and, most commonly, the fingers (herpetic whitlow).

Herpes Simplex Virus Infection During Pregnancy. Pregnant women with a primary episode of HSV near the time of delivery have the highest risk of transmitting genital herpes to the neonate (Stephenson-Famy & Gardella, 2014). The risk for transmission is lowest for women who acquire HSV early in the pregnancy or have a history of recurrent HSV. An active genital lesion at the time of delivery is usually an indication for Caesarean section delivery because most infections in neonates occur during birth (Su & McKay, 2012).

Diagnostic Studies and Collaborative Care

A diagnosis of genital herpes is usually based on the patient's symptoms and history. The diagnosis can be confirmed through isolation of the virus from active lesions by means of tissue culture, and this is the most common method currently used in Canada (PHAC, 2013a). Polymerase chain reaction assay is four times more sensitive than HSV culture and is 100% specific; however, it has not yet replaced the culture for routine screening in Canada (PHAC, 2013a). Other techniques to detect HSV include direct immuno-fluorescence, enzyme immunoassay, and DNA amplification. These tests enable more rapid identification of HSV than a culture does. Highly accurate serological methods for

FIGURE 55-8 Unruptured vesicles of herpes simplex virus type 2 (HSV-2). **A,** Vulvar area. **B,** Perianal area. **C,** Penile herpes simplex, ulcerative stage. Sources: **A** and **C,** From the Centers for Disease Control and Prevention; courtesy Susan Lindsley. **B,** From Morse, S., Moreland, A., & Holmes, K. (Eds.). (1996). *Atlas of sexually transmitted diseases and AIDS,* London: Mosby-Wolfe.

FIGURE 55-9 Autoinoculation of herpes simplex virus (HSV) to the lips. Source: Centers for Disease Control and Prevention public image library. Retrieved from *http://phil.cdc.gov/phil/quicksearch.asp* (image #5434).

detecting the HSV type are available. The Tzanck smear, with a low sensitivity, is no longer considered a reliable test to confirm diagnosis (PHAC, 2013a).

It is important to encourage symptomatic treatment, such as using good genital hygiene and wearing loose-fitting cotton undergarments. The lesions should be kept clean and dry. To ensure complete drying of the perineal area, women may use a hair dryer set on a cool setting. Frequent sitz baths may soothe the area and reduce inflammation. Drying agents such as colloidal oatmeal (Aveeno) and aluminum salts (Burow solution) may provide some relief from the burning and itching. Techniques to reduce pain on urination include pouring a pitcher of water onto the perineal area while voiding to dilute the urine, and voiding in a warm tub of water or shower. Pain may require a local anesthetic such as lidocaine (Xylocaine) or systemic analgesics such as codeine and acetylsalicylic acid (ASA; Aspirin).

Sexual transmission of HSV can occur during asymptomatic periods so the use of barrier methods, especially condoms, should be encouraged. When lesions are present, the patient should avoid sexual activity altogether because even barrier protection is not satisfactory in eliminating infection transmission.

Drug Therapy. Three antiviral agents are available for the treatment of HSV: acyclovir (Zovirax), valacyclovir (Valtrex), and famciclovir (Famvir). These drugs inhibit herpetic viral replication and are prescribed for primary and recurrent infections (Table 55-7). Acyclovir, valacyclovir, and famciclovir are also used to suppress frequent recurrences (more than six episodes per year). Although not a cure, these drugs shorten the duration of viral shedding and the healing time of genital lesions and reduce outbreaks by 62% (Barnabas, Baeten, Lingappa, et al., 2015). Continued use of oral acyclovir as suppressive therapy for up to 6 years is safe and effective. Adverse reactions are mild and include headache, occasional nausea and vomiting, and diarrhea. The safety of these drugs for treatment of pregnant women has not been established. Acyclovir ointment appears to have no clinical benefit in the treatment of recurrent lesions, either in speed of healing or in resolution of pain, and is not commonly recommended. IV acyclovir is reserved for severe or life-threatening infections in which hospitalization is required for the treatment of disseminated infections, CNS infections (meningitis), or pneumonitis. Nephrotoxicity has been observed with high-dose IV administration. Clinical trials are examining the effectiveness of a vaccine for HSV-2 (Johnston, Koelle, & Wald, 2011).

GENITAL HUMAN PAPILLOMA VIRUS INFECTIONS

Human papilloma virus (HPV) causes skin and mucosal infections and has a strong affinity for the moist mucosa of the anal, genital, and aerodigestive tracts. There are more than 130 types of the virus, many of which are sexually transmitted. Most types do not cause any symptoms and go away on their own. The most common low-risk genotypes are 6 and 11, which cause condylomata acuminata (genital warts), and the most common high-risk genotypes are 16 and 18, predisposing to precancerous or cancerous lesions (PHAC, 2014). HPV infection is a highly contagious STI and is the most common viral STI; it is frequently observed in young, sexually active adults. Risk factors include young age, lower level of education, lower consumption of vegetables, more sexual partners, young age at first sexual experience, more pregnancies, and high alcohol consumption (Bell, Schmidt-Grimminger, Jacobsen, et al., 2011). Of the adult

---

TABLE 55-7   COLLABORATIVE CARE

Genital Herpes

Diagnostic
- History and physical examination
- Antibody assay for specific HSV viral type
- Viral isolation by tissue culture

Collaborative Therapy
Treatment for First Episode
- For severe primary disease, IV acyclovir 5 mg/per kg over 60 min every 8 hours with later conversion to oral drug therapy
- Acyclovir (Zovirax) 200 mg PO five times daily for 5–10 days; or famciclovir (Famvir) 250 mg PO three times daily for 5 days; or valacyclovir (Valtrex) 1 000 mg PO twice daily for 10 days; or acyclovir 400 mg PO three times daily for 7–10 days (recommended by Centers for Disease Control and Prevention).

Treatment for Recurrent Episodes
- Acyclovir (Zovirax) 200 mg PO five times daily for 5 days or 800 mg PO three times daily for 2 days
- Valacyclovir (Valtrex) 500 mg PO twice daily or 1 g daily for 3 days; or famciclovir (Famvir) 125 mg PO twice daily for 5 days

Suppressive Therapy for Frequent Recurrence in Nonpregnant Patients
Any of the treatments listed below:
- Acyclovir (Zovirax) 200 mg PO 3–5 times daily or 400 mg PO twice daily
- Famciclovir (Famvir) 250 mg PO twice daily
- Valacyclovir (Valtrex) 500 mg PO daily (patients with ≤9 recurrences per year) or 1 000 mg PO daily (patients with >9 recurrences per year)

Other Considerations
- Abstinence from sexual contact while lesions are present; however, virus may be shed without lesions
- Annual Pap smear
- Confidential counselling and testing for HIV
- Identify trigger mechanisms
- Symptomatic care

HIV, human immunodeficiency virus; *HSV,* herpes simplex virus; *IV,* intravenously; *Pap,* Papanicolaou; *PO,* by mouth (per os).
Source: Modified from Public Health Agency of Canada. (2013a). *Canadian guidelines on sexually transmitted infections. Section 5: Genital herpes simplex virus (HSV) infections.* Ottawa: Author. Retrieved from *http://www.phac-aspc.gc.ca/std-mts/sti-its/cgsti-ldcits/section-5-4-eng.php.*

---

population in Canada, 75% have at least one genital HPV infection over their lifetime (PHAC, 2014).

Minor trauma during intercourse can cause abrasions that allow HPV to enter the body. The incubation period of the virus is generally 3 to 4 months but may be longer. Prevention is hampered by a high proportion of asymptomatic infections and lack of curative treatment. In Canada, the reporting of HPV infection is not required.

Clinical Manifestations and Complications

The discussion of clinical manifestations, complications, and care focuses on the low-risk HPV genotypes resulting in genital warts; cervical cancer is discussed in Chapter 56. Genital warts are discrete single or multiple papillary growths that are white to grey and flesh-pink. They may grow and coalesce to form large, cauliflower-like masses. Most affected patients have from 1 to 10 genital warts. In men, the warts may occur on the penis and the scrotum, around the anus, or in the urethra. In women, the warts may be located on the vulva, in the vagina or the cervix,

FIGURE 55-10 Genital warts. **A,** Severe vulvar warts. **B,** Perineal wart. **C,** Multiple genital warts of the glans penis. Source: **A,** From the Centers for Disease Control and Prevention, courtesy Joe Millar. **B,** From the Centers for Disease Control and Prevention, courtesy Dr. Wiesner. **C,** From the Centers for Disease Control and Prevention, courtesy Susan Lindsley.

and in the perianal area (Figure 55-10). There are usually no other signs or symptoms. Itching may occur with anogenital warts. Bleeding on defecation may occur with anal warts.

During pregnancy, genital warts tend to grow rapidly and there is recent evidence that mild local hyperthermia may be a promising method for treating genital warts in pregnant women (Huo, Di, Xiao, et al., 2014). An infected mother may transmit the condition to her newborn (Nigam & Mishra, 2011). Caesarean delivery is not routinely indicated unless the birth canal becomes blocked by massive warts.

Diagnostic Studies and Collaborative Care

Up to two-thirds of the early lesions caused by HPV are undetectable by visual examination. Genital warts can be diagnosed on the basis of the gross appearance of the lesions. However, the warts may be confused with condylomata lata of secondary syphilis, carcinoma, or benign neoplasms. The HPV DNA test is recommended with women who have abnormal Papanicolaou (Pap) test results (PHAC, 2014). The HPV DNA test can identify women who are infected with the high-risk HPV strains (types 16 and 18), associated with cervical cancer. At present, access to HPV DNA tests in Canada is limited to a small number of jurisdictions, and HPV cannot be confirmed by culture (PHAC, 2014).

The primary goal in treating visible genital warts is the removal of symptomatic warts. The removal may or may not decrease infectivity. Genital warts are difficult to treat and often necessitate multiple office visits with a variety of treatment modalities. The therapy should be modified if a patient has not experienced improvement after three treatments or if after six treatments the warts have not completely disappeared. Treatment consists of chemical or ablative (removal with laser or electrocautery) methods. One common treatment is the use of 50% to 80% trichloroacetic acid (TCA) or bichloroacetic acid (BCA) solutions in 70% alcohol, applied directly to the wart surface. Petroleum jelly is applied to the surrounding normal skin to minimize irritation before a small amount of TCA is applied to the wart with a cotton swab. A sharp stinging pain is often felt with initial acid contact, but this quickly subsides. TCA is not washed off after treatment and is safe for use during pregnancy.

Topical treatments include imiquimod, podofilox/podophyllo-toxin, podophyllin, sinecatechins, and trichloroacetic acid (TCA) (PHAC, 2014). With topical treatments it is important to avoid contact with mucosal tissue, eyes, tongue, lips, broken skin, and surrounding healthy skin, and patients should be instructed to refrain from sexual activity while undergoing treatment (PHAC, 2014). Treatment may cause skin reactions such as itching, tenderness, erythema, and ulceration. TCA is the only treatment that is to be used with pregnant, and lactating women (PHAC, 2014). If topical treatments are not effective, over-the-counter, self-applied cryotherapy kits are available (PHAC, 2014). Because treatment does not destroy the virus, merely the infected tissue, recurrences and reinfection are possible, and careful long-term follow-up is advised.

Human Papilloma Virus Immunization

HPV infection has been linked to cervical and anogenital cancers, as well as certain cancers of the head and neck (PHAC, 2013c). HPV vaccines include Gardasil (HPV4) and Cervarix (HPV2). HPV2 or HPV4 vaccine is recommended for women 9 to 26 years of age and HPV4 vaccine is recommended for men aged 9 to 26 years (PHAC, 2013c). The most commonly reported adverse events following HPV vaccination are injection site pain, swelling or redness, and syncope (PHAC, 2013c). These vaccines do not treat active HPV infections. Ideally, they should be administered before the start of sexual activity, but people who are sexually active, as well as those infected, would still obtain protection from the HPV types not already acquired.

NURSING MANAGEMENT
SEXUALLY TRANSMITTED INFECTIONS

NURSING ASSESSMENT

Subjective and objective data that should be obtained from a person with an STI are presented in Table 55-8.

NURSING DIAGNOSES

Nursing diagnoses for the patient with an STI include, but are not limited to, the following:

- *Risk for infection* as evidenced by *insufficient knowledge to avoid exposure to pathogens* (STI transmission, engaging in high-risk behaviours)
- *Anxiety* related to *stressors, threat to current status* (impact of condition on relationships, long-term effects of infection)
- *Ineffective health maintenance* related to *insufficient resources* (lack of knowledge about disease process and transmission)

EVIDENCE-INFORMED PRACTICE
Translating Research Into Practice

Francis Ceres is a 19-yr-old man who is being seen in the health care centre for signs and symptoms of a urinary tract infection. When asked, he shares with the nurse that he is sexually active. After reviewing his health history, the nurse learns that he has not received the human papilloma virus (HPV) vaccine. The nurse discusses the risks and benefits of the vaccine and suggests that he consider getting it.

Best Available Evidence	Clinician Expertise	Patient Preferences and Values
Males ages 9–26 years, including males who have sex with males, are advised to be vaccinated with one of the HPV vaccines available to reduce the incidence of penile, anal, and oropharyngeal cancers as well as genital warts. The majority of all HPV–associated cancers are caused by HPV 16 or 18. Approximately 64% of invasive HPV-associated cancers are attributable to HPV 16 or 18.	Approximately 90% of anal cancers have been linked to HPV infection. Males may be unaware of the expanded recommendations for HPV vaccines, which were originally approved to prevent cervical, vulvar, and vaginal cancer caused by HPV types 6, 11, 16, and 18 in females ages 9 through 26.	Mr. Ceres states that he never has unprotected sex and does not like injections.

Decision and Action
After listening carefully, Mr. Ceres decides to talk to a few of his friends before making a decision about the vaccine. He tells the nurse that he had no idea that he could get HPV infections. If he decides to get the vaccine, he will be back. The nurse documents the discussion in his chart.

Reference for Evidence
Petrosky, E., Bocchini, J. A., Jr., Hariri, S., et al. (2015). Use of 9-valent human papillomavirus (HPV) vaccine: Updated HPV vaccination recommendations of the advisory committee on immunization practices. *MMWR. Morbidity and Mortality Weekly Report, 64*(1), 300–304. Retrieved from *http://www.cdc.gov/mmwr/pdf/wk/mm6411.pdf#page=12*; National Advisory Committee on Immunization (NACI). (February 2015). *Update on the recommended human papillomavirus (HPV) vaccine immunization schedule.* Retrieved from *http://www.phac-aspc.gc.ca/naci-ccni/acs-dcc/2015/hpv-vph_0215-eng.php.*

PLANNING
The overall goals are that the patient with an STI will (a) demonstrate understanding of the mode of transmission of STIs and the risk posed by STIs, (b) complete treatment and return for appropriate follow-up, (c) notify or assist in notification of sexual contacts about their need for testing and treatment, (d) abstain from intercourse until the infection is resolved, and (e) demonstrate knowledge of safer sex practices.

NURSING IMPLEMENTATION
HEALTH PROMOTION. Many approaches to curtailing the spread of STIs have been advocated and have met with varying degrees of success. Nurses should be prepared to discuss "safe" sex practices with all patients, not only those who are perceived to

TABLE 55-8   NURSING ASSESSMENT
Sexually Transmitted Infections

Subjective Data
Important Health Information
Past health history: Contact with individuals with STIs, multiple sexual partners, pregnancy, shared needles during IV drug use, previous vaccination against HPV
Medications: Oral contraceptives; allergy to any antibiotics, especially penicillin

Symptoms
- Alopecia
- Arthralgia, headache
- Dyspareunia; vaginal discharge, menstrual abnormalities; presence of painful, burning genital or perianal lesions
- Dysuria, urinary frequency, retention; urethral discharge; tenesmus, proctitis
- Itching at infected site; lesions that cause pain or burning sensation
- Malaise; chills
- Nausea, vomiting, anorexia, pharyngitis, oral lesions

Objective Data
General
Fever, lymphadenopathy (generalized or inguinal)

Integumentary
Syphilis:
- *Primary:* painless, indurated genital, oral, or perianal lesions
- *Secondary:* bilateral, symmetrical rash on palms, soles, or entire body; mucous patches on mouth or tongue; alopecia
Genital herpes: Painful genital or anal vesicular lesions
Genital warts: Single or multiple grey or white genital or anal warts (possibly becoming massive)

Gastro-Intestinal
Purulent rectal discharge (indicator of gonorrhea), rectal lesions, proctitis

Urinary
Urethral discharge, erythema

Reproductive
Cervical discharge, lesions, inflamed Bartholin glands

Possible Diagnostic Findings
- *Chlamydial infection:* Positive culture or DNA amplification for *Chlamydia*
- *Genital herpes:* Positive tissue culture for HSV-1 or HSV-2; positive HSV-1 or HSV-2 antibody titre
- *Gonorrhea:* Positive Gram stain, smears, cultures, and DNA amplification for *Neisseria gonorrhoeae*
- *Syphilis:* Positive findings on VDRL and RPR tests, spirochetes on dark-field microscopy

HPV, human papilloma virus; *HSV-2,* herpes simplex virus type 2; *IV,* intravenous; *RPR,* rapid plasma reagin; *STI,* sexually transmitted infection; *VDRL,* Venereal Disease Research Laboratory.

be at risk. These practices include abstinence, monogamy with an uninfected partner, avoidance of certain high-risk sexual practices, and use of barriers (e.g., dental dams, condoms) to limit contact with potentially infectious body fluids or lesions. Limiting sexual intimacies outside of a well-established monogamous relationship can reduce the risk of contracting an STI. A patient and caregiver teaching guide related to the patient with an STI is presented in Table 55-9.

All sexually active women should be screened for cervical cancer using a Pap test. Women with a history of STIs are at

TABLE 55-9 PATIENT & CAREGIVER TEACHING GUIDE

Sexually Transmitted Infections

When teaching the patient with sexually transmitted infections, the nurse should carry out the following steps:

1. Instruct patient in hygienic measures, such as washing and urinating after intercourse to flush out some of the causative organisms.
2. Explain the importance of taking all antibiotics or antiviral agents (or both) as prescribed. Symptoms improve after 1 to 2 days of therapy but organisms may still be present.
3. Teach patient about the need for treatment of sexual partners to prevent transmission of disease.
4. Instruct patient to abstain from sexual intercourse during treatment and to use condoms when sexual activity is resumed to prevent spread of infection and prevent reinfection.
5. Explain the importance of follow-up examination and repeated culture at least once after treatment if appropriate, to confirm complete cure and prevent relapse.
6. Allow patient and partner to verbalize concerns to clarify areas that need explanation.
7. Instruct patient about symptoms of complications and need to report problems to ensure proper follow-up and early treatment of reinfection.
8. Explain precautions to take, such as being monogamous; asking potential partners about sexual history; avoiding sex with partners who use intravenous drugs or who have visible oral, inguinal, genital, perineal, or anal lesions; using male or female condoms or dental dams; and voiding and washing genitalia after intercourse to reduce the occurrence of reinfection.
9. Inform patient regarding state of infectivity to prevent a false sense of security, which might result in careless sexual practices and poor personal hygiene.
10. Provide information related to HPV vaccination.

HPV, human papilloma virus.

greater risk for cervical cancer than women without this history are. Anal Pap tests should also be done for all individuals who are recipients of anal sex. (Pap smears are discussed in Chapter 56.)

Measures to Prevent Infection. An inspection of the sexual partner's genitalia before coitus is recommended. Discharge, sores, blisters, or rash should be viewed with concern. A person who is aware of specific signs and symptoms of infection can intelligently make the decision to continue the sexual interaction with modifications or elect not to have sexual relations. The person should remember that, when engaging in sex, there is exposure to the infections of everyone with whom the partner has ever had sex. Men should be told that some protection is provided if they void immediately after intercourse and wash their genitalia and the adjacent areas with soap and water. Women may also benefit from postcoital voiding and washing. However, it is important to emphasize that this does not provide adequate protection against STIs after exposure to infection.

Vaginal microbicides, topical gels, or creams that contain tenofovir may reduce HIV and HSV-2 acquisition in heterosexual women, but there is no evidence that other kinds of vaginal microbicides have an effect in reducing acquisition of HIV, HSV-2, or any other STI (Obiero, Mwethera, & Wiysonge, 2012). These gels or creams can serve as supplementary lubrication, thereby decreasing irritation and friction and chances for development of a minor laceration that could serve as an entry point for the organism. Proper use of a condom is a highly effective mechanical barrier to infection—the condom should be undamaged and correctly in place throughout all phases of sexual activity. A deterrent to condom usage is alcohol and drug use (Davis, Jacques-Tiura, Stappenbeck, et al., 2015). Use of barrier contraceptives requires planning and motivation, both of which are impaired with alcohol or drug ingestion. The patient should be given specific verbal and written instructions on the proper use of condoms (see Chapter 17, Table 17-19). The objections to condom usage, such as interference with spontaneity and the presence of a barrier, should be discussed by the partners. Information about the mechanics of sexual arousal and incorporating the use of a condom into lovemaking can help in overcoming resistance to its use. Female condoms are lubricated polyurethane sheaths with a ring at each end designed for vaginal use but are considerably more expensive than male condoms (see Chapter 17, Table 17-20).

Among couples with one infected partner, consistent and scrupulous barrier use can reduce transmission to the uninfected partner. Unprotected anal intercourse and other high-risk behaviours should be eliminated, and condoms should be used if sexual contact continues.

The nurse should initiate a discussion to assess the patient's risk of contracting an STI. Questions to ask include number of partners, type of birth control used, use of condoms and dental dams, use of intravenous drugs, history of STIs, and sexual preference. Although the majority of STIs are transmitted between men having sex with men and heterosexual contact, it is possible to transmit an STI between women (Ripley, 2011). The nurse should plan patient education based on the response to these questions. Interpersonal skills necessary for this interview include respect, compassion, and a nonjudgemental attitude. Counselling should be tailored to the individual patient. The nurse should not assume that older people are not at risk; an increasing number of older people are acquiring STIs.

Screening Programs. Screening programs can help prevent certain STIs. For many years, there have been various screening programs to identify cases of syphilis. With the increase of infection rates across Canada, more stringent screening and follow-up treatment are required. Many institutions offer voluntary prenatal HIV and syphilis testing and counselling for pregnant women.

Screening programs have also been developed and implemented for detection of gonorrhea and chlamydial infection. These programs are targeted to women because women are more likely to have asymptomatic gonorrhea and thereby serve as sources of infection. Gonorrheal and chlamydial testing during pelvic examinations and prenatal visits is becoming a major routine part of these programs. Mass application of screening programs for genital chlamydial infections, genital herpes, and HPV infections may also be possible with the advent of rapid, cost-effective tests.

Case Finding. Interviewing and case finding are other processes used to control STIs. These activities are directed toward locating and examining all contacts of each known patient with an STI as soon after sexual exposure as possible so that effective treatment can be initiated. Trained interviewers may often find cases even if they are supplied with only limited information. The caseworkers, who are often nurses, are aware of the social implications of these diseases and the need for discretion. Often, sexual contacts are not informed about the origin of the information naming them as a contact, so that greater cooperation and privacy is ensured. (See the "Ethical Dilemmas" box on confidentiality.) Although still controversial, *expedited partner therapy (EPT)* allows a health care provider to provide prescriptions to a patient to take to his or her partner, without examining the partner; this method may be beneficial in high-risk and hard-to-reach populations (PHAC, 2013a).

ETHICAL DILEMMAS
Confidentiality

Situation

A nurse in a clinic gives the positive results of a test for *Chlamydia* infection to a patient and advises her to tell her sexual partners that she has this infection. The patient refuses to tell her boyfriend because he will then know that she has had sex with another partner. Should the nurse contact the boyfriend?

Important Points for Consideration

• Nurses and other health care providers have both a legal and an ethical obligation to maintain confidentiality of patient information. If confidentiality is violated, trust is eroded and patients may not share privileged information that is essential to plan effective care.
• Nurses have a legal responsibility to report three STIs in Canada: chlamydia, syphilis, and gonorrhea.
• The nurse must assess if giving the patient the option to tell his or her partner is responsible, accountable, ethical nursing practice, as this may put the patient at risk for intimate partner violence.
• Health care providers have an obligation to maintain confidentiality unless there is a risk to the health or life of innocent third parties.
• The nurse's primary obligation is to the patient seeking care. However, there are long-term health consequences for this patient, as well as for the public in general.
• Patient teaching is one way to establish a partnership with this woman. Information should be shared about the effects of the infection being untreated, the risks for and consequences of re-infection, and the results that the infection may have on others who may not know they are infected. The patient can then be encouraged to inform her partners of the diagnosis for the good of everyone.

Clinical Decision-Making Questions

1. What are the provincial or territorial requirements for reportable conditions?
2. What information should the nurse share with this patient regarding the transmission of chlamydial infection so that she may be more willing to discuss the results with her boyfriend?
3. What is the best way to balance the needs of an individual patient with those of the general public?

Educational and Research Programs. Nurses should actively encourage those in their community to provide better education about STIs for its citizens. Teenagers, who are known to have a high incidence of infection, should be a prime target for such educational programs. STI rates are on the rise among older adults (Jeffers & DiBartolo, 2011); they are less likely to use condoms and in general have a harder time initiating discussion of sexual health issues. Hotline services, reliable Internet sites, school nurses, nurse practitioners, nurse midwives, and outreach programs sponsored by Canada's Health Protection Branch are effective means of providing educational programs.

Knowledge and understanding can decrease the STI epidemic. The HPV vaccine that protects against genital warts and cervical cancer should be encouraged before the start of sexual activity. Accurate and current information may help reduce parental fears related to the vaccine. Nurses should consider stressing the prevention of cancer as a reason for the vaccine, which may be more productive and less controversial, thus making the parent and adolescent more receptive. Efforts are being made to develop

vaccines for syphilis, gonorrhea, genital herpes, and HIV. The development of effective vaccines is viewed by many clinicians as a prerequisite for eradication of STIs.

Harm Reduction. Behavioural interventions to promote condom use, to modify HIV sexual risk behaviours, or both include individual counselling, skills training, coping strategies, peer education, and social and educational support (Carvalho, Goncalves, Faria, et al., 2011) and should be integrated in harm-reduction programs and health care settings to prevent STIs and reduce HIV transmission. For individuals identified as being at ongoing risk for STIs, screening is recommended at 3-month intervals for HIV, gonorrhea, syphilis, and chlamydial infection. Ongoing contact with a health care provider is an opportunity for reinforcement of safer sex practices. Canada has an annual Sexual and Reproductive Health week, which occurs in February. (Harm reduction is discussed in Chapter 11.)

ACUTE INTERVENTION

Psychological Support. The diagnosis of an STI may be met with a variety of emotions, such as shame, guilt, anger, and a desire for vengeance. Nurses should provide counselling and encourage the patient to verbalize feelings. Couples in marital or committed relationships are confronted with an added problem when an STI is diagnosed because they must face the implication of sexual activity outside the relationship. Support and counselling for the couple are needed.

A patient who has genital herpes is faced with the fact that infections can recur and that no cure is available. This can be frustrating and disruptive to the patient's physical, emotional, social, and sexual life. The nurse should help the patient identify and avoid any factors that may precipitate the condition and inform the patient that the frequency and severity of recurrences may decrease over time.

HPV infections involve a prolonged course of treatment. The patient can become frustrated and distressed because of frequent office visits, associated costs, potential for unpleasant adverse effects as a result of treatment, and effects of the infection on future health and sexual relationships. Tremendous support and a willingness to listen to the patient's concerns are needed. Support groups are also available.

Follow-Up. A nurse working in public health facilities, clinics, or other outpatient settings may care for patients with STIs more often than a nurse in a hospital. This nurse is in a position to explain and interpret treatment measures such as the purpose and possible adverse effects of prescribed drugs and the need for follow-up care.

Single-dose treatment for gonococcal infection, chlamydial infection, and syphilis helps prevent the problems associated with nonadherence to drug therapy. Patients who require multiple-dose therapy should be given special instructions in completing the prescribed regimen and should be informed about problems resulting from nonadherence. All patients should return to the treatment centre for a repeat culture from the infected sites or for serological testing at designated times to determine the effectiveness of the treatment. Explaining to the patient that cures are not always obtained on the first treatment can reinforce the need for a follow-up visit. The patient should also be advised to inform sexual partners of the need for testing and treatment, regardless of whether they are free of symptoms or are experiencing symptoms.

Hygiene Measures. The nurse must emphasize certain hygiene measures to patients with an STI. An important measure is frequent handwashing and bathing. Bathing and cleaning of the involved areas can provide local comfort and prevent secondary infection. Douching may spread the infection or undermine local immune responses and is therefore contraindicated. The synthetic materials used in most undergarments frequently increase or exacerbate local irritations by trapping moisture. Cotton under-garments provide better absorption and are cooler and more comfortable for the patient with an STI.

Sexual Activity. Sexual abstinence is indicated during the communicable phase of the infection. If sexual activity occurs before treatment of the patient has been completed, the use of condoms may prevent the spread of infection and reinfection. Condom usage after treatment should be encouraged to prevent future exposure to infection. The patient can also choose to relate to a partner in an intimate way that avoids both coitus and oral-genital contact. It is important to note that even single-dose treatments can take up to 1 week to be effective, and the patient is infectious during this period.

AMBULATORY AND HOME CARE. Because many STIs are cured with a single dose or short course of antibiotic therapy, many people are casual about the outcome of these diseases. The consequences of this attitude can include delays in treatment, nonadherence to instructions, and subsequent development of complications. The complications are serious and costly; they can result in disfigurement and destruction of important tissues and organs.

Surgery and prolonged therapy are indicated for many patients with infection-related complications. Major surgical procedures such as resection of an aneurysm or aortic valve replacement may be necessary to treat cardiovascular problems caused by syphilis. Pelvic surgery and procedures to correct fertility problems secondary to an STI may include lysis of adhesions, dilation of strictures, reconstructive tuboplasty, and in vitro fertilization.

EVALUATION

Expected outcomes for a patient with an STI are that the patient will do the following:

- Describe modes of transmission
- Use appropriate hygienic measures
- Experience no reinfection
- Demonstrate adherence to a follow-up protocol

CASE STUDY

Chlamydial Infection and Gonorrhea

Source: lukas_zb/ Shutterstock.

Patient Profile

Cynthia Raeburn is a 23-yr-old woman who is seen at the outpatient clinic with complaints of a purulent yellow-white discharge and frequent urination over the past 2 weeks. She is sexually active with a new partner after breaking up with a long-term boyfriend. She was treated in the past for chlamydia at age 20.

Subjective Data

- Did not use condom or spermicide
- Her sexual partner was recently treated for epididymitis
- Last menstrual period was 3 weeks ago
- Appears very nervous

Objective Data

- Cervical ectopy noted during Pap test
- Mucopurulent cervical discharge
- Nucleic acid amplification test is positive for *Neisseria gonorrhoeae* and *Chlamydia trachomatis*
- Urine pregnancy test is negative
- Patient crying and very upset when informed of positive test results

Collaborative Care

- Doxycycline, 100 mg PO twice a day for 7 days
- Ceftriaxone, 250 mg intramuscularly once

Discussion Questions

1. What were Ms. Raeburn's risk factors for acquiring chlamydial and gonococcal infections?
2. What complications could occur if Ms. Raeburn's infections are not treated?
3. *Priority decision:* What is the priority of care for Ms. Raeburn?
4. What instructions should Ms. Raeburn receive to ensure successful treatment? To prevent reinfection? To prevent further transmission of the infection?
5. What impact is her diagnosis likely to have on Ms. Raeburn's self-image? On her relationship with her sexual partner?
6. *Priority decision:* Based on the assessment data presented, what are the priority nursing diagnoses? Are there any collaborative problems?
7. *Evidence-informed practice:* Ms. Raeburn asks if she should use the spermicide nonoxynol-9 (N-9) to protect herself against STIs. How should the nurse advise her?

ⓔvolve

Answers are available at *http://evolve.elsevier.com/Canada/Lewis/medsurg*.

REVIEW QUESTIONS

The number of the question corresponds to the same-numbered objective at the beginning of the chapter.

1. Using which of the following methods will a woman have the lowest risk for sexually transmitted pelvic inflammatory disease?
   a. Oral contraceptives
   b. Barrier methods of contraception
   c. An intrauterine device for contraception
   d. A Norplant implant or injectable Depo-Provera for contraception

2. The nurse is obtaining subjective assessment data from a woman reported as a sexual contact of a man with chlamydial infection. The nurse understands which of the following about symptoms of chlamydial infection in women?
   a. They are frequently absent.
   b. They are similar to those of genital herpes.
   c. They include a macular palmar rash in later stages.
   d. They may involve chancres hidden inside the vagina.

3. In which way(s) does a primary HSV infection differ from recurrent HSV episodes? *(Select all that apply)*
   a. Symptoms are less severe during recurrent episodes.
   b. Only primary infections are sexually transmissible.
   c. Systemic manifestations such as fever and myalgia are more common in primary infection.
   d. Transmission of the virus to a fetus is less likely during primary infection.
   e. Lesions from recurrent HSV are more likely to transmit the virus than lesions from primary HSV.

4. Why should the nurse explain to a client with gonorrhea that treatment will include both ceftriaxone and doxycycline?
   a. Most clients need both drugs to eradicate the organism.
   b. Coverage with more than one antibiotic will prevent reinfection.
   c. No single agent successfully eradicates both primary and recurrent infections.
   d. The high rate of coexisting chlamydial infection and gonorrhea indicates coverage with both drugs.

5. In assessing clients for STIs, the nurse needs to know that many STIs can be asymptomatic. Which of the following STIs can be asymptomatic? *(Select all that apply)*
   a. Syphilis
   b. Gonorrhea
   c. Genital warts

   d. Genital herpes
   e. Chlamydial infection

6. To prevent infection and the transmission of STIs, the nurse's teaching plan would include an explanation of which of the following?
   a. The appropriate use of oral contraceptives
   b. Sexual positions that can be used to avoid infection
   c. The necessity of annual Pap smears for clients with HPV
   d. Sexual practices that are considered high-risk behaviours

7. Which of the following is an appropriate nursing intervention to provide emotional support to a client with an STI?
   a. Offering information on how safe sexual practices can prevent STIs
   b. Showing concern when listening to the client who expresses negative feelings
   c. Reassuring the client that the disease is highly curable with appropriate treatment
   d. Helping the client who received an STI from his or her sexual partner in forgiving the partner

1. b; 2. a; 3. a, c; 4. d; 5. a, b, c, d; 6. d, e; 7. b.

⊝volve

For even more review questions, visit *http://evolve.elsevier.com/Canada/ Lewis/medsurg.*

REFERENCES

Barnabas, R., Baeten, J., Lingappa, J., et al. (2015). Acyclovir prophylaxis reduces the incidence of herpes zoster among HIV-infected individuals: Results of a randomized clinical trial. *The Journal of Infectious Diseases, 212*(11), 1–5. doi:10.1093/infdis/jiv318.

Bell, M., Schmidt-Grimminger, D., Jacobsen, C., et al. (2011). Risk factors for HPV infection among American Indian and white women in the Northern Plains. *Gynecologic Oncology, 121*(3), 532–536. doi:10.1016/j.ygyno.2011.02.032.

Bender, N., Hermann, B., Anderson, B., et al. (2011). *Chlamydia* infection, pelvic inflammatory disease, ectopic pregnancy and infertility: A cross national study. *Sexually Transmitted Infections, 87*(7), 601–608. doi:10.1136/sextrans-2011-050205.

Borhart, J., & Birnbaumer, D. (2011). Emergency department management of sexually transmitted infections. *Emergency Medicine Clinics of North America, 29*(3), 587–603. doi:10.1016/j.emc.2011.04.008.

Carvalho, F., Goncalves, T., Faria, E., et al. (2011). Behavioural interventions to promote condom use among women living with HIV. *The Cochrane Database of Systematic Reviews,* (9), CD007844, doi:10.1002/14651858.CD007844.pub2.

Centers for Disease Control and Prevention (CDC). (2015). *Genital herpes: CDC fact sheet.* Retrieved from *http://www.cdc.gov/std/ herpes/stdfact-herpes.htm.*

Champion, J., & Collins, J. (2012). Reducing STIs: Screening, treatment, and counseling. *The Nurse Practitioner, 37*(4), 40–46. doi:10.1097/01.NPR.0000412894.04686.d0.

Da Silva Carneiro, S. C., Pirmez, R., de Hollanda, T. R., et al. (2013). Syphilis mimicking other dermatological diseases: Reactive arthritis and Mucha-Habermann disease. *Case Reports in Dermatology, 5*(1), 15–20. doi.org/10.1159/000346745.

Davis, K., Jacques-Tiura, A., Stappenbeck, C., et al. (2015). Men's condom use resistance: Alcohol effects on theory of planned behaviour constructs. *Health Psychology, 35*(2), 178–186. doi:10.1037/hea0000269.

Government of Canada. (2013). *Chlamydia.* Ottawa, ON: Author. Retrieved from *http://healthycanadians.gc.ca/diseases-conditions -maladies-affections/disease-maladie/chlamyd-eng.php?_ga =1.159094714.1853370565.1458502526.*

Hawkes, S., Matin, N., Broutet, N., et al. (2011). Effectiveness of interventions to improve screening for syphilis in pregnancy: A systematic review and meta-analysis. *The Lancet Infectious Diseases, 11*(9), 684–691. doi:10.1016/S1473-3099(11)70104-9.

Huo, W., Di, Z.-H., Xiao, B.-H., et al. (2014). Clearance of genital warts in pregnant women by mild local hyperthermia: A pilot report. *Dermatologic Therapy, 27*(2), 109–112. doi:10.1111/dth.12066.

Jeffers, L., & DiBartolo, M. (2011). Raising health care provider awareness of sexually transmitted disease in patients over age 50. *Medsurg Nursing, 20*(6), 285–289.

Johnston, C., Koelle, D. M., & Wald, A. (2011). HSV-2: In pursuit of a vaccine. *Journal of Clinical Investigation, 121*(12), 4600–4609. doi:10.1172/JCI57148.

Lin, L., Zheng, W., Tong, M., et al. (2011). Further evaluation of the characteristics of *Treponema pallidum*–specific IgM antibody in syphilis serofast reaction patients. *Diagnostic Microbiology and Infectious Disease, 71*(3), 201–207. doi:10.1016/j.diagmicrobio .2011.07.005.

Mehrabian, S., Raycheva, M., Traykova, M., et al. (2012). Neurosyphilis with dementia and bilateral hippocampal atrophy on brain magnetic resonance imaging. *BMC Neurology, 12,* 96. doi:10.1186/1471-2377-12-96.

Newman, L., Kamb, M., Hawkes, S., et al. (2013). Global estimates of syphilis in pregnancy and associated adverse outcomes: Analysis of multinational antenatal surveillance data. *PLoS Medicine, 10*(2), e1001396. doi:10.1371/journal.pmed.1001396.

Nigam, A., & Mishra, A. (2011). Condyloma acuminatum: Atypical presentation during pregnancy. *International Journal of STD & AIDS, 22*(9), 534–535. doi:10.1258/ijsa.2009.009114.

Obiero, J., Mwethera, P. G., & Wiysonge, C. S. (2012). Topical microbicides for prevention of sexually transmitted infections. *The Cochrane Database of Systematic Reviews*, No. 6, Article CD007961.

Perry, S. E., Hockenberry, M. J., Lowdermilk, D. L., et al. (2017). *Maternal child nursing care in Canada*. Toronto: Mosby Canada.

Public Health Agency of Canada. (2012). *Report on sexually transmitted infections in Canada: 2012*. Retrieved from *http:// www.phac-aspc.gc.ca/sti-its-surv-epi/rep-rap-2012/sum-som-eng .php#tblSum*.

Public Health Agency of Canada. (2013a). *Canadian guidelines on sexually transmitted infections* (Updated 2016 Edition). Ottawa: Author. Retrieved from *http://www.phac-aspc.gc.ca/std-mts/sti-its/ index-eng.php*.

Public Health Agency of Canada. (2013b). *The chief public health officer's report on the state of public health in Canada, 2013— Infectious disease—The never-ending threat*. Ottawa, ON: Author. Retrieved from *http://www.phac-aspc.gc.ca/cphorsphc-respcacsp/ 2013/sti-its-eng.php*.

Public Health Agency of Canada. (2013c). *Canadian immunization guide*. Ottawa, ON: Author. Retrieved from *http://www.phac-aspc .gc.ca/publicat/cig-gci/index-eng.php*.

Public Health Agency of Canada. (2014). *Canadian guidelines on sexually transmitted infections. HPV infections: Revised October 2014*. Ottawa: Author. Retrieved from *http://www.phac-aspc.gc.ca/ std-mts/sti-its/cgsti-ldcits/section-5-5-eng.php*.

Ripley, V. (2011). Promoting sexual health in women who have sex with women. *Nursing Standard, 25*(51), 41–46. doi: *http:// dx.doi.org/10.7748/ns2011.08.25.51.41.c8660*.

Roett, M., Mayor, M., & Uduhiri, K. (2012). Diagnosis and management of genital ulcers. *American Family Physician, 85*(3), 254–262.

Statistics Canada. (2015). *Canadian community health survey: Combined data, 2013/2014*. Ottawa, ON: Author. Retrieved from *http://www.statcan.gc.ca/daily-quotidien/150624/dq150624b -eng.htm*.

Stephenson-Famy, A., & Gardella, C. (2014). Herpes simplex virus infection during pregnancy. *Obstetrics and Gynecology Clinics of North America, 41*(4), 601–614. doi:10.1016/j.ogc.2014.08.006.

Su, C., & McKay, B. (2012). Treatment of HSV infection in late pregnancy. *American Family Physician, 85*(4), 390–393.

RESOURCES

Action Canada for Sexual Health & Rights
http://www.sexualhealthandrights.ca/

CATIE: Canada's Source for HIV and Hepatitis C Information
http://www.catie.ca/en/home

Health Canada: Sexually Transmitted Infections
http://www.hc-sc.gc.ca/hc-ps/dc-ma/sti-its-eng.php

International Herpes Resource Center
http://www.herpesresourcecenter.com/

Phoenix Association—Toronto Help
http://www.torontoherpes.com/

Public Health Agency of Canada
Sexual Health Promotion/Education: FAQs on Emergency Contraception
http://www.phac-aspc.gc.ca/std-mts/ec_cu-eng.php
Sexual Health and Sexually Transmitted Infections
http://www.phac-aspc.gc.ca/std-mts
Canadian Guidelines for Sexual Health Education
http://www.phac-aspc.gc.ca/publicat/cgshe-ldnemss/index-eng.php

Sex Information and Education Council of Canada
http://www.sieccan.org

SexualityandU.ca
http://www.sexualityandu.ca/

Teaching Sexual Health
http://www.teachingsexualhealth.ca/

For additional Internet resources, see the website for this book at *http://evolve.elsevier.com/Canada/Lewis/medsurg*.

Nursing Management

Female Reproductive Problems

Written by: Amy McKeever and Kim K. Choma
Adapted by: Maureen A. Barry

evolve WEBSITE

http://evolve.elsevier.com/Canada/Lewis/Canada/medsurg

- Review Questions (Online Only)
- Key Points
- Answer Guidelines for Case Study
- Student Case Study
- Endometrial Cancer and Blood Transfusion
- Customizable Nursing Care Plan
- Abdominal Hysterectomy
- Conceptual Care Map Creator
- Audio Glossary
- Content Updates

LEARNING OBJECTIVES

1. Summarize the etiologies of infertility and the strategies for diagnosis and treatment of women who are infertile.
2. Describe the etiology, clinical manifestations, and nursing and collaborative management of menstrual problems and abnormal vaginal bleeding.
3. Identify the risk factors, clinical manifestations, and collaborative care of ectopic pregnancy.
4. Discuss the changes related to menopause and the nursing and collaborative management of patients with menopausal symptoms.
5. Differentiate among the common problems that affect the vulva, vagina, and cervix and related nursing and collaborative management.
6. Describe the assessment, collaborative care, and nursing management of women with pelvic inflammatory disease and endometriosis.
7. Explain the clinical manifestations, diagnostic studies, collaborative care, and surgical therapy for cervical, endometrial, ovarian, and vulvar cancers.
8. Summarize the preoperative and the postoperative nursing management for the patient requiring surgery of the female reproductive system.
9. Differentiate among the common problems that occur with cystoceles, rectoceles, and fistulas and the related nursing and collaborative management.

KEY TERMS

abortion, p. 1392
amenorrhea, p. 1395
cystocele, p. 1415
dysmenorrhea, p. 1394
ectopic pregnancy, p. 1397
endometriosis, p. 1404

hysterectomy, p. 1396
infertility, p. 1390
leiomyomas, p. 1405
menopause, p. 1398
pelvic inflammatory disease (PID), p. 1402
perimenopause, p. 1397

postmenopause, p. 1398
premenstrual syndrome (PMS), p. 1393
rectocele, p. 1415
uterine prolapse, p. 1415

INFERTILITY

Infertility is the inability to achieve a pregnancy after at least 1 year of regular unprotected intercourse (Sabanegh & Agarwal, 2011). Current evidence indicates that approximately 16% of couples (one in six) in Canada experience infertility (Government of Canada, 2013). Assessment and therapy measures can be invasive, expensive, and lengthy. Understandably, infertility can be both a physical and emotional crisis.

Etiology and Pathophysiology

Infertility may be caused by either female, male, or combined factors. (Conditions that cause male infertility are discussed

in Chapter 57.) In some cases, the cause of infertility may not be identified.

The factors usually causing female infertility include problems with ovulation (anovulation or inadequate corpus luteum), tubal obstruction or dysfunction (endometriosis or damage from pelvic infection), and uterine or cervical factors (fibroid tumours or structural anomalies). Risk factors for infertility include tobacco and illicit drug use and being obese or thin. In women, the risk for infertility starts at about age 30 and increases after age 40 (Schmidt, Sobotka, Bentzen, et al., 2012).

Diagnostic Studies

A detailed history and general physical examination of the woman and her partner provide the basis for selecting diagnostic

TABLE 56-1   COLLABORATIVE CARE

Infertility

Diagnostic
- History and physical examination of both partners, including psychosocial functioning
- Assessment of possible sexually transmitted infections
- Genetic screening
- Hormone levels
  - Serum hormone levels (e.g., FSH, LH, prolactin)
  - Urinary LH
- Ovulatory study
- Pap test
- Pelvic ultrasonography
- Postcoital test
  - Cervical mucus
  - Semen analysis
  - Sperm penetration assay
- Review of menstrual and gynecological history
- Tubal patency study
  - Hystero-salpingogram

Collaborative Therapy
- Assisted reproductive technologies (ARTs)
- Drug therapy (see Table 56-2)
- Hormone supplement therapy
- Intrauterine insemination

FSH, follicle-stimulating hormone; *LH,* luteinizing hormone.

FIGURE 56-1 Basal body temperature chart. **A,** Typical biphasic temperature curve indicative of ovulation and normal progesterone effect. **B,** Irregular monophasic curve characteristic of anovulatory cycles. **C,** Ovulatory curve with sustained temperature elevation following conception and the first missed period.

studies (Table 56-1). The possibility of medical, genetic, or gynecological diseases is explored before tests are performed to determine problems affecting general health as well as fertility. These tests include hormonal levels, ovulatory studies, tubal patency studies, and postcoital studies. Other screening tests for infertility include semen analysis and pelvic ultrasound.

Ovulatory Studies. A basal body temperature record is kept to determine whether there is regular ovulation (Figure 56-1). The woman is instructed to take and graph her temperature, referred to as *basal body temperature,* on awakening, before any activity. As ovulation approaches, the production of estrogen increases, which may cause a drop in temperature. When ovulation occurs, progesterone is produced, causing a rise in temperature. Thus a temperature graph helps detect ovulation and suggests the timing of intercourse if pregnancy is desired. Ovulation prediction kits are now available for use by women at home. Other tests for ovulation include cervical and vaginal smears, endometrial biopsy, and plasma progesterone levels.

Tubal Patency Studies. Tubal factors (occlusion or deformity) are assessed most commonly by means of hystero-salpingogram. This procedure consists of the radiographic visualization of the uterus and tubes by injecting a radiopaque dye through the cervix. Tubal patency, shape, and position and any distortions of the endometrial cavity can be determined. Laparoscopy may be used when a hystero-salpingogram is contraindicated or other pathological pelvic conditions appear likely.

Postcoital Studies. A postcoital test can determine whether the cervical environment is favourable for the sperm. The couple is asked to have intercourse about the time ovulation is expected and 2 to 12 hours before the office visit. Douching or bathing should be avoided before the test. The cervical and vaginal secretions are aspirated and examined for the number and the motility of sperm present.

NURSING AND COLLABORATIVE MANAGEMENT INFERTILITY

The management of infertility problems depends on the cause. If infertility is secondary to an alteration in ovarian function, supplemental hormone therapy to restore and maintain ovulation may be attempted. Drug therapy used to treat infertility is presented in Table 56-2. Chronic cervicitis and inadequate estrogenic stimulation are cervical factors causing infertility. Antibiotic therapy is indicated for cervicitis. Inadequate estrogenic stimulation is treated using estrogen.

When a couple has not succeeded in conceiving during infertility management, an option is intrauterine insemination (IUI) with sperm from the partner or a donor. If this technique does not succeed, assisted reproductive technologies (ARTs) may be used. ARTs include in vitro fertilization (IVF), gamete intrafallopian transfer (GIFT), zygote intrafallopian transfer (ZIFT), donor gametes, and embryo cryopreservation. IVF is the removal of mature oocytes from the woman's ovarian follicle via laparoscopy, followed by IVF of the ova with the partner's or donor's sperm. When fertilization and cleavage have occurred, the resulting embryos are transferred into the woman's uterus. The procedure requires 2 to 3 days to complete and is used in cases of fallopian tube obstruction, diminished sperm count, and unexplained infertility. Frequently, multiple attempts are needed for successful implantation. IVF is costly and emotionally stressful (Nachtigall, MacDougall, Davis, et al., 2012).

Nurses can assist women experiencing infertility by providing information about the physiology of reproduction and infertility evaluation and addressing the psychological and social distress that can accompany infertility. There is some evidence that psychological stress can have a negative effect on fertility, especially during the time of ovulation (Akhter, Marcus, Kerber, et al., 2016).

TABLE 56-2   DRUG THERAPY

Infertility

Drug	Mechanism of Action
Menotropin (Human Menopausal Gonadotropin)	
Repronex	Product made of equal amounts of FSH and LH that promotes the development and maturation of follicles in the ovaries.
Follicle-Stimulating Hormone Agonists	
Follitropin alpha (Gonal-F & Gonal-F pen)	Stimulate follicle growth and maturation by mimicking the actions of the body's natural FSH.
GnRH Antagonists	
Cetrorelix (Cetrotide) Ganirelix (Orgalutran)	Prevent premature LH surges and premature ovulation in women undergoing ovarian stimulation.
GnRH Agonists	
Leuprolide (Lupron, Eligard) Nafarelin (Synarel)	Suppress release of LH and FSH with continuous use. May also be used in the treatment of endometriosis.
Human chorionic gonadotropin hCG (Pregnyl)	Induce ovulation by stimulating the release of eggs from follicles.

FSH, follicle-stimulating hormone; *GnRH*, gonadotropin-releasing hormone; *hCG*, human chorionic gonadotropin; *LH*, luteinizing hormone.

The nurse has a major responsibility for teaching and providing emotional support throughout infertility testing and treatment. Feelings of anger, frustration, grief, and helplessness may heighten as additional diagnostic tests are performed. Infertility can generate great tension in a marriage as the couple exhausts financial and emotional resources. Few insurance carriers cover the high cost of infertility testing and treatment. Couples should be encouraged to participate in a support group for infertile couples as well as individual therapy.

ABORTION

An **abortion** is the loss or termination of a pregnancy before the fetus has developed to a state of viability. Abortions are classified as *spontaneous* (those occurring naturally) or *induced* (those occurring as a result of mechanical or medical intervention). *Miscarriage* is the common term for the unintended loss of a pregnancy or spontaneous abortion.

Spontaneous Abortion

Spontaneous abortion is the natural loss of pregnancy before 20 weeks of gestation. Fetal chromosomal anomalies may account for many miscarriages before 8 weeks of gestation. Other causes of spontaneous abortions include endocrine abnormalities, maternal infection, acquired anatomical abnormalities (e.g., uterine fibroids, endometriosis), immunological factors, and environmental factors. About 10% to 15% of all clinically recognized pregnancies end as a result of spontaneous abortion (Davidson, London, & Ladewig, 2014).

Uterine cramping coupled with vaginal bleeding often indicates a spontaneous abortion. Cramping is usually absent if the vaginal bleeding is caused by other conditions, such as polyps. Serial measurements of serum β-human chorionic gonadotropin (β-hCG) hormone and vaginal ultrasonography examination of the pelvis are the most reliable indicators of viability of the pregnancy.

Treatment to prevent a possible spontaneous abortion is limited. Although bed rest and avoiding vaginal intercourse are often recommended, there is no evidence that these measures improve the outcome. The woman is advised to report any bleeding to her health care provider. Most women proceed to abortion regardless of treatment. If the products of conception do not pass completely or bleeding becomes excessive, a *dilation and curettage* (D & C) procedure is generally performed (Williams & Pridjian, 2011). The D & C involves dilating the uterine cervix and scraping the endometrium of the uterus to empty the contents of the uterus.

Women who are experiencing bleeding and cramping during pregnancy may be admitted to the hospital. Vital signs and estimated blood loss are monitored. Arranging for someone to stay with the patient provides important emotional support. The nurse should be aware of the grieving process that results from pregnancy loss.

Induced Abortion

Induced abortion is an intentional or elective termination of a pregnancy. Induced abortion is done for personal reasons (at the request of the woman) or for medical reasons. The number of induced abortions performed in Canada in 2014 was approximately 81 897 (Canadian Institute for Health Information [CIHI], 2014). Induced abortions continue to be most common among women in their early 20s (Sabourin & Burnett, 2012).

Several techniques are used to induce abortion, including menstrual evacuation, suction curettage, dilation and evacuation (D & E), and drug therapy. Deciding which technique to use to terminate a pregnancy depends on the gestational age (length of the pregnancy) and the woman's condition and preference. Suction curettage may be performed up to 14 weeks of gestation and accounts for more than 90% of abortion procedure. D & E is conducted in the second semester. Table 56-3 lists current methods for induced abortion available in Canada.

Drug therapy is another method to induce abortion (medical abortion) early in pregnancy. These agents must be given within the first 49 days of pregnancy (day 1 being the first day of the last menstrual period).

Once the decision is made to have an abortion, the woman and her significant others need support and acceptance. The patient should be prepared for what to expect both emotionally and physically. For some women, grief and sadness can be normal emotions after an abortion. The patient needs to understand the procedure, including instructions prior to the procedure as well as afterwards. The nurse's caring, nonjudgemental attitude can be a positive factor in the patient's experience.

Follow-up care includes instructions on signs and symptoms of possible complications, including abnormal vaginal bleeding, severe abdominal cramping, fever, and foul drainage. The need to avoid intercourse, tampons, and douching until re-examination in 2 weeks should be stressed. Contraception can be started the day of the procedure or during the patient's return visit, in accordance with her needs and desires.

PROBLEMS RELATED TO MENSTRUATION

The normal menstrual cycle is discussed in Chapter 53. The hormonal influences related to the menstrual cycle are shown

TABLE 56-3   METHODS FOR INDUCING ABORTION

Method	Length of Pregnancy	Description
Early Abortion		
Methotrexate with misoprostol	≤7 wk	Methotrexate is administered intramuscularly. Misoprostol is given intravaginally, 5–7 days later.
Menstrual extraction	Usually up to 2nd wk after first missed period	Catheter is inserted through cervix into uterus, and suction is applied. Endometrium and contents of uterus aspirated.
Suction aspiration (curettage)	≤14 wk	Cervix is usually dilated, uterine aspirator is introduced, and suction is applied, removing endometrial tissue and implanted pregnancy.
Dilation and evacuation (D & E)	10–16 wk (approximate)	Cervix is dilated, and products of conception are removed by vacuum cannula and use of other instruments as needed.
Late Abortion		
After 20 weeks, late abortion is available in Canada only under special circumstances, such as risk to the health of the mother or serious fetal abnormalities.		

ETHICAL DILEMMAS

Abortion

Situation

A recently married, 39-year-old woman is informed that the results of her amniocentesis indicate that her fetus has major chromosomal abnormalities and is expected to have severe physical and intellectual disabilities. The patient has no children, but her husband has three children from a previous marriage. She asks the nurse what she should do. How would the nurse respond?

Important Points for Consideration

- Decisions about whether to continue a pregnancy with a child who has severe disabilities are extremely personal and emotional. The woman and her husband will need support and information to explore their options and their values.
- Pregnancy counselling is warranted about the woman's choices, her feelings about the pregnancy, her desire to have a child with her husband, her concerns about raising a child with severe disabilities, her feelings about abortion, and concerns about possible future pregnancies.
- Patient autonomy ensures that a woman decide for herself whether or not to continue a pregnancy.
- Abortion is legal in Canada. Canada is one of a small number of countries without a law restricting abortion. Abortion is governed by provincial or territorial and medical regulations and treated like any other medical procedure. In the first trimester, abortion is a private matter between a woman and her physician. An abortion can be obtained in a clinic or hospital in many, but not all, provinces and territories.
- The role of the health care provider in these difficult situations is to provide education and support in order to facilitate a decision consistent with the patient's values.
- Nurses are bound by core nursing values and ethical responsibilities such as providing safe, compassionate, competent, and ethical care; promoting health and well-being; promoting and respecting informed decision making; honouring dignity; maintaining privacy and confidentiality; promoting justice; and being accountable (Canadian Nurses Association, 2017).

Clinical Decision-Making Questions

1. How would the nurse's feelings about abortion affect her or his ability to care for this patient?
2. What type of counselling and genetic testing are available to the patient regarding genetic abnormalities?

duration, amount, and character of the menstrual flow (see Table 53-2).

PREMENSTRUAL SYNDROME

Premenstrual syndrome (PMS) is a symptom complex related to the luteal phase of the menstrual cycle that resolves with menstruation (Davidson et al., 2014). The symptoms can be severe enough to impair interpersonal relationships or interfere with usual activities. Because many symptoms are associated with PMS, it is difficult to concisely define. However, PMS symptoms always occur cyclically, during the luteal phase before the onset of menstruation, and are not present at other times of the month. About 40% of all women have been significantly affected by PMS during their lifetime (Lentz, 2013).

Etiology and Pathophysiology

The etiology and pathophysiology of PMS are not well understood. It may have a biological trigger with compounding psychosocial factors. Neurotransmitters, such as serotonin, could also be involved. Some women may have a genetic predisposition to PMS. Other proposed causes include hormone imbalance and nutritional deficiencies. It occurs in 20% to 30% of women who are premenopausal. *Premenstrual dysphoric disorder* (PMDD) is the term applied to a type of PMS that affects 3% to 8% of women who are premenopausal (Biggs & Demuth, 2011). Women with PMDD have a severe mood disorder (marked depression and anxiety) in addition to PMS (National Library of Medicine, 2015).

Clinical Manifestations

PMS is extremely variable in its clinical manifestations between women and, for an individual woman, from one cycle to another. Common physical symptoms include breast discomfort, peripheral edema, abdominal bloating, sensation of weight gain, episodes of binge eating, and migraine headache. Abdominal bloating and breast swelling are caused by fluid shifts because total body weight does not generally change. Anxiety, depression, irritability, and mood swings are some of the emotional symptoms that women may experience.

Diagnostic Studies and Collaborative Care

PMS can be diagnosed only when other possible causes for the symptoms have been ruled out. A focused health history and physical examination are done to identify any underlying conditions, such as thyroid dysfunction, uterine fibroids, or depression, that may account for the symptoms. No definitive

in Figure 53-9. Menstruation may be irregular during the first few years after menarche and the years preceding menopause. Once established, a woman's menstrual cycles usually have a predictable pattern. However, considerable normal variation exists among women in cycle length as well as in the

---

TABLE 56-4   COLLABORATIVE CARE

Premenstrual Syndrome (PMS)

Diagnostic
- History and physical examination
- Symptom diary

Collaborative Therapy
- Aerobic exercise
- Drug therapy
  - Combined oral contraceptives
  - Diuretics
  - Prostaglandin inhibitors (e.g., ibuprofen [Advil])
  - Selective serotonin reuptake inhibitors (e.g., sertraline [Zoloft])
- Nutritional therapy
- Stress management and relaxation therapy

---

diagnostic test is available for PMS. When PMS or PMDD is a possible diagnosis, a woman is given a symptom diary to record her symptoms prospectively for two or three menstrual cycles. Diagnosis is based on an evaluation of the woman's symptoms.

Nonpharmacological and pharmacological strategies can relieve some PMS symptoms (Table 56-4). However, no single treatment is available. The goal of treatment is to reduce the severity of symptoms and enhance the woman's sense of control and quality of life.

Several conservative approaches to managing the symptoms are considered helpful, including stress management, diet changes, exercise, education, and counselling. Techniques for stress reduction include yoga, meditation, imagery, and biofeedback (see Chapter 12). To decrease autonomic nervous system arousal, women should avoid caffeine, reduce dietary intake of refined carbohydrates, exercise on a regular basis, and practise relaxation techniques. Eating complex carbohydrates with high fibre, foods rich in vitamin B_6, and sources of tryptophan (dairy and poultry) is thought to promote serotonin production, which improves the symptoms. Vitamin B_6 may be found in such foods as pork, milk, egg yolk, and legumes.

Exercise results in a release of endorphins, leading to mood elevation. Aerobic exercise can also have a relaxing effect. Because fatigue tends to exaggerate the symptoms of PMS, adequate rest in the premenstrual period is a priority.

Explanations about PMS help the woman understand the complexity of the disorder and ways that she can regain a better sense of control. The patient needs to be assured that her symptoms are real, PMS exists, and she is not imagining the problem. Acknowledgement of having PMS can itself be therapeutic. Teaching the woman's partner about the nature of PMS assists the partner to better understand the disorder and its effects.

Drug Therapy. Drug therapy is considered when symptoms persist or interfere with daily functioning. At present, no single drug can treat all the symptoms associated with PMS. One therapy may be tried for a time, and if no improvement is observed, another approach is tried. Many treatments are symptom specific. For fluid retention, diuretics such as spironolactone (Aldactone) are used. For reducing cramps, backache, and headache, prostaglandin inhibitors such as ibuprofen (Advil) are used. To improve negative mood, vitamin B_6 supplementation (50 mg daily) may be used. Calcium and magnesium supplementation may also be effective in alleviating psychological and physiological symptoms. For anxiety, buspirone taken during the luteal phase has helped some women. Women with PMDD may benefit from

antidepressants, including fluoxetine HCl (Prozac) and tricyclic antidepressants (e.g., amitriptyline).

Other pharmacological treatments are directed at PMS in general. Selective serotonin reuptake inhibitors (SSRIs) (e.g., sertraline [Zoloft]) have provided significant relief to women with severe PMS. Other general treatments include oral contraceptives containing estrogen and progesterone. Evening primrose oil may help some women.

DRUG ALERT—Oral Contraceptives (Both Estrogen and Progesterone)
- May increase the risk for cervical, liver, and perhaps breast cancer
- May elevate blood pressure and cholesterol (related to estrogen)
- Increase risk for cardiac disease if patient is also smoking
- May have impaired effectiveness if used concurrently with certain antibiotics
- Are contraindicated in patients with migraine headaches and depression

DYSMENORRHEA

Dysmenorrhea is abdominal cramping pain or discomfort associated with menstrual flow. The degree of pain and discomfort varies with the individual. The two types of dysmenorrhea are primary (no pathology exists) and secondary (pelvic disease is the underlying cause) (Lentz, 2013). Dysmenorrhea is one of the most common gynecological problems, affecting approximately 50% of all women.

Etiology and Pathophysiology

Primary dysmenorrhea is not a disease. It is caused by an excess of prostaglandin $F_{2\alpha}$ ($PGF_{2\alpha}$), an increased sensitivity to it, or both. Stimulation of the endometrium by estrogen followed by progesterone results in a dramatic increase in prostaglandin production by the endometrium. With the onset of menses, degeneration of the endometrium releases prostaglandin. Locally, prostaglandins increase myometrial contractions and constriction of small endometrial blood vessels. This causes tissue ischemia and increased sensitization of the pain receptors, resulting in menstrual pain. Primary dysmenorrhea begins in the first few years after menarche, typically with the onset of regular ovulatory cycles.

Secondary dysmenorrhea is acquired usually after adolescence, occurring most commonly at 30 to 40 years of age. Common pelvic conditions that cause secondary dysmenorrhea include endometriosis, chronic pelvic inflammatory disease (PID), and uterine fibroids. Because secondary dysmenorrhea is caused by multiple conditions, symptoms vary. However, painful menses are present in all situations.

Clinical Manifestations

Primary dysmenorrhea starts 12 to 24 hours before the onset of menses. The pain is most severe the first day of menses and rarely lasts more than 2 days. Characteristic manifestations include lower abdominal pain that is colicky in nature, frequently radiating to the lower back and upper thighs. The abdominal pain is often accompanied by nausea, diarrhea, loose stools, fatigue, and headache.

Secondary dysmenorrhea occurs usually after the woman has experienced problem-free periods for some time. The pain may be unilateral and it is generally more constant and continues longer than in primary dysmenorrhea. Depending on the cause, symptoms such as *dyspareunia* (painful intercourse), painful defecation, or irregular bleeding may occur at times other than menstruation.

NURSING AND COLLABORATIVE MANAGEMENT DYSMENORRHEA

Evaluation begins with distinguishing primary from secondary dysmenorrhea. A complete health history with special attention to menstrual and gynecological history should be obtained. A pelvic examination is also performed. The probable diagnosis is primary dysmenorrhea if the history reveals an onset shortly after menarche, symptoms are associated only with menses, and the pelvic examination is normal. If any specific cause of dysmenorrhea is evident, the diagnosis is secondary dysmenorrhea.

Treatment for primary dysmenorrhea includes heat, exercise, and drug therapy. Heat is applied to the lower abdomen or back. Regular exercise is thought to be beneficial because it may reduce endometrial hyperplasia and subsequently reduce prostaglandin production. The primary drug therapy is nonsteroidal anti-inflammatory drugs (NSAIDs) such as naproxen (Naprosyn, Aleve), which has antiprostaglandin activity. NSAIDs should be started at the first sign of menses and continued every 4 to 8 hours to maintain a sufficient level of the drug to inhibit prostaglandin synthesis for the usual duration of discomfort.

Oral contraceptives may also be used. They decrease dysmenorrhea by reducing endometrial hyperplasia. Acupuncture and transcutaneous nerve stimulation may be used for women who have inadequate relief from medications or who prefer not to take medications. Patients who are unresponsive to these treatments should be evaluated for chronic pelvic pain (discussed later in this chapter).

Treatment of secondary dysmenorrhea depends on the cause. Some individuals with secondary dysmenorrhea will be helped by the approaches used for primary dysmenorrhea.

Women should be taught why dysmenorrhea occurs as well as how to treat it. Teaching and supportive therapy can provide women with a foundation for coping with this common occurrence and increase feelings of control and self-reliance.

Women often ask what can be done for minor discomforts associated with menstrual cycles. Women should be advised that, during acute pain, relief may be obtained by applying heat to the abdomen or the back and taking NSAIDs for analgesia. The nurse can also suggest noninvasive pain-relieving practices such as relaxed breathing and guided imagery.

Other health care measures to reduce the discomfort of dysmenorrhea include regular exercise and proper nutritional habits. Avoiding constipation, maintaining good body mechanics, and eliminating stress and fatigue, particularly during the time preceding menstrual periods, can also decrease discomfort. Staying active and interested in activities may also help.

ABNORMAL VAGINAL BLEEDING

Abnormal vaginal or uterine bleeding is a common gynecological concern. Irregularities include *oligomenorrhea* (long intervals between menses, generally longer than 35 days), amenorrhea (absence of menstruation), *menorrhagia* (excessive or prolonged menstrual bleeding), and *metrorrhagia* (irregular uterine bleeding or bleeding between menses). The cause of abnormal bleeding may vary from anovulatory menstrual cycles to more serious causes such as ectopic pregnancy or endometrial cancer.

TABLE 56-5	CAUSES OF AMENORRHEA	
Natural Amenorrhea		**Hormonal Imbalance**
• Breastfeeding		• Pituitary tumours
• Menopause		• Polycystic ovary syndrome
• Pregnancy		• Premature menopause
Medications		**Structural Problems**
• Antidepressants		• Damage to ovaries or uterus from radiation
• Antipsychotics		• Structural abnormalities of vagina
• Chemotherapy		• Uterine scarring
Lifestyle		
• Acute and chronic illness		
• Excessive exercise		
• Low body weight		
• Stress		

The woman's age provides direction for identifying the cause of bleeding. For example, a woman who is postmenopausal with abnormal bleeding must always be evaluated for endometrial cancer but does not need to be evaluated for possible pregnancy. For a 20-year-old woman with abnormal bleeding, the possibility of pregnancy must always be considered, and the possibility of endometrial cancer would be unlikely.

Abnormal bleeding may be caused by dysfunction of the hypothalamic-pituitary-ovarian axis, such as a pituitary adenoma. Another cause may be infection. Changes in lifestyle such as marriage, recent moves, a death in the family, financial stress, and other emotional crises can also cause irregular bleeding. Because psychological factors can influence endocrine function, they should be considered when the patient is evaluated.

Types of Irregular Bleeding

Oligomenorrhea and Amenorrhea. Once pregnancy has been ruled out, anovulation is the most common cause for missing menses. Additional causes of amenorrhea are listed in Table 56-5. *Primary amenorrhea* refers to the failure of menstrual cycles to begin by age 16 years or by age 14 years if secondary sex characteristics are present. *Secondary amenorrhea* refers to cessation of menstrual cycles once established. Women who are pregnant, breastfeeding, or in menopause are not considered to have secondary amenorrhea.

Ovulation is often erratic for several years following menarche and before menopause. Thus, oligomenorrhea owing to anovulation is common for women at the beginning and end of menstruation. In anovulatory cycles, the corpus luteum that produces progesterone does not form. This may result in a situation referred to as *unopposed estrogen*. When unopposed by progesterone, estrogen can cause excessive build-up of the endometrium. Persistent overgrowth of the endometrium increases a woman's risk for endometrial cancer. To reduce this risk, progesterone or oral contraceptives are prescribed to ensure that the patient's endometrial lining will be shed at least four to six times per year.

Menorrhagia. The excessive bleeding associated with menorrhagia can be characterized as an increased duration (>7 days), increased amount (>80 mL), or both. Menorrhagia is a common condition that affects 20% to 30% of all women in the reproductive age (Roa, 2011). Anovulatory uterine bleeding is the most common cause of menorrhagia. An unopposed estrogen state continues to build up the endometrium until it becomes unstable, resulting in menorrhagia. For young women with excessive bleeding, clotting disorders must be considered. Uterine fibroids (also called *leiomyomas*) and endometrial polyps are a common cause of menorrhagia for women in their 30s and 40s.

Metrorrhagia. Metrorrhagia, also referred to as spotting or breakthrough bleeding, is bleeding between menstrual periods. For all women of reproductive age, pregnancy complications such as spontaneous abortion or ectopic pregnancy must be considered as a possible cause. Other causes include cervical or endometrial polyps, infection, and carcinoma. Spotting is common during the first three cycles of oral contraceptives. If spotting continues beyond that, a different pill formulation can be prescribed once other causes of metrorrhagia have been ruled out. Spotting with long-acting progestin therapy (e.g., Mirena intrauterine device [IUD]) or progestin-only pills (Depo-Provera) is also common. For women who are postmenopausal, endometrial cancer must be considered whenever spotting is experienced. In women who are postmenopausal, exogenous estrogen administration during hormone therapy is a common cause of metrorrhagia.

Diagnostic Studies and Collaborative Care

Because abnormal vaginal bleeding has multiple causes, the diagnostic and collaborative care varies. A health history and physical examination directed at the most likely causes of vaginal bleeding for the woman's age group is the first step. These findings will provide the basis for selecting the necessary laboratory tests and diagnostic procedures. Treatment depends on the etiology of the problem (e.g., menorrhagia, amenorrhea), the degree of threat to the patient's health, and whether the patient wishes to preserve her fertility.

Combined oral contraceptives may be prescribed for a woman with amenorrhea to ensure regular shedding of endometrium if she also wants contraception. Tranexamic acid (Cyklokapron) may be used to treat heavy menstrual bleeding. This drug stabilizes a protein that helps blood to clot. Adverse effects may include headache, back pain, abdominal pain, muscle and joint pain, anemia, and fatigue. Women using hormonal contraception should take tranexamic acid only if there is a strong medical need, since there is an increased risk for blood clots and stroke. Estradiol valerate/dienogest (Natazia) may be given to women with heavy menstrual bleeding who desire an oral contraceptive to prevent pregnancy.

The treatment goal for women with menorrhagia is to minimize further blood loss. If menorrhagia is the result of anovulatory cycles, the endometrium must be stabilized by a combination of oral estrogen and progesterone.

Balloon thermotherapy is a technique for menorrhagia that involves the introduction of a soft, flexible balloon into the uterus. The balloon is inflated with sterile fluid (Figure 56-2). The fluid in the balloon is heated and maintained for 8 minutes, then causing ablation (removal) of the uterine lining. When the treatment is completed, the fluid is withdrawn from the balloon and the catheter is removed from the uterus. The uterine lining sloughs off in the following 7 to 10 days. Uterine balloon thermotherapy is contraindicated for women desiring to maintain their fertility and for women with any suspected uterine abnormalities such as fibroids, suspected endometrial cancer, prior Caesarean section, or myomectomy. With severe bleeding, hospitalization is indicated.

FIGURE 56-2 Balloon thermotherapy for treatment of menorrhagia. A balloon-tipped catheter is inserted into the uterus through the vagina and cervix. The balloon is inflated with a sterile fluid that expands to fit the size and shape of the uterus. The fluid is heated to 87°C and maintained for 8 minutes while the uterine lining is treated. The fluid is then withdrawn from the balloon and the catheter is removed. Source: Nucleus Medical Media Inc./Alamy Stock Photo.

All patients with menorrhagia should be evaluated for anemia and treated as indicated.

Surgical Therapy. Surgery may be indicated, depending on the underlying cause of the abnormal vaginal bleeding. D & C is used only in cases of acute excess bleeding or for older-adult women when endometrial biopsy and ultrasonography have not provided the necessary diagnostic information. Endometrial ablation for menorrhagia may be done by laser, thermal balloon, cryotherapy, or microwave energy for patients who do not want to maintain their fertility.

If menorrhagia is caused by uterine fibroids, a **hysterectomy** (surgical removal of the uterus) may be performed. A *myomectomy* (removal of fibroids without removal of the uterus) may be performed if the patient wants to preserve her uterus. The myomectomy is done via laparotomy, laparoscopy, or hysteroscopy. Hormonal regimens and embolization of blood vessels supplying the fibroids are other treatment options.

NURSING MANAGEMENT
ABNORMAL VAGINAL BLEEDING

Teaching women about the characteristics of the menstrual cycle will assist them to identify normal variations. Table 53-2 in Chapter 53 includes characteristics of the menstrual cycle and related patient teaching. This knowledge can diminish apprehension and dispel misconceptions about the menstrual cycle. If the patient's menstrual cycle pattern does not fall within the normal range, the nurse should urge her to visit her health care provider.

The selection of internal or external sanitary protection is a matter of personal preference. Tampons are convenient and make menstrual hygiene easier, whereas pads may provide better protection. Using a combination of tampons and pads and avoiding prolonged use of superabsorbent tampons may decrease the risk for *toxic shock syndrome* (TSS). TSS is an acute condition caused by a toxin from *Staphylococcus aureus*. Symptoms of TSS may initially include flulike symptoms such as high fever, nausea, vomiting, diarrhea, dizziness, fainting, and disorientation. Other symptoms may include low blood pressure, shock, dehydration,

Fetus

Fallopian tube

Uterus

FIGURE 56-3 Ectopic pregnancy occurring in the fallopian tube.

sore throat, muscle pain, peeling skin, and a sunburn-like rash (Government of Canada, 2015).

Whenever excessive, the amount of the patient's vaginal bleeding should be assessed as accurately as possible. The patient should record and report the number and size of pads or tampons used and the degree of saturation. The patient's fatigue level, along with variations in blood pressure and pulse, should be monitored because anemia and hypovolemia may be present. If a surgical procedure is indicated, the nurse should provide appropriate preoperative and postoperative care.

ECTOPIC PREGNANCY

An **ectopic pregnancy** is the implantation of the fertilized ovum anywhere outside the uterine cavity (Figure 56-3). Approximately 3% of all pregnancies are ectopic, and approximately 98% of these occur in the fallopian tube (McQueen, 2011). The remaining 2% to 3% may be ovarian, abdominal, or cervical (McQueen, 2011).

Ectopic pregnancy is a life-threatening condition. Earlier identification has contributed to decreased mortality rates.

Etiology and Pathophysiology

Any blockage of the fallopian tube or reduction of tubal peristalsis that impedes or delays the zygote passing to the uterine cavity can result in tubal implantation. After implantation, the growth of the gestational sac expands the tubal wall. Eventually, the tube ruptures, causing acute peritoneal symptoms. Less acute symptoms usually begin within 6 to 8 weeks after the last normal menstrual period and weeks before rupture would occur.

Risk factors for ectopic pregnancy include a history of PID, prior ectopic pregnancy, current progestin-releasing IUD, progestin-only birth control failure, and prior pelvic or tubal surgery. Additional risk factors for ectopic pregnancy include procedures used in infertility treatment, including in IVF, embryo transfer, and ovulation induction.

Clinical Manifestations

The classic manifestations of ectopic pregnancy are abdominal or pelvic pain, missed menses, and irregular vaginal bleeding. Other manifestations include morning sickness, breast tenderness, gastro-intestinal disturbance, malaise, and syncope. Pain is almost always present and is caused by distension of the fallopian tube. It may start unilaterally and then spread to become bilateral. The character of the pain varies among women and can be colicky or vague. If tubal rupture occurs, the pain is intense and may be referred to the shoulder as a result of irritation of the diaphragm

by blood released into the abdominal cavity. Symptom severity does not necessarily correlate with the extent of external (vaginal) bleeding present. With rupture, the risk for hemorrhage and hypovolemic shock is present. Suspected rupture is treated as an emergency.

The vaginal bleeding that may accompany ectopic pregnancy is usually described as spotting. However, it is also possible that bleeding may be heavier and can be confused with menses.

Diagnostic Studies

Ectopic pregnancy can be a diagnostic challenge because of its similarity to other pelvic and abdominal disorders, such as salpingitis, spontaneous abortion, ruptured ovarian cyst, appendicitis, and peritonitis. A serum (radioimmunoassay) pregnancy test should be performed. If the test is negative, an ectopic pregnancy is not likely. If ectopic pregnancy cannot be excluded by the pregnancy test, further evaluation is warranted. If the patient is in a stable condition, a combination of serial β-hCG and vaginal ultrasonography is used (Givens & Lipscomb, 2012).

Absence of a normal intrauterine pregnancy means that the diagnosis is probably spontaneous abortion or ectopic pregnancy. With a spontaneous abortion, serial β-hCG levels will decrease over time. A complete blood cell count is obtained when there is any concern regarding the amount of blood loss or if surgery is contemplated.

NURSING AND COLLABORATIVE MANAGEMENT ECTOPIC PREGNANCY

Surgery remains the primary approach for treating ectopic pregnancies and should be performed immediately. However, medical management with intramuscular injection of methotrexate is being used with increasing success and safety in patients who are hemodynamically stable and where the size of gestation is smaller than 3 cm (Sitka, 2012). A conservative surgical approach limits damage to the reproductive system as much as possible. Removal of the fetus from the tube is preferred to removing the tube. Laparoscopy is preferable to laparotomy because it decreases blood loss and the length of the hospital stay. If the tube ruptures, conservative surgical approaches may not be possible. The patient may need a blood transfusion and supplemental intravenous (IV) fluid therapy to relieve shock and restore a satisfactory blood volume for safe anaesthesia and surgery. The use of laparoscopy has resulted in fewer repeated ectopic pregnancies and a higher rate of future successful pregnancies.

Nursing care depends on the patient's condition. Before the diagnosis has been confirmed, the nurse should be alert to signs of increasing pain and vaginal bleeding, which may indicate that rupture of the tube has occurred. Vital signs are monitored closely, along with observation for signs of shock. Explanations and preparation for diagnostic procedures are given when appropriate. Preparation of the patient for abdominal surgery may follow rapidly. The patient's emotional status should be assessed. Reassurance and support for the surgery should be given to the patient and her family. Postoperatively, the patient may express a fear of future ectopic pregnancies and have many questions about the impact of this experience on her future fertility.

PERIMENOPAUSE AND POSTMENOPAUSE

Perimenopause is a normal life transition that begins with the first signs of change in menstrual cycles and ends after cessation of menses. Menopause is the physiological cessation of menses associated with declining ovarian function. It is made retrospectively after 1 year of *amenorrhea* (absence of menstruation). Menopause starts gradually and is usually associated with changes in menstruation, including menstrual flows that are increased, decreased, irregular, or some combination of these changes and ends with the cessation of menses. Postmenopause is a term that refers to the time in a woman's life after menopause.

The age at which menopause occurs ranges from 44 to 55 years, with the average being 51 years. Menopause may occur earlier as a result of illness; surgical removal of the uterus or both ovaries; or the adverse effects of radiation therapy, chemotherapy, or drugs. The age at which menopause occurs is not affected by age at menarche, physical characteristics, number of pregnancies, date of last pregnancy, or oral contraceptive use. However, genetic factors, autoimmune conditions, cigarette smoking, and racial or ethnic factors have been linked to earlier age at menopause.

Changes within the ovary start the cascade of events that finally result in menopause. The regression of the follicles within each ovary begins at puberty and accelerates after age 35. With age, fewer follicles remain that are responsive to follicle-stimulating hormone (FSH). FSH normally stimulates the dominant follicle to secrete estrogen. When the follicles can no longer respond to FSH, ovarian production of estrogen and progesterone declines. However, women who are perimenopausal can get pregnant until menopause has occurred, since many women have long anovulatory cycles interspersed with shorter, ovulatory cycles.

With decreased ovarian function, decreased levels of estrogen cause a gradual increase in FSH and luteinizing hormone (LH) as a result of the negative feedback process. By the time menopause occurs, there is a ten- to twenty-fold increase in FSH. The elevated FSH level may take several years to return to the premenopausal level. The reduced estrogen level also causes a decrease in the frequency of ovulation and results in changes in the reproductive organs and tissues (e.g., atrophy of vaginal tissue).

Clinical Manifestations

Clinical manifestations of perimenopause and postmenopause are presented in Table 56-6. Perimenopause is a time of erratic hormonal fluctuation. Irregular vaginal bleeding is common. With decreasing estrogen, hot flashes and other symptoms begin. The signs and symptoms of diminished estrogen are listed in Table 56-7. The loss of estrogen plays a significant role in the cause of age-related alterations. Changes most critical to a woman's well-being are the increased risks for coronary artery disease (CAD) and osteoporosis (secondary to bone density loss). Other

changes include a redistribution of fat, a tendency to gain weight more easily, muscle and joint pain, loss of skin elasticity, changes in hair amount and distribution, and atrophy of external genitalia and breast tissue.

Hallmarks of perimenopause include *vasomotor instability* (hot flashes) and irregular menses. A hot flash (occurs in up to 80% of all women) is described as a sudden sensation of intense heat along with perspiration and flushing (University of California–Berkeley, 2011). These sensations last from several seconds to 5 minutes and occur most often at night, thereby disturbing sleep. The cause of hot flashes, or vasomotor instability, is not clearly understood. It has been theorized that temperature regulators in the brain are in proximity to the area where gonadotropin-releasing hormone (GnRH) is released. The lowered estrogen levels are correlated with dilation of cutaneous blood vessels, resulting in hot flashes and increased sweating. The more sudden the withdrawal of estrogen (e.g., surgical removal of the ovaries), the more likely the symptoms will be severe if no hormone replacement is provided. Symptoms usually subside over time and typically last from 5 to 10 years with or without treatment (Roush, 2012). Hot flashes can be triggered by situations that affect body temperature, such as eating a hot meal, hot weather, drinking an alcoholic beverage, stress, or warm clothing. Women who smoke are at higher risk for hot flashes because smoking affects estrogen metabolism. In the United States, Black women report the highest incidence of hot flashes, whereas Asian women report the lowest number (Roush, 2012).

Atrophic vaginal changes secondary to decreased estrogen include thinning of the vaginal mucosa and disappearance of rugae. Vaginal secretions also decrease and become more alkaline. As a result of these changes, the vagina is easily traumatized and more susceptible to infection, including a higher risk for human immunodeficiency virus (HIV) infection if exposed. *Dyspareunia* (painful intercourse) may also occur. This can lead to unnecessary

---

TABLE 56-7	SIGNS AND SYMPTOMS OF ESTROGEN DEFICIENCY

Vasomotor
- Hot flashes
- Night sweats

Genito-Urinary
- Atrophic vaginitis
- Dyspareunia secondary to poor lubrication
- Incontinence

Psychological
- Change in sleep pattern
- Decreased REM sleep
- Emotional lability

Skeletal
- Increased fracture rate, especially of vertebral bodies but also of humerus, distal radius, and upper femur

Cardiovascular
- Decreased high-density lipoproteins (HDLs)
- Increased low-density lipoproteins (LDLs)

Dermatological
- Breast tissue changes
- Diminished collagen content of skin

REM, rapid eye movement.

TABLE 56-6	CLINICAL MANIFESTATIONS OF PERIMENOPAUSE AND POSTMENOPAUSE

Perimenopause	Postmenopause
• Atrophy of genito-urinary tissue with decreased support	• Atrophy of genito-urinary tissue (e.g., vaginal epithelium)
• Irregular menses	• Breast tenderness
• Mood changes	• Cessation of menses
• Occasional vasomotor symptoms	• Stress and urge incontinence
• Osteoporosis	• Vasomotor instability (hot flashes and night sweats)
• Stress and urge incontinence	

and premature cessation of sexual activity. Dryness is a problem that can be easily corrected with water-soluble lubricants or, if needed, with hormonal creams or systemic HT.

Atrophic changes in the lower urinary tract also occur with a decrease in estrogen. Bladder capacity decreases, and the bladder and urethral tissue lose tone. These changes can cause symptoms that mimic a bladder infection (e.g., dysuria, urgency, frequency) when no infection is present.

Whether decreasing estrogen is responsible for the psychological changes associated with perimenopause is unclear. Depression, irritability, and cognitive problems, which are often attributed to menopause, could result from life stressors or sleep deprivation from hot flashes. Depressive symptoms appear to improve when hormone levels stabilize.

Collaborative Care

The diagnosis of perimenopause should be made only after careful consideration of other possible causes for the woman's symptoms. Depression, thyroid dysfunction, anemia, or anxiety could be responsible for the same symptoms. An accurate history of menstrual patterns should be reviewed as part of establishing the diagnosis. Because of the hormonal fluctuations that occur before menopause, routine testing of the serum FSH level is not indicated.

Drug Therapy. Hormone therapy (HT) was once standard therapy in Canada for treating menopausal symptoms. HT includes estrogen for women without ovaries or estrogen and progesterone for women with a uterus. Findings from the Women's Health Initiative (WHI) clinical trials led to changes in this practice. (National Institutes of Health [NIH], 2015). The data showed that women who had taken estrogen plus progestin had an increased risk for breast cancer, stroke, heart disease, and emboli. However, these women had fewer hip fractures and a lower risk of developing colorectal cancer. Women who took only estrogen (Premarin) had an increased risk for stroke and emboli. However, these women had decreased risk for fractures with no increased risk for heart disease or breast or colorectal cancer. A recent systematic review has updated and validated the results of the WHI trials (Nelson, Walker, Zakher, et al., 2012).

If women wish to consider taking HT for the short-term treatment (less than 5 years) of menopausal symptoms, the risks and benefits of therapy (e.g., minimizes bone loss, hot flashes, vaginal atrophic changes) should be considered carefully. The woman and her health care provider should thoroughly discuss the decision to take HT. If a woman chooses to use HT, the lowest effective dose should be used for the shortest amount of time to manage menopausal symptoms (Stuenkel, Gass, Manson, et al., 2012). Estrogen-alone HT may decrease the risk for coronary heart disease and decrease mortality in women younger than 60 years and within 10 years of menopause (de Villiers, Gass, Haines, et al., 2013; Sood, Faubion, Kuhle, et al., 2014).

The adverse effects of estrogen include nausea, fluid retention, headache, and breast enlargement. Adverse effects of progesterone include increased appetite, weight gain, irritability, depression, spotting, and breast tenderness. A commonly used estrogen preparation is 0.625 mg of conjugated estrogen (Premarin) daily. For symptom relief, a higher dose may be needed. To receive the protective benefit of progesterone, 5 to 10 mg of medroxyprogesterone (Provera) is indicated for 12 days of each month on a cyclical regimen or 2.5 mg if on a continuous regimen. If the estrogen is to be increased for symptom relief, the progesterone should also be increased. Other forms of progesterone include

norethindrone-ethinyl estradiol (Brevicon, Synphasic) and micronized progesterone creams, dermal patches, gels, and lotions; rings placed around the cervix; and subcutaneous pellets. Vaginal creams are especially useful for urogenital symptoms (e.g., dryness). Transdermal estrogen (skin patch or spray) has the advantage of bypassing the liver but has the disadvantage of causing skin irritation.

> **DRUG ALERT—Medroxyprogesterone (Depo-Provera, Provera)**
> • Report immediately the development of sudden loss of vision, severe headache, chest pain, hemoptysis, pain in calves (especially with swelling, redness), numbness in arm or leg, and abdominal pain or tenderness.

SSRI antidepressants, including paroxetine (Paxil), fluoxetine (Prozac), and venlafaxine (Effexor XR), are an effective alternative to HT in reducing hot flashes. This effect is noted even if the user is not depressed. The mechanism of action is unknown. In randomized control trials (RCTs), gabapentin (Neurontin), an anticonvulsant drug, has also been shown to relieve hot flashes (Kaunitz & Manson, 2015).

Selective estrogen receptor modulators (SERMs), such as raloxifene (Evista), are also used in treating menopausal problems. These drugs have some of the positive benefits of estrogen, such as preventing bone loss, without the negative effects, such as endometrial hyperplasia. Raloxifene competes with estrogen for estrogen receptor sites (American Cancer Society, 2014). It decreases bone loss and serum cholesterol but has minimal effects on breast and uterine tissue.

Bisphosphonates, including alendronate (Fosamax) and risedronate (Actonel/Actonel DR), are also used to decrease the risk for osteoporosis in women who are postmenopausal. These drugs enhance bone mineral density by suppressing resorption. SERMs and bisphosphonates are discussed further in Chapter 66 with respect to their role in the management of osteoporosis.

Nonhormonal Therapy. Because of the risks associated with HT, many women try other therapies to relieve menopausal symptoms. Paroxetine (Paxil) is a newer nonhormonal treatment that may be used for moderate to severe hot flashes associated with menopause. This drug is an SSRI.

Hot flash frequency and severity can be reduced through measures that lead to a decrease in heat production and an increase in heat loss. Keeping a cool environment and limiting caffeine and alcohol intake lower heat production. Relaxation techniques (e.g., relaxation breathing, imagery) may also help. To promote heat loss at night when hot flashes can disrupt sleep, increase air circulation in the room and avoid bedding that traps the heat (e.g., heavy quilts). Loose-fitting clothes do not retain body heat, whereas clothes with tight necks and wrists do. Cool cloths applied to flushed areas also aid in heat loss.

Daily intake of vitamin E in doses up to 800 IU may also help reduce hot flashes in some women. Changing sleep patterns may be helped by avoiding alcohol and controlling hot flashes. Relaxation techniques can promote a better night's sleep by decreasing anxiety. A regular, moderate program (three to four times per week) of aerobic and weight-bearing exercises can slow the process of bone loss and a tendency toward weight gain.

Nutritional Therapy. Good nutrition can decrease the risk for cardiovascular disease and osteoporosis in addition to assisting with vasomotor symptoms. A daily intake of about 30 kcal/kg of body weight is recommended. A decrease in metabolic rate and careless eating habits can cause the weight gain and fatigue often attributed to menopause. An adequate intake of calcium and vitamin D helps maintain healthy bones and counteracts loss of bone density. Women who are postmenopausal and are not receiving supplemental estrogen should have a daily calcium intake of at least 1 500 mg, whereas those taking estrogen replacement need at least 1 000 mg/day. Calcium supplements are best absorbed when taken with meals. Either dietary calcium or calcium supplements may be used (see Chapter 66, Tables 66-12 and 66-13).

The diet should be high in complex carbohydrates and vitamin B complex, especially B6. Phytoestrogens (soy, tofu, chickpeas, sunflower seeds) may reduce menopausal symptoms. Herbal remedies, such as black cohosh, have become popular in treating menopausal symptoms (see the "Complementary & Alternative Therapies" box). Consultation with an experienced herbal practitioner is recommended before initiating therapy.

🌿 COMPLEMENTARY & ALTERNATIVE THERAPIES

Herbs and Supplements for Menopause*

Herb	Scientific Evidence	Nursing Implications
Black cohosh	Mixed evidence for use in the treatment of menopausal symptoms†	Generally well tolerated in recommended doses for ≤6 months to relieve symptoms such as hot flashes Should not be used in people with a liver disorder Should not be combined with birth control pills, hormone therapy, or tamoxifen or used by women who are allergic to acetylsalicylic acid (ASA; Aspirin)
Soy	Mixed evidence for treatment of menopausal symptoms‡	Soy isoflavone (rather than soy protein) has shown the most promise for treatment of hot flashes The long-term effects of a high soy diet have not been well-researched. High soy intake can't be considered safe until more studies are done. In some women, soy causes digestive upset.

*In general, the evidence for use of these herbs as treatments for menopause symptoms is limited by a lack of well-designed, controlled trials.
†HealthLinksBC. (2015). Black cohosh for menopause symptoms. Retrieved from *http://www.healthlinkbc.ca/healthtopics/content.asp?hwid=tn9522.*
‡HealthLinksBC. (2015). Soy for Menopause Symptoms. Retrieved from *http://www.healthlinkbc.ca/healthtopics/content.asp?hwid=tn9521.*

CULTURALLY COMPETENT CARE

MENOPAUSE

Although all women experience menopause, the perception of menopause varies by culture. Different ethnic groups have different traditions and beliefs regarding menopause, including the use of complementary and alternative therapies to manage symptoms (Im, Ko, Hwang, et al., 2012). In many cultures, menopause is considered a normal part of aging, and little emphasis is placed on the physical and emotional symptoms that accompany the loss of fertility. In cultures in which older adults are revered,

menopause is often seen as a liberating transition to a state of being a "wise woman."

North American culture is generally negative toward aging and places a high value on youth. Menopause is often considered a disorder that requires treatment. Menopausal symptoms may be viewed as troublesome, with a strong need to treat hot flashes and mood swings. Numerous substances, from HT to herbal preparations, are often used to treat menopausal symptoms.

Although menopause is experienced by all women, its meaning and symptoms vary. Menopause is a milestone in a woman's life that is embedded in her own personality and culture. Approaching women who are menopausal with this understanding is important to provide culturally competent care.

NURSING MANAGEMENT
PERIMENOPAUSE AND POSTMENOPAUSE

Nurses can play a key role in helping women to understand perimenopausal changes and options to minimize unwanted symptoms that are bothersome (see Table 56-7). Nurses can foster a positive image of perimenopause as a time of vitality and attractiveness. Perimenopause can provide women with a renewed incentive to enhance self-care and well-being. It is important to provide teaching and reassurance to women who are perimenopausal who experience difficulty in managing their symptoms. The fact that symptoms are normal and only temporary should be discussed. Nonpharmacological approaches to managing symptoms should also be reviewed with women who are perimenopausal.

Dry skin can be improved by the use of moisturizing soaps and body lotions. Kegel exercises may help decrease stress incontinence (see Table 48-19). Sexual function can continue with little change in the vast majority of women who are postmenopausal. Cessation of menstruation and ability to bear children should not be equated with cessation of sexual capability.

Femininity and libido do not disappear with menopause. A water-soluble lubricant (e.g., Replens, Astroglide, K-Y Jelly) is often effective in managing atrophic changes in vaginal epithelium. An active sex life helps increase lubrication and maintains the pliability of vaginal tissues. The nurse should provide the patient with an opportunity to candidly discuss concerns related to sexual functioning.

CONDITIONS OF VULVA, VAGINA, AND CERVIX

Etiology and Pathophysiology

Infection and inflammation of the vagina, the cervix, and the vulva tend to occur when the natural defences of the acid vaginal secretions (maintained by sufficient estrogen levels) and the presence of *Lactobacillus* are disrupted. Women's resistance may also be decreased as a result of aging, poor nutrition, and the use of drugs that alter the bacterial flora or mucosa. Organisms gain entrance to the areas through contaminated hands, clothing, douching, and intercourse. Table 56-8 presents the causes, manifestations and diagnostic methods, and collaborative care of common inflammations and infections.

Most lower genital tract infections are related to sexual intercourse. Intercourse can transmit organisms, injure tissues, and alter the acid–base balance of the vagina. Vulvar infections caused by viruses such as herpes and genital warts can be sexually transmitted when no lesions are apparent. Oral contraceptives, antibiotics, and corticosteroids may produce changes in the vaginal

TABLE 56-8   INFECTIONS OF THE LOWER GENITAL TRACT

Infection/Etiology	Manifestations and Diagnostic Methods	Drug Therapy
Vulvo-Vaginal Candidiasis (VVC) (Monilial Vaginitis)		
Candida albicans (fungus)	Commonly found in mouth, gastro-intestinal tract, and vagina; pruritus, thick white, curdlike discharge; KOH microscopic examination—pseudohyphae; pH 4–4.7	Antifungal agents, over-the-counter vaginal suppository and creams (e.g., clotrimazole [Canesten], miconazole [Micozole]) Fluconazole (Diflucan)
Trichomoniasis Vaginitis		
Trichomonas vaginalis (protozoa)	Sexually transmitted; pruritus; frothy greenish or grey discharge; hemorrhagic spots on cervix or vaginal walls; saline microscopic examination—swimming trichomonads; pH >4.5	Metronidazole (Flagyl) for patient and partner
Bacterial Vaginosis		
Gardnerella vaginalis Corynebacterium vaginale	Mode of transmission unclear; watery discharge with fishy odour; may or may not have symptoms; saline microscopic examination—epithelial cells; pH >4.5	Oral or vaginal metronidazole (Flagyl) or clindamycin (Dalacin C) cream 2% Lactobacillus acidophilus taken orally by diet (e.g., yogourt, fermented soy products) or supplements can decrease unwanted vaginal bacteria Examine and treat partner
Cervicitis		
Chlamydia trachomatis Neisseria gonorrhoeae	Sexually transmitted; mucopurulent discharge with postcoital spotting from cervical inflammation; culture for Chlamydia trachomatis and Neisseria gonorrhoeae	Combination gonorrhea infection therapy (e.g., Azithromycin [Zithromax] and cephalosporins [e.g., cefixime and ceftriaxone]) should be used due to increasing antimicrobial resistance. Treat partners with same drugs
Severe Recurrent Vaginitis		
C. albicans (most often)	May be indicative of HIV infection; all women who are unresponsive to first-line treatment should be offered HIV testing	Drug appropriate to opportunistic organism

HIV, human immunodeficiency virus; KOH, potassium hydroxide.
Source: Adapted from Public Health Agency of Canada [PHAC]. (2015). *Canadian guidelines on sexually transmitted infections*. Ottawa: Author. Retrieved from *http://www. phac-aspc.gc.ca/std-mts/sti-its/cgsti-ldcits/index-eng.php*.

pH and trigger an overgrowth of the organisms present. For example, *Candida albicans* may be present in small numbers in the vagina. An overgrowth of this organism causes vulvo-vaginitis.

Clinical Manifestations

Abnormal vaginal discharge and reddened vulvar lesions are common clinical manifestations. In addition to a thick, white, curdlike discharge, women with vulvo-vaginal candidiasis (VVC) often experience intense itching and dysuria, which is the result of urine coming into contact with fissures and irritated areas on the vulva. The hallmark of bacterial vaginosis is the fishy odour of the discharge. Women with cervicitis may notice spotting after intercourse.

Common vulvar lesions include herpes infection and genital warts. Initial or primary herpes infections may be extremely painful. Herpes begins as a small vesicle followed by a superficial red ulcer. Most herpes lesions are painful. Genital warts, caused by the human papilloma virus (HPV), vary in appearance. Irregularly shaped "cauliflower" lesions are common. Genital warts are painless unless traumatized. (Herpes infection and genital warts are discussed in Chapter 55.)

Women who are postmenopausal may develop gynecological problems such as *lichen sclerosis* (Stiles, Redmer, Paddock, et al., 2012). This chronic inflammatory condition is associated with intense itching in the genital skin area (e.g., labia minora, clitoris). The lesions are white with a "tissue paper" appearance initially, although scratching produces changes in the appearance. The

cause is unknown. High-potency topical corticosteroid ointment such as clobetasol propionate (Clobex) helps relieve itching.

Collaborative Care

Genital problems are evaluated by taking a history, performing a physical examination, and obtaining the appropriate laboratory and diagnostic studies. Because many problems relate to sexual activity, a sexual history is essential. The nature of the problem determines the extent of the evaluation. Ulcerative lesions should be cultured for herpes. A blood test for syphilis may be done when ulcerative lesions are present. Genital warts are usually identified by their clinical appearance. Vulvar dystrophies may be examined via colposcopy with a biopsy taken for diagnosis.

Problems involving vaginal discharge are evaluated by microscopy and cultures. The most common vaginal conditions (i.e., bacterial vaginosis, VVC, and trichomoniasis) are diagnosed by a procedure called a *wet mount*. The findings that are characteristic of each condition are shown in Table 56-8. To assess for cervicitis, endocervical cultures are obtained for *Chlamydia* and gonorrhea. If purulent discharge is observed coming from the cervix, a sample of endocervical cells may be taken to be evaluated by Gram staining. The Gram-stained slide is examined with a microscope to identify white blood cells and Gram-negative diplococci (indicative of gonorrhea). (Sexually transmitted infections [STIs] are discussed in Chapter 55.)

Drug therapy is based on the diagnosis and is shown in Table 56-8. Antibiotics taken as directed will cure bacterial infections.

Treatment duration and medications vary with specific STIs. Teach patients how to properly take their medications and to follow up to verify a cure. Partners should be treated so that reinfection does not occur.

Women with vaginal conditions or cervical infection should abstain from intercourse for at least 1 week. Douching should be avoided because it has been adversely linked to PID, STIs, and ectopic pregnancy. Sexual partners must be evaluated and treated if the patient is diagnosed with trichomoniasis, chlamydial infection, gonorrhea, syphilis, or HIV.

Treatment of vulvar dystrophies is symptomatic because no cures are available. Treatment involves controlling the itching and the scratching. Interrupting the "itch–scratch cycle" prevents further secondary damage to the skin.

NURSING MANAGEMENT
CONDITIONS OF VULVA, VAGINA, AND CERVIX

Nurses have the opportunity to teach women about common genital conditions and how to reduce their risks. The ability to recognize symptoms that indicate a problem helps women seek care in a timely manner. Discussing problems concerning one's genitals or sexual intercourse is frequently difficult. The nurse's nonjudgemental attitude makes women feel more comfortable and empowers them to ask questions and seek accurate information.

When a woman is diagnosed with a genital condition, the nurse should ensure that she fully understands the directions for treatment. Taking the full course of medication is especially important to decrease the chance of relapse. Because genitalia are such a private area, use of graphs and models is especially helpful for patient teaching. When a woman will be using a vaginal medication for the first time, showing her the applicator and how to fill it is important. The woman should be taught where and how the applicator should be inserted, using visual aids or models. Vaginal creams should be inserted before going to bed so that the medication will remain in the vagina for a long time. Women using vaginal creams or suppositories may wish to use panty liners during the day, when the residual medication may drain out.

PELVIC INFLAMMATORY DISEASE

Pelvic inflammatory disease (PID) is an infectious condition of the pelvic cavity that may involve the fallopian tubes (salpingitis), ovaries (oophoritis), and pelvic peritoneum (peritonitis). A tubo-ovarian abscess may also form (Figure 56-4). There are about 100 000 cases of symptomatic PID annually in Canada, but precise numbers are not known as PID is not reportable nationally (Public Health Agency of Canada [PHAC], 2013). PID is referred to as "silent" when women do not perceive any symptoms; other women with PID will be in acute distress.

Etiology and Pathophysiology

PID is often the result of untreated cervicitis. The organism infecting the cervix ascends higher into the uterus, fallopian tubes, ovaries, and peritoneal cavity. *C. trachomatis* and *N. gonorrhoeae* are the most common causative organisms of PID. These organisms, as well as anaerobes, mycoplasma, streptococci, and enteric Gram-negative rods, gain entrance during sexual intercourse or after pregnancy termination, pelvic surgery, or childbirth. It is important to remember that not all cases of PID are the result of an STI.

FIGURE 56-4 Pelvic inflammatory disease. Acute infection of the fallopian tubes and ovaries. The tubes and ovaries have become an inflamed mass attached to the uterus. A tubo-ovarian abscess is also present. Source: Kumar, V., Abbas, A. K., Fausto, N., et al. (2010). *Robbins and Cotran pathologic basis of disease* (8th ed., p. 1010, Figure 22-4A). Philadelphia: Saunders.

Women at increased risk for chlamydial infections (younger than 24 years of age, with multiple sex partners, or with a new sex partner) should be routinely tested for *C. trachomatis*. Chlamydial infections can be asymptomatic and unknowingly transmitted during intercourse. Silent PID is a major cause of female infertility.

Clinical Manifestations

Women with PID usually go to a health care provider because they are experiencing lower abdominal pain. The pain typically starts gradually and then becomes constant. The intensity may vary from mild to severe. Movement such as walking can increase the pain; pain is also frequently associated with intercourse. Spotting after intercourse and purulent cervical or vaginal discharge may also be noted. Fever and chills may also be present. Women with less acute symptoms notice increased cramping pain with menses, irregular bleeding, and some pain with intercourse. Women who have mild symptoms may go untreated either because they did not seek care or the health care provider misdiagnosed their complaints.

A pelvic examination assists in the diagnosis of PID. Women with PID have pelvic organ tenderness, as indicated by adnexal tenderness (tenderness of uterine appendages such as fallopian tubes, ovaries, and ligaments that hold the uterus in place), positive cervical motion tenderness or uterine compression tenderness during bimanual examination (Brunham, Gottlieb, & Paavonen, 2015). Additional criteria useful for diagnosis include fever and abnormal discharge (vaginal or cervical) as well as lower genital tract inflammation. Cultures for *N. gonorrhoeae* and *C. trachomatis* are also obtained, and a pregnancy test should be done to rule out ectopic pregnancy. Drug therapy begins when minimal diagnostic criteria are met. Thus, treatment is not delayed for culture results. When the patient's pain or obesity compromises the pelvic examination and a tubo-ovarian abscess may be present, vaginal ultrasonography is indicated.

Complications

Immediate complications of PID include septic shock and *Fitz–Hugh–Curtis syndrome*, which occurs when PID spreads to the liver and causes acute perihepatitis. The patient has symptoms of right upper quadrant pain, but liver function tests are normal. Tubo-ovarian abscesses may "leak" or rupture, resulting in pelvic or generalized peritonitis. As the general circulation is flooded with bacterial endotoxins from the infected areas, septic shock may result. Embolisms may occur as the result of thrombophlebitis of the pelvic veins.

PID can cause adhesions and strictures to develop in the fallopian tubes. Ectopic pregnancy may result when a tube is partially obstructed because the sperm can pass through the stricture but the fertilized ovum cannot reach the uterus. After one episode of PID, the risk of having an ectopic pregnancy increases ten-fold. Further damage can obstruct the fallopian tubes and cause infertility.

Collaborative Care

PID is usually treated on an outpatient basis. The patient is given a combination of antibiotics such as cefoxitin and doxycycline to provide broad coverage against the causative organisms. With effective antibiotic therapy, the pain should subside. The patient must have no intercourse for 3 weeks. Her partner(s) must be examined and treated. An important part of care is physical rest and oral fluids. Re-evaluation in 48 to 72 hours, even if symptoms are improving, is an essential part of outpatient care.

If outpatient treatment is unsuccessful or if the patient is acutely ill or in severe pain, admission to hospital is indicated. If a tubo-ovarian abscess is present, hospitalization is necessary. Maximum doses of parenteral antibiotics are given in hospital. Corticosteroids may be added to the antibiotic regimen to reduce inflammation, allowing for faster recovery and improvement in subsequent fertility. Application of heat to the lower abdomen or sitz baths may be used to improve circulation and decrease pain. Bed rest in the semi-Fowler's position promotes drainage of the pelvic cavity by gravity and may prevent the development of abscesses high in the abdomen. Analgesics to relieve pain and IV fluids to prevent dehydration are also used.

Surgery is indicated for abscesses that fail to resolve with IV antibiotics. The abscess may be drained by laparoscopy or laparotomy. In extreme cases of infection or severe chronic pelvic pain, a hysterectomy may be performed. When surgery is necessary, every attempt is made to preserve fertility in women of child-bearing age.

NURSING MANAGEMENT
PELVIC INFLAMMATORY DISEASE

Subjective and objective data that should be obtained from women with PID are presented in Table 56-9. Prevention, early recognition, and prompt treatment of vaginal and cervical infections can help prevent PID and its serious complications. Nurses should urge women to seek medical attention for any unusual vaginal discharge or possible infection of their reproductive organs. Women should be helped to understand that not all discharge is indicative of infection, but that early diagnosis and treatment of an infection, if present, can prevent serious complications. Women should be informed of the methods to decrease the risk of getting STIs and to recognize the signs of infection in their partner(s).

The patient may have guilt feelings about having PID, especially if it was associated with an STI. She may also be concerned about the complications associated with PID, such as adhesions and strictures of the fallopian tubes, infertility, and the increased incidence of ectopic pregnancy. Discussion with the patient

---

TABLE 56-9   NURSING ASSESSMENT

Pelvic Inflammatory Disease

Subjective Data

Important Health Information

Past health history: use of IUD; previous PID, gonorrhea, or chlamydial infection; multiple sexual partners; exposure to partner with urethritis; infertility

Medications: Use of and allergy to any antibiotics

Surgery or other treatments: Recent abortion or pelvic surgery

Symptoms

- Abnormal vaginal bleeding and menstrual irregularity; vaginal discharge
- Lower abdominal and pelvic pain; low back pain; pain on fundal palpation and cervical motion; onset of pain just after a menstrual cycle; dysmenorrhea, dyspareunia, dysuria, vulvar pruritus
- Malaise
- Nausea, vomiting; chills; fever
- Urinary frequency, urgency

Objective Data

General

Fever

Reproductive

Mucopurulent cervicitis, vulvar maceration, vaginal discharge (from heavy and purulent to thin and mucoid), tenderness on motion of cervix and uterus; presence of inflammatory masses on palpation

Possible Findings

Leukocytosis; ↑ erythrocyte sedimentation rate; positive culture of secretions or endocervical fluid; pelvic inflammation and positive endometrial biopsy on laparoscopic examination; abscess or inflammation on ultrasonography

IUD, intrauterine device; *PID,* pelvic inflammatory disease.

---

regarding her feelings and concerns can assist her to cope more effectively with them.

For patients requiring hospitalization, nurses have an important role in implementing drug therapy, monitoring the patient's health status, and providing symptom relief and patient teaching. Vital signs and character, amount, colour, and odour of the vaginal discharge should be recorded. Explanations about the need for limited activity, maintaining a semi-Fowler's position, and increased fluid intake should increase patient cooperation. Assessing the degree of abdominal pain will provide information about the effectiveness of drug therapy.

CHRONIC PELVIC PAIN

Chronic pelvic pain refers to pain in the pelvic region (below the umbilicus and between the hips) that lasts 6 months or longer (Shin & Howard, 2011). It accounts for 10% of all visits to gynecologists and is the reason for 20% to 30% of all laparoscopies. Up to one-third of women who have PID have chronic pelvic pain (Apte, Nelson, & Brisme, et al., 2012).

The cause of chronic pelvic pain is often hard to find. Many different conditions can cause pelvic pain. Gynecological etiologies include dysmenorrhea, endometriosis, PID, ovarian cysts, uterine fibroids, pelvic adhesions, and ectopic pregnancies. Abdominal etiologies include irritable bowel syndrome, interstitial cystitis, appendicitis, and colitis. Psychological factors (e.g., depression, chronic stress, history of sexual or physical abuse) may increase the risk of developing chronic pelvic pain. Emotional distress makes pain worse, and living with chronic pain contributes to emotional distress.

Chronic pelvic pain has many different clinical manifestations, including severe and steady pain, intermittent pain, dull and achy pain, pelvic pressure or heaviness, and sharp pain or cramping. In addition, pain may occur during intercourse or while having a bowel movement.

Determining the cause of chronic pelvic pain often involves a process of elimination. In addition to a detailed history and physical examination (including a pelvic examination), the patient may be asked to keep a journal of the onset of symptoms and any precipitating factors.

Diagnostic tests may include cultures from cervix or vagina (used to detect STIs), ultrasound, computed tomographic (CT) scan, or magnetic resonance imaging (MRI) to detect abnormal structures or growths. Laparoscopy may be used to visualize the pelvic organs. This procedure is especially useful in detecting endometriosis and chronic PID.

If the cause of chronic pelvic pain is found, treatment focuses on that cause. If no cause can be found, treatment involves managing the pain. Over-the-counter pain medications (e.g., acetylsalicylic acid [ASA: Aspirin], ibuprofen, acetaminophen) may provide some relief. Sometimes, stronger pain drugs may be needed. Birth control pills or other hormonal medications may help relieve cyclic pelvic pain related to menstrual cycles. If an infection is the source of the problem, antibiotics are used.

Tricyclic antidepressants (e.g., amitriptyline, nortriptyline) have pain-relieving and antidepressant effects. These drugs may help improve chronic pelvic pain even in women who do not have depression. The patient may be encouraged to get counselling for any emotional issues.

Laparoscopic surgery may be used to remove pelvic adhesions or endometrial tissue. As a last resort, a hysterectomy may be done.

ENDOMETRIOSIS

Endometriosis is the presence of endometrial epithelial cells in sites outside the uterine cavity (Donegan, 2012). The most frequent sites are in or near the ovaries, uterosacral ligaments, and utero-vesical peritoneum (Figure 56-5). However, endometrial tissues can be in many other locations, such as the stomach, the lungs, the intestines, and the spleen. The tissue responds to the hormones of the ovarian cycle and undergoes a "mini-menstrual cycle" similar to the uterine endometrium.

The typical patient with endometriosis is in her late twenties or early thirties and has never had a full-term pregnancy. Although it is not a life-threatening condition, endometriosis can cause considerable pain. It is also a common cause of infertility and increases the risk for ovarian cancer. Endometriosis is one of the most common gynecological problems, but is it difficult to know the number of women with the condition as many do not have symptoms. Current estimates suggest that 6% to 10% of women in the reproductive years have endometriosis (National Institute for Child Health and Development [NICHD], 2013).

Etiology and Pathophysiology

Although the etiology of endometriosis is poorly understood, many theories have been proposed. A widely held view is that retrograde menstrual flow passes through the fallopian tubes carrying viable endometrial tissues into the pelvis (Mayo Clinic, 2013). The tissue attaches to various sites, as shown in Figure 56-6.

FIGURE 56-5 Common sites of endometriosis.

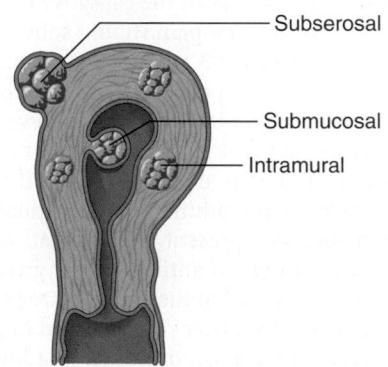

FIGURE 56-6 Leiomyomas. Uterine section shows the whorl-like appearance and locations of leiomyomas, which are also called *uterine fibroids*. Source: McCance, K. L., Huether, S. E., Brashers, V. L., et al. (2014). *Pathophysiology: The biologic basis for disease in adults and children* (7th ed., p. 823, Figure 24-15A). St. Louis: Mosby.

Another theory suggests that undifferentiated embryonic peritoneal cavity cells remain dormant in the pelvic tissue until the ovaries produce sufficient hormones to stimulate their growth. Other proposed causes are a genetic predisposition and altered immune function.

Clinical Manifestations

Patients with endometriosis have a wide range of clinical manifestations and severity. The magnitude of a woman's symptoms does not necessarily correlate with the clinical extent of her endometriosis. Dysmenorrhea after years of relatively pain-free menses and infertility may serve as a clue to the presence of endometriosis. The most common manifestations are secondary dysmenorrhea, infertility, pelvic pain, dysparcunia, and irregular bleeding. Less common manifestations include backache, painful bowel movements, and dysuria. With menopause, estrogen is no longer produced in the ovaries, and the symptoms may disappear.

When the ectopic endometrial tissues "menstruate," the blood collects in cystlike nodules that have a characteristic bluish-black colour. Nodules in the ovaries are sometimes called *chocolate cysts* because of the thick, chocolate-coloured material they contain. When a cyst ruptures, the pain may be acute, and the resulting irritation promotes the formation of adhesions, which fix the affected area to another pelvic structure. Endometrial adhesions may become severe enough to cause a bowel obstruction or painful micturition.

TABLE 56-10 **TABLE 56-10 COLLABORATIVE CARE**

Endometriosis

Diagnostic
- History and physical examination
- Laparoscopy
- MRI
- Pelvic examination
- Pelvic ultrasonography

Collaborative Therapy
- Conservative therapy (watch and wait)

Drug Therapy
- Danazol (Cyclomen)
- GnRH agonists (e.g., leuprolide [Lupron])
- Nonsteroidal anti-inflammatory drugs
- Oral contraceptives

Surgical Therapy
- Laparotomy to remove implants and adhesions
- Total abdominal hysterectomy and bilateral salpingo-oophorectomy (TAH-BSO)

GnRH, gonadotropin-releasing hormone; *MRI,* magnetic resonance imaging.

Collaborative Care

Endometriosis may be suspected from a woman's history of the characteristic symptoms and the health care provider's palpation of firm nodular lumps in the adnexa on bimanual examination. However, laparoscopy is necessary for a definitive diagnosis. The treatment of endometriosis is influenced by the patient's age, desire for pregnancy, symptom severity, and the extent and the location of the disease. When symptoms are not disruptive, a "watch-and-wait" approach is used (Table 56-10). When endometriosis is identified as a probable cause of infertility, therapy proceeds more rapidly.

Drug Therapy. Drug therapy is used to reduce symptoms. Pain may be relieved with NSAIDs such as ibuprofen (Advil) and diclofenac (Voltaren). Drugs to inhibit estrogen production by the ovaries are often given to shrink the endometrial tissue. Ovulation is suppressed by progestin agents such as medroxyprogesterone. Another approach to hormonal treatment is danazol (Cyclomen), a synthetic androgen that inhibits the anterior pituitary. This drug causes atrophy of ectopic endometrial tissue. Subjective relief of symptoms is noted within 6 weeks of danazol use. The adverse effects of weight gain, acne, hot flashes, and hirsutism and the expense of this drug restrict its use.

Another class of drugs used is gonadotropin-releasing hormone (GnRH) agonists (e.g., leuprolide [Lupron], nafarelin [Synarel]). These drugs result in amenorrhea. Adverse effects are usually the same as those of menopause (hot flashes, vaginal dryness, emotional lability). Loss of bone density has also been reported in women who remain on the therapy longer than 6 months. Endometriosis is controlled but not cured by HT. Persistent lesions give rise to subsequent recurrences once the menstrual cycle is re-established.

DRUG ALERT—Leuprolide (Lupron)
- Assess patient for pregnancy before initiating therapy
- Monitor patient for dysrhythmias, palpitations
- Instruct patient to use nonhormonal contraceptive measures during therapy

Surgical Therapy. The only cure for endometriosis is surgical removal of all the endometrial implants. Surgical therapy may be conservative or definitive. Conservative surgery is done to confirm the diagnosis or to remove implants. It involves removal or destruction of endometrial implants and lysing or excision of adhesions by means of laparoscopic laser surgery or laparotomy. GnRH agonist therapy (e.g., leuprolide) can be administered for 4 to 6 months to reduce the size of the lesions before surgery. By reducing the extent of the surgery, this preoperative drug treatment helps reduce the development of adhesions that may further threaten fertility. Definitive surgery involves removal of the uterus, fallopian tubes, ovaries, and as many endometrial implants as possible.

For women wishing to get pregnant, conservative surgical therapy is used to remove implants blocking the fallopian tube. Adhesions are removed from the tubes, the ovaries, and the pelvic structures. Efforts are made to conserve all tissues necessary to maintain fertility.

The woman should be actively involved in making the decision about preserving part or all of her ovaries if surgically possible. Her feelings about maintaining her cyclical ovarian function must be explored. The health care provider should assess the woman's risk for ovarian cancer and provide this information for her consideration.

NURSING MANAGEMENT ENDOMETRIOSIS

Education of the patient and reassurance that a life-threatening situation does not exist may permit her to accept a conservative and progressive treatment. When the symptoms are less severe, teaching about nondrug comfort measures may be helpful. Nurses must assist patients to understand the drugs that have been ordered to treat their condition. The action of the prescribed drug should be explained as well as the possible adverse effects. Psychological support may be needed for women experiencing severe disabling pain, sexual difficulties secondary to dyspareunia, and infertility.

If conservative surgery is the treatment selected, the nursing care is similar to the general preoperative and postoperative care of a patient undergoing laparotomy (see Nursing Care Plan [NCP] 45-2 for the patient following laparotomy, available on the Evolve website). If definitive surgery is planned, the nursing care is similar to care for the patient undergoing an abdominal hysterectomy (NCP 56-1). The nurse must know the extent of the procedure so that appropriate preoperative teaching can be done.

BENIGN TUMOURS OF THE FEMALE REPRODUCTIVE SYSTEM

LEIOMYOMAS

Etiology and Pathophysiology

Leiomyomas (uterine fibroids) are benign smooth muscle tumours that occur most commonly within the uterus (see Figure 56-6). Estimates of the prevalence of fibroids in women range from 20% to 77%, but the literature provides weak evidence of the overall burden of disease posed by uterine fibroids (Munro, 2011). The cause of leiomyomas is unknown. They appear to depend on ovarian hormones because they grow slowly during the reproductive years and undergo atrophy after menopause.

Clinical Manifestations

The majority of women with leiomyomas do not have any symptoms. When present, the most common symptoms include abnormal uterine bleeding, pain, and symptoms associated with pelvic pressure. Increased bleeding is thought to be associated with the increased endometrial surface area that is associated with leiomyomas. Pain is associated with infection or twisting of the pedicle from which the tumour is growing. Devascularization and blood vessel compression may also contribute to pain. Pressure on surrounding organs may result in rectal, bladder, and lower abdominal discomfort. Large tumours may cause a general enlargement of the lower abdomen. These tumours are sometimes associated with miscarriage and infertility.

Collaborative Care

Clinical diagnosis is based on the characteristic pelvic findings of an enlarged uterus distorted by nodular masses. Treatment depends on the symptoms, the patient's age, her desire to preserve her fertility, and the location and size of the tumour or tumours. If the symptoms are minimal, the health care provider may elect to follow the patient closely for a time.

Persistent, heavy menstrual bleeding causing anemia and large or rapidly growing tumours are indications for surgery. The leiomyomas are removed by hysterectomy or myomectomy for women who wish to maintain their fertility. In this case, only the fibroids are removed to preserve the uterus. Small tumours may be removed using a hysteroscope and laser resection instruments.

Uterine artery embolization is an increasingly used alternative treatment for uterine fibroids (Gupta, Sinha, Lumsden, et al., 2012). Embolic material (small plastic or gelatin beads) is injected into the uterine artery and carried to the fibroid branches.

Cryosurgery is another option. In cases of large leiomyomas, a GnRH agonist (e.g., leuprolide [Lupron]) may be used preoperatively to shrink the size of the tumour. However, the risks and benefits of this drug should be fully discussed, including the potential for irreversible loss of bone mass. The treatment should not be used on women who wish to preserve their fertility.

Another treatment option uses MRI-guided focused ultrasonography to target and destroy uterine fibroids. Treatment requires repeated targeting and heating of the fibroid tissue while the patient lies inside the MRI machine. The procedure can last as long as 3 hours.

CERVICAL POLYPS

Cervical polyps are benign pedunculated lesions that generally arise from the endocervical mucosa and are seen protruding through the cervical os during a speculum examination. Polyps are a characteristic bright cherry red and are soft and fragile in consistency. They are generally small, measuring less than 3 cm in length, and may be single or multiple. Their cause is unknown. Symptoms are usually not present, but metrorrhagia and bleeding after straining for a bowel movement and coitus can occur. Polyps are prone to infection. When the polyp is small, it can be excised in an outpatient procedure. If the point of attachment of the polyp cannot be identified and is not accessible to cautery, a polypectomy is performed in an operating room. All tissue removed is sent for pathological review because polyps occasionally undergo malignant changes.

FIGURE 56-7 Large ovarian cyst. Source: Symonds, E. M., & MacPherson, M. B. A. (1994). *Colour atlas of obstetrics and gynecology.* London: Mosby.

BENIGN OVARIAN TUMOURS

There are many different types of benign tumours. The cause of most of them is unknown. They can be divided into cysts and neoplasms. *Cysts* are usually soft, are surrounded by a thin capsule, and may be detected during the reproductive years. Follicle and corpus luteum cysts are common ovarian cysts (Figure 56-7). Multiple small ovarian follicles may occur in a condition called *polycystic ovary syndrome* (PCOS) (discussed in the next section). Epithelial ovarian neoplasms may be cystic or solid, small or extremely large. Cystic teratomas, or dermoid cysts, originate from germ cells and can contain bits of any type of body tissue, such as hair or teeth.

Ovarian masses are often asymptomatic until they are large enough to cause pressure in the pelvis. Constipation, menstrual irregularities, urinary frequency, a full feeling in the abdomen, anorexia, and peripheral edema may occur, depending on the size and the location of the tumour. There may be an increase in abdominal girth. Pelvic pain may be present if the tumour is growing rapidly. Severe pain results when the cyst twists on its pedicle (ovarian torsion).

In some cases, an ovarian cyst can rupture. A ruptured ovarian cyst is not only extremely painful, but it can lead to serious complications, such as hemorrhage and infection.

Pelvic examination reveals a mass or an enlarged ovary that demands further investigation. If the mass is cystic and smaller than 8 cm, the patient is asked to return for re-examination in 4 to 6 weeks. If the mass is cystic and greater than 8 cm or is solid, laparoscopic surgery or laparotomy is performed. Immediate surgery is necessary if ovarian torsion occurs, causing the ovary to rotate and cutting off circulation. Surgical techniques are used to save as much of the ovary as possible.

Polycystic Ovary Syndrome

PCOS is a chronic disorder in which many benign cysts form on the ovaries. It most commonly occurs in women younger than 30 years and is a cause of infertility. It affects about 5% to 10% of women of reproductive age (Lobo, 2013). PCOS is caused by hormonal abnormalities in which the ovaries produce estrogen and excess testosterone but not progesterone. Fluid-filled cysts develop from mature ovarian follicles that fail to rupture (thereby releasing an egg) each month (Figure 56-8). This problem affects both ovaries.

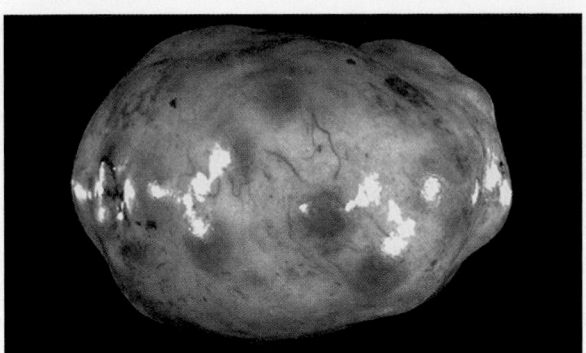

FIGURE 56-8 Polycystic ovary syndrome. Multiple fluid-filled cysts in the ovary. Source: Patton, K. T. & Thibodeau, G. (2013). *Anatomy and physiology* (8th ed., p. 1089, Figure 35-23). St Louis: Mosby.

FIGURE 56-9 Cervical cancer. View through a speculum inserted into the vagina. Source: Drake, R. L., Vogl, W., & Mitchell, A. W. M. (2010). *Gray's anatomy for students* (2nd ed., p. 457, Figure 5.55). Edinburgh: Churchill Livingstone.

Clinical manifestations include irregular menstrual periods, amenorrhea, hirsutism, and obesity. Of these manifestations, obesity in particular has been associated with severe symptoms such as excess androgens, oligomenorrhea, amenorrhea, and infertility. Many women start with normal menstrual periods that, after 1 to 2 years, become irregular and then infrequent. If PCOS is left untreated, cardiovascular disease and abnormal insulin resistance with type 2 diabetes mellitus may develop (Toulis, Goulis, Mintziori, et al., 2011; Androgen Excess and PCOS Society [AE-PCOS], 2012).

Pelvic ultrasonography will reveal enlarged ovaries with multiple small cysts. Successful management includes early diagnosis and treatment to improve quality of life and decrease the risk for complications. Oral contraceptives are useful in regulating menstrual cycles. Hirsutism may be treated with spironolactone (Aldactone). Hyperandrogenism can be treated with flutamide and a GnRH agonist such as leuprolide (Lupron). Metformin (Glucophage) reduces hyperinsulinemia and has been shown to improve hyperandrogenism and restore ovulation. For women desiring to become pregnant, fertility drugs may be used to induce ovulation. If all other treatments are unsuccessful, a hysterectomy with bilateral salpingo-oophorectomy may be performed.

Patient teaching for the patient with PCOS includes the importance of weight management and exercise to decrease insulin resistance. Obesity exacerbates the problems related to PCOS. Lipid profile and fasting glucose levels should be monitored. Hirsutism is cosmetically distressing for many women. It is important to support the patient as she explores measures to remove unwanted hair (e.g., depilating agents, electrolysis). Regular follow-up care is important to monitor the effectiveness of therapy and to detect any complications.

CANCER OF THE FEMALE REPRODUCTIVE SYSTEM

CERVICAL CANCER

Cervical cancer is the second most common cancer affecting women in the world, with 80% to 85% of these cases occurring in under-resourced countries. Noninvasive cervical cancer is about four times more common than invasive cervical cancer. Based on 2012 estimates, the lifetime probability of a woman developing cervical cancer in Canada is 1 in 152, and the lifetime probability of dying from cervical cancer is 1 in 426 (Canadian Cancer Society's Advisory Committee on Cancer Statistics, 2017). An increased risk for cervical cancer is associated with low socioeconomic status, early sexual activity (before 17 years of age), multiple sexual partners, infection with HPV, immunosuppression, and smoking.

The number of deaths from cervical cancer in women who undergo regular screening and follow-up has fallen steadily since the 1950s. This is attributable to better and earlier diagnosis with the widespread use of the Papanicolaou (Pap) test. In addition to being used to detect cancer, the Pap test is also used to detect precancerous changes. By treating precancerous lesions, progression to cervical cancer can be prevented.

Etiology and Pathophysiology

The progression from normal cervical cells to dysplasia and then to cervical cancer appears to be related to repeated injuries to the cervix. The progression occurs slowly over years. A strong relationship exists between dysplasia and HPV infections. Cancer rates are expected to decline further with vaccines (e.g., Gardasil, Cervarix) now being used for the prevention of HPV (NIH, 2014).

Clinical Manifestations

Precancerous changes are asymptomatic. This highlights the importance of routine screening. The peak incidence of noninvasive cervical cancer is in women in their early 30s. The average age for women with invasive cervical cancer is 50 (Figure 56-9). Early cervical cancer is generally asymptomatic, but leukorrhea (also called *leucorrhea*) and intermenstrual bleeding (abnormal vaginal bleeding between menstrual periods) eventually occur. The discharge is usually thin and watery but becomes dark and foul smelling as the disease advances, suggesting the presence of an infection. The vaginal bleeding is initially only spotting. As the tumour enlarges, the bleeding becomes heavier and more frequent. Pain is a late symptom and is followed by weight loss, anemia, and cachexia.

Diagnostic Studies

Cervical cancer screening is recommended in Canada for sexually active women between the ages of 21 and 69. Some provinces or territories may offer screening at earlier or later ages. The Canadian Cancer Society (CCS, 2016a) recommends that women have a Pap test every 1 to 3 years, depending on the screening guidelines in their province or territory and depending on their previous test results. After age 69, women should talk to their health care provider about the possibility of stopping the Pap test following two or three previously normal (negative) Pap results. Women who have sex with women, women who are no longer sexually active, women who have had a partial hysterectomy and transgender men who are sexually active should follow the same cervical screening guidelines. Women with previous abnormal Pap tests may be screened more often (CCS, 2016a). Women who have had a total hysterectomy do not need to be screened for cervical cancer, unless the surgery was done for cervical precancer or cancer.

EVIDENCE-INFORMED PRACTICE

Translating Research Into Practice

Hanna Khan is a 38-yr-old woman who had a tubal ligation in the outpatient surgery unit. She had a kidney transplant less than a year ago and is taking immuno-suppressant medications to prevent rejection. In preparing Ms. Khan for discharge, the nurse reminds her that she needs to have regular Pap tests to screen for cervical cancer. She expresses concern over the distance she has to travel to see her family doctor. She does not drive and is a single mother with three young children at home. She tells the nurse that she does not remember when she last had a Pap test done.

Best Available Evidence	Clinician Expertise	Patient Preferences and Values
For women after age 21 who have had three normal Pap tests, the Canadian Cancer Society recommends screening every 1 to 3 years.	The nurse knows that she is at higher risk for cervical cancer due to the immuno-suppression drugs that she is taking for her recent kidney transplant.	Ms. Khan is concerned about the difficulty getting to see her family doctor. She adds that no one in her family has ever had cervical cancer.

Decision and Action

Her nurse explains the Canadian Cancer Society recommendations and her increased risk for cervical cancer. She tells the nurse that she understands and will schedule a follow-up appointment, but unless she gets some help with child care and travel costs, she will probably not be able to get yearly Pap tests.

Reference for Evidence

Canadian Cancer Society. (2016). *Screening for cervical cancer*. Retrieved from *http://www.cancer.ca/en/cancer-information/cancer-type/cervical/screening/?region=on*.

Women with a history of cervical cancer should continue with screening for at least 20 years, as recommended by their health care provider. A woman who has been vaccinated against HPV needs to continue following the screening guidelines for her age group.

The two types of HPV that have been associated with most cases of cervical cancer (types 16 and 18) can be identified through deoxyribonucleic acid (DNA) testing. HPV DNA tests help to determine if women with abnormal Pap test results need further follow-up. Women aged 30 to 65 who have the HPV DNA test

and the Pap test (co-testing) can be screened every 5 years rather than every 3 years.

Pap tests are less than 100% accurate. There are problems with both false-positive and false-negative reports. ThinPrep, a newer, liquid-based technique for Pap tests, has reduced the number of inaccurate Pap test results.

The finding of an abnormal Pap smear indicates the need for follow-up. Women with minor changes may be followed with a repeated Pap test in 4 to 6 months for 2 years. Up to 80% of abnormal Pap tests may revert to normal results spontaneously. Women with more prominent changes will receive additional procedures, such as colposcopy and biopsy, before a definitive diagnosis can be made. Colposcopy helps identify possible epithelial abnormalities and suggests areas for biopsy. Biopsies are sent for pathology evaluation. Colposcopy and biopsy have improved diagnosis and allow more focused treatments.

The type and the extent of the biopsy vary with the abnormality seen. A punch biopsy may be done on an outpatient basis with special punch biopsy forceps. The excision of a cone-shaped section of the cervix may be used for both diagnosis and treatment. Conization is accomplished using one of several techniques, depending on the health care provider's experience and the availability of equipment. *Cryotherapy* (freezing) and laser cone vaporization destroy the tissue. Laser cone excision and *loop electrosurgery excision procedure* (LEEP) remove the identified tissue and allow for histological examination to ensure that all microinvasive tissue has been removed. These procedures can be performed as outpatient procedures with mild analgesics or sedation. Complications of these procedures include excessive bleeding and possible cervical stenosis after healing.

Collaborative Care

Vaccines against HPV (e.g., Gardasil, Cervarix) reduce the incidence of both cervical-related neoplasia and cervical cancer caused by infection from HPV types 16 and 18. HPV types 16 and 18 together cause 70% of cervical cancers (Maine, Hurlburt, & Greeson, 2011; CCS, 2016b). According to the National Advisory Committee on Immunization (NACI, 2012), the primary group recommended for vaccination is females aged 9 to 13. Gardasil is also recommended in males between 9 and 26 years of age, and in males ≥9 years of age who have sex with males (PHAC, 2017). Since the fall of 2008, all provinces and territories have introduced or announced HPV immunization programs into their routine immunization schedules for young girls (NACI, 2012). (HPV vaccines are discussed further in Chapter 55.)

The treatment of cancer of the cervix is guided by the stage of the tumour and the patient's age and general state of health (Table 56-11). There are four procedures in which fertility can be preserved. Conization may be the only type of therapy needed for noninvasive cervical cancer if analysis of removed tissue demonstrates that a wide area of normal tissue surrounds the excised tissue. Laser treatments can be used in which a directed infrared beam is employed to destroy abnormal tissue. Cautery and cryosurgery may also be used.

Invasive cancer of the cervix is treated with surgery, irradiation, and chemotherapy as single treatments or in combination. Surgical procedures include hysterectomy, radical hysterectomy (involving adjacent structures), and rarely, pelvic exenteration. (Surgical therapy is discussed earlier in this chapter; pelvic exenteration is discussed later in the chapter.) Radiation may be external (e.g., cobalt) or internal implants (e.g., cesium, radium) may be used. Standard radiation treatment is 4 to 6 weeks of external radiation

TABLE 56-11	STAGING AND TREATMENT OF CERVICAL CANCER	
Stage	Extent	Treatment
0	In situ	Cervical conization, hysterectomy, cryosurgery, laser surgery
I	Confinement to cervix	Radiation, radical hysterectomy
II	Spread beyond cervix to upper two-thirds of vagina but not to tissues around uterus	Radiation, cisplatin-based chemotherapy, radical hysterectomy
III	Spread to pelvic wall, involvement of lower third of vagina, or has caused kidney problems (or both of the latter two)	Radiation, cisplatin-based chemotherapy
IV	Spread to other parts of the body such as bladder, rectum, liver, lungs, and bones	Radiation, surgery (e.g., pelvic exenteration), cisplatin-based chemotherapy

Source: Modified from National Cancer Institute (NCI). (2016). *Cancer cervical treatment: Stages of cervical cancer.* Retrieved from *www.cancer.gov/cancertopics/pdq/treatment/cervical/Patient/page2.*

followed with one or two treatments with internal implants (brachytherapy). (Radiation therapy is discussed in Chapter 18 and in NCP 18-1, available on the Evolve website.) Cisplatin-based chemotherapy regimens benefit patients with cancer that has spread beyond the cervix.

ENDOMETRIAL OR UTERINE CANCER

Cancer of the endometrium is the most common gynecological malignancy, accounting for nearly 50% of female genital tract neoplasms. The probability of a Canadian woman developing uterine cancer in her lifetime is 1 in 40. In 2015, it was estimated that there would be 6 300 new cases of endometrial cancer in Canada and that 1 050 women would die from the condition (Canadian Cancer Society's Advisory Committee on Cancer Statistics, 2015). Endometrial cancer has a relatively low mortality rate, since most cases are diagnosed early. The survival rate is 95% if the cancer has not spread at the time of diagnosis.

Etiology and Pathophysiology

The major risk factor for endometrial cancer is estrogen, especially unopposed estrogen (Arora & Quinn, 2012). Additional risk factors include increasing age, nulliparity (women who have never been pregnant), late menopause, obesity, smoking, diabetes mellitus, and having a personal or family history of hereditary nonpolyposis colorectal cancer (HNPCC) (see the "Genetics in Clinical Practice" box on HNPCC in Chapter 45). Obesity is a risk factor because adipose cells store estrogen, thus increasing endogenous estrogen. Pregnancy and oral contraceptives are protective factors.

Endometrial cancer arises from the lining of the endometrium. Most tumours are adenocarcinomas. The precursor may be a hyperplasic state that progresses to invasive carcinoma. Hyperplasia occurs when estrogen is not counteracted by progesterone. The cancer extends directly into the cervix and through the uterine serosa. As invasion of the myometrium occurs, regional lymph nodes, including the paravaginal and para-aortic, become

involved. Hematogenous metastases develop concurrently. The usual sites of metastases are the lung, bones, the liver, and eventually, the brain. Malignant cells can be found in the peritoneal cavity, probably having arrived by transport through the fallopian tubes.

Prognostic factors include histological differentiation, myometrial invasion, peritoneal cytology, lymph node and adnexal metastases, and tumour size. Endometrial cancer grows slowly, metastasizes late, and is amenable to therapy if diagnosed early.

Clinical Manifestations

The first sign of endometrial cancer is abnormal uterine bleeding, usually in women who are postmenopausal. Because women who are perimenopausal have sporadic periods for a time, it is important that this sign not be ignored or attributed to menopause.

Pain occurs late in the disease process. Other manifestations that may arise are related to metastasis to other organs. Metastatic spread occurs in a characteristic pattern. Spread to the pelvic and para-aortic nodes is common. When distant metastasis occurs, it most commonly involves the lungs, liver, bones, brain, and vagina.

Collaborative Care

Endometrial biopsy is the primary diagnostic procedure for endometrial cancer. Endometrial biopsy is done on an outpatient basis. Any abnormal or unexpected bleeding in a postmenopausal woman requires obtaining a tissue sample to exclude endometrial cancer. It is recommended that an endometrial biopsy be performed at menopause and then periodically in women who are at risk. The Pap test is not a reliable diagnostic tool for endometrial cancer, but it can rule out cervical cancer.

Most cases of endometrial cancer are diagnosed at an early stage, when surgery alone may result in cure. Treatment of endometrial cancer is a total abdominal hysterectomy and bilateral salpingo-oophorectomy (TAH-BSO) with lymph node biopsies. The lack of estrogen and progesterone receptors is a poor prognostic indicator. Surgery may be followed by radiation, either to the pelvis or the abdomen, externally or intravaginally, to decrease local recurrence.

No tumour markers with high sensitivity and high specificity for endometrial cancer are known at present, although CA-125 is often used in clinical practice. CA-125 has been used in surveillance of advanced endometrial cancer. In patients who have increased CA-125 values pretreatment, this test might prove useful in post-treatment surveillance.

Treatment of advanced or recurrent disease is difficult. Progesterone HT (e.g., megestrol [Megace OS]) is the treatment of choice when the progesterone receptor status is positive and the tumour is well differentiated (Jelovac & Armstrong, 2011). Tamoxifen (Nolvadex-D), either alone or in combination with progesterone therapy, is also effective in women with advanced or recurrent endometrial cancer. Chemotherapy is considered when progesterone therapy is unsuccessful. The most common agents used are doxorubicin, cisplatin (Cisplatin), carboplatin, and paclitaxel.

Ovarian Cancer

Ovarian cancer is a malignant neoplasm of the ovaries. In 2015, it was estimated that there would be 2 800 new cases of ovarian cancer in Canada and that 1 750 women would die from the condition (Canadian Cancer Society's Advisory Committee on

Cancer Statistics, 2015). Ovarian cancer has the highest mortality rate of all gynecological cancers because most women have advanced disease at diagnosis (Jelovac & Armstrong, 2011). In Canada, the lifetime probability of a woman dying from ovarian cancer is 1 in 91 (Canadian Cancer Society's Advisory Committee on Cancer Statistics, 2015). It occurs most frequently in women between 55 and 65 years of age.

Etiology and Pathophysiology

The cause of ovarian cancer is not known. Women who have mutations of the *BRCA* genes have increased susceptibility for ovarian and breast cancer (Jelovac & Armstrong, 2011). The *BRCA* genes are tumour suppressor genes that inhibit tumour growth when functioning normally. When they mutate, they lose their tumour suppressor ability. This loss results in an increased risk for women to develop ovarian or breast cancer (see the "Genetics in Clinical Practice" box).

🧬 GENETICS IN CLINICAL PRACTICE

Ovarian Cancer

Genetic Basis
- Mutations in genes *BRCA1* and *BRCA2*
- Autosomal dominant transmission
- Mutations can be passed down from either mother or father

Incidence
- About 10% of cases of ovarian cancer are related to hereditary factors.
- Women with *BRCA1* mutations have a 25% to 40% lifetime risk of developing ovarian cancer.
- Women with *BRCA2* mutations have a 10% to 20% lifetime risk of developing ovarian cancer.
- Family history of both breast and ovarian cancer increases the risk of having a *BRCA* mutation.
- *BRCA* mutations occur in 10% to 20% of patients with ovarian cancer who have no family history of breast or ovarian cancer.

Genetic Testing
- DNA testing is available for *BRCA1* and *BRCA2* genetic mutations.

Clinical Implications
- Bilateral oophorectomy reduces the risk for ovarian cancer in women with *BRCA1* and *BRCA2* mutations.
- Genetic counselling and testing for *BRCA* mutations should be considered for women whose personal or family history puts them at high risk for a genetic predisposition to ovarian cancer.

The major risk factor for ovarian cancer is family history (one or more first-degree relatives with ovarian cancer). A family history of breast or colon cancer is also a risk factor. Other risk factors include a personal history of breast or colon cancer and HNPCC (see the "Genetics in Clinical Practice" box on HNPCC in Chapter 45).

Nulliparity also places women at higher risk. Other risk factors include increasing age, high-fat diet, increased number of ovulatory cycles (usually associated with early menarche and late menopause), HT, and possibly the use of infertility drugs. Breastfeeding, multiple pregnancies, oral contraceptive use (>5 years), and early age at first birth seem to reduce the risk for ovarian cancer. These factors may have a protective effect because they reduce the number of ovulatory cycles and, thus, reduce the exposure to estrogen.

About 90% of ovarian cancers are epithelial carcinomas that arise from malignant transformation of the surface epithelial cells. Epithelial ovarian cancer is primarily a disease of women who are postmenopausal and in the sixth or seventh decade of life (Jelovac & Armstrong, 2011). Germ cell tumours account for the other 10%. Histological grading is an important prognostic determinant. Tumours are graded according to the level of differentiation, ranging from *well differentiated* (grade I), *moderately well differentiated* (grade II), and *poorly differentiated* (grade III) to *undifferentiated* (grade IV). Grade IV lesions carry a poorer prognosis than the other grades.

Intraperitoneal dissemination is a common characteristic of ovarian cancer. It metastasizes to the uterus, bladder, bowel, and omentum. In advanced disease, it can spread to the stomach, colon, liver, and other parts of the body.

Clinical Manifestations

Nonspecific symptoms that warrant further evaluation include pelvic or abdominal pain, bloating, urinary urgency or frequency, and difficulty eating or feeling full quickly (Jelovac & Armstrong, 2011). Women who have one or more of these symptoms, especially if they are new, persistent (occur at least 12 days per month), or worsening, need to see their health care provider. Vaginal bleeding rarely occurs, and pain is not an early symptom. Later signs are increased abdominal girth, unexplained weight loss or gain, and menstrual changes.

Diagnostic Studies

No screening test exists for ovarian cancer. Because early ovarian cancer has vague symptoms, yearly bimanual pelvic examinations should be performed to identify the presence of an ovarian mass (Table 56-12). Women who are postmenopausal should not have palpable ovaries, so a mass of any size should be suspected as possible ovarian cancer. An abdominal or transvaginal ultrasonography can be used to detect ovarian masses. An exploratory laparotomy may be used to establish the diagnosis and stage the disease.

A test called OVA1 can help detect whether a pelvic mass is benign or malignant before it is surgically removed. OVA1 uses a blood sample to test for levels of five proteins that change due

---

TABLE 56-12 COLLABORATIVE CARE

Ovarian Cancer

Diagnostic
- History and physical examination
- Abdominal and transvaginal ultrasonography
- CA 125 levels
- Laparotomy for diagnostic staging
- Pelvic examination

Collaborative Therapy
- Surgery
  - Abdominal hysterectomy and bilateral salpingo-oophorectomy with pelvic lymph node biopsies
  - Debulking for advanced disease
- Chemotherapy
  - Adjuvant and palliative
- Radiation therapy
  - Adjuvant and palliative

CA, carbohydrate antigen.

to ovarian cancer. It is not intended for ovarian cancer screening or for a definitive diagnosis of ovarian cancer.

For women with a high risk for ovarian cancer, screening using a combination of the tumour marker (carbohydrate antigen-125 [CA-125]) and ultrasonography is recommended in addition to a yearly pelvic examination. CA-125 is positive in 80% of women with epithelial ovarian cancer and is used to monitor the course of the disease. However, levels of CA-125 may be elevated with other malignancies (e.g., pancreatic cancer) or with benign conditions such as fibroids or endometriosis. A large, recent clinical trial has reported that screening by CA-125 and ultrasound did not result in fewer deaths from ovarian cancer (Buys, Partridge, Black, et al., 2011). Currently only 20% of ovarian cancers are diagnosed at an early stage.

Collaborative Care

Women identified as being at high risk based on family and health history may require counselling regarding options such as prophylactic oophorectomy and oral contraceptives. It is important to note that, although oophorectomy will significantly reduce the risk for ovarian cancer, it will not completely eliminate the possibility of the disease.

Ovarian cancer staging is critical for guiding treatment decisions. Stage I describes disease limited to the ovaries; stage II, disease limited to the true pelvis; stage III, disease limited to the abdominal cavity; and stage IV, distant metastatic disease. The overall survival rate is 90% with early disease, 36% with local spread, and 20% with distant metastases.

Most patients with ovarian cancer have widespread disease at presentation. The initial treatment for all stages of ovarian cancer is surgery, which is usually a total abdominal hysterectomy (TAH) and bilateral salpingo-oophorectomy (BSO) with omentectomy and removal of as much of the tumour as possible (i.e., tumour debulking). Surgery facilitates chemotherapy by reducing the number of cells that the chemotherapy has to kill.

Depending on the differentiation of the cells and the stage of cancer, other treatment options include intraperitoneal and systemic chemotherapy, intraperitoneal instillation of radioisotopes, and external abdominal and pelvic radiation therapy. If a patient is clinically free of symptoms after completing treatment, a "second-look" surgical procedure is often performed to determine whether there is any evidence of disease. If no disease is found, the patient is monitored for recurrent disease.

Chemotherapy usually consists of a combination of a platinum compound, such as cisplatin or carboplatin, and a taxane, such as paclitaxel or docetaxel (Taxotere). The typical course of chemotherapy involves three to six cycles. A cycle is a schedule that allows regular doses of a drug, followed by a rest period.

Other chemotherapy drugs used include topotecan (Hycamtin), etoposide (Vepesid), gemcitabine, and oxaliplatin (Eloxatin). These drugs may be used to treat recurrent disease or as a palliative measure to shrink the tumour to relieve pressure and pain.

VAGINAL CANCER

Primary vaginal cancers are rare. The peak incidence is between 50 and 70 years of age. Vaginal tumours are usually secondary sites or metastases of other cancers such as cervical or endometrial carcinomas. The most common type of vaginal cancer is squamous cell carcinoma. Intrauterine exposure to DES (a synthetic form of estrogen no longer in use) places a woman at risk for clear cell adenocarcinoma of the vagina.

Treatment of vaginal cancer depends on the type of cells involved and the stage of the disease, the size of the tumour, and the location of the tumour. Squamous cell carcinomas can be treated with both surgery and radiation.

VULVAR CANCER

Cancer of the vulva is relatively rare. Similarly to cervical cancer, preinvasive lesions, referred to as *vulvar intraepithelial neoplasia* (VIN), precede invasive vulvar cancer. The invasive form occurs mainly in women older than 60 years, with the highest incidence being in women in their 70s.

Patients with vulvar neoplasia may have symptoms of vulvar itching or burning, pain, bleeding, or discharge. Women who are immuno-suppressed or have diabetes mellitus, hypertension, or chronic vulvar dystrophies are at a higher risk of developing vulvar cancers. Several subtypes of HPV have been identified in some but not all vulvar cancers. Vaccines (Gardasil, Cervarix) are now available to protect against some vaginal and vulvar cancers that are caused by these HPV subtypes. (HPV vaccines are discussed further in Chapter 55.)

Diagnosis of vulvar cancer is determined by the pathology report on the biopsy of the suspicious lesion. VIN can be treated topically with imiquimod cream (Aldara) or surgery.

Laser therapy may be used to kill cancer cells. Surgery is the most common treatment for cancer of the vulva. The goal of surgery is to remove all the cancer without any loss of the woman's sexual function. A local excision with removal of the lesion and surrounding tissue may be done. For more extensive lesions, vulvectomy may be done (various types of vulvectomies are presented in Table 56-13). If the cancer is extensive, a pelvic exenteration may be done. The patient may have chemotherapy or radiation therapy after surgery, as adjuvant measures.

SURGICAL PROCEDURES: FEMALE REPRODUCTIVE SYSTEM

A variety of surgical procedures are performed when benign or malignant tumours of the genital tract are found (Table 56-13). A *hysterectomy* (removal of the uterus) is the type of surgery performed for excision of cancerous tumours of the female reproductive system. A hysterectomy may be done abdominally, vaginally, or laparoscopically. The abdominal route is used when large tumours are present and the pelvic cavity is to be explored or when the tubes and ovaries are to be removed at the same time (Figure 56-10). The abdominal route can present more postoperative problems because it involves an incision and the opening of the abdominal cavity.

A vaginal route is often used when vaginal repair is done in addition to removal of the uterus. In both vaginal and abdominal hysterectomies, the ligaments that support the uterus are attached to the vaginal cuff to maintain the normal depth of the vagina. Laparoscopic procedures have the advantage of quicker recovery time and fewer complications (Koehler, Gottschalk, Chiantera, et al., 2013).

RADIATION THERAPY: CANCERS OF THE FEMALE REPRODUCTIVE SYSTEM

Radiation is used to cure or control or as a palliative measure for cancers of the female reproductive system, either alone or in combination with other treatments. The goal of radiation

TABLE 56-13	SURGICAL PROCEDURES INVOLVING THE FEMALE REPRODUCTIVE SYSTEM
Type of Surgery	**Description**
Abdominal Hysterectomy	
Total hysterectomy	Uterus and cervix removed using large abdominal incision (bikini cut)
Total abdominal hysterectomy and bilateral salpingo-oophorectomy (TAH-BSO)	Uterus, cervix, fallopian tubes, and ovaries removed using large abdominal incision
Radical hysterectomy	Panhysterectomy, partial vaginectomy, and dissection of lymph nodes in pelvis
Vaginal Hysterectomy	Uterus and cervix removed through a cut in the top of vagina
Laparoscopic Hysterectomy	Laparoscope (video camera and small surgical instruments)
Laparoscopic-assisted vaginal hysterectomy (LAVH)	Incision made at top of vagina; uterus and cervix removed through the vagina; laparoscope inserted into abdomen to assist in the procedure
Laparoscopic supracervical hysterectomy	Uterus removed using only laparoscopic instruments; cervix is left intact
Robot-Assisted Surgery	Robot (special machine) used to do surgery through small abdominal incisions; most often used when a patient has cancer or is very overweight and vaginal surgery is not safe
Vulvectomy	Surgical procedure to remove part or all of the vulva
Skinning vulvectomy	Removal of top layer of vulvar skin where the cancer is found; skin grafts from other parts of the body may be needed to cover the area
Simple vulvectomy	Entire vulva is removed
Radical vulvectomy	Entire vulva, including clitoris, labia majora and minora, and nearby tissue, is removed; nearby lymph nodes may also be removed
Vaginectomy	Removal of vagina
Pelvic Exenteration	Radical hysterectomy, total vaginectomy, removal of bladder with diversion of urinary system and resection of colon and rectum with colostomy

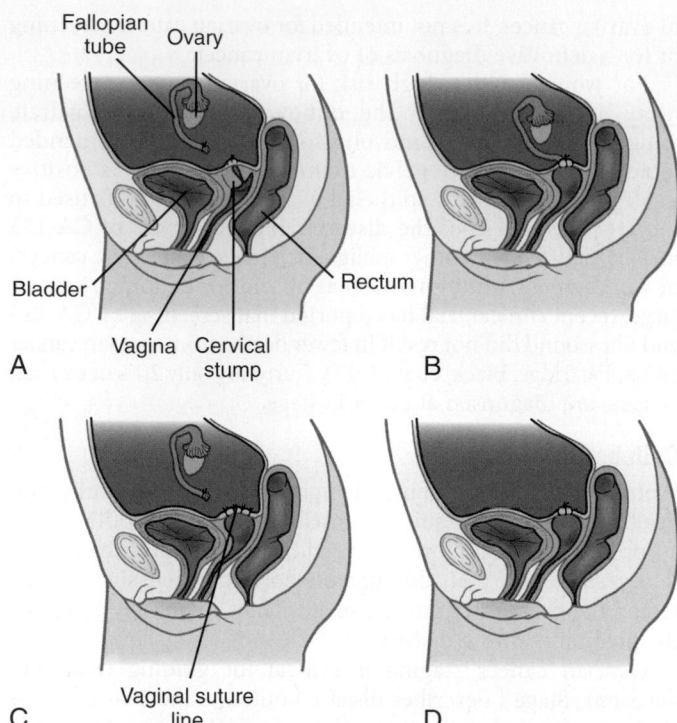

FIGURE 56-10 A, Cross-section of subtotal hysterectomy. Note that the cervical stump, fallopian tubes, and ovaries remain. **B,** Cross-section of total hysterectomy. Note that the fallopian tubes and ovaries remain. **C,** Cross-section of vaginal hysterectomy. Note that the fallopian tubes and ovaries remain. **D,** Total hysterectomy, salpingectomy, and oophorectomy. Note that the uterus, fallopian tubes, and ovaries are completely removed.

therapy is to deliver a specific amount of high-energy (or ionizing) radiation to the cancer with minimal damage to the normal surrounding tissue. Radiation therapy may be external or internal (brachytherapy).

External Radiation Therapy

With external radiation therapy, a source outside of the body delivers electromagnetic radiation in the form of waves. (External radiation therapy and related nursing care are discussed in Chapter 18 and in NCP 18-1, available on the Evolve website.)

Internal Radiation Therapy (Brachytherapy)

Brachytherapy allows the radiation to be placed near or into the tumour. This method can deliver a high dose of radiation directly to the tumour (Viswanathan, 2012). The dose decreases sharply as distance from the source increases, causing less damage to the surrounding normal tissue. A variety of forms are used to deliver the therapy, including wires, capsules, needles, tubes, and seeds. Brachytherapy is used in the management of cervical and endometrial cancer because of the accessibility of these body parts and the favourable results obtained. Radium and cesium are two commonly used isotopes.

To prepare the patient for the treatment, the nurse gives a cleansing enema to prevent straining at stool, which could cause displacement of the isotope. An indwelling catheter is inserted to prevent a distended bladder from coming into contact with the radioactive source.

A variety of applicators have been developed for intrauterine treatment. Applicators are inserted into the endometrial cavity and the vagina in the operating room. When the applicator contains the radioactive material, this is known as *preloading*. In *afterloading*, the applicator is implanted in the operating room but is not loaded with the radioactive material until its correct placement is verified and the patient has been returned to her room.

Radiation exposure to the patient is precisely controlled. The radiation exposure to the physician and other personnel involved in the implantation is reduced when the afterload technique is used. The applicator is secured with vaginal packing and is left in place for 24 to 72 hours.

During the treatment, the patient is placed in a lead-lined private room, on absolute bed rest. She may be turned from side to side. The presence of an intrauterine applicator produces uterine contractions that may require analgesics. The destruction of cells results in a foul-smelling vaginal discharge, and a deodorizer is helpful. Nausea, vomiting, diarrhea, and malaise may develop as a systemic reaction to the radiation.

At the end of the prescribed period of radiation, the radioactive material and the catheter are removed. The patient is allowed off bed rest and is discharged from the hospital when stable. Late complications that may arise include fistulas (vesico-vaginal, uretero-vaginal), cystitis, phlebitis, hemorrhage, and fibrosis. If fibrosis occurs, the vaginal wall becomes smaller in diameter and shorter. Dilation of the vagina through intercourse or the use of sequentially sized dilators may be indicated. The patient is urged to report any unusual symptoms or complaints to her physician. (Brachytherapy and related nursing care are discussed in Chapter 18.)

NURSING MANAGEMENT
CANCERS OF THE FEMALE REPRODUCTIVE SYSTEM

NURSING ASSESSMENT

Malignant tumours of the female reproductive system can be found in the cervix, endometrium, ovaries, vagina, and vulva. The patient with any of these malignant tumours may experience a variety of clinical manifestations, including leukorrhea, other types of vaginal discharge, irregular vaginal bleeding, increase in abdominal pain and pressure, bowel and bladder dysfunction, and vulvar itching and burning. Assessment for these signs and symptoms is an important nursing responsibility.

NURSING DIAGNOSES

Nursing diagnoses for the female patient with cancer of the reproductive system include, but are not limited to, the following:

- *Anxiety* related to *threat to current status, threat of death* (cancer diagnosis)
- *Acute pain* related to *biological injury agent* (enlarging tumour)
- *Disturbed body image* related to *alteration in self-perception* (loss of body part, loss of good health)
- *Ineffective sexuality pattern* related to *insufficient knowledge about alternatives related to sexuality* (physiological limitations, fatigue)
- *Grieving* (related to poor prognosis of advanced disease)

PLANNING

The overall goals are that the patient with cancer of the female reproductive system will (1) actively participate in treatment decisions, (2) achieve satisfactory pain and symptom management, (3) recognize and report problems promptly, (4) maintain preferred lifestyle as long as possible, and (5) continue to practise cancer detection strategies.

NURSING IMPLEMENTATION

HEALTH PROMOTION. Through their contact with women in a variety of settings, nurses can teach women the importance of routine screening for cancers of the reproductive system. Cancer may be prevented when screening reveals precancerous conditions of the vulva, cervix, endometrium, and rarely, the ovaries. Also, routine screening increases the chance that a cancer will be identified in its early stage. When cancer is identified

earlier, treatment can be more conservative and the woman's prognosis improves. Regular pelvic examinations and Pap tests (as indicated) will allow the health care provider to detect lesions on the vulva or any uterine or ovarian irregularities and screen for cervical cancer. Nurses can assist women to view routine cancer screening and vaccination against cervical cancer as important self-care activities.

Educating women about risk factors for cancers of the reproductive system is also important. Limiting sexual activity during adolescence, using condoms, having fewer sexual partners, and not smoking reduce the risk for cervical cancer. When high-risk behaviours are identified, nurses should assist women to identify lifestyle changes to decrease risk.

ACUTE INTERVENTION RELATED TO SURGERY. All patients experience a degree of anxiety when surgery is contemplated, but the prospect of major gynecological surgery increases these concerns. Some women may experience guilt, anger, or embarrassment. Still others may focus on the effect the surgery will have on their reproductive and sexual functions. Some women view the whole process as annoying, whereas others are relieved by the thought of no longer having menstrual periods or becoming pregnant. The nurse should try to understand the patient's fears and concerns. Each patient needs to be assessed as an individual. Being willing to listen can provide considerable psychological support for patients.

Physically, the patient is prepared preoperatively for surgery with the standard perineal or abdominal preparation. A vaginal douche and enemas may be given (based on the surgeon's preference). The bladder should be emptied before the patient is sent to the operating room. An indwelling catheter is sometimes inserted preoperatively (see Chapter 20 for discussion of general preoperative patient care).

Hysterectomy. Postoperatively, the patient who has had a hysterectomy will have an abdominal dressing (abdominal hysterectomy) or a sterile perineal pad (vaginal hysterectomy). (See NCP 56-1 for care of the patient after a total abdominal hysterectomy. See Chapter 22 for potential surgical complications, wound care, and other postoperative care.) The dressing should be observed frequently for any sign of bleeding during the first 8 hours after surgery.

The patient may experience urinary retention postoperatively because of temporary bladder atony resulting from edema or nerve trauma. At times, an indwelling catheter is used for 1 to 2 days postoperatively to maintain constant drainage of the bladder and prevent strain on the suture line. If an indwelling catheter is not used, catheterization may be necessary if the patient has not urinated for 8 hours postoperatively. If residual urine is suspected after the removal of an indwelling catheter, intermittent catheterization is done to prevent bladder infection caused by pooling of urine. Accidental ligation of a ureter is a serious surgical complication. Report any complaint of backache or decreased urine output to the surgeon.

Abdominal distension may develop from the sudden release of pressure on the intestines when a large tumour is removed or from paralytic ileus secondary to anaesthesia and manipulation of the bowel. Food and fluids may be restricted if the patient is nauseated. Early ambulation is encouraged to relieve abdominal pain related to flatus and to prevent abdominal distension.

Special care must be taken to prevent the development of deep venous thrombosis (DVT). Frequent changes of position, avoidance of the high Fowler's position, and avoidance of pressure under the knees minimize stasis and pooling of blood. Leg exercises should be encouraged to promote circulation.

The loss of the uterus may bring about a grief response in some women, similar to any significant personal loss. The ability to bear children may be associated with her perception of womanhood. Grief from this loss is normal. Eliciting the woman's feelings and concerns about her surgery will provide the needed information to give understanding care.

When surgery removes the ovaries as well, women experience surgical menopause. Estrogen is no longer available from the ovaries, so symptoms of estrogen deficiency will arise. To counter this, HT may be initiated in the early postoperative period.

Discharge teaching should prepare the patient for what to expect following surgery (e.g., she will not menstruate). Teaching should include specific activity restrictions. Intercourse should be avoided until the wound is healed (~4 to 6 weeks). If a vaginal hysterectomy is performed, the woman needs to know that there may be a temporary loss of vaginal sensation. She should be reassured that sensation will return in several months.

Physical restrictions are limited for a short time. Heavy lifting should be avoided for 6 to 8 weeks. The patient should be assured that once healing is complete, all previous activity can be resumed.

Salpingectomy and Oophorectomy. Postoperative care of the woman who has undergone removal of a fallopian tube (salpingectomy) or an ovary (oophorectomy) is similar to that for any patient having abdominal surgery. However, if a large ovarian cyst is removed, there may be abdominal distension caused by the sudden release of pressure in the intestines. An abdominal binder may provide relief until the distension subsides.

When both ovaries are removed (bilateral oophorectomy), surgical menopause results. The symptoms are similar to those of regular menopause but may be more severe because of the sudden withdrawal of hormones. Attempts may be made to leave at least a portion of an ovary.

Vulvectomy. Although cancer of the vulva is relatively uncommon, it is important that the nurse recognize the extent of the vulvectomy and the significant effect it is likely to have on the patient's life. An honest, open attitude with the patient and her partner preoperatively can be most helpful in the postoperative period.

After a vulvectomy (see Table 56-13), the patient returns to the unit with a wound in the perineal area extending to the groin. The wound may be covered or left exposed and frequently has drains attached to portable suction (e.g., Hemovac, Jackson-Pratt). Often, a heavy pressure dressing is in place for the first 24 to 48 hours. The wound is cleaned with normal saline solution, twice daily. The normal saline can be applied with an aseptic bulb syringe or a Water Pik machine. A heat lamp or a hair dryer may be used to dry the area. Wound care must be meticulous to prevent infection, which results in delayed healing.

Special attention to bowel and bladder care is needed. A low-residue diet and stool softeners prevent straining and wound contamination. An indwelling catheter is used to provide urinary drainage. Great care is taken not to dislodge the catheter because extensive edema makes its reinsertion difficult. Heavy, taut sutures are often used to close the wounds, resulting in severe discomfort for the patient. In other instances, the wound may be allowed to heal by granulation. Analgesics may be required frequently to control pain. Careful positioning of the patient through the use of strategically placed pillows provides comfort. Anticoagulant therapy to prevent DVT is common.

Because the surgery causes mutilation of the perineal area and the healing process is slow, the patient is likely to become discouraged. Opportunities for the patient to express her feelings

and concerns about the operation should be provided. The patient needs specific instructions in self-care before she is discharged. She should be told to report any unusual odour, fresh bleeding, breakdown of incision, or perineal pain. Home care nursing can benefit the patient during her adjustment period.

Sexual function is often retained. Whether clitoral sensation is retained may be critical to some women, particularly if it was a primary source of orgasmic satisfaction. A discussion of alternative methods of achieving sexual satisfaction may also be indicated.

Pelvic Exenteration. When other forms of therapy fail to control the spread of cancer and no metastases have been found outside of the pelvis, pelvic exenteration may be performed. This radical surgery usually involves removal of the uterus, ovaries, fallopian tubes, vagina, bladder, urethra, and pelvic lymph nodes. In some situations, the descending colon, rectum, and anal canal may also be removed. Candidates for this procedure are selected on the basis of their likelihood of surviving the surgery and their ability to adjust to and accept the resulting limitations.

Postoperative care is similar to that of a patient who has had a radical hysterectomy, an abdominal perineal resection, and an ileostomy or colostomy. The physical, emotional, and social adjustments to life on the part of the woman and her family are great. There are urinary or fecal diversions in the abdominal wall, a reconstructed vagina, and the onset of menopausal symptoms.

The patient's rehabilitative process should keep pace with her acceptance of the situation. Much understanding and support is needed from the nursing staff during a long recovery period. The patient should be gently encouraged to regain her independence. She needs to verbalize her feelings about her altered body structure. Inclusion of the family in the plan of care is important.

The patient will need to return to her health care provider at specified intervals. Early recurrence of the cancer may be identified and treated. At this time, the patient's physical and emotional adjustment to the changes in body image produced by the surgery and her ability to carry out any treatment measures can also be assessed. Additional teaching and counselling can then be provided.

ACUTE INTERVENTION WITH RADIATION THERAPY. When the patient is to receive external radiation, she should be told to urinate immediately before the treatment to minimize radiation exposure to the bladder. She should be advised about radiation adverse effects, including enteritis and cystitis. These are natural reactions to radiotherapy and do not indicate an overdose. The patient should be fully informed of the possible adverse effects and measures to use to reduce their impact.

Nursing management of the patient receiving brachytherapy requires special considerations. Efficient organization of nursing care is essential so that the nurse does not stay in the immediate area of the patient any longer than is necessary to give proper care and attention. No individual nurse should attend the patient for more than 30 minutes per day. The nurse should stay at the foot of the bed or at the entrance to the room to minimize radiation exposure. Visitors need to be told to stay about 2 m away from the bed and limit visits to less than 3 hours a day. The reasons for these precautions must be explained fully to the patient and her visitors. (A more detailed discussion of nursing care of the patient receiving brachytherapy is given in Chapter 18.)

EVALUATION

The expected outcomes are that the patient with cancer of the female reproductive system will do the following:

- Actively participate in treatment decisions
- Achieve satisfactory pain and symptom management
- Recognize and report problems promptly
- Maintain preferred lifestyle as long as possible
- Continue to practise cancer-detection strategies

PROBLEMS WITH PELVIC SUPPORT

The most commonly occurring problems with pelvic support are uterine prolapse, cystocele, and rectocele. Pelvic organ prolapse (POP) is a common condition involving the loss of fibromuscular support of the pelvic viscera, causing the descent or herniation of the pelvic organs into the vagina. The general prevalence of POP is thought to be 41% of parous women, with the prevalence of cystocele varying from 25% to 34%, rectocele varying from 13% to 19%, and uterine prolapse varying from 4% to 14% (Ciangola, Perrone, & Franceschilli, 2014).

Although vaginal birth increases the risk for these problems, these conditions can occur in women who have never experienced childbirth. Obesity, chronic coughing, and straining during bowel movements can increase the likelihood of these problems. The decreased estrogen that normally accompanies perimenopause also reduces some connective tissue support.

UTERINE PROLAPSE

Uterine prolapse is the downward displacement of the uterus into the vaginal canal as a result of impaired pelvic support (Prasad & Alvero, 2013) (Figure 56-11). Prolapse is rated by degrees. In first-degree prolapse, the cervix rests in the lower part of the vagina. Second-degree prolapse means the cervix is at the vaginal opening. Third-degree prolapse means the uterus protrudes through the introitus (entrance to the vaginal canal).

Symptoms vary with the degree of prolapse. The patient may describe a feeling of "something coming down." She may have dyspareunia, a dragging or heavy feeling in the pelvis, backache, and bowel or bladder problems if cystocele or rectocele is also present. Stress incontinence is a common and troubling problem.

When third-degree uterine prolapse occurs, the protruding cervix and vaginal walls are subjected to constant irritation, and tissue changes may occur.

Therapy depends on the degree of prolapse and how much the woman's daily activities have been affected. Pelvic floor muscle training (PFMT) or Kegel exercises may be effective for some women (Hagen & Thakar, 2015) (see Chapter 48, Table 48-19). There is some evidence that proper training and consistent interpersonal support from health care providers increases the effectiveness of PFMT (Hagen & Thakar, 2015). If PFMT does not provide improvement, a pessary may be used. A *pessary* is a device that is placed in the vagina to help support the uterus (Figure 56-12). The pessary can help prevent worsening of the POP, decrease the frequency or severity of symptoms, and delay need for surgical intervention. A wide variety of pessary shapes exist, including rings, arches, and balls. They can be made from materials such as rubber, clear plastic, soft plastic with metal reinforcements, or silicone. When a woman first receives a pessary, she needs instructions for its cleaning and for follow-up. Pessaries that are left in place for long periods are associated with erosion, fistulas, and an increased incidence of vaginal carcinoma.

If more conservative measures are not successful, surgery is indicated. Surgery generally involves a vaginal hysterectomy with anterior and posterior repair of the vagina and the underlying fascia.

CYSTOCELE AND RECTOCELE

Cystocele or anterior wall prolapse occurs when support between the vagina and the bladder is weakened (Figure 56-13). Similarly, a rectocele or posterior wall prolapse results from weakening between the vagina and the rectum (see Figure 56-13). Cystocele and rectocele are common problems, and in many women they are asymptomatic. With large cystoceles, complete emptying of the bladder can be difficult, predisposing women to bladder infections. A woman with a large rectocele may not be able to completely empty her rectum when defecating unless she helps push the stool out by putting her fingers in her vagina.

As with uterine prolapse, pelvic floor muscle training (PFMT) or Kegel exercises (see Chapter 48, Table 48-19) may be used to

FIGURE 56-11 Uterine prolapse. **A,** First-degree prolapse. **B,** Second-degree prolapse. **C,** Third-degree prolapse.

FIGURE 56-12 Various types of pessaries. Source: Huckfinne/Wikimedia Commons.

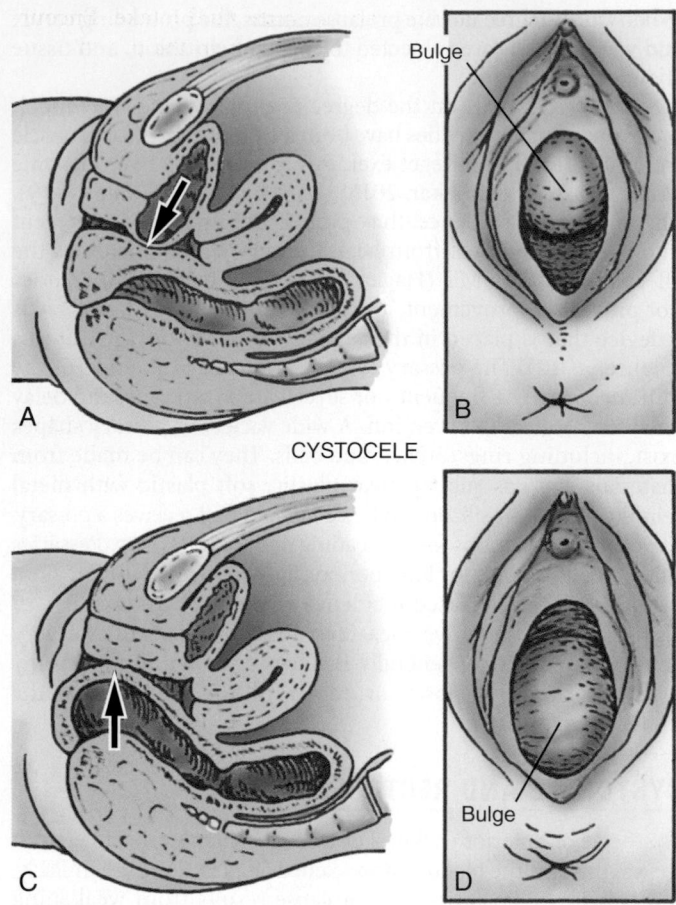

CYSTOCELE

RECTOCELE

FIGURE 56-13 A, Cystocele. Note the bulging of the anterior vaginal wall. The urinary bladder is displaced downward. **B,** The cystocele pushes the anterior vaginal wall downward into the vagina. **C,** Rectocele. Note the bulging of the posterior vaginal wall. **D,** The rectocele pushes the posterior vaginal wall into the vagina. Source: Black, J. M., & Hawks, J. H. (2009). *Medical-surgical nursing: Clinical management for positive outcomes* (8th ed., p. 930, Figure 39-7). St. Louis: Saunders.

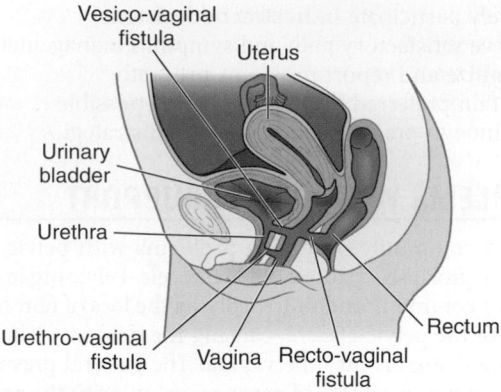

FIGURE 56-14 Common fistulas involving the vagina.

strengthen the weakened perineal muscles if the cystocele or rectocele is not too problematic. A pessary may be helpful for cystoceles. Surgery designed to tighten the vaginal wall is generally the method of treatment. A cystocele is corrected with a procedure called an *anterior colporrhaphy,* whereas a *posterior colporrhaphy* is done for a rectocele. If further surgery is needed to relieve stress incontinence, procedures to support the urethra and restore the proper angle between the urethra and the posterior bladder wall are used.

NURSING MANAGEMENT
PROBLEMS WITH PELVIC SUPPORT

Nurses can assist women to avoid or decrease problems with pelvic support by teaching them how to do PFMT or Kegel exercises. Women of all ages can benefit from these exercises. However, the exercises are especially important following childbirth or whenever women begin to have incontinence. To instruct a patient in this exercise, she should be told to pull in or contract her muscles as if she were trying to stop the flow of urine. She should hold the contraction for several seconds and

then relax. Sets of 5 to 10 contractions each should be done, several times daily.

If vaginal surgery is necessary, the preoperative preparation may include a cleansing douche the morning of surgery. A cathartic and a cleansing enema are usually given when a rectocele repair is scheduled.

In the postoperative period, the goals of care are to prevent wound infection and pressure on the vaginal suture line. This necessitates perineal care at least two to three times per day and after each urination or defecation. An ice pack applied locally may relieve the initial perineal discomfort and swelling. Later, sitz baths may be used.

After an anterior colporrhaphy, often, an indwelling catheter is left in the bladder for 2 to 3 days to allow the local edema to subside. Alternatively, a suprapubic catheter can be inserted at the time of surgery. The catheter keeps the bladder empty, preventing strain on the sutures. The amount of urine left in the bladder after voiding is checked for the first few voidings to make sure it is less than 150 mL. This is checked by intermittent catheterization after the patient has voided (postresidual) or by using a bladder scanner or by opening the valve on the suprapubic catheter. After posterior colporrhaphy, straining at stool is avoided by means of a low-residue diet and daily stool softeners to prevent constipation.

Discharge instructions should be reviewed before the patient leaves the hospital. They include the use of a mild laxative as needed; restriction of heavy lifting and prolonged standing, walking, or sitting; and avoidance of intercourse until the physician gives permission. There may be a temporary loss of vaginal sensation, which can last for several months.

FISTULA

A *fistula* is an abnormal opening between internal organs or between an organ and the exterior of the body (Figure 56-14). Gynecological procedures cause most urinary tract fistulas. Other causes include injury during childbirth and disease processes, such as cancer. Fistulas may develop between the vagina and the bladder, the urethra, the ureter, or the rectum. When *vesico-vaginal* fistulas (between the bladder and the vagina) develop, some urine leaks into the vagina, whereas with recto-vaginal fistulas (between the rectum and the vagina), flatus and feces escape into the vagina. In both instances, excoriation and irritation of the vaginal and vulvar tissues occur and may lead to severe infections.

In addition to wetness, offensive odours may develop, causing embarrassment and severely limiting socialization.

Because small fistulas may heal spontaneously within a matter of months, treatment may not be needed. If the fistula does not heal, surgical excision is required. Inflammation and tissue edema must be eliminated before surgery is attempted. This may involve a wait of up to 6 months for the surgery. The fistulectomy may result in the patient's having an ileal conduit or temporary colostomy.

NURSING MANAGEMENT
FISTULAS

Perineal hygiene is of great importance, both preoperatively and postoperatively. The perineum should be cleansed every 4 hours. Warm sitz baths should be taken three times daily if possible. Perineal pads should be changed frequently. The patient should be encouraged to maintain an adequate fluid intake. Encouragement and reassurance are needed to help the patient cope with her problems.

Postoperatively, nursing care emphasis is on avoidance of stress on the repaired areas and prevention of infection. Care should be taken so that the indwelling catheter, usually in place for 7 to 10 days, is draining at all times. Oral fluids should be urged to provide for internal catheter irrigation. Minimal pressure and strict asepsis are used if catheter irrigation becomes necessary. The first stool after bowel surgery may be purposely delayed to prevent contamination of the wound. Later, stool softeners or mild laxatives may be given. (See Chapter 48 and NCP 48-3, available on the Evolve website, for care of a patient with an ileal conduit and Chapter 45 and NCP 45-4 for care of a patient with a colostomy.) Surgical repair of fistulas is not always effective, even in the best conditions. Therefore, supportive nursing care for the patient and her significant others is especially important.

CASE STUDY

Uterine Prolapse and Vaginal Hysterectomy

Source: Billon Photos/ Shutterstock.

Patient Profile

Thérèse Pelletier is a 62-year-old woman who has developed lower pelvic discomfort and stress incontinence. She has type 2 diabetes and hypertension. She is the mother of four children. A second-degree uterine prolapse is diagnosed. She was treated conservatively with a pessary, but her symptoms did not improve. She comes to the hospital for a vaginal hysterectomy and anteroposterior vaginal repair.

Subjective Data
• Was initially reluctant about surgery
• Concerned about her dyspareunia and her husband's reaction to the surgery
• Concerned she may have uterine cancer
• States that she has stress incontinence and pelvic discomfort

Objective Data
Physical Examination
• Second-degree uterine prolapse on vaginal examination
• Blood pressure (BP) 150/100 mm Hg, pulse 110 beats/min, respirations 20 breaths/min

Laboratory Studies
• Hemoglobin 100 g/L
• Hemoglobin A$_{1c}$ 9%

Postoperative Status
• Returned to room with suprapubic urinary catheter in place
• Vaginal packing in place
• Sequential compression devices on lower extremities
• Patient-controlled analgesia (PCA) pump for pain management

Discussion questions
1. What are the common causes of uterine prolapse?
2. Ms. Pelletier asks about the effect of the surgery on her sexuality. How would the nurse respond?
3. **Priority decision:** What are the priorities of care for Ms. Pelletier?
4. What possible complications (including reasons for their development) can arise after vaginal hysterectomy?
5. What does Ms. Pelletier need to be taught before discharge related to her diabetes and hypertension?
6. **Priority decision:** Based on the assessment data presented, what are the priority nursing diagnoses? Are there any collaborative problems?

*e*volve
Answers are available at *http://evolve.elsevier.com/Canada/Lewis/medsurg.*

REVIEW QUESTIONS

The number of the question corresponds to the same-numbered objective at the beginning of the chapter.

1. A couple will be undergoing infertility assessment. Which of the following facts should the nurse mention when discussing what the couple should expect during the assessment?
   a. Ovulatory studies can help determine tube patency.
   b. A hystero-salpingogram is a common diagnostic study.
   c. The cause will remain unexplained for 40% of couples.
   d. If postcoital studies are normal, tests for infection will be done.

2. Which of the following is the most appropriate question to ask the client with painful menstruation to differentiate primary from secondary dysmenorrhea?
   a. "Does your pain become worse with activity or overexertion?"
   b. "Have you had a recent personal crisis or change in your lifestyle?"
   c. "Is your pain relieved by nonsteroidal anti-inflammatory medications?"
   d. "When in your menstrual history did the pain with your period begin?"

3. The nurse is caring for a client after an ectopic pregnancy was surgically removed. What should the nurse advise the recovering client?
   a. She has an increased risk for salpingitis.
   b. Bed rest must be maintained for 12 hours to assist healing.
   c. Having one ectopic pregnancy increases her risk for another.
   d. Intrauterine devices and infertility treatments should be avoided.

4. The nurse is teaching a client who chooses not to take hormone therapy how to prevent or decrease age-related changes that occur after menopause. Which of the following is the most important self-care measure that the nurse should teach?
   a. Maintaining usual sexual activity
   b. Increasing the intake of dairy products
   c. Performing regular aerobic, weight-bearing exercise
   d. Taking vitamin E and B-complex vitamin supplements

5. The client has a history indicating thick, white, and curdlike vaginal discharge and vulvar pruritus. What are these symptoms most consistent with?
   a. Trichomoniasis
   b. Monilial vaginitis
   c. Bacterial vaginosis
   d. Chlamydial cervicitis

6. Why does the nurse caring for a client with pelvic inflammatory disease place her in a semi-Fowler's position?
   a. To relieve severe pain
   b. To promote drainage to prevent abscesses
   c. To improve circulation and promote healing
   d. To prevent complication of bowel obstruction

7. Which of the following is a nursing responsibility related to the care of the client receiving brachytherapy for endometrial cancer?
   a. Maintaining absolute bed rest
   b. Keeping the client in high Fowler's position
   c. Allowing visitors to stay if they remain 1 m from the bed
   d. Limiting direct nurse-to-client contact to 30 minutes per shift

8. Postoperative goals in caring for the client who has undergone an abdominal hysterectomy include which of the following? *(Select all that apply)*
   a. Monitoring urine output
   b. Changing position frequently
   c. Restricting all food for 24 hours
   d. Observing perineal pad for bleeding
   e. Encouraging leg exercises to promote circulation

9. Which of the following are included in the postoperative nursing care for the woman with a gynecological fistula? *(Select all that apply)*
   a. Ambulation
   b. Bladder training
   c. Warm sitz baths
   d. Perineal hygiene
   e. Use of stool softeners

1. b, 2. d, 3. c, 4. c, 5. b, 6. b, 7. a, 8. a, b, e, 9. c, d.

 evolve

For even more review questions, visit *http://evolve.elsevier.com/Canada/Lewis/medsurg.*

REFERENCES

Akhter, S., Marcus, M., Kerber, R. A., et al. (2016). The impact of periconceptional maternal stress on fecundability. *Annals of Epidemiology, 26*(10), 710–716e7. doi:10.1016/j.annepidem.2016.07.015.

American Cancer Society. (2014). *Tamoxifen and ralozifene.* Retrieved from *http://www.cancer.org/cancer/breastcancer/moreinformation/medicinestoreducebreastcancer/medicines-to-reduce-breast-cancer-risk-tamoxifen-raloxifene.*

Androgen Excess and PCOS Society [AE-PCOS]. (2012). *Polycystic ovary syndrome.* Retrieved from *http://www.ae-society.org/poly_syndrome.*

Apte, G., Nelson, P., Brisme, J. M., et al. (2012). Chronic female pelvic pain. Part 1: Clinical pathoanatomy and examination of the pelvic region. *Pain Practice, 12*(2), 88–110. doi:10.1111/j.1533-2500.2011.00465.x.

Arora, V., & Quinn, M. A. (2012). Endometrial cancer. *Best Practice & Research. Clinical Obstetrics & Gynaecology, 26*(3), 311–324. doi:10.1016/j.bpobgyn.2011.12.007.

Biggs, W. S., & Demuth, R. H. (2011). Premenstrual syndrome and premenstrual dysphoric disorder. *American Family Physician, 84*(8), 918–924.

Brunham, R. C., Gottlieb, S. L., & Paavonen, J. (2015). Pelvic inflammatory disease. *The New England Journal of Medicine, 372*(21), 2039–2048. doi:10.1056/NEJMra1411426.

Buys, S., Partridge, E., Black, A., et al. (2011). Effect of screening on ovarian cancer mortality: The prostate, lung, colorectal and ovarian (PLCO) cancer screening randomized controlled trial. *JAMA: The Journal of the American Medical Association, 305*(22), 2295–2303. doi:10.1001/jama.2011.766.

Canadian Cancer Society (CCS). (2016a). *Screening for cervical cancer.* Retrieved from *http://www.cancer.ca/en/cancer-information/cancer-type/cervical/screening/?region=on.*

Canadian Cancer Society (CCS). (2016b). *HPV vaccines.* Retrieved from *http://www.cancer.ca/en/cancer-information/cancer-101/what-is-a-risk-factor/viruses-bacteria-and-other-infectious-agents/hpv-vaccines/?region=on.*

Canadian Cancer Society (CCS). (2017). *Canadian cancer statistics 2017.* Retrieved from *http://www.cancer.ca/~/media/cancer.ca/CW/cancer%20information/cancer%20101/Canadian%20cancer%20statistics/Canadian-Cancer-Statistics-2017-EN.pdf?la=en.*

Canadian Cancer Society's Advisory Committee on Cancer Statistics. (2015). *Canadian Cancer Statistics 2015.* Toronto, ON: Canadian Cancer Society. Retrieved from *http://www.cancer.ca/en/cancer-information/cancer-type/cervical/statistics/?region=on.*

Canadian Institute for Health Information [CIHI]. (2014). *Induced abortions reported in Canada in 2014.* Retrieved from *https://www.cihi.ca/sites/default/files/document/induced_abortion_can_2014_en_web.xlsx.*

Canadian Nurses Association [CNA]. (2017). *Code of ethics for registered nurses.* Retrieved from *https://www.cna-aiic.ca/html/en/Code-of-Ethics-2017-Edition/files/assets/basic-html/page-1.html#.*

Ciangola, C. I., Perrone, F., & Franceschilli, L. (2014). Epidemiology and prevalence of pelvic floor disorders. In A. L. Gaspari & P. Sileri (Eds.), *Pelvic floor disorders: Surgical approach.* Milan, Italy: Springer.

Davidson, M. R., London, M. L., & Ladewig, P. A. (2014). *Maternal-newborn nursing and women's health across the lifespan* (10th ed.). Upper Saddle River, NJ: Pearson Prentice Hall.

de Villiers, T. J., Gass, M. L., Haines, C. J., et al. (2013). Global consensus statement on menopausal hormone therapy.

Climacteric: The Journal of the International Menopause Society, 16(2), 203–204. doi:10.3109/13697137.2013.771520.

Donegan, C. (2012). Caring for women with endometriosis. *Practice Nurse,* 42(4), 24–28.

Givens, M., & Lipscomb, G. (2012). Diagnosis of ectopic pregnancy. *Clinical Obstetrics and Gynecology,* 55(2), 387–394. doi:10.1097/GRF.0b013e31824e3618.

Government of Canada. (2013). *Fertility.* Retrieved from *http:// healthycanadians.gc.ca/healthy-living-vie-saine/pregnancy-grossesse/ fertility-fertilite/fert-eng.php.*

Government of Canada. (2015). *Menstrual tampons: Toxic shock syndrome (TSS).* Retrieved from *http://healthycanadians.gc.ca/ drugs-products-medicaments-produits/buying-using-achat -utilisation/products-canada-produits/drugs-devices-medicaments -instruments/tampons-eng.php.*

Gupta, J., Sinha, A., Lumsden, M., et al. (2012). Uterine artery embolization for symptomatic uterine fibroids. *The Cochrane Database of Systematic Reviews,* No. 5, Article CD005073. doi:10.1002/14651858.CD005073.pub3. Retrieved from *http:// www.cochrane.org/CD005073/MENSTR_uterine-artery -embolization-for-symptomatic-uterine-fibroids.*

Hagen, S., & Thakar, R. (2015). Conservative management of pelvic organ prolapse. *Obstetrics, Gynaecology and Reproductive Medicine,* 25(4), 91–95. *http://dx.doi.org/10.1016/j.ogrm.2015 .01.006.*

Im, E., Ko, Y., Hwang, H., et al. (2012). "Symptom-specific or holistic": Menopausal symptom management. *Health Care for Women International,* 33(6), 575–592. doi:10.1080/07399332 .2011.646371.

Jelovac, D., & Armstrong, D. K. (2011). Recent progress in the diagnosis and treatment of ovarian cancer. *CA: A Cancer Journal for Clinicians,* 61(3), 183–203. doi:10.3322/caac.20113.

Kaunitz, A. M., & Manson, F. E. (2015). Management of menopausal symptoms. *Obstetrics and Gynecology,* 126(4), 859–876. doi:10.1097/AOG.0000000000001058.

Koehler, C., Gottschalk, E., Chiantera, V., et al. (2013). From laparoscopic assisted radical vaginal hysterectomy to vaginal assisted laparoscopic radical hysterectomy. *BJOG: An International Journal of Obstetrics and Gynaecology,* 119(2), 254–262. doi:10.1111/j.1471-0528.2011.03202.x.

Lentz, G. (2013). Premenstrual syndrome and premenstrual dysphoric disorder. In G. M. Lentz, R. Lobo, D. Gershenson, et al. (Eds.), *Comprehensive gynecology* (6th ed.). St Louis: Mosby.

Lobo, R. (2013). Hyperandrogenism. In G. M. Lentz, R. Lobo, D. Gershenson, et al. (Eds.), *Comprehensive gynecology* (6th ed.). St Louis: Mosby.

Maine, D., Hurlburt, S., & Greeson, D. (2011). Cervical cancer prevention in the 21st century: Cost is not the only issue. *American Journal of Public Health,* 101(9), 1549–1555. doi:10.2105/AJPH.2011.300204.

Mayo Clinic. (2013). *Endometriosis: Causes.* Retrieved from *http:// www.mayoclinic.org/diseases-conditions/endometriosis/basics/ causes/con-20013968.*

McQueen, A. (2011). Ectopic pregnancy: Risk factors, diagnostic procedures and treatment. *Nursing Standard,* 25(37), 49–56. doi:10.7748/ns2011.05.25.37.49.c8521.

Munro, M. (2011). Uterine leiomyomas, current concepts: Pathogenesis, impact on reproductive health, and medical, procedural, and surgical management. *Obstetrics and Gynecology Clinics of North America,* 38(4), 703–731. doi:10.1016/j.ogc.2011.09.006.

Nachtigall, R., MacDougall, K., Davis, A., et al. (2012). Expensive but worth it: Older parents' attitudes and opinions about the costs and insurance coverage for in vitro fertilization. *Fertility and Sterility,* 97(1), 82–87. doi:10.1016/j.fertnstert.2011.10.019.

National Advisory Committee on Immunization [NACI]. (2012). *Update on Human Papillomavirus (HPV) vaccines.* Retrieved from *http://www.phac-aspc.gc.ca/publicat/ccdr-rmtc/12vol38/acs-dcc-1/ index-eng.php.*

National Institute for Child Health and Development [NICHD]. (2013). *How many people are affected by or at risk for endometriosis?* Retrieved from *https://www.nichd.nih.gov/health/ topics/endometri/conditioninfo/Pages/at-risk.aspx.*

National Institutes of Health [NIH]. (2015). *Menopausal hormone therapy information—Women's health initiative hormone therapy study.* Retrieved from *http://www.nih.gov/health-information/ menopausal-hormone-therapy-information.*

National Institutes of Health [NIH]—National Cancer Institute. (2014). *A snapshot of cervical cancer.* Retrieved from *http:// www.cancer.gov/research/progress/snapshots/cervical.*

National Library of Medicine (NLM). (2015). *Premenstrual dysphoric disorder (PMDD).* Retrieved from *http://www.ncbi.nlm.nih.gov/ pubmedhealth/PMHT0024721/.*

Nelson, H. D., Walker, M., Zakher, B., et al. (2012). *Menopausal hormone therapy for the primary prevention of chronic conditions: A systematic review to update the U.S. Preventive Services Task Force Recommendations,* AHRQ Pub No 12-05168-EF-1, Washington, DC: Agency for Healthcare Research and Quality, Department of Health and Human Services.

Prasad, A., & Alvero, R. (2013). Uterine prolapse. In F. Ferri (Ed.), *Ferri's clinical advisor 2013.* Philadelphia: Mosby.

Public Health Agency of Canada [PHAC]. (2017 on website now). *Human papillomavirus (HPV)—Prevention and HPV vaccines: Questions and answers—Who should get the vaccine?* Retrieved from *http://www.phac-aspc.gc.ca/std-mts/hpv-vph/hpv-vph-vaccine -eng.php.*

Public Health Agency of Canada [PHAC]. (2013). *Pelvic inflammatory disease (PID). Canadian guidelines on sexually transmitted infections. Section 4—Management and treatment of specific syndromes.* Retrieved from *http://www.phac-aspc.gc.ca/ std-mts/sti-its/cgsti-ldcits/section-4-4-eng.php.*

Roa, S. (2011). Menorrhagia. *Obstetrics, Gynaecology and Reproductive Medicine,* 21(9), 254–256. doi:10.1016/j .ogrm.2011.06.003.

Roush, K. (2012). Managing menopausal symptoms. *The American Journal of Nursing,* 112(6), 28–35. doi:10.1097/01.NAJ.0000415120 .76982.7a.

Sabanegh, E., & Agarwal, A. (2011). Definition and demographics of infertility. In A. Wien (Ed.), *Campbell-Walsh urology* (10th ed.). St Louis: Saunders.

Sabourin, J. N., & Burnett, M. (2012). A review of therapeutic abortions and related areas of concern in Canada. *Journal of Obstetrics and Gynaecology Canada,* 34(6), 532–542.

Schmidt, L., Sobotka, T., Bentzen, B., et al. (2012). Demographic and medical consequences of the postponement of parenthood. *Human Reproduction Update,* 18(1), 29–43. doi:10.1093/humupd/ dmr040.

Shin, J., & Howard, F. (2011). Management of chronic pelvic pain. *Current Pain and Headache Reports,* 15(5), 377–385. doi:10.1007/ s11916-011-0204-4.

Sitka, C. (2012). Methotrexate: The pharmacology behind medical treatment for ectopic pregnancy. *Clinical Obstetrics and Gynecology,* 55(2), 433–439. doi:10.1097/GRF.0b013e3182510a35.

Sood, R., Faubion, S. S., Kuhle, C. L., et al. (2014). Prescribing menopausal hormone therapy: An evidence-based approach.

International Journal of Women's Health [Electronic Resource],
6, 47–57. doi:10.2147/IJWH.S38342.

Stiles, M., Redmer, J., Paddock, E., et al. (2012). Gynecologic issues
in geriatric women. *Journal of Women's Health, 21*(1), 4–6.
doi:10.1089/jwh.2011.2803.

Stuenkel, C. A., Gass, M. L., Manson, J. E., et al. (2012). A decade
after the Women's Health Initiative—the experts do agree.
Menopause (New York, N.Y.), 19(8), 846–847. doi:10.1097/
gme.0b013e31826226f2.

Toulis, K., Goulis, D., Mintziori, G., et al. (2011). Meta-analysis of
cardiovascular disease risk markers in women with polycystic
ovary syndrome. *Human Reproduction Update, 17*(6), 741–760.
doi:10.1093/humupd/dmr025.

University of California–Berkeley. (2011). *Living with hot flashes.*
Retrieved from *http://www.berkeleywellness.com/self-care/
preventive-care/over-counter-products/article/living-hot-flashes.*

Viswanathan, A. N. (2012). Advances in the use of radiation for
gynecologic cancers. *Hematology/Oncology Clinics of North
America, 26*(1), 157–168. doi:10.1016/j.hoc.2011.11.004.

Williams, D., & Pridjian, G. (2011). Obstetrics. In R. Rakel & D.
Rakel (Eds.), *Textbook of family medicine* (8th ed.). St Louis:
Saunders.

RESOURCES

Canadian Cancer Society
http://www.cancer.ca

Canadian Fertility and Andrology Society
http://www.cfas.ca/

endometriosisinfo.ca: The facts of endometriosis
http://endometriosisinfo.ca/index_e.aspx

myfertility.ca
http://www.myfertility.ca/

National Ovarian Cancer Coalition (NOCC)
http://www.ovarian.org/about_us.php

Ovarian Cancer Canada
http://www.ovariancanada.org

SexualityandU.ca
http://www.sexualityandu.ca/

Society of Obstetricians and Gynaecologists of Canada
https://sogc.org/index.html

Women's Health Matters
http://www.womenshealthmatters.ca/

American Cancer Society
http://www.cancer.org

American Congress of Obstetricians and Gynecologists
http://www.acog.org

American Urological Association
http://www.auanet.org

**Hysterectomy Educational Resources and Services (HERS)
Foundation**
http://www.hersfoundation.com/

North American Menopause Society
http://www.menopause.org

**Sexuality Information and Education Council of the United
States (SIECUS)**
http://www.siecus.org

For additional Internet resources, see the website for this book
at *http://evolve.elsevier.com/Canada/Lewis/medsurg.*

Nursing Management
Male Reproductive Problems

Written by: Susanne A. Quallich
Adapted by: Shelley L. Cobbett

evolve WEBSITE

http://evolve.elsevier.com/Canada/Lewis/medsurg

- Review Questions (Online Only)
- Key Points
- Answer Guidelines for Case Study

- Student Case Study
  - Benign Prostatic Hyperplasia
- Customizable Nursing Care Plan
  - Prostate Surgery

- Conceptual Care Map Creator
- Audio Glossary
- Content Updates

LEARNING OBJECTIVES

1. Describe the pathophysiology, clinical manifestations, and collaborative care of benign prostatic hyperplasia.
2. Discuss the nursing management of benign prostatic hyperplasia.
3. Describe the pathophysiology, clinical manifestations, and collaborative care of prostate cancer.
4. Explain the nursing management of prostate cancer.
5. Specify the pathophysiology, clinical manifestations, and nursing and collaborative management of prostatitis and problems of the penis and scrotum.

6. Explain the clinical manifestations and collaborative care of testicular cancer.
7. Describe the pathophysiology, clinical manifestations, and nursing and collaborative management of problems related to male sexual function.
8. Summarize the psychological and emotional implications related to male reproductive problems.

KEY TERMS

benign prostatic hyperplasia (BPH), p. 1421
epididymitis, p. 1436
epispadias, p. 1436
erectile dysfunction (ED), p. 1439
hydrocele, p. 1437
hypospadias, p. 1436

orchitis, p. 1437
paraphimosis, p. 1436
phimosis, p. 1436
prostate-specific antigen (PSA), p. 1423
prostatitis, p. 1434
radical prostatectomy, p. 1430

spermatocele, p. 1437
testicular torsion, p. 1438
transurethral resection of the prostate (TURP), p. 1426
varicocele, p. 1437
vasectomy, p. 1439

Problems of the male reproductive system can involve a variety of structures, including the prostate, the penis, the urethra, the ejaculatory duct, the scrotum, the testes, the epididymis, the vas deferens, and the rectum (Figure 57-1).

PROBLEMS OF THE PROSTATE GLAND

BENIGN PROSTATIC HYPERPLASIA

Benign prostatic hyperplasia (BPH) is a benign, noninflammatory enlargement of the prostate gland. It is the most common urological problem in male adults (National Institute of Health, 2014). About 50% of all men in their lifetime will develop BPH. Of these men, almost half of them will have bothersome lower urinary tract symptoms (Rosenberg, Witt, Miner, et al., 2014).

Research is not clear about whether having BPH leads to an increased risk of developing prostate cancer (Weight, Kim, Jacobson, et al., 2013; Ørsted & Bojesen, 2013).

Etiology and Pathophysiology

Although the cause of BPH is not completely understood, it is thought that BPH results from hormonal changes associated with the aging process (Rosenberg, Witt, Miner, et al., 2014). Possible causes include excessive accumulation of dihydroxytestosterone (DHT) (the principal intraprostatic androgen), stimulation by estrogen, and local growth hormone action.

Typically, BPH develops in the inner part of the prostate. (Prostate cancer is most likely to develop in the outer part.) This enlargement gradually compresses the urethra, eventually leading to partial or complete obstruction (Figure 57-2). The

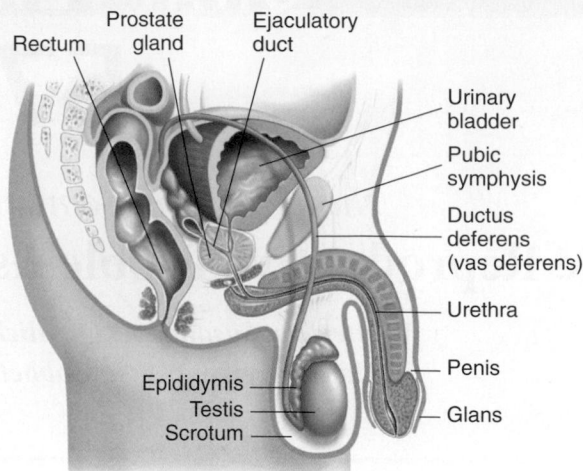

FIGURE 57-1 Areas of the male reproductive system in which problems are likely to develop.

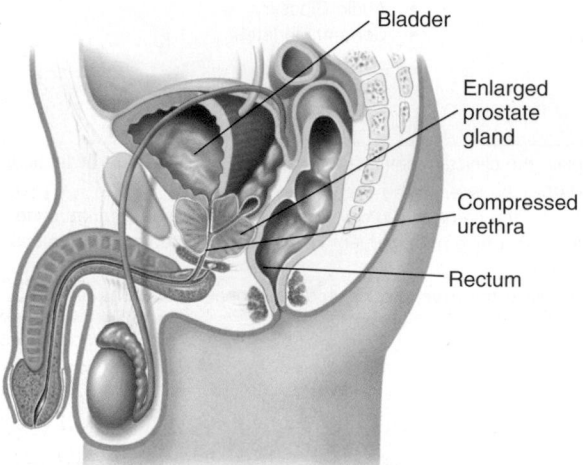

FIGURE 57-2 Benign prostatic hyperplasia. The enlarged prostate compresses the urethra.

FIGURE 57-3 Views of the prostate by cystoscopy. **A,** Normal appearance. **B,** Moderate benign prostatic hyperplasia with urethral obstruction. Source: Townsend, C. M., Beauchamp, R. D., Evers, B. M., et al. (2012). *Sabiston textbook of surgery* (19th ed.). Philadelphia: Saunders.

compression of the urethra ultimately leads to the development of clinical symptoms. There is no direct relationship between the size of the prostate and the severity of symptoms or degree of obstruction. The location of the enlargement is most significant in the development of obstructive symptoms (Figure 57-3). For example, it is possible for mild hyperplasia to cause severe obstruction; likewise, it is possible for extreme hyperplasia to cause few obstructive symptoms.

Risk factors for BPH include aging, obesity (in particular, large waist circumference), lack of physical activity, smoking, and diabetes (Trumble, Stieglitz, Eid Rodriguez, et al., 2015). A positive family history of BPH in first-degree relatives may also be a risk factor.

Clinical Manifestations

Manifestations of BPH mainly result from urinary obstruction. Symptoms are usually gradual in onset and may not be noticed until prostatic enlargement has been present for some time. Early symptoms are usually minimal because the bladder can compensate for a small amount of resistance to urine flow. The

symptoms gradually worsen as the degree of urethral obstruction increases.

Symptoms can be divided into two groups: obstructive and irritative. *Obstructive symptoms* include a decrease in the calibre and force of the urinary stream, difficulty in initiating voiding, intermittency (stopping and starting stream several times while voiding), and dribbling at the end of urination. *Irritative symptoms*, which include urinary frequency, urgency, dysuria, bladder pain, nocturia, and incontinence, are associated with inflammation or infection. Nocturia is often the first symptom that the patient notices. The American Urological Association (AUA) Symptom Index for BPH (Table 57-1) is a widely used tool to assess voiding symptoms associated with obstruction (Barry, Fowler, O'Leary, et al., 1992). Although this tool is not diagnostic, it is useful in determining the degree of symptoms. Higher scores on this tool indicate greater symptom severity.

Complications

Complications of urinary obstruction are relatively uncommon in BPH. Acute urinary retention is a complication that is manifested by the sudden and painful inability to urinate. Treatment involves the insertion of a catheter to drain the bladder. Surgery may also be indicated.

Another common complication is urinary tract infection (UTI) and, potentially, sepsis secondary to UTI. Incomplete bladder emptying (associated with partial obstruction) results in residual urine, providing a favourable environment for bacterial growth. Calculi may develop in the bladder because of the alkalinization of the residual urine. Although bladder stones are more common in men with BPH, the risk for renal calculi is not significantly increased. Additional complications include renal failure caused by *hydronephrosis* (distension of the pelvis and the calyces of the kidney by urine that cannot flow through the ureter to the bladder), pyelonephritis, and bladder damage if treatment for acute urinary retention is delayed.

Diagnostic Studies

The primary methods used to diagnose BPH include a history and physical examination (See Table 57-2). The prostate can be palpated by digital rectal examination (DRE) to estimate its size, symmetry, and consistency. In BPH, the prostate is symmetrically enlarged, firm, and smooth.

Additional diagnostic tests may be indicated, depending on the type and the severity of symptoms and clinical findings. A urinalysis with culture is routinely done to determine the presence

TABLE 57-1 AMERICAN UROLOGICAL ASSOCIATION SYMPTOM INDEX TO DETERMINE SEVERITY OF PROSTATIC PROBLEMS

	American Urological Association (AUA) Symptom Score*					
	(Circle one number on each line.)					
Questions to Be Answered	**Not at All**	**Less Than 1 Time in 5**	**Less Than Half the Time**	**About Half the Time**	**More Than Half the Time**	**Almost Always**
Over the past month:	0	1	2	3	4	5
1. How often have you had a sensation of not emptying your bladder completely after you finished urinating?						
2. How often have you had to urinate again <2 hr after you finished urinating?	0	1	2	3	4	5
3. How often have you found you stopped and started again several times when you urinated?	0	1	2	3	4	5
4. How often have you found it difficult to postpone urination?	0	1	2	3	4	5
5. How often have you had a weak urinary stream?	0	1	2	3	4	5
6. How often have you had to push or strain to begin urination?	0	1	2	3	4	5
7. How many times did you most typically get up to urinate from the time you went to bed at night until the time you got up in the morning?	0 (None)	1 (1 time)	2 (2 times)	3 (3 times)	4 (4 times)	5 (≥5 times)
Sum of circled numbers (AUA Symptom Score):* _____						

*Score is interpreted as 0–7, mild; 8–19, moderate; 20–35, severe.

Source: Reprinted from *Journal of Urology*, 148(5), Barry, M. J., Fowler, F. J., Jr., O'Leary, M. P., et al., The American Urological Association symptom index for benign prostatic hyperplasia, pp. 1549–1557, Copyright 1992, with permission from Elsevier.

TABLE 57-2 COLLABORATIVE CARE

Benign Prostatic Hyperplasia

Diagnostic
- History and physical examination
- Digital rectal examination (DRE)
- Urinalysis with culture
- Serum creatinine
- Prostate-specific antigen (PSA)
- Postvoid residual
- Uroflowmetry
- Transrectal ultrasonography (TRUS)
- Cysto-urethroscopy

Collaborative Therapy
- Conservative therapy (active surveillance or "watchful waiting")

Drug Therapy
- 5α-Reductase inhibitors
- α-Adrenergic receptor blockers
- Erectogenic drugs

Invasive Therapy*
- Open prostatectomy
- Transurethral incision of the prostate (TUIP)
- Transurethral resection of the prostate (TURP)

Minimally Invasive Therapy*
- Intraprostatic urethral stents
- Laser prostatectomy
- Transurethral electrovaporization of the prostate (TUVP)
- Transurethral microwave thermotherapy (TUMT)
- Transurethral needle ablation (TUNA)

*See Table 57-3.

of infection. Bacteria, white blood cells, or microscopic hematuria indicate infection or inflammation.

A blood test for **prostate-specific antigen (PSA)**, a glycoprotein found only in the epithelial cells of the prostate, may be done to rule out prostate cancer. Elevated PSA levels indicate a pathological condition of the prostate, although not necessarily prostate cancer. PSA levels may be slightly elevated in patients with BPH. Serum creatinine levels may be ordered to rule out

renal insufficiency. Because symptoms of BPH are similar to those of a neurogenic bladder, a neurological examination may also be performed.

In patients with an abnormal DRE and elevated PSA, a *transrectal ultrasonography* (TRUS) scan is typically indicated. This examination allows for accurate assessment of prostate size and is helpful in differentiating BPH from prostate cancer. Biopsies can be taken during the ultrasonography procedure. *Uroflowmetry*, a study that measures the volume of urine expelled from the bladder per second, is helpful in determining the extent of urethral blockage and thus the type of treatment needed. Postvoid residual urine volume is often measured to determine the degree of urine flow obstruction. *Cysto-urethroscopy*, a procedure allowing internal visualization of the urethra and the bladder, is performed if the diagnosis is uncertain and in patients scheduled for prostatectomy.

Collaborative Care

The goals of collaborative care are to restore bladder drainage, relieve the patient's symptoms, and prevent or treat the complications of BPH. Treatment is generally based on the degree to which the symptoms bother the patient or the presence of complications rather than the size of the prostate. Alternatives to surgical intervention for some patients now include drug therapy and minimally invasive procedures, for example, holmium laser enucleation (Lingeman, 2011).

The most conservative initial treatment for BPH is referred to as *active surveillance* or *watchful waiting*. When there are no symptoms or only mild ones (AUA symptom scores <7), a wait-and-see approach is taken. Because symptoms may come and go, a conservative approach has value. Dietary changes (decreasing intake of caffeine, artificial sweeteners, and spicy or acidic foods), avoiding medications such as decongestants and anticholinergics, and restricting evening fluid intake may improve symptoms. A timed voiding schedule may reduce or eliminate symptoms, thus negating the need for further intervention. If the patient begins to have signs or symptoms that indicate an increase in obstruction, further treatment is indicated.

Drug Therapy. Drugs that have been used to treat BPH with variable degrees of success include 5α-reductase inhibitors and α-adrenergic receptor blockers. Combination therapy has been shown to be more effective in reducing symptoms than using one medication alone (Ismaila et al., 2013).

5α-Reductase Inhibitors. These drugs work by reducing the size of the prostate gland. Finasteride (Proscar) blocks the enzyme 5α-reductase, which is necessary for the conversion of testosterone to DHT, the principal intraprostatic androgen. This medication causes regression of hyperplastic tissue through suppression of androgens. Finasteride is an appropriate treatment option for individuals who score between 12 and 26 on the AUA Symptom Index (see Table 57-1). Although more than 50% of men who are treated with the medication show symptom improvement, it takes about 6 months to be effective, and the medication must be taken on a continuous basis to maintain therapeutic results. Serum PSA levels decrease by almost 50% when taking finasteride. Therefore, PSA levels should be doubled when comparing the patient's current levels to premedication levels.

Dutasteride (Avodart) is a dual inhibitor of 5α-reductase types 1 and 2 isoenzymes. (Finasteride inhibits only the type 2 isoenzyme.) The combination of a 5α-reductase inhibitor (dutasteride) and an α-adrenergic receptor blocker (tamsulosin) is now available in a single oral medication (Jalyn). Adverse effects of 5α-reductase inhibitors include decreased libido, decreased volume of ejaculate, and erectile dysfunction (ED).

> **DRUG ALERT—Finasteride (Proscar)**
> - Patient should be aware of the increased risk for orthostatic hypotension with concomitant use of ED drugs.
> - Women who may be or are pregnant should not handle finasteride tablets due to potential risk to male fetus (anomaly).

α-Adrenergic Receptor Blockers. α-Adrenergic receptor blockers are another drug treatment option for BPH. These agents selectively block $α_1$-adrenergic receptors, which are abundant in the prostate and are increased in hyperplastic prostate tissue. Although α-adrenergic blockers are more commonly used for treatment of hypertension, these drugs promote smooth muscle relaxation in the prostate, facilitating urinary flow through the urethra. These agents demonstrate a 50% to 60% efficacy in improvement of symptoms, which occurs within 2 to 3 weeks.

Several α-adrenergic blockers, including silodosin (Rapaflo), alfuzosin (Xatral), prazosin, doxazosin (Cardura), terazosin, and tamsulosin, are currently being used. Adverse effects include postural hypotension, dizziness, fatigue, retrograde ejaculation, and nasal congestion. It must be pointed out that, although these drugs offer symptomatic relief of BPH, they do not treat hyperplasia.

Erectogenic Drugs. Tadalafil (Cialis) has been used in men who have symptoms of BPH alone or in combination with ED. The drug has shown effectiveness in reducing symptoms for both these conditions (Roehrborn, Casabé, Glina, et al., 2015) (see "Erectile Dysfunction" later in this chapter).

Herbal Therapy. Herbal extracts have been used in the management of lower urinary symptoms associated with BPH. In particular, some patients take plant extracts such as saw palmetto (*Serenoa repens*). However, research indicates that saw palmetto has no benefit over a placebo (Barry, Cantor, Roehrborn, et al., 2013; Andriole, McCullum-Hill, Sandhu, et al., 2013). ProstateEZE Max, an oral herbal preparation containing *Cucurbita*

🌿 COMPLEMENTARY & ALTERNATIVE THERAPIES

ProstateEZE Max

Clinical Uses
Benign prostatic hyperplasia (BPH); physical symptoms of BPH

Effects
Appears to have a significant positive effect on the physical symptoms of BPH including a decrease in urinary frequency, urgency, dysuria, and nocturia.

Nursing Implications
Generally well tolerated. No adverse reactions were reported in this trial. No known drug interactions. Patient should be advised to consult a physician for the correct diagnosis of BPH.

Source: Coulson, S., Rao, A., Beck, S., et al. (2013). A phase II randomised double-blind placebo-controlled clinical trial investigating the efficacy and safety of ProstateEZE Max: A herbal medicine preparation for the management of symptoms of benign prostatic hypertrophy. *Complementary Therapies in Medicine, 21*(3), 172–179. doi:10.1016/j.ctim.2013.01.007

pepo, Epilobium parviflorum, lycopene, *Pygeum africanum*, and *Serenoa repens*, is being considered in the management of symptoms of BPH (see the Complementary & Alternative Therapies box on ProstateEZE Max).

Minimally Invasive Therapy. Minimally invasive therapies are becoming more common as an alternative to watchful waiting and invasive treatment (Table 57-3). They generally do not require hospitalization or catheterization and are associated with few adverse events.

Transurethral Microwave Thermotherapy. *Transurethral microwave thermotherapy* (TUMT) is an outpatient procedure that involves the delivery of microwaves directly to the prostate through a transurethral probe to raise the temperature of the prostate tissue to about 45°C. The heat causes death of tissue, thus relieving the obstruction. A rectal temperature probe is used during the procedure to ensure that the temperature is kept below 43.5°C to prevent rectal tissue damage. The procedure takes about 90 minutes.

Postoperative urinary retention is a common complication. Thus the patient is generally sent home with an in-dwelling catheter for 2 to 7 days to maintain urinary flow and to facilitate the passing of small clots or necrotic tissue. Antibiotics, pain medication, and bladder antispasmodic medications are used to treat and prevent postprocedure problems. The procedure is not appropriate for men with rectal problems. Anticoagulant therapy should be stopped 10 days before treatment. Mild adverse effects include occasional problems of bladder spasm, hematuria, dysuria, and retention.

Transurethral Needle Ablation. *Transurethral needle ablation* (TUNA) is another procedure that increases the temperature of prostate tissue, causing localized necrosis. TUNA differs from TUMT in that low-wave radiofrequency is used to heat the prostate. Only prostate tissue in direct contact with the needle is affected, thus allowing greater precision in removal of the target tissue. The extent of tissue removed by this process is determined by the amount of tissue contact (needle length), amount of energy delivered, and duration of treatment. The majority of the patients undergoing TUNA have an improvement in symptoms.

This procedure is performed in an outpatient unit or physician's office using local anaesthesia and IV or oral sedation. The TUNA procedure lasts approximately 30 minutes. The patient typically experiences little pain with an early return to regular activities.

TABLE 57-3   TREATMENT FOR BENIGN PROSTATIC HYPERPLASIA

Description	Advantages	Disadvantages
Minimally Invasive		
Transurethral Microwave Thermotherapy (TUMT)		
Use of microwave radiating heat to produce coagulative necrosis of the prostate	Outpatient procedure Erectile dysfunction, urinary incontinence, and retrograde ejaculation are rare	Potential for damage to surrounding tissue Urinary catheter needed after procedure
Transurethral Needle Ablation (TUNA)		
Low-wave radiofrequency used to heat the prostate, causing necrosis	Outpatient procedure Erectile dysfunction, urinary incontinence, and retrograde ejaculation are rare Precise delivery of heat to desired area Very little pain experienced	Urinary retention common Irritative voiding symptoms Hematuria
Laser Prostatectomy		
Use of a laser beam to cut or destroy part of the prostate Techniques available: • Visual laser ablation of prostate (VLAP) • Contact laser • Photovaporization of prostate (PVP) • Interstitial laser coagulation (ILC)	Short procedure Comparable results to TURP Minimal bleeding Fast recovery time Rapid symptom improvement Very effective	Catheter (up to 7 days) needed after procedure due to edema and urinary retention Delayed sloughing of tissue Takes several weeks to reach optimal effect Retrograde ejaculation
Transurethral Electrovaporization of Prostate (TUVP)		
Electrosurgical vaporization and desiccation used together to destroy prostatic tissue	Minimal risks Minimal bleeding and sloughing	Retrograde ejaculation Intermittent hematuria
Intraprostatic Urethral Stents		
Insertion of self-expandable metallic stent into the urethra, where enlarged area of prostate occurs	Safe and effective Low risk	Stent may move Long-term effect unknown
Invasive (Surgery)		
Transurethral Resection of Prostate (TURP)		
Use of excision and cauterization to remove prostate tissue cystoscopically Remains the standard for treatment of BPH	Erectile dysfunction unlikely	Bleeding Retrograde ejaculation
Transurethral Incision of Prostate (TUIP)		
Involves transurethral incisions into prostatic tissue to relieve obstruction Effective for men with small to moderate prostates	Outpatient procedure Minimal complications Low occurrence of erectile dysfunction or retrograde ejaculation	Urinary catheter needed after procedure
Open Prostatectomy		
Surgery of choice for men with large prostates, bladder damage, or other complicating factors Involves external incision with two possible approaches (see Figure 57-6)	Complete visualization of prostate and surrounding tissue	Erectile dysfunction Bleeding Postoperative pain Risk for infection

Complications include urinary retention, UTI, and irritative voiding symptoms (e.g., frequency, urgency, dysuria). Some patients require a urinary catheter for a short time. Patients often have hematuria for up to a week.

Laser Prostatectomy. The use of laser therapy through visual or ultrasound guidance is an effective alternative to transurethral resection of the prostate (TURP) in treating BPH. The laser beam is delivered transurethrally through a fibre instrument and is used for cutting, coagulation, and vaporization of prostatic tissue. There are a variety of laser procedures using different sources, wavelengths, and delivery systems. Retreatment rates are comparable to those of a TURP (Chughtai, Simma-Chiang, Lee, et al., 2015).

One common procedure is *visual laser ablation of the prostate* (VLAP), which uses the laser beam to produce deep coagulation necrosis. The affected prostate tissue gradually sloughs in the urinary stream. It takes several weeks before the patient reaches optimal results after this type of laser therapy. At the completion of VLAP, a urinary catheter is inserted to allow for drainage.

Contact laser techniques involve the direct contact of the laser with the prostate tissue, producing an immediate vaporization of the tissue. Blood vessels near the laser tip are immediately cauterized. Thus bleeding during the procedure is rare. A three-way catheter with slow-drip irrigation is placed immediately after the procedure for a short time. Typically, the catheter is removed within 6 to 8 hours after the procedure. Advantages of this procedure over TURP include minimal bleeding both during and after the procedure, faster recovery time, and ability to perform the surgery on patients taking anticoagulants.

Photovaporization of the prostate (PVP) uses a high-powered green laser light to vaporize prostate tissue. Improvements in urine flow and symptoms are almost immediate after the procedure. Bleeding is minimal, and a catheter is usually inserted for 24 to 48 hours afterward. PVP works well for larger prostate glands.

Another approach to laser prostatectomy is *interstitial laser coagulation* (ILC). The prostate is viewed through a cystoscope. A laser is used to treat precise areas of the enlarged prostate quickly by placement of interstitial light guides directly into the prostate tissue.

Intraprostatic Urethral Stents. Symptoms from obstruction in patients who are poor surgical candidates can be relieved with intraprostatic urethral stents. The stents are placed directly into the prostatic tissue. Complications include chronic pain, infection, and encrustation. The long-term effects are not known.

Invasive Therapy (Surgery). Invasive treatment of symptomatic BPH involves surgery. The choice of the treatment approach depends on the size and location of the prostatic enlargement and patient factors such as age and surgical risk. Invasive treatments are summarized in Table 57-3.

Invasive therapy is indicated when the decrease in urine flow is sufficient to cause discomfort, persistent residual urine, acute urinary retention because of obstruction with no reversible precipitating cause, or hydronephrosis. Intermittent catheterization or insertion of an in-dwelling catheter can temporarily reduce symptoms and bypass the obstruction. However, long-term catheter use should be avoided because of the increased risk for infection.

Transurethral Resection of the Prostate. Transurethral resection of the prostate (TURP) is a surgical procedure involving the removal of prostate tissue using a resectoscope inserted through the urethra. TURP has long been considered the "gold standard" surgical treatment for obstructing BPH. Although it remains the most common operation performed, there has been a decrease in the number of TURP procedures in recent years owing to the development of less invasive technologies (Herrmann, Liatsikos, Nagele, et al., 2012).

TURP is performed under a spinal or general anaesthetic. No external surgical incision is made. Instead, a resectoscope is inserted through the urethra to excise and cauterize obstructing prostatic tissue (Figure 57-4). A large three-way in-dwelling catheter with a 30-mL balloon is inserted into the bladder after the procedure to provide hemostasis and to facilitate urinary drainage. Usually for the first 24 hours, the bladder is irrigated, either continuously or intermittently, to prevent obstruction from mucus and blood clots.

The outcome for 80% to 90% of patients is excellent, with marked improvements in symptoms and urinary flow rates. TURP is a surgical procedure with relatively low risk. Postoperative complications include bleeding, clot retention, bladder spasms, and dilutional hyponatremia associated with irrigation. Because bleeding is a common complication, patients taking acetylsalicylic acid (ASA; Aspirin) or warfarin (Coumadin) or other anticoagulants must discontinue these medications several days before surgery.

Transurethral Incision of the Prostate. Transurethral incision of the prostate (TUIP) is a surgical procedure that is indicated for men with moderate to severe symptoms and small prostates who are poor surgical candidates. It is done under local anaesthesia and is as effective as TURP in symptom relief.

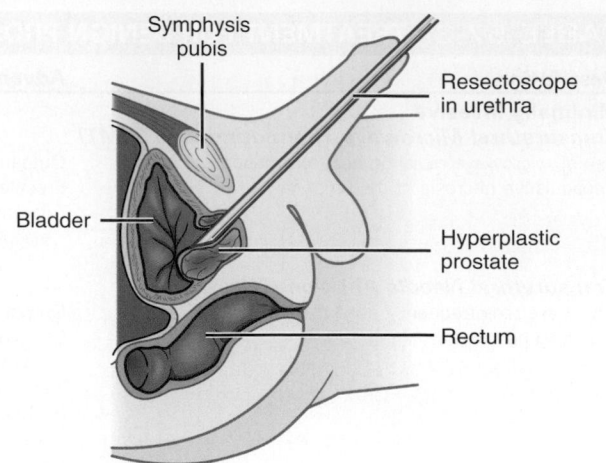

FIGURE 57-4 Transurethral resection of the prostate.

Prostatectomy. Prostatectomy is the surgery of choice for large prostates and is discussed later in this chapter.

NURSING MANAGEMENT
BENIGN PROSTATIC HYPERPLASIA

Because the nurse is most directly involved in the care of patients with BPH who are having invasive procedures, the focus of nursing management in this section is on preoperative and postoperative care.

NURSING ASSESSMENT

Subjective and objective data that should be obtained from a patient with BPH are presented in Table 57-4.

NURSING DIAGNOSES

Nursing diagnoses for a patient with BPH preoperatively may include but are not limited to the following:

- *Acute pain* related to *biological injury agent* (bladder distention secondary to enlarged prostate)
- *Risk for infection* as evidenced by *insufficient knowledge to avoid pathogens, stasis of body fluid* (indwelling catheter, urinary stasis)

Nursing diagnoses for a patient with BPH who has invasive therapy (surgery) are presented in Nursing Care Plan (NCP) 57-1, available on the Evolve website.

PLANNING

The overall preoperative goals for patients having invasive procedures are (a) restoration of urinary drainage; (b) treatment of any UTI; and (c) an understanding of the upcoming procedure, the implications for sexual functioning, and urinary control. The overall postoperative goals are (a) no complications, (b) restoration of urinary control, (c) complete bladder emptying, and (d) the ability for satisfying sexual expression.

NURSING IMPLEMENTATION

HEALTH PROMOTION. The cause of BPH is largely attributed to the aging process. Health promotion focuses on early detection and treatment. The Canadian Task Force on Preventive Health Care (Bell, Connor Gorber, Shane, et al., 2014) recommends that men not be screened for prostate cancer with the PSA test,

TABLE 57-4 NURSING ASSESSMENT

Benign Prostatic Hyperplasia

Subjective Data
Important Health Information
Past health history: Family history of BPH; obesity; diet high in fat or zinc
Medications: Estrogen or testosterone supplementation
Surgeries or other treatments: Previous treatment for BPH

Symptoms
- Voluntary fluid restriction; urinary urgency; urinary dysuria; diminution in calibre and force of urinary stream; hesitancy in initiating voiding; postvoiding dribbling; urinary retention; incontinence; nocturia; bladder discomfort; anxiety about sexual functioning

Objective Data
General
Older-adult male

Urinary
Distended bladder on palpation; smooth, firm, elastic enlargement of prostate on rectal examination

Possible Findings
Enlarged prostate on ultrasonography; vesicle neck obstruction on cysto-urethroscopy; residual urine with postvoiding catheterization; presence of WBCs, bacteria, or microscopic hematuria with infection; ↑ serum creatinine levels with renal involvement

BPH, benign prostatic hyperplasia; *WBCs,* white blood cells.

because available evidence does not support PSA screening as a means of reducing prostate cancer, and it clearly shows an increased risk for harm (e.g., bleeding, infection, incontinence, a false-positive result and the possibility of overdiagnosis). Some men may be interested in PSA screening despite the advice of their health care provider about their personal risk of developing prostate cancer and the benefits and risks of having a PSA test. PSA is indicated as a surveillance test for men with prostate cancer. The Canadian Cancer Society (2017a) recommends a yearly medical history and DRE for men over 50 years of age in an effort to detect prostate problems early. When symptoms of prostatic hyperplasia become evident, further diagnostic screening may be necessary (see Table 57-2).

Some men find that the ingestion of alcohol and caffeine increases prostatic symptoms because the diuretic effect of these substances increases bladder distension. Compounds found in common cough and cold remedies such as pseudoephedrine (e.g., Sudafed) and phenylephrine (e.g., Dimetapp) often worsen the symptoms of BPH. These drugs are α-adrenergic agonists that cause smooth muscle contraction.

Patients with obstructive symptoms should be advised to urinate every 2 to 3 hours and when first feeling the urge. Doing so will minimize urinary stasis and acute urinary retention. Fluid intake should be maintained at a normal level to prevent dehydration or fluid overload. The patient may believe that, if he restricts his fluid intake, symptoms will be less severe, but this only increases the chances of an infection. However, if the patient increases his intake too rapidly, bladder distension can develop because of the prostatic obstruction.

ACUTE INTERVENTION. The following discussion focuses on preoperative and postoperative care for the patient undergoing a TURP.

Preoperative Care. Urinary drainage must be restored before surgery. Prostatic obstruction may result in acute retention or inability to void. A urethral catheter such as a coudé (curved-tip) catheter may be needed to restore drainage. In many health care settings, 10 mL of sterile 2% lidocaine gel is injected into the urethra before insertion of the catheter. The lidocaine gel not only acts as a lubricant but also provides local anaesthesia and helps open the urethral lumen. If a sizable obstruction of the urethra exists, the urologist may insert a filiform catheter with sufficient rigidity to pass the obstruction. Aseptic technique is important at all times to avoid introducing bacteria into the bladder. (Urinary catheters are discussed in Chapter 48.)

Antibiotics are usually administered before any invasive procedure. Any infection of the urinary tract must be treated before surgery. Restoring urine drainage and encouraging a high fluid intake (2 to 3 L/day unless contraindicated) are also helpful in managing the infection.

Patients are often concerned about the impact of the impending surgery on sexual functioning. Patients and their partners should be provided an opportunity to express their concerns. They should be informed that surgery may affect sexual function and that most types of prostatic surgery result in some degree of retrograde ejaculation. The patient should know that the amount of ejaculate may decrease or be totally absent. As a result, orgasmic sensations felt during ejaculation may decrease. Retrograde ejaculation is not harmful because the semen is eliminated during the next urination.

Postoperative Care. The main complications following surgery are hemorrhage, bladder spasms, urinary incontinence, and infection. The plan of care should be adjusted to the type of surgery, the reasons for surgery, and the patient's response to surgery.

After surgery, the patient will have a standard catheter or a triple-lumen catheter. Bladder irrigation is typically done to remove clotted blood from the bladder and to ensure drainage of urine. The bladder is irrigated either manually on an intermittent basis or, more commonly, as continuous bladder irrigation (CBI) with sterile normal saline solution or another prescribed solution. If manual irrigation of the bladder is ordered, instill 50 mL of irrigating solution (commonly normal saline) and then withdraw with a syringe to remove clots that may be in the bladder and catheter. Painful bladder spasms often occur as a result of manual irrigation. With CBI, irrigating solution is continuously infused and drained from the bladder. The rate of infusion is based on the colour of drainage. Ideally, the urine drainage should be light pink without clots. The inflow and outflow of irrigant must be continuously monitored. If outflow is less than inflow, the bladder should be assessed immediately and the catheter patency checked. If the outflow is blocked and patency cannot be re-established by manual irrigation, the CBI must be stopped and the health care provider notified.

Careful aseptic technique is essential when irrigating the bladder because bacteria can easily be introduced into the urinary tract. Proper care of the catheter is also important. To prevent urethral irritation and minimize the risk for bladder infection, the nurse should secure the catheter to the leg with tape or a catheter strap. The catheter should be connected to a closed drainage system and should not be disconnected unless it is being removed, changed, or irrigated. The secretions that accumulate around the meatus can be cleansed daily with soap and water.

Blood clots are expected for the first 24 to 36 hours after prostate surgery. However, large amounts of bright-red blood in the urine can indicate hemorrhage. Postoperative hemorrhage may occur from displacement of the catheter, dislodgement of a large clot, or increases in abdominal pressure. Release or displacement of the catheter dislodges the balloon that provides counter-pressure on the operative site. Traction on the catheter may be applied to provide counter-pressure (tamponade) on the bleeding site in the prostate, thereby decreasing bleeding. Such traction can result in local necrosis if pressure is applied for too long. Therefore, pressure should be relieved on a scheduled basis by qualified personnel. Activities that increase abdominal pressure, such as sitting or walking for prolonged periods and straining to have a bowel movement (Valsalva manoeuvre), should be avoided in the postoperative recovery period.

Bladder spasms are a distressing complication for patients after transurethral procedures. They occur as a result of irritation of the bladder mucosa from the insertion of the resectoscope, presence of a catheter, or clots leading to obstruction of the catheter. Patients should be instructed not to urinate around the catheter because it increases the likelihood of spasm. If bladder spasms develop, the catheter should be checked for clots. Any clots discovered should be removed by irrigation so that urine can flow freely. Antispasmodics (e.g., belladonna and opium suppositories, oxybutynin [Oxytrol]), along with relaxation techniques, are used to relieve the pain and decrease spasm. The catheter is often removed 2 to 4 days after surgery. The patient should urinate within 6 hours after catheter removal. If he cannot, a catheter is reinserted for a day or two. If the problem continues, the nurse may need to instruct the patient in clean intermittent self-catheterization (see Chapter 48).

Sphincter tone may be poor immediately after catheter removal, resulting in urinary incontinence or dribbling. This is a common but distressing situation for patients. Sphincter tone can be strengthened with Kegel exercises (pelvic floor muscle technique) practised 10 to 20 times per hour while awake (see Table 48-19 in Chapter 48). Patients should be encouraged to practise starting and stopping the stream several times during urination. This facilitates learning of the pelvic floor exercises. It usually takes several weeks to achieve urinary continence. In some instances, control of urine may never be fully regained. Continence can improve for up to 12 months. If continence has not been achieved by that time, patients may be referred to a continence clinic. A variety of methods, including biofeedback, have been used to achieve positive results. Patients can also be instructed to use a penile clamp, condom catheter, or incontinence pads or briefs to avoid embarrassment from dribbling. In severe cases, an occlusive cuff that serves as an artificial sphincter can be surgically implanted to restore continence. The nurse should assist the patient in finding ways to manage the problem that will allow him to continue socializing and interacting with others.

Patients should be observed for signs of postoperative infection. If an external wound is present (from an open prostatectomy), the nurse should assess the area for redness, heat, swelling, and purulent drainage. Special care must be taken if a perineal incision is present because of the proximity of the anus. Rectal procedures, such as taking rectal temperatures and administering enemas, should be avoided. The insertion of well-lubricated belladonna and opium suppositories is acceptable.

Dietary intervention and stool softeners are important in the postoperative period to prevent patients from straining while having bowel movements. Straining increases the intra-abdominal pressure, which can lead to bleeding at the operative site. Adequate fluid intake and a diet high in fibre facilitate the passage of stool.

AMBULATORY AND HOME CARE. Discharge planning and home care issues are important aspects of care after prostate surgery. Instructions patients will need include those for (a) caring for an in-dwelling catheter (if one is left in place); (b) managing urinary incontinence; (c) maintaining oral fluids between 2 000 and 3 000 mL/day; (d) observing for signs and symptoms of UTI and wound infection; (e) preventing constipation; (f) avoiding heavy lifting (>4.5 kg); and (g) refraining from driving or having intercourse after surgery as directed by the physician.

Patients may experience a change in sexual functioning following surgery, for example, retrograde ejaculation or physiological ED (if the nerves are cut or damaged during surgery). Patients may experience anxiety over the change because of a perceived loss of sex role, lower self-esteem, or perceived decrease in the quality of sexual interaction with a partner. The nurse should discuss these changes with the patient and his partner and allow them to ask questions and express their concerns. Sexual counselling and treatment options may be necessary if ED becomes a chronic or permanent problem. (ED is discussed later in this chapter.) Although some patients experience concerns regarding change in sexual functioning, this is not a universal concern. It may take up to 1 year for complete sexual functioning to return.

The bladder may take up to 2 months to return to its normal capacity. Patients should be instructed to drink at least 2 to 3 L of fluid per day and to urinate every 2 to 3 hours to flush the urinary tract. The nurse should also teach the patient to avoid or limit the intake of bladder irritants such as caffeine products, citrus juices, and alcohol. Because the patient may be experiencing incontinence or dribbling, he may incorrectly believe that decreasing fluid intake will relieve this problem. Urethral strictures may result from instrumentation or catheterization. Treatment may include intermittent clean self-catheterization (which will need to be taught to the patient) or a urethral dilation.

Patients who have had any procedure other than complete removal of the prostate will need to continue having yearly DREs because hyperplasia or cancer can occur in the remaining prostatic tissue.

EVALUATION

Expected outcomes for a patient with BPH are presented in NCP 57-1, available on the Evolve website.

PROSTATE CANCER

Prostate cancer is a malignant tumour of the prostate gland. In 2017, it was estimated that 21 300 new cases of prostate cancer would be diagnosed in Canada that year and that 4 100 men would die of it (Canadian Cancer Society's Advisory Committee on Cancer Statistics, 2017), meaning that, on average, 59 Canadians are diagnosed with prostate cancer each day and 11 men die from it. Prostate cancer is the most common cancer among men, excluding skin cancer. The majority (>75%) of cases occur in men older than age 65. However, many cases occur in younger men, who sometimes have a more aggressive type of cancer.

There were peaks in the incidence of newly diagnosed cases of prostate cancer in 1993 and 2001. These peaks were followed by a decline. These increases were attributed to the widespread use of PSA as a screening procedure and were in fact linked to two waves of intense screening. The age-standardized incidence rate has been in decline since 2001 (1.6% per year) (Canadian Cancer Society's Advisory Committee on Cancer Statistics, 2017).

Etiology and Pathophysiology

Prostate cancer is an androgen-dependent adenocarcinoma that is usually slow growing. It can spread by three routes: (a) through direct extension, (b) through the lymph system, or (c) through the bloodstream. Spread by direct extension involves the seminal vesicles, the urethral mucosa, the bladder wall, and the external sphincter. The cancer later spreads through the lymphatic system to the regional lymph nodes. The veins from the prostate seem to be the mode of spread to the pelvic bones, the head of the femur, the lower lumbar spine, the liver, and the lungs.

Age, ethnicity, and family history are three nonmodifiable risk factors for prostate cancer. The incidence of prostate cancer rises markedly after age 50 with a median age at diagnosis of 67 years old (Siegel, DeSantis, Virgo, et al., 2012). Men of Asian ancestry have lower rates of prostate cancer, while men of African ancestry have a higher risk of developing prostate cancer (Canadian Cancer Society, 2017b). See the "Determinants of Health" box for other risk factors. Research suggests that consumption of tomatoes and tomato-based products may protect patients against prostate cancer (Zu, Mucci, Rosner, et al., 2014).

Clinical Manifestations and Complications

Prostate cancer is usually asymptomatic in the early stages. Eventually, the patient may have symptoms similar to those of BPH, including dysuria, hesitancy, dribbling, frequency, urgency, hematuria, nocturia, retention, interruption of urinary stream, and inability to urinate. Pain in the lumbosacral area that radiates down to the hips or the legs, when coupled with urinary symptoms, may indicate metastasis.

Early recognition and treatment are required to control growth, prevent metastasis, and preserve quality of life. The tumour can spread to pelvic lymph nodes, bones, bladder, lungs, and liver. Once the tumour has spread to distant sites, the major problem becomes the management of pain. As the cancer spreads to the bones (a common site of metastasis), pain can become severe, especially in the back and the legs because of compression of the spinal cord and destruction of bone (Figure 57-5).

Diagnostic Studies

The primary screening tool for prostate cancer is a digital rectal examination (DRE). On DRE, an abnormal prostate may feel hard, nodular, and asymmetrical. The DRE, however, is not a definitive diagnostic test for prostate cancer. If the DRE is abnormal, biopsy of the prostate tissue is indicated and necessary to confirm the diagnosis of prostate cancer. The biopsy is typically done using TRUS because it allows the physician to visualize the prostate and pinpoint abnormalities. When a suspicious area is located, a biopsy needle is inserted into the prostate to obtain a tissue sample. A pathological examination of the specimen is done to assess for malignant changes.

The PSA test is no longer recommended as the risks may outweigh the benefits (Bell, Connor Gorber, Shane, et al., 2014). Although specific recommendations regarding PSA screening vary, there is general agreement that men should talk to their health care provider about their personal risk of developing prostate cancer and the potential risks (e.g., subsequent evaluation and treatment that may be unnecessary) and benefits (early detection of prostate cancer) of PSA screening before being tested.

FIGURE 57-5 Metastasis *(arrows)* of prostate cancer to the pelvis and lumbar spine. Source: Mettler, F. (2004). *Essentials of radiology* (2nd ed.). Philadelphia: Saunders.

DETERMINANTS OF HEALTH

Prostate Cancer

Biology, Genetic Endowment, and Culture
- Canadian men of African descent have the highest rates of prostate cancer, while Canadians of Asian descent have the lowest rates.
- Men of African descent are diagnosed at a younger age, have more aggressive tumours, and are diagnosed at a more advanced stage than White men.
- Prostate cancer is one of the most commonly occurring cancers in First Nations men.*
- There is a genetic link to the development of prostate cancer, especially if a first-degree relative has a history of the disease.
- The *BRCA2* gene, which is linked with breast cancer, is also linked with prostate cancer.
- Long-term exposure to high levels of testosterone DHT may increase the risk for prostate cancer.

Personal Health Practices and Coping Skills
- Eating a diet high in fat increases the risk for prostate cancer.
- Consuming large amounts of dairy products increases the risk, as calcium is linked to prostate cancer.
- Consuming red meat (e.g., beef, pork) cooked at high temperatures and processed meat (e.g., bacon, hot dogs) increases the risk for prostate cancer.
- Being overweight or obese is linked to being diagnosed with advanced or aggressive prostate cancer.

Physical Environment; Employment/Working Conditions
- Occupational exposure to chemical carcinogens such as insecticides, cadmium, or rubber manufacturing is linked to prostate cancer.

References

Canadian Cancer Society. (2017). *Risk factors for prostate cancer*. Retrieved from *http://www.cancer.ca/en/cancer-information/cancer-type/prostate/risks/?region=on*; except *Moore, S., Antoni, A., Colquhoun, A., et al. (2015). Cancer incidence in indigenous people in Australia, New Zealand, Canada, and the USA: A comparative population-based study. *The Lancet Oncology*, 16(15), 1483–1492. doi:10.1016/S1470-2045(15)00232-6.

TABLE 57-5 WHITMORE–JEWETT STAGING CLASSIFICATION OF PROSTATE CANCER

Stage A: Clinically Unrecognized
A_1 <5% of prostatic tissue neoplastic
A_2 >5% of prostatic tissue neoplastic, all high-grade tumours

Stage B: Clinically Intracapsular
B_1 Nodule <2 cm and surrounded by palpably normal tissue
B_2 Nodule >2 cm or multiple nodules

Stage C: Clinically Extracapsular
C_1 Minimal extracapsular extension
C_2 Large tumours involving seminal vesicles, adjacent structures, or both

Stage D: Metastatic Disease
D_1 Pelvic lymph node metastases or ureteral obstruction causing hydronephrosis
D_2 Distant metastases to bone, viscera, or other soft tissue structures

TABLE 57-6 COLLABORATIVE CARE

Prostate Cancer

Diagnostic
- History and physical examination
- Digital rectal examination
- Prostatic acid phosphatase
- Transrectal ultrasonography
- Biopsy of prostate and lymph nodes
- CT scan, MRI, bone scan (to evaluate for metastatic disease)

Collaborative Therapy
Active Surveillance
- Watchful waiting with annual physical exam including DRE

Surgery
- Radical prostatectomy
- Cryotherapy
- Orchiectomy (for metastatic disease)

Radiation Therapy
- External beam for primary, adjuvant, and recurrent disease
- Brachytherapy

Drug Therapy
- Androgen deprivation therapy
- Chemotherapy for metastatic disease

CT, computed tomography; *MRI*, magnetic resonance imaging.

PSA is, however, used to monitor the success of treatment. When treatment for prostate cancer has been successful, PSA levels should fall to undetectable levels. Regular measurement of PSA levels following treatment is important to evaluate the continuing effectiveness of treatment and the possible recurrence of prostate cancer.

Elevated levels of prostatic isoenzyme of serum acid phosphatase (prostatic acid phosphatase [PAP]) is an indicator of prostate cancer, especially if there is extracapsular spread. In advanced prostate cancer, serum alkaline phosphatase is increased as a result of bone metastasis.

A recent development in the diagnosis of prostate cancer is the discovery of the gene—*Prostate Cancer Associated 3* (non–protein coding) (*PCA3*)—that is specific to prostate cancer cells and, if present in the urine, indicates prostate cancer. The *PCA3* test is more accurate than the PSA test because benign enlargement of the prostate will not cause an increase in *PCA3*, whereas it can cause an increase in the PSA test. The *PCA3* test offers a potential solution to the clinical diagnostic challenge posed by the PSA test.

Once a diagnosis of prostate cancer is confirmed, other tests used to determine the location and the extent of the spread of the cancer may include bone scan, computed tomography (CT), and magnetic resonance imaging (MRI) using an endorectal probe.

Collaborative Care

Early-stage prostate cancer is a curable disease in most men. The prostate cancer is staged and graded based on findings from diagnostic studies. Two common classification systems for staging prostate cancer, the Whitmore–Jewett and tumour–nodes–metastasis (TNM) systems, are both based on the size (volume) of the tumour and spread (Table 57-5). Both classification systems are used in Canada, with description and treatment based upon the Whitmore–Jewett classification (i.e., stage A, B, C, or D) and description of the extent of the cancer based upon the TNM system. Approximately 80% of patients with prostate cancer are initially diagnosed when the cancer is in either a local or a regional stage. The lifetime probability of a man developing prostate cancer

in Canada is 1 in 7 (Canadian Cancer Society's Advisory Committee on Cancer Statistics, 2017).

Grading of the tumour is done based on tumour histology using the Gleason scale. With this scale, tumours are graded from 1 to 5 based on the degree of glandular differentiation. Grade 1 represents the most well differentiated (most like the original cells), and grade 5 represents the most poorly differentiated (undifferentiated). Gleason grades are given to the two most commonly occurring patterns of cells and added together. The Gleason score is a number from 2 to 10. This scale is used to predict how quickly the cancer will progress.

The collaborative care of the patient with prostate cancer depends on the stage of the cancer and the overall health of the patient. At all stages, there is more than one possible treatment option. The decision of which treatment course to pursue is made jointly by the patient and the health care team based on a careful analysis of the facts and the patient's preference (Canadian Cancer Society, 2017b). Table 57-6 summarizes the various treatment options available.

Conservative Therapy. Prostate cancer is relatively slow growing, and an active surveillance approach to the management of prostate cancer is indicated. This strategy is appropriate when the patient has (a) a life expectancy of less than 10 years (low risk of dying of the disease), (b) serious coexisting medical conditions, and (c) a low-grade, low-stage tumour. These patients are typically followed with frequent PSA measurements, along with DRE, to monitor the progress of the disease. A significant change in either PSA or DRE or the development of symptoms warrants a re-evaluation of treatment options.

Surgical Therapy

Radical Prostatectomy. With **radical prostatectomy,** the entire prostate gland, the seminal vesicles, and part of the bladder neck (ampulla) are surgically removed. The entire prostate is removed because the cancer tends to be in many different locations within the gland. In addition, a retroperitoneal lymph node dissection is usually done as a separate procedure. Surgery is usually not considered an option for advanced stage disease (except to relieve

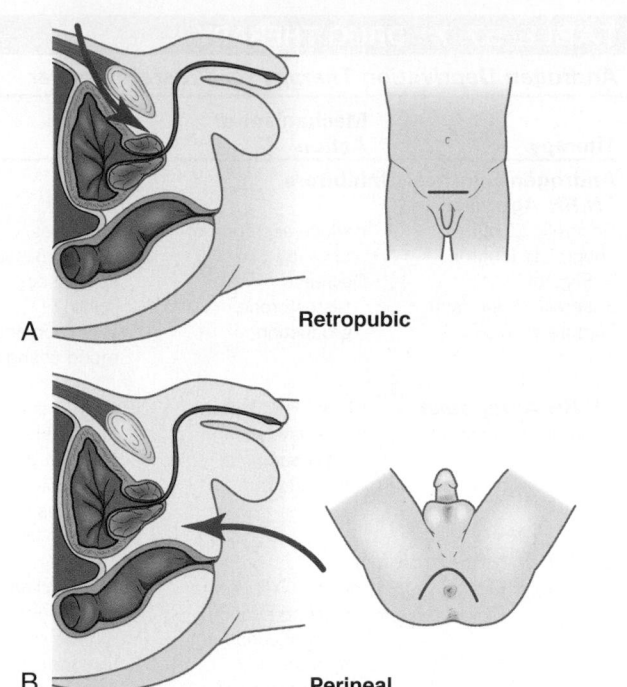

FIGURE 57-6 Common approaches used to perform a prostatectomy. **A,** Retropubic approach involves a midline abdominal incision. **B,** Perineal approach involves an incision between the scrotum and the anus.

symptoms associated with obstruction) because metastasis has already occurred. The two most common approaches for radical prostatectomy are retropubic and perineal resection (Figure 57-6). With the *retropubic* approach, a low midline abdominal incision is made to access the prostate gland, and the pelvic lymph nodes then can be dissected. With the *perineal* resection, an incision is made between the scrotum and the anus.

A *laparoscopic* approach to prostatectomy is being used in some settings. In this method, four small incisions are made into the abdomen. It results in less bleeding, less pain, and a faster recovery compared with other approaches.

A *robotic-assisted* (e.g., da Vinci system) prostatectomy is a type of laparoscopy in which the surgeon sits at a computer console while controlling high-resolution cameras and micro-surgical instruments. Robotics is being used more, since it allows for increased precision, visualization, and dexterity by the surgeon when removing the prostate gland. Compared with traditional approaches, robotic-assisted radical prostatectomy has resulted in similar surgical outcomes with improved recovery time (Trinh, Sammon, Sun, et al., 2012).

After surgery, the patient has a large in-dwelling catheter with a 30-mL balloon placed in the bladder via the urethra. This catheter is typically left in place for 1 to 2 weeks. A drain is left in the surgical site to aid in the removal of drainage from the area. This drain is typically removed after a couple of days. Because the perineal approach has a higher risk for postoperative infection (owing to the location of the incision related to the anus), careful dressing changes and perineal care after each bowel movement are important to promote comfort and prevent infection. Depending on the type of surgery, the length of hospital stay postoperatively ranges from 1 to 3 days.

Two major adverse outcomes following a radical prostatectomy are ED and urinary incontinence (Boorjian, Eastham, Graefen, et al., 2012). The incidence of ED is dependent on the patient's age, preoperative sexual functioning, whether nerve-sparing surgery was performed, and the surgeon's expertise. Problems with urinary control occur in nearly all men for the first few months following surgery because the bladder must be reattached to the urethra after the prostate is removed. Over time, the bladder adjusts, and most men regain control (Gandaglia, Gallina, Suardi, et al., 2014). Kegel exercises strengthen the urinary sphincter and may help improve incontinence. Other common complications associated with surgery include hemorrhage, urinary retention, infection, wound dehiscence, deep-vein thrombosis, and pulmonary emboli.

Nerve-Sparing Procedure. In proximity to the prostate gland are neuro-vascular bundles that maintain erectile functioning. The preservation of these bundles during a prostatectomy is possible while still removing all of the cancer. This procedure is not indicated for patients with cancer outside of the prostate gland. Although the risk for ED is significantly reduced with this procedure, there is no guarantee that potency will be maintained. However, most men younger than 50 years with good preoperative erectile function and low-stage prostate cancer can expect a return of potency after nerve-sparing prostatectomy.

Cryosurgery. *Cryotherapy* (cryoablation) is a surgical technique for prostate cancer that destroys cancer cells by freezing the tissue. It has been used both as an initial treatment and as a second-line treatment after radiation treatment failures. A TRUS probe is inserted to visualize the prostate gland. Probes containing liquid nitrogen are then inserted into the prostate. Liquid nitrogen delivers freezing temperatures, destroying the tissue. The treatment takes about 2 hours under general or spinal anaesthesia and does not involve an abdominal incision. Possible complications of prostatic cryosurgery include damage to the urethra and, in rare cases, a urethro-rectal fistula (an opening between the urethra and the rectum) or a urethro-cutaneous fistula (an opening between the urethra and the skin). Tissue sloughing, ED, urinary incontinence, prostatitis, and hemorrhage have also been reported.

Radiation Therapy. Radiation therapy is a common treatment option for prostate cancer, especially for men older than 70, patients who are poor surgical risks, or those who wish to avoid surgery. Radiation therapy may be offered as the only treatment, or it may be offered in combination with surgery or with hormonal therapy. Salvage radiation therapy given for cancer recurrence after a radical prostatectomy may improve survival in some men.

External Beam Irradiation. External beam is the most widely used method of delivering radiation treatments in those with prostate cancer. This therapy can be used to treat patients with prostate cancer confined to the prostate or surrounding tissue. Patients are treated on an outpatient basis 5 days a week for 4 to 8 weeks. Each treatment lasts only a few minutes. Adverse effects from radiation can be acute (occurring during treatment or within 90 days following) or delayed (occurring months or years after treatment). Common adverse effects involve the skin (dryness, redness, irritation, pain), gastro-intestinal (GI) tract (diarrhea, abdominal cramping, bleeding), urinary tract (dysuria, frequency, hesitancy, urgency, nocturia), sexual functioning (ED), fatigue, and bone marrow suppression (Cameron, Springer, Fox-Wasylyshyn, et al., 2012). These problems usually resolve 2 to 3 weeks after the completion of radiation therapy. In patients with localized prostate cancer, cure rates using external beam radiation are comparable with those using radical prostatectomy.

Brachytherapy. *Brachytherapy* involves the implantation of radioactive seeds into the prostate gland, allowing higher radiation

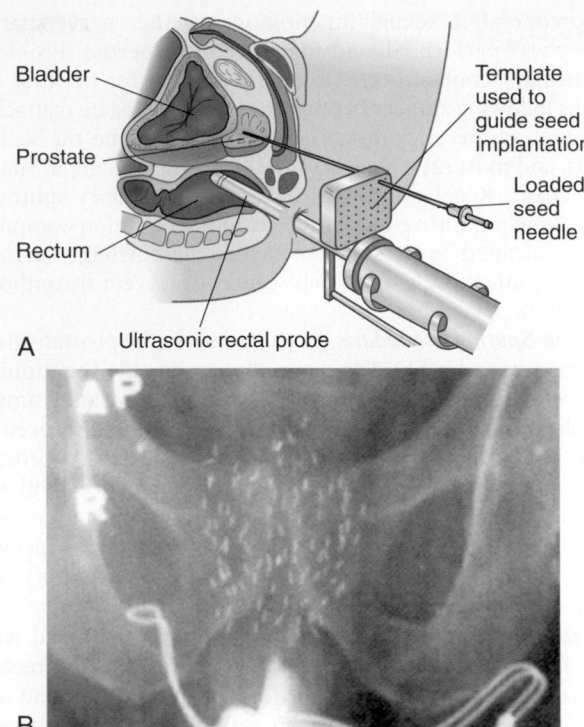

FIGURE 57-7 A, Prostate brachytherapy. Implantation of seeds with a needle guided by ultrasonography and a template grid. **B,** Radioactive seeds. Source: **B,** Abeloff, M., Armitage, J. O., Niederhuber, J. D., et al. (Eds.). (2008). *Abeloff's clinical oncology* (4th ed., Figure 88-12A). Edinburgh: Churchill Livingstone.

doses directly in the tissue while sparing the surrounding tissue (rectum and bladder). The radioactive seeds are placed in the prostate gland with a needle through a grid template guided by TRUS (Figure 57-7). The grid template and ultrasonography ensure accurate placement of the seeds. Because brachytherapy is a one-time outpatient procedure, many patients find it more convenient than external beam radiation treatment. Brachytherapy is best suited for patients with early-stage prostate cancer. The most common adverse effect is the development of urinary irritative or obstructive problems. The AUA Symptom Index (see Table 57-1) can be used to measure urinary function for patients undergoing brachytherapy and can be incorporated into postoperative nursing management. For those with more advanced tumours, brachytherapy may be offered in combination with external beam radiation treatment (Pieters, Rezaie, Geijsen, et al., 2011). (Brachytherapy is discussed further in Chapter 18.)

Drug Therapy. The forms of drug therapy available for the treatment of prostate cancer are androgen deprivation (hormone) therapy, chemotherapy, or a combination of both.

Androgen Deprivation Therapy. Prostate cancer growth is largely dependent on the presence of androgens. *Androgen deprivation therapy* (ADT) reduces the levels of circulating androgens to diminish the tumour's growth. Androgen deprivation can be produced by inhibiting androgen production or blocking androgen receptors (Table 57-7). One of the biggest challenges with ADT is that almost all tumours treated become resistant to this therapy *(hormone refractory)* within a few years. An elevated PSA level is often the first sign that this therapy is no longer effective. Osteoporosis and fractures may occur in prostate cancer patients receiving ADT. Drugs recommended to reduce bone mineral

TABLE 57-7   DRUG THERAPY

Androgen Deprivation Therapy for Prostate Cancer

Therapy	Mechanism of Action	Adverse Effects
Androgen Synthesis Inhibitors		
LH-RH Agonists		
Goserelin (Zoladex)	Reduce secretion of LH and FSH	Hot flashes, gynecomastia,
Leuprolide (Lupron, Eligard)	Decrease	decreased
Buserelin (Suprefact)	testosterone	libido, ED
Triptorelin (Trelstar)	production	Depression and mood changes
LH-RH Antagonist		
Degarelix (Firmagon)	Block LH receptors Immediately suppress testosterone	Pain, redness, and swelling at injection site Elevated liver enzymes
CYP17 Enzyme Inhibitor		
Abiraterone (Zytiga)	Inhibits CYP17, an enzyme needed for production of testosterone Inhibits testosterone synthesis from the testes, adrenal glands, and prostate cancer cells	Joint swelling, fluid retention, muscle discomfort, hot flashes, diarrhea
Androgen Receptor Blockers		
Bicalutamide (Casodex)	Block the action of testosterone by competing with receptor sites	Loss of libido, ED, and hot flashes
Flutamide		
Nilutamide (Anandron)		Breast pain and
Enzalutamide (Xtandi)		gynecomastia may also occur

CYP17, cytochrome P450 17α–hydroxy/17,20-lyase; *ED,* erectile dysfunction; *FSH,* follicle-stimulating hormone; *LH,* luteinizing hormone; *LH-RH,* luteinizing hormone–releasing hormone.

loss in these patients include zoledronic acid (Aclasta) and raloxifene (Evista) (VanderWalde & Hurria, 2011).

Androgen Synthesis Inhibitors. Luteinizing hormone–releasing hormone (LH-RH) is released from the hypothalamus to stimulate the anterior pituitary to produce luteinizing hormone (LH) and follicle-stimulating hormone (FSH). LH stimulates the testicular Leydig cells to produce testosterone. LH-RH agonists super-stimulate the pituitary, ultimately resulting in down-regulation of the LH-RH receptors, leading to a refractory condition in which the anterior pituitary is unresponsive to LH-RH. These drugs cause an initial transient increase in LH and testosterone called a "flare," and a worsening of symptoms may occur during this time. However, with continued administration, LH and testosterone levels decrease. LH-RH agonists include leuprolide (Lupron, Eligard), goserelin (Zoladex), buserelin (Suprefact) and triptorelin (Trelstar). These medications essentially produce a chemical castration similar to the effects of an orchiectomy. They are administered by subcutaneous or intramuscular injections on a regular basis, and they must be taken indefinitely. Leuprolide acetate implant (Viadur) is a subcutaneous implant that delivers leuprolide continuously for 1 year (Warlick, Weight, & Konety, 2014).

Degarelix (Firmagon) is an LH-RH antagonist that lowers testosterone levels. Unlike the LH-RH agonists, degarelix does not cause a testosterone flare because it acts directly to block LH and FSH receptors. It is given as a subcutaneous injection.

Abiraterone (Zytiga) works by inhibiting an enzyme, CYP17, which is needed for the production of testosterone. This medication is given orally.

Androgen Receptor Blockers. Another classification of antiandrogens is drugs that compete with circulating androgens at the receptor sites. Flutamide, nilutamide (Anandron), enzalutamide (Xtandi), and bicalutamide (Casodex) are androgen receptor blockers. They are often used in combination with an LH-RH agonist (e.g., goserelin, leuprolide), resulting in a combined androgen blockade.

Orchiectomy. Testosterone, produced by the testes, stimulates growth of the prostate cancer. A bilateral orchiectomy is the surgical removal of the testes that may be done alone or in combination with prostatectomy. An orchiectomy is one treatment option for cancer control in patients in an advanced stage of prostate cancer. Another possible benefit of this procedure is the rapid relief of bone pain associated with advanced tumours. Orchiectomy may also induce sufficient shrinkage of the prostate to relieve urinary obstruction in later stages of disease when surgery is not an option.

Adverse effects of orchiectomy include hot flashes, ED, loss of sex drive, osteoporosis, and irritability. Weight gain and loss of muscle mass, which are also common, can alter a man's physical appearance, possibly affecting self-esteem and leading to grief and depression. Because this procedure is permanent, many men prefer drug therapy to orchiectomy.

Chemotherapy. The use of chemotherapy has primarily been limited to treatment for those with hormone-resistant prostate cancer (HRPC) in late-stage disease. In HRPC the cancer progresses despite treatment. This progression occurs in patients who have taken an antiandrogen for a certain period of time. The goal of chemotherapy is mainly palliation. Some of the more commonly used chemotherapeutic drugs include docetaxel (Taxotere), mitoxantrone, cyclophosphamide (Procytox), idarubicin, cabazitaxel (Jevtana), and paclitaxel (Abraxane).

Radiotherapy. Radium-223 dichloride (Xofigo) can be used in the treatment of patients with castration-resistant prostate cancer, symptomatic bone metastases, and no known visceral metastatic disease. It is an alpha particle–emitting radiotherapy drug that mimics calcium and forms complexes with hydroxyapatite at areas of increased bone turnover, such as bone metastases.

CULTURALLY COMPETENT CARE

PROSTATE CANCER
Nurses need to be aware of ethnic and cultural considerations when providing information about the risk for prostate cancer and screening recommendations. They must consider not only the ethnic differences in the incidence of prostate cancer but also differences in health-promotion practices.

Despite the importance of annual checkups and a DRE, individuals in lower socioeconomic groups frequently do not use such services. Although exposure to electronic and print media is successful in informing some men about prostate cancer, significant differences of effectiveness exist based on demographic variables such as ethnicity, age, education level, and socioeconomic level. Nurses should consider patients individually and determine the best method to communicate this information to each in

order to achieve the greatest degree of understanding and participation in prostate cancer screening.

NURSING MANAGEMENT
PROSTATE CANCER

NURSING ASSESSMENT
Subjective and objective data that should be obtained from a patient with prostate cancer are presented in Table 57-8.

NURSING DIAGNOSES
Nursing diagnoses for the patient with prostate cancer depend on the stage of the cancer. General nursing diagnoses may include the following.

- *Decisional conflict* related to *conflicting information sources, inexperience with decision-making* (numerous alternative treatment options)
- *Acute pain* related to *biological injury agent, physical injury agent* (prostatic enlargement, surgery)
- *Impaired urinary elimination* related to *multiple causality* (obstruction of the urethra by the prostate, loss of bladder tone)
- *Sexual dysfunction* related to *vulnerability* (effects of treatment)
- *Anxiety* related to *threat to current status, threat of death* (effect of treatment on sexual function, uncertain outcome of disease process)

TABLE 57-8 NURSING ASSESSMENT

Prostate Cancer

Subjective Data
Important Health Information
Past health history: Family history of prostate cancer; diet high in fat
Medications: Use of testosterone supplements or any other medications affecting urinary tract such as morphine, anticholinergics, monoamine oxidase inhibitors, and tricyclic antidepressants
Surgeries or other treatments: History of urinary tract infections or prostate problems

Symptoms
- *Urinary:* Hesitancy or straining to start stream; weak stream; urinary urgency or frequency; dysuria; retention with dribbling; hematuria; nocturia
- *Other:* Low back pain radiating to legs or pelvis; bone pain (possible indicators of metastasis); anorexia, weight loss (possible indicators of metastasis); increasing fatigue and malaise; anxiety related to self-concept or sexuality

Objective Data
General
Older-adult male; pelvic lymphadenopathy (late sign)

Urinary
Distended bladder on palpation; unilaterally hard, enlarged, fixed prostate on rectal examination

Musculo-Skeletal
Pathological fractures (metastasis)

Possible Findings
↑ Serum PSA; ↑ serum PAP (metastasis); nodular and irregular prostate on ultrasonography, positive biopsy results; anemia

PAP, prostatic acid phosphatase; *PSA,* prostate-specific antigen.

PLANNING

The overall goals are that the patient with prostate cancer will (a) be an active participant in the treatment plan, (b) have satisfactory pain control, (c) follow the therapeutic plan, (d) understand the effect of the therapeutic plan on sexual function, and (e) find a satisfactory way to manage the impact on bladder or bowel function.

NURSING IMPLEMENTATION

HEALTH PROMOTION. One of the nurse's most important roles in relation to prostate cancer is to encourage patients, in consultation with their health care providers, to have annual health checkups, including a DRE, starting at age 50 (or younger if risk factors are present).

⟳ EVIDENCE-INFORMED PRACTICE

Translating Research Into Practice

George Nandi is a 56-year-old man who has gone to the occupational health nurse at his place of employment in a manufacturing company for his regular blood pressure check. His father and uncle have a history of prostate cancer. He tells the nurse that he has heard "all over the news" about screening for prostate cancer. He has been getting a blood test for prostate-specific antigen (PSA) yearly and asks if he needs to continue.

Best Available Evidence	Clinician Expertise	Patient Preferences and Values
PSA screening saves lives when performed appropriately in men at *high risk* of developing prostate cancer.	The nurse knows that Mr. Nandi is in a high-risk category for prostate cancer. He has African ancestry. He is more than 50 yr old, and he has first-degree relatives with prostate cancer. Based on these risk factors, the nurse encourages him to have an annual health examination, including DRE and a *PCA3* urine test.	Mr. Nandi wants the best preventive measures to screen for prostate cancer. He was involved in the care of both his father and uncle when they were sick, and he does not want what happened to them to happen to him.

Decision and Action

The nurse encourages Mr. Nandi to discuss his concerns about annual PSA testing with his primary health care provider and for him to have a thorough discussion about the use of *PCA3* testing to screen for prostate cancer. The nurse also discusses the potential influence of risk factors and diet on developing prostate cancer and teaches him about food to avoid or limit (e.g., red meat, high-fat dietary products) and those to increase (e.g., vegetables, fruits).

Reference for Evidence

Canadian Cancer Society. (2017). *Finding prostate cancer early*. Retrieved from *http://www.cancer.ca/en/cancer-information/cancer-type/prostate/finding-cancer-early/?region=on*; Bell, N., Connor Gorber, S., Shane, A., et al. (2014). Guidelines. Recommendations on screening for prostate cancer with the prostate-specific antigen test. *Canadian Medical Association Journal, 186*(16), 1225–1234. doi:10.1503/cmaj.140703.

ACUTE INTERVENTION. Preoperative and postoperative phases of radical prostatectomy are similar to surgical procedures for BPH (see pp. 1426–1428). Nursing interventions for a patient who undergoes radiation therapy and chemotherapy are discussed in Chapter 18. An additional consideration is the psychological response of the patient to a diagnosis of cancer. The nurse should provide sensitive, caring support for the patient and his family to help them cope with the diagnosis of cancer. Prostate support groups are available for men and their families to encourage them to be active, informed participants in their own care.

AMBULATORY AND HOME CARE. The nurse should teach appropriate catheter care if the patient is discharged with an in-dwelling catheter. The patient should be instructed to clean the urethral meatus with soap and water once a day; maintain a high fluid intake; keep the collecting bag lower than the bladder at all times; keep the catheter securely anchored to the inner thigh or the abdomen; and report any signs of bladder infection, such as bladder spasms, fever, or hematuria. If urinary incontinence is a problem, patients should be encouraged to practise pelvic floor muscle exercises (Kegel exercises) at every urination and throughout the day. Continuous practice during the 4- to 6-week healing process improves the success rate. Products for incontinence specifically designed for men are available through home care product catalogues and many retail stores.

Palliative and end-of-life care are often appropriate and beneficial to the patient and family (see Chapter 13). Common problems experienced by patients with advanced prostate cancer include fatigue, bladder outlet obstruction and ureteral obstruction (caused by compression of the urethra or ureters or both from tumour mass or lymph node metastasis), severe bone pain and fractures (caused by bone metastasis), spinal cord compression (from spinal metastasis), and leg edema (caused by lymphedema, deep-vein thrombosis, or another medical condition). Nursing interventions must focus on all of these problems. However, management of pain is one of the most important aspects of nursing care for these patients. Pain control involves ongoing pain assessment, administration of prescribed medications (both opioid and nonopioid agents), and nonpharmacological methods of pain relief (e.g., relaxation breathing). (Pain management is discussed further in Chapter 10.)

EVALUATION

The outcomes for the patient with prostate cancer are that he will:

- Be an active participant in the treatment plan
- Have satisfactory pain control
- Follow the therapeutic plan
- Understand the effect of the treatment on sexual function
- Find a satisfactory way to manage the impact on bladder or bowel function

PROSTATITIS

Etiology and Pathophysiology

Prostatitis is a broad term that describes a group of acute or chronic inflammatory conditions affecting the prostate gland, usually as a result of infection. It is the most common urological problem in men younger than 50 years, and nearly 50% of men will have some form of prostatitis in their lifetime (Canadian Cancer Society, 2017c). Classifications for prostatitis include four categories: (a) acute bacterial prostatitis, (b) chronic bacterial prostatitis, (c) chronic prostatitis–chronic pelvic pain syndrome, and (d) asymptomatic inflammatory prostatitis (Anothaisintawee, Attia, Nickel, et al., 2011).

Both acute and chronic bacterial prostatitis generally result from organisms reaching the prostate gland by one of the following routes: ascending from the urethra, descending from the bladder, or invading via the bloodstream or the lymphatic channels. Common causative organisms are *Escherichia coli, Klebsiella, Pseudomonas, Enterobacter, Proteus, Chlamydia trachomatis, Neisseria gonorrhoeae,* and group D streptococci. Chronic bacterial prostatitis differs from acute prostatitis in that it involves recurrent episodes of infection.

Chronic prostatitis–chronic pelvic pain syndrome describes a syndrome with prostate and urinary pain in the absence of an obvious infectious process. The etiology of this syndrome is not known. It may occur after a viral illness, or it may be associated with sexually transmitted infections, particularly in younger adults. A culture reveals no causative organisms. However, leukocytes may be found in prostatic secretions.

Asymptomatic inflammatory prostatitis is usually diagnosed in individuals who have no symptoms but are found to have an inflammatory process in the prostate. These patients are usually diagnosed during the evaluation of other genito-urinary tract problems. Leukocytes are present in the seminal fluid from the prostate, but the cause of this process is unclear.

Clinical Manifestations and Complications

Common clinical manifestations of acute bacterial prostatitis include fever, chills, back pain, and perineal pain, along with acute urinary symptoms such as dysuria, urinary frequency, urgency, and cloudy urine (Anothaisintawee, Attia, Nickel, et al., 2011). The patient may also have acute urinary retention caused by prostatic swelling. With DRE, the prostate is extremely swollen, very tender, and firm. The complications of prostatitis are epididymitis and cystitis. Sexual functioning may be affected as evidenced by postejaculation pain, libido problems, and ED. Prostatic abscess is also a potential but uncommon complication.

Chronic bacterial prostatitis and chronic prostatitis–pelvic pain syndrome manifest with similar symptoms that are generally milder than those associated with acute bacterial prostatitis. These include irritative voiding symptoms (frequency, urgency, dysuria), backache, perineal or pelvic pain, and ejaculatory pain. Obstructive symptoms are uncommon unless the patient has coexisting BPH. With DRE, the prostate feels enlarged and firm (often described as "boggy") and is slightly tender with palpation. Chronic prostatitis can predispose the patient to recurrent UTIs.

The clinical features of prostatitis can mimic those of a UTI. However, acute cystitis (inflammation of the bladder associated with bacterial infection) is not common in men.

Diagnostic Studies

Because patients with prostatitis have urinary symptoms, a urinalysis and urine culture are indicated; often white blood cells and bacteria are present. If the patient has a fever, white blood cell count and blood cultures are also indicated. The PSA test may be done to rule out prostate cancer. However, PSA levels are often elevated with prostatic inflammation. Thus the test is not considered diagnostic in itself.

Microscopic evaluation and culture of expressed prostate secretion are considered useful in the diagnosis of prostatitis. Expressed prostate secretion is obtained using a premassage and postmassage test (HealthLinkBC, 2016). The patient is asked to void into a specimen cup just before and just after a vigorous prostate massage. Prostatic massage (for expressed prostate secretion) should be avoided if acute bacterial prostatitis is suspected because compression is extremely painful and can increase the risk for bacteria spread. TRUS has not been particularly useful in the diagnosis of prostatitis. However, transabdominal ultrasonography or MRI may be done to rule out an abscess on the prostate.

NURSING AND COLLABORATIVE MANAGEMENT PROSTATITIS

Antibiotics commonly used for acute and chronic bacterial prostatitis include trimethoprim–sulfamethoxazole and ciprofloxacin (Cipro). Doxycycline or tetracycline may be prescribed for patients who have multiple sex partners. Antibiotics are usually given orally for up to 4 weeks for acute bacterial prostatitis. However, if the patient has high fever or other signs of impending sepsis, hospitalization and intravenous antibiotics are prescribed. Patients with chronic bacterial prostatitis are given oral antibiotic therapy for 4 to 12 weeks. A short course of oral antibiotics is usually prescribed for those with chronic prostatitis–chronic pelvic pain syndrome. However, antibiotic therapy often is ineffective for patients whose prostatitis is not caused by bacteria.

Although patients with acute and chronic bacterial prostatitis tend to experience a great amount of discomfort, the pain resolves as the infection is treated. Pain management for patients with chronic prostatitis–chronic pelvic pain syndrome is more difficult because the pain persists for weeks to months. Anti-inflammatory agents are the most common agents used for pain control in prostatitis, but these provide only moderate pain relief. Opioid pain medications can be used, but if the pain is chronic in nature, multimodal therapies should be considered. Relaxation of muscle tissue in the prostate using α-adrenergic blockers has been shown to be effective in reducing discomfort for some men (Azoulay, Eberg, Benayoun, et al., 2015).

Acute urinary retention can develop in acute prostatitis, necessitating bladder drainage with suprapubic catheterization. Passage of a catheter through the inflamed urethra in acute prostatitis is contraindicated. Repetitive prostatic massage may be recommended as adjunct therapy for prostatitis for men. This measure relieves congestion within the prostate by squeezing out excess prostatic secretions, thus providing pain relief. Prostatic massage is performed by using the index finger of a gloved hand and pressing down on the prostate, covering the entire gland's surface in longitudinal strokes. Measures to stimulate ejaculation (masturbation and intercourse) help drain the prostate and provide some relief.

Because the prostate can serve as a source of bacteria, patients experiencing prostatitis should maintain a high fluid intake. The nurse should therefore encourage the patient to drink plenty of fluids. This is especially important for those with acute bacterial prostatitis because of the increased fluid needs associated with fever and infection. Management of fever is also an important nursing intervention.

PROBLEMS OF THE PENIS

Health problems of the penis are rare if sexually transmitted infections are excluded (see Chapter 55). Problems of the penis may be classified as congenital, problems of the prepuce, problems with the erectile mechanism, and cancer.

CONGENITAL PROBLEMS

Hypospadias is a urological abnormality in which the urethral meatus is located on the ventral surface of the penis anywhere from the corona to the perineum. Hormonal influences in utero, environmental factors, and genetic factors are possible causes. Surgical repair of hypospadias may be necessary if it is associated with *chordee* (a painful downward curvature of the penis during erection) or if it prevents intercourse or normal urination. Surgery may also be done for cosmetic reasons or emotional well-being.

Epispadias, an opening of the urethra on the dorsal surface of the penis, is a complex birth defect that is usually associated with other genito-urinary tract defects. Corrective surgery to place the urethra in a normal position in the penis is usually done in early childhood.

PROBLEMS OF THE PREPUCE

Problems of the prepuce are rare in Canada because, up until the 1990s, circumcision was a routine procedure for most male infants. Circumcision, the surgical removal of the foreskin of the penis, is a procedure done to male infants for religious or cultural reasons.

Phimosis is a constriction of the uncircumcised foreskin around the head of the penis, making retraction over the glans penis difficult. It is caused by edema or inflammation of the foreskin, usually associated with poor hygiene techniques that allow bacterial and yeast organisms to become trapped under the foreskin (Figure 57-8, *A*). The goal of treatment is to return the foreskin to its natural position over the glans penis through manual reduction. One strategy involves pushing the glans back through the prepuce by applying constant thumb pressure while the index fingers pull the prepuce over the glans. Ice, hand compression, or both on the foreskin, glans, and penis may be used before this technique to reduce edema. Topical corticosteroid cream applied two or three times daily to the exterior and interior of the tip of the foreskin may also be effective.

Paraphimosis is narrowing or edema of the retracted uncircumcised foreskin, preventing normal return over the glans and causing strangulation. This can occur when the foreskin is pulled back for cleansing, for the use of a urinary catheter, or during intercourse and is not returned to the forward position. Antibiotics, warm soaks, and sometimes circumcision or dorsal slitting of the prepuce may be required. Careful cleaning followed by replacement of the foreskin generally prevents these problems (see Figure 57-8, *B*).

FIGURE 57-8 A, Phimosis: inability to retract the foreskin due to secondary lesions on the prepuce. **B,** Paraphimosis: ulcer with edema from foreskin remaining contracted over the prepuce.

PROBLEMS OF ERECTILE MECHANISM

Priapism is a painful erection lasting longer than 4 hours and may constitute a medical emergency (Song & Moon, 2013). Causes of priapism include thrombosis of the corpus cavernosal veins, leukemia, sickle cell anemia, diabetes mellitus, degenerative lesions of the spine, neoplasms of the brain or spinal cord, prolonged foreplay, injection of vasoactive medications into the corpus cavernosa, and use of certain medications and cocaine. Treatment may include sedatives, injection of smooth muscle relaxants directly into the penis, aspiration and irrigation of the corpora cavernosa with a large-bore needle, and the surgical creation of a shunt to drain the corpora. Complications may include penile tissue necrosis caused by lack of blood flow or hydronephrosis from bladder distension. With immediate medical treatment, the risk for permanent ED is low.

Peyronie's disease, sometimes referred to as *curved* or *crooked penis,* is caused by plaque formation in one of the corpora cavernosa of the penis. The palpable, nontender, hard plaque formation is usually found on the posterior surface. It may result from trauma to the penile shaft or may occur spontaneously. The plaque prevents adequate blood flow into the spongy tissue, which results in a curvature during erection. The condition is not dangerous but can result in painful erections, ED, or embarrassment. Patients may improve over time, stabilize, or need surgery.

CANCER OF THE PENIS

Cancer of the penis is rare. Major risk factors include human papilloma virus infection, smoking, and psoriasis (Latendresse & McCance, 2011), as well as not having been circumcised as an infant (Lawindy, Rodriguez, Horenblas, et al., 2011). The tumour may appear as a superficial ulceration or a pimple-like nodule. The nontender warty lesion may be mistaken for a venereal wart. The majority of malignancies (95%) are well-differentiated squamous cell carcinomas. Treatment in the early stages is laser removal of the growth. A radical resection of the penis may be done if the cancer has spread. Surgery, radiation, or chemotherapy may be tried, depending on the extent of the disease, lymph node involvement, or metastasis.

▌PROBLEMS OF THE SCROTUM AND TESTES

INFLAMMATORY AND INFECTIOUS PROBLEMS

Skin Problems

The skin of the scrotum is susceptible to a number of common skin diseases. The most common conditions of the scrotal skin are fungal infections, dermatitis (neurodermatitis, contact dermatitis, seborrheic dermatitis), and parasitic infections (scabies, lice). These conditions involve discomfort for the patient but are associated with few, if any, severe complications (see Chapter 26).

Epididymitis

Epididymitis is an inflammation of the epididymis (Figure 57-9), usually secondary to an infectious process (sexually or nonsexually transmitted) and rarely as a result of trauma or urinary reflux down the vas deferens from the urethra. Swelling may progress to the point that the epididymis and the testis

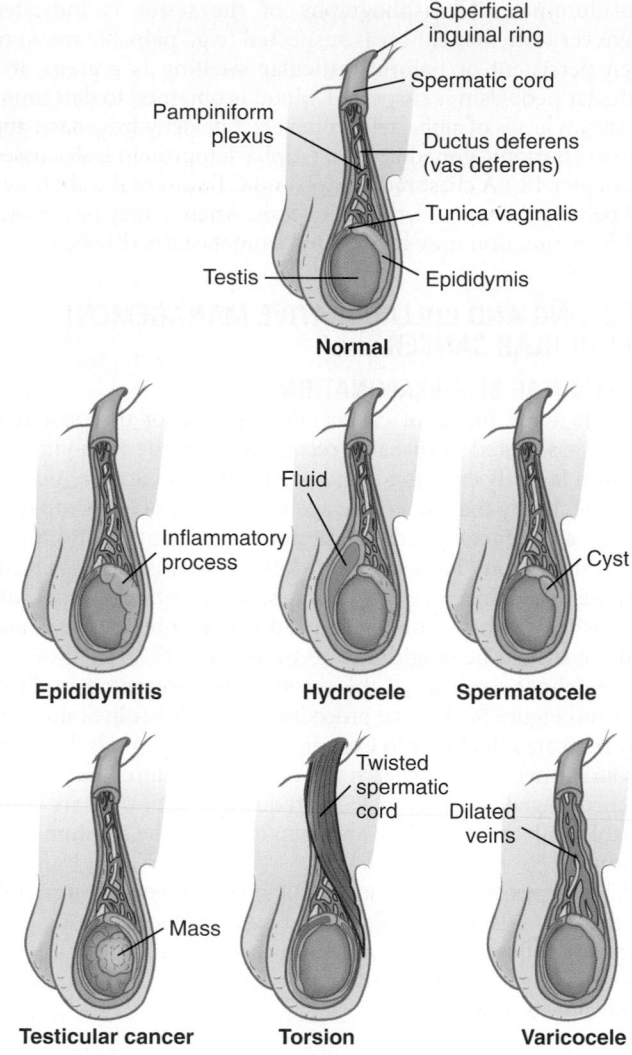

Superficial
inguinal ring

Spermatic cord

Pampiniform
plexus

Ductus deferens
(vas deferens)

Tunica vaginalis

Testis

Epididymis

Normal

Inflammatory
process

Fluid

Cyst

Epididymitis

Hydrocele

Spermatocele

Twisted
spermatic
cord

Dilated
veins

Mass

Testicular cancer

Torsion

Varicocele

FIGURE 57-9 Scrotal masses.

FIGURE 57-10 Hydrocele. Source: Swartz, M. H. (2010). *Textbook of physical diagnosis: History and examination* (6th ed., p. 537, Figure 18-28). Philadelphia: Saunders.

known), pain medications, or bed rest with the scrotum elevated on an ice pack.

CONGENITAL PROBLEMS

Cryptorchidism (undescended testes) is failure of the testes to descend into the scrotal sac before birth. It is the most common congenital testicular condition. It may occur bilaterally or unilaterally and may be the cause of infertility if corrective surgery is not done by 2 years of age. The incidence of testicular cancer is also higher if the condition is not corrected before puberty. Surgery is performed to locate and suture the testis or testes to the scrotum.

Maternal use of acetaminophen during pregnancy may increase the risk of male offspring being born with cryptorchidism; however, there is little evidence that implicates maternal use of ibuprofen or acetylsalicylic acid (Jensen, Henriksen, Rebordosa, et al., 2011).

ACQUIRED PROBLEMS

Hydrocele

A **hydrocele** is a nontender, fluid-filled mass that results from interference with lymphatic drainage of the scrotum and swelling of the tunica vaginalis that surrounds the testis (Figure 57-10; see also Figure 57-9). Diagnosis is fairly simple because the mass can be seen by shining a flashlight through the scrotum (transillumination). No treatment is indicated unless the swelling becomes very large and uncomfortable, in which case aspiration or surgical drainage of the mass is performed.

Spermatocele

A **spermatocele** is a firm, sperm-containing, painless cyst of the epididymis that may be visible with transillumination (see Figure 57-9). The cause is unknown, and surgical removal is the treatment. It is important for men to see their doctor if they feel any scrotal lumps. Patients would be unable to distinguish this cyst from cancer when performing self-examination.

Varicocele

A **varicocele** is a dilation of the veins that drain the testes (see Figure 57-9). The scrotum feels wormlike when palpated. The cause of the problem is unknown. The varicocele is usually located on the left side of the scrotum as a consequence of retrograde blood flow from the left renal vein. Surgery is indicated for patients who are infertile because persistent varicoceles are associated

are indistinguishable. In men younger than 40 years of age, the most common cause is gonorrhea or chlamydial infection. UTI and prostatitis are common causes in older men. The use of antibiotics is important for both partners if the transmission is through sexual contact. Patients should be encouraged to refrain from sexual intercourse during the acute phase. If they do engage in intercourse, a condom should be used. Conservative treatment consists of bed rest with elevation of the scrotum, use of ice packs, and analgesics. Ambulation places the scrotum in a dependent position and increases pain. Most tenderness subsides within 1 week, although swelling may last for weeks or months.

Orchitis

Orchitis refers to an acute inflammation of the testis. In orchitis, the testis is painful, tender, and swollen. It generally occurs after an episode of bacterial or viral infections such as mumps, pneumonia, tuberculosis, or syphilis. It can also be caused by epididymitis, prostatectomy, trauma, infectious mononucleosis, influenza, catheterization, or complicated UTI. Mumps orchitis is a condition contributing to infertility, and its incidence could easily be decreased by childhood vaccination against mumps. Treatment involves the use of antibiotics (if the organism is with 40% to 50% of cases of infertility. Repair of the varicocele may be through injection of a sclerosing agent or by surgical ligation of the spermatic vein.

Testicular Torsion

Testicular torsion involves a twisting of the spermatic cord that supplies blood to the testes and epididymis, causing an interruption to the blood supply (see Figure 57-9). It is most commonly seen in males younger than age 20. The patient experiences severe scrotal pain, tenderness, swelling, nausea, and vomiting. Urinary symptoms, fever, and white blood cells or bacteria in the urine are absent. The pain does not usually subside with rest or elevation of the scrotum. Nuclear technetium scan of the testes or Doppler ultrasonography is typically performed to assess blood flow within the testicle. The cremasteric reflex is absent on the side of the swelling, and a decrease in or absence of blood flow confirms the diagnosis. Unless the torsion resolves spontaneously, surgery to untwist the cord and restore the blood supply must be performed immediately. Torsion constitutes a surgical emergency because, if the blood supply to the affected testicle is not restored within 4 to 6 hours, ischemia to the testis will occur, leading to necrosis and the possible need for removal.

TESTICULAR CANCER

Etiology and Pathophysiology

Testicular cancer is relatively rare, accounting for less than 1% of all cancers found in males. It has a 5-year survival rate of 96% (Canadian Cancer Society, 2017d). Testicular cancer is the most common type of cancer in young men between 15 and 29 years of age (Canadian Cancer Society, 2017e). Testicular cancer occurs more commonly in the right testicle than in the left (Latendresse & McCance, 2011). Testicular tumours are also more common in males who have had undescended testes (cryptorchidism), a family history of testicular cancer or anomalies, or Klinefelter's syndrome (Canadian Cancer Society, 2017f). Other predisposing factors include orchitis, human immunodeficiency virus infection, maternal exposure to diethylstilbestrol, and testicular cancer in the contralateral testis.

Most testicular cancers develop from embryonic germ cells. The two types of germ cell cancers are seminomas and nonseminomas. Although seminoma germ cell cancers are the most common, they are the least aggressive. Nonseminoma testicular germ cell tumours are rare but are very aggressive. Non–germ cell tumours arise from other testicular tissue and include Leydig cell and Sertoli cell tumours. These account for less than 10% of testicular cancers.

Clinical Manifestations and Complications

Testicular cancer may have a slow or rapid onset depending on the type of tumour. The patient may notice a painless lump in his scrotum as well as scrotal swelling and a feeling of heaviness. The scrotal mass usually is nontender and very firm. Some patients complain of a dull ache or heavy sensation in the lower abdomen, the perianal area, or the scrotum. Acute pain is the presenting symptom in about 10% of patients. Manifestations associated with advanced disease are varied and include lower back or chest pain, cough, and dyspnea.

Diagnostic Studies

Palpation of the scrotal contents is the first step in diagnosing testicular cancer. A cancerous mass is firm and does not transilluminate. Ultrasonography of the testes is indicated whenever testicular cancer is suspected (e.g., palpable mass) or when persistent or painful testicular swelling is present. If a testicular neoplasm is suspected, blood is obtained to determine the serum levels of alpha-fetoprotein, lactate dehydrogenase, and human chorionic gonadotropin. (Alpha-fetoprotein is discussed in Chapter 18.) A chest radiograph and CT scan of the abdomen and pelvis are done to detect metastasis. Anemia may be present, and liver function may be elevated in metastatic disease.

NURSING AND COLLABORATIVE MANAGEMENT TESTICULAR CANCER

TESTICULAR SELF-EXAMINATION

As with many forms of cancer, the survival of the patient is closely associated with early recognition of the tumour. The scrotum is easily examined, and beginning tumours are usually palpable. Every male from the age of 15 years of age should be taught and encouraged to perform a monthly testicular self-examination (TSE) so that he knows what is normal for his testicles and can notice any changes. Male patients, especially those with a history of undescended testis or a previous testicular tumour, should be taught how to perform TSE.

Guidelines for TSE of the scrotum are presented in Table 57-9 and Figure 57-11. The procedure is not difficult. Some men may indicate reluctance to examine their own genitals, but with encouragement, they can learn this simple procedure. They should be encouraged to perform TSEs frequently until they are comfortable with the procedure and then examine the scrotum once a month.

Videotapes and illustrations on shower hangers are available as teaching aids and ideally should be introduced during high school or college physical education classes. Free information is available through the Canadian Cancer Society and on various medical websites.

COLLABORATIVE CARE

Collaborative care of testicular cancer generally involves an orchiectomy or a radical orchiectomy (surgical removal of the affected testis, the spermatic cord, and regional lymph nodes).

TABLE 57-9	PATIENT & CAREGIVER TEACHING GUIDE

Testicular Self-Examination

The nurse should include the following instructions when teaching a patient how to perform testicular self-examination:

1. Just after a shower or bath is the best time to examine the testes. Warm temperatures make the testes hang lower in the scrotum.
2. Stand in front of a mirror. Look for any swelling on the skin of the scrotum.
3. Hold your scrotum in the palms of your hands so that you can feel the size and weight of each testicle. It is normal for one testicle to be larger and hang lower than the other.
4. Gently roll each testicle between your thumb and your fingers (see Figure 57-11, *A*). Feel for lumps or bumps. If you feel a soft, tender tube cord leading upward from the back of each testicle, that is normal (see Figure 57-11, *B*).
5. Notify the health care provider at once if any abnormalities are found.

Source: Adapted from Canadian Cancer Society. (2016). *Testicular cancer: Finding testicular cancer early.* Retrieved from http://www.cancer.ca/en/cancer-information/cancer-type/testicular/finding-cancer-early/?region=on.

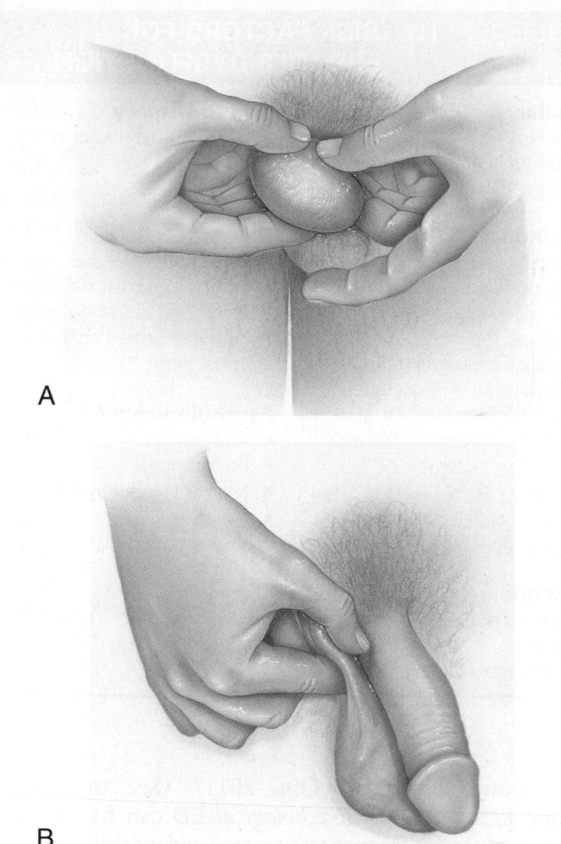

FIGURE 57-11 Testicular self-examination. **A,** The testicle is checked for smoothness by rolling it between the thumb and the fingers. **B,** The spermatic cord or vas deferens can be felt toward the back of the testicle and should feel soft and tender. Source: *The wellness way: Testicular examination.* Copyright 1987, 1994, 2000, 2001, 2002. The StayWell Company.

FIGURE 57-12 Vasectomy procedure. The vas deferens is ligated or resected for the purpose of sterilization.

SEXUAL FUNCTIONING

VASECTOMY

Vasectomy is the bilateral surgical ligation or resection of the vas deferens performed for the purpose of sterilization (Figure 57-12). The procedure requires only 15 to 30 minutes and is usually performed on an outpatient basis with the patient under local anaesthesia. Vasectomy is considered a permanent form of sterilization, although some successful reversals *(vasovasotomy)* have been reported.

After vasectomy, the patient should not notice any difference in the look or feel of the ejaculate because its major component is seminal and prostatic fluid. The patient will need to use an alternative form of contraception until semen examination reveals no sperm. This usually requires at least 10 ejaculations or 6 weeks, until sperm distal to the surgical site are evacuated. Sperm cells continue to be produced by the testes but are absorbed by the body rather than being passed through the vas deferens. Occasionally, postoperative hematoma and swelling of the scrotum occur.

Vasectomy does not affect the production of hormones, the ability to ejaculate, or the physiological mechanisms related to erection or orgasm. Psychological adjustment may be a problem after surgery. It may be difficult for the patient to separate vasectomy from castration at a subconscious level. Some men may develop ED or may feel the need to prove their masculinity by becoming much more sexually active than they were in the past. Careful discussion of the procedure and its outcome before the surgery can be helpful in detecting patients who may have problems with psychological adjustment. Surgery should be delayed for these patients. (The Ethical Dilemmas box discusses sterilization.)

ERECTILE DYSFUNCTION

Erectile dysfunction (ED) is the inability to attain or maintain an erect penis that allows satisfactory sexual performance. Although sexual function is a topic that many individuals are uncomfortable discussing, health care providers must be able and willing to address ED. Treatment may include phosphodiesterase type 5 inhibitors, a class of medications used to treat

Postorchiectomy treatment involves surveillance, radiation therapy, or chemotherapy, depending on the stage of the cancer. Chemotherapy protocols use combination therapy: bleomycin, etoposide (Vepesid), and cisplatin; or etoposide (Vepesid), ifosfamide (Ifex), and cisplatin. (Testicular germ cell tumours are more sensitive to systemic chemotherapy than any other adult solid tumour.)

Of patients with testicular cancer, 97% obtain complete remission if the disease is detected in the early stages (Canadian Cancer Society, 2017d). As a result of treatment successes, the majority of men with testicular cancer become long-term survivors. Treatment-related toxicity, however, is a significant issue. All patients with testicular cancer, regardless of pathological condition or stage, require meticulous follow-up and regular physical examinations, chest radiographic examinations, CT scans, and assessment of human chorionic gonadotropin and alpha-fetoprotein. The goal is to detect relapse when the tumour burden is minimal. Secondary malignancies that occur as a result of chemotherapy and radiation are described in Chapter 18 and in the NCPs 18-1 and 18-2, available on the Evolve website.

Men with testicular cancer should have the opportunity to discuss fertility and sperm banking before any treatment. The nurse should be sensitive to any psychosocial problems this type of cancer can have on a man's feelings of self-worth or sexual performance. Treatment has the potential to interfere with both erections and fertility.

ETHICAL DILEMMAS
Sterilization

Situation

A 43-year-old male patient is requesting a vasectomy and informs the nurse that he does not wish to discuss it with his wife. The physician's policy is to have the spouse or partner sign a form acknowledging the patient's desire to be sterilized. This patient explains that, although his wife wants to have more children, the one they already have is all he wants.

Important Points for Consideration

- Patient autonomy suggests that matters of reproduction are left to the privacy and discretion of the individual. Competent adults may legally choose to be sterilized for medical reasons or for convenience.
- To prevent possible future harm, this man should include his wife in the decision to permanently eliminate his ability to procreate.
- In most provinces and territories, women can terminate a pregnancy without proof that their partners are aware of their intentions. Sterilization, conversely, can be considered a more permanent decision that has consequences for both parties in the relationship.
- This physician's standard is to have evidence of the spouse's or significant other's knowledge of the intent for sterilization. The nurse should inform the man of the standard in this particular physician's practice and the benefits to the integrity of his marriage.
- If the patient is still unwilling to discuss the matter with his wife, either the nurse or the physician should inform the man that they will not participate in deception and he is free to select another physician to perform the procedure.

Clinical Decision-Making Questions

1. How should the nurse approach this situation?
2. Should the nurse tell the wife of her husband's plans?
3. Are there ever circumstances in which deception of a patient or family would be justified?

TABLE 57-10 RISK FACTORS FOR ERECTILE DYSFUNCTION

Vascular • Atherosclerosis • Hypertension • Peripheral vascular disease	**Genito-Urinary** • Radical prostatectomy • Prostatitis • Renal failure
Drug-Induced • Alcohol • Antiandrogens • Antilipidemic agents • Antihypertensives • Diuretics (chlorothiazide, spironolactone [Aldactone]) • Major tranquilizers (diazepam [Valium], alprazolam [Xanax]) • Marijuana, cocaine • Nicotine • Tricyclic antidepressants (e.g., amitriptyline [Elavil])	**Neurological** • Parkinson's disease • Cerebro-vascular disease • Trauma to the spinal cord • Tumours or transection of spinal cord **Psychological** • Anxiety • Depression • Fear of failure to perform • Stress
Endocrine • Diabetes mellitus • Obesity • Testosterone deficiency	**Other** • Aging

---

ED, including tadalafil (Cialis), vardenafil (Levitra), and sildenafil (Viagra).

The effects of ED can lead to anxiety and depression as well as potentially interfere with a man's self-esteem, confidence, relationships, and overall sense of well-being. ED is a condition that is significant because of its prevalence; it is estimated that its prevalence among men in Canada aged 40 to 88 is 49.4%, with estimates that approximately 3 million Canadians over the age of 40 years are affected by ED (Bella, Lee, Carrier, et al., 2015). The problem is increasing in all segments of the sexually active male population and affects both the man and his partner. In younger men, the increase is attributed to substance use, such as recreational drugs and alcohol. Middle-aged men are affected by medical conditions such as diabetes, hypertension, renal disease, organ transplants, coronary artery bypass graft surgeries, and cancer or the therapy for these problems. Men are living longer and expect to remain sexually active, regardless of any existing medical conditions.

Etiology and Pathophysiology

ED can result from a number of factors in two general categories: physiological (organic) and psychological. Common causes of *physiological ED* (Table 57-10) include vascular disease (most common cause), diabetes mellitus, adverse effects from medications, result of surgery (such as prostatectomy), trauma, chronic illness, and decreased gonadal hormone secretion (Elliott, 2011). Although studies suggest a link between cardiovascular disease (CVD) and ED, whether ED is a risk factor for CVD is contro-

versial (Dong, Zhang, & Qin, 2011). (See the Evidence-Informed Practice box.) *Psychological ED* can be caused by a number of issues but is most often associated with stress, difficulty in a relationship, depression, or low self-esteem.

Normal physiological age-related changes are associated with changes in erectile function and may be an underlying cause of ED for some men. Table 53-4 in Chapter 53 lists age-related changes in sexual function. The nurse should be able to explain these age-related changes if necessary to reassure an anxious older man regarding normal changes in his sexual abilities. (The male sexual response is discussed in Chapter 53.)

Clinical Manifestations and Complications

The typical symptom of ED is a patient's self-report of problems associated with sexual performance. He usually describes an inability to attain or maintain an erection. The symptoms may occur only occasionally, may be continual with a gradual onset, or may occur with a sudden onset. A gradual onset of symptoms is usually associated with physiological factors, whereas a sudden or rapid onset of symptoms may be associated with psychological issues.

A man's inability to perform sexually can cause great distress in his interpersonal relationships and may interfere with his concept of himself as a man. It can also affect the relationship between the man and his partner. Problems with ED can lead to a number of personal issues, including anger, anxiety, and depression.

Diagnostic Studies

The first step in diagnosis and management of ED begins with a thorough sexual, health, and psychosocial history. Self-administered assessment and treatment-related questionnaires have been developed and may prove useful as primary screening tools, for example, the Erection Quality Scale (Rosen, Wincze, Mollen, et al., 2007). Second, a physical examination should be performed that focuses on secondary sexual characteristics,

EVIDENCE-INFORMED PRACTICE

Research Highlight

Do Lifestyle Changes and Cardiovascular Medication Improve Erectile Dysfunction?

Clinical Question
For patients with erectile dysfunction (P), what is the effect of lifestyle modifications and drugs for cardiovascular risk factors (I) on severity of dysfunction (O)?

Best Available Evidence
Systematic review and meta-analysis of randomized controlled trials (RCTs)

Critical Appraisal and Synthesis of Evidence
- Six RCTs (*n*=740, mean age of 55 yr old) that examined the effect of lifestyle interventions and drugs targeting cardiovascular (CV) risk factors on erectile dysfunction (ED).
- Interventions lasting at least 6 weeks included diet, exercise, maintenance of an active lifestyle, and drugs to reduce CV risk factors (i.e., statins to lower cholesterol).
- Changes in lifestyle with improved lipid values were related to a decrease in the severity of ED.

Conclusion
- Sexual function was significantly improved in men with ED through lifestyle modification and drugs for CV risk factors.

Implications for Nursing Practice
- Emphasis on the importance of a healthy diet and regular physical activity for men experiencing ED.
- Counselling that declining sexual health should be brought to the attention of the health care provider for early identification of CV risk factors.

Reference for Evidence
Gupta, B. P., Murad, M. H., Clifton, M. M., et al. (2011). The effect of lifestyle modification and cardiovascular risk factor reduction on erectile dysfunction: A systematic review and meta-analysis. *Archives of Internal Medicine, 171*(20), 1797–1803. doi:10.1001/archinternmed.2011.440.

P, Patient population of interest; *I,* intervention or area of interest; *O,* outcomes of interest (see Chapter 1).

including pubic hair distribution, size and appearance of the penis and scrotum, and rectal examination. A DRE should be done to assess prostate size, consistency, and presence of nodules. Assessment of blood pressure, palpation of peripheral pulses, and sensation of the genitalia should also be included.

Further examination or diagnostic testing is typically based on findings from the history and physical examination. Serum glucose and lipid profile bloodwork is recommended to rule out diabetes mellitus. Hormonal levels for testosterone, prolactin, LH, and thyroid may help identify endocrine-related problems, and a complete blood count may be helpful in identifying unrecognized systemic diseases.

Other diagnostic tests may be conducted to diagnose ED. Nocturnal penile tumescence and rigidity testing is a noninvasive method that involves the continuous measurement of penile circumference and axial rigidity during sleep. Such measurements are used to differentiate between physiological and psychological causes of ED as well as to evaluate the effectiveness of drug therapy. Vascular studies, including penile arteriography, penile blood flow study, and duplex Doppler ultrasonography studies, are used to assess penile blood inflow and outflow. Such studies help assess vascular problems interfering with erection.

TABLE 57-11   COLLABORATIVE CARE

Erectile Dysfunction

Diagnostic	Collaborative Therapy
• History and physical examination	• Drug therapy [sildenafil (Viagra), vardenafil (Levitra), tadalafil (Cialis)]
• Nocturnal penile tumescence and rigidity testing	• Intracavernosal self-injection
• Serum glucose and lipid profile	• Intraurethral medication pellet
• Sexual history	• Modify reversible causes
• Testosterone, prolactin, and thyroid hormone levels	• Penile implants
• Vascular studies	• Sexual counselling
	• Topical gels
	• Vacuum constriction device (VCD)

Collaborative Care

The goal of ED therapy is for the patient and his partner to achieve a satisfactory sexual relationship. The treatment for ED is based on the underlying cause. A variety of treatment options are available (Bella, Lee, Carrier, et al., 2015) (Table 57-11). The results of these interventions are usually most satisfactory when both partners are involved in the decision-making process and have realistic expectations of the treatment.

It is important to determine whether ED is reversible before treatment is started. For example, if ED appears to be an adverse effect of prescribed drugs, alternative agents or treatments should be explored. When there is an established diagnosis of testicular failure (hypogonadism), androgen replacement therapy may sometimes be effective in improving erectile function. For individuals who have ED that is psychological in nature, counselling should be provided by a qualified therapist for the patient (and possibly his partner).

Erectogenic Drugs. Sildenafil (Viagra), tadalafil (Cialis), and vardenafil (Levitra) are erectogenic drugs (Lee, 2011). These drugs are phosphodiesterase type 5 (PDE5) inhibitors that cause smooth muscle relaxation and increased blood flow into the corpus cavernosum, thus promoting penile erection. They are taken orally about 30 to 60 minutes before sexual activity, but not more than once a day. These drugs have been found to be generally safe and effective for the treatment of most types of ED.

Adverse effects include headaches, dyspepsia, flushing, and nasal congestion. Additional rare adverse effects are blurred or blue-green visual disturbances, sudden hearing loss, and priapism. The patient should be instructed to seek immediate medical attention if any of these rare reactions occur. Because these drugs may potentiate the hypotensive effect of nitrates (e.g., nitroglycerin), they are contraindicated for individuals taking nitrates.

DRUG ALERT—Sildenafil (Viagra)
- Should not be used with nitrates (nitroglycerin) in any form
- Can potentiate hypotensive effects of nitrates

Vacuum Constriction Devices. Vacuum constriction devices (VCDs) are suction devices that can be applied to the flaccid penis to produce an erection by pulling blood up into the corporeal bodies. A penile ring or constrictive band is placed around the base of the penis to retain venous blood, thereby preventing the erection from subsiding. Special care must be taken in using these devices to prevent tissue bruising.

Vasoactive Drugs. Vasoactive drugs can be administered as a topical gel, by injection into the penis (intracavernosal self-injection), or by insertion of a medicated pellet (alprostadil)

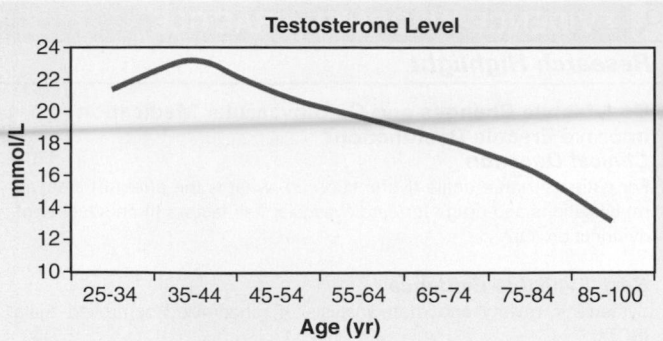

FIGURE 57-14 Changes in testosterone plasma level in men as they age.

FIGURE 57-13 Penile implants. **A,** A malleable implant is always erect but can be bent close to the body for concealment. **B,** An inflatable implant consists of cylinders in the penis, a small pump in the scrotum, and a reservoir in the lower abdomen. When activated, the pump fills the cylinders with fluid from the reservoir. A small release valve permits the fluid to drain back into the reservoir after intercourse.

into the urethra using an intraurethral device. These vasoactive drugs enhance blood flow into the penile arteries. Current vasoactive medications include papaverine, alprostadil (Caverject), and phentolamine.

Penile Implants. Surgical implantation of semirigid or inflatable penile prostheses is shown in Figure 57-13. These surgical procedures are highly invasive and associated with potential complications. Thus, they are usually indicated only for men with severe ED for which other interventions are ineffective.

The devices are implanted into the corporeal bodies to provide an erection firm enough for penetration. The semirigid malleable implant is displayed in Figure 57-13, A. The inflatable implant consists of cylinders in the penis, a small pump in the scrotum, and a reservoir in the lower abdomen (Figure 57-13, B). The main problems associated with penile prostheses are mechanical failure, infection, and erosions.

Sexual Counselling. Sexual counselling is often recommended before and after treatment. It should address psychological or interpersonal factors that may enhance sexual expression as well as other factors that are of concern. Counselling can be effective for the individual patient, but it is typically preferred to include his partner, particularly if he is involved in a long-term relationship. The ability for both partners to be pleased enhances a patient's satisfaction levels. Counselling should begin after the start of medical treatment for ED.

NURSING MANAGEMENT ERECTILE DYSFUNCTION

Patients experiencing ED require a great deal of emotional support for both themselves and their partners. Men often do not feel comfortable discussing these types of problems with others because of society's expectations of a man's sexual abilities. They need reassurance that confidentiality will be maintained. Men may experience and demonstrate isolation from support systems, and they may also lose self-esteem. In conjunction with medical treatment, counselling and therapy may be necessary for couples to establish realistic expectations and develop meaningful communication patterns.

The majority of men delay seeking medical assistance. Once they do, they are often highly motivated and expect immediate solutions to their problems. The health care team should provide a support system and accurate information as soon as possible. Nurses are in a unique position of conducting routine health assessments on men seeking any form of medical treatment. These assessments provide an opportunity to ask questions pertaining to general health as well as sexual health and function. Given the opportunity and recognition that someone cares and can provide them with answers, men are less hesitant to answer these questions.

ANDROPAUSE

Andropause is a gradual decline in androgen secretion that occurs in most men as they age and can begin as early as age 40. The primary male androgen that is reduced is testosterone. Factors that determine the rate of decline are not clearly known. Signs and symptoms associated with a lowered level of testosterone include loss of libido, fatigue, ED, depression and mood swings, and sleep disturbances. Symptoms are often attributed to normal aging and frequently are not reported by the patient (Figure 57-14). The long-term effects, including a loss of muscle mass and strength, may contribute to an increased risk for falls and fractures (LeBlanc, Wang, Lee, et al., 2011).

INFERTILITY

Infertility in a couple is defined as the inability to conceive after 1 year of frequent, unprotected intercourse. Infertility is a disorder of a couple, not of one individual. For this reason, both partners must be involved in determining the cause of infertility. In about 33% of the cases, the cause primarily involves the man. Male infertility can be caused by disorders of the hypothalamic–pituitary system, disorders of the testes, and abnormalities of the ejaculatory system.

The physical causes are generally divided into three categories: pretesticular, testicular, and post-testicular. The *pretesticular or endocrine causes* occur in only about 3% of the cases and can generally be treated with medication or surgery. Seventy-five percent of all male infertility factors are attributable to primary *testicular causes,* with genetic factors identified in about 15% of these cases (Krausz, 2011). Other factors that influence the testes include infection (e.g., mumps virus, sexually transmitted infections, bacterial infections), congenital anomalies, medications, radiation, substance use (alcohol, nicotine, drugs), and environmental hazards. *Post-testicular causes* account for approximately 5% to 7% of the cases, with obstruction, infection, or the result of a surgical procedure being the primary causes. The remaining 40% are classified as *idiopathic,* or of unknown cause.

A careful health history and examination may reveal the cause of a patient's infertility. Thus, the history is a starting point for determining cause and treatment. The history should include age; occupation; past injury, surgery, or infections to the genital tract; lifestyle issues such as use of hot tubs, weight training, or wearing of tight undergarments; sexual practices; frequency of intercourse; and emotional factors such as stress levels and the desire for children. The use of drugs, such as chemotherapeutic drugs, anabolic steroids (testosterone), sulphasalazine, cimetidine, and recreational drugs, should be documented because these can reduce sperm count. A physical examination can disclose a varicocele, Peyronie's disease, or other physical abnormalities.

The first test in an infertility study is a semen analysis. The test determines the sperm concentration (count >20 million/mL), forward progressive motility (at least 60% with a grade >2), and morphology (at least 60% have a normal oval head and long tail). Additional tests that may be helpful in determining the etiology include plasma testosterone and serum LH and FSH measurements. A test for sperm penetration abilities may also be done. The specific cause of infertility is often not determined.

Nurses should be concerned and tactful in dealing with male patients undergoing infertility studies. Many men equate fertility and masculinity. The nurse must be sensitive to the problem of gender identity in the infertile man.

Treatment options for men include medications, conservative lifestyle changes (e.g., avoidance of scrotal heat, substance abuse, high stress), in vitro fertilization techniques, and corrective surgery. Infertility can seriously strain a marriage, and the couple may require counselling and discussion of alternatives if conception is not achieved. (Female infertility is discussed in Chapter 56.)

CASE STUDY

Benign Prostatic Hyperplasia

Patient Profile

LeRon Wilson, a 60-year-old married man, comes to the primary health outpatient clinic because of an inability to void for the past 13 hours and pain in the lower abdomen.

Subjective Data

- Complains of urge to void
- Is very restless, anxious, and agitated

Source: sirtravelalot/ Shutterstock .com

Objective Data

- Has prostate enlargement on digital rectal examination
- Has hematuria, bacteria, and white blood cells in urine
- Has a tender and palpable bladder above umbilicus

Collaborative Care

- In-dwelling catheter inserted by a urology resident
- Admitted to hospital

Discussion Questions

1. What risk factors for prostate problems are present in Mr. Wilson?
2. Explain the etiology of the objective symptoms Mr. Wilson exhibited.
3. Discuss the drug options available to Mr. Wilson.
4. Discuss the invasive options available to Mr. Wilson.
5. Mr. Wilson asks about the effect of the various treatment options on his ability to have sex. How should the nurse respond?
6. ***Priority decision:*** What are the priority nursing diagnoses based on the assessment data presented? Are there any collaborative problems?
7. ***Priority decision:*** What is the priority nursing intervention for Mr. Wilson?
8. On further assessment, the nurse notes that Mr. Wilson has a nursing diagnosis of *decisional conflict.* How should the nurse help him resolve this conflict related to treatment options?
9. ***Evidence-informed practice:*** What information should the nurse offer to Mr. Wilson when he asks if he should start taking saw palmetto to prevent future UTIs?

⊝volve

Answers are available at *http://evolve.elsevier.com/Canada/Lewis/medsurg.*

REVIEW QUESTIONS

The number of the question corresponds to the same-numbered objective at the beginning of the chapter.

1. An older male client is experiencing difficulty in initiating voiding and a feeling of incomplete bladder emptying. What are these symptoms of BPH primarily caused by?
   a. Obstruction of the urethra
   b. Untreated chronic prostatis
   c. Decreased bladder compliance
   d. Excessive secretion of testosterone

2. Postoperatively, a client who has had a laser prostatectomy has continuous bladder irrigation with a three-way urinary catheter with a 30-mL balloon. When he complains of bladder spasms with the catheter in place, what should the nurse do?

   a. Deflate the catheter balloon to 10 mL to decrease bulk in the bladder.
   b. Deflate the catheter balloon and then reinflate to ensure that it is patent.
   c. Encourage the client to try to have a bowel movement to relieve colon pressure.
   d. Explain that this feeling is normal and that he should not try to urinate around the catheter.

3. Which factors would place a client at higher risk for prostate cancer? *(Select all that apply)*
   a. Older than 65 years
   b. Asian or Indigenous Canadian
   c. Long-term use of an in-dwelling urethral catheter

    d. Father diagnosed and treated for early-stage prostate cancer

    e. Previous history of undescended testicle and testicular cancer

4. A client scheduled for a prostatectomy for prostate cancer expresses the fear that he will have erectile dysfunction (ED). In responding to this client, what should the nurse keep in mind?

    a. ED can occur even with a nerve-sparing procedure.

    b. Retrograde ejaculation affects sexual function more frequently than erectile dysfunction.

    c. The most common complication of this surgery is postoperative bowel incontinence.

    d. Preoperative sexual function is the most important factor in determining postoperative erectile dysfunction.

5. What should the nurse explain to the client with chronic bacterial prostatitis who is undergoing antibiotic therapy? *(Select all that apply)*

    a. All clients require hospitalization.

    b. Pain will lessen once the infection is resolved.

    c. Course of treatment is generally 4 to 12 weeks.

    d. Long-term therapy may be indicated in immuno-compromised clients.

    e. If the condition is unresolved and untreated, he is at risk for prostate cancer.

6. Which manifestations of testicular cancer would the nurse observe for when assessing a client for this disease?

    a. Acute back spasms and testicular pain

    b. Rapid onset of scrotal swelling and fever

    c. Fertility problems and bilateral scrotal tenderness

    d. Painless mass and sensation of heaviness in the scrotal area

7. What should the nurse explain to the client who has had a vasectomy?

    a. The procedure blocks the production of sperm.

    b. ED is temporary and will return with continued sexual activity.

    c. The ejaculate will be about half the volume it was before the procedure.

    d. An alternative form of contraception will be necessary for 6 to 8 weeks.

8. What measure should the nurse use to decrease the client's discomfort over care related to his reproductive organs?

    a. Relate his sexual concerns to his sexual partner.

    b. Arrange to have only male nurses care for the client.

    c. Maintain a nonjudgemental attitude toward his sexual practices.

    d. Use only technical terminology when discussing reproductive function.

1. b; 2. d; 3. a; 4. a; 5. b, c, d; 6. d; 7. d; 8. c.

⊜volve

For even more review questions, visit *http://evolve.elsevier.com/Canada/Lewis/medsurg*.

REFERENCES

Andriole, G., McCullum-Hill, C., Sandhu, G., et al. (2013). The effect of increasing doses of saw palmetto fruit extract on serum prostate specific antigen: Analysis of the CAMUS randomized trial. *Journal of Urology, 189*(2), 486–492.

Anothaisintawee, T., Attia, J., Nickel, J., et al. (2011). Management of chronic prostatitis/chronic pelvic pain syndrome: A systematic review and network meta-analysis. *JAMA: The Journal of the American Medical Association, 305*(1), 78–86. doi:10.1001/jama.2010.1913.

Azoulay, L., Eberg, M., Benayoun, S., et al. (2015). 5α-reductase inhibitors and the risk of cancer-related mortality in men with prostate cancer. *Journal of the American Medical Association Oncology, 1*(3), 314–320. doi:10.1001/jamaoncol.2015.0387.

Barry, M., Cantor, A., Roehrborn, C., et al. (2013). Relationships between participants' International Prostate Symptom Score and BPH Impact Index changes and global ratings of change in a trial of phytotherapy for men with lower urinary tract symptoms. *Journal of Urology, 189*(3), 987–992.

Barry, M., Fowler, F., O'Leary, M., et al. (1992). The American Urologic Association symptom index for benign prostatic hyperplasia. *Journal of Urology, 148*(5), 1549–1557. (Seminal).

Bell, N., Connor Gorber, S., Shane, A., et al. (2014). Guidelines. Recommendations on screening for prostate cancer with the prostate-specific antigen test. *Canadian Medical Association Journal, 186*(16), 1225–1234. doi:10.1503/cmaj.140703.

Bella, A. J., Lee, J. C., Carrier, S., et al. (2015). 2015 CUA Practice guidelines for erectile dysfunction. *Canadian Urological Association Journal, 9*(1–2), 23–29. doi:10.5489/cuaj.2699.

Boorjian, S., Eastham, J., Graefen, M., et al. (2012). A critical analysis of the long-term impact of radical prostatectomy on cancer control and function outcomes. *European Urology, 61*(4), 664–675. doi:10.1016/j.eururo.2011.11.053.

Cameron, S., Springer, C., Fox-Wasylyshyn, S., et al. (2012). A descriptive study of functions, symptoms, and perceived health state after radiotherapy for prostate cancer. *European Journal of Oncology Nursing, 16*(3), 310–314. doi:10.1016/j.ejon.2011.07.007.

Canadian Cancer Society. (2017a). *Finding prostate cancer*. Retrieved from *http://www.cancer.ca/en/prevention-and-screening/early-detection-and-screening/finding-cancer-early/finding-prostate-cancer/?region=on*.

Canadian Cancer Society. (2017b). *Risk factors for prostate cancer*. Retrieved from *http://www.cancer.ca/en/cancer-information/cancer-type/prostate/risks/?region=on*.

Canadian Cancer Society. (2017c). *Prostatitis*. Retrieved from *http://www.cancer.ca/en/cancer-information/cancer-type/prostate/prostate-cancer/prostatitis/?region=on*.

Canadian Cancer Society. (2017d). *Survival statistics for testicular cancer*. Retrieved from *http://www.cancer.ca/en/cancer-information/cancer-type/testicular/prognosis-and-survival/survival-statistics/?region=on*.

Canadian Cancer Society. (2017e). *Risk factors for testicular cancer*. Retrieved from: *http://www.cancer.ca/en/cancer-information/cancer-type/testicular/risks/?region=on*.

Canadian Cancer Society. (2017f). *Risk factors for testicular cancer*. Retrieved from *http://www.cancer.ca/en/cancer-information/cancer-type/testicular/risks/?region=on*.

Canadian Cancer Society's Advisory Committee on Cancer Statistics. (2017). *Canadian cancer statistics 2017*. Toronto: Canadian Cancer Society. Retrieved from *http://www.cancer.ca/~/media/*

cancer.ca/CW/cancer%20information/cancer%20101/Canadian%20 cancer%20statistics/Canadian-Cancer-Statistics-2017-EN.pdf?la=en.

Chughtai, B., Simma-Chiang, V., Lee, R., et al. (2015). Trends and utilization of laser prostatectomy in ambulatory surgical procedures for the treatment of benign prostatic hyperplasia in New York State (2000–2011). *Journal of Endourology*, 29(6), 700–706.

Dong, J., Zhang, Y., & Qin, L. (2011). Erectile dysfunction and risk of cardiovascular disease: Meta-analysis of prospective cohort studies. *Journal of American College of Cardiology*, 58(13), 1378–1385. doi:10.1016/j.jacc.2011.06.024.

Elliott, S. (2011). Hot topics in erectile dysfunction. *BC Medical Journal*, 53(9), 480–486.

Gandaglia, G., Gallina, A., Suardi, N., et al. (2014). Preoperative erectile function is the only predictor of the use of a high number of phosphodiesterase type-5 inhibitors after bilateral nerve-sparing radical prostatectomy. *International Journal of Impotence Research*, 26(6), 201–204. doi:10.1038/ijir.2014.10.

HealthLinkBC. (2016). *Prostatitis: Pre- and post-massage test.* Retrieved from *https://www.healthlinkbc.ca/health-topics/aa134353.*

Herrmann, T. R., Liatsikos, E., Nagele, U., et al. (2012). EAU guidelines on laser technologies. *European Urology*, 61(4), 783–795. doi:10.1016/j.eururo.2012.01.010.

Jensen, M. S., Henriksen, T. B., Rebordosa, C., et al. (2011). Analgesics during pregnancy and cryptorchidism: Additional analyses. *Epidemiology (Cambridge, Mass.)*, 22(4), 610–612. doi:10.1097/EDE.0b013e31821eca69.

Krausz, C. (2011). Male infertility: Pathogenesis and clinical diagnosis. *Best Practice & Research Clinical Endocrinology & Metabolism*, 25(2), 271–285. doi:10.1016/j.beem.2010.08.006.

Latendresse, G., & McCance, K. L. (2011). Alterations of the reproductive systems, including sexually transmitted infections. In S. E. Huether & K. L. McCance (Eds.), *Understanding pathophysiology* (5th ed., pp. 799–870). St. Louis: Mosby.

Lawindy, S. M., Rodriguez, A. R., Horenblas, S., et al. (2011). Current and future strategies in the diagnosis and management of penile cancer. *Advances in Urology*, 2011, doi:10.1155/2011/593751. Article No. 593751.

LeBlanc, E. S., Wang, P. Y., Lee, C. G., et al. (2011). Higher testosterone levels are associated with less loss of lean body mass in older men. *Journal of Clinical Endocrinology and Metabolism*, 96(12), 3855–3863. doi:10.1210/jc.2011-0312.

Lee, M. (2011). Focus on phosphodiesterase inhibitors for the treatment of erectile dysfunction in older men. *Clinical Therapeutics*, 33(11), 1590–1608. doi:10.1016/j.clinthera .2011.09.029.

Lingeman, J. (2011). Holmium laser enucleation of the prostate— If not now, when? *Journal of Urology*, 186(5), 1762–1763. doi:10.1016/j.juro.2011.08.020.

National Institute of Health. (2014). Prostate enlargement: Benign prostatic hyperplasia. *National Kidney and Urologic Diseases Information Clearinghouse, Pub. No. 14-3012.* Bethesda, MD: Author.

Ørsted, D., & Bojesen, S. (2013). The link between benign prostatic hyperplasia and prostate cancer. *Nature Reviews Urology*, 10, 49–54.

Pieters, B., Rezaie, E., Geijsen, E., et al. (2011). Development of late toxicity and International Prostate Symptom Score resolution after external-beam radiotherapy combined with pulse dose rate brachytherapy for prostate cancer. *International Journal of Radiation Oncology, Biology, Physics*, 81(3), 758–764. doi:10.1016/j.ijrobp.2010.05.044.

Roehrborn, C., Casabé, A., Glina, S., et al. (2015). Treatment satisfaction and clinically meaningful symptom improvement in men with lower urinary tract symptoms and prostatic enlargement secondary to benign prostatic hyperplasia: Secondary results from a 6-month, randomized, double-blind study comparing finasteride plus tadalafil with finasteride plus placebo. *International Journal of Urology*, 22(6), 582–587. doi:10.1111/iju.12741.

Rosen, R., Wincze, J., Mollen, M., et al. (2007). Responsiveness and minimum important differences for the erection quality scale. *Journal of Urology*, 178(5), 2076–2081. doi:10.1016/j.juro .2007.07.019. (Seminal).

Rosenberg, M., Witt, E., Miner, M., et al. (2014). A practical primary care approach to lower urinary tract symptoms caused by benign prostatic hyperplasia (BPH-LUTS). *The Canadian Journal of Urology*, 21(Suppl. 2), 12–24.

Schenk, J., Kristal, A., Arnold, B., et al. (2011). Association of symptomatic benign prostatic hyperplasia and prostate cancer: Results from the prostate cancer prevention trial. *American Journal of Epidemiology*, 173(12), 1419–1428. doi:10.1093/aje/ kwq493.

Siegel, R., DeSantis, C., Virgo, K., et al. (2012). Cancer treatment and survivorship statistics. *CA: A Cancer Journal for Clinicians*, 62(5), 220–241. doi:10.3322/caac.21149.

Song, P. H., & Moon, K. H. (2013). Priapism: Current updates in clinical management. *Korean Journal of Urology*, 54(12), 816–823. doi:10.4111/kju.2013.54.12.816.

Trinh, Q. D., Sammon, J., Sun, M., et al. (2012). Perioperative outcomes of robot-assisted radical prostatectomy compared with open radical prostatectomy: Results from the nationwide inpatient sample. *European Urology*, 61(4), 679–685. doi:10.1016/j .eururo.2011.12.027.

Trumble, B., Stieglitz, J., Eid Rodriguez, D., et al. (2015). Challenging the inevitability of prostate enlargement: Low levels of benign prostatic hyperplasia among Tsimane forager-horticulturalists. *Journals of Gerontology. Series A: Biological Sciences & Medical Sciences*, 70(10), 1262–1268. doi:10.1093/gerona/glv051.

VanderWalde, A., & Hurria, A. (2011). Aging and osteoporosis in breast and prostate cancer. *CA: A Cancer Journal for Clinicians*, 61(3), 139–156. doi:10.3322/caac.20103.

Warlick, C., Weight, C., & Konety, B. (2014). Prostate cancer in older adults. In T. L. Griebling (Ed.), *Geriatric Urology* (pp. 273–288). New York: Springer.

Weight, C., Kim, S., Jacobson, D., et al. (2013). The effect of benign lower urinary tract symptoms on subsequent prostate cancer testing and diagnosis. *European Urology*, 63(6), 1021–1027.

Zu, K., Mucci, L., Rosner, B. A., et al. (2014). Dietary lycopene, angiogenesis, and prostate cancer: A prospective study in the prostate-specific antigen era. *Journal of the National Cancer Institute*, 106(2), djt430. doi:10.1093/jnci/djt430.

RESOURCES

Canadian Cancer Society
http://www.cancer.ca

Canadian Urological Association
http://www.cua.org

Dr. Ernest W. Ramsey Manitoba Prostate Centre— CancerCare Manitoba
http://www.cancercare.mb.ca/home/patients_and_family/about_ your_cancer/manitoba_prostate_centre

Ontario Men's Health: Erectile Dysfunction
http://www.ontariomenshealth.ca/erectile-dysfunction

Prostate Cancer Canada
http://www.prostatecancer.ca

Prostate Cancer Centre
http://www.prostatecancercentre.ca

Vancouver Prostate Centre
http://www.prostatecentre.com

National Cancer Institute
https://www.cancer.gov/types/prostate

Prostate Calculator: Forecasting the Course of Disease (Artificial Neural Networks in Prostate Cancer Project)
http://prostatecalculator.org

For additional Internet resources, see the website for this book at *http://evolve.elsevier.com/Canada/Lewis/medsurg.*

Problems Related to Movement and Coordination

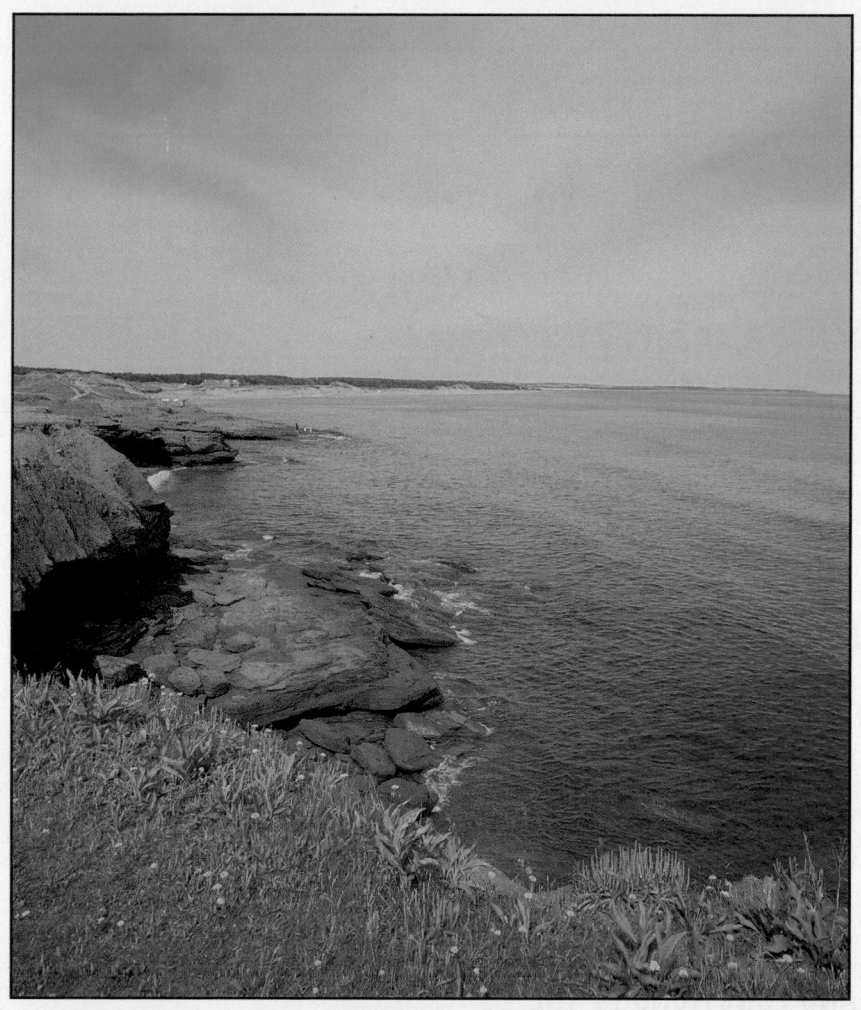

Source: Takuji Oishi/Shutterstock.com.

Nursing Assessment

Nervous System

Written by: Linda Littlejohns
Adapted by: Jana Lok

evolve WEBSITE

http://evolve.elsevier.com/Canada/Lewis/medsurg

- Review Questions (Online Only)
- Key Points
- Answers Guidelines for Case Study
- Conceptual Care Map Creator

- Audio Glossary
- Supporting Media—Animations
  - Motor Pathways and Clinical Evaluation of the Central Nervous System

- Reflex Arc
- Sensory Pathways and Clinical Evaluation of the Central Nervous System
- Content Updates

LEARNING OBJECTIVES

1. Describe the functions of neurons and glial cells.
2. Explain the electrochemical aspects of nerve impulse transmission.
3. Explain the anatomical location and functions of the cerebrum, brain stem, cerebellum, spinal cord, peripheral nerves, and cerebro-spinal fluid.
4. Identify the major arteries supplying the brain.
5. Describe the functions of the 12 cranial nerves.
6. Compare the functions of the two divisions of the autonomic nervous system.
7. Describe age-related changes in the neurological system and differences in assessment findings.
8. Identify the significant subjective and objective data related to the nervous system that should be obtained from a patient.
9. Select appropriate techniques in the physical assessment of the nervous system.
10. Differentiate normal from common abnormal findings of a physical assessment of the nervous system.
11. Describe the purpose, the significance of results, and the nursing responsibilities related to diagnostic studies of the nervous system.

KEY TERMS

autonomic nervous system (ANS), p. 1456
blood–brain barrier, p. 1459
central nervous system (CNS), p. 1448
cerebro-spinal fluid (CSF), p. 1453
cranial nerves (CNs), p. 1456

dermatome, p. 1455
glial cells, p. 1449
lower motor neurons (LMNs), p. 1451
meninges, p. 1459
neurons, p. 1448

neurotransmitter, p. 1450
peripheral nervous system (PNS), p. 1448
reflex, p. 1452
synapse, p. 1450
upper motor neurons (UMNs), p. 1452

STRUCTURES AND FUNCTIONS OF THE NERVOUS SYSTEM

The human nervous system is a highly specialized system responsible for the control and integration of the body's many activities. The nervous system has two main divisions: the **central nervous system (CNS)** and the **peripheral nervous system (PNS).** The CNS consists of the brain, the spinal cord, and cranial nerves I and II. The PNS consists of cranial nerves III to XII, the spinal nerves, and the peripheral components of the autonomic nervous system (ANS).

Cells of the Nervous System

The nervous system is made up of two types of cells: neurons and glial cells. **Neurons** are the primary functional unit of the nervous system. Glial cells provide structural support and are more numerous than neurons.

Neurons. Neurons come in many different shapes and sizes, but they share three characteristics: (a) *excitability,* or the ability to generate a nerve impulse; (b) *conductivity,* or the ability to transmit an impulse; and (c) the ability to *influence* other neurons, muscle cells, and glandular cells by transmitting nerve impulses to them.

A typical neuron consists of a cell body, an axon, and several dendrites (Figure 58-1). The cell body, which contains the nucleus and the cytoplasm, is the metabolic centre of the neuron. *Dendrites* are short processes extending from the cell body. They receive nerve impulses from the axons of other neurons and conduct impulses toward the cell body. The nerve *axon* projects varying distances from the cell body, ranging from

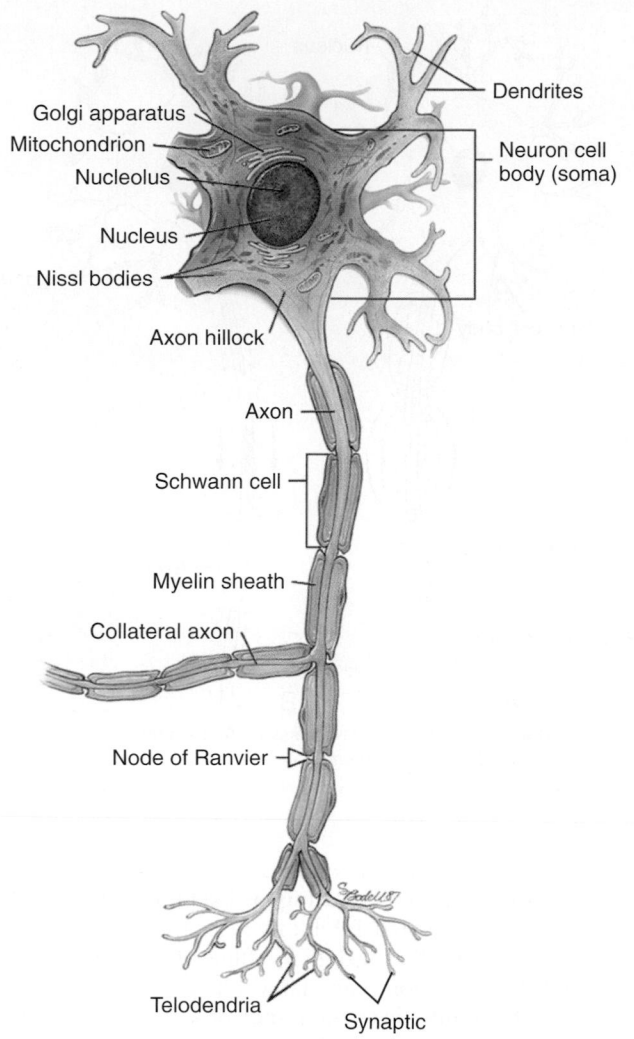

Golgi apparatus
Mitochondrion
Nucleolus
Nucleus
Nissl bodies
Axon hillock
Axon
Schwann cell
Myelin sheath
Collateral axon
Node of Ranvier
Telodendria
Dendrites
Neuron cell body (soma)
Synaptic knobs

FIGURE 58-1 Structural features of neurons: dendrites, cell body, and axons. Source: Adapted from Patton, K. T., & Thibodeau, G. A. (2010). *Anatomy and physiology* (7th ed., p. 379, Figure 12-5). St. Louis: Mosby.

several micrometres to more than a metre. Its function is to carry nerve impulses to other neurons or to end organs. The end organs are smooth and striated muscles and glands. Axons may be myelinated or unmyelinated. Many axons present in the CNS and the PNS are covered by a segmentally interrupted myelin sheath composed of a white lipid substance that acts as an insulator for the conduction of impulses. In general, the smaller fibres are unmyelinated.

Glial Cells. Glial cells provide support, nourishment, and protection to neurons. They constitute almost half the brain and spinal cord mass and are five to ten times more numerous than neurons. Different types of glial cells include astrocytes (most abundant), oligodendrocytes, ependymal cells, and microglia. *Astrocytes* provide structural support to neurons and their delicate processes, form the blood–brain barrier with the endothelium of the blood vessels, and play a role in synaptic transmission (conduction of impulses between neurons). They are found primarily in grey matter. When the brain is injured, astrocytes act as phagocytes for neuronal debris. They help restore the neurochemical milieu and provide support for repair. Proliferation

of astrocytes contributes to the formation of scar tissue (gliosis) in the CNS.

Oligodendrocytes are specialized cells that produce the myelin sheath of nerve fibres in the CNS and are found primarily in the white matter of the CNS. (Schwann cells myelinate the nerve fibres in the periphery.)

Ependymal cells line the brain ventricles and aid in the secretion of cerebro-spinal fluid. *Microglia*, a type of macrophage, are relatively rare in normal CNS tissue. They are phagocytes and are important in host defence.

Neurogenesis

Neurons have long been thought to be nonmitotic—that is, after being damaged, neurons could not be replaced. The discovery of neuronal stem cells now demonstrates that neurogenesis can occur in adult brains after cerebral injury (Gopurappilly, Pal, Krishna Mamidi, et al., 2011). Neuroglia are mitotic and can replicate. In general, when neurons are destroyed, the tissue is replaced by the proliferation of neuroglial cells. Most primary CNS tumours involve glial cells. Primary malignancies involving neurons are rare.

If the axon of a nerve cell is damaged, the cell attempts to repair itself. Damaged nerve cells attempt to grow back to their original destinations by sprouting many branches from the damaged ends of their axons. Unfortunately, axons in the CNS are less successful than peripheral axons in regenerating. Endogenous inhibitors (e.g., neurite outgrowth inhibitor, myelin-associated glycoprotein) decrease axon regeneration.

In the PNS (outside the brain and the spinal cord), injured nerve fibres can successfully regenerate by growing within the protective myelin sheath of the supporting Schwann cells if the cell body is intact. The final result of nerve regeneration depends on the number of axon sprouts that join with the appropriate Schwann cell columns and re-innervate appropriate end organs.

Nerve Impulse

The function of a neuron is to initiate, receive, and process messages about events both within and outside the body. The initiation of a neuronal message *(nerve impulse)* involves the generation of an action potential. An *action potential* is a rapid, self-propagating and transient change in the voltage across a cell membrane (caused by the influx of Na^+ followed by an efflux of K^+). An action potential is generated when a stimulus causes the resting membrane potential (-70 mV) to depolarize (to about $+30$ mV) within a short time period (1–2 ms). Once an action potential is initiated, a series of action potentials travel along the axon. When the impulse reaches the end of the nerve fibre, it is transmitted across the junction between nerve cells *(synapse)* by a chemical interaction involving neurotransmitters. This chemical interaction generates another set of action potentials in the next neuron. These events are repeated until the nerve impulse reaches its destination.

Because of its insulating capacity, myelination of nerve axons facilitates the conduction of an action potential. Many peripheral nerve axons have gaps, termed *nodes of Ranvier*, at regular intervals in the myelin sheath surrounding them. An action potential travelling down one of these axons hops from node to node without traversing the insulated membrane segment between nodes, which makes the action potential travel much faster than it would otherwise. This process is called *saltatory* (hopping) conduction. In an unmyelinated fibre, the wave of depolarization traverses the entire length of the axon, and each portion of the

🔍 **EVIDENCE-INFORMED PRACTICE**

Research Highlight

Can Enteric Glia Regenerate Axons Following Spinal Cord Injury?

Clinical Question

Following spinal cord injuries (P), can transplanted enteric glia (I) promote axonal regeneration (O)?

Best Available Evidence

- Dr. Shucui Jiang and her research team at McMaster University, Ontario, are developing a new therapy that harvests enteric (intestinal) glia cells and transplants them to sites of injury to promote regeneration of injured spinal cord nerve fibres.

Critical Appraisal and Synthesis of Evidence

- This research is still in its experimental stage. Research using animal models has shown that enteric glial cells induce regeneration of damaged spinal cords, reduce tissue damage, and promote functional recovery.

Conclusion

- Research has shown that transplanting enteric glial cells can promote axonal regeneration following spinal cord injury. Current studies are exploring the mechanisms through which enteric glia mediate neuronal regeneration as well as trying to isolate and obtain human enteric glia.

Implications for Nursing Practice

1. Damage to the spinal cord is one of the most traumatic events that affect an individual's life. Unfortunately, there are few viable treatment options.
2. This research provides new insight into future treatment options for spinal cord injuries.

Reference for Evidence

Hansebout, C. R., Su, C., Reddy, K., et al. (2012). Enteric glia mediate neuronal outgrowth through release of neurotrophic factors. *Neural regeneration research, 7*(28), 2165.

P, Patient population of interest; *I*, intervention or area of interest; *O*, outcomes of interest (see Chapter 1).

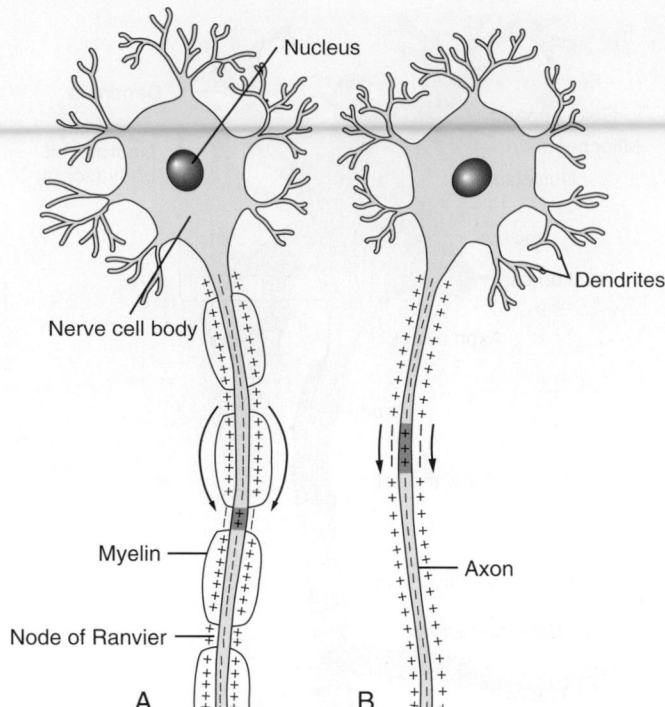

FIGURE 58-2 Nerve impulse transmission. **A,** Saltatory conduction in a myelinated nerve. **B,** Depolarization in an unmyelinated fibre.

membrane becomes depolarized in turn. Figure 58-2 depicts a comparison of nerve impulse transmission of myelinated and unmyelinated fibres.

Synapse. A synapse is the structural and functional junction between two neurons. It is the point at which the nerve impulse is transmitted from one neuron to another or from a neuron to glands or muscles. The essential structures of synaptic transmission are a presynaptic terminal, a synaptic cleft, and a receptor site on the postsynaptic cell (Figure 58-3). There are two types of synapses: electrical and chemical. In an electrical synapse, an action potential moves from neuron to neuron directly, by allowing electrical current to flow between neurons. In a chemical synapse, an action potential reaches the end of the axon (presynaptic terminal); then it causes release of a chemical substance (neurotransmitter) from tiny vesicles within the axon terminal. The neurotransmitter then crosses the microscopic space (synaptic cleft) between the two neurons and attaches to receptor sites of the receiving (postsynaptic) neuron. Parts of the synapse include the neurotransmitters, the inactivators, and the receptors (see Figure 58-3).

Neurotransmitters. A neurotransmitter is a chemical agent that affects the transmission of an impulse across the synaptic cleft. Examples of neurotransmitters are presented in Table 58-1.

Excitatory neurotransmitters activate postsynaptic receptors, causing an influx of Na^+, increasing the likelihood that an action potential will be generated. Inhibitory neurotransmitters activate postsynaptic receptors, causing an efflux of K^+, inhibiting the likelihood that an action potential will be generated.

Each of the hundreds to thousands of synaptic connections of a single neuron has an influence on that neuron. The net effect of the input is sometimes excitatory and sometimes inhibitory. In general, the net effect depends on the number of presynaptic neurons that are releasing neurotransmitters on the postsynaptic cell. A presynaptic cell that releases an excitatory neurotransmitter does not always cause the postsynaptic cell to depolarize enough to generate an action potential. However, when many presynaptic cells release excitatory neurotransmitters on a single neuron, the sum of their input is enough to generate an action potential.

Neurotransmitters continue to combine with the receptor sites at the postsynaptic membrane until they are inactivated by enzymes, are taken up by the presynaptic endings, or diffuse away from the synaptic region. In addition, the action of neurotransmitters can be affected by drugs and toxins, which can modify their function or block their attachment to receptor sites on the postsynaptic membrane.

Central Nervous System

The major structural components of the CNS are the cerebrum (cerebral hemispheres), brain stem, cerebellum, and spinal cord.

Spinal Cord. The spinal cord is continuous with the brain stem and exits from the cranial cavity through the foramen magnum. A cross-section of the spinal cord reveals grey matter that is centrally located in an H-shape and is surrounded by white matter (Figure 58-4). The grey matter contains the cell bodies of voluntary motor neurons and preganglionic autonomic motor neurons, as well as

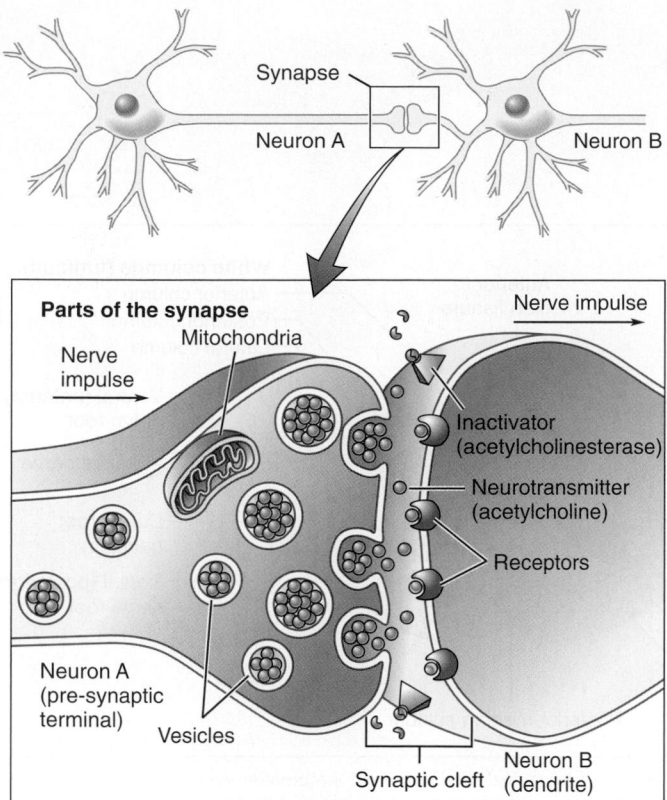

Parts of the synapse

Nerve impulse

Mitochondria

Nerve impulse

Inactivator (acetylcholinesterase)

Neurotransmitter (acetylcholine)

Receptors

Neuron A (pre-synaptic terminal)

Vesicles

Synaptic cleft

Neuron B (dendrite)

Synapse

Neuron A

Neuron B

FIGURE 58-3 The synapse is located in the space between neuron A and neuron B. Parts of the synapse include the neurotransmitters, the inactivators, and the receptors. The neurotransmitters are located in the vesicles of neuron A. The inactivators are located on the membrane of neuron B. The receptors are located on the membrane of neuron B. Source: Adapted from Herlihy, B. (2007). *The human body in health and illness* (3rd ed., p. 170, Figure 10-9). Philadelphia: W. B. Saunders.

TABLE 58-1	**EXAMPLES OF NEUROTRANSMITTERS**
Substance	**Clinical Relevance***
Acetylcholine	The number of acetylcholine-secreting neurons decreases in Alzheimer's disease; myasthenia gravis results from a reduction in acetylcholine receptors.
Amines	
Epinephrine	Acts as a hormone when secreted by the neurosecretory cells of the adrenal medulla.
Norepinephrine	Cocaine and amphetamines increase the release and block the reuptake of norepinephrine, resulting in overstimulation of postsynaptic neurons.
Serotonin	Involved in moods, emotions, and sleep.
Dopamine	Involved in emotions and moods and regulating motor control. Parkinson's disease results from destruction of dopamine-secreting neurons.
Amino Acids	
γ-Aminobutyric acid (GABA)	Drugs that increase GABA function have been used to treat seizure disorders.
Glutamate and aspartate	Sustained release of glutamate triggers neuronal apoptosis.
Neuropeptides	
Endorphins and enkephalins	The opioids morphine and heroin bind to endorphin and enkephalin receptors on presynaptic neurons and reduce pain by blocking the release of neurotransmitter (see Chapter 10).
Substance P	A neurotransmitter in pain transmission pathways; morphine blocks its release.

*These are examples only; most of the neurotransmitters are also found in other locations and may have additional functions.

cell bodies of association neurons (interneurons). The white matter contains the axons of the ascending sensory and the descending (suprasegmental) motor fibres. The myelin surrounding these fibres gives them their white appearance. Specific ascending and descending pathways in the white matter can be identified. The spinal pathways or tracts are named for the point of origin and the point of destination (e.g., spino-cerebellar tract [ascending], cortico-spinal tract [descending]).

Ascending Tracts. In general, the ascending tracts carry specific sensory information to higher levels of the CNS. This information comes from special sensory endings (receptors) in the skin, the muscles and joints, the viscera, and the blood vessels and enters the spinal cord by way of the dorsal roots of the spinal nerves. The fasciculus gracilis and the fasciculus cuneatus (together, commonly called the *dorsal* or *posterior column*) carry information and transmit impulses concerned with touch, deep pressure, vibration, position sense, and kinesthesia (appreciation of movement, weight, and body parts). The *spino-cerebellar tracts* carry information about muscle tension and body position to the cerebellum for coordination of movement. The *spino-thalamic tracts* carry pain and temperature sensations. Thus, the ascending tracts are organized by sensory modality as well as by anatomy.

Other ascending tracts may also participate in transmission of sensory information. The symptoms of various neurological diseases suggest the existence of alternative pathways for touch, position sense, and vibration.

Descending Tracts. Descending tracts carry impulses that are responsible for muscle movement. Among the most important descending tracts are the cortico-bulbar and cortico-spinal tracts, collectively termed the *pyramidal tract*. These tracts carry volitional (voluntary) impulses from the cortex to the cranial and the peripheral nerves. Another group of descending motor tracts carries impulses from the extrapyramidal system, which includes all motor systems (except the pyramidal system) concerned with voluntary movement. It includes descending pathways originating in the brain stem, basal ganglia, and cerebellum. The motor output exits the spinal cord by way of the ventral roots of the spinal nerves.

Lower Motor Neurons. Lower motor neurons (LMNs) are the final common pathway through which descending motor tracts influence skeletal muscle, the effector organ for movement. The cell bodies of LMNs, which send axons to innervate the skeletal muscles of arms, trunk, and legs, are located in the anterior horn of the corresponding segments of the spinal cord (e.g., cervical segments contain LMNs for the arms). LMNs for skeletal muscles of eyes, face, mouth, and throat are located in the corresponding segments of the brain stem. These cell bodies and their axons make up the somatic motor components of the cranial nerves. LMN lesions generally cause weakness or paralysis, denervation

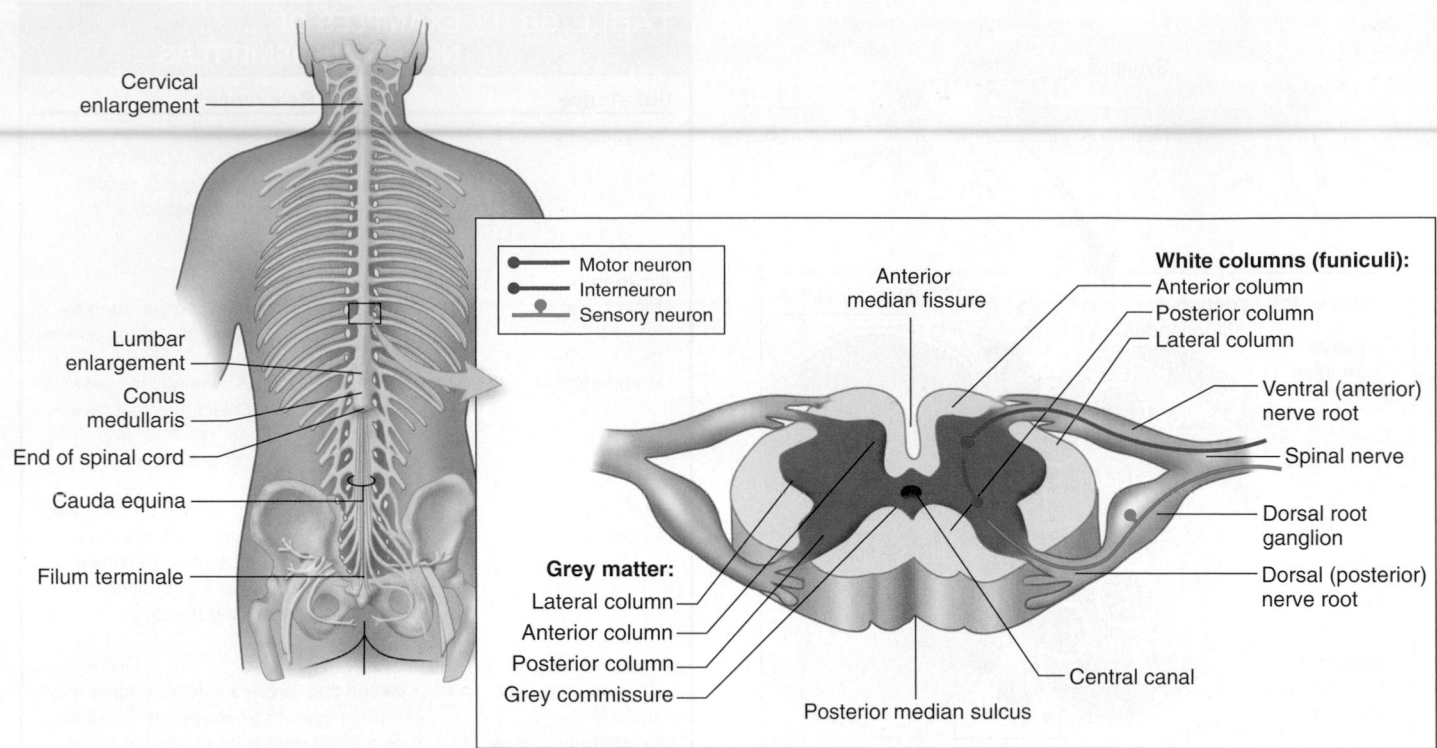

FIGURE 58-4 Spinal cord. The inset illustrates a transverse section of the spinal cord shown in the broader view. Source: Adapted from Patton, K. T., & Thibodeau, G. A. (2013). *Anatomy and physiology* (8th ed., p. 426, Figure 14-6). St. Louis: Mosby.

atrophy, hyper-reflexia or areflexia, and decreased muscle tone (flaccidity).

Upper Motor Neurons. Upper motor neurons (UMNs) originate in the cerebral cortex and project downward. The cortico-bulbar tract ends in the brain stem, and the cortico-spinal tract descends into the spinal cord. These neurons influence skeletal muscle movement. UMN lesions generally cause weakness or paralysis, disuse atrophy, hyper reflexia, and increased muscle tone (spasticity).

Reflex Arc. A **reflex** is defined as an involuntary response to a stimulus. The components of a monosynaptic reflex arc (the simplest kind of reflex arc) are a receptor organ, an afferent neuron, an effector neuron, and an effector organ (e.g., skeletal muscle). The afferent neuron synapses with the efferent neuron in the grey matter of the spinal cord. A reflex arc is shown in Figure 58-5. In more complex (polysynaptic) reflex arcs, the effector neuron is influenced by other neurons (interneurons) in addition to the afferent neuron. In the spinal cord, reflex arcs play an important role in maintaining muscle tone, which is essential for body posture.

Brain. The brain can be divided into three major components: cerebrum, brain stem, and cerebellum.

Cerebrum. The *cerebrum* is composed of the right and left cerebral hemispheres and divided into four major lobes: frontal, temporal, parietal, and occipital (Figure 58-6).

The functions of the cerebrum are multiple and complex. Specific areas of the cerebral cortex are associated with specific functions. Table 58-2 summarizes the location and function of the parts of the cerebrum. The *frontal lobe* controls higher cognitive function, memory, voluntary eye movements, voluntary movements, and, usually in the left hemisphere, expressive speech

and language in Broca's area. The *temporal lobe* contains integration of somatic, visual, and auditory data and, usually in the left hemisphere, Wernicke's area, which is responsible for receptive language. The *parietal lobe* is composed of the sensory cortex and controlling and interpreting spatial information. Processing of visual data takes place in the *occipital lobe.*

The basal ganglia, the thalamus, the hypothalamus, and the limbic system are also located in the cerebrum. The basal ganglia are a group of paired structures located centrally in the cerebrum and the midbrain; most of them are on both sides of the thalamus. The function of the basal ganglia is to modulate initiation, execution, and completion of voluntary movements and automatic movements associated with skeletal muscle activity, such as swinging of the arms during walking, swallowing saliva, and blinking.

The *thalamus* (part of the diencephalon) lies directly above the brain stem (Figure 58-7) and is the major relay centre for sensory and other afferent (e.g., cerebellar) inputs to the cerebral cortex. The *hypothalamus* is located just inferiorly to the thalamus and slightly in front of the midbrain. It regulates the ANS and the endocrine system. The limbic system is located near the inner surfaces of the cerebral hemispheres (Figure 58-8) and is concerned with emotion, aggression, feeding behaviour, and sexual response.

Brain Stem. The *brain stem* includes the midbrain, the pons, and the medulla (see Figure 58-7). Ascending and descending fibres pass through the brain stem between the cerebrum and the cerebellum. The cell bodies, or nuclei, of cranial nerves III through XII are in the brain stem. Also located in the brain stem is the *reticular formation,* a diffusely arranged group of neurons and their axons that extends from the medulla to the thalamus

FIGURE 58-5 Basic diagram of the patellar "knee-jerk" reflex arc. The impulse travels through the (1) sensory stretch receptor and (2) afferent sensory neuron, through the (3) interneuron, and back through the (4) efferent motor neuron and to the (5) quadriceps muscle (effector organ). Source: Adapted from Thibodeau, G. A., & Patton, K. T. (2008). *Structure and function of the body* (13th ed., p. 192, Figure 8-5). St. Louis: Mosby.

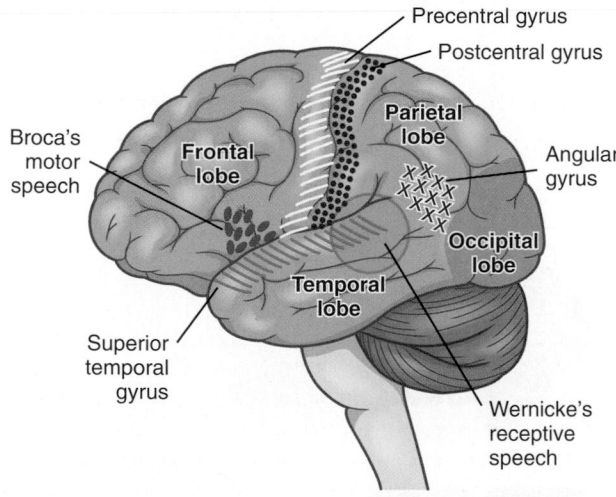

FIGURE 58-6 Left hemisphere of cerebrum, lateral surface, showing major lobes and areas of the brain.

and the hypothalamus. The functions of the reticular formation include relaying sensory information, influencing excitatory and inhibitory control of spinal motor neurons, and controlling vasomotor and respiratory activity. The reticular activating system is part of the reticular formation and is the regulatory system for arousal, a component of consciousness.

The vital centres concerned with respiratory, vasomotor, and cardiac function are located in the medulla. The brain stem also contains the centres for sneezing, coughing, hiccupping, gagging, vomiting, sucking, and swallowing.

Cerebellum. The *cerebellum* is located in the posterior part of the cranial fossa, inferior to the occipital lobe. The cerebellum coordinates voluntary movement and maintains trunk stability and equilibrium. To perform these functions, the cerebellum

receives information from the cerebral cortex, the muscles, the joints, and the inner ear. It influences motor activity through its axonal connections to the motor cortex, the brain stem nuclei, and their descending pathways.

Ventricles and Cerebro-Spinal Fluid. The ventricles are four cavities within the brain, filled with cerebro-spinal fluid (CSF), that connect with one another and with the spinal canal. The lower portion of the fourth ventricle becomes the central canal in the lower part of the brain stem. The spinal canal is located in the centre of the spinal cord and extends the full length of the spinal cord. Figure 58-9 depicts the ventricles and the flow of cerebro-spinal fluid in the CNS.

Cerebro-Spinal Fluid. Cerebro-spinal fluid (CSF) is a clear, colourless fluid similar to blood plasma and interstitial fluid (McCance & Huether, 2014). CSF circulates within the subarachnoid space that surrounds the brain, the brain stem, and the spinal cord; provides cushioning for the brain and the spinal cord; allows fluid shifts from the cranial cavity to the spinal cavity; and carries nutrients. CSF is produced primarily by the choroid plexus in the lateral, third, and fourth ventricles. It flows from the lateral ventricles to the third ventricle via the interventricular foramen and then moves from the third to the fourth ventricle through the cerebral aqueduct. Finally, CSF flows into the subarachnoid space through the lateral and median foramen (see Figure 58-9). It is absorbed primarily through the *arachnoid villi* (tiny projections into the subarachnoid space), into the intradural venous sinuses, and eventually into the venous system. Although CSF is continually being formed, many physiological factors influence its rate of absorption and formation. The ventricles and the central canal are normally filled with an average of 135 mL of CSF. A disturbance in the formation, flow, or absorption of CSF can lead to hydrocephalus.

The analysis of CSF composition provides useful diagnostic information relating to certain nervous system diseases. CSF

TABLE 58-2   LOCATION AND FUNCTION OF THE PARTS OF THE CEREBRUM

Part	Location	Function	Part	Location	Function
Cortical Areas *Motor*			**Language**		
Primary	Precentral gyrus	Facilitates motor control and movement on the opposite side of the body	Comprehension	Wernicke's area, usually in the left hemisphere	Integrates auditory language (understanding of spoken words)
Supplemental	Anterior to precentral gyrus	Facilitates proximal muscle activity, including activity for stance and gait, spontaneous movement, and coordination	Expression	Broca's area, usually in the left hemisphere	Regulates verbal expression
Sensory			**Other Functions**		
Somatic	Postcentral gyrus	Processes sensory response from the opposite side of body	Basal ganglia	Near lateral ventricles of both cerebral hemispheres	Control and facilitate learned and automatic movements
Visual	Occipital lobe	Registers visual images	Thalamus	Below basal ganglia	Relays sensory and motor inputs to cortex and other parts of cerebrum
Auditory	Superior temporal gyrus	Registers auditory inputs			
Association areas	Parietal lobe	Integrates somatic and sensory inputs	Hypothalamus	Below thalamus	Regulates endocrine and autonomic functions (e.g., feeding, sleeping, emotional and sexual responses)
	Posterior temporal lobe	Integrates visual and auditory inputs for language comprehension			
	Anterior temporal lobe	Integrates past experiences	Limbic system	Lateral to hypothalamus	Influences affective (emotional) behaviour and basic drives such as feeding and sexual behaviour
	Anterior frontal lobe	Controls higher-order processes (e.g., judgement, insight, reasoning, problem solving, planning)			

FIGURE 58-7 The central nervous system. **A,** Side view of major divisions. **B,** Coronal overview of the components of the basal ganglia. Source: **B,** Based on Nieuwenhuys, Voogd, and van Huijzen, 1981.

pressure is often measured in patients with actual or suspected intracranial diseases. Increases in intracranial pressure, indicated by increased CSF pressure, can lead to herniation of the brain and compression of vital brain stem structures. The signs marking this event are part of the herniation (see Chapter 59).

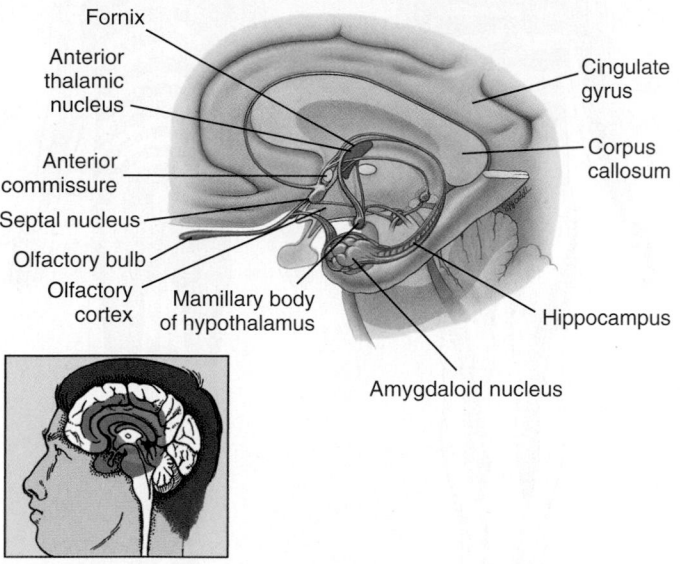

FIGURE 58-8 Structures of the limbic system. Source: Adapted from Patton, K. T., & Thibodeau, G. A. (2010). *Anatomy and physiology* (7th ed., p. 436, Figure 13-22). St. Louis: Mosby.

Peripheral Nervous System

The PNS includes all of the neuronal structures that lie outside the CNS. It consists of the spinal and cranial nerves, their associated ganglia (groupings of cell bodies), and portions of the ANS.

Spinal Nerves. The spinal cord is a series of spinal segments, one on top of another. In addition to the cell bodies, each segment contains a pair of dorsal (afferent) sensory nerve fibres or roots and ventral (efferent) motor fibres or roots, which innervate a specific region of neck, trunk, or limbs. This combined motor–sensory nerve is called a *spinal nerve* (Figure 58-10). The cell bodies of the voluntary motor system are located in the anterior horn of the spinal cord grey matter. The cell bodies of the autonomic (involuntary) motor system are located in the anterolateral portion of spinal cord grey matter. The cell bodies of sensory fibres are located in the dorsal root ganglia just outside the spinal cord. On exiting the spinal column, each spinal nerve divides into ventral and dorsal rami, a collection of motor and sensory fibres that eventually extend to peripheral structures (e.g., skin, muscles, viscera).

A **dermatome** is the area of skin innervated by the sensory fibres of a single dorsal root of a spinal nerve. The locations of dermatomes indicate the general pattern of somatic sensory innervation by spinal segments. A *myotome* is a muscle group innervated by the primary motor neurons of a single ventral root. The dermatomes and myotomes of a given spinal segment overlap with those of adjacent segments because of the development of ascending and descending collateral branches of nerve fibres (Figure 58-11).

FIGURE 58-9 Flow of cerebro-spinal fluid (CSF). The fluid produced by filtration of blood by the choroid plexus of each ventricle flows inferiorly through the lateral ventricles, the interventricular foramen, the third ventricle, the cerebral aqueduct, the fourth ventricle, and the subarachnoid space and to the blood. Source: Adapted from Patton, K. T., & Thibodeau, G. A. (2010). *Anatomy and physiology* (7th ed., p. 417, Figure 13-5). St. Louis: Mosby.

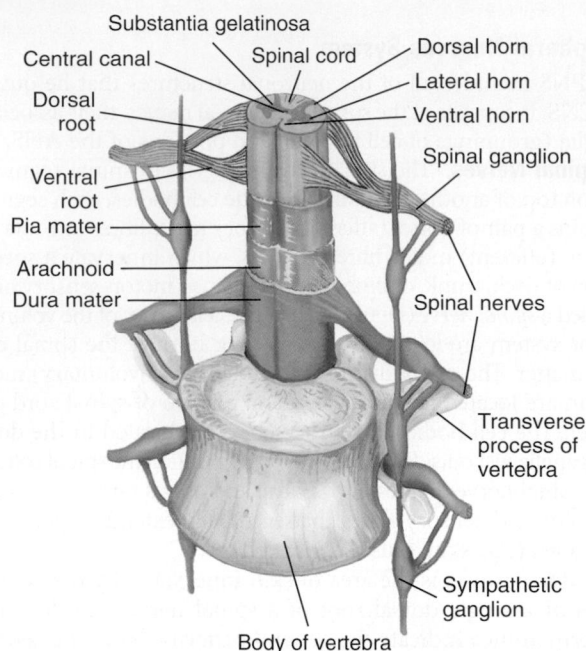

FIGURE 58-10 Illustration of a cross-section of spinal cord, showing attachments of spinal nerves and coverings of the spinal cord. Source: Adapted from Thibodeau, G. A., & Patton, K. T. (2008). *Structure and function of the body* (13th ed., p. 205, Figure 8-13). St. Louis: Mosby.

Cranial Nerves. The cranial nerves (CNs) are the 12 paired nerves composed of cell bodies with fibres that exit from the cranial cavity. Unlike the spinal nerves, which always have both afferent sensory and efferent motor fibres, some CNs are only sensory, some only motor, and some both. Figure 58-12 summarizes the cranial nerves and their functions and position in relation to the brain and the spinal cord. Just as the cell bodies of the spinal nerves are located in specific segments of the spinal cord, the cell bodies (nuclei) of the cranial nerves are located in specific segments of the brain. Exceptions are the nuclei of the olfactory and optic nerves. The primary cell bodies of the olfactory nerve are located in the nasal epithelium, and those of the optic nerve are in the retina.

Autonomic Nervous System. The autonomic nervous system (ANS) governs involuntary functions of cardiac muscle, smooth (involuntary) muscle, and glands.

The ANS is divided into two components, sympathetic and parasympathetic, that are anatomically and functionally different. These two systems function together to maintain a relatively balanced internal environment. The ANS is both an efferent and an afferent system. It consists of preganglionic nerves and postganglionic nerves.

The preganglionic cell bodies of the *sympathetic nervous system* (SNS) are located in spinal segments T1 through L2. The major neurotransmitter released by the postganglionic fibres of the SNS is norepinephrine, and the neurotransmitter released by the preganglionic fibres is acetylcholine.

In contrast, the preganglionic cell bodies of the *parasympathetic nervous system* (PSNS) are located in the brain stem and in the sacral spinal segments (S2 through S4). Acetylcholine is the neurotransmitter released at both preganglionic and postganglionic nerve endings.

The ANS provides dual and often reciprocal innervation to many structures. For example, the SNS increases the rate and force of the heart contraction, and the PSNS decreases the rate and force. Table 58-3 lists the effects of the SNS and PSNS.

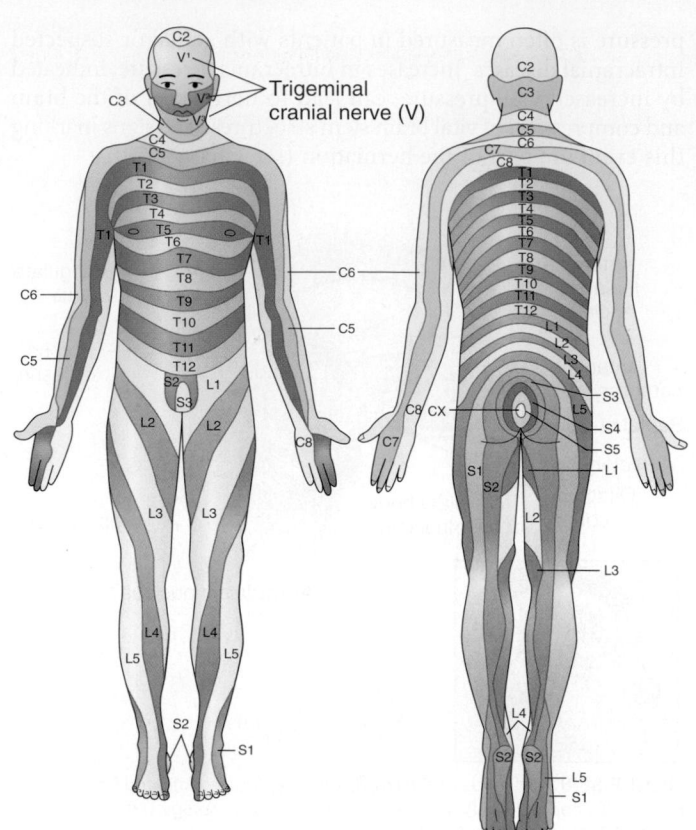

FIGURE 58-11 Dermatome distribution of front and back of body surface. Source: McCance, K. L., & Huether, S. E. (2014). *Pathophysiology: The biologic basis for disease in adults and children* (7th ed., p. 471, Figure 15-24). St. Louis: Mosby.

The result of SNS stimulation is activation of mechanisms required for the "fight or flight" response that occurs throughout the body. In contrast, the PSNS is geared to act in localized and discrete regions. It serves to conserve and restore the energy stores of the body.

Cerebral Circulation

Knowledge of the distribution of the major arteries of the brain and the area supplied is essential for understanding and evaluating the signs and symptoms of cerebro-vascular disease and trauma. The blood supply of the brain arises from the internal carotid arteries (anterior circulation) and the vertebral arteries (posterior circulation) (see Figure 58-13).

The internal carotid arteries provide blood flow to the anterior and middle portions of the cerebrum. The vertebral arteries join to form the basilar artery and provide blood flow to the brain stem, cerebellum, and posterior cerebrum. The *circle of Willis* arises from the basilar artery and the two internal carotid arteries (Figure 58-14). This vascular circle may act as a safety valve when differential pressures are present in these arteries. It also may function as an anastomotic pathway when a major artery on one side of the brain becomes occluded. Superior to the circle of Willis, three pairs of arteries supply blood to the left and right hemispheres. The anterior cerebral artery feeds the medial and anterior portions of the frontal lobes. The middle cerebral artery feeds the outer portions of the frontal, parietal, and superior temporal lobes. The posterior cerebral artery feeds the medial portions of the occipital and inferior temporal lobes. Venous blood drains from the brain through the dural sinuses, which form channels that drain into the two jugular veins.

CRANIAL NERVES

I Olfactory
II Optic
III Oculomotor
IV Trochlear
VI Abducens
V Trigeminal
VII Facial
VIII Acoustic
IX Glossopharyngeal
X Vagus
XII Hypoglossal
XI Spinal (accessory)

—— SENSORY
—— MOTOR

Cranial Nerve	Type	Function
I: Olfactory	Sensory	Smell
II: Optic	Sensory	Vision
III: Oculomotor	Mixed*	Motor—most EOM movement, opening of eyelids
		Parasympathetic—pupil constriction, lens shape
IV: Trochlear	Motor	Down and inward movement of eye
V: Trigeminal	Mixed	Motor—muscles of mastication
		Sensory—sensation of face and scalp, cornea, mucous membranes of mouth and nose
VI: Abducens	Motor	Lateral movement of eye
VII: Facial	Mixed	Motor—facial muscles, close eye, labial speech, close mouth
		Sensory—taste (sweet, salty, sour, bitter) on anterior two-thirds of tongue
		Parasympathetic—saliva and tear secretion
VIII: Acoustic	Sensory	Hearing and equilibrium
IX: Glossopharyngeal	Mixed	Motor—pharynx (phonation and swallowing)
		Sensory—taste on posterior one third of tongue, pharynx (gag reflex)
		Parasympathetic—parotid gland, carotid reflex
X: Vagus	Mixed	Motor—pharynx and larynx (vocalizing and swallowing)
		Sensory—general sensation from carotid body, carotid sinus, pharynx, viscera
		Parasympathetic—carotid reflex
XI: Spinal (accessory)	Motor	Movement of trapezius and sternocleidomastoid muscles
XII: Hypoglossal	Motor	Movement of tongue

*Mixed refers to a nerve carrying a combination of fibres: motor + sensory; motor + parasympathetic; or motor + sensory + parasympathetic.

FIGURE 58-12 The cranial nerves and their functions. Source: Jarvis, C. (2014). *Physical examination & health assessment* (2nd Canadian ed., p. 662, Figure 25-7). (A. J. Brown, J. MacDonald-Jenkins, & M. Luctkar-Flude). Toronto: Saunders/Elsevier.

TABLE 58-3 EFFECTS OF SYMPATHETIC AND PARASYMPATHETIC NERVOUS SYSTEMS

Visceral Effector	Effect of Sympathetic Nervous System*	Effect of Parasympathetic Nervous System†
Heart	Increase in rate and strength of heartbeat (β-receptors)	Decrease in rate and strength of heartbeat
Smooth muscle of blood vessels		
• Skin blood vessels	Constriction (α-receptors)	No effect
• Skeletal muscle blood vessels	Dilation (β-receptors)	No effect
• Coronary blood vessels	Dilation (β-receptors), constriction (α-receptors)	Dilation (β-receptors)
• Abdominal blood vessels	Constriction (α-receptors)	No effect
• Blood vessels of external genitals	Ejaculation (contraction of smooth muscle in male ducts [e.g., epididymis, ductus deferens])	Dilation of blood vessels, causing penile erection
Smooth muscle of hollow organs and sphincters		
• Bronchi	Dilation (β-receptors)	Constriction (α-receptors)
• Digestive tract, except sphincters	Decrease in rate of peristalsis (β-receptors)	Increase in rate of peristalsis
• Sphincters of digestive tract	Contraction (α-receptors)	Relaxation
• Urinary bladder	Relaxation (β-receptors)	Contraction
• Urinary sphincters	Contraction (α-receptors)	Relaxation
Eye		
Iris	Contraction of radial muscle, dilation of pupil	Contraction of circular muscle, constriction of pupil
• Ciliary	Relaxation, accommodation for far vision	Contraction, accommodation for near vision
Hairs (pilomotor muscles)	Contraction producing goose pimples or piloerection (α-receptors)	No effect
Glands		
• Sweat	Increase in sweat (neurotransmitter, acetylcholine)	No effect
Digestive (e.g., salivary, gastric)	Decrease in secretion of saliva; not known for others	Increase in secretion of saliva and gastric hydrochloric acid (HCl)
• Pancreas, including islets	Decrease in secretion	Increase in secretion of pancreatic juice and insulin
• Liver	Increase in glycogenolysis (β-receptors), increase in blood glucose level	No effect
Adrenal medulla‡	Increase in epinephrine secretion	No effect

*Neurotransmitter is norepinephrine unless otherwise stated.
†Neurotransmitter is acetylcholine unless otherwise stated.
‡Sympathetic preganglionic axons terminate in contact with secreting cells of the adrenal medulla. Thus, the adrenal medulla functions as what is sometimes called a *giant sympathetic postganglionic neuron.*
Source: Adapted from Patton, K. T., & Thibodeau, G. A. (2010). *Anatomy and physiology* (7th ed., p. 483, Table 14-6). St. Louis: Mosby.

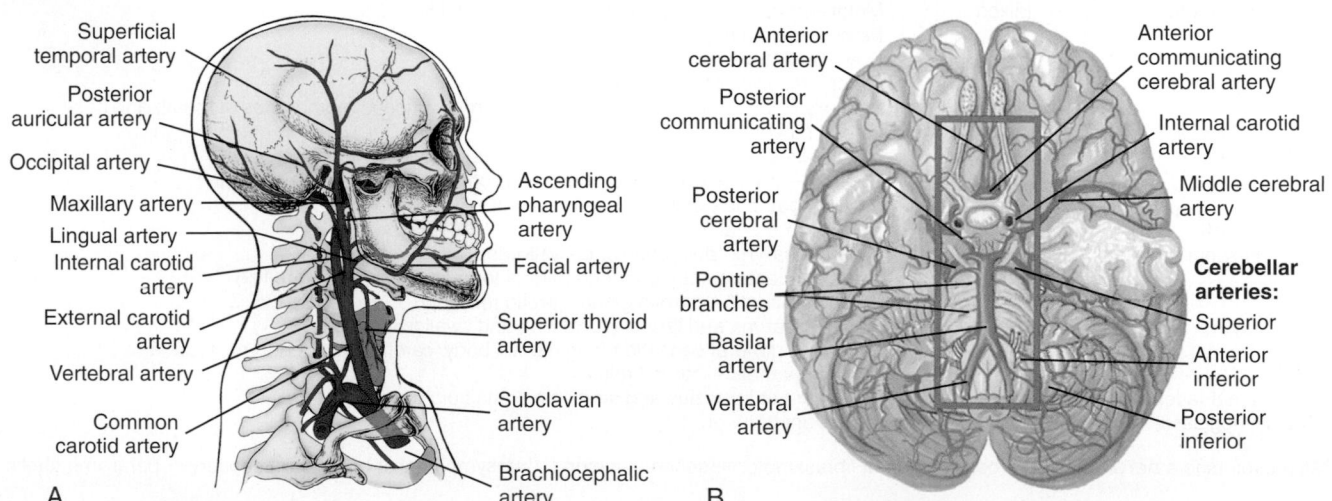

FIGURE 58-13 Arteries of the head and neck. **A,** Right lateral view: brachiocephalic artery, right common carotid artery, right subclavian artery, and their branches. The major arteries to the head are the common carotid and vertebral arteries. **B,** Inferior view of the brain, showing the vertebral, basilar, and internal carotid arteries and their branches. Source: Adapted from Patton, K. T., & Thibodeau, G. A. (2010). *Anatomy and physiology* (7th ed., p. 633, Figure 18-19). St. Louis: Mosby.

Blood–Brain Barrier. The **blood–brain barrier** is a physiological barrier between blood capillaries and brain tissue (McCance & Huether, 2014). This barrier protects the brain from certain potentially harmful agents, while allowing nutrients and gases to enter. Because the blood–brain barrier affects the penetration of drugs, only certain ones can enter the CNS from the bloodstream. Lipid-soluble compounds enter the brain quickly, whereas water-soluble and ionized drugs enter the brain and spinal cord slowly. Damage to the blood–brain barrier results in the penetration of drugs and other substances into brain tissue.

Protective Structures

Meninges. The **meninges** are three layers of protective membranes that surround the brain and the spinal cord: dura mater, arachnoid, and pia mater (see Figure 58-9). The thick *dura mater* forms the outermost layer. The *falx cerebri* is a fold of the dura that separates the two cerebral hemispheres and

prevents expansion of brain tissue in situations such as the presence of a rapidly growing tumour or acute hemorrhage. The *tentorium cerebelli* is a fold of dura that separates the cerebral hemispheres from the posterior fossa, which contains the brain stem and the cerebellum. Expansion of mass lesions in the cerebrum forces the brain to herniate through the opening created by the brain stem. This condition is termed *tentorial herniation* (see Chapter 59).

The *arachnoid layer* is a delicate, impermeable membrane that lies between the thick dura mater and the pia mater (the delicate, innermost layer of the meninges). The area between the arachnoid layer and the pia mater is the *subarachnoid space* and is filled with CSF. Structures such as arteries, veins, and cranial nerves passing to and from the brain and the skull must pass through the subarachnoid space. A larger subarachnoid space in the region of the third and fourth lumbar vertebrae is the area used to obtain CSF during a lumbar puncture. (The spinal cord itself ends between the first and second lumbar vertebrae.)

Skull. The bony skull protects the brain from external trauma. It is composed of 8 cranial bones and 14 facial bones. Although the top and the sides of the inside of the skull are relatively smooth, the bottom surface is uneven; it has many ridges, prominences, and foramina (holes through which blood vessels and nerves enter the intracranial vault). The largest hole is the foramen magnum, through which the brain stem extends to the spinal cord. This foramen is the only major space for the expansion of brain contents when increased intracranial pressure occurs.

Vertebral Column. The vertebral column protects the spinal cord, supports the head, and provides flexibility. The vertebral column is made up of 33 individual vertebrae: 7 cervical, 12 thoracic, 5 lumbar, 5 sacral (fused into one, the sacrum), and 4 coccygeal (fused into one, the coccyx). Each vertebra has a central opening through which the spinal cord passes. The vertebrae are held together by a series of ligaments. Intervertebral discs occupy the spaces between vertebrae. Figure 58-15 depicts the vertebral column in relation to the trunk.

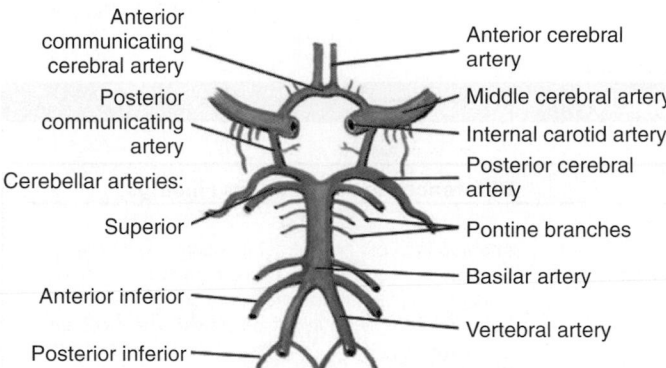

FIGURE 58-14 Arteries at the base of the brain. The arteries that compose the circle of Willis are the two anterior cerebral arteries, joined to each other by the anterior communicating cerebral artery and to the posterior cerebral arteries by the posterior communicating arteries. Source: Adapted from Patton, K. T., & Thibodeau, G. A. (2010). *Anatomy and physiology* (7th ed., p. 634, Figure 18-20). St. Louis: Mosby.

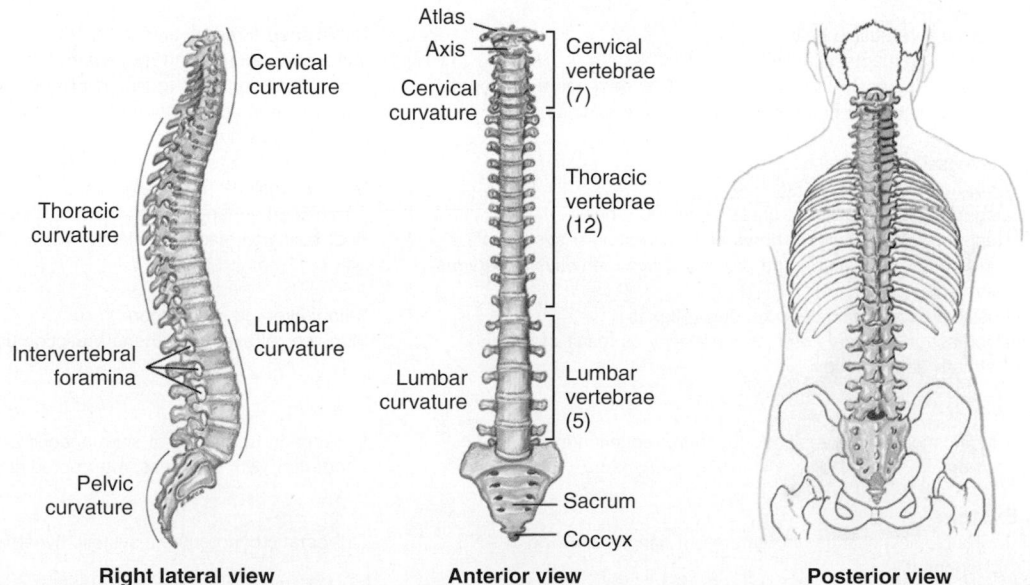

FIGURE 58-15 Vertebral column (three views). Source: Adapted from Patton, K. T., & Thibodeau, G. A. (2010). *Anatomy and physiology* (7th ed., p. 237, Figure 8-13). St. Louis: Mosby.

AGE-RELATED CONSIDERATIONS

EFFECTS OF AGING ON THE NERVOUS SYSTEM

Several parts of the nervous system are affected by aging. In the CNS, neurons are lost in certain areas of the brain stem, the cerebellum, and the cerebral cortex. This loss is a gradual process that begins in early adulthood. With loss of neurons, the ventricles widen. Brain weight also decreases by 10% to 15% between the second and ninth decades of life (Porter & Kaplan, 2011). Cerebral blood flow decreases, and CSF production declines. Changes in neurotransmitters of the dopaminergic and cholinergic systems result in decreasing amounts of acetylcholine, serotonin, and catecholamines.

In the PNS, degenerative changes in myelin cause a decrease in nerve conduction. Coordinated neuro-muscular activity, such as the maintenance of blood pressure in response to changing from a lying to a standing position, is altered with aging. As a result, older adults are more likely to experience orthostatic hypotension. Similarly, coordination of neuro-muscular activity to maintain body temperature is also less efficient with aging, making older adults less able to adapt to extremes in environmental temperature and more vulnerable to both hypothermia and hyperthermia.

In general, the intellectual performance of older adults who do not have brain dysfunction remains fairly consistent. A slowdown in central processing may result in needing longer to perform certain tasks. Sensory changes, including decreases in taste and smell perception, may result in decreased dietary intake in older adults. Changes in pain perception may occur. Decline in visual and auditory acuity can result in perceptual challenges. Problems with balance and coordination can increase older adults' risk for falls and subsequent fractures.

Changes in assessment findings result from age-related alterations in the various components of the nervous system. Age-related changes in the nervous system and differences in assessment findings are presented in Table 58-4.

TABLE 58-4   AGE-RELATED DIFFERENCES IN ASSESSMENT

Nervous System

Component	Changes	Differences in Assessment Findings
Central Nervous System		
Brain	Reduction in cerebral blood flow and metabolism	Alterations in certain mental functions
	Decrease in efficiency of temperature-regulating mechanism	Decrease in body temperature, impairment of ability to adapt to environmental temperature
	Decrease in neurotransmitter volume, disruption in integration as result of loss of neurons	Conduction of nerve impulses slowed, response time slowed
	Decrease in oxygen supply, changes in basal ganglia caused by vascular changes	Changes in gait and ambulation; diminished kinesthetic sense
	Cerebral tissue atrophy and increased size of ventricles	Altered balance, vertigo, syncope; increased postural hypotension; decreased proprioception; decreased sensation
Peripheral Nervous System		
Cranial and spinal nerves	Loss of myelin and decrease in conduction time in some nerves	Decrease in reaction time in specific nerves
	Cellular degeneration, death of neurons	Decrease in speed and intensity of neuronal reflexes
Functional Divisions		
Motor	Decrease in muscle bulk	Diminished strength and agility
	Decrease in electrical activity	Increased reaction and movement time
Sensory*	Decrease in sensory receptors caused by degenerative changes and involution of fine corpuscles of nerve endings	Diminished sense of touch; inability to localize stimuli; decrease in appreciation of touch, temperature, and peripheral vibrations
	Decrease in electrical activity	Slowing of or alteration in sensory reception
	Atrophy of taste buds	Signs of malnutrition, weight loss
	Degeneration and loss of fibres in olfactory bulb	Diminished sense of smell
	Degenerative changes in nerve cells in vestibular system of inner ear, cerebellum, and proprioceptive pathways in nervous system	Poor ability to maintain balance, widened gait
Reflexes	Possible decrease in deep tendon reflexes	Below-average reflex score
	Decrease in sensory conduction velocity as result of myelin sheath degeneration	Sluggish reflexes, lengthened reaction time
Reticular Formation		
Reticular activating system	Modification of hypothalamic function, reduction in stage IV sleep	Increase in frequency of spontaneous awakening, together with tiredness, interrupted sleep, insomnia
Autonomic Nervous System		
SNS and PSNS	Morphological changes in features of ganglia, slowing of ANS responses	Orthostatic hypotension, systolic hypertension

ANS, autonomic nervous system; *PSNS,* parasympathetic nervous system; *SNS,* sympathetic nervous system.
*Specific changes related to the eye and the ear are described in Chapter 24.

ASSESSMENT OF THE NERVOUS SYSTEM

Because of the complexity of the nervous system, neurological assessment is challenging and lengthy. Involving family members in the assessment is critical because patients with neurological problems often experience cognitive, emotional, and motivational deficits. Careful observation is an especially important nursing skill because many neurological changes are subtle.

Subjective Data

The history should begin with an open-ended and indirect inquiry that allows the patient to describe the chief complaint and current health (Jarvis, 2014). Three points should be considered in documenting the history of a patient with neurological problems. First, questions about symptoms should be open-ended. It is better to ask, "What is your headache like?" rather than "Do you experience headaches?" It is also better to allow the patient to provide the details, for example, "Is there anything about your right side that bothers you?" than to ask leading questions like, "Is your headache throbbing?" or "Are you weak on the right side?" Second, the mode of onset and the course of the illness are especially important aspects of the history. The nature of a neurological disease process can often be described by these facts alone, and the nurse should obtain all pertinent data in the history of the present illness, especially data related to the characteristics and progression of the symptoms. Third, because many neurological diseases affect a patient's mental functioning, mental status must be assessed accurately before the nurse assumes that the history is factual. If the patient is not considered a reliable historian, the history should be obtained from a person who has first-hand knowledge of the patient's problems and complaints. In many cases, a complete health history cannot be obtained, and the nurse must proceed with only objective data.

Important Health Information

Past Health History. The health history helps guide the approach for the neurological examination; that is, it can direct the nurse toward the parts of the nervous system that must be closely assessed. If the patient's primary complaint is dizziness, the examination may be focused on visual, vestibular, and cerebellar functions rather than on somatic motor and sensory functions.

Medications. Special attention should be given to obtaining a careful medication history, especially the use of sedatives, opioids, tranquilizers, mood-elevating drugs, over-the-counter medications, and herbal remedies. Many drugs can cause adverse neurological effects.

Surgery or Other Treatments. The nurse should inquire about any surgery involving any part of the nervous system, such as the head or brain, the spine or spinal cord, or the sensory organs. If a patient has had surgery, the date, the cause, the procedure, the recovery, and the current status should be investigated.

The perinatal history may reveal exposure to toxic agents such as viruses, alcohol, tobacco, drugs, and radiation, which are known to adversely influence the development of the nervous system. The history may reveal a difficult labour and delivery, which can cause brain damage as a result of hypoxia, forceps delivery, or Rh incompatibility.

Growth and developmental history can be important in ascertaining whether nervous system dysfunction was present at an early age. The nurse should specifically inquire about major developmental tasks such as walking and talking. Successes at school or identified problems in an educational setting are other

---

CASE STUDY

Patient Introduction

Evelyn Jones is a 66-year-old woman who arrives in the emergency department after falling in the middle of the night when she tried to get up to go to the bathroom. She states that she fell because she could not control her left leg. Her husband brought her to the hospital but states that he had a really hard time getting her to the car.

Source: Jeanette Dietl/ Shutterstock .com.

Critical Thinking

Throughout this assessment chapter, think about Ms. Jones's concerns, with the following questions in mind:

1. What are the possible causes for her acute leg weakness?
2. What type of assessment would be most appropriate for Ms. Jones: comprehensive, focused, or emergency? What would the priority assessment be?
3. What questions should the nurse ask Ms. Jones?
4. What should be included in the physical assessment? What should the nurse be looking for?
5. What diagnostic studies might be ordered?
   See pp. 1463, 1467, and 1468 for more information on Ms. Jones.

evolve

Answers are available at *http://evolve.elsevier.com/Canada/Lewis/medsurg.*

---

important developmental data to gather. Often, this information is not available when an older patient is interviewed.

Health Status. Key questions to ask a patient with a neurological problem are presented in Table 58-5.

General Health Practices. The nurse should ask about the patient's general health practices that may affect the nervous system, such as substance use and smoking, nutrition, participation in physical and recreational activities, use of seat belts and helmets, and control of hypertension. The nurse should ask about previous hospitalizations for neurological problems. A careful family history may determine whether the neurological problem has a hereditary or congenital background.

GENETICS IN CLINICAL PRACTICE

- Huntington's disease is a genetically transmitted, autosomal dominant disorder.
- Major neurological disorders that may have a genetic basis are multiple sclerosis, headaches, Parkinson's disease, and Alzheimer's disease. The presence of these problems in a family history increases the likelihood of similar problems occurring in the patient.
- A careful family history may determine whether a neurological problem has a genetic basis.

If the patient has an existing neurological problem, the nurse should ask about how it affects daily living and the ability to carry out self-care. After a careful review of information, and with the patient's permission, the nurse may find it helpful to ask someone who knows the patient well whether any mental or physical changes have been noticed in the patient. The patient with a neurological problem may not be aware of it or may be unable to provide enough specific data to aid in the diagnosis.

Nutritional Problems. Neurological problems can result in inadequate nutrition. Problems related to chewing, swallowing,

TABLE 58-5 HEALTH HISTORY

Nervous System

Headaches
- Have you had any unusually frequent or severe headaches?
- When did this start? How often does this happen?
- Show me where you feel the pain in your head.
- What do you think the headaches are caused by?

Head Injury
- Please describe any head injuries you have had.
- Which part of your head was injured?
- Did you lose consciousness? For how long?

Dizziness or Vertigo
- Have you ever felt light-headed or faint?
- When does this feeling occur? Do activity or change in position bring this on?
- Do you ever feel something called *vertigo* (a spinning sensation)? Does the room spin (objective vertigo)? Do you feel you are spinning (subjective vertigo)?

Seizures
- Have you ever had seizures or convulsions? When did they start? How often did they or do they occur?
- When a seizure starts, do you have any warning? What do you experience?
- Where in your body do the seizures begin? On one side or both? Do they travel through your body? Are your muscles tense or limp?
- Are there other signs that go along with the seizures (loss of consciousness, colour change in face or lips, eyelid fluttering, eye-rolling, lip smacking, or incontinence)?
- After the seizure, are you told that you fall asleep or experience confusion, weakness, headache, or muscle ache?
- What seems to bring on the seizures (activity, discontinuing medications, fatigue, stress)?
- Are you taking medication for the seizures?
- How have the seizures affected your daily life?

Tremors
- Have you experienced any shaking or tremors in the hands or the face? When did these start?
- Are the tremors worse with anxiety? With deliberate movement? With rest?
- Are the tremors better with rest? With activity? With alcohol?
- Do the tremors affect your daily activity?

Weakness
- Do you have any weakness or problem moving any body part? Is the weakness just in one body part or everywhere?
- Does this occur with any particular movement? (Example: difficulty getting out of a chair may signal proximal or large muscle weakness, whereas distal or small muscle weakness makes it difficult to open a jar or write.)

Coordination
- Do you have any problems with coordination or balance when walking?
- Do you lean to one side?
- Do you have any problems with falling? Which way?
- Do your legs give out from under you?
- Do you have any clumsy movement?

Numbness or Tingling
- Have you experienced any numbness or tingling? Does it feel like pins and needles? When did this start? Is it worse with activity?
- Show me where you feel this.

Difficulty Swallowing
- Do you have any difficulty swallowing? Does this occur with solids or liquids?
- Have you experienced excessive salivation or drooling?

Difficulty Speaking
- Have you had any problems with forming words or with saying what you meant to say?
- When did this start? How long did it last?

Significant Past History
- Have you ever had a stroke, a spinal cord or head injury, or meningitis or encephalitis?
- Do you have any congenital defects?
- Have you had past problems with alcohol or drug use?

Environmental and Occupational Hazards
- Are you exposed to any environmental or occupational hazards such as insecticides, lead, or organic solvents?
- Are you taking any medications now, including pain medications?
- How much alcohol do you drink? Each day? Each week?
- Do you use any mood-altering drugs: marijuana, barbiturates, tranquilizers?

Additional History for Older Adults
- Have you had any increase in falls? Is this related to dizziness? Does this occur with movement (e.g., change of position) or after taking medications?
- Have you had any changes in memory or mental function? Have you felt any confusion? Has it come on suddenly or gradually?
- Have you noticed any tremors? Are they in your hands or face? Do they change with activity, rest, use of alcohol? Do they interfere with your daily life?
- Have you had any sudden vision changes? Did this occur with weakness or loss of consciousness?

Source: Adapted from Jarvis, C. (2014). *Physical examination & health assessment* (2nd Canadian ed., pp. 666–668). (A. J. Brown, J. MacDonald-Jenkins, & M. Luctkar-Flude, Canadian Eds.). Toronto: Saunders/Elsevier.

facial nerve paralysis, or muscle coordination could make it difficult for affected patients to ingest adequate nutrients. Also, certain vitamins, such as thiamine (B_1), niacin (B_3), and pyridoxine (B_6), are essential for the maintenance and health of the CNS. Deficiencies in one or more of these vitamins could result in such nonspecific complaints as depression, apathy, neuritis, weakness, mental confusion, and irritability. Risk for cobalamin (vitamin B_{12}) deficiency is higher in older adults because they may have problems with vitamin absorption. Untreated, this deficiency may cause a decline in mental function (Lachner, Steinle, & Regenold, 2014).

Bowel and Bladder Problems. Bowel and bladder problems are often associated with neurological conditions, such as stroke, head injury, spinal cord injury, multiple sclerosis, and dementia. To plan appropriate interventions, it is important to determine whether the bowel or bladder problem was present before or after the neurological event. Incontinence of urine and feces and urinary retention are the most common elimination problems associated with a neurological problem or its treatment (Coggrave, Norton, & Cody, 2014; Panicker, Fowler, & Kessler, 2015). For example, nerve root compression leads to a sudden onset of incontinence. The details of the problem—such as number of episodes, accompanying sensations or lack of sensations, and measures taken to control the problem—must be documented carefully.

Motor Problems. Many neurological disorders can cause problems in the patient's mobility, strength, and coordination. Neurological problems can result in changes in the patient's usual activity and exercise patterns. These problems can also result in falls (Homann, Plaschg, Grunder, et al., 2013). Many activities of daily living, such as getting out of a bed or chair, ambulating, preparing meals, and performing personal hygiene, can be affected and should be assessed. The ability to perform fine motor tasks may be affected, which increases the possibility of personal injury.

Sleep Problems. Sleep pattern disruptions can be both a cause of and a response to many neurologically related concerns. Discomfort from pain and inability to move and change to a position of comfort because of muscle weakness and paralysis could interfere with sound sleep. Hallucinations resulting from dementia or drugs can also interrupt sleep. The nurse should carefully document the sleep problem and the patient's methods of dealing with the problem.

Cognition and Sensory Problems. Because the nervous system controls cognition and sensory integration, many neurological disorders affect these functions. The nurse should assess orientation, memory, language, calculation ability, problem-solving ability, insight, and judgement. A structured mental status questionnaire is often used to evaluate these functions and provide baseline data.

Information about sensory changes related to hearing, sight, and touch should be sought. The patient should be questioned about problems with vertigo and sensitivity to heat and cold.

Ability to both use and understand language is a cognitive function that the nurse should assess. Appropriateness of responses is a useful indicator of cognitive and perceptual ability, but it is culturally determined.

Pain is a common event associated with many health problems. Pain is often the reason why patients seek health care. A patient's pain should be assessed carefully (see Chapter 10).

Emotional Problems. Neurological disease can drastically alter control over one's life and create dependency on others for daily needs. A patient's physical appearance and emotional control can be affected. The nurse should ask in a sensitive manner about the patient's evaluation of self-worth, perception of abilities, body image, and general emotional pattern. The physical sequelae of a neurological problem can seriously strain the patient's coping abilities. The nurse should determine whether coping abilities are sufficient to meet the challenges faced by the patient.

Relationship Problems. The patient should be asked whether a neurological problem has resulted in changes to roles such as spouse, parent, or breadwinner. Physical impairments such as weakness and paralysis can alter or limit participation in usual roles and activities. Cognitive changes, however, can permanently change a person's ability to maintain previous roles. These changes can dramatically affect both the patient and significant others. Dependent relationships can develop.

Sexual Problems. Because many nervous system disorders can affect sexual functioning, sexual health may be an important part of the assessment for some patients. Cerebral lesions may inhibit the desire phase or the reflex responses of the excitement phase. Brain stem and spinal cord lesions may partially or completely interrupt the connections between the brain and the effector systems necessary for intercourse.

Neuropathies and spinal cord lesions that affect sensation, especially in the erotic zones, may decrease desire. Autonomic neuropathies and lesions of the sacral cord and the cauda equina may prevent reflex activities of the sexual response. The nurse should determine whether the patient and the partner are satisfied with their sexual activity. The use or need for alternative methods of achieving sexual satisfaction should be explored. Despite neurologically related changes in sexual functioning, many people can achieve satisfying expression of intimacy and affection.

CASE STUDY

Subjective Data

A subjective assessment of Ms. Jones revealed the following information:

History of Current Illness. States that she fell due to sudden weakness in her left leg. States that she had a brief episode of left-sided weakness and tingling of the face, arm, and hand, 3 months ago. The symptoms totally resolved and she did not seek treatment. Denies dizziness, change in hearing, or memory deficits. Has never been hospitalized for a neurologic problem. Is depressed and fearful. Concerned she is having a stroke.

Source: Jeanette Dietl/ Shutterstock .com.

Past Health History: Hyperlipidemia, hypertension.

Medications: Pravastatin 40 mg/day PO; lisinopril 10 mg/day PO.

Functional Assessment: Has smoked one pack of cigarettes per day since she was 28 years old. Drinks alcohol occasionally. Hypertension controlled when on medication but has not taken her lisinopril for a few weeks because she did not have enough money for the refill and was waiting for her next Social Assistance cheque. Ms. Jones is 160 cm tall and weighs 73 kg. States that up until tonight she was able to walk slowly, but her knees and hips hurt.

See pp. 1461, 1467, and 1468 for more information on Ms. Jones.

Objective Data

Physical Examination. The standard neurological examination helps determine the presence, the location, and the nature of disease of the nervous system. In this examination, six categories of functions are assessed: mental status, function of cranial nerves, motor function, cerebellar function, sensory function, and reflex function. The choice of particular parts of the examination depends on what information is needed. The nurse should develop a systematic and consistent approach to assessment.

Mental Status. Assessment of mental status (cerebral functioning) gives an indication of how the patient is functioning. It involves determination of complex and high-level cerebral functions that are governed by many areas of the cerebral cortex. Much of the mental status examination can be conducted during the routine history and may not need to be evaluated further. For example, language and memory can be assessed when the patient is asked for details of the illness and significant past events. The patient's cultural and educational background should be taken into account when mental status is evaluated.

The components of the mental status examination are as follows:

- *General appearance and behaviour:* This component includes motor activity, body posture, dress and hygiene, facial expression, and speech.
- *Level of consciousness (LOC):* This is the most sensitive indicator of changes in neurological status (McCance & Huether, 2014). LOC concerns arousal and wakefulness and the ability to

respond to the environment. The Glasgow Coma Scale is often used to assess a patient's response to stimuli (see Chapter 59 and Table 59-5).

- *Cognition:* The nurse should note the patient's orientation to time, place, person, and situation. Further assessment of memory, intellectual ability, insight, judgement, problem solving, and calculation may be warranted (see Chapter 62). The nurse should consider whether the patient's plans and goals match the patient's physical and mental capabilities. Problems with memory may have implications for retention of new information, and impaired judgement and insight may jeopardize the patient's safety.

- *Mood and affect:* The nurse should note restlessness, agitation, anger, depression, or euphoria and the appropriateness of these states. The nurse should also note whether the patient's affect is appropriate for the situation.

- *Thought content:* The nurse should note the presence or report of illusions, hallucinations, delusions, or paranoia.

Function of Cranial Nerves. Testing of each cranial nerve (CN) is an essential component of the neurological examination (see Figure 58-12).

Olfactory Nerve. After determining that both nostrils are patent, the olfactory nerve (CN I) is tested by asking the patient to close one nostril, close both eyes, and sniff from a bottle containing coffee, spice, soap, or some other readily recognized odour. The same procedure is done for the other nostril. In general, olfaction is not tested unless the patient has some disturbance with smell. Chronic rhinitis, sinusitis, and heavy smoking can often decrease the sense of smell. Disturbance in ability to smell may be associated with a tumour involving the olfactory bulb, or it may be the result of a basilar skull fracture that has damaged the olfactory fibres as they pass through the delicate cribriform plate of the skull.

Optic Nerve. Visual fields and visual acuity are assessed to test the function of the optic nerve (CN II). Visual fields are assessed by gross confrontation. The nurse, positioned directly opposite the patient, asks the patient to close one eye, look directly at the bridge of the nurse's nose, and indicate when an object (finger, pencil tip, head of pin) presented from the periphery of each of the four visual field quadrants becomes visible (Figure 58-16). The same test is repeated for the other eye. The nurse is used as a control because both nurse and patient are sharing the

same visual field. It is important to remember that the nasal side of the visual field is narrower because of the nasal bridge. Visual field defects may arise from lesions of the optic nerve, the optic chiasm, or the tracts that extend through the temporal, parietal, and occipital lobes. Visual field changes resulting from brain lesions are usually a *hemianopia* (one-half of the visual field is affected), a *quadrantanopsia* (one-fourth of the visual field is affected), or monocular (one eye is affected).

To test visual acuity, the patient reads a Snellen chart from 6 metres away. The nurse records the number of the lowest line that the patient can read accurately. The patient who wears glasses should wear them during testing, unless they are used only for reading. The eyes should be tested individually and together. If a Snellen chart is not available, the patient should be asked to read newsprint for a gross assessment of acuity. The distance from the patient to the newsprint required for accurate reading should be recorded. Acuity may not be testable by these means if the patient does not read English or has aphasia (a language disorder).

Funduscopy reveals the physical condition of the optic disc (head of the optic nerve), as well as that of the retina and the blood vessels. This procedure is routinely performed when the optic nerve is tested. Optic nerve atrophy and papilledema can be detected by this method.

Oculomotor, Trochlear, and Abducens Nerves. Because the oculomotor (CN III), trochlear (CN IV), and abducens (CN VI) nerves all help move the eye, they are tested together for what are termed *extraocular movements* (EOMs). The patient is asked to keep the head steady and to follow the nurse's finger only with the eyes. The nurse should keep the finger back about 30 cm so that the patient can focus on it comfortably. The nurse moves the finger to each of the six positions (right and up, right, right and down, left and up, left, left and down), holds it momentarily, and then moves back to the centre (Figure 58-17). A normal response is parallel tracking of the object with both eyes. If weakness or paralysis is present in one of the eye muscles, the eyes do not move together, and the patient has a *disconjugate gaze.* The presence and direction of *nystagmus* (fine, rapid jerking movements of the eyes) are observed at this time, even though this condition most often indicates vestibulo-cerebellar problems.

Other functions of the oculomotor nerve are tested by checking for pupillary constriction and for *convergence* (eyes turning

FIGURE 58-16 Assessment of visual fields by gross confrontation. In gross confrontation, the target is moved in a flat plane between the nurse and the patient. The nurse's own monocular field is compared with that of that patient.

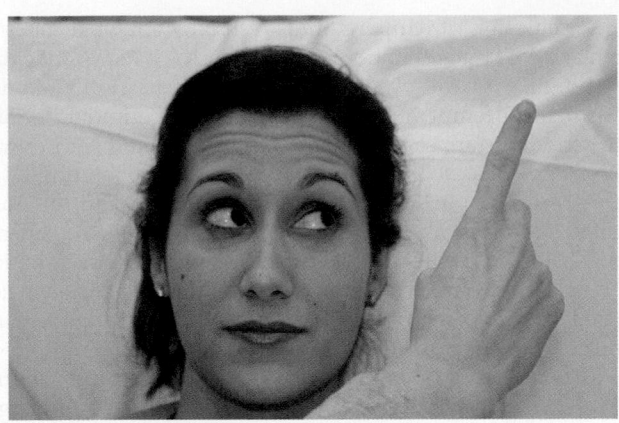

FIGURE 58-17 Nurse checking extraocular movement. Normally, both eyes move together. Eye movements should be smooth and coordinated.

inward) and *accommodation* (pupils constricting with near vision). To test pupillary constriction, the nurse shines a light into the pupil of one eye and looks for ipsilateral (same side) constriction of the same pupil and contralateral (consensual) constriction of the opposite eye. The size and shape of the pupils are also noted. For this reflex to occur, the optic nerve must be intact. Testing for papillary constriction is an important component of the neurological assessment of patients at risk for herniation (see Chapter 59). Because the oculomotor nerve exits at the top of the brain stem at the tentorial notch, it can be easily compressed by expanding mass lesions in the cerebral hemispheres. The result is that the pupil does not constrict in response to light; it may become dilated because the sympathetic input to the pupil acts unopposed. To test convergence and accommodation, the patient focuses on the nurse's finger as it moves toward the patient's nose. Another function of the oculomotor nerve is to keep the eyelid open. Damage to the nerve can cause *ptosis* (drooping eyelid), pupillary abnormalities, and eye muscle weakness.

Trigeminal Nerve. To test the sensory component of the trigeminal nerve (CN V), the patient is asked to identify light touch (cotton) and pinprick in each of the three divisions (ophthalmic, maxillary, and mandibular) of the nerve on both sides of the face. The patient's eyes should be closed during this part of the examination. To test the motor component, the patient clenches the teeth, and the masseter muscles, just above the mandibular angle, are palpated. The corneal reflex test, in which CN V and CN VII are evaluated simultaneously, involves applying a cotton wisp strand to the cornea. The sensory component of this reflex (corneal sensation) is innervated by the ophthalmic division of CN V. The motor component (eye blink) is innervated by the facial nerve (CN VII). This reflex is not normally tested in patients who are awake and alert because other tests are used to evaluate these two nerves. However, for patients with a decreased level of consciousness, the corneal reflex test provides an opportunity to evaluate the integrity of the brain stem at the level of the pons because the fibres of CN V and CN VII have connections in this area.

Facial Nerve. The facial nerve (CN VII) innervates the muscles of facial expression. To test its function, the patient raises the eyebrows, closes the eyes tightly, purses the lips, draws back the corners of the mouth in an exaggerated smile, and frowns. The nurse should note any asymmetry in the facial movements because this can indicate damage to the facial nerve. Although taste discrimination of salt and sugar in the anterior two-thirds

of the tongue is a function of this nerve, it is not routinely tested unless a peripheral nerve lesion is suspected.

Vestibulo-cochlear Nerve. To test the cochlear portion of the acoustic (vestibulo-cochlear) nerve (CN VIII), the patient closes the eyes and indicates when a ticking watch or the rustling of the nurse's fingertips is heard as the stimulus is brought closer to the patient's ear. Each ear is tested individually, and the distance from the patient's ear to the sound source when first heard is recorded. This test identifies only gross deficits in hearing. For more precise assessment of hearing, an audiometer (or tuning forks) can be used (see Chapter 23). The vestibular portion of this nerve is not routinely tested unless the patient complains of dizziness, vertigo, or unsteadiness or has auditory dysfunction. In a patient who is unconscious, the oculo-cephalic reflex (movement of the eyes when the head is briskly turned to the side) may be assessed.

Glossopharyngeal and Vagus Nerves. The glossopharyngeal and vagus nerves are tested together because both innervate the pharynx. The glossopharyngeal nerve (CN IX) is primarily sensory. In the gag reflex (bilateral contraction of the palatal muscles initiated by stroking or touching either side of the posterior pharynx or soft palate with a tongue blade), the sensory component is mediated by CN IX and the major motor component by the vagus nerve (CN X). It is important to assess the gag reflex in patients who have a decreased level of consciousness, a brain stem lesion, or a disease involving the throat musculature. If the reflex is weak or absent, the patient may be at risk of aspirating food or secretions. The strength and efficiency of swallowing are important to test in these patients for the same reason. In another test for an awake, cooperative patient, the patient phonates by saying "ah" and the nurse notes the bilateral symmetry of elevation of the soft palate. Any asymmetry can indicate weakness or paralysis. To assess swallowing, the nurse's hands are held lightly on either side of the patient's throat while the patient swallows. Any asymmetry is noted. If the patient is endotracheally intubated, the cough reflex (elicited when the suction catheter contacts the carina of the respiratory tree) is a method of assessing cranial nerve X.

Spinal Accessory Nerve. To test the spinal accessory nerve (CN XI), the patient shrugs the shoulders against resistance and turns the head to either side against resistance. The contraction of the sternocleidomastoid and trapezius muscles should be smooth. Symmetry, atrophy, or fasciculation of the muscle should also be noted. A *fasciculation* is a small, local involuntary muscular contraction.

Hypoglossal Nerve. To test the hypoglossal nerve (CN XII), the patient sticks out the tongue. It should protrude in the midline. The patient should also be able to push the tongue to either side against the resistance of a tongue blade. Again, any asymmetry, atrophy, or fasciculation should be noted.

Motor Function. The motor system examination includes assessment of bulk, tone, and power of the major muscle groups of the body, as well as assessment of balance and coordination. To test strength, the patient pushes and pulls against the resistance of the nurse's arm as it opposes flexion and extension of the patient's muscle. The patient should be asked to offer resistance at the shoulders, elbows, wrists, hips, knees, and ankles. The patient's grip strength can also be tested. To test for mild weakness of the upper extremities, the patient extends both arms forward at shoulder height with palms up while the eyes are closed. Mild weakness of the arm is demonstrated by downward drifting of the arm or pronation of the palm *(pronator drift)*. Any weakness or asymmetry of strength between the same muscle groups of the right and left side should be noted.

To test tone, the limbs are passively moved through their range of motion; there should be a slight resistance to these movements. Abnormal tone is described as *hypotonia* (flaccidity) or *hypertonia* (spasticity). Involuntary movements—such as tics, tremor, *myoclonus* (spasm of muscles), *athetosis* (slow, writhing, involuntary movements of extremities), *chorea* (involuntary, purposeless, rapid motions), and *dystonia* (impairment of muscle tone)—should be noted.

To test cerebellar function, balance and coordination are assessed. A good screening test for both balance and muscle strength is to observe the patient's stance (posture while standing) and gait. The nurse should note the pace and rhythm of the gait and observe the arm swing. (The arms should move symmetrically and in the opposite direction of the leg on the same side.) The patient's ability to ambulate is a key factor in determining the amount of nursing care that is needed and the risk for injury from falling. A patient with cerebellar disease may have an *ataxic* or *staggering gait*, in which the feet are placed wide apart and the steps are unsteady.

Coordination can be easily tested in several ways. In the finger-to-nose test, the patient alternately touches the nose with the index finger and then touches the nurse's finger. The nurse repositions the finger while the patient is touching the nose so that the patient must adjust to a new distance each time the nurse's finger is touched. These movements should be performed smoothly and accurately. Other tests include asking the patient to pronate and supinate both hands rapidly and to perform a shallow knee bend, first on one leg and then on the other. Dysarthria or slurred speech should be noted because it is a sign of incoordination of the speech muscles.

In the heel-to-shin test, the patient places one heel on the opposite shin below the knee and moves the heel down the shin to the ankle. This procedure is repeated for the other leg. These movements should flow smoothly without jerking or hesitation.

Sensory Function. Several modalities are tested in the somatic sensory examination. Each modality is carried by a specific ascending pathway in the spinal cord before it reaches the sensory cortex.

There are some general guidelines for performing the sensory examination. The patient should always have the eyes closed to avoid visual clues. The nurse should avoid giving verbal cues such as, "Is this sharp?" The sensory stimulus should be applied in such a way that the patient does not expect it; that is, the nurse should avoid rhythmic application of the stimulus. In the routine neurological examination, sensory testing of the four extremities is sufficient. However, if a disturbance in sensory function of the skin is identified, the boundaries of that dysfunction should be carefully delineated along the dermatome.

Light Touch. The sensation of light touch is usually tested first. The nurse gently strokes each of the four extremities with a cotton wisp and asks the patient to indicate when the stimulus is felt by saying "touch." (The sensory examination of the trigeminal nerve may be delayed until this time because the same material for testing sensation is used.)

Pain and Temperature. Pain is tested by touching the skin with the sharp end of a safety pin. This stimulus is irregularly alternated with a simple touch stimulus with the dull end of the pin to determine whether the patient can distinguish the two stimuli.

The sensation of temperature is tested by applying tubes of warm and cold water to the skin and asking the patient to identify the stimuli with the eyes closed. If pain sensation is intact, assessment of temperature sensation may be omitted because both sensations are carried by the same ascending pathways.

Vibration Sense. To assess vibration sense, a vibrating C128 tuning fork is applied to the patient's fingernails and the bony prominences of the hands, the legs, and the feet while the patient's eyes are closed. The nurse asks the patient whether the vibration or "buzz" is felt. The nurse then asks the patient to indicate when the vibration ceases. The nurse stops the vibration with the hand as desired.

Position Sense. To assess position sense, the nurse's thumb and forefinger are placed on either side of the patient's forefinger or great toe and gently move the patient's digit up or down. The patient is asked to indicate the direction in which the digit is moved.

Another test of position sense of the lower extremities is the *Romberg test*. The patient is asked to stand with the feet together and then to close his or her eyes. If the patient is able to maintain balance with the eyes open but sways or falls with the eyes closed (i.e., a positive result of the Romberg test), disease may be present in the posterior columns of the spinal cord or the cerebellum. It is important for the nurse to ensure the patient's safety during this test.

Cortical Sensory Functions. Several tests are used to evaluate cortical integration of sensory perceptions (which occurs in the parietal lobes). The patient's eyes should remain closed during these assessments. To assess two-point discrimination, the two points of a calibrated compass are placed on the tips of the patient's fingers and toes. The minimum recognizable separation is 4 to 5 mm in the fingertips and a greater degree of separation elsewhere. This test is important in diagnosing diseases of the sensory cortex and the PNS.

To test *graphesthesia* (ability to feel writing on skin), the patient is asked to identify numbers traced on the palm of the hands. To test *stereognosis* (ability to perceive the form and nature of objects), the patient is asked to identify the size and shape of easily recognized objects (e.g., coins, keys, a safety pin) placed in the hands. To evaluate sensory extinction or inattention, the nurse touches both sides of the patient's body simultaneously. An abnormal response occurs when the patient perceives the stimulus only on one side. The other stimulus is "extinguished."

Reflex Function. Tendons attached to skeletal muscles have receptors that are sensitive to stretch. A reflex contraction of the skeletal muscle occurs when the tendon is stretched. A simple muscle stretch reflex is initiated by briskly tapping the tendon of a stretched muscle, usually with a reflex hammer (Figure 58-18). The response (muscle contraction of the corresponding muscle) is measured as follows:

0	Absence of response—always abnormal
1+	Slight but definitely present response—may or may not be normal
2+	Brisk response—normal
3+	Very brisk response—may or may not be normal
4+	Repeating reflex (clonus)—always abnormal

Clonus is a continued rhythmic contraction of the muscle with continuous application of the stimulus.

In general, the biceps, triceps, brachioradialis, and patellar and Achilles tendon reflexes are tested. The nurse elicits the biceps reflex by placing his or her thumb over the patient's biceps tendon in the antecubital space and striking the thumb with a hammer. The nurse should support the patient's forearm so that it is partially

FIGURE 58-18 The nurse strikes a swift blow over a stretched tendon to elicit a stretch reflex. **A,** Biceps reflex. **B,** Patellar reflex.

flexed at the elbow, with the palm up and relaxed. The normal response is flexion of the arm at the elbow or contraction of the biceps muscle that can be felt by the nurse's thumb.

To elicit the triceps reflex, the nurse should support the patient's upper arm (to let the arm hang limply) and then strike the patient's triceps tendon above the elbow. The normal response is extension of the arm or visible contraction of the triceps.

To elicit the brachioradialis reflex, the nurse strikes the patient's radius 3 to 5 cm above the wrist while the patient's arm is relaxed. The normal response is flexion and supination at the elbow or visible contraction of the brachioradialis muscle.

To elicit the patellar reflex, the nurse strikes the patient's patellar tendon just below the patella. The patient can be sitting or lying as long as the leg being tested hangs freely. The normal response is extension of the leg with contraction of the quadriceps.

To elicit the Achilles tendon reflex, the nurse strikes the patient's Achilles tendon while the patient's leg is flexed at the knee and the foot is dorsiflexed at the ankle. The normal response is plantar flexion at the ankle.

A focused assessment (see Table 3-6) is used to evaluate the status or previously identified neurological problems and to monitor for signs of new problems. A focused assessment of the neurological system is presented in the "Focused Assessment" box.

Table 58-6 is a listing of normal findings in a neurological assessment. Abnormal assessment findings of the neurological system are presented in Table 58-7.

Diagnostic Studies of the Nervous System

Numerous diagnostic studies are available to assess the nervous system. Table 58-8 presents the most commonly encountered studies.

Cerebro-Spinal Fluid Analysis. CSF analysis provides information about a variety of CNS diseases. Normal CSF fluid is clear, colourless, and free of red blood cells and contains little protein. Normal CSF values are listed in Table 58-9.

FOCUSED ASSESSMENT
Neurological System

Use this checklist to make sure the key assessment steps have been performed.

Subjective
Ask the patient about any of the following, and note responses:

Blackouts or loss of memory	Y	N
Weakness, numbness, tingling sensation in arms or legs	Y	N
Headaches, especially of new onset	Y	N
Loss of balance or coordination	Y	N
Orientation to person, place, and time	Y	N

Objective: Diagnostic
Check the following laboratory results for critical values:

Lumbar puncture	✓
CT or MRI of brain	✓
EEG	✓

Objective: Physical Examination
Inspect or observe the following:

General level of consciousness and orientation	✓
Oropharynx for gag reflex and soft palate movement	✓
Peripheral sensation of light touch and pinprick (face, hands, feet)	✓
Sense of smell with an alcohol wipe	✓
Eyes for extraocular movements, PERRLA, peripheral vision, nystagmus	✓
Gait for smoothness and coordination	✓

Palpate for the following:

Strength of neck, shoulders, arms, and legs; full and symmetrical	✓

Percuss for the following:

Reflexes	✓

CT, computed tomographic (scan); *EEG,* electroencephalogram; *MRI,* magnetic resonance imaging; *PERRLA,* pupils equal, round, and reactive to light and accommodation.

CASE STUDY
Objective Data: Physical Examination

A physical examination findings of Ms. Jones reveals the following:
- Alert, oriented, and able to answer questions appropriately but mild slowness in responding
- BP 180/110, HR 94, RR 22, T 37°C
- CNS (Canadian Neurological Scale) (see Chapter 60, Figure 60-11) score is 10
- Left-sided arm weakness (3/5) and leg weakness (4/5)

Source: Jeanette Dietl/Shutterstock.com.

Throughout this chapter, consider diagnostic studies that may be ordered for Ms. Jones.

See pp. 1461, 1463, and 1468 for more information on Ms. Jones.

Lumbar Puncture. Lumbar puncture is the most common method of obtaining CSF for analysis. It is contraindicated in the presence of increased intracranial pressure or infection at the site of puncture.

Nurses often assist in this procedure because it is usually performed in the patient's room. Before the procedure, the patient

TABLE 58-6   NORMAL PHYSICAL ASSESSMENT OF THE NERVOUS SYSTEM*

Mental Status
Alert and oriented, orderly thought processes, appropriate mood and affect

Cranial Nerves†
Sense of smell intact for soap and coffee; visual fields full to confrontation; visual acuity 20/20 in both eyes; intact extraocular movements; no nystagmus; pupils equal, round, reactive to light and accommodation; intact facial sensation for touch and pinprick; facial movements full; intact gag and swallow reflexes; symmetrical elevation of soft palate; full strength with head turning and shrugging of shoulders against resistance; midline protrusion of tongue

Motor System
Normal gait and station; normal tandem walk; negative result of Romberg test; normal and symmetrical muscle bulk, tone, strength; smooth performance of finger–nose, heel–shin movements

Sensory System
Intact sensation to light touch, position sense, vibration, pinprick, heat and cold, two-point discrimination; intact stereognosis and graphesthesia

Reflexes‡
Biceps, triceps, brachioradialis, patellar, and Achilles tendon reflexes 2+ bilaterally; downward-pointing toes with plantar stimulation

*If some portion of the neurological examination was not performed, this should be indicated (e.g., "Smell not tested").
†May also be recorded as "CNs [cranial nerves] I to XII intact."
‡May also be recorded as drawing of stick figure indicating reflex strength at appropriate sites.

should empty the bladder. The patient should lie in the lateral recumbent position, with the back as near as possible to the edge of the bed. The nurse should assist the patient in drawing up the knees to the abdomen and flexing the head to the chest. This helps separate the vertebrae so that the needle can be inserted more easily.

Using strict sterile technique, the physician inserts a long needle below the third lumbar vertebra. This may cause some local discomfort. There is no danger of injuring the spinal cord because the cord terminates between the first and second lumbar vertebrae. However, the patient may experience some pain radiating down the leg or muscle twitching if the needle irritates the spinal root. The nurse can assure the patient that this is temporary and that the patient is not in danger of being paralyzed.

A manometer is attached to the needle, and CSF pressure is determined after the patient is asked to relax and extend the legs. If the patient does not relax and extend the legs, the pressure reading is abnormally high. Normal CSF pressure is approximately 9 to 14 mm Hg (McCance & Huether, 2014). CSF is withdrawn in a series of tubes and sent for analysis. Some examiners believe that the patient should be kept lying flat for at least a few hours after the procedure to avoid a spinal headache, which is presumably caused by loss of the cushioning effect of CSF as a result of leakage at the puncture site. The prone position may be effective in preventing CSF leakage. Other examiners do not believe that the lying position is necessary because headache seems to develop in some patients despite precautions. Meningeal irritation (nuchal

FIGURE 58-19 Cerebral angiogram illustrating an arteriovenous malformation *(arrow)*. Source: From Chipps, E., Clanin, N., & Campbell, V. (1992). *Neurologic disorders*. St. Louis: Mosby.

rigidity) or signs and symptoms of local trauma (e.g., hematoma, pain) may develop in some patients.

Radiological Studies

Cerebral Angiography. Cerebral angiography is indicated when vascular lesions or tumours are suspected. A catheter is inserted into the femoral (sometimes brachial) artery. It is then passed up the artery to the aortic arch and into the base of a carotid or a vertebral artery for injection of radiopaque contrast medium. Radiographs are taken in a timed sequence so that pictures of the arteries, smaller vessels, and veins can be obtained (Figure 58-19). This study can help localize and determine the presence of abscesses, aneurysms, hematomas, arteriovenous malformations, arterial spasm, and certain tumours.

Because this is an invasive procedure, adverse reactions may occur. The patient may have an allergic (anaphylactic) reaction to the contrast medium. When this reaction occurs, it is usually immediately after injection of the contrast medium and may necessitate emergency resuscitation measures in the procedure room. The most common precaution for nurses to take in caring for the patient after the return to the room is observation for bleeding at the catheter puncture site (usually the groin). A pressure dressing and ice are usually placed on the site to promote hemostasis and prevent swelling.

CASE STUDY

Objective Data: Diagnostic Studies

The emergency department physician immediately orders a stat CT scan of the head. The CT scan rules out a hemorrhagic stroke. Stat laboratory test results include a blood glucose of 7.5 mmol/L and a PT/INR of 12.0/1.1.

This case study is continued in Chapter 60.

See pp. 1461, 1463, and 1468 for more information on Ms. Jones.

Source: Jeanette Dietl/ Shutterstock.com.

TABLE 58-7 ASSESSMENT ABNORMALITIES

Nervous System

Finding	Description	Possible Etiology and Significance
Agnosia	Inability to determine meaning or significance of sensory stimulus	Cerebral cortex lesion
Altered consciousness	Inability to speak, obey commands, open eyes appropriately with verbal or painful stimulus	Intracranial lesions, metabolic disorder, psychiatric disorders
Anaesthesia	Absence of sensation	Lesions in spinal cord, thalamus, sensory cortex, or peripheral sensory nerve
Analgesia	Loss of pain sensation	Lesion in spino-thalamic tract or thalamus, lack of or damage to sensory nerve endings
Anisocoria	Unequal pupil size	Lesion, injury, or intracranial pressure in area of midbrain; can also be normal
Anosognosia	Inability to recognize bodily defect or disease	Lesions in right parietal cortex, common in right-sided brain stroke
Aphasia	Loss of language faculty (language comprehension, language expression, or both)	Cerebral cortex lesion
Apraxia	Inability to perform learned movements; defect in motor planning	Cerebral cortex lesion
Astereognosis	Inability to recognize form of object by touch	Lesions in parietal cortex
Ataxia	Lack of coordination of movement	Lesions of sensory or motor pathways, cerebellum; anticonvulsant drug, sedative, or hypnotic drug toxicity (including alcohol)
Bladder dysfunction		
• Atonic (autonomous)	Absence of muscle tone and contractility, enlarged capacity, no discomfort, overflow with large residual, inability to voluntarily empty or empty by reflex	Early stage of spinal cord injury
• Hypotonic	More ability to empty by reflex than with atonic bladder but less than normal	Interruption of afferent pathways from bladder
• Hypertonic	Increase in muscle tone, diminished capacity, reflex emptying, dribbling, incontinence	Lesions in pyramidal tracts (efferent pathways)
Diplopia	Double vision	Lesions affecting nerves of extraocular muscles, cerebellar damage
Dysarthria	Lack of coordination in articulating speech	Lesions in cerebellum or pathway of cranial nerves (including brain stem); anticonvulsant drug, sedative, or hypnotic drug toxicity (including alcohol)
Dyskinesia	Impaired power of voluntary movement, resulting in fragmentary or incomplete movements	Disorders of basal ganglia, idiosyncratic reaction to psychotropic drugs
Dysphagia	Difficulty in swallowing	Lesions involving motor pathways of cranial nerves IX and X (including lower brain stem)
Extensor plantar response (Babinski sign)	Upward-pointing toes with plantar stimulation	Suprasegmental or upper motor neuron lesion
Hemiplegia	Paralysis on one side	Stroke and other lesions involving motor cortex
Homonymous hemianopia	Loss of vision in one side of visual field	Injury or lesions in area of optic tract or its radiations to occipital cortex
Hyperaesthesia	Increase in sensation	Shingles, nerve compression, stress, or chronic pain
Hypoaesthesia	Decrease in sensation	Impingement or damage of a nerve (e.g., peripheral neuropathy in diabetes)
Muscle atrophy (disuse or denervation atrophy)	Wasting away or diminution in size of muscle	Suprasegmental (upper motor neuron) lesions, segmental (lower motor neuron) lesions
Nystagmus	Jerking or bobbing of eyes as they track moving object	Lesions in cerebellum, brain stem, vestibular system; toxic effects of anticonvulsants, sedatives, hypnotics (including alcohol)
Ophthalmoplegia	Paralysis of eye muscles	Lesions in brain stem or cranial nerves III, IV, and VI
Opisthotonus	Extreme arching of back with retraction of head	Meningitis, tonic phase of grand mal seizure
Papilledema	Swelling of optic disk	Increase in intracranial pressure
Paraplegia	Paralysis of lower extremities	Spinal cord transection or mass lesion (thoracolumbar region)
Tetraplegia (quadriplegia)	Paralysis of all extremities	Spinal cord transection or mass lesion (cervical region or brain stem)

Computed Tomography. Computed tomography (CT) is a noninvasive procedure, although intravenous injection of contrast medium may be used to enhance visualization of the blood vessels and identify disruptions in the blood–brain barrier. A number of radiographic scans of different levels of the brain are compiled with computer assistance and presented in a series of black-and-white pictures. These pictures, which illustrate "slices" of the brain (Figure 58-20, *A*), can show hemorrhages, tumours, cysts, edema, infarction, brain atrophy, and hydrocephalus. CT does not illustrate structures in the posterior fossa and the base of the brain as clearly as magnetic resonance imaging (MRI) does.

Magnetic Resonance Imaging. Magnetic resonance imaging (MRI) provides greater detail than CT and improved resolution (detail) of the intracranial structures (see Figure 58-20, *B*).

FIGURE 58-20 Normal images of the brain. **A,** Computed tomography. **B,** Magnetic resonance imaging. Source: From Fuller, G., & Manford, M. (2006). *Neurology: An illustrated colour text.* Edinburgh: Churchill Livingstone.

TABLE 58-8   DIAGNOSTIC STUDIES

Nervous System

Study	Description and Purpose	Nursing Responsibility
Cerebro-Spinal Fluid Analysis		
Lumbar puncture	CSF is aspirated by needle insertion in L3–4 or L4–5 interspace to assess many CNS diseases (see Table 58-9).	Help patient assume and maintain lateral recumbent position with knees flexed. Ensure maintenance of strict aseptic technique. Ensure labelling of CSF specimens in proper sequence. Encourage patient to drink fluids. Monitor neurological and VS. Administer analgesia as needed.
Radiological		
Cerebral angiography	Serial radiographic visualization of intracranial and extracranial blood vessels can help detect vascular lesions and tumours of brain. Contrast medium is used (Figure 58-19).	Assess for risk for stroke because thrombi may be dislodged during procedure. Withhold preceding meal. Explain that patient will experience hot flush of head and neck when contrast medium is injected. Explain need to be absolutely still during procedure. Monitor neurological and VS every 15–30 min for first 2 hr, every hour for next 6 hr, then every 2 hr for 24 hr. Maintain pressure dressing and ice on injection site. Maintain bed rest until patient is alert and VS are stable. Report any signs of change in neurological status.
Computed tomography (CT)	Computer-assisted radiographic views of several levels or thin cross-sections of body parts can help detect problems such as hemorrhage, space-occupying lesions, cerebral edema, brain atrophy, and other abnormalities (Figure 58-20, *A*).	Explain that procedure is noninvasive (if no contrast medium is used). Observe for allergic reaction, and note puncture site (if contrast medium is used). Explain appearance of scanner. Instruct patient to remain absolutely still during procedure.
Magnetic resonance angiography (MRA)	Differential signal characteristics of flowing blood are studied to evaluate extracranial and intracranial blood vessels. Test provides both anatomical and hemodynamic information. MRA can be used in conjunction with contrast medium (contrast-enhanced MRA [cMRA]). MRA is rapidly replacing cerebral angiography for use in diagnosing cerebro-vascular diseases.	Nursing responsibilities are similar to those for MRI.
Magnetic resonance imaging (MRI)	Imaging of brain, spinal cord, and spinal canal by means of magnetic energy helps detect infarctions, multiple sclerosis, tumours, trauma, herniation, and seizures. No invasive procedures are required (Figure 58-20, *B*).	Screen patient for joint replacements and pacemaker in body. Instruct patient to lie very still for up to 1 hr. Sedation may be necessary if patient is claustrophobic.
Positron emission tomography (PET)	Metabolic activity of brain regions is measured to assess cell death or damage. Test involves the use of radioactive material that shows up as a bright spot on the image.	Explain procedure to patient. Explain that two IV lines will be inserted. Instruct patient not to take sedatives or tranquilizers and to empty bladder before procedure. Patient may be asked to perform different activities during test.

TABLE 58-8   DIAGNOSTIC STUDIES

Nervous System—cont'd

Study	Description and Purpose	Nursing Responsibility
Single-photon emission computed tomography (SPECT)	This method of scanning is similar to PET, but more stable substances and different detectors are used. Radiolabelled compounds are injected, and their photon emissions can be detected. Images made are an accumulation of labelled compound. SPECT is used to visualize blood flow or oxygen or glucose metabolism in the brain. It is useful in diagnosing strokes, brain tumours, and seizure disorders.	Nursing responsibilities are similar to those for PET.
Skull and spine radiographs	Simple radiographs of skull and spinal column can help detect fractures, spinal misalignment, bone erosion, calcifications, or abnormal vascularity.	Explain that procedure is noninvasive. Explain positions to be assumed.
Electrographic		
Electroencephalography (EEG)	Electrical activity of brain is recorded by scalp electrodes to evaluate cerebral disease, CNS effects of systemic diseases, and brain death.	Inform patient that procedure is painless and without danger of electric shock. Withhold stimulants. Inform patient that he or she may be asked to perform various activities such as hyperventilation during test. Determine whether any medications (e.g., tranquilizers, anticonvulsant drugs) should be withheld. Resume medications after test. Assist patient in washing electrode paste out of hair.
Electromyography (EMG) and nerve conduction	Electrical activity associated with nerve and skeletal muscle is recorded by insertion of needle electrodes to detect muscle and peripheral nerve disease.	Inform patient of slight discomfort associated with insertion of needles.
Evoked potentials	Electrical activity associated with nerve conduction along sensory pathways is recorded by electrodes placed on skin and scalp. Stimulus generates the impulse. Procedure is used to diagnose disease, locate nerve damage, and monitor function intraoperatively.	Explain procedure to patient. Avoid hair spray, gel, or other hair care products and sedative drugs such as benzodiazepines and barbiturates.
Magnetoencephalography (MEG)	A sensitivity machine called a *biomagnetometer* is used to detect very small magnetic fields generated by neural activity. It can accurately pinpoint the part of the brain involved in a stroke, seizure, or other disorder or injury. Extracranial magnetic fields, as well as scalp electrical field (EEG), are measured.	MEG, a passive sensor, does not make physical contact with patient. Explain procedure to patient.
Ultrasonography		
Carotid duplex studies	Sound waves are used to determine blood flow velocity, which may indicate presence of occlusive vascular disease.	Explain procedure to patient.
Transcranial Doppler ultrasonography	Technology is the same as that for carotid duplex studies, but intracranial vessels are evaluated.	Explain procedure to patient.

CNS, central nervous system; *CSF*, cerebro-spinal fluid; *IV*, intravenous; *VS*, vital signs.

TABLE 58-9   NORMAL CEREBRO-SPINAL FLUID VALUES

Parameter	Normal Value
Appearance	Clear, colourless
Glucose	2.8–4.2 mmol/L
Microorganisms	None
pH	7.33
Pressure	9–14 mm Hg
Protein	
• Cisternal	0.15–0.25 g/L
• Lumbar	0.15–0.45 g/L
• Ventricular	0.05–0.15 g/L
RBCs	None
Specific gravity	1.007
WBCs	Adult: $0–5 \times 10^9$ WBCs/L

RBCs, red blood cells; *WBCs*, white blood cells.

However, MRI requires a longer time to complete and may not be appropriate in life-threatening emergencies. Techniques of functional MRI (fMRI) provide time-related (temporal) images that can be used to evaluate how the brain responds to various stimuli.

MRI is useful in evaluating brain and spinal cord edema, hemorrhage, infarction, blood vessels, tumours, herniation, and bone lesions. It is used in the detection of early strokes and multiple sclerosis. Intravenous injection of gadolinium-containing contrast agents can enhance the images obtained with MRI. Because the images of soft tissue structures have greater contrast with MRI than with CT, MRI is the diagnostic test of choice for many neurological conditions and diseases.

Positron Emission Tomography. *Positron emission tomography* (PET) is used to determine regional metabolism in the brain. PET provides a noninvasive means of determining biochemical processes that occur in the brain. PET is increasingly used to monitor patients with stroke, Alzheimer's disease, seizure disorders, epilepsy, tumours, and Parkinson's disease.

Electrographic Studies

Electroencephalography. *Electroencephalography* (EEG) is the recording of the electrical activity of the surface cortical neurons of the brain, using 8 to 16 electrodes placed on specific areas of the scalp. This test is done to evaluate not only cerebral disease but also the CNS effects of many metabolic and systemic diseases and to determine brain death. Among the cerebral diseases and other conditions assessed with EEG are epilepsy, mass lesions (e.g., tumour, abscess, hematoma), cerebro-vascular lesions, and brain injury. The procedure is noninvasive. Patients sometimes have the misconception that the recording electrodes will give them an electric shock. They should be assured that this idea is not true and that the procedure is similar to electrocardiography.

Electromyography and Nerve Conduction Studies. *Electromyography* (EMG) is the recording of electrical activity associated with innervation of skeletal muscle. The recording is displayed on a computer screen and may be played on a loudspeaker for simultaneous analysis. Needle electrodes are inserted into the muscle to record specific motor units because recording from the skin is not sufficient. Normal muscle at rest shows no electrical activity. Typical electrical activity occurs when the muscle contracts. This activity may be altered in diseases of muscle itself (e.g., myopathic conditions) or in disorders of muscle innervation (e.g., segmental or LMN lesions, peripheral neuropathic conditions). *Fibrillations* are spontaneous, independent contractions of individual muscle fibres that can be detected only by EMG. They appear on EMG 1 to 3 weeks after a muscle has lost its nerve supply.

In *nerve conduction studies,* a brief electrical stimulus is applied to a distal portion of a sensory or mixed nerve, and the resulting wave of depolarization is recorded at some point proximal to the stimulation. For example, a stimulus can be applied to the forefinger and a recording electrode placed over the median nerve at the wrist. The time between the onset of the stimulus and the initial wave of depolarization at the recording electrode is measured. The speed of this response is termed *nerve conduction velocity*. Damaged nerves have slower conduction velocities.

Evoked Potentials. *Evoked potentials* are recordings of electrical activity associated with nerve conduction along sensory pathways. The activity is generated by a specific sensory stimulus related to the type of study (e.g., checkerboard patterns for visual evoked potentials, clicking sounds for auditory evoked potentials, mild electrical pulses for somatosensory evoked potentials). Electrodes placed on specific areas of the skin and scalp record the electrical activity, and these data are stored and averaged by a computerized instrument. A wave pattern appears on a screen and is printed on paper. Peaks in the wave pattern correspond to conduction of the stimulus through certain points along the sensory pathway (e.g., peripheral nerve, brain stem, cortical areas). Increases in the time from stimulus onset to a given peak (latency) indicate slowed nerve conduction or nerve damage. This technique is useful in diagnosing abnormalities of the visual or auditory systems because it reveals whether a sensory impulse is reaching the appropriate part of the brain. Purposes for these tests include evaluation of the optic nerve in conditions such as multiple sclerosis (optic neuritis) and the vestibulo-cochlear nerve in acoustic neuroma.

Combined Doppler and Ultrasound (Duplex) Studies

Carotid Duplex. In a duplex study, ultrasonography and pulsed Doppler technology are combined. A technician places a probe on the patient's skin over the carotid artery and slowly moves the probe along the course of the common carotid artery to the bifurcation of the external and internal carotid arteries. The ultrasound signal emitted from the probe reflects off the moving blood cells within the vessel. The frequency of the reflected signal corresponds to the blood flow velocity. This response is amplified and is registered on a graphic record and also as sound. The graphic record registers blood flow velocity. Increases in blood flow velocity can indicate stenosis of a vessel. Duplex scanning is a noninvasive study in which the degree of stenosis of the carotid and vertebral arteries is evaluated.

Transcranial Doppler Sonography. The same technology used in duplex studies is used in transcranial Doppler sonography, except that blood flow velocities of the intracranial blood vessels are recorded. The probe is placed on the patient's skin at various "windows" in the skull (areas in the skull that have only a thin bony covering) to register velocities of the middle cerebral artery, anterior cerebral artery, posterior cerebral artery, terminal carotid artery, and occasionally the anterior and posterior communicating arteries. The temporal, orbital, and suboccipital sites are used. The ultrasound signal received is recorded graphically as a waveform. Peak blood flow velocities and systolic–diastolic ratios can be calculated from this information. Transcranial Doppler sonography is a noninvasive technique that is useful in assessing vasospasm associated with subarachnoid hemorrhage, altered intracranial blood flow dynamics associated with occlusive vascular disease, presence of emboli, and cerebral autoregulation.

▌ REVIEW QUESTIONS

The number of the question corresponds to the same-numbered objective at the beginning of the chapter.

1. In a client with a disease that affects the myelin sheath of nerves, such as multiple sclerosis, which glial cells are affected?
   a. Microglia
   b. Astrocytes
   c. Oligodendrocytes
   d. Ependymal cells

2. A state of hypoxia alters the repeated action potentials necessary for transmission of nerve impulses. Which of the following requires energy?

   a. Repolarization of the cell membrane
   b. Creation of cell membrane permeability
   c. Movement of sodium into the nerve cell
   d. Maintenance of the resting membrane potential

3. Drugs or diseases that impair the function of the extrapyramidal system may cause the loss of which of the following?
   a. Sensations of pain and temperature
   b. Regulation of the ANS
   c. Integration of somatic and special sensory inputs
   d. Automatic movements associated with skeletal muscle activity

4. Which of the following will be affected by an obstruction of the anterior cerebral arteries?
   a. Visual imaging
   b. Balance and coordination
   c. Judgement, insight, and reasoning
   d. Visual and auditory integration for language comprehension
5. Data regarding mobility, strength, coordination, and activity tolerance are important for the nurse to obtain for which of the following reasons?
   a. Many neurological diseases affect one or more of these abilities.
   b. Clients are less able to identify other neurological impairments.
   c. These are the first functions to be lost in neurological disease.
   d. Aspects of movement are the most important function of the nervous system.
6. Which of the following is a result of stimulation of the parasympathetic nervous system? *(Select all that apply)*
   a. Constriction of the bronchi
   b. Increase in rate of peristalsis
   c. Increased secretion of insulin
   d. Increased blood glucose levels
   e. Relaxation of the urinary sphincters
7. Why should the muscle strength of older adults not be compared with that of younger adults?
   a. Stroke is more common in older adults.
   b. Nutritional status is better in young adults.
   c. Most young people exercise more than older adults.
   d. Aging leads to a decrease in muscle bulk and strength.
8. A lesion of which cranial nerve would cause paralysis of the lateral gaze?
   a. Cranial nerve II
   b. Cranial nerve III
   c. Cranial nerve IV
   d. Cranial nerve VI
9. During neurological testing, the client is able to perceive pain elicited by pinprick. On the basis of this finding, which of the following tests may the nurse omit?
   a. Position sense
   b. Patellar reflexes
   c. Temperature perception
   d. Heel-to-shin movements
10. A client's eyes jerk as they follow the nurse's moving finger. How would the nurse record this finding?
    a. Nystagmus
    b. Normal tracking
    c. Ophthalmoplegia
    d. Ophthalmic dyskinesia
11. Which of the following are nursing responsibilities for lumbar puncture?
    a. Ensuring the client has a full bladder
    b. Placing the client in the lateral recumbent position
    c. Straightening the client's legs just before the puncture
    d. Having the client cough when the needle has been inserted

1. c; 2. d; 3. d; 4. c; 5. a; 6. a, b, c, e; 7. d; 8. d; 9. c; 10. a; 11. b.

⊜volve

For even more review questions, visit *http://evolve.elsevier.com/Canada/Lewis/medsurg.*

REFERENCES

Coggrave, M., Norton, C., & Cody, J. D. (2014). Management of faecal incontinence and constipation in adults with central neurological diseases. *The Cochrane Database of Systematic Reviews*, No. 1, Article CD002115. doi:10.1002/14651858. CD002115.pub5.

Gopurappilly, R., Pal, R., Krishna Mamidi, M., et al. (2011). Stem cells in stroke repair: Current success & future prospects. *CNS & Neurological Disorders—Drug Targets (Formerly Current Drug Targets—CNS & Neurological Disorders)*, 10(6), 741–756. doi:10.2174/187152711797247894.

Homann, B., Plaschg, A., Grundner, M., et al. (2013). The impact of neurological disorders on the risk for falls in the community dwelling elderly: A case-controlled study. *BMJ Open*, 3(11), e003367. doi:10.1136/bmjopen-2013-003367.

Jarvis, C. (2014). A. J. Brown, J. MacDonald-Jenkins, & M. Luctkar-Flude (Canadian Eds.), *Physical examination & health assessment* (2nd Canadian ed.). Toronto: Saunders/Elsevier.

Lachner, C., Steinle, N. I., & Regenold, W. T. (2014). The neuropsychiatry of vitamin B12 deficiency in elderly patients. *The Journal of Neuropsychiatry and Clinical Neurosciences*, 24(1), 5–15. doi:10.1176/appi.neuropsych.11020052.

McCance, K. L., & Huether, S. E. (2014). *Pathophysiology: The biologic basis for disease in adults and children* (7th ed.). St. Louis: Mosby.

Panicker, J. N., Fowler, C. J., & Kessler, T. M. (2015). Lower urinary tract dysfunction in the neurological patient: Clinical assessment and management. *The Lancet. Neurology*, 14(7), 720–732. doi:10.1016/S1474-4422(15)00070-8.

Porter, R. S., & Kaplan, J. L. (2011). *Merck manual of diagnosis and therapy* (19th ed.). West Point, PA: Merck & Co.

RESOURCES

Resources for this chapter are listed in Chapters 59 to 63.

Nursing Management

Acute Intracranial Problems

Written by: Linda Littlejohns
Adapted by: Sarah L. Johnston

evolve WEBSITE

http://evolve.elsevier.com/Canada/Lewis/medsurg

- Review Questions (Online Only)
- Key Points
- Answer Guidelines for Case Study
- Student Case Studies
  - Meningitis
- Customizable Nursing Care Plans
  - Bacterial Meningitis
  - Increased Intracranial Pressure
  - Cranial Surgery
- Conceptual Care Map Creator
- Audio Glossary
- Supporting Media Animations
  - Functional Areas of the Brain
- Content Updates

LEARNING OBJECTIVES

1. Explain the physiological mechanisms that maintain normal intracranial pressure.
2. Describe the common etiologies, clinical manifestations, and collaborative care of the patient with increased intracranial pressure.
3. Describe the collaborative care and nursing management of the patient with increased intracranial pressure.
4. Differentiate between the types of head injury by mechanism of injury and clinical manifestations.
5. Describe the collaborative care and nursing management of the patient with a head injury.
6. Explain the types, clinical manifestations, and collaborative care of brain tumours.
7. Discuss the nursing management of the patient with a brain tumour.
8. Discuss the nursing management of the patient undergoing cranial surgery.
9. Compare the primary causes, collaborative care, and nursing management of meningitis, encephalitis, and brain abscess.

KEY TERMS

brain abscess, p. 1503
cerebral edema, p. 1476
coma, p. 1477
concussion, p. 1488
contusion, p. 1489
diffuse axonal injury (DAI), p. 1488
encephalitis, p. 1502

epidural hematoma, p. 1489
Glasgow Coma Scale (GCS), p. 1483
head injury, p. 1486
intracranial pressure (ICP), p. 1475
intraparenchymal or intracerebral
  hematoma, p. 1490
meningitis, p. 1500

nuchal rigidity, p. 1500
subdural hematoma, p. 1489
unconsciousness, p. 1478

Acute intracranial problems include diseases and disorders that can increase intracranial pressure (ICP). This chapter discusses the mechanisms that maintain normal ICP, increased ICP, head injuries, brain tumours, and cerebral inflammatory disorders.

INTRACRANIAL PRESSURE

Understanding the mechanisms associated with ICP is important in caring for patients with many different neurological problems. The skull is like a closed box, with three essential components constituting its volume: brain tissue, blood, and cerebro-spinal fluid (CSF) (Figure 59-1). The brain compartment, made up of neurons, neuroglial cells, and intracellular and extracellular fluids of brain tissue, makes up approximately 78% of this volume. Blood in the arterial, the venous, and the capillary networks makes up 12% of the volume, and the remaining 10% is the volume of the CSF. Under normal conditions, the volume of these three compartments is relatively stable, maintaining ICP within normal limits. Factors that influence ICP under normal circumstances are changes in (1) blood pressure (BP), (2) cardiac function, (3) intra-abdominal and intrathoracic pressure, (4) body position, (5) temperature, and (6) blood

Cerebro-spinal fluid: 10%

Intravascular blood: 12%

Brain tissue: 78%

FIGURE 59-1 Components of the brain.

gases, particularly CO_2 levels. The degree to which these factors increase or decrease the ICP depends on the ability of the brain to accommodate to the changes.

Primary versus secondary injury is another important concept in understanding ICP. *Primary injury* occurs at the initial time of an injury (e.g., impact of motor vehicle accident, blunt-force trauma) that results in displacement, bruising, or damage of the three components. *Secondary injury* is the resulting hypoxia, ischemia, hypotension, edema, or increased ICP that follows the primary injury. Secondary injury, which could occur several hours to days after the initial injury, is a primary concern when managing brain injury. Nursing management of the patient with an acute intracranial problem must include management of secondary injury, and thus increased ICP.

Regulation and Maintenance of Intracranial Pressure

Normal Intracranial Pressure. Intracranial pressure (ICP) is the pressure exerted because of the combined total volume of the three components within the skull: brain tissue, blood, and CSF. The modified Monro–Kellie doctrine describes how a state of dynamic equilibrium is maintained by the volume relationship of these three components within the rigid skull structure. If the volume in any one of the three components increases within the cranial vault and the volume from another component is displaced, the total intracranial volume will not change (Cushing, 1925). If the volume of any one of these three components increases without a corresponding decrease in another component, the result is an elevated ICP. This hypothesis is not applicable in situations in which the skull is not rigid (e.g., in neonates, in adults with unfused skull fractures).

ICP can be measured in the ventricles, subarachnoid space, subdural space, epidural space, or brain tissue, using a pressure transducer (Kawoos, McCarron, Auker, et al., 2015). Normal ICP ranges from 5 to 15 mm Hg. A sustained pressure greater than 20 mm Hg is considered abnormal and must be treated.

Normal Compensatory Adaptations. Intrinsic compensatory mechanisms exist to resist increases in ICP. A major compensatory mechanism involves changes in the CSF volume. These changes are achieved primarily by the displacement of CSF into the spinal subarachnoid space or the basal subarachnoid cisterns and, to a lesser degree, by altering CSF production and absorption rates. Alterations in intracranial blood volume occur through the compression of cerebral veins and dural sinuses, regional cerebral vasoconstriction or dilation, and changes in venous outflow.

Brain tissue volume compensates through distension of the dura or compression of brain tissue. Initially, an increase in volume produces no increase in ICP as a result of these compensatory mechanisms. However, compensatory adaptations are finite, and progressive increases in volume eventually exhaust compensatory mechanisms (Cushing, 1925). The result is increased ICP, neuronal compression, and ischemia.

Cerebral Blood Flow

Cerebral blood flow (CBF) is the amount of blood in millilitres (mL) passing through 100 grams (g) of brain tissue per minute. In adults, this equates to approximately 50 mL of blood/min/100 g of brain tissue or approximately 750 mL/min. Unlike other organs, the brain lacks the ability to store oxygen or glucose, and therefore the maintenance of adequate blood flow to the brain is critical for neuronal functioning and survival. Although the brain accounts for only about 2% of body weight, it uses 20% of the body's oxygen and 25% of its glucose.

Autoregulation of Cerebral Blood Flow. The brain's intrinsic ability to regulate its own blood flow in response to its metabolic needs in spite of wide fluctuations in systemic arterial pressure is termed *autoregulation*. Autoregulation is the automatic alteration in the diameter of the cerebral blood vessels to maintain a constant blood flow to the brain during changes in BP. The purpose of autoregulation is to ensure adequate CBF to meet the metabolic needs of brain tissue and to maintain cerebral perfusion pressure within normal limits.

In healthy individuals, autoregulation operates within limited parameters. In cases of extreme hypotension or hypertension, autoregulation fails. If mean arterial pressure (MAP) is less than 50 mm Hg, CBF is decreased and symptoms of cerebral ischemia may occur. If MAP is greater than 150 mm Hg, the cerebral vessels are maximally constricted and further vasoconstrictor response is lost; CBF increases and intracranial hypertension may occur.

Other Factors Affecting Cerebral Blood Flow. Carbon dioxide, oxygen, and hydrogen ion concentration affect cerebral vessel tone. The partial pressure of arterial carbon dioxide ($PaCO_2$) is a potent factor in vasoactive reactivity. An increase in $PaCO_2$ relaxes smooth muscle, dilates cerebral vessels, decreases cerebro-vascular resistance, and increases CBF. Alternately, a decrease in $PaCO_2$ reverses this process and decreases CBF. Cerebral oxygen tension (PaO_2) below 50 mm Hg results in cerebral vascular dilation. This dilation decreases cerebral vascular resistance and increases CBF. If PaO_2 is not raised, anaerobic metabolism begins, resulting in an accumulation of lactic acid. As lactic acid increases and hydrogen ions accumulate, the cerebral environment becomes more acidic. Within this acidic environment, further vasodilation occurs in a continued attempt to increase blood flow. The combination of a severely low arterial oxygen pressure (PaO_2) and an elevated hydrogen ion concentration (acidosis), which are both potent cerebral vasodilators, may produce a state wherein autoregulation is lost and compensatory mechanisms fail to meet tissue metabolic demands (Cushing, 1925).

CBF can be globally affected by cardiac or respiratory arrest, systemic hemorrhage, and other pathophysiological states (e.g., diabetic coma, encephalopathies, infections, toxicities). Regional CBF can also be affected by trauma, tumours, cerebral hemorrhage, or stroke. When regional or global autoregulation is lost, CBF is no longer maintained at a constant level but is directly influenced by changes in systemic BP, $PaCO_2$ levels, or catecholamine levels. CBF can be indirectly reflected by calculating *cerebral*

TABLE 59-1	CALCULATION OF CEREBRAL PERFUSION PRESSURE

$$CPP = MAP - ICP$$

$$MAP = DBP + \tfrac{1}{3}(SBP - DBP) \quad \text{or} \quad \frac{SBP + 2(DBP)}{3}$$

Example: Systemic blood pressure = 122/84 mm Hg

MAP = 97 mm Hg

ICP = 12 mm Hg

CPP = 85 mm Hg

CPP, cerebral perfusion pressure; *DBP*, diastolic blood pressure; *ICP*, intracranial pressure; *MAP*, mean arterial pressure; *SBP*, systolic blood pressure.

FIGURE 59-2 Intracranial pressure–volume curve. (See text for descriptions of *1*, *2*, *3*, and *4*.)

perfusion pressure (CPP). CPP is the pressure needed to ensure adequate brain tissue perfusion. CPP is equal to the MAP minus the ICP (CPP = MAP − ICP) (see example in Table 59-1). If CPP is inadequate, brain perfusion can be improved by either decreasing ICP or increasing MAP.

As the CPP decreases, autoregulation fails and CBF decreases. Normal CPP is 70 to 100 mm Hg, and a minimum of 50 to 60 mm Hg is necessary for adequate cerebral perfusion. CPP less than 50 mm Hg is associated with cerebral ischemia. A CPP below 30 mm Hg results in cellular ischemia and is incompatible with life. Under normal circumstances, autoregulation maintains an adequate CBF and perfusion pressure primarily by cerebral vasoreactivity and metabolic adjustments that affect ICP. It is of paramount importance to maintain MAP when ICP is elevated. It should be remembered that CPP does not reflect perfusion pressure in all parts of the brain. There may be local areas of swelling and compression limiting regional perfusion pressure. Thus, for patients with these symptoms, a higher CPP may be needed to prevent localized tissue damage.

Pressure Changes. The relationship of pressure to volume is depicted in the pressure–volume curve (Figure 59-2). The curve is affected by the brain's compliance. *Compliance* is the expandability of the brain. It is represented as the volume increase for each unit increase in pressure. With low compliance, small increases in volume result in greater increases in pressure.

The pressure–volume curve can be used to represent the stages of increased ICP (see Figure 59-2). At stage 1 on the curve, there is high compliance. The brain is in total compensation, with accommodation and autoregulation intact. An increase in volume

(in brain tissue, blood, or CSF) does not increase the ICP. At stage 2, the compliance is lessening, and an increase in volume places the patient at risk for increased ICP. At stage 3, there is low compliance as compensatory mechanisms are becoming exhausted. Any small addition of volume causes a great increase in ICP. As compensatory mechanisms fail, there is a loss of autoregulation, and the patient may exhibit symptoms indicating increased ICP, such as headache, changes in level of consciousness, or pupil responsiveness.

As the patient enters stage 4, the ICP rises to lethal levels with even slight increases in volume. Here the patient is at significant risk for hypoperfusion and brain herniation and death. *Herniation* occurs as the brain tissue is forcibly shifted from the compartment of greater pressure to a compartment of lesser pressure. In this situation, intense pressure is placed on the brain stem, and if herniation continues, brain stem death is imminent.

INCREASED INTRACRANIAL PRESSURE

Increased ICP is a life-threatening situation resulting from an increase in any or all of the three components (brain tissue, blood, CSF) of the skull. Elevated ICP (above the threshold of 20 mm Hg) is clinically significant because it diminishes CPP, increasing risk for brain ischemia and infarction, and is associated with a poor prognosis (Kawoos et al., 2015).

Mechanisms of Increased Intracranial Pressure

The brain tissue component of ICP can be increased by cerebral neoplasm, contusion, abscess, or cerebral edema. Conditions that increase the cerebral blood volume include intracranial hematomas or hemorrhages, metabolic and physiological factors (e.g., CO_2, O_2, fever, pain), and vascular anomalies. Increases in the CSF volume can result from CSF-secreting tumours or hydrocephalus. These cerebral insults may result in hypercapnia, cerebral acidosis, impaired autoregulation, and systemic hypertension, which promote the formation and spread of cerebral edema. This edema distorts brain tissue, further increasing the ICP, which leads to even more tissue hypoxia and acidosis. Figure 59-3 illustrates the progression of increased ICP.

Crucial to preservation of tissue is maintenance of CBF. Elevations in pressure that are more evenly distributed throughout the brain or slow increases in ICP (e.g., an enlarging brain lesion) preserve blood flow better than a rapid increase, as in primary brain injury. Sustained increases in ICP result in brain stem compression and herniation of the brain from one compartment to another.

Displacement and herniation of brain tissue cause a potentially reversible pathophysiological process to become irreversible. Ischemia and edema are further increased, compounding the pre-existing problem. Herniations force the cerebellum and the brain stem downward through the foramen magnum. If compression of the brain stem is unrelieved, respiratory arrest may occur. Compression of brain tissue, brain stem structures, cranial nerves, and vessels may be fatal. Figure 59-4 illustrates herniation. (Herniation is further described in the later section of this chapter on complications of ICP.)

Cerebral Edema

As shown in Table 59-2, there are a variety of causes of **cerebral edema** (increased accumulation of fluid in the extravascular spaces of brain tissue). Regardless of the cause, cerebral edema results in an increase in tissue volume that carries the potential

PATHOPHYSIOLOGY MAP

FIGURE 59-3 Progression of increased intracranial pressure (ICP).

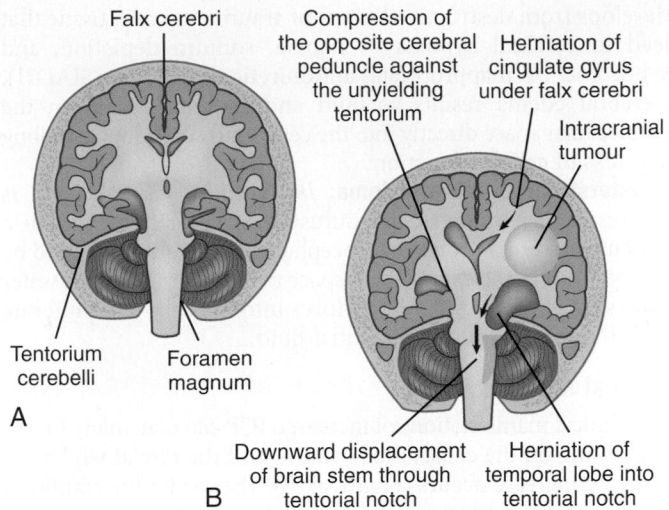

Falx cerebri

Compression of the opposite cerebral peduncle against the unyielding tentorium

Herniation of cingulate gyrus under falx cerebri

Intracranial tumour

Tentorium cerebelli

Foramen magnum

A

Downward displacement of brain stem through tentorial notch

Herniation of temporal lobe into tentorial notch

B

FIGURE 59-4 Herniation. **A,** Normal relationship of intracranial structures. **B,** Shift of intracranial structures. Source: Adapted from McCance, K. L., & Huether, S. E. (2010). *Pathophysiology: The biologic basis for disease in adults and children* (6th ed., p. 558, Figure 16-16). St. Louis: Mosby.

TABLE 59-2 CAUSES OF CEREBRAL EDEMA

- Mass lesions
  - Brain abscess
  - Brain tumour (primary or metastatic)
  - Hematoma (intracerebral, subdural, epidural)
  - Hemorrhage (intracerebral, cerebellar, brain stem)
- Head injuries
  - Contusion
  - Diffuse axonal injury
  - Hemorrhage
  - Post-traumatic brain swelling
- Brain surgery
- Cerebral infections
  - Meningitis
  - Encephalitis
- Vascular insult
  - Anoxic and ischemic episodes
  - Cerebral infarction (thrombotic or embolic)
  - Venous sinus thrombosis
- Toxic or metabolic encephalopathic conditions
  - Hepatic encephalopathy
  - Lead or arsenic intoxication
  - Uremia

for increased ICP. Factors that contribute to the degree of cerebral edema are the extent and the severity of the original insult as well as the cascade of secondary cellular events that occur in the hours and days following insult or injury.

Three types of cerebral edema have been distinguished: vasogenic, cytotoxic, and interstitial. More than one type may result from a single insult in the same patient. Regardless of the cause of cerebral edema, manifestations of increased ICP result, unless compensation is adequate.

Vasogenic Cerebral Edema. *Vasogenic cerebral edema,* the most common type of edema, occurs mainly in the white matter and is attributed to changes in the endothelial lining of cerebral capillaries. These changes allow leakage of macromolecules from the capillaries into the surrounding extracellular space, resulting in an osmotic gradient that favours the flow of water from the intravascular to the extravascular space. A variety of insults,

such as brain tumours, head trauma, abscesses, and ingested toxins, may cause an increase in the permeability of the blood–brain barrier and produce an increase in the extracellular fluid volume. The speed and extent of the spread of the edema fluid are influenced by the systemic BP, the site of the brain injury, and the extent of the blood–brain barrier defect. This edema may produce a continuum of symptoms, ranging from headache and focal neurological deficits to disturbances in consciousness, including **coma** (profound state of unconsciousness). It is important to recognize that although a headache may seem to be a benign symptom, in cases of cerebral edema it can quickly progress to coma and death; therefore vigilant assessment is key.

Cytotoxic Cerebral Edema. *Cytotoxic cerebral edema* results from local disruption of the functional or morphological integrity of cell membranes and occurs most often in the grey matter. It develops from destructive lesions or trauma to brain tissue that lead to cerebral hypoxia or anoxia, sodium depletion, and syndrome of inappropriate antidiuretic hormone (SIADH). Cerebral edema results as fluid and protein shift from the extracellular space directly into the cells, with subsequent swelling and loss of cellular function.

Interstitial Cerebral Edema. *Interstitial cerebral edema is* the result of periventricular diffusion of ventricular CSF in a patient with uncontrolled hydrocephalus. It can also be caused by enlargement of the extracellular space as a result of systemic water excess (hyponatremia). Fluid moves into the cells to equilibrate with the hypo-osmotic interstitial fluid.

Clinical Manifestations

The clinical manifestations of increased ICP can take many forms, depending on the cause, the location, and the rate at which the pressure increase occurs (Figure 59-5). The earlier the condition is recognized and treated, the better the prognosis.

Change in Level of Consciousness. *Level of consciousness* (LOC) is a sensitive and early indicator of the patient's neurological status. Changes in LOC are a result of impaired CBF, which deprives the cells of the cerebral cortex and the reticular activating system (RAS) of oxygen. The RAS is located in the brain stem, with neural connections to many parts of the nervous system. An intact RAS can maintain a state of wakefulness even in the absence of a functioning cerebral cortex. Interruptions of impulses from the RAS or alteration of the functioning of the cerebral hemispheres can cause unconsciousness (an abnormal state of complete or partial unawareness of self or environment).

The patient's state of consciousness is defined by both the behaviour and the pattern of brain activity recorded by an electroencephalogram (EEG). The change in consciousness may be subtle, such as a flattening of affect, confusion, or decrease in level of attention. A decrease in consciousness may be dramatic, as in coma—the deepest state of unconsciousness, when the patient does not respond to sensory stimuli. The EEG pattern demonstrates decreased neuronal activity.

Changes in Vital Signs. Changes in vital signs are caused by increasing pressure on the thalamus, the hypothalamus, the pons, and the medulla. Manifestations such as Cushing's triad, consisting of increasing systolic pressure (widening pulse pressure), bradycardia with a full and bounding pulse, and irregular respiratory pattern, may be present but often do not appear until ICP has been increased for some time or suddenly and markedly increases (e.g., head trauma). (Pulse pressure is discussed in Chapter 34.) Always recognize Cushing's triad as a medical emergency, since this is a sign of brain stem compression and impending death. A change in body temperature may also be noted and is caused by associated pressure on the hypothalamus.

Ocular Signs. Compression of the oculomotor nerve (cranial nerve [CN] III) results in dilation of the pupil *ipsilateral* to (same side as) the mass or lesion, sluggish or no response to light, inability to move the eye upward, and ptosis of the eyelid. These signs can be the result of a shifting of the brain from the midline, a process that compresses the trunk of CN III, paralyzing the pupil sphincter. A fixed (unresponsive), unilaterally dilated pupil is a neurological emergency that indicates herniation of the brain.

Other cranial nerves may also be affected, such as the optic (CN II), trochlear (CN IV), and abducens (CN VI) nerves. Signs of dysfunction of these cranial nerves include blurred vision, diplopia, and changes in extraocular eye movements. Central herniation may initially manifest as sluggish but equal pupil responses. Lateral herniation of the uncus, the innermost part of the temporal lobe, may cause a dilated unilateral pupil.

FIGURE 59-5 Clinical manifestations of increased intracranial pressure. *LOC,* level of consciousness.

Papilledema, an edematous optic disc seen on retinal examination, is also noted and is a nonspecific sign associated with swelling of the optic nerve related to increased ICP.

Decrease in Motor Function. As the ICP continues to rise, the patient manifests changes in motor ability. A *contralateral* (opposite side of the mass lesion) hemiparesis or hemiplegia may be seen, depending on the location of the source of the increased ICP. If painful stimuli are used to elicit a motor response, the patient may exhibit localization to the stimuli or a withdrawal from the stimuli. Decorticate (flexor) and decerebrate (extensor) posturing may also be elicited by noxious stimuli (Figure 59-6). *Decorticate posture* consists of internal rotation and adduction of the arms, with flexion of elbows, wrists, and fingers as a result of interruption of voluntary motor tracts. Extension of the legs may also be seen. A *decerebrate posture* may indicate more serious damage and results from disruption of motor fibres in the midbrain and brain stem. In this position, the arms are stiffly extended, adducted, and hyperpronated. There is also hyperextension of the legs, with plantar flexion of the feet.

Headache. Although the brain itself is insensitive to pain, compression of other intracranial structures, such as the walls of arteries and veins and the cranial nerves, can produce headache. Headaches associated with increased ICP are often continuous. Straining, agitation, or movement may accentuate the pain.

Vomiting. Vomiting, usually not preceded by nausea, is often a nonspecific sign of increased ICP. This is related to direct pressure on the vomiting centre, located on the floor of the fourth ventricle in the medulla. Vomiting associated with increased ICP is often described as *projectile,* owing to the force of vomitus ejection.

Complications

The major complications of uncontrolled, increased ICP are inadequate cerebral perfusion and cerebral herniation (see Figure 59-4). To better understand cerebral herniation, three important structures in the brain must be described. The *falx cerebri* is a thin wall of dura that folds down between the cortex separating the two cerebral hemispheres. The *tentorium cerebelli* is a rigid fold of dura that separates the cerebral hemispheres from the cerebellum (see Figure 59-4). There is a central opening in the tentorium cerebelli called the *tentorial incisura,* from which the brain stem emerges. This is a common site of herniation related to increased ICP.

Cingulate herniation occurs when there is lateral displacement of brain tissue beneath the falx cerebri. *Tentorial herniation* occurs when a mass lesion in the cerebrum forces the brain to herniate downward through the tentorial incisura. *Cerebellar tonsillar herniation* occurs when there is lateral and downward herniation

of the cerebellar tonsils through the foramen magnum. This herniation results in medullary compression and is often fatal.

Diagnostic Studies

Diagnostic studies can identify the underlying cause of increased ICP (Table 59-3). Magnetic resonance imaging (MRI) and computed tomography (CT) have revolutionized the diagnosis of acute intracranial events. Significant technological advancement in these modalities now offers enhanced evaluation of the brain's vasculature utilizing magnetic resonance angiography (MRA) and computed tomographic angiography (CTA). All of these tests are used to differentiate the many conditions that can cause increased ICP and to evaluate therapeutic options. Other diagnostic tests that may be used include conventional cerebral angiography, EEG, ICP measurement, brain tissue oxygenation measurement via the Licox catheter (described later in this chapter), transcranial Doppler studies, and evoked potential

---

TABLE 59-3 COLLABORATIVE CARE
Increased Intracranial Pressure

Diagnostic Tests and Neuromonitoring
- History and physical examination
- Cerebral oxygenation monitoring (Licox catheter, $SjvO_2$)
- ECG
- Infrascanner
- Laboratory studies, including CBC; coagulation profile; electrolytes; creatinine; BUN; ABGs; ammonia level; general drug and toxicology screen; CSF analysis for protein, cells, glucose*
- MRI, CT scan, MRA, CTA, EEG, angiography, EP studies, PET
- Skull and facial radiographic studies
- Transcranial Doppler studies
- Vital signs, neurological assessments, ICP measurements

Collaborative Therapy
- Cerebral oxygenation monitoring ($PbtO_2$, $SjvO_2$)
- Drug therapy
  - Anticonvulsant drugs (e.g., phenytoin [Dilantin])
  - Antipyretics
  - Corticosteroids (dexamethasone) (for brain tumours, bacterial meningitis)
  - Histamine H_2-receptor antagonist (e.g., ranitidine [Zantac]) or proton pump inhibitor (e.g., pantoprazole [Pantoloc]) to prevent gastro-intestinal ulcers and bleeding
  - Hypertonic saline
  - Nutritional support
  - Osmotic diuretics (mannitol)
  - Stool softeners
- Elevation of head of bed to 30 degrees with head in a neutral position
- ICP monitoring
- Intubation and mechanical ventilation
- Maintenance of CPP >60 mm Hg
- Maintenance of fluid balance and assessment of osmolality
- Maintenance of PaO_2 at ≥100 mm Hg
- Maintenance of systolic arterial pressure between 100 and 160 mm Hg
- Reduction of cerebral metabolism (e.g., high-dose barbiturates)

ABGs, arterial blood gases; *BUN,* blood urea nitrogen; *CBC,* complete blood count; *CPP,* cerebral perfusion pressure; *CSF,* cerebro-spinal fluid; *CT,* computed tomography; *CTA,* computed tomography angiography; *ECG,* electrocardiogram; *EEG,* electroencephalogram; *EP,* evoked potential; *ICP,* intracranial pressure; *MAP,* mean arterial pressure; *MRA,* magnetic resonance angiography; *MRI,* magnetic resonance imaging; *PaO₂,* partial pressure of arterial oxygen; *PbtO₂,* pressure of oxygen in brain tissue; *SjvO₂,* jugular venous oxygen saturation.
*CSF sampling via lumbar puncture is contraindicated if there is suspected raised ICP because there is a possibility of cerebral herniation and death.

FIGURE 59-6 Decorticate and decerebrate posturing. **A,** Decorticate response. Flexion of arms, wrists, and fingers with adduction in upper extremities. Extension, internal rotation, and plantar flexion in lower extremities. **B,** Decerebrate response. All four extremities in rigid extension, with hyperpronation of forearms and plantar flexion of feet.

studies. Positron emission tomography (PET) can also be used to diagnose the cause of increased ICP. In general, a lumbar puncture is not performed when increased ICP is suspected because of the possibility of cerebral herniation from the sudden release of the pressure in the skull from the area above the lumbar puncture.

A hand-held device called an Infrascanner can be used to detect life-threatening intracranial bleeding. The scanner directs a wavelength of light that can penetrate tissue and bone. Blood from intracranial hematomas absorbs the light differently from other areas of the brain.

Neuromonitoring

Measurement of Intracranial Pressure. ICP may become elevated because of head trauma, stroke, subarachnoid hemorrhage, brain tumour, inflammation or infection, hydrocephalus, or brain tissue damage from other causes. Patients with or at risk for elevated ICP usually receive invasive ICP monitoring in an intensive care unit (ICU), except those with irreversible problems or advanced neurological disease. Goals for nursing management of elevated ICP include preservation of cerebral oxygenation and perfusion, early identification of neurological

FIGURE 59-7 Coronal section of the brain shows potential sites for placement of intracranial pressure monitoring devices.

changes, and prevention of complications secondary to intracranial hypertension.

ICP monitoring is used to guide clinical care when the patient is at risk for or has elevations in ICP. ICP should be monitored in patients admitted with a Glasgow Coma Scale (GCS) score of 8 or less and an abnormal CT scan or MRI (hematomas, contusion, edema). (The GCS is presented in Table 59-5.) Multiple methods and devices are available to monitor ICP (Figure 59-7).

The "gold standard" for monitoring ICP is the *ventriculostomy,* whereby a catheter is inserted into the lateral ventricle and coupled to an external transducer. This technique directly measures the pressure within the ventricles and facilitates removal or sampling (or both) of CSF. Significant consideration in caring for a patient with a ventriculostomy is the constant positioning of the external transducer relative to the position of the patient's head to maintain consistent measurements. The transducer should be level with the foramen of Monro (intraventricular foramen); the reference point for this on the patient is the tragus of the ear (Figure 59-8, *A*). When repositioning a patient with a ventriculostomy, the system may need to be rezeroed to maintain the level of the transducer. Another device used for monitoring ICP is the *fibre-optic catheter,* the tip of which is placed directly into the ventricle or the brain tissue. A sensor transducer located in the catheter tip provides measurement of the pressure in the brain. Lastly, the *subarachnoid bolt* or *screw* may be placed through the skull between the arachnoid membrane and the cerebral cortex to measure ICP; this method does not allow for drainage of CSF but can be converted into a ventriculostomy if the patient's clinical condition changes to require that intervention.

Infection is a serious consideration with ICP monitoring. Prophylactic systemic antibiotics may be administered to reduce the chances of infection. Factors that contribute to the development of infection include ICP monitoring for longer than 5 days, use of a ventriculostomy, the presence of a CSF leak, a concurrent systemic infection, and improper aseptic technique during manipulation by health care team members. Routine care may include regular diagnostic testing for CSF organism growth.

The ICP waveform is derived from the arterial pulsations of the choroids plexus in the lateral ventricles. A normal ICP waveform has a diastolic and a systolic component and correlates

FIGURE 59-8 A, Levelling a ventriculostomy. **B,** Cerebro-spinal fluid is drained into a drainage system. Source: Courtesy Meg Zomorodi.

with the cardiac cycle. When the waveform is monitored so that components in synchrony with the cardiac cycle can be visualized, the normal ICP waveform has three phases (Table 59-4).

It is important to monitor the ICP waveform and the CPP (Figure 59-9). It has been noted that, when the height of P2 is higher than P1, this represents low *compliance* and the patient is at risk for development of elevated ICP. It is important to consider both the rate at which changes occur and the patient's clinical condition. Neurological deterioration might not occur until ICP elevation is pronounced and sustained. Any indication of ICP elevation, either as a mean increase in pressure or as an abnormal waveform configuration, should be reported to the physician immediately.

Inaccurate ICP readings can be caused by CSF leaks around the monitoring device, obstruction of the intraventricular catheter or bolt (from tissue or blood clot), a difference between the

height of the bolt and the transducer, kinks in the tubing, and incorrect height of the drainage system relative to the patient's reference point. Bubbles or air in the tubing can also dampen the waveform.

Cerebro-Spinal Fluid Drainage. With the ventricular catheter and certain fibre-optic systems, it is possible to control elevations in ICP by removing CSF. Using a closed system (Figure 59-10), CSF is removed by gravity drainage and by adjusting the height of the drip chamber and drainage bag relative to the patient's ventricular reference point. Typically, a point 15 cm above the ear is selected (see Figure 59-8, *B*). Raising the system diminishes drainage, whereas lowering the system increases drainage volume. The physician orders the level of the ICP indicating that drainage should be initiated, the amount of fluid to be drained, the height of the system, and the frequency of drainage (intermittent or continuous).

The two options for CSF drainage are intermittent and continuous. If intermittent drainage is ordered, the ventriculo-stomy system is opened at the indicated ICP and CSF is allowed to drain for 2 to 3 minutes. Then the stopcock is closed to return the ventriculostomy to a closed system. If continuous ICP drainage is ordered, careful monitoring of the volume of CSF drained is essential, keeping in mind that normal CSF production is about 20 to 30 mL/hr, with a total CSF volume of 90 to 150 mL within the ventricles and subarachnoid space.

Prevention of infection is imperative by use of strict aseptic technique during dressing changes or sampling of CSF. The system must remain intact to ensure that the ICP readings are accurate because treatment is initiated and evaluated on the basis of the readings. It is also recommended that a sign be posted above

TABLE 59-4	NORMAL INTRACRANIAL PRESSURE WAVEFORMS*
Waveform	**Meaning**
P1 Percussion wave	Represents arterial pulsations; normally the highest of the three waveforms
P2 Rebound wave	Reflects intracranial compliance or relative brain volume. When P2 is higher than P1, intracranial compliance is compromised
P3 Dicrotic wave	Follows dicrotic notch; represents venous pulsations; normally, the lowest waveform

*See Figure 59-9.

FIGURE 59-9 Intracranial pressure (ICP) monitoring can be used to continuously measure ICP. The ICP tracing shows normal, elevated, and plateau waves. At high ICP, the P2 peak is higher than the P1 peak, and the peaks become less distinct and plateau. Source: Copstead-Kirkhorn, L. C., & Banasik, J. L. (2010). *Pathophysiology* (4th ed., p. 1043, Figure 44-7). St Louis: Mosby.

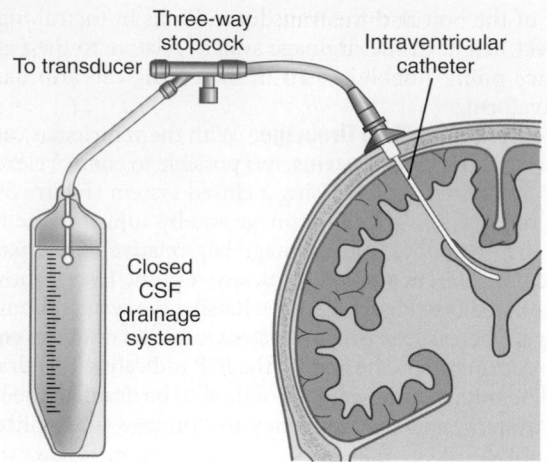

FIGURE 59-10 Intermittent drainage system. Cerebro-spinal fluid (CSF) is drained via a ventriculostomy when intracranial pressure (ICP) exceeds the upper pressure parameter set by the physician. Intermittent drainage involves opening the three-way stopcock to allow CSF to flow into the draining bag for brief periods (≤5 min) until the pressure is below the upper pressure parameters.

the patient's bed to notify anyone before turning, moving, or suctioning the patient to prevent the removal of too much CSF, which can result in complications such as ventricular collapse, herniation, or subdural hematoma from rapid decompression. Although it is generally recognized that CSF removal decreases ICP and improves CPP, guidelines for CSF removal are not universally accepted but are typically based on institution or physician preference.

Cerebral Oxygenation Monitoring. Failure to adequately deliver oxygenated blood to an injured brain is a major contributor to poor outcomes. Technology is available to measure cerebral oxygenation and cerebral perfusion. Two such devices are currently being used in intensive care settings: the *Licox brain tissue oxygenation catheter* and the *jugular venous bulb catheter*. The Licox catheter is placed in the healthy white matter of the brain and provides continuous monitoring of the pressure of oxygen in brain tissue ($PbtO_2$); the normal range for $PbtO_2$ is 20 to 40 mm Hg. A lower-than-normal $PbtO_2$ level is indicative of ischemia.

The jugular venous bulb catheter is placed in the internal jugular vein and positioned so that the catheter tip is located in the jugular bulb; placement is confirmed by radiographic study. This catheter provides a measurement of jugular venous oxygen saturation ($SjvO_2$), which indicates total venous brain tissue extraction of oxygen as a measure of cerebral oxygen supply and demand. The normal $SjvO_2$ range is 55% to 75%. Values less than 50% demonstrate impaired cerebral oxygenation. With the use of either device, interventions can be specifically focused to improve brain tissue oxygen levels. The Licox catheter has the ability to also measure brain temperature; neither device has the capability of monitoring ICP, and therefore, an ICP monitoring device may be placed for this purpose.

Collaborative Care

The goals of collaborative care (see Table 59-3) are to identify and treat the underlying cause of increased ICP and to support brain function. A careful history is an important diagnostic aid that can direct the search for the underlying cause of increased ICP (usually an increase in blood [hemorrhage],

brain tissue [tumour or edema], or CSF [hydrocephalus] in the brain).

Ensuring adequate oxygenation to support brain function is the first step in the management of increased ICP. An endotracheal tube or tracheostomy may be necessary to maintain adequate ventilation. Arterial blood gas (ABG) analysis guides the oxygen therapy. The goal is to maintain the PaO_2 at 100 mm Hg or greater. It may be necessary to maintain the patient on a mechanical ventilator to ensure adequate oxygenation.

If the condition is caused by a mass lesion, such as a tumour or hematoma, surgical removal of the mass is the best management (see the Brain Tumours and Cranial Surgery sections, later in this chapter). Nonsurgical intervention for the reduction of tissue volume related to cerebral tissue swelling and cerebral edema includes the use of osmotic diuretics, hypertonic saline, and corticosteroids.

Drug Therapy. Drug therapy plays an important role in the management of increased ICP. Frequently, mannitol (Osmitrol), an osmotic diuretic given intravenously, is used to decrease the ICP in acute situations. Mannitol acts to decrease ICP in two ways: plasma expansion and osmotic effect. There is an immediate plasma-expanding effect that reduces the hematocrit and blood viscosity, thereby increasing CBF and cerebral oxygen delivery. A vascular osmotic gradient is created by mannitol. Thus, fluid moves from the tissues into the blood vessels. ICP is reduced by the decrease in the total brain fluid content. Fluid and electrolyte status must be closely monitored when osmotic diuretics are used as multiple administrations can increase serum sodium levels and osmolality (Shawkat, Westwood, & Mortimer, 2012).

DRUG ALERT—Mannitol (Osmitrol)
- Careful monitoring of patients is required due to the adverse effect of fluid shift and the potential for fluid overload and pulmonary congestion.
- Mannitol may crystallize at lower temperatures; administer intravenously using a filter.

Hypertonic saline is another drug therapy used to manage increased ICP. It reduces swelling and improves CBF, drawing water out of the brain tissue. A patient receiving hypertonic saline infusion must also be monitored closely; blood pressure and serum sodium levels can be affected by intravascular fluid volume excess as a result of treatment. Hypertonic saline offers effective first-line treatment for elevated ICP when compared with mannitol (Kamel, Navi, Nakagawa, et al., 2011).

Corticosteroids (e.g., dexamethasone) are used to treat vasogenic edema surrounding tumours and abscesses but appear to have limited value in the management of patients with head injuries and are not recommended for those patients. Corticosteroids act by stabilizing the cell membrane and inhibiting the synthesis of prostaglandins (see Chapter 14), thus preventing the formation of proinflammatory mediators. Corticosteroids are also thought to improve neuronal function by improving CBF and restoring autoregulation.

Complications associated with the use of corticosteroids include hyperglycemia, increased incidence of infections, gastro-intestinal (GI) bleeding, and hyponatremia. Fluid intake and sodium and glucose levels should be monitored regularly. Patients receiving corticosteroids should concurrently be given antacids or histamine (H_2)-receptor blockers (e.g., ranitidine [Zantac]) or proton pump inhibitors (e.g., omeprazole [Losec], pantoprazole [Pantoloc]) to prevent GI ulcers and bleeding.

Drug therapy for reducing cerebral metabolism may be an effective strategy to control ICP. Sedation with propofol [Diprivan] and analgesia, along with the treatments described above, can be used to manage elevated ICP (Oddo, Crippa, Mehta, et al., 2016). (The discussion of drug therapy used in the management of patients with increased ICP is continued on pages 1482–1483 of this chapter.) The decision may be made to use high-dose barbiturates (e.g., pentobarbital sodium [Somnotol]) in patients with increased ICP that is refractory to all other treatments (Dinsmore, 2013). Barbiturates dampen the effects of environmental stimuli on patients, thereby decreasing cerebral metabolism and subsequently ICP. Capabilities to monitor the patient's ICP, blood flow, EEG, and metabolism should be available when this treatment is used; hypotension as a result of treatment is a concern. There is not sufficient evidence to suggest that outcomes for patients with acute traumatic brain injuries are improved with this treatment (Roberts & Sydenham, 2012). Anticonvulsant drugs such as phenytoin (Dilantin) may be used because seizures can further increase ICP (seizures are discussed in greater detail in Chapter 61).

Nutritional Therapy. All patients must have their nutritional needs met, regardless of their state of consciousness or health. The patient with increased ICP is in a hypermetabolic and hypercatabolic state that increases the need for glucose to provide the necessary fuel for metabolism of the injured brain. If the patient cannot maintain an adequate oral intake, other means of meeting the nutritional requirements, such as enteral feedings or parenteral nutrition, should be initiated. Early feeding after brain injury may improve outcomes (Wang, Dong, Han, et al., 2013). Because malnutrition promotes continued cerebral edema, maintenance of optimal nutrition is imperative. (Nutritional therapy is discussed in Chapter 42.) Feedings or supplements should be guided by the patient's fluid and electrolyte status as well as the patient's metabolic needs.

Therapy is directed at keeping patients normovolemic. Intravenous (IV) 0.9% sodium chloride is the preferred solution for administration of piggyback medications because a lowering of serum osmolarity and an increase in cerebral edema occur if 5% dextrose in water is used.

Supportive Therapy. Metabolic demands such as fever (38°C), agitation or shivering, pain, and seizures can also increase ICP. The health care team should plan to reduce these metabolic demands to lower the ICP in patients who are at risk. Patients should be monitored for seizure activity. Fever should be well controlled to maintain a temperature of 36° to 37°C by using antipyretics (e.g., acetaminophen [Tylenol]), cool baths, cooling blankets, ice packs, or intravascular cooling devices, as necessary. However, patients should be kept from shivering or shaking, since this increases the metabolic workload on the brain. If shivering or shaking occurs, sedatives may be needed or a different cooling method selected.

Pain should be managed while being careful not to oversedate or overmedicate. Finally, the patient should remain in a quiet, calm environment with minimal noise and interruptions. The patient should be observed for signs of agitation, irritation, or frustration. Also the caregiver and the family should be taught about decreasing stimulation, and the health care team should coordinate to minimize procedures that may produce agitation.

NURSING MANAGEMENT
INCREASED INTRACRANIAL PRESSURE

NURSING ASSESSMENT

Subjective data about the patient with increased ICP can be obtained from the patient or family members or other persons who are familiar with the patient. The nurse must learn appropriate assessment techniques and describe the LOC by noting the specific behaviours observed. When a deviation from the normal state of consciousness occurs, a more structured method of observation should be initiated. Adequate circulation and respiration are the most vital body functions and should always be the first ones assessed.

GLASGOW COMA SCALE. The Glasgow Coma Scale (GCS), developed in 1974, is a quick, practical, and standardized system for assessing the degree to which consciousness is impaired. It provides a universal language for describing altered states of consciousness. The three areas assessed in the GCS correspond to the definition of coma as the inability of a patient to speak, obey commands, or open the eyes when a verbal or painful stimulus is applied (Jennett & Teasdale, 1977). Specific assessments evaluate the patient's response to varying degrees of stimuli. Three indicators of response are evaluated: (1) eye opening, (2) best verbal response, and (3) best motor response (see Table 59-5). Specific behaviours that are seen as responses to the testing stimulus in each of these three areas are given a numeric value and can be plotted on a graph. The nurse's responsibility is to elicit the best response on each of the scales; the higher the scores, the higher the level of brain functioning. A graph can be used to determine whether the patient's condition is stable, improving, or deteriorating. The subscale scores are particularly important if a patient is untestable in one area. For example, severe periorbital edema may make eye opening impossible. The total GCS score is a sum of the numeric values assigned to each of the three areas evaluated. The highest GCS score is 15 for a fully alert person, and the lowest possible score is 3. A GCS score of 8 or less is generally indicative of coma (Teasdale & Jennett, 1974).

The GCS offers several advantages in the assessment of the unconscious patient. It is specific and structured, allowing different health care providers to arrive at the same conclusion regarding the patient's status. It saves time for the assessor because the ratings are done with numbers rather than with lengthy descriptions.

The GCS is also specific enough to discriminate between different or changing states. It is used to assess the arousal aspect of consciousness. Other components of the neurological assessment include pupillary checks, extremity strength testing, vital signs, and if appropriate, testing of the function of specific cranial nerves.

NEUROLOGICAL ASSESSMENT. The pupils are compared with one another for size, movement, and response (Figure 59-11). If the oculomotor nerve is compressed, the pupil on the affected side (ipsilateral) becomes larger until it fully dilates. If ICP continues to increase, both pupils dilate. Pupil size is measured in millimetres before assessing the pupil response to light.

Pupillary reaction is tested with a penlight. The normal reaction is brisk constriction when the light is shone directly into the eye. A consensual response (a slight constriction in the opposite pupil) should also be noted at the same time. A sluggish reaction can indicate early pressure on CN III. A fixed pupil shows no response to light stimulus, which usually indicates increased ICP. However, there are other causes of a fixed pupil, including direct injury to CN III, previous eye surgery, administration of atropine, and use of mydriatic eye drops.

Evaluation of other cranial nerves can be included in the neurological assessment. Eye movements controlled by CNs III, IV, and VI can be examined in the patient who is awake and can be used to assess the function of the brain stem. In patients

TABLE 59-5   GLASGOW COMA SCALE

Appropriate Stimulus	Response	Score
Eyes Open		
Approach to bedside	Spontaneous response	4
Verbal command	Opening of eyes to name or command	3
Pain	Lack of opening of eyes to previous stimuli but opening to pain	2
	Lack of opening of eyes to any stimulus	1
	Untestable* (e.g., swollen)	U
Best Verbal Response		
Verbal questioning with maximum arousal	Appropriate orientation, conversant; correct identification of self, place, year, and month	5
	Confusion; conversant, but disorientation in one or more spheres	4
	Inappropriate or disorganized use of words (e.g., cursing), lack of sustained conversation	3
	Incomprehensible words, sounds (e.g., moaning)	2
	Lack of sound, even with painful stimuli	1
	Untestable* (e.g., endotracheal tube)	U
Best Motor Response		
Verbal command (e.g., "raise your arm, hold up two fingers")	Obedience of command	6
Pain applied centrally (e.g., sternal rub, pinching of upper third of trapezius, or supraorbital pressure)	Localization of pain, lack of obedience but presence of attempts to remove offending stimulus—purposeful movement	5
	Flexion withdrawal, flexion of arm in response to pain without abnormal flexion posture—nonpurposeful movement	4
	Abnormal flexion, flexing of arm at elbow and pronation, making a fist	3
	Abnormal extension, extension of arm at elbow usually with adduction and internal rotation of arm at shoulder	2
	Lack of response	1
	Untestable*	U

*Added to the original scale by many centres.

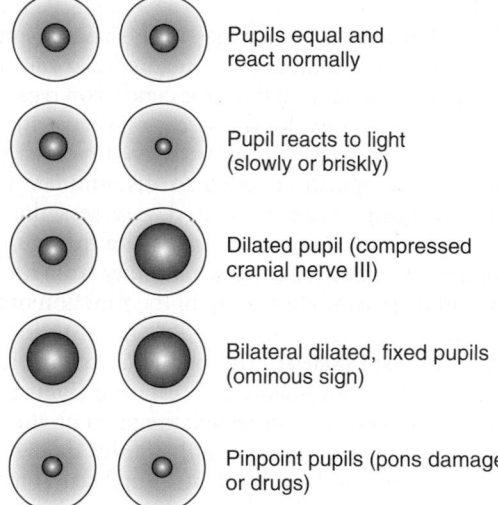

FIGURE 59-11 Pupillary check for size and response.

- Pupils equal and react normally
- Pupil reacts to light (slowly or briskly)
- Dilated pupil (compressed cranial nerve III)
- Bilateral dilated, fixed pupils (ominous sign)
- Pinpoint pupils (pons damage or drugs)

who are unconscious, eye movements can be elicited by reflex with the use of head movements (oculo-cephalic) and caloric stimulation (oculo-vestibular). (Chapters 23 and 24 discuss assessment and problems of the eye and ear.) Testing the corneal reflex provides clinical information regarding the function of CNs V and VII. If corneal reflexes are absent, routine eye care should be initiated to prevent corneal abrasion.

For the patient who is awake, motor strength is tested by asking the patient to squeeze the nurse's hands to compare strength in the hands. The palmar (or pronator) drift test is an excellent measure of strength in the upper extremities. With eyes closed, the patient raises the arms in front of the body with the palmar surface facing upward. If there is any weakness in the upper extremity, the palmar surface rotates inward and the arm may drift downward. The patient keeps the eyes closed to prevent being able to see the palmar drift and trying to correct the rotating hand position. Detection of a palmar drift is an early indicator of cortico-spinal tract compression and possible increased ICP. Asking the patient to raise the foot from the bed or to bend the knees up in bed is a good assessment of lower extremity strength. All four extremities should be tested for strength and evaluated for any asymmetry in strength or movement.

For patients who are unconscious or uncooperative, motor strength can be assessed by observation of their spontaneous movement. If no spontaneous movement is possible, a pain stimulus should be applied to the patient, and the response should be noted. Resistance to movement during passive range of motion exercises is another measure of strength.

Vital signs, including BP, pulse, respiratory rate, and temperature, should also be systematically recorded. Cushing's triad is a triad of changes to vital signs (increased BP with a widening pulse pressure, bradycardia, and irregular respiratory pattern). This triad indicates severe increased ICP and impending cerebral herniation. Specific respiratory patterns are associated with severely increased ICP (Figure 59-12).

NURSING DIAGNOSES

Nursing diagnoses for the patient with increased ICP include, but are not limited to, the following:

- *Decreased intracranial adaptive capacity* (related to decreased cerebral perfusion or increased ICP)

Pattern	Location of Lesion	Description
1. Cheyne–Stokes	Bilateral hemispheric disease or metabolic brain dysfunction	Cycles of hyperventilation and apnea
2. Central neurogenic hyperventilation	Brain stem between lower midbrain and upper pons	Sustained, regular rapid and deep breathing
3. Apneustic breathing	Mid or lower pons	Prolonged inspiratory phase or pauses alternating with expiratory pauses
4. Cluster breathing	Medulla or lower pons	Clusters of breaths follow each other with irregular pauses between
5. Ataxic breathing	Reticular formation of the medulla	Completely irregular with some breaths deep and some shallow. Random, irregular pauses, slow rate

FIGURE 59-12 Common abnormal respiratory patterns associated with coma.

- *Risk for ineffective cerebral tissue perfusion* as evidenced by *brain injury, brain neoplasm, cerebral aneurysm*
- *Risk for disuse syndrome* as evidenced by *alteration in level of consciousness, mechanical immobility, paralysis*

Additional information on nursing diagnoses for patients with increased ICP is presented in Nursing Care Plan (NCP) 59-1, available on the Evolve website.

PLANNING

The overall goals are that the patient with increased ICP will (1) maintain a patent airway, (2) have ICP within normal limits, (3) have normal fluid and electrolyte balance, and (4) have no complications secondary to immobility and decreased LOC.

NURSING IMPLEMENTATION
ACUTE INTERVENTION

Respiratory Function. Maintenance of a patent airway is critical in the patient with increased ICP and is a primary nursing responsibility. As the LOC decreases, the patient is at increased risk for airway obstruction from the tongue dropping back and occluding the airway or from accumulation of secretions. Altered breathing patterns may become evident. Airway patency can be aided by keeping the patient lying on one side, with frequent position changes.

SAFETY ALERT
- Be alert to altered breathing patterns.
- Snoring sounds indicate obstruction and require immediate intervention.

Accumulated secretions should be removed by suctioning, as needed. An oral airway facilitates breathing and provides an easier suctioning route in the patient who is comatose. Any patient with altered LOC who is unable to maintain a patent airway or effective ventilation requires intubation and mechanical ventilation.

The nurse must use measures to prevent hypoxia and hypercapnia. Proper positioning of the head is important. Elevation of the head of the bed by 30 degrees enhances respiratory exchange and aids in decreasing cerebral edema. Suctioning and coughing can cause transient decreases in the PaO_2 and increases in the ICP. Suctioning should be less than 10 seconds in duration, with administration of 100% oxygen before and after to prevent decreases in the PaO_2. To avoid cumulative increases in the ICP, suctioning should be limited to two passes per suction procedure. Patients with elevated ICP are at risk for lower CPP during suctioning. Abdominal distension can interfere with respiratory function and should be prevented. Increased intra-abdominal or intrathoracic pressures can contribute to elevated ICP by impeding cerebral venous drainage. Insertion of a nasogastric tube to aspirate the stomach contents can prevent distension, vomiting, and possible aspiration. However, in patients with facial and skull fractures, a nasogastric tube is contraindicated, and oral insertion of a gastric tube is preferred.

Pain, anxiety, and fear from the initial injury, therapeutic procedures, or noxious stimuli can increase ICP and BP, complicating the management and the recovery of the patient with a brain injury. The appropriate choice or combination of sedatives, paralytics, and analgesics for symptom management presents a challenge to the ICU team. Administration of these agents may alter the neurological state, masking true neurological changes. It may be necessary to temporarily suspend pharmacological therapy to appropriately assess neurological status. The choice, the dosage, and the combination of agents may vary depending on the patient's history, neurological state, and overall clinical presentation.

The IV anaesthetic sedative propofol (Diprivan) has gained popularity in the management of pain and anxiety in the ICU because of its rapid onset, short half-life, and oxygen-saving properties. It has been shown to depress cerebral metabolism and oxygen consumption, offering neuroprotective benefits, and is a drug of choice for sedation and elevated ICP in the ICU setting (Oddo et al., 2016).

Dexmedetomidine (Precedex), an α_2-adrenergic agonist, is used for continuous IV sedation of patients who are intubated and mechanically ventilated in the ICU setting for up to 24 hours. It is another ideal agent for patients with neurological conditions because of the ease in obtaining a neurological assessment without altering the dose because of its anxiolytic properties. The benzodiazepine midazolam can be used for sedation and management of ICP as well (Oddo et al., 2016). When using continuous IV sedatives, be aware of the adverse effects of these drugs, especially hypotension, since this can result in a lower CPP value.

Non-depolarizing neuromuscular blocking agents (e.g., cisatracurium) are useful for ventilatory management and treatment of refractory intracranial hypertension. Because these agents paralyze muscles without blocking pain or noxious stimuli, they are used in combination with sedatives, analgesics, or benzodiazepines. Opioids, such as morphine sulphate and fentanyl, are rapid-onset analgesics with minimal effect on CBF or oxygen metabolism.

ABGs should be measured and evaluated regularly (see Chapter 28). The nurse should frequently monitor the ABG values and maintain the levels within prescribed or acceptable parameters. The appropriate ventilatory support can be ordered on the basis of the PaO_2 and $PaCO_2$ values.

Fluid and Electrolyte Balance. Fluid and electrolyte disturbances can have an adverse effect on ICP. IV fluids should be closely monitored with the use of a limited-volume device or a volume-control apparatus for accuracy. Intake and output, with insensible losses and daily weights taken into account, are important parameters in the assessment of fluid balance.

Electrolyte determinations should be made daily, and any abnormal values should be discussed with the physician. It is especially important to monitor serum glucose, sodium, potassium, and osmolality. Urinary output is monitored to detect problems related to *diabetes insipidus* (DI) (e.g., increased urinary output related to a decrease in antidiuretic hormone secretion); SIADH, which results in decreased urinary output; and cerebral salt wasting, a form of hyponatremia caused by excessive renal sodium excretion associated with cerebral insult. Besides urinary output, the serum and urine sodium and osmolality are also used to diagnose DI, SIADH, and cerebral salt wasting. DI may result in severe dehydration unless treated. The usual treatment is fluid replacement, vasopressin, or desmopressin acetate (DDAVP). SIADH results in a dilutional hyponatremia that may produce cerebral edema, changes in LOC, seizures, and coma. (Treatment of SIADH is described in Chapter 51.) Treatment of cerebral salt wasting consists of aggressive sodium (Na^+) and volume replacement.

Monitoring Intracranial Pressure. ICP monitoring is used in combination with other physiological parameters to guide the care of the patient and assess the patient's response to routine care. The Valsalva manoeuvre, coughing, sneezing, hypoxemia, pain, fever, and environmental stimuli are factors that can increase ICP. Nurses should be alert to these factors and should attempt to keep them to a minimum.

Body Position. The patient with increased ICP should be maintained in the head-up position. The nurse must take care to prevent extreme neck flexion, which can cause venous obstruction and contribute to elevated ICP. The body position should be adjusted to decrease the ICP as much as possible and to improve the CPP. Traditional practice has been to elevate the head of the bed to 30 degrees, unless a concurrent cervical neck injury has been identified, in which case a reverse Trendelenburg position may be indicated to elevate the head while keeping the spine aligned. Elevation of the head of the bed reduces sagittal sinus pressure, promotes venous drainage from the head via the valveless jugular system, and decreases the vascular congestion that can produce cerebral edema. However, raising the head of the bed above 30 degrees may decrease the CPP. Careful evaluation of the effects of elevation of the head of the bed on both the ICP and the CPP is required—the bed should be positioned so that it lowers the ICP while maintaining the CPP and other indices of cerebral oxygenation.

Care should be taken to turn the patient with slow, gentle movements because rapid changes in position may increase the ICP. Caution should be used to prevent discomfort in turning and positioning the patient because pain or agitation also increases ICP. Increased intra-abdominal and intrathoracic pressure contribute to increased ICP by impeding the venous return. Thus, coughing, straining, and the Valsalva manoeuvre should be avoided. Extreme hip flexion should be prevented to decrease the risk of raising the intra-abdominal pressure. The patient should be turned at least every 2 hours.

Decorticate or decerebrate posturing is a reflex response in some patients with increased ICP (see Figure 59-6). Turning, skin care, and even passive range of motion can elicit the posturing reflexes. Attempts should be made to provide needed physical care activities to minimize complications of immobility, such as

atelectasis and contractures. In cases of severe posturing reflexes, these activities may have to be done less frequently because posturing can cause increases in ICP.

Protection From Injury. The patient with increased ICP and a decreased LOC needs protection from self-injury. Confusion, agitation, and the possibility of seizures can put the patient at risk for injury. In these cases, environmental, chemical, or physical restraints may be considered to protect the patient from harm (e.g., removing tubes, wandering). A least-restraint approach should be used and considered only after all possible alternative interventions are exhausted. Specific employer policies and procedures should help guide restraint practice. The need for restraints should be reassessed daily. If restraints are necessary, they should be secure enough to be effective, and the area under the restraints should be observed regularly for skin irritation and adequate blood circulation. Restrained extremities should be assessed at least every 2 hours for colour, warmth, sensation, and movement. Agitation may increase with the use of restraints, which indicates the need for other measures to protect the patient from injury. Light sedation with agents such as haloperidol (Haldol) or lorazepam (Ativan) may be needed. Patient history and clinical presentation may be used to guide drug choice. Having a family member stay with the patient may have a calming effect. For the patient with seizures or the patient at risk for seizure activity, seizure precautions should be instituted. These include padded side rails, an airway at the bedside, accurate and timely administration of anticonvulsant drugs, and close observation (see Chapter 61). The patient can benefit from a quiet, nonstimulating environment. The nurse should always use a calm, reassuring approach. Touching and talking to the patient, even one who is in a coma, is always appropriate care. The nurse must create a balance between sensory deprivation and overload for the patient with increased ICP.

Psychological Considerations. In addition to providing carefully planned physical care to patients with increased ICP, the nurse must also be aware of the psychological well-being of patients and their families. Anxiety over the diagnosis and the prognosis for patients with neurological problems can be distressing to patients and their families. The nurse's competent and assured manner in performing the care patients need is reassuring to everyone involved. Short, simple explanations are appropriate and allow patients and their families to acquire the amount of information they desire. There is a need for support, information, and education of patients, families, and caregivers. The nurse should assess the family members' desire to assist in providing care for the patient and allow for their participation as appropriate. Encourage interdisciplinary management (social work, chaplain, etc.) of the patient and family in decision making as much as possible.

EVALUATION

The expected outcomes for the patient with ICP are addressed in NCP 59-1, available on the Evolve website.

HEAD INJURY

Head injury includes any trauma to the scalp, the skull, or the brain. The term *head trauma* is used primarily to signify cranio-cerebral trauma, which includes an alteration in consciousness, no matter how brief.

Statistics for head injuries are incomplete because many victims die at the scene of the accident or because the condition is considered minor and health care services are not sought. Approximately 160 000 Canadians sustain a head injury annually, and over 1 million live with the effects of an acquired brain injury (Brain Injury Association of Canada, n.d.). Traumatic brain injury (TBI) continues to be one of the leading causes of death and the leading cause of disability after trauma. In Canada, the most common causes of TBI requiring hospitalizations are motor vehicle accidents and falls (Fu, Jing, McFaull, et al., 2015). Other causes include assaults, sports-related injuries, and recreational accidents.

Head trauma has a high potential for poor outcome. Death from head trauma occurs at three time periods following an injury: immediately after the injury, within 2 hours after the injury, and approximately 3 weeks after injury. Factors associated with a poor outcome include the increasing age of the patient, lower Glasgow Coma Scale (GCS) scores, impaired or absent eye movements or pupil light reflexes, hypoxemia, intracranial edema and intraventricular hemorrhage, and ICP levels higher than 20 mm Hg (Badri, Chen, Barber, et al., 2012). The majority of deaths after a head injury occur immediately after the injury, either from the direct head trauma or from massive hemorrhage and shock. Deaths occurring within a few hours of the trauma are caused by progressive worsening of the head injury or from internal bleeding. An immediate note of changes in neurological status and surgical intervention are critical in the prevention of deaths at this point. Deaths occurring 3 weeks or longer after injury result from multisystem failure. Expert nursing care in the weeks following the injury is crucial in decreasing mortality and optimizing patient outcomes.

Types of Head Injuries

Scalp Lacerations. *Scalp lacerations* are the most minor type of head trauma. Because the scalp contains many blood vessels with poor constrictive abilities, most scalp lacerations are associated with profuse bleeding. The major complications associated with scalp laceration are blood loss and infection.

Skull Fractures. *Skull fractures* frequently occur with head trauma. There are several ways to describe skull fractures: (1) linear or depressed; (2) simple, comminuted, or compound; and (3) closed or open (Table 59-6). Fractures may be closed or open, depending on the presence of a scalp laceration or extension of the fracture into the air sinuses or the dura. The type and severity of a skull fracture depend on the velocity, the momentum, the direction of the injuring agent, and the site of impact.

The location of the fracture alters the presentation of the manifestations (Table 59-7). For example, a specialized type of linear fracture is seen when the fracture occurs at the base of the skull—a basilar skull fracture. Manifestations include *Battle sign* (postauricular ecchymosis) (Figure 59-13) and *bilateral periorbital ecchymosis* (raccoon eyes). This fracture generally crosses a sinus and tears the dura (e.g., the frontal or temporal dura) and is associated with cranial nerve damage and leakage of CSF. *CSF rhinorrhea* (CSF leakage from the nose) or *CSF otorrhea* (CSF leakage from the ear) generally confirms that the fracture has traversed the dura (Figure 59-14). The CSF leak places these patients at high risk for meningitis.

Two methods of testing can be used to determine whether the fluid leaking from the nose or ear is CSF. The first method is to test the leaking fluid with a Dextrostix or Tes-Tape strip to determine whether glucose is present. CSF gives a positive reading for glucose. If blood is present in the fluid, testing for the presence of glucose is unreliable because blood contains glucose. In this

event, the nurse should look for the *halo* or *ring* sign (see Figure 59-14, *C*). To perform this test, the nurse allows the leaking fluid to drip onto a white pad (4×4) or towel and observes the drainage. Within a few minutes, the blood coalesces into the centre, and a yellowish ring encircles the blood if CSF is present. The colour, the appearance, and the amount of leaking fluid must be noted because both tests can give false-positive results.

TABLE 59-6	TYPES OF SKULL FRACTURES
Description	**Cause**
Linear	
Break in continuity of bone without alteration of relationship of parts	Low-velocity injuries
Depressed	
Inward indentation of skull	Powerful blow
Simple	
Linear or depressed skull fracture without fragmentation or communicating lacerations	Low-to-moderate impact
Comminuted	
Multiple linear fractures with fragmentation of bone into many pieces	Direct, high-momentum impact
Compound	
Depressed skull fracture and scalp laceration with communicating pathway to intracranial cavity	Severe head injury

TABLE 59-7	CLINICAL MANIFESTATIONS OF DIFFERENT TYPES OF SKULL FRACTURES
Location	**Clinical Manifestations**
Frontal fracture	Exposure of brain to contaminants through frontal air sinus, possible association with air in forehead tissue, CSF rhinorrhea, or pneumocranium (air between the cranium and dura mater)
Orbital fracture	Periorbital ecchymosis (raccoon eyes), optic nerve injury
Temporal fracture	Boggy temporalis muscle because of extravasation of blood, oval bruise behind ear in mastoid region (Battle sign), CSF otorrhea, middle meningeal artery disruption, epidural hematoma
Parietal fracture	Deafness, CSF or brain otorrhea, bulging of tympanic membrane caused by blood or CSF, facial paralysis, Battle sign
Posterior fossa fracture	Occipital bruising resulting in cortical blindness, visual field defects; rare appearance of ataxia or other cerebellar signs
Basilar skull fracture	Otorrhea, bulging of tympanic membrane caused by blood or CSF, Battle sign, tinnitus or hearing difficulty, rhinorrhea, facial paralysis, conjugate deviation of gaze, vertigo, bilateral raccoon eyes

CSF, cerebro-spinal fluid.

FIGURE 59-13 Battle sign. Source: Bingham, B. J. G., Hawke, M., & Kwok, P. (1992). *Clinical atlas of otolaryngology*. St. Louis: Mosby.

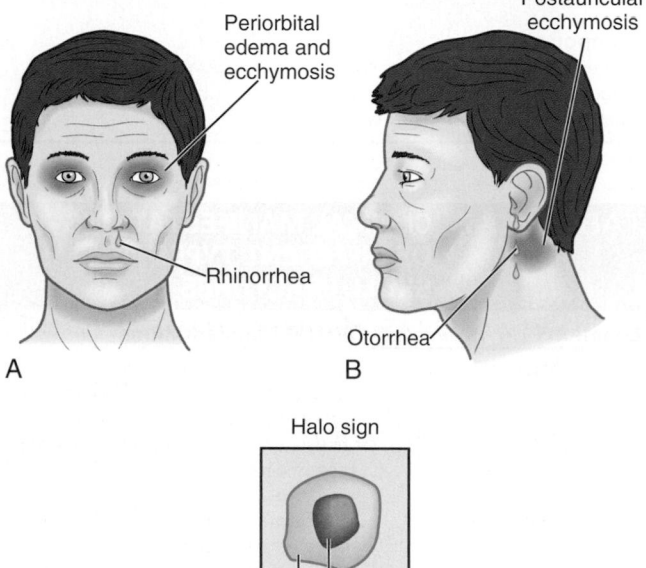

FIGURE 59-14 A, Raccoon eyes and rhinorrhea. **B,** Battle sign (postauricular ecchymosis) with otorrhea. **C,** Halo or ring sign (see text).

The major potential complications of skull fractures are intracranial infections and hematoma, as well as meningeal and brain tissue damage.

Head Trauma. Brain injuries are categorized as diffuse (generalized) or focal (localized). In a *diffuse* injury (e.g., concussion, diffuse axonal injury), damage to the brain cannot be localized to one particular area. In a *focal injury* (e.g., contusion, hematoma), damage can be localized to a specific area of the brain. Brain injury can be classified as *mild* (GCS score of 13 to 15), *moderate* (GCS score of 9 to 12), and *severe* (GCS score of 3 to 8).

Diffuse Injury. Concussion (a sudden, transient, mechanical head injury with disruption of neural activity and a change in the LOC) is considered a mild brain injury. The patient may or may not lose total consciousness with this injury.

Signs of concussion may include a brief disruption in LOC, amnesia regarding the event (retrograde amnesia), and headache. The manifestations are generally of short duration. If the patient has not lost consciousness, or if the loss of consciousness lasts less than 5 minutes, the patient is usually discharged to the care of a responsible adult with instructions to notify the health care provider if symptoms persist or if behavioural changes are noted. Mild TBI is significantly underdiagnosed, and the societal impact is great.

Postconcussion syndrome is seen anywhere from 2 weeks to 2 months after the concussion. Symptoms include persistent headache, lethargy, personality and behavioural changes, shortened attention span, decreased short-term memory, and changes in intellectual ability. This syndrome can significantly affect the patient's abilities to perform the activities of daily living.

Although concussion is generally considered benign and usually resolves spontaneously, the symptoms may be the beginning of a more serious, progressive problem that can continue for years following the injury. At the time of discharge, it is important to give the patient and the family instructions for observation and accurate reporting of symptoms or changes in neurological status.

Individuals with mild or moderate, sports-related concussions are more likely to have future concussive injuries. Recurrent concussions are also associated with slower recovery and may have long-term effects. Patients should be instructed to avoid contact sports until all symptoms have subsided. In addition, return to play should be gradual.

Chronic traumatic encephalopathy (CTE) is the term used to describe degeneration in the brain from repeated concussions, including those sustained during sports. Research is ongoing to examine the link between repeated concussions and brain degeneration (Canadian Concussion Centre, 2017).

Diffuse Axonal Injury. Diffuse axonal injury (DAI) is widespread axonal damage occurring after a mild, moderate, or severe TBI. The damage occurs primarily around axons in subcortical white matter of the cerebral hemispheres, the basal ganglia, the thalamus, and the brain stem. Initially, DAI was believed to occur from the tensile forces of trauma that sheared axons, resulting in axonal disconnection. There is increasing evidence that axonal damage is not preceded by an immediate tearing of the axon from the traumatic impact, but rather that the trauma changes the function of the axon, resulting in axon swelling (axonal ballooning) and disconnection. This process takes approximately 12 to 24 hours to develop and may persist longer. The clinical signs and symptoms include a decreased LOC, increased ICP, decerebration or decortication, and global cerebral edema. Approximately 90% of patients with severe DAI remain in a persistent vegetative state (Wasserman, Koenigsberg, & Feldman, 2014).

Focal Injury. Focal injury can be mild to severe and is localized to an area of injury. Focal injury consists of lacerations, contusions, hematomas, and cranial nerve injuries.

Lacerations involve actual tearing of the brain tissue and often occur in association with depressed and compound fractures and penetrating injuries. Tissue damage is severe, and surgical repair of the laceration is impossible because of the texture of the brain tissue.

When major head trauma occurs, many delayed responses are seen, including hemorrhage, hematoma formation, seizures, and cerebral edema. Intracerebral hemorrhage is generally associated with cerebral laceration. This hemorrhage manifests as a space-occupying lesion accompanied by unconsciousness, hemiplegia on the contralateral side, and a dilated pupil on the ipsilateral side. As the hematoma expands, symptoms of increased

FIGURE 59-15 Coup–contrecoup injury. After the head strikes the wall, a coup injury occurs as the brain strikes the skull (primary impact). The contrecoup injury (the secondary impact) occurs when the brain strikes the skull surface opposite to the site of the original impact.

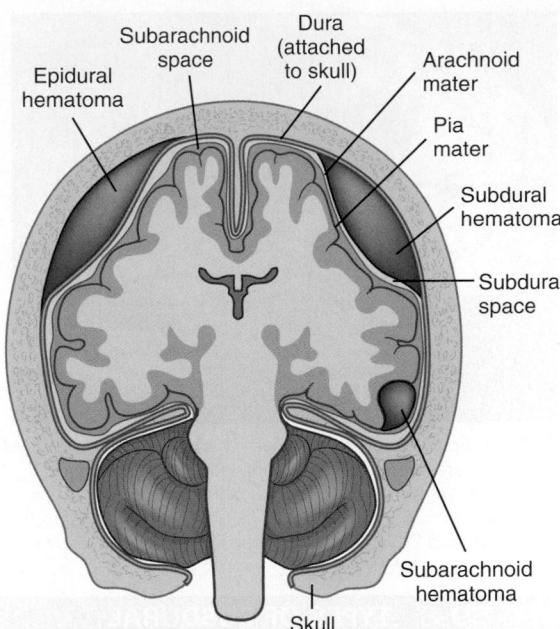

FIGURE 59-16 Locations of epidural, subdural, and subarachnoid hematomas. Source: Copstead, L. C., & Banaski, J. L. (2010). *Pathophysiology* (4th ed., p. 1051, Figure 44-13). Philadelphia: Saunders.

ICP become more severe. Prognosis is generally poor for the patient with a large intracerebral hemorrhage. Subarachnoid hemorrhage and intraventricular hemorrhage can also occur secondary to head trauma. The "Ethical Dilemmas" box considers a case of brain death due to severe brain injury.

A **contusion**, frequently occurring near the site of a skull fracture, is the bruising of the brain tissue within a focal area. A contusion often develops in areas of hemorrhage, infarction, necrosis, and edema. With contusion, the phenomenon of *coup–contrecoup injury* is often noted (Figure 59-15). Damage from coup–contrecoup injury occurs because of mass movement of the brain inside the skull. Contusions or lacerations occur both at the site of the direct impact of the brain on the skull *(coup)* and at a secondary area of damage on the opposite side away from the injury *(contrecoup)*, leading to multiple contused areas. Patient prognosis is dependent upon the amount of bleeding around the contusion sites, which can range from minimal to severe. Contusions may continue to bleed or rebleed and appear to evolve on subsequent CT scans of the brain. Contusions that continue to evolve have a poorer prognosis. Neurological assessment demonstrates focal findings and a generalized disturbance in the LOC. Seizures are a common complication of brain contusion.

Complications

Epidural Hematoma. An **epidural hematoma** is a collection of blood that results from bleeding between the dura and the inner surface of the skull (Figure 59-16); it produces compression of the dura mater and thus of the brain. Epidural hematomas that are a result of a torn artery and are under the influence of a high-pressure arterial system form rapidly. An arterial epidural hematoma is a neurological emergency (Figure 59-17) and is usually associated with a linear fracture to the thin squamous portion of the temporal bone and laceration of the middle meningeal artery or one of its branches. Venous epidural hematomas are less common, are associated with a tear of the dural venous sinus, and develop slowly. Symptoms typically include unconsciousness at the scene, with a brief lucid interval followed by a decrease in LOC. Other symptoms may be a headache, nausea and vomiting, or focal findings. Rapid surgical intervention to prevent cerebral herniation dramatically improves outcomes.

Subdural Hematoma. A **subdural hematoma** is a collection of blood that results from bleeding between the dura mater and the arachnoid layer of the meningeal covering of the brain. A

ETHICAL DILEMMAS

Brain Death

Situation

The emergency nurse receives a radio call from emergency medical services (EMS) personnel about a young man who has been involved in a motorcycle crash. The patient was not wearing a helmet and has a large, open-skull fracture with obvious grey matter oozing from the area. Transport from the accident scene was delayed by 45 minutes as a result of a severe thunderstorm and traffic congestion. On the way to the hospital, the patient has fixed, dilated pupils and a cardiac arrest. Estimated time of arrival at the hospital is still an additional 45 minutes as a result of the severe weather. EMS personnel request permission to stop cardiopulmonary resuscitation (CPR) efforts.

Important Points for Consideration

- Death by neurological criteria occurs when the cerebral cortex stops functioning or is irreversibly destroyed.
- Because technology has been developed that assists in supporting life, controversies have arisen related to an exact definition of *death*.
- Criteria for brain death include coma or unresponsiveness, absence of brain stem reflexes, and apnea. Specific assessments by a physician are required to validate each of the criteria.
- The patient's clinical manifestations indicate that brain death has occurred.
- Although there is a slight chance that the patient's heart function could be resuscitated and supported with mechanical ventilation, there is no obligation to provide medically futile care for a patient with brain death.
- Brain death criteria do not address patients in a permanent vegetative state because the brain stem activity in these patients is adequate to maintain heart and lung function.

Critical Thinking Questions

1. What are the nurse's feelings about cessation of brain function versus cessation of heart and lung function as the criteria for death of a patient?
2. What legislation or practices are there in the nurse's province or territory about EMS personnel stopping CPR efforts in the field?

FIGURE 59-17 Epidural hematoma covering a portion of the dura. Multiple small contusions are seen in the temporal lobe. Source: Kumar, V., Abbas, A. K., Fausto, N., et al. (2010). *Robbins and Cotran: Pathologic basis of disease* (8th ed., p. 1289, Figure 28-11). Philadelphia: Saunders. Courtesy the late Dr. Raymond D. Adams, Massachusetts General Hospital, Boston.

TABLE 59-8 TYPES OF SUBDURAL HEMATOMAS

Occurrence After Injury	Progression of Symptoms	Treatment
Acute Up to 48 hr after severe trauma	Immediate deterioration	Craniotomy, evacuation, and decompression
Subacute 48 hr to 2 wk after severe trauma	Alteration in mental status as hematoma develops; progression dependent on size and location of hematoma	Evacuation and decompression
Chronic Weeks, months, usually >20 days after injury; often, injury seemed trivial or is forgotten by patient	Nonspecific, nonlocalizing progression; progressive alteration in LOC	Evacuation and decompression, membranectomy

LOC, level of consciousness.

subdural hematoma usually results from injury to the brain substance and its parenchymal vessels (see Figure 59-16). The bridging veins that drain from the surface of the brain into the sagittal sinus are the source of most subdural hematomas. Because a subdural hematoma is usually venous in origin, the hematoma is much slower to develop into a mass large enough to produce symptoms. However, a subdural hematoma may also be caused by tearing of small cortical arteries, in which case it develops more rapidly. Subdural hematomas may be acute, subacute, or chronic (Table 59-8).

An *acute subdural hematoma* manifests signs within 48 hours of the injury. The size of the hematoma determines the patient's clinical presentation as well as prognosis. The signs and symptoms are similar to those associated with brain tissue compression in increased ICP and include decreasing LOC and headache. The patient can range from being drowsy and confused to being unconscious. The ipsilateral pupil may dilate and become fixed

if ICP is sufficiently increased. Acute subdural hematoma is most often associated with traumatic injury, and underlying brain injury may result in cerebral edema, worsening the neurological assessment. The subsequent cerebral edema contributes to increased morbidity and mortality despite surgical intervention to evacuate the hematoma.

A *subacute subdural hematoma* usually occurs within 2 to 14 days of the injury. Failure to regain consciousness may point to this possibility. After the initial bleeding, a subdural hematoma may appear to enlarge over time as the breakdown products of the blood draw fluid into the subdural space to reach isotonicity.

A *chronic subdural hematoma* develops over weeks or months after a seemingly minor head injury. The peak incidence of chronic subdural hematoma occurs to those in their 50s and 60s, when a potentially larger subdural space is available as a result of brain atrophy. With atrophy, the brain remains attached to the supportive structures, but tension to the bridging veins is increased and the bridging veins are subject to tearing. The larger size of the subdural space also accounts for the presenting complaint being the focal symptoms, rather than the signs of increased ICP. People with chronic alcoholism are also prone to cerebral atrophy and subsequent development of subdural hematoma.

Delay in diagnosis of a subdural hematoma in older adults can be attributed to symptoms that mimic other health problems in people of this age group, such as vascular disease and dementia. Somnolence, confusion, lethargy, and memory loss are also associated with health problems other than subdural hematoma.

Intraparenchymal Hematoma. Intraparenchymal or intracerebral hematoma is a collection of blood within the parenchyma that results from bleeding within the brain tissue itself and occurs in approximately 16% of head injuries. Usually, it occurs within the frontal and temporal lobes, possibly from the rupture of intracerebral vessels at the time of injury. The size and location of the hematoma are key determinants of patient outcome.

Traumatic Subarachnoid Hemorrhage. Traumatic subarachnoid hemorrhage is a result of traumatic forces damaging the superficial vascular structures in the subarachnoid space. The presence of a *traumatic subarachnoid hemorrhage* may predispose the patient to cerebral vasospasm and diminished CBF, increasing the risk for ischemic damage following brain injury.

Diagnostic Studies and Collaborative Care

CT scan is considered the best diagnostic test to determine cranio-cerebral trauma because it allows for rapid diagnosis and intervention. An MRI scan is more sensitive in detecting small DAI lesions than a CT scan because of the lack of gross pathological changes in brain tissue. Transcranial Doppler studies allow for the measurement of CBF velocity. A cervical spine radiographic study is indicated because cervical spine trauma often occurs concomitantly with head injury. In general, the diagnostic studies are similar to those used for a patient with increased ICP (see Table 59-3).

Emergency management of the patient with a head injury is presented in Table 59-9. In addition to measures to prevent secondary injury by treating cerebral edema and managing increased ICP, the principal treatment of head injuries is timely diagnosis and surgery if necessary. For the patient with concussion and contusion, observation and management of increased ICP are the primary management strategies.

The treatment of skull fractures is usually conservative. For depressed fractures and fractures with loose fragments, a craniotomy is necessary to elevate the depressed bone and remove

✚ TABLE 59-9 EMERGENCY MANAGEMENT

Head Injury

Etiology	Assessment Findings	Interventions
Blunt	**Surface Findings**	**Initial**
• Assault	• Bruises or contusions on face, Battle sign (bruising behind ears)	• Ensure patent airway.
• Fall		• Stabilize cervical spine.
• Motor vehicle accident	• Fracture or depressions in skull	• Administer O$_2$ via nasal cannula or nonrebreather mask.
• Pedestrian event	• Raccoon eyes (dependent bruising around eyes)	
• Sports injury		• Establish IV access with two large-bore catheters to infuse normal saline or lactated Ringer's solution.
	• Scalp lacerations	
Penetrating		• Control external bleeding with sterile pressure dressing.
• High-velocity projectile (e.g., gunshot wound)	**Respiratory**	
• Low-velocity projectile (e.g., knife, bone fragments from skull fracture)	• Abnormal respiratory patterns (e.g., Cheyne–Stokes respirations)	• Assess for rhinorrhea, otorrhea, scalp wounds.
	• Central neurogenic hyperventilation	• Remove patient's clothing.
	• Decreased O$_2$ saturation	
	• Pulmonary edema	**Ongoing Monitoring**
		• Administer fluids cautiously to prevent fluid overload and increasing ICP.
	Central Nervous System	• Anticipate need for intubation for ineffective breathing patterns or absent gag reflex.
	• Asymmetrical facial movements	
	• Bowel and bladder incontinence	• Assume cervical spine injury until proven otherwise.
	• Combativeness	
	• Confusion	• Maintain patient warmth using blankets; warm IV fluids; overhead warming lights; warm, humidified O$_2$.
	• CSF leaking from ears or nose	
	• Decerebrate or decorticate posturing	
	• Decreased level of consciousness	• Monitor frequently for signs and symptoms of increased ICP or decreased cerebral perfusion.
	• Depressed or hyperactive reflexes	
	• Flaccidity	• Monitor vital signs, level of consciousness, O$_2$ saturation, cardiac rhythm, Glasgow Coma Scale score, pupil size and reactivity.
	• Glasgow Coma Scale score <12	
	• Incomprehensible speech, abusive speech	
	• Involuntary movements	
	• Seizures	
	• Unequal or dilated pupils	

CSF, cerebro-spinal fluid; *ICP,* intracranial pressure; *IV,* intravenous.

the free fragments. If large amounts of bone are destroyed, the bone may be removed *(craniectomy)* and a cranioplasty will be needed at a later time (see the Cranial Surgery section later in this chapter).

In cases of clinically large subdural and epidural hematomas, or those associated with significant neurological impairment, the blood must be removed surgically through either a craniotomy or a burr-hole approach.

NURSING MANAGEMENT HEAD INJURY

NURSING ASSESSMENT

The patient with a head injury is always considered to have the potential for developing increased ICP. The most important aspects of the objective data are noting the GCS score (see Table 59-5), assessing and monitoring the neurological status (see Figure 59-11), and determining whether a CSF leak has occurred. (See the Nursing Assessment section for Increased Intracranial Pressure earlier in this chapter.)

NURSING DIAGNOSES

Nursing diagnoses and potential complications for the patient who has sustained a head injury may include, but are not limited to, the following:

• *Risk for ineffective cerebral tissue perfusion* as evidenced by *brain injury, brain neoplasm, cerebral aneurysm*
• *Hyperthermia* related to *increased metabolic rate*

• *Impaired physical mobility* related to *physical deconditioning* (decreased level of consciousness)
• *Anxiety* related to *threat to current status, threat of death* (abrupt change in health status)
• Potential complication: Increased ICP related to cerebral edema and hemorrhage

PLANNING

The overall goals are that the patient with an acute head injury will (1) maintain adequate cerebral perfusion; (2) remain normothermic; (3) be free from pain, discomfort, and infection; and (4) attain maximal cognitive, motor, and sensory function.

NURSING IMPLEMENTATION

HEALTH PROMOTION. One of the best ways to prevent head injuries is to prevent motor vehicle accidents. The nurse can be active in campaigns that promote driving safety and can speak to driver education classes regarding the dangers of unsafe driving and of driving after drinking alcohol or using drugs. The use of seat belts in cars and of helmets for riding on motorcycles are the most effective measures for increasing survival after accidents. It is also recommended that lumberjacks, construction workers, miners, horseback riders, bicycle riders, snowboarders, and skydivers wear protective helmets. The use of helmets when cycling can significantly reduce serious head injury, but not all provinces and territories in Canada have legislation for helmet use (Parachute, n.d.). Nurses can become involved with organizations such as Parachute that attempt to reduce the incidence of injuries among Canadian youth through education, community awareness, and healthy public policy initiatives.

ACUTE INTERVENTION. Management at the scene of the accident can have a significant impact on the outcome of a head injury. Emergency management of head injury is discussed in Table 59-9. The general goal of nursing management of the patient with a head injury is to maintain cerebral oxygenation and perfusion and prevent secondary cerebral ischemia. Surveillance or monitoring for changes in neurological status is critically important because the patient's condition may deteriorate rapidly, necessitating emergency surgery. Appropriate preoperative and postoperative nursing interventions are initiated if surgery is anticipated. Because of the close association between hemodynamic status and cerebral perfusion, the nurse must be aware of any coexisting injuries or conditions. In the acute injury period, treating other life-threatening conditions (e.g., hemorrhage, hypoxia) may take initial priority in nursing care.

The nurse should explain the need for frequent neurological assessments to both the patient and the caregivers. Behavioural manifestations associated with head injury can result in patients who may be frightened and disoriented, may be combative, and may resist help. The nurse's approach should be calm and gentle. A family member may be available to stay with the patient and thus prevent increasing anxiety and fear. Nursing research also validates that one of the most pressing needs for family members in the acute injury phase of care is for information about the patient's diagnosis, the treatment plan, and the rationale for the interventions (Coco, Tossavainen, Jaaskelainen, et al., 2011).

The nurse should perform neurological assessments at intervals based on the patient's condition. The GCS is useful in assessing the level of arousal (see Table 59-5). Indications of a deteriorating neurological state, such as a decreasing LOC, increasingly impaired motor strength, or pupillary changes, should be reported to a physician, and the patient's condition should be closely monitored.

The major focus of nursing care for patients with brain injuries relates to increased ICP (see NCP 59-1 on the Evolve website). However, there may be specific problems that require nursing intervention.

Eye problems may include loss of the corneal reflex, periorbital ecchymosis and edema, and diplopia. Loss of the corneal reflex may necessitate administering lubricating eye drops, taping the eyes shut, or suturing the eyelids closed to prevent abrasion. Periorbital ecchymosis and edema disappear spontaneously, but cold and, later, warm compresses provide comfort and hasten the process. Diplopia can be relieved by use of an eye patch.

Hyperthermia may occur in relation to an infectious process or from injury to or inflammation of the hypothalamus. Elevations in body temperature can result in increased cerebral metabolic rate, CBF, cerebral blood volume, and ICP. Pyrexia increases cerebral metabolic rate, which increases CBF, which in turn can further increase ICP. The nurse should attempt to control hyperthermia and maintain normothermia (goal temperature of 36° to 38°C) in patients with head injuries using strategies previously discussed (see section on Supportive Therapy).

If CSF rhinorrhea or otorrhea occurs, the nurse should inform the physician immediately. The head of the bed may be raised to decrease the CSF pressure so that a dural tear can seal. A loose collection pad may be placed under the nose or over the ear. No dressing should be placed into the nasal cavity or ear canal. The patient should be cautioned not to sneeze or blow the nose. Nasogastric tubes should not be used, and nasotracheal

suctioning should not be performed on these patients because of the high risk for meningitis.

Nursing measures specific to the care of patients who are immobilized—such as those related to bladder and bowel function, skin care, and infection—are also indicated. Nausea and vomiting may be a problem and can be alleviated by antiemetic drugs. Headache can usually be controlled with acetaminophen or small doses of codeine.

If the patient's condition deteriorates, urgent intracranial surgery may be necessary (see the Cranial Surgery section later in this chapter). A burr-hole opening or craniotomy may be indicated, depending on the underlying injury causing the symptoms.

The patient is often unconscious before surgery, making it necessary for a family member to sign the consent form for surgery. This is a difficult and frightening time for the patient's family, and the situation requires sensitive nursing management. The suddenness of the situation makes it especially difficult for the family to cope.

AMBULATORY AND HOME CARE. Once the condition has stabilized, the patient is usually transferred for acute rehabilitation management to prepare the patient for re-entry into the community. As with any cranio-cerebral problem, there may be chronic problems related to motor and sensory deficits, communication, memory, and cognitive functioning. Many of the principles of nursing management of patients with a stroke are appropriate (see Chapter 60). Conditions that may require nursing and collaborative management include poor nutritional status, bowel and bladder management, spasticity, dysphagia, deep venous thrombosis, and hydrocephalus. The patient's outward appearance is not a good indicator of how well the patient will ultimately function in the home or work environment given recovery time and rehabilitation.

Post-traumatic seizure (PTS) disorders are seen in approximately 5% of patients with a nonpenetrating head injury. The time when the patient is most vulnerable to the development of PTS is during the first week after the head injury, though some patients may not develop a PTS disorder until years after the initial injury. Anticonvulsant drugs may be used to decrease the risk for early PTS within 7 days of injury (Thompson, Pohlmann-Eden, Campbell, et al., 2015). Phenytoin (Dilantin) is the anticonvulsant drug of choice to use with post-traumatic seizure activity.

The cognitive and emotional sequelae of brain trauma are often the most incapacitating problems. Many patients with head injuries who have been comatose for more than 6 hours undergo some personality change. They may suffer loss of concentration and memory and defective memory processing. Personal drive may decrease; apathy and apparent laziness may increase. Euphoria and mood swings, along with a seeming lack of awareness of the seriousness of the injury, may occur. The patient's behaviour may indicate a loss of social restraint, judgement, tact, and emotional control.

Progressive recovery may continue for 6 months or more before a plateau is reached and a prognosis for recovery can be made. Specific nursing management in the post-traumatic phase depends on specific residual deficits.

In all cases, the family must be given special consideration. They need to be helped to understand what is happening and be taught appropriate interaction patterns. The nurse must give guidance and referrals for financial aid, child care, and other personal needs and must assist the family in involving the patient in family activities whenever possible. Community referrals for support should be offered. Assisting the patient and family in developing and maintaining hope and keeping communication open are strategies perceived as supportive by families (Coco et al., 2011).

The family often has unrealistic expectations of the patient as the coma begins to recede. The family expects full return to pretrauma status. In reality, the patient experiences a reduced awareness and ability to interpret environmental stimuli. The nurse must prepare the family for the emergence of the patient from coma and must explain that the process of awakening often takes several weeks.

When the time for discharge planning arrives, the family and the patient may benefit from very specific posthospital instructions to avoid family–patient friction. Special "no" policies that may be appropriately suggested by the neurosurgeon, neuropsychologist, and nurse include no drinking of alcoholic beverages, no driving, no work with hazardous implements and machinery, and no unsupervised smoking. Family members, particularly spouses, go through role transition as the role changes from spouse to caregiver.

EVALUATION

The following are expected outcomes for the patient with a head injury:

- The patient will maintain normal CPP.
- The patient will achieve maximal cognitive, motor, and sensory function.
- The patient will experience no infection or hyperthermia.
- The patient will achieve pain control.

BRAIN TUMOURS

It is estimated that 55 000 Canadians are surviving with a brain tumour, and that every day, 27 Canadians are diagnosed with one (Brain Tumour Foundation of Canada [BTFC], 2017a). The brain is a frequent site for metastasis from other sites, as well. The 5-year relative survival rate for brain tumours in Canada is approximately 25% (Canadian Cancer Society, 2017).

Types

Brain tumours can occur in any part of the brain or spinal cord. Tumours of the brain may be *primary*, arising from tissues within the brain, or *secondary*, resulting from a metastasis from a malignant neoplasm elsewhere in the body. Secondary brain tumours are the most common type. Brain tumours are generally classified according to the tissue from which they arise. Meningiomas represent 34% of all primary brain tumours, making them the most common primary brain tumour (BTFC, 2017b). Most meningiomas are benign. Gliomas (a group of tumour types including astrocytoma and glioblastoma multiforme) account for 60% of all primary intracranial brain tumours and are frequently malignant. Glioblastoma multiforme is the most common form of glioma (BTFC, 2017a).

More than half of all brain tumours are malignant; they infiltrate the brain parenchyma and are not amenable to complete surgical removal. Other tumours may be histologically benign, but their location is such that complete removal is not possible. Brain tumours are more commonly seen in middle-aged persons, but they may occur at any age.

Unless treated, all brain tumours eventually cause death from increasing tumour volume leading to increased ICP. Brain tumours rarely metastasize outside the central nervous system (CNS) because they are contained by structural (meninges) and

TABLE 59-10	TYPES OF BRAIN TUMOURS	
Type	**Tissue of Origin**	**Characteristics**
Gliomas		
• Astrocytoma	Supportive tissue, glial cells and astrocytes	Can range from low-grade to moderate-grade malignancy
• Ependymoma	Ependymal epithelium	Range from benign to highly malignant; most are benign and encapsulated
• Glioblastoma multiforme	Primitive stem cell (glioblast)	Highly malignant and invasive; among the most devastating of primary brain tumours
• Medulloblastoma	Primitive neuroectodermal cell	Highly malignant and invasive; metastatic to spinal cord and remote areas of brain
• Oligodendroglioma	Oligodendrocytes	Benign (encapsulation and calcification)
Meningioma	Meninges	Can be benign or malignant; most are benign
Acoustic neuroma (Schwannoma)	Cells that form myelin sheath around nerves; commonly affects cranial nerve VIII	Many grow on both sides of the brain; usually benign or low-grade malignancy
Pituitary adenoma	Pituitary gland	Usually benign
Hemangioblastoma	Blood vessels of brain	Rare and benign; surgery is curative
Primary central nervous system lymphoma	Lymphocytes	Increased incidence in transplant recipients and patients with acquired immune deficiency syndrome (AIDS)
Metastatic tumours	Lungs, breast, kidney, thyroid, prostate	Malignant

physiological (blood–brain) barriers. Table 59-10 compares the major brain tumours. A glioblastoma and a meningioma are depicted in Figure 59-18.

Clinical Manifestations

The clinical manifestations of brain tumours depend mainly on the location, the rate of growth, and the size of the tumour. Figure 59-19 illustrates the functional areas of the cerebral cortex and can be used as a guide to correlate manifestations with the location of the tumour. Some tumours have aggressive mitotic rates and are associated with a rapid onset of symptoms. Tumours such as meningiomas are slow growing and can become quite large before clinical symptoms are noted. The rate of growth depends on the location and size of the tumour and the mitotic rate of the cells of the tissue of origin.

Wide ranges of possible clinical manifestations are associated with brain tumours. Headache is a common problem. Tumour-related headaches tend to be worse at night and may awaken the patient. The headaches are usually dull and constant but occasionally throbbing. Seizures are common in gliomas and brain metastases. Brain tumours can cause nausea and vomiting from increased ICP. Cognitive dysfunction, including memory

FIGURE 59-18 A, Glioblastoma. A large glioblastoma (G) arises from one cerebral hemisphere and has grown to fill the ventricular system. **B,** Meningioma. These two different sections from different levels in the same brain show a meningioma (M) compressing the frontal lobe and distorting the underlying brain. Source: Stevens, A., & Lowe, J. (2000). *Pathology: Illustrated review in colour* (2nd ed.). London: Mosby.

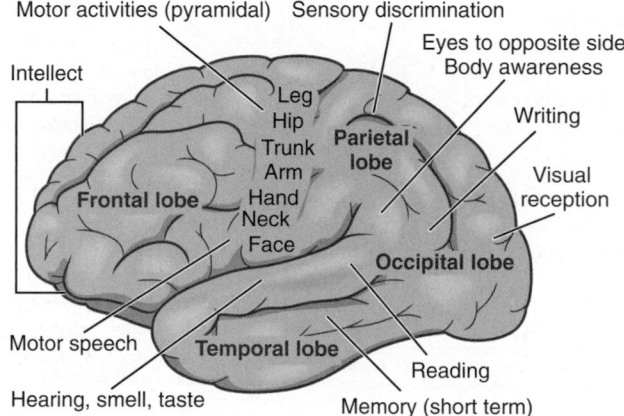

FIGURE 59-19 Each area of the brain controls a particular activity.

TABLE 59-11	BRAIN TUMOUR LOCATIONS AND PRESENTING MANIFESTATIONS
Tumour Location	**Clinical Manifestations**
Cerebral hemisphere	
• Frontal lobe (unilateral)	Unilateral hemiplegia, seizures, memory deficit, personality and judgement changes, visual disturbances
• Frontal lobe (bilateral)	Symptoms associated with unilateral frontal lobe tumours; ataxic gait
• Occipital lobe	Vision deficits and seizures
• Parietal lobe	Speech disturbance (if tumour is in the dominant hemisphere: inability to write, spatial disorders, and unilateral neglect)
• Temporal lobe	Few symptoms; seizures, impaired speech, and memory difficulty
Subcortical	Hemiplegia; other symptoms may depend on area of infiltration.
Meningeal tumours	Symptoms are associated with compression of the brain and depend on tumour location.
Metastatic tumours	Headache, nausea, or vomiting because of ↑ ICP; other symptoms depend on tumour location
Thalamus and sellar tumours	Headache, nausea, vision disturbances, papilledema, and nystagmus occur from ↑ ICP; diabetes insipidus may occur.
Fourth ventricle and cerebellar tumours	Headache, nausea, and papilledema from ↑ ICP; ataxic gait and changes in coordination
Cerebellopontine tumours	Tinnitus and vertigo, deafness
Brain stem tumours	Headache on awakening, drowsiness, vomiting, ataxic gait, facial muscle weakness, hearing loss, dysphagia, dysarthria, "crossed eyes" or other visual changes, hemiparesis

ICP, intracranial pressure.

problems and mood or personality changes, is another common manifestation, especially in patients with brain metastases. Muscle weakness, sensory losses, aphasia, and visuospatial dysfunction are further manifestations of brain tumours. As the brain tumour expands, it may also produce global signs of increased ICP, cerebral edema, or obstruction of the CSF pathways. Manifestations may clearly indicate the location of the tumour by an alteration in the function controlled by the affected area (Table 59-11).

Complications

If the tumour mass obstructs the ventricles or occludes the outlet, ventricular enlargement (hydrocephalus) can occur. As a tumour expands, patients may develop manifestations of increased ICP, cerebral edema, or obstruction of the CSF pathways. Unless treated, all brain tumours eventually cause death from increasing tumour volume leading to increased ICP.

Diagnostic Studies

An extensive history and a comprehensive neurological examination must be done in the workup of a patient with a suspected brain tumour. A careful history and physical examination may provide data concerning location. Diagnostic studies are similar to those used for a patient with increased ICP (see Table 59-3). The sensitivity of techniques such as MRI and PET scans allows for detection of very small tumours and may provide more reliable diagnostic information. CT and brain scanning are used to diagnose the location of the lesion. Other tests include magnetic resonance spectroscopy, functional MRI, and single-photon emission computed tomography (SPECT). The EEG is useful but of less importance. A lumbar puncture is seldom diagnostic and carries with it the risk for cerebral herniation. Angiography can be used to determine blood flow to the tumour and further localize the tumour. Other studies are done to rule out a primary lesion elsewhere in the body. Endocrine studies are helpful when a pituitary adenoma is suspected (see Chapter 51).

The correct diagnosis of a brain tumour can be made by obtaining tissue for histological study. In most patients, tissue is obtained at the time of surgery. Computer-guided stereotactic biopsy is also an option if surgical intervention does not appear to be the most advantageous treatment option. A smear or frozen section can be performed in the operating room for a preliminary interpretation of the histological type. With this information, the neurosurgeon can make a better decision about the extent of surgery. In some cases, immunohistochemical stains or electron microscopy may be necessary to ascertain the correct diagnosis.

Collaborative Care

Treatment goals are aimed at (1) identifying the tumour type and location, (2) removing or decreasing tumour mass, and (3) preventing or managing increased ICP.

Drug Therapy. Corticosteroids (dexamethasone, prednisone, or methylprednisolone [Solu-Medrol]) are useful in reducing cerebral edema associated with neoplasms. Corticosteroids are often prescribed at diagnosis and continued following surgery, until radiation and chemotherapy have been completed.

Surgical Therapy. Surgical removal is the preferred treatment for brain tumours (see Cranial Surgery, later in this chapter). Stereotactic surgical techniques are used with increasing frequency to perform a biopsy and remove small brain tumours. The outcome of surgical therapy depends on the type, size, and location of the tumour. Meningiomas and oligodendrogliomas can usually be completely removed, whereas the more invasive gliomas and medulloblastomas can be only partially removed. Computer-guided stereotactic biopsy, ultrasound, functional MRI, and cortical mapping can be used to localize brain tumours intraoperatively. Complete surgical removal is not always possible because the tumour is not always accessible and sometimes involves vital parts of the brain. Surgery can reduce tumour mass, which decreases ICP and provides relief of symptoms with an extension of survival time.

Ventricular Shunts. Hydrocephalus can be treated with the placement of a ventricular shunt. A catheter with one-way valves is placed in the lateral ventricle and then tunnelled through the skin to drain CSF into the right atrium or the peritoneum. Rapid decompression of ICP can cause total body collapse and weakness, including a headache that may be prevented by gradually introducing the patient to the upright position.

Manifestations of shunt malfunction, which are related to increased ICP, include decreasing LOC, restlessness, headache, blurred vision, or vomiting. This may necessitate shunt revision or replacement. Infection may also occur, as exhibited by high fever, persistent headache, and stiff neck. Antibiotics are used to treat the infection. In some situations the shunt must be replaced.

Radiation Therapy and Radiosurgery. Radiation therapy may be used as a follow-up measure after surgery. Radiation seeds can also be implanted into the brain. Cerebral edema and rapidly increasing ICP may be a complication of radiation therapy, but they can be managed with high doses of corticosteroids (dexamethasone, prednisone, or methylprednisolone). (Radiation therapy is discussed in Chapter 18 and in NCP 18-1, available on the Evolve website.)

Stereotactic radiosurgery is a method of delivering a high, concentrated dose of radiation precisely directed at a location within the brain and may be used when conventional surgery has failed or is not an option because of the tumour location. (Radiosurgery is discussed later in this chapter.)

Chemotherapy and Targeted Therapy. The effectiveness of chemotherapy has been limited by difficulty getting drugs across the blood–brain barrier, tumour cell heterogeneity, and tumour cell drug resistance. A group of chemotherapeutic drugs called the *nitrosoureas* (e.g., carmustine [BiCNU], lomustine [CeeNU]) are particularly effective in treating brain tumours. Normally, the blood–brain barrier prohibits the entry of most drugs into the brain. However, the most malignant tumours cause a breakdown of the blood–brain barrier in the area of the tumour, allowing chemotherapeutic agents to be used to treat the malignancy. Chemotherapy-laden biodegradable wafers implanted at the time of surgery can deliver chemotherapy directly to the tumour site. Other drugs being used include methotrexate and procarbazine (Matulane). Chemotherapeutic drugs can be administered intrathecally via an Ommaya reservoir (see Chapter 18).

Temozolomide (Temodal) is the first oral chemotherapeutic agent found to cross the blood–brain barrier. In contrast with many traditional chemotherapies, which require metabolic activation to exert their effects, temozolomide has the ability to convert spontaneously to a reactive agent that directly interferes with tumour growth. It does not interact with other drugs commonly taken by patients with brain tumours, such as anticonvulsant drugs, corticosteroids, and antiemetics.

Bevacizumab (Avastin) is used to treat patients with glioblastoma multiforme that continues to progress after standard therapy. Bevacizumab is a targeted therapy that inhibits the action of vascular endothelial growth factor, which helps form new blood vessels. These vessels can feed a tumour, helping it to grow, and can also provide a pathway for cancer cells to circulate in the body. (Targeted therapy is discussed in Chapter 18 and Table 18-16.)

Other Therapies. A medical device system, NovoTTF-100A System, is used to treat glioblastoma multiforme that recurs or progresses after receiving chemotherapy and radiation therapy. With this system, electrodes are placed on the surface of the patient's scalp to deliver low-intensity, changing electrical fields called *tumour treatment fields* (TTFs) to the tumour site.

Many techniques to control and treat brain tumours are currently under investigation. These include local hyperthermia and biological therapy. Although progress in treatment has increased the length and quality of survival of patients with gliomas, outcomes still remain poor (Preusser, de Ribaupierre, Wohrer, et al., 2011).

NURSING MANAGEMENT
BRAIN TUMOURS

NURSING ASSESSMENT

The initial assessment should be structured to provide baseline data of the neurological status and the information needed to design a realistic, individualized care plan. Areas to be assessed include the LOC and cognitive function, motor abilities, sensory perception, integrated function (including bowel and bladder function), balance and proprioception, and the coping abilities of the patient and family. Watching a patient perform activities of daily living and listening to the patient's conversation are possible ways to perform part of the neurological assessment.

Having the patient or the family explain the problem can be helpful in determining the patient's limitations and can also provide the nurse with information about the patient's insight into the problems. All initial data should be accurately recorded to provide a baseline for comparison to determine whether the patient's condition is improving or deteriorating.

Interview data are as important as the actual physical assessment. Questions should be asked concerning medical history, intellectual abilities and educational level, and history of nervous system infections and trauma. Determination of the presence of seizures, syncope, nausea and vomiting, pain, headaches, and physical limitations is important in planning care for the patient.

NURSING DIAGNOSES

Nursing diagnoses and potential complications for the patient with a brain tumour may include, but are not limited to, the following:

- *Risk for ineffective cerebral tissue perfusion* as evidenced by *brain injury* (cerebral edema)
- *Acute pain* related to *biological injury agent, physical injury agent* (cerebral edema, increased intracranial pressure)
- *Anxiety* related to *threat to current status, threat of death* (diagnosis and treatment)
- Potential complications: seizures related to abnormal electrical activity of the brain and increased ICP related to tumour and failure of normal compensatory mechanisms

PLANNING

The overall goals are that the patient with a brain tumour will (1) maintain normal ICP, (2) maximize neurological functioning, (3) be free from pain and discomfort, and (4) be aware of the long-term implications with respect to prognosis and cognitive and physical functioning.

NURSING IMPLEMENTATION

A primary or metastatic tumour of the frontal lobe can cause behavioural and personality changes. Loss of emotional control, confusion, disorientation, memory loss, and depression may be signs of a frontal lobe lesion. These behavioural changes are often not perceived by the patient but can be disturbing and even frightening to the family. These changes can also cause a distancing to occur between the family and the patient. The nurse has an important role in assisting the family in understanding what is happening to the patient and emotionally supporting the family.

The patient who is confused and has behavioural instability can be a challenge. Protecting the patient from self-harm is an important part of nursing care. At times when the patient manifests rage and aggression, the nurse must also be concerned about self-protection. Close supervision of activity; use of side rails; use of restraints; padding of the rails and the area around the bed; and a calm, reassuring approach to care are all essential techniques for the care of these patients.

Perceptual problems associated with frontal lobe and parietal lobe tumours contribute to a patient's disorientation and confusion. Minimization of environmental stimuli, creation of a routine, and use of reality orientation can be incorporated into the care plan for the patient experiencing confusion.

Seizures often occur with brain tumours. These are managed with anticonvulsant drugs. Seizure precautions should be instituted for the protection of the patient. Some behavioural changes seen in the patient with a brain tumour are a result of seizure disorders and can improve with control of the seizures by means of drugs (see Chapter 61 for more information regarding seizures and anticonvulsant drug therapy).

Motor and sensory dysfunctions are problems that interfere with the activities of daily living. Alterations in mobility must be managed, and the patient should be encouraged to provide as much self-care as physically possible. Self-image often depends on the patient's ability to participate in care within the limitations of the physical deficits.

Language deficits can also occur in patients with brain tumours. Motor (expressive) or sensory (receptive) aphasia may occur (see Chapter 60). The disturbance in communication can be frustrating for the patient and may interfere with the nurse's ability to meet the patient's needs. Attempts should be made to establish a communication system that can be used by both the patient and the staff.

Nutritional intake may be decreased because of the patient's inability to eat, loss of appetite, or loss of desire to eat. Assessing the patient's nutritional status and ensuring adequate nutritional intake are important aspects of care. The patient may need encouragement to eat or, in some cases, may have to be fed nonorally, by gastrostomy or nasogastric tube, or by parenteral nutrition. The patient with a brain tumour who undergoes cranial surgery requires complex nursing care. This care is discussed in the next section.

EVALUATION

The following are expected outcomes for the patient with a brain tumour:

- The patient will achieve control of pain, vomiting, and other discomforts.
- The patient will maintain ICP within normal limits.
- The patient will demonstrate maximal neurological function (cognitive, motor, sensory) in regard to the location and extent of the tumour.
- The patient will maintain optimal nutritional status.
- The patient will accept the long-term consequences of the tumour and its treatment.

CRANIAL SURGERY

The cause or indication for cranial surgery may be related to a brain tumour, CNS infection (e.g., abscess), vascular abnormalities, cranio-cerebral trauma, seizure, or intractable pain (Table 59-12).

Types

Various types of cranial surgical procedures are presented in Table 59-13.

Stereotactic Surgery. Stereotactic surgery is a precision apparatus (often computer-guided) that assists the surgeon to target a very precise area of the brain (Figure 59-20).

Stereotactic biopsy can be performed to obtain tissue samples for histological examination. CT scanning and MRI are used to image the targeted tissue. With the patient under general or local anaesthesia, the surgeon drills a burr hole or creates a bone flap for an entry site and then introduces a probe and biopsy needle. Stereotactic procedures are used for removal of small brain tumours and abscesses, drainage of hematomas, ablative procedures for extrapyramidal diseases (e.g., Parkinson's disease), and repair of arteriovenous malformations. A major advantage of the stereotactic approach is a reduction in damage to surrounding tissue.

TABLE 59-12 INDICATIONS FOR CRANIAL SURGERY

Cause	Manifestations	Procedure
Brain Abscess Bacteria that caused intracranial infection	*Early findings:* stiff neck, headache, fever, weakness, seizures *Later findings:* seizures, hemiplegia, speech disturbances, ocular disturbances, change in LOC	Excision or drainage of abscess
Hydrocephalus Overproduction of CSF, obstruction to flow, defective reabsorption	*Early findings:* mental changes, disturbances in gait *Later findings:* memory impairment, urinary incontinence, increased tendon reflexes	Placement of ventriculo-atrial or ventriculo-peritoneal shunt
Brain Tumours Benign or malignant cell growth	Change in LOC, pupillary changes, sensory or motor deficit, papilledema, seizures, personality changes	Excision or partial resection of tumour
Intracranial Bleeding Rupture of cerebral vessels because of trauma or stroke	*Epidural:* momentary unconsciousness; lucid period, then rapid deterioration *Subdural:* headache, seizures, pupillary changes	Surgical evacuation through burr holes or craniotomy
Skull Fractures Trauma to skull	Headache, CSF leakage, cranial nerve deficit	Debridement of fragments and necrotic tissue, elevation and realignment of bone fragments
Arteriovenous Malformation (AVM) Congenital tangle of arteries and veins (frequently in middle cerebral artery)	Headache, intracranial hemorrhage, seizures, mental deterioration	Excision of malformation
Aneurysm Repair Dilation of weak area in arterial wall (usually near anterior portion of circle of Willis)	*Before rupture:* headache, lethargy, visual disturbance *After rupture:* violent headache, decreased LOC, visual disturbances, motor deficit	Dissection and clipping or coiling of aneurysm

CSF, cerebro-spinal fluid; *LOC,* level of consciousness.

TABLE 59-13 TYPES OF CRANIAL SURGERY

Type	Description
Burr hole	Opening into the cranium made with a drill; used to remove localized fluid and blood beneath the dura
Craniotomy	Opening into the cranium with removal of a bone flap and opening the dura to remove a lesion, repair a damaged area, drain blood, or relieve increased ICP
Craniectomy	Excision into the cranium to cut away a bone flap
Cranioplasty	Repair of a cranial defect resulting from trauma, malformation, or previous surgical procedure; artificial material used to replace damaged or lost bone
Stereotaxis	Precision localization of a specific area of the brain using a frame or a frameless system based on three-dimensional coordinates; procedure is used for biopsy, radiosurgery, or dissection
Shunt procedures	Alternate pathway created to redirect cerebro-spinal fluid from one area to another using a tube or implanted device; examples include ventriculo-peritoneal shunt and Ommaya reservoir

ICP, intracranial pressure.

FIGURE 59-20 A, Stereotactic frame. **B,** Brain surgery using stereotactic frame. Sources: *A,* Rodw. This file is licensed under the Creative Commons Attribution-Share Alike 4.0 International license, *https://creativecommons.org/licenses/by-sa/4.0/deed.en. B,* Dake. This file is licensed under the Creative Commons Attribution-Share Alike 2.5 Generic license, *https://creativecommons.org/licenses/by-sa/2.5/deed.en.*

Stereotactic radiosurgery is a procedure that involves closed-skull destruction of an intracranial target using ionizing radiation, focused with the assistance of an intracranial guiding device. A sophisticated computer program is used while the patient's head is held still in a stereotactic frame. Radiosurgical techniques can use linear accelerator or a gamma knife. In the gamma-knife procedure, a high dose of cobalt radiation is delivered to precisely targeted tumour tissue. The dose of radiation can be delivered in a few minutes or may take up to an hour or more, depending on the size and shape of the tumour. In some situations, tumours are treated over several weeks.

In combination with stereotactic procedures to identify and localize tumour sites, surgical lasers can be used to destroy tumours. Stereotactic procedures are used to identify the tumour site. Three surgical lasers currently used include the carbon dioxide, argon, and neodymium:yttrium–aluminum–garnet (Nd:YAG) lasers. All three work by creating thermal energy, which destroys the tissue on which it is focused. Laser therapy also provides the benefit of reducing damage to surrounding tissue.

Craniotomy. Depending on the location of the pathological condition, a craniotomy may be frontal, parietal, occipital, temporal, or a combination of any of these. A set of burr holes is drilled, and a saw is used to connect the holes to remove the bone flap. Sometimes operating microscopes are used to magnify the site. After surgery, the bone flap is wired or sutured. Sometimes drains are placed to remove fluid and blood. Patients are usually cared for in an ICU until stable.

In certain cases, a tumour may be infiltrating brain tissue that is involved in essential functions such as language. In these cases, an *awake craniotomy* may be performed. The patient is fully anaesthetized during the opening of the cranial vault and then brought to consciousness once the brain is exposed. Relevant areas of the brain are stimulated to assess function and determine what tissue can and cannot be safely resected. Although keeping the patient awake adds to the complexity and length of the surgery, it enhances the safety of the procedure.

NURSING MANAGEMENT
CRANIAL SURGERY

NURSING ASSESSMENT

The nursing assessment of the patient undergoing cranial surgery is similar to that for the patient with increased ICP.

NURSING DIAGNOSES

Nursing diagnoses for the patient undergoing cranial surgery are similar to those for the patient with increased ICP and may include, but are not limited to, the following:

- *Acute pain* related to *physical injury agent, biological injury agent* (tissue injury, inflammation)
- *Risk for surgical site infection* as evidenced by *invasive procedure*
- *Risk for infection* as evidenced by *invasive procedure* (venous or urinary catheters)

Additional information on nursing diagnoses for the patient undergoing cranial surgery are presented in NCP 59-3, available on the Evolve website.

PLANNING

The overall goals are that the patient with cranial surgery will (1) return to normal consciousness, (2) be free from pain and discomfort, (3) have maximal neuromuscular functioning, and (4) be rehabilitated to their maximal ability.

NURSING IMPLEMENTATION

ACUTE INTERVENTION. Nursing management is presented in NCP 59-1. The patient facing cranial surgery (if conscious and coherent), the caregiver, and the family will be gravely concerned about the potential physical and emotional problems that can result from surgery. The uncertainty regarding prognosis and outcome necessitates compassionate nursing care in the preoperative period.

Preoperative teaching is important in allaying the fears of the patient and the family and also in preparing them for the postoperative period. The patient and the family should be given information regarding the operative procedure and what can be expected immediately after the surgery. Explaining that some hair may be shaved may help alleviate the patient's concern. The family should also be informed that the patient will be taken to an ICU or to a special care unit after the operation.

The primary goal of care after cranial surgery is prevention of increased ICP. (Nursing management of the patient with increased ICP is presented on pp. 1483–1486.) Frequent assessment of the patient's neurological status is essential during the first 48 hours. In addition to the neurological functions, fluids, electrolyte levels, and osmolality are monitored closely to detect changes in sodium regulation, the onset of diabetes insipidus, or severe hypovolemia. The turning and positioning of the patient sometimes depend on the site of the operation. To lessen postoperative cerebral edema, the patient is cared for with the head of the bed elevated 30 to 45 degrees (see the "Evidence-Informed Practice: Research Highlight" box). Maximum swelling in the operative area usually occurs within 24 to 48 hours after the surgery. If a bone flap has been removed (craniectomy), care should be taken not to have the patient positioned on the operative side.

The surgical dressing should be observed for colour, odour, and amount of drainage. The health care provider should be notified immediately of any excessive bleeding or clear drainage. Checking drains for placement and assessing the area around the dressing are also important. Scalp care should include meticulous care of the incision to prevent wound infection. The area should be cleansed and treated in accordance with hospital protocol. Once the dressing is removed, use of an antiseptic soap for washing the scalp may also be beneficial. Sutures or staples may be removed after 7 days. Incisions to the posterior fossa require sutures or staples to remain in situ for a minimum of 10 days.

Monitor the patient for pain and nausea. Although the brain itself does not possess pain receptors, patients often report headache caused by edema or pain at the incision site. Control pain with short-acting opioids and monitor neurological status. Nausea and vomiting are common after surgery and are usually treated with antiemetics.

The psychological impact of hair removal can be alleviated by the use of a wig, a turban, scarves, or a cap after the incision has completely healed. For the patient who is receiving radiation, use of a sunblock and head covering should be advocated if any exposure to the sun is anticipated.

AMBULATORY AND HOME CARE. The rehabilitative potential for a patient after cranial surgery depends on the reason for the surgery, the postoperative course, and the patient's general state of health. Nursing interventions must be based on a realistic appraisal of these factors. An overall goal for the nurse is to

EVIDENCE-INFORMED PRACTICE

Research Highlight

What Is the Optimal Head Elevation to Decrease ICP After Craniotomy?

Clinical Question

In patients who have undergone craniotomy (P), does elevation of the head (I) versus no elevation (C) decrease ICP (O)?

Best Available Evidence

Meta-analysis of interrupted-time-series and randomized crossover experimental designed studies.

Critical Appraisal and Synthesis of Evidence

- 10 (*n* >237) eligible studies were identified that met the following criteria:
  - The study compared different elevations with ICP changes in patients who were postcraniotomy.
  - The study participants had a subarachnoid, subdural, or interventricular monitor.
  - The data included measures of ICP and standard ICP differences (or values could be calculated).
- Interrupted-time-series studies (data are collected at time points before and after an intervention) were used in the analysis as controlled trials were not available.
- Previously published studies demonstrate a decrease in ICP with head elevation; however, most have small sample sizes, and results vary. This is the first published meta-analysis of the optimal degree of head elevation in patients postcraniotomy.

Conclusions

- ICP is significantly decreased when the head is elevated to 45, 30, 15 and 10 degrees when compared with no head elevation (0 degrees).
- 30 and 45 degrees of elevation results in lower ICP than 15 degrees of elevation.
- No significant difference in ICP decrease was noted between elevations of 30 and 45 degrees.
- 30 or 45 degrees is the optimal head elevation to reduce ICP in patients who are postcraniotomy.

Implications for Nursing Practice

- This review provides an evidence base for the standard nursing intervention of patient positioning.
- Nurses can use this information when positioning the head of the bed for patients who are postcraniotomy.

Reference for Evidence

Jiang, Y., Zeng, Y., You, C., et al. (2015). Systematic review of decreased intracranial pressure with optimal head elevation in postcraniotomy patients: A meta-analysis. *Journal of Advanced Nursing, 71*(10), 2237–2246. doi:10.1111/jan.12679.

P, patient population of interest; *I*, intervention or area of interest; *C*, comparison of interest or comparison group; *O*, outcome(s) of interest (see Chapter 1).

ETHICAL DILEMMAS

Withholding Treatment

Situation

A 26-year-old patient in a persistent vegetative state is diagnosed with her fifteenth bladder infection. Her home care nurse must determine whether or not to seek antibiotics for this infection. The family members have expressed a concern that no heroic measures be used to extend the biological life of their daughter and sister, but they have been unwilling to withdraw the existing treatment, which is enteral nutrition through a gastrostomy tube. Should antibiotics be withheld?

Important Points for Consideration

- Patients in a persistent vegetative state do not recover.
- Providing nutrition and hydration, even if by artificial means, can have significant cultural, religious, and psychological meaning to patients and families.
- It is imperative to clarify with the family about the goals of treatment and the patient's wishes, when she was competent and if they are known. It is important to know whether treatment for an infection would be considered heroic based on the family's perspective of what the patient would want.
- The family's concerns about pain, suffering, and quality of life for the patient must be explored within the context of the overall plan of care.
- Withholding treatment is morally acceptable when a competent patient consents to it, if there is no medical benefit to the patient, if the treatment merely prolongs life, or if the burden of treatment outweighs the benefit to the patient.

Clinical Decision-Making Questions

1. How would the nurse approach the patient's family?
2. What might the nurse be feeling about providing nutrition, hydration, and treatments that will prolong life in a patient for whom there is no hope of recovery?
3. What options are available to the family for the care of their daughter once a decision is made about withholding antibiotics?

Mental and physical deterioration of the patient, including seizures, personality disorganization, apathy, and wasting, is difficult for both family and health care providers to endure. Cognitive and emotional residual deficits are often more difficult for the patient and the family to accept than are motor and sensory losses. Although progress is continually being made to help the patient with a brain tumour by means of chemotherapy, conventional and interstitial radiation, and biological therapies, prognosis has not changed. The nurse can provide much help and support during the adjustment phase and in long-range planning.

EVALUATION

The following are expected outcomes for the patient who has had cranial surgery:

- The patient will regain cognitive, motor, and sensory function to the fullest possible extent.
- The patient will be free of infection.
- The patient's pain and discomfort will be alleviated.
- The patient will be free of seizures.
- The patient will have optimal nutritional intake.

INFLAMMATORY CONDITIONS OF THE BRAIN

Meningitis, encephalitis, and brain abscesses are the most common inflammatory conditions of the brain and spinal cord.

---

foster independence for as long as possible and to the highest degree possible.

Specific rehabilitation potential cannot be determined until cerebral edema and increased ICP subside postoperatively. Care must be taken to maintain as much function as possible through measures such as careful positioning, meticulous skin and mouth care, regular range of motion exercises, bowel and bladder care, and adequate nutrition.

Referrals may be made to other specialists on the health care team. For example, the speech pathologist may be helpful to the patient who has speech and language or swallowing deficits or the physiotherapist may provide an exercise plan to regain functional deficits. The needs and problems of each patient should be addressed individually because many variables affect the plan.

TABLE 59-14 COMPARISON OF CEREBRAL INFLAMMATORY CONDITIONS

	Meningitis	Encephalitis	Brain Abscess
Causative organisms	Bacteria (*Streptococcus pneumoniae, Neisseria meningitidis,* group B streptococcus, viruses, fungi)	Bacteria, fungi, parasites, herpes simplex virus (HSV), other viruses (e.g., West Nile virus)	Streptococci, staphylococci through bloodstream
CSF			
• Pressure (normal, <20 cm H$_2$O, same as SI units)	Increased	Normal to slightly increased	Increased
• WBC count (normal, 0–5 × 10^6/L or 0–5 cells/mcL	*Bacterial:* >1 000/mcL (mainly PMN) *Viral:* 25–500/mcL (mainly lymphocytes)	500/mcL, PMN (early), lymphocytes (later)	25–300/mcL (PMN)
• Protein (normal, 0.15–0.45 g/L)	*Bacterial:* >5 g/L *Viral:* 0.5–5 g/L	Slightly increased	Normal
• Glucose (normal, 2.8–4.2 mmol/L)	*Bacterial:* decreased *Viral:* normal or low	Normal	Low or absent
• Appearance	*Bacterial:* turbid, cloudy *Viral:* clear or cloudy	Clear	Clear
Diagnostic studies	CT scan, Gram stain, smear, culture, PCR*	CT Scan, EEG, MRI, PET, PCR, IgM antibodies to virus in serum or CSF	CT scan, skull radiograph, MRI
Treatment	Antibiotics, dexamethasone, supportive care, prevention of ↑ ICP	Supportive care, prevention of ↑ ICP, acyclovir (Zovirax) for HSV	Antibiotics, incision and drainage, supportive care

CSF, cerebro-spinal fluid; *CT,* computed tomography; *EEG,* electroencephalogram; *ICP,* intracranial pressure; *IgM,* immunoglobulin M; *MRI,* magnetic resonance imaging; *PCR,* polymerase chain reaction; *PET,* positron emission tomography; *PMN,* polymorphonuclear cell; *WBC,* white blood cell.
*PCR is used to detect viral RNA or DNA.

Inflammation can be caused by bacteria, viruses, fungi, and chemicals (e.g., contrast media used in diagnostic tests or blood in the subarachnoid space) (Table 59-14). CNS infections may occur via the bloodstream (e.g., insect bites), by extension from a primary site (e.g., ear infection, sinusitis, open skull fracture), or along cranial, spinal, and peripheral nerves (e.g., rabies).

BACTERIAL MENINGITIS

Etiology and Pathophysiology

Meningitis is an acute inflammation of meningeal tissues (the pia mater, arachnoid mater, and dura mater) surrounding the brain and the spinal cord. Bacterial meningitis is considered a medical emergency, and untreated meningitis has a mortality rate approaching 100%. The organisms usually gain entry to the CNS through the upper respiratory tract or the bloodstream, but they may enter by direct extension from penetrating wounds of the skull or through fractured sinuses in basal skull fractures. Cases most often occur in infants, older adults, and members of certain high-risk groups.

Meningitis usually occurs in winter or early spring and is often secondary to viral respiratory disease. *Streptococcus pneumoniae* (pneumococcus meningitis) and *Neisseria meningitidis* (meningococcal meningitis) are the leading causes of bacterial meningitis in adults. *Haemophilus influenzae* was once the most common cause. However, the use of *H. influenzae* vaccine has resulted in a significant decrease in meningitis related to this organism.

Other causes of meningitis are *Listeria monocytogenes* (commonly called *Listeria*), a bacteria found in food that can cause a rare and potentially fatal disease called *listeriosis*. In Canada, listeriosis is a relatively rare disease, with only a few cases each year (Meningitis Research Foundation of Canada, n.d.).

The inflammatory response to the infection of the meninges and CSF (whatever the cause) may increase CSF production, while exudate accumulation leads to blockage of the arachnoid villi, causing obstruction of CSF absorption. The resulting hydrocephalus may cause an increase in ICP. The purulent secretions that are produced spread quickly to other areas of the brain through the CSF. If this process extends into the brain parenchyma or if concurrent encephalitis is present, cerebral edema and increased ICP become more of a problem. All patients with meningitis must be observed closely for manifestations of increased ICP, which is thought to be a result of swelling around the dura, and increased CSF volume.

Clinical Manifestations

Fever, severe headache, nausea, vomiting, and **nuchal rigidity** (resistance to flexion of the neck) are key signs of meningitis. A positive Kernig sign (flexion of the patient's hip 90 degrees and extension of the knee cause pain), a positive Brudzinski sign (flexion of the patient's neck causes flexion of the patient's hips and knees), photophobia, a decreased LOC, and signs of increased ICP may also be present. Coma is associated with a poor prognosis and occurs in 5% to 10% of patients with bacterial meningitis. Seizures occur in one-third of all cases. With meningitis, the headache becomes progressively worse and may be accompanied by vomiting and irritability. If the infecting organism is a meningococcus, early symptoms may include chills, fever, headache, malaise, rash, and petechial hemorrhage on skin and mucous membranes.

Complications

The most common acute complication of bacterial meningitis is increased ICP. Most patients with the infection will have increased ICP, and it is the major cause of altered mental status. Another complication of bacterial meningitis is residual neurological dysfunction. Cranial nerve dysfunction in bacterial meningitis often occurs with cranial nerves III, IV, VI, VII, or VIII. The dysfunction usually disappears within a few weeks. However, hearing loss may be permanent after bacterial meningitis.

Cranial nerve irritation can have serious sequelae. The optic nerve (CN II) is compressed by increased ICP. Papilledema is often present, and blindness may occur. When the oculomotor (CN III), trochlear (CN IV), and abducens (CN VI) nerves are irritated, ocular movements are affected. Ptosis, unequal pupils, and diplopia are common. Irritation of the trigeminal nerve (CN V) is evidenced by sensory losses and loss of the corneal reflex, and irritation of the facial nerve (CN VII) results in facial paresis. Irritation of the vestibulo-cochlear nerve (CN VIII) causes tinnitus, vertigo, and deafness.

Hemiparesis, aphasia, and hemianopia may also occur. These signs usually resolve over time. If resolution does not occur, the presence of a cerebral abscess, subdural empyema, subdural effusion, or persistent meningitis is suggested. Acute cerebral edema may occur with bacterial meningitis, causing seizures, CN III palsy, bradycardia, hypertensive coma, and death.

A noncommunicating hydrocephalus may occur if the exudate causes adhesions that prevent the normal flow of CSF from the ventricles. CSF reabsorption by the arachnoid villi may also be obstructed by the exudate. In these cases, surgical implantation of a shunt may be necessary.

Headaches may occur for months after the diagnosis of meningitis until the irritation and inflammation have completely resolved. It is important to implement pain management for chronic headaches.

Waterhouse–Friderichsen syndrome is a complication of meningococcal meningitis. The syndrome is manifested by petechiae, disseminated intravascular coagulation (DIC), adrenal hemorrhage, and circulatory collapse. DIC and shock, which are some of the most serious complications of meningitis, are associated with meningococcemia. (DIC is discussed in detail in Chapter 33.)

Diagnostic Studies

When a patient is seen with manifestations suggestive of bacterial meningitis, a blood culture and CT scan should be done. Diagnosis is usually verified by doing a lumbar puncture and analysis of the CSF. Variations in the CSF depend on the causative organism. Protein levels in the CSF are usually elevated and are higher in bacterial than in viral meningitis. Decreased CSF glucose concentration is common in bacterial meningitis; the glucose level may be normal in viral meningitis. The CSF is purulent and turbid in bacterial meningitis; it may be the same or clear in viral meningitis. The predominant white blood cell type in the CSF during bacterial meningitis is polymorphonuclear cells (see Table 59-14). Specimens of CSF, sputum, and nasopharyngeal secretions are taken for culture before the start of antibiotic therapy to identify the causative organism. A Gram stain is done to detect bacteria. Variations in the CSF depend on the causative organism (bacterial or viral); see Table 59-14.

Radiographic studies of the skull may demonstrate infected sinuses. CT scans and MRI may be normal in uncomplicated meningitis. In other cases, CT scans may reveal evidence of increased ICP or hydrocephalus.

Collaborative Care

Rapid diagnosis based on history and physical examination is crucial because the patient is usually in a critical state when health care is sought. When meningitis is suspected, antibiotic therapy is instituted after the collection of specimens for cultures, even before the diagnosis is confirmed (Table 59-15).

TABLE 59-15 COLLABORATIVE CARE
Bacterial Meningitis

Diagnostic
- History and physical examination
- Analysis of CSF for protein, glucose, WBC; Gram stain; culture
- Blood culture
- CBC, coagulation profile, electrolyte levels, glucose, platelet count
- CT scan, MRI
- Skull radiograph studies

Collaborative Therapy
- Acetaminophen (Tylenol) for temperature >38.5°C
- Clear liquids as desired or tolerated
- Codeine for headache
- Dexamethasone
- Hypothermia
- IV antibiotics
  - Ampicillin, penicillin
  - Cephalosporin (e.g., ceftriaxone)
- IV fluids
- IV furosemide (Lasix) or mannitol (Osmitrol) for diuresis
- IV phenytoin (Dilantin)
- Rest

CBC, complete blood cell count; *CSF,* cerebro-spinal fluid; *CT,* computed tomography; *IV,* intravenous; *MRI,* magnetic resonance imaging; *WBC,* white blood cell.

Ampicillin, vancomycin, cefotaxime (Claforan), and ceftriaxone (Moayedi & Gold, 2012) are the drugs of choice for treating meningitis. The corticosteroid dexamethasone may also be prescribed before or with the first dose of antibiotics. Although data are limited, administration of dexamethasone appears to be associated with a reduced incidence of hearing loss in patients with bacterial meningitis (Brouwer, McIntyre, Prasad, et al., 2015).

NURSING MANAGEMENT
BACTERIAL MENINGITIS

NURSING ASSESSMENT
Initial assessment should include vital signs, neurological evaluation, assessment of fluid intake and output, and evaluation of the lungs and skin (see Figure 59-10).

NURSING DIAGNOSES
Nursing diagnoses for the patient with bacterial meningitis may include, but are not limited to, the following:
- *Decreased intracranial adaptive capacity* (related to decreased cerebral perfusion or increased ICP)
- *Risk for ineffective cerebral tissue perfusion* as evidenced by *brain injury* (reduction of blood flow, cerebral edema)
- *Hyperthermia* related to *increase in metabolic rate* (infection)
- *Acute pain* related to *biological injury agent* (headache, muscle aches)

Additional information on nursing diagnoses for the patient with bacterial meningitis is presented in NCP 59-2, available on the Evolve website.

PLANNING
The overall goals are that the patient with bacterial meningitis will have (1) return to maximal neurological functioning, (2) resolution of infection, and (3) control of pain and discomfort.

NURSING IMPLEMENTATION
HEALTH PROMOTION. Prevention of respiratory infections through vaccination programs for pneumococcal pneumonia and influenza should be supported by nurses. Several meningococcal

vaccine preparations are available in Canada and are recommended to protect against developing bacterial meningitis. The schedule varies by province and territory. In addition, early and vigorous treatment of respiratory and ear infections is important. People who have close contact with anyone who has bacterial meningitis should be given prophylactic antibiotics. In Canada, cases of pneumococcal meningitis must be reported to the Public Health Agency of Canada.

ACUTE INTERVENTION. The patient with bacterial meningitis is usually acutely ill. The fever is high, and headache is severe. Irritation of the cerebral cortex may result in seizures. The changes in mental status and LOC depend on the degree of increased ICP. Assessment of vital signs, neurological evaluation, monitoring of fluid intake and output, and evaluation of lung fields and skin should be performed at regular intervals, based on the patient's condition, and recorded carefully.

Head pain and neck pain secondary to movement require attention. Codeine provides some pain relief without undue sedation for most patients. The patient should be assisted to a position of comfort, often curled up with the head slightly extended. The head of the bed should be slightly elevated, when permitted after lumbar puncture. A darkened room and a cool cloth over the eyes may relieve the discomfort of photophobia.

For the patient who is delirious, additional low lighting may be necessary to decrease hallucinations. All patients with bacterial meningitis suffer some degree of mental distortion and hypersensitivity and may be frightened and misinterpret the environment. Every attempt should be made to minimize environmental stimuli and prevent injury. The presence of a familiar person at the bedside often has a calming effect. The nurse must be efficient with care but also should project an attitude of caring and of unhurried gentleness. The use of touch and a soothing voice to give simple explanations of activities is helpful. If seizures occur, appropriate observations should be made and protective measures should be taken. Anticonvulsant drugs such as phenytoin (Dilantin) are administered as ordered. Problems associated with increased ICP are also managed (see the "Increased Intracranial Pressure" section, earlier in this chapter).

Fever must be vigorously managed because it increases cerebral edema and the frequency of seizures. In addition, neurological damage may result from an extremely high temperature over a prolonged time. If the fever is resistant to antipyretics, more vigorous means may be necessary, such as an automatic cooling blanket. Care should be taken not to reduce the temperature too rapidly because shivering may result, causing a rebound effect and increasing the temperature. The extremities should be wrapped in soft towels or covered with a thin blanket to protect them from "frostbite." Skin assessment and care should be meticulous. If a cooling blanket is not available or desirable, tepid sponge baths with water may be effective in lowering the temperature. The skin must be protected from excessive drying and injury.

Because high fever greatly increases the metabolic rate and thus insensible fluid loss, the patient should be assessed for dehydration and adequacy of fluid intake. Diaphoresis further increases fluid losses, which should be estimated and included in an intake and output record. Replacement fluids should be calculated as 800 mL/day for respiratory losses plus 100 mL for each degree of temperature above 38°C. Supplemental feeding to maintain adequate nutritional intake via tube or oral feedings may be necessary. The designated antibiotic schedule must be followed to maintain therapeutic blood levels. Observations should be made for adverse effects of the drugs used.

In most cases, patients with meningitis are placed in respiratory isolation for up to 48 hours of appropriate antibiotic therapy. Meningococcal meningitis is highly contagious, whereas other causes of meningitis may pose minimal to no infection risk with patient contact. Routine practices (also called *Standard Precautions*) are essential to protect the patient and the nurse.

AMBULATORY AND HOME CARE. After the acute period has passed, the patient requires several weeks of convalescence before normal activities can be resumed. In this period, good nutrition should be stressed, with an emphasis on a high-protein, high-calorie diet in small, frequent feedings.

Muscle rigidity may persist in the neck and the backs of the legs. Progressive range of motion exercises and warm baths are useful. Activity should be gradually increased as tolerated, but adequate bed rest and sleep should be encouraged.

Residual effects are uncommon in meningococcal meningitis, but pneumococcal meningitis can result in sequelae such as dementia, seizures, deafness, hemiplegia, and hydrocephalus. Vision, hearing, cognitive skills, and motor and sensory abilities should be assessed after recovery, with appropriate referrals as indicated. Throughout the acute and convalescent periods, the nurse should be aware of the anxiety and stress experienced by individuals close to the patient.

| EVALUATION

The expected outcomes for the patient with bacterial meningitis are addressed in NCP 59-2, available on the Evolve website.

VIRAL MENINGITIS

The most common causes of viral meningitis are enteroviruses, arboviruses, human immunodeficiency virus (HIV), and herpes simplex virus (HSV). Viral meningitis usually presents as a headache, fever, photophobia, and nuchal rigidity. The fever may be moderate or high. There are usually no symptoms of brain involvement.

The most important diagnostic test is examination of the CSF obtained via a lumbar puncture. The CSF can be clear or cloudy, and the typical finding is lymphocytosis (see Table 59-14). Organisms are not seen on Gram stain or acid-fast smears. Polymerase chain reaction used to detect viral-specific deoxyribonucleic acid (DNA) or ribonucleic acid (RNA) is a highly sensitive method for diagnosing CNS viral infections. Viral meningitis is managed symptomatically because the disease is self-limiting. Antiviral therapy is not used. Full recovery from viral meningitis is expected. Rare sequelae include persistent headaches, mild mental impairment, and incoordination.

ENCEPHALITIS

Etiology and Pathophysiology

Encephalitis, an acute inflammation of the brain, is a serious and sometimes fatal disease. Encephalitis is usually caused by a virus. Many different viruses have been implicated in encephalitis, some associated with seasons of the year or endemic to certain geographic areas. Ticks and mosquitoes transmit epidemic encephalitis. Examples include La Crosse encephalitis, St. Louis encephalitis, West Nile virus, and Western equine encephalitis. Nonepidemic encephalitis may occur as a complication of measles, chicken pox, or mumps. HSV encephalitis is the most common form of acute, nonepidemic, viral encephalitis. Cytomegalovirus encephalitis is one of the common complications in patients with acquired immune deficiency syndrome (AIDS).

West Nile virus was first identified in Uganda in 1937. The first human case of West Nile virus in Canada occurred in summer–fall 2001. Since that time, the number of cases annually has fluctuated. In 2014, only 21 cases were reported in Canada. (Public Health Agency of Canada [PHAC], 2015a). Advanced age is the primary risk factor for encephalitis and mortality associated with this virus. The incubation period is from 3 to 14 days. Most cases involve mild, flulike symptoms, but about 1 in 150 will result in severe neurological disease, with encephalitis more commonly seen than meningitis.

Clinical Manifestations and Diagnostic Studies

The onset of infection is typically nonspecific, with fever, headache, nausea, and vomiting. It can be acute or subacute. Signs of encephalitis appear on day 2 or 3 and may vary from minimal alterations in mental status to coma. Virtually any CNS abnormality can occur, including hemiparesis, tremors, seizures, cranial nerve palsies, personality changes, memory impairment, amnesia, and aphasia.

Early diagnosis and treatment of viral encephalitis are essential for favourable outcomes. Diagnostic findings related to viral encephalitis are shown in Table 59-14. Brain imaging techniques include CT, MRI, and PET. Polymerase chain reaction tests for HSV DNA and RNA levels in CSF allow for early detection of HSV viral encephalitis. West Nile virus should be strongly considered in adults older than 50 years who develop encephalitis or meningitis in summer or early fall. The best diagnostic test for West Nile virus is a blood test that detects viral RNA. This test is also used in screening blood, organs, cells, and tissues that have been donated.

NURSING AND COLLABORATIVE MANAGEMENT VIRAL ENCEPHALITIS

To prevent encephalitis, mosquito control should be practised, including cleaning rain gutters, removing old tires, draining bird baths, and removing water where mosquitoes can breed. In addition, insect repellent should be used during mosquito season.

Collaborative and nursing management of encephalitis, including West Nile virus infection, is symptomatic and supportive. Treatment for mild cases consists mainly of rest, adequate nutrition and fluids, acetaminophen for fever and headaches, and anticonvulsant drugs for seizures, if necessary. Generally, encephalitis does not respond to antiviral medications; however, the HSV and varicella-zoster virus respond to antiviral drugs such as acyclovir (Zovirax) or ganciclovir (Cytovene), and these have been shown to reduce mortality rates. For maximal benefit, antiviral agents should be started before the onset of coma. Current research is investigating the use of interferon therapy as a treatment for encephalitis caused by West Nile and St. Louis viruses; however, more studies are needed. In the initial stages, many patients require intensive care.

Seizure disorders should be treated with anticonvulsant drugs (see Chapter 61, Table 61-10). Prophylactic treatment with anticonvulsant drugs may be used in severe cases of encephalitis. Treatment of cytomegalovirus encephalitis in patients with AIDS is discussed in Chapter 17.

RABIES

Rabies has been a threat to humans since ancient times. Between 30 000 and 70 000 people die each year from rabies worldwide; however, only 24 people have died in Canada from rabies since reporting started in 1924 (PHAC, 2015b). Louis Pasteur developed the first rabies vaccine in 1885, which drastically reduced the risk for disease transmission from domestic animals to humans, particularly in developed countries where vaccine programs were effectively implemented. The threat is much greater in developing countries. Rabies vaccine is encouraged for individuals who travel globally, since it remains a serious public health concern.

The etiology of rabies is an RNA virus that produces an acute, progressive viral encephalitis. Although rabies is generally transmitted via saliva from the bite of an infected animal, it can also be spread by scratches, mucous membrane contact with infected secretions, and inhalation of aerosolized virus into the respiratory tract. Any warm-blooded mammal can carry rabies, including livestock. Throughout the world, rabid dogs are the most common disease vector. In developed countries, raccoons, skunks, bats, and foxes are the primary animal carriers.

The rabies virus spreads from the contact site through the CNS via peripheral nerves and possibly muscle fibres. During this time (2 to 14 days after exposure), patients experience flulike symptoms, and pain, paresthesias, or numbness at the bite site. An acute neurological syndrome then occurs 2 to 7 days later and is manifested by agitation, hypersalivation, hydrophobia, dysarthria, vertigo, diplopia, hallucinations, and other neurological sequelae (e.g., hyperactive reflexes, nuchal rigidity, and a positive Babinski sign). Coma develops within 7 to 10 days of the neurological syndrome. Death ensues as a result of respiratory and cardiovascular collapse within a few days after the onset of coma. Treatment is a vaccine series to induce active immunity. Because rabies is nearly always fatal, management efforts are directed at preventing the transmission and onset of the disease.

BRAIN ABSCESS

Brain abscess is an accumulation of pus within the brain tissue that can result from a local or systemic infection. Direct extension from ear, tooth, mastoid, or sinus infection is the primary cause. Other causes for brain abscess formation include spread from a distant site (e.g., pulmonary infection, bacterial endocarditis), skull fracture, and a prior brain trauma or surgery. *Streptococci* and *Staphylococcus aureus* are the primary infective organisms.

Manifestations are similar to those of meningitis and encephalitis and include headache, fever, and nausea and vomiting. Signs of increased ICP may include drowsiness, confusion, and seizures. Focal symptoms may be present and reflect the local area of the abscess. For example, visual field defects or psychomotor seizures are common with a temporal lobe abscess, whereas an occipital abscess may be accompanied by visual impairment and hallucinations. CT and MRI are used to diagnose a brain abscess.

Antimicrobial therapy is the primary treatment for brain abscess. Depending on the size and response of the abscess to antimicrobial treatment, the patient may require surgery to drain or remove the abscess if it is encapsulated. Other manifestations are treated symptomatically. In untreated cases, the mortality rate approaches 100%. Nursing measures are similar to those for management of meningitis or increased ICP. However, the distinct difference is the requirement of longer term (6 weeks or possibly longer) antibiotic therapy (either IV or oral) (Brouwer, Tunkel, McKhann, et al., 2014). If surgical drainage or removal is the treatment of choice, nursing care is similar to that described under cranial surgery. Some patients may be clinically well enough after the acute surgical phase to be discharged home. The nurse must be aware of the additional discharge planning requirements of a patient going home with IV antibiotic therapy, if indicated.

CASE STUDY

Head Injury

Source: Andriy
Solovyov/
Shutterstock.com.

Patient Profile

George Roustas is a 33-year-old driver of a motorcycle that ran into an automobile broadside at a high rate of speed. He was sedated, paralyzed, and intubated by emergency medical personnel (EMS) at the scene before transport by helicopter. He was brought to the emergency department with a prehospital report of multiple trauma and an open skull fracture. Paramedics also reported that he was not wearing a helmet.

Subjective Data

He was reportedly unresponsive at the scene, with a Glasgow Coma Scale (GCS) score of 3, hypotension, tachycardia, and shallow, irregular respirations.

Objective Data

At the Scene
- Was unresponsive, with obvious deformity to the left side of the skull
- Respirations were shallow and irregular
- O_2 saturations ranged from 88% to 90%
- Systolic BP ranged from 50 to 80 mm Hg
- Heart rate ranged from 100 to 130 beats/min

In the Emergency Department
- Right pupil, 4 mm nonreactive; left pupil, 3 mm nonreactive
- GCS score = 3
- Hypotension and tachycardia continued in spite of fluid resuscitation

Diagnostic Studies
- Computed tomography (CT) of the head showed left skull fracture, left subdural hematoma, bilateral intraventricular and subarachnoid hemorrhage, and cerebral edema.
- CT of the abdomen and pelvis showed a lacerated liver, multiple infarcts to the right kidney, fluid around the duodenum and pancreas, and multiple left pelvic fractures.
- C-spine radiograph series was negative.
- Chest radiograph showed a right lung contusion and pneumomediastinum and subcutaneous emphysema.

Discussion Questions
1. What could be the cause of Mr. Roustas's hypoxia, hypotension, and tachycardia?
2. How could the injuries affect his neurological condition?
3. What area of the brain do Mr. Roustas's clinical manifestations suggest may be injured?
4. **Priority decision:** What are the priority nursing interventions that should be implemented?
5. **Priority decision:** Based on the assessment data presented, what are the priority nursing diagnoses? Are there any collaborative problems?

⊝volve

Answers are available at *http://evolve.elsevier.com/Canada/Lewis/medsurg*.

■ REVIEW QUESTIONS

The number of the question corresponds to the same-numbered objective at the beginning of the chapter.

1. Vasogenic cerebral edema increases intracranial pressure by which of the following effects?
   a. Shifting fluid in the grey matter
   b. Altering the endothelial lining of cerebral capillaries
   c. Leaking molecules from the intracellular fluid to the capillaries
   d. Altering the osmotic gradient flow into the intravascular component

2. A client with ICP monitoring has pressure of 12 mm Hg. The nurse understands that this pressure reflects which of the following?
   a. A severe decrease in cerebral perfusion pressure
   b. An alteration in the production of cerebro-spinal fluid (CSF)
   c. The loss of autoregulatory control of intracranial pressure
   d. A normal balance between brain tissue, blood, and cerebro-spinal fluid

3. A nurse caring for a client with increased intracranial pressure knows that the best way to position the client is which of the following?
   a. Keep the head of the bed flat.
   b. Elevate the head of the bed to 30 degrees.
   c. Maintain the client on the left side with head supported on a pillow.
   d. Use a continuous-rotation bed to continuously change the client's position.

4. The nurse is alerted to a possible acute subdural hematoma in the client who has which of the following symptoms?
   a. A linear skull fracture crossing a major artery
   b. Focal symptoms of brain damage with no recollection of a head injury
   c. Decreased level of consciousness and a headache within 48 hours of a head injury
   d. An immediate loss of consciousness with a brief lucid interval followed by decreasing level of consciousness

5. During admission of a client with a severe head injury to the emergency department, the nurse places the highest priority on assessment for which of the following?
   a. Patency of the airway
   b. Presence of a neck injury
   c. Neurological status according to the Glasgow Coma Scale
   d. Cerebro-spinal fluid leakage from the ears or nose

6. A client is suspected of having an intracranial tumour. The signs and symptoms include memory deficits, visual disturbances, weakness of right upper and lower extremities, and personality changes. The nurse recognizes that the tumour is most likely located in which of the following areas?
   a. The frontal lobe
   b. The parietal lobe
   c. The occipital lobe
   d. The temporal lobe

7. Nursing management of a client with a brain tumour includes which of the following? *(Select all that apply)*
   a. Discussing with the client methods to control inappropriate behaviour
   b. Using diversion techniques to keep the client stimulated and motivated
   c. Assisting and supporting the family in understanding any changes in behaviour
   d. Limiting self-care activities until the client has regained maximum physical functioning
   e. Planning for seizure precautions and teaching the patient and the caregiver about anticonvulsant drugs
8. The nurse on the clinical unit is assigned to four clients. Which client should the nurse assess first?
   a. The client with a skull fracture whose nose is bleeding
   b. The older adult client with a stroke who is confused and whose daughter is present
   c. The client with meningitis who is suddenly agitated and reporting a headache of 10 on a 0–10 scale
   d. The client who had a craniotomy for a brain tumour who is now 3 days postoperative and has had continued emesis

9. Which of the following nursing measures is indicated to reduce the potential for seizures and increased intracranial pressure in the client with bacterial meningitis?
   a. Administering codeine for relief of head and neck pain
   b. Controlling fever with prescribed drugs and cooling techniques
   c. Keeping the room darkened and quiet to minimize environmental stimulation
   d. Maintaining the client on strict bed rest with the head of the bed slightly elevated

1. b; 2. d; 3. b; 4. c; 5. a; 6. a; 7. c, e; 8. c; 9. b.

⊜volve

For even more review questions, visit *http://evolve.elsevier.com/Canada/ Lewis/medsurg.*

REFERENCES

Badri, S., Chen, J., Barber, J., et al. (2012). Mortality and long-term functional outcome associated with intracranial pressure after traumatic injury. *Intensive Care Medicine, 38,* 1800–1809. doi:10.1007/s00134-012-2655-4.

Brain Injury Association of Canada (BIAC). (n.d.). *About acquired brain injury (ABI).* Retrieved from *http://braininjurycanada.ca/ acquired-brain-injury/.*

Brain Tumour Foundation of Canada (BTFC). (2017a). *Brain tumour facts.* Retrieved from *http://www.braintumour.ca/2494/ brain-tumourfacts.*

Brain Tumour Foundation of Canada (BTFC). (2017b). *Meningioma.* Retrieved from *http://www.braintumour.ca/4879/meningioma.*

Brouwer, M. C., McIntyre, P., Prasad, K., et al. (2015). Corticosteroids for acute bacterial meningitis. *The Cochrane Database of Systematic Reviews,* No. 9, Article CD004405. doi:10.1002/14651858.CD004405.pub.5.

Brouwer, M. C., Tunkel, A. R., McKhann, G. M., et al. (2014). Brain abscess. *The New England Journal of Medicine, 371,* 447–456. doi:10.1056/NEJMra1301635.

Canadian Cancer Society. (2017). *Brain and spinal tumours.* Retrieved from *http://www.cancer.ca/en/cancer-information/ cancer-type/brain-spinal/prognosis-and-survival/ survival-statistics/?region=on.*

Canadian Concussion Centre. (2017). *Research details of the Chronic Traumatic Encephalopathy (CTE) Study at the Canadian Concussion Centre.* Retrieved from *http://www.uhn.ca/ KNC/Research/Projects/Canadian_Concussion_Centre/ Pages/research.aspx.*

Coco, K., Tossavainen, K., Jaaskelainen, J. E., et al. (2011). Support for traumatic brain injury patients' family members in neurosurgical nursing: A systematic review. *Journal of Neuroscience Nursing, 43*(6), 337–348. doi:10.1097/ JNN.0b013e318234ea0b.

Cushing, H. (1925). *Studies in intracranial physiology and surgery.* London: Oxford University Press. (Seminal.)

Dinsmore, J. (2013). Traumatic brain injury: An evidence-based review of management. *Continuing Education in Anaesthesia, Critical Care & Pain, 13*(6), 189–195. doi:10.1093/bjaceaccp/ mkt010.

Fu, T. S., Jing, R., McFaull, S. R., et al. (2015). Recent trends in hospitalization and in-hospital mortality associated with traumatic brain injury in Canada: A nationwide, population-based study. *The Journal of Trauma and Acute Care Surgery, 79*(3), 449–455. doi:10.1097. TA.0000000000000733.

Jennett, B., & Teasdale, G. (1977). Aspects of coma after severe head injury. *Lancet, 1*(8017), 878–881. doi:10.1016/S0140-6736(77) 91201-6. (Seminal.)

Kamel, H., Navi, B. B., Nakagawa, K., et al. (2011). Hypertonic saline versus mannitol for the treatment of elevated intracranial pressure: A meta-analysis of randomized clinical trials. *Critical Care Medicine, 39*(3), 554–559. doi:10.1097/CCM .0b013e318206b9be.

Kawoos, U., McCarron, R. M., Auker, C. R., et al. (2015). Advances in intracranial pressure monitoring and its significance in managing traumatic brain injury. *International Journal of Molecular Science, 16*(12), 28979–28997. doi:10.3390/ ijms161226146.

Meningitis Research Foundation of Canada (n.d.). *Bacterial.* Retrieved from *http://www.meningitis.ca/en/Bacterial.*

Moayedi, Y., & Gold, W. L. (2012). Acute bacterial meningitis in adults. *Canadian Medical Association Journal, 184*(9), 1060. doi:10.1503/cmaj.111304.

Oddo, M., Crippa, I. A., Mehta, S., et al. (2016). Optimizing sedation in patients with acute brain injury. *Critical Care: The Official Journal of the Critical Care Forum, 20*(128), doi:10.1186/s130 -54-016-1294-5.

Parachute (n.d.). *Helmet Safety.* Retrieved from *http://www .parachutecanada.org/policy/item/helmet-safety.*

Preusser, M., de Ribaupierre, S., Wohrer, A., et al. (2011). Current concepts and management of glioblastoma. *Annals of Neurology, 70*(1), 9–21. doi:10.1002/ana.22425.

Public Health Agency of Canada (PHAC). (2015a). *West Nile virus and other mosquito-borne diseases national surveillance report 2014-Final.* Retrieved from *http://healthycanadians.gc.ca/ publications/diseases-conditions-maladies-affections/west-nile -2014-nil-occidental/alt/west-nile-2014-nil-occidental-eng.pdf.*

Public Health Agency of Canada (PHAC). (2015b). *Canadian immunization guide: Rabies Vaccine.* Retrieved from *http:// www.phac-aspc.gc.ca/publicat/cig-gci/p04-rabi-rage-eng.php#epi.*

Roberts, I., & Sydenham, E. (2012). Barbiturates for acute traumatic brain injury. *The Cochrane Database of Systematic Reviews,* No. 12, Article CD000033. doi:10.1002/14651858.CD000033.pub2.

Shawkat, H., Westwood, M., & Mortimer, A. (2012). Mannitol: A review of its clinical uses. *Continuing Education in Anaesthesia, Critical Care & Pain, 12*(2), 82–85. doi:10.1093/bjaccp/mkr063.

Teasdale, G., & Jennett, B. (1974). Assessment of coma and impaired consciousness: A practical scale. *Lancet, 2*(7872), 81–84. doi:10.1016/S0140-6736(74)91639-0. (Seminal.)

Thompson, K., Pohlmann-Eden, B., Campbell, L. A., et al. (2015). Pharmacological treatments for preventing epilepsy following traumatic head injury. *The Cochrane Database of Systematic Reviews,* No. 8, Article CD009900. doi:10.1002/14651858. CD009900.pub2.

Wang, X., Dong, Y., Han, X., et al. (2013). Nutritional support for patients sustaining traumatic brain injury: A systematic review and meta-analysis of prospective studies. *PLoS ONE, 8*(3). doi:10.1371/journal.pone.0058838.

Wasserman, J., Koenigsberg, R. A., & Feldman, R. S. (2014). *Diffuse axonal injury imaging.* Retrieved from *http://emedicine.medscape .com/article/339912-overview.*

RESOURCES

Acquired Brain Injury Network
http://www.abinetwork.ca

Brain Injury Association of Canada
http://www.biac-aclc.ca

Brain Tumour Foundation of Canada
http://www.braintumour.ca

Canadian Cancer Society
http://www.cancer.ca

Parachute Leaders in Injury Prevention
http://www.parachutecanada.org

Encephalitis Global Support Group and Discussion Community
http://www.inspire.com/groups/encephalitis-global/

National Brain Tumor Foundation
http://www.braintumor.org

For additional Internet resources, see the website for this book at *http://evolve.elsevier.com/Canada/Lewis/medsurg.*

Nursing Management
Stroke

Written by: Meg Zomorodi
Adapted by: Denise Elliott

evolve WEBSITE

http://evolve.elsevier.com/Canada/Lewis/medsurg

- Review Questions
  (Online Only)
- Key Points
- Answer Guidelines for Case Study
- Student Case Study
  - Stroke

- Customizable Nursing Care Plan
  - Stroke
- Conceptual Care Map Creator
  - Conceptual Care Map for Textbook Case Study
- Audio Glossary
- Content Updates

LEARNING OBJECTIVES

1. Describe the incidence of and risk factors for stroke.
2. Explain mechanisms that affect cerebral blood flow.
3. Differentiate the etiology and pathophysiology of ischemic and hemorrhagic strokes.
4. Correlate the clinical manifestations of stroke with the underlying pathophysiology.
5. Identify diagnostic studies performed for a patient with a stroke.

6. Describe the collaborative care, drug therapy, and nutritional therapy for a patient with a stroke.
7. Describe the acute nursing management of a patient with a stroke.
8. Discuss the rehabilitative nursing management of a patient with a stroke.
9. Explain the psychosocial impact of a stroke on the patient, caregiver, and family.

KEY TERMS

aneurysm, p. 1512
aphasia, p. 1507
cerebro-vascular accident (CVA), p. 1507
dysarthria, p. 1511
dysphasia, p. 1513

embolic stroke, p. 1511
hemorrhagic strokes, p. 1511
intracerebral hemorrhage, p. 1511
ischemic strokes, p. 1510
stroke, p. 1507

subarachnoid hemorrhage (SAH), p. 1512
thrombotic stroke, p. 1511
transient ischemic attack (TIA), p. 1510

Stroke, or cerebro-vascular accident (the medical term for *stroke*), occurs when there is *ischemia* (inadequate blood flow) to a part of the brain or hemorrhage into the brain that results in death of brain cells. Functions such as movement, sensation, or emotions that were controlled by the affected area of the brain are lost or impaired. The severity of the loss of function varies according to the location and extent of the brain involved. Early recognition of the clinical manifestations associated with the onset of a stroke is vital to ensure that immediate medical attention is sought, which is crucial in reducing disability and preventing death.

Stroke is a major public health concern. Each year 62 000 persons in Canada experience a stroke (Heart and Stroke Foundation of Canada, 2016). Over 13 000 Canadians die from stroke annually, making it the third most common cause of

death in Canada, behind cancer and heart disease (Statistics Canada, 2017). More than 400 000 Canadians are currently living with the effects of stroke, and it is the leading cause of adult disability (Ontario Stroke Network, 2016; Heart and Stroke Foundation of Canada, 2017a). Common long-term disabilities include *hemiparesis* (paralysis of one side of the body), inability to walk, complete or partial dependence in activities of daily living (ADLs), aphasia (total loss of comprehension and use of language or total inability to communicate), and depression. In addition to the physical, cognitive, and emotional impact of a stroke on stroke survivors and their families, stroke also has an enormous financial impact. The direct and indirect costs of strokes are estimated to be greater than $3.6 billion per year in Canada (Public Health Agency of Canada, 2011).

PATHOPHYSIOLOGY OF A STROKE

Anatomy of Cerebral Circulation

Blood is supplied to the brain by two major pairs of arteries: the internal carotid arteries (anterior circulation) and the vertebral arteries (posterior circulation). The carotid arteries branch to supply most of the frontal, parietal, and temporal lobes; the basal ganglia; and part of the diencephalon (thalamus and hypothalamus). The major branches of the carotid arteries are the middle cerebral and anterior cerebral arteries. The vertebral arteries join to form the basilar artery, which branches to supply the middle and lower part of the temporal lobes, the occipital lobes, the cerebellum, the brain stem, and part of the diencephalon. The main branch of the basilar artery is the posterior cerebral artery. The anterior and posterior cerebral circulation is connected at the circle of Willis by the anterior and posterior communicating arteries (Figure 60-1). (See Chapter 58, Figure 58-14, for an illustration of the arteries at the base of the brain.) Genetic variations in this area are common, and some connecting vessels may not be present.

Regulation of Cerebral Blood Flow

The brain requires a continuous supply of blood to provide the oxygen and glucose that neurons need to function. Blood flow must be maintained at 750 to 1000 mL/min (55 mL/100 g of brain tissue), or 20% of the cardiac output, for optimal brain functioning. If blood flow to the brain is totally interrupted (e.g., cardiac arrest), neurological metabolism is altered in 30 seconds, metabolism stops in 2 minutes, and cellular death occurs in 5 minutes.

The brain is normally well protected from changes in blood pressure (BP) by a mechanism known as *cerebral autoregulation* (see Chapter 59). Factors that affect blood flow to the brain include systemic BP, cardiac output, and blood viscosity. During normal activity, oxygen requirements vary considerably, but changes in cardiac output, vasomotor tone, and distribution of blood flow normally maintain adequate blood flow to the head. Cardiac output has to be reduced by one-third before cerebral blood flow is reduced. Changes in blood viscosity affect cerebral blood flow, with decreased viscosity increasing flow.

Collateral circulation may develop to compensate for a decrease in cerebral blood flow. Because of the connections between arteries at the circle of Willis, an area of the brain can potentially receive blood supply from another blood vessel if its original blood supply is cut off (e.g., because of thrombosis). Individual differences in collateral circulation partly determine the degree of brain damage and functional loss when a stroke occurs.

Intracranial pressure (ICP) also influences cerebral blood flow (see Chapter 58). Increased ICP within the fixed space of the skull may cause reduced cerebral blood flow as a compensatory mechanism.

Atherosclerosis

Atherosclerosis (hardening and thickening of arteries) is a major cause of stroke. It can lead to thrombus formation and contribute to emboli. (The role of atherosclerosis in thrombosis and emboli development is discussed in Chapter 36.) Initially, there is abnormal infiltration of lipids in the intimal layer of the artery. This fatty streak further develops into a plaque. Plaques often develop in areas of increased turbulence of the blood, such as at the bifurcation of an artery or a tortuous area (Figure 60-2). Calcified, brittle plaques may rupture or fissure, leading to an inflammatory response. Platelet and fibrin are released and stick to the roughened plaque surface. Plaque may narrow or occlude the artery. Also, parts of the plaque or thrombus can break off and travel to a narrower distal artery. Cerebral infarction occurs when a cerebral artery becomes blocked and blood supply to the brain beyond the blockage is occluded.

In response to ischemia, a series of metabolic events, termed the *ischemic cascade,* occur, including inadequate adenosine triphosphate production, loss of ion homeostasis, release of excitatory amino acids (e.g., glutamate), free radical formation, and cell death. Around the core area of ischemia is a border zone of reduced blood flow called the *penumbra,* where ischemia

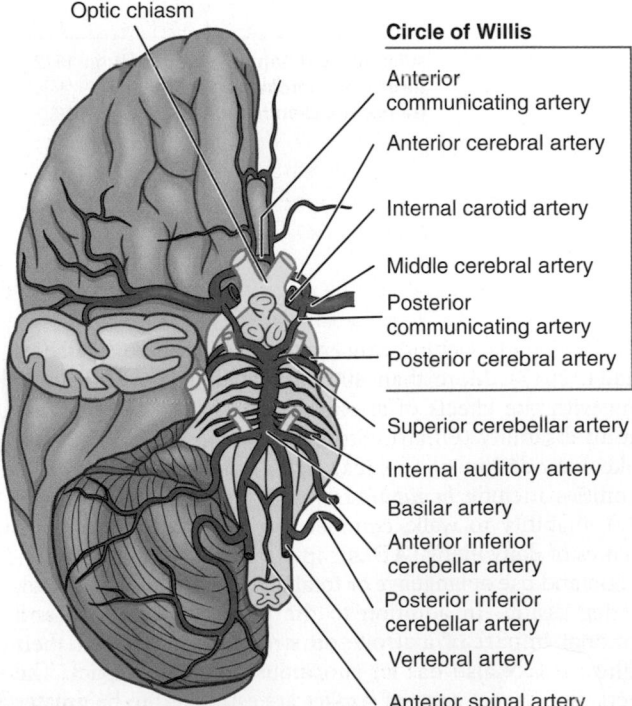

Optic chiasm

Circle of Willis

Anterior communicating artery

Anterior cerebral artery

Internal carotid artery

Middle cerebral artery

Posterior communicating artery

Posterior cerebral artery

Superior cerebellar artery

Internal auditory artery

Basilar artery

Anterior inferior cerebellar artery

Posterior inferior cerebellar artery

Vertebral artery

Anterior spinal artery

FIGURE 60-1 Cerebral arteries and the circle of Willis. The tip of the temporal lobe has been removed to show the course of the middle cerebral artery.

Internal carotid artery

External carotid artery

Vertebral artery

Right subclavian artery

Left and right common carotid arteries

Innominate artery

Left subclavian artery

Aortic arch

FIGURE 60-2 Common sites for the development of atherosclerosis in extracranial and intracranial arteries. The main locations are just above the common carotid bifurcation (most common site) and the start of the branches from the aorta and the innominate and subclavian arteries.

is potentially reversible. If adequate blood flow can be restored early (i.e., within 3 hours) and the ischemic cascade can be interrupted, brain damage may be minimized and less neurological function lost. Research is ongoing to identify thrombolytic and neuroprotective therapies to re-establish blood flow and protect neurons from further ischemic damage.

RISK FACTORS FOR STROKE

The most effective way to decrease the burden of and reduce the incidence of stroke is prevention through awareness and control of modifiable risk factors. Stroke risk increases considerably in the presence of multiple risk factors. The "Determinants of Health" box offers more specific information on nonmodifiable and modifiable risk factors within the Canadian population.

Nonmodifiable Risk Factors

Nonmodifiable risk factors include age, gender, ethnicity and race, family history and heredity, and low birth weight (Meschia, Bushnell, Boden-Albala, et al., 2014; Heart and Stroke Foundation, 2016). Stroke risk increases with age, doubling each decade after age 55. Two-thirds of all strokes occur in individuals older than 65 years, but a stroke can occur at any age. Strokes are more common in men, but more women than men die from them (Ontario Stroke Network, 2016). Because women tend to live longer than men, they have more opportunity to suffer a stroke. A family history of stroke, a prior TIA, or a prior stroke also increases the risk for stroke.

DETERMINANTS OF HEALTH

Stroke

Gender
- Men have a slightly higher risk for stroke than women, although the mortality rates are higher for women than for men.

Biology and Genetic Endowment
- Individuals from African, Latin American, or South Asian descent and Indigenous people are at increased risk for stroke due to underlying risk factors (e.g., hypertension, diabetes).
- Risk for stroke increases with a family history (first-generation) prior to age 65.

Personal Health Practices and Coping Skills
- Illicit drug use (e.g., cocaine, crack cocaine) can lead to stroke.
- Central obesity (waist circumference >84 cm) is linked to a higher risk for stroke.
- Physical inability, excessive alcohol consumption, smoking, and unhealthy diet increase stroke risk.
- Heart healthy diets can reduce stroke risk by up to 80%.
- Stress is associated with increased risk for stroke.

Reference

Ontario Stroke Network. (2015). *Stroke stats and facts*. Retrieved from *http:// ontariostrokenetwork.ca/information-about-stroke/stroke-stats-and-facts/*.

Modifiable Risk Factors

Modifiable risk factors are those that can potentially be altered through lifestyle changes and medical treatment, thus reducing the risk for stroke (Table 60-1).

Hypertension is the single most important, well-documented modifiable risk factor for stroke. Five million Canadian adults, approximately 22.6% of the population, have diagnosed hypertension (Padwal, Bienek, McAlister, et al., 2015). Increases in

---

TABLE 60-1	MODIFIABLE RISK FACTORS FOR STROKE

- Asymptomatic carotid stenosis
- Arteriovenous malformation (in brain)
- Diabetes mellitus
- Heart disease; atrial fibrillation
- Alcohol use
- Hypercoagulability
- Illicit drugs
- Dyslipidemia
- Hypertension
- Obesity and body fat distribution
- Oral contraceptive use
- Physical inactivity
- Sleep apnea
- Smoking

---

systolic and diastolic BP independently increase the risk for stroke. Stroke risk can be significantly reduced through the adequate treatment and early diagnosis of hypertension (Coutts, Wein, Lindsay, et al., 2014).

Heart disease, including atrial fibrillation (AF), myocardial infarction (MI), cardiomyopathy, cardiac valve abnormalities, and congenital defects, is also a risk factor for stroke. Of these, AF is the most important modifiable cardiac-related risk factor, controlled through the use of anticoagulants. The incidence of AF increases with age. Approximately 15% of all strokes are caused by AF, and this risk is greater after the age of 60, when 33% of strokes are caused by atrial fibrillation (Heart and Stroke Foundation of Canada, 2017b).

Diabetes mellitus is a significant risk factor for ischemic stroke. The risk for stroke in people with diabetes mellitus is four to five times higher than in the general population. Although tight control of hypertension in diabetics significantly decreases stroke risk, achieving a hemoglobin A_{1c} less than or equal to 7% and treatment with a "statin" and, if appropriate, a low dose of acetylsalicylic acid (ASA; Aspirin), have been proved to be beneficial (Coutts, Wein, Lindsay, et al., 2014).

Increased serum cholesterol and carotid stenosis are both other risk factors for ischemic stroke. Smoking increases the risk for ischemic stroke two to four times. Fortunately, the risk associated with smoking decreases over time after quitting smoking and, in 5 to 10 years, is reduced to that of nonsmokers (Centers for Disease Control and Prevention, 2017).

The effect of alcohol on stroke risk appears to depend on the amount consumed. Light to moderate use of alcohol, in particular wine, has been linked to reduced risk for ischemic stroke. Heavier use of alcohol does increase risk for stroke. Heavy drinking is defined as >4 drinks per day or 14 drinks a week in men; and >3 drinks per day or 7 drinks per week in women (Meschia, Bushnell, Boden-Albala, et al., 2014).

About 54% of adults ages 18 and older, or 14.2 million Canadians, self-reported being overweight or obese in 2014 (Statistics Canada, 2016). An association between physical inactivity and increased ischemic stroke risk is present in both men and women, regardless of ethnicity. Benefits of physical activity can occur with even light to moderate regular activity and may be in part related to the beneficial effect of exercise on other risk factors. Nutrition teaching is important for individuals at risk for stroke, since a diet high in fat and low in fruits and vegetables may increase stroke risk (Coutts, Wein, Lindsay, et al., 2014). Use of illicit drugs, notably the herbal stimulant khat, cocaine, methamphetamine, and heroin, has been associated with increased stroke risk (Meschia, Bushnell, Boden-Albala, et al., 2014).

An *arteriovenous malformation* (AVM) is an abnormal group of tangled arteries and veins. AVMs can occur anywhere in the body; however, they pose the greatest risk in the brain as these vessels are more likely than others to bleed. Based on the location and size of the AVM, treatment options can include embolization, radiation, or surgery (Toronto Brain Vascular Malformation Study Group, 2012).

The early forms of birth control pills that contained high levels of progestin and estrogen increased a woman's chance of experiencing a stroke, especially if the woman also smoked heavily. Newer, low-dose oral contraceptives have lower risks for stroke except in those individuals who are hypertensive and smoke. Women also face higher risk for stroke during pregnancy and when taking hormone therapy, so their other risk factors should be assessed by a health care provider (Rantanen & Tatlisumak, 2013). Other conditions that may increase stroke risk include migraines, metabolic syndrome, sleep-disordered breathing, inflammation and infection, hypercoagulability, and hyperhomocysteinemia.

TYPES OF STROKE

Strokes are classified as ischemic or hemorrhagic based on the underlying pathophysiological findings (Figure 60-3 and Table 60-2).

Ischemic Stroke

Ischemic strokes result from inadequate blood flow to the brain from partial or complete occlusion of an artery; these account for approximately 87% of all strokes (American Heart Association, 2017). Ischemic strokes are further divided by their causality into *thrombotic* and *embolic*. A TIA is usually a precursor to ischemic stroke.

Transient Ischemic Attack. A transient ischemic attack (TIA) is a temporary episode of neurological dysfunction caused by focal brain, spinal cord, or retinal ischemia but without acute infarction of the brain. Clinical symptoms typically last less than 1 hour. In the past, TIAs were operationally defined as any focal cerebral ischemic event with symptoms lasting less than 24 hours. However, it has been demonstrated that this arbitrary time

threshold was too broad because over 30% of classically defined TIAs show brain infarction on magnetic resonance imaging (MRI) (Souillard-Scemama, Tisserand, Calvet, et al., 2015). Patients experiencing TIAs with imaging that demonstrates tissue damage can have a 20 times higher risk for stroke than patients experiencing TIA without brain injury on MRI (Sorenson & Ay, 2011).

Most TIAs resolve. However, once a TIA starts, it is not possible to know whether it will persist and become a true stroke or resolve. Stroke risk following TIA is greatest immediately after the event; therefore, it is urgent that individuals seek medical attention immediately upon symptom onset (Sorenson & Ay, 2011).

TABLE 60-2	**TYPES OF STROKE**	
Gender/Age	**Warning/Onset**	**Course**
Ischemic		
Thrombotic	*Warning:* TIA	Stepwise progression,
Men more than women	(30%–50% of cases)	signs and symptoms develop slowly, usually
Oldest median age	*Onset:* Often during or after sleep	some improvement, recurrence in 20%–25% of survivors
Embolic	*Warning:* TIA	Single event, signs and
Men more than women	uncommon	symptoms develop
	Onset: Lack of relationship to activity, sudden onset	quickly, usually some improvement, recurrence common without aggressive treatment of underlying disease
Hemorrhagic		
Intracerebral	*Warning:* Headache	Progression over 24
Slightly higher in women	(25% of cases)	hours; fatality more likely with presence of
	Onset: Activity (often)	coma
Subarachnoid	*Warning:* Headache	Acute onset, usually
Higher in women	(common)	single sudden event
Youngest median age	*Onset:* Activity (often), sudden onset	described as the "worst headache of the patient's life," fatality more likely with presence of coma

TIA, transient ischemic attack.

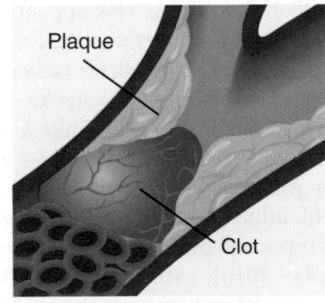

Thrombotic stroke. Cerebral thrombosis is a narrowing of the artery by fatty deposits called *plaque.* Plaque can cause a clot to form, which blocks the passage of blood through the artery.

Embolic stroke. An embolus is a blood clot or other debris circulating in the blood. When it reaches an artery in the brain that is too narrow to pass through, it lodges there and blocks the flow of blood.

Hemorrhagic stroke. A burst blood vessel may allow blood to seep into and damage brain tissues until clotting shuts off the leak.

A   **B**   **C**

FIGURE 60-3 A to **C,** Major types of stroke.

TIAs may be caused by microemboli or plaque that temporarily block the blood flow. TIAs are a warning sign of progressive cerebro-vascular disease (Heart and Stroke Foundation of Canada, 2017c). The signs and symptoms of a TIA depend on the blood vessel that is involved and the area of the brain that is ischemic. If the carotid system is involved, patients may have a temporary loss of vision in one eye *(amaurosis fugax)*, a transient hemiparesis, numbness or loss of sensation, or a sudden inability to speak. Signs of a TIA involving the vertebrobasilar system may include tinnitus, vertigo, darkened or blurred vision, *diplopia* (double vision), *ptosis* (drooping eyelid), dysarthria (a disturbance in the muscular control of speech), *dysphagia* (difficulty swallowing), *ataxia* (loss of muscle control), and unilateral or bilateral numbness or weakness.

Thrombotic Stroke. A thrombotic stroke occurs when a blood clot forms in a diseased and narrowed blood vessel in the brain (see Figure 60-3, *A*). If the narrowed lumen of the blood vessel becomes occluded, infarction occurs. Thrombosis develops readily where atherosclerotic plaques have already narrowed blood vessels. Thrombotic stroke is the most common type of ischemic stroke. Two-thirds of thrombotic strokes are associated with hypertension or diabetes mellitus, both of which accelerate atherosclerosis. Patients experiencing a TIA have symptoms that resolve without interventions, whereas patients suffering a thrombotic stroke have symptoms that will continue to evolve if treatment is not received quickly. In 30% to 50% of individuals, TIAs have preceded thrombotic strokes.

The extent of the stroke depends on the rapidity of onset, the size of the lesion, and the presence of collateral circulation. Most patients with ischemic stroke do not have a decreased level of consciousness (LOC) in the first 24 hours, unless it is owing to a brain stem stroke or other conditions such as seizures, increased ICP, or hemorrhage. Ischemic stroke symptoms may progress in the first 72 hours as infarction and cerebral edema increase.

A *lacunar stroke* refers to a stroke from occlusion of a small penetrating artery that supplies blood to tissues deep within the brain. This most commonly occurs in the basal ganglia, thalamus, internal capsule, or pons. Although many lacunar strokes are asymptomatic, when present, symptoms can cause considerable deficits. These include pure motor *hemiplegia* (paralysis of one side of the body), pure sensory stroke (contralateral loss of all sensory modalities), contralateral leg and face weakness with arm and leg ataxia, and isolated motor or sensory stroke. Multiple small vessel infarcts may also result in a decrease in vascular function (e.g., vascular dementia) (see Chapter 62).

Embolic Stroke. Embolic stroke occurs when an embolus lodges in and occludes a cerebral artery, resulting in infarction and edema of the area supplied by the involved vessel (see Figure 60-3, *B*). Embolism is the second most common cause of stroke, accounting for about 24% of strokes. The majority of emboli originate in the endocardial (inside) layer of the heart, with plaque breaking off from the endocardium and entering the circulation. The embolus travels upward to the cerebral circulation and lodges where a vessel narrows or bifurcates. Heart conditions associated with emboli include valvular heart disease and valvular prosthesis MI, infective endocarditis, rheumatic heart disease, and intracardiac congenital defects such as atrial septal defects and patent foramen ovale. In addition, AF is associated with a four- to five-fold increased risk for ischemic stroke owing to embolism of stasis-induced

thrombi in the left atrium (Meschia, Bushnell, Boden-Albala, et al., 2014). Less common triggers of emboli include air and fat from long bone (femur) fractures.

The patient with an embolic stroke commonly has a rapid occurrence of severe clinical symptoms, but warning signs are less common than with thrombotic stroke. The onset of an embolic stroke is usually sudden and may or may not be related to activity. The patient usually remains conscious and may or may not experience a headache. Prognosis is related to the amount and location of brain tissue deprived of its blood supply. The effects of the emboli are initially characterized by severe neurological deficits, which can be temporary if the clot breaks up and allows blood to flow. Smaller emboli then continue to obstruct smaller vessels, which in turn involve smaller portions of the brain with fewer deficits noted. The embolic stroke often occurs rapidly, and the body does not have time to accommodate by developing collateral circulation. Recurrence of embolic stroke is common unless the underlying cause is aggressively treated.

Hemorrhagic Stroke

Hemorrhagic strokes account for approximately 15% of all strokes; they result from bleeding into the brain tissue itself (intracerebral or intraparenchymal hemorrhage) or into the subarachnoid space or the ventricles (subarachnoid hemorrhage [SAH] or intraventricular hemorrhage).

Intracerebral Hemorrhage. Intracerebral hemorrhage is bleeding within the brain caused by a rupture of a vessel; it accounts for about 10% of all strokes (see Figure 60-3, *C*). Hypertension is the most important risk factor for intracerebral hemorrhage (Figure 60-4). Other causes include cerebral amyloid angiopathy, vascular malformations, coagulation disorders, anticoagulant and thrombolytic drugs, trauma, brain tumours, and ruptured aneurysms. Hemorrhage commonly occurs during periods of activity. There is most often a sudden onset of symptoms, with progression over minutes to hours because of ongoing bleeding. Symptoms include neurological deficits, headache, nausea, vomiting, decreased LOC (in about 50% of patients), and hypertension. The extent of the symptoms varies depending on the amount, location, and duration of the bleeding. A blood clot within the closed skull can result in a mass that causes pressure on brain tissue, displaces brain tissue, and decreases cerebral blood flow, leading to ischemia and infarction.

Approximately 50% of intracerebral hemorrhages occur in the putamen and the internal capsule, central white matter, thalamus, cerebellar hemispheres, and pons. Initially, patients experience a severe headache with nausea and vomiting. Clinical manifestations of bleeding within the putamen and internal capsule include weakness of one side (including face, arm, and leg), slurred speech, and deviation of the eyes. Progression of symptoms related to a severe hemorrhage includes hemiplegia, fixed and dilated pupils, abnormal body posturing, and coma. Thalamic hemorrhage results in hemiplegia with more sensory than motor loss. Bleeding into the subthalamic areas of the brain leads to problems with vision and eye movement. Cerebellar hemorrhages are characterized by severe headache, vomiting, loss of ability to walk, dysphagia, dysarthria, and eye movement disturbances. Hemorrhage in the pons is the most serious because basic life functions (e.g., respiration) are rapidly affected. Hemorrhage in the pons can be characterized by hemiplegia leading to complete paralysis, coma, abnormal body posturing, fixed pupils (small in size), hyperthermia, and death. It is difficult to predict the prognosis of patients with intracerebral hemorrhage. Early

FIGURE 60-4 Massive hypertensive hemorrhage rupturing into a lateral ventricle of the brain. Source: Kumar, V., Abbas, A. K., Fausto, N., et al. (2010). *Robbins and Cotran pathologic basis of disease* (8th ed., p. 1296, Figure 28-18). Philadelphia: Saunders.

recognition and aggressive medical management are associated with improved outcomes. Factors such as the patient's age, initial Glasgow Coma Scale (GCS) score, and location and volume of hemorrhage play a role in decision making and prognostication (Hemphill, Greenberg, Anderson, et al., 2015).

Subarachnoid Hemorrhage. Subarachnoid hemorrhage (SAH) occurs when there is intracranial bleeding into the cerebro-spinal fluid (CSF)–filled space between the arachnoid and the pia mater membranes on the surface of the brain. SAH is commonly caused by rupture of a cerebral aneurysm (congenital or acquired permanent, localized outpouching or dilation of the blood vessel wall). Aneurysms may vary in shape and can be described as saccular or berry aneurysms, ranging from a few millimetres to 20 to 30 mm in size, or fusiform atherosclerotic aneurysms. The majority of aneurysms are in the circle of Willis. Other causes of SAH include AVMs, trauma, and illicit drug (cocaine) use. About 25% of people who have a hemorrhagic stroke owing to a ruptured aneurysm die, and 50% of survivors have persistent neurological deficits. The incidence of SAH caused by a ruptured aneurysm increases with age and is higher in women than in men (Connolly, Rabinstein, Carhuapoma, et al., 2012).

The patient may have warning symptoms if the ballooning artery applies pressure to brain tissue or if an aneurysm leaks before major rupture. Overall, cerebral aneurysms are viewed as a "silent killer" because individuals usually do not have warning signs of an aneurysm until rupture has occurred.

SAFETY ALERT

Sudden onset of a severe headache that is different from a previous headache and typically the "worst headache of one's life" is characteristic of a ruptured aneurysm, and individuals experiencing it should seek medical attention immediately.

Loss of consciousness may or may not occur. The patient's LOC may range from alert to comatose, depending on the severity of the bleed. Other symptoms include focal neurological deficits (including cranial nerve deficits), nausea, vomiting, seizures, and stiff neck. Improvements in surgical techniques and aggressive medical management of complications have led to better outcomes; however, many patients are left with significant morbidity, including cognitive difficulties.

Complications of aneurysmal SAH include rebleeding before surgery or other therapy is initiated and cerebral vasospasm (narrowing of the large blood vessels at the base of the brain), which can result in cerebral infarction. Cerebral vasospasm is most likely owing to an interaction between the metabolites of blood and the vascular smooth muscle. During the lysis of subarachnoid blood clots, metabolites are released. These metabolites can cause endothelial damage and vasoconstriction. In addition, release of endothelin (a potent vasoconstrictor) may play a major role in the induction of cerebral vasospasm after SAH. Peak time for vasospasm to occur is 7 to 10 days after the initial bleed.

Clinical Manifestations of Stroke

The neurological manifestations do not significantly differ between ischemic and hemorrhagic stroke. The reason for this is that destruction of neural tissue is the basis for neurological dysfunction caused by both types of stroke. The clinical manifestations are related to location of the stroke. Specific manifestations related to the type of stroke are discussed in the previous section on types of stroke.

The general clinical manifestations of ischemic and hemorrhagic stroke are discussed together in this section. A stroke can have an effect on many body functions, including motor activity, bladder and bowel elimination, intellectual function, spatial–perceptual alterations, personality, affect, sensation, and communication. The functions affected are directly related to the artery involved and the area of the brain it supplies (Table 60-3). Manifestations related to right- and left-brain damage differ somewhat and are shown in Figure 60-5.

Motor Function. Motor deficits are the most obvious effect of stroke. Motor deficits include impairment of (a) mobility, (b) respiratory function, (c) swallowing and speech, (d) gag reflex, and (e) self-care abilities. Symptoms are caused by the destruction of motor neurons in the pyramidal pathway (nerve fibres from the brain and passing through the spinal cord to the motor cells). The characteristic motor deficits include loss of skilled voluntary movement *(akinesia),* impairment of integration of movements, alterations in muscle tone, and alterations in reflexes. The initial *hyporeflexia* (depressed reflexes) progresses to *hyperreflexia* (hyperactive reflexes) for most patients.

Motor deficits after a stroke follow certain specific patterns. A lesion on one side of the brain affects facial features on the same side as the lesion *(ipsilateral);* however, because the pyramidal pathway crosses at the level of the medulla, motor function on the opposite side of the brain lesion becomes impaired *(contralateral).* The arms and legs of the affected side may be weakened or paralyzed to different degrees depending on which part of and to what extent the cerebral circulation was compromised. A stroke

TABLE 60-3 STROKE MANIFESTATIONS RELATED TO ARTERY INVOLVEMENT

Artery	Deficit or Syndrome
Anterior cerebral	Motor or sensory deficit (contralateral) or both, sucking or rooting reflex, rigidity, gait problems, loss of proprioception, fine touch
Middle cerebral	*Dominant side:* Aphasia, motor and sensory deficit, *hemianopia* (blindness over half the field of vision)
	Nondominant side: Neglect, motor and sensory deficit, hemianopia
Posterior cerebral	Hemianopia, visual hallucination, spontaneous pain, motor deficit
Vertebral	Cranial nerve deficits, diplopia, dizziness, nausea, vomiting, dysarthria, dysphagia, coma

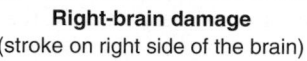

Right-brain damage (stroke on right side of the brain)	Left-brain damage (stroke on left side of the brain)
• Paralyzed left side: hemiplegia	• Paralyzed right side: hemiplegia
• Left-sided neglect	• Impaired speech–language (aphasias)
• Spatial–perceptual deficits	• Impaired right–left discrimination
• Tends to deny or minimize problems	• Slow performance, cautious
• Rapid performance, short attention span	• Aware of deficits: depression, anxiety
• Impulsive; safety problems	• Impaired comprehension related to language, math
• Impaired judgement	
• Impaired time concepts	

FIGURE 60-5 Manifestations of right-brain and left-brain stroke.

affecting the middle cerebral artery leads to a greater weakness in the upper extremity than the lower extremity. The affected shoulder tends to rotate internally and the hip rotates externally. The affected foot is plantar flexed and inverted. An initial period of flaccidity may last from days to several weeks and is related to nerve damage. Spasticity of the muscles follows the flaccid stage and is related to interruption of upper motor neuron influence.

Communication. The left hemisphere is dominant for language skills in right-handed persons and in most left-handed persons. Language disorders involve expression and comprehension of written and spoken words. The patient may experience aphasia affecting the comprehension of language, the ability to speak, or both. It occurs when a stroke damages the dominant hemisphere of the brain. **Dysphasia** refers to impaired ability to communicate. However, in most settings, the terms *aphasia* and *dysphasia* are used interchangeably to mean the same thing, with *aphasia* often being the more common term used.

According to the National Institute of Neurological Disorders and Stroke (NINDS, 2017), there are four categories of aphasia: (a) *Expressive aphasia* (also called *Broca's aphasia*) is difficulty in expressing thoughts through speech or writing. The patient cannot find the words needed but does know what he or she wants to say. The stroke survivor's speech is reduced often to fewer than four words. (b) *Receptive aphasia* (also called *Wernicke's aphasia*) is difficulty understanding spoken or written language. These patients are difficult to understand. They speak without hesitation, but words may be used incorrectly and sentences may be ungrammatical. (c) *Anomic* or *amnesic aphasia* is the least severe form of aphasia and involves problems finding the correct names for specific objects, people, places, or events. (d) *Global aphasia* results in loss of all expressive and receptive function. It is usually caused by a massive stroke. Some aphasia is mixed, with impairment in both expression and understanding.

Many stroke patients also experience dysarthria, a disturbance in the muscular control of speech. Impairments may involve pronunciation, articulation, and phonation (use of the voice). Dysarthria does not affect the meaning of communication or the comprehension of language, but it does affect the mechanics of speech. Some patients experience a combination of aphasia and dysarthria.

Affect. Patients who have had a stroke may have difficulty controlling their emotions, and so emotional responses may be exaggerated or unpredictable. Depression, common in the first year following a stroke (National Stroke Association, 2017), and feelings associated with changes in body image and loss of function can make this worse. Patients may also be frustrated by mobility and communication problems.

Intellectual Function. Both memory and judgement may be impaired as a result of stroke. These impairments can occur with strokes affecting either side of the brain. A left-brain stroke is more likely to result in memory problems related to language. Patients with a left-brain stroke often are very cautious in making judgements. The patient with a right-brain stroke tends to be impulsive and to move quickly. An example of behaviour with right-brain stroke is the patient who tries to rise quickly from the wheelchair without locking the wheels or raising the foot rests. The patient with a left-brain stroke would move slowly and cautiously from the wheelchair. Patients with either type of stroke may have difficulty making generalizations, which interferes with their ability to learn.

Spatial–Perceptual Alterations. A stroke on the right side of the brain is more likely to cause problems in spatial–perceptual orientation, although these issues can also occur with left-brain stroke. Spatial–perceptual problems may be divided into four categories:

1. The patient's incorrect perception of self and illness. This deficit follows damage to the parietal lobe. Patients may deny their illnesses or their own body parts *(anosognosia).*
2. The patient's erroneous perception of self in space. The patient may neglect all input from the affected side. This may be worsened by *homonymous hemianopia,* in which blindness occurs in the same half of the visual fields of both eyes. The

patient also has difficulty with spatial orientation, such as judging distances.

3. *Agnosia,* the inability to recognize an object by sight, touch, or hearing.
4. *Apraxia,* the inability to carry out learned sequential movements on command.

Patients may or may not be aware of their spatial–perceptual alterations.

Elimination. Fortunately, most problems with urinary and bowel elimination that occur initially are temporary. When a stroke affects one hemisphere of the brain, the prognosis for normal bladder function is excellent. At least partial sensation for bladder filling remains, and voluntary urination is present. Initially, the patient may experience frequency, urgency, and incontinence. Although motor control of the bowel is usually not a problem, patients frequently become constipated. Constipation is associated with immobility, weak abdominal muscles, dehydration, and diminished response to the defecation reflex. Urinary and bowel elimination problems may also be related to inability to express needs and to manage clothing.

Diagnostic Studies

When manifestations of a stroke occur, diagnostic studies are done to (a) confirm that it is a stroke and not another brain lesion, such as a subdural hematoma, and (b) identify the likely cause of the stroke (Table 60-4). Tests also guide decisions about therapy to prevent a secondary stroke. The single most important timely primary assessment tool for a stroke patient is brain imaging—either MRI or noncontrast computed tomographic (CT) scan (Casaubon, Boulanger, Blacquiere, et al., 2015). The CT scan is quick and easy to access in most facilities. It should optimally be obtained within 25 minutes and read within 45

TABLE 60-4   DIAGNOSTIC STUDIES

Stroke

Diagnosis of Stroke (Including Extent of Involvement) • Computed tomographic (CT) scan • CT angiography (CTA) • Magnetic resonance angiography (MRA) • Magnetic resonance imaging (MRI) **Cerebral Blood Flow** • Carotid angiography • Carotid duplex scanning • Cerebral angiography • Digital subtraction angiography • Transcranial Doppler ultrasonography **Cardiac Assessment** • Cardiac markers (troponin, creatine kinase–MB) • Chest radiograph	• Echocardiography (transthoracic, transesophageal) • Electrocardiogram **Additional Studies** • Cerebro-spinal fluid (CSF) analysis* • Coagulation studies: prothrombin time/international normalized ratio (INR), activated partial thromboplastin time (aPTT) • Complete blood cell count (CBC) including platelets • Electrolytes, blood glucose; hemoglobin A_{1c} (Hb A_{1c}) • Lipid profile • Renal and hepatic studies

*A lumbar puncture to obtain CSF is avoided if increased intracranial pressure is suspected because this procedure can cause a low-pressure shunt, drawing the CSF fluid down the spinal column. As the CSF pressure decreases, CSF and brain mass may shift toward the lower pressure area, causing herniation of the brain (see Chapter 58).

minutes of arrival at the emergency department. The CT scan indicates the size and location of the lesion and helps to differentiate between ischemic and hemorrhagic stroke. Serial CT scans may be used to assess the effectiveness of treatment and to evaluate recovery.

Computed tomographic angiography (CTA) provides visualization of cerebral vasculature and can be performed after or at the same time as the noncontrast CT scan. CTA can provide an estimate of perfusion and detect defects in the cerebral arteries.

MRI is used to determine the extent of brain injury and has greater specificity than CT in determining the location of vascular lesions and blockages. Patient preparation and access to an MRI scanner can be delayed for many reasons but should not delay the patient having alternative diagnostic studies performed. Magnetic resonance angiography can detect vascular lesions and blockages, similar to CTA.

Angiography can identify cervical and cerebro-vascular occlusion, atherosclerotic plaques, and malformation of vessels. Cerebral angiography is a definitive study to identify the source of SAH. Risks of angiography include dislodging an embolus, vasospasm, inducing further hemorrhage, and allergic reaction to contrast media.

Intra-arterial digital subtraction angiography uses a smaller dose of contrast material, uses smaller catheters, and is a shorter procedure compared with conventional angiography. Digital subtraction angiography involves the injection of a contrast agent to visualize blood vessels in the neck and the large vessels of the circle of Willis. It is considered safer than cerebral angiography because less vascular manipulation is required.

Transcranial Doppler ultrasonography is a noninvasive study that measures the velocity of blood flow in the major cerebral arteries. Transcranial Doppler has been shown to be effective in detecting microemboli and vasospasm and is ideal for patients confirmed to have SAH. Carotid duplex scanning is used not only to detect the cause of the stroke but also to stratify patients for either medical management or carotid intervention if they have carotid stenosis.

If the suspected cause of the stroke includes emboli from the heart, diagnostic cardiac tests should be done (see Table 60-4). Blood tests are also done to help identify conditions contributing to stroke and to guide treatment (see Table 60-4).

Collaborative Care

Prevention Therapy. Primary prevention is a priority for decreasing morbidity and mortality from stroke (Table 60-5). The goals of stroke prevention include health management for the well individual and education and management of modifiable risk factors to prevent a primary or secondary stroke. Health management focuses on (a) BP control, (b) blood glucose control, (c) diet and exercise, (d) smoking cessation, (e) limiting alcohol consumption, and (f) routine health assessments. Patients with known risk factors such as diabetes mellitus, hypertension, smoking, high serum lipids, or cardiovascular dysfunction require close management.

Drug Therapy. Measures to prevent the development of a thrombus or embolus are used in patients with TIAs because they are at risk for stroke. Antiplatelet drugs are usually the chosen treatment to prevent stroke in patients who have had a TIA. ASA (Aspirin) is the most frequently used antiplatelet agent, commonly at a dose of 81 to 325 mg/day. Drug therapy may also include clopidogrel (Plavix). Oral anticoagulation using apixaban (Eliquis), dabigatran (Pradaxa), or rivaroxaban (Xarelto)

TABLE 60-5 COLLABORATIVE CARE

Stroke

Diagnostic
- History and physical examination
- See Table 60-4

Collaborative Therapy
Prevention
- Control of hypertension
- Control of diabetes mellitus
- Treatment of underlying cardiac problem

Lifestyle Modifications
- Limiting of alcohol intake
- Increase in exercise
- Weight loss to normalize BMI
- Reduction of sodium intake
- Smoking cessation

Drug Therapy
- Anticoagulation therapy for patients with atrial fibrillation (if indicated by use of the CHADS2 classification)
- Platelet inhibitors (e.g., acetylsalicylic acid [ASA; Aspirin])

Surgical Therapy
- Carotid endarterectomy (see Figure 60-6)

- Extracranial–intracranial bypass
- Stenting of carotid artery
- Surgical interventions for aneurysms at risk of bleeding
- Transluminal angioplasty

Acute Care
- DVT prevention with LMWH
- Fluid therapy
- Maintenance of airway
- Prevention of secondary injury
- Treatment of cerebral edema

Ischemic Stroke
- Endovascular treatment
- Tissue plasminogen activator (tPA)

Hemorrhagic Stroke
- Clipping or coiling of aneurysm
- Surgical decompression if indicated

Embolic Stroke
- Treatment of underlying cause (usually cardiac related)

BMI, body mass index; *CHADS2,* clinical prediction rule used to estimate the risk for stroke in patients with atrial fibrillation and to determine the degree of anticoagulation required; *DVT,* deep-vein thrombosis; *LMWH,* low-molecular-weight heparin.

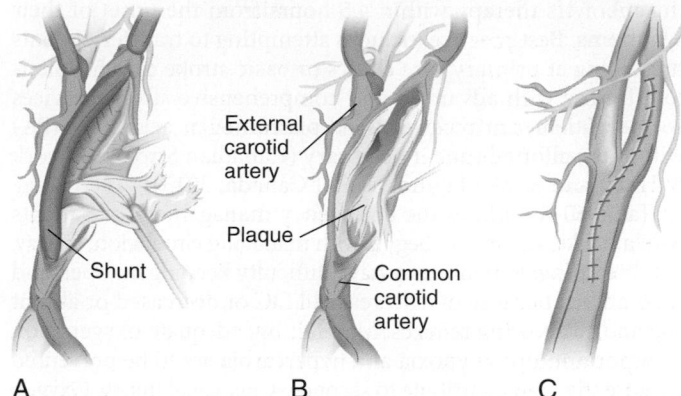

FIGURE 60-6 Carotid endarterectomy is performed to prevent impending cerebral infarct. **A,** A tube is inserted above and below the blockage to reroute the blood flow. **B,** Atherosclerotic plaque in the common carotid artery is removed. **C,** Once the artery is stitched closed, the tube can be removed. A surgeon may also perform the technique without rerouting the blood flow.

FIGURE 60-7 Brain stent used to treat blockages in cerebral blood flow. **A,** A balloon catheter is used to implant the stent into an artery of the brain. **B,** The balloon catheter is moved to the blocked area of the artery and then inflated. The stent expands due to inflation of the balloon. **C,** The balloon is deflated and withdrawn, leaving the stent permanently in place holding the artery open and improving the flow of blood.

is the treatment of choice for individuals with AF who have had a TIA. Patients using these anticoagulation drugs need to have their renal function regularly monitored and doses adjusted accordingly. Statins (simvastatin [Zocor], lovastatin) have also been shown to be effective in the prevention of stroke for individuals who have experienced a TIA (Coutts, Wein, Lindsay, et al., 2014).

DRUG ALERT—Clopidogrel (Plavix)
- All health care providers and dentists must be informed that this medication is being taken, especially before scheduling surgery or major dental procedures.
- Medication may need to be discontinued 10 to 14 days before surgery if antiplatelet effect is not desired.

Surgical Therapy. Surgical interventions for the patient with TIAs from carotid disease are outlined in Table 60-5. Figure 60-6 demonstrates one intervention, carotid endarterectomy.

Transluminal angioplasty is the insertion of a balloon to open a stenosed artery and improve blood flow. The balloon is threaded up to the carotid artery via a catheter inserted in the femoral artery. Stenting involves intravascular placement of a stent in an attempt to maintain patency of the artery (Figure 60-7). The stent can be inserted during an angioplasty. Once in place, the system can be used with a tiny filter that opens like an umbrella. The filter catches and removes the debris that is stirred up during the stenting procedure so that it does not float to the brain, where it can trigger a stroke. Patients' comorbidities should be carefully considered as carotid stenting is associated with a higher

risk for stroke, whereas carotid endarterectomy has an increased risk for MI (Liu, Fu, Guo, et al., 2012).

Extracranial-to-intracranial artery bypass involves anastomosing (surgically connecting) a branch of an extracranial artery to an intracranial artery (most commonly, superficial temporal to middle cerebral artery) beyond an area of obstruction with the goal of increasing cerebral perfusion. This procedure is generally reserved for those patients who do not benefit from other forms of therapy.

Collaborative Acute Care for Ischemic Stroke. The goals for collaborative care during the acute phase are preserving life, preventing further brain damage, and reducing disability. During initial evaluation, the single most important point in the patient's history is the time of onset. Fifty-four percent of patients who seek acute care for stroke present at the emergency department, and the rest seek out their primary health care physicians. The current standard for acute care treatment of stroke is that all patients with possible stroke will be assessed, have their acute health needs addressed, undergo diagnostic studies, and receive thrombolytic therapy within 4.5 hours from the onset of their symptoms. Best practice includes attempting to transfer patients presenting at primary care clinics or basic stroke care hospitals to a facility with advanced and comprehensive stroke services so the patient can receive tissue plasminogen activator (tPA) within the allotted time if necessary (Canadian Stroke Network & Heart and Stroke Foundation of Canada, 2013).

Table 60-6 outlines the emergency management of patients with a stroke. Acute care begins with managing circulation, airway, and breathing. Patients may have difficulty keeping an open and clear airway because of a decreased LOC or decreased or absent gag and swallowing reflexes. Maintaining adequate oxygenation is important. Both hypoxia and hypercarbia are to be prevented because they can contribute to secondary neuronal injury. Oxygen administration, artificial airway insertion, intubation, and mechanical ventilation may be required. Baseline neurological assessment is carried out, and patients are monitored closely for signs of increasing neurological deficit. About 25% of patients will worsen in the first 24 to 48 hours. It is recommended that acute care facilities have designated protocols in place to ensure stroke patients receive timely access to care and have interprofessional stroke teams in place in a geographically dedicated unit to improve outcomes (Canadian Stroke Network & Heart and Stroke Foundation of Canada, 2013).

Elevated BP is common immediately after a stroke and may be a protective response to maintain cerebral perfusion. Immediately following ischemic stroke, use of drugs to lower BP is recommended only if BP is markedly increased (mean arterial pressure >130 mm Hg or systolic BP >220 mm Hg). Intravenous (IV) antihypertensive drugs such as labetalol are used in the acute phase. Although low BP immediately following stroke is uncommon, hypotension and hypovolemia should be corrected if present.

Fluid and electrolyte balance must be controlled carefully. The goal generally is to keep the patient adequately hydrated to promote perfusion and decrease further brain injury. Overhydration may compromise perfusion by increasing cerebral edema. Adequate fluid intake during acute care via oral, IV, or tube feedings should be 1 500 to 2 000 mL/day. Urine output should be closely monitored. If secretion of antidiuretic hormone increases in response to the stroke, urine output decreases and fluid is retained. Low serum sodium (hyponatremia) may occur. IV solutions with glucose and water are avoided because they are hypotonic and may further increase cerebral edema and ICP. In addition, hyperglycemia may be associated with further brain damage and should be treated. In general, decisions regarding individualized fluid and electrolyte replacement therapy are based on the extent of intracranial edema, symptoms of increased ICP, central venous pressure levels, laboratory values for electrolytes, and intake and output.

Increased ICP is more likely to occur with hemorrhagic strokes but can occur with ischemic strokes. Increased ICP from cerebral edema usually peaks in 72 hours and may cause brain herniation. Management of increased ICP includes practices that improve venous drainage, such as elevating the head of the bed, maintaining head and neck in alignment, and avoiding hip flexion. Hyperthermia, which is seen commonly following stroke, is associated with poorer outcome, and should be prevented if possible (Campos, Sobrino, Vieites-Prado, et al., 2013). Increased temperature contributes to increased cerebral metabolism. Drug

✚ TABLE 60-6 EMERGENCY MANAGEMENT

Stroke

Etiology	Assessment Findings	Interventions

• Aneurysm
• Arteriovenous malformation
• Embolism
• Hemorrhage
• Sudden vascular compromise causing disruption of blood flow to the brain
• Thrombosis
• Trauma
	• Altered level of consciousness
	• Bladder or bowel incontinence
	• Difficulty swallowing
	• Facial drooping on affected side
	• Hypertension
	• Increased or decreased heart rate
	• Nausea and vomiting
	• Respiratory distress
	• Seizures
	• Severe headache
	• Speech or visual disturbances
	• Unequal pupils
	• Vertigo
	• Weakness, numbness, or paralysis of portion of body
		Initial Care
		• Ensure patent airway.
		• Call a stroke code or the stroke team.
		• Remove dentures.
		• Perform pulse oximetry.
		• Maintain adequate oxygenation (SaO$_2$ >95%) with supplemental O$_2$, if necessary.
		• Establish IV access with normal saline.
		• Maintain BP according to guidelines (e.g., advanced cardiac life support).
		• Remove clothing.
		• Insert Foley catheter.
		• Obtain CT scan immediately.
		• Perform baseline laboratory tests (including blood glucose) immediately, and treat if hypoglycemic.
		• Position head midline.
		• Elevate head of bed 30 degrees if no symptoms of shock or suspicion of spinal cord injury.
		• Institute seizure precautions.
		  • Anticipate thrombolytic therapy for ischemic stroke.
		  • Keep patient NPO until swallow reflex evaluated.
		
		Ongoing Monitoring
		• Monitor vital signs and neurological status, including level of consciousness (e.g., Glasgow Coma Scale or Canadian Neurological Scale or NIH Stroke Scale), motor and sensory function, pupil size and reactivity, SaO$_2$, and cardiac rhythm.
		• Educate and update patient and family/caregiver.

BP, blood pressure; *CT*, computed tomography; *IV*, intravenous; *NIH*, National Institutes of Health; *NPO*, nothing by mouth; *O₂*, oxygen; *SaO₂*, arterial oxygen saturation.

therapies to treat hyperthermia include acetaminophen (Tylenol) or indomethacin. A temperature elevation of even 1°C can increase brain metabolism by 10% and contribute to further brain damage. Cooling blankets or intravenous cooling methods may be used to lower temperature. The nurse must closely monitor the patient's temperature. Aggressive management of temperature during the first 24 hours after a stroke is most effective in preventing detrimental outcomes.

Seizures occur in 5% to 7% of stroke patients in the first 24 hours. Anticonvulsant drugs, such as phenytoin (Dilantin) or levetiracetam (Keppra), are given if a seizure occurs. There is varying research that supports and opposes the prophylactic use of anticonvulsant drugs in patients who have not had a seizure (Sykes, Wood, & Kwan, 2014).

Other measures include pain management, avoidance of hypervolemia, and management of constipation. CSF drainage may be used in some patients to reduce ICP or manage hydrocephalus. Osmotic agents, such as mannitol (Osmitrol) or hypertonic saline (3% saline), may be used to decrease cerebral edema. Current research shows that both agents are successful in lowering ICP (Rickard, Smith, Newell, et al., 2014).

As a last resort in the management of increased ICP, a bone flap may be removed to allow for cerebral edema without increases in ICP. Additional strategies for managing ICP are found in Chapter 59.

Drug Therapy for Ischemic Stroke. Recombinant tPA is administered intravenously to re-establish blood flow through a blocked artery to prevent cell death in patients with the acute onset of ischemic stroke symptoms. Patients are screened carefully before tPA can be given. Screening includes a noncontrast CT or MRI to rule out hemorrhagic stroke; blood tests for coagulation disorders; and screening for recent history (past 3 months) of gastro-intestinal bleeding, stroke, or head trauma or major surgery within previous 14 days. Intra-arterial infusion of tPA remains an option for a subgroup of patients with large vessel occlusions primarily in the middle cerebral artery. Thrombolytic drugs, such as tPA, produce localized fibrinolysis by binding to the fibrin in the thrombi. The fibrinolytic action of tPA occurs as the plasminogen is converted to plasmin, whose enzymatic action digests fibrin and fibrinogen and thus lyses the clot. Because it is clot specific in its activation of the fibrinolytic system, tPA is the only treatment indicated for acute ischemic stroke. tPA must be administered within 3 to 4.5 hours of the onset of clinical signs of ischemic stroke. The door-to-needle time for tPA remains less than 60 minutes whether the patient arrives at the hospital at 3 hours or 1 hour after the onset of clinical signs. Thrombolytics given in this time frame reduce disability, but at the expense of an increase in deaths within the first 7 to 10 days and an increase in the incidence of intracranial hemorrhage (Heart and Stroke Foundation of Canada, 2015; Grotta, 2014). (Thrombolytic therapy is further discussed in Chapter 36.)

During infusion of the drug, the patient's vital signs and neurological status are monitored closely to assess for improvement or for potential deterioration related to intracerebral hemorrhage. Control of BP is critical during treatment and for 24 hours afterward. No anticoagulant or antiplatelet drugs are given for 24 hours after tPA treatment because of the risk for intracranial hemorrhage.

Surgical Therapy for Ischemic Stroke. Endovascular treatment (Figure 60-8) during cerebral ischemia allows physicians to go inside the blocked artery of patients who are experiencing ischemic strokes. The retriever goes to the artery that is blocked,

FIGURE 60-8 Endovascular treatment removes blood clots in patients who are experiencing ischemic strokes. The retriever is a long, thin wire that is threaded through a catheter into the femoral artery. The wire is pushed through the end of the catheter up to the carotid artery. The wire reshapes itself into tiny loops that latch onto the clot, and the clot can then be pulled out. To prevent the clot from breaking off, a balloon at the end of the catheter inflates to stop blood flow through the artery.

directly to the site of the problem, and pulls the clot out. The retriever is a tiny corkscrew device that uses a microcatheter inserted through a femoral artery balloon catheter. Once the corkscrew device reaches the clot in the brain, the device penetrates the clot, allowing it to be removed. Under radiographic guidance, the balloon catheter is manoeuvred up to the carotid artery in the neck; a guide wire and the microcatheter are deployed through the balloon catheter and then placed just beyond the clot. The physician then deploys the retriever device to engage and ensnare the clot. Once the clot is captured, the balloon catheter is inflated to temporarily arrest forward flow while the clot is being withdrawn. The clot is pulled into the balloon catheter and completely out of the body. The balloon is then deflated, and blood flow is restored. Research has shown that endovascular treatment reduces mortality and increases functional outcomes (Goyal, Demchuk, Menon, et al., 2015).

Collaborative Acute Care for Hemorrhagic Stroke

Drug Therapy. Anticoagulants and platelet inhibitors are contraindicated in patients with acute hemorrhagic strokes. The main drug therapy for patients with hemorrhagic stroke is the management of hypertension. Oral and IV agents may be used to maintain BP within a normal to high-normal range (systolic BP <160 mm Hg). Once BP is stabilized, low-dose anticoagulation can be initiated for DVT prophylaxis (Hemphill, Greenberg, Anderson, et al., 2015). Patients who are on blood thinners and experience a hemorrhagic stroke should be given reversal agents (if available) as soon as possible to reduce the risk for further bleeding.

Seizure prophylaxis in the acute period after intracerebral hemorrhages and SAHs may be used. Limited research has been conducted to strongly support or oppose the use of antiepileptic drugs in this patient population (Connolly, Rabinstein, Carhuapoma, et al., 2012).

Surgical Therapy. Surgical interventions for hemorrhagic stroke include immediate evacuation of aneurysm-induced hematomas or cerebellar hematomas larger than 3 cm. Individuals who have an AVM may experience a hemorrhagic stroke if the AVM ruptures. The treatment of AVM is surgical resection, radiosurgery (e.g., Gamma Knife), or both. Either may be preceded by interventional neuroradiology to embolize the blood vessels that supply the AVM.

SAH is usually caused by a ruptured aneurysm. Approximately 20% of patients will have multiple aneurysms. Treatment of an aneurysm involves coiling or clipping the aneurysm to prevent

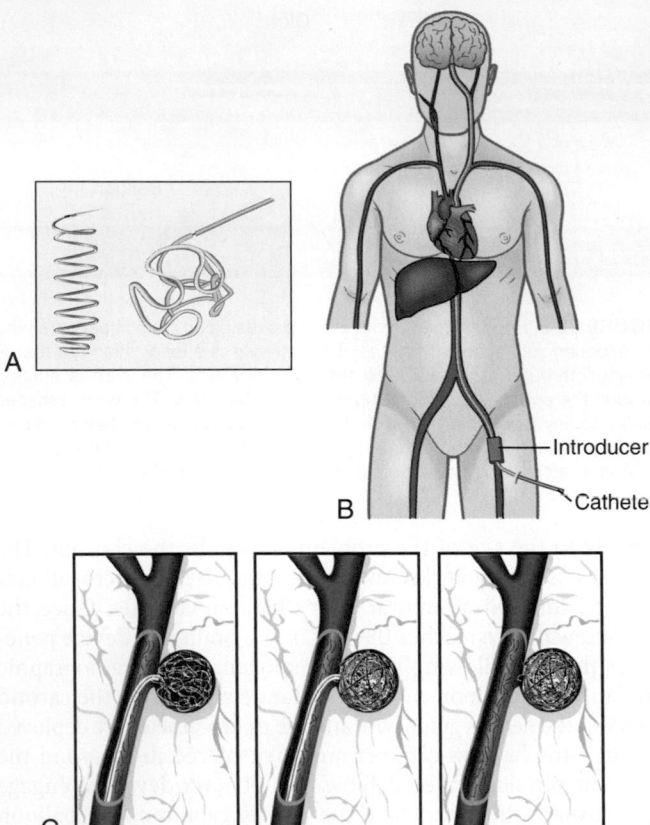

FIGURE 60-9 Guglielmi detachable coil. **A,** A coil is used to occlude an aneurysm. Coils are made of soft, springlike platinum. The softness of the platinum allows the coil to assume the shape of irregularly shaped aneurysms while posing little threat of rupture of the aneurysm. **B,** A catheter is inserted through an introducer (small tube) in an artery in the leg. The catheter is threaded up to the cerebral blood vessels. **C,** Platinum coils attached to a thin wire are inserted into the catheter and then placed in the aneurysm until the aneurysm is filled with coils. Packing the aneurysm with coils prevents the blood from circulating through the aneurysm, reducing the risk for rupture.

FIGURE 60-10 Clipping of aneurysms.

rebleeding (Figures 60-9 and 60-10). In the endovascular procedure known as *coiling*, a metal coil is inserted into the lumen of the aneurysm via interventional neuroradiology (see Figure 60-9). Guglielmi detachable coils provide immediate protection against hemorrhage by reducing the blood pulsations within the aneurysm. Eventually, a thrombus forms within the aneurysm and the aneurysm becomes sealed off from the parent vessel by the formation of an endothelialized layer of connective tissue. Guglielmi detachable coils provide a less invasive therapy than the traditional surgical clipping of aneurysms (see Figure 60-10).

The calcium channel blocker nimodipine (Nimotop) is given every 2 or 4 hours from the time of aneurysmal rupture (SAH) for 21 days to decrease the effects of vasospasm and minimize cerebral damage. Nimodipine restricts the influx of calcium ions into cells by reducing the number of open calcium channels. Although nimodipine is a calcium channel blocker, its exact mechanism of action in reducing vasospasm is not well understood.

Slight neurological decline or pronator drift is an indicator of vasospasm. Assessment for these complications is important. Once vasospasm is confirmed by a CTA, the goals of therapy are to use IV milrinone to promote cerebral vasodilation and to maintain homeostasis by replacing fluid losses, targeting normal parameters for glucose, electrolytes, and temperature (Lannes, Teitelbaum, del Pilar Cortés, et al., 2012).

> **DRUG ALERT—Nimodipine (Nimotop)**
> • Assessment of BP and apical pulses before administration.
> • If pulse ≤60 beats/min or systolic BP <90 mm Hg, medication should be held and the physician contacted.

SAH and intracerebral hemorrhage can involve bleeding into the ventricles of the brain. This situation produces hydrocephalus (enlarged ventricles), which further damages brain tissue from increased ICP. Insertion of an external ventricular drain (EVD) for CSF drainage in patients with hydrocephalus can drain excess CSF that is not draining due to lack of absorption or obstruction. CSF drainage can reduce ICP, and the patient may have an improved neurological examination.

Rehabilitation Care. After the acute stroke patient has stabilized for 12 to 72 hours, collaborative care shifts from preserving life to lessening disability and attaining optimal function. The patient may be evaluated by a physiatrist (a physician who specializes in physical medicine and rehabilitation). It is important to remember that some aspects of rehabilitation actually begin in the acute care phase as soon as the patient is stabilized. Depending on the patient's status, other medical conditions, rehabilitation potential, and available resources, the patient may be transferred to a rehabilitation unit. Other options for rehabilitation include outpatient therapy and home care–based rehabilitation (Canadian Stroke Network & Heart and Stroke Foundation of Canada, 2013).

As part of the long-term collaborative care after a stroke, various members of the health care team may be involved in the effort to promote optimal function of the patient and family. The composition of the interdisciplinary team depends on patient and family or caregiver needs and rehabilitation facility resources. The "Evidence-Informed Practice" box discusses how health care providers can assist family caregivers. It highlights family caregivers' changes in support needs as the patient transitions through the health care system.

NURSING MANAGEMENT
STROKE

NURSING ASSESSMENT

Subjective and objective data that should be obtained from a person who has had a stroke are presented in Table 60-7. Primary assessment focuses on cardiac status and respiratory and neurological assessment. If the patient's condition is stable, the nursing history is obtained as follows: (a) description of the current illness with attention to initial symptoms, including onset and duration, nature (intermittent or continuous), and changes; (b) history of similar symptoms previously experienced; (c) current medications; (d) history of risk factors and other illnesses such as hypertension; and (e) family history of stroke or cardiovascular diseases. This information is gained through an interview of the patient, family members, significant others, or caregiver.

EVIDENCE-INFORMED PRACTICE

Research Highlight

How Can Nurses Support Stroke Patients and Their Caregivers?

Clinical Question

What kinds of support do family caregivers of stroke survivors (P) need from health care providers (E) across the continuum from acute care to the community (O)?

Best Available Evidence

Qualitative study within a large Canadian city

Critical Appraisal and Synthesis of Evidence

- 38 interviews conducted (24 caregivers and 14 health care providers).
- Three themes emerged: (a) the type and intensity of support, (b) who provides the support and how it is provided, and (c) the primary focus of care.
- Caregivers and health care providers have similar outlooks regarding caregivers' need for support during the acute phase and in preparing for transition into the community. Caregivers of stroke survivors with communication difficulties or high cognitive or physical disability or both require long-term support.
- The patient was the primary focus of the support; however, caregivers had more needs than were being addressed. Since caregivers often come to facilities after hours and on weekends, they have limited time to receive education and support from rehabilitation therapists in order to prepare them for the patient's transition into the community.

Conclusion

- Be aware of caregivers' needs for education.

Implications for Nursing Practice

- Caregivers should be offered frequent opportunities to ask questions in an unhurried atmosphere. This is most effectively done well in advance of discharge.
- Active patient involvement has greater impact on improving mood than passive receipt of information.

Reference for Evidence

Cameron, J. I., Naglie, G., Silver, F. L., et al. (2013). Stroke family caregivers' support needs change across the care continuum: A qualitative study using the Timing It Right framework. *Disability and Rehabilitation, 35*(4), 315–324. doi:10.3109/09638288.2012.691937.

P, population and their problem; *E*, exposure; *O*, outcomes/themes of interest (see Chapter 1).

Secondary assessment should include a comprehensive neurological examination of the patient. This includes (a) LOC, using the Canadian Neurological Scale (Figure 60-11) (or a similar tool), (b) cognition, (c) motor abilities, (d) cranial nerve function, (e) sensation, (f) proprioception, (g) cerebellar function, and (h) deep tendon reflexes. Clear documentation of initial and ongoing neurological examinations is essential to note changes in patient status. The Registered Nurses' Association of Ontario (2005) and the Canadian Stroke Strategy (Heart and Stroke Foundation of Canada, 2017d) have also developed best-practice guidelines and recommendations for stroke care across the continuum.

NURSING DIAGNOSES

Nursing diagnoses for a person with a stroke may include but are not limited to the following:

- *Decreased intracranial adaptive capacity* (related to decreased cerebral perfusion pressure of ≤50 to 60 mm Hg, baseline ICP ≥15 mm Hg, elevated systolic BP, bradycardia, widened pulse pressure, and decreasing Canadian Neurological Scale score)

TABLE 60-7 NURSING ASSESSMENT

Stroke

Subjective Data
Important Health Information

Past health history: Hypertension; previous stroke, TIA, aneurysm, trauma, cardiac disease (including recent MI), dysrhythmias, heart failure, valvular disease, infective endocarditis, polycythemia, dyslipidemia, smoking, kidney disease, diabetes, gout, family history of hypertension, diabetes, deep-vein thrombosis, stroke, or coronary artery disease

Medications: Use of hormone therapy or oral contraceptives; use of and compliance with antihypertensive and diabetes regimen, antiplatelet therapy, and anticoagulant drugs; use of illegal substances (e.g., cocaine)

Symptoms

- Anorexia, nausea, vomiting; dysphagia, altered sensation of taste and smell
- Change in bowel and bladder patterns
- Loss of movement and sensation; syncope; weakness on one side; mouth droop, half smile; generalized weakness, easy fatigability
- Numbness, tingling of one side of the body; loss of memory; alteration in speech, language, problem-solving ability
- Pain; headache, possibly sudden and severe (hemorrhage); visual disturbances; denial of illness

Objective Data
General

Emotional lability, lethargy, apathy or combativeness, fever

Respiratory

Loss of cough reflex, laboured or irregular respirations, tachypnea, wheezing (aspiration), airway occlusion (tongue), apnea, coughing when eating or delayed coughing

Cardiovascular

Hypertension, tachycardia, carotid bruit

Gastro-Intestinal

Loss of gag reflex, bowel incontinence, decreased or absent bowel sounds, constipation

Urinary

Frequency, urgency, incontinence

Neurological

Contralateral motor and sensory deficits, including weakness, paresis, paralysis, anaesthesia; unequal pupils, hand grasps; akinesia, aphasia (expressive, receptive, global), dysarthria (slurred speech), agnosias, apraxia, visual deficits, perceptual or spatial disturbances, altered level of consciousness (drowsiness to deep coma) and Babinski reflex, ↓followed by ↑deep tendon reflexes, flaccidity followed by spasticity, amnesia, ataxia, personality change, nuchal rigidity, seizures

Possible Findings

Positive CT, CTA, MRI, MRA, or other neuroimaging scans showing size, location, and type of lesion; positive Doppler ultrasonography and angiography indicating stenosis

CT, computed tomography; *CTA*, computed tomographic angiography; *MI*, myocardial infarction; *MRA*, magnetic resonance angiography; *MRI*, magnetic resonance imaging; *TIA*, transient ischemic attack.

- *Risk for aspiration* related to as evidenced by *barrier to elevating upper body, decrease in level of consciousness, depressed gag reflex*
- *Impaired physical mobility* related to *decrease in muscle control, decrease in muscle strength, physical deconditioning*

CANADIAN NEUROLOGICAL SCALE

Assess: Vital Signs and Pupils   **Vital Signs:** BP, Temp, Pulse, Respirations, Oximetry   **Pupils:** Size and reaction to light

Section A: MENTATION: LOC, Orientation, Speech

LEVEL OF CONSCIOUSNESS:
CNS (Alert, Drowsy) GCS (Stuporous, Comatose)

ORIENTATION:
Place (city or hospital), Time (month and year)
*Patient can speak, write, or gesture their responses.
SCORE: Patient is Oriented, score 1.0, if they correctly state both place and correct month and year. If dysarthric, speech must be intelligible. If patient cannot state both. Disoriented, score 0.0

SPEECH:
RECEPTIVE: Ask patient the following separately (do not prompt by gesturing):

1. Close your eyes
2. "Does a stone sink in water?"
3. Point to the ceiling

SCORE: If patient is unable to do all three, Receptive Deficit, score 0.0, go to A2.

EXPRESSIVE:

1. Show patient 3 items separately (pencil, watch, key) and ask patient to name each object.
2. Ask patient what each object is used for while holding each up again, i.e. "What do you do with a pencil?"

SCORE: If patient is able to state the name and use of all 3 objects, Normal Speech, score 1.0.

If patient is unable to state the name and use of all 3 objects, Expressive Deficit, score 0.5.

*If patient answers all questions correctly but speech is slurred and intelligible, score Normal Speech and record "SL" along with the score.

Section A1: MOTOR FUNCTION

NO RECEPTIVE DEFICIT

FACE: Ask patient to smile/grin, note weakness in mouth or nasal/labial folds.
SCORE: None/no weakness = 0.5 or Present/weakness = 0.0 Test both limbs and always record the side with the WORST deficit and indicate side by entering a R/L.

None 1.5	no weakness present
Mild 1.0	mild weakness present, full ROM, cannot withstand resistance
Significant 0.5	moderate weakness, some movement, not full ROM
Total 0.0	complete loss of movement, total weakness

SCORE:
Arm: Proximal Ask patient to lift arm 45-90 degrees. Apply resistance between shoulder and elbow.
Arm: Distal Ask patient to make fist and flex wrist backwards, apply resistance between wrist and knuckles.
Leg: Proximal In supine, ask patient to flex hip to 90 degrees, apply pressure to mid thigh.
Leg: Distal Ask patient to dorsiflex foot, apply resistance to top of foot.

Section A2: MOTOR RESPONSE

RECEPTIVE DEFICIT PRESENT
FACE: Have patient mimic your smile. If unable, note facial expression while applying sternal pressure.
ARMS: Demonstrate or lift patient's arms to 90 degrees, score ability to maintain equal levels (>5 secs). If unable to maintain raised arms, apply nail bed pressure to assess reflex response.
LEGS: Lift patient's hip to 90 degrees, score ability to maintain equal levels (>5 secs), If unable to maintain raised position, apply nail bed pressure to assess reflex response.

FIGURE 60-11 Canadian Neurological Scale. *CNS,* central nervous system; *GCS,* Glasgow Coma Scale; *LOC,* level of consciousness; *R/L,* right/left; *ROM,* range of motion. Source: Heart and Stroke Foundation of Canada. (2015). *Stroke nurse pocket guide.* Ottawa: Author. Used by permission of Dr. Robert Côté, MD.

- *Unilateral neglect* (related to visual field cut and sensory loss on one side of body and brain injury from cerebro-vascular problems)
- *Impaired urinary elimination* related to *multiple causality* (impaired impulse to void, inability to reach toilet, manage tasks of voiding)
- *Impaired swallowing* related to *behavioural feeding problem* (weakness, paralysis of affected muscles)
- *Situational low self-esteem* related to *alteration in body image, decreased control over environment*

Additional information on nursing diagnoses for the patient with stroke is presented in Nursing Care Plan (NCP) 60-1.

PLANNING

The patient, the family, and the nurse establish the goals of nursing care in a cooperative manner. Typical goals are that the patient will (a) maintain a stable or improved LOC, (b) attain maximum physical functioning, (c) attain maximum self-care abilities and skills, (d) maintain stable body functions (e.g., bladder control), (e) maximize communication abilities, (f) maintain adequate nutrition, (g) avoid complications of stroke, and (h) maintain effective personal and family coping.

NURSING IMPLEMENTATION

HEALTH PROMOTION. In any health care setting and for the population as a whole, nurses can play a major role in the promotion of a healthy lifestyle. To reduce the incidence of stroke, the nurse should focus teaching efforts toward stroke prevention, particularly for persons with known risk factors (see Table 60-1). Measures to reduce risk factors for stroke are similar to those for coronary artery disease (see Table 36-2 and surrounding discussion of health promotion in Chapter 36).

Stroke

NURSING DIAGNOSIS	***Decreased intracranial adaptive capacity*** (related to decreased cerebral perfusion pressure of ≤50–60 mm Hg, baseline ICP ≥15 mm Hg, elevated systolic BP, bradycardia, widened pulse pressure, and decreasing Canadian Neurological Scale score)

Expected Patient Outcome	Nursing Interventions and *Rationales*
• Demonstrates signs of stable or improved cerebral perfusion	*Cerebral Perfusion Promotion* • Consult with physician *to determine hemodynamic parameters, and maintain hemodynamic parameters within this range.* • Monitor neurological status *to detect changes indicative of worsening or improving condition.* • Calculate and monitor CPP *to detect change in condition.* • Monitor respiratory status (e.g., rate, rhythm, and depth of respirations; PaO_2, $PaCO_2$, pH, and bicarbonate levels) *because high $PaCO_2$ and a high hydrogen ion concentration (acidosis) are potent vasodilators that increase cerebral blood flow.* • Monitor patient's ICP and neurological responses to care activities *because changes in positioning and movement can increase ICP.* • Monitor determinants of tissue oxygen delivery (e.g., $PaCO_2$, SaO_2, hemoglobin levels, and cardiac output) *to ensure adequate cerebral oxygenation.* • Administer and titrate vasoactive drugs, as ordered, *to maintain hemodynamic parameters.* • Avoid neck flexion or extreme hip or knee flexion *to avoid obstruction of arterial and venous blood flow.*

NURSING DIAGNOSIS	***Risk for aspiration*** as evidenced by *decreased level of consciousness, depressed gag reflex, impaired ability to swallow*

Expected Patient Outcomes	Nursing Interventions and *Rationales*
• Demonstrates ability to swallow oral foods without aspiration • Maintains a clear airway	*Aspiration Precautions* • Monitor level of consciousness, cough reflex, gag reflex, and swallowing ability *to determine patient's ability to swallow food without aspiration.* • Avoid liquids or use thickening agent *to facilitate swallowing.* • Feed in small amounts *to reduce risk for aspiration.* • Offer foods or liquids that can be formed into a bolus before swallowing. *Airway Management* • Auscultate breath sounds, noting areas of decreased or absent ventilation and presence of adventitious sounds *to identify airway obstruction and accumulation of secretions.* • Remove secretions by encouraging coughing or by suctioning *to clear airway.* • Encourage slow, deep breathing; turning; and coughing *to increase airway clearance without increasing ICP.* • Assist with incentive spirometer *to open collapsed alveoli, promote deep breathing, and prevent atelectasis.*

NURSING DIAGNOSIS	***Impaired physical mobility*** related to *decrease in muscle control, decrease in muscle strength, physical deconditioning* as evidenced by *neuro-muscular impairment, sensory-perceptual impairment*

Expected Patient Outcomes	Nursing Interventions and *Rationales*
• Demonstrates increased muscle strength and ability to move • Uses adaptive equipment to increase mobility	*Exercise Therapy: Muscle Control* • Collaborate with physical, occupational, and recreational therapists in developing and executing exercise program *to determine extent of problem and plan appropriate interventions.* • Determine patient's readiness to engage in activity or exercise protocol *to assess expected level of participation.* • Apply splints to achieve stability of proximal joints involved with fine motor skill activities *to prevent contractures.* • Encourage patient to practise exercises independently *to promote patient's sense of control.* • Reinforce instructions provided to patient about the proper way to perform exercises *to minimize injury and maximize effectiveness.* • Provide restful environment for patient after periods of exercise *to facilitate recuperation.*

NURSING DIAGNOSIS	***Impaired verbal communication*** related to *central nervous system impairment* as evidenced by *difficulty speaking*

Expected Patient Outcomes	Nursing Interventions and *Rationales*
• Uses effective oral and written communication techniques • Demonstrates congruency of verbal and nonverbal communication	*Communication Enhancement: Speech Deficit* • Provide alternative methods of speech communication (e.g., writing tablet, flash cards, eye blinking, communication board with pictures and letters, hand signals or other gestures, and computer) *to aid and promote patient communication.* • Provide positive reinforcement *to build self-esteem and confidence.* • Adjust communication style (e.g., stand in front of patient when speaking, listen attentively, present one idea or thought at a time, speak slowly while avoiding shouting, use written communication, or solicit caregiver's or family's assistance in understanding patient's speech) *to meet patient's needs.* • Maintain structured environment and routines (e.g., ensure consistent daily schedules, provide frequent reminders, and provide calendars and other environmental cues) *to promote patient's independence and self-care.* • Collaborate with caregiver, family, or both and speech–language pathologist or therapist *to develop a plan for effective communication.*

Continued

◎ **NURSING CARE PLAN 60-1**

Stroke—cont'd

NURSING DIAGNOSIS	**Unilateral neglect** (related to visual field cut and sensory loss on one side of body and brain injury from cerebro-vascular problems as evidenced by consistent inattention to stimuli on affected side)

Expected Patient Outcomes	**Nursing Interventions and *Rationales***
• Cares for both sides of the body appropriately • Uses strategies to minimize unilateral neglect	*Unilateral Neglect Management* • Monitor for abnormal responses to three types of stimuli—sensory, visual, and auditory—*to determine the presence of and degree to which unilateral neglect exists* (e.g., inability to see objects on affected side, leaving food on a plate that corresponds to affected side, lack of sensation on affected side). • Instruct patient to scan from left to right *to visualize the entire environment.* • Position bed in room so that individuals approach and care for patient on unaffected side. • Rearrange the environment to use the right or left visual field; position personal items, television, or reading materials within view on unaffected side *to compensate for visual field deficits.* • Touch unaffected shoulder when initiating conversation *to attract patient's attention.* • Gradually move personal items and activity to affected side as patient demonstrates an ability to compensate for neglect. • Include caregiver(s), family member(s), or both in rehabilitation process *to support the patient's efforts and assist with care to promote reintegration with the whole body.*

NURSING DIAGNOSIS	**Impaired urinary elimination** related to *multiple causality* (impaired impulse to void, inability to reach toilet or manage tasks of voiding) as evidenced by *sensory motor impairment*

Expected Patient Outcomes	**Nursing Interventions and *Rationales***
• Perceives impulse to void, removes clothing for toileting, and uses toilet • Demonstrates ability to urinate when the urge arises or with a timed schedule	*Urinary Habit Training* • Keep a continence specification record for 3 days *to establish voiding pattern and plan appropriate interventions.* • Establish interval of initial toileting schedule (based on voiding pattern and usual routine) *to initiate process of improving bladder functioning and increased muscle tone.* • Assist patient to toilet and prompt to void at prescribed intervals *to assist patient in adapting to new toileting schedule.* • Discuss daily record of continence with staff *to provide reinforcement and encourage compliance with toileting schedule.* • Give positive feedback or positive reinforcement to patient when he or she voids at scheduled toileting times, and make no comment when patient is incontinent, *to reinforce desired behaviour.*

NURSING DIAGNOSIS	**Impaired swallowing** related to *behavioural feeding problem* (weakness, paralysis of affected muscles) as evidenced by *brain injury* (difficulty swallowing, choking).

Expected Patient Outcome	**Nursing Interventions and *Rationales***
• Demonstrates effective swallowing without choking, coughing, or aspiration	*Swallowing Therapy* • Collaborate with other members of health care team (e.g., occupational therapist, speech–language pathologist, dietitian) *to provide continuity in patient's rehabilitative plan.* • Assist patient to sit in an erect position (as close to 90 degrees as possible) for feeding and exercise *to provide optimal position for chewing and swallowing without aspirating.* • Assist patient to position head in forward flexion in preparation for swallowing ("chin tuck"). • Assist patient to maintain sitting position for 30 minutes after completing meal *to prevent regurgitation of food.* • Instruct patient or caregiver on emergency measures for choking *to prevent complications in the home setting.* • Check mouth for pocketing of food after eating *to prevent collection and putrefaction of food or aspiration.* • Provide mouth care as needed *to promote comfort and oral health.* • Monitor body weight *to determine adequacy of nutritional intake.*

NURSING DIAGNOSIS	**Situational low self-esteem** related to *decreased control over environment, alteration in body image* as evidenced by *helplessness, purposelessness, indecisive behaviour, self-negating verbalizations.*

Expected Patient Outcomes	**Nursing Interventions and *Rationales***
• Expresses positive feelings of self-worth • Participates in self-care of affected body parts	*Self-Esteem Enhancement* • Monitor patient's statements of self-worth *to determine effect of stroke on self-esteem.* • Encourage patient to identify strengths *to facilitate patient's recognition of intrinsic value.* • Assist in setting realistic goals *to achieve higher self-esteem.* • Reward or praise patient's progress toward reaching goals. • Encourage increased responsibility for self *to promote sense of satisfaction, independence, and control and to reduce frustrations.* • Monitor levels of self-esteem over time *to determine stressors or situations that trigger low self-esteem and to teach coping mechanisms.*

BP, blood pressure; *CPP,* cerebral perfusion pressure; *ICP,* intracranial pressure; *PaCO₂,* partial pressure of carbon dioxide in arterial blood; *PaO₂,* partial pressure of oxygen in arterial blood; *SaO₂,* saturation of oxygen in arterial blood.

One of the nurse's major roles is education about hypertension control and maintaining adherence with antihypertensive medications. Uncontrolled hypertension is the primary cause of stroke.

The nurse needs to be an advocate for the monitoring and management of hypertension, including assessing financial need and prescription coverage. For patients with diabetes, it is very important that the blood glucose level be well controlled. For patients with AF, an anticoagulant such as apixaban (Eliquis), dabigatran (Pradaxa), or rivaroxaban (Xarelto) may be used to treat the problem to prevent the risk for stroke. Because smoking is a major risk factor for stroke, the nurse needs to be actively involved in helping patients to stop smoking (see Chapter 11).

Another very important aspect of health promotion is teaching patients and families about early symptoms associated with stroke or TIA. Table 60-8 presents information on when to seek health care for these symptoms.

ACUTE INTERVENTION FOR ALL STROKE PATIENTS. Acute intervention for the stroke patient includes care of the respiratory, neurological, cardiovascular, musculo-skeletal, integumentary, gastro-intestinal, and urinary systems, as well as attention to the patient's nutrition.

Respiratory System. During the acute phase following a stroke, management of the respiratory system is a nursing priority. Stroke patients are particularly vulnerable to respiratory problems as it has been shown that respiratory muscle strength decreases following stroke. Advancing age and immobility increase the risk for atelectasis and pneumonia (Pollock, Rafferty, Moxham, et al., 2013).

Risk for aspiration pneumonia may be high because of impaired consciousness or dysphagia. Dysphagia after stroke is common. Airway obstruction can occur because of problems with chewing and swallowing, food pocketing (food remaining in the buccal cavity of the mouth), and the tongue falling back. Some patients with stroke, especially those with brain stem or hemorrhagic stroke, may require endotracheal intubation and mechanical ventilation initially or with increasing cerebral edema or ICP. Enteral tube feedings also place the patient at risk for aspiration pneumonia. All patients should be screened for their ability to swallow and kept on nothing-by-mouth status until dysphagia has been ruled out (Daniels, Anderson, & Willson, 2012).

Nursing interventions to support adequate respiratory function are individualized to meet the needs of the patient. An oropharyngeal airway may be used in comatose patients to prevent the tongue from falling back and obstructing the airway and to provide access for suctioning. Alternatively, a nasopharyngeal airway may be used to provide airway protection and access. When an artificial airway will be required for a prolonged time, a tracheostomy may be performed. Nursing interventions include frequent assessment of airway patency and function, oxygenation, suctioning, patient mobility, positioning of the patient to prevent aspiration, and encouraging deep breathing. Patients who have an unclipped or uncoiled aneurysm may experience rebleeding and the possibility of further ICP increases with coughing exercises.

Interventions related to maintenance of airway function are described in NCP 60-1.

Neurological System. The patient's neurological status must be monitored closely to detect slight changes suggesting extension of the stroke, increased ICP, vasospasm, or recovery from stroke symptoms. There are many neurological assessment tools, such as the Glasgow Coma Scale (GCS), National Institutes of Health Stroke Scale, and the Canadian Neurological Scale, that can be used to assist in the monitoring of a patient's neurological status. The GCS measures LOC, mental status, pupillary responses, and extremity movement and strength. (The GCS is shown in Chapter 59, Table 59-5.) The GCS might not be sensitive enough for use with stroke patients who have cognitive and communication deficits (rather than impaired LOC), which would not be detected using this scale. The Canadian Neurological Scale was designed specifically for evaluating and monitoring the neurological status of patients with acute stroke (see Figure 60-11). It is an assessment tool that measures LOC, orientation, speech, and motor responses of the face, arms, and legs and takes into account if the patient has a receptive deficit.

Additional neurological assessment includes mental status, pupillary responses, checking for pronator drift, and extremity movement and strength. Also, vital signs need to be monitored closely. A decreasing LOC may indicate increasing ICP. ICP and cerebral perfusion pressure may be monitored as well if the patient is in an intensive care environment. Data from the nursing assessment are recorded on flow sheets to compare the trends over time and to communicate the evaluation of neurological status to the interdisciplinary team.

Cardiovascular System. Nursing goals for the cardiovascular system are aimed at maintaining homeostasis. Many patients with stroke have decreased cardiac reserves from the secondary

---

TABLE 60-8 PATIENT & CAREGIVER TEACHING GUIDE

Warning Signs of Stroke

Learn the signs of stroke

Face is it drooping?

Arms can you raise both?

Speech is it slurred or jumbled?

Time to call 9-1-1 right away.

Act **F A S T** because the quicker you act, the more of the person you save.

© Heart and Stroke Foundation of Canada, 2017

Source: © 2017, Heart and Stroke Foundation of Canada. Reproduced with the permission of the Heart and Stroke Foundation of Canada. *www.heartandstroke.ca.*

diagnoses of cardiac diseases. Cardiac efficiency may be further compromised by fluid retention, overhydration, dehydration, BP variations, or a combination of these. Fluids are retained if there is increased production of antidiuretic hormone and aldosterone secondary to stress. Fluid retention plus overhydration can result in fluid overload. It can also increase cerebral edema and ICP. At the same time, dehydration can add to the morbidity and mortality associated with stroke, especially in patients with vasospasm. IV therapy should be carefully regulated. The nurse should closely monitor intake and output. Central venous pressure, pulmonary artery pressure, or hemodynamic monitoring may be used as indicators of fluid balance or cardiac function in the intensive care unit.

Nursing interventions include (a) monitoring vital signs frequently; (b) monitoring cardiac rhythms; (c) calculating intake and output, noting imbalances; (d) regulating IV infusions; (e) adjusting fluid intake to the individual needs of the patient; (f) monitoring lung sounds for indications of pulmonary congestion; and (g) monitoring heart sounds for murmurs or for third (S_3) or fourth (S_4) heart sounds. Bedside monitors or telemetry may record cardiac rhythms. Hypertension is sometimes seen following a stroke as the body attempts to increase cerebral blood flow. It is important to monitor for orthostatic hypertension before ambulating the patient for the first time. Neurological changes can occur with a sudden decrease in BP.

After a stroke, the patient is at risk for deep-vein thrombosis (DVT), especially in the weak or paralyzed lower extremity. This complication is related to immobility, loss of venous tone, and decreased muscle pumping activity in the leg. The most effective prevention is to keep the patient moving. Active range-of-motion exercises should be taught if the patient has voluntary movement in the affected extremity. For the patient with hemiplegia, passive range-of-motion exercises should be done several times a day. Additional measures to prevent DVT include positioning to minimize the effects of dependent edema and the use of elastic gradient compression stockings or support hose. Sequential compression devices may be ordered for bedridden patients. DVT prophylaxis may include low-molecular-weight heparin (e.g., dalteparin [Fragmin]). The nursing assessment for DVT includes measuring the calf and the thigh daily, observing for swelling or colour changes of the extremities, noting unusual warmth of the leg, and asking the patient about pain in the limbs.

Musculo-Skeletal System. The nursing goal for the musculo-skeletal system is to maintain optimal function. This is accomplished by preventing joint contractures and muscular atrophy. In the acute phase, range-of-motion exercises and positioning are important nursing interventions. Passive range-of-motion exercise is begun on the first day of hospitalization. If the stroke is caused by SAH, the movement is limited to the extremities. The patient is taught to actively exercise as soon as possible. Muscle atrophy secondary to lack of innervation and activity can develop within 1 month following stroke.

The paralyzed or weak side needs special attention when the patient is positioned. Each joint should be positioned higher than the joint proximal to it to prevent dependent edema. Specific deformities on the weak or paralyzed side that may be present in patients with stroke include internal rotation of the shoulder; flexion contractures of the hand, wrist, and elbow; external rotation of the hip; and plantar flexion of the foot. Subluxation of the shoulder on the affected side is common. Careful positioning and moving of the affected arm may prevent the development of a painful shoulder condition; immobilization of the affected upper extremity may precipitate a painful shoulder–hand syndrome.

Nursing interventions to optimize musculo-skeletal function include (a) placing a trochanter roll at the hip to prevent external rotation; (b) using hand splints (not rolled washcloths) to prevent hand contractures; (c) providing arm supports with slings and lap boards to prevent shoulder displacement; (d) avoiding pulling the patient by the arm to prevent shoulder displacement; (e) using posterior leg splints, footboards, or high-topped tennis shoes to prevent foot drop; and (f) using hand splints to reduce spasticity. The early use of splints in hemiplegic patients has been associated with improved mobility and strength in the extremities following rehabilitation (Chang & Lai, 2015; Tyson, Sadeghi-Demneh, & Nestor, 2013).

Integumentary System. The skin of the patient with stroke is particularly susceptible to breakdown related to loss of sensation, decreased circulation, and immobility. This complication is compounded by patient age, poor nutrition, dehydration, edema, and incontinence. The nursing plan for prevention of skin breakdown includes (a) relieving pressure through position changes, special mattresses, or wheelchair cushions; (b) providing good skin hygiene; (c) applying emollients to dry skin; and (d) promoting early mobility. The ideal position change schedule is side–back–side with a maximum duration of 2 hours for any position. Nurses should position the patient on the weak or paralyzed side for only 30 minutes. If an area of redness develops and does not return to normal colour within 15 minutes of pressure relief, the epidermis and dermis are damaged. The damaged area should not be massaged because massage may cause additional damage. Pressure relief is the single most important factor in both the prevention and the treatment of skin breakdown. Pillows can be used under lower extremities to reduce pressure on the heels. Vigilance and good nursing care are required to prevent pressure injuries.

Gastro-Intestinal System. The most common bowel problem for patients who have experienced a stroke is constipation. Patients may be prophylactically placed on stool softeners or fibre (psyllium [Metamucil]) or both. The patient who has liquid stools should also be checked for stool impaction. Depending on the patient's fluid balance status and swallowing ability, fluid intake should be 1 800 to 2 000 mL/day, and fibre intake up to 25 g/day. Physical activity also promotes bowel function. Laxatives, suppositories, or additional stool softeners may be ordered if the patient does not respond to increased fluid and fibre. Similarly, enemas are used only if suppositories and digital stimulation are ineffective because they cause vagal stimulation and increase ICP.

Urinary System. In the acute stage of stroke, the primary urinary problem is poor bladder control, resulting in incontinence. Efforts should be made to promote normal bladder function and avoid the use of in-dwelling catheters. If an in-dwelling catheter must be used initially, it should be removed as soon as the patient is medically and neurologically stable. Long-term use of an in-dwelling catheter is associated with urinary tract infections and delayed bladder retraining. An alternative to intermittent catheterizations is offering the opportunity for frequent toileting to patients with urinary incontinence. Male patients with urinary incontinence also have the alternative of using an external catheter.

A bladder retraining program consists of (a) adequate fluid intake with the majority given between 0800 and 1900 hours; (b) scheduled toileting every 2 hours using bedpan, urinal, commode, or bathroom; and (c) noting signs of restlessness, which may indicate the need for urination.

Nutrition. The nutritional needs of patients require quick assessment and treatment. Patients may initially receive IV infusions to maintain fluid and electrolyte balance as well as for administration of drugs. Patients with severe impairment may require enteral or parenteral nutrition support. Individual assessment and planning for nutrition are necessary, and patients' needs will depend on the severity of the stroke.

SAFETY ALERT

The first oral feeding should be approached carefully because dysphagia may be present following a stroke. A swallowing screen should be performed prior to administering any food or drink.

Speech–language pathologists (SLPs) (if available) can perform a swallowing evaluation before patients are started on oral intake. The first oral feeding should be approached carefully because dysphagia may be present. The majority of patients will experience dysphagia after a stroke (Daniels, Anderson, & Willson, 2012). Before initiation of feeding, the gag reflex may be assessed by gently stimulating the back of the throat with a tongue blade. If a gag reflex is present, the patient will gag spontaneously. If it is absent, feeding should be deferred, and exercises to stimulate swallowing should be started. The SLP or occupational therapist is usually responsible for designing this program. However, in some clinical settings, the nurse may be called on to develop the program.

To screen for swallowing ability, the nurse should elevate the head of the bed to an upright position (unless contraindicated) and do a bedside trial of fluid (e.g., Toronto Bedside Swallowing Screening Test [TOR-BSST] or Burke test), giving the patient at least 3 tsp of water before proceeding to 50 mL of water by cup. Because of the dangers of silent aspiration, the nurse should not use any other liquid but water for this screening. If problems are experienced, the patient is not allowed anything orally and is referred to an SLP. If no problems are experienced, the patient should be placed on a modified diet and monitored during meals (Daniels, Anderson, & Willson, 2012).

After careful assessment of swallowing, chewing, gag reflex, and pocketing, oral feedings can be initiated. Mouth care before feeding helps stimulate sensory awareness and salivation and can facilitate swallowing. The patient should remain in a high Fowler's position, preferably in a chair with the head flexed forward for the feeding and for 30 minutes afterward. Various dietary items may be recommended by the SLP. Foods should be easy to swallow and provide enough texture, temperature (warm or cold), and flavour to stimulate a swallow reflex. Crushed ice can be used as a stimulant. The patient should be instructed to swallow and then swallow again. Puréed foods are not usually the best choice because they are often bland and too smooth. Thin liquids are often difficult to swallow and may promote coughing. Thin fluids can be thickened through the use of a commercially available thickening agent (e.g., Thick-It). Milk products should be avoided because they tend to increase the viscosity of mucus and increase salivation.

Food should be placed on the unaffected side of the mouth. The nurse should ensure an unrushed, nonstressful atmosphere. Feedings must be followed by scrupulous oral hygiene because food may collect on the affected side of the mouth.

Communication. During the acute stage of stroke, the nurse's role in meeting the psychological needs of the patient is primarily supportive. An alert patient is usually anxious because of lack of understanding about what has happened and because communication is difficult. The patient is assessed for the ability to both speak and understand. The patient's response to simple

TABLE 60-9	COMMUNICATION WITH A PATIENT EXPERIENCING APHASIA

1. Environmental stimuli that may distract and disrupt communication efforts should be avoided.
2. When speaking, the nurse should look in the patient's direction because observance of facial expression may help the patient with aphasia to understand what the nurse is saying.
3. The nurse should speak with normal volume and in a tone of voice suitable for communicating with an adult rather than a child.
4. The nurse should present one thought or idea at a time.
5. Writing out key words or drawing instructions using a thick black marker and large printed letters can help the patient to follow along.
6. Questions should be kept simple and preferably be able to be answered with "yes" or "no."
7. The nurse should let the patient speak and not interrupt, allowing the patient time to complete thoughts.
8. Mimicking or making use of gestures or demonstration is an acceptable alternative form of communication. The nurse can encourage this by saying, "Show me …" or "Point to what you want."
9. If the nurse does not understand the patient, the nurse should calmly express the lack of understanding and encourage the use of nonverbal communication or ask the person to write out what he or she wants.
10. The patient should be given time to process information and generate a response before a question or statement is repeated.
11. The nurse should allow body contact (e.g., the clasp of a hand, touching) as much as possible. Touching may be the only way the patient can express feelings.
12. The more familiar a routine, the easier it will be, so the nurse should organize the patient's day by preparing and following a schedule.
13. The nurse should not push communication if the patient is tired or upset. Aphasia worsens with fatigue.

questions can give the nurse a guideline for structuring explanations and instructions. If the patient cannot understand words, gestures may be used to support verbal cues. It is helpful to speak slowly and calmly, using simple words or sentences to enhance communication. The nurse must give the patient extra time to comprehend and respond to communication. The stroke patient with aphasia may be easily overwhelmed by verbal stimuli. (Guidelines for communicating with a patient who has aphasia are presented in Table 60-9.) Evaluation and treatment of language and communication deficits are often done by the SLP once the patient has stabilized.

Sensory–Perceptual Alterations. Homonymous hemianopia (blindness in the same half of each visual field) is a common problem after a stroke (Figure 60-12, *B*). Persistent disregard of objects in part of the visual field should alert the nurse to this possibility. Initially, the nurse helps the patient to compensate by arranging the environment within the patient's perceptual field, such as arranging the food tray so that all foods are on the right side or the left side to accommodate for field of vision (see Figure 60-12, *B*). Later, the patient learns to compensate for the visual defect by consciously attending or scanning the neglected side (see Figure 60-12, *A*). The weak or paralyzed extremities are carefully checked for adequacy of dressing, for hygiene, and for trauma.

In the clinical situation, it is often difficult to distinguish between a visual field cut and a neglect syndrome. Both problems may occur with strokes affecting either the right or the left side

A   **B**

FIGURE 60-12 Spatial and perceptual deficits in stroke. **A,** The patient is instructed to look toward the affected side when walking to avoid bumping into things. **B,** With homonymous hemianopia, the patient is unable to see the left side of the tray and may ignore items on that side. Source: Monahan, F. D., Neighbors, M., Sands, J. K., et al. (2007). *Phipps' medical-surgical nursing: Health and illness perspectives* (8th ed., p. 1437, Figure 49-10). St. Louis: Mosby.

of the brain. A person may be unfortunate enough to have both homonymous hemianopia and a neglect syndrome, a combination that increases the inattention to the weak or paralyzed side. A neglect syndrome results in decreased safety awareness and thereby places the patient at high risk for injury. Immediately after the stroke, the nurse must anticipate potential safety hazards and provide protection from injury. Safety measures can include close observation of the patient, use of a sitter or family member, a lower bed height, and video monitors. The use of restraints and soft vests is avoided as they may agitate the patient.

Other visual problems may include diplopia, loss of the corneal reflex, and ptosis, especially if the area of stroke is in the vertebrobasilar distribution. Diplopia is often treated with an eye patch. If the corneal reflex is absent, the patient is at risk for corneal abrasion and should be observed closely and protected against eye injuries. Corneal abrasion can be prevented with artificial tears or gel to keep the eyes moist and an eye shield (especially at night). Ptosis is generally not treated because it usually does not inhibit vision.

Coping. A stroke is usually a sudden, extremely stressful event for the patient, family members, and significant others. A stroke is often a family disease, affecting the family emotionally, socially, and financially as well as changing roles and responsibilities within the family. An older couple may perceive the stroke as a very real threat to life and to accustomed lifestyle. Reactions to this threat vary considerably but may involve fear, apprehension, denial of the severity of stroke, depression, anger, and sorrow. During the acute phase of caring for the stroke patient and the family, nursing interventions designed to facilitate coping involve providing information and emotional support.

Explanations to the patient and family about what has happened and about diagnostic and therapeutic procedures should be clear, detailed, and understandable. However, if the family is extremely anxious and upset during the acute phase, explanations may need to be repeated at a later time. Because family members usually have not had time to prepare for the illness, they may need assistance in arranging care for family members or pets and for transportation and finances. A social services referral is often helpful.

The patient's decision making and health care providers' commitment to uphold the patient's wishes during this challenging time are of utmost importance. Advance directives should be honoured and family meetings or updates should be held regularly in regard to feeding tube placement or tracheotomy.

It is particularly challenging to keep the aphasic patient adequately informed. Tone, demeanour, and touch may help to convey support. When communicating with a patient who has a communication deficit, the nurse should speak with normal volume and tone, keep questions simple, and present one thought or idea at a time. To decrease the patient's frustration, the nurse should always let the patient speak without interruption and use gestures. It is important, too, to make use of writing and communication boards (Burns, Baylor, Dudgeon, et al., 2015).

AMBULATORY AND HOME CARE: STROKE RECOVERY. The patient is usually discharged from the acute care setting to home, an intermediate- or long-term care facility, or a rehabilitation facility. Ideally, discharge planning with the patient and family or caregiver starts early in the hospitalization and promotes a smooth transition from one care setting to another. The interdisciplinary team provides the guidance for the appropriate care required after discharge. If the patient requires a short- or long-term health care facility, the team can make appropriate referrals that allow time for the family to select and arrange care. A critical factor in discharge planning is the patient's level of independence in performing ADLs. If the patient is returning home, the team can make referrals for needed equipment and services in preparation for discharge.

Nurses have an excellent opportunity to prepare the patient and family or caregiver for discharge through education, demonstration and return demonstration, practice, and evaluation of self-care skills before discharge. Total care is considered in discharge planning: medications, nutrition, mobility, exercises, hygiene, and toileting. Follow-up care is carefully planned to permit continuing nursing care, physiotherapy, occupational therapy, and speech therapy, as well as medical care. Community resources should be identified to provide recreational activities, group support, spiritual assistance, respite care, adult day care, and home assistance based on the individual patient's needs.

Rehabilitation is the process of maximizing the patient's capabilities and resources to promote optimal functioning related to physical, mental, and social well-being. The goals of rehabilitation are to prevent deformity and maintain and improve function. Regardless of the care setting, ongoing rehabilitation is essential to maximize the patient's abilities. Most patients will see the maximum benefit in the first year of recovery following a stroke (Pollock, Baer, Campbell, et al., 2014).

Rehabilitation requires a team approach so the patient and family can benefit from the combined, expert care of an interdisciplinary team. The team must communicate and coordinate care to achieve the patient's and family's goals. There is strong evidence that organized post-acute inpatient stroke care delivered within the first 4 weeks by an interdisciplinary team of health care providers can result in a reduction in the number of deaths related to stroke. The stroke rehabilitation team generally consists of a rehabilitation nurse, neuropsychologist, occupational therapist, certified rehabilitation counsellor, physiotherapist, physician, recreational therapist, social worker, and SLP. The nurse is in a good position to facilitate rehabilitation and is often key to successful rehabilitation efforts. Physiotherapy focuses on mobility, progressive ambulation, transfer techniques, and equipment needed for mobility (Pollock, Baer, Campbell, et al., 2014). Occupational therapy emphasizes retraining for ADLs such as eating, dressing, hygiene, and cooking. Occupational therapists are also skilled in cognitive and perceptual evaluation and training. Speech–language pathology focuses on speech, communication, cognition, and swallowing abilities.

Many of the nursing interventions outlined in NCP 60-1 for the patient with a stroke are initiated in the acute phase of care and continue throughout rehabilitation. Some of the interventions are independent nursing actions, whereas others involve the entire rehabilitation team.

The rehabilitation nurse assesses the patient, caregiver, and family with attention to the (a) rehabilitation potential of the patient, (b) physical status of all body systems, (c) presence of complications caused by the stroke or other chronic conditions, (d) cognitive status of the patient, (e) family resources and support, and (f) expectations of the patient and family related to the rehabilitation program.

Musculo-Skeletal Function. The nurse initially emphasizes the musculo-skeletal functions of eating, toileting, and walking for the rehabilitation of the patient. Initial assessment consists of determining the stage of recovery of muscle function. If the muscles are still flaccid several weeks after the stroke, the prognosis for regaining function is poor, and the focus of care is on preventing additional loss. Most patients begin to show signs of spasticity with exaggerated reflexes within 48 hours following the stroke. Spasticity at this phase of the stroke denotes progress toward recovery. As improvement continues, small voluntary movements of the hip or the shoulder may be accompanied by involuntary movements in the rest of the extremity (*synergy*). The final stage of recovery occurs when the patient has voluntary control of isolated muscle groups.

Interventions for the musculo-skeletal system advance in a manner of progressive activity. Balance training is the initial step and begins with the patient sitting up in bed or dangling the legs from the edge of the bed. The nurse evaluates tolerance by noting dizziness or syncope caused by vasomotor instability. Loss of postural stability is common after a stroke. When the nondominant hemisphere is involved, walking apraxia and loss of postural control are usually apparent. Assess whether patients autocorrect their posture when sitting on the edge of the bed. If the patient can straighten her or his posture instead of leaning to the weaker side, the patient may be ready for the next step of transferring from the bed to a chair. The chair is placed beside the bed so that the patient can lead with the stronger arm and leg. The patient sits on the side of the bed, stands, places the strong hand on the far wheelchair arm, and sits down. The nurse may either supervise the transfer or provide minimal assistance by guiding the patient's strong hand to the wheelchair arm, standing in front of the patient and blocking the patient's knees with his or her own knees to prevent knee buckling, and guiding the patient into a sitting position.

A more recent approach to stroke rehabilitation is constraint-induced movement therapy. Constraint-induced movement therapy encourages the patient to use the weakened extremity by restricting movement of the unaffected extremity. This approach

INFORMATICS IN PRACTICE

Video Games for Stroke Recovery

Patients dealing with the effects of a stroke often have difficulty performing ADLs. Playing active video games, like Nintendo Wii or Xbox Kinect, brings some fun into stroke recovery and may get patients to spend more time in therapy.

Gaming helps patients regain lost strength, improve motor skills, and improve problem solving and short- and long-term memory.

Patients can play with their families, including children, making gaming a way to involve others in rehabilitation.

has demonstrated improved mobility in patients following stroke; however, research is still being conducted to determine the best protocol. Movement training, skill acquisition, splinting, and exercise are additional therapies offered for the rehabilitation of stroke patients (Peurala, Kantanen, Sjögren, et al., 2011). Supportive or assistive equipment, such as canes, walkers, and leg braces, may be needed on a short- or long-term basis for mobility. The physiotherapist usually selects the most appropriate supportive device(s) to meet individual needs and instructs the patient regarding use. The nurse should incorporate physiotherapy activities into the patient's daily routine for additional practice and repetition of rehabilitation efforts.

Nutritional Therapy. After the acute phase, a dietitian can assist in determining the appropriate daily caloric intake based on the patient's size, weight, and activity level. If the patient is unable to take in an adequate oral diet, a percutaneous endoscopic gastrostomy (see Chapter 42, Figure 42-8) may be used for nutritional support if dysphagia persists. Most commercially prepared formulas provide about 1 cal/mL. (Enteral feedings are described in Chapter 42.)

The nurse and the SLP must assess the ability of the patient to swallow solids and fluids and adjust the diet appropriately. The dietitian plans the diet type, texture, calorie count, and fluids to meet the patient's nutritional needs. The occupational therapist and the nurse must evaluate the patient's ability to feed himself or herself and recommend assistive devices to allow for independent eating.

The inability to feed oneself can be frustrating and may result in malnutrition and dehydration. Interventions to promote self-feeding include using the unaffected upper extremity to eat; employing assistive devices such as rocker knives, plate guards, and nonslip pads for dishes (Figure 60-13); removing unnecessary items from the tray or table, which can reduce spills; and providing a nondistracting environment to decrease sensory overload and distraction. The effectiveness of the dietary program is evaluated in terms of maintenance of weight, adequate hydration, and patient satisfaction.

Bowel Function. A bowel management program is implemented for problems with bowel control, constipation, or incontinence. A high-fibre diet (see Chapter 45, Table 45-9) and adequate fluid intake (2 500–3 000 mL) are usually recommended. Patients with stroke frequently have constipation, which responds to the following dietary management:

- Fluid intake of 2 500 to 3 000 mL daily unless contraindicated
- Prune juice (120 mL) or stewed prunes daily
- Cooked vegetables or fruit three times daily
- Whole-grain cereal or bread three to five times daily

The bowel management program for incontinence consists of placing the patient on the bedpan or bedside commode or taking

FIGURE 60-13 Assistive devices for eating. **A,** The curved fork fits over the hand. The rounded plate helps keep food on the plate. Special grips and swivel handles are helpful for some persons. **B,** Knives with rounded blades are rocked back and forth to cut food. The person does not need a fork in one hand and a knife in the other. **C,** Plate guards help keep food on the plate. **D,** Cup with special handle. Source: Courtesy Sammons Preston, Bolingbrook, Illinois.

the patient to the bathroom at a regular time daily to re-establish bowel regularity. A good time for the bowel program is 30 minutes after breakfast because eating stimulates the gastrocolic reflex and peristalsis. The time can be adjusted for individual bowel habits and preferred timing. Sitting on the commode or toilet promotes bowel elimination through both gravity and increased abdominal pressure. Stool softeners or suppositories may be ordered if the bowel program is ineffective in re-establishing bowel regularity. A glycerin suppository can be inserted 15 to 30 minutes before evacuation time to stimulate the anorectal reflex. A bisacodyl (Dulcolax) suppository is a chemical stimulant to the bowel and is used when other measures are ineffective. Ideally, suppository use is for short-term management.

Bladder Function. The nurse assists the patient with urinary difficulties or incontinence that may follow a stroke. Often the patient with stroke has functional incontinence, which is associated with communication difficulties, mobility problems, and dressing or undressing difficulties. Nursing interventions focused on urinary continence include (a) assessing for bladder distension by palpation; (b) offering the bedpan, urinal, commode, or toilet every 2 hours during waking hours and every 3 to 4 hours at night; (c) focusing the patient on the need to urinate with direct command; (d) assisting with clothing and mobility; (e) scheduling the majority of fluid intake between 0700 and 1900 hours; and (f) encouraging the usual position for urinating (standing for men and sitting for women).

Short-term interventions for urinary incontinence may include in-dwelling catheters, intermittent catheterization, frequent toileting, or incontinence briefs. These are not long-term solutions for urinary incontinence because complications such as urinary infections or skin irritation may occur.

Nurses often assess postvoid residual volume using bladder ultrasonography. The ultrasonogram measures how much urine is in the bladder after voiding. If urine remains in the bladder, incomplete emptying is a problem and may cause urinary tract infections. A coordinated program by the entire nursing staff is needed to achieve urinary continence.

Sensory–Perceptual Function. Patients who have had a stroke frequently have perceptual deficits. Patients with a stroke on the right side of the brain usually have difficulty in judging position, distance, and rate of movement. These patients are often impulsive and impatient and tend to deny problems related to strokes. They may fail to correlate spatial–perceptual problems with the inability to perform activities, such as guiding a wheelchair through the doorway. The patient with a right-brain stroke (left hemiplegia) is at higher risk for injury because of mobility difficulties. Directions for activities are best given verbally for comprehension. The task should be broken down into simple steps for ease of understanding. Environmental control, such as removing clutter and obstacles and providing good lighting, aids in concentration and helps provide safer mobility. The patient should wear nonslip socks at all times. One-sided neglect is common for people with right-brain stroke, so the nurse may assist or remind the patient to dress the weak or paralyzed side or shave the forgotten side of the face.

Patients with a left-brain stroke (right hemiplegia) commonly are slower in organization and performance of tasks. They tend to have impaired spatial discrimination. These patients usually admit to deficits and have a fearful, anxious response to a stroke. Their behaviours are slow and cautious. Nonverbal cues and instructions are helpful for comprehension with patients who have had a left-brain stroke.

Affect. Patients who have had strokes often exhibit emotional responses that are not appropriate or typical for the situation. Patients may appear apathetic, depressed, fearful, anxious, weepy, frustrated, or angry. Some patients, especially those with a stroke on the left side of the brain, exhibit exaggerated mood swings. The patient may be unable to control emotions and may suddenly burst into tears or laughter. This behaviour is out of context and often is unrelated to the underlying emotional state of the patient. Nursing interventions for atypical emotional response are to (a) distract the patient who suddenly becomes emotional, (b) explain to the patient and family that emotional outbursts may occur after a stroke, (c) maintain a calm environment, and (d) avoid shaming or scolding the patient during emotional outbursts.

Coping. The patient with a stroke may experience many losses, including those that are sensory, intellectual, communicative, functional, role behaviour, emotional, social, and vocational. The patient, caregiver, and family often go through the process of grief and mourning associated with the losses. Some patients experience long-term depression, exhibiting symptoms such as anxiety, weight loss, loss of energy, poor appetite, and sleep disturbances. In addition, the time and energy required to perform previously simple tasks can arouse anger and frustration.

The patient, caregiver, and family need help with coping with the losses associated with stroke. The nurse may assist the coping by (a) supporting communication between the patient and the family; (b) discussing lifestyle changes resulting from stroke deficits; (c) discussing changing roles and responsibilities within the family; (d) being an active listener to allow the expression of fear, frustration, and anxiety; (e) including the family and patient in short- and long-term goal planning and patient care; and (f) supporting family conferences. Maladjusted dependence with inadequate coping occurs when the patient does not maintain optimal functioning for self-care, family responsibilities, decision making, or socialization. This situation can cause resentment from both the patient and the family with a negative cycle of interpersonal dependency and control. *Maladjusted independence* occurs when the patient overestimates personal cognitive or physical capabilities and energy levels. These patients are at risk for injury.

Family members must cope with three aspects of the patient's behaviour: (a) recognition of behavioural changes resulting from neurological deficits that are not changeable, (b) responses to multiple losses by both the patient and the family, and (c) behaviours that may have been reinforced during the early stages of stroke as continued dependency. The patient, caregiver, and family may express feelings of guilt over not living healthy lifestyles or not seeking professional help sooner. Family therapy is a helpful adjunct to rehabilitation. Open communication, information regarding the total effects of stroke, education regarding stroke treatment, and therapy are helpful. Stroke support groups within rehabilitation facilities and in the community are helpful in terms of mutual sharing, education, coping, and understanding.

Sexual Function. A patient who has had a stroke may be concerned about the loss of sexual function. Many patients are comfortable talking about their anxieties and fears regarding sexual function if the nurse is comfortable and open to the topic. The nurse may initiate the topic with the patient and spouse or significant other. Common concerns about sexual activity among patients with stroke are impotence and the occurrence of another stroke during sex. Nursing interventions for sexual activity include education on (a) optimal positioning of partners, (b) timing for peak energy times, and (c) patient and partner counselling.

Community Reintegration. Traditionally, successful community integration following stroke has been difficult for the patient because of persistent problems with cognition, coping, physical deficits, and emotional lability that interfere with functioning. Older patients who have had a stroke often have more severe deficits and frequently experience multiple health problems. Failure to continue the rehabilitation regimen at home may result in deterioration and further complications.

Improved outcomes have been noted in patients suffering from severe stroke who have received inpatient rehabilitation. Results showed these patients had lower mortality rates, stayed in hospital for shorter lengths, and were more likely to return home than those receiving rehab in other facilities. Best results were seen in patients treated in units that were designated as specialized stroke units (Pereira, Graham, Shahabaz, et al., 2012).

Community resources can be an asset to patients and their families. The Heart and Stroke Foundation of Canada is a great resource for anyone who has been affected by or had a family member affected by a stroke. The Canadian Stroke Network provides newsletters on stroke, and Stroke Recovery Canada offers support to stroke survivors. Other local groups can offer more daily assistance, such as provision of meals and transportation. These resources can be identified by nurse case managers, advanced-practice nurses, community health nurses, discharge planners, and social workers. (Resources are listed at the end of the chapter.)

AGE-RELATED CONSIDERATIONS

STROKE

Stroke is a significant cause of death and disability. The highest incidence of stroke occurs among older adults. Stroke can result in a profound disruption in the life of an older person. The magnitude of disability and changes in total function can leave patients wondering if they can ever return to their prestroke life, and loss of independence may be a major concern. Performing ADLs may require many adaptive changes because of physical, emotional, perceptual, and cognitive deficits. Home management may be a particular challenge if the patient has an elderly spouse caretaker who also has health problems. There may be limited family members (including adult children) living nearby to provide help.

Assisting the older patient through the rehabilitative phase and to deal with the residual deficits of stroke, as well as aging, can provide a challenging nursing experience. Patients may become fearful and depressed because of the possibility of another attack or death. The fear can become immobilizing and interfere with effective rehabilitation.

Changes may occur in the patient–spouse relationship. The dependency resulting from a stroke can be threatening to the relationship. Some spouses may also have chronic medical problems that affect their ability to take care of the stroke survivor. The patient may not want anyone other than the spouse to provide care, putting a significant burden on the spouse.

The nurse has the opportunity to assist the patient and family in the transition through acute hospitalization, rehabilitation, long-term care, and home care. The needs of the patient and the family require ongoing nursing assessment, and interventions must be adapted in response to changing needs to optimize quality of life for both the patient and the family.

CASE STUDY

Stroke

Patient Profile

Ms. Evelyn Jones, a 66-year-old woman, awoke in the middle of the night and fell when she tried to get up to go to the bathroom (see the Chapter 58 case study). She fell because she was not able to control her left leg. Her husband took her to the hospital, where she was diagnosed with an acute right-sided ischemic stroke (right middle cerebral artery stroke). Because she had awakened with symptoms, the actual time of onset was unknown, and she was not a candidate for tissue plasminogen activator (tPA).

Source: Jeanette Dietl/ Shutterstock .com.

Subjective Data

- Left arm, leg, and face are weak and feel numb
- Feeling depressed and fearful
- Requires help with activities of daily living
- Is concerned about having another stroke
- Says she has not taken her drugs for high cholesterol for many weeks
- Has history of a brief episode of left-sided weakness and tingling of face, arm, and hand 3 months earlier, which totally resolved and for which she did not seek treatment

Objective Data

- BP: 180/110 mm Hg
- ECG is as follows:

- Left-sided arm weakness (3/5) and leg weakness (4/5)
- Decreased sensation on the left side, particularly the hand

- Left homonymous hemianopsia
- 160 cm tall and weighs 73 kg; body mass index = 28.5
- Alert, oriented, and able to answer questions appropriately but has mild slowness in responding

Past Medical History

- Migraines
- Hyperlipidemia
- Hypertension
- Smoking

Discussion Questions

1. How does Ms. Jones's health history and current findings put her at risk for a stroke?
2. How can the nurse address Ms. Jones's concerns regarding having another stroke?
3. Why would Ms. Jones's ability to drive be affected after the stroke?
4. What strategies might the nurse use to help Ms. Jones and her family cope with her feeling depressed?
5. **Priority decision:** What priority lifestyle changes should Ms. Jones make to reduce the likelihood of another stroke?
6. How will homonymous hemianopia affect Ms. Jones's hygiene, eating, driving, and community activities?
7. What factors should the nurse assess for related to outpatient rehabilitation for Ms. Jones?
8. **Priority decision:** What are the priority nursing interventions for Ms. Jones?
9. **Priority decision:** Based on the assessment data provided, what are the priority nursing diagnoses? Are there any collaborative problems?
10. **Evidence-informed practice:** Ms. Jones's family wants to know if her atrial flutter caused her stroke and, if so, what she can do to prevent additional problems with her atrial flutter.

ⓔvolve

Answers are available at *http://evolve.elsevier.com/Canada/Lewis/medsurg*.

REVIEW QUESTIONS

The number of the question corresponds to the same-numbered objective at the beginning of the chapter.

1. Which health condition(s) can increase an individual's risk for stroke? *(Select all that apply)*
   a. Pneumonia
   b. Atrial fibrillation
   c. Previous TIA
   d. Hypertension
   e. Migraines

2. Which of the following factors related to cerebral blood flow most often determines the extent of cerebral damage from a stroke?
   a. Amount of cardiac output
   b. Oxygen content of the blood
   c. Degree of collateral circulation
   d. Level of carbon dioxide in the blood

3. Which of the following pieces of information provided by the client would help differentiate a hemorrhagic stroke from an ischemic stroke?
   a. Sensory disturbance
   b. A history of hypertension
   c. Presence of motor weakness
   d. Sudden onset of severe headache

4. A client with right-sided hemiplegia and aphasia resulting from a stroke most likely has involvement of which of the following?
   a. Brain stem
   b. Vertebral artery
   c. Left middle cerebral artery
   d. Right middle cerebral artery

5. A client with a stroke is scheduled for angiography. Which of the following can this test detect?
   a. Presence of increased intracranial pressure
   b. Site and size of the infarction
   c. Patency of the cerebral blood vessels
   d. Presence of blood in the cerebro-spinal fluid

6. A client experiencing transient ischemic attacks is scheduled for a carotid endarterectomy. What does the nurse explain to the client about the purpose of this procedure?
   a. To decrease cerebral edema
   b. To reduce the brain damage that occurs during a stroke in evolution
   c. To prevent a stroke by removing atherosclerotic plaques blocking cerebral blood flow
   d. To provide a circulatory bypass around thrombotic plaques obstructing cranial circulation

7. For a client who is suspected to have had a stroke, what is one of the most important pieces of information that the nurse can obtain?
   a. Time of the client's last meal
   b. Time at which stroke symptoms first appeared
   c. Client's hypertension history and management
   d. Family history of stroke and other cardiovascular diseases
8. What does bladder training in a male client who has urinary incontinence after a stroke include?
   a. Limiting fluid intake
   b. Keeping a urinal in place at all times
   c. Assisting the client to stand to void
   d. Catheterizing the client every 4 hours

9. What is the most common response of a client who sustained a stroke regarding the change in body image?
   a. Denial
   b. Depression
   c. Dissociation
   d. Intellectualization

1. b, c, d; 2. c; 3. d; 4. c; 5. c; 6. c; 7. b; 8. c; 9. b.

⊝volve

For even more review questions, visit *http://evolve.elsevier.com/Canada/Lewis/medsurg*.

REFERENCES

American Heart Association. (2017). *Types of stroke*. Retrieved from *http://www.strokeassociation.org/STROKEORG/AboutStroke/TypesofStroke/Types-of-Stroke_UCM_308531_SubHomePage.jsp*.

Burns, M., Baylor, C., Dudgeon, B. J., et al. (2015). Asking the stakeholders: Perspectives of individuals with aphasia, their family members, and physicians regarding communication in medical interactions. *American Journal of Speech-Language Pathology, 24*(3), 341–357. doi:10.1044/2015_AJSLP-14-0051.

Campos, F., Sobrino, T., Vieites-Prado, A., et al. (2013). Hyperthermia in human ischemic and hemorrhagic stroke: Similar outcome, different mechanisms. *PLoS ONE, 8*(11), e78429. doi:10.1371/journal.pone.0078429.

Canadian Stroke Network & Heart and Stroke Foundation of Canada. (2013). *Canadian best practices recommendations for stroke care*. Retrieved from *http://www.strokebestpractices.ca/wp-content/uploads/2013/05/CSBP-Taking-Action-Resource-OVERVIEW_EN_22May13F.pdf*.

Casaubon, L. K., Boulanger, J. M., Blacquiere, D., et al. (2015). *Canadian stroke best practice recommendations: Hyperacute stroke care guidelines, update 2015*. Retrieved from *http://onlinelibrary.wiley.com/doi/10.1111/ijs.12551/full*.

Centers for Disease Control and Prevention. (2017). *Health effects of cigarette smoking*. Retrieved from *https://www.cdc.gov/tobacco/data_statistics/fact_sheets/health_effects/effects_cig_smoking*.

Chang, W. D., & Lai, P. T. (2015). New design of home-based dynamic hand splint for hemiplegic hands: A preliminary study. *Journal of Physical Therapy Science, 27*(3), 829–831. doi:10.1589/jpts.27.829.

Connolly, E. S., Rabinstein, A. A., Carhuapoma, J. R., et al. (2012). Guidelines for the management of aneurysmal subarachnoid hemorrhage. *Stroke; a Journal of Cerebral Circulation, 43*, 1711–1737. doi:10.1161/STR.0b013e3182587839.

Coutts, S. B., Wein, T. H., Lindsay, M. W., et al. (2014). Canadian stroke best practice recommendations: Secondary prevention of stroke guidelines, update 2014. *International Journal of Stroke: Official Journal of the International Stroke Society, 10*(3), 282–291. doi:10.1111/ijs.12439.

Daniels, S. K., Anderson, J. A., & Willson, P. C. (2012). Valid items for screening dysphagia risk in patients with stroke: A systematic review. *Stroke; a Journal of Cerebral Circulation, 43*, 892–897. doi:10.1161/STROKEAHA.111.640946.

Goyal, M., Demchuk, A. M., Menon, B. K., et al. (2015). Randomized assessment of rapid endovascular treatment of ischemic stroke. *The New England Journal of Medicine, 372*(11), 1019–1030. doi:10.1056/NEJMoa1414905.

Grotta, J. C. (2014). tPA for Stroke: Important progress in achieving faster treatment. *Journal of the American Medical Association, 311*(16), 1615–1617. doi:10.1001/jama.2014.3322.

Heart and Stroke Foundation of Canada. (2015). Acute inpatient stroke care. *Canadian stroke best practices* (5th ed.). Retrieved from *http://www.strokebestpractices.ca/acute-stroke-management*.

Heart and Stroke Foundation of Canada. (2016). *Mind the connection: Preventing stroke and dementia*. Retrieved from *https://www.heartandstroke.ca/-/media/pdf-files/canada/stroke-report/hsf-stroke-report-2016.ashx?la=en&hash=B84FFD2C434B4E3F5CF4585D9CB35713E6C406E5*.

Heart and Stroke Foundation of Canada. (2017a). *Different strokes: Recovery triumphs and challenges at any age*. Retrieved from *https://www.heartandstroke.ca/-/media/pdf-files/canada/stroke-report/strokereport2017en.ashx?la=en&hash=67F86E4C3338D5A7FE7862EA5D0DD57CA8539847*.

Heart and Stroke Foundation of Canada. (2017b). *Atrial fibrillation*. Retrieved from *https://www.heartandstroke.ca/heart/conditions/atrial-fibrillation*.

Heart and Stroke Foundation of Canada. (2017c). *Types of stroke*. Retrieved from *https://www.heartandstroke.ca/stroke/what-is-stroke/types-of-stroke*.

Heart and Stroke Foundation of Canada. (2017d). *Canadian stroke best practice recommendations: About us*. Retrieved from *http://www.strokebestpractices.ca/about-us*.

Hemphill, J. C., Greenberg, S. M., Anderson, C. S., et al. (2015). Guidelines for the management of spontaneous intracerebral hemorrhage. *Stroke; a Journal of Cerebral Circulation, 46*(7), 1–30. doi:10.1161/STR.0000000000000069.

Lannes, M., Teitelbaum, J., del Pilar Cortés, M., et al. (2012). Milrinone and homeostasis to treat cerebral vasospasm associated with subarachnoid hemorrhage: The Montreal Neurological Hospital protocol. *Neurocritical Care, 16*, 354–362. doi:10.1007/s12028-012-9701-5.

Liu, Z., Fu, W., Guo, Z., et al. (2012). Updated systematic review and meta-analysis of randomized clinical trials comparing carotid artery stenting and carotid endarterectomy in the treatment of carotid stenosis. *Annals of Vascular Surgery, 26*(4), 576–590. doi:10.1016/j.avsg.2011.09.009.

Meschia, J. F., Bushnell, C., Boden-Albala, B., et al. (2014). Guidelines for the primary prevention of stroke: A statement for healthcare professionals from the American Heart Association/American Stroke Association. *Stroke, 45*, 3754–3832. doi:10.1161/STR.0000000000000046.

National Institute of Neurological Disorders and Stroke (NINDS). (2017). *Aphasia information page*. Retrieved from *https://www.ninds.nih.gov/Disorders/All-Disorders/Aphasia-Information-Page*.

National Stroke Association. (2017). *Emotional.* Retrieved from *http://www.stroke.org/we-can-help/survivors/stroke-recovery/post -stroke-conditions/emotional.*

Ontario Stroke Network. (2016). *Stroke stats & facts.* Retrieved from *https://ontariostrokenetwork.ca/information-about-stroke/stroke -stats-and-facts/.*

Padwal, R. S., Bienek, A., McAlister, F. A., et al. (2015). Epidemiology of hypertension in Canada: An update. *The Canadian Journal of Cardiology.* Retrieved from *http://dx.doi.org/10.1016/j.cjca.2015 .07.734.*

Pereira, S., Graham, J. R., Shahabaz, A., et al. (2012). Rehabilitation of individuals with severe stroke: Synthesis of best evidence and challenges in implementation. *Topics in Stroke Rehabilitation, 19*(2), 122–131. doi:10.1310/tsr1902-122.

Peurala, S. H., Kantanen, M. P., Sjögren, T., et al. (2011). Effectiveness of constraint-induced movement therapy on activity and participation after stroke: A systematic review and meta-analysis of randomized control trials. *Clinical Rehabilitation, 26*(3), 209–223. doi:10.1177/0269215511420306.

Pollock, A., Baer, G., Campbell, P., et al. (2014). Physical rehabilitation approaches for the recovery of function and mobility following stroke. *Stroke; a Journal of Cerebral Circulation, 45*(10), e202. doi:10.1161/STROKEAHA.114.006275.

Pollock, R. D., Rafferty, G. F., Moxham, J., et al. (2013). Respiratory muscle strength and training in stroke and neurology: A systematic review. *International Journal of Stroke : Official Journal of the International Stroke Society, 8*(2), 124–130. doi:10.1111/j .1747-4949.2012.00811.x.

Public Health Agency of Canada. (2011). *Tracking heart disease and stroke in Canada: Stroke highlights 2011.* Retrieved from *http:// www.phac-aspc.gc.ca/cd-mc/cvd-mcv/sh-fs-2011/index-eng.php.*

Rantanen, K., & Tatlisumak, T. (2013). Stroke in women—Oral contraception, pregnancy, and hormone replacement therapy. *Current Vascular Pharmacology, 11*(1), 58–73. doi:10.2174/157016113804547638.

Registered Nurses' Association of Ontario. (2005). *Stroke assessment across the continuum of care.* Toronto: Author. (Seminal).

Rickard, A. C., Smith, J. E., Newell, P., et al. (2014). Salt or sugar for your injured brain? A meta-analysis of randomized controlled trials of mannitol versus hypertonic sodium solutions to manage raised intracranial pressure in traumatic brain injury. *Emergency Medicine Journal, 31*, 679–683. doi:10.1136/emermed-2013-202679.

Sorenson, A. G., & Ay, H. (2011). Transient ischemic attack definition, diagnosis, and risk stratification. *Neuroimaging Clinics of North America, 21*(2), 303–313. doi:10.1016/j.nic.2011.01.013.

Souillard-Scemama, R., Tisserand, M., Calvet, D., et al. (2015). An update on brain imaging in transient ischemic attack. *Journal of Neuroradiology, 42*(1), 3–11. doi:10.1016/j.neurad.2014.11.001.

Statistics Canada. (2016). *Body mass index, overweight or obese, self-reported, adult, by sex, provinces and territories.* Retrieved from *https://www.statcan.gc.ca/tables-tableaux/sum-som/l01/cst01/ health82b-eng.htm?sdi=body%20mass%20index.*

Statistics Canada. (2017). *The 10 leading causes of death, 2013.* Retrieved from *http://www.statcan.gc.ca/pub/82-625-x/2017001/ article/14776-eng.htm.*

Sykes, L., Wood, E., & Kwan, J. (2014). Antiepileptic drugs for the primary and secondary prevention of seizures after stroke. *The Cochrane Database of Systematic Reviews*, No. 1, Article CD005398. doi:10.1002/14651858.CD005398.pub3.

Toronto Brain Vascular Malformation Study Group. (2012). *Brain arteriovenous malformations (AVM).* Retrieved from *http:// brainavm.oci.utoronto.ca/malformations/brain_avm_index.htm.*

Tyson, S. F., Sadeghi-Demneh, E., & Nestor, C. J. (2013). A systematic review and meta-analysis of the effect of an ankle-foot orthosis on gait biomechanics after stroke. *Clinical Rehabilitation, 27*(10), 879–891. doi:10.1177/0269215513486497.

RESOURCES

Aphasia Institute
http://www.aphasia.ca

Canadian Association of Neuroscience Nurses (CANN)
http://www.cann.ca

Canadian Lung Association: Smoking Cessation Resource
http://www.lung.ca/quit

Canadian Stroke Best Practice Recommendations (developed by the Heart and Stroke Foundation of Canada)
http://www.strokebestpractices.ca

Canadian Stroke Network
http://www.canadianstrokenetwork.ca

Diabetes Canada
http://www.diabetes.ca

Heart and Stroke Foundation of Canada
http://www.heartandstroke.com

Hypertension Canada
http://www.hypertension.ca

Montreal Cognitive Assessment (MoCA)
http://www.mocatest.org

Registered Nurses' Association of Ontario: Smoking Cessation Resource
http://rnao.ca/bpg/guidelines/integrating-smoking-cessation -daily-nursing-practice

Registered Nurses' Association of Ontario: Stroke Assessment Across the Continuum of Care
http://rnao.ca/bpg/guidelines/stroke-assessment-across -continuum-care

Stroke Recovery Canada
http://www.strokerecoverycanada.com

Thrombosis Canada
http://thrombosiscanada.ca

American Association of Neuroscience Nurses (AANN)
http://www.aann.org

American Heart Association: Stroke Journal
http://stroke.ahajournals.org

American Stroke Association
http://www.strokeassociation.org

Association of Rehabilitation Nurses (ARN)
http://www.rehabnurse.org

DASH Diet: DASH Eating Plan (pp. 8–11)
http://www.nhlbi.nih.gov/health/public/heart/hbp/dash/new _dash.pdf

The Internet Stroke Center
http://www.strokecenter.org

National Institute of Neurological Disorders and Stroke
http://www.ninds.nih.gov

National Stroke Association
http://www.stroke.org

Society for Neuroscience
http://www.sfn.org

World Health Organization: Stroke
http://www.who.int/topics/cerebrovascular_accident/en

For additional Internet resources, see the website for this book at *http://evolve.elsevier.com/Canada/Lewis/medsurg*.

CHAPTER

61

Nursing Management
Chronic Neurological Problems

Written by: Dottie Roberts and Madona Plueger
Adapted by: Denise Ouellette

evolve WEBSITE

LEARNING OBJECTIVES

1. Compare and contrast the etiology, clinical manifestations, collaborative care, and nursing management of tension-type, migraine, and cluster headaches.
2. Differentiate the etiology, clinical manifestations, diagnostic studies, collaborative care, and nursing management of seizure disorders, multiple sclerosis, Parkinson's disease, myasthenia gravis, and normal pressure hydrocephalus.

3. Describe the clinical manifestations and the nursing and collaborative management of restless legs syndrome, amyotrophic lateral sclerosis, and Huntington's disease.
4. Explain the potential impact of chronic neurological disease on physical, emotional, and psychological well-being.
5. Outline the major goals of treatment for the patient with a chronic, progressive neurological disease.

KEY TERMS

absence seizure, p. 1540
amyotrophic lateral sclerosis (ALS), p. 1560
aura, p. 1535
cluster headaches, p. 1536
epilepsy, p. 1539
focal seizures, p. 1541
generalized seizures, p. 1540

headache, p. 1534
Huntington's disease (HD), p. 1560
migraine headache, p. 1534
multiple sclerosis (MS), p. 1546
myasthenia gravis (MG), p. 1557
myasthenic crisis, p. 1558
normal pressure hydrocephalus (NPH), p. 1561

Parkinson's disease (PD), p. 1552
prodrome, p. 1535
restless legs syndrome (RLS), p. 1559
seizure, p. 1539
status epilepticus, p. 1541
tension-type headache, p. 1535
tonic–clonic seizure, p. 1540

HEADACHE

Headache is probably the most common type of pain that humans experience. The majority of people have functional headaches, such as migraine or tension-type headaches. Others have organic headaches caused by intracranial or extracranial disease.

Not all tissues of the head are sensitive to pain. Pain-sensitive cranial structures include the venous sinuses, the dura, cranial blood vessels, the three divisions of the trigeminal nerve, the facial nerve, the glossopharyngeal nerve, the vagus nerve, and the first three cervical spinal nerves.

Headaches are classified as either primary or secondary. Primary headaches have no organic cause and include tension-type,

migraine, and cluster headaches. The type of primary headache is determined using the International Headache Society (IHS) guidelines, based on characteristics of the headache (Table 61-1). Secondary headaches are caused by another condition or disorder, such as sinus infection or stroke. A patient may have more than one type of headache. The history and neurological examination are keys to determining the type of headache.

MIGRAINE HEADACHE

Migraine headache (MH) is characterized by unilateral throbbing pain, a triggering event or factor, and manifestations associated with neurological and autonomic nervous system dysfunction. The effects of MH pain are dramatic, often causing

TABLE 61-1 COMPARISON OF MIGRAINE, TENSION-TYPE, AND CLUSTER HEADACHES

	Migraine Headache	Tension-Type Headache	Cluster Headache
Site (see Figure 61-1)	Unilateral (in 60%), may switch sides, commonly anterior	Bilateral, bandlike pressure at base of skull	Unilateral, radiating up or down from one eye
Quality	Throbbing, synchronous with pulse	Constant, squeezing tightness	Severe, "bone-crushing"
Frequency	Periodic, cycles of several months to years	Cycles for many years	May have months or years between attacks
			Attacks occur in clusters: once every second day to eight times a day over a period of 4 to 8 weeks
Duration	4–72 hours	30 minutes–7 days	15–180 minutes
Time and mode of onset	May be preceded by prodrome Onset after awakening Gets better with sleep	Not related to time	Nocturnal, commonly awakens patient from sleep
Associated symptoms	Nausea; vomiting; edema; irritability; sweating; photophobia; phonophobia; prodrome of sensory, motor, or psychic phenomena	Palpable neck and shoulder muscle tension, stiff neck, tenderness	Facial flushing or pallor, unilateral lacrimation, ptosis, and rhinitis

both physical and emotional disability. In Canada, the lifetime prevalence of MH is 24% of females and 9% of males (Pringsheim, Davenport, Mackie, et al., 2012).

Etiology and Pathophysiology

Although many theories have addressed the cause of MHs, the exact etiology is unknown. The current theory is that a complex series of neuro-vascular events initiates an MH (Cecil, Goldman, & Schafer, 2012). People with migraines have a state of neuronal hyper-excitability in the cerebral cortex, especially in the occipital cortex. Approximately 70% of those with migraine have a first-degree relative who also had MHs. Migraine is associated with seizure disorders, ischemic stroke, asthma, depression, anxiety, myocardial infarction, Raynaud's syndrome, and irritable bowel syndrome (Cecil et al., 2012). In many cases, MHs have no known precipitating events; however, for some patients, specific factors may trigger a headache. These may include dietary factors, menstruation, head trauma, physical exertion, fatigue, stress, weather, and drugs. Food triggers include chocolate, cheese, oranges, tomatoes, onions, monosodium glutamate, aspartame, and alcohol (particularly red wine).

Clinical Manifestations

MHs are subdivided by the IHS into categories, including those without **aura** and those with aura (Headache Classification Committee of the International Headache Society [HCCIHS], 2013). Auras are the neurological symptoms such as visual field defects, tingling or burning sensations, paresthesias, motor dysfunction (e.g., weakness, paralysis), dizziness, confusion, and even loss of consciousness that usually precede the onset of migraine pain (HCCIHS, 2013). Clinical manifestations that might occur in MH without and with aura are generalized edema, irritability, pallor, nausea and vomiting, and sweating. In MH without and with aura, the **prodrome** is not sharply defined. Prodrome signs or symptoms are those that may precede a MH, including psychic disturbances, gastro-intestinal upset, and changes in fluid balance.

During the headache phase, some patients with MH may seek shelter from noise, light, odours, people, and problems. The headache is described as a steady, throbbing pain that is synchronous with the pulse. However, the presentation of MH is varied in its severity. Although the headache is usually unilateral,

it may switch to the opposite side in another episode. Not all MHs are disabling, and many patients do not seek health care treatment for them. In some patients, the symptoms of MHs may become worse over time.

Diagnostic Studies

Usually, the diagnosis of MH is made based on patient history. Neurological and other diagnostic examinations are often normal. There are no specific laboratory or radiological tests used to diagnose MHs. Neuroimaging techniques (e.g. computed tomographic [CT] scan or magnetic resonance imaging [MRI]) of the head are not recommended for routine evaluation of headache unless there are abnormal findings on the neurological examination. If atypical features are present, secondary headaches must be ruled out.

TENSION-TYPE HEADACHE

Tension-type headache (TTH), also called *stress headache*, is the most common type of primary headache. These headaches are characterized by their bilateral location and pressing or tightening quality. TTHs are usually of mild or moderate intensity and can last from minutes to days. TTHs are divided by frequency into episodic and chronic types (HCCIHS, 2013).

Etiology and Pathophysiology

It was originally thought that TTHs were the result of sustained and painful contraction of the muscles of the scalp and the neck. However, research has shown it is likely that neuro-vascular factors similar to those involved in MH play a role in the development of TTH, including central neurological disturbances (Tfelt-Hansen & Koehler, 2011; HCCIHS, 2013).

Clinical Manifestations

Patients usually present with a bilateral frontal–occipital headache described as a constant, dull pressure, or bandlike headache associated with neck pain and increased muscle tension. The headache may involve sensitivity to light or sound but does not involve nausea or vomiting. There is no prodrome, and physical activity does not aggravate symptoms. The headaches may occur intermittently for weeks, months, or even years. Many patients can have a combination of migraine and TTHs, with features of both occurring simultaneously. Patients with MHs may experience

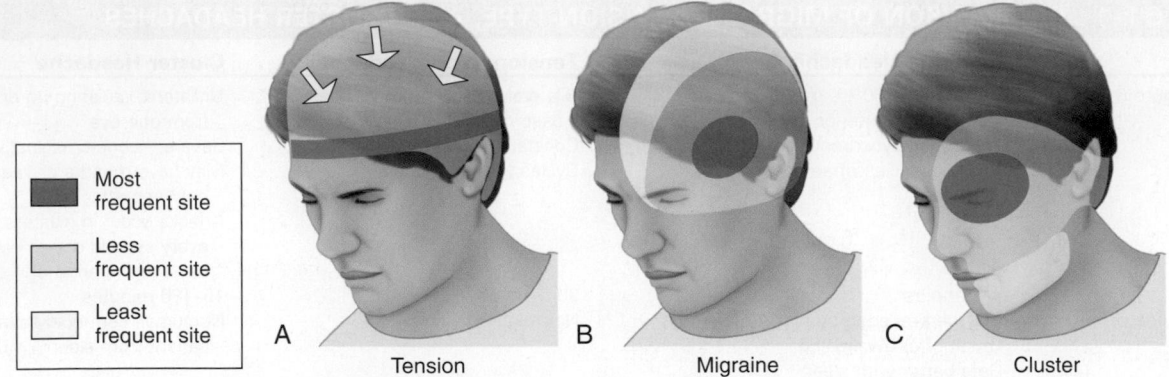

FIGURE 61-1 Location of pain for common headache syndromes. **A,** Tension headache is often described as the feeling of a weight in or on the head or a band squeezing the head (or both). **B,** Migraine headache is described as an intense, throbbing, or pounding pain that involves one temple. The pain is usually unilateral, although it can be bilateral. **C,** Cluster headache pain is focused in and around one eye and is often described as sharp, penetrating, or burning.

TTHs between migraine attacks. Figure 61-1 shows the location of pain for common headache syndromes.

Diagnostic Studies

If a patient meets TTH criteria, further diagnostic tests are not always conclusive, but they may be done to rule out secondary headache disorders. If TTH is present during physical examination, increased resistance to passive movement of the head, and tenderness of the head and neck may be present.

CLUSTER HEADACHE

Cluster headaches (CHs) are a rare form of headache, affecting less than 0.1% of the population (Costa, Antonaci, Ramusino, et al., 2015). CHs involve repeated headaches that can occur for weeks to months at a time, followed by periods of remission.

Etiology and Pathophysiology

Neither the cause nor the pathophysiological mechanism of CH is fully known. The trigeminal nerve is implicated in the production of pain, but CHs also involve dysfunction of intracranial blood vessels, the sympathetic nervous system, and pain modulation systems. Imaging studies show hypothalamic activation at the onset of CH (Goldman & Schafer, 2012). Common triggers include beer, caffeine, histamines, nicotine, and bright lights (Rozen & Fishman, 2012).

Clinical Manifestations

The CH is one of the most severe forms of headache and is characterized by intense, stabbing pain that is ipsilateral in nature and lasts an average of 97 minutes per attack (Gaul, Diener, & Müller, 2011). Other manifestations may include swelling around the eye, lacrimation (tearing), facial flushing or pallor, rhinitis, and constriction of the pupil (Gaul et al., 2011). During the headache, the patient is often agitated and restless, unable to sit still or relax. The headaches occur with regularity, usually occurring at the same time each day, during the same seasons of the year. Clusters typically last 2 weeks to 3 months and then go into remission for months to years (HCCIHS, 2013).

Diagnostic Studies

The diagnosis of CH is based primarily on the patient history. Asking patients to keep a headache diary can be useful. CT scan, MRI, or magnetic resonance angiography (MRA) may rule out an aneurysm, a tumour, or an infection. A lumbar puncture may rule out other disorders that may cause similar symptoms.

OTHER TYPES OF HEADACHES

The inability to diagnose a headache as MH, TTH, or CH may indicate that the pain is a symptom of a more serious illness. Headache can accompany subarachnoid hemorrhage; brain tumours; other intracranial masses; arteritis; vascular abnormalities; trigeminal neuralgia (tic douloureux); diseases of the eyes, nose, and teeth; and systemic illness (e.g., bacteremia, carbon monoxide poisoning, mountain sickness, polycythemia vera). The symptoms vary greatly. Because of the variety of causes of headache, clinical evaluation must be thorough. It should include an evaluation of personality, life adjustment, environment, and family situation as well as a comprehensive evaluation of neurological and physical status.

COLLABORATIVE CARE FOR HEADACHES

If no systemic underlying disease is the cause, the type of headache guides therapy. Table 61-2 outlines the general workup for a patient with headache to rule out any intracranial or extracranial disease. Table 61-3 summarizes the current therapies for prophylaxis and symptom relief of common headaches. These therapies include drugs, meditation, yoga, biofeedback, cognitive behavioural therapy, and relaxation training.

Drug Therapy

Migraine Headache. Drug treatment of the acute MH attack is aimed at terminating or decreasing the symptoms of the attack. Many people with mild or moderate MH can obtain relief with nonsteroidal anti-inflammatory drugs (NSAIDs), acetylsalicylic acid (ASA: Aspirin), or caffeine-containing combination analgesics. For moderate to severe headaches, the triptans have become the first line of therapy. Triptans are drugs that affect selected serotonin receptors and treat the primary cause of MH. These drugs reduce neurogenic inflammation of the cerebral blood vessels and produce vasoconstriction. Because these drugs cause constriction of coronary arteries, they must be avoided in patients with heart disease. Triptans should be taken at the first symptom of MH.

DRUG ALERT—Sumatriptan (Imitrex)
- Should not be given to patients with the following:
  - History or manifestations of ischemic cardiac, cerebro-vascular, or peripheral vascular problems
  - Uncontrolled hypertension since it may increase blood pressure
- Excess dosage may produce tremor and decrease respirations.

Tension-type Headache. Drug treatment for TTH usually involves ASA (Aspirin), acetaminophen (Tylenol), or NSAIDs used alone or in combination with a sedative, caffeine, or antidepressants; however, many of these drugs have serious adverse effects. Caution the patient about the long-term use of ASA (Aspirin) and ASA (Aspirin)-containing drugs because they can cause gastric bleeding and coagulation abnormalities in susceptible patients. Drugs containing acetaminophen (Tylenol) can cause kidney damage with chronic use and liver damage when taking large doses or when combined with alcohol. To decrease the recurrence of TTH, the patient may receive preventive therapy with amitriptyline (Elavil), venlafaxine (Effexor), or mirtazapine (Remeron).

DRUG ALERT—Topiramate (Topamax)
Instruct patient to do the following:
- Not abruptly discontinue drug since this may cause seizures
- Avoid tasks that require alertness until response to drug is established
- Take adequate fluids to decrease risk for development of renal stones

Cluster Headache. Because CHs occur suddenly, often at night, and are not long-lasting, they are extremely hard to treat. Acute treatment of CH is inhalation of 100% oxygen delivered at a rate of 8 to 12 L/minute for 15 minutes (Gaul et al., 2011), which may relieve headache by causing vasoconstriction and increasing synthesis of serotonin in the central nervous system. Prophylactic drugs may include calcium channel blockers, steroids, topiramate (Topamax), melatonin, NSAIDs, and inhaled dihydro-ergotamine (DHE).

Other Headaches. Patients with frequent headaches may overuse analgesic drugs. Such overuse can lead to chronic daily headache, also called *analgesic rebound headache* or *drug-induced headache*. Drugs known to cause this problem are acetaminophen

---

TABLE 61-2 DIAGNOSTIC STUDIES

Headaches

- History and physical examination
  - Neurological examination (often negative)
  - Inspection for local infections
  - Palpation for tenderness, bony swellings
  - Auscultation for bruits over major arteries
- Routine laboratory studies
  - CBC
  - Electrolytes
  - Urinalysis
- CT scan of sinuses
- Special studies (e.g., CT scan of brain, angiography, EEG, EMG, MRA, MRI, lumbar puncture)

CBC, complete blood cell count; *CT*, computed tomographic (scan); *EEG*, electroencephalography; *EMG*, electromyography; *MRA*, magnetic resonance angiography; *MRI*, magnetic resonance imaging.

TABLE 61-3 COLLABORATIVE CARE

Headaches

	Migraine Headache	Tension-Type Headache	Cluster Headache
Diagnostic	• History*	• History*	• History*
Collaborative Therapy			
Symptomatic	• Anti-emetic: metoclopramide Prokinetics: domperidone • Nonopioid analgesics: acetylsalicylic acid (ASA; Aspirin), acetaminophen (Tylenol), ibuprofen (Advil), naproxen (Naprosyn) • Sympatholytic (adrenergic blocking) agent: dihydroergotamine (DHE) via inhalation or intravenous • Triptans: sumatriptan (Imitrex), zolmitriptan (Zomig)	• Analgesic combinations: acetaminophen with caffeine, ibuprofen with caffeine • Nonopioid analgesics: acetylsalicylic acid (ASA; Aspirin), ibuprofen (Advil), acetaminophen (Tylenol), nonsteroidal anti-inflammatory drug: naproxen (Naprosyn)	• Oxygen • Sympatholytic (adrenergic blocking) agent: dihydroergotamine (DHE) via inhalation or intravenous • Triptans: sumatriptan (Imitrex), zolmitriptan (Zomig)
Prophylactic	• β-Adrenergic blockers: propranolol (Inderal), metoprolol (Lopresor), nadolol • Acupuncture • Anticonvulsant: valproic acid (Depakene), divalproex sodium (Epival), gabapentin (Neurontin), topiramate (Topamax) • Antidepressants: amitriptyline (Elavil), nortriptyline (Aventyl), venlafaxine (Effexor) • Biofeedback • Cognitive behavioural therapy • Relaxation therapy	• Acupuncture • Antidepressants: amitriptyline (Elavil), mirtazapine (Remeron), venlafaxine (Effexor) • Biofeedback • Cognitive behavioural therapy • Muscle relaxation training • Physiotherapy • Psychotherapy • Relaxation therapy	• Anticonvulsant: topiramate (Topamax) • Antimanic agent: lithium • Biofeedback • Calcium channel blocker: verapamil (Isoptin) • Corticosteroid: prednisone (Apo-prednisone) • Melatonin • Physiotherapy

*Magnetic resonance imaging (MRI) should be considered in patients with nonacute headache who have an unexplained abnormal neurological examination, an atypical headache or headache features, or an additional risk factor, such as immune deficiency.

(Tylenol), ASA (Aspirin), NSAIDs (e.g., ibuprofen [Advil]), triptans, and opioids. Treatment can be difficult and involves gradual withdrawal, possible hospitalization, and initiation of prophylactic drugs such as amitriptyline (Elavil).

NURSING MANAGEMENT HEADACHES

NURSING ASSESSMENT

Data that should be obtained from a patient with headache are presented in Table 61-4. Because the history provides the key to assessment of headache, it should include specific details of the headache itself, such as the location and type of pain, onset, frequency, duration, relation to events (emotional, psychological, physical), and time of day of the occurrence. Information should also be obtained about previous illnesses, surgery, trauma, allergies, family history, and response to medication. The nurse should suggest that the patient keep a diary of headache episodes with specific details. This type of record can be of great help in determining the type of headache and the precipitating events. If the patient has a history of MH, TTH, or CH, it is important to determine if the character, intensity, or location of the headache has changed. This may be an important clue about the cause of the headache (Table 61-5).

NURSING DIAGNOSES

Nursing diagnoses for the patient with headache may include, but are not limited to, the following:
* *Acute pain* related to *biological injury agent* (headache)
* *Ineffective health management* related to *difficulty managing complex treatment regimen* (drug therapy, lifestyle adjustment)

Additional information on nursing diagnoses for the patient with headache is presented in NCP 61-1, Patient With Headache, available on the Evolve website.

PLANNING

The overall goals are that the patient with a headache will (1) have reduced or no pain, (2) experience increased comfort and decreased anxiety, (3) demonstrate understanding of triggering events and treatment strategies, (4) use positive coping strategies to deal with chronic pain, and (5) experience increased quality of life and decreased disability.

NURSING IMPLEMENTATION

Patients with chronic headache present a challenge to nurses. Headaches may be related to an inability to cope with daily stresses. The most effective therapy may be to help patients examine their lifestyle, recognize stressful situations, and learn to cope with them more appropriately. Encouraging the patient to keep a journal may aid in identifying precipitating factors and developing ways of avoiding them. Daily exercise, relaxation periods, and socializing can be encouraged because each can help decrease the recurrence of headache. The nurse can suggest alternative ways of handling the pain of headache.

In addition to using analgesics for the symptomatic relief of headache, patients should be encouraged to use relaxation techniques because they are effective in relieving TTH and MH. People with MHs often need a quiet, dimly lit environment. Massage and moist hot packs to the neck and head can help a patient with TTH. Patients should learn about the drugs prescribed for prophylactic and symptomatic treatment of headache and should be able to describe the purpose, action, dosage, and

---

TABLE 61-4 NURSING ASSESSMENT

Headaches

Subjective Data
Important Health Information
Current health history: Pain assessment including location, characteristics, onset and duration, frequency, quality, intensity or severity of pain, and precipitating factors (nurse should use a pain scale and observation of actions for cognitively impaired individual); positive family history of headaches; history of recent ingestion of alcohol, caffeine, cheese, chocolate, monosodium glutamate, aspartame, lunch meats (nitrites in cured meats), sausage, hot dog, onion, avocado; level of hydration
Past health history: Seizures, cancer, recent fall or trauma, cranial infection, stroke; asthma or allergies; mental health disorder; relationship of headache to overwork, stress, menstruation, sexual activity, travel, bright lights, disruptions in sleep, or noxious environmental stimuli
Medications: Use of hydralazine, bromides, nitroglycerin, ergotamine (withdrawal), nonsteroidal anti-inflammatory drugs, estrogen preparations, oral contraceptives, over-the-counter or prescription remedies
Surgery or other treatments: Craniotomy, sinus surgery, facial surgery, dental surgery

Symptoms
* Anorexia, nausea, vomiting (migraine prodrome)
* Vertigo, fatigue, weakness, paralysis, fainting, malaise
* *Migraine:* aura; unilateral, severe, throbbing (possible switching of side) headache; visual disturbances; photophobia; phonophobia; dizziness; tingling or burning sensations
* *Tension-type:* bilateral, bandlike, dull and persistent, base-of-skull headache, neck tenderness
* *Cluster:* unilateral and severe, nocturnal headaches; nasal stuffiness, unilateral lacrimation

Objective Data
General
Anxiety, apprehension

Integumentary
Cluster: Forehead diaphoresis, pallor, unilateral facial flushing with cheek edema, conjunctivitis
Migraine: Generalized edema (prodrome), pallor, diaphoresis

Neurological
Horner syndrome (results from damage to sympathetic nerves, and is signified by the following ipsilateral signs: pupillary contraction, ptosis, and a lack of facial sweating), restlessness (*cluster*), hemiparesis (*migraine*)

Musculo-Skeletal
Neck stiffness (or nuchal rigidity) resulting from impaired neck flexion secondary to muscle spasms of the neck (*meningeal, tension-type*), palpable neck and shoulder muscles (*tension-type*)

Possible Findings
Possible evidence of disease, deformity, or infection on brain imaging, cerebral angiogram, lumbar puncture, EEG, EMG; nonspecific brain imaging or laboratory tests

CT, computed tomographic (scan); *EEG,* electroencephalography; *EMG,* electromyography; *MRA,* magnetic resonance angiography; *MRI,* magnetic resonance imaging.

---

adverse effects of the drug. To prevent accidental overdose, patients should make a written note of each dose of drug taken.

For patients whose headaches are triggered by food, dietary counselling may be provided. Patients are encouraged to eliminate foods that may provoke headaches. Active challenge and

TABLE 61-5 COMMON SCREENING ASSESSMENT QUESTIONS TO DETERMINE TYPE OF HEADACHE

- When do the headaches occur?
- How frequent are the headaches?
- What is the duration of the headache(s)?
- Are there any known triggers for the headaches, such as environmental, food, or alcohol?
- Where do you feel the headache pain? Does the pain radiate?
- Do you experience any visual changes such as blurring or double vision?
- Do you experience any other symptoms, such as nausea, vomiting, dizziness, weakness, changes in speech, swallowing difficulty?
- What relieves the headache pain?

TABLE 61-6 PATIENT & CAREGIVER TEACHING GUIDE

Headaches

The following information should be included when teaching the caregiver about headaches.
1. Keep a diary or calendar of headaches and possible precipitating events.
2. Avoid factors that can trigger a headache:
   - Foods containing amines (cheese, chocolate), nitrites (meats such as hot dogs), vinegar, onions, or monosodium glutamate
   - Fermented or marinated foods
   - Caffeine
   - Nicotine
   - Ice cream
   - Alcohol (particularly red wine)
   - Emotional stress
   - Fatigue
   - Drugs such as those containing ergot and monoamine oxidase inhibitors
3. Describe the purpose, action, dosage, and adverse effects of drugs taken.
4. Be able to self-administer sumatriptan (Imitrex) subcutaneously if prescribed.
5. Use stress-reduction techniques such as relaxation.
6. Participate in regular exercise.
7. Contact the health care provider if any of the following occur:
   - Symptoms become more severe, last longer than usual, or are resistant to medication.
   - Nausea and vomiting (if severe or not typical), change in vision, or fever occurs with the headache.

provocative testing with specific foods may be necessary to determine the specific causative agents. However, food triggers may change over time. Patients should avoid smoking and exposure to triggers such as strong perfumes, volatile solvents, and gasoline fumes. CH attacks may occur at high altitudes with low oxygen levels, such as during air travel. Inhaled DHE may decrease the likelihood of these attacks. A teaching guide for patients with headaches is presented in Table 61-6. The "Evidence-Informed Practice" box looks at evidence related to the efficacy of botulinum toxin A (Botox) in headache prevention.

EVALUATION

Expected outcomes for the patient with headache are addressed in the Nursing Care Plan (NCP) 61-1, available on the Evolve website.

🔍 EVIDENCE-INFORMED PRACTICE

Research Highlight

Can Botulinum Toxin A Prevent Headaches?
Clinical Question
For adults with chronic headaches (P), does prophylactic botulinum toxin A (I) versus placebo versus medication (C) decrease headache frequency or severity (O)?

Best Available Evidence
Meta-analysis of randomized controlled trials (RCTs) and comparative effectiveness trials

Critical Appraisal and Synthesis of Evidence
- Twenty-seven RCTs (n = 5313) comparing botulinum toxin A (Botox) with placebo, and four trials comparing botulinum toxin A (Botox) with medication (amitriptyline [Elavil], topiramate [Topamax], valproic acid (Depakene).
- Headaches assessed were migraine or tension, episodic (<15 headaches per month) or chronic (>15 headaches per month), or a chronic daily headache.
- Botulinum toxin A (Botox) resulted in decreased frequency of chronic daily and chronic migraine headaches. It had no effect on episodic migraine or chronic tension-type headaches.
- Botulinum toxin A (Botox) was not related to fewer migraine headaches when compared with valproic acid (Depakene), topiramate (Topamax), or amitriptyline (Elavil).

Conclusion
Botulinum toxin A (Botox) is beneficial for chronic daily headaches and chronic migraine headaches.

Implications for Nursing Practice
- Inform patients that botulinum toxin A (Botox) can prevent some types of headaches.
- Advise patients of botulinum toxin A (Botox) adverse effects, including blepharoptosis (drooping upper eyelid), paresthesia, neck stiffness and pain, and muscle weakness.

Reference for Evidence
Jackson, J. L., Kuriyama, A., & Hayashino, Y. (2012). Botulinum toxin A for prophylactic treatment of migraine and tension headaches in adults: A meta-analysis. *JAMA: The Journal of the American Medical Association*, *307*(16), 1736–1745.

P, Patient population of interest; *I*, intervention or area of interest; *O*, outcomes of interest (see Chapter 1).

CHRONIC NEUROLOGICAL DISORDERS

SEIZURE DISORDERS AND EPILEPSY

Seizure is transient, uncontrolled electrical discharge of neurons in the brain that interrupts normal function. Often, seizures are symptoms of an underlying illness. They may accompany a variety of disorders, or they may occur spontaneously without apparent cause. Seizures resulting from systemic and metabolic disturbances are not considered epilepsy if the seizures cease when the underlying problem is corrected. In adults, metabolic disturbances that cause seizures include acidosis, electrolyte imbalances, hypoglycemia, hypoxia, alcohol and barbiturate withdrawal, dehydration, and water intoxication. Extracranial disorders that can cause seizures are heart, lung, liver, or kidney diseases; systemic lupus erythematosus; diabetes mellitus; hypertension; and septicemia.

Epilepsy is a condition in which at least two spontaneous seizures occur more than 24 hours apart and is caused by a chronic underlying pathology (Cavazos, 2012). Epilepsy affects approximately 0.6% of Canadians, with 75% to 85% of people with epilepsy receiving a diagnosis before age 18. Epilepsy is more prevalent in developing countries. The incidence rates are high during the first year of life, decline through childhood and adolescence, plateau in middle age, and rise sharply again among older adults.

Etiology and Pathophysiology

The most common causes of seizures during the first 6 months of life are severe birth injury, central nervous system (CNS) congenital defects, infections, and inborn errors of metabolism. In patients between 2 and 20 years of age, the primary causative factors are birth injury, infection, trauma, and genetic factors. In individuals between 20 and 30 years of age, seizure disorder usually occurs as the result of structural lesions, such as trauma, brain tumours, or vascular disease. After 50 years of age, primary causes of seizure disorders are cerebro-vascular lesions and metastatic brain tumours. Although many causes of seizure disorders have been identified, 50% to 60% of all people with seizure disorders cannot be attributed to a specific cause (Epilepsy Canada, 2016). The role of heredity in seizure disorders has been difficult to determine because of the problem of separating hereditary from environmental or acquired influences. Furthermore, some families carry a predisposition to seizure disorders in the form of an inherently low threshold to seizure-producing stimuli, such as trauma, disease, and high fever. The etiology of recurring seizures (epilepsy) has long been attributed to a group of abnormal neurons (seizure focus) that seem to undergo spontaneous firing. This firing spreads by physiological pathways to involve adjacent or distant areas of the brain. If this activity spreads to involve the whole brain, a generalized seizure occurs. The factor responsible for this abnormal firing is not clear. Any stimulus that causes the cell membrane of the neuron to depolarize induces a tendency to spontaneous firing. Scar tissue (gliosis) is often found in the area of the brain from which the epileptic activity arises. Scarring is believed to interfere with the normal chemical and structural environment of neurons, making them more likely to fire abnormally. In addition to neuronal alterations, changes in the function of astrocytes may play several key roles in recurring seizures. Activation of astrocytes by hyperactive neurons is one of the crucial factors that predispose neurons nearby to the generation of an epileptic discharge. Previously, epilepsy research focused on neuronal causes. However, there is now evidence that dysfunctional astrocytes may play a key role in recurring seizures; therefore, therapies targeting astrocytic dysfunction could prove promising (Seifert & Steinhäuser, 2013).

Clinical Manifestations

The specific clinical manifestations of a seizure are determined by the site of the electrical disturbance. The preferred method of classifying recurring seizures is the International League Against Epilepsy (ILAE) Classification System (Fisher, Cross, French, et al., 2017) (Table 61-7). Revised in 2017, this system is based on the clinical and electroencephalographic manifestations of seizures. In this system, seizures are divided into three major classes: generalized onset, focal onset, and unknown onset, with each of these classes further subdivided according to motor or non-motor presentation (Fisher et al., 2017). Depending on the type, a seizure may progress through several phases, which include (1) the prodrome phase, with signs or activities that precede a seizure; (2) the aural phase, with a sensory warning; (3) the ictal

TABLE 61-7 INTERNATIONAL CLASSIFICATION OF SEIZURE TYPES

Focal Onset	Generalized Onset	Unknown Onset
Aware or impaired awareness Motor or non-motor onset	Motor or non-motor onset	Motor or non-motor onset
Motor onset type examples: • Automatisms • Atonic • Clonic • Epileptic spasms • Hyperkinetic • Myoclonic • Tonic	Motor onset type examples: • Atonic • Epileptic spasms • Clonic • Myoclonic • Tonic • Tonic–clonic	Motor onset type examples: • Epileptic spasms • Tonic–clonic
Non-motor onset type examples: • Autonomic • Behaviour arrest • Cognitive • Emotional • Sensory	Non-motor (absence) onset type examples: • Atypical • Eyelid myoclonia • Myoclonic • Typical	Non-motor onset type examples: • Behaviour arrest

Source: Adapted from Fisher, R. S., Cross, J. H., French, J. A., et al. (2017). Operational classification of seizure types by the International League Against Epilepsy: Position Paper of the ILAE Commission for Classification and Terminology. *Epilepsia, 58*(4), 522–530.

phase, with full seizure; and (4) the postictal phase, which is the period of recovery after the seizure.

Generalized Seizures. Generalized seizures are characterized by bilateral synchronous epileptic discharges in the brain from the onset of the seizure. Because the entire brain is affected at the onset of the seizures, there is no warning or aura. In most cases, the patient loses consciousness for a few seconds to several minutes. There are a number of generalized seizure types. Some of the more common ones are discussed below.

Tonic–Clonic Seizures. The most common generalized seizure is the generalized tonic–clonic seizure. Tonic–clonic seizure is characterized by loss of consciousness and falling to the ground if the patient is upright, followed by stiffening of the body (tonic phase) for 10 to 20 seconds and subsequent jerking of the extremities (clonic phase) for another 30 to 40 seconds. Cyanosis, excessive salivation, tongue or cheek biting, and incontinence may accompany the seizure.

In the postictal phase, the patient usually has muscle soreness, is very tired, and may sleep for several hours. Some patients may not feel normal for several hours or days after a seizure. The patient has no memory of the seizure.

Typical Absence Seizures. Usually, the absence seizure occurs only in children and rarely continues beyond adolescence. This type of seizure may cease altogether as the child matures, or it may evolve into another type of seizure. The typical clinical manifestation is a brief staring spell that lasts only a few seconds, so it often occurs unnoticed. There may be an extremely brief loss of consciousness. When untreated, the seizures may occur up to 100 times a day.

The electroencephalogram (EEG) demonstrates a 3-Hz (cycles/sec) spike-and-wave pattern that is unique to this type of seizure. Absence seizures can often be precipitated by hyperventilation and flashing lights.

Atypical Absence Seizures. Another type of generalized seizure is atypical absence seizure, which is characterized by a staring spell accompanied by other signs and symptoms, including brief warnings, peculiar behaviour during the seizure, or confusion after the seizure. The EEG demonstrates atypical spike-and-wave patterns.

Other Types of Generalized Seizures. Other types of generalized seizures are myoclonic, atonic, tonic, and clonic seizures. A myoclonic seizure is characterized by a sudden, excessive jerk of the body or the extremities. The jerk may be forceful enough to hurl the person to the ground. These seizures are very brief and may occur in clusters.

An atonic ("drop attack") seizure involves either a tonic episode or a paroxysmal loss of muscle tone and begins suddenly with the person falling to the ground. Usually, consciousness returns by the time the person hits the ground, and normal activity can be resumed immediately. Patients with this type of seizure are at a great risk for head injury and often have to wear protective helmets. A tonic seizure involves a sudden onset of sustained increased tone in the extensor muscles. These patients often fall. Clonic seizures begin with loss of consciousness and sudden loss of muscle tone, followed by limb jerking that may or may not be symmetrical.

Focal Seizures. Focal seizures (previously known as *partial seizures*) are one of the other major classes of seizures in the ILAE classification system. They are caused by electrical activity that is focal to a particular area of the brain, resulting in unilateral manifestations. Focal seizures begin in a specific region of the cortex, as indicated by the EEG and the clinical manifestations. For example, if the discharging focus is located in the medial aspect of the postcentral gyrus, the patient may experience numbness and tingling in the leg on the side opposite the focus. If the discharging focus is located in the part of the brain that governs a particular function, manifestations of those functions—for example, sensory, motor, cognitive, or emotional—may occur.

Focal seizures may be confined to one side of the brain and remain partial, or focal, in nature, or they may spread to involve the entire brain, culminating in a generalized tonic–clonic seizure. Any tonic–clonic seizure that is preceded by an aura is a focal seizure that generalizes secondarily. Many tonic–clonic seizures that appear to be generalized from the outset may actually be secondary generalized seizures, but the preceding partial component may be so brief that it is undetected by the patient, by an observer, or even on the EEG. Unlike the primary generalized tonic–clonic seizure, the secondary generalized seizure may result in a transient residual neurological deficit postically. This phenomenon is called *Todd paralysis* (focal weakness), which resolves after varying lengths of time.

As per the ILAE's updated classification system, focal seizures are further divided into (1) focal aware seizures (those with simple motor or sensory phenomena) and (2) focal impaired awareness seizures (those with complex symptoms).

Focal Aware Seizures. Focal aware seizures (formerly known as *simple partial seizures*) with elementary symptoms do not involve loss of consciousness and rarely last longer than one minute. They may involve motor, sensory, or autonomic phenomena, or a combination of these. The terms *focal motor, focal sensory,* and *jacksonian* have been used to describe seizures of the focal aware type.

Focal Impaired Awareness Seizures. Focal impaired awareness (FIA) seizures (formerly called *complex partial seizures*) can involve behavioural, emotional, affective, sensory, and cognitive functions. The location of the discharging focus is usually in the temporal lobe; hence the seizure is often termed a *temporal lobe seizure.* Usually, these seizures last longer than one minute, and they are frequently followed by a period of postictal confusion. FIA seizures are distinct from focal aware seizures in that they involve alterations in consciousness. The sole manifestation of FIA seizures may be a confused state without any motor or sensory components. This type of attack is sometimes termed *temporal lobe absence.* There is rarely the complete loss of consciousness that is typical of the generalized absence attack, and the patient does not snap back to the preseizure state as occurs in the patient who has had a generalized absence attack.

Most commonly, FIA seizures involve lip smacking and automatisms (repetitive movements that may not be appropriate). These are often called *psychomotor seizures.* The patient may continue an activity that was initiated before the seizure, such as counting out change or picking items from a grocery shelf but after the seizure does not remember the activity performed during the seizure. Other automatisms are less organized, such as picking at clothing, fumbling with objects (real or imaginary), or simply walking away.

A variety of psychosensory symptoms may occur during a FIA seizure, including distortions of visual or auditory sensations and vertigo. There may be alterations in memory, such as a feeling of having experienced an event before (déjà vu) or alterations in thought processes. Alterations in sexual functioning can vary from hyposexuality to hypersexuality. Many patients with temporal lobe seizures have decreased sexual drive or erectile dysfunction. However, some may experience sexual sensations during their seizures. This is because the abnormal electrical activity arises from the brain centres responsible for these sensations. Some experience increased sexual drive just after a seizure. In addition, some anticonvulsant drugs can cause a decrease in sexual drive because of sedation. Others can cause erectile dysfunction.

Complications

Physical. Status epilepticus is a state of continuous seizure activity in which seizures recur in rapid succession without return to consciousness between seizures. Status epilepticus is a neurological emergency and can involve any type of seizure. During repeated seizures, the brain uses more energy than can be supplied. Permanent brain damage may result. Tonic–clonic status epilepticus is the most dangerous type because it can cause ventilatory insufficiency, hypoxemia, cardiac dysrhythmias, hyperthermia, and systemic acidosis, all of which can be fatal. Airway securement via medical intervention using sedation and endotracheal intubation may be necessary to avoid life-threatening complications. Patients who lose consciousness during a seizure are at greatest risk. Death can result from head injury incurred during a fall, from drowning, or from severe burns. Perinatal seizures are associated with acute and long-term adverse outcomes to pregnant women and their babies (Hart & Sibai, 2013).

Psychosocial. Seizure disorders place many limitations on a patient's lifestyle. Epilepsy generally carries a social stigma, and patients diagnosed with seizure disorders may experience depression, anxiety, or anger, and relationships are often affected. The patient with epilepsy may experience discrimination in employment and educational opportunities. Obtaining a driver's license may be difficult because of legal sanctions against driving (Epilepsy Canada, 2016).

Depression is common among people with epilepsy (Zamani, Mehdizadeh, & Sadeghi, 2012). Not only can depression impair daily functioning, but it can also lead to increased seizure

TABLE 61-8 COLLABORATIVE CARE

Diagnosis of Seizure Disorders and Epilepsy

Diagnostic
- History and physical examination
  - Birth and development history
  - Comprehensive neurological assessment
  - Family history
  - Febrile seizures
  - Significant illnesses and injuries
- Seizure history
  - Antecedent events
  - Precipitating factors
  - Seizure description (including onset, duration, frequency, postictal state)

- Diagnostic studies
  - CBC, urinalysis, electrolytes, creatinine, fasting blood glucose
  - CT, MRI, MRA, MRS, PET scan
  - EEG
  - Lumbar puncture

Collaborative Therapy
- Anticonvulsant drugs (see Table 61-10)
- Psychosocial counselling
- Surgery (see Table 61-11)
- Vagal nerve stimulation

CBC, complete blood cell count; *CT,* computed tomographic (scan); *EEG,* electroencephalography; *MRA,* magnetic resonance angiography; *MRI,* magnetic resonance imaging; *MRS,* magnetic resonance spectroscopy; *PET,* positron emission tomography.

frequency through sleep deprivation and its role as an emotional stressor. Treatment for depression among patients with epilepsy should focus first on seizure control, and if depression persists in spite of the latter, antidepressant medication and psychological therapy may be necessary (McLaughlin & McFarland, 2011).

Diagnostic Studies

The most useful diagnostic tools are accurate and comprehensive description of the seizures and the patient's health history (Table 61-8). The EEG is a useful diagnostic adjuvant to the history but only if it shows abnormalities. Abnormal findings help determine the type of seizure and help pinpoint the seizure focus. Unfortunately, only a small percentage of patients with seizure disorders have abnormal findings on the EEG the first time the test is done. EEGs may need to be repeated often, or continuous EEG monitoring may be needed to detect abnormalities. Abnormal discharges may not occur during the 30 to 40 minutes of sampling during EEG, and the test may be negative. It is not a definitive test because some patients who do not have seizure disorders have abnormal patterns on their EEGs, whereas many patients with seizure disorders have normal EEGs between seizures. Magnetoencephalography may be done in conjunction with the EEG. This test has greater sensitivity in detecting small magnetic fields generated by neuronal activity. Video-EEG can give definitive diagnosis of seizures with impairment of consciousness.

A complete blood cell count, serum chemistries, studies of liver and kidney function, and urinalysis should be done to rule out metabolic disorders. A CT or MRI scan should be done with any new-onset seizure to rule out structural abnormalities (Cavazos, 2012). Cerebral angiography, single-photon emission computed tomography, magnetic resonance spectroscopy, magnetic resonance angiography, and positron emission tomography may be used in selected situations.

Collaborative Care

Most seizures do not require professional emergency medical care because they are self-limiting and rarely cause bodily injury. However, if status epilepticus occurs, if significant bodily harm occurs, or if the event is a first-time seizure, medical care should be sought immediately. Table 61-9 summarizes emergency care

of the patient with a generalized tonic–clonic seizure, the seizure most likely to warrant professional emergency medical care. The diagnostic studies and collaborative care of seizure disorders are summarized in Table 61-8.

Drug Therapy. Seizure disorders are treated primarily with anticonvulsant drugs (Table 61-10). Therapy is aimed at preventing seizures because a cure is not possible. Drugs generally act by stabilizing nerve cell membranes and preventing spread of the epileptic discharge. Anticonvulsant drugs offer seizure control in approximately 50% of patients; 30% have a reduction in both the intensity and frequency of seizures; and 20% of patients have seizures that are resistant to medication (Epilepsy Ontario, 2016).

The primary goal of anticonvulsant drug therapy is to obtain maximum seizure control with minimal toxic adverse effects. The principle of drug therapy is to begin with a single drug and increase the dosage until seizures are controlled or toxic adverse effects occur (Epilepsy Foundation, 2013a). Serum levels of the drug should be monitored if seizures continue to occur, if seizure frequency increases, or if drug compliance is questioned. The therapeutic range for each drug indicates the serum level above which most patients experience toxic adverse effects and below which most continue to have seizures. Therapeutic ranges are only guides for therapy. If the patient's seizures are well controlled with a subtherapeutic level, the drug dose need not be increased. Likewise, if a drug level is above the therapeutic range and the patient has good seizure control without toxic adverse effects, the drug dose need not be decreased. Many of the newer drugs do not require drug-level monitoring because the therapeutic range is very large. If seizure control is not achieved with a single drug, the drug dosage or the timing of administration may be changed, or a second drug may be added.

DRUG ALERT—Carbamazepine (Tegretol)

Patients taking carbamazepine should be instructed as follows:
- Do not take with grapefruit juice.
- Report visual abnormalities.
- Be aware that abrupt withdrawal after long-term use may precipitate seizures.

For many years, the primary drugs for treatment of generalized tonic–clonic and focal seizures were sodium channel blockers. Barbiturates, such as phenobarbital, also have a long history of use. Both sodium channel blockers and benzodiazepines are effective in the treatment of absence, akinetic, and myoclonic seizures.

Treatment of status epilepticus requires immediate initiation of a rapid-acting anticonvulsant drug that can be given intravenously. The drugs most commonly used are lorazepam (Ativan) and diazepam (Valium). Because these are short-acting drugs, they must be followed by administration of long-acting drugs such as phenytoin (Dilantin) or phenobarbital (Epilepsy Ontario, 2011).

Current drugs used in seizure management are shown in Table 61-10. Because many of these drugs (e.g., phenytoin [Dilantin], phenobarbital, ethosuximide [Zarontin], lamotrigine [Lamictal], topiramate [Topamax]) have a long half-life, they can be given in once- or twice-daily doses. This increases the patient's compliance with taking the drug by simplifying the drug regimen and avoiding the need to take it at work or school.

DRUG ALERT—Phenytoin (Dilantin)
- IV phenytoin (Dilantin) should be administered slowly to prevent acute hypotension.
- Serum albumin levels should be considered along with serum phenytoin levels during therapeutic monitoring.
- Phenytoin (Dilantin) should be discontinued at the first sign of rash and anticonvulsive treatment therefore re-assessed.
- Alcoholic intake (acute and chronic) may affect phenytoin serum levels

✚ TABLE 61-9 EMERGENCY MANAGEMENT

Tonic–Clonic Seizures

Etiology	Assessment Findings	Interventions
Head Trauma • Epidural hematoma • Subdural hematoma • Intracranial hematoma • Cerebral contusion • Traumatic birth injury **Drug-Related Processes** • Overdose • Withdrawal of alcohol, opioids, anticonvulsant drugs • Ingestion, inhalation **Infectious Processes** • Meningitis • Septicemia • Encephalitis **Intracranial Events** • Brain tumour • Subarachnoid hemorrhage • Stroke • Neurodegenerative diseases • Hypertensive crisis • Increased ICP secondary to clogged shunt **Metabolic Imbalances** • Fluid and electrolyte imbalance • Hypoglycemia **Medical Disorders** • Heart, liver, lung, or kidney disease • Systemic lupus erythematosus **Other** • Cardiac arrest • Idiopathic • Psychiatric disorders • High fever • Autoimmune disease • Genetic diseases	• Aura—peculiar sensations that precede seizure • Loss of consciousness • Bowel and bladder incontinence • Tachycardia • Diaphoresis • Warm skin • Pallor, flushing, or cyanosis • *Tonic phase:* continuous muscle contractions • *Hypertonic phase:* extreme muscular rigidity lasting 5–15 sec • *Clonic phase:* rigidity and relaxation alternate in rapid succession • *Postictal phase:* lethargy, altered level of consciousness • Confusion and headache • Repeated tonic–clonic seizures for several minutes	**Initial** • Ensure patent airway (sedation may be required if teeth are clenched). • Apply oxygen as needed. • Assist ventilations if patient does not breathe spontaneously after seizure. Anticipate need for intubation if gag reflex absent. • Suction as needed. • Stay with patient until seizure has passed. • Ensure safety at all times and protect patient from injury during seizure. *Do not restrain.* Pad side rails. • Establish IV access. • Anticipate administration of phenobarbital, phenytoin (Dilantin), or benzodiazepines (diazepam [Valium], midazolam, lorazepam [Ativan]) to control seizures. • Reposition to side lying position when possible to avoid aspiration if patient vomits. • Remove or loosen tight clothing. **Ongoing Monitoring** • Monitor vital signs, level of consciousness, oxygen saturation, Glasgow Coma Scale score, pupil size and reactivity. • Reassure and orient the patient after seizure. • Never force an airway between a patient's clenched teeth. • Give IV dextrose for hypoglycemia.

ICP, intracranial pressure; *IV,* intravenous.

Adverse effects of anticonvulsant drugs primarily involve the CNS and include diplopia, drowsiness, ataxia, and mental slowing. Neurological assessment for dose-related toxicity involves testing the eyes for nystagmus, hand and gait coordination, cognitive functioning, and general alertness. Anticonvulsant drugs should not be discontinued abruptly because this can precipitate seizures or status epilepticus and can be life-threatening (Epilepsy Canada, 2009).

DRUG ALERT—Anticonvulsant Drugs
• Abrupt withdrawal after long-term use may precipitate seizures.
• If weaning is to occur, the patient must be seizure free for a prolonged period (e.g., 2 to 5 years) and have a normal neurological examination and EEG.

Idiosyncratic adverse effects involve organs outside the CNS, including skin (rashes), gingiva (hyperplasia), bone marrow (blood dyscrasias), liver, and kidneys. Nurses should teach patients about these adverse effects. A common adverse effect of phenytoin is gingival hyperplasia (excessive growth of gingival tissue), especially in children and young adults. This can be limited by good dental hygiene. If gingival hyperplasia is extensive, the hyperplastic tissue may have to be surgically removed (gingivectomy), and phenytoin may have to be replaced by another drug. Because phenytoin can also cause hirsutism in young people, other drugs are often used first.

Medication nonadherence can be a problem in people with epilepsy, owing to the aforementioned adverse effects. Therefore, measures should be taken to increase adherence to the prescribed drug regimens. If made aware of the issue, health care providers can work with the patient to find an acceptable drug regimen to prevent many of these undesirable adverse effects.

Surgical Therapy. A significant number of patients whose epilepsy cannot be controlled with drug therapy are candidates for surgical intervention to remove the epileptic focus or prevent spread of epileptic activity in the brain (Table 61-11).

TABLE 61-10 **DRUG THERAPY**

Epilepsy

Drug	Average Adult Daily Dosage	Possible Adverse Effects
carbamazepine (Tegretol)	800–1 200 mg	Dizziness, drowsiness, blurred or double vision, nausea, skin rashes, blood abnormalities
clobazam (Frisium)	30–40 mg	Drowsiness, dizziness, fatigue
clonazepam (Rivotril)	8–10 mg	Drowsiness, clumsiness, behaviour changes, tremor, appetite loss
divalproex sodium (Epival)	1 750–3 000 mg	Upset stomach, altered bleeding time, liver toxicity (rare), hair loss, weight gain, tremor
ethosuximide (Zarontin)	500 mg	Appetite loss, nausea, drowsiness, headache, dizziness, fatigue
gabapentin (Neurontin)	900–2 400 mg	Somnolence, fatigue, dizziness
lamotrigine (Lamictal)	100–500 mg	Headache, fatigue, nausea, dizziness, clumsiness, serious and life-threatening rash (rare), double or blurred vision
levetiracetam (Keppra)	1 000–3 000 mg	Dizziness, somnolence, asthenia (weakness), low hematocrit and leukocyte count (rare), depression and mood swings
oxcarbazepine (Trileptal)	1 200–2 400 mg	Somnolence, diplopia, rash, hyponatremia, ataxia and staggering gait
phenobarbital	30–600 mg	Drowsiness, irritability, hyperactivity, somnolence
phenytoin (Dilantin)	300 mg	Clumsiness, drowsiness, nausea, rash, gum overgrowth, hairiness, thickening of features
primidone	250–1 000 mg	Clumsiness, dizziness, appetite loss, fatigue, drowsiness, hyperirritability
topiramate (Topamax)	200–600 mg	Drowsiness, dizziness, weight loss, tingling, decreased alertness, kidney stones (rare)
vigabatrin (Sabril)	1 000–4 000 mg	Drowsiness, weight gain, headache, dizziness, decreased peripheral vision, depression
valproic acid (Depakene)	1 750–3 000 mg	Upset stomach, altered bleeding time, liver toxicity

Source: Adapted from Epilepsy Canada. (1987 [revised 2009]). *Your medication for epilepsy.* (pp. 12–13). Toronto: Author. Retrieved from *http://www.epilepsy.ca/ uploads/7/0/8/6/70868839/medication-new.pdf.*

TABLE 61-11 **SURGICAL PROCEDURES FOR SEIZURE DISORDERS AND EPILEPSY**

Type of Seizure	Surgical Procedure	Results
Focal impaired awareness seizures of temporal lobe origin	Resectioning of epileptogenic tissue	Absence of seizures 5 yr postoperatively in 55%–70% of patients
Focal seizures of frontal lobe origin	Resectioning of epileptogenic tissue (if in resectable area)	Absence of seizures 5 yr postoperatively in 30%–50% of patients
Generalized seizures (Lennox–Gastaut syndrome or drop attacks)	Sectioning of corpus callosum	Persistence of seizures; less violent, less frequent, less disabling events
Intractable, unilateral multifocal epilepsy associated with infantile hemiplegia	Hemispherectomy or callosotomy	Reduction in seizure frequency and type, improvement in behaviour

Surgical interventions include resections or lobectomies, and disconnection procedures such as corpus callosotomies (Epilepsy Foundation, 2013b).

The benefits of surgery include cessation or reduction in frequency of the seizures, but not all types of epilepsy benefit from surgery. An extensive preoperative evaluation is important, including continuous EEG monitoring and other specific tests to ensure precise localization of the focal point. Before surgery is performed, three requirements must be met: (1) the diagnosis of epilepsy must be confirmed, (2) there must have been an adequate trial with drug therapy without satisfactory results, and (3) the electroclinical syndrome (type of seizure disorder) must be defined.

Alternate Therapies. Vagal nerve stimulation is used as an adjunct to medications when surgery is not feasible. The exact mechanism of action is unknown, but it is thought to interrupt the synchronization of epileptic brain wave activity and stop excessive discharge of neurons. A surgically implanted electrode in the neck is programmed to deliver the electrical impulse to the vagus nerve. The patient can activate it with a magnet when he or she senses a seizure is imminent. Vagal nerve stimulation can cause adverse effects such as coughing, hoarseness, dyspnea, and tingling in the neck. Battery replacement is required via surgery about every 5 years.

The ketogenic diet is a special high-fat, low-carbohydrate diet that has been used to control seizures in some people with epilepsy. When a person is on this diet, ketones are produced and pass into the brain and replace glucose as an energy source. The diet may be effective for some patients with drug-resistant epilepsy, but the long-term effects of the diet are not clear. Current literature suggests that this diet is not without adverse effects and that there may be risks with long-term adherence to it (Southern, Fitzsimmons, & Cross, 2015). Patients on this diet who use anticoagulants need close monitoring for bleeding (Payne, Cross, Sander, et al., 2011).

Biofeedback to control seizures is aimed at teaching the patient to maintain a certain brain wave frequency that is refractory to seizure activity. Further trials are needed to assess the effectiveness of biofeedback for seizure control.

NURSING MANAGEMENT
SEIZURE DISORDERS AND EPILEPSY

NURSING ASSESSMENT

Data that should be obtained from a patient with a seizure disorder are presented in Table 61-12. Data related to a specific seizure episode can be obtained from a witness.

NURSING DIAGNOSES

Nursing diagnoses for the patient with seizure disorders and epilepsy may include, but are not limited to, the following:

TABLE 61-12 NURSING ASSESSMENT

Seizure Disorders and Epilepsy

Subjective Data

Important Health Information

Past health history: Previous seizures, birth defects, or injuries; anoxic episodes; CNS trauma, tumours, or infections; stroke; metabolic disorders; alcoholism; exposure to metals and carbon monoxide; hepatic or renal failure; fever; pregnancy; systemic lupus erythematosus; positive family history of seizure disorders or epilepsy

Medications: Compliance with anticonvulsant drugs; barbiturate or alcohol withdrawal; use of cocaine, amphetamines, lidocaine, theophylline (Theo-Dur, Uniphyl), penicillins, lithium, phenothiazines, tricyclic antidepressants, benzodiazepines

Symptoms

- Headaches, aura, mood or behavioural changes before seizure; mentation changes; abdominal pain, muscle pain (postictal)
- Anxiety, depression; loss of self-esteem, social isolation
- Decreased sexual drive, erectile dysfunction; increased sexual drive (postictal)

Objective Data

General

Precipitating factors, including severe metabolic acidosis or alkalosis, hyperkalemia, hypoglycemia, dehydration, or water intoxication

Integumentary

Bitten tongue, soft tissue damage, cyanosis, diaphoresis (postictal)

Respiratory

Abnormal respiratory rate, rhythm, or depth; apnea (ictal); absent or abnormal breath sounds, possible airway occlusion

Cardiovascular

Hypertension, tachycardia, or bradycardia (ictal)

Gastro-Intestinal

Bowel incontinence; excessive salivation

Urinary

Incontinence

Neurological

Generalized

Tonic–clonic: Loss of consciousness, muscle tightening, then jerking; dilated pupils; hyperventilation, then apnea; postictal somnolence

Absence: Altered consciousness (5–30 sec), minor facial motor activity

Focal

Simple: Aura; consciousness; focal sensory, motor, cognitive, or emotional phenomena (focal motor); unilateral "marching" motor seizure (jacksonian)

Complex: Altered consciousness with inappropriate behaviours, automatisms, amnesia of event

Musculo-Skeletal

Weakness, paralysis, ataxia (postictal)

Possible Findings

Positive toxicology screen or alcohol level; altered serum electrolytes, acidosis or alkalosis, very low blood glucose level, ↑ blood urea nitrogen or creatinine, liver function tests, ammonia; abnormal CT scan or MRI of head, abnormal findings from lumbar puncture; abnormal discharges on EEG

CNS, central nervous system; *CT,* computed tomographic (scan); *EEG,* electroencephalography; *MRI,* magnetic resonance imaging.

- *Ineffective breathing pattern* related to *body position that inhibits lung expansion* (neuro-muscular impairment)
- *Ineffective health management* related to *difficulty managing complex treatment regimen* (drug therapy and lifestyle adjustment)
- *Risk for injury* as evidenced by *alteration in cognitive functioning, alteration in psychomotor functioning* (seizure)

Additional information on nursing diagnoses for the patient with a seizure disorder is presented in Nursing Care Plan (NCP) 61-2, available on the Evolve website.

PLANNING

The overall goals are that the patient with seizures will (1) be free from injury during a seizure, (2) have optimal mental and physical functioning while taking anticonvulsant drugs, and (3) have satisfactory psychosocial functioning.

NURSING IMPLEMENTATION

HEALTH PROMOTION. Complications such as head injury related to seizure disorders can be prevented through general safety measures such as the wearing of helmets. Optimal perinatal care facilitates reduced fetal trauma and hypoxia, and therefore, reduced brain damage leading to seizure disorders.

The patient with a seizure disorder should practise good general health habits (e.g., maintaining a proper diet, getting adequate rest, exercising). The nurse should help the patient identify events or situations that precipitate the seizures and provide suggestions for avoiding them or handling them better. The patient should be taught to avoid excessive alcohol intake, fatigue, and loss of sleep and be helped to handle stress constructively.

ACUTE INTERVENTION. The nurse caring for a patient who is hospitalized with seizures involves several responsibilities, including observation and treatment of the seizure, education, and psychosocial intervention.

When a seizure occurs, the nurse should carefully observe and record details of the event because the diagnosis and subsequent treatment often rest solely on the seizure description. All aspects of the seizure should be noted. What events preceded the seizure? When did the seizure occur? How long did each phase last? What occurred during each phase?

Both subjective and objective data are important. Objective data should include the exact time of seizure onset; the course and nature of the seizure activity (loss of consciousness, tongue biting, automatisms, stiffening, jerking, total lack of muscle tone); the body parts involved and their sequence of involvement; and the presence of autonomic signs, such as dilated pupils, excessive salivation, altered breathing, cyanosis, flushing, diaphoresis, or incontinence. Assessment of the postictal period should include a detailed description of level of consciousness, vital signs, memory loss, muscle soreness, speech disorders (aphasia, dysarthria), weakness or paralysis, sleep period, and the duration of each sign or symptom.

SAFETY ALERT

During a seizure, the nurse should do the following:

- Maintain a patent airway for the patient. This may be facilitated by turning the patient to the side and ensuring the tongue falls forward so as not to block the patient's airway.
- Protect the patient's head, turn the patient to the side, loosen constrictive clothing, ease patient to the floor (if seated).
- Do not restrain the patient.
- Do not place any objects in the patient's mouth.

After the seizure, the patient may require suctioning, and oxygen may be needed; therefore, the nurse should ensure that oxygen and suction equipment are available and in working order for patients with a history of seizures. A seizure can be a frightening experience for the patient and for others who may witness it. The nurse should assess their level of understanding and provide information about how and why the event occurred. This is an excellent opportunity for the nurse to dispel many common misconceptions about seizures.

AMBULATORY AND HOME CARE. Prevention of recurring seizures is the major goal in the treatment of epilepsy. Because many seizure disorders cannot be cured, drugs must be taken regularly, often for life. The nurse should ensure that the patient knows this, as well as the specifics of the drug regimen and what to do if a dose is missed. Usually, the dose should be made up if the omission is remembered within 24 hours. The patient should be cautioned not to adjust drug doses without professional guidance because this can increase seizure frequency and even cause status epilepticus. The patient should be encouraged to report any adverse effects and to keep regular appointments with a health care provider.

Nurses play an important role in teaching the patient and caregivers. Guidelines for teaching are shown in Table 61-13. Nurses should teach family members and significant others the emergency management of tonic–clonic seizures (see Table 61-9). They should be reminded that it is not necessary to call an ambulance or send a person to the hospital after a single seizure unless it is the first seizure, it is prolonged, it is immediately followed by another seizure, or extensive injury has occurred.

Patients with a seizure disorder also experience concerns or fears related to recurrent seizures, incontinence, and loss of self-control. The nurse provides support for the patient through education and by helping to identify coping mechanisms.

Perhaps the greatest challenge that a seizure disorder presents to the patient is adjusting to the personal limitations imposed by the illness. Discrimination in employment is the most serious problem facing the person with a seizure disorder. For issues relating to job discrimination, patients can be referred to the Canadian Human Rights Commission through its national or regional offices.

A variety of other resources can be offered to the patient with a seizure disorder. Patients should be informed that medical alert bracelets, necklaces, and identification cards are available through a number of North American companies specializing in identification devices (e.g., MedicAlert; see Figure 52-11). If the nurse believes that associating with others who have a seizure disorder would be beneficial, the patient can be referred to Epilepsy Canada, a voluntary agency with local members' associations across the country that offer a variety of services to patients with epilepsy. Patients who are eligible veterans can be referred to Veterans Affairs Canada to explore services for which they may qualify.

Social workers and welfare agencies can help with financial problems and living arrangements. Provincial and territorial services for individuals with developmental disabilities include assistance with vocational assessment and training, sheltered housing, funding for special needs, and placement for patients whose seizures are not well controlled. They can also offer financial assistance for transportation and medical costs that are necessary for vocational rehabilitation or job maintenance. If intensive psychological counselling is needed, the nurse can refer the patient to a community mental health centre.

Patients should be encouraged to learn more about epilepsy through self-education materials. Epilepsy Canada provides information pamphlets and may facilitate support groups. Many agencies that offer services to people with epilepsy, as well as many locally based epilepsy associations, have these services available.

EVALUATION
Expected outcomes for patients with seizures are addressed in NCP 61-2.

MULTIPLE SCLEROSIS
Multiple sclerosis (MS) is a chronic, progressive, degenerative, autoimmune disorder of the CNS characterized by disseminated demyelination of nerve fibres of the brain, the spinal cord, and the optic nerves. Canadians have one of the highest rates of MS in the world, and an estimated 55 000 to 75 000 Canadians have MS (Government of Canada, 2016). Across the country, prevalence rates range from 1 case per 500 to 1 000 people. More than three Canadians a day are diagnosed with MS (Multiple Sclerosis Society of Canada, 2014). On a global scale (Figure 61-2), MS has relatively high prevalence rates (>33 cases per 100 000 people) in areas with temperate climates (like those found in large areas of Europe [including Russia], Canada, northern United States, southeastern Australia, and New Zealand), and relatively low prevalence rates (<5 cases per 100 000 people) in warmer climates (like those found in large areas of Asia, Africa, and northern South America) (Multiple Sclerosis International Federation, 2013). MS is considered a disease of young to middle-aged adults, with an average age of onset of 30 years (Multiple Sclerosis International Federation, 2013). Women are affected more often than men, with a ratio of 3:1 (Multiple Sclerosis Society of Canada, 2016a). Chao, Ramagopalan, Herrera, and colleagues (2011) suggest that MS may be triggered by environmental factors in individuals, with genetic susceptibility seen more commonly in females.

TABLE 61-13 PATIENT & CAREGIVER TEACHING GUIDE

Seizure Disorders and Epilepsy

The following information should be included when teaching the patient and caregiver about seizure disorders and epilepsy.
1. Drugs must be taken as prescribed. Adverse effects of drugs should be reported to the health care provider. When necessary, blood work may be drawn to ensure that therapeutic drug levels are maintained.
2. Use of nonpharmacological techniques, such as diet and biofeedback training, to potentially reduce the number of seizures.
3. Availability of community resources.
4. Need to wear a medical alert bracelet or necklace and carry an identification card.
5. Avoidance of excessive alcohol intake, fatigue, and loss of sleep.
6. Regular meals and snacks in between if feeling shaky, faint, or hungry.

Caregivers should be taught the following:
1. For first aid treatment of tonic–clonic seizure, it is not necessary to call an ambulance or send the patient to the hospital after a single seizure unless the seizure is prolonged, another seizure immediately follows, or extensive injury has occurred.
2. During an acute seizure, it is important to protect the patient from injury. This may involve supporting and protecting the head, turning the patient to the side, loosening constrictive clothing, and easing the patient to a lying position on the floor, if seated.

People per
100 000 with MS

■ >100

■ 60.01–100

■ 20.01–60

■ 5.01–20

□ 0–5

□ Data not provided

FIGURE 61-2 Prevalence of MS. Source: Multiple Sclerosis International Federation. (2013). Atlas of MS 2013. p. 8. Retrieved from *http://www.msif.org/about-us/advocacy/atlas/*. Reprinted with permission.

Etiology and Pathophysiology

The cause of MS is unknown, although research findings suggest that MS may be related to environmental, infectious (viral), and vascular factors, and to a vitamin D deficiency (Bernstein, 2012; Mokry, Ross, Ahmad, et al., 2015; Guo, He, Zhang, et al., 2012). The susceptibility to MS appears to be inherited. First-, second-, and third-degree relatives of patients with MS are at a slightly increased risk.

The role of precipitating factors, such as exposure to pathogenic agents, in the etiology of MS is controversial. It is possible that their association with MS is random and that there is no cause-and-effect relationship. Possible precipitating factors include infection, trauma, emotional stress, excessive fatigue, pregnancy, and a state of poor health.

MS is characterized by chronic inflammation, demyelination, and gliosis (scarring) in the CNS. The primary neuropathological condition is an autoimmune disease orchestrated by autoreactive T cells (lymphocytes). This process may be initially triggered by a virus in genetically susceptible individuals. The activated T cells in the systemic circulation migrate to the CNS, causing blood–brain barrier disruption. This is likely the initial event in the development of MS. Subsequent antigen–antibody reaction within the CNS results in activation of the inflammatory response and, through multiple effector mechanisms, leads to demyelination of axons. The disease process consists of loss of myelin, disappearance of oligodendrocytes, and proliferation of astrocytes. These changes result in characteristic plaque formation, or sclerosis, with plaques scattered throughout multiple regions of the CNS.

Initially, the myelin sheaths of the neurons in the brain and spinal cord are attacked (Figure 61-3, *A* and *B*). Early in the

FIGURE 61-3 Pathogenesis of multiple sclerosis. **A,** Normal nerve cell with myelin sheath. **B,** Normal axon. **C,** Myelin breakdown. **D,** Myelin totally disrupted; axon not functioning.

disease, the myelin sheath is damaged, but the nerve fibre is not affected and nerve impulses are still transmitted (see Figure 61-3, *C*). At this point, the patient may complain of a noticeable impairment of function (e.g., weakness). However, the myelin can regenerate, and the symptoms disappear, resulting in a remission.

In addition to myelin disruption, the axon also becomes involved (see Figure 61-3, *D*). Myelin is replaced by glial scar

FIGURE 61-4 Chronic multiple sclerosis. Demyelination plaque (P) at grey-white junction and adjacent partially remyelinated shadow plaque (V). Source: Stevens, A., & Lowe, J. (2000). *Pathology: Illustrated review in colour* (2nd ed.). London: Mosby.

TABLE 61-14	CLINICAL COURSES OF MULTIPLE SCLEROSIS (MS)
Category	**Characteristics**
Clinically isolated syndrome (CIS)	CIS is defined by a single episode of neurological symptoms reminiscent of MS.
Relapsing–remitting MS (RRMS)	Clearly defined relapses with full recovery or sequelae and residual deficit on recovery. This is the most common form of MS.
Primary-progressive MS (PPMS)	Slow and steady disease progression from onset with occasional plateaus and temporary minor improvements; no clear relapses or remissions
Secondary-progressive MS (SPMS)	A relapsing–remitting initial course, followed by progression with or without occasional relapses, minor remissions, and plateaus; disability generally accumulates over time.
Progressive–relapsing MS (PRMS)	Progressive disease from onset, with clear acute relapses, with or without full recovery; periods between relapses are characterized by continuing progression, occurring in approximately 5% of cases of MS.

Source: Adapted from Multiple Sclerosis Society of Canada. (2016). *Types of MS.* Retrieved from *https://mssociety.ca/about-ms/types.*

tissue, which forms hard, sclerotic plaques in multiple regions of the CNS (Figure 61-4). Without myelin, nerve impulses slow down, and with destruction of nerve axons, impulses are totally blocked, resulting in permanent loss of function. In many chronic lesions, demyelination continues with progressive loss of nerve function.

Clinical Manifestations

The onset of MS is often insidious, with vague symptoms that occur intermittently over months or years. As a result, the disease may not be diagnosed until long after the onset of the first symptom. The disease process has a spotty distribution in the CNS, so the signs and symptoms vary over time. MS is characterized by chronic, progressive deterioration in some people and by remissions and exacerbations in others. With repeated exacerbations, the overall trend is progressive deterioration in neurological function resulting in disability (Shirani, Zhao, Karim, et al., 2012).

The clinical manifestations vary according to the areas of the CNS involved. Some patients have severe, long-lasting symptoms early in the course of the disease. Others may experience only occasional and mild symptoms for several years after onset. A classification scheme that identifies the various courses of MS has been developed (Multiple Sclerosis Society of Canada, 2016b) (Table 61-14 and Figure 61-5).

Common signs and symptoms of MS include motor, sensory, cerebellar, and emotional problems. Motor symptoms include weakness or paralysis of the limbs, the trunk, or the head; diplopia; scanning speech (spoken words are unintentionally slowed or injected with pauses between syllables and may be accompanied by involuntary variations in vocal tone); and spasticity of the muscles that are chronically affected. Patients with MS experience a variety of sensory abnormalities, including numbness, tingling and other paresthesias, patchy blindness (scotomas), blurred vision, vertigo, tinnitus, decreased hearing, and chronic neuropathic pain. Radicular (nerve root) pains may be present, particularly in the low thoracic and abdominal regions. Lhermitte sign is a transient sensory symptom described as an electric shock radiating down the spine or into the limbs with flexion of the neck. Cerebellar signs include nystagmus, ataxia, dysarthria,

and dysphagia. Severe fatigue is present in many patients with MS, and it causes significant disability for some patients. The fatigue is usually associated with increased energy needs, deconditioning, depression, and medication adverse effects (Multiple Sclerosis International Federation, 2011).

Bowel and bladder function can be affected if the sclerotic plaque is located in areas of the CNS that control elimination. Problems with defecation usually involve constipation rather than fecal incontinence. Urinary problems are variable. A common problem in patients with MS is a spastic (uninhibited) bladder. This indicates a lesion above the second sacral nerve, which cuts off suprasegmental inhibiting influences on bladder contractility. As a result, the bladder has a small capacity for urine, and its contractions are unchecked. This problem is accompanied by urinary urgency and frequency and results in dribbling or incontinence. A flaccid (hypotonic) bladder indicates a lesion in the reflex arc governing bladder function. The bladder has a large capacity for urine because there is no sensation or desire to void, no pressure, and no pain. Generally, there is urinary retention, but urgency and frequency may also occur with this type of lesion. Another urinary problem is a combination of the previous two problems. Urinary problems cannot be adequately diagnosed and treated unless urodynamic studies are done.

Sexual dysfunction occurs in many people with MS and may stem from anatomical, physiological, psychological, and medical factors (Guo et al., 2012). Physiological erectile dysfunction may result from spinal cord involvement in men. Women may experience decreased libido, difficulty with orgasmic response, painful intercourse, and decreased vaginal lubrication. Diminished sensation can prevent a normal sexual response in both sexes.

MS has no apparent effect on the course of pregnancy, labour, delivery, or lactation. Some women with MS who become pregnant experience remission or an improvement in their symptoms during the gestation period. The hormonal changes associated with pregnancy appear to affect the immune system. However, during the postpartum period, women are at greater risk for remission relapses (Houtchens & Kolb, 2013).

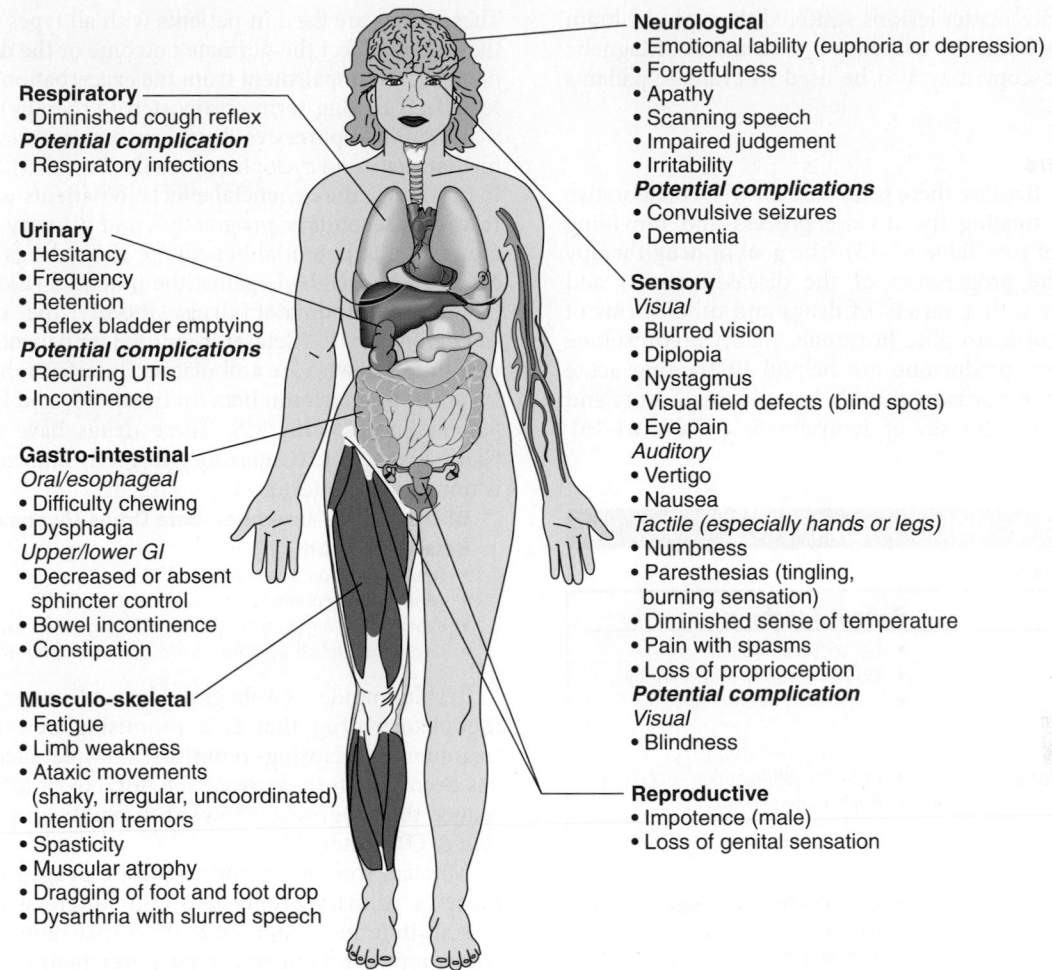

Respiratory
- Diminished cough reflex
Potential complication
- Respiratory infections

Urinary
- Hesitancy
- Frequency
- Retention
- Reflex bladder emptying
Potential complications
- Recurring UTIs
- Incontinence

Gastro-intestinal
Oral/esophageal
- Difficulty chewing
- Dysphagia
Upper/lower GI
- Decreased or absent
  sphincter control
- Bowel incontinence
- Constipation

Musculo-skeletal
- Fatigue
- Limb weakness
- Ataxic movements
  (shaky, irregular, uncoordinated)
- Intention tremors
- Spasticity
- Muscular atrophy
- Dragging of foot and foot drop
- Dysarthria with slurred speech

Neurological
- Emotional lability (euphoria or depression)
- Forgetfulness
- Apathy
- Scanning speech
- Impaired judgement
- Irritability
Potential complications
- Convulsive seizures
- Dementia

Sensory
Visual
- Blurred vision
- Diplopia
- Nystagmus
- Visual field defects (blind spots)
- Eye pain
Auditory
- Vertigo
- Nausea
Tactile (especially hands or legs)
- Numbness
- Paresthesias (tingling,
  burning sensation)
- Diminished sense of temperature
- Pain with spasms
- Loss of proprioception
Potential complication
Visual
- Blindness

Reproductive
- Impotence (male)
- Loss of genital sensation

FIGURE 61-5 Multisystem effects of multiple sclerosis. UTIs, urinary tract infections. Source: *LEMONE, PRISCILLA T; BURKE, KAREN M.; BAULDOFF, GERENE, MEDICAL-SURGICAL NURSING: CRITICAL THINKING IN PATIENT CARE, 5th Ed., ©2011.* Reprinted by permission of Pearson Education, Inc., New York, New York.

Although intellectual functioning generally remains intact, emotional stability may be affected. Cognitive sequelae can produce significant disability for some patients with MS. They may experience anger, depression, or euphoria. Signs and symptoms of MS are aggravated or triggered by physical and emotional trauma, fatigue, and infection.

The average life expectancy after the onset of symptoms is more than 25 years. Usually, death occurs because of infective complications (e.g., pneumonia) of immobility or because of an unrelated disease.

Diagnostic Studies

Because there is no definitive diagnostic test for MS, diagnosis is based primarily on history, clinical manifestations, and the presence of multiple lesions over time as measured by MRI (Table 61-15). Certain laboratory tests are currently used as adjuncts to clinical examination. In some patients, cerebro-spinal fluid (CSF) analysis may show an increase in oligoclonal immunoglobulin G. The CSF also contains a high number of lymphocytes, monocytes, and protein. Evoked responses are often delayed in people with MS because of decreased nerve conduction from the eye and the ear to the brain. MRI scan may be helpful because sclerotic plaques as small as 3 to 4 mm in diameter can be detected.

TABLE 61-15 COLLABORATIVE CARE

Multiple Sclerosis

Diagnostic	Collaborative Therapy
• History and physical examination • CSF analysis • CT scan • Evoked response testing (also called *evoked potential testing,* e.g., somatosensory evoked potential [SSEP], auditory evoked potential [AEP], visual evoked potential [VEP]) • MRI, MRS	**Drug Therapy*** • Anticholinergics • Cholinergics • Corticosteroids • Immuno-modulators • Immuno-suppressants • Muscle relaxants **Surgical Therapy** • Neurectomy, rhizotomy, cordotomy (unmanageable spasticity) • Thalamotomy (unmanageable tremor)

CSF, cerebro-spinal fluid; CT, computed tomographic (scan); MRI, magnetic resonance imaging; MRS, magnetic resonance spectroscopy.
*See Table 61-16.

Characteristic white-matter lesions scattered through the brain or spinal cord (or both) are evident on such a scan. Magnetic resonance spectroscopy may also be used to evaluate patients with MS.

Collaborative Care

Drug Therapy. Because there is no cure for MS, collaborative care is aimed at treating the disease process and providing symptomatic relief (see Table 61-15). The goal of drug therapy is to decrease the progression of the disease process and control symptoms with a variety of drugs and other forms of therapy. Adrenocorticotrophic hormone, methylprednisolone (Solu-Medrol), and prednisone are helpful in treating acute exacerbations of the disease, probably by reducing edema and acute inflammation at the site of demyelination (Table 61-16).

TABLE 61-16 DRUG THERAPY

Multiple Sclerosis

Drug	Patient Teaching
Corticosteroids ACTH, prednisone, methylprednisolone (Solu-Medrol)	• Restrict salt intake. • Do not abruptly stop therapy. • Know drug interactions.
Immuno-modulators Interferon beta (Betaseron, Avonex, Rebif) glatiramer acetate (Copaxone)	• Perform self-injection techniques. • Report adverse effects.
Cholinergics bethanechol (Duvoid) neostigmine	• Consult with health care provider before using other drugs, including over-the-counter drugs.
Anticholinergics oxybutynin (Ditropan)	• Consult health care provider before using other drugs, especially sleeping aids, antihistamines (possibly leading to potentiated effect).
Muscle Relaxants diazepam (Valium) baclofen (Lioresal) dantrolene (Dantrium) tizanidine	• Avoid driving and similar activities because of sedative effects. • Do not abruptly stop therapy. • Avoid use with tranquilizers and alcohol.
Acetylcholinesterase Inhibitor donepezil (Aricept)	• Maintain adequate hydration of 2–3 L of fluid per day. • Rise slowly when getting up from a sitting or lying position. • Report persistent abdominal discomfort, increased salivation, unresolved diarrhea, increased muscle pain, visual changes, or shortness of breath.
Nerve Conduction Enhancer fampridine (Fampyra)	• Be aware that drug may cause seizures, especially at higher doses.
Sphingosine-1-Phosphate Receptor Modulator fingolimod (Gilenya)	• May increase risk for infections and reduce effectiveness of influenza and tetanus boosters (Absher, 2015)

ACTH, adrenocorticotrophic hormone.

These drugs are used in patients with all types of MS; however, they do not affect the ultimate outcome or the degree of residual neurological impairment from the exacerbation (See Chapter 51 for effects of long-term corticosteroid therapy).

Immuno-suppressive drugs, such as azathioprine (Imuran), methotrexate, and cyclophosphamide (Procytox), have been shown to produce some beneficial effects in patients with progressive–relapsing, secondary-progressive, and primary-progressive MS. However, the potential benefits of these drugs in patients with MS must be weighed against the potential risks.

Immuno-modulator drugs modify the disease process. Interferon beta-1b (Betaseron) is used for patients with relapsing–remitting MS who are ambulatory. Interferon beta-1a (Avonex) is similar to interferon beta-1b in efficacy and is used in similar patient groups with MS. These drugs have antiviral effects. Glatiramer acetate (Copaxone), formerly known as copolymer-1, is unrelated to interferon.

> **DRUG ALERT—Interferon Beta Drugs (Avonex, Betaseron, Rebif)**
> • Rotate injection sites with each dose.
> • Assess for depression, suicidal ideation.
> • Wear sunscreen and protective clothing while exposed to sun.
> • Know that flulike symptoms are common after initiation of therapy.

Teriflunomide (Aubagio) is an emerging immuno-modulatory drug that is a promising new therapy for the treatment of relapsing–remitting multiple sclerosis (RRMS). It has been shown to decrease the number of MS relapses and to reduce the progression toward disability in patients with MS (Oh & O'Connor, 2014).

Mitoxantrone is an antineoplastic drug used for the treatment of primary-progressive and progressive–relapsing MS. It is an immuno-suppressant drug that reduces both B and T lymphocytes and impairs antigen presentation. Unlike the other disease-modifying drugs, it has a lifetime dose limit because of cardiac toxicity. Therefore, it cannot be used for more than 2 to 3 years.

Many other drugs are used to treat the symptoms of MS. Antispasmodics are used for spasticity. Amantadine and CNS stimulants such as methylphenidate (Ritalin) and modafinil (Alertec) are used for fatigue. Anticholinergics are used to treat bladder symptoms. Tricyclic antidepressants and anticonvulsant drugs are used for chronic pain. Dopamine (DA) agonists may be effective in the treatment of erectile dysfunction, while hormone therapy has shown efficacy in increasing libido (Guo et al., 2012). Cannabinoids have also been used to treat both pain and spasticity, with mild adverse effects (Corey-Bloom, Wolfson, Gamst, et al., 2012).

Alternate Therapies. A variety of alternate therapies have been utilized, aiming to minimize MS symptoms and decrease exacerbations. Surgical intervention may include neurectomy, rhizotomy, cordotomy, dorsal-column electrical stimulation, or use of an intrathecal baclofen (Lioresal) pump may be required to manage spasticity. Tremors that become unmanageable with drugs are sometimes treated by thalamotomy or deep brain stimulation.

Neurological dysfunction may improve with physiotherapy and speech therapy. Exercise improves the daily functioning for patients with MS not experiencing an exacerbation. Exercise decreases spasticity, increases coordination and muscle strength, and improves mobilization, gait, fatigue, and quality of life for patients with MS (Motl & Pilutti, 2012). The Canadian Physical Activity Guidelines for Adults With MS (Multiple Sclerosis

Society of Canada, 2016c) is a useful document that outlines recommendations for adults with mild to moderate disability related to MS. An especially beneficial type of physical therapy is water exercise. Water gives buoyancy to the body and allows the patient to perform activities that would normally be too difficult because the patient has more control over the body. Other therapies may include the use of heat therapy, massage, acupuncture, bee stings, and aromatherapy. The effectiveness of these therapies requires more research.

In recent years, media attention has emerged surrounding the controversial MS treatment of chronic cerebro-spinal venous insufficiency (CCSVI). Zamboni, Galeotti, Menegatti, and associates (2008) first proposed the theory that CCSVI may be a contributing factor in the pathology of MS. These researchers suggest that MS may be related to an immune or inflammatory reaction to iron accumulation in the CNS relating to drainage impairment of the cerebro-spinal vessels. This accumulation was detected via the use of cranial ultrasound. Patients with MS have undergone endovascular CCSVI procedures such as angioplasty or stent placement in jugular and azygos veins to improve venous drainage (Figure 61-6). The safety and efficacy of these procedures is unknown and they are not without risk (Awad, Marder, Milo, et al., 2011; Burton, Alikhani, Goyal, et al., 2011; Lazzaro, Zaidat, Mueller-Kronast, et al., 2011). In 2010, the American and Canadian Multiple Sclerosis Societies contributed to the funding of seven studies to investigate the link between CCSVI and MS (Multiple Sclerosis Society of Canada, 2017). At the time of writing, four of the seven studies presented no relationship between CCSVI and MS, and CCSVI surgery for patients with MS remained unavailable in Canada (Multiple Sclerosis Society of Canada, 2017).

Nutritional Therapy. Various nutritional measures have been used in the management of MS, including megavitamin therapy (cobalamin [vitamin B_{12}], vitamin C), supplemental vitamin D, and diets consisting of low-fat, gluten-free food and raw vegetables. Particular dietary measures are not widely recommended, owing to insufficient evidence supporting their effectiveness.

A nutritious, well-balanced diet is essential. Although there is no standard prescribed diet, a high-protein, high roughage diet with supplementary vitamins is often advocated. Vitamins are merely supplemental and not curative. Nutrition therapy must be adapted, depending on the patient's ability to chew and swallow.

NURSING MANAGEMENT
MULTIPLE SCLEROSIS

NURSING ASSESSMENT

Subjective and objective data that should be obtained from a patient with MS are presented in Table 61-17.

NURSING DIAGNOSES

Nursing diagnoses for patients with MS may include, but are not limited to, the following:

- *Impaired physical mobility* related to *decrease in muscle strength, decrease in muscle control, physical deconditioning*
- *Overflow urinary incontinence* related to *detrusor hypocontractility*

FIGURE 61-6 Cerebro-spinal vessels of interest in chronic cerebro-spinal venous insufficiency (CCSVI). Source: Lazzaro, M. A., Zaidat, O. O., Mueller-Kronast, N., et al. (2011). Endovascular therapy for chronic cerebrospinal venous insufficiency in multiple sclerosis. *Frontiers in Neurology, 2*(44), 1–7. doi:10.3389/fneur.2011.00044

TABLE 61-17 NURSING ASSESSMENT

Multiple Sclerosis

Subjective Data

Important Health Information

Past health history: Recent or past viral infections or vaccinations, other recent infections, residence in cold or temperate climates, recent physical or emotional stress, pregnancy, exposure to extremes of heat and cold; positive family history

Medications: Use of and compliance in taking corticosteroids, immuno-modulators, immuno-suppressants, selective adhesion molecule inhibitor cholinergics, anticholinergics, antispasmodics, antivirals

Symptoms

- Weight loss; difficulty chewing, dysphagia
- Urinary frequency, urgency, dribbling or incontinence, retention; constipation
- Generalized muscle weakness, muscle fatigue; tingling and numbness, ataxia (clumsiness), malaise
- Eye, back, leg, joint pain; painful muscle spasms; vertigo; blurred or lost vision; diplopia; tinnitus
- Erectile and sexual dysfunction; decreased libido
- Anger, depression, euphoria, social isolation, cognitive changes, memory loss

Objective Data

General

Apathy, inattentiveness

Neurological

Scanning speech, nystagmus, ataxia, tremor, spasticity, hyper-reflexia, decreased hearing

Musculo-Skeletal

Muscular weakness, paresis, paralysis, spasms, foot dragging, dysarthria (may be unilateral or bilateral changes)

Possible Findings

↓ T suppressor cells, demyelinating lesions on MRI or MRS scans, increased IgG or oligoclonal banding in cerebro-spinal fluid, delayed evoked potential

IgG, immunoglobulin G; *MRI,* magnetic resonance imaging; *MRS,* magnetic resonance spectroscopy.

- *Ineffective health management* related to *difficulty managing complex treatment regimen* (knowledge deficit regarding management of MS)

Additional information on nursing diagnoses for the patient with MS is presented in NCP 61-3, available on the Evolve website.

▌PLANNING

The overall goals are that the patient with MS will (1) maximize neuro-muscular function, (2) maintain independence in activities of daily living for as long as possible, (3) manage disabling fatigue, (4) optimize psychosocial well-being, (5) adjust to the illness, and (6) reduce factors that precipitate exacerbations.

▌NURSING IMPLEMENTATION

Patients with MS should be aware of triggers that may cause exacerbations or worsening of the disease. Exacerbations of MS may be triggered by infection (especially upper respiratory and urinary tract infections), trauma, immunization, childbirth, stress, and change in climate. Each person responds differently to these triggers. The nurse should help the patient identify particular triggers and develop ways to avoid them or minimize their effects.

INFORMATICS IN PRACTICE

Phone Applications in Multiple Sclerosis

- Patients with multiple sclerosis (MS), especially those who are newly diagnosed, might feel overwhelmed at the thought of living with a chronic disease and managing multiple medications.
- Smartphone applications can improve the lives of patients with MS by helping them manage their health care.
- Applications are available that send medication reminders by text message or email, track injection site rotation, and email medication reports to the health care provider. Patients can keep track of their medication inventory and be reminded to order refills.

The most common reasons for hospitalization of the patient with MS are for a diagnostic workup and for treatment of an acute exacerbation. During the diagnostic phase, the patient needs reassurance that, even though there is a tentative diagnosis of MS, certain diagnostic studies must be done to rule out other neurological disorders. The nurse should assist the patient in dealing with the anxiety caused by a diagnosis of a disabling illness. Patients with recently diagnosed MS may need assistance with the grieving process.

During an acute exacerbation, the patient may be immobile and bedridden. The focus of nursing intervention at this phase is to prevent major complications of immobility, such as respiratory and urinary tract infections and pressure injuries.

Patient teaching should focus on building general resistance to illness, including avoiding fatigue, extremes of heat and cold, and exposure to infection. It is also important to teach the patient to achieve a good balance of exercise and rest, eat nutritious and well-balanced meals, and avoid the hazards of immobility (e.g., contractures, pressure injuries). Patients should know their treatment regimens, the adverse effects of drugs and how to watch for them, and drug interactions with over-the-counter medications. The patient should consult a health care provider before taking nonprescription drugs.

Bladder control is a major problem for many patients with MS. Although anticholinergics may be beneficial for some patients to decrease spasticity, other patients may need to be taught self-catheterization (see Chapter 48). Bowel problems, particularly constipation, occur frequently in patients with MS. Increasing dietary fibre intake may help some patients achieve regularity in bowel habits.

Patients with MS and their families must make many emotional adjustments because of the unpredictability of the disease, the need to change lifestyles, and the challenge of avoiding or decreasing precipitating factors. The Multiple Sclerosis Society of Canada and its local chapters can offer a variety of services to meet the needs of patients with MS and their families.

▌EVALUATION

Expected outcomes for patients with MS are addressed in NCP 61-3, available on the Evolve website.

PARKINSON'S DISEASE

Parkinson's disease (PD) is a progressive, neurodegenerative disease of the CNS (basal ganglia) characterized by a slowing down in the initiation and the execution of movement (bradykinesia), increased muscle tone (rigidity), tremor at rest, and impaired postural reflexes. It is the most common form of parkinsonism (a syndrome characterized by similar symptoms). PD is named after James Parkinson, who in 1817 wrote a classic essay on "shaking palsy," a disease whose cause is still unknown and for which no cure exists.

Etiology and Pathophysiology

PD is the second most common neurodegenerative disease. As of 2011, approximately 55 000 living adults have been diagnosed with PD, a movement disorder (Statistics Canada, 2015). This number is expected to rise dramatically as the population ages because the average age of diagnosis is 60 years (Parkinson Society Canada, 2015). Research has shown that many forms of PD have a genetic component, and the field continues to grow and evolve as new genes are identified and mutations in known genes are discovered (Singleton, Farrer, & Bonifati, 2013). PD is more common in men than in women, by a ratio of 3 : 2.

There are many forms of parkinsonism other than PD. Parkinsonism-like symptoms have occurred after intoxication with a variety of chemicals, including carbon monoxide and manganese (among copper miners) and the product of meperidine-analogue synthesis, 1-methyl-4-phenyl-1,2,3,6-tetrahydropyridine (MPTP). Drug-induced parkinsonism can sometimes follow the use of medications within the antipsychotic, other neuroleptic, and calcium-channel entry-blocking classes (Bohlega & Al-Foghom, 2013). Parkinsonism can also be seen following the use of illicit drugs, including amphetamine and methamphetamine. Other causes of parkinsonism include encephalitis, vascular parkinsonism, normal pressure hydrocephalus, progressive supranuclear palsy, multiple system atrophy, and dementia with Lewy bodies (National Institute for Neurological Disorders and Stroke, 2016).

The pathological process of PD involves degeneration of the DA-producing neurons in the substantia nigra of the midbrain (Figures 61-7 and 61-8), which in turn disrupts the normal balance between DA and acetylcholine (ACh) in the basal ganglia. DA is a neurotransmitter that is essential for normal functioning of the extrapyramidal motor system, including control of posture, support, and voluntary motion. Manifestations of PD do not occur until 80% of neurons in the substantia nigra are lost.

Clinical Manifestations

The onset of PD is gradual and insidious, with an ongoing progression. It may involve only one side of the body, initially. The classic manifestations of PD are a triad of tremor, rigidity,

and bradykinesia (Figure 61-9). In the beginning stages, only a mild tremor, a slight limp, or a decreased arm swing may be evident. Later in the disease, the patient may have a shuffling, propulsive gait with arms flexed and loss of postural reflexes. Some patients have a slight change in speech patterns. None of these manifestations alone is sufficient evidence for a diagnosis of the disease.

Tremor. Tremor, often the first sign, may be minimal initially, so the patient is the only one who notices it. This tremor can affect handwriting, causing it to trail off, particularly toward the ends of words. Parkinsonian tremor is more prominent at rest and is aggravated by emotional stress or increased concentration. The hand tremor is described as "pill rolling" because the thumb and forefinger appear to move in a rotary fashion, as if rolling

FIGURE 61-8 Dopaminergic synaptic activity is mediated by dopamine. Cholinergic synaptic activity is mediated by acetylcholine. A balance between the two kinds of activity produces normal motor function. A relative excess of cholinergic activity produces akinesia and rigidity. A relative excess of dopaminergic activity produces involuntary movements. Neurons in the caudate nucleus contain γ-aminobutyric acid (GABA) and possibly control dopaminergic neurons in the substantia nigra through a feedback pathway. Source: McCance, K. L., & Huether, S. E. (2006). *Pathophysiology: The biologic basis for disease in adults and children* (5th ed., p. 537, Figure 16-23, B). St. Louis: Mosby.

FIGURE 61-7 Nigrostriatal disorders produce parkinsonism. Left-sided view of the human brain shows the substantia nigra and the corpus striatum (shaded area) lying deep within the cerebral hemisphere. Nerve fibres extend upward from the substantia nigra, divide into many branches, and carry dopamine to all regions of the corpus striatum.

FIGURE 61-9 Characteristic appearance of a patient with Parkinson's disease.

a pill, coin, or other small object. Tremor can also involve the diaphragm, tongue, lips, and jaw but rarely causes shaking of the head.

Unfortunately, in many people, a benign essential tremor is mistakenly diagnosed as PD. Essential tremor occurs during voluntary movement, has a more rapid frequency than parkinsonian tremor, and is often familial.

Rigidity. Rigidity, the second sign of the triad, is the increased resistance to passive motion when the limbs are moved through their range of motion. Parkinsonian rigidity is typified by cogwheel rigidity, or a jerky quality, as if there were intermittent catches in the movement of a cogwheel, when the joint is moved passively. Sustained muscle contraction causes the rigidity and consequently elicits complaints of muscle soreness; feeling tired and achy; or pain in the head, the upper body, the spine, or the legs. Another consequence of rigidity is slowness of movement because it inhibits the alternating of contraction and relaxation in opposing muscle groups (e.g., biceps and triceps).

Bradykinesia. Bradykinesia is particularly evident in the loss of automatic movements, which is secondary to the physical and chemical alteration of the basal ganglia and related structures in the extrapyramidal portion of the CNS. In the unaffected patient, automatic movements are involuntary and occur subconsciously. They include blinking of the eyelids, swinging of the arms while walking, swallowing of saliva, self-expression with facial and hand movements, and minor movements of postural adjustment. Patients with PD do not execute these movements and lack spontaneous activity. These factors account for the stooped posture, masked face (deadpan expression), drooling of saliva, and shuffling gait (festination) that are characteristic of a person with this disease. The posture is that of a slowed "old man" image, with the head and trunk bent forward and the legs constantly flexed (Figure 61-9). Postural instability is common. Patients may complain of being unable to stop themselves from going forward or backward. Assessment of postural instability includes the "pull test," in which the examiner stands behind the patient and gives a tug backward on the shoulder, causing the patient to lose his or her balance and fall backward. In addition to the motor signs of PD, many non-motor symptoms are common. They include depression, anxiety, apathy, fatigue, pain, constipation, impotence, and short-term memory impairment. Sleep problems are common in patients with PD and include difficulty staying asleep, restless sleep, nightmares, and drowsiness or sudden sleep onset during the day (National Institute of Neurological Disorders and Stroke, 2016).

Complications

As the disease progresses, complications increase. These include motor symptoms (e.g., dyskinesias [spontaneous, involuntary movements], weakness, akinesia [total immobility]), neurological problems (e.g., dementia), and neuropsychiatric problems (e.g., depression, hallucinations, psychosis). As PD progresses, it often results in severe dementia, which is associated with an increase in mortality. As swallowing becomes more difficult (dysphagia), malnutrition or aspiration may result. General debilitation may lead to pneumonia, urinary tract infections, and skin breakdown. Orthostatic hypotension may occur in some patients and, along with loss of postural reflexes, may result in falls or other injuries.

Diagnostic Studies

Because there is no specific diagnostic test for PD, the diagnosis is based on the history and clinical features. A firm diagnosis

TABLE 61-18 COLLABORATIVE CARE

Parkinson's Disease

Diagnostic	Collaborative Therapy
• History and physical examination	• Antiparkinsonian drugs*
• Bradykinesia	• Ablation surgery
• MRI	• Deep brain stimulation
• Positive response to antiparkinsonian drugs*	
• Rigidity	
• Rule out adverse effects of phenothiazines, benzodiazepines, haloperidol	
• Tremor	

MRI, magnetic resonance imaging.
*See Table 61-19.

can be made only when at least two of the three signs of the classic triad are present: tremor, rigidity, and bradykinesia. The ultimate confirmation of PD is a positive response to antiparkinsonian drugs. Research is ongoing regarding the role of genetic testing and MRI in diagnosing patients with PD (Chahine & Stern, 2011).

Collaborative Care

Because there is no cure for PD, collaborative management (Table 61-18) is focused on symptom management.

Drug Therapy. Drug therapy for PD is aimed at correcting an imbalance of neurotransmitters within the CNS. Antiparkinsonian drugs either enhance the release or supply of DA (dopaminergic) or antagonize or block the effects of the overactive cholinergic neurons in the striatum (anticholinergic). Levodopa (L-dopa) with carbidopa (Sinemet) is often the first drug used. L-Dopa is a precursor of DA and can cross the blood–brain barrier. It is converted to DA in the basal ganglia. Sinemet is the preferred drug because it also contains carbidopa, an agent that inhibits the enzyme dopa decarboxylase in the peripheral tissues. This enzyme breaks down L-dopa before it reaches the brain. The net result of the combination of L-dopa and carbidopa is that more L-dopa reaches the brain, and therefore less drug is needed.

DRUG ALERT—Carbidopa–Levodopa (Sinemet)
• The patient should be monitored for signs of dyskinesia.
• Effects may be delayed for several weeks to months.
• The patient or caregiver should be instructed to report any uncontrolled movement of the face, eyelids, mouth, tongue, arms, hands, or legs; mental changes; palpitations; severe nausea and vomiting; and difficulty urinating.

Many patients are given Sinemet early in the disease course. However, some health care providers believe that after a few years of therapy, the effectiveness of Sinemet wears off. Instead, these providers may prefer to initiate therapy with a dopaminergic drug that directly stimulates DA receptors. When more moderate-to-severe symptoms become present, L-dopa with carbidopa (Sinemet) is added to the drug regimen.

Anticholinergic drugs are also used to manage PD. These drugs act by decreasing the activity of ACh, thus providing balance between cholinergic and dopaminergic actions. Antihistamines (e.g., diphenhydramine [Benadryl]) with anticholinergic properties or a β-adrenergic blocker (e.g., propranolol [Inderal]) is used to manage tremors. The antiviral agent amantadine is also an effective antiparkinsonian drug. Although its exact mechanism of action is not known, amantadine promotes the release of DA from neurons.

Selegiline is a monoamine oxidase inhibitor that is sometimes used in combination with Sinemet. By inhibiting monoamine oxidase, the degradative enzyme for DA, levels of DA are increased. Rasagiline (Azilect), a type B monoamine oxidase inhibitor, is used as an initial drug therapy in early PD and as an addition to L-dopa in patients with more advanced disease.

Entacapone (Comtan) blocks the enzyme catechol-O-methyltransferase, which breaks down L-dopa in the peripheral circulation, thus prolonging the effect of Sinemet. These drugs are used only as adjuncts to L-dopa (Lindahl & MacMahon, 2011).

Table 61-19 summarizes the drugs commonly used in PD. The use of only one drug is preferred because there are fewer adverse effects and the drug dosage is easier to adjust than when several drugs are used. However, as the disease progresses, combination therapy is often required. Excessive amounts of dopaminergic drugs can lead to paradoxical intoxication (aggravation rather than relief of symptoms).

Surgical Therapy. Surgical procedures are aimed at relieving symptoms of PD and are usually used in patients who are unresponsive to drug therapy or who have developed severe motor complications. Surgical procedures fall into three categories: ablation (destruction), deep brain stimulation (DBS), and transplantation.

Ablation surgery involves stereotactic ablation of areas in the thalamus (thalamotomy), globus pallidus (pallidotomy), and subthalamic nucleus (subthalamic nucleotomy). Ablative procedures have been used for PD for over 50 years, but they have been replaced recently by DBS. DBS involves placing an electrode in the thalamus, the globus pallidus, or the subthalamic nucleus and connecting it to a generator placed in the upper chest (like a pacemaker). The device is programmed to deliver a specific current to the targeted brain location. Unlike ablation procedures, DBS can be adjusted to control symptoms better and is reversible (the device is removable). These ablative and DBS procedures work by blocking the neuronal impulses that lead to the motor symptoms seen in PD (National Institute of Neurological Disorders and Stroke, 2016).

Transplantation of fetal neural tissue into the basal ganglia is designed to provide DA-producing cells in the brains of patients with PD. Currently, it is the only therapy that allows patients full functional restoration. Aside from the ethical dilemma of

TABLE 61-19 DRUG THERAPY

Parkinson's Disease

Drug	Symptoms Relieved	Adverse Effects and Precautions
Dopaminergic		
levodopa (L-dopa)	Bradykinesia, tremor, rigidity	Nausea, dyskinesia, hypotension, palpitations, dysrhythmias; agitation, hallucinations, confusion (in older-adult patient)
		Avoidance of multivitamin pills and diet high in vitamin B_6 (reversal of effect of levodopa); contraindicated in narrow-angle glaucoma
levodopa–carbidopa (Sinemet)	Same as above	Less nausea but greater chance of dyskinesia, confusion, hallucinations
		Periodic check of BUN, AST, WBCs, Hct
		Contraindicated in melanoma; narrow-angle glaucoma; combination with MAO inhibitors, methyldopa, antipsychotics
bromocriptine mesylate	Same as above	Orthostatic hypotension, nausea, vomiting, toxic psychosis, limb edema, phlebitis, dizziness, headache, insomnia
pramipexole (Mirapex)	Same as above	
ropinirole (Requip)	Same as above	
amantadine	Rigidity, akinesia	Nervousness, insomnia, confusion, hallucinations, dry mouth, nausea, edema, orthostatic hypotension
Anticholinergic		
benztropine	Tremor	Dry mouth, blurred vision, constipation, delirium, anxiety, agitation, hallucinations
procyclidine		
trihexyphenidyl		Avoidance of drugs with similar actions, including over-the-counter drugs containing scopolamine or antihistamines, antispasmodics (e.g., Bellergal), tricyclic antidepressants (e.g., amitriptyline [Elavil])
Antihistamine		
diphenhydramine (Benadryl)	Tremor, rigidity	Sedation, same precautions as for anticholinergic drugs
orphenadrine		
Monoamine Oxidase Inhibitor		
selegiline	Bradykinesia, rigidity, tremor	Similar to dopaminergic drugs
Catechol-O-Methyltransferase (COMT) Inhibitor		
entacapone (Comtan)	By blocking COMT, this drug slows down the breakdown of levodopa, thus prolonging the action of levodopa	Similar to dopaminergic drugs; works only when used in combination with Sinemet

AST, aspartate aminotransferase; *BUN,* blood urea nitrogen; *Hct,* hematocrit; *MAO,* monoamine oxidase; *WBCs,* white blood cells.

using fetal tissue as a treatment, this therapy has many limitations and is still in experimental stages. Stem cell transplantation is an alternative therapy showing some promise. Both epithelial and bone marrow cells are currently being studied. Clinical trial outcomes related to stem cell transplantation have been inconsistent (Politis & Lindvall, 2012).

Nutritional Therapy. Diet is important for patients with PD because malnutrition and constipation can be serious consequences of inadequate nutrition. Patients who have dysphagia and bradykinesia need appetizing foods that are easily chewed and swallowed. The diet should contain adequate roughage and fruit to avoid constipation. Food should be cut into bite-sized pieces before it is served, and hot food should be served on a warmed plate to preserve its appeal. Eating six small meals a day may be less exhausting than eating three large meals a day. Ample time should be planned for eating to avoid frustration and encourage independence. In addition, absorption of L-dopa can be impaired by ingestion of protein and of vitamin B_6. Some patients are advised to limit their protein intake to the evening meal to decrease this problem and to consult with their health care provider regarding vitamin B_6 in their multivitamins and fortified cereals.

NURSING MANAGEMENT
PARKINSON'S DISEASE

NURSING ASSESSMENT

Subjective and objective data that should be obtained from a patient with PD are presented in Table 61-20.

NURSING DIAGNOSES

Nursing diagnoses for patients with PD may include, but are not limited to, the following:

- *Impaired physical mobility* related to *decrease in muscle control, decrease in muscle strength, physical deconditioning*
- *Imbalanced nutrition: less than body requirements* related to *insufficient dietary intake* (difficulty ingesting food)
- *Impaired swallowing* related to *behavioural feeding problem* (neuro-muscular impairment)

Additional information on nursing diagnoses for the patient with PD is presented in NCP 61-4, available on the Evolve website.

PLANNING

The overall goals are that the patient with PD will (1) experience a lower intensity and frequency of distressing symptoms, (2) maximize neurological function, (3) maintain independence in activities of daily living for as long as possible, and (4) optimize psychosocial well-being.

NURSING IMPLEMENTATION

Because PD is a chronic, degenerative disorder with no acute exacerbations, patient teaching and nursing care should include the assessment and management of medications (Magennis, Lynch, & Corry, 2014), maintenance of good health, encouragement of independence, and avoidance of complications such as contractures. Problems secondary to bradykinesia can be alleviated by relatively simple measures.

Promotion of physical exercise and a well-balanced diet are major concerns for nursing care. Exercise can limit the consequences of decreased mobility, such as muscle atrophy, contractures, and constipation. Parkinson Canada (see Resources section at the end of this chapter) publishes a series of booklets and

TABLE 61-20 NURSING ASSESSMENT
Parkinson's Disease

Subjective Data
Important Health Information
Past health history: CNS trauma, cerebro-vascular disorders, exposure to metals or carbon monoxide, encephalitis; positive family history
Medications: Use of major tranquilizers, especially haloperidol and phenothiazines, methyldopa, amphetamines

Symptoms
- Excessive salivation, dysphagia; weight loss
- Constipation, incontinence; excessive sweating
- Fatigue, sleep disturbance, difficulty initiating movements; postural instability; frequent falls; loss of dexterity; micrographia (handwriting deterioration)
- Diffuse headache; pain in shoulders, neck, back, legs, and hips; muscle soreness and cramping; difficulty concentrating
- Depression, mood swings, hallucinations

Objective Data
General
Blank (masked) facies, slow and monotonous speech, infrequent blinking

Integumentary
Seborrhea, dandruff; ankle edema

Cardiovascular
Postural hypotension

Gastro-Intestinal
Drooling

Neurological
Tremor at rest, first in hands (pill rolling), later in legs, arms, face, and tongue; aggravation of tremor with anxiety, absence in sleep; poor coordination; subtle dementia, impaired postural reflexes

Musculo-Skeletal
Cogwheel rigidity, dysarthria, bradykinesia, contractures, stooped posture, shuffling gait

Possible Findings
Lack of specific tests; diagnosis on basis of history and physical findings and ruling out of other diseases

CNS, central nervous system.

videos with helpful exercises that can be used by family members and health care professionals.

A physiotherapist may be consulted to design an exercise program aimed at strengthening, muscle tone, and stretching specific muscles. A speech–language pathologist may be consulted to strengthen the muscles involved with speaking and swallowing. Although exercise will not halt the progress of the disease, it will enhance the patient's functional ability. An occupational therapist can also assist the patient with strategies to increase self-care abilities, including eating and dressing.

SAFETY ALERT
Have patients who are at risk for falling and tend to "freeze" while walking do the following:
- Consciously think about stepping over imaginary or real lines on the floor.
- Drop grains of rice and step over them.
- Rock from side to side.
- Lift the toes when stepping.
- Take one step backward and two steps forward.

The nurse should work closely with the patient's caregiver and family in exploring creative adaptations that allow maximal independence and self-care. The patient can facilitate getting out of a chair by using an upright chair with arms and placing the back legs of the chair on small (2-inch) blocks. Encourage environmental alterations, such as removing rugs and excess furniture to avoid stumbling, using an elevated toilet seat to facilitate getting on and off the toilet, and elevating the legs on an ottoman to decrease dependent ankle edema. Clothing can be simplified by the use of slip-on shoes and Velcro hook-and-loop fasteners or zippers on clothing, instead of buttons and hooks.

Effective management of sleep problems can greatly improve the quality of life for patients with PD. Some patients with PD find the use of satin nightwear or satin sheets beneficial. Information on teaching regarding sleep hygiene practices is presented in Chapter 9.

In the early stages of PD, many patients experience depression and anxiety. Patients need to adjust their lifestyle, including work and home responsibilities. As the disease progresses, the impact on the patient's psychological well-being also increases. The nurse can assist the patient by listening, providing teaching, challenging distorted thoughts, and encouraging social interactions. Psychotherapy and counselling can also be helpful.

In the early stage of the disease, the patient has subtle changes in cognitive function, which may progress to dementia. This progression results in increased caregiver burden and the potential for long-term care placement. Information on care of the patient with dementia is provided in Chapter 62.

The majority of patients with PD are cared for by family caregivers. As the disease progresses, the caregiver burden increases, often while the caregiver's physical and mental health decline. Strategies to reduce caregiver stress are described in Chapter 62, Table 62-15. Other interventions for the patient with PD are presented in NCP 61-4 (available on the Evolve website).

EVALUATION

The expected outcomes are that the patient with PD will:
- Perform physical exercise to deter muscle atrophy and joint contractures.
- Use assistive devices appropriately for ambulation and mobility.
- Maintain nutritional intake adequate for metabolic needs.
- Experience safe passage of fluids and solids from the mouth to the stomach.
- Use methods of communication that meet needs for interaction with others.

Additional information on expected outcomes for the patient with PD is presented in NCP 61-4 (available on the Evolve website).

MYASTHENIA GRAVIS

Myasthenia gravis (MG) is an autoimmune disease of the neuro-muscular junction characterized by fluctuating weakness of certain skeletal muscle groups. MG can occur at any age. The mean age at time of diagnosis is 60.2 years plus or minus 17.1 years, with the incidence of MG reportedly higher in younger women and older men (Breiner et al., 2015). In 2013, there were approximately 32 cases of MG per 100 000 population in Ontario (Breiner, Widdifield, Katzberg, et al., 2015); however, MG is thought to be underdiagnosed and the prevalence is likely higher.

Etiology and Pathophysiology

MG is caused by an autoimmune process in which antibodies attack ACh receptors, resulting in a decreased number of ACh receptor (AChR) sites at the neuro-muscular junction (Figure 61-10). This prevents ACh molecules from attaching and stimulating muscle contraction. Anti-AChR antibodies are detectable in the serum of patients with generalized MG. In patients who lack autoantibodies to AChR, their muscular weakness may be related to autoantibodies to the muscle-specific receptor tyrosine kinase, although other autoantibodies may also be involved (Guptill, Soni, & Meriggioli, 2016). Thymic tumours are found in about 15% of patients, and abnormal thymus tissue is found in most others.

Clinical Manifestations and Complications

The primary feature of MG is fluctuating weakness of skeletal muscle. Strength is usually restored after a period of rest. The muscles most often involved are those used for moving the eyes and eyelids, chewing, swallowing, speaking, and breathing. The muscles are generally the strongest in the morning and become exhausted with continued activity. Consequently, by the end of the day, muscle weakness is prominent (Myasthenia Gravis Coalition of Canada, 2017) (Table 61-21).

The course of this disease is variable. Some patients may have short-term remissions, others may stabilize, and others may have severe, progressive involvement. Restricted ocular myasthenia, usually seen only in men, has a good prognosis.

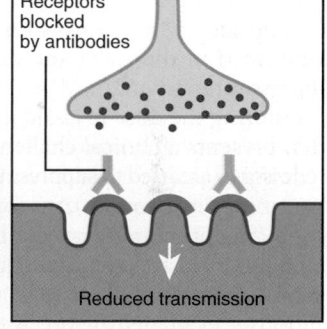

Normal neuro-muscular junction

Neuro-muscular junction in myasthenia gravis

FIGURE 61-10 Neuromuscular junction in myasthenia gravis. *ACh,* acetylcholine. Source: Myasthenia Gravis Coalition of Canada. (2017). *What is MG?* Retrieved from *http://www.mgcc-ccmg.org/about.asp.*

TABLE 61-21	CLINICAL MANIFESTATIONS OF MYASTHENIA GRAVIS

- A change in facial expression
- Chronic muscle fatigue
- Difficulty breathing
- Difficulty chewing or swallowing
- Drooping eyelid(s) (ptosis)
- Impaired or slurred speech
- Unstable or unusual gait
- Vision changes (blurred or double)
- Weakness in arms, hands, fingers, legs, and neck

Source: National Institute of Neurological Disorders and Stroke. (2015). *Myasthenia fact sheet.* Retrieved from *http://www.ninds.nih.gov/disorders/myasthenia_gravis/detail_myasthenia_gravis.htm?css=print#3153_4.*

Exacerbations of MG can be precipitated by stress, pregnancy, menses, secondary illness, trauma, temperature extremes, and hypokalemia. Ingestion of drugs including chlorpromazine, haloperidol, amitriptyline (Elavil), lithium, carbamazepine (Tegretol), and quetiapine have also been associated with worsening of MG (Wilson & Ferguson, 2013).

Myasthenic crisis is an acute exacerbation of muscle weakness triggered by infection, surgery, emotional distress, or overdose of or inadequate drugs in a person with MG. Generally, it occurs in the first 2 years after diagnosis. The major complications of MG result from muscle weakness in areas that affect swallowing and breathing. This weakness results in aspiration, respiratory insufficiency, and respiratory infection.

Diagnostic Studies

The diagnosis of MG can be made on the basis of history, physical examination, and diagnostic testing. Diagnostic testing would include a routine electromyography (EMG) (to rule out other possible causes of the symptoms) as well as repetitive nerve stimulation. In addition, single-fibre EMG is done to show the muscles' response to electrical shocks, and antibody testing is done to detect acetylcholine receptor antibodies.

Collaborative Care

Drug Therapy. Drug therapy for MG includes anticholinesterase drugs, alternate-day corticosteroids, and immunosuppressants (Table 61-22). Anticholinesterase drugs are aimed at enhancing function of the neuro-muscular junction. Acetylcholinesterase is the enzyme that breaks down ACh in the synaptic cleft. Thus, inhibition of this enzyme by an anticholinesterase inhibitor will prolong the action of ACh and facilitate transmission of impulses at the neuro-muscular junction. Pyridostigmine (Mestinon) is the most successful drug of this group in the long-term treatment of MG.

Tailoring the dose to avoid a myasthenic or cholinergic crisis often presents a clinical challenge. Corticosteroids (specifically prednisone) are used to suppress the immune response. Drugs such as azathioprine (Imuran), mycophenolate (CellCept), and cyclosporin (Sandimmune) may also be used for immuno-suppression.

Many drugs are contraindicated for use or must be used with caution in patients with MG. Classes of drug that should be cautiously evaluated before use include anaesthetics, antidysrhythmics, antibiotics, quinine, antipsychotics, barbiturates and sedative–hypnotics, cathartics, diuretics, opioids, muscle relaxants, thyroid preparations, and tranquilizers.

Surgical Therapy. Because the presence of the thymus gland in patients with MG appears to enhance the production of ACh

TABLE 61-22   COLLABORATIVE CARE
Myasthenia Gravis

Diagnostic	Collaborative Therapy
• History and physical examination	• Drugs
• Acetylcholine receptor antibodies	• Anticholinesterase agents
• EMG	• Corticosteroids
• Fatigability when upward gaze is prolonged (2–3 min)	• Immuno-suppressive agents
• Muscle weakness	• Plasmapheresis
	• Surgery (thymectomy)

EMG, electromyography.

receptor antibodies, removal of the thymus gland results in improvement in most patients. Thymectomy is indicated for all patients with thymoma, for patients with generalized MG between puberty and about age 65 years, and for patients with purely ocular MG.

Other Therapies. Plasmapheresis and IV immunoglobulin G (IVIG) can yield a short-term improvement in symptoms and are indicated for patients in myasthenic crisis or in preparation for surgery when corticosteroids must be avoided. Plasmapheresis directly removes circulating AChR antibodies, leading to a decrease in symptoms. (Plasmapheresis is discussed in Chapter 16.) Some evidence has shown that IVIG is just as effective as plasmapheresis in the treatment of MG (Dhawan, Goodman, Harper, et al., 2015). Treatment decisions should be based on the patient's unique clinical presentation.

NURSING MANAGEMENT
MYASTHENIA GRAVIS

NURSING ASSESSMENT

The nurse can assess the severity of MG by asking the patient about fatigability, what body parts are affected, and how severely he or she is affected. The patient's coping abilities and understanding of the disorder should also be assessed. Some patients become so fatigued that they are no longer able to ambulate.

Objective data should include respiratory rate and depth, oxygen saturation, arterial blood gas analyses, pulmonary function tests, and evidence of respiratory distress in patients with acute myasthenic crisis. Muscle strength of all face and limb muscles should be assessed, as should swallowing, speech (dysarthria) and voice (volume and clarity), cough and gag reflexes, and bladder function.

NURSING DIAGNOSES

Nursing diagnoses for patients with MG may include, but are not limited to, the following:

- *Ineffective airway clearance* related to *excessive mucus, retained secretions* (intercostal muscle weakness, impaired cough and gag reflexes)
- *Activity intolerance* related to *immobility, physical deconditioning* (muscle weakness, fatigue)
- *Disturbed body image* related to *alteration in self-perception* (inability to maintain usual lifestyle and role responsibility)

PLANNING

The overall goals are that the patient with MG will have a return of normal muscle endurance, avoid complications, and maintain a quality of life appropriate to disease course.

NURSING IMPLEMENTATION

The patient with MG who is admitted to the hospital usually has a respiratory tract infection or is in an acute myasthenic crisis. Nursing care is aimed at maintaining adequate ventilation, continuing drug therapy, and watching for adverse effects of therapy. The nurse must be able to distinguish cholinergic from myasthenic crisis (Table 61-23) because the causes and treatment of the two conditions differ greatly.

As with other chronic illnesses, care focuses on the neurological deficits and their impact on daily living. A balanced diet, with food that can be chewed and swallowed easily, should be prescribed. Semisolid foods may be easier to eat than solids or liquids. Scheduling doses of drugs so that peak action is

TABLE 61-23	COMPARISON OF MYASTHENIC CRISIS AND CHOLINERGIC CRISIS	
Myasthenic Crisis	**Cholinergic Crisis**	
Causes		
Exacerbation of myasthenia following precipitating factors or failure to take drug as prescribed or drug dose too low	Overdose of anticholinesterase drugs resulting in increased ACh at the receptor sites, remission (spontaneous or after thymectomy)	
Differential Diagnosis		
Improved strength after IV administration of anticholinesterase drugs	Weakness within 1 hour after ingestion of anticholinesterase	
Increased weakness of skeletal muscles manifesting as ptosis, bulbar signs (e.g., difficulty in swallowing, difficulty in articulating words), or dyspnea	Increased weakness of skeletal muscles manifesting as ptosis, bulbar signs, dyspnea	
	Effects on smooth muscle, include papillary miosis, salivation, diarrhea, nausea or vomiting, abdominal cramps, increased bronchial secretions, sweating, or lacrimation	

ACh, acetylcholine; *IV*, intravenous.

reached at mealtime may make eating less difficult. Teaching should focus on the importance of following the medical regimen, potential adverse reactions to specific drugs, planning activities of daily living to avoid fatigue, the availability of community resources, and the complications of the disease and therapy (crisis conditions) and what to do about them. Contact with the Myasthenia Gravis Coalition of Canada or an MG support group may be helpful.

EVALUATION

The following are overall expected outcomes for the patient with MG:
- The patient will maintain optimal muscle function.
- The patient will be free from adverse effects of drugs.
- The patient will not experience complications from the disease, in particular, myasthenic or cholinergic crisis.
- The patient will maintain a quality of life appropriate to the disease course.

RESTLESS LEGS SYNDROME

Etiology and Pathophysiology

Restless legs syndrome (RLS) (also known as Willis–Ekbom disease) is characterized by unpleasant sensory (paresthesias) and motor abnormalities of one or both legs. RLS is more common in older adults, and prevalence rates range from 5% to 15% (Yeh, Walters, & Tsuang, 2012); however, the numbers may be higher because the condition is often underdiagnosed. There are two distinct types of RLS: primary (idiopathic) and secondary. The majority of cases are primary, and many patients with this type of RLS report a positive family history. Secondary RLS can occur with metabolic abnormalities associated with iron deficiency, renal failure, hypertension, diabetes mellitus, or rheumatoid arthritis. Conditions such as anemia, pregnancy, and certain medications can cause or worsen symptoms. Although the exact pathophysiology of primary RLS is unknown, it is believed that RLS is related to a dysfunction in the brain's basal ganglia circuits that use the neurotransmitter DA, which controls movement. In RLS, this dysfunction causes the urge to move the legs. Abnormal iron metabolism or brain iron deficiencies may result in abnormalities of the DA system, thus leading to RLS (National Institute for Disorders and Stroke, 2015c).

Clinical Manifestations

The severity of RLS sensory symptoms ranges from infrequent minor discomfort (paresthesias, including numbness and tingling) to severe pain. Sensory symptoms often appear first. Patients describe annoying and uncomfortable (but usually not painful) sensations in the legs. Some describe the sensations like bugs crawling on the legs. The leg pain is localized within the calf muscles. Patients can also experience pain in the upper extremities and the trunk. The discomfort occurs when the patient is sedentary and is most common in the evening or at night, resulting in sleep disruption. In severe cases, patients sleep only a few hours at night, resulting in daytime fatigue and disruption of the daily routine. Physical activity, such as walking or stretching, often relieves the pain. The motor abnormalities associated with RLS consist of voluntary restlessness and stereotyped, periodic, involuntary movements (National Institute for Neurological Disorders and Stroke, 2015c). Fatigue further aggravates symptoms. Over time, RLS advances to more frequent and severe episodes.

Diagnostic Studies

RLS is a clinical diagnosis and is based in large part on the patient's history or the report of the bed partner related to nighttime activities. The International Restless Legs Study Group proposed five minimum diagnostic criteria. They are (1) desire to move the limbs, not necessarily in relation to, or accompanied by, pain or discomfort, (2) desire to move limbs, and any accompanying discomfort begins or worsens at rest, (3) desire to move limbs, and any accompanying discomfort is relieved with continuous activity, (4) desire to move limbs, and any accompanying discomfort begins or worsens at night, and (5) the presence of any of the above criteria are not uniquely attributable to a medical or psychological condition (International Restless Legs Syndrome Study Group, 2015). Generally, the patient history clearly suggests a diagnosis of RLS (Restless Legs Syndrome Foundation, 2015a). If the patient has a history of diabetes mellitus, its management may provide information to determine whether paresthesias are caused by peripheral neuropathy or RLS.

NURSING AND COLLABORATIVE MANAGEMENT RESTLESS LEGS SYNDROME

The goal of collaborative management is to reduce patient discomfort and distress and to improve sleep quality. When RLS is secondary to uremia or iron deficiency, correction of these conditions will decrease symptoms. Nonpharmacological approaches to RLS management include establishing regular sleep habits, encouraging exercise, and eliminating aggravating factors such as certain activities, alcohol, caffeine, and certain drugs (i.e., neuroleptics, lithium, antihistamines, and antidepressants) (Restless Legs Syndrome Foundation, 2015b).

If nonpharmacological measures fail to provide symptom relief, drug therapy may be started. The main drugs used in RLS are dopaminergic agents, opioids, and benzodiazepines. Dopaminergic agents such as carbidopa–levodopa (Sinemet) and DA agonists (bromocriptine, pramipexole [Mirapex]) are preferred for treating RLS. These agents are effective in managing sensory and motor symptoms.

Other agents that may be used include anticonvulsant drugs such as gabapentin (Neurontin), divalproex (Epival), lamotrigine (Lamictal), and carbamazepine (Tegretol). Clonidine and propranolol (Inderal) are also effective in some patients. While quinine sulphate has been used prophylactically and as a treatment for RLS, its use is not recommended as it has been linked with serious adverse reactions such as life-threatening hematological reactions and chronic renal failure. Opioids are usually reserved for those patients with severe symptoms who fail to respond to other drugs. When used, opioids given in low doses have also been found to be effective in reducing the symptoms associated with RLS.

AMYOTROPHIC LATERAL SCLEROSIS

Amyotrophic lateral sclerosis (ALS) is a rare progressive neurological disorder that is characterized by loss of motor neurons and by weakness and atrophy of the muscles of the hands, the forearms, and the legs, spreading to involve most of the body and the face. ALS became known as Lou Gehrig's disease when the famous baseball player was stricken with it in the 1940s.

The Canadian incidence of ALS is about 2 of every 100 000 per year, and approximately 2 500 to 3 000 Canadians are currently living with it (Amyotrophic Lateral Sclerosis [ALS] Society of Canada, 2015). The mortality rate of ALS is approximately 2 per 100 000 per year (ALS Society of Canada, 2015). ALS usually leads to death within 2 to 6 years after diagnosis.

For unknown reasons, motor neurons in the brain stem and spinal cord gradually degenerate in ALS. Dead motor neurons cannot produce or transport vital signals to muscles. Consequently, electrical and chemical messages originating in the brain do not reach the muscles to activate them.

The typical symptoms of ALS are limb weakness, dysarthria, and dysphagia. Muscle wasting and fasciculations result from the denervation of the muscles and lack of stimulation and use. Other symptoms include pain, sleep disorders, spasticity, drooling, emotional lability, depression, constipation, and esophageal reflux. Death usually results from respiratory tract infection secondary to compromised respiratory function. Unfortunately, there is no cure for ALS. Riluzole (Rilutek) slows the progression of ALS. This drug works to decrease the amount of glutamate (an excitatory neurotransmitter) in the brain.

The illness trajectory for ALS is devastating because the patient remains cognitively intact while wasting away. The nurse guides the patient in the use of moderate-intensity, endurance-type exercises for the trunk and limbs since this may help reduce ALS spasticity. Nursing interventions include facilitating communication, reducing risk for aspiration, facilitating early identification of respiratory insufficiency, decreasing pain secondary to muscle weakness, decreasing risk for injury related to falls, and providing diversional activities such as reading and companionship.

The patient's cognitive and emotional functions are supported, and the patient and family are helped to manage the disease process, including grieving related to the loss of motor function and ultimately death. The nurse discusses with the patient and caregiver issues such as artificial methods of ventilation and advance directives.

HUNTINGTON'S DISEASE

Huntington's disease (HD) is a genetically transmitted, autosomal dominant disorder that affects both men and women of all races.

It is characterized by chronic, devastating loss of all neurological function, resulting in a movement disorder and dementia. The offspring of a person with this disease have a 50% risk of inheriting it (see the "Genetics in Clinical Practice" box). The onset of HD is usually between 30 and 50 years of age. Often, the diagnosis is made after the affected individual has had children. The estimated prevalence rate of HD is at 13.7 per 100 000 in the general population (Fisher & Hayden, 2013).

The diagnostic process for HD begins with a review of the family history and clinical symptoms. Genetic testing confirms the disease in a person with symptoms. People who are asymptomatic but who have a positive family history of HD face the dilemma of whether to be genetically tested. If the test is positive, the person will develop HD, but when and to what extent the disease develops cannot be determined.

Like PD, the pathological process of HD involves the basal ganglia and the extrapyramidal motor system. However, instead of a deficiency of DA, HD involves a deficiency of the neurotransmitters ACh and γ-aminobutyric acid. The net effect is an

---

🧬 GENETICS IN CLINICAL PRACTICE

Huntington's Disease

Genetic Basis
- Autosomal dominant disorder
- Caused by HTT gene, located on chromosome 4

Incidence
- 1 in 10 000
- Higher incidence in people of European ancestry
- With each pregnancy, heterozygous affected parent has a 5% chance of having a child with HD

Genetic Testing
- DNA testing is available
- DNA testing can be done on fetal cells obtained by amniocentesis or chorionic villus sampling
- Preimplantation genetic diagnosis can be done on embryos before implantation and pregnancy
- One copy of altered gene is sufficient to cause HD
- No test is available to predict when symptoms will develop

Clinical Implications
- HD is a progressive, degenerative brain disorder
- Onset of disease usually occurs between 30 and 50 years of age
- No cure is available
- Drugs are available to control movements and behavioural problems
- Genetic counselling may be considered if there is a family history of HD
- Because HD is an autosomal dominant disorder, individuals who are at risk have a strong motivation to seek genetic testing
- A positive result is not considered a diagnosis, since it may be obtained decades before the symptoms begin
- A negative test means that the individual does not carry the mutated gene and will not develop HD

Social Networking in Huntington's Disease
- Many patients with Huntington's disease experience social isolation and depression.
- The patient should be encouraged to participate in an online community where people who have Huntington's disease discuss their condition.
- Social contact and a social network with others who have Huntington's disease will help patients deal better with their illness and improve their quality of life.

excess of DA, which leads to symptoms that are the opposite of those of parkinsonism.

The clinical manifestations are characterized by abnormal and excessive involuntary movements (chorea) as well as psychiatric abnormalities. The chorea involves writhing, twisting movements of the face, the limbs, and the body. The movements worsen as the disease progresses. Facial movements used for speech, chewing, and swallowing are affected and may cause aspiration and malnutrition. The gait deteriorates, and ambulation eventually becomes impossible.

Psychiatric symptoms are frequently present in the early stage of the disease, often before the onset of motor symptoms. Depression is common. Other psychiatric symptoms include anxiety, agitation, impulsivity, apathy, social withdrawal, and obsessiveness. Cognitive deterioration is more variable and involves perception, memory, attention, and learning. Eventually, all psychomotor processes, including the ability to eat and talk, are impaired.

Death usually occurs within 15 years after the onset of symptoms (Huntington Society of Canada, 2013). The most common causes of death related to HD are pneumonia and suicide; however, injuries related to a fall or other complications have also been attributed to HD-related mortality (National Institute of Neurological Disorders and Stroke, 2015a).

Because there is no cure, collaborative care is palliative. The first drug of any kind approved specifically for HD is tetrabenazine (Nitoman). It is used to treat the chorea and works to decrease the amount of DA available at synapses in the brain and thus decreases the involuntary movements of chorea.

Other medications used for the movement disorder include neuroleptics such as haloperidol and risperidone (Risperdal), benzodiazepines such as diazepam (Valium) and clonazepam (Rivotril), and DA-depleting agents. Cognitive disorders are treated as needed with nondrug therapies (e.g., counselling, memory books). The psychiatric disorders can be treated with selective serotonin reuptake inhibitors such as sertraline

(Zoloft) and paroxetine (Paxil). Antipsychotic medication, such as haloperidol or risperidone (Risperdal), may also be needed. Because of the choreic movements, caloric requirements are high. Patients may require as many as 5 000 calories per day to maintain body weight. As the disease progresses, meeting caloric needs becomes more challenging as the patient has difficulty swallowing and holding the head still. Depression and mental deterioration can also compromise nutritional intake. Alternative sources of nutrition may be indicated as the disease progresses.

HD presents a great challenge to health care providers. The goal of nursing management is to provide the most comfortable environment possible for the patient and the family by maintaining physical safety, treating physical symptoms, and providing emotional and psychological support. End-of-life issues should be discussed with the patient and caregiver. These include care in the home or long-term care facility, artificial methods of feeding, advance directives and cardiopulmonary resuscitation (CPR), use of antibiotics to treat infections, and guardianship. These topics should be readdressed throughout the course of the disease as the patient and caregiver adapt to increasing disability.

NORMAL PRESSURE HYDROCEPHALUS

Normal pressure hydrocephalus (NPH) is an abnormal increase of CSF characterized by an obstruction in the normal flow of CSF throughout the brain, spinal cord, and ventricles. NPH is a relatively uncommon disorder, and symptoms of the condition include mental impairment, dementia, urinary incontinence, and gait and balance disturbances. Meningitis, encephalitis, or head injury may cause the condition. NPH can occur at any age, although it is most common in older adults. If diagnosed early in the disease, NPH is treatable by surgery that involves a shunt insertion to divert the fluid away from the brain into the abdomen to help resolve the symptoms (National Institute of Neurological Disorders and Stroke, 2015b).

CASE STUDY

Parkinson's Disease

Source: Air Images/ Shutterstock .com.

Patient Profile

Mr. Jean Dufresne, a 79-year-old retiree, was diagnosed with Parkinson's disease 3 years ago after experiencing months of progressive tremor, rigidity, and bradykinesia. He has been taking L-dopa with carbidopa (Sinemet) since then, and his symptoms had been improving until recently. When his daughter was visiting, she noticed that he had lost considerable weight over the past month, and his speech had become slower and difficult to understand.

Subjective Data
- Reports increasing difficulty with speech and swallowing
- Dietary intake has decreased
- Reports being constipated for 2 weeks

Objective Data
Physical Examination
- Body weight has decreased by 5 kg in 1 month.
- Gait has developed a mild shuffling and propulsive quality.

- "Pill rolling" motion and tremor are observed in both hands at rest.
- "Cogwheel rigidity" is encountered during passive range of motion exercises.

Discussion Questions
1. What is the pathogenesis of Parkinson's disease?
2. What is the likely explanation for the progression of Mr. Dufresne's condition?
3. What teaching plan should be developed for Mr. Dufresne?
4. **Priority decision:** What are the priority nursing interventions for Mr. Dufresne?
5. **Priority decision:** What are the priority nursing diagnoses based on the assessment data presented for Mr. Dufresne?

Answers are available at *http://evolve.elsevier.com/Canada/Lewis/medsurg*.

▮ REVIEW QUESTIONS

The number of the question corresponds to the same-numbered objective at the beginning of the chapter.

1. What of the following is the nurse most likely to recognize as a symptom of a client with a migraine headache?
   a. Withdraws from stimuli
   b. Acts out with bizarre behaviour
   c. Seeks out the company of others
   d. Experiences painful facial spasms and tearing
2. What is the triad of symptoms the nurse would expect to find during assessment of the client with Parkinson's disease?
   a. Spasticity, diplopia, tremor
   b. Tremor, rigidity, bradykinesia
   c. Ataxia, drowsiness, dysarthria
   d. Diplopia, tremor, bradykinesia
3. What would the nurse expect to find during an assessment of the client with amyotrophic lateral sclerosis?
   a. Emotional lability
   b. Mental deterioration
   c. Muscle weakness and wasting
   d. Sensory loss in the extremities

4. Social effects of a chronic neurological disease include which of the following? *(Select all that apply)*
   a. Divorce
   b. Job loss
   c. Depression
   d. Role changes
   e. Loss of self-esteem
5. What is a major goal of treatment for the client with a chronic, progressive neurological disease?
   a. Reversal of pathophysiological features
   b. Total remission of the disease
   c. Continuation of usual lifestyle
   d. Adaptation by client and family to the disease

1. a; 2. b; 3. c; 4. a, b, c, d, e; 5. d.

℮volve

For even more review questions, visit *http://evolve.elsevier.com/Canada/Lewis/medsurg*.

REFERENCES

Absher, J. R. (2015). In multiple sclerosis, use of fingolimod reduced immune responses to influenza and tetanus booster vaccines. ACP Journal Club. *Annals of Internal Medicine, 162*(12), doi:10.7326/ACPJC-2015-162-12-008.

Amyotrophic Lateral Sclerosis Society of Canada. (2015). *ALS quick facts.* Retrieved from *http://als.ca/en/publications/als-fact-sheets*.

Awad, A., Marder, E., Milo, R., et al. (2011). Multiple sclerosis and chronic cerebrospinal venous insufficiency: A critical review. *Therapeutic Advances in Neurological Disorders, 4*(4), 231–253. doi:10.1177/1756285611405565.

Bernstein, S. (2012). Does a virus help trigger MS? *Momentum (19403410), 6*(1), 57–60.

Bohlega, S. A., & Al-Foghom, N. B. (2013). Drug-induced Parkinson's disease: A clinical review. *Neurosciences (Riyadh), 18*(3), 215–221.

Breiner, A., Widdifield, J., Katzberg, H. D., et al. (2015). Epidemiology of myasthenia gravis in Ontario, Canada. *Neuromuscular Disorders : NMD, 26*(1), 41–46. doi:10.1016/j.nmd.2015.10.009.

Burton, J. M., Alikhani, K., Goyal, M., et al. (2011). Complications in MS patients after CCSVI procedures abroad (Calgary, AB). *Canadian Journal of Neurosciences, 38*(5), 741–746. doi:10.1017/S0317167100054123.

Cavazos, J. E. (2012). *Epilepsy and seizures.* Retrieved from *http://emedicine.medscape.com/article/1184846-overview*.

Cecil, R. L. F., Goldman, L., & Schafer, A. I. (2012). *Goldman's Cecil Medicine, Expert Consult Premium Edition—Enhanced Online Features and Print, Single Volume, 24: Goldman's Cecil Medicine* (Vol. 2). Philadelphia: Elsevier Health Sciences.

Chahine, L. M., & Stern, M. B. (2011). Diagnostic markers for Parkinson's disease. *Current Opinion in Neurology, 24*(4), 309–317. doi:10.1097/WCO.0b013e3283461723.

Chao, M. J., Ramagopalan, S. V., Herrera, B. M., et al. (2011). MHC transmission: Insights into gender bias in MS susceptibility. *Neurology, 76*(3), 242–246. doi:10.1212/WNL.0b013e318207b060.

Corey-Bloom, J., Wolfson, T., Gamst, A., et al. (2012). Smoked cannabis for spasticity in multiple sclerosis: A randomized, placebo-controlled trial. *Canadian Medical Association Journal, 184*(10), 1143–1150. doi:10.1503/cmaj.110837.

Costa, A., Antonaci, F., Ramusino, M. C., et al. (2015). The neuropharmacology of cluster headache and other trigeminal autonomic cephalalgias. *Current Neuropharmacology, 13*(3), 304–323. doi:10.2174/1570159X13666150309233556.

Dhawan, P. S., Goodman, B. P., Harper, C. M., et al. (2015). IVIG versus PLEX in the treatment of worsening myasthenia gravis: What is the evidence? A critically appraised topic. *The Neurologist, 19*(5), 145–148. doi:10.1097/NRL.0000000000000026.

Epilepsy Canada. (2016). *Epilepsy facts.* Retrieved from *http://www.epilepsy.ca/epilepsy-facts.html*.

Epilepsy Canada. (2009). *Your medication for epilepsy.* Retrieved from *http://www.epilepsy.ca/uploads/7/0/8/6/70868839/medication-new.pdf*.

Epilepsy Foundation. (2013a). *Finding the best dosage.* Retrieved from *http://www.epilepsy.com/learn/treating-seizures-and-epilepsy/seizure-and-epilepsy-medicines/finding-best-dosage*.

Epilepsy Foundation. (2013b). *Types of surgeries.* Retrieved from *http://www.epilepsy.com/learn/treating-seizures-and-epilepsy/surgery/types-surgeries*.

Epilepsy Ontario. (2011). *Status epilepticus.* Retrieved from *http://epilepsyontario.org/status-epilepticus/*.

Epilepsy Ontario. (2016). *Medications.* Retrieved from *http://epilepsyontario.org/about-epilepsy/treatments/medications/*.

Fisher, E. R., & Hayden, M. R. (2013). Multisource ascertainment of Huntington disease in Canada: Prevalence and population at risk. *Movement Disorders: Official Journal of the Movement Disorder Society, 29*(1), 105–114. doi:10.1002/mds.25717.

Fisher, R. S., Cross, J. H., French, J. A., et al. (2017). Operational classification of seizure types by the International League Against Epilepsy: Position Paper of the ILAE Commission for Classification and Terminology. *Epilepsia, 58*(4), 522–530.

Gaul, C., Diener, H. C., & Müller, O. M. (2011). Cluster headache: Clinical features and therapeutic options. *Deutsches Ärzteblatt International, 108*(33), 543. doi:10.3238/arztebl.2011.0543.

Goldman, L., & Schafer, A. I. (2012). *Goldman's Cecil Medicine* (24th ed.). Philadelphia: Elsevier Health Sciences.

Government of Canada. (2016).*What is multiple sclerosis?* Retrieved from *https://www.canada.ca/en/public-health/services/chronic -diseases/multiple-sclerosis.html.*

Guo, Z. N., He, S. Y., Zhang, H. L., et al. (2012). Multiple sclerosis and sexual dysfunction. *Asian Journal of Andrology, 14*(4), 530. doi:10.1038/aja.2011.110.

Guptill, J. T., Soni, M., & Meriggioli, M. N. (2016). Current treatment, emerging translational therapies, and new therapeutic targets for autoimmune myasthenia gravis. *Neurotherapeutics, 13*(1), 118–131. doi:10.1007/s13311-015-0398-y.

Hart, L. A., & Sibai, B. M. (2013). Seizures in pregnancy: Epilepsy, eclampsia, and stroke. *Seminars in Perinatology, 37*(4), 207–224. doi:10.1053/j.semperi.2013.04.001.

Headache Classification Committee of the International Headache Society (HCCIHS). (2013). The international classification of headache disorders, (beta version). *Cephalalgia: An International Journal of Headache, 33*(9), 629–808. doi:10.1177/ 0333102413485658.

Houtchens, M. K., & Kolb, C. M. (2013). Multiple sclerosis and pregnancy: Therapeutic considerations. *Journal of Neurology, 260*(5), 1202–1214. doi:10.1007/s00415-012-6653-9.

Huntington Society of Canada. (2013). *Learn About HD.* Retrieved from *http://www.huntingtonsociety.ca/learn-about-hd/what-is -huntingtons/.*

International Restless Legs Syndrome Study Group. (2015). *Diagnostic Criteria.* Retrieved from *http://irlssg.org/diagnostic -criteria/.*

Lazzaro, M., Zaidat, O. O., Mueller-Kronast, N., et al. (2011). Endovascular therapy for chronic cerebrospinal venous insufficiency in multiple sclerosis. *Frontiers in Neurology, 2*(44), 1–7. doi:10.3389/fneur.2011.00044.

Lindahl, A., & MacMahon, D. (2011). Parkinson's: Treating the symptoms. *British Journal of Nursing, 20*(14), 852–857.

Magennis, B., Lynch, T., & Corry, M. (2014). Current trends in the medical management of Parkinson's disease: Implications for nursing practice. *British Journal of Neuroscience Nursing, 10*(2), 67–74.

McLaughlin, D., & McFarland, K. (2011). A randomized trial of a group-based cognitive behavior therapy program for older adults with epilepsy: The impact on seizure frequency, depression and psychosocial well-being. *Journal of Behavioral Medicine, 34*(3), 201–207. doi:10.1007/s10865-010-9299-z.

Mokry, L. E., Ross, S., Ahmad, O. S., et al. (2015). Vitamin D and risk of multiple sclerosis: A Mendelian randomization study. *PLoS Medicine, 12*(8), e1001866. doi:10.1371/journal.pmed.1001866.

Motl, R. W., & Pilutti, L. A. (2012). The benefits of exercise training in multiple sclerosis. *Nature Reviews. Neurology, 8*(9), 487–497. doi:10.1038/nrneurol.2012.136.

Multiple Sclerosis International Federation. (2011). Pharmacological treatments in MS. *MS in Focus, 18,* 1–7.

Multiple Sclerosis International Federation. (2013). *Atlas of MS.* Retrieved from *http://www.msif.org/about-us/advocacy/atlas/.*

Multiple Sclerosis Society of Canada. (2014). *Newly diagnosed with multiple sclerosis—The facts.* Retrieved from *https://mssociety.ca/ uploads/files/infosheetnewlydiagnosed24jan2014.pdf.*

Multiple Sclerosis Society of Canada. (2016a). *What is MS?* Retrieved from *https://mssociety.ca/about-ms/what-is-ms.*

Multiple Sclerosis Society of Canada. (2016b). *Types of MS.* Retrieved from *https://mssociety.ca/about-ms/types.*

Multiple Sclerosis Society of Canada. (2016c). *Physical activity.* Retrieved from *http://csep.ca/CMFiles/Guidelines/specialpops/ CSEP_MS_PAGuidelines_adults_en.pdf.*

Multiple Sclerosis Society of Canada. (2017). *Chronic cerebrospinal venous insufficiency (CCSVI).* Retrieved from *https://mssociety.ca/ hot-topics/chronic-cerebrospinal-venous-insufficiency-ccsvi.*

Myasthenia Gravis Coalition of Canada. (2017). *Signs and symptoms of MG.* Retrieved from *http://mgcc-ccmg.org/about.asp.*

National Institute of Neurological Disorders and Stroke. (2015a). *Huntington's disease: Hope through research.* Retrieved from *http:// www.ninds.nih.gov/disorders/huntington/detail_huntington .htm#3137_4.*

National Institute of Neurological Disorders and Stroke. (2015b). *Normal pressure hydrocephalus information page.* Retrieved from *https://www.ninds.nih.gov/Disorders/All-Disorders/Normal-Pressure -Hydrocephalus-Information-Page.*

National Institute of Neurological Disorders and Stroke. (2015c). *Restless legs syndrome fact sheet.* Retrieved from *http://www .ninds.nih.gov/disorders/restless_legs/detail_restless_legs.htm.*

National Institute of Neurological Disorders and Stroke. (2016). *Parkinson's disease: Hope through research.* Retrieved from *https:// www.ninds.nih.gov/Disorders/All-Disorders/Parkinsons-Disease -Information-Page.*

Oh, J., & O'Connor, P. W. (2014). Teriflunomide in the treatment of multiple sclerosis: Current evidence and future prospects. *Therapeutic advances in neurological disorders, 7*(5), 239–252. doi:10.1177/1756285614546855.

Parkinson Society Canada. (2015). *A Parkinson's diagnosis at any age has unique challenges.* Retrieved from *http://www.parkinson.ca/ site/c.kgLNIWODKpF/b.9275285/k.A1FD/A_Parkinson8217s _diagnosis_at_any_age_has_unique_challenges.htm.*

Payne, N. E., Cross, J. H., Sander, J. W., et al. (2011). The ketogenic and related diets in adolescents and adults—A review. *Epilepsia, 52*(11), 1941–1948. doi:10.1111/j.1528-1167.2011.03287.x.

Politis, M., & Lindvall, O. (2012). Clinical application of stem cell therapy in Parkinson's disease. *BMC Medicine, 10*(1), 1. doi:10.1186/1741-7015-10-1.

Pringsheim, T., Davenport, W., Mackie, G., et al. (2012). Canadian Headache Society guideline for migraine prophylaxis. *Canadian Journal of Neurological Sciences, 39*(2 Suppl. 2), S1–S59.

Restless Legs Syndrome Foundation. (2015a). *Diagnostic criteria for RLS.* Retrieved from *http://www.rls.org/about-rls/diagnosis.*

Restless Legs Syndrome Foundation. (2015b). *Treatment Options.* Retrieved from *http://www.rls.org/about-rls/treatment-options.*

Rozen, T. D., & Fishman, R. S. (2012). Cluster headache in the United States of America: Demographics, clinical characteristics, triggers, suicidality, and personal burden. *Headache. The Journal of Head and Face Pain, 52,* 99–113. doi:10.1111/j.1526-4610.2011 .02028.x.

Seifert, G., & Steinhäuser, C. (2013). Neuron–astrocyte signaling and epilepsy. *Experimental Neurology, 244,* 4–10. doi:10.1016/j .expneurol.2011.08.024.

Shirani, A., Zhao, Y., Karim, M. E., et al. (2012). Association between use of interferon beta and progression of disability in patients with relapsing-remitting multiple sclerosis. *Journal of the American Medical Association, 308*(3), 247–256. doi:10.1001/jama.2012.7625.

Singleton, A. B., Farrer, M. J., & Bonifati, V. (2013). The genetics of Parkinson's disease: Progress and therapeutic implications. *Movement Disorders: Official Journal of the Movement Disorder Society, 28*(1), 14–23. doi:10.1002/mds.25249.

Southern, L., Fitzsimmons, G., & Cross, H. (2015). The ketogenic diet in drug-resistant epilepsies. *British Journal of Neuroscience Nursing, 11*(3), 137–141.

Statistics Canada. (2015). *Parkinson's disease: Prevalence, diagnosis and impact.* Retrieved from *http://www.statcan.gc.ca/pub/82-003 -x/2014011/article/14112-eng.htm.*

Tfelt-Hansen, P., & Koehler, P. (2011). One hundred years of migraine research: Major clinical and scientific observations from 1910 to 2010. *Headache: Journal of Head and Face Pain, 51*(5), 752–778. doi:10.111/j.1526-4610.2011.01892.x.

Wilson, C. L., & Ferguson, J. (2013). Myasthenia gravis unmasked by antipsychotic medication. *Progress in Neurology and Psychiatry, 17*(1), 17–19. doi:10.1002/pnp.264.

Yeh, P., Walters, A. S., & Tsuang, J. W. (2012). Restless legs syndrome: A comprehensive overview on its epidemiology, risk factors, and treatment. *Sleep and Breathing, 16*(4), 987–1007. doi:10.1007/s11325-011-0606-x.

Zamani, G., Mehdizadeh, M., & Sadeghi, P. (2012). Attempt to suicide in young ages with epilepsy. *Iranian Journal of Pediatrics, 22*(3), 404–407.

Zamboni, P., Galeotti, R., Menegatti, E., et al. (2008). Chronic cerebrospinal venous insufficiency in patients with multiple sclerosis. *Journal of Neurology, Neurosurgery, and Psychiatry, 80*(4), 392–399. doi:10.1136/jnnp.2008.157164. (Seminal).

RESOURCES

Amyotrophic Lateral Sclerosis Society of Canada
http://www.als.ca

Canadian Association of Neuroscience Nurses (CANN)
http://www.cann.ca

Canadian Human Rights Commission
http://www.chrc-ccdp.ca

Canadian Institute of Health Research
http://www.cihr irsc.gc.ca

CCSVI Foundation of Canada
http://ccsvifoundationcanada.org

Epilepsy Canada
http://www.epilepsy.ca

Huntington Society of Canada
http://www.hsc-ca.org

Multiple Sclerosis Society of Canada
http://www.mssociety.ca

Myasthenia Gravis Coalition of Canada
http://www.mgcc-ccmg.org

Parkinson Canada
General: http://www.parkinson.ca
Exercises for People with Parkinson's: http://www.parkinson.ca/atf/cf/%7B9ebd08a9-7886-4b2d-a1c4-a131e7096bf8%7D/EXERCISEMAR2012_EN.PDF

Veterans Affairs Canada
http://www.vac-acc.gc.ca

American Council for Headache Education (ACHE)
http://www.achenet.org

Association of Rehabilitation Nurses (ARN)
http://www.rehabnurse.org

Myasthenia Gravis Foundation of America
http://www.myasthenia.org

National Headache Foundation
http://www.headaches.org

National Institute of Neurological Disorders and Stroke (NINDS)
http://www.ninds.nih.gov

Willis–Ekbom Disease Foundation, formerly Restless Legs Syndrome Foundation
http://www.rls.org

For additional Internet resources, see the website for this book at *http://evolve.elsevier.com/Canada/Lewis/medsurg.*

Nursing Management

Delirium, Alzheimer's Disease, and Other Dementias

Written by: Sharon L. Lewis
Adapted by: Lynn McCleary

evolve WEBSITE

http://evolve.elsevier.com/Canada/Lewis/medsurg

- Review Questions
  (Online Only)
- Key Points
- Answer Guidelines for Case Study
- Student Case Study
  - Alzheimer's Disease

- Customizable Nursing Care Plans
  - Dementia
  - Family Caregivers of the Patient With Dementia
- Conceptual Care Map Creator
- Audio Glossary
- Content Updates

LEARNING OBJECTIVES

1. Describe the etiology, the pathophysiology, and the clinical manifestations of delirium.
2. Describe the diagnostic studies and the collaborative management of delirium.
3. Define dementia, and describe its effect on society.
4. Compare and contrast etiologies of different types of dementia.
5. Describe the clinical manifestations, the diagnostic studies, and the collaborative management of dementia.
6. Describe the clinical manifestations of mild cognitive impairment.
7. Describe the nursing management of patients with dementia.

KEY TERMS

amyloid plaques, p. 1569
Alzheimer's disease (AD), p. 1569
behavioural and psychological symptoms
  of dementia (BPSDs), p. 1572
Confusion Assessment Method, p. 1566
Creutzfeldt–Jakob disease (CJD), p. 1569

delirium, p. 1565
dementia, p. 1568
dementia with Lewy bodies (DLB), p. 1570
familial Alzheimer's disease, p. 1569
frontotemporal dementia (FTD), p. 1570
mild cognitive impairment (MCI), p. 1570

neurofibrillary tangles, p. 1569
responsive behaviours, p. 1572
self-protective behaviours, p. 1572
sundowning, p. 1578
vascular dementia, p. 1570

The three most common cognitive problems in adults are delirium, dementia, and depression. These problems often manifest with overlapping clinical features and may coexist in an older adult (O'Sullivan, Inouye, & Meagher, 2014; Gauthier, Patterson, Chertkow, et al., 2012). It is important to identify the distinguishing characteristics because the treatment for each problem is different. This chapter focuses on delirium and dementia. The reader should consult a mental health nursing textbook for additional information about depression.

DELIRIUM

Delirium, a state of acute mental confusion, is a medical emergency. It is one of the most common life-threatening conditions in older individuals. It is preventable in 30% to 40% of cases (Inouye, Westendorp, & Saczynski, 2014). Nurses are at the front line for prevention and early detection of delirium. However, like other health care providers, nurses often fail to recognize delirium. The prevalence of delirium is highest among hospitalized older adults. More than half of hospitalized older adults develop delirium, with rates of up to 50% after fractures or surgery and 82% in the critical care unit. Rates are even higher among patients with pre-existing dementia (Inouye, Westendorp, & Saczynski, 2014). Delirium is associated with longer hospitalizations, loss of brain function, higher rates of institutionalization, and higher rates of mortality (Gage & Hogan, 2014; Inouye, Westendorp, & Saczynski, 2014).

Etiology and Pathophysiology

The pathophysiology of delirium is poorly understood and is related to multiple mechanisms. Inflammation, hypoxia, and other biological and physiological factors are thought to cause neurotransmitter imbalance, particularly acetylcholine deficiency and dopamine excess (Chaput & Bryson, 2012; Inouye, Westendorp, & Saczynski, 2014).

Delirium is usually the result of interaction between the patient's underlying condition and a precipitating event. Delirium can occur after a relatively minor insult in a vulnerable patient. For example, patients with underlying health problems such as heart failure, cognitive impairment, or sensory limitations may develop delirium after a relatively minor change (e.g., a single dose of a sleeping medication). In less vulnerable patients, it may take a combination of factors (e.g., anaesthesia, major surgery, infection, prolonged sleep deprivation) to precipitate delirium (Inouye, Westendorp, & Saczynski, 2014). Delirium can also be a symptom of a serious medical illness such as bacterial meningitis.

Knowing which factors increase vulnerability to delirium (predisposing factors) or precipitate delirium (precipitating factors) facilitates prevention of delirium and effective intervention. These factors are listed in Table 62-1.

Delirium occurs in children and adults, but older adults are at higher risk. They are more likely to have one of more of the risk factors for delirium. Normal age-related changes (see Chapter 7) limit older adults' abilities to compensate for physiological insults such as hypoxia, hypoglycemia, and dehydration and increase their susceptibility to medication-induced delirium. Patients with dementia are at risk on two fronts: Their risk for developing delirium is higher, and the probability that the delirium will be identified is lower (Morandi, Lucchi, Turco, et al., 2015).

Clinical Manifestations

The core features of delirium are as follows: (a) Disturbance of attention and of awareness of the environment; (b) a change in cognition (such as memory deficit, disorientation, language disturbance, perceptual disturbance) that is not due to neurocognitive disorder such as dementia; and (c) development of the disturbance over a short time (usually hours to days) and a tendency for it to fluctuate during the course of the day (American Psychiatric Association, 2013, p. 596).

There are three subtypes of delirium: hyperactive delirium, which is characterized by restlessness, psychomotor agitation, and hypervigilance; hypoactive delirium, which is characterized by lethargy, drowsiness, and decreased motor activity; and mixed delirium, which has features of both hypoactive and hyperactive delirium. Other common symptoms include hallucinations, illusions, disturbed sleep–wake cycle, and labile emotions (Inouye, Westendorp, & Saczynski, 2014). Hypoactive delirium is more common in older adults and is potentially more serious, because this form is often not identified. It may be overlooked because the patient is quiet, or it may be mistaken for depression.

Delirium is often mistaken for dementia. A key distinction between delirium and dementia is the *sudden* development of symptoms of delirium over a short time period. (A comparison of delirium and dementia is presented in Table 62-2.) To distinguish between dementia and delirium superimposed on dementia, the nurse may need collateral information from a reliable informant about baseline mental status and changes in cognition.

When effectively treated, delirium usually resolves within 4 to 7 days. However, it can recur, and it may persist for weeks to months after hospital discharge. Discharge planning should account for the safety of patients who have had an episode of delirium.

Diagnostic Studies

Delirium is diagnosed based on behavioural observation and the results of mental status examination. The **Confusion Assessment**

TABLE 62-1 RISK FACTORS FOR DELIRIUM

Predisposing Factors
- Age over 75 years
- Alcohol misuse
- Comorbid or severe illness
- Dementia
- Depression
- Functional impairment
- History of cerebro-vascular incident
- History of delirium
- Pain
- Sensory impairment

Precipitating Factors
- Abnormal physiological indices (i.e., electrolytes, BUN, serum urea, serum albumin)
- Bladder catheter
- Coma
- Drugs
  - Multiple drugs prescribed
  - Psychoactive drugs
  - Sedatives or hypnotics
- Iatrogenic event
- Infection
- Metabolic disturbance
- Overstimulating or understimulating environment
- Physical restraints
- Surgery
- Trauma
- Urgent admission

Source: Adapted from in Inouye, S. K., Westendorp, R. G. J., & Saczynski, J. S. (2014). Delirium in elderly people [Table 2]. *Lancet, 383*, 911–922. doi:10.1016/S0140-6736(13)60688-1; and Tullmann, D. F., Fletcher, K., & Foreman, M. D. (2012). *Nursing standard of practice protocol: Delirium.* Retrieved from *https://consultgeri.org/geriatric-topics/delirium.*
BUN, blood urea nitrogen.

TABLE 62-2 COMPARISON OF THE CLINICAL FEATURES OF DELIRIUM, DEMENTIA, AND DEPRESSION

Feature	Delirium	Dementia	Depression
Onset	Acute	Insidious	Variable
Duration	Days to weeks	Months to years	Variable
Course	Fluctuating	Slowly progressive	Diurnal variation (worse in morning, improves during day)
Consciousness	Impaired, fluctuating	Clear until late in the course of the illness	Unimpaired
Attention and memory	Inattentiveness Poor memory	Poor memory without marked inattention	Difficulty concentrating: memory intact/minimally impaired
Affect	Variable	Variable	Depressed; loss of interest and pleasure in usual activities

Source: Canadian Coalition for Seniors' Mental Health (CCSMH). (2006). *National guidelines for seniors' mental health: The assessment and treatment of delirium* (p. 23, Table 1.1). Toronto: Author.

Method is a widely used, validated screening instrument and diagnostic aid that is effective in identifying the presence of delirium. This 5- to 10-minute assessment provides a standardized method of identification of delirium (Inouye, van Dyck, Alessi, et al., 1990). Evaluation with the Confusion Assessment Method can be incorporated into routine nursing assessment. Ratings may be based on findings from a brief mental status assessment such as the Mini-Mental State Examination (MMSE; Folstein, Folstein, & McHugh, 1975, and see Table 62-9) or the Mini-Cog (Borson, Scanlan, Brush, et al., 2000). The Mini-Cog takes 3 minutes to administer. Patients repeat three words, draw a clock, and recall the three words. The ConsultGeriRN.org website includes guides for using the Confusion Assessment Method and the Mini-Cog, in addition to streaming videos demonstrating their use (see the Resources at the end of this chapter).

When delirium is diagnosed, identification and treatment of the underlying causes is urgent. The patient's history and physical examination findings, medication history, laboratory test results, additional diagnostic investigation as indicated, and environmental risk factors must be evaluated. Usual investigations include complete blood cell count; biochemistry evaluations (measurements of calcium, albumin, magnesium, phosphate, creatinine, urea, electrolytes, and glucose levels; liver function tests); thyroid function tests; blood, urine, and sputum cultures; oxygen saturation measurement; urinalysis; chest radiography; and electrocardiography (Inouye, Westendorp, & Saczynski, 2014). If meningitis or encephalitis is suspected, a lumbar puncture may be performed (see Chapter 59). If the patient's history includes head injury, appropriate radiographic examinations or scans may be ordered. Brain imaging studies such as computed tomography and magnetic resonance imaging are performed if the patient has a known or suspected head injury or brain lesion.

NURSING AND COLLABORATIVE MANAGEMENT DELIRIUM

The priority for nursing care is prevention of delirium. The priorities for nursing care are to identify and treat underlying cause or causes, to maintain physiological stability, and to ensure the patient's safety (Canadian Coalition for Seniors' Mental Health [CCSMH], 2006; Tullmann, Fletcher, & Foreman, 2012). Prevention involves recognition of patients at high risk for delirium (see Table 62-1) and providing care that targets each patient's risk factors. Among older adults, the five precipitating factors that are most predictive of delirium in the first 9 days of hospitalization are influenced by nursing interventions (Inouye & Charpentier, 1996):

- Use of physical restraints
- Low serum albumin levels, indicative of malnutrition
- Prescription of more than three new medications
- Use of a urinary catheter
- An iatrogenic event (e.g., cardiopulmonary complications, infections, injury, and complications caused by medications or diagnostic or therapeutic procedures)

There is strong research evidence that proactive multicomponent interventions reduce incidence of new cases of delirium and improve outcomes for patients with delirium (Tullmann, Fletcher, & Foreman, 2012). The Canadian Patient Safety Institute (2013) recommended that hospitals develop delirium management protocols and enable staff to follow them. The Hospital Elder Life Program (HELP) is a well-researched multicomponent program. It has been implemented in more than 600 hospitals, including 10 Canadian hospitals (Agency for Healthcare Research and Quality, 2014). Components of the program are listed in Table 62-3. Details about the program are available on the HELP website (see the Resources at the end of this chapter).

Additional strategies to eliminate or minimize risk factors are listed in Table 62-4. It is important to maintain physiological stability. Many drugs can contribute to delirium. Categories of drugs to use with caution are neuroleptic antipsychotics, anticholinergics, H_2-blocking agents, analgesics, sedative hypnotics, antipsychotics, and dihydropyridine calcium channel blockers (Clegg & Young, 2011; Inouye, Westendorp, & Saczynski, 2014). The publication concerning inappropriate use of medication in older patients (American Geriatrics Society 2015 Beers Criteria Update Expert Panel, 2015) is a good tool for reviewing medications. Resources for using it are available on the American Geriatrics Society website (see the Resources at the end of this chapter).

TABLE 62-3	COMPONENTS OF THE HOSPITAL ELDER LIFE PROGRAM (HELP)

1. Systematic screening to identify patients at risk for developing delirium
2. Tailored interventions developed by an interdisciplinary team that consists of a geriatric nurse specialist, elder life specialist, and trained volunteers. Interventions include the following:
   - Daily visit and orientation
   - Sleep deprivation prevention
   - Ambulation three times a day and minimization of immobilizing equipment (e.g., bladder catheters)
   - Visual aids
   - Hearing support
   - Avoiding dehydration
   - Preventing falls
3. Interdisciplinary rounds twice a week
4. Geriatrician and interdisciplinary team consultations
5. Community liaison and postdischarge telephone follow-up

Source: Agency for Healthcare Research and Quality. (2014). *Hospital-based program proactively identifies, addresses delirium risk factors in elderly, leading to less cognitive/functional decline and lower nursing home costs.* Retrieved from *https:// innovations.ahrq.gov/profiles/hospital-based-program-proactively-identifies-addresses -delirium-risk-factors-elderly.*

TABLE 62-4	STRATEGIES TO ELIMINATE OR MINIMIZE RISK FACTORS FOR DELIRIUM

- Adequate nutrition
- Assessment and treatment of pain
- Judicious use of medication, elimination of nonessential medication, use of the lowest possible dose, avoidance of medications that contribute to delirium
- Maximal oxygen delivery
- Prevention and prompt treatment of dehydration and electrolyte imbalance
- Prevention and prompt treatment of infections
- Regulation of bowel and bladder function
- Use of sensory aids

Source: Adapted from Tullmann, D. F., Fletcher, K., & Foreman, M. D. (2012). *Nursing standard of practice protocol: Delirium.* Retrieved from *https://consultgeri.org/ geriatric-topics/delirium;* and Regional Geriatric Program of Toronto. (2014). *Preventing and managing delirium.* Retrieved from *https://consultgeri.org/geriatric-topics/ delirium.*

Adequate pain management is important because undertreated pain significantly increases risk for delirium. However, analgesics, too, can increase risk for delirium. Thus interventions that minimize the use of opioids are recommended; these interventions include the following (Barr, Fraser, Puntillo, et al., 2013):

- Use of nonpharmacological pain management approaches
- Use of nonopioid analgesics as an adjunct to reduce the dose of opioids
- When opioids are needed, use of the minimum effective dose for the shortest appropriate time

Strategies to provide a therapeutic environment for patients with delirium or who are at risk for delirium are provided in Table 62-5. Frequent assessment is required. Mental status should be assessed every shift for patients who have delirium or are at risk for delirium. Close observation is required, especially for

TABLE 62-5 THERAPEUTIC ENVIRONMENT FOR PATIENTS WITH DELIRIUM OR RISK FOR DELIRIUM

Strategy	Examples
Foster orientation	• Explanation of all activities • Frequent reassurance and orientation (unless this causes agitation), avoiding confrontation about delusional beliefs • Use of hearing aids and glasses • Visible calendars, clocks, and staff identification
Provide appropriate stimulation	• Adequate light • Music as preferred by the patient • Noise reduction • One task at a time • Quiet room
Facilitate sleep	• Back massage, warm milk, or herbal tea at bedtime • Noise reduction strategies (e.g., vibrating beepers) • Plan care to avoid waking the patient • Provide light during the day and reduce light at night • Relaxation music
Foster familiarity	• Bring familiar objects from home • Encourage family or friends to stay with patient • Minimize relocation • Provide consistent nursing staff
Maximize mobility	• Ambulate or provide range-of-motion exercises three times a day • Avoid bladder catheters • Avoid restraints
Communicate clearly	• Convey warmth, kindness, and calmness • One question or direction at a time • Simple explanations
Reassure and educate patient and family	• Acknowledge emotions • Manage stigma • Provide post-delirium education • Provide written and verbal information and education about delirium and family role in management • Use distraction

Sources: Adapted from Canadian Coalition for Seniors' Mental Health. (2006). *National guidelines for seniors' mental health: The assessment and treatment of delirium.* Toronto: Author; and Tullmann, D. F., Fletcher, K., & Foreman, M. D. (2012). *Nursing standard of practice protocol: Delirium.* Retrieved from *https://consultgeri.org/geriatric-topics/delirium.*

patients with hyperactive delirium. Invasive procedures should be minimized (Tullmann, Fletcher, & Foreman, 2012).

Drug Therapy

Drug therapy is reserved for patients with severe agitation, especially when agitation interferes with needed medical therapy (e.g., fluid replacement, intubation) or presents a danger. Antipsychotics (neuroleptic agents) are the recommended drug therapy. Haloperidol, the first-line treatment, is started with low doses (0.25–0.5 mg once or twice a day) and slowly titrated upwards if necessary. Adverse effects of haloperidol include sedation; hypotension; extrapyramidal drug effects, including tardive dyskinesia (involuntary muscle movements of face, trunk, and arms) and athetosis (involuntary writhing movements of the limbs); muscle tone changes; and anticholinergic effects. Newer antipsychotics, including risperidone (Risperdal), olanzapine (Zyprexa), and quetiapine (Seroquel), may be used. Although these drugs produce fewer adverse effects than does haloperidol, the adverse effects are significant; antipsychotics may worsen the delirium. Close monitoring is required. Drug therapy should be limited to the shortest time needed to manage the symptoms. Benzodiazepines (e.g., lorazepam [Ativan]) are contraindicated, except for treatment of delirium caused by withdrawal from either alcohol or sedative-hypnotics (Gage & Hogan, 2014).

DEMENTIA

Dementia is a collection of symptoms caused by various diseases affecting the brain. Cognitive functioning in multiple areas declines progressively. In addition to impairing memory, dementia affects the individual's judgement, reasoning, and abilities to communicate, to carry out purposeful movements, and to recognize common objects and familiar people. Mood and behaviour are commonly affected. Ultimately, these problems lead to inability to work, carry out social and family responsibilities, and perform activities of daily living (ADLs). The multiple effects on cognition and slow gradual decline differentiate dementia from delirium, which has a sudden onset.

In Canada, approximately 564000 people are living with dementia, and this number is expected to nearly double in the next 15 years (Alzheimer Society of Canada, 2017). Dementia occurs most often in older adults. Among those between the ages of 65 and 69 years, the prevalence is 2.4%. Prevalence rises with increasing age, up to 21.7% of people older than 85 (Prince, Bryce, & Albanese, 2013).

The cost of dementia in Canada is high. In 2011, family members and friends provided approximately 19.2 million hours of informal unpaid caregiver time to people with dementia, and this number is expected to double by 2031 (Alzheimer Society of Canada, 2016a). The estimated economic value of informal care is almost $1.2 billion per year. The economic burden of dementia, including health care costs and indirect costs (e.g., lost wages and lost productivity) is approximately $33 billion per year (Alzheimer Society of Canada, 2016a).

As the average human lifespan increases and the baby boom generation ages, the number of people affected with dementia is growing. By 2040, the total annual cost of dementia is projected to be $293 billion (Senate Canada, 2016).

The four most common types of dementia are Alzheimer's disease (approximately 60% to 80% of cases), vascular dementia (approximately 10% of cases), dementia with Lewy bodies, and frontotemporal dementia (Alzheimer's Association, 2015). Mixed dementia, in which more than one type of dementia is present, occurs in approximately 10% of cases of dementia (Chertkow, 2008). Dementia is also part of the later stages of Parkinson's disease and Huntington's disease. Moreover, in individuals with Down syndrome, the incidence of Alzheimer's disease is three to five times greater than in the general population (Alzheimer Society of Canada, 2016b). Another type of dementia is caused by Creutzfeldt–Jakob disease (CJD), a very rare, fatal, infectious brain disorder thought to be caused by accumulation in the brain of an abnormally folded prion protein.

Etiology and Pathophysiology

In a small number of patients, dementia symptoms are secondary to a treatable condition such as delirium, depression, subdural hematoma, cerebral tumours, normal-pressure hydrocephalus, heavy metal neurotoxicity, Wilson's disease, and infections such as bacterial meningitis and viral encephalitis. The diagnostic workup for dementia includes ruling out other causes of cognitive impairment (Lee, Weston, Heckman, et al., 2013).

Dementia is not a normal part of aging. Old age and family history are risk factors for the four most common types of irreversible dementias. There are more women than men who have dementia because women have a longer life expectancy and may have different gender-related protective factors, such as access to education (Mielke, Vemuri, & Rocca, 2014). Indigenous Canadians are at higher risk for dementia than are non-Indigenous Canadians, and they are likely to be younger when they develop dementia. This may be related to social determinants of health and to physiological risk factors such as diabetes and hypertension. Among Indigenous Canadians, men are more likely than women to have dementia (Jacklin, Walker, & Shawande, 2013). Etiology and pathophysiology of each of the most common types of dementia are described separately as follows.

Alzheimer's Disease. Alzheimer's disease (AD) is a chronic, progressive, degenerative disease of the brain. The exact etiology of AD is unknown. As in other forms of dementia, age is the most important risk factor for developing AD. Only a small percentage of people younger than 60 years develop AD. When AD develops in someone younger than 60 years old, it is referred to as familial Alzheimer's disease (also known as *early-onset AD*). AD that begins after age 60 is called *late-onset AD*. Early-onset AD has a stronger genetic basis than does late-onset AD (see the Genetics in Clinical Practice box). The pathogenesis is similar in both forms of AD.

Knowing the modifiable risk factors for AD means that nurses can advise individuals about how to reduce their risk of developing AD. Table 62-6 lists risk factors for AD. Mild cognitive impairment, discussed later in this chapter, is a risk factor for developing AD. More research is needed about the following possible risk factors: low education level, low socioeconomic status, smoking, and excessive alcohol consumption (Alzheimer Society of Canada, 2014). More information is available in the *Brain Health* section of the Alzheimer Society of Canada website (listed in the Resources at the end of this chapter).

Characteristic findings of AD are related to changes in the brain's structure and function: (a) amyloid plaques, (b) neurofibrillary tangles, and (c) loss of connections between cells, as well as cell death (National Institute on Aging, 2017). Figure 62-1 depicts the pathological changes in AD.

In AD, amyloid plaques are present in the brain in abnormal quantities. These plaques consist of clusters of insoluble deposits of a protein called *beta-amyloid,* other proteins, remnants of

GENETICS IN CLINICAL PRACTICE
Alzheimer's Disease (AD)

Genetic Basis
Early Onset (Familial; Age <60 Years at Onset)
- Autosomal dominant disorder
- Various mutations in the following genes:
  - Amyloid precursor protein gene on chromosome 21
  - Presenilin-1 *(PSEN1)* gene on chromosome 14
  - Presenilin-2 *(PSEN2)* gene on chromosome 1

Late Onset (Sporadic; Age >60 Years at Onset)
- Genetically more complex than early-onset form
- Apolipoprotein E-4 *(ApoE-4)* allele on chromosome 19 increases the likelihood of developing AD.
- Presence of apolipoprotein E-2 allele is associated with a lower risk of AD

Incidence
Early Onset
- Rare form of AD, accounting for <5% of cases
- Fifty percent risk of disease for children of affected parents
- May occur in people as young as 30 years old

Late Onset
- *ApoE-4* is present in approximately 40% of people with late-onset AD. (It is present in 25%–30% of normal population.)
- Many people with *ApoE-4* do not develop AD, and many people without *ApoE-4* people do.

Genetic Testing
Early Onset
- Genetic screening for mutations on chromosomes 1, 14, and 21 is available.

Late Onset
- Blood test can identify which *ApoE* allele a person has but cannot predict whether the person will develop the disease.*
- *ApoE* testing is used mainly in research to identify people who may have an increased risk of developing AD.

Clinical Implications
- Genetic testing and counselling for family members of patients with early-onset AD may be appropriate.
- If the test for *ApoE-4* yields positive results, it does not mean that the person will develop AD.

ApoE testing is useful for studying AD risk in large groups of people but not for determining an individual's specific risk.

neurons, non-nerve cells such as microglia (cells that surround and digest damaged cells or foreign substances), and other cells, such as astrocytes. Beta-amyloid is cleaved from amyloid precursor protein, which is associated with the cell membrane (Figure 62-2). The normal function of amyloid precursor protein is unknown. In AD, plaques develop first in areas of the brain used for memory and cognitive function, including the hippocampus (a structure that is important in forming and storing short-term memories). Eventually, AD attacks the cerebral cortex, especially the areas responsible for language and reasoning.

Neurofibrillary tangles are abnormal collections of twisted protein threads inside nerve cells seen in the areas of the brain most affected by AD. The main component of these structures is a protein called *tau*. Tau proteins in the central nervous system are involved in intracellular structure through their support of microtubules. Tau proteins hold the microtubules together. In AD, the tau protein is altered in a way that causes the microtubules to twist together in a helical manner (see Figure 62-2). This

TABLE 62-6   ALZHEIMER'S DISEASE

Modifiable Risk Factors	Reducing Risk
Medical conditions • Type 2 diabetes • Stroke and transient ischemic attack • Hyperlipidemia • Hypertension • Obesity • Chronic inflammatory conditions (e.g., arthritis)	• Healthy lifestyle choices to reduce the risk of developing these conditions (maintaining healthy weight, regular physical activity, healthy balanced diet, not smoking, stress management) • Appropriate treatment when such conditions are present
Head injury	• Use of recreational/sport helmets
History of clinical depression	• Identification and appropriate treatment of depression • Healthy lifestyle choices and appropriate support for traumatic experiences and stressful life events (may reduce risk for depression)
Inadequate intellectual stimulation	• Active social life • Participation in intellectual activities (reading, playing cards, solving puzzles, playing chess, learning new skills, hobbies)

Sources: Alzheimer Society of Canada. (2014). *Risk factors*. Retrieved from *http://www.alzheimer.ca/en/About-dementia/Alzheimer-s-disease/Risk-factors*; and Alzheimer Society of Canada. (2017). *Brain health*. Retrieved from *http://www.alzheimer.ca/en/About-dementia/Brain-health*.

Amyloid plaques

Neurofibrillary tangles

Neuron

FIGURE 62-1 Pathological changes in Alzheimer's disease. **A,** Senile plaque with central amyloid core *(white arrow)* next to a neurofibrillary tangle *(red arrow)* on the histological specimen from a brain autopsy. **B,** Schematic representation of neuritic plaque and neurofibrillary tangle. Source: **A,** From Damjanov, I., & Linder, J. (Eds.). (1996). *Anderson's pathology* (10th ed.). St. Louis: Mosby.

twisting ultimately forms the neurofibrillary tangles observed in the neurons of persons with AD.

Plaques and neurofibrillary tangles are not unique to patients with AD. They are also found in the brains of individuals without evidence of cognitive impairment. However, they are more plentiful in the brains of individuals with AD.

The third feature of AD is the gradual loss of connections between neurons. This process leads to damage and then death of the neurons. Affected parts of the brain begin to shrink in a process called *brain atrophy*. By the final state of AD, brain tissue has shrunk significantly (Figure 62-3).

A short video, *How Alzheimer's Changes the Brain*, illustrating and explaining the pathology of AD, is available at the National Institute on Aging website (see the Resources at the end of this chapter).

Cholinergic neurons are lost in people with AD, particularly in regions essential for memory and cognition. Other neurotransmitter systems, including serotonin and norepinephrine, also show losses over time in patients with AD. Such neurotransmitter changes are the basis of current drug therapies for AD.

Genetic factors may play a critical role in how the brain processes the beta-amyloid protein. Overproduction of beta-amyloid appears to be an important risk factor for AD. Abnormally high levels of beta-amyloid cause cell damage either directly or by eliciting an inflammatory response and ultimately neuron death. Understanding why neurons produce beta-amyloid led researchers to examine the enzymes (and their genes) that are responsible for both the synthesis and processing of amyloid precursor protein. In patients with early-onset AD, mutations in three genes have been identified as causing brain cells to overproduce beta-amyloid (Wu, Rosa-Neto, & Hsiung, et al., 2012). (See the Genetics in Clinical Practice box on Alzheimer's disease, earlier in this chapter.)

Vascular Dementia. Vascular dementia, also called *multi-infarct dementia,* is a type of dementia that results from ischemic, ischemic-hypoxic, or hemorrhagic brain damage caused by cardiovascular disease. When these events occur, blood and oxygen supply to brain tissues is blocked, which results in cell death. Vascular dementia may be caused by a single stroke (infarct) or by multiple strokes. As with AD, risk for vascular dementia increases with older age. Other risk factors are smoking, hypertension, cardiac diseases, diabetes mellitus, hypercholesterolemia, coronary artery disease, and atrial fibrillation.

Dementia With Lewy Bodies. Dementia with Lewy bodies (DLB) is characterized by the presence of Lewy bodies (deposits of alpha-synuclein protein) in the brainstem, amygdala, and cortex. The alpha-synuclein protein is also linked to dementia in Parkinson's disease. DLB has features of both AD and Parkinson's disease (changes in thinking and reasoning, confusion, memory loss, balance problems, and muscle rigidity). Men are at higher risk for developing it than are women (Alzheimer Society of Canada, 2016c).

Frontotemporal Dementia. Frontotemporal dementia (FTD) is characterized by degeneration of the frontal lobe, temporal lobe, or both. Nerve cells die because of abnormal accumulation of proteins in the neurons. The proteins most commonly found are ubiquitin and transactive response DNA binding protein 43 (TDP-43). Tau proteins are present in approximately 40% of cases. Approximately 10% of patients with FTD have an inherited form of the disorder, and 40% have a family history of FTD. The typical age at onset is between 50 and 60 years (Association for Frontotemporal Degeneration, 2012).

Clinical Manifestations

The onset of symptoms of dementia is usually insidious and gradual, with progressive deterioration. Vascular dementia, however, may have a sudden onset after a cerebro-vascular event. In vascular dementia, mental decline is typically stepwise: Deterioration is followed by stabilization, then deterioration again. The rate of deterioration in AD is highly variable from individual to individual, and the course ranges in duration from 3 to 20 years.

AD may be preceded by mild cognitive impairment (MCI). MCI is cognitive decline that is not severe enough to interfere with ADLs. The diagnosis of MCI is made in the presence of several conditions: (a) evidence of change in cognition; (b) objective evidence of impairment in memory or another cognitive domain; (c) preservation of the ability to independently perform ADLs and instrumental ADLs; and (d) the absence of dementia or medical

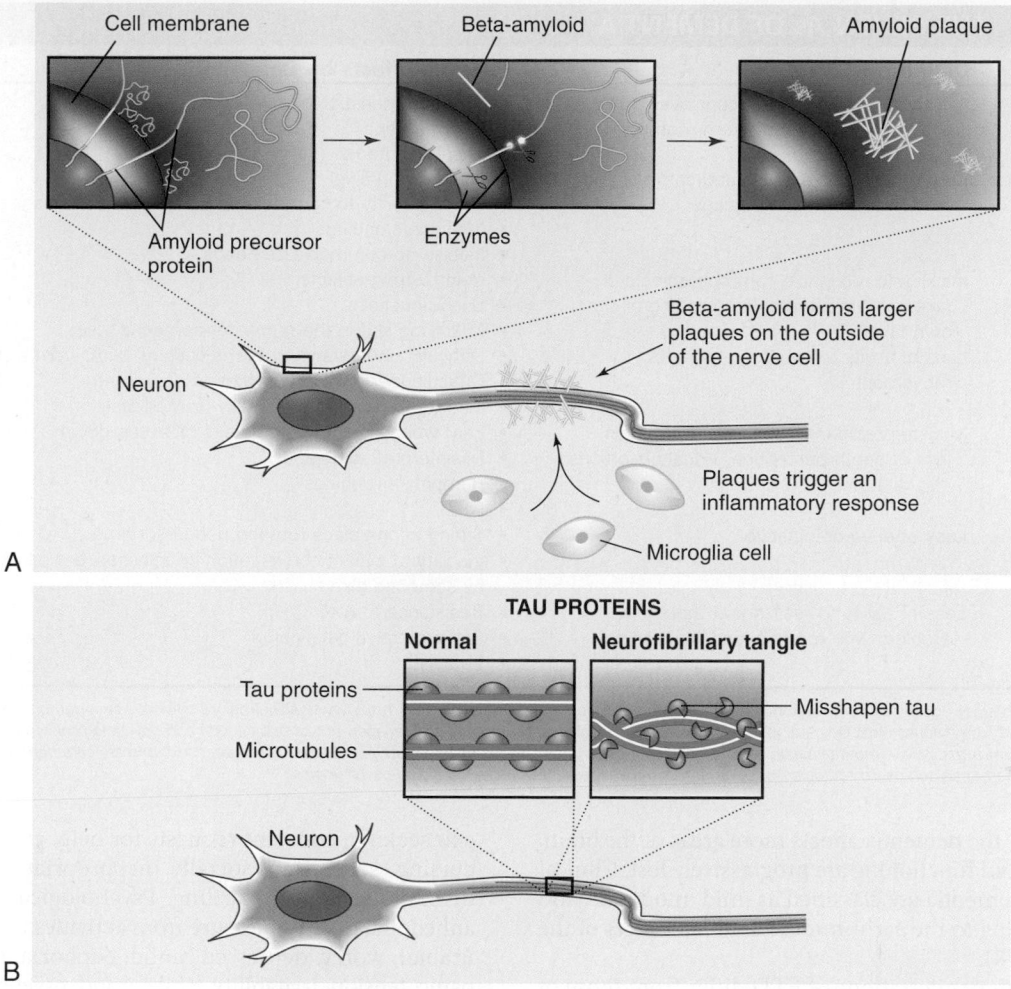

FIGURE 62-2 Current etiological theories for the development of Alzheimer's disease. **A,** Abnormal amounts of beta-amyloid are cleaved from the amyloid precursor protein (APP) and released into the circulation. The beta-amyloid fragments clump together to form plaques that attach to the neuron. Microglia react to the plaque, and an inflammatory response results. **B,** Tau proteins provide structural support for the neuron microtubules. Chemical changes in the neuron produce structural changes in tau proteins. This results in twisting and tangling of the microtubules (neurofibrillary tangles).

FIGURE 62-3 The effects of Alzheimer's disease on the brain, shown by positron emission tomography (PET). In PET, radioactive fluorine is applied to glucose (fluorodeoxyglucose), and the yellow areas indicate metabolically active cells. **A,** A normal brain. **B,** Advanced AD, evidenced by hypometabolism that indicates cell death in many areas of the brain. Source: From Stuart, G. W. (2009). *Principles and practice of psychiatric nursing* (9th ed., p. 398, Figure 22-4, *A* & *D*). St. Louis: Mosby.

condition that explains the symptoms (Albert, DeKosky, Dickson, et al., 2011). The origin of MCI—whether it is a precursor to AD, a heterogeneous condition with several possible causes, including AD, or a separate clinical condition—is a subject of controversy. Many patients with MCI eventually develop dementia. Between 5% and 10% of people who have MCI develop dementia within a year of the onset of MCI (Peterson, 2011).

The symptoms of dementia can be classified according to the *seven As of dementia* (Alzheimer Society of York Region, 2016): **a**nosognosia, **a**gnosia, **a**phasia, **a**praxia, **a**ltered perception, **a**mnesia, and **a**pathy (Table 62-7). By recognizing these symptoms, the nurse can understand why and how dementia affects the patient's ability to function. These symptoms are common, but patients with dementia do not necessarily exhibit all of them.

The initial changes of dementia may be difficult to recognize. Many people mistakenly think that they are part of normal aging. It can take up to 4 years after the onset of symptoms until patients and their family members seek health care. Reasons for this delay include lack of knowledge about dementia, lack of knowledge about services for dementia, attributing the changes to normal aging, and stigma (McCleary, Persaud, Hum, et al., 2012).

TABLE 62-7 THE SEVEN As OF DEMENTIA

Deficit	Definition	Possible Effects on Behaviour
Amnesia	Initially loss of recall of recent events but eventually loss of long-term memory	• Repeated questions • Disorientation • Misplaces items
Aphasia	Loss of ability to express and comprehend spoken and written language	• Social withdrawal • Loss of ability to communicate in a second language • Misunderstandings • Inability to communicate needs
Agnosia	Inability to recognize common objects or faces of familiar people (including one's own face)	• Using wrong objects • Suspiciousness • Mistaking self in the mirror for someone else
Apraxia	Loss of ability to initiate purposeful movement	• Difficulty understanding terms such as *back, front, up,* and *down* • Difficulty performing activities of daily living • Inability to perform previously learned tasks
Altered perception	Misinterpretation of sensory information, loss of depth perception, visual distortions	• Fear when walking down stairs or sitting down • Misinterpreting objects • Bumping into things • Falls
Apathy	Loss of drive or initiative	• Sitting in one place for long periods of time • Inability to initiate conversation or activities, but participation when invited by someone else
Anosognosia	Loss of ability to realize that there is a problem with memory and functioning	• Resistance to care • Self-protective behaviours • Irritability

Source: Adapted from Alzheimer Society of York Region. (2016). *Seven A's of dementia.* Retrieved from *http://www.alzheimer.ca/en/york/About-dementia/What-is-dementia/Seven-A-s-of-dementia;* and from Mount Sinai Hospital. (2013). *Non-pharmacological assessment and management of behavioural and psychological symptoms of dementia in primary care.* Retrieved from *https://www.mountsinai.on.ca/care/psych/patient-programs/geriatric-psychiatry/prc-dementia-resources-for-primary-care/dementia-toolkit-for-primary-care/responsive-behaviours-in-dementia/non-pharmacological-assessment-and-management-of-behavioural-and-psychological.*

As time goes on, the dementia affects more areas of the brain. Cognitive abilities and functioning are progressively lost. Clinical manifestations of dementia are classified as mild, moderate, and severe, corresponding to the early, middle, and late stages of the disorder (Table 62-8).

The early clinical manifestations of FTD differ from those of AD because FTD initially affects the frontal lobe, temporal lobe, or both lobes of the brain. Eventually, all areas of the brain are involved diffusely, and the symptoms resemble those of AD. Early in the course of FTD, social conduct and personality are profoundly altered, but little memory loss is evident (UCSF Memory and Aging Center, 2016). Behavioural symptoms include personality changes, blunted emotions, lack of insight, apathy, hyperorality (putting objects in the mouth), hoarding, compulsions and complex rituals, disinhibition, and socially inappropriate behaviour. If the temporal lobe is affected first, the patient experiences problems with speech and language, including loss of knowledge of the meanings of words and objects (Bott, Radke, Stephens, et al., 2014).

Like those of FTD, the early clinical manifestations of DLB differ from those of AD. Patients with DLB have symptoms of Parkinson's disease: In addition to symptoms of dementia, they have least two of the following symptoms: (a) extrapyramidal signs such as bradykinesia, rigidity, and postural instability, but not always a tremor; (b) fluctuating cognitive ability; and (c) hallucinations (McKeith, Dickson, Lowe, et al., 2005). Swallowing problems can lead to impairment in nutrition. Affected patients are at risk for falls because of impaired mobility and balance. Pneumonia is a common complication.

Behavioural and Psychological Symptoms of Dementia. Some of the clinical manifestations of dementia are called **behavioural and psychological symptoms of dementia (BPSDs).** Behavioural symptoms include appetite changes, slowed or excessive movements and speech, agitation, pacing, wandering,

exit seeking, constant requests for help, grabbing on to people, cursing, screaming, socially inappropriate behaviours, sexual disinhibition, and hoarding. Psychological symptoms include anhedonia (loss of pleasure from activities that are usually pleasurable), worry, depressed mood, euphoria, fear, apprehension, panic, tension, irritability, labile mood, psychosis (hallucinations, delusions, illusions), and sleep disturbances (Cerejeira, Lagarto, & Mukaetova-Ladinska, 2012; Murray Alzheimer Research and Education Program [MAREP] & Alzheimer Societies of Hamilton & Halton, Brant, Haldimand-Norfolk, & Niagara Regions, 2006). BPSDs cause distress to patients and negatively affect their functioning. BPSDs are caused by a combination of biological factors (e.g., changes in brain functioning, medical conditions, pain, adverse effects of medication, hearing or visual impairment), environmental factors (e.g., changes in routine, changes in environment), and social factors (e.g., inadequate support for the patient or family caregiver). These behaviours may be mistakenly interpreted. For example, the grasp reflex may appear in patients in middle to late stages because of frontal lobe damage. Reflexive grasping of care providers or objects on contact may be misinterpreted as intentional. Dementia affects patients' abilities to communicate. Sometimes, BPSDs are the only way in which the affected person can communicate an unmet need. These behaviours are often responses to something in the patient's environment (**responsive behaviours**) or to a perceived threat (**self-protective behaviours**; MAREP et al., 2006; Pizzacalla, Montemuro, Coker, et al., 2015).

SAFETY ALERT
A sudden change in behaviour should trigger a search for underlying causes, including possible delirium.

Diagnostic Studies

Canadian Consensus Conferences on the Diagnosis and Treatment of Dementia produced comprehensive recommendations

TABLE 62-8 CLINICAL MANIFESTATIONS OF DEMENTIA

Early (Mild)
- Anxiety
- Confusion about location of familiar places (may become lost)
- Difficulty finding the right word
- Difficulty recognizing what numbers mean, trouble handling money and paying bills
- Loss of initiative and interests
- Mild forgetfulness and misplacing items
- Poor judgement
- Short-term memory impairment, especially for learning new information
- Taking longer than usual to accomplish daily tasks

Middle (Moderate)
- Anxiety, mood swings, suspiciousness, jealousy, irritability
- Difficulty completing tasks that involve a sequence of steps; interference with activities of daily living
- Difficulty learning new things or coping in new and unexpected situations
- Difficulty recognizing family members and friends
- Difficulty with language and understanding, and problems with reading, writing, and working with numbers
- Difficulty with logic and organizing thoughts
- Flat affect
- Hallucinations and delusions
- Impaired attention
- Increasing memory loss, including some loss of remote memory
- Loss of impulse control (e.g., undressing at inappropriate times or places, vulgar language)

- Loss of interest in hygiene
- Loss of remote memory
- Poor insight and decision making, need for supervision and cuing
- Sleep disturbances
- Wandering, getting lost

Late (Severe)
- Behaviours that may appear aggressive (verbal [e.g., swearing, screaming, shouting, making threats] or physical [e.g., hitting, pinching, scratching hair-pulling, biting]) but are communicating a need (relief from, e.g., physical discomfort, social isolation, lack of stimulation, emotional distress, confusion, frustration)
- Difficulty eating, swallowing
- Hallucinations, delusion, agitation
- Inability to perform self-care activities
- Inability to understand words
- Incontinence
- Loss of appetite and weight loss
- Loss of most memories, inability to process new information
- Loss of social skills
- Progression to loss of facial expression, primitive reflexes, loss of voluntary movement, loss of speech, recurrent infections
- Repetitious words or sounds
- Responding to short, simple communication
- Seizures
- Sexual disinhibition

Source: Adapted from National Institute on Aging. (2017). *What are the signs of Alzheimer's disease?* Retrieved from *https://www.nia.nih.gov/health/what-are-signs-alzheimers-disease;* and from Vancouver Health Authority. (2010). *Clinical stages of Alzheimer disease.* Retrieved from *http://geropsychiatriceducation.vch.ca/docs/edu-downloads/dementia/clinical_stages_CPS-MMSE_comparison.pdf.*

for diagnosis of dementia (Feldman, Jacova, Robillard, et al., 2008; Gauthier, Patterson, Chertkow, et al., 2012). The process includes making a clinical diagnosis based on the history, interviews with the patient and a caregiver or family member, physical examination, and brief cognitive tests. The next step in the process is laboratory tests to identify treatable medical conditions. Neuropsychological testing and neuroimaging are performed only when certain symptoms are present. Routine laboratory tests include complete blood cell count and measurements of thyroid-stimulating hormone; serum electrolytes; and serum calcium, serum fasting glucose, and serum vitamin B_{12} levels. Measurements of serum folic acid or red blood cell folate levels are optional. Neuropsychological testing may assist with differentiating among normal aging, MCI, and dementia (Feldman, Jacova, Robillard, et al., 2008). Neuroimaging studies (computed tomography or magnetic resonance imaging) are recommended if the patient has one or more of the following characteristics: age younger than 60 years; rapid decline in cognition over 1 to 2 months; less than 2 years' duration of symptoms; recent head trauma; unexplained neurological symptoms; history of cancer that could metastasize to the brain; use of anticoagulants or bleeding disorder; urinary incontinence and gait disorder early in the course of the dementia; localizing neurological signs (e.g., hemiparesis); atypical cognitive symptoms; or gait disturbance. None of the diagnostic procedures can identify whether the underlying pathological change in the brain is present (e.g., plaques and tangles in AD). This determination can be made only by microscopic examination of brain tissue after the person dies. If MCI is diagnosed, annual monitoring of symptoms and

functioning is recommended (Gauthier, Patterson, Chertkow, et al., 2012).

Related Assessments. Mental status testing is an important component of assessment. Patients with mild dementia may be able to compensate, which makes it difficult to evaluate cognitive function through conversation alone. Cognitive testing is focused on evaluating memory, attention, ability to perform calculations, language, visuospatial skills, and degree of alertness. The Mini-Mental State Examination (MMSE; Folstein, Folstein, & McHugh, 1975) is the most commonly used tool for brief assessment of cognitive functioning (Table 62-9). It cannot be used to diagnose dementia, but it is useful for monitoring change over time. However, the MMSE is not sensitive to very early stages of dementia and MCI. The Montreal Cognitive Assessment (MoCA) is a brief cognitive screening tool that has good sensitivity for detecting early dementia (Nasreddine, Phillips, Bédirian, et al., 2005).

The ConsultGeriRN.org website includes two-page *Try This* summaries of research about three additional mental status assessment tools for nurses, copies of the tools, articles about how to use them, and videos that demonstrate and explain how to use them. These tools include the Mini-Cog (Borson, Scanlan, Brush, et al., 2000), a brief screening tool for dementia; the Brief Evaluation of Executive Dysfunction (Kennedy, 2012); and the Recognition of Dementia in Hospitalized Older Adults tool (Mezey & Maslow, 2016).

Depression is often mistaken for dementia in older adults, and conversely, dementia for depression. Manifestations of depression include excessive sadness, difficulty thinking and concentrating,

TABLE 62-9 MINI MENTAL STATE EXAMINATION (MMSE): SAMPLE ITEMS

Orientation to Time
"What is the date?"

Naming
"What is this?" (Point to a pencil or pen.)

Reading
"Please read this and do what it says." (Show examinee the words on the stimulus form) CLOSE YOUR EYES

Source: Reproduced by special permission of the Publisher, Psychological Assessment Resources, Inc., 16204 North Florida Avenue, Lutz, Florida 33549, from the Mini Mental State Examination, by Marshal Folstein and Susan Folstein, Copyright 1975, 1998, 2001, by Mini Mental LLC, Inc. Published 2001 by Psychological Assessment Resources, Inc. Further reproduction is prohibited without permission of PAR, Inc. The MMSE can be purchased from PAR, Inc. by calling (813) 968-3003.

TABLE 62-10 DRUG THERAPY
Alzheimer's Disease

Problem	Drugs
Decreased memory and cognition	Cholinesterase inhibitors • Donepezil (Aricept) • Galantamine (Reminyl) • Rivastigmine (Exelon) N-Methyl-D-aspartate (NMDA) receptor antagonist • Memantine (Ebixa)
Depression	Selective serotonin reuptake inhibitors • Citalopram (Celexa) • Sertraline (Zoloft) Serotonin modulator • Trazodone
Behavioural symptoms	Atypical antipsychotics (neuroleptic agents) • Olanzapine (Zyprexa) • Risperidone (Risperdal) • Aripiprazole (Abilify)

fatigue, apathy, feelings of despair, and inactivity. When the depression is severe, concentration and attention may be poor, which manifests as memory and functional impairment. When dementia and depression do occur together (which may be the situation in as many as 40% of dementia cases), the intellectual deterioration may be more extreme. Depression, alone or in combination with dementia, is treatable. The challenge is to make an early assessment. Information about how to use the Geriatric Depression Scale (Sheikh & Yesavage, 1986), a short screening instrument for depression in older adults, is available on the ConsultGeriRN.org website (see the Resources at the end of this chapter).

Risk Modification

Many of the risk factors for AD and vascular dementia are modifiable. Individuals who reduce their risk for cardiovascular disease also reduce their risk for vascular dementia. Table 62-6 lists strategies to reduce risk for AD. In a landmark report titled *Rising Tide*, the Alzheimer Society of Canada (2010) showed that national programs to reduce risk of developing dementia are needed. Preventing dementia or delaying its onset would reduce the economic burden of dementia. The *Rising Tide* report demonstrated that a program to increase physical activity in older Canadians would reduce the incidence of dementia and reduce the total economic burden of dementia by $5.6 billion over 10 years and $51.8 billion over 30 years. The report also recommended implementing a comprehensive prevention program targeting all Canadians aged 65 and older. This could reduce risk of developing dementia by 23%, which would result in fewer new cases of dementia, delayed onset of dementia, and lower prevalence of dementia. It would reduce the economic burden of dementia by $24.2 billion over 10 years and $218.6 billion over 30 years.

Collaborative Care

There is no cure for any of the forms of dementia. The goals of collaborative management of dementia are to slow decline in cognition; to maintain and maximize functioning and quality of life of the person with dementia; and to support family caregivers.

Drug Therapy. Drugs used for dementia do not cure or reverse the progression of the disease. They may slow decline, but the

FIGURE 62-4 Mechanism of action of cholinesterase inhibitors. Acetylcholine **(A)** is released from the nerve synapses and carries a message across the synapse. Cholinesterase **(B)** breaks down acetylcholine. Cholinesterase inhibitors **(C)** block cholinesterase, which gives acetylcholine more time to transmit the message.

effects are modest (Lee, Hsiung, Seitz, et al., 2011). AD is the only form of dementia for which drugs that affect cognitive decline are approved by Health Canada. However, some experts recommend prescribing these drugs for dementia associated with Parkinson's disease as well (Gauthier, Patterson, Chertkow, et al., 2012). There are no medications that slow cognitive decline in other types of dementia. Drug therapy for AD is listed in Table 62-10.

Cholinesterase inhibitors block cholinesterase, the enzyme responsible for the breakdown of acetylcholine in the synaptic cleft (Figure 62-4). Cholinesterase inhibitors include donepezil (Aricept), rivastigmine (Exelon), and galantamine (Reminyl). These drugs may stabilize or improve cognitive function in AD and enhance the patient's functional abilities. Cholinesterase inhibitors increase risk for bradycardia and syncope—and associated falls (Herrmann, Black, Li, et al., 2011). The bradycardia may be difficult to detect because it is often transient.

DRUG ALERT—Galantamine
The extended-release formulation of galantamine (Reminyl) may cause severe skin reactions. Its use should be discontinued if skin rash is observed.

DRUG ALERT—Cholinesterase Inhibitors
Fall risk assessment and interventions should be part of care for patients taking cholinesterase inhibitors.

Memantine (Ebixa), an *N*-methyl-D-aspartate (NMDA) receptor antagonist, may be prescribed if cholinesterase inhibitors are ineffective. Memantine appears to protect the brain's nerve cells against excess amounts of glutamate, which is released in large amounts by cells damaged by AD. The attachment of glutamate to NMDA receptors enables calcium to flow freely into the cell, which in turn may lead to cell degeneration. Memantine may prevent this destructive sequence by adjusting the activity of glutamate. It may reduce behavioural and psychological symptoms in later stages of AD. Memantine is recommended for severe AD. Drugs for AD are prescribed until their clinical benefit can no longer be demonstrated. They are discontinued in very late stages of AD, when patients are bedridden and noncommunicative and cannot perform ADLs (Gauthier, Patterson, Chertkow, et al., 2012).

Antipsychotic drugs should be used for the management of the BPSDs only when nonpharmacological approaches alone are not successful and the patient is experiencing severe psychosis, aggression, or agitation. Even in that case, adverse effects and risk of adverse events may outweigh the benefits of these drugs. Pharmacological therapy for BPSDs begins with the lowest possible dose, with slow increases, if necessary. Patients should be monitored carefully for effectiveness and adverse effects, and routine assessment must be conducted to taper and discontinue the drug (CCSMH, 2006).

Conventional antipsychotic drugs (e.g., haloperidol) should not be administered because of extrapyramidal and anticholinergic adverse effects. The atypical antipsychotic agents reduce aggression and psychosis (see Table 62-10). Adverse drug effects include cardiac and metabolic disturbance, extrapyramidal adverse effects, gait disturbance, sedation, and anticholinergic effects. The risk of cerebro-vascular events and mortality is increased, especially in patients with forms of dementia other than AD. Antipsychotic agents are not used in patients with DLB because they produce severe adverse effects (CCSMH, 2006).

DRUG ALERT—Risperidone

Risperidone (Risperdal) is not recommended for patients with dementia other than AD.

BPSDs without psychosis can be treated with atypical antipsychotic agents and selective serotonin reuptake inhibitors such as such as sertraline (Zoloft), fluvoxamine (Luvox), and citalopram (Celexa). Benzodiazepines are generally not recommended because they produce adverse effects such as disinhibition and increase the risk for falls. In urgent situations, very low doses of short-acting benzodiazepines such as lorazepam (Ativan) may be used with caution. Valproate should not be used (Gauthier, Patterson, Chertkow, et al., 2012).

DRUG ALERT

- Do not give antipsychotics to patients who have dementia with Lewy bodies.
- Psychiatric medications increase the risk of delirium.

For patients who have depression in addition to dementia, the depression should be treated with a combination of pharmacological and nonpharmacological approaches. The first choice of drugs is selective serotonin reuptake inhibitors such as venlafaxine (Effexor), mirtazapine (Remeron), or bupropion (Wellbutrin; Herrmann, Lactôt & Hogan, 2013). Tricyclic antidepressants are not recommended because of negative effects on cognition associated with anticholinergic adverse effects (Herrmann, Lactôt & Hogan, 2013). The patient must be carefully monitored for effectiveness and adverse effects.

NURSING MANAGEMENT DEMENTIA

Nursing care for patients with dementia is based on four principles (Registered Nurses' Association of Ontario [RNAO], 2004/2010):
1. Knowing the person beyond the symptoms.
2. Recognizing retained abilities.
3. Manipulating the social and physical environment to meet the patient's unique needs.
4. Relating effectively, in ways that enable the patient to feel supported, valued, and confident.

NURSING ASSESSMENT

Comprehensive assessment is necessary to provide patient-centred care. Assessment should focus on the patient, his or her family or caregivers, and the physical and social environment. Assessment includes mental status, cognition, neurological symptoms, psychiatric symptoms, and functional assessment of ADLs and instrumental ADLs. Many patients with dementia lack awareness of their condition, and communication deficits are frequent. Thus collateral information should be obtained from people who know the patient well. Assessment of communication abilities helps the nurse adapt assessment approaches to the patient's abilities. Objective data from observation are important.

Data that should be obtained are listed in Table 62-11. In addition to cognitive assessment tools described earlier in this chapter, the ConsultGeriRN.org website provides standardized assessment tools, including tools specific to patients with dementia (Table 62-12). The CCSMH's pocket tool for assessment and treatment of behavioural symptoms is useful and can be

---

TABLE 62-11 NURSING ASSESSMENT

Patient With Dementia

Subjective Data
Important Information
Past health history: Head trauma, falls, history of previous delirium or psychiatric illness
Medications: All drugs, including cholinesterase inhibitors, psychotropic drugs, and nonprescription drugs

Symptoms
- Activities of daily living (e.g., dressing, feeding, using the toilet, performing personal hygiene)
- Instrumental activities of daily living (e.g., managing money, performing household chores, cooking, using transportation)
- Mental status examination (mood, perceptions and beliefs, thinking, orientation, memory and recall, concentration, insight, hallucinations, delusions, apathy)
- Pain
- Response to stressful situations
- Strength and mobility
- Symptoms according to mild, moderate, and severe stages of dementia (see Table 62-8)

Objective Data
- Appearance and behaviour
- Neurological symptoms (tremors, gait, tone, akathisia, dystonia)
- Symptoms according to mild, moderate, and severe stages of dementia
- Behavioural changes

TABLE 62-12	EVIDENCE-INFORMED DEMENTIA CARE RESOURCES: *TRY THIS:* TOOLS*

Amella, E. J., & Lawrence, J. F. Eating and feeding issues with older adults with dementia: Part II: Interventions (Issue D11.2).

Conedera, F., & Kingston, L. Therapeutic activity kits (Issue D4).

Cotter, V. T., & Evans, L. K. Avoiding restraints in patients with dementia (Issue D1).

Debrzuski, C. Communication difficulties: Assessment and interventions (Issue D7).

Maslow, K. Working with families of hospitalized older adults with dementia (Issue D10).

Silverstein, N. M., & Flaherty, G. Wandering in the hospitalized older adult (Issue D6)

Try This tools are a collaboration of The Hartford Institute for Geriatric Nursing, New York University, College of Nursing, and the Alzheimer's Association and are available at *https://consultgeri.org/tools/try-this-series.*

downloaded from its website (see the Resources at the end of this chapter). A number of assessment tools are provided as appendices to the RNAO's (2004/2010) nursing best practice guideline, *Caregiving Strategies for Older Adults with Delirium, Dementia, and Depression.*

NURSING DIAGNOSES

Nursing diagnoses for dementia may include, but are not limited to, the following:

- *Self-neglect* related to *deficient executive function* (memory deficit, cognitive impairment)
- *Risk for injury* as evidenced by *alteration in cognitive functioning* (impaired judgement, gait instability, sensory/perceptual alteration)
- *Wandering* related to *physiological state* (cognitive impairment)

Additional information on nursing diagnoses for the patient with dementia is presented in Nursing Care Plan (NCP) 62-1, available on the Evolve website.

PLANNING

The overall goal is that patients with dementia will have a dignified quality of life. Specific goals are (a) enhancement of ADLs and instrumental ADLs (retaining functional abilities as long as possible), (b) enhancement or stabilization of cognition, (c) elimination of pain, (d) prevention or minimization of behaviours that adversely affect functioning, and (e) enhancement of emotional well-being (RNAO, 2004/2010). The goals for the family caregiver of a patient with dementia are to (1) reduce caregiver stress, and (2) maintain personal health. A nursing goal is to developing partnerships with families (RNAO, 2004/2010).

NURSING IMPLEMENTATION

HEALTH PROMOTION. Strategies to prevent dementia are described earlier in this chapter. The Alzheimer Society of Canada's *Brain Health* Web page provides helpful information about healthy lifestyle choices for long-term brain health (see the Resources at the end of this chapter).

Dementia must be recognized early so that patients with dementia and their families can have time to make treatment decisions and plan for the future. Sometimes dementia is first identified when patients are admitted to an acute care facility for another condition (McCleary, Persaud, Hum, et al., 2012). Nurses who recognize signs of undiagnosed dementia can help patients access appropriate health care resources. Useful information for

patient and family health teaching about early signs of dementia is available on the Alzheimer Society of Canada website.

Health promotion can improve quality of life for patients with dementia and for family caregivers. Exercise programs for patients with dementia may improve the patient's ability to perform ADLs and reduce caregiver burden (Forbes, Forbes, Blake, et al., 2015). Yoga may improve physical health, mental health, and behaviours for patients with dementia (Fan & Chen, 2011).

ACUTE INTERVENTION. The diagnosis of dementia can be traumatic for both the patient and the family. It is not unusual for patients to respond with depression, denial, anxiety and fear, isolation, and grieving. The nurse is in an important position to assess for depression and suicidal ideation. Antidepressant drugs and counselling may be appropriate interventions. The nurse must assess the abilities of family members to accept and cope with the diagnosis.

Ongoing assessment of the patient and caregiver is required as the dementia progresses and the patient's functioning changes. An important nursing responsibility is to work in partnership with the caregiver to effectively manage clinical manifestations as they change over time. Effective partnership is enhanced when the nurse provides support, education, and collaboration with a focus on enabling meaningful caregiving roles in all settings (RNAO, 2004/2010). The nurse must consider both the patient with dementia and the caregiver as having overlapping but unique problems. To aid in identifying challenges the caregiver may experience, see NCP 62-2, Family Caregivers of the Patient with Dementia, available on the Evolve website.

Patients with dementia may be hospitalized for other health care problems. Approximately 25% of older patients in hospitals have dementia. This dementia is not necessarily documented on their health record (Russ, Shenkin, Reynish, et al., 2012). They are at higher risk than other older patients for negative outcomes, including delirium, avoidable functional decline, longer admissions, and death (Mukadam & Sampson, 2011; Russ, Shenkin, Reynish, et al., 2012). Access to rehabilitation after acute care is an issue for patients with dementia. The following "Evidence-Informed Practice" box describes a program to improve access to rehabilitation after hip fracture.

SAFETY ALERT

Patients with dementia who are admitted to hospitals are at risk for delirium, falls, dehydration, inadequate nutrition, untreated pain, drug-related problems, wandering, behavioural symptoms, and functional decline, and the use of restraints is more likely to be necessary.

Patients' inability to communicate symptoms of health problems places the responsibility for assessment and diagnosis on caregivers and health care providers. Patients with dementia who are hospitalized in acute care settings should be observed more closely because of concerns for safety. Consistent assignment of nursing staff, frequent reassurance, and orientation to place and time may reduce anxiety and prevent behavioural symptoms. See the preceding "Evidence-Informed Practice" box.

AMBULATORY AND HOME CARE. Most persons with dementia live in their homes, supported and cared for by family members or friends. The most typical caregiver is a spouse or an adult daughter. Depending on care needs, safety, availability of family caregivers, finances, and availability of formal programs, patients with dementia may eventually move to assisted-living facilities or long-term care homes.

Patients with dementia progress through the stages at variable rates. Nursing care needs of patients with dementia change as the disease progresses. Thus regular assessment, monitoring, and

EVIDENCE-INFORMED PRACTICE

Translating Research Into Practice

Rehabilitation After Hip Fracture for Patients With Cognitive Impairment

Clinical Question

In patients with cognitive impairment, after hip fracture surgery (P), does an interdisciplinary patient-centred model of rehabilitation (I), in comparison with routine rehabilitation (C), improve functional gain, cognitive gain, rehabilitation efficiency, and discharge location (O)?

Best Available Evidence

Quasi-experimental study

Critical Appraisal and Synthesis of Evidence

- Participants were patients with and without cognitive impairment who were admitted to a specialized inpatient rehabilitation unit after hip fracture surgery; their outcomes were compared.
- A new interdisciplinary model provided individualized rehabilitation care based on patient- and family-driven goals, with care strategies to minimize BPSDs.
- Participants were patients with cognitive impairment (*n* = 47) and patients without cognitive impairment (*n* = 102). Of the total of 149 patients, 73 (including 24 with cognitive impairment) received the new model of care, and their outcomes were compared with those of the patients who did not receive this intervention (*n* = 76).
- Patients with cognitive impairment had greater functional dependence at baseline.
- Both patients with and without cognitive impairment had significant gains in motor functioning, and 82% were discharged to the community
- Living alone, longer length of stay, and having cognitive impairment were associated with not being discharged to home.

Conclusions

- Patients with dementia benefit from rehabilitation after hip fracture.

Implications for Nursing Practice

- Support of staff to provide appropriate individualized care to patients with dementia was an essential part of the program.
- Nursing and interdisciplinary staff should receive education about dementia and effective dementia care strategies.
- A gerontological advanced practice nurse supported staff to implement the program.

Reference for Evidence

McGilton, K. S., Davis, A. M., Mahomed, N., et al. (2013). Evaluation of patient-centred rehabilitation model targeting older persons with a hip fracture, including those with cognitive impairment. *BMC Geriatrics, 13,* 135. doi:10.1186/1471-2318-13-136.

BPSDs, behavioural and psychological symptoms of dementia; *P*, patient population of interest; *I*, intervention or area of interest; *C*, comparison of interest or comparison group; *O*, outcome(s) of interest (see Chapter 1).

support are necessary. Regardless of the setting, cognition and functioning decline, and the amount of care required intensifies over time. The specific manifestations of the disease depend on the areas of the brain involved.

In the phase of MCI, memory aids (e.g., calendars) may be beneficial. Patients may develop depression in this phase. Depression may occur because of the neurochemical changes in the brain. Depression may be related to adjusting to a diagnosis of an incurable disorder, as well as the effect of dementia on the person's life (e.g., driving, socializing with friends, participating in hobbies or recreational activities). Drug therapy with cholinesterase inhibitors may be effective. However, adverse effects may deter some people from continuing with the drugs. Adherence

to the regimen may be challenging when dementia affects the patient's ability to remember to take drugs.

After the initial diagnosis, patients need to be aware that the progression of the disease is variable. Effective management of the disease can enhance quality of life of the patient and family and may slow the progress of the disease. The patient, family members, and the health care team should collaborate in making decisions related to care early in the disease. The nurse has a role in advising the patient and the family to discuss decision making for health care and planning for advanced care while the patient still has the capacity to do so.

Adult day care programs are an option for patients with dementia. The goals of adult day care programs are to provide respite for the family and to support the patient in the community for as long as possible. During the early and middle stages of dementia, patients benefit from therapeutic activities in a safe environment that support functioning. Services that may be provided at adult day care programs include assistance with ADLs, therapeutic recreation, cognitive stimulation, and transportation to the program. Patients return home more relaxed, content, less frustrated, and ready to be with the family. The respite from the demands of care allows the caregiver to be more responsive to the patient's needs. Other respite options include home visits from community respite workers, overnight care provided by community nursing services, and short-term (1–2 weeks) admission to a respite bed in a long-term care home. In many provinces and territories, this service is subsidized by government funding.

As the disease progresses, the demands on the caregiver may eventually exceed the resources, and the person with dementia may have to move to a long-term care home (Rockwood, Richard, Garden, et al., 2014). Dementia care units are becoming increasingly common in long-term care homes. Patients in the final stages of dementia require total care. Family caregiving responsibility continues when the person moves to a long-term care home. Family caregivers continue to provide personal care, preserve the dignity of the person with dementia, share their unique knowledge of the person with staff, and monitor quality of care.

There are specific issues related to the care of the patient with dementia that span all phases of the disease. Brief, evidence-informed guides to effective nursing intervention help with care planning (Table 62-12). These issues are described in the following sections.

Behavioural Changes. BPSDs occur in approximately 50% to 60% of patients with dementia. BPSDs are more common in middle and late stages, and most patients with dementia demonstrate BPSDs at some time. Often, the behaviours are not persistent. Caregivers need to be aware that these behaviours are not intentional. Behaviours are a way of communicating. It is up to the nurse to try to understand the meaning of the behaviour and what is being communicated. Behaviours may communicate emotions. By responding to these emotions, the nurse validates the patient's feelings (Pizzacalla, Montemuro, Coker, et al., 2015). BPSDs may worsen in acute care settings when behaviour is influenced by delirium, pain, changes in routine, and the unfamiliar environment. BPSDs often contribute to the decision to move patients to a long-term care home. See the following "Evidence-Informed Practice" box, which describes how training nurses on orthopaedic units to use gentle-persuasive approaches can be helpful to patients.

Behaviours do not occur in a vacuum; they are often in response to a precipitating factor (e.g., pain, frustration, temperature

🔍 EVIDENCE-INFORMED PRACTICE

Research Highlight

What Is the Effect of Training Nurses on Orthopaedic Units to Use Gentle-Persuasive Approaches?

Clinical Question
In nursing staff working on orthopaedic surgery units (P), does education and training to use gentle-persuasive approaches (I), in comparison with no training (C), increase competencies in behavioural management with cognitively impaired patients (O)?

Best Available Evidence
One quasi-experimental study.

Critical Appraisal and Synthesis of Evidence
- Staff and leaders identified distress related to responsive and self-protective behaviours on postoperative patients.
- One-day workshops on the principles of gentle-persuasive approaches (an approach that had been previously shown to be effective in long-term care settings) was provided to 82% of the multidisciplinary staff on the unit.
- The training focused on the following:
  - Person-centred care and understanding the meaning of behaviour as communication
  - Effect of dementia and delirium on the brain and how that relates to behaviour
  - Communication techniques to use with patients with delirium or dementia
  - Respectful self-protective techniques to use when encountering responsive behaviours
- The staff who received this training noted that their confidence in working with patients was significantly improved after the training.
- Most participants recommended training for colleagues.
- Success on one unit led other units in the hospital to adopt the training.

Conclusions
- Staff who receive training and education to understand the reasons for responsive behaviours improve their competence to provide effective safe care to patients with delirium and dementia.

Implications for Nursing Practice
- Hospital administrators should provide education to staff members who work with patients with dementia or delirium and should support them in using their learning in practice.
- Further examination of effects for patients is needed.

Reference for Evidence
Pizzacalla, A., Montemuro, M., Coker, E., et al. (2014). Gentle persuasive approaches introducing an educational program on an orthopaedic unit for staff caring for patients with dementia and delirium. *Orthopaedic Nursing, 34*(2), 101–107. doi:10.1097/NOR.0000000000000127.

P, patient population of interest; *I*, intervention or area of interest; *C*, comparison of interest or comparison group; *O*, outcome(s) of interest (see Chapter 1).

extremes, anxiety, perceived danger). The first step to identifying precipitating factors is for to assess the patient's physical status. Physical assessment includes checking for changes in vital signs, urinary and bowel patterns, and pain that could contribute to behavioural changes. Environmental assessment to identify factors that could trigger behaviours is the next step. Extremes in temperature, as well as excessive noise, may result in behaviour change. When the patient is agitated by the environment, either the patient or the stimulus should be moved. The patient can be assisted to call family members if this is reassuring. When a patient resists or pulls at tubes or dressings, these items can be covered with stretch tube gauze or removed from the visual field. The

patient should be reassured that the nurse is present to provide safety and protection. Orientation to place and person can be used, depending on the patient's cognitive abilities. Allowing the patient to live in his or her memories is often more appropriate and provides comfort and reassurance. Avoid challenging "why" questions when the patient is anxious or agitated. If the patient cannot verbalize distress, his or her mood should be validated. The patient's statement can be rephrased to validate its meaning. The patient's emotional state should be closely observed.

When nurses communicate effectively with patients during care, patients are less anxious and agitation is reduced. To communicate effectively, it is important that the nurse (a) stay near the patient during care, sit beside the patient, and use touch as appropriate; (b) recognize the patient's rhythm and adapt the pace of care to it; and (c) focus on care beyond the task by acknowledging the personal experience and providing reassurance (RNAO, 2004/2010).

Other strategies to manage behaviour include redirection, distraction, and reassurance. For a patient who is restless or agitated, redirecting would involve changing the patient's focus by having him or her perform activities such as sweeping, raking, or dusting. Effective strategies to distract the agitated patient might include snacks, car rides, favourite music, looking at family photographs, or walking. Repetitive activities, songs, poems, massage, aromas, or a favourite object can be soothing to some patients.

When nonpharmacological therapies are ineffective and patient safety is of concern, drugs may be used with caution (see Table 62-10). However, the drugs do not treat the unmet needs such as pain, social isolation, or boredom that are often the underlying cause of symptoms such as agitation (Voyer, McCusker, Cole, et al., 2015). Adverse effects should be monitored carefully.

Resources about assessment and treatment of behavioural symptoms are available on the CCSMH website (see the Resources at the end of this chapter). These resources include a practice guideline (CCSMH, 2006), a guide for patients and families, and a pocket tool for clinicians.

Some patients have a pattern of behavioural disturbance that occurs in the late afternoon. This is often referred to as **sundowning**. However, there is controversy about whether sundowning exists. According to some experts, there is no change in behaviour; rather, BPSDs are more disruptive to staff when they occur in the evening and are thus more noticeable to them. Others point out that the symptoms are characteristic of delirium. Possible causes include fatigue, unfamiliar environment, noise (especially in an acute care setting or during shift changes), medications, reduced lighting, restraint use, and sleep fragmentation. Behaviour should be assessed for underlying cause. Maximizing exposure to light during the day, ensuring quiet and uninterrupted nighttime sleep, implementing other sleep hygiene interventions (see Chapter 9), and engaging the patient in activities during the day may be helpful (Yevchak, Steis, & Evans, 2012).

Safety. The person with dementia is at risk for a number of problems related to personal safety. These problems include injury from falls, wandering in unsafe areas, injury to others and self with sharp objects or from fire and other heat sources, and impaired judgement and decision making. These concerns necessitate careful attention to the home environment to minimize risk and provide supervision. As cognitive function declines over time, patients with dementia may have difficulty navigating physical spaces and interpreting environmental cues. The Alzheimer Society of Canada website (see the Resources at the end of this chapter) has a home safety checklist that nurses can assist families to use. Environmental modifications include improving lighting; removing tripping hazards; stairway handrails, with the end of rail shaped differently to alert the patient that it is the end of the stairway; wiping wet areas on the floors; removing snow and ice; and grip bars and nonskid surfaces in showers and bathtubs (Alzheimer Society of Canada, 2015; RNAO, 2011).

In hospitals, the risk of falling is 2.6 to 6 times higher in patients with dementia than in patients who do not have dementia (RNAO, 2011). Nursing assessment should include fall risk assessment. Effective fall prevention programs include multiple components such as staff training, environmental modification, and exercises (RNAO, 2011).

Wandering is a major safety concern. Wandering may be the expression of a physical or emotional need or may result from cognitive loss, adverse effects of drugs, restlessness, curiosity, or stimuli that trigger memories of earlier routines. The nurse should observe for factors or events that may precipitate wandering. For example, patients may be sensitive to stress and tension in the environment. In such cases, wandering may reflect an attempt to leave the environment. Patients with dementia can be registered with the Alzheimer Society of Canada's MedicAlert Safely Home Registry. The registry includes identification products (e.g., bracelets, necklaces, watches) that allow police and emergency responders to identify the person quickly and return him or her home (Alzheimer Society of Canada, 2016d).

Pain Management. Pain management is complex. Often, pain in persons with dementia is not recognized by health professionals. Because of dementia-associated difficulties with oral and written language, affected patients may have difficulty expressing physical complaints, including pain. The nurse must rely on other behavioural clues or distress such as resistance to care, agitation, pacing, grimacing, withdrawal, increased vocalization, and changes in function. If nurses cannot determine the reasons for such behaviours, they should suspect and treat pain and monitor the patient's response. Nonpharmacological approaches such as massage may provide relief. Patients with dementia may not be able to tolerate therapeutic doses of analgesics. Low doses of long-acting opioids with slow titration to higher doses is recommended when trials of acetaminophen [Tylenol] are ineffective (Flegel, 2013; Gallagher, 2013). The *Try This* series on the ConsultGeriRN.org website includes tools for pain assessment with older adults and patients who have dementia. See Chapter 10 for information about pain assessment and management.

Eating and Swallowing Difficulties. Loss of interest in food and decreased ability to feed oneself *(feeding apraxia)*, as well as comorbid conditions, can result in significant nutritional deficits and possible dehydration in patients with dementia. In long-term care and acute care settings, inadequate assistance with eating may further add to the problem.

Individualized nursing interventions should be based on assessment of the patient's needs and abilities (see Table 62-13). Puréed foods, thickened liquids, and nutritional supplements can be used when chewing and swallowing become problematic for patients. Patients may need to be reminded to chew their food and to swallow. A quiet and unhurried environment for eating is essential. Distractions at mealtimes, including television, should be avoided. Creation of a normal social environment for meals provides supportive cues for patients with dementia. If self-feeding is difficult, finger foods, verbal cuing, demonstrating eating motions, and hand-over-hand techniques can initiate self-feeding. Liquids should be offered frequently.

TABLE 62-13 **STANDARDIZED NURSING ASSESSMENT TOOLS**
Amella, E. J., & Lawrence, J. F. Eating and feeding issues in older adults with dementia: Part I: Assessment. *Try This Series: Dementia,* Issue D11.1.
Boltz, M. Assessing family preferences for participation in care in hospitalized older adults. *Try This Series: General Assessment,* Issue 22.
Debrzuski, C. Communication difficulties: Assessment and interventions. *Try This Series: Dementia,* Issue D7.
Fick, D., & Mion, L. Assessing and managing delirium in persons with dementia. *Try This Series: Dementia,* Issue D8.
Graf, C. The Lawton Instrumental Activities of Daily Living Scale. *Try This Series: General Assessment,* Issue 23.
Horgas, A. L. Assessing pain in persons with dementia. *Try This Series: Dementia,* Issue D2.
Mezey, M., & Maslow, K. Recognition of dementia in hospitalized older adults. *Try This Series: Dementia,* Issue D5.
Onega, L. L. The Modified Caregiver Strain Index (MCSI). *Try This Series: General Assessment,* Issue 14.
Shelkey, M. Katz Index of Independence in Activities of Daily Living. *Try This Series: General Assessment,* Issue 2.
Silverstein, N. M., & Flaherty, G. Wandering in the hospitalized older adult. *Try This Series: Dementia,* Issue D6.
Zwicker, D. Preparedness for Caregiving Scale. *Try This Series: General Assessment,* Issue 28.

Source: These tools are available at *https://consultgeri.org/tools/try-this-series.* This website includes demonstrations of how to use many of the tools.

When oral feeding is not possible, alternative routes may be explored. Nutritional support therapies are described in Chapter 42.

Oral Care. Ability to perform oral self-care declines as dementia progresses. With decreased toothbrushing and flossing, dental problems are likely to occur. Food may become lodged in pockets in the mouth because of swallowing difficulties, which increases the potential for tooth decay. Dental caries and tooth abscesses cause discomfort and pain, potentially increasing responsive behaviours. The mouth should be inspected regularly and mouth care provided for patients unable to perform self-care. Pocket tools about providing oral care to patients with dementia are available in the resources section of the Regional Geriatric Program Central website (see the Resource at the end of this chapter).

Infection Prevention. Urinary tract infection and pneumonia are the most common infections in patients with dementia. Such infections are ultimately the cause of death in many patients with dementia. Patients with dementia are at risk for aspiration pneumonia because of feeding and swallowing problems. See Chapters 30 and 48 for additional information about these infections. Manifestations of infection—including changes in behaviour, delirium, fever, cough (pneumonia), and pain on urination (bladder)—are evaluated and appropriately treated. See Chapter 7 for information about normal changes of aging that diminish signs of infection.

Skin Care. It is important to monitor the patient's skin. Rashes, areas of redness, and skin breakdown should be noted and treated appropriately. In the late stages of dementia, incontinence along with immobility and undernutrition can increase patients' risk for skin breakdown. The nurse must keep the patient's skin dry and clean and change the patient's position regularly to prevent the creation of pressure areas over bony prominences.

Elimination Problems. During the middle and late stages of dementia, urinary and fecal incontinence become more common.

Multifaceted individualized nursing care to reduce incontinence should include regular toileting (with prompting and reminders if necessary), changing incontinence products, increasing fluid and fibre intake, and ensuring that the toilet is accessible.

Constipation is also a common problem. Causes may include immobility, dietary intake (e.g., reduced fibre intake), and decreased fluid intake. Management of constipation is discussed in Chapter 45.

Caregiver Support. Dementia is a disease that disrupts all aspects of personal and family life. Individuals caring for the person with dementia frequently describe such care as stressful. Caregivers of patients with dementia often experience negative effects on their work and family roles and on their mental and physical health. Caregiver strain is common. Actions that caregivers may take are suggested in Table 62-14. Strategies for reducing caregiver stress are listed in Table 62-15.

As the disease progresses, the relationship of the caregiver to the patient changes. Family roles may be altered or reversed (e.g., child caring for parent). Decisions that must be made include when the patient must stop driving or performing activities that might be dangerous, when to ask for assistance, and when to use respite care services or long-term care homes. With early-onset dementia and FTD, the person is often affected during the most productive working years. The financial consequences can be devastating for the individual and the family.

Sexual relations for couples are also seriously affected by dementia. As dementia progresses, sexual interest may decline for both the patient and the partner. A number of reasons account for this, including caregiver fatigue (when the partner is the caregiver), as well as memory impairment, apraxia, and episodes of incontinence in the patient with AD. It is also possible for patients to become sexually disinhibited as the disease progresses.

The nurse works with the caregiver to identify stressors and determine coping strategies to reduce the burden of caregiving. For example, the nurse should ask which behaviours are most disruptive to family life and remind the caregiver that this is likely to change over time as the disease progresses. Establishing what the caregiver views as most disruptive or distressful can help in identifying priorities for care. Risk to the safety of the patient and the caregiver is given high priority. It is also important to assess the caregiver's expectations regarding the patient's behaviour: are the expectations reasonable in view of the progression of the disease? The nurse must work with the caregiver to identify risk factors for complications, including behavioural problems.

Support groups for caregivers and family members (Figure 62-5) provide emotional support and information about dementia and related topics such as safety, legal, ethical, and financial issues. These groups are often facilitated by nurses, social workers, or occupational therapists. The Alzheimer Society of Canada has many educational and support systems available to help family caregivers. Other strategies related to stress management are discussed in Chapters 8 and 12.

Legal Matters and Personal Care Planning. In the early stage of dementia, while the patient is still capable of making decisions and signing legal papers, it is important for the patient to be part of the decision making about his or her financial and legal affairs. Some important legal documents that must be put in

---

TABLE 62-14 PATIENT & CAREGIVER TEACHING GUIDE

Dementia Caregiving

The following information should be included when teaching the caregiver about dementia.

1. Adapt communication to the person with dementia's abilities (e.g., read verbal and nonverbal cues, interpret what the person is trying to communicate). Know that communication is possible at all stages of dementia. Nonverbal communication is important in later stages of dementia.
2. Try to remain positive and encouraging. Avoid criticism and corrections. Focus on abilities.
3. Accept the reality of the person with dementia, and interact with him or her in that reality. Do not correct misstatements or faulty memory.
4. Assess and ensure home safety.
5. Monitor driving ability and discuss with the person with dementia and health care providers.
6. Encourage activities such as household chores, listening to music, reminiscence, exercising, hobbies, and visiting with friends and relatives.
7. Establish routines and simplify tasks (e.g., wearing clothing that is easy to put on, simplifying the table setting, breaking tasks down into small steps).
8. Register with the Alzheimer Society MedicAlert® Safely Home® program.

Source: Alzheimer Society of Canada. (2014). *Day to day living.* Retrieved from *http://www.alzheimer.ca/en/Living-with-dementia/Day-to-day-living.*

TABLE 62-15 TEN WAYS TO REDUCE CAREGIVER STRESS

1. Learn about the disease.
2. Be realistic about the disease.
3. Be realistic about how much you can do.
4. Accept your feelings.
5. Share information and feelings with others.
6. Be positive.
7. Look for humour.
8. Take care of yourself.
9. Get help, both practical help and support.
10. Plan for the future.

Source: Alzheimer Society of Canada. (2015). *Reducing caregiver stress.* Retrieved from *http://www.alzheimer.ca/en/Living-with-dementia/Caring-for-someone/Self-care-for-the-caregiver/Reducing-caregiver-stress.*

FIGURE 62-5 Support groups are an effective way to help caregivers cope. Source: Pressmaster/Shutterstock.com.

place as soon as possible are a will; an enduring power of attorney (a document naming a substitute decision maker) for financial and legal matters, as well as for future health care decisions; and an advance directive. The names and the required content of these documents vary among the provinces and territories, and the local chapter of the Alzheimer Society of Canada can help locate this information for persons with dementia and their families. Chapters 7 and 13 provide more information about these documents.

EVALUATION

Expected outcomes for patients with dementia are addressed in NCP 62-1, available on the Evolve website. See NCP 62-2 for expected outcomes for the caregiver of a patient with dementia.

CASE STUDY

Alzheimer's Disease

Source: Nadino/ Shutterstock .com.

Patient Profile

Mr. Yves Bédard, an 80-year-old man, received a diagnosis of AD 3 years ago. Today, his 78-year-old wife brings him to the emergency department because he wandered from his home, fell, and injured his left hip.

Subjective Data
- Can state his name
- Is disoriented regarding place and time
- Cannot recall wandering or falling
- Is agitated, trying to get up
- Denies pain

Objective Data
Physical Examination
- Left leg shorter than right leg
- Patient is tense and anxious
- Grimacing

Diagnostic Studies
- Radiographic study of left hip indicates a fracture.
- Mini-Mental State Examination shows cognitive impairment.

Discussion Questions
1. What is the pathogenesis of AD?
2. What precipitating factors may have resulted in Mr. Bédard's fall?
3. **Priority decision:** What are the priority nursing interventions for Mr. Bédard?
4. What precautions must be taken regarding the inpatient care of Mr. Bédard?
5. What teaching plan should be developed for Mr. Bédard and his wife?
6. **Priority decision:** Based on the assessment data presented, what are the priority nursing diagnoses? Are there any collaborative problems?
7. **Evidence-informed practice:** Mr. Bédard's wife asks whether she should give her husband ginkgo to help his memory. How should the nurse respond?

evolve

Answers are available at *http://evolve.elsevier.com/Canada/Lewis/medsurg.*

REVIEW QUESTIONS

The number of the question corresponds to the same-numbered objective at the beginning of the chapter.

1. Which of the following clients is most at risk for developing delirium?
   a. A 50-year-old woman with cholecystitis
   b. A 19-year-old man with a fractured femur
   c. A 42-year-old woman having an elective hysterectomy
   d. A 78-year-old man admitted to the medical unit with complications related to congestive heart failure

2. Which of the following symptoms are the hallmarks of delirium?
   a. Inattention, fluctuating course, hyperactivity, and altered level of consciousness
   b. Disorganized thinking, insidious onset, inattention, and altered level of consciousness
   c. Acute onset, fluctuating course, memory loss, and altered level of consciousness
   d. Acute onset, fluctuating course, inattention or disorganized thinking, and altered level of consciousness

3. Which of the following descriptions best characterizes dementia?
   a. Syndrome that results only in memory loss
   b. Disease associated with abrupt changes in behaviour
   c. Disease that is always due to reduced blood flow to the brain
   d. Syndrome characterized by cognitive dysfunction and loss of memory

4. Which of the following is associated with vascular dementia?
   a. Transient ischemic attacks
   b. Bacterial or viral infection of neuronal tissue
   c. Cognitive changes secondary to cerebral ischemia
   d. Abrupt changes in cognitive function that are irreversible

5. On which of the following findings is the clinical diagnosis of dementia based?
   a. Brain biopsy
   b. Electroencephalography
   c. Patient history and cognitive assessment
   d. Computed tomography or MRI

6. Which statement(s) accurately describe(s) mild cognitive impairment? *(Select all that apply)*
   a. Always progresses to AD
   b. Caused by variety of factors and may progress to AD
   c. Should be aggressively treated with acetylcholinesterase drugs
   d. Caused by vascular infarcts that, if treated, will delay progression to AD
   e. Client is usually not aware that there is a problem with his or her memory

7. What is a major goal of treatment for the client with dementia?
   a. Maintain safety
   b. Maintain or increase body weight
   c. Return to a higher level of self-care
   d. Enhance functional ability over time

evolve

1. d, 2. d, 3. d, 4. c, 5. c, 6. b, 7. a.

For even more review questions, visit *http://evolve.elsevier.com/Canada/Lewis/medsurg.*

REFERENCES

Agency for Healthcare Research and Quality. (2014). *Hospital-based program proactively identifies, addresses delirium risk factors in elderly, leading to less cognitive/functional decline and lower nursing home costs.* Retrieved from *https://innovations.ahrq.gov/profiles/hospital-based-program-proactively-identifies-addresses-delirium-risk-factors-elderly.*

Albert, M. S., DeKosky, S. T., Dickson, D., et al. (2011). The diagnosis of mild cognitive impairment due to Alzheimer's disease: Recommendations from the National Institute on Aging-Alzheimer's Association workgroups on diagnostic guidelines for Alzheimer's disease. *Alzheimer's & Dementia, 7,* 270–279. doi:10.1016/j.jalz.2011.03.008.

Alzheimer's Association. (2015). *Alzheimer's disease: Facts and figures.* Retrieved from *https://www.alz.org/facts/downloads/facts_figures_2015.pdf.*

Alzheimer Society of Canada. (2010). *Rising tide: The impact of dementia on Canadian society.* Toronto: Author. Retrieved from *http://www.alzheimer.ca/~/media/Files/national/Advocacy/ASC_Rising_Tide_Full_Report_e.pdf.* (Seminal).

Alzheimer Society of Canada. (2014). *Risk factors.* Retrieved from *http://www.alzheimer.ca/en/About-dementia/Alzheimer-s-disease/Risk-factors.*

Alzheimer Society of Canada. (2015). *Safety in the home.* Retrieved from *http://www.alzheimer.ca/en/Living-with-dementia/Day-to-day-living/Safety/Safety-in-the-home.*

Alzheimer Society of Canada. (2016a). *Prevalence and cost of dementia in Canada.* Retrieved from *http://www.alzheimer.ca/sites/default/files/Files/national/Statistics/PrevalenceandCostsofDementia_EN.pdf.*

Alzheimer Society of Canada. (2016b). *Down syndrome and Alzheimer's disease.* Retrieved from *http://www.alzheimer.ca/sites/default/files/Files/national/Other-dementias/down_syndrome_e.pdf.*

Alzheimer Society of Canada. (2016c). *Lewy body dementia.* Retrieved from *http://www.alzheimer.ca/en/About-dementia/Dementias/Lewy-Body-Dementia.*

Alzheimer Society of Canada. (2016d). *MedicAlert® Safely Home®.* Retrieved from *http://www.alzheimer.ca/en/Living-with-dementia/Day-to-day-living/Safety/Safely-Home.*

Alzheimer Society of Canada. (2017). *Dementia numbers in Canada.* Retrieved from *http://www.alzheimer.ca/en/About-dementia/What-is-dementia/Dementia-numbers.*

Alzheimer Society of York Region. (2016). *Seven A's of dementia.* Retrieved from *http://www.alzheimer.ca/en/york/About-dementia/What-is-dementia/Seven-A-s-of-dementia.*

American Geriatrics Society 2015 Beers Criteria Update Expert Panel. (2015). American Geriatrics Society 2015 updated Beers criteria for potentially inappropriate medication use in older adults. *Journal of the American Geriatric Society, 63,* 2227–2246. doi:10.1111/jgs.13702.

American Psychiatric Association. (2013). *Diagnostic and statistical manual of mental disorders* (5th ed.). Washington, DC: Author.

Association for Frontotemporal Degeneration. (2012). *Understanding the genetics of FTD.* Retrieved from *http://www.theaftd.org/wp-content/uploads/2009/03/Final-FTD-Genetics-Brochure-with-Cover-8.2.2012.pdf.*

Barr, J., Fraser, G. L., Puntillo, K., et al. (2013). Clinical practice guidelines for the management of pain, agitation, and delirium in adult patients in the intensive care unit: Executive summary. *American Journal of Health-System Pharmacy, 70,* 53–58. doi:10.1097/CCM.0b013e3182783b72.

Borson, S., Scanlan, J., Brush, M., et al. (2000). The Mini-Cog: A cognitive "vital signs" measure for dementia screening in multi-lingual elderly. *International Journal of Geriatric Psychiatry, 15,* 1021–1027. doi:10.1002/1099-1166(200011)15:11<1021::AID-GPS234>3.0.CO;2-6. (Seminal).

Bott, N. T., Radke, A., Stephens, M. L., et al. (2014). Frontotemporal dementia: Diagnosis, deficits and management. *Neurodegenerative Disease Management, 4(6),* 439–454.

Canadian Coalition for Seniors' Mental Health. (2006). *National guidelines for seniors' mental health: The assessment and treatment of delirium.* Toronto: Author. (Seminal).

Canadian Patient Safety Institute. (2013). *Prevention and management of delirium (delirium): Getting started kit.* Retrieved from *http://www.patientsafetyinstitute.ca/en/toolsResources/Pages/Delirium-Resources-%E2%80%8BGetting-Started-Kit.aspx.*

Cerejeira, J., Lagarto, L., & Mukaetova-Ladinska, E. B. (2012). Behavioral and psychological symptoms of dementia. *Frontiers in Neurology, 3,* 1–21. doi:10.3389/fneur.2012.00073.

Chaput, A. J., & Bryson, G. L. (2012). Postoperative delirium: Risk factors and management: Continuing professional development. *Canadian Journal of Anesthesia, 59,* 304–320. doi:10.1007/s12630-011-9658-4.

Chertkow, H. (2008). Diagnosis and treatment of dementia: Introduction. *Canadian Medical Association Journal, 178,* 316–321. doi:10.1503/cmaj.070795. (Seminal).

Clegg, A., & Young, J. B. (2011). Which medications to avoid in people at risk of delirium: A systematic review. *Age and Ageing, 40,* 23–29. doi:10.1093/ageing/afq140.

Fan, J. T., & Chen, K. M. (2011). Using silver yoga exercises to promote physical and mental health of elders with dementia in long-term care facilities. *International Psychogeriatrics, 23,* 1222–1230. doi:10.1017/S1041610211000287.

Feldman, H. H., Jacova, C., Robillard, A., et al. (2008). Diagnosis and treatment of dementia: 2. Diagnosis. *Canadian Medical Association Journal, 178,* 825–836. doi:10.1503/cmaj.070798. (Seminal).

Flegel, K. (2013). People with dementia need better pain management. *Canadian Medical Association Journal, 185,* 1195. doi:10.1503/cmaj.131296.

Folstein, M. F., Folstein, S. E., & McHugh, P. R. (1975). "Mini-mental state": A practical method for grading the cognitive state of patients for the clinician. *Journal of Psychiatric Research, 12,* 189–198. doi:10.1016/0022-3956(75)90026-6. (Seminal).

Forbes, D., Forbes, S. C., Blake, C. M., et al. (2015). Exercise programs for people with dementia. *The Cochrane Database of Systematic Reviews,* No. 4, Article CD006489. doi:10.1002/14651858.CD006489.pub4.

Gage, L., & Hogan, D. B. (2014). *2014 CCSM guideline update: The assessment and treatment of delirium.* Toronto: Canadian Coalition for Seniors' Mental Health. Retrieved from *http://ccsmh.ca/wp-content/uploads/2016/03/2014-ccsmh-Guideline-Update-Delirium.pdf.*

Gallagher, R. (2013). Practical and strategic pain management in residential care. *BC Medical Journal, 55,* 85–89. Retrieved from *http://bcmj.org/articles/practical-and-strategic-pain-management-residential-care.*

Gauthier, S., Patterson, C., Chertkow, H., et al. (2012). Recommendations of the 4th Canadian Consensus Conference on the Diagnosis and Treatment of Dementia (CCCDTD4). *Canadian Geriatrics Journal, 15(4),* 120–126. doi:10.5770/cgj.15.49.

Herrmann, N., Black, S. E., Li, A., et al. (2011). Discontinuing cholinesterase inhibitors: Results of a survey of Canadian dementia experts. *International Psychogeriatrics, 23,* 539–545. doi:10.1017/S1041610210001535.

Herrmann, N., Lanctôt, K. L., & Hogan, D. B. (2013). Pharmacological recommendations for the symptomatic treatment of dementia: The Canadian Consensus Conference on the Diagnosis and Treatment of Dementia 2012. *Alzheimer's Research & Therapy, 5*(Suppl. 1), S5. doi:10.1186/alzrt201.

Inouye, S. K., & Charpentier, P. A. (1996). Precipitating factors for delirium in hospitalized elderly persons: Predictive model and interrelationship with baseline vulnerability. *Journal of the American Medical Association, 275,* 852–857. doi:10.1001/jama.275.11.852. (Seminal).

Inouye, S. K., van Dyck, C. H., Alessi, C. A., et al. (1990). Clarifying confusion: The Confusion Assessment Method, a new method for detecting delirium. *Annals of Internal Medicine, 113,* 941–948. doi:10.7326/0003-4819-113-12-941. (Seminal).

Inouye, S. K., Westendorp, R. G. J., & Saczynski, J. S. (2014). Delirium in elderly people. *Lancet, 383,* 911–922. doi:10.1016/S0140-6736(13)60688-1.

Jacklin, K. M., Walker, J. D., & Shawande, M. (2013). The emergence of dementia as a health concern among First Nations populations in Alberta, Canada. *Canadian Journal of Public Health, 104*(1), e39–e44. doi:10.17269/cjph.104.3348.

Kennedy, G. J. (2012). Brief Evaluation of Executive Dysfunction: An essential refinement in the assessment of cognitive impairment. *Try This Series: Dementia,* (No. D3). Retrieved from *https://consultgeri.org/try-this/dementia/issue-d3.pdf.*

Lee, L., Weston, W. W., Heckman, G., et al. (2013). Structured approach to patients with memory difficulties in family practice. *Canadian Family Physician, 59,* 249–254. Retrieved from *http://www.cfp.ca/content/59/3/249.full.*

Lee, P., Hsiung, G. R., Seitz, D., et al. (2011). Cholinesterase inhibitors. *BC Medical Association Journal, 53,* 404–408. Retrieved from *http://www.bcmj.org/sites/default/files/BCMJ_53_Vol8_cholinesterase.pdf.*

McCleary, L., Persaud, M., Hum, S., et al. (2012). Pathways to dementia diagnosis among South Asian Canadians. *Dementia (London, England), 12*(6), 769–789. doi:10.1177/1471301212444806.

McKeith, I. G., Dickson, D. W., Lowe, J., et al. (2005). Diagnosis and management of dementia with Lewy bodies: Third report of the DLB consortium. *Neurology, 65,* 1863–1872. doi:10.1212/01.wnl.0000187889.17253.b1. (Seminal).

Mezey, M., & Maslow, K. (2016). Recognition of dementia in hospitalized older adults. *Try This Series: Dementia,* (D5). Retrieved from *https://consultgeri.org/try-this/dementia/issue-d5.pdf.*

Mielke, M. M., Vemuri, P., & Rocca, W. A. (2014). Clinical epidemiology of Alzheimer's disease: Assessing sex and gender differences. *Clinical Epidemiology, 6,* 37–48. doi:10.2147/CLEP.S37929.

Morandi, A., Lucchi, E., Turco, R., et al. (2015). Delirium superimposed on dementia: A quantitative and qualitative evaluation of informal caregivers and health care staff experience. *Journal of Psychosomatic Research, 79,* 272–280. doi:10.1016/j.jpsychores.2015.06.012.

Mukadam, N., & Sampson, E. L. (2011). A systematic review of the prevalence, associations and outcomes of dementia in older general hospital inpatients. *International Psychogeriatrics, 23,* 344–355. doi:10.1017/S1041610210001717.

Murray Alzheimer Research and Education Program & Alzheimer Societies of Hamilton & Halton, Brant, Haldimand-Norfolk, & Niagara Regions. (2006). *Managing and accommodating responsive behaviours in dementia care: A resource guide for long-term care.* Waterloo, ON: University of Waterloo. (Seminal).

Nasreddine, Z. S., Phillips, N. A., Bédirian, V., et al. (2005). The Montreal Cognitive Assessment, MoCA: A brief screening tool for mild cognitive impairment. *Journal of the American Geriatrics Society, 53,* 695–699. doi:10.1111/j.1532-5415.2005.53221.x. (Seminal).

National Institute on Aging. (2017). *What happens to the brain in Alzheimer's disease?* Retrieved from *https://www.nia.nih.gov/health/what-happens-brain-alzheimers-disease.*

O'Sullivan, R., Inouye, S. K., & Meagher, D. (2014). Delirium and depression: Inter-relationship and clinical overlap in elderly people. *Lancet Psychiatry, 1,* 303–311. doi:10.1016/S2215-0366(14)70281-0.

Peterson, R. C. (2011). Mild cognitive impairment. *The New England Journal of Medicine, 364,* 2227–2234. doi:10.1056/NEJMcp0910237.

Pizzacalla, A., Montemuro, M., Coker, E., et al. (2014). Gentle persuasive approaches introducing an educational program on an orthopaedic unit for staff caring for patients with dementia and delirium. *Orthopaedic Nursing, 34*(2), 101–107. doi:10.1097/NOR.0000000000000127.

Prince, M., Bryce, R., Albanese, E., et al. (2013). The global prevalence of dementia: A systematic review and metaanalysis. *Alzheimer's & Dementia, 9,* 63–76. doi:10.1016/j.jalz.2012.11.007.

Registered Nurses' Association of Ontario. (2004/2010). *Nursing best practice guideline: Caregiving strategies for older adults with delirium, dementia, and depression.* Toronto: Author. (Seminal).

Registered Nurses' Association of Ontario. (2011). *Nursing best practice guideline: Prevention of falls and fall injuries in the older adult.* Toronto: Author.

Rockwood, J. K. H., Richard, M., Garden, K., et al. (2014). Precipitating and predisposing events and symptoms for admission to assisted living or nursing home care. *Canadian Geriatrics Journal, 17,* 16–21. doi:10.5770/cgj.17.92.

Russ, T. C., Shenkin, S. D., Reynish, E., et al. (2012). Dementia in acute hospital inpatients: The role of the geriatrician. *Age and Ageing, 41,* 282–284. doi:10.1093/ageing/afs048.

Senate Canada. (2016). *Dementia in Canada: A national strategy for dementia-friendly communities.* Retrieved from *http://www.alzheimer.ca/sites/default/files/Files/national/Advocacy/SOCI_6thReport_DementiaInCanada-WEB_e.pdf.*

Sheikh, J. I., & Yesavage, J. A. (1986). Geriatric Depression Scale (GDS). Recent evidence and development of a shorter version. In T. L. Brink (Ed.), *Clinical gerontology: A guide to assessment and intervention* (pp. 165–173). New York: Haworth. (Seminal).

Tullmann, D. F., Fletcher, K., & Foreman, M. D. (2012). *Nursing standard of practice protocol: Delirium.* Retrieved from *https://consultgeri.org/geriatric-topics/delirium.*

UCSF Memory and Aging Center. (2016). *FTD misdiagnosis.* Retrieved from *http://memory.ucsf.edu/ftd-misdiagnosis.*

Voyer, P., McCusker, J., Cole, M. G., et al. (2015). Behavioral and psychological symptoms of dementia: How long does every behavior last, and are particular behaviors associated with PRN antipsychotic agent use? *Journal of Gerontological Nursing, 41,* 23–37. doi:10.3928/00989134-20141030-01.

Wu, L., Rosa-Neto, P., Hsiung, G. Y., et al. (2012). Early-Onset Familial Alzheimer's Disease (EAFAD). *Canadian Journal of Neurological Science, 39,* 436–445. doi:10.1017/S0317167100013949.

Yevchak, A. M., Steis, M. R., & Evans, L. K. (2012). Sundown syndrome: A systematic review of the literature. *Research in Gerontological Nursing, 5,* 294–303. doi:10.3928/19404921-20120906-04.

RESOURCES

Acute Care Geriatric Nurse Network
http://www.acgnn.ca

Alzheimer Society of Canada
http://www.alzheimer.ca

Alzheimer Society of Canada: "Brain Health"
http://www.alzheimer.ca/en/About-dementia/About-the-brain/
Brain-health

Alzheimer Society of Canada: "Safety in the Home"
http://www.alzheimer.ca/en/Living-with-dementia/
Day-to-day-living/Safety/Safety-in-the-home

BrainXchange
http://brainxchange.ca/public/home.aspx

Canadian Academy of Geriatric Psychiatry (CAGP)
http://www.cagp.ca

Canadian Association of Retired Persons
http://www.carp.ca

Canadian Coalition for Seniors' Mental Health
General website: *http://www.ccsmh.ca*
Tool on the Assessment and Treatment of Behavioural Symptoms of
Older Adults Living in Long Term Care Facilities: http://ccsmh.
ca/wp-content/uploads/2016/03/MHI-in-LTC-Final.pdf

Canadian Geriatrics Society
http://www.canadiangeriatrics.ca

Canadian Gerontological Nursing Association (CGNA)
http://www.cgna.net

Canadian Study of Health and Aging
http://www.csha.ca

Carers Canada
http://www.carerscanada.ca/

National Initiative for the Care of the Elderly (NICE)
http://www.nicenet.ca

Regional Geriatrics Programs of Ontario
http://www.rgps.on.ca
Pocket tools for providing oral care to patients with dementia:
http://www.rgpc.ca/resources/

Murray Alzheimer Research & Education Program,
University of Waterloo
http://www.marep.uwaterloo.ca

Registered Nurses' Association of Ontario (RNAO):
Nursing Best Practice Guidelines (BPG)
http://www.rnao.org/bestpractices

Vancouver Island Health Authority: Delirium Resources
http://www.viha.ca/mhas/resources/delirium/tools.htm

Work Safe BC
Working with Dementia: Safe Work Practices for Caregivers
https://www.worksafebc.com/en/resources/health-safety/
books-guides/working-with-dementia-safe-work-practices
-for-caregivers

American Geriatrics Society 2015 Updated Beers Criteria
for Potentially Inappropriate Medication Use in Older
Adults
http://onlinelibrary.wiley.com/doi/10.1111/jgs.13702/pdf

Confusion Assessment Method Training Manual
https://innovations.ahrq.gov/qualitytools/confusion-assessment
-method-cam-training-manual-and-coding-guide

Hartford Institute for Geriatric Nursing: ConsultGeriRN
.org
http://www.consultgerirn.org

Hospital Elder Life Program (HELP) for Prevention of
Delirium
http://www.hospitalelderlifeprogram.org/public/public-main.php

National Institute on Aging
http://www.nia.nih.gov
"How Alzheimer's Changes the Brain" (video): *https://*
www.nia.nih.gov/health/what-happens-brain-alzheimers
-disease?sort_by=totalcount

National Institute of Neurological Disorders and Strokes
http://www.ninds.nih.gov

For additional Internet resources, see the website for this book
at *http://evolve.elsevier.com/Canada/Lewis/medsurg*

Nursing Management

Peripheral Nerve and Spinal Cord Problems

Written by: Cindy M. Sullivan
Adapted by: Angela Sarro

⊘volve WEBSITE

http://evolve.elsevier.com/Canada/Lewis/medsurg

- Review Questions
  (Online Only)
- Key Points
- Answer Guidelines for Case Study

- Customizable Nursing Care Plan
  - Spinal Cord Injury
- Student Case Study
  - Spinal Cord Injury

- Audio Glossary
- Content Updates

LEARNING OBJECTIVES

1. Explain the etiology, clinical manifestations, collaborative care, and nursing management of trigeminal neuralgia and Bell's palsy.
2. Explain the etiology, clinical manifestations, collaborative care, and nursing management of Guillain-Barré syndrome, botulism, tetanus, and neuro-syphilis.
3. Describe the classification of spinal cord injuries and associated clinical manifestations.
4. Describe the clinical manifestations, collaborative care, and nursing management of spinal cord injury.
5. Explain the correlation between the severity and location of spinal cord injury and disruption of bodily function and the functional goals for rehabilitation.

6. Describe the nursing management of the major physical and psychological problems of patients with a spinal cord injury.
7. Describe the effects of spinal cord injury on the older-adult population.
8. Explain the types, clinical manifestations, collaborative care, and nursing management of spinal cord tumours.
9. Describe the pathophysiology, clinical manifestations, and the nursing and collaborative management of postpolio syndrome.

KEY TERMS

autonomic dysreflexia, p. 1605	Guillain-Barré syndrome (GBS), p. 1590	paraplegia, p. 1594	tetanus, p. 1592
Bell's palsy, p. 1588		poikilothermism, p. 1599	tetraplegia, p. 1594
botulism, p. 1592	neurogenic bladder, p. 1606	postpolio syndrome (PPS), p. 1612	trigeminal neuralgia (TN), p. 1585
Brown-Séquard syndrome, p. 1596	neurogenic shock, p. 1594	spinal shock, p. 1594	
	neuro-syphilis, p. 1593		

CRANIAL NERVE DISORDERS

Cranial nerve disorders are commonly classified as peripheral neuropathies. The 12 pairs of cranial nerves are considered the peripheral nerves of the brain. The disorders usually involve the motor or sensory (or both) branches of a single nerve *(mononeuropathies)*. Causes of cranial nerve problems include tumours, trauma, infections, inflammatory processes, and idiopathic (unknown) causes. Two cranial nerve disorders that will be discussed are trigeminal neuralgia and Bell's palsy.

TRIGEMINAL NEURALGIA

Etiology and Pathophysiology

Trigeminal neuralgia (TN), also known as *tic douloureux,* is a relatively uncommon cranial nerve disorder. The annual incidence of TN is 5 in 100 000 in Canada (Kastanias, Buzon, & Sarro, 2012). The average age of onset is 60 years; it is rarely diagnosed in individuals under 40 and develops slightly more often in women than men (Larsen, Piepgras, Chyatte, et al., 2011).

The trigeminal nerve is the fifth cranial nerve (cranial nerve V) and has both motor and sensory branches (Boyd & Tymianski, 2012). In TN, the sensory, or afferent, branches, primarily the maxillary and mandibular branches, are involved (Figure 63-1).

The pathophysiology of TN is not fully understood. One theory is that blood vessels, the superior cerebellar artery in particular, are compressed. This compression results in chronic irritation of the trigeminal nerve at the root entry zone. This irritation results in increased firing of the afferent or sensory fibre, commonly referred to as *classical TN*. Symptomatic TN is typically caused by a structural, nonvascular lesion (benign tumours, aneurysms, multiple sclerosis) (Al-Quliti, 2015). Other factors that may result in neuralgia include herpesvirus infection, infection of gums and jaw, and a brain stem infarct. The effectiveness of anticonvulsant drug therapy in reducing pain may be related to the ability of these drugs to stabilize the neuronal membrane and decrease paroxysmal afferent impulses of the nerve (Al-Quliti, 2015).

Clinical Manifestations

The classic feature of trigeminal neuralgia is an abrupt onset of paroxysms of flashing, stabbing pain radiating along the course of a branch of the trigeminal facial nerve from the angle of the jaw, described as a burning, knifelike, or lightning-like shock in the lips, the upper or lower gums, the cheek, the forehead, or the side of the nose. Intense pain, twitching, grimacing, and frequent blinking and tearing of the eye occur during the acute attack (hence the term *tic douloureux*). Some patients may experience facial sensory loss. The attacks are usually brief, lasting only seconds to 2 or 3 minutes, and are generally unilateral. Recurrences are unpredictable; they may occur several times a day or weeks or months apart. After the refractory (pain-free) period, a phenomenon known as *clustering* can occur. Clustering is characterized by a cycle of pain and refractoriness that continues for hours.

The painful episodes are usually initiated by a triggering mechanism of light cutaneous stimulation at a specific point (*trigger zone*) along the distribution of the nerve branches. Precipitating stimuli include chewing, brushing teeth, a hot or cold blast of air on the face, washing the face, yawning, and even talking. Touch and tickle seem to predominate as causative triggers, rather than pain or changes in temperature. As a result, the patient may eat improperly, neglect hygienic practices, wear a cloth over the face, and withdraw from interaction with other individuals. The patient may sleep excessively as a means of coping with the pain.

Although this condition is considered benign, the severity of the pain and the disruption of lifestyle can result in almost total physical and psychological dysfunction or even suicide.

Diagnostic Studies

It is important to rule out other problems with similar manifestations, such as other forms of facial and cephalic neuralgias and pain arising from the sinuses, the gums, and the jaws. In young adults with bilateral facial pain, magnetic resonance imaging (MRI) is performed to rule out lesions, vascular abnormalities, and multiple sclerosis (Zakrzewska, 2014). A complete neurological assessment is performed, including audiological evaluation, although results are usually normal. Electromyography (EMG) can be performed to help distinguish between symptomatic and classical trigeminal neuralgia. Once the diagnosis is made, the goal of treatment is relief of pain by either medical or surgical intervention (Table 63-1).

Collaborative Care

Drug Therapy. Carbamazepine (Tegretol) is considered the first-line therapy in patients with newly diagnosed trigeminal

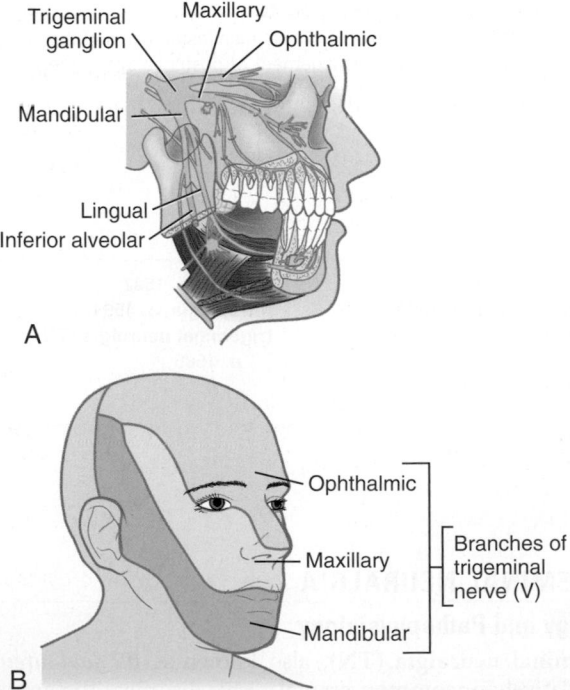

FIGURE 63-1 A, Trigeminal nerve (fifth cranial nerve) and its three main divisions: the ophthalmic, maxillary, and mandibular nerves. **B,** Sensory fibres of the trigeminal nerve for three branch nerves (ophthalmic, maxillary, and mandibular nerves), each of which conducts information from a different region of the face. Source: Modified from Patton, K. T., & Thibodeau, G. A. (2016). *Anatomy and physiology* (9th ed., p. 491, Figure 21-11). St. Louis: Mosby.

TABLE 63-1 COLLABORATIVE CARE

Clinical Management of Trigeminal Neuralgia

Diagnostic
- EMG studies
- Evaluation for symptomatic TN
- MRI of brain to assess for secondary causes
- Normal neurological examination
- Paroxysmal lancinating facial pain in distribution of trigeminal nerve (classic TN)

Collaborative Therapy
Drug Therapy
- First line: carbamazepine (Tegretol), oxcarbazepine (Trileptal)
- Second line: baclofen (Lioresal), lamotrigine (Lamictal)
- Third line: gabapentin (Neurontin), pregabalin (Lyrica), topiramate (Topamax)

Surgical Options
- Percutaneous
  - Glycerol rhizotomy
  - Radiofrequency rhizotomy
- Intracranial
  - Gamma Knife radiosurgery
  - Microvascular decompression

EMG, electromyography; *MRI,* magnetic resonance imaging.

neuralgia (Zakrzewska, 2014). By acting on sodium channels, carbamazepine and other anticonvulsant drugs lengthen the time needed for neuron repolarization, which results in decreased neuron firing. Adverse effects of carbamazepine may include bone marrow suppression, which leads to blood abnormalities. Therefore, routine complete blood cell (CBC) counts are required. Baclofen (Lioresal), an antispasmodic agent, has demonstrated efficacy in reducing pain from trigeminal neuralgia. Baclofen works synergistically with carbamazepine and can therefore be used as a monotherapy or in conjunction with carbamazepine if pain relief is incomplete. Other anticonvulsant medications that may be used in the management of trigeminal neuralgia are listed in Table 63-1. These anticonvulsant drugs may prevent an acute attack or promote a remission of symptoms. Because drug therapy may not provide permanent pain relief, some patients may seek continued help and make numerous visits to otolaryngologists for assessment or may attempt alternative therapies such as acupuncture and megavitamins.

Conservative Therapy. Local anaesthetics can be used to block nerves. Local nerve blocking results in complete anaesthesia of the area supplied by the injected branches. Relief of pain is temporary, lasting from 6 to 18 months.

Biofeedback is another strategy that may be helpful for some patients. In addition to controlling the pain, the patient may experience a strong sense of personal control by mastering the technique and altering certain body functions. (Biofeedback is discussed in Chapter 12.)

Surgical Therapy. If a conservative approach, including drug therapy, is not effective, surgical therapy is available. *Glycerol rhizotomy* is a percutaneous procedure that consists of an injection of glycerol through the foramen ovale into the trigeminal cistern (Figure 63-2). Glycerol injections produce immediate pain relief in 90% of patients, but by 5 years, approximately 50% experience recurrence of pain (Al-Quliti, 2015; Zakrzewska, 2014).

Percutaneous radiofrequency rhizotomy (electrocoagulation) and microvascular decompression provide the greatest relief of pain. In *percutaneous radiofrequency rhizotomy,* a needle is inserted into the trigeminal rootlets that are adjacent to the pons, and the area is destroyed by means of a radiofrequency current. This can result in facial numbness (although some degree of sensation may be retained), corneal anaesthesia, and trigeminal motor weakness. This procedure is easily performed with few complications and minimal risk to the patient and essentially exchanges pain for numbness. It is usually performed on an outpatient basis. It is tolerated well by older adults and avoids a major operative procedure, which is beneficial for patients at high risk for surgical complications (Al-Quliti, 2015; Zakrzewska, 2014).

Microvascular decompression of the trigeminal nerve, another commonly used procedure, is accomplished by displacing and repositioning blood vessels that appear to be compressing the nerve at the root entry zone where it exits the pons. This procedure relieves pain without residual sensory loss. Microvascular decompression has a long-term success rate equal or superior to that of percutaneous procedures, and the rate of permanent neurological outcomes such as numbness is lower (Al-Quliti, 2015; Zakrzewska, 2014). *Gamma Knife radiosurgery* is another surgical treatment that is used to alleviate trigeminal neuralgia. Radiosurgery with the Gamma Knife provides precise radiation of the proximal trigeminal nerve identified on high-resolution imaging. This approach has been useful both for patients with persistent pain after other surgical procedures and as a primary surgical option (Al-Quliti, 2015; Zakrzewska, 2014).

NURSING MANAGEMENT
TRIGEMINAL NEURALGIA

NURSING ASSESSMENT

Assessment of the attacks—including triggering factors, characteristics, frequency, and pain management techniques—helps the nurse plan for patient care. The nursing assessment should include examination of the patient's nutritional status, hygiene (especially oral), and behaviour (including withdrawal). The degree of pain and its effects on the patient's lifestyle, drug history, emotional state, and depression and suicidal ideation are other important factors to assess.

NURSING DIAGNOSES

Nursing diagnoses for the patient with trigeminal neuralgia include but are not limited to the following:

- *Acute pain* related to *physical injury agent* (inflammation or compression of the trigeminal nerve)
- *Imbalanced nutrition: less than body requirements* related to *insufficient dietary intake* (fear of triggering pain by eating or chewing)
- *Anxiety* related to *threat to current status* (uncertainty of timing and initiating event of pain)
- *Impaired oral mucous membrane integrity* related to *inadequate oral hygiene* (potential for initiating pain)
- *Social isolation* related to *social behaviour incongruent with norms* (anxiety over pain attacks, desire to maintain non-stimulating environment)

PLANNING

The overall goals are that the patient with trigeminal neuralgia will (a) be free of pain, (b) maintain adequate nutritional and oral hygiene status, (c) have minimal to no anxiety, and (d)

FIGURE 63-2 Glycerol rhizotomy. **A,** Needle placed in face of patient with trigeminal neuralgia. **B,** Physician injecting glycerol. Source: Courtesy Joe Rothrock, Media, PA.

return to normal or previous socialization and occupational activities.

NURSING IMPLEMENTATION

HEALTH PROMOTION. Because the etiology of trigeminal neuralgia remains unknown, health promotion is directed at reducing recurrent episodes in patients who have trigeminal neuralgia. Awareness and reduction of triggering events may be possible in some patients.

ACUTE INTERVENTION. Patients with trigeminal neuralgia are usually treated on an outpatient basis. Pain relief is obtained primarily by the administration of the recommended drug therapy. The nurse monitors the patient's response to therapy and notes any adverse effects. Alternative pain relief measures, such as biofeedback, should be explored for patients who are not surgical candidates and whose pain is not controlled by other therapeutic measures. A thorough assessment of pain with a valid and reliable tool, which includes the history of the pain problem and effectiveness of pain relief measures, can assist in selecting appropriate pain management interventions.

The nurse should review with the patient the importance of nutrition, hygiene, and oral care and teach methods to achieve all of this if neglect is apparent. For cleansing the face, the nurse should provide lukewarm water and soft cloths or cotton saturated with solutions that do not necessitate rinsing. A small, soft-bristled toothbrush or a warm mouthwash assists in promoting oral care. Hygiene activities are best performed when pain is managed and analgesic effectiveness is at its peak. Environmental management is essential during an acute period to lessen triggering stimuli.

Food should be high in protein and calories and easy to chew. It should be served lukewarm and offered frequently. When oral intake is sharply reduced and the patient's nutritional status is compromised, a nasogastric tube can be inserted on the unaffected side for enteral feedings.

The patient will probably not engage in extensive conversation during the acute period. Alternative communication methods, such as paper and pencil, should be provided.

The nurse should provide information or instructions related to diagnostic studies used to rule out other problems—such as multiple sclerosis, dental or sinus problems, and neoplasms—and for preoperative teaching if surgery is planned. The nurse may also have to clarify expectations related to postoperative outcomes. Appropriate teaching related to postoperative activities depends on the type of procedure planned (e.g., percutaneous, intracranial). The patient needs to know that he or she will be awake during local procedures so that he or she can cooperate when corneal and ciliary reflexes and facial sensations are checked. Patients are informed about the potential risk of postoperative facial numbness.

After the procedure, the patient's pain is compared with the preoperative level. The corneal reflex, extraocular muscles, hearing, sensation, and facial nerve function are evaluated frequently (see Chapter 58). If the corneal reflex is impaired, special attention must be paid to eye protection. This includes the use of artificial tears or eye shields. General postoperative nursing care after a craniotomy is appropriate if intracranial surgery is performed. (Nursing care related to craniotomy is discussed in Chapter 59.) Caloric intake and ambulation should be increased according to the patient's progress or specific orders.

After a percutaneous radiofrequency electrocoagulation procedure, an ice pack is applied to the jaw on the operative side for 3 to 5 hours. To avoid injuring the mouth, the patient should not chew on the operative side until sensation has returned.

AMBULATORY AND HOME CARE. Regular follow-up care should be planned. The patient needs instruction regarding the dosage and adverse effects of medications. Although relief of pain may be complete, the patient should be encouraged to keep environmental stimuli to a moderate level and to use stress-reduction methods. The patient may have developed protective practices to prevent pain and may need counselling or psychiatric assistance in the readjustment, especially in re-establishing personal relationships. Herpes simplex infection (cold sores) can occur as a result of manipulation of the gasserian ganglion. Treatment consists of antiviral agents such as acyclovir (Zovirax) (see Chapter 26).

Long-term management after surgical intervention depends on the residual effects of the type of procedure. If hypesthesia (decreased sensitivity to stimulation, excluding the special senses) is present or the corneal reflex is altered, the patient should be taught to (a) chew on the unaffected side; (b) avoid hot foods or beverages, which can burn the mucous membranes; (c) check the oral cavity after meals to remove food particles; (d) practise meticulous oral hygiene and continue with semiannual dental visits; (e) protect the face against extremes of temperature; (f) use an electric razor; and (g) wear a protective eye shield.

EVALUATION

The following are expected outcomes for patients with trigeminal neuralgia:

- Relief or decreased pain
- Appearing more comfortable and less anxious
- Normal facial sensation or expected paresthesias and anaesthesias
- Return to previous socialization, or improved socialization, and occupational activities

BELL'S PALSY

Etiology and Pathophysiology

Bell's palsy (peripheral facial paralysis, acute benign cranial polyneuritis) is a disorder characterized by a disruption of the motor branches of the facial nerve (cranial nerve VII) on one side of the face in the absence of any other disease such as a stroke. Bell's palsy is an acute, peripheral facial paresis of unknown cause. Average annual incidence rates of Bell's palsy are similar throughout the world, ranging between 11.5 and 40.2 per 100 000. It affects males and females equally and has slightly higher incidence in mid- to later life. (Eviston, Croxson, Kennedy, et al., 2015).

Although the exact etiology is not known, there is evidence associating immune, infective, and ischemic mechanisms as potential contributors. The reactivation of the herpes simplex virus infection is one example. The reactivation causes an inflammatory response with subsequent demyelination of the nerve, causing alterations in motor and sensory function (Eviston, Croxson, Kennedy, et al., 2015). Bell's palsy is considered benign; the majority of patients make a complete recovery. Improvement in facial function occurs in 85% of people within 3 weeks of onset. Patients with complete facial paralysis at onset who have not experienced some recovery within the first 3 to 4 months are more likely to have incomplete recovery. Chronic facial palsy can be a disabling condition that has an impact on social function, emotional expression, and quality of life (Eviston, Croxson, Kennedy, et al., 2015).

Clinical Manifestations

The characteristic findings of Bell's palsy are acute onset of unilateral facial paralysis affecting muscles of the upper and

FIGURE 63-3 Facial characteristics of Bell's palsy. **A,** At rest the face may look almost normal, but the patient is not able to wrinkle her forehead on the affected (right) side, and the right corner of the mouth droops. **B,** When she tries to close her eyes and show her teeth, the differences between the affected and unaffected sides become more obvious. Source: Forbes, C. D., & Jackson, W. F. (2003). *Color atlas and text of clinical medicine* (3rd ed., p. 453, Figures 11.15 and 11.16). London: Mosby.

lower face reaching a peak within 72 hours, resulting in facial drooping, an inability to close the eyelid, or an inability to frown or smile (Figure 63-3). Decreased muscle movement may alter chewing ability. Some patients may experience a loss of or excessive tearing. The muscle weakness causes the lower eyelid to turn out, allowing overflow of normal tear production. These symptoms are frequently accompanied by neck, mastoid, or ear pain; distortion in sense of taste; and altered facial sensation.

Diagnostic Studies

The diagnosis of Bell's palsy is based on clinical presentation. The diagnosis and prognosis are indicated by observation of the typical pattern of onset of symptoms. In situations with complete facial paralysis, neuro-physiological testing (EMG studies) is helpful in predicting potential nerve recovery. Computed tomographic (CT) scan or MRI may be performed to rule out stroke or other neurological disease (Eviston, Croxson, Kennedy, et al., 2015).

Collaborative Care

Nonpharmacological treatments for Bell's palsy include eye protection for those with incomplete closure of their eyes. Prolonged irritation and drying can cause keratitis and ulceration and potentially impair eyesight. Eye protection includes barrier protection, lubrication, and taped closure at night. Oral care may include use of a straw for drinking. A change in diet texture toward soft foods may be necessary, and mastication techniques may need to adapt to avoid mucous membrane trauma (Eviston, Croxson, Kennedy, et al., 2015).

Drug Therapy. Treatment with corticosteroids (prednisone) should be commenced within 72 hours of onset of symptoms. Steroids are given over a 2- to 3-week period with tapering doses after approximately 10 days (Eviston, Croxson, Kennedy, et al., 2015). Usually, the corticosteroid treatment decreases the edema and pain, but analgesics can be used if necessary to manage pain. Combining prednisone with an antiviral drug such as acyclovir (Zovirax) or valacyclovir (Valtrex) can improve the rate of recovery given that the herpes simplex virus can be a causal factor (Eviston, Croxson, Kennedy, et al., 2015). The length of treatment with antiviral medications is usually between 5 and 10 days. It is important to review with the patient and the family the medications that have been prescribed for the treatment of Bell's palsy, including any potential adverse effects.

NURSING MANAGEMENT
BELL'S PALSY

NURSING ASSESSMENT

Early recognition of the possibility of Bell's palsy is important. Because herpes simplex virus is a possible etiological factor, any person who is prone to herpes simplex should be alerted to seek health care if pain occurs in or around the ear. A complete assessment of cranial nerve VII, which includes the facial muscles should be completed, carefully assessing for any signs of weakness; patients should be asked to close their eyes, show their teeth, puff their cheeks and smile (Boyd & Tymianski, 2012).

NURSING DIAGNOSES

The nursing diagnoses for the patient with Bell's palsy may include but are not limited to the following:
- *Acute pain* related to *physical injury agent* (inflammation of cranial nerve VII—facial nerve)
- *Imbalanced nutrition: less than body requirements* related to *insufficient dietary intake* (inability to ingest food secondary to muscle weakness)
- *Risk for corneal injury* as evidenced by *blinking < 5 times per minute*
- *Disturbed body image* related to *alteration in self-perception* (change in facial appearance)

PLANNING

The overall goals are that the patient with Bell's palsy will (a) be pain free or be able to manage pain, (b) maintain adequate nutritional status, (c) maintain appropriate oral hygiene, (d) not experience injury to the eye, (e) return to normal or previous perception of body image, and (f) be optimistic about disease outcome.

NURSING IMPLEMENTATION

Bell's palsy is treated on an outpatient basis. The following interventions are used throughout the course of the disease. Mild analgesics can relieve pain. Hot wet packs can reduce the discomfort of herpetic lesions if present, aid circulation, and relieve pain. The face should be protected from cold and drafts because trigeminal *hyperesthesia* (increased sensitivity to stimulation such as touch) may accompany the syndrome. Maintenance of good nutrition is important. The patient should be taught to chew on the unaffected side of the mouth to avoid trapping food and to enjoy the taste of food. Thorough oral hygiene must be carried out after each meal to prevent the development of parotitis, caries, and periodontal disease from accumulated residual food.

Dark glasses may be worn for protective and cosmetic reasons. Artificial tears (methyl cellulose) should be instilled frequently during the day to prevent drying of the cornea. The eye should be inspected for the presence of eyelashes. Ointment and an impermeable eye shield can be used at night to retain moisture. In some patients, taping the lids closed at night may be necessary to provide protection. The patient is taught to report ocular pain, drainage, or discharge.

A facial sling may be helpful to support affected muscles, improve lip alignment, and facilitate eating. The facial sling is usually made and fitted by a physical or occupational therapist. Vigorous massage can break down tissues, but gentle upward massage has psychological benefits even if physical effects, other than the maintenance of circulation, are questionable. When function begins to return, active facial exercises are performed several times a day.

The change in physical appearance as a result of Bell's palsy can be devastating. Affected patients must be reassured that a stroke did not occur and that chances for a full recovery are good. A patient's need for privacy should be respected, especially during meals, but the nurse's assistance in the patient's adjustment to the physical changes should not be delayed. Enlisting support from family and friends is important. It is important to inform the patient that most patients with Bell's palsy recover within about 6 weeks of the onset of symptoms.

EVALUATION

The following are expected outcomes for the patient with Bell's palsy:

- Freedom from pain
- No complications (e.g., corneal abrasion)
- Appropriate nutritional intake
- Minimal adverse effects associated with corticosteroid treatment
- Return to previous perception of body image

POLYNEUROPATHIES

GUILLAIN-BARRÉ SYNDROME

Etiology and Pathophysiology

Guillain-Barré syndrome (GBS), also known as *Landry–Guillain-Barré–Strohl syndrome, postinfectious polyneuropathy,* and *ascending polyneuropathic paralysis,* is an acute, rapidly progressing, and potentially fatal form of polyneuritis. GBS affects the peripheral nervous system and results in loss of myelin (segmental demyelination), edema, and inflammation of the affected nerves. GBS manifests as a symmetrical ascending paralysis. The incidence is 1 to 2 per 100 000 per year. The disease is present worldwide and affects individuals of all age groups (Koopman & Shcharinsky, 2012).

The etiology of this disorder is unknown, but it is believed to be a cell-mediated immunological reaction directed at the peripheral nerves. It is typically preceded by either an upper respiratory (58%) or a gastro-intestinal infection (22%) (Ansar & Valadi, 2015). A possible link between vaccinations and the occurrence of GBS has been proposed, although the evidence for this link is not strong. *Campylobacter jejuni* is the organism most recognized to be associated with GBS (Ansar & Valadi, 2015). Other potential pathogens include *Mycoplasma pneumoniae,* cytomegalovirus, Epstein-Barr virus, varicella-zoster virus, and vaccines (rabies, swine influenza). These stimuli are thought to cause an alteration in the immune system, resulting in sensitization of T lymphocytes to the patient's myelin and, ultimately, myelin damage. Demyelination occurs, and the transmission of nerve impulses is stopped or slowed down. The muscles innervated by the damaged peripheral nerves undergo denervation and atrophy. In the recovery phase, remyelination occurs slowly, and neurological function returns in a proximal-to-distal pattern.

Clinical Manifestations

GBS symptoms range from mild to severe and typically progress over the course of hours to several days. GBS is characterized by relatively symmetrical muscle weakness, mild distal sensory symptoms of paresthesias (first in the feet, then in the hands) with absent or depressed deep tendon reflexes. Weakness develops classically in an ascending pattern involving the lower limbs first, then the upper extremities, followed by the face and respiratory muscle; weakness may progress to complete paralysis (Koopman & Shcharinsky, 2012).

Four main subtypes of GBS include (a) acute inflammatory demyelinating polyneuropathy (AIDP) (80%–90%); (b) acute motor axonal neuropathy and acute sensorimotor axonal neuropathy (5%–10%); and (c) Miller Fisher syndrome (5%), a rare disorder characterized by ataxia, areflexia, and ophthalmoplegia (weakness or paralysis of the muscles controlling eye movements). In GBS, autonomic nervous system dysfunction results from alterations in both the sympathetic and the parasympathetic nervous systems. Autonomic disturbances are usually observed in patients with severe muscle involvement and respiratory muscle paralysis. The most dangerous autonomic dysfunctions include orthostatic hypotension, hypertension, and abnormal vagal responses (bradycardia, heart block, asystole). Other autonomic dysfunctions include bowel and bladder dysfunction, facial flushing, and diaphoresis (Koopman & Shcharinsky, 2012). Affected patients may also have the syndrome of inappropriate antidiuretic hormone secretion (SIADH, discussed in Chapter 51). Progression of GBS to include the lower brain stem involves the facial, abducens, oculomotor, hypoglossal, trigeminal, and vagus nerves (cranial nerves VII, VI, III, XII, V, and X, respectively). This involvement manifests itself through facial weakness, difficulties with extraocular eye movement, dysphagia, and paresthesia of the face.

Pain is a common symptom in patients with GBS secondary to the neuropathy that is occurring. The pain can be categorized as neuropathic pain and is described as prickling (paresthesia), burning, shooting, or stabbing. Pain appears to be worse at night. Pain may lead to a decrease in appetite and may interfere with sleep. Management of pain can include the use of analgesics such as nonsteroidal anti-inflammatory drugs, opioids, and drugs used to treat neuropathic pain (gabapentin, pregabalin, and carbamazepine). Nonpharmacological measures such as positioning, range-of-motion exercises, massage, and distraction can also be used to help manage pain. Pain management measures should be adapted based on assessment findings and evaluation of the pain management plan.

Complications. The most serious complication of this syndrome is respiratory failure, which occurs as the paralysis progresses to the nerves that innervate the thoracic area. Constant monitoring of the respiratory system by checking respiratory rate, depth, forced vital capacity, and negative inspiratory force provides information about the need for immediate intervention, including intubation and mechanical ventilation. Urinary tract infections (UTIs) or respiratory tract infections may occur. Fever is generally the first sign of infection, and treatment is directed at the infecting organism. Immobility from the paralysis can cause problems such as paralytic ileus, muscle atrophy, contractures, deep-vein thrombosis (DVT), pulmonary emboli (PEs), skin breakdown, orthostatic hypotension, and nutritional deficiencies.

Diagnostic Studies

Diagnosis is based primarily on the patient's history and clinical signs. Cerebro-spinal fluid (CSF) is normal or has a low protein content initially, but after 7 to 10 days, the protein level is elevated and the white cell count is normal. Results of EMG and nerve conduction studies are markedly abnormal and show evidence of demyelination (Koopman & Shcharinsky, 2012).

Collaborative Care

Management is aimed at supportive care, particularly ventilatory support, during the acute phase. Prevention of DVT and PE through prophylactic anticoagulation with heparin or low-molecular-weight heparin (LMWH) is routine. Practice guidelines endorse the use of plasma exchange or intravenous administration of immune globulin (IVIG) within 4 weeks of symptom onset in nonambulatory patients and within 2 weeks in ambulatory patients (Ansar & Valadi, 2015). Treatment results in distinct reductions in the length of hospital stay, length of time on a ventilator, and time required to resume walking. IVIG has also been shown to be as effective as plasma exchange (plasmapheresis) and has the advantage of immediate availability and greater safety. However, patients receiving IVIG need to be well hydrated and have adequate renal function. (Plasmapheresis is discussed in Chapter 16.) Once 3 weeks pass after disease onset, plasma exchange and IVIG therapies have little value. A review of the use of corticosteroids in the treatment of GBS has not shown them to be of any benefit (Ansar & Valadi, 2015).

Nutritional Therapy. Nutritional intake can be compromised in patients with GBS. During the acute phase, patients may experience difficulty swallowing because of cranial nerve involvement. Mild dysphagia can be managed by placing patients in an upright position and flexing the head forward during feeding. For more severe dysphagia, tube feedings may be required. Patients who experience paralytic ileus or intestinal obstruction may require total parenteral nutrition. Later in the course of the disease, motor paralysis or weakness continues to affect the ability to self-feed. Patients' nutritional status, including body weight, serum albumin levels, and calorie counts, must be evaluated at regular intervals.

NURSING MANAGEMENT
GUILLAIN-BARRÉ SYNDROME

NURSING ASSESSMENT

Assessment of patients with GBS is the most important aspect of nursing care during the acute phase. The nurse must monitor for ascending paralysis; assess respiratory function; monitor arterial blood gas (ABG) levels; and assess the gag, corneal, and swallowing reflexes during the routine assessment. Reflexes are usually decreased or absent.

Monitoring blood pressure and cardiac rate and rhythm is also important during the acute phase because transient cardiac dysrhythmias may occur as a result of autonomic dysfunction. Orthostatic hypotension secondary to muscle atony may occur in severe cases. Vasopressor agents and volume expanders may be needed to treat the low blood pressure. However, if SIADH is present, fluid restriction may be required.

NURSING DIAGNOSES

Nursing diagnoses for patients with GBS may include but are not limited to the following:

- *Impaired spontaneous ventilation* related to *respiratory muscle fatigue*
- *Risk for aspiration* as evidenced by *depressed gag reflex, impaired ability to swallow*
- *Acute pain* related to *physical injury agent* (paresthesias, muscle aches and cramps, hyperesthesias)
- *Impaired verbal communication* related to *environmental barrier* (intubation)
- *Anxiety* related to *threat to current status* (uncertain outcome and seriousness of the disease)
- *Self-care (bathing, dressing, feeding, toileting) deficits* related to fatigue, weakness, pain
- *Risk for impaired skin integrity* related to pressure over bony prominences (decreased mobility)

PLANNING

The overall goals are that the patient with GBS will (a) maintain adequate ventilation, (b) be free from aspiration, (c) be able to manage pain, (d) maintain an acceptable method of communication, (e) maintain adequate nutritional intake, and (f) return to usual physical functioning.

NURSING IMPLEMENTATION

The objective of therapy is to support body systems until the patient recovers. In the acute phase, patients are often cared for in the intensive care unit (ICU). Respiratory failure and infection are serious threats. Monitoring the vital lung capacity and ABG values is essential. If the vital capacity drops to less than 800 mL (15 mL/kg, or two-thirds of the patient's normal vital capacity) or the ABG levels deteriorate, endotracheal intubation or tracheostomy may be performed so that the patient can be mechanically ventilated (see Chapter 70). Meticulous suctioning technique is needed to prevent infection if the patient has an endotracheal tube or tracheostomy. Thorough bronchial hygiene and chest physiotherapy help clear secretions and prevent respiratory deterioration. If fever develops, sputum cultures should be obtained to identify the pathogen. Appropriate antibiotic therapy is then initiated.

Fear and anxiety are common feelings for both the patient and the family. These feelings often result from lack of knowledge regarding the disease progression. Answering the patient's and family's questions, clarifying misconceptions, and keeping the patient and the family informed help reduce this fear. Collaboration with other members of the interdisciplinary team, including occupational therapists and speech–language pathologists, is essential. At the peak of a severe episode, the patient may be incapable of communicating, and this can add to the patient's fear. A communication system must be established according to the patient's available abilities. Communication, however, remains extremely difficult if the disease progresses to involve the cranial nerves. The nurse must explain all procedures before performing them and reassure the patient that muscle function will return.

Urinary retention is common for a few days. Intermittent catheterization is preferred to an in-dwelling catheter to decrease the incidence of UTIs. However, for acutely ill patients receiving a large volume of fluids (>2.5 L/day), in-dwelling catheterization may be safer because it reduces overdistension of a temporarily flaccid bladder and prevents vesico-ureteral reflux. Physiotherapy is indicated early to help prevent problems related to immobility. Passive range-of-motion exercises and attention to body position help maintain function and prevent contractures. Patients who develop facial paralysis must receive meticulous eye care to prevent corneal irritation or damage (*exposure keratitis*). Artificial tears should be instilled frequently during the day to prevent drying of the cornea. The eyes should be inspected for the presence of eyelashes. Ointment and an impermeable eye shield can be used at night to retain moisture.

Nutritional needs must be met despite possible problems associated with delayed gastric emptying, paralytic ileus, and potential for aspiration if the gag reflex is lost. In addition to checking for the gag reflex, nurses should note drooling and other difficulties with secretions, which may be more indicative of an inadequate gag reflex. Initially, tube feedings or parenteral nutrition may be used to ensure adequate caloric intake. Because of delayed gastric emptying, residual volumes of the feedings should be assessed at regular intervals or before feedings (see Chapter 42). Fluid and electrolyte therapy must be monitored carefully to prevent electrolyte imbalances. A bowel program should be initiated because constipation is a common problem related to diet changes, immobility, and decreased gastro-intestinal motility.

Pain assessment should be completed at least daily with a valid and reliable tool and the patient's self-report. A method of assessing pain without the patient's self-report may have to be established if the patient is unable to communicate verbally.

Patients with GBS who are experiencing paralysis are prone to skin breakdown as a result of immobility and decreased sensation. Patients should be assisted or encouraged to turn frequently; a turning schedule can be helpful in this regard. Skin and wound assessment should be performed daily. Specialty pressure-relieving beds can be used to decrease the potential for skin breakdown in these patients.

Throughout the course of the illness, the nurse must provide support and encouragement to the family and the patient. Residual problems and relapses are uncommon except in the chronic form of the disease. Complete recovery can be anticipated, although many patients continue to have a degree of residual pain and fatigue requiring them to change their work and daily activities. Recovery is a slow process that takes months (3–6 on average), with the majority of recovery occurring within the first year. Further recovery can be seen even up to 3 years (Willison, Jacobs, & van Doorn, 2016).

EVALUATION

The following are expected outcomes for the patient with GBS:
- Return to usual level of physical functioning
- Freedom from pain and discomfort
- Maintenance of nutritional status

BOTULISM

Etiology and Pathophysiology

Botulism is an acute neurological disorder that causes potentially life-threatening neuroparalysis due to a neurotoxin produced by the spore-forming bacterium *Clostridium botulinum,* which is present naturally throughout the environment and can be found in soil, water, and household dust and on surfaces of many foods. There are three main clinical presentations: foodborne botulism, infant botulism, and wound botulism. Botulism, a reportable disease, is rare in Canada. All forms of botulism can cause paralysis and be fatal. It is thought that the botulism neurotoxin destroys or inhibits the neurotransmission of acetylcholine at the myoneural junction, resulting in disturbed muscle innervation. The classic syndrome of botulism is a symmetrical, descending motor paralysis in an alert patient, with no sensory deficits (Public Health Agency of Canada, 2012).

Clinical Manifestations

Symptoms of foodborne botulism generally begin 12 to 36 hours after ingesting contaminated food; however, onset can begin as soon as 6 hours after exposure, or as long as 10 days later. Neurological manifestations develop rapidly over 2 to 4 days. Early symptoms for all types of botulism include fatigue, weakness, dizziness, double or blurred vision, difficulty speaking and swallowing, dry mouth, and headache. Symptoms associated with foodborne botulism include nausea, vomiting, and abdominal cramps. Paralysis typically starts in the shoulders and arms and progresses down the body. The course of the disease depends on the amount of toxin absorbed. If only a small amount is absorbed, symptoms are mild and recovery is complete. When large amounts are absorbed, death may occur from circulatory failure, respiratory paralysis, or development of pulmonary complications. With proper early treatment, the fatality rate of botulism cases in Canada is as low as 5% to 10% (Public Health Agency of Canada, 2012).

Drug Therapy

The initial treatment of botulism is intravenous administration of botulinum antitoxin. Botulism antitoxin may be readministered in 2 to 4 hours if symptoms persist and again at 12- to 24-hour intervals if required.

The gastro-intestinal tract is purged by high colonic enemas, gastric lavage, and laxatives that do not contain magnesium to decrease the absorption of the toxin. Magnesium is contraindicated because it worsens toxin-induced neuro-muscular blockade.

Most people recover if diagnosed and treated quickly. Recovery can take several weeks to months. Severe botulism can require intensive medical and nursing care. If not diagnosed and treated, botulism can lead to death from respiratory failure within 3 to 10 days.

TETANUS

Etiology and Pathophysiology

Tetanus (lockjaw) is an extremely severe polyradiculitis (inflammation of the nerve roots) and polyneuritis (inflammation of nerves) affecting spinal and cranial nerves. It results from the effects of a potent neurotoxin produced by *Clostridium tetani*. The toxin interferes with the function of the reflex arc by blocking inhibitory transmitters at the presynaptic sites in the spinal cord and the brain stem. The spores of the bacillus are present in soil, garden mould, and manure. Thus *C. tetani* enters the body through contamination of a traumatic wound that provides an appropriate low-oxygen environment for the organisms to mature and produce toxin. The incubation period for tetanus is usually 3 to 21 days, with a range of 1 day to several months.

Tetanus is very rare in Canada thanks to routine immunizations. Over the years, the death rate has fallen to almost zero. Only six deaths had been reported in Canada between 2000 and 2014, with the last death reported in 2010 (Public Health Agency of Canada, 2014).

Clinical Manifestations

Initial manifestations of generalized tetanus include a feeling of stiffness in the jaw *(trismus)* or the neck, fever, and other symptoms of general infection; these symptoms then descend. Generalized tonic spasms occur because of the lack of reciprocal innervation. As the disease progresses, the neck muscles, the back, the abdomen, and the extremities become progressively rigid. In severe forms, continuous tonic convulsions may occur with *opisthotonos* (extreme arching of the back and retraction of the head). Laryngeal and respiratory spasms cause apnea and anoxia. Additional effects are manifested by overstimulation of the sympathetic nervous system, including profuse diaphoresis, labile hypertension, episodic tachycardia, hyperthermia, and dysrhythmias. The slightest noise, jarring motion, or bright light can set off a seizure. These seizures are agonizing. Mortality rates are highest in infants and older adults, and death is usually attributable to asphyxia or heart failure resulting from constantly recurring spasms. Residual injury—such as vertebral fracture, muscle contracture, and brain damage secondary to hypoxia—may be long-term consequences.

Drug Therapy. The management of tetanus includes administration of tetanus and diphtheria toxoid booster and tetanus immune globulin (TIG) before the onset of symptoms to neutralize circulating toxins (see Chapter 71, Table 71-6). A much larger dose of TIG is administered to patients with manifestations of clinical tetanus. Control of spasms is essential and is managed by deep sedation and skeletal muscle relaxation, usually with diazepam (Valium), barbiturates, and, in severe cases, neuro-muscular blocking agents such as rocuronium (Zemuron) that act to paralyze skeletal muscles. Opioid analgesics such as morphine or fentanyl are also indicated for pain management. A 10- to 14-day course of penicillin, metronidazole, tetracycline, or doxycycline is recommended to inhibit further growth of *C. tetani.*

Because of laryngospasm and the potential need for neuro-muscular blocking drugs, a tracheostomy is usually performed early, and the patient is maintained on mechanical ventilation. Sedative agents and opioid analgesics are given concomitantly to all patients who are pharmacologically paralyzed. Any recognized wound should be debrided, and any abscess drained. Antibiotics may be given to prevent secondary infections. Nutrition is maintained through parenteral nutrition or nasogastric feeding. The mortality rate associated with tetanus is declining. For patients who recover, convalescence is long and includes extensive physiotherapy.

NURSING MANAGEMENT
TETANUS

Health teaching is aimed at ensuring tetanus prophylaxis, which is the most important factor influencing the incidence of this disease. Tetanus prevention and immunization protocols are summarized in Table 71-6 in Chapter 71. Adults should receive a tetanus and diphtheria toxoid booster every 10 years. The patient should be taught that immediate, thorough cleansing of all wounds with soap and water is important to the prevention of tetanus. If a patient sustains an open wound and has not been immunized within the previous 5 years, the health care provider should be contacted so that the patient can receive a tetanus booster.

The acute nursing management of the patient with tetanus is aimed at supportive care based on the treatment of clinical manifestations. The patient should be placed in a quiet, darkened room that is insulated against noise. Sedation should be induced judiciously. Nursing care should be administered with the utmost caution to avoid triggering spasms. Nursing care related to tracheostomy and mechanical ventilation is given as appropriate. An in-dwelling urinary catheter may be used to prevent bladder distension and urinary reflux in the presence of spasms in the muscles of the pelvic floor. Attention is also given to skin care. The patient needs emotional support during the acute phase because of the fear of death. The family also needs support and education.

NEURO-SYPHILIS

Neuro-syphilis is an infection of any part of the nervous system by the organism *Treponema pallidum* (see Chapter 55). The organism can invade the central nervous system within a few months of the original infection, and the disease can be fatal if not treated. Neuro-syphilis is often referred to incorrectly as "tertiary syphilis," but it can occur at any time in the course of syphilis and occurs in about 30% of untreated cases (Marra, 2015). Except for causing some changes in the CSF, including increases in the white blood cell count and protein levels and positive serological reaction, *T. pallidum* lies dormant for years. Late neuro-syphilis results from degenerative changes in the spinal cord *(tabes dorsalis)* and the brain stem *(general paresis)*. *Tabes dorsalis* (progressive locomotor ataxia) is characterized by vague, sharp pains in the legs; ataxia; "slapping" gait; loss of proprioception and deep tendon reflexes; and zones of hyperesthesia. *Charcot joints,* which are characterized by enlargement, bone destruction, and hypermobility, also occur as a result of joint effusion and edema. Other manifestations of neuro-syphilis include seizures and problems with vision and hearing.

Neurological symptoms associated with neuro-syphilis are numerous and, in many cases, nonspecific. Neuro-syphilis is a differential diagnosis for patients with neurological and psychiatric symptoms. *Dementia paralytica* is an ongoing spirochetal meningo-encephalitis that causes a general dissolution of mental and physical capabilities. It may mimic a number of major or minor psychoses. Management includes treatment with penicillin, symptomatic care, and protection from physical injury.

SPINAL CORD PROBLEMS

SPINAL CORD INJURY

Spinal cord injuries (SCIs) have a devastating effect on health and well-being. The physical effects of SCI, as well as the complications and comorbid conditions associated with SCI, significantly affect quality of life and can even be life-threatening. Associated economic burdens result not only from health care costs but also from physical morbidity and premature mortality that affect productivity at a societal level. SCI is divided into traumatic (result of external physical impact) and nontraumatic (result of disease, infection, or tumour) categories.

The incidence of SCIs in Canada in 2010, based on discharge incidence (those discharged into the community), was reported to be 1 389 cases per year for traumatic SCI and 2 286 per year for nontraumatic SCI (Noonan, Fingas, Farry, et al., 2012). The overall prevalence of SCI in Canada is 85 586 persons (51% traumatic SCI and 49% nontraumatic SCI) (Noonan, Fingas, Farry, et al., 2012). Projected prevalence of SCI by 2025 is estimated to be 121 000 people living with SCI in Canada, with the greatest increase being individuals in the nontraumatic category (Farry & Baxter, 2010). The predicted increase in nontraumatic SCI is due to the aging population, which will result in a greater number of older individuals (60 years and older) living with SCI in the community. Traumatic SCI typically occurs in a younger age group, 20 to 30 years of age, with male-to-female ratio of 4:1, with the next largest group being those in the age range of 60 to 70 years of age, with male-to-female ratio of 2:1 (Noonan, Fingas, Farry, et al., 2012).

Older adults with traumatic injuries experience more complications, are hospitalized longer, and have a higher rate of mortality. Injuries are most common in the cervical spine, and such injuries are associated with the most devastating neurological impairments. In comparison with the general population, an individual with a traumatic SCI has a shorter life expectancy (15–30 years less), requires 2.7 times more contact with a physician, requires 30 times more hours of home care services, and is rehospitalized 2.6 times more often (Farry & Baxter, 2010).

The most common causes of premature death in the patient with **tetraplegia** (formerly called *quadriplegia* and used interchangeably; paralysis of both arms and legs and the trunk, which occurs with spinal cord damage at C8 or above) are usually related to compromised respiratory function (pneumonia), impaired renal function (UTI), and impaired skin integrity (pressure injuries). Any combination of these will certainly increase risk for mortality.

Because of the potential for disruption of individual growth and development, altered family dynamics, economic loss in terms of absence from work, and the high cost of rehabilitation and long-term health care, spinal cord trauma is a major problem. Lifetime economic burden of SCI is substantial. For individuals with traumatic SCI, the estimates range from $1.5 million for incomplete **paraplegia** (paralysis and loss of sensation in the lower limbs and the trunk) to a cost of $3.0 million for complete tetraplegia (Krueger, Noonan, Trenaman, et al., 2013). Although many people with SCIs can care for themselves independently, those with the highest level of injury may require round-the-clock care at home or in a long-term care facility.

Etiology and Pathophysiology

Common causes of traumatic SCI include motor vehicle and motorcycle crashes, which account for 50%, and falls and work-related injuries (30%–40%). Falls are more typically causes of SCI in the older adult while motor vehicle crashes are a more common cause among young adults. The most common anatomical region affected by injury is the cervical spine (Singh, Tetreault, Kalsi-Ryan, et al., 2014).

Initial Injury. SCI can result from cord compression by bone displacement, tumour, or abscess or from interruption of blood supply to the cord. The spinal cord is wrapped in tough layers of dura and is rarely torn or transected by direct trauma. Penetrating trauma, such as gunshot and stab wounds, can result in tearing and transection. The pathophysiology of SCI is best described as *biphasic*. The initial mechanical injury *(primary injury)* with failure of the spinal column (fracture or dislocation) imparts force to the spinal cord, disrupting axons, blood vessels, and cell membranes. This process is followed by a second phase *(secondary injury)* involving vascular dysfunction, edema, ischemia, electrolyte shifts, inflammation, free radical production, and apoptotic cell death (Witiw & Fehlings, 2015).

At the molecular level, *apoptosis* (cell death) occurs and may continue for weeks or months after the initial injury. Thus the complete cord damage in severe trauma is related to autodestruction of the cord. This autodestruction is confirmed by observations that, shortly after the injury, petechial hemorrhages occur in the central grey matter of the cord. This hemorrhaging further leads to microvascular disruption and hemorrhage in surrounding white matter. Cord ischemia develops and may extend for many segments above and below the injury (Witiw & Fehlings, 2015). By 24 hours or less after injury, the development of edema above and below the level of injury as a result of ischemic damage may cause permanent cord damage. This ongoing destructive process is dominant early on, and it is therefore crucial that the initial care and management of the patient with an SCI limit further activation of these processes.

Figure 63-4 illustrates the cascade of events causing secondary injury after traumatic SCI. The resulting hypoxia reduces the oxygen tension below the level that meets the metabolic

PATHOPHYSIOLOGY MAP

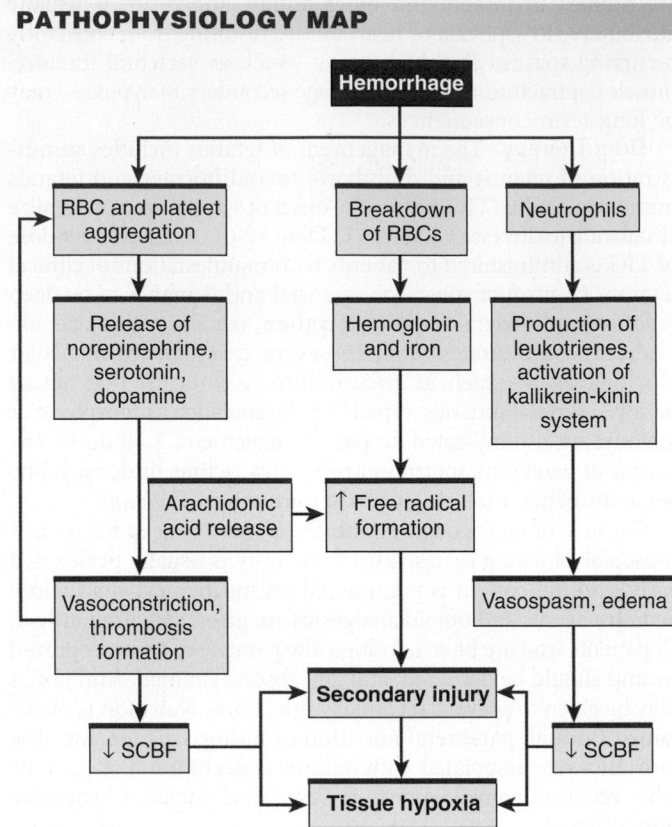

FIGURE 63-4 Cascade of metabolic and cellular events that leads to spinal cord ischemia and the hypoxia of secondary injury. *RBC,* red blood cell; *SCBF,* spinal cord blood flow. Source: Redrawn from Marciano, F. F., Greene, K., Apostolides, P. J., et al. (1995). Pharmacologic management of spinal cord injury. *BNI Quarterly, 11*(2), 6; and from McCance, K. L., & Huether, S. E. (2006). *Pathophysiology: The biologic basis for disease in adults and children* (5th ed.). St. Louis: Mosby.

needs of the spinal cord. Lactate metabolites and an increase in vasoactive substances—including norepinephrine, serotonin, and dopamine—are noted. At high levels, these vasoactive substances cause vasospasms and hypoxia, leading to subsequent necrosis. Unfortunately, the spinal cord has minimal ability to adapt to vasospasm.

The extent of the neurological damage caused by an SCI results both from primary injury or damage (actual physical disruption of axons) and from secondary injury damage (ischemia, hypoxia, microhemorrhage, and edema) (Witiw & Fehlings, 2015). Because secondary injury processes occur over time, the extent of injury and the prognosis for recovery are most accurately determined at 72 hours or longer after injury.

Spinal and Neurogenic Shock. About 50% of people with acute SCI experience a temporary neurological syndrome known as **spinal shock** that is characterized by decreased reflexes, loss of sensation, and flaccid paralysis below the level of the injury (Chin, 2015). This syndrome lasts days to months and may mask post-injury neurological function. Active rehabilitation may begin in the presence of spinal shock.

Neurogenic shock, in contrast, is caused by SCI at the fifth thoracic (T5) vertebra or above. It is a hemodynamic syndrome of massive vasodilation without compensation that results from the loss of sympathetic nervous system vasoconstrictor tone caused by spinal cord injury. Neurogenic shock is characterized

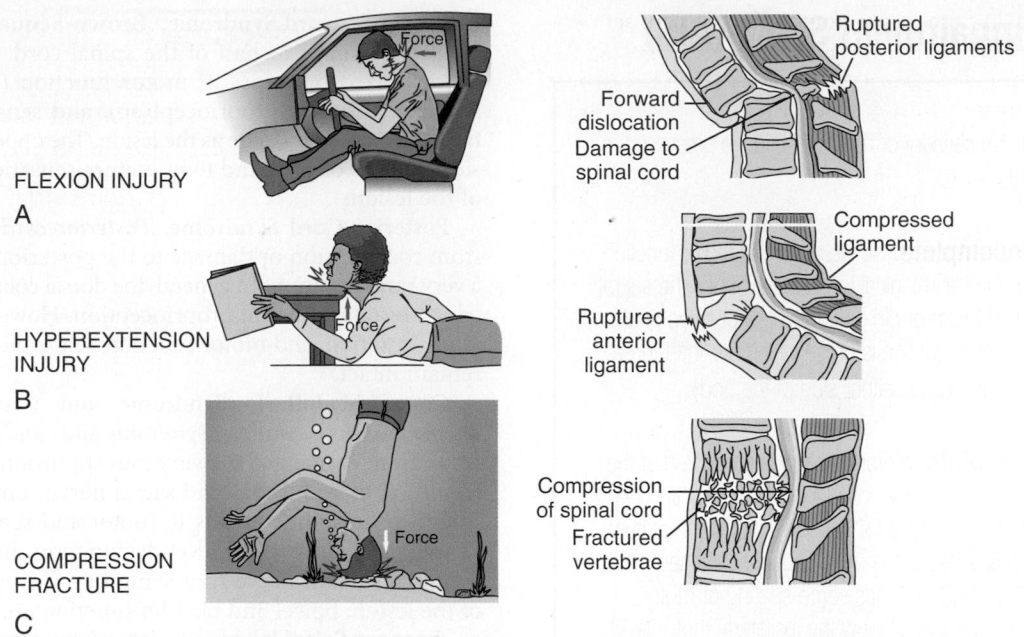

FLEXION INJURY
A

HYPEREXTENSION INJURY
B

COMPRESSION FRACTURE
C

Ruptured posterior ligaments

Forward dislocation
Damage to spinal cord

Compressed ligament

Ruptured anterior ligament

Compression of spinal cord
Fractured vertebrae

FIGURE 63-5 Mechanisms of spinal cord injury. Many situations can produce these injuries. This figure shows only some examples. **A,** Flexion injury of the cervical spine ruptures the posterior ligaments. **B,** Hyperextension injury of the cervical spine ruptures the anterior ligaments. **C,** Compression fractures crush the vertebrae and force bony fragments into the spinal canal. Source: Copstead-Kirkhorn, L. C., & Banasik, J. L. (2014). *Pathophysiology* (5th ed., p. 937, Figure 45-12). Philadelphia: W. B. Saunders.

by hypotension, bradycardia, and loss of sympathetic innervation, which produces peripheral vasodilation, venous pooling, and a decreased cardiac output (Chin, 2015).

Classification of Spinal Cord Injury. SCIs are classified according to the mechanism of injury, the skeletal and neurological level of injury, and the completeness or degree of injury.

Mechanisms of Injury. The major mechanisms of injury are flexion, hyperextension, flexion-rotation, extension-rotation, and compression (Figure 63-5). The flexion-rotation injury is the most unstable of all injuries because the ligamentous structures that stabilize the spine are torn. This injury is most often implicated in severe neurological deficits.

Level of Injury. The *skeletal level* of injury is the vertebral level where damage to vertebral bones and ligaments is most extensive. The *neurological level* of injury is the lowest segment of the spinal cord at which sensory and motor function on both sides of the body are normal. The level of injury may be cervical, thoracic, or lumbar. Cervical and lumbar injuries are most common because these levels are associated with the greatest flexibility and movement. If the cervical cord is involved, paralysis of all four extremities (tetraplegia) occurs. If the thoracic cord or conus in the lumbar spine is damaged, the result is paraplegia. Figure 63-6 shows affected structures and functions at different levels of cord injury.

Degree of Injury. The degree of spinal cord involvement may be either complete or incomplete (partial). *Complete cord involvement* (American Spinal Injury Association [ASIA] grade A) results in total loss of sensory and motor function below the level of the lesion (injury). *Incomplete cord involvement* (ASIA grades B–D) results in a mixed loss of motor and sensory function (Figure 63-7). The degree of sensory and motor loss varies depending on the level of the lesion and reflects the specific nerve tracts damaged. Six syndromes are associated with incomplete lesions: central cord syndrome, anterior cord syndrome,

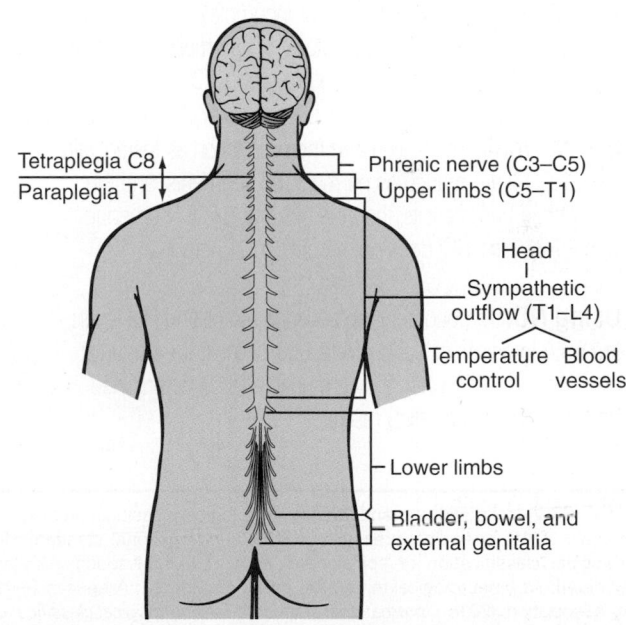

Tetraplegia C8
Paraplegia T1

Phrenic nerve (C3–C5)
Upper limbs (C5–T1)

Head
Sympathetic outflow (T1–L4)

Temperature control   Blood vessels

Lower limbs

Bladder, bowel, and external genitalia

FIGURE 63-6 Results of spinal cord injury, depending on location. Symptoms, degree of paralysis, and potential for rehabilitation depend on the level of the lesion.

Brown-Séquard syndrome, posterior cord syndrome, cauda equina syndrome, and conus medullaris syndrome.

Central Cord Syndrome. Damage to the central spinal cord is termed *central cord syndrome*. It occurs most commonly in the cervical cord region and is common with hyperextension injuries. Motor weakness and sensory loss are present in both the upper and the lower extremities; the upper extremities are more affected than the lower ones.

ASIA Impairment Scale (AIS)

A = Complete. No sensory or motor function is preserved in the sacral segments S4-5.

B = Sensory Incomplete. Sensory but not motor function is preserved below the neurological level and includes the sacral segments S4-5 (light touch or pin prick at S4-5 or deep anal pressure) AND no motor function is preserved more than three levels below the motor level on either side of the body.

C = Motor Incomplete. Motor function is preserved at the most caudal sacral segments for voluntary anal contraction (VAC) OR the patient meets the criteria for sensory incomplete status (sensory function preserved at the most caudal sacral segments (S4-S5) by LT, PP or DAP), and has some sparing of motor function more than three levels below the ipsilateral motor level on either side of the body.
(This includes key or non-key muscle functions to determine motor incomplete status.) For AIS C – less than half of key muscle functions below the single NLI have a muscle grade ≥3.

D = Motor Incomplete. Motor incomplete status as defined above, with at least half (half or more) of key muscle functions below the single NLI having a muscle grade ≥3.

E = Normal. If sensation and motor function as tested with the ISNCSCI are graded as normal in all segments, and the patient had prior deficits, then the AIS grade is E. Someone without an initial SCI does not receive an AIS grade.

Using ND: To document the sensory, motor and NLI levels, the ASIA Impairment Scale grade, and/or the zone of partial preservation (ZPP) when they are unable to be determined based on the examination results.

FIGURE 63-7 International standards for neurological classification of spinal cord injury. *DAP,* deep anal pressure; *ISNCSCI,* international standards for neurological classification of spinal cord injury; *LT,* light touch; *ND,* not determined; *NLI,* neurological injury; *PP,* pin prick. Source: American Spinal Injury Association. (2015). *International standards for neurological classification of spinal cord injury.* Retrieved from *http://asia-spinalinjury.org/wp-content/uploads/2016/02/International_Stds_Diagram_Worksheet.pdf.* © 2011 American Spinal Injury Association. Reprinted with permission.

Anterior Cord Syndrome. *Anterior cord syndrome* is caused by damage to the anterior spinal artery. It typically results from acute compression of the anterior portion of the spinal cord, often from a flexion injury. Manifestations include motor paralysis and loss of pain and temperature sensation below the level of injury. Because the posterior cord tracts are not injured, sensations of touch, position, vibration, and motion remain intact.

Brown-Séquard Syndrome. Brown-Séquard syndrome is a result of damage to half of the spinal cord. This syndrome is characterized by a loss of motor function (spastic paralysis), sense of position (proprioception), and sense of vibration on the same *(ipsilateral)* side as the lesion. The opposite *(contralateral)* side has loss of pain and temperature sensation below the level of the lesion.

Posterior Cord Syndrome. *Posterior cord syndrome* results from compression or damage to the posterior spinal artery. It is a very rare condition. In general, the dorsal columns are damaged, which results in loss of proprioception. However, pain, temperature sensation, and motor function below the level of the lesion remain intact.

Conus Medullaris Syndrome and Cauda Equina Syndrome. *Conus medullaris syndrome* and *cauda equina syndrome* result from damage to the very lowest portion of the spinal cord *(conus)* and the lumbar and sacral nerve roots *(cauda equina).* Injury to the conus results in motor and sensory impairment, as well as bladder and bowel dysfunction. Injury to the cauda equina results in nerve root symptoms dependent on the level of the lesion; bowel and bladder function are typically affected.

American Spinal Injury Association Impairment Scale. The ASIA Impairment Scale is the "gold standard" assessment scale used for classifying the severity of impairment resulting from SCI. It combines assessments of motor and sensory function of various myotomes and dermatomes to determine neurological level and completeness of injury. The strength of key muscle groups is graded on a scale of 0 to 5 and is tested bilaterally. Sensation is documented as *absent, impaired,* or *normal.* An ASIA grade (A–E) is then determined based on the assessment findings (Figure 63-8). This grading establishes whether the findings indicate complete or incomplete SCI or are normal. Various incomplete cord syndromes are also defined with this classification system and have been discussed previously. In addition, this scale is useful for recording changes in neurological status and identifying appropriate functional goals for rehabilitation.

Clinical Manifestations

The manifestations of SCI are generally the direct result of trauma that causes cord compression, ischemia, edema, and, rarely, cord transection. Manifestations of SCI are related to the level and the degree of injury. A patient with an incomplete lesion may demonstrate a mixture of symptoms. The higher the injury, the more serious the sequelae because of the proximity of the cervical cord to the medulla and the brain stem. Movement and functional goals related to specific locations of the SCI are described in Table 63-2. In general, sensory function closely parallels motor function at all levels.

Immediate post-injury care includes maintaining patency of the airway, adequate ventilation, and adequate circulating blood volume and blood pressure to minimize extension of spinal cord damage (secondary injury).

Respiratory System. Respiratory complications closely correspond to the level of the injury (Grossman, Frankowski, Burau, et al., 2012). Cervical injury above the level of C4 presents special problems because of the total loss of respiratory muscle function. Mechanical ventilation is required to keep the patient alive. At one time, most patients with these injuries died at the scene of the injury, but with improved emergency medical services, more such patients are surviving the initial events of the SCI. Injury or fracture below the level of C4 spares diaphragmatic breathing if the phrenic nerve is functioning. Even if the injury is below C4,

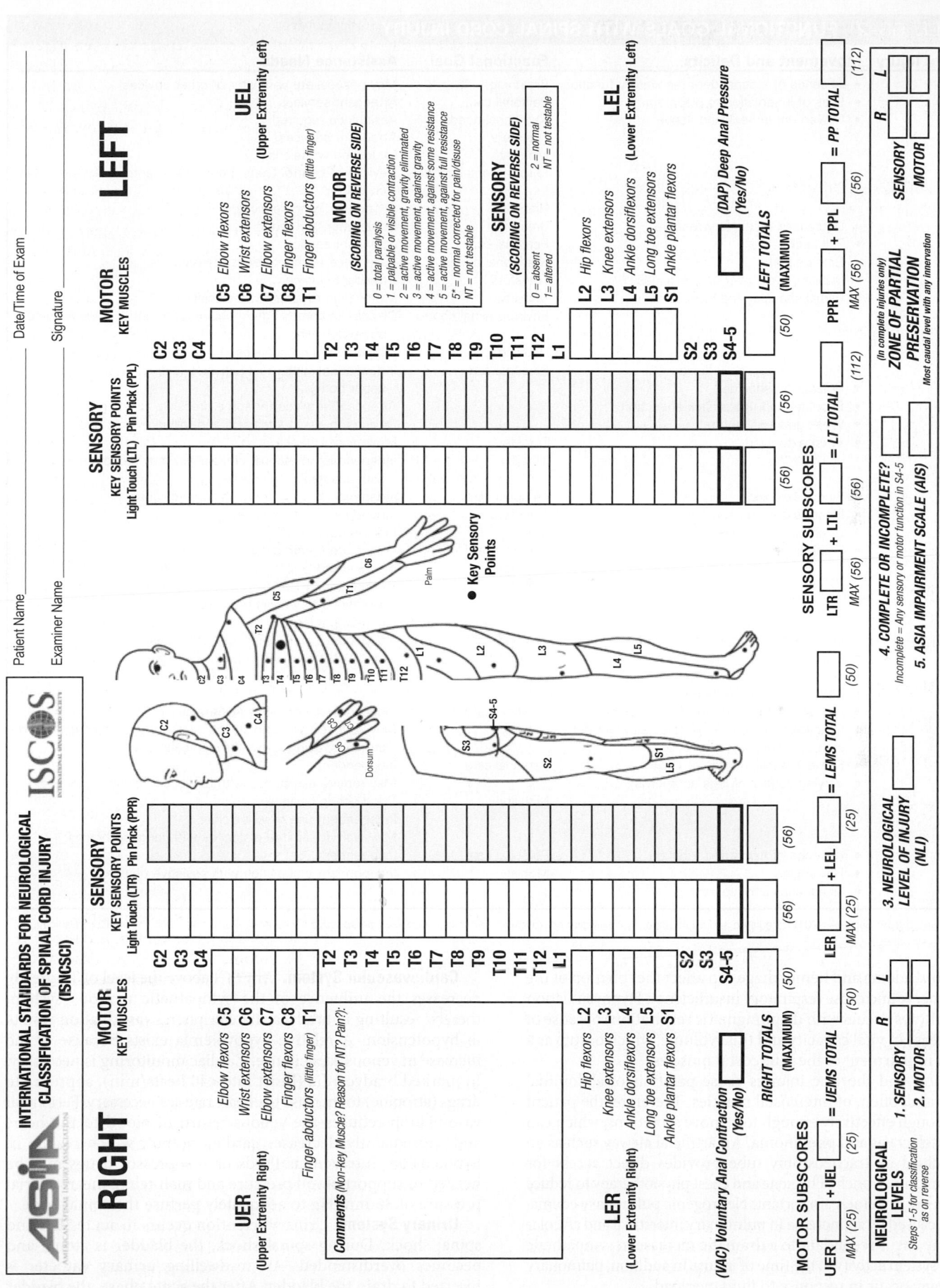

FIGURE 63-8 International standards for neurological classification of spinal cord injury. Source: American Spinal Injury Association. (2015). *International standards for neurological classification of spinal cord injury.* Retrieved from http://asia-spinalinjury.org/wp-content/uploads/2016/02/International_Stds_Diagram_Worksheet.pdf. © 2011 American Spinal Injury Association. Reprinted with permission.

TABLE 63-2   FUNCTIONAL GOALS WITH SPINAL CORD INJURY

Level of Injury	Movement and Deficits	Functional Goal	Assistance Needs
C1–4	• Absence of independent respiratory function • Loss of innervation to diaphragm • Movement in neck and above	Breathing Personal care Nutritional needs Transfers Mobility Environmental control Housing	May necessitate ventilator or other devices Attendant services Assistance required Attendant services Motorized wheelchair Devices to control lights, phone, door entry, voice-activated computer Supportive living services
C5	• Decreased respiratory reserve • Full neck • Gross elbow • Inability to roll over or use hands • Partial shoulder and biceps	Breathing Personal care Nutritional needs Transfers Mobility Environmental control Housing	No assistance needed Attendant services Assistance to meet needs (devices) Attendant services Motorized or manual wheelchair Devices to control lights, phone, door entry, voice-activated computer Supportive living services
C6	• Full biceps to elbow flexion • Rotation at shoulder • Shoulder and upper back abduction • Weak grasp of thumb • Wrist extension	Personal care Transfers Mobility	Independent with most activities (eating, washing, dressing upper body) Attendant services for some dressing, toileting Devices to assist sitting up and rolling over in bed Minimal assistance Independent in manual wheelchair; may be able to drive with adaptation to vehicle
C7	• Elbow extension • Finger extensors and flexors • Good grasp with some decreased strength	Personal care Transfers Mobility	Independent with most self-care activities Independent with transfers Independent in wheelchair
C8–T1	• Same as for C7	Personal care Transfers Mobility Driving Housing	Independent with all self-care activities Independent Independent Adaptations to vehicle required Independent living
T2–6	• Decreased trunk stability • Full movement of upper extremities • Full strength and dexterity of grasp • Intrinsic muscles of hand	Personal care Mobility	Independent with all self-care activities May be able to stand in long leg braces with supports
T7–12	• Full, stable thoracic muscles and upper back • Functional intercostal muscles and therefore increased respiratory reserve	Personal care Mobility	Independent with all self-care activities May walk for limited distances with long leg braces and crutches, using swing-through gait
1 1–2	• Some instability of lower back • Varying control of legs and pelvis	Personal care Mobility	Independent May require assistance with bowel and bladder functioning Good sitting balance Independent use of wheelchair May walk for limited distances with long leg braces
L3–4	• Absence of hamstring function • Flail ankles • Quadriceps and hip flexors	Personal care Mobility	Independent Independent ambulation with assistive devices

Source: Adapted from Sarro, A. (2012). Pediatric and adult spine. In *Navigating neuroscience nursing: A Canadian perspective* (Chapter 4). Pembroke, ON: Pappin Communications.

spinal cord edema and hemorrhage can affect the function of the phrenic nerve and cause respiratory insufficiency. Hypoventilation almost always occurs with diaphragmatic respirations because of the decrease in vital capacity and tidal volume, which occurs as a result of impairment of the intercostal muscles.

Cervical and thoracic injuries cause paralysis of abdominal muscles and, often, of intercostal muscles. Therefore, the patient cannot cough effectively enough to remove secretions, which can lead to atelectasis and pneumonia. An artificial airway such as an endotracheal or tracheostomy tube provides direct access for pathogens; thus bronchial hygiene and chest physiotherapy to reduce infection are extremely important. Neurogenic pulmonary edema, which is caused by an increase in pulmonary interstitial and alveolar fluid, may occur secondary to a dramatic increase in sympathetic nervous system activity at the time of injury. In addition, pulmonary edema may occur in response to fluid overload.

Cardiovascular System.   Any SCI above the level of T6 greatly decreases the influence of the sympathetic nervous system, thereby resulting in bradycardia. Peripheral vasodilation results in hypotension. A relative hypovolemia exists because of the increase in venous capacitance. Cardiac monitoring is necessary. In marked bradycardia (heart rate <40 beats/min), appropriate drugs (atropine) to increase the heart rate are necessary. Peripheral vasodilation reduces the venous return of blood to the heart and subsequently decreases cardiac output, which results in hypotension. Intravenous fluids or vasopressor drugs may be needed to support blood pressure and maintain a mean arterial pressure of 85 mm Hg to adequately perfuse the spinal cord.

Urinary System.   Urinary retention occurs in acute SCIs and spinal shock. During spinal shock, the bladder is atonic and becomes overdistended. An in-dwelling urinary catheter is inserted to drain the bladder. After the acute phase, the bladder may become hyperirritable, with a loss of inhibition from the brain, which results in reflex emptying. Once the patient is medically and hemodynamically stable and large quantities of intravenous fluids are no longer required, the in-dwelling catheter should be removed and intermittent catheterization should begin as early as possible. Removal of the in-dwelling catheter helps to maintain bladder tone and decrease the risk for infection. (Intermittent catheterization is discussed later on in this chapter and in Chapter 48.)

Gastro-Intestinal System. If the cord injury has occurred above the level of T5, the primary gastro-intestinal problems are related to hypomotility. Decreased gastro-intestinal motor activity contributes to the development of paralytic ileus and gastric distension. A nasogastric tube for intermittent suctioning may relieve the gastric distension. Metoclopramide may be used to treat delayed gastric emptying. The development of stress ulcers is common because of excessive release of hydrochloric acid in the stomach. Histamine H_2-receptor blockers (such as ranitidine [Zantac] and famotidine [Pepcid AC]) and proton pump inhibitors (e.g., omeprazole [Losec] or lansoprazole [Prevacid]) are frequently administered to prevent the occurrence of stress ulcers during the initial phase. Intra-abdominal bleeding may occur and is difficult to diagnose because the patient exhibits no subjective signs such as pain, tenderness, or guarding. Continued hypotension, despite vigorous treatment and decreased hemoglobin and hematocrit, may be indications of bleeding. The girth of the abdomen may also expand.

Loss of neurological control over the bowel results in a *neurogenic bowel*. In the early period after injury when spinal shock is present and for patients with an injury level of T12 or below, the bowel is areflexic and sphincter tone is decreased. As reflexes return, the bowel becomes reflexic, sphincter tone is enhanced, and reflex emptying occurs. Both types of neurogenic bowel can be managed successfully with a regular bowel program coordinated with the gastrocolic reflex to minimize untimely incontinence.

Integumentary System. A major consequence of lack of movement is the potential for skin breakdown over bony prominences in areas of decreased or no sensation. Pressure injuries can occur quickly and can lead to major infection or sepsis. See Chapter 14 for further information on pressure injuries.

Thermoregulation. Poikilothermism is the adjustment of the body temperature to the room temperature. It occurs in patients with SCIs because the interruption of the sympathetic nervous system prevents peripheral temperature sensations from reaching the hypothalamus. The ability to sweat or shiver is also decreased below the level of the lesion, which affects the ability to regulate body temperature. The degree of poikilothermism depends on the level of injury. Patients with high cervical injuries have a greater loss of the ability to regulate temperature than do those with thoracic or lumbar injuries.

Metabolic Needs. Nasogastric suctioning may lead to metabolic alkalosis, and decreases in tissue perfusion may lead to acidosis. Electrolyte levels can be altered by gastric suctioning and must be monitored until suctioning is discontinued and normal nutritional requirements are met. Loss of body weight (10% or more) is common, and nitrogen excretion mirrors weight loss (Fraser, McIntyre, Thompson, et al., 2014). Nutritional needs are much greater than what would be expected for an immobilized person. A positive nitrogen balance, which may not occur for more than 2 months after the injury, and a high-protein diet help prevent skin breakdown and infections and decrease the rate of muscle atrophy.

Peripheral Vascular Problems. DVT is a common problem accompanying SCI during the first 3 months (Chung, Lee, Kim, et al., 2011). It is more difficult to detect a DVT in a person with an SCI because the patient does not exhibit the usual signs and symptoms, such as pain and tenderness. PE is one of the leading causes of death in patients with SCI. Techniques for assessment of DVT include Doppler ultrasound examination and measurement of leg and thigh girth.

Diagnostic Studies

Complete spine radiography may be performed initially to assess for vertebral fracture. However, MRI has become the "gold standard" for imaging neurological tissues, including the spinal cord. It is recommended that MRI be used to direct clinical decision making. An MRI is performed to assess spinal cord compression and damage, ligamentous injury, and soft tissue changes (Morais, de Melo Neto, Meguins, et al., 2014). CT may be used to assess the degree of bony injury and the degree of spinal canal compromise. A comprehensive neurological examination is performed, along with assessment of head, chest, and abdomen for additional injuries or trauma. In patients with cervical injuries who demonstrate altered mental status, vertebral angiography may also be needed to rule out vertebral artery damage.

Collaborative Care

The initial goals for the patient with an SCI are to sustain life and prevent further cord damage. Table 63-3 outlines the emergency management of a patient with an SCI. Systemic and neurogenic shock must be treated to maintain blood pressure. For injury at the cervical level, all body systems must be maintained until the full extent of the damage can be evaluated.

Collaborative care during the acute phase for a patient with a cervical injury is described in Table 63-4. The systemic support required by the patient is less intense for SCIs of the thoracic and lumbar vertebrae. Respiratory compromise is not as severe, and bradycardia is not a problem. Specific problems are treated symptomatically. After stabilization at the injury scene, the patient is transferred to a medical facility, where further assessment, both clinical and radiological, is completed. A thorough assessment is performed to specifically evaluate the degree of deficit and to establish the level and the degree of injury. A history is obtained, with emphasis on how the accident occurred and the extent of injury as perceived by the patient immediately after the accident. Assessment involves testing muscle groups rather than individual muscles. Muscle groups should be tested with and against gravity, alone and against resistance, and on both sides of the body. Spontaneous movement should be noted. The patient should be asked to move legs and then hands, spread fingers, extend wrists, and shrug shoulders. After assessment of motor status, a sensory examination, including assessment of touch and pain, should be carried out, starting at the toes and working upward. If time and conditions permit, position sense can also be assessed.

The types of injury mechanisms that cause spinal cord trauma, especially those involving the cervical cord, may also result in brain injury. The patient should therefore be assessed for history of unconsciousness, signs of concussion, and increased intracranial pressure (see Chapter 59). In addition, a careful assessment for musculo-skeletal injuries and trauma to internal organs should be performed. Because the patient may have no muscle, bone, or visceral sensations, the only clue to internal trauma with hemorrhage may be rapidly falling hematocrit levels or persistent

✚ TABLE 63-3 EMERGENCY MANAGEMENT

Spinal Cord Injury

Etiology
Blunt Injury
- Compression, flexion, extension, or rotational injuries to spinal column
- Diving
- Falls
- Motor vehicle accidents
- Pedestrian accidents

Penetrating Injury
- Gunshot
- Stab wounds
- Stretched, torn, crushed, or lacerated spinal cord

Assessment Findings
- Alterations in sensation: temperature, light touch, deep pressure, proprioception
- Bowel and bladder incontinence
- Cuts; bruises; open wounds over head, face, neck, or back
- Difficulty breathing
- Diminished rectal sphincter tone
- Neurogenic shock: hypotension; bradycardia; dry, flushed skin
- Numbness, paresthesias
- Pain, tenderness, deformities, or muscle spasms adjacent to vertebral column
- Priapism
- Spinal shock
- Urinary retention
- Weakness or heaviness in limbs
- Weakness, paralysis, or flaccidity of muscles

Interventions
Initial
- Administer oxygen via nasal cannula or nonrebreather mask.
- Assess for other injuries.
- Control external bleeding.
- Ensure patency of airway.
- Establish intravenous access with two large-bore catheters to infuse normal saline or lactated Ringer's solution as appropriate.
- Insert Foley catheter.
- Stabilize cervical spine with hard collar or sandbags.

Ongoing Monitoring
- Anticipate need for intubation if gag reflex is absent or respiratory function declines.
- Keep patient warm.
- Monitor vital signs, level of consciousness, oxygen saturation, cardiac rhythm, and urine output.

TABLE 63-4 COLLABORATIVE CARE

Cervical Cord Injury

Diagnostic
- History and physical examination, including complete neurological examination
- Anteroposterior, lateral, and odontoid spinal radiographs
- Arterial blood gas measurements
- CT, MRI
- Electrolyte measurements, glucose level, coagulation studies, hemoglobin and hematocrit levels
- Serial bedside pulmonary function testing
- Urinalysis

Collaborative Therapy
Acute Care
- Administration of intravenous fluids
- Administration of O_2 by high-humidity mask
- Bowel and bladder monitoring and initiation of training when hemodynamically stable
- High-dose methylprednisolone therapy if ordered
- Insertion of nasogastric tube and attachment to suction
- Intubation if indicated
- Maintenance of heart rate (e.g., with atropine) and blood pressure (e.g., with dopamine)
- Placement and maintenance of halo traction if necessary
- Placement of in-dwelling urinary catheter
- Prophylaxis for deep-vein thrombosis
- Prophylaxis for stress ulcers
- Use of pressure-relieving surface

Rehabilitation and Home Care
- Bowel and bladder training
- Occupational therapy (activities of daily living training)
- Patient and caregiver education
- Physiotherapy
  - Chest physiotherapy
  - Mobility training
  - Muscle strengthening
  - Range-of-motion exercises
- Prevention of autonomic dysreflexia
- Prevention of pressure injuries
- Recreation therapy

CT, computed tomography; *MRI*, magnetic resonance imaging; *O₂*, oxygen.

hypotension. Urinary output is examined for volume and hematuria, another indication of internal injuries.

To prevent further injury, the patient must be moved in alignment as a unit, as in log-rolling, during transfers and when repositioned. Respiratory, cardiac, urinary, and gastro-intestinal functions should be monitored closely. The patient may undergo surgery directly after initial immobilization and stabilization or be taken to the ICU for monitoring and management.

Nonoperative Stabilization. Nonoperative treatments focus on stabilization and realignment of the injured spinal segment through traction. Stabilization methods eliminate damaging motion at the injury site. They are intended to prevent secondary spinal cord damage caused by repeated contusion or compression.

Surgical Therapy. The decision to perform surgery on a patient with an SCI often depends on the preference of the

physician and the availability of surgical services. Surgery stabilizes, realigns, and decompresses the spinal column. There is evidence that early surgical intervention is safe and feasible and that it can improve clinical and neurological outcomes and reduce health care costs (see the "Evidence-Informed Practice: Research Highlight" box). Other criteria used in the decision for early surgery include (a) evidence of cord compression, (b) progressive neurological deficit, (c) compound fracture of the vertebrae, (d) bony fragments (may dislodge and penetrate the cord), and (e) penetrating wounds of the spinal cord or surrounding structures.

The more common surgical procedures include decompression, realignment, and stabilization with instrumentation. These procedures are performed either posteriorly or anteriorly, depending on the level of injury and the area of cord compression (i.e., anterior versus posterior). If instability is considered severe enough, both anterior and posterior stabilization may be considered.

Drug Therapy. Clinical trials (National Acute Spinal Cord Injury Studies [NASCIS] I, II, and III) have provided conflicting evidence about steroid treatment in acute SCI (Hurlbert, Hadley,

🔍 **EVIDENCE-INFORMED PRACTICE**

Research Highlight

What Is the Effect of Early Versus Delayed Surgery for Patients With Traumatic Spinal Cord Injury?

Clinical Question

In patients with traumatic spinal cord injury *(P)*, what is the effect of early *(I)* versus delayed *(C)* decompressive surgery on patient grades on the ASIA Impairment Scale *(O)?*

Best Available Evidence

A multicentre, international, prospective cohort study was conducted in adults aged 16 to 80 with SCI. Primary outcome was a change in ASIA Impairment Scale grade at the 6-month follow-up visit.

Clinical Appraisal and Synthesis of Evidence

Results of previous studies in the laboratory supported the theory that decompressive surgery of the spinal cord within 24 hours of SCI reduced secondary injury and improved neurological outcome.
- 313 patients with SCI were enrolled
- 182 underwent early surgical decompression
- At 6-month follow-up after the injury, those who underwent early surgery showed an improvement of ≥2 grades on the ASIA Impairment Scale
- Complications occurred in 24.2% of patients who underwent early surgery and in 30.5% of those who underwent late surgery

Conclusions

- Surgical decompression within 24 hours after SCI can be performed safely and is associated with improved neurological outcome (defined as at least a 2-grade improvement on the ASIA Impairment Scale at the 6-month follow-up visit).

Implications for Nursing Practice

- It is important for nurses working in emergency and acute care to realize the effect of early surgical treatment for SCI and advocate for the transfer of the patient to a tertiary care facility that offers specialized care in SCI. A change in grade on the ASIA Impairment Scale for patients with SCI can indicate a huge effect on functional gain and can mean the difference between dependence and independence.

Reference for Evidence

Fehlings, M. G., Vaccaro, A., Wilson, J. R., et al. (2012). Early versus delayed decompression for traumatic cervical spinal cord injury: Results of the Surgical Timing in Acute Spinal Cord Injury Study (STASCIS). *PLoS ONE*, *7*(2), e32037. doi:10.1371/journal.pone.0032037.

P, patient population of interest; *I*, intervention or areas of interest; *C*, comparison of interest; *O*, outcomes of interest (see Chapter 1).

Walters, et al., 2013). Steroid therapy is not without risk. Most patients with acute SCI are treated in ICUs, have polytrauma and impaired lung capacity, and are vulnerable to sepsis. Use of steroids superimposes risks on these compromised patients. The current medical opinion around the use of high-dose steroids is that it should be considered neither a standard treatment nor a guideline for treatment but, rather, a treatment option. If steroid use is considered, the protocol to be followed must be initiated within 8 hours of the SCI. It begins with a loading dose of 30 mg/kg intravenous (IV) over 15 minutes, followed by 5.4 mg/kg IV over the next 23 hours (Bracken, 2012).

Other neuroprotective drugs are being tested, and more treatment options may be available in the near future. Researchers are examining regeneration and repair strategies to induce axonal sprouting and promote remyelination of spared axons. Some of these approaches include anti-Nogo antibodies, BA-210 (Cethrin), bone marrow and stem cell implantation, and various cellular approaches (Wilson, Forgione, & Fehlings, 2013).

Vasopressor agents such as dopamine and norepinephrine are administered in the acute phase as adjuvants to treatment. These agents are used to maintain the mean arterial pressure at a level greater than 85 mm Hg so that perfusion to the spinal cord is improved (Hawryluk, Whetstone, Saigal, et al., 2015).

Pharmacological agents are administered to treat specific autonomic dysfunctions such as bradycardia, orthostatic hypotension, gastro-intestinal hypoactivity, inadequate emptying of the bladder, and autonomic dysreflexia (discussed later in this chapter). The nurse must know the intended effects of such agents, observe responses, and provide specific interventions when adverse reactions are seen.

NURSING MANAGEMENT SPINAL CORD INJURY

NURSING ASSESSMENT

Subjective and objective data that should be obtained from a patient with a recent SCI are presented in Table 63-5.

NURSING DIAGNOSES

Nursing diagnoses for patients with an SCI depend on the severity of the injury and the level of dysfunction. The nursing diagnoses for patients with an SCI may include but are not limited to the following:
- *Ineffective breathing pattern* related to *respiratory muscle fatigue, body position that inhibits lung expansion, fatigue*
- *Imbalanced nutrition: less than body requirements* related to *insufficient dietary intake* (paralytic ileus, metabolic demands of body)
- *Ineffective peripheral tissue perfusion* related to *sedentary lifestyle* (lack of mobility)
- *Impaired skin integrity* related to *pressure over bony prominence* (immobility)
- *Impaired urinary elimination* related to *multiple causality* (spinal injury, limited fluid intake)
- *Constipation* related to *irregular defecation habits* (neurogenic bowel, immobility)

Additional information on nursing diagnoses for the patient with SCI is presented in Nursing Care Plan (NCP) 63-1, available on the Evolve website.

PLANNING

The overall goals are that the patient with an SCI will (a) maintain optimal level of neurological functioning; (b) have minimal or no complications of immobility; (c) learn new skills, gain new knowledge, and acquire new behaviours to be able to care for self or successfully direct others to do so; and (d) return to home and the community at an optimal level of functioning.

NURSING IMPLEMENTATION

HEALTH PROMOTION. Nursing interventions for injury prevention include identification of at-risk populations, counselling, and education. Support of local legislation related to seat belt use in cars, helmets for motorcyclists and bicyclists, child safety seats, and tougher penalties for drunk driving offences is a professional responsibility. Parachute Canada is a national charitable organization that is dedicated to preventing injuries and saving lives. It has partnered with organizations including ThinkFirst Canada, Safe Communities Canada, SMARTRISK, and Safe Kids Canada to develop injury-prevention programs.

TABLE 63-5   NURSING ASSESSMENT

Spinal Cord Injury

Subjective Data
Important Health Information
Past health history: Motor vehicle accident, sports injury, industrial accident, gunshot or stabbing injury, falls
Current medical history: Use of alcohol or recreational drugs; risk-taking behaviours

Symptoms
* Dyspnea, inability to breathe adequately ("air hunger")
* Fear, denial, anger, depression
* Loss of strength, movement, and sensation below level of injury
* Presence of tenderness, pain at or above level of injury; numbness, tingling sensation, burning sensation, twitching of extremities

Objective Data
General
Poikilothermism (inability to regulate body heat)

Integumentary
Warm, dry, flushed extremities below level of injury (neurogenic shock)

Respiratory
Lesions at C1–3: apnea, inability to cough
Lesions at C4: poor cough, diaphragmatic breathing, hypoventilation
Lesions at C5–T6: decreased respiratory reserve

Cardiovascular
Lesions above T5: bradycardia, hypotension, postural hypotension, absence of vasomotor tone

Gastro-Intestinal
Decreased or absent bowel sounds (paralytic ileus in lesions above T5), abdominal distension, constipation, fecal incontinence, fecal impaction

Urinary
Retention (for lesions between T1 and L2); flaccid bladder (acute stages); spasticity with reflex bladder emptying (later stages)

Reproductive
Priapism, loss of sexual function

Neurological
Complete: Flaccid paralysis and anaesthesia below level of injury that results in tetraplegia (for lesions above C8) or paraplegia (for lesions below C8); hyperactive deep tendon reflexes; bilaterally positive response to Babinski test (after resolution of spinal shock)
Incomplete: Mixed loss of voluntary motor activity and sensation

Musculo-Skeletal
Muscle atony (in flaccid state), contractures (in spastic state)

Possible Findings
Spinal radiography: location of level and type of bony involvement
CT: bony destruction and compression
MRI: lesions and edema

CT, computed tomography; *MRI,* magnetic resonance imaging.

It is important that the nurse emphasize the importance of other health promotion and health screening in addition to SCI care. After injury, health-promoting behaviours can have a significant effect on the health and well-being of the individual with SCI. Nursing interventions include education; counselling and referral to programs such as smoking cessation classes,

recreation and exercise programs, and alcohol treatment programs; and maintenance of routine physical examinations for non-neurological problems. Outpatient health care requires that screening and prevention programs be accessible to people with SCIs. Nurses in these settings should facilitate the availability of wheelchair-accessible examination rooms, adjustable-height examination tables, and scheduling that allows extra time if needed.

ACUTE INTERVENTION. Regardless of the mechanism of injury and resultant spinal column damage, care of patients with SCIs is similar. Interventions for care are discussed in this section and may need to be modified on an individual basis.

Immobilization. Proper immobilization of the neck involves the maintenance of a neutral position. A blanket or rolled towel, a hard cervical collar, and a backboard can be used to stabilize the neck to prevent lateral rotation of the cervical spine. The body should always be correctly aligned, and turning should be performed so that the patient is moved as a unit (e.g., log-rolling) to prevent movement of the spine.

SAFETY ALERT
* A hard cervical collar and a backboard to stabilize the neck should be used to prevent lateral rotation of the cervical spine.
* The body should always be correctly aligned.
* The patient should be moved as a unit (i.e., log-rolling) when turned to prevent movement of the spine.

For cervical injuries, cervical traction is used less frequently. Traction should not be used unless the patient can communicate any changes in clinical status during application and subsequent assessments. When cervical traction is used, realignment or reduction of the injury is the goal. Halo traction involves the placement of a halo ring or crown, secured into the skull with four pins, with subsequent additions of weight to aid in spinal realignment. Traction is provided by a rope that is extended from the centre of the halo crown over a pulley and has weights attached at the end. Traction must be maintained at all times. The initial weight is typically 4.5 to 6.8 kg and thereafter approximately 2.2 kg per level of SCI (e.g., 2.2 kg for C1, 4.4 kg for C2, 6.6 kg for C3) with continual neurological monitoring. Additional weights are added until alignment is achieved, neurological changes occur, or overdistraction within the disc space is noted. Once proper alignment has been established, a halo vest is applied to provide ongoing immobilization of the cervical spine (Sarro, Anthony, Magtoto, et al., 2010). The halo vest stabilizes the injured area and allows ambulation if the patient is neurologically intact (Figure 63-9). Special care of the halo pin sites and halo vest is important for preventing infection and skin breakdown (Sarro, Anthony, Magtoto, et al., 2010) (Table 63-6).

Infection at the sites of pin insertion is a potential problem. Preventive care includes cleansing the sites twice a day with normal saline solution. The development of redness or crusting could indicate looseness of pins, and the physician or designate should be informed. The preventive care of insertion sites may vary, depending on individual hospital standards of care (Sarro, Anthony, Magtoto, et al., 2010).

Specialized beds or mattresses are often used in the management of patients with SCIs to help prevent pressure injury development. Many products are available and are often institution dependent. Mattress overlays often use gel as mediums. Specialized beds are typically dynamic and use a power source to alternate air currents and pressure against the body (Kruger, Pires, Ngann, et al., 2013).

FIGURE 63-9 Halo vest. The halo traction brace immobilizes the cervical spine, which allows the patient to ambulate and perform self-care. Source: Urden, L. D., Stacy, K. M., & Lough, M. E. (2012). *Priorities in critical care nursing* (6th ed., p. 525, Figure 25-6). St. Louis: Mosby.

TABLE 63-6 PATIENT & CAREGIVER TEACHING GUIDE

Halo Vest Care

The following are teaching guidelines for a patient with a halo vest:

1. Visually inspect the pin sites on the halo ring on a regular basis. Report to the health care provider if pins are loose or if there are signs of infection, including redness, tenderness, swelling, or drainage at the insertion sites.
2. Clean pin sites daily with a clean cotton tip applicator or gauze soaked with normal saline for each individual pin site. If crusting or drainage is present, increase the frequency of cleansing to three times a day or as needed.
3. If crusting is present, wrap the pin site with normal saline–soaked gauze for 15–20 minutes and then remove. Using a gentle rolling motion, the crust can then be removed with a cotton-tipped applicator that has been soaked in normal saline.
4. To provide skin care, have the patient lie down on a bed on his or her side. Loosen one side of the vest, and place a towel against the sheepskin to protect it from getting wet. Assess skin for redness or areas of potential skin breakdown. Wash the patient's chest and back with soap and water. Dry the skin thoroughly, and resecure buckle straps. Do not use lotions or powders underneath the vest. Turn the patient onto the opposite side and repeat the steps.
5. A cotton T-shirt can be worn under the sheepskin for comfort and absorption of perspiration.
6. In case of an emergency, keep a wrench taped to the halo vest at all times.

Source: Based on Sarro, A., Anthony, T., Magtoto, R., et al. (2010). Developing a standard of care for halo vest and pin site care including patient and family education: A collaborative approach among three Greater Toronto Area teaching hospitals. *Journal of Neuroscience Nursing, 42*, 169–175. doi:10.1097/JNN.0b013e3181d4a3be.

Cervical collars for postsurgical stabilization are used on the basis of the surgeon's preference. With new techniques and better surgical stabilization, a collar is not required postoperatively. Patients with thoracic or lumbar spine injuries are stabilized with a custom thoraco-lumbar-sacral orthosis (TLSO brace), which controls spinal flexion, extension, and rotation, or with a Jewett brace, which restricts forward flexion.

Immobilization of the neck of a patient with SCI prevents further injury, but the effects of immobility are profound. Meticulous skin care is critical because decreased sensation and circulation render the patient particularly susceptible to skin breakdown. Patients should be removed from backboards as soon as possible to prevent coccygeal and occipital area skin breakdown. Cervical collars should be properly fitted or replaced with other forms of stabilization. It is important that areas under the halo vest, braces, and orthoses be inspected regularly to assess skin condition.

Respiratory Dysfunction. Patients should be monitored in a special care unit to minimize pulmonary complications. During the first 48 hours after injury, spinal cord edema may increase the level of spinal cord dysfunction, and respiratory distress may occur. If the injury is at or above C3, if the patient is exhausted from laboured breathing, or if ABG levels deteriorate (indicating inadequate oxygenation or ventilation), endotracheal intubation and mechanical ventilation should be initiated. Respiratory arrest is a possibility that necessitates careful monitoring of the respiratory system and prompt action. Pneumonia and atelectasis are potential problems because of reduced vital capacity and the loss of intercostal and abdominal muscle function, which can result in diaphragmatic breathing, pooling of secretions, and ineffectiveness of cough (Ryken, Hurlbert, Hadley, et al., 2013). In addition to the neurological injury, predictive factors of potential respiratory complications include tachypnea on admission, older age, and previous respiratory disease. Older adults have a more difficult time responding to hypoxia and hypercapnia and are extremely intolerant of hypoxia caused by lack of reserve. Therefore, aggressive chest physiotherapy, adequate oxygenation, and proper pain management are essential for maximizing respiratory function and gas exchange. Other problems include nasal stuffiness and bronchospasm.

The nurse must regularly assess (a) breath sounds, (b) ABG levels, (c) tidal volume, (d) vital capacity, (e) skin colour, (f) breathing patterns (especially the use of accessory muscles), (g) subjective comments about the ability to breathe, and (h) the amount and colour of sputum. Partial pressure of oxygen in arterial blood (PaO_2) above 60 mm Hg and partial pressure of carbon dioxide in arterial blood ($PaCO_2$) below 45 mm Hg are acceptable values in a patient with uncomplicated tetraplegia. A patient who is unable to count to 10 out loud without taking a breath needs immediate attention.

In addition to monitoring, the nurse can intervene in maintaining ventilation. Oxygen is administered until ABG levels stabilize. Chest physiotherapy and assisted coughing facilitate the expulsion of secretions. Assisted or augmented coughing simulates the action of the ineffective abdominal muscles during the expiratory phase of a cough. The nurse places the heels of both hands just below the patient's xiphoid process and exerts firm upward pressure to the area, timed with the patient's efforts to cough (see discussion of augmented coughing in Chapter 70). Tracheal suctioning should be performed if crackles or wheezes are present. Incentive spirometry is an additional technique that can be used to improve the patient's respiratory status.

Cardiovascular Instability. Because of unopposed vagal response, the heart rate slows, often to less than 60 beats per minute. Any increase in vagal stimulation, such as turning or suctioning, can result in cardiac arrest. Loss of sympathetic tone in peripheral vessels results in chronic low blood pressure with potential postural hypotension. Lack of muscle tone to aid venous return can result in sluggish blood flow and predispose the patient to venous thrombo-embolism (VTE), DVT, or PE.

Vital signs should be assessed frequently. If bradycardia is symptomatic, an anticholinergic drug such as atropine is administered. A temporary pacemaker may be inserted. Hypotension is managed with a vasopressor agent, such as dopamine or norepinephrine (Levophed), and fluid replacement.

In older adults, the presence of cardiovascular disease must be considered. The cardiovascular system becomes less able to handle the stress of traumatic injury because heart contractions weaken, and cardiac output decreases. Maximum heart rate is also reduced.

Gradient compression stockings can be used to prevent thrombo-emboli and to promote venous return. The stockings must be removed every 8 hours for skin care. The use of pneumatic compression devices for the calves is advocated, and they must be applied as soon as possible after injury and maintained throughout the hospitalization. Venous duplex studies may be performed before compression devices are applied. The nurse should also help the patient perform range-of-motion exercises and stretch regularly. The thighs and calves of the legs should be assessed every shift for signs of DVT.

Administration of LMWH within 72 hours of injury and for a 3-month duration is recommended to minimize the occurrence of DVT or PE. Furthermore, when surgical intervention is required, LMWH therapy should be withheld the morning of surgery and resumed within 24 hours postoperatively. LMWH is preferable to unfractionated heparin in patients with SCI because of its longer half-life, lower risk for bleeding complications, and more predictable dose effect in comparison with unfractionated heparin (Dhall, Hadley, Aarabi, et al., 2013).

If blood loss has resulted from other injuries, hemoglobin and hematocrit levels should be monitored, and blood should be administered according to protocol. The nurse should also monitor the patient for indications of hypovolemic shock secondary to hemorrhage.

Fluid and Nutritional Maintenance. During the first 48 to 72 hours after the injury, the gastro-intestinal tract may stop functioning (paralytic ileus), and a nasogastric tube must be inserted. Because the patient cannot have oral intake, fluid and electrolyte needs must be carefully monitored. Specific solutions and additives are ordered based on individual requirements. Once bowel sounds are present or flatus is passed, oral food and fluids can gradually be introduced. Because of severe catabolism, a high-protein, high-calorie diet is necessary for energy and tissue repair. In patients with cervical cord injuries, swallowing must be evaluated before oral feedings are started. Enteral feeding is the optimal route after SCI. When oral feeding is not possible, nasogastric, followed by nasojejunal and then percutaneous, endoscopic gastrostomy is suggested. The acute stage of injury is characterized by a reduction in metabolic activity, as well as a negative nitrogen balance that cannot be corrected, even with aggressive nutritional support. Metabolic demands need to be accurately monitored to avoid overfeeding (Fraser, McIntyre, Thompson, et al., 2014).

Some patients experience anorexia, which can result from psychological depression, boredom with institutional food, or discomfort with being fed. Some patients have a normally small appetite. On occasion, refusal to eat is used as a means of maintaining control over the environment because of diminished or absent control over one's body (see the "Ethical Dilemmas" box). If the patient is not eating adequately, the cause should be thoroughly assessed. On the basis of this assessment, a contract may be made in which the patient and the nurse set mutual goals regarding the diet. This gives the patient increased control

of the situation and often results in improved nutritional intake. General measures such as providing a pleasant eating environment, allowing adequate time to eat (including any self-feeding that the patient can achieve), encouraging the family to bring in special foods, and planning social rewards for eating may be useful. A calorie count should be kept, and the patient's daily weight recorded as a means of evaluating progress. If feasible, the patient should participate in recording calorie intake. Dietary supplements may be necessary to meet nutritional needs. Increased dietary fibre should be included to promote bowel function. The nurse should avoid allowing the patient's nutritional intake to become a basis for a power struggle.

EVIDENCE-INFORMED PRACTICE

Translating Research Into Practice

A nurse working in the rehabilitation unit for patients recovering from SCIs is assigned to Kelvin Tran, a 26-year-old man who suffered an SCI after his 4-wheeler overturned. Mr. Tran has an areflexic bladder. The nurse has discussed with him the various options for bladder management. He tells the nurse that he would prefer the in-dwelling catheter because he thinks that it would be the least disruptive to his daily schedule of activities.

Best Available Evidence	Clinician Expertise	Patient Preferences and Values
Patients using in-dwelling catheters, compared with those using intermittent catheters, have similar satisfaction with life and perceived health status. There may be more complications associated with an in-dwelling catheter (e.g., urinary tract infections) than with intermittent catheterization.	The nurse knows that an areflexic bladder is best managed with either an in-dwelling catheter or intermittent catheterization. The nurse also knows that patients may hesitate to select intermittent catheterization for a variety of reasons (e.g., they believe the procedure is painful, they are afraid of performing the procedure incorrectly and possibly hurting themselves, they do not want their lives interrupted by the need to drain their bladder 5–6 times per day).	After reviewing all the information, Mr. Tran indicates that he would prefer an in-dwelling catheter to intermittent catheterization as the method to self-manage his bladder.

Decision and Action
His nurse respects and supports his decision and plans to teach Mr. Tran and his caregiver how to obtain the necessary supplies and how to care for the catheter once discharged.

References for Evidence
Akkoç, Y., Ersöz, M., Yildiz, N., et al. (2013). Effects of different bladder management methods on the quality of life in patients with traumatic spinal cord injury. *Spinal Cord, 51*(3), 226–231. doi:10.1038/sc.2012.131.
Cameron, A. P., Wallner, L. P., Forchheimer, M. B., et al. (2011). Medical and psychosocial complications associated with method of bladder management after traumatic spinal cord injury. *Archives of Physical Medicine and Rehabilitation, 92*(3), 449–456. doi:10.1016/j.apmr.2010.06.028.

ETHICAL DILEMMAS

Right to Refuse Treatment

Situation

A 25-year-old man suffered an SCI to C7–T1 after a motorcycle accident. Anterior cord syndrome was diagnosed, and he has motor paralysis, which may prevent him from riding motorcycles again. He has become extremely depressed and no longer wishes to live. Because of his emotional state, he is now refusing to eat. Can the patient be forced to receive enteral nutrition (tube feeding)?

Important Points for Consideration

- Withholding treatment in a newly injured but otherwise healthy young adult may present an ethical dilemma for health care providers.
- Approximately 20% to 30% of people with a new SCI experience a major depressive disorder as a result of the sudden loss of bodily control and feelings of helplessness.
- A thorough mental health and psychological evaluation is warranted; treatment of depression is necessary before determining the patient's capacity to make decisions.
- Most people (more than 90%) with an SCI who receive health care and have access to appropriate resources report a good quality of life. Therefore, requests to withhold treatment soon after SCI should be scrutinized.
- If, after adequate treatment for pain, depression, or other medical conditions, the patient persists in requests to withhold treatment, his ability to make an informed choice must be reassessed.
- A competent adult can decide to withhold treatment. If possible, action on the request should be delayed to ensure adequate informed consent and to determine whether quality of life is adequate.

Clinical Decision-Making Questions

1. How might the nurse feel about requests to withhold treatment for a young person with a newly acquired disability?
2. What resources are available to help the patient and the staff work through this emotionally charged and ethically complex situation?

Bladder and Bowel Management. Immediately after injury, urine is retained because of the loss of autonomic and reflex control of the bladder and the sphincter. Because the patient has no sensation of fullness, overdistension of the bladder can result in reflux into the kidneys, with eventual renal failure. Bladder distension may even result in rupture of the bladder. Consequently, an in-dwelling catheter is usually inserted as soon as possible after injury. Its patency must be ensured by frequent inspection and irrigation if necessary. Strict aseptic technique for catheter care is essential to avoid introducing infection.

After patients are stabilized, the best means of managing urinary function is assessed. Usually, an intermittent catheterization program is started. As well as having been shown to reduce UTIs in comparison with use of an in-dwelling catheter, intermittent catheterization is the safest method of bladder management for protecting the kidneys. Many patients are maintained on fluid restriction of 1 800 to 2 000 mL/day to facilitate a bladder training program, and urinary output is monitored closely.

UTIs are a common problem. The best method for preventing UTIs is regular and complete bladder drainage. Catheterization should be performed to prevent bladder volume from exceeding 500 mL. A typical regimen would be to catheterize every 4 hours for volumes of 300 to 500 mL, every 3 hours for volumes greater than 500 mL, and every 6 hours for volumes less than 300 mL. If the appearance or odour of the urine is suspect or if the patient develops symptoms of a UTI (e.g., chills, fever, malaise), a urine specimen is sent for culture.

Age-related changes in renal function should be considered. Older adults are more likely to develop renal calculi, and older men may have prostatic hyperplasia, which may interfere with urinary flow and complicate management of urinary problems.

Constipation is generally a problem during spinal shock because no voluntary or involuntary (reflex) evacuation of the bowels occurs. A bowel program should be started during acute care. This consists of a rectal stimulant (suppository or mini-enema) to be inserted daily at a regular time of day, followed by gentle digital stimulation or manual evacuation performed by the nurse until evacuation is complete. Initially, the program may be performed in bed in the side-lying position, but as soon as the patient has resumed sitting, it should be performed in the upright position on a padded bedside commode chair.

Temperature Control. Temperature control is largely external to the patient because there is no vasoconstriction, piloerection, or heat loss through perspiration below the level of injury. The nurse must monitor the environment closely to maintain an appropriate temperature. Body temperature should be monitored regularly. The patient should not be overloaded with covers or unduly exposed (such as during bathing). If an infection with high fever develops, more extensive means of temperature control, such as a cooling blanket, may be necessary.

Stress Ulcers. Stress ulcers are a problem for the patient with an SCI because of the physiological response to severe trauma, psychological stress, and high-dose corticosteroids if used. The incidence of ulcers peaks 6 to 14 days after injury. Histamine H_2-receptor blockers, such as ranitidine (Zantac) and famotidine (Pepcid AC), or proton pump inhibitors, such as omeprazole (Losec) or pantoprazole (Prevacid), may be given prophylactically to decrease the secretion of hydrochloric acid.

Sensory Deprivation. To prevent sensory deprivation, the nurse must compensate for the patient's absence of sensations by stimulating the patient above the level of injury. Conversation, music, strong aromas, and interesting flavours should be a part of the nursing care plan. Every effort should be made to prevent the patient from withdrawing from the environment.

Patients with SCIs often report altered sensorium and vivid dreams during the acute phase of their treatment. Whether this is caused by drugs used to manage pain and anxiety is not known. Patients may also experience disrupted sleep patterns as a result of the hospital environment or post-traumatic stress disorder.

Reflexes. Once spinal cord shock is resolved, the return of reflexes may complicate rehabilitation. In the absence of control from the higher brain centres, reflexes are often hyperactive, and responses may be exaggerated. Penile erections can result from a variety of stimuli, causing embarrassment and discomfort. Spasms ranging from mild twitches to convulsive movements below the level of the lesion may also occur. This reflex activity may be interpreted by the patient or family as a return of function, and the nurse must tactfully explain the reason for the activity. The patient may be informed of the positive use of these reflexes in sexual, bowel, and bladder retraining. Spasms may be controlled with the use of antispasmodic drugs. Most commonly prescribed are baclofen (Lioresal), dantrolene (Dantrium), and tizanidine. Botulism toxin injections may also be given to treat severe spasticity.

Autonomic Dysreflexia. The return of reflexes after the resolution of spinal shock means that patients with an injury level at T6 or higher may develop autonomic dysreflexia. **Autonomic dysreflexia** (also known as *autonomic hyper-reflexia*) is a massive, uncompensated cardiovascular reaction mediated by the sympathetic nervous system. It occurs in response to visceral stimulation once spinal shock is resolved in patients with spinal cord lesions. This condition is a life-threatening situation that necessitates immediate resolution. If resolution does not occur, this condition can lead to status epilepticus, stroke, myocardial infarction, or even death.

The most common precipitating cause is distension of the bladder or rectum, although any sensory stimulation may cause autonomic dysreflexia. Contraction of the bladder or the rectum, stimulation of the skin, or stimulation of the pain receptors may also cause autonomic dysreflexia. Manifestations include hypertension (up to 300 mm Hg systolic), throbbing headache, marked diaphoresis or flushing of skin above the level of the lesion, bradycardia (30 to 40 beats per minute), piloerection (erection of body hair) as a result of pilomotor spasm, blurred vision or spots in the visual fields, nasal congestion, anxiety, and nausea. It is important to measure blood pressure when a patient with an SCI complains of a headache (Krassioukov, Blackmer, Teasell, et al., 2014). A normal blood pressure for a patient with tetraplegic SCI is a systolic blood pressure of 90 to 100 mm Hg. Any pressure higher than this should be considered hypertensive.

The pathology of autonomic dysreflexia involves the stimulation of sensory receptors below the level of the cord lesion. The intact autonomic nervous system below the level of the lesion responds to the stimulation with a reflex arteriolar vasoconstriction that increases blood pressure. Baroreceptors in the carotid sinus and the aorta detect the hypertension and stimulate the parasympathetic system. This stimulation results in a decrease in heart rate, but the visceral and peripheral vessels do not dilate because efferent impulses cannot pass through the cord lesion.

In this serious emergency, nursing interventions include elevating the head of the bed 45 degrees or sitting the patient upright, notifying the physician, and assessing the patient to determine the cause. The most common cause is bladder distension. Immediate catheterization to relieve bladder distension may be necessary. Lidocaine jelly should be instilled in the urethra before catheterization. If a catheter is already in place, it should be checked for kinks or folds. If it is plugged, small-volume irrigation should be performed slowly and gently to open the catheter, or a new catheter may be inserted. Stool impaction can also result in autonomic dysreflexia. A digital rectal examination should be performed only after application of an anaesthetic ointment to decrease rectal stimulation and to prevent an increase of symptoms. If neither bladder nor bowel distension is determined to be causative, the nurse should remove all skin stimuli, such as constrictive clothing, tight shoes, and splints. Blood pressure should be monitored frequently during the episode. If symptoms persist after the source has been relieved, an α-adrenergic blocker or an arteriolar vasodilator (e.g., nifedipine) is administered. Careful monitoring must continue until the vital signs stabilize.

The patient and caregivers should be taught the causes and symptoms of autonomic dysreflexia (Table 63-7). They must understand the life-threatening nature of this dysfunction and know how to relieve the cause.

REHABILITATION AND HOME CARE. The physiological and psychological rehabilitation of patients with SCIs is complex and involved. With physical and psychological care and intensive and specialized rehabilitation, patients with SCIs learn to function at the highest level of wellness. It is recommended that all patients with a new SCI receive comprehensive inpatient rehabilitation in a rehabilitation unit or centre that specializes in SCIs.

TABLE 63-7 **PATIENT & CAREGIVER TEACHING GUIDE**

Autonomic Dysreflexia

The following information should be included in the teaching plan for a patient at risk for autonomic dysreflexia:

1. Signs and symptoms
   - Sudden onset of acute headache
   - Elevation in blood pressure, reduction in pulse rate, or both
   - Flushed face and upper chest (above the level of the lesion) and pale extremities (below the level of the lesion)
   - Sweating above the level of the lesion
   - Nasal congestion
   - Feeling of apprehension
2. Immediate interventions
   - Raise the patient to a sitting position.
   - Remove the stimulus (fecal impaction, distended bladder, tight clothing).
   - Call the health care provider if these actions do not relieve the signs and symptoms.
3. Measures to suppress the incidence of autonomic dysreflexia
   - Maintain regular bladder and bowel function.
   - If manual rectal stimulation is used to promote bowel function, local anaesthetics may prevent autonomic dysreflexia from occurring.
   - Wear a medical alert bracelet indicating a history of autonomic dysreflexia.

Many of the problems identified in the acute period become chronic and continue throughout life. Rehabilitation focuses on refined retraining of physiological processes and extensive patient and caregiver teaching about how to manage the physiological and life changes resulting from injury.

Rehabilitation is a multidisciplinary endeavour carried out through a team approach. Team members include rehabilitation nurses, physicians, physiotherapists, occupational therapists, speech–language pathologists, vocational counsellors, psychologists, therapeutic recreation specialists, prosthetists, orthotists, and dietitians. Rehabilitation care is organized around the individual patient's goals and needs. During rehabilitation, patients are expected to be involved in therapies and learn self-care for several hours each day. Such intensive work at a time when the patient is dealing with the sudden change in health and functional status can be very stressful. Progress may be slow, and frequent encouragement may be required. The rehabilitation nurse has a pivotal role in providing encouragement, specialized nursing care, and patient and caregiver teaching and in helping to coordinate the efforts of the rehabilitation team.

Respiratory Rehabilitation. The patient with high cervical SCI may have greatly increased mobility with phrenic nerve stimulators or electronic diaphragmatic pacemakers. These devices are not appropriate for all ventilator-dependent patients but may be helpful for those with an intact phrenic nerve. Today, ventilators are also reasonably portable, and ventilator-dependent tetraplegic patients can be mobile and somewhat independent. Patients and caregivers should be taught all aspects of home ventilator care, and referrals should be made to appropriate community agencies. Patients with injuries at the cervical level who are not ventilator dependent should be taught assisted coughing and regular use of incentive spirometry or deep-breathing exercises.

Neurogenic Bladder. A **neurogenic bladder** is any type of bladder dysfunction related to abnormal or absent bladder innervation. After spinal cord shock resolves, depending on the completeness of

TABLE 63-8   TYPES OF NEUROGENIC BLADDER

Type	Characteristics	Causes	Clinical Manifestations
Reflexic (spastic, uninhibited, upper motor neuron)	No inhibitions influence time and place of voiding; bladder empties in response to stretching of bladder wall	Cortico-spinal tract lesion; observed in spinal cord injury, stroke, multiple sclerosis, brain tumour, brain trauma	Incontinence, frequency, urgency; voiding is unpredictable and incomplete
Areflexic (autonomous, flaccid, lower motor neuron)	Bladder acts as if all motor functions are paralyzed, fills without emptying	Lower motor neuron lesion caused by trauma involving S2–4; observed in lesions of cauda equina, pelvic nerves	If sensory function intact, patient feels bladder distension and hesitancy; no control of micturition results in overdistension of bladder and overflow incontinence
Sensory	Lack of sensation of need to urinate	Damage to sensory limb of bladder spinal reflex arc; observed in multiple sclerosis, diabetes mellitus	Poor bladder sensation, infrequent voiding of large residual volume

TABLE 63-9   COLLABORATIVE CARE

Neurogenic Bladder

Diagnostic
- History and physical examination, including neurological examination
- Urodynamic testing
- Urine culture

Collaborative Therapy
- Drug therapy
  - Relaxation of urethral sphincter (α-adrenergic blockers)
  - Suppression of bladder contractions (anticholinergics)
  - Suppression of pelvic floor spasticity (baclofen [Lioresal])
- Fluid intake of 1 800–2 000 mL/day
- Surgery
  - Electrical stimulation
  - Sphincterotomy
  - Urinary diversion
- Urine drainage
  - In-dwelling catheter
  - Intermittent catheterization
  - Voluntary or reflex voiding

the SCI, patients usually have some degree of neurogenic bladder. Normal voiding requires nervous system coordination of urethral and pelvic floor relaxation with simultaneous contraction of the detrusor muscle. Depending on the lesion, a neurogenic bladder may have no reflex detrusor contractions (areflexic, flaccid), may have hyperactive reflex detrusor contractions (hyper-reflexic, spastic), or may lack coordination between detrusor contraction and urethral relaxation (dyssynergia). Common problems with a neurogenic bladder include urgency, frequency, incontinence, inability to void, and high bladder pressures that cause reflux of urine into the kidneys.

Neurogenic bladder can be classified according to reflex detrusor activity, intravesical filling pressure, and continence function. Types of neurogenic bladder are outlined in Table 63-8. Diagnostic and collaborative care of neurogenic bladder is described in Table 63-9. Patients with SCI and a neurogenic bladder require a comprehensive program to manage bladder function.

After the patient's overall condition is stable and there is evidence of neurological reflexes, urodynamic testing and a urine culture are performed to aid in determining the type of neurogenic

bladder dysfunction experienced. The method used for urinary drainage depends on the type of neurogenic bladder dysfunction, the preference of the patient, and availability of a family member or caregiver, the physician, and the nursing staff. Numerous drainage methods are possible. Surgical options include sphincterectomy, implantation of a functional electrical stimulation device, and urinary diversion.

Many factors are considered when a bladder management strategy is selected: upper extremity function, caregiver burden, and lifestyle choices. The type of bladder dysfunction also defines treatment goals and management options. For a reflexic bladder with detrusor and sphincter dyssynergia, interventions must enable low-pressure storage, low-pressure voiding, and adequate emptying. Anticholinergic drugs (e.g., oxybutynin [Oxytrol], tolterodine [Detrol]) may be used to suppress bladder contraction. α-Adrenergic blockers (e.g., terazosin, alfuzosin, doxazosin [Cardura]) may be used to decrease outflow resistance at the bladder neck, and antispasmodic drugs (e.g., baclofen [Lioresal]) may be used to decrease spasticity of pelvic floor muscles.

Drainage options include intermittent catheterization, placement of an external catheter (condom catheter), or placement of an in-dwelling catheter. A reflexic bladder with detrusor hyper-reflexia may be treated with anticholinergic drugs, intravesical capsaicin, or botulinum A toxin. An areflexic bladder is usually managed with intermittent catheterization or an in-dwelling catheter.

The long-term use of an in-dwelling catheter should be carefully evaluated because of the associated high incidence of UTI, fistula formation, and diverticula. However, for some patients, it is the best option. Adequate fluid intake and patency of the catheter should be ensured. The frequency of routine catheter changes ranges from 1 week to 1 month, depending on the type of catheter used and institutional policy.

Intermittent catheterization is the most commonly recommended method of bladder management (see Chapter 48). Nursing assessment is important in selecting the time interval between catheterizations. Catheterization should be performed to prevent bladder volume from exceeding 500 mL. A typical regimen would be to catheterize every 4 hours for volumes of 300 to 500 mL, every 3 hours for volumes greater than 500 mL, and every 6 hours for volumes less than 300 mL. An overdistended bladder can cause ischemia of the bladder wall, which may predispose tissues to bacterial invasion and infection. Patients often experience diuresis at a regular time during a 24-hour period. The number of intermittent catheterizations per day is usually five or six.

TABLE 63-10	PATIENT & CAREGIVER TEACHING GUIDE

Bowel Management After Spinal Cord Injury

The following information should be included when teaching the caregiver and patient with a spinal cord injury:

1. Optimal nutritional intake includes three well-balanced meals each day in accordance with the recommended number of servings from *Eating Well With Canada's Food Guide.* *
2. Daily fibre intake should be approximately 20 to 30 g. The amount of fibre eaten should be increased gradually over 1 to 2 weeks.
3. Three litres of fluid per day should be consumed, unless contraindicated. Water or fruit juices should be used, and caffeinated beverages such as coffee, tea, and cola should be avoided. Fluid softens hard stools; caffeine stimulates fluid loss through urination.
4. Foods that produce gas (e.g., beans) or upper gastro-intestinal upset (spicy foods) should be avoided.
5. *Timing:* A regular schedule for bowel evacuation should be established. A good time is 30 minutes after the first meal of the day.
6. *Position:* If possible, an upright position with feet flat on the floor or on a step stool enhances bowel evacuation. Staying on the toilet, commode, or bedpan for longer than 20 to 30 minutes may cause skin breakdown. Depending on the patient's stability, someone may need to stay with the patient.
7. *Activity:* Exercise is important for bowel function. In addition to improving muscle tone, it increases gastro-intestinal transit time and increases appetite. Muscles should be exercised. Exercise includes stretching, range of motion, position changing, and functional movement.
8. *Drug treatment:* Suppositories may be necessary to stimulate a bowel movement. Manual stimulation of the rectum may also be helpful in initiating defecation. Stool softeners and oral laxatives may be used as needed to regulate stool consistency.

*Health Canada. (2011). *Eating Well With Canada's Food Guide.* Retrieved from http://www.hc-sc.gc.ca/fn-an/alt_formats/hpfb-dgpsa/pdf/food-guide-aliment/view_eatwell_vue_bienmang-eng.pdf.

Urinary diversion surgery may be necessary if a patient has repeated UTIs with renal involvement or repeated stones or if therapeutic intervention has been unsuccessful (see Chapter 48). Surgical treatment of neurogenic bladder includes bladder neck revision (sphincterotomy), bladder augmentation (augmentation cystoplasty), penile prosthesis, artificial sphincter, perineal ureterostomy, cystotomy, vesicotomy, and anterior urethral transplantation.

Regardless of which bladder management strategy is selected, the nurse must teach the patient and the family or caregivers about how to accomplish successful self-management, including management techniques, how to obtain necessary supplies, care of supplies and equipment, and when to seek health care. Resources and referrals for supplies and ongoing care must be arranged.

Neurogenic Bowel. Careful management of bowel evacuation is necessary in patients with SCIs because voluntary control of this function may be lost. The usual measures for preventing constipation include a high-fibre diet and adequate fluid intake (see Chapter 45, Table 45-9). Patient and caregiver teaching guidelines related to bowel management are presented in Table 63-10. However, these measures by themselves may not be adequate to stimulate evacuation. In addition, suppositories (bisacodyl [Dulcolax] or glycerin) or small-volume enemas and digital stimulation by the nurse or patient may be necessary. In patients with an upper motor neuron lesion, digital stimulation

is necessary to relax the external sphincter to promote defecation. A stool softener such as docusate sodium (Colace) can be used to regulate stool consistency. Oral stimulant laxatives should be used only if absolutely necessary for a day or two and not on a regular basis.

Valsalva manoeuvre and manual stimulation are useful in patients with lower motor neuron lesions. Valsalva manoeuvre requires intact abdominal muscles, and so it is used in patients with injuries below T12.

In general, a bowel movement every other day is considered adequate. However, preinjury patterns should be considered. Incontinence can result from too much stool softener or fecal impaction.

Careful recording of bowel movements, including amount, time, and consistency, is important to overall success. Timing of defecation may also be an important factor. If bowel evacuation is planned for 30 to 60 minutes after the first meal of the day, success may be enhanced by taking advantage of the gastrocolic reflex induced by eating. Again, patient and family education is required to promote successful independent bowel management.

Neurogenic Skin. Prevention of pressure injuries and other types of injury to insensitive skin is essential for every patient with SCI. The 2013 *Canadian Best Practice Guidelines for the Prevention and Management of Pressure Ulcers in People with Spinal Cord Injury* (Houghton, Campbell, & CPG Panel, 2013) provides an updated resource for health care providers and considers the unique challenges of pressure injury management. The guidelines take a comprehensive approach to pressure management, including self-management and telehealth approaches. Nurses in rehabilitation are responsible for teaching these skills and providing patients information about daily skin care. A comprehensive visual and tactile examination of the skin should be performed twice daily, with special attention to areas over bony prominences. The areas most vulnerable to breakdown include the ischia, the trochanters, the heels, and the sacrum. Careful positioning and repositioning should be performed every 2 hours, with gradual increases in the times between turns if no redness over bony prominences is apparent at the time of turning. Pressure-relieving cushions must be used in wheelchairs, and special mattresses may also be needed. Movement during turns and transfers should be performed carefully to avoid shear (stretching and folding of soft tissues), friction, or abrasion (Houghton, Campbell, & CPG Panel, 2013).

Nutritional status should be assessed regularly. Both loss and gain in body weight can contribute to skin breakdown. Adequate intake of protein is essential for skin health. Measurement of total protein and albumin can help identify inadequate protein intake. The importance of nutrition to skin health should be stressed to the patient and caregivers.

Protection of the skin also requires avoidance of thermal injury. Burns can be caused by hot food or liquids, bath or shower water that is too warm, radiators, heating pads, and uninsulated plumbing. Thermal injury also can result from extreme cold (frostbite). Injuries may not be noticed until severe damage is done. Anticipatory guidance about potential risks is essential. Patient and caregiver education related to skin care is provided in Table 63-11.

Sexuality. The effects of a SCI on sexual functioning, ability to engage in sexual activities, sexual intimacy and relationships, sexual self-view, and fertility and reproductive health vary with each individual. Sexual health is a significant component of a

TABLE 63-11	PATIENT & CAREGIVER TEACHING GUIDE

Skin Care for Patients With Spinal Cord Injury

Skin breakdown is a potential problem after spinal cord injury. The following information should be included when teaching the caregiver how to decrease this possibility:

Frequent Change of Position
- Patient in a wheelchair: lift self up and shift weight every 15 to 30 minutes.
- Patient in a bed: follow a regular turning schedule (at least every 2 hours) that includes sides, back, and abdomen.
- Use special mattresses and wheelchair cushions.
- Use pillows to protect bony prominences when in bed.

Monitor Skin Condition
- Inspect skin frequently for areas of redness, swelling, and breakdown.
- Keep fingernails trimmed to avoid scratches and abrasions.
- If a wound develops, follow standard wound care management procedures.

person's overall health and well-being. Both men and women retain desire for sexual activity following SCI.

Male fertility after SCI is often compounded by the difficulties of erectile dysfunction, as well as retrograde ejaculation or anejaculation. Erectile dysfunction often causes erections unreliable or inadequate for sexual intercourse due to difficulties in maintaining an erection. Medications or surgical procedures are available to help overcome this issue. Few men with SCI are able to ejaculate with partner sexual practices alone and require medical assistance to obtain sperm. This sperm is then used for intravaginal/intrauterine insemination or other assisted reproductive technology. Fertility rates resulting in pregnancy are generally lower than those among the general population as a result of the decline in semen quality following SCI (Elliott & McBride, 2014).

Female fertility appears to be unaffected by SCI. Amenorrhea can occur following SCI and last from 4 to 5 months. Women are still able to conceive, carry, and deliver a baby, although they tend to have more complications during pregnancy, labour, and delivery than women in the general population. Bladder problems, spasticity, pressure sores, autonomic dysreflexia, and problems with mobility can pose a threat to the pregnant woman with SCI. A pre-emptive epidural prior to delivery is used to manage autonomic dysreflexia, which otherwise can become uncontrolled. Breastfeeding can also be difficult secondary to possible autonomic dysreflexia and inhibition of milk ejection reflexes (Elliott & McBride, 2014).

Sexual rehabilitation for both men and women should begin informally after the acute phase of the injury has passed. Questions such as "Have you had an erection since your accident?" and "Have your menstrual periods continued since the accident?" are nonthreatening ways to introduce the topic of sexual functioning. The male patient may pose a question such as "Can I ever be a man again?"

Open discussion with the patient is essential. This important aspect of rehabilitation should be handled by someone specially trained in sexual counselling. A nurse or other rehabilitation professional with such expertise works with the patient and partner to provide support with an emphasis on open communication. The nurse's educational role requires respect for

every couple's religious beliefs and cultural norms. Alternative methods of obtaining sexual satisfaction such as oral–genital sex (cunnilingus and fellatio) may be suggested. Explicit video material may also be used, such as a movie demonstrating the sexual activities of a patient with paraplegia with a nondisabled partner. Graphic materials should be used cautiously because they may be too limiting or focus too much on the mechanics of sex rather than on the relationship.

Sexual activities may require more planning and be less spontaneous than before the injury. For example, an attendant may have to undress the patient and remove equipment. A relaxed atmosphere with music and perfume may create an attractive environment. Ample time for caressing, fondling, and kissing is essential. The partners should be encouraged to explore each other's erogenous areas, such as lips, neck, and ears, which can arouse psychogenic erection or orgasm. Few demands should be made initially.

Care should be taken not to dislodge an in-dwelling catheter during sexual activity. If an external catheter is used, it should be removed before sexual activity, and the patient should refrain from drinking fluids. The bowel program should include evacuation the morning after sexual activity. The partner should be informed that incontinence is always possible. The woman with an SCI may need a water-soluble lubricant to supplement diminished vaginal secretions and facilitate vaginal penetration.

Grief and Depression. Patients with SCI may feel an overwhelming sense of loss. They may temporarily lose control over everyday life activities and must depend on others for activities of daily living and for life-sustaining measures. Patients may believe that they are useless and burdens to their families. At a stage when independence is often of the greatest importance, they may be totally dependent on others.

The patient's response and recovery differ in some important aspects from those of patients experiencing loss from amputation or terminal illness. First, regression can and does occur at different stages. Working through grief is a difficult, lifelong process for which the patient needs support and encouragement. With advances in rehabilitation, it is usual for the patient to be independent physically and discharged from the rehabilitation centre before completion of the grief process. The goal of recovery is related more to adjustment than to acceptance. Adjustment implies the ability to go on living with certain limitations. Although patients who are cooperative and accepting are easier to treat, the nurse should expect a wide fluctuation of emotions from all patients with SCIs. Depression may not be a component of the recovery process. Societal norms allow depression after severe loss, and persons confronted with death or radical lifestyle changes are almost expected to become depressed. However, not every patient may experience depression.

The nurse's role in grief work is to allow mourning as a component of the rehabilitation process. Table 63-12 summarizes the mourning process and appropriate nursing interventions. Maintaining hope is an important strategy during the grieving process and should not be interpreted as denial (Krause & Edles, 2014). During the shock and denial stage, the nurse reassures the patient and stresses the expertise of the entire health care team. During the anger stage, the nurse assists the patient in achieving control over the environment, particularly by allowing the patient's input into the plan of care. The nurse should not respond to anger or manipulation or become involved in a power struggle with the patient. As self-care abilities increase, the patient's independence increases.

TABLE 63-12	**MOURNING PROCESS AND NURSING INTERVENTIONS IN SPINAL CORD INJURY**
Patient Behaviour	**Nursing Intervention**
Shock and Denial	
Struggle for survival, complete dependence, excessive sleep, withdrawal, fantasies, unrealistic expectations	• Employ meticulous nursing care. • Provide honest information. • Use simple diagrams to explain injury. • Encourage patient to begin process of recovery. • Establish agreement to use and improve all current abilities while not denying the possibility of future improvement.
Anger	
Refusal to discuss paralysis, decreased self-esteem, manipulation, hostile and abusive language	• Coordinate care with patient and encourage self-care. • Support family members; prevent them from alleviating their guilt by supporting the patient's dependency. • Use humour liberally. • Allow patient outbursts. • Do not allow fixation on injury.
Depression	
Sadness, pessimism, anorexia, nightmares, insomnia, agitation, psychomotor retardation, "blues," suicidal preoccupation, refusal to participate in any self-care activities	• Encourage family involvement and resources. • Plan graded steps in rehabilitation to give success with minimal opportunity for frustration. • Give cheerful and willing assistance with activities of daily living. • Avoid expressing sympathy. • Use firm kindness.
Adjustment	
Planning for future, active participation in therapy, finding of personal meaning in experience and continuation of growth, return to preinjury personality	• Remember that patients have individual personalities. • Balance support systems to encourage independence. • Set goals with the patient's input. • Emphasize potentials.

Peer support groups can be helpful in helping individuals and their families begin to cope with injury and help them adjust to life with a spinal cord injury. Spinal Cord Injury Ontario connects people living with spinal cord injuries to fully trained volunteers who can share their experience and knowledge. They can also connect family members with others who have gone through this journey. They complement professional services provided in acute hospitals, rehabilitation centres, and community-based health and social service agencies.

The patient's caregiver and family also require counselling to avoid promoting dependency in the patient through guilt or misplaced sympathy. The family and caregiver are also experiencing an intense grieving process. A support group of family members and friends of patients with SCIs can help increase family members' knowledge and participation in the grieving process, physical difficulties, the rehabilitation plan, and the meaning of the disability in society (Krause & Edles, 2014).

During the stage of depression, the nurse must be patient and persistent and maintain a sense of humour. Sympathy is not helpful. The patient should be treated in an adult manner and be involved in decision making about care, but the nurse must insist that the care be performed. A primary nurse relationship is helpful. Staff planning and sessions in which staff members can express their feelings are helpful in providing consistency of care. To achieve the stage of adjustment, the patient needs continual support throughout the rehabilitation process in the forms of acceptance, affection, and caring. The nurse must be attentive when the patient needs to talk and sensitive to needs at the various stages of the grief process (Krause & Edles, 2014).

Although the stage of depression during the grief process usually lasts days to weeks, some individuals may become clinically depressed and require treatment for depression. Evaluation by a psychiatric nurse or psychiatrist is recommended. Treatment may include drugs and psychotherapy.

EVALUATION

Expected outcomes for patients with SCIs are presented in NCP 63-1, available on the Evolve website.

AGE-RELATED CONSIDERATIONS

SPINAL CORD INJURY

The demographics of patients living with SCI are changing. The fact that persons with SCI now have longer lifespans has contributed to the increasing number of older adults living with SCI. Moreover, increasing numbers of older adults sustain SCIs later in life as a result of falls. Aging is also associated with an increased likelihood of other chronic illnesses that may have a serious effect on older adults with SCI. As patients with SCI age, both individual aging changes and duration since injury affect functional ability. For example, bowel and bladder dysfunction can increase with duration and severity of SCI.

Health promotion and screening are important for older patients with SCI. Daily skin inspections, UTI prevention measures, monthly breast examinations for women, and regular prostate cancer screening for men are recommended. Cardiovascular disease is the most common cause of morbidity and mortality among persons with SCIs. The lack of sensation, including that of angina, in patients with high-level injuries may mask acute myocardial ischemia. Altered autonomic nervous system function and decreases in physical activity can increase the risk for cardiovascular problems, including hypertension.

At the same time, because of increased work and recreational activities of older adults, an increasing number of older adults are experiencing SCI. Health promotion to decrease injury risk includes fall prevention strategies (e.g., using a stepstool or a grab bar to reach high shelves, handrails on stairs). Rehabilitation for older persons who have SCIs may take longer because of other pre-existing illnesses and poorer health status at the time of the initial injury. Studies show that older persons with SCIs can gain the same degree of neurological recovery as those who are younger at the time of injury, but this does not necessarily translate into meaningful functional outcomes. An interdisciplinary team approach to tailored rehabilitation to match specific needs of older individuals is needed to maximize their potential for recovery and reintegration into the community (Hsieh, DeJong, Groah, et al., 2013).

SPINAL CORD INJURY RESEARCH IN CANADA

The Rick Hansen Institute is a Canadian organization committed to accelerating the translation of discoveries and best practices into improved treatments for individuals with SCIs. Its four distinct programs focus on *cure, care, commercialization,* and *consumers* and support research from the lab to clinical application in an effort to improve the lives of individuals with SCI (see Resources at the end of this chapter).

SPINAL CORD TUMOURS

Etiology and Pathophysiology

Spinal cord tumours account for 0.5% to 1% of all neoplasms. These tumours are classified as primary (arising from some component of cord, dura, nerves, or vessels) or secondary (from primary growths in other places in the body that have metastasized to the spinal cord). Spinal cord tumours are further classified as *extradural* (outside the spinal cord), *intradural extramedullary* (within the dura but outside the actual spinal cord), and *intradural intramedullary* (within the spinal cord itself). Intradural intramedullary tumours are usually astrocytomas or ependymomas (Figure 63-10 and Table 63-13). Approximately 90% of all spinal tumours are extradural. Extradural tumours are usually metastatic and most often arise in the vertebral bodies. These metastatic lesions can invade intradurally and compress the spinal cord. Tumours that commonly metastasize to the spinal epidural space are those that spread to bone, such as prostate, breast, lung, and kidney cancer. Spinal intradural extramedullary tumours account for two-thirds of all intraspinal neoplasms and consist mainly of meningiomas and schwannomas.

Because many of these tumours are slow growing, their symptoms stem from the mechanical effects of bone destruction, slow compression and irritation of nerve roots, displacement of the cord, or gradual obstruction of the vascular supply. The slow growth does not cause autodestruction (secondary injury), as occurs with traumatic lesions. Therefore, partial to complete functional restoration may be possible when the tumour is removed.

Clinical Manifestations

Both sensory and motor deficits may result; the location and extent of the tumour determine the severity and the distribution of the problem. The most common early symptom of an extradural spinal cord tumour is back pain. Radicular pain may occur as the tumour compresses nerve roots. The location of the pain depends on the level of compression. The pain worsens with activity, coughing, and straining. Some relief may occur with lying down, but there is usually a baseline of pain even in this position secondary to the inflammatory changes within the bone structure. Sensory disruption is manifested by pain, coldness sensation, numbness, and tingling sensation in the dermatomal distribution of the lesion. Motor weakness accompanies the sensory disturbances and consists of slowly increasing clumsiness, weakness, and spasticity, which can lead to paralysis. The sensory and motor disturbances are ipsilateral to the lesion. Bladder dysfunction, if present, is marked by urgency with difficulty in starting the flow and progresses to retention with overflow incontinence.

Manifestations of intradural spinal tumours develop as damage to the long spinal tracts progresses, producing paralysis, sensory loss, and bladder dysfunction. Pain can be severe as a result of compression of spinal roots or vertebrae.

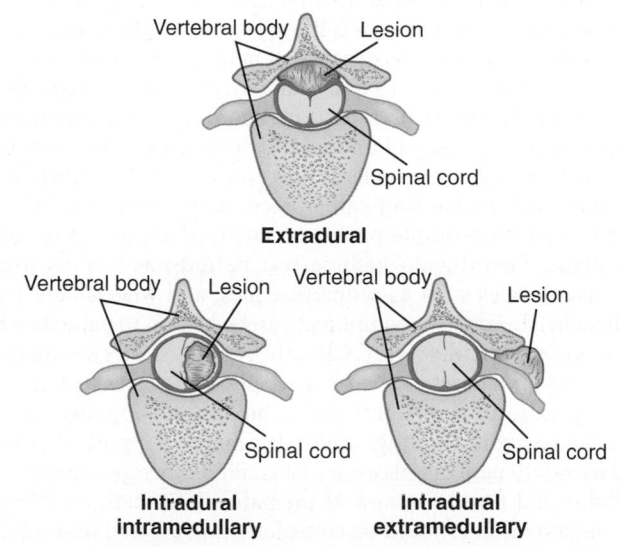

FIGURE 63-10 Types of spinal cord tumours.

NURSING AND COLLABORATIVE MANAGEMENT SPINAL CORD TUMOURS

Extradural, intradural, and intramedullary tumours are best detected with MRI. CT may be performed to determine amount of bone destruction. More than 85% of primary neoplasms are benign and can be completely resected; 90% of such patients recover without residual problems.

Compression of the spinal cord is an emergency. Relief of the ischemia related to the compression is the goal of therapy. Dexamethasone is usually used to treat edema, often in large doses (100 mg as a bolus dose). Surgical decompression can involve various approaches (anterior, posterior, or a combination

TABLE 63-13	CLASSIFICATION OF SPINAL CORD TUMOURS		
Type	**Incidence**	**Treatment**	**Prognosis**
Extradural: from bones of spine, in extradural space, or in paraspinal tissue	20%–50% of all intraspinal tumours; mostly malignant metastatic lesions	Relief of cord pressure by surgical laminectomy, radiation, chemotherapy, or combination approach	Dependent on tumour type and stage
Intradural extramedullary: within dura mater, outside spinal cord	Most frequent of intradural tumours (40%), mostly benign meningiomas and neurofibromas	Complete surgical removal of tumour (if possible), partial removal followed by radiation	Usually very good if no damage to cord from compression
Intradural intramedullary: within spinal cord	Least frequent of intradural tumours (5%–10%)	Partial surgical removal, radiation therapy (resulting in only temporary improvement)	Dependent on neurological function before and after decompression

of both), followed by reconstruction and stabilization. In a randomized control study, Patchell, Tibbs, Regine, and colleagues (2005) compared direct decompressive therapy followed by radiotherapy with radiotherapy alone; they demonstrated better patient outcomes in patients receiving both therapies in regard to neurological recovery, decreased postoperative morbidity, and long-term survival. They concluded that the best treatment for spinal cord compression caused by metastatic cancer is surgery as initial treatment, followed by radiotherapy (Patchell, Tibbs, Regine, et al., 2005).

Treatment for nearly all spinal cord tumours is surgical removal. The exception is the metastatic tumour that is sensitive to chemotherapy or radiation and that has caused only minimal neurological deficits (e.g., multiple myeloma). In general, extra-dural and intradural extramedullary tumours can be completely removed surgically. Intradural intramedullary tumours have a less favourable prognosis. However, exploration and removal are usually attempted.

Standard radiation therapy after surgical decompression is considered if the tumour is radiosensitive. Treatment is started approximately 3 to 4 weeks after surgery and usually consists of five doses. In a newer therapy, intensity-modulated radiotherapy, higher doses of radiation are delivered to the tumour site, which minimizes injury to surrounding normal spinal and paraspinal tissues. Chemotherapy has also been used in conjunction with radiation therapy.

Relief of pain and prevention of continued neurological decline are the ultimate goals of treatment. Nurses must be aware of the neurological status of the patient before and after treatment. Ensuring that the patient receives analgesics to manage pain is an important nursing responsibility. Depending on the amount of neurological dysfunction exhibited, the patient may need to be cared for as though he or she were recovering from an SCI. Rehabilitation of patients with spinal cord tumours is similar to rehabilitation of patients with SCIs.

POSTPOLIO SYNDROME

Polio, also known as *poliomyelitis,* is an infectious viral disease transmitted through the oral route by ingestion of contaminated water or food or by contact with infected sources such as unwashed hands. The virus is shed in the feces of infected individuals for as long as 6 weeks. The disease produces a range of manifestations from influenza-like symptoms (abortive poliomyelitis) that resolve in 24 to 36 hours (nonparalytic) to paralytic poliomyelitis that attacks the motor neurons in the anterior horn of the spinal cord, the brain stem, or both. Polio ravaged North American communities during the 1930s, 1940s, and 1950s. Polio was effectively eradicated in North America by the development of the Salk injectable polio vaccine in 1954 and the Sabin oral polio vaccine in 1961. It is still a threat in developing countries because of a lack of effective immunization programs. Polio survivors who recovered from the disease decades ago, notably those who had paralytic poliomyelitis, are now experiencing a recurrence of neuro-muscular symptoms as they age. These late effects of polio are collectively referred to as postpolio syndrome (PPS). On the basis of criteria for diagnosis of PPS, the incidence and prevalence can range from 10% to 40% (Kedlaya, 2017).

Etiology and Pathophysiology

The etiology of PPS is not completely clear. The most commonly accepted theory is that enlarged distal motor neurons that had recovered after polio degenerate and subsequently begin to fail (Kedlaya, 2017). It appears that cellular damage caused by the effects of the polio virus may lead to exhaustion and premature failure of the motor neurons. The result is slowly progressive muscle weakness and fatigue. Factors thought to contribute to PPS include age-related motor neuron loss, musculo-skeletal overuse and disuse, weight gain, pain, and other neuro-muscular or systemic illnesses. There is no evidence to support the theory that PPS is caused by reactivation of the original polio virus.

Clinical Manifestations and Diagnostic Studies

PPS is manifested by a new onset of joint and muscle weakness, easy fatigability, generalized fatigue, and pain. In uncommon cases, individuals may also exhibit speech, swallowing, and respiratory difficulties. Patients should undergo thorough diagnostic testing to rule out other medical conditions that may produce similar symptoms. Criteria used to establish the diagnosis of PPS include a history of polio in the abortive, nonparalytic, or paralytic forms; recovery from polio; a lengthy period of stability of at least 10 to 20 years' duration; and clinical manifestations of PPS that are not associated with other medical disorders. Disabilities caused by PPS can have a significant effect on the patient's quality of life.

NURSING AND COLLABORATIVE MANAGEMENT POSTPOLIO SYNDROME

Management approaches for PPS are targeted at controlling symptoms, particularly fatigue, weakness, and pain. An interdisciplinary team approach is essential for management of the patient. The cornerstone of management is lifestyle modification to conserve energy and support performance of activities of daily living.

During the polio epidemic, polio victims were subjected to rigorous therapy to regain muscle function. A particular challenge may be helping the patient understand that aggressive or strenuous therapy to strengthen muscles is now considered counterproductive and that overexertion can worsen fatigue and weakness. It is important to promote pacing of activities to prevent feelings of fatigue. Planning to include rest periods, as well as using assistive devices such as scooters, canes, and wheelchairs may be beneficial. Adaptive equipment can be helpful to patients who experience difficulty with self-care. Other strategies include arranging for a handicapped licence plate or sticker to facilitate parking close to shops and public buildings, shopping on the Internet to avoid walking, and enlisting the support of family and friends to perform necessary tasks. Physiotherapy can support mobility and fitness in view of the patient's limitations. Weight loss interventions should be considered for affected individuals who are overweight.

Effective pain management through both pharmacological and nonpharmacological approaches with the health care provider or pain management team can enable an individual to remain active and achieve a greater sense of well-being. Nonpharmacological measures include massage, relaxation strategies, and guided imagery (see Chapter 12). Protection from the cold can also aid in pain relief since the individual with PPS may be especially sensitive to a cold environment. For affected individuals with speech, swallowing, or respiratory difficulties, it is important to take measures to prevent aspiration, maintain airway patency, and promote optimal nutrition. Nursing interventions for these problems are similar to those described for patients with GBS and SCI.

Experiencing the re-emergence of symptoms related to polio can have a devastating effect on a patient's psychosocial well-being. Memories of paralysis and the challenges of recovery can cause fear when PPS is diagnosed. Anxiety and depression can occur, as can difficulties with coping. The nurse can assist the individual by actively listening to concerns, providing information about PPS and available resources, and referring the patient to support groups or counselling when necessary. Gaining a sense of control through active participation in lifestyle modifications and therapy may improve the patient's ability to cope with PPS.

CASE STUDY

Spinal Cord Injury

Source: Joana Lopes/ Shutterstock .com.

Patient Profile: Acute Phase

Sal Diaz, a 24-year-old man, is admitted to the emergency department with the diagnosis of a cervical SCI. Mr. Diaz was swimming at a neighbour's backyard pool. He dove into the shallow end, striking his head on the bottom of the pool. His friends noticed that he did not resurface. They rescued him and brought him to the side of the pool. They maintained neck immobilization until the rescue crews arrived.

Subjective Data
- Is awake and alert
- Has complaints of neck pain
- Is anxious and asking why he cannot move his legs and has weak arms
- Is asking to see his family

Objective Data
Physical Examination
- Weak biceps movement bilaterally
- No triceps movement bilaterally
- Gross elbow movement present bilaterally
- No movement bilaterally in lower extremities
- Decreased sensation from the shoulders down
- Loss of anal sphincter contraction
- BP: 85/50 mm Hg; pulse: 56; respirations: 32 and laboured

Diagnostic Studies
- CT of cervical spine shows subluxation and compression fracture at C5–6
- MRI of cervical spine shows a severe spinal cord compression at C5–6

Collaborative Care
- Intubated in the emergency department
- Started on mechanical ventilation
- Placed in halo traction on arrival in the ICU
- Further went on to have surgical decompression and stabilization

Discussion Questions: Acute Phase
1. **Priority decision:** What nursing activities would be a priority on Mr. Diaz's arrival in the ICU?
2. What physiological problems are causing Mr. Diaz to have hypotension and bradycardia?

3. What would the first line of treatment be for Mr. Diaz's hypotension and bradycardia?
4. What signs and symptoms would indicate respiratory distress, and what physiological problem would cause respiratory distress in Mr. Diaz's injury state?
5. What can the nurse do to decrease Mr. Diaz's anxiety?
6. **Priority decision:** Based on the assessment data provided, what are the priority nursing diagnoses or problem statements? Are there any collaborative problems?

Patient Profile: Rehabilitation Phase
One month after the injury, Mr. Diaz is at a local inpatient SCI rehabilitation facility. He has since been extubated and uses a wheelchair to mobilize. He eats three meals a day with assistance and is on a strict bowel and bladder program.

Subjective Data
- Awake and alert but anxious
- Complaining of severe headache, blurred vision, and nausea

Objective Data
Physical Examination
- Flushed and diaphoretic above the level of injury
- No bowel movement for 2 days
- BP: 180/90 mm Hg; pulse: 32 beats/min; respirations: 30 breaths/min and laboured

Discussion Questions: Rehabilitation Phase
1. **Priority decision:** What initial priority nursing interventions would be appropriate?
2. What physiological problem is causing Mr. Diaz's hypertension and bradycardia?
3. Once the physician has been notified, what other interventions would be appropriate?
4. **Priority decision:** Based on the assessment data provided, what are the priority nursing diagnoses?
5. **Evidence-informed practice:** Mr. Diaz and his family are concerned about the risk for autonomic dysreflexia. What effective strategies to prevent autonomic dysreflexia could the nurse discuss with the patient and family?

evolve

Answers are available at *http://evolve.elsevier.com/Canada/Lewis/medsurg*

REVIEW QUESTIONS

The number of the question corresponds to the same-numbered objective at the beginning of the chapter.

1. What should the nurse do during assessment of a client with trigeminal neuralgia?
   a. Inspect all aspects of the mouth and teeth.
   b. Lightly palpate the affected side of the face for edema.
   c. Test for temperature and sensation perception on the face.
   d. Ask the client to describe factors that initiate an episode.

2. During routine assessment of a client with GBS, the nurse finds the client to be short of breath. What is the cause of the client's respiratory distress?
   a. Elevated protein levels in the CSF
   b. Immobility resulting from ascending paralysis
   c. Degeneration of motor neurons in the brain stem and the spinal cord
   d. Paralysis ascending to the nerves that stimulate the thoracic area

3. A client is admitted to the ICU with a C7 SCI, and Brown-Séquard syndrome is diagnosed. What would the nurse probably find on physical examination?
   a. Upper extremity weakness only
   b. Complete motor and sensory loss below C7
   c. Loss of position sense and vibration in both lower extremities
   d. Ipsilateral motor loss and contralateral sensory loss below C7

4. A client is admitted to the hospital with SCI after an automobile accident. The nurse recognizes that the pathophysiology of secondary SCI involves which of the following?
   a. Initial infarction of the white matter of the spinal cord
   b. Mechanical transection of the cord by the trauma
   c. Necrotic destruction of the cord from hemorrhage and edema
   d. Release of epinephrine leading to massive vasodilation of spinal cord vessels

5. Goals of rehabilitation for the client with an injury at the C6 level include which of the following? *(Select all that apply)*
   a. Stand erect with leg brace
   b. Feed self with hand devices
   c. Drive a motorized wheelchair
   d. Assist with transfer activities
   e. Control bowel and bladder function

6. A client with a C7 SCI undergoing rehabilitation tells the nurse he must have the flu because he has a bad headache and nausea. What should the nurse's initial action be?
   a. Call the physician.
   b. Check the client's temperature.
   c. Take the client's blood pressure.
   d. Elevate the head of the bed to 90 degrees.

7. For a 65-year-old female client who has lived with a T1 SCI for 20 years, what health teaching information would the nurse emphasize?
   a. A mammogram is needed every 2 years.
   b. Bladder function tends to improve with age.
   c. Heart disease is not common in persons with SCI.
   d. As a person ages, the need to change body position is less important.

8. What is the most common early symptom of a spinal cord tumour?
   a. Urinary incontinence
   b. Back pain that worsens with activity
   c. Paralysis below the level of involvement
   d. Impaired sensation of pain, temperature, and light touch

9. Which of the following descriptions best characterizes PPS?
   a. Autoimmune disease of motor neurons triggered by polio virus
   b. Reactivation of poliomyelitis resulting in acute musculo-skeletal disease
   c. Degeneration of enlarged motor neurons many years after poliomyelitis
   d. Disorder characterized by active viral destruction of the upper motor neurons

1. d; 2. d; 3. d; 4. c; 5. b, c, d; 6. c; 7. a; 8. b; 9. c.

⊜volve

For even more review questions, visit *http://evolve.elsevier.com/Canada/Lewis/medsurg.*

REFERENCES

Al-Quliti, K. W. (2015). Update on neuropathic pain treatment for trigeminal neuralgia. The pharmacological and surgical options. *Neurosciences, 20*(2), 107–114. doi:10.17712/nsj.2015.2.20140501.

Ansar, V., & Valadi, N. (2015). Guillain-Barré syndrome. *Primary Care: Clinics in Office Practice, 42*(2), 189–193. doi:10.1016/j.pop.2015.01.001.

Boyd, J., & Tymianksi, D. (2012). Neurological assessment for the nurse. In *Navigating neuroscience nursing: A Canadian perspective.* Pembroke, ON: Pappin Communications.

Bracken, M. B. (2012). Steroids for acute spinal cord injury. *The Cochrane Database of Systematic Reviews*, No. 1, Article CD001046. doi:10.1002/14651858.CD001046.pub2.

Chin, L. (2015). *Spinal cord injuries.* Retrieved from *http://emedicine.medscape.com/article/793582-overview#a4.*

Chung, S. B., Lee, S. H., Kim, E. S., et al. (2011). Incidence of deep vein thrombosis after spinal cord injury: A prospective study in 37 consecutive patients with traumatic or nontraumatic spinal cord injury treated by mechanical prophylaxis. *The Journal of Trauma and Acute Care Surgery, 71*(4), 867–871. doi:10.1097/TA.0b013e31822dd3be.

Dhall, S. S., Hadley, R. J., Aarabi, B., et al. (2013). Deep venous thrombosis and thromboembolism in patients with cervical spinal cord injuries. *Neurosurgery, 72*(Suppl. 2), 244–254. doi:10.1227/NEU.0b013e31827728c0.

Elliott, S., & McBride, K. (2014). Sexual and reproductive health following spinal cord injury. In J. J. Eng, R. W. Teasell, W. C. Miller, et al. (Eds.), *Spinal cord injury rehabilitation evidence* (version 5.0, pp. 1–84). Retrieved from *https://scireproject.com/evidence/rehabilitation-evidence/sexual-and-reproductive-health/.*

Eviston, T., Croxson, G., Kennedy, P., et al. (2015). Bell's palsy: Aetiology, clinical features and multidisciplinary care. *Journal of Neurology, Neurosurgery, and Psychiatry, 86*(12), 1356–1361. doi:10.1136/jnnp-2014-309563.

Farry, A., & Baxter, D. (2010). *The incidence and prevalence of spinal cord injury in Canada: Overview and estimates based on current evidence.* Richmond, BC: Rick Hansen Institute & Urban Futures. Retrieved from *http://fecst.inesss.qc.ca/fileadmin/documents/photos/LincidenceetlaprevalencedestraumamedullaireauCanada.pdf.* (Seminal).

Fraser, C., McIntyre, A., Thompson, S., et al. (2014). Nutrition issues following spinal cord injury. In J. J. Eng, R. W. Teasell, W. C. Miller, et al. (Eds.), *Spinal cord injury rehabilitation evidence* (version 6.0, pp. 1–52). Retrieved from *https://scireproject.com/wp-content/uploads/nutrition-v6.pdf*.

Grossman, R. G., Frankowski, R. F., Burau, K. D., et al. (2012). Incidence and severity of acute complications after spinal cord injury. *Journal of Neurosurgery. Spine, 17*(Suppl. 1), 119–128. doi: 10.3171/2012.5.AOSPINE12127.

Hawryluk, G., Whetstone, W., Saigal, R., et al. (2015). Mean arterial blood pressure correlates with neurological recovery after human spinal cord injury: Analysis of high frequency physiologic data. *Journal of Neurotrauma, 32*(24), 1958–1967. doi:10.1089/neu.2014.3778.

Houghton, P. E., Campbell, K. E., & Panel, C. P. G. (2013). *Canadian best practice guidelines for the prevention and management of pressure ulcers in people with spinal cord injury: A resource handbook for clinicians.* Retrieved from *http://onf.org/system/attachments/168/original/Pressure_Ulcers_Best_Practice_Guideline_Final_web4.pdf*.

Hsieh, C. H., DeJong, G., Groah, S., et al. (2013). Comparing rehabilitation services and outcomes between older and younger people with spinal cord injury. *Archives of Physical Medicine and Rehabilitation, 94*(4 Suppl. 4), S175–S186. doi:10.1016/j.apmr.2012.10.038.

Hurlbert, R. J., Hadley, M. N., Walters, B. C., et al. (2013). Pharmacological therapy for acute spinal cord injury. *Neurosurgery, 72*(Suppl. 2), 93–105. doi:10.1227/NEU.0b013e31827765c6.

Kastanias, P., Buzon, A., & Sarro, A. (2012). Pain assessment and management in adults. In *Navigating neuroscience nursing: A Canadian perspective.* Pembroke, ON: Pappin Communications.

Kedlaya, D. (2017). *Postpolio syndrome.* Retrieved from *http://emedicine.medscape.com/article/306920-overview*.

Koopman, W., & Shcharinsky, A. (2012). Neuromuscular disorders. In *Navigating neuroscience nursing: A Canadian perspective.* Pembroke, ON: Pappin Communications.

Krassioukov, A., Blackmer, J., Teasell, R. W., et al. (2014). Autonomic dysreflexia following spinal cord injury. In J. J. Eng, R. W. Teasell, W. C. Miller, et al. (Eds.), *Spinal cord injury rehabilitation evidence* (version 5.0, pp. 1–35). Retrieved from *https://scireproject.com/wp-content/uploads/autonomic_dysreflexia-1.pdf*.

Krause, J., & Edles, P. A. (2014). Injury perceptions, hopes for recovery and psychological status after spinal cord injury. *Rehabilitation Psychology, 59*(2), 176–182. doi:10.1037/a0035778.

Krueger, H., Noonan, V. K., Trenaman, L. M., et al. (2013). The economic burden of traumatic spinal cord injury in Canada. *Chronic Diseases and Injuries in Canada, 33*(3), 113–122.

Kruger, E. A., Pires, M., Ngann, Y., et al. (2013). Comprehensive management of pressure ulcers in spinal cord injury: Current concepts and future trends. *The Journal of Spinal Cord Medicine, 36*(6), 572–585. doi:10.1179/2045772313Y.0000000093.

Larsen, A., Piepgras, D., Chyatte, D., et al. (2011). Trigeminal neuralgia: Diagnosis and medical and surgical management. *Journal of the American Academy of Physician Assistants, 24*(7), 20–25.

Marra, C. M. (2015). Neurosyphilis. *Neuroinfectious Diseases, 21*(6), 1714–1728. doi:10.1212/CON.0000000000000250.

Morais, D. F., de Melo Neto, J. S., Meguins, L. C., et al. (2014). Clinical applicability of magnetic resonance imaging in acute spinal cord trauma. *European Spine Journal, 23*(7), 1457–1463. doi:10.1007/s00586-013-3047-3.

Noonan, V. K., Fingas, M., Farry, A., et al. (2012). Incidence and prevalence of spinal cord injury in Canada: A national perspective. *Neuroepidemiology, 38*(4), 219–226. doi:10.1159/000336014.

Patchell, R. A., Tibbs, P. A., Regine, W. F., et al. (2005). Direct decompressive surgical resection in the treatment of spinal cord compression caused by metastatic cancer: A randomised trial. *Lancet, 366*, 643–648. doi:10.1016/S0140-6736(05)66954-1. (Seminal).

Public Health Agency of Canada. (2012). *Botulism.* Retrieved from *http://www.phac-aspc.gc.ca/fs-sa/fs-fi/botulism-eng.php*.

Public Health Agency of Canada. (2014). *Tetanus.* Retrieved from *http://www.phac-aspc.gc.ca/im/vpd-mev/tetanus-tetanos-eng.php*.

Ryken, T. C., Hurlbert, R. J., Hadley, M. N., et al. (2013). The acute cardiopulmonary management of patients with cervical spinal cord injuries. *Neurosurgery, 72*(Suppl. 3), 84–92. doi:10.1227/NEU.0b013e318276ee16.

Sarro, A., Anthony, T., Magtoto, R., et al. (2010). Developing a standard of care for halo vest and pin site care including patient and family education: A collaborative approach among three Greater Toronto Area teaching hospitals. *The Journal of Neuroscience Nursing, 42*(3), 169–175. doi:10.1097/JNN.0b013e3181d4a3be. (Seminal).

Singh, A., Tetreault, L., Kalsi-Ryan, S., et al. (2014). Global prevalence and incidence of traumatic spinal cord injury. *Clinical Epidemiology, 2014*(6), 309–331. doi:10.2147/CLEP.S68889.

Willison, H., Jacobs, B. C., & van Doorn, P. A. (2016). Guillain-Barré syndrome. *The Lancet, 388*(10045), 717–727. doi:10.1016/S0140-6736(16)00339-1.

Wilson, J. R., Forgione, N., & Fehlings, M. G. (2013). Emerging therapies for acute spinal cord injury. *Canadian Medical Association Journal, 185*(6), 485–492. doi:10.1503/cmaj.121206.

Witiw, C. D., & Fehlings, M. G. (2015). Acute spinal cord injury. *Journal of Spinal Disorders & Techniques, 28*(6), 202–210. doi:10.1097/BSD.0000000000000287.

Zakrzewska, J. M. (2014). Clinical review: Trigeminal neuralgia. *British Medical Journal, 348*(7946), doi:10.1136/bmj.g474.

RESOURCES

Canadian Association of Neuroscience Nurses (CANN)
http://www.cann.ca

Canadian Paraplegic Association (Manitoba)
http://www.cpamanitoba.ca

Canadian Spinal Research Organization (CSRO)
http://www.csro.com

Canadian Spine Society
http://www.spinecanada.ca

Parachute Canada
http://parachutecanada.org

Rick Hansen Institute
http://www.rickhanseninstitute.org

SCI Action Canada
http://www.sciactioncanada.ca

Spinal Cord Injury Alberta
http://www.sci-ab.ca

Spinal Cord Injury Canada
http://sci-can.ca

Spinal Cord Injury Ontario
http://www.sciontario.org

Spinal Cord Injury PEI
http://www.sci-pei.ca

Spinal Cord Injury Research Evidence
http://www.scireproject.com

Trigeminal Neuralgia Association of Canada
http://www.tnac.org

Academy of Spinal Cord Injury Professionals
http://test.academyscipro.org/aboutscin

Christopher and Dana Reeve Foundation
http://www.crpf.org

Guillain-Barré Syndrome–Chronic Inflammatory Demyelinating Polyneuropathy Foundation International
http://gbs-cidp.org

National Institute of Neurological Disorders and Stroke (NINDS)
http://www.ninds.nih.gov

National Rehabilitation Information Center (NARIC)
http://www.naric.com

For additional Internet resources, see the website for this book at *http://evolve.elsevier.com/Canada/Lewis/medsurg*.

Nursing Assessment

Musculo-Skeletal System

Written by: Michael E. Zychowicz
Adapted by: Jana Lok

⊖volve WEBSITE

http://evolve.elsevier.com/Canada/Lewis/medsurg

- Review Questions
  (Online Only)
- Key Points
- Answer Guidelines for Case Study

- Supporting Media—Animations:
  - Classification of Joints: Condyloid Joint
  - Classification of Joints: Gliding Joint—Hand
  - Classification of Joints: Hinge Joint

- Conceptual Care Map Creator
- Audio Glossary
- Content Updates

LEARNING OBJECTIVES

1. Describe the gross anatomical and microscopic composition of bone.
2. Explain the classification system of joints and movements at diarthroidal joints.
3. Describe the types and structure of muscle tissue.
4. Describe the functions of cartilage, muscles, ligaments, tendons, fascia, and bursae.
5. Describe age-related changes in the musculo-skeletal system and differences in assessment findings.
6. Identify the significant subjective and objective data related to the musculo-skeletal system that should be obtained from a patient.
7. Describe the appropriate techniques used in the physical assessment of the musculo-skeletal system.
8. Differentiate normal from abnormal findings of a physical assessment of the musculo-skeletal system.
9. Describe the purpose, significance of results, and nursing responsibilities related to diagnostic studies of the musculo-skeletal system.

KEY TERMS

ankylosis, p. 1626, Table 64-6
arthrocentesis, p. 1630
arthroscopy, p. 1629
atrophy, p. 1626, Table 64-6

contracture, p. 1626, Table 64-6
crepitation, p. 1626, Table 64-6
isometric contractions, p. 1619
isotonic contractions, p. 1619

kyphosis, p. 1626, Table 64-6
lordosis, p. 1626, Table 64-6
scoliosis, p. 1626, Table 64-6

The unique structures of the musculo-skeletal system allow human beings to complete complex movements. The dexterity of the upper extremities enables an individual to perform complicated technical tasks, whereas stronger lower extremities enable mobility for varied activities. The musculo-skeletal system is composed of voluntary muscle and five types of connective tissue: bones, cartilage, ligaments, tendons, and fascia (Roberts, 2016). Resilient bone and cartilage absorb energy from any impact, minimizing the risk of injury to other body structures. However, this characteristic ability makes the musculo-skeletal system itself particularly vulnerable to injury from external forces. Any damage to bone and related soft tissues can cause functional disruption for an individual. Deformity, alteration in body image, alteration in mobility, pain, or permanent disability may result from musculo-skeletal injury.

STRUCTURES AND FUNCTIONS OF THE MUSCULO-SKELETAL SYSTEM

Bone

Function. The main functions of bone are support, movement, protection of the body's internal structures, blood cell production, and mineral storage (McCance & Huether, 2014). Bones provide the supporting framework that keeps the body from collapsing and allow the body to bear weight. Bones serve as a point of attachment for muscles, which are connected to bones by tendons. Bones act as a lever for muscles, and movement occurs as a result of muscle contractions applied to these levers. Bones also protect underlying vital organs and tissues. For example, the skull encloses the brain, the vertebrae surround the spinal cord, and the rib cage covers the lungs and heart. Bones contain hematopoietic tissue for the production of red and white blood cells. Bones also serve as a site for storage of inorganic minerals such as calcium and phosphorus.

Bone is a dynamic tissue that continually changes form and composition. It contains both organic material (i.e., collagen) and inorganic material (i.e., calcium, phosphate). The internal and external growth and remodelling of bone are ongoing processes.

Microscopic Structure. Bone is classified according to structure as *cortical* (compact and dense) or *cancellous* (spongy). In *cortical bone,* cylinder-shaped structural units called *osteons* (Haversian systems) fit closely together to form a dense bone structure (Figure 64-1, *B*). Within the systems, the Haversian canals run parallel to the bone's long axis and contain the blood vessels that travel to the bone's interior from the periosteum.

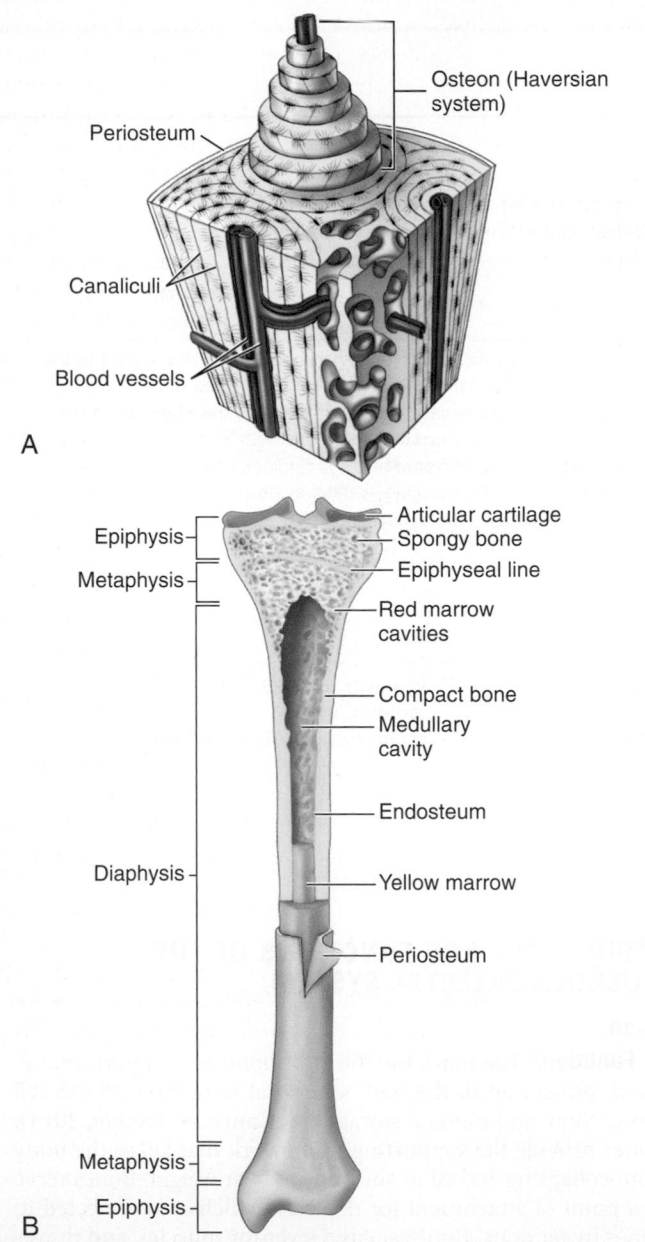

FIGURE 64-1 Illustrations of bone structure. **A,** Cortical (compact) bone showing numerous structural units called *osteons.* **B,** Anatomy of a long bone (tibia), showing cancellous and compact bone. Sources: *A,* Herlihy, B. (2011). *The human body in health and illness* (4th ed.). Philadelphia: Saunders. *B,* From Patton, K. T., & Thibodeau, G. A. (2013). *Anatomy and physiology* (8th ed.). St Louis: Mosby.

Surrounding each *osteon* are concentric rings known as *lamellae,* which characterize mature bone. Smaller canals (*canaliculi*) extend from the Haversian canals to the *lacunae,* where mature bone cells are embedded. Cancellous (spongy) bone lacks the organized structure of cortical (compact) bone. The lamellae are arranged not in concentric rings but rather along the lines of maximum stress placed on the bone. Cancellous bone tissue is filled with red or yellow marrow, and blood reaches the bone cells by passing through spaces in the marrow.

The three types of bone cells are osteoblasts, osteocytes, and osteoclasts (McCance & Huether, 2014). *Osteoblasts* synthesize organic bone matrix (collagen) and are the basic bone-forming cells. *Osteocytes* are the mature bone cells. *Osteoclasts* participate in bone remodelling by assisting in the breakdown of bone tissue. *Bone remodelling* is the removal of old bone by osteoclasts (*resorption*) and the deposition of new bone by osteoblasts (*ossification*). The inner layer of bone is primarily made up of osteoblasts with a few osteoclasts.

Gross Structure. The anatomical structure of bone is best represented by a typical long bone such as the tibia (see Figure 64-1, *A*). Each long bone consists of the epiphysis, the diaphysis, and the metaphysis. The *epiphysis,* the widened area found at each end of a long bone, is composed primarily of cancellous bone. The width of the epiphysis allows for greater weight distribution and provides stability for the joint. The epiphysis is also the location of muscle attachment. Articular cartilage covers the ends of the epiphysis to provide a smooth surface for joint movement. The *diaphysis* is the main shaft of the bone. It provides structural support and is composed of compact bone. The tubular structure of the diaphysis allows it to more easily withstand bending and twisting forces. The *metaphysis* is the flared area between the epiphysis and the diaphysis. Like the epiphysis, it is composed of cancellous bone. The *epiphyseal plate,* or growth plate, is the cartilaginous area between the epiphysis and the metaphysis. It actively produces bone to allow longitudinal growth in children. Injury to the epiphyseal plate in a growing child can lead to development of a shorter extremity, which can cause significant functional problems. In the adult, the metaphysis and the epiphysis become joined as this plate hardens to become mature bone.

The *periosteum* is composed of fibrous connective tissue that covers the bone. Tiny blood vessels penetrate the periosteum to provide nutrition to underlying bone. Musculotendinous fibres anchor to the outer layer of the periosteum. The inner layer of the periosteum is attached to the bone by bundles of collagen. No periosteum exists on the articular surfaces of long bones. These bone ends are covered by articular cartilage.

The *medullary* (marrow) cavity is in the centre of the diaphysis and contains either red or yellow bone marrow (Thibodeau & Patton, 2016). In a growing child, red bone marrow is actively involved in blood cell production (hematopoiesis). In the adult, the medullary cavity of long bones contains yellow bone marrow, which is mainly adipose tissue. Yellow marrow is involved in hematopoiesis only in times of great blood cell need. In adults, red marrow is found mainly in the flat bones, such as the pelvis, skull, sternum, cranium, ribs, vertebrae, and scapulae and in the cancellous (spongy) material at the epiphyseal ends of long bones such as the femur and the humerus.

Types. The skeleton consists of 206 bones, which are classified according to shape as long, short, flat, or irregular.

Long bones are characterized by a central shaft (diaphysis) and two widened ends (epiphyses) (see Figure 64-1, *B*). Examples include the femur, humerus, and radius. *Short bones* are composed of cancellous bone covered by a thin layer of compact bone. Examples include the carpals in the hand and the tarsals in the foot.

Flat bones have two layers of compact bone separated by a layer of cancellous bone. Examples include the ribs, skull, scapula, and sternum. The spaces in the cancellous bone contain bone marrow. *Irregular bones* appear in a variety of shapes and sizes. Examples include the vertebrae, sacrum, and ear ossicles.

Joints

A *joint* (articulation) is a place where the ends of two bones are in proximity and move in relation to each other. Joints are classified according to the degree of movement that they allow.

The most common joint is the freely movable *diarthrodial* (synovial) type. Each joint is enclosed in a capsule of fibrous connective tissue that joins the two bones together to form a cavity (Figure 64-2). The capsule is lined by a synovial membrane, which secretes thick synovial fluid to lubricate the joint and reduce friction. The end of each bone is covered with articular (hyaline) cartilage. Supporting structures (i.e., ligaments, tendons) reinforce the joint capsule and provide limits to joint movement (National Association of Orthopaedic Nurses, 2013). Types of diarthrodial joints are shown in Figure 64-3.

Cartilage

Cartilage is a rigid connective tissue that serves as a support for soft tissue and provides the articular surface for joint movement. It protects underlying tissues. The cartilage in the epiphyseal plate is also involved in the growth of long bones before physical maturity is reached. Because articular cartilage is relatively avascular, it must receive nourishment by the diffusion of material from the synovial fluid. The lack of a direct blood supply contributes to the slow metabolism of cartilage cells, which is the reason why cartilage tissue heals slowly.

Hyaline cartilage, containing a moderate amount of collagen fibres, is the most common type of cartilage. It is found in the trachea, bronchi, nose, epiphyseal plate, and articular surfaces of bones. *Elastic cartilage,* which contains both collagen and elastic fibres, is more flexible than hyaline cartilage. It is found in the ear, epiglottis, and larynx. *Fibrocartilage* consists mostly of collagen fibres and is a tough tissue that often functions as a shock absorber. It is found between the vertebral discs and also forms a protective cushion between the bones of the pelvic girdle, knee, and shoulder.

Muscle

Types. The three types of muscle tissue are *cardiac* (striated, involuntary), *smooth* (nonstriated, involuntary), and *skeletal* (striated, voluntary) muscle. Cardiac muscle is found in the heart. Its spontaneous contractions propel blood through the circulatory system. Smooth muscle occurs in the walls of hollow structures such as airways, arteries, gastro-intestinal tract, urinary bladder, and uterus. Smooth muscle contraction is modulated by neuronal and hormonal influences. Skeletal muscle, which requires neuronal stimulation for contraction, accounts for about half of a human being's body weight. It is the focus of the following discussion.

Structure. The skeletal muscle is enclosed by the *epimysium,* a continuous layer of deep fascia. The epimysium helps muscles slide over nearby structures. Connective tissue surrounding and extending into the muscle can be subdivided into fibre bundles, or fasciculi. These bundles are covered by perimysium and an innermost connective tissue layer called the *endomysium* that surrounds each fibre (Figure 64-4).

The structural unit of muscle is the muscle cell or muscle fibre, which is highly specialized for contraction. Skeletal muscle fibres are long, multinucleated cylinders that contain many mitochondria to support their high metabolic activity. Muscle fibres are composed of *myofibrils,* which in turn are made up of contractile filaments (protein).

The *sarcomere* is the contractile unit of the myofibrils (McCance & Huether, 2014). Each sarcomere consists of myosin (thick) filaments and actin (thin) filaments. The arrangement of the thick and thin filaments accounts for the characteristic banding of muscle when it is seen under a microscope. Muscle contraction occurs as thick and thin filaments slide past each other, causing the sarcomeres to shorten.

Contractions. Skeletal muscle contractions enable posture maintenance, movement, and facial expressions. Isometric contractions increase the tension within a muscle but do not produce movement. Repeated isometric contractions make muscles grow larger and stronger. Isotonic contractions shorten a muscle to produce movement. Most contractions are a combination of tension generation (isometric) and shortening (isotonic). Muscle *atrophy* (wasting of muscle and subsequent decrease in its size) occurs with the absence of contraction that results from immobility, whereas increased muscular activity leads to *hypertrophy* (increase in size).

Skeletal muscle fibres are divided into two groups according to the type of activity they demonstrate. *Slow-twitch muscle fibres* support prolonged muscle activity such as marathon running. Because they also support the body against gravity, they assist in posture maintenance. *Fast-twitch muscle fibres* are used for rapid muscle contraction required for activities such as blinking the eye, jumping, or sprinting. Fast-twitch fibres tend to tire more quickly than slow-twitch fibres.

Neuro-muscular Junction. Skeletal muscle fibres require a nerve impulse to contract. A nerve fibre and the skeletal muscle fibres it stimulates are called a *motor end plate*. The junction

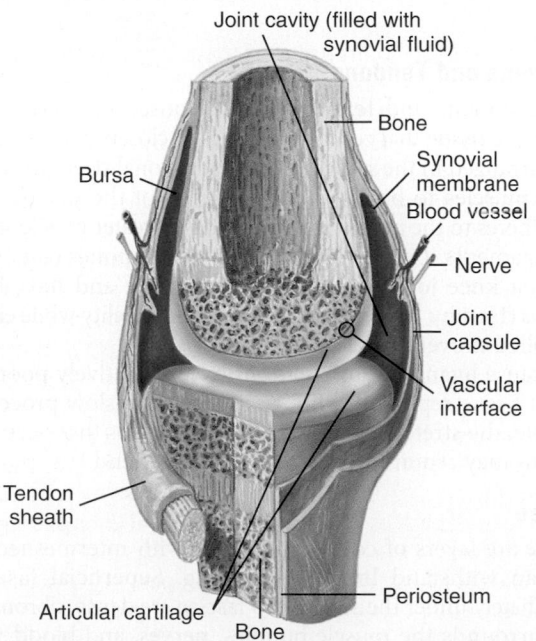

FIGURE 64-2 Structure of a diarthrodial (synovial) joint.

Joint	Movement	Examples	Illustration
Hinge joint	Flexion, extension	Elbow joint (shown), interphalangeal joints, knee joint	
Ball and socket (spheroidal)	Flexion, extension; adduction, abduction; circumduction	Shoulder (shown), hip	
Pivot (rotary)	Rotation	Atlas-axis, proximal radioulnar joint (shown)	
Condyloid	Flexion, extension; abduction, adduction; circumduction	Wrist joint (between radial and carpals) (shown)	
Saddle	Flexion, extension; abduction, adduction; circumduction, thumb-finger opposition	Carpometacarpal joint of thumb (shown)	
Gliding	One surface moves over another surface	Between tarsal bones, sacroiliac joint, between articular processes of vertebrae, between carpal bones (shown)	

FIGURE 64-3 Types of diarthrodial (synovial) joints.

between the axon of the nerve cell and the adjacent muscle cell is called the *myoneural* or *neuro-muscular junction* (Figure 64-5).

Acetylcholine is released from the motor end plate of the neuron and diffuses across the neuro-muscular junction to bind with receptors on the muscle fibre. In response to this stimulation, the sarcoplasmic reticulum releases calcium ions into the cytoplasm which triggers the contraction in the myofibrils. When calcium is low, *tetany* (involuntary contractions of skeletal muscle) can occur.

Energy Source. The direct energy source for muscle fibre contractions is adenosine triphosphate (ATP). ATP is synthesized by cellular oxidative metabolism in numerous mitochondria located close to the myofibrils. It is rapidly depleted through conversion to adenosine diphosphate and must be rephosphorylated. Phosphocreatine provides a rapid source for the resynthesis of ATP, but it is in turn converted to creatine and must be recharged. Glycolysis can serve as a source of ATP when the oxygen supply is inadequate for the metabolic needs of the muscle tissue. Glucose is broken down to pyruvic acid, which can be further converted to lactic acid to make more oxygen available. An accumulation of lactic acid in tissues leads to fatigue and pain.

Ligaments and Tendons

Both ligaments and tendons are composed of dense, fibrous connective tissue that contains bundles of closely packed collagen fibres arranged in the same plane for additional strength. *Tendons* attach muscles to bones as an extension of the muscle sheath that adheres to the periosteum. They have greater tensile strength than ligaments. *Ligaments* connect bones to bones (e.g., tibia to femur at knee joint). They are more elastic and flexible than tendons (Herlihy, 2011). Ligaments provide stability while enabling controlled movement at the joint.

Because ligaments and tendons have a relatively poor blood supply, tissue repair after injury to them is a slow process. For example, the stretching or tearing of ligaments that occurs with a sprain may require weeks to months to mend.

Fasciae

Fasciae are layers of connective tissue with intermeshed fibres that can withstand limited stretching. Superficial fasciae lie immediately under the skin. Deep fasciae are dense, fibrous tissue that surrounds the muscle bundles, nerves, and blood vessels. Deep fasciae also enclose individual muscles, allowing them to act independently and to glide over each other during contraction. In addition, they provide strength to muscle tissues.

Bursae

Bursae are small sacs of connective tissue lined with synovial membrane and containing synovial fluid. They are typically located at bony prominences or joints to relieve pressure and prevent friction between moving parts (Jarvis, Browne, MacDonald-Jenkins, et al., 2014). For example, bursae are found between the patella and the skin *(prepatellar bursa)* and between the greater trochanter of the proximal femur and the skin *(trochanteric bursa)*. *Bursitis* is an inflammation of a bursa sac.

AGE-RELATED CONSIDERATIONS

THE MUSCULO-SKELETAL SYSTEM

Many of the functional problems experienced by older adults are related to changes in the musculo-skeletal system. Although some changes begin in early adulthood, obvious signs of musculo-skeletal impairment may not appear until later adulthood. Alterations may affect an older adult's ability to complete self-care tasks and pursue other usual activities. Effects of musculo-skeletal changes may range from mild discomfort and decreased ability to perform activities of daily living to severe, chronic pain and immobility. The risk for falls also increases in older adults as a result of a loss of strength, change in balance, and change in *proprioception* (awareness of self in relation to the environment).

The bone remodelling process changes as adults age. Bone resorption increases and bone formation decreases; these events cause a loss of bone density, contributing to development of osteopenia and osteoporosis (see Chapter 66). Muscle mass and strength also decrease with aging. Tendons and ligaments become less flexible, and joints and limbs become more rigid. Joints in aging adults are also more likely to be affected by osteoarthritis (see Chapter 67).

In addition to the usual musculo-skeletal assessment with an emphasis on functional and activity status, the nurse should also determine the effect of age-related musculo-skeletal changes on an older patient's psychosocial well-being and quality of life.

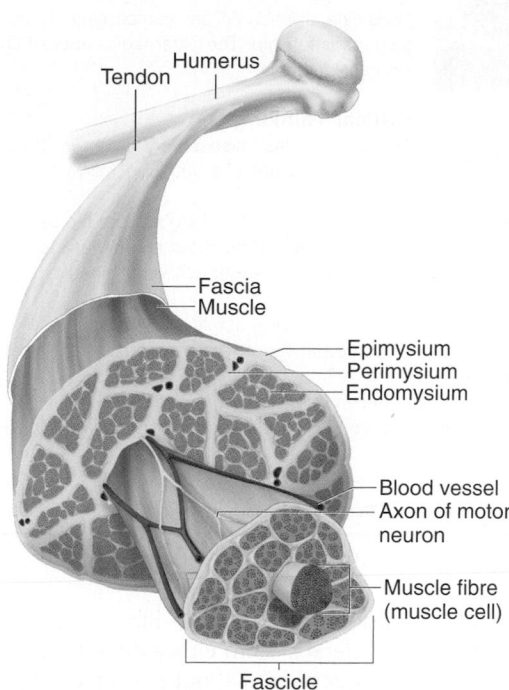

FIGURE 64-4 Structure of a muscle. Source: Patton, K. T., Thibodeau, G. A., & Douglas, M. (2012). *Essentials of anatomy and physiology*. St Louis: Mosby.

FIGURE 64-5 Neuro-muscular junction. Illustration of a side view of the neuro-muscular junction. Note how the distal end of a motor neuron fibre forms a synapse, or "chemical junction," with an adjacent muscle fibre. Neuro-transmitter molecules (specifically, acetylcholine [ACh]) are released from the neuron's synaptic vesicles and diffuse across the synaptic cleft. There they stimulate receptors in the motor end plate region of the sarcolemma. Source: Patton, K. T., & Thibodeau, G. A. (2013). *Anatomy and physiology* (8th ed., p. 353, Figure 12-7). St. Louis: Mosby.

TABLE 64-1 AGE-RELATED DIFFERENCES IN ASSESSMENT

Musculo-Skeletal System

Changes	Differences in Assessment Findings
Muscle	
Decreased number and diameter of muscle cells, replacement of muscle cells by fibrous connective tissue	Decreased muscle strength and bulk, abdominal protrusion, flabby muscle
Loss of elasticity in ligaments and cartilage	Decreased fine motor dexterity, decreased agility
Reduced ability to store glycogen; decreased ability to release glycogen as quick energy during stress	Slowed reaction times and reflexes as a result of slowing of impulse conduction along motor units; earlier fatigue with activity
Joints	
Increased risk for cartilage disruption that contributes to direct contact between bone ends and overgrowth of bone around joint margins	Joint stiffness, possible crepitation on movement; pain with motion, weight bearing, or both
Loss of water from discs between vertebrae; narrowing of intervertebral spaces	Loss of height from disc compression; posture change
Bone	
Decrease in bone density	Loss of height from vertebral compression, back pain; deformity such as kyphosis (dowager's hump) caused by vertebral compression

Older adults can use various strategies to prevent musculo-skeletal problems (see Chapter 65, Table 65-1).

Diseases such as osteoarthritis and osteoporosis are not the normal consequences of growing old; rather, they are the effects of disease in an aging adult. Symptoms of disease can be treated in many cases, helping the older adult to return to a higher functional level. Age-related changes in the musculo-skeletal system and differences in assessment findings are presented in Table 64-1.

ASSESSMENT OF THE MUSCULO-SKELETAL SYSTEM

Correct diagnosis of any complaint depends on a complete patient history and a thorough physical examination. Musculo-skeletal assessment focuses on good analyses of symptoms, functional assessment, medical history specific to the musculo-skeletal system, family history, and personal and social history. The most common symptoms of musculo-skeletal impairment include pain, weakness, deformity, limitation of movement, stiffness, and joint crepitation (described in Table 64-6). Neuro-vascular structures are often affected by musculo-skeletal problems, and muscular disorders may be manifestations of neurological problems. A neurological system assessment (discussed in Chapter 58) and head-to-toe physical assessment are often conducted simultaneously.

Subjective Data

Important Health Information. Appropriate questions to ask during a musculo-skeletal assessment are listed in Table 64-2.

CASE STUDY

Patient Introduction

Terry King is a 78-year-old man brought to the emergency department by ambulance after he fell on a patch of ice outside his home. He is accompanied by his wife, who was asleep when he fell. He lay outside in the cold for 2 hours before neighbours found him. He is pale, diaphoretic, and complaining of excruciating pain in his left hip. The paramedics applied O_2 at 2 L via nasal cannula.

Source: And-One/ Shutterstock .com.

Critical Thinking

Throughout this assessment chapter, think about Mr. King's symptoms with the following questions in mind:

1. What is the most likely cause for Mr. King's acute hip pain?
2. What type of assessment would be most appropriate for Mr. King: comprehensive, focused, or emergency? What should the nurse's priority assessment(s) be?
3. What questions should the nurse ask Mr. King?
4. What should be included in the physical assessment? What would the nurse be looking for?
5. What diagnostic studies might the nurse be ordered?
   See pp. 1624, 1625, and 1630 for more information on Mr. King.

ⓔvolve

Answers available at *http://evolve.elsevier.com/Canada/Lewis/medsurg.*

Past Health History. Because certain illnesses are known to affect the musculo-skeletal system either directly or indirectly, the patient should be questioned about past medical problems; questions should concern specifically tuberculosis, poliomyelitis, diabetes mellitus, parathyroid problems, hemophilia, rickets, soft tissue infection, and neuro-muscular disabilities. In addition, past or developing musculo-skeletal problems can affect the patient's overall health. Trauma to the musculo-skeletal system is a common reason for seeking medical evaluation. The nurse should record details of emergency treatment for any musculo-skeletal injuries. Questions should also focus on symptoms of arthritic and connective tissue diseases (e.g., gout, psoriatic arthritis, systemic lupus erythematosus), osteomalacia, osteomyelitis, and fungal infection of the bones or joints. The nurse should ask the patient about possible sources of a secondary bacterial infection, such as the ears, tonsils, teeth, sinuses, lungs, or genito-urinary tract. These infections can enter the bones, resulting in osteomyelitis or joint destruction. Obtain a detailed account of the course and treatment of any of these problems.

Medications. The nurse should carefully question the patient about use of prescription drugs, over-the-counter drugs, herbal products, and nutritional supplements (especially calcium and vitamin D; refer to Chapter 12, Tables 12-7 and 12-8, for commonly used herbs and dietary supplements). Detailed information should be obtained about each treatment, including its name, the dose and frequency, the length of time it was taken, its effects, and any possible adverse effects. The nurse should inquire specifically about use of any skeletal muscle relaxants, opioids, nonsteroidal anti-inflammatory drugs, and systemic and topical corticosteroids. A patient who has taken anti-inflammatory drugs should be questioned about gastro-intestinal distress or signs of bleeding.

In addition to drugs taken for treatment of a musculo-skeletal problem, the patient should be questioned about drugs that can have detrimental effects on this system. Such drugs and their

TABLE 64-2   HEALTH HISTORY

Musculo-Skeletal System: Questions for Obtaining Subjective Data

Joints
- Do you have any problems with your joints?*
- Do you have any pain?* (If so, ask patient to describe location, quality, severity, onset, timing, frequency; aggravating/relieving factors; refer to Chapter 10 for pain assessment.)
- Is the joint pain associated with fever, recent infection, trauma, or repetitive activity?*
- Have you noticed any stiffness, swelling, heat, or redness in your joints?*
- Do you have any limitations in movement or function of any joint?* Which activities give you problems?

Muscles
- Do you have any problems with your muscles (pain, cramping)?* Is the pain widespread and associated with fatigue?
- Do you have any pain in your calf muscles?* With walking? Does it go away with rest?
- Are your muscle aches associated with fever, chills, or the "flu"?
- Do you have any muscular weakness?* Where? How long have you noticed the weakness? Do the muscles look smaller there?

Bones
- Do you have any bone pain?* Is it affected by movement? How do you manage the pain?
- Do you have any deformity of any bone or joint? What is the cause? Does it affect range of motion?*
- Have any accidents or trauma ever affected your bones or joints? When? What was the treatment? Have any ongoing limitations resulted?*

Functional Assessment (Activities of Daily Living)
- Do your joint, muscle, or bone problems limit any of your usual daily activities?*
  - Bathing: getting in and out of tub, turning faucets
  - Toileting: voiding, defecating, getting on or off toilet, wiping self
- Dressing: fastening buttons, zippers, pulling clothes over head, pulling up pants or skirt, tying shoes
- Grooming: shaving, brushing teeth, fixing hair, applying makeup
- Eating: preparing meals, pouring liquids, cutting up foods, bringing food to mouth, drinking
- Mobility: walking up and down stairs, getting in and out of bed, getting out of the house
- Communicating: talking, using phone, writing

Self-Care Behaviours
- Are there any occupational hazards that could affect your muscles and joints? Does your work involve heavy lifting or repetitive motion?*
- Do you use any mechanical assistive devices or prosthetic or orthotic devices?*
- Describe your exercise pattern (frequency, warm-up, type of exercise, any pain).
- Have you had any recent weight gain or loss?* What is your usual daily diet? What dietary supplements do you take? (Ask specifically about calcium, vitamin D supplements, and herbal products.) Are you taking any medications for the musculo-skeletal system (anti-inflammatory, pain reliever)?*
- How do you deal with problems (such as pain or immobility) that have resulted from your musculo-skeletal problem?
- Has your illness affected your interaction with friends, family, or the way you view yourself?

Additional History for the Aging Adult
- Have you noticed any change in strength or weakness over the past weeks or months?*
- Have you been falling or stumbling more often over the past weeks or months?*
- Do you use any mobility aids to help you get around (cane, walker)?*

Source: Based on Jarvis, C., Browne, A. J., MacDonald-Jenkins, J., et al. (Eds.). (2014). *Physical examination and health assessment* (2nd Canadian ed., pp. 610–612). Toronto: Elsevier.
*If yes, ask patient to describe.

GENETICS IN CLINICAL PRACTICE

Autoimmune Diseases
- Many autoimmune diseases of the musculo-skeletal system have a genetic basis involving human leukocyte antigens.
- Autoimmune diseases include ankylosing spondylitis, rheumatoid arthritis, and systemic lupus erythematosus.

Osteoporosis
- Genetic factors contribute to osteoporosis by influencing not only bone mineral density but also bone size, bone quality, and bone turnover.

Osteoarthritis, Gout, and Scoliosis
- A genetic predisposition is a contributing risk factor in all these diseases.

Muscular Dystrophy
- The most common types of muscular dystrophy are X-linked recessive disorders.

Obtain a family history related to rheumatoid arthritis, systemic lupus erythematosus, ankylosing spondylitis, osteoarthritis, gout, osteoporosis, and scoliosis because a patient may have a genetic predisposition to these or other musculo-skeletal disorders.

potential adverse effects include anticonvulsant drugs (osteomalacia), phenothiazines (gait disturbances), corticosteroids (avascular necrosis, decreased bone and muscle mass), and potassium-depleting diuretics (muscle cramps and weakness). Women should be questioned about their menstrual history; episodes of amenorrhea can contribute to early development of osteoporosis. The nurse should ask postmenopausal women about their use of hormone therapy.

Surgery or Other Treatments. Information about past hospitalizations related to a musculo-skeletal problem should be obtained. The nurse documents the reason for hospitalization; the date and the duration; and the treatment, including ongoing rehabilitation. The nurse should obtain specific information about any surgical procedure and the postoperative course. If the patient experienced a period of prolonged immobilization, the development of osteoporosis and muscle atrophy should be considered.

Objective Data

Physical Examination. Examination of the musculo-skeletal system involves inspection, palpation, motion, and muscular assessment. The nurse should conduct a general overview, while

CASE STUDY

Subjective Data

Source: And-One/ Shutterstock .com.

A focused subjective assessment of Terry King revealed the following information:

History of Current Illness: Rates left hip pain at a 9 on a scale of 0–10. Describes pain as sharp spasms that increase in intensity with any movement. Is asking for pain medicine "as strong as you can give me." Denies any history of musculo-skeletal problems.

Past Health: Type 2 diabetes for 11 yr. COPD for 15 yr; 40 pack-year smoking history.

Medications: Metformin (Glucophage), 500 mg PO bid; glyburide (DiaBeta), 5 mg/day PO; fluticasone and salmeterol combination (Advair), 250/50 mcg, 1 inhalation bid; salbutamol (Ventolin), 2 puffs q4h PRN as rescue inhaler.

Functional Assessment: Until this current fall, has been able to perform ADLs without assistance. Currently smokes 2 to 3 packs of cigarettes per day. Is trying to quit but finding it difficult. Drinks alcohol at night. Is 188 cm tall and weighs 88 kg. Does not take any nutritional supplements and tends to shy away from milk and other dairy products because they make him "gassy." Leads a sedentary lifestyle because of dyspnea on exertion.

See pp. 1622, 1625, and 1630 for more information on Mr. King.

ADLs, activities of daily living; *COPD,* chronic obstructive pulmonary disease.

FIGURE 64-6 Measurement of joint motion with a goniometer. Source: **A,** Wilson, S. F., & Giddens, J. F. (2013). *Health assessment for nursing practice* (5th ed., p. 34, Figure 3-23). St. Louis: Mosby; **B,** From Patton, K. T., & Thibodeau, G. A. (2013). *Anatomy and physiology* (8th ed., p. 286, Figure 10-15). St. Louis: Mosby.

obtaining data in a careful health history to provide guidance in choosing areas on which to concentrate during the local examination. Specific measurements should be taken as indicated by the results of the local examination.

Inspection. Inspection begins during the nurse's initial contact with the patient. The nurse notes the use of an assistive device such as a walker or cane. The nurse also observes general body build, muscle configuration, and symmetry of joint movement. If the patient is able to move independently, the nurse should assess posture and gait by watching the patient walk, stand, and sit. Musculo-skeletal and neurological problems can result in changes from a normal gait.

A systematic inspection is performed, starting at the head and neck and proceeding to the upper extremities, lower extremities, and trunk. The skin is inspected for general colour, scars, or other overt signs of previous injury or surgery. The nurse notes any swelling, deformity, nodules or masses, and discrepancies in limb length or muscle size. The patient's opposite-side body part is observed for comparison when an abnormality is suspected.

Palpation. Any area that has aroused concern because of a subjective complaint or appears abnormal on inspection should be carefully palpated. Palpation usually proceeds from head to toe to examine neck, shoulders, elbows, wrists, hands, back, hips, knees, ankles, and feet. Both superficial and deep palpation are usually performed, one after the other. The nurse's hands should be warm to prevent muscle spasm, which can interfere with identification of essential landmarks or soft tissue structures. Palpation allows for evaluation of skin temperature, local tenderness, swelling, crepitation, and presence of nodules. Muscles are palpated during active and passive motion for tone, strength, and ease of movement.

Motion. When assessing the patient's joint mobility, the nurse must carefully evaluate both passive and active ranges of joint motion. Measurements should be similar for both. *Active range of motion* means the patient takes his or her own joints through

all movements without assistance. *Passive range of motion* occurs when someone else moves the patient's joints without the patient's participation. The nurse should be cautious in performing passive range of motion because of the risk of injury to underlying structures. Manipulation must cease immediately if pain or resistance is encountered. If deficits in active or passive range of motion are noted, the nurse must also assess functional range of motion to determine whether performance of activities of daily living has been affected by joint changes. In this assessment, the patient is asked whether activities such as eating and bathing must be performed with assistance or cannot be done at all.

Range of motion is most accurately assessed with a goniometer, which measures the angle of the joint (Figure 64-6). Specific degrees of range of motion of all joints are usually not measured unless a musculo-skeletal problem has been identified. A less exact but valuable assessment method is to compare the range of motion of one extremity with the range of motion on the opposite side. The most common movements that occur at the diarthrodial joints are described in Table 64-3.

Muscle Strength Testing. The nurse grades the strength of individual muscles or groups of muscles during contraction (Table 64-4). The patient should be instructed to apply resistance to the force exerted by the nurse. For example, if the examiner tries to pull the patient's bent arm down, the patient tries to raise it. Muscle strength should also be compared with the strength of the opposite extremity. Subtle variations in muscle strength may be noted when the patient's dominant side is compared with the nondominant side.

Measurement. When length discrepancies or subjective problems are noted, the nurse obtains limb length and circumferential muscle mass measurements. For example, leg length

TABLE 64-3 MOVEMENT AT DIARTHROIDAL JOINTS

Movement	Description
Abduction	Movement of part away from midline of body
Adduction	Movement of part toward midline of body
Circumduction	Combination of flexion, extension, abduction, and adduction that results in circular motion of a body part
Dorsiflexion	Flexing of toes and foot upward
Eversion	Turning of sole outward away from midline of body
Extension	Straightening of joint that increases angle between two bones
External rotation	Movement along longitudinal axis away from midline of body
Flexion	Bending of joint that results in decreased angle between two bones
Hyperextension	Extension in which angle exceeds 180 degrees or beyond a joint's normal range of motion
Internal rotation	Movement along longitudinal axis toward midline of body
Inversion	Turning of sole inward toward midline of body
Opposition	Moving the thumb tip to meet the tip of each finger
Plantar flexion	Flexing toes and foot downward
Pronation	Turning of palm downward
Supination	Turning of palm upward

TABLE 64-4 MUSCLE STRENGTH SCALE

0	No detection of muscular contraction
1	A barely detectable flicker or trace of contraction with observation or palpation
2	Active movement of body part with elimination of gravity
3	Active movement against gravity only and not against resistance
4	Active movement against gravity and some resistance
5	Active movement against full resistance without evident fatigue (normal muscle strength)

should be measured when gait disorders are observed. The affected limb is measured between two bony prominences, and that measurement is compared with the corresponding measurement of the opposite extremity. Muscle mass is measured circumferentially at the largest area of the muscle. When recording measurements, the nurse documents the exact location at which the measurements were obtained (e.g., the quadriceps muscle is measured 15 cm above the patella). This informs the next examiner of the exact area to be measured and ensures consistency during reassessment.

Other. Assessment of reflexes is discussed in Chapter 58. Table 64-5 lists the elements of a normal physical assessment of the musculo-skeletal system. Abnormal assessment findings of the musculo-skeletal system are presented in Table 64-6.

DIAGNOSTIC STUDIES OF THE MUSCULO-SKELETAL SYSTEM

Diagnostic studies provide important objective data that aid the nurse in monitoring the patient's condition and planning appropriate interventions. Table 64-7 lists diagnostic studies commonly used to evaluate the musculo-skeletal system. Tests must be carefully chosen to enhance or clarify information gained from the patient's history and physical examination.

TABLE 64-5 EXAMPLE OF A NORMAL PHYSICAL ASSESSMENT OF THE MUSCULO-SKELETAL SYSTEM

- Full range of motion of all joints without pain or laxity (hypermobility)
- No joint swelling, deformity, or crepitation
- Normal spinal curvatures
- No tenderness on palpation of spine
- No muscle atrophy or asymmetry
- Muscle strength of 5

FOCUSED ASSESSMENT
Musculo-Skeletal System

Use this checklist to ensure that the key assessment steps have been done.

Subjective
Ask the patient about any of the following and note responses:

Joint pain or stiffness	Y	N
Muscle weakness	Y	N
Bone pain	Y	N

Objective: Diagnostic
Check the following laboratory results for critical values:

Radiograph results	✓
Bone scans	✓
Erythrocyte sedimentation rate	✓

Objective: Physical Examination
Inspect and palpate:

Skeleton and extremities (and compare sides) for alignment, contour, symmetry, size, and gross deformities	✓
Joints for range of motion, tenderness/pain, heat, crepitus, and swelling	✓
Muscles (and compare sides) for size, symmetry, tone, and tenderness/pain	✓
Bones for tenderness or pain	✓

CASE STUDY
Objective Data: Physical Examination

A physical examination of Terry King reveals the following:
- BP, 166/94; heart rate, 98; respiratory rate, 36; temperature, 35.8°C; O₂ saturation rate, 91% on 2 L of O₂.
- Alert and oriented × 3.
- Left leg shortened and externally rotated. No external bruising noted.
- + 1 Pedal pulses bilaterally. Lungs with bibasilar crackles and expiratory wheezing.

Source: And-One/Shutterstock.com

In continuing to read this chapter, consider diagnostic studies the nurse would anticipate being performed for Mr. King. See pp. 1622, 1624, and 1630 for more information on Mr. King.

BP, blood pressure.

TABLE 64-6 ASSESSMENT ABNORMALITIES

Musculo-Skeletal System

Finding	Description	Possible Etiology
Achilles tendinitis	Pain in posterior leg initially during running or walking; can progress to pain at rest	Cumulative stress on Achilles tendon, resulting in inflammation
Ankylosis	Stiffness or fixation of a joint, usually resulting from destruction of articular cartilage and subchondral bone with subsequent tissue scarring	Chronic joint inflammation
Antalgic gait	Shortened stride with as little weight bearing as possible on the affected side	Pain or discomfort in the lower extremity on weight bearing; can be related to trauma or other disorders
Ataxic gait	Staggering, uncoordinated gait, often with sway	Neurogenic disorders (e.g., spinal cord lesion)
Atrophy	Decrease in the size of a tissue or organ caused by a reduction in the number or size of the individual cells; characterized by decreased circumference and flabby appearance and leading to decreased function and tone	Muscle denervation, contracture, and prolonged disuse as a result of immobilization
Contracture	Abnormal, usually permanent flexion and fixation of a muscle or joint; resistance to movement is a result of fibrosis of supporting soft tissues	Shortening of muscle or ligaments, tightness of soft tissue, incorrect positioning of immobilized extremity
Crepitation (crepitus)	Crackling sound or grating sensation as a result of friction between bones, broken bone, or cartilage bits in joint	Fracture, dislocation, chronic inflammation, osteoarthritis
Dislocation	Displacement of bone from its normal joint	Trauma, disorders of surrounding soft tissues
Hypertrophy	Increase in size of muscle as a result of enlargement of existing cells	Exercise or other increased stimulation, increased androgens
Kyphosis (dowager's hump)	Forward bending of thoracic spine: exaggerated thoracic curvature	Poor posture, tuberculosis, arthritis, osteoporosis, growth disturbance of vertebral epiphyses
Limited range of motion (ROM)	Failure of joint to achieve the expected degrees of motion	Injury, inflammation, contracture
Lordosis (swayback)	Lumbar spinal deformity that results in exaggerated lumbar curvature	Secondary to other spinal deformities, muscular dystrophy, obesity, flexion contracture of hip, congenital dislocation of hip
Muscle spasticity	Increased muscle tone (rigidity) with sustained muscle contractions (spasms); stiffness or tightness may interfere with gait, movement, speech	Neuro-muscular disorders such as multiple sclerosis or cerebral palsy
Myalgia	General muscle tenderness and pain	Chronic rheumatic syndromes (e.g., fibromyalgia)
Paresthesia	Numbness and tingling, often described as a "pins and needles" sensation	Compromised sensory nerves, often owing to edema in a closed space such as a cast or bulky dressing
Pes planus (flatfoot)	Abnormal flatness of the sole and arch of the foot	Hereditary, muscle paralysis, mild cerebral palsy, early muscular dystrophy, injury to posterior tibial tendon
Plantar fasciitis	Burning, sharp pain on sole of foot; worse in the morning	Chronic degenerative–reparative cycle that results in inflammation
Scoliosis	Deformity resulting from lateral S-shaped curvature of the thoracic and lumbar spine	Idiopathic or congenital condition, fracture or dislocation, osteomalacia
Subluxation	Partial dislocation of joint	Instability of joint capsule and supporting ligaments (e.g., as a result of trauma, arthritis)
Swan neck deformity	Hyperextension of the PIP joint with flexion of the MCP and DIP joints of the fingers (see Chapter 67, Figure 67-4)	Deformity typical of rheumatoid and psoriatic arthritis, caused by contracture of muscles and tendons
Swelling	Enlargement, often of a joint, owing to fluid collection; generally leads to pain, stiffness	Trauma or inflammation
Torticollis (wry neck)	Twisting of neck in unusual position to one side	Prolonged contraction of neck muscles, congenital or acquired
Ulnar deviation (ulnar drift)	Displacement of fingers to ulnar side of forearm (see Chapter 67, Figure 67-4)	Typical deformity of rheumatoid arthritis owing to tendon contracture
Valgum deformity (genu valgum; knock knees)	Condition in which the space between the medial malleoli > 2.5 cm when knees are together	Poliomyelitis, congenital deformity, arthritis
Varum deformity (genu varum; bowleg)	Condition in which the space between the knees > 2.5 cm when the medial malleoli are together	Arthritis, congenital deformity

DIP, distal interphalangeal; *MCP,* metacarpophalangeal; *PIP,* proximal interphalangeal.

Radiography

The *radiograph* is the diagnostic study most commonly used to assess musculo-skeletal problems and to monitor the effectiveness of treatment. The x-ray beam produces an image on a photographic film; the image appears dark if the x-rays penetrate the body tissues (e.g., lungs) and white if the transmission is partially blocked (e.g., by bones). Radiographs are two-dimensional, and multiple views may be necessary to facilitate diagnosis (e.g., anteroposterior [front-to-back], lateral [side], oblique [45-degree angle]). The contours and shades of the structures on these images provide useful information, such as showing the presence of deformity, joint congruity, calcification in soft tissue, and bone fractures. Radiographs are also useful in the

TABLE 64-7 DIAGNOSTIC STUDIES

Musculo-Skeletal System

Study	Description and Purpose	Nursing Responsibility
Radiological Studies		
Standard radiography (x-ray study)	• Helps determine density of bone • Used to evaluate structural or functional changes of bones and joints • One-dimensional image provided by anteroposterior view because x-ray beam passes from front to back • Two-dimensional image provided by lateral position	• Instruct patient to avoid excessive exposure of patient and self to radiation. • Remove any radiopaque objects that can interfere with results. • Explain procedure to patient. • Instruct the patient to remain still. • Pregnancy is a contraindication to x-ray studies; however, sometimes the benefits outweigh the risks.
Computed tomography (CT)	• Three-dimensional radiography provided by use of an x-ray beam with a computer • Used to identify soft tissue abnormalities, bony abnormalities, and various musculo-skeletal trauma • Iodinated dye often used for better visualization	• Same as for radiography. • Also, assess for adverse reactions to iodinated dye. • Patients with kidney disease or diabetes require adequate hydration to flush out the dye.
Magnetic resonance imaging (MRI)	• Viewing of soft tissue with use of radiofrequency waves and magnetic field • Especially useful in the diagnosis of avascular necrosis, disc disease, tumours, osteomyelitis, ligament tears, and cartilage tears • Patient placed inside scanning chamber • Gadolinium-based contrast dyes used to enhance visualization of the structures, may be injected into a vein • In open MRI, no requirement for placing the patient inside a chamber	• MRI is contraindicated in patients with metallic implants. • Ensure that patient has no metal on clothing (e.g., snaps, zippers, jewellery, credit cards). • Inform patient that procedure is painless, and emphasize importance of remaining still throughout examination. • Claustrophobic patients may require antianxiety agents if indicated and ordered. • Open MRI may be indicated for patients with large chest and abdominal girth or severe claustrophobia.
Arthrography	• Radiography in which contrast medium or air is injected into joint cavity, enabling visualization of joint structures • Joint movement assessed with series of radiographic images	• Same as for radiography. • Assess patient for possible allergy to contrast medium. • Inform patient that procedure is painless.
Discography	• Radiography of cervical or lumbar intervertebral disc, performed after injection of contrast dye into nucleus pulposus • Enables visualization of intervertebral disc abnormalities	• Same as for arthrography.
Bone Mineral Density (BMD) Measurements		
Dual-energy x-ray absorptiometry (DEXA)	• Used to measure bone mass of spine, femur, forearm, and total body • Allows assessment of bone density with minimal radiation exposure • Used to diagnose metabolic bone disease and to monitor changes in bone density with treatment • Widely available; free screening test	• Same as for radiography. • Inform patient that procedure is painless.
Quantitative ultrasonography (QUS)	• Helps evaluate density, elasticity, and strength of bone through the use of ultrasound waves rather than radiation	• Inform patient that procedure is painless.
Radioisotope Studies		
Bone scan	• Radiography in which radioisotope (usually technetium-99m) is injected and taken up by bone • Isotope uptake uniform when bones are normal • Uptake increased in osteomyelitis, osteoporosis, primary and metastatic malignant lesions of bone, and certain fractures • Uptake decreased uptake in areas of avascular necrosis	• Pregnancy and lactation are usually contraindicated. • The technician gives a calculated dose of radioisotope 2 hr before procedure. • The patient's bladder is emptied before the procedure. • The procedure requires 1 hr while patient lies supine. • Increase patient's fluid intake after the examination. • The isotopes are excreted from the body within 6–24 hr.
Endoscopy		
Arthroscopy	• Procedure in which an arthroscope is inserted into the joint (usually knee) for visualization of structure and contents • Can be used for exploratory surgery (removal of loose bodies and biopsy) and for diagnosing abnormalities of meniscus, articular cartilage, ligaments, or joint capsule • Other structures that can be visualized through the arthroscope: shoulder, elbow, wrist, jaw, hip, and ankle	• Inform patient that procedure can be performed in outpatient setting and that local or general anaesthesia may be used. • Patient is on NPO status after midnight on the day of the test. • After procedure, cover wound with sterile dressing. • Explain postprocedure care.

Continued

TABLE 64-7 DIAGNOSTIC STUDIES

Musculo-Skeletal System—cont'd

Study	Description and Purpose	Nursing Responsibility
Mineral Metabolism		
Alkaline phosphatase (ALP)	• Enzyme produced by osteoblasts of bone; needed for mineralization of organic bone matrix • Levels elevated in healing fractures, bone cancers, osteoporosis, osteomalacia, and Paget's disease • *Normal:* 35–120 units/L (age dependent) • Blood samples obtained by venipuncture	• Inform patient that fasting is preferred but not required. • Note any medications that may affect test results.* • Observe venipuncture site for bleeding or hematoma formation.
Calcium	• Stored primarily in bone • Provides bone with rigid consistency • Serum level decreased in osteomalacia, renal disease, and hypoparathyroidism • Level increased in hyperparathyroidism, some bone tumours; varies with level of albumin • *Normal:* 2.25–2.75 mmol/L (age dependent)	• Inform patient that fasting is not required. • Note any medications that may affect test results. • Excessive milk ingestion and prolonged tourniquet application may increase calcium levels.*
Phosphate (phosphorus)	• Amount that is present indirectly related to calcium metabolism • Level decreased in osteomalacia • Level increased in chronic renal disease, healing fractures, osteolytic metastatic tumour • *Normal:* 0.97–1.45 mmol/L (age dependent)	• Recent carbohydrate intake (including IV glucose) causes decrease in phosphorus levels. • Patient should be on NPO status after midnight on the day of the test. • Note any medications that may affect test results. • Avoid hemolysis of the blood sample because this can elevate phosphate levels.*
Serological Studies		
Rheumatoid factor (RF)	• Study to assess presence of autoantibody (RF) in serum • Factor not specific for rheumatoid arthritis; present in other connective tissue diseases, as well as in a small percentage of normal population • *Normal:* negative or <60 units/mL by nephelometric method	• Inform patient that fasting is not required. • In older adults, results are often falsely positive. • False-positive results also occur with hemolysis or lipemia.*
Erythrocyte sedimentation rate (ESR)	• Nonspecific index of inflammation • Used to measure rapidity with which red blood cells settle out of unclotted blood in 1 hr • Results influenced by physiological factors as well as by diseases • Levels elevated with any inflammatory process (especially rheumatoid arthritis, rheumatic fever, osteomyelitis, and respiratory infections) • *Normal:* male, <15 mm/hr; female, ≤20 mm/hr (age dependent).	• Numerous interfering factors can affect test results (e.g., pregnancy, menstruation, anemias, medications). • Withhold medications that may affect results, if indicated.*
Antinuclear antibody (ANA)	• Used to assess presence of antibodies capable of destroying nucleus of body's tissue cells. • Finding positive in 95% of patients with systemic lupus erythematosus and may also be positive in individuals with systemic sclerosis (scleroderma) or rheumatoid arthritis and in a small percentage of normal population • *Normal:* negative at 1:40 dilution	• Inform patient that fasting is not required. • Note any medications that may affect test results. • Assess for signs of infection at the venipuncture site in patients with autoimmune diseases.*
C-reactive protein (CRP)	• Used to diagnose inflammatory diseases, infections, and active widespread malignancy. • CRP synthesized by the liver and present in large amounts in serum 18–24 hr after onset of tissue damage • *Normal:* negative or ≤10 mg/L	• Fasting may sometimes be required (laboratory specific). • Note any medications that may affect test results.*
Uric acid	• End product of purine metabolism that is normally excreted in urine • Levels not specific to gout but are usually elevated in patients with gout • *Normal:* male, 240–501 mcmol/L; female, 160–430 mcmol/L (age dependent)	• Fasting may sometimes be required (laboratory specific).*
Human leukocyte antigen–B27 (HLA-B27)	• Antigen present in disorders such as ankylosing spondylitis and rheumatoid arthritis.	• Inform patient that fasting or other preparation is not needed.*

TABLE 64-7 DIAGNOSTIC STUDIES
Musculo-Skeletal System—cont'd

Study	Description and Purpose	Nursing Responsibility
Muscle Enzymes		
Creatine kinase (CK)	• Concentration highest in skeletal muscle • Values increased in progressive muscular dystrophy, polymyositis, and traumatic injuries • *Normal:* men, 55–170 units/L; women, 30–135 units/L	• Obtain blood samples by venipuncture. • Observed venipuncture site for bleeding or hematoma formation. • Inform patient that procedure does not necessitate fasting. • Values can be increased after strenuous exercise, recent surgery, and intramuscular injections and with certain medications.*
Serum potassium (K⁺)	• Values sometimes increased with muscle trauma because cell destruction releases this electrolyte into the serum (depends on renal function) • *Normal:* 3.5–5.0 mmol/L	• Monitor patients in trauma unit for cardiac dysrhythmias related to hypokalemia or hyperkalemia. • Note any medications that may affect test results. • Hemolysis of the blood sample and prolonged tourniquet application can elevate potassium levels.*
Invasive Procedures		
Arthrocentesis	• Procedure in which a needle is inserted into the joint cavity to aspirate synovial fluid, blood, or pus or to instill medications • Local anaesthesia and aseptic technique required • Useful in diagnosis of joint inflammation, infection, and subtle fractures	• Inform patient that procedure is usually done at bedside or in examination room. • Send samples of synovial fluid to laboratory for examination (if indicated). • After procedure, apply pressure dressing. • Observe dressing for leakage of blood or fluid.
Electromyography (EMG)	• Used to evaluate electrical potential associated with skeletal muscle contraction • Involves insertion of small-gauge needles into certain muscles • Needle probes attached to leads that feed information to EMG machine; recordings of electrical activity of muscle traced on audio transmitter, as well as on oscilloscope and recording paper • Study useful in providing information related to lower motor neuron dysfunction and primary muscle disease	• Inform patient that procedure is usually done in EMG laboratory while patient lies supine on special table. • Keep patient awake to cooperate with voluntary movement. • Inform patient that procedure involves some discomfort from needle insertion. • Contraindications include anticoagulant therapy and extensive skin infection. • Fasting is not required, but some laboratories may restrict intake of stimulants (e.g., coffee, cigarettes) 2–3 hr before procedure.
Miscellaneous		
Thermography	• Infrared detector used to measure degree of heat radiating from skin surface • Useful in investigation of cause of joint inflammation and in following up patient's response to anti-inflammatory drug therapy	• Inform patient that procedure is painless and noninvasive.
Somatosensory evoked potential (SEP)	• Used to evaluate evoked potential of muscle contractions • Electrodes placed on skin and provide recordings of electrical activity of muscle • Useful in identifying subtle dysfunction of lower motor neuron and primary muscle disease • Possible to measure nerve conduction along pathways not accessible by EMG	• Inform patient that procedure is similar to EMG but does not involve needles. • Electrodes are applied to the skin.

*Blood samples are obtained by venipuncture. The nurse should observe venipuncture site for bleeding or hematoma formation.
IV, intravenous; *NPO,* nothing by mouth.

evaluation of hereditary, developmental, infectious, inflammatory, neoplastic, metabolic, and degenerative disorders.

Magnetic Resonance Imaging

Magnetic resonance imaging (MRI) can be useful for the early diagnosis of soft tissue disorders, including cartilage or ligament tears and herniated discs, as well as bone disorders such as avascular necrosis, tumours, and multiple myeloma. The body is composed primarily of hydrogen, which possesses magnetic properties that can be scanned by the powerful magnetic fields and radiofrequency waves. Contrast material may be necessary to enhance the images. MRI is contraindicated in patients who have implanted metal objects (e.g., pacemaker, aneurysm clips, prosthesis, implanted cardioverter–defibrillator, electronic devices, hearing aids, shrapnel).

Arthroscopy

A small fibre optic tube called an *arthroscope* is inserted into a joint and used to directly examine or operate on the interior of the joint cavity in a procedure known as **arthroscopy** (see Table 64-7). Arthroscopy is performed under sterile conditions. After local anaesthetic has been administered, a large-bore needle is inserted into the joint, and the joint is distended with fluid or air (Figure 64-7). The arthroscope enables extensive, accurate visualization of the joint cavity. Photographs or videotapes can

FIGURE 64-7 Knee arthroscopy in progress. Notice the monitor in the background. Source: From Miller, M. D., Howard, R. F., & Plancher, K. D. (2003). *Surgical atlas of sports medicine*. Philadelphia: Saunders.

be made through the arthroscope, and a biopsy of the synovium or cartilage can be obtained. Torn tissue can be repaired through arthroscopic surgery, which eliminates the need for a larger incision and greatly decreases the recovery time.

Arthrocentesis and Synovial Fluid Analysis

Arthrocentesis, or joint aspiration, is a procedure in which an incision or puncture is made in a joint capsule, usually to obtain samples of synovial fluid from within the joint cavity for a synovial fluid analysis. It may also be used to instill medications for a patient with septic arthritis or to remove excess fluid from joints to relieve pain. After the skin has been cleaned, a local anaesthetic is instilled. An 18-gauge or larger needle is inserted into the joint, and fluid is withdrawn. The appropriate sterile container should be readily available to receive the aspirated fluid, which must be transported immediately to the laboratory. The fluid is examined grossly for volume, colour, clarity, viscosity, and *mucin clot formation*. Normal synovial fluid is transparent, colourless (or straw-coloured), scant in amount, and of low viscosity. Fluid from an infected joint may be purulent and thick or grey and thin. In gout, the fluid may be whitish yellow. Blood may be aspirated in cases of hemarthrosis because of injury or a bleeding disorder. The mucin clot test indicates the character of the protein

portion of the synovial fluid. Normally a white, ropelike mucin clot is formed. In the presence of an inflammatory process, the clot breaks apart and easily fragments. The fluid is examined grossly for floating fat globules, which indicate bone injury.

The fluid is examined microscopically for cell count and identification. Infection would be suspected with an elevated white blood cell count and an increase in polymorphonuclear cells (i.e. neutrophils). Protein content is elevated, and the glucose level is considerably decreased in septic arthritis. The presence of uric acid crystals suggests a diagnosis of gout (Pagana & Pagana, 2013). Specimens for a Gram stain and culture may also be obtained in arthrocentesis.

Muscle Enzymes

Muscle enzymes are released from injured or dead muscle cells. Determinations of muscle enzyme values are used to distinguish between muscle weakness caused by innervation problems and that caused by dystrophic disease of the muscle itself. The level of enzymes reflects the progress of the disorder and the effectiveness of treatment. Creatine kinase is a reliable measure of muscle damage.

Serological Studies

In approximately 80% of people with rheumatoid arthritis and related diseases, an autoantibody known as rheumatoid factor (RF) is present in the serum. RF is an autoantibody directed against immunoglobulin G. RF titres are higher during periods of increased disease activity. Elevated erythrocyte sedimentation rate and C-reactive protein level are nonspecific indicators of active inflammation.

CASE STUDY

Diagnostic Studies

Source: And-One/ Shutterstock .com.

The emergency department physician immediately orders the following diagnostic studies for Terry King:
- Radiograph of left hip
- Chest radiograph
- CBC, electrolytes, aPTT, PT/INR
- Arterial blood gases (ABGs)

The radiograph of the left hip reveals an extracapsular fracture. The chest radiographic findings are consistent with COPD without any evidence of pneumonia at present. Hematocrit is 43%; hemoglobin, 140 mmol/L; and WBC is 15.1 × 10⁹/L. The remainder of CBC, electrolytes, aPTT, and PT/INR are WNL. The ABGs demonstrate compensated respiratory acidosis.

See pp. 1622, 1624, and 1625 in this chapter for more information on Mr. King. This case is continued in Chapter 65.

aPTT, activated partial thromboplastin time; *CBC*, complete blood cell count; *COPD*, chronic obstructive pulmonary disease; *INR*, international normalized ratio; *PT*, prothrombin time; *WNL*, within normal limits.

▌ REVIEW QUESTIONS

The number of the question corresponds to the same-numbered objective at the beginning of the chapter.

1. What are the bone cells that function in the breakdown of bone tissue (resorption) called?
   a. Osteoids
   b. Osteocytes
   c. Osteoclasts
   d. Osteoblasts

2. While performing passive range-of-motion exercises for a client, the nurse puts the ankle joint through the movements of which of the following? (*Select all that apply*)
   a. Flexion and extension
   b. Inversion and eversion
   c. Pronation and supination
   d. Flexion, extension, abduction, and adduction
   e. Pronation, supination, rotation, and circumduction

3. To prevent muscle atrophy, the nurse teaches the client with a leg immobilized in traction to perform which of the following manoeuvres? *(Select all that apply)*
   a. Flexion contractions
   b. Tetanic contractions
   c. Isotonic contractions
   d. Isometric contractions
   e. Extension contractions

4. A client with bursitis of the shoulder asks the nurse what the bursa does. What does the nurse tell the client about the function of the bursa?
   a. Bursae connect bone to bone.
   b. Bursae separate muscle from muscle.
   c. Bursae lubricate joints with synovial fluid.
   d. Bursae relieve friction between moving parts.

5. Why are many older adults at increased risk for falls?
   a. Changes in balance
   b. Decrease in bone mass
   c. Loss of ligament elasticity
   d. Erosion of articular cartilage

6. While the nurse is obtaining subjective assessment data related to the musculo-skeletal system, which of the following conditions requires the nurse to ask about family history?
   a. Osteomyelitis
   b. Osteomalacia
   c. Low back pain
   d. Rheumatoid arthritis

7. When a nurse grades muscle strength with a score of 2, what does that indicate?
   a. Active movement against gravity
   b. A barely detectable flicker of contraction
   c. Active movement with elimination of gravity
   d. Active movement against full resistance without evident fatigue

8. Which of the following is a normal finding in the assessment of the musculo-skeletal system?
   a. Muscle strength of 4
   b. A lateral curvature of the spine
   c. Angulation of bone toward midline
   d. Full range of motion of all joints without pain

9. Which of the following are nursing considerations for a client undergoing magnetic resonance imaging (MRI)? *(Select all that apply)*
   a. Ensuring that the client has no metal on clothing
   b. Informing the client that the procedure is painless
   c. Checking for history of claustrophobia
   d. Ensuring that the client is on NPO status at least 8 hours before the study
   e. Administering a fluid bolus immediately before the study

1. c; 2. a, b; 3. d, d; 4. d; 5. a; 6. d; 7. c; 8. d; 9. a, b, c.

⊜volve

For even more review questions, visit *http://evolve.elsevier.com/Canada/ Lewis/medsurg.*

REFERENCES

Herlihy, B. (2014). *The human body in health and illness* (5th ed.). St. Louis: Saunders.

Jarvis, C., Browne, A. J., MacDonald-Jenkins, J., et al. (2014). *Physical examination and health assessment* (2nd Canadian ed.). Toronto: Elsevier.

McCance, K. L., & Huether, S. E. (2014). *Pathophysiology: The biologic basis for disease in adults and children* (7th ed.). St. Louis: Mosby.

National Association of Orthopaedic Nurses. (2013). *NAON core curriculum for orthopaedic nursing* (7th ed.). Boston: Pearson.

Pagana, K. D., & Pagana, T. J. (2013). *Mosby's Canadian manual of diagnostic and laboratory tests* (1st Canadian ed.). St. Louis: Elsevier Mosby.

Roberts, D. (2016). The musculoskeletal system. In H. Craven (Ed.), *Core curriculum for medical-surgical nursing* (5th ed.). Pitman, NJ: Academy of Medical-Surgical Nurses.

Thibodeau, G. A., & Patton, K. T. (2016). *Structure and function of the body* (15th ed.). St. Louis: Mosby.

RESOURCES

Resources for this chapter are listed in Chapters 65 to 67.

Nursing Management

Musculo-Skeletal Trauma and Orthopaedic Surgery

Written by: Mary K. Wollan
Adapted by: Maureen A. Barry

evolve WEBSITE

http://evolve.elsevier.com/Canada/Lewis/medsurg

- Review Questions (Online Only)
- Key Points
- Answer Guidelines for Case Study
- Student Case Studies
  - Musculo-Skeletal Trauma
  - Parkinson's Disease and Hip Fracture

- Customizable Nursing Care Plans
  - Patient With a Fracture
  - Patient Having Orthopaedic Surgery
- Conceptual Care Map Creator
- Audio Glossary
- Content Updates

LEARNING OBJECTIVES

1. Explain the etiology, pathophysiology, clinical manifestations, and collaborative care of soft tissue injuries, including strains; sprains; dislocations; subluxations; bursitis; repetitive strain injury; carpal tunnel syndrome; and injuries to the rotator cuff, meniscus, and anterior cruciate ligament.
2. Relate the sequential events involved in fracture healing.
3. Compare closed reduction, cast immobilization, open reduction, and traction regarding purpose, complications, and nursing management.
4. Describe a neuro-vascular assessment for a patient with an injured extremity.

5. Explain common complications associated with a fracture and fracture healing.
6. Describe the collaborative care and nursing management of patients with specific fractures.
7. Describe the indications for and the collaborative care and nursing management of the patient with an amputation.
8. Describe the types of joint replacement surgery associated with arthritis and connective tissue diseases.
9. Identify the preoperative and postoperative management of the patient having joint replacement surgery.

KEY TERMS

arthrodesis, p. 1663
arthroplasty, p. 1662
avascular necrosis (AVN), p. 1635
bursitis, p. 1638
carpal tunnel syndrome (CTS), p. 1636
compartment syndrome, p. 1649

dislocation, p. 1635
fat embolism syndrome (FES), p. 1650
fracture, p. 1639
osteotomy, p. 1661
phantom limb sensation, p. 1659
repetitive strain injury (RSI), p. 1636

sprain, p. 1634
strain, p. 1634
subluxation, p. 1635
synovectomy, p. 1661
traction, p. 1641

Musculo-skeletal problems resulting from trauma, along with common orthopaedic surgical procedures, are discussed in this chapter. The nurse's role in the prevention of complications and promotion of function in patients with fractures and orthopaedic surgery is emphasized. The most common cause of musculo-skeletal injuries is a traumatic event resulting in fracture, dislocation, and associated soft tissue injury. Although most of these injuries are not fatal, the cost in terms of pain, disability, medical expense, and lost wages is enormous. Injury is a serious public health issue with a major impact on the

lives of Canadians. In 2009, the most recent date for which data are available, injury was the leading cause of death for Canadians between the ages of 1 and 34 and an important cause of hospitalization. Injury is also a major cause of both short- and long-term impairment and disability in children, young adults, and older adults (Statistics Canada, 2015a). Adolescent males were the age group injured most frequently, mainly while participating in sports. In the working-age adult population, overexertion was the most common cause of injury. Older adults were most often injured from falls while doing household chores or walking (Statistics Canada, 2015a). For all ages, accidents were exceeded only by cancer, heart disease, stroke, and chronic lower respiratory disease as a cause of death (Statistics Canada, 2015b).

The nurse has an important role in educating the public about the basic principles of safety and accident prevention. The morbidity associated with accidents can be significantly reduced if people are aware of environmental hazards, use existing safety equipment, and apply safety and traffic rules. In the occupational and industrial setting, the nurse should teach employees and employers about the use of proper safety equipment and avoidance of hazardous working situations.

SAFETY ALERT
- Falls account for many musculo-skeletal injuries, particularly in older adults.
- Preventive teaching should be provided to high-risk individuals (e.g., people with gait instability or visual or cognitive impairment).
- The nurse should stress the importance of wearing shoes with functional soles and heels, avoidance of wet or slippery surfaces, and removing throw rugs from the home.

Ways to prevent common musculo-skeletal problems in the older adult are listed in Table 65-1.

SOFT TISSUE INJURIES

Soft tissue injuries include sprains, strains, dislocations, and subluxations. These common injuries are usually caused by trauma. Sprains and strains are the most common injury (51%), with fractures and broken bones accounting for 17% of injuries (Statistics Canada, 2015a).

The increasing number of people involved in a fitness program or participating in sports has contributed to the increased incidence of soft tissue injuries. Common sports-related injuries are summarized in Table 65-2. In Canada, 35% of injuries occurred during participation in sports or exercise (Statistics Canada, 2015a).

Sprains and Strains

Sprains and strains are common injuries from abnormal stretching or twisting forces that may occur during vigorous activities.

TABLE 65-1 PATIENT & CAREGIVER TEACHING GUIDE

Prevention of Musculo-Skeletal Problems in the Older Adult

The following instructions should be included when teaching older adults and their caregivers how to prevent musculo-skeletal problems.
- Use ramps in buildings and at street corners instead of steps to prevent falls.
- Eliminate scatter rugs in the home.
- Treat pain and discomfort from osteoarthritis.
  - Rest in a reclining position to decrease discomfort.
  - Discuss use of medication for pain with health care provider.
- Use a walker or cane to help with walking to prevent falls.
- Eat the amount and the kind of foods needed to prevent excess weight gain because obesity adds stress to joints, which may predispose to osteoarthritis.
- Get regular and frequent exercise.
  - ADLs provide ROM exercises. Tai chi may also be helpful.
  - Hobbies (e.g., jigsaw puzzles, needlework, model building) exercise finger joints and prevent stiffness.
  - Performing weight-bearing exercise (e.g., walking) is essential and should be done on a daily basis.
- Use shoes with good support to provide for safety and promote comfort.
- Gradually initiate activities to promote optimal coordination. Rise slowly to a standing position to prevent dizziness, falls, and fractures.
- Avoid walking on uneven surfaces and wet floors.

ADLs, activities of daily living; *ROM,* range of motion.

TABLE 65-2 SPORTS-RELATED INJURIES

Injury	Definition	Treatment
Anterior cruciate ligament tear	Traumatic tearing of ligament by deceleration forces together with pivoting or odd positions of the knee or leg.	• Physiotherapy with rehabilitation, knee brace. • If knee instability or continued injuries, reconstructive surgery may be done.
Impingement syndrome	Entrapment of soft tissue structures under coraco-acromial arch of shoulder.	• NSAIDs; rest until symptoms decrease, and then gradual ROM and strengthening exercises.
Ligament injury	Tearing or stretching of ligament; usually occurs as a result of inversion, eversion, shearing, or torque applied to a joint. Characterized by sudden pain, swelling, and instability.	• Rest, ice, elevation of extremity if possible, NSAIDs; protection of affected extremity by use of brace. • If symptoms persist, surgical repair may be necessary.
Meniscus injury	Injury to fibrocartilage of the knee, characterized by popping, clicking, tearing sensation, effusion, and swelling.	• Rest, ice, elevation of extremity if possible, NSAIDs; gradual return to regular activities. • If symptoms persist, MRI to diagnose meniscal injury and possible arthroscopic surgery.
Rotator cuff tear	Tear within muscle or tendino-ligamentous structures around shoulder.	• *If minor tear:* rest, NSAIDs, and gradual mobilization with ROM and strengthening exercises. • *If major tear:* surgical repair.
Shin splints	Inflammation along anterior aspect of calf from periostitis caused by improper shoes, overuse, or running on hard pavement.	• Rest, ice, NSAIDs, proper shoes; gradual increase in activity. • If pain persists, radiographic study to rule out stress fracture of tibia.
Tendinitis	Inflammation of tendon as a result of overuse or incorrect use.	• Rest, ice, NSAIDs; gradual return to sport activity; protective brace (orthosis) may be necessary if symptoms recur.

MRI, magnetic resonance imaging; *NSAIDs,* nonsteroidal anti-inflammatory drugs; *ROM,* range of motion.

These injuries tend to occur around joints and in the spinal musculature.

A *sprain* is an injury related to the ligamentous structures surrounding a joint, usually caused by a wrenching or twisting motion. Most sprains occur in the ankles, knees, or wrists (American Academy of Orthopedic Surgeons [AAOS], 2015). A sprain is classified according to the degree of tearing in the ligament fibres. A *first-degree (mild) sprain* involves tears in only a few fibres, resulting in mild tenderness and minimal swelling. A *second-degree (moderate) sprain* is a partial tearing of the ligament, with more swelling and tenderness. A *third-degree (severe) sprain* is a complete tearing of the ligament in association with moderate to severe swelling. A gap in the muscle may be apparent or palpated through the skin if the muscle is torn. Because areas around joints are rich in nerve endings, the injury can be extremely painful.

A *strain* is an excessive stretching of a muscle, a muscle's fascial sheath, or a tendon. Most strains occur in the foot, leg (typically hamstrings), or back (AAOS, 2015). Strains may also be classified as first-degree (mild or slightly pulled muscle), second-degree (moderate or moderately torn muscle), and third-degree (severely torn or ruptured muscle).

The clinical manifestations of sprains and strains are similar and include pain, edema, decrease in function, and bruising. Pain aggravated by continued use is common. Edema develops in the injured area because of the local inflammatory response.

Mild sprains and strains are usually self-limiting, with full function returning within 3 to 6 weeks. A severe sprain can result in a concomitant *avulsion fracture,* in which the ligament pulls loose a fragment of bone. Alternatively, the joint structure may become unstable and result in subluxation or dislocation. At the time of injury, *hemarthrosis* (bleeding into a joint space or cavity) or disruption of the synovial lining may occur.

Radiographs of the affected part are usually made to rule out a fracture or widening of the joint structure. However, some health care providers use an assessment protocol called the "Ottawa Rules" (or "Ottawa Guidelines") for the examination of an injured ankle or knee before ordering radiographs (Woods, 2011). These rules specify radiographic studies for a patient, based on age, capability of flexion, location of tenderness, and ability to bear weight immediately after the injury or when examined. Surgical repair may be necessary if the injury is significant enough to produce severe disruption of ligamentous or muscle structures, fracture, or dislocation.

NURSING MANAGEMENT SPRAINS AND STRAINS

NURSING IMPLEMENTATION

HEALTH PROMOTION. Warm-up exercises before exercising and vigorous activity, followed by stretching, significantly reduce the risk for sprains and strains. Strength, balance, and endurance exercises are also important. Strengthening exercises involve working against resistance. These exercises build up muscle strength and bone density. Balance exercises, which may overlap with some strengthening exercises, help to prevent falling. Endurance exercises should start at a low level of effort and progress gradually to a moderate level of activities. Patients should try to build up to 30 minutes of moderate-intensity endurance activity on most or all days of the week (National Institute on Aging, 2015). Exercise instructions for these types of physical activity are available online at the National Institute of Aging website (see the Resources at the end of this chapter).

ACUTE INTERVENTION. If an injury occurs, the immediate care focuses on (1) stopping the activity and limiting movement, (2) application of ice compresses to the injured area, (3) compression of the involved extremity, (4) elevation of the extremity, and (5) providing analgesia as necessary (Table 65-3).

RICE (**R**est, **I**ce, **C**ompression, **E**levation) have been found to decrease local inflammation and pain for most musculo-skeletal injuries. Movement should be limited and the extremity rested as soon as pain is felt. Unless the injury is severe, prolonged rest is usually not necessary.

Cold *(cryotherapy)* in several forms can be used to produce hypothermia in the involved part. The cold induces physiological changes in soft tissue, including vasoconstriction and reduction

✚ TABLE 65-3 EMERGENCY MANAGEMENT

Acute Soft Tissue Injury

Etiology	Assessment Findings	Interventions
• Falls • Crush injury • Direct blows • Motor vehicle accidents • Sports injuries	• Decreased movement • Decreased pulse, coolness, and capillary refill >2 sec • Decreased sensation with severe edema • Ecchymosis, contusion • Edema • Inability to bear weight when lower extremity involved • Limited or decreased function with upper extremity involvement • Muscle spasms • Pain, tenderness • Pallor • Shortening or rotation of extremity	**Initial** • Ensure airway, breathing, and circulation. • Assess neuro-vascular status of involved limb. • Elevate involved limb. • Apply compression bandage unless dislocation present. • Apply ice packs to affected area. • Immobilize affected extremity in the position found. Do not attempt to realign or reinsert protruding bones. • Anticipate radiographs of injured extremity. • Give analgesia as necessary. • Administer tetanus prophylaxis if skin integrity breached or open fracture. • Administer antibiotic prophylaxis for open fracture, large tissue defects, or mangled extremity injury. **Ongoing Monitoring** • Monitor for changes in neuro-vascular status. • Eliminate weight bearing when lower extremity involved. • Anticipate compartment pressure monitoring if neuro-vascular status changes and compartment syndrome suspected.

in the transmission and perception of nerve pain impulses. In addition to pain relief, these changes reduce muscle spasms, inflammation, and edema. Cold is most useful when applied immediately after the injury has occurred. Ice applications should not exceed 20 to 30 minutes per application and ice should not be applied directly to the skin.

An elastic compression bandage can be wrapped around the injured part. To prevent edema and encourage fluid return, the bandage should be wrapped starting distally (at the point farthest from the midline of the body), and progress proximally (toward the midline of the body). If numbness is felt below the area of compression or if there is additional pain or swelling beyond the edge of the bandage, the bandage is too tight. The bandage can be left in place for 30 minutes and then removed for 15 minutes. However, some elastic bandages are left on during training, athletic, and occupational activities.

The injured part should be elevated above the heart level to help mobilize excess fluid from the area and impede further edema. The injured part should be elevated even during sleep. Mild analgesics such as nonsteroidal anti-inflammatory drugs (NSAIDs) may be necessary to manage patient discomfort.

After the acute phase (usually lasting 24 to 48 hours), warm, moist heat can be applied to the affected part to reduce swelling and provide comfort. Heat applications should not exceed 20 to 30 minutes, allowing a "cool-down" time between applications. NSAIDs may be recommended to decrease edema and pain. The patient is encouraged to use the limb, provided that the joint is protected by means of casting, bracing, taping, or splinting. Movement of the joint maintains nutrition to the cartilage, and muscle contraction improves circulation and resolution of the contusion and swelling.

AMBULATORY AND HOME CARE. Most sprains and strains are treated in an outpatient setting. The patient should be instructed in the use of ice and elevation for 24 to 48 hours after the injury to reduce edema. The use of mild analgesics to promote comfort should be encouraged. Use of an elastic bandage may provide additional support during activity. The patient should learn proper measures of strengthening and conditioning to prevent reinjury.

The physiotherapist may help to provide pain relief by means of modalities such as ultrasonography. The therapist may also teach the patient exercises to perform for flexibility and strength.

DISLOCATION AND SUBLUXATION

A dislocation is a severe injury of the ligamentous structures around a joint that results in the complete displacement of the bone from its normal position. A subluxation is a partial or incomplete displacement of the joint surface. The clinical manifestations of a subluxation are similar to those of a dislocation, but they are less severe. Treatment of a subluxation is similar to that of a dislocation, but a subluxation may require less healing time.

Dislocations characteristically result from overwhelming forces transmitted to the joint that cause a disruption of the soft tissue support structure surrounding the joint. The joints most frequently dislocated in the upper extremity include the thumb, elbow, and shoulder. In the lower extremity, the hip is vulnerable to dislocation occurring as a result of severe trauma, often associated with motor vehicle accidents (Figure 65-1). The patella may dislocate because of a sharp blow to the kneecap or after a sudden twisting inward motion while the planted foot is pointed outward (Buttarovoli & Leffler, 2012).

FIGURE 65-1 Soft tissue injury of the hip, causing subluxation or dislocation. **A,** Normal (before injury). **B,** Subluxation (partial dislocation). **C,** Dislocation.

The most obvious clinical manifestation of a dislocation is deformity. For example, if a hip is dislocated in a posterior (or backward) direction, the limb can be shorter and is often internally rotated on the affected side. Additional manifestations include local pain, tenderness, loss of function of the injured part, and swelling of the soft tissues in the region of the joint. The major complications of a dislocated joint are open joint injuries, intra-articular fractures, fractures, avascular necrosis (AVN) (bone cell death as a result of inadequate blood supply), and damage to adjacent neuro-vascular tissue.

Radiographic studies are performed to determine the extent of displacement of the involved structures. The joint may also be aspirated to determine the presence of hemarthrosis or fat cells. Fat cells in the aspirate indicate a probable intra-articular fracture.

NURSING AND COLLABORATIVE MANAGEMENT DISLOCATION

A dislocation requires prompt attention and is considered an orthopaedic emergency. The longer the joint remains unreduced, the greater the possibility of AVN. Compartment syndrome (discussed on pp. 1649–1650) may also occur after dislocation, and dislocation is often associated with significant vascular injury. The hip joint is particularly susceptible to AVN. Neuro-vascular assessment is critical (see Neuro-Vascular Assessment on pp. 1644–1645).

The first goal of management is to realign the dislocated portion of the joint in its original anatomical position. This can be accomplished by a closed reduction, which may be performed under local or general anaesthesia or intravenous conscious sedation. Anaesthesia is often necessary to produce muscle relaxation so that the bones can be manipulated. In some situations, surgical open reduction may be necessary. After reduction, the extremity is usually immobilized by bracing, splinting, taping, or using a sling to allow the torn ligaments and capsular tissue time to heal.

Nursing management of subluxation or dislocation is directed toward relief of pain and support and protection of the injured joint. After the joint has been reduced and immobilized, motion is usually restricted. A carefully regulated rehabilitation program can prevent fracture instability and joint dysfunction. Gentle range of motion (ROM) may be started if the joint is stable and the affected joint is well supported. An exercise program slowly restores the joint to its original ROM without causing another dislocation. The patient should gradually return to normal activities.

A patient who has dislocated a joint may be at greater risk for repeated dislocations because of loose ligaments. Activity restrictions of the affected joint may be imposed to decrease the risk for repeated dislocation.

REPETITIVE STRAIN INJURY

Repetitive strain injury (RSI) and *cumulative trauma disorder* are terms used to describe injuries resulting from prolonged force or repetitive movements and awkward postures. RSI is also reported as *repetitive trauma disorder, nontraumatic musculo-skeletal injury, overuse syndrome* (sports medicine), *regional musculo-skeletal disorder,* and *work-related musculo-skeletal disorder.* The exact cause of these disorders is unknown. There are no specific diagnostic tests, and diagnosis is often difficult.

In 2013–2014, 15% of Canadians (an estimated 4.5 million people) reported having had an RSI (males and females in equal proportions) (Statistics Canada, 2015c). In Canada, RSI most often affects the upper body: 22.6% of cases occur in the shoulders, 15% in the elbows, 14% in the wrists, 12.8% in the knees, and 12.4% in the lower back (Statistics Canada, 2015c). People at risk for RSI include musicians, dancers, butchers, grocery clerks, vibratory tool workers, and those who frequently use a computer mouse and keyboard. Competitive athletes and poorly trained athletes may also develop RSI. Swimming, overhead throwing (e.g., baseball), weightlifting, gymnastics, tennis, skiing, and kicking sports (e.g., soccer) require repetitive motion, and overtraining compounds the effects of RSI.

In addition to the repetitive movements, other factors related to RSI include poor posture and positioning, poor work space ergonomics, badly designed workplace equipment (e.g., computer keyboard), and repetitive lifting of heavy workloads without sufficient muscle rest. The result may be inflammation, swelling, and pain in the muscles, tendons, and nerves of the neck, shoulder, forearm, and hand. Symptoms of RSI include pain, weakness, numbness, or impairment of motor function. RSI can be prevented through education and *ergonomics* (the science that promotes efficiency and safety in the interaction of humans and their work environment). Ergonomic considerations for people who work at a desk and use a computer include keeping the hips and knees flexed to 90 degrees with the feet flat, keeping the wrist straight to type, having the top of the monitor even with the forehead, and taking at least hourly stretch breaks. Once RSI is diagnosed, treatment consists of identification of the precipitating activity; modification of equipment or activity; pain management, including heat or cold application and NSAIDs; rest; physiotherapy for strengthening and conditioning exercises; and lifestyle changes.

CARPAL TUNNEL SYNDROME

Carpal tunnel syndrome (CTS) is a condition caused by compression of the median nerve, which enters the hand through the narrow confines of the carpal tunnel (see Figure 65-2). The carpal tunnel is formed by ligaments and bones in the wrist. CTS is the most common compression neuropathy in the upper extremity. This syndrome is associated with hobbies or occupations that require continuous wrist movement (e.g., musicians, painters, carpenters, computer operators).

This condition often is caused by pressure from trauma or edema caused by inflammation of a tendon (tenosynovitis), neoplasm, rheumatoid arthritis (RA), or soft tissue masses such as ganglia. Hormones may be involved as initial manifestations often occur during the premenstrual period, pregnancy, and menopause. People with diabetes mellitus or other metabolic disorders have a higher incidence of CTS (National Institute of Neurological Disorders and Stroke [NINDS], 2012). Women are

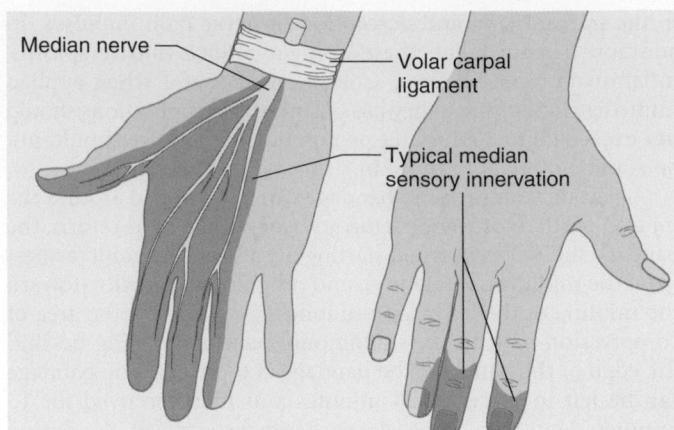

FIGURE 65-2 Wrist structures involved in carpal tunnel syndrome. Median nerve distribution. *Shaded areas* depict the locations of pain in carpal tunnel syndrome. Source: Buttaravoli, P. (2012). *Minor emergencies.* (3rd ed.). Philadelphia: Saunders.

more likely than men to develop CTS, possibly owing to a smaller carpal tunnel.

The clinical manifestations of CTS are weakness (especially of the thumb), burning pain (causalgia), and numbness, or impaired sensation in the distribution of the median nerve and clumsiness in performing fine hand movements. Numbness and tingling may be present, which awaken the patient at night. Shaking the hands will often relieve these symptoms.

Manifestations of CTS include a positive Tinel sign and Phalen sign. The *Tinel sign* can be elicited by tapping over the median nerve as it passes through the carpal tunnel in the wrist (Figure 65-2). A positive response is a sensation of tingling in the distribution of the median nerve over the hand. The *Phalen sign* can be elicited by allowing the wrists to fall freely into maximum flexion and maintaining the position for longer than 60 seconds. A positive response is a sensation of tingling in the distribution of the median nerve over the hand. In late stages, there is atrophy of the thenar muscles around the base of the thumb, resulting in recurrent pain and eventual dysfunction of the hand.

NURSING AND COLLABORATIVE MANAGEMENT CARPAL TUNNEL SYNDROME

Prevention of CTS involves educating employees and employers to identify risk factors. Adaptive devices such as wrist splints may be worn to hold the wrist in slight extension to relieve pressure on the median nerve. Special keyboard pads and mice that help prevent repetitive pressure on the median nerve are available for use at computers. Other ergonomic changes include workstation modifications, change in body positions, and frequent breaks from work-related activities.

Collaborative care of the patient with CTS is directed toward relieving the underlying cause of the nerve compression. The early symptoms associated with CTS can usually be relieved by stopping the aggravating movement and by placing the hand and wrist at rest by immobilizing them in a hand splint. Splints worn at night help keep the wrist in a neutral position and may reduce night pain and numbness. Physiotherapy with hand and wrist exercises may lessen symptom severity. Injection of a corticosteroid drug directly into the carpal tunnel may provide short-term relief. The patient may need to consider a change in occupation because of discomfort and sensory changes.

Carpal tunnel release is generally recommended if symptoms last for more than 6 months. Surgery involves severing the band of tissue around the wrist to reduce pressure on the median nerve (see Figure 65-2). Surgery is done under local anaesthesia and does not require an overnight hospital stay. The types of carpal tunnel release surgery include open release and endoscopic surgery (Middleton & Anakwe, 2014). In *open release surgery,* an incision is made in the wrist and then the carpal ligament is cut to enlarge the carpal tunnel. *Endoscopic carpal tunnel release* is performed through one or more small puncture incisions in the wrist and palm. A camera is attached to a tube, and the carpal ligament is cut. The endoscopic approach may allow faster functional recovery and less postoperative discomfort than traditional open release surgery.

Although symptoms may be relieved immediately after surgery, full recovery may take months. After surgery, the neuro-vascular status of the hand is assessed before discharge. The patient is instructed about wound care and the appropriate assessments to perform at home.

ROTATOR CUFF INJURY

The rotator cuff is a complex of four muscles in the shoulder: the supraspinatus, infraspinatus, teres minor, and subscapularis muscles. These muscles act to stabilize the humeral head in the glenoid fossa while assisting with ROM of the shoulder joint and rotation of the humerus.

A tear in the rotator cuff may occur as a gradual, degenerative process resulting from aging, repetitive stress (especially overhead arm motions), or injury to the shoulder while falling. The rotator cuff can tear as a result of sudden adduction forces applied to the cuff while the arm is held in abduction. In sports, repetitive overhead motions, such as in swimming, weightlifting, and swinging a racquet (e.g., tennis, racquetball) often cause injury. Other causative factors include (1) falling onto an outstretched arm and hand, (2) a blow to the upper arm, (3) heavy lifting, or (4) repetitive work motions.

Manifestations of a rotator cuff injury include shoulder weakness and pain and decreased ROM. The patient usually experiences severe pain when the arm is abducted between 60 and 120 degrees (the painful arc). The *drop arm test,* in which the arm falls suddenly after the patient is asked to slowly lower the arm to the side after it has been abducted 90 degrees, is another sign of rotator cuff injury. A radiograph alone is usually not beneficial in the diagnosis. A tear can be confirmed by magnetic resonance imaging (MRI).

The patient with a partial tear or cuff inflammation may be treated conservatively with rest, ice and heat, NSAIDs, corticosteroid injections into the joint, and physiotherapy. If the patient does not respond to conservative treatment in 3 to 6 months or if a complete tear is present, a surgical repair may be necessary. Most surgical repairs are performed through an arthroscope (Figure 65-3). If an extensive tear is present, *acromioplasty* (surgical removal of part of the acromion to relieve compression of the rotator cuff during movement) may be necessary. A sling or, more commonly, a shoulder immobilizer may be used immediately after surgery. However, the shoulder should not be immobilized for too long a period because "frozen" shoulder or arthrofibrosis may occur. Pendulum exercises and physiotherapy begin the first postoperative day. Restrictions for lifting weights are usually given, with full recovery taking up to 6 months.

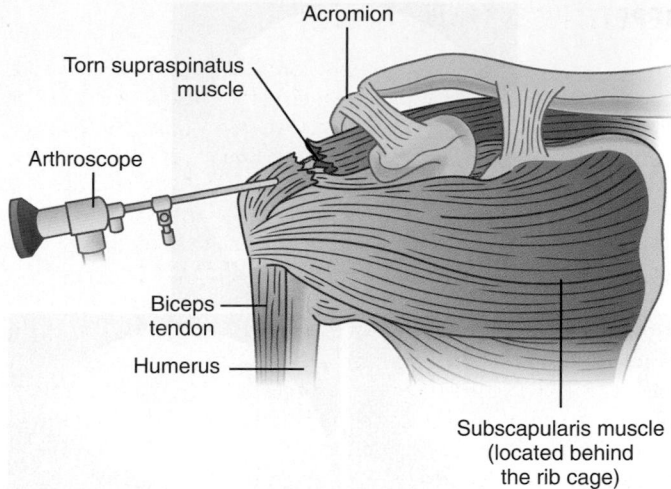

FIGURE 65-3 A torn rotator cuff is repaired using arthroscopic surgery.

MENISCUS INJURY

The menisci are crescent-shaped pieces of fibrocartilage in the knee. Menisci are also found in other joints. Meniscus injuries are closely associated with ligament sprains, commonly occurring in athletes engaged in sports such as basketball, football, soccer, and hockey. These activities produce rotational stress when the knee is in varying degrees of flexion and the foot is planted or fixed. A blow to the knee can cause the meniscus to be sheared between the femoral condyles and the tibial plateau, resulting in a torn meniscus. Individuals in occupations that require squatting or kneeling, as well as older adults, may be at higher risk for meniscus injuries.

Meniscus injuries alone do not usually cause significant edema because most of the cartilage is avascular. However, an acutely torn meniscus may be suspected when localized tenderness, pain, and effusion are noted (Figure 65-4). Pain is elicited by flexion, internal rotation, and then extension of the knee (called the *McMurray test*). The usual clinical picture is the patient feeling that the knee is unstable and a report that the knee may "click," "pop," "lock," or "give way." Quadriceps atrophy may be evident if the injury has been present for some time. Traumatic arthritis may occur from repeated meniscal injury and chronic inflammation.

MRI is beneficial for confirming the diagnosis before arthroscopy. The degree of knee pain and dysfunction, occupation, sport activities, and age may affect the patient's decision to have or postpone surgery.

NURSING AND COLLABORATIVE MANAGEMENT MENISCUS INJURY

Because meniscal injuries are commonly caused by sports-related activity, athletes should be taught to do warm-up activities. Examination of the acutely injured knee should occur within 24 hours of injury. Initial care of this type of injury involves application of ice, immobilization, and partial weight bearing with crutches. Most meniscal injuries are treated in an outpatient setting. Use of a knee brace or immobilizer during the first few days after the injury protects the knee and offers some pain relief. After acute pain has decreased, physiotherapy can help the patient regain knee flexion and muscle strength to assist in

FIGURE 65-4 Arthroscopic views of the meniscus. **A,** Normal meniscus. **B,** Torn meniscus. **C,** Surgically repaired meniscus. Source: **A,** David Lintner, MD, Houston. Retrieved from *http://www.drlintner.com;* **B** and **C,** Courtesy Peter Bonner, San Antonio, TX.

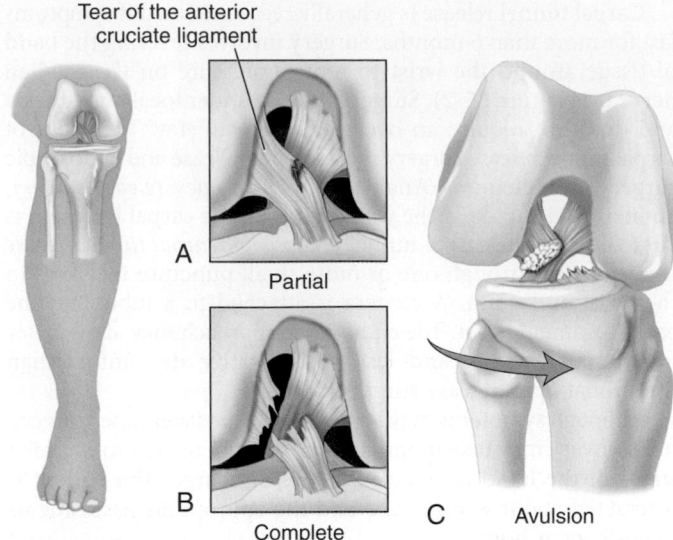

FIGURE 65-5 Anterior cruciate ligament injury. **A,** Partial tear. **B,** Complete tear. **C,** Avulsion.

returning to full function. In older adults with degenerative meniscus tears, progressive exercise therapy may improve neuro-muscular function and muscle strength (Stensrud, Roos, & Risberg, 2012).

Surgical repair or excision of part of the meniscus (meniscectomy) may be necessary. Meniscal surgery is performed by arthroscopy. Pain relief may include NSAIDs or other analgesics. Rehabilitation starts soon after surgery, including quadriceps- and hamstring-strengthening exercises and ROM. When the patient's strength is back to its preinjury level, normal activities may be resumed.

ANTERIOR CRUCIATE LIGAMENT INJURY

Knee injuries account for over 50% of all sport injuries. The most commonly injured knee ligament is the anterior cruciate ligament (ACL). ACL injuries usually occur from noncontact when the athlete pivots, lands from a jump, or slows down when running. Patients often report coming down on the knee, twisting, and hearing a pop, followed by acute knee pain and swelling. Athletes usually cannot continue playing, and the knee may feel unstable. An injury to the ACL can result in a partial tear, a complete tear, or an *avulsion* (tearing away) from the bone attachments that form the knee (Figure 65-5).

Examination of the knee with an ACL tear may produce a positive *Lachman test* (Meuffels, Poldervaart, Diercks, et al., 2012). This test is performed by flexing the knee 15 to 30 degrees and pulling the tibia forward while the femur is stabilized. The test is considered positive for an ACL tear if there is forward motion of the tibia with the feeling of a soft or indistinct end point. MRI is often used to diagnose coexisting conditions, including a fracture, meniscus tear, and collateral ligament injuries.

NURSING AND COLLABORATIVE MANAGEMENT ACL INJURY

Prevention programs have been shown to significantly reduce ACL injuries in athletes (Sadoghi von Keudell & Vavken, 2012). Conservative treatment for an intact ACL injury includes rest, ice, NSAIDs, elevation, and ambulation as tolerated with crutches. If there is a tight, painful effusion, it may be aspirated. A knee immobilizer or hinged knee brace may be helpful in supporting the knee. Often, physiotherapy assists the patient in maintaining knee joint motion and muscle tone.

Reconstructive surgery is usually recommended in physically active patients who have sustained severe injury to the ligament and meniscus. In reconstruction, the torn ACL tissue is removed and replaced with autologous or allograft tissue (Shea, Carey, Richmond, et al., 2015). ROM exercises are encouraged soon after surgery and the knee is placed in a brace or immobilizer. Rehabilitation with physiotherapy is critical, with progressive weight bearing determined by the degree of surgical repair. A safe return to the patient's prior level of physical functioning may take 6 to 8 months.

BURSITIS

Bursae are closed sacs that are lined with synovial membrane and contain a small amount of synovial fluid. They are located at sites of friction, such as between tendons and bones and near the joints. Bursitis (inflammation of a bursa) results from repeated or excessive trauma or friction, gout, RA, or infection.

The primary clinical manifestations of bursitis are warmth, pain, swelling, and limited ROM in the affected part. Sites at which bursitis commonly occurs include the hand, knee, greater trochanter of the hip, shoulder, and elbow. Improper body mechanics, repetitive kneeling (e.g., in carpet layers, coal miners, gardeners), jogging in worn-out shoes, and prolonged sitting with crossed legs are common precipitating activities.

Attempts are made to determine and correct the cause of the bursitis. Rest is often the only treatment needed. Icing the area will decrease pain and may reduce inflammation. The affected

FIGURE 65-6 Fracture classification according to communication with the external environment.

part may be immobilized in a compression dressing or splint. NSAIDs may be used to reduce inflammation and pain (Aaron, Patel, Kayiaros, et al., 2011). Aspiration of the bursal fluid and intra-articular injection of a corticosteroid may be necessary. If the bursal wall has become thickened and continues to interfere with normal joint function, surgical excision (bursectomy) may be necessary. Septic bursae usually require surgical incision and drainage.

FRACTURES

Classification

A **fracture** is a disruption or break in the continuity of the structure of bone. Although traumatic injuries account for the majority of fractures, some fractures are secondary to a disease process (pathological fractures from cancer or osteoporosis).

Fractures can be classified as *open* (formerly called *compound*) or *closed* (formerly called *simple*) depending on communication or noncommunication with the external environment (Figure 65-6). In an *open fracture,* the skin is broken, exposing the bone and causing soft tissue injury. In a *closed fracture,* the skin has not been ruptured and remains intact.

Fractures can also be classified as complete or incomplete. Fractures are termed *complete* if the break is completely through the bone and described as *incomplete* if the fracture occurs partly across a bone shaft but the bone is still in one piece. An incomplete fracture is often the result of bending or crushing forces applied to a bone.

Fractures are also described and classified according to the direction of the fracture line. Types include linear, oblique, transverse, longitudinal, and spiral fractures (see Figure 65-7 for selected fracture types).

Fractures can also be classified as displaced or nondisplaced. In a *displaced* fracture, the two ends of the broken bone are separated from one another and out of their normal positions. Displaced fractures are usually *comminuted* (more than two fragments) or *oblique* (see Figure 65-7). In a *nondisplaced fracture,* the periosteum is intact across the fracture and the bone is still in alignment. Nondisplaced fractures are usually transverse, spiral, or greenstick (see Figure 65-7).

Clinical Manifestations

The clinical manifestations of a fracture include immediate localized pain, decreased function, and inability to bear weight on or use the affected part (Table 65-4). The patient guards and protects the extremity against movement. Obvious bone deformity

FIGURE 65-7 Types of fractures. **A,** Transverse fracture: the line of the fracture extends across the bone shaft at a right angle to the longitudinal axis. **B,** Spiral fracture: the line of the fracture extends in a spiral direction along the shaft of the bone. **C,** Greenstick fracture: an incomplete fracture with one side splintered and the other side bent. **D,** Comminuted fracture: fracture with more than two fragments. The smaller fragments appear to be floating. **E,** Oblique fracture: the line of the fracture extends in an oblique direction. **F,** Pathological fracture: a spontaneous fracture at the site of a bone disease. **G,** Stress fracture: occurs in normal or abnormal bone that is subject to repeated stress, such as from jogging or running.

may not be present. If a fracture is suspected, the extremity is immobilized in the position in which it is found. Unnecessary movement increases soft tissue damage and may convert a closed fracture to an open fracture or create further injury to adjacent neuro-vascular structures.

Fracture Healing

It is important to understand the principles of fracture healing (Figure 65-8) to provide appropriate therapeutic interventions. Bone goes through a remarkable reparative process of self-healing (termed *union*) that occurs in the following stages (Fazzalari, 2011):

1. *Fracture hematoma.* When a fracture occurs, bleeding creates a hematoma, which surrounds the ends of the fragments. The hematoma is extravasated blood that changes from a liquid to a semisolid clot. This hematoma formation occurs in the initial 72 hours after injury.
2. *Granulation tissue.* During this stage, active phagocytosis absorbs the products of local necrosis. The hematoma converts to granulation tissue. Granulation tissue (consisting of new blood vessels, fibroblasts, and osteoblasts) produces the basis for new bone substance called *osteoid* during days 3 to 14 after injury.
3. *Callus formation.* As minerals (calcium, phosphorus, and magnesium) and new bone matrix are deposited in the osteoid, an unorganized network of bone is formed that is woven about the fracture parts. Callus is composed primarily of cartilage, osteoblasts, calcium, and phosphorus. It usually appears by the end of the second week after injury. Evidence of callus formation can be verified by radiography.

TABLE 65-4   CLINICAL MANIFESTATIONS OF FRACTURE

Manifestation	Significance
Edema and Swelling Disruption and penetration of bone through skin or soft tissues, or bleeding into surrounding tissues	Unchecked bleeding, swelling, and edema in closed space can occlude circulation and damage nerves (i.e., risk for compartment syndrome).
Pain and Tenderness Muscle spasm as a result of involuntary reflex action of muscle, direct tissue trauma, increased pressure on nerves, movement of fracture parts	Pain and tenderness encourage splinting of musculature around the fracture, with reduction in motion of injured area.
Muscle Spasm Irritation of tissues and protective response to injury and fracture	Muscle spasms may displace nondisplaced fracture or prevent it from reducing spontaneously.
Deformity Abnormal position of extremity or part as result of original forces of injury and action of muscles pulling fragment into abnormal position; seen as a loss of normal bony contours	Deformity is cardinal sign of fracture; if uncorrected, it may result in problems with bony union and restoration of function of injured part.
Ecchymosis or Contusion Discoloration of skin as a result of extravasation of blood into subcutaneous tissues	Ecchymosis may appear immediately after injury and may appear distal to injury. Patient should be reassured that process is normal and that discoloration will eventually resolve.
Loss of Function Disruption of bone or joint, preventing functional use of limb or part	Fracture must be managed properly to ensure restoration of function to limb or part.
Crepitation Grating or crunching together of bony fragments, producing palpable or audible crunching or popping sensation	Crepitation may increase chance for nonunion if bone ends are allowed to move excessively. Micromovement of bone-end fragments (postfracture) assists in osteogenesis (new bone growth).

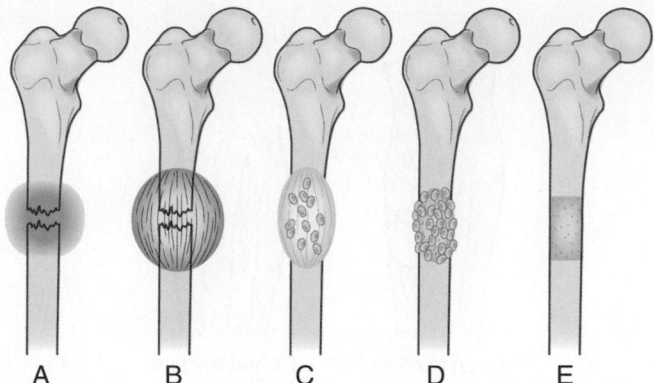

FIGURE 65-8 Bone healing (schematic representation). **A,** Bleeding at broken ends of the bone with subsequent hematoma formation. **B,** Organization of hematoma into fibrous network. **C,** Invasion of osteoblasts, lengthening of collagen strands, and deposition of calcium. **D,** Callus formation: new bone is built up as osteoclasts destroy dead bone. **E,** Remodelling is accomplished as excess callus is reabsorbed and trabecular bone is laid down.

evidence of complete bony union. This phase can occur up to one year following injury.

6. *Remodelling.* Excess bone tissue is reabsorbed in the final stage of bone healing, and union is completed. Gradual return of the injured bone to its preinjury structural strength and shape occurs. Bone remodels in response to physical loading stress, or *Wolff's law.* Initially, stress is provided through exercise. Weight bearing is gradually introduced. New bone is deposited in sites subjected to stress and resorbed at areas where there is little stress.

Many factors influence the time required for complete fracture healing, including displacement and site of the fracture, blood supply to the area, immobilization, and internal fixation devices (e.g., screws, pins). The ossification process may be arrested by inadequate reduction and immobilization, excessive movement of the fracture fragments, infection, poor nutrition, and systemic disease. Healing time for fractures increases with age. For example, an uncomplicated midshaft fracture of the femur heals in 3 weeks in a newborn and in 20 weeks in an adult. Smoking also increases fracture healing time. Fracture healing may not occur in the expected time *(delayed union)* or may not occur at all *(nonunion).* Table 65-5 summarizes complications of fracture healing.

Collaborative Care

The overall goals of fracture treatment are (1) anatomical realignment of bone fragments (reduction), (2) immobilization to maintain realignment, and (3) restoration of normal or near-normal function of the injured part. Table 65-6 summarizes the collaborative care of fractures.

Fracture Reduction

Closed Reduction. *Closed reduction* is a nonsurgical, manual realignment of bone fragments to their previous anatomical position. Traction and countertraction are manually applied to the bone fragments to restore position, length, and alignment. Usually, closed reduction is performed with the patient under local or general anaesthesia. After reduction, traction, casting, external fixation, splints, or orthoses (braces), the injured part is immobilized to maintain alignment until healing occurs.

Open Reduction. *Open reduction* is the correction of bone alignment through a surgical incision. It often includes internal fixation of the fracture with the use of wire, screws, pins, plates,

4. *Ossification.* Ossification of the callus occurs from 3 weeks to 6 months after the fracture and continues until the fracture has healed. Callus ossification is sufficient to prevent movement at the fracture site when the bones are gently stressed. However, the fracture is still evident on a radiograph. During this stage of *clinical union,* the patient may be allowed limited mobility or the cast may be removed.

5. *Consolidation.* As callus continues to develop, the distance between bone fragments diminishes and eventually closes. During this stage, ossification continues. It can be equated with *radiological union,* which occurs when there is radiographic

TABLE 65-5 COMPLICATIONS OF FRACTURE HEALING

Problem	Description
Delayed union	Fracture healing progresses more slowly than expected; healing eventually occurs
Nonunion	Fracture fails to heal properly despite treatment; no radiographic evidence of callus formation
Malunion	Fracture heals in expected time but in unsatisfactory position, possibly resulting in deformity or dysfunction
Angulation	Fracture heals in abnormal position in relation to midline of structure (type of malunion)
Pseudoarthrosis	Type of nonunion occurring at fracture site in which a false joint is formed with abnormal movement at site
Refracture	New fracture occurs at original fracture site
Myositis ossificans	Deposition of calcium in muscle tissue at the site of significant blunt muscle trauma or repeated muscle injury

TABLE 65-6 COLLABORATIVE CARE

Fractures

Diagnostic	***Fracture Immobilization***
• History and physical examination	• Casting or splinting
• CT scan, MRI	• External fixation
• Radiographs	• Internal fixation
	• Traction
Collaborative Therapy ***Fracture Reduction***	***Open Fractures***
• Closed reduction	• Immobilization
• Manipulation	• Prophylactic antibiotic therapy
• Open reduction	• Surgical debridement and irrigation
• Skeletal traction	• Tetanus and diphtheria immunization
• Skin traction	

CT, computed tomographic (scan); MRI, magnetic resonance imaging.

FIGURE 65-9 Buck traction is most commonly used for fractures of the hip and femur. Source: Courtesy Mary Wollan, RN, BAN. Spring Park, MN.

pathological joint condition (e.g., tumour, infection). Traction is also indicated to (1) provide immobilization to prevent soft tissue damage, (2) promote active and passive exercise, (3) expand a joint space during arthroscopic procedures, and (4) expand a joint space before major joint reconstruction.

Traction devices apply a pulling force on a fractured extremity to attain realignment, while countertraction pulls in the opposite direction. The two most common types of traction are skin traction and skeletal traction. *Skin traction* is generally used for short-term treatment (48–72 hours) until skeletal traction or surgery is possible. Tape, boots, or splints are applied directly to the skin to maintain alignment, assist in reduction, and help diminish muscle spasms in the injured extremity. The traction weights are usually limited to 2.3 to 4.5 kg. A Buck traction boot is a type of skin traction used to immobilize a fracture, prevent hip flexion contractures, and reduce muscle spasms (Figure 65-9). Pelvic or cervical skin traction may require heavier weights applied intermittently. In skin traction, assessment of the skin is a priority, since pressure points and skin breakdown may develop quickly. Key pressure points are assessed every 2 to 4 hours.

Skeletal traction, generally in place for longer periods than skin traction, is used to align injured bones and joints or to treat joint contractures and congenital hip dysplasia. It provides a long-term pull that keeps the injured bones and joints aligned. To apply skeletal traction, the physician inserts a pin or wire into the bone, either partially or completely, to align and immobilize the injured body part (Marshall & Browner, 2012). Weight for skeletal traction ranges from 2 to 20 kg. The use of too much weight can result in delayed union or nonunion. The major disadvantages of skeletal traction are risk for infection in the area of the bone where the skeletal pin has been inserted and the consequences of prolonged immobility.

When traction is used to treat fractures, the forces are usually exerted on the distal fragment to obtain alignment with the proximal fragment. Several types of traction can be used for this purpose. One of the more common types of skeletal traction is balanced suspension traction (Figure 65-10). Fracture alignment depends on the correct positioning and alignment of the patient while the traction forces remain constant. For extremity traction to be effective, forces must be pulling in the opposite direction (countertraction). Countertraction is commonly supplied by the patient's body weight or by weights pulling in the opposite direction and may be augmented by elevating the end of the bed. It is imperative to maintain traction continuously and keep the weights off the floor and moving freely through the pulleys.

intramedullary rods, or nails. The type and location of the fracture, patient age, and the presence of concurrent disease may influence the decision to use open reduction. The main disadvantages of this form of fracture management are the possibility of infection, the complications associated with anaesthesia, and the effect of pre-existing medical conditions (e.g., diabetes).

If open reduction with internal fixation (ORIF) is used for intra-articular fractures, early initiation of active ROM of the joint is indicated. Machines that provide continuous passive motion (CPM) to various joints (e.g., knee, shoulder) are used to prevent extra-articular and intra-articular adhesions. The use of CPM results in faster reconstruction of the subchondral (beneath cartilage) bone plate, more rapid healing of the articular cartilage, and decreased incidence of post-traumatic arthritis. ORIF facilitates early ambulation, thus decreasing the risk for complications related to prolonged immobility.

Traction. Traction is the application of a pulling force to an injured or diseased part of the body or extremity. *Countertraction* pulls in the opposite direction. Traction is used to (1) prevent or reduce pain and muscle spasm associated with low back pain or cervical sprain (e.g., whiplash), (2) immobilize a joint or part of the body, (3) reduce a fracture or dislocation, and (4) treat a

FIGURE 65-10 Balance suspension skeletal traction. Most commonly used for fractures of the femur, hip, and lower leg. Source: Courtesy Zimmer, Inc.

FIGURE 65-11 Common types of casts.

Fracture Immobilization. Fracture immobilization can be done using casts (including air casts), braces, splints, immobilizing devices, and external and internal fixation devices.

Casts. A *cast* is a temporary circumferential immobilization device. Casting is a common treatment following closed reduction. It allows the patient to perform many normal activities of daily living (ADLs) while providing sufficient immobilization to ensure stability. Cast materials are natural (plaster of Paris) or synthetic acrylic; fibreglass-free, latex-free polymer; or a hybrid of materials. A cast generally incorporates the joints above and below a fracture. Immobilization above and below a joint restricts tendon and ligament movement, thus assisting with joint stabilization while the fracture heals.

To apply a plaster cast on an extremity, the affected part is first covered with a stockinette that is cut longer than the extremity (Satryb, Wilson, & Patterson, 2011). Then, padding is placed over the stockinette with the bony prominences given extra padding. If plaster of Paris casting material is used, it is usually immersed in warm water, then wrapped and moulded around the affected part. The number of layers of plaster bandage and the technique of application determine the strength of the cast. Plaster sets within 15 minutes, so patients may soon move around without difficulty. However, the cast is not strong enough for weight bearing until about 24 to 72 hours after application. (The decision about weight bearing is determined by the physician.)

A fresh plaster cast should never be covered because air cannot circulate, heat builds up in the cast that may cause a burn, and drying is delayed. Direct pressure on the cast should be avoided during the drying period. The cast should be handled gently with an open palm to avoid denting it. Once the cast is thoroughly dry, the edges may have to be *petalled* to prevent skin irritation from rough edges and to prevent plaster of Paris debris from falling into the cast and causing irritation or pressure necrosis. Several strips (petals) of tape are placed by the health care provider over the rough areas to ensure a smooth cast edge.

Casts made of fibreglass are being used more often than those made of plaster because they are lightweight, relatively waterproof, stronger and faster-drying than plaster, porous (less risk for skin problems), and allow for almost immediate mobilization (Satryb et al., 2011). Synthetic casting materials (thermolabile plastic, thermoplastic resins, polyurethane, and fibreglass) are activated by submersion in cool or tepid water. Then they are moulded to fit the torso or the extremity.

Upper Extremity Injuries. Immobilization of an acute fracture or soft tissue injury of the upper extremity is often accomplished by use of a (1) sugar-tong splint, (2) posterior splint, (3) short arm cast, or (4) long arm cast (Figure 65-11). The sugar-tong splint is typically used for acute wrist injuries or injuries that may result in significant swelling. Plaster splints are applied over a well-padded forearm, beginning at the phalangeal joints of the hand, extending up the dorsal aspect of the forearm around the distal humerus, and then extending down the volar aspect of the forearm to the distal palmar crease. The splinting material is wrapped with either elastic bandage or bias stockinette. The sugar-tong posterior splint accommodates for postinjury swelling in the fractured extremity.

The *short arm cast* is often used for the treatment of stable wrist or metacarpal fractures. An aluminum finger splint can be fabricated into the short arm cast for concurrent treatment of phalangeal injuries. The short arm cast is a circular cast extending from the distal palmar area to the proximal forearm. This cast provides wrist immobilization and permits unrestricted elbow motion.

The *long arm cast* is commonly used for stable forearm or elbow fractures and unstable wrist fractures. It is similar to the short arm cast but extends to the proximal humerus, restricting motion in the wrist and the elbow. Nursing measures should be directed toward supporting the extremity and reducing the effects of edema by maintaining extremity elevation with a sling. However, when a hanging arm cast is used for a proximal humerus fracture, elevation or a supportive sling is contraindicated because hanging provides traction and maintains fracture alignment.

When a sling is used, the nurse must ensure that the axillary area is well padded to prevent skin excoriation and maceration associated with direct skin-to-skin contact. Placement of the sling should not put undue pressure on the posterior neck. Movement of the fingers (unless contraindicated) should be encouraged to enhance the pumping action of vascular and soft tissue structures to decrease edema. The nurse should also encourage the patient to actively move nonimmobilized joints of the upper extremity to prevent stiffness and contractures.

Vertebral Injuries. The *body jacket* brace is often used for immobilization and support for stable spine injuries of the thoracic or lumbar spine. This brace goes around the chest and abdomen and extends from above the nipple line to the pubis. After application of the cast, the nurse must assess the patient for the development of superior mesenteric artery syndrome *(cast syndrome)*. This condition occurs if the body cast is applied too tightly and compresses the superior mesenteric artery against the duodenum. The patient generally complains of abdominal pain, abdominal pressure, nausea, and vomiting. The abdomen should be assessed for decreased bowel sounds (a window in the brace may be left over the umbilicus). Treatment includes gastric decompression with a nasogastric tube and suction. Nursing assessment also includes observation of respiratory status, bowel and bladder function, and areas of pressure over the bony prominences, especially the iliac crest. The brace may need to be adjusted or removed if any complications occur.

Lower Extremity Injuries. Injuries to the lower extremity are often immobilized by a long leg cast, short leg cast, cylinder cast, Jones dressing, or prefabricated splint or immobilizer. The usual indications for applying a long leg cast are an unstable ankle fracture, soft tissue injuries, a fractured tibia, and knee injuries. The cast usually extends from the base of the toes to the groin and the gluteal crease. The short leg cast can be used for a variety of conditions, but primarily for stable ankle and foot injuries. A cylinder cast, which is used for knee injuries or fractures, extends from the groin to the malleoli of the ankle. A Jones dressing is composed of bulky padding materials (absorption dressing and cotton sheet wadding), splints, and an elastic wrap or bias-cut stockinette.

After application of a lower extremity cast or dressing, the extremity should be elevated on pillows above the heart level for the first 24 hours. After the initial phase, the casted extremity should not be placed in a dependent position because of the possibility of excessive edema. After cast application, the patient should be observed for signs of compartment syndrome (discussed on pp. 1649–1650 later in this chapter) and increased pressure, especially in the heel, anterior tibia, head of the fibula, and malleoli. This increased pressure is manifested by pain or a burning feeling in these areas.

Prefabricated knee and ankle splints and immobilizers are being used in many settings. This type of immobilization is easy to apply and remove, which permits close observation of the affected joint for signs of swelling and skin breakdown (Figure 65-12). Depending on the injury, removal of the splint or immobilizer facilitates ROM of the affected joint and a faster return to function.

The *hip spica cast* is now used mainly for femur fractures in children. The purpose of the hip spica cast is to immobilize the affected extremity and the trunk. The cast extends from above the nipple line to the base of the foot (single spica) and may include the opposite extremity up to an area above the knee (spica and a half) or both extremities (double spica). Assess the patient with a hip spica cast for the same problems that are associated with the body jacket brace.

FIGURE 65-12 Knee immobilizer. Source: Maher, A. B., Salmond, S. W., & Pellino, T. A. (Eds.). (2002). *Orthopaedic nursing* (3rd ed.). Philadelphia: Saunders.

External Fixation. An external fixator is a metallic device composed of metal pins that are inserted into the bone and attached to external rods to stabilize the fracture while it heals. It can be used to apply traction or to compress fracture fragments and to immobilize reduced fragments when the use of a cast or other traction is not appropriate. The external device holds fracture fragments in a manner similar to a surgically implanted internal device. The external fixator is attached directly to the bones by percutaneous transfixing pins or wires (Figure 65-13). External fixation is indicated in closed fractures, complex fractures with extensive soft tissue damage, correction of bony defects (congenital), nonunion or malunion, and limb lengthening.

Often, external fixation is used in an attempt to salvage extremities that otherwise might require amputation. Because the use of an external device is a long-term process, assessment for pin loosening and infection is critical. Infection—signalled by exudate, erythema, tenderness, and pain—may necessitate removal of the device. The nurse should instruct the patient and caregivers about meticulous pin care. Although each health care provider has a protocol for pin care cleaning, half-strength hydrogen peroxide with normal saline is often used.

Internal Fixation. Internal fixation devices (pins, plates, intramedullary rods, and metal and bioabsorbable screws) are surgically inserted at the time of realignment (Figure 65-14). These metal devices are biologically inert and made from stainless steel, vitallium, or titanium. Proper alignment is evaluated by radiographs at regular intervals.

Electrical Bone Growth Stimulation. Electrical bone growth stimulation is used to facilitate the healing process for certain types of fractures, especially those with nonunion or delayed healing. The mechanism of action of electrical bone growth stimulation may include (1) increasing the calcium uptake of bone, (2) activating intracellular calcium stores, and (3) increasing the production of bone growth factors (e.g., bone morphogenic protein).

Noninvasive, semi-invasive, and invasive methods of electrical bone growth stimulation are used. Noninvasive stimulators use direct current or pulsed electromagnetic fields (PEMFs) to

FIGURE 65-13 External fixators. Stabilization of a tibial fracture. Source: Canale, S.T., &, Beatty, J. H. (2013). *Campbell's operative orthopaedics*. (12th ed.). Philadelphia: Mosby.

FIGURE 65-14 Views of internal fixation devices to stabilize a fractured tibia and fibula. Source: Courtesy and © *www.rehabmypatient.com.*

generate a weak electrical current. Electrodes are placed over the patient's skin or cast and are used 10 to 12 hours each day, usually while the patient is sleeping. Semi-invasive or percutaneous bone growth stimulators use an external power supply and electrodes that are inserted through the skin and into the bone. Invasive stimulators require surgical implantation of a current generator in an intramuscular or subcutaneous space. An electrode is implanted in the bone fragments.

Drug Therapy. Patients with fractures often experience varying degrees of pain associated with muscle spasms. Involuntary reflexes that result from edema following muscle injury cause these spasms. Central and peripheral muscle relaxants, such as cyclobenzaprine or methocarbamol (Robaxin), may be prescribed for relief of pain associated with muscle spasms.

Acute pain management for the patient with a fracture is presented in Nursing Care Plan (NCP) 65-1, available on the Evolve website.

In an open fracture, the threat of tetanus occurring can be reduced with tetanus and diphtheria toxoid or tetanus immunoglobulin for the patient who has not been previously immunized (see Table 65-6). Bone-penetrating antibiotics (such as cefazolin) are used prophylactically before surgery.

Nutritional Therapy. Proper nutrition is an essential component of the reparative process in injured tissue. An adequate energy source is needed to promote muscle strength and tone,

build endurance, and enhance ambulation and gait-training skills. The patient's dietary intake must include ample protein (e.g., 1 g/kg of body weight); vitamins (especially B, C, and D); and calcium, phosphorus, and magnesium to ensure optimal soft tissue and bone healing. Low serum protein levels and vitamin C deficiencies interfere with tissue healing. Immobility and callus formation increase calcium needs.

Three well-balanced meals a day will usually provide the necessary nutrients. The well-balanced meal should be supplemented by a fluid intake of 2 000 to 3 000 mL/day to promote optimal bladder and bowel function. Adequate fluid and a high-fibre diet with fruits and vegetables will prevent constipation. If immobilized in bed with skeletal traction or in a body jacket brace, the patient should be instructed to eat six small meals to avoid overeating and thus abdominal pressure and cramping.

NURSING MANAGEMENT
FRACTURES

NURSING ASSESSMENT

A brief history of the traumatic episode, the mechanism of injury, and the position in which the patient was found can be obtained from the patient or witnesses. As soon as possible, the patient should be transported to an emergency department, where a thorough assessment and treatment can be initiated (Table 65-7). Subjective and objective data that should be obtained from an individual with a fracture are presented in Table 65-8.

Special emphasis must be placed on the region distal to the site of injury. Clinical findings must be documented before fracture treatment is initiated to prevent doubts about whether a problem discovered later was missed during the original examination or was caused by the treatment.

NEURO-VASCULAR ASSESSMENT. Musculo-skeletal injuries have the potential to cause changes in the neuro-vascular status of an injured extremity. With musculo-skeletal trauma, application of a cast or constrictive dressing, poor positioning, and the physiological response to the traumatic injury can cause nerve or vascular damage, usually distal to the injury.

The neuro-vascular assessment should consist of a *peripheral vascular assessment* (colour, temperature, capillary refill, peripheral pulses, and edema) and a *peripheral neurological assessment* (sensation, motor function, and pain). Throughout the neuro-vascular assessment, both extremities are compared to obtain an accurate assessment.

✚ TABLE 65-7 EMERGENCY MANAGEMENT

Fractured Extremity

Etiology	Assessment Findings	Interventions
Blunt • Motor vehicle accident • Pedestrian event **Falls** • Direct blows • Forced flexion or hyperextension • Twisting forces **Penetrating** • Blast • Gunshot **Other** • Crush injury • Pathological conditions • Violent muscle contractions (seizures)	• Deformity (loss of normal bony contours) or unnatural position of affected limb • Edema and ecchymosis • Grating (crepitus) • Loss of function • Muscle spasm • Numbness, tingling, loss of distal pulses • Open wound over injured site, exposure of bone • Tenderness and pain • Warmth at site	**Initial** • Treat life-threatening injuries first. • Ensure airway, breathing, and circulation. • Control external bleeding with direct pressure or sterile pressure dressing and elevation of the limb. • Check neuro-vascular status distal to injury before and after splinting. • Elevate injured limb if possible. • Do *not* attempt to straighten fractured or dislocated joints. • Do *not* manipulate protruding bone ends. • Apply ice packs to affected area. • Obtain radiographs of affected limb. • Administer tetanus and diphtheria prophylaxis if there is a break in skin integrity. • Mark location of pulses to facilitate repeat assessment. • Splint fracture site, including joints above and below fracture site. **Ongoing Monitoring** • Monitor vital signs, level of consciousness, oxygen saturation, peripheral pulses, and pain. • Monitor for compartment syndrome, characterized by excessive pain, pain with passive stretch of the affected extremity muscles, pallor, paresthesia, and late signs of paralysis and pulselessness. • Monitor for signs and symptoms of a fat embolism (e.g., dyspnea, chest pain, temperature elevation).

An extremity's colour (pink, pale, cyanotic) and temperature (hot, warm, cool, cold) in the area of the affected extremity are assessed. Pallor or a cool to cold extremity below the injury could indicate arterial insufficiency. A warm, cyanotic extremity could indicate poor venous return. A capillary refill (blanching of the nail bed) of less than 3 seconds indicates good arterial perfusion.

Pulses on both the unaffected and the injured extremity are compared to identify differences in rate or quality. Pulses are described as strong, diminished, audible by hand-held Doppler transducer, or absent. A diminished or absent pulse distal to the injury can indicate vascular dysfunction and insufficiency. However, up to 12% of healthy adults do not have a palpable dorsalis pedis or posterior tibial pulse (Roberts & Hedges, 2014). Peripheral edema is also assessed, and pitting edema may be present with severe injury.

Sensation and motor innervation in the upper extremity are assessed by evaluating the ulnar, median, and radial nerves. Neuro-vascular status can be assessed by abduction and adduction of the fingers, opposition of the fingers, and supination and pronation of the hand. In the lower extremity, dorsiflexion and plantar flexion provide information about motor function of the peroneal and tibial nerves. Sensory innervation is evaluated for the peroneal nerve on the dorsal part of the foot between the web space of the great and the second toes. Tibial nerve assessment is performed by stroking the plantar surface (sole) of the foot. Contralateral evaluation is critical. The patient may report paresthesia (abnormal sensation [e.g., numbness,

tingling]) and hyperesthesia (hypersensation). Partial or full loss of strength or movement (paresis or paralysis) may be a late sign of neuro-vascular damage. Reduced motion or strength in an injured extremity can alert the nurse to potential limb-threatening complications or disability.

Pain is the final element of the neuro-vascular assessment. The nurse must carefully assess the location, quality, and intensity of the pain (see Chapter 10). Current best practice in pain management is to ask the patient to rate his or her level of pain on a scale of 0 to 10, with 0 being no pain and 10 being the worst pain ever experienced. Increasing pain unrelieved by drugs and out of proportion to the injury can be an indication of compartment syndrome.

Patients should be instructed to report any changes in their neuro-vascular status. Patients must verbalize and demonstrate a thorough understanding of all elements before they are discharged from the treatment setting.

NURSING DIAGNOSES

Nursing diagnoses for the patient with a fracture may include, but are not limited to, the following:

- *Impaired physical mobility* related to *joint stiffness, pain*
- *Risk for peripheral neuro-vascular dysfunction* as evidenced by *fracture* (vascular insufficiency and nerve compression, mechanical compression by traction, splints, or casts)
- *Acute pain* related to *physical injury agent* (edema, movement of bone fragments, muscle spasms)
- *Readiness for enhanced health management*

TABLE 65-8 NURSING ASSESSMENT

Fracture

Subjective Data
Important Health Information

Past health history: Traumatic injury; long-term repetitive forces (stress fracture); bone or systemic diseases, prolonged immobility (pathological fracture), osteopenia, osteoporosis

Medications: Corticosteroids (osteoporotic fractures), analgesics, hormone therapy, calcium supplementation

Surgery or other treatments: First aid treatment of fracture, previous musculo-skeletal surgeries

Symptoms
- Loss of motion or weakness of affected part; muscle spasms
- Sudden and severe pain in affected area; numbness, tingling, loss of sensation distal to injury; chronic pain that increases with activity (stress fracture)

Objective Data
General

Apprehension, guarding of injured site

Integumentary
Skin lacerations, pallor and cool skin or bluish and warm skin distal to injury; ecchymosis, hematoma, edema at site of fracture

Cardiovascular
Reduced or absent pulse distal to injury, decreased skin temperature, delayed capillary refill

Neurological
Paresthesias, decreased or absent sensation, hypersensation

Musculo-Skeletal
Restricted or lost function of affected part; local bony deformities; abnormal angulation; shortening, rotation, or crepitation of affected part; muscle weakness

Possible Findings
Identification and extent of fractures on radiograph, bone scan, CT scan, or MRI

CT, computed tomographic (scan); *MRI,* magnetic resonance imaging.

🔍 EVIDENCE-INFORMED PRACTICE

Research Highlight

Do Vitamin D Supplements Improve Strength in Older Adults?
Clinical Question

In older adults (P) does vitamin D supplementation (I) improve strength, balance, and gait (O)?

Best Available Evidence
Systematic review of randomized controlled trials (RCTs)

Critical Appraisal and Synthesis of Evidence
- Thirteen RCTs (*n* = 2268) of older adults (mainly women) were done to determine the effect of supplemental vitamin D without an exercise intervention on muscle strength, gait, and balance.
- Supplemental vitamin D with daily doses of 800 to 1000 IU consistently demonstrated beneficial effects on strength and balance. An effect on gait was not demonstrated, although further evaluation is recommended.
- Increasing serum vitamin D to normal levels resulted in better muscle strength.

Conclusion
Supplemental vitamin D has beneficial effects on strength and balance in older adults.

Implications for Nursing Practice
- Patients should be assessed for vitamin D deficiencies and strategies offered to improve nutritional uptake, brief sunlight exposure, and supplementation.
- The importance of vitamin D in reducing the risk for falls should be discussed.

Reference for Evidence

Muir, S. W., & Montero-Odasso, M. (2011). Effect of vitamin D supplementation on muscle strength, gait and balance in older adults: A systematic review and meta-analysis. *Journal of American Geriatrics Society, 59*(12), 2291–2300. doi:10.1111/j.1532-5415.2011.03733.x.

P, Patient population of interest; *I,* intervention or area of interest; *O,* outcomes of interest (see Chapter 1).

Additional information on nursing diagnoses for the patient with a fracture is presented in Nursing Care Plan 65-1 (on the Evolve website).

▌PLANNING
The overall goals are that the patient with a fracture will (1) have healing with no associated complications, (2) obtain satisfactory pain relief, and (3) achieve maximal rehabilitation potential.

▌NURSING IMPLEMENTATION
HEALTH PROMOTION. The public should be taught to take appropriate safety precautions to prevent injuries while at home, at work, when driving, and when participating in sports. Nurses should be advocates for personal actions known to reduce injuries such as regular use of seat belts, driving within posted speed limits, stretching and warming up muscles before exercise, use of protective athletic equipment (helmets and knee, wrist, and elbow pads), use of safety equipment at work, and not driving under the influence of alcohol or illicit drugs.

Individuals (especially older adults) should be encouraged to participate in moderate exercise to aid in the maintenance of muscle strength and balance. To reduce falls, they should wear adequate footwear and assess their living environment for safety (e.g., remove scatter rugs, maintain good lighting, clear paths to the bathroom for nighttime use) (see Table 65-1). The nurse should also stress the importance of adequate calcium and vitamin D intake.

ACUTE INTERVENTION. Patients with fractures may be treated in an emergency department or a physician's office and discharged to home care, or they may require hospitalization for varying amounts of time. Specific nursing measures depend on the setting and type of treatment used.

Preoperative Management. If surgical intervention is required to treat the fracture, patients will need preoperative preparation. In addition to the usual preoperative nursing measures (see Chapter 20), the nurse should inform patients of the type of immobilization and assistive devices that will be used and the expected activity limitations after surgery. Assurance that pain medication will be available, if needed, is often beneficial.

Postoperative Management. In general, postoperative nursing care and management are directed toward monitoring vital signs and applying the general principles of postoperative nursing care (see Chapter 22). Frequent neuro-vascular assessments of the affected extremity are necessary to detect early and subtle neuro-vascular changes. Any limitations of movement or activity related to turning, positioning, and extremity support should be monitored closely. Pain and discomfort can be minimized through proper alignment and positioning. Dressings or casts should be carefully observed for any overt signs of bleeding or drainage. A significant increase in size of the drainage area should be reported. If a wound drainage system is in place, the volume of drainage should be regularly measured and the patency of the system assessed, using aseptic technique to avoid contamination.

Additional nursing responsibilities depend on the type of immobilization used. A blood salvage and reinfusion system that allows for recovery and reinfusion of the patient's own blood may be used. The blood is retrieved from a joint space or cavity, and the patient receives this blood in the form of an autotransfusion. (Autotransfusion is discussed in Chapter 33.) Additional nursing measures for the patient who has had orthopaedic surgery are discussed in NCP 65-2, available on the Evolve website.

Other Measures. Patients often have reduced mobility as a result of the fracture. The nurse must plan care to prevent the many complications associated with immobility. Constipation can be prevented by activity and maintenance of a high-fluid intake (>2 500 mL/day unless contraindicated by the patient's health status) and a diet high in bulk and roughage (fresh fruit and vegetables). If these measures are not effective in maintaining the patient's normal bowel pattern, warm fluids, stool softeners, laxatives, or suppositories may be necessary. Maintaining a regular time for elimination helps to promote regularity.

Renal calculi can develop as a result of bone demineralization. The hypercalcemia from demineralization causes a rise in urine pH and stone formation resulting from the precipitation of calcium. Unless contraindicated, a fluid intake of 2 500 mL/day is recommended. (Renal calculi are discussed in Chapter 48.)

Rapid deconditioning of the cardiopulmonary system can occur as a result of prolonged bed rest, resulting in orthostatic hypotension and decreased lung capacity. Unless contraindicated, these effects can be diminished by permitting the patient to sit on the side of the bed, allowing the patient's lower limbs to dangle over the bedside, and having the patient perform standing transfers. When the patient is allowed to increase activity, careful evaluation should be made to assess for orthostatic hypotension. Patients must also be assessed for deep venous thrombosis (DVT) and pulmonary emboli. (DVT and pulmonary embolism are discussed in Chapter 40 and pulmonary embolism is discussed in Chapter 30.)

Traction. When slings are used with traction, the nurse should inspect exposed skin areas regularly. Pressure over a bony prominence created by the wrinkling of sheets or bedclothes may cause pressure necrosis. Persistent skin pressure may impair blood flow, causing injury to the peripheral neuro-vascular structures. Skeletal traction pin sites must be observed for signs of infection. Pin-site care varies but usually includes regular removal of exudates with half-strength hydrogen peroxide, rinsing pin sites with sterile saline, and drying of the area with sterile gauze.

External rotation of the hip can occur when skin traction is used on the lower extremity. The nurse can correct this position by placing a pillow or rolled-up towels (called a *trochanter roll*) along the greater trochanteric region of the femur. Generally, the patient should be in the centre of the bed, in a supine position. Incorrect alignment can result in increased pain, nonunion, or malunion.

To offset some of the problems associated with prolonged immobility, the nurse should discuss activity of a specific patient with the health care provider. If exercise is permitted, the nurse should encourage the patient's participation in a simple exercise regimen within activity restrictions. Activities that the patient should participate in include frequent position changes, ROM exercises of unaffected joints, deep-breathing exercises, isometric exercises, and use of the trapeze bar (if permitted) to raise himself or herself off the bed for linen changes and use of the bedpan. These activities should be performed several times each day. The nurse should encourage and help the hospitalized patient to stay connected with friends and family through social media resources (see the "Informatics in Practice" box).

INFORMATICS IN PRACTICE

Staying Connected While Immobilized

A patient in traction or other immobilization devices for a long period may feel lonely or isolated.

There are a number of ways to use a computer or smartphone to ease separation anxiety and help the patient reconnect with family and friends.

The patient can set up a video chat. The nurse should encourage the patient to maintain personal contact through text messaging and email and have the patient catch up on the latest news and blogs on social networking sites.

AMBULATORY AND HOME CARE

Cast Care. Because many fractures are treated in an outpatient setting, the patient often requires only a short hospitalization or none at all. Regardless of the type of cast material, a cast can interfere with circulation and nerve function from being applied too tightly or because of excessive edema after application. Thus, frequent neuro-vascular assessments of the immobilized extremity are critical. The patient must be taught about signs of cast complications so that they can be reported promptly. Elevation of the extremity above the level of the heart to promote venous return, and applications of ice to control or prevent edema, are frequently used measures during the initial phase. (If compartment syndrome is suspected, the extremity should not be elevated above the heart.) The nurse should instruct the patient to exercise joints above and below the cast. Pulling out cast padding and scratching or placing foreign objects inside the cast is forbidden because it predisposes the patient to skin breakdown and infection. For itching, instruct the patient that a hair dryer set on a cool setting can be directed under the cast.

Patient and caregiver teaching is an important nursing responsibility to prevent complications. In addition to providing specific instructions for cast care and recognition of complications, the nurse should encourage the patient to contact the clinic or health care provider if questions arise. Table 65-9 summarizes patient and caregiver instructions for cast care. The nurse should validate the patient's and caregivers' understanding of these instructions before discharging the patient from inpatient and ambulatory settings. Follow-up phone contact is appropriate, and home care nursing visits are warranted, especially with body or spica casts.

Cast removal is done in the outpatient setting. Patients often fear being cut by the oscillating blade of the cast saw. The nurse should reassure the patient. More importantly, the nurse should educate the patient about possible alterations in the appearance of the extremity (e.g., dry, wrinkled skin, atrophied muscle) that

TABLE 65-9	PATIENT & CAREGIVER TEACHING GUIDE

Cast Care

After a cast is applied, include the following instructions when teaching the patient and the caregiver about cast care.

Do
- Apply ice directly over fracture site for first 24 hr (avoid getting cast wet by keeping ice in plastic bag and protecting cast with cloth).
- Check with health care provider before getting fibreglass cast wet.
- Dry cast thoroughly after exposure to water.
  - Blot dry with towel.
  - Use hair dryer on low setting until cast is thoroughly dry.
- Elevate extremity above level of heart for first 48 hr.
- Move joints above and below cast regularly.
- Use hair dryer on cool setting for itching.
- Report signs of possible problems to health care provider:
  - Increasing pain despite elevation, ice, and analgesia
  - Swelling associated with pain and discoloration of toes or fingers
  - Pain during movement
  - Burning or tingling under cast
  - Sores or foul odour under cast
- Keep appointment to have fracture and cast checked.

Do Not
- Get plaster cast wet.
- Remove any padding.
- Insert any objects inside cast.
- Bear weight on new cast for 48 hr (not all casts are made for weight bearing; check with health care provider if unsure).
- Cover cast with plastic if it will be wet for long periods of time.

has been beneath the cast. The patient may also have anxiety related to using the injured extremity after the cast is removed.

Psychosocial Problems. Short-term rehabilitative goals are directed toward the transition from dependence to independence in performing simple ADLs and preserving or increasing strength and endurance. Long-term rehabilitative goals are aimed at preventing problems associated with musculo-skeletal injury (Table 65-10). An important part of nursing care during the rehabilitative phase is assisting the patient to adjust to any problems caused by the injury (e.g., separation from family, financial impact of medical care, loss of income from inability to work, potential for lifetime disability). The nurse has an important role in offering support and encouragement while actively listening to the patient's and the caregiver's concerns.

Ambulation. The nurse must know the overall goals of physiotherapy in relation to the patient's abilities, needs, and tolerance. Mobility training and instruction in the use of assistive aids (cane, crutches, walker) constitute major areas of responsibility of the physiotherapist. The patient with lower extremity dysfunction is usually started in mobility training when able to sit in bed and dangle the feet over the side. This activity should be done two or three times a day for 10 to 15 minutes, with the nurse assisting as necessary. Collaboration of the nurse and physiotherapist to coordinate pain management and thus increase patient participation at therapy sessions is critical.

When the patient begins to ambulate, the nurse should know the patient's weight-bearing status and the correct technique if the patient is using an assistive device. Weight-bearing ambulation occurs in different degrees: (1) non–weight-bearing [NWB] ambulation (no weight on affected leg), (2) touch-down weight-bearing ambulation [TDWB] or toe-touch weight-bearing

ambulation [TTWB] (contact with floor only for balance; no weight on affected leg), (3) partial weight-bearing ambulation [PWB] (directions given by physician), (4) weight bearing as tolerated [WBAT] (dictated by patient's pain and tolerance), and (5) full weight-bearing [FWB] ambulation (no limitations) (University of Pittsburgh Medical Center, 2016).

Assistive Devices. Devices for ambulation range from a cane, which can relieve up to 40% of the weight normally borne by a lower limb, to a walker or crutches, which may allow for complete non–weight-bearing ambulation. The decision about which device is appropriate for a patient involves weighing the need for maximum stability and safety versus manoeuvrability, which is required in small spaces such as bathrooms. It is essential to discuss with patients the requirements of their lifestyles and determining the device with which each patient feels most secure and independent.

The technique for using assistive devices varies. The involved limb is usually advanced at the same time or immediately after the advance of the device. The uninvolved limb is advanced last. In almost all cases, canes are held in the hand opposite the involved extremity.

A transfer belt can be placed around the patient's waist to provide stability during the learning stages. The nurse should discourage the patient from reaching for furniture or relying on another person for support. When there is inadequate upper limb strength or poorly fitted crutches, the patient bears weight at the axilla rather than at the hands, endangering the neuro-vascular bundle that passes across the axilla. If verbal coaching does not correct the problem, the patient should be instructed in another form of ambulation until strength is adequate (e.g., platform crutches, walker).

Patients who must ambulate without weight bearing require sufficient upper limb strength to lift their own weight at each step. Because the muscles of the shoulder girdle are not accustomed to this work, they require vigorous and diligent training in preparation for this task. Push-ups, pull-ups using the overhead trapeze bar, and lifting weights develop the triceps and biceps. Straight-leg raises and quadriceps-setting exercises strengthen the quadriceps.

Counselling and Referrals. During the rehabilitative process, the patient's caregiver assumes an important role in the provision and follow-through of long-term care plans. The caregiver should be instructed in the techniques of strength and endurance exercises, assistance with mobility training, and promotion of activities that enhance the quality of daily living. The nurse should also evaluate patients for post-traumatic stress disorder. This is especially important if significant injury to others or fatalities were associated with the patient's injuries.

EVALUATION

The following are expected outcomes for the patient with a fracture:
- Report satisfactory relief of pain
- Demonstrate appropriate care of cast or immobilizer
- Experience no peripheral neuro-vascular dysfunction
- Experience uncomplicated bone healing

COMPLICATIONS OF FRACTURES

The majority of fractures heal without complications. If death occurs after a fracture, it is usually the result of damage to underlying organs and vascular structures or from complications of the fracture or immobility. Complications of fractures

TABLE 65-10	PROBLEMS ASSOCIATED WITH MUSCULO-SKELETAL INJURIES	
Problem	**Description**	**Nursing Considerations**
Muscle atrophy	• Decreased muscle mass normally occurs as a result of disuse following prolonged immobilization. • Loss of nerve innervation can precipitate muscle atrophy.	• Isometric muscle-strengthening exercise regimen within the confines of the immobilization device assists in reducing the amount of atrophy. • Muscle atrophy interferes with and prolongs the rehabilitation process.
Contracture	• Abnormal condition of joint characterized by flexion and fixation. • Caused by atrophy and shortening of muscle fibres or by loss of normal elasticity of skin over a joint.	• Can be prevented by frequent position change, correct body alignment, and active and passive range of motion exercises several times a day. • Intervention requires gradual and progressive stretching of the muscles or ligaments in the region of the joint.
Footdrop	• Plantar-flexed position of the foot (footdrop) occurs when the Achilles tendon in the ankle shortens because it has been allowed to assume an unsupported position. • Peroneal nerve palsy (a compression neuropathy) also causes footdrop.	• Management of the patient with long-term injuries must include supporting the foot in a neutral position. • Once footdrop has developed, ambulation and gait training may be significantly hindered. • The patient may require a splint to keep the foot or feet in a neutral position. • High-top athletic shoes may also help.
Pain	• Frequently associated with fractures, edema, and muscle spasm. • Pain varies in intensity from mild to severe and is usually described as aching, dull, burning, throbbing, sharp, or deep.	• Causes of pain include incorrect positioning and alignment of the extremity, incorrect support of the extremity, sudden movement of the extremity, and immobilization devices that are applied too tightly or in an incorrect position, constrictive dressings, and motion occurring at the fracture site. • Determine causes of pain so that corrective nursing action can be taken.
Muscle spasms	• Caused by involuntary muscle contraction after fracture, muscle strain, or nerve injury, these may last as long as several weeks. • Pain associated with muscle spasms is often intense and can last from several seconds to several minutes.	• Measures to reduce the intensity of the muscle spasms are similar to the corrective actions for pain control. • Do not massage muscle spasms. • Thermotherapy, especially heat, may reduce muscle spasm.

can be either direct or indirect. *Direct complications* include problems with bone infection, bone union, and AVN. *Indirect complications* are associated with blood vessel and nerve damage resulting in conditions such as compartment syndrome, venous thrombo-embolism, fat embolism, rhabdomyolysis (breakdown of skeletal muscle), and hypovolemic shock. Although most musculo-skeletal injuries are not life-threatening, open fractures, fractures accompanied by severe blood loss, and fractures that damage vital organs (e.g., lung, heart) are medical emergencies requiring immediate attention.

Infection

Open fractures and soft tissue injuries have a high incidence of infection. An open fracture usually results from high-energy trauma and can lead to significant long-term morbidity and disability (Halawi & Morwood, 2015). Massive or blunt soft tissue injury often has more serious consequences than the fracture. Devitalized and contaminated tissue is an ideal medium for many common pathogens, including gas-forming (anaerobic) bacilli such as *Clostridium tetani*. Treatment of infection is costly in terms of extended nursing and medical care, time for treatment, and loss of patient income. Osteomyelitis can become chronic (Patrice & Hatch, 2011b). (See Chapter 66 for a discussion of osteomyelitis.)

Collaborative Care. Open fractures require aggressive surgical debridement. The wound is initially cleansed with a sterile saline solution via low-pressure lavage, in the operating room. Gross contaminants are irrigated or mechanically removed. Contused, contaminated, and devitalized tissue such as muscle, subcutaneous fat, skin, and fragments of bone are surgically excised (*debridement*). The extent of the soft tissue damage determines whether the wound is closed at the time of surgery and whether

it requires repeat debridement, closed suction drainage, and skin grafting. Depending on the location and the extent of the fracture, reduction may be maintained by external fixation or traction. During surgery, the open wound may be irrigated with antibiotic solution. Antibiotic-impregnated beads may also be placed in the surgical site. During the postoperative phase, the patient will have antibiotics administered intravenously for 3 to 7 days. Antibiotics, in conjunction with aggressive surgical management, have greatly reduced the occurrence of infection.

Compartment Syndrome

Compartment syndrome is a condition in which swelling and increased pressure within a limited space (a compartment) press on and compromise the function of blood vessels, nerves, and tendons that run through that compartment. Compartment syndrome causes capillary perfusion to be reduced below a level necessary for tissue viability. It is classified as acute, subacute, or chronic (Ali, Santy-Tomlinson, & Watson, 2014). Compartment syndrome usually involves the leg but can also occur in the arm, shoulder, and buttock.

Thirty-eight compartments are located in the upper and lower extremities. Two basic causes of compartment syndrome are (1) decreased compartment size resulting from restrictive dressings, splints, casts, excessive traction, or premature closure of fascia and (2) increased compartment contents related to bleeding, edema, chemical response to snakebite, or intravenous infiltration.

Edema can create sufficient pressure to obstruct circulation and cause venous occlusion, which further increases edema. Eventually, arterial flow is compromised, resulting in inadequate arterial circulation (*ischemia*) to the extremity. As ischemia continues, muscle and nerve cells are destroyed over time, and fibrotic tissue replaces the healthy tissue. Contracture, disability, and loss of function can occur. Delay in diagnosis and treatment can result in irreversible muscle and nerve ischemia, resulting in a functionally useless or severely impaired extremity.

Compartment syndrome is usually associated with trauma, fractures (especially of the long bones), extensive soft tissue damage, and crush injury. Fractures of the distal humerus and proximal tibia are the most common fractures associated with compartment syndrome. Compartment injury can also occur following knee or leg surgery. Prolonged pressure on a muscle compartment may occur when someone is trapped under a heavy object or a person's limb is trapped beneath the body because of an obtunded state such as drug or alcohol overdose. In the upper extremity, this condition is referred to as *Volkmann ischemic contracture,* and in the lower extremity, it is known as *anterior tibial compartment syndrome,* although the underlying patho-physiological mechanism is similar.

Clinical Manifestations. Compartment syndrome may occur initially from the body's physiological response to the injury, or it may be delayed for several days after the original insult or injury. Ischemia can occur within 4 to 8 hours after the onset of compartment syndrome.

The "six Ps" are a neuro-vascular assessment mnemonic that can be used to assess for impending compartment syndrome: (1) *pain* distal to the injury that is not relieved by opioid analgesics and pain on passive stretch of muscle travelling through the compartment; (2) increasing *pressure* in the compartment; (3) *paresthesia* (numbness and tingling); (4) *pallor,* coolness, and loss of normal colour of the extremity; (5) *paralysis* or loss of function; and (6) *pulselessness* or diminished or absent peripheral pulses.

Collaborative Care. Prompt, accurate diagnosis of compartment syndrome is critical. Prevention or early recognition is the key. Regular neuro-vascular assessments should be performed and documented on all patients with fractures but especially those with injury of the distal humerus or proximal tibia or soft tissue disruption in these areas.

Carefully assess the location, quality, and intensity of the pain (see Chapter 10). Evaluate the pain on a scale of 0 to 10. Pain unrelieved by drugs and out of proportion to the level of injury and pain on passive muscle stretch appear to be the most effective clinical observations (Ali et al., 2014) and some of the first indications of impending compartment syndrome. Pulselessness and paralysis (in particular) are later signs of compartment syndrome. The health care provider should be notified immediately of a patient's changing condition.

Because of the possibility of muscle damage, urine output should be assessed. Myoglobin released from damaged muscle cells precipitates as a gel-like substance and causes obstruction in renal tubules. This condition results in acute tubular necrosis and acute kidney injury. Common signs are dark, reddish-brown urine and clinical manifestations associated with acute kidney injury (see Chapter 49).

Elevation of the extremity may lower venous pressure and slow arterial perfusion; thus, the extremity should not be elevated above heart level. Similarly, the application of cold compresses may result in vasoconstriction and exacerbate compartment syndrome. It may also be necessary to remove or loosen the bandage and bivalve or split the cast in half. A reduction in traction weight may also decrease external circumferential pressures.

Surgical decompression (e.g., fasciotomy) of the involved compartment may be necessary (Figure 65-15). The fasciotomy site is left open for several days to ensure adequate soft tissue

FIGURE 65-15 Fasciotomy associated with compartment syndrome. Stabilization of fracture with external fixator. Source: Browner, B. D., Jupiter, J. B., Levine, A. M., et al. (2009). *Skeletal trauma: Fractures, dislocations, ligamentous injuries.* (4th ed.). Philadelphia: Saunders.

decompression. Infection resulting from delayed wound closure is a potential problem following a fasciotomy. In severe cases of compartment syndrome, an amputation may be required.

Venous Thrombo-Embolism

The veins of the lower extremities and the pelvis are highly susceptible to thrombus formation after fracture, especially a hip fracture. Venous thrombo-embolism may also occur after total hip or total knee replacement surgery (Welle, 2012). In patients with limited mobility, venous stasis is aggravated by inactivity of the muscles that normally assist in the pumping action of venous blood returning to the extremities.

Because of the high risk for venous thrombo-embolism in the orthopaedic surgical patient, prophylactic anticoagulant drugs such as warfarin, low–molecular weight heparin (LMWH) (e.g., enoxaparin [Lovenox]), or fondaparinux (Arixtra) or rivaroxaban (Xarelto) may be ordered. In addition to wearing compression gradient stockings (antiembolism hose) and using sequential compression devices, the patient should be instructed to move (dorsiflex and plantar flex) the fingers or toes of the affected extremity against resistance and to perform ROM exercises on the unaffected lower extremities. (Assessment and management of venous thrombo-embolism are discussed in Chapter 40.)

Fat Embolism Syndrome

Fat embolism syndrome (FES) is characterized by the presence of systemic fat globules from fractures that are distributed into tissues and organs after a traumatic skeletal injury. FES is fatal in 5% to 15% of patients (Carlson & Pfadt, 2011). The fractures that most often cause FES are those of the long bones, ribs, and pelvis. FES has also been known to occur following total joint replacement, spinal fusion, liposuction, crush injuries, and bone marrow transplantation. Two theories about fat embolism exist. The mechanical theory is that fat is released from the marrow of injured bone and enters the systemic circulation, where the fat embolizes to other organs such as the brain (Tzioupis & Giannoudis, 2011). Microvascular lodging of droplets produces local ischemia and inflammation. The biochemical theory is that hormonal changes caused by trauma or sepsis stimulate the systemic release of free fatty acids such as chylomicrons, which form the fat emboli.

Clinical Manifestations. Early recognition of FES is crucial in preventing a potentially lethal course. Most patients manifest symptoms within 24 to 48 hours after injury. Severe forms have occurred within hours of injury. The fat emboli in the lungs cause a hemorrhagic interstitial pneumonitis that produces signs and symptoms of acute respiratory distress syndrome (ARDS), such as chest pain, tachypnea, cyanosis, dyspnea, apprehension, tachycardia, and decreased partial pressure of arterial oxygen (PaO_2). All of these symptoms are caused by poor oxygen exchange. Because they are frequently the first symptoms to manifest, changes in the mental status as a result of hypoxemia are important to recognize. Memory loss, restlessness, confusion, elevated temperature, and headache prompt further investigation so that central nervous system involvement is not mistaken for alcohol withdrawal or acute head injury. The continued change in level of consciousness and petechiae located around the neck, anterior chest wall, axilla, buccal membrane, and eye conjunctiva help distinguish fat emboli from other problems. Petechiae result from intravascular thromboses caused by decreased oxygenation.

The clinical course of a fat embolus may be rapid and acute. Frequently, the patient expresses a feeling of impending disaster. In a short time, skin colour changes from pallid to cyanotic, and the patient may become comatose. No specific laboratory examinations are available to aid in the diagnosis (Tzioupis & Giannoudis, 2011). However, certain diagnostic abnormalities may be present. These include fat cells in the blood, urine, or sputum; a decrease of the PaO_2 to less than 60 mm Hg; ST-segment changes on the electrocardiogram; a decrease in the platelet count and hematocrit levels; and a prolonged prothrombin time resulting from hemorrhaging into the lungs. A chest radiograph may reveal areas of pulmonary infiltrate or multiple areas of consolidation. This appearance is sometimes referred to as the "white-out effect."

Collaborative Care. Treatment for fat embolism is directed at prevention. Careful immobilization of a long bone fracture is probably the most important element in the prevention of fat embolism. Management of FES is essentially symptom related and supportive. Treatment includes fluid resuscitation to prevent hypovolemic shock, correction of acidosis, and replacement of blood loss. Coughing and deep breathing should be encouraged. The patient should be repositioned as little as possible before fracture immobilization or stabilization because of the danger of dislodging more fat droplets into the general circulation.

Use of corticosteroids to prevent or treat fat embolism is controversial. Oxygen is administered to treat hypoxia. Intubation or intermittent positive-pressure breathing may be considered if a satisfactory PaO_2 cannot be obtained with supplemental oxygen alone. Some patients may develop pulmonary edema, ARDS, or both, leading to an increased mortality rate. Most patients survive FES with few sequelae.

TYPES OF FRACTURES

COLLES FRACTURE

A *Colles fracture* is a fracture of the distal radius and is one of the most common fractures in adults (Figure 65-16). The styloid process of the ulna may be involved as well. Usually, the injury occurs when the patient attempts to break a fall with an outstretched hand. This type of fracture most often occurs in patients over 50 years old whose bones are osteoporotic. A younger person with a Colles fracture caused by a low-energy force should be referred for an osteoporosis evaluation.

The clinical manifestations of a Colles fracture are pain in the immediate area of injury, pronounced swelling, and dorsal displacement of the distal fragment (silver-fork deformity). This may appear as an obvious deformity on the wrist. The major complication associated with a Colles fracture is vascular insufficiency as a result of edema. CTS can be a later complication.

FIGURE 65-16 Colles fracture. Fracture of the distal radius (R) and ulnar (U) styloid from patient falling on the outstretched hand. Source: Mettler, F.A. (2005). *Essentials of radiology.* (2nd ed.). Philadelphia: Saunders.

A Colles fracture is usually managed by closed manipulation of the fracture and immobilization by either a splint or a cast or, if displaced, by external fixation. The wrist must be immobilized to prevent wrist supination and pronation. Nursing management should include frequent neuro-vascular assessments and measures to prevent or reduce edema. Support and protection of the extremity should be provided, along with encouragement of active movement of the thumb and fingers. This type of movement helps reduce edema and increases venous return. The patient should be instructed to perform active movements of the shoulder to prevent stiffness or contracture.

FRACTURE OF THE HUMERUS

Fractures involving the shaft of the humerus are a common injury among young and middle-aged adults. The most common clinical manifestations are an obvious displacement of the humerus shaft, shortened extremity, abnormal mobility, and pain. The major complications associated with fracture of the humerus are radial nerve injury and vascular injury to the brachial artery as a result of laceration, transection, or muscle spasm.

The treatment for a fracture of the humerus depends on the location and displacement of the fracture. Nonoperative treatment may include a hanging arm cast, a shoulder immobilizer, or the sling and swathe, which is a type of immobilization that prevents glenohumeral movement. The swathe encircles the trunk and the humerus as an additional binder. It is often used for surgical repairs and shoulder dislocation.

When these devices are used, the head of the bed should be elevated to assist gravity in reducing the fracture. The arm should be allowed to hang freely when the patient is sitting and standing. Nursing care should include measures to protect the axilla and prevent skin maceration by placing absorbable composite dressing pads (i.e., ABD pads) in the axilla and change them twice daily or as needed. Skin or skeletal traction may be used for purposes of reduction and immobilization.

During the rehabilitative phase, an exercise program geared toward improving strength and motion of the injured extremity is extremely important. This program should include assisted motion of the hand and fingers. The shoulder can also be exercised if the fracture is stable. This helps prevent stiffness secondary to frozen shoulder or fibrosis of the shoulder capsule.

FRACTURE OF THE PELVIS

Pelvic fractures range from benign to life-threatening, depending on the mechanism of injury and associated vascular insult. Although only a small percentage of all fractures are pelvic fractures, this type of injury is associated with the highest mortality rate. Preoccupation with more obvious injuries at the time of a traumatic event may result in an oversight of pelvic injuries.

Pelvic fractures may cause serious intra-abdominal injury, such as paralytic ileus; hemorrhage; and laceration of the urethra, the bladder, or the colon. Pelvic fractures can cause acute pelvic compartment syndrome (Ojike, Robers, & Giannoudis, 2012). Patients may survive the initial pelvic injury, only to die from sepsis, FES, or DVT complications.

Physical examination of the abdomen demonstrates local swelling, tenderness, deformity, unusual pelvic movement, and ecchymosis. The neuro-vascular status of the lower extremities and manifestations of associated injuries should be assessed. Pelvic fractures are diagnosed by radiography and computed tomographic (CT) scan (Walker, 2011).

Treatment of a pelvic fracture depends on the severity of the injury. Stable, nondisplaced fractures require limited intervention, and early mobilization is encouraged. Bed rest for stable pelvic fractures is maintained from a few days to 6 weeks. More complex fractures may be treated with pelvic sling traction, skeletal traction, external fixation, open reduction, or a combination of these methods. ORIF of a pelvic fracture may be necessary if the fracture is displaced. Extreme care in handling and moving the patient is important to prevent serious injury from a displaced fracture fragment. The patient should be turned only when ordered by the health care provider. Because a pelvic fracture can lead to damage to other organs, assessment of bowel and urinary tract function and distal neuro-vascular status are important nursing measures. Back care should be provided while the patient is raised from the bed either by independent use of the trapeze or with adequate assistance. Pelvic fractures can be extremely painful and require the appropriate assessment and management of pain to promote recovery and participation in rehabilitation.

FRACTURE OF THE HIP

Hip fractures are common in older adults and are serious injuries. There are approximately 30 000 hip fractures per year in Canada and 70% to 90% of them are caused by osteoporosis (Osteoporosis Canada, 2017). Ninety-five percent of hip fractures result from a fall (Centers for Disease Control and Prevention [CDC], 2015). Women older than 75 years are the most likely to have a fractured hip (Moja, Piatti, Pecoraro, et al., 2012). Hip fractures require one of the longest hospital stays, averaging more than 19 days. Of older adults hospitalized with hip fracture, 10% die within 1 month, 20% at 4 months, and 30% at 1 year (Moja et al., 2012).

Patients with hip fractures are "the frailest among those who are admitted to hospital, and their outcomes are likely to depend closely on how their care is managed" (Moja et al., 2012). Timely access to care is critical as longer wait times have been associated with a higher risk for mortality, especially in the older-adult population (Canadian Institute for Health information [CIHI], 2016). Wait times for hip fracture repair are improving in Canada. In 2015, 87% of patients were treated within the benchmark time of 48 hours (8% higher than in 2011) (CIHI, 2016).

A *fracture of the hip* (Figure 65-17) refers to a fracture of the proximal third of the femur, which extends up to 5 cm below

FIGURE 65-17 Femur with location of various types of fracture.

the lesser trochanter. Fractures that occur within the hip joint capsule are called *intracapsular fractures*. Intracapsular (femoral neck) fractures are further identified by a name derived from specific locations: (1) *capital* (fracture of the head of the femur), (2) *subcapital* (fractures just below the head of the femur), and (3) *transcervical* (fractures of the neck of the femur). These fractures are often associated with osteoporosis and minor trauma. *Extracapsular fractures* occur outside the joint capsule. They are termed (1) *intertrochanteric* if they occur in a region between the greater and the lesser trochanter or (2) *subtrochanteric* if they occur in the region below the lesser trochanter. Extracapsular fractures are usually caused by severe direct trauma or a fall.

Clinical Manifestations

The clinical manifestations of hip fractures are external rotation, muscle spasm, shortening of the affected extremity, and severe pain and tenderness in the region of the fracture site. Displaced femoral neck fractures cause serious disruption of the blood supply to the femoral head, which can result in AVN of the femoral head.

Collaborative Care

Initially, the affected extremity may be temporarily immobilized by Buck traction (see Figure 65-9) until the patient's physical condition is stabilized and surgery can be performed. Buck traction relieves painful muscle spasms and is used for up to 24 to 48 hours.

Surgical treatment of hip fractures permits early mobilization and decreases the risk for major complications. The type of surgery depends on the location and severity of the fracture and the person's age. Surgical options include (1) repair with internal fixation devices (e.g., hip compression screw, intramedullary devices) (Figure 65-18), (2) replacement of part of the femur with a prosthesis (partial hip replacement) (see Figure 65-18), and (3) total hip replacement (involves both the femur and acetabulum) (see Figures 65-18 and 65-19).

NURSING MANAGEMENT
HIP FRACTURE

NURSING IMPLEMENTATION

PREOPERATIVE MANAGEMENT. The majority of people with hip fractures are older adults. When planning treatment of the hip fracture, consider the patient's chronic health problems (e.g., diabetes mellitus, cardiac disease, and pulmonary disease). Surgery

Hip compression screw   Partial hip replacement   Total hip replacement

FIGURE 65-18 Types of surgical repair for a hip fracture.

FIGURE 65-19 Total hip replacement (arthroplasty) with a cementless femoral prosthesis of metal alloy with a plastic acetabular socket.

may be delayed for a brief time until the patient's general health is stabilized (Hung, Egol, Zuckerman, et al., 2012).

Before surgery, severe muscle spasms may increase pain. Appropriate analgesics or muscle relaxants, comfortable positioning (unless contraindicated), and properly adjusted traction (if used) can help in managing the spasms.

Often, teaching is done in the emergency department because quick surgical intervention is the standard of care today. Many patients will not have an overnight preoperative period in which to receive instructions, or the patient may not have the cognitive abilities to retain this important patient education.

When possible, the patient can be taught the method and frequency for exercising the unaffected leg and both arms. The patient should also be encouraged to use the overhead trapeze bar and the opposite side rail to assist in changing positions. A physiotherapist can begin to teach out-of-bed and chair transfers. The family or caregiver must also be informed about the patient's weight-bearing status after surgery. Plans for discharge begin as the patient enters the hospital because the length of stay postoperatively will be only a few days.

POSTOPERATIVE MANAGEMENT. The initial postoperative management of a patient following ORIF of a hip fracture is similar to that for any older-adult patient undergoing surgery.

TABLE 65-11	PATIENT & CAREGIVER TEACHING GUIDE

Femoral Head Prosthesis*

The following information should be included when teaching the patient and caregiver about a femoral head prosthesis.

Do

- Use an elevated toilet seat.
- Place chair inside shower or tub and remain seated while washing.
- Use pillow between legs for first 8 wk after surgery when lying on the side recommended by surgeon or when supine.
- Keep hip in neutral, straight position when sitting, walking, or lying.
- Notify surgeon if severe pain, deformity, or loss of function occurs.
- Inform dentist of presence of prosthesis before dental work so that prophylactic antibiotics can be given if indicated.

Do Not

- Force hip into greater than 90 degrees of flexion (e.g., sitting in low chairs or on low toilet seats).
- Force hip into adduction.
- Force hip into internal rotation.
- Cross legs at knees.
- Put on own shoes or stockings without adaptive device (e.g., long-handled shoehorn or stocking-helper) until 8 wk after surgery.
- Sit on chairs without arms. They are needed to aid rising to a standing position.

*For patients having surgery by a posterior approach.

The nurse must monitor vital signs, intake, and output; supervise respiratory activities, such as deep breathing and coughing; administer pain medication; and observe the dressing and incision for signs of bleeding and infection. Care for the patient undergoing orthopaedic surgery is presented in Nursing Care Plan 65-2, available on the Evolve website.

In the early postoperative period, there is a potential for neuro-vascular impairment. The nurse assesses the patient's extremity for (1) colour, (2) temperature, (3) capillary refill, (4) distal pulses, (5) edema, (6) sensation, (7) motor function, and (8) pain. Edema is alleviated by elevation of the leg whenever the patient is in a chair. The pain resulting from poor alignment of the affected extremity can be reduced by keeping pillows (or an abductor splint) between the patient's knees when turning to either side.

If the hip fracture has been treated by insertion of a femoral head prosthesis with a *posterior approach* (accessing the hip joint from the back), measures to prevent dislocation must always be used (Table 65-11). Avoid extremes in flexion initially after prosthetic replacement from a posterior approach. The patient and the caregiver must be fully aware of positions and activities that predispose the patient to dislocation (more than 90 degrees of flexion, adduction across the midline [crossing of legs and ankles], internal rotation). Many daily activities may reproduce these positions, including putting on shoes and socks; crossing the legs or feet while seated; assuming the side-lying position incorrectly; standing up or sitting down while the body is flexed more than 90 degrees relative to the chair; and sitting on low seats, especially low toilet seats. The patient should be taught to avoid these activities until the soft tissue capsule surrounding the hip has healed sufficiently to stabilize the prosthesis (usually for at least 6 weeks).

Elevated toilet seats and chair alterations (e.g., raising the seat with pillows, maintaining a straight back) are necessary. Towel rolls (i.e., trochanter rolls) or pillows placed on the lateral side of

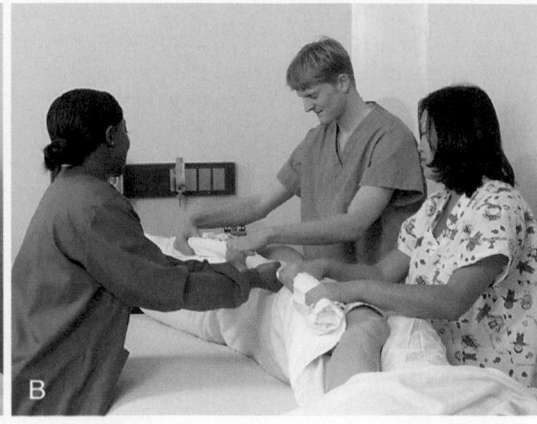

FIGURE 65-20 Log rolling a patient. Source: Perry, A. G., Potter, P. A., & Ostendorf, W. R. (2016). *Nursing interventions and clinical skills.* (6th ed., p. 418). St. Louis: Elsevier.

the leg are also used to prevent external rotation. If a foam abduction pillow is used, it should be placed between the legs to prevent dislocation of the new joint (see Figure 65-20). The nurse should ensure that the top straps are above the knee to avoid placing pressure on the peroneal nerve at the lateral tibial tubercle.

In addition to teaching the patient and caregiver how to prevent prosthesis dislocation, the nurse should also (1) place an abductor pillow or several pillows between the patient's legs when turning and (2) avoid turning the patient on the affected side until this has been approved by the surgeon. Also, some health care providers prefer that the patient keep the leg abductor pillow on except when bathing.

Taking a tub bath and driving a car are not allowed for 4 to 6 weeks. An occupational therapist may teach the patient to use assistive devices, such as reachers or grabbers, to avoid bending over to pick something off the floor; long-handled shoehorns; or sock assists. The knees must be kept apart. Instruct the patient to never cross the legs or twist to reach behind.

When the hip fracture is accessed during surgery with an *anterior* or *anterolateral approach* (joint reached from front of body), the hip muscles are left intact. This approach generally results in a more stable hip in the postoperative period, with a lower rate of complications (e.g., infection, dislocation) (Ferguson & Eastman, 2011). Precautions for the patient related to motion and weight bearing are few and may include instructions to avoid hyperextension.

Usually, the physiotherapist supervises exercises for the affected extremity and ambulation when the surgeon permits it. The patient is usually out of bed on the first postoperative day. In collaboration with the physiotherapist, the nurse monitors the patient's ambulation status for proper use of crutches or a walker. For the patient to be discharged home, the nurse should have the patient demonstrate the proper use of crutches or a walker, the ability to transfer into and from a chair and bed, and the ability to ascend and descend stairs.

Weight bearing on the involved extremity varies. Weight bearing of especially fragile fractures may be restricted until radiological examination indicates adequate healing, usually 6 to 12 weeks.

Complications associated with femoral neck fracture include nonunion, AVN, dislocation, and degenerative arthritis. As a result of an intertrochanteric fracture, the affected leg may be shortened. A cane or built-up shoe may be required for safe ambulation.

Sudden, severe pain; a lump in the buttock; limb shortening; and external rotation indicate prosthesis dislocation. Dislocation requires a closed reduction with conscious sedation or open reduction to realign the femoral head in the acetabulum. If it occurs (regardless of the setting), the patient should be kept on nothing-by-mouth status in anticipation of a possible surgical intervention.

The nurse assists both the patient and caregiver in adjusting to the restrictions and dependence imposed by the hip fracture. Anxiety and depression can easily occur, but creative nursing care and awareness of potential problems can help to prevent them. The nurse should inform the patient and caregiver about community referral services that can assist in the postdischarge rehabilitation phase.

AMBULATORY AND HOME CARE. Hospitalization averages 3 or 4 days. Patients frequently require care in a subacute unit, at a skilled nursing facility, or in a rehabilitation facility for a few weeks before returning home. Regular follow-up care should be arranged for after discharge, including home health nursing.

Home care considerations include ongoing assessment of pain management, monitoring for infection, and prevention of DVT. The incision may be closed with metal staples, which are removed at the surgeon's office. If warfarin is used to decrease the high risk for thrombo-embolism, prothrombin times are determined weekly and anticoagulation adjusted accordingly. Alternatives to warfarin include enoxaparin (Lovenox), fondaparinux (Arixtra), and rivaroxaban (Xarelto). These newer anticoagulants require less monitoring than warfarin does. The patient is who is receiving an anticoagulant should be taught to immediately report signs of bleeding to the health care provider.

Exercises designed to restore strength and muscle tone in the quadriceps and muscles of the hip area are essential to improve function and ROM. These exercises include quadriceps setting (e.g., tightening the kneecap), gluteal muscle setting (e.g., tightening the buttocks), leg raises in supine and prone positions, and abduction exercises from the supine and standing positions (e.g., swinging the leg out but never crossing midline). The patient continues these exercises for many months after discharge. It is important to teach the exercise program to the caregiver who will be encouraging the patient at home.

A physiotherapist assesses ROM, ambulation, and compliance with the exercise regimen. The patient gradually increases the number of repetitions of exercises, adds weights to ankles, may swim, and may eventually use a stationary bicycle to tone quadriceps and improve cardiovascular fitness. High-impact exercises and sports, such as jogging and tennis, may loosen the implant and should be avoided.

EVALUATION

The following are expected outcomes for the patient with a fracture of the hip:

- Report satisfactory pain relief
- Participate in exercise therapy
- Understand prescribed treatment plan

AGE-RELATED CONSIDERATIONS

HIP FRACTURE

Factors that increase the risk for a hip fracture in older adults include a tendency to fall, inability to correct a postural imbalance, inadequacy of local tissue shock absorbers (e.g., fat, muscle bulk), and reduced skeletal strength. Factors that increase the older adult's risk of falling include gait and balance problems, decreased vision and hearing, slowed reflexes, orthostatic hypotension, and medication use. Leading hazards of falls in the home include "throw rugs and loose, worn or deep pile carpets; electrical cords in walkways; raised door sills; cluttered floors; poor lighting; slippery floors; poorly designed tubs, toilets and fixtures in the bathroom; no aids or poorly installed aids such as grab bars or hand rails; and pets that get under foot" (Public Health Agency of Canada [PHAC], 2014).

Many falls are associated with getting in or out of a chair or bed. Falls to the side, the most common type seen in frail older adults, are more likely to result in a hip fracture than a forward fall (CDC, 2015). External hip protectors may help prevent hip fractures in the frail older-adult patient (Juby, 2009). Older-adult women often have osteoporosis and accompanying low bone density, which increases their risk for hip and other types of fractures.

Calcium and vitamin D supplementation, estrogen replacement, and bisphosphonate drug therapy decrease bone loss or increase bone density and thus reduce the likelihood of fracture, especially in patients with osteoporosis. (Osteoporosis is discussed in Chapter 66.) Nurses must be vigilant in planning interventions for the older adult that are known to reduce the incidence of falls and hip fractures (Registered Nurses' Association of Ontario [RNAO], 2005, rev. 2011).

FEMORAL SHAFT FRACTURE

Femoral shaft fracture occurs with a severe direct force because the femur can bend slightly before an actual fracture occurs. Young adults have a higher incidence of this type of fracture. The force exerted to cause the fracture, such as from a motor vehicle accident or gunshot wound, frequently damages the adjacent soft tissue structures. These injuries may be more serious than the bone injury.

Displacement of the fracture fragments often results in open fracture and increased soft tissue damage. This injury can lead to considerable blood loss (1 to 1.5 L). The most common types of femoral shaft fracture include transverse, spiral, comminuted, oblique, and open (see Figures 65-6 and 65-7).

The clinical manifestations of a femoral shaft fracture are usually obvious. They include marked deformity and angulation, shortening of the extremity, inability to move either the hip or

the knee, and pain. The common complications associated with fracture of the femoral shaft include fat embolism; nerve and vascular injury; and problems associated with bone union, open fracture, and soft tissue damage.

Initial management of a femoral shaft fracture is directed toward stabilization of the patient and immobilization of the fracture. Traction may be used as a temporary measure before surgical treatment or in patients unable to undergo surgery. The method of treatment most often used for a femoral shaft fracture is *intramedullary nailing* (Faucett, Collinge, & Koval, 2012). A metal rod is placed into the marrow canal of the femur. The rod passes across the fracture to keep it in position. Internal fixation is preferred because it reduces the hospital stay and the complications associated with prolonged bed rest.

In the postoperative period, the patient should be taught to carefully follow the health care provider's instructions for weight bearing. Promotion and maintenance of strength in the affected extremity usually include gluteal and quadriceps isometric exercises. The nurse should ensure that the patient performs ROM and strengthening exercises for all uninvolved extremities in preparation for ambulation. The patient may be allowed to begin non–weight-bearing activities with an ambulatory assistive device (e.g., walker, crutches). Full weight bearing is usually restricted until there is radiological evidence of union of the fracture fragments.

FRACTURE OF THE TIBIA

Although the tibia is vulnerable to injury because it lacks anterior muscle covering, strong force is required to produce a fractured tibia. As a result, soft tissue damage, devascularization, and open fracture are frequent. The tibia is one of the more common sites of a stress fracture. Complications associated with tibial fractures are compartment syndrome, FES, problems associated with bony union, and possible infection associated with open fracture.

The recommended management for closed tibial fracture is closed reduction followed by immobilization in a long leg cast. ORIF with intramedullary rods, plate fixation, or external fixation is indicated for complex fractures and those with extensive soft tissue damage. Locking plates (screw and plate system) are another type of surgical device. In both types of reduction, emphasis is placed on maintaining the strength of the quadriceps.

The neuro-vascular status of the affected extremity must be assessed at least every 2 hours during the first 48 hours. Patients are instructed to perform active ROM exercises with all uninvolved extremities, as well as exercises for the upper extremities, to build the strength required for crutch walking. When the health care provider has determined that the patient is ready for gait training, the patient is instructed in the principles of crutch walking. The patient may be on non–weight-bearing status for 6 to 12 weeks, depending on healing. Home nursing visits can be initiated to augment outpatient appointments and monitor the patient's progress.

STABLE VERTEBRAL FRACTURES

Stable fractures of the vertebral column are usually caused by motor vehicle accidents, falls, diving, or other athletic injuries. A *stable fracture* is one in which the fracture or the fragment is not likely to move or cause spinal cord damage. This type of injury is frequently confined to the anterior element (vertebral body) of the spinal column in the lumbar region and involves the cervical and thoracic regions less frequently. The vertebral bodies are usually protected from displacement by the intact spinal ligaments.

Most patients with spinal fractures have stable fractures and experience only brief periods of disability. However, if the ligamentous structures are significantly disrupted, dislocation of the vertebral structures may occur, resulting in instability and injury to the spinal cord *(unstable fracture)*. These injuries generally necessitate surgery. The most serious complication of vertebral fractures is fracture displacement, which can cause damage to the spinal cord (see Chapter 63). Although stable vertebral fractures are not associated with pathological spinal cord conditions, all spinal injuries should initially be considered unstable and potentially serious until diagnostic tests are done and the physician determines that the fracture is stable.

Usually, the patient complains of pain and tenderness in the affected region of the spine. Sudden loss of function below the level of the fracture indicates spinal cord impingement and paraplegia. Stable compression fractures are associated with a *kyphotic deformity* (flexion angulation of several vertebrae). This deformity may be noted during the physical examination. In patients with a stable vertebral fracture secondary to osteoporosis, several vertebral levels may be involved, as evidenced by a *dowager's hump* (abnormal curvature of the thoracic spine) or *lumbar lordosis* (extreme inward curve). The cervical spine may also be involved. Bowel and bladder dysfunction may be an indication of an interruption of the autonomic nervous system or injury to the spinal cord.

The overall goal in management of stable vertebral fractures is to keep the spine in good alignment until union has been accomplished. Many nursing interventions are aimed at assessing for the possibility of spinal cord trauma. Vital signs and bowel and bladder function should be evaluated regularly. The nurse should also monitor the motor and sensory status of the peripheral nerves distal to the injured region. Any deterioration in the patient's neuro-vascular status should be promptly reported.

Treatment includes pain medication followed by early mobilization and bracing. If hospitalized, the patient is usually placed in a standard hospital bed with firm support from the mattress. The aim is to support the spinal column, relax muscles, and prevent any potential compression on nerve roots. When turning, the patient should be taught to keep the spine straight by turning shoulders and pelvis together. Nursing assistance is necessary for the patient to learn the technique of "log rolling" (Figure 65-20). Several days after the initial injury, the physician may apply a specially constructed orthotic device (e.g., Milwaukee, Jewett, or Taylor brace), a jacket cast, or a removable corset if there is no evidence of neurological deficit.

Vertebral compression fractures (which are often caused by osteoporosis) can be treated with two outpatient procedures: vertebroplasty or kyphoplasty. *Vertebroplasty* uses radioimaging to guide the injection of bone cement into the fractured vertebral body. The cement (when hardened) serves to stabilize and prevent further vertebral compression. *Kyphoplasty* initially involves inserting a balloon into the vertebral body and then inflating it. This procedure creates a cavity that is filled with bone cement under low pressure. Kyphoplasty results in a lower leakage of bone cement when compared with vertebroplasty and helps restore the height of the vertebral body. Vertebroplasty and kyphoplasty result in improved healing, better pain relief, and decreased complications compared to conservative treatment (Asenjo & Rossel, 2012).

If the fracture is in the cervical spine, the patient may wear a hard cervical collar. Some cervical fractures are immobilized by use of a halo vest (see Chapter 63, Figure 63-9). The halo vest consists of a plastic jacket or cast fitted around the chest and attached to a halo that is held in place by skeletal pins inserted into the cranium. These devices immobilize the spine in the fracture area but allow patient mobility.

The patient is discharged after (1) regaining ambulation skills, (2) learning care of the cast or orthotic device, and (3) learning how to cope with the safety and security imposed by injury and treatment. Unstable vertebral fractures and spinal cord injuries are discussed in Chapter 63.

FACIAL FRACTURES

Any bone of the face can be fractured as a result of trauma, such as a motor vehicle accident, assault, or fall (Smith, Peek-Asa, Nesheim, et al., 2012). The primary concern after facial injury is to establish and maintain a patent airway and to provide adequate ventilation. Suctioning may be necessary. An alternative airway (tracheostomy) may be needed if a patent airway cannot be maintained.

Concurrent facial fractures and cervical spine injuries are common. All patients with facial injuries should be treated as if they have a cervical injury until proven otherwise by examination and imaging studies (e.g., CT scan, radiographs). Table 65-12 describes the clinical manifestations of common facial fractures.

Associated soft tissue injury often makes assessment of a facial injury difficult. Oral and facial examinations are performed after the patient has been stabilized and any life-threatening situations have been treated. Careful assessment is made of the ocular muscles and cranial nerve involvement (cranial nerves III, IV, and VI) (Patrice & Hatch, 2011a). Radiographs are used to determine the extent of the injury. CT scanning helps differentiate between bone and soft tissue.

Injury to the eye should be suspected when a facial injury occurs, particularly if the injury is near the orbit. If an eye-globe rupture is suspected, the examination should be stopped and a protective shield should be placed over the eye. Signs of globe rupture include the extrusion of vitreous humor or brown tissue (iris or ciliary body) on the surface of the globe or penetrating through a laceration with an eccentric or teardrop-shaped pupil.

Specific treatment depends on the site and extent of the facial fracture and the associated soft tissue injury. Immobilization or surgical stabilization may be necessary. A patent airway

TABLE 65-12	MANIFESTATIONS OF FACIAL FRACTURES
Fracture	**Clinical Manifestation**
Frontal bone	Rapid edema that may mask underlying fractures
Mandible	Tooth fractures, bleeding, limited motion of mandible
Maxilla	Segmental motion of maxilla and alveolar fracture of teeth
Nasal bone	Displacement of nasal bones, epistaxis
Periorbital bone	Possible frontal sinus involvement, entrapment of ocular muscles
Zygomatic arch	Depression of zygomatic arch and entrapment of ocular muscles

and adequate nutrition must be maintained throughout the recovery period.

The nurse needs to be sensitive about the alterations in the patient's appearance that may occur after a facial fracture. The changes may be drastic. Edema and discoloration subside with time, but concurrent soft tissue injuries may result in permanent scarring.

Mandible Fracture

A fracture of the mandible may result from trauma to the face or the jaws. Maxillary fractures may also occur, but they are less common than mandibular fractures. The fracture may be closed, with no bone displacement, or it may involve loss of tissue and bone. The fracture may require immediate and sometimes long-term treatment to ensure survival and restore satisfactory appearance and function.

A mandibular fracture may also be therapeutically performed to correct an underlying malocclusion problem that cannot be corrected by orthodontic procedures alone. The mandible is resected during surgery and manipulated forward or backward, depending on the occlusion problem.

Surgery consists of immobilization, usually by wiring the jaws (*intermaxillary fixation*). Internal fixation may be done with screws and plates. In a closed fracture with no loss of teeth, the lower jaw is wired to the upper jaw. Wires are placed around the teeth, and then cross-wires or rubber bands are used to hold the lower jaw tight against the upper jaw (Figure 65-21). Arch bars may be placed on the maxillary and mandibular arches of the teeth. Vertical wires are placed between the arch bars holding the jaws together. If teeth are missing or bone is displaced, other forms of fixation, such as metal arch bars in the mouth or insertion of a pin in the bone, may be needed. Bone grafting may also be required. Immobilization is usually necessary for only 4 to 6 weeks because the fractures often heal rapidly.

NURSING MANAGEMENT
MANDIBULAR FRACTURE

NURSING IMPLEMENTATION

PREOPERATIVE MANAGEMENT. The patient undergoing mandibular surgery should be told preoperatively about the surgical procedure, including what it involves, how the face will look, and alterations caused by the surgery. The patient must be reassured about the ability to breathe normally, speak, and swallow liquids. Usually, hospitalization is brief unless there are other injuries or problems.

FIGURE 65-21 Intermaxillary fixation. Source: Courtesy Weinstein, R. A., Denver, CO.

POSTOPERATIVE MANAGEMENT. Postoperative care should focus on a patent airway, oral hygiene, communication, pain management, and adequate nutrition. Two major potential problems in the immediate postoperative period are airway obstruction and aspiration of vomitus. Because the patient cannot open the jaws, measures to ensure an airway are essential. The nurse must observe for signs of respiratory distress (e.g., dyspnea; alterations in rate, quality, and depth of respirations). The patient should be placed on the side with the head slightly elevated immediately after surgery.

Wire cutters or scissors (for rubber bands) must be taped to the head of the bed and sent with the patient on all appointments and examinations away from the bedside. The wire cutter or scissors may be used to cut the wires or elastic bands in case of an emergency (e.g., cardiac arrest or respiratory distress) requiring access to the pharynx or lungs. Information, including a picture showing the appropriate wires to cut, should be included in the care plan. In some cases, cutting the wires may cause the entire facial and upper jaw structure to shift or collapse and worsen the problem. A tracheostomy or endotracheal tray should always be available.

If the patient begins to vomit or choke, the nurse should try to clear the mouth and airway either by (1) having the patient bend his or her head over or to the side to allow the vomitus to flow out of the mouth and nose or (2) using a suction catheter to clear the mouth and nose. When suctioning is necessary, it can be performed by the nasopharyngeal or oral route, depending on the extent of injury and the type of repair. A nasogastric tube may be used for decompression to remove fluids and gas from the stomach in an effort to help prevent aspiration. This technique also helps prevent vomiting. Antiemetic medications may also be administered.

Oral hygiene is an important part of the nursing care. The mouth should be rinsed frequently, particularly after meals and snacks, to remove food debris. Warm normal saline solution or water may be used. A soft, rubber catheter or a Water-Pik is effective for a thorough oral cleansing. The nurse should inspect the mouth several times a day to see that it is clean. A flashlight is necessary, and a tongue depressor is used to retract the cheeks. The lips and corners of the mouth as well as the buccal mucosa should be kept moist. Dental wax may be used to cover any sharp edges of the wires to prevent irritation of the buccal mucosa.

Communication may be a problem, particularly in the early postoperative period. An effective way of communicating must be established preoperatively (e.g., use of dry erase board, pad and pencil). Usually, the patient can speak well enough to be understood, especially after the first few postoperative days.

Ingestion of sufficient nutrients poses a challenge because the diet must be liquid. The patient easily tires of sucking through a straw or laboriously using a spoon. The diet must be planned to include adequate calories, protein, and fluids. Liquid protein supplements may be helpful for improving the nutritional status. The nurse works with the dietitian and the patient to ensure adequate nutrition. The low-bulk, high-carbohydrate diet and the intake of air through the straw create a problem with constipation and flatus. Ambulation, prune juice, and bulk-forming laxatives may help relieve these problems.

Usually, the patient is discharged with the wires in place. The nurse should allow the patient to verbalize feelings about the altered appearance. Discharge teaching should include oral care, techniques of handling secretions, diet, how and when to use wire cutters, and when to notify the health care provider about concerns and problems.

AMPUTATION

Major advances in surgical amputation techniques, prosthetic design, and rehabilitation programs are enabling people with amputations to return to productive and satisfying social roles. People in the middle and older-adult age groups have the highest incidence of amputation because of the effects of peripheral vascular disease (PVD), atherosclerosis, and vascular changes related to diabetes mellitus. Amputation in the younger population is usually secondary to trauma (e.g., motor vehicle accidents, land mines, farming-related injuries).

Clinical Indications

Most amputations are performed due to PVD, especially in older-adult patients with diabetes mellitus. These patients often experience peripheral neuropathy that progresses to trophic ulcers and subsequent gangrene. Fifty percent of lower limb amputations in Ontario are related to diabetes (Canadian Association of Wound Care [CAWC], 2016). More than 4 000 individuals with diabetes had a limb amputation in 2006 (CAWC, 2016). Other common reasons for amputation are trauma and thermal injuries, tumours, osteomyelitis, and congenital limb disorders. Although pain is often present, it is not usually the primary reason for an amputation.

Diagnostic Studies

The types of diagnostic studies performed depend on the underlying problem that makes the amputation necessary (Table 65-13). Test results that show an elevated white blood cell count with abnormal differential may indicate infection. Vascular studies such as arteriography, Doppler studies, and venography provide information about the circulatory status of the extremity.

Collaborative Care

If amputation is to be considered "elective," the patient's general health is carefully assessed. Chronic illnesses and the presence of infection are important considerations. The patient and family should be helped to understand the need for the amputation and be assured that rehabilitation can result in an active, useful life. If the amputation is done on an emergency basis as a result of trauma, the management is physically and emotionally more complicated.

The goal of amputation surgery is to preserve extremity length and function while removing all infected, pathological, or ischemic tissue. (Levels of amputation of upper and lower extremities are illustrated in Figure 65-22.) The type of amputation depends on the reason for the surgery. A closed amputation is performed to create a weight-bearing *residual limb*. An anterior skin flap with dissected soft tissue padding covers the bony part of the residual limb. The skin flap is sutured posteriorly so that it will not be positioned in a weight-bearing area. Special care is necessary to prevent accumulation of drainage, which can produce pressure and harbour bacteria that may cause infection.

Disarticulation is an amputation performed through a joint. A *Syme amputation* is a form of disarticulation at the ankle. An open amputation leaves a surface on the residual limb that is not covered with skin. This type of surgery is generally indicated for control of actual or potential infection. The wound is usually closed later by a second surgical procedure or by skin traction surrounding the residual limb. This type of amputation is often called a "guillotine amputation."

NURSING MANAGEMENT
AMPUTATION

NURSING ASSESSMENT

Pre-existing illnesses must be adequately assessed because most amputations are performed as a result of vascular problems. Assessment of the vascular and neurological status is an important part of this assessment process (see Chapters 34 and 58).

TABLE 65-13 **COLLABORATIVE CARE**	
Amputation	
Diagnostic	**Collaborative Therapy**
• History and physical examination	***Medical***
• Physical appearance of soft tissues	• Appropriate management of underlying disease
• Presence of peripheral pulses	• Stabilization of patient with trauma
• Sensory function	
• Skin temperature	***Surgical***
• Arteriography	• Selective type of amputation
• Plethysmography	• Residual limb management
• Transcutaneous ultrasonic Doppler recordings	• Immediate prosthetic fitting
• Venography	• Delayed prosthetic fitting
	Rehabilitation
	• Coordination of prosthesis-fitting and gait-training activities
	• Coordination of muscle-strengthening and physiotherapy regimens

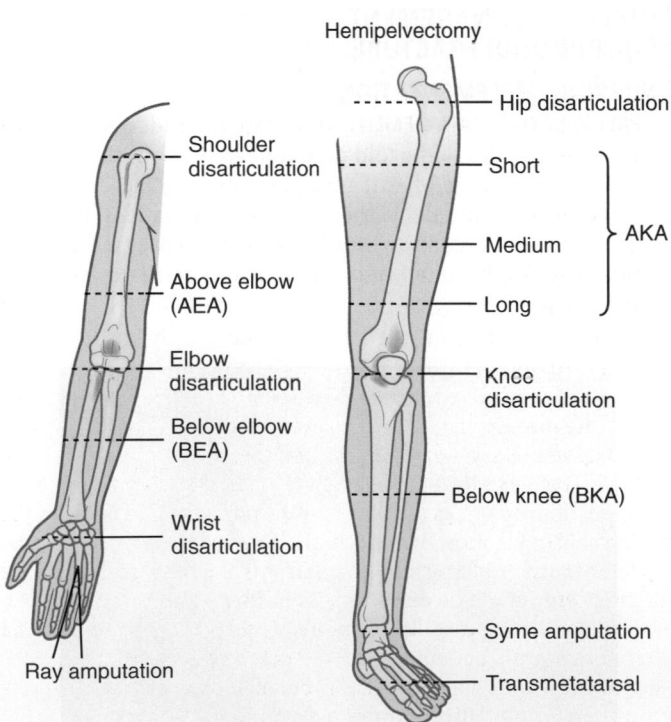

FIGURE 65-22 Location and description of amputation sites of the upper and lower extremities. *AKA*, above-the-knee amputation.

NURSING DIAGNOSES

Nursing diagnoses for the patient with an amputation may include, but are not limited to, the following:

- *Disturbed body image* related to *alteration in self-perception* (amputation, impaired mobility)
- *Impaired skin integrity* related to *pressure over bony prominence* (improperly fitted prosthesis)
- *Chronic pain* related to *emotional distress, nerve compression* (phantom limb sensation/pain)
- *Impaired physical mobility* related to *pain, physical deconditioning* (amputation of lower limb)

PLANNING

The overall goals are that the patient with an amputation will (1) have adequate relief from the underlying health problem, (2) have satisfactory pain control, (3) reach maximum rehabilitation potential with the use of a prosthesis (if indicated), (4) cope with the body image changes, and (5) make satisfying lifestyle adjustments.

NURSING IMPLEMENTATION

HEALTH PROMOTION. Control of causative illnesses such as PVD, diabetes mellitus, chronic osteomyelitis, and pressure injuries can eliminate or delay the need for amputation. Patients with these problems should be taught to carefully examine their lower extremities daily for signs of potential problems. If the patient cannot assume this responsibility, a caregiver should be instructed in the procedure. Patients and their caregiver should be instructed to report problems such as a change in skin colour or temperature, decrease or absence of sensation, tingling, pain, or the presence of a lesion to the health care provider.

Instruction in proper safety precautions in recreation and in the performance of hazardous work is an important nursing responsibility, especially for occupational health nurses.

ACUTE INTERVENTION. The nurse must recognize the tremendous psychological and social implications of an amputation for the patient. The disruption in body image caused by an amputation often causes a patient to go through psychological stages similar to the grieving process (see Chapter 13). Allowing the patient to go through a grieving process or period of depression and recognizing it as a normal consequence may do much to aid the patient's acceptance of the amputation. The patient's family must also be helped to work through the process to arrive at a realistic and positive attitude about the future. The reasons for an amputation and the rehabilitation potential depend on age, diagnosis, occupation, personality, resources, and support systems.

Preoperative Management. Before surgery, the nurse should reinforce information that the patient and family have received about the reasons for the amputation, the proposed prosthesis, and the mobility training program. To meet the patient's educational needs, the nurse must know the level of amputation, the type of postsurgical dressing to be applied, and the type of prosthesis to be utilized. The patient should receive instruction in the performance of upper extremity exercises such as push-ups in bed or the wheelchair to promote arm strength. This instruction is essential for later crutch walking and gait training. General postoperative nursing care should be discussed, including positioning, support, and residual limb care. If a compression bandage is to be used after surgery, the patient should be instructed about its purpose and how it will be applied. If an immediate prosthesis is planned, the general ambulation program should be discussed.

The patient should be warned that she or he may feel as though the amputated limb is still present after surgery. This phenomenon is termed **phantom limb sensation** (any sensation of the missing limb except pain). Different sources have reported the incidence of phantom limb sensation as anywhere between 60% and 100% of individuals with amputations (Jerath, Crawford, & Jenson, 2015). This sensation can cause patients grave concern unless they are forewarned. It can take various forms, such as the feeling that someone is touching the missing limb, pressure on the missing limb, cold, wetness, itching, tickle, or fatigue (Magee, 2013). Recent studies suggest that 60% to 80% of people with amputations may also experience *phantom limb pain* (any painful sensations that are referred to the absent limb), which often begins immediately after surgery. The pain can be described as shooting, burning, crushing, or severe and agonizing (Chapman, 2011). It is more common for the pain to be intermittent, with short episodes (seconds to minutes) of severe pain occurring several times a day. There is some evidence that the pain present preoperatively may be mimicked in the phantom limb. Often, the patient may be extremely anxious about this pain because the patient knows the limb is gone but still feels pain in it. As recovery and ambulation progress, phantom limb sensation and pain usually subside, although the pain may become chronic.

Postoperative Management. General postoperative care for the patient who has had an amputation depends largely on the patient's general state of health, the reason for the amputation, and the patient's age. Individuals who undergo amputation as a result of a traumatic injury need to be monitored for post-traumatic stress disorder because they had no time to prepare or perhaps even participate in the decision to have a limb amputated.

Prevention and detection of complications are important nursing responsibilities during the postoperative period. Careful monitoring of the patient's vital signs and dressing can alert the nurse to hemorrhage in the operative area. Careful attention to sterile technique during dressing changes reduces the potential for wound infection.

If an *immediate* postoperative prosthesis has been applied, the nurse must monitor vital signs carefully because the surgical site is heavily covered and may not be visible. A surgical tourniquet must always be available for emergency use. If excessive bleeding occurs, the surgeon should be notified immediately.

The *delayed* prosthetic fitting may be the best choice for patients who have had amputations above the knee or below the elbow, older adults, individuals who are debilitated, and those with infection. The appropriate time for use of a prosthesis depends on satisfactory healing of the residual limb as well as on the general condition of the patient. A temporary prosthesis may be used for partial weight bearing once the sutures are removed. Barring any problems, patients can bear full weight on permanent prostheses by approximately 3 months after their amputation.

Not all patients are candidates for a prosthesis. People who are seriously ill or debilitated may not have the upper body strength and energy required to use a lower extremity prosthesis. Mobility with a wheelchair may be the most realistic goal for patients who are not candidates for prostheses.

Often, patients may be extremely anxious about phantom limb sensation because they still perceive pain in the missing portion of the limb. As recovery and ambulation progress, phantom limb sensation and pain usually subside, although the pain may become chronic. The patient may also complain of shooting, burning, or crushing pain and feelings of coldness, heaviness, and cramping,

Mirror therapy reduces phantom limb sensation and pain in some patients (Rothgangel, Brau, Beurskens, et al., 2011)

FIGURE 65-23 A physiotherapist demonstrates mirror therapy, a type of treatment that may reduce phantom limb sensation and pain. Source: U.S. Navy photo courtesy Mass Communication Specialist Seaman Joseph A. Boomhower.

(Figure 65-23). The mirror is thought to provide visual information to the brain, replacing the sensory feedback expected from the missing limb. However, it is unknown why looking in the mirror at the unaffected limb would decrease phantom limb sensation and pain. Mirror therapy may also improve patient functioning after a stroke.

Success of the rehabilitative program depends on the physical and emotional health of the patient. Chronic illness and deconditioning complicate aggressive rehabilitation efforts. Both physiotherapy and occupational therapy must be an integral component of the patient's overall plan of care.

Flexion contractures may delay the rehabilitation process. The most common and debilitating contracture is hip flexion. Hip adduction contracture is rare. Patients should avoid sitting in a chair for more than 1 hour with hips flexed, or having pillows under the surgical extremity, to prevent flexion contractures. Unless specifically contraindicated, patients should lie on their abdomen for 30 minutes, three to four times each day, and position the hip in extension while prone.

Proper residual limb bandaging fosters shaping and moulding for eventual prosthesis fitting (Figure 65-24). The physician usually orders a compression bandage to be applied immediately after surgery to support the soft tissues, reduce edema, hasten healing, minimize pain, and promote residual limb shrinkage and maturation. This bandage may be an elastic roll applied to the residual limb or a residual limb shrinker, which is an elastic stocking that fits tightly over the residual limb and lower trunk area.

The compression bandage is initially worn at all times except during physiotherapy and bathing. The bandage is taken off and reapplied several times daily, and care is taken so that it is applied snugly but not so tightly as to interfere with circulation. Shrinker bandages should be washed and changed daily. After healing has occurred, the residual limb is bandaged only when the patient is not wearing the prosthesis. The patient should be instructed to avoid dangling the residual limb over the bedside to minimize edema formation.

As the patient's overall condition improves, an exercise regimen is normally started under the supervision of the health care provider and the physiotherapist. Active ROM exercises of all joints should be started as soon after surgery as the patient's

FIGURE 65-24 Bandaging for the above-the-knee amputation residual limb. Figure-of-eight style covers progressive areas of the residual limb. Two elastic wraps are required.

pain level and medical status permit. In preparation for mobility, the patient should increase triceps and shoulder strength and lower limb support and learn balance of the altered body. The loss of the weight of a limb necessitates adaptation of the patient's proprioceptive and coordination mechanisms to prevent falls and injury.

Crutch walking is started as soon as patients are physically able. After an immediate postsurgical fitting, orders related to weight bearing must be carefully followed to avoid injury to the skin flap and delay of the healing process. Before discharge, the patient and caregiver need careful instruction related to residual limb care, ambulation, prevention of contractures, recognition of complications, exercise, and follow-up care. Table 65-14 outlines patient and caregiver teaching following an amputation.

AMBULATORY AND HOME CARE. When healing has occurred satisfactorily and the residual limb is well moulded, the patient is ready for fitting of a prosthesis. A prosthetist initially makes a mould of the residual limb and measures landmarks for fabrication of the prosthesis. The moulded limb socket allows the residual limb to fit snugly into the prosthesis. The limb is covered with a stocking to ensure good fit and prevent skin breakdown. The limb may continue to shrink, causing a loose fit, in which case a new socket has to be fabricated. The patient may need to have the prosthesis adjusted to prevent rubbing and friction between the residual limb and the socket. Excessive movement of a loose prosthesis can cause severe skin irritation and breakdown.

Artificial limbs become an integral part of the patient's body image. Proper care ensures their long life and useful functioning. The patient should be instructed to clean the prosthesis socket daily with a mild soap and rinse thoroughly to remove irritants.

TABLE 65-14   PATIENT & CAREGIVER TEACHING GUIDE

Following an Amputation

After an amputation, patient and caregiver teaching should include the following information.

- Inspect the residual limb daily for signs of skin irritation, especially erythema, excoriation, and odour. Pay particular attention to areas prone to pressure.
- Discontinue use of the prosthesis if an irritation develops. Have the area checked before resuming use of the prosthesis.
- Wash residual limb thoroughly each night with warm water and a bacteriostatic soap. Rinse thoroughly and dry gently. Expose the residual limb to air for 20 min.
- Do not use any substance such as lotions, alcohol, powders, or oil on the residual limb unless prescribed by the health care provider.
- Wear only a residual limb sock that is in good condition and supplied by the prosthetist.
- Change residual limb sock daily. Launder in a mild soap, squeeze, and lay flat to dry.
- Use prescribed pain management techniques.
- Perform ROM to all joints daily. Perform general strengthening exercises, including the upper extremities, daily.
- Do not elevate the residual limb on a pillow.
- Lay prone with hip in extension for 30 min., three to four times daily.

ROM, range of motion.

The leather and metal parts of the prosthesis should not get wet. The patient should be encouraged to have regular maintenance of the prosthesis. Consideration of the condition of the shoe is also necessary. A badly worn shoe alters the gait and may cause damage to the prosthesis.

SPECIAL CONSIDERATIONS IN UPPER-LIMB AMPUTATION. The emotional implications of an upper limb amputation are often more devastating than those for lower limb amputation. The enforced dependency brought about by one-handedness may be both frustrating and humiliating to the patient. Because most upper extremity amputations result from trauma, often, the patient has not had the opportunity to adjust psychologically to an amputation or to participate in the decision-making process about amputation.

Both immediate and delayed prosthetic fittings are possible for the person with a below-the-elbow amputation. Prosthetic fitting is delayed for the person with an above-the-elbow amputation. The usual functional prosthesis is the arm and hook. A cosmetic hand is available but has limited functional value. As with the lower limb prosthesis, patient motivation and endurance are major factors contributing to a satisfactory outcome. Technological advances to improve the functionality of upper limb prostheses are an active area of research (Velez & Dellefield, 2011). Many companies are also experimenting with 3D printing to make less expensive prosthetic limbs that also take less time to develop and produce.

EVALUATION

The following are expected outcomes for the patient with an amputation:

- Accept changed body image and integrate changes into his or her lifestyle
- Have no evidence of skin breakdown
- Have reduction or absence of pain
- Become mobile within limitations imposed by amputation

AGE-RELATED CONSIDERATIONS

AMPUTATION

If a lower limb amputation has been performed on an older adult, the patient's previous ability to ambulate may affect the extent of recovery. Use of a prosthesis requires a significant amount of energy for ambulation. Walking with a below-the-knee prosthesis requires 40% additional energy, and an above-the-knee prosthesis requires 60% more energy than walking on two legs. Older adults whose general health is weakened by disorders such as cardiac or pulmonary problems may not be candidates for prosthesis use. These patients' ability to ambulate will be limited. If possible, this should be discussed with patients and their families before surgery so that realistic expectations can be set.

COMMON JOINT SURGICAL PROCEDURES

Surgery plays an important role in the treatment and rehabilitation of patients with various forms of joint disease. Surgery is aimed at relieving chronic pain, improving joint motion, correcting deformity and malalignment, and removing intra-articular erosion. Joint replacement surgery is the most common orthopaedic operation performed on older adults. If decreased functional ability of the joint is not corrected, contractures with permanent limitation of motion often occurs. Limitation of motion at the joint can be demonstrated on physical examination and by joint-space narrowing on radiological examination.

Indications for hip or knee arthroplasty include arthritis, connective tissue disease, failed prior procedures, sepsis, tumours, Paget's disease, congenital hip dysplasia, severe varus or valgus deformity, and spondyloarthropathies.

TYPES OF JOINT SURGERIES

Synovectomy

Synovectomy (removal of synovial membrane) is used as a prophylactic measure and as a palliative treatment of RA. Removal of the synovial membrane, thought to be the location of the basic pathological changes in joint destruction, helps prevent further progression of joint damage. A synovectomy is best performed early in the disease process to prevent serious destruction of joint surfaces. Removal of the thickened synovium prevents extension of the inflammatory process into the adjacent cartilage, ligaments, and tendons.

It is impossible to surgically remove all the synovium in a joint. The underlying disease process is still present and will again affect the regenerating synovium. However, the disease appears to be milder after synovectomy, and definite improvement in pain, weight bearing, and ROM can be expected. Common sites for this surgery include the elbow, wrist, and fingers. Synovectomy in the knee is done less frequently because knee joint replacement techniques are usually performed.

Osteotomy

An osteotomy is performed by removing or adding a wedge or slice of bone to change alignment (joint and vertebral) and to shift weight bearing, thereby correcting deformity and relieving pain. Cervical osteotomy may be used to correct deformity in some patients with ankylosing spondylitis. Halo and body jackets are worn until fusion occurs (at 3–4 months). Subtrochanteric or femoral osteotomy may provide some relief of pain and improve motion in selected patients with hip osteoarthritis (OA).

Osteotomy has proved ineffective in patients with inflammatory joint disease. Osteotomy of the knee (tibia) provides relief of pain in selected patients, but advanced joint destruction is usually corrected by joint replacement surgery.

The postoperative care for osteotomy is similar to the treatment of an internal fixation of a fracture at a comparable site (see pp. 1644–1648). Internal wires, screws and plates, bone grafts, or an external fixator usually fix the bone in place.

Debridement

Debridement is the removal of degenerative debris such as loose bodies, osteophytes, joint debris, and degenerated menisci from a joint. This procedure is usually performed on the knee or the shoulder, using a fibreoptic arthroscope. Usually, the procedure is done on an outpatient basis. A compression dressing is applied postoperatively. Weight bearing is permitted following knee arthroscopy. Patient education includes monitoring for signs of infection, managing pain, and restricting excessive activity for 24 to 48 hours.

Arthroplasty

Arthroplasty is the reconstruction or replacement of a joint to relieve pain, improve or maintain ROM, and correct deformity. There were 49 503 hip and 60 136 knee replacements in Canada for 2013–2014 (a 19.1% increase in hip replacements and a 22.9% increase in knee replacements since 2009–2010) (CIHI, 2015).

Reducing wait times for hip and knee replacement surgeries is a top health care priority in Canada. All provinces are now collecting and reporting wait time data for joint replacements through the Canadian Joint Replacement Registry (CIHI, 2016). In 2015, at least three out of four patients received their hip and knee replacement surgery within the benchmark time frame (182 days or 26 weeks). The median wait time in Canada for a knee replacement was 104 days and for hip replacement, 86 days, compared to 157 and 121 days, respectively, using international comparative data. Wait times across Canada for hip and knee replacements were stable from 2011 to 2015, but wait times varied considerably among provinces and territories (CIHI, 2016).

The most common uses of arthroplasty are for patients with OA, RA, AVN, congenital deformities or dislocations, and other systemic problems. There are several types of arthroplasty, including surgical reshaping of the bones of the joints, replacement of part of a joint *(hemiarthroplasty),* and total joint replacement. Replacement arthroplasty is available for elbow, shoulder, phalangeal joints of the fingers, wrist, hip, knee, ankle, and foot.

Minimally invasive surgery is available in many centres in Canada for hip and knee replacements. Minimally invasive surgery involves less dissection and smaller incisions (5 to 10 cm in the hip and 10 to 12.7 cm in the knee) and a shorter hospital stay. It is technically demanding and requires extra training for the surgeon. There is an initial quicker recovery with less rehabilitation and a quicker return to ADLs for the patient. Minimally invasive surgery also results in less blood loss and less need for transfusions.

Hip Arthroplasty. Total hip arthroplasty (THA) provides significant relief of pain and improvement of function for patients with OA, RA, and other conditions. Partial and total hip replacements are also used to treat hip fractures.

In THA, the prosthesis (implant) replaces the ball and socket joint and upper shaft of the femur (see Figure 65-19). The socket can be "cemented" in place with polymethyl methacrylate, which bonds to the bone. The socket may also be inserted and not cemented ("cementless"). Cementless THAs may provide longer-term prosthesis stability by facilitating biological ingrowth of new bone tissue into the porous surface coating of the prosthesis. Although some surgeons use cementless devices for all patients, they are most often recommended for younger, more active patients and patients with good bone quality, where bone ingrowth into the components can be readily achieved.

The nursing care for a patient who has a THA is discussed in the section on nursing management of a patient with a hip fracture, on pp. 1652–1655.

Hip Resurfacing. An alternative to hip replacement is hip resurfacing, which allows the femoral head to be preserved and reshaped rather than replaced. (In contrast, in a THA, the prosthesis replaces the femoral head.) The resurfaced femoral head (ball) is then capped by a metal prosthesis. The metal appears to have a lower rate of wear, and thus the prosthesis may have a longer lifetime. Hip resurfacing is a more favourable option for younger, active patients. After surgery, there is generally a 6-month waiting period before strenuous activity, until strong muscles are built around the joint. Patients receiving a smaller femoral head (including many women) have a higher failure rate with a resurfaced implant when compared with patients receiving a THA (Smith, Dieppe, & Howard, et al., 2012).

Knee Arthroplasty. Unremitting pain and instability as a result of severe destructive deterioration of the knee joint is the main indication for total knee arthroplasty (TKA) or total knee replacement (TKR) (Bartlett, 2012). Osteoporosis may necessitate bone grafting to augment defects and to correct bone deficiencies. Either part or all of the knee joint may be replaced with a metal and plastic prosthetic device. A compression dressing is used to immobilize the knee in extension immediately after the operation. This is usually removed within 24 hours and may be replaced with a knee immobilizer such as a Zimmer immobilizer splint or posterior plastic shell, which stabilizes the knee and maintains extension during ambulation and at rest for about 4 weeks. Knee immobilizers are removed for various portions of physiotherapy. Dislocation is not typical with TKA.

After surgery, an emphasis is placed on physiotherapy. Isometric quadriceps setting begins the first day after surgery. The patient progresses to straight-leg raises and gentle ROM to increase muscle strength and obtain 90-degree knee flexion. Active flexion exercises or passive flexion exercises through the use of a continuous passive motion (CPM) machine postoperatively may promote joint mobility. Full weight bearing is begun before discharge. An active home-exercise program involves progressive ROM with muscle strengthening, and flexibility exercises. Following TKA, many older-adult patients with advanced OA have shown significant improvement in mobility, motor function tests, and ability to complete daily tasks.

Finger Joint Arthroplasty. A silicone rubber arthroplastic device is used to help restore function in the fingers of the patient with RA. Ulnar deviation is often present, which results in severe functional limitations of the hand. The goal of hand surgery is primarily to restore function related to grasp, pinch, stability, and strength rather than to correct cosmetic deformity. Before surgery, the patient is instructed in hand exercises, including flexion, extension, abduction, and adduction of the fingers.

Postoperatively, the hand is kept elevated with a bulky dressing in place. Neuro-vascular assessment is conducted postoperatively, and the nurse assesses for signs of infection. The success of the surgery depends largely on the postoperative treatment plan, which is often carried out under the direction of an occupational therapist. Once the dressing is removed, a guided splinting program is initiated. The patient is discharged with splints to use while sleeping and hand exercises to perform for 10 to 12 weeks, at least three or four times a day. The patient is also instructed to avoid lifting heavy objects.

Elbow and Shoulder Arthroplasty. Although available, total replacement of elbow and shoulder joints is not as common as other forms of arthroplasty. Shoulder replacements are used in patients with severe pain because of RA, OA, AVN, or a previous trauma. The shoulder replacement is usually considered if the patient has adequate surrounding muscle strength and bone stock. If joint replacement is necessary for both elbow and shoulder, the elbow is usually done first because a severely painful elbow interferes with the shoulder rehabilitation program.

Significant pain relief has been achieved following arthroplasty, with most patients having no pain at rest or minimal pain with activity. Functional improvements have resulted in better hygiene and increased ability to perform ADLs in most patients. Rehabilitation is longer and more difficult than with other joint surgeries.

Ankle Arthroplasty. Total ankle arthroplasty (TAA) is indicated for RA, OA, AVN, and trauma. Although the use of TAA is not widespread, it is becoming a viable alternative to fusion for the treatment of advanced ankle arthritis in selected patients. Devices available include several fixed-bearing devices and a mobile-bearing "cementless" prosthesis. This device more closely imitates natural ankle function.

Ankle fusion is often selected over arthroplasty, although TAA volume has increased dramatically over the past decade (Marx & Mizel, 2015). However, the patient is left with a stiff foot and the inability to change heel height. TAA is advantageous because it achieves a more normal gait pattern (Marx & Mizel, 2015). Postoperatively, the patient may not bear weight for 6 weeks, must elevate the extremity to reduce and prevent edema, must be extremely careful to prevent postoperative infection, and must maintain immobilization as directed by the physician.

Arthrodesis

Arthrodesis is the surgical fusion of a joint. This procedure is indicated only if articular surfaces are too severely damaged or infected to allow joint replacement or if reconstructive surgery fails. Arthrodesis relieves pain and provides a stable but immobile joint. The fusion is usually accomplished by removal of the articular hyaline cartilage and the addition of bone grafts across the joint surface. The affected joint must be immobilized until bone healing has occurred. Common areas of fusion are wrist, ankle, cervical spine, lumbar spine, and metatarsophalangeal (MTP) joint of the great toe.

Complications of Joint Surgery

Infection is a serious complication of joint surgery, particularly joint replacement surgery (Bartlett, 2012). The most common causative organisms are Gram-positive aerobic streptococci and staphylococci. Infection almost always leads to pain and loosening of the prosthesis, generally necessitating extensive surgery. Efforts to reduce the incidence of infection include the use of specially designed self-contained operating suites, operating rooms with laminar airflow, and prophylactic antibiotic administration. Current recommendations for perioperative antibiotic prophylaxis in elective joint arthroplasty include stopping therapy after 24 hours (Gutowski, Parvizi, & Purtill, 2014).

Thrombo-embolism is another potentially serious complication after joint surgeries, particularly those involving the lower extremities. Prophylactic measures such as warfarin, LMWH, and sequential compression devices of the legs are usually instituted. Patients may be followed postoperatively with venous Doppler ultrasonography to detect DVT, the source of most pulmonary emboli.

Collaborative Care

Preoperative Management. The primary goal of preoperative assessment is to identify risk factors associated with postoperative complications so that nursing strategies can be implemented to promote optimal positive outcomes. A careful history will include previous medical diagnoses and complications such as diabetes and thrombo-phlebitis, pain tolerance and management preferences, current functional status and expectations following surgery, and level of social support and home care needs after discharge. The patient should be free from evidence of infection and acute joint inflammation.

If lower extremity surgery is planned, upper extremity muscle strength and joint function are assessed to determine the type of assistive devices needed postoperatively for ambulation and ADLs. Preoperative teaching informs the patient and family of the expected hospital course and postoperative management at home. In addition, it prepares them to maximize the usefulness and longevity of the prosthesis. Patients also need to realize that recovery does not happen quickly. Both patients and their families or significant others need to speak with individuals who have had a total joint arthroplasty to better understand the reality of rehabilitation.

Postoperative Management. Postoperatively, neuro-vascular assessment is performed to assess nerve function and circulatory status. Anticoagulation therapy, analgesia, and parenteral antibiotics are administered. In general, the affected joint is exercised, and ambulation is encouraged as early as possible to prevent complications of immobility. Specific protocols vary according to patient, type of prosthesis, and surgeon preference. Pain management postoperatively may use epidural or intrathecal analgesia, femoral nerve block (knee only), patient-controlled analgesia (PCA), intravenous injections, and oral opioids or NSAIDs.

The hospital stay after arthroplasty is 3 to 5 days, depending on the patient's course and need for physiotherapy. Physiotherapy and ambulation enhance mobility, build muscle strength, and reduce the risk for thrombus formation. If the patient is taking warfarin, therapy starts on the day of surgery and continues for 3 weeks with an international normalized ratio (INR) done on a regular basis. For those taking LMWH (e.g., enoxaparin), therapy starts after surgery and continues for 2 weeks postoperatively. Daily monitoring of the patient's coagulation status is not necessary with LMWH.

NURSING MANAGEMENT
JOINT SURGERY

The nursing management of the patient undergoing joint surgery begins with preoperative teaching and realistic goal setting. It is important that the patient understands and accepts the limitations of the proposed surgery and realizes that in some cases surgery will not remove or treat the underlying disease. Postoperative procedures such as turning, deep breathing, use of a bedpan and high bedside commode, and use of abductor pillows should be explained and opportunities for practice provided. The patient should be reassured that pain relief will be available.

PCA can be helpful. A preoperative visit from a physiotherapist allows practice of postoperative exercises and measurement for crutches or other assistive devices.

Discharge planning begins immediately on admission to the hospital. The duration of the hospital stay and the expected postoperative events should be discussed because the patient and caregiver must prepare ahead. The home environment must be assessed for safety (e.g., presence of scatter rugs and electrical cords) and accessibility. Are the bathroom and bedroom on the first floor? Are door frames wide enough to accommodate a walker? Social support must also be assessed. Is a friend or family member available to assist the patient in the home, or will the patient need extra assistance? Will the patient require

a homemaker or meal services? The older-adult patient may need the rehabilitation services of a subacute or long-term care facility for a few weeks postoperatively to progressively develop independent living skills. Specific nursing interventions related to the patient having orthopaedic surgery are summarized in NCP 65-2, available on the Evolve website.

Patient teaching includes instructions on reporting complications, including infection (e.g., fever, increased pain, drainage) and dislocation of the prosthesis (e.g., pain, loss of function, shortening or misalignment of an extremity). The home care nurse acts as the liaison between the patient and the surgeon, monitoring for postoperative complications, assessing comfort and ROM, and facilitating improvements in functional performance.

CASE STUDY

Hip Fracture Surgery

Source: And-One/
Shutterstock.com.

Patient Profile

Terry King is a 78-year-old man admitted to the hospital through the emergency department. It appears that he may have sustained a fracture to his left hip (see Chapter 64 case study). He is scheduled for a surgical hip repair in the morning.

Subjective Data

See the case study in Chapter 64.

Collaborative Care
Preoperative
- Pain not relieved by morphine.
- Accompanying Mr. King is his wife of 40 years, who is crying and anxious. Her anxiety is also causing Mr. King to become anxious.

Operative Procedure

Left hip repair using hip compression plate and bone screws

Postoperative
- Cefazolin 1g IV q8hr
- Intake and output for 48 hr
- Morphine via patient-controlled analgesia (PCA) pump

Discussion Questions
1. How do Mr. King's pre-existing medical conditions predispose him to postoperative complications?

2. What actions could be taken to help decrease his wife's anxiety?
3. *Priority decision:* As care is planned for Mr. King, what are the preoperative and postoperative priority nursing interventions?
4. What are the most likely postoperative complications that Mr. King could develop?
5. *Priority decision:* On assessment of Mr. King on the second postoperative day, an irregular pulse is noted, which is a new finding. The pulse rate is 66 and the ECG tracing is shown below. Which dysrhythmia is this? What is the priority action at this time?

6. *Priority decision:* What are the priority teaching interventions that should be done before discharge?
7. *Evidence-informed practice:* Why is satisfactory pain relief an important nursing goal in the postoperative period for Mr. King?

⊖volve
Answers are available at *http://evolve.elsevier.com/Canada/Lewis/medsurg.*

▮ REVIEW QUESTIONS

The number of the question corresponds to the same-numbered objective at the beginning of the chapter.
1. When would the nurse suspect an ankle sprain for the client being seen at the urgent care centre?
   a. Client was hit by another soccer player on the field.
   b. Client has ankle pain after sprinting around the track.
   c. Client dropped a 4.5-kg weight on his lower leg at the health club.
   d. Client had a twisting injury while running bases during a baseball game.
2. The nurse explains to a client with a distal tibial fracture returning for a 3-week checkup that healing is indicated by which of the following?

   a. Callus formation
   b. Complete bony union
   c. Hematoma at the fracture site
   d. Presence of granulation tissue
3. A client with a comminuted fracture of the femur is to have an open reduction with internal fixation (ORIF) of the fracture. In which of the following situations is an ORIF indicated?
   a. The client is able to tolerate prolonged immobilization.
   b. The client cannot tolerate the surgery for a closed reduction.
   c. A temporary cast would be too unstable to provide normal mobility.
   d. Adequate alignment cannot be obtained by other nonsurgical methods.

4. Which of the following indicates a neuro-vascular problem during the nurse's assessment of a client with a fracture?
   a. Exaggeration of extremity movement
   b. Increased redness and heat below the injury
   c. Decreased sensation distal to the fracture site
   d. Purulent drainage at the site of an open fracture
5. A client with a stable, closed fracture of the humerus caused by trauma to the arm has a temporary splint with bulky padding applied with an elastic bandage. For which of the following symptoms would the nurse suspect compartment syndrome and notify the physician?
   a. Increasing edema of the limb
   b. Muscle spasms of the lower arm
   c. Rebounding pulse at the fracture site
   d. Pain when passively extending the fingers
6. Which of the following symptoms should the nurse be monitoring for, in a client with pelvic fracture?
   a. Changes in urinary output
   b. Petechiae on the abdomen
   c. A palpable lump in the buttock
   d. Sudden increase in blood pressure
7. During the postoperative period, what should the client with an above-the-knee amputation be told about the problem of routinely elevating the residual limb?
   a. The flexed position can promote hip flexion contracture.
   b. This position reduces the development of phantom pain.

c. This position promotes clot formation at the incision site and thigh.
   d. Unnecessary movement of the extremity can cause wound dehiscence.
8. A client with rheumatoid arthritis is scheduled for an arthroplasty. How should the nurse explain the purpose of this procedure? *(Select all that apply)*
   a. To fuse the joint
   b. To replace the joint
   c. To prevent further damage
   d. To improve or maintain ROM
   e. To decrease the amount of destruction in the joint
9. What should the nurse teach a client recovering from a total hip replacement to avoid?
   a. Sleeping on the abdomen
   b. Sitting with the legs crossed
   c. Abduction exercises of the affected leg
   d. Bearing weight on the affected leg for 6 weeks

1. d; 2. a; 3. d; 4. c; 5. d; 6. a; 7. a; 8. b, b, d; 9. b.

⊖volve

For even more review questions, visit *http://evolve.elsevier.com/Canada/ Lewis/medsurg.*

REFERENCES

Aaron, D. L., Patel, A., Kayiaros, S., et al. (2011). Four common types of bursitis: Diagnosis and management. *Journal of American Academy of Orthopedic Surgeons, 19*(6), 359–367.

Ali, P., Santy-Tomlinson, J., & Watson, R. (2014). Assessment and diagnosis of acute limb compartment syndrome: A literature review. *International Journal of Orthopaedic & Trauma Nursing, 18*, 180–190. doi:10.1016/j.ijotn.2014.01.002.

American Academy of Orthopedic Surgeons. (AAOS). (2015). *Sprains, strains, and other soft- tissue injuries.* Retrieved from *http://www.orthoinfo.org/topic.cfm?topic=A00111.*

Asenjo, J., & Rossel, F. (2012). Vertebroplasty and kyphoplasty: New evidence adds heat to the debate. *Current Opinion in Anesthesiology, 25*(5), 577–583. doi:10.1097/ACO.0b013e328357a2c7.

Bartlett, D. (2012). What you need to know about total knee arthroplasty. *OR Nurse, 6*(1), 16–25. *http://dx.doi.org/10.1097/ 01.orn.0000407780.43380.20.*

Buttarovoli, P., & Leffler, S. (2012). Patellar dislocation. In P. Buttavarovoli (Ed.), *Minor emergencies* (3rd ed.). St Louis: Saunders.

Canadian Association of Wound Care (CAWC). (2016). *Statistics: Diabetic foot ulcers.* Retrieved from *http://cawc.net/index.php/ public/facts-stats-and-tools/statistics/.*

Canadian Institute for Health Information (CIHI) (2015). *Hip and knee replacements in Canada: Canadian Joint Replacement Registry (CJRR) 2015 annual report.* Ottawa: CIHI. Retrieved from *https://secure.cihi.ca/estore/productFamily.htm?locale=en &pf=PFC2945&lang=en.*

Canadian Institute for Health Information (CIHI). (2016). *Wait times for priority procedures in Canada, 2016.* Retrieved from *https:// secure.cihi.ca/free_products/wait_time_report2016_en.pdf.*

Carlson, D. S., & Pfadt, E. (2011). Action STAT. Fat embolism syndrome. *Nursing, 41*(4), 72. doi:10.1097/01.NURSE.0000395312 .91409.7f.

Centers for Disease Control and Prevention (CDC). (2015). *Hip fractures among older adults.* Retrieved from *http://www.cdc.gov/ HomeandRecreationalSafety/Falls/adulthipfx.html.*

Chapman, S. (2011). Pain management in patients following limb amputation. *Nursing Standard, 25*(19), 35–40. doi:10.7748/ ns2011.01.25.19.35.c8269. *http://dx.doi.org/.*

Faucett, S., Collinge, C., & Koval, K. J. (2012). Is reconstruction nailing of all femoral shaft fractures cost effective? A decision analysis. *Journal of Orthopaedic Trauma, 26*(11), 624–632. doi:10.1097/BOT.0b013e318246dfd9.

Fazzalari, N. (2011). Bone fracture and bone fracture repair. *Osteoporosis International, 22*(6), 2003–2006. doi:10.1007/ s00198-011-1611-4.

Ferguson, T. A., & Eastman, J. A. (2011). Anterior approach hip arthroplasty: A novel technique in the management of femoral neck fractures. *Current Orthopedic Practice, 22*(1), 39–45. doi:10.1097/BCO.0b013e3182059ba6.

Gutowski, C. J., Parvizi, J., & Purtill, J. J. (2014). Protocol-based arthroplasty: Less is more. *Orthopedics, 38*(10), 631–638. doi:10.3928/01477447-20151002-06.

Halawi, M. J., & Morwood, M. P. (2015). Acute management of open fractures: An evidence-based review. *Orthopedics, 38*(11), e1025–e1033. doi:10.3928/01477447-20151020-12.

Hung, W., Egol, K., Zuckerman, J. D., et al. (2012). Hip fracture management: Tailoring care for the older patient. *JAMA: The Journal of the American Medical Association, 307*(20), 2185–2194. doi:10.1001/jama.2012.4842.

Jerath, R., Crawford, M., & Jenson, M. (2015). Etiology of phantom limb syndrome: Insights from a 3D default space consciousness model. *Medical Hypotheses, 85*(2015), 153–159. doi:10.1016/j .mehy.2015.04.025.

Juby, A. G. (2009). The challenges of interpreting efficacy of hip protector pads in fracture prevention in high-risk seniors. *Clinical Rheumatology, 28*(6), 723–727. doi:10.1007/s10067-009-1115-1. (Seminal).

Magee, D. (2013). *Orthopedic physical assessment.* St Louis: Saunders.

Marshall, S., & Browner, B. (2012). Emergency care of musculoskeletal injuries. In C. Townsend, R. Beauchamp, M. Evers, et al. (Eds.), *Sabiston textbook of surgery: The biological basis of modern surgical practice* (19th ed.). St Louis: Saunders.

Marx, R. C., & Mizel, M. S. (2015). What's new in foot and ankle surgery. *Journal of Bone & Joint Surgery, 97*(10), 862–868. doi:10.2106/JBJS.O.00126.

Meuffels, D. E., Poldervaart, M. T., Diercks, R. L., et al. (2012). Guideline on anterior cruciate ligament injury. *Acta Orthopaedica, 83*(4), 379–386. doi:10.3109/17453674.2012.704563.

Middleton, S. D., & Anakwe, R. E. (2014). Carpal tunnel syndrome. *British Medical Journal, 349,* g6437. doi:10.1136/bmj.g6437.

Moja, L., Piatti, A., Pecoraro, V., et al. (2012). Timing matters in hip fracture surgery: Patients operated within 48 hours have better outcomes. A meta-analysis and meta-regression of over 190 000 patients. *PLoS ONE, 7*(10), e46175. doi:10.1371/journal.pone .0046175.

National Institute of Neurological Disorders and Stroke. (2012). *Carpal tunnel syndrome.* Retrieved from http://www.ninds.nih.gov/ disorders/carpal_tunnel/detail_carpal_tunnel.htm.

National Institute on Aging. (2015). *Exercise & physical activity: Your everyday guide from the National Institute on Aging.* Retrieved from https://www.nia.nih.gov/health/publication/exercise-physical -activity/introduction.

Ojike, N., Robers, C. S., & Giannoudis, P. V. (2012). Pelvic compartment syndrome: A systematic review. *Acta Orthopaedica Belgica, 78*(1), 6–10.

Osteoporosis Canada. (2017). *Osteoporosis facts & statistics.* Retrieved from http://www.osteoporosis.ca/osteoporosis-and-you/ osteoporosis-facts-and-statistics/.

Patrice, M., & Hatch, R. (2011a). General principles of fracture care. In M. Patrice & R. Hatch (Eds.), *Fracture management for primary care* (3rd ed.). St Louis: Mosby.

Patrice, M., & Hatch, R. (2011b). Facial and skull fractures. In M. Patrice & R. Hatch (Eds.), *Fracture management for primary care* (3rd ed.). St Louis: Mosby.

Public Health Agency of Canada (PHAC). (2014). *Seniors' falls in Canada: Second report.* Retrieved from http://www.phac-aspc .gc.ca/seniors-aines/publications/public/injury-blessure/seniors _falls-chutes_aines/assets/pdf/seniors_falls-chutes_aines-eng.pdf.

Registered Nurses' Association of Ontario (RNAO). (2005, rev. 2011). *Prevention of falls and fall injuries in the older adult. Best Practice Guidelines.* Retrieved from http://rnao.ca/sites/rnao-ca/files/ Prevention_of_Falls_and_Fall_Injuries_in_the_Older_Adult.pdf.

Roberts, J., & Hedges, J. (2014). Arterial puncture and cannulation. In J. Roberts & J. Hedges (Eds.), *Roberts and Hedges' clinical procedures in emergency medicine* (6th ed.). Philadelphia: Saunders.

Rothgangel, A., Brau, S., Beurskens, A., et al. (2011). The clinical aspects of mirror therapy in rehabilitation: A systematic review of the literature. *International Journal of Rehabilitation Research, 34*(1), 1–13. doi:10.1097/MRR.0b013e3283441e98.

Sadoghi, P., von Keudell, P., & Vavken, P. (2012). Effectiveness of anterior cruciate ligament injury prevention training programs. *Journal of Bone and Joint Surgery, 94*(9), 769–776. doi:10.2106/ JBJS.K.00467.

Satryb, S. A., Wilson, T. J., & Patterson, M. M. (2011). Casting: All wrapped up. *Orthopaedic Nursing, 30*(1), 37–41. doi:10.1097/ NOR.0b013e31820574f9.

Shea, K. G., Carey, J. L., Richmond, J., et al. (2015). The American Academy of Orthopaedic Surgeons evidence-based guideline on management of anterior cruciate ligament injuries. *Journal of Bone and Joint Surgery, 97*(8), 672–674. doi:10.2106/JBJS.N.01257.

Smith, A., Dieppe, P., Howard, P., et al. (2012). Failure rates of metal-on-metal hip resurfacings: Analysis of data from the National Joint Registry for England and Wales. *Lancet, 380*(9855), 1759–1766. doi:10.1016/S0140-6736(12)60989-1.

Smith, H., Peek-Asa, C., Nesheim, D., et al. (2012). Etiology, diagnosis, and characteristics of facial fracture at a Midwestern level I trauma center. *Journal of Trauma Nursing, 19*(1), 57–65. doi:10.1097/JTN.0b013e31823a4c0e.

Statistics Canada. (2015a). *Health at a glance. Injuries in Canada: Insights from the Canadian Community Health Survey.* Retrieved from http://www.statcan.gc.ca/pub/82-624-x/2011001/article/ 11506-eng.htm.

Statistics Canada. (2015b). *Table 102-0561—Leading causes of death, total population, by age group and sex, Canada, annual, CANSIM* (database). Retrieved from http://www5.statcan.gc.ca/cansim/ a26?lang=eng&id=1020561.

Statistics Canada. (2015c). *Canadian Community Health Survey: Combined data, 2013/2014.* Retrieved from http://www.statcan .gc.ca/daily-quotidien/150624/dq150624b-eng.htm.

Stensrud, S., Roos, E., & Risberg, M. (2012). A 12-week exercise therapy program in middle-aged patients with degenerative meniscus tears: A case series with 1-year follow-up. *Journal of Orthopaedic Sports Physical Therapy, 42*(1), 919–931. doi:10.2519/ jospt.2012.4165.

Tzioupis, C. C., & Giannoudis, P. V. (2011). Fat embolism syndrome: What have we learned over the years? *Trauma, 13,* 259–281. doi:10.1177/1460408610396026.

University of Pittsburgh Medical Center [UPMC]. (2016). *Patient education materials: Weight bearing.* Retrieved from http:// www.upmc.com/patients-visitors/education/rehab/Pages/weight -bearing.aspx.

Velez, D., & Dellefield, M. (2011). Provide a helping hand to patients with upper extremity prostheses. *Nursing, 41*(1), 49–51. doi:10.1097/01.NURSE.0000391403.05698.fa.

Walker, J. A. (2011). Pelvic fractures: Classification and nursing management. *Nursing Standard, 26*(10), 49–57. doi:10.7748/ ns2011.11.26.10.49.c8816.

Welle, M. (2012). Understanding the new emerging oral anticoagulants for venous thromboembolism prophylaxis. *Orthopedic Nursing, 31*(5), 265–278. doi:10.1097/NOR .0b013e31826649a0.

Woods, S. (2011). Sprains and strains. *Practice Nurse, 41*(19), 33–36.

RESOURCES

About Face
http://www.aboutface.ca

Amputee.ca
http://www.amputee.ca/

The Arthritis Society
http://www.arthritis.ca

Canadian Academy of Sport and Exercise Medicine
http://www.casm-acms.org

Canadian Arthritis Network
http://www.arthritisnetwork.ca

Canadian Centre for Occupational Health and Safety
http://www.ccohs.ca

Canadian Orthopedic Association
http://www.coa-aco.org

Canadian Orthopedic Foundation
http://www.canorth.org

Canadian Orthopedic Nurses Association
http://www.cona-nurse.org

GTA Rehab Network
http://www.gtarehabnetwork.ca/

myJointReplacement.ca
http://myjointreplacement.ca/

Osteoporosis Society of Canada
http://www.osteoporosis.ca

War Amps of Canada
http://www.waramps.ca/home/

American Academy of Orthopedic Surgeons (AAOS)
http://www.aaos.org

American Association for Hand Surgery
http://www.handsurgery.org

American College of Sports Medicine (ACSM)
http://www.acsm.org

Amputee Coalition of America (ACA)
http://www.amputee-coalition.org

National Association of Orthopaedic Nurses, Inc. (NAON)
http://www.orthonurse.org

National Center on Physical Activity and Disability (NCPAD)
http://www.ncpad.org

National Institute on Aging: Exercise & Physical Activity: Your Everyday Guide from the National Institute on Aging
http://www.nia.nih.gov/health/publication/exercise-physical-activity -your-everyday-guide-national-institute-aging

National Institute of Arthritis and Musculoskeletal and Skin Diseases (NIAMS)
http://www.niams.nih.gov/

OrthoInfo
http://orthoinfo.aaos.org/

For additional Internet resources, see the website for this book at *http://evolve.elsevier.com/Canada/Lewis/medsurg.*

Nursing Management

Musculo-Skeletal Problems

Written by: Matthew C. Price
Adapted by: Jacqueline Klemann

℮volve WEBSITE

http://evolve.elsevier.com/Canada/Lewis/medsurg

- Review Questions (Online Only)
- Key Points
- Answer Guidelines for Case Study

- Customizable Nursing Care Plans
- Low Back Pain
- Osteomyelitis

- Conceptual Care Map Creator
- Audio Glossary
- Content Updates

LEARNING OBJECTIVES

1. Describe the pathophysiology, clinical manifestations, collaborative care, and nursing management of patients with osteomyelitis.
2. Describe the types, pathophysiology, clinical manifestations, and collaborative care of patients with bone cancer.
3. Differentiate between the causes and characteristics of acute and chronic low back pain.
4. Explain the conservative and surgical therapy of patients with herniated intervertebral disc.

5. Describe the postoperative nursing management of a patient who has undergone spinal surgery.
6. Explain the etiology and the nursing management of patients with common foot disorders.
7. Describe the etiology, pathophysiology, clinical manifestations, and collaborative and nursing management of patients with osteoporosis and Paget's disease.

KEY TERMS

degenerative disc disease (DDD), p. 1676
Ewing sarcoma family of tumours (ESFT), p. 1673

herniated intervertebral disc, p. 1677
low back pain (LBP), p. 1674
osteoclastoma, p. 1672

osteomyelitis, p. 1668
osteoporosis, p. 1682
osteosarcoma, p. 1672

Paget's disease of the bone, p. 1686
sarcoma, p. 1672

Acute and chronic musculo-skeletal problems are a common source of pain and disability. A variety of problems unrelated to trauma that affect the musculo-skeletal system are presented in this chapter, including osteomyelitis, bone cancer, foot disorders, and metabolic bone diseases. Management of the patient with both acute and chronic low back pain is addressed, and spinal surgery is discussed as an intervention for a herniated disc. Throughout the discussion of all of these problems, the nurse's role in prevention of injury and maintenance of mobility is emphasized.

OSTEOMYELITIS

Etiology and Pathophysiology

Osteomyelitis is a severe infection of the bone, bone marrow, and surrounding soft tissue. The most common infecting

microorganism is *Staphylococcus aureus.* A variety of microorganisms can cause osteomyelitis (Matteson & Osmon, 2016) (Table 66-1). Aerobic Gram-negative bacteria, alone or mixed with Gram-positive organisms, are often found. The widespread use of antibiotics in conjunction with surgical treatment has significantly reduced the mortality rate and complications associated with osteomyelitis.

The infecting microorganisms can invade by indirect or direct entry. The *indirect (hematogenous) entry* of microorganisms most frequently affects children because the metaphyseal (growing) regions of long bones are highly vascular and susceptible to even minor trauma. Adults with vascular insufficiency disorders (e.g., caused by diabetes mellitus), genito-urinary or respiratory infections are at higher risk for a primary infection to spread via the blood to the bone. The pelvis and the vertebrae, which consist of vascular-rich bone, are the most common sites of infection.

Direct-entry osteomyelitis can occur at any age, when there is an open wound (e.g., fractures, penetrating wounds) and microorganisms gain entry to the body. Osteomyelitis may also occur in the presence of a foreign body such as an implant or an orthopaedic prosthetic device (e.g., plate, total joint prosthesis). After gaining entrance to the bone by way of the blood, the microorganisms then lodge in an area of the bone where circulation slows, usually the metaphysis. The microorganisms grow, resulting in an increase in pressure because of the nonexpanding nature of most bone. This increasing pressure within the rigid bone structure leads to ischemia and vascular compromise of the periosteum. Eventually, the infection spreads through the bone cortex and the marrow cavity, ultimately resulting in cortical devascularization and necrosis. Once ischemia occurs, the bone dies. The area of devitalized bone eventually separates from the surrounding living bone, forming *sequestra* (sing., *sequestrum*). The part of the periosteum that continues to have a blood supply forms new bone, called *involucrum* (Figure 66-1).

Once formed, a sequestrum continues to be an infected island of dead bone surrounded by purulent drainage. It is difficult for bloodborne antibiotics or white blood cells to reach the sequestrum. A sequestrum may serve as a reservoir for microorganisms that spread to other sites, including the lungs and brain. The sequestrum can move out of the bone and into the soft tissue.

Once outside of the bone, the sequestrum may revascularize and then undergo removal by the body's normal immune processes. Another possibility is that the sequestrum can be surgically removed through debridement of the necrotic bone. If the necrotic sequestrum is not resolved naturally or surgically, it may develop a sinus tract, resulting in a chronic, purulent cutaneous drainage (see Figure 66-1).

Despite advances in identification of pathogens, current use of antibiotics, and surgical debridement, acute osteomyelitis becomes chronic in 10% to 30% of cases and it is difficult to treat. In recent years, our understanding of bacterial virulence and host defence has improved due to emerging research of bacterial biofilm models (Sanchez, Mende, Beckius, et al., 2013). A biofilm is a cluster of bacterial cells that form a matrix (three-dimensional structure) that requires necrotic tissue and bone. This matrix functions as a barrier, offering the bacteria protection from mechanical influences, antibiotics, and the host's defence cells (Chen & Wen, 2011). The pathogens pass from planktonic phase to maturation. The biofilm essentially functions as a permanent source of virulent pathogens insensitive to the body's own immune system and antibiotics. Surgical excision of sequestrum and biofilm is required.

Clinical Manifestations

Acute osteomyelitis refers to the initial infection or an infection of less than 1 month in duration. The clinical manifestations of acute osteomyelitis are both systemic and local. Systemic manifestations include fever, night sweats, chills, restlessness, nausea, and malaise. Local manifestations include constant bone pain that is unrelieved by rest and worsens with activity; swelling, tenderness, and warmth at the infection site; and restricted movement of the affected part. Later signs include drainage from sinus tracts to the skin or the fracture site.

Chronic osteomyelitis refers to a bone infection that persists for longer than 1 month or an infection that has failed to respond to the initial course of antibiotic therapy. Chronic osteomyelitis is either a continuous, persistent problem (a result of inadequate acute treatment) or a process of exacerbations and remissions (Figure 66-2). Systemic signs may be diminished; local signs of infection, including constant bone pain and swelling, tenderness, and warmth at the infection site, are more common. Over time, granulation tissue turns to scar tissue. This avascular scar tissue provides an ideal site for continued microorganism growth and is impenetrable by antibiotics. Long-term and rare complications

TABLE 66-1	ORGANISMS CAUSING OSTEOMYELITIS
Organism	**Predisposing Problem**
Staphylococcus aureus	Pressure injury, penetrating wound, open fracture, orthopaedic surgery, vascular insufficiency disorders (e.g., atherosclerosis; diabetes)
Staphylococcus epidermidis	Indwelling prosthetic devices (e.g., joint replacements, fracture fixation devices)
Streptococcus viridans	Abscessed tooth, gingival disease
Escherichia coli	Urinary tract infection
Mycobacterium tuberculosis	Tuberculosis
Neisseria gonorrhoeae	Gonorrhea
Pseudomonas species	Puncture wounds, intravenous drug use
Salmonella species	Sickle cell disease
Fungi, Mycobacteria species	Immuno-compromised host

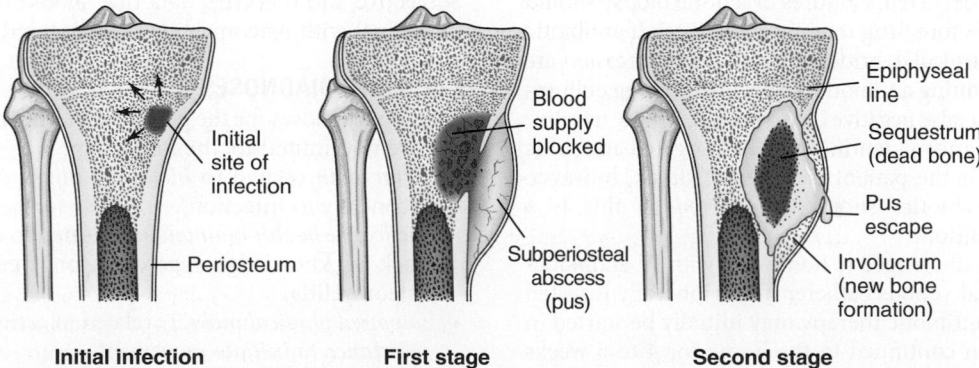

FIGURE 66-1 Development of osteomyelitis infection with involucrum and sequestrum. Source: McCance, K. L., Huether, S. E., Brashers, V. L., et al. (2014). *Pathophysiology: The biologic basis for disease in adults and children* (7th ed., p. 1559, Figure 44-15). St. Louis: Mosby.

FIGURE 66-2 Resection of femur owing to osteomyelitis. Source: Patton, K. T., & Thibodeau, G. A. (2014). *The human body in health and disease.* (6th ed., p. 199, Figure 8-34). St. Louis: Mosby.

of osteomyelitis include septicemia, septic arthritis, pathological fractures and amyloidosis (condition where abnormal protein called amyloid builds up in tissues and organs and can cause organ failure).

Diagnostic Studies

A bone or soft tissue biopsy is the definitive way to determine the causative microorganism. Once the causative organism is identified, antibiotic treatment can be adjusted. The patient's blood, wound cultures, or both are frequently positive for the presence of microorganisms. An elevated white blood cell and erythrocyte sedimentation rate may also be found. Radiological signs suggestive of osteomyelitis usually do not appear until 10 days to weeks after the appearance of clinical symptoms, by which time the disease will have progressed. Radionuclide bone scans (gallium and indium) are helpful in diagnosis and are usually positive in the area of infection. Magnetic resonance imaging (MRI) and computed tomographic (CT) scans may be used to help identify the extent of the infection, including soft tissue involvement.

Collaborative Care

Vigorous and prolonged intravenous (IV) antibiotic therapy is the treatment of choice for acute osteomyelitis, provided bone ischemia has not yet occurred. Cultures or a bone biopsy should be done, if possible, before drug therapy is initiated. If antibiotic therapy is delayed, surgical debridement and decompression are often necessary. Beginning antibiotics prior to obtaining cultures or biopsy can lead to a false negative culture result. A false negative culture (no microorganism identified) makes targeted antibiotic therapy impossible. If the patient is in septic shock, however, broad spectrum antibiotics should be started as this is a life-threatening condition.

Often, patients are discharged to home care with IV antibiotics delivered via a central venous catheter or peripherally inserted central catheter. IV antibiotic therapy may initially be started in the hospital and then continued in the home for 4 to 6 weeks or for as long as 3 to 6 months. A variety of antibiotics may be prescribed, depending on the microorganism. These drugs include penicillin, cefazolin, gentamicin, and vancomycin.

DRUG ALERT—Gentamicin
- Patients should be assessed for dehydration before starting therapy.
- Renal function testing must be done before starting therapy, especially in older-adult patients.
- Peak and trough levels must be monitored for therapeutic effect and to minimize renal and inner ear toxicity (Burchurn & Rosenthal, 2015).
- Patients should be instructed to notify the health care provider if any visual, hearing, or urinary problems develop.

In adults with chronic osteomyelitis, the choice between a palliative and a curative approach should be considered. Surgery is necessary in most cases to cure the infection, but this may not always be the best option (Lima, Oliveira, Carvalho, et al., 2014). Oral antibiotic therapy may also be given after acute IV therapy is complete to ensure resolution of the infection. The patient's response to drug therapy is monitored through various imaging methods (bone scan, CT, MRI) and by monitoring erythrocyte sedimentation rate and C-reactive protein.

Treatment of chronic osteomyelitis includes surgical removal of the poorly vascularized tissue and dead bone and the extended use of antibiotics. Palacos spacers with or without added antibiotics, along with antibiotic-impregnated bead chains or cement, may be implanted at this time to aid in combating the infection (Walter, Kemmerer, Kappler, et al., 2012). After debridement of the devitalized and infected tissue, the wound may be closed and a suction irrigation system inserted. Intermittent surgical irrigation and debridement of the affected bone may continue. Negative pressure over the site of the infection may be used (vacuum-assisted closure). (Negative-pressure wound therapy is presented in Chapter 14). The limb or surgical site may be protected with a cast or brace during this time.

Hyperbaric oxygen therapy with 100% oxygen may be administered as an adjunct therapy in refractory cases of chronic osteomyelitis. This therapy is thought to stimulate circulation and healing in the infected tissue (see Chapter 14). Orthopaedic prosthetic devices, if a source of chronic infection, must be removed. Muscle flaps or skin grafting provide wound coverage over the dead space (cavity) in the bone. Bone grafts may help to restore blood flow. Amputation of the extremity may be indicated in order to preserve an individual's life or improve quality of life when there is extensive bone destruction due to chronic osteomyelitis.

NURSING MANAGEMENT
OSTEOMYELITIS

NURSING ASSESSMENT

Subjective and objective data that should be obtained from an individual with osteomyelitis are presented in Table 66-2.

NURSING DIAGNOSES

Nursing diagnoses for the patient with osteomyelitis may include, but are not limited to, the following:
- *Acute pain* related to *biological injury agent* (inflammation secondary to infection)
- *Ineffective health maintenance* related to *insufficient resources* (lack of knowledge regarding long term management of osteomyelitis)
- *Impaired physical mobility* related to *activity intolerance, pain, reluctance to initiate movement*

Additional information on nursing diagnoses for the patient with osteomyelitis is presented in Nursing Care Plan (NCP) 66-2 on the Evolve website.

TABLE 66-2 NURSING ASSESSMENT

Osteomyelitis

Subjective Data

Important Health Information

Past health history: Bone trauma, open fracture, open or puncture wounds, other infections (e.g., genito-urinary and respiratory infections); vascular insufficiency disorders (e.g., arising from diabetes mellitus); adults who are immuno-compromised

Medications: Analgesics or antibiotics

Surgery or other treatments: Bone surgery, especially implantation of an orthopaedic prosthetic device (e.g., plate, total joint prosthesis)

Symptoms

Constant bone pain that is unrelieved by rest and worsens with activity; restricted movement of the affected part; malaise

Objective Data

General

Restlessness; fever, chills, night sweats

Integumentary

Diaphoresis; erythema, warmth, edema at infected bone

Later signs include drainage from sinus tracts to the skin or the fracture site

Musculo-Skeletal

Restricted movement; wound drainage; spontaneous fractures

Possible Findings

Leukocytosis, positive blood or wound cultures, ↑ erythrocyte sedimentation rate; presence of sequestrum and involucrum on radiographs, radionuclide bone scans, CT, and MRI

CT, computed tomography; *MRI,* magnetic resonance imaging.

PLANNING

The overall goals are that the patient with osteomyelitis will (1) have satisfactory pain and fever control, (2) not experience any complications associated with osteomyelitis, (3) cooperate with the treatment plan, and (4) maintain a positive outlook on the outcome of the disease.

NURSING IMPLEMENTATION

HEALTH PROMOTION. The control of infections already in the body (e.g., urinary, respiratory tract) is important in preventing osteomyelitis. Individuals susceptible to osteomyelitis are those who (alone or in combination) are immuno-compromised, have orthopaedic prosthetic devices, or have vascular insufficiencies. These patients should be instructed regarding the local and systemic manifestations of osteomyelitis. Families should also be aware of their role in monitoring the patient's health. Symptoms of bone pain, fever, swelling, and restricted limb movement should be reported immediately to the health care provider.

ACUTE INTERVENTION. Some immobilization of the affected limb (e.g., splint) is usually indicated to decrease pain. The involved limb should be handled carefully and excessive manipulation avoided as it increases pain and may cause pathological fracture. An important nursing responsibility is to assess the patient's pain. Nonsteroidal anti-inflammatory drugs (NSAIDs), opioid analgesics, and muscle relaxants may be prescribed to provide patient comfort. Nonpharmacological approaches to pain management (e.g., guided imagery, relaxation breathing) should be encouraged (see Chapters 10 and 12).

Dressings are used to absorb the exudate from draining wounds. Soiled dressings should be handled carefully to prevent cross-contamination of the wound or spread of the infection to other patients. Sterile technique should be practised when changing the dressing.

If the patient is on bed rest, proper body alignment and frequent position changes prevent complications associated with immobility and promote comfort. Flexion contracture, especially of the hip or knee, is a common sequela of osteomyelitis of the lower extremity because the patient frequently positions the affected extremity in a flexed position to promote comfort. Footdrop can develop quickly if the foot is not correctly supported in the neutral position by a splint or if there is excessive pressure on the peroneal nerve, which can occur with an improperly fitted splint. The patient should be instructed to avoid any activities, such as exercise or heat application, that increase circulation and serve as stimuli to the spread of infection. Uninvolved joints and muscles should continue to be exercised.

The patient should be taught about potential adverse and toxic reactions associated with prolonged and high-dose antibiotic therapy. These reactions include hearing deficit, fluid retention, and neurotoxicity—which can occur with the aminoglycosides (e.g., tobramycin)—and jaundice, colitis, and photosensitivity from the extended use of the cephalosporins (e.g., cefazolin). Tendon rupture (especially the Achilles tendon) can occur with use of the fluoroquinolones (e.g., ciprofloxacin, levofloxacin). Peak and trough blood levels of most antibiotics must be carefully monitored throughout the course of therapy to prevent these adverse effects. Lengthy antibiotic therapy can also result in an overgrowth of *Candida albicans* and *Clostridium difficile* in the genito-urinary tract and oral cavities, especially in patients who are immuno-suppressed and in older-adult patients. The nurse should instruct the patient to report any whitish, yellowish, curdlike lesions or frequent, watery diarrhea to the health care provider. The patient and family are often frightened and discouraged because of the serious nature of the disease, the uncertainty of the outcome, and the lengthy course of treatment. Continued psychological and emotional support is an integral part of the nursing management for patients with osteomyelitis.

AMBULATORY AND HOME CARE. With the introduction of various intermittent venous access devices, IV antibiotics today can be administered to the patient in his or her home setting. The patient and family should be instructed on the proper care and management of the venous access device, the antibiotic schedule, antibiotic administration, and the need for follow-up laboratory testing. The importance of taking antibiotics even after the symptoms have subsided should be stressed.

If there is an open wound, dressing changes are often necessary. The patient and family may require supplies and instruction in the technique. If the osteomyelitis becomes chronic, patients need physical and psychological support for a prolonged period. Periodic home nursing visits for IV medication administration or dressing changes provide the family with support, which helps to reduce anxiety.

EVALUATION

The expected outcomes are that the patient with osteomyelitis will:

- Have satisfactory pain relief
- Follow the recommended treatment regimen
- Verbalize confidence in the ability to implement the treatment regimen at home
- Demonstrate a consistent increase in mobility and range of motion

BONE TUMOURS

Primary benign and malignant bone tumours are rare in adults and occur most often during childhood through young adulthood. Metastatic bone cancer, in which the cancer has spread from another site, is a more common problem. The name given to a bone tumour is based on the area of the bone and surrounding tissue that is affected and on the type of cells forming the tumour. In 2010, 340 new cases of bone cancer occurred in Canada, and there were 185 related deaths (Canadian Cancer Society's Advisory Committee on Cancer Statistics, 2015).

Clinical Manifestations

Persistent nonmechanical bone pain in any bone lasting more than a few weeks is cause for concern and should undergo further evaluation and investigation. Diagnosis of a suspected bone tumour is related to age, family history, presence and location of swelling, patient's mobility, and the presence of regional or local lymph nodes (The European Sarcoma Network Working Group [ESMO], 2012). Recent injury does not rule out a tumour, and the patient should undergo the appropriate diagnostic procedures.

Diagnostic Studies

Conventional radiographs should always be the first investigation when a patient presents with bone pain. If the diagnosis of tumour cannot be excluded with certainty, the next step is to arrange an MRI. A CT scan is helpful in visualizing calcification, periosteal bone formation, cortical destruction, or soft tissue involvement. In order to definitely identify and characterize the tumour, a biopsy for histology and pathology needs to be obtained by either a radiologist (radiology-guided biopsy) or surgeon (open-surgical biopsy). Once the biopsy material has been reviewed and identified, discussions about diagnosis, staging assessment, and treatment can occur with the patient and family.

BENIGN TUMOURS

Benign bone tumours are more common than primary malignant tumours. The main types of benign bone tumours are osteochondroma, osteoclastoma, and endochroma. These types of tumours are often removed by surgery.

Osteochondroma

Osteochondroma is the most common primary benign bone tumour. It is characterized by an overgrowth of cartilage and bone near the end of the bone, at the growth plate. It is more commonly found in the long bones of the leg, pelvis, or scapula.

Clinical manifestations include a painless, hard, immobile mass; lower-than-normal height for age; soreness of muscles in close proximity to the tumour; one leg or arm longer than the other; and pressure or irritation with exercise. Patients may also be asymptomatic. No treatment is necessary for asymptomatic osteochondroma. If the tumour is causing pain or neurological symptoms because of compression, surgical resection is usually done. Patients should have regular screening examinations for early detection of malignant transformation.

Osteoclastoma

Osteoclastoma (*giant-cell tumour*) is a destructive tumour that arises in the cancellous ends of long bones in young adults. Most

(98%) of these variant, giant-cell tumours are benign, but about 10% of the time they can be locally aggressive and spread to the lungs. Giant-cell tumours most commonly occur in women between the ages of 20 and 35. Common tumour sites are in the epiphysis of the distal femur, the proximal tibia, and the distal radius. Clinical manifestations are usually swelling, local pain, and some disturbances in joint function. Radiographic evidence of giant-cell tumours usually reveals local areas of bone destruction and eventual expansion of the bone ends (Figure 66-4).

After diagnosis, surgical curettage of the tumour is usually done, followed by bone grafting or bone cement; however, this treatment has been associated with high recurrence rates. Additional treatments with adjuvants such as zinc chloride, bisphosphonates, phenol, liquid nitrogen, and alcohol are often used to reduce recurrence (Hakim, Pelly, Kulendran, et al., 2015). Recurrent giant-cell tumours may have to be treated with amputation and prosthesis.

MALIGNANT BONE TUMOURS

A sarcoma is a malignant tumour in the connective tissues of the body (fat, muscles, blood vessels, nerves, bones, or cartilage). The most common types of malignant bone tumours are osteosarcoma, chondrosarcoma (see Figure 66-3B), and Ewing sarcoma. Primary malignant tumours occur most often during childhood and young adulthood. They are characterized by their rapid metastasis and bone destruction.

Osteosarcoma

Osteosarcoma is a malignant primary bone tumour that is extremely aggressive and is characterized by rapid growth and metastasis. It usually occurs in the metaphyseal region of the long bones of the extremities, particularly in the regions of the distal femur, proximal tibia, and proximal humerus as well as the pelvis (Figure 66-3A). Osteosarcoma is the most common malignant bone tumour affecting children and young adults; the highest incidence is in boys and men in the 10- to 25-year-old age group. Secondary osteosarcoma is known to occur in adults older than age 60 and is most commonly associated with Paget's disease.

FIGURE 66-3 A, Osteosarcoma. **B,** Chondrosarcoma. Source: Damjanov, I., & Linder, J. (1996). *Anderson's Pathology.* (10th ed.). St. Louis: Mosby.

FIGURE 66-4 Osteoclastoma (giant-cell tumour) in a long bone. Source: Damjanov, I., & Linder, J. (1996). *Anderson's pathology* (10th ed.). St Louis: Mosby.

Clinical manifestations of osteosarcoma are usually associated with a gradual onset of pain and swelling, especially around the knee. The neoplasm grows rapidly and can restrict joint motion if the tumour is close to a joint structure. Metastasis is present in 10% to 20% of individuals on diagnosis, with the lung being the most frequent site.

Canadian Terry Fox was diagnosed with osteosarcoma at 18 years of age and underwent an above-knee amputation in early 1977. Influenced by his experience, Terry decided in 1980 to run across Canada to raise money and awareness about cancer. Since then, more than $550 million has been raised worldwide for cancer research in Terry's name, through the annual Terry Fox Run held across Canada and around the world (Terry Fox Foundation, 2015). Fortunately, major advances continue to be made in the treatment of osteosarcoma.

Preoperative chemotherapy is used to decrease tumour size, and limb-salvage procedures (e.g., wide surgical resection of the tumour) are being used more often. Limb salvage is contraindicated if there is major neurovascular involvement, pathological fracture, infection, skeletal immaturity, or extensive muscle involvement. Quality-of-life considerations also factor into the decision regarding limb salvage compared with amputation. The introduction of multiagent chemotherapy has improved the outcomes for these patients. Chemotherapeutic agents used include methotrexate, doxorubicin, cisplatin, dactinomycin (Cosmegen), and ifosfamide (Ifex).

Ewing Sarcoma Family of Tumours

Ewing sarcoma family of tumours (ESFT) is one of the most common primary malignant neoplasms of bone and soft tissue. It occurs most often in adolescents or young adults, the majority of whom are younger than 30 years of age.

ESFT is characterized by rapid growth within the medullary cavity of long bones, especially the femur, humerus, pelvis, and tibia. Metastasis occurs early, and the most frequent site is the lungs. Common manifestations are progressive local pain, swelling, palpable soft tissue mass, noticeable increase in size of the affected part, fever, and leukocytosis. Multimodal treatment strategies combining local therapy (radiotherapy, surgery) and systemic chemotherapy have improved survival rates; however, for those with disseminated disease or recurrent disease, prognosis is still unfavourable. Chemotherapeutic agents commonly used are vincristine, ifosfamide (Ifex), doxorubicin, and etoposide (VePesid). The 5-year disease-free survival rate for localized Ewing sarcoma treated with radiation, surgical resection, and

multiagent chemotherapy is 65% to 76%. Hopefully, as new biology-driven treatment options emerge, the odds of survival can begin to improve (Potratz, Dirksen, Jürgens, et al., 2012).

METASTATIC BONE CANCER

The most common type of malignant bone tumour occurs as a result of metastasis from a primary tumour located at another site. Common sites for the primary tumour include breast, prostate, gastro-intestinal tract, lungs, kidney, ovary, and thyroid. The bone is the third-most common site for metastatic disease. Metastatic cancer cells travel from the primary tumour via the lymph and blood supply to other sites in the body. Metastatic bone lesion(s) are commonly found in vertebrae, pelvis, femur, humerus, or ribs. Pathological fractures at the site of metastasis are common because of weakening of the involved bone. High serum calcium levels result as calcium is released from damaged bones.

Once a primary lesion has been identified, often, radionuclide bone scans are done to detect the presence of metastatic lesions before they are visible on radiography. It is important to note that metastatic bone lesions may occur at any time (even years later) following diagnosis and treatment of the primary tumour. Metastasis to the bone should be suspected in any patient who has local bone pain and a past history of cancer. Treatment may be palliative and consists of pain management and radiation (see Chapter 18). Neurosurgical or orthopaedic surgical interventions may include prophylactic fixation at sites of impeding fracture, stabilization after pathological fracture, and stabilization or decompression of spinal cord and nerve roots for spinal instability (Khodabukus, Debattista, Reynolds, et al., 2015). Prognosis depends on the primary type of cancer and the extent of metastasis throughout the body.

NURSING MANAGEMENT
BONE CANCER

Patients with bone cancer should be assessed for location and severity of pain. The tumour site is also assessed for swelling, changes in circulation, and joint function, movement, and sensation. The patient is monitored for weakness caused by anemia and decreased mobility.

The overall goals are that the patient with bone cancer will (1) have satisfactory pain relief; (2) maintain preferred activities as long as possible; (3) demonstrate acceptance of body image changes resulting from chemotherapy, radiation, and surgery; (4) remain free from injury; and (5) verbalize a realistic idea of disease progression and prognosis.

Nursing care of the patient with a malignant bone neoplasm does not differ significantly from the care given to the patient with a malignant disease of any other body system (see Chapter 18). These patients are at high risk for injury due to the nature of their disease as well as the medications they may be taking so they require special attention and safety precautions while in hospital. Careful handling and support of the affected extremity, and logrolling for those on bed rest, are important to prevent pathological fractures Often, patients suffer from fatigue and weakness. As such, they are often reluctant to participate in activities based on fear of pain and of falling and fracturing a bone. Regular rest periods should be provided between activities. Plans should be discussed for home safety, including wearing nonslip footwear, ensuring a well-lit environment, and removing throw rugs and cords from the floor (Monczewski, 2013).

The pain associated with bone cancer can be severe. Often, the pain is caused by the tumour pressing against nerves and other organs near the bone. The patient's pain should be carefully monitored and the nurse should ensure that the patient has adequate pain medication. Sometimes, radiation therapy is used as a palliative therapy to shrink the tumour and decrease the pain.

The patient and family should be assisted in accepting the guarded prognosis associated with bone neoplasms. Inability to accomplish age-specific developmental tasks can increase the frustrations with this condition. General principles related to cancer nursing are applicable (see Chapter 18 and NCPs 18-1 and 18-2, available on the Evolve website). Special attention is necessary for the problems of pain and disability, chemotherapy, adverse effects of chemotherapy, and postoperative care after surgery such as spinal cord decompression or amputation. As with all types of cancer, the nurse should stress the importance of follow-up examinations.

LOW BACK PAIN

Etiology and Pathophysiology

Chronic back pain is a prevalent and a costly public health issue. The incidence of back pain does not differ significantly across social or demographic groups. Back pain continues to be the leading overall cause of lost productivity in the workplace (National Institute of Neurological Disorders and Stroke [NINDS], 2014). In Canada, it is estimated that medical expenditures for investigation and treatment of lower back pain are between $6 and $12 billion annually (Bone and Joint Canada, 2014).

Low back pain (LBP) is a common problem because the lumbar region (1) bears most of the weight of the body, (2) is the most flexible region of the spinal column, (3) contains nerve roots that are vulnerable to injury or disease, and (4) has an inherently poor biomechanical structure. Several risk factors are associated with LBP, including lack of muscle tone and excess body weight, poor posture, cigarette smoking, and stress. Jobs that require repetitive heavy lifting, operation of vibrating machinery, or prolonged periods of sitting are also associated with LBP. In Canada, those living in more rural and geographically remote areas are more likely than urban dwellers to have LBP (Bath, Trask, McCrosky, et al., 2014).

The causes of LBP of musculo-skeletal origin include (a) acute lumbosacral strain, (b) instability of the lumbosacral bony mechanism, (c) osteoarthritis of the lumbosacral vertebrae, (d) degenerative disc disease (DDD), and (e) herniation of an intervertebral disc.

According to Yassi & Lockhart (2013), international studies have shown a higher prevalence of nonspecific LBP in nurses than in the general population. Overall nursing activities increased the "risk for and were associated with back disorders regardless of nursing technique, personal characteristics, and non-work-related factors" with patient handling conferring the highest risk (Yassi & Lockhart, 2013, p. 223).

ACUTE LOW BACK PAIN

Acute low back pain usually lasts 6 weeks or less. Most LBP is caused by trauma or some type of activity that causes undue stress (often hyperflexion) of the lower back. Often, symptoms of LBP do not appear at the time of injury but develop later because of a gradual increase in pressure on the nerve by an intervertebral disc. Symptoms may range from muscle ache to shooting or stabbing pain, limited flexibility or range of motion, or an inability to stand straight.

Few definitive diagnostic abnormalities are present with nerve irritation and muscle strain. Diagnostic imaging, including radiography, MRI, and CT scans, are generally not done unless there are red flags, such as focal neurological deficits, trauma, or systemic disease (e.g., cancer, spinal infection) (Chou, Qaseem, Owens, et al., 2011).

Collaborative Care

If the acute muscle spasms and accompanying pain are not severe and debilitating, the patient is treated with analgesics such as NSAIDs or muscle relaxants. Severe pain may require a short course of opioid analgesics. A brief period (1 to 2 days) of rest at home may be necessary for some people, but most do better with a continuation of their regular activities (Nicholas & George, 2011). Bed rest provides no benefit to patients who have acute LBP, with or without sciatica (see "Evidence-Informed Practice" box). Evidence suggests that to stay active rather than rest in

---

🔍 EVIDENCE-INFORMED PRACTICE

Research Highlight

Should Patients With Acute Low Back Pain Do Motor Control Exercises?
Clinical Question
In patients with acute low back pain (P), do motor control exercises (I) as compared to other forms of exercise or doing nothing (C) improve recovery (O)?

Best Available Evidence
Systematic review of randomized controlled trials (RCTs)

Critical Appraisal and Synthesis of Evidence
- 29 randomized trials ($n = 2431$); the impact of using motor control exercises as a treatment for lower back pain was compared to other forms of exercise or doing nothing.
- Acute LBP was defined as pain lasting <6 wk.
- People that used motor control exercises for 20 days to 12 weeks, 1–5 days per week, experienced improvements, especially in pain and disability.
- Targeting the strength and coordination of muscles that support the spine through motor control exercise provided an alternative treatment for lower back pain. It is unclear how motor control exercise compares with other forms of exercise long term.

Conclusions
- Motor exercises are as effective as other types of exercise, so the choice of exercise should account for factors such as patient or therapist preferences, cost, and availability.
- There is no evidence that staying active is harmful.

Implications for Nursing Practice
- Patients with acute LBP should be encouraged to continue daily activities and use motor control exercises within their limitations of pain.
- Patients should be instructed on the potential harm of extended bed rest.
- Research on the effects of staying active for chronic LBP is needed.

Reference for Evidence
Saragiotto, B. T., Maher, C. G., Yamato, T. P., et al. (2016). Motor control exercise for chronic non-specific low back pain. *The Cochrane Database of Systematic Reviews*, (1), CD012004, doi:10.1002/14651858.CD012004.

P, patient population of interest; *I*, intervention or area of interest; *C*, comparison of interest or comparison group; *O*, outcome(s) of interest (see Chapter 1).

bed means the patient will return to work sooner, improve functional status, and have less pain. Patients who are unable to return to normal activities may have short-term benefits from spinal manipulation, but it may be no more effective than usual care. Multidisciplinary rehabilitation programs in occupational settings may be an option for workers with sick leave of more than 4 to 8 weeks.

The effectiveness of invasive treatments, such as epidural corticosteroid injections and implanted devices that deliver pain medication, remains controversial. The latest research evidence suggests that transcutaneous electrical nerve stimulation (TENS) and traction are not effective for the treatment of LBP. Although it is important that the patient remains active and fit, the current scientific evidence does not support the use of specific exercises (e.g., strengthening, stretching, flexion, and extension exercises) as a treatment for acute nonspecific LBP (Hayden, van Tulder, Malmivaara, et al., 2011). Patients experiencing acute nonspecific LBP should avoid bed rest for prolonged periods and activities that aggravate the pain, including lifting, bending, twisting, and prolonged sitting. Most cases spontaneously improve within 2 to 6 weeks.

CHRONIC LOW BACK PAIN

Chronic low back pain is low back pain that lasts more than 3 months or is a repeated incapacitating episode. Causes include (1) degenerative conditions such as arthritis or disc disease; (2) osteoporosis or other metabolic bone diseases; (3) prior injury (scar tissue weakens the back); (4) chronic strain on the lower back muscles from obesity, pregnancy, or job-related stooping, bending, or other stressful postures; and (5) congenital abnormalities in the spine.

Spinal Stenosis

Spinal stenosis is a narrowing of the vertebral canal or nerve root canals caused by encroachment of bone on the space. The stenosis may be inherited or acquired through degenerative or traumatic changes to the spine. Common acquired causes include osteo-arthritis, rheumatoid arthritis, spinal tumours, Paget's disease, and trauma. Inherited conditions that lead to spinal stenosis include congenital spinal stenosis and scoliosis.

Arthritic changes (bone spurs, calcification of spinal ligaments, degeneration of discs) narrow the space around the spinal canal and nerve roots, eventually leading to compression. Inflammation caused by the compression results in pain, weakness, and numbness.

The pain associated with lumbar spinal stenosis often starts in the low back and then radiates to the buttock and the leg. It worsens with walking and particularly when standing without walking. Numbness, tingling, weakness, and heaviness in the legs and buttocks may also be present. In most cases, the stenosis slowly progresses and does not cause paralysis.

NURSING AND COLLABORATIVE MANAGEMENT CHRONIC LOW BACK PAIN

Chronic LBP is not a clinical entity but a symptom in patients with very different stages of impairment, disability, and chronicity. Treatment for chronic LBP is much the same as for acute LBP. Epidural injections have been used since 1901 in managing chronic lower back pain, but their effectiveness is still unclear (Kaye,

Manchikanti, Abdi, et al., 2015). Cold, damp weather aggravates back pain, but this can be relieved with rest and local heat application. Relief of pain and stiffness by the use of mild analgesics, such as NSAIDs, is integral to the daily comfort of people with chronic LBP. Weight reduction, sufficient rest periods, local heat or cold application, and exercise and activity throughout the day help to keep the muscles and joints mobilized. Tricyclic antidepressants (e.g., amitriptyline [Elavil]) and selective serotonin reuptake inhibitors (e.g., sertraline) have been shown to improve the chronic symptoms of LBP.

Surgical intervention may be indicated in patients with severe chronic LBP who do not respond to conservative care or have continued neurological deficits. (Surgery for low LBP is discussed on p. 1679.)

NURSING MANAGEMENT NONSPECIFIC LOW BACK PAIN

NURSING ASSESSMENT

Subjective and objective data that should be obtained from the patient with LBP are summarized in Table 66-3.

TABLE 66-3 NURSING ASSESSMENT

Low Back Pain

Subjective Data
Important Health Information
Past health history: Acute or chronic lumbosacral strain or trauma, osteoarthritis, degenerative disc disease, obesity; metabolic, circulatory, gynecological, or urological problems
Occupation requiring heavy lifting, vibrations, or extended driving
Medications: Opioid and nonopioid analgesics; muscle relaxants; NSAIDs; corticosteroids; antidepressants; anticonvulsant drugs; over-the-counter remedies, including herbal products and nutritional supplements
Surgery or other treatments: Previous back surgery, epidural corticosteroid injections

Symptoms
- Pain in back, buttocks, or leg, associated with walking, turning, straining, coughing, leg raising
- Numbness or tingling of legs, feet, toes; muscle spasms
- Activity intolerance
- Interrupted sleep

Objective Data
General
Guarded movement

Neurological
Depressed or absent Achilles tendon reflex or patellar tendon reflex; positive straight leg–raising test, positive cross-over straight leg–raising test, positive Trendelenburg test

Musculo-Skeletal
Tense, tight paravertebral muscles on palpation, decreased range of motion of spine; poor posture

Possible Findings
Localization of site of lesion or disorder on myelogram, CT scan, or MRI; determination of nerve root impingement on electromyography

CT, computed tomography; *MRI,* magnetic resonance imaging; *NSAIDs,* nonsteroidal anti-inflammatory drugs.

NURSING DIAGNOSES

Nursing diagnoses for the patient with LBP may include, but are not limited to, the following list.

- *Acute pain* related to *physical injury agent* (mechanical disorders or nonmechanical diseases and ineffective comfort measures)
- *Impaired physical mobility* related to *pain*
- *Chronic pain* related to *injury agent* (progressive degenerative changes of the muscles and skeletal structures of the back)
- *Ineffective coping* related to *insufficient sense of control* (chronic pain)
- *Ineffective health management* related to *insufficient knowledge of therapeutic regimen*

Additional information on nursing diagnoses for the patient with LBP is presented in NCP 66-1, available on the Evolve website.

PLANNING

The overall goals are that the patient with LBP will (1) have satisfactory pain relief, (2) avoid constipation secondary to medication and immobility, (3) learn back-sparing practices, and (4) return to the previous level of activity within prescribed restrictions.

NURSING IMPLEMENTATION

HEALTH PROMOTION. Patients should also be advised to maintain appropriate body weight. Excess body weight places extra stress on the lower back and weakens the abdominal muscles that support the lower back. Flat shoes or shoes with low heels (<2.5 cm) and shock-absorbing shoe inserts are recommended for women.

The position assumed while sleeping is also important in preventing LBP. Sleeping in a prone position should be avoided because it produces excessive lumbar lordosis, placing excessive stress on the lower back. A firm mattress is recommended. The patient should sleep in either a supine or a side-lying position, with the knees and hips flexed to prevent unnecessary pressure on support muscles, ligamentous structures, and lumbosacral joints. Patients should be educated about the necessity to avoid or cease smoking. Nicotine has been shown to decrease circulation to the vertebral discs, and a causal relationship exists between smoking and some types of LBP.

ACUTE INTERVENTION. The primary nursing responsibilities in acute LBP are to assist the patient to maintain activity limitations, promote comfort, and educate the patient about the health problem and appropriate exercises. Other nursing interventions are summarized in NCP 66-1 on the Evolve website. The use of analgesics, NSAIDs, muscle relaxants, antidepressants, anticonvulsant drugs, and thermotherapy (ice and heat), while avoiding continued bed rest, is incorporated into the plan of care.

Muscle stretching and strengthening exercises may be part of the management plan. Exercises can help to strengthen the back as a preventive measure, but there is no evidence to support their effectiveness as treatment for LBP. Although the actual exercises are often taught by a physiotherapist, it is the nurse's responsibility to ensure that the patient understands the type and the frequency of exercise prescribed as well as the rationale for the program.

As a role model, the nurse should use proper body mechanics at all times. The nurse should assess the patient's use of body mechanics and offer advice when activities that could produce back strain are performed (Table 66-4).

AMBULATORY AND HOME CARE. The goal of management is to make an episode of acute LBP an isolated incident. If the lumbosacral mechanism is unstable, repeated episodes can be

---

TABLE 66-4 PATIENT & CAREGIVER TEACHING GUIDE

Low Back Problems

The following instructions should be included when teaching the patient how to manage low back problems.

Do

- Prevent lower back from straining forward by placing a foot on a step or stool during prolonged standing.
- Sleep in a side-lying position with knees and hips bent.
- Sleep on back with a lift under knees and legs or on back with 25-cm–high pillow under knees to flex hips and knees.
- Exercise 15 minutes in the morning and 15 minutes in the evening, regularly; begin exercises with a 2- or 3-minute warm-up period by moving arms and legs; alternate relaxing and tightening muscles; exercise slowly, with smooth movements, as directed by a physiotherapist.
- Carry light items close to your body.
- Maintain appropriate body weight.
- Use local heat and cold application.
- Use a lumbar roll or pillow for sitting.
- Use proper body mechanics to avoid low back strain (e.g., when lifting objects, bend at the knees, not at the waist; stand up slowly with the object close to your body).

Do Not

- Lean forward without bending knees.
- Lift anything above level of your elbows.
- Stand in one position for prolonged time.
- Sleep on abdomen or on back or side with legs out straight.
- Exercise without consulting your health care provider, if having severe pain.
- Exceed prescribed amount and type of exercises without consulting your health care provider.

---

anticipated. The lumbosacral spine may be unable to meet the demands placed on it without strain because of factors such as obesity, poor posture, poor muscular support, advancing age, or local trauma. Intervention is aimed at strengthening the supporting muscles through exercise. A corset limits extremes of movement and may be useful in decreasing pain and the use of pain medication.

Persistent use of poor body mechanics may also result in repeated episodes of LBP. If the strain is work related, occupational counselling may be necessary. The frustration, pain, and disability imposed on the patient with LBP require emotional support and understanding care by the nurse.

EVALUATION

The expected outcomes for the patient with LBP are presented in NCP 66-1 (available on the Evolve website.)

INTERVERTEBRAL DISC DISEASE

Etiology and Pathophysiology

An intervertebral disc is interposed between the vertebrae from the cervical axis to the sacrum. Structural degeneration of the lumbar disc is often caused by **degenerative disc disease (DDD)**. This progressive degeneration is a normal process of aging and results in the intervertebral discs losing their elasticity, flexibility, and shock-absorbing capabilities. Thinning of the discs occurs as the nucleus pulposus (gelatinous centre of the disc) starts to dry out and shrink. These changes limit the ability of the discs to distribute pressure loads between the vertebrae. The once normal central loading of the intervertebral discs then changes, and the load now is transferred to the annulus fibrosis (strong outside portion of the intervertebral disc), causing structural deterioration. The annulus is now torn or stretched, which allows the nucleus pulposus to herniate or bulge outward between the vertebrae. This phenomenon is called a herniated intervertebral disc (slipped disc) (Figure 66-5).

An acute herniated intervertebral disc (slipped disc) can be the result of natural degeneration with age or repeated stress and trauma to the spine. Herniation of the nuclear material from the intervertebral disc may compress or place tension on a cervical, lumbar, or sacral spinal nerve root, causing acute back pain. The most common sites of rupture are the lumbosacral discs, specifically, L4–5 and L5–S1. Disc herniation may also occur at C5–6 and C6–7.

The spinal nerves emerge from the spinal column through an opening (*intervertebral foramen*) between adjacent vertebrae. Herniated discs can press against these nerves ("pinched nerve"), causing *radiculopathy* (radiating pain, numbness, tingling, and diminished strength or range of motion). Additionally, nerve and vascular ingrowth into the disk and exposure of these nerves to inflammatory mediators contribute to lower back pain (Simon, McAuliffe, Shamim, et al., 2014).

Osteoarthritis of the spine is associated with DDD and the stresses placed on the vertebrae. The joints, which are not adequately lubricated, rub against each other, leading to damage of the protective cartilage and the formation of painful bone spurs, which are one of the changes found in osteoarthritis.

Clinical Manifestations

The most common clinical manifestation of *lumbar disc disease* is LBP. Radicular pain that radiates down the buttock and below the knee, along the distribution of the sciatic nerve, generally indicates disc herniation. (Specific manifestations for lumbar disc herniation are summarized in Table 66-5). The straight leg raise test may be positive, indicating nerve root irritation. Back or leg pain may be reproduced by raising the leg and flexing the foot at 90 degrees. LBP from other causes may not be accompanied by leg pain. Reflexes may be depressed or absent, depending on the spinal nerve root involved. Paresthesia or muscle weakness in the legs, feet, or toes may be reported by the patient. Multiple nerve root (*cauda equina*) compression from a herniated disk, a tumour, or an epidural access may be manifested as bowel and bladder incontinence or erectile dysfunction. This condition is a medical emergency.

In *cervical disc disease*, there is often pain radiating into the arms and hands, following the pattern of the nerve involved. Reflexes may or may not be present, and there is often weakness of the hand grips.

Diagnostic Studies

Radiographic studies are done to note any structural defects. A myelogram, MRI, or CT scan is helpful in localizing the damaged site. An epidural venogram or discogram may be necessary if other methods of diagnosis are unsuccessful. An electromyogram of the extremities can be performed to determine the severity of nerve irritation or to rule out other pathological conditions, such as peripheral neuropathy.

Collaborative Care

The patient with suspected disc damage is usually managed first with conservative therapy (Table 66-6). This includes limitation of extremes of spinal movement (brace, corset, or belt), local heat or ice, ultrasonography and massage, traction, and TENS. Drug therapy includes NSAIDs, short-term opioids, muscle relaxants, anticonvulsant drugs, and antidepressants (Cepoiu-Martin, Faris, Lorenzetti, et al., 2011). Epidural corticosteroid injections may be effective in reducing inflammation and relieving acute pain. If the underlying cause remains, the pain tends to recur. Once the symptoms subside, back-strengthening exercises are done twice a day and are encouraged for a lifetime. The patient is taught the principles of good body mechanics. Extremes of flexion and torsion are strongly discouraged. Most patients heal with a conservative (nonoperative) plan after 6 months.

Surgical Therapy. If conservative treatment is unsuccessful, radiculopathy becomes progressively worse, or loss of bowel or

Normal disc

Degenerated disc

Bulging disc

Herniated disc

Thinning disc

Disc degeneration with osteophyte formation

FIGURE 66-5 Common causes of degenerative disc damage.

Intervertebral Level	Subjective Pain	Affected Reflex	Motor Function	Sensation
TABLE 66-5	**CLINICAL MANIFESTATIONS BASED ON LEVEL OF DISC HERNIATION***			
L3–4	Back to buttocks to posterior thigh to inner calf	Patellar	Quadriceps, anterior tibialis	Inner aspect of lower leg, anterior part of thigh
L4–5	Back to buttocks to dorsum of foot and big toe	None	Anterior tibialis, extensor hallucis longus, gluteus medius	Dorsum of foot and big toe
L5–S1	Back to buttocks to sole of foot and heel	Achilles	Gastrocnemius, hamstring, gluteus maximus	Heel and lateral foot

*A disc herniation can involve pressure on more than one nerve root.

| TABLE 66-6   **COLLABORATIVE CARE** |

Intervertebral Disc Disease

Diagnostic	**Surgical**

• History and physical examination
• Radiography
• CT scan
• MRI
• Myelogram
• Discogram
• EMG
 	
Collaborative Therapy
Conservative
• Restricted activity for several days, limit total bed rest
• Medication
  • Analgesics
  • Muscle relaxants
  • NSAIDs
• Local ice or heat
• Physiotherapy
• Epidural corticosteroid injections
	• Intradiscal electrothermoplasty (IDET)
	• Radiofrequency discal nucleoplasty
	• Interspinous process decompression system (X Stop)
	• Laminectomy with or without spinal fusion
	• Discectomy
	• Percutaneous laser discectomy
	• Artificial disc replacement
	• Spinal fusion with or without instrumentation (e.g., plates, screws)

CT, computed tomography; *EMG,* electromyogram; *MRI,* magnetic resonance imaging; *NSAIDs,* nonsteroidal anti-inflammatory drugs.

FIGURE 66-6 The Charité artificial disc used in degenerative disc disease to replace a damaged intervertebral disc. The Charité artificial disc consists of two cobalt-chromium alloy end plates sandwiched around a movable high-density plastic core. The design of the disc helps align the spine and preserve its natural ability to move.

bladder control (cauda equina) occurs, surgery may then be indicated. Surgery for a damaged disc is generally performed when diagnostic tests indicate the problem is not responding to conservative treatment and the patient is in constant pain or has a persistent neurological deficit. Surgery should be carefully considered because some patients, for unknown reasons, do not improve and symptoms may actually worsen after surgery.

An *intradiscal electrothermoplasty* (IDET) is a minimally invasive outpatient procedure that may help in treating back and sciatica pain. The procedure involves the insertion of a needle into the affected disc with radiological guidance. A wire is then threaded down through the needle and into the disc. The wire is then heated, which denervates the small nerve fibres that have grown into the cracks and invaded the degenerating disc. The heat also partially melts the annulus fibrosus, which triggers the body to generate new reinforcing proteins in the fibres of the annulus.

Another outpatient technique is *radiofrequency discal nucleoplasty* (coblation nucleoplasty). A needle is inserted into the disc similar to IDET. Instead of a heating wire, a special radiofrequency probe is used. The probe generates energy that breaks up the molecular bonds of the gel in the nucleus. The result is that up to 20% of the nucleus is removed, which decompresses the disc and reduces the pressure on both the disc and the surrounding nerve roots. Relief from pain varies among patients.

A third procedure is the use of an *interspinous process decompression system* (X Stop). This device is made of titanium and fits onto a mount that is placed on vertebrae in the lower back. The X Stop is used in patients with pain owing to lumbar spinal stenosis. The device works by lifting the vertebrae off the pinched nerve. The effect is similar to and less invasive than a laminectomy.

The most common surgical procedure for lumbar disc disease is a *laminectomy*. It involves the surgical excision of part of the posterior arch of the vertebra (referred to as the *lamina*) to gain access to the protruding disc to remove it. A minimal hospital stay is usually required after the procedure. Laminectomy is a safe and viable option when compared with decompression and fusion for older-adult patients who have failed conservative therapy and those with significant comorbidities.

A *discectomy* is another common type of surgical procedure that may be performed to decompress the nerve root. Microsurgical discectomy is a version of the standard discectomy in which the surgeon uses a microscope to allow better visualization of the disc and disc space during surgery to aid in the removal of the damaged portion. This procedure helps maintain the bony stability of the spine.

A *percutaneous discectomy* is an outpatient surgical procedure using a tube that passes through the retroperitoneal soft tissues to the disc with local anaesthesia and the aid of fluoroscopy. A laser is then used on the damaged portion of the disc. Small stab wounds are used, and minimal blood loss occurs during the procedure. The procedure is effective and safe, and it decreases rehabilitation time.

Total disc replacement is used in patients with disc damage associated with DDD. This artificial disc is made up of a high-density core sandwiched between two cobalt-chromium end plates (Figure 66-6). This device is surgically placed in the spine through a small incision below the umbilicus after the damaged disc is removed. The disc allows for movement at the level of the implant. When considering long-term benefits of total disc replacement versus nonsurgical options, long-term outcomes are unclear. There is a significant difference in functional outcome immediately postoperatively. However, when considering long-term outcomes (>2 years), there is only a modest difference between total disc replacement and nonsurgical treatment (Hellum, Johnsen, Storheim, et al., 2011).

A *spinal fusion* may be performed if the spine is unstable. Spinal stabilization is created by an *ankylosis* (fusion) of contiguous vertebrae with a bone graft from the patient's fibula or iliac crest or from donated cadaver bone. Metal fixation with rods, plates, or screws may be implanted at the time of spinal surgery to provide more stability and decrease vertebral motion. A posterior lumbar interbody fusion may be performed in patients to provide extra support for bone grafting or a prosthetic device.

Bone morphogenetic protein (BMP), a genetically engineered protein, may be used to stimulate bone growth of the graft in spinal fusions (Deyo, Ching, Matsen, et al., 2012). A dissolvable sponge soaked with BMP is implanted into the spine. The protein on the sponge stimulates the body's own cells to become active and produce bone. BMP begins the process of fusion, which continues even after the protein and sponge dissolve, leaving living bone behind.

NURSING MANAGEMENT SPINAL SURGERY

Postoperative nursing interventions focus on maintaining proper alignment of the spine at all times until healing has occurred. Depending on the type and extent of surgery, and the surgeon's preference, the patient may be able to dangle the legs at the side of the bed, stand, or even ambulate the first day after surgery.

Pillows can be used under the thighs of each leg when the patient is supine and between the legs when in side-lying positions to provide comfort and ensure alignment. Often, the patient fears turning or any movement that increases pain by straining the surgical area. The patient should be reassured that the proper technique is being used to maintain body alignment. Sufficient staff should be available to move the patient without undue pain or strain on staff members or the patient.

Postoperatively, most patients will require opioids such as morphine, intravenously, for 24 to 48 hours. Patient-controlled analgesia (PCA) allows for optimal analgesic levels and is the preferred method of continued pain management during this time. Once fluids are being taken, the patient may be switched to oral drugs such as acetaminophen with codeine or oxycodone. Medications may be prescribed for muscle relaxation. Pain management and its effectiveness should be monitored and documented.

The spinal canal may be entered during surgery so there is potential for cerebrospinal fluid leakage. Severe headache or leakage of cerebrospinal fluid on the dressing should be reported immediately. Cerebrospinal fluid appears as clear or slightly yellow drainage on the dressing. It has a high glucose concentration and will be positive for glucose when a dipstick test is done. The amount, colour, and characteristics of drainage should be noted.

The patient's peripheral neurological signs should be monitored frequently after spinal surgery. Movement of the arms and legs and assessment of sensation should be unchanged when compared with the preoperative status. Table 66-7 summarizes a lumbar laminectomy assessment appropriate for the patient who has undergone back surgery. These assessments are repeated every 2 to 4 hours during the first 48 hours after surgery, and findings are compared with the preoperative assessment. Paresthesias, such as numbness and tingling, may not be relieved immediately after surgery. Any new muscle weakness or paresthesias should be documented and reported to the surgeon immediately. Extremity circulation should be assessed by temperature, capillary refill, and pulses.

Paralytic ileus and interference with bowel function may occur for several days and may manifest as nausea, abdominal distension, and constipation. The nurse should assess whether the patient is passing flatus, has bowel sounds in all quadrants, and has a flat, soft abdomen. A bowel protocol should be initiated to prevent constipation.

Adequate bladder emptying may be altered because of activity restrictions, opioids, or anaesthesia. If allowed by the surgeon,

TABLE 66-7 POSTOPERATIVE ASSESSMENT FOLLOWING LUMBAR SURGERY

Sensation*
Assess sensation of extremities for paresthesia in all appropriate dermatomes.

Movement*
Assess ability to move all extremities.

Muscle Strength*
Assess for any weakness of the extremities.

Wound
Assess dressing for drainage, and note amount, colour, and characteristics.

Pain
- Document location of the pain.
- Ask patient to rate the pain on a scale of 0 to 10, with 0 being no pain and 10 being the worst pain.
- Evaluate pain after analgesia has been administered.

*Postoperative findings should be compared with preoperative assessments. It is not unusual for the patient to continue to experience these symptoms after surgery. Symptoms gradually decrease over several months.

men should be encouraged to dangle their legs or stand to urinate. Patients should use the commode or ambulate to the bathroom when allowed, to promote adequate emptying of the bladder. Ensure that privacy is maintained. Intermittent catheterization or an indwelling catheter may be necessary for patients who have difficulty urinating.

Loss of sphincter tone or bladder tone may indicate nerve damage. Incontinence or difficulty evacuating the bowel or bladder must be monitored closely and reported to the surgeon.

In addition to the nursing care appropriate for a patient who has had a laminectomy, there are other nursing responsibilities if the patient has also had a spinal fusion. A bone graft is usually involved, so postoperative healing time maybe prolonged in comparison to a laminectomy. Reduced activity for an extended time may be necessary. A rigid orthosis (thoraco-lumbar-sacral orthosis or chairback brace) is often used during this period. Some surgeons require that the patient be taught to put the orthosis on and take it off by logrolling in bed, whereas others allow their patients to apply the brace in a sitting or standing position. The nurse should verify the preferred method before initiating this activity.

In addition to the primary surgical site, the donor site for the bone graft must be regularly assessed. The posterior iliac crest is the most commonly used donor site, although the fibula may also be used. The donor site usually causes greater postoperative pain than the fused area. The donor site is bandaged with a pressure dressing to prevent excessive bleeding. If the donor site is the fibula, neurovascular assessments of the extremity are a postoperative nursing responsibility.

After a spinal fusion, the patient may experience some immobility of the spine at the fusion site. Instruction in proper body mechanics is essential and should be evaluated during the hospital stay. The patient should be instructed to avoid sitting or standing for prolonged periods. Activities that should be encouraged include walking, lying down, and shifting weight from one foot to the other when standing. The patient should learn to mentally think through an activity before starting any potentially injurious task such as bending, lifting, or stooping. Any twisting movement of the spine is contraindicated. The thighs and knees, rather than the back, should be used to absorb the shock of activity and movement. A firm mattress or bed board is essential.

NECK PAIN

Neck pain may occur almost as frequently as LBP. Neck pain may be the result of many conditions, both benign (e.g., poor posture) and serious (e.g., traumatic injury).

Cervical neck sprains and strains occur from hyperflexion and hyperextension injuries. Patients have symptoms of stiffness and neck pain and possible pain radiating into the arm and hand. Pain may also radiate into the head, anterior chest, thoracic spine region, and shoulders. Cervical nerve root compression from stenosis, DDD, or herniation may be indicated by weakness or paresthesia of the arm and hand. Diagnosing the cause of neck pain is done by history, physical examination, radiography, MRI, CT scan, and electromyography. An electromyogram of the upper extremities is done to diagnose cervical radiculopathy.

Conservative treatment for neck pain that commonly occurs in patients without an underlying disorder includes head support via soft cervical collars, heat and ice applications, massage, rest until symptoms subside, physiotherapy, ultrasound, and NSAIDs. Therapeutic neck exercises and acupuncture may also be used for pain relief. Most neck pain resolves without surgical intervention. Indications for cervical spine surgery are similar to those for the lower back. Types of surgery are also similar, including discectomy, laminectomy, and spinal fusion. If surgery is done on the cervical spine, the nurse must be alert for symptoms of spinal cord edema, such as respiratory distress and a worsening neurological status of the upper extremities. An orthosis or halo may be necessary after surgery, depending on the degree of spine stabilization. After surgery, the patient's neck is immobilized in either a soft or a hard cervical collar.

Preventing benign neck pain that occurs owing to everyday activities such as prolonged sitting at a computer or television, sleeping in nonalignment spinal positions, or jarring movements during exercise is important. Preventive strategies can begin by encouraging patients to practise good posture and maintain neck flexibility (Table 66-8).

FOOT DISORDERS

The foot is the platform that provides support for the weight of the body and absorbs considerable shock in ambulation. It is a complicated structure, composed of bony structures, muscles, tendons, and ligaments. It can be affected by (1) congenital conditions, (2) structural weakness, (3) traumatic injuries, and (4) systemic conditions such as diabetes mellitus and rheumatoid arthritis. Abnormalities of the foot affect millions of Canadians. Much of the pain, deformity, and disability associated with foot disorders can be directly attributed to or accentuated by improperly fitting shoes, which cause crowding and angulation of the toes and inhibition of the normal movement of foot muscles.

The purposes of footwear are to (1) provide support, foot stability, protection, shock absorption, and a foundation for orthoses; (2) increase friction with the walking surface; and (3) treat foot abnormalities. Table 66-9 summarizes common foot disorders. One of the most common forefoot disorders is a bunion

TABLE 66-8	**PATIENT & CAREGIVER TEACHING GUIDE**

Neck Exercises

The following instructions should be included when teaching the patient about neck exercises.
- Bend your head backward until you are looking up at the ceiling. Repeat slowly five times. Stop if experiencing dizziness.
- Bring your head forward so that your chin touches your chest and your face is looking down at the floor. Repeat slowly five times.
- Keep your head facing forward, and bend your ear down toward one shoulder. Alternate this movement with your other ear. Repeat slowly five times on each side.
- Turn your head slowly around to one side as far as it will go. Repeat toward the other side. Repeat exercise five times on each side.
- Without tipping your head in any direction, pull your chin and head straight back. Relax the chin forward to its neutral position. Repeat slowly five times.

FIGURE 66-7 A, Severe hallux valgus with bursa formation. **B,** Postoperative correction. Source: Canale, S., & Beaty, J. (Eds). (2013). *Campbell's operative orthopaedics.* (12th ed.). Philadelphia: Saunders.

(Figure 66-7). A lateral deviation of the great toe, termed *hallux valgus,* occurs with a bunion (Aly, Mousa, & Elsallakh, 2011).

NURSING MANAGEMENT
FOOT DISORDERS

NURSING IMPLEMENTATION

HEALTH PROMOTION. Well-constructed and properly fitting shoes are essential for healthy, pain-free feet. Instead of considerations of comfort and support, fashion styles, especially for women, often influence selection of footwear. Patient teaching should stress the importance of wearing shoes that conform to the foot rather than to current fashion trends. Shoes must be long enough and wide enough to prevent crowding of the toes and forcing of the great toe into a position of hallux valgus. At the metatarsal head, the width of shoes should be sufficient to allow free movement of the foot muscles and permit bending of the toes. The shank (narrow part of sole under the instep) of the shoes should be rigid enough to give optimal support. The height of the heels should be realistic in relation to the purpose for which the shoes are worn. Ideally, the heels of the shoes should not rise more than 2.5 cm higher than the forefoot support.

TABLE 66-9   COMMON FOOT DISORDERS

Disorder	Description	Treatment
Forefoot		
Hallux valgus (bunion)	Painful deformity of great toe consisting of lateral angulation of great toe toward second toe, bony enlargement of medial side of first metatarsal head, swelling of bursa and formation of callus over bony enlargement (see Figure 66-7)	Conservative treatment includes wearing shoes with wide forefoot or "bunion pocket" and use of bunion pads to relieve pressure on bursal sac. Surgical treatment is removal of bursal sac and bony enlargement and correction of lateral angulation of great toe; may include temporary or permanent internal fixation.
Hallux rigidus	Painful stiffness of first MTP joint, caused by osteoarthritis or local trauma	Conservative treatment includes intra-articular corticosteroids and passive manual stretching of first MTP joint. A shoe with a stiff sole decreases pain in the joint during walking. Surgical treatment is joint fusion or arthroplasty with silicone rubber implant.
Hammer toe	Deformity of second through fifth toes, including dorsiflexion of MTP joint, plantar flexion of PIP joint, and callus on dorsum of PIP joint and end of involved toe; complaints related to hammertoe include burning on bottom of foot and pain and difficulty in walking when wearing shoes	Conservative treatment consists of passive manual stretching of PIP joint and use of metatarsal arch support. Surgical correction consists of resection of base of middle phalanx and head of proximal phalanx and bringing raw bone ends together. Kirschner wire maintains straight position.
Morton's neuroma (Morton's toe or plantar neuroma)	Neuroma in web space between third and fourth metatarsal heads, causing sharp, sudden attacks of pain and burning sensations	Surgical excision is the usual treatment.
Midfoot		
Pes planus (flatfoot)	Loss of metatarsal arch, causing pain in foot or leg	Symptoms are relieved by use of resilient, longitudinal arch supports. Surgical treatment consists of triple arthrodesis or fusion of subtalar joint.
Pes cavus	Elevation of longitudinal arch of foot resulting from contracture of plantar fascia or bony deformity of arch	Treatment is manipulation and casting (in patients <6 yr of age); surgical correction is necessary if it interferes with ambulation (in patients ≥6 yr of age).
Hindfoot		
Painful heels	Complaint of heel pain with weight bearing; common causes include plantar bursitis, plantar fasciitis, or bone spur in adults	Corticosteroids are injected locally into inflamed bursa, and sponge rubber heel cushion is used; surgical excision of bursa or spur is performed. For plantar fasciitis, stretching exercises, NSAIDs, and corticosteroids are used.
Other Problems		
Corn	Localized thickening of skin caused by continual pressure over bony prominences, especially metatarsal head, frequently causing localized pain	Corn is softened with warm water or preparations containing salicylic acid and trimmed with razor blade or scalpel. Pressure on bony prominences caused by shoes is relieved.
Soft corn	Painful lesion caused by bony prominence of one toe pressing against adjacent toe; usual location in web space between toes; softness caused by secretions keeping web space relatively moist	Pain is relieved by placing cotton between toes to separate them. Surgical treatment is excision of projecting bone spur (if present).
Callus	Similar formation to corn but covers wider area and usual location is on weight-bearing part of foot	Same as for corn.
Plantar wart	Painful papillomatous growth caused by virus that may occur on any part of skin on sole of foot, tend to cluster on pressure points	Remedies containing salicylic acid; liquid nitrogen; excision with electrocoagulation or surgical removal; ultrasonography may also be used. Many disappear without treatment.

MTP, metatarso-phalangeal; *NSAIDs*, nonsteroidal anti-inflammatory drugs; *PIP*, proximal interphalangeal.

Effective strategies for preventing foot injuries are also required at the workplace. Prolonged standing, especially on hard, unyielding floors, can cause the joints of bones of the feet to become misaligned and inflamed. Special antislip flooring or matting can reduce slipping accidents that can result in sprained ankles or broken foot bones. All jurisdictions in Canada mandate that workers wear adequate protection against workplace hazards. Workers who are exposed to high foot-hazard risk (e.g., those in the construction industry) are required to use footwear certified by the Canadian Standards Association.

ACUTE INTERVENTION. Many foot problems require referral to a podiatrist. Depending on the problem, conservative therapies are usually tried first (see Table 66-9). These therapies include NSAIDs, icing, physiotherapy, alterations in footwear, stretching, warm soaks, orthotics, ultrasonography, and corticosteroid injections. If these methods do not offer relief, surgery may then be recommended.

Depending on the type of surgery, pins or wires (hardware) may extend through the toes, or a protective splint that extends over the end of the foot may be in place. Postoperatively, the foot is usually immobilized by a bulky dressing, short leg cast, slipper (plaster) cast, or a platform "shoe" that fits over the dressing and has a rigid sole (known as a *bunion boot*). The foot should be elevated with the heel off the bed to help reduce discomfort and prevent edema. Neurovascular status should be assessed frequently during the immediate postoperative period. Care must be taken to protect hardware as impact or movement cause pain. The hardware may interfere with or preclude assessment for movement. Sensation may be difficult to evaluate because postoperative pain can interfere with the patient's ability to differentiate pain caused by the surgical procedure from pain resulting from nerve pressure or circulatory impairment.

The type and the extent of surgery determine the degree of ambulation allowed. Crutches, a walker, a kneeler scooter, or a cane may be necessary. The patient may experience pain or a throbbing sensation when starting ambulation. The nurse should reinforce instructions given by the physiotherapist and ensure that the patient does not develop a faulty gait pattern, such as walking on the heels, in an attempt to avoid excessive pain or pressure. The nurse also ensures that the patient walks with an erect posture and with proper weight distribution. Dysfunction of gait or continued pain should be reported to the physician. The patient should be instructed on the importance of frequent rest periods with the foot elevated.

AMBULATORY AND HOME CARE. Foot care should include carrying out daily hygienic care and wearing clean socks, which should be long enough to prevent wrinkling and the development of pressure areas. Trimming toenails straight across helps prevent ingrown toenails and reduces the possibility of infection. People with impaired circulation or diabetes mellitus require detailed instruction to prevent serious complications associated with blisters, pressure areas, and infections. (See Chapter 52, Table 52-20 for guidelines on foot care.)

AGE-RELATED CONSIDERATIONS

FOOT PROBLEMS

The older adult is prone to developing foot problems because of poor circulation, atherosclerosis, and decreased sensation in the lower extremities. This problem is especially true for older-adult patients with diabetes mellitus (Turns, 2012). A patient may develop an open wound but not feel it because of altered sensation. This may be the result of peripheral vascular disease or diabetic neuropathy. Older-adult patients should be instructed to inspect their feet daily and report any open wounds or breaks in the skin to their health care provider (Stolt, Suhonen, Puukka, et al., 2012). If left untreated, wounds may become infected, lead to osteomyelitis, and require surgical debridement. If the infection becomes widespread, lower limb amputation may be necessary. The caregiver of the older adult who needs assistance with hygiene practices should be taught the importance of carefully assessing the feet at regular intervals.

METABOLIC BONE DISEASES

Normal bone metabolism is affected by hormones, nutrition, and hereditary factors. When there is dysfunction in any of these factors, a generalized reduction in bone mass and strength may result. Examples of metabolic bone diseases include osteoporosis and Paget's disease.

OSTEOPOROSIS

Osteoporosis, or porous bone (Figure 66-8), is a chronic, progressive metabolic bone disease. It is characterized by low bone mass and structural deterioration of bone tissue, leading to

FIGURE 66-8 A, Normal bone. **B,** Osteoporotic bone. Source: Patton, K. T., & Thibodeau, G. A. (2016). *Anatomy and physiology* (7th ed., p. 277, Figure 11-25, *B* and *C*). St. Louis: Mosby.

increased bone fragility, which predisposes the individual to bone fractures at the hip, wrist, and spine. Osteoporosis is known as the "silent thief" because it slowly and insidiously, over many years, robs the skeleton of its banked resources. Fractures from osteoporosis are more common than heart attack, stroke, and breast cancer combined (Osteoporosis Canada, 2017a).

Osteoporotic fractures occur in at least 1 in 3 Canadian women and 1 in 5 Canadian men (Osteoporosis Canada, 2017a). Approximately 30 000 Canadians will suffer a hip fracture, annually. From 70% to 90% of these hip fractures are due to osteoporosis (Osteoporosis Canada, 2017b).

Osteoporotic fractures result in significant morbidity and mortality. It is estimated that 28% of women and 37% of men will suffer a hip fracture due to osteoporosis and die within the following year (Osteoporosis Canada, 2017a). The cost of treating osteoporosis and related fractures is estimated to be $2.3 billion each year, but this cost increases to $3.9 billion as many of the fractures occur in individuals in long-term care facilities (Tarride, Hopkins, Leslie, et al., 2012).

Residents of long-term care facilities need special considerations as many are frail, suffer from dementia, and are at high risk for delirium. They have a fracture rate two to four times greater than that of similar-aged adults living in the community, and one-third of patients with hip fractures are long-term care residents (Papaioannou, Santesso, Morin, et al., 2015). They also have a 30% rate of moderate to severe vertebral fractures. Papaioannou, Santesso, Morin, et al. (2015) developed Fracture Prevention for Long-Term Care Residents, which includes osteoporosis prevention, assessment, and nutritional and drug therapy recommendations.

Secondary prevention through the development of Osteoporosis Canada's Fracture Liaison Services (FLS) and Fracture Registry has proven to decrease the number of subsequent fractures and decrease the associated economic burden to the health care system (Marsh, Akesson, Beaton, et al., 2011). The International Osteoporosis Foundation took the Osteoporosis Canada recommendations and developed a global campaign to facilitate and implement FLS (International Osteoporosis Foundation [IOF], 2015). The FLS is a world class, cost-effective model of postfracture care that ensures that patients over the age of 50 are assessed and treated for osteoporosis (Osteoporosis Canada, n.d.). Canada now has FLS material online, and several provinces have or are in the process of developing and implementing FLS.

Osteoporosis is more common in women than in men for several reasons: (1) women tend to have lower calcium intake than men (men between 15 and 50 years of age consume twice

DETERMINANTS OF HEALTH

Osteoporosis

Culture

- There is a higher risk for osteoporosis development in immigrants (especially Asian Canadians) due to differences in nutritional intake (i.e., less calcium, protein, iron).*

Gender

- One in three women and one in five men will develop an osteoporosis-related fracture in their lifetime.†
- Women and men begin to lose bone mass in their mid-thirties†. Women tend to lose bone at a younger age and faster pace than men.‡

Healthy Child Development

- Strong bone formation during childhood reduces the likelihood of osteoporosis in adulthood.†
- Optimal bone mass is developed during adolescence and early adulthood (ages 16–20 in females; ages 20–25 in males).†

References

*Sanou, D., O'Reilly, E., Ngnie-Teta, I., et al. (2014). Acculturation and nutritional health of immigrants in Canada: A scoping review. *Journal of Immigrant and Minority Health, 16*(1), 24–34. doi:10.1007/s10903-013-9823-7.

†Osteoporosis Canada. (2017). *Fast facts*. Retrieved from *https://osteoporosis .ca/about-the-disease/fast-facts/*.

‡Alswat, K. A. (2017). Gender disparities in Osteoporosis. *Journal of Clinical Medicine Research, 9*(5), 382–287.

TABLE 66-10 INDICATIONS FOR MEASURING BONE MINERAL DENSITY

Older Adults (Age ≥50 yr)	Younger Adults (Age <50 yr)
• Age ≥65 yr (both women and men)	• Fragility fracture
• Clinical risk factors for fracture (menopausal women, men age 50–64 yr)	• Prolonged use of glucocorticoids*
• Fragility fracture after age 40 yr	• Use of other high-risk medications†
• Prolonged use of glucocorticoids*	• Hypogonadism or premature menopause (age <45 yr)
• Use of other high-risk medications†	• Malabsorption syndrome
• Parental hip fracture	• Primary hyperparathyroidism
• Vertebral fracture or osteopenia identified on radiography	• Other disorders strongly associated with rapid bone loss, fracture, or both
• Current smoking	
• High alcohol intake	
• Low body weight (<60 kg) or major weight loss (>10% of body weight at age 25 yr)	
• Rheumatoid arthritis	
• Other disorders strongly associated with osteoporosis	

*At least 3 months cumulative therapy in the previous year at a prednisone-equivalent dose ≥7.5 mg daily.

†steoporosis Canada. (2017). Fast facts. Retrieved from https://osteoporosis.ca/about-the-disease/fast-facts/

Source: Papaioannou, A., Morin, S., Cheung, A. M., et al. (2010). 2010 clinical practice guidelines for the diagnosis and management of osteoporosis in Canada: Summary. *Canadian Medical Association Journal 182*(17), 1864–1873, Table 1, p. 1865. doi: 10.1503/cmaj.100771. Copied under licence from Access Copyright. Further reproduction, distribution or transmission is prohibited except as otherwise permitted by law.

as much calcium as women); (2) women have less bone mass because of their generally smaller frame; (3) bone resorption begins at an earlier age in women and is accelerated at menopause; (4) pregnancy and breastfeeding deplete a woman's skeletal reserve unless calcium intake is adequate; and (5) longevity increases the likelihood of osteoporosis, and women live longer than men. The "Determinants of Health" box lists other factors that contribute to risk for osteoporosis.

Etiology and Pathophysiology

Evaluation of assessment of osteoporosis has shifted from simply treating low bone mineral density to that of an integrated approach of patients with certain clinical factors at increased risk for a fragility fracture. As such, indications for measuring bone mineral density have shifted slightly, as shown in Table 66-10. Decreased risk is associated with regular weight-bearing exercise and calcium and vitamin D ingestion. Low testosterone levels are a risk factor in men.

Peak bone mass (maximum bone tissue) is mainly achieved before age 20 and is determined by a combination of four major factors: heredity, nutrition, exercise, and hormone function. Heredity may be responsible for up to 70% of a person's peak bone mass. Bone loss from midlife (age 35–40 years) onward is inevitable, but the rate of loss varies. At menopause, women experience rapid bone loss when the decline in estrogen production is the sharpest. This rate of loss then slows, and eventually matches the rate of bone lost by men at 65 to 70 years old.

Bone is continually being deposited by osteoblasts and resorbed by osteoclasts, a process called *remodelling*. Normally, the rates of bone deposition and resorption are equal to each other so that the total bone mass remains constant (Armas & Recker, 2012). In osteoporosis, bone resorption exceeds bone deposition. Although resorption affects the entire skeletal system, osteoporosis occurs most commonly in the bones of the spine, hips, and wrists. Over time, wedging and fractures of the vertebrae produce gradual loss of height and a humped back, known as *dowager's*

hump, or *kyphosis* (Figure 66-9). The usual first signs of osteoporosis are back pain or spontaneous fractures. The loss of bone substance causes the bone to become mechanically weakened and prone to either spontaneous fractures or fractures from minimal trauma. Specific diseases and conditions associated with osteoporosis include inflammatory bowel disease, intestinal malabsorption, kidney disease, rheumatoid arthritis, hyperthyroidism, chronic alcoholism, cirrhosis of the liver, hypogonadism, and diabetes mellitus.

Many drugs can interfere with bone metabolism, including corticosteroids, anticonvulsant drugs (e.g., phenytoin [Dilantin]), aluminum-containing antacids, heparin, certain cancer treatments, and excessive thyroid hormones. At the time a drug is prescribed, the patient should be informed of this possible adverse effect. Long-term corticosteroid use is a major contributor to osteoporosis. When a corticosteroid is taken, there is a disproportionate loss of bone, resulting from the inhibition of new bone formation.

Clinical Manifestations

Osteoporosis is often called the "silent disease" because bone loss occurs slowly, without symptoms. People may not know they have osteoporosis until their bones become so weak that a sudden strain, bump, or fall causes a hip, vertebra, or wrist fracture. Collapsed vertebrae may initially be manifested as back pain, loss of height, or spinal deformities such as kyphosis or severely stooped posture.

Diagnostic Studies

Osteoporosis often goes unnoticed because it cannot be detected by conventional radiography until more than 25% to 40% of calcium in the bone is lost. Serum calcium, phosphorus, and

FIGURE 66-9 The effects of osteoporosis. **A,** Comparison of a young woman with an older-adult woman. **B,** Severe fixed kyphosis, producing a question-mark appearance. Source: *A,* From Phillips, N. (2013). *Berry & Kohn's operating room technique.* (12th ed.). St. Louis: Mosby. *B,* Courtesy of Mir, M. A. In J. J. Kanski. (2006). *Clinical diagnosis in ophthalmology* (8th ed., p. 405, Figure 11.10). St. Louis: Mosby.

alkaline phosphatase levels usually are normal, although alkaline phosphatase may be elevated after a fracture.

Bone mineral density (BMD) measurements are typically used to measure bone density. BMD assesses the mass of bone per unit volume, or how tightly the bone is packed. (BMD measurements are presented in Chapter 64, Table 64-7.) Quantitative ultrasonography measures bone density with sound waves in the heel, kneecap, or shin. One of the most common BMD studies is dual-energy X-ray absorptiometry (DEXA), which measures bone density in the spine, hips, and forearm (the most common sites of fractures resulting from osteoporosis). DEXA studies are also useful to evaluate changes in bone density over time and to assess the effectiveness of treatment.

The World Health Organization (2007) released a fracture risk assessment system called FRAX. FRAX tools have been individualized by each country as fracture rates are different. FRAX calculates the 10-year risk for hip fracture and the 10-year risk for a major osteoporotic fracture (spine, forearm, hip, or shoulder). Osteoporosis Canada Best Practice Guidelines (Papaioannou, Morin, Cheung, et al., 2010) included the FRAX as a tool to assess for osteoporosis. The tool can be completed by the health care practitioner or the individual as it includes personal risk factors (e.g., smoking, fracture history) as well as bone mineral density at the hip.

DEXA results are frequently reported as T-scores. A T-score of −1 or higher indicates normal bone density. Osteoporosis is quantitatively defined as a BMD T-score at least 2.5 or more below the mean BMD of young adults. *Osteopenia* is defined as bone loss that is greater than normal (a T-score greater than a range of −1 to −2.5 standard deviations [SDs] below the mean), but not yet at the level for a diagnosis of osteoporosis. In addition to the BMD T-score, the patient's risk factors are included in determining a 10-year absolute fracture risk. This risk changes with advancing age and the development of new risk factors. Those patients with low risk are assessed in 5 to 10 years, whereas those with moderate risk are assessed in 1 to 5 years. Quantitative ultrasonography may be considered for fracture risk assessment when DEXA is not available, but it is not precise enough to be used for follow-up BMD testing.

TABLE 66-11	**COLLABORATIVE CARE**

Osteoporosis

Diagnostic
- History and physical examination
- Serum calcium, phosphorus, and alkaline phosphatase levels
- Bone mineral densitometry
- Dual-energy X-ray absorptiometry (DEXA)
- Quantitative ultrasonography (QUS)

Collaborative Therapy
- Diet high in calcium (see Table 66-12)

- Calcium supplements (see Table 66-13)
- Vitamin D supplements
- Exercise program
- Estrogen replacement therapy
- Bisphosphonates
  - Alendronate (Fosamax)
  - Etidronate
  - Risedronate (Actonel)
  - Zoledronic Acid (Aclasta)
- Selective estrogen receptor modulator (SERM)
  - Raloxifene (Evista)
- Teriparatide (Forteo)
- Salmon calcitonin (Calcimar)

NURSING AND COLLABORATIVE MANAGEMENT OSTEOPOROSIS

The reduced quality of life for those with osteoporosis can be enormous. Osteoporosis can result in disfigurement, lowered self-esteem, reduction in or loss of mobility, and decreased independence. Collaborative care of osteoporosis focuses on proper nutrition, calcium supplementation, exercise, prevention of fractures, and medications (Table 66-11). The National Osteoporosis Foundation (2014) recommends that women who are postmenopausal and men age 50 or older should be considered for treatment of osteoporosis if presenting with any of the following: (1) a hip or vertebral fracture; (2) a DEXA hip (femoral neck) or spine T-score of 1.0 to -2.5; or (3) a FRAX score of 3% or higher at the hip or 20% or higher at other sites.

Prevention and treatment of osteoporosis focus on adequate calcium intake (1 000 mg/day in women between the ages 19 and 50 and men between the ages 19 and 70; and 1 200 mg in women >50 years of age and men >70 years of age). If dietary intake of calcium is inadequate, supplemental calcium should be taken (Health Canada, 2012). Foods that are high in calcium content

TABLE 66-12   NUTRITIONAL THERAPY

Sources of Calcium

Food	Calcium (mg)
250 mL (1 cup) milk	
Whole	291
Low-fat	300
Skim	302
30 g (1 oz) cheese	
Processed	174
Cheddar	130
Cottage	130
Mozzarella	207
Parmesan	390
Swiss	272
250 mL (1 cup) yogourt	415
250 mL (1 cup) ice cream	
Hard	176
Soft-serve	272
90 g (3 oz) seafood	
Salmon	167
Sardines with bones	372
Shrimp	98
Oysters	113
1 medium stalk cooked broccoli	158
250 g (1 cup) cooked spinach	200
250 g (1 cup) almonds	304

TABLE 66-13   ELEMENTAL CALCIUM CONTENT OF VARIOUS ORAL CALCIUM PREPARATIONS

Calcium Preparation	Elemental Calcium Content
Calcium carbonate (Tums 500)	500 mg/tablet
Calcium carbonate + 5 mcg vitamin D2 (Os-Cal 250)	250 mg/tablet
Calcium gluconate	40 mg/500 mg
Calcium carbonate	400 mg/g
Calcium lactate	80 mg/600 mg
Calcium citrate	40 mg/300 mg

include whole and skim milk, yogourt, cottage cheese, ice cream, spinach, almonds, and sardines (Table 66-12). The amount of elemental calcium varies in different calcium preparations (Table 66-13). Calcium supplementation inhibits age-related bone loss; however, it does not stimulate the formation of new bone.

Vitamin D is important in calcium absorption and function and may have a role in bone formation. Most Canadians do not get enough vitamin D from their diet or naturally through synthesis in the skin from exposure to sunlight. Supplemental vitamin D, for all adults, year round, is recommended by Osteoporosis Canada (2017c). For adults who are healthy and between 19 and 50 years of age, 400–1000 IU of vitamin D daily are required. For adults over 50 years of age and for those younger adults at high risk (e.g., with osteoporosis, multiple fractures, or conditions affecting vitamin D absorption), 800–2000 IU daily is recommended (Osteoporosis Canada, 2017c).

Regular physical activity is important to build up and maintain bone mass. Exercise also increases muscle strength, coordination, and balance. The best exercises are weight-bearing exercises that force an individual to work against gravity. These include walking, hiking, weight training, stair climbing, tennis, and dancing. Walking is preferred to high-impact aerobics or running, both of which may put too much stress on the bones, resulting in stress fractures. Walking for 30 minutes, three times a week, is recommended.

Cigarette smoking and excess alcohol intake are risk factors for osteoporosis. Regular consumption of 60 to 90 mL of alcohol a day may increase the degree of osteoporosis, even in young men and women. Patients should be instructed to quit smoking and cut down on alcohol intake to decrease the likelihood of losing bone mass.

Although loss of bone cannot be significantly reversed, further loss can be prevented if the patient follows a regimen of calcium and vitamin D supplementation, exercise, estrogen replacement, and alendronate (Fosamax) or raloxifene (Evista), if indicated. Efforts should be made to keep patients with osteoporosis ambulatory to prevent further loss of bone substance as a result of immobility.

DRUG THERAPY

Hormone therapy should be considered as first-line therapy for preventing bone loss and fractures in early menopausal women who are symptomatic (e.g., have vasomotor, urogenital, and psychological symptoms). It is believed that estrogen inhibits osteoclast activity, leading to decreased bone resorption and preventing both cortical and trabecular bone loss. Estrogen therapy (for women who have had a hysterectomy) and estrogen–progesterone therapy (for women who have not had a hysterectomy) provide significant protection against osteoporotic fractures. Despite earlier concerns raised by a number of studies, it now seems that women who are younger and recently postmenopausal do not have an increased cardiovascular risk with estrogen or estrogen–progesterone therapy. Considering the risk–benefit profile of hormone therapy, the North American Menopause Society states that the extended use of hormone therapy is suitable for women at risk for osteoporotic fractures who also have moderate to severe menopausal symptoms. As with any drug therapy, doses and regimens must be individualized according to the patient's needs. (See Chapter 56 for further discussion of hormone therapy.)

Calcitonin is secreted by the thyroid gland and inhibits osteoclastic bone resorption by directly interacting with active osteoclasts. Salmon calcitonin (Calcimar) is available in intramuscular, subcutaneous, and intranasal forms. The nasal form is easy to administer, and patients should be taught to alternate nostrils daily. Nasal dryness and irritation are the most frequent adverse effects. Administration of the intramuscular or subcutaneous form of the drug at night has been shown to decrease the adverse effects of nausea and facial flushing. Nausea does not occur with the nasal spray. When calcitonin is used, calcium supplementation is necessary to prevent secondary hyperparathyroidism.

Bisphosphonates inhibit osteoclast-mediated bone resorption, thereby increasing BMD and total bone mass. This group of drugs has been shown to increase BMD by 5%. Common adverse effects are anorexia, weight loss, and gastritis. Effective osteoporosis treatment has been shown to reduce mortality in older adults and individuals who are frail and at high risk for a fracture. The most commonly used bisphosphonate drug in treating osteoporosis is alendronate (Fosamax). Patients should be instructed on the proper administration of alendronate to aid in its absorption. It should be taken with a full glass of water after rising in the morning. The patient should not eat or drink anything for 30 minutes after taking it. The patient should also be instructed not to lie down after taking the drug. These precautions have been shown to decrease gastro-intestinal adverse effects (especially esophageal irritation) and increase absorption. Alendronate is also available as a once-per-week oral tablet. Zoledronic acid (Aclasta) is approved for a once-yearly IV infusion and can prevent osteoporosis for 2 years after a single infusion. One potential adverse effect of bisphosphonates is atypical femur fractures and osteonecrosis of the jaw.

DRUG ALERT—Bisphosphonates

Patients should be instructed to do the following:
- Take with full glass of water
- Take 30 min before food or other medications
- Remain upright for at least 30 min after taking

Another type of drug used in treating osteoporosis is raloxifene (Evista), a selective estrogen receptor modulator. This drug mimics the effect of estrogen on bone by reducing bone resorption without stimulating the tissues of the breast or uterus. Raloxifene in women who are postmenopausal significantly increases BMD. The most commonly reported adverse effects are leg cramps, hot flashes, and blood clots. Raloxifine may decrease breast cancer risk. Similar to tamoxifen, it blocks the estrogen receptor sites of cancer sites.

Teriparatide (Forteo) is used for the treatment of osteoporosis in men and in women who are postmenopausal and at high risk for fractures. Teriparatide is a recombinant form of human parathyroid hormone and works by increasing the action of osteoblasts. It is the first drug approved for the treatment of osteoporosis that stimulates new bone formation. Most drugs used to treat osteoporosis prevent further bone loss. Teriparatide is administered by subcutaneous injection, once a day. Adverse effects include leg cramps and dizziness. Denosumab (Prolia) may be used for women with osteoporosis who are postmenopausal and at high risk for fractures. It is a monoclonal antibody that binds to a protein (RANKL) involved in the formation and function of osteoclasts. Denosumab is given as a subcutaneous injection every 6 months.

Current guidelines clearly advocate for pharmacological treatment in patients who are at high risk for fractures and are diagnosed with osteoporosis; however, there is no clear guidance about when treatment should be stopped (Lewiecki, Cummings, & Cosman, 2013).

Medical management of patients receiving corticosteroids includes prescribing the lowest possible dose of the drug as well as calcium and vitamin D supplementation. If osteopenia is evident on bone densitometry, treatment with bisphosphonate agents, such as alendronate (Fosamax), should be considered.

PAGET'S DISEASE

Paget's disease of the bone (*osteitis deformans*) is a chronic skeletal bone disorder in which there is excessive bone resorption followed by replacement of normal marrow by vascular, fibrous connective tissue. The new bone is larger, disorganized, and structurally weaker. The regions of the skeleton commonly affected are the pelvis, long bones, spine, ribs, sternum, and cranium. The etiology of Paget's disease is unknown, although there is evidence that the rate of Paget's disease is influenced by genetic and environmental factors (Singer, 2015). Up to 40% of all patients with Paget's disease have at least one relative with the disorder. Men are affected at a rate of 2 : 1 compared to women, and Paget's disease is rarely seen in people younger than 40 years. Viral

EVIDENCE-INFORMED PRACTICE

Translating Research Into Practice

Rita Farrouk is a 76-yr-old woman who fell in her home and sustained a hip fracture. Her recent laboratory work shows a vitamin D deficiency. The nurse discusses her options for improving this deficiency. She tells the nurse that she is moving to Arizona to be with her daughter and is planning to spend "many hours in the sun" every day.

Best Available Evidence	Clinician Expertise	Patient Preferences and Values
Women who are postmenopausal should receive 1 200 mg of calcium and 800 IU of vitamin D daily. Dietary sources and supplements should be used to meet these requirements.	The nurse has worked with many patients recovering from fractures related to osteoporosis. The nurse reviews Ms. Farrouk's usual diet and determines that it is deficient in calcium and vitamin D.	Patient prefers sun exposure over changing her diet (she is a vegetarian) or taking supplements.

Action and Decision

The nurse discusses the risks associated with daily sun exposure and points out that sun exposure will not correct a calcium deficiency. Ms. Farrouk tells the nurse she understands but wants to try before taking "any more pills." The nurse explains the importance of adding foods high in calcium to her diet. The nurse provides her with a list of some choices that meet her vegetarian diet restrictions.

Reference for Evidence

Statistics Canada. (2013). *Health at a glance—Vitamin D blood levels of Canadians*. Retrieved from *http://www.statcan.gc.ca/pub/82-624-x/2013001/article/11727-eng.htm*; Mangels, R. (2014). *Calcium in the vegan diet*. Retrieved from *http://www.vrg.org/nutrition/calcium.php*.

etiology remains controversial as no specific virus has been isolated thus far.

In milder forms of Paget's disease, patients may remain free of symptoms, and the disease may be discovered incidentally on radiography or serum chemistry. The initial clinical manifestations are usually insidious development of bone pain (which may progress to severe, intractable pain), fatigue, and progressive development of a waddling gait. Patients may complain that they are becoming shorter or that their heads are becoming larger. Headaches, dementia, visual deficits, and loss of hearing can result, with an enlarged, thickened skull. Increased bone volume in the spine can cause spinal cord or nerve root compression. Pathological fracture is the most common complication of Paget's disease and may be the first indication of the disease. Other complications include osteosarcoma, fibrosarcoma, and osteoclastoma (giant cell) tumours.

SAFETY ALERT

The risk for patient harm resulting from falls can be reduced as follows:
- Patients should be evaluated for fall risk.
- High-risk factors should be identified, including medications that increase risk for falls.
- Action should be taken to address any identified risks.
- Patients at risk should be encouraged to attend a fall-prevention class.

Serum alkaline phosphatase levels are markedly elevated (indicating high bone turnover) in advanced forms of the disease. Radiographs may demonstrate that the normal contour of the affected bone is curved and the bone cortex is thickened and irregular, especially the weight-bearing bones and cranium. Bone scans using a radiolabelled biphosphate demonstrate increased uptake in the skeletal areas affected.

Collaborative care of Paget's disease is usually limited to symptomatic and supportive care and correction of secondary deformities by either surgical intervention or braces. Bisphosphonate drugs are the preferred treatment in individuals at risk for pathological fracture(s) since bisphosphonates reduce bone turnover (Singer, Bone, Hosking, et al., 2014). Often, calcium and vitamin D are given to decrease hypocalcemia, a common adverse effect with these drugs. Drug effectiveness may be monitored by serum alkaline phosphatase levels.

Calcitonin therapy is recommended for patients who cannot tolerate bisphosphonate drugs. Human calcitonin inhibits osteoclastic activity, prevents bone resorption, relieves acute symptoms, and lowers the serum alkaline phosphatase levels. This drug is available as a subcutaneous injection. Salmon calcitonin can also be used as a subcutaneous or intramuscular injection for treating Paget's disease. Salmon calcitonin has a longer half-life and greater milligram potency than human calcitonin. Response to calcitonin therapy is not permanent and often stops when therapy is discontinued. Pain from Paget's disease is usually managed by NSAIDs or acetaminophen. Orthopaedic surgery for fractures, hip and knee replacements, and knee realignment may be necessary.

A firm mattress should be used to provide back support and to relieve pain. The patient may be required to wear a corset or light brace to relieve back pain and provide support when in the upright position. The patient should be proficient in the correct application of such devices and know how to regularly examine areas of the skin for friction damage. Activities such as lifting and twisting should be discouraged. Physiotherapy may increase muscle strength. Good body mechanics are essential. A properly balanced nutritional program is important in the management of metabolic disorders of bone, especially pertaining to vitamin D, calcium, and protein, which are necessary to ensure the availability of the components for bone formation. Prevention measures such as patient education, use of an assistive device, and environmental changes should be actively pursued to prevent falls and subsequent fractures.

AGE-RELATED CONSIDERATIONS

METABOLIC BONE DISEASES

Osteoporosis and Paget's disease are common in older adults. Patients should be instructed in proper nutritional management to prevent further bone loss such as that occurring from osteoporosis.

Since metabolic bone disorders increase the possibility of pathological fractures, extreme caution should be used when turning or moving the patient. Hip fractures in particular can adversely affect quality of life and may lead to admission to a long-term care facility. It is important to keep the patient as active as possible to slow demineralization of bone resulting from disuse or extended immobilization. A supervised exercise program is an essential part of the treatment program. If the patient's condition permits, ambulation without causing fatigue must be encouraged.

Protection from falls is paramount for prevention of osteoporotic fracture among older adults. Osteoporosis-related fractures cause considerable morbidity and an enormous financial burden through the use of health services. In Canada, 1 in 3 older adults will experience a fall each year, and half of those will fall more than once. Falls are the leading cause of injury among older Canadians and the cause of 95% of all hip fractures; also, 85% of falls are the cause of injury-related hospitalizations (Public Health Agency of Canada [PHAC], 2015). The frequency of falls increases dramatically with age, with women being more likely to fall than men.

Medical conditions, medications, and environmental factors have been implicated as predisposing factors to injurious falls among older adults. Best practice guidelines (Registered Nurses' Association of Ontario [RNAO], 2017) should be implemented to prevent falls and fall injuries in older adults, who may already have bone mass below the threshold for fracture. Fall prevention could have a significant impact on the incidence of fracture in this susceptible population.

CASE STUDY

Osteoporosis

Source: Blaj Gabriel/
Shutterstock.com.

Patient Profile

Antonija Roncevic is a 56-year-old retired librarian who had a total hysterectomy and salpingo-oophorectomy for removal of a benign ovarian cyst, 4 years ago. She also has a history of a seizure disorder since childhood, and Addison's disease.

Subjective Data

- Acute, severe lumbar pain and tenderness that radiate to her right hip and lateral thigh after falling and landing on her buttocks last week
- Walking and bending increases pain
- Stress fracture in wrist 6 months ago
- Reports no noticeable loss of height
- Maternal history of osteoporosis
- Taking corticosteroids and mineralocorticoids for past 6 years for Addison's disease
- Taking phenytoin (Dilantin) every evening
- Drinks two alcoholic beverages every evening
- Dislikes dairy products

Objective Data

- 167 cm tall, 72 kg

Diagnostic Studies

- Bone mass measurement tests show decreased bone mineral density at spine and hip
- Lumbar spine radiographs reveal a slightly displaced L4 compression fracture
- Normal serum calcium, phosphorus, and alkaline phosphatase levels

Collaborative Care

- L4 vertebroplasty
- Thoraco-lumbar-sacral orthosis (TLSO) brace postoperatively
- Alendronate (Fosamax) 70 mg once weekly PO
- Total calcium intake of 1 200 mg/day PO (supplement + dietary intake)
- High-calcium diet
- Reduction in alcohol intake
- Regular, low-impact weight-bearing exercise program

Continued

CASE STUDY

Osteoporosis—cont'd

Discussion Questions

1. What factors place Ms. Roncevic at risk of developing osteoporosis?
2. Why does walking and bending increase Ms. Roncevic's pain?
3. What is the purpose of the TLSO brace prescribed for Ms. Roncevic?
4. *Priority decision:* What are the priority teaching needs for Ms. Roncevic?
5. How might the nurse assist Ms. Roncevic in increasing her intake of calcium?
6. Why would regular exercise be important for Ms. Roncevic?

7. *Priority decision:* Based on the assessment data presented, what are the priority nursing diagnoses? Are there any collaborative problems?
8. *Evidence-informed practice:* Ms. Roncevic asks why taking corticosteroids increases her risk of developing osteoporosis. How should the nurse respond to her?

⊝volve

Answers are available at *http://evolve.elsevier.com/Canada/Lewis/medsurg.*

REVIEW QUESTIONS

The number of the question corresponds to the same-numbered objective at the beginning of the chapter.

1. A client with osteomyelitis is treated with surgical debridement with implantation of antibiotic beads. When the client asks why the beads are used, what should the nurse answer? *Select all that apply.*
   a. "The beads are used to directly deliver antibiotics to the area of the infection."
   b. "There are no effective oral or IV antibiotics to treat most cases of bone infection."
   c. "This is the safest method of delivering long-term antibiotic therapy for a bone infection."
   d. "The beads are used for deep infections in addition to removing the damaged tissue and oral and IV antibiotics."
   e. "The lack of blood flow and bone death that occur with osteomyelitis make IV antibiotics less effective."

2. A client has been diagnosed with osteosarcoma of the humerus. Which of the following statements would indicate that he has an understanding of his treatment options?
   a. "I accept that I have to lose my arm with surgery."
   b. "The chemotherapy before surgery will shrink the tumour."
   c. "This tumour is related to the melanoma I had 3 years ago."
   d. "I'm glad they can take out the cancer with such a small scar."

3. Which of the following individuals does the nurse identify as being high risk for low back pain? *Select all that apply.*
   a. A 63-year-old man who is a long-distance truck driver
   b. A 36-year-old construction worker who is 190 cm tall and weighs 118 kg
   c. A 28-year-old female yoga instructor who is 170 cm tall and weighs 59 kg
   d. A 30-year-old male nurse who works on an orthopaedic unit and smokes
   e. A 44-year-old female chef with prior compression fracture of the spine

4. What is the primary nursing responsibility in caring for a client with a suspected disc herniation who is experiencing acute pain and muscle spasms?
   a. Encourage total bed rest for several days.
   b. Teach the principles of back strengthening exercises.
   c. Stress the importance of straight-leg raises to decrease pain.
   d. Promote the use of cold and hot compresses and pain medication.

5. When caring for a client after a spinal fusion, which of the following symptoms would the nurse immediately report to the physician?
   a. The client experiences a single episode of emesis.
   b. The client is unable to move the lower extremities.
   c. The client is nauseated and has not voided in 4 hours.
   d. The client complains of pain at the bone graft donor site.

6. What instructions should the nurse give the client who is being discharged from same-day surgery after surgical correction of bilateral hallux valgus?
   a. Rest frequently, with the feet elevated.
   b. Soak the feet in warm water several times a day.
   c. Expect the feet to be numb for several days postoperatively.
   d. Expect continued pain in the feet, since this is not uncommon.

7. The nurse is teaching a client with osteopenia. What is important to include in the teaching plan?
   a. Lose weight.
   b. Stop smoking.
   c. Eat a high-protein diet.
   d. Start swimming for exercise.

1.a,d, 2. b, 3. a, b, d, e, 4. d, 5. b, 6. a, 7. b.

⊝volve

For even more review questions, visit *http://evolve.elsevier.com/Canada/Lewis/medsurg.*

REFERENCES

Aly, T. A., Mousa, W., & Elsallakh, S. (2011). Evaluation of scarf osteotomy for management of hallux valgus deformity. *Orthopaedics, 34*(2), 95. doi:10.3928/01477447-20101221-08.

Armas, L., & Recker, R. (2012). Pathophysiology of osteoporosis. *Endocrinology and Metabolism Clinics of North America, 41*(3), 475–486. doi:10.1016/j.ecl2012.04.006.

Bath, B., Trask, C., McCrosky, J., et al. (2014). Demographic and health characteristics of rural- and urban-dwelling Canadians with chronic back disorders. *Spine, 39*(23), 1960–1968. doi:10.1097/BRS.0000000000000561.

Bone and Joint Canada. (2014). *Low back pain.* Retrieved from *http://boneandjointcanada.com/low-back-pain/*

Burchurn, J., & Rosenthal, L. (2015). *Lehne's Pharmacology for Nursing Care* (9th ed.). Philadelphia: Saunders.

Canadian Cancer Society's Advisory Committee on Cancer Statistics (2015). *Canadian Cancer Statistics 2015.* Toronto, ON: Canadian Cancer Society. Retrieved from *http://www.cancer.ca/en/cancer-information/cancer-101/canadian-cancer-statistics-publication/?region=on.*

Cepoiu-Martin, M., Faris, P., Lorenzetti, D., et al. (2011). Artificial cervical disc arthroplasty: A systemic review. *Spine, 36*(25), 1623–1633. doi:10.1097/BRS.0b013e3182163814.

Chen, L., & Wen, Y. (2011). The role of bacterial biofilm in persistent infections and control strategies. *Int J Oral Sci, 3*(2), 66–73. doi:10.4248/IJOS11022.

Chou, R., Qaseem, A., Owens, D. K., et al. (2011). Diagnostic imaging for lower back pain: Advice for high value health care from the American College of Physicians. *Annals of Internal Medicine, 154*(3), 181–189. doi:10.7326/0003-4819-154-3-201102010-00008.

Deyo, R., Ching, A., Matsen, L., et al. (2012). Use of bone morphogenetic proteins in spinal fusion surgery for older adults with lumbar stenosis. *Spine, 37*(3), 222–230. doi:10.1097/BRS.0b013e31821bfa3a.

European Sarcoma Network Working Group (ESMO). (2012). Bone sarcomas: ESMO clinical practice guidelines for diagnosis, treatment and follow-up. *Annals of Oncology, 23*(7), vii100–vii109. doi:10.1093/annonc/mds254.

Hakim, D. N., Pelly, T., Kulendran, M., et al. (2015). Benign tumors of the bone: A review. *J Bone Oncol, 4*, 37–41. doi:10.1016/j.jbo.2015.02.001.

Hayden, J., van Tulder, M. W., Malmivaara, A., et al. (2011). Exercise therapy for treatment of non-specific low back pain. *The Cochrane Database of Systematic Reviews*, (3), CD000335, doi:10.1002/14651858.CD000335.pub2.

Health Canada. (2012). *Vitamin D and calcium: Updated dietary reference intakes.* Retrieved from *http://www.hc-sc.gc.ca/fn-an/nutrition/vitamin/vita-d-eng.php.*

Hellum, C., Johnsen, L. G., Storheim, K., et al. (2011). Surgery with disc prosthesis versus rehabilitation in patients with low back pain and degenerative disc: Two-year follow-up of randomised study. *British Medical Journal, 342.* doi:10.1136/bmj.d2786. Retrieved from *http://www.bmj.com/content/342/bmj.d2786.*

International Osteoporosis Foundation. (IOF). (2015). *Capture the fracture.* Retrieved from *http://www.iofbonehealth.org/capture-fracture.*

Kaye, A. D., Manchikanti, L., Abdi, S., et al. (2015). Efficacy of epidural injections in managing chronic spinal pain: A best evidence synthesis. *Pain Physician, 18*, E939–E1004.

Khodabukus, A. F., Debattista, M., Reynolds, J., et al. (2015). *Guidelines for the prevention of pathological fractures in palliative care.* Cheshire & Merseyside Palliative & End of Life Care Strategic Clinical Network. Retrieved from: *www.cmscnsenate.nhs.uk/files/2514/2789/9749/Guidelines_for_the_Prevention_of_Pathological_Fracture_in_Palliative_Care_Final_March_30_2015.pdf.*

Lewiecki, E. M., Cummings, S. R., & Cosman, F. (2013). Treat-to-target for osteoporosis: Is now the time? *Journal of Clinical Endocrinology and Metabolism, 98*(3), 946–953. doi:10.1210/jc2012-3680.

Lima, A. L. L., Oliveira, P. R., Carvalho, V. C., et al. (2014). Recommendations for the treatment of osteomyelitis. *The Brazilian Journal of Infectious Diseases, 18*(5), 526–534. doi:10.1016/j.bjid.2013.12.005.

Marsh, D., Akesson, K., Beaton, D. E., et al. (2011). Coordinator-based systems for secondary prevention in fragility fracture patients. *Osteoporosis International, 22*(7), 2051–2065. doi:10.1007/s00198-011-1642-x.

Matteson, E., & Osmon, D. (2016). Infections of the bursae, joints, and bones. In L. Goldman & A. Schafer (Eds.), *Goldman: Goldman–Cecil Medicine* (25th ed.). Philadelphia: Saunders.

Monczewski, L. (2013). Managing bone metastasis in the patient with advanced cancer. *Orthopaedic Nursing, 32*(4), 209–214. doi:10.1097/NOR.0b013e31829a4da3.

National Institute of Neurological Disorders and Stroke (NINDS). (2014). *Low back pain fact sheet.* Retrieved from *http://www.ninds.nih.gov/disorders/backpain/detail_backpain.htm.*

National Osteoporosis Foundation. (NOF). (2014). *NOF Clinician's guide to prevention and treatment of osteoporosis.* Retrieved from *https://my.nof.org/bone-soruce/education/clinicians-guide-to-the-prevention-and-treatment-of-osteoporosis.*

Nicholas, M. K., & George, S. Z. (2011). Psychologically informed interventions for low back pain: An update for physical therapists. *Physical Therapy, 91*(5), 765–776. doi:10.2522/ptj.20100278.

Osteoporosis Canada. (n.d.). *Fracture liaison service (FLS).* Retrieved from *http://fls.osteoporosis.ca/what-is-fls/.*

Osteoporosis Canada. (2017a). *About the disease.* Retrieved from *https://osteoporosis.ca/about-the-disease/.*

Osteoporosis Canada. (2017b). *Fast facts.* Retrieved from *https://osteoporosis.ca/about-the-disease/fast-facts/.*

Osteoporosis Canada. (2017c). *Calcium and vitamin D.* Retrieved from *https://osteoporosis.ca/bone-health-osteoporosis/calcium-and-vitamin-d/.*

Papaioannou, A., Morin, S., Cheung, A. M., et al. (2010). 2010 clinical practice guidelines for the diagnosis and management of osteoporosis in Canada: Summary. *Canadian Medical Association Journal, 182*(17), 1864–1873. doi:10.1503/cmaj.100771.

Papaioannou, A., Santesso, N., Morin, S. N., et al. (2015). Recommendations for preventing fracture in long-term care. *Canadian Medical Association Journal, 187*(15), 1135–1144. doi:10.1503/cmaj.141331.

Potratz, J., Dirksen, U., Jürgens, H., et al. (2012). Ewing sarcoma: Clinical state-of-the-art. *Pediatric Hematology and Oncology, 29*(1), 1–11. doi:10.3109/08880018.2011.622034.

Public Health Agency of Canada (PHAC). (2015). *You CAN prevent falls!* Retrieved from *http://www.phac-aspc.gc.ca/seniors-aines/alt-formats/pdf/publications/public/injury-blessure/prevent-eviter/prevent-eviter-e.pdf.*

Registered Nurses' Association of Ontario (RNAO). (2017). *Preventing falls and reducing injury from falls* (3rd ed.). Clinical Best Practice Guideline. Toronto: Author. Retrieved from *http://rnao.ca/bpg/guidelines/prevention-falls-and-fall-injuries.*

Sanchez, C. J., Jr., Mende, K., Beckius, M. L., et al. (2013). Biofilm formation by clinical isolates and the implications in chronic infections. *BMC Infectious Diseases, 13*(47), doi:10.1186/1471-2334-13-47.

Simon, J., McAuliffe, M., Shamim, F., et al. (2014). Discogenic low back pain. *Physical Medicine and Rehabilitation Clinics of North America, 25*(2), 305–317.

Singer, F. R. (2015). Paget's disease of bone—genetic and environmental factors. *Nature Reviews. Endocrinology, 11*(11), 662–671. doi:10.1038/nrendo.2015.138.

Singer, F. R., Bone, H. G., Hosking, D. J., et al. (2014). Paget's disease of bone: An Endocrine Society clinical practice guideline. *The Journal of Clinical Endocrinology and Metabolism, 99*(12), 4408–4422. doi:10.1210/jc.2014-2910.

Stolt, M., Suhonen, R., Puukka, P., et al. (2012). Foot health and self-care activities of older people in home care. *Journal of Clinical Nursing, 21*(1), 3082–3095. doi:10.1111/j.1365-2702.2012.04223.x.

Tarride, J. E., Hopkins, R. B., Leslie, W. D., et al. (2012). The burden of illness of osteoporosis in Canada. *Osteoporosis International, 23*(11), 2591–2600.

Terry Fox Foundation. (2015). *Terry Fox and the Foundation.* Retrieved from *http://www.terryfox.org/TerryFox/.*

Turns, M. (2012). The diabetic foot: An overview for community nurses. *British Journal of Community Nursing, 17*(9), 422, 424–427, 430–433. doi:10.12968/bjcn.2012.17.9.422.

Walter, G., Kemmerer, M., Kappler, C., et al. (2012). Treatment algorithms for chronic osteomyelitis. *Deutsches Ärzteblatt International, 109*(14), 257–264. doi:10.3238/arztebl.2012.0257.

World Health Organization. (WHO). (2007). *WHO scientific group on the assessment of osteoporosis at primary health care level.* Retrieved from: *www.who.int/chp/topics/Osteoporosis.pdf.* (Seminal).

Yassi, A., & Lockhart, K. (2013). Work-relatedness of low back pain in nursing personnel: A systematic review. *International Journal of Occupational and Environmental Health, 19*(3), 223–244. doi: 10.1179/2049396713Y.0000000027.

RESOURCES

Canadian Academy of Exercise and Sport Medicine
http://www.casm-acms.org

Canadian Cancer Society—National Office
http://www.cancer.ca/

Canadian Centre for Occupational Health and Safety
http://www.ccohs.ca

The Canadian Orthopaedic Association
http://www.coa-aco.org

The Canadian Orthopaedic Foot & Ankle Society
http://www.coa-aco.org/cofas/cofas-main

Canadian Orthopaedic Nurses Association
http://www.cona-nurse.org/

Canadian Podiatric Medical Association
http://www.podiatrycanada.org

Easter Seals Canada
http://www.easterseals.ca

International Osteoporosis Foundation: Capture the Fracture
www.capturethefracture.org

Osteoporosis Canada
http://www.osteoporosis.ca

National Association of Orthopaedic Nurses (NAON)
http://www.orthonurse.org

NIH Osteoporosis and Related Bone Diseases—National Resource Center
http://www.niams.nih.gov/Health_Info/Bone

Older Women's League
http://www.owl-national.org

For additional Internet resources, see the website for this book at *http://evolve.elsevier.com/Canada/Lewis/medsurg.*

Nursing Management

Arthritis and Connective Tissue Diseases

Written by: Dottie Roberts
Adapted by: Erica Cambly

evolve WEBSITE

http://evolve.elsevier.com/Canada/Lewis/medsurg

- Review Questions
  (Online Only)
- Key Points
- Student Case Studies
  - Obesity and Osteoarthritis
  - Rheumatoid Arthritis
  - Systemic Lupus Erythematosus

- Customizable Nursing Care Plans
  - Rheumatoid Arthritis
  - Systemic Lupus Erythematosus
- Conceptual Care Map Creator
  - Conceptual Care Map for Textbook Case Study
- Audio Glossary
- Content Updates

LEARNING OBJECTIVES

1. Compare and contrast the sequence of events leading to joint destruction in osteoarthritis and rheumatoid arthritis.
2. Detail the clinical manifestations, collaborative care, and nursing management of osteoarthritis and rheumatoid arthritis.
3. Describe the pathophysiology, clinical manifestations, and collaborative care of gout, Lyme disease, and septic arthritis.
4. Summarize the pathophysiology, clinical manifestations, collaborative care, and nursing management of ankylosing spondylitis, psoriatic arthritis, and reactive arthritis.

5. Differentiate the pathophysiology, clinical manifestations, collaborative care, and nursing management of systemic lupus erythematosus, scleroderma, polymyositis, dermatomyositis, and Sjögren syndrome.
6. Explain the drug therapy and related nursing management associated with arthritis and connective tissue diseases.
7. Compare and contrast the possible etiologies, clinical manifestations, collaborative care, and nursing management of fibromyalgia and systemic exertion tolerance disease.

KEY TERMS

ankylosing spondylitis (AS),
    p. 1710
arthritis, p. 1691
CREST, p. 1717
dermatomyositis, p. 1719
fibromyalgia syndrome (FMS),
    p. 1721

gout, p. 1707
Lyme disease, p. 1709
myofascial pain syndrome,
    p. 1720
osteoarthritis (OA), p. 1691
polymyositis, p. 1719
psoriatic arthritis, p. 1711

Raynaud's phenomenon,
    p. 1717
rheumatoid arthritis (RA),
    p. 1700
scleroderma, p. 1717
septic arthritis, p. 1710
Sjögren syndrome, p. 1720

spondyloarthropathies,
    p. 1710
systemic exertion intolerance
    disease (SEID), p. 1722
systemic lupus erythematosus
    (SLE), p. 1712

This chapter discusses *rheumatic diseases*, which primarily affect body joints, tendons, ligaments, muscles, and bones. These diseases are often characterized by inflammation. Rheumatic diseases result from the loss of function in one or more of the connective or bone structures of the body. There are more than 100 kinds of rheumatic diseases, affecting millions of Canadians.

ARTHRITIS

Arthritis, a type of rheumatic disease, involves inflammation of a joint or joints. Most forms of arthritis affect women more frequently than men (Arthritis Society, 2017a). The most common types of arthritis are osteoarthritis, rheumatoid arthritis, and gout.

OSTEOARTHRITIS

Osteoarthritis (OA), the most common form of joint (articular) disease in North America, is a slowly progressive noninflammatory disorder of the diarthrodial (synovial) joints. Currently, more than 3 million Canadians are affected by OA, and the numbers are expected to increase greatly as the population ages (Arthritis Society, 2017b).

Etiology and Pathophysiology

OA involves the formation of new joint tissue in response to cartilage destruction (Sovani & Grogan, 2013). OA is not considered a normal part of the aging process, but aging is one risk factor for disease development (Arthritis Society, 2017b). Cartilage destruction may begin between ages 20 and 30 and the majority of adults are affected by age 40. Few patients experience symptoms until after age 50 or 60, but more than half of those older than 65 years have radiographic evidence of the disease in at least one joint. Women are affected by OA more often than men (Arthritis Society, 2017b).

OA is usually caused by a known event or condition that directly damages cartilage or causes joint instability (Table 67-1). The increased incidence of OA in older-adult women is believed to be due to estrogen reduction at menopause. Modifiable risk factors for OA have been identified, including obesity, which contributes to hip and knee OA. Regular moderate exercise, which also helps with weight control, has been shown to decrease the likelihood of disease development and progression. Anterior cruciate ligament injury, which is associated with quick stops and pivoting as in football and soccer, has been linked to an increased risk for knee OA (Sovani & Grogan, 2013). Occupations that require frequent kneeling and stooping are also linked to a higher risk for knee OA.

The pathogenesis of OA is complex, with genetic, metabolic, and local factors that interact and cause a process of cartilage deterioration. OA results from cartilage damage that triggers a metabolic response at the level of the chondrocytes (Figure 67-1). Progression of OA causes the normally smooth, white, translucent articular cartilage to become dull, yellow, and granular. Affected cartilage gradually becomes softer, less elastic, and less able to resist wear with heavy use.

The body's attempts at cartilage repair cannot keep up with the destruction that is occurring. Continued changes in the collagen structure of the cartilage lead to fissuring and erosion of the articular surfaces. As the central cartilage becomes thinner, cartilage and bony growth *(osteophytes)* increase at the joint margins. The resulting incongruity in joint surfaces creates an uneven distribution of stress across the joint and contributes to a reduction in motion.

Although inflammation is not characteristic of OA, a secondary synovitis may result when phagocytic cells try to rid the joint of small pieces of cartilage torn from the joint surface. These inflammatory changes contribute to the pain and stiffness of early OA. The pain of later disease results from contact between exposed bony joint surfaces after the articular cartilage has deteriorated completely.

Clinical Manifestations

Systemic. Systemic manifestations, such as fatigue, fever, and organ involvement, are not present in OA. This is an important distinction between OA and inflammatory joint disorders such as rheumatoid arthritis.

Joints. Manifestations of OA range from mild discomfort to significant disability. Joint pain is the predominant symptom and the typical reason that affected patients seek medical attention. Pain generally worsens with joint use. In the early stages of OA, joint pain is relieved by rest. However, in advanced disease, patients may complain of pain with rest or experience sleep disruptions caused by increasing joint discomfort. Pain may also become worse as the barometric pressure falls before inclement weather. As OA progresses, increasing pain can contribute significantly to disability and loss of function. The pain of OA may be referred to the groin, the buttock, or the medial side of the thigh or knee. Sitting down becomes difficult, as does rising from a chair when the hips are lower than the knees. As OA develops in the intervertebral (apophyseal) joints of the spine, localized pain and stiffness are common.

Unlike pain, which is typically provoked by activity, joint stiffness occurs after periods of rest or static position. Early morning stiffness is common but generally resolves within 30 minutes, a factor distinguishing OA from inflammatory arthritic disorders such as rheumatoid arthritis. Overactivity can cause a mild joint effusion that temporarily increases stiffness. *Crepitation,* a grating sensation caused by loose particles of cartilage in the joint cavity, can also contribute to stiffness. Crepitation is a common sign in patients with knee OA.

OA usually affects joints asymmetrically. The most commonly involved joints are the distal interphalangeal (DIP) and proximal interphalangeal (PIP) joints of the fingers, the metacarpophalangeal (MCP) joint of the thumb, weight-bearing joints (hips, knees), the metatarso-phalangeal (MTP) joint of the foot, and the cervical and lower lumbar vertebrae (Figure 67-2).

Deformity. Deformity or instability associated with OA is specific to the involved joint. For example, *Heberden nodes* occur on the DIP joints as an indication of osteophyte formation and loss of joint space (see Figure 67-1). They can appear in patients with OA as early as age 40 and tend to be seen in family members. *Bouchard nodes* on the PIP joints indicate similar disease involvement. Heberden and Bouchard nodes are often red, swollen, and tender. Although these bony enlargements do not usually cause significant loss of function, patients may be distressed by the visible disfigurement.

Knee OA often leads to joint malalignment as a result of cartilage loss in the medial compartment. Affected patients have a characteristic bow-legged appearance, and may develop an altered gait in response to the obvious deformity. In advanced

TABLE 67-1	CAUSES OF OSTEOARTHRITIS
Cause	**Effects on Joint Cartilage**
Drugs	Drugs such as indomethacin, colchicine, and corticosteroids can stimulate collagen-digesting enzymes in joint synovium.
Hematological or endocrine disorders	Chronic hemarthrosis (e.g., hemophilia) can contribute to cartilage deterioration.
Inflammation	Release of enzymes in response to local inflammation can affect cartilage integrity.
Joint instability	Damage to supporting structures causes instability, placing uneven stress on articular cartilage.
Mechanical stress	Repetitive physical activities (e.g., sports) cause cartilage deterioration.
Neurological disorders	Pain and loss of reflexes from neurological disorders, such as diabetic neuropathy, and in Charcot's joint cause abnormal movements that contribute to cartilage deterioration.
Skeletal deformities	Congenital or acquired conditions such as Legg–Calvé–Perthes disease or dislocated hip contribute to cartilage deterioration.
Trauma	Dislocations or fractures may lead to avascular necrosis or uneven stress on cartilage.

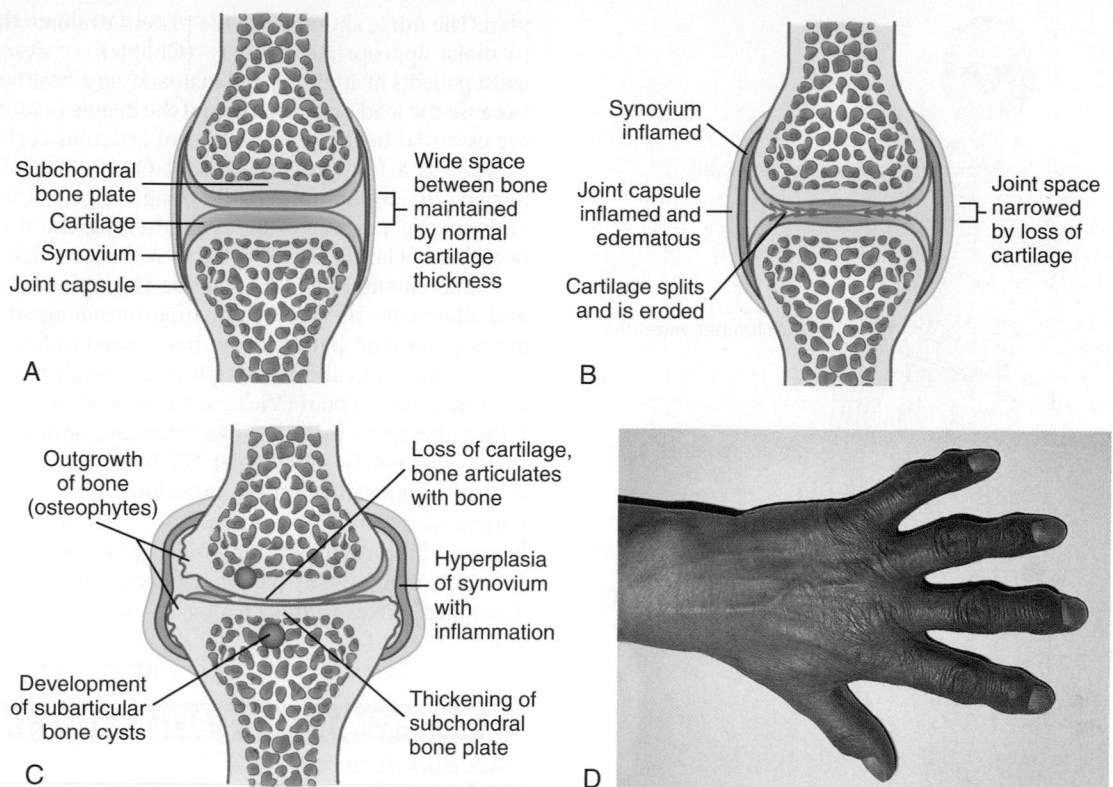

FIGURE 67-1 Pathological changes in osteoarthritis. **A,** Normal synovial joint. **B,** Early change in osteoarthritis is destruction of articular cartilage and narrowing of the joint space. Inflammation and thickening of the joint capsule and synovium occur. **C,** With time, thickening of subarticular bone is caused by constant friction of the two bone surfaces. Osteophytes form around the periphery of the joint by irregular outgrowths of bone. **D,** In osteoarthritis of the hands, osteophytes on the interphalangeal joints of the fingers, termed *Heberden nodes,* appear as small nodules. Source: **D,** Stevens, A., & Lowe, J. (2000). *Pathology: Illustrated review in colour* (2nd ed.). London: Mosby.

hip OA, one of the patient's legs may become shorter as a result of a loss of joint space.

Diagnostic Studies

A bone scan, computed tomographic (CT) scan, or magnetic resonance imaging (MRI) may be useful for diagnosing OA because of the sensitivity of these tests in detecting early joint changes. Radiological studies are helpful in confirming disease and staging the progression of joint damage. As OA progresses, radiographs typically show joint space narrowing, bony sclerosis, and osteophyte formation. However, these changes do not always correlate with the degree of pain that the patient experiences. Despite significant radiological indications of disease, patients may be relatively free of symptoms. Conversely, other patients may have severe pain with only minimal radiographic changes.

No laboratory abnormalities or biomarkers have been identified that are specific diagnostic indicators of OA. The erythrocyte sedimentation rate (ESR) is normal except in instances of acute synovitis, when minimal elevations may be noted. Other routine blood tests (e.g., complete blood cell count [CBC], kidney and liver function tests) are useful only in screening for related conditions or for establishing baseline values before the initiation of therapy. Synovial fluid analysis allows differentiation between OA and other forms of inflammatory arthritis. In OA, the fluid remains clear yellow with little or no sign of inflammation.

Collaborative Care

Because OA has no cure, collaborative care focuses on managing pain and inflammation, preventing disability, and maintaining and improving joint function (Table 67-2). Nonpharmacological interventions are the foundation for OA management and should be maintained throughout a patient's treatment period. Drug therapy serves as an adjunct to nonpharmacological treatments.

Rest and Joint Protection. The patient with OA must understand the importance of a balance between rest and activity. The affected joint(s) should be rested during any periods of acute inflammation and maintained in a functional position with splints or braces if necessary. However, immobilization should not exceed 1 week because of the risk for joint stiffness with inactivity. Patients may need to modify their usual activities to decrease stress on affected joints. Teach patients with knee OA to avoid prolonged periods of standing, kneeling, or squatting. Using an assistive device such as a cane, walker, or crutches can also help decrease stress on arthritic joints.

Heat and Cold Applications. Applications of heat and cold may help reduce complaints of pain and stiffness. Although ice is not used as often as heat in the treatment of OA, it can be appropriate if patients experience acute inflammation. Heat therapy—including hot packs, whirlpool baths, ultrasound, and paraffin wax baths—is especially helpful for stiffness.

Nutritional Therapy and Exercise. If a patient is overweight, a weight-reduction program is a critical part of the total treatment

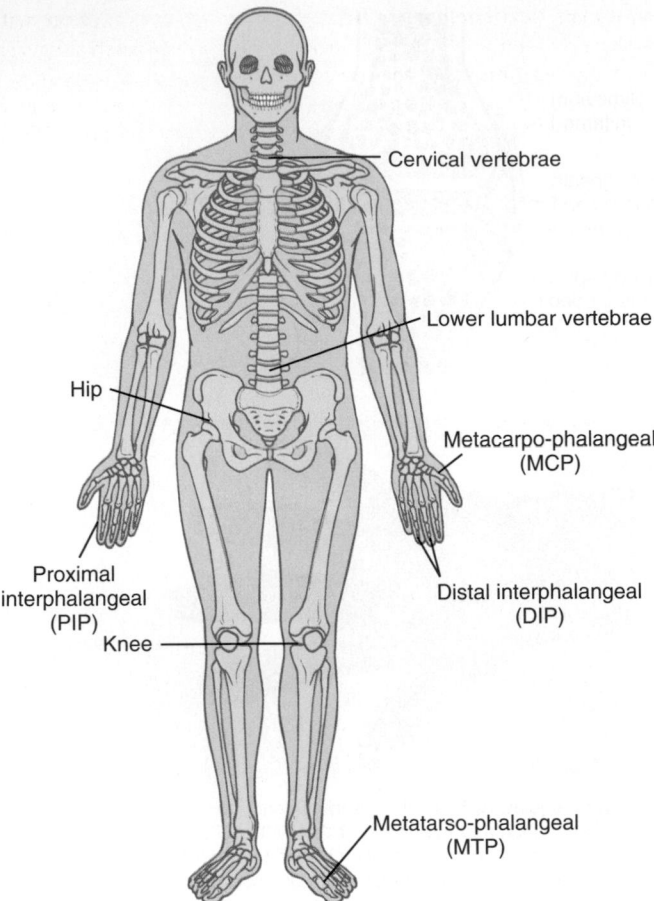

Cervical vertebrae

Lower lumbar vertebrae

Hip

Metacarpo-phalangeal
(MCP)

Proximal
interphalangeal
(PIP)

Distal interphalangeal
(DIP)

Knee

Metatarso-phalangeal
(MTP)

FIGURE 67-2 Joints most frequently involved in osteoarthritis.

plan. The nurse should help the patient evaluate the current diet to make appropriate changes. (Chapter 42 describes ways to assist patients in attaining and maintaining a healthy body weight.) Because the load on the joints and the degree of joint mobilization are essential to the preservation of articular cartilage integrity, exercise is a fundamental part of OA management (Arthritis Society, 2017b). Aerobic conditioning, range-of-motion exercises, and specific programs for strengthening the quadriceps have been beneficial for many patients with knee OA.

Complementary and Alternative Therapies. Complementary and alternative therapies for symptom management of arthritis are popular with patients who have failed to find relief through traditional medical care. Acupuncture is effective in decreasing chronic arthritis pain (Vickers, Cronin, Maschino, et al., 2012). Other therapies include yoga, massage, guided imagery, and therapeutic touch (see Chapter 12). Nutritional supplements such as glucosamine and chondroitin sulphate may be helpful in some patients for relieving moderate to severe arthritis pain in the knees and improving joint mobility (Hochberg, Martel-Pelletier, Monfort, et al., 2016) (see the "Complementary & Alternative Therapies" boxes in this chapter).

COMPLEMENTARY & ALTERNATIVE THERAPIES

Acupuncture

Acupuncture is a traditional Chinese medical practice of inserting very fine needles into the skin to stimulate specific anatomical points in the body (called *acupoints*) for therapeutic purposes.

Scientific Evidence*
The evidence is moderately strong for reducing chronic pain from osteoarthritis; chronic headache; and back, neck, and shoulder pain.

Nursing Implications
- Acupuncture is an effective treatment to suggest to patients with chronic pain.
- Refer interested patients to a practitioner who is appropriately trained and licensed (see Chapter 12).

*Source: Vickers, A., Cronin, A., Maschino, A., et al. (2012). Acupuncture for chronic pain: Individual patient data meta-analysis. *Archives of Internal Medicine, 172*(19), 1444–1453.

TABLE 67-2 COLLABORATIVE CARE

Osteoarthritis

Diagnostic
- History and physical examination
- Radiological studies of involved joints (e.g. radiographs, CT scan, MRI, bone scan)
- Synovial fluid analysis

Collaborative Therapy
- Nutritional and weight management counselling
- Rest and joint protection, use of assistive devices
- Therapeutic exercise
- Heat and cold applications
- Complementary and alternative therapies
  - Herbs and nutritional supplements (e.g., glucosamine)
  - Movement therapies (e.g., yoga, tai chi)
  - Transcutaneous electrical nerve stimulation (TENS)
  - Acupuncture

- Drug therapy*
  - Acetaminophen
  - Nonsteroidal anti-inflammatory drugs
  - Antibiotics
  - Intra-articular hyaluronic acid
  - Intra-articular corticosteroids
  - Opioid analgesics
- Reconstructive joint surgery

*See Table 67-3.
CT, computed tomographic (scan); *MRI,* magnetic resonance imaging.

COMPLEMENTARY & ALTERNATIVE THERAPIES

Glucosamine and Chondroitin

Scientific Evidence*
Both glucosamine and chondroitin provide some relief for moderate to severe arthritic pain but not for mild arthritic pain. Pain outcomes over 2 years were similar to those of patients taking celecoxib (Celebrex) or placebo.

Nursing Implications
- Can be suggested to patients who are unable to take celecoxib or other nonsteroidal anti-inflammatory drugs (NSAIDs).
- Discontinue if no effects after consistent use over 90–120 days.
- May decrease effectiveness of insulin or other drugs used to control blood glucose.
- May increase the risk of bleeding.

*Source: Hochberg, M., Martel-Pelletier, J., Monfort, J., et al. (2016). Combined chondroitin sulfate and glucosamine for painful knee osteoarthritis: A multicenter, randomized, double-blind, non-inferiority trial versus celecoxib. *Annals of Rheumatic Diseases, 75*(1), 37–44. doi:10.1136/annrheumdis-2014-206792

Drug Therapy. Drug therapy is based on the severity of the patient's symptoms (Table 67-3). Patients with mild to moderate joint pain may get relief from acetaminophen (Tylenol). The patient may receive up to 1 000 mg every 6 hours, with the daily dose not to exceed 4 g. A topical agent such as capsaicin cream may also be beneficial, either alone or in conjunction with acetaminophen. It blocks pain by locally interfering with substance P, which is responsible for the transmission of pain impulses. A concentrated product is available by prescription, but creams of 0.025% to 0.075% capsaicin are available over the counter (OTC).

TABLE 67-3 DRUG THERAPY

Arthritis and Connective Tissue Disorders

Drug	Mechanism of Action	Adverse Effects	Nursing Considerations
Salicylates			
ASA (Aspirin, Asaphen)	Analgesic Anti-inflammatory Antipyretic Inhibits prostaglandin synthesis	Exacerbation of asthma (ASA [Aspirin]-sensitive asthma) GI irritation (dyspepsia, nausea, ulcer, hemorrhage) Prolonged bleeding time Tinnitus, dizziness with repeated large doses	Administer drug with food, milk, antacids as prescribed, or full glass of water; enteric-coated ASA (Aspirin) may be administered. Report signs of bleeding (e.g., tarry stools, bruising, petechiae, nosebleeds).
Nonsteroidal Anti-Inflammatory Drugs (NSAIDs)			
Celecoxib (Celebrex) Diclofenac (Voltaren) Ibuprofen (Motrin, Advil) Indomethacin Ketoprofen Ketorolac tromethamine (Toradol) Meloxicam (Mobicox) Nabumetone (Apo-Nabumetone) Naproxen (Naprosyn, Aleve) Piroxicam (Teva-Piroxicam) Sulindac (Teva-Sulindac)	Analgesic Anti-inflammatory Antipyretic Inhibits prostaglandin synthesis	Acute renal insufficiency and other renal medullary changes Exacerbation of asthma (cross-reactivity with ASA [Aspirin]) GI irritation (dyspepsia, nausea, ulcer, hemorrhage) Headache, tinnitus Prolonged bleeding time Rash	Administer drug with food, milk, or antacids as prescribed. Report signs of bleeding (e.g., tarry stools, bruising, petechiae, nosebleeds), edema, skin rashes, persistent headaches, visual disturbances. Monitor BP for elevations related to fluid retention. Drug must be administered regularly for maximal effect.
Antibiotics			
Doxycycline Minocycline	Antirheumatic effect, possibly related to immuno-modulatory or anti-inflammatory properties Decreases action of enzymes on cartilage degradation	Dizziness GI effects (nausea and vomiting, diarrhea, stomach cramps) Monilial vaginitis, sensitivity to direct sunlight or ultraviolet light, nonspecific GI irritation Photosensitivity (severe)	This is a possible treatment alternative for mild disease.
Topical Analgesics			
Capsaicin cream	Depletes substance P from nerve endings, interrupting pain signals to the brain	Erythema Localized burning sensation Rash Urticaria	Drug must be administered regularly over time for maximal effect. Aloe vera cream may modify burning sensation. Advise patient not to use cream with external heat source (heating pad) because of risk for burns. Available in OTC and prescriptive strengths.
Diclofenac diethylamine (Voltaren Emulgel)	Anti-inflammatory Analgesic	Adverse GI effects similar to those of systemic NSAIDs Skin irritation	Advise patient to avoid sun and ultraviolet exposure. Drug should not be used in combination with other oral NSAIDs or ASA (Aspirin) because of potential for increased adverse effects.
Corticosteroids *Intra-Articular Injections*			
Methylprednisolone acetate (Depo-Medrol) Triamcinolone	Analgesic Anti-inflammatory Inhibit synthesis and release of mediators of inflammation	Dermal or subdermal changes leading to depression at injection site Local osteoporosis Neuropathic arthropathy from frequent injection Possibility of local infection Tendon rupture	Use strict aseptic technique for joint fluid aspiration or corticosteroid injection. Inform patient that joint may feel worse immediately after injection. Inform patient that improvement lasts weeks to months after injection. Advise patient to avoid overusing affected joint after injection.

Continued

TABLE 67-3 DRUG THERAPY

Arthritis and Connective Tissue Disorders—cont'd

Drug	Mechanism of Action	Adverse Effects	Nursing Considerations
Systemic			
Dexamethasone (Apo-dexamethasone) Hydrocortisone sodium succinate (Cortef) Methylprednisolone sodium succinate (Solu-Medrol) Prednisone Triamcinolone	Analgesic Anti-inflammatory Inhibit synthesis and release of mediators of inflammation	Acne Bruising Cushing's syndrome (including fluid retention) Diabetes mellitus GI irritation Hirsutism Hypertension Insomnia Menstrual irregularities Osteoporosis Risk for antibiotic-resistant infection Steroid psychosis	Use only in life-threatening exacerbation or when symptoms persist after treatment with less potent anti-inflammatory drugs. Administer for limited time only, tapering dose slowly. Be aware that symptom exacerbation occurs with abrupt withdrawal of drug. Monitor BP, weight, CBC, and potassium level. Limit sodium intake. Have patient report signs of infection to health care provider.
Disease-Modifying Antirheumatic Drugs (DMARDs)			
Methotrexate	Antimetabolite Inhibits DNA, RNA, and protein synthesis	Hepatotoxicity (occurs more often with frequent small doses than with large intermittent doses); symptoms related to drug's antineoplastic activity (e.g., GI and skin toxicity, bone marrow depression, neuropathy); smaller dose and different administration schedule for RA decrease likelihood that these adverse effects will develop	Monitor CBC and hepatic and renal function. Advise patient to report signs of anemia (fatigue, weakness). Keep patient well hydrated. Because of teratogenic potential, drug should not be administered to children or women of child-bearing age. Inform patient that contraception should be used during and for 3 months after treatment.
Sulphasalazine (Salazopyrin)	Anti-inflammatory Blocks prostaglandin synthesis Sulphonamide	Bleeding, bruising, jaundice GI effects (anorexia, nausea and vomiting) Headache Rash, urticaria, pruritus	Advise patient that drug may cause orange-yellow discoloration of urine or skin. Space doses evenly around the clock, administering drug with 250 mL water after meals. Treatment may be continued even after symptoms are relieved. Monitor CBC.
Leflunomide (Arava)	Anti-inflammatory Immuno modulatory agent that inhibits proliferation of lymphocytes	Alopecia Diarrhea Hepatotoxicity (especially if patient is also taking methotrexate or has history of prior alcohol abuse) Nausea Rash Respiratory tract infection	Evaluate for relief of pain, swelling, and stiffness and for increase in joint mobility. Advise women of child-bearing age to avoid pregnancy.
D-penicillamine (Cuprimine)	Anti-inflammatory Exact mechanism of action in RA unknown, but may suppress cell-mediated immune response	GI irritation (nausea and vomiting, anorexia, diarrhea) Iron deficiency (especially in menstruating women) Proteinuria, hematuria Rash Reduced or altered taste	Monitor WBCs, platelets, urinalysis. Advise patient to take medication 1 hr before or 2 hr after meals or at least 1 hr before or after any other drug, food, or milk. Advise women of child-bearing age to avoid pregnancy.
Gold Compounds			
Oral (auranofin [Ridaura]) Parenteral (gold sodium aurothiomalate [Myochrysine])	Alters immune responses, suppressing synovitis of active RA Antirheumatic	Decreased hemoglobin Leukopenia, thrombo-cytopenia Proteinuria, hematuria Stomatitis	Rule out pregnancy before beginning treatment. Monitor CBC, urinalysis, and hepatic and renal function. Advise patient that therapeutic response may not occur for 3 to 6 mo. Advise patient to immediately report pruritus, rash, sore mouth, indigestion, or metallic taste.

TABLE 67-3 DRUG THERAPY

Arthritis and Connective Tissue Disorders—cont'd

Drug	Mechanism of Action	Adverse Effects	Nursing Considerations
Antimalarials			
Hydroxychloroquine (Plaquenil)	Antirheumatic action unknown, but may suppress formation of antigens	Ocular toxicity (retinopathy) may progress even after drug is discontinued Ototoxicity Peripheral neuritis, neuromyopathy, hypotension, electrocardiographic changes with prolonged therapy	Monitor CBC and hepatic function. Advise patient that therapeutic response may not occur for up to 6 mo. Advise patient to immediately report visual difficulties, muscular weakness, and decreased hearing or tinnitus.
Immuno-suppressants			
Azathioprine (Imuran) Cyclophosphamide (Procytox)	Inhibit DNA, RNA, and protein synthesis	GI irritation (nausea and vomiting; anorexia with large doses) Rash	Evaluate for relief of pain, swelling, and stiffness and for increase in joint mobility. Advise patient to immediately report unusual bleeding or bruising. Advise patient that therapeutic response may take up to 12 wk. Advise women of child-bearing age to avoid pregnancy.
JAK (Janus Kinase) Inhibitors			
Tofacitinib (Xeljanz)	Inhibits the action of the JAK enzymes, which are signalling pathways inside the cell and have an important role in the inflammation involved in RA		Patients are at increased risk for serious infections, including opportunistic infections. Monitor patient for any sign or symptom of infection so it can be treated early.
Biological and Targeted Therapies *Tumour Necrosis Factor (TNF) Inhibitors*			
Adalimumab (Humira) Certolizumab (Cimzia) Etanercept (Enbrel) Golimumab (Simponi) Infliximab (Remicade)	Binds to TNF, blocking its interaction with TNF cell surface receptors to decrease inflammatory and immune responses	Abdominal pain, vomiting Dizziness, headache Injection site reaction including erythema, pain, itching, swelling Rhinitis, pharyngitis, cough	Evaluate for relief of pain, swelling, and stiffness and for increase in joint mobility. Advise patient of increased risk for tuberculosis. Advise patient to have yearly TB skin test. Monitor for infection, bleeding, and emergence of malignancies. Advise patient that psoriasis may worsen. Advise patient that injection site reaction generally occurs in first month of treatment and decreases with continued therapy. Advise patient not to receive live virus vaccines during treatment.
Interleukin-1 Receptor Antagonist			
Anakinra (Kineret)	Blocks the action of interleukin-1 and thus decreases the inflammatory response	Abdominal pain Headache Injection site reaction Leukopenia Rash	Evaluate for relief of pain, swelling, and stiffness and for increase in joint mobility. Advise patient that injection site reaction generally occurs during first month of treatment and decreases with continued therapy. Evaluate renal function. Monitor for infection. Do not administer drug with other TNF inhibitors.
Interleukin-6 Receptor Antagonist			
Tocilizumab (Actemra)	Blocks action of interleukin-6	↑ BP ↑ liver enzyme levels Headache Inflammation of nose or nasal passage Upper respiratory tract infections	Administered to patients with RA in whom other therapies have failed. Monitor BP and for infection. Advise patient of adverse GI effects (e.g., perforation). Monitor liver enzyme and LDL levels.

Continued

TABLE 67-3 DRUG THERAPY

Arthritis and Connective Tissue Disorders—cont'd

Drug	Mechanism of Action	Adverse Effects	Nursing Considerations
T-Cell Activation Inhibitor			
Abatacept (Orencia)	Modulates T-cell activation; suppresses immune response	Headache Injection site reaction Nausea Sore throat Upper respiratory infection	Not recommended for concomitant use with TNF inhibitors. Evaluate for relief of pain, swelling, and stiffness and for increase in joint mobility.
B-Cell Depleting Agent			
Rituximab (Rituxan)	Monoclonal antibody that targets B cells	Difficulty breathing Dizziness Fever Itching Palpitations Sore throat	Administer in combination with methotrexate. Monitor for infection and bleeding. Advise patient to not receive live virus vaccines during treatment. Monitor for low BP if patient is also taking antihypertensives.
Tocilizumab (Actemra)	Blocks action of interleukin-6	↑ BP ↑ liver enzyme levels Headache Inflammation of nose or nasal passage Upper respiratory tract infections	Administered to patients with RA in whom other therapies have failed. Monitor BP and for infection. Advise patient of adverse GI effects (e.g., perforation). Monitor liver enzyme and LDL levels.

BP, blood pressure; *CBC,* complete blood cell count; *GI,* gastro-intestinal; *LDL,* low-density lipoprotein; *NSAIDs,* nonsteroidal anti-inflammatory drugs; *OTC,* over-the-counter; *RA,* rheumatoid arthritis; *TNF,* tumour necrosis factor; *TNF-α,* tumour necrosis factor–alpha; *WBC,* white blood cell.

Other OTC products that contain camphor, eucalyptus oil, and menthol (e.g., BenGay, Arthricare) may also provide temporary pain relief. Topical salicylates (e.g., Aspercreme) that can be absorbed into the blood are an alternative for patients who are able to take acetylsalicylic acid (ASA; Aspirin)–containing medication. Because effects of topical agents are not sustained, several applications daily may be needed.

For patients who do not obtain adequate pain management with acetaminophen or for patients with moderate to severe OA pain or signs of joint inflammation, an NSAID may be more effective for pain treatment. NSAID therapy is typically initiated in low-dose OTC strengths (e.g., ibuprofen [Motrin, Advil]) of 200 mg, up to four times daily, with the dosage increased as the patient's symptoms indicate. If a patient is at risk for or experiences adverse gastro-intestinal (GI) effects with a conventional NSAID, supplemental treatment with a protective agent such as miso-prostol may be indicated. Arthrotec, a combination of misoprostol and the NSAID diclofenac, is also available. Diclofenac gel may be applied to the affected joint.

Because traditional NSAIDs block the production of prosta-glandins from arachidonic acid by inhibiting the production of cyclo-oxygenase–1 (COX-1) and cyclo-oxygenase–2 (COX-2), the risk for GI erosion and bleeding is increased. Traditional NSAIDs affect platelet aggregation, which prolongs bleeding time. Patients taking both warfarin (Coumadin) and an NSAID are at high risk of bleeding. Concerns have also been raised regarding the possible negative effects of long-term NSAID treatment on cartilage metabolism, particularly in older-adult patients, in whom cartilage integrity may already be diminished. As an alternative to traditional NSAIDs, treatment with the COX-2 inhibitor celecoxib (Celebrex) may be considered in selected patients.

When given in equivalent anti-inflammatory dosages, all NSAIDs are considered comparable in efficacy but vary widely in cost. Individual responses to the NSAIDs are also variable.

Some patients still prefer ASA (Aspirin), but it is no longer a common treatment and should not be used in combination with NSAIDs because both inhibit platelet function and prolong bleeding time. Intra-articular injections of corticosteroids may be appropriate for older adults with local inflammation and effusion. Four or more injections without relief suggest the need for additional intervention. Systemic use of corticosteroids is not indicated and may actually accelerate the disease process.

Another treatment for mild to moderate OA is hyaluronic acid (HA) injection, a type of viscosupplementation. HA is found in normal joint fluid and articular cartilage. It contributes to both the viscosity and the elasticity of synovial fluid, and its degradation can result in joint damage. Synthetic and naturally occurring HA derivatives (e.g., NeoVisc, OrthoVisc, Synvisc-One) are administered in three injections, a week apart, directly into the joint space. Synvisc-1, a newer, single-injection HA drug, may offer pain relief for up to 6 months. HA may also be added to oral supplements of glucosamine, chondroitin, and methyl-sulphonylmethane (MSM). Few adverse effects have been reported with HA.

Medications thought to slow the progression of OA or support joint healing are known as *disease-modifying osteoarthritis drugs (DMOADs)*. To date, no drugs have been approved to modify OA progression, despite numerous clinical trials. A variety of molecular targets are under investigation, including the use of anticatabolic agents to stimulate new cartilage growth and slow OA progression (Le Graverand-Gastineau, 2010).

Surgical Therapy. Symptoms of disease are often managed conservatively for many years, but the patient's loss of joint function, unrelieved pain, and diminished ability to independently perform self-care may prompt a recommendation for surgery. In patients less than 55 years of age, arthroscopic surgery for knee OA may delay the need for more serious surgery, such as knee replacement. The main indication for arthroscopic surgery for OA is to remove debris (i.e., bits of cartilage known as *loose* *bodies*) that may be causing problems with joint motion. Reconstructive surgical procedures (e.g., hip and knee replacements) are discussed in Chapter 65.

NURSING MANAGEMENT OSTEOARTHRITIS

NURSING ASSESSMENT

The nurse should carefully assess and document the type, location, severity, frequency, and duration of the patient's joint pain and stiffness and the extent to which these symptoms affect his or her ability to perform activities of daily living (ADLs). The nurse should note pain management practices and question the patient about the duration and success of each treatment. Physical examination of the affected joint or joints includes assessment of tenderness, swelling, limitation of movement, and crepitation. An involved joint should be compared with the contralateral joint if it is not affected.

NURSING DIAGNOSES

Nursing diagnoses for patients with OA may include, but are not limited to, the following:

- *Acute pain* related to *physical injury agent* (painful physical activity)
- *Impaired physical mobility* related to *activity intolerance, decrease in muscle strength, joint stiffness*
- *Obesity* related to *average daily physical activity is less than recommended for gender and age*
- *Ineffective coping* related to *inadequate confidence in ability to deal with a situation*

PLANNING

The overall goals are that patients with OA will (a) maintain or improve joint function through a balance of rest and activity, (b) use joint protection measures (Table 67-4) to improve activity tolerance, (c) achieve independence in self-care and maintain optimal role function, and (d) use pharmacological and non-pharmacological strategies to manage pain satisfactorily.

NURSING IMPLEMENTATION

HEALTH PROMOTION. Prevention of primary OA is possible in many cases. Community education should focus on altering modifiable risk factors through weight loss and the reduction of occupational and recreational hazards. Athletic instruction and physical fitness programs should include safety measures

that protect and reduce trauma to the joints. Traumatic joint injuries should be treated promptly to prevent the development of OA.

ACUTE INTERVENTION. Patients with OA most often complain of pain, stiffness, limitation of function, and the frustration of coping with these physical difficulties on a daily basis. Older adults may believe that OA is an inevitable part of the aging process and that nothing can be done to ease the discomfort and related disability.

Patients with OA are usually treated on an outpatient basis, often by an interdisciplinary team of health care providers that includes a family health care provider, a rheumatologist, a nurse, an occupational therapist, and a physiotherapist. Often, health assessment questionnaires are used to pinpoint areas of decreased function. Questionnaires are repeated at regular intervals to document disease and treatment progression. Treatment goals can be developed on the basis of data from the questionnaires and the physical examination, with specific interventions to target identified problems. Usually, patients are hospitalized only if joint surgery is planned (see Chapter 65).

Medications are administered for the treatment of pain and inflammation. Nonpharmacological strategies to decrease pain and disability may include gentle exercise, the application of heat (thermal packs) or cold (ice packs), relaxation, and yoga (Arthritis Society, 2017b). Splints may be prescribed to rest and stabilize painful or inflamed joints.

Once an acute flare has subsided, a physiotherapist can provide valuable assistance in planning an exercise program. Therapists often recommend tai chi as a low-impact form of exercise. Tai chi can be performed by patients of all ages and may be practised in a wheelchair. The nurse should emphasize the importance of warming up before practice to prevent stretch injuries.

Patient and caregiver teaching related to OA is an important nursing responsibility. Teaching should include information about the nature and the treatment of the disease, pain management, correct posture and body mechanics, correct use of assistive devices such as a cane or walker, principles of joint protection and energy conservation (see Table 67-4), nutritional choices and weight and stress management, and an exercise program.

Patients should be assured that OA is a localized disease and that severe deforming arthritis is not the usual course. Patients can also obtain support and understanding of the disease process through community resources such as the Arthritis Self-Management Courses (Arthritis Society, 2017c).

AMBULATORY AND HOME CARE. Home management goals should be individualized to meet the patient's needs. The caregiver, family members, and significant others should be included in goal setting and teaching. Home and work environment modification is essential for the patient's safety, accessibility, and self-care. Measures include removing scatter rugs, providing rails at the stairs and in the bathtub, using nightlights, and wearing well-fitting supportive shoes. Assistive devices such as canes, walkers, elevated toilet seats, and grab bars also reduce the load on the affected joint(s) and promote safety. Patients should be urged to continue all prescribed therapies at home and also be open to new approaches to symptom management.

Sexual counselling may help the patient and significant other enjoy physical closeness by introducing the idea of alternate positions and timing for sexual activity. Discussion also increases awareness of each partner's needs. The nurse should encourage the patient to take analgesics or a warm bath to decrease joint stiffness before sexual activity.

TABLE 67-4	PATIENT & CAREGIVER TEACHING GUIDE

Joint Protection and Energy Conservation

The following should be included when teaching patients with arthritis to protect joints and conserve energy:
- Avoid forceful repetitive movements.
- Avoid positions of joint deviation and stress.
- Develop organizing and pacing techniques for routine tasks.
- Maintain appropriate weight.
- Modify home and work environment to create less stressful ways to perform tasks.
- Seek assistance with necessary tasks that may cause pain.
- Use assistive devices, if indicated.
- Use good posture and proper body mechanics.

EVALUATION

The expected outcomes for patients with OA are as follows:

- Experience adequate amounts of rest and activity.
- Achieve satisfactory pain management.
- Maintain joint flexibility and muscle strength through joint protection and therapeutic exercise.
- Verbalize acceptance of OA as a chronic disease and collaborate with health care providers in disease management.

RHEUMATOID ARTHRITIS

Rheumatoid arthritis (RA) is a chronic, systemic autoimmune disease characterized by inflammation of connective tissue in the diarthrodial (synovial) joints, typically with periods of remission and exacerbation. RA is frequently accompanied by extra-articular manifestations.

RA occurs globally, affecting all ethnic groups. It can occur at any time of life, but the incidence increases with age, peaking between 30 and 50 years old. An estimated 300 000 Canadians are affected by RA. Women are more likely than men to have the disease (Arthritis Society, 2017d).

Etiology and Pathophysiology

Although the exact cause of RA is unknown, it probably results from a combination of genetics and environmental triggers. An autoimmune etiology that is currently the most widely accepted theory suggests that changes associated with RA begin when a genetically susceptible person has an initial immune response to an antigen. Although a bacterium or virus has been proposed as a possible antigen, to date, no infection or organism has been identified as the cause.

The antigen, which is probably not the same in all affected patients, triggers the formation of an abnormal immunoglobulin G (IgG). RA is characterized by the presence of autoantibodies against this abnormal IgG. The autoantibodies, known as *rheumatoid factor* (RF), combine with IgG to form immune complexes that initially deposit on synovial membranes or superficial articular cartilage in the joints. Immune complex formation leads to the activation of complement, and an inflammatory response results. (Complement activation is discussed in Chapter 14, and immune complex formation is discussed in Chapter 16.)

Neutrophils are attracted to the site of inflammation, where they release proteolytic enzymes that can damage articular cartilage and cause the synovial lining to thicken (Figure 67-3). Other inflammatory cells include T helper (CD4) cells, which are the primary orchestrators of cell-mediated immune responses. Activated CD4 cells stimulate monocytes, macrophages, and synovial fibroblasts to secrete the proinflammatory cytokines interleukin-1 (IL-1), interleukin-6 (IL-6), and tumour necrosis

FIGURE 67-3 Rheumatoid arthritis. **A,** Early pathological change in rheumatoid arthritis is rheumatoid synovitis. The synovium is inflamed. Lymphocytes and plasma cells increase greatly. **B,** With time, articular cartilage destruction occurs, vascular granulation tissue grows across the surface of the cartilage (pannus) from the edges of the joint, and the articular surface shows loss of cartilage beneath the extending pannus, most marked at the joint margins. **C,** Inflammatory pannus causes focal destruction of bone. At the edges of the joint, there is osteolytic destruction of bone, responsible for erosions seen on radiographs. This phase is associated with joint deformity. **D,** Multiple deformities of the foot associated with rheumatoid arthritis. Source: **D,** Canale, S. T., & Beaty, J. H. (2013). *Campbell's operative orthopaedics* (12th ed.). Philadelphia: Mosby.

TABLE 67-5 ANATOMICAL STAGES OF RHEUMATOID ARTHRITIS

Stage I: Early
No destructive changes visible on radiograph; possible radiographic evidence of osteoporosis

Stage II: Moderate
Radiographic evidence of osteoporosis, with or without slight bone or cartilage destruction; no joint deformities (although possibly limited joint mobility); adjacent muscle atrophy; possible presence of extra-articular soft-tissue lesions (e.g., nodules, tenosynovitis)

Stage III: Severe
Radiographic evidence of cartilage and bone destruction in addition to osteoporosis; joint deformity, such as subluxation, ulnar deviation, or hyperextension, without fibrous or bony ankylosis; extensive muscle atrophy; possible presence of extra-articular soft-tissue lesions (e.g., nodules, tenosynovitis)

Stage IV: Terminal
Fibrous or bony ankylosis; stage III criteria

Source: American College of Rheumatology. (2012). *Classification criteria for determining progression of rheumatoid arthritis.* Retrieved from http://www.hopkins -arthritis.org/physician-corner/education/acr/acr.html#class_rheum. Originally from Steinbrocker, O., Traeger, C. H., & Batterman, R. C. (1949). Therapeutic criteria in rheumatoid arthritis. *Journal of American Medical Association, 140*(8), 659–662.

TABLE 67-6 COMPARISON OF RHEUMATOID ARTHRITIS AND OSTEOARTHRITIS

Parameter	Rheumatoid Arthritis	Osteoarthritis
Affected joints	Small joints first (PIP, MCP, and MTP joints), wrists, elbows, shoulders, knees; usually bilateral, symmetrical joint involvement	Weight-bearing joints (knees, hips); small joints (MCP, DIP, and PIP); cervical and lumbar spine; often asymmetrical
Age at onset	Young to middle age	Usually >40 yr of age
Disease	Systemic disease with exacerbations and remissions	Localized disease with variable, progressive course
Effusions	Common	Uncommon
Gender	Female-to-male ratio is 2:1 or 3:1; less marked difference after age 60	Before age 50, more men than women; after age 50, more women than men
Laboratory findings	RF positive in 80% of patients; Elevated ESR and CRP level indicative of active inflammation	RF negative; Transient elevation in ESR related to synovitis
Nodules	Present, especially on extensor surfaces	Heberden nodes (DIP joints) and Bouchard nodes (PIP joints)
Pain characteristics	Stiffness lasts from 1 hr to all day and may decrease with use; pain is variable, may disrupt sleep	Stiffness occurs on arising but usually subsides after 30 min; pain gradually worsens with joint use and disease progression, relieved with rest
Radiographs	Joint space narrowing, erosion, subluxation with advanced disease; osteoporosis related to corticosteroid use	Joint space narrowing, osteophytes, subchondral cysts, sclerosis
Synovial fluid	WBC count >2×10⁹/L with mostly neutrophils	WBC count <2×10⁹/L (mild leukocytosis)
Weight	Lost or maintained weight	Often overweight

CRP, C-reactive protein; *DIP,* distal interphalangeal; *ESR,* erythrocyte sedimentation rate; *MCP,* metacarpo-phalangeal; *MTP,* metatarso-phalangeal; *PIP,* proximal interphalangeal; *RF,* rheumatoid factor; *WBC,* white blood cell.

factor (TNF). These cytokines are the primary factors that drive the inflammatory response in RA. If unarrested, the disease progresses through four stages, which are identified in Table 67-5.

Genetic Factors. Genetic predisposition is important in the development of RA. For example, a higher concurrence of RA has been noted in identical twins compared with fraternal twins (Firestein, 2012). The strongest evidence for a familial influence is the increased occurrence of a human leukocyte antigen (HLA) known as HLA-DR4 and HLA-DR1 antigens. Smoking increases the risk for RA for people who are genetically predisposed to the disease and makes successful treatment more difficult.

Clinical Manifestations

Joints. The onset of RA is typically insidious. Nonspecific manifestations such as fatigue, anorexia, weight loss, and generalized stiffness may precede the onset of arthritic complaints. The stiffness becomes more localized in the following weeks to months. Some patients report a history of a precipitating stressful event such as infection, work stress, physical exertion, childbirth, surgery, or emotional upset. However, researchers have been unable to correlate such events directly with the onset of RA.

Specific articular involvement is manifested clinically by pain, stiffness, limitation of motion, and signs of inflammation such as heat, swelling, and tenderness. Joint symptoms occur symmetrically and frequently affect the small joints of the hands (PIP and MCP joints) and feet (MTP joints). Larger peripheral joints such as wrists, elbows, shoulders, knees, hips, ankles, and the jaw may also be involved. The cervical spine may be affected, but the axial skeleton (the spine and the bones connected to it) is generally spared. In Table 67-6, the manifestations of RA and OA are compared.

Patients characteristically experience joint stiffness after periods of inactivity. Morning stiffness may last from 60 minutes to several hours or more, depending on disease activity. MCP and PIP joints are typically swollen. In early disease, the fingers may become spindle-shaped from synovial hypertrophy and thickening

of the joint capsule (see Figure 67-3). Joints become tender, painful, and warm to the touch. Joint pain increases with motion, varies in intensity, and may not be proportional to the degree of inflammation. Tenosynovitis frequently affects the extensor and flexor tendons around the wrists, producing manifestations of carpal tunnel syndrome and making it difficult for patients to grasp objects.

As disease activity progresses, inflammation and fibrosis of the joint capsule and supporting structures may lead to deformity and disability. Atrophy of muscles and destruction of tendons around the joint cause one articular surface to slip past the other *(subluxation).* Metatarsal head dislocation and subluxation in the feet may cause pain and walking disability. Typical distortions of the hand include ulnar drift ("zigzag deformity"), swan-neck deformity, and boutonnière deformity (Figure 67-4).

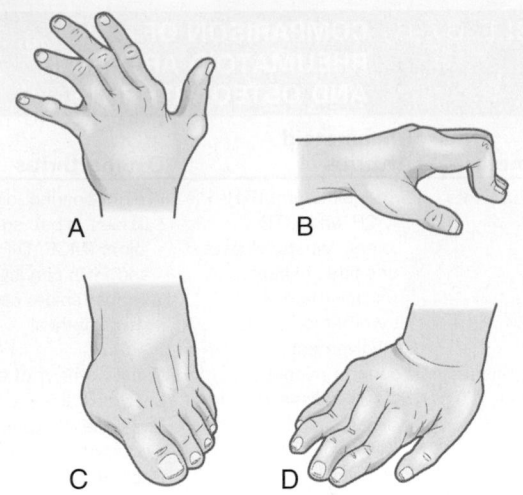

FIGURE 67-4 Typical deformities of rheumatoid arthritis. **A,** Ulnar drift. **B,** Boutonnière deformity. **C,** Hallux valgus. **D,** Swan-neck deformity.

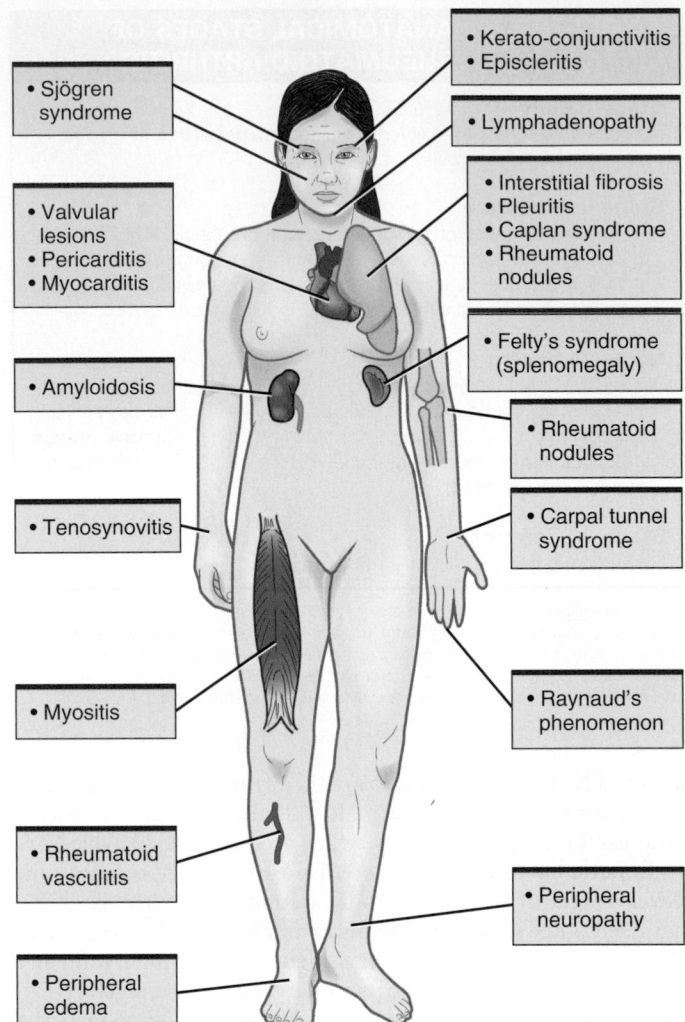

- Kerato-conjunctivitis
- Episcleritis

- Sjögren syndrome

- Lymphadenopathy

- Valvular lesions
- Pericarditis
- Myocarditis

- Interstitial fibrosis
- Pleuritis
- Caplan syndrome
- Rheumatoid nodules

- Felty's syndrome (splenomegaly)

- Amyloidosis

- Rheumatoid nodules

- Tenosynovitis

- Carpal tunnel syndrome

- Myositis

- Raynaud's phenomenon

- Rheumatoid vasculitis

- Peripheral neuropathy

- Peripheral edema

FIGURE 67-5 Extra-articular manifestations of rheumatoid arthritis.

Extra-Articular Manifestations. RA can affect nearly every system in the body. Extra-articular manifestations of RA are depicted in Figure 67-5. Extra-articular manifestations are more likely to occur in people with high levels of biomarkers such as RF.

Rheumatoid nodules develop in 20% of all patients with RA (Arthritis Society, 2017d). Those affected with nodules usually have high titres of RF. Rheumatoid nodules appear subcutaneously as firm, nontender, granuloma-type masses and are usually over the extensor surfaces of joints such as those of the fingers and elbows. Nodules at the base of the spine and the back of the head are common in older adults. On the skin, these nodules can ulcerate, similar to pressure injuries. In later disease, cardiopulmonary effects may occur. These may include pleurisy, pleural effusion, pericarditis, pericardial effusion, and cardiomyopathy.

Sjögren syndrome is seen in 10% to 15% of patients with RA. Sjögren syndrome can occur by itself or in conjunction with other arthritic disorders such as RA and systemic lupus erythematosus. Affected patients have diminished lacrimal and salivary gland secretion, leading to a dry mouth; burning, itchy eyes with decreased tearing; and photosensitivity.

Felty's syndrome occurs most commonly in patients with severe, nodule-forming RA. It is characterized by splenomegaly and leukopenia.

Flexion contractures and hand deformities cause diminished grasp strength and affect the patient's ability to perform self-care tasks. Nodular myositis and muscle fibre degeneration can lead to pain similar to that of vascular insufficiency. Cataract development and loss of vision can result from scleral nodules. Depression may occur and is often related to the chronic pain associated with RA (Durham, Fowler, Donato, et al., 2015).

Diagnostic Studies

An accurate diagnosis is essential to the initiation of appropriate treatment and the prevention of unnecessary disability. A diagnosis is often based on history and physical findings, but some laboratory tests are useful for confirmation and to monitor disease progression (see Table 67-7). Positive RF occurs in approximately 80% of adult patients, and titres rise during active disease. Elevations in ESR and C-reactive protein (CRP) levels are general indicators of active inflammation. Antinuclear

antibody (ANA) titres are also present in some patients with RA. Testing for the anti-citrullinated protein antibody (ACPA) is another important diagnostic test for RA. Levels of ACPA are more specific than those of RF for RA and in some cases may allow for an earlier and more accurate diagnosis (Durham, Fowler, Donato, et al., 2015).

Synovial fluid analysis early in the course of the disease often reveals a straw-coloured fluid with many fibrin flecks. The enzyme MMP-3 is increased in the synovial fluid of patients with RA and may be a marker of progressive joint damage. The white blood cell (WBC) count of synovial fluid is elevated (up to 25×10^9/L). Inflammatory changes in the synovium can be confirmed by tissue biopsy.

Radiological studies are not specifically diagnostic of RA. The findings may be inconclusive during early stages of the disease, revealing only soft-tissue swelling and possible bone demineralization. In later stages of the disease, narrowing of the joint space, destruction of articular cartilage, erosion, subluxation, and deformity are seen. Malalignment and ankylosis are often evident in advanced disease. Baseline radiographs may be useful in monitoring disease progression and treatment effectiveness. Bone scans are more useful in detecting early joint changes and confirming a diagnosis so that RA treatment can be initiated.

TABLE 67-7 DIAGNOSTIC CRITERIA FOR RHEUMATOID ARTHRITIS

Patients should be tested for RA if they are initially seen with the following signs:
- At least one joint with definite clinical synovitis
- Synovitis not better explained by another disease

Criterion	Score
A. Joint Involvement	
1 large joint	0
2–10 large joints	1
1–3 small joints (with or without involvement of large joints)	2
4–10 small joints (with or without involvement of large joints)	3
>10 joints (at least 1 small joint)	5
B. Serology (at Least One Test Result Needed)	
Negative RF and negative ACPA	0
Low-positive RF or low-positive ACPA	2
High-positive RF or high-positive ACPA	3
C. Acute-Phase Reactants (at Least One Test Result Needed)	
Normal CRP and normal ESR	0
Abnormal CRP or abnormal ESR	1
D. Duration of Symptoms	
<6 weeks	0
≥6 weeks	1

Source: Aletaha, D., Neogi, T., Silman, A., et al. (2010). 2010 rheumatoid arthritis classification criteria. *Arthritis and Rheumatism, 62*(9), 2569–2581. doi:10.1002/art.27584. Copyright © 2010 by the American College of Rheumatology.
Scoring: Add score of categories A–D. Possible scores range from 0–10. A score of ≥6 indicates the definitive presence of RA.
ACPA, anti-citrullinated peptide antibodies; *CRP,* C-reactive protein; *ESR,* erythrocyte sedimentation rate; *RF,* rheumatoid factor.

TABLE 67-8 COLLABORATIVE CARE

Rheumatoid Arthritis

Diagnostic
- History and physical examination
- Laboratory studies
  - Complete blood cell (CBC) count
  - Erythrocyte sedimentation rate (ESR)
  - Rheumatoid factor (RF)
  - Anti-citrullinated protein antibody (ACPA)
  - Antinuclear antibody (ANA)
  - C-reactive protein (CRP)
- Radiological studies of involved joints
- Analysis of synovial fluid

Collaborative Therapy
- Nutritional and weight management counselling
- Therapeutic exercise
- Psychological support
- Rest, joint protection, and use of assistive devices
- Heat and cold applications
- Complementary and alternative therapies
  - Herbal products
  - Acupuncture
  - Movement therapies
- Drug therapy (see Table 67-3)
  - Disease-modifying antirheumatic drugs (DMARDs)
  - Intra-articular or systemic corticosteroids
  - Nonsteroidal anti-inflammatory drugs (NSAIDs)
  - Biological and targeted therapy
- Reconstructive surgery (e.g., arthroplasty)

Criteria for the diagnosis of RA in a newly presenting patient are described in Table 67-7.

Collaborative Care

Care of patients with RA begins with a comprehensive program of education and drug therapy. Education regarding drug therapy includes correct administration, reporting of adverse effects, and frequent medical and laboratory follow-up visits. Patients and caregivers should be taught about the disease process and home management strategies. NSAIDs are prescribed to promote physical comfort. Physiotherapy helps patients maintain joint motion and muscle strength. Occupational therapy helps to develop upper extremity function and encourages joint protection through the use of splints or other assistive devices and strategies for activity pacing.

An individualized treatment plan accounts for the nature of the disease activity, joint function, age, gender, family and social roles, and response to previous treatment (Table 67-8). A caring, long-term relationship with an arthritis health care team can promote the patient's self-esteem and positive coping.

Drug Therapy

Disease-Modifying Antirheumatic Drugs. Drugs remain the cornerstone of RA treatment (see Table 67-3). Because irreversible joint changes can occur as early as the first year of RA, health care providers now aggressively prescribe disease-modifying antirheumatic drugs (DMARDs). These drugs have the potential to lessen the permanent effects of RA, such as joint erosion and deformity. The choice of drug is based on disease activity, the patient's level of function, and lifestyle considerations, such as the desire to bear children.

Treatment of early RA often involves DMARD therapy with methotrexate (Durham, Fowler, Donato, et al., 2015). The rapid anti-inflammatory effect of methotrexate reduces clinical symptoms in days to weeks. It has a lower toxicity compared to other drugs. Adverse effects include bone marrow suppression and hepatotoxicity. Methotrexate therapy necessitates frequent laboratory monitoring, including CBC and chemistry panel.

Sulphasalazine (Salazopyrin) and the antimalarial drug hydroxychloroquine (Plaquenil) may be effective DMARDs for mild to moderate disease. They are rapidly absorbed, relatively safe, and well tolerated. The synthetic DMARD leflunomide (Arava) blocks immune cell overproduction. Its efficacy and adverse effects are similar to those of methotrexate and sulphasalazine. Because the drug is teratogenic, the possibility of pregnancy must be excluded before therapy is initiated.

Tofacitinib (Xeljanz) is a new drug used to treat moderate to severe active RA. This drug is from a new class of medications called JAK (Janus kinase) inhibitors. The drug interferes with the JAK enzymes that contribute to joint inflammation in RA.

Biological and Targeted Therapies. Biological or targeted drug therapies are also used to slow disease progression in RA. These drugs can be categorized based on their mechanism of action (see Table 67-3). They can be used to treat patients with moderate to severe disease who have not responded to DMARDs or in combination therapy with an established DMARD such as methotrexate.

Tumour necrosis factor inhibitors include etanercept (Enbrel), infliximab (Remicade), adalimumab (Humira), certolizumab (Cimzia), and golimumab (Simponi). Etanercept is a biologically engineered copy (using recombinant deoxyribonucleic acid [DNA] technology) of the TNF cell receptor. This soluble TNF receptor binds to TNF in circulation before TNF can bind to the cell surface receptor. By inhibiting binding of TNF, etanercept inhibits the inflammatory response. This drug is given as a subcutaneous injection.

DRUG ALERT—Etanercept (Enbrel)
- Increased risk for serious infection and heart failure is a concern.
- Persistent fever, bruising, bleeding, or other signs of infection should be reported.

Infliximab and adalimumab are monoclonal antibodies that bind to TNF, thus preventing it from binding to TNF receptors on cells. Infliximab is given by intravenous (IV) in combination with methotrexate. Adalimumab is administered subcutaneously.

Certolizumab and golimumab are TNF inhibitors that improve symptoms in patients with moderate to severe RA. Both drugs are given in combination with methotrexate. When compared to other biological and targeted therapy, certolizumab stays in the system longer and may also show a more rapid (1 to 2 weeks) and significant reduction in RA symptoms. Certolizumab is also used in treating Crohn's disease.

DRUG ALERT—Tumour Necrosis Factor Inhibitors
- Tuberculin test and chest radiograph should be administered before initiation of therapy.
- The patient should be monitored for signs of infection and the drug stopped if acute infection develops.
- Patients should be instructed to avoid live vaccination while taking the drug.

Anakinra (Kineret) is a recombinant version of IL-1 receptor antagonist (IL-1Ra). It blocks the biological activity of IL-1 by competitively inhibiting the binding of IL-1 to the IL-1 receptor. It is given as a subcutaneous injection. Anakinra is used to reduce the pain and swelling associated with moderate to severe RA. It can be used in combination with DMARDs but not with TNF inhibitors. Concurrent use of anakinra and TNF inhibitors can cause serious infection and neutropenia.

Tocilizumab (Actemra) blocks the action of IL-6, a proinflammatory cytokine. It is used to treat patients who have moderate to severe RA and have not adequately responded to or cannot tolerate other drugs for RA.

Abatacept (Orencia) blocks T-cell activation. It is recommended for patients who have an inadequate response to DMARDS and TNF inhibitors. It is given IV. Like anakinra, it should not be used concomitantly with TNF inhibitors.

Rituximab (Rituxan) is a monoclonal antibody that targets B cells. It may be used in combination with methotrexate for patients with moderate to severe RA not responding to TNF inhibitors (e.g., etanercept, infliximab). It is given IV.

Other Drug Therapy. Additional medications used infrequently for treating RA include antibiotics (minocycline), immunosuppressants (azathioprine [Imuran]), D-penicillamine (Cuprimine), and gold preparations (auranofin [Ridaura], gold sodium thiomalate [Myochrysine]).

Corticosteroid therapy can be used for symptom control. Intra-articular injections may temporarily reduce the pain and inflammation associated with disease flare-ups. Long-term use of oral corticosteroids should not be a mainstay of RA treatment because of the risk for complications, including osteoporosis and avascular necrosis. However, low-dose prednisone may be used for a limited time with select patients to decrease disease activity until DMARD therapy is effective.

Various NSAIDs and salicylates continue to be included in the drug regimen to treat arthritis pain and inflammation. Enteric-coated ASA (Aspirin) is often used in high dosages of 3.2 to 5.4 g/day (10 to 18 tablets). NSAIDs have anti-inflammatory, analgesic, and antipyretic properties. Some relief may be noted within days of the start of treatment with NSAIDs, but full effectiveness may take 2 to 3 weeks. NSAIDs may be used when patients cannot tolerate high doses of ASA (Aspirin). Anti-inflammatory drugs that are taken only once or twice a day may improve the patient's ability to follow the treatment regimen (see Table 67-3). The newer generation NSAIDs, the COX-2 inhibitors, are effective in RA as well as OA. Celecoxib (Celebrex) is currently the only available COX-2 inhibitor.

Nutritional Therapy. Although there is no special diet for RA, balanced nutrition is important. Fatigue, pain, depression, limited endurance, and mobility deficits often accompany RA and may cause a loss of appetite or interfere with the patient's ability to shop for and prepare food. Weight loss may result. An occupational therapist may help the patient modify the home environment and use assistive devices to make food preparation easier.

Corticosteroid therapy or immobility secondary to pain may result in unwanted weight gain. A sensible weight loss program, consisting of balanced nutrition and exercise, reduces stress on affected joints. Corticosteroids also increase the appetite, which results in a higher caloric intake. In addition, patients may become distressed as signs and symptoms of Cushing's syndrome—including moon facies and the redistribution of fatty tissue to the trunk—change the physical appearance. Patients must be encouraged to continue to eat a balanced diet and not to alter the corticosteroid dose or stop therapy abruptly. Weight slowly adjusts to normal several months after cessation of therapy.

Surgical Therapy. Occasionally, surgery is needed to relieve severe pain and improve the function of severely deformed joints. Removal of the joint lining (synovectomy) is one type of surgical therapy. Total joint replacement (arthroplasty) can be done for many different joints in the body. Joint surgery is discussed in Chapter 65.

NURSING MANAGEMENT
RHEUMATOID ARTHRITIS

NURSING ASSESSMENT
Subjective and objective data that should be obtained from patients with RA are presented in Table 67-9.

NURSING DIAGNOSES
Nursing diagnoses for patients with RA may include, but are not limited to, the following:
- *Impaired physical mobility* related to *pain* (joint pain, stiffness and deformity)
- *Chronic pain* related to *injury agent* (joint inflammation, overuse of joints, and ineffective pain or comfort measures)
- *Disturbed body image* related to *alteration in self-perception* (chronic disease activity, long term treatment, deformities, stiffness, and inability to perform usual activities)

Additional information on nursing diagnoses for the patient with RA is presented in Nursing Care Plan (NCP) 67-1, available on the Evolve website.

PLANNING
The overall goals are that patients with RA will (a) have satisfactory pain management, (b) have minimal loss of functional ability of the affected joints, (c) participate in planning and carrying out the therapeutic regimen, (d) maintain a positive self-image, and (e) perform self-care to the maximum extent possible.

TABLE 67-9   NURSING ASSESSMENT

Rheumatoid Arthritis

Subjective Data

Important Health Information

Past health history: Recent infections; precipitating factors such as emotional upset, infections, overwork, childbirth, surgery; pattern of remissions and exacerbations

Family history: Family history of rheumatoid arthritis or other autoimmune diseases

Medications: Use of ASA (Aspirin), NSAIDs, corticosteroids, DMARDs

Surgery or other treatments: Any joint surgery

Symptoms

- Symmetrical joint pain and aching that increases with motion or stress on joint; stiffness and joint swelling; muscle weakness, difficulty walking; paresthesias of hands and feet; numbness, tingling, loss of sensation
- Dry mucous membranes of mouth and pharynx; anorexia, weight loss; fatigue, malaise

Objective Data

General

Lymphadenopathy, fever

Integumentary

Kerato-conjunctivitis; subcutaneous rheumatoid nodules on forearm, elbows; skin ulcers; shiny, taut skin over involved joints; peripheral edema

Cardiovascular

Symmetrical pallor and cyanosis of fingers (Raynaud's phenomenon); distant heart sounds, murmurs, dysrhythmias

Respiratory

Chronic bronchitis, tuberculosis, histoplasmosis, fibrosing alveolitis

Gastro-Intestinal

Splenomegaly (Felty's syndrome)

Musculo-Skeletal

Symmetrical joint involvement with swelling, erythema, heat, tenderness, and deformities; enlargement of proximal phalangeal and MCP joints; limitation of joint movement; muscle contractures, muscle atrophy

Possible Diagnostic Findings

Positive rheumatoid factor, ↑ ESR, anemia; ↑ WBC count in synovial fluid; evidence of joint space narrowing and of bone erosion and deformity on radiograph (osteoporosis with advanced disease)

DMARDs, disease-modifying antirheumatic drugs; *ESR,* erythrocyte sedimentation rate; *MCP,* metacarpo-phalangeal; *NSAIDs,* nonsteroidal anti-inflammatory drugs; *WBC,* white blood cell.

NURSING IMPLEMENTATION

HEALTH PROMOTION. Prevention of RA is not possible based on the current state of knowledge. However, early treatment can help prevent further joint damage. Community education programs should focus on symptom recognition to promote early diagnosis and treatment of RA. The Arthritis Society offers many publications, classes, and support activities to assist people who are affected (see the Resources at the end of this chapter).

ACUTE INTERVENTION. The primary goals in the management of RA are reduction of inflammation, management of pain, maintenance of joint function, and prevention or minimization of joint deformity. Goals may be met through a comprehensive program of drug therapy, balance of rest and activity with joint

TABLE 67-10   PATIENT & CAREGIVER TEACHING GUIDE

Protection of Small Joints

The following instructions should be included when teaching the patient with arthritis how to protect small joints.

1. Maintain joint in neutral position to minimize deformity.
   - Press water from a sponge instead of wringing.
2. Use strongest joint available for any task.
   - When rising from chair, push with palms rather than fingers.
   - Carry laundry basket in both arms rather than with fingers.
3. Distribute weight over many joints instead of stressing a few.
   - Slide objects instead of lifting them.
   - Hold packages close to body for support.
4. Change positions frequently.
   - Do not hold a book or grip a steering wheel for long periods without resting.
   - Avoid grasping pencils or cutting vegetables with a knife for extended periods.
5. Avoid repetitive movements.
   - Do not knit for long periods.
   - Rest between rooms when vacuuming.
   - Modify home environment to include faucets and doorknobs that are pushed rather than turned.
6. Modify chores to avoid stress on joints.
   - Avoid heavy lifting.
   - Sit on stool instead of standing during meal preparation.

protection, heat and cold applications, exercise, and patient and caregiver teaching. The nurse works closely with other health care providers to restore function and to help patients make appropriate lifestyle adjustments to chronic illness.

Patients who are newly diagnosed with RA are usually treated on an outpatient basis. Hospitalization may be necessary for patients with extra-articular complications or advancing disease that necessitates reconstructive surgery for disabling deformities.

Intervention begins with a careful physical assessment (e.g., joint pain, swelling, range of motion [ROM], and general health status). The nurse must also evaluate psychosocial needs (e.g., family support, sexual satisfaction, emotional stress, financial constraints, vocational and career limitations) and environmental concerns (e.g., transportation, home or work modifications). After problem identification, a carefully planned program for rehabilitation and education can be coordinated by the nurse for the interdisciplinary health care team.

Suppression of inflammation is achieved most effectively through the administration of NSAIDs, DMARDs, and biological and targeted therapies. Careful attention to timing of drug administration is crucial to sustain a therapeutic drug level and reduce early morning stiffness. The nurse should discuss the action and adverse effects of each prescribed drug and the importance of necessary laboratory monitoring. Because many patients with RA take several different drugs, the drug regimen must be as easy as possible to understand. The nurse should encourage patients to develop a method for remembering to take their medications (e.g., pill container).

Nonpharmacological management may include the use of therapeutic heat and cold, rest, relaxation techniques, joint protection (Table 67-10; see also Table 67-4), biofeedback (see Chapter 12), transcutaneous electrical nerve stimulation (TENS; see Chapter 10), and hypnosis. The nurse should help the patient and family choose therapies that promote optimal comfort within the parameters of their lifestyle.

Lightweight splints may be prescribed to rest an inflamed joint and prevent deformity from muscle spasms and contractures. Splints should be removed at regular intervals to give skin care and perform ROM exercises. After assessment has been completed and supportive care has been given, the splints should be reapplied as prescribed. The occupational therapist may help identify additional self-help devices for ADLs.

Care and procedures should be scheduled around the patient's morning stiffness. Sitting or standing in a warm shower, sitting in a tub with warm towels around the shoulders, or simply soaking the hands in a basin of warm water may help relieve joint stiffness and allow the patient to perform ADLs more comfortably.

AMBULATORY AND HOME CARE

Rest. Alternating scheduled rest periods with activity throughout the day helps relieve fatigue and pain. The amount of rest needed varies according to the severity of the disease and the patient's limitations. Patients should rest before becoming exhausted. Total bed rest is rarely necessary and should be avoided, to prevent stiffness and other effects of immobility. However, even a patient with mild disease may require daytime rest in addition to 8 to 10 hours of sleep at night. The nurse should help patients identify ways to modify daily activities to avoid overexertion that can lead to fatigue and an exacerbation of disease activity. For example, a patient may tolerate meal preparation more easily while sitting on a high stool in front of the sink.

Good body alignment during rest can be maintained through use of a firm mattress or bed board. Positions of extension should be encouraged, and positions of flexion should be avoided. To decrease the risk for joint contracture, pillows should never be placed under the knees. A small, flat pillow may be used under the head and shoulders.

Joint Protection. Protecting joints from stress is important. The nurse can help patients identify ways to modify tasks to put less stress on joints during routine activities (see Table 67-10). Energy conservation requires careful planning. The emphasis is on work simplification techniques. Work should be done in short periods with scheduled rest breaks to avoid fatigue (pacing). Activities should be organized to avoid going up and down stairs repeatedly. Carts should be used to carry supplies, and materials that are used often can be stored in a convenient, easily reached area. Time-saving joint protective devices (e.g., electric can opener) should be used whenever possible. Tasks can also be delegated to other family members.

The patient's independence may be increased by occupational therapy training with assistive devices that help simplify tasks, such as built-up utensils, buttonhooks, modified drawer handles, lightweight plastic dishes, and raised toilet seats. Wearing shoes with Velcro fasteners and clothing with snaps or a zipper down the front makes dressing easier. A cane or a walker offers support and relief of pain when walking.

Heat and Cold Therapy and Exercise. Heat and cold applications can help relieve stiffness, pain, and muscle spasm. Application of ice is especially beneficial during periods of disease exacerbation, whereas moist heat appears to offer better relief of chronic stiffness. Superficial heat sources such as heating pads, moist hot packs, paraffin baths, and warm baths or showers can relieve stiffness to allow participation in therapeutic exercises. Plastic bags of frozen vegetables (peas or corn), which can easily mould around the shoulder, wrists, or knees, are an effective home treatment. Patients can also use ice cubes or small paper cups of frozen water to massage areas proximal or distal to a painful joint. Heat and cold can be used as often as desired. However,

heat application should not exceed 20 minutes at one time, and the cold application should not exceed 10 to 15 minutes at one time. The nurse should alert patients to the possibility of a burn and advise them to avoid the use of a heat-producing cream (e.g., capsaicin) with another external heat device.

Individualized exercise is an integral part of the treatment plan. Usually, a physiotherapist develops a therapeutic exercise program to improve the flexibility and strength of the affected joints and the patient's overall endurance. The nurse should reinforce program participation and ensure that the exercises are being performed correctly. Inadequate joint movement can result in progressive joint immobility and muscle weakness, and overaggressive exercise can result in increased pain, inflammation, and joint damage. It should be emphasized that participating in a recreational exercise program (e.g., walking, swimming) or performing usual daily activities docs not eliminate the patient's need for therapeutic exercise to maintain adequate joint motion.

Gentle ROM exercises are usually performed daily to keep the joints functional. Patients should have the opportunity to practise the exercises with supervision. Aquatic exercises in warm water (25°C to 30°C) allow easier joint movement because of the buoyancy and warmth of the water. At the same time, although movement seems easier, water provides two-way resistance that makes muscles work harder than they would in the air. During acute inflammation, exercises should be limited to one or two repetitions.

Psychological Support. Self-management and adherence to an individualized home treatment program can be accomplished only if the patient has a thorough understanding of RA, the nature and course of the disease, and the goals of therapy. In addition, the patient's value system and perception of the disease must be considered.

The patient is constantly challenged by problems of limited function and fatigue, loss of self-esteem, altered body image, and fear of disability and deformity. Alterations in sexuality should be discussed. Chronic pain or loss of function may make the patient vulnerable to believing the claims of false advertising and attempting unproven or even dangerous remedies. The nurse can help patients recognize fears and concerns that are faced by all people who live with chronic illness.

Evaluation of the family support system is important. Financial planning may be necessary. Community resources such as a home care nurse, homemaker services, and vocational rehabilitation may be considered. Self-help groups are beneficial for some patients.

The presence of chronic pain may lead to depression. Strategies that may help to decrease depressive symptoms include listening to music, reading, exercising, and counselling. Hypnosis and biofeedback may also be of value.

AGE-RELATED CONSIDERATIONS

ARTHRITIS
The prevalence of arthritis among older adults is high, and the disease is accompanied by problems unique to this age group. The most problematic areas related to connective tissue disease in older adults include the following:

- Because of the high incidence of OA expected in older adults, health care providers often do not consider the presence of other types of arthritis.
- Age alone causes changes in serological profiles, which makes interpretation of laboratory values such as RF and ESR more

difficult. Medications taken for comorbid conditions can also affect laboratory values.

- Polypharmacy in older adults can result in iatrogenic arthritis.
- Nonorganic musculo-skeletal pain syndromes and weakness may be related to depression and physical inactivity.
- Diseases such as systemic lupus erythematosus (SLE), which commonly occurs in younger adults, can develop in a milder form in older adults.

Aging brings many physical and metabolic changes that may increase older-adult patients' sensitivity to both the therapeutic and the toxic effects of some drugs. Older adults who take NSAIDs have an increased risk for adverse effects, particularly GI bleeding and renal toxicity. The use of NSAIDS with a shorter half-life may require more frequent dosing but may also produce fewer adverse effects in older-adult patients with altered drug metabolism.

The common occurrence of polypharmacy in the older adult makes the use of additional drugs for RA treatment particularly problematic because of the increased likelihood of untoward drug interactions. The drug regimen should be simplified as much as possible to increase adherence (e.g., limited number of drugs with decreased frequency of administration), particularly for patients who don't receive regular assistance.

A major concern of treatment in older-adult patients relates to the use of corticosteroid therapy. Corticosteroid-induced osteopenia can add to the problem of decreased bone density related to age and inactivity. It can also increase the occurrence of pathological fractures, especially compression fractures of vertebrae. Corticosteroid-induced myopathy can be minimized or prevented by an age-appropriate exercise program. Although important for all age groups, an adequate support system for older adults is a critical factor in the ability to follow a treatment regimen that includes nutritional planning, exercise, general health maintenance, and appropriate therapy.

GOUT

Gout is a type of recurring acute arthritis characterized by the accumulation of uric acid crystals in one or more joints. Characteristic deposits of sodium urate crystals occur in articular, periarticular, and subcutaneous tissues. Gout occurs more frequently in men than in women and affects up to 2% of Canadians (Arthritis Society, 2015a).

Gout may be classified as primary or secondary. In *primary gout,* a hereditary error of purine metabolism leads to the overproduction or retention of uric acid. Primary gout, which accounts for 90% of cases, occurs primarily in middle-aged men.

Secondary gout may be related to another acquired disorder or may be the result of drugs known to inhibit uric acid excretion. Secondary gout may also be caused by drugs that increase the rate of cell death, such as the chemotherapeutic agents used in treating leukemia. Hyperuricemia may also develop in patients taking thiazide diuretics, women who are postmenopausal, and organ transplant recipients who are receiving immuno-suppressive agents.

Obesity in men has been shown to increase the risk for gout. Hypertension, diuretic use, and excessive alcohol consumption are additional risk factors. A diet high in purine-rich foods (e.g., shellfish such as crab and shrimp; vegetables such as lentils, asparagus, and spinach; meats such as beef, chicken, and pork) will not cause gout but can trigger an acute attack if a person is susceptible to gout.

Etiology and Pathophysiology

Uric acid is the major end product of purine catabolism and is excreted primarily by the kidneys. Gout is caused by (1) an increase in uric acid production; (2) underexcretion of uric acid by the kidneys; or (3) increased intake of foods containing purines, which are metabolized to uric acid by the body. Underexcretion of uric acid is believed to be the major cause of hyperuricemia in 80% to 90% of people who are affected. High dietary intake of purine alone has relatively little effect on the uric acid levels. Hyperuricemia may result from prolonged fasting or excessive alcohol drinking because of the increased production of keto acids, which then inhibit uric acid excretion.

Clinical Manifestations and Complications

In the acute phase, gouty arthritis may occur in one or more joints but usually fewer than four. Affected joints may appear dusky or cyanotic and are extremely tender. Inflammation of the great toe *(podagra)* is the most common initial problem. Other affected joints may include the midtarsal area of the foot, the ankle, the knee, and the wrist. Olecranon (bony tip of the elbow) bursae may also be involved. Acute gouty arthritis is usually precipitated by trigger events such as trauma, surgery, alcohol ingestion, or systemic infection. Symptoms typically begin at night, with sudden swelling and excruciating pain; peak within several hours; and are often accompanied by low-grade fever. Individual attacks usually subside, treated or untreated, in 2 to 10 days. The affected joint returns entirely to normal, and patients are often free of symptoms between attacks.

Chronic gout is characterized by multiple joint involvement and visible deposits of sodium urate crystals, called *tophi.* These are typically noted in the synovium, the subchondral bone, the olecranon bursae, and the vertebrae; along tendons; and in the skin and cartilage (Figure 67-6). Tophi are rarely present at the time of the initial attack and are generally noted only many years after the onset of disease.

The severity of gouty arthritis varies. The clinical course may consist of infrequent mild attacks or multiple severe episodes (up to 12 per year) associated with a slowly progressive disability. In general, the higher the serum uric acid level, the earlier the appearance of tophi and the greater the tendency toward more frequent, severe episodes of acute gout. Chronic inflammation may result in joint deformity, and cartilage destruction may

FIGURE 67-6 Tophi associated with chronic gout. Nodules are painless and filed with uric acid crystals. Source: Courtesy of John Cook, MD. From Goldstein, B. G., & Goldstein, A. E. (1997). *Practical dermatology.* (2nd ed.). St Louis: Mosby.

predispose the joint to secondary OA. Large and unsightly tophaceous deposits may perforate overlying skin, producing draining sinuses that often become infected.

Excessive uric acid excretion may lead to kidney or urinary tract stone formation. Pyelonephritis associated with intrarenal sodium urate deposits and obstruction may contribute to renal disease.

Diagnostic Studies

In gout, serum uric acid levels are usually elevated as high as 0.51 mmol/L. However, hyperuricemia is not specifically diagnostic of gout because increased levels may be related to a variety of drugs or may exist as an asymptomatic abnormality in the general population. Specimens for 24-hour urine uric acid values may be obtained to determine if the disease is caused by decreased renal excretion or overproduction of uric acid.

Synovial fluid aspiration is a controversial part of patient evaluation because an accurate diagnosis of gout is possible in 80% of patients on the basis of clinical symptoms alone. However, aspiration may have therapeutic value by decompressing a swollen joint capsule. Joint aspiration is also the only reliable method to distinguish gout from septic arthritis and *pseudogout* (calcium phosphate crystals are formed). Affected fluid characteristically contains needle-like monosodium urate crystals (Saccomano & Ferrera, 2015). Radiographic studies appear normal in the early stages of gout. In chronic disease, tophi may appear as eroded areas in the bone.

Collaborative Care

Goals for care of patients with gout (Table 67-11) include termination of an acute attack through use of an anti-inflammatory agent such as colchicine. Drug therapy is the primary therapy used in treating acute and chronic gout. In addition, weight reduction (as needed) and possible avoidance of alcohol and foods high in purine (red and organ meats) are recommended.

Drug Therapy. Acute gout is treated with colchicine and NSAIDs. Because colchicine has anti-inflammatory effects but no analgesic properties, an NSAID is added to the treatment regimen for pain management. Oral administration of colchicine generally produces dramatic pain relief when given within 12 to 24 hours of an attack (Hardy, 2011). Colchicine also has diagnostic merit in that a good response to this drug offers further evidence for the diagnosis of gout.

Future attacks of gout are prevented in part by a maintenance dose of urate-lowering drugs such as a xanthine oxidase inhibitor (allopurinol [Zyloprim]) or a uricosuric drug (probenecid [Benuryl]). Febuxostat (Uloric), a selective inhibitor of xanthine oxidase, is given for long-term management of hyperuricemia in people with chronic gout.

Corticosteroids, given either orally or by intra-articular injection, can be helpful in treating acute attacks of gout. Systemic corticosteroids may be used only if routine therapies are contraindicated or ineffective. Adrenocorticotrophic hormone (ACTH) may also be used for treating acute gout.

For many years, the standard therapy for hyperuricemia caused by urate underexcretion has been uricosuric drugs such as probenecid, which inhibit renal tubular reabsorption of urates. However, these drugs are ineffective when creatinine clearance is reduced, as can occur in patients older than 60 years and those with renal impairment. ASA (Aspirin) inactivates the effect of uricosurics, resulting in urate retention, and should be avoided while patients are taking uricosuric drugs. Acetaminophen can be used safely if analgesia is required.

Adequate urine volume with normal renal function (2 to 3 L/day) must be maintained to prevent precipitation of uric acid in the renal tubules. Allopurinol, which blocks the production of uric acid, is particularly useful in patients with uric acid stones or renal impairment, in whom uricosuric drugs may be ineffective or dangerous. The angiotensin II receptor antagonist losartan (Cozaar) may be especially useful in the treatment of older-adult patients with both gout and hypertension. Losartan promotes urate diuresis and may normalize serum urate levels. Combination therapy with losartan and allopurinol may also be given. Regardless of which drugs are prescribed, serum uric acid levels must be checked regularly to monitor treatment effectiveness.

Nutritional Therapy. Dietary restrictions that limit alcohol and foods high in purine help minimize uric acid production (see Chapter 48, Table 48-13). Patients who are obese should be instructed to follow a carefully planned weight-reduction program.

NURSING MANAGEMENT
GOUT

Nursing interventions for patients with an acute episode of gout include supportive care for the inflamed joints. The nurse must avoid causing pain to an inflamed joint by careless handling. Bed rest may be appropriate, with affected joints properly immobilized. Involvement of a lower extremity may require use of a cradle or footboard to protect the painful area from the weight of bed linens. The nurse should assess the limitation of motion and degree of pain and document treatment effectiveness.

The nurse should help patients and their families understand that hyperuricemia and gouty arthritis are chronic problems that can be controlled with careful adherence to a treatment program (Saccomano & Ferrera, 2015). The importance of drug therapy and the need for periodic determination of serum uric acid levels should be explained thoroughly. Patients should be able to demonstrate knowledge of precipitating factors that may cause an attack, including excessive caloric intake or overindulgence in purine-containing foods and alcohol; starvation (fasting); drug use (e.g., niacin, ASA [Aspirin], diuretics); and major medical events (e.g., surgery, myocardial infarction).

TABLE 67-11 COLLABORATIVE CARE

Gout

Diagnostic
- History and physical examination
- Elevated serum uric acid levels
- Elevated uric acid levels in 24-hr urine collection
- Family history of gout
- Presence of sodium urate crystals in synovial fluid
- Radiographic studies

Collaborative Therapy
- Dietary avoidance of food and fluids with high purine content (e.g., anchovies, liver, wine, beer)
- Joint aspiration and intra-articular corticosteroids

- Drug therapy
  - Adrenocorticotrophic hormone (ACTH)
  - Allopurinol (Zyloprim)
  - Colchicine
  - Corticosteroids (prednisone)
  - Febuxostat (Uloric)
  - Intra-articular corticosteroids (methylprednisolone acetate)
  - Nonsteroidal anti-inflammatory drugs (e.g., naproxen [Naprosyn])
  - Probenecid (Benuryl)
- Joint immobilization
- Local application of heat or cold

LYME DISEASE

Lyme disease is a spirochetal infection caused by *Borrelia burgdorferi* and transmitted by the bite of an infected deer tick. It was first identified in 1975 in Lyme, Connecticut, after an unusual clustering of arthritis in children. The tick typically feeds on mice, dogs, cats, cows, horses, deer, and humans. Wild animals do not exhibit the illness, but clinical Lyme disease does occur in domestic animals. Person-to-person transmission does not occur.

The peak season for infection in humans is from spring and summer. The number of infected ticks continues to rise in Canada. The most prevalent areas in Canada include southern British Columbia; southeastern and south-central Manitoba; southern, eastern, and northwestern Ontario; southern Quebec; southern New Brunswick and Grand Manan Island; and parts of Nova Scotia (Public Health Agency of Canada, 2016).

Symptoms of Lyme disease can mimic those of other diseases, such as multiple sclerosis, mononucleosis, and meningitis. The most characteristic clinical symptom of early localized disease is erythema migrans (EM), a skin lesion at the site of the tick bite that occurs in 70% to 80% of people who are infected, within 3 to 30 days after exposure (Figure 67-7). The lesion begins as a red macule or papule that slowly expands to form a large round lesion of up to 30 cm with a bright red border and central clearing ("bull's eye rash"). The EM lesion is often accompanied by acute flulike symptoms, such as low-grade fever, chills, headache, stiff neck, fatigue, swollen lymph nodes, and migratory joint and muscle pain. Of note, loss of tone in facial muscles can manifest as Bell's palsy. Symptoms usually occur within a week but may be delayed for up to 30 days. The flulike symptoms generally resolve over a period of weeks or months, even if untreated.

If not treated, the spirochete can disseminate within several weeks or months to the heart, joints, and central nervous system (CNS). Carditis may occur (Bockenstedt, 2012). About 60% of people with untreated infection develop chronic arthritic pain and swelling in the large joints. Nervous system problems may include severe headaches or poor motor coordination. One neurological condition, tertiary neuroborreliosis, results in confusion and forgetfulness.

A diagnosis of Lyme disease is often based on clinical manifestations, particularly the EM lesion, and a history of exposure in an endemic area. CBC count and ESR are usually normal. A two-step laboratory testing process is recommended to confirm diagnosis (Government of Canada, 2015). The first step is the enzyme immunoassay (EIA), a test that yields positive results for most people with Lyme disease. If the EIA result is positive or inconclusive, a Western blot test is done to confirm the infection. Cerebro-spinal fluid should be examined in individuals with neurological involvement.

Active lesions can be treated with oral antibiotic therapy. Doxycycline, cefuroxime (Ceftin), and amoxicillin are often effective in early stages of infection and in prevention of later stages of the disease. Doxycycline prevents Lyme disease when given within 3 days after the bite of a deer tick. Short-term therapy for 2 to 3 weeks is usually effective for solitary EM, but patients with neurological or cardiac complications may require IV therapy with ceftriaxone or penicillin. In most cases, people with Lyme disease are treated successfully with antibiotics. Approximately 10% to 20% of people treated with antibiotics for Lyme disease may experience lingering fatigue or joint and muscle pain. This condition, known as post–Lyme disease syndrome, may result from residual damage to tissues and the immune system (Bockenstedt, 2012).

Reducing exposure to ticks is the best way to prevent Lyme disease. Teaching of patients and caregivers who live in endemic areas is outlined in Table 67-12. No vaccine is available for Lyme disease.

FIGURE 67-7 Erythema migrans of Lyme disease. Source: Swartz, M. H. (2010). *Textbook of physical diagnosis: History and examination* (6th ed., p. 186, Figure 8-112). Philadelphia: W. B. Saunders.

TABLE 67-12   PATIENT & CAREGIVER TEACHING GUIDE

Prevention and Early Treatment of Lyme Disease

The following instructions should be included when teaching patients and caregivers how to prevent Lyme disease.

- Avoid walking through tall grasses and low brush and sitting on logs.
- Mow grass. Remove brush around paths, buildings, and campsites to create "tick-safe zones."
- Move woodpiles and bird feeders away from house. Discourage deer (main source of food for adult ticks) from being in the area.
- Wear long pants or nylon tights of tightly woven, light-coloured fabric so that ticks can be easily seen.
- Tuck pants into boots or long socks, tuck long-sleeved shirts into pants, and wear closed shoes when hiking.
- Check often for ticks crawling from pant legs to open skin.
- Thoroughly inspect and wash clothes. Placing clothing in dryer on high heat effectively kills ticks.
- Spray insect repellent containing DEET sparingly on skin or apply permethrin to boots and clothes (especially on lower extremities) and camping gear.
- Have pets wear tick collars, inspect them often, and do not allow pets on furniture or beds.

The following instructions should be included when teaching patients and caregivers living in endemic areas.

- Remove attached ticks with tweezers (not fingers). Grasp tick's mouth parts as close to skin as possible and gently pull straight out. Do not twist or jerk. Avoid folk solutions such as painting the tick with nail polish or petroleum jelly.
- Wash bitten area with soap and water and apply antiseptic. Wash hands.
- See a health care provider immediately if flulike symptoms or a bull's eye rash appears within 3 to 30 days after removal of tick.

DEET, diethyltoluamide.
Source: Adapted from Centers for Disease Control and Prevention. (2015). *It's spring: Time to prevent Lyme disease.* Retrieved from *http://www.cdc.gov/features/lymedisease;* and Centers for Disease Control and Prevention. (2015). *Tick removal.* Retrieved from *www.cdc.gov/lyme/removal/index.html.*

SEPTIC ARTHRITIS

Septic arthritis (infectious or bacterial arthritis) is caused by microorganisms invading the joint cavity. Bacteria can travel through the bloodstream from another site of active infection, resulting in hematogenous seeding of the joint. Organisms can also be introduced directly through trauma or surgical incision.

Any bacteria can cause the infection, including nonpathogenic bacteria in patients who are immuno-compromised. *Staphylococcus aureus* and *Streptococcus hemolyticus* are the most common causative organisms. *Neisseria gonorrhoeae* is the most common cause in sexually active young adults. Factors that increase the risk for infection include diseases in which host resistance is decreased (e.g., leukemia, diabetes mellitus); treatment with corticosteroids or immuno-suppressive drugs; and debilitating chronic illness.

Large joints such as the knee and the hip are most frequently involved. Inflammation of the joint cavity causes severe pain, erythema, and swelling. Because infection has often spread from a primary site elsewhere in the body, fever or shaking chills often accompany articular manifestations. A diagnosis may be made by aspiration of the joint (arthrocentesis) and culture of the synovial fluid. However, WBC counts may be low early in the infectious process, and diagnosis is not possible based solely on WBC counts. Blood cultures for aerobic and anaerobic organisms should also be obtained.

Septic arthritis requires prompt treatment to prevent joint destruction and bone loss. Broad-spectrum antibiotics against Gram-negative organisms, pneumococci, and staphylococci are often started before the causative organism is identified. Once the organism is determined, the treatment can become specific. Infections may respond to treatment within 2 weeks or may take as long as 4 to 8 weeks, depending on the causative organism. Local aspiration and surgical drainage may be required. If diagnosis and treatment are delayed, destruction of articular cartilage can occur, followed by loss of joint function. Chronic infection can also develop. Septic arthritis of the hip can contribute to development of avascular necrosis.

Nursing intervention includes assessment and monitoring of joint inflammation, pain, and fever. To control pain, use resting splints or traction to immobilize affected joints. Local hot compresses can also help relieve pain. Gentle ROM exercises should be initiated as soon as tolerated to prevent muscle atrophy and joint contractures. The nurse should explain the need for antibiotics and the importance of their continued use until the infection is resolved. The nurse should offer support to a patient who requires arthrocentesis or operative drainage. Strict aseptic technique should be used in assisting with joint aspiration procedures.

SPONDYLOARTHROPATHIES

The spondyloarthropathies are a group of interrelated multisystem inflammatory disorders that affect the spine, the peripheral joints, and periarticular structures. These disorders are all negative for rheumatoid factor (RF) and thus are often referred to as seronegative arthropathies.

Inheritance of HLA-B27 is strongly associated with these diseases. Both genetic and environmental factors play a role in the development of this group of diseases, which includes ankylosing spondylitis, psoriatic arthritis, and reactive arthritis.

(HLAs and their relationship to autoimmune diseases are discussed in Chapter 16.)

The spondyloarthropathies share clinical and laboratory characteristics that make it difficult to distinguish among them in early stages of disease. These characteristics include absence of antibodies in the serum, inflammatory arthritis of the spine, peripheral joint involvement predominantly of the lower extremities, sacroiliitis, uveitis, enteric mucosal lesions, and skin lesions (Robinson & Benham, 2015).

ANKYLOSING SPONDYLITIS

Ankylosing spondylitis (AS) is a chronic inflammatory disease that affects primarily the axial skeleton, including the sacroiliac joints, the intervertebral disc spaces, and the costovertebral articulations. HLA-B27 antigen is found in approximately 90% of people with AS. Individuals with the antigen have a significantly greater risk of developing a spondyloarthropathy than those who do not. As many as 150 000 to 300 000 Canadians are affected by AS (Arthritis Society, 2015b). The usual age at onset is 15 to 30 years, and three times more men than women develop AS (Arthritis Society, 2015b).

Etiology and Pathophysiology

Genetic predisposition appears to play an important role in the disease pathogenesis, but the precise mechanisms are unknown. Aseptic synovial inflammation in joints and adjacent tissue causes the formation of granulation tissue *(pannus)* and dense fibrous scars that lead to fusion of articular tissues. Extra-articular inflammation can affect the eyes, the lungs, the heart, the kidneys, and the peripheral nervous system.

Clinical Manifestations and Complications

AS is characterized by symmetrical sacroiliitis and progressive inflammatory arthritis of the axial skeleton. Symptoms of inflammatory spine pain are the first clues to the diagnosis. Affected patients typically complain of low back pain, stiffness, and limitation of motion that is worse during the night and in the morning but improves with mild activity. In affected women, early symptoms of disease may be pain and stiffness in the neck rather than the lower back. General symptoms such as fever, fatigue, anorexia, and weight loss are rarely present. Uveitis (intraocular inflammation) is the most common nonskeletal symptom. It can appear as an initial manifestation of the disease years before arthritic symptoms develop. Patients with AS may also experience chest pain and sternal or costal cartilage tenderness that can be distressing.

Severe postural abnormalities and deformity can lead to significant disability for patients with AS (Figure 67-8). Impaired spinal ROM and fixed kyphosis contribute to altered visual function, which raises concerns about safe ambulation. Aortic insufficiency and pulmonary fibrosis are frequent complications. Cauda equina syndrome can also result, contributing to lower extremity weakness and bladder dysfunction. In addition, affected patients are at risk for spinal fracture because of associated osteoporosis.

Diagnostic Studies

Radiological studies are essential for the diagnosis and follow-up of AS. However, radiographs are limited in detecting early sacroiliitis or subtle changes in posterior vertebrae. MRI can be useful in assessing early cartilage abnormalities, while CT scan

FIGURE 67-8 Advanced ankylosing spondylitis. Kyphotic posture causes many patients to have a protuberant abdomen secondary to pulmonary restriction. Source: Kim, D. H., Henn, J., Vaccaro, A. R., et al. (Eds.). (2006). *Surgical anatomy and techniques to the spine.* Philadelphia: W. B. Saunders.

is appropriate in specific situations (e.g., cases with subtle radiographic changes). Changes on later spinal radiographs include the appearance of "bamboo spine," which is the result of calcifications *(syndesmophytes)* that bridge from one vertebra to another.

Laboratory testing is not specific, but ESR may be elevated and mild anemia may be present. When the suspicion of AS is high, the presence of HLA-B27 antigen increases the likelihood of this diagnosis.

Collaborative Care

Prevention of AS is not possible. However, families with other diagnosed HLA-B27–positive rheumatic diseases (e.g., acute anterior uveitis, juvenile spondyloarthritis) should be alert to signs of low back pain for early identification and treatment of AS.

Care of the patient with AS is aimed at maintaining maximal skeletal mobility while decreasing pain and inflammation. Heat applications can help in the relief of local symptoms. NSAIDs and salicylates are commonly prescribed. DMARDs such as sulphasalazine (Salazopyrin) or methotrexate have little effect on spinal disease but may help with peripheral joint disease. Local corticosteroid injections may be beneficial in relieving symptoms.

TNF, which promotes inflammation, is found in elevated levels in the blood and certain tissues of patients with AS. Etanercept (Enbrel), a biological and targeted therapy drug, binds TNF and inhibits its action. Etanercept reduces active inflammation and improves spinal mobility. Additional anti-TNF inhibitors (infliximab, adalimumab, golimumab) may also be effective.

Once pain and stiffness are managed, exercise is essential. Postural control is important for minimizing spinal deformity. The exercise regimen should include back, neck, and chest stretches. Hydrotherapy has also been shown to decrease pain and facilitate spinal extension. Surgery may be indicated for severe deformity and mobility impairment. Spinal osteotomy

🧬 **GENETICS IN CLINICAL PRACTICE**

Ankylosing Spondylitis

Genetic Basis
Inheritance of human leukocyte antigen HLA-B27 increases susceptibility to development of ankylosing spondylitis (AS).

Incidence
- About 80% to 90% of White patients with ankylosing spondylitis (AS) have HLA-B27 antigen.
- Inheriting HLA-B27 does not mean that a person will develop the disease. Of children who inherit HLA-B27 from a parent with AS, 80% do not develop the disease.
- AS is three times more common in men than in women.
- It occurs more often in White people than in other ethnic groups.
- It affects 7 per 100 000 people.

Genetic Testing
- Testing for HLA-B27 antigen is available.

Clinical Implications
- Diagnosis of AS usually occurs between ages 18 and 30.
- Multiple genetic and environmental factors play a role in the pathogenesis of the disease.
- It is not known how HLA-B27 increases the risk for AS.
- AS is present in about 3% to 10% of patients with inflammatory bowel disease (IBD).
- About 50% to 70% of patients with both AS and IBD have the HLA-B27 antigen.

HLA, human leukocyte antigen.

and total joint replacement are the most commonly performed procedures (see Chapter 65).

NURSING MANAGEMENT ANKYLOSING SPONDYLITIS

The key nursing responsibility for patients with AS is education about the disease and principles of therapy. The home management program should include regular exercise and attention to posture, local moist heat applications, and knowledgeable use of drugs.

The nurse's baseline ROM assessment should include chest expansion (using breathing exercises). Smoking cessation must be encouraged to decrease the risk for lung complications in patients with reduced chest expansion. Ongoing physiotherapy includes gentle, graded stretching and strengthening exercises to preserve ROM and improve thoracolumbar flexion and extension.

The nurse should discourage excessive physical exertion during flare-ups of the disease. Proper positioning at rest is essential. The mattress should be firm, and patients should sleep on the back with a flat pillow, avoiding positions that encourage flexion deformity. Postural training emphasizes avoiding spinal flexion (e.g., leaning over a desk); heavy lifting; and prolonged walking, standing, or sitting. Participation in sports that facilitate natural stretching, such as swimming and racquet games, should be encouraged. Family counselling and vocational rehabilitation are important.

PSORIATIC ARTHRITIS

Psoriatic arthritis (PsA) is a progressive inflammatory disease that affects approximately 10% to 30% of people with psoriasis (Arthritis Society, 2017e). *Psoriasis* is a common, benign, inflammatory skin disorder characterized by red, irritated, and scaly patches. Both PsA and psoriasis appear to have a genetic link with the HLA antigens in many patients. Although the exact cause of PsA is unknown, a combination of immune, genetic, and environmental factors is suspected.

PsA can occur in different forms. These include (1) arthritis involving primarily the small joints of the hands and feet (DIP), (2) asymmetric arthritis involving joints of the extremities, (3) symmetric polyarthritis resembling RA, and (4) arthritis of the sacroiliac joints and spine (psoriatic spondylitis) (Arthritis Society, 2017e).

On radiographs, the cartilage loss and erosion resemble those of RA. Many patients with advanced cases of PsA have widened joint spaces. A "pencil-in-cup" deformity is common at the DIP joints as a result of osteolysis. In this deformity, the narrowed end(s) of the metacarpals or phalanges insert into the expanded end of the other (adjacent) bone sharing the joint. Elevated ESR, mild anemia, and elevated blood uric acid levels are present in some patients; therefore, gout must be ruled out.

Treatment includes splinting, joint protection, and physiotherapy. NSAIDs given early in the course of the disease may help with inflammation. Drug therapy also includes DMARDs such as methotrexate, which are effective for both cutaneous and articular manifestations. Sulphasalazine (Salazopyrin) and cyclosporin may be used for treating PsA. In addition, biological and targeted therapy, such as etanercept, golimumab, adalimumab, and infliximab, may also be used.

REACTIVE ARTHRITIS

Reactive arthritis *(Reiter's syndrome)* occurs more commonly in young men than in young women. It is associated with a symptom complex that includes urethritis, conjunctivitis, and mucocutaneous lesions. Although the exact etiology is unknown, reactive arthritis appears to occur after exposure to specific genito-urinary or GI tract infections. *Chlamydia trachomatis* is most often implicated in sexually transmitted reactive arthritis (Arthritis Society, 2017f). Reactive arthritis is also associated with GI infections with *Shigella, Salmonella, Campylobacter,* or *Yersinia* species and other microorganisms.

Individuals who are positive for HLA-B27 are at increased risk of developing reactive arthritis after sexual contact or exposure to certain enteric pathogens. This finding supports the likelihood of a genetic predisposition.

Urethritis develops within 1 to 2 weeks after sexual contact or GI infection. In women, symptoms include cervicitis. Low-grade fever, conjunctivitis, and arthritis may occur over the next several weeks. This type of arthritis tends to be asymmetrical, frequently involving the large joints of the lower extremities and the toes. Lower back pain may occur with severe disease. Mucocutaneous lesions commonly manifest as small, painless, superficial ulcerations on the tongue, the oral mucosa, and the glans penis. Soft-tissue manifestations commonly include Achilles tendinitis or plantar fasciitis. Few laboratory findings are abnormal, although the ESR may be elevated.

Prognosis is favourable; most patients recover after 2 to 16 weeks. Because reactive arthritis is often associated with *C. trachomatis* infection, treatment of patients and their sexual partners with doxycycline is widely recommended. Conjunctivitis and lesions require no treatment, but topical ophthalmic corticosteroids are typically prescribed for treatment of uveitis. Drug therapy may also include NSAIDs, methotrexate, and sulphasalazine. Physiotherapy may be helpful during disease recovery.

Most patients have complete remission with restoration of full joint function. Up to 30% may develop chronic or recurring disease, which can result in major disability (Hill, 2012). Radiographic changes in chronic disease closely resemble those of AS. Treatment of chronic reactive arthritis is based on symptoms.

OTHER CONNECTIVE TISSUE DISORDERS

SYSTEMIC LUPUS ERYTHEMATOSUS

Systemic lupus erythematosus (SLE) is a multisystem, inflammatory, autoimmune disease. It is a complex disorder of multifactorial origin resulting from interactions among genetic, hormonal, environmental, and immunological factors. SLE typically affects the skin, the joints, and serous membranes (pleura, pericardium), along with the renal, hematological, and neurological systems. SLE is characterized by a chronic, unpredictable course marked by alternating periods of exacerbation and remission.

The overall incidence of SLE in Canada is approximately 1 per 2 000 people. Most cases occur in women during their child-bearing years. Approximately 90% of people with SLE are women (Arthritis Society, 2017g).

Etiology and Pathophysiology

The etiology of the abnormal immune response in SLE is unknown. Because of the high prevalence of SLE among family members, a genetic influence is suspected. Multiple susceptibility genes from the HLA complex, including HLA-DR3, show associations with SLE.

Hormones are also known to play a role in the etiology of SLE. Onset or exacerbation of disease symptoms sometimes occurs after the onset of menarche, with the use of oral contraceptives, and during and after pregnancy. The disease tends to worsen in the immediate postpartum period.

Environmental factors are believed to contribute to the occurrence of SLE; sun exposure and burns are the most common environmental triggers. Infectious agents may serve as a stimulus for immune hyperactivity. SLE may also be precipitated or aggravated by certain drugs, such as procainamide, hydralazine (Apresoline), and a number of anticonvulsant agents.

SLE is characterized by the production of a large variety of autoantibodies against nucleic acids (e.g., single- and double-stranded DNA), erythrocytes, coagulation proteins, lymphocytes, platelets, and many other self-proteins. Autoimmune reactions characteristically are directed against constituents of the cell nucleus (antinuclear antibodies [ANAs]), particularly DNA.

Circulating immune complexes containing antibodies against DNA are deposited in the basement membranes of capillaries in the kidneys, the heart, the skin, the brain, and the joints. Complement is activated and inflammation occurs. The over-aggressive antibody response is also related to activation of B and T cells. The specific manifestations of SLE depend on which cell types or organs are involved. (SLE is a type III hypersensitivity response [see Chapter 16].)

Clinical Manifestations and Complications

The severity of SLE is extremely variable, ranging from relatively mild to rapidly progressive and affecting many organ systems (Figure 67-9). The progressive organ involvement of SLE has no characteristic pattern. Any organ can be affected by an accumulation of circulating immune complexes. The most commonly

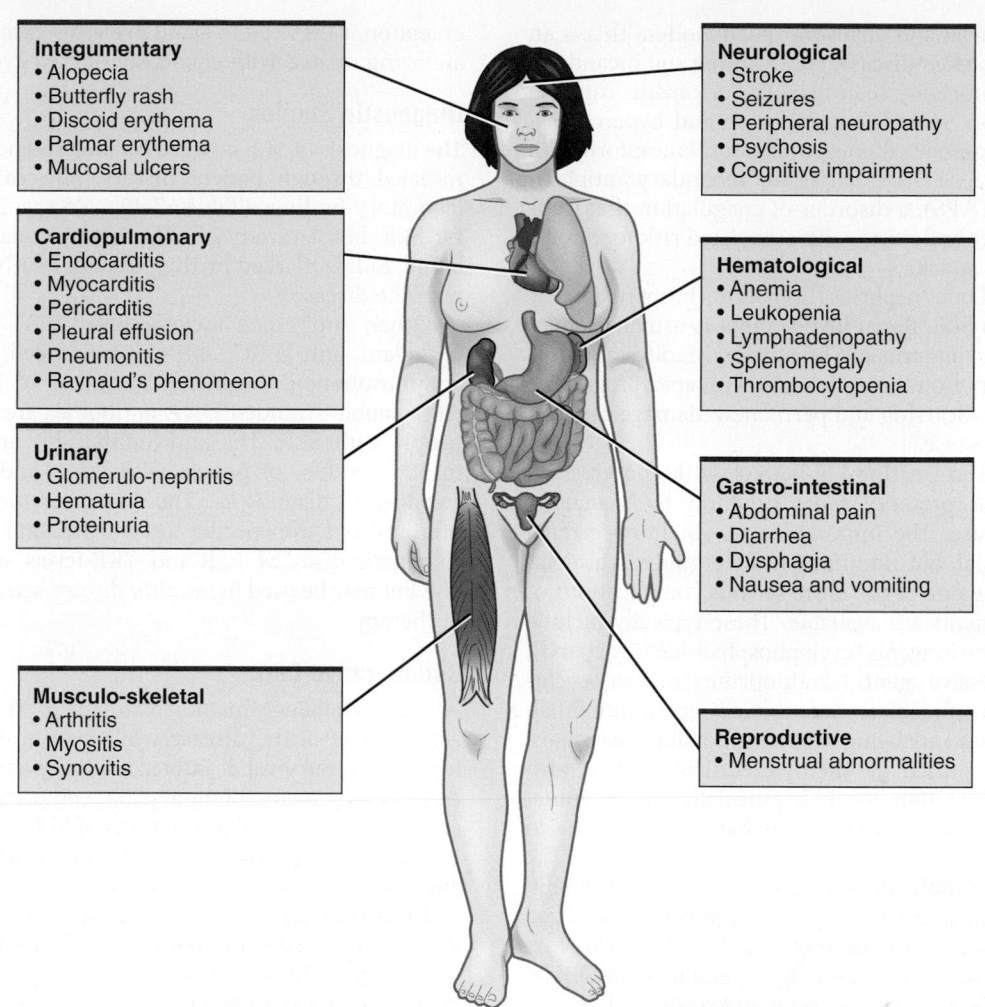

Integumentary
• Alopecia
• Butterfly rash
• Discoid erythema
• Palmar erythema
• Mucosal ulcers

Cardiopulmonary
• Endocarditis
• Myocarditis
• Pericarditis
• Pleural effusion
• Pneumonitis
• Raynaud's phenomenon

Urinary
• Glomerulo-nephritis
• Hematuria
• Proteinuria

Musculo-skeletal
• Arthritis
• Myositis
• Synovitis

Neurological
• Stroke
• Seizures
• Peripheral neuropathy
• Psychosis
• Cognitive impairment

Hematological
• Anemia
• Leukopenia
• Lymphadenopathy
• Splenomegaly
• Thrombocytopenia

Gastro-intestinal
• Abdominal pain
• Diarrhea
• Dysphagia
• Nausea and vomiting

Reproductive
• Menstrual abnormalities

FIGURE 67-9 Multisystem involvement in systemic lupus erythematosus.

affected tissues are the skin and muscle, the lining of the lungs, the heart, nervous tissue, and the kidneys. Generalized complaints such as fever, weight loss, arthralgia, and excessive fatigue may precede an exacerbation of disease activity.

Dermatological Manifestations. Cutaneous vascular lesions can appear in any location but are most likely to develop in sun-exposed areas. Severe skin reactions can occur in people who are photosensitive. The classic "butterfly rash" over the cheeks and bridge of the nose occurs in 50% of patients with SLE (Figure 67-10). About 20% of patients have *discoid* (round, coin-shaped) lesions. A small number of patients have persistent lesions, photosensitivity, and mild systemic disease, in a syndrome referred to as *subacute cutaneous lupus.*

Ulcers of the oral or the nasopharyngeal membranes occur in up to one-third of patients with SLE. Alopecia is also common, with or without underlying scalp lesions. The hair may grow back during remission, but hair loss may be permanent over lesions. The scalp becomes dry and scaly and atrophied.

Musculo-Skeletal Problems. Arthritis occurs in more than 90% of patients with SLE. Polyarthralgia with morning stiffness is often the patient's first complaint and may precede the onset of multisystem disease by many years. Diffuse swelling is accompanied by joint and muscle pain, and some stiffness may be experienced. Lupus-related arthritis is generally nonerosive, but it may cause deformities such as swan-neck appearance of the fingers (see Figure 67-4, *D*), ulnar deviation, and subluxation

FIGURE 67-10 Butterfly rash manifestation of systemic lupus erythematosus. Source: Kliegman, R. M., Stanton, B. F., St. Geme III, J. W., et al. (Eds.). (2011). *Nelson textbook of pediatrics* (19th ed., Figure 152-1, A). Philadelphia: W. B. Saunders.

with hyperlaxity of the joints. Patients with SLE have an increased risk for bone loss and fracture.

Cardiopulmonary Problems. Tachypnea and cough in patients with SLE are suggestive of lung disease. Pleurisy is also possible. Cardiac involvement may include dysrhythmias that result from fibrosis of the sinoatrial and atrioventricular nodes. This is an ominous sign of advanced disease, contributing significantly to the morbidity and mortality seen in SLE. Pericarditis can also occur. Clinical factors such as hypertension and hypercholesterolemia require aggressive therapy and careful monitoring. In addition, people with SLE are at risk for secondary antiphospholipid syndrome (APS), a disorder of coagulation that leads to clots in the arteries and veins, with associated risk for stroke, gangrene, and heart attack.

Renal Problems. Lupus nephritis (LN) occurs in approximately 40% of patients with SLE. Renal involvement is usually evident within 5 years after symptoms of SLE appear. Manifestations of renal involvement vary from mild proteinuria to rapid, progressive glomerulo-nephritis. Scarring and permanent damage can lead to end-stage renal disease.

The primary goal in treating LN is to slow the progression of nephropathy and preserve renal function by managing the underlying disease. The importance of obtaining a renal biopsy is controversial, but findings can help guide treatment. Although LN may be one of the more serious complications of SLE, effective treatments are available. These typically include corticosteroids, cytotoxic agents (cyclophosphamide [Procytox]), and immuno-suppressive agents (azathioprine [Imuran], cyclosporin [Neoral], mycophenolate mofetil [CellCept]). Rituximab and eculizumab (Soliris) are being studied as possible treatments. Oral prednisone or pulsed IV methylprednisolone may also be used as an intervention for LN, especially in the initial treatment period, when cytotoxic agents have not had time to take effect.

Nervous System Problems. Along with renal involvement, neuro-psychiatric manifestations are prevalent in SLE. Generalized or focal seizures are the most common manifestation involving the CNS and occur in as many as 15% of patients with SLE by the time of diagnosis. Seizures are generally controlled by corticosteroids or anticonvulsant drugs. Peripheral neuropathy can also occur, leading to sensory and motor deficits.

Cognitive dysfunction, recognized as a CNS manifestation of SLE, may result from the deposition of immune complexes within brain tissue. It is characterized by disordered thought processes, disorientation, memory deficits, and psychiatric symptoms such as severe depression and psychosis. Occasionally, a stroke or aseptic meningitis may be attributable to SLE. Headaches are also common and can become severe during exacerbation of the disease.

Hematological Problems. The formation of antibodies against blood cells, such as erythrocytes, leukocytes, and thrombocytes, and against coagulation factors, is also a common feature of SLE (Tsokos, 2011). Anemia, mild leukopenia, and thrombo-cytopenia are often present in SLE. Some patients develop a tendency toward coagulopathy, involving either excessive bleeding or blood clot development. A manifestation of antiphospholipid antibody syndrome is a common cause of hypercoagulability in patients with SLE, many of whom benefit from high-intensity treatment with warfarin (Coumadin).

Infection. Patients with SLE appear to have increased susceptibility to infections, possibly in relation to defects in the ability to phagocytize invading bacteria, deficiencies in production of antibodies, and the immuno-suppressive effect of many anti-inflammatory drugs. Infection is a major cause of death, with pneumonia being the most common infection. Fever may indicate an underlying infectious process rather than lupus activity alone. Vaccinations are generally safe for patients with SLE. The exception is the need to avoid live virus vaccines in patients who are being treated with corticosteroids or cytotoxic agents.

Diagnostic Studies

The diagnosis of SLE is based on the presence of distinct criteria revealed through patient history, physical examination, and laboratory findings (Table 67-13). No specific test is diagnostic for SLE, but a variety of abnormalities may be present in the blood. SLE is marked by the presence of ANA in 97% of people with the disease.

Other antibodies include anti-DNA, antineuronal, anti-coagulant, anti-WBC, anti–red blood cell (RBC), antiplatelet, antiphospholipid, and anti–basement membrane antibodies. Anti-double-stranded DNA antibodies are found in half of all people with SLE. The anti-Smith (Sm) antibodies are found in 30% to 40% of people with lupus and are almost always considered diagnostic. The lupus erythematosus (LE) cell prep test is a nonspecific test for SLE and is positive in other rheumatic diseases. ESR and CRP levels are not diagnostic of SLE but may be used to monitor disease activity and effectiveness of therapy.

Collaborative Care

A major challenge in the treatment of SLE is to manage the active phase of the disease while preventing complications of treatments. Survival is influenced by several factors, including age, race, sex, socioeconomic status, comorbid conditions, and the severity of disease. The prognosis of SLE can be improved with early diagnosis, prompt recognition of serious organ involvement, and effective therapeutic regimens.

Drug Therapy. NSAIDs continue to be an important intervention, especially for patients with mild polyarthralgias or polyarthritis. Because prolonged therapy is likely, patients must be monitored carefully for GI and renal effects from NSAID use.

TABLE 67-13   CRITERIA FOR DIAGNOSIS OF SYSTEMIC LUPUS ERYTHEMATOSUS*

- Antinuclear antibodies
- Arthritis: nonerosive, involvement of two or more joints characterized by tenderness, swelling, and effusion
- Discoid rash
- Hematological disorder: hemolytic anemia, leukopenia, lymphopenia, or thrombo-cytopenia
- Immunological disorder: positive result of LE preparation; anti-DNA antibody or antibody to Sm nuclear antigen; or false-positive result of serological tests for syphilis
- Malar rash
- Neurological disorder: seizures or psychosis
- Oral ulcers
- Photosensitivity
- Renal disorder: persistent proteinuria or cellular casts in urine
- Serositis: pleuritis or pericarditis

LE, lupus erythematosus; *Sm,* Smith.
*SLE is diagnosed if four or more of the criteria are present, serially or simultaneously, during any interval of observation. Revised criteria by a subcommittee of the American College of Rheumatology are used for the purpose of classification in population surveys, not for the diagnosis in individual patients.
Sources: Tan, E. M., Cohen, A. S., Fries, J. F., et al. (1982). The 1982 revised criteria for the classification of systemic lupus erythematosus. *Arthritis and Rheumatism, 25*(11), 1271–1277. doi:10.1002/art.1780251101; and Hochberg, M. C. (1997). Updating the American College of Rheumatology revised criteria for the classification of systemic lupus erythematosus [Letter]. *Arthritis and Rheumatism, 40*(9), 1725. doi:10.1002/art.1780400928.

Antimalarial agents such as hydroxychloroquine (Plaquenil) and chloroquine are often used to treat fatigue and moderate skin and joint problems. Unlike the rapid response noted with corticosteroids, effects of antimalarial therapy may not be noticed for several months. Flares may also be prevented with these drugs. Funduscopic and visual field examinations must be performed by an ophthalmologist every 6 to 12 months when patients are on hydroxychloroquine. Retinopathy can develop with high-dosage use of these drugs, but it generally reverses when they are discontinued. If patients cannot tolerate an antimalarial agent, an antileprosy drug such as dapsone may be used.

The use of corticosteroids should be limited. However, tapering doses of IV methylprednisolone may be useful in controlling severe exacerbations of polyarthritis. Steroid-sparing immuno-suppressants such as methotrexate can serve as an alternative treatment and are prescribed in combination with folic acid to decrease the adverse effects of corticosteroids. However, high doses of corticosteroids may be especially appropriate for patients with very severe cutaneous SLE.

Immuno-suppressive drugs such as azathioprine (Imuran) and cyclophosphamide (Procytox) may be prescribed to reduce the need for long-term corticosteroid therapy. Close monitoring is necessary to minimize drug toxicity and other adverse effects. Azathioprine or cyclophosphamide is also appropriate for treatment of severe organ-system disease, especially LN. Close monitoring is necessary to minimize drug toxicity and adverse effects. Because blood clots can be a life-threatening complication of SLE, anticoagulants such as warfarin or heparin may be prescribed.

Clinical trials are currently investigating the effect of various medications on SLE management. These include biological and targeted therapy agents that interfere with the immune response, such as abatacept (Orencia). Thalidomide as a second-line therapy has been shown to improve cutaneous lupus even in people who have not responded to other therapies.

When teaching patients about their prescribed drugs, the nurse should include the indications for use, proper administration, and possible adverse effects. Patients should understand that abrupt cessation may exacerbate disease activity.

Disease management is most appropriately monitored by serial anti-DNA titres and serum complement levels (Table 67-14). Simpler and less costly tests such as ESR or CRP measurement may also help in monitoring treatment effectiveness.

TABLE 67-14 COLLABORATIVE CARE

Systemic Lupus Erythematosus

Diagnostic	Collaborative Therapy
• History and physical examination	• Antimalarials (e.g., hydroxychloroquine [Plaquenil])
• Antibody titres (e.g., anti-DNA, anti-Sm, ANA)	• Corticosteroids for exacerbations and severe disease
• Chest radiograph	
• Complete blood cell count	• Immuno-suppressive drugs (e.g., cyclophosphamide [Procytox], mycophenolate [CellCept])
• ECG to determine extra-articular involvement	
• LE cell prep	
• Radiographic examination of affected joints	• NSAIDs for mild disease
• Serum complement levels	• Steroid-sparing drugs (e.g., methotrexate)
• Urinalysis	

ANA, antinuclear antibody; *DNA,* Deoxyribonucleic acid; *ECG,* electrocardiogram; *LE,* lupus erythematosus; *NSAIDs,* nonsteroidal anti-inflammatory drugs; *Sm,* Smith.

NURSING MANAGEMENT
SYSTEMIC LUPUS ERYTHEMATOSUS

NURSING ASSESSMENT

Subjective and objective data that should be obtained from patients with SLE are presented in Table 67-15. In particular, the extent to which pain and fatigue influence ADLs must be evaluated.

NURSING DIAGNOSES

Nursing diagnoses for the patient with SLE may include, but are not limited to, the following:

- *Fatigue* related to *physical deconditioning* (chronic inflammation and altered immunity)
- *Impaired comfort* related to *insufficient situational control* (symptoms of illness, treatment adverse effects, variable and unpredictable disease progression)

Additional information on nursing diagnoses for patients with SLE is presented in NCP 67-2, available on the Evolve website.

PLANNING

The overall goals are that patients with SLE will (1) have satisfactory pain management, (2) adhere to the therapeutic regimen to achieve maximum symptom management, (3) demonstrate awareness of and avoid activities that cause disease exacerbation, and (4) maintain optimal role function and a positive self-image.

NURSING IMPLEMENTATION

HEALTH PROMOTION. Prevention of SLE is not possible at this time. However, education of health care providers and the community should promote a clear understanding of the disease and the need for early diagnosis and treatment.

ACUTE INTERVENTION. As in the majority of rheumatic diseases, the unpredictable nature of SLE presents many challenges to the patient and caregiver. The physical, psychological, and socio-cultural problems associated with the long-term management of SLE require the varied approaches and skills of the multidisciplinary health care team.

During an exacerbation of SLE, a patient may become abruptly and dramatically ill. Nursing interventions include accurately recording the severity of symptoms and documenting the response to therapy. The nurse should assess fever pattern, joint inflammation, limitation of motion, location and degree of discomfort, and fatigue. The nurse should also monitor the patient's weight and fluid intake and output if corticosteroids are prescribed because of the fluid-retention effect of these drugs and the possibility of acute kidney injury. Collection of 24-hour urine samples for protein and creatinine clearance may be ordered. The nurse should observe for signs of bleeding that result from drug therapy, such as pallor, skin bruising, petechiae, or tarry stools.

Careful assessment of neurological status includes observation for visual disturbances, headaches, personality changes, seizures, and forgetfulness. Psychosis may indicate CNS disease or may be an adverse effect of corticosteroid therapy. Irritation of the nerves of the extremities (peripheral neuropathy) may produce numbness, tingling sensation, and weakness of the hands and feet.

The nurse should also explain the nature of the disease, modes of therapy, and all diagnostic procedures. Emotional support for the patient and family is essential, especially during an exacerbation.

AMBULATORY AND HOME CARE. Nursing interventions must emphasize the importance of patient cooperation for successful

TABLE 67-15 NURSING ASSESSMENT

Systemic Lupus Erythematosus

Subjective Data
Important Health Information
Past health history: Exposure to ultraviolet radiation, drugs, chemicals, viral infections; stress (physical or psychological); states of increased estrogen activity (including early onset of menarche; pregnancy and postpartum period); pattern of remissions and exacerbations

Medications: Oral contraceptives, procainamide, hydralazine (Apresoline), isoniazid (INH), anticonvulsant drugs, antibiotics (possibly precipitating symptoms of SLE), corticosteroids, NSAIDs

Symptoms
- Weight loss; nausea and vomiting; xerostomia (salivary gland dryness); oral and nasal ulcers; dysphagia; diarrhea or constipation; decreased urine output.
- Morning stiffness; joint swelling and deformity; polyarthralgia; painful, throbbing cold fingers with numbness and tingling; photosensitivity with rash; chest pain (pericardial, pleuritic); abdominal pain; shortness of breath, dyspnea
- Visual disturbances: vertigo; headache; excessive fatigue, insomnia
- Amennorrhea; irregular menstrual periods; frequent infections
- Depression; withdrawal

Objective Data
General
Fever, lymphadenopathy, periorbital edema

Integumentary
Alopecia; dry, scaly scalp; kerato-conjunctivitis, malar "butterfly" rash, palmar or discoid erythema, urticaria, periungual erythema, purpura, or petechiae; leg ulcers

Respiratory
Pleural friction rub, decreased breath sounds

Cardiovascular
Vasculitis; pericardial friction rub; hypertension, edema, dysrhythmias, murmurs; bilateral, symmetrical pallor and cyanosis of fingers (Raynaud's phenomenon)

Gastro-Intestinal
Oral and pharyngeal ulcers; splenomegaly

Neurological
Facial weakness, peripheral neuropathies, papilledema, dysarthria, confusion, hallucination, disorientation, psychosis, seizures, aphasia, hemiparesis

Musculo-Skeletal
Myopathy, myositis, arthritis

Urinary
Proteinuria

Possible Findings
Presence of anti-DNA, anti-Sm, and antinuclear antibodies; anemia, leukopenia, thrombo-cytopenia; ↑ ESR; positive result of LE cell prep; ↑ serum creatinine; microscopic hematuria, cellular casts in urine; pericarditis or pleural effusion evident on chest radiograph

DNA, deoxyribonucleic acid; *ESR,* erythrocyte sedimentation rate; *LE,* lupus erythematosus; *NSAIDs,* nonsteroidal anti-inflammatory drugs; *SLE,* systemic lupus erythematosus; *Sm,* Smith.

TABLE 67-16 PATIENT & CAREGIVER TEACHING GUIDE

Systemic Lupus Erythematosus

The following instructions should be included in the teaching plan for a patient with systemic lupus erythematosus and the caregiver.
- Avoidance of drying soaps, powders, household chemicals
- Avoidance of exposure to individuals with infection
- Avoidance of physical and emotional stress
- Community resources and health care agencies
- Disease process
- Energy conservation and pacing techniques
- Marital and pregnancy counselling as needed
- Names of drugs, actions, adverse effects, dosage, administration
- Pain management strategies
- Regular medical and laboratory follow-up
- Therapeutic exercise, use of heat therapy (for arthralgia)
- Use of sunscreen protection (at least SPF 15), with minimal sun exposure between the hours of 1100 and 1500

SPF, sun protection factor.

home management. The nurse should help patients understand that even strong adherence to the treatment plan is not a guarantee against exacerbation because the course of the disease is unpredictable. A variety of factors may increase disease activity, such as fatigue, sun exposure, emotional stress, infection, drugs, and surgery. Nursing interventions should be directed toward assisting patients and their families in eliminating or minimizing exposure to precipitating factors (Table 67-16).

Lupus and Pregnancy. Because SLE is most common in women of child-bearing age, treatment during pregnancy must be considered. The woman's primary health care provider (or rheumatologist) and obstetrician should thoroughly discuss with the woman her desire to become pregnant. Infertility may have already resulted from renal involvement and the use of high-dose corticosteroid and chemotherapy drugs. Patients with SLE should understand that spontaneous abortion, stillbirth, and intrauterine growth retardation are common problems during pregnancy. They occur because of deposits of immune complexes in the placenta and because of inflammatory responses in the placental blood vessels.

The renal, cardiovascular, and pulmonary systems and the CNS may be especially affected during pregnancy. Women who already demonstrate serious SLE involvement in these systems should be counselled against pregnancy. For the best outcome, pregnancy should be planned at a time when the disease activity is minimal. Exacerbation is common during the postpartum period. Therapeutic abortion offers the same risk for postdelivery exacerbation as does carrying the fetus to term.

Psychosocial Issues. Patients with SLE confront many psychosocial issues. Disease onset and symptoms may be vague, and SLE may remain undiagnosed for a long period. Supportive therapies may become as important as medical treatment in helping patients cope with the disease. The nurse should inform patients and their families that the prognosis for the majority of people with SLE is good.

Families worry about hereditary aspects, and patients with SLE want to know whether their children will also have SLE. Many couples require pregnancy and sexual counselling. Individuals making decisions about marriage and careers worry about how SLE will interfere with their plans. The nurse may have to educate teachers, employers, and co-workers.

The obvious physical effects of skin rashes, discoid lesions, and alopecia may cause social isolation for a patient with SLE, affecting the individual's self-esteem and body image (Jolly, Pickard, Mikolaitis, et al., 2012). Consultation with a dermatologist may be recommended for appropriate treatment and cosmetic products to conceal the rash.

Pain and fatigue may interfere with quality of life. Pacing techniques and relaxation therapy can help the patient remain involved in day-to-day activities. The nurse should stress the importance of planning both recreational and occupational activities. Young adults may find physical limitations and restrictions of sun exposure particularly difficult to follow. Nursing interventions should assist patients in developing and accomplishing reasonable goals for improving or maintaining mobility, energy levels, and self-esteem.

EVALUATION

Following are the expected outcomes for the patient with SLE:
- Use energy conservation techniques
- Adapt lifestyle to energy level
- Maintain skin integrity with the use of topical treatments
- Prevent exacerbations with the use of sunscreens and limited sun exposure

Additional information on expected outcomes for patients with SLE is presented in NCP 67-2 on the Evolve website.

SCLERODERMA

Scleroderma, or *systemic sclerosis,* is a disorder of connective tissue characterized by fibrotic, degenerative, and occasionally inflammatory changes in skin, blood vessels, synovium, skeletal muscle, and internal organs.

Although symptoms may begin at any time, the usual age at onset is between 30 and 50 years. Scleroderma affects up to five times more women than men (Arthritis Society, 2017h).

Two types of disease exist: limited cutaneous scleroderma, which is the more common type (80%), and diffuse scleroderma. Both forms are systemic, with distinct degrees and types of organ involvement and disease progression. The prognosis for patients with limited disease is generally better than for those with diffuse disease.

Etiology and Pathophysiology

The exact cause of scleroderma is unknown. Immunological dysfunction and vascular abnormalities are believed to play a role in the development of widespread systemic disease. Other risk factors associated with skin thickening include environmental occupational exposure to coal, plastics, and silica dust.

In scleroderma, collagen—the protein that gives normal skin its strength and elasticity—is overproduced (Figure 67-11). Excessive production of collagen leads to progressive tissue fibrosis and occlusion of blood vessels. Proliferation of collagen disrupts the normal functioning of internal organs, such as the lungs, the kidneys, the heart, and the GI tract.

The vascular alterations, which primarily involve the small arteries and arterioles, are almost always present in scleroderma. These changes are some of the earliest alterations in scleroderma.

Clinical Manifestations

Manifestations of scleroderma range from a diffuse cutaneous thickening with rapidly progressive and widespread organ involvement to the more benign limited cutaneous form. The

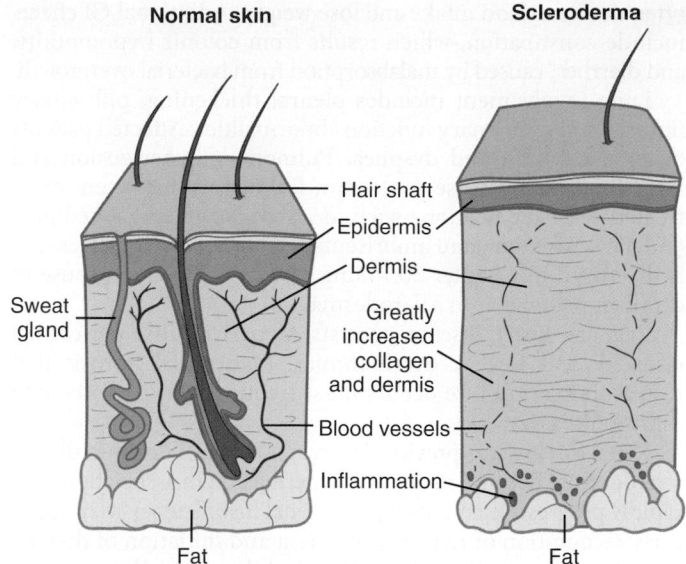

FIGURE 67-11 Skin changes in scleroderma.

signs of limited disease appear on the face and the hands, whereas diffuse disease initially involves the trunk and extremities. Clinical manifestations can be described by the acronym **CREST**:

Calcinosis: painful deposits of calcium in the skin
Raynaud's phenomenon: abnormal blood flow in response to cold or stress
Esophageal dysfunction: difficulty with swallowing, caused by internal scarring
Sclerodactyly: tightening of the skin on the fingers and toes
Telangiectasia: red spots on the hands, the forearms, the palms, the face, and the lips

Raynaud's Phenomenon. Raynaud's phenomenon (an episodic vasospastic disorder of small cutaneous arteries, most frequently involving the fingers and toes) is the most common initial complaint in limited scleroderma. Blood flow to these extremities is diminished on exposure to cold (blanching or white phase), followed by cyanosis as hemoglobin releases oxygen to the tissues (blue phase) and then erythema during rewarming (red phase). The colour changes are often accompanied by numbness and tingling. Raynaud's phenomenon may precede the onset of systemic disease by months, years, or even decades. (Raynaud's phenomenon is described in more detail in Chapter 40.)

Skin and Joint Changes. Symmetrical, painless swelling or thickening of the skin of the fingers and hands may progress to diffuse scleroderma of the trunk. In limited disease, skin thickening does not generally extend above the elbow or above the knee, although in some individuals the face is affected. In more diffuse disease, the skin loses elasticity and becomes taut and shiny, producing the typical expressionless facies with tightly pursed lips. Skin changes in the face may also contribute to reduction in ROM in the temporo-mandibular joint. The hands may be affected by *sclerodactyly,* in which the fingers are in a semiflexed position, with tightened skin up to the wrist. Reduced peripheral joint function may occur as an early symptom of polyarthritis.

Internal Organ Involvement. About 20% of people with scleroderma develop secondary Sjögren syndrome, a condition associated with dry eyes and mouth. Dysphagia, gum disease, and dental caries can result. Frequent reflux of gastric acid can result from esophageal fibrosis. If swallowing becomes difficult, patients often decrease food intake and lose weight. Additional GI effects include constipation, which results from colonic hypomotility, and diarrhea, caused by malabsorption from bacterial overgrowth.

Lung involvement includes pleural thickening, pulmonary fibrosis, and pulmonary function abnormalities. Affected patients develop a cough and dyspnea. Pulmonary hypertension and interstitial lung disease can occur. Pulmonary hypertension is treated with medications such as extended-release nifedipine (Adalat), bosentan, and ambrisentan. (Pulmonary hypertension is discussed in Chapter 30.) Lung disease is the main cause of death in patients with scleroderma.

Primary heart disease consists of pericarditis, pericardial effusion, and cardiac dysrhythmias. Myocardial fibrosis that results in heart failure occurs most frequently in patients with diffuse disease.

Renal disease was previously a major cause of death in diffuse scleroderma. Because malignant hypertension in association with rapidly progressive and irreversible renal insufficiency may occur, early recognition of renal involvement and initiation of therapy are critical. Improvements in dialysis, bilateral nephrectomy in patients with uncontrollable hypertension, and kidney transplantation have offered some hope to patients with renal failure. In particular, use of angiotensin-converting enzyme (ACE) inhibitors (e.g., lisinopril [Prinivil]) has markedly improved the treatment of renal disease.

Diagnostic Studies

Laboratory findings in scleroderma are relatively normal. Blood studies may reveal a mildly elevated ESR and mild hemolytic anemia as a result of RBC damage from diseased small vessels. ANAs are found in most patients (Varga, 2011). The scleroderma antibody SCL-70 is found in about 30% of patients with diffuse disease, and serum RF is found in 30% of affected patients. An anticentromere antibody is seen in many patients with CREST. If renal involvement is present, urinalysis may reveal proteinuria, microscopic hematuria, and casts. Serum levels of creatinine may be elevated. Radiographic evidence of subcutaneous calcification, distal esophageal hypomotility, or bilateral pulmonary fibrosis is diagnostic of scleroderma. Pulmonary function studies reveal decreased vital capacity and lung compliance.

Collaborative Care

The collaborative care of scleroderma (Table 67-17) offers no specific long-term treatment. Supportive care is directed toward attempts to prevent or treat secondary complications of involved organs. Physiotherapy helps maintain joint mobility and preserve muscle strength. Occupational therapy assists patients in maintaining functional abilities.

Drug Therapy. No specific drug or combination of drugs has been proven effective in the treatment of scleroderma. Vasoactive agents are often prescribed for early stages of the disease, and calcium channel blockers (nifedipine [Adalat] and diltiazem) are now a common treatment choice for Raynaud's phenomenon. Prazosin, an α-adrenergic blocking agent, increases blood flow to the fingers. Bosentan (Tracleer), an endothelin-receptor antagonist, and epoprostenol (Flolan), a vasodilator, may assist in preventing and treating digital ulcers while improving exercise capacity and heart and lung dynamics. Losartan (Cozaar), an angiotensin II blocker, may also be used to treat Raynaud's phenomenon.

Corticosteroids may have little effect on scleroderma. Topical agents may provide some relief from joint pain. Capsaicin cream

TABLE 67-17 COLLABORATIVE CARE

Scleroderma

Diagnostic	Collaborative Therapy

• History and physical examination
• Anticentromere antibody titre
• Antinuclear antibody titre
• Electrocardiography
• Microscopic study of nail bed capillaries
• Pulmonary function test
• Radiographic studies of chest and hands
• Skin or visceral biopsy
• Urinalysis (proteinuria, hematuria, casts)
	• Physiotherapy and occupational therapy
	• Drug therapy
	  • Angiotensin-converting enzyme (ACE) inhibitors (lisinopril [Prinivil])
	  • Calcium channel blockers (diltiazem [Cardizem], nifedipine [Adalat])
	  • Immuno-suppressive drugs (e.g., cyclophosphamide [Procytox]; mycophenolate mofetil [CellCept])
	  • Vasoactive agents: bosentan (Tracleer); epoprostenol (Flolan)

may be useful, not only as a local analgesic, but also as a vasodilator. Other therapies are prescribed to address specific systemic problems, such as tetracycline for diarrhea caused by bacterial overgrowth, histamine H_2-receptor blockers (e.g., cimetidine) and proton pump inhibitors (e.g., omeprazole [Losec]) for esophageal symptoms, antihypertensive agents (e.g., captopril, propranolol [Inderal]), methyldopa for hypertension with renal involvement, and immuno-suppressive drugs (e.g., cyclophosphamide [Procytox]; mycophenolate mofetil [CellCept]).

NURSING MANAGEMENT
SCLERODERMA

Prevention of scleroderma is not possible. Nursing intervention often begins during a hospitalization for diagnostic purposes. The nurse assesses vital signs, weight, intake and output, respiratory and bowel function, and joint ROM at regular intervals, as indicated by specific symptoms, to plan appropriate care. Emotional stress and cold ambient temperatures may aggravate Raynaud's phenomenon. Patients with scleroderma should not undergo finger-stick blood testing because of compromised circulation and poor healing of the fingers.

Health teaching is an important nursing intervention as patients and their families begin to live with this disease. Obvious changes in the face and the hands often lead to poor self-image and the loss of mobility and function. Patients must actively complete therapeutic exercises at home to prevent skin retraction and promote vascularization. Mouth excursion (opening the mouth widely, as in yawning) is a good exercise to help with temporo-mandibular joint function. Isometric exercises are most appropriate if the patient has arthropathy (disease of the joint) because no joint movement occurs. The nurse should encourage the use of moist heat applications or paraffin baths to promote skin flexibility in the hands and feet. Patients should use assistive devices as appropriate and organize activities to preserve strength and reduce disability.

Hands and feet should be protected from cold exposure and possible burns or cuts that might heal slowly. Smoking should be avoided because of its vasoconstricting effect. Signs of infection should be promptly reported. Lotions may help alleviate skin dryness and cracking, but they must be rubbed in for an unusually long time because of the thickness of the skin.

Dysphagia may be reduced by eating small, frequent meals, chewing carefully and slowly, and drinking fluids with food. Heartburn may be minimized with the use of antacids 45 to 60 minutes after each meal and by sitting upright for at least 2 hours after eating. Using additional pillows or raising the head of the bed on blocks may help reduce nocturnal gastro-esophageal reflux.

Job modifications are often necessary because stair climbing, using a computer, writing, and cold exposure may pose particular problems. Patients may become socially withdrawn as skin tightening alters the appearance of the face and the hands. Dining out may become a socially embarrassing event because of the patient's restricted opening of the mouth, difficulty swallowing, and reflux. Some individuals with scleroderma wear gloves to protect fingertip ulcers and to provide extra warmth. Daily oral hygiene must be emphasized; neglect may lead to increased tooth and gingival problems. Patients need a dentist who is familiar with scleroderma and can deal with a small mouth opening.

Psychological support, biofeedback training, and relaxation techniques can reduce stress and improve sleeping habits. Sexual dysfunction resulting from body changes, pain, muscular weakness, limited mobility, decreased self-esteem, erectile dysfunction, and decreased vaginal secretions may necessitate sensitive counselling.

POLYMYOSITIS AND DERMATOMYOSITIS

Polymyositis (PM) refers to diffuse, idiopathic, inflammatory myopathies of the connective tissues, especially striated muscle, that produce bilateral weakness, usually most severe in the proximal or limb-girdle muscles. When muscle changes associated with PM are accompanied by characteristic skin changes, the disorder is called dermatomyositis (DM) (Arthritis Society, 2017i).

Although these relatively rare disorders can be similar in signs, symptoms, and treatment, PM and DM are two distinct diseases. They are most common in children and adults over 50 years. (Arthritis Society, 2017i). Both diseases occur twice as often in women as in men. Patients with PM generally have more severe disease than those with DM.

Etiology and Pathophysiology

The exact cause of PM and DM is unknown. Theories include an infectious agent, neoplasms, drugs or vaccinations, and stress. Because T cytotoxic cells and macrophages have been found near the damaged muscle fibres of patients with PM, this disease is believed to be caused by cell-mediated injury. In contrast, DM has been associated with B cells (humoral immunity) and destruction of the muscle microvasculature. An autoimmune response to nuclear and cytoplasm self-antigens has also been noted in many people with these disorders (von Mühlen & Nakamura, 2011).

Clinical Manifestations and Complications
Muscular. Patients with DM and PM experience weight loss and increasing fatigue, with gradually developing weakness of the muscles, that leads to difficulty in performing routine activities. The muscles most commonly affected are those of the shoulders, the legs, the arms, and the pelvic girdle. Patients may have difficulty rising from a chair or bathtub, climbing stairs, combing the hair, or reaching into a high cupboard. Neck muscles may become so weak that patients are unable to raise the head

FIGURE 67-12. Dermatomyositis skin changes. Gottron papules. Source: Firestein, G. S., Budd, R. C., Gabriel, S. E. et al. (2012). *Kelley's textbook of rheumatology.* (9th ed.). Philadelphia: Saunders.

from the pillow. Muscle discomfort or tenderness is uncommon. Muscle examination reveals an inability to move against resistance or even gravity. Weakness of the pharyngeal muscles may result in dysphagia and dysphonia (nasal or hoarse voice).

Dermal. Skin changes of DM include a classic violet-coloured, cyanotic, or erythematous symmetrical rash *(heliotrope rash)* with edema around the eyelids. Violet-coloured or erythematous papules (Gottron papules) and small plaques develop over the DIP or MCP areas and at elbow or knee joints in about 70% of patients with DM (Figure 67-12). Because of these early skin changes, DM is usually recognized earlier than PM, in which a rash does not appear. Reddened, smooth, or scaly patches appear with the same symmetrical distribution but sparing the interphalangeal spaces (Gottron sign); they can be confused with psoriasis or seborrheic dermatitis. An erythematous scaling rash (poikiloderma) may develop as a late finding on the back, buttocks, and a V-shaped area of the anterior neck and chest. Hyperemia and telangiectasias are often present at the nail beds. Calcium nodules (calcinosis cutis), which can develop throughout the skin, are especially common in long-standing DM.

Other Manifestations. Joint redness, pain, and inflammation often occur and contribute to limitations in joint ROM in DM and PM. Contractures and muscle atrophy may occur with advanced disease. Weakening of the pharyngeal muscles can lead to a poor cough effort, difficulty swallowing, and increased risk for aspiration pneumonia in both disorders. Interstitial lung disease occurs in up to 65% of all affected patients. People with DM also have an increased risk for cancer, which may be present at time of diagnosis. Both diseases may be associated with other connective tissue disorders (e.g., scleroderma).

Diagnostic Studies

Diagnosis of DM or PM is confirmed by MRI, electromyographic (EMG) findings, muscle biopsy, and serum enzyme levels. An EMG suggestive of PM shows bizarre, high-frequency discharges and spontaneous fibrillation, with positive spikes at rest. Muscle biopsy reveals necrosis, degeneration, regeneration, and fibrosis with pathological findings distinct for DM or PM. Markers such as creatinine kinase and myoglobin are elevated. Elevation of the ESR or CRP is also expected with active disease. In addition, more than 50% of people with PM have positive RF. The skin rash typical of DM is not commonly found with other disorders.

NURSING AND COLLABORATIVE MANAGEMENT POLYMYOSITIS AND DERMATOMYOSITIS

PM and DM are initially treated with high-dose corticosteroids. Improvement is generally achieved if corticosteroid therapy is promptly instituted, and the dosage can typically be reduced as improvement is noted. Long-term corticosteroid therapy may often be required because relapses are common when the drug is withdrawn. If corticosteroids are ineffective after 4 weeks of treatment or organ involvement is occurring (or both), immunosuppressive drugs (methotrexate, azathioprine [Imuran], cyclophosphamide [Procytox]) may be administered.

DM has been shown to improve with high doses of IV immunoglobulin. Topical corticosteroids and hydroxychloroquine (Plaquenil) may also be prescribed to treat the skin rash.

The role of newer medications such as TNF inhibitors remains unclear, although their use in refractory cases has shown some success.

Physiotherapy can be helpful and should be tailored to the activity of the disease. Massage and passive movement are appropriate during active disease. More aggressive exercises should be reserved for periods when disease activity is minimal, as evidenced by low serum enzyme levels.

Nursing interventions should include a thorough explanation of the disease, the prescribed therapies, all diagnostic tests, and the importance of regular medical care. It is important for patients to understand that the benefits of therapy are often delayed. For example, weakness may increase during the first few weeks of corticosteroid therapy. Special attention is paid to patient safety. Use of assistive devices should be encouraged as a fall prevention strategy. To prevent aspiration, patients should be encouraged to rest before meals, maintain an upright position when eating, and choose a diet of easily swallowed foods.

The nurse should assist patients in organizing activities and using pacing techniques to conserve energy. The nurse should encourage the patient to perform daily ROM exercises to prevent contractures. When active inflammation is not evident, muscle-strengthening (repetitive) exercises may be started. Home care and bed rest may become necessary during the acute phase of PM because profound muscle weakness renders patients unable to carry out ADLs.

MIXED (OVERLAPPING) FORMS OF CONNECTIVE TISSUE DISEASE

Patients with a combination of clinical features of several rheumatic diseases are described as having *mixed* or *overlapping connective tissue disease.* The term is used to describe a disorder with features of SLE, Sjögren syndrome, and PM. Approximately 80% of people with this disease are women.

SJÖGREN SYNDROME

Sjögren syndrome is a relatively common autoimmune disease that targets moisture-producing exocrine glands, leading to the common symptoms of *xerostomia* (dry mouth) and *kerato-conjunctivitis sicca* (dry eyes) (Jonsson, Vogelsang, Volchenkov, et al., 2011). The nose, the throat, the airways, and the skin can also become dry. The disease can affect other glands as well, including those in the stomach, the pancreas, and the intestines (extraglandular involvement). The disease is usually diagnosed in people older than 40, and 90% of them are women.

In primary Sjögren syndrome, symptoms can be traced to problems with the lacrimal and the salivary glands. Patients with primary disease are likely to have antibodies against the cytoplasmic antigens SS-A (or Ro) and SS-B (or La), as well as ANA. Patients with secondary Sjögren syndrome typically had another autoimmune disease (e.g., RA, SLE) before Sjögren syndrome developed.

Sjögren syndrome appears to be caused by genetic and environmental factors. Several genes seem to be involved. The trigger may be a viral or bacterial infection that adversely stimulates the immune system. In Sjögren syndrome, lymphocytes attack and damage the lacrimal and salivary glands.

Dry eyes are characterized by decreased tearing, which leads to a "gritty" sensation in the eyes, burning sensation, blurred vision, and photosensitivity. Dry mouth leads to buccal membrane fissures, altered sense of taste, dysphagia, and increased frequency of mouth infections or dental caries. Dry skin and rashes, joint and muscle pain, and thyroid problems may also be present. Other exocrine glands can be affected. For example, vaginal dryness may lead to dyspareunia (painful intercourse).

Autoimmune thyroid disorders, including Graves' disease and Hashimoto thyroiditis, are common with Sjögren syndrome. Histological study reveals lymphocyte infiltration of salivary and lacrimal glands. The disease may become more generalized and involve the lymph nodes, the bone marrow, and the visceral organs (pseudolymphoma). Lymphoma develops in about 5% of patients with Sjögren syndrome (Covelli, Lanciano, Tartaglia, et al., 2012).

Ophthalmological examination (Schirmer test for tear production), measures of salivary gland function, and lower lip biopsy of minor salivary glands aid in the diagnosis. The treatment for Sjögren syndrome is based on symptoms, including (a) instillation of preservative-free artificial tears as necessary to maintain adequate hydration and lubrication, (b) surgical punctal occlusion, and (c) increased fluids with meals. Dental hygiene is also important.

Pilocarpine (Salagen) can be used to treat symptoms of dry mouth. Increased humidity in the home may reduce respiratory infections. Vaginal lubrication with a water-soluble product may increase comfort during intercourse.

SOFT-TISSUE RHEUMATIC SYNDROMES

MYOFASCIAL PAIN SYNDROME

Myofascial pain syndrome is a chronic form of muscle pain. It is characterized by musculo-skeletal pain and tenderness, typically in the chest, neck, shoulders, hips, and lower back. Referred pain from these muscle groups can also travel to the head, causing severe headaches, as well as to the buttocks and hands.

Temporo-mandibular joint pain may also originate in myofascial pain. Regions of pain are often within the taut bands and fascia of skeletal muscles. When activated by pressure, trigger points are thought to activate a characteristic pattern of pain that can worsen with activity or stress.

Myofascial pain syndrome occurs most often in middle-aged adults and more often in women than in men. Affected patients describe the pain as deep and aching, accompanied by a sensation of burning, stinging, and stiffness. Examples of this syndrome include fibromyalgia, myalgia, and myositis (Belden, DeFriez, & Huether, 2012).

Physiotherapy is one treatment used for myofascial pain syndrome. A typical exercise is the "spray and stretch" method, in which the painful area is iced or sprayed with a coolant such as ethyl chloride and then stretched. Positive results have been achieved by injection of the trigger points with a local anaesthetic (e.g., 1% lidocaine). Massage, acupuncture, biofeedback, and ultrasound therapy have also been shown to benefit some patients.

FIBROMYALGIA

Fibromyalgia syndrome (FMS) is a chronic disorder characterized by widespread, nonarticular musculo-skeletal pain and fatigue with multiple tender points. People with fibromyalgia also typically experience nonrestorative sleep, morning stiffness, irritable bowel syndrome, and anxiety. Fibromyalgia is a commonly diagnosed musculo-skeletal disorder and a major cause of disability that affects approximately 2% of Canadians, with 80% to 90% being women (Arthritis Society, 2017j). Fibromyalgia and systemic exertion intolerance disease (SEID) share many commonalities (Table 67-18).

Etiology and Pathophysiology

Research continues to focus on identifying the underlying causes and the pathophysiological mechanisms of fibromyalgia. There is general agreement that fibromyalgia is a disorder involving neuroendocrine or neurotransmitter dysregulation. The pain amplification experienced by the affected patient is caused by abnormal sensory processing in the CNS.

Multiple physiological abnormalities have been found. They include increased levels of substance P in the spinal fluid, low levels of blood flow to the thalamus, dysfunction of the hypothalamic-pituitary-adrenal (HPA) axis, low levels of serotonin and tryptophan, and abnormalities in cytokine function. Serotonin and substance P play a role in mood regulation, sleep, and pain perception. Changes in the HPA axis can also negatively affect

TABLE 67-18	COMMONALITIES BETWEEN FIBROMYALGIA AND SYSTEMIC EXERTION INTOLERANCE DISEASE
Commonality	**Description**
Clinical manifestations	Generalized musculo-skeletal pain, malaise and fatigue, cognitive dysfunction, headaches, sleep disturbances, depression, anxiety, fever.
Collaborative therapy	Treatment is symptomatic and may include antidepressant drugs such as amitriptyline (Elavil) and fluoxetine (Prozac). Other measures are heat, massage, regular stretching, biofeedback, stress management, and relaxation training. Patient and caregiver teaching is essential.
Course of disease	Variable intensity of symptoms; fluctuates over time.
Diagnosis	No definitive laboratory tests or joint and muscle examinations; mainly a diagnosis of exclusion.
Etiology (theories)	Infectious trigger, dysfunction in HPA axis, alteration in CNS.
Occurrence	Previously healthy, young, and middle-aged women.

HPA, hypothalamic-pituitary-adrenal; *CNS,* central nervous system.

a person's physical and mental health, leading to an increased incidence of depression and a decreased response to stress. Genetic factors also contribute to the etiology of fibromyalgia, as a familial tendency exists. A recent illness or trauma may serve as a trigger in susceptible people.

Clinical Manifestations and Complications

Patients with fibromyalgia experience a widespread burning pain that worsens and improves through the course of a day. It is often difficult for patients to discriminate whether pain occurs in the muscles, the joints, or soft tissues. Head or facial pain often results from stiff or painful neck and shoulder muscles. The pain can accompany temporo-mandibular joint dysfunction, which affects an estimated one-third of patients with fibromyalgia.

Physical examination characteristically reveals point tenderness at 11 or more of 18 identified sites (Figure 67-13). Patients with fibromyalgia are sensitive to painful stimuli throughout the body and not merely at the identified tender sites. In addition, point tenderness can vary from day to day. On some occasions, the patient may respond to fewer than 11 tender points. At other times, palpation of all sites may elicit pain.

Cognitive effects range from difficulty concentrating to memory lapses and a feeling of being overwhelmed when dealing with multiple tasks. Many individuals report migraine headaches. Depression and anxiety often occur and may necessitate drug therapy. Stiffness, nonrefreshing sleep, fatigue, and numbness or tingling sensation in the hands or feet (paresthesia) often accompanies fibromyalgia. Restless legs syndrome is also typical, with patients describing an irresistible urge to move the legs when at rest or lying down.

Irritable bowel syndrome with manifestations of constipation, diarrhea, or both; abdominal pain; and bloating is common. Patients with fibromyalgia may also experience difficulty swallowing, perhaps because of abnormalities in esophageal smooth-muscle function. Increased frequency of urination and urinary urgency, in the absence of a bladder infection, are typical complaints. Women with fibromyalgia may experience more difficult menstruation, with a worsening of disease symptoms during this time.

Diagnostic Studies

A definitive diagnosis of fibromyalgia is often difficult to establish. Lack of knowledge among health care providers may also cause delays in diagnosis and treatment.

Laboratory results in most cases serve to rule out other disorders suspected on the basis of the patient's history and physical examination. On occasion, a low ANA titre is present, but it is not considered diagnostic. Muscle biopsy may reveal a nonspecific moth-eaten appearance or fibre atrophy. The American College of Rheumatology classifies an individual as having fibromyalgia if the following two criteria are met: (a) pain is experienced in 11 of the 18 tender points on palpation (see Figure 67-13) and (b) a history of widespread pain for at least 3 months is documented (Wolfe, Clauw, Fitzcharles, et al., 2010). *Widespread pain* is defined as occurring on both sides of the body and above and below the waist. In addition, fatigue, cognitive symptoms, and extensive somatic symptoms are considered in establishing a diagnosis.

Collaborative Care

The treatment of fibromyalgia is symptomatic and requires a high level of patient motivation. The nurse can play a key role

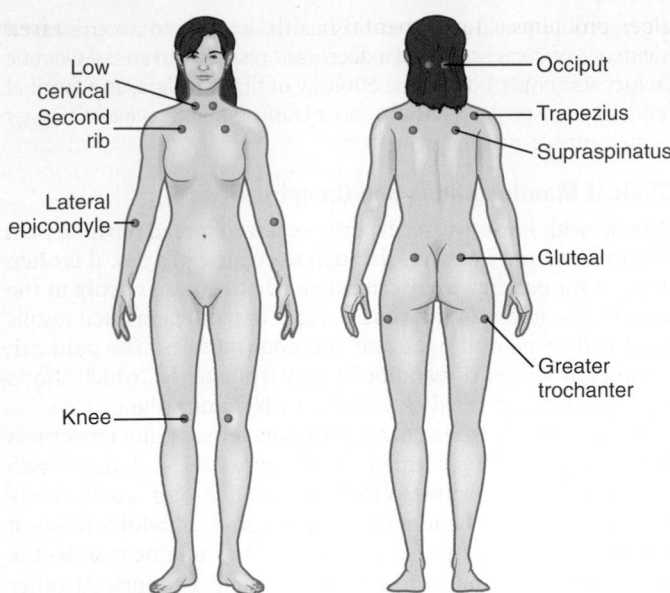

Low
cervical
Second
rib

Lateral
epicondyle

Knee

Occiput

Trapezius

Supraspinatus

Gluteal

Greater
trochanter

FIGURE 67-13 Tender points in fibromyalgia.

in teaching patients to be active participants in the therapeutic regimen. Rest can help pain, aching, and tenderness.

Drug treatment for the chronic widespread pain associated with fibromyalgia includes pregabalin (Lyrica) and duloxetine (Cymbalta). Low-dose tricyclic antidepressants, selective serotonin reuptake inhibitors (SSRIs), or benzodiazepines (e.g., diazepam [Valium]) may also be prescribed. If the tricyclic antidepressant amitriptyline (Elavil) is not well tolerated, similar drugs can be substituted (e.g., doxepin [Sinequan], imipramine, trazodone). SSRI antidepressants (e.g., sertraline [Zoloft], paroxetine [Paxil]) tend to be reserved for affected patients who also have depression. SSRIs may need to be prescribed at higher doses than when used to treat depression. Both antidepressants and muscle relaxants have sedative effects that can help in improving nighttime rest for patients with fibromyalgia.

Long-acting opioids are generally not recommended unless fibromyalgia is refractory to other therapies. In some patients, pain may be managed with OTC analgesics such as acetaminophen (Tylenol), ibuprofen (Motrin, Advil), or naproxen (Aleve).

NURSING MANAGEMENT
FIBROMYALGIA

Because of the chronic nature of fibromyalgia, patients need consistent support from the nurse and other members of the health care team. Massage is often combined with ultrasound therapy or the application of alternating heat and cold packs to soothe tense, sore muscles and increase blood circulation. Gentle stretching can be performed by a physiotherapist or practised by the patient at home to relieve muscle tension and spasm. Yoga and tai chi are often appropriate. Low-impact aerobic exercise, such as walking, can help prevent muscle atrophy.

Often, dietitians urge patients with fibromyalgia to limit their consumption of sugar, caffeine, and alcohol because these substances have been shown to be muscle irritants. Vitamin and mineral supplements may be appropriate to combat stress, correct deficiencies, and support the immune system. However, unproven "miracle diets" or supplements should be carefully investigated by patients and discussed with the health care provider before

any of them is used. Patients should understand that some foods and supplements may cause serious and even dangerous adverse effects when taken along with certain drugs.

Pain and the related symptoms of fibromyalgia can cause significant stress. Patients with fibromyalgia may not deal effectively with stress. Effective relaxation strategies include biofeedback, mindfulness meditation, and cognitive behavioural therapy. Patients need to receive initial training for these interventions, but they can then continue to practise them on their own. Psychological counselling (individual or group) may also prove beneficial for patients. (Stress and stress management are discussed in Chapter 8.)

SYSTEMIC EXERTION INTOLERANCE DISEASE

Systemic exertion intolerance disease (SEID), also known as *chronic fatigue syndrome (CFS) or myalgic encephalomyelitis,* is a serious, complex, multisystem disease in which exertion of any sort (physical, emotional, cognitive) can adversely affect multiple organs in a person (Institute of Medicine, 2015). SEID is a poorly understood condition that can have a devastating effect on the lives of patients and their families. More women are affected than men. SEID occurs in all ethnic and socioeconomic groups. The true prevalence of SEID is unknown because many people with the disease have not been diagnosed.

Etiology and Pathophysiology

Despite efforts to determine the etiology and the pathology of SEID, the precise mechanisms remain unknown. However, there are many theories about the cause of SEID. Neuroendocrine abnormalities that have been implicated involve a hypofunction of the HPA axis and the hypothalamic-pituitary-gonadal (HPG) axis, which together regulate the stress response and reproductive hormone levels. Several microorganisms have been investigated as etiological agents, including herpes viruses (e.g., Epstein Barr virus [EBV], cytomegalovirus [CMV]), retroviruses, enteroviruses, *Candida albicans,* and mycoplasma. Because many patients with the disease have cognitive deficits (e.g., decreased memory, attention, concentration), changes in the CNS have been suggested as the cause of SEID.

Clinical Manifestations

Diagnosis of SEID requires that the patient have the following three symptoms:
1. Profound fatigue lasting at least 6 months
2. Postexertional malaise: total exhaustion after even minor physical or mental exertion that patients sometimes describe as a "crash"
3. Unrefreshing sleep

At least one of the following two manifestations is also required:
1. Cognitive impairment ("brain fog")
2. Worsening of symptoms upon standing (orthostatic intolerance)

SEID is often difficult to distinguish from fibromyalgia because many clinical features are similar (Table 67-18). In about half the cases, SEID develops insidiously, or patients may have intermittent episodes that gradually become chronic. Severe fatigue is the most common symptom of SEID and causes patients to seek health care.

In other situations, SEID arises suddenly in a previously active, healthy individual. An unremarkable influenza-like illness or other acute stress is often identified as a triggering event. Associated symptoms may fluctuate in intensity over time.

Patients may become angry and frustrated with the inability of health care providers to diagnose a problem. The disorder may have a major effect on work and family responsibilities. Some patients may need help with ADLs.

Diagnostic Studies

Physical examination and diagnostic studies can be used to rule out other possible causes of a patient's symptoms. No laboratory test can diagnose SEID or measure its severity. SEID generally remains a diagnosis of exclusion.

NURSING AND COLLABORATIVE MANAGEMENT SEID

Because there is no definitive treatment for SEID, supportive management is essential. Patients should be informed about what is known about the disease, and all complaints should be taken seriously.

NSAIDs can be used to treat headaches, muscle and joint aches, and fever. Because many patients with SEID also have allergies and sinusitis, antihistamines and decongestants can be used to treat allergic symptoms. Tricyclic antidepressants (e.g., doxepin [Sinequan], amitriptyline [Elavil]) and SSRIs (e.g., fluoxetine [Prozac], paroxetine [Paxil]) can improve mood and

sleep problems. Clonazepam (Rivotril) can also be used to treat sleep disturbances and panic disorders. The use of low-dose hydrocortisone to decrease fatigue and disability is being studied.

Total rest is not advised because it can potentiate the self-image of being an invalid. On the other hand, strenuous exertion can exacerbate the exhaustion. Therefore, it is important to plan a carefully graduated exercise program. A well-balanced diet that includes fibre and fresh, dark-coloured fruits and vegetables for antioxidant action is essential in treatment. Behavioural therapy may be used to promote a positive outlook, as well as improve overall disability, fatigue, and other symptoms.

One of the major problems facing many patients with SEID is loss of livelihood and economic security. When the illness strikes, they cannot work or must decrease the amount of time working. Obtaining disability benefits can be frustrating because of the difficulty in establishing a diagnosis of SEID. Patients with SEID may experience substantial occupational and psychosocial impairments and loss, including the social pressure and isolation from being characterized as lazy or having a mental illness.

SEID does not appear to progress. Although most patients recover or experience at least gradual improvement over time, some do not show substantial improvement. Recovery is more common in individuals with a sudden onset of SEID.

CASE STUDY

Rheumatoid Arthritis

Source: Blend Images/ Shutterstock.com.

Patient Profile

Grace Kim, a 42-year-old married woman, is seen at the rheumatology clinic because she is experiencing swelling and stiffness in the small joints of her hands.

Subjective Data
- Is a concert pianist
- Experiencing joint pain and stiffness in both hands for the past 6 weeks
- Experiencing fatigue, anorexia, and morning stiffness
- Gave birth to her first child 2 months ago

Objective Data
Physical Examination
- Swelling and tenderness of third and fourth MCP joints of both hands
- Mild pain with neck motion

Diagnostic Studies
- Elevated ESR, positive RF and ACPA
- Evidence of moderate bone demineralization on bilateral hand radiographs

Collaborative Care
- Diagnosis: RA
- Therapy: started on methotrexate, 7.5 mg PO once per week; etanercept (Enbrel), 50 mg subcutaneously once per week; and prednisone, 10 mg daily

Discussion Questions
1. How might the nurse explain the pathophysiology of RA to Ms. Kim?
2. How might the recent childbirth have influenced the symptoms that she is currently experiencing?
3. What are some home and work modifications that the nurse can suggest to Ms. Kim that will reduce her symptoms?
4. What suggestions can the nurse make to Ms. Kim about coping with fatigue?
5. *Priority decision:* On the basis of the assessment data presented, what are the priority nursing diagnoses? Are there any collaborative problems?
6. *Evidence-informed practice:* Why is an exercise program important in the treatment plan for Ms. Kim?

evolve

Answers are available at *http://evolve.elsevier.com/Canada/Lewis/medsurg*

REVIEW QUESTIONS

The number of the question corresponds to the same-numbered objective at the beginning of the chapter.

1. Which of the following would the nurse understand as causing damage to the joints of a client with rheumatoid arthritis?
   a. The development of Heberden nodes in the joint capsule
   b. The deterioration of cartilage by the enzyme hyaluronidase
   c. Invasion of pannus into the joint capsule and subchondral bone
   d. Bony ankylosis after inflammation of the joints in HLA-B27– positive individuals

2. A client with rheumatoid arthritis is experiencing articular involvement of the joints. The nurse recognizes that these characteristic changes include which of the following? (*Select all that apply*)
   a. Bamboo-shaped fingers
   b. Metatarsal head dislocation in feet
   c. Noninflammatory pain in large joints
   d. Asymmetric involvement of small joints
   e. Morning stiffness lasting 60 minutes or more

3. Which of the following would the nurse teach to a client with ankylosing spondylitis?
   a. Avoid extremes in environmental temperatures.
   b. Continue with physical activity during flare-ups.
   c. Apply cool compresses for relief of local symptoms.
   d. Maintain proper posture and engage in regular exercise.

4. When the nurse administers medications to clients with gout, which of the following would the nurse recognize as a treatment for acute disease?
   a. Colchicine
   b. Sulphasalazine
   c. Allopurinol
   d. Cyclosporin

5. The nurse is teaching a client with SLE about the disorder. The nurse understands that the pathophysiology of SLE includes which of the following?
   a. Circulating immune complexes formed from IgG autoantibodies reacting with IgG
   b. An autoimmune T-cell reaction that results in destruction of the deep dermal skin layer
   c. Immunological dysfunction leading to chronic inflammation in the cartilage and bones
   d. The production of a variety of autoantibodies directed against constituents of the cell nucleus

6. The nurse is caring for a client with Sjögren syndrome. Which of the following autoimmune disorders may the client also develop?
   a. Uveitis
   b. Ulcerative colitis
   c. Glomerulo-nephritis
   d. Hashimoto thyroiditis

7. Which of the following should be considered in the management of systemic exertion intolerance disease (SEID)? *(Select all that apply)*
   a. Dark green vegetables in diet
   b. DMARDs to reduce symptoms
   c. Total rest during acute exacerbations
   d. SSRIs or tricyclic antidepressants
   e. Behavioural therapy

1. c, 2. b, e; 3. d; 4. a; 5. d; 6. d; 7. a, d, e.

⊝volve

For even more review questions, visit *http://evolve.elsevier.com/Canada/Lewis/medsurg.*

REFERENCES

Arthritis Society. (2015a). *Gout*. Retrieved from *https://arthritis.ca/understand-arthritis/types-of-arthritis/gout.*

Arthritis Society. (2015b). *Ankylosing spondylitis.* Retrieved from *https://www.arthritis.ca/about-arthritis/types-of-arthritis-(a-z)/types/ankylosing-spondylitis.*

Arthritis Society. (2017a). *About arthritis.* Retrieved from *https://www.arthritis.ca/about-arthritis.*

Arthritis Society. (2017b). *Osteoarthritis.* Retrieved from *https://www.arthritis.ca/about-arthritis/types-of-arthritis-(a-z)/types/osteoarthritis.*

Arthritis Society. (2017c). *Online arthritis self-management courses.* Retrieved from *http://education.arthritis.ca/landing.aspx.*

Arthritis Society. (2017d). *Rheumatoid arthritis.* Retrieved from *https://arthritis.ca/understand-arthritis/types-of-arthritis/rheumatoid-arthritis.*

Arthritis Society. (2017e). *Psoriatic arthritis.* Retrieved from *https://www.arthritis.ca/about-arthritis/types-of-arthritis-(a-z)/types/psoriatic-arthritis.*

Arthritis Society. (2017f). *Reactive arthritis.* Retrieved from *https://www.arthritis.ca/about-arthritis/types-of-arthritis-(a-z)/types/reactive-arthritis.*

Arthritis Society. (2017g). *Systemic lupus erythematosus.* Retrieved from *https://www.arthritis.ca/about-arthritis/types-of-arthritis-(a-z)/types/systemic-lupus-erythematosus.*

Arthritis Society. (2017h). *Scleroderma.* Retrieved from *https://www.arthritis.ca/about-arthritis/types-of-arthritis-(a-z)/types/scleroderma.*

Arthritis Society. (2017i). *Myositis (dermatomyositis, polymyositis).* Retrieved from *https://www.arthritis.ca/about-arthritis/types-of-arthritis-(a-z)/types/myositis-(dermatomyositis,-polymyositis).*

Arthritis Society. (2017j). *Fibromyalgia.* Retrieved from *https://www.arthritis.ca/about-arthritis/types-of-arthritis-(a-z)/types/myositis-(dermatomyositis,-polymyositis).*

Belden, J., DeFriez, C., & Huether, S. (2012). Pain, temperature, sleep, and sensory function. In S. Huether & K. McCance (Eds.), *Understanding pathophysiology* (5th ed.). St. Louis: Mosby.

Bockenstedt, L. (2012). Lyme disease. In G. Firestein, R. Budd, S. Gabriel, et al. (Eds.), *Kelley's textbook of rheumatology* (9th ed.). Philadelphia: Saunders.

Covelli, M., Lanciano, P., Tartaglia, M., et al. (2012). Rituximab treatment for Sjögren syndrome–associated non-Hodgkin's lymphoma: Case series. *Rheumatology International, 32*(10), 3281–3284. doi:10.1007/s00296-011-2036-2.

Durham, C., Fowler, T., Donato, A., et al. (2015). Pain management in patients with rheumatoid arthritis. *The Nurse Practitioner, 40*(5), 38–45. doi:10.1097/01.NPR.0000463784.36883.23.

Firestein, G. (2012). Etiology and pathogenesis of rheumatoid arthritis. In G. Firestein, R. Budd, S. Gabriel, et al. (Eds.), *Kelley's textbook of rheumatology* (9th ed.). Philadelphia: Saunders.

Government of Canada. (2015). *Information for health professionals on Lyme Disease.* Retrieved from *http://www.healthycanadians.gc.ca/diseases-conditions-maladies-affections/disease-maladie/lyme/professionals-professionnels/index-eng.php#a4.*

Hardy, E. (2011). Gout diagnosis and management: What NPs need to know. *The Nurse Practitioner, 36*(6), 14–19. doi:10.1097/01.NPR.0000397909.52327.8b.

Hill, G. (2012). Reactive arthritis and undifferentiated spondyloarthritis. In G. Firestein, R. Budd, S. Gabriel, et al. (Eds.), *Kelley's textbook of rheumatology* (9th ed.). Philadelphia: Saunders.

Hochberg, M., Martel-Pelletier, J., Monfort, J., et al. (2016). Combined chondroitin sulfate and glucosamine for painful knee osteoarthritis: A multicenter, randomized, double-blind, non-inferiority trial versus celecoxib. *Annals of the Rheumatic Diseases, 75*(1), 37–44. doi:10.1136/annrheumdis-2014-206792.

Institute of Medicine. (2015). *Beyond myalgic encephalopathy/chronic fatigue syndrome: Redefining an illness.* Retrieved from *http://www.nationalacademies.org/hmd/~/media/Files/Report%20Files/2015/MECFS/MECFSclinciansguide.pdf.*

Jolly, M., Pickard, A. S., Mikolaitis, R. A., et al. (2012). Body image in patients with systemic lupus erythematosus. *International Journal of Behavioural Medicine, 19*(2), 157–164. doi:10.1007/s12529-011-9154-9.

Jonsson, R., Vogelsang, P., Volchenkov, R., et al. (2011). The complexity of Sjögren's syndrome: Novel aspects on pathogenesis. *Immunology Letters, 141*(1), 1–9. doi:10.1016/j.imlet.2011.06.007.

Le Graverand-Gastineau, M. (2010). Disease-modifying osteoarthritis drugs: Facing development challenges and choosing molecular targets. *Current Drug Targets, 11*(5), 528–535. doi:10.2174/45010791011893.

Public Health Agency of Canada (PHAC). (2016). *Public health reminder: Lyme disease.* Retrieved from *http://www.phac-aspc .gc.ca/phn-asp/2015/lyme-eng.php.*

Robinson, P., & Benham, H. (2015). Advances in classification, basic mechanisms and clinical science in ankylosing spondylitis and axial spondyloarthritis. *Internal Medicine Journal, 45*(2), 127–133. doi:10.1111/imj.12544.

Saccomano, S., & Ferrera, L. (2015). Treatment and prevention of gout. *The Nurse Practitioner, 40*(8), 24–30. doi:10.1097/01 .NPR.0000469254.90496.ab.

Sovani, S., & Grogan, S. (2013). Osteoarthritis: Detection, pathophysiology, and current/future treatment strategies. *Orthopaedic Nursing, 32*(1), 25–36. doi:10.1097/NOR .0b013e31827d96da.

Tsokos, G. (2011). Systemic lupus erythematosus. *The New England Journal of Medicine, 365*(22), 2110–2121. doi:10.1056/ NEJMra1100359.

Varga, J. (2011). Systemic sclerosis (scleroderma). In L. Goldman & A. Schafer (Eds.), *Goldman: Goldman's Cecil Medicine* (24th ed.). Philadelphia: Saunders.

Vickers, A., Cronin, A., Maschino, A., et al. (2012). Acupuncture for chronic pain: Individual patient data meta-analysis. *Archives of Internal Medicine, 172*(19), 1444–1453. doi:10.1001/ archinternmed.2012.3654.

von Mühlen, C., & Nakamura, R. (2011). Clinical and laboratory evaluation of systemic rheumatic diseases. In R. McPherson & M. Pincus (Eds.), *McPherson: Henry's clinical diagnosis and management by laboratory methods* (22nd ed.). Philadelphia: Saunders.

Wolfe, F., Clauw, D., Fitzcharles, M., et al. (2010). The American College of Rheumatology criteria for fibromyalgia and measurement of symptom severity. *Arthritis Care and Research, 62*(5), 600–610. doi:10.1002/acr.20140.

RESOURCES

Arthritis Research Centre of Canada
http://www.arthritisresearch.ca

The Arthritis Society
http://www.arthritis.ca

Canadian Arthritis Network (CAN)
http://www.arthritisnetwork.ca

Canadian Lyme Disease Foundation (CanLyme)
http://www.canlyme.com

Canadian Organization for Rare Disorders (CORD)
http://www.raredisorders.ca

Canadian Rheumatology Association (CRA)
http://www.rheum.ca

Canadian Spondylitis Association
http://www.spondylitis.ca

FM-CFS Canada
http://www.fm-cfs.ca/

Lupus Canada
http://www.lupuscanada.org

National ME/FM Action Network
http://www.mefmaction.net

Scleroderma Society of Canada
http://www.scleroderma.ca

For additional Internet resources, see the website for this book at *http://evolve.elsevier.com/Canada/Lewis/medsurg.*

Nursing Care in Specialized Settings

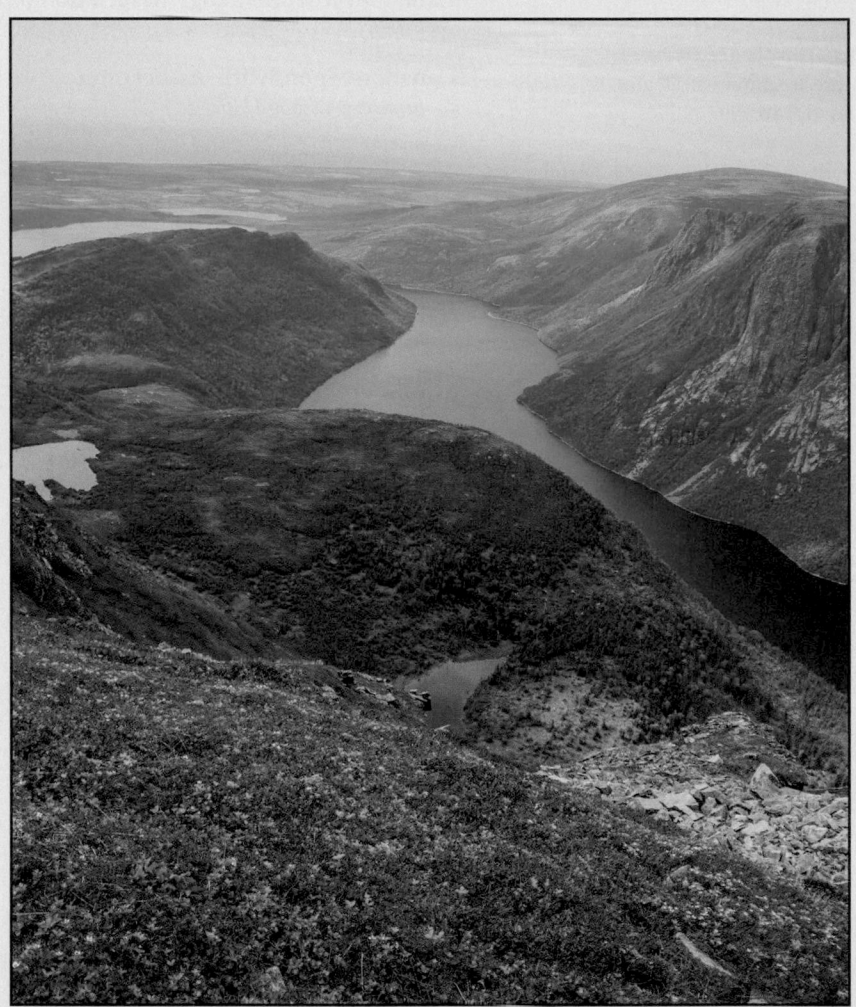

Source: RuthChoi/Shutterstock.com.

Nursing Management
Critical Care Environment

Written by: Maureen A. Seckel and Linda Bucher
Adapted by: Sandra Goldsworthy

evolve WEBSITE

http://evolve.elsevier.com/Canada/Lewis/medsurg

- Review Questions (Online Only)
- Key Points
- Answer Guidelines for Case Study
- Student Case Study
  - Pulmonary Embolism and Respiratory Failure
- Customizable Nursing Care Plan:
  - Mechanical Ventilation
- Conceptual Care Map Creator
- Audio Glossary
- Content Updates

LEARNING OBJECTIVES

1. Describe the critical care certification process available to critical care nurses in Canada as well as advanced-practice roles such as the clinical nurse specialist and the acute care nurse practitioner.
2. Select appropriate nursing interventions to manage common problems and needs of critically ill patients.
3. Develop effective strategies to manage issues related to the families and caregivers of critically ill patients.
4. Apply the principles of hemodynamic monitoring and the collaborative care and nursing management of the patient receiving this intervention.
5. Differentiate the purpose of, indications for, and function of circulatory assist devices and related collaborative care and nursing management.
6. Differentiate the indications for and contrast the modes of mechanical ventilation.
7. Select appropriate nursing interventions related to the care of an intubated patient.
8. Relate the principles of mechanical ventilation to the collaborative care and nursing management of patients receiving this intervention.

KEY TERMS

arterial pressure–based cardiac output (APCO), p. 1735
assist-control ventilation (ACV), p. 1748
circulatory assist devices (CADs), p. 1739
continuous positive airway pressure (CPAP), p. 1750
endotracheal (ET) intubation, p. 1742
hemodynamic monitoring, p. 1731

high-frequency oscillatory ventilation (HFOV), p. 1750
intra-aortic balloon pump, p. 1739
mechanical ventilation, p. 1747
negative-pressure ventilation, p. 1747
phlebostatic axis, p. 1733
positive end-expiratory pressure (PEEP), p. 1749

positive-pressure ventilation (PPV), p. 1747
pressure-support ventilation (PSV), p. 1749
ventricular assist device (VAD), p. 1741
volume ventilation, p. 1747
weaning, p. 1753

CRITICAL CARE NURSING

Critical Care Units

According to the Canadian Association of Critical Care Nurses (CACCN, 2017), critical care nursing is "a specialty which exists to care for patients who are experiencing life-threatening health crises within a patient-/family-centred model of care." Critical care nurses care for patients with acute and unstable physiological problems, as well as their caregivers. Their role involves assessing life-threatening conditions, initiating appropriate interventions, and evaluating the outcomes of the interventions.

Critical care units, also called *intensive care units (ICUs)*, are designed to meet the special needs of critically ill patients.

In many acute care settings, the concept of critical care has expanded from delivering care in a standard unit to bringing critical care to patients wherever they might be. The electronic or virtual ICU is designed to augment the bedside critical care team by monitoring the patient from a remote location (Figure 68-1). Similarly, a rapid response team provides advanced care by specialized health care providers, usually including a critical care nurse, a respiratory therapist, and a critical care physician. The team ensures immediate care to unstable patients in noncritical units. Patients often exhibit subtle early signs of deterioration (e.g., mild confusion) 6 to 8 hours before cardiac or respiratory arrest, and early critical care intervention has made significant contributions to

FIGURE 68-1 Electronic intensive care unit control room. Source: Frownfelter, D., & Dean, E. (2012). *Cardiovascular and pulmonary physical therapy: Evidence and practice* (5th ed., p. 562, Figure 34-2). St. Louis: Mosby Elsevier.

FIGURE 68-2 Typical critical care unit. Source: Amélie Benoist/Science Source.

reducing mortality rates in these patients (Maharaj, Raffaele, & Wendon, 2015).

The technology available in the ICU is extensive and always evolving. It is possible to continuously monitor the electrocardiogram (ECG), blood pressure (BP), oxygen (O_2) saturation, cardiac output (CO), intracranial pressure, and temperature. More advanced monitoring devices measure cardiac index (CI), stroke volume (SV), stroke volume variation (SVV), ejection fraction, end-tidal carbon dioxide (CO_2), and tissue O_2 consumption. Patients may receive ongoing support from mechanical ventilators, intra-aortic balloon pumps (IABPs), circulatory assist devices (CADs), or dialysis machines. Figure 68-2 shows a typical ICU.

Progressive-care units (PCUs), also called *intermediate-care units* or *step-down units,* provide a transition between the ICU and the general care unit or discharge (Prin & Wunsch, 2014).

Generally, PCU patients are at risk for serious complications, but their risk is lower than that of ICU patients. Examples of patients found in PCUs include those scheduled for interventional cardiac procedures (e.g., stent placement), awaiting heart transplant, receiving stable doses of vasoactive intravenous (IV) drugs, or being weaned from prolonged mechanical ventilation. Monitoring capabilities in these units include continuous ECG, arterial BP, O_2 saturation, and end-tidal CO_2. PCUs provide critical care nursing for an at-risk population in a more cost-effective environment.

Critical Care Nurse

A critical care nurse has in-depth knowledge of anatomy, physiology, pathophysiology, pharmacology, and advanced assessment skills as well as the ability to use advanced technology. Critical care nurses perform frequent assessments to monitor trends (patterns) in the patient's physiological parameters (e.g., BP, ECG). This level of observation allows the nurse to rapidly recognize and manage complications while fostering healing and recovery. The nurse also provides psychological support to the patient and caregiver(s). To be effective, the critical care nurse must be able to communicate and collaborate with all members of the multidisciplinary health care team (e.g., physician, dietitian, social worker, respiratory therapist, and occupational therapist).

Critical care nurses face ethical dilemmas related to the care of patients. Moral distress over perceived issues of delivering futile or nonbeneficial care can lead to emotional exhaustion or burnout. Consequently, it is important that all members of the health care team coexist in a healthy work environment.

Specialization in critical care nursing usually initially requires comprehensive theoretical preparation and a preceptored orientation or internship. New innovations for preparing nurses to practise in critical care settings include educational opportunities to participate in cases that mimic the critical care environment in the human simulation laboratory (Alberta Health Services, 2016).

The Canadian Nurses Association offers critical care certification (CNCC[C]) in critical care nursing. The designation requires that a registered nurse have practice experience in critical care nursing and successfully complete a comprehensive written examination set to national standards. Continued critical care practice and retesting or continuing education is required for recertification at 5-year intervals. CNCC(C) certification validates knowledge of critical care nursing. In Canada, registered nurses may also choose to complete a critical care certificate through classroom or online education, typically combined with preceptored clinical experience.

Advanced-practice critical care nurses have a graduate degree (master's or doctorate). These nurses are employed in a variety of roles: patient and staff educators, consultants, administrators, researchers, or expert practitioners. The advanced-practice critical care nurse who is a clinical nurse specialist typically functions in one or more of these roles. Typically, a clinical nurse specialist has graduate preparation as well as expertise in critical care. Another advanced-practice role is the acute care nurse practitioner (ACNP). ACNPs provide comprehensive care to select critically ill patients and their families. They conduct comprehensive assessments, order and interpret diagnostic tests, manage health problems and disease-related symptoms, prescribe treatments, and coordinate care during transitions in settings. ACNPs may practise independently (e.g., providing comprehensive care to the chronically critically ill) or collaboratively (e.g., providing symptom management in conjunction with physicians). In Canada, ACNPs are prepared at the graduate level.

Critical Care Patient

A patient is generally admitted to the ICU for one of three reasons. First, the patient may be physiologically unstable, requiring advanced and sophisticated clinical judgements by a nurse or physician. Second, the patient may be at risk for serious complications and require frequent and often invasive interventions. Third, the patient may require intensive and complicated nursing support related to the use of IV polypharmacy (e.g., neuro-muscular blockade, thrombolytics, drugs requiring titration) and advanced technology (e.g., mechanical ventilation, intracranial pressure monitoring, continuous renal replacement therapy, hemodynamic monitoring).

ICU patients can be clustered by disease condition (e.g., neurology, pulmonary) or age group (e.g., neonatal, pediatrics). ICU patients are sometimes clustered by acuity (e.g., acute and unstable as opposed to technology-dependent but stable). Patients commonly treated in the ICU include those with respiratory distress, myocardial ischemia or infarction, or acute neurological impairment or those receiving care after cardiac surgery or major organ transplantation. The care of critically injured patients is provided in trauma and burn ICUs. Patients with medical emergencies (e.g., septic shock, drug overdoses, or diabetic ketoacidosis) are often treated in a medical ICU. Patients who are not expected to recover from an illness are usually not admitted to an ICU. For example, the ICU is not used to manage a patient in a persistent coma or to prolong the natural process of death.

Common Problems of Critical Care Patients.

Patients admitted to the ICU are at risk for numerous complications and special problems. Critically ill patients are usually immobile and at risk for venous thrombo-embolism and skin problems (see Chapter 26). The use of multiple invasive devices predisposes patients to health care–associated infections (HAIs). Sepsis and multiple-organ dysfunction syndrome may follow (see Chapter 69).

Nutrition. Patients are often admitted to ICUs with conditions that result in either hypermetabolic states (e.g., burns, trauma, sepsis) or catabolic states (e.g., acute kidney injury). Other times, patients may be admitted in severely malnourished states (e.g., chronic heart, pulmonary, or liver disease). In general, malnutrition has been linked to increases in mortality and morbidity.

Whom to feed, what to feed, when to feed, and how to feed (e.g., route of administration) are crucial questions that the nurse must ask when caring for a critically ill patient. The nurse must collaborate with the physician and the dietitian to determine how best to meet the nutritional needs of ICU patients.

The primary goal of nutritional support is to prevent or correct nutritional deficiencies. This is usually accomplished by the early provision of enteral nutrition (i.e., delivery of calories via the gastro-intestinal [GI] tract) or parenteral nutrition (i.e., delivery of calories intravenously). Enteral nutrition preserves the structure and function of the gut mucosa and prevents the movement of gut bacteria across the intestinal wall and into the bloodstream. In addition, early enteral nutrition is associated with fewer complications and shorter hospital stays and is less expensive than parenteral nutrition (McClave, Taylor, Martindale, et al., 2016). (Enteral and parenteral nutrition are discussed in Chapter 42.)

Parenteral nutrition is used when the enteral route cannot provide adequate nutrition or is contraindicated. Examples of these conditions include paralytic ileus, diffuse peritonitis, intestinal obstruction, pancreatitis, GI ischemia, intractable vomiting, and severe diarrhea.

Anxiety. Anxiety is a common problem for ICU patients. The primary sources of anxiety include the perceived or anticipated threat to physical health, actual loss of control of body functions, and placement in a foreign environment. Many patients and caregivers feel uncomfortable in the ICU environment with its complex equipment, high noise and light levels, isolation from family, and intense pace of activity. Pain and sleeplessness enhance anxiety, as do immobilization, loss of control, and impaired communication.

To help reduce anxiety, the nurse should encourage patients and caregivers to express concerns, ask questions, and state their needs. Patients and caregivers should be included in all conversations and have the purpose of equipment and procedures explained to them. The nurse should structure the patient's environment in such a way as to decrease anxiety if possible and encourage caregivers to bring in photographs and personal items. Appropriate use of antianxiety drugs (e.g., lorazepam [Ativan]) and relaxation techniques (e.g., music therapy) may reduce the stress response that can be triggered by anxiety (Chlan, Weinert, Heiderscheit, et al., 2013).

Pain. The control of pain in an ICU patient is paramount. Pain management is a significant issue among critically ill patients and with poor assessment can result in serious physical and psychological consequences (Georgiou, Hadjibalassi, Lambrinou, et al., 2015). Inadequate pain control is often linked to agitation and anxiety and is known to contribute to the stress response. Critically ill patients at high risk for pain include patients who (a) have medical conditions that include ischemic, infectious, or inflammatory processes; (b) are immobilized; (c) have invasive monitoring devices, including endotracheal (ET) tubes; and (d) are scheduled for any invasive or noninvasive procedures.

For some critically ill patients, continuous IV sedation (e.g., propofol [Diprivan]) and an analgesic agent (e.g., fentanyl) are a practical and effective strategy for sedation and pain control. However, patients receiving deep sedation are unresponsive, which prevents the nurse and other health care providers from properly assessing the patient's neurological status. To address this limitation, guidelines that include a daily, scheduled interruption of sedation, or "drug holiday," have been developed. Daily sedative interruption allows the patient to awaken and the health care provider to conduct a neurological examination and assess readiness for weaning from the mechanical ventilator (Safer Health Care Now, 2012). (Chapter 10 has more detailed information on pain management.) The most current guidelines for pain, agitation, and delirium in the ICU include an analgesia-first approach, with lighter sedation so that patients can report their pain scale (Barr, Fraser, Puntillo, et al., 2013).

INFORMATICS IN PRACTICE

Smart Infusion Pumps

Smart infusion pumps, with preprogrammed drug libraries and wireless technology, calculate medication dose and delivery rates to help prevent IV medication errors and reduce the risk for patient harm.

Smart pumps provide information used in ensuring safe practices, such as how many infusions were programmed using the drug library, how many times pumps were manually overridden, and how often an alert resulted in reprogramming an infusion.

Remember, if a nurse enters incorrect data, there will be incorrect results. Some drugs (e.g., heparin) require that a second nurse confirm the pump settings. Nurses must use their best judgement when using smart infusion pumps or any other technology and follow employer policy.

Impaired Communication. Inability to communicate is a distressing problem for patients who are unable to speak because of the use of sedative or paralyzing drugs or an ET tube. As part of any procedure, the nurse should explain what will happen or is happening to the patient. When the patient cannot speak, the nurse should explore alternative methods of communication, including the use of devices such as picture boards, notepads, magic slates, tablets, cellphones (instant messaging applications), or computer keyboards. When speaking with the patient, the nurse should look directly at the patient and use hand gestures when appropriate. For patients who do not speak English, an approved interpreter must be used (see Chapter 2, Tables 2-5 and 2-6).

Nonverbal communication is also important. A large amount of procedure-related touch and much less comfort-related touch often characterize the ICU environment. Patients have different levels of tolerance for being touched, usually related to cultural background and personal history. It may be appropriate to provide comforting touch with ongoing evaluation of the patient's response. If appropriate, the nurse can encourage caregivers to touch and talk with the patient even if the patient is unresponsive or comatose.

Sensory-Perceptual Problems. Acute and reversible sensory-perceptual changes are common in ICU patients. The combination of alterations in mentation (e.g., delusions, short attention span, loss of recent memory), psychomotor behaviour (e.g., restlessness, lethargy), and sleep–wake cycle (e.g., daytime sleepiness, nighttime agitation) has been inappropriately labelled *ICU psychosis.* The patient experiencing these alterations is not psychotic but is suffering from delirium. Delirium has been found to be common in mechanically ventilated patients in the ICU and can lead to increased length of hospital stay and increased length of mechanical ventilation (Mehta, Cook, Devlin, et al., 2015).

Demographic factors predisposing the patient to delirium include advanced age, pre-existing cognitive impairment (e.g., dementia), vision or hearing impairments, and a history of drug or alcohol use. Environmental factors that can contribute to delirium include sleep deprivation, anxiety, sensory overload, and immobilization. Physical conditions such as hemodynamic instability, hypoxemia, hypercarbia, electrolyte disturbances, and severe infections can precipitate delirium. As well, certain drugs (e.g., sedatives [benzodiazepines], furosemide [Lasix], antimicrobials [aminoglycosides]) have been associated with the development of delirium (Barr, Fraser, Puntillo, et al., 2013). (Delirium is discussed in Chapter 62.)

The nurse should monitor the patient for delirium and mental clarity. Tools to assess for delirium include the Confusion Assessment Method (CAM) for the ICU and the Intensive Care Delirium Screening Checklist (ICDSC) (see the Resources at the end of the chapter). It is critical that physiological factors be addressed (e.g., correction of oxygenation, perfusion, and electrolyte problems). The use of clocks and calendars can help orient the patient. In addition, the presence of a caregiver may help orient the patient and reduce agitation.

Sensory overload can also result in patient distress and anxiety. Environmental noise levels are particularly high in the ICU. One study in the United Kingdom found that sounds in the five ICUs studied peaked above 85 dBA and that all sites consistently had noise levels greater than the limit of 35 dB recommended by the World Health Organization (WHO; Darbyshire & Young, 2013). The nurse can limit noise and assist the patient in understanding noises that cannot be prevented. Conversation is a particularly stressful noise, especially when the discussion concerns the patient

and is held in the presence of, but without participation from, the patient. The nurse can eliminate this source of stress by finding suitable places for patient-related discussions and, when possible, including the patient in the discussion.

The nurse can also limit noise levels directly by muting phones, setting alarms appropriate to the patient's condition, and eliminating unnecessary alarms. For example, the nurse can silence the BP alarms when manipulating invasive lines and then reactivate the alarms when done. Similarly, the nurse can silence ventilator alarms during ET suctioning. Finally, the nurse can limit overhead paging and all unnecessary noise in patient care areas.

Sleep Problems. Nearly all ICU patients experience sleep disturbances. Patients may have difficulty falling asleep or have disrupted sleep because of noise, anxiety, pain, frequent monitoring, or treatment procedures. Sleep disturbance is a significant stressor in the ICU, contributing to delirium and possibly affecting recovery (Delaney, Van Haren, & Lopez, 2015). The nurse can structure the environment to promote the patient's sleep–wake cycle. Strategies for achieving this include clustering activities, scheduling rest periods, dimming lights at nighttime, opening curtains during the daytime, obtaining physiological measurements without disturbing the patient, limiting noise, and providing comfort measures (e.g., back rubs). If necessary, pharmacological therapy may be needed to induce and maintain sleep. (Sleep and sleep disorders are discussed in Chapter 9.)

Issues Related to Caregivers. When a person becomes critically ill, care extends beyond the patient to the patient's caregivers because they are intimately involved. Caregivers play a valuable role in the patient's recovery and are members of the health care team. They contribute to the patient's well-being by:

- Providing a link to the patient's personal life (e.g., news of family, job)
- Advising the patient in health care decisions or functioning as the decision maker when the patient cannot
- Helping with activities of daily living (e.g., bathing, oral suctioning)
- Providing positive, loving, and caring support

To be effective in caring for their loved one, caregivers need the nurse's guidance and support. The experience of having a friend or family member as a patient in the ICU is physically and emotionally difficult, often to the point of exhaustion. Anxiety regarding the patient's condition and prognosis and concerns regarding the patient's pain and other discomforts are some of the issues caregivers confront. In addition, it is common for caregivers to experience anxiety regarding the financial issues related to the provision of care during a critical illness. Consulting with the case manager or social worker is helpful in these instances.

Caregivers typically experience disruption of their daily routines to support the patient. They may be far from their own home and supportive friends and family members. Ultimately, caregivers of the critically ill are considered to be in crisis, and family-centred care is essential. To provide family-centred care effectively, the nurse must be skilled in crisis intervention. The nurse should conduct a family assessment and intervene as necessary. Interventions can include active listening, reduction of anxiety, and support of those who become upset or angry (Davidson, 2016).

The nurse should acknowledge the caregivers' feelings and accept and support their decisions. The nurse should consult other health care team members (e.g., chaplains, psychologists, patient representatives) as necessary to assist caregivers to adjust. The extent to which family-centred care is provided can affect the patient's clinical course in the ICU. The nurse can identify a spokesperson for the family so that information between the health care team and the family is coordinated.

The caregiver needs reassurance regarding the way in which the patient's care is managed and decisions are made. To this end, the nurse can invite the caregiver to meet the health care team members and also evaluate the appropriateness of including caregivers in multidisciplinary rounds and patient care conferences. The nurse should provide the caregiver with the opportunity to participate in decision making. When patients are incapable of making their own health care decisions, they may have designated a durable power of attorney for health care, and this person also should be involved in the patient's plan of care. If the patient has an advance directive or a living will, the caregiver will need to see that the patient's wishes are followed.

Caregivers are better able to accept and cope with problems if they observe that the health care team is hopeful, caring, and competent; decisions are deliberate; and their input is valued. Caregivers of critically ill patients need the convenience of access to the patient. Limiting visitation does not protect the patient from adverse physiological consequences (Davidson, 2016). In addition, flexible visiting hours for family align with a family-centred approach. The first time that caregivers visit, it is important for the nurse to prepare them for the experience by briefly describing the patient's appearance and the physical environment (e.g., equipment, noise). The nurse should accompany the caregivers as they enter the room and observe the responses of both the patient and the caregivers and invite the caregivers to participate in the patient's care if they desire. In some ICUs, visitation includes animal-assisted therapy or pet visitation. The positive benefits of these interventions (e.g., decreases in BP and anxiety) far outweigh the risks (e.g., transmission of infection from animal to patient), and they should be a part of the visitation policy.

In addition to traditional visiting, research has shown that caregivers of patients undergoing invasive procedures (e.g., central line insertion) and cardiopulmonary resuscitation want the option of being present at the bedside during these events. Even when the outcomes were not favourable, being present helped caregivers remove doubts about the patient's condition, decreased their anxiety and fear, facilitated the need to be together and to support their loved one, and facilitated the grief process when death occurred. The Canadian Critical Care Society encourages ICUs to develop policies and procedures that provide for the option of family presence during invasive procedures and cardiopulmonary resuscitation (Oczkowski, Mazzetti, Cupido, et al., 2015).

CULTURALLY COMPETENT CARE

CRITICAL CARE PATIENTS

Providing culturally competent care to critically ill patients and families is challenging. Often, the nurse is focused on meeting the physiological needs of the patient and may not appreciate the influence of the patient's culture on the illness experience. However, the cultural dimensions of the meaning of sickness and health, pain, dying and death, and grief need to be considered when caring for critically ill patients and their families. (Chapter 2 discusses cultural issues.)

Cultural perspectives on dying and death are complex. For example, telling some patients that they are dying as a way of letting them prepare for death may be considered an infringement on the role of the family. Others view a discussion about advance

directives as a legal device to deny care. Customs surrounding dying and death vary widely, from leaving a window open to allow the spirit of the dead person to leave to providing the final bath for the deceased. The nurse caring for the dying patient must make every attempt to understand and accommodate the family's cultural traditions.

The expressions of grief that follow the loss of a loved one are highly individualized and influenced by several variables. These include the relationship between the grieving person and the deceased, whether the loss is sudden or anticipated, the support systems available to the grieving person, the person's past experiences with loss, and the person's religious and cultural beliefs. It is of utmost importance that the critical care nurse proceed cautiously with patients facing death and their families. Asking patients "What do you want to know?" and "Who do you want with you when discussing options?" is a good starting point (CACCN, 2011). (Chapter 13 provides additional information about end-of-life care.)

HEMODYNAMIC MONITORING

Hemodynamic monitoring is the measurement of pressure, flow, and oxygenation within the cardiovascular system. Both invasive (internally placed devices) and noninvasive (external devices) hemodynamic measurements are made in the ICU. Values commonly measured include systemic arterial pressure and pulmonary artery pressure (PAP), central venous pressure (CVP), pulmonary artery occlusive pressure (PAOP), CO and CI, SV/ stroke volume index (SVI), and oxygen saturation of the hemoglobin of arterial blood (SaO_2) and mixed venous blood (SvO_2). From these measurements, the clinician calculates several values, including the resistance of the systemic and pulmonary arterial vasculature as well as oxygen content, delivery, and consumption. When these data are integrated with clinical assessment data, the nurse can derive a picture of the patient's hemodynamic status and the effect of therapy. All measures need to be made with attention to technical accuracy. False or inaccurate data can result in unnecessary and inappropriate treatment.

Hemodynamic Terminology

Cardiac Output and Cardiac Index. *Cardiac output* (CO) is the volume of blood pumped by the heart in 1 minute. *Cardiac index* (CI) is the measurement of the CO adjusted for body size, and it is a more precise measurement of the efficiency of the pumping action of the heart. Although minor beat-to-beat changes may occur, generally the left and right ventricles pump the same volume. The volume pumped with each heartbeat is the SV. Like CI, SVI is the measurement of SV adjusted for body size. CO and the forces opposing blood flow determine BP, the force exerted by blood on the vessel wall. The opposition to blood flow offered by the vessels is called *systemic vascular resistance* (SVR) or *pulmonary vascular resistance*. Preload, afterload, and contractility (see Chapter 34) determine SV (and thus CO and BP). Understanding these concepts and relationships is essential for the critical care nurse. In addition, the nurse must understand the effects of manipulation of each of these variables. The formulas and normal values for common hemodynamic parameters are given in Table 68-1.

Preload. *Preload* is the volume within a cardiac chamber at the end of diastole. Unfortunately, chamber volume measurements are difficult to obtain. Instead, various pressures are used to estimate volume. Left ventricular preload is called *left ventricular*

TABLE 68-1   RESTING HEMODYNAMIC PARAMETERS

Indicators	Normal Range
Preload	
Right atrial pressure (RAP) or central venous pressure (CVP)	2–8 mm Hg
Pulmonary artery wedge pressure (PAWP) or left atrial pressure (LAP)	6–12 mm Hg
Pulmonary artery diastolic pressure (PADP)	4–12 mm Hg
Right ventricular end-diastolic volume $(RVEDV) = \dfrac{\text{Stroke volume (SV)}}{\text{Right ventricular ejection fraction (RVEF)}}$	100–160 mL
Afterload	
Pulmonary vascular resistance $(PVR) = \dfrac{(\text{Pulmonary artery mean pressure [PAMP]} - \text{PAWP}) \times 80}{\text{Cardiac output (CO)}}$	<250 dynes/sec/cm^{-5}
Pulmonary vascular resistance index $(PVRI) = \dfrac{(\text{PAMP} - \text{PAWP}) \times 80}{\text{Cardiac index (CI)}}$	160–380 dynes/sec/cm^{-5}/m^2
Systemic vascular resistance $(SVR) = \dfrac{(\text{Mean arterial pressure [MAP]} - \text{CVP}) \times 80}{\text{CO}}$	800–1200 dynes/sec/cm^{-5}
Systemic vascular resistance index $(SVRI) = \dfrac{(\text{MAP} - \text{CVP}) \times 80}{\text{CI}}$	1970–2390 dynes/sec/cm^{-5}/m^2
*MAP $= \dfrac{\text{Systolic blood pressure} + 2\,(\text{Diastolic blood pressure}}{3}$	70–105 mm Hg
*PAMP $= \dfrac{\text{Pulmonary artery systolic pressure (PASP)} + 2\,\text{PADF}}{3}$	10–20 mm Hg
Other	
Stroke volume $= \dfrac{\text{CO}}{\text{Heart rate}}$	60–150 mL/beat
Stroke volume index $(SVI) = \dfrac{\text{CI}}{\text{Heart rate}}$	30–65 mL/beat/m^2
Stroke volume variation $(SVV) = \dfrac{SV_{max} - SV_{min}}{SV_{mean}}$	<13%
Heart rate (HR)	60–100 beats/min
CO $= $ SV $\times$ HR	4–8 L/min
CI $= \dfrac{\text{CO}}{\text{Body surface area (BSA)}}$	2.2–4 L/min/m^2
RVEF $= \dfrac{\text{SV}}{\text{RVEDV} \times 100}$	40%–60%
Arterial hemoglobin O$_2$ saturation	95%–100%
Mixed venous homoglobin O$_2$ saturation	60%–80%
Venous hemoglobin O$_2$ saturation	70%

*These formulas are approximations because they do not take into consideration the heart rate. The monitor looks at the area under the pressure curve, as well as the heart rate, to calculate MAP and PAMP.

end-diastolic pressure. PAOP, a measure of pulmonary occlusive pressure, reflects left ventricular end-diastolic pressure under normal conditions (i.e., when there is no mitral valve pathological condition, intracardiac defect, or dysrhythmia). CVP, measured in the right atrium or in the vena cava close to the heart, is the right ventricular preload or right ventricular end-diastolic pressure when there is no tricuspid valve pathological condition, intracardiac defect, or dysrhythmia.

The effects of preload are explained by *Starling's law,* which states that the more a myocardial fibre is stretched during filling, the more it shortens during systole and the greater the force of the contraction to a physiological limit. As preload increases, force generated in the following contraction increases; thus, SV and CO increase. The greater the preload, the greater the myocardial (heart muscle) stretch and the greater the oxygen requirement of the myocardium. Hence, increases in CO via increased preload require increased delivery of oxygen to the myocardium. It should be remembered that the change in SV with preload comes about because of stretching of the heart muscle. However, the clinical measurement made is not a direct measurement of the muscle length; the measurement made is pressure at the time of the peak stretch (end diastole) (see Table 68-1). This pressure indirectly indicates the amount of stretch and the volume. This pressure is also important because it indicates pressure in the blood vessels of the lung or in the blood returning to the heart. Preload can be increased by fluid administration and decreased by diuresis.

Afterload. *Afterload* refers to the forces opposing ventricular ejection. These forces include systemic arterial pressure, the resistance offered by the aortic valve, and the mass and density of the blood to be moved. Clinically, although the measures fail to include all the components of afterload, SVR and arterial pressure are indexes of left ventricular afterload. Similarly, pulmonary vascular resistance and PAP are indexes of right ventricular afterload. Increased afterload often results in a decreased CO. CO can be restored by decreasing afterload (i.e., decreasing forces opposing contraction). When afterload is reduced, myocardial oxygen needs are decreased. Thus, when CO is increased, myocardial oxygen requirements are decreased. Drug therapy directed at reducing afterload (e.g., nitroglycerine or nitroprusside) is often used in the management of heart failure (see Chapter 37).

Vascular Resistance. *Systemic vascular resistance* (SVR) is the resistance of the systemic vascular bed. *Pulmonary vascular resistance* is the resistance of the pulmonary vascular bed. Both of these measures reflect afterload as described earlier and can be adjusted for body size (see Table 68-1).

Contractility. *Contractility* describes the strength of contraction. Contractility is said to increase when preload is not changed yet the heart contracts more forcefully. Epinephrine, norepinephrine, isoproterenol, dopamine, dobutamine, digitalis-like drugs, calcium, and milrinone (Primacor) increase contractility. These agents are termed *positive inotropes*. Contractility is diminished by *negative inotropes*, such as acidosis and certain drugs (e.g., barbiturates, alcohol, procainamide, calcium channel blockers, β-adrenergic blockers). Increased contractility results in increased SV and increased myocardial oxygen requirements. There are no direct clinical measures of cardiac contractility. To indirectly determine contractility, the nurse measures the patient's preload (PAOP or wedge) and CO and graphs the results. If preload, heart rate, and afterload remain constant yet CO changes, contractility is altered. Contractility diminishes in the failing heart.

Principles of Invasive Pressure Monitoring

Invasive lines are commonly used in the ICU to measure systemic and pulmonary BPs. Components of a typical invasive arterial pressure monitoring system are illustrated in Figure 68-3. The catheter, pressure tubing, flush system, and usually the transducer are disposable.

To accurately measure pressure, equipment must be referenced and zero-balanced, and dynamic response characteristics optimized. *Levelling* means positioning the transducer so that the zero reference point is at the level of the atria of the heart. The stopcock nearest the transducer is usually the zero reference for the transducer. To place this level with the atria, the nurse uses an external landmark, the phlebostatic axis. To identify the **phlebostatic axis**, two imaginary lines are drawn with the patient supine (Figure 68-4, *A*). The first line, a horizontal line, is drawn through the midchest, halfway between the outermost anterior and the outermost posterior surfaces. The second line, a vertical line, is drawn through the fourth intercostal space at the sternum. The phlebostatic axis is the intersection of the two imaginary lines. Once the phlebostatic axis is identified, it should be marked on the patient's chest with a permanent marker. The port of the stopcock nearest the transducer must be positioned level with the phlebostatic axis.

Zeroing confirms that when pressure within the system is zero, the equipment reads zero. This is accomplished by opening the reference stopcock to room air and observing the monitor for a reading of zero. Most transducers in current use are disposable and have little zero drift. Zeroing the transducer is recommended during initial setup, immediately after insertion of the arterial line, when the transducer has been disconnected from the pressure cable or the pressure cable has been disconnected from the monitor, and when the accuracy of the measurements is questioned, and it should be done according to the manufacturer's guidelines. Optimizing dynamic response characteristics involves checking that the equipment reproduces without distortion a signal that changes rapidly. A *dynamic response test (square wave test)* is performed every 8 to 12 hours and when the system is opened to air, or if the accuracy of the measurements is questioned. It

FIGURE 68-3 Components of a pressure monitoring system. The cannula, shown entering the radial artery, is connected via pressure (nondistensible) tubing to the transducer. The transducer converts the pressure wave into an electronic signal. The transducer is wired to the electronic monitoring system, which amplifies, conditions, displays, and records the signal. Stopcocks are inserted into the line for specimen withdrawal and for referencing and zero-balancing procedures. A flush system, consisting of a pressurized bag of intravenous fluid, tubing, and a flush device, is connected to the system. The flush system provides continuous slow (≈3 mL/hr) flushing and provides a mechanism for fast flushing of lines.

involves checking that the equipment reproduces a distortion-free signal (Figure 68-5).

Steps in obtaining BP measurements with an invasive line are given in Table 68-2. Pressure measurements can be obtained from both digital and printed analogue outputs, but accurate readings are best obtained from a printed pressure tracing at the end of expiration. Initial readings are made with the patient flat. Unless the patient's BP is extremely sensitive to orthostatic changes, values at modest degrees of backrest elevation (≤45 degrees) are generally equivalent to measurements with the patient flat. Studies have not demonstrated the accuracy of readings obtained for patients in the lateral position but do support the accuracy of readings in the prone position. It is not necessary to reposition the patient for each pressure reading. However, it is necessary to move the zero reference stopcock to keep it positioned at the phlebostatic axis (see Figure 68-4, *B*).

Types of Invasive Pressure Monitoring

Arterial Blood Pressure. Continuous arterial pressure monitoring is indicated for patients in many situations, including acute

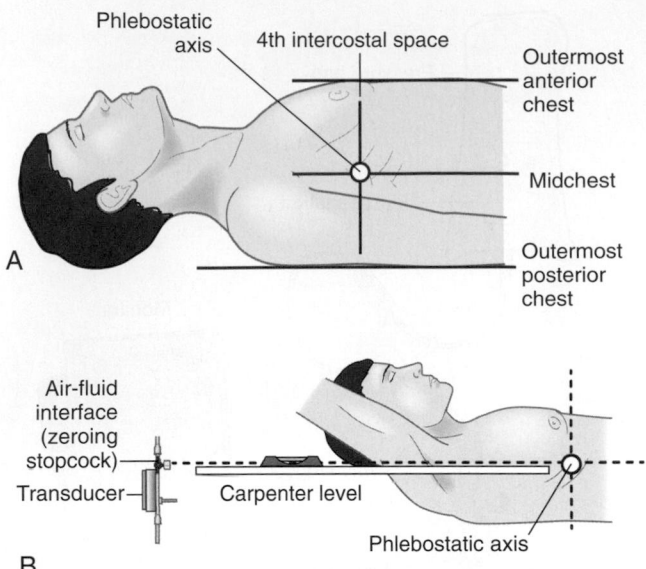

FIGURE 68-4 Identification of the phlebostatic axis. **A,** Phlebostatic axis is an external landmark used to identify the level of the atria in the supine patient. It is defined as the intersection of two imaginary lines: one drawn horizontally from the midchest, midway between the anterior and posterior chest walls, and the other drawn vertically through the fourth intercostal space along the lateral chest wall. **B,** Air–fluid interface (zeroing the stopcock) is level with the phlebostatic axis using a carpenter's or laser level.

Square wave test configuration

Observed waveform

When the fast flush of the continuous flush system is activated and quickly released, a sharp upstroke terminates in a flat line at the maximal indicator on the monitor and hard copy. This is then followed by an immediate rapid downstroke extending below baseline with just 1 or 2 oscillations within 0.12 second (minimal ringing) and a quick return to baseline. The patient's pressure waveform is also clearly defined with all components of the waveform, such as the dicrotic notch on an arterial waveform, clearly visible.

FIGURE 68-5 Optimally damped system. Dynamic response test (square wave test) using the fast-flush system: normal response. No adjustment in the monitoring system is required. Source: Darovic, G. O. (1995). *Hemodynamic monitoring* (2nd ed.). Philadelphia: Saunders.

hypertension and hypotension, respiratory failure, shock, neurological injury, coronary interventional procedures, continuous infusion of vasoactive drugs, and frequent arterial blood gas (ABG) sampling. A 20-gauge, 5.1-cm, nontapered Teflon over-the-needle cannula is typically used to cannulate a peripheral artery, such as the radial, brachial, or femoral, using a percutaneous approach.

FIGURE 68-6 A, Simultaneously recorded electrocardiogram (ECG) tracing. **B,** Systemic arterial pressure tracing. Systolic pressure is the peak pressure. The dicrotic notch indicates aortic valve closure. Diastolic pressure is the lowest value before contraction. Mean pressure is the average pressure over time calculated by the monitoring equipment. Source: Adapted from Urden, L. D., Stacy, K. M., & Lough, M. E. (2010). *Critical care nursing: Diagnosis and management* (6th ed., p. 333, Figure 18-8). St. Louis: Mosby.

TABLE 68-2	MEASUREMENT OF BLOOD PRESSURE WITH INVASIVE LINES

1. The nurse explains the procedure to the patient.
2. The nurse positions the patient supine and flat or, if appropriate, with the head of the bed elevated up to 45 degrees.
3. The nurse confirms that the zero reference (port of the stopcock nearest the transducer) is placed at the level of the phlebostatic axis (see Figure 68-4). If the reference stopcock is not taped to the patient's chest, a carpenter's level should be used to position the stopcock on a bedside pole at the point level with the phlebostatic axis.
4. The nurse observes the monitor tracing, assesses the quality of the tracing, and performs a dynamic response test (see Figure 68-5).
5. The nurse obtains an analogue printout, if available, and measures the systolic and diastolic pressures at end-expiration (see Figure 68-6). If no printout is available, the nurse freezes the tracing on the oscilloscope screen and uses the cursor to measure the pressures at end-expiration.
6. The nurse records the pressure measurements promptly, including (if available) the printout marked to identify the points read.

It is important that the insertion site be immobilized so that the catheter line is not dislodged and lines do not become kinked.

Measurements. The nurse can use the arterial line to obtain systolic, diastolic, and mean BPs (Figure 68-6). High- and low-pressure alarms should be set, based on the patient's current status, and activated. Measurements are obtained at end-expiration to limit the effect of the respiratory cycle on arterial pressure (Shaffer, 2011). In patients with heart failure, the systolic upstroke may be slower. In patients with volume depletion, systolic pressure varies greatly with mechanical ventilation, diminishing during inspiration. In the case of severe heart failure, systolic amplitude does not vary with ventilation. With dysrhythmias, it is useful to observe simultaneous ECG and pressure tracings. Dysrhythmias that significantly diminish arterial pressure are more urgent than those that cause only a slight decrease in systolic amplitude.

Complications. Arterial lines carry a risk for hemorrhage, infection, thrombus formation, and neuro-vascular impairment. Hemorrhage is most likely to occur when the catheter becomes dislodged or the line becomes disconnected. To avoid this serious complication, the nurse uses Luer-Lok connections and always checks the arterial waveform and ensures that the alarms are activated. If the pressure in the line falls (e.g., when the line is disconnected), the low-pressure alarm sounds immediately, allowing prompt correction of the problem. Pressure is always monitored when an arterial line is in place, even if the line was placed for ABG sampling.

Infection is a risk with any invasive line. The nurse should inspect the insertion site for local signs of inflammation and monitor the patient for signs of systemic infection. To limit the risk for contamination and catheter-related infection, the pressure tubing and transducer should be changed every 72 hours. As well, the pressure bag should be changed every 24 hours.

Circulatory impairment can result from formation of a thrombus around the catheter, release of an embolus, spasm, or occlusion of the circulation by the catheter. Before inserting a line into the radial artery, an Allen test should be performed to confirm that ulnar circulation is sufficient to sustain the hand. In this test, pressure is applied to the radial and ulnar arteries simultaneously. The patient is instructed to open and close the hand repeatedly. The hand should blanch. The nurse then releases the pressure on the ulnar artery while compressing the radial artery. If pinkness fails to return within 6 seconds, the ulnar artery is insufficient, indicating that the radial artery should not be used for line insertion.

To maintain line patency and limit thrombus formation, assess the continuous flush system every 1 to 4 hours to determine that (a) the pressure bag is inflated to 300 mm Hg, (b) the flush bag contains fluid, and (c) the system is delivering 3 to 6 mL/hr. Because of the risk for heparin-induced thrombo-cytopenia, heparinized saline should not be routinely used for the flush solution (Shaffer, 2011). Once the catheter is inserted, the nurse should evaluate the neuro-vascular status distal to the arterial insertion site hourly. The limb with compromised arterial flow will be cool and pale, with capillary refill time longer than 3 seconds. There may be symptoms of neurological impairment (e.g., paresthesia, pain, paralysis). Neuro-vascular impairment can result in loss of a limb and is an emergency.

Arterial Pressure–Based Cardiac Output. Arterial pressure–based cardiac output (APCO) monitoring is a minimally invasive technique to determine *continuous CO (CCO)/continuous CI (CCI)*, in order to assess a patient's ability to respond to fluids by increasing stroke volume (*preload responsiveness*). This assessment is determined by using SVV or by measuring the percentage of increase in SV after a fluid bolus (Edwards Lifesciences, 2006; see Table 68-1). This technology uses a specialized sensor that attaches to a standard arterial pressure line and a monitor (Figure 68-7).

SVV is the variation of the arterial pulsation caused by the heart–lung interaction. It is a sensitive indicator of preload responsiveness when used on select patients. SVV is used only for patients on controlled mechanical ventilation with a fixed respiratory rate and a fixed tidal volume (V_T) of 8 mL/kg. Also, the APCO monitor may not be able to filter certain dysrhythmias—specifically atrial fibrillation—limiting the use of SVV in these patients. These limitations apply only to SVV, not to the use of APCO for CO monitoring.

Measurements. Arterial pressure is the force generated by the ejection of blood from the left ventricle into the arterial

FIGURE 68-7 FloTrac sensor and Vigileo monitor. Source: Courtesy Edwards Lifesciences LLC, Irvine, CA. FloTrac, Vigileo and Swan Ganz are trademarks of Edwards Lifesciences.

TABLE 68-3	CLINICAL INDICATIONS FOR PULMONARY ARTERY CATHETERIZATION

- Acute respiratory distress syndrome
- Acute respiratory failure in patients with chronic obstructive pulmonary disease
- Cardiac tamponade
- Complex fluid imbalance (e.g., trauma, burns, sepsis)
- Evaluation of circulatory syndromes (e.g., heart failure, mitral valve regurgitation, intraventricular shunts)
- Intra-aortic balloon pump therapy
- Myocardial infarction with complications (e.g., left ventricular failure, cardiogenic shock, ventricular septal rupture)
- Perioperative fluid imbalance in high-risk patients (e.g., cardiac history)
- Shock states (e.g., cardiogenic, septic, hypovolemic)
- Vasoactive drug therapy support

circulation. Pulsatile pressure waves are produced by the heart's contractions (systole). The specialized sensor measures the arterial pulse pressure, which is proportional to SV. APCO monitoring uses the arterial waveform characteristics along with patient demographic data (i.e., gender, age, height, and weight) to calculate SV and pulse rate (PR) to calculate CCO/CCI and SV/SVI every 20 seconds. CO is calculated by multiplying the PR and SV and is displayed on a continuous basis (Kern, 2011). APCO monitoring is frequently used in conjunction with a central venous oximetry catheter. Together, these allow for continuous monitoring of central venous oxygen saturation ($ScvO_2$) and SVR that is derived from the CVP.

APCO is indicated only in adult patients and cannot be used in patients who are on IABP therapy (Kern, 2011).

Pulmonary Artery Flow-Directed Catheter. PAP monitoring is used to guide acute-phase management of patients with complicated cardiac, pulmonary, or intravascular volume problems (Table 68-3). Pulmonary artery (PA) diastolic pressure and PAOP are sensitive indicators of fluid volume status and cardiac function. PA diastolic pressure and PAOP are increased in patients with fluid volume overload and heart failure and are decreased in patients with volume deficit. Fluid therapy based on PAP allows restoration of fluid balance while avoiding overcorrection of the problem. Monitoring PAPs can allow precise therapeutic manipulation of preload, which allows CO to be maintained without placing the patient at risk for pulmonary edema.

A PA flow-directed catheter is used to measure PAPs, including PAOP. The standard PA catheter is number 7.5 French, 110 cm long, with four or five lumens (Figure 68-8). When properly positioned, the distal lumen port (catheter tip) is within the PA (Figure 68-9). This port is used to monitor PAPs and withdraw mixed venous blood specimens (e.g., to evaluate oxygen saturation). A balloon connected to an external valve via the second lumen surrounds the distal lumen port. Balloon inflation has two purposes: (a) to allow moving blood to float the catheter forward and (b) to allow PAOP measurement. There will be one

FIGURE 68-8 Pulmonary artery (PA) catheter. **A,** Illustrated catheter has five lumens. When properly positioned, the distal lumen port is in the PA, and the proximal lumen ports are in the right atrium and the right ventricle. The distal port and one of the proximal ports are used to measure PA and central venous pressures, respectively. A balloon surrounds the catheter near the distal end. The balloon inflation valve is used to inflate the balloon with air to allow reading of the pulmonary artery wedge pressure. A thermistor located near the distal tip senses PA temperature and is used to measure thermodilution cardiac output when solution cooler than body temperature is injected into a proximal port. **B,** Photograph of a catheter. Source: *B,* Courtesy Edwards Lifesciences LLC, Irvine, CA. Edwards Critical Care Division, Baxter Healthcare Corporation, Santa Ana, California. FloTrac, Vigileo and Swan Ganz are trademarks of Edwards Lifesciences.

FIGURE 68-9 Position of the pulmonary artery flow-directed catheter during progressive stages of insertion with corresponding pressure waveforms. Source: Adapted from Urden, L. D., Stacy, K. M., & Lough, M. E. (2010). *Critical care nursing: Diagnosis and management* (6th ed., p. 348, Figure 18-18). St. Louis: Mosby.

or two proximal lumens, with exit ports in the right atrium (if only one) or the right atrium and the right ventricle (if two). The right atrium port is used for measurement of CVP, injection of fluid for CO determination, and withdrawal of blood specimens. If a second proximal port is available, it is used for infusion of fluids and drugs or blood sampling. A thermistor lumen port located near the distal tip is wired to an external connector. This port is used for monitoring blood or core temperature and for measuring CO using the thermodilution method.

In addition to these standard features, PA catheters with specialized features are available. One modification is the inclusion of an atrial electrode, useful in recording the atrial ECG or pacing the heart. Another common modification is inclusion of a fibre-optic sensor in the distal tip that detects SvO_2. Another type of PA catheter provides continuous measurement of right ventricular volume and ejection fraction, and some catheters provide continuous CO monitoring. The PA catheter sheath (introducer) usually has a side port that serves as a large-bore IV line. Most catheters have a plastic "sleeve" connected to the sheath, which allows the catheter to be advanced or pulled back while maintaining sterility. The physician or other qualified health care provider (e.g., ACNP) usually manipulates the PA catheter, but this practice varies by institution.

Pulmonary Artery Catheter Insertion. Before PA catheter insertion, the nurse should note the patient's electrolyte, acid–base, oxygenation, and coagulation status. Imbalances such as hypokalemia, hypomagnesemia, hypoxemia, or acidosis can make the heart more irritable and increase the risk for ventricular dysrhythmia during catheter insertion. Coagulopathy increases the risk for hemorrhage.

Preparation for the procedure includes arranging the monitor, cables, and infusion and pressurized flush solutions. The system is zero-referenced to the phlebostatic axis. The physician or other health care provider explains the procedure to the patient and obtains informed consent. The patient is positioned supine and flat. The PA catheter is inserted through a sheath percutaneously into the internal jugular, subclavian, antecubital, or femoral vein using surgical asepsis. Venous cutdown is rarely required. The catheter is advanced through the venous system to the right side of the heart.

The nurse must continuously observe the characteristic waveforms on the monitor as the catheter is moved through the heart to the PA (see Figure 68-9). When the tip reaches the right atrium, the balloon is inflated. Inflation of the balloon should not exceed the balloon's capacity (usually 1–1.5 mL of air). The catheter is then "floated" through the tricuspid valve into the right ventricle and then through the pulmonic valve to the PA. It is necessary to monitor the ECG continuously during insertion because of the risk for dysrhythmias, particularly when the catheter reaches the right ventricle. Once a typical PAOP tracing is observed, the balloon is deflated, and the PA waveform should return on the monitor. Following insertion, a chest radiograph confirms the catheter's position. To maintain the catheter in its proper position, it is secured at the point of entry into the skin. The nurse should note and record the measurement at the exit point. At the procedure's end, an occlusive dressing is applied and then is changed according to institution policy.

Recently, the use of PA catheters has decreased dramatically. This decrease is due in part to the risks associated with the technology (e.g., infection, PA rupture, and infarction) and the development of less invasive techniques (e.g., APCO monitoring).

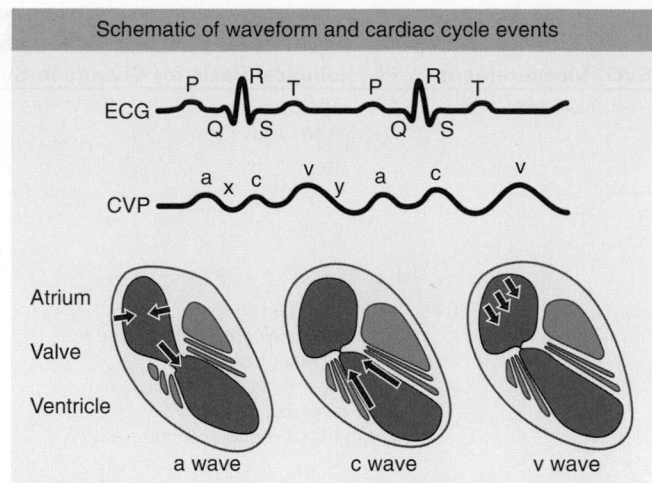

FIGURE 68-10 Cardiac events that produce the central venous pressure (CVP) waveform with *a*, *c*, and *v* waves. *a* wave represents atrial contraction. *x* descent represents atrial relaxation. *c* wave represents the bulging of the closed tricuspid valve into the right atrium during ventricular systole. *v* wave represents atrial filling. *y* descent represents opening of the tricuspid valve and filling of the ventricle. *ECG*, electrocardiogram. Source: Adapted from Urden, L. D., Stacy, K. M., & Lough, M. E. (2010). *Critical care nursing: Diagnosis and management* (6th ed., p. 338, Figure 18-11). St. Louis: Mosby.

Central Venous or Right Atrial Pressure Measurement. CVP is a measurement of right ventricular preload. It can be measured with a PA catheter using one of the proximal lumens or with a central venous catheter placed in the internal jugular or subclavian vein. CVP is measured as a mean pressure at the end of expiration. CVP waveforms (Figure 68-10) are similar to PAOP waveforms. Although the PA diastolic pressure and the wedge pressure are more sensitive indicators of fluid volume status, CVP also reflects fluid volume problems. An elevated CVP indicates right ventricular failure or volume overload. A low CVP indicates hypovolemia.

Noninvasive Hemodynamic Monitoring: Impedance Cardiography. *Impedance cardiography* (ICG) is a continuous or intermittent, noninvasive method of obtaining CO and assessing thoracic fluid status. Based on the concepts of impedance (the resistance to the flow of electric current [Ω]), ICG uses four sets of external electrodes to deliver a high-frequency, low-amplitude current similar to that used in apnea monitors. Blood is an excellent conductor of electricity (lower impedance), and pulsatile blood flow generates electrical impedance changes. ICG measures the change in impedance ($d\Omega$) in the ascending aorta and left ventricle over time (dt) and is represented as $d\Omega/dt$. Ωo is the measurement of the average impedance of the fluid in the thorax. Impedance-based hemodynamic parameters (CO, SV, and SVR) are calculated from Ωo, $d\Omega/dt$, mean arterial pressure, CVP, and the ECG.

Major indications for ICG include early signs and symptoms of pulmonary or cardiac dysfunction, differentiation of cardiac or pulmonary cause of shortness of breath, evaluation of etiology and management of hypotension, monitoring after discontinuing a PA catheter or justification for insertion of a PA catheter, evaluation of pharmacotherapy, and diagnosis of rejection following cardiac transplantation. ICG is not recommended in patients who have generalized edema or third spacing because the excess volume interferes with accurate signals.

TABLE 68-4	CLINICAL INTERPRETATION OF SVO₂ MEASUREMENTS	
SvO₂ Measurement	**Physiological Basis for Change in SvO₂**	**Clinical Diagnosis and Rationale**
High SvO₂ (80%–95%)	Increased oxygen supply Decreased oxygen demand	• Patient receiving more oxygen than required by clinical condition • Anaesthesia, which causes sedation and decreased muscle movement • Hypothermia, which lowers metabolic demand (e.g., with cardiopulmonary bypass) • Sepsis caused by decreased ability of tissues to use oxygen at the cellular level • False high-positive because pulmonary artery catheter is wedged in a pulmonary capillary
Normal SvO₂ (60%–80%) Low SvO₂ (<60%)	Normal oxygen supply and metabolic demand Decreased oxygen supply caused by: • Low hemoglobin • Low arterial saturation (SaO₂) • Low cardiac output • Increased oxygen consumption (VO₂)	• Balanced oxygen supply and demand • Anemia or bleeding with compromised cardiopulmonary system • Hypoxemia resulting from decreased oxygen supply or lung disease • Cardiogenic shock caused by left ventricular pump failure • Metabolic demand exceeds oxygen supply in conditions increasing metabolic rate, including physiological states such as shivering, seizures, and hyperthermia and nursing interventions that increase muscle movement, such as obtaining bed scale weight and repositioning

Source: Urden, L. D., Stacy, K. M., & Lough, M. E. (2010). *Critical care nursing: Diagnosis and management* (6th ed., p. 362, Table 18-8). St. Louis: Mosby.

Venous Oxygen Saturation. Both CVP and PA catheters can include sensors to measure O₂ saturation of hemoglobin of venous blood. Either ScVO₂ (O₂ saturation of venous blood from the CVP catheter) or SvO₂ (O₂ saturation from the PA catheter) is useful in determining the adequacy of tissue oxygenation. ScvO₂/SvO₂ reflects the dynamic balance between oxygenation of the arterial blood, tissue perfusion, and tissue oxygen consumption. ScvO₂/SvO₂ is useful in assessing hemodynamic status and response to treatments or activities when considered in conjunction with arterial O₂ saturation (Table 68-4). Normal ScvO₂/SvO₂ at rest is 60% to 80%.

Sustained decreases and increases in ScvO₂/SvO₂ must be analyzed carefully. Decreased SvO₂ may indicate (a) decreased arterial oxygenation, (b) low CO, (c) low hemoglobin, or (d) increased O₂ consumption. If the ScvO₂/SvO₂ falls, the nurse determines which of these four factors has changed. The nurse observes for changes in arterial oxygenation by monitoring pulse oximetry results or ABGs. By noting any changes in level of consciousness, strength and quality of peripheral pulses, urine output, and skin colour and temperature, the nurse can grossly assess CO and tissue perfusion. If arterial oxygenation, CO, and hemoglobin are unchanged, a fall in SvO₂ indicates increased O₂ consumption, which could result from an increased metabolic rate, pain, movement, or fever. If O₂ consumption increases without a comparable increase in O₂ delivery, more O₂ is extracted from the blood, and ScvO₂/SvO₂ will continue to fall.

Increased ScvO₂/SvO₂ is also clinically significant and may indicate a clinical improvement (e.g., increased SaO₂, improved perfusion, decreased metabolic rate) or problems (e.g., sepsis, ventricular septal defect). In sepsis, O₂ may not be extracted properly at the tissue level, resulting in increased mixed venous O₂ saturation.

Nursing interventions may be guided by changes in ScvO₂/SvO₂. The nurse might note that the patient's heart rate increased moderately during repositioning but that the ScvO₂/SvO₂ remained stable. In this case, the nurse might conclude that the position change was tolerated. A drop in the ScvO₂/SvO₂ would be an indication to stop the activity until the SvO₂ returns to the previous level.

In many cases, as activity or metabolism increases, heart rate and CO increase, and SvO₂ remains constant or varies slightly.

However, it is not uncommon for critically ill patients to have conditions that prevent substantial increases in CO. For example, such an increase could occur in the patient with heart failure, shock, dysrhythmias, or cardiac transplantation. In these cases, ScvO₂/SvO₂ can provide a useful indicator of the balance between O₂ delivery and consumption.

Noninvasive Arterial Oxygenation Monitoring. *Pulse oximetry* is a noninvasive and continuous method of determining arterial oxygenation (SpO₂), and monitoring SpO₂ may reduce how often ABG sampling is needed (see Chapter 28). SpO₂ is normally 95% to 100%. A common use for pulse oximetry is to evaluate the effectiveness of O₂ therapy. Decreased SpO₂ indicates inadequate oxygenation of the blood in the pulmonary capillaries. This may be corrected by increasing the fraction of inspired oxygen (FiO₂) and evaluating the patient's response. Similarly, the nurse uses SpO₂ to monitor how the patient tolerates decreases in FiO₂ and responds to changes in position and treatments. For example, the nurse might note that SpO₂ falls when the patient is positioned in a left lateral recumbent position. The nurse could then plan position changes that pose less risk for the patient.

Accurate SpO₂ measurements may be difficult to obtain on patients who are hypothermic, receiving IV vasopressor therapy (e.g., norepinephrine [Levophed]), or experiencing hypoperfusion (e.g., shock). The usual location for placement of the oximetry probe is a finger; alternative locations for probe placement may have to be considered (e.g., forehead, earlobe) during periods of hypoperfusion.

NURSING MANAGEMENT
HEMODYNAMIC MONITORING

Assessment of hemodynamic status requires integration of data from many sources and comparison of the data over time. Thorough, basic nursing observations provide important clues about the patient's hemodynamic status. The nurse should begin by obtaining baseline data regarding the patient's general appearance, level of consciousness, skin colour and temperature, vital signs, peripheral pulses, and urine output. Does the patient appear tired, weak, exhausted? There may be too little cardiac reserve to sustain even minimal activity. Pallor, cool skin, and diminished pulses may indicate decreased CO. Changes in mental clarity may reflect problems with cerebral perfusion or oxygenation. Monitoring urine output reflects the adequacy of perfusion to the kidneys. The patient with diminished perfusion to the GI tract may develop hypoactive or absent bowel sounds. If the patient is bleeding and developing shock, BP might initially be relatively stable, yet the patient may become increasingly pale and cool from peripheral vasoconstriction. Conversely, the patient experiencing septic shock may remain warm and pink yet develop tachycardia and BP instability. Although heart rates of 100 beats per minute are common among stressed, compromised, critically ill patients, sustained tachycardia greatly increases myocardial oxygen demand and may result in diminished CO.

The critical care nurse correlates observational data with data obtained from biotechnology (e.g., ECG; arterial pressure, PAP, PAOP; SvO$_2$). Single hemodynamic values are rarely significant. The nurse must evaluate the whole clinical picture with the goals of recognizing early clues and intervening before problems escalate.

CIRCULATORY ASSIST DEVICES

Mechanical **circulatory assist devices (CADs)**, such as the IABP and the left ventricular assist device (VAD), are used to decrease cardiac work and improve organ perfusion in patients with heart failure when conventional drug therapy is no longer adequate. The type of device used depends on the extent and the nature of the myocardial problem and the capabilities of the institution and staff. CADs provide interim support in three types of situations: (a) the left ventricle requires support while recovering from acute injury; (b) the heart requires surgical repair (e.g., a ruptured septum), but the patient's condition must be stabilized; and (c) the heart has failed, and the patient is awaiting cardiac transplantation. All CADs decrease left ventricular workload, increase myocardial perfusion, and augment circulation. The most commonly used CAD is the IABP. Several types of VADs are available, and additional devices are under development.

Intra-Aortic Balloon Pump

The **intra-aortic balloon pump (IABP)** provides temporary circulatory assistance to the compromised heart by reducing afterload (via reduction in systolic pressure) and augmenting the aortic diastolic pressure. Table 68-5 lists clinical conditions for which the IABP is used. The IABP consists of a sausage-shaped balloon, a pump that inflates and deflates the balloon, control devices for synchronizing the balloon inflation to the cardiac cycle, and fail-safe devices (Figure 68-11). Under strict aseptic technique, the balloon is inserted percutaneously or surgically into the femoral artery, advanced toward the heart, and positioned in the descending thoracic aorta just below the left subclavian artery (Figure 68-12). Following placement of the balloon, the position is confirmed radiologically. A pneumatic device cyclically fills the balloon with helium at the start of diastole (immediately after aortic valve closure) and deflates it just before systole. The ECG is the primary trigger used to initiate the deflation on the R wave (of the QRS) and the inflation on the T wave, and the dicrotic notch of the arterial pressure tracing is used to refine timing. IABP support is referred to as *counter-pulsation* because the timing of balloon inflation is opposite to ventricular contraction. The IAPB assist ratio is 1 : 1 in the acute phase of treatment, that is, one IABP cycle of inflation and deflation for every heartbeat.

Effects of Counter-Pulsation.
In late diastole, when the balloon is totally inflated, blood is forcibly displaced distally to the

TABLE 68-5	INDICATIONS AND CONTRAINDICATIONS FOR THE INTRA-AORTIC BALLOON PUMP

Indications
- Acute myocardial infarction with any of the following:*
  - Acute mitral valve dysfunction
  - Acute ventricular septal defect
  - Cardiogenic shock
  - High-risk interventional cardiology procedures
  - Preoperative, intraoperative, and postoperative cardiac surgery (e.g., prophylaxis before surgery, failure to be weaned from cardiopulmonary bypass, left ventricular failure after cardiopulmonary bypass)
  - Recurrent chest pain with or without ventricular dysrhythmias
- Ventricular aneurysm accompanied by ventricular dysrhythmias
- Refractory unstable angina (when drugs have failed)
- Short-term bridge to cardiac transplantation

Contraindications
- Abdominal aortic and thoracic aneurysms
- Generalized peripheral vascular disease†
- Irreversible brain damage
- Moderate to severe aortic insufficiency
- Terminal or untreatable diseases of any major organ system

*Allows time for emergent angiography and corrective cardiac surgery to be performed.
†May inhibit placement of balloon and is considered a relative contraindication; sheathless insertion may be used.

FIGURE 68-11 Intra-aortic balloon pump machine. Source: © Ivan Stojanovic/ Dreamstime.

extremities and proximally to the coronary arteries and the main branches of the aortic arch. Diastolic arterial pressure rises (diastolic augmentation), increasing coronary artery perfusion pressure and perfusion of vital organs. The rise in coronary artery perfusion pressure causes an increase in blood flow to the

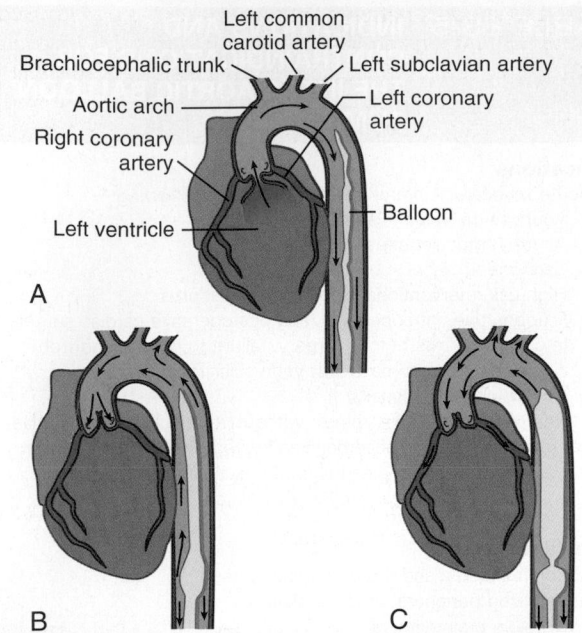

FIGURE 68-12 Intra-aortic balloon pump. **A,** During systole, the balloon is deflated, which facilitates ejection of the blood into the periphery. **B,** In early diastole, the balloon begins to inflate. **C,** In late diastole, the balloon is totally inflated, which augments aortic pressure and increases the coronary perfusion pressure, with the end result of increased coronary and cerebral blood flow.

TABLE 68-6	HEMODYNAMIC EFFECTS OF INTRA-AORTIC BALLOON PUMPS

Effects of Inflation During Diastole
- Improved oxygen delivery to the myocardium
  - Decreased angina pain
  - Decreased electrocardiographic evidence of ischemia
  - Decreased ventricular ectopy
- Increased diastolic pressure (may exceed systolic pressure)
- Increased pressure in the aortic root during diastole
- Increased coronary perfusion pressure

Effects of Deflation During Systole
- Decreased afterload
- Decreased myocardial oxygen consumption
- Decreased peak systolic pressure
- Increased forward flow of blood, decreasing preload
  - Decreased crackles
  - Decreased PA pressures, including PAOP
- Increased stroke volume, possibly associated with the following:
  - Decreased heart rate
  - Improved sensorium
  - Increased urine output
  - Warmed skin

PA, pulmonary artery; *PAOP,* pulmonary artery occlusive pressure.

myocardium. The balloon is rapidly deflated just before systole. The suddenly created vacuum causes aortic pressure to drop. With aortic resistance to left ventricular ejection reduced (reduced afterload), the left ventricle empties more easily and completely. As with other types of afterload reduction, the SV increases, yet the myocardial oxygen consumption decreases. Hemodynamic effects of the IABP are summarized in Table 68-6.

Complications With IABP Therapy. Vascular injuries such as dislodgment of plaque, aortic dissection, and compromised

TABLE 68-7	NURSING MANAGEMENT: POTENTIAL COMPLICATIONS OF THE INTRA-AORTIC BALLOON PUMP

Potential Complication	Nursing Management
Site infection from invasive lines	• Use strict aseptic technique for insertion and dressing changes for all lines. • Cover all insertion sites with occlusive dressings. • Administer prescribed prophylactic antibiotic for entire course of therapy.
Pneumonia associated with immobilization	• Reposition patient q2h, being careful not to displace balloon. • If patient with pneumonia requires physiotherapy of the chest, avoid introducing an ECG artifact.
Arterial trauma caused by insertion or displacement of balloon	• Evaluate and mark peripheral pulses before insertion of balloon to use as baseline for assessing pulses after insertion. • After insertion of balloon, evaluate perfusion to both extremities at least every hour. • Measure urine output at least every hour (occlusion of renal arteries causes severe decrease in urine output). • Observe arterial waveforms for sudden changes. • Keep head of bed <45 degrees. • Do not flex cannulated leg at the hip. • Immobilize cannulated leg to prevent flexion using a draw sheet tucked under the mattress, a soft ankle restraint, or a knee immobilizer.
Thrombo-embolism caused by trauma, balloon obstruction of blood flow distal to catheter	• Administer prophylactic heparin if ordered. • Evaluate pulses, urine output, and level of consciousness at least every hour. • Check circulation, sensation, and movement in both legs at least every hour.
Hemorrhage from insertion site	• Check site for bleeding at least every hour. • Observe vital signs for hypovolemia.

ECG, electrocardiogram.

distal circulation are common with IABP therapy. Thrombus and embolus formation add to the risk for circulatory compromise to the extremity. The action of the IABP can also destroy platelets and cause thrombo-cytopenia. Peripheral nerve damage can occur, particularly when a cutdown is performed for insertion. Movement of the balloon can block the left subclavian, renal, or mesenteric arteries, in turn resulting in a weak or absent radial pulse, decreased urine output, and reduced or absent bowel sounds. Patients receiving IABP therapy are prone to infection. Local or systemic signs of infection require catheter removal (Castellucci, 2011). To reduce these complications, the nurse should perform cardiovascular, neuro-vascular, and hemodynamic assessments every 15 to 60 minutes, depending on the patient's status (Table 68-7).

Mechanical complications from IABP are rare but can occur. Improper timing of balloon inflation may cause increased afterload, decreased CO, myocardial ischemia, and increased myocardial O_2 demand. These complications must be recognized immediately. If the balloon develops a leak, the pump will automatically stop. The catheter must be promptly removed to avoid an embolus. Signs of a leak include less effective augmentation, repeated alarms for gas loss, and blood backing up into the catheter. A malfunction of the balloon or console triggers fail-safe alarms and automatically shuts down the unit.

The patient with an IABP is relatively immobile, limited to side-lying or supine positions with the head of the bed (HOB) elevated less than 45 degrees. The patient may be receiving ventilatory support and will likely have multiple invasive lines that increase the challenge of comfortable positioning. The patient may experience sleeplessness and anxiety. Adequate sedation, pain relief, skin care, and comfort measures are essential.

As the patient improves, circulatory support provided by the IABP is gradually reduced. Weaning involves reducing the IABP assist ratio from 1:1 to 1:2 and assessing the patient's response. If hemodynamic parameters remain stable, the ratio can be changed from 1:2 to 1:3 until the IABP catheter is removed. Pumping is continued until the line is removed even if the patient is stable. This reduces the risk for thrombus formation around the catheter.

Ventricular Assist Devices

The **ventricular assist device (VAD)** provides short- and long-term support for the failing heart and allows more mobility than the IABP. VADs are inserted into the path of flowing blood to augment or replace the action of the ventricle. Some VADs are implanted internally (e.g., peritoneum), and others are positioned externally. A typical VAD shunts blood from the left atrium or ventricle to the device and then to the aorta. Some VADs provide right ventricular or biventricular support (Figure 68-13).

Failure to wean a patient from cardiopulmonary bypass (CPB) after surgery is a primary indicator for VAD support. VADs are also used to support patients with ventricular failure caused by myocardial infarction and patients awaiting heart transplantation. A VAD is a temporary device that can partially or totally support circulation until the heart recovers or a donor heart is obtained. Cannula sites depend on the type of device used. For support of the right side of the heart, the right atrium and PA are cannulated. The left ventricular apex can be cannulated for left VADs. Direct cannulation of the atria and great vessels occurs in the operating room through a sternotomy.

Appropriate patient selection for VAD therapy is critical. Indications include (a) failure to be weaned from CPB or post-cardiotomy cardiogenic shock, (b) a bridge to recovery or heart transplantation, and (c) patients with New York Heart Association class IV heart disease (see Table 37-4 in Chapter 37) who have failed medical therapy. Relative contraindications for VAD therapy include (a) body surface area less than manufacturer's limit (i.e., 1.3 m^2), (b) renal or liver failure unrelated to a cardiac event, and (c) comorbidities that would limit life expectancy to less than 3 years (Puhlman & Fleck, 2011).

Implantable Artificial Heart

In 2013, 142 patients in Canada received cardiac transplants (Canadian Institute for Health Information, 2017), yet the demand for donor hearts far exceeds the supply. Research on mechanical CADs has led to the development of a fully implantable artificial heart that can sustain the body's circulatory system. This device is used to replace the hearts of patients who are not eligible for a transplantation and have no other treatment alternative. One major advantage of the artificial heart compared with heart transplantation is decreased costs for implantation and drug therapies.

NURSING MANAGEMENT
CIRCULATORY ASSIST DEVICES

The patient with an IABP requires highly skilled nursing care. The nurse must perform frequent and thorough cardiovascular assessments. These include measurement of hemodynamic parameters (e.g., arterial BP, CO/CI, SVR), auscultation of the heart and lungs, and evaluation of the ECG (e.g., rate, rhythm). The nurse must also assess for adequate tissue perfusion (e.g., skin colour and temperature, mental status, capillary refill, peripheral pulses, urine output, bowel sounds) at regular intervals. It is expected that IABP therapy will improve these findings.

Nursing care of the patient with a VAD is similar to that of the patient with an IABP. The nurse must observe the patient for bleeding, cardiac tamponade, ventricular failure, infection, dysrhythmias, renal failure, hemolysis, and thrombo-embolism. Unlike the patient with an IABP, who must remain in bed with limited position changes, the patient with VAD may be mobile and require an activity plan. In some cases, patients with VADs may go home. Preparation for discharge is complex and requires in-depth teaching about the device and support equipment (e.g., battery chargers). A competent caregiver must be present at all times once the patient is discharged home.

Ideally, patients with CADs will recover through ventricular improvement, heart transplantation, or artificial heart implantation. However, many patients die, or the decision to terminate the device is made, and death follows. Both the patient and caregiver require emotional support. Other members of the health care team, such as social workers or clergy, should be consulted as appropriate.

FIGURE 68-13 Schematic diagram of a biventricular assist device (BVAD).

ARTIFICIAL AIRWAYS

Patients in the ICU often need mechanical assistance to maintain airway patency. Inserting a tube into the trachea, bypassing upper airway and laryngeal structures, creates an artificial airway. The tube is placed into the trachea via the mouth or nose past the larynx (**endotracheal [ET] intubation**) or through a stoma in the neck *(tracheostomy)*. ET intubation is more common than a tracheostomy in ICU patients. It is performed quickly and safely at the bedside. Indications for ET intubation include (a) upper airway obstruction (e.g., secondary to burns, tumour, bleeding), (b) apnea, (c) high risk for aspiration, (d) ineffective clearance of secretions, and (e) respiratory distress. Figure 68-14 shows the parts of an ET tube.

A *tracheotomy* is a surgical procedure that is performed when the need for an artificial airway is expected to be long term. There is ongoing debate regarding the timing of a tracheotomy in the patient requiring an ET tube. Research suggests that early tracheotomy (2 to 10 days) may have advantages over delayed tracheotomy, particularly when mechanical ventilation is predicted to be needed for longer than 10 to 14 days (Villwock & Jones, 2014). The situation varies with the patient, physician, and institution. Chapter 29 discusses tracheostomy tubes and related nursing management.

Endotracheal Tubes

In *oral intubation*, the ET tube is passed through the mouth and vocal cords and into the trachea with the aid of a laryngoscope or a bronchoscope. In *nasal ET intubation*, the ET is placed blindly (i.e., without seeing the larynx) through the nose, nasopharynx, and vocal cords. Oral ET intubation is preferred for most emergencies because the airway can be secured rapidly and a larger-diameter tube is used. A larger-bore ET tube reduces the *work of breathing* (WOB) because of less airway resistance. It is easier to remove secretions and perform fibre-optic bronchoscopy if needed. Nasal ET intubation is rarely used but may be needed when head and neck movement is risky.

There are risks associated with oral ET intubation. It is difficult to place an oral tube if head and neck mobility is limited (e.g.,

🔍 **EVIDENCE-INFORMED PRACTICE**

Research Highlight

Does Timing of Tracheotomy Affect Critically Ill Patient Outcomes?
Clinical Question
In critically ill patients (P), what is the effect of an early tracheotomy (I) versus late tracheotomy (C) on short-term mortality and incidence of ventilator-assisted pneumonia (O)?

Best Available Evidence
Systematic review of randomized controlled trials (RCTs)

Critical Appraisal and Synthesis of Evidence
- In seven RCTs ($n = 1044$) of critically ill adult patients requiring prolonged mechanical ventilation, early tracheotomy was compared with either late tracheotomy or prolonged endotracheal intubation.
- Primary outcomes were short-term mortality and ventilator-assisted pneumonia (VAP).
- Secondary outcomes were long-term mortality, duration of ventilation and sedation, length of stay in ICU and hospital, and complications.
- Early tracheotomy did not significantly reduce short-term or long-term mortality or rate of VAP. Tracheotomy timing was not related to reductions in duration of mechanical ventilation or sedation, shorter stays in ICU or hospital, or more complications.

Conclusion
- Clinically significant outcomes are not affected by timing of a tracheotomy.

Implications for Nursing Practice
- The optimal tracheotomy timing (early vs. late) for patients on prolonged mechanical ventilation is not really known.
- Benefits of tracheotomy (e.g., increased patient comfort, improved oral hygiene) and the risks and complications (e.g., bleeding, wound infection, tracheal stenosis) need to be considered and weighed against the risks and benefits of prolonged endotracheal intubation.

Reference for Evidence
Wang, F., Wu, Y., Bo, L., et al. (2011). The timing of tracheotomy in critically ill patients undergoing mechanical ventilation: A systematic review and meta-analysis of randomized controlled trials. *Chest, 140*(6), 1456–1465.

P, Patient population of interest; *I*, intervention or area of interest; *C*, comparison of interest or comparison group; *O*, outcomes of interest (see Chapter 1).

15-mm connector to oxygen source
Cuff inflation line
Pilot balloon
Spring-loaded cuff inflation valve

Tube cuff

A

B — Tube / Trachea / Deflated cuff

C — Tube / Trachea / Inflated cuff

D

FIGURE 68-14 Endotracheal tube. **A,** Parts of an endotracheal tube. **B,** Tube in place with the cuff deflated. **C,** Tube in place with the cuff inflated. **D,** Photograph of the tube before placement. Source: *A,* Beare, P. G., & Myers, J. L. (1998). *Adult health nursing* (3rd ed.). St. Louis: Mosby.

suspected spinal cord injury). Teeth can be chipped or accidentally removed during the procedure. Salivation is increased and swallowing is difficult. Patients can obstruct the ET tube by biting down on it. Sedation along with a bite block or oropharyngeal airway may be used to avoid this. The ET tube and bite block (if used) should be secured (separately) to the face. Mouth care is a challenge because of limited space in the oral cavity. Using smaller or pediatric-sized oral products for tooth brushing, cleaning, and suctioning may be necessary.

Nasal intubation is contraindicated in patients with facial fractures or suspected fractures at the base of the skull and postoperatively after cranial surgeries. The WOB is greater because the longer, narrower tube offers more airflow resistance and may kink. Suctioning and secretion removal are more difficult.

Endotracheal Intubation Procedure

Unless ET intubation is emergent, consent for the procedure is obtained. The patient and caregiver must be told the reason for ET intubation, the steps in the procedure, and the patient's role in the procedure (if indicated). It should also be explained that, while intubated, the patient will not be able to speak but that other means of communication will be provided. The patient should also be informed that his or her hands may briefly be restrained for safety purposes.

A self-inflating *bag–valve–mask* (BVM) (e.g., Ambu bag) should be available and attached to O_2, suctioning equipment ready at the bedside, and IV access. The BVM contains a reservoir that is filled with O_2 so that concentrations of 90% to 95% are delivered. The slower the bag is deflated and inflated, the higher the O_2 concentration that is delivered. The nurse should assemble and check the equipment to be used, remove the patient's dentures or partial plates (for oral intubation), and administer medications as ordered. Premedication varies depending on the patient's level of consciousness (e.g., awake, obtunded) and the nature of the procedure (e.g., emergent, nonemergent).

Rapid-sequence intubation (RSI) is the rapid, concurrent administration of both a sedative and a paralytic agent during emergency airway management to decrease the risks for aspiration and injury to the patient. RSI is not indicated in patients who are in cardiac arrest or are known to have a difficult airway (Stollings, Diedrich, Oyen, et al., 2014). A sedative–hypnotic–amnesic (e.g., midazolam, etomidate) is used to induce unconsciousness, along with a rapid-onset opioid (e.g., fentanyl) to blunt the pain of the procedure. A paralytic drug (e.g., succinylcholine) is then given to produce skeletal muscle paralysis. The patient's oxygenation status must be monitored during the procedure using pulse oximetry.

For oral intubation, place the patient supine with the head extended and the neck flexed ("sniffing position"). This position permits visualization of the vocal cords. For nasal intubation, the nasal passages may be sprayed with a local anaesthetic and vasoconstrictor (e.g., lidocaine [Xylocaine] with epinephrine) to reduce trauma and bleeding. Before intubation is started, the patient should be preoxygenated using the BVM and 100% O_2 for 3 to 5 minutes. Each intubation attempt is limited to less than 30 seconds, and the patient should be ventilated between successive attempts using the BVM and 100% O_2.

After intubation, the cuff should be inflated and the placement of the ET tube confirmed while the patient is manually ventilated using the BVM with 100% O_2. An end-tidal CO_2 detector is used to confirm proper placement by noting the presence of exhaled CO_2 from the lungs. The detector should be placed between the

BVM and the ET tube, and the nurse should observe for either a colour change (indicating the presence of CO_2) or a number. If no CO_2 is detected, the tube is in the esophagus and needs to be reinserted (Walsh, Crotwell, & Restrepo, 2011) The lungs must be auscultated for bilateral breath sounds, and the epigastrium for the absence of air sounds. The nurse should observe the chest for symmetric chest wall movement. In addition, SpO_2 should be stable or improved.

If the findings support proper ET tube placement, the tube is then connected to an O_2 source and secured per employer policy (Figure 68-15). The nurse should suction the ET tube and pharynx and insert a bite block as needed. A chest radiograph is done immediately to confirm tube location (2 to 6 cm above the carina in the adult). This position allows the patient to move the neck without moving the tube or causing it to enter the right mainstem bronchus. Once proper positioning is confirmed with radiography, the nurse should record and mark the position of the tube at the lip or teeth (usually 21 cm for women and 23 cm for men) or nose. Excess tubing is cut to reduce dead air space.

The ET tube is connected to either humidified air, O_2, or a mechanical ventilator. ABGs are obtained immediately after intubation to determine baseline oxygenation and ventilation status. ABG values are reviewed and used to guide oxygenation and ventilation changes. Continuous pulse oximetry and end-tidal CO_2 monitoring provide valuable data related to arterial oxygenation and ventilation.

NURSING MANAGEMENT
ARTIFICIAL AIRWAY

Management of a patient with an artificial airway is often a shared responsibility between the nurse and the respiratory therapist, with specific management tasks determined by employer policy. Nursing responsibilities for the patient with an artificial airway may include some or all of the following: (a) maintaining correct tube placement, (b) maintaining proper cuff inflation, (c) monitoring oxygenation and ventilation, (d) maintaining tube patency, (e) assessing for complications, (f) providing oral care

FIGURE 68-15 Closed tracheal suction system.

and maintaining skin integrity, and (g) fostering comfort and communication.

MAINTAINING CORRECT TUBE PLACEMENT

The patient with an ET tube should be continuously monitored to ensure the tube remains in place. A tube that is dislodged could end up in the pharynx or enter the esophagus or the right mainstem bronchus (thus ventilating only the right lung).

> **SAFETY ALERT—Endotracheal Tube Placement**
> - Proper ET tube position can be maintained by placing an "exit mark" on the tube.
> - The mark must remain constant while the patient is at rest and during patient care, repositioning, and transport.

The chest wall must be observed for symmetrical movement and auscultated to confirm bilateral breath sounds. If the ET tube is not positioned properly, it is an emergency. The nurse should stay with the patient, maintain the airway, support ventilation, and call for the appropriate help to immediately reposition the tube. It may be necessary to ventilate the patient with a BVM and 100% O_2. If a dislodged tube is not repositioned, minimal or no O_2 is delivered to the lungs or the entire V_T is delivered to one lung. This places the patient at risk for pneumothorax.

MAINTAINING PROPER CUFF INFLATION

The cuff is an inflatable, pliable sleeve encircling the outer wall of the ET tube (see Figure 68-14). The high-volume, low-pressure cuff stabilizes and "seals" the ET tube within the trachea and prevents escape of ventilating gases. However, excess volume in the cuff can damage the tracheal mucosa. To avoid this, once the cuff is inflated with air, the cuff pressure should be measured and monitored. To ensure adequate tracheal perfusion, cuff pressure should be maintained at 20 to 25 cm H_2O (Lorente, Lecuona, Jiménez, et al., 2014). It will need to be measured and recorded after intubation and on a routine basis (e.g., every 8 hours) using the *minimal occluding volume (MOV) technique* or *the minimal leak technique* (MLT).

The steps in the MOV technique for cuff inflation are as follows: (a) for the mechanically ventilated patient, a stethoscope is placed over the trachea and the cuff inflated to MOV by adding air until no air leak is heard at peak inspiratory pressure (end of ventilator inspiration); (b) for the spontaneously breathing patient, the cuff is inflated until no sound is heard after a deep breath or after inhalation with a BVM; (c) a manometer is used to verify that cuff pressure is between 20 and 25 cm H_2O; and (d) cuff pressure is recorded in the chart. If adequate cuff pressure cannot be maintained or larger volumes of air are needed to keep the cuff inflated, there could be a leak in the cuff or tracheal dilation at the cuff site. In these situations, the nurse should notify the physician to reposition or change the ET tube.

The procedure for MLT is similar with one exception: a small amount of air is removed from the cuff until a slight air leak is auscultated at peak inflation. Both techniques aim to prevent the risk for tracheal damage from high cuff pressures. The use of continuous cuff measurement is being studied (Sole, Su, Talbert, et al., 2011).

MONITORING OXYGENATION AND VENTILATION

The patient with an ET tube is vigilantly monitored for adequate oxygenation through assessments of clinical findings, ABGs, SpO_2, and, if available, $ScvO_2/SvO_2$. The nurse should assess for signs of hypoxemia such as a change in mental status (e.g.,

confusion), anxiety, dusky skin, and dysrhythmias. Periodic ABGs (specifically partial pressure of oxygen in arterial blood [PaO_2]) and continuous SpO_2 provide objective data regarding oxygenation. Lower values are expected in patients with some disease states, such as chronic obstructive pulmonary disease (COPD).

Indicators of ventilation include clinical findings, partial pressure of carbon dioxide in arterial blood ($PaCO_2$), and continuous partial pressure of end-tidal CO_2 ($PETCO_2$). The nurse should assess the patient's respirations for rate, rhythm, and use of accessory muscles. The patient who is hyperventilating will be breathing rapidly and deeply and may experience circumoral and peripheral numbness and tingling. The patient who is hypoventilating will be breathing shallowly or slowly and may appear dusky. $PaCO_2$ is the best indicator of alveolar hyperventilation (e.g., decreased $PaCO_2$, increased pH indicate respiratory alkalosis) or hypoventilation (e.g., increased $PaCO_2$, decreased pH indicate respiratory acidosis).

$PETCO_2$ monitoring *(capnography)* is done by analyzing exhaled gas directly at the ventilator circuit *(mainstream sampling)* or by transporting a sample of gas via small-bore tubing to a bedside monitor *(sidestream sampling)*. Continuous $PETCO_2$ monitoring can assess the patency of the airway and the presence of breathing. In addition, gradual changes in $PETCO_2$ values may accompany an increase in CO_2 production (e.g., sepsis, hypoventilation, neuro-muscular blockade) or a decrease in CO_2 production (e.g., hypothermia, decreased CO, metabolic acidosis). In patients with normal ventilation-to-perfusion ratios (see Chapter 70), $PETCO_2$ can be used as an estimate of $PaCO_2$, with $PETCO_2$ generally 1 to 5 mm Hg lower than $PaCO_2$.

MAINTAINING TUBE PATENCY

A patient should not be routinely suctioned; rather, the nurse should assess the patient regularly to determine if suctioning is needed. Indications for suctioning include (a) visible secretions in the ET tube, (b) sudden onset of respiratory distress, (c) suspected aspiration of secretions, (d) increase in peak airway pressures, (e) auscultation of adventitious breath sounds over the trachea or bronchi, (f) increase in respiratory rate or sustained coughing, and (g) sudden or gradual decrease in PaO_2 or SpO_2.

Table 68-8 describes two recommended suctioning methods: the closed-suction technique (CST) and the open-suction technique (OST). The CST uses a suction catheter that is enclosed in a plastic sleeve connected directly to the ventilator circuit (see Figure 68-15). With the CST, oxygenation and ventilation are maintained during suctioning, and exposure to the patient's secretions is reduced. The CST should be used for patients who (a) require high levels of positive end-expiratory pressure (PEEP) (greater than 10 cm H_2O), (b) have high levels of FiO_2, (c) have bloody or infected pulmonary secretions, (d) require frequent suctioning, or (e) experience clinical instability with the OST (Seckel, 2017).

Potential complications associated with suctioning include hypoxemia, bronchospasm, increased intracranial pressure, dysrhythmias, hypertension, hypotension, mucosal damage, pulmonary bleeding, pain, and infection. The patient must be assessed closely before, during, and after the suctioning procedure. If the patient does not tolerate suctioning (e.g., decreased SpO_2, increased or decreased BP, sustained coughing, development of dysrhythmias), the procedure should be stopped and the patient hyperoxygenated until equilibration occurs before attempting another suction pass. Hypoxemia can be prevented

TABLE 68-8 SUCTIONING PROCEDURES FOR A PATIENT ON A MECHANICAL VENTILATOR

General Measures

1. Gather all equipment.
2. Wash hands and don personal protective equipment.
3. Explain procedure and patient's role in assisting with secretion removal by coughing.
4. Monitor patient's cardiopulmonary status (e.g., vital signs, SpO_2, SvO_2, $ScvO_2$, ECG, level of consciousness) before, during, and after the procedure.
5. Turn on suction and set vacuum to 100 to 120 mm Hg.
6. Pause ventilator alarms.

Open-Suction Technique

1. Open sterile catheter package using the inside of the package as a sterile field. *Note:* Suction catheter should be no wider than half the diameter of the ET tube (e.g., for a 7-mm ET tube, select a 10-French suction catheter).
2. Fill the sterile solution container with sterile normal saline or water.
3. Don sterile gloves.
4. Pick up sterile suction catheter with the dominant hand. Using the nondominant hand, secure the connecting tube (to suction) to the suction catheter.
5. Check equipment for proper functioning by suctioning a small volume of sterile saline solution from the container. (Go to step 7.)

Closed-Suction Technique

6. Connect the suction tubing to the closed-suction port.
7. Hyperoxygenate the patient for 30 sec using one of the following methods:

- Activate the suction hyperoxygenation setting on the ventilator using the nondominant hand.
- Increase FiO_2 to 100%. *Note:* FiO_2 must be returned to baseline level at the completion of the procedure if not done automatically after preset time by ventilator.
- Disconnect the ventilator tubing from the ET tube and manually ventilate the patient with 100% O_2 using a BVM device.* Administer 5 or 6 breaths over 30 sec. *Note:* Use of a second person to deliver the manual breaths will significantly increase the tidal volume delivered.

8. With suction off, gently and quickly insert the catheter using the dominant hand. When resistance is met, pull back 1 cm.
9. Apply continuous or intermittent suction using the nondominant thumb. Withdraw the catheter within 10 sec or less.
10. Hyperoxygenate for 30 sec as described in step 7.
11. If secretions remain and the patient has tolerated the procedure, perform two to three suction passes as described in steps 8 and 9. *Note:* Rinse the suction catheter with sterile saline solution between suctioning passes as needed.
12. Reconnect patient to ventilator (open-suction technique).
13. At the completion of ET tube suctioning, rinse the catheter and connecting tubing with the sterile saline solution.
14. Suction oral pharynx. *Note:* A separate catheter must be used for this step when using the closed-suction technique.
15. Discard the suction catheter, and rinse the connecting tubing with the sterile saline solution (open-suction technique).
16. Reset FiO_2 (if necessary) and ventilator alarms.
17. Reassess patient for signs of effective suctioning.

BVM, bag–valve–mask; *ECG,* electrocardiogram; *ET,* endotracheal; *FiO₂,* fraction of inspired oxygen; *PEEP,* positive end-expiratory pressure; *ScvO₂,* central venous oxygen saturation; *SpO₂,* oxygen saturation; *SvO₂,* venous oxygen saturation.
*Attach a PEEP valve to the BVM for patients on >5 cm H₂O PEEP.
Source: Adapted from Seckel, M. A. (2017). Suctioning: Endotracheal or tracheostomy tube. In D. L. Wiegand (Ed.), *AACN procedure manual for critical care* (7th ed.). St. Louis: Elsevier.

by hyperoxygenating the patient before and after each suctioning pass and limiting each pass to 10 seconds or less (see Table 68-8). Both the ECG and SpO_2 should be assessed before, during, and after the suctioning procedure.

Causes of dysrhythmias during suctioning include (a) hypoxemia resulting in myocardial ischemia; (b) vagal stimulation caused by tracheal irritation; and (c) sympathetic nervous system stimulation caused by anxiety, discomfort, or pain. Dysrhythmias include tachydysrhythmias and bradydysrhythmias, premature beats, and asystole. If any new dysrhythmias develop, suctioning should be stopped. Excessive suctioning must be avoided in patients with severe hypoxemia or bradycardia.

Tracheal mucosal damage may occur because of excessive suction pressures (greater than 120 mm Hg), overly vigorous catheter insertion, or the characteristics of the suction catheter itself. Blood streaks or tissue shreds in aspirated secretions may indicate that mucosal damage has occurred. Mucosal damage increases the risk for infection and bleeding, particularly if the patient is receiving anticoagulants (Seckel, 2017). Trauma to the mucosa can be prevented by following the steps described in Table 68-8.

Secretions may be thick and difficult to suction because of inadequate hydration, inadequate humidification, infection, or inaccessibility of the left mainstem bronchus or lower airways. Adequately hydrating the patient (e.g., oral or IV fluids) and providing supplemental humidification of inspired gases may assist in thinning secretions. Instillation of normal saline into the ET tube is discouraged and may be harmful. If infection is the cause of thick secretions, the patient must receive appropriate antibiotics. Mobilization, postural drainage, percussion, and turning of the patient every 2 hours may help move secretions into larger airways.

PROVIDING ORAL CARE AND MAINTAINING SKIN INTEGRITY

When an oral ET tube is in place, the patient's mouth is always open. The nurse should moisten the lips, tongue, and gums with saline or water swabs to prevent mucosal drying. Proper oral care provides comfort and prevents injury to the gums and plaque formation (Table 68-9). Meticulous care is required to prevent skin breakdown on the face, lips, tongue, and nares because of pressure from the ET tube or bite block or the method used to secure the ET tube to the patient's face. The ET tube should be repositioned and retaped every 24 hours and as needed. This practice may be shared between the nurse and respiratory therapist or limited to the respiratory therapist.

For the nasally intubated patient, the nurse should remove the old tape or ties and clean the skin around the ET tube with saline-soaked gauze or cotton swabs. For the orally intubated patient, the nurse should remove the bite block (if present) and the old tape or ties. After providing oral hygiene, the nurse repositions the ET tube to the opposite side of the mouth, replaces

TABLE 68-9 ORAL CARE PROCEDURES FOR A PATIENT ON A MECHANICAL VENTILATOR—GENERAL MEASURES

1. Gather all equipment.
2. Wash hands and don personal protective equipment.
3. Explain procedure to the patient and the family, if present.
4. Perform oral care using pediatric or adult soft toothbrushes at least twice a day by gently brushing to clean and remove plaque.
5. Use oral swabs with a 1.5% hydrogen peroxide solution q2–4h. *Note:* Postoperative cardiac surgery patients are the only population in which use of 2% chlorhexidine gluconate is recommended twice a day.
6. Apply a mouth moisturizer to oral mucosa and lips with each cleaning.
7. Suction oral cavity and pharynx frequently. See Figure 68-16 for an example of an endotracheal tube that can provide continuous subglottic suctioning.

Note
- All oral suction equipment and suction tubing should be changed q24h.
- The nondisposable oral suction apparatus should be rinsed with sterile normal saline after each use and placed on a dry paper towel.

Source: Adapted from Vollman, K. M., & Sole, M. L. (2011). Endotracheal tube and oral care. In D. L. Wiegand (Ed.), *AACN procedure manual for critical care* (6th ed., pp. 33–37). St. Louis: Elsevier.

FIGURE 68-16 Continuous subglottal suctioning can be provided by the Hi-Lo Evac Tube. A dorsal lumen above the cuff allows for suctioning of secretions from the subglottic area. Source: © 2017 Medtronic. All rights reserved. Used with the permission of Medtronic.

the bite block (if appropriate), and reconfirms proper cuff inflation and tube placement. The ET tube is then secured again per employer policy. If a manufactured tube holder is used, the straps should be loosened, the area under the straps massaged, and then the straps reapplied. Two staff members should perform the repositioning procedure to prevent accidental dislodgement.

The patient must be monitored for any signs of respiratory distress throughout the procedure.

FOSTERING COMFORT AND COMMUNICATION

Intubation is a major stressor for the patient (Wade, Hardy, Howell, et al., 2013). The intubated patient may experience anxiety from not being able to talk or not knowing what to expect.

The physical discomfort associated with ET intubation and mechanical ventilation often requires sedating the patient and giving an analgesic until the ET tube is no longer required. The patient may need morphine, lorazepam, propofol, or other sedatives to blunt the anxiety and discomfort related to intubation. The nurse should evaluate the drugs' effectiveness in achieving an acceptable level of patient comfort. In addition, relaxation techniques (e.g., music therapy) should be considered to complement drug therapy.

COMPLICATIONS OF ENDOTRACHEAL INTUBATION

Two major complications of ET intubation are unplanned extubation and aspiration. Unplanned *extubation* (i.e., removal of the ET tube from the trachea) can be a catastrophic event and usually complicates the patient's recovery. Unplanned extubations can be due to patient removal of the ET tube or accidental removal during movement or a procedure. Usually the unplanned extubation is obvious (the patient is holding the ET tube). Other times, the tip of the ET tube is in the hypopharynx or esophagus and the extubation is not so obvious.

SAFETY ALERT—Unplanned Extubation
The nurse should observe for signs of unplanned extubation, which can be a life-threatening event:
- Patient talking
- Activation of the low-pressure ventilator alarm
- Diminished or absent breath sounds
- Respiratory distress
- Gastric distension

The nurse is responsible for preventing unplanned extubation by ensuring that the ET tube is secured and observing and supporting the ET tube during repositioning, procedures, and patient transfers.

Should an unplanned extubation occur, the nurse should stay with the patient and call for help. Interventions are aimed at maintaining the patient's airway, supporting ventilation (e.g., manually ventilating the patient with a BVM and 100% O_2), securing the appropriate assistance to immediately reintubate the patient (if necessary), and providing psychological support to the patient.

Aspiration is another potential hazard for the patient with an ET tube. The ET tube passes through the epiglottis, splinting it in an open position. Thus the intubated patient cannot protect the airway from aspiration. The high-volume, low-pressure ET or tracheal cuff cannot totally prevent the trickle of oral or gastric secretions into the trachea. Further, secretions collect above the cuff. When the cuff is deflated, those secretions can move into the lungs. Some ET tubes provide continuous suctioning of secretions above the cuff.

Oral intubation increases salivation, yet swallowing is difficult, so the nurse should suction the patient's mouth frequently using a tonsil-tip (Yankauer) suction catheter or a sterile single-use catheter. Other factors contributing to aspiration include improper cuff inflation, patient positioning, and tracheo-esophageal fistula. Patients with an ET tube are at risk for aspiration of gastric contents. Even when the cuff is properly inflated, precautions should be taken to prevent vomiting, which can lead to aspiration. Often, a nasogastric (NG) or an orogastric (OG) tube is inserted and connected to low, intermittent suction when a patient is first intubated. An OG tube is preferred over an NG tube to reduce the risk for sinusitis. All patients who are intubated or receiving enteral feedings must have the HOB elevated a minimum of 30 to 45 degrees unless medically contraindicated.

MECHANICAL VENTILATION

Mechanical ventilation is the process by which the FiO_2 (21% [room air] or more) is moved in and out of the lungs by a machine. Mechanical ventilation is not curative. It is a means of supporting patients until they recover the ability to breathe independently. It can also serve as a bridge to long-term mechanical ventilation or to a decision being made to withdraw ventilatory support.

Indications for mechanical ventilation include (a) apnea or impending inability to breathe or protect the airway, (b) acute respiratory failure (see Chapter 70), (c) severe hypoxia, and (d) respiratory muscle fatigue (Burns, 2011a). Patients with chronic pulmonary disease and their caregivers should be given the opportunity to discuss mechanical ventilation before end-stage respiratory disease develops. The nurse should encourage all patients, particularly those with chronic illnesses, to discuss the subject with their families and health care providers. Patients should then record and place the results of these discussions in an advance directive. The decision to use, withhold, or withdraw mechanical ventilation must be made carefully, respecting the wishes of the patient and caregiver. When the health care team, patient, and caregiver disagree over the plan of care, the employer's ethics committee must be consulted for assistance.

Types of Mechanical Ventilation

The two major types of mechanical ventilation are negative-pressure and positive-pressure ventilation.

Negative-Pressure Ventilation. Negative-pressure ventilation involves the use of chambers that encase the chest or body and surround it with intermittent subatmospheric (or negative) pressure. The "iron lung," developed during the polio epidemic, was the first form of negative-pressure ventilation. Intermittent negative pressure around the chest wall causes the chest to be pulled outward, reducing intrathoracic pressure. Air rushes in via the upper airway, which is outside the sealed chamber. Expiration is passive. The machine cycles off, allowing chest retraction. This type of ventilation is similar to normal ventilation in that decreased intrathoracic pressures produce inspiration, and expiration is passive. Negative-pressure ventilation is delivered by noninvasive ventilation and does not require an artificial airway.

Positive-Pressure Ventilation. Positive-pressure ventilation (PPV) is the primary method used with acutely ill patients (Figure 68-17). During inspiration, the ventilator pushes air into the lungs under positive pressure. Unlike spontaneous ventilation, intrathoracic pressure is raised during lung inflation rather than lowered. Expiration occurs passively as in normal expiration. Modes of PPV are categorized into two groups: volume and pressure ventilation (Goldsworthy & Graham, 2014).

Volume Ventilation. With volume ventilation, a predetermined V_T is delivered with each inspiration, and the amount of pressure needed to deliver the breath varies based on compliance and resistance factors of the patient–ventilator system. Consequently, the V_T is consistent from breath to breath, but airway pressures vary.

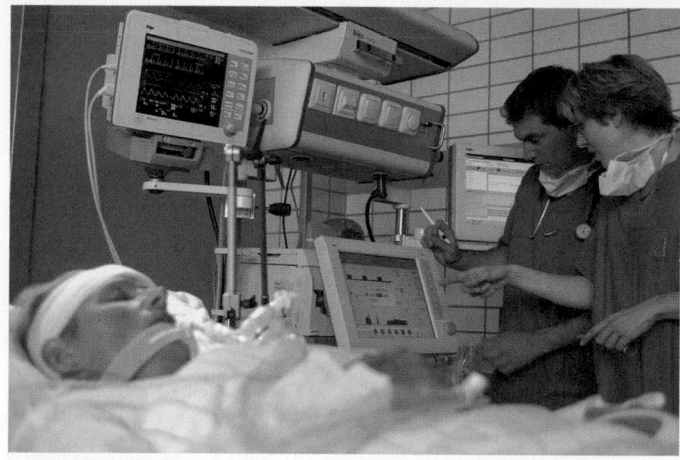

FIGURE 68-17 Patient receiving mechanical ventilation. Source: Courtesy Draeger Medical.

Pressure Ventilation. With *pressure ventilation*, the peak inspiratory pressure is predetermined, and the V_T delivered to the patient varies based on the selected pressure and compliance and resistance factors of the patient–ventilator system. With this understanding, careful attention must be given to the V_T to prevent unplanned hyperventilation or hypoventilation. For example, when the patient breathes out of synchrony with the ventilator, the pressure limit may be reached quickly, and the volume of gas delivered may be small. Initially, pressure ventilation was used only in stable patients being weaned from the ventilator. Today, pressure ventilation is frequently used to treat critically ill patients.

Settings of Mechanical Ventilators

Mechanical ventilator settings regulate rate, depth, and other characteristics of ventilation (Table 68-10). Settings are based on the patient's status (e.g., ABGs, ideal body weight, level of consciousness, muscle strength). The ventilator is tuned as finely as possible to match the patient's ventilatory pattern. Settings are evaluated and adjusted frequently until the patient achieves optimal ventilation. Some settings serve as a fail-safe mechanism, alerting staff to problems with ventilation. It is important that the nurse check that all ventilator alarms are always on. Alarms alert the staff to potentially dangerous situations such as mechanical malfunction, apnea, unplanned extubation, or patient asynchrony with the ventilator (Table 68-11). On many ventilators, the alarms can be temporarily suspended or silenced for up to 2 minutes for suctioning or testing while a staff member is in the room. After that time, the alarm system automatically becomes functional again.

Modes of Volume Ventilation

The variable methods by which the patient and ventilator interact to deliver effective ventilation are called *ventilator modes*. The selected ventilator mode is based on how much WOB the patient should or can perform. *WOB* refers to inspiratory effort needed to overcome the elasticity and viscosity of the lungs along with the airway resistance. The mode is determined by the patient's ventilatory status, respiratory drive, and ABGs. Generally, ventilator modes are controlled or assisted.

With controlled ventilatory support, the ventilator does all of the WOB. With assisted ventilatory support, the ventilator and patient share the WOB. Historically, volume modes such as

TABLE 68-10 SETTINGS OF MECHANICAL VENTILATION

Parameter	Description
High-pressure limit	Regulates the maximal pressure the ventilator can generate to deliver the V_T; when the pressure limit is reached, the ventilator terminates the breath and spills the undelivered volume into the atmosphere; usual setting is 10–20 cm H_2O above peak inspiratory pressure
I : E ratio	Duration of inspiration (I) to duration of expiration (E); usual setting is 1 : 2 to 1 : 1.5 unless IRV is desired
Inspiratory flow rate and time	Speed with which the V_T is delivered; usual setting is 40–80 L/min and time is 0.8–1.2 sec
Oxygen concentration	Fraction of inspired oxygen (FiO_2) delivered to patient; may be set between 21% (essentially room air) and 100%; usually adjusted to maintain PaO_2 level >60 mm Hg or SpO_2 level >90%
Positive end-expiratory pressure (PEEP)	Positive pressure applied at the end of expiration of ventilator breaths; usual setting is 5 cm H_2O
Pressure support	Positive pressure used to augment patient's inspiratory pressure; usual setting is 6–18 cm H_2O
Respiratory rate (f)	Number of breaths the ventilator delivers per minute; usual setting is 6–20 breaths/min
Sensitivity	Determines the amount of effort the patient must generate to initiate a ventilator breath; it may be set for pressure triggering or flow triggering; usual setting for a pressure trigger is 0.5–1.5 cm H_2O below baseline pressure and for a flow trigger is 1–3 L/min below baseline flow
Tidal volume (V_T)	Volume of gas delivered to patient during each ventilator breath; usual volume is 6–10 mL/kg

IRV, inverse ratio ventilation; *PaO₂,* partial pressure of oxygen in arterial blood; *SpO₂,* oxygen saturation value obtained by pulse oximetry.
Source: Urden, L. D., Stacy, K. M., & Lough, M. E. (2010). *Critical care nursing: Diagnosis and management* (6th ed., p. 655, Table 25-6). St. Louis: Mosby.

controlled mandatory ventilation (CMV), assist-control ventilation (ACV), and synchronized intermittent mandatory ventilation (SIMV) have been used to treat critically ill patients. More recently, pressure modes such as pressure-support ventilation (PSV) and pressure-control inverse ratio ventilation (PC-IRV) have become more widespread (Burns, 2011a). Table 68-11 describes these ventilator modes.

Assist-Control Ventilation. With **assist-control ventilation (ACV),** the ventilator delivers a preset V_T at a preset frequency. When the patient initiates a spontaneous breath, the ventilator senses a decrease in intrathoracic pressure and then delivers the preset V_T. The patient can breathe faster than the preset rate but not slower. This mode has the advantage of allowing the patient some control over ventilation while providing some assistance. ACV is used in patients with a variety of conditions, including neuro-muscular disorders (e.g., Guillain-Barré syndrome), pulmonary edema, and acute respiratory failure.

In the ACV mode, the patient has the potential for hypoventilation and hyperventilation. The spontaneously breathing patient can easily be overventilated, resulting in hyperventilation. If the volume or minimum rate is set low and

TABLE 68-11 MODES OF MECHANICAL VENTILATION

Volume Modes
Controlled Mandatory Ventilation (CMV) or Control Ventilation (CV)
In this mode, the ventilator provides all of the patient's minute ventilation. The clinician sets rate, tidal volume (V_T), inspiratory time, and positive end-expiratory pressure (PEEP). Generally, *PEEP* is used to describe those situations in which the patient is chemically relaxed or is paralyzed from a spinal cord or neuro-muscular disease and is therefore unable to initiate spontaneous breaths. The ventilator may be set on CMV, assist-control (AC), or synchronized intermittent mandatory ventilation (SIMV)—all these options provide volume breaths at the clinician-selected rate.

Assist-Control (ACV) or Assisted Mandatory Ventilation (AMV)
This option requires that a rate, V_T, inspiratory time, and PEEP be set for the patient. The ventilator sensitivity is also set, and when the patient initiates a spontaneous breath, a full-volume breath is delivered.

Intermittent Mandatory Ventilation (IMV) and Synchronized Intermittent Mandatory Ventilation (SIMV)
This mode requires that rate, V_T, inspiratory time, sensitivity, and PEEP be set by the clinician. In between "mandatory breaths," patients can spontaneously breathe at their own rates and V_T. With SIMV, the ventilator synchronizes the mandatory breaths with the patient's own inspirations.

Pressure Modes
Pressure-Support Ventilation (PSV)
This mode provides an augmented inspiration to a spontaneously breathing patient. With PSV, the clinician selects an inspiratory pressure level, PEEP, and sensitivity. When the patient initiates a breath, a high flow of gas is delivered to the preselected pressure level, and pressure is maintained throughout inspiration. The patient determines the parameters of V_T, rate, and inspiratory time.

Pressure-Controlled Inverse Ratio Ventilation (PC-IRV)
This mode combines pressure-limited ventilation with an inverse ratio of inspiration to expiration. The clinician selects the pressure level, the rate, the inspiratory time (1 : 1, 2 : 1, 3 : 1, 4 : 1), and the PEEP level. With the prolonged inspiratory times, auto-PEEP may result. The auto-PEEP may be a desirable outcome of the inverse ratios. Some clinicians use PC without IRV. Conventional inspiratory times are used, and rate, pressure level, and PEEP are selected.

Positive End-Expiratory Pressure (PEEP) and Continuous Positive Airway Pressure (CPAP)
PEEP
This ventilatory option creates positive pressure at end-exhalation. PEEP restores functional residual capacity (FRC). The term *PEEP* is used when end-expiratory pressure is provided during ventilator positive-pressure breaths.

CPAP
Similar to PEEP, CPAP restores FRC. This pressure is continuous during spontaneous breathing; no positive-pressure breaths are present.

Source: Modified from Burns, S. M. (2011). Ventilatory management: Volume and pressure modes. In D. L. Wiegand (Ed.), *AACN procedure manual for critical care* (6th ed., p. 266, Table 35-2). St. Louis: Mosby.

the patient is apneic or weak, the patient will be hypoventilated. Thus these patients require vigilant assessment and monitoring of ventilatory status, including respiratory rate, ABGs, SpO_2, and $ScvO_2/SvO_2$. It is also important that the sensitivity or amount of negative pressure required to initiate a breath is appropriate to the patient's condition. For example, if it is too difficult for the patient to initiate a breath, the WOB is increased and the patient may tire or develop ventilator asynchrony (i.e., the patient "fights" the ventilator).

Synchronized Intermittent Mandatory Ventilation. With *synchronized intermittent mandatory ventilation* (SIMV), the ventilator delivers a preset V_T at a preset frequency in synchrony with the patient's spontaneous breathing. Between ventilator-delivered breaths, the patient is able to breathe spontaneously through the ventilator circuit. Thus the patient receives the preset FiO_2 during the spontaneous breaths but self-regulates the rate and volume of those breaths. This mode of ventilation differs from ACV, in which all breaths are of the same preset volume. It is used during continuous ventilation and during weaning from the ventilator. SIMV may also be combined with PSV (described below). Potential benefits of SIMV include improved patient–ventilator synchrony, lower mean airway pressure, and prevention of muscle atrophy, as the patient takes on more of the WOB.

SIMV also has disadvantages. If spontaneous breathing decreases when the preset rate is low, ventilation might not be adequately supported. Only patients with regular, spontaneous breathing should use low-rate SIMV. Weaning with SIMV demands close monitoring and may take longer because the rate of breathing is gradually reduced. Patients being weaned from SIMV may also have increased muscle fatigue associated with spontaneous breathing efforts.

Modes of Pressure Ventilation

Pressure-Support Ventilation. With pressure-support ventilation (PSV), positive pressure is applied to the airway only during inspiration and is used in conjunction with the patient's spontaneous respirations. The patient must be able to initiate a breath for this modality to be used. The level of positive airway pressure is preset so that the gas flow rate is greater than the patient's inspiratory flow rate. As the patient initiates a breath, the machine senses the spontaneous effort and supplies a rapid flow of gas at the initiation of the breath and variable flow throughout the breath. With PSV, the patient determines inspiratory length, V_T, and respiratory rate. V_T depends on the pressure level and airway compliance.

PSV is used with continuous ventilation and during weaning. PSV may also be used with SIMV during weaning. PSV is not used as a sole ventilatory support during acute respiratory failure because of the risk for hypoventilation. Advantages of PSV include increased patient comfort, decreased WOB (because inspiratory efforts are augmented), decreased O_2 consumption (because inspiratory work is reduced), and increased endurance conditioning (because the patient is exercising respiratory muscles).

Pressure-Control Inverse Ratio Ventilation. *Pressure-control inverse ratio ventilation* (PC-IRV) combines pressure-limited ventilation with an inverse ratio of inspiration (I) to expiration (E). Some clinicians use PC without IRV. The I/E ratio is the ratio of duration of inspiration to the duration of expiration. This value is normally a ratio of 1:2. With IRV, the I/E ratio begins at 1:1 and may progress to 4:1. Prolonged positive pressure is applied, increasing inspiratory time. IRV progressively expands collapsed alveoli. The short expiratory time has a PEEP-like effect, preventing alveolar collapse. Because IRV imposes a nonphysiological breathing pattern, the patient requires sedation with or without paralysis. PC-IRV is indicated for patients with acute respiratory distress syndrome (ARDS) who continue to have

refractory hypoxemia despite high levels of PEEP. Not all patients with poor oxygenation respond to PC-IRV.

Airway Pressure Release Ventilation. *Airway pressure release ventilation* (APRV) permits spontaneous breathing at any point during the respiratory cycle with a preset continuous positive airway pressure (CPAP) with short timed pressure releases. The CPAP level (pressure high, pressure low) is adjusted to maintain oxygenation goals while the timed releases (time high, time low) are increased or decreased to meet ventilation goals. V_T is not a set variable and depends on the CPAP level, the patient's compliance and resistance, and spontaneous breathing effort. The mode is designed for patients with ARDS who need high pressure levels for alveolar recruitment (open collapsed alveoli). One advantage of this mode is the ability to permit spontaneous respirations, which may reduce the need for deep sedation or paralytics.

Other Modes. Improvements in ventilator technology have led to the development of additional pressure modes. However, because of the nonstandardization of these options, the names and features are manufacturer specific. The superiority of these modes has not been established. Some examples include *volume-assured pressure ventilation* and *adaptive support ventilation*.

Other Ventilatory Manoeuvres

Positive End-Expiratory Pressure. Positive end-expiratory pressure (PEEP) is a ventilatory manoeuvre in which positive pressure is applied to the airway during exhalation. Normally during exhalation, airway pressure drops to zero, and exhalation occurs passively. With PEEP, exhalation remains passive, but pressure falls to a preset level, often 3 to 20 cm H_2O. Lung volume during expiration and between breaths is greater than normal with PEEP. This increases functional residual capacity (FRC) and often improves oxygenation with restoration of lung volume that normally remains at the end of passive exhalation. The mechanisms by which PEEP increases FRC and oxygenation include increased aeration of patent alveoli, aeration of previously collapsed alveoli, and prevention of alveolar collapse throughout the respiratory cycle.

PEEP is titrated to the point that oxygenation improves without compromising hemodynamics. This setting is termed *best* or *optimal PEEP*. Often, 5 cm H_2O PEEP (referred to as *physiological PEEP*) is used prophylactically to replace the glottic mechanism, help maintain a normal FRC, and prevent alveolar collapse. PEEP of 5 cm H_2O is also used for patients with a history of alveolar collapse during weaning. PEEP improves gas exchange, vital capacity, and inspiratory force when used during weaning.

In contrast, *auto-PEEP* is not purposely set on the ventilator but is a result of inadequate exhalation time. Auto-PEEP is additional PEEP over what is set by the health care provider. This additional PEEP may result in increased WOB, barotrauma, and hemodynamic instability. However, during some ventilator modes (e.g., PC-IRV), auto-PEEP may be desirable. Interventions to limit auto-PEEP include sedation and analgesia, large-diameter ET tube, bronchodilators, short inspiratory times, and decreased respiratory rates. Reducing water accumulation in the ventilator circuit by frequent emptying or use of heated circuits also limits auto-PEEP. In patients with short exhalation times and early airway closure (e.g., asthma), setting PEEP can offset auto-PEEP by splinting the airway open during exhalation and preventing "air trapping."

In general, the major purpose of PEEP is to maintain or improve oxygenation while limiting risk for O_2 toxicity. FiO_2 can often be reduced when PEEP is used. PEEP is indicated in lungs with diffuse disease, severe hypoxemia unresponsive to FiO_2 greater than 50%, and loss of compliance or stiffness. It is used in pulmonary edema to provide a counter-pressure opposing fluid extravasation. The classic indication for PEEP therapy is ARDS (see Chapter 70). PEEP is contraindicated or used with extreme caution in patients with highly compliant lungs (e.g., COPD), unilateral or nonuniform disease, hypovolemia, and low CO. In these cases, the adverse effects of PEEP may outweigh any benefits.

Continuous Positive Airway Pressure. Continuous positive airway pressure (CPAP) restores FRC and is similar to PEEP. However, the pressure in CPAP is delivered continuously during spontaneous breathing, thus preventing the patient's airway pressure from falling to zero. For example, if CPAP is 5 cm H_2O, airway pressure during expiration is 5 cm H_2O. During inspiration, 1 to 2 cm H_2O of negative pressure is generated, thus reducing airway pressure to 3 or 4 cm H_2O. The patient receiving SIMV with PEEP receives CPAP when breathing spontaneously. CPAP is commonly used in the treatment of severe obstructive sleep apnea or hypopnea (Burns, 2011b). A nasal mask attached to a high-flow blower is applied to maintain pressure in the airway and prevent airway collapse. An ET or tracheal tube can be used in place of the nasal mask. CPAP increases WOB because the patient must forcibly exhale against the CPAP. Therefore, it must be used with caution in patients with myocardial compromise.

Bilevel Positive Airway Pressure. In addition to O_2, *bilevel positive airway pressure* (BiPAP) provides two levels of positive-pressure support: higher inspiratory positive airway pressure and lower expiratory positive airway pressure. It is a noninvasive modality and is delivered through a tight-fitting face mask, nasal mask, or nasal pillows. As with PSV delivered through an artificial airway, the patient must be able to spontaneously breathe and cooperate with this treatment (Burns, 2011b). BiPAP is used for COPD patients with heart failure and acute respiratory failure and for patients with sleep apnea. BiPAP may also be used after extubation to prevent reintubation. Patients with shock, altered mental status, or increased airway secretions are not candidates for BiPAP because of the risk for aspiration and the inability to remove the mask.

High-Frequency Oscillatory Ventilation. High-frequency oscillatory ventilation (HFOV) involves delivery of a small V_T (usually 1 to 5 mL/kg of body weight) at a rapid respiratory rate (100 to 300 breaths/min) in an effort to recruit and maintain lung volume and reduce intrapulmonary shunting. One benefit of HFOV is the ability to support gas exchange at a fixed mean airway pressure while limiting the risk for ventilator-induced lung injury. HFOV has been widely accepted in neonatal and pediatric ICUs. It is used in adults for the treatment of refractory hypoxemia and ARDS (Ali & Ferguson, 2011). Patients receiving HFOV must be sedated and may be paralyzed to suppress spontaneous respiration. All patients must receive concurrent sedation and analgesia if using a paralytic drug.

Nitric Oxide. *Nitric oxide* (NO) is a gaseous molecule that is made intravascularly and participates in the regulation of pulmonary vascular tone. Inhibition of NO production results in pulmonary vasoconstriction, and administration of continuous inhaled NO results in pulmonary vasodilation. NO may be administered via an ET tube, a tracheostomy, or a face mask. Currently, NO is used in ARDS, as a diagnostic screening tool for pulmonary hypertension during a cardiac catheterization, and during or after cardiac surgery.

Prone Positioning. *Prone positioning* is the repositioning of a patient from a supine or lateral position to a prone position (on the stomach, face down). This repositioning improves lung recruitment (re-expansion) through various mechanisms. Gravity reverses the effects of fluid in the dependent parts of the lungs as the patient is moved from supine to prone. The heart rests on the sternum, away from the lungs, contributing to an overall uniformity of pleural pressures. The prone position is a relatively safe (although nurse-intensive), supportive therapy used to improve oxygenation in critically ill patients with acute lung injury or ARDS (Henderson, Griesdale, Dominelli, et al., 2014).

Extracorporeal Membrane Oxygenation. *Extracorporeal membrane oxygenation* (ECMO) is an alternative form of pulmonary support for the patient with severe respiratory failure. It is used more frequently in the pediatric and neonatal populations but is increasingly being used in adults. ECMO is a modification of cardiac bypass and involves partially removing blood from a patient with large-bore catheters, infusing O_2, removing CO_2, and returning the blood to the patient. This intensive therapy requires systemic anticoagulation and is a time-limited intervention. A skilled team of specialists, including a perfusionist, is required continuously at the bedside (Combes, Brodie, Bartlett, et al., 2014).

Complications of Positive-Pressure Ventilation

Although PPV may be essential to maintain ventilation and oxygenation, it can cause adverse effects. It is often difficult to distinguish complications of mechanical ventilation from the underlying disease.

Cardiovascular System. PPV can affect circulation because of the transmission of increased mean airway pressure to the thoracic cavity. With increased intrathoracic pressure, thoracic vessels are compressed. This compression results in decreased venous return to the heart, decreased left ventricular end-diastolic volume (preload), decreased CO, and hypotension. Mean airway pressure is further increased if titrating PEEP (greater than 5 cm H_2O) to improve oxygenation.

If the lungs are noncompliant (e.g., ARDS), airway pressures are not as easily transmitted to the heart and blood vessels. Thus effects of PPV on CO are reduced. Conversely, with compliant lungs (e.g., emphysema), there is increased danger of transmission of high airway pressures and negative effects on hemodynamics.

Compromised venous return by PPV is worsened by hypovolemia (e.g., hemorrhage) and decreased venous tone (e.g., sepsis, spinal shock). Restoration and maintenance of the circulating blood volume are important in minimizing cardiovascular complications.

Pulmonary System. Complications of PPV affecting the pulmonary system include barotrauma, volutrauma, alveolar hypoventilation and hyperventilation, and ventilator-associated pneumonia.

Barotrauma. As lung inflation pressures increase, risk of *barotrauma* increases. Patients with compliant lungs (e.g., COPD) are at greater risk for barotrauma, which results when the increased airway pressure distends the lungs and possibly ruptures fragile alveoli or emphysematous blebs. Patients with stiff lungs (e.g., ARDS) who are given high inspiratory pressures and high levels of PEEP (greater than 5 cm H_2O) and patients with lung abscesses resulting from necrotizing organisms (e.g., staphylococci) are also susceptible to barotrauma.

Air can escape into the pleural space from alveoli or interstitium and become trapped. Pleural pressure increases and collapses the lung, causing pneumothorax. (Chapter 30 discusses the clinical manifestations of pneumothorax.) The lungs receive air during inspiration but cannot expel it during expiration. Respiratory bronchioles are larger on inspiration than expiration. They may close on expiration, and air becomes trapped. With PPV, a simple pneumothorax can become a life-threatening tension pneumothorax. The mediastinum and contralateral lung are compressed, reducing CO. Immediate treatment of the pneumothorax is required. For some patients, chest tubes are placed prophylactically.

Pneumomediastinum usually begins with rupture of alveoli into the lung interstitium. Progressive air movement occurs into the mediastinum and subcutaneous neck tissue, and a pneumothorax often follows. New, unexplained subcutaneous emphysema is an indication for immediate chest radiography. Pneumomediastinum and subcutaneous emphysema may be too small to detect on a radiograph or to appear clinically before the development of a pneumothorax.

Volutrauma. The concept of *volutrauma* in PPV relates to the lung injury that occurs when a large V_T is used to ventilate noncompliant lungs. Volutrauma results in alveolar fractures and movement of fluids and proteins into the alveolar spaces. Low-volume ventilation rather than pressure ventilation should be used in ARDS patients to protect the lungs.

Alveolar Hypoventilation. *Alveolar hypoventilation* can be caused by inappropriate ventilator settings, leakage of air from the ventilator tubing or around the ET tube or tracheostomy cuff, lung secretions or obstruction, and low ventilation/perfusion ratio. A low V_T or respiratory rate decreases minute ventilation. This decrease results in hypoventilation and leads to respiratory acidosis. A leaking cuff or tubing that is not secured may cause air leakage, lowering the delivered V_T. Excess lung secretions can cause hypoventilation. Mobilizing the patient, turning the patient every 1 to 2 hours, providing chest physiotherapy to lung areas with increased secretions, encouraging deep breathing and coughing, and suctioning (as needed) may limit hypoventilation. Atelectasis may develop. Increasing the V_T, adding small increments of PEEP, and adding a preset number of sighs to the ventilator settings reduce the risk for atelectasis.

Alveolar Hyperventilation. Respiratory alkalosis can occur if the respiratory rate or V_T is set too high *(mechanical overventilation)* or if the patient receiving assisted ventilation is *hyperventilating*. It is easy to overventilate a patient on PPV. Particularly at risk are patients with chronic alveolar hypoventilation and CO_2 retention. For example, the patient with COPD may have a chronic $PaCO_2$ elevation (acidosis) and compensatory bicarbonate retention by the kidneys. When the patient is ventilated, the patient's "normal baseline" rather than the standard normal values is the therapeutic goal. If the COPD patient is returned to a standard normal $PaCO_2$, the patient will develop alkalosis because of the retained bicarbonate. Such a patient could move from compensated respiratory acidosis to serious metabolic alkalosis. The presence of alkalosis makes weaning from the ventilator difficult. Alkalosis, especially if the onset is abrupt, can have additional serious consequences, including hypokalemia, hypocalcemia, and dysrhythmias. Neuro-muscular irritability, seizures, coma, and death can occur. Usually the patient with COPD who is supported on the ventilator does better with a short inspiratory and longer expiratory time.

If hyperventilation is spontaneous, it is important to determine the cause and treat it. Possible causes include hypoxemia, pain, fear, anxiety, or compensation for metabolic acidosis. Patients who fight the ventilator or breathe out of synchrony may be anxious or in pain. If the patient is anxious and fearful, the nurse can help by sitting with the patient and verbally coaching the patient to breathe with the ventilator. If these measures fail, manually ventilating the patient slowly with a BVM and 100% O_2 may slow breathing enough to bring it in synchrony with the ventilator.

Ventilator-Associated Pneumonia. The risk for health care–associated pneumonia is highest in patients requiring mechanical ventilation because the ET or tracheostomy tube bypasses normal upper airway defences. In addition, a poor nutritional state, immobility, and the underlying disease process (e.g., immuno-suppression, organ failure) make the patient more prone to infection. *Ventilator-associated pneumonia* (VAP) is pneumonia that occurs 48 hours or more after ET intubation (Safer Healthcare Now, 2012). It occurs in 9% to 27% of all intubated patients, with half of the cases developing within the first 4 days of mechanical ventilation. In addition, patients who develop VAP have significantly longer hospital stays and higher mortality rates than those who do not.

In patients with early VAP (within 96 hours of mechanical ventilation), sputum cultures often grow Gram-negative bacteria (e.g., *Escherichia coli*, *Klebsiella*, *Streptococcus pneumoniae*, *Haemophilus influenzae*). Organisms associated with late VAP include antibiotic-resistant organisms such as *Pseudomonas aeruginosa* and oxacillin-resistant *Staphylococcus aureus*. These organisms are abundant in the hospital environment. They can spread in a number of ways, including contaminated respiratory equipment, inadequate handwashing, adverse environmental factors such as poor room ventilation and high traffic flow, and decreased patient ability to cough and clear secretions. Colonization of the oropharynx tract by Gram-negative organisms predisposes the patient to Gram-negative pneumonia.

Clinical evidence suggesting VAP includes fever, elevated white blood cell count, purulent or odorous sputum, crackles or rhonchi on auscultation, and pulmonary infiltrates noted on chest radiograph. The patient is treated with antibiotics after appropriate cultures are taken by tracheal suctioning or bronchoscopy and when infection is evident.

Guidelines on VAP prevention include (a) elevating the HOB a minimum of 30 to 45 degrees unless medically contraindicated, (b) avoiding routine changes of the patient's ventilator circuit tubing, and (c) using an ET tube with a dorsal lumen above the cuff to allow continuous suctioning of secretions in the subglottic area (Canadian Patient Safety Institute, 2016; Safer Healthcare Now, 2012). Prevention also includes strict handwashing before and after suctioning, after touching ventilator equipment, and after contact with any respiratory secretions (see "Nursing Management: Artificial Airway," earlier in this chapter). Always wear gloves when in contact with the patient and change gloves between activities (e.g., emptying urinary catheter drainage, hanging an IV drug). Finally, always drain the water as it collects in the ventilator tubing, keeping it away from the patient.

Sodium and Water Imbalance. Progressive fluid retention often occurs after 48 to 72 hours of PPV, especially PPV with PEEP. Fluid retention is associated with decreased urine output and increased sodium retention. Fluid balance changes may be due to decreased CO, which in turn results in diminished renal perfusion. Consequently, renin release is stimulated with subsequent production of angiotensin and aldosterone (see Chapter 47, Figure 47-6). This process results in sodium and water retention. It is also possible that pressure changes within the thorax are associated with decreased release of atrial natriuretic peptide, which also causes sodium retention. Mild water retention is also associated with PPV. Less insensible water loss occurs via the airway because ventilated delivered gases are humidified with body-temperature water. In addition, as a part of the stress response, the release of antidiuretic hormone and cortisol contributes to sodium and water retention.

Neurological System. In patients with head injury, PPV (especially with PEEP) can impair cerebral blood flow. The increased intrathoracic positive pressure impedes venous drainage from the head, resulting in jugular venous distension. The patient may exhibit increases in intracranial pressure because of the impaired venous return and increase in cerebral volume. Elevating the HOB and keeping the patient's head in alignment may decrease the harmful effects of PPV on intracranial pressure.

Gastro-Intestinal System. Patients receiving PPV are stressed because of the serious illness, immobility, or discomforts associated with the ventilator. This places the ventilated patient at risk for developing stress ulcers and GI bleeding. Patients with a pre-existing ulcer or those receiving corticosteroids are at an increased risk. Any kind of circulatory compromise, including reduction of CO caused by PPV, may contribute to ischemia of the gastric and intestinal mucosa and possibly increase the risk for translocation of GI bacteria.

To decrease the risk for VAP, guidelines support the use of routine peptic ulcer prophylaxis in mechanically ventilated patients (Plummer, Blaser, & Deane, 2014). Peptic ulcer prophylaxis includes the administration of histamine (H_2)-receptor blockers (e.g., ranitidine [Zantac]), proton pump inhibitors (PPIs) (e.g., esomeprazole [Nexium]), and enteral nutrition to decrease gastric acidity and diminish the risk for stress ulcer and hemorrhage.

Gastric and bowel dilation may occur because of gas accumulation in the GI tract from swallowed air. The irritation of an artificial airway may cause excessive air swallowing and subsequent gastric dilation. Gastric or bowel dilation may put pressure on the vena cava, decrease CO, and prohibit adequate diaphragmatic excursion during spontaneous breathing. Elevation of the diaphragm as a result of paralytic ileus or bowel dilation leads to compression of the lower lobes of the lungs. This compression may cause atelectasis and compromise respiratory function. Decompression of the stomach is done by inserting an OG or NG tube (Plummer, Blaser, & Deane, 2014).

Immobility, sedation, circulatory impairment, decreased oral intake, use of opioid pain medications, and stress contribute to decreased peristalsis. The patient's inability to exhale against a closed glottis may make defecation difficult. As a result, the ventilated patient is at risk for constipation, so a bowel regimen should be initiated.

Musculo-Skeletal System. Maintenance of muscle strength and prevention of the problems associated with immobility are important. Adequate analgesia and nutrition can enhance exercise tolerance. Plans should be made for early and progressive mobility of appropriate patients receiving PPV. In collaboration with physiotherapists and occupational therapists, the nurse should perform passive and active exercises to maintain muscle tone in the upper and lower extremities. Simple manoeuvres such as leg lifts, knee bends, quadriceps setting, or arm circles are appropriate. Contractures, pressure ulcers, foot drop, and external rotation of the hip and legs can be prevented by proper positioning and the use of specialized mattresses or beds. For ventilating the patient during ambulation, a portable ventilator or manual ventilation with a BVM and 100% O_2 is appropriate.

Psychosocial Needs. The patient receiving mechanical ventilation often experiences physical and emotional stress. In addition to the problems related to critical care patients discussed at the beginning of this chapter, the patient supported by a mechanical ventilator is unable to speak, eat, move, or breathe normally. Tubes and machines cause pain, fear, and anxiety. Usual activities of daily living such as eating, elimination, and coughing are extremely complicated. The nurse should involve patients and caregivers in decision making as much as possible.

Patients receiving PPV usually require sedation (e.g., propofol), analgesia (e.g., fentanyl), or both to facilitate optimal ventilation. Before initiating sedation or analgesia in the mechanically ventilated patient who is agitated or anxious, the nurse should identify the cause of distress. Common problems that can result in patient agitation or anxiety include PPV, nutritional deficits, pain, hypoxemia, hypercapnia, drugs, and environmental stressors (e.g., sleep deprivation). Delirium is an acute change in mental status. It is a marker of cerebral insufficiency and is associated with longer hospital stays and higher mortality rates. ICU patients are particularly vulnerable to delirium, and the nurse must make every effort to assess and treat it (Barr, Fraser, Puntillo, et al., 2013).

In some situations, the decision is made to paralyze the patient with a neuro-muscular blocking agent (e.g., cisatracurium) to provide more effective synchrony with the ventilator and improve oxygenation. Health care providers should remember that the paralyzed patient can hear, see, think, and feel. It is important to administer IV sedation and analgesia concurrently when the patient is paralyzed. Monitoring patients receiving these medications is challenging. Assessment of the patient should include train-of-four (TOF) testing, clinical assessment for physiological signs of pain or anxiety (changes in heart rate and BP), and ventilator synchrony. The TOF assessment involves using a peripheral nerve stimulator to deliver four successive stimulating currents to elicit muscle twitches (Figure 68-18). The number of twitches varies with the percentage of neuro-muscular blockade. The usual goal is one or two twitches out of four. Noninvasive electroencephalogram-based technology can also help guide sedative and analgesic therapy in these patients. Excessive administration of neuro-muscular blocking agents may predispose the patient to prolonged paralysis and muscle weakness even after these agents are stopped.

FIGURE 68-18 Placement of electrodes along ulnar nerve.

Many patients have few memories of their time in the ICU, whereas others remember vivid details. Although appearing to be asleep, sedated, or paralyzed, patients may be aware of their surroundings, so health care providers should always address them as if they were awake and alert (Desai, Law, & Needham, 2011).

Machine Disconnection or Malfunction. Mechanical ventilators may become disconnected or malfunction. When turned on and operative, alarms alert the nurse to problems (Table 68-12). Most deaths from accidental ventilator disconnection occur while the alarm is off, and most accidental disconnections in critical care settings are discovered by low-pressure alarms. The most frequent site for disconnection is between the tracheal tube and the adapter. Connections should be pushed together and then twisted to ensure they are secure. Alarms should be set at all times, and the nurse should chart that this is the case. Alarms can be paused (not inactivated) during suctioning or removal from the ventilator but must be reactivated before the nurse leaves the patient's bedside.

Ventilator malfunction may occur due to several factors. Although most institutions have emergency generators in the event of a power failure and newer ventilators may have battery backup, power failure is always a possibility. A plan should be in place for manually ventilating all patients who depend on a ventilator. If, at any time, the ventilator is determined to be malfunctioning (e.g., failure of O_2 supply), the patient should be disconnected from the machine and manually ventilated with a BVM and 100% O_2 until the ventilator is fixed or replaced.

Weaning From Positive-Pressure Ventilation and Extubation

Weaning is the process of reducing ventilator support and resuming spontaneous ventilation. The weaning process differs for patients requiring short-term ventilation (up to 3 days) than for those requiring long-term ventilation (longer than 3 days). Patients requiring short-term ventilation (e.g., after cardiac surgery) experience a linear weaning process. Patients likely to require prolonged PPV (e.g., patients with COPD who develop respiratory failure) often experience a weaning process that consists of peaks and valleys. Preparation for weaning begins when PPV is initiated and involves a team approach (e.g., nurse, physician, patient, caregiver, dietitian, respiratory therapist, physiotherapist).

Weaning generally consists of three phases: the *preweaning phase*, the *weaning process*, and the *outcome phase*. The preweaning, or assessment, phase determines the patient's ability to breathe spontaneously. Assessment in this phase depends on a combination of respiratory (Table 68-13) and nonrespiratory factors. Weaning assessment parameters should include criteria to assess muscle strength (negative inspiratory force) and endurance (spontaneous V_T, vital capacity, minute ventilation, and rapid shallow breathing index). In addition, the patient's lungs should be reasonably clear on auscultation and chest radiograph. Nonrespiratory factors include the patient's neurological status; hemodynamics; fluid, electrolytes, and acid–base balance; nutrition; and hemoglobin. It is important to have an alert, well-rested, and well-informed patient relatively free from pain and anxiety who can cooperate with the weaning plan. This does not mean complete withdrawal from sedatives or analgesics. Instead, drugs should be titrated to achieve comfort without causing excessive drowsiness.

A *spontaneous breathing trial* (SBT) is recommended for patients who demonstrate weaning readiness (Burns, 2011c). An SBT should be at least 30 minutes but no more than 120 minutes. It may be done with low levels of CPAP, low levels of PSV, or a T-piece. Tolerance of the trial may lead to extubation. Failure to tolerate an SBT should prompt a search for reversible or complicating factors and a return to a nonfatiguing ventilator modality for the patient. The SBT should be reattempted the next day.

The use of a weaning protocol decreases ventilator days. The parts of a protocol are not as important as the use of a protocol to prevent delays in weaning. Patients receiving SIMV can have the ventilator breaths gradually reduced as their ventilatory status permits. CPAP or PSV can be added to SIMV. PSV is thought to provide gentle, slow respiratory muscle conditioning. It may be especially beneficial for patients who are deconditioned or have heart problems. Some patients may be weaned by simply providing humidified oxygen (T-piece or flow-by method).

Weaning may be tried at any time of day, although it is usually done during the day, with the patient ventilated at night in a rest mode. The rest mode should be a stable, nonfatiguing, and comfortable form of support for the patient. Regardless of the weaning mode selected, all health care team members should be familiar with the weaning plan. Additionally, it is important

TABLE 68-12	INTERPRETING MECHANICAL VENTILATION ALARMS
Alarm	**Possible Causes**
Apnea	Change in patient condition
	Loss of airway (e.g., total or partial extubation)
	Oversedation
	Respiratory arrest
High tidal volume, minute ventilation, or respiratory rate	Change in patient condition
	Excess condensate (water) in tubing (i.e., false reading)
	Pain, anxiety
High-pressure limit	Condensate in tubing
	Decreased compliance (e.g., pulmonary edema, pneumothorax)
	Increased resistance (e.g., bronchospasm)
	Kinked or compressed tubing (e.g., patient biting on ET tube)
	Patient fighting ventilator (ventilator asynchrony)
	Secretions, coughing, or gagging
Low tidal volume or minute ventilation	Change in patient's breathing efforts (e.g., rate and volume)
	ET tube or tracheal cuff leak (e.g., patient speaking, grunting)
	Insufficient gas flow
	Patient disconnection, loose connection, or leak in circuit
Low-pressure limit	ET tube or tracheal cuff leak (e.g., patient speaking, grunting)
	Loss of airway (e.g., total or partial extubation)
	Total or partial ventilator disconnect
Ventilator inoperative or low battery	Machine malfunction
	Unplugged, power failure, or internal battery not charged

ET, endotracheal.
Source: Adapted from Pierce, L.N. (2007). *Management of the mechanically ventilated patient* (2nd ed.). St. Louis: Saunders.

TABLE 68-13 INDICATORS FOR WEANING

Weaning Readiness

Patients receiving mechanical ventilation for respiratory failure should undergo a formal assessment of weaning potential if the following are satisfied:*

1. Reversal of the underlying cause of respiratory failure
2. Adequate oxygenation:
   PaO_2 >80–100
   FiO_2 ≤40%–50%
   PEEP ≤5–8 cm H_2O
   pH ≥7.25
3. Hemodynamic stability:
   Absence of clinically significant hypotension (low-dose or no vasopressor therapy)
   Absence of myocardial ischemia
4. Patient ability to initiate an inspiratory effort

Weaning Assessment

Measurement	Significance	Normal Values	Indices for Weaning
Compliance, rate, oxygenation, and pressure (CROP) index	Combined index that is complex to calculate C_{Dyn}=Compliance $C_{Dyn} \times NIF \times (PaO_2/PAO_2)/f$ PaO_2/PAO_2=Oxygenation ratio of arterial O_2/alveolar O_2	Not applicable	>13
Minute ventilation (V_E)	Tidal volume (V_T) multiplied by respiratory rate over 1 min For example: 0.350 (V_T)×28 (f)=8.8 L/min	5–10 L/min	≤10 L/min
Negative inspiratory force (NIF) or pressure (NIP)	Amount of negative pressure that a patient is able to generate to initiate spontaneous respirations Measured by clinician: After complete occlusion of inspiratory valve, a pressure manometer is attached to airway or mouth for 10–20 sec while negative inspiratory efforts are noted	−75 to −100 cm H_2O	>−20 cm H_2O The more negative the number, the better indication for weaning.
Positive expiratory pressure (PEP)	Measure of expiratory muscle strength and ability to cough. Measured by clinician: After complete occlusion of expiratory valve, a pressure manometer is attached to the airway or mouth for 10–20 sec while positive expiratory efforts are noted	60–85 cm H_2O	≥30 cm H_2O
Rapid shallow breathing index (f/V_T)	Spontaneous respiratory rate over 1 min divided by tidal volume (in L) Easier calculation and more widely used For example: 30 (f)/0.400 (V_T)=75/L	60–105/L	<105/L
Spontaneous respiratory rate (f)	Respiratory rate and frequency >1 min	12–20 min	<38 min
Spontaneous tidal volume (V_T)	Amount of air exchanged during normal breathing at rest; measure of muscle endurance	7–9 mL/kg	≥5 mL/kg
Vital capacity (VC)	Maximum inspiration and then measurement of air during maximal forced expiration; measure of respiratory muscle endurance or reserve or both; requires patient cooperation	65–75 mL/kg	≥10–15 mL/kg

*The decision to use these criteria must be individualized to the patient.

C_{Dyn}, dynamic compliance; (f), spontaneous respiratory rate; FiO_2, fraction of inspired oxygen; NIF, negative inspiratory force; PaO_2, partial pressure of oxygen in arterial blood; PAO_2; PEEP, positive end-expiratory pressure.

Sources: Adapted from MacIntyre, N. R., Cook, D. J., Ely E. W., Jr., et al. (2001). Evidence-based guidelines for weaning and discontinuing ventilatory support. *Chest, 120*(6 Suppl), 375S–395S; and Burns, S. M. (2011). Weaning process. In D. L. Wiegand (Ed.), *AACN procedure manual for critical care* (6th ed., pp. 291–300). St. Louis: Elsevier.

to permit the patient's respiratory muscles to rest between weaning trials. Once the respiratory muscles become fatigued, they may require 12 to 24 hours to recover.

The patient being weaned and the caregiver need ongoing emotional support. The nurse should explain the weaning process to them and keep them informed of progress. For the weaning trial, the patient should be in a comfortable sitting or semirecumbent position. Baseline vital signs and respiratory parameters are obtained, and, during the trial, the nurse closely monitors the patient for signs and symptoms that may signal intolerance and a need to end the trial (e.g., tachypnea, dyspnea, tachycardia, dysrhythmias, sustained desaturation [SpO_2 less than 91%], hypertension or hypotension, agitation, diaphoresis, anxiety, sustained V_T less than 5 mL/kg, changes in mentation). The patient's tolerance throughout the weaning process should be documented, including statements regarding the patient's and the caregiver's perceptions.

The *weaning outcome phase* is the period when the patient is extubated or weaning is stopped because no further progress is being made. The patient who is ready for extubation should receive hyperoxygenation and suctioning (e.g., oropharynx, ET tube). For extubation, the nurse instructs the patient to take a deep breath and, at the peak of inspiration, deflates the cuff and removes the tube in one motion. After the tube has been removed, the nurse encourages the patient to deep-breathe and cough and suctions the oropharynx as needed. Supplemental O_2 should be administered, and naso-oral care provided. The patient's vital signs, respiratory status, and oxygenation must be carefully monitored immediately after extubation, within 1 hour, and per institution policy. If the patient does not tolerate extubation, immediate reintubation or a trial of noninvasive ventilation may be necessary.

Chronic Mechanical Ventilation

Mechanical ventilators are no longer limited to the ICU but are now a part of long-term and home care. In some instances, terminally ill, ventilated patients may be discharged to hospice. The success of home mechanical ventilation depends, in part, on careful predischarge assessment and planning for both the patient and caregivers.

Both negative-pressure and positive-pressure ventilators are used in the home. Negative-pressure ventilators do not require an artificial airway and are less complicated to use. Several types of small, portable (battery-powered) positive-pressure ventilators are available and can be attached to a wheelchair or placed on a bedside table. Settings and alarms on these ventilators are simpler to use than on standard ICU ventilators.

Home mechanical ventilation has advantages and disadvantages. Having the patient in the home eliminates the strain that the hospital setting imposes on family dynamics. Caregivers' feelings of helplessness when they first hear about the necessity for long-term mechanical ventilation is frequently balanced by the opportunity to participate in the patient's care in the home setting. At home, the patient may be able to take part in more activities of daily living around an individualized schedule and, because of the smaller size of the home ventilator, be more mobile. Another advantage of home mechanical ventilation is the reduced risk for HAIs.

Disadvantages of home mechanical ventilation include problems related to equipment, reimbursement, caregiver stress and fatigue, and the patient's complex needs. Ventilated patients are usually dependent, requiring extensive nursing care, at least initially. Disposable products may not be reimbursable. Financial resources must be carefully assessed when arranging home mechanical ventilation. A meeting with the discharge team should be scheduled before a teaching plan for discharge is initiated.

Another disadvantage of home mechanical ventilation is its potential impact on the family. Caregivers may seem enthusiastic about caring for their loved one in the home but may be motivated by numerous, complex factors. They may not understand the sacrifices they may have to make financially and in personal time and commitment. Caregivers should be encouraged to consider respite care to periodically relieve their stress and fatigue.

NURSING MANAGEMENT
MECHANICAL VENTILATION

Nursing Care Plan (NCP) 68-1 for the patient receiving mechanical ventilation is available on the Evolve website for this chapter.

OTHER CRITICAL CARE CONTENT

Table 68-14 lists additional critical care content presented in other chapters of this book.

TABLE 68-14	CROSS-REFERENCES TO OTHER CRITICAL CARE CONTENT
Topic	**Discussed in Chapter**
Acute coronary syndrome	36
Acute heart failure	37
Acute respiratory distress syndrome	70
Acute respiratory failure	70
Burns	27
Cardiac dysrhythmias	38
Cardiac pacemakers	38
Cardiac surgery	36
Central venous access device	19
Continuous renal replacement therapy	49
Delirium	62
Emergencies	71
End-of-life care	13
Enteral nutrition	42
Head injury, including ICP monitoring	59
Multiple-organ dysfunction syndrome	69
Myocardial infarction	36
Oxygen delivery	31
Pain management	10
Pulmonary edema	37
Renal dialysis	49
Shock	69
Stroke	60
Systemic inflammatory response syndrome	69
Parenteral nutrition	42
Tracheostomy	29
Trauma	71

ICP, intracranial pressure.

CASE STUDY

Critical Care and Mechanical Ventilation

Source: Kulniz/Shutterstock.com.

Patient Profile

Richard Kincaid is a 72-year-old man who collapsed on the street. He was unresponsive on admission and remains in the same state. He has an oral ET tube in place and is receiving mechanical ventilation. He weighs 90 kg. A subclavian central line was placed to monitor CVP and administer fluids.

Subjective Data

None; patient is unresponsive to painful stimuli.

Objective Data
Physical Examination

- Noninvasive BP is 100/75 mm Hg; heart rate is 128 (atrial fibrillation with a rapid ventricular response); temperature is 38.8°C; SpO$_2$ is 98%.
- Purulent secretions from ET tube.
- Breath sounds: rhonchi bilaterally, decreased breath sounds on the right.

Diagnostic Studies

- Chest radiography reveals right lower lung consolidation.
- ABGs: pH 7.48; PaO$_2$: 94 mm Hg; PaCO$_2$: 30 mm Hg; bicarbonate (HCO$_3$) 34 mmol/L.
- Computed tomography (CT) scan is positive for massive cerebro-vascular accident.

Continued

CASE STUDY

Critical Care and Mechanical Ventilation—cont'd

Collaborative Care

- Positive-pressure ventilation settings: assist-control mode
- Settings: FiO_2 70%, V_T 700 mL, respiratory rate 16 breaths/min, PEEP 5 cm H_2O
- Enteral feeding at 25 mL/hr via small-bore feeding tube
- In-dwelling urinary catheter to bedside drainage
- HOB elevated at 40 degrees
- Position change every 2 hours
- Chest physical therapy performed every 2 to 4 hours
- Azithromycin (Zithromax) 500 mg intravenously q24h
- Cefotaxime (Claforan) 2 g intravenously q6h
- 5% dextrose in normal saline (D5NS) with potassium chloride (KCl) 20 mmol/L at 100 mL/hr

Discussion Questions

1. Identify two reasons for intubating and providing mechanical ventilation for Mr. Kincaid.
2. What do Mr. Kincaid's ABGs indicate, and which ventilator setting(s) should be changed?
3. What is his PaO_2/FiO_2 ratio and what does it signify?
4. Mr. Kincaid's BP drops to 80 mm Hg, and he remains in atrial fibrillation with a ventricular rate of 158. A PA catheter is inserted for further hemodynamic monitoring. What would be the purpose of hemodynamic monitoring (in addition to CVP monitoring) in this patient?

5. *Priority decision:* What are the two priority nursing considerations for a patient with a PA catheter?
6. Mr. Kincaid's initial PAOP is 14 mm Hg, CI is 2 L/min/m², and systemic vascular resistance index (SVRI) is 2667 dynes/sec/cm⁻⁵/m². How would the nurse interpret these values? What medical interventions would the nurse anticipate?
7. Mr. Kincaid's pulmonary condition deteriorates. PaO_2 drops to 70 mm Hg, and SpO_2 is 89%. PEEP is increased to 7.5 cm H_2O. What implications does this have for Mr. Kincaid given his hemodynamic status?
8. Based on the data presented, what are the actual and potential problems that the nurse can identify with this patient?
9. *Evidence-informed practice:* Mr. Kincaid's family wants to know why he is getting tube feedings. What should the nurse tell the family? What is the evidence to support the use of tube feedings?
10. After 4 days, Mr. Kincaid remains unresponsive and has developed renal failure. The physician believes the patient will not recover and wishes to discuss goals of care with the patient's caregiver. What would be the nurse's role in this meeting?

ⓔvolve
Answers are available at *http://evolve.elsevier.com/Canada/Lewis/medsurg*.

REVIEW QUESTIONS

The number of the question corresponds to the same-numbered objective at the beginning of the chapter.

1. What does a certification in critical care by the Canadian Nurses Association indicate?
   a. Has earned a master's degree in the field of providing advanced critical care nursing
   b. Is an advanced-practice nurse in the care of acutely ill clients
   c. May practise independently to provide symptom management for the critically ill
   d. Has practised in critical care and successfully completed a test of critical care knowledge

2. What are the appropriate nursing interventions for the client with delirium in the ICU? *(Select all that apply)*
   a. Use clocks and calendars to maintain orientation.
   b. Encourage round-the-clock presence of caregivers at the bedside.
   c. Sedate the client with appropriate drugs to protect the client from harmful behaviours.
   d. Silence all alarms, reduce overhead paging, and avoid conversations around the client.
   e. Identify physiological factors that may be contributing to the client's confusion and irritability.

3. What is the most ideal plan for family involvement in the ICU?
   a. Having a family member at the bedside at all times
   b. Allowing family at the bedside at brief intervals
   c. Devising an individual plan with family involved with care and comfort measures
   d. Restricting visitation in the ICU because the environment is overwhelming to visitors

4. In hemodynamic monitoring, what does zeroing refer to, and which one of the following does the nurse zero to?
   a. Cardiac output (CO) monitoring system to the level of the left ventricle
   b. Pressure monitoring system to the level of the catheter tip located in the client
   c. Pressure monitoring system to the level of the atrium, identified as the midaxillary line
   d. Pressure monitoring system to the level of the atrium, identified as the phlebostatic axis

5. What hemodynamic changes should the nurse expect to find after successful initiation of intra-aortic balloon pump use in a client in cardiogenic shock?
   a. Decreased wedge and increased CO
   b. Decreased systemic vascular resistance and decreased stroke volume
   c. Increased diastolic blood pressure (BP) and decreased systolic BP
   d. Decreased central venous pressure and increased right atrial pressure

6. What nursing management should be included for the client with an artificial airway?
   a. Routine suctioning of the tube at least every 2 hours
   b. Observing for cardiac dysrhythmias during suctioning
   c. Maintaining endotracheal tube cuff pressure at 30 cm H_2O
   d. Preventing tube dislodgement by limiting mouth care to lubrication of the lips

7. What is the purpose of adding positive end-expiratory pressure to positive-pressure ventilation?
   a. To increase functional residual capacity and improve oxygenation
   b. To increase fraction of inspired oxygen in an attempt to wean the client and avoid oxygen toxicity
   c. To determine whether the client is able to be weaned and avoid the risk of pneumomediastinum
   d. To determine whether the client is in synchrony with the ventilator or needs to be paralyzed
8. For what should the nurse monitor the client with positive-pressure mechanical ventilation?
   a. Paralytic ileus because pressure on the abdominal contents affects bowel motility
   b. Diuresis and sodium depletion because of increased release of atrial natriuretic peptide

   c. Signs of cardiovascular insufficiency because pressure in the chest impedes venous return
   d. Respiratory acidosis in a client with chronic obstructive pulmonary disease because of alveolar hyperventilation and increased arterial partial pressure of oxygen levels

1. d; 2. a, c; 3. c; 4. d; 5. a; 6. b; 7. a; 8. c.

🅔volve

For even more review questions, visit *http://evolve.elsevier.com/Canada/Lewis/medsurg.*

REFERENCES

Alberta Health Services. (2016). *Alberta's strategic clinical networks: Orientation program for adult critical care in Alberta (OPACCA).* Retrieved from *http://www.albertahealthservices.ca/assets/about/scn/ahs-scn-sb-cc-opacca.pdf.*

Ali, S., & Ferguson, M. (2011). High frequency oscillatory ventilation in ALI/ARDS. *Critical Care Clinics, 27,* 487.

Barr, J., Fraser, G. L., Puntillo, K., et al. (2013). Clinical practice guidelines for management of pain, agitation and delirium in adult patients in the intensive care unit. *Critical Care Medicine, 41*(1), 263–306. doi:10.1097/CCM.0b013e3182783b72.

Burns, S. M. (2011a). Invasive mechanical ventilation: Volume and pressure modes. In D. L. Wiegand (Ed.), *AACN procedure manual for critical care* (6th ed., pp. 262–284). St. Louis: Elsevier.

Burns, S. M. (2011b). Noninvasive positive pressure ventilation: Continuous positive airway pressure (CPAP) and bilevel positive airway pressure (BiPap). In D. L. Wiegand (Ed.), *AACN procedure manual for critical care* (6th ed., pp. 225–234). St. Louis: Elsevier.

Burns, S. M. (2011c). Weaning process. In D. L. Wiegand (Ed.), *AACN procedure manual for critical care* (6th ed., pp. 291–302). St. Louis: Elsevier.

Canadian Association of Critical Care Nurses (CACCN). (2011). *Providing end of life care in the ICU.* Retrieved from *http://www.caccn.ca/en/publications/position_statements/providing_end_of_life_care_in_the_icu.html.*

Canadian Association of Critical Care Nurses (CACCN). (2017). *Philosophy statement.* Retrieved from *https://www.caccn.ca/en/about/caccn_philosophy_statement.html.*

Canadian Institute for Health Information. (2017). *CORR annual report: Treatment of end-stage organ failure in Canada, 2004 to 2013.* Retrieved from *https://www.cihi.ca/en/types-of-care/specialized-services/organ-replacements/report-page-corr-2015.*

Canadian Patient Safety Institute. (2016). *Latest updates to the Canadian VAP guidelines.* Retrieved from *http://www.patientsafetyinstitute.ca/en/toolsResources/Presentations/2014Webinars/Pages/Latest-Updates-to-the-Canadian-VAP-Guidelines—What's-New.aspx.*

Castellucci, D. (2011). Intraaortic balloon pump management. In D. L. Wiegand (Ed.), *AACN procedure manual for critical care* (6th ed., pp. 443–463). St. Louis: Elsevier.

Chlan, L. L., Weinert, C. R., Heiderscheit, A., et al. (2013). Effects of patient-directed music intervention on anxiety and sedative exposure in critically ill patients receiving mechanical-ventilatory support: A randomized clinical trial. *Journal of the American Medical Association, 309*(22), 2335–2344.

Combes, A., Brodie, D., Bartlett, R., et al. (2014). Position paper for the organization of extracorporeal membrane oxygenation programs for acute respiratory failure in adult patients. *American Journal of Respiratory and Critical Care Medicine, 190*(5), 488–496. doi:10.1164/rccm.201404-0630CP.

Darbyshire, J., & Young, J. (2013). An investigation of sound levels on intensive care with reference to the WHO guidelines. *Critical Care: The Official Journal of the Critical Care Forum, 17*(5), R187. doi:10.1186/cc12870.

Davidson, J. (2016 in press). Family-centered care in the ICU. In *International best practices for critical care.* New York: Springer Publishing.

Delaney, L., Van Haren, F., & Lopez, V. (2015). Sleeping on a problem: The impact of sleep disturbance on ICU patients—A clinical review. *Annals of Intensive Care, 5,* 3. doi:10.1186/s13613-015-0043-2.

Desai, S., Law, T., & Needham, D. (2011). Long-term complications of critical care. *Critical Care Medicine, 39*(2), 371–379. doi:10.1097/CCM.0b013e3181fd66e5.

Edwards Lifesciences. (2006). *Edwards FloTrac Sensor and Edwards Vigileo Monitor: Understanding stroke volume variation and its clinical application.* Retrieved from *http://ht.edwards.com/presentationvideos/powerpointslides/strokevolumevar/strokevolumevariation.pdf.* (Seminal).

Georgiou, E., Hadjibalassi, M., Lambrinou, E., et al. (2015). The impact of pain assessment on critically ill patient outcomes: A systematic review. *BioMed Research International.* doi:10.1155/2015/503830.

Goldsworthy, S., & Graham, L. (2014). *Compact clinical guide to mechanical ventilation: Foundations of practice for critical care nurses.* New York: Springer Publishing.

Henderson, W. R., Griesdale, D. E., Dominelli, P., et al. (2014). Does prone positioning improve oxygenation and reduce mortality in patients with acute respiratory distress syndrome? *Canadian Respiratory Journal, 21*(4), 213–215.

Kern, M. (2011). Arterial pressure-based cardiac output monitoring. In D. L. Wiegand (Ed.), *AACN procedure manual for critical care* (6th ed., pp. 548–554). St. Louis: Elsevier.

Lorente, L., Lecuona, M., Jiménez, A., et al. (2014). Continuous endotracheal tub cuff pressure control system protects against ventilator-associated pneumonia. *Critical Care: The Official Journal of the Critical Care Forum, 18*(2), R77. doi:10.1186/cc13837.

Maharaj, R., Raffaele, I., & Wendon, J. (2015). Rapid response systems: A systematic review and meta-analysis. *Critical Care: The Official Journal of the Critical Care Forum, 19*, 254. doi:10.1186/s13054-015-0973-y.

McClave, S. A., Taylor, B. E., Martindale, R. G., et al. (2016). Guidelines for the provision and assessment of nutrition support therapy in the adult critically ill patient: Society of Critical Care Medicine (SCCM) and American Society for Parenteral and Enteral Nutrition (A.S.P.E.N.). *Journal of Parenteral and Enteral Nutrition, 40*(2), 159–211.

Mehta, S., Cook, D., Devlin, J. W., et al. (2015). Prevalence, risk factors, and outcomes of delirium in mechanically ventilated adults. *Critical Care Medicine, 43*(3), 557–566. doi:10.1097/CCM.0000000000000727.

Oczkowski, S. J., Mazzetti, I., Cupido, C., et al. (2015). Family presence during resuscitation: A Canadian Critical Care position paper. *Canadian Respiratory Journal, 22*(4), 201–205.

Plummer, M. P., Blaser, A. R., & Deane, A. M. (2014). Stress ulceration: Prevalence, pathology and association with adverse outcomes. *Critical Care: The Official Journal of the Critical Care Forum, 18*(2), 213. doi:10.1186/cc13780.

Prin, M., & Wunsch, H. (2014). The role of stepdown beds in hospital care. *American Journal of Respiratory and Critical Care Medicine, 190*(11), 1210–1216. doi:10.1164/rccm.201406-1117PP.

Puhlman, M., & Fleck, D. A. (2011). Ventricular assist devices. In D. L. Wiegand (Ed.), *AACN procedure manual for critical care* (6th ed., pp. 464–489). St. Louis: Elsevier.

Safer Healthcare Now! (2012). *Prevent ventilator associated pneumonia: Getting started kit.* Retrieved from *http://www.patientsafetyinstitute.ca/en/toolsResources/Documents/Interventions/Ventilator-Associated%20Pneumonia/VAP%20Getting%20Started%20Kit.pdf*.

Seckel, M. A. (2017). Suctioning: Endotracheal or tracheostomy tube. In D. L. Wiegand (Ed.), *AACN procedure manual for critical care* (7th ed.). St. Louis: Elsevier.

Shaffer, R. B. (2011). Arterial catheter insertion (assist), care, and removal. In D. L. Wiegand (Ed.), *AACN procedure manual for critical care* (6th ed., pp. 534–547). St. Louis: Elsevier.

Sole, M. L., Su, X., Talbert, S., et al. (2011). Evaluation of an intervention to maintain endotracheal cuff pressure within therapeutic range. *American Journal of Critical Care, 20*(2), 109–117. doi:10.4037/ajcc2011661.

Stollings, J. L., Diedrich, D. A., Oyen, L. J., et al. (2014). Rapid-sequence intubation: A review of the process and considerations when choosing medications. *Annals of Pharmacotherapy, 48*(1), 62–76. doi:10.1177/1060028013510488.

Villwock, J. A., & Jones, K. (2014). Outcomes of early versus late tracheostomy: 2008–2010. *The Laryngoscope, 124*(8), 1801–1806. doi:10.1002/lary.24702.

Wade, D., Hardy, R., Howell, D., et al. (2013). Identifying clinical and acute psychological risk factors for PTSD after critical care: A systematic review. *Minerva Anestesiologica, 79*(8), 944–963.

Walsh, B., Crotwell, D., & Restrepo, R. (2011). Capnography/capnometry during mechanical ventilation: 2011. *Respiratory Care, 56*(4), 503–509. doi:10.4187/respcare.01175.

RESOURCES

Canadian Association of Critical Care Nurses (CACCN)
http://www.caccn.ca

Canadian Critical Care Society
http://www.canadiancriticalcare.org

Canadian Patient Safety Institute: Safer Healthcare Now!
http://www.patientsafetyinstitute.ca/en/About/Programs/SHN/Pages/default.aspx

American Association of Critical-Care Nurses (AACN)
http://www.aacn.org

Australian College of Critical Care Nurses (ACCCN)
http://www.acccn.com.au

Confusion Assessment Method for the ICU (CAM–ICU)
https://consultgeri.org/try-this/general-assessment/issue-25.pdf

ICU Delirium and Cognitive Impairment Study Group
http://www.icudelirium.org/delirium/monitoring.html

Intensive Care Delirium Screening Checklist (ICDSC)
http://www.lhsc.on.ca/Health_Professionals/CCTC/elearning/bedside_sheets_CCTC_icdsc.pdf

Society of Critical Care Medicine (SCCM)
http://www.sccm.org

World Federation of Critical Care Nurses (WFCCN)
http://wfccn.org

For additional Internet resources, see the website for this book at *http://evolve.elsevier.com/Canada/Lewis/medsurg*.

Nursing Management
Shock, Systemic Inflammatory Response Syndrome, and Multiple-Organ Dysfunction Syndrome

Written by: Maureen A. Seckel
Adapted by: Janet A. Piper

evolve WEBSITE

http://evolve.elsevier.com/Canada/Lewis/medsurg

- Review Questions (Online Only)
- Key Points
- Answer Guidelines for Case Study

- Student Case Studies
  - Cardiogenic Shock
  - Sepsis
  - Acute Pancreatitis and Septic Shock

- Customizable Nursing Care Plan
  - Shock
- Conceptual Care Map Creator
- Audio Glossary
- Content Updates

LEARNING OBJECTIVES

1. Relate the pathophysiology to the clinical manifestations of the different types of shock: cardiogenic, hypovolemic, distributive, and obstructive.
2. Compare the effects of shock, systemic inflammatory response syndrome (SIRS), and multiple-organ dysfunction syndrome (MODS) on the major body systems.

3. Compare the collaborative care, drug therapy, and nursing management of patients experiencing different types of shock.
4. Describe the nursing management of a patient experiencing multiple-organ dysfunction syndrome (MODS).

KEY TERMS

anaphylactic shock, p. 1764
cardiogenic shock, p. 1760
hypovolemic shock, p. 1760
multiple-organ dysfunction syndrome (MODS), p. 1777
neurogenic shock, p. 1763

sepsis, p. 1764
septic shock, p. 1764
severe sepsis, p. 1764
shock, p. 1759
systemic inflammatory response syndrome (SIRS), p. 1777

Shock, systemic inflammatory response syndrome (SIRS), and multiple-organ dysfunction syndrome (MODS) are serious and interrelated problems. Figure 69-1 shows the relationship of how shock can lead to the development of SIRS and then MODS. This chapter provides an overview and related management of shock, SIRS, and MODS.

SHOCK

Shock is a syndrome characterized by decreased tissue perfusion and impaired cellular metabolism. This condition results in an imbalance between the supply of and the demand for oxygen and nutrients. The exchange of oxygen and nutrients at the cellular level is essential for life. When cells experience hypoperfusion, the demand for oxygen and nutrients exceeds the supply at the microcirculatory level.

Classification of Shock

Although the cause, the initial presentation, and the management strategies of the various types of shock differ, the physiological responses of the cell to hypoperfusion are similar. Shock may be classified as *low flow*—cardiogenic and hypovolemic

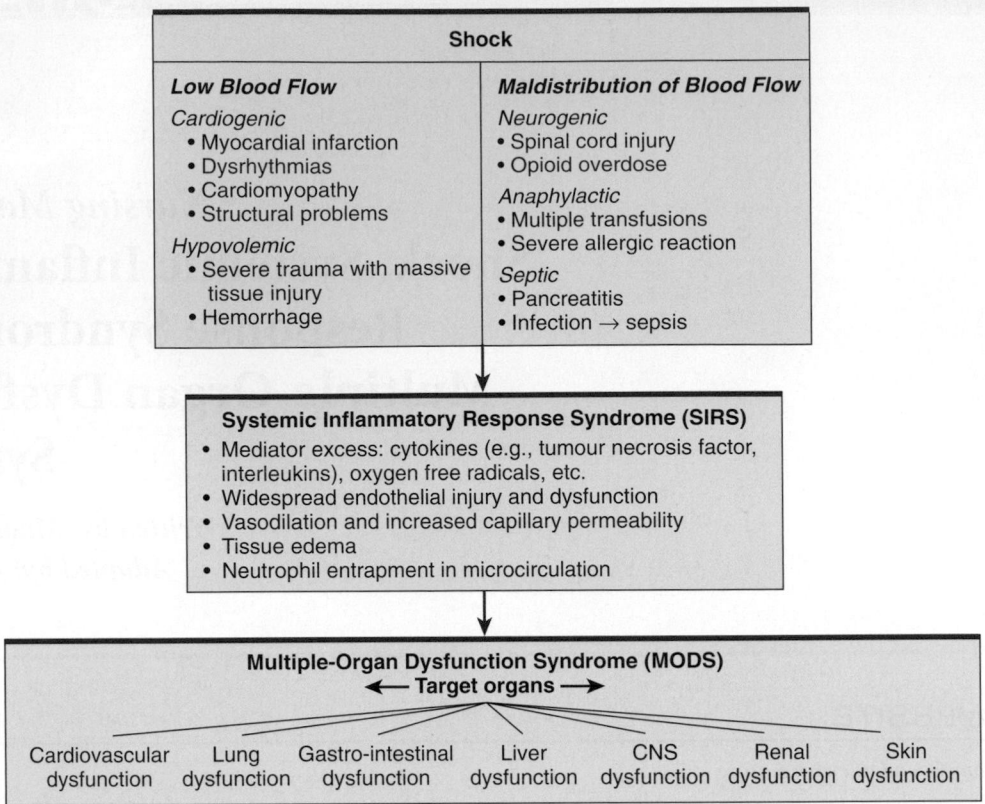

FIGURE 69-1 Relationship of shock, systemic inflammatory response syndrome, and multiple-organ dysfunction syndrome. *CNS,* central nervous system.

shock—or *distributive*—neurogenic, anaphylactic, and septic shock (Lawrence, 2011). Classification details are listed in Table 69-1.

Shock Caused by Low Blood Flow

Cardiogenic Shock. Cardiogenic shock occurs when either systolic or diastolic dysfunction of the pumping action of the heart results in compromised cardiac output (CO). Causes of cardiogenic shock are listed in Table 69-1. Mortality rates for patients with cardiogenic shock approach 60% (Patel & Hollenberg, 2011).

The heart's inability to pump the blood forward is classified as *systolic dysfunction*. Systolic dysfunction affects primarily the left ventricle because systolic pressure and tension are greater in the left chambers of the heart. When systolic dysfunction affects the right chambers of the heart, blood flow through the pulmonary circulation is compromised. Extensive left ventricular infarction and subsequent ventricular failure account for more than 75% of all cases of cardiogenic shock, and the prognosis is extremely poor. *Diastolic dysfunction* impairs the ability of the right or left ventricle to fill during diastole. Decreased filling of the ventricle results in decreased stroke volume (McAtee, 2011).

Figure 69-2 describes the pathophysiology of cardiogenic shock. Whether the initiating event is myocardial dysfunction, a structural problem (e.g., valvular abnormality, ventricular septal rupture, tension pneumothorax), or dysrhythmias, the physiological responses are similar—both tissue perfusion and cellular metabolism are impaired.

The early clinical presentation of cardiogenic shock is similar to that of a patient with acute decompensated heart failure (see Chapter 37). An increase in systemic vascular resistance (SVR) increases the workload of the heart, thus increasing the myocardial

oxygen consumption. The heart's inability to pump blood forward results in low CO (<4 L/min) and low cardiac index (<2.1 L/min/m²). On examination, the patient may exhibit tachycardia, hypotension, and narrowed pulse pressure. Pulmonary congestion may be present, as evidenced by tachypnea and lung crackles. The hemodynamic profile demonstrates increases in the pulmonary artery occlusive (or wedge) pressure (PAOP) and pulmonary vascular resistance (Table 69-2). Signs of peripheral hypoperfusion (e.g., cyanosis, pallor, cool and clammy skin, decreased capillary refill time) are apparent. Decreased renal blood flow results in sodium and water retention and decreased urine output. Anxiety, confusion, and agitation may develop as cerebral perfusion is impaired. Diagnostic workup for cardiogenic shock will include laboratory studies, electrocardiography (ECG), chest radiography, and echocardiography (Table 69-3). The overall clinical presentation of a patient with cardiogenic shock is described in Table 69-4.

Hypovolemic Shock. Hypovolemic shock occurs when intravascular fluid volume is lost and the remaining volume is inadequate to fill the vascular space. The volume loss may be either an absolute or a relative volume loss. *Absolute hypovolemia* results when fluid is lost through hemorrhage, gastro-intestinal (GI) loss (e.g., through vomiting, diarrhea), fistula drainage, diabetes insipidus, hyperglycemia, or diuresis. *Relative hypovolemia* develops when fluid volume moves out of the vascular space into the extravascular space (e.g., interstitial or intracavitary space). This type of fluid shift is called *third spacing*. One mechanism of relative volume loss is leakage of fluid from the vascular space to the interstitial space from increased capillary permeability, as occurs in sepsis or burns (see Chapter 27). Table 69-1 provides other examples of hypovolemic shock.

TABLE 69-1 CLASSIFICATION OF SHOCK STATES

Types and Causes	Examples
Cardiogenic Shock	
Diastolic dysfunction: inability of the heart to fill	Cardiac tamponade, ventricular hypertrophy, cardiomyopathy
Dysrhythmias	Bradydysrhythmias, tachydysrhythmias
Structural factors	Valvular stenosis or regurgitation, ventricular septal rupture, tension pneumothorax
Systolic dysfunction: inability of the heart to pump blood forward	Myocardial infarction, cardiomyopathy, blunt cardiac injury, severe systemic or pulmonary hypertension, myocardial depression from metabolic problems
Hypovolemic Shock	
Absolute Hypovolemia	
External loss of whole blood	Hemorrhage from trauma, surgery, gastro-intestinal bleeding
Loss of other body fluids	Vomiting, diarrhea, excessive diuresis, diabetes insipidus, diabetes mellitus
Relative Hypovolemia	
Fluid shifts	Burn injuries, ascites
Internal bleeding	Fracture of long bones, ruptured spleen, hemothorax, severe pancreatitis
Massive vasodilation	Sepsis
Pooling of blood or fluids	Bowel obstruction
Distributive Shock	
Neurogenic Shock	
Hemodynamic consequence of spinal cord injury or disease at or above T5	Severe pain, drugs, hypoglycemia, injury
Spinal anaesthesia	
Vasomotor centre depression	
Anaphylactic Shock	
Hypersensitivity (allergic) reaction to a sensitizing substance	Contrast media, blood or blood products, drugs, insect bites, anaesthetic agents, food or food additives, vaccines, environmental agents, latex
Septic Shock	
At-risk patients	Older adults, patients with chronic diseases (e.g., diabetes mellitus, chronic kidney disease, heart failure), patients receiving immuno-suppressive therapy or who are malnourished or debilitated
Infection	Pneumonia, peritonitis, urinary tract, invasive procedures, indwelling lines and catheters

In hypovolemic shock, the size of the vascular compartment remains unchanged, but the volume of blood or plasma decreases. Whether the loss of intravascular volume is absolute or relative, the physiological consequences are similar. A reduction in intravascular volume results in a decreased venous return to the heart, decreased preload, decreased stroke volume, and decreased CO (see Table 69-2). A cascade of events results in decreased

PATHOPHYSIOLOGY MAP

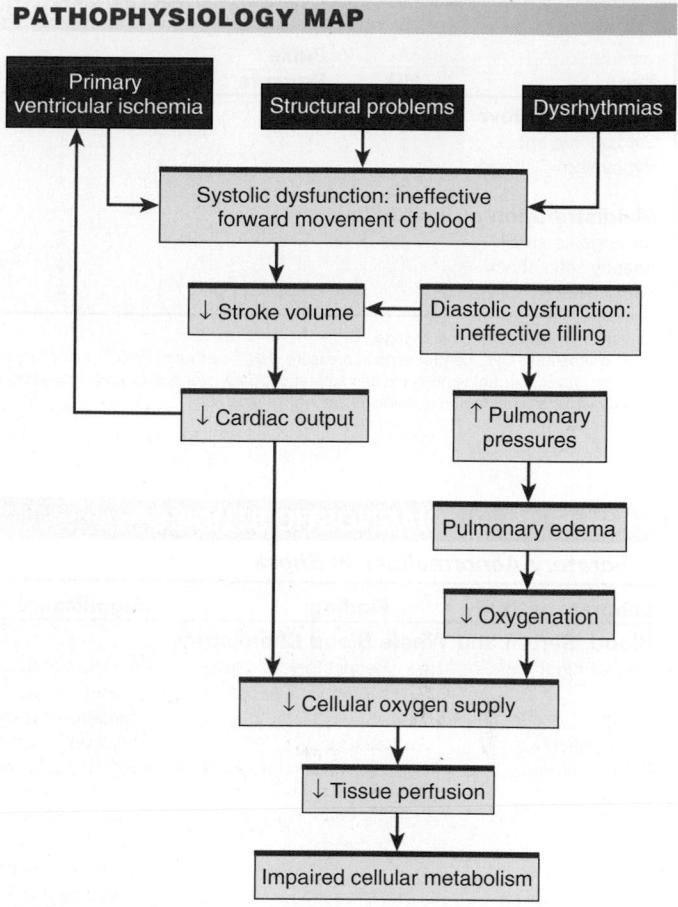

FIGURE 69-2 The pathophysiology of cardiogenic shock. Source: Urden, L. D., Stacy, K. M., & Lough, M. E. (2010). *Critical care nursing: Diagnosis and management* (6th ed., p. 984, Figure 39-2). St. Louis: Mosby.

tissue perfusion and impaired cellular metabolism, the hallmarks of shock (Figure 69-3).

The patient's response to low blood flow as a result of acute volume loss is dependent on a number of factors, including the extent of the injury or insult, the patient's age, and the patient's general state of health; however, the clinical presentations of hypovolemic shock are similar (see Table 69-4). An overall assessment of physiological reserves may indicate the patient's ability to compensate. A patient may compensate for a loss of up to 15% of the total blood volume (approximately 750 mL). Further loss of volume (15% to 30%) results in a sympathetic nervous system (SNS)–mediated response. This response results in increases in heart rate, CO, and respiratory rate and depth. The stroke volume and PAOP are decreased because of the decreased circulating blood volume.

The patient may appear anxious, and urine output begins to decrease. If hypovolemia is corrected by crystalloid fluid replacement at this time, tissue dysfunction is generally reversible. If volume loss is greater than 30%, compensatory mechanisms may begin to fail, and replacement with blood or blood products should be initiated immediately. With loss of more than 40% of the total blood volume, autoregulation in the microcirculation is lost, and irreversible tissue destruction occurs (Hall, 2016). Laboratory studies that may be helpful include serial measurements of hemoglobin and hematocrit levels, urine specific gravity, serum electrolytes, blood gases, and lactic acid (see Table 69-3).

TABLE 69-2 EFFECTS OF SHOCK ON HEMODYNAMIC PARAMETERS*

Type	HR	Pulse Pressure	BP	SVR	PVR	CVP	PAP	PAOP	CO	$S_vO_2/S_{cv}O_2$
Low Blood Flow										
Cardiogenic shock	↑	↓	↓	↑	↑	≈, ↑	↑	↑	↓	↓
Hypovolemic shock	↑	↓	↓	↑	↑	↓	↓	↓	↓	↓
Maldistribution of Blood Flow										
Neurogenic shock	↓	↓	↓	↓	≈	↓	↓	↓	↓	↓
Anaphylactic shock	↑	↓	↓	↓	≈, ↑	↓	↓	↓	↓	↓
Septic shock	↑	↓	↓	↓	≈, ↑	↓	↑, ≈, ↓	↓	↑, ≈, ↓	↑, ≈, ↓

↓, decrease; ↑, increase; ≈, no change.
BP, blood pressure; *CVP*, central venous pressure; *HR*, heart rate; *PAOP*, pulmonary artery occlusive pressure; *PAP*, pulmonary artery pressure; *PVR*, pulmonary vascular resistance; *ScvO₂*, central venous oxygen saturation; *SvO₂*, venous oxygen saturation; *SVR*, systemic vascular resistance.
*Hemodynamic effects in some illnesses are highly variable.

TABLE 69-3 DIAGNOSTIC STUDIES

Laboratory Abnormalities in Shock

Laboratory Study	Finding	Significance of Finding
Blood, Serum and Whole Blood Chemistries		
Arterial blood gases	Respiratory alkalosis	In early shock, occurs secondary to hyperventilation
	Metabolic acidosis	In later shock, occurs when organic acids, such as lactic acid, accumulate in blood as a result of anaerobic metabolism
Base deficit	≥6	Indicates acid production secondary to hypoxia
Blood cultures	Growth of organisms	May occur in patients who are in septic shock
BUN	Increased	Indicates impaired kidney function as a result of hypoperfusion caused by severe vasoconstriction, or occurs secondary to catabolism of cells (e.g., in trauma, infection)
Creatinine	Increased	Indicates impaired kidney function as a result of hypoperfusion caused by severe vasoconstriction; is more sensitive indicator of renal function than BUN
Creatine kinase	Increased	In trauma and MI, increases in response to cellular damage or hypoxia
DIC screen		Acute DIC can develop within hours to days after an initial assault on the body (e.g., shock)
D-dimer	Increased	
Fibrin split products	Increased	
Fibrinogen level	Decreased	
Platelet count	Decreased	
PTT and INR	Prolonged	
Thrombin time	Increased	
Glucose	Increased	In early shock, increases because of release of liver glycogen stores in response to SNS stimulation and cortisol; insulin insensitivity develops
	Decreased	Decreases because of depleted glycogen stores, with hepatocellular dysfunction as shock progresses
Lactic acid	Increased	Usually increases once significant hypoperfusion and impaired oxygen use at the cellular level have occurred; by-product of anaerobic metabolism
Liver enzymes (ALT, AST, GGT)	Increased	Elevations indicate liver cell destruction in progressive stage of shock
Potassium	Increased	Increases when cellular death liberates intracellular potassium; in AKI; and in the presence of acidosis
	Decreased	In early shock, decreases because of increased secretion of aldosterone, which causes renal excretion of potassium
RBC count, hematocrit, hemoglobin	Normal	Remains within normal limits (a) in shock because of relative hypovolemia and pump failure and (b) in hemorrhagic shock before fluid resuscitation
	Decreased	In hemorrhagic shock, decreases after fluid resuscitation when fluids other than blood are used
	Increased	In nonhemorrhagic shock, increases as a result of actual hypovolemia because fluid lost does not contain erythrocytes
Sodium	Increased	In early shock, increases because of increased secretion of aldosterone, causing renal retention of sodium
	Decreased	May occur iatrogenically when excessive hypotonic fluid is administered after fluid loss
Troponin	Increased	In MI
Urine		
Specific gravity	Increased	Occurs secondary to the action of ADH
	Fixed at 1.010	Occurs in renal failure

ADH, antidiuretic hormone; *AKI*, acute kidney injury; *ALT*, alanine aminotransferase; *AST*, aspartate aminotransferase; *BUN*, blood urea nitrogen; *DIC*, disseminated intravascular coagulation; *GGT*, γ-glutamyl transferase; *INR*, international normalized ratio; *MI*, myocardial infarction; *PTT*, partial thromboplastin time; *RBC*, red blood cell; *SNS*, sympathetic nervous system.

TABLE 69-4 CLINICAL PRESENTATION IN THE MAJOR TYPES OF SHOCK

Low Blood Flow		Maldistribution of Blood Flow		
Cardiogenic Shock	**Hypovolemic Shock**	**Neurogenic Shock**	**Anaphylactic Shock**	**Septic Shock**
Cardiovascular System (see Table 69-2 for complete hemodynamic profile)				
↓ Capillary refill time Chest pain may or may not be present ↑ MVO₂	↓ Capillary refill time ↓ Preload ↓ Stroke volume	Bradycardia ↓ or ↑ Temperature	Chest pain Third spacing of fluid	Biventricular dilation: ↓ ejection fraction ↓ or ↑ Temperature
Gastro-Intestinal System				
↓ Bowel sounds Nausea and vomiting	Absence of bowel sounds	Bowel dysfunction	Abdominal pain Cramping Diarrhea Nausea Vomiting	GI bleeding Paralytic ileus
Neurological System				
↓ Cerebral perfusion: anxiety, confusion, agitation	Agitation Anxiety Confusion	Flaccid paralysis below level of lesion Loss of reflex activity	Anxiety Confusion ↓ LOC Metallic taste Sensation of impending doom	Agitation Alteration in mental status (e.g., confusion) Coma (late)
Pulmonary System				
Crackles Cyanosis Tachypnea Wheezes	Tachypnea, progressing to bradypnea (late)	Dysfunction related to level of injury	Edema of larynx and epiglottis Rhinitis Shortness of breath Stridor Swelling of lips and tongue Wheezing	ARDS Crackles Hyperventilation Hypoxemia Pulmonary hypertension Respiratory alkalosis, progressing to respiratory acidosis Respiratory failure
Renal System				
↑ Na⁺ and H₂O retention ↓ Renal blood flow ↓ Urine output	↓ Urine output	Bladder dysfunction		↓ Urine output
Skin				
Cool, clammy Pallor	Cool, clammy Pallor	Cool or warm Dry ↓ Skin perfusion	Angioedema Flushing Pruritus Urticaria	Warm and flushed (early), becoming cool and mottled (late)
Other Diagnostic Findings (also see Table 69-3)				
↑ Blood glucose ↑ BUN ↑ Cardiac markers Chest radiographic (e.g., pulmonary infiltrates) Echocardiographic (e.g., left ventricular dysfunction) Electrocardiographic (e.g., dysrhythmias)	↓ Hematocrit ↓ Hemoglobin ↑ Lactate ↑ Urine specific gravity Changes in electrolytes		History of allergies History of exposure to contrast media Sudden onset	↑ Glucose ↑ Lactate ↓ Platelets Positive blood cultures ↓ Urine Na⁺ ↑ Urine specific gravity ↑ or ↓ WBC count

ARDS, acute respiratory distress syndrome; *BUN*, blood urea nitrogen; *GI*, gastro-intestinal; *LOC*, level of consciousness; *MVO₂*, myocardial oxygen consumption; *WBC*, white blood cell.

Distributive Shock: Shock Caused by Maldistribution of Blood Flow

Neurogenic Shock. Neurogenic shock is a hemodynamic phenomenon that can occur within 30 minutes of a spinal cord injury at the fifth thoracic (T5) vertebra or above and lasts up to 6 weeks. The injury results in a massive vasodilation without compensation that is caused by the loss of SNS vasoconstrictor tone. This massive vasodilation leads to a pooling of blood in the blood vessels, tissue hypoperfusion, and, ultimately, impairment of cellular metabolism (Figure 69-4).

In addition to spinal cord injury, spinal anaesthesia can block transmission of impulses from the SNS. Depression of the vasomotor centre of the medulla from drugs (e.g., benzodiazepines, opioids) also can result in decreased vasoconstrictor tone of the peripheral blood vessels, which leads to neurogenic shock (see Table 69-1).

PATHOPHYSIOLOGY MAP

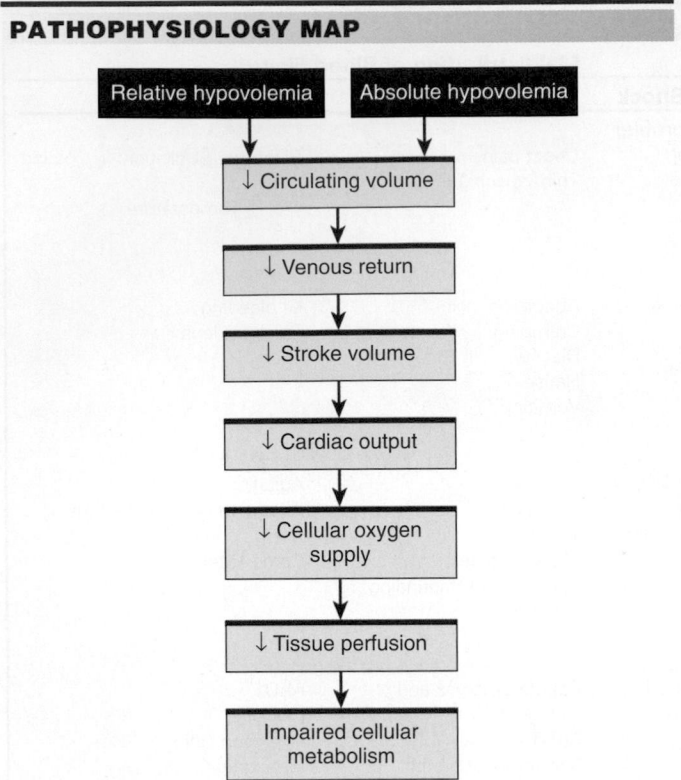

FIGURE 69-3 The pathophysiology of hypovolemic shock. Source: Urden, L. D., Stacy, K. M., & Lough, M. E. (2010). *Critical care nursing: Diagnosis and management* (6th ed., p. 982, Figure 39-1). St. Louis: Mosby.

PATHOPHYSIOLOGY MAP

FIGURE 69-4 The pathophysiology of neurogenic shock. *BP,* blood pressure. Source: Urden, L. D., Stacy, K. M., & Lough, M. E. (2010). *Critical care nursing: Diagnosis and management* (6th ed., p. 990, Figure 39-4). St. Louis: Mosby.

Classic clinical manifestations in neurogenic shock are hypotension (from the massive vasodilation) and bradycardia (from unopposed parasympathetic stimulation) (Casha & Christie, 2011). A patient in neurogenic shock may be unable to regulate temperature, and in combination with massive vasodilation, severe heat loss can result. Initially, the patient's skin is warm as a result of the massive dilation without compensation. As the heat dissipates, the risk for hypothermia escalates. Later, the patient's skin may be cool or warm, depending on the ambient temperature (*poikilothermia,* the taking on of the temperature of the environment). In either case, the skin is usually dry. Tables 69-2, 69-3, and 69-4 further describe the clinical presentation of a patient with neurogenic shock.

Although spinal shock and neurogenic shock often occur in the same patient, they are not the same disorder. *Spinal shock* is a transient condition that is present after an acute spinal cord injury (see Chapter 63). A patient with spinal shock experiences the absence of all voluntary and reflex neurological activity below the level of the injury (Casha & Christie, 2011).

Anaphylactic Shock. Anaphylactic shock is an acute, life-threatening hypersensitivity (allergic) reaction to a sensitizing substance (e.g., drug, chemical, vaccine, food, insect venom). Usually an immediate reaction causes massive vasodilation, release of vasoactive mediators, and an increase in capillary permeability. As capillary permeability increases, fluid leaks from the vascular space into the interstitial space. Anaphylactic shock can lead to airway swelling (pharyngeal and laryngeal edema, stridor, hoarse voice), breathing problems (shortness of breath, increased respirations, fatigue, confusion as a result of hypoxia), and circulation problems (hypotension; tachycardia; pale, clammy skin; faintness;

and even loss of consciousness). The patient becomes anxious and experiences a sense of impending doom. Without prompt treatment, respiratory or cardiac arrest may develop.

A patient can develop a severe allergic reaction, which possibly leads to anaphylactic shock, after contact, inhalation, ingestion, or injection of an antigen (allergen) to which the person has previously been sensitized (see Table 69-1). Parenteral administration of the antigen (allergen) is the route most likely to cause anaphylaxis; however, oral, topical, and inhalation routes can also cause anaphylactic reactions. Tables 69-2, 69-3, and 69-4 describe the clinical presentation of anaphylactic shock. Quick and decisive action by the nurse is crucial for preventing the progression of an anaphylactic reaction to anaphylactic shock. (Anaphylaxis is discussed in Chapter 16.)

Septic Shock. Sepsis is a systemic inflammatory response to a documented or suspected infection. Severe sepsis is defined as sepsis complicated by organ dysfunction, hypoperfusion, or hypotension. Septic shock develops when hypotension cannot be reversed with fluid resuscitation and tissue perfusion abnormalities are present (Dellinger, Levy, Rhodes, et al., 2013). Recent statistics indicate that, in 2011, 1 in 18 deaths involved sepsis, and it was the 12th leading cause of all deaths in Canada (Navaneelan, Alam, Peters, et al., 2016).

PATHOPHYSIOLOGY MAP

FIGURE 69-5 The pathophysiology of septic shock. *CNS,* central nervous system. Source: Urden, L. D., Stacy, K. M., & Lough, M. E. (2010). *Critical care nursing: Diagnosis and management* (6th ed., p. 992, Figure 39-5). St. Louis: Mosby.

In Canada, mortality rates in the period 2008 to 2009 were 30% among patients with sepsis, 45.2% among patients with severe sepsis, and 20.9% among patients in whom sepsis did not worsen from the initial state (Canadian Institute for Health Information [CIHI], 2009). In as many as 30% of patients with sepsis, the causative organism is not identified (CIHI, 2009). The primary organisms that do cause sepsis are Gram-negative and Gram-positive bacteria. The morbidity and mortality rates from infections with Gram-negative organisms are higher than those with Gram-positive organisms. Parasites, fungi, and viruses can also lead to the development of sepsis and septic shock (CIHI, 2009). The pathogenesis of septic shock is complex (Figure 69-5).

When an antigen (microorganism) enters the body, the normal immune or inflammatory cascade responses are initiated and work together to destroy the antigen; however, in severe sepsis and septic shock, the response initiated by the body to an antigen is exaggerated. Inflammation and coagulation are increased, and fibrinolysis is decreased. Endotoxins from the microorganism cell wall stimulate the release of cytokines, including tumour necrosis factor (TNF) and interleukin-1 (IL-1), as well as other proinflammatory mediators that act through secondary mediators such as platelet-activating factor XII and interleukin-6 (Fry, 2012). (See Chapter 14 for a discussion of the inflammatory response.) The release of platelet-activating factor XII results in the formation of microthrombi and obstruction of the microvasculature. The combined effects of the mediators result in damage to the endothelium due to neutrophils and aggregated platelets adhering to the endothelium (Lawrence, 2011). With increased capillary permeability to fluid, the intravascular volume leaks into the interstitial space, further reducing SVR. This response results in vasodilation. If CO cannot increase further to compensate, septic shock develops (Lawrence, 2011).

The clinical presentation of sepsis is complex, and no single symptom or group of symptoms is specific to the diagnosis (Table 69-5). Affected patients usually experience an initial hyperdynamic state, characterized by increased CO and decreased SVR, which stresses the myocardium, causing tachycardia and tachypnea (Fry, 2012). Initially, the skin is warm and flushed. Persistence of high CO and low SVR beyond 24 hours is an ominous finding and is often associated with an increased development of hypotension leading to MODS. Skin then becomes cool and clammy.

In addition to the cardiovascular dysfunction that accompanies sepsis, respiratory failure is common. Affected patients initially hyperventilate as a compensatory mechanism, which results in respiratory alkalosis. Once the patient can no longer compensate, respiratory acidosis develops. Respiratory failure develops in 85% of patients with sepsis, and acute respiratory distress syndrome (ARDS) develops in 40%. Other clinical signs of septic shock include alteration in neurological status, decreased urine output, and GI dysfunction, such as GI bleeding and paralytic ileus. Tables 69-2 and 69-4 further delineate the clinical presentation of septic shock.

Stages of Shock

The health care provider must understand the underlying pathogenesis of the type of shock the patient is experiencing,

TABLE 69-5 DIAGNOSTIC CRITERIA FOR SEPSIS

Infection, documented or suspected, as well as one or more of the following:

General Variables
- Altered mental status
- Fever (temperature >38.3°C)
- Heart rate >90 beats/min
- Hyperglycemia (blood glucose >7.77 mmol/L) in the absence of diabetes
- Hypothermia (core temperature <36°C)
- Significant edema or positive fluid balance (>20 mL/kg over 24 hr)
- Tachypnea

Inflammatory Variables
- Elevated C-reactive protein
- Elevated procalcitonin
- Leukocytosis (WBC count >12 × 10⁹/L)
- Leukopenia (WBC count <4 × 10⁹/L)
- Normal WBC count with >10% immature forms

Hemodynamic Variables
- Arterial hypotension (SBP <90 mm Hg, MAP <70 mm Hg, or a decrease in SBP >40 mm Hg)

Organ Dysfunction Variables
- Acute oliguria (urine output <0.5 mL/kg/hr for at least 2 hr despite adequate fluid resuscitation)
- Arterial hypoxemia (PaO₂/FIO₂ <300)
- Coagulation abnormalities (INR >1.5 or PTT >60 sec)
- Hyperbilirubinemia (total bilirubin >68.4 mcmol/L)
- Ileus (absent bowel sounds)
- Serum creatinine increase >44.2 mcmol/L
- Thrombo-cytopenia (platelet count <100 × 10⁹/L)

Tissue Perfusion Variables
- Decreased capillary refill or mottling
- Hyperlactatemia (>1 mmol/L)

FIO₂, fraction of inspired oxygen; *INR*, international normalized ratio; *MAP*, mean arterial pressure; *PaO₂*, partial pressure of arterial oxygen; *PTT*, partial thromboplastin time; *SBP*, systolic blood pressure.
Source: Dellinger, R. P., Levy, M. M., Rhodes, A., et al. Surviving Sepsis Campaign guidelines committee including the pediatric subgroup. (2013). Surviving sepsis campaign: International guidelines for management of severe sepsis and septic shock, 2012. *Critical Care Medicine 41*(2), 580.

but monitoring and management are also guided by knowing which stage of the shock "continuum" the patient is in. This continuum begins with the initial stage of shock, which occurs at a cellular level and is usually not clinically apparent. Metabolism changes at the cellular level from aerobic to anaerobic, causing lactic acid build-up. Lactic acid is a waste product and must be removed by the liver. However, this process requires oxygen, which is unavailable because of the decrease in tissue perfusion. This stage is followed by the three clinically apparent but overlapping stages of shock: the compensatory stage, the progressive stage, and the refractory (irreversible) stage (Hall, 2016).

Compensatory Stage. In the *compensatory stage,* the body activates neural, hormonal, and biochemical compensatory mechanisms in an attempt to overcome the increasing consequences of anaerobic metabolism and to maintain homeostasis. The clinical presentation begins to reflect the body's responses to the imbalance in oxygen supply and demand (Table 69-6).

One of the first clinical signs of shock is hypotension, which occurs because of a decrease in CO and a narrowing of the pulse pressure. The baroreceptors in the carotid and aortic bodies immediately respond by activating the SNS. The SNS stimulates vasoconstriction and the release of the potent vasoconstrictors epinephrine and norepinephrine. Blood flow to the most vital organs (the heart and the brain) is maintained, whereas blood flow to the nonvital organs, such as the kidneys, the GI tract, the skin, and the lungs, is diverted or shunted (Hall, 2016).

Decrease in blood flow to the kidneys activates the renin–angiotensin system. Renin is released, which activates angiotensinogen to produce angiotensin I, which is then converted to angiotensin II (see Chapter 47, Figure 47-6). Angiotensin II is a potent vasoconstrictor that causes both arterial and venous vasoconstriction. The net result is an increase in venous return to the heart and an increase in blood pressure (BP). Angiotensin II also stimulates the adrenal cortex to release aldosterone, which results in sodium and water reabsorption and in potassium excretion by the kidneys. The increase in sodium reabsorption raises the serum osmolality and stimulates the release of antidiuretic hormone (ADH) from the posterior pituitary gland. ADH works by increasing water reabsorption by the kidneys, thus further increasing blood volume. The increase in total circulating volume results in increases in CO and BP (Hall, 2016).

Shunting of blood from the GI tract leads to decreased motility and paralytic ileus. The skin is then cold and clammy from low distribution of blood flow.

Shunting blood away from the lungs increases the patient's physiological dead space—the amount of air that does not reach gas-exchanging units and any inspired air that cannot participate in gas exchange. The clinical result of an increase in dead space is a ventilation–perfusion mismatch. Some areas of the lungs participating in ventilation are not perfused because of the decrease in blood flow to the lungs. Arterial oxygen levels decrease, and the rate and depth of respirations increase to compensate.

The myocardium responds to the SNS stimulation and the increase in oxygen demand by increasing the heart rate and contractility. However, increased contractility increases myocardial oxygen consumption (MVO₂). The coronary arteries dilate in an attempt to meet the increased oxygen demands of the myocardium.

A multisystem response to decreasing tissue perfusion is initiated in the compensatory stage of shock. At this stage, the body is able to compensate for the changes in tissue perfusion. If the perfusion deficit is corrected, the patient recovers with few or no residual consequences. If the perfusion deficit is not corrected and the body is unable to compensate, the patient enters the progressive stage of shock.

Progressive Stage. The *progressive stage* of shock begins as compensatory mechanisms fail. In this stage, aggressive interventions are necessary to prevent the development of MODS. Continued decreased cellular perfusion and resulting altered capillary permeability are the distinguishing features of this stage. As a result of altered capillary permeability, fluid and protein leak out of the vascular space into the surrounding interstitial space. In addition to the decrease in circulating volume, systemic interstitial edema increases. The patient may have *anasarca* (diffuse, profound edema). Fluid leakage from the vascular space also affects the solid organs (e.g., liver, spleen, GI tract, lungs) and peripheral tissues by further decreasing perfusion.

The pulmonary system is often the first to display signs of critical dysfunction as blood flow to the lungs is already reduced. In response to the decreased blood flow and the SNS stimulation,

TABLE 69-6 CLINICAL MANIFESTATIONS OF THE STAGES OF SHOCK

Compensatory Stage	Progressive Stage	Refractory Stage
Cardiovascular System		
BP adequate to perfuse vital organs (heart, brain)	↑ Capillary permeability → systemic interstitial edema	↓ BP inadequate to perfuse vital organs
Coronary artery dilation	↓ CO → ↓ BP and ↑ HR	Bradycardia; irregular rhythm
Narrowed pulse pressure	Loss of autoregulation in microcirculation	↓ CO
SNS response:	MAP <60 mm Hg (or 40 mm Hg drop in BP from baseline)	Profound hypotension
• Release of epinephrine and norepinephrine, which promotes vasoconstriction	↓ Coronary perfusion →	
• ↑ Contractility	• Dysrhythmias	
• ↑ HR	• Myocardial ischemia	
• ↑ MVO$_2$	• MI	
	• Myocardial dysfunction → impaired CO	
	↓ Peripheral perfusion → ischemia of distal extremities, diminished pulses, ↓ capillary refill	
Gastro-Intestinal System		
↓ Blood supply	Vasoconstriction and ↓ perfusion → ischemic gut (e.g., stomach, small and large intestines, gallbladder, pancreas)	Ischemic gut
Hypoactive bowel sounds	• Erosive ulcers	
Possible ileus	• GI bleeding	
	• Translocation of GI bacteria	
	• Impaired absorption of nutrients	
Hematological System	DIC	DIC
	• Thrombin clots in microcirculation	
	• Consumption of clots in microcirculation	
Hepatic System	Failure to metabolize drugs and waste products	Metabolic changes from accumulation of waste products (e.g., NH$_3$, lactate, CO$_2$)
	Jaundice (decreased clearance of bilirubin)	
	↑ NH$_3$ and lactate	
Neurological System		
Change in level of consciousness	↓ Cerebral blood flow	Unresponsive
Changes in Glasgow Coma Scale score	↓ Cerebral perfusion pressure	Areflexia (loss of reflexes)
Oriented to person, place, time	Listless or agitated	Pupils unreactive and dilated
Restless, apprehensive, confused	↓ Responsiveness to stimuli	
Renal System		
↑ Aldosterone level, resulting in Na$^+$ and H$_2$O reabsorption	↑ BUN/creatinine ratio	Anuria
	Metabolic acidosis	
↑ ADH level, resulting in H$_2$O reabsorption ↓ Renal blood flow	Renal tubules become ischemic → ATN	
	↓ Urine output	
↑ Renin level, resulting in release of angiotensin II (vasoconstrictor)	↑ Urine Na$^+$	
	↓ Urine osmolarity and specific gravity	
	↓ Urine K$^+$	
Respiratory System		
↓ Blood flow to the lungs	Acute respiratory distress syndrome (ARDS)	Respiratory failure
Hyperventilation	• ↑ Capillary permeability	Severe refractory hypoxemia
↑ Minute ventilation (V$_E$)	• Pulmonary vasoconstriction	
↑ Physiological dead space	• Pulmonary interstitial edema	
↑ Ventilation–perfusion mismatch	• Alveolar edema	
	• ↓ Compliance	
	• Diffuse infiltrates	
	• ↑ Respiratory rate	
	Moist crackles	
Skin		
Warm and flushed	Cold and clammy	Mottled, cyanotic
Temperature		
Normal or abnormal	Hypothermia	Hypothermia
	Sepsis: hypothermia or hyperthermia	

Continued

TABLE 69-6   CLINICAL MANIFESTATIONS OF THE STAGES OF SHOCK—cont'd

Compensatory Stage	Progressive Stage	Refractory Stage
Key Laboratory Findings		
↑ Blood glucose	↑ Bleeding times	↓ Blood glucose
↓ PaO₂	↑ Liver enzymes: ALT, AST, GGT	Metabolic acidosis
↓ PaCO₂	Thrombo-cytopenia	↑ NH₃, lactate, and K⁺
↑ pH		

ADH, antidiuretic hormone; *ALT,* alanine aminotransferase; *AST,* aspartate aminotransferase; *ATN,* acute tubular necrosis; *BP,* blood pressure; *BUN,* blood urea nitrogen; *CO,* cardiac output; *DIC,* disseminated intravascular coagulation; *GGT,* γ-glutamyl transferase; *GI,* gastro-intestinal; *HR,* heart rate; *K⁺,* potassium ions; *MAP,* mean arterial pressure; *MI,* myocardial infarction; *MVO₂,* myocardial oxygen consumption; *Na⁺,* sodium ions; *NH₃,* ammonia; *PaCO₂,* partial pressure of arterial carbon dioxide; *PaO₂,* partial pressure of arterial oxygen; *SNS,* sympathetic nervous system.

the pulmonary arterioles constrict, resulting in increased pulmonary artery (PA) pressure. As the pressure within the pulmonary vasculature increases, blood flow to the pulmonary capillaries decreases, and ventilation–perfusion mismatch worsens. Another key response in the lungs is the movement of fluid from the pulmonary vasculature into the interstitial space. As capillary permeability increases, the movement of fluid to the interstitial spaces results in interstitial edema, bronchoconstriction, and a decrease in functional residual capacity. With further increases in capillary permeability, the fluid moves to the alveoli, with resultant alveolar edema and a decrease in surfactant production. The combined effects of pulmonary vasoconstriction and bronchoconstriction are impaired gas exchange, decreased compliance, and worsening ventilation–perfusion mismatch. Clinical manifestations are tachypnea, crackles, and overall increased work of breathing.

The cardiovascular system is profoundly affected. CO begins to fall, resulting in hypotension and markedly decreased coronary artery, cerebral artery, and peripheral artery perfusion. Changes in the patient's mental status become apparent in this stage. Capillary permeability continues to increase, enhancing the movement of fluid from the vascular space into the interstitial space. Sustained hypoperfusion results in weakening of peripheral pulses and ischemia of the distal extremities. Myocardial dysfunction from decreased perfusion results in dysrhythmias, myocardial ischemia, and potentially myocardial infarction (MI). The effect of prolonged hypoperfusion on the kidneys is renal tubular ischemia. The resulting acute tubular necrosis (ATN) may lead to the development of acute kidney injury (AKI), which can be worsened by nephrotoxic drugs, including certain antibiotics, anaesthetics, and diuretics (see Chapter 49). Renal function is markedly impaired during the progressive stage of shock. The urine output is decreased, and blood urea nitrogen (BUN) and serum creatinine (Cr) levels are elevated. Metabolic acidosis results from an inability to excrete acids and reabsorb bicarbonate.

The GI system is also affected as the blood supply to the GI tract is decreased. The normally protective mucosal barrier becomes ischemic. This ischemia predisposes the patient to erosive ulcers and GI bleeding (see Chapter 44), thus increasing the potential risk for bacterial translocation from the GI tract to the blood. The decrease in perfusion to the GI tract also leads to a decrease in the ability to absorb nutrients (Miller, Kiraly, Lowen, et al., 2011).

Other systems are also affected by the sustained hypoperfusion in the progressive stage of shock. The loss of the functional ability of the liver leads to a failure of the liver to metabolize drugs and waste products such as ammonia (NH₃) and lactate.

Jaundice results from an accumulation of bilirubin. As the liver cells die, enzyme levels become elevated, particularly alanine aminotransferase (ALT), aspartate aminotransferase (AST), and γ-glutamyl transferase (GGT). The liver also loses its ability to function as an immune organ. Bacteria that may translocate from the GI system cannot be scavenged by Kupffer cells. Instead, they are released into the bloodstream, which increases the possibility of the development of bacteremia.

Dysfunction of the hematological system adds to the complexity of the clinical picture. The patient is at risk for the development of disseminated intravascular coagulation (DIC). In DIC, the platelets and the clotting factors are consumed, and secondary fibrinolysis develops. This situation results in clinically significant bleeding from many orifices, including, but not limited to, the GI tract, the lungs, and puncture sites (see Chapter 33). Numerous blood laboratory values are altered (see Chapter 33, Table 33-21; Table 69-3; Table 69-6).

Refractory Stage. In the final stage of shock, the *refractory stage,* decreased perfusion from peripheral vasoconstriction and decreased CO exacerbate anaerobic metabolism. The accumulation of lactic acid contributes to an increased capillary permeability and dilation of the capillaries. Because capillary permeability is increased, fluid and plasma proteins leave the vascular space and move to the interstitial space. Blood pools in the capillary beds as a result of constriction of the venules and dilation of the arterioles. The loss of intravascular volume worsens hypotension and tachycardia and decreases coronary blood flow. Decreases in coronary blood flow lead to worsening myocardial depression and a further decline in CO. Cerebral blood flow cannot be maintained, and cerebral ischemia results.

Patients in this stage of shock demonstrate profound hypotension and hypoxemia. The failure of the liver, the lungs, and the kidneys results in an accumulation of waste products, such as lactate, urea, ammonia, and carbon dioxide. The failure of one organ system has an effect on several other organ systems. In this final stage, recovery is unlikely. The organs are in failure, and the body's compensatory mechanisms are overwhelmed (see Table 69-6).

Diagnostic Studies

Prompt and accurate diagnosis is crucial. Establishing a diagnosis begins with a physical examination, a thorough medical and surgical history, and findings of recent events (e.g., upper respiratory tract infection, surgery, chest pain, trauma). Numerous laboratory studies must be collected initially and serially.

Decreased tissue perfusion in shock initially leads to an elevation of lactate levels (>4 mmol/L) and a high base deficit (the amount needed to bring the pH back to normal). These laboratory changes reflect an undesirable increase in anaerobic metabolism. Other laboratory values found in shock are summarized in Table 69-3.

Additional diagnostic studies include 12-lead ECG, continuous cardiac monitoring, chest radiography, continuous pulse oximetry, and hemodynamic monitoring (e.g., arterial pressure monitoring, central venous or PA pressure monitoring). (Chapter 68 discusses hemodynamic monitoring.)

TABLE 69-7 SURVIVING SEPSIS CAMPAIGN CARE BUNDLES

To Be Completed Within 3 Hours
1. Measure lactate level.
2. Obtain blood cultures before administering antibiotics.
3. Administer broad-spectrum antibiotics.
4. Administer 30 mL/kg crystalloid for hypotension or lactate level ≥4 mmol/L.

To Be Completed Within 6 Hours
5. Apply vasopressors (for hypotension that does not respond to initial fluid resuscitation) to maintain a mean arterial pressure (MAP) ≥65 mm Hg.
6. In the event of persistent arterial hypotension despite volume resuscitation (septic shock) or initial lactate level ≥4 mmol/L (36 mg/dL):
   - Measure central venous pressure (CVP).*
   - Measure central venous oxygen saturation ($S_{cv}O_2$).*
7. Remeasure lactate level if initial lactate level was elevated.*

*Targets for quantitative resuscitation included in the guidelines are CVP of ≥8 mm Hg, $S_{cv}O_2$ of ≥70%, and normalization of lactate.
Source: Dellinger, R. P., Levy, M. M., Rhodes, A., et al. (2013). Surviving Sepsis Campaign guidelines committee including the pediatric subgroup. Surviving sepsis campaign: International guidelines for management of severe sepsis and septic shock, 2012, *Critical Care Medicine 41*(2), 580.

Collaborative Care: General Measures

Critical factors in the successful management of a patient experiencing shock are early recognition and prompt intervention. Astute assessment skills and urgent communication with a rapid response team may prevent the decline to the progressive or the refractory stage. Successful management likely requires quick transfer to a critical care unit; however, nurses in non–critical care settings should institute physician's orders and bundles, even before transfer to the critical care unit (Aitken, Williams, Harvey, et al., 2011). *Bundles* are collections of, generally, three to five evidence-informed practices that, when combined, improve patient outcomes [Institute for Healthcare Improvement (IHI), 2017]. Table 69-7 provides the international guidelines for the 3-hour Resuscitation Bundle and the 6-hour Septic Shock Bundle.

Table 69-8 provides an overview of the initial assessment findings and interventions for the emergency care of patients in shock. The nurse must ensure that the patient's airway is patent. Once the airway is established, either as a natural airway or with an endotracheal tube, oxygen should be delivered to maintain an arterial oxygen saturation (SaO_2) of 90% or higher (partial pressure of arterial oxygen [PaO_2] >60 mm Hg) to avoid hypoxemia (see Chapter 68). Mechanical ventilation may be necessary. The mean arterial pressure (MAP) and the circulating blood volume are optimized with fluid replacement and drug therapy.

Oxygen and Ventilation. Oxygen delivery is dependent on CO, available hemoglobin, and SaO_2. Methods to optimize oxygen delivery are directed at increasing supply and decreasing demand. Supply can be increased by (a) optimizing CO with drug therapy or fluid replacement, (b) increasing hemoglobin by the transfusion

---

✚ TABLE 69-8 EMERGENCY MANAGEMENT

Shock

Etiology*	Assessment Findings	Interventions
Surgical • Aortic dissection • Gastro-intestinal bleeding • Postoperative bleeding • Rupture from ectopic pregnancy or of ovarian cyst • Rupture of organ or vessel • Vaginal bleeding **Medical** • Addisonian crisis • Dehydration • Diabetes insipidus • Diabetes mellitus • MI • Pulmonary embolus • Sepsis **Trauma** • Burns • Fractures, spinal injury • Multisystem or multiorgan injury • Rupture or laceration of vessel or organ (e.g., spleen)	• Anxiety • Chills • Confusion • Cool, clammy skin (warm skin in early stages of septic and neurogenic shock) • Cyanosis • Decreased level of consciousness • Decreased O_2 saturation • Dysrhythmias • Extreme thirst • Hypotension • Narrowed pulse pressure • Nausea and vomiting • Obvious hemorrhage or injury • Pallor • Rapid, weak, thready pulses • Restlessness • Sensation of impending doom • Tachypnea, dyspnea, or shallow, irregular respirations • Temperature dysregulation • Weakness	**Initial** • Administer humidified, high-flow oxygen (100%) by nonrebreather mask or bag–valve–mask device. • Anticipate need for intubation and mechanical ventilation. • Assess for life-threatening injuries (e.g., pericardial tamponade, liver laceration, tension pneumothorax). • Collect blood for laboratory studies (e.g., blood cultures, lactate measurement, WBC count). • Consider vasopressor therapy only after hypovolemia has been corrected. • Control any external bleeding with direct pressure or pressure dressing. • Establish and maintain patency of airway. • Establish IV access with two large-bore catheters, and begin fluid resuscitation with isotonic or hypertonic crystalloids (e.g., normal saline solution). • Insert an indwelling bladder catheter and nasogastric tube. • Institute antibiotic therapy if sepsis is suspected. • Stabilize cervical spine as appropriate. • Treat dysrhythmias. **Ongoing Monitoring** • Cardiac rhythm • Level of consciousness • Respiratory status • Urine output • Vital signs, including pulse oximetry, peripheral pulses, capillary refill

IV, intravenous; *MI*, myocardial infarction; *WBC*, white blood cell.
*See Table 69-1 for additional causes of shock.

of blood or packed red blood cells (RBCs), (c) increasing the SaO_2 with supplemental oxygen and mechanical ventilation, or some combination of these.

Care should be planned to avoid disrupting the balance of oxygen supply and demand. Activities that increase oxygen consumption (e.g., endotracheal suctioning, position changes) should be appropriately spaced for oxygen conservation. Continuous monitoring of central venous oxygen saturation ($ScvO_2$) by a central venous catheter or of mixed venous oxygen saturation (SvO_2) by a PA catheter is helpful. Both values reflect the dynamic balance between oxygen supply and demand. These values are considered in conjunction with the SaO_2, CO, hemoglobin, and oxygen consumption to evaluate the patient's response to treatments or activities (see Chapter 68).

Fluid Resuscitation. The cornerstone of therapy for septic, hypovolemic, and anaphylactic shock is volume expansion with prompt and aggressive fluid resuscitation to restore tissue perfusion and improve hemodynamic status. However, fluid is given cautiously for cardiogenic and neurogenic shock. Before fluid resuscitation begins, two large-bore intravenous (IV) catheters must be inserted peripherally, or preferably, a central venous catheter. Both crystalloids and colloids may have a role in fluid resuscitation (Table 69-9; see Chapter 19).

Crystalloids (e.g., N/S 0.9%, lactated Ringer's solution) are the initial fluid of choice for severe hypovolemia to achieve at least 30 ml/kg and may increase the amount and rate of administration in more patients who are compromised (Dellinger et al., 2013). Lactated Ringer's solution should be used judiciously in all shock situations because the failing liver cannot convert lactate to bicarbonate, increasing serum lactate levels further.

Colloids (e.g., albumin) are effective volume expanders as they require less volume to improve hemodynamic effect (Rochwerg, Alhazzani, Sindi, et al., 2014). Albumin, a natural compound, is recommended when the patient requires substantial amounts of crystalloids (Dellinger et al., 2013). Albumin 5% is used in patients who are hypovolemic and 25% is used in patients with fluid and sodium restrictions. Synthetic colloids (e.g., hydroxyethyl starch [HES], gelatin, or dextran) are not recommended due to possible development of AKI and coagulation disorders (Dellinger et al., 2013; Rochwerg et al., 2014).

TABLE 69-9 FLUID THERAPY FOR SHOCK

Fluid Type	Mechanism of Action	Type of Shock	Nursing Implications
Crystalloids *Isotonic* 0.9% NaCl (N/S) most commonly used Lactated Ringer's solution	Fluid remains primarily in the intravascular space, increasing intravascular volume.	Used cautiously for initial volume replacement in most types of shock	Patient is monitored closely for circulatory overload. Lactated Ringer's solution is contraindicated for patients with liver failure.
Hypertonic 1.8%, 3%, or 5% NaCl	Fluid remains in the intravascular space, producing rapid volume expansion.	May be used for initial volume expansion in hypovolemic shock	Patient is monitored closely for signs of hypernatremia (e.g., disorientation, convulsions). Central line is required to limit damage to veins.
Blood/Blood Products Whole blood or packed RBCs Fresh-frozen plasma	These replace blood loss and increase oxygen-carrying capability. They also replace coagulation factors.	All types of shock if hemoglobin is <120 g/L or if the patient does not respond to crystalloids	Same precautions as for any blood administration (see Chapter 33).
Colloids Hetastarch	This is made from starch and acts as volume expander; it is at least as effective as albumin; it can exert osmotic effect for up to 36 hr.	All types of shock except cardiogenic and neurogenic shock NOT recommended with severe sepsis and septic shock*	Use cautiously in patients with heart failure, renal failure, or bleeding disorders (because of antiplatelet effect).
Human serum albumin (5%, 25%), plasma protein fraction (5% albumin in 500 mL of N/S)	This can increase plasma colloid osmotic pressure and produces rapid volume expansion.	All types of shock except cardiogenic and neurogenic shock	Patient is monitored for circulatory overload. Mild adverse effects of chills, fever, and urticaria may develop. Use 5% for hypovolemia. Use 25% for patients with fluid and sodium restrictions.
Dextran; dextran 40; dextran 70	This is a hyperosmotic glucose polymer; similar degrees of volume expansion are achieved with dextran, dextran 40, and dextran 70; duration of action is longer with dextran 70.	Limited use because of adverse effects, including reducing platelet adhesion, diluting clotting factors	Increases risk of bleeding. Patient is monitored for allergic reactions and AKI.

AKI, acute kidney injury; *N/S*, normal saline solution; *RBCs*, red blood cells.
*Dellinger, R. P., Levy, M. M., Rhodes, A., et al. (2013). Surviving Sepsis Campaign: International guidelines for management of severe sepsis and septic shock, 2012. *Intensive Care Medicine*, 39(2), 165–228. doi:10.1007/s00134-012-2769-8.

Serial BP measurements with an automatic BP cuff or an intra-arterial catheter can be used to monitor the patient's response. An indwelling bladder catheter to monitor urine output also assists in monitoring the patient's fluid status. Hemodynamic improvement may be *dynamic* (e.g., change in pulse pressure or stroke volume), or *static* (e.g., arterial pressure, heart rate) (Dellinger et al., 2013).

The doctor should choose the type of fluid that will best restore intravascular volume with the least untoward metabolic or systemic effects (Pavlik, Simpson, Horn, et al., 2015). When large amounts of fluids are required, the patient must be protected against complications—hypothermia and coagulopathy. Hypothermia can be prevented by warming both crystalloid and colloid solutions used during massive fluid resuscitation. If the patient is receiving large volumes of packed RBCs, it is important to remember that they do not contain clotting factors. Therefore, clotting factors must be replaced on the basis of the clinical situation and results of blood studies. If the patient has chronic hypotension after adequate fluid resuscitation, the physician may consider vasoactive drug therapy. Decisions about which drug to use should be based on the physiological goal. Although BP helps determine whether the patient's CO is adequate, an assessment of end-organ perfusion (e.g., urine output, neurological function, peripheral pulses) provides more relevant information.

SAFETY ALERT
- Warm crystalloid and colloid solutions during massive fluid resuscitation.
- When administering large volumes of packed RBCs, remember that they do not contain clotting factors. Replace these factors based on the clinical situation and results of laboratory studies.

Drug Therapy. The primary goal of drug therapy for shock is the correction of decreased tissue perfusion. Ideally, medications are administered intravenously via an infusion pump through a central venous catheter instead of a peripheral site as these drugs are quite viscous and may cause IV complications (e.g., extravasation) (Table 69-10).

Sympathomimetic Drugs. Many of the drugs used in the treatment of shock have an effect on the SNS. Drugs that mimic the action of the SNS are termed *sympathomimetic*. The effects of these drugs are mediated through their binding to α-adrenergic or β-adrenergic receptors. The various drugs have different relative α-adrenergic and β-adrenergic effects (see Chapter 35, Table 35-1). Many of the sympathomimetic drugs cause peripheral vasoconstriction and are referred to as *vasopressor drugs* (e.g., epinephrine [Adrenalin], dopamine, norepinephrine [Levophed]). These drugs have the potential to cause severe peripheral vasoconstriction and an increase in SVR. This response further jeopardizes tissue perfusion, either directly or indirectly. The increased SVR increases the workload of the heart and can be detrimental to a patient in cardiogenic shock by causing further myocardial damage. Use of vasopressor drugs is generally reserved for patients who have been unresponsive to other therapies. Adequate fluid resuscitation must be achieved before the use of any vasopressor drug because peripheral vasoconstrictor effects in patients with low blood volume cause further reduction in tissue perfusion.

The goal of vasopressor therapy is to achieve and maintain a MAP of at least 65 mm Hg (Dellinger et al., 2013). The nurse must continuously monitor end-organ perfusion (e.g., urine output, SvO_2, serum lactate levels) to ensure that tissue perfusion is adequate.

Vasodilator Drugs. Some patients in shock show evidence of excessive vasoconstriction and poor tissue perfusion in spite of

TABLE 69-10 DRUG THERAPY

Shock*

Mechanism of Action	Hemodynamic Effects	Type of Shock	Nursing Implications
Dobutamine			
↑ Myocardial contractility ↓ Ventricular filling pressures	↑ CO, stroke volume, and CVP ↑ ↓ HR ↓ SVR and PAOP	Used for cardiogenic shock with severe systolic dysfunction Used for septic shock with normal CO that is not meeting metabolic demands	Hypovolemia is corrected. Should not be administered in same catheter with $NaHCO_3$. Administration via central catheter is recommended (infiltration leads to tissue sloughing). HR and BP are monitored (hypotension may worsen, necessitating addition of a vasopressor). Patient is monitored for tachydysrhythmias.
Dopamine			
Precursor to epinephrine and norepinephrine Hemodynamic effects from release of norepinephrine Positive inotropic effects: • ↑ Myocardial contractility • ↑ Automaticity • ↑ Atrioventricular conduction Low doses: ↑ blood flow to renal, mesenteric, and cerebral circulation High doses: can cause progressive vasoconstriction	↑ BP ↑ CO ↑ HR	Cardiogenic shock: • ↑ HR • ↑ Mean arterial pressure • ↑ MVO_2	Hypovolemia is corrected. Administer via central catheter (infiltration leads to tissue sloughing); should not be administered in same catheter with $NaHCO_3$. Patient is monitored for tachydysrhythmias. Patient is monitored for peripheral vasoconstriction at moderate to high doses (e.g., paresthesias, coldness in extremities).

Continued

TABLE 69-10 DRUG THERAPY

Shock—cont'd

Mechanism of Action	Hemodynamic Effects	Type of Shock	Nursing Implications
Epinephrine (Adrenalin)			
Low doses: β-adrenergic agonist (cardiac stimulation, bronchial dilation, peripheral vasodilation)	↑ HR, contractility, and CO ↓ SVR	Cardiogenic shock combined with afterload reduction Anaphylactic shock	Hypovolemia is corrected if necessary. Patient is monitored for HR >110 beats/min. Patient is monitored for dyspnea and pulmonary edema.
High doses: α-adrenergic agonist (peripheral vasoconstriction)	↑ Stroke volume ↑ SVR ↑ Systolic BP, ↓ diastolic BP, widened pulse pressure ↑ CVP, PAOP	Cardiac arrest, pulseless ventricular tachycardia, ventricular fibrillation, asystole	Patient is monitored for renal failure secondary to ischemia. Patient is monitored for chest pain, dysrhythmias secondary to ↑ MVO₂.
Hydrocortisone (Solu-Cortef)			
Decreases inflammation; reverses increased capillary permeability	↑ BP, HR	Septic shock necessitating vasopressor therapy, despite fluid resuscitation, to maintain adequate BP Anaphylactic shock if hypotension persists past initial therapy	Patient is monitored for hypokalemia and hyperglycemia.
Norepinephrine (Levophed)			
β₁-Adrenergic agonist (cardiac stimulation) α-Adrenergic agonist (peripheral vasoconstriction) Renal and splanchnic vasoconstriction	↑ BP, MAP ↑ CVP, PAOP ↑ SVR ↑ or ↓ CO	Cardiogenic shock after MI Septic shock: works by increasing vascular tone	Used for hypotension unresponsive to adequate fluid resuscitation. Administered via a central catheter (infiltration leads to tissue sloughing). Patient is monitored for dysrhythmias secondary to ↑ MVO₂ requirements.
Phenylephrine (Neo-Synephrine)			
α-Adrenergic agonist Vasoconstriction: renal, mesenteric, splanchnic, cutaneous, and pulmonary vessels	↑ HR ↑ BP ↑ SVR ↑↓ CO	Neurogenic shock	Patient is monitored for reflex bradycardia, headache, restlessness. Patient is monitored for renal failure secondary to ↓ renal blood flow. Administered via central catheter (infiltration leads to tissue sloughing).
Nitroglycerin			
Venodilation Dilates coronary arteries ↓ Preload ↓ MVO₂	↓ SVR ↓ BP	Cardiogenic shock	Patient is continuously monitored for BP and for reflex tachycardia. Use glass bottles for storage of drug.
Sodium Nitroprusside (Nipride)			
Arterial and venous vasodilation ↓ Preload, afterload	↓ BP ↑↓ CO ↓ CVP, PAOP	Cardiogenic shock with ↑ SVR	BP is continuously monitored. Solution should be protected from light; infusion bottle should be wrapped with opaque covering. Administered with D₅W only. Patient is monitored for cyanide toxicity (e.g., tinnitus, hyper-reflexia, confusion, seizures).
Vasopressin			
ADH, nonadrenergic vasoconstrictor	↑ MAP ↓ Need for other vasopressors ↑ Urine output	Shock states (most commonly septic shock) refractory to other vasopressors	Low dose usually administered. Hemodynamic pressures and urine output are monitored.

ADH, antidiuretic hormone; *BP,* blood pressure; *CO,* cardiac output; *CVP,* central venous pressure; *D₅W,* 5% dextrose in water; *HR,* heart rate; *INR,* international normalized ratio; *MAP,* mean arterial pressure; *MI,* myocardial infarction; *MVO₂,* myocardial oxygen consumption; *PAOP,* pulmonary artery occlusive pressure; *PTT,* partial thromboplastin time; *SVR,* systemic vascular resistance.

*Individual facility's guidelines, pharmacist, pharmacology references, and drug manufacturer's administration materials should be consulted for additional information and dosage recommendations.

fluid replacement and normal or even high systemic BP. This is especially true of patients in cardiogenic shock. Although generalized sympathetic vasoconstriction is a useful compensatory mechanism for maintaining systemic pressure, excessive constriction can reduce tissue blood flow and increase the workload of the heart. The rationale for using vasodilator therapy for a patient in shock is to break the deleterious cycle in which widespread vasoconstriction causes a decrease in CO and BP, resulting in further SNS-induced vasoconstriction.

The goal of vasodilator therapy, as in vasopressor therapy, is to maintain a MAP greater than 65 mm Hg. Other hemodynamic pressures are also monitored so that fluids can be increased or the dose of the vasodilator decreased if CO or BP falls dramatically. The vasodilator agent most often used in cardiogenic shock is nitroglycerin. Vasodilation may be enhanced with nitroprusside (Nipride) in non-cardiogenic shock.

Nutritional Therapy. Protein–calorie malnutrition is one of the primary manifestations of hypermetabolism in shock. Nutrition is vital in decreasing morbidity. Enteral nutrition to enhance perfusion of the GI tract and help maintain the integrity of the gut mucosa should be initiated within the first 24 hours (Aitken et al., 2011; Dellinger et al., 2013; Miller et al., 2011). Slow continuous enteral feedings are started for the first week and advanced only as tolerated (Dellinger et al., 2013).

Parenteral nutrition is often required when enteral nutrition is contraindicated or not meeting nutritional needs; however, it must be used with caution because the dextrose can cause hyperglycemia and the lipids can have an immuno-suppressive effect (Miller et al., 2011) (see Chapter 42).

Patients should be weighed on the same scale at the same time of day. If significant weight loss is noted, dehydration should be ruled out before additional calories are provided. Large weight gains are common because of third spacing of fluids. Therefore, daily weight measurements may function better as an indicator of fluid status than caloric needs and balance do. Serum protein, nitrogen balance, BUN, serum glucose level, and serum electrolyte values are all used to assess nutritional status.

Collaborative Care: Specific Measures

Cardiogenic Shock. For the patient in cardiogenic shock, the overall goal is to restore blood flow to the myocardium by restoring the balance between oxygen supply and demand. Specific measures to restore blood flow include thrombolytic therapy, angioplasty with stent implantation, emergency revascularization, and valve replacement (see Chapter 36). Cardiac catheterization should be performed as soon as possible after the initial insult. Coronary angioplasty with or without stent implantation may be performed during the cardiac catheterization. Until these interventions can be performed, stroke volume and CO must be optimized in an effort to facilitate optimal perfusion (Table 69-11; see also Table 69-10).

Hemodynamic management aims to decrease the workload of the heart through reperfusion, drug therapy, or mechanical interventions. Early recognition and prompt revascularization by means of percutaneous coronary intervention or coronary artery bypass graft (CABG) substantially improves survival rates. Fibrinolytic therapy is another option for reperfusion. Inotropes and vasopressors in low doses are effective pharmacological agents. Dopamine is the first drug of choice because it is both an inotrope and a vasopressor. Dobutamine is an effective inotrope for mild hypotension and can improve CO when combined with a vasopressor, such as norepinephrine or vasopressin. Patients

with pulmonary edema should receive diuretics. Acetylsalicylic acid (ASA; Aspirin) is given to patients with acute MI. Amiodarone is used to treat arrhythmias. β-Blockers and nitrates should be given with caution and avoided in the acute stage (Patel & Hollenberg, 2011).

Patients may also benefit from a circulatory assist device such as an intra-aortic balloon pump (IABP) or a ventricular assist device (VAD) (see Chapter 68). The IABP is inserted into the femoral artery and placed in the aorta just distal to the aortic arch. The goal of this intervention is to increase coronary blood flow and thus decrease left ventricular workload. The VAD is used when cardiogenic shock is refractory to the IABP or fibrinolytic therapy. It is a temporary measure for patients who are in cardiogenic shock or awaiting cardiac transplantation. Cardiac transplantation is an option for a small and select group of patients with cardiogenic shock.

Hypovolemic Shock. The underlying principles of managing hypovolemic shock focus on stopping the loss of fluid and restoring the circulating volume. Fluid resuscitation in hypovolemic shock initially is calculated according to a 3:1 rule (3 mL of isotonic crystalloid for every 1 mL of estimated blood loss). Table 69-9 delineates the different types of fluid used for volume resuscitation, the mechanisms of action, and specific nursing implications for each fluid type.

Septic Shock. Patients in septic shock require large amounts of fluid replacement to achieve hemodynamic improvement (Dellinger et al., 2013). Predetermined end points of fluid resuscitation are suggested in Table 69-11. To optimize and evaluate large-volume fluid resuscitation, hemodynamic monitoring with a PA catheter or central venous catheter (target central venous pressure [CVP] of 8 to 12 mm Hg) and arterial pressure monitoring (target MAP of >65 mm Hg) may be necessary. If fluid resuscitation is unsuccessful, vasopressor drug therapy may be added. Vasodilation and low CO, or vasodilation alone, can cause low BP in spite of adequate volume resuscitation. Norepinephrine is the first-choice vasopressor to initially target a MAP of 65 mm Hg (Dellinger et al., 2013). Vasopressin, an antidiuretic hormone, may be given for patients whose condition is refractory to norepinephrine (Dellinger et al., 2013). Exogenous vasopressin is used to replace the stores of physiological vasopressin that are often depleted in septic shock.

DRUG ALERT—Vasopressin
- Infuse at low doses (e.g., 0.03 U/min)
- Do not titrate infusion
- Use cautiously in patients with coronary artery disease

Vasopressor drugs may increase BP but may also decrease stroke volume. Often, an inotropic agent (e.g., dobutamine) is added to offset the decrease in stroke volume (see Table 69-10). Corticosteroids are not recommended; however, IV corticosteroids (e.g., hydrocortisone 200 mg/day) may be used only when hemodynamic status is not improving despite fluid resuscitation attempts and vasopressor therapy (Dellinger et al., 2013). In an attempt to meet the increasing tissue demands coupled with a low SVR, the patient initially demonstrates normal or high CO. If the patient is unable to achieve and maintain adequate CO and has unmet tissue oxygen demands, CO may have to be increased through drug therapy (e.g., dopamine) (Dellinger et al., 2013). The adequacy of CO can be assessed with SvO_2 monitoring. The SvO_2 (normal, 65%–75%) is a reflection of the balance between oxygen delivery and consumption (see Chapter 68). If the balance is maintained, the tissue demands are met.

TABLE 69-11 COLLABORATIVE CARE

Specific Strategies for the Treatment of Shock

Cardiogenic Shock	Hypovolemic Shock	Septic Shock	Neurogenic Shock	Anaphylactic Shock
Oxygenation				
Supplemental O₂ (e.g., via nasal cannula, non-rebreather mask) provided Intubation and mechanical ventilation, initiated, if necessary SvO₂ or ScvO₂ monitored	Supplemental O₂ provided SvO₂ or ScvO₂ monitored	Supplemental O₂ provided Intubation and mechanical ventilation initiated, if necessary SvO₂ or ScvO₂ monitored	Patency of airway maintained Supplemental O₂ provided Intubation and mechanical ventilation initiated, if necessary	Patency of airway maintained Oxygenation optimized with supplemental O₂ Intubation and mechanical ventilation initiated, if necessary
Circulation				
Blood flow restored with thrombolytics, angioplasty with stent implantation, emergency coronary revascularization Workload of the heart reduced with circulatory assist devices (IABP, VAD)	Fluid volume restored (e.g., blood or blood products, crystalloids) Rapid fluid replacement provided via two large-bore (14- to 16-gauge) peripheral IV lines End points of fluid resuscitation accomplished: • CVP of 15 mm Hg • PAOP of 10–12 mm Hg	Aggressive fluid resuscitation provided End points of fluid resuscitation accomplished: • CVP of 15 mm Hg • PAOP of 10–12 mm Hg	Fluids administered with caution	Aggressive fluid resuscitation provided with colloids
Drug Therapies				
Nitrates (e.g., nitroglycerin) Inotropes (e.g., dobutamine) Diuretics (e.g., furosemide) β-Adrenergic blockers (contraindicated with ↓ ejection fraction)	No specific drug therapies	Antibiotics as ordered Vasopressors (e.g., dopamine) Inotropes (e.g., dobutamine) Anticoagulants (e.g., low-molecular-weight heparin)	Vasopressors (e.g., phenylephrine) Atropine (for bradycardia)	Antihistamines (e.g., diphenhydramine) Epinephrine (subQ, IV, with nebulizer) Bronchodilators: with nebulizer (e.g., albuterol) Corticosteroids (if hypotension persists)
Supportive Therapies				
Dysrhythmias corrected	Cause corrected (e.g., stop bleeding, GI losses) Warmed fluids used	Cultures obtained (e.g., blood, wound) before beginning antibiotics Temperature monitored Blood glucose level controlled Stress ulcers prevented	Spinal cord trauma minimized with stabilization Temperature monitored	Offending cause identified and removed Prevented by avoidance of known allergens Patient premedicated according to history of prior sensitivity (e.g., contrast media)

CVP, central venous pressure; *GI,* gastro-intestinal; *IABP,* intra-aortic balloon pump; *IV,* intravenously; *PAOP,* pulmonary artery occlusive pressure; *subQ,* subcutaneously; *ScvO₂,* central venous oxygen saturation; *SvO₂,* venous oxygen saturation; *VAD,* ventricular assist device.

Antimicrobial therapy is an important and early component of therapy. Outcomes are improved if administered within the first 45 minutes or at least the first 3 hours (Dellinger et al., 2013). Before definitive treatment for the infection begins, the cause of the infection must be identified. Cultures (e.g., blood, wound exudate, urine, stool, sputum) are obtained before antimicrobial medications are started. Broad-spectrum antimicrobials (e.g., antibiotics, antifungals, antivirals) are given initially, followed by more specific medication once the organism has been identified (Dellinger et al., 2013).

Glucose levels should be monitored every 1 to 2 hours and maintained at less than 10 mmol/L (Dellinger et al., 2013). Stress ulcer prophylaxis with histamine H₂-receptor blockers (e.g., famotidine [Pepcid]) or proton pump inhibitors (e.g., pantoprazole) are recommended for patients with risk of bleeding (Dellinger et al., 2013). Deep venous thrombosis prophylaxis using low-dose unfractionated heparin or low-molecular-weight heparin (e.g., enoxaparin [Lovenox]) is also recommended, in combination with intermittent pneumatic compressions devices (Dellinger et al., 2013).

Neurogenic Shock. The specific treatment of neurogenic shock is dependent on the cause. If the cause is spinal cord injury, general measures to promote spinal stability (e.g., spinal precautions, cervical stabilization with a collar) are initially used. Once the spine is stabilized, definitive treatment of the hypotension and bradycardia is essential to prevent further spinal cord damage. Hypotension, which occurs as a result of a loss of sympathetic tone, is associated with peripheral vasodilation and decreased venous return. Treatment involves the use of vasopressors (e.g., phenylephrine [Neo-Synephrine]) to maintain BP and organ perfusion (see Table 69-10). Bradycardia may be treated with atropine. Fluids are administered cautiously because the cause of the hypotension is not related to fluid loss (Casha & Christie, 2011).

The patient with a spinal cord injury also needs to be monitored for hypothermia because of hypothalamic dysfunction (see Table 69-11). Although corticosteroids do not have an effect in neurogenic shock, methylprednisolone (Solu-Medrol) is used for patients with a spinal cord injury to prevent secondary spinal cord damage caused by the release of chemical mediators (see Chapter 63).

Anaphylactic Shock. Anaphylaxis can quickly progress to anaphylactic shock within minutes if not treated immediately. Triggers of anaphylaxis are foods (peanuts, shellfish, soy), stinging insect venoms (honeybee and yellow jacket), and drugs (nonsteroidal anti-inflammatory drugs [NSAIDs], antibiotics, and neuro-muscular blocking agents) (see Table 69-1).

World Allergy Organization anaphylaxis guidelines (2015) recommend epinephrine as the first line of treatment. Ideally, an intramuscular (IM) epinephrine auto-injector dose is self-administered at the onset of an event, prior to hospitalization. IV epinephrine is used with anaphylactic shock and must not be delayed. Overdosing of epinephrine can lead to detrimental cardiovascular effects, such as hypertension, stroke, and even death; however the benefits far outweigh the risks.

The second line of treatment includes H_1-antihistamines (e.g., diphenhydramine hydrochloride [Benadryl]), and H_2-antihistamines (e.g., Zantac) which block the histamine receptors. IV glucocorticoids are used to prevent further episodes or anaphylaxis. These drugs should be used in combination with epinephrine (Simons, Ebisawa, Sanchez-Borges, et al., 2015).

Maintaining patency of the airway is important because the patient can quickly develop airway compromise from laryngeal edema or bronchoconstriction. Nebulized bronchodilators are highly effective. Aerosolized epinephrine can also be used to treat laryngeal edema. Endotracheal intubation or cricothyroidotomy may be necessary to secure and maintain airway patency. Aggressive fluid resuscitation, predominantly with colloids, is necessary (see Tables 69-10 and 69-11).

Methylene blue can rapidly reverse anaphylaxis refractory to epinephrine, oxygen, and IV fluid resuscitation. It works by reversing vasodilation, thus improving hypotension and improving cerebral blood flow (Zheng, Barthel, Collange, et al., 2013).

NURSING MANAGEMENT
SHOCK

NURSING ASSESSMENT

The initial assessment should be focused on the ABCs: **a**irway, **b**reathing, and **c**irculation. Further assessment should focus on tissue perfusion and includes evaluation of vital signs, level of consciousness, peripheral pulses, capillary refill, skin (e.g., temperature, colour, moisture), and urine output. As shock progresses, the patient's skin becomes cooler and mottled, urine output decreases, peripheral pulses diminish, and neurological status continues to deteriorate.

To understand the complexity of the patient's clinical status, the nurse must integrate all the assessment data. As care is initiated (see Tables 69-7 and 69-11), it is essential for the nurse to obtain a brief history from the patient or substitute decision maker. This information should include a description of the events leading to the shock condition, time at onset and duration of symptoms,

and a health history (e.g., medications, allergies, date of last tetanus vaccination, recent travel). In addition, details should be obtained regarding any care that the patient received before hospitalization.

NURSING DIAGNOSES

Nursing diagnoses for the patient in shock may include, but are not limited to, the following:

* *Ineffective peripheral tissue perfusion, risk for decreased cardiac tissue perfusion, ineffective cerebral tissue perfusion, and risk for impaired liver function*
* *Anxiety* related to *threat of death, threat to current status (severity of condition)*

Additional information on nursing diagnoses for the patient with shock is presented in Nursing Care Plan (NCP) 69-1, available on the Evolve website. Many other diagnoses are relevant, and examples appear in other chapters.

PLANNING

The overall goals for patients in shock include (a) restoration of adequate tissue perfusion, (b) normal vital signs, specifically, MAP greater than 65 mm Hg, (c) recovery of organ function, and (d) prevention of progression toward further complications related to prolonged states of hypoperfusion.

NURSING IMPLEMENTATION

HEALTH PROMOTION. In order to prevent shock, the nurse must identify patients at risk. In general, patients who are older, those with debilitating illnesses, and those who are immuno-compromised are at increased risk. Any person who sustains surgical or accidental trauma is at high risk for shock as a result of hemorrhage, spinal cord injury, and other conditions (see Table 69-1). Any patient who is at risk for decreased oxygen delivery or tissue hypoxia is also at risk for the development of shock. Planning is essential to help prevent shock after a susceptible individual has been identified. For example, a patient diagnosed with an acute anterior MI is at risk for cardiogenic shock. The primary goal in this scenario is to limit the size of the infarction. The infarct size can be limited by restoring coronary blood flow through thrombolytic therapy, percutaneous coronary intervention, or surgical revascularization. Rest, analgesics, sedatives, and judicious use of paralytic agents (if the patient is intubated) can reduce the myocardial demand for oxygen. The nurse can modify the patient's environment to provide care intermittently so to not increase the patient's oxygen demand. For example, if the patient becomes fatigued or anxious during bathing, that activity can be planned at a time so as not to interfere with tests or other activities that may also increase oxygen demand.

A person with a severe allergy to such substances as drugs, shellfish, and insect bites is at increased risk of developing anaphylactic shock. The risk for anaphylactic shock can be decreased if the patient is carefully questioned about allergies before a drug is administered or before the patient undergoes diagnostic procedures involving the use of contrast media. If a patient's condition warrants receiving a medication to which he or she is at high risk for an allergic reaction (e.g., contrast media), the patient should receive a premedication such as diphenhydramine or methylprednisolone. Patients with severe allergies should wear a medical alert tag that identifies their allergies. Patients and those close to them should always have an epinephrine EpiPen auto-injector ready.

Careful monitoring of fluid balance can help prevent hypovolemic shock. Ongoing monitoring of intake and output and daily weight measurements are important. In addition, monitoring the patient's clinical status is essential because trends in clinical findings are more meaningful than any single piece of clinical information.

All patients should be carefully monitored for the development of infection. Progression from an infection to sepsis and septic shock is dependent on the patient's host defence mechanisms. Patients who are immuno-compromised or immuno-suppressed are at especially high risk of developing an opportunistic infection. These patients may be ventilated or have numerous invasive lines. Strategies to decrease the risk for health care–associated infections (HAIs) include decreasing the number of indwelling catheters (e.g., central lines, urinary catheters), using aseptic technique during invasive procedures, and paying strict attention to handwashing. In addition, all equipment must be changed according to institutional policy or thoroughly cleaned or discarded (if disposable) before use with another patient. The use of standardized bundles, such as the central line bundle or the ventilator bundle should be considered (see the Resources at the end of Chapter 71).

ACUTE INTERVENTION. The nurse's role with patients in shock involves (a) monitoring the patient's ongoing physical and emotional status to detect subtle changes in the patient's condition, (b) planning and quickly implementing nursing interventions and therapy, (c) evaluating the patient's response to therapy, (d) providing emotional support to the patient and family, and (e) collaborating with other members of the health team to coordinate care (see NCP 69-1 on the Evolve website).

Neurological Status. Neurological status, including orientation and level of consciousness, should be assessed every hour or more often. The patient's neurological status is the best indicator of cerebral blood flow. The nurse should be aware of neurological clinical manifestations such as changes in behaviour, restlessness, hyperalertness, blurred vision, confusion, and paresthesias. Note any subtle changes in the patient's mental status (e.g., mild agitation).

The patient should be oriented to time, place, person, and events. If the patient is in a critical care unit, orientation to the environment is particularly important. Measures such as minimizing noise and light levels should be taken to control sensory input. A day–night cycle of activity and rest should be maintained as much as possible. Sensory overload and disruption of the patient's diurnal cycle may contribute to delirium (see Chapter 68).

Cardiovascular Status. Most therapy for shock is based on information about the patient's cardiovascular status. If the patient is unstable, careful assessment of the heart rate, the BP, the CVP, and the PA pressures, including continuous CO (if available), should be completed at least every 15 minutes. PAOP should be measured every 1 to 2 hours. (Hemodynamic monitoring is discussed in Chapter 68.) Monitoring trends in hemodynamic parameters yields more important information than individual numbers. Integration of hemodynamic data with physical assessment data is essential in planning strategies to manage the patient with shock.

Patients in shock classically exhibit hypotension, which should be treated with fluid resuscitation, medications, or a combination of these, after the type of shock has been identified. Trendelenburg position should be avoided as the patient could experience compromised pulmonary function and increased intracranial pressure.

The patient's ECG should be monitored continuously to detect dysrhythmias. Heart sounds should be assessed for the presence of an S_3 or S_4 sound or new murmurs. The presence of an S_3 sound in an adult may indicate heart failure. The frequency of monitoring is decreased as the patient's condition improves.

In addition to monitoring the patient's cardiovascular status, the nurse must administer the prescribed therapy to correct the dysfunctions of the cardiovascular system. The patient's response to fluid and medication administration is assessed and titrated as often as every 5 to 15 minutes. Once tissue perfusion is restored and the patient is stabilized, the frequency of monitoring is decreased, and the patient is slowly weaned off medications that support BP and tissue perfusion.

Respiratory Status. The respiratory status of the patient in shock must be frequently assessed to ensure adequate oxygenation, detect complications early, and provide data regarding the patient's acid–base status. The rate, the depth, and the rhythm of respirations are initially monitored as frequently as every 15 to 30 minutes. Increased rate and depth provide information regarding the patient's attempts to correct metabolic acidosis. Breath sounds should be assessed every hour for any changes that may indicate fluid overload or accumulation of secretions.

Pulse oximetry is used to continuously monitor oxygen saturation. Pulse oximetry using a patient's finger or toe may not be accurate in an advanced shock state because of poor peripheral circulation. In this situation, the probe should be attached to the nose, the ear, or the forehead (according to the manufacturer's guidelines) to increase accuracy. Levels of ABGs provide definitive information on ventilation and oxygenation status and acid–base balance. Initial interpretation of ABGs is often the nurse's responsibility. A PaO_2 below 60 mm Hg (in the absence of chronic lung disease) indicates the presence of hypoxemia and the need for the administration of higher oxygen concentrations or for a different mode of oxygen administration. Low partial pressure of arterial carbon dioxide ($PaCO_2$) in the presence of a low pH and low bicarbonate level may indicate that the patient is attempting to compensate for metabolic acidosis. A rising $PaCO_2$ in the presence of a persistently low pH and PaO_2 may indicate the need for intubation and mechanical ventilation.

Most patients in shock are intubated and on mechanical ventilation. Maintaining airway patency and monitoring for ventilator-related complications are critical. (Artificial airways and mechanical ventilation are discussed in Chapter 68.)

Renal Status. Hourly measurements of urinary output are essential in the assessment of the adequacy of renal perfusion. An indwelling bladder catheter is inserted to facilitate measurements. Urine output of less than 0.5 mL/kg/hr may indicate inadequate perfusion of the kidneys. BUN and serum creatinine values are additional indicators used to assess renal function. Serum creatinine is a better indicator of renal function because BUN levels can be influenced by the catabolic state of the patient.

Body Temperature and Skin Changes. When temperature is normal, it should be monitored every 4 hours. If it is elevated or subnormal, tympanic or pulmonary arterial temperatures should be monitored hourly. If the temperature rises above 38.6°C and the patient becomes uncomfortable or experiences cardiovascular compromise, the fever may be managed with NSAIDs (e.g., ibuprofen [Motrin]), with acetaminophen (Tylenol), or by removing some of the patient's covers.

The patient's skin should be monitored for temperature, pallor, flushing, cyanosis, diaphoresis, and piloerection. In addition, capillary refill should be assessed as an indicator of peripheral perfusion.

Gastro-Intestinal Status. Bowel sounds should be auscultated at least every 4 hours, and abdominal distension should be assessed. If a nasogastric tube is inserted, drainage should be measured and checked for occult blood. Stools should also be checked for occult blood.

Personal Hygiene. Hygiene is especially important for patients in shock because impaired tissue perfusion predisposes the skin to breakdown and infection. However, bathing and other nursing measures must be carried out judiciously due to problems with oxygen delivery to tissues. The nurse must use clinical judgement to determine priorities of care in order to limit the demands for increased oxygen.

Oral care is essential because mucous membranes may become dry and fragile in the state of volume depletion. In addition, patients who are intubated usually have difficulty swallowing, which results in pooled secretions in the mouth. A water-soluble lubricant applied to the lips prevents drying and cracking. Moist swabbing of the tongue and oral mucosa with saline solution or diluted mouthwash is also beneficial.

Passive range of motion (ROM) should be performed three to four times per day to maintain joint mobility. The patient should be turned at least every 1 to 2 hours and positioned in good body alignment to help prevent pressure injuries. A pressure-relieving mattress or a specialty bed may also be needed. If possible, oxygen consumption (e.g., SvO_2 or $ScvO_2$) should be monitored during all nursing interventions to monitor the patient's tolerance of activity.

Emotional Support and Comfort. The nurse must recognize that the patient and family are faced with a critical, life-threatening situation and may experience problems such as anxiety, fear, and pain (see Chapter 68). The nurse should address these responses because such symptoms may aggravate respiratory distress and increase the release of catecholamines. Medications to decrease anxiety and pain are common modes of therapy. Continuous infusions of a benzodiazepine (e.g., lorazepam [Ativan]), an opioid or anaesthetic (e.g., morphine, propofol [Diprivan]), and occasionally a neuro-muscular blocking agent (e.g., cisatracurium) are extremely helpful in decreasing anxiety, pain, and oxygen demand. Goals of care and prognosis should be discussed as early as feasible, considering end-of-life care planning and palliative care principles where appropriate (Dellinger et al., 2013).

AMBULATORY AND HOME CARE. Rehabilitation involves ensuring that the precipitating cause is corrected, preventing or treating complications, and providing education focused on disease management or prevention of recurrence. A collaborative approach involving allied health services on discharge is necessary for success (e.g., transitional and rehabilitation units, home health care, occupational therapists, physiotherapists, and dietitians, to name a few).

Rehabilitation of the patient who has experienced critical illness must be monitored for indications of complications throughout the recovery period. Complications may include decreased ROM, decreased physical endurance, renal failure after ATN (see Chapter 49), and the development of fibrotic lung disease as a result of ARDS (see Chapter 70). Thus, patients recovering from shock may require diverse services on discharge. These can include admission to transitional care units (e.g., for weaning from mechanical ventilation), rehabilitation centres (inpatient or outpatient), or home health care agencies. The nurse should begin to anticipate and facilitate a safe transition from the hospital to home when the patient is admitted.

EVALUATION

Expected outcomes for the patient with shock are addressed in NCP 69-1, available on the Evolve website.

SYSTEMIC INFLAMMATORY RESPONSE SYNDROME AND MULTIPLE-ORGAN DYSFUNCTION SYNDROME

Etiology and Pathophysiology

Systemic inflammatory response syndrome (SIRS) is a systemic inflammatory response to a variety of insults, including infection, ischemia, infarction, and injury (see Table 69-5). SIRS is characterized by at least two of the following: fever, edema, hypotension, tachycardia, impaired oxygenation, and elevated white blood cell (WBC) count (Moser, 2014).

A systemic inflammatory response can be triggered by many mechanisms. Examples are as follows:

- *Abscess formation:* intra-abdominal, on extremities
- *Endotoxin release:* Gram-negative bacteria
- *Global perfusion deficits:* after cardiac resuscitation, in shock states
- *Ischemic or necrotic tissue:* pancreatitis, vascular disease, MI
- *Mechanical tissue trauma:* burns, crush injuries, surgical procedures
- *Microbial invasion:* bacteria, viruses, fungi, parasites
- *Regional perfusion deficits:* distal perfusion deficits

It is important to determine if SIRS is caused by an infection, as early treatment is crucial to deter sepsis from advancing to severe sepsis or septic shock (Moser, 2014).

To differentiate between SIRS and sepsis, a useful biomarker is to check serum procalcitonin (PCT) levels, as well as other diagnostic criteria (see Table 69-5) (Meynaar, Droog, Batstra, et al., 2011).

Supportive measures, such as mechanical ventilation, aggressive fluid resuscitation, nutritional support, cardiac pharmacology, and broad-spectrum antibiotics can assist to survive the acute hypoperfusion state of SIRS; however, many patient progress to multiple-organ dysfunction syndrome (MODS) (Fry, 2012).

Multiple-organ dysfunction syndrome (MODS) is the failure of two or more organ systems in a patient who is acutely ill to such a degree that homeostasis cannot be maintained without intervention. MODS is a progression from SIRS. The mortality rate is 70% when three or more organs fail (Dellinger et al., 2013; see Figure 69-1).

Organ and Metabolic Dysfunction. When the inflammatory response is not controlled, the consequences that occur include activation of inflammatory cells and release of mediators, direct damage to the endothelium, and hypermetabolism. Vasodilation becomes excessive and leads to decreased SVR and hypotension. In addition, vascular permeability increases, which allows mediators and protein to leak out of the endothelium and into the interstitial space. The WBCs begin to phagocytize the foreign debris, and the coagulation cascade is activated (see Chapter 32). Organ perfusion may be compromised because of hypotension, decreased perfusion, microemboli, and redistributed or shunted blood flow.

The respiratory system is most commonly affected in MODS (Aitken et al., 2011; Dellinger et al., 2013). Inflammatory mediators have a direct effect on the pulmonary vasculature. The endothelial damage from the release of inflammatory mediators results in an increase in capillary permeability and facilitates movement of proteinaceous fluid from the pulmonary vasculature into the pulmonary interstitial spaces. The fluid then moves to the alveoli, causing alveolar edema. Type I pneumocytes (alveolar cells) are destroyed. Type II pneumocytes become dysfunctional, and surfactant production decreases. The alveoli collapse, which leads to an increase in shunt (blood flow to the lungs that does not participate in gas exchange) and a worsening of the ventilation–perfusion mismatch. The end result is ARDS. Patients with ARDS require aggressive pulmonary management with mechanical ventilation. (See Chapter 70 for more on ARDS and mechanical ventilation.)

Cardiovascular changes in MODS include myocardial depression and massive vasodilation in response to increasing tissue demands. Vasodilation results in decreased SVR and BP. The baroreceptor reflex causes release of *inotropic* factors (which increase force of contraction) and *chronotropic* factors (which increase heart rate) that enhance CO. To compensate for hypotension, CO rises by means of an increase in heart rate and stroke volume. Increases in capillary permeability cause a shift of albumin and fluid out of the vascular space, further diminishing venous return and thus preload. The patient becomes warm and tachycardic, with a high CO and a low SVR. Other signs of MODS include decreased capillary refill, skin mottling, increases in CVP and PAOP, and dysrhythmias. SvO$_2$ may be abnormally high because areas not consuming much oxygen (e.g., skin, nonworking muscle) are being perfused but other areas may have blood shunted away from them. Eventually, either perfusion of vital organs becomes insufficient, or the cells are unable to use oxygen and their function is further compromised.

Neurological dysfunction with SIRS and MODS commonly manifests as mental status changes. Acute alteration in mental status can be an early sign of MODS. The patient may become confused and agitated, combative, disoriented, lethargic, or comatose. These changes may be caused by hypoxemia, the direct effect of the inflammatory mediators, or impaired perfusion. AKI is frequent in SIRS and MODS. AKI can be caused not only by hypoperfusion but also by the effects of the mediators. When kidney perfusion is decreased, the SNS and the renin–angiotensin system are activated. The stimulation of the renin–angiotensin system results in systemic vasoconstriction and aldosterone-mediated sodium and water reabsorption. Another risk factor for the development of AKI is the use of nephrotoxic drugs. Antibiotics commonly used to treat Gram-negative bacteria, such as aminoglycosides, can be nephrotoxic. Careful monitoring of drug levels is essential to avoid the nephrotoxic effects.

The GI tract also plays a key role in the development of MODS. GI motility is often decreased in critical illness, and this condition results in abdominal distension and paralytic ileus. In the early stages of SIRS and MODS, blood also is shunted away from the GI mucosa; thus the mucosa is highly vulnerable to ischemic injury. Decreased perfusion leads to a breakdown of this normally protective mucosal barrier, thus increasing the risk for ulceration and GI bleeding. The breakdown of the mucosal barrier of the gut increases the potential for bacterial translocation from the GI tract into the systemic circulation, which provides a pathway to the lungs, liver, and kidneys (Miller et al., 2011).

Metabolic changes are pronounced in SIRS and MODS. Both syndromes trigger a hypermetabolic response. Glycogen stores are rapidly converted to glucose (glycogenolysis). Once glycogen is depleted, amino acids are converted to glucose (gluconeogenesis), which reduces protein stores. Fatty acids are mobilized for fuel. Catecholamines and glucocorticoids are released, which results in hyperglycemia and insulin resistance. The net result is a catabolic state, and lean body mass (muscle) is lost.

The hypermetabolism associated with SIRS and MODS may last for several days and results in liver dysfunction. Liver dysfunction in MODS may exist long before it is clinically evident. The liver is unable to synthesize albumin, one of the key proteins that has an essential role in maintaining plasma oncotic pressure. Consequently, plasma oncotic pressure is altered, and fluid and protein leak from the vascular spaces to the interstitial space. Administration of albumin does not normalize oncotic pressure in this situation.

As the state of hypermetabolism persists, the patient becomes unable to convert lactate to glucose, and lactate accumulates (lactic acidosis). Despite increases in glycogenolysis and gluconeogenesis, the liver eventually becomes unable to maintain a glucose level, and the patient becomes hypoglycemic.

DIC, or simultaneous microvascular clotting and bleeding, may occur because of the depletion of clotting factors and platelets in addition to excessive fibrinolysis. (DIC is discussed in Chapter 33.)

Electrolyte imbalances are common and result from hormonal and metabolic changes and fluid shifts. These changes exacerbate mental status changes, neuro-muscular dysfunction, and dysrhythmias. The release of ADH and aldosterone results in sodium and water retention. Aldosterone increases urinary potassium loss, and catecholamines cause potassium to move into the cell, which results in hypokalemia. Hypokalemia is associated with dysrhythmias and muscle weakness. Metabolic acidosis results from impairment in tissue perfusion, hypoxia, and a shift to anaerobic metabolism with a resultant increase in hydrogen ion production. Progressive renal dysfunction also contributes to metabolic acidosis. Hypocalcemia, hypomagnesemia, and hypophosphatemia are common.

Clinical Manifestations

The clinical manifestations of MODS are presented in Table 69-12.

NURSING AND COLLABORATIVE MANAGEMENT SIRS AND MODS

Without early, goal-directed therapy, the prognosis for patients with SIRS and MODS is poor. Mortality rates have been as high as 70% to 80% when three or more organs are involved (Dellinger et al., 2013). A critical component of the nursing role is vigilant assessment and ongoing monitoring to detect early signs of deterioration or organ dysfunction. Collaborative care for patients with MODS focuses on (a) prevention and treatment of infection, (b) maintenance of tissue oxygenation, (c) nutritional and metabolic support, and (d) appropriate support of individual failing organs. Table 69-12 summarizes the management for patients with MODS.

PREVENTION AND TREATMENT OF INFECTION

Aggressive infection control strategies are essential to decrease the risk for HAIs. Strict asepsis can decrease infections related to intra-arterial lines, endotracheal tubes, urinary catheters, IV lines, and other invasive devices or procedures. Daily assessment of the ongoing need for invasive lines is an important strategy to prevent or limit HAIs.

TABLE 69-12 MULTIPLE-ORGAN DYSFUNCTION SYNDROME: CLINICAL MANIFESTATIONS AND MANAGEMENT

Clinical Manifestations of Organ Failure	Management	Clinical Manifestations of Organ Failure	Management
Cardiovascular System Biventricular failure ↓ Ejection fraction, contractility ↑ HR, ↑ SVR, ↓ CO ↓ MAP ↓ Stroke volume Myocardial depression Systolic, diastolic dysfunction	Balancing O₂ supply and demand • Supplemental O₂ • Continuous SvO₂ monitoring Circulatory assist devices • Intra-aortic balloon pump • Ventricular assist devices Continuous ECG monitoring Hemodynamic monitoring • Arterial pressure catheter • Central venous or PA catheter • PAOP readings • Maintaining MAP >65 mm Hg Maintaining CO • Volume management • Vasopressors, inotropes, vasodilators VTE prophylaxis	**Hematological System** ↑ Bleeding times, ↑ PT, ↑ PTT, ↑ INR ↑ D-dimer test results ↑ Fibrin split products ↓ Platelet count (thrombocytopenia)	Minimizing traumatic interventions (e.g., intramuscular injections, multiple venipunctures) Observation for bleeding from obvious and occult sites Replacement of factors being lost (e.g., platelets)
		Hepatic System Bilirubin >34 mcmol/L ↑ Liver enzymes (ALT, AST, GGT) ↑ Serum NH₃ ↓ Serum albumin, prealbumin, transferrin Jaundice Hepatic encephalopathy	Maintenance of adequate tissue perfusion Nutritional support (e.g., enteral feedings) Judicious use of hepatically metabolized drugs
Central Nervous System Acute change in neurological status Confusion, disorientation Failure to wean, prolonged rehabilitation Fever Hepatic encephalopathy Seizures	Evaluation for hepatic and metabolic encephalopathy Optimization of cerebral blood flow ↓ Cerebral oxygen requirements Prevention of secondary tissue ischemia • Calcium channel blockers (reduce cerebral vasospasm) Prevention of further compromise	**Renal System** Prerenal: renal hypoperfusion • BUN/creatinine ratio >20:1 • ↓ Urine Na⁺ level to <40 mmol/L • ↑ Urine specific gravity to >1.020 • ↑ Urine osmolality Intrarenal: ATN BUN/creatinine ratio <10:1–15:1 • ↑ Urine Na⁺ level to >40 mmol/L • ↓ Urine osmolality • Urine specific gravity (≈1.010)	Diuretics • Loop diuretics (e.g., furosemide [Lasix]) • May need to increase dose owing to ↓ glomerular filtration rate Dopamine (Intropin) • Enhances renal blood flow • Improves renal perfusion • Increases urine output (if volume resuscitated) • May work synergistically with diuretics Continuous renal replacement therapy (see Chapter 49)
Endocrinological System Hyperglycemia → hypoglycemia	Continuous infusion of insulin and glucose to maintain blood glucose at <8.33 mmol/L		
Gastro-Intestinal System Mucosal ischemia • ↓ Intramucosal pH • Potential translocation of gut bacteria Hypoperfusion → ↓ peristalsis, paralytic ileus Mucosal ulceration on endoscopy GI bleeding	Dietary consultation Enteral feedings • Provide essential nutrients and optimal calories • Stimulate mucosal activity Stress ulcer prophylaxis • Antacids (e.g., Maalox) • Histamine H₂-receptor blockers (e.g., famotidine [Pepcid]) • Proton pump inhibitors (e.g., omeprazole) • Sucralfate	**Respiratory System** Development of ARDS (see Chapter 70): • Severe dyspnea • PaO₂/FiO₂ ratio <200 • Bilateral fluffy infiltrates on chest radiograph • PAOP <18 mm Hg • Ventilation–perfusion mismatch • Pulmonary hypertension • Increased minute ventilation • Increased respiratory rate • Decreased compliance • Refractory hypoxemia	Prevention Optimizing oxygen delivery, minimizing oxygen consumption Mechanical ventilation (see Chapter 68) • Positive end-expiratory pressure • Lung protective modes (e.g., pressure control or inverse ratio ventilation, low tidal volumes) • Permissive hypercapnia Positioning (e.g., continuous lateral rotation therapy, prone positioning)

ALT, alanine aminotransferase; *ARDS,* acute respiratory distress syndrome; *AST,* aspartate aminotransferase; *ATN,* acute tubular necrosis; *BUN,* blood urea nitrogen; *CO,* cardiac output; *FiO₂,* fraction of inspired oxygen; *ECG,* electrocardiograph; *GGT,* γ-glutamyl transferase; *GI,* gastro-intestinal; *HR,* heart rate; *INR,* international normalized ratio; *MAP,* mean arterial pressure; *PA,* pulmonary artery; *PaO₂,* partial pressure of arterial oxygen; *PAOP,* pulmonary artery occlusive pressure; *PT,* prothrombin time; *PTT,* partial thromboplastin time; *SvO₂,* venous oxygen saturation; *SVR,* systemic vascular resistance; *VTE,* venous thrombo-embolism.

Despite these strategies, host dysfunction may lead to the development of an infection. Once an infection is suspected, interventions to control the source must be instituted. Appropriate cultures should be taken, and broad-spectrum antibiotic therapy should be initiated. Early, aggressive surgery is recommended to remove necrotic tissue (e.g., early debridement of burn tissue) that may provide a culture medium for microorganisms. Once a specific organism is identified, therapy should be modified if necessary. Aggressive pulmonary management, including early ambulation, can reduce the risk for infection devices or procedures.

MAINTENANCE OF TISSUE OXYGENATION

Hypoxemia frequently occurs in patients with SIRS and MODS. These patients have greater oxygen needs and decreased oxygen supply to the tissues. Interventions that decrease oxygen demand and increase oxygen delivery are essential. Sedation, mechanical ventilation, analgesia, paralysis, and rest may decrease oxygen demand and should be considered. Oxygen delivery may be optimized by maintaining normal levels of hemoglobin (e.g., transfusion of packed RBCs) and PaO_2 (80 to 100 mm Hg), using individualized tidal volumes with positive end-expiratory pressure (PEEP), increasing preload or myocardial contractility to enhance CO, or reducing afterload to increase CO.

NUTRITIONAL AND METABOLIC NEEDS

Hypermetabolism in SIRS or MODS can result in profound weight loss, cachexia, and further organ failure. Protein–calorie malnutrition is one of the primary manifestations of hypermetabolism and MODS. Total energy expenditure is often increased to 1.5 to 2.0 times the normal metabolic rate. Because of their relatively short half-life, plasma transferrin and prealbumin levels are monitored to assess hepatic protein synthesis.

The goal of nutritional support is to preserve organ function. Providing early and optimal nutrition decreases morbidity and mortality rates in patients with SIRS and MODS (Dellinger et al., 2013). Ideally, the patient consumes intake orally. If the patient

is unable to do so, the enteral route is initiated slowly and increased as tolerated (Dellinger et al., 2013). If enteral nutrition is not meeting caloric needs, parenteral nutrition should be initiated or added. (Enteral and parenteral nutrition are discussed in Chapter 42.) Attention to tight glycemic control (blood glucose level of <10 mmol/L) with the use of insulin protocols is important in these patients (Dellinger et al., 2013).

SUPPORT OF FAILING ORGANS

Support of any failing organs is a primary goal of therapy. For example, the patient with ARDS requires aggressive oxygen therapy and mechanical ventilation (see Chapter 70). DIC should be treated appropriately (e.g., blood products; see Chapter 33). Renal failure may necessitate dialysis. Continuous renal replacement therapy (CRRT) is better tolerated than hemodialysis, especially in a patient with hemodynamic instability (see Chapter 49).

Given the poor prognosis for MODS, withdrawal of life support may need to be considered when all resuscitative attempts fail. It is important to ensure that advance directives are clearly indicated and that the nurse follows the patient's wishes regarding end-of-life care.

CASE STUDY

Shock

Source: Scott Dumas/ Shutterstock .com.

Patient Profile

Ken Masaki, a 25-year-old male patient, was not wearing his seat belt when the car he was driving was involved in a motor vehicle accident. The windshield was broken, and Mr. Masaki was found 5 metres from his car. He was face down, conscious, and moaning. His wife and daughter were found in the car with their seat belts on. They sustained no serious injuries but were upset. All passengers were taken to the emergency department (ED). The following information pertains to Mr. Masaki.

Subjective Data

- States, "I can't breathe"
- Cries out when abdomen is palpated

Objective Data
Physical Examination

- Abdomen: slightly distended and left upper quadrant painful on palpation
- Cardiovascular: BP 80/56 mm Hg; apical pulse 138 but no palpable radial or pedal pulses; carotid pulse present but weak
- ECG as follows:

- Lungs: respiratory rate 38 breaths/min; laboured breathing with shallow respirations; asymmetric chest wall movement; absence of breath sounds on left side
- Musculo-skeletal: open compound fracture of the lower left leg
- Trachea deviated slightly to the right

Diagnostic Studies

Chest radiograph: Hemothorax and six rib fractures on left side
Hematocrit: 0.28 volume fraction

Collaborative Care (in the ED)

- Left chest tube placed, draining bright red blood
- IV access obtained via one peripheral line and right subclavian central line
- Fluid resuscitation started with crystalloids
- High-flow O_2 via nonrebreather mask

Surgical Procedure

- Repair of compound fracture
- Repair of torn intercostal artery
- Splenectomy

Discussion Questions

1. What types of shock is Mr. Masaki experiencing? What clinical manifestations did he display that support this answer?
2. What were the causes of Mr. Masaki's shock states? What are other causes of these types of shock?
3. *Priority decision:* What are the priority nursing responsibilities for Mr. Masaki?
4. *Priority decision:* What ongoing nursing assessment parameters are essential for this patient?
5. What are his potential complications?
6. *Priority decision:* Based on the assessment data presented, what are the priority nursing diagnoses?
7. *Evidence-informed practice:* The nurse is orienting a new graduate RN. He asks why crystalloids are used instead of colloids for fluid resuscitation. What should the nurse's response be?

evolve
Answers are available at *http://evolve.elsevier.com/Canada/Lewis/medsurg.*

REVIEW QUESTIONS

The number of the question corresponds to the same-numbered objective at the beginning of the chapter.

1. A client has a spinal cord injury at T4. Vital signs include falling blood pressure with bradycardia. The nurse recognizes that the client is experiencing which of the following?
   a. A relative hypervolemia
   b. An absolute hypovolemia
   c. Neurogenic shock from low blood flow
   d. Neurogenic shock from massive vasodilation

2. A 78-year-old man has confusion and temperature of 40°C. He has diabetes with purulent drainage from his right heel. After an infusion of 3 L of normal saline solution, his assessment findings are BP 84/40 mm Hg; heart rate 110; respiratory rate 42 and shallow; CO 8 L/min; and PAOP 4 mm Hg. This client's symptoms are most likely indicative of which of the following?
   a. Sepsis
   b. Septic shock
   c. Multiple-organ dysfunction syndrome
   d. Systemic inflammatory response syndrome

3. Appropriate treatment modalities for the management of cardiogenic shock include which of the following? *(Select all that apply)*
   a. Dobutamine to increase myocardial contractility
   b. Vasopressors to increase systemic vascular resistance
   c. Circulatory assist devices such as an intra-aortic balloon pump
   d. Corticosteroids to stabilize the cell wall in the infarcted myocardium
   e. Trendelenburg positioning to facilitate venous return and increase preload

4. The most accurate assessment parameters for the nurse to use to determine adequate tissue perfusion in the client with MODS are which of the following?
   a. Blood pressure, pulse, and respirations
   b. Breath sounds, blood pressure, and body temperature
   c. Pulse pressure, level of consciousness, and pupillary response
   d. Level of consciousness, urine output, and skin colour and temperature

1. d, 2. b, 3. a, c, 4. d.

ⓔvolve

For even more review questions, visit *http://evolve.elsevier.com/Canada/Lewis/medsurg*.

REFERENCES

Aitken, L. M., Williams, G., Harvey, M., et al. (2011). Nursing considerations to complement the Surviving Sepsis Campaign guidelines. *Critical Care Medicine, 39*(7), 1800–1817.

Canadian Institute for Health Information. (2009). *In focus: A national look at sepsis*. Ottawa: Author. Retrieved from *https://secure.cihi.ca/free_products/HSMR_Sepsis2009_e.pdf*. (Seminal).

Casha, S., & Christie, S. (2011). A systematic review of intensive cardiopulmonary management after spinal cord injury. *Journal of Neurotrauma, 28*(8), 1479–1495. doi:10.1089/neu.2009.1156.

Dellinger, R. P., Levy, M. M., Rhodes, A., et al. (2013). Surviving Sepsis Campaign: International guidelines for management of severe sepsis and septic shock, 2012. *Intensive Care Medicine, 39*(2), 165–228. doi:10.1007/s00134-012-2769-8.

Fry, D. E. (2012). Sepsis, systemic inflammatory response, and multiple organ dysfunction: The mystery continues. *The American Surgeon, 78*(1), 1–8.

Hall, J. E. (2016). Circulatory shock and its treatment. In *Guyton and Hall textbook of medical physiology* (13th ed.). Philadelphia: Elsevier.

Institute for Healthcare Improvement. (2017). *Bundles*. Retrieved from *http://www.ihi.org/Topics/Bundles/Pages/default.aspx*.

Lawrence, K. (2011). Pediatric sepsis and multiorgan dysfunction syndrome: Progress and continued challenges. *Critical Care Nursing Clinics of North America, 23*(2), 323–337. doi:10.1016/j.ccell.2011.02.005.

McAtee, M. E. (2011). Cardiogenic shock. *Critical Care Nursing Clinics of North America, 23*(4), 607–615. doi:10.1016/j.ccell.2011.09.001.

Meynaar, I. A., Droog, W., Batstra, M., et al. (2011). In critically ill patients, serum procalcitonin is more useful in differentiating between sepsis and SIRS than CRP, Il-6, or LBP. *Critical Care Research and Practice, 2011*, 1–6. doi:10.1155/2011/594645.

Miller, K. R., Kiraly, L. N., Lowen, C. C., et al. (2011). "Can we feed?" A mnemonic to merge nutrition and intensive care assessment of the critically ill patient. *Journal of Parenteral and Enteral Nutrition, 35*(5), 643. doi:10.1177/0148607111414136.

Moser, H. (2014). Early recognition and rapid intervention of sepsis: Implementation of a focused educational initiative emphasizing early goal-directed therapy in the emergency department. *Journal of Nursing Education and Practice, 4*(6), 23–29. doi:10.5430/jnep.v4n6p23.

Navaneelan, T., Alam, S., Peters, P. A., et al. (2016). *Health at a glance: Deaths involving sepsis in Canada*. Retrieved from *http://www.statcan.gc.ca/pub/82-624-x/2016001/article/14308-eng.htm*.

Patel, A. K., & Hollenberg, S. M. (2011). Cardiovascular failure and cardiogenic shock. *Seminars in Respiratory and Critical Care Medicine, 32*(5), 598. doi:10.1055/s-0031-1287869.

Pavlik, D. J., Simpson, R. W., Horn, E. T., et al. (2015). Pharmacotherapy of sepsis. *Critical Care Nursing Quarterly, 38*(2), 121–136. doi:10.1097/CNQ.0000000000000053.

Rochwerg, B., Alhazzani, W., Sindi, A., et al. (2014). Fluid resuscitation in sepsis: A systematic review and network meta-analysis. *Annals of Internal Medicine, 161*(5), 347–355. doi:10.7326/M14-0178.

Simons, F. E. R., Ebisawa, M., Sanchez-Borges, M., et al. (2015). 2015 update of the evidence base: World Allergy Organization anaphylaxis guidelines. *World Allergy Organization Journal, 8*(1), 32. doi:10.1186/s40413-015-0080-1.

Zheng, F., Barthel, G., Collange, O., et al. (2013). Methylene blue and epinephrine: A synergetic association for anaphylactic shock treatment. *Critical Care Medicine, 41*(1), 195–204. doi:10.1097/CCM.0b013e318267667b.

RESOURCES

Additional resources for this chapter are listed in Chapter 71.

Nursing Management

Respiratory Failure and Acute Respiratory Distress Syndrome

Written by: Richard Arbour
Adapted by: Debbie Rickeard

---

evolve WEBSITE

http://evolve.elsevier.com/Canada/Lewis/medsurg

- Review Questions (Online Only)
- Key Points
- Answer Guidelines for Case Study

- Student Case Studies
  - Acute Respiratory Failure and Ventilatory Management
  - Pulmonary Embolism and Respiratory Failure

- Customizable Nursing Care Plan
  - Acute Respiratory Failure
- Conceptual Care Map Creator
- Audio Glossary
- Content Updates

LEARNING OBJECTIVES

1. Compare the pathophysiological mechanisms that result in hypoxemic and hypercapnic respiratory failure.
2. Differentiate between early and late clinical manifestations of acute respiratory failure.
3. Describe the nursing and collaborative management of a patient with hypoxemic or hypercapnic respiratory failure.
4. Explain how the pathophysiological mechanisms that result in acute respiratory distress syndrome are related to the clinical manifestations of this syndrome.

5. Describe the nursing and collaborative management of a patient with acute respiratory distress syndrome.
6. Identify complications that may result from acute respiratory failure or acute respiratory distress syndrome and measures to prevent or reverse these complications.

KEY TERMS

acute respiratory distress syndrome (ARDS), p. 1794
alveolar hypoventilation, p. 1785
diffusion limitation, p. 1785

hypercapnia, p. 1783
hypercapnic respiratory failure, p. 1783
hypoxemia, p. 1783
hypoxemic respiratory failure, p. 1783

hypoxia, p. 1788
refractory hypoxemia, p. 1795

The normal function of the respiratory system is to facilitate gas exchange. Without an adequate exchange of oxygen (O_2) and carbon dioxide (CO_2), the metabolic demands of the tissues would not be met, and body systems would begin to rapidly fail. The management of patients in acute respiratory distress or failure revolves around the improvement of oxygenation and ventilation, treatment of the underlying disease state, reduction of anxiety, and prevention and management of complications. Acute respiratory failure and acute respiratory distress syndrome (ARDS) represent important and costly public health problems. The global effect of ARDS is difficult to estimate. The in-hospital rate of mortality from ARDS has remained high since it was first described; current mortality

rates range from 40% to 50% (Villar, Blanco, & Kacmarck, 2016). Patients with ARDS require critical nursing assessments and collaborative management to improve their outcomes, which is the focus of this chapter.

ACUTE RESPIRATORY FAILURE

The major function of the respiratory system is gas exchange, which involves the transfer of O_2 and CO_2 between the atmosphere and the blood (Figure 70-1; Urden, Stacy, & Lough, 2014). *Respiratory failure* is the state in which one or both gas-exchanging functions are inadequate: Either the amount of O_2 transferred to the blood is insufficient or the amount of CO_2 removed from

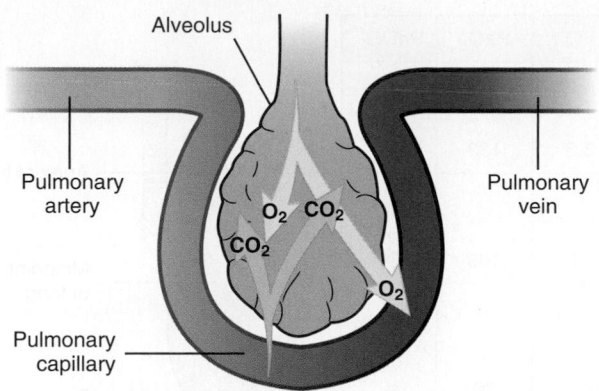

FIGURE 70-1 Normal gas-exchange unit in the lung.

FIGURE 70-2 Classification of respiratory failure. *PaCO₂*, partial pressure of carbon dioxide in arterial blood; *PaO₂*, partial pressure of oxygen in arterial blood.

the lungs is inadequate. Clinical states that interfere with O_2 transfer result in **hypoxemia**—a state of low oxygen tension in the blood (partial pressure of oxygen in arterial blood [PaO_2] <60 mm Hg), characterized by a variety of nonspecific clinical signs and symptoms—and a decrease in arterial oxygen saturation (SaO_2) as determined by measurements of arterial blood gases (ABGs). Insufficient CO_2 removal results in **hypercapnia**, the presence of excessive amounts of CO_2 in the blood; also called *hypercarbia,* it is manifested by an increase in partial pressure (or tension) of carbon dioxide in arterial blood ($PaCO_2$; Brashers & Huether, 2014; Fournier, 2014). ABGs can be measured to intermittently assess changes in pH, PaO_2, $PaCO_2$, bicarbonate, and SaO_2; and oxygen saturation can be assessed intermittently or continuously with pulse oximetry (SpO_2). Pulse oximetry offers advantages of noninvasiveness and real-time values; however, the accuracy of readings depends on correct application of the sensor to a well-perfused digit, usually a middle or ring finger. When the SpO_2 is 90%, the PaO_2 is approximately 60 mm Hg, if factors such as temperature, $PaCO_2$ and pH are normal (Brashers & Huether, 2014; Fournier, 2014). Data should be interpreted alongside clinical assessment findings and the patient's baseline values. For example, an individual with chronic lung disease may have a baseline $PaCO_2$ higher than what is considered the "normal" range. (To assist the reader, Table 70-1 summarizes abbreviations used in this chapter.)

Respiratory failure is not a disease; it is a condition that occurs as a result of one or more diseases involving the lungs or other body systems (see Tables 70-2 and 70-3). It is classified as hypoxemic or hypercapnic (Figure 70-2). *Hypoxemic respiratory failure* is also referred to as *oxygenation failure* because the primary problem is inadequate O_2 transfer between the alveoli and the pulmonary capillary bed (Fournier, 2014). Although no universal definition exists, **hypoxemic respiratory failure** is commonly defined as a PaO_2 of 60 mm Hg or less when the patient is receiving inspired oxygen at a fractional concentration (FiO_2) of 60% or greater. This definition incorporates two important concepts: (1) the PaO_2 level indicates inadequate O_2 saturation of hemoglobin; and (2) this PaO_2 level exists despite administration of supplemental O_2 at a percentage (60%) that is three times that in room air (21%). Disorders that interfere with O_2 transfer into the blood include pneumonia, pulmonary edema, pulmonary emboli, alveolar injury related to inhalation of toxic gases (e.g., smoke inhalation), and ventilator-induced lung injury. In addition, states of low cardiac output (e.g., heart failure, shock) can also cause hypoxemic respiratory failure (Urden, Stacy, & Lough, 2014).

TABLE 70-1	ABBREVIATIONS OF COMMON PULMONARY TERMS
Arterial Blood Monitoring	
ABGs	Arterial blood gases
pH	Negative log of the free hydrogen ion [H⁺]
PaO_2	Partial pressure of oxygen in arterial blood
$PaCO_2$	Partial pressure of carbon dioxide in arterial blood
SaO_2	Oxygen saturation in arterial blood as measured by ABGs
SpO_2	Oxygen saturation in arterial blood as measured by pulse oximetry
Oxygen and Lung Function Monitoring	
FiO_2	Fraction of inspired oxygen concentration
FRC	Functional residual capacity (volume of air in lung at end of expiration)
PEEP	Positive end-expiratory pressure (pressure in lungs at end of expiration)
PEFR	Peak expiratory flow rate (maximum airflow during a forced expiration)
VQ	Ventilation–perfusion ratio (relationship of ventilation to perfusion in the lungs)
V_E	Minute ventilation (tidal volume × respiratory rate)
V_T	Tidal volume (volume of air inspired with each breath)

Hypercapnic respiratory failure is referred to as *ventilatory failure* because the primary problem is insufficient CO_2 removal. **Hypercapnic respiratory failure** is commonly defined as a $PaCO_2$ above normal (>45 mm Hg) in combination with acidemia (arterial pH <7.35). This definition incorporates three important concepts: (1) the $PaCO_2$ is higher than normal; (2) there is evidence of the body's inability to compensate for this increase (acidemia); and (3) the pH is at a level at which a further decrease may lead to severe acid–base imbalance. (See Chapter 19 for a discussion of acid–base balance.) Conditions that compromise lung ventilation and subsequent CO_2 removal include drug overdoses with central nervous system (CNS) depressants, neuro-muscular diseases (e.g., myasthenia gravis), and trauma or diseases involving the spinal cord and its role in lung ventilation. Many patients experience both hypoxemic and hypercapnic respiratory failure.

TABLE 70-2	**TYPES OF RESPIRATORY FAILURE AND COMMON CAUSES***

Hypoxemic Respiratory Failure

Respiratory system	Acute respiratory distress syndrome
	Pneumonia
	Toxic inhalation (smoke inhalation)
	Hepatopulmonary syndrome (low-resistance flow state, ventilation–perfusion [VQ] mismatch)
	Massive pulmonary embolism (e.g., thrombus emboli, fat emboli)
Cardiac system	Anatomical shunt (e.g., ventricular septal defect)
	Cardiogenic pulmonary edema
	Shock (decreasing blood flow through pulmonary vasculature)

Hypercapnic Respiratory Failure

Respiratory system	Asthma
	Chronic obstructive pulmonary disease
	Cystic fibrosis
Central nervous system	Brainstem infarction
	Sedative and opioid overdose
	Spinal cord injury
	Severe head injury
Chest wall	Thoracic trauma (e.g., flail chest)
	Kyphoscoliosis
	Pain
	Morbid obesity
Neuro-muscular system	Myasthenia gravis
	Critical illness polyneuropathy
	Acute myopathy
	Toxic ingestion (e.g., tree tobacco)
	Amyotrophic lateral sclerosis
	Phrenic nerve injury
	Guillain-Barré syndrome
	Poliomyelitis
	Muscular dystrophy
	Multiple sclerosis

*This list is not all-inclusive.

Etiology and Pathophysiology

Hypoxemic Respiratory Failure. Common diseases and conditions that cause hypoxemic respiratory failure are listed in Table 70-2. Four physiological mechanisms may cause hypoxemia and subsequent hypoxemic respiratory failure: (1) mismatch between ventilation (V) and perfusion (Q), commonly referred to as *VQ mismatch*; (2) shunting; (3) diffusion limitation; and (4) hypoventilation. The most common causes are VQ mismatch and shunting (Urden, Stacy, & Lough, 2014).

Ventilation–Perfusion Mismatch. In normal lungs, the volume of blood perfusing the lungs each minute (4 to 5 L) approximates the amount of fresh gas that reaches the alveoli each minute (4 to 5 L). In a perfectly matched system, each portion of the lung would receive approximately 1 mL of air for each 1 mL of blood flow. This match of ventilation and perfusion would result in a VQ ratio of 1:1 (e.g., 1 mL of air per 1 mL of blood), which is expressed as VQ = 1; thus ventilation volume would be identical to perfusion volume. Although this example implies that the ideal situation is that ventilation and perfusion are matched in all areas of the lung, this situation does not normally exist. In reality, there is some regional mismatch even under normal conditions. At the lung apex, VQ ratios are greater than 1 (more

VQ	PaO$_2$	PaCO$_2$
3.3	132	28
1.0	108	39
0.63	89	42

FIGURE 70-3 Regional ventilation–perfusion (VQ) differences in the normal lung. At the lung apex, the VQ ratio is 3.3; at the midpoint, it is 1.0; and at the base, it is 0.63. This difference causes the arterial partial pressure of oxygen (PaO$_2$) to be higher at the apex of the lung and lower at the base. Values for arterial partial pressure of carbon dioxide (PaCO$_2$) are the opposite (i.e., lower at the apex and higher at the base). Blood that exits the lung has a mixture of these values.

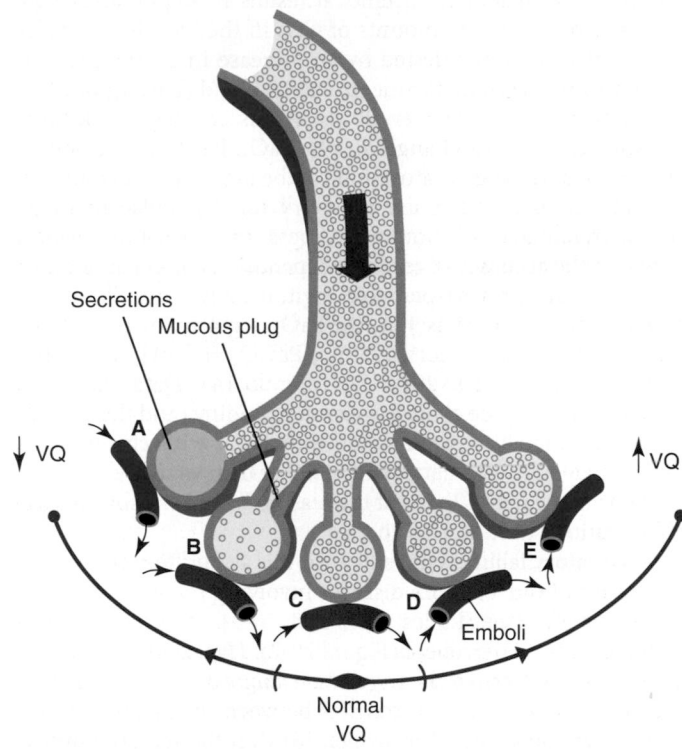

FIGURE 70-4 Range of ventilation–perfusion (VQ) relationships. **A,** Absolute shunt: no ventilation as a result of fluid filling the alveoli. **B,** VQ mismatch in which ventilation partially compromised by secretions in the airway. **C,** Normal lung unit. **D,** VQ mismatch in which perfusion is partially compromised by emboli obstructing blood flow. **E,** Dead space: no perfusion as a result of obstruction of the pulmonary capillary.

ventilation than perfusion). At the lung base, VQ ratios are less than 1 (less ventilation than perfusion). Because changes at the lung apex balance changes at the base, the net effect is a close overall match (Figure 70-3).

Many diseases and conditions alter overall VQ matching and thus cause VQ mismatch (Figure 70-4). The most common are those in which increased secretions are present in the airways (as in chronic obstructive pulmonary disease [COPD]) or the alveoli (as in pneumonia) and when bronchospasm is present (as in asthma). VQ mismatch may also result from alveolar collapse (atelectasis) or from pain. Uncontrolled pain interferes with chest and abdominal wall movement, compromising lung ventilation. In addition, pain increases muscle and motor tension, which leads to generalized muscle rigidity; causes systemic vasoconstriction and activation of the stress response; and increases O_2 consumption and CO_2 production (Brashers & Huether, 2014; Fournier, 2014). All of these conditions may increase both metabolic demands (for O_2) and ventilatory demands, and, at the same time, airflow (ventilation) to alveoli is limited. Because no effect on blood flow (perfusion) to the gas-exchange units is exerted to balance the equation, the consequence is VQ mismatch. A pulmonary embolus affects the perfusion portion of the VQ relationship. The embolus limits blood flow but has no effect on airflow to the alveoli, which again causes VQ mismatch (see Figure 70-4).

Oxygen therapy is an appropriate first step to reverse hypoxemia caused by VQ mismatch because not all gas-exchange units are affected. Oxygen therapy increases the PaO_2 in blood leaving normal gas-exchange units, thus causing the PaO_2 to be higher than normal. The well-oxygenated blood mixes with poorly oxygenated blood, which raises the overall PaO_2 of blood leaving the lungs. Optimal treatment for hypoxemia caused by VQ mismatch is directed at the cause.

Shunt. Shunting is the situation in which blood exits the heart without having participated in gas exchange. A shunt can be viewed as an extreme VQ mismatch (see Figure 70-4). There are two types of shunts: In an *anatomical shunt,* blood passes through an anatomical channel in the heart (e.g., ventricular septal defect), bypassing the lungs. In an *intrapulmonary shunt,* blood flows through the pulmonary capillaries without participating in gas exchange. Intrapulmonary shunt occurs in conditions in which alveoli fill with fluid (e.g., ARDS, pneumonia, pulmonary edema). In hypoxemia due to shunt, O_2 therapy alone may not effectively increase the PaO_2 because (a) blood passes from the right side of the heart to the left side without passing through the lungs (anatomical shunt) or (b) the alveoli are filled with fluid, which prevents gas exchange (intrapulmonary shunt). Patients with such shunts are usually more hypoxemic than patients with VQ mismatch, and they may require both mechanical ventilation and a high FiO_2 to improve gas exchange.

Diffusion Limitation. Diffusion limitation is the decrease in gas exchange across the alveolar–capillary membrane by processes that thicken or destroy the membrane (Figure 70-5). Conditions that affect the pulmonary vascular bed, such as severe emphysema or recurrent pulmonary emboli, can worsen diffusion limitation. Some diseases (e.g., pulmonary fibrosis, interstitial lung disease, ARDS) cause the alveolar–capillary membrane to become thicker (fibrotic), which slows gas transport. Diffusion limitation is more likely to cause hypoxemia during exercise than at rest. During exercise, blood moves more rapidly through the lungs. Because the transit rate is increased, red blood cells are in the lungs for a shorter time, limiting opportunity for diffusion of O_2 across the alveolar–capillary membrane. The classical sign of diffusion limitation is hypoxemia that is present during exercise but not at rest.

Alveolar Hypoventilation. Alveolar hypoventilation is a decrease in ventilation that results in an increase in $PaCO_2$ and a consequent decrease in PaO_2. Alveolar hypoventilation may result from restrictive lung disease, CNS disease, chest wall

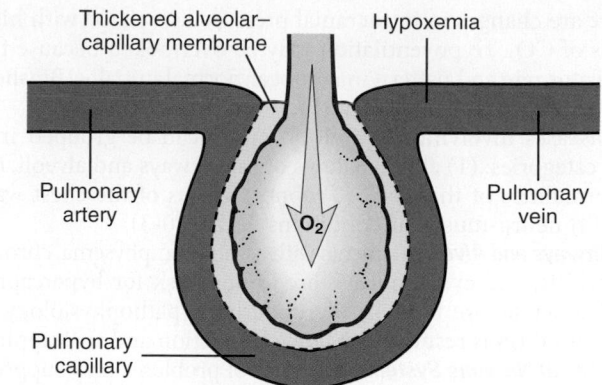

FIGURE 70-5 Diffusion limitation. Exchange of CO_2 and O_2 cannot occur because of the thickened alveolar–capillary membrane.

dysfunction, or neuro-muscular disease. Although primarily a mechanism of hypercapnic respiratory failure, alveolar hypoventilation is mentioned here because it also causes hypoxemia.

Interrelationship of Mechanisms. Frequently, hypoxemic respiratory failure is caused by a combination of two or more of the following: VQ mismatch, shunting, diffusion limitation, and hypoventilation. Patients with acute respiratory failure secondary to pneumonia may have a combination of VQ mismatch and shunting because inflammation, edema, and the hypersecretion of exudate within the bronchioles and the terminal respiratory units obstruct the airways (VQ mismatch) and fill the alveoli with exudate (shunt). In addition, shunting may be increased because of improper positioning (affected lung down). Patients with cardiogenic pulmonary edema or ARDS may have a combination of shunting and VQ mismatch because some alveoli are completely filled with fluid from edema (shunting) and others are partially filled with fluid (VQ mismatch).

Hypoxemia resulting from shunting does not respond to increases in supplemental oxygen because the capillary bed surrounding the affected alveoli is never exposed to oxygen-rich gas. As a result, hypoxemia that results from shunting is difficult to treat (Brashers & Huether, 2014; Fournier, 2014).

Hypercapnic Respiratory Failure. Hypercapnic respiratory failure results from an imbalance between ventilatory supply and ventilatory demand. *Ventilatory supply* is the maximum ventilation (gas flow in and out of the lungs) that the patient can sustain without developing respiratory muscle fatigue. *Ventilatory demand* is the amount of ventilation needed to keep the $PaCO_2$ normal. Normally, ventilatory supply far exceeds ventilatory demand. As a consequence, individuals with normal lung function can engage in strenuous exercise, which increases CO_2 production without an elevation in $PaCO_2$. Patients with pre-existing lung disease (e.g., severe emphysema) do not have this advantage and cannot effectively increase lung ventilation in response to exercise or metabolic demands. Typically, considerable dysfunction is present before ventilatory demand exceeds supply.

When ventilatory demand does exceed supply, a normal $PaCO_2$ cannot be sustained, and hypercapnia occurs, which reflects substantial lung dysfunction. Hypercapnic respiratory failure is sometimes called *ventilatory failure* because it represents primarily an inability of the respiratory system to clear sufficient CO_2 and maintain a normal $PaCO_2$.

The associated respiratory acidosis that accompanies hypercapnia can result in dysrhythmias, somnolence, and even coma.

There are changes in intracranial pressure associated with high levels of CO_2. Hypoventilation may be overlooked because the ventilator rate and pattern may appear normal initially (Brashers & Huether, 2014; Fournier, 2014).

Diseases involving respiratory failure can be grouped into four categories: (1) abnormalities of the airways and alveoli, (2) abnormalities of the CNS, (3) abnormalities of the chest wall, and (4) neuro-muscular conditions (Table 70-3).

Airways and Alveoli. Patients with asthma, emphysema, chronic bronchitis, and cystic fibrosis are at high risk for hypercapnic respiratory failure because the underlying pathophysiology of these conditions results in airflow obstruction and air trapping.

Central Nervous System. A variety of problems may suppress the drive to breathe. Commonly, overdose of an opioid or other CNS depressant drug decreases CO_2 reactivity in the brainstem, which allows arterial CO_2 levels to rise. A brainstem infarction or severe head injury may also interfere with normal function of the respiratory centre in the medulla. Affected patients are at risk for respiratory ailure because the medulla does not alter the respiratory rate in response to changes in $PaCO_2$. Independent of direct brainstem dysfunction, brain injury resulting in significant CNS depression or loss of consciousness may impair the patient's ability to protect the airway. CNS dysfunction may also include high-level spinal cord injuries that limit innervation of the respiratory muscles.

Chest Wall. Various conditions prevent normal chest wall movement, thereby limiting lung expansion. In patients with flail chest, the rib cage cannot expand normally because of painful fractures, mechanical restriction, and muscle spasm. In patients with kyphoscoliosis, changes in spinal configuration compress the lungs, preventing normal chest wall expansion. In patients with massive obesity, the weight of the chest and abdominal contents may limit lung expansion. Patients with these conditions are at risk for respiratory failure because these dysfunctions limit lung expansion or diaphragmatic movement and, consequently, gas exchange.

TABLE 70-3 PREDISPOSING FACTORS FOR ACUTE RESPIRATORY FAILURE

Predisposing Factors	Mechanisms of Respiratory Failure
Airways and Alveoli	
Acute respiratory distress syndrome • *Direct lung injury:* Aspiration; severe, disseminated pulmonary infection; near-drowning; toxic gas inhalation; airway contusion • *Indirect lung injury:* Sepsis or septic shock, severe nonthoracic trauma, cardiopulmonary bypass	Fluid enters the interstitial space and the alveoli, markedly impairing gas exchange. The result is an initial ↓ in PaO_2 and a later ↑ in $PaCO_2$. A low-flow state to pulmonary capillaries can result in ischemic injury to lung tissues with loss of integrity of the alveolar–capillary membrane.
Asthma	Bronchospasm escalates in severity rather than responding to therapy. Bronchospasm, edema of the bronchial mucosa, and plugging of small airways with secretions greatly reduce airflow. Work of breathing increases, causing respiratory muscle fatigue. ↓ in PaO_2 and ↑ in $PaCO_2$ (see Chapter 31).
Chronic obstructive pulmonary disease (COPD)	Alveoli are destroyed by protease–antiprotease imbalance or respiratory infection, or an exacerbation of COPD escalates in severity rather than responding to therapy. Secretions obstruct airflow. Work of breathing increases and causes respiratory muscle fatigue. ↓ in PaO_2 and ↑ in $PaCO_2$.
Cystic fibrosis	Abnormal Na^+ and Cl^- transport results in secretions that are viscous, poorly cleared, and therefore foci for infection. Over time, the airways become clogged with copious, purulent sputum. Secretions obstruct airflow. Repeated infections destroy alveoli. Work of breathing increases, causing respiratory muscle fatigue. ↓ in PaO_2 and ↑ in $PaCO_2$.
Central Nervous System	
Overdose of opioid or other CNS depressant	Respirations are slowed by drug effect. Insufficient CO_2 is excreted, resulting in ↑ $PaCO_2$.
Brainstem infarction, head injury	Medulla cannot alter respiratory rate in response to changes in $PaCO_2$.
Chest Wall	
Severe soft tissue injury, flail chest, rib fracture, pain	Structural dysfunction and pain prevent normal rib cage expansion, resulting in inadequate gas exchange.
Kyphoscoliosis	Change in spinal configuration compresses the lungs and prevents normal expansion of the chest wall, resulting in inadequate gas exchange.
Morbid obesity	Weight of the chest and abdominal contents prevents normal rib cage movement, resulting in inadequate gas exchange.
Neuro-Muscular Conditions	
Cervical cord injury, phrenic nerve injury	Neural control is lost, preventing use of the diaphragm, the major muscle of respiration. Consequently, the patient inspires a smaller tidal volume, which predisposes to an ↑ in $PaCO_2$.
Amyotrophic lateral sclerosis (ALS), Guillain-Barré syndrome, muscular dystrophy, multiple sclerosis, poliomyelitis, myasthenia gravis, myopathy, critical illness polyneuropathy, prolonged use of neuro-muscular blocking agents	Respiratory muscle weakness or paralysis occurs, preventing normal CO_2 excretion. Dysfunction may be progressive (muscular dystrophy, multiple sclerosis), progressive with no potential of recovery (ALS), rapid with good expectation of recovery (Guillain-Barré), or stable for extended periods (poliomyelitis, myasthenia gravis).

CNS, central nervous system; *$PaCO_2$*, partial pressure of carbon dioxide in arterial blood; *PaO_2*, partial pressure of oxygen in arterial blood.

Neuro-muscular Conditions. Various types of neuro-muscular diseases may result in respiratory muscle weakness or paralysis (see Table 70-2). For example, patients with Guillain-Barré syndrome, muscular dystrophy, myasthenia gravis (acute exacerbation), or multiple sclerosis are at risk for respiratory failure because the respiratory muscles are weakened or paralyzed. Therefore, they are unable to maintain normal $PaCO_2$ levels.

Note that respiratory failure occurs in three of these categories (CNS, chest wall, neuro-muscular conditions) even if the lungs are normal. Affected patients may have no damage to lung tissue but are unable to inspire sufficient tidal volume to expel CO_2 from the lungs.

Tissue Oxygen Needs. Even though respiratory failure is determined by the PaO_2 and $PaCO_2$, the major threat is the inability of the lungs to meet the oxygen demands of the tissues, whether as a result of inadequate O_2 delivery or because the tissues are unable to use the O_2 delivered to them. Respiratory failure may also occur as a result of the stress response and dramatic increases in tissue oxygen consumption (Brashers & Huether, 2014; Fournier, 2014). Tissue O_2 delivery is determined by the amount of O_2 carried in the hemoglobin, as well as by cardiac output. Therefore, respiratory failure increases risk if the patient has coexisting cardiac problems or anemia. Failure of O_2 utilization most commonly occurs as a result of septic shock. In this situation, adequate O_2 may be delivered to the tissues, but an abnormally high amount of O_2 returns in the venous blood, which indicates that it is not being extracted and used at the tissue level. (Shock is discussed in Chapter 69.) Acid–base alterations (e.g., alkalosis, acidosis) may also interfere with oxygen delivery to peripheral tissues (see Chapter 28).

Clinical Manifestations

Respiratory failure may develop suddenly or gradually over several days or longer. A sudden decrease in PaO_2 or a rapid rise in $PaCO_2$ implies a serious condition, which can rapidly become a life-threatening emergency. An example is the development of severe bronchospasm and a marked decrease in airflow in a patient with asthma, which can result in respiratory arrest. A more gradual change in PaO_2 and $PaCO_2$ is better tolerated because compensation can occur. An example is the development of a progressive increase in $PaCO_2$ over several days after the onset of a respiratory infection in a patient with COPD. Because the change occurs gradually over several days, there is time for renal compensation (e.g., retention of bicarbonate), which minimizes the change in arterial pH. The patient has compensated respiratory acidosis (Urden, Stacy, & Lough, 2014). (See Chapter 19 for a discussion of renal compensation for acid–base disorders.)

Manifestations of respiratory failure are related to the extent of change in PaO_2 or $PaCO_2$, the rapidity of change (acute versus chronic), and the ability to compensate or overcome this change. When the patient's compensatory mechanisms fail, respiratory failure occurs. Because clinical manifestations are variable, it is important to monitor trends in ABGs and pulse oximetry to evaluate the extent of change. These measurements cannot substitute for clinical assessment and should be interpreted within the context of clinical assessment findings. Frequently, the initial indication of respiratory failure is a change in the patient's mental status. The cerebral cortex is very sensitive to variations in oxygenation and acid–base balance, and mental status changes occur early and frequently before ABG results show change. Restlessness, confusion, agitation, and combative behaviour suggest inadequate delivery of O_2 to the brain and should be investigated.

The nurse may detect manifestations of respiratory failure that are specific (arise from the respiratory system) or nonspecific (arise from other body systems; Table 70-4). An understanding of these manifestations is critical for detecting the onset of respiratory failure and effective treatment.

Tachycardia and mild hypertension can also be early signs of respiratory failure. They may indicate an attempt by the heart to compensate for decreased O_2 delivery. A severe morning headache may suggest that hypercapnia occurred during the night, increasing cerebral blood flow by vasodilation. At night, the respiratory rate is slower, and the lungs of patients at risk for respiratory failure may remove less $PaCO_2$. Rapid, shallow breaths suggest that the tidal volume may be inadequate to remove CO_2 from the lungs. Cyanosis is an unreliable indicator of hypoxemia and is a late sign of respiratory failure because it does not occur until hypoxemia is severe ($PaO_2 \leq 45$ mm Hg).

TABLE 70-4	**CLINICAL MANIFESTATIONS OF HYPOXEMIA AND HYPERCAPNIA***
Specific	**Nonspecific**
Hypoxemia	
Respiratory	Cerebral
• ↓ SpO_2 (<80%)	• Agitation
• Dyspnea	• Coma (late)
• Intercostal muscle retraction	• Confusion
• Prolonged expiration (ratio of length of inspiration to that of expiration: 1:3, 1:4)	• Delirium
	• Disorientation
	• ↓ Level of consciousness
• Tachypnea	• Restlessness, combativeness
• Use of accessory muscles in respiration	Cardiac
	• Dysrhythmias (late)
• Cyanosis (late)	• Hypertension
• Paradoxical chest or abdominal wall movement with respiratory cycle (late)	• Hypotension (late)
	• Skin cool, clammy, and diaphoretic
	• Tachycardia
	Other
	• Fatigue
	• Inability to speak without pausing to breathe
Hypercapnia	
Respiratory	Cerebral
• Dyspnea	• Coma (late)
• ↓ Minute ventilation	• Disorientation
• ↓ Respiratory rate or ↑ rate with shallow respirations	• Morning headache
	• Progressive somnolence
• ↓ Tidal volume	Cardiac
	• Bounding pulse
	• Dysrhythmias
	• Hypertension
	• Tachycardia
	Neuro-muscular
	• ↓ Deep tendon reflexes
	• Muscle weakness
	• Tremor, seizures (late)
	Other
	• Pursed-lip breathing

*This list is not all-inclusive.
SpO_2, oxygen saturation in arterial blood as measured by pulse oximetry.

Consequences of Hypoxemia and Hypoxia. *Hypoxemia* occurs when the amount of O_2 in arterial blood is less than the normal value (see Chapter 28). **Hypoxia** is the condition in which the PaO_2 has fallen sufficiently to cause signs and symptoms of inadequate oxygenation (see Table 70-4). Hypoxemia can lead to hypoxia if not corrected. If hypoxia or hypoxemia is severe, cell metabolism shifts from aerobic to anaerobic. Anaerobic metabolism entails the use of more fuel, produces less energy, and is less efficient than aerobic metabolism. The waste product of anaerobic metabolism, lactic acid, is more difficult to remove from the body than CO_2 because lactic acid must be buffered with sodium bicarbonate. When the body does not have adequate sodium bicarbonate to buffer the lactic acid produced by anaerobic metabolism, metabolic acidosis and cell death may result.

Hypoxia and metabolic acidosis have adverse effects on the vital organs and systems, especially the heart and the CNS. To compensate for decreased O_2 in the blood, the heart rate and cardiac output increase. A cardiovascular hyperdynamic state may also occur as a result of catecholamine release in association with the physiological stress response. This response can occur fairly rapidly. As the PaO_2 decreases and acidosis increases, the heart muscle may become dysfunctional, and cardiac output may decrease. In addition, angina and dysrhythmias may occur. All of these consequences result in a further decrease in oxygenation. Permanent brain damage may occur because of O_2 deprivation. Renal function may also be impaired, and sodium retention, edema formation, acute tubular necrosis, and uremia may occur. Gastro-intestinal system alterations include tissue ischemia, increased permeability of the intestinal wall, and possible translocation of bacteria from the gastro-intestinal tract into the circulation.

Specific Clinical Manifestations. A patient in respiratory failure may have several clinical findings indicating distress, such as rapid, shallow breathing or a respiratory rate slower than normal. Both changes predispose to insufficient CO_2 removal. The patient may increase the respiratory rate in an effort to blow off accumulated CO_2. This breathing pattern requires a substantial amount of work and predisposes to respiratory muscle fatigue. A change from a rapid rate to a slower rate in a patient in acute respiratory distress suggests extreme fatigue and possible impending respiratory arrest.

The position that the patient assumes is an indication of the effort associated with breathing. The patient may be able to lie down (mild distress), be able to lie down but prefer to sit (moderate distress), or be unable to breathe unless sitting upright (severe distress). A common position is to sit with the arms propped on the overbed table. This position, called the *tripod position*, helps decrease the work of breathing because propping the arms increases the anterior–posterior diameter of the chest and changes pressure in the thorax. The patient may use pursed-lip breathing (see Chapter 31) because it increases SaO_2 by slowing respirations, allowing more time for expiration, and preventing the small bronchioles from collapsing, thus facilitating air exchange. Another assessment parameter is the number of pillows the patient requires in order to breathe comfortably when resting. The degree of dyspnea that the patient experiences when lying flat is termed *orthopnea*, documented as one-, two-, three-, or four-pillow orthopnea.

A person experiencing dyspnea is working hard to breathe and may be able to speak only a few words between breaths. The degree to which the patient is able to speak without pausing to breathe is an indication of the severity of dyspnea. The patient may speak in sentences (mild or no distress), phrases (moderate distress), or words (severe distress). The patient may have "two-word" or "three-word" dyspnea, signifying that only two or three words can be said before pausing to breathe. When walking, the patient may also experience earlier onset of fatigue. An additional assessment parameter is how far the patient is able to walk without stopping to rest.

There may be a change in the *inspiratory-to-expiratory (I:E) ratio*. Normally, the I:E ratio is 1:2, meaning expiration is twice as long as inspiration. In respiratory distress, the ratio may increase to 1:3 or 1:4, which signifies airflow obstruction, and more time is necessary to empty the lungs.

The nurse may observe *retraction* (inward movement) of the intercostal spaces or the supraclavicular area and use of the accessory muscles during inspiration or expiration, which signifies moderate distress. Paradoxical breathing indicates severe distress. Normally, the thorax and the abdomen move outward on inspiration and inward on exhalation. During *paradoxical breathing,* the abdomen and the chest move in the opposite manner: outward during exhalation and inward during inspiration. Paradoxical breathing results from maximal use of the accessory muscles of respiration. The patient may also be diaphoretic from the work associated with breathing.

Auscultation should be performed in order to assess the patient's baseline breath sounds, as well as any changes from baseline. The nurse should note the presence and the location of any adventitious breath sounds. Crackles and wheezes may indicate pulmonary edema or emphysema. Absence of or diminished breath sounds may indicate atelectasis or pleural effusion. Bronchial breath sounds over the lung periphery often result from lung consolidation, as occurs with pneumonia. A pleural friction rub may also be heard in the presence of pneumonia that has involved the pleura.

A thorough nursing assessment may result in early detection of manifestations associated with respiratory insufficiency, which allows therapy to be instituted before the patient experiences respiratory failure. Patients with end-stage (severe) chronic lung disease may have low PaO_2 values or elevated $PaCO_2$ values and crackles as their "normal" baseline. It is especially important to monitor specific and nonspecific signs of respiratory failure in patients with COPD or other pre-existing chronic diseases because a small change can cause significant decompensation (see Table 70-4). Any deterioration in mental status, such as agitation, combative behaviour, confusion, or decreased level of consciousness, should be reported immediately because this may indicate deterioration in clinical status and the need for mechanical ventilation.

Diagnostic Studies

After physical assessment, the diagnostic studies most commonly used to determine respiratory failure are ABG analysis and chest radiographic studies. ABG measurements are used to determine the levels of $PaCO_2$, PaO_2, bicarbonate, and pH. An indwelling catheter may be inserted into a peripheral artery for monitoring systemic blood pressure and obtaining ABGs measurements. Pulse oximetry is used for monitoring oxygenation but reveals little about ventilation. In respiratory failure, ABG measurements are necessary to determine both oxygenation (PaO_2) and ventilation ($PaCO_2$) status, as well as obtain information related to acid–base balance (Burns, 2014). Chest radiographic examination helps identify possible causes of respiratory failure (e.g., atelectasis, pneumonia). In patients with respiratory failure that does not necessitate acute intervention, pulmonary function tests may be performed.

Other diagnostic studies that may be done include a complete blood cell count (CBC), serum electrolyte measurements, urinalysis, and electrocardiography. Sputum and blood cultures are obtained if infection is likely. If pulmonary embolus is suspected, a VQ lung scan or pulmonary angiography may be done. For a patient requiring endotracheal intubation, end-tidal CO_2 is measured to assess tube placement immediately after intubation and during ventilator management to assess trends in lung ventilation.

In severe respiratory failure, a pulmonary artery catheter may be inserted to measure pressures on the right side of the heart and cardiac output, as well as mixed venous oxygen saturation. This information is helpful in determining the adequacy of tissue perfusion and the patient's response to treatment. Pulmonary artery, pulmonary artery wedge (occlusion), and left atrial pressures are monitored to determine whether the accumulation of fluid in the lungs is the result of cardiac or pulmonary problems. These parameters are also monitored to determine the response of the lungs and heart to hypoxemia and the patient's response to therapy. Pulmonary arterial pressure monitoring can also provide feedback about the physiological effects of mechanical ventilation on hemodynamic status. (See Chapter 68 for a discussion of hemodynamic monitoring.)

NURSING AND COLLABORATIVE MANAGEMENT ACUTE RESPIRATORY FAILURE

Because many different problems cause respiratory failure, care of affected patients varies. This section is a discussion of general assessment and collaborative treatments that apply to patients with acute respiratory failure. In acute care settings, there is often an overlap of function between nursing and other members of the health care team. Aside from the multidisciplinary health care team, family members play a valuable role in the patient's care and recovery. Further discussion of issues related to the family and caregivers can be found in Chapter 68.

Nursing Assessment

Subjective and objective data that should be obtained from patients with acute respiratory failure are listed in Table 70-5.

NURSING DIAGNOSES

Nursing diagnoses for the patient with acute respiratory failure include, but are not limited to, the following:

- *Impaired gas exchange* (related to alveolar hypoventilation, intrapulmonary shunting, VQ mismatch, and diffusion impairment)
- *Ineffective airway clearance* related to *excessive mucus, retained secretions*

TABLE 70-5   NURSING ASSESSMENT

Acute Respiratory Failure

Subjective Data
Important Health Information
Past health history: Chronic lung disease; potential occupational exposures to lung toxins; smoking (pack-years); childhood illnesses, previous hospitalizations related to lung disease; thoracic or spinal cord trauma; extreme obesity; altered consciousness; age (physiological and chronological); use or abuse of alcohol, other drugs; drug allergies, recent travel, SARS
Medications: Use of oxygen, inhalers (bronchodilators), home nebulization, over-the-counter medications; immuno-suppressant (corticosteroid) therapy, CNS depressants; vitamin and herbal supplements
Surgery or other treatments: Previous intubation and mechanical ventilation; recent thoracic or abdominal surgery

Symptoms
- Anorexia, bloatedness, heartburn; weight gain or loss; decreased appetite
- Anxiety, depression
- Changes in sleep pattern
- Dyspnea at rest or with activity; wheezing or cough (productive or nonproductive); sputum (volume, colour, viscosity)
- Fatigue, dizziness; diaphoresis
- Headache, chest pain or tightness
- Palpitations, swollen feet

Objective Data
General
Restlessness, agitation

Integumentary
Pale, cool, clammy skin or warm flushed skin; peripheral and central cyanosis; peripheral dependent edema

Respiratory
Shallow, increased respiratory rate progressing to decreased rate; use of accessory muscles with evidence of retractions, altered I : E ratio; increased diaphragmatic excursion or asymmetrical chest expansion; asynchronous respirations; tactile fremitus, crepitus, or deviated trachea on palpation; resonant, hyper-resonant, or dull percussion note; absence of, diminished, or adventitious breath sounds; bronchial or bronchovesicular sounds heard in other than normal location, inspiratory stridor, pleural friction rub

Cardiovascular
Tachycardia progressing to bradycardia, dysrhythmias, extra heart sounds (S_3, S_4); bounding pulse; hypertension progressing to hypotension; pulsus paradoxus; jugular vein distension; pedal edema

Gastro-Intestinal
Abdominal distension with tympany; ascites, epigastric tenderness, hepatojugular reflex

Neurological
Somnolence, confusion, slurred speech, restlessness, delirium, agitation, tremors, seizures, coma; asterixis, decreased deep tendon reflexes; papilledema

Possible Laboratory Findings
↑ or ↓ pH, ↑ or ↓ $PaCO_2$, ↓ PaO_2, ↑ or ↓ bicarbonate, ↓ SaO_2, ↓ PEFR, ↓tidal volume, ↓ forced vital capacity, ↓ minute ventilation, ↓ negative inspiratory force; altered serum electrolyte values, hemoglobin, white blood cells, and hematocrit; abnormal findings on chest radiograph; abnormal pulmonary artery and pulmonary artery wedge pressures

CNS, central nervous system; *I : E,* inspiratory to expiratory; *$PaCO_2$,* partial pressure of carbon dioxide in arterial blood; *PaO_2,* partial pressure of oxygen in arterial blood; *PEFR,* peak expiratory flow rate; *SaO_2,* oxygen saturation in arterial blood as measured by arterial blood gases; *SARS,* severe acute respiratory syndrome.

- *Ineffective breathing pattern* related to *neuro-muscular impairment of respirations, pain, anxiety, decreased level of consciousness, respiratory muscle fatigue, and bronchospasm*

Additional information on nursing diagnoses for the patient with acute respiratory failure is presented in Nursing Care Plan (NCP) 70-1, available on the Evolve website.

PLANNING

The overall goals for patients in acute respiratory failure are to restore baseline (a) ABG values, (b) breath sounds, (c) breathing patterns, and (d) ability to clear secretions.

PREVENTION

Prevention and early recognition of respiratory distress are important aspects of care for any patient at risk for respiratory failure. Prevention involves a thorough physical assessment and history (to identify patients at risk for respiratory failure) followed by appropriate nursing interventions. For example, a patient at risk for respiratory failure should receive teaching regarding coughing, deep breathing, incentive spirometry, and ambulation as appropriate. Prevention of atelectasis, pneumonia, and complications of immobility, as well as optimizing hydration and nutrition, can potentially decrease the risk of respiratory failure in acute or critically ill patients.

RESPIRATORY THERAPY

The major goals of care for acute respiratory failure include maintaining adequate oxygenation and ventilation. This is accomplished by collaboration among the nursing, medical, and respiratory care teams. The interventions used include O$_2$ therapy, mobilization of secretions, and positive-pressure ventilation (Table 70-6).

OXYGEN THERAPY. The primary goal of O$_2$ therapy is to correct hypoxemia. If hypoxemia is secondary to VQ mismatch, supplemental O$_2$ administered at 1 to 3 L/min by nasal cannula or at 24% to 32% by simple face mask or Venturi mask should improve the PaO$_2$ and SaO$_2$. Hypoxemia secondary to intrapulmonary shunt is usually not responsive to high O$_2$ concentrations, and affected patients usually require positive-pressure ventilation (PPV). PPV helps provide O$_2$ therapy and humidification, decrease the work of breathing, and reduce respiratory muscle fatigue. In addition, the positive pressure may assist in opening collapsed airways and decreasing shunting. PPV may be provided via an endotracheal tube (most frequently) or noninvasively by means of a tight-fitting mask (Messika, Ahmed, Gaudry, et al., 2015). (See Chapter 68 for a detailed discussion of mechanical ventilation.)

The type of O$_2$ delivery system chosen for a patient in acute respiratory failure should (a) be tolerated by the patient, inasmuch as feelings of claustrophobia related to the face mask may prompt the patient to remove it, and (b) maintain PaO$_2$ at 55 to 60 mm Hg or more and SaO$_2$ at 90% or more at the lowest O$_2$ concentration possible. High O$_2$ concentration is associated with adverse effects. Intubated patients who receive more than 50% FiO$_2$ for more than 24 hours are at greatest risk to develop O$_2$ toxicity (Urden, Stacy, & Lough, 2014). Toxic O$_2$ free radicals are a metabolite of O$_2$ metabolism; in the setting of extended exposure to high concentrations, the supply of enzymes responsible for neutralizing those radicals is exhausted, which results in in acute lung injury. Absorption atelectasis can also occur when excess O$_2$ displaces the nitrogen normally present in alveoli, causing alveolar collapse (Brashers & Huether, 2014; Fournier, 2014). The effects of prolonged exposure to high levels of O$_2$ include increased pulmonary microvascular permeability, decreased

TABLE 70-6 **COLLABORATIVE CARE**	
Acute Respiratory Failure	
Diagnostic • History and physical examination • ABG measurements • Blood and sputum cultures (if indicated) • Chest radiography • Complete blood cell count • Electrocardiography • O$_2$ saturation • Pulmonary artery pressure, pulmonary artery occlusive (wedge) pressure, and left atrial pressure • Serum electrolyte mesurements and urinalysis	• Noninvasive positive-pressure ventilation • O$_2$ therapy • Positive-pressure ventilation **Drug Therapy** • Reduction of airway inflammation (corticosteroids) • Reduction of anxiety and restlessness (e.g., lorazepam [Ativan]) • Reduction of pulmonary congestion (e.g., furosemide [Lasix]) • Relief of bronchospasm (e.g., salbutamol) • Treatment of pulmonary infections (e.g., antibiotics)
Collaborative Therapy **Respiratory Therapy** • Airway suctioning • Chest physiotherapy • Effective coughing • Hydration and humidification • Incentive spirometry • Intubation with mechanical ventilation • Mobilization of secretions	**Medical Supportive Therapy** • Maintenance of adequate cardiac output • Maintenance of adequate hemoglobin concentration • Management of the underlying cause of respiratory failure **Nutritional Therapy** • Enteral nutrition support • Parenteral nutrition support

ABG, arterial blood gas.

surfactant production and surfactant inactivation, and fibrotic changes in the alveoli. (Oxygen delivery devices are discussed in Chapter 31.)

Additional risks of O$_2$ therapy are specific to patients with chronic hypercapnia, such as those with COPD. Chronic hypercapnia may blunt the response of chemoreceptors in the medulla. In this situation, respirations are stimulated by hypoxia. If the PaO$_2$ is suddenly increased, the patient is no longer hypoxemic, the stimulus to breathe is decreased, and respiratory arrest may occur. Patients with chronic hypercapnia should receive O$_2$ through a low-flow device such as a nasal cannula at 1 to 2 L/min or a Venturi mask at a volume of 24% to 28%. Close monitoring for changes in mental status and of respiratory rate and ABG results is essential until PaO$_2$ levels have reached their baseline value.

MOBILIZATION OF SECRETIONS. Retained pulmonary secretions may cause or exacerbate acute respiratory failure by blocking both movement of O$_2$ into the alveoli and the pulmonary capillary blood and removal of CO$_2$ during the respiratory cycle. Secretions can be mobilized through effective coughing, adequate hydration and humidification, chest physiotherapy, and tracheal suctioning.

Effective Coughing and Positioning. If secretions are obstructing the airway, the patient should be encouraged to cough. Patients with a neuro-muscular weakness from a disease or exhaustion may not be able to generate sufficient airway pressures to produce an effective cough. *Augmented coughing (quad coughing)* may be of benefit to such patients. Augmented coughing is performed by placing the palm of the hand or hands on the abdomen below

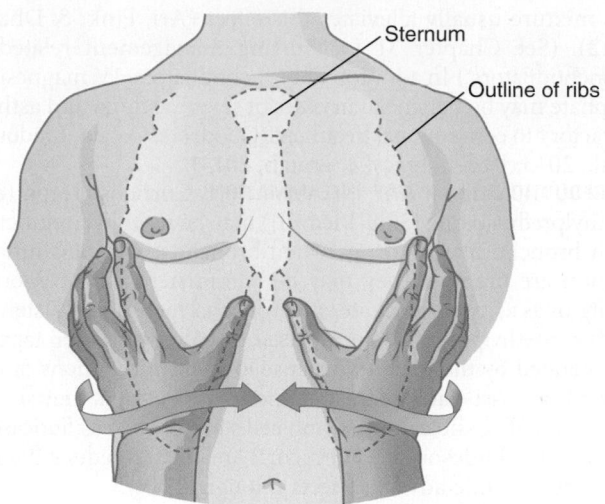

Sternum

Outline of ribs

FIGURE 70-6 Augmented coughing is performed by placing one or both hands over the anterolateral base of the lungs. After the patient takes a deep inspiration and at the beginning of expiration, the hand or hands are moved forcefully upward. This increases abdominal pressure and aids in producing a forceful cough.

the xiphoid process (Figure 70-6). As the patient ends a deep inspiration and begins the expiration, the hands should be moved forcefully upward, increasing abdominal pressure and facilitating the cough. This measure helps increase expiratory flow and thereby facilitates secretion clearance. Health care providers need to receive appropriate training before using augmented coughing techniques.

Some patients may benefit from therapeutic cough techniques. *Huff coughing* is a series of coughs performed while saying the word "huff." This technique prevents the glottis from closing during the cough. Patients with COPD generate higher flow rates with a huff cough than they can with a normal cough. The huff cough is effective in clearing only the central airways, but it may assist in moving secretions upward. The *staged cough* also assists secretion mobilization. To perform the staged cough, the patient sits in a chair, breathes three or four times in and out through the mouth, and coughs while bending forward and pressing a pillow inward against the diaphragm.

Positioning the patient either by elevating the head of the bed at least 45 degrees or with a reclining chair or chair bed may help maximize thoracic expansion, thereby decreasing dyspnea and improving secretion mobilization. A sitting position improves pulmonary function and assists in venous pooling in dependent body areas such as the lower extremities. When lungs are upright, ventilation and perfusion are best in the lung bases. Lateral or side-lying positioning, termed *good lung down,* may be used in patients with disease involving only one lung and allows for improved VQ matching in the affected lung. Pulmonary blood flow and ventilation are optimal in dependent lung areas. This positioning also allows for secretions to drain out of the affected lung to the point at which they may be removed by suctioning. For example, in patients with significant right-sided pneumonia, optimal positioning would be to place them on their left side to maximize ventilation and perfusion in the "good" lung and facilitate secretion removal from the affected lung (postural drainage). All patients should be lying on the side if there is any possibility that the tongue will obstruct the airway or that aspiration may occur. Equipment to create

an oral or nasal airway should be kept at the bedside for use if necessary.

Hydration and Humidification. Thick and viscous secretions should be thinned to facilitate removal. Adequate fluid intake (2 to 3 L/day) is necessary to keep secretions thin and easy to expel. If a patient is unable to take sufficient fluids orally, intravenous (IV) hydration is used. Thorough assessment of the patient's cardiac and renal status determines whether he or she can tolerate the intravascular volume and avoid heart failure and pulmonary edema. Assessment for signs of fluid overload (e.g., crackles, dyspnea, and increased central venous pressure) at regular intervals is essential. These considerations would also apply to patients with renal dysfunction.

An appropriate humidification device is an adjunct in secretion management. Aerosols of sterile normal saline, administered by a nebulizer, may be used to liquefy secretions. Oxygen may also be administered by aerosol mask to thin secretions and facilitate their removal. Aerosol therapy may induce bronchospasm and severe coughing, causing a decrease in PaO$_2$. In such cases, frequent assessment of the patient's tolerance of therapy is paramount (Ari, Fink, & Dhand, 2012). Mucolytic agents such as nebulized acetylcysteine (Mucomyst) mixed with a bronchodilator may be used to thin secretions; however, as an adverse effect, such mixtures may also cause airway erythema and bronchospasm. Therefore, they are used only in special situations (e.g., during bronchoscopy to remove thick, copious secretions).

Chest Physiotherapy. Chest physiotherapy is indicated in patients who produce more than 30 mL of sputum per day or have evidence of severe atelectasis or pulmonary infiltrates. If tolerated, postural drainage, percussion, and vibration to the affected lung segments may assist in moving secretions to the larger airways, where they may be removed by coughing or suctioning. Because positioning may affect oxygenation, patients may not tolerate head-down or lateral positioning as a result of extreme dyspnea or hypoxemia caused by VQ mismatch. (Chest physiotherapy is discussed in Chapter 31.)

Airway Suctioning. If the patient is unable to expectorate secretions, then nasopharyngeal, oropharyngeal, or nasotracheal suctioning (blind suctioning without a tracheal tube in place) is indicated. Suctioning through an artificial airway, such as endotracheal or tracheostomy tubes, may also be performed (see Chapters 29 and 68). A mini-tracheostomy (commonly called a "mini-trach") may be used to perform suction in patients who have difficulty mobilizing secretions and when blind suctioning is difficult or ineffective. The *mini-tracheostomy* is a 4-mm indwelling plastic cuffless cannula inserted through the cricothyroid membrane. It is used to instill sterile normal saline solution to elicit a cough and to perform suctioning with a size 10 or smaller French catheter. Contraindications for a mini-tracheostomy include absence of the gag reflex, a history of aspiration, and the need for long-term mechanical ventilation.

POSITIVE-PRESSURE VENTILATION. If intensive measures fail to improve ventilation and oxygenation and the patient continues to exhibit acute respiratory failure, ventilatory assistance may be initiated. PPV may be provided invasively through endotracheal or nasotracheal intubation or noninvasively through a nasal or face mask. Patients who require PPV are typically cared for in an intensive care unit. (See Chapter 68 for a discussion of artificial airways and mechanical ventilation.)

Noninvasive positive-pressure ventilation (NIPPV) may be used to treat patients with acute or chronic respiratory failure. During NIPPV, a mask is placed over the patient's nose or nose

FIGURE 70-7 Noninvasive bilevel positive airway pressure ventilation. A mask is placed over the nose or the nose and mouth. Positive pressure from a mechanical ventilator assists the patient's breathing efforts, decreasing the work of breathing. Source: Courtesy Richard Arbour, RN, MSN, CCRN, CNRN, CCNS, FAAN, and Anna Kirk, RN, MSN.

and mouth while the patient breathes spontaneously (Figure 70-7). With NIPPV, it is possible to decrease the work of breathing without the use of invasive endotracheal intubation. Bilevel positive airway pressure ventilation is a form of NIPPV in which different positive-pressure levels are set for inspiration and expiration (see Figure 70-7). In continuous positive airway pressure, another form of NIPPV, the positive pressure delivered to the airway is constant during inspiration and expiration (Urden, Stacy, & Lough, 2014).

NIPPV is most useful in managing chronic respiratory failure in patients with chest wall and neuro-muscular disease (see Table 70-3). NIPPV has been used in patients with hypoxemic respiratory failure (e.g., those with ARDS, cardiogenic pulmonary edema) but with less success (Luo, Wang, Zhu, et al, 2014; Wang, Singh, Tian, et al., 2013). NIPPV may also be used for patients who refuse endotracheal intubation but still desire some palliative ventilatory support (e.g., patients with end-stage COPD). NIPPV is not appropriate for the patient who has no spontaneous respirations, excessive secretions, decreased level of consciousness, high O_2 requirements, facial trauma, or hemodynamic instability (Urden, Stacy, & Lough, 2014).

DRUG THERAPY

Goals of drug therapy for patients in acute respiratory failure include relief of bronchospasm, reduction of airway inflammation and pulmonary congestion, treatment of pulmonary infection, and reduction of severe anxiety and restlessness.

RELIEF OF BRONCHOSPASM. Alveolar ventilation will be increased with relief of bronchospasm. To reverse bronchospasm, short-acting *bronchodilators,* such as fenoterol hydrobromide and salbutamol, are frequently administered through either a hand-held nebulizer or a metered-dose inhaler with a spacer (Ari, Fink, & Dhand, 2012). For acute bronchospasm, these drugs may be given at 15- to 30-minute intervals until a response can be determined. If severe bronchospasm continues, IV aminophylline may be administered. The bronchodilator effects of all of these medications can sometimes cause a worsening of arterial hypoxemia by redistributing the inspired gas to areas of decreased perfusion. Administering the bronchodilator with an O_2-enriched

gas mixture usually alleviates this effect (Ari, Fink, & Dhand, 2012). (See Chapter 31 for nursing management related to bronchodilators.) In addition to bronchodilators, IV magnesium sulphate may be beneficial in cases of severe asthma and asthma refractory to conventional treatment (Goodacre, Cohen, Bradburn, et al., 2013; Urden, Stacy, & Lough, 2014).

REDUCTION OF AIRWAY INFLAMMATION. Corticosteroids (e.g., methylprednisolone [Solu-Medrol]) may be used in conjunction with bronchodilating drugs when bronchospasm and inflammation are present. They may be administered intravenously, orally, or as aerosols. In acute exacerbations, high-dose IV steroids such as methylprednisolone are used. The dosage is then tapered as tolerated by the patient. Because long-term regimens of oral steroids are associated with systemic adverse effects, they should be avoided if possible. Instead, inhaled steroids such as fluticasone (Flovent) or budesonide (Pulmicort) are used to reduce the risk of those systemic adverse effects (Hough, 2014).

REDUCTION OF PULMONARY CONGESTION. Pulmonary interstitial fluid can accumulate as a consequence of direct or indirect injury to the alveolar capillary membrane (as in ARDS) or from right- or left-sided heart failure and can therefore be either cardiac or noncardiac in origin. The result is decreased alveolar ventilation and hypoxemia. IV diuretics (e.g., furosemide [Lasix]) and nitroglycerine are used to decrease the pulmonary congestion caused by heart failure. If atrial fibrillation is also present, calcium channel blockers (e.g., diltiazem) and β-adrenergic blockers (e.g., metoprolol) may be used to decrease heart rate and improve cardiac output. (See Chapter 37 for discussion of heart failure.)

TREATMENT OF PULMONARY INFECTIONS. Pulmonary infections (pneumonia, acute bronchitis) result in excessive mucus production, fever, and increased oxygen consumption, and alveoli become inflamed or fluid filled or collapse. Alveoli that are fluid filled or collapsed cannot participate in gas exchange. Pulmonary infections can either cause or exacerbate acute respiratory failure. IV antibiotics, such as vancomycin (Vancocin) or ceftriaxone, are frequently administered to inhibit bacterial growth. Chest radiographic examinations are performed to determine the location and the extent of a suspected infectious process. Sputum cultures are used to determine the type of organisms causing the infection and their sensitivity to antimicrobial medications.

REDUCTION OF SEVERE ANXIETY, PAIN, AND AGITATION. Anxiety, restlessness, and agitation result from cerebral hypoxia. In addition, fear caused by the inability to breathe and a sense of loss of control may exacerbate anxiety. Anxiety, pain, and agitation increase O_2 consumption, which may worsen the degree of hypoxemia. Increase in anxiety and agitation can affect ventilator management. Administration of sedatives, opioids, or muscle relaxants may be necessary to provide adequate oxygenation and ventilation. Several nursing strategies can assist the patient in reducing the level of anxiety and pain (see NCP 70-1, available on the Evolve website).

Sedation and analgesia with drug therapy such as benzodiazepines (e.g., lorazepam [Ativan], midazolam) and opioids (e.g., morphine, fentanyl) may decrease anxiety, agitation, and pain. Continued agitation increases the patient's work of breathing, O_2 consumption, CO_2 production, and risk of injury (e.g., accidental extubation). In the intensive care setting, sedatives and analgesics are commonly administered, and patients must be monitored closely for cardiovascular and respiratory depression. Of importance is that agitation is best characterized as a symptom and may be caused by pain, hypoxemia, electrolyte imbalance, evolution of structural or metabolic brain injury, and adverse drug reactions;

therefore, potentially reversible causes should always be assessed and treated. Sedative and analgesic drugs may have prolonged duration of action in critically ill patients. This may contribute to increased length of stay and prolonged time on a ventilator (Mendez, Lazar, Digiovine, et al., 2013). Patients receiving these drugs are best managed with a research-based, protocol-driven plan of care (Mendez, Lazar, Digiovine, et al., 2013).

Sedation protocols can be used to guide the level of sedation. Most patients in whom oxygenation is difficult require heavy sedation (4 to 5 on the Richmond Agitation Sedation Scale). Patients who breathe asynchronously with mechanical ventilation may also benefit from titration of ventilator settings, as well as addressing underlying causes of agitation.

Once complete sedation is achieved, if the patient is still hypoxic, the use of neuro-muscular blockade may be indicated with agents such as vecuronium or cisatracurium (Nimbex). Neuro-muscular blockade produces skeletal muscle relaxation and synchrony with mechanical ventilation. These drugs may also decrease the patient's risk of lung injury related to excessive intrathoracic pressures and promote optimal ventilatory support. Patients receiving neuro-muscular blockade should receive sedation and analgesia to the point of unconsciousness for comfort, pain relief, and elimination of the awareness of being paralyzed, which is a terrifying experience (Hraiech, Yoshida, & Papazian, 2015). The level of pharmacological paralysis is monitored with a peripheral nerve stimulator and clinical correlation to achieve absence of respiratory effort. Daily interruption of sedative drug infusions decreases the duration of mechanical ventilation and length of stay in the intensive care unit (Mendez, Lazar, Digiovine, et al., 2013).

MEDICAL SUPPORTIVE THERAPY

Interventions to maximize O_2 delivery and treat the underlying cause of respiratory failure are essential for improving the patient's oxygenation and ventilation status. The primary goal is to treat the underlying cause of the respiratory failure. Other goals include maintaining an adequate cardiac output and hemoglobin concentration.

TREATING THE UNDERLYING CAUSE. Interventions are directed toward reversing the disease process that resulted in the development of acute respiratory failure. Patients with hypoventilation can be diagnosed and treated rapidly. Patients with VQ mismatch, shunting, or diffusion limitation are managed differently depending on the underlying cause. In all patient situations, monitoring treatment effects, including trends in ABGs and changes in respiratory status, is a continuous process.

MAINTAINING ADEQUATE CARDIAC OUTPUT. Cardiac output reflects the blood flow reaching the tissues. Blood pressure and mean arterial pressure are important indicators of the adequacy of cardiac output and should be interpreted within the context of the overall assessment to determine adequacy of cardiac output and tissue perfusion. Usually, a systolic blood pressure of 90 mm Hg or higher and a mean arterial pressure of 60 mm Hg or higher is adequate to maintain perfusion to the vital organs; therefore, changes in mental status can usually be attributed to the level of O_2 and CO_2, rather than to decreased cerebral perfusion, when these pressures are maintained. Patients with chronic, uncontrolled hypertension may require higher systemic arterial pressures and mean arterial pressures to prevent episodes of brain ischemia.

Decreased cardiac output is treated by administration of IV fluids, medications, or both. (See Chapter 69 for a discussion of drugs used to treat decreased cardiac output and shock.) Cardiac output may also be decreased by changes in intrathoracic or intrapulmonary pressures from PPV. Patients experiencing exacerbation of COPD or asthma and those receiving controlled ventilation are at risk of alveolar hyperinflation, increased right ventricular afterload, and excessive intrathoracic pressures. These alterations in thoracic pressure dynamics may cause an increase in right ventricular afterload, which limits blood flow from the right side of the heart through the pulmonary vasculature to the left side of the heart; dramatic hemodynamic compromise may result. In addition, blood return from the systemic circulation to the right side of the heart may be impaired, decreasing preload (Urden, Stacy, & Lough, 2014). Each of these physiological consequences can potentially compromise hemodynamics. Consequently, clinical indicators of adequate cardiac output and tissue perfusion should be monitored alongside initiation or titration of mechanical ventilation by mask or endotracheal intubation.

MAINTAINING ADEQUATE HEMOGLOBIN CONCENTRATION. Hemoglobin is the primary carrier when blood delivers O_2 to the tissues. In patients who are anemic, tissue O_2 delivery is compromised. A hemoglobin concentration of 6 mmol/L or greater typically ensures adequate O_2 saturation of the hemoglobin. Patients should be monitored for sites of blood loss and receive transfusions of packed red blood cells if an adequate hemoglobin concentration cannot be maintained.

NUTRITIONAL THERAPY

Maintenance of protein and energy stores is especially important in patients with acute respiratory failure because nutritional depletion causes loss of muscle mass, including the respiratory muscles, and may prolong recovery. During the acute manifestations of respiratory failure, the risk of aspiration typically prevents oral intake; therefore, enteral or parenteral nutrition may be administered until symptoms subside and the patient tolerates oral intake. A multitude of nutritional supplements are available (Matos, Manzanares, & Nava, 2015). The prescription of a high-carbohydrate diet should be based on individual patient needs (Taylor, McClave, Martindale, et al., 2016), It may be avoided in patients who retain CO_2 because carbohydrates metabolize into CO_2, further increasing CO_2 load. However, the hypermetabolic state present in critical illness can dramatically increase caloric requirements.

EVALUATION

The expected outcomes for the patient with acute respiratory failure are presented in NCP 70-1, on the Evolve website.

AGE-RELATED CONSIDERATIONS

RESPIRATORY FAILURE

The older adult population is the fastest growing age group in North America, and this trend is reflected within acute and intensive care settings. Of importance is that older adults are more vulnerable to delirium, hospital-acquired infections, and medication effects. Multiple factors contribute to an increased risk of respiratory failure in older adults, including the reduction in ventilatory capacity that accompanies aging, especially if risk factors are present. Physiological aging of the lung may produce alveolar dilation, diminish elastic recoil within the airways, decrease chest wall compliance, and decrease respiratory muscle strength. In older adults, the PaO_2 falls further and the $PaCO_2$ rises to a higher level before the respiratory system is stimulated to alter the rate and the depth of breathing. This delayed response can contribute to the development of respiratory failure. In addition, smoking is a risk factor that accelerates age-related respiratory changes. Poor nutritional status predisposes to decreased muscle mass, and less physiological reserve in cardiovascular, respiratory, and autonomic nervous systems increases the risk of additional diseases such as pneumonia and cardiac disease that may compromise respiratory function and precipitate respiratory failure (Schmidt, Balzer, Pille, et al., 2013; Urden, Stacy, & Lough, 2014).

Assessment parameters should be adjusted for age. For example, heart rate and blood pressure generally increase with age and with changes in the cardiovascular system. Therefore, determination of baseline vital signs and using them as a basis for comparison of physical assessment findings is most appropriate in evaluating changes in cardiopulmonary function in older adults.

ACUTE RESPIRATORY DISTRESS SYNDROME

Acute respiratory distress syndrome (ARDS) is a sudden and progressive form of acute respiratory failure in which the alveolar–capillary membrane becomes damaged and more permeable by intravascular fluid (Figure 70-8). The alveoli fill with fluid, which results in severe dyspnea, hypoxemia refractory to supplemental O_2, reduced lung compliance, and diffuse pulmonary infiltrates (Fournier, 2014; Urden, Stacy, & Lough, 2014). Despite the fact that ARDS has been the focus of extensive clinical research, survival rates have not significantly improved (Grek, Booth, Festic, et al., 2017; Schell-Chaple, Puntillo, Matthay, et al., 2015). Despite supportive therapy, the rate of mortality from ARDS is approximately 50% (Villar, Blanco, & Kacmarek, 2016). Patients who have both Gram-negative septic shock and ARDS have a significantly higher rate of mortality (Fratantoro, 2015).

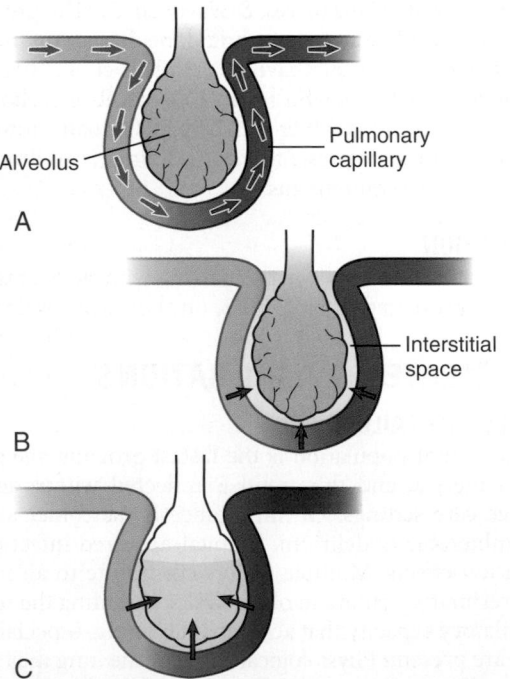

Alveolus

Pulmonary capillary

A

Interstitial space

B

C

FIGURE 70-8 Stages of edema formation in acute respiratory distress syndrome. **A,** Normal alveolus and pulmonary capillary. **B,** Interstitial edema occurs with increased flow of fluid into the interstitial space. **C,** Alveolar edema occurs when the fluid crosses the blood–gas barrier.

Etiology and Pathophysiology

Table 70-7 lists conditions that predispose patients to the development of ARDS. The most common cause of ARDS is sepsis. Patients with multiple risk factors are three to four times more likely to develop ARDS than are those without risk factors. Community-acquired pneumonia is another common cause of ARDS that develops outside of the hospital community. Common pathogens include *Streptococcus pneumoniae, Legionella pneumophila,* and a variety of respiratory viruses. Nosocomial (health care–related) pneumonias, including ventilator-associated pneumonia, can also progress to ARDS (see Chapter 68).

Patients may develop ARDS in the setting of influenza infection. ARDS is a fatal complication of influenza infection (Töpfer, Menk, Weber-Carstens, et al., 2014).

Direct lung injury may cause ARDS (Figure 70-9), or ARDS may develop as a consequence of the systemic inflammatory response syndrome (see Chapter 69, Figure 69-1). This syndrome may have an infectious or a noninfectious etiology and is characterized by widespread inflammation or clinical responses to inflammation after a variety of physiological insults, including severe trauma, gut ischemia, lung injury, and sepsis (Urden, Stacy, & Lough, 2014). ARDS may also develop as a consequence of multiple-organ dysfunction syndrome, which results from organ system dysfunction that progressively increases in severity and ultimately results in multisystem organ failure. (Systemic inflammatory response syndrome and multiple-organ dysfunction syndrome are discussed in Chapter 69.)

In the initial injury to the lungs, the alveolar–capillary membrane is damaged. This activates complement and stimulates platelet aggregation and intravascular thrombus formation. Platelets release substances that attract and activate neutrophils (Brashers & Huether, 2014; Fournier, 2014). The neutrophils cause a release of biochemical, humoral, and cellular mediators (Table 70-8) that produce changes in the lung, including increased pulmonary capillary membrane permeability, destruction of elastin and collagen, formation of pulmonary microemboli, and pulmonary artery vasoconstriction (see Figure 70-9). (Mediators are discussed in Chapters 14 and 16.) The pathophysiological changes in ARDS are divided into three phases: (1) injury or

TABLE 70-7	CONDITIONS PREDISPOSING TO ACUTE RESPIRATORY DISTRESS SYNDROME
Direct Lung Injury	**Indirect Lung Injury**
Common Causes	
• Aspiration	• Sepsis (especially Gram-negative infection)
• Viral or bacterial pneumonia	• Severe massive trauma
Less Common Causes	
• Chest trauma	• Acute pancreatitis
• Embolism: fat, air, amniotic fluid	• Anaphylaxis
	• Blood transfusions
• Inhalation of toxins	• Cardiopulmonary bypass
• Near-drowning	• Disseminated intravascular coagulation
• O_2 toxicity	
• Radiation pneumonitis	• Opioid overdose (e.g., heroin)
	• Nonpulmonary systemic diseases
	• Severe head injury
	• Shock

PATHOPHYSIOLOGY MAP

FIGURE 70-9 Pathophysiology of acute respiratory distress syndrome (ARDS). *ALI*, acute lung injury.

TABLE 70-8   **MEDIATORS OF ACUTE LUNG INJURY**
• Arachidonic acid metabolites, including prostaglandins and leukotrienes
• Coagulation products, including kallikreins, kinins, fibrin degradation products, and plasminogen-activating factor
• Collagenase
• Complement component C5a
• Elastase
• Histamine
• Monocyte and macrophage products, including tumour necrosis factor, interleukin-1, and colony-stimulating factor
• Neutrophil products, including proteases and O_2 radicals
• Serotonin endotoxin

exudative phase, (2) reparative or proliferative phase, and (3) fibrotic phase.

Injury or Exudative Phase. The *injury or exudative phase* occurs approximately 1 to 7 days (usually 24 to 48 hours) after the initial direct lung injury or host insult. Neutrophils adhere to the pulmonary microcirculation, causing damage to the vascular endothelium and increased capillary permeability. In the earliest phase of injury, the peribronchial and perivascular interstitial spaces become engorged with fluid, which produces interstitial edema. Next, fluid from the interstitial space crosses the alveolar epithelium and enters the alveolar space. Intrapulmonary shunting

develops because the alveoli fill with fluid, and blood passing through them cannot be oxygenated (see Figures 70-4 and 70-8).

Type I and type II alveolar cells (which produce surfactant) are damaged by the changes caused by ARDS. This damage, in addition to further fluid and protein accumulation, results in surfactant dysfunction. The function of *surfactant* is to maintain alveolar stability by decreasing alveolar surface tension and preventing alveolar collapse. Decreased synthesis of surfactant and inactivation of existing surfactant cause the alveoli to become unstable and collapse (atelectasis). Widespread atelectasis further decreases lung compliance, compromises gas exchange, and contributes to hypoxemia (Urden, Stacy, & Lough, 2014).

Also during this stage, hyaline membranes begin to line the alveoli. These membranes are composed of necrotic cells, protein, and fibrin, and they lie adjacent to the alveoli wall. They are thought to result from the exudation of high-molecular-weight substances (particularly fibrinogen) in the edematous fluid. Hyaline membranes contribute to the development of fibrosis and atelectasis, which lead to a decrease in gas-exchange capability and lung compliance.

The primary pathophysiological changes that characterize the injury or exudative phase of ARDS are interstitial and alveolar edema (noncardiogenic pulmonary edema) and atelectasis (Brashers & Huether, 2014; Modrykamien & Gupta, 2015). Severe VQ mismatch and shunting of pulmonary capillary blood result in hypoxemia unresponsive to increasing concentrations of O_2 (termed **refractory hypoxemia**). Diffusion limitation, caused by hyaline membrane formation, further contributes to the severity of the hypoxemia. As the lungs become less compliant ("stiffer") because of decreased surfactant, pulmonary edema, and atelectasis, the patient must generate higher airway pressures to inflate them. Reduced lung compliance greatly increases the patient's work of breathing. During ventilator management at this stage, a progressive increase in plateau and inspiratory pressures may be noted as lung compliance worsens.

Hypoxemia and the stimulation of juxtacapillary receptors in the stiff lung parenchyma (the juxtacapillary [J] reflex) initially cause an increase in respiratory rate and a decrease in tidal volume. This breathing pattern increases CO_2 removal, which leads to respiratory alkalosis. Cardiac output increases in response to hypoxemia, a compensatory effort to increase pulmonary blood flow. However, as atelectasis, pulmonary edema, and pulmonary shunting increase, compensation fails, and hypoventilation, a decrease in cardiac output, and a decrease in tissue O_2 perfusion eventually occur.

Reparative or Proliferative Phase. The *reparative or proliferative phase* of ARDS begins 1 to 2 weeks after the initial lung injury. During this phase the inflammatory response includes an influx of neutrophils, monocytes, and lymphocytes, together with fibroblast proliferation. The injured lung has an immense regenerative capacity after acute lung injury. The proliferative phase is complete when the diseased lung becomes characterized by dense, fibrous tissue. Increased pulmonary vascular resistance and pulmonary hypertension may occur in this stage because fibroblasts and inflammatory cells destroy the pulmonary vasculature. Lung compliance continues to decrease as a result of interstitial fibrosis. Hypoxemia worsens because of the thickened alveolar membrane, causing diffusion limitation and shunting. If the reparative phase persists, widespread fibrosis results. If the reparative phase is arrested, the lesions resolve (Brashers & Huether, 2014; Meduri & Eltorky, 2015; Urden, Stacy, & Lough, 2014).

Fibrotic Phase. The *fibrotic phase* of ARDS, also called the *chronic* or *late phase,* occurs approximately 2 to 3 weeks after the initial lung injury. During this time, the lung is completely remodelled by sparsely collagenous and fibrous tissues. Diffuse scarring and fibrosis further decrease lung compliance. In addition, the surface area for gas exchange is significantly reduced because the interstitium is fibrotic, and therefore, hypoxemia continues. Pulmonary hypertension results from pulmonary vascular destruction and fibrosis.

Clinical Progression

Progression of ARDS varies among patients. Some people survive the acute phase of lung injury; pulmonary edema resolves, and complete recovery occurs in a few days. The chance for survival is poor in patients who enter the fibrotic (chronic or late) phase, which necessitates long-term mechanical ventilation. It is not known why injured lungs repair and recover in some patients whereas ARDS progresses in others. Several factors seem to be important in determining the course of ARDS, including the nature of the initial injury, the extent and the severity of coexisting diseases, and pulmonary complications (Koh, 2014; Kress, 2015).

Clinical Manifestations

The initial presentation of ARDS is often insidious. At the time of the initial injury, and up to 48 hours afterward, the patient may exhibit only dyspnea, tachypnea, cough, and restlessness. Chest auscultation may be normal or reveal fine, scattered crackles.

ABG measurements usually indicate mild hypoxemia and respiratory alkalosis caused by hyperventilation. Respiratory alkalosis results from tachypnea, hypoxemia, and the stimulation of juxtacapillary receptors. The chest radiograph may be normal or exhibit evidence of minimal scattered interstitial infiltrates. Bilateral infiltrates become visible the radiographs as ARDS progresses. As ARDS progresses, symptoms worsen because of increased fluid accumulation and decreased lung compliance. Respiratory distress becomes evident as the work of breathing increases. Tachypnea and intercostal and suprasternal retractions may be present. Pulmonary function tests in ARDS reveal decreased compliance and decreased lung volumes, particularly a decreased functional residual capacity. Tachycardia, diaphoresis, changes in sensorium with decreased mentation, cyanosis, and pallor may be present. Chest auscultation usually reveals scattered to diffuse crackles and wheezes. Chest radiographs demonstrate diffuse and extensive bilateral interstitial and alveolar infiltrates. A pulmonary artery catheter may need to be inserted. Pulmonary artery wedge pressure does not increase in ARDS because the cause is noncardiogenic (not related to cardiac function).

Hallmarks of ARDS include hypoxemia and a PaO_2/FiO_2 ratio below 200 despite increased FiO_2 by mask, cannula, or endotracheal tube. ABG measurements may initially demonstrate a normal or decreased $PaCO_2$ despite severe dyspnea and hypoxemia. Hypercapnia signifies that hypoventilation is occurring and the patient is no longer able to maintain the level of ventilation needed to provide optimum gas exchange.

As ARDS progresses, it is associated with profound respiratory distress that necessitates endotracheal intubation and PPV. The chest radiograph (Figure 70-10) shows what is often termed *whiteout* or *white lung* because consolidation and coalescing infiltrates are widespread throughout the lungs, leaving few recognizable air spaces. Pleural effusions may also be present. Severe hypoxemia, hypercapnia, and metabolic acidosis, with

FIGURE 70-10 Chest radiograph of a patient with acute respiratory distress syndrome. The image shows new, bilateral diffuse, homogeneous pulmonary infiltrates without cardiac failure, fluid overload, chest infection, or chronic lung disease. Source: Cohen, J., & Powderly, W. G. (2004). *Infectious diseases* (2nd ed.). St. Louis: Mosby.

symptoms of target organ or tissue hypoxia, may ensue if therapy is not instituted promptly.

No precise criteria define ARDS. ARDS is considered to be present if (a) the patient has refractory hypoxemia, (b) a chest radiograph shows new bilateral interstitial or alveolar infiltrates, (c) the pulmonary artery wedge pressure is 18 mm Hg or less with no evidence of heart failure, and (d) a predisposing condition for ARDS develops within 48 hours of clinical manifestations (Table 70-9).

Complications

Complications may develop as a result of ARDS or its treatment. (Table 70-10 lists the common complications of ARDS.) The major cause of death in ARDS is multiple-organ dysfunction

TABLE 70-9 DIAGNOSTIC FINDINGS IN ACUTE RESPIRATORY DISTRESS SYNDROME

Chest radiograph	New bilateral interstitial and alveolar infiltrates
Predisposing condition	Identification of a predisposing condition for ARDS within 48 hr of clinical manifestations
Pulmonary artery wedge pressure	≤18 mm Hg and no evidence of heart failure
Refractory hypoxemia	PaO_2 <50 mm Hg, with an FiO_2 >40% and with PEEP >5 cm H_2O PaO_2/FiO_2 ratio <200

ARDS, acute respiratory distress syndrome; *FiO₂*, fraction of inspired oxygen; *PaO₂*, partial pressure of oxygen in arterial blood; *PEEP*, positive end-expiratory pressure.

TABLE 70-10 COMPLICATIONS ASSOCIATED WITH ACUTE RESPIRATORY DISTRESS SYNDROME

Cardiac complications	Decreased cardiac output Dysrhythmias
Endotracheal intubation complications	Laryngeal ulceration Tracheal malacia Tracheal stenosis Tracheal ulceration
Gastro-intestinal complications	Hypermetabolic state, dramatically increased nutritional requirements Paralytic ileus Pneumoperitoneum Stress ulceration and hemorrhage
Hematological complications	Anemia Disseminated intravascular coagulation Thrombo-cytopenia
Infection	Catheter-related infection Hospital-acquired pneumonia Sepsis (bacteremia)
Renal complications	Acute kidney injury
Respiratory complications	O₂ toxicity Pulmonary barotraumas (e.g., pneumothorax, pneumomediastinum, subcutaneous emphysema) Pulmonary emboli Pulmonary fibrosis Ventilator-associated pneumonia

syndrome, often accompanied by sepsis. The vital organs most commonly involved are the kidneys, liver, and heart. The organ systems most often involved are the CNS and the hematological and gastro-intestinal systems.

Hospital-Acquired Pneumonia. A frequent complication of ARDS is hospital-acquired pneumonia, occurring in as many as 68% of patients with ARDS. Risk factors include impaired host defences, contaminated medical equipment, invasive monitoring devices, aspiration of gastro-intestinal contents, and prolonged mechanical ventilation as well as colonization of the respiratory tract. Strategies to prevent hospital-acquired pneumonia include infection control measures (e.g., strict handwashing and sterile technique during endotracheal suctioning) and elevating the head of the bed 45 degrees or more to prevent aspiration (Moazed & Calfee, 2014; Urden, Stacy, & Lough, 2014). (See Chapter 30 for discussion of pneumonia.)

Barotrauma. *Barotrauma* may result from rupture of overdistended alveoli during mechanical ventilation. The high airway pressures necessary to ventilate patients with ARDS predispose to this complication. Barotrauma results in the presence of alveolar air in locations where it is not usually found. This can lead to pulmonary interstitial emphysema, pneumothorax, subcutaneous emphysema, pneumoperitoneum, pneumomediastinum, and tension pneumothorax. (See Chapter 30 for discussion of pneumothorax.)

To avoid barotrauma, patients with ARDS are ventilated with smaller tidal volumes. Different approaches to lung-protective ventilation are in current clinical use. Ventilation protocol include the use of small tidal volumes (e.g., 6 mL/kg) and varying amounts of positive end-expiratory pressure (PEEP) while the $PaCO_2$ gradually rises above normal *(permissive hypercapnia)*, with the pH supported at 7.2 to 7.25 or above (Marhong & Fan, 2014). Permissive hypercapnia is commonly accepted as a consequence of lung-protective ventilation in ARDS (Marhong & Fan, 2014). High-frequency oscillation uses a constant mean airway pressure to maintain the alveoli in a recruited state while low tidal volumes are oscillated at a fast rate. Ventilation is achieved by the generation of extremely rapid pressure oscillations, usually in the range of 300 to 900 cycles/minute (Koh, 2014).

Volutrauma. *Volutrauma*, or *volupressure trauma*, can occur in patients with ARDS when large tidal volumes (10 to 15 mL/kg) are used to ventilate noncompliant lungs. Volutrauma results in alveolar fractures and movement of fluids and proteins into the alveolar spaces. To limit this complication, it is recommended that smaller (lower) tidal volumes or pressure ventilation be used in patients with ARDS (Bein, Weber-Carstens, Goldmann, et al., 2013; see Chapter 68). Ventilation with low tidal volume reduces the damaging, excessive stretch of lung tissue that results in volutrauma.

Stress Ulcers. Critically ill patients with acute respiratory failure are at high risk for stress ulcers. Bleeding from stress ulcers occurs in 30% of patients with ARDS who require PPV, a higher incidence than those with other causes of acute respiratory failure. Management strategies include correction of predisposing conditions such as hypotension, shock, and acidosis. Prophylactic management includes antiulcer agents (e.g., famotidine [Pepcid], omeprazole [Losec], sucralphate [Sulcrate]) and early initiation of enteral nutrition (see Chapters 42 and 68).

Renal Failure. Renal failure results from decreased renal tissue oxygenation owing to hypotension, hypoxemia, or hypercapnia and from administration of nephrotoxic drugs (e.g., aminoglycosides).

NURSING AND COLLABORATIVE MANAGEMENT ACUTE RESPIRATORY DISTRESS SYNDROME

The collaborative care for acute respiratory failure (see Table 70-6) and the nursing care plan for acute respiratory failure (see NCP 70-1, available on the Evolve website) are applicable to ARDS. The following section is a discussion of additional collaborative care measures for patients with ARDS (Table 70-11). Patients with ARDS are commonly cared for in intensive care units.

NURSING ASSESSMENT

Because ARDS causes acute respiratory failure, the subjective and objective data that should be obtained from a patient with ARDS are the same as that for acute respiratory failure (see Table 70-5). Abnormal findings on physical examination are indications that ARDS has progressed beyond the initial stages.

NURSING DIAGNOSES

Nursing diagnoses for patients with ARDS may include, but are not limited to, those described for acute respiratory failure (see also NCP 70-1, available on the Evolve website).

PLANNING

With appropriate therapy, the overall goals for the patient with ARDS are a PaO_2 of at least 60 mm Hg and adequate lung ventilation to maintain normal pH. After recovery from ARDS, (a) the patient's PaO_2 should be within normal limits for age or baseline values on room air (FiO_2 of 21%), (b) the SaO_2 should be greater than 90%, (c) the patient's airway should be patent, and (d) on auscultation, the lungs should sound clear.

RESPIRATORY THERAPY

OXYGEN ADMINISTRATION. The primary goal of O_2 therapy is to correct hypoxemia. Use of a simple face mask or nasal cannula is usually inadequate to treat refractory hypoxemia associated with ARDS. Masks with high-flow systems that deliver higher O_2 concentrations are initially used to maximize O_2 delivery, and O_2 saturation is monitored continuously to assess their effectiveness. The standard for O_2 administration is to administer the lowest concentration that results in a PaO_2 of 60 mm Hg or higher so as to minimize the risk of O_2 toxicity.

Early noninvasive ventilation application may be extremely helpful in immuno-compromised patients with pulmonary infiltrates, in whom intubation dramatically increases the risk of infection, pneumonia, and death. Overall, because of the high

rate of failure with noninvasive ventilation, noninvasive ventilation should be used with caution in patients with acute lung injury/ARDS. Prompt intubation is required if signs of noninvasive ventilation failure emerge (Wang, Singh, Tian, et al., 2013). Patients with ARDS commonly need intubation with mechanical ventilation because the PaO_2 cannot otherwise be maintained at acceptable levels.

MECHANICAL VENTILATION. Endotracheal intubation and mechanical ventilation provide additional respiratory support. However, FiO_2 of 50% or greater may still be necessary to maintain the PaO_2 at 60 mm Hg or higher. During mechanical ventilation, it is common to apply PEEP at 5 cm H_2O to compensate for loss of glottic function caused by the presence of the endotracheal tube. In patients with ARDS, higher levels of PEEP (e.g., 10–20 cm H_2O) may be used to increase functional residual capacity and recruit (open up) collapsed alveoli. PEEP is typically applied in increments of 3 to 5 cm H_2O until oxygenation is adequate with FiO_2 of 60% or lower. PEEP may improve VQ in respiratory units that collapse at low airway pressures, thus allowing the FiO_2 to be lowered.

PEEP, however, is not a benign therapy. The additional intra-thoracic and intrapulmonic pressures can compromise venous return to the right side of the heart, thereby decreasing preload, cardiac output, and blood pressure. PEEP can also cause hyper-inflation of the alveoli, compression of the pulmonary capillary bed, a reduction in blood return to the left side of the heart, and a dramatic reduction in blood pressure. In addition, PEEP and excessive inspiratory pressures can contribute to barotrauma and volutrauma (Retamal, Bugedo, Larsson, et al., 2015).

If hypoxemia persists despite high PEEP, alternative modes and therapies may be used. These include pressure-support ventilation, pressure-release ventilation, pressure-control ventilation, inverse-ratio ventilation, high-frequency oscillation, and permissive hypercapnia. (Additional information on mechanical ventilation and PEEP is provided in Chapter 68.)

In extracorporeal membrane oxygenation and extracorporeal carbon dioxide removal, blood passes across an external gas-exchanging membrane, is oxygenated, and returns to the body. Although extracorporeal membrane oxygenation has not clearly been demonstrated to be better than the standard of care for ARDS, referral to a specialized centre with extracorporeal membrane oxygenation experience should be considered early after the initiation of high-level ventilator support (Papazian & Herridge, 2013).

POSITIONING STRATEGIES. Some patients with ARDS demonstrate an improvement in PaO_2 when turned from supine to prone position with no change in FiO_2. The response may be sufficient to allow a reduction in FiO_2 or PEEP.

In early ARDS, fluid moves freely throughout the lung. Because of gravity, this fluid pools in dependent lung regions in such a way that some alveoli are fluid filled (dependent areas), whereas others are air filled (nondependent areas). In addition, when the patient is supine, the mediastinal contents place more pressure on the lungs than in the prone position, which changes pleural pressure and predisposes to atelectasis. If the patient is turned to the prone position, air-filled, nonatelectic alveoli in the ventral (anterior) lung become dependent. Perfusion may be better matched to ventilation, causing less VQ mismatch. Prone positioning is typically reserved for patients with refractory hypoxemia, but not all respond with an increase in PaO_2. When prone positioning is used, there must be a plan for immediate repositioning for cardiopulmonary resuscitation in the event of a cardiac arrest (Kallet, 2015; Koh, 2014). The RotoProne

TABLE 70-11   COLLABORATIVE CARE

Acute Respiratory Distress Syndrome

Diagnostic	Supportive Therapy
See Table 70-9.	• Diuretics
	• Dobutamine
Collaborative Therapy	• Dopamine
Respiratory Therapy	• Hemodynamic monitoring
• High-frequency oscillation	• Identification and treatment of underlying cause
• Lateral rotation therapy	
• Mechanical ventilation with PEEP	• Inotropic or vasopressor medications
• O_2 administration	• IV fluid administration (fluid resuscitation early and less fluid later)
• Prone positioning	

IV, intravenous; *PEEP,* positive end-expiratory pressure.

FIGURE 70-11 RotoProne bed. The RotoProne Delta Therapy System allows clinicians to place patients in the prone position, safely and effectively. This product is not specifically indicated for the treatment of acute respiratory distress syndrome or ventilator-associated pneumonia (VAP). Source: Photo courtesy Arjo Inc.

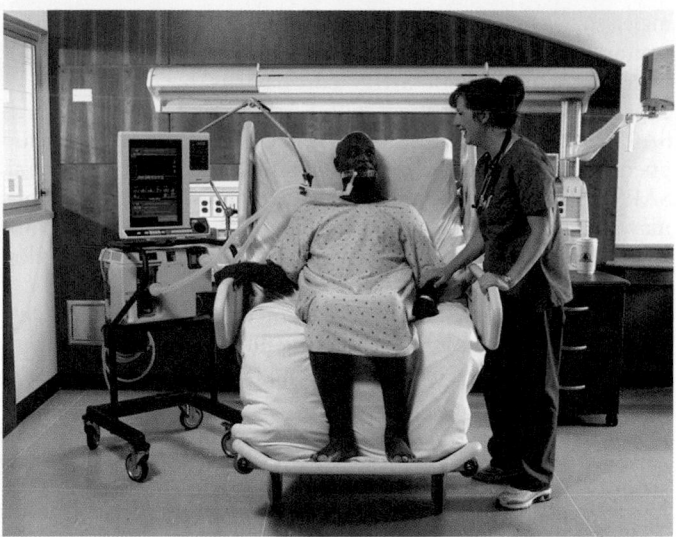

FIGURE 70-12 TotalCare SpO₂RT Bed System offers continuous lateral rotation therapy and percussion and vibration therapies. Patients can be repositioned easily and quickly. Source: © 2006 Hill-Rom Services, Inc. Reprinted with permission. All rights reserved.

Therapy System (Figure 70-11) is a bed that is designed for a patient placed in the prone position and provides kinetic therapy in which the patient is turned side to side to any angle between 40 and 62 degrees (Jackson, Verano, Fry, et al., 2012).

Other positioning strategies used in ARDS are lateral rotation therapy and kinetic therapy (Kallet, 2015; Koh, 2014). The purpose of this therapy is to provide continuous, slow, side-to-side turning of the patient by rotation of the bed frame. Lateral movement of the bed is maintained for 18 hours daily to simulate postural drainage and help mobilize secretions. In addition, the bed may also contain a vibrator pack that can provide chest physiotherapy to further assist with secretion removal (Figure 70-12). The patient's pulmonary status (e.g., respiratory rate and rhythm, breath sounds, ABGs, SpO₂) should be assessed before initiation of the therapy and continued throughout.

MEDICAL SUPPORTIVE THERAPY

MAINTENANCE OF CARDIAC OUTPUT AND TISSUE PERFUSION. Patients receiving PPV and PEEP frequently experience decreased cardiac output in relation to impaired contractility, decreased preload, decreased venous return, or some combination, as a result of PEEP-induced increases in intrathoracic pressure. Continuous hemodynamic monitoring is essential for detecting changes and titrating therapy. An arterial catheter is inserted for continuous blood pressure monitoring and ABG sampling. A pulmonary artery catheter enables monitoring of pulmonary artery pressures, pulmonary artery wedge pressures (which reflect the fluid status of the left side of the heart), mixed venous oxygen saturation, and cardiac output. If the cardiac output falls, it may be necessary to administer fluids or to lower the PEEP. Use of inotropic drugs such as dobutamine or dopamine may also be necessary. (See Chapter 68 for discussion of hemodynamic monitoring.)

The hemoglobin is usually kept above 6 mmol/L with an O₂ saturation of 90 or higher (when PaO₂ ≥60 mm Hg). Packed red blood cells may be administered to increase hemoglobin and thus the O₂-carrying capacity of the blood.

MAINTENANCE OF NUTRITION AND FLUID BALANCE. Maintenance of nutrition and fluid balance is challenging in patients with ARDS. Nutrition consultations determine optimal caloric needs. Attaining access and initiating enteral nutrition should be considered as soon as fluid resuscitation is completed and the patient is hemodynamically stable. A "window of opportunity" exists in the first 24 to 72 hours after the patient's admission or the onset of a hypermetabolic insult. However, current research has shown that the use of enteral omega-3 fatty acids did not significantly reduce all-cause 28-day mortality rates (Zhu, Zhang, Li, et al., 2014).

Increased pulmonary capillary permeability results in pulmonary edema. However, the patient may be volume depleted, hypotensive, and prone to decreased cardiac output from mechanical ventilation and PEEP. Pulmonary artery wedge pressures, daily weights, and intake and output are monitored to assess fluid status. Fluid replacement with crystalloids or colloids is controversial. Critics of colloids believe that proteins in colloid solutions leak into the pulmonary interstitium, exacerbating the movement of proteinaceous fluid into the alveoli (Kallet, 2015). Advocates of colloids as replacement believe that colloids help keep fluid from leaking into the alveoli (Neamu & Martin, 2013). The pulmonary artery wedge pressure is kept as low as possible without impairing cardiac output in order to limit pulmonary edema. Fluids are usually restricted mildly, with diuretics administered as needed (Urden, Stacy, & Lough, 2014).

EVALUATION
The expected outcomes for patients with ARDS are similar to those for patients with acute respiratory failure and are presented in NCP 70-1, available on the Evolve website.

SEVERE ACUTE RESPIRATORY SYNDROME

Severe acute respiratory syndrome (SARS) is a serious, acute respiratory infection caused by a coronavirus. The virus spreads by close contact between people. The SARS coronavirus is probably spread via droplets in the air. It is possible that SARS coronavirus may also be spread more broadly through the air or from touching contaminated objects.

Most patients with SARS coronavirus have a history of exposure to another patient with SARS or to a setting in which SARS coronavirus transmission is occurring, and they develop pneumonia (Khandelwal, Hough, Bansal, et al., 2014). In general, SARS begins with a fever greater than 38°C. Other manifestations may include sore throat, headache, chills, generalized discomfort, and muscle aches. After 2 to 7 days, affected patients may develop a dry cough and dyspnea.

Because the disease is severe, treatment is started immediately on the basis of symptoms, before the illness is confirmed. First, patients with suspected SARS should be placed in isolation

to protect others. There is no definitive treatment for SARS, but antiviral medications (such as ribavirin) and cortico-steroids may be used. Although antibiotics do not help with SARS (because it is believed to be caused by a virus), they may be used in cases in which the patient also has a bacterial infection.

Approximately 80% to 90% of infected people start to recover after 6 to 7 days. However, 10% to 20% go on to develop severe breathing problems and may need mechanical ventilation. The risk of death is higher among such patients and appears to be linked to pre-existing health conditions. People older than 40 years are more likely than those younger to develop severe breathing problems (Khandelwal, Hough, Bansal, et al., 2014).

CASE STUDY

Acute Respiratory Distress Syndrome

Source: Phovoir/ Shutterstock .com.

Patient Profile

Farid Habib is a 55-year-old man who was admitted to a surgical intensive care unit (ICU) 72 hours ago after bowel resection. The surgery was extensive to repair a perforated colon, irrigate the abdominal cavity, and provide hemostasis. During surgery, his systolic blood pressure (BP) dropped to 70 mm Hg. Seven units of packed red blood cells and 4 L of normal saline were administered to restore blood loss and circulating volume. He is currently receiving 60% FiO$_2$ through an aerosol face mask and has continuous cardiac monitoring and O$_2$ saturation in place. He is receiving 0.9% normal saline at 125 mL/hr through a central line. A urinary catheter is in place.

Subjective Data

- He complains of shortness of breath, inability to lie flat, and diffuse abdominal pain.
- His wife and two adult children are at the bedside voicing concerns and asking questions about his condition.

Objective Data
Physical Assessment

- *General:* Alert, well nourished, appears restless and anxious; head of bed elevated 30 degrees; skin cool, moderate diaphoresis
- *Respiratory:* No accessory muscle use, retractions, or paradoxical breathing; respiration rate, 28 breaths/min; SpO$_2$, 85%; fine crackles at lung bases
- *Cardiovascular:* BP, 90/60 mm Hg; sinus tachycardia at 130 beats/min; equal apical–radial pulse; temperature, 38°C orally

- *Gastro-intestinal:* No bowel sounds heard; surgical dressing dry and intact
- *Urological:* Catheter draining concentrated urine at <30 mL/hr

Diagnostic Findings

- ABG results: pH, 7.35; PaO$_2$, 55 mm Hg; PaCO$_2$, 27 mm Hg; bicarbonate level, 16 mmol/L; SaO$_2$, 86%
- Chest radiograph: new scattered interstitial infiltrates compatible with ARDS

Discussion Questions

1. How does the pathophysiology of ARDS predispose to the development of refractory hypoxemia?
2. What clinical manifestations does Mr. Habib exhibit that support a diagnosis of ARDS?
3. What are the possible causes of ARDS in Mr. Habib?
4. What are the possible complications that Mr. Habib is at risk for developing secondary to ARDS?
5. *Evidence-informed practice:* A new nurse who is being oriented asks why Mr. Habib's family was offered the opportunity to stay at the bedside while the chest tube was placed. How should the nurse respond?
6. *Priority decision:* What priority interventions should be implemented to improve Mr. Habib's respiratory status and hypoxemia?
7. *Priority decision:* On the basis of the assessment data presented, what are the priority nursing diagnoses?
8. What information should the nurse provide to the caregivers, in view of Mr. Habib's decline in cardiopulmonary function?

ⓔvolve
Answers are available at *http://evolve.elsevier.com/Canada/Lewis/medsurg*

▌ REVIEW QUESTIONS

The number of the question corresponds to the same-numbered objective at the beginning of the chapter.

1. Which signs and symptoms differentiate hypoxemic respiratory failure from hypercapnic respiratory failure? *(Select all that apply)*
   a. Cyanosis
   b. Tachypnea
   c. Morning headache
   d. Paradoxical breathing
   e. Use of pursed-lip breathing
2. What is an early sign of acute respiratory failure?
   a. Coma
   b. Cyanosis
   c. Restlessness
   d. Paradoxical breathing

3. Which type of oxygen delivery system should be chosen for clients in acute respiratory failure?
   a. Always use a low-flow device, such as a nasal cannula
   b. One that should correct the partial pressure of oxygen in arterial blood (PaO$_2$) to a normal level as quickly as possible
   c. Positive-pressure ventilation to prevent CO$_2$ narcosis
   d. One that should maintain the PaO$_2$ at 60 mm Hg or higher at the lowest fraction of inspired oxygen (FiO$_2$) possible
4. What are the early clinical manifestations of ARDS?
   a. Dyspnea and tachypnea
   b. Cyanosis and apprehension
   c. Hypotension and tachycardia
   d. Respiratory distress and frothy sputum

5. How is fluid balance maintained in clients with ARDS?
   a. Hydration with colloids
   b. Administration of surfactant
   c. Mild fluid restriction and diuretics as necessary
   d. Keeping the hemoglobin at levels of 9.5 mmol/L (15 g/dL)
6. Which of the following is designed to prevent barotrauma in clients with ARDS?
   a. Increasing positive end-expiratory pressure (PEEP)
   b. Increasing the tidal volume

c. Permissive hypercapnia
d. Pressure support ventilation

1. a, b, d. 2. c. 3. d. 4. a. 5. c. 6. c.

⊖volve

For even more review questions, visit *http://evolve.elsevier.com/Canada/Lewis/medsurg*.

REFERENCES

Ari, A., Fink, J. B., & Dhand, R. (2012). Inhalation therapy in patients receiving mechanical ventilation: An update. *Journal of Aerosol Medicine and Pulmonary Drug Delivery, 25*(6), 319–332.

Bein, T., Weber-Carstens, S., Goldmann, A., et al. (2013). Lower tidal volume strategy combined with extracorporeal CO2 removal in severe ARDS. *Intensive Care Medicine, 39*(5), 847–856. doi:*http://dx.doi.org/10.1007/s00134-012-2787-6*.

Brashers, V., & Huether, S. E. (2014). Alterations of pulmonary function. In K. L. McCance & S. E. Huether (Eds.), *Pathophysiology: The biologic basis for disease in adults and children* (7th ed., pp. 1248–1289). St. Louis: Elsevier Mosby.

Burns, S. M. (Ed.), (2014). *AACN essentials of critical care nursing* (3rd ed.). New York: McGraw-Hill.

Fournier, M. (2014). Caring for patients in respiratory failure. *American Nurse Today, 9*(11), 18–23.

Fratantoro, M. (2015). New drug being developed to fight sepsis and ARDS. *RT: The Journal for Respiratory Care Practitioners, 28*(9), 4.

Goodacre, S., Cohen, J., Bradburn, M., et al. (2013). Intravenous or nebulised magnesium sulphate versus standard therapy for severe acute asthma (3Mg trial): A double-blind, randomised controlled trial. *The Lancet Respiratory Medicine, 1*(4), 293–300.

Grek, A., Booth, S., Festic, E., et al. (2017). Sepsis and shock response team: Impact of a multidisciplinary approach to implementing Surviving Sepsis Campaign guidelines and surviving the process. *American Journal of Medical Quality, 32*(5), 500–507. doi:10.1177/1062860616676887.

Hough, C. L. (2014). Steroids for acute respiratory distress syndrome? *Clinics in Chest Medicine, 35*(4), 781–795. doi:10.1016/j.ccm.2014.08.014.

Hraiech, S., Yoshida, T., & Papazian, L. (2015). Balancing neuromuscular blockade versus preserved muscle activity. *Current Opinion in Critical Care, 21*(1), 26–33. doi:10.1097/MCC.0000000000000175.

Jackson, M. E., Verano, J. X., Fry, J. E., et al. (2012). Skin preparation process for the prevention of skin breakdown in patients who are intubated and treated with RotoProne. *Respiratory Care, 57*(2), 311–314. doi:10.4187/respcare.01235.

Kallet, R. H. (2015). A comprehensive review of prone position in ARDS. *Respiratory Care, 60*(11), 1660–1687. doi:10.4187/respcare.0427.

Khandelwal, N., Hough, C. L., Bansal, A., et al. (2014). Long-term survival in patients with severe acute respiratory distress syndrome and rescue therapies for refractory hypoxemia. *Critical Care Medicine, 42*(7), 1610–1618. doi:10.1097/CCM.0000000000000322.

Koh, Y. (2014). Update in acute respiratory distress syndrome. *Journal of Intensive Care, 2*(2), 1–6.

Kress, J. P. (2015). Mortality is the only relevant outcome in ARDS: No. *Intensive Care Medicine, 41*(1), 144–146.

Luo, J., Wang, M., Zhu, H., et al. (2014). Can non-invasive positive pressure ventilation prevent endotracheal intubation in acute lung injury/acute respiratory distress syndrome? A meta-analysis. *Respirology (Carlton, Vic.), 19*(8), 1149–1157. doi:10.1111/resp.12383.

Marhong, J., & Fan, E. (2014). Carbon dioxide in the critically ill: Too much or too little of a good thing? *Respiratory Care, 59*(10), 1597–1605 9p. doi:10.4187/respcare.03405.

Matos, A. A., Manzanares, W., & Nava, V. S. (2015). Nutrition support for pulmonary failure. In G. A. Cresci (Ed.), *Nutrition support for the critically ill patient: A guide to practice* (pp. 467–482). Boca Raton, FL: CRC Press.

Meduri, G. U., & Eltorky, M. A. (2015). Understanding ARDS-associated fibroproliferation. *Intensive Care Medicine, 41*(3), 517–520. doi:10.1007/s00134-014-3613-0.

Mendez, M. P., Lazar, M. H., Digiovine, B., et al. (2013). Dedicated multidisciplinary ventilator bundle team and compliance with sedation vacation. *American Journal of Critical Care, 22*(1), 54–60. doi:10.4037/ajcc2013873.

Messika, J., Ahmed, K. B., Gaudry, S., et al. (2015). Use of high-flow nasal cannula oxygen therapy in subjects with ARDS: A 1-year observational study. *Respiratory Care, 60*(2), 162–169. doi:10.4187/respcare.03423.

Moazed, F., & Calfee, C. S. (2014). Environmental risk factors for acute respiratory distress syndrome. *Clinics in Chest Medicine, 35*(4), 625–637. doi:10.1016/j.ccm.2014.08.003.

Modrykamien, A. M., & Gupta, P. (2015). The acute respiratory distress syndrome. *Baylor University Medical Center Proceedings, 28*(2), 163–171.

Neamu, R., & Martin, G. (2013). Fluid management in acute respiratory distress syndrome. *Current Opinion in Critical Care, 19*(1), 24–30. doi:10.1097/MCC.0b013e32835c285b.

Papazian, L., & Herridge, M. (2013). Outcomes and risk stratification for severe ARDS treated with ECMO. *Intensive Care Medicine, 39*(10), 1857–1860. doi:*http://dx.doi.org/10.1007/s00134-013-3067-9*.

Retamal, J., Bugedo, G., Larsson, A., et al. (2015). High PEEP levels are associated with overdistension and tidal recruitment/derecruitment in ARDS patients. *Acta Anaesthesiologica Scandinavica, 59*(9), 1161–1169. doi:10.1111/aas.12563.

Schell-Chaple, H. M., Puntillo, K. A., Matthay, M. A., et al. (2015). Body temperature and mortality in patients with acute respiratory distress syndrome. *American Journal of Critical Care, 24*(1), 15–23. doi:10.4037/ajcc2015320.

Schmidt, M., Balzer, F., Pille, C., et al. (2013). Higher age in ARDS predicts mortality in severe ARDS and older age starts in the fourth decade. In *Intensive Care Medicine* (Vol. 39, pp. s373–s374). New York: Springer.

Taylor, B. E., McClave, S. A., Martindale, R. G., et al. (2016). Guidelines for the provision and assessment of nutrition support therapy in the adult critically ill patient: Society of Critical Care Medicine (SCCM) and American Society for Parenteral and Enteral Nutrition (A.S.P.E.N.). *Critical Care Medicine, 44*(2), 390–438. doi:10.1097/CCM.0000000000001525.

Töpfer, L., Menk, M., Weber-Carstens, S., et al. (2014). Influenza A (H1N1) vs non-H1N1 ARDS: Analysis of clinical course. *Journal of Critical Care, 29*(3), 340–346. doi:10.1016/j.jcrc.2013.12.013.

Urden, L. D., Stacy, K. M., & Lough, M. E. (2014). *Critical care nursing: Diagnosis and management* (7th ed.). St. Louis: Mosby.

Villar, J., Blanco, J., & Kacmarek, R. M. (2016). Current incidence and outcome of the acute respiratory distress syndrome. *Current Opinion in Critical Care, 22*(1), 1–6.

Wang, S., Singh, B., Tian, L., et al. (2013). Epidemiology of noninvasive mechanical ventilation in acute respiratory failure—A retrospective population-based study. *BMC Emergency Medicine, 13*(1), 6. doi:10.1186/1471-227X-13-6.

Zhu, D., Zhang, Y., Li, S., et al. (2014). Enteral omega-3 fatty acid supplementation in adult patients with acute respiratory distress syndrome: A systematic review of randomized controlled trials with meta-analysis and trial sequential analysis. *Intensive Care Medicine, 40*(4), 504–512. doi:*http://dx.doi.org/10.1007/s00134 -014-3244-5.*

RESOURCES

Resources for this chapter are listed in Chapter 71.

Nursing Management
Emergency Care Situations

Written by: Linda Bucher
Adapted by: Jane Tyerman

℮volve WEBSITE

http://evolve.elsevier.com/Canada/Lewis/medsurg

- Review Questions (Online Only)
- Key Points
- Answer Guidelines for Case Study
- Student Case Study
  - Musculo-Skeletal Trauma
- Conceptual Care Map Creator
- Audio Glossary
- Content Updates

LEARNING OBJECTIVES

1. Apply the sequential steps in the primary and secondary surveys to assess a patient in an emergency situation.
2. Describe the pathophysiology, the assessment, and the collaborative care of select environmental emergencies, including hyperthermia, hypothermia, submersion injury, bites, and stings.
3. Discuss the assessment and the collaborative care of select toxicological emergencies.
4. Discuss the nurse's role in the process of organ and tissue donations.

5. Recognize the nurse's role in assessing and caring for survivors of domestic violence in the emergency department and in the mandatory reporting of abuse and weapon-related injuries.
6. Summarize the clinical manifestations of sexual assault and the appropriate nursing and collaborative management of the patient who has been sexually assaulted.

KEY TERMS

domestic violence, p. 1819
frostbite, p. 1813
heat cramps, p. 1811
heat exhaustion, p. 1811

heatstroke, p. 1812
hypothermia, p. 1813
jaw-thrust manoeuvre, p. 1805
primary survey, p. 1804

rapid-sequence intubation, p. 1805
secondary survey, p. 1806
sexual assault, p. 1820

submersion injury, p. 1814
triage system, p. 1804

Most patients with life-threatening problems arrive at the hospital through the emergency department (ED). According to the National Trauma Registry of the Canadian Institute for Health Information (CIHI, 2013), there were 15 190 major-injury cases in 2010 and 2011. The leading causes of injury were unintentional falls and motor vehicle collisions, each responsible for 39% of the identified cases. Blunt trauma was the most common injury (95%), followed by penetrating injuries (4%) and burn injuries (1%). Intentional injuries, both self-inflicted and through assaults, accounted for 10% of injuries (CIHI, 2013).

Many patients report to the ED for less urgent conditions, often because they do not have access to a health care provider. Emergency nurses care for patients of all ages and with a variety of problems, especially in the areas of health promotion and prevention and chronic disease management. Some EDs specialize in certain patient populations, such as pediatric patients, or certain conditions, such as trauma.

Nursing roles within the ED include patient care, research, and management. The National Emergency Nurses Association (NENA) is the Canadian specialty nursing organization aimed at advancing emergency nursing practice. NENA publishes standards of care for nurses working in the ED and endorses the Canadian Nurses Association (CNA) certification process to become a certified emergency nurse, ENC(C). This certification validates the knowledge and skills that a nurse needs to provide competent care in emergency settings (CNA, 2018; NENA, 2016).

Specific emergency management of patients with various medical, surgical, and traumatic emergencies is described throughout this book (Table 71-1).

This chapter focuses on initial assessment and management of patients with trauma and emergency conditions not addressed elsewhere in this book. These include heat- and cold-related emergencies, submersion injuries, bites, stings, poisonings, abuse, and violence.

CARE OF THE EMERGENCY PATIENT

A **triage system** identifies and categorizes patients' conditions so that those in most critical condition are treated first. The process is based on the premise that patients who have a threat to life, limb, or vision should be treated before other patients. Unique to the ED, the triage nurse performs a brief patient assessment to categorize and prioritize the needs of each patient seeking care. This categorization is facilitated through the Canadian Triage and Acuity Scale (CTAS). CTAS is used in the ED and by community paramedics to define the urgency of a patient's presenting problem (Bullard, Chan, Brayman, et al., 2014; Bullard, Unger, Spence, et al., 2008).

✚ TABLE 71-1   EMERGENCY MANAGEMENT

Emergency Management Tables

Subject	Chapter
Abdominal trauma	45
Acute abdominal pain	45
Acute soft-tissue injury	65
Anaphylactic shock	16
Chemical burns	27
Chest pain	36
Chest trauma	30
Cocaine and amphetamine toxicity	11
Depressant drugs, overdose of	11
Diabetic ketoacidosis	52
Electrical burns	27
Eye injury	24
Fractured extremity	65
Head injury	59
Hyperthermia	71
Hypothermia	71
Inhalation injury	27
Sexual assault	71
Shock	69
Spinal cord injury	63
Stroke	60
Submersion injuries	71
Thermal burns	27
Thoracic injuries	30
Tonic–clonic seizures	61

The CTAS is a five-level scale consisting of the following categories: resuscitation, emergency, urgent, less urgent, and nonurgent (Table 71-2). Patients who are assigned a high triage level (level I: resuscitation) are allocated the most health care resources and are assessed immediately. Those assigned to a low triage level (e.g., level V: nonurgent) wait longer for nurse and physician assessment unless they experience a deterioration in clinical status while they wait (Bullard, Chan, Brayman, et al., 2014). The CTAS has four major components: (1) five *triage levels* (ranging from nonurgent to resuscitation); (2) a *time to nurse and physician assessment*, which is based on the assigned triage level; (3) *usual presentation of the patient* (e.g., head injury, alert, with no vomiting; sore throat with no respiratory symptoms), which is based on the patient's complaints and presentation; and (4) a *sentinel diagnosis* (e.g., head injury; upper respiratory infection).

The emergency nurse must complete an initial assessment to determine the presence of actual or potential threats to life and then rapidly initiate interventions appropriate for the patient's condition. Simultaneously, the nurse collects a history. A systematic approach to the initial assessment of the patient decreases the time required to identify potential threats and keeps to a minimum the risk of missing a life-threatening condition. Two systematic approaches initially developed for use with patients with trauma, a primary and a secondary survey, can be applied to emergency assessment.

PRIMARY SURVEY

The **primary survey** (Table 71-3) focuses on *a*irway, *b*reathing, *c*irculation, and *d*isability (ABCDs) and serves to identify life-threatening conditions so that appropriate interventions can be initiated. Life-threatening conditions related to airway, breathing, circulation, and disability (Table 71-4) may be identified during the primary survey, and the nurse starts interventions immediately before proceeding to the next step of the survey.

A=Airway With Cervical Spine Stabilization or Immobilization

Nearly all immediate deaths from trauma occur because of airway obstruction. Saliva, bloody secretions, vomitus, laryngeal trauma, facial trauma, fractures, and the tongue can obstruct the airway. Patients at risk for airway compromise include those who have

TABLE 71-2   THE CANADIAN EMERGENCY DEPARTMENT TRIAGE AND ACUITY SCALE

Consideration	Resuscitation (Level I)	Emergency (Level II)	Urgent (Level III)	Less Urgent (Level IV)	Nonurgent (Level V)
Condition	Threat to life or limb; immediate assessment required. Example: cardiac or respiratory arrest, major trauma, shock state	Potential threat to life, limb, or function. Example: altered mental state, head injury, cardiac chest pain, stroke	Potential to progress to serious problem. Example: asthma, GI bleed, acute pain	May progress to urgent status. Example: headache, corneal foreign body, chronic back pain	Acute or chronic but nonurgent. Example: sore throat, mild abdominal pain that is chronic or recurring
Time to nurse and physician assessment	Immediate	15 min	30 min	60 min	120 min
Recommended re-evaluation	Continuous	Every 15 min	Every 30 min	Every 60 min	Every 120 min

GI, gastro-intestinal.

Source: Adapted from Bullard, M. J., Unger, B., Spence, J., et al. (2008). Revisions to the Canadian Triage and Acuity Scale (CTAS) adult guidelines. *Canadian Journal of Emergency Medicine, 10*(2), 137.

TABLE 71-3 PRIMARY SURVEY OF A PATIENT IN AN EMERGENCY

Assessment	Interventions
Airway With Simultaneous Cervical Spine Stabilization and Immobilization	
• Assessment of airway for patency • Assessment for respiratory distress • Check for loose teeth and foreign objects • Assessment for bleeding, vomitus, or edema	• Open airway. • Perform jaw-thrust manoeuvre. • Remove or suction any foreign objects. • Insert oropharyngeal or nasopharyngeal airway, endotracheal tube, cricothyroidectomy. • Immobilize cervical spine with collar, backboard, or soft rolls; tape forehead to board.
Breathing	
• Assessment of ventilation • Chest scan for signs of breathing • Observation for paradoxical movement of the chest wall during inspiration and expiration • Observation for use of accessory muscles or abdominal muscles • Observation and count of respiratory rate • Colour of nail beds, mucous membranes, and skin • Auscultation of lungs • Assessment for jugular venous distension and position of trachea	• Administer supplemental O_2 via appropriate delivery system (e.g., nonrebreather mask) • Ventilate with bag–valve–mask device with 100% O_2 if respirations are inadequate or absent. • Prepare to intubate if respiratory distress is severe (e.g., agonal breaths, respiratory arrest). • Have suction available. • If breath sounds are absent, prepare for needle thoracostomy and chest tube insertion.
Circulation	
• Check of carotid or femoral pulse • Palpation of pulse for quality and rate • Assessment of skin colour, temperature, and moisture • Check of capillary refill • Assessment for external bleeding • Measurement of blood pressure	• If pulse is absent, initiate cardiopulmonary resuscitation and advanced life-support measures. • If shock symptoms are present, insert two large-bore (14- to 16-gauge) intravenous catheters and initiate infusions of normal saline or lactated Ringer's solution. • Control bleeding with direct pressure. • Administer blood products, if ordered. • Consider autotransfusion if chest trauma is isolated. • Obtain blood samples for type and crossmatch.
Disability: Brief Neurological Assessment	
• Assessment of level of consciousness by determining response to verbal stimuli, painful stimuli, and motor response (e.g., Glasgow Coma Scale) • Assessment of pupils for size, shape, equality, and response to light	• Periodically reassess level of consciousness. • Consider the possibility of hyperventilation if signs of brain herniation are present (e.g., motor posturing).

TABLE 71-4 CAUSES OF LIFE-THREATENING CONDITIONS IDENTIFIED DURING THE PRIMARY SURVEY*

Airway
• Inhalation injury
• Obstruction, partial or complete, by foreign bodies, debris (e.g., vomitus), or tongue
• Penetrating wounds, blunt trauma, or both to the upper airway structures

Breathing
• Anaphylaxis
• Flail chest with pulmonary contusion
• Hemothorax
• Pneumothorax (e.g., open, tension)

Circulation
• Direct cardiac injury (e.g., myocardial infarction, trauma)
• Pericardial tamponade
• Shock (e.g., massive burns, hypovolemia)
• Uncontrolled external hemorrhage
• Hypothermia

Disability
• Head injury
• Stroke

*This list is not all-inclusive.

seizures, near-drowning, anaphylaxis, foreign body obstruction, or cardiopulmonary arrest. If an airway is not maintained, airflow is obstructed, and hypoxia, acidosis, and death result.

Primary signs and symptoms in a patient with a compromised airway include dyspnea, inability to vocalize, presence of a foreign body in the airway, and trauma to the face or neck. Airway maintenance should progress rapidly from the least to the most invasive method. One treatment method is to open the airway by means of the **jaw-thrust manoeuvre,** in which the rescuer uses forearms to stabilize the patient's head (while avoiding neck hyperextension) and then applies pressure with the index fingers to push the patient's jaw forward (Figure 71-1). Other treatment methods include suctioning and removal of foreign objects; insertion of a nasopharyngeal or oropharyngeal airway (which causes a conscious patient to gag); and endotracheal intubation. If the patient cannot be intubated because of airway obstruction, an emergency cricothyroidotomy or tracheotomy should be performed (Chapter 29). Patients should be ventilated with 100% oxygen (O_2) through a bag–valve–mask (BVM) device before intubation or cricothyroidotomy (Bair, Walls, & Grayzel, 2017).

Rapid-sequence intubation is the preferred procedure for securing an unprotected airway in the ED. The patient is given a rapid-acting sedative (e.g., midazolam) and a paralyzing neuro-muscular blocking agent (e.g., succinylcholine) to facilitate

FIGURE 71-1 The jaw-thrust manoeuvre is the only widely recommended procedure for use on an unconscious patient with possible neck or spinal injuries. The patient should be lying supine, and the rescuer should kneel at the top of the patient's head. The rescuer carefully reaches forward and gently places one hand on each side of the patient's chin at the lateral angles of the lower jaw. The patient's head should be stabilized by the rescuer's forearms; then the rescuer applies pressure with the index fingers to push the patient's jaw forward.

intubation and minimize the risk for aspiration and airway trauma (Stollings, Diedrich, Oyen, et al., 2013; Patanwala, Stahle, Sakles, et al., 2011).

The nurse should suspect cervical spine trauma in any patient with significant injuries to the upper torso or trauma to the face, head, or neck. The cervical spine should be stabilized with the head maintained in a neutral position. At the scene of the injury, the cervical spine is immobilized with a rigid cervical collar or an immobilization device such as head blocks or towel rolls that are secured to a backboard on either side of the head. The patient's forehead then is taped to the backboard.

B=Breathing

Adequate airflow through the upper airway does not ensure adequate ventilation. Breathing alterations are caused by many conditions, including fractured ribs, pneumothorax, penetrating injuries, allergic reactions, pulmonary emboli, and asthma attacks. Patients may exhibit a variety of signs and symptoms, including dyspnea (e.g., pulmonary emboli), stridor, accessory muscle use, paradoxical or asymmetrical chest wall movement (e.g., flail chest), decreased or absent breath sounds on the affected side (e.g., pneumothorax), visible wound to chest wall (e.g., penetrating injury), cyanosis (e.g., asthma), tachycardia, and hypotension.

Every critically injured or ill patient has increased metabolic and oxygen demands and should receive supplemental O_2. The nurse should administer high-flow O_2 (100%) via a nonrebreather mask and monitor the patient's response. Life-threatening conditions, (e.g., tension pneumothorax, flail chest) can severely compromise ventilation. Interventions in these situations include BVM ventilation with 100% O_2, intubation, needle decompression, and treatment of the underlying cause. In patients with established chronic obstructive pulmonary disease, carbon dioxide retention and level of consciousness must be monitored.

C=Circulation

An effective circulatory system includes the heart, intact blood vessels, and adequate blood volume. Uncontrolled internal or external bleeding increases the risk for hemorrhagic shock (Chapter 69). Because peripheral pulses may be absent as a result of direct injury or vasoconstriction, the central (e.g., carotid) pulse should be checked. Palpating the pulse allows for assessment of the quality, rate, and regularity. The nurse should also assess skin for colour, temperature, and moisture. A capillary refill delay longer than 3 seconds and altered mental status are the most

significant signs of shock. Care must be taken when capillary refill is evaluated in cold environments because the cold can cause vasoconstriction, which delays refill.

Two large-bore (14- to 16-gauge) intravenous (IV) catheters should be inserted into veins in the upper extremities unless this location is contraindicated, for example, due to a massive fracture or an injury that affects limb circulation, and aggressive fluid resuscitation initiated with lactated Ringer's solution or normal saline. The nurse should apply direct pressure with a sterile dressing to obvious bleeding sites. Blood samples should be obtained for typing to determine ABO and Rh group and then type-specific packed red blood cells administered. In an emergency (life-threatening) situation, blood that is not cross-matched may be given if immediate transfusion is warranted.

D=Disability

A brief neurological examination completes the primary survey. The degree of disability is measured by level of consciousness, which is assessed by determining the patient's alertness and response to verbal and painful stimuli with the following scale:

A Alert
V Responsive to voice
P Responsive to pain
U Unresponsive

The Glasgow Coma Scale (GCS) and the Canadian Neurological Scale are used to further assess the arousal aspect of the patient's consciousness (The GCS is further discussed in Chapter 59, and the Canadian Neurological Scale is discussed in Chapter 60). Pupils should be also assessed for size, shape, equality, and response or reactivity to light.

SECONDARY SURVEY

After each step of the primary survey is addressed and any necessary life-saving interventions are initiated, the secondary survey begins. The secondary survey is a brief, systematic process that is aimed at identifying *all* injuries and continues the ABCD mnemonic through EFGHI: *e*xposure and *e*nvironmental control; *f*ull set of vital signs/*f*ive interventions/*f*acilitating family presence; *g*iving comfort measures; *h*istory and *h*ead-to-toe assessment; and *i*nspection of the posterior surfaces (Table 71-5).

E=Exposure and Environmental Control

Any patient who has suffered trauma should have clothes removed so that a thorough physical assessment can be performed. Once the patient is exposed, it is important to limit heat loss and prevent hypothermia by using warming blankets, overhead warmers, and warmed IV fluids. The nurse should observe for medical alert bracelets or necklaces, tattoos, or wallet cards for ongoing health illnesses. Any faith-based objections to blood transfusions should be ascertained.

F=Full Set of Vital Signs/Five Interventions/Facilitating Family Presence

A complete set of vital signs, including blood pressure (BP), heart rate, respiratory rate, and temperature, should be measured after the patient's clothes are removed. BP should be obtained in both arms if the patient has sustained or is suspected of having chest trauma.

At this point, it must be determined whether to proceed with the secondary survey or to perform additional interventions. The availability of other team members often influences this

TABLE 71-5   SECONDARY SURVEY OF A PATIENT IN AN EMERGENCY

Parameter	Assessment
Exposure and environmental control	Removal of clothing for adequate examination; keeping patient warm with blankets, IV fluids, and overhead lights
Full set of vital signs	Obtainment of vital signs: temperature, heart rate, respiratory rate, and blood pressure bilaterally
Five interventions	(a) Monitoring and recording of heart rhythm; (b) monitoring of O_2 saturation; (c) insertion of a urinary catheter (if not contraindicated); (d) insertion of a gastric tube; and (e) obtainment of specimens for laboratory studies
Facilitating family presence	Determining family's desire to be present during resuscitation
Giving comfort measures	Addressing patient's level of pain and anxiety
History and head-to-toe assessment	
• History	Documentation of details of the incident or illness, mechanism and pattern of injury, length of time since incident occurred, injuries suspected, treatment provided and patient's response, and patient's level of consciousness
	Assessment for allergies
	Documentation of medication history
	Documentation of past health history (e.g., pre-existing medical conditions, most recent menstrual period)
	Determination of the patient's most recent meal
	Documentation of events and environment preceding illness or injury
• Head, neck, face	Notation of general appearance, skin, and colour
	Examination of face and scalp for lacerations, bone or soft-tissue deformity, tenderness, bleeding, and foreign bodies
	Examination of eyes, ears, nose, and mouth for bleeding, foreign bodies, drainage, pain, deformity, ecchymosis, and lacerations
	Examination of head for depressions of cranial or facial bones, contusions, hematomas, areas of softness, and bony crepitus
	Examination of neck for stiffness, pain in cervical vertebrae, tracheal deviation, distended neck veins, bleeding, edema, difficulty swallowing, bruising, subcutaneous emphysema, and bony crepitus
• Chest	Observation of rate, depth, and effort of breathing, including chest wall movement
	Palpation for bony crepitus and subcutaneous emphysema
	Observation for use of accessory muscles
	Auscultation of breath sounds
	Obtainment of ECG
	Documentation of external signs of injury: petechiae, bleeding, cyanosis, bruises, abrasions, lacerations, or scars
• Abdomen and flanks	Assessment of symmetry of external abdominal wall and bony structures
	Observation for external signs of injury: bruising, abrasions, lacerations, or punctures
	Assessment for masses, notation of guarding, and checking of femoral pulses
	Documentation of type and location of pain, rigidity, or distension of abdomen
	Assessment of bowel sounds
• Pelvis and perineum	Assessment of genitalia for blood at meatus and for priapism, ecchymosis, rectal bleeding, and anal sphincter tone
• Extremities	Documentation of signs of external injury: deformity, ecchymosis, abrasions, lacerations, or swelling
	Assessment for pain
	Evaluation of movement and strength in arms and legs
	Assessment of sensation in each limb
	Evaluation of colour of skin
	Documentation of presence and quality of peripheral pulses
Inspection of posterior surfaces	Inspection and palpation of back for deformity, bleeding, lacerations, or bruising (performed by log-rolling patient)

ECG, electrocardiogram; *IV,* intravenous; O_2, oxygen.

decision. For patients who have sustained significant trauma and have required life-saving interventions during the primary and secondary surveys, the following five interventions should be performed next:

1. The patient should be monitored by electrocardiography for heart rate and rhythm.
2. Pulse oximetry and O_2 saturation monitoring are initiated.
3. An in-dwelling catheter should be inserted to monitor urine output and to check for hematuria, unless a urethral tear is suspected. Patients with pelvic injuries or blood at the meatus, and men with a high-riding prostate gland (detected on digital rectal examination), are at risk for a urethral tear or transection. Urethrography should be performed before a catheter is inserted.
4. An orogastric or nasogastric tube should be inserted to provide gastric decompression and emptying to reduce the risk for aspiration and to test contents for blood. A nasogastric tube

should not be placed in the nares in a patient suspected of having facial fractures or a basilar skull fracture because the tube could enter the brain through the cribriform plate; it should be placed orally.

5. Laboratory studies should be performed for typing and crossmatching, hematocrit, hemoglobin, blood urea nitrogen, creatinine, blood alcohol level, toxicology screening, arterial blood gases (ABGs), electrolytes, coagulation profile, liver enzymes, cardiac enzymes, and pregnancy.

Facilitating *family presence* completes this step of the secondary survey. Although research findings support the positive benefits of family presence during invasive procedures and cardiopulmonary resuscitation (CPR), it is not a widely accepted practice (Jabre, Tazarourte, Azoulay, et al., 2013; NENA, 2014a). The most significant barrier to family presence during CPR was the concern that conflicts may occur within the emergency team. If family presence during CPR is allowed, written policies, guidelines, and education on the practice need to be developed (Edwards, Despotopulos, & Carroll, 2013; Porter, Cooper, & Sellick, 2014). It is essential that a member of the team explain to the family the care delivered and be available to answer their questions.

G = Giving Comfort Measures

Provision of comfort measures is of paramount importance during care for patients in the ED. It has been reported that pain (both acute and chronic) is the primary complaint of all patients who come to the ED (Iyer, 2011). Many EDs have developed pain management guidelines to treat pain early, beginning at triage. Pain management strategies should include a combination of pharmacological (e.g., opioids) and nonpharmacological (e.g., imagery) measures (Kahan, Mailis-Gagnon, Wilson, et al., 2011). Emergency nurses play a pivotal role in pain management because of their frequent contact with patients. General comfort measures such as offering verbal reassurance, listening, reducing stimuli (e.g., dimming lights), and developing a trusting relationship with the patient and family should be provided in the ED. Additional measures include splinting, elevating, and icing injured extremities as appropriate.

H = History and Head-to-Toe Assessment

The history of the incident, injury, or illness provides clues to the cause of the crisis and suggests specific assessment and intervention needs. The patient may be unable to provide a history; however, family, friends, witnesses, and personnel involved before arrival at the hospital can frequently provide important information. Prehospital information should focus on the mechanism and the pattern of injury, injuries suspected, vital signs, treatment initiated, and the patient's responses.

Details of the incident are extremely important because the mechanism of injury and injury patterns can help predict specific injuries. For example, a front-seat passenger with a seat belt may have a head injury from hitting the steering wheel; knee, femur, or hip fractures or dislocation from striking the dashboard; and an abdominal injury from the seat belt. If other victims were dead at the scene, the patient has a high chance of significant injury.

Patients who jump from buildings or bridges may have bilateral calcaneal (heel) fractures, wrist fractures, or lumbar spine compression fractures, and they may be at risk for aortic tears. In older patients who have climbed ladders and fallen, a stroke or myocardial infarction may have led to the fall.

Prehospital personnel often provide a detailed description of the patient's general condition, level of consciousness, and apparent injuries. An experienced ED team can complete a history within 5 minutes of the patient's arrival. If the patient's condition is classified by triage as resuscitative, a thorough history is obtained from family or friends after the patient is taken to the treatment area. The history should include the following questions:

1. What is the chief complaint? What caused the patient to seek attention?
2. What are the patient's subjective complaints?
3. What is the patient's description of pain (e.g., location, duration, quality, character)?
4. What are witnesses' (if any) descriptions of the patient's behaviour since the onset?
5. What is the patient's health care history? The mnemonic AMPLE helps:

A	Allergies
M	Medication history
P	Past health history (e.g., pre-existing medical conditions, previous hospitalizations and surgeries, smoking history, recent use of drugs or alcohol, tetanus immunization, most recent menstrual period)
L	Last meal
E	Events or environment preceding illness or injury

Head, Neck, and Face. The patient should be assessed for general appearance, skin colour, and temperature, and the eyes should be checked for extraocular movements. A disconjugate gaze is an indication of neurological damage. Periorbital ecchymosis ("raccoon eyes") is usually caused by a basilar skull fracture. The tympanic membranes and the external canals are checked for blood and cerebro-spinal fluid. Cerebro-spinal fluid is allowed to flow freely because the leak usually resolves in 2 to 10 days (Chapter 59).

The nurse should assess the airway for foreign bodies, bleeding, edema, and loose or missing teeth; check for the ability to open the mouth and swallow; examine the neck for bruising, edema, bleeding, pain, or distended neck veins; and palpate the trachea to determine whether it is in the midline. A deviated trachea may signal a life-threatening tension pneumothorax. Subcutaneous emphysema may indicate laryngotracheal disruption. A stiff or painful cervical spine area may signify a fracture of a cervical vertebra. The cervical spine should be protected with a rigid collar and supine positioning, and patients with cervical spine injuries must be log-rolled when movement is necessary.

Chest. The chest should be inspected for paradoxical chest movements and large, sucking chest wounds and assessed for pain on palpation, respiratory distress, decreased breath sounds, distant or muffled heart sounds (e.g., pericardial tamponade), and distended neck veins. Palpation of the sternum, the clavicles, and the ribs can reveal any deformity or point tenderness. In addition to tension and open pneumothorax, the patient should be evaluated for rib fractures, pulmonary contusion, blunt cardiac injury, and simple pneumothorax. A 12-lead ECG should be obtained to detect dysrhythmias and evidence of ischemia or infarction, particularly for an older patient or a patient with suspected heart disease.

Abdomen and Flanks. Assessment of the abdomen and the flanks is more difficult. Frequent evaluation for subtle changes in the abdominal examination is essential. Motor vehicle collisions and assaults can cause blunt trauma. Penetrating trauma tends to injure specific organs. Decreased bowel sounds may indicate a temporary paralytic ileus. Bowel sounds in the chest may indicate a diaphragmatic rupture. The abdomen is percussed for distension (e.g., tympany [excessive air] and dullness [excessive fluid]) and palpated for peritoneal irritation.

If intra-abdominal hemorrhage is suspected, diagnostic peritoneal lavage may be performed to determine the presence of blood in the peritoneal space (hemoperitoneum) (Harris, 2013). Before the procedure, a gastric tube and a bladder catheter must be inserted to decompress these organs and reduce the possibility of perforation. An alternative to diagnostic peritoneal lavage that is gaining support is bedside ultrasonography: *focused abdominal sonography for trauma (FAST)*. This procedure is noninvasive and can be performed quickly.

Pelvis and Perineum. The pelvis is gently palpated. If pain is elicited, the patient may have a pelvic fracture. The genitalia are inspected for bleeding and obvious injuries. A rectal examination is performed to check for blood, a high-riding prostate gland, and loss of sphincter tone. The examiner should assess for bladder distension, hematuria, dysuria, or the inability to void.

Extremities. The upper and the lower extremities are assessed for point tenderness, crepitus, and deformities. Injured extremities are splinted above and below the injury to decrease the occurrence of further soft-tissue injury and pain. Grossly deformed, pulseless extremities should be realigned and splinted. Pulses are checked before and after movement or splinting. A pulseless extremity represents a time-critical vascular or orthopedic emergency.

Injured extremities should be elevated, and ice applied. Fractures necessitate splinting, and patients may need pain control with analgesics. Prophylactic antibiotics are administered for open fractures.

I=Inspect the Posterior Surfaces

All patients who have suffered trauma should be turned using spinal precautions to inspect the posterior surfaces. The back is inspected for ecchymosis, abrasions, puncture wounds, cuts, and obvious deformities. The entire spine is palpated for misalignment, deformity, and pain.

INTERVENTION AND EVALUATION

Once the secondary survey is complete, all findings are recorded. Patients should be evaluated to determine their need for tetanus prophylaxis. It is not uncommon for older adults to have an outdated tetanus status. Information is needed about previous vaccinations and the condition of any wounds to make an appropriate decision (Table 71-6).

Regardless of the patient's chief complaint, ongoing monitoring and evaluation are critical in an emergency situation. The nurse is responsible for providing appropriate interventions and assessing the patient's response. The evaluation of airway patency and the effectiveness of breathing always assume highest priority. The nurse monitors O_2 saturation and ABGs to help determine the patient's progress. Level of consciousness, vital signs, quality of peripheral pulses, urine output, and skin temperature, colour, and moisture provide key information about circulation and perfusion.

Depending on the patient's injuries or illness, the patient may be (a) transported for diagnostic tests such as a computed tomographic (CT) scan, radiography, or magnetic resonance imaging (MRI); (b) admitted to a general or critical care unit; or (c) transferred to another facility. The emergency nurse is responsible for monitoring the patient during transport and notifying the team if the patient's condition changes from baseline. Nurses accompanying critically ill patients must be competent in advanced life-support measures.

Mandatory Reporting of Gunshot and Stab Wounds

Most provinces have legislation that requires mandatory reporting of gunshot and stab wounds by health care agencies. Emergency staff must be familiar with their specific provincial law.

Reporting of Abuse of Children

Mandatory reporting of suspected or confirmed child abuse and maltreatment is a strategy to address violence against children. Therefore, health professionals must be aware of the legislation that governs their jurisdiction. In Canada, the Canadian Child Welfare Research Portal website (see the Resources at the end of the chapter) provides provincial and territorial policies and legislation. Professional organizations collaborate to align reporting policies for health care providers. For example, the Ontario Association of Children's Aid Societies and the College

---

TABLE 71-6   PROPHYLAXIS AGAINST TETANUS IN WOUND MANAGEMENT

Vaccination History	Type of Wound	
	Clean, Minor Wounds	**All Other Wounds**
Age 11–64 Yr*		
Unknown or <3 doses of tetanus toxoid–containing vaccine	Tdap and recommend catch-up vaccination	Tdap and recommend catch-up vaccination TIG
≥3 doses of tetanus toxoid–containing vaccine *and* <5 yr since last dose	No indication	No indication
≥3 doses of tetanus toxoid–containing vaccine *and* 5–10 yr since last dose	No indication	Tdap preferred (if not yet received) or Td
≥3 doses of tetanus toxoid–containing vaccine *and* >10 yr since last dose	Tdap preferred (if not yet received) or Td	Tdap preferred (if not yet received) or Td
Age ≥65 Yr		
Unknown or <3 doses of tetanus toxoid–containing vaccine	Td or Tdap and recommend catch-up vaccination. Tdap preferred if patient has close contact with children <12 mo of age	Td or Tdap and recommend catch-up vaccination. Tdap preferred if patient has close contact with children <12 mo of age TIG
≥3 doses of tetanus toxoid–containing vaccine *and* <5 yr since last dose	No indication	No indication
≥3 doses of tetanus toxoid–containing vaccine *and* 5–10 yr since last dose	No indication	Td or Tdap. Tdap preferred if patient has close contact with children <12 mo of age
≥3 doses of tetanus toxoid–containing vaccine *and* >10 yr since last dose	Tdap preferred (if not yet received) or Td	Td or Tdap. Tdap preferred if patient has close contact with children <12 mo of age

TD, tetanus–diphtheria toxoid absorbed (adult use); *Tdap*, tetanus toxoid, reduced diphtheria toxoid, and acellular pertussis vaccine; *TIG*, tetanus immune globulin (human).
*Pregnant women: As part of standard wound management care to prevent tetanus, a tetanus toxoid–containing vaccine might be recommended for wound management in a pregnant woman if ≥5 yr has elapsed since last receiving Td. If a tetanus booster is indicated for a pregnant woman who previously has not received Tdap, Tdap should be administered (at any gestational age).
Source: Centers for Disease Control and Prevention. (2015). *Natural disasters and severe weather: Tetanus prevention after a disaster.* Retrieved from *https://www.cdc.gov/disasters/disease/tetanus.html*.

of Nurses of Ontario mandate that nurses be vigilant and accountable in reporting abuse concerns:

1. If the nurse suspects that a child is being abused or neglected, it is the nurse's legal duty to report the situation to the local Children's Aid Society.
2. Maltreatment may be in the form of physical or sexual abuse. It can also be in the form of neglect: failure to meet a child's basic needs for food, clothing, shelter, sleep, medical attention, education, and protection from harm.
3. Unexplained injuries, fear of a specific adult, difficulty trusting others or making friends, sudden changes in eating or sleeping patterns, poor hygiene, secrecy, and inappropriate sexual behaviour may be signs of abuse.

DEATH IN THE EMERGENCY DEPARTMENT

Unfortunately, a number of patients in the ED do not survive, despite the skill, expertise, and technology available in the ED. It is important for the emergency nurse to be able to deal with his or her own feelings about sudden death so that the nurse can help families and significant others begin the grieving process. The nurse may require debriefing when dealing with traumatic deaths.

The emergency nurse should recognize the importance of rituals in preparing the bereaved to grieve, such as multicultural differences, the collection of belongings, coroner considerations, arranging for autopsy, viewing of the body, and the making of mortuary arrangements. The emergency nurse plays a significant role in providing comfort to and advocacy for the surviving loved ones after a death. Collaborations with clergy and social workers are valued enhancements to the team's crisis management and grief work.

Organ and Tissue Donation

Transplantation is a critical component of the health care system. Many patients who die in the ED are potential candidates for tissue and organ donation. Over 1600 Canadians are added to organ wait lists yearly (Canadian Transplant Society, 2014). The solid organs that can be procured include the heart, lungs, liver, pancreas, and kidney. Certain tissues and organs, including corneas, heart valves, skin, bone, and kidneys, can be harvested from patients after death. Everyone is a potential donor, regardless of age, if the organs and the tissue are healthy at the time of death. Organ and tissue recovery is carried out with confidentiality, respect, and dignity and does not interfere with funeral practices.

Approaching families about donation after an unexpected death is distressing to both the staff and the family. For many families, however, the act of donation may be the first positive step in the grieving process. Studies show that donating the organs and tissue of a loved one who has died can provide immediate comfort and lasting consolation to family members in their grieving (Trillium Gift of Life Network, 2017). Before families are made aware of the option for donation, they must be told that the patient has died, and they must accept the fact that death has occurred. Once the family has accepted the patient's death, then the nurse can provide the family with the choice to donate, offer information, and support the family's decision.

Careful assessment of patients with standardized criteria is necessary to make an accurate determination of death. Neurological determination of death is defined as "a permanent loss of all brain function" (BC Transplant, 2017). Once this determination is complete, the donor is screened to ensure that only viable organs are recovered for transplantation. *Organ donor coordinators* are available in most institutions to assist in the process of screening potential donors, counselling donor families, obtaining informed consent, and retrieving organs from patients who have died in the ED.

The organ donor who is on a mechanical ventilator is often hemodynamically unstable, with many fluid and electrolyte imbalances. The nurse carries out interventions in an attempt to stabilize the patient's condition until the organs can be retrieved. Nursing care may consist of administration of fluids (crystalloids and colloids) and medications (vasopressors and hormones); promotion of normothermia; maintenance of ventilation and oxygenation through ventilator manipulation; and review of laboratory values such as electrolytes, blood urea nitrogen, creatinine, hematological studies, ABGs, liver function studies, and cardiac enzymes. (Transplantation is discussed in Chapter 16.)

Emergency Department Wait Times. In the period 2014 to 2015, Canadians made more than 10 million visits to EDs (CIHI, 2015). Of these visits, 21.7% were for trauma (CIHI, 2015). The amount of time that people spent in the ED varied according to the severity of their illness, the patient's age, how many other patients were being cared for, and the time of day the visit took place. Admitted patients spent almost five times longer in the ED (30.5 hours/visit) than patients not admitted (6.5 hours/visit). While the decision to admit was usually reached within 11.9 hours, the remaining time involved waiting for an inpatient bed to become available (CIHI, 2015). Individuals aged 65 years and older spent more time in the ED and were more likely to be admitted (CIHI, 2015).

AGE-RELATED CONSIDERATIONS

EMERGENCY CARE

The proportion of the population older than 65 is growing; most older adults lead active lives. Regardless of a patient's age, aggressive interventions are warranted for all injuries or illnesses, unless the patient is known to have a pre-existing terminal illness, an extremely low probability of survival, or an advance directive indicating a different course of action.

The older population is at high risk for injury because of many anatomical and physiological changes that occur with aging (e.g., reduced visual acuity, limited neck rotation, slower gait, reduced reaction time).

Of the injury-related admissions of people aged 65 or older, many are for fractures resulting from falls. Age-related decline in balance and gait stability, as well as in cardiovascular function, increases the risk of falling (Kiel, 2016). When assessing a patient who has experienced a fall, the nurse must determine whether the physical findings may have caused the fall or may have been caused by the fall. For example, a patient may exhibit acute confusion (delirium). The confusion may be the result of an acute myocardial infarction that caused the patient to lose consciousness and fall, or the patient may have suffered a head injury as a result of a fall from tripping.

Knowledge of the concepts of aging improves the care delivered to older adults in the ED (Chapter 7). Older adults and their conditions must be fully investigated because of atypical presentations and comorbid conditions. The expertise of advanced-practice nurses, such as nurse practitioners or clinical nurse specialists, should be put to use in caring for this complex population to improve access to care. In Ontario, geriatric emergency medicine (GEM) nurse clinicians target the older population in the ED and have been found to improve care and clinical outcomes (Wilding, Gilsenan, Dalziel, et al., 2015).

The Triage Risk Screening Tool is a brief screening tool that can identify older patients as being at high risk and can predict adverse health outcomes (Foo, Sui, Ang, et al., 2014). The results enable GEM nurses to deliver targeted interventions. It is a risk stratification tool used to predict functional decline. The six-item questionnaire is completed by registered nurses to identify older patients at risk for repeat ED visits, hospitalization, and nursing home placement after an index ED visit. Risk factors include being 75 years of age or older when discharged home; having cognitive impairment; living alone; having difficulty transferring or a history of falling; taking five or more medications (polypharmacy); and having used the ED recently (previous 30 days) or having been hospitalized recently (previous 90 days). Other risk factors are identified by registered nurses' recommendation for issues such as malnutrition, depression, and failure to cope. Patients are considered at high risk if cognitive impairment or two or more other risk factors are present, and the GEM nurse is consulted.

ENVIRONMENTAL EMERGENCIES

Increased interest in outdoor activities such as running, hiking, cycling, skiing, sailing, and swimming has resulted in more environmental emergencies seen in the ED. Illness or injury may be caused by the activity, exposure to weather, or attack from various animals or humans. Specific environmental emergencies discussed in this section include heat-related emergencies, cold-related emergencies, submersion injuries, bites, and stings.

HEAT-RELATED EMERGENCIES

Brief exposure to intense heat or prolonged exposure to less intense heat leads to heat stress. Thermoregulatory mechanisms such as sweating, vasodilation, and increased respirations cannot compensate for such exposure to increased ambient temperatures (Atha, 2013; Krau, 2013). Ambient temperature is a product of environmental temperature and humidity. Strenuous activities in hot or humid environments, clothing that interferes with perspiration, high fevers, and pre-existing illnesses predispose individuals to heat stress (Table 71-7). Effects can be mild (heat rash and heat edema) or severe (heat exhaustion and heatstroke). The management of heat-related emergencies is summarized in Table 71-8.

Heat rash (miliaria or prickly heat) is a fine, red, papular rash that occurs on the torso and the neck and in skin folds. The rash occurs when sweat ducts are obstructed and become inflamed so that sweat excretion does not occur. The rash usually occurs in warm weather, but it has also been reported in cold weather as a result of clothing.

Heat syncope is associated with prolonged standing and heat exposure. Manifestations include dizziness, orthostatic hypotension, and syncope. Inadequate vasomotor tone associated with aging increases older adults' risk for heat syncope.

Heat edema is characterized by swelling of the hands, the feet, and the ankles, usually in nonacclimatized individuals as a result of prolonged standing or sitting. Swelling usually resolves in days with rest, elevation, and support hose. Diuretics are not

TABLE 71-7	RISK FACTORS FOR HEAT-RELATED EMERGENCIES
Age • Extremely young age • Older age **Environmental Conditions** • High environmental temperature • High relative humidity • Low wind **Pre-Existing Illness** • Cardiovascular disease • Cystic fibrosis • Diabetes • Obesity • Previous stroke or other central nervous system lesion • Skin disorders (e.g., large burn scars)	**Prescription Drugs** • Anticholinergics • Antihistamines • Antiparkinsonian drugs • Antispasmodics • β-Adrenergic blockers • Butyrophenones • Diuretics • Phenothiazines • Tricyclic antidepressants **Street Drugs** • Amphetamines • Jimson weed • Lysergic acid diethylamide (LSD) • 3,4-Methylenedioxy-methamphetamine (MDMA, Ecstasy) • Phencyclidine (PCP)
Alcohol	

Source: Emergency Nurses Association. (2010). *Sheehy's emergency nursing: Principles and practice* (6th ed., p. 537, Box 40-1) (L. Newberry, Ed.). St. Louis: Mosby.

recommended because this condition is self-limiting and necessitates no additional treatment.

Heat Cramps

Heat cramps are severe cramps in large muscle groups fatigued by heavy work. Cramps are brief and intense and tend to occur during rest after exercise or heavy labour. Nausea, tachycardia, pallor, weakness, and profuse diaphoresis are often present. The condition occurs most often in healthy, acclimated athletes with inadequate fluid intake. Cramps resolve rapidly with rest and oral or parenteral replacement of sodium and water. Elevation, gentle massage, and analgesia keep pain to a minimum. The patient should avoid strenuous activity for at least 12 hours after the development of heat cramps. Education should emphasize salt replacement during strenuous exercise in hot, humid environments. Commercially prepared electrolyte solutions and sports drinks are recommended.

Heat Exhaustion

Prolonged exposure to heat over hours or days leads to **heat exhaustion**, a clinical syndrome characterized by fatigue, light-headedness, nausea, vomiting, diarrhea, and a sensation of impending doom (see Table 71-8). Tachypnea, hypotension, tachycardia, elevated body temperature, dilated pupils, mild confusion, ashen colour, and profuse diaphoresis are also present. Hypotension and mild to severe temperature elevation (37.5°–40°C) are caused by dehydration (Becker & Stewart, 2011). Heat exhaustion usually occurs in individuals engaged in strenuous activity in hot, humid weather, but it also occurs in sedentary individuals.

Treatment begins with placing the patient in a cool area and removing constrictive clothing. The patient is monitored for airway, breathing, and circulation (ABCs), including cardiac dysrhythmias. Oral and parenteral fluid replacement should correspond to clinical and laboratory parameters. Salt

✚ TABLE 71-8   EMERGENCY MANAGEMENT

Hyperthermia

Etiology	Assessment Findings	Interventions
Environmental • Lack of acclimatization • Physical exertion, especially during hot weather • Prolonged exposure to extreme temperatures **Trauma** • Head injury • Spinal cord injury **Metabolic** • Dehydration • Diabetes • Thyrotoxicosis **Drugs** • Antihistamines • Cocaine • Diuretics • Ethanol • Phenothiazines • Tricyclic antidepressants	**Heat Cramps** • Excessive thirst • Severe muscle contractions in muscles subjected to exertion **Heat Exhaustion** • Altered mental status (e.g., irritability) • Fatigue, weakness • Hypotension • Pale, ashen complexion • Profuse sweating • Tachycardia • Temperature >37.8°C but <40°C • Weak, thready pulse **Heatstroke** • Altered mental status (e.g., ranging from confusion to coma) • Hot, dry skin • Hypotension • Tachycardia • Temperature >40°C • Weakness	**Initial** • Manage and maintain ABCs. • Provide high-flow O_2 via nonrebreather mask or BVM device. • Establish IV access, and begin fluid replacement for significant heat injury. • Place patient in a cool environment. • For patient with heatstroke, initiate rapid cooling measures: remove patient's clothing, place wet sheets over patient, and place patient in front of fan; immerse in ice-water bath; administer cool IV fluids or perform lavage with cool fluids. • Obtain ECG. • Obtain blood specimens for electrolytes and CBC. • Insert urinary catheter. **Ongoing Monitoring** • Monitor ABCs, vital signs, level of consciousness. • Monitor cardiac rhythm, O_2 saturation, electrolyte levels, and urinary output. • Monitor clotting studies for development of disseminated intravascular coagulation. • Monitor urine for development of myoglobinuria.

ABCs, airway, breathing, and circulation; BVM, bag–valve–mask; CBC, complete blood cell count; ECG, electrocardiogram; IV, intravenous; O_2, oxygen.

tablets are not recommended because of potential gastric irritation and hypernatremia. A 0.9% normal saline solution is initiated intravenously when oral solutions are not tolerated. An initial fluid bolus may be used to correct hypotension. Admission is considered for affected older adults, chronically ill patients, and those whose condition does not improve within 4 hours.

Heatstroke

Heatstroke, the most serious form of heat stress, results from failure of the central thermoregulatory mechanisms and is considered a medical emergency. Table 71-7 lists risk factors for heat-related emergencies. Increased sweating, vasodilation, and increased respiratory rate, which occur in an attempt to lower temperature, deplete fluids and electrolytes. Eventually, sweat glands stop functioning, and so core temperature increases rapidly. The patient exhibits a core temperature higher than 40°C, altered mentation, absence of perspiration, and circulatory collapse. The skin is hot, dry, and ashen. Because the brain is extremely sensitive to thermal injuries, a range of neurological symptoms occur, such as hallucinations, combativeness, and loss of muscle coordination. Cerebral edema and hemorrhage may occur as a result of direct thermal injury to the brain and decreased cerebral blood flow.

The development of heatstroke is a potentially fatal disorder that directly relates to the amount of time that the patient's core body temperature remains elevated from either activity or the external environment (Crawford Mechem, 2017; Epstein & Roberts, 2011; Hammond & Zimmermann, 2013). Prognosis is affected by age, baseline health status, and length of exposure. Older adults and individuals with diabetes mellitus, chronic renal disease, cardiovascular disease, pulmonary disease, or other physiological compromise are vulnerable.

Collaborative Care. Treatment of heatstroke focuses on stabilizing the patient's ABCs and rapidly reducing the core temperature. Administration of 100% O_2 compensates for the patient's hypermetabolic state. Ventilation with a BVM device or intubation and mechanical ventilation may be required. Fluid and electrolyte imbalances are corrected, and continuous cardiac monitoring for dysrhythmias is initiated.

Various cooling methods are available, such as removing clothing, covering with wet sheets, and placing the patient in front of a large fan (evaporative cooling); immersing the patient in cold water (conductive cooling); and administering cool fluids or performing lavage with cool fluids (Hammond & Zimmermann, 2013; Crawford Mechem, 2017). Whatever method is selected, the nurse is responsible for closely monitoring the patient's temperature and controlling shivering. Shivering increases core temperature and is associated with heat generated by muscle activity, which complicates cooling efforts. Aggressive temperature reduction should continue until core temperature reaches 38.9°C. Antipyretics are not recommended because they have no effect on the nonfunctioning thermoregulatory mechanisms.

The patient is also monitored for signs of *rhabdomyolysis*, a fatal disease characterized by the breakdown of skeletal muscle. Muscle breakdown leads to myoglobinuria, which increases the risk for acute kidney injury or failure. Therefore, urine should be carefully monitored for colour, amount, pH, and myoglobin. Finally, clotting studies are performed to monitor the patient for signs of disseminated intravascular coagulation (clotting studies are discussed in Chapter 32, and DIC is discussed in Chapter 33).

Patient and caregiver teaching focuses on how to avoid future problems. Providing essential information regarding proper hydration during hot weather and physical exercise is imperative. Patients should also be instructed on the early signs of and interventions for heat-related stress.

COLD-RELATED EMERGENCIES

Cold-related injuries may be localized (frostbite) or systemic (hypothermia). Contributing factors include age, duration of exposure, environmental temperature, homelessness, pre-existing conditions (e.g., diabetes), medications that suppress shivering (opioids, heroin, psychotropic agents, and antiemetics), and alcohol intoxication, which causes peripheral vasodilation, increases sensations of warmth, and depresses shivering. People who smoke have an increased risk for cold-related injury as a result of the vasoconstrictive effects of nicotine.

Frostbite

Frostbite can be described as "true tissue freezing," which results in the formation of ice crystals in the tissues and cells. Peripheral vasoconstriction is the initial response to cold stress and results in a decrease in blood flow and vascular stasis. As cellular temperature decreases and ice crystals form in intracellular spaces, intracellular sodium and chloride levels increase, the cell membrane is destroyed, and organelles are damaged. These alterations result in edema. The depth of frostbite is the result of ambient temperature, length of exposure, type and condition of clothing (wet or dry), and contact with metal surfaces. Other factors that affect severity include skin colour (dark-skinned people are more prone to frostbite), lack of acclimatization, previous episodes, exhaustion, and poor peripheral vascular status.

Superficial frostbite involves skin and subcutaneous tissue, usually the ears, the nose, the fingers, and the toes. The skin appearance ranges from pale and blue to mottled, and the skin feels crunchy and frozen. The patient may complain of tingling, numbness, or a burning sensation. Injured tissue is easily damaged, and so the area should be handled carefully and never squeezed, massaged, or scrubbed. Clothing and jewellery should be removed because they may constrict the extremity and decrease circulation. The affected area should be immersed in a water bath of 37° to 39°C (Hammond & Zimmermann, 2013; Crawford Mechem & Zafren, 2017). Warm soaks may be used for the face. The patient often experiences a warm, stinging sensation as tissue thaws. Blisters form within a few hours (Figure 71-2). Nonhemorrhagic blisters should be drained, debrided, and covered with a sterile dressing. Heavy blankets and clothing should be avoided because friction and weight can lead to sloughing of damaged tissue. Rewarming is extremely painful. Residual pain may last for weeks or even years. Analgesics should be administered, and tetanus prophylaxis should be provided as appropriate (see Table 71-6). The patient should be evaluated for systemic hypothermia.

Deep frostbite involves muscle, bone, and tendon. The skin is white, hard, and insensitive to touch and involves complete tissue necrosis. The area has the appearance of deep thermal injury with mottling gradually progressing to gangrene (see Figure 14-1 in Chapter 14). Significant edema may begin within 3 hours, with blistering in 6 hours to days. Intravenous analgesia is always

FIGURE 71-2 Edema and blister formation 24 hours after frostbite injury occurring in an area covered by a tightly fitted boot. Source: Courtesy Cameron Bangs, MD. From Auerbach, P. S., Donner, H. J., & Weiss, E. A. (2007). *Wilderness medicine* (5th ed., p. 201, Figure 8-2, *A*). St. Louis: Mosby.

required in severe frostbite because of the pain associated with tissue thawing. Tetanus prophylaxis should be given (see Table 71-6), and the patient should be evaluated for systemic hypothermia. Amputation may be required if the injured area is untreated or if treatment is unsuccessful. Thrombolytic agents have been shown to reduce the need for amputation when used within the first 24 hours of injury. The use of thrombolytic agents may be considered if there are no contraindications (Crawford Mechem & Zafren, 2017; Gross & Moore, 2012). The patient may be admitted to the hospital, with bed rest and elevation of the injured part. Prophylactic antibiotics are used if the wound is at risk for infection.

Hypothermia

Hypothermia, defined as a core temperature lower than 35°C, occurs when heat loss exceeds production. Up to 60% of all body heat is lost as radiant energy; the loss is greatest from the head, the thorax, and the lungs (with each breath). Wet clothing increases evaporative heat loss five times greater than normal; immersion in cold water (e.g., near-drowning) increases evaporative heat loss 25 times greater than normal. Environmental exposure to freezing temperatures, cold winds, and wet, damp terrain in the presence of physical exhaustion, inadequate clothing, or inexperience predisposes individuals to hypothermia (Crawford Mechem & Zafren, 2017). Near-drowning and water immersion are also associated with hypothermia.

Older adults are more prone to hypothermia because of decreased body fat, diminished energy reserves, decreased basal metabolic rate, decreased shivering response, decreased sensory perception, chronic medical conditions, and medications that alter body defences. In addition, certain drugs, alcohol, and diabetes are considered risk factors for hypothermia.

Hypothermia mimics cerebral or metabolic disturbances, causing ataxia, confusion, and withdrawal, and so the condition may be misdiagnosed. Peripheral vasoconstriction is the body's first attempt to conserve heat. As cold temperatures persist, shivering and movement are the body's only mechanisms for producing heat. Death usually occurs when core temperature falls below 25.6°C.

Core temperature below 30.6°C is severe and potentially life-threatening. Assessment findings in hypothermia are variable and dependent on core temperature (Table 71-9). Patients with *mild hypothermia* (34°–36°C) exhibit shivering, increased heart rate, slurred speech, and incoordination. *Moderate hypothermia* (30°–34°C) causes decreased shivering, bradycardia, slowed respiratory rate, and lethargy. *Severe hypothermia* (≤30°C) causes coma, hypotension, arrhythmias, and muscle rigidity (Zafren & Crawford Mechem, 2017).

As core temperature drops, basal metabolic rate decreases to 50% or 25% of normal. The cold myocardium is extremely irritable, making it vulnerable to dysrhythmias (e.g., atrial and ventricular fibrillation). Decreased renal blood flow decreases glomerular filtration rate, which impairs water reabsorption and leads to dehydration. Hematocrit increases as intravascular volume decreases. Cold blood becomes viscous and acts as a thrombus, increasing the patient's risk for stroke, myocardial infarction, pulmonary emboli, acute tubular necrosis, and renal failure. Decreased blood flow leads to lactic acid accumulation from anaerobic metabolism and subsequent metabolic acidosis.

In *severe hypothermia* (≤30°C), the person appears dead. Metabolic rate, heart rate, and respirations are so slow that they may be difficult to detect. Reflexes are absent, and the pupils are

---

✚ TABLE 71-9   EMERGENCY MANAGEMENT

Hypothermia*

Etiology	Assessment Findings	Interventions

Environmental
• Inadequate clothing for environmental temperature
• Prolonged exposure to cold
• Prolonged submersion
	• Altered mental status (ranging from confusion to coma)
	• Areflexia (absence of reflexes)
	• Blue, white, or frozen extremities
	• Core body temperature:
	  • Mild hypothermia: 34°–36°C
	  • Moderate hypothermia: 30°–34°C
	  • Severe hypothermia: ≤30°C
	• Dysrhythmias: bradycardia, atrial fibrillation, ventricular fibrillation, asystole
	• Fixed, dilated pupils
	• Hypotension
	• Hypoventilation
	• Pale, cyanotic skin
	• Shivering (diminished or absent at core body temperature ≤30°C)
		Initial
		• Remove patient from cold environment.
		• Manage and maintain ABCs.
		• Provide high-flow O$_2$ via nonrebreather mask or BVM device.
		• Anticipate intubation if gag reflex is diminished or absent.*
		• Rewarm patient:
		  • *Passive external warming:* Remove wet clothing, apply dry clothing and warm blankets, and administer warm fluids.
		  • *Active external warming:* Use body-to-body contact; apply heating devices (e.g., air-filled warming blankets) or radiant lights.
		  • *Active core warming:* Administer warmed IV fluids; heated, humidified O$_2$; and peritoneal, gastric, or colonic lavage with warmed fluids.
		• Anticipate the need for hemodialysis or cardiopulmonary bypass.
		• Obtain 12-lead ECG.
		• Warm central trunk first in patients with moderate, severe, or profound hypothermia to prevent aftershock.
		• Establish IV access with two large-bore catheters for fluid resuscitation.
		• Assess for other injuries.
		• Keep patient's head covered with warm, dry towels, or stocking cap, to limit loss of heat.
		• Treat patient gently to avoid increased cardiac irritability.
		
		Ongoing Monitoring
		• Monitor ABCs, level of consciousness, temperature, and vital signs.
		• Monitor O$_2$ saturation and cardiac rhythm.
		• Monitor electrolyte and glucose levels.

ABCs, airway, breathing, and circulation; *BVM*, bag–valve–mask; *ECG*, electrocardiogram; *IV*, intravenous; *O$_2$*, oxygen.
*NOTE: Medications and defibrillation may not be effective with core temperatures <30°C.

---

fixed and dilated. Profound bradycardia, asystole, or ventricular fibrillation may be present. Every effort is made to warm the patient to at least 32°C before the person is pronounced dead. The cause of death is usually refractory ventricular fibrillation.

Collaborative Care. Treatment of hypothermia focuses on managing and maintaining ABCs, rewarming the patient, correcting dehydration and acidosis, and treating cardiac dysrhythmias. Passive or active external rewarming is used for mild hypothermia. *Passive external rewarming* involves moving the patient to a warm, dry place; removing damp clothing; and placing warm blankets on the patient. Gentle handling is essential to prevent stimulation of the cold myocardium. *Active external rewarming* involves body-to-body contact (when the patient cannot access health care), fluid- or air-filled warming blankets, or radiant heat lamps. The patient should be closely monitored for marked vasodilation and hypotension during rewarming.

Active core rewarming is used for moderate to profound hypothermia and involves heat applied directly to the core. Techniques include the use of heated, humidified O$_2$; warmed intravenous fluids; and peritoneal, gastric, or colonic lavage with warmed fluids. Hemodialysis or cardiopulmonary bypass may also be considered for profound hypothermia (Rahman, Rubinstein, Singh, et al., 2012).

Core temperature should be carefully monitored during rewarming procedures. Warming places the patient at risk for *afterdrop*, a further drop in core temperature, which occurs when cold peripheral blood returns to the central circulation. Rewarming shock can produce hypotension and dysrhythmias. Thus, in patients with moderate to profound hypothermia, the core should be warmed before the extremities.

Patient teaching should focus on how to avoid future cold-related problems. Essential education includes dressing in layers for cold weather, covering the head, carrying high-carbohydrate foods for extra calories, and developing a plan for survival should an injury occur.

SUBMERSION INJURIES

Submersion injury results when a person becomes hypoxic as a result of submersion in a substance, usually water. The primary risk factors for submersion injury include inability to swim, risk taking, inadequate adult supervision, use of alcohol or drugs, trauma, seizures, and hypothermia (Chandy & Weinhouse, 2017).

Drowning is death from suffocation after submersion in water or other fluid medium. *Near-drowning* is defined as survival from potential drowning. *Immersion syndrome* occurs with immersion in cold water, which leads to stimulation of the vagus nerve and potentially fatal dysrhythmias (e.g., bradycardia).

Death from a submersion injury is caused by hypoxia secondary to aspiration and swallowing of fluid. Swallowed water may cause vomiting and additional aspiration. The majority of all drowning victims aspirate water into the pulmonary tree and develop pulmonary edema. Victims who do not aspirate fluid develop intense laryngospasm and airway obstruction; the cause of death is "dry drowning." The osmotic gradient that results from aspirated fluid causes fluid imbalances. Hypotonic fresh water is rapidly absorbed into the circulatory system through the alveoli. Fresh water may be contaminated with chlorine, mud, and algae, which cause the breakdown of lung surfactant, fluid seepage, and pulmonary edema. Hypertonic salt water draws protein-rich fluid from the vascular space into the alveoli, impairing alveolar ventilation and resulting in hypoxia. Figure 71-3 shows the pulmonary effects of salt water and fresh water aspiration.

The body attempts to compensate for hypoxia by shunting blood to the lungs. As a result, pulmonary pressures increase and respiratory status deteriorates. Blood is shunted through the alveoli; however, it is not adequately oxygenated, and so the hypoxemia worsens. Anaerobic metabolism occurs, which leads to lactic acidosis.

The assessment findings of a patient with a submersion injury are listed in Table 71-10. Aggressive resuscitation efforts and the mammalian diving reflex improve survival of near-drowning victims even after submersion in cold water for long periods (Chandy & Weinhouse, 2017). Cold water lowers the body's metabolic rate and O$_2$ demand. The mammalian diving reflex causes apnea, bradycardia, and peripheral vasoconstriction and further decreases the metabolic rate. Blood flow is redistributed to the most vital organs (i.e., heart, lungs, and brain).

Collaborative Care

Treatment of submersion injuries includes aggressive resuscitation efforts that focus on correcting hypoxia and acid–base and fluid imbalances; support of basic physiological functions; and rewarming when hypothermia is present. Initial evaluation and interventions involve assessment of airway, cervical spine, breathing, and circulation (see Table 71-10).

Mechanical ventilation with positive end-expiratory pressure or continuous positive airway pressure may be used to improve gas exchange across the alveolar–capillary membrane when significant pulmonary edema is present. Ventilation and oxygenation are the primary techniques used to treat acidosis. Mannitol or furosemide (Lasix) may be used with caution to decrease the amount of free water and treat cerebral edema.

PATHOPHYSIOLOGY MAP

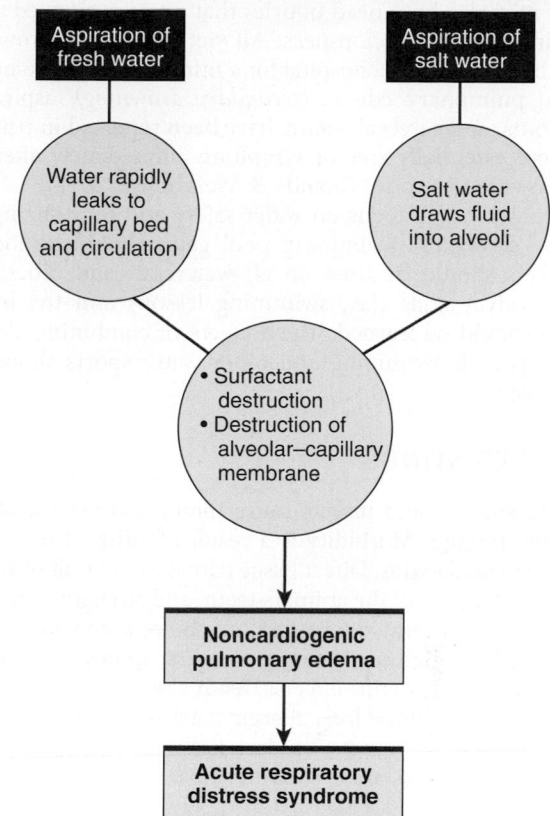

FIGURE 71-3 Pathophysiology of submersion injury.

TABLE 71-10 EMERGENCY MANAGEMENT

Submersion Injuries

Etiology	Assessment Findings	Interventions
• Inability to swim or exhaustion while swimming • Entrapment in or entanglement with objects in water • Loss of ability to move secondary to trauma, stroke, hypothermia, acute MI • Poor judgement as a result of alcohol or drugs • Seizure while in water	**Pulmonary** • Cough with pink, frothy sputum • Crackles, wheezes • Cyanosis • Dyspnea • Ineffective breathing • Respiratory distress/arrest **Cardiac** • Bradycardia • Cardiac arrest • Dysrhythmia • Hypotension • Tachycardia **Other** • Coexisting illness (e.g., MI) or injury (e.g., cervical spine injury) • Coma • Core temperature slightly elevated or below normal depending on water temperature and length of submersion • Exhaustion • Panic	**Initial** • Manage and maintain ABCs. • Assume cervical spine injury in all drowning victims, and stabilize or immobilize cervical spine. • Provide 100% O$_2$ via nonrebreather mask or BVM device. • Anticipate need for intubation if gag reflex is absent. • Establish IV access with two large-bore catheters for fluid resuscitation and infuse warmed fluids if appropriate. • Assess for other injuries. • Remove wet clothing and cover with warm blankets. • Measure temperature, and begin rewarming if needed. • Obtain cervical spine and chest radiographs. • Insert gastric tube. **Ongoing Monitoring** • Monitor ABCs, vital signs, and level of consciousness. • Monitor O$_2$ saturation and cardiac rhythm. • Monitor temperature, and maintain normothermia. • Monitor for signs of acute respiratory failure. • Monitor for signs of secondary drowning.

ABCs, airway, breathing, and circulation; *BVM*, bag–valve–mask; *IV*, intravenous; *MI*, myocardial infarction; *O$_2$*, oxygen.

Deterioration of neurological status is suggestive of cerebral edema, increased hypoxia, or profound acidosis. Near-drowning victims may also have head injuries that cause prolonged alterations in level of consciousness. All victims of near-drowning should be observed in a hospital for a minimum of 4 to 6 hours. Delayed pulmonary edema *(secondary drowning)*, aspiration pneumonia, and cerebral edema have been reported in patients who were essentially free of symptoms immediately after the near-drowning episode (Chandy & Weinhouse, 2017).

Teaching should focus on water safety and minimizing the risks for drowning. Swimming pool gates should be locked; life jackets should be used on all watercraft and tubes; and water survival skills (i.e., swimming lessons and the buddy system) should be learned. The dangers of combining alcohol and drugs with swimming and other water sports should be emphasized.

BITES AND STINGS

Animals, spiders, and insects cause injury and even death by biting or stinging. Morbidity is a result of either direct tissue damage or lethal toxins. Direct tissue damage is a result of animal size, characteristics of the animal's teeth, and strength of the jaw. Tissue may be lacerated, crushed, or chewed, and toxins that are released through teeth, fangs, stingers, spines, or tentacles provoke local or systemic effects. Death associated with animal bites is caused by blood loss, allergic reactions, or lethal toxins. Injuries caused by insects, spiders, ticks, snakes, dogs, cats, rodents, and humans are described below.

Hymenopteran Stings

The Hymenoptera order includes bees, yellow jackets, hornets, and wasps. Stings can cause reactions ranging from mild discomfort to life-threatening anaphylaxis (Chapters 16 and 69). Venom may be cytotoxic, hemolytic, allergenic, or vasoactive. Symptoms may begin immediately or may be delayed up to 48 hours. Reactions are more severe with multiple stings. Most hymenopterans sting repeatedly. However, the honeybee stings only once, usually leaving the stinger in the skin so that the release of venom continues. A scraping motion with a fingernail, knife, or needle is recommended for removing the stinger. Tweezers squeeze the stinger and may cause more venom release. However, the fastest method of removing the stinger is ultimately the best, so if tweezers are available, they can be used.

Manifestations vary and range from stinging, burning sensation, swelling, and itching to edema, headache, fever, syncope, malaise, nausea, vomiting, wheezing, bronchospasm, laryngeal edema, and hypotension. Treatment depends on the severity of the reaction. Mild reactions are treated with elevation, cool compresses, antipruritic lotions, and oral antihistamines. Rings, watches, and restrictive clothing must be removed. More severe reactions necessitate intramuscular or intravenous antihistamines (diphenhydramine [Benadryl]), subcutaneous epinephrine, and corticosteroids. Allergic reactions and anaphylaxis are discussed in Chapter 16.

Spider Bites (Arachnid)

Although there are 20 000 species of venomous spiders in the world, only 50 species cause illness. The venomous black widow spider is found in southern parts of Canada and also has been found in imported grapes. The venom can provoke responses ranging from a localized reaction to systemic anaphylaxis.

Tarantulas look more dangerous than they actually are; their bite causes only localized stinging and pain. Other types of spiders release venom when they bite and may cause allergic reactions in some individuals, but they are not considered poisonous.

Black Widow Spiders. Black widow spiders are the most feared of all spiders. The female's venom is especially poisonous. Both the female and the male are black. The fully grown female is about 1.2 cm long and is jet black, with an hourglass-shaped red mark on the underside of the abdomen (Figure 71-4). Males are only about half as long and usually have four pairs of red dots along the sides of the abdomen. Males are rarely seen and are generally harmless. The female rarely leaves the web, biting defensively if disturbed. Black widow spiders are found among fallen branches and firewood and under objects such as furniture, outhouse seats, and garbage.

The black widow spider's venom is neurotoxic. When bitten, the patient feels a pinprick-like sensation, and a tiny, red bite mark appears. Approximately 15 to 60 minutes later, the patient experiences severe pain that increases over the next 12 to 48 hours. Systemic symptoms develop 30 minutes after *envenomation* (introduction of poisonous venom into the body by a bite or sting). These symptoms can include nausea, vomiting, abdominal cramping, hypertension, dyspnea, paresthesias, and tachycardia. Symptoms usually peak 2 to 3 hours after onset; however, muscle spasms and hypertension can recur for 12 to 24 hours. Chest and abdominal pain, seizures, and shock can also occur. Bites on the lower body cause abdominal rigidity, whereas bites on the upper body lead to chest, back, and shoulder rigidity. A black widow spider bite is not prominent and can be easily missed. In patients not aware of the bite, the envenomation can be misdiagnosed because symptoms mimic those of a perforated ulcer, appendicitis, pancreatitis, or other abdominal emergency.

Treatment includes IV access and O_2 administration as needed. The wound should be cleaned and tetanus prophylaxis given as appropriate. Muscle spasms are treated with benzodiazepines such as lorazepam. Pain medication may be required either orally or parentally. Antivenin may be used to reduce the duration of symptoms (Vetter, Swanson, & White, 2017).

FIGURE 71-4 Female black widow spider. Source: Auerbach, P. S., Donner, H. J., & Weiss, E. A. (2003). *Field guide to wilderness medicine* (2nd ed.). St. Louis: Mosby.

Tick Bites

Ticks are found in various parts of Canada. Emergencies associated with tick bites include Rocky Mountain spotted fever, Lyme disease, and tick paralysis. Disease is caused by an infected tick or by the release of neurotoxin. Ticks release a neurotoxic venom for the duration that the tick head is attached to the body (Hammond & Zimmermann, 2013). Early removal of the attached tick is essential for effective treatment, ideally within less than 24 hours as it greatly reduces the risk for tickborne illness transmission. Forceps may be used to safely remove the tick by grasping at the point of entry and pulling upward in a steady motion (Figure 71-5). Additional information and instructional videos can be found on the Canadian Lyme Disease Foundation website (see the Resources at the end of this chapter).

Lyme disease, an arthropod-borne disease, is becoming more prevalent in Canada. Most of the reported Canadian cases have occurred in Ontario and Quebec (Government of Canada, 2017; Public Health Agency of Canada & Health Canada, 2017). It develops from a bite from the *Ixodes* tick and results from exposure to the spirochete *Borrelia burgdorferi*, which is found on the tick. Symptoms range from mild to severe and can occur in overlapping stages: early localized Lyme disease, early disseminated Lyme disease, and late Lyme disease. The initial stage of this disease is characterized by nonspecific influenza-like symptoms (e.g., headache, stiff neck, fatigue) and a characteristic bull's-eye rash—an expanding circular area of redness that is 5 cm in diameter or more. Monoarticular arthritis, meningitis, and neuropathies occur days or weeks after the initial symptoms. Chronic arthritis and myocarditis characterize the later stage of the disease, which can develop several months to 2 years after the initial skin lesion. When symptoms include a bull's-eye rash, oral antibiotic treatment is recommended. (Lyme disease is discussed in Chapter 67.)

Rocky Mountain spotted fever caused by *Rickettsia rickettsii* has an incubation period of 2 to 14 days. A pink, macular rash appears on palms, wrists, soles, feet, and ankles within 10 days of exposure. Other symptoms include fever, chills, malaise, myalgias, and headache. Treatment is antibiotic therapy.

Within 5 to 7 days after exposure to a wood or dog tick, tick paralysis occurs. Classic symptoms are flaccid ascending paralysis, which develops over 1 to 2 days. Without tick removal, the patient dies as respiratory muscles become paralyzed. Tick removal leads to return of muscle movement, usually within 48 to 72 hours.

Animal and Human Bites

Children are at greatest risk for animal bites. The most significant associated problems are infection and mechanical destruction of skin, muscle, tendons, blood vessels, and bone. The bite may cause a simple laceration or be associated with a crush injury, puncture wound, or tearing or avulsion of tissue. The severity of injury depends on animal size, victim size, and anatomical location of the bite. Animal bites from cats and dogs are common; dog bites account for the majority of the bite injuries that are treated in the ED. Wild or domestic rodents are ranked behind dogs and cats as the third most frequent offenders in reported animal bites (Ricci & Rizzolo, 2011). All animal bites should be reported to the local public health unit.

Dog bites usually occur on the extremities; however, facial bites are common in small children. Most victims own the dogs that bite them. Dog bites may involve significant tissue damage, and fatalities have been reported, usually in children. Skull fractures with intracranial injury and death may occur in children younger than 2 years. Disfiguring wounds of the face should be evaluated by a plastic surgeon.

Cat bites cause deep puncture wounds that can involve tendons and joint capsules and result in a greater incidence of infection (Enzler, Berbari, & Osmon, 2011). The most common causative organisms of infections from cat and dog bites are from species of the genus *Pasteurella* (e.g., *P. canis*). This organism is found in the mouths of most healthy cats and dogs (Ricci & Rizzolo, 2011). Septic arthritis, osteomyelitis, and tenosynovitis have been reported as a result of cat bites.

Human bites also cause puncture wounds or lacerations and carry a high risk for infection from oral bacterial flora, most commonly *Staphylococcus aureus*, streptococci, and hepatitis virus. The hands, fingers, ears, nose, vagina, and penis are the most common sites of human bites and are frequently a result of violence or sexual activity. Boxer's fracture of the fifth metacarpal is often associated with an open wound when knuckles strike teeth. The human jaw has great crushing ability, causing laceration, puncture, crush injury, soft-tissue tearing, and even amputation. More than 40 potential pathogens found in the human mouth account for an infection rate of approximately 50% in cases in which victims do not seek medical intervention within 24 hours of injury.

Collaborative Care. Initial treatment for animal and human bites includes cleaning with copious irrigation, debridement, tetanus prophylaxis, and analgesics as needed. Prophylactic antibiotics are used for animal and human bites at risk for infection such as wounds over joints, wounds more than 6 to 12 hours old, puncture wounds, and bites of the hand or foot. Individuals at greatest risk for infection are infants, older adults, immuno-suppressed patients, people with alcohol use disorder, people with diabetes, and people taking corticosteroids (Ricci & Rizzolo, 2011).

Puncture wounds are left open, whereas lacerations are loosely sutured. Wounds over joints are splinted. Initial closure is reserved only for facial wounds. The patient may require intravenous antibiotic therapy when an infection is present because of an increased incidence of cellulitis, osteomyelitis, and septic arthritis.

Consideration of rabies prophylaxis is an essential component in management of animal bites. A neurotoxic virus found in the saliva of some mammals causes rabies. If untreated, the condition is fatal in humans. Rabies exposure should be considered if an animal attack was not provoked, involved a wild animal, or involved a domestic animal not immunized against rabies. Rabies prophylaxis is always given when the animal cannot be found or when a carnivorous wild animal causes the bite. The prophylaxis regimen begins with an injection of rabies immune globulin to

FIGURE 71-5 Tick removal. **A,** Use tweezers to grasp the tick close to the skin. **B,** With a steady motion, pull the tick's body up and away from the skin. Do not be alarmed if the tick's mouthparts remain in the skin. Once the mouthparts are removed from the rest of the tick, it can no longer transmit disease.

provide passive immunity. This is followed by a series of five injections of human diploid cell vaccine on days 0, 3, 7, 14, and 28 to provide active immunity. Dosage is based on the patient's weight.

POISONINGS

A poison is any chemical that harms the body. Poisoning is the third leading cause of unintentional death in Canada (Chen, Mo, Yi, et al., 2013). Poisonings can be accidental, occupational, recreational, or intentional. Natural or manufactured toxins can be ingested, inhaled, injected, splashed in the eye, or absorbed through the skin. Common poisons are reviewed in Table 71-11. Other poisonings related to the use of illegal drugs such as amphetamines, opioids, and hallucinogens are discussed in Chapter 11. Poisoning may also be caused by toxic plants or contaminated foods. (Food poisoning is discussed in Chapter 44.)

The severity of the poisoning depends on type, concentration, and route of exposure. Toxins can affect every tissue of the body, and so symptoms can be manifested by any body system. Specific management of toxins involves decreasing absorption, enhancing elimination, and implementing toxin-specific interventions. Local poison control centres are available 24 hours a day and should be consulted for the most current treatment-specific protocols.

Options for decreasing absorption of poisons include emesis, gastric lavage, activated charcoal, dermal cleansing, and eye irrigation. Gastric lavage involves oral insertion of a large-diameter (36- to 40-French) gastric tube for instillation of copious amounts of saline. The head of the bed should be elevated or the patient placed in the side-lying position to prevent aspiration. Patients with an altered level of consciousness or diminished gag reflex are intubated before lavage. Lavage is contraindicated in patients who ingested caustic agents, sharp objects, or nontoxic substances. Otherwise, gastric lavage must be performed within 1 hour of ingestion of most poisons to be effective (Denke, 2010; Burchum

TABLE 71-11 COMMON POISONS

Substance	Manifestations	Treatment
Acetaminophen (Tylenol)	*Phase 1* (within 24 hr of ingestion): malaise, diaphoresis, nausea, and vomiting *Phase 2* (24–28 hr): right upper quadrant pain, decreased urine output, diminished nausea; increase in LFTs *Phase 3* (72–96 hr): nausea and vomiting; malaise; jaundice; hypoglycemia; enlarged liver; possible coagulopathies, including DIC *Phase 4* (7–8 days after ingestion): recovery, resolution of symptoms; results of LFTs return to normal	Activated charcoal *N*-acetylcysteine (oral form may cause vomiting; IV form can be used)
Acetylsalicylic acid (ASA; Aspirin) and ASA-containing medications	Tachypnea, tachycardia, hyperthermia, seizures, pulmonary edema, occult bleeding or hemorrhage, metabolic acidosis	Gastric lavage, activated charcoal, urine alkalinization, hemodialysis for severe acute ingestion, intubation and mechanical ventilation, supportive care
Acids and alkalis • *Acids:* toilet bowl cleaners, antirust compounds • *Alkalis:* drain cleaners, dishwashing detergents, ammonia	Excess salivation, dysphagia, epigastric pain, pneumonitis; burns of mouth, esophagus, and stomach	Immediate dilution (water, milk); corticosteroids (for alkali burns) Induced vomiting is contraindicated
Alcohol, barbiturates, benzodiazepines, cocaine, hallucinogens, stimulants	See Chapter 11	See Chapter 11
Bleaches	Irritation of lips, mouth, and eyes; superficial injury to esophagus; chemical pneumonia and pulmonary edema	Washing of exposed skin and eyes, dilution with water and milk, gastric lavage, prevention of vomiting and aspiration
Carbon monoxide	Dyspnea, headache, tachypnea, confusion, impaired judgement, cyanosis, respiratory depression	Removal from source; administration of 100% O_2 via nonrebreather mask, BVM device, or intubation and mechanical ventilation; hyperbaric oxygen therapy a consideration
Cyanide	Almond odour to breath, headache, dizziness, nausea, confusion, hypertension, bradycardia followed by hypotension and tachycardia, tachypnea followed by bradypnea and respiratory arrest	Amyl nitrate (nasally), IV sodium nitrate, supportive care
Ethylene glycol	Sweet aromatic odour to breath, nausea and vomiting, slurred speech, ataxia, lethargy, respiratory depression	Gastric lavage, activated charcoal, supportive care
Iron	Vomiting (often bloody), diarrhea (often bloody), fever, hyperglycemia, lethargy, hypotension, seizures, coma	Gastric lavage, chelation therapy (deferoxamine [Desferal])
Nonsteroidal anti-inflammatory drugs	Gastro-enteritis, abdominal pain, drowsiness, nystagmus, hepatic and renal damage	Gastric lavage, activated charcoal, cathartics, supportive care
Tricyclic antidepressants (e.g., amitriptyline [Elavil])	In low doses: anticholinergic effects, agitation, hypertension, tachycardia In high doses: central nervous system depression, dysrhythmias, hypotension, respiratory depression	Multidose activated charcoal, gastric lavage, serum alkalinization with sodium bicarbonate, intubation and mechanical ventilation, supportive care Never induce vomiting

BVM, bag–valve–mask; *DIC,* disseminated intravascular coagulation; *IV,* intravenous; *LFTs,* liver function tests; O_2, oxygen.

& Rosenthal, 2016). Problems associated with lavage include epistaxis, esophageal perforation, and aspiration.

The most effective intervention for management of poisonings is administration of activated charcoal orally or via a gastric tube. Toxins adhere to charcoal and are excreted through the gastro-intestinal (GI) tract rather than absorbed into the portal circulation. Adults receive 50 to 100 g of charcoal. Activated charcoal can absorb a number of poisons from the GI tract, but it does not absorb ethanol, alkali, iron, boric acid, lithium, methanol, or cyanide. For some toxins (e.g., phenobarbital), multiple doses of charcoal may be required (Burchum & Rosenthal, 2016; Hammond & Zimmermann, 2013). Contra-indications to charcoal administration are diminished bowel sounds, ileus, ingestion of a substance poorly absorbed by charcoal, or previous administration of *N*-acetylcysteine because charcoal inactivates oral *N*-acetylcysteine, the antidote used for acetaminophen toxicity.

Skin and ocular decontamination involves copious amounts of water or saline. With the exception of mustard gas, most toxins can be safely removed with water or saline (Hammond & Zimmermann, 2013). Water mixes with mustard gas and releases chlorine gas. As a general rule, dry substances should be brushed from the skin and clothing before water is used. Powdered lime should not be removed with water; it should just be brushed off. Health care providers should wear personal protective equipment (gloves, gowns, goggles, and respirators) for decontamination to prevent secondary exposure. Decontam-ination procedures are usually performed by professionals specially trained in hazardous material decontamination before the patient arrives at the hospital. Decontamination takes priority over all interventions except basic life-support techniques. Resources such as the Workplace Hazardous Materials Information System are part of mandatory orientation.

Elimination of poisons is increased through administration of cathartics, whole-bowel irrigation, hemodialysis, hemoperfusion, urine alkalinization, chelating agents, and antidotes. Cathartics such as sorbitol, magnesium citrate, and magnesium sulphate are administered with activated charcoal to stimulate intestinal motility and increase elimination. The use of cathartics is contro-versial, and multiple doses should be avoided because they can induce potentially fatal electrolyte abnormalities. Whole-bowel irrigation is controversial and involves administration of a nonabsorbable bowel evacuant solution (e.g., GoLYTELY). The solution is administered every 4 to 6 hours until stools are clear. This process can be effective for swallowed objects such as cocaine-filled balloons or condoms. There is a high risk for electrolyte imbalance from fluid and electrolyte losses with this intervention (Burchum & Rosenthal, 2016).

Hemodialysis and hemoperfusion are reserved for patients who develop severe acidosis from ingestion of toxic substances (e.g., acetylsalicylic acid [ASA; Aspirin]). Other interventions include alkalinization and chelation therapy. Sodium bicarbonate administration raises the pH (to >7.5), which is particularly effective for phenobarbital and salicylate poisoning. Vitamin C may be added to IV fluids to enhance excretion of amphetamines and quinidine. Chelation therapy may be considered for heavy-metal poisoning (e.g., edetate calcium disodium [calcium EDTA] for lead poisoning). A limited number of true antidotes are available, and many are themselves toxic (Burchum & Rosenthal, 2016).

Education for toxic emergencies focuses on how the poisoning occurred. Patients who experience poisoning because of a suicide attempt or related to substance abuse should be evaluated by a mental health care provider and referred for alcohol or drug detoxification if required. Patients who have been exposed to poison in their jobs should be made aware of Canadian Centre for Occupational Health and Safety measures for a safe work environment.

VIOLENCE

Violence is the acting out of the emotions of fear or anger to cause harm to someone or something. It may be the result of organic disease (e.g., temporal lobe epilepsy), psychosis (e.g., schizophrenia), or antisocial behaviour (e.g., assault, murder). The patient cared for in the ED may be the victim or the perpe-trator of violence. Violence can take place in a variety of settings, including the home, community, and workplace.

EDs have been identified as high-risk areas for *workplace violence* (NENA, 2014b). Violence within the ED that puts staff, patients, and visitors at risk for harm includes physical attacks, verbal abuse, and intimidating behaviour. Violent incidents are often under-reported by nurses; however, without reports being made, the implementation of safe policies and practices can hindered.

Domestic Violence

Domestic violence, or intimate partner violence, is a pattern of coercive behaviour in a relationship that involves fear; humiliation; intimidation; neglect; intentional physical, emotional, financial, or sexual injury or assault; or a combination of these (sexual assault is discussed separately). It occurs in all professions, cultures, and socioeconomic groups. People of all ages and of either gender may be victims, although most victims are women, children, and older adults. Domestic violence is often hidden and undiagnosed (Halter, 2014).

It is recommended that all patients arriving at the ED be screened to determine whether they are victims of domestic violence. Barriers to conducting effective screening include limited privacy for screening, lack of time, and lack of knowledge about how to inquire about domestic violence. The development and implementation of policies, procedures, and education programs can improve the practices of ED staff in screening for domestic violence. Screening should begin by creating a safe and supportive environment in which to talk with the patient. Privacy must be provided, and the patient should not be questioned in the presence of the possible abuser. Several instruments have been developed for screening, but research has shown that a few short questions are the most realistic for health care providers (Nelson, Bougatsos, & Blazina, 2012). The Partner Violence Screen includes the following three questions:

1. Have you been hit, kicked, punched, or otherwise hurt by someone within the past year? If so, by whom?
2. Do you feel safe in your current relationship?
3. Is there a partner from a previous relationship who is making you feel unsafe?

In addition to questioning the patient, the nurse must assess for risk factors such as injuries consistent with abuse; fearfulness of caregivers, including health care providers; withdrawn behaviour; regular ED use; and mental health and sleep disorders (Hammond & Zimmermann, 2013). If the assessment reveals physical and behavioural findings suggestive of abuse, a more detailed assessment should be completed. A caring, nonjudgemental, and respectful approach should be used to facilitate patient disclosure. Detailed documentation and preservation of forensic evidence may be necessary, and appropriate interventions should be initiated, such as making referrals, providing emotional support, and informing victims about their options (e.g., safe plan, safe house, legal rights). Some EDs have an affiliated sexual assault care centre or domestic violence centre to facilitate ED and community referrals and linkages and to support discharges into the community.

Elder Abuse. *Elder abuse* (physical, psychological, and financial) is any action by someone in a relationship of trust that causes harm or distrust in an older adult (Government of Canada, 2016). Because the older adult rarely self-reports abuse, it is often identified, reported, and reported by health care providers (Bond & Butler, 2013). (See Chapter 7 for a discussion of elder abuse.)

Sexual Assault

In Canada, **sexual assault** is the legal term used to refer to any form of sexual contact imposed on another person without that person's voluntary consent. Kissing; fondling; and vaginal, oral, or anal intercourse are all examples of sexual assault if done without voluntary consent.

The large majority of sexual assault crimes (91%) are not reported to authorities, so the prevalence of sexual assault is hard to quantify (Statistics Canada, 2013). According to the most recent data from Statistics Canada (2017), women self-reported 555 000 sexual assaults in 2014 while men reported 80 000.

Sexual assault may be committed by a stranger or by an intimate partner. Intimate partner violence (IPV) is defined as "violence perpetrated against spouses and dating partners, either in current or former relationships" (Sinha, 2013, p. 38). Survivors can suffer physical trauma and mental health consequences. Pregnancy, sexually transmitted infections (STIs), and gynecological problems can also result from IPV. More than half of all female sexual assault survivors were assaulted by an intimate partner. Female survivors of IPV frequently report chronic pain, sleep disturbances, poor physical health, and activity limitations. According to Sinha (2013), in 2011, there were approximately 97 500 survivors of IPV, representing a rate of 341 survivors per 100 000 population (p. 38).

Clinical Manifestations

Physical. Many women and men who seek help immediately will not have any evidence of physical trauma. Evidence of trauma may be limited because survivors do not resist for fear of physical danger and injury. When present, physical injuries may include bruising and lacerations to perineum, hymen, vulva, vagina, cervix, and anus. Fractures, subdural hematomas, cerebral concussions, and intra-abdominal injuries have resulted in the need for hospitalization. Sexual assault also places survivors at risk for STIs and pregnancy in the case of women survivors.

Psychological. Immediately after the assault, survivors may show shock, numbness, denial, or withdrawal. Some may seem unnaturally calm; others may cry or express anger. Feelings of humiliation, degradation, embarrassment, anger, self-blame, and fear of another assault are commonly expressed. These symptoms usually decrease after 2 weeks, and survivors may appear to have adjusted. Yet, any time from 2 to 3 weeks to months to years after the assault, symptoms may return and become more severe. *Rape trauma syndrome* is a classification of post-traumatic stress disorder. Flashbacks, intrusive recall, sleep disturbances, gastro-intestinal symptoms, and numbing of feelings are common initial symptoms. Survivors of assault will feel embarrassment, self-blame, and powerlessness. Later symptoms include mood swings, irritability, and anger. Feelings of despair, shame, and hopelessness are often the cause of the anger. These feelings may be internalized and expressed as depression. Suicidal ideations may also occur.

Collaborative Care

In the acute care of an assault survivor, ensuring the patient's emotional and physical safety has the highest priority. Table 71-12 outlines the emergency management of the patient who has been sexually assaulted. Most EDs have identified personnel who have received special training in order to work with people who have been assaulted.

Each province and territory has created the position of sexual assault nurse examiner (SANE). The SANE is a registered nurse who is certified to provide care to survivors of sexual assault while ensuring evidence is safeguarded. Special procedures are followed in taking the history and conducting the examination in order to preserve all evidence in case of future prosecution.

When the survivor of an assault is admitted to the ED or clinic, a specific chain of events occurs (Table 71-13). A signed informed consent is obtained before any data are collected. All materials gathered are well documented, labelled, and given to the appropriate person, such as a pathologist or a police officer. The materials are handled by as few people as possible, and signatures of all responsible for keeping and handling the data are obtained. Many items can be used as evidence if the survivor chooses to file a complaint. Consequently, the integrity of the material must be maintained. The nurse's involvement in the medicolegal process depends on the policies of the individual institution and provincial or territorial law.

A gynecological and sexual history and an account of the assault (who, what, when, and where), as well as a general physical and pelvic examination, add further information about the incident. In the case of female survivors, laboratory tests are done primarily to look for sperm in the vagina and to identify any existing STIs or pregnancy.

Follow-up physical and psychological care is essential. Survivors of assault should return weekly for the first month following the assault. This time period is when psychological reactions may be the most severe. Health care providers should have the telephone numbers and names of contact people for local resources for sexual assault survivors, including rape crisis centres, legal and law enforcement authorities, and human services.

NURSING MANAGEMENT
SEXUAL ASSAULT

Nurses can assist people to become aware of prevention tactics (Table 71-14). They should also be encouraged to learn some basic self-defence techniques. Local high schools and the YWCA usually have self-defence classes for formal instruction. Practising the various techniques with a friend builds a person's confidence in his or her ability to fight back. Learning self-defence can make a person less vulnerable and more self-reliant.

When a sexual assault survivor is brought to the clinic or ED, a quiet, private area should be used for the initial assessment and the examinations that follow. The patient should not be left alone. Whenever possible, the same nurse should remain with the person throughout the hospital stay and provide needed emotional support. The patient's actions and words while describing the incident may be inconsistent, confused, and inappropriate. The nurse should maintain a nonjudgemental attitude.

The patient usually has many feelings and thoughts about the assault and generally wants to talk about them. Talking may help

✚ TABLE 71-12 EMERGENCY MANAGEMENT

Sexual Assault

Etiology	Assessment Findings	Interventions
• Assault involving genitalia (male or female) without consent • Sexual molestation • Sodomy	• Agitation • Anger • Crying • Decreased level of consciousness • Emotional or physical manifestations of shock • Extragenital injuries • Hyperventilation • Hysteria • Oral, vaginal, and rectal injuries • Pain in genital area or extragenital area • Silence	**Initial** • Treat shock and other urgent medical problems (e.g., head injury, hemorrhage, wounds, fractures). • Assess emotional state. • Contact support person (e.g., social worker, rape advocate, sexual assault nurse examiner). • Do *not* clean the patient until all evidence is collected. Make sure the patient does not wash, douche, urinate, brush teeth, or gargle. • Place sheet on floor. Then have patient stand on sheet to remove clothing. Place sheet with clothing in paper bag. • SANE will collect forensic evidence per local protocol (i.e., body hair, nail scrapings, tissue, dried semen, vaginal washing, blood samples). • Maintain chain of evidence for all legal specimens. Clearly label evidence and keep in locked cabinet until given to law enforcement agency. • Obtain baseline HIV, syphilis, and other STI screening. • Obtain toxicology sample to evaluate drug-facilitated sexual assault. • Determine method of contraception, date of last menstrual period, and date of last tetanus immunization. • Consider tetanus prophylaxis if lacerations contain soil or dirt. • Vaccinate for hepatitis B if not already done. **Ongoing Monitoring** • Monitor vital signs and emotional status. • Provide clothing as needed. • Counsel patient regarding confidential HIV and STI testing.

HIV, human immunodeficiency virus; *SANE*, sexual assault nurse examiner; *STI*, sexually transmitted infection.

TABLE 71-13 EVALUATION OF ALLEGED SEXUAL ASSAULT

1. Medicolegal
• Valid written consent for examination, photographs, laboratory tests, release of information, and laboratory samples
• Appropriate "chain of evidence" documentation

2. History
• Activities since assault (e.g., changed clothes, bathed, douched)
• Current symptoms
• Emotional status
• History of assault (who, what, when, where)
• Inquiries about safety
• Medical history
• Menstrual and contraceptive history
• Penetration, ejaculation, extragenital acts

3. General Physical Examination
• Cuts, bruises, scratches (photographs taken)
• Extragenital trauma—mouth, breasts, neck
• Vital signs and general appearance

4. Pelvic Examination (Females)
• Adnexa, especially hematomas
• Matted hairs or free hairs
• Uterine size
• Vaginal examination with unlubricated speculum for discharge, blood, lacerations
• Vulvar trauma, erythema; hymen, anal, and rectal status

5. Laboratory Samples
• Blood samples—VDRL serology, pregnancy test; serological testing for HIV and hepatitis B infection
• Clipping of matted pubic hairs
• Cultures—cervix and other areas (if indicated) for gonorrhea and chlamydial infection
• Fingernail scrapings
• Serum sample frozen for later testing
• Oral or rectal swabs and smears, if indicated
• Pubic hair scrapings
• Vaginal smears—microscope evaluation for trichomonads and semen
• Vaginal vault content sampling

6. Treatment
• Care of injuries and emotional trauma
• Prophylaxis for STIs, tetanus, and hepatitis B (see Chapters 55, 63, and 46, respectively)
• If appropriate, consider levonorgestrel (Plan B) emergency contraceptive pill up to 72 hr after assault; follow-up for pregnancy test in 2–3 wk
• Follow-up for pregnancy test in 2–3 wk (if appropriate)
• Testing for HIV, syphilis, and hepatitis B may be done at 6–8 wk
• Protection of legal rights
• Recommendation of continued follow-up and services of rape crisis centre

HIV, human immunodeficiency virus; *STIs*, sexually transmitted infections; *VDRL*, venereal disease research laboratory.

the patient feel better and gain an understanding of her or his reactions to the incident. When the nurse listens carefully, the patient feels less alone and is better able to gain control over the situation.

The nurse should assess the patient's stress before preparing him or her for the various procedures that will follow. The patient's coping mechanisms are supported when he or she knows what to expect and what is expected as well as why the particular procedure must be done. Because the pelvic examination may trigger a flashback of the attack for female survivors, the nurse should answer all related questions before the examination and be a supportive presence during the examination.

After the examinations, the patient's physical comfort needs should be considered. The patient will need a change of clothing because original garments may have been torn or soiled or may need to be kept as evidence. Most people who have been sexually assaulted feel dirty and would appreciate a place to wash as well as to use a mouthwash, especially if oral sex was involved. Food and drink may also provide comfort to the survivor.

For female survivors of sexual assault, the possibility of pregnancy should be discussed and the patient can be offered emergency contraception (sold as levonorgestrel [Plan B or Option 2] in Canada) to prevent an unintended pregnancy. It is similar to birth control pills but taken in different doses and can be used up to 3 to 5 days after unprotected sex, reducing the risk of getting pregnant by approximately 75% to 89% (Dunn & Guilbert, 2012). The effectiveness of emergency contraception (EC) is highest when taken within 24 hours after unprotected sexual intercourse and declines over time. EC pills might be less effective in women weighing 75 to 80 kg, and are not effective in women over 80 kg (Government of Canada, 2014).

Many sexual assault survivors are unaware of the availability of compensation or financial assistance programs and appreciate information about the application process. All provinces and territories except Newfoundland and Labrador, Yukon, and Nunavut have financial compensation programs for victims and survivors of violent crime such as sexual assault to cover some, but not all, expenses incurred as the direct result of a violent crime (Canadian Resource Centre for Victims of Crime, 2016). The programs were created to recognize the harm done to innocent people and to ease the financial burden that often accompanies victimization. All other coverage must be exhausted before claims for compensation are considered (Canadian Resource Centre for Victims of Crime, 2016).

When the patient is discharged, the nurse should make certain the patient has transportation home. If friends or family members are not available, the hospital or clinic should make arrangements with an appropriate community resource. The patient should not be sent home alone. The survivor's partner and family have a tremendous potential for both negative and positive influence. If the partner is the perpetrator of the assault, consultation with the risk management department and law enforcement is necessary to protect the patient.

Many communities today have crisis centres. These public service organizations have trained professional and nonprofessional volunteers who provide an emotional support system for survivors on request. Their programs provide advocacy to ensure dignified treatment throughout the medical and police procedures, short-term counselling for survivors and their families, and court assistance and public education on rape-related issues.

TABLE 71-14 PATIENT & CAREGIVER TEACHING GUIDE

Sexual Assault Prevention

The following suggestions should be included when discussing ways to prevent sexual assault.

- Avoid walking alone in deserted areas. Walk to the parking lot with a friend; be sure you see each other leave.
- Be aware of date-rape drugs (e.g., gamma-hydroxybutyrate [GHB], flunitrazepam [Rohypnol], ketamine). Do not leave your beverage unattended or accept a drink from an open container.
- Be proactive and take a self-defence class.
- Carry a loud whistle and use it when you think you are in danger.
- Consume alcohol in moderation if you drink. Many sexual assaults involve the use of alcohol by the offender, the survivor, or both.
- Do not advertise that you live alone. List only your initials with your last name in the telephone directory or on the mailbox. Never reveal to a caller that you are home alone.
- Have your keys ready as you approach your car or home.
- Keep all doors locked and windows up when driving.
- Keep your residence doors locked, and do not open them to a stranger; ask for identification if a service person comes to the door.
- Never get on an elevator with a person behaving suspiciously or furtive. Pretend you have forgotten something and get off.
- Place and maintain lights at all entrances to your home.
- Proceed with caution in online correspondence.
- Say what you mean in social situations. Be sure your voice and body language reflect your response.
- Yell "fire" if you are attacked, and run toward a lighted area.

CASE STUDY

Trauma

Source: Monkey Business Images/ Shutterstock .com.

Patient Profile

Lian Wu, a 20-year-old woman, is brought to the ED in an ambulance. She was the driver in a motor vehicle collision and was not wearing a seat belt. Two children in the car were pronounced dead at the scene. The paramedics stated that there was significant damage to the car on the driver's side.

Subjective Data

- Ms. Wu asks, "What happened? Where are the children?"
- Complains of shortness of breath and abdominal pain

Objective Data
Physical Examination

- Asymmetrical chest movement
- Badly deformed right lower leg with a pedal pulse detectable only by Doppler ultrasonography
- Decreased breath sounds on left side of chest
- Glasgow Coma Score of 14; unequal pupils

- O₂ saturation, 82%
- One 4-cm head laceration
- Vital signs: blood pressure, 90/40 mm Hg; heart rate, 130 beats/min; respiratory rate, 36 breaths/min

Discussion Questions

1. What life-threatening injury does Ms. Wu probably have?
2. *Priority decision:* What is the priority of care for Ms. Wu?
3. *Priority decision:* What interventions are needed immediately?
4. What other interventions should the nurse consider?
5. Several family members have arrived in the ED, including the mother of one of the children who died. The second child who died was Ms. Wu's child. How should the nurse approach the family of the first child?
6. *Priority decision:* Based on the assessment data presented, what are the priority nursing diagnoses? Are there any collaborative problems?

℮volve
Answers are available at *http://evolve.elsevier.com/Canada/Lewis/medsurg.*

REVIEW QUESTIONS

The number of the question corresponds to the same-numbered objective at the beginning of the chapter.

1. An older man arrives at the ED disoriented and breathing rapidly. He has hot, dry skin. What is the priority for treatment at this point?
   a. To assess his airway, breathing, and circulation
   b. To obtain a detailed medical history from his family
   c. To determine that he has his health card before treating him
   d. To start oxygen administration and have the ED physician see him

2. A client has a core temperature of 32°C. Which of the following is the most appropriate rewarming technique?
   a. Passive rewarming with body-to-body contact
   b. Active core rewarming using warmed IV fluids
   c. Passive rewarming using air-filled warming blankets
   d. Active external rewarming by submersion in a warm bath

3. Effective interventions to decrease absorption or increase elimination of an ingested poison include which of the following? (Select all that apply)
   a. Hemodialysis
   b. Milk dilution
   c. Eye irrigation
   d. Gastric lavage
   e. Activated charcoal

4. Of clients who die in the ED, whom should the nurse regard as potential organ donors?
   a. Those who were young and strong
   b. Victims of accidents who were otherwise disease free
   c. Clients who can be kept on life support until the transplantation team is ready
   d. Anyone whose organs and tissues were healthy at the time of death

5. An older-adult client arrives in the ED with his son. The older man is in no apparent physical distress, although his clothes are soiled with urine and feces and he is tearful. Which of the following should the nurse consider?
   a. Cancer
   b. Stroke
   c. Neglect
   d. Depression

6. Which of the following would be the first nursing intervention for the client who has been sexually assaulted?
   a. Treat urgent medical problems.
   b. Contact a support person for the client.
   c. Provide supplies for the client to cleanse himself or herself.
   d. Document bruises and lacerations of the perineum and the cervix.

1. a; 2. b; 3. a, d, e; 4. d; 5. c, 6. a.

⊜volve

For even more review questions, visit *http://evolve.elsevier.com/Canada/ Lewis/medsurg.*

REFERENCES

Atha, W. F. (2013). Heat-related illness. *Emergency Medicine Clinics of North America, 31*(4), 1097–1108. doi:10.1016/j .emc.2013.07.012.

Bair, A. E., Walls, R. M., & Grayzel, J. (2017). *Rapid sequence intubation for adults outside the operating room.* Retrieved from *https://www.uptodate.com/contents/rapid-sequence-intubation-for-adults-outside-the-operating-room.*

BC Transplant. (2017). *Organ donation after brain death (neurological determination of death).* Retrieved from *http:// www.transplant.bc.ca/Documents/BCT%20NDD%202012 %20FINAL.pdf.*

Becker, J. A., & Stewart, L. K. (2011). Heat-related illness. *American Family Physician, 83*(11), 1325.

Bond, M. C., & Butler, K. H. (2013). Elder abuse and neglect: Definitions, epidemiology, and approaches to emergency department screening. *Clinics in Geriatric Medicine, 29*(1), 257–273. doi:10.1016/j.cger.2012.09.004.

Bullard, M. J., Chan, T., Brayman, C., et al. (2014). Revisions to the Canadian emergency department triage and acuity scale (CTAS) guidelines. *Canadian Journal of Emergency Medicine, 16*(06), 485–489.

Bullard, M. J., Unger, B., Spence, J., et al. (2008). Revisions to the Canadian Triage and Acuity Scale (CTAS) adult guidelines. *Canadian Journal of Emergency Medicine, 10*, 136–151. (Seminal).

Burchum, J. R., & Rosenthal, L. D. (2016). *Lehne's pharmacology for nursing care* (9th ed.). St. Louis, MO: Elsevier Saunders.

Canadian Institute for Health Information (CIHI). (2013). *National Trauma Registry report 2013: Hospitalizations for major injury in Canada, 2011–2012 data.* Ottawa: Author. Retrieved from *https:// secure.cihi.ca/estore/productSeries.htm?pc=PCC46.*

Canadian Institute for Health Information (CIHI). (2015). *Emergency department visits in 2014–2015.* Retrieved from *https://secure .cihi.ca/free_products/NACRS_ED_QuickStats_Infosheet_2014-15 _ENweb.pdf.*

Canadian Nurses Association (CNA). (2018). *CNA certification: Commit to excellence.* Retrieved from *https://cna-aiic.ca/~/media/ cna/page-content/pdf-en/certifcation-brochure-2018_en.pdf?la=en.*

Canadian Resource Centre for Victims of Crime. (2016). *Navigating the Canadian criminal justice system: A guide for victims.* Retrieved from *https://crcvc.ca/wp-content/uploads/2016/05/ A-Victims-Guide_Jan2016.pdf.*

Canadian Transplant Society. (2014). *Home page.* Retrieved from *http://www.cantransplant.ca/home.*

Chandy, D., & Weinhouse, G. (2017). *Drowning (submersion injuries).* Retrieved from *http://www.uptodate.com/contents/drowning -submersion-injuries.*

Chen, Y., Mo, F., Yi, Q. L., et al. (2013). Unintentional injury mortality and external causes from 2001 to 2007. *Chronic Diseases and Injuries in Canada, 33*(2), 95–102.

Crawford Mechem, C. (2017). *Severe nonexertional hyperthermia (heat stroke) in adults.* Retrieved from *http://www.uptodate.com/ contents/severe-nonexertional-hyperthermia-classic-heat-stroke-in-adults.*

Crawford Mechem, C., & Zafren, K. (2017). *Frostbite.* Retrieved from *http://www.uptodate.com/contents/frostbite.*

Denke, N. J. (2010). Wound management. In P. K. Howard & R. A. Steinmann (Eds.), *Sheehy's emergency nursing* (6th ed.). St Louis: Mosby. (Seminal).

Dunn, S., & Guilbert, E. (2012). Emergency contraception. *Journal of Obstetrics and Gynaecology Canada, 34*(9), 870–878. doi:10.1016/S1701-2163(16)35387-7.

Edwards, E., Despotopulos, L., & Carroll, D. (2013). Changes in provider perceptions of family presence during resuscitation. *Clinical Nurse Specialist CNS, 27*(5), 239–244. doi:10.1097/NUR.0b013e3182a0ba13.

Enzler, M., Berbari, E., & Osmon, D. (2011). Antimicrobial prophylaxis in adults. *Mayo Clinic Proceedings, 86*(7), 686–701. doi:10.4065/mcp.2011.0012.

Epstein, Y., & Roberts, W. O. (2011). The pathophysiology of heat stroke: An integrative view of the final common pathway. *Scandinavian Journal of Medicine & Science in Sports, 21*(6), 742–748. doi:10.1111/j.1600-0838.2011.01333.x.

Foo, C. L., Siu, V. W., Ang, H., et al. (2014). Risk stratification and rapid geriatric screening in an emergency department—A quasi-randomised controlled trial. *BMC Geriatrics, 14*(1), 98–107. doi:10.1186/1471-2318-14-98.

Government of Canada. (2014). *Emergency contraceptive pills to carry warnings for reduced effectiveness in women over a certain body weight.* Retrieved from *http://healthycanadians.gc.ca/recall-alert-rappel-avis/hc-sc/2014/38701a-eng.php.*

Government of Canada. (2016). *Elder abuse: It's time to face the reality.* Retrieved from *https://www.canada.ca/en/employment-social-development/campaigns/elder-abuse/reality.html.*

Government of Canada. (2017). *Surveillance of Lyme disease.* Retrieved from *http://healthycanadians.gc.ca/diseases-conditions-maladies-affections/disease-maladie/lyme/surveillance-eng.php.*

Gross, E. A., & Moore, J. C. (2012). Using thrombolytics in frostbite injury. *Journal of Emergencies, Trauma, and Shock, 5*(3), 267. doi:10.4103/0974-2700.99709.

Halter, M. J. (2014). *Varcarolis' foundations of psychiatric mental health nursing* (7th ed.). St. Louis: Elsevier Saunders.

Hammond, B. B., & Zimmermann, P. G. (Eds.), (2013). *Sheehy's manual of emergency care* (7th ed.). St. Louis: Mosby.

Harris, C. (2013). Abdominal trauma. In B. B. Hammond & P. G. Zimmermann (Eds.), *Sheehy's manual of emergency care* (7th ed.). St Louis: Mosby.

Iyer, I. G. (2011). Pain documentation and predictors of analgesic prescribing for elderly patients during emergency department visits. *Journal of Pain and Symptom Management, 41*(2), 364–373. doi:10.1016/j.jpainsymman.2010.04.023.

Jabre, P., Tazarourte, K., Azoulay, E., et al. (2013). Family presence during cardiopulmonary resuscitation. *New England Journal of Medicine, 368*(11), 1008–1018. doi:10.1056/NEJMoa1203366.

Kahan, M., Mailis-Gagnon, A., Wilson, L., et al. (2011). Canadian guideline for safe and effective use of opioids for chronic noncancer pain: Clinical summary for family physicians. Part 1: General population. *Canadian Family Physician, 57*(11), 1257–1266.

Kiel, D. P. (2016). *Falls in older persons: Risk factors and patient evaluation.* Retrieved from *http://www.uptodate.com/contents/falls-in-olderpersons-risk-factors-and-patient-evaluation.*

Krau, S. D. (2013). Heat-related illness: A hot topic in critical care. *Critical Care Nursing Clinics of North America, 25*(2), 251–262. doi:10.1016/j.ccell.2013.02.012.

National Emergency Nurses Affiliation (NENA). (2014a). *Position statement: Family-PSU presence during resuscitation.* Retrieved from *http://nena.ca/w/wp-content/uploads/2014/11/Family PrimarySupport.pdf.*

National Emergency Nurses Association (NENA). (2014b). *Position statement: Violence in the emergency department.* Retrieved from *http://nena.ca/w/wp-content/uploads/2015/11/Violence-in-the-ED.pdf.*

National Emergency Nurses Association (NENA). (2016). *Certification.* Retrieved from *http://nena.ca/courses.*

Nelson, H. D., Bougatsos, C., & Blazina, I. (2012). Screening women for intimate partner violence: A systematic review to update the U.S. Preventive Services Task Force recommendation. *Annals of Internal Medicine, 156*(11), 796–808. doi:10.7326/0003-4819-156-11-201206050-00447.

Patanwala, A. E., Stahle, S. A., Sakles, J. C., et al. (2011). Comparison of succinylcholine and rocuronium for first-attempt intubation success in the emergency department. *Academic Emergency Medicine: Official Journal of the Society for Academic Emergency Medicine, 18*(1), 10–14. doi:10.1111/j.1553-2712.2010.00954.x. (Seminal).

Porter, J. E., Cooper, S. J., & Sellick, K. (2014). Family presence during resuscitation (FPDR): Perceived benefits, barriers and enablers to implementation and practice. *International Emergency Nursing, 22*(2), 69–74.

Public Health Agency of Canada & Health Canada. (2017). *Lyme disease.* Retrieved from *https://www.canada.ca/en/public-health/services/diseases/lyme-disease.html.*

Rahman, S., Rubinstein, S., Singh, J., et al. (2012). Early use of hemodialysis for active rewarming in severe hypothermia: A case report and review of literature. *Renal Failure, 34*(6), 784–788.

Ricci, N., & Rizzolo, P. (2011). Laceration repair: Avoid infection, optimize healing, minimize scarring. *Journal of the American Academy of Physician Assistants, 24*(9), 29–33.

Sinha, M. (2013). *Family violence in Canada: A statistical profile, 2011* (Statistics Canada Catalogue no. 85-002-X). *Juristat.* Retrieved from *http://www.statcan.gc.ca/pub/85-002-x/2013001/article/11805-eng.pdf.*

Statistics Canada. (2013). *Trends in sexual offences.* Retrieved from *http://www.statcan.gc.ca/pub/85f0033m/2008019/findings-resultats/trends-tendances-eng.htm.*

Statistics Canada. (2017). *Self-reported sexual assault in Canada, 2014.* Retrieved from *http://www.statcan.gc.ca/pub/85-002-x/2017001/article/14842-eng.htm.*

Stollings, J. L., Diedrich, D. A., Oyen, L. J., et al. (2013). Rapid-Sequence Intubation: A review of the process and considerations when choosing medications. *The Annals of Pharmacotherapy, 48*(1), 62–76. doi:10.1177/1060028013510488.

Trillium Gift of Life Network. (2017). *Caring for families.* Retrieved from *https://www.giftoflife.on.ca/en/professionals.htm.*

Vetter, R. S., Swanson, D. L., & White, J. (2017). *Management of widow spider bites.* Retrieved from *http://www.uptodate.com/contents/management-of-widow-spider-bites.*

Wilding, L., Gilsenan, R., Dalziel, B., et al. (2015). Promising best practice: The champlain geriatric emergency management plus (GEM Plus) program. *Canadian Geriatric Journal of CME, 5*(1), 6–9.

Zafren, K., & Crawford Mechem, C. (2017). *Accidental hypothermia in adults.* Retrieved from *http://www.uptodate.com/contents/accidental-hypothermia-in-adults.*

RESOURCES

ARDS Foundation Canada
http://www.ardscanada.org/

Canadian Association of Emergency Physicians
http://www.caep.ca

Canadian Association of Poison Control Centres
http://www.capcc.ca/en

Canadian Centre for Abuse Awareness (CCAA)
https://abusehurts.com

Canadian Centre for Occupational Health and Safety
http://www.ccohs.ca

Canadian Child Welfare Research Portal
http://cwrp.ca/policy-legislation

Canadian Forensic Nurses Association
http://forensicnurse.ca

Canadian Institute for Health Information
http://www.cihi.ca

Canadian Lyme Disease Foundation: Tick Removal
http://canlyme.com/lyme-basics/tick-removal

Canadian Nurses Association
http://www.cna-aiic.ca

Canadian Red Cross
http://www.redcross.ca

Centre for Research & Education on Violence Against Women & Children
http://learningtoendabuse.ca

Health Canada
https://www.canada.ca/en/health-canada.html

National Emergency Nurses Association (NENA)
http://www.nena.ca

National Trauma Registry Metadata
https://www.cihi.ca/en/national-trauma-registry-metadata

Parachute: Preventing Injuries, Saving Lives
http://parachutecanada.org

Public Health Agency of Canada
https://www.canada.ca/en/public-health.html

Public Health Agency of Canada: Stop Family Violence
*https://www.canada.ca/en/public-health/services/health-promotion/
stop-family-violence.html*

Safe Kids Canada
http://www.safekidscanada.ca

St. John Ambulance Canada
http://www.sja.ca

Trauma Association of Canada
http://www.traumacanada.org

Centers for Disease Control and Prevention: Emergency Preparedness and Response
https://emergency.cdc.gov

Institute for Healthcare Improvement: Evidence-Based Care Bundles
http://www.ihi.org/Topics/Bundles/Pages/default.aspx

NOLS Wilderness Medicine
https://www.nols.edu/en/courses/wilderness-medicine

For additional Internet resources, see the website for this book at *http://evolve.elsevier.com/Canada/Lewis/medsurg*.

CHAPTER

72

Emergency Management and Disaster Planning

Written by: Karen Baguley

evolve WEBSITE

http://evolve.elsevier.com/Canada/Lewis/medsurg

- Review Questions (Online Only)
- Key Points
- Answer Guidelines for Case Study
- Conceptual Care Map Creator
- Audio Glossary
- Content Updates

LEARNING OBJECTIVES

1. Differentiate between an emergency and a disaster situation.
2. Identify the roles and responsibilities of individuals, communities, and select provincial or territorial and federal agencies in emergency planning and disaster management.
3. Define and describe the characteristics of disaster nursing.
4. Outline the components of a comprehensive emergency management program.
5. Describe the four phases of disaster management and the nursing role in each phase.
6. Describe the application of the Incident Management System and the roles of command centre team members.
7. Describe the differences between daily emergency department triage and triage in disaster situations.
8. Outline the components of START triage and its application in disaster situations.
9. Classify the major types of disasters based on their characteristics and describe their consequences.
10. Identify those agents most likely to be used in a terrorist attack and their health impact.
11. Describe key differences between chemical, biological, radiological, nuclear, and explosive (CBRNE) events and the relevance of casualty decontamination in health care settings.
12. Describe the difference between epidemics and pandemics and discuss the importance of pandemic planning.

KEY TERMS

bioterrorism, p. 1835
CBRNE event, p. 1835
critical incident stress management (CISM) or debriefing, p. 1834
decontamination, p. 1836
disaster, p. 1827
disaster nursing, p. 1843

emergency, p. 1827
emergency/disaster management, p. 1828
emergency management and disaster planning, p. 1827
epidemic, p. 1840
hazards, p. 1827
outbreak management, p. 1840

pandemic, p. 1840
pandemic influenza, p. 1841
quarantine, p. 1841
terrorism, p. 1835
triage, p. 1833

Daily media coverage has allowed the world to witness first-hand the depth and overwhelming impact of natural and human-made or human-induced disasters. The increasing frequency of disasters globally emphasizes the pivotal need for advanced planning and collaboration to effectively mitigate and manage the outcomes. Disasters have extensive history within the human experience, resulting in premature death, diminished quality of life, and altered health status (Veenema & Woolsey, 2013). Hurricane Katrina (2005), the earthquakes in Haiti (2010) and in Great East Japan (2011), and more recently the Fort McMurray forest fires (2016), coupled with the images of the Paris (2015), Orlando (2016), and Nice (2016) terrorist attacks, and the Las Vegas (2017) mass shooting reflect the far-reaching impact of disasters and the critical need for broad-scale planning, prevention, response, and recovery mechanisms.

Nurses, as the largest sector of the health care workforce in Canada, can expect to be on the front lines of an emergency at some point in their careers. In recent years, nurses have played a pivotal role in responding to emergency situations nationally and internationally, contributing to large-scale health surveillance, education, and the assessment of health needs and service and resource allocation (Canadian Nurses Association [CNA], 2012). According to the World Health Organization and the International Council of Nurses (WHO & ICN, 2009), the unique knowledge, skills, and abilities possessed by nurses allow them to support humanitarian efforts and positively contribute to disaster response. It is an expectation that all nurses demonstrate an awareness of the impact of emergency planning on disaster response and that they work collaboratively to implement strategies to prevent illness and injuries that are a result of community disasters and global health issues (CNA, 2012; College of Nurses of Ontario, 2014; WHO & ICN, 2009).

EMERGENCY MANAGEMENT AND DISASTER PLANNING

Emergency management and disaster planning involve advanced preparation for a variety of potential situations, including mass casualty incidents, natural or biological events, technological failures, human conflicts, and acts of terrorism. Advanced planning, when done in a comprehensive and diligent manner, decreases the impact that an emergency or disaster situation has on individuals, organizations, and communities. When discussing emergency management and disaster planning, it is important to differentiate between the terms. According to WHO and ICN (2009), no single, agreed-upon definition of the term *disaster* exists. Disasters are often defined by governments, humanitarian groups, and other agencies, reflecting the mission and needs of that agency. While events may be labelled as "disasters," by the communities affected and by the media, many events are more accurately classified as emergencies.

An emergency may be described as a present or imminent event that requires a rapid and skilled response to protect the health, safety, and wellness of individuals and to limit damage to property or the environment (Public Safety Canada [PSC], 2015a). Emergency situations are typically able to be quickly managed without requiring the support and resources of other communities but require urgent intervention to prevent worsening of the situation. A disaster is the outcome of a natural hazard or event (e.g., hurricane, flood, earthquake) or a result of human action or error, whether malicious (e.g., terrorist attacks, use of biological warfare) or unintentional (e.g., an accidental chemical spill), that seriously disrupts the functioning of a community or society (PSC, 2015a). Disasters typically occur suddenly and can result in mass casualties (i.e., large numbers of people injured); loss of human life and materials; and significant destruction of property, the environment, and critical infrastructure (e.g., government, water, power, food supply) (Veenema & Woolsey, 2013). A disaster, owing to its scale and impact, exceeds the capacity of a community to cope and respond with existing resources, requiring "outside" assistance from trained responders, government, nongovernmental organizations, humanitarian relief agencies, or some combination of all of these (WHO & ICN, 2009; PSC, 2015b).

Two approaches are used in disaster planning initiatives: an *agent specific approach,* in which planning efforts are directed at those threats most likely to take place within a single geographical location (e.g., earthquakes in California); and more commonly, an *all-hazards approach,* a comprehensive strategy, where vulnerabilities to both natural and human-induced hazards are considered to be potential possibilities even if they have never happened or are unlikely to ever occur (PSC, 2015b; Veenema & Woolsey, 2013). An all-hazards approach to emergency management is used across all jurisdictions in Canada and helps to ensure that managing one type of risk does not increase vulnerability to other risks. Hazards are defined as anything that has the potential to cause harm or loss. Hazards can be substances, human activities, or physical events that may cause injury or loss of life, threaten the delivery of critical services, cause social and economic disruption, or cause property or environmental damage (PSC, 2015a). Disasters occur when a hazard interacts with a vulnerable area to produce serious adverse

consequences that may exceed a community's or society's ability to cope for an unknown period of time.

Individual, Local–Municipal, Provincial–Territorial, and Federal and First Nations Responsibilities

To be successful, emergency and disaster planning initiatives must be done at a variety of levels, specifically the individual and family; local, community, or municipal; provincial or territorial; and federal levels. *Emergency management and disaster planning* involves having plans of action, supplies, and resources in place to respond in a timely and efficient manner to inevitable events.

Preparedness starts at an individual level and requires that individuals and families assume responsibility for taking appropriate steps to ensure that they have the basics of what might be required for short-term survival. This level of preparation requires stockpiling items that would be needed to be self-sufficient for a period of at least 72 hours and a detailed plan, considering risks to the region, knowledge of safe exits and evacuation routes, advanced identification of emergency contacts and meeting places for reunification, and an awareness of where to find household fire extinguishers, water and gas valves, floor drains, and electrical control panels (Canadian Red Cross, 2016a; Government of Canada, 2015a). Emergency workers focus on community members with the most urgent needs, and search and rescue efforts for casualties take precedence in the first 72 hours of an emergency event. Critical infrastructure (e.g., water and power) could potentially be interrupted for an extended period of time, reflecting the need for advanced planning and availability of basic survival resources. Table 72-1 details items that should be included in an individual or family emergency preparedness kit.

Most emergencies in our country are local in nature and are managed by municipalities and, when required, with provincial or territorial support. Accountability for emergency planning and response in Canada is held by individual municipalities, the underlying principle being that communities possess the greatest knowledge of their individual needs and, thus, are in a strategic position to most effectively plan for and manage local events (PSC, 2015b; PSC, 2015c). Local first responders (fire, police, and paramedics) are typically the first to respond to an emergency as a component of the municipal emergency plan. While most situations can be effectively handled by a community, different levels of organizations are introduced progressively if the situation escalates and as additional help and resources are needed. When a community is unable to provide required response efforts because of the scope of the situation or because of inadequate personnel or equipment, a "community emergency" is declared and the province or territory is contacted for support (PSC, 2015a).

The *Emergency Management Act* (EMA) was developed with the goal of strengthening emergency management efforts in this country. The Act sets out clear roles and responsibilities for all stakeholders within Canada's emergency management system and is directed at ensuring that our country and its jurisdictions are engaged in disaster mitigation and response activities (PSC, 2015b). All provinces and territories have an *Emergency Management Organization* (EMO) that is responsible for the development, coordination, training, and response operations in their jurisdiction. EMOs typically manage large-scale emergencies, providing assistance to municipal or community response teams (PSC, 2015a; 2015b). Recognizing the potential for emergencies to escalate rapidly in scope and severity, cross jurisdictional lines, and have an international impact, the provincial–territorial EMO

TABLE 72-1	INDIVIDUAL OR FAMILY EMERGENCY PREPAREDNESS KIT

Meeting Places

Safe meeting place near home: _____

Safe meeting place outside immediate neighbourhood: _____

Evacuation routes from neighbourhood: _____

Basic Emergency Kit Items to Include

Food and drinking water: Have at least a 3-day (72-hr) supply of food and water on hand

Food: Ready-to-eat foods that will not spoil, such as canned food, energy bars, and dried foods (replace food and water once per year)

Drinking water: At least two litres of water per person per day (include small water bottles that can be carried easily)

Equipment for Emergency Survival

☐ A copy of emergency plan and contact information and numbers

☐ Cash (include smaller bills, such as $10 bills and change for pay phones)

☐ Extra keys for car and house

☐ First-aid kit

☐ Wind-up or battery-powered flashlight (with extra batteries)

☐ Wind-up or battery-powered radio (with extra batteries)

Additional Supplies That Should Be Considered

☐ Additional bottles of water (2 L per person) for cooking and cleaning

☐ Backpack or duffel bag (in case of evacuation)

☐ Blankets or sleeping bags for each household member

☐ Candles in a deep can; matches or lighter

☐ Change of clothing and footwear (one change of clothes per person)

☐ Duct tape and basic tools (hammer, pliers, wrench, screwdriver, pocket knife)

☐ Garbage bags

☐ Important papers (identification, personal documents)

☐ Manual can opener, bottle opener

☐ Playing cards and games

☐ Small, fuel-operated stove and fuel

☐ Toiletries, hand sanitizer

☐ Utensils, disposable cups and plates

☐ Warning light or road flares

☐ Whistle (to attract attention)

Any Special Needs Family Members Might Have

☐ Equipment for people with disabilities

☐ Infant formula, diapers

☐ Personal prescription medications, including allergy medications

☐ A record of details about medical conditions, allergies, medication, family medical history, recent vaccinations, health screenings, and surgeries

☐ Pet food

Source: Adapted from: Government of Canada. (2015). Get Prepared: Your emergency preparedness guide. Retrieved from *http://www.getprepared.gc.ca/cnt/rsrcs/pblctns/yprprdnssgd/index-en.aspx*.

will notify the federal government for assistance when required. Federal assistance is most commonly dispatched in disaster situations—for example, in those involving mass casualties or in areas under federal authority, such as nuclear safety, national defence, and border security (PSC 2015a; 2015b; 2015c).

Public Safety Canada (PSC) is the department of the federal government accountable for Canadian safety and protection. Created after the events of September 11, 2001, PSC plays a role in the development of national policy, response systems, and standards and is responsible for providing guidance to federal government institutions on the development of emergency management plans.

This approach strengthens the Canadian government's capacity to prevent, protect against, respond to, and recover from major disasters and other emergencies (PSC, 2015b; 2015c; 2015d).

PSC also plays a critical role by establishing partnerships across sectors with key organizations, like the provincial–territorial EMOs, Canadian Security Intelligence Services, the Royal Canadian Mounted Police, and the United States Department of Homeland Security, as a means of managing national risks, reducing vulnerabilities to hazards, and strengthening the resilience of critical infrastructure (PSC, 2015b; 2015c; 2015d). *Critical infrastructure* consists of physical and information technology facilities, networks, services, and assets that are considered to be essential to the health, safety, security, and economic well-being of Canadians and to the continued functioning of the country as a whole. Examples of critical infrastructure include power, water, government, and sewage services. Several federal departments work alongside PSC to provide emergency response resources. For example, Health Canada plays a role in implementing strategies aimed at reducing risks to individual health and the overall environment. The Department of National Defence administers the Canadian Forces Disaster Assistance Response Team (DART), a multidisciplinary military organization designed to deploy on short notice anywhere in the world in response to situations ranging from natural disasters to complex humanitarian emergencies (Government of Canada, 2015b).

Around the world, many government and nongovernmental organizations deliver expert humanitarian aid programs and services. *Nongovernmental organizations* (NGOs) are an important component of the emergency response system. These nonprofit agencies offer assistance with disaster prevention and preparedness, response, and recovery. The Canadian Red Cross, St. John Ambulance, and the Salvation Army are examples of NGOs that provide resources that support emergency response (equipment, supplies, and human resources) and that address basic human needs (food, clothing, shelter, emotional support, and family reunification) in times of disaster (Canadian Red Cross, 2016b; St. John Ambulance, 2016).

Disaster Response in First Nations Communities

First Nations are responsible for developing and implementing emergency plans that address the needs of their communities. When an emergency occurs in a First Nations community, it is the responsibility of the chief and council to use all available resources to respond to the situation. As is true of other communities, if the situation extends beyond the capacity and resources available to respond, additional support is requested. Disaster response in First Nations communities involves a collaborative agreement between Indigenous and Northern Affairs Canada (INAC) and provincial–territorial governments, ensuring community access to comparable emergency assistance services available to other residents in their respective provinces or territories. Through these agreements, INAC provides funding to cover eligible costs related to emergency assistance, while the provincial or territorial government provides the service (INAC, 2017). INAC also collaborates with provinces and territories to manage situations on reserves that have the potential to affect communities, lands, assets, and the environment (INAC, 2017).

EMERGENCY/DISASTER MANAGEMENT

Emergency/disaster management is a process that includes a series of steps, from the anticipation of a hazardous event, to

FIGURE 72-1 Disaster management continuum. Source: World Health Organization and International Council of Nurses (2009). ICN Framework of Disaster Nursing Competencies (p. 40, Figure 1). Retrieved from *http://www.icn .ch/images/stories/documents/networks/DisasterPreparednessNetwork/Disaster_Nursing_Competencies_lite.pdf.*

minimizing the risks from such an event, to responding to and recovering from an emergency or disaster. The life cycle of a disaster is commonly referred to as the *disaster management continuum* and is accepted globally as the method for addressing all aspects of a disaster (WHO & ICN, 2009) (Figure 72-1). This cycle is characterized by three major phases that provide the disaster timeline: (1) pre-incident (before the event); (2) incident (during the event); and (3) post-incident (after the event) (WHO & ICN, 2009; Veenema & Woolsey, 2013). Within each phase of the disaster management continuum are activities that include the following: (1) pre-incident: activities designed to plan, prevent or mitigate, and prepare for the potential impact of an emergency or disaster; (2) incident: all activities involved in the response to and management of an emergency or disaster situation; and (3) post-incident: recovery or rehabilitation from said situation with evaluation of efforts (WHO & ICN, 2009; Moore, Geller, & Clark, 2015). Actions taken at each phase aim to reduce harm to populations and critical infrastructure and to build community resilience. The nature and scope of planning will influence the extent of illness, injury, and death that occur following a disaster. The use of an all-hazards approach to planning, multilevel partnerships to respond to emergency and disaster situations, and integration of activities outlined in each phase together comprise a *comprehensive emergency and disaster management program.*

Mitigation

Mitigation, also called *prevention,* is a critical first step to emergency management that occurs in the pre-incident phase of the disaster management continuum. Mitigation involves reducing the impact of disasters on communities, helps to reduce financial costs of disaster response and recovery (PSC, 2015b), and starts with an assessment of potential risks. A *risk* is defined as the combination of the likelihood that a hazard or event will occur and the consequences that may result if it does (PSC, 2015a). Emergency management is a *risk-based* process, meaning that decisions and activities are based on an assessment, understanding, and evaluation of hazards, risks, and vulnerabilities. *Vulnerabilities* are conditions that increase the susceptibility of communities to the negative impact of a hazard and are a measure of how prepared a community is to cope with the impact of a hazard (PSC, 2015a). Examples of vulnerabilities include poor construction and design of buildings, lack of public information, and inadequate preparation. Mitigation, therefore, involves the identification of potential hazards faced by an organization or a community and the minimization of possible consequences from those hazards.

The goal of mitigation is to identify and implement in advance long-term strategies to reduce, deflect, or altogether avoid the consequences a hazard might have on human health, organiza-

tional or community function, and critical infrastructure (PSC, 2015a; 2015c). Examples of mitigation strategies within a community include flood mapping; the use of water-resistant building materials to decrease the effects of floods and hurricanes; and the development of public warning systems to assist with evacuation in times of emergency (PSC, 2015a). In the hospital setting, mitigation might include ensuring the availability of essential equipment (e.g., portable medical gases) that does not require the use of electricity, or availability of backup emergency generators for critical equipment, thereby decreasing the impact on patients should critical infrastructure fail (Markenson, 2013; Veenema & Landesman, 2013). Nurses play a pivotal role in mitigation activities across acute care and community settings. Nurses' knowledge of community needs, available resources, populations at risk, and workforce issues is essential in preparing an organization or a community for emergency situations (WHO & ICN, 2009).

Preparedness

Preparedness is a proactive activity that occurs in the pre-incident phase and that involves preplanning for emergency situations that could occur within an organization, a community, or a jurisdiction. Preparedness is closely tied to emergency response and involves delineation of "what should happen, when" and "who does what, where," at the time of an emergency. Preparedness includes the knowledge and capacity developed by individuals, organizations, communities, governments, and response organizations to anticipate, respond to, and recover from the impact of a hazard (PSC, 2015a). Nurses play an important role in preparedness by educating individuals and communities on disaster preparedness; working to reduce hazards in the home, in work settings, and within communities; by participating in drills and training exercises; and through the development of emergency operations plans and protocols (WHO & ICN, 2009). Within the hospital setting, the nursing role is one of leadership and advocacy, through participation on unit- and corporate-based committees and task forces and in the development of disaster protocols and exercises.

Health Care Emergency Operations Plans. An *emergency operations plan* (EOP) is a comprehensive document that describes strategies and frameworks for how emergencies or disasters will be planned for and managed and that delineates training requirements with the goal of increasing resilience. Accreditation Canada requires health care organizations to have policies and processes in place to respond to internal emergencies as well as those arising external to the organization that, owing to their size and impact, have the potential of affecting day-to-day operations and patient care.

Internal and External Disasters. *Internal disasters* refer to any situation that threatens or disrupts the daily, routine services of a health care facility. These situations present a potential danger to patients and staff and may or may not occur at the same time as an external event (Veenema & Woolsey, 2013). Some of the causes of internal disasters include bomb threats, chemical or radiological accidents, fire, spills, power and water loss, unavailability of staff, outbreaks of communicable disease, and violence. Internal disasters have the potential to result in a series of outcomes, including patient and staff evacuation, decreased levels of service, diversion of transportation (e.g., ambulance and air transport), and reallocation of patient care (Gebbie & Qureshi, 2013; Veenema & Woolsey, 2013).

External disasters are a result of events that originate outside of a health care organization. This type of disaster has the potential to threaten a facility when the consequences of the event create a demand for service that exceeds what is routinely available (Gebbie & Qureshi, 2013). External disasters may be the result of *mass casualty incidents*, which involve an influx of patients from a single incident and that exceed the capacity of a system to manage within its current resources. A health care organization can also experience an external disaster during an influx of patients who have been exposed to a hazardous material, or *chemical-biological-radiological-nuclear-explosive* (CBRNE) *event*.

Combined external–internal disasters occur as a result of external situations or events that trigger a response within the internal environment of a health care facility (Gebbie & Qureshi, 2013). In Canada, severe weather conditions (e.g., snowstorms) can result in a combined external–internal disaster. For example, the inability of staff to travel to work, coupled with an increased volume of trauma patients due to a winter storm, can precipitate a staffing crisis in the internal hospital setting. Consequently, remaining staff resources may be unable to address demands due to increased volumes and acuity in patients needing care.

Contents of Health Care Emergency Operations Plans. Most disaster response activities occur in the hospital setting. An effective EOP uses an all-hazards approach to ensure preparedness for any event and is able to be implemented almost automatically in an emergency or disaster situation (Markenson, 2013). A hospital EOP must be flexible and scaleable to the situation and consider actions required for emergencies that are a result of internal, external, or a combination of external–internal circumstances. Some plans further delineate disaster responses according to the level or to the organization's ability to respond. Furin (2016) describes a three-phase classification system that reflects the magnitude of a disaster relative to an organization's ability to respond:

Level 1 Disaster: The organization or community is able to effectively respond to the event utilizing its own resources.

Level II Disaster: The emergency or disaster situation requires support and assistance from sources external to the organization that can be attained through nearby agencies or communities.

Level III Disaster: The emergency or disaster situation exceeds the ability and resources available in the community, requiring support from provincial–territorial or federal-level organizations.

The EOP starts with a risk assessment that evaluates the likelihood of disasters for the organization or community. Potential hazards to consider include weather patterns; geographical location, age, and condition of the facility; industries in close proximity (nuclear plants or factories); and large-scale public events (Gebbie & Qureshi, 2013). The assessment also includes an evaluation of staffing resources needed under various situations and supplies considered to be essential. Stockpiles of medications

(analgesics, sedatives, vaccines, and antidotes); required personal protective equipment (PPE) (masks, splash suits, chemical-resistant gloves); and medical supplies (stretchers, ventilators, bandages, dressings) to support patient care should be identified, with processes for acquisition developed. Information technology requirements may include computers (for documentation and patient registration); televisions and radios (for external coverage of emergency events); telephones, two-way radios, and fax machines. Space and needed resources for emergency response (emergency operations centre, media centre, staffing and patient–family information centres, and patient surge locations) should also be included in the plan. Basic human-needs requirements (nonperishable food, water, accommodations, and rest areas) for staff and family members who stay and work for prolonged periods should be identified as essential resources.

Numerous challenges have been identified in the management of disaster situations. These include communication difficulties; lack of leadership, planning, and clear lines of accountability; inadequate surge capacity, casualty triage, transportation, and evacuation processes; poor safety, security, and control of entry points; patient identification and data tracking processes; management of resources; and resistance to planning initiatives (Andress, 2010a). Addressing these challenges in advance in the EOP will facilitate effective management. Components of a health care EOP are as follows:

1. *Activation of Emergency Status.* The EOP should outline how emergency or disaster notification is received. Notification of an internal event normally comes from an inpatient unit or department, based on staff observation and escalation; whereas, in an external disaster situation, notification may come from emergency medical services or the media. The EOP must describe how notification and escalation of emergency status occurs, when, and to whom.

2. *Communication Plan.* This portion of the EOP provides details highlighting internal and external communication processes that should take place between first responders and the hospital; among staff members (front-line and management staff); and between the hospital and family members of casualties. It is essential that response activities also include a designated individual who is prepared and able to effectively communicate with the public and the media (Nacos, 2013), through a *media communication plan.* Documentation tools and tracking forms are of assistance in enhancing communication between departments and with family members. Communication of decisions made, requests for support, and initiation and setup of emergency response centres follow a hierarchical process and this communication is a component of the Incident Management System (California Emergency Medical Services Authority [CEMSA], 2014; Gebbie & Qureshi, 2013).

3. *Plan for the Coordination of Patient Care.* This section of the EOP outlines processes for managing patient care with a specific focus on the area(s) most affected by the event; this might be the emergency department as the portal of entry for those injured or, in the case of an internal disaster, those areas directly affected by the situation. *Surge capacity* reflects an organization's ability to manage an unanticipated increase in patient numbers, with higher demands on the skills of the staff involved (Veenema, 2013a). Surge planning involves a calculation of the number of available beds and potential care locations (including potential transfers and discharges) and access to and availability of multidisciplinary staff and

supplies (backboards, ventilators, medications) (Lentz, Reid, & Primomo, 2013). A process for the suspension of normal daily services (e.g., elective surgeries, outpatient clinics) should be included in the plan, with triggers, should it be required.

4. *Staffing Plan.* This plan provides a detailed process for calling in additional staff when required (a process referred to as *fan-out*) to support surges in patient volumes and acuity and delineates processes for staff reassignment to areas with the highest volume, acuity level, and patient concentration. Staffing needs are determined based on the total number of care areas, the size of the disaster and anticipated number of patients, the type of event, and the medical problems that are anticipated to be seen relative to the incident (Veenema, 2013a). An inventory of staff skill sets across the facility assists with this process. Reassignment of staff is typically coordinated via the facility's emergency operations centre, through use of a *labour pool and staffing centre.*

5. *Equipment and Supply Plan.* This plan includes tracking of equipment and supplies that will be needed in an emergency response. These inventories should include medical (e.g., PPE, medications) and nonmedical (e.g., food, linen, water, fuel) supplies. Storage for the stockpiling of equipment and supplies should be considered and a process outlined for accessing additional resources from suppliers. Access to equipment and supplies is of particular importance in situations involving exposure to hazardous materials, as safe patient care cannot be provided without immediate access to PPE. The availability of equipment required in an emergency situation must be assessed on a regular basis, and a process for monitoring expiration dates and ensuring circulation of supplies before their expiration should be a component of planning activities (Markenson, 2013).

6. *Security Plan.* This plan outlines procedures for ensuring a secure work and patient care environment and is key to supporting safe response. This response includes procedures for instating *lockdown status* within the organization. Lockdown, a process that involves restricting access to entry points to a health care facility, should ideally be an instantaneous process (CEMSA, 2014). This process is of particular importance to control flow through the organization, accounting for patients and staff should evacuation be required; to prevent acts of violence or terrorism; and to avert entry of potentially contaminated patients to the hospital (Markenson, 2013). For example, in cases in which there is chemical, biological, radiological, or nuclear exposure, lockdown will assist in redirecting contaminated patients to a single designated point of entry, where decontamination can occur before entry to common areas.

7. *Documentation and Data Management Strategy.* This component of the EOP outlines how patients will be rapidly identified (also called *banded*) and tracked when moving within and across departments or institutions. Standard medical record items requiring documentation in a disaster include demographic data, brief medical history, medications and allergies, type of illness or injury, treatment provided, and patient disposition (Veenema, 2013a). Detailed records of the sickest patients, who are unable to self-identify, includes documenting characteristics (age, gender, clothing, tattoos, and piercings) to assist with identification and reunification. Due to the potential for loss of critical infrastructure (e.g., power, communication) during an emergency, backup paper-based systems should be created. Hand-held devices and smartphones may enhance and expedite documentation in the medical record (Veenema, 2013a).

8. *Deactivation and Recovery Process.* Deactivation and recovery processes should be outlined in the EOP, describing how emergency status will be terminated. Clear delineation as to who is able to deactivate disaster response activities, how this is to be done and when, as well as next steps to restore core services and operations is included.

9. *Post-Incident Debriefing Plan.* This plan provides guidelines as to when debriefing of individuals involved in emergency response will occur and in what format. Health care providers involved in disaster response are at high risk for stress, due not only to extended periods of demanding workload, but by the need to respond to families and the media while bearing witness to pain and suffering. Because stress on workers may continue for some time after the event, early debriefing will support coping and a return to normalcy. Debriefing also assists in improving components of the emergency plan and future response activities (Grigg & Hughes, 2010; Coyne-Plum & Meeker, 2013).

10. *Educational Plan.* An educational plan for emergency drills and training exercises should be outlined in the EOP and include dates, times, frequency, and format for testing the plan (Andress, 2010).

Testing of Emergency Plans. Organizations and staff respond to and recover from disaster situations based on their level of preparation, the culture of the organization, past experiences in dealing with emergencies, and the nature or scale of the situation (Veenema, 2013a; Markenson, 2013). Testing exercises are a key component of emergency management and are done to promote preparation, evaluate an organization's level of readiness, identify process gaps and alternate strategies, and assist in training staff in understanding and enacting response roles. While the most effective form of testing an EOP is its use in an actual disaster situation, other strategies, including traditional educational formats (e.g., lectures, case studies) and hands-on learning (e.g., tabletop exercises, computer simulations, role-play, drills), complement and enhance individual and organizational response (Andress, 2010a). Responders require an understanding of the core competencies of emergency preparedness, incident command, risk communication, and roles relative to other responders (WHO & ICN, 2009).

Response

Response occurs in the incident phase of the disaster management continuum, either on impact of an event (e.g., explosion, fire) or upon an imminent event (e.g., hurricane, tornado). The EOP is critical in this stage because it provides details and information as to how response initiatives should occur. Response involves execution of the plan, where trained and exercised staff are in place, possessing the knowledge of where they need to be and the skill to do what they need to do when confronted with an emergency situation. The goal of response is to save lives, reduce health impacts, ensure public safety, and meet the needs of individuals affected by the event (Gebbie & Qureshi, 2013). It is in the response phase that the Incident Management System is enacted and triage of patients occurs.

The nursing role is most visible in the response phase of a disaster. Nurses provide care in a variety of areas, including patient triage, emergency and trauma care, critical care, infection control and occupational health and safety, supportive and palliative care, and public health. Nurses are also pivotal in acute care, inpatient settings in disaster response because they receive the casualties who may require care on a longer-term basis as they recover from their injuries. Nurses may be required to work in a variety of alternate settings during the response phase, such as emergency aid shelters, homes, mass immunization sites, shelters, mortuaries, or makeshift clinics (WHO & ICN, 2009).

The Incident Management System. The Incident Management System (IMS) used in Canada is based on the incident command system that was developed as a result of mass wildfires that took place in California in the 1970s. These incidents were poorly managed as a result of competition for supplies and equipment between response agencies, precipitating the need for a systematic and coordinated process (Menzel & White, 2015). IMS is used by police, fire, emergency medical services, health care organizations, power utilities, and government agencies, as well as in many areas of the private sector.

IMS, an integrated and flexible framework that identifies disaster response roles, ensures that effective communication, incident command, and control are maintained during disaster response (Figure 72-2). Communication and teamwork between groups of people and departments that do not usually work together are emphasized (CEMSA, 2014). IMS in the hospital setting, also referred to as the *hospital incident command system (HICS)*, enables quick action, provides access to needed resources,

and ensures continuation of essential services through all phases of a disaster (Gebbie & Qureshi, 2013; DeAtley, 2010).

IMS is a modular organizational structure that can be used in small- and large-scale emergency situations. All directives, information, and requests flow up or down the hierarchical structure through a chain of command. Using this structure, organizations identify problems and develop and coordinate plans of action by delegated positions (CEMSA, 2014; DeAtley, 2010). Each position in the IMS structure has an accompanying job action, accountabilities, and a set of tasks and responsibilities that must be fulfilled. Typically, the role of *incident manager* is held by an individual with sound knowledge of the organization and of disaster management processes. The incident manager is in charge of the mission, directs response processes, and monitors and oversees deviations from the EOP. The incident manager appoints other command staff and establishes the emergency operations centre, which serves as the control point for disaster oversight (DeAtley, 2010; Gebbie & Qureshi, 2013).

IMS command roles are filled by individuals possessing knowledge of the tasks required to successfully address the emergency situation and include the following: (1) a *public information officer,* who is responsible for coordinating and overseeing public affairs. This includes providing information to the public and media, helping to create media releases,

FIGURE 72-2 Incident Management System. *IS,* information services; *IT,* information technology; *VP,* vice-president. Source: California Emergency Medical Services Authority. (2014). *Hospital incident command system guidebook* (Appendix D, p. D-2). Retrieved from *http://hicscenter.org/Shared%20Documents/Appendices/Appendix%20D%20 Potential%20Candidates_3.pdf.*

coordinating interviews and media tours, and developing question-and-answer sheets or other resources required; (2) a *safety officer,* whose role is to ensure the safety of staff, patients, visitors, and the facility during the emergency operation; (3) a *liaison officer,* who serves as a link to external agencies and emergency response services, and (4) a *medical–technical specialist,* who possesses the specific knowledge required (e.g., legal affairs, risk management, ethics, infectious diseases) to guide decision making and response actions (CEMSA, 2014; DeAtley, 2010).

Additional positions in the IMS structure include (1) a *logistics section chief,* who ensures that resources—including staff, fuel, and services to support staff (equipment, supplies, and food)—are available as needed; (2) a *finance section chief,* whose role is to monitor financial assets used; (3) a *planning section chief,* who is accountable for gathering information (data and research) and assisting with planning decisions; and (4) an *operations section chief,* who directs patient care activities and is responsible for work direction of staff at the scene of the incident (CEMSA, 2014; DeAtley, 2010; Gebbie & Qureshi, 2013). Unit-specific supervisors oversee activities at the ground or unit level and are required to report progress and difficulties in emergency response activities to people in the IMS structure if and when these arise.

Triage. Triage involves the sorting or ranking of casualties to prioritize health care needs and to allocate resources. It is a process that ensures "the right patient is in the right place, at the right time, so he/she may receive the right level of care" (Rice & Abel, 1992, p. 67). The Canadian Triage and Acuity Scale (CTAS) is used in emergency departments (EDs) in nonemergency or nondisaster situations (see Chapter 71, Table 71-2). Using this five-level scale, care providers assign high priority to those who are most critically ill, according to the seriousness of their condition, reported signs, and symptoms (CAEP, 2016; Bullard, Chan, Brayman, et al., 2014). Daily ED triage is described with greater detail in Chapter 71.

Triage in Disaster Situations. Effective and timely prehospital triage is pivotal to human survival, helping to ensure equitable distribution of patients to appropriate services and facilities through the health system. Although several mass casualty triage systems exist, one of the more common types, *simple triage and rapid treatment* (START), offers a systematic approach to triage that may be used to rank the seriousness of casualty injuries in a mass casualty incident (MCI) (Table 72-2). MCIs can be as simple as an overturned bus with five passengers or as severe as a collapsed building, a terrorist explosion, or a chemical or

biological event (Critical Illness and Trauma Foundation [CITF], 2001). This process, used at the disaster scene by first responders, involves rapid assessment and sorting of casualties by a *triage officer.* The START system is based on five clinical observations: (1) the person's ability to ambulate; (2) the presence of spontaneous breathing; (3) the respiratory rate (greater or less than 30 breaths per min); (4) perfusion and circulation (i.e., palpable radial pulse or visible capillary refill rate); and (5) mental status (as assessed by an ability to obey commands) (U.S. Department of Health and Human Services [USDHHS], 2016a). These parameters are referred to as *RPM* (respirations, perfusion, and mental status) (CITF, 2001; Romig, 2013).

Triage is followed by tagging and transportation to a medical facility or the provision of lifesaving interventions (e.g., intubation, defibrillation) by members of the first-response team. *Patient tagging* involves a system of coloured tags (see Figure 72-3) that

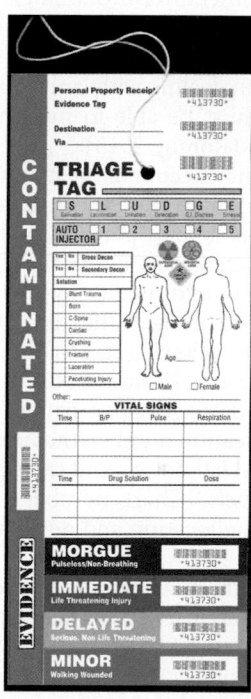

FIGURE 72-3 Triage tag. Source: Copyright © 2004, Steve Mann. This picture is released under the Shared Experience License, *http://eyetap.org/sel.txt.*

TABLE 72-2	SIMPLE TRIAGE AND RAPID TREATMENT (START)		
START Category/ Triage Tag Colour	**Type of Injury**	**Patient Condition and Examples of Presenting Features**	**Clinical Indicators**
Green "MINOR"	MINOR injuries Walking wounded; minor injuries	Sprains Lacerations	Able to ambulate
Yellow "DELAYED"	DELAYED Transport can be delayed; non–life-threatening	Open fractures Soft tissue wounds	Respiration rate: <30 breaths/min Perfusion: <2 sec Mental status: Follows commands
Red "IMMEDIATE"	Unstable; immediate transport needed; life-threatening, requiring immediate intervention	Shock Airway obstruction Unstable wounds	Respiration rate: >30 breaths/min Perfusion: capillary refill >2 sec Mental status: Does not follow commands
Black "EXPECTANT"	Deceased or expected to die owing to injuries	Massive head trauma Profound shock with multiple injuries	Respirations/spontaneous breathing: not breathing/apnea

Source: Adapted from: Romig, L. (2013). Disaster triage. In T. G. Veenema (Ed.), *Disaster nursing and emergency preparedness for chemical, biological, and radiological terrorism and other hazards* (3rd ed.). New York: Springer; U.S. Department of Health and Human Services (USDHHS). (2016). *START adult triage algorithm.* Retrieved from *http://www.remm.nlm.gov/startadult.htm;* and Critical Illness and Trauma Foundation (CITF). (2001). *START Simple triage and rapid treatment.* Retrieved from *http://citmt.org/Start/default.htm.*

are used to designate both the seriousness of the injury and the likelihood of survival (Romig, 2013; USDHHS, 2016a; CITF, 2001). A green tag using the START approach indicates a *minor* injury (i.e., walking wounded: sprains, lacerations), and is used for patients who may be able to assist with their own care. A yellow tag indicates a non–life-threatening injury where transport can be delayed (e.g., open fractures, soft tissue wounds). A red tag is used to indicate a life-threatening injury requiring immediate intervention (e.g., shock, airway obstruction, unstable wounds). These patients require immediate intervention and transport for survival. A black tag is used to identify those casualties who are deceased or who are unlikely to survive as a result of their injuries (e.g., profound shock with multiple injuries) (Markenson, 2013; Romig, 2013; USDHHS, 2016a). Triage of children, or people who look like children, is done using the *JumpSTART* framework, which addresses the physiological differences between children and adults (USDHHS, 2016b; Romig, 2008).

Disaster Triage in the Hospital Setting. Triage of casualties in a disaster situation differs from routine emergency triage processes. Disaster response is dependent on the size of the organization, the number of staff and amount of resources available, and past experience in dealing with large-scale events. All health care organizations must be able to implement disaster triage with minimal notice (Romig, 2013).

When an emergency occurs in the community, hospitals are typically notified by emergency medical services in the field, and the facility prepares for a potential influx of patients. This preparation includes gathering necessary equipment, including first-aid supplies, PPE, and medications (e.g., analgesics, antidotes). As patients are triaged, they are given a pre-assigned medical record number, allowing care to be provided immediately, without formal registration (Romig, 2013). Disaster charts should include a prestamped triage slip, a patient identification band with medical identification number, medical and nursing documentation forms, and laboratory and radiographic examination requisitions and labels. Chart numbers should be entered onto a log so patient allocation and destination can be tracked (Romig, 2013).

As patients enter the ED, they are greeted by a triage team. In mass-casualty incidents, several triage teams may be used, usually consisting of one to two experienced triage nurses, a physician (the triage officer), a porter (who assists with patient transportation), and a registration clerk (who assists with patient banding and data entry on the tracking form) (Romig, 2013). Disaster triage in the hospital setting must be rapid and should be conducted in less than 15 seconds per patient. Following this rapid assessment, patients assigned with higher levels of acuity are directed to a treatment location in the ED. In situations in which patient volume is high and ED space is limited, another predesignated area of the facility to accommodate surge may be used for the care of less-acute casualties.

Recovery and Rehabilitation

Recovery and rehabilitation takes place in the post-incident phase of the disaster management continuum (WHO & ICN, 2009) and is the process through which staff, an organization, or a community regains the ability to function after a disaster. Services have typically been disrupted during the disaster response, and the goal is to return to a state of "normal." This includes the restoration of vital services normally provided by an organization, within a community, or by local government, rebuilding infrastructure and meeting the needs of the population served (WHO

& ICN, 2009; Markenson, 2013). Nurses are critical in the recovery and rehabilitation phase and in re-establishing health care infrastructure and must consider the psychosocial impact of a disaster on its survivors. Nursing functions related to the care and coordination of health care services, case management, identification, and implementation of casualty referrals (e.g., social services) are essential for return to normal activities. Nurses play a key role in the documentation, review, and evaluation of the disaster response as well as in championing changes to EOPs and to corporate, municipal, and provincial or territorial policy (WHO & ICN, 2009).

Critical Incident Stress Management. The massive effort put forth by health care workers in response to a catastrophic event is critical to a community's recovery. Health care workers, who are already at risk of experiencing high levels of stress and burnout, are at increased risk following participation in a disaster event (Public Health Agency of Canada [PHAC], 2011). A critical incident is a situation faced by individuals involved in a disaster that causes them to experience strong emotional reactions that have the potential to interfere with their ability to return to a normal state of functioning at work and at home during or after the event (McMahon, 2010; PHAC, 2011). Multiple deaths; inadvertent exposure to hazardous materials; exposure to shocking sights, sounds, or smells; and incidents with high media coverage are examples of critical incidents. Challenging triage decisions, the volume of seriously injured people, limited resources, ethical issues that accompany disasters, concern for personal safety and liability, lack of sleep, heavy workload, time pressures and unmet basic needs, and political and organizational pressures also significantly contribute to the stress and an individual's resilience in the aftermath of a disaster event (Coyne-Plum & Meeker, 2013; McMahon, 2010; PHAC, 2011).

All disasters have the potential to cause psychological stress to the individuals involved. This stress can persist for an extended period and is influenced in part by the nature of the event and the individual's age, pre-existing coping mechanisms, role in the event, and prior medical and psychological history (Coyne-Plum & Meeker, 2013). Although the psychological trauma that results from involvement in a critical incident varies, common symptoms range from insomnia to excessive sleeping, from loss of appetite to overeating, and a loss of interest in activities normally considered pleasurable (PHAC, 2011). Post-traumatic stress disorder (PTSD) is a response to a specific, identifiable stressor that severely affects an individual's ability to function at a normal level. The diagnosis is given to individuals who have experienced or witnessed situations involving death or serious injury or a threat to self or others. PTSD can result in the development of symptoms in the first few weeks or months, or up to years following an event, that include avoidance, numbing, or the individual re-experiencing the event, causing significant impairment in function (McMahon, 2010; Coyne-Plum & Meeker, 2013). PTSD requires ongoing psychological counselling, psychiatric support, or both.

Critical incident stress management (CISM) or debriefing is a comprehensive approach to preventing and managing the emotional trauma that can be a result of involvement in a disaster response. Strategies may include pre-incident education; individual crisis intervention and on-the-scene support; defusing and debriefing sessions; support services for families and children; and follow-up professional intervention (Meeker, Coyne-Plum, & Veenema, 2013; McMahon, 2010). Debriefing occurs as a part of the incident review within the first 24 to 72 hours, particularly among police officers, firefighters, and medical teams. *Defusing sessions* occur within a few hours of the incident and may be offered as a group discussion prior to staff going off duty. This process involves brief discussion of the incident and assistance with stress management (Meeker, Coyne-Plum, & Veenema, 2013).

THE ROLE OF NURSING LEADERSHIP IN DISASTER PREPAREDNESS AND RESPONSE

Leadership at all levels is essential for a positive outcome after a disaster event. However, nurses who hold formal leadership roles have extended responsibilities to ensure the delivery of safe care at all stages of the disaster management continuum. Leadership in times of disaster involves recognition of the uncertainty created during the response and requires open, consistent communication, flexibility, and creative problem solving (Druce, 2009). Clear communication of expectations and goals, and a commitment to cause with an expectation of success, is an antecedent to a positive outcome. Nursing leadership plays a role in advocating for individual and community needs and services in the recovery and rehabilitation stage and ensuring that staff have the emotional support needed (WHO & ICN, 2009; Druce, 2009). At the executive level, nurse leaders play a key role in ensuring organizations are prepared for response; providing oversight for recovery processes; creating safe work environments; influencing policy and financial decisions; and ensuring that needed resources and supports are available and accessible before, during, and following a disaster event (Fahlgren & Drenkard, 2002).

NATURAL AND HUMAN-MADE OR INDUCED DISASTERS

A *disaster* can be defined in numerous ways, but the term is generally interpreted to mean a destructive event that disrupts the normal functioning of a community. There are two general classifications of disasters: *natural disaster* and *human-made or human-induced disasters*. Disease outbreaks and epidemics are usually considered to be "natural" events, but they can also be classified as "human-made" disasters when disease-causing organisms are used as an agent of terrorism with the goal of inducing large-scale epidemics. Because of these variations, disease outbreaks and epidemics are described in a separate section of this chapter. Table 72-3 presents a timeline of notable disasters in Canadian history.

Natural Disasters

Due to its size and geographical location, our country poses a host of threats. Its landforms and variation in weather patterns makes severe weather and the threat of natural hazards a significant reality for Canadians. *Natural disasters* are caused by nature or the environment, are often unpredictable, and can happen at a rapid or slow rate. Natural disasters include extreme natural events such as forest fires, avalanches, landslides, storm surges, cold or heat waves, hurricanes, tsunamis, floods, drought, earthquakes, and volcanic eruptions (PSC, 2015a). Human-caused damage to the environment and the resultant climate change has also altered the intensity, pattern, and distribution of natural forces, contributing to an increase in the number of natural disasters (Veenema & Landesman, 2013).

Human-Made or Human-Induced Disasters

Human-made, also referred to as *human-induced disasters*, can be accidental or deliberate and can cause injuries, deaths, and long-term consequences for individuals and communities. *Accidental human-made disasters* include industrial accidents, chemical spills, inadvertent release of nuclear energy, explosions (e.g., from hazardous materials such as chemicals, nuclear materials, fuel), contamination, fires, structural collapse, large transportation accidents, and power outages. *Deliberate human-made disasters* include warfare, civil unrest, and acts of terrorism. Computer viruses or cyber-attacks are classified as human-made disasters because of their cost and potential impact on critical infrastructure.

Natural and human-made disasters can trigger one another, with both having the ability to elicit secondary disasters. These events, referred to as *synergistic disasters*, often occur simultaneously. As an example, an earthquake causes an explosion at a nuclear plant, requiring large-scale evacuation and causing illness and population displacement. The synergistic effects are exacerbated by death and devastation created by each event (Veenema & Woolsey, 2013).

Terrorism. September 11, 2001, marks a tragic day of death and destruction, when two of four hijacked planes crashed into the Twin Towers in New York City, the others crashing into the Pentagon in Washington, DC, and a field near Shanksville, Pennsylvania. More recently, terrorist attacks across several public sites in Paris, France, (2015) and in a nightclub in Orlando, Florida, (2016) further illustrate the far-reaching impact of terrorism and the critical need for emergency planning.

Terrorism involves intentional and overt actions that are committed to cause fear, panic, destruction, injury, and death in service of political, religious, or ideological goals. The intent of a terrorist event is to intimidate the public or to compel a specific person, government, or international organization to take specific action. Terrorist events include threats, assassinations, kidnappings, hijackings, bomb scares and bombings, and computer cyber-attacks. The use of chemical or biological agents as the element of a terrorist attack is referred to as *chemical terrorism* or bioterrorism, respectively (Croddy & Ackerman, 2013). In both cases, the terms refer to a type of terrorist event involving the deliberate spreading of microbes or chemical toxins with the intent of causing disease or death in animals, plants, or humans (Croddy & Ackerman, 2013). Plans for dealing with each type of event, coupled with advanced training exercises and availability of necessary protective personal equipment, are essential to a safe, expedient response.

Chemical–Biological–Radiological–Nuclear–Explosive Events. A *CBRN event* refers to any situation in which weapons of a *chemical, biological, radiological,* or *nuclear* nature are used with the goal of causing harm. A CBRN event can also be the result of a civilian or military accident. More recently, the term CBRNE event has been used, with "E" representing situations in which an *explosive or incendiary device* is used. *Weapons of mass destruction* refers to a broad range of weapons that have the potential to affect the health and the well-being of a large population.

Under ideal circumstances, decontamination following a CBRNE event will occur in the field, prior to the casualties' arrival to hospital. A response in the field may not occur when exposure is a result of a terrorist event as casualties are likely to flee the site, not knowing they have been contaminated, and pose a risk to others. People may arrive at health care facilities

TABLE 72-3 BEST-KNOWN CANADIAN DISASTERS

Year	Disaster and Place	Approximate # of Fatalities	Injured/Infected	Evacuated
1862	Smallpox epidemic (nationwide)	20 000		0
1885	Smallpox epidemic, Montreal, Quebec	6 000	9 600	0
1903	Rock slide in town of Frank (Frank Slide), Turtle Mountain, Alberta	70	23	0
1910	Avalanche, Rogers Pass, Bear Creek, British Columbia	62	0	0
1912	Tornado, Regina, Saskatchewan	28	100	2 500
1917	Harbour explosion, Halifax, Nova Scotia	2 000	9 000	6 000
1918	Spanish influenza pandemic (Spanish flu) across Canada	50 000	2 000 000	0
1922	Wildfire, Timiskaming District, Ontario	43	0	11 000
1942	Building fire, Knights of Columbus hostel, St. John's, Newfoundland	100	100	0
1954	Hurricane Hazel, Ontario	81	0	7 472
1958	Mining accident, Springhill, Nova Scotia	75	99	0
1971	Landslide, St-Jean-Vianney, Quebec	31	99	1 500
1974	Airplane crash, Rea Point, Northwest Territories	32	0	0
1978	Soviet satellite, COSMOS 954, came down in the Northwest Territories, scattering 65 kg of radioactive material over a wide area	0	0	0
1985	Airplane crash, Gander, Newfoundland	256	0	0
1986	Train derailment, Hinton, Alberta	23	71	0
1987	Tornado, Edmonton, Alberta	27	600	1 700
1992	Westray mining accident, Plymouth, Nova Scotia	26	0	0
1996	Floods, Saguenay, Quebec	10	0	15 825
1997	Bus crash, St. Joseph de la Rive, Quebec	43	0	0
1998	Plane crash, Peggy's Cove, Nova Scotia	230	0	0
1998	Ice storm, Eastern Ontario, Quebec, Maritimes	35	0	0
2000	Contaminated water, Walkerton, Ontario	7	2 300	0
2000	Tornado, Pine Lake, Alberta	12	140	1 000
2003	Severe acute respiratory syndrome (SARS), Toronto, Ontario	44	375	0
2005	Legionnaire's disease outbreak, Toronto, Ontario	23	112	0
2008	Listeriosis outbreak across Canada	22	57	0
2009–2010	New strain of pandemic influenza	425	8 582	0
2010	Hurricane Igor, Cape Race, Newfoundland	1	0	300
2011	Slave Lake Wildfire, Slave Lake, Alberta	1	0	12 055
2011	First Air Flight 6560 crash near Resolute Bay, Nunavut	12	0	3
2012	Wildfire, Timmins, Ontario	0	0	1 000
2012	Legionnaire's disease epidemic, Quebec, Quebec	13	180	0
2012	Train derailment, Burlington, Ontario	3	45	0
2013	Alberta floods, Calgary, Alberta	4	0	100 000
2013	Rail disaster, Lac-Mégantic, Quebec	47	0	2 000
2014	Nursing home fire, near L'Isle-Verte, Quebec	32	15	0
2014	Terrorist shooting, Ottawa, Ontario	2	0	0
2014	Wildfire due to heatwave, British Columbia	0	0	4 500
2016	School shooting, La Loche, Saskatchewan	4	0	0
2016	Forest fire, Fort McMurray, Alberta	0	0	90 000
2017	Quebec City, Mosque shooting	6	19	0

Sources: Adapted from Stanhope, M., Lancaster, J., Jessup-Falcioni, H., et al. (2011). *Community health nursing in Canada* (Table 16-2, p. 506). Toronto: Mosby; and PSC. (2015e). *The Canadian Disaster Database*. Retrieved from *http://www.publicsafety.gc.ca/cnt/rsrcs/cndn-dsstr-dtbs/index-eng.aspx*.

in large or small numbers and without advanced notice or may delay seeking treatment until they become symptomatic or once public information has been shared about potential exposure (Crowe, 2010; Holland & Cawthon, 2015). Consequently, CBRNE events have significant implications for the health and safety of those who come into contact with casualties and, to ensure public safety, health care staff should assume, until it has been proven otherwise, that all individuals presenting to hospital have *not* undergone adequate decontamination (Koenig, Boatright, Hancock, et al., 2008; Veenema, 2013b). Hospitals must have plans in place to address CBRNE exposure, which requires advanced planning and input from nurses, physicians, medical toxicologists, hazardous materials (HAZMAT) teams, and health and safety team members (Moore, Geller, & Clark, 2015). The use of evidence-informed protocols and systems for triage and decontamination, combined with the application of appropriate PPE, is essential for safe response, not only for first responders

in the field but also for health care workers in hospital settings (Veenema, 2013b; Holland & Cawthon, 2015). Despite significant focus over the last decade on emergency planning and preparation, there is still broad discomfort across the health care sector with addressing and responding to these types of events (Moore, Geller, & Clark, 2015).

Early identification, diagnosis, and treatment of people exposed to CBRNE substances is essential to preventing secondary injury and avoiding contamination of the public, staff, and the health care facility (Croddy & Ackerman, 2013; Rihl-Pryor, 2013), requiring people to be decontaminated *before* medical care or surgical intervention is provided. **Decontamination** is the process of removing or neutralizing a hazardous agent from the environment, property, equipment, or a life form, through the use of water, cleansers, or neutralizers (Veenema, 2013b; Moore, Geller, & Clark, 2015). Decontamination accomplishes the following: (1) decreases absorption and toxicity of the agent; (2) reduces contamination of other people and equipment by substances on casualties' bodies, clothing, or belongings; and (3) prevents potential closure of a health care organization where people who have been contaminated may seek care (Koenig et al., 2008). The degree of casualty contamination is affected by four factors: (1) the contact time with the agent; (2) the concentration of the agent; (3) temperature, which affects the agent's permeative characteristics; and (4) the physical state of the agents (i.e., liquids, solids, vapours) (Koenig et al., 2008).

For a safe response in the hospital setting, it is necessary to have decontamination teams and advanced preparation for activation of a decontamination area complete with showers, scrubbing instruments, and ventilation (Moore, Geller, & Clark, 2015; Holland & Cawthon, 2015). Decontamination is a multi-disciplinary strategy that includes participation from a team of trained and prepared nursing and physician staff, security and housekeeping, engineering and occupational health and safety members, and porters. Participation in casualty decontamination requires significant education and training before a potential event on the application and use of PPE, activation of decontamination equipment (showers, tents, etc.), setup of operation zones, and decontamination and scrubbing processes, through regular, full-scale hospital drills (Koenig et al., 2008; Moore, Geller, & Clark, 2015). Hospitals are to ensure they have adequate amounts of antidotes, adequate numbers of showers and decontamination tents, appropriate availability of PPE, and staff trained to participate in response (Veenema, 2013b). Triage will require, when possible, identification of the contaminant and an assessment of the degree of contamination and casualty distress. Information about the event and the casualties is to be provided on an ongoing basis to the Incident Command Centre, which will oversee operations and decision making for response efforts.

Casualties should be segregated from other patient populations until appropriate decontamination takes place, and security must be in place to prevent inadvertent contamination (Holland & Cawthon, 2015). Similar to decontamination in the field, decontamination in hospital settings requires activation of *Operation or Decontamination Zones.* Typically, these zones are created through the use of barricades to determine points of entry from one area to the next. Crowd control, safety, and security are of primary concern—first responders, health care workers, and other patients who have physical contact with contaminated casualties, their belongings, or both without appropriate protection may also require decontamination (Koenig et al., 2008; Holland & Cawthon, 2015). Lockdown of entry points to a health care facility, with the exception of a designated access point for those who require decontamination, is one strategy to prevent inadvertent exposure of patients and staff to the contaminant (Markenson, 2013).

Three operation zones—*hot, warm,* and *cold*—support triage and decontamination activities. The *hot zone* is the area farthest from hospital entry and requires all responders to don full PPE. Minimal triage is provided in this area and is limited to life-saving measures and administration of antidotes. The *warm zone* is typically adjacent to the ED and is the location where staff in full PPE provide decontamination of casualties (Veenema, 2013b). Nonambulatory patients will be scrubbed by staff through the use of hoses, trailers, or tents, using conveyor belts and trolley systems, whereas ambulatory patients will be directed to remove contaminated clothing and then assist with personal scrubbing and decontamination, using hoses and warm showers. Patients with the most severe symptoms receive priority

for decontamination. The *cold zone* is the treatment location adjacent to the warm zone and is the location where patients, once decontaminated, enter. All staff who have worked in hot or warm zones also require decontamination prior to entering the cold zone. A more thorough triage occurs in the cold zone, following which people are directed to treatment areas (Veenema, 2013b).

The health and safety of health care providers is essential in a CBRNE event. A combination of respirators and protective gear (goggles, boots, full-facepiece respirators, protective suits, chemically resistant gloves) must be used (Holland & Cawthon, 2015; Veenema, 2013b). Because of the equipment that is required to be worn, workers must undergo medical screening or surveillance (including a full set of vital signs) before donning and after removing protective gear. Staff also need to be monitored by a designated surveyor while involved in the decontamination process (Koenig et al., 2008). Staff who have higher-than-normal blood pressure; rashes, open sores, or wounds; a previous history of nausea, vomiting, or diarrhea; an upper respiratory infection or history of respiratory illness (e.g., asthma); allergies; sensitivities or phobias (e.g., claustrophobia); or who are potentially or known to be pregnant may not participate in the decontamination process. Time in decontamination gear is usually limited to 30 minutes or less because extreme heat, poor ventilation, and the heavy weight of the suit cause fatigue and other common adverse effects (Veenema, 2013b). These risks also make it necessary to monitor hydration status before and after protective gear is donned.

Biological Agents of Terrorism. Biological terrorism involves the deliberate use of microbial pathogens or toxins, the effects of which may not be known until many hours or days after exposure. Terrorist attacks using biological agents represent challenges for health care providers because they can be difficult to detect and can have a prolonged impact on health care facilities. Contaminants can range from accidental releases of biohazardous waste to intentional exposure from bioweapons (Koenig et al., 2008; Rihl-Pryor, 2013). People exposed in a bioterrorist attack typically do not require decontamination (the exception being exposure to anthrax spores), and most agents are noncontagious (Croddy & Ackerman, 2013). Hospitals should have access to a variety of antidotes for biological agents and should have plans that include means for urgent acquisition of antidotes from other sources (Moore, Geller, & Clark, 2015). Table 72-4 summarizes general information regarding biological agents of terrorism. The pathogens most likely to be used as biological weapons include anthrax, smallpox, botulism, plague, tularemia, and hemorrhagic fever. Anthrax, plague, and tularemia can be treated effectively with antibiotics if the organisms are not resistant and if there is an available and sufficient quantity of the appropriate drug. Smallpox can be prevented or ameliorated by vaccination, even if it is first given after initial exposure. Botulism can be treated with antitoxin. In most cases, supportive treatment is the primary mode of care for viruses that cause hemorrhagic fever (Centers for Disease Control and Prevention [CDC], 2013a).

Chemical Agents of Terrorism. Typically, a chemical event is overt, with a sudden onset in a localized area, and has potential for vast spread, making rapid containment and decontamination essential (Rihl-Pryor, 2013; Koenig et al., 2008). Chemically exposed individuals are more likely to seek care in large numbers and to have early, external evidence of contamination (Powers, 2010). These events are most likely to cause significant limitations of health care personnel, time, equipment, and space and have potential to cause major disruptions in clinical care due to their rarity and the psychological impact on both casualties and

TABLE 72-4   BIOLOGICAL AGENTS OF TERRORISM

Pathogen and Description	Clinical Manifestations	Transmissibility	Treatment
Anthrax (Bacillus anthracis) ***Inhalation*** • Bacterial spores multiply in the alveoli • High mortality rate • Toxins cause hemorrhage and destruction of lung tissue	• Incubation period: 1–7 days; can be delayed up to 60 days (2 months) • Abrupt onset • Dyspnea • Diaphoresis • Fever • Cough • Chest pain • Septicemia • Shock • Meningitis • Respiratory failure • Widened mediastinum (seen on chest radiograph)	• No person-to-person spread • Found in nature; most commonly infects wild and domestic hoofed animals • Spread through direct contact with bacterium and its spores • Spores are dormant, encapsulated bacteria that become active when they enter a living host	• Antibiotics prevent systemic manifestations • Effective only if treated early • Ciprofloxacin (Cipro) is the treatment of choice • Penicillin • Doxycycline • Post-exposure prophylaxis for 30 days (if vaccine available) or 60 days (if vaccine not available) • Vaccine has limited availability
Cutaneous • 95% of anthrax infections • Least lethal form • Spores enter skin through cuts or abrasions • Handling of contaminated animal skin products • Toxins destroy surrounding tissue	• Incubation period: 2–6 days • Small papule resembles an insect bite • Advances to a depressed, black ulcer • Swollen lymph nodes in adjacent areas • Edema	—	—
Gastro-Intestinal • Ingestion of contaminated, undercooked meat • Intestinal lesions in ileum or cecum • Acute inflammation of intestines	• Abdominal pain • Anorexia • Ascites • Diarrhea • Hematemesis • Incubation period: 3–7 days • Nausea • Sepsis • Vomiting	—	—
Smallpox (Variola Major and Minor Viruses) • Canada ended routine vaccination in 1972 • Global eradication declared in 1980	• Incubation period: 7–17 days • Sudden onset of symptoms • Fever • Headache • Myalgia • Lesions that progress from macules to papules to pustular vesicles • Malaise • Back pain	• Direct person-to-person spread • Highly contagious • Transmitted by handling contaminated materials • Transmitted in air droplets	• Cidofovir (Vistide) under testing • Isolation for containment • No known cure • Vaccine available for those exposed • Vaccinia immune globulin (VIG) available
Botulism (Clostridium botulinum) • Spore-forming anaerobe • Found in soil • Seven different toxins • Lethal bacterial neurotoxin • Can die within 24 hr	• Incubation period: 12–36 hr • Abdominal cramps • Diarrhea • Nausea • Vomiting • Cranial nerve palsies (diplopia, dysarthria, dysphonia, dysphagia) • Skeletal muscle paralysis • Respiratory failure	• Spread through air or food • No person-to-person spread • Improperly canned foods • Contaminated wound	• Induce vomiting • Enemas • Antitoxin • Mechanical ventilation • Penicillin • No vaccine available • Toxin can be inactivated by heating food or drink to 100°C for at least 10 min

TABLE 72-4 BIOLOGICAL AGENTS OF TERRORISM—cont'd

Pathogen and Description	Clinical Manifestations	Transmissibility	Treatment
Plague (Yersinia pestis) • Bacteria found in rodents and fleas **Forms** • Bubonic (most common) • Pneumonic • Septicemic (most deadly)	• Incubation period: 2–4 days • Hemoptysis • Cough • High fever • Chills • Myalgia • Headache • Respiratory failure • Lymph node swelling	• Direct person-to-person spread • Transmitted through flea bites • Ingestion of contaminated meat	• Antibiotics only effective if administered immediately • Drug of choice: streptomycin or gentamicin • Vaccine under development • Hospitalization • Isolation for containment
Tularemia (Francisella tularensis) • Bacterial infectious disease of animals • Mortality rate about 35% without treatment	• Incubation period: 3–10 days • Sudden onset • Fever • Swollen lymph nodes • Fatigue • Sore throat • Weight loss • Pneumonia • Pleural effusion • Ulcerated sore from tick bite	• No person-to-person spread • Aerosol or intradermal route • Spread by rabbits and ticks • Contaminated food, air, water	• Gentamicin treatment of choice • Streptomycin, doxycycline, and ciprofloxacin are alternatives • Vaccine in developmental stage
Hemorrhagic Fever • Caused by several viruses, including Marburg, Ebola, Lassa fever, yellow fever, and Rift Valley fever	• Fever • Conjunctivitis • Headache • Malaise • Prostration • Hemorrhage of tissues and organs • Nausea • Vomiting • Hypotension • Organ failure	• Carried by rodents and mosquitoes • Direct person-to-person spread by body fluids • Virus can be aerosolized	• No intramuscular injections • No anticoagulants • Isolation for containment • Ribavirin (Virazole) effective in some cases • Supportive treatment only, for most • Vaccine available for yellow fever only

Source: Adapted from Lewis, S. L., Heitkemper, M. M., Dirksen, S. R., et al. (2011). *Medical-surgical nursing: Assessment and management of clinical problems* (8th ed., Table 69-12). St. Louis: Mosby.

TABLE 72-5 CHEMICAL AGENTS OF TERRORISM BY TARGET ORGAN OR EFFECT

Nerve	Blood	Pulmonary	Blister or Vesicants
• Sarin (isopropyl methylphosphonofluoridate) • Tabun (ethyl N,N-dimethylphosphoramidocyanidate) • Soman (pinacolyl methylphosphonofluoridate) • GF (cyclohexylmethylphosphonofluoridate) • VX (O-ethyl S-[2-diisopropylaminoethyl] methylphosphonothiolate)	• Hydrogen cyanide • Cyanogen chloride	• Phosgene • Chlorine • Vinyl chloride	• Nitrogen and sulphur mustards • Lewisite (an aliphatic arsenic compound, 2-chlorovinyldichloroarsine) • Phosgene oxime

responders (Croddy & Ackerman, 2013; Moore, Geller, & Clark, 2015).

Certain chemicals may be used as agents of terrorism because their toxic properties produce significant physiological and psychological effects. Chemical agents are categorized according to their target organ or effect (Andress, 2010b). For example, sarin, a highly toxic nerve gas that enters the body through the eyes and the skin, acts by paralyzing the respiratory muscles, potentially causing death within minutes of exposure. Phosgene, a colourless gas normally used in chemical manufacturing, can cause severe respiratory distress, pulmonary edema, and death when it is inhaled at high concentrations for a long enough time (Andress, 2010b). Mustard gas, an agent used during World War I, is yellow to brown in colour and has a garlic-like odour and acts by irritating the eyes and causing skin burns and blisters.

Protocols to treat people with chemical exposure are varied but are specific for the causative agent (Croddy & Ackerman, 2013). Table 72-5 details the effects chemical agents have on various human organs.

Radiological and Nuclear Agents of Terrorism. Radiological and nuclear substances can also be categorized as agents of terrorism. Radiological dispersal devices (RDDs), or "dirty bombs," consists of chemical explosives mixed with radioactivity (Karam, 2013). When an RDD is detonated, the blast is likely to lead to widespread radioactive contamination through dispersed dust, smoke, and other material into the surrounding environment (CDC, 2013b). Uranium and iodine-131, the radioactive materials used in RDDs, typically generate only enough radiation to cause immediate serious illness to those in close proximity to the explosion. Health care personnel will confront large volumes of patients, some with high levels of radioactivity contamination and many others with high levels of anxiety without presenting illness from exposure (Karam, 2013). The main danger of an RDD results from the explosion itself, with those patients suffering traumatic injury combined with significant exposure to radiation having substantially worse prognosis (Karam, 2013). Because radiation cannot be seen, has no scent, and is unable to be felt or tasted, measures to limit contamination, like covering the patient's nose and mouth and prompt decontamination (e.g., through the use of a decontamination shower), are best initiated in a timely manner (CDC, 2013b). Ionizing radiation, which comes from a nuclear bomb or damage to a nuclear reactor, represents a serious threat to the health and safety of casualties and the environment. Although exposure to ionizing radiation may or may not include skin contamination, decontamination procedures should be initiated immediately in circumstances in which radioactive contaminants are present (Andress, 2010b).

Explosive Agents of Terrorism. MCIs involving explosives have occurred globally, with the most known examples being in London, Madrid, Oklahoma City, Brussels, Burkina Faso, and Mogadishu. Compared to other events, injuries that are a result of terrorist attacks with explosives typically involve younger civilian casualties, with critical severity, requiring longer hospitalization and surgical interventions, and result in higher mortality rates (Sacco, 2013). Whether the result of an accident or terrorist event, the use of explosion devices (TNT, dynamite) in acts of terrorism results in blunt, crush, penetrating, and burn injuries as well as injuries from the blast itself (Sacco, 2013). *Blast injuries* occur from the supersonic overpressurization shock wave that results from the explosion, having the potential to cause mass injury to multiple body systems (Plurad, 2011). This shock wave primarily causes damage to the lungs, gastro-intestinal tract, and middle ear; the injuries are the result of casualties being blown by the blast wind against objects and structures. *Crush injuries* (i.e., blunt trauma) often ensue from explosions that occur in confined spaces and result from structural collapse (e.g., falling debris). Some explosive devices contain materials that are projected during the explosion (e.g., shrapnel), leading to *penetrating injuries* (Plurad, 2011).

EPIDEMICS AND PANDEMICS

Nurses are required to have an understanding of the etiology and impact of communicable disease, whether a consequence of a natural disaster (e.g., contaminated water during flooding) or a result of a deliberate act (e.g., bioterrorism) (CNA, 2012). Morbidity, mortality, and disruption from an infectious disease epidemic overwhelm a community and its infrastructure. Lessons learned as a result of SARS (2003) and the H1N1 (2009) infectious disease outbreaks highlight the enormous toll on individuals, communities, and health care workers and the need for advanced planning.

Communicable diseases may occur in an individual or a group of individuals. The term *outbreak* refers to an illness occurring amongst a cluster of individuals. When the number of cases of a communicable disease exceeds the normal expected occurrence during a given period, it is referred to as an **epidemic.** If transmission of the disease is widespread and affects large numbers of people across several countries or continents or globally, it is considered to be a **pandemic** (Slepski, 2010). The investigation and management of an outbreak requires recognition; investigation of the source, mode of transmission, and risk factors for

infection; and implementation of appropriate control measures (Veenema & Woolsey, 2013).

Severe Acute Respiratory Syndrome

Severe acute respiratory syndrome, also known as *SARS,* refers to an outbreak that occurred primarily in Canada and Asia in 2003. SARS is a contagious, severe, febrile respiratory illness caused by a coronavirus and characterized by a fever of 38°C or higher; myalgia; headache; malaise; chills; a dry, nonproductive cough; and shortness of breath (Farquharson & Baguley, 2003). The illness is spread through close contact with someone who is infected with the virus, such as those living in the same household, providing unprotected care to someone with SARS, or having direct contact with respiratory secretions of someone affected by SARS.

The SARS outbreak was a critical juncture in Canadian emergency management because it demonstrated the tremendous impact a communicable disease outbreak could have on individuals, communities, and the economy (PSC, 2015e). SARS cost billions of dollars across Asia and Canada as a result of its impact on health care, critical infrastructure, trade, and tourism and served as a wake-up call for health care institutions, governments, and health care providers, highlighting Canada's inadequacies in responding to public health threats. Since 2003, our country has recognized the central role of health care services in disaster mitigation and response, resulting in enhanced planning initiatives. Stockpiles of medications and PPE, and mobile hospital response teams have been put in place in anticipation of future communicable disease outbreaks (Amaratunga, Carter, O'Sullivan, et al., 2008).

Outbreak Management

Studies of the SARS outbreak across numerous countries have provided insight into the need for diligent infection control practices and disease monitoring. The effects of globalization and the ease of air travel have led not only to the "shrinking" of the world but also to the global mobility of people, food, viruses, and bacteria. In the Middle Ages, cities and towns could close their gates and erect high walls to keep out disease; now, our global problems demand a global response. The strategies used to prevent and contain communicable diseases are fundamental, and nurses play an essential role in understanding common outbreak management strategies. This knowledge helps nurses working in acute and chronic care and within community settings to implement containment interventions and to understand how best to protect themselves and their patients.

Outbreak Management Strategies. Outbreak management refers to the strategies used to prevent the spread of communicable disease among clusters of people. Management of outbreaks within health care facilities begins with recognition of potentially exposed patients by trained staff or through public health notification. Case-finding, early-detection, and treatment strategies not only improve the health of the infected individuals but also prevent transmission to others.

Surveillance is the ongoing and systematic process of gathering, analyzing, and disseminating data on communicable diseases or events to detect changes in trends or distribution of diseases. In the case of disease outbreaks, surveillance processes gather the data that epidemiologists analyze to determine the *who, what, when, where, and why* behind the outbreak (Stanhope, Lancaster, Jessup-Falcioni, et al., 2017). There have been major efforts across our country to develop and strengthen early-warning mechanisms

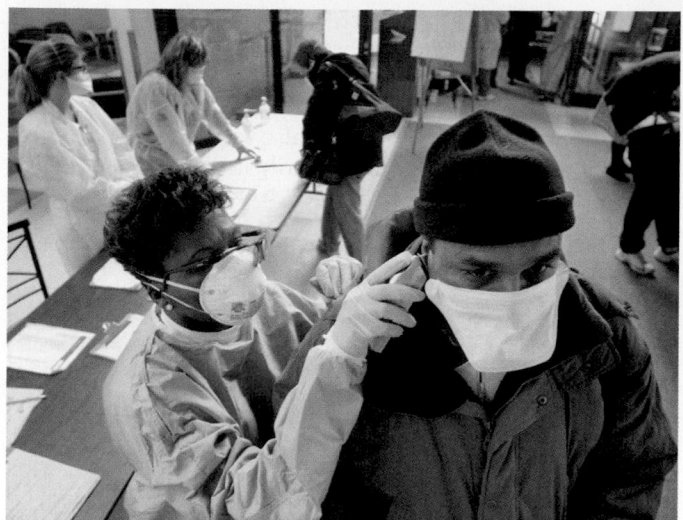

FIGURE 72-4 A critical strategy in managing the severe acute respiratory syndrome (SARS) outbreak was screening patients for possible signs of the disease. Source: CP PHOTO/J.P. Moczulski.

FIGURE 72-5 Particle mist created upon sneezing. Source: Photo by Andrew Davidhazy/RIT.

at local and global levels. The Public Health Agency of Canada (PHAC) operates a number of national surveillance systems on health problems that range from chronic diseases and congenital anomalies to the *Respiratory Virus Detection Surveillance System* and *FluWatch*. These systems are in place to observe and scrutinize changes in the number of febrile and respiratory illnesses across the country. Many communicable diseases are considered to be reportable or notifiable diseases and must be reported to local public health units (PHAC, 2017). Nurses are often involved, both formally and informally, in different levels of the surveillance system, being the first to detect an outbreak through abnormal clusters of illness among populations, for example, in a school setting.

Isolation is an outbreak management strategy that separates infected people from those assumed to be unaffected during a period of the disease's communicability (Figure 72-4). In Toronto, the SARS epidemic demonstrated how rapidly airborne diseases can spread through crowded spaces, EDs, or shared rooms (Varia, Wilson, Sarwal, et al., 2003). Infected individuals may be confined to a hospital room or unit or to their home. There are varying types of isolation, depending on the disease, its route of transmission, and the period of communicability.

Quarantine involves the isolation of people who have been exposed, or potentially exposed, to an infection or contagious disease but who are not yet sick or showing signs of illness. These individuals are assumed to be incubating the disease and may be infectious to other people before they display symptoms. The quarantine period is the longest usual incubation period for the disease (Richter, 2010). During the SARS outbreak, thousands of people, mostly in the Toronto area, were quarantined at home for 10-day periods, the incubation period for SARS (Farquharson & Baguley, 2003). Although most people complied voluntarily during the SARS event, all provinces and territories have public health legislation that enforces compliance with a quarantine order. Owing to circumstances and the number of staff potentially infected with the virus, a special form of quarantine, called *work quarantine,* was used for health care workers during the SARS outbreak. This level of quarantine allowed health care workers who may have been exposed to SARS to continue working as

long as they followed certain requirements, including wearing N95 respirators at work and on any public commute; home confinement when not at work; and self-monitoring for temperature and signs and symptoms of SARS.

Pandemic Planning

Pandemic influenza is a highly infectious outbreak of influenza that spreads rapidly around the world, with much more serious consequences than the usual effects of seasonal influenza. There are two primary routes by which the influenza virus exits the respiratory tract of an infected person: (1) expulsion of the virus into the air through sneezing (Figure 72-5), coughing, speaking, or breathing, or through aerosol-generating medical procedures and (2) by direct transfer of respiratory secretions to another person or surface. Coupled with the short incubation period (from 1 to 3 days) and the fact that the virus can be transmitted before an infected person is symptomatic, it is essential that nurses use appropriate infection control techniques to prevent the spread of influenza (see the "Evidence-Informed Practice" box, "Influenza Transmission and the Role of Personal Protective Respiratory Equipment").

In June 2009, the beginning of a global influenza pandemic was confirmed as the illness was identified across 74 countries, raising the WHO alert from a "5" (widespread human transmission) to a "6" (pandemic phase) (Slepski, 2010). The impact of pandemic influenza is vast and far-reaching. Owing to this concern and the need for vigilant monitoring of this illness in humans, the WHO monitors the risk as determined by its experts and an analysis of the situation in countries around the world. For further information about the current phase of pandemic influenza alert and a detailed explanation of the phases of pandemic alert, follow the WHO link in the Resources at the end of this chapter.

Faced with the demands of a novel H1N1 pandemic, in recent years, hospitals and communities have shifted much of their focus in emergency planning to pandemic planning. In the hospital setting, inpatient areas and critical services are key to an effective pandemic response (Hota, Fried, Burry, et al., 2010). The duration and acuity of patient illness, impact on hospital systems, and prior experiences with the H1N1 pandemic reflect a need for advanced surge capacity planning across clinical settings. H1N1 brings a surge in patient volume, affecting a

EVIDENCE-INFORMED PRACTICE
Research Highlight

Influenza Transmission and the Role of Personal Protective Respiratory Equipment: An Assessment of the Evidence

The following are the consensus findings of the Expert Panel on Influenza and Personal Protective Respiratory Equipment (PPRE).

Conclusions on the Modes of Influenza Transmission

1. Ballistic-, nasopharyngeal-, tracheo-bronchial–, and alveolar-sized particles are all emitted from the human respiratory tract.
2. Evidence about the relative contributions of the different modes of transmission to the spread of influenza is sparse and inconclusive.
3. There is evidence that influenza is transmitted primarily at short range.
4. There is evidence that influenza can be transmitted via inhalation of tracheo-bronchial– and alveolar-sized particles at short range.
5. There is evidence that deposition of nasopharyngeal-sized particles in the upper respiratory tract can cause infection.
6. There is evidence that contact transmission can occur. The current weight of evidence suggests that transmission of influenza by inhalation is more probable than by indirect contact.
7. The evidence is lacking to determine whether long-range transmission of influenza occurs, but it cannot be ruled out.

Conclusions on Protective Measures Against Influenza Transmission

1. The primary elements of protection against influenza transmission are engineering and administrative controls. When exposure to an infected person is required or unavoidable, PPRE is the final layer of protection.
2. N95 respirators protect against the inhalation of nasopharyngeal-, tracheo-bronchial–, and alveolar-sized particles.
3. Surgical masks worn by an infected person may play a role in the prevention of influenza transmission by reducing the amount of infectious material that is expelled into the environment.
4. Both surgical masks and N95 respirators offer a physical barrier to contact with contaminated hands and ballistic trajectory particles.
5. The efficiency of the filters of surgical masks to block penetration of alveolar- and tracheo-bronchial–sized particles is highly variable. When combined with the inability of these masks to ensure a sealed fit, these factors suggest that surgical masks offer no significant protection against the inhalation of alveolar- and tracheo-bronchial–sized particles.
6. The efficiency of the filters of surgical masks to block penetration of nasopharyngeal-sized particles is unknown. The lack of a sealed fit on a surgical mask will allow for the inhalation of an unknown quantity of nasopharyngeal-sized particles.

Reference for Evidence

Council of Canadian Academies. (2007). *Influenza transmission and the role of personal protective respiratory equipment (PPRE): An assessment of the evidence* (pp. 5, 8). Ottawa: Council of Canadian Academies. Retrieved from *http://www.scienceadvice.ca/uploads/eng/assessments%20and%20 publications%20and%20news%20releases/flu/(2007-12-19)_influenza_ ppre_final_report.pdf.*

ETHICAL DILEMMAS
Duty to Provide Care During a Pandemic

Situation

A senior undergraduate nursing student is in the last semester of her program. The Centre for Emergency Preparedness and Response, part of the Public Health Agency of Canada, has declared that areas in her province are in the midst of the initial wave of a pandemic influenza. Because the university she attends is in a city that has not yet had any reported cases of pandemic influenza, her university is open, and both her classes and her clinical practice placements are continuing. Her parents are worried about her safety and are urging her to return home to her rural community, 200 kilometres north of the city. She does not know what to do because she wants to finish her program.

Important Points for Consideration

There will be a massive need for health care workers during a pandemic owing to the number of people who are ill and in need of care; health care workers will also be ill. Many provincial and territorial pandemic influenza plans discuss the utilization of health science students in response to the overwhelming health human resource requirements. Universities are preparing pandemic influenza plans and have developed contingency plans for students who live in residence or cannot travel to their home communities during a pandemic. Nursing programs have begun developing specific guidelines and decision-making protocols for use during a pandemic because nursing students participate in the health care system.

Clinical Decision-Making Questions

1. What guidance is provided by the Canadian Nurses Association (CNA) *Code of Ethics* to help nurses address their ethical dilemmas about providing care during a pandemic?
2. The student is not yet a registered nurse. What are the legal obligations for her, as a student, during a pandemic?
3. What is the registered nurse's duty to provide care during a pandemic? What are the ethical considerations?

---

younger population of individuals, many with severe lung injury as a result of the illness. Prolonged ventilation resulting in an extended surge situation has a significant impact on the health care system as a whole (Hota et al., 2010). With a pandemic wave that typically lasts 8 to 10 weeks, consideration of staff, patient triage, equipment and supplies, space to accommodate patients, and systems to respond to the pandemic event are key to preparedness and response activities (Hota et al., 2010).

Ethical Issues During a Disaster or Pandemic. Either in connection with experiences with SARS or in anticipation of a major health disaster such as a pandemic, nurses have raised tough ethical questions. These include questions like, who gets access to critical care unit services, ventilators, and respiratory support in hospital and which sectors of the population should be given priority to receive vaccines and antivirals during a pandemic? During a disaster situation, the primary health focus shifts from obtaining the best possible health outcomes for the individual patient to protecting the health and safety of the population as a whole, which is both the moral and the legal mandate of public health (Gostin, Bayer, & Fairchild, 2003). Many of these ethical dilemmas are about balancing the best interests of the entire population, which is referred to as the "public good," with the rights of the individual. The duty to provide care, when care poses a risk to self and loved ones, highlights the ethical implications for all health care providers (see the "Ethical Dilemmas" box). Nurses and other health care workers have expressed the conflict they feel between their professional and legal obligations to their patients and their responsibilities to themselves and their families (CNA, 2017). Since the SARS outbreak, there have been a number of ethical frameworks, articles, and resources created to provide guidance for nurses, other health care workers, and decision makers in health care and government settings. Many of these resources can be found in the Resources list at the end of this chapter.

Vulnerable Individuals and Populations. Special attention, in all the phases of a disaster or emergency, must be given to vulnerable individuals and marginalized groups. Failure to address the physical and psychological impact of a disaster in a timely and comprehensive manner can lead to long-term challenges and mental health issues. Individuals with pre-existing health conditions, disabilities, and mental health issues; women; people who are frail; people who are homeless; recent immigrants; children; and older adults are among the more vulnerable of the population and are at higher risk for the negative impacts of a disaster (WHO & ICN, 2009; Slepski, 2010). Where possible, these populations should be pre-identified as a part of emergency preparation, with the creation of specific plans to address their unique needs. Vulnerable populations often have limited resources, and their ability to recover is affected by their culture, support systems, and previous experiences. In the aftermath of a disaster, nurses are key to offering reassurance, education, and referral to needed resources to these higher-risk populations. An understanding of stress and the impact of stress, while offering strategies to cope, is a key component of the nursing role.

DISASTER NURSING

With an increasing number of global disasters has come recognition of the need for increased health care preparedness. **Disaster nursing** involves the provision of nursing care, advocacy, and health promotion within the context of a disaster situation. Nurses, owing to their position and numbers, are essential in disaster mitigation, preparedness, response, and recovery (CNA, 2012; WHO & ICN, 2009). Nurses fill a variety of roles throughout the disaster management continuum. Eric Laroche, former WHO assistant director general for Health Action in Crises, states, "Nurses are often the first medical personnel on site after disaster strikes. In disaster situations, nurses are called upon to take roles as first responder, direct care provider, on-site coordinator of care, information provider or educator, mental health counsellor or triage officer" (WHO & ICN, 2009, pp. 5–6). Therefore, the need for nurses to develop competencies in this growing field is vital.

When disaster strikes, the demand for nurses is much greater than for other health care providers. Opportunities for nursing abroad in countries affected by disaster also exist through humanitarian networks and volunteer agencies. Disaster nursing, irrespective of the location of the disaster, requires application of basic nursing knowledge and skills in difficult environments with scarce resources, rapidly changing conditions, and large volumes of patients. Disaster nursing involves collaboration with other health care providers, first responders, and individuals not commonly worked with, requiring an ability to shift focus in care while working within the parameters of the laws in place in the area of work (WHO & ICN, 2009). The International Council of Nurses (ICN) has a mission to advance nurses and to bring nursing together worldwide (ICN, 2006; WHO & ICN, 2009). Recognizing the valuable role that nurses play in disaster responses, the ICN believes that "nurses with their technical skills and knowledge of epidemiology, physiology, pharmacology, cultural familial structures, and psychological issues can assist in disaster preparedness programs, as well as during disasters" (ICN, 2006, p. 2). The *ICN Framework of Disaster Nursing Competencies* (WHO & ICN, 2009) was created as an underpinning for the development of additional advanced competencies among nurses, globally. These competencies have been included in the Resources section at the end of this chapter.

CASE STUDY

Pepper Spray

Profile

It is 1636 hours on a Thursday in the month of May, in the emergency department of a downtown hospital in a major Canadian city. It has been an extremely busy day, and the triage nurse is working with the corridors fully occupied by patients, many of whom have been waiting a day or longer for inpatient beds. Several ambulances are waiting to off-load their patients from stretchers. The nurse receives a call from emergency medical services informing her of the need to be prepared for the potential arrival of patients from a nearby protest rally. She is told that the protesters breached the security fences and the police intervened by using significant amounts of pepper spray. On-site first responders (emergency medical services) have conducted some decontamination on site; however, many of the protesters fled on foot before decontamination.

Source: thomas koch/Shutterstock.com.

Subjective Data

- Patients arrive within 6 minutes, with the following complaints:
  - Eye burning; some patients have temporary blindness
  - "Skin is burning"

Objective Data

- High levels of panic and anxiety
- Runny nose and watery eyes
- Severe coughing; some patients with shortness of breath

Collaborative Care

Decontamination shower and scrubbing are ordered before any medical intervention.

Discussion Questions

1. What risk factors do patients who require decontamination pose to an emergency department?
2. ***Priority decision:*** Identify priority actions the nurse will need to take in order to prepare for potential patient arrival.
3. Who should the nurse inform regarding the potential arrival of these patients?
4. What actions must be taken to manage patients who have been contaminated?
5. What equipment might be needed to care for contaminated patients?
6. ***Priority decision:*** What are the primary concerns of a triage nurse in this situation?
7. What information will the nurse need to obtain from contaminated patients?
8. What actions should the nurse take to ensure the safety of staff and patients currently in the emergency department?

evolve

Answers are available at *http://evolve.elsevier.com/Canada/Lewis/medsurg.*

REVIEW QUESTIONS

The number of the question corresponds to the same-numbered objective at the beginning of the chapter.

1. A chemical spill has occurred at a nearby industrial site. The first responders report that approximately 20 casualties need to be transported to the emergency department after decontamination at the site. What is this scenario an example of?
   a. An emergency
   b. A natural disaster or hazard
   c. A human-made or human-induced disaster
   d. An emergency response plan

2. Individuals and families must assume responsibility for taking appropriate steps to ensure they have the basics of what might be required following an emergency or disaster. Which list of items should be included in an individual emergency preparedness kit?
   a. Batteries, fresh fruits and vegetables, cups and plates
   b. Canned soups and stews, can opener, 2 L of water per day per person
   c. Fresh bread, frozen vegetables, lighter or matches
   d. 1 L of water per day per person, utensils, blankets, and sleeping bags

3. Which of the following statements *best* describes disaster nursing?
   a. Provision of nursing care, advocacy, and health promotion
   b. Provision of medical care and teaching
   c. Development and review of emergency operations plan and policy
   d. Provision of nursing care and coordination of health care interventions

4. Which of the following is a component of a comprehensive emergency operations plan?
   a. A closure strategy
   b. A documentation and data management strategy
   c. A pandemic plan
   d. A transfer policy

5. Which activity is correlated with the recovery and rehabilitation phase?
   a. Development of an emergency plan
   b. Conducting emergency exercises and drills
   c. Conducting critical incident debriefing with responders
   d. Completing construction to build a flood-resistant emergency department

6. Which of the following statements best describes the Incident Management System (IMS)?
   a. IMS is an administrative structure that can be used in large-scale emergency situations.
   b. IMS involves a circular organizational structure where all participants are interlinked.
   c. IMS involves a modular organizational structure that can be used in small- and large-scale situations.
   d. IMS may be activated only by municipal or federal agencies.

7. Which of the following statements related to disaster triage in hospitals is correct?
   a. Hospital and emergency department disaster triage is conducted by first responders.

b. The Canadian Triage and Acuity Scale was specifically designed for disaster triage.
   c. Disaster triage should be done in 2 minutes or less.
   d. Disaster triage involves a triage team composed of one to two nurses, a physician, a porter, and a registration clerk.

8. A nurse is assisting first responders during a mass casualty incident involving a bus rollover in an isolated rural community. Using the colour triage codes outlined in the START algorithm, place the following casualties in order of highest to lowest priority:
   a. A 38-year-old female who is obese and dyspneic and has an upper thigh deformity
   b. A 40-year-old male, minimally responsive, with shallow respirations, bleeding from the mouth
   c. An older adult female, unresponsive, with a large scalp wound and a large amount of blood noted
   d. A 14-year-old female, screaming, with lower back pain
   e. An 8-year-old male, crying, with bloody gauze to the forehead

9. Which of the following is an example of a human-made disaster?
   a. A terrorist attack
   b. A pandemic
   c. A hurricane
   d. A severe ice storm

10. Which of the following biological agents of bioterrorism has no effective treatment?
   a. Anthrax
   b. Botulism
   c. Smallpox
   d. Hemorrhagic fever

11. Which of the following situations is an example of a chemical-biological-radiological-nuclear-explosive (CBRNE) event?
   a. Dissemination of anthrax spores to a department in an office building
   b. A train derailment
   c. An outbreak of seasonal influenza
   d. Forest fires

12. Which of the following examples meets the criteria for a pandemic?
   a. A cluster of clients on an inpatient unit with diarrhea
   b. Acquired immune deficiency syndrome (AIDS)
   c. A school that has been closed as a result of flulike symptoms in children in three classrooms
   d. Sudden acute respiratory syndrome (SARS) in Asia and Toronto

1. c; 2. b; 3. a; 4. b; 5. c; 6. c; 7. d; 8. b, c, a, e, d; 9. a; 10. d; 11. a; 12. b.

© evolve

For even more review questions, visit *http://evolve.elsevier.com/Canada/Lewis/medsurg.*

REFERENCES

Amaratunga, C., Carter, M., O'Sullivan, T., et al. (2008). *Caring for nurses in public health emergencies: Enhancing capacity for gender-based support mechanisms in emergency preparedness planning.* Ottawa: Canadian Policy Research Networks. Retrieved from *http://www.cprn.org/documents/49473_EN.pdf.* (Seminal).

Andress, K. (2010a). Healthcare facility preparedness. In R. Powers & E. Daly (Eds.), *International disaster nursing.* Cambridge, UK: Cambridge University Press. (Seminal).

Andress, K. (2010b). Nuclear, biologic and chemical agents of mass destruction. In P. K. Howard & R. A. Steinmann (Eds.), *Sheehy's emergency nursing* (6th ed.). St. Louis: Mosby. (Seminal).

Bullard, M. J., Chan, T., Brayman, C., et al. (2014). Revisions to the Canadian emergency department triage and acuity scale (CTAS) guidelines. *Canadian Journal of Emergency Medicine, 16*(06), 485–489. doi:10.2310/8000.2014.012014.

California Emergency Medical Services Authority (CEMSA). (2014). *Hospital incident command guidebook* (5th ed.). Retrieved from *http://www.emsa.ca.gov/media/default/HICS/HICS_Guidebook_2014_10.pdf.*

Canadian Association of Emergency Physicians. (2016). *CTAS: Implementation Guidelines.* Retrieved from *http://caep.ca/resources/ctas/implementation-guidelines.*

Canadian Nurses Association (CNA). (2012). *Position statement: Emergency preparedness and response.* Retrieved from *https://cna-aiic.ca/~/media/cna/page-content/pdf-fr/ps119_emergency_preparedness_2012_e.pdf?la=en.*

Canadian Nurses Association. (2017). *Code of ethics for registered nurses.* Retrieved from *https://www.cna-aiic.ca/html/en/Code-of-Ethics-2017-Edition/files/assets/basic-html/page-1.html#.*

Canadian Red Cross. (2016a). *Make a plan.* Retrieved from *http://www.redcross.ca/how-we-help/emergencies-and-disasters-in-canada/for-home-and-family/make-a-plan.*

Canadian Red Cross. (2016b). *Emergencies and disasters in Canada.* Retrieved from *http://www.redcross.ca/how-we-help/emergencies-and-disasters-in-canada.*

Centers for Disease Control and Prevention (CDC). (2013a). *Viral hemorrhagic fevers.* Retrieved from *www.cdc.gov/ncidod/dvrd/spb/mnpages/dispages/vhf.htm.*

Centers for Disease Control and Prevention (CDC). (2013b). *Frequently asked questions (FAQs) about dirty bombs.* Retrieved from *https://emergency.cdc.gov/radiation/dirtybombs.asp.*

College of Nurses of Ontario (CNO). (2014). *Competencies for entry-level registered nurses.* Retrieved from *http://www.cno.org/globalassets/docs/reg/41037_entrytopracitic_final.pdf.*

Coyne-Plum, K. C., & Meeker, E. C. (2013). Understanding the psychosocial impact of disasters. In T. G. Veenema (Ed.), *Disaster nursing and emergency preparedness for chemical, biological, and radiological terrorism and other hazards* (3rd ed.). New York: Springer.

Critical Illness and Trauma Foundation (CITF). (2001). *START Simple triage and rapid treatment.* Retrieved from *http://citmt.org/Start/default.htm.* (Seminal).

Croddy, E., & Ackerman, G. (2013). Biological and chemical terrorism: A unique threat. In T. G. Veenema (Ed.), *Disaster nursing and emergency preparedness for chemical, biological, and radiological terrorism and other hazards* (3rd ed.). New York: Springer.

Crowe, A. (2010). Biological preparedness and response. In R. Powers & E. Daly (Eds.), *Disaster nursing international.* Cambridge, UK: Cambridge University Press.

DeAtley, C. (2010). Healthcare facilities incident command. In R. Powers & E. Daly (Eds.), *International disaster nursing.* Cambridge, UK: Cambridge University Press. (Seminal).

Druce, S. (2009). Leadership and management in a disaster. In D. S. Adelman & T. J. Legg (Eds.), *Disaster nursing: A handbook for practice.* Sudbury, MA: Jones & Bartlett. (Seminal).

Fahlgren, T. L., & Drenkard, K. N. (2002). Healthcare system disaster preparedness, part 2: Nursing executive role in leadership. *Journal of Nursing Administration, 32*(1), 531–537. (Seminal).

Farquharson, C., & Baguley, K. (2003). Responding to the severe acute respiratory syndrome (SARS) outbreak: Lessons learned in a Toronto emergency department. *Journal of Emergency Nursing, 29*(3), 222–228. doi:10.1067/men.2003.109. (Seminal).

Furin, M. A. (2016). *Disaster Planning: Categorizing Disasters.* Retrieved from *https://emedicine.medscape.com/article/765495-overview#a2.*

Gebbie, K. M., & Qureshi, K. (2013). Disaster management. In T. G. Veenema (Ed.), *Disaster nursing and emergency preparedness for chemical, biological, and radiological terrorism and other hazards* (3rd ed.). New York: Springer.

Gostin, L. O., Bayer, R., & Fairchild, A. L. (2003). Ethical and legal challenges posed by SARS: Implications for the control of severe infectious disease threats. *Journal of the American Medical Association, 290*(24), 3229–3237. doi:10.1001/jama.290.24.3229. (Seminal).

Government of Canada (2015a). *Get Prepared: Your emergency preparedness guide.* Retrieved from *http://www.getprepared.gc.ca/cnt/rsrcs/pblctns/yprprdnssgd/index-en.aspx.*

Government of Canada. (2015b). *The Disaster Assistance Response Team (DART).* Retrieved from *http://www.forces.gc.ca/en/operations-abroad-recurring/dart.page.*

Grigg, M., & Hughes, F. (2010). Disaster mental health. In R. Powers & E. Daly (Eds.), *International disaster nursing.* Cambridge, UK: Cambridge University Press. (Seminal).

Holland, M. G., & Cawthon, D. (2015). Personal protective equipment and decontamination of adults and children. *Emergency Medicine Clinics of North America, 33*(1), 51–68. doi:10.1016/j.emc.2014.09.006.

Hota, S., Fried, E., Burry, L., et al. (2010). Preparing your intensive care unit for the second wave of H1N1 and future surges. *Critical Care Medicine, 38*(4), e110–e115. doi:10.1097/CCM.0b013e3181c66940. (Seminal).

Indigenous and Northern Affairs Canada. (2017). *Indigenous and Northern Affairs Canada (INAC) National On-reserve Emergency Management Plan.* Retrieved from *https://www.aadnc-aandc.gc.ca/eng/1324572607784/1324572653216#chp8.*

International Council of Nurses (ICN). (2006). *Position statement: Nurses and disaster preparedness.* Retrieved from *http://www.icn.ch/images/stories/documents/publications/position_statements/A11_Nurses_Disaster_Preparedness.pdf.* (Seminal).

Karam, A. (2013). Radiological incidents and emergencies. In T. G. Veenema (Ed.), *Disaster nursing and emergency preparedness for chemical, biological, and radiological terrorism and other hazards* (3rd ed.). New York: Springer.

Koenig, K. L., Boatright, C. J., Hancock, J. A., et al. (2008). Health care facility–based decontamination of victims exposed to chemical, biological and radiological materials. *American Journal of Emergency Medicine, 26*(1), 71–80. doi:10.1016/j.ajem.2007.07.004. (Seminal).

Lentz, C., Reid, D., & Primomo, B. (2013). Management of burn mass casualty incidents. In T. G. Veenema (Ed.), *Disaster nursing and emergency preparedness for chemical, biological, and radiological terrorism and other hazards* (3rd ed.). New York: Springer.

Markenson, D. (2013). Hospital and emergency department preparedness. In T. G. Veenema (Ed.), *Disaster nursing and emergency preparedness for chemical, biological, and radiological terrorism and other hazards* (3rd ed.). New York: Springer.

McMahon, M. M. (2010). Hospital impact: Emergency Department. In R. Powers & E. Daly (Eds.), *International disaster nursing.* Cambridge, UK: Cambridge University Press. (Seminal).

Meeker, E. C., Coyne-Plum, K., & Veenema, T. G. (2013). Management of the psychosocial effects of disasters. In T. G. Veenema (Ed.), *Disaster nursing and emergency preparedness for chemical, biological, and radiological terrorism and other hazards* (3rd ed.). New York: Springer.

Menzel, D. C., & White, H. L. (Eds.), (2015). *The state of public administration: Issues, challenges, and opportunities.* New York: Routledge.

Moore, B. L., Geller, R. J., & Clark, C. (2015). Hospital preparedness for chemical and radiological disasters. *Emergency Medicine Clinics of North America, 33*(1), 37–49. doi:10.1016/j.emc.2014.09.005.

Nacos, B. L. (2013). Crisis communication: The role of the media. In T. G. Veenema (Ed.), *Disaster nursing and emergency preparedness for chemical, biological, and radiological terrorism and other hazards* (3rd ed.). New York: Springer.

Plurad, D. S. (2011). Blast injury. *Military Medicine, 176*(3), 276–282.

Powers, R. (2010). Decontamination. In R. Powers & E. Daly (Eds.), *International disaster nursing.* Cambridge, UK: Cambridge University Press. (Seminal).

Public Health Agency of Canada (PHAC). (2011). *Self-care for caregivers.* Retrieved from *http://www.phac-aspc.gc.ca/publicat/oes-bsu-02/caregvr-eng.php.*

Public Health Agency of Canada (PHAC). (2017). *Infectious diseases.* Retrieved from *https://www.canada.ca/en/public-health/services/infectious-diseases.html.*

Public Safety Canada (PSC). (2015a). *An emergency management framework for Canada: Ministers responsible for emergency management* (2nd ed.). Retrieved from *http://www.publicsafety.gc.ca/cnt/rsrcs/pblctns/mrgnc-mngmnt-frmwrk/index-eng.aspx.*

Public Safety Canada (PSC). (2015b). *Emergency management.* Retrieved from *http://www.publicsafety.gc.ca/cnt/mrgnc-mngmnt/index-eng.aspx.*

Public Safety Canada (PSC). (2015c). *Canada's national disaster mitigation strategy.* Retrieved from *http://www.publicsafety.gc.ca/cnt/rsrcs/pblctns/mtgtn-strtgy/index-eng.aspx.*

Public Safety Canada (PSC). (2015d). *Emergency management planning.* Retrieved from *http://www.publicsafety.gc.ca/cnt/mrgnc-mngmnt/mrgnc-prprdnss/mrgnc-mngmnt-plnnng-eng.aspx.*

Public Safety Canada (PSC). (2015e). *The Canadian disaster database.* Retrieved from *https://www.publicsafety.gc.ca/cnt/rsrcs/cndn-dsstr-dtbs/index-en.aspx.*

Rice, M., & Abel, C. (1992). S. B. Sheehy (Ed.), *Emergency nursing: Principals and practice.* St. Louis, MO: Mosby Year Book. (Seminal).

Richter, J. E. V. (2010). Public health response. In R. Powers & E. Daly (Eds.), *International disaster nursing.* Cambridge, UK: Cambridge University Press. (Seminal).

Rihl-Pryor, E. (2013). Early recognition and detection of biological events. In T. G. Veenema (Ed.), *Disaster nursing and emergency preparedness for chemical, biological, and radiological terrorism and other hazards* (3rd ed.). New York: Springer.

Romig, L. (2008). *The JumpSTART pediatric MCI triage tool: Principles of multicasualty triage.* Retrieved from *http://www.jumpstarttriage.com/JumpSTART_and_MCI_Triage.php.* (Seminal).

Romig, L. (2013). Disaster triage. In T. G. Veenema (Ed.), *Disaster nursing and emergency preparedness for chemical, biological, and radiological terrorism and other hazards* (3rd ed.). New York: Springer.

Sacco, T. L. (2013). Traumatic injury due to explosives and blast effects. In T. G. Veenema (Ed.), *Disaster nursing and emergency preparedness for chemical, biological, and radiological terrorism and other hazards* (3rd ed.). New York: Springer.

Slepski, L. A. (2010). Pandemic planning. In R. Powers & E. Daly (Eds.), *International Disaster Nursing.* Cambridge, UK: Cambridge University Press. (Seminal).

St. John Ambulance. (2016). *Emergency preparedness information.* Retrieved from *http://www.sja.ca/English/Community-Services/Pages/Emergency%20Response/Emergency-Response-Services-Home.aspx.*

Stanhope, M., Lancaster, J., Jakubec, S. L., et al. (2017). *Community health nursing in Canada* (3rd ed.). Toronto: Elsevier.

U.S. Department of Health and Human Services: Radiation Emergency Medical Management (USDHHS-REMM). (2016a). *START adult triage algorithm.* Retrieved from *http://www.remm.nlm.gov/startadult.htm.*

U.S. Department of Health and Human Services: Radiation Emergency Medical Management (USDHHS-REMM). (2016b). *JumpSTART pediatric triage algorithm.* Retrieved from *http://www.remm.nlm.gov/startpediatric.htm.*

Varia, M., Wilson, S., Sarwal, S., et al. (2003). Investigation of a nosocomial outbreak of severe acute respiratory syndrome (SARS) in Toronto, Canada. *Canadian Medical Association Journal, 169*(4), 285–292. (Seminal).

Veenema, T. G. (2013a). Emergency medical consequence planning for special events, mass gatherings, and mass casualty incidents. In T. G. Veenema (Ed.), *Disaster nursing and emergency preparedness for chemical, biological, and radiological terrorism and other hazards* (3rd ed.). New York: Springer.

Veenema, T. G. (2013b). Decontamination and personal protective equipment. In T. G. Veenema (Ed.), *Disaster nursing and emergency preparedness for chemical, biological, and radiological terrorism and other hazards* (3rd ed.). New York: Springer.

Veenema, T. G., & Landesman, L. Y. (2013). Natural disasters. In T. G. Veenema (Ed.), *Disaster nursing and emergency preparedness for chemical, biological, and radiological terrorism and other hazards* (3rd ed.). New York: Springer.

Veenema, T. G., & Woolsey, C. (2013). Essentials of disaster planning. In T. G. Veenema (Ed.), *Disaster nursing and emergency preparedness for chemical, biological, and radiological terrorism and other hazards* (3rd ed.). New York: Springer.

World Health Organization and International Council of Nurses (WHO & ICN). (2009). *ICN framework of disaster nursing competencies.* Retrieved from *http://www.icn.ch/images/stories/documents/networks/DisasterPreparednessNetwork/Disaster_Nursing_Competencies_lite.pdf.* (Seminal).

RESOURCES

Canadian Disaster Database (Public Safety Canada)
http://www.publicsafety.gc.ca/index-eng.aspx

Canadian Pandemic Influenza Plan for the Health Sector
http://www.phac-aspc.gc.ca/cpip-pclcpi/

Canadian Red Cross
http://www.redcross.ca/

Government of Canada—Get Prepared
http://www.GetPrepared.ca

**Government of Canada—Emergency Management
Organizations**
*http://www.getprepared.gc.ca/cnt/rsrcs/mrgnc-mgmt-rgnztns
-eng.aspx*

**Ontario Ministry of Health and Long-Term Care:
Ontario Health Plan for an Influenza Pandemic 2013**
*http://www.health.gov.on.ca/en/pro/programs/emb/pan_flu/
pan_flu_plan.aspx*

Public Health Agency of Canada
http://www.phac-aspc.gc.ca/index-eng.php

**Public Health Agency of Canada: Chemical, Biological,
Radiological and Nuclear Resource Links**
*http://www.phac-aspc.gc.ca/cepr-cmiu/ophs-bssp/links_
index-eng.php*

Public Safety Canada
http://www.publicsafety.gc.ca

Salvation Army
http://www.salvationarmy.ca

St. John Ambulance
http://www.sja.ca/
*http://www.sja.ca/English/Community-Services/Pages/Emergency
%20Response/Emergency-Response-Services-Home.aspx*

Centers for Disease Control and Prevention
http://www.cdc.gov/

Federal Emergency Management Agency (FEMA)
http://www.fema.gov/

Simple Triage and Rapid Treatment (START) Triage
http://www.start-triage.com/

World Health Organization
http://www.who.int/en/

**World Health Organization and International Council of Nurses
Framework of Disaster Nursing Competencies**
*http://www.icn.ch/images/stories/documents/networks/
DisasterPreparednessNetwork/Disaster_Nursing_Competencies_
lite.pdf*

For additional Internet resources, see the website for this book
at *http://evolve.elsevier.com/Canada/Lewis/medsurg.*

APPENDIX

A

Nursing Diagnoses

Domain Label	Class Label	Diagnosis Code	Diagnosis Label
Health promotion	Health awareness	00097	Decreased diversional activity engagement
	Health awareness	00262	Readiness for enhanced health literacy
	Health awareness	00168	Sedentary lifestyle
	Health management	00257	Frail elderly syndrome
	Health management	00231	Risk for frail elderly syndrome
	Health management	00215	Deficient community health
	Health management	00188	Risk-prone health behaviour
	Health management	00099	Ineffective health maintenance
	Health management	00078	Ineffective health management
	Health management	00162	Readiness for enhanced health management
	Health management	00080	Ineffective family health management
	Health management	00043	Ineffective protection
Nutrition	Ingestion	00002	Imbalanced nutrition: less than body requirements
	Ingestion	00163	Readiness for enhanced nutrition
	Ingestion	00216	Insufficient breast milk production
	Ingestion	00104	Ineffective breastfeeding
	Ingestion	00105	Interrupted breastfeeding
	Ingestion	00106	Readiness for enhanced breastfeeding
	Ingestion	00269	Ineffective adolescent eating dynamics
	Ingestion	00270	Ineffective child eating dynamics
	Ingestion	00271	Ineffective infant feeding dynamics
	Ingestion	00107	Ineffective infant feeding pattern
	Ingestion	00232	Obesity
	Ingestion	00233	Overweight
	Ingestion	00234	Risk for overweight
	Ingestion	00103	Impaired swallowing
	Metabolism	00179	Risk for unstable blood glucose level
	Metabolism	00194	Neonatal hyperbilirubinemia
	Metabolism	00230	Risk for neonatal hyperbilirubinemia
	Metabolism	00178	Risk for impaired liver function
	Metabolism	00263	Risk for metabolic imbalance syndrome
	Hydration	00195	Risk for electrolyte imbalance
	Hydration	00025	Risk for imbalanced fluid volume
	Hydration	00027	Deficient fluid volume
	Hydration	00028	Risk for deficient fluid volume
	Hydration	00026	Excess fluid volume
Elimination and exchange	Urinary function	00016	Impaired urinary elimination
	Urinary function	00020	Functional urinary incontinence
	Urinary function	00176	Overflow urinary incontinence
	Urinary function	00018	Reflex urinary incontinence
	Urinary function	00017	Stress urinary incontinence
	Urinary function	00019	Urge urinary incontinence
	Urinary function	00022	Risk for urge urinary incontinence
	Urinary function	00023	Urinary retention
	Gastrointestinal function	00011	Constipation
	Gastrointestinal function	00015	Risk for constipation
	Gastrointestinal function	00012	Perceived constipation
	Gastrointestinal function	00235	Chronic functional constipation
	Gastrointestinal function	00236	Risk for chronic functional constipation
	Gastrointestinal function	00013	Diarrhea

NANDA International, Inc.: Nursing Diagnoses—Definitions and Classification 2018–2020 © 2017 NANDA International, ISBN 978-1-62623-929-6. Used by arrangement with the Thieme Group, Stuttgart/New York.

Domain Label	Class Label	Diagnosis Code	Diagnosis Label
	Gastrointestinal function	00196	Dysfunctional gastrointestinal motility
	Gastrointestinal function	00197	Risk for dysfunctional gastrointestinal motility
	Gastrointestinal function	00014	Bowel incontinence
	Respiratory function	00030	Impaired gas exchange
Activity/rest	Sleep/rest	00095	Insomnia
	Sleep/rest	00096	Sleep deprivation
	Sleep/rest	00165	Readiness for enhanced sleep
	Sleep/rest	00198	Disturbed sleep pattern
	Activity/exercise	00040	Risk for disuse syndrome
	Activity/exercise	00091	Impaired bed mobility
	Activity/exercise	00085	Impaired physical mobility
	Activity/exercise	00089	Impaired wheelchair mobility
	Activity/exercise	00237	Impaired sitting
	Activity/exercise	00238	Impaired standing
	Activity/exercise	00090	Impaired transfer ability
	Activity/exercise	00088	Impaired walking
	Energy balance	00273	Imbalanced energy field
	Energy balance	00093	Fatigue
	Energy balance	00154	Wandering
	Cardiovascular/pulmonary responses	00092	Activity intolerance
	Cardiovascular/pulmonary responses	00094	Risk for activity intolerance
	Cardiovascular/pulmonary responses	00032	Ineffective breathing pattern
	Cardiovascular/pulmonary responses	00029	Decreased cardiac output
	Cardiovascular/pulmonary responses	00240	Risk for decreased cardiac output
	Cardiovascular/pulmonary responses	00033	Impaired spontaneous ventilation
	Cardiovascular/pulmonary responses	00267	Risk for unstable blood pressure
	Cardiovascular/pulmonary responses	00200	Risk for decreased cardiac tissue perfusion
	Cardiovascular/pulmonary responses	00201	Risk for ineffective cerebral tissue perfusion
	Cardiovascular/pulmonary responses	00204	Ineffective peripheral tissue perfusion
	Cardiovascular/pulmonary responses	00228	Risk for ineffective peripheral tissue perfusion
	Cardiovascular/pulmonary responses	00034	Dysfunctional ventilatory weaning response
	Self-care	00098	Impaired home maintenance
	Self-care	00108	Bathing self-care deficit
	Self-care	00109	Dressing self-care deficit
	Self-care	00102	Feeding self-care deficit
	Self-care	00110	Toileting self-care deficit
	Self-care	00182	Readiness for enhanced self-care
	Self-care	00193	Self-neglect
Perception/cognition	Attention	00123	Unilateral neglect
	Cognition	00128	Acute confusion
	Cognition	00173	Risk for acute confusion
	Cognition	00129	Chronic confusion
	Cognition	00251	Labile emotional control
	Cognition	00222	Ineffective impulse control
	Cognition	00126	Deficient knowledge
	Cognition	00161	Readiness for enhanced knowledge
	Cognition	00131	Impaired memory
	Communication	00157	Readiness for enhanced communication
	Communication	00051	Impaired verbal communication
Self-perception	Self-concept	00124	Hopelessness
	Self-concept	00185	Readiness for enhanced hope
	Self-concept	00174	Risk for compromised human dignity
	Self-concept	00121	Disturbed personal identity
	Self-concept	00225	Risk for disturbed personal identity
	Self-concept	00167	Readiness for enhanced self-concept
	Self-esteem	00119	Chronic low self-esteem
	Self-esteem	00224	Risk for chronic low self-esteem
	Self-esteem	00120	Situational low self-esteem
	Self-esteem	00153	Risk for situational low self-esteem
	Body image	00118	Disturbed body image
Role relationship	Caregiving roles	00061	Caregiver role strain
	Caregiving roles	00062	Risk for caregiver role strain
	Caregiving roles	00056	Impaired parenting
	Caregiving roles	00057	Risk for impaired parenting
	Caregiving roles	00164	Readiness for enhanced parenting
	Family relationships	00058	Risk for impaired attachment
	Family relationships	00063	Dysfunctional family processes
	Family relationships	00060	Interrupted family processes

Continued

Domain Label	Class Label	Diagnosis Code	Diagnosis Label
	Family relationships	00159	Readiness for enhanced family processes
	Role performance	00223	Ineffective relationship
	Role performance	00229	Risk for ineffective relationship
	Role performance	00207	Readiness for enhanced relationship
	Role performance	00064	Parental role conflict
	Role performance	00055	Ineffective role performance
	Role performance	00052	Impaired social interaction
Sexuality	Sexual function	00059	Sexual dysfunction
	Sexual function	00065	Ineffective sexuality pattern
	Reproduction	00221	Ineffective childbearing process
	Reproduction	00227	Risk for ineffective childbearing process
	Reproduction	00208	Readiness for enhanced childbearing process
	Reproduction	00209	Risk for disturbed maternal-fetal dyad
Coping/stress tolerance	Post-trauma responses	00260	Risk for complicated immigration transition
	Post-trauma responses	00141	Post-trauma syndrome
	Post-trauma responses	00145	Risk for post-trauma syndrome
	Post-trauma responses	00142	Rape-trauma syndrome
	Post-trauma responses	00114	Relocation stress syndrome
	Post-trauma responses	00149	Risk for relocation stress syndrome
	Coping responses	00199	Ineffective activity planning
	Coping responses	00226	Risk for ineffective activity planning
	Coping responses	00146	Anxiety
	Coping responses	00071	Defensive coping
	Coping responses	00069	Ineffective coping
	Coping responses	00158	Readiness for enhanced coping
	Coping responses	00077	Ineffective community coping
	Coping responses	00076	Readiness for enhanced community coping
	Coping responses	00074	Compromised family coping
	Coping responses	00073	Disabled family coping
	Coping responses	00075	Readiness for enhanced family coping
	Coping responses	00147	Death anxiety
	Coping responses	00072	Ineffective denial
	Coping responses	00148	Fear
	Coping responses	00136	Grieving
	Coping responses	00135	Complicated grieving
	Coping responses	00172	Risk for complicated grieving
	Coping responses	00241	Impaired mood regulation
	Coping responses	00125	Powerlessness
	Coping responses	00152	Risk for powerlessness
	Coping responses	00187	Readiness for enhanced power
	Coping responses	00210	Impaired resilience
	Coping responses	00211	Risk for impaired resilience
	Coping responses	00212	Readiness for enhanced resilience
	Coping responses	00137	Chronic sorrow
	Coping responses	00177	Stress overload
	Neurobehavioural stress	00258	Acute substance withdrawal syndrome
	Neurobehavioural stress	00259	Risk for acute substance withdrawal syndrome
	Neurobehavioural stress	00009	Autonomic dysreflexia
	Neurobehavioural stress	00010	Risk for autonomic dysreflexia
	Neurobehavioural stress	00049	Decreased intracranial adaptive capacity
	Neurobehavioural stress	00264	Neonatal abstinence syndrome
	Neurobehavioural stress	00116	Disorganized infant behaviour
	Neurobehavioural stress	00115	Risk for disorganized infant behaviour
	Neurobehavioural stress	00117	Readiness for enhanced organized infant behaviour
Life principles	Beliefs	00068	Readiness for enhanced spiritual well-being
	Value/belief/action congruence	00184	Readiness for enhanced decision-making
	Value/belief/action congruence	00083	Decisional conflict
	Value/belief/action congruence	00242	Impaired emancipated decision-making
	Value/belief/action congruence	00244	Risk for impaired emancipated decision-making
	Value/belief/action congruence	00243	Readiness for enhanced emancipated decision-making
	Value/belief/action congruence	00175	Moral distress
	Value/belief/action congruence	00169	Impaired religiosity
	Value/belief/action congruence	00170	Risk for impaired religiosity
	Value/belief/action congruence	00171	Readiness for enhanced religiosity
	Value/belief/action congruence	00066	Spiritual distress
	Value/belief/action congruence	00067	Risk for spiritual distress

Domain Label	Class Label	Diagnosis Code	Diagnosis Label
Safety/protection	Infection	00004	Risk for infection
	Infection	00266	Risk for surgical site infection
	Physical injury	00031	Ineffective airway clearance
	Physical injury	00039	Risk for aspiration
	Physical injury	00206	Risk for bleeding
	Physical injury	00048	Impaired dentition
	Physical injury	00219	Risk for dry eye
	Physical injury	00261	Risk for dry mouth
	Physical injury	00155	Risk for falls
	Physical injury	00245	Risk for corneal injury
	Physical injury	00035	Risk for injury
	Physical injury	00250	Risk for urinary tract injury
	Physical injury	00087	Risk for perioperative positioning injury
	Physical injury	00220	Risk for thermal injury
	Physical injury	00045	Impaired oral mucous membrane integrity
	Physical injury	00247	Risk for impaired oral mucous membrane integrity
	Physical injury	00086	Risk for peripheral neurovascular dysfunction
	Physical injury	00038	Risk for physical trauma
	Physical injury	00213	Risk for vascular trauma
	Physical injury	00249	Risk for pressure ulcer
	Physical injury	00205	Risk for shock
	Physical injury	00046	Impaired skin integrity
	Physical injury	00047	Risk for impaired skin integrity
	Physical injury	00156	Risk for sudden infant death
	Physical injury	00036	Risk for suffocation
	Physical injury	00100	Delayed surgical recovery
	Physical injury	00246	Risk for delayed surgical recovery
	Physical injury	00044	Impaired tissue integrity
	Physical injury	00248	Risk for impaired tissue integrity
	Physical injury	00268	Risk for venous thromboembolism
	Violence	00272	Risk for female genital mutilation
	Violence	00138	Risk for other-directed violence
	Violence	00140	Risk for self-directed violence
	Violence	00151	Self-mutilation
	Violence	00139	Risk for self-mutilation
	Violence	00150	Risk for suicide
	Environmental hazards	00181	Contamination
	Environmental hazards	00180	Risk for contamination
	Environmental hazards	00265	Risk for occupational injury
	Environmental hazards	00037	Risk for poisoning
	Defensive processes	00218	Risk for adverse reaction to iodinated contrast media
	Defensive processes	00217	Risk for allergy reaction
	Defensive processes	00041	Latex allergy reaction
	Defensive processes	00042	Risk for latex allergy reaction
	Thermoregulation	00007	Hyperthermia
	Thermoregulation	00006	Hypothermia
	Thermoregulation	00253	Risk for hypothermia
	Thermoregulation	00254	Risk for perioperative hypothermia
	Thermoregulation	00008	Ineffective thermoregulation
	Thermoregulation	00274	Risk for ineffective thermoregulation
Comfort	Physical comfort	00214	Impaired comfort
	Physical comfort	00183	Readiness for enhanced comfort
	Physical comfort	00134	Nausea
	Physical comfort	00132	Acute pain
	Physical comfort	00133	Chronic pain
	Physical comfort	00255	Chronic pain syndrome
	Physical comfort	00256	Labour pain
	Environmental comfort	00214	Impaired comfort
	Environmental comfort	00183	Readiness for enhanced comfort
	Social comfort	00214	Impaired comfort
	Social comfort	00183	Readiness for enhanced comfort
	Social comfort	00054	Risk for loneliness
	Social comfort	00053	Social isolation
Growth/development	Development	00112	Risk for delayed development

B

Laboratory Values

Adapted by Jana Lok

The tables in this appendix list some of the most common tests, their normal values, and possible etiologies of abnormal values. Laboratory values are expressed in the Système International d'Unités (SI) units, which are used in Canada. Conventional units, used in the United States, are presented after the SI units in parentheses. Laboratory values may vary with different techniques and in different laboratories. Possible etiologies are presented in alphabetical order. SI abbreviations and other symbols appearing in the tables are defined as follows:

<	=	less than
>	=	greater than
≥	=	greater than or equal to
≤	=	less than or equal to
AU	=	arbitrary unit
cm H$_2$O	=	centimetres of water
dL	=	decilitre
EU	=	Ehrlich unit
fL	=	femtolitre
g	=	gram
IU	=	international unit
kPa	=	kilopascal
kU	=	kilounit
L	=	litre
mcg	=	microgram (one millionth [10^{-6}] of a gram)
mcIU	=	micro–international unit (one millionth [10^{-6}] of an international unit)

mcL	=	microlitre
mcmol	=	micromole
mEq	=	milliequivalent
mg	=	milligram (one thousandth [10^{-3}] of a gram)
microkat	=	microkatal
microU	=	microunit
mL	=	millilitre
mm	=	millimetre
mm Hg	=	millimetre of mercury
mmol	=	millimole
mOsm	=	milliosmole
mU	=	milliunit (one hundredth [10^{-2}] of a unit)
nmol	=	nanomole (one billionth [10^{-9}] of a mole)
ng	=	nanogram (one billionth [10^{-9}] of a gram)
pg	=	picogram (one trillionth [10^{-12}] of a gram)
pmol	=	picomole (one trillionth [10^{-12}] of a mole)
U	=	unit

TABLE B-1 SERUM, PLASMA, AND WHOLE BLOOD CHEMISTRIES

Test	Normal Values (SI Units [Conventional Units])	Possible Etiology Higher Values	Lower Values
Acetone		Diabetic ketoacidosis, high-fat diet, low-carbohydrate diet, starvation	—
• Quantitative	<200 mcmol/L (<1.16 mg/dL)		
• Qualitative	Negative (negative)		
Alanine aminotransferase (ALT; formerly known as serum glutamate pyruvate transferase [SGPT])	4–36 U/L (same as in SI units)	Liver disease, shock	—
Albumin	35–50 g/L (3.5–5 g/dL)	Dehydration	Burns, chronic liver disease, inflammatory disease, malabsorption, malnutrition, nephrotic syndrome, pregnancy
Aldolase	<8.0 mU/L (3–8.2 Sibley-Lehninger U/dL)	Infection, hepato-cellular disease, MI, muscle trauma, skeletal muscle disease	Hereditary fructose intolerance, late muscular dystrophy, renal disease
α$_1$-Antitrypsin	0.85–2.13 g/L (85–213 mg/dL)	Acute and chronic inflammation and infection, arthritis, malignancy, stress, thyroid infections	Chronic lung disease (early onset of emphysema), end-stage cancer, malnutrition, nephrotic syndrome

TABLE B-1 SERUM, PLASMA, AND WHOLE BLOOD CHEMISTRIES—cont'd

Test	Normal Values (SI Units [Conventional Units])	Possible Etiology	
		Higher Values	Lower Values
Alpha-fetoprotein	0–40 mcg/L (<40 ng/mL)	Cancers of testes, lymphoma, stomach, colon, breasts and ovaries; carcinoma of liver; fetal death; fetal distress or congenital abnormalities; neural tube defects or multiple pregnancies in pregnant women	In pregnant women, fetal trisomy 21 or fetal wastage
Ammonia	6–47 mcmol/L (10–80 mcg/dL)	GI bleeding, hepatic encephalopathy, portal hypertension, Reye syndrome, severe liver disease, severe heart failure or congestive hepatomegaly	Essential or malignant hypertension, hyperornithinemia
Amylase	100–300 U/L (60–120 Somogyi units/dL)	Acute and chronic pancreatitis, mumps (salivary gland disease), perforated ulcers	Acute alcoholism, cirrhosis of liver, extensive destruction of pancreas
Ascorbic acid	23–85 mcmol/L (0.4–1.5 mg/dL)	Excessive ingestion of vitamin C	Connective tissue disorders, hepatic disease, renal disease, rheumatic fever, vitamin C deficiency
Aspartate aminotransferase (AST) (formerly known as serum glutamic oxaloacetic transferase [SGOT])	0–35 U/L (same as SI units)	Acute hepatitis, liver disease, MI, pulmonary infarction, skeletal muscle disease	Acute renal disease, chronic renal dialysis, diabetic ketoacidosis, pregnancy
B-type (brain-type) natriuretic peptide	<100 mcg/L (<100 ng/mL)	Cor pulmonale, heart failure, hypertension, MI	—
Beta-carotene	1.4–4.7 mcmol/L (75–253 mcg/dL)	Cystic fibrosis, hypothyroidism, pancreatic insufficiency	Dietary deficiency, malabsorption disorders
Bicarbonate	21–28 mmol/L (21–28 mEq/L)	Chronic use of loop diuretics, compensated respiratory acidosis, metabolic alkalosis	Acute kidney injury, compensated respiratory alkalosis, diarrhea, metabolic acidosis
Bilirubin		Biliary obstruction, Dubin-Johnson syndrome, hemolytic anemia, hepatitis, impaired liver function, pernicious anemia, prolonged fasting, sickle cell anemia, sepsis	—
• Total	5.1–17 mcmol/L (0.3–1.0 mg/dL)		
• Indirect	3.4–12 mcmol/L (0.2–0.8 mg/dL)		
• Direct	1.7–5.1 mcmol/L (0.1–0.3 mg/dL)		
Blood gases*			
• Arterial pH	7.35–7.45 (same as SI units)	Alkalosis	Acidosis
• Venous pH	7.31–7.41 (same as SI units)	Alkalosis	Acidosis
• Partial pressure of carbon dioxide in arterial blood (PaCO$_2$)	35–45 mm Hg (same as SI units)	Compensated metabolic alkalosis, respiratory acidosis	Compensated metabolic acidosis, respiratory alkalosis
• Partial pressure of oxygen in arterial blood (PaO$_2$)	80–100 mm Hg (same as SI units)	Administration of high concentration of oxygen	Chronic lung disease, decreased cardiac output
• Partial pressure of oxygen in venous blood (PvO$_2$)	40–50 mm Hg (same as SI units)		
Calcium	2.25–2.75 mmol/L (9–10.5 mg/dL)	Acute osteoporosis, hyperparathyroidism, multiple myeloma, vitamin D intoxication	Acute pancreatitis, hypoparathyroidism, liver disease, malabsorption syndrome, renal failure, vitamin D deficiency
Calcium, ionized	1.05–1.30 mmol/L (4.5–5.6 mg/dL)	—	—
Carbon dioxide (CO$_2$ content)	21–28 mmol/L (21–28 mEq/L)	COPD, metabolic alkalosis, severe vomiting	Chronic use of loop diuretics, DKA, metabolic acidosis, renal failure, shock, starvation
Chloride	98–106 mmol/L (98–106 mEq/L)	Corticosteroid therapy, dehydration, excessive infusion of normal saline, metabolic acidosis, respiratory alkalosis, uremia	Addison's disease, diarrhea, heart failure, metabolic alkalosis, overhydration, respiratory acidosis, SIADH, vomiting
Cholesterol	<5 mmol/L (<200 mg/dL) age dependent	Biliary obstruction, cirrhosis hyperlipidemia, hypothyroidism, idiopathic hypercholesterolemia, renal disease, uncontrolled diabetes	Corticosteroid therapy, extensive liver disease, hyperthyroidism, malnutrition
• High-density lipoproteins (HDL)	>1.55 mmol/L (>60 mg/dL)		
• Low-density lipoproteins (LDL)	<2.59 mmol/L (<100 mg/dL)		
Cholinesterase (RBC)	5–10 U/L (same as SI units)	Exercise, sickle cell disease	Acute infections, insecticide intoxication, liver disease, muscular dystrophy

Continued

TABLE B-1   SERUM, PLASMA, AND WHOLE BLOOD CHEMISTRIES—cont'd

Test	Normal Values (SI Units [Conventional Units])	Possible Etiology Higher Values	Lower Values
Copper	11–22 mcmol/L (70–140 mcg/dL)	Cirrhosis, contraceptive use by female patient	Wilson's disease
Cortisol		Adrenal adenoma, Cushing's syndrome, hyperthyroidism, pancreatitis, stress	Addison's disease, adrenal insufficiency, hypopituitary states, hypothyroidism, liver disease
• 0800 hours	138–635 nmol/L (5–23 mcg/dL)		
• 1600 hours	<83–359 nmol/L (3–13 mcg/dL)		
Creatine	15.3–76.3 mcmol/L (0.2–1.0 mg/dL)	Active rheumatoid arthritis, biliary obstruction, hyperthyroidism, renal disease, severe muscle disease	Diabetes mellitus
Creatine kinase (CK)		Brain damage, exercise, musculo-skeletal injury or disease, MI, numerous intramuscular injections, severe myocarditis	—
• Male	55–170 U/L (same as SI units)		
• Female	30–135 U/L (same as SI units)		
Creatine kinase isozyme of heart (CK-MB [CK-2])		Acute MI	—
• Male	2–6 mcg/L (2–6 ng/mL)		
• Female	2–5 mcg/L (2–5 ng/mL)		
Creatine kinase mass fraction	<5% fraction of total CK	—	—
Creatinine		Severe renal disease	Diseases with decreased muscle mass (e.g. muscular dystrophy, myasthenia gravis)
• Male	53–106 mcmol/L (0.6–1.2 mg/dL)		
• Female	44–97 mcmol/L (0.5–1.1 mg/dL)		
Ferritin (serum)		Anemia of chronic disease (infection, inflammation, liver disease), sideroblastic anemia	Iron-deficiency anemia, severe protein deficiency
• Male	26–674 pmol/L (12–300 ng/mL)		
• Female	22–337 pmol/L (10–150 ng/mL)		
Folic acid (folate)	11–57 mmol/L (5–25 ng/mL)	Hypothyroidism, pernicious anemia	Alcoholism, hemolytic anemia, inadequate diet, malabsorption syndrome, malnutrition, megaloblastic anemia
Gamma-glutamyltranspeptidase (GGT)		Cholestasis, cytomegalovirus infection, Epstein-Barr, liver disease, MI, pancreatitis	—
• Male	8–38 U/L (same as SI units)		
• Female	5–27 U/L (same as SI units)		
Glucose, fasting	4–6 mmol/L (70–110 mg/dL)	Acute stress, cerebral lesions, Cushing's syndrome, diabetes mellitus, hyperthyroidism, pancreatic insufficiency	Addison's disease, hepatic disease, hypothyroidism, insulin overdosage, pancreatic tumour, pituitary hypofunction, postdumping syndrome
Glucose, 2-hr oral glucose tolerance testing (OGTT)		Diabetes mellitus	Hyperinsulinism
• Fasting	4–6 mmol/L (70–110 mg/dL)		
• 1 hr	<11.1 mmol/L (<200 mg/dL)		
• 2 hr	<7.8 mmol/L (<140 mg/dL)		
Haptoglobin	0.5–2.2 g/L (50–220 mg/dL)	Acute MI, infectious and inflammatory processes, malignant neoplasms	Chronic liver disease, hemolytic anemia, mononucleosis, systemic lupus erythematosus, toxoplasmosis, transfusion reactions
Homocysteine		Cardiovascular disease, cerebro-vascular disease, cystinuria, folate deficiency, malnutrition, peripheral vascular disease, vitamin B_6 or B_{12} deficiency	—
• 0–30 years	4.6–8.1 mcmol/L (same as SI units)		
• 30–59 years			
• Male	6.13–11.2 mcmol/L (same as SI units)		
• Female	4.5–7.9 mcmol/L (same as SI units)		
• >59 years	5.8–11.9 mcmol/L (same as SI units)		
Insulin	43–186 pmol/L (6–26 microU/mL)	Acromegaly, adenoma of islet cells, obesity, untreated mild case of type 2 diabetes mellitus	Diabetes mellitus, obesity

TABLE B-1   SERUM, PLASMA, AND WHOLE BLOOD CHEMISTRIES—cont'd

Test	Normal Values (SI Units [Conventional Units])	Possible Etiology Higher Values	Lower Values
Iron		Excessive RBC destruction, hemochromatosis, massive transfusion	Anemia of chronic disease, iron-deficiency anemia
• Male	14–32 mcmol/L (80–180 mcg/dL)		
• Female	11–29 mcmol/L (60–160 mcg/dL)		
Total iron-binding capacity (TIBC)	45–82 mcmol/L (250–460 mcg/dL)	Iron-deficiency state, oral contraceptive use, polycythemia	Cancer, chronic infections, pernicious anemia, uremia
Lactic acid (venous blood)	0.6–2.2 mmol/L (5–20 mg/dL)	Acidosis, heart failure, severe liver disease, shock, tissue ischemia	—
Lactic dehydrogenase (LDH)	100–190 U/L (same as SI units)	Heart failure, hemolytic disorders, hepatitis, metastatic cancer of liver, MI, pernicious anemia, pulmonary embolus and infarction, skeletal muscle damage	—
Lactic dehydrogenase isoenzymes			
• LDH$_1$	0.17–0.27 (17%–27%)	MI, pernicious anemia, strenuous exercise	—
• LDH$_2$	0.27–0.37 (27%–37%)	Exercise, pulmonary embolus, sickle cell crisis	—
• LDH$_3$	0.18–0.25 (18%–25%)	Malignant lymphoma, pulmonary embolus	—
• LDH$_4$	0.03–0.08 (3%–8%)	Systemic lupus erythematosus, pancreatitis, pulmonary infarction, renal disease	—
• LDH$_5$	0.0–0.05 (0%–5%)	Heart failure, hepatitis, pulmonary embolus and infarction, skeletal muscle damage, strenuous exercise	—
Lipase	0–160 U/L (same as SI units)	Acute and chronic pancreatitis, hepatic disorders, pancreatic disorder (cancer, pseudocyst), perforated peptic ulcer, salivary gland inflammation or tumour	—
Magnesium	0.74–1.07 mmol/L (1.8–2.6 mEq/L)	Addison's disease, hypothyroidism, renal failure	Chronic alcoholism, hyperparathyroidism, hyperthyroidism, hypoparathyroidism, malnutrition, severe malabsorption
Myoglobin	1.0–5.3 nmol/L (<90 ng/mL)	MI, myositis, malignant hyperthermia, muscular dystrophy, skeletal muscle ischemia or trauma, rhabdomyolysis, seizures	Polymyositis
Osmolality	280–300 mmol/kg (280–300 mOsm/kg)	Chronic renal disease, dehydration, diabetes mellitus, hypernatremia, shock	Addison's disease, diuretic therapy, hyponatremia, overhydration
Oxygen saturation		Increased inspired oxygen, polycythemia vera	Anemia, cardiac decompensation, decreased inspired oxygen, respiratory disorders
• Arterial	95%–100% (same as SI units)		
• Venous	60%–80% (same as SI units)		
pH	See Blood gases		
Phenylalanine	0–121 mcmol/L (0–2 mg/dL)	Phenylketonuria	—
Phosphatase, acid	2.2–10.5 U/L (0.13–0.63 U/L)	Advanced Paget's disease, cancer of prostate, hyperparathyroidism	—
Phosphatase, alkaline (ALP)	35–120 U/L (0.5–2.0 mckat/L)	Bone diseases, cirrhosis, malignancy of liver/bone, marked hyperparathyroidism, obstruction of biliary system, rickets	Excessive vitamin D ingestion, hypothyroidism, milk-alkali syndrome
Phosphorus, phosphate	0.97–1.45 mmol/L (3.0–4.5 mg/dL)†	Bone metastasis, healing fractures, hypocalcemia, hypoparathyroidism, renal disease, vitamin D intoxication	Chronic alcoholism, diabetes mellitus, hypercalcemia, hyperparathyroidism, vitamin D deficiency
Potassium	3.5–5.0 mmol/L (3.5–5.0 mEq/L)	Acute or chronic renal failure, Addison's disease, dehydration, diabetic ketosis, excessive dietary or IV intake, massive tissue destruction, metabolic acidosis	Burns, Cushing's syndrome, deficient dietary or IV intake, diarrhea (severe), diuretic therapy, GI fistula, insulin administration, pyloric obstruction, starvation, vomiting

Continued

TABLE B-1   SERUM, PLASMA, AND WHOLE BLOOD CHEMISTRIES—cont'd

Test	Normal Values (SI Units [Conventional Units])	Possible Etiology Higher Values	Lower Values
Prostate-specific antigen (PSA)	<4 mcg/L (<4 ng/mL)	Benign prostatic hypertrophy, prostate cancer, prostatitis	—
Proteins		Burns, cirrhosis (globulin fraction), dehydration	Congenital agammaglobulinemia, increased capillary permeability, inflammatory disease, liver disease, malabsorption, malnutrition
• Total	64–83 g/L (6.4–8.3 g/dL)		
• Albumin	35–50 g/L (3.5–5 g/dL)		
• Globulin	23–34 g/L (2.3–3.4 g/dL)		
• Albumin/globulin ratio	1.5:1–2.5:1 (same as SI units)	Multiple myeloma (globulin fraction), shock, vomiting	Malnutrition, nephrotic syndrome, proteinuria, renal disease, severe burns
Pseudocholinesterase (serum)	8–18 U/mL (same as SI units)	—	—
Renin		Renal hypertension, salt-losing GI disease (vomiting/diarrhea), volume decrease (e.g., hemorrhage)	Increased salt intake, primary aldosteronism
• Upright position	0.03–1.2 ng/L/sec (0.1–4.3 mg/mL/hr)		
Sodium	135–145 mmol/L (135–145 mEq/L)	Corticosteroid therapy, dehydration, impaired renal function, increased dietary or IV intake, primary aldosteronism	Addison's disease, decreased dietary or IV intake, diabetic ketoacidosis, diuretic therapy, excessive loss from GI tract, excessive perspiration, water intoxication
Testosterone		Adrenal hyperplasia, adrenal or pituitary tumours, testicular tumours	Hypofunction of testes
• Male	174–729 pmol/L (50–120 pg/mL)		
• Female	3.5–29.5 pmol/L (1.0–8.5 pg/mL)	Polycystic ovary, virilizing tumours	—
Thyroxine (T₄), total	64–154 nmol/L (5–12 mcg/dL)	Hyperthyroidism, thyroiditis	Cretinism, hypothyroidism, myxedema
Thyroxine (T₄), free	10–36 pmol/L (0.8–2.8 ng/dL)	Hyperthyroidism, metastatic neoplasms	Hypothyroidism, pregnancy
Thyroid-stimulating hormone (TSH)	2–10 mIU/L (2–10 mcIU/mL)	Graves' disease, myxedema, primary hypothyroidism	Secondary hypothyroidism
Triglycerides		Diabetes mellitus, hyperlipidemia, hypothyroidism, liver disease	Hyperthyroidism, malabsorption syndrome, malnutrition
• Male	0.45–1.81 mmol/L (40–160 mg/dL)		
• Female	0.40–1.52 mmol/L (35–135 mg/dL)		
Triiodothyronine (T₃) uptake	24–34 AU (24%–34%)	—	—
Triiodothyronine (T₃)	1.7–5.2 pmol/L (110.4–337.7 ng/dL)	Hyperthyroidism	Hypothyroidism
Troponin T (cTnT)	<0.1 mcg/L (<0.1 ng/mL)	Cardiac muscle damage (resulting from MI, myocarditis, or pericarditis), chronic renal failure, multiorgan failure, severe heart failure	—
Troponin I (cTnI)	<0.35 mcg/L (<0.35 ng/mL)		—
Urea nitrogen, blood (blood urea nitrogen [BUN], serum urea nitrogen)	3.6–7.1 mmol/L (10–20 mg/dL)	Burns, dehydration, GI bleeding, increase in protein catabolism (fever, stress), renal disease, shock, urinary tract infection	Fluid overload, malnutrition, severe liver damage, SIADH
Uric acid		Alcoholism, eclampsia, gout, gross tissue destruction, high-protein weight reduction diet, leukemia, multiple myeloma, renal failure	Administration of uricosuric drugs
• Male	240–501 mcmol/L (4.0–8.5 mg/dL)		
• Female	160–430 mcmol/L (2.7–7.3 mg/dL)		
Vitamin A	0.52–2.09 mcmol/L (15–60 mcg/dL)	Excess ingestion of vitamin A	Vitamin A deficiency
Vitamin B₁₂	118–701 pmol/L (160–950 pg/mL)	Chronic myeloid leukemia	Malabsorption syndrome, pernicious anemia, strict vegetarianism, total or partial gastrectomy
Zinc	11.5–18.5 mcmol/L (75–120 mcg/dL)	—	Alcoholic cirrhosis

*Because arterial blood gases are influenced by altitude, the values for PaCO₂, PaO₂, and PvO₂ decrease as altitude increases. The lower values are normal for an altitude of 1.6 km (1 mile).

†Values for older adults are significantly lower than those for younger adults.

COPD, chronic obstructive pulmonary disease; *DKA,* diabetic ketoacidosis; *GI,* gastro-intestinal; *IV,* intravenous; *MI,* myocardial infarction; *RBC,* red blood cell; *SIADH,* syndrome of inappropriate antidiuretic hormone.

TABLE B-2 HEMATOLOGY

Test	Normal Values (SI Units [Conventional Units])	Possible Etiology	
		Higher Values	Lower Values
Activated coagulation time or automated clotting time (ACT)	70–120 sec (same as SI units)	Same as for aPTT	—
Activated partial thromboplastin time (aPTT)	30–40 sec* (same as SI units)	Deficiency of one or more of the following: factor I, II, V, or VIII; factors IX and X; factor XI; and factor XII Hemophilia; heparin therapy; liver disease	—
Bleeding time (Ivy method)	1–9 min	Acetylsalicylic acid (ASA; Aspirin) ingestion, clotting factor deficiency, defective platelet function, thrombocytopenia, vascular disease, von Willebrand's disease	—
D-dimer	<3.0 mmol/L (<50 ng/mL)	Deep-vein thrombosis, DIC, myocardial infarction, unstable angina	—
Erythrocyte count† (RBC count [altitude dependent])		Dehydration, high altitudes, polycythemia vera, severe diarrhea	Anemia, leukemia, posthemorrhage
• Male	$4.7–6.1 \times 10^{12}$/L		
• Female	$4.2–5.4 \times 10^{12}$/L		
Erythrocyte sedimentation rate (ESR), Westergren Method		*Moderate increase:* acute hepatitis, myocardial infarction, rheumatoid arthritis	Malaria, severe liver disease, sickle cell anemia
• Male	≤15 mm/hr (same as SI units)	*Marked increase:* acute and severe bacterial infections, malignancies, pelvic inflammatory disease	
• Female	≤20 mm/hr (same as SI units)		
Fibrin split (degradation) products	<10 mg/L (<10 mcg/mL)	Acute DIC, massive hemorrhage, massive trauma, primary fibrinolysis	—
Fibrinogen	2.0–5.0 g/L (60–100 mg/dL)	Burns (after first 36 hr), inflammatory disease	Burns (during first 36 hr), DIC, severe liver disease
Hematocrit (altitude dependent)†		Dehydration, high altitudes, polycythemia	Anemia, bone marrow failure, hemorrhage, leukemia, overhydration
• Male	0.42–0.52 volume fraction (42%–52%)		
• Female	0.37–0.47 volume fraction (37%–47%)		
Hemoglobin (altitude dependent)†		Chronic obstructive pulmonary disease, high altitudes, polycythemia	Anemia, hemorrhage
• Male	140–180 g/L (14–18 g/dL)		
• Female	120–160 g/L (12–16 g/dL)		
Hemoglobin, glycosylated or glycated (hemoglobin A_{1c} [HbA_{1c}])	<6% (adult without diabetes)	Nondiabetic hyperglycemia, poorly controlled diabetes mellitus	Chronic blood loss, chronic renal failure, pregnancy, sickle cell anemia
International normalized ratio (INR)	0.81–1.20 (same as SI units)	Same as for PT	—
Mean corpuscular hemoglobin (MCH) [Hb/RBC]	27–31 pg (same as SI units)	Macrocytic anemia	Microcytic anemia
Mean corpuscular hemoglobin concentration (MCHC) [Hb/Hct]	32–36 g/dL (32%–36%)	Intravascular hemolysis, spherocytosis	Hypochromic anemia
Mean corpuscular volume (MCV) [Hct/RBC]	80–95 fL (80–95 mm³)	Folic acid and vitamin B_{12} deficiency, liver disease, macrocytic anemia	Microcytic anemia
Partial thromboplastin time (PTT)	60–70 sec (same as SI units)	Same as for aPTT	—
Platelet count (thrombocytes)	$150–400 \times 10^9$/L (150,000–400,000/mm³)	Acute infections, chronic granulocytic leukemia, chronic pancreatitis, cirrhosis, collagen disorders, polycythemia, post-splenectomy	Acute leukemia, cancer chemotherapy, DIC, hemorrhage, infection, systemic lupus erythematosus, thrombocytopenic purpura
Prothrombin time (PT; Protime)	11–12.5 sec* (same as SI units)	Deficiency of one or more of the following: factor I, II, V, VII, or X Liver disease; vitamin K deficiency; warfarin therapy	—

Continued

TABLE B-2 HEMATOLOGY—cont'd

Test	Normal Values (SI Units [Conventional Units])	Possible Etiology	
		Higher Values	Lower Values
Red cell distribution width (RDW)	11%–14.5% (same as SI units)	—	Anisocytosis, macrocytic anemia, microcytic anemia
Reticulocyte count (manual)	0.5%–2% total number of RBC	Hemolytic anemia, polycythemia vera	Hypoproliferative anemia, macrocytic anemia, microcytic anemia
Sickle cell solubility	Negative (negative)	Sickle cell anemia	—
Thrombin time	8–12 sec (same as SI units)	DIC, increased tendency to bleed	—
WBC count†	5–10 × 10^9/L (5000–10,000/mm³)	Inflammatory and infectious processes, leukemia	Aplastic anemia, autoimmune diseases, overwhelming infection, side effects of chemotherapy and irradiation
WBC differential			
• Band neutrophils	0–1 × 10^9/L (0%–9%)	Acute infections	—
• Basophils	0.02–0.05 × 10^9/L (15–50/mm³; 0.5%–1%)	Hypothyroidism, myeloproliferative diseases, ulcerative colitis	Hyperthyroidism, stress
• Eosinophils	0.00–0.5 × 10^9/L (50–500/mm³; 1%–4%)	Allergic reactions, eosinophilic and chronic granulocytic leukemia, Hodgkin's disease, parasitic disorders	Corticosteroid therapy
• Lymphocytes	1.0–4.0 × 10^9/L (1000–4000/mm³; 20%–40%)	Chronic infections, lymphocytic leukemia, mononucleosis, viral infections	Corticosteroid therapy, whole body irradiation
• Monocytes	0.1–0.7 × 10^9/L (100–700/mm³; 2%–8%)	Acute infections, chronic inflammatory disorders, Hodgkin's disease, malaria, monocytic leukemia	—
• Segmented neutrophils	2.5–7.5 × 10^9/L (62%–68%)	Bacterial infections, collagen diseases, Hodgkin's disease	Aplastic anemia, viral infections

*For patients receiving anticoagulant therapy, aPTT is 1.5–2.5 times control value in seconds; PT is 1.5–2.0 times control value in seconds.
†Components of complete blood count (CBC).
DIC, disseminated intravascular coagulation; *RBC*, red blood cell; *WBC*, white blood cell.

TABLE B-3 SEROLOGY–IMMUNOLOGY

Test	Normal Values (SI Units [Conventional Units])	Possible Etiology	
		Higher Values	Lower Values
Antinuclear antibody (ANA)	Negative at 1:40 dilution (same as SI units)	Chronic hepatitis, rheumatoid arthritis, scleroderma, systemic lupus erythematosus (SLE)	—
Anti-DNA antibody	Negative <70 U/mL (same as SI units)	SLE	—
Anti-RNP (ribonucleoprotein)	Negative (negative)	Mixed connective tissue disease, rheumatoid arthritis, scleroderma, Sjögren's syndrome, SLE	—
Anti-Sm (Smith)	Negative (negative)	SLE	—
Antistreptolysin-O (ASO)	≤160 Todd units/mL (same as SI units)	Acute glomerulo-nephritis, rheumatic fever, streptococcal infection	—
C-reactive protein (CRP)	<10 mg/L (<1.0 mg/dL)	Acute infections, any inflammatory condition (e.g., acute rheumatic fever/arthritis), widespread malignancy	—
Carcinoembryonic antigen (CEA)	<5 mcg/L (5 ng/mL)	Carcinomas of colon, liver, pancreas; chronic cigarette smoking; inflammatory bowel disease; other cancers	—
Complement assay components		—	Acute glomerulo-nephritis, rheumatoid arthritis, serum sickness, SLE, subacute bacterial endocarditis
• Total	75–160 kU/L (75–160 U/mL)		
• C3	0.55–1.2 g/L (55–120 mg/dL)		
• C4	0.2–0.5 g/L (20–50 mg/dL)		

TABLE B-3 SEROLOGY–IMMUNOLOGY—cont'd

Test	Normal Values (SI Units [Conventional Units])	Possible Etiology Higher Values	Possible Etiology Lower Values
Direct antihuman globulin test (DAT) or direct Coombs' test	Negative (negative) (no agglutination)	Acquired hemolytic anemia, drug reactions, hemolytic disease of the newborn, transfusion reactions	—
Fluorescent treponemal antibody absorption (FTAAbs)	Negative (nonreactive)	Syphilis	—
Hepatitis A antibody	Negative (negative)	Hepatitis A	—
Hepatitis B surface antigen (HBsAg)	Negative (negative)	Hepatitis B	—
Hepatitis C antibody	Negative (negative)	Hepatitis C	—
Immunoglobulins			
• IgA	0.85–3.85 g/L (85–385 mg/dL)	Autoimmune disorders, chronic infection, chronic liver disease, IgA myeloma, rheumatoid arthritis	Burns, hereditary telangiectasia, malabsorption syndromes
• IgD	Minimal	Chronic infection, connective tissue disease	—
• IgE	24–400 mcg/L	Anaphylactic shock, atopic disease (allergies), parasite infections	—
• IgG	5.65–17.65 g/L (565–1765 mg/dL)	Hepatitis, IgG monoclonal gammopathy, infections—acute and chronic, SLE	Acquired deficiencies, burns, congenital deficiencies, immuno-suppression, nephrotic syndromes
• IgM	0.55–3.75 g/L (55–375 mg/dL)	Acute infections, liver disease, rheumatoid arthritis	Congenital and acquired antibody deficiencies, lymphocytic leukemia, protein-losing enteropathies
Monospot or Mono-Test	Negative (<1:28 titre)	Infectious mononucleosis,	—
Rheumatoid factor (RA factor)	Negative or <60 IU/mL by nephelometric method	Rheumatoid arthritis, Sjögren's syndrome, SLE	—
RPR (rapid plasma reagin) test	Negative or nonreactive (same as SI units)	Febrile diseases, IV drug abuse, leprosy, malaria, rheumatoid arthritis, syphilis, SLE	—
VDRL (Venereal Disease Research Laboratory) test	Negative or nonreactive (same as SI units)	Syphilis	—
Thyroid antibodies	Titre <1:100 (same as SI units)	Early hypothyroidism, Graves' disease, Hashimoto's thyroiditis, pernicious anemia, SLE, thyroid carcinoma	—

IV, intravenous.

TABLE B-4 URINE CHEMISTRY

Test	Specimen	Normal Values (SI Units [Conventional Units])	Possible Etiology Higher Values	Possible Etiology Lower Values
Acetone (ketones)	Random	Negative (negative)	Diabetes mellitus, high-fat and low-carbohydrate diets, starvation states	—
Aldosterone	24 hr	17–70 nmol/24 hr (2–26 mcg/24 hr)	*Primary aldosteronism:* Adrenocortical tumours *Secondary aldosteronism:* Cardiac failure, cirrhosis, large dose of ACTH, salt depletion	Addison's disease, adrenocorticotrophic hormone (ACTH) deficiency, corticosteroid therapy
Amylase	24 hr	100–300 U/L (60–120 Somogyi units/dL)	Acute pancreatitis	—
Bence Jones protein	Random	Negative (negative)	Biliary duct obstruction, multiple myeloma	—
Bilirubin	Random	5.1–16 mcmol/L (0.3–1.0 mg/dL)	Gallstones, Dubin-Johnson syndrome, Rotor syndrome	—
Calcium	24 hr	2.25–2.75 mmol/day (9.0–10.5 mg/dL)	Bone tumour, hyperparathyroidism, milk-alkali syndrome, lymphoma, Addison's disease	Hypoparathyroidism, malabsorption of calcium and vitamin D, renal failure, pancreatitis

Continued

TABLE B-4 URINE CHEMISTRY—cont'd

Test	Specimen	Normal Values (SI Units [Conventional Units])	Possible Etiology Higher Values	Lower Values
Catecholamines	24 hr		Heart failure, pheochromocytoma, progressive muscular dystrophy	
• Epinephrine		<109 nmol/day (<20 mcg/24 hr)		
• Norepinephrine		<590 nmol/day (<100 mcg/24 hr)		
Chloride	24 hr	110–250 mmol/day (110–250 mEq/day)	Dehydration, Cushing's syndrome, eclampsia, kidney dysfunction	Addison's disease, burns, diarrhea, excess perspiration, heart failure, menstruation, vomiting
Copper	24 hr	0.6 mcmol/day (<40 mcg/day)	Cirrhosis, Wilson's disease	—
Coproporphyrin	24 hr	<300 nmol/day (<200 mcg/day)	Lead poisoning, oral contraceptive use, poliomyelitis	—
Creatine	24 hr		Acromegaly, diabetic nephropathy, disease affecting renal function	Decrease muscle mass (e.g., muscular dystrophy, myasthenia gravis)
• Male		53–106 mcmol/day (0.6–1.2 mg/dL)		
• Female		44–97 mcmol/L (0.6–1.2 mg/dL)		
Creatinine	24 hr		Anemia, leukemia, muscular atrophy, salmonellosis	Renal disease
• Male		53–106 mcmol/L (0.6–1.2 mg/dL)		
• Female		44–97 mcmol/L (0.5–1.1 mg/dL)		
Creatinine clearance	24 hr	1.42–2.25 mL/sec (85–135 mL/min)	—	Renal disease
• Male		1.78–2.32 mL/sec (107–139 mL/min)		
• Female		1.45–1.78 mL/sec (87–107 mL/min)		
Estriol	24 hr		Gonadal or adrenal tumour	
• Female				Agenesis of ovaries, endocrine disturbance, menopause, ovarian dysfunction
• Ovulatory phase		28–100 mcg/24 hr (104–370 nmol/L)		
• Luteal phase		22–80 mcg/24 hr (81–296 nmol/L)		
• Pregnancy		≤166,455 nmol/day (≤45,000 mcg/day)		
• Menopause		1.4–19.6 mcg/24 hr (5.2–72.5 nmol/L)		
• Male		5–18 mcg/24 hr (18–67 nmol/L)	—	—
Glucose	Random	Random: negative; 24-hour: <2.78 mmol/24 hr (<0.5 g/24 hr)	Diabetes mellitus, low renal threshold for glucose resorption, physiological stress, pituitary disorders	—
Hemoglobin	Random		Extensive burns, glomerulo-nephritis, hemolytic anemias, hemolytic transfusion reaction	—
• Male		140–180 mmol/L (14–18 g/dL)		
• Female		120–160 (12–16 g/dL)		
5-Hydroxyindole-acetic acid (5-HIAA)	24 hr	10–40 mcmol/day (2–8 mg/24 hr)	Malignant carcinoid syndrome	—
Ketone bodies	Random	Negative (negative)	Alcoholism, fasting, high-protein diets, marked ketonuria, poorly controlled diabetes mellitus, starvation	—
Lead	24 hr	<0.40 mcmol/day (<80 mcg/day)	Lead poisoning	—
Metanephrine	24 hr	12–60 pg/mL	Pheochromocytoma	—
Myoglobin	Random	1.0–5.3 nmol/L (<90 ng/mL)	Crushing injuries, electric injuries, extreme physical exertion	—
pH	Random	4.6–8.0 (average, 6.0)	Chronic renal failure, compensatory phase of alkalosis, salicylate intoxication, vegetarian diet	Compensatory phase of acidosis, dehydration, emphysema
Phenylpyruvic acid	Random	Negative (negative)	Phenylketonuria	—
Phosphorus, inorganic	24 hr	0.97–1.45 mmol/L (3.0–4.5 mg/dL)	Fever, hypoparathyroidism, nervous exhaustion, rickets, tuberculosis	Acute infections, nephritis
Porphobilinogen	Random 24 hr	Negative (negative) 0–6.6 mg/24 hr (0–2 mg/24 hr)	Acute intermittent porphyria, liver disorders	—
Potassium	24 hr	25–100 mmol/day (25–100 mEq/L/day)	Alkalosis, chronic renal failure, Cushing's syndrome, diuretic therapy, hyperaldosteronism, starvation,	Acute kidney injury, Addison's disease, dehydration, diarrhea, malnutrition, reduced intake, vomiting
Protein (dipstick)	Random	Negative (negative)	Heart failure, nephritis, nephrosis, physiological stress	—
Protein (quantitative)	24 hr	<0.15 g/day (<150 mg/day)	Cardiac failure, inflammatory processes of urinary tract, nephritis, nephrosis, toxemia of pregnancy	—
• At rest		0.05–0.08 g/day (<50–80 mg/day)		
• During exercise		<0.25 g/day (<250 mg/day)		
Sodium	24 hr	40–250 mmol/day (40–250 mEq/day)	Acute tubular necrosis	Hyponatremia

TABLE B-4 URINE CHEMISTRY—cont'd

Test	Specimen	Normal Values (SI Units [Conventional Units])	Possible Etiology Higher Values	Possible Etiology Lower Values
Specific gravity	Random	1.005–1.030 (usually, 1.010–1.025)*	Albuminuria, dehydration, fever, GI losses (vomiting/diarrhea), glycosuria, SIADH	Diabetes insipidus, diuresis, overhydration
Titratable acidity	24 hr	20–50 mEq/day (same as SI units)	Metabolic acidosis	Metabolic alkalosis
Uric acid	24 hr	1.48–4.43 mmol/day (250–750 mg/24 hr)	Gout, leukemia	Nephritis
Urobilinogen	24 hr	0.5–4.0 mg/24 hr (0.5–4.0 Ehrlich units/24 hr)	Hemolytic disease, hepatic parenchymal cell damage, liver disease	Complete obstruction of bile duct
Uroporphyrins	24 hr		Lead poisoning, liver disease, porphyria	—
• Male		10–53 nmol/24 hr (8–44 mcg/24 hr)		
• Female		10–26 nmol/24 hr (4–22 mcg/24 hr)		
Vanillylmandelic acid	24 hr	<35 mcmol/day (<6.8 mg/24 hr)	Pheochromocytoma, neuroblastomas	—

*Values decrease with age.
GI, gastro-intestinal; *SIADH,* syndrome of inappropriate antidiuretic hormone.

TABLE B-5 GASTRIC ANALYSIS

Test	Normal Values (SI Units [Conventional Units])	Possible Etiology Higher Values	Possible Etiology Lower Values
Basal			
Free hydrochloric acid	0.3 mmol/L (0.3 mEq/L)	Hypermotility of stomach	Pernicious anemia
Total acidity	15–45 mmol/L (15–45 mEq/L)	Gastric and duodenal ulcers, Zollinger-Ellison syndrome	Gastric carcinoma, severe gastritis
Post-stimulation			
Free hydrochloric acid	10–130 mmol/L (10–130 mEq/L)	—	—
Total acidity	20–150 mmol/L (20–150 mEq/L)	—	—

TABLE B-6 FECAL ANALYSIS

Test	Normal Values (SI Units [Conventional Units])	Possible Etiology Higher Values	Possible Etiology Lower Values
Blood*	Negative (negative)	Anal fissures, hemorrhoids, inflammatory bowel disease, malignant tumour, peptic ulcer	—
Colour			
• Brown		Various shades, depending on diet	—
• Clay		Biliary obstruction or presence of barium sulphate	—
• Tarry		More than 100 mL of blood in GI tract	—
• Red		Blood in large intestine	—
• Black		Blood in upper GI tract or iron medication	—
Fecal fat	7–21mmol/day (2–6 g/24 hr)	Chronic pancreatic disease, cystic fibrosis, malabsorption syndrome, obstruction of common bile duct, short gut syndrome	—
Mucus	Negative (negative)	Mucous colitis, spastic constipation	—
Pus	Negative (negative)	Chronic bacillary dysentery, chronic ulcerative colitis, localized abscesses	—
Urobilinogen	51–372 mcmol/100 g of stool (30–220 mg/100 g of stool)	Hemolytic anemias	Complete biliary obstruction

*Ingestion of meat may produce false-positive results. Patient may be placed on a meat-free diet for 3 days before the test.
GI, gastro-intestinal.

TABLE B-7 CEREBRO-SPINAL FLUID ANALYSIS

Test	Normal Values (SI Units [Conventional Units])	Possible Etiology	
		Higher Values	Lower Values
Blood	Negative (negative)	Intracranial hemorrhage	—
Cell count (age dependent)			
• White blood cells (WBCs)	$0-5 \times 10^6$ WBCs/L (0–5 WBCs/mcL)	Inflammation or infections of CNS	—
• Red blood cells (RBCs)	Negative (negative)		—
Chloride	116–122 mmol/L of CSF (116–122 mEq/L of CSF)	Uremia	Bacterial infections of CNS (meningitis, encephalitis)
Glucose	2.8–4.2 mmol/L (50–75 mg/dL)	Diabetes mellitus, viral infections of CNS	Bacterial infections and tuberculosis of CNS
Protein			
• Lumbar	0.15–0.45 g/L (15–45 mg/dL)	Guillain-Barré syndrome, poliomyelitis, traumatic tap	—
• Cisternal	0.15–0.25 g/L (15–25 mg/dL)	Syphilis of CNS	—
• Ventricular	0.05–0.15 g/L (5–15 mg/dL)	Acute meningitis, brain tumour, chronic CNS infections, multiple sclerosis	—
Pressure	<20 cm H_2O (same as SI units)	Hemorrhage, intracranial tumour, meningitis	Head injury, spinal tumour, subdural hematoma

NB: All of the changes are based on the values presented in the Pagana & Pagana textbook.
CNS, central nervous system; *CSF,* cerebro-spinal fluid.

abortion   The loss or termination of a pregnancy before the fetus has developed to a state of viability. Ch. 56

absence seizure   Type of seizure typically characterized by a brief staring spell that lasts only a few seconds; there may be an extremely brief loss of consciousness. Occurs most commonly in children and may cease altogether or evolve into another type of seizure as the child matures. Ch. 61

absorption   Transfer of food products into circulation. Ch. 41

absorption atelectasis   Absorption of oxygen into the bloodstream and collapse of the alveoli as a result of airway obstruction. Ch. 31

accommodation   The convergence of the eyes and the constriction of the pupils when the eyes focus from a far to near object. Ch. 23

acculturation   A multidimensional process in which individuals and groups undergo stages of adjustment, as well as changes in several domains, such as language, socioeconomic status, values, and attitudes, that result in increased similarity between two cultures. Ch. 2

achalasia   Absence of peristalsis of the lower two-thirds smooth muscle of the esophagus. Ch. 44

acidosis   A condition in which the blood pH drops below 7.35. Ch. 19

acne vulgaris   An inflammatory disorder of the sebaceous glands most common in teenagers. Noninflammatory lesions include open comedones (blackheads) and closed comedones (whiteheads); inflammatory lesions include papules, pustules, and cysts. Ch. 26

acoustic neuroma   A unilateral benign tumour that occurs where the vestibulo-cochlear nerve (cranial nerve [CN] VIII) enters the internal auditory canal. Ch. 24

acquired immune deficiency syndrome (AIDS) End stage of chronic HIV infection; a syndrome involving a defect in cell-mediated immunity that has a long incubation period and is manifested by various opportunistic infections and cancers. Ch. 17

acromegaly   A condition caused by excessive secretion of growth hormone and characterized by an overgrowth of the bones and soft tissues in the hands, feet, and face; occurs most often as a result of a benign pituitary tumour (adenoma). Ch. 51

actinic keratosis   Hyperkeratotic papules and plaques occurring on sun-exposed areas; also known as *solar keratosis*. Ch. 26

action potential   The electrical impulse created and transported by the conduction system (specialized nerve tissue). Ch. 34

active transport   A process requiring energy in which molecules move against the concentration gradient. Ch. 19

acupuncture   The insertion of fine needles into the circulation of qi underneath the skin's surface to correct disruptions in the flow of qi. Ch. 12

acute arterial ischemia   A sudden interruption in the arterial blood supply to a tissue, organ, or extremity that, if left untreated, can result in tissue death. Ch. 40

acute bronchitis   An inflammation of the bronchi in the lower respiratory tract that is usually caused by infection. Ch. 30

acute coronary syndrome (ACS)   Condition encompassing unstable angina, non–ST-segment elevation myocardial infarction, and ST-segment elevation myocardial infarction; develops when myocardial ischemia is prolonged and not immediately reversible. Ch. 36

acute illness   Illness typically characterized by a sudden onset, with signs and symptoms related to the disease process itself. Ch. 5

acute kidney injury (AKI)   An abrupt decline in kidney function, leading to a rise in serum creatinine or a reduction in urine output or both; the severity of dysfunction can range from a small increase in serum creatinine or reduction in urine output to the development of azotemia. (Previously known as *acute renal failure [ARF].*) Ch. 49

acute liver failure (ALF)   A clinical condition characterized by rapid deterioration of liver function resulting in encephalopathy and coagulopathy in persons with no known history of liver disease. Ch. 46

acute pancreatitis   An acute inflammation of the pancreas, ranging from mild edema to severe hemorrhagic necrosis. Ch. 46

acute renal failure (ARF)   Former term for *acute kidney injury (AKI)*. Ch. 49

acute respiratory distress syndrome (ARDS)   A sudden and progressive form of acute respiratory failure in which the alveolar–capillary membrane becomes damaged and more permeable by intravascular fluid. Ch. 70

acute retroviral syndrome   A flulike syndrome of fever, swollen lymph glands, sore throat, headache, malaise, nausea, muscle and joint pain, diarrhea, or a diffuse rash, or some combination of these. Ch. 21

acute rheumatic fever (ARF)   A complication that occurs as a delayed sequela (usually after 2–3 wk) of group A streptococcal pharyngitis. Ch. 39

acute tubular necrosis (ATN)   Necrosis of the renal tubular cells caused by ischemia, nephrotoxins, or sepsis; the most common intrarenal cause of AKI. Ch. 49

Addison's disease   A disease that causes adrenocortical insufficiency (hypofunction of the adrenal cortex) and in which the supply of all three classes of adrenal corticosteroids (glucocorticoids, mineralocorticoids, and androgens) is reduced. Ch. 51

adhesions   Bands of scar tissue that form between or around organs. Ch. 14

advance care planning   A process of thinking about and sharing one's wishes for future health and personal care; a means by which an individual can tell others what would be important if he or she were ill and unable to communicate. Ch. 13

advance directives   Legal documents specifying an individual's decisions regarding end-of-life care and specifying alternative decision makers as required. Ch. 13

advanced nursing practice   Clinical nursing practice at a level that requires graduate education and attainment and advancement of in-depth nursing knowledge and expertise. Ch. 1

adventitious sounds   Extra breath sounds that are abnormal. Ch. 28

adverse event   An event that results in unintended harm to the patient and is related to the care and/or services provided to the patient rather than to the patient's underlying medical condition, p. 4

afterload   The peripheral resistance against which the left ventricle must pump. Ch. 34

ageism   Negative attitude based on age, leading to discrimination and disparities in the care of older people. Ch. 7

age-related macular degeneration (AMD)   An eye disease that begins after age 60 that progressively destroys the macula (the central portion of the retina), causing irreversible central vision loss. Ch. 24

airway obstruction   A blockage of the patient's airway, most commonly caused by the patient's tongue. Ch. 22

alarm reaction   First stage of the stress response, in which the individual perceives a stressor physically or mentally and the fight-or-flight response is initiated. Ch. 8

aldosterone   A potent mineralocorticoid that maintains extracellular fluid volume. Ch. 50

alkalosis   A condition in which the blood pH is greater than 7.45. Ch. 19

allele   One of two or more alternative forms of a gene that can occupy a particular chromosomal locus. Ch. 15

allergic rhinitis   The reaction of the nasal mucosa to a specific allergen. Ch. 29

allostasis   The process of achieving homeostasis in the presence of a challenge. Ch. 8

alopecia   Partial or complete lack of hair resulting from normal aging, endocrine disorder, drug reaction, anticancer medication, or skin disease. Ch. 25

alternative therapies   Therapies used as the primary treatment instead of traditional Western health practices. Ch. 12

alveolar hypoventilation   A decrease in ventilation that results in an increase in partial pressure of arterial carbon dioxide ($PaCO_2$) and a consequent decrease in partial pressure of arterial oxygen (PaO_2). Ch. 70

Alzheimer's disease (AD)   A chronic, progressive, degenerative disease of the brain. Ch. 62

amblyopia   Reduced or no vision in an affected eye; also termed "lazy eye." Ch. 24

ambulatory surgery   Also called *same-day surgery*; refers to surgery conducted in emergency departments, endoscopy clinics, doctors' offices, and outpatient surgery units in hospitals, after which the patient can be discharged on the same day. Ch. 20

amenorrhea Absence of menstruation. Chs. 53, 56

amniocentesis Transabdominal puncture of the amniotic sac under ultrasound guidance using a needle and syringe in order to remove amniotic fluid to detect genetic and biochemical disorders. Ch. 15

amyloid plaques Clusters of insoluble deposits of a protein called *beta-amyloid*, other proteins, remnants of neurons, non-nerve cells such as microglia (cells that surround and digest damaged cells or foreign substances), and other cells, such as astrocytes; present in abnormal quantities in the brains of persons with Alzheimer's disease. Ch. 62

amyotrophic lateral sclerosis (ALS) A rare, progressive neurological disorder characterized by loss of motor neurons and by weakness and atrophy of the muscles of the hands, the forearms, and the legs, spreading to involve most of the body and the face. Ch. 61

anaesthesia care team An anaesthesiologist-led care model in which anaesthesiologists practise among a team of other professionals such as nurse practitioners—anaesthesia, anaesthesia assistants, registered nurses, and respiratory therapists. Ch. 21

anaesthesiologist Physician who is an expert in administering potent drugs used to deliver general and regional anaesthesia and in ensuring absence of pain during surgery. Ch. 21

anal fissure A skin ulcer or a crack in the lining of the anal wall that is caused by trauma, local infection, or inflammation. Ch. 45

anal fistula An abnormal tunnel leading out from the anus or the rectum, which may extend to the outside of the skin, the vagina, or the buttocks. Ch. 45

analgesic ceiling A dosage at which no additional analgesia is produced regardless of further dosage increases. Ch. 10

anaphylactic shock An acute, life-threatening hypersensitivity (allergic) reaction to a sensitizing substance, such as a drug, chemical, vaccine, food, or insect venom. Ch. 69

anaplasia Cell differentiation to a more immature or embryonic form. Ch. 14

andragogy The theoretical basis of adult learning. Ch. 4

anemia A deficiency in the number of erythrocytes (red blood cells), the quantity or quality of hemoglobin, the volume of packed RBCs (hematocrit), or a combination of these. Ch. 33

anergy Immunodeficient condition characterized by lack of or diminished reaction to an antigen or a group of antigens. Ch. 16

aneurysm A permanent, localized outpouching or dilation of the blood vessel wall (either congenital or acquired). Chs. 40, 60

angina Chest pain that is the clinical manifestation of reversible myocardial ischemia. Ch. 36

anions Negatively charged ions. Ch. 19

ankylosing spondylitis (AS) A chronic inflammatory disease that affects primarily the axial skeleton, including the sacroiliac joints, intervertebral disc spaces, and costovertebral articulations. Ch. 67

ankylosis Stiffness or fixation of a joint, usually resulting from destruction of articular cartilage and subchondral bone with subsequent scarring. Ch. 64

anorexia nervosa A serious, often chronic, and life-threatening eating disorder characterized by self-imposed weight loss, endocrine dysfunction, and a distorted psychopathological attitude toward weight and eating. Ch. 42

antidiuretic hormone (ADH) A potent vasoconstrictor whose major physiological role is the regulation of fluid volume by stimulating reabsorption of water in the renal tubules; also called *vasopressin*. Ch. 50

antigen A substance that elicits an immune response. Ch. 16

aortic dissection Not a type of aneurysm; rather, a dissection that results from the creation of a false lumen (between the intima and the media) through which blood flows. Ch. 40

aortic stenosis A narrowing or stricture of the aortic valve resulting in obstruction of the blood flow from the left ventricle to the aorta during systole; causes left ventricular hypertrophy and increased myocardial oxygen consumption. Ch. 39

aortic valve regurgitation (AR) Retrograde blood flow from the ascending aorta into the left ventricle when the valve should be closed, resulting in volume overload. Ch. 39

aphasia Total loss of comprehension and use of language or total inability to communicate. Ch. 60

apheresis A procedure in which components of the blood are separated and then one or more of those components is removed. Ch. 16

aplastic anemia A disease in which the patient has peripheral blood pancytopenia (decrease of all blood cell types—red blood cells, white blood cells, and platelets) and hypocellular bone marrow. Ch. 33

apoptosis Programmed cell death. Ch. 14

appendicitis An inflammation of the appendix. Ch. 45

aqueous humor A clear, watery fluid that fills the anterior and posterior chambers of the anterior cavity of the eye. Ch. 23

arterial blood pressure (BP) A measure of the pressure exerted by blood against the walls of the arterial system. Ch. 34

arterial pressure–based cardiac output (APCO) A technique for determining continuous cardiac output/continuous cardiac index, used to assess a patient's ability to respond to fluids by increasing stroke volume (preload responsiveness). Ch. 68

arteriovenous fistula (AVF) The preferred hemodialysis access, created by the surgical connection of a vein and an artery, usually in the forearm. Ch. 49

arteriovenous graft (AVG) A hemodialysis access created with a synthetic graft that is attached to an artery and vein; used for people who do not have suitable vessels for an AVF. Ch. 49

arthritis A type of rheumatic disease involving inflammation of a joint or joints; the most common types are osteoarthritis, rheumatoid arthritis, and gout. Ch. 67

arthrocentesis A procedure in which an incision or puncture is made in a joint capsule, usually to obtain samples of synovial fluid from within the joint cavity for a synovial fluid analysis. Ch. 64

arthrodesis The surgical fusion of a joint. Ch. 65

arthroplasty The reconstruction or replacement of a joint to relieve pain, improve or maintain range of motion, and correct deformity. Ch. 65

arthroscopy A procedure in which a small fibre-optic tube called an *arthroscope* is inserted into a joint and used to directly examine or to operate on the interior of the joint cavity. Ch. 64

Aschoff bodies Tiny, rounded or spindle-shaped nodules formed by a reaction to myocardial inflammation with accompanying swelling and fragmentation of collagen fibres. Ch. 39

ascites The accumulation of serous fluid in the peritoneal or the abdominal cavity. Ch. 46

assessment The collection of subjective and objective information about the patient. Ch. 1

assist-control ventilation (ACV) The ventilator delivery of a preset tidal volume at a preset frequency; when the patient initiates a spontaneous breath, the preset tidal volume is delivered. Ch. 68

assisted-living facilities (ALFs) Residential care facilities that provide housing and personal care. Ch. 7

asterixis Flapping tremors (liver flap) commonly affecting the arms and hands; a manifestation of hepatic encephalopathy. Ch. 46

asthma A chronic inflammatory disorder of the airways; inflammation causes varying degrees of obstruction, which leads to recurrent episodes of wheezing, breathlessness, chest tightness, and cough, particularly at night and in the early morning. Ch. 31

astigmatism A visual distortion caused by an unevenness in the cornea. Ch. 23

asystole The total absence of ventricular electrical activity. Ch. 38

atelectasis A complete or partial collapse of a lung or segment of a lung that occurs when the alveoli become deflated. Chs. 22, 30

atherosclerosis A disease characterized by deposits of lipids within the intima of the artery; major cause of coronary artery disease. Ch. 36

atrial fibrillation A cardiac dysrhythmia characterized by a total disorganization of atrial electrical activity resulting in loss of effective atrial contraction. Ch. 38

atrial flutter An atrial tachydysrhythmia identified by recurring, regular, sawtooth-shaped flutter waves. Ch. 38

atrophy Decrease in the size of a tissue or organ caused by a reduction in the number or size of the individual cells; characterized by decreased circumference and flabby appearance, leading to decreased function and tone. Ch. 14

aura Neurological symptoms such as visual field defects, tingling or burning sensations, paresthesias, motor dysfunction (e.g., weakness, paralysis), dizziness, confusion, and even loss of consciousness that usually precede the onset of migraine pain. Ch. 61

auscultation The act of listening for sounds produced by the body to assess normal conditions and deviations from normal; particularly useful in evaluating the heart, lungs, abdomen, and vascular system. Ch. 3

autoimmunity An immune reaction to self-proteins: the immune system no longer differentiates self from nonself. Ch. 16

automated peritoneal dialysis (APD) A popular form of peritoneal dialysis that is done while the patient sleeps, using a device called a cycler. (Also called *continuous cycling peritoneal dialysis*.) Ch. 49

automatic external defibrillators (AEDs) Defibrillators that have rhythm detection capability and the ability to advise the operator to deliver a shock with hands-free defibrillator pads. Ch. 38

automaticity A property of specialized cells of the heart found in the sinoatrial (SA) node, parts of the atria, the atrioventricular (AV) node, and the His–Purkinje system that are able to discharge spontaneously. Ch. 38

autonomic dysreflexia A massive, life-threatening, uncompensated cardiovascular reaction mediated by the sympathetic nervous system that occurs in patients with spinal cord lesions in response to visceral stimulation. Ch. 63

autonomic nervous system (ANS) The division of the nervous system that governs involuntary functions of cardiac muscle, smooth (involuntary) muscle, and glands. Ch. 58

autosome Any chromosome that is not a sex chromosome. Ch. 15

avascular necrosis (AVN) Bone cell death as a result of inadequate blood supply. Ch. 65

azotemia An accumulation of nitrogen waste products (urea nitrogen, creatinine) in the blood. Ch. 49

B

bacteria One-celled microorganisms that are found virtually everywhere on earth and are involved in fermentation, putrefaction, infectious diseases, and nitrogen fixation. Ch. 17

bariatric surgery An invasive procedure used to treat morbid obesity. Ch. 43

baroreceptors Specialized nerve cells located in the carotid sinus and in the arch of the aorta that are sensitive to stretching and, when stimulated by an increase in blood pressure, send inhibitory impulses to the sympathetic vasomotor centre in the brain stem. Ch. 35

Barrett's esophagus A condition in which the normal squamous epithelium of the esophagus is replaced with columnar epithelium. Ch. 44

basal cell carcinoma (BCC) A locally invasive malignancy arising from epidermal basal cells; the most common type of skin cancer but the least deadly. Ch. 26

behavioural and psychological symptoms of dementia (BPSDs) The behavioural manifestations (e.g., appetite changes, slowed or excessive movements and speech, agitation, pacing, wandering) and psychological manifestations (e.g., anhedonia, worry, depressed mood, euphoria, fear) of dementia. Ch. 62

Bell's palsy A disorder characterized by the disruption of the motor branches of the facial nerve (cranial nerve VII) on one side of the face in the absence of any other disease. Ch. 63

benign neoplasms Well-differentiated tumours that are usually encapsulated, do not metastasize, have slight vascularity, and rarely recur. Ch. 18

benign paroxysmal positional vertigo (BPPV) A common cause of vertigo in which free-floating debris ("ear rocks") in the semicircular canal produces symptoms of dizziness, vertigo, light-headedness, loss of balance, and nausea with specific head movements. Ch. 24

benign prostatic hyperplasia (BPH) A nonmalignant, noninflammatory enlargement of the prostate gland thought to be caused by an excessive accumulation of dihydroxytestosterone, stimulation by estrogen, or local growth hormone action. Ch. 57

bereavement The period after the death of a loved one during which grief is experienced and mourning occurs. Ch. 13

best buys Actions that should be undertaken immediately to produce accelerated results in terms of lives saved, diseases prevented, and heavy costs avoided. Ch. 5

bilirubin A pigment derived from the breakdown of aged red blood cells. Ch. 41

biological therapy Treatment involving the use of biological agents such as interferons, interleukins, monoclonal antibodies, and growth factors to modify the relationship between the host and the tumour. Ch. 18

bioterrorism The use of biological agents as the element of a terrorist attack; involves the deliberate spreading of microbes or toxins with the intent of causing disease or death in animals, plants, or humans. Ch. 72

blebs Air-filled alveolar dilations less than 1 cm in diameter on the edge of the lung at the apex of the upper lobe or superior segment of the lower lobe. Ch. 30

blood–brain barrier A physiological barrier between blood capillaries and brain tissue that protects the brain from certain potentially harmful agents while allowing nutrients and gases to enter. Ch. 58

blood pressure (BP) The force exerted by the blood against the walls of blood vessels; must be adequate for tissue perfusion to be maintained during activity and rest. Ch. 35

body mass index (BMI) A ratio of weight to height calculated by dividing weight (in kilograms) by height (in metres squared); higher ranges are associated with increased health risk. Ch. 43

bone marrow transplantation Life-saving procedure for a number of nonmalignant diseases; cells are allogeneic (from non-monozygotic twin donor), autologous (from self), or synegeneic (from healthy monozygotic twin). Ch. 18

botulism An acute neurological disorder that causes potentially life-threatening neuroparalysis due to a neurotoxin produced by *Clostridium botulinum*. Ch. 63

brachytherapy "Closed" radiation delivery system in which "radioactive materials are implanted or inserted directly into the tumour or close to the tumour." Ch. 18

brain abscess An accumulation of pus within the brain tissue that can result from a local or systemic infection. Ch. 59

brain reward system A system involving the mesolimbic and mesocortical pathways; responsible for creating the sensation of pleasure in reaction to certain behaviours that are required for survival of the human species. Ch. 11

breakthrough pain Moderate to severe pain that occurs despite treatment. Ch. 10

bronchiectasis A condition of the lungs characterized by permanent, abnormal dilation of one or more large bronchi. Ch. 30

bronchospasm The result of an increase in bronchial smooth muscle tone with resultant closure of small airways. Ch. 22

Brown-Séquard syndrome A syndrome resulting from damage to half of the spinal cord; characterized by a loss of motor function, sense of position, and sense of vibration on the same side as the lesion. Ch. 63

buffers Fast-acting regulatory mechanisms that act chemically to change strong acids into weaker acids or to bind acids to neutralize their effect. Ch. 19

bulimia nervosa An eating disorder characterized by frequent binge eating, self-induced vomiting associated with loss of control over eating, and a persistent concern with body image. Ch. 42

burn An injury to the tissues of the body caused by heat, chemicals, electric current, or radiation. Ch. 27

bursitis Inflammation of a bursa. Ch. 65

C

calculus An abnormal stone formed in body tissues by an accumulation of mineral salts. Ch. 48

cancer A group of more than 200 diseases characterized by uncontrolled and unregulated growth of cells. Ch. 18

carcinogens Cancer-causing agents capable of producing cellular alterations. Ch. 18

carcinoma in situ A lesion with all the histological features of cancer except invasion; becomes invasive if left untreated. Ch. 18

carcinomas Malignant tumours that originate from embryonal ectoderm (skin and glands) and endoderm (mucous membrane linings of the respiratory, gastro-intestinal, and genito-urinary tracts). Ch. 18

cardiac index A measure of the cardiac output divided by the body mass index. Ch. 34

cardiac output (CO) The volume of blood ejected from the heart per minute; can be described as the stroke volume (SV, or amount of blood pumped out of the left ventricle per beat [~70 mL]) multiplied by the heart rate (HR) over 1 minute. Chs. 34, 35

cardiac pacemaker An electronic device used to pace the heart when the normal conduction pathway is damaged or diseased. Ch. 38

cardiac reserve The ability of the heart to respond to increased demands on the cardiovascular system by increasing cardiac output as much as three-fold or four-fold. Ch. 34

cardiac tamponade A condition that develops as fluid accumulates in the pericardial sac (pericardial effusion), causing an increase in intrapericardial pressure and producing compression of the heart. Ch. 39

cardiac transplantation Transfer of a heart from one person to another. Ch. 37

cardiogenic shock Shock occurring when either systolic or diastolic dysfunction of the pumping action of the heart results in compromised cardiac output. Ch. 69

cardiomyopathy A group of diseases that directly affect the structural or functional ability of the myocardium. Ch. 39

caregiver burden The overall physical, emotional, and financial costs of caregiving. Ch. 5

carpal tunnel syndrome (CTS) A condition caused by compression of the median nerve, which enters the hand through the narrow confines of the carpal tunnel, located in the wrist. Ch. 65

carrier An individual who carries a copy of a mutated gene for a recessive disorder. Ch. 15

cataplexy A brief and sudden loss of skeletal muscle tone or muscle weakness. Manifestations range from a brief episode of muscle weakness to complete postural collapse and falling to the ground. Ch. 9

cataract An area of opacity within the lens. Ch. 24

catecholamines Substances that are usually considered neurotransmitters but are hormones when secreted by the adrenal medulla; they include epinephrine, norepinephrine, and dopamine. Catecholamines are an essential part of the body's response to stress. Ch. 50

cations Positively charged ions. Ch. 19

CBRNE event Any situation in which weapons of a **c**hemical, **b**iological, **r**adiological, **n**uclear, or **e**xplosive nature are used with the goal of causing harm. Ch. 72

ceiling effect A phenomenon in which increasing the dose of a given medication beyond an upper limit provides no greater analgesia. Ch. 10

celiac disease An autoimmune disease characterized by damage to the small intestinal mucosa from the ingestion of wheat, barley, and rye in genetically susceptible individuals. Ch. 45

cell-mediated immunity Immune responses that are initiated through specific antigen recognition by T cells. Ch. 16

cellulitis An inflammation of subcutaneous tissues. Ch. 26

central nervous system (CNS) The division of the nervous system that consists of the brain, the spinal cord, and cranial nerves I and II. Ch. 58

cerebral edema Increased accumulation of fluid in the extravascular spaces of brain tissue. Ch. 59

cerebro-spinal fluid (CSF) A clear, colourless fluid that provides cushioning for the brain and the spinal cord, allows fluid shifts from the cranial cavity to the spinal cavity, and carries nutrients. Ch. 58

cerebro-vascular accident (CVA) The medical term for *stroke*. Ch. 60

certification of death A written formal statement that the patient is dead, which is usually required within 24 hours of a death. Ch. 13

chancre A painless, indurated lesion found on the penis, vulva, lips, mouth, vagina, or rectum; a primary manifestation of syphilis. Ch. 55

chemical burns Burns that result from contact with acids, alkalis, and organic compounds. Ch. 27

chemoreceptor A receptor in the medulla that responds to a change in the chemical composition (partial pressure of arterial carbon dioxide [$PaCO_2$] and pH) of the fluid around it. Ch. 28

chest physiotherapy Airway clearance technique for reducing mucus; consists of percussion, vibration, and postural drainage. Ch. 31

Cheyne–Stokes respiration A pattern of breathing characterized by alternating periods of apnea and deep, rapid breathing. Ch. 13

chlamydial infections A superficial mucosal infection, caused by *Chlamydia trachomatis*, that can be transmitted during vaginal, anal, or oral sex; the most prevalent bacterial sexually transmitted infection in Canada today. Ch. 55

cholecystitis Inflammation of the gallbladder. Ch. 46

cholelithiasis Stones in the gallbladder. Ch. 46

chorionic villus sampling (CVS) Aspiration of fetal trophoblastic tissue (chorionic villi) by either transcervical or transabdominal approach for prenatal evaluation of the chromosomal, enzymatic, and DNA status of the fetus. Ch. 15

chronic bronchitis The presence of chronic productive cough for 3 months in 2 successive years. Ch. 31

chronic disease management The use of elements and tools within the health care system (e.g., information systems, decision support tools, self-management promotion, and realignment of health services) and within the community (e.g., a supportive environment, health policy, and strengthened community action) to help patients living with chronic diseases. Ch. 6

chronic illness Health problems that persist over extended periods and that are often (but not always) associated with participation and activity limitations (disability). Ch. 5

chronic kidney disease (CKD) The progressive, irreversible destruction of the nephrons in both kidneys, leading to loss of kidney function; classified at one of five stages, depending on level of severity based on glomerular filtration rate. Ch. 49

chronic kidney disease–mineral and bone disorder (CKD–MBD) A clinical syndrome with systemic components that include characteristic bone abnormalities, changes in mineral balance, and vascular and other soft tissue calcification. Ch. 49

chronic obstructive pulmonary disease (COPD) A preventable disease characterized by persistent airflow limitation that is usually progressive; associated with enhanced chronic inflammatory response in the airways and lungs, caused primarily by cigarette smoking and other noxious particles and gases. Ch. 31

chronic pancreatitis Progressive destruction of the pancreas as it is replaced with fibrotic tissues. Ch. 46

chronic stable angina Chest pain that occurs intermittently over a long period with the same pattern of onset, duration, and intensity of symptoms. Ch. 36

chronic venous insufficiency (CVI) A condition in which leg veins and valves fail to keep blood moving forward. Ch. 40

chylothorax Presence of lymphatic fluid in the pleural space caused by a leak in the thoracic duct. Ch. 30

circadian rhythms The biological rhythms of behaviour and physiology that fluctuate within a 24-hour period. Ch. 9

circadian rhythm sleep–wake disorders (CRSWDs) A group of sleep disorders that result in a person having good quality sleep at the wrong time of day. Ch. 9

circulating nurse A perioperative nurse who is not scrubbed, gowned, or gloved and remains in an unsterile field. Ch. 21

circulatory assist devices (CADs) Devices that are used to decrease cardiac work and improve organ perfusion in patients with heart failure. Ch. 68

cirrhosis The final stage of chronic liver disease; a diffuse pathological process characterized by fibrosis and conversion of normal liver architecture to abnormal nodules. Ch. 46

clinical (critical) pathway A plan outlining daily care goals for select health care problems; includes a nursing care plan, specific interventions for each day of hospitalization, and a documentation tool. Ch. 1

clitoris Erectile tissue in women that lies anterior to the urethral meatus and the vaginal orifice and becomes engorged during sexual excitation. Ch. 53

cluster headaches A rare form of headache that involves repeated headaches that can occur for weeks to months at a time, followed by periods of remission; characterized by intense, stabbing pain that is ipsilateral in nature and lasts an average of 97 minutes per attack. Ch. 61

collaborative problems Potential or actual complications of disease or of treatment that nurses manage together with other health care providers. Ch. 1

collateral circulation Arterial connections within the coronary circulation; development depends on (a) the inherited predisposition to develop new blood vessels and (b) the presence of chronic ischemia. Ch. 36

colorectal cancer A malignant disease of the colon, the rectum, or both; the second-most common cause of cancer death in Canada. Ch. 45

coma A profound state of unconsciousness. Ch. 59

community-acquired pneumonia (CAP) A lower respiratory tract infection of the lung parenchyma with onset in the community or during the first 2 days of hospitalization. Ch. 30

comorbidity The presence of two or more chronic illnesses that are not directly related to each other in a person at the same time. Ch. 5

compartment syndrome A condition in which swelling and increased pressure within a limited space (a compartment) press on and compromise the function of blood vessels, nerves, and tendons that run through that compartment. Ch. 65

complementary therapies Therapies that accompany traditional Western health practices. Ch. 12

complete heart block A type of heart block in which no impulses from the atria are conducted to the ventricles; also called *third-degree AV heart block*. Ch. 38

compliance A measure of the elasticity of the lungs and thorax. Ch. 28

concussion A sudden, transient, mechanical head injury, with disruption of neural activity and a change in the level of consciousness; considered a mild brain injury. Ch. 59

Confusion Assessment Method A widely used, validated screening instrument and diagnostic aid that is effective in identifying the presence of delirium. Ch. 62

conjunctiva A transparent mucous membrane that covers the inner surfaces of the eyelids (the palpebral conjunctiva) and extends over the sclera (the bulbar conjunctiva), forming a "pocket" under each eyelid. Ch. 23

conjunctivitis An infection or inflammation of the conjunctiva caused by bacteria, viruses, allergies, or chemical irritants. Ch. 24

constipation A decrease in frequency of bowel movements from what is "normal" for the individual; hard, difficult-to-pass stools; a decrease in stool volume; and retention of feces in the rectum; or some combination of these symptoms. Ch. 45

continuing competence The ongoing ability to perform one's duties skillfully, safely, and ethically. Ch. 1

continuous ambulatory peritoneal dialysis (CAPD) A type of peritoneal dialysis that is done during the day and consists of a minimum of four exchanges of dialysis fluid over a 24-hour period. Ch. 49

continuous positive airway pressure (CPAP) A treatment for severe apnea or hypopnea in which a nasal mask attached to a high-flow blower is applied to maintain pressure in the airway and prevent airway collapse. Ch. 9

continuous renal replacement therapy (CRRT) An alternative or adjunctive method for treating acute kidney injury that provides a means by which uremic toxins and fluids are removed from patients who are hemodynamically unstable, while acid–base status and electrolytes are adjusted slowly and continuously. Ch. 49

contracture An abnormal, usually permanent condition of a muscle or joint, characterized by flexion and fixation. Chs. 27, 64

contusion Bruising of the brain tissue within a focal area. Ch. 59

coping A person's cognitive and behavioural efforts to manage specific external or internal stressors that seem to exceed available resources. Ch. 8

coping resources Internal or external assets, characteristics, or actions that a person draws upon to manage stress. Ch. 8

cor pulmonale A hypertrophy of the right side of the heart, with or without heart failure, resulting from pulmonary hypertension. Diseases of the lung or thorax or changes in pulmonary circulation can lead to pulmonary hypertension. Chs. 30, 31

coronary angiography Imaging with left-sided heart catheterization in which the catheter is positioned at the origin of the coronary arteries and contrast medium is injected into the arteries; images identify the location and severity of any coronary blockages. Ch. 34

coronary artery disease (CAD) An abnormal condition that may affect the heart's arteries and produce various pathological effects, especially the reduced flow of oxygen and nutrients to the myocardium. Ch. 36

coronary revascularization An intervention that restores blood flow to the affected myocardium. Ch. 36

corticosteroid Any of the hormones synthesized by the adrenal cortex (excluding androgens). Ch. 50

cortisol The most abundant and potent glucocorticoid; one of its major functions is the regulation of blood glucose concentration. Ch. 50

costovertebral angle A physical examination landmark used to locate the kidneys, formed by the rib cage and the vertebral column. Ch. 47

cough variant asthma A type of asthma in which cough is the only symptom. Ch. 31

crackles Short, low-pitched sounds caused by the passage of air through an airway intermittently occluded by mucus, unstable bronchial wall, or fold of mucosa. Ch. 28

cranial nerves (CN) The 12 paired nerves composed of cell bodies with fibres that exit from the cranial cavity. Ch. 58

creatinine A waste product produced by protein breakdown (primarily body muscle mass); clearance of creatinine by the kidney approximates the glomerular filtration rate. Ch. 47

crepitation Crackling sound or grating sensation as a result of friction between bones, broken bone, or cartilage bits in joint. Ch. 64

CREST An acronym used to describe the clinical manifestations of systemic sclerosis (scleroderma): **c**alcinosis, **R**aynaud's phenomenon, **e**sophageal dysfunction, **s**clerodactyly, and **t**elangiectasia. Ch. 67

cretinism Hypothyroidism that develops in infancy, caused by thyroid hormone deficiencies during fetal or early neonatal life. Ch. 50

Creutzfeldt–Jakob disease (CJD) A very rare, fatal, infectious brain disorder thought to be caused by accumulation in the brain of an abnormally folded prion protein. Ch. 62

critical incident stress management (CISM) or debriefing A comprehensive approach to preventing and managing the emotional trauma that can be a result of involvement in a disaster response. Ch. 72

critical limb ischemia A condition characterized by chronic ischemic rest pain lasting more than 2 weeks, arterial leg ulcers, or gangrene of the leg as a result of peripheral artery disease. Ch. 40

critical thinking The art of analyzing and evaluating thinking with a view to improving it. Ch. 1

Crohn's disease A chronic, inflammatory bowel disease of unknown origin that can affect any part of the gastro-intestinal tract, from the mouth to the anus. Ch. 45

cross-tolerance The development of resistance to one or more effects of a drug as a result of tolerance developed to a similar drug. Ch. 11

cryosurgery The use of subfreezing temperatures to destroy epidermal lesions. Ch. 26

cultural competence The application of knowledge, attitudes, and skills that enhance cross-cultural communication and foster meaningful, respectful interactions with others. Ch. 2

cultural imposition The situation in which a person's own cultural beliefs and practices are, intentionally or unintentionally, imposed on another person or group of people. Ch. 2

cultural safety A concept that focuses on the power imbalances that lead to a disregard for health and illness beliefs of the Indigenous people and to a privileging of the dominant cultural values. Ch. 2

culture A way of life characterized by dimensions such as ethnicity, language, religion, sex, socio-economic class, professional status, age, sexual orientation, group history, and life experiences. Ch. 2

cultured epithelial autograft Skin grafts grown from biopsy specimens obtained from the patient's own skin. Ch. 27

curettage The removal and scooping away of tissue using an instrument with a circular cutting edge attached to a handle. Ch. 26

Cushing's syndrome A spectrum of clinical abnormalities caused by excess levels of corticosteroids, particularly glucocorticoids; most common causes are iatrogenic administration of exogenous corticosteroids (e.g., prednisone) in large doses for several weeks or longer and excessive production of cortisol by the adrenal cortex. Ch. 51

cyst Palpable, fluid-filled mass. Ch. 54

cystic fibrosis An autosomal recessive, multisystem disease characterized by altered function of the exocrine glands, involving primarily the lungs, the pancreas, and the sweat glands. Ch. 31

cystitis An inflammatory condition of the urinary bladder, characterized by pain, urgency and frequency of urination, and hematuria. Ch. 48

cystocele Herniation or protrusion of the urinary bladder through the wall of the vagina; occurs when support between the vagina and the bladder is weakened; also known as *anterior wall prolapse*. Ch. 56

cystometrography A urodynamic study used to evaluate the compliance (elastic property) and stability of the detrusor muscle of the bladder and to evaluate bladder tone, sensations of filling, and bladder (detrusor) stability. Ch. 47

cystoscopy A radiological bladder procedure in which contrast material is instilled into the bladder to allow inspection of the interior of the bladder and evaluation of the vesico-ureteral reflux using a tubular lighted instrument called a cystoscope. Ch. 47

cytokines Soluble factors secreted by white blood cells and a variety of other cells in the body. Ch. 16

D

database All the health information about a patient, including the data from the nursing history and physical examination, the data from the medical history and physical examination, results of laboratory and diagnostic tests, and information contributed by other health care providers. Ch. 3

death The permanent loss of capacity for consciousness and all brain stem functions. Ch. 13

death rattle Noisy, wet-sounding respirations caused by mouth breathing and accumulation of mucus in the airways. Ch. 13

debridement Removal of necrotic tissue from a wound to prevent infection and promote healing. Ch. 27

decontamination The process of removing or neutralizing a hazardous agent from the environment, property, equipment, or a life form, through the use of water, cleansers, or neutralizers. Ch. 72

deep-vein thrombosis (DVT) A disorder involving a thrombus in a deep vein, most commonly the iliac and femoral veins. Ch. 40

defecation The discharge of feces from the rectum. Ch. 41

degenerative disc disease (DDD) Progressive degeneration that results in intervertebral discs' losing their elasticity, flexibility, and shock-absorbing capabilities; thinning of the discs also occurs. A normal process of aging. Ch. 66

deglutition The process of swallowing. Ch. 41

dehiscence Separation and disruption of previously joined wound edges. Ch. 14

delayed awakening Longer-than-expected duration of postoperative unconsciousness, usually caused by prolonged drug action or, rarely, by neurological injury. Ch. 22

delayed sleep phase disorder (DSPD) Difficulty falling asleep (staying awake until 0100–0300 hours) and typically sleeping later into the morning. Ch. 9

delirium A state of acute mental confusion. Ch. 62

dementia A collection of symptoms caused by various diseases affecting the brain. Ch. 62

dementia with Lewy Bodies (DLB) A type of dementia characterized by the presence of Lewy bodies (deposits of alpha-synuclein protein) in the brain stem, amygdala, and cortex. Ch. 62

deoxyribonucleic acid (DNA) A nucleic acid that forms the chromosomes in human cells. Ch. 15

dermatomes Areas on the skin that are innervated primarily by a single spinal cord segment. Chs. 10, 58

dermatomyositis An inflammatory myopathy that presents with characteristic skin changes along with the symptoms of polymyositis (diffuse, idiopathic, inflammatory myopathies of the connective tissues, especially striated muscle, that produce bilateral weakness, usually most severe in the proximal or the limb-girdle muscles). Ch. 67

dermis Connective tissue below the epidermis. Ch. 25

determinants of health Factors that influence the health of individuals and groups. Ch. 1

deviated septum A deflection of the normally straight nasal septum. Ch. 29

diabetes insipidus (DI) A group of conditions associated with a deficiency of production or secretion of antidiuretic hormone (ADH) or with a decreased renal response to ADH; caused by injury to the neurohypophyseal system. Ch. 51

diabetes mellitus (DM) A multisystem disease related to abnormal insulin production, impaired insulin utilization, or both. Ch. 52

diabetic ketoacidosis (DKA) An acute metabolic complication of diabetes mellitus occurring when fats are metabolized in the absence of insulin; caused by a profound deficiency of insulin and characterized by hyperglycemia, ketosis, metabolic acidosis, and dehydration (volume depletion). Ch. 52

diabetic nephropathy A microvascular complication of diabetes mellitus associated with damage to the small blood vessels that supply the glomeruli of the kidney; the leading cause of end-stage renal disease in Canada. Ch. 52

diabetic neuropathy Nerve damage that occurs because of the metabolic derangements associated with diabetes mellitus. Ch. 52

dialysis A clinical technique, used to correct fluid and electrolyte imbalances and to remove waste products in renal failure, in which substances move from the blood through a semipermeable membrane (dialyzer/peritoneal membrane) and into a dialysis solution (dialysate). Ch. 49

diarrhea The frequent passage of loose, watery stools; a symptom, not a disease. Ch. 45

diastole Relaxation of the myocardium. Ch. 34

diastolic blood pressure (DBP) The residual pressure of the arterial system during ventricular relaxation. Ch. 34

diffuse axonal injury (DAI) Widespread axonal damage occurring after a mild, moderate, or severe traumatic brain injury. Ch. 59

diffusion The movement of molecules from an area of high concentration to one of low concentration. Ch. 19

diffusion limitation Decrease in gas exchange across the alveolar–capillary membrane caused by processes that thicken or destroy the membrane. Ch. 70

digestion The process by which food is broken down in the gastro-intestinal tract in order to be converted into a substance suitable for absorption and assimilation into the body; involves both mechanical digestion (mastication) and chemical digestion. Ch. 41

dilated cardiomyopathy A disease characterized by a diffuse inflammation and rapid degeneration of myocardial fibres that result in ventricular dilation, impairment of systolic function, atrial enlargement, and stasis of blood in the left ventricle. Ch. 39

disability Any of a range of mental or physical impairments that limit one's functioning in society. Ch. 5

disaster The outcome of a natural hazard or event (e.g., hurricane, flood, earthquake) or a result of human action or error, whether malicious (e.g., terrorist attacks, use of biological warfare) or unintentional (e.g., an accidental chemical spill) that seriously disrupts the functioning of a community or society. Ch. 72

disaster nursing The provision of nursing care, advocacy, and health promotion within the context of a disaster situation. Ch. 72

disease A condition that a practitioner views from a pathophysiological model. Ch. 5

dislocation A severe injury of the ligamentous structures that surround a joint, resulting in the complete displacement of the bone from its normal position. Ch. 65

disseminated intravascular coagulation (DIC) A serious bleeding and thrombotic disorder resulting from the abnormally initiated and accelerated clotting and anticlotting processes that occur in response to disease or injury. Ch. 33

diversity Presence of persons with differences from the majority or dominant group that is assumed to be the norm. Ch. 2

diverticulum An outpouching of the mucosa through the circular smooth muscle of the intestinal wall; may occur at any point within the gastro-intestinal tract but is most commonly found in the sigmoid colon. Ch. 45

domestic violence A pattern of coercive behaviour in a relationship that involves fear; humiliation; intimidation; neglect; intentional physical, emotional, financial, or sexual injury or assault; or a combination of these. Ch. 71

dry gangrene Necrosis of an appendage as a result of degenerative changes that occur with chronic diseases such as atherosclerosis or diabetes, when the blood supply to the lower extremities is gradually reduced. Ch. 14

ductus deferens (or vas deferens) A long, thick tube through which sperm exit the epididymis. Ch. 53

dysarthria A disturbance in the muscular control of speech. Ch. 60

dysmenorrhea Abdominal cramping pain or discomfort associated with menstrual flow. Ch. 56

dyspareunia Abnormal pain during sexual intercourse. Ch. 53

dysphagia Difficulty swallowing. Ch. 44

dysphasia Impaired ability to communicate; often used interchangeably with *aphasia*. Ch. 60

dysplasia Abnormal differentiation of dividing cells that results in changes in their size, shape, and appearance. Ch. 14

dysplastic nevi Atypical moles that are larger than usual and have irregular borders and various shades of colour. Ch. 26

dyspnea Shortness of breath. Ch. 28

dysrhythmias Abnormal cardiac rhythms. Ch. 38

E

ecchymosis Bruising. Ch. 32

ectopic pregnancy The implantation of the fertilized ovum anywhere outside the uterine cavity. Ch. 56

eHealth The use of communication and information technologies in order to support the delivery and integration of clinical care within and across settings. Ch. 1

ejection fraction (EF) The percentage of end-diastolic blood volume that is ejected during systole. Ch. 34

elastic recoil The tendency for the lungs to recoil after being stretched or expanded. Ch. 28

elder abuse A single or repeated act, or lack of appropriate action, occurring within a relationship in which there is an expectation of trust, which causes harm or distress to an older person. Ch. 7

elder mistreatment An act of commission (elder abuse) or omission (elder neglect) that harms or threatens to harm an older adult's health or welfare. Ch. 7

elder neglect An act of omission that harms or threatens to harm an older adult's health or welfare. Ch. 7

elective surgery Surgery that is planned. Ch. 20

electrical burns Burns that result from intense heat generated from an electric current. Ch. 27

electrocardiogram (ECG) A graphic tracing of the electrical impulses produced in the heart. Ch. 38

electrolytes Substances whose molecules dissociate or split into ions when placed in solution. Ch. 19

electronic health records (EHRs) Computerized records of patient information that are shared among all health care team members involved in a patient's care and that moves with the patient to other providers and across care settings. Ch. 1

embolic stroke A stroke that occurs when an embolus lodges in and occludes a cerebral artery, resulting in infarction and edema of the area supplied by the involved vessel. Ch. 60

emergence delirium A neurological alteration that occurs in some patients awakening from anaesthesia after surgery, manifesting as restlessness, agitation, disorientation, thrashing, and shouting; also called *violent emergence*. Ch. 22

emergency A present or imminent event that requires a rapid and skilled response to protect the health, safety, and wellness of individuals and to limit damage to property or the environment. Ch. 72

emergency management and disaster planning Advanced preparation for a variety of potential situations, including mass casualty incidents, natural or biological events, technological failures, human conflicts, and acts of terrorism. Ch. 72

emergency surgery Surgery that is unexpected and urgent. Ch. 20

emerging infectious disease An infectious disease whose incidence has recently increased or threatens to increase in the immediate future. Ch. 17

emotion-focused coping A coping strategy that concentrates on methods of managing the emotional response to a stressful event (e.g., discussing feelings with a friend, relaxing in a hot bath). Ch. 8

empathy The quality that allows one person to enter into the world of another so as not to judge, sympathize, or correct but to establish mutual understanding. Ch. 4

emphysema Destruction of the alveoli. Ch. 31

empirical therapy Therapy based on observation and experience, implemented when the condition's exact cause is not known. Ch. 30

empyema A pleural effusion that contains pus. Ch. 30

encephalitis Acute inflammation of the brain. Ch. 59

end-of-life care Care given during the last months, weeks, or days of a patient's life. Ch. 13

endometriosis The presence of endometrial epithelial cells in sites outside the uterine cavity. Ch. 56

endomyocardial biopsy (EMB) A technique that involves removing several small pieces of myocardial tissue percutaneously from the right ventricle and microscopically examining the samples. Ch. 39

endoscopy The direct visualization of a body structure through a lighted fibre-optic instrument (endoscope). Ch. 41

endotracheal (ET) intubation Insertion of a tube into the trachea, bypassing the upper airway and laryngeal structures, to create an artificial airway. Ch. 68

end-stage renal disease (ESRD) Advanced kidney disease with glomerular filtration rate <15 mL/min, when most patients with chronic kidney disease require some form of renal replacement therapy; also referred to as *stage 5 CKD*. Ch. 49

enteral nutrition (EN) Nutrition (e.g., a nutritionally balanced liquefied food or formula) delivered through the gastro-intestinal tract distal to the oral cavity via a tube, catheter, or stoma. Ch. 42

enucleation Removal of the eye. Ch. 24

epidemic An occurrence of the number of cases of a communicable disease exceeding the normal expected occurrence during a given period. Ch. 72

epidermis The thin avascular superficial layer of the skin; made up of an outer dead portion that serves as a protective barrier and a deeper, living portion that folds into the dermis. Ch. 25

epididymis A comma-shaped structure located on posterior-superior aspect of each testis within the scrotum; transports the sperm as they mature. Ch. 53

epididymitis An inflammation of the epididymis, usually secondary to an infectious process and rarely as a result of trauma or urinary reflux down the vas deferens from the urethra. Ch. 57

epidural analgesia The infusion of pain-relieving medications through a catheter placed into the epidural space surrounding the spinal cord. Ch. 22

epidural block Injection of a local anaesthetic into the epidural (extradural) space via either a thoracic or a lumbar approach. Ch. 21

epidural hematoma A collection of blood that results from bleeding between the dura mater and the inner surface of the skull; produces compression of the dura mater and thus of the brain. Ch. 59

epilepsy A condition in which at least two spontaneous seizures occur more than 24 hours apart; caused by a chronic underlying pathology. Ch. 61

epispadias A congenital opening of the urethra on the dorsal surface of the penis; usually associated with other genito-urinary tract defects. Ch. 57

epistaxis Nosebleed. Ch. 29

equianalgesic dose A dose of one analgesic that produces pain-relieving effects equivalent to those of another analgesic. Ch. 10

erectile dysfunction (ED) The inability to attain or maintain an erect penis that allows satisfactory sexual performance. Ch. 57

erythema Skin redness occurring in patches of variable size and shape, caused by heat, certain drugs, alcohol, ultraviolet rays, and other problems. Ch. 25

erythropoiesis The process of red blood cell production. Ch. 32

escharotomy Scalpel or electrocautery incision into necrotic tissue from a severe burn; performed when circulation to extremities is compromised. Ch. 27

esophageal cancer A rare malignant neoplasm of the esophagus; the two main types are squamous cell carcinoma and adenocarcinoma. Ch. 44

esophageal diverticula Saclike outpouchings of one or more layers of the esophagus. Ch. 44

esophageal speech A method of swallowing air, trapping it in the esophagus, and releasing it to create sound. Ch. 29

esophageal varices Complexes of tortuous veins at the lower end of the esophagus; they are enlarged and swollen as a result of portal hypertension. Ch. 46

esophagitis Inflammation of the esophagus. Ch. 44

essential data Clinical and other information about a patient that must be included in the patient's records (e.g., level of distress). Ch. 13

ethnicity The common social, cultural, linguistic, or religious heritage of a group of people. Ch. 2

ethnocentrism A tendency of people to believe that their way of viewing and responding to the world is the most correct, natural, and superior one. Ch. 2

ethnogeriatrics A specialty area of culturally competent care for older people who are identified with a particular ethnic group. Ch. 7

eustress Stress associated with positive events such as the birth of a baby, going for a run, falling in love, or attending a much-anticipated event. Ch. 8

evaluation Process of determining whether identified outcomes have been met. Ch. 1

evidence-informed nursing Nursing that employs best practices as determined by the most current reliable research. Ch. 1

evisceration Protrusion of intestines through a wound when wound edges separate to a certain extent. Ch. 14

Ewing sarcoma family of tumours (ESFT) One of the most common primary malignant neoplasms of bone and soft tissue; characterized by rapid growth within the medullary cavity of long bones, especially the femur, humerus, pelvis, and tibia. Ch. 66

excision and grafting Procedure during which eschar is removed down to the subcutaneous tissue or fascia, depending on the degree of injury, and a graft is then placed on clean, viable tissue to achieve good adherence. Ch. 27

exophthalmos A protrusion of the eyeballs from the orbits; a type of infiltrative ophthalmopathy that results from impairment of venous drainage from the orbit, which causes increased fat deposits and fluid (edema) in the retro-orbital tissues. Ch. 51

expected patient outcomes Goals that articulate what is desired or expected as a result of care. Ch. 1

explanatory model Set of beliefs regarding what causes the disease or illness and the methods that would potentially best treat the condition. Ch. 2

external otitis Inflammation or infection of the epithelium of the auricle and ear canal. Ch. 24

extravasation The infiltration of drugs into tissues surrounding the infusion site. Ch. 18

F

facilitated diffusion Diffusion that involves the use of a protein carrier in the cell membrane (e.g., glucose transport into cell). Ch. 19

facilitator Someone who helps a group of people share insights about a common problem and keeps information moving among group members. Ch. 4

familial Alzheimer's disease Alzheimer's disease that develops in someone younger than 60 years old. Ch. 62

family-centred care An approach to nursing care that involves patients and families in the planning, delivery, and evaluation of health care and emphasizes dignity and respect, information sharing, participation, and collaboration. Ch. 6

family conference A meeting of the patient, caregivers, and members of the interdisciplinary health care team to identify needs for information and assistance with health care matters. Ch. 4

fat embolism syndrome (FES) A syndrome characterized by the presence of systemic fat globules that are distributed into tissues and organs after a traumatic skeletal injury involving fractures. Ch. 65

fatigue A subjective and complex condition that prevents functioning at normal capacity due to a feeling of exhaustion. Ch. 5

fecal impaction An accumulation of hardened feces in the rectum or the sigmoid colon that the individual is unable to move. Ch. 45

fecal incontinence The involuntary passage of stool. Ch. 45

fetor hepaticus A musty, sweet odour of the patient's breath resulting from the accumulation of digestive by-products that the liver is unable to degrade. Ch. 46

fibrinolysis A means of maintaining blood in its fluid form; a continual process that results in the dissolution of fibrin and thus clots. Ch. 32

fibroadenoma A common cause of discrete benign breast lumps in young women; painless, round, well delineated, and very mobile. Ch 54

fibroblasts Immature connective tissue cells that migrate into the healing site and secrete collagen. Ch. 14

fibrocystic changes A benign condition of the breasts characterized by development of excess fibrous tissue, hyperplasia of the epithelial lining of the mammary ducts, proliferation of mammary ducts, and cyst formation. Ch. 54

fibromyalgia syndrome (FMS) A chronic disorder characterized by widespread, nonarticular musculo-skeletal pain and fatigue with multiple tender points. Ch. 67

fistula An abnormal passage that forms between organs or between a hollow organ and the skin. Ch. 14

flail chest A condition resulting from multiple rib fractures, causing instability of the chest wall. Ch. 30

fluid spacing Distribution of body water in different body compartments. Ch. 19

focal seizures One of the major classes of seizures; caused by electrical activity that is focal to a particular area of the brain, resulting in unilateral manifestations. (Previously known as *partial seizures*.) Ch 61

food security The ready availability of enough nutritious food to meet the daily requirements for health and well-being. Ch. 42

fracture A disruption or break in the continuity of the structure of bone. Ch. 65

frail older adults Older adults who, because of declining resources and physical health (e.g., as evidenced by unplanned weight loss, weakness, poor endurance and energy, slowness, or low activity), are most vulnerable to poor outcomes. Ch. 7

fremitus An abnormal, palpable vibration in the chest wall that is produced during vocalization and caused by the passage of air past thick bronchial mucus. Ch. 28

frontotemporal dementia (FTD) A type of dementia characterized by degeneration of the frontal lobe, temporal lobe, or both. Ch. 62

frostbite True tissue freezing, which results in the formation of ice crystals in the tissues and cells. Ch. 71

full-thickness burn Destruction of all skin elements and subcutaneous tissues, with possible involvement of muscles, tendons, and bones. Ch. 27

fulminant hepatitis An acute clinical syndrome that results in severe impairment or necrosis of liver cells and potential liver failure. Ch. 46

fungi Organisms similar to plants but lacking in chlorophyll. Ch. 17

G

galactorrhea A milky secretion from the nipple caused by inappropriate lactation. Ch. 54

gastric cancer Adenocarcinoma of the stomach wall; the second-most frequent cause of cancer death worldwide. Ch. 44

gastritis Inflammation of the gastric mucosa. Ch. 44

gastro-enteritis An inflammation of the mucosa of the stomach and the small intestine. Ch. 45

gastro-esophageal reflux disease (GERD) A syndrome presenting as any clinically significant symptomatic condition or histopathological alteration presumed to be secondary to reflux of gastric contents into the lower esophagus. Ch. 44

gene therapy An experimental technique that is used to replace or functionally repair defective or missing genes with normal genes. Ch. 15

general adaptation syndrome The three stages of physiological response pattern to stress proposed by Hans Selye: alarm reaction, stage of resistance, and stage of exhaustion. Ch. 8

general anaesthesia An altered physiological state characterized by reversible loss of consciousness, skeletal muscle relaxation, amnesia, and analgesia. Ch. 21

general survey statement Statement of the health care provider's general impression of a patient, including behavioural observations. Ch. 3

generalized seizures Seizures characterized by bilateral synchronous epileptic discharges in the brain from the onset, with no warning or aura; in most cases, the patient loses consciousness for a few seconds to several minutes. Ch. 61

genetics The study of inheritance. Ch. 15

genital herpes A sexually transmitted infection caused by the herpes simplex virus (HSV), usually HSV-2; results in painful genital or anal vesicular lesions. Ch. 55

genotype An individual's heritable collection of genetic material. Ch. 15

gerontological nursing A nursing specialty focused on the care of older adults. Ch. 7

Glasgow Coma Scale (GCS) A quick, practical, and standardized system for assessing the degree to which consciousness is impaired. Ch. 59

glaucoma A group of disorders characterized by elevated intraocular pressure and the consequences of elevated pressure, optic nerve atrophy, and peripheral visual field loss. Ch. 24

glial cells The cells in the nervous system that provide support, nourishment, and protection to neurons. Ch. 58

glomerular filtration rate (GFR) The amount of blood filtered by the glomeruli in a given time. Ch. 47

glomerulo-nephritis An immune-related inflammation of the glomeruli characterized by protein-uria, hematuria, decreased urine production, and edema. Ch. 48

glomerulus A capillary network within the kidneys that comprises up to 50 capillaries. Ch. 47

glucagon A hormone synthesized and released from pancreatic alpha cells in response to low levels of blood glucose, to protein ingestion, and to exercise; increases blood glucose levels by stimulating glycogenolysis, gluconeogenesis, and ketogenesis. Ch. 50

glycemic index (GI) The rise in blood glucose levels after a person has consumed carbohydrate-containing food. Ch. 52

goitre An enlarged thyroid gland; the thyroid cells are stimulated to grow, which may result in an overactive thyroid (hyperthyroidism) or an underactive one (hypothyroidism). Ch. 51

gonads The primary reproductive organs (i.e., ovaries in the female and testes in the male). Ch. 53

gonorrhea The second-most frequently occurring sexually transmitted infection, caused by *Neisseria gonorrhoeae*, which spreads by direct physical contact with an infected host, usually during sexual activity (vaginal, oral, or anal). Ch. 55

Goodpasture's syndrome An autoimmune disease characterized by the presence of circulating antibodies against the glomerular and alveolar basement membranes. Ch. 48

gout A type of recurring, acute arthritis characterized by the accumulation of uric acid crystals in one or more joints; characteristic deposits of sodium urate crystals occur in articular, periarticular, and subcutaneous tissues. Ch. 67

Graves' disease An autoimmune disease of unknown etiology marked by diffuse thyroid enlargement and excessive thyroid hormone secretion. Ch. 51

grief A normal reaction to loss that may manifest in both psychological and physiological ways. Ch. 13

growth hormone (GH) A hormone that affects the growth and development of skeletal muscles and long bones, thereby affecting a person's size and height; also has a role in the metabolism of protein, fat, and carbohydrate. Ch. 50

Guillain-Barré syndrome An acute, rapidly progressing, and potentially fatal form of polyneuritis believed to be caused by a cell-mediated immunological reaction directed at the peripheral nerves. Ch. 63

gummas Chronic, destructive lesions associated with late syphilis and affecting any organ of the body, especially the skin, bones, liver, and mucous membranes. Ch. 55

gynecomastia A transient, noninflammatory enlargement of one or both breasts in men. Ch. 54

H

hazards Anything that has the potential to cause harm or loss; can be substances, human activities, or physical events that may cause injury or loss of life, threaten the delivery of critical services, cause social and economic disruption, or cause property or environmental damage. Ch. 72

head injury Any trauma to the scalp, the skull, or the brain. Ch. 59

headache Probably the most common type of pain that humans experience. The majority of people have functional headaches, such as migraine or tension-type headaches; others have organic headaches caused by intracranial or extracranial disease. Ch. 61

healing touch A biofield therapy that encompasses a group of noninvasive techniques that use the hands to clear, energize, and balance the human and environmental energy fields. Ch. 12

health A state encompassing the biopsychosocial and spiritual aspects of well-being rather than one solely defined by the absence of disease. Ch. 5

health equity A situation in which all people have the opportunity to achieve their full health potential through fair and just access to resources for health. Ch. 2

health inequality Differences in the health status of individuals and groups as a result of factors such as biological and genetic makeup, physical environments, actions of the health care system, and broad social and economic issues. Ch. 2

health inequity Disparities in health that are a result of factors that are generally considered to be unfair or unjust and modifiable. Ch. 2

health literacy Ability to access, understand, and act on information regarding health. Ch. 2

health-related hardiness (HRH) A personality resource characterized by a sense of control, commitment, and challenge and an ability to withstand a high degree of stress without falling ill. Ch. 5

health-related quality of life (HRQL) At an individual level, perceptions of physical and mental health status; at a community level, resources, conditions, policies, and practices that influence a populations health perceptions and functional status. Ch. 5

heart failure (HF) An abnormal clinical syndrome involving impaired cardiac pumping or filling or both. Ch. 34

heart failure with preserved ejection fraction (HF-PEF) The inability of the ventricles to relax and fill during diastole; often referred to as diastolic HF. Ch. 37

heart failure with reduced ejection fraction (HF-REF) Heart failure that results from an inability of the heart to pump blood effectively; the most common form of HF. Ch. 37

heat cramps Severe cramps in large muscle groups fatigued by heavy work. Ch. 71

heat exhaustion A clinical syndrome characterized by fatigue, light-headedness, nausea, vomiting, diarrhea, and a sensation of impending doom, caused by prolonged exposure to heat over hours or days. Ch. 71

heatstroke The most serious form of heat stress, resulting from failure of the central thermoregulatory mechanisms. Ch. 71

heaves Sustained lifts of the chest wall in the precordial area that can be seen or palpated. Ch. 34

hematemesis Vomiting of blood, which indicates bleeding in the upper gastro-intestinal tract. Ch. 41

hematopoiesis Blood cell production. Ch. 32

hemochromatosis An iron overload disorder caused primarily by a genetic defect or occurring secondary to diseases such as sideroblastic anemia or liver disease. Ch. 33

hemodialysis (HD) A type of dialysis that uses a machine to remove waste products and excess fluid from the blood by pumping the blood

through an artificial semipermeable membrane. Ch. 49

hemodynamic monitoring The measurement of pressure, flow, and oxygenation within the cardiovascular system. Ch. 68

hemoglobin A complex compound composed of heme (an iron compound) and globin (a simple protein) that binds with oxygen and carbon dioxide. Ch. 32

hemolysis Destruction of erythrocytes. Ch. 32

hemolytic anemia A condition caused by the destruction or hemolysis of red blood cells at a rate that exceeds production. Ch. 33

hemophilia An X-linked recessive genetic disorder caused by defective or deficient coagulation factor. Ch. 33

hemorrhagic stroke A stroke that results from bleeding into the brain tissue itself or into the subarachnoid space or the ventricles. Ch. 60

hemorrhoids Varicosities in the lower rectum or the anus caused by congestion in the veins of the hemorrhoidal plexus. Ch. 45

hemothorax An accumulation of blood in the intrapleural space. Ch. 30

hepatic encephalopathy A neuropsychiatric manifestation of advanced liver disease, resulting from ammonia crossing the blood–brain barrier; manifested as changes in neurological and mental responsiveness, ranging from sleep disturbances to deep coma. Ch. 46

hepatitis Inflammation of the liver. Ch. 46

hepatocytes Specialized hepatic cells. Ch. 41

hepatorenal syndrome (HRS) A serious complication of decompensated cirrhosis; a type of kidney failure with advancing azotemia, oliguria, and intractable ascites. Ch. 46

herbal therapy The use of individual herbs or combinations of herbs for therapeutic benefit to treat, prevent, or cure disease. Ch. 12

hernia A protrusion of a viscus through an abnormal opening or a weakened area in the wall of the cavity in which it is normally contained. Ch. 45

herniated intervertebral disc Herniation of nuclear material from the intervertebral disc that may compress or place tension on a cervical, lumbar, or sacral spinal nerve root, causing acute back pain; also called a *slipped disc*. Ch. 66

herpes zoster Varicella-zoster virus infection, characterized by an eruption of grouped vesicles on erythematous base; usually unilateral on trunk, face, and lumbosacral areas. Also called *shingles*. Ch. 26

heterozygous Having two different alleles for one given gene. Ch. 15

hiatal hernia Herniation of a portion of the stomach into the esophagus through an opening, or hiatus, in the diaphragm. Ch. 44

high-frequency oscillatory ventilation (HFOV) A ventilator that delivers a small tidal volume (usually 1 to 5 mL/kg of body weight) at a rapid respiratory rate (100 to 300 breaths/min) in an effort to recruit and maintain lung volume and reduce intrapulmonary shunting. Ch. 68

hirsutism Male-pattern distribution of hair in women, caused by an abnormality of ovaries or adrenal glands, decrease in estrogen level, or a familial trait. Ch. 25

histological grading A categorization of tumours in which the appearance of cells and the degree of differentiation are evaluated pathologically. Ch. 18

Hodgkin's lymphoma A malignant condition characterized by proliferation of abnormal, giant, multinucleated cells, called *Reed–Sternberg cells*, which are located in lymph nodes. Ch. 33

holding area Also called the *preoperative holding area*; an admission and waiting area inside or adjacent to the surgical suite. Ch. 21

holistic nursing Nursing practice that incorporates mind–body–spirit principles into the development of a caring–healing relationship with patients. Ch. 12

home health nursing A specialized area of nursing practice rooted in community health nursing in which nursing care is delivered in the residence of the patient or where the patient works or attends school. Ch. 6

homeostasis The state of equilibrium in the internal environment of the body, naturally maintained by adaptive responses that promote healthy survival. Ch. 19

homozygous Having two identical alleles for one given gene. Ch. 15

hordeolum An infection of the sebaceous glands in the eyelid margin; commonly called a *sty*. Ch. 24

hormone A chemical substance synthesized and secreted by a specific organ or tissue; most hormones have common characteristics, including (a) secretion in small amounts at variable but predictable rates, (b) circulation through the blood, and (c) binding to specific cellular receptors either in the cell membrane or within the cell wall. Ch. 50

hospice A paradigm of care for patients with advanced malignant disease; end-of-life services. Ch. 13

hospice palliative care Care aimed at improving the quality of life of patients with life-threatening illness and of their families through the relief of pain and suffering. Chs. 6, 13

hospital-acquired pneumonia (HAP) Pneumonia occurring 48 hours or longer after hospital admission and not incubating at the time of hospitalization. Ch. 30

human immunodeficiency virus (HIV) Retrovirus that causes AIDS. Ch. 17

human leukocyte antigen (HLA) system A series of linked genes that occur together on the sixth chromosome in humans that plays an important part in the body's immune response to foreign substances. Ch. 16

humoral immunity Antibody-mediated immunity. Ch. 16

Huntington's disease (HD) A genetically transmitted, autosomal dominant disorder that affects both men and women of all races; characterized by chronic, devastating loss of all neurological function, resulting in a movement disorder and dementia. Ch. 61

hydrocele A nontender, fluid-filled mass that results from interference with lymphatic drainage of the scrotum and swelling of the tunica vaginalis that surrounds the testis. Ch. 57

hydronephrosis Dilation or enlargement of the renal pelvis and the calyces resulting from increased bladder pressure and backflow of urine to the kidney caused by obstruction in the lower urinary tract. Ch. 48

hydrostatic pressure The force within a fluid compartment. Ch. 19

hydroureter Dilation of the renal pelvis caused by backflow of urine. Ch. 48

hyperaldosteronism A condition characterized by excessive aldosterone secretion. Ch. 51

hypercapnia The presence of greater than normal amounts of carbon dioxide in the blood; also called *hypercarbia*. Ch. 70

hypercapnic respiratory failure A partial pressure of arterial carbon dioxide above normal (>45 mm Hg) in combination with acidemia (arterial pH <7.35). Ch. 58

hyperopia A condition in which an affected person can see distant objects clearly (farsightedness) but close objects appear blurred. Ch. 23

hyperosmolar hyperglycemic state (HHS) A life-threatening syndrome that can occur in the patient with diabetes who is able to produce enough insulin to prevent diabetic ketoacidosis but not enough to prevent severe hyperglycemia, osmotic diuresis, and extracellular fluid depletion. Ch. 52

hyperparathyroidism A condition involving increased secretion of parathyroid hormone (PTH). Ch. 51

hyperplasia Multiplication of cells resulting from increased cellular division. Ch. 14

hypersensitivity reaction An overreactive immune response against foreign antigens or a reaction against one's own tissue that may result in tissue damage. Ch. 16

hypertension Sustained elevation of systemic arterial blood pressure; in adults, exists when systolic blood pressure (SBP) is equal to or greater than 140 mm Hg or diastolic blood pressure (DBP) is equal to or greater than 90 mm Hg. Ch. 35

hypertensive crisis A severe and abrupt elevation in blood pressure, arbitrarily defined as a diastolic blood pressure above 120 to 130 mm Hg. Ch. 35

hyperthyroidism Hyperactivity of the thyroid gland with sustained increase in synthesis and release of thyroid hormones. Ch.51

hypertonic Solutions in which solutes are more concentrated than they are in cells. Ch. 19

hypertrophic cardiomyopathy (HCM) Asymmetrical left ventricular hypertrophy without ventricular dilation. Ch. 39

hypertrophic scar Inappropriately large, red, raised, and hard scar. Ch. 14

hypertrophy Expansion in the size of cells, which results in increased tissue mass without cell division. Ch. 14

hypoparathyroidism An uncommon condition associated with inadequate levels of circulating parathyroid hormone (PTH); characterized by hypocalcemia that results from a lack of PTH to maintain serum calcium levels. Ch. 51

hypopituitarism A rare disorder that involves a decrease in one or more of the pituitary hormones. Ch. 51

hypospadias A urological abnormality in which the urethral meatus is located on the ventral surface of the penis anywhere from the corona to the perineum. Ch. 57

hypothermia A core temperature of less than 35°C; occurs when heat loss exceeds heat production. Chs. 22, 71

hypothyroidism Insufficient circulation of thyroid hormone as a result of various abnormalities; can be primary or secondary. Ch. 51

hypotonic Solutions in which solutes are less concentrated than they are in cells. Ch. 19

hypoventilation Deficient ventilation of the lungs, characterized by a decreased respiratory rate or effort, hypoxemia, and an increasing arterial partial pressure of carbon dioxide ($PaCO_2$). Ch. 22

hypovolemic shock Shock that occurs when intravascular fluid volume is lost, and the remaining volume is inadequate to fill the vascular space. Ch. 69

hypoxemia Low oxygen tension in the blood (partial pressure of oxygen in arterial blood [PaO_2] <60 mm Hg), characterized by a variety of nonspecific clinical signs and symptoms. Chs. 22, 70

hypoxemic respiratory failure A condition in which the partial pressure of oxygen in arterial blood (PaO_2) is 60 mm Hg or less when the patient is receiving inspired oxygen at a fractional concentration (FiO_2) of 60% or greater. Ch. 70

hypoxia The condition in which the partial pressure of oxygen in arterial blood (PaO_2) has fallen sufficiently to cause signs and symptoms of inadequate oxygenation. Ch. 70

hysterectomy Surgical removal of the uterus. Ch. 56

I

ileal conduit Urinary diversion procedure; ureters are anastomosed into a segment of ileum that is converted into a conduit for urinary drainage; the other end of the bowel is brought out through the abdominal wall to form a stoma. Ch. 48

illness The human experience of symptoms and suffering; specifically, how the disease is perceived, lived with, and responded to by individuals and their families. Ch. 5

illness behaviour The varying ways individuals respond to physical symptoms: how they monitor internal states, define and interpret symptoms, make attributions, take remedial actions, and use various sources of informal and formal care. Ch. 5

illness trajectory A pathway along which the person with an illness progresses; it includes three phases: crisis phase, chronic phase, and terminal phase. Ch. 5

imagery The use of the mind to generate images that have a calming effect on the body. Ch. 8

immunity The body's ability to resist disease. Ch. 16

immuno-competence The ability of the body's immune system to identify and inactivate or destroy foreign substances. Ch. 16

immunodeficiency The inability of the immune system to protect the body adequately. Ch. 16

immunological surveillance The response of the immune system to antigens of the malignant cells. Ch.18

immuno-suppressive therapy Therapy with the goal of adequately suppressing the immune response to prevent rejection of a transplanted organ and yet maintain sufficient immunity to prevent overwhelming infection; also used to treat autoimmune disorders. Ch. 16

impetigo A condition caused by Group A β-hemolytic streptococci, staphylococci, or a combination of both and characterized by pruritus and an eruption of vesiculo-pustular lesions with a honey-coloured crust surrounded by erythema. Ch. 26

implementation The use of nursing interventions to carry out the nursing care plan. Ch. 1

infective endocarditis (IE) An infection of the heart valves or the endocardial surface of the heart; previously called *bacterial endocarditis*. Ch. 39

infertility The inability to achieve a pregnancy after at least 1 year of regular unprotected intercourse. Ch. 56

inflammatory bowel disease (IBD) An autoimmune disease characterized by idiopathic inflammation and ulceration; includes two disorders of the gastro-intestinal tract—Crohn's disease and ulcerative colitis. Ch. 45

inflammatory response A biological response to cell injury that neutralizes and dilutes the inflammatory agent, removes necrotic materials, and establishes an environment suitable for healing and repair. Ch. 14

informal caregiver A person who provides care without pay and who usually has personal ties to the care recipient. Ch. 5

information and communication technologies (ICT) The tools and applications that support the management of clinical data, information, and knowledge. Ch. 1

informed consent An active, shared decision-making process between the provider and the recipient of health care; this process protects the patient, the surgeon, the hospital, and its employees. Ch. 20

ingestion The intake of food. Ch. 41

insomnia Difficulty falling asleep, difficulty staying asleep, waking up too early, or poor quality of sleep. Ch. 9

inspection The visual examination of a part or region of the body to assess normal conditions or deviations. Ch. 3

insulin The principal regulator of the metabolism and storage of ingested carbohydrates, fats, and proteins; facilitates glucose transport across cell membranes in most tissues. Ch. 52

insulin resistance A condition in which body tissues do not respond to the action of insulin; caused by insulin receptors that are unresponsive to the action of insulin, insufficient in number, or both. Ch. 52

integrated palliative approach A approach to care that focuses on meeting a person's and family's full range of needs—physical, psychosocial, and spiritual—at all stages of illness, not just at the end of life. Ch. 13

integrins Cell receptors that mediate attachment between endothelial cells and surrounding tissues; involved in leukocyte extravasation during the immune response. Ch. 14

intermittent claudication An ischemic muscle ache or pain that is precipitated by a consistent level of exercise, resolves within 10 minutes or less with rest, and is reproducible. Ch. 40

intersectionality A framework for understanding how multiple social identities such as race, gender, sexual orientation, and economic status interact with each other to reflect interlocking systems of privilege and oppression. Ch. 2

interstitial cystitis (IC) A chronic, painful inflammatory disease of the bladder believed to be associated with an autoimmune or allergic response. Ch. 48

intertriginous Describing an area where opposing skin surfaces overlap and rub on each other, such as skin folds of groin, axilla, abdomen, or breast. Ch. 25

intestinal obstruction Partial or complete obstruction of the intestine, preventing intestinal contents from passing through the gastro-intestinal tract; may be classified as mechanical or nonmechanical. Ch. 45

intra-aortic balloon pump Device that provides temporary circulatory assistance to the compromised heart by reducing afterload (via reduction in systolic pressure) and augmenting the aortic diastolic pressure. Ch. 68

intracerebral hemorrhage A type of hemorrhagic stroke in which bleeding occurs within the brain, caused by a rupture of a blood vessel. Ch. 60

intracranial pressure (ICP) Pressure exerted because of the combined total volume of the three components within the skull: brain tissue, blood, and cerebro-spinal fluid. Ch. 59

intraparenchymal or intracerebral hematoma A collection of blood within the parenchyma that results from bleeding within the brain tissue itself and occurs in approximately 16% of head injuries. Ch. 59

intravenous pyelography (IVP) A diagnostic study in which an intravenous contrast medium circulates in the blood and is excreted through the urinary system; used to evaluate the presence, position, size, and shape of the kidneys, ureters, and bladder. Ch. 47

ions Electrically charged atoms or molecules. Ch. 19

iron-deficiency anemia A microcytic hypochromic anemia caused by inadequate supplies of the iron needed to synthesize hemoglobin. Ch. 33

irritable bowel syndrome (IBS) A chronic functional disorder characterized by intermittent and recurrent abdominal pain associated with an alteration in bowel function (diarrhea, constipation, or both). Ch. 45

ischemic strokes Strokes that result from inadequate blood flow to the brain from partial or complete occlusion of an artery. Ch. 60

islets of Langerhans The hormone-secreting portion of the pancreas. Ch. 50

isolated systolic hypertension (ISH) A sustained elevation in systolic blood pressure equal to or greater than 140 mm Hg with a diastolic blood pressure less than 90 mm Hg. Ch. 35

isometric contractions Muscular contractions that increase tension within a muscle but do not produce movement. Ch. 64

isotonic State in which the fluid that surrounds a cell has the same osmolality as the cell interior. Ch. 19

isotonic contractions Muscular contraction that shortens a muscle to produce movement. Ch. 64

J

Janeway's lesions Flat, painless, small, red spots that may be found on the palms and the soles in patients with infective endocarditis. Ch. 39

jaundice A yellowish discoloration of body tissues resulting from an abnormal increase in the concentration of bilirubin in the blood. Ch. 46

jaw-thrust manoeuvre A technique for establishing a clear airway, in which the rescuer uses forearms to stabilize the patient's head (while avoiding neck hyperextension) and then applies pressure with the index fingers to push the patient's jaw forward. Ch. 71

K

keloid A protrusion of scar tissue that extends beyond the wound edges and may form tumour-like masses. Ch. 14

keratinocytes Cells synthesized from epidermal cells in the basal layer; they produce a fibrous protein, called *keratin*, which is vital to the skin's protective barrier function. Ch. 25

keratitis An inflammation or infection of the cornea that can be caused by a variety of microorganisms or by other factors. Ch. 24

Korotkoff sounds Sounds of turbulent blood flow through a compressed artery. Ch. 34

Korsakoff syndrome An irreversible form of amnesia caused by thiamine deficiency and characterized by loss of short-term memory and an inability to learn. Ch. 11

Kupffer cells A type of macrophage found in the liver that removes bacteria and toxins from the blood. Ch. 41

kyphosis Forward bending of thoracic spine: exaggerated thoracic curvature. Ch. 64

L

lactase deficiency A condition in which the lactase enzyme is deficient or absent. Ch. 45

lapses Very short periods of substance use followed by quick return to maintaining nonuse. Ch. 11

laryngeal mask airway (LMA) A supraglottic airway device that is easily placed and used as a method of elective ventilation. Ch. 21

learning A cognitive ability that is reflected by a change in behaviour (knowledge, attitudes, or skills or a combination of these) that can be observed and measured. Ch. 4

learning needs The new knowledge and skills that an individual must acquire to be able to meet an objective or a goal. Ch. 4

learning outcomes The competencies and the knowledge that the patient has achieved and can demonstrate successfully. Ch. 4

learning style The way in which each individual understands and responds to a learning situation; may be visual, auditory, or physical. Ch. 4

leiomyomas Benign smooth muscle tumours that occur most commonly within the uterus; also known as *uterine fibroids*. Ch. 56

lens A biconvex structure located behind the iris and supported in place by small fibres, collectively called the *suspensory ligament* (also called the *zonule*), that connect the lens to the ciliary body; the primary function of the lens is to bend light rays, which enables them to fall onto the retina. Ch. 23

lethal injury Irreversible cell injury that causes cell death. Ch. 14

leukemia A broad term given to a group of malignant diseases that affect the blood and

blood-forming tissues of the bone marrow, lymph system, and spleen. Ch. 33

leukopenia An abnormal decrease in the total white blood cell count to less than 4×10^9/L. Ch. 32

leukoplakia A whitish precancerous lesion on the mucosa of the mouth or tongue that results from chronic irritation, especially from smoking. Ch. 44

lichenification A thickening of epidermis with exaggerated markings resembling a washboard, caused by chronic scratching or rubbing of the skin. Ch. 26

lifestyle The health choices made by individuals, which are influenced by social, economic, and environmental factors. Ch. 5

lipectomy Procedure performed to remove unsightly loose folds of adipose tissue for cosmetic reasons; also called *adipectomy*. Ch. 43

lipodystrophy A condition that produces lumps and dents in the skin—hypertrophy or atrophy of subcutaneous tissue; caused by repeated injection in the same spot. Ch. 52

lithotripsy The use of sound waves to break renal stones into small particles that can be eliminated from the urinary tract. Ch. 48

local anaesthesia The loss of sensation without loss of consciousness; induced topically or via intracutaneous or subcutaneous infiltration. Ch. 21

long-term care (LTC) facilities A placement alternative for adults who can no longer live alone, who need continuous supervision, who have three or more disabilities involving activities of daily living or who are frail. Ch. 7

lordosis Lumbar spinal deformity resulting in exaggerated lumbar curvature; also called *swayback*. Ch. 64

low back pain (LBP) A condition most often owing to a musculo-skeletal problem caused by (a) acute lumbosacral strain, (b) instability of the lumbosacral bony mechanism, (c) osteoarthritis of the lumbosacral vertebrae, (d) degenerative disc disease, or (e) herniation of an intervertebral disc. Ch. 66

lower motor neurons (LMNs) The final common pathway through which descending motor tracts influence skeletal muscle, the effector organ for movement. Ch. 58

lumpectomy Breast-conserving surgery that involves the removal of the entire tumour along with a margin of normal surrounding tissue. Ch. 54

lung abscess A pus-containing lesion of the lung parenchyma that gives rise to a cavity. Ch. 30

Lyme disease A spirochetal infection caused by *Borrelia burgdorferi* and transmitted by the bite of an infected deer tick; the most characteristic clinical symptom of early localized disease is migrans, a skin lesion at the site of the tick bite that occurs within 3 to 30 days in 70% to 80% of people who are infected. Ch. 67

lymphedema Accumulation of lymph in soft tissue that results from the excision or irradiation of lymph nodes. Ch. 54

lymphomas Malignant neoplasms originating in the bone marrow and lymphatic structures resulting in the proliferation of lymphocytes. Ch. 33

M

malabsorption syndrome The impaired absorption of nutrients from the gastro-intestinal tract. Ch. 42

malignant hyperthermia A rare, potentially fatal metabolic disease characterized by hyperthermia with rigidity of skeletal muscles. Ch. 21

malignant melanoma A tumour arising in melanocytes, the cells producing melanin. Ch. 26

malignant neoplasms Tumours that have the ability to invade and metastasize; can be undifferentiated or well differentiated. Ch. 18

Mallory–Weiss tear A tear in the mucosa near the esophagogastric junction; usually caused by severe retching and vomiting. Ch. 44

malnutrition A deficit, excess, or imbalance of the essential components of a balanced diet. Ch. 42

mammoplasty Surgical change in the size or shape of the breast. Ch. 54

massage therapy Therapy involving the manipulation of soft tissues and joints of the body to improve health and promote healing. Ch. 12

mastalgia Breast pain; most common breast-related complaint in women. Ch. 54

mastectomy Surgical removal of all or a portion of a breast. Ch. 54

mastitis An inflammatory condition of the breast that occurs most frequently in lactating women; usually caused by staphylococcal infection. Ch. 54

mean arterial pressure A measurement related to BP; calculated by adding the diastolic pressure to one-third of the pulse pressure. Ch. 34

mechanical receptors Receptors located in the lungs, upper airways, chest wall, and diaphragm that are stimulated by a variety of physiological factors, such as irritants, muscle stretching, and alveolar wall distortion. Ch. 28

mechanical ventilation The process by which the fraction of inspired oxygen is moved in and out of the lungs by a machine. Ch. 68

medical-surgical nursing A type of nursing that involves caring for acutely ill adults experiencing complex variations in health. Ch. 1

megaloblastic anemias A group of disorders caused by impaired DNA synthesis and characterized by the presence of large RBCs. Ch. 33

melanocytes Cells contained in the deep, basal layer *(stratum germinativum)* of the epidermis that contain melanin, a pigment that gives colour to the skin and hair and protects the body from damaging ultraviolet sunlight. Ch. 25

melena Abnormal, black, tarry stool containing digested blood. Ch. 41

menarche The first episode of menstrual bleeding; indicates that a girl has reached puberty. Ch. 53

Ménière's disease A condition characterized by symptoms of inner ear disease, including episodic vertigo, tinnitus, fluctuating sensorineural hearing loss, and a sense of aural fullness; results in an excessive accumulation of endolymph in the membranous labyrinth; also called *endolymphatic hydrops*. Ch. 24

meninges Three layers of protective membranes that surround the brain and the spinal cord: dura mater, arachnoid, and pia mater. Ch. 58

meningitis An acute inflammation of meningeal tissues (the pia mater, arachnoid mater, and dura mater) surrounding the brain and the spinal cord. Ch. 59

menopause The physiological cessation of menses associated with declining ovarian function. Ch. 53, 56

menstrual cycle A monthly process mediated by the hormonal activity of the hypothalamus, the pituitary gland, and the ovaries (during which the major functions of the ovaries are ovulation and the secretion of hormones). Ch. 53

metabolic syndrome A collection of risk factors that increase an individual's chance of developing cardiovascular disease and diabetes mellitus. Ch. 43

metaplasia Transformation of one cell type into another in response to a change in physiological condition or to an external irritant. Ch. 14

metastasis Spread of the cancer to a distant site. Ch. 18

migraine headache A type of headache characterized by unilateral throbbing pain, a triggering event or factor, and manifestations associated with neurological and autonomic nervous system dysfunction; the effects of migraine headache pain are dramatic, often causing both physical and emotional disability. Ch. 61

mild cognitive impairment (MCI) A state of cognitive decline that is not severe enough to interfere with activities of daily living. Ch. 62

mitral valve prolapse (MVP) A structural abnormality of the mitral valve leaflets and the papillary muscles or chordae that allows the leaflets to prolapse, or buckle, back into the left atrium during ventricular systole. Ch. 39

modifiable risk factors Factors such as behaviour that can be changed to reduce the risk of developing an illness. Ch. 5

modulation The activation of descending pathways that exert inhibitory or facilitatory effects on the transmission of pain. Ch. 10

mole (nevus) Benign overgrowth of melanocytes, occurring as a defect of development; excessive numbers of large, irregular moles are often familial. Ch. 25

monoclonal antibodies Homogeneous populations of identical antibody molecules produced by specialized tissue cell culture lines. Ch. 16

mons pubis A fatty layer lying over the pubic bone that is covered in coarse hair after puberty (in a triangular pattern in women and a diamond pattern in men). Ch. 53

morbidity Rates of disease in a population. Ch. 5

morbidly obese Classification describing individuals with a body mass index greater than 40 kg/m^2. Ch. 43

mortality Rates of death in a population. Ch. 5

motivational interviewing A collaborative, person-centred counselling approach aimed at changing a patient's ambivalence and, ultimately, the patient's behaviour. Ch. 11

multimorbidity The simultaneous occurrence of several chronic medical conditions in the same person. Ch. 5

multiple myeloma A condition in which neoplastic plasma cells infiltrate the bone marrow and destroy bone. Ch. 33

multiple-organ dysfunction syndrome (MODS) In a patient who is acutely ill, the failure of two or more organ systems to such a degree that homeostasis cannot be maintained without intervention. Ch. 69

multiple sclerosis (MS) A chronic, progressive, degenerative autoimmune disorder of the central nervous system characterized by disseminated demyelination of nerve fibres of the brain, the spinal cord, and the optic nerves. Ch. 61

murmurs Sounds produced by turbulent blood flow through the heart or the walls of large arteries. Ch. 34

mutation A change in the DNA sequence of a gene, affecting the original expression of the gene. Ch. 15

myasthenia gravis (MG) An autoimmune disease of the neuro-muscular junction characterized by fluctuating weakness of certain skeletal muscle groups. Ch. 61

myasthenic crisis An acute exacerbation of muscle weakness triggered by infection, surgery, emotional distress, overdose of drugs, or inadequate drugs in a person with myasthenia gravis. Ch. 61

myelodysplastic syndrome (MDS) A group of related hematological disorders characterized by a change in the quantity and the quality of bone marrow elements. Ch. 33

myocardial infarction (MI) Irreversible myocardial cell death (necrosis) caused by sustained ischemia. Ch. 36

myocarditis A focal or diffuse inflammation of the myocardium. Ch. 39

myofascial pain syndrome A chronic form of muscle pain; characterized by musculo-skeletal pain and tenderness, typically in the chest, neck, shoulders, hips, and lower back. Ch. 67

myopia A condition in which an affected person can see near objects clearly (nearsightedness) but objects in the distance appear blurred. Ch. 23

myxedema The accumulation of hydrophilic mucopolysaccharides in the dermis and other tissues; causes the characteristic facies of hypothyroidism (i.e., puffiness, periorbital edema, and masklike affect). Ch. 51

myxedema coma A medical emergency in which the mental sluggishness, drowsiness, and lethargy of hypothyroidism progresses gradually or suddenly to a notable impairment of consciousness or coma. Ch. 51

nadir The lowest level of the peripheral blood cell counts that occurs secondary to bone marrow depression. Ch. 18

narcolepsy A chronic degenerative neurological disorder caused by the brain's inability to regulate sleep–wake cycles normally. Ch. 9

nasal polyps Benign mucous membrane masses that form slowly in response to repeated inflammation of the sinus or the nasal mucosa. Ch. 29

nausea A feeling of discomfort in the epigastrium with a conscious desire to vomit. Ch. 44

necrosis Tissue death that occurs as a result of a traumatic injury, infection, or exposure to a toxic chemical that causes a local inflammatory response. Ch. 14

negative feedback A highly specialized mechanism in the regulation of hormone levels; the most common type of feedback system, in which the gland responds by increasing or decreasing the secretion of a hormone on the basis of feedback from various factors. Ch. 50

negative-pressure ventilation Noninvasive ventilation (i.e., not requiring an artificial airway) delivered through the use of chambers that encase the chest or body and surround it with intermittent subatmospheric (or negative) pressure. Ch. 68

nephrolithiasis The formation of stones in the urinary tract. Ch. 48

nephron The functional unit of the kidney; each kidney has 800 000 to 1.2 million nephrons. Ch. 47

nephrosclerosis A vascular disease of the kidney characterized by sclerosis of the small arteries and arterioles of the kidney, resulting in renal tissue destruction. Ch. 48

nephrotic syndrome A clinical course associated with a number of disease conditions of the kidney; characterized by peripheral edema, massive proteinuria, dyslipidemia, and hypoalbuminemia. Ch. 48

neuraxial blocks Regional anaesthesia (epidural or spinal) that blocks pain transmission during surgery. Ch. 21

neurofibrillary tangles Abnormal collections of twisted protein threads inside nerve cells seen in the areas of the brain most affected by Alzheimer's disease. Ch. 62

neurogenic bladder A bladder dysfunction related to abnormal or absent bladder innervation. Ch. 63

neurogenic shock A hemodynamic syndrome of massive vasodilation without compensation that results from the loss of sympathetic nervous system vasoconstrictor tone caused by spinal cord injury; characterized by hypotension, bradycardia, and hypothermia. Chs. 63, 69

neurons The primary functional units of the nervous system; share three characteristics: excitability, conductivity, and the ability to influence other neurons, muscle cells, and glandular cells. Also called *nerve cells*. Ch. 58

neuropathic pain Pain caused by damage to nerve cells or changes in spinal cord processing, typically described as burning, shooting, stabbing, or electrical in nature. Ch. 10

neuro-syphilis An infection of any part of the nervous system by the organism *Treponema pallidum*. Ch. 63

neurotransmitter A chemical agent that affects the transmission of an impulse across the synaptic cleft. Ch. 58

neutropenia An abnormal reduction of the neutrophil count to less than 1×10^9/L to 1.5 × 10^9/L. Chs. 32, 33

nociception The activation of the primary afferent nociceptors with peripheral terminals (free nerve endings) that respond differently to noxious (tissue-damaging) stimuli. Ch. 10

nociceptive pain Pain caused by damage to somatic or visceral tissue. Ch. 10

nonalcoholic fatty liver disease (NAFLD) A spectrum of disease that ranges from simple fatty liver that causes no hepatic inflammation to severe liver scarring; characterized by accumulation of fat in hepatocytes not associated with alcohol. Ch. 46

nonalcoholic steatohepatitis (NASH) A condition characterized by the accumulation of fat in the liver cells, causing inflammation and liver cell injury; occurs in people who drink little or no alcohol. Ch. 46

non-Hodgkin's lymphomas (NHLs) A heterogeneous group of malignant neoplasms of primarily B-, T-, or natural killer cell origin that can affect people of all ages. Ch. 33

nonmodifiable risk factors Factors such as age and sex that contribute to the development of an illness but cannot be changed. Ch. 5

normal pressure hydrocephalus (NPH) An abnormal increase of cerebro-spinal fluid, characterized by an obstruction in the normal flow of cerebro-spinal fluid throughout the brain, spinal cord, and ventricles; a relatively uncommon disorder. Ch. 61

nuchal rigidity Resistance to flexion of the neck. Ch. 59

nulliparous Never pregnant. Ch. 53

nurse practitioners (NPs) Registered nurses with advanced education; NPs' scope of practice may include ordering and interpreting diagnostic tests, prescribing medications, and performing procedures beyond the scope of practice of registered nurses. Ch. 6

NurseONE A Web-based information portal for nurses that provides access to libraries and information related to evidence-informed practice and clinical practice issues. Ch. 1

nursing diagnosis The process of the nurse's identifying and labelling human responses to actual or potential health problems; also, the product of this process as articulated in standard terminology. Ch. 1

nursing history Information used to determine the patient's strengths and responses to a health problem that is diagnosed and treated by nurses. Ch. 3

nursing informatics The integration of nursing science, computer science, and information technology to manage and communicate data, information, and knowledge in nursing practice. Ch. 1

nursing intervention Any treatment, based on clinical judgement and knowledge that a nurse performs to enhance patient outcomes. Ch. 1

nursing leadership An attitude and approach in which lifelong learning and a commitment to excellence in practice are valued. Ch. 1

nursing process An assertive, problem-solving approach to the identification and treatment of patient health problems; a framework to organize the knowledge, judgements, and actions that nurses supply in patient care. Ch. 1

nursing-sensitive outcomes Empirical-based indicators linking nursing interventions to problem or symptom resolution. Ch. 6

nutrition The process by which the body uses food for energy, growth, maintenance, and repair of body tissues. Ch. 42

nystagmus Abnormal eye movements that may be observed by other people as twitching of the eyeball or may be described by the patient as a blurring of vision with head or eye movement. Ch. 23

O

obese Classification used to describe individuals with body mass index value of 30 to 40 kg/m² or more. Ch. 43

obesity A complex, chronic, multifactorial disease that develops from the interaction between genetics and the environment; manifests as an abnormal increase in the proportion of fat cells in the body. Ch. 43

objective data Data relating to the patient's condition that can be observed and measured; also called *signs*. Ch. 3

obstructive sleep apnea (OSA) Partial or complete obstruction of the upper airway during sleep. Ch. 9

oliguria A urine output of less than 400 mL in 24 hours. Ch. 49

oncogenes Tumour-inducing genes that interfere with normal cell expression under some conditions, causing the cell to become malignant. Ch. 18

oncotic pressure Osmotic pressure exerted by colloids in solution. Ch. 19

operating room (OR) A unique acute care setting specially designed for surgery that, in a hospital, is usually adjacent to the postanaesthesia care unit and the surgical intensive care unit. Ch. 21

opiates Substances that are directly derived from the opium poppy, such as opium, morphine, and codeine. Ch. 11

opioids Umbrella term that includes both the opiates and the many semisynthetic and synthetic narcotic agents used as analgesics. Ch. 11

opportunistic diseases Infections and cancers that occur in immuno-suppressed patients that can lead to disability, disease, and death. Ch. 17

optimal nutritional status State achieved when nutrients consumed meet daily requirements and metabolic demands. Ch. 42

oral hairy leukoplakia An Epstein-Barr virus infection that causes painless, white, raised lesions on the lateral aspect of the tongue. Ch. 17

orchitis An acute inflammation of the testis. Ch. 57

organ transplantation The transfer of a whole or partial organ from one individual to another for the purpose of replacing the recipient's damaged or failing organ with a working one from the donor. Ch. 16

orthostatic hypotension A decrease of 20 mm Hg (or more) in systolic blood pressure or a decrease of 10 mm Hg (or more) in diastolic blood pressure that occurs when an individual assumes a standing position. Ch. 35

Osler's nodes Painful, tender, red or purple, pea-size lesions that may be found on the fingertips or the toes in patients with infective endocarditis; last only 1 or 2 days. Ch. 39

osmolality A measure of the osmotic force of solute per unit of weight of solvent. Ch. 19

osmolarity A measure of the total milliosmoles of solute per unit of total volume of solution. Ch. 19

osmosis The movement of water between two compartments separated by a semipermeable membrane, one that allows the movement of water but not solute. Ch. 19

osmotic pressure The amount of pressure necessary to stop the osmotic flow of water. Ch. 19

osteoarthritis (OA) A slowly progressive, noninflammatory disorder of the diarthrodial (synovial) joints; the most common form of joint (articular) disease in North America. Ch. 67

osteoclastoma A destructive tumour that arises in the cancellous ends of long bones in young adults; also called a *giant-cell tumour*. Ch. 66

osteomyelitis A severe infection of the bone, bone marrow, and surrounding soft tissue, most commonly caused by *Staphylococcus aureus*. Ch. 66

osteoporosis A chronic, progressive metabolic bone disease characterized by low bone mass and structural deterioration of bone tissue, leading to increased bone fragility, which predisposes the individual to bone fractures at the hip, wrist, and spine. Ch. 66

osteosarcoma A malignant primary bone tumour that is extremely aggressive and is characterized by rapid growth and metastasis. Ch. 66

osteotomy Surgery to remove or add a wedge or slice of bone to change alignment (joint and vertebral) and to shift weight bearing, thereby correcting a deformity and relieving pain. Ch. 65

ostomy A surgical procedure in which an opening is made to allow passage of urine from the bladder, or intestinal contents from the bowel, to an incision or stoma surgically created in the wall of the abdomen. Ch. 45

otosclerosis A hereditary autosomal dominant disease in which spongy bone develops from the bony labyrinth, causing immobilization of the footplate of the stapes in the oval window; most common cause of hearing loss in young adults. Ch. 24

outbreak management Strategies used to prevent the spread of communicable disease among a cluster of people. Ch. 72

overnutrition A state that results from the consumption of nutrients—most frequently, calories, sodium, and fat—in excess of requirements. Ch. 42

overweight Classification used to describe individuals with a body mass index value of 25 to 29.9 kg/m². Ch. 43

oxygen toxicity A condition of oxygen overdosage. Ch. 31

P

Paget's disease of the bone A chronic skeletal bone disorder in which there is excessive bone resorption followed by replacement of normal marrow by vascular, fibrous connective tissue and new bone that is larger, disorganized, and structurally weaker; also called *osteitis deformans*. Ch. 66

Paget's disease of the breast A rare breast malignancy characterized by a persistent lesion of the nipple and areola with or without a palpable mass. Ch. 54.

pain A subjective and unpleasant sensation caused by actual or potential tissue damage. Ch. 10

pain perception Recognition of, definition of, and response to pain by the individual experiencing it. Ch. 10

paired organ donation An option for organ donation that allows a living donor to donate an organ (e.g., kidney) to a different compatible recipient, with the intent that another donor will donate to the first donor's designated recipient. Ch. 49

palliative Relieving pain without attempting to treat the cause; originates from the Latin word *palliaire*, which means "to cloak." Ch. 13

palpation Examination of the body through the use of touch. Ch. 3

pancytopenia Marked decrease in the number of red blood cells, white blood cells, and platelets. Ch. 32

pandemic The occurrence of a communicable disease being widespread and affecting large numbers of people across several countries or continents or globally. Ch. 72

pandemic influenza A highly infectious outbreak of influenza that spreads rapidly around the world, with much more serious consequences than the usual effects of seasonal influenza. Ch. 72

paracentesis A needle puncture of the abdominal cavity performed to remove ascitic fluid or to test the fluid for infection. Ch. 46

paralytic ileus Impairment of intestinal motility (ileus that persists for more than 2 to 3 days) postoperatively. Ch. 22

paraphimosis Narrowing or edema of the retracted uncircumcised foreskin, preventing normal return over the glans and causing strangulation. Ch. 57

paraplegia Paralysis and loss of sensation in the lower limbs and the trunk. Ch. 63

parasomnias Unusual and often undesirable behaviours that occur during sleep or during arousal from sleep (e.g., abnormal movements; dream-related behaviours, emotions, and perceptions). Ch. 9

parenteral nutrition (PN) The administration of nutrients by a route other than the gastro-intestinal tract (e.g., the bloodstream). Ch. 42

Parkinson's disease (PD) A progressive neurodegenerative disease of the central nervous system (basal ganglia) characterized by a slowing down in the initiation and the execution of movement (bradykinesia), increased muscle tone (rigidity), tremor at rest, and impaired postural reflexes. Ch. 61

paroxysmal nocturnal dyspnea A disorder that occurs when the patient is asleep; characterized by awakening in a panic with feelings of suffocation and a strong desire to sit or stand up; caused by the reabsorption of fluid from dependent body areas when the patient is flat. Ch. 37

partial-thickness burn Varying degrees of epidermal and dermal skin injury, with some skin elements remain viable for regeneration. Ch. 27

patient-centred approach An approach that focuses on the patient as a multifaceted person and not just on the condition. Ch. 1

patient-controlled analgesia (PCA) An infusion system that allows the patient to self-administer a dose of opioid through a pump when needed. Ch. 10

patient safety A cornerstone of nursing practice. Ch. 1

peer teaching Teaching that is conducted within the setting of a peer group, such as a self-help or support group. Ch. 4

pelvic inflammatory disease (PID) An infectious condition of the pelvic cavity that may involve the fallopian tubes (*salpingitis*), ovaries (*oophoritis*), and pelvic peritoneum (*peritonitis*). Ch. 56

peptic ulcer disease (PUD) A condition characterized by erosion of the gastro-intestinal mucosa that results from the digestive action of hydrochloric acid and pepsin. Ch. 44

percussion Technique in physical examination of tapping the body directly or indirectly with the fingertips or fist to produce a sound and vibration to obtain information about the underlying area. Ch. 3

percutaneous coronary intervention (PCI) An intervention to treat coronary artery disease in which a catheter equipped with an inflatable balloon tip is inserted into a narrowed coronary artery and the balloon is inflated; common elective procedure and also used in emergent situations. Ch. 36

pericardial effusion An accumulation of excess fluid in the pericardium. Ch. 39

pericardial friction rub A scratching, grating, high-pitched sound believed to arise from friction between the roughened pericardial and the epicardial surfaces. Ch. 39

pericardiocentesis Procedure in which a 16- to 18-gauge needle is inserted into the pericardial space to remove fluid for analysis and to relieve cardiac pressure. Ch. 39

pericarditis A condition caused by inflammation of the pericardial sac. Ch. 39

perimenopause A normal life transition that begins with the first signs of change in menstrual cycles and ends after cessation of menses. Ch. 56

peripheral artery disease (PAD) A condition that involves thickening of artery walls, which results in a progressive narrowing of the arteries of the upper and lower extremities. Ch. 40

peripheral nervous system (PNS) The division of the nervous system that consists of cranial nerves III to XII, the spinal nerves, and the peripheral components of the autonomic nervous system. Ch. 58

peritoneal dialysis (PD) A type of dialysis that uses a natural semipermeable membrane, the peritoneum; dialysis fluid is infused into the peritoneal cavity, and excess fluid and waste products pass across the membrane into the fluid, which is then drained and discarded. Ch. 49

peritonitis A localized or generalized inflammatory process of the peritoneum. Ch. 45

pernicious anemia A disease in which the gastric mucosa does not secrete intrinsic factor (IF) because of either gastric mucosal atrophy or autoimmune destruction of parietal cells and possibly also because of IF itself. Ch. 33

PERRLA Acronym that stands for "**p**upils are **e**qual, **r**ound, and **r**eactive to **l**ight and **a**ccommodation" (a description of normal pupil function). Ch. 23

petechiae Small purplish-red lesions. Ch. 32

pH H⁺ concentration, usually expressed as a negative logarithm. Ch. 19

phagocytosis A process by which white blood cells ingest or engulf an unwanted organism and then digest and kill it. Ch. 32

phantom limb sensation Phenomenon whereby the patient feels as though the amputated limb is still present after surgery to remove it; describes any sensation of the missing limb except pain. Ch. 65

pheochromocytoma A rare condition characterized by a tumour of the adrenal medulla that produces excessive amounts of catecholamines (epinephrine, norepinephrine), resulting in severe hypertension. Ch. 51

phimosis A constriction of the uncircumcised foreskin around the head of the penis, making retraction over the glans penis difficult. Ch. 57

phlebostatic axis A landmark used to establish the zero reference point at the level of the atria of the heart for positioning the stopcock nearest the transducer; located at the intersection of two imaginary lines, one through the fourth intercostal space at the sternum and one through midchest, halfway between the outermost anterior and the outermost posterior surfaces. Ch. 68

physical dependence Physiological adaptation to ongoing exposure to pharmacological agents such that use and cessation of use cause an expected physiological response. Ch. 10

physical examination The systematic assessment of a patient's physical status. Ch. 3

pilonidal sinus A small tract under the skin between the buttocks, in the sacrococcygeal area; may have several openings and is lined with epithelium and hair. Ch. 45

planning Setting goals and expected outcomes with the patient and, when feasible, the patient's family and determining strategies for accomplishing the goals. Ch. 1

pleural effusion A collection of fluid in the pleural space. Ch. 30

pleural friction rub A creaking or grating sound that occurs when roughened, inflamed surfaces of the pleura rub together; evident during inspiration, expiration, or both; does not change with coughing. Ch. 28

pleurisy (pleuritis) Inflammation of the pleura. Ch. 30

pneumoconiosis A general term for lung diseases caused by the inhalation and retention of dust particles, literally meaning "dust in the lungs." Ch. 30

pneumonia Acute inflammation of the lung parenchyma caused by a microbial agent. Ch. 30

pneumothorax Presence of air in the pleural space. Ch. 30

poikilothermism The adjustment of the body temperature to the room temperature. Ch. 63

point of maximal impulse (PMI) The site of strongest pulsation; lies within the midclavicular line in the fifth intercostal space. Ch. 34

polycystic kidney disease (PKD) A genetic kidney disorder in which the cortex and the medulla are filled with thin-walled cysts that enlarge and destroy surrounding tissue by compression. Ch. 48

polycythemia An abnormal condition characterized by increased red blood cells. Chs. 32, 33

polymyositis Diffuse, idiopathic, inflammatory myopathies of the connective tissues, especially striated muscle, that produce bilateral weakness, usually most severe in the proximal or the limb-girdle muscles. Ch. 67

polypharmacy Use of multiple medications by a patient who has more than one health problem. Ch. 7

portal hypertension Hypertension characterized by increased venous pressure in the portal circulation, as well as by splenomegaly, large collateral veins, ascites, systemic hypertension, and esophageal varices. Ch. 46

positive end-expiratory pressure (PEEP) A ventilatory manoeuvre in which positive pressure is applied to the airway during exhalation. Ch. 68

positive feedback A second method of regulation of hormone secretion; increases the target organ action beyond normal. Ch. 50

positive-pressure ventilation (PPV) A ventilatory mode in which the ventilator pushes air into the lungs under positive pressure; the primary method used with acutely ill patients. Ch. 68

postmenopause The time in a woman's life after menopause. Ch. 56

postpolio syndrome (PPS) Recurrence of neuromuscular symptoms of polio in disease survivors as they age. Ch. 63

post-thrombotic syndrome (PTS) A condition that results in chronic venous hypertension caused by valvular destruction (from inflammation and scarring); stiffness and noncompliance of vein walls; and persistent venous obstruction; occurs in 20% to 50% of patients with venous thrombo-embolism. Ch. 40

postural drainage An airway clearance technique in which gravity is used to assist in bronchial drainage. Ch. 31

potentiation A drug interaction causing a response greater than the sum of the individual responses to each drug. Ch. 11

prayer A form of communication or fellowship with a divine entity or the sacred. Ch. 12

prediabetes A condition in which a fasting or a 2-hour plasma glucose level is higher than normal but lower than that considered diagnostic for diabetes mellitus; places the individual at risk of developing diabetes mellitus and its complications. (Also known as *impaired glucose tolerance [IGT]* or *impaired fasting glucose [IFG]*). Ch. 52

preload The volume of blood in the ventricles at the end of diastole, before the next contraction. Ch. 34

premature atrial contraction (PAC) Contraction originating from an ectopic focus in the atrium in a location other than the sinus node. Ch. 38

premature ventricular contraction (PVC) A contraction originating in an ectopic focus in the ventricles. Ch. 38

premenstrual syndrome (PMS) A symptom complex related to the luteal phase of the menstrual cycle that resolves with menstruation. Ch. 56

presbycusis Hearing loss associated with aging; includes the loss of peripheral auditory sensitivity, a decline in word recognition ability, and associated psychological and communication issues. Ch. 24

presbyopia A form of hyperopia, or farsightedness, that occurs as a normal process of aging, usually beginning around age 40. Ch. 23

pressure injury A localized injury to the skin or underlying soft tissue, usually over a bony prominence or related to a medical or other device, as a result of pressure or pressure in combination with shear, friction, or both. Ch. 14

primary care A facet of primary health care that focuses on aspects of health care such as health promotion, illness prevention, diagnosis, and treatment. Ch. 6

primary (essential) hypertension Elevated blood pressure without an exact identified cause but considered to be due to a complex interaction between genes and the environment; accounts for about 90% to 95% of all cases of hypertension. Ch. 35

primary health care A philosophy and an approach to health care that focuses on a system-wide partnership between health, social services, housing, and the environment. Ch. 6

primary survey A systematic approach to emergency assessment that focuses on airway, breathing, circulation, and disability (ABCDs) and serves to identify life-threatening conditions. Ch. 71

Prinzmetal's angina Angina that occurs at rest, usually in response to spasm of a major coronary artery; also called *variant angina*. Ch. 36

problem-focused coping A cognitive approach that focuses on finding solutions to the problems causing stress (e.g., setting priorities, collecting information, seeking advice). Ch. 8

procedural sedation Mild depression of consciousness that results from administration of IV sedatives, analgesics, or both so patients can tolerate minor procedures yet still maintain airway control and protective airway reflexes. Ch. 21

prodrome Signs or symptoms that may precede a migraine headache, including psychic disturbances, gastro-intestinal upset, and changes in fluid balance. Ch. 61

pronouncement of death Verification of the absence of an apical pulse and respirations and that the pupils are fixed and dilated. Ch. 13

prostate-specific antigen (PSA) A glycoprotein found only in the epithelial cells of the prostate that, when elevated, indicates a pathological condition of the prostate, although not necessarily prostate cancer. Ch. 57

prostatitis An acute or chronic inflammatory condition affecting the prostate gland, usually as a result of infection. Ch. 57

protein–calorie malnutrition (PCM) The most common form of undernutrition. Ch. 42

proto-oncogenes Normal genes that are regulators of normal cellular processes; promote growth. Ch. 18

protozoa Single-cell, animal-like microorganisms that normally live in soil and bodies of water but, when introduced into the human body, can cause infection; include amoebas, ciliates, flagellates, and sporozoa. Ch. 17

pruritus Itching. Ch. 25

pseudocyst A cavity continuous with or surrounding the outside of the pancreas. Ch. 46

pseudo-obstruction An apparent mechanical obstruction of the intestine without demonstration of obstruction by radiological methods. Ch. 45

psoriasis A common inherited benign disorder that is characterized by the eruption of reddish, silver-scaled maculopapules, predominantly on the elbows, knees, scalp, and trunk. Ch. 26

psoriatic arthritis A progressive inflammatory disease that affects approximately 10% to 30% of people with psoriasis (a skin disorder); has a genetic link with the HLA antigens in many patients. Ch. 67

psychological dependence Emotional and mental reliance on a substance because of the pleasurable and reinforcing effects of the substance. Ch. 11

psychoneuroimmunology Interdisciplinary science in which investigators seek to understand the interactions among psychological, neurological, and immune responses. Ch. 8

public health nursing A specialized area of nursing practice in which the nurse combines knowledge from public health science, primary health care, nursing science, and the social sciences and focuses on promoting, protecting, and preserving the health of populations. Ch. 6

pulmonary edema An abnormal, life-threatening accumulation of fluid in the alveoli and the interstitial spaces of the lungs. Chs. 30, 37

pulmonary embolism (PE) The blockage of pulmonary arteries by a thrombus, fat or air embolus, or tumour tissue. Ch. 30

pulmonary hypertension Elevated pulmonary pressure resulting from an increase in pulmonary vascular resistance to blood flow through small arteries and arterioles. Ch. 30

pulse pressure The difference between the systolic blood pressure and the diastolic blood pressure. Ch. 34

purpura Purplish-red rash. Ch. 32

pursed-lip breathing A breathing exercise (breathing in through the nose and then breathing out through pursed lips); used to prolong exhalation, prevent bronchiolar collapse and air trapping, and assist with dyspnea. Ch. 31

pyelonephritis Inflammation (usually caused by infection) of the renal parenchyma and the collecting system. Ch. 48

pyrosis Heartburn; burning in epigastric or substernal area. Ch. 41

Q

quality of life A subjective evaluation of both the positive and negative aspects of life. Ch. 5

quarantine The isolation of people who have been exposed, or potentially exposed, to an infection or contagious disease but who are not yet sick or showing any signs of illness. Ch. 72

R

race A group characterized by specific biological and physical traits, such as skin colour, bone structure, or blood group. Ch. 2

racialization Social processes of categorization or differentiation of groups according to race. Ch. 2

radiation The emission and distribution of energy through space or a material medium. Ch. 18

radical prostatectomy Surgical removal of the entire prostate gland, the seminal vesicles, and part of the bladder neck (ampulla). Ch. 57

rapid-sequence intubation The preferred procedure for securing an unprotected airway; the patient is given a sedative and a neuro-muscular blocking agent to facilitate intubation and minimize the risk for aspiration and airway trauma. Ch. 71

Raynaud's phenomenon An episodic vaso-spastic disorder of small cutaneous arteries, most frequently involving the fingers and toes. Ch. 40

recessive allele An allele that has no noticeable effect on the phenotype in a heterozygous individual. Ch. 15

rectocele Herniation or protrusion of the rectum through the wall of the vagina; occurs when support between the vagina and the rectum is weakened; also known as *posterior wall prolapse*. Ch. 56

reflex An involuntary response to a stimulus. Ch. 58

refractive error A defect in which light rays focus either in front of or behind the eye, causing images to be out of focus. Ch. 24

refractory hypoxemia Hypoxemia unresponsive to increasing concentrations of oxygen. Ch. 70

regeneration Replacement of lost cells and tissues with cells of the same type. Ch. 14

regional anaesthesia Reversible loss of sensation to a region of the body without loss of consciousness, achieved by blocking nerve fibres with the administration of a local anaesthetic. Ch. 21

regulated health care providers Paid workers who meet certain requirements that allow them to legally use a specific title and to undertake a specific type of work. Ch. 1

regurgitation Incomplete closure of the valve leaflets, resulting in the backward flow of blood. Ch. 39

relapse A return to substance use after a period of abstinence. Ch. 11

relief craving The intense desire for a substance, usually experienced after decreased use, resulting from the memory aspect related to the brain reward pathway. Ch. 11

renal arteriography A radiological study performed by injecting contrast material into the renal artery via a catheter inserted into the femoral artery; the purpose is to visualize renal blood vessels. Ch. 47

renal artery stenosis A partial occlusion of one or both renal arteries and their major branches; a major cause of abrupt-onset hypertension. Ch. 48

renal biopsy Procedure to obtain renal tissue for examination to establish a diagnosis or to follow progress of renal disease; may be an open biopsy or, more commonly, a skin (percutaneous) biopsy conducted through needle insertion into the lower lobe of the kidney. Ch. 47

renal osteodystrophy A disorder of the bones associated with chronic kidney disease that includes a number of skeletal disorders: osteitis fibrosa, osteomalacia, adynamic bone disorder, and mixed osteodystrophy. Ch. 49

renal replacement therapy (RRT) All forms of life-supporting therapies for renal failure, including hemodialysis, peritoneal dialysis, hemofiltration, and renal transplantation. Ch. 49

renal vein thrombosis An embolus occurring in the renal vein. Ch. 48

repair Healing as a result of lost cells' being replaced by connective tissue. Ch. 14

repetitive strain injury (RSI) Injury resulting from prolonged force or repetitive movements and awkward postures; also called *cumulative trauma disorder, repetitive trauma disorder, nontraumatic musculo-skeletal injury, overuse syndrome* (sports medicine), *regional musculo-skeletal disorder*, and *work-related musculo-skeletal disorder*. Ch. 65

resilience The ability to be resourceful, be flexible, and recover from stressful situations and return to prior levels of functioning. Ch. 8

responsive behaviours In patients with dementia, behaviours that are responses to something in the patient's environment. Ch. 62

restless legs syndrome (RLS) Syndrome characterized by unpleasant sensory (paresthesias) and motor abnormalities of one or both legs; also known as *Willis–Ekbom disease*. Ch. 61

retina The innermost layer of the eye that extends and gives rise to the optic nerve; responsible for converting images into a form that the brain can understand and process as vision. Ch. 23

retinal detachment A separation of the sensory retina and the underlying pigment epithelium, with fluid accumulation between the two layers. Ch. 24

retinopathy The process of microvascular damage to the retina. Ch. 24

retrograde pyelography Radiographic visualization of the kidneys, the ureter, and the bladder after direct injection of a contrast material into the kidney. Ch. 47

retroviruses Viruses that replicate in a "backward" manner (transcribing their RNA and DNA after entering a cell). Ch. 17

reverse transcriptase An enzyme made by HIV and other retroviruses that helps transcribe viral RNA into a double strand of viral DNA. Ch. 17

reward craving A craving that occurs when in the presence of people, places, or things that were previously associated with taking the substance. Ch. 11

rheumatic fever A disease that causes inflammation in connective tissues; commonly affects the heart, the brain, the joints, or the skin. Ch. 39

rheumatic heart disease A chronic condition resulting from rheumatic fever that is characterized by scarring and deformity of the heart valves. Ch. 39

rheumatoid arthritis (RA) A chronic, systemic autoimmune disease characterized by inflammation of connective tissue in the diarthrodial (synovial) joints, typically with periods of remission and exacerbation. Ch. 67

rhinoplasty Surgical reconstruction of the nose, performed for cosmetic reasons or to improve airway function when trauma or developmental deformities result in nasal obstruction. Ch. 29

ribonucleic acid (RNA) A single-stranded nucleic acid that translates DNA genetic information into protein. Ch. 15

S

same-day admission Admission to hospital on the day that surgery will take place. Ch. 20

sarcoma A malignant tumour in the connective tissue of the body (fat, muscles, blood vessels, nerves, bones, or cartilage). Chs. 18, 66

SBAR (situation, background, assessment, and recommendation) A means for members of the health care team to talk about a patient's condition in a predictable, structured manner. Ch. 1

sclera The bulbar conjunctiva, composed of collagen fibres meshed together to form an opaque structure commonly referred to as the "white" of the eye; helps protect the intraocular structures. Ch. 23

scleroderma A disorder of connective tissue characterized by fibrotic, degenerative, and occasionally inflammatory changes in skin, blood vessels, synovium, skeletal muscle, and internal organs; also called *systemic sclerosis*. Ch. 67

scoliosis A deformity resulting from lateral S-shaped curvature of the thoracic and lumbar spine. Ch. 64

scrub nurse A perioperative nurse who performs surgical hand asepsis, is gowned and gloved in sterile attire, and remains in the sterile field assisting the surgical team. Ch. 21

sebaceous glands Oil-producing glands that secrete sebum, which waterproofs and lubricates the skin and hair. Ch. 25

secondary hypertension Elevated blood pressure with a specific cause that often can be identified and corrected; accounts for about 5% to 10% of hypertension in adults and more than 80% of hypertension in children. Ch. 35

secondary survey A brief, systematic process that is aimed at identifying all injuries (follows primary survey and life-saving interventions). Ch. 71

seizure A transient uncontrolled electrical discharge of neurons in the brain that interrupts normal function. Often, seizures are symptoms of an underlying illness. Ch. 61

selectins Cell surface carbohydrate-binding proteins that mediate cell adhesion; involved in leukocyte extravasation during the immune response. Ch. 14

self-efficacy A person's sense of confidence in his or her ability to perform a set of actions. Ch. 4

self-management A person's ability to manage symptoms, treatments, and the various consequences of an illness. Ch. 5

self-protective behaviours In patients with dementia, behaviours that are responses to a perceived threat. Ch. 62

sense of coherence An optimistic view of the world and perceived ability to function optimally in that world. Ch. 8

sepsis A systemic inflammatory response to a documented or suspected infection. Ch. 69

septic arthritis An infection caused by microorganisms that invade the joint cavity; also called *infectious* or *bacterial arthritis*. Ch. 67

septic shock A condition in which hypotension cannot be reversed with fluid resuscitation; tissue perfusion abnormalities are present. Ch. 69

severe sepsis Sepsis complicated by organ dysfunction, hypoperfusion, or hypertension. Ch. 69

sex-linked gene A gene located on a sex chromosome. Ch. 15

sexual assault The legal term used to refer to any form of sexual contact imposed on another person without that person's voluntary consent. Ch. 71

sexually transmitted infections (STIs) Infectious diseases that are commonly acquired through sexual contact but may also be contracted by other routes, such as through blood, blood products, perinatal transmission, and autoinoculation; can be bacterial, viral, or both. Ch. 55

shared decision making A decision-making process engaged in jointly by patients and their health care providers. Ch. 5

shearing force Pressure exerted on the skin when it adheres to the bed and the underlying skin layers slide in the direction of body movement. Ch. 14

shift work sleep disorder Insomnia, sleepiness, and fatigue often experienced by people who work a permanent night shift or rapidly rotating shifts. Ch. 9

shock A syndrome characterized by decreased tissue perfusion and impaired cellular metabolism that results in an imbalance between the supply of and the demand for oxygen and nutrients. Ch. 69

short bowel syndrome (SBS) Syndrome resulting from extensive resection of the small intestine and characterized by rapid intestinal transit, impaired digestive and absorption processes, and fluid and electrolyte losses. Ch. 45

sickle cell disease (SCD) A group of inherited, autosomal recessive disorders characterized by the presence of an abnormal form of hemoglobin in the red blood cell. Ch. 33

signs Objective manifestations of a condition. Ch. 5

silent ischemia Ischemia that occurs in the absence of clinical symptoms such as chest pain. Ch. 36

Sjögren syndrome A relatively uncommon autoimmune disease that targets moisture-producing exocrine glands, leading to the common symptoms of xerostomia (dry mouth) and kerato-conjunctivitis sicca (dry eyes). Ch. 67

sleep A state during which an individual lacks conscious awareness of environmental surroundings and from which the individual can be easily aroused. Ch. 9

sleep disorder A condition that specifically affects the quality of sleep and wake behaviour. Ch. 9

sleep-disordered breathing Abnormal respiratory patterns associated with sleep, such as snoring, apnea, and hypopnea, characterized by increased respiratory effort that leads to frequent arousals. Ch. 9

sleep disturbances Situations of poor quality sleep. Ch. 9

sleep hygiene A variety of different practices that are important for normal, quality nighttime sleep and daytime alertness. Ch. 9

sleep terrors A sudden awakening from sleep along with a loud cry and signs of panic; includes an intense autonomic response, including increased heart rate, increased respiration, and diaphoresis. Ch. 9

smoke and inhalation injuries Damage to the tissues of the respiratory tract as a result of the inhalation of hot air or noxious chemicals. Ch. 27

Somogyi effect An effect characterized by wide differences in early-morning (low) and fasting (high) glucose levels. Usually occurs during the hours of sleep and produces a decline in blood glucose level in response to too much insulin; counter-regulatory hormones are released, stimulating lipolysis, gluconeogenesis, and glycogenolysis, which in turn produce rebound hyperglycemia and ketosis. Ch. 52

spermatocele A firm, sperm-containing, painless cyst of the epididymis. Ch. 57

spermatogenesis The process of sperm production. Ch. 53

spider angiomas Small, dilated blood vessels of the skin that have a bright-red centre and spider-like branches; occur on nose, cheeks, upper trunk, neck, and shoulders. Ch. 46

spinal anaesthesia The injection of a local anaesthetic into the cerebro-spinal fluid found in the subarachnoid space, usually below the level of L2. Ch. 21

spinal shock A temporary neurological syndrome experienced after spinal cord injury and characterized by decreased reflexes, loss of sensation, and flaccid paralysis below the level of the injury. Ch. 63

spirituality Beliefs, values, and practices that relate to the search for existential meaning and purpose; may or may not include belief in a higher power. Ch. 13

spondyloarthropathies A group of interrelated, multisystem inflammatory disorders that affect the spine, the peripheral joints, and the periarticular structures. Ch. 67

sprain An injury related to the ligamentous structures surrounding a joint, usually caused by a wrenching or twisting motion. Ch. 65

squamous cell carcinoma (SCC) A malignant neoplasm of keratinizing epidermal cells that frequently occurs on sun-exposed skin. Ch. 26

stage of exhaustion Final stage of general adaptation syndrome, which occurs when all of the energy for adaptation has been expended; usually results in illness and can result in death without external sources of adaptive energy, such as medication or psychotherapy. Ch. 8

stage of resistance Second stage of general adaptation syndrome, in which physiological reserves are mobilized to increase the resistance to stress. Ch. 8

stages of behavioural change The six stages of change identified by Prochaska and Velicer (1997) in their transtheoretical model of behaviour change: precontemplation, contemplation, preparation, action, maintenance, and termination. Ch. 4

staging Classifying the extent and spread of disease. Ch. 18

standard of practice An authoritative statement outlining the legal and professional foundation for nursing practice and the expected level of performance. Ch. 1

status epilepticus A state of continuous seizure activity, in which seizures recur in rapid succession without the person returning to consciousness between seizures. It is a neurological emergency and can involve any type of seizure. Ch. 61

steatorrhea Passage of large amounts of fat as bulky, fatty, frothy, foul-smelling, yellow-grey, greasy stools with putty-like consistency; results from failure to digest and absorb the fat. Ch. 41

stem cell An immature blood cell that is able to self-renew and to differentiate into hematopoietic progenitor cells. Ch. 32

stereotyping The assumption that members of a specific culture, race, or ethnic group have certain characteristics associated with that group, without further exploration of what the individuals are actually like. Ch. 2

stigmatization Being regarded by others as unworthy or disgraceful. Ch. 5

strabismus A condition in which the patient cannot consistently focus both eyes simultaneously on the same object. Ch. 24

strain An excessive stretching of a muscle, a muscle's fascial sheath, or a tendon; most occur in the foot, leg (typically hamstring), or back. Ch. 65

stress The inability to cope with perceived (real or imagined) demands or threats to an individual's mental, emotional, or spiritual well-being. Ch. 8

stressors Stress-inducing demands on a person. Ch. 8

stricture An abnormal temporary or permanent narrowing of the lumen of a hollow organ such as the ureter or the urethra. Ch. 48

stroke Death of brain cells as a result of ischemia to a part of the brain or hemorrhage into the brain. Ch. 60

subarachnoid hemorrhage (SAH) A stroke resulting from intracranial bleeding into the cerebro-spinal fluid–filled space between the arachnoid and the pia mater membranes on the surface of the brain. Ch. 60

subdural hematoma A collection of blood that results from bleeding between the dura mater and arachnoid layer of the meningeal covering of the brain; usually results from injury to the brain substance and its parenchymal vessels. Ch. 59

subjective data What the person tells the nurse either spontaneously or in response to a direct question; also called *symptoms*. Ch. 3

sublethal injury Cell injury that alters function without causing cell destruction. Ch. 14

subluxation A partial or incomplete displacement of the joint surface. Ch. 65

submersion injury Injury resulting when a person becomes hypoxic as a result of submersion in a substance, usually water. Ch. 71

substance use disorder Problematic use of a substance resulting from the prolonged effects of the substance on the brain. Ch. 11

sudden cardiac death (SCD) Unexpected death resulting from various causes, including cardiac arrest. Ch. 36

suffering Distress that occurs when stressors threaten the biopsychosocial integrity of an individual. Ch. 10

sun protection factor (SPF) A method of measuring the effectiveness of a sunscreen in filtering and absorbing ultraviolet B light (UVB) radiation. Ch. 26

sundowning A pattern of behavioural disturbance that occurs in the late afternoon. Ch. 62

superficial vein thrombosis (SVT) The formation of a thrombus in a superficial vein, usually the greater or lesser saphenous vein. Ch. 40

surfactant A lipoprotein that lowers the surface tension in the alveoli, reduces the amount of pressure needed to inflate the alveoli, and decreases the tendency of the alveoli to collapse. Ch. 28

surgeon A physician who performs surgical procedures. Ch. 21

surgical suite A controlled environment designed to maximize infection control and provide a seamless flow of patients, personnel, and operative instruments, equipment, and supplies; it is divided into unrestricted, semirestricted, and restricted areas. Ch. 21

symptoms The subjective reports of the patient. Ch. 5

synapse The structural and functional junction between two neurons; the point at which the nerve impulse is transmitted from one neuron to another or from a neuron to glands or muscles. Ch. 58

syncope Fainting that may occur with decreased cardiac output, fluid deficits, or defects in cerebral perfusion. Ch. 22

syndrome of inappropriate antidiuretic hormone (SIADH) A condition in which there is overproduction or oversecretion of antidiuretic hormone; characterized by fluid retention, serum hypo-osmolality, dilutional hyponatremia, hypochloremia, concentrated urine in the presence of normal or increased intravascular volume, and normal renal function. Ch. 51

synovectomy Removal of the synovial membrane; used as a prophylactic measure or as a palliative treatment for rheumatoid arthritis. Ch. 65

syphilis A sexually transmitted infection caused by *Treponema pallidum*; may also be spread through contact with infectious lesions and sharing of needles among people who use intravenous drugs. Ch. 55

systemic exertion intolerance disease (SEID) A serious, complex, multisystem disease in which exertion of any sort (physical, emotional, cognitive) can adversely affect multiple organs in a person; also known as *chronic fatigue syndrome (CFS)*. Ch. 67

systemic inflammatory response syndrome (SIRS) A systemic inflammatory response to a variety of insults, including infection, ischemia, infarct, and injury; characterized by at least two of the following: fever, edema, hypotension, tachycardia, impaired oxygenation, and elevated white blood cell count. Ch. 69

systemic lupus erythematosus (SLE) A multisystem, inflammatory disease that typically affects the skin, the joints, and the serous membranes (pleura, pericardium), along with the renal, hematological, and neurological systems. Ch. 67

systemic vascular resistance (SVR) The force opposing the movement of blood within the blood vessels; the radius of the small arteries and arterioles is the principal factor determining vascular resistance. Ch. 35

systole Contraction of the myocardium. Ch. 34

systolic blood pressure (SBP) The peak pressure exerted against the arteries when the heart contracts. Ch. 34

T

teaching A process of deliberately planning experiences and sharing knowledge to meet learner outcomes in the cognitive, affective, and psychomotor domains. Ch. 4

teaching plan A learner-centred approach for action to achieve the goals and learning outcomes agreed upon by the patient and nurse. Ch. 4

teaching process The development and implementation of a plan that includes assessment, diagnosis, the setting of patient outcomes or objectives, intervention, and evaluation. Ch. 4

tenesmus Spasmodic contraction of the anal sphincter with pain and persistent desire to empty the bowel; painful and ineffective straining at stool. Ch. 41

tension pneumothorax A pneumothorax with rapid accumulation of air in the pleural space, causing severely high intrapleural pressures with resultant tension on the heart and great vessels. Ch. 30

tension-type headache The most common type of primary headache, characterized by bilateral location and pressing or tightening quality; usually of mild or moderate intensity and lasting from minutes to days. (Also called *stress headache*.) Ch. 61

terrorism Intentional and overt actions that are committed to cause fear, panic, destruction, injury, and death in service of political, religious, or ideological goals. Ch. 72

testicular torsion A condition involving a twisting of the spermatic cord that supplies blood to the testes and epididymis, causing an interruption to the blood supply. Ch. 57

tetanus An extremely severe polyradiculitis and polyneuritis affecting spinal and cranial nerves that results from the effects of a potent neurotoxin released by the anaerobic bacillus *Clostridium tetani*; also called *lockjaw*. Ch. 63

tetany Condition of sustained muscle contraction. Ch. 19

tetraplegia Paralysis of the arms, the legs, and the trunk occurring with spinal cord damage at the eighth cervical (C8) vertebra or above; formerly called *quadriplegia*. Ch. 63

thalassemia A group of diseases involving inadequate production of normal hemoglobin; caused by an absent or reduced globulin protein. Ch. 33

therapeutic touch A method of detecting, balancing, and repatterning the human energy field. Ch. 12

thermal burns Burns caused by flame, flash fire, scald, or contact with hot objects. Ch. 27

thoracentesis A procedure to remove fluid from the pleural space. Ch. 30

thoracotomy Surgical opening into the thoracic cavity. Ch. 30

thromboangiitis obliterans (Buerger's disease) A nonatherosclerotic, segmental, recurrent inflammatory disorder of the small and medium-sized arteries and veins of the upper and lower extremities. Ch. 40

thrombo-cytopenia A reduction of platelets to an amount below 150×10^9/L. Chs. 32, 33

thrombo-cytosis A condition characterized by excessive levels of platelets; a disorder that occurs with inflammation and some malignant diseases. Ch. 32

thrombotic stroke A stroke resulting from the formation of a blood clot in a diseased and narrowed blood vessel in the brain. Ch. 60

thyroiditis An inflammation of the thyroid gland; can have several causes. Ch. 51

thyrotoxicosis The clinical syndrome of hypermetabolism caused by excess circulating levels of thyroxine, triiodothyronine, or both. Ch. 51

thyroxine (T_4) The most abundant hormone produced by the thyroid gland and the precursor to triiodothyronine. Ch. 50

tidal volume Volume of air exchanged with each breath. Ch. 28

tinnitus The perception of ringing in the ears. Ch. 23

titration Dosage adjustment based on assessment of the adequacy of analgesic effect versus the adverse effects produced. Ch. 10

tolerance The need for a larger dose of a drug to obtain the original euphoria. Ch. 11

tonic–clonic seizure The most common type of generalized seizure, characterized by loss of consciousness and falling to the ground if the patient is upright, followed by stiffening of the body (tonic phase) for 10 to 20 seconds and subsequent jerking of the extremities (clonic phase) for another 30 to 40 seconds. Ch. 61

tracheostomy A stoma (opening) that results from a tracheotomy. Ch. 29

tracheotomy A surgical incision into the trachea for the purpose of establishing an airway. Ch. 29

traction The application of a pulling force to an injured or diseased part of the body or extremity while counter-traction pulls in the opposite direction. Ch. 65

traditional Chinese medicine (TCM) A group of treatment modalities used to replenish and smooth the flow of qi, or the fundamental life force; interventions include acupressure, acupuncture, Chinese massage, cupping, moxibustion, nutrition counselling, and meditative physical exercise. Ch. 12

transcription The process through which RNA is synthesized from the DNA template. Ch. 15

transduction The conversion of a mechanical, thermal, or chemical stimulus to a neuronal action potential. Ch. 10

transient ischemic attack (TIA) A temporary episode of neurological dysfunction caused by focal brain, spinal cord, or retinal ischemia but without acute infarction of the brain. Ch. 60

translation The process through which the codon sequence is converted into amino acids. Ch. 15

transmission The movement of pain impulses from the site of transduction to the brain. Ch. 10

transtheoretical model of change A framework of behaviour change that provides a contextual approach for clinicians; the stages of change include precontemplation, contemplation, preparation, action, maintenance, and termination, Ch. 11

transurethral resection of the prostate (TURP) A surgical procedure involving the removal of prostate tissue using a resectoscope inserted through the urethra. Ch. 57

triage The sorting or ranking of casualties to prioritize health care needs and to allocate resources. Ch. 72

trigeminal neuralgia (TN) Uncommon cranial nerve disorder affecting cranial nerve V; characterized by paroxysms of flashing, stabbing pain radiating along the course of a branch of the trigeminal facial nerve from the angle of the jaw; also called *tic douloureux*. Ch. 63

trigger point A circumscribed hypersensitive area within a tight band of muscle that is caused by acute or persistent muscle strain. Ch. 10

triiodothyronine (T_3) A potent hormone produced by the thyroid gland that regulates the metabolic rate of all cells and processes of cell growth and tissue differentiation. Ch. 50

tropic hormones Several hormones secreted by the anterior pituitary gland that control the secretion of hormones by other glands. Ch. 50

tuberculosis An infectious disease caused by *Mycobacterium tuberculosis*; usually involves the lungs but also occurs in the larynx, the kidneys, the bones, the adrenal glands, the lymph nodes, and the meninges and can be disseminated throughout the body. Ch. 30

tumour angiogenesis The process of the formation of blood vessels within the tumour itself. Ch. 18

tumour-associated antigens Cell surface antigens on some cancer cells that have changes as a result of malignant transformation. Ch. 18

tumour suppressor genes Normal genes that are regulators of normal cellular processes; suppress growth. Ch. 18

U

ulcerative colitis (UC) A chronic inflammatory bowel disease characterized by inflammation and ulceration of the rectum and colon. Ch. 45

unconsciousness An abnormal state of complete or partial unawareness of self or environment. Ch. 59

undernutrition A state that occurs when nutritional reserves become depleted or when nutrient intake is inadequate to meet daily requirements or metabolic demands. Ch. 42

unregulated care providers Paid employees who are not licensed or registered by a regulatory body, who have no legally defined scope of practice, who may or may not have mandatory education or practice standards, who provide care under the direct or indirect supervision of a nurse, and who are accountable for their own actions and decisions. Ch. 1

unstable angina (UA) Angina that is new in onset, occurs at rest, or has a worsening pattern. Ch. 36

upper motor neurons (UMNs) The classification of motor pathways that originate in the cerebral cortex and project downward; the cortico-bulbar tract ends in the brain stem, and the cortico-spinal tract descends into the spinal cord. Ch. 58

uremia A constellation of signs and symptoms resulting from the buildup of waste products and excess fluid associated with kidney failure; these signs and symptoms may include but are not limited to elevated serum creatinine and blood urea nitrogen, abnormal electrolytes, acidosis, anemia, fluid volume excess, nausea, loss of appetite, fatigue, decreased cognition, pruritus, and neuropathy. Ch. 49

urethritis Inflammation of the urethra. Ch. 48

urinalysis A general examination of urine for routine and microscopic findings; may establish baseline information, provide information about possible abnormalities, indicate what further studies need to be done, and supply information on the progression of a diagnosed disorder. Ch. 47

urinary incontinence (UI) An uncontrolled leakage loss of urine that is of sufficient magnitude to be a problem, p. 1315. Ch. 48

urinary retention The inability to empty the bladder despite micturition, or the accumulation of urine in the bladder because of an inability to urinate. Ch. 48

urodynamics testing A set of studies designed to measure urinary tract function—the storage of urine within the bladder and the flow of urine through the urinary tract to the outside of the body. Ch. 47

urticaria An eruption of spontaneously occurring, raised or irregularly shaped wheals; usually allergic phenomenon. Ch. 26

uterine prolapse The downward displacement of the uterus into the vaginal canal as a result of impaired pelvic support. Ch. 56

V

valence The electrical charge of an ion. Ch. 19

Valsalva manoeuvre A manoeuvre that involves contraction of the chest muscles on a closed glottis with simultaneous contraction of the abdominal muscles; used during straining. Ch. 41

varicocele A dilation of the veins that drain the testes. Ch. 57

varicose veins Dilated, tortuous subcutaneous veins most commonly found in the saphenous vein system. Ch. 40

vascular dementia A form of dementia that results from ischemic, ischemic–hypoxic, or hemorrhagic brain damage caused by cardiovascular disease; also called *multi-infarct dementia*. Ch. 62

vasectomy The bilateral surgical ligation or resection of the vas deferens performed for the purpose of sterilization. Ch. 57

venous thrombo-embolism (VTE) Condition in which a thrombus forms in association with inflammation of the vein. Ch. 40

ventilation Inspiration (movement of air into the lungs) and expiration (movement of air out of the lungs). Ch. 28

ventricular assist device (VAD) An internally implanted or externally positioned device that provides short- and long-term support for the failing heart; inserted into the path of flowing blood to augment or replace the action of the ventricle. Ch. 68

ventricular fibrillation A severe derangement of the heart rhythm characterized by irregular undulations of varying shapes and amplitude on the ECG. Ch. 38

ventricular tachycardia (VT) The occurrence of three or more PVCs in succession; occurs when an ectopic focus or foci fire repetitively and the ventricle takes control as the pacemaker. Ch. 38

vertigo A sense that the person or objects around the person are moving or spinning; usually stimulated by movement of the head. Ch. 23

vesicants Drugs that cause severe local tissue breakdown and necrosis when accidentally infiltrated into the skin. Ch. 18

villi Minute, finger-like projections in the mucous membrane of the small intestine, containing goblet cells that secrete mucus and epithelial cells that produce the intestinal digestive enzymes. Ch. 41

viral load The number of HIV (or other virus) particles in the blood. Ch. 17

Virchow's triad Three important factors in the etiology of venous thrombosis: (a) venous stasis, (b) damage of the endothelium (inner lining of the vein), and (c) hypercoagulability of the blood. Ch. 40

viremia Large amounts of virus in the blood. Ch. 17

viruses Infectious agents consisting of either RNA or DNA and a protein envelope; can reproduce only in the cells of a living organism. Ch. 17

vitiligo Complete absence of melanin (pigment) resulting in a chalky white patch of skin. Ch. 25

volume ventilation A predetermined tidal volume is delivered to the patient with each inspiration, and the amount of pressure needed to deliver the breath varies. Ch. 68

vomiting   The forceful ejection of partially digested food and secretions *(emesis)* from the upper gastro-intestinal tract. Ch. 44

waist-to-hip ratio (WHR)   A method of describing the distribution of both subcutaneous and visceral adipose tissue; calculated by dividing the waist measurement by the hip measuremen. Ch. 43

wake behaviour   Behaviour associated with an activated cortical brain wave (EEG) pattern. Ch. 9

weaning   The process of reducing ventilator support and resuming spontaneous ventilation. Ch. 68

Wernicke's encephalopathy   An inflammatory, hemorrhagic, degenerative condition of the brain associated with long-term alcohol abuse. Ch. 11

wet gangrene   Ischemic necrosis of an appendage as a result of a sudden, rapid elimination of blood flow, such as that seen in a severe burn or traumatic crash injury. Ch. 14

wheezes   Continuous high-pitched squeaking sounds caused by rapid vibration of bronchial walls. Ch. 28

window period   The time between exposure to HIV infection and when the test yields an accurate result. Ch. 17

windup   A pain process that results in an increase in the firing of specialized dorsal horn neurons and that is dependent on the activation of N-methyl-D-aspartate receptors. Ch. 10

withdrawal   Constellation of physiological and psychological responses that occur upon abrupt cessation or reduced intake of a substance on which an individual is dependent. Ch. 11

withdrawal management   Interventions and processes aimed at addressing the physiological and psychological symptoms that occur in response to stopping a substance on which physiological and psychological dependence has developed. Ch. 11

world view   A paradigm or a set of assumptions, values, concepts, and practices that influences how people perceive, interpret, and relate to the world around them. Ch. 2

α_1-antitrypsin (AAT) deficiency   The only known genetic abnormality that leads to chronic obstructive pulmonary disease; AAT, the major antiprotease in plasma, inhibits neutrophil elastase and the action of proteolytic enzymes from neutrophils and macrophages. Ch. 31

A

ABCDEs of cultural competence, 26, 26f
ABCDs of primary survey, 1804
Abdomen
  emergency assessment of, 1808
  inflammatory disorders of, 1068–1069
  physical examination of, 44, 957–959, 959f
  quadrants of, 957f, 958t
  structures of, 958t
Abdominal aortic aneurysms (AAAs), 924–925, 926f, 927–928. *See also* Aortic aneurysms
Abdominal pain. *See* Acute abdominal pain; Chronic abdominal pain
Abdominal paradox, 570t–571t
Abdominal trauma, 1067–1068, 1067t
Abdominal ultrasonography, 962t–966t, 966, 966f
Abducens nerve (VI), 1457f, 1464–1465
ABO blood groups, 708, 709t
Aboriginal Canadians. *See* Indigenous Canadians
Aboriginal Navigators, 211
Abortion, 1392, 1393b, 1393t
Absence seizures, 1540
Absorption, 948, 951
Absorption atelectasis, 676
Accommodation, 441, 461
Acculturation, 24
Achalasia, 1029–1030, 1030f
Achilles tendinitis, 1626t
Acid, 370t
Acid–base imbalances
  assessment of, 374–375
  causes of, 369–370, 372t
  kinds of, 371f
  respiratory acidosis, 371–372
  ROME mnemonic for, 374t
Acid–base regulation, 370–371
Acidemia, 370t
Acid-fast smear and culture, 572t–573t
Acidosis, 370, 370t, 562. *See also* Metabolic acidosis; Respiratory acidosis
Acne (comedone), 501t
Acne vulgaris, 519t, 520f
Acoustic (vestibulocochlear) nerve (VIII), 1457f, 1465
Acoustic neuroma (Schwannoma), 484, 1493t
Acquired hemolytic anemia, 727–728. *See also* Anemia
Acquired immunity, 261, 261t

Acquired immunodeficiency syndrome (AIDS). *See* AIDS (acquired immunodeficiency syndrome)
Acquired thrombo-cytopenia, 734
Acrochordons (skin tags), 496, 509, 519t
Acromegaly, 1256–1258, 1257f
ACTH. *See* Adrenocorticotrophic hormone (ACTH)
Actigraphy, 128, 128f
Actinic keratosis (solar keratosis), 496, 499f, 506, 510, 511t
Action potential, 142, 143f, 767, 867, 867f, 1449
Active acquired immunity, 261, 261t
Active listening, 51, 215
Active transport, 354
Activities of daily living (ADL), 80–81, 100
Activity–exercise pattern, 41
Acupressure, 197
Acupuncture, 130, 197, 197t, 1016b, 1694b
Acute abdominal pain, 1063–1064, 1065t–1066t
Acute angle-closure glaucoma, 476, 476t–478t, 478. *See also* Glaucoma
Acute arterial ischemia, 921–922
Acute blood loss, 723–724
Acute bronchitis, 601
Acute chest syndrome, 726
Acute coronary syndrome (ACS)
  overview of, 827–842
  acute intervention for, 835–838
  assessment of, 835t
  collaborative care for, 825f
  drug therapy for, 826t
  electrocardiographic changes with, 884–885, 885f, 885t
  emotional and behavioural responses to, 838, 838t
  nursing care plan for, 836b–837b
  patient teaching for, 839–841, 840t
  rehabilitation after, 837t
Acute decompensated heart failure (ADHF), 848–849, 850f, 859b. *See also* Heart failure (HF)
Acute exacerbation of chronic bronchitis (AECB), 601
Acute exacerbations of COPD (AECOPD), 669–670
Acute gastritis, 1032. *See also* Gastritis
Acute illness, characteristics of, 64, 64t
Acute infectious diarrhea, 1057t
Acute kidney injury (AKI)
  overview of, 1202–1206, 1203t, 1206t
  age-related considerations with, 1208–1215
  chronic kidney disease (CKD) vs, 1202t
  collaborative care for, 1205–1206, 1205t

Acute kidney injury (AKI) *(Continued)*
  diagnostic studies for, 1205, 1205t
  fluid and electrolyte imbalances in, 1204
  infection risk with, 1207
  RIFLE Criteria for, 1202, 1202f
Acute liver failure, 1123
Acute low back pain, 1674–1675, 1674b
Acute lung injury, 1795f, 1795t
Acute lymphocytic leukemia (ALL), 745, 745t, 747t. *See also* Leukemia
Acute myelogenous leukemia (AML), 744–745, 745f, 745t, 747t, 761b. *See also* Leukemia
Acute otitis media (AOM), 481
Acute pain, 146t, 147, 174–175
Acute pain services (APS), 163
Acute pancreatitis, 1126–1128, 1126f, 1127t–1128t
Acute pericarditis, 894–897, 895f, 896t. *See also* Pericarditis
Acute pharyngitis, 587
Acute poststreptococcal glomerulo-nephritis (APSGN), 1172–1173
Acute pyelonephritis, 1168–1169, 1168f, 1169t. *See also* Pyelonephritis
Acute rejection, 279
Acute renal failure (ARF). *See* Acute kidney injury (AKI)
Acute respiratory distress syndrome (ARDS)
  overview of, 1794–1797, 1794f–1796f, 1794t, 1797t
  case study, 1800b
  collaborative care for, 1798–1799, 1798t
  diagnostic findings for, 1797t
  lung injury and, 1794t–1795t
  MODS and, 1779t
  phases of, 1795–1796
  restrictive lung disease and, 633t
  sepsis and, 1765
  shock and, 1763t, 1767t–1768t
Acute respiratory failure. *See also* Respiratory failure
  overview of, 670, 1782–1789
  assessment of, 1789t
  collaborative care for, 1789–1793, 1790t
  drug therapy for, 1792–1793
  predisposing factors for, 1786t
Acute retroviral syndrome, 297
Acute rheumatic fever (ARF)
  overview of, 898–899
  collaborative care for, 899–900, 900t
  diagnostic criteria for, 899, 899t
  diagnostic studies for, 899
Acute thyrotoxicosis, 1268–1269
Acute tubular necrosis (ATN), 532–533, 1203, 1203f

Page numbers followed by "*f*" indicate figures, "*t*" indicate tables, and "*b*" indicate boxes.

CASE STUDIES

Assessment

COLLABORATIVE CARE TABLES

COMPLEMENTARY & ALTERNATIVE THERAPIES BOXES

DETERMINANTS OF HEALTH BOXES

DIAGNOSTIC STUDIES TABLES

DRUG THERAPY TABLES

✚ EMERGENCY MANAGEMENT TABLES

ETHICAL DILEMMAS BOXES

🔍 EVIDENCE-INFORMED PRACTICE BOXES

Research Highlight

EVIDENCE-INFORMED PRACTICE BOXES

Translating Research Into Practice

Topic	Chapter	Page
Adverse Effects of Hypertension Medication	35	807
Annual PSA Screening	57	1434
Extreme Exercise and Chemotherapy	33	754
Heart Failure: Hawthorn Versus Biventricular Pacing	37	859
HIV and Unprotected Sex	17	304
Human Papilloma Vaccine	55	1384
Importance of Yearly Pap Tests	56	1408
Location for Enoxaparin Injections	40	937
NPO Order for Preoperative Patient	20	393
Patient Reluctant to Take Warfarin	38	876
Physical Activity and COPD	31	672
Post-Bariatric Surgery Support Groups	43	1009
Radiation Therapy for Breast Cancer	54	1361
Rehabilitation After Hip Fracture for Patients With Cognitive Impairment	62	1577
Skin Cancer and Indoor Tanning	26	508
Spinal Cord Injury and Bladder Management	63	1604
Stage 1 Pressure Injury	14	243
Vitamin D Deficiency	66	1686

FOCUSED ASSESSMENT BOXES

Box Title	Chapter	Page
Auditory System	23	455
Cardiovascular System	34	777
Endocrine System	50	1247
Gastro-Intestinal (GI) System	41	960
Hematological System	32	705
Integumentary System	25	502
Musculo-Skeletal System	64	1625
Neurological System	58	1467
Reproductive System	53	1340
Respiratory System	28	570
Urinary System	47	1154
Visual System	23	449

GENETICS IN CLINICAL PRACTICE BOXES

Box Title	Chapter	Page
Alzheimer's Disease	62	1569
α_1-Antitrypsin (AAT) Deficiency	31	665
Ankylosing Spondylitis	67	1711
Autoimmune Diseases	64	1623
Breast Cancer	54	1355
Familial Adenomatous Polyposis	45	1084
Familial Hypercholesterolemia	36	815
Genetics in Clinical Practice Boxes Throughout This Text	15	253
Hemochromatosis	33	729
Hemophilia A and B	33	736
Hereditary Nonpolyposis Colorectal Cancer	45	1085
Huntington's Disease	58, 61	1461, 1560
Ovarian Cancer	56	1410
Polycystic Kidney Disease	48	1182
Sickle Cell Disease	33	728
Skin Malignancies	25	498
Types 1 and 2 Diabetes Mellitus	52	1291

HEALTH HISTORY TABLES

Table Title	Table Number	Page
Auditory System	Table 23-8	453
Cardiovascular System	Table 34-2	773
Endocrine System	Table 50-6	1244
Gastro-Intestinal System	Table 41-8	957
Hematological System	Table 32-5	702
Integumentary System	Table 25-3	497
Musculo-Skeletal System	Table 64-2	1623
Nervous System	Table 58-5	1462
Patient About to Undergo Surgery	Table 20-3	390
Reproductive System	Table 53-6	1337
Respiratory System	Table 28-5	564
Urinary System	Table 47-4	1150
Visual System	Table 23-2	444

INFORMATICS IN PRACTICE

Box Title	Chapter	Page
Bar-coding in Medication Administration	20	397
Chest Drainage System	30	627
Communication Devices for Patient With Laryngectomy	29	592
Computer Monitoring of Antibiotic Safety	49	1207
Digital Images	14	243
Discharge Teaching	22	434
Heart Surgery DVD or CD	39	905
Managing Symptoms of Cancer	18	327
Monitoring Blood Pressure	35	807
Patient Teaching Using Gaming	52	1311
Phone Applications in Multiple Sclerosis	61	1552
Responsible Use of Social Media	1	9
Sleep Apnea Diagnosis and Monitoring	9	134
Smart Infusion Pumps	68	1729
Staying Connected While Immobilized	65	1647
Texting for Patients With Chronic Obstructive Pulmonary Disease (COPD)	31	678
Use of Internet to Access Information on Unfamiliar Diseases	33	744
Use of Internet and Mobile Devices to Manage Human Immunodeficiency Virus Infection	17	306
Video Games for Stroke Recovery	60	1527
Wireless ECG Monitoring	38	869

NURSING ASSESSMENT TABLES

NURSING CARE PLANS*

*All plans are available in customizable format from the Evolve website at *http://evolve.elsevier.com/Canada/Lewis/medsurg.* Seven plans are also provided in this text at the page numbers listed in this table.

NUTRITIONAL THERAPY TABLES

PATIENT & CAREGIVER TEACHING GUIDES